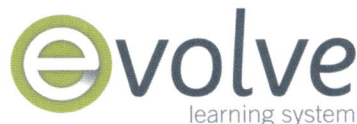
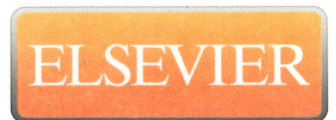

YOU'VE JUST PURCHASED

MORE THAN A TEXTBOOK

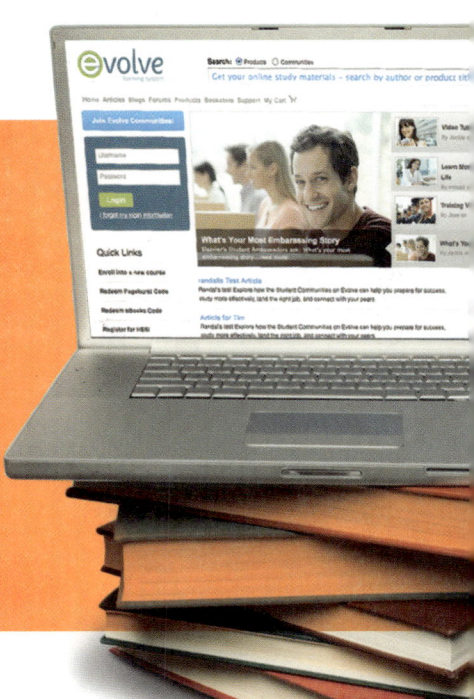

ACTIVATE THE COMPLETE LEARNING EXPERIENCE THAT COMES WITH YOUR BOOK BY REGISTERING AT

http://evolve.elsevier.com/Sanders/Paramedic

Evolve Student Learning Resources for Sanders: Mosby's Paramedic Textbook, Fourth Edition offers the following features:

- Prepare for Class, Clinical, or Lab
  Video Clips, English/Spanish Audio Glossary, Audio Summaries, Competency Checklists, Fluids & Electrolytes Tutorial, Crossword Puzzles, Content Updates

- Prepare for Exams
  Review Questions with Answers and Rationales, Critical Thinking Questions with Answers and Rationales

- Additional Resources
  Appendices

REGISTER TODAY!

Mosby's

Paramedic Textbook

ABOUT THE AUTHOR AND CONTRIBUTORS

Mick J. Sanders, EMT-P, MSA, received his paramedic training in 1978 from St. Louis University Hospitals. He earned a Bachelor of Science degree and a Master of Science degree from Lindenwood University in St. Charles, Missouri. He has worked in various health care systems as a field paramedic, emergency department paramedic, and EMS instructor. For 12 years, Mr. Sanders served as Training Specialist with the Bureau of Emergency Medical Services, Missouri Department of Health, where he oversaw EMT and paramedic training and licensure in St. Louis city and the surrounding metropolitan areas.

Kim D. McKenna, MEd, RN, CEN, EMT-P is the Director of Education for the St. Charles County Ambulance District and Adjunct Professor at Lindenwood University, located in the metropolitan St. Louis, Missouri area. There she is primary instructor for the paramedic program, program director for the district's emergency medical technician programs, and leads a training staff that provides education for district paramedics and for firefighters and emergency personnel within St. Charles County. Kim has been teaching in EMS for more than 25 years. She formerly worked as an emergency and intensive care nurse, and served as Chief Medical Officer for the Florissant Valley Fire Protection District for 6 years. Kim was the EMR Project Level Leader for the National EMS Education Standards project and is currently a Board of Director for the National Association of EMS Educators.

Lawrence M. Lewis, MD, FACEP, is Professor of Emergency Medicine in Medicine at Washington University School of Medicine and Barnes-Jewish Hospital in St. Louis, Missouri. He completed his medical school training at the University of Miami School of Medicine before attending a residency at Washington University. Dr. Lewis is an active researcher in emergency medicine with more than 60 publications and serves on several national and state emergency medicine committees.

Gary Quick, MD, FACEP retired as Medical Director at Southwestern Medical Center, Lawton, Oklahoma in December, 2010. Previously he served as an Associate Professor and Chair of the Department of Emergency Medicine at the University of Oklahoma Health Sciences Center in Oklahoma City, Oklahoma. Dr. Quick is a career emergency physician with 40 years in clinical practice, as well as extensive educational and research experience. He is widely published with more than 100 articles and book chapters to his credit. Before his retirement, he served the specialty of emergency medicine in several capacities at the national and state level for the American College of Emergency Physicians..

Mosby's Paramedic Textbook

FOURTH EDITION
MICK J. SANDERS, EMT-P, MSA

PHYSICIAN ADVISERS

Lawrence M. Lewis, MD, FACEP
Professor of Emergency Medicine
Washington University School of Medicine/Barnes-Jewish Hospital
St. Louis, Missouri

Gary Quick, MD, FACEP
Attending Emergency Physician
Oklahoma Heart Hospital
Prior Associate Professor and Chief of Emergency Medicine
University of Oklahoma
Oklahoma City, Oklahoma

CONTRIBUTING EDITOR

Kim D. McKenna, MED, RN, CEN, EMT-P
Director of Education
St. Charles County Ambulance District
Adjunct Professor, Lindenwood University
St. Charles, Missouri

With more than 1500 illustrations

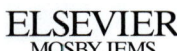

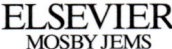

3251 Riverport Lane
St. Louis, Missouri 63043

MOSBY'S PARAMEDIC TEXTBOOK, FOURTH EDITION   978-0-323-07275-5

The Publisher
Previous editions copyrighted 1994, 2001, 2007

Managing Editor: Laura Bayless
Associate Developmental Editor: Mary Jo Adams
Publishing Services Manager: Julie Eddy
Project Manager: Rich Barber
Designer: Paula Catalano

Printed in the United States

Last digit is the print number: 9 8 7 6 5 4 3 2 1

To my family,
and
in loving memory of my father,
James H. Sanders

Preface

As a paramedic student, you have chosen to work in an exciting and rewarding area of health care prehospital emergency care. Few professions can provide the same type of opportunities that lie before you. Through your training, you will meet the educational demands of a profession that requires knowledge in anatomy and physiology, mathematics, pharmacology, advanced education in the health sciences, and physical skills in using highly technical and sophisticated equipment. You will have an opportunity to play an important role in injury prevention, to participate in research, and to be a role model in your community. And most importantly, you will be entrusted with the lives of the people you serve. This describes today's paramedic–a member of a unique profession composed of highly trained men and women dedicated to making a difference in people's lives.

CONTENT AND ORGANIZATION

The fourth edition of *Mosby's Paramedic Textbook* has been extensively reviewed by physicians, nurses, paramedics, educators, and national and international experts in the field of emergency care people who know and value the important role of the paramedic in health care delivery. The text was developed from the 2008 National Highway Traffic Safety Administration's National EMS Education Standards Instructional Guidelines for Paramedics. Every effort was made to meet *all* educational components as defined in that document. The fourth edition has also been enhanced to address recent advances and important issues in emergency medical services (EMS), including new equipment and procedures; critical care transport (CCT); and special considerations for dealing with bioterrorism and weapons of mass destruction (WMD).

Part One explains the paramedic's role and the unique aspects of the profession, such as an overview of EMS systems and the importance of personal well-being. It also introduces the paramedic student to medical/legal issues, ethics, documentation, and EMS communications. New chapters included in this section include Injury Prevention and Public Health (Chapter 3) and Research Principles and Evidence-Based Practice (Chapter 8). Personal safety is emphasized in Part One and throughout the text.

Part Two provides a review of human systems and is an easily located reference for anatomical structures and their functions. This section begins with a new chapter to explain Medical Terminology (Chapter 9). The general principles of pathophysiology lay the foundation for the textbook and are presented here as well. Chapters that map lifespan development and special considerations for specific age groups are included in this section.

Part Three introduces the paramedic student to pharmacology, methods of venous access, and medication administration. The pharmacology chapter has been enhanced to include new emergency drugs. It also has an expanded appendix on herbal products, their common uses, indications, and possible interactions with medications.

Part Four is devoted to airway management and ventilation. The physiology of the respiratory system is presented in depth, and basic and advanced methods of managing a patient's airway with new equipment and techniques are illustrated in this chapter.

Part Five focuses on patient assessment and the importance of caring for both the physical and emotional needs of the patient. New chapters devoted to Scene Size-Up (Chapter 16), Primary Assessment (Chapter 19), and Secondary Assessment (Chapter 20) are included in this edition. Separate chapters address therapeutic communications, history taking, and clinical decision making.

Part Six covers cardiology in detail. Electrophysiology of the heart and electrocardiogram (ECG) interpretation is presented first and is followed by cardiovascular emergencies such as cardiac rhythm disturbances, myocardial infarction, and stroke. Techniques in managing cardiac emergencies, including basic and advanced cardiac life support, follow the 2010 guidelines established by the American Red Cross (ARC) and the American Heart Association (AHA).

Part Seven addresses the many types of medical conditions that can lead to an emergency response. New chapters to this edition are Diseases of the Eyes, Ears, Nose, and Throat (Chapter 23), Immunology (Chapter 27), and Nontraumatic Musculoskeletal Disorders (Chapter 33). Separate chapters are included for disorders of specific body systems. Discussed in depth here are respiratory, neurology, endocrinology, gastrointestinal, genitourinary, gynecology, and hematology disorders. In addition, infectious and communicable diseases, toxicology, and behavioral and psychiatric disorders are covered in detail.

Part Eight is a complete discussion of the Pathophysiology and Management of Shock, a complicated disease process that can affect both medical and trauma patients.

Part Nine is devoted to a thorough presentation of trauma. It begins with a discussion of trauma systems and mechanism of injury. This is followed by separate chapters on bleeding and soft tissue trauma; burns; head, face, and neck trauma; and injury to the spine, chest, abdomen, and musculoskeletal system. A separate chapter on Environmental Conditions (Chapter 45) describes illness and injury that can result from exposure to elements in the environment.

Part Ten describes special considerations for select patient groups such as pregnant women, neonates, pediatrics, and geriatrics. It also addresses the needs of patients who have been victims of abuse and neglect, those with special challenges, and home care patients who may require acute interventions.

Part Eleven deals with the various aspects of advanced EMS systems, such as ambulance operations, medical incident command, rescue operations, crime scene awareness, and hazardous materials incidents. A separate chapter that provides an overview of bioterrorism and weapons of mass destruction is included here, reflecting the hazards and responsibilities important to today's paramedic. The last chapter in this section (Chapter 59) "puts it all together" for the student. It serves as a review of the important concepts in providing emergency care that have been presented throughout the text. Finally, a new appendix has been included to provide an overview of advanced practice procedures for the critical care paramedic.

Each chapter of *Mosby's Paramedic Textbook* begins with an introduction and a list of objectives that provide an overview of the material to be presented. This allows the student to review the content and progression of each chapter in an easy-to-follow format. Key terms are included to highlight terminology and concepts critical to providing emergency care, and boldfaced items identify terms that are included in the glossary. Each chapter concludes with current references that can be used as a resource for supplemental reading and a bulleted summary that reviews the most important material presented in the chapter. The textbook also is accompanied by a student workbook to help measure understanding of the core material. Included in the workbook are questions, activities, and case studies designed to enhance understanding, promote reflection on learning, and integrate key concepts and knowledge.

The fourth edition of *Mosby's Paramedic Textbook* also includes the following features that help make this textbook a leader in EMS education:

- Emergency Drug Index. The Emergency Drug Index (EDI) details specific information on more than 70 emergency drugs. It provides a quick source of reference for a drug's description, onset and duration, indications, contraindications, adverse reactions, drug interactions, packaging, dosage and administration for adult and pediatric patients, and special considerations. Drugs in the textbook that are found in the EDI are denoted with a bold italic font as a reminder to the reader of their importance and easy location of reference.

- Critical Thinking Questions. Critical thinking questions are found in each chapter to aid in understanding concepts and how information presented in the text can impact day-to-day activities and "real life" patient care.

- Advanced ECG Rhythm Interpretation. All cardiac rhythms and dysrhythmias are presented in lead I, II, III, and MCL_1 to enhance assessment of the cardiac patient. In addition, the text includes advanced electrophysiology, 12-lead monitoring, fibrinolytic therapy, and current treatment modalities as recommended by the American Heart Association.

- Full-Color Illustrations. More than 1500 tables, charts, line drawings, and photographs are included in the text to illustrate anatomy, physiology, and patient management guidelines. State-of-the-art equipment and step-by-step demonstrations of practical skills also are presented in full color to demonstrate emergency care procedures.

- "Did You Know?" The new "Did You Know?" boxes are included throughout the text to expand on interesting and relevant information, such as unusual facts and figures, "nice-to-know" data, and "need-to-know" material, such as the rights of terminally ill patients and the possible effects of biological terrorism.

- Box Notes. Box notes are presented in each chapter to highlight vital information and words of warning.

- "Look Again." The new "Look Again" feature prevents text information from being repeated in numerous chapters. This feature directs the student to the chapters and page numbers where the material was first presented for easy reference and review.

- "Show Me the Evidence." Each new "Show Me the Evidence" feature summarizes a research study related to the chapter content. This feature familiarizes the paramedic with the research process, its language, and its findings. "Show me the Evidence" will encourage students to look for information throughout their careers to promote evidence-based practice.

- Expanded Glossary. The glossary has been expanded to include definitions on hundreds of medical terms and key terms presented in the textbook chapters.

- Index. The thorough and detailed index makes it easy to find information that was presented in the text.

I hope reading this preface reinforces the decision you made to choose this textbook. Whether you're a paramedic student, practicing paramedic, nurse, physician, administrator, or educator, I think you will find this textbook to be a valuable EMS resource.

Mick J. Sanders

Author Acknowledgments

The fourth edition of *Mosby's Paramedic Textbook* resulted from the combined efforts of many talented and dedicated people. In addition to my physician advisers, Larry Lewis and Gary Quick, and the many experts who reviewed the manuscript, I would like to acknowledge a few others who helped make this textbook possible:

Kim McKenna, my friend, colleague, contributor, and the author of the workbook. She's been my "can't-do-without" partner since the first edition of the text. Her devotion, her contributions, and her handling of the art program in this edition have been invaluable. (Kim, I owe you—big time!)

Laura Bayless, my managing editor. Mary Jo Adams, my developmental editor. Rich Barber, my project manager. Together, their support and daily emails helped remind me that there was light at the end of the tunnel. Kim and I are grateful for their involvement. These are the people who made the book "come to life."

Don McKenna and Rick Brady, who supplied the excellent photography. Ray Kemp who provided many of the scene photos for this edition. The paramedics and paramedic students from St. Charles County Ambulance District and their family members who were models in this edition (especially my nephew, Dusty Sanders). The McKenna family (Don, Becky, Ginny, Grant, Kim, Maggie, and Bill). St. Louis City EMS (especially Monroe Yancie), O'Fallon Fire Protection District, and the many equipment manufacturers who supplied photos and illustrations to accompany the text. And of course, a special thanks to the many others who were instrumental in the success of previous editions. Their contributions remain an important part of this project.

Finally, I want to mention a few special people whose interest in me and whose support of this project was something I could always count on: Dixie Allen (my mother), Randy Sanders (my brother), and Will Denney (a great friend).

Mick J. Sanders

Publisher Acknowledgments

The editors wish to acknowledge and thank the many reviewers of this book, who devoted countless hours to intensive review. Their comments were invaluable in helping to develop and fine tune the revision of this textbook.

Organizations and individuals who took part in this extensive project were:

Mark "Sharky" Alexander, EMTP, ACLS, PALS, DMT
EMT-P, PHTLS-Instructor/ Chamber Operator, USCG Master Captain, TDI Closed Circuit Rebreather Instructor and Mixed Gas Diver, PADI Master Instructor,
St. Charles Ambulance District/ Sharky's Underwater Expedition, LCC
St. Charles, Missouri

David S. Becker, MA, EMT-P, EFO
Sanford-Brown College
St. Louis, Missouri

Kristen D. Borchelt, RN, NREMTP
Cincinnati Children's Hospital
Cincinnati, Ohio

Robert P. Breese, EMT-P, MICP, CCEMTP, FP-C
Flight Paramedic, Paramedic Instructor
Monroe Community College
Rochester, New York

Helen E. Burkhalter, BAS, NREMT-P/RN
Chairperson of Public Safety Technology
Atlanta Technical College
Atlanta, Georgia

Peter Connick, EMT-P, EMT I/C
Captain-Chatham Fire Rescue
Chatham, Massachusetts
Adjunct Faculty
Cape Cod Community College
West Barnestable, Maryland

Jon S. Cooper, Paramedic, NCEE
Lieutenant
Baltimore City Fire Department
Baltimore, Maryland

Thomas Czerniak, EMT-Basic, MS in Teaching, BS in Biology
Instructor/Coordinator
Gateway Technical College
Burlington, Wisconsin

Carolyn V Daigneau, BSN, MSN ANCC Certification, RN, PNP-BC
The University of Texas Health Science Center at Houston
Division of Pediatrics
Department of Gastroenterology, Nutrition and Hepatology: Texas Liver Center
Pediatric Hepatology and Liver Transplant
Houston, Texas

Ken Davis, BA, EMT-P
Outreach Coordinator
Eastern New Mexico University- Roswell
Roswell, New Mexico

John A. DeArmond, NREMT-P
Half Moon, Bay, California

Steven Dralle, MBA, LP
San Antonio, Texas

Dennis Edgerly, AAS, EMTP
Program Coordinator
Health One EMS
Englewood, Colorado

Harold C. Etheridge, Lic-P, NREMT-P
Lifecare EMS
Weatherford, Texas

James M. Farmer, EMT-P, AOS, FF
Lead Instructor
IHM- Health Studies Center
St. Louis, Missouri

Janet Fitts, RN, BSN, CEN, TNS, EMT-P
Training Officer
New Haven Ambulance District
New Haven, Missouri

Jeffery S. Force, BA, NREMT-P
Pikes Peak Community College
Penrose-St. Frances Health Services
Colorado Springs, Colorado

Scott Gilmore, M.D., EMT-P
Clinical Instructor
Washington University School of Medicine
Assistant Medical Director, Saint Louis Fire Department
St. Louis, Missouri

Mark Goldstein, RN, MSN, EMT-P I/C
Emergency Services Clinical Nurse Specialist and EMS
    Coordinator
William Beaumont Hospital
Grosse Pointe, Michigan

Lynn Pierzchalski-Goldstein, RPH, BS Pharm, Pharm D
Penrose St. Francis Health System
Colorado Springs, Colorado

**Wes Hamilton, BSN, CCRN, CFRN, CTRN,
    NREMT-P, FP-C**
Clinical Development Specialist
Air Evac EMS
West Plains, Missouri

Seth C. Hawkins, MD, FACEP, FAAEM, FAWM
Medical Director and Chair
Grace Hospital Emergency Department
Medical Director
Burke County EMS
Assistant Professor, Emergency Medical Care Program
Western Carolina University
Morganton, North Carolina

Gary Hoertz, NREMT-P
EMS Division Chief
Kootenai County Fire & Rescue
Post Falls, Idaho

Julie C. Leonard, MD, MPH
Assistant Professor, Pediatric Emergency Medicine
Washington University in St. Louis School of Medicine
St. Louis, Missouri

Reylon Meeks, RN, PhD
Clinical Nurse Specialist/Fire Chief
Blank Children's Hospital/Pleasant Hill Fire
    Department
Pleasant Hill, Iowa

Laraine Moody, MSN, RN, CPNP-AC/PC
Pediatric Nurse Practitioner
Children's Hospital of Michigan
Detroit, Michigan

Ruth Novitt-Schumacher, RN, MSN
Pediatric Nursing Instructor
UIC College of Nursing
Chicago, Illinois

Joanne Onderko, RN, MA, CEN, CFN
Senior Education Specialist- Emergency Services
Providence Park Hospital
Novi, Michigan

Dennis Parker, MA, EMT-P, I/C
EMS Program Coordinator
Tennessee Tech University
Cookeville, Tennessee

Deborah L. Petty, BS, CICP, EMT-P
Paramedic Training Officer
St. Charles County Ambulance District
St. Peters, Missouri

Gary Quick, MD, Fellow of ACEP
Education Medical Director
Southwestern Hospital
Lawton, Oklahoma

Larry Richmond, AS, NREMT-P, CCEMT-P
EMS Coordinator
Rapid City HIS Hospital
Rapid City, South Dakota

Randy L. Sanders
Deputy Fire Chief of Operations
O'Fallon Fire Protection District
IAFC-Disaster Go Team-International Association of Fire
    Chiefs
O'Fallon, Missouri

Kimberly Schmitzer, NREMT-P, MA
Century College
White Bear Lake, Minnesota

**Michael E. Scott, BAS, Firefighter Paramedic
    IC Adjunct Faculty, Paramedic Instructor
    Coordinator**
Bloomfield Township Fire Department
Bloomfield Township, Michigan

**Heather Seemann, NREMT-P, FP-C, CCP-C, MLT
    (ASCP), BA**
Paramedic
North Slope Search and Rescue
Barrow, Alaska

Gale P. Sewell, RN, MSN, CNE
Assistant Professor
Indiana Wesleyan University
Marion, Indiana

David M. Stamey, CCEMT-P
Flight Paramedic
STAT Med Evac
West Mifflin, Pennsylvania
ALS Faculty
University of Maryland Fire/Rescue Institute
College Park, Maryland

Sara Stewart, RN, EMT-P
Supervisor
St. Charles County Ambulance District

David L. Sullivan, PhD, NREMT-P
EMS/CME Program
St. Petersburg College
Pinellas Park, Florida

David K. Tan, M.D., FAAEM, EMT-T
Medical Director
St. Charles County Sheriff's Department
Assistant Professor and EMS Chief
Washington University School of Medicine
St. Louis, Missouri

David M. Tauber, NREMT-P, CCEMT-P, FP-C, NCEE
Education Coordinator/Executive Director
New Haven Sponsor Hospital Program/Advanced Life
   Support Institute
New Haven, Connecticut/Conway, New Hampshire

Mark A. Trueman, BS, NREMT-P
Director, Paramedic Technology
Pennsylvania College of Technology
Williamsport, Pennsylvania

Keith Widmeier, NREMT-P, CCEMT-P
Training Officer
Wayne County EMS
Monticello, Kentucky

Brian J. Williams, BS, NREMT-P, CCEMT-P
EMS Chief
Pembina Ambulance
Pembina, North Dakota

And we offer a special thanks to those who helped on the current and previous editions of this text:

Julie Long, Claire Merrick, Nancy Peterson, Mark Weiber, Barb Aehlert, Rich Barber, Catherine Parvenski Barwell, Amy Buxton, Lin Dempsey, Jen Etling, Janet Fitts, William Greenblatt, Larry Hatfield, Jon King, Dana Knighten, Tina Kult, Christa Lenk, Yavilah McCoy, Linda McKinley, Gayle Morris, Ronald Olshwanger, Darrell Paranich, Janice Ratchie Saia, James Silvernail, Karen Snyder, Nadine Sokol, Rob Theriault, Derril and Kelly Trakalo, Elaine Steinborn, Lana VanLaningham, and Kellie White. The McKenna family (Don, Becky, Ginny, Grant, Kim, Maggie, and Bill), Dan Peters, Steve Sanneman, John Taylor, Lance Varga, Joel Vanderploeg, and Monroe Yancie. Creve Coeur Fire Protection District, Eureka Fire Protection District, Tom Fitts (Alliance Medical), Chris Shanks (Armstrong Medical), Rob Kuchick (Medtronic-PhysioControl), St. Charles County Ambulance, St. John's Mercy Medical Center, St. Louis City EMS. Photo shoot models Mark Alexander, Dixie Allen, Chris Arter, Larry Ashby, Drew Bass, Timothy Bobbitt,

Jason Bostic, Amy Cameron, Tim Cooper, Noah Cutshall, Tim Dorsey, Mark Flauter, Rosalyn Golden, Adams Hager, Chad Heflin, Jason Herin, Scott Herin, Jeremy Hollreh, Julie Hull, Amy Jennings, Diane Kaatman, Rick Lane, Sue Lakebrink, Kurt Limpert, Frank Lipski, Morgan Luter, Bill Lowe, Beth Maddock, Mindy McCoy, Gerard Orf, John Romeo, Dusty Sanders, Ann Schneider, Timothy D. Sebert, Lori Sizer, Ashley Smith, Daniel Swofford, Brian Webb. Any other physicians, hospitals, and equipment manufacturers who supplied illustrations and scene photos to accompany the text.

First edition reviewers: National Association of EMTs Society of Paramedics Instructor/Coordinators Society; National Council of State EMS Training Coordinators; National Association of EMS Physicians; Thomas F. Anderson, PhD, RRT; Doug Austin, Jr.; Vatche H. Ayvazian, MD; John Barrett, MD; David S. Becker; John E. Blue, II, EMTP, BS; Chip Boehm, RN, EMT-P; Kevin Brown, MD, MPH; Jeffrey A. Crill, RN, EMT-P; David DaBell, MD; Alice "Twink" Dalton; Theodore R. Delbridge, MD; Linda D. Dodge; Robert Elling, MPA, NREMT-P; Franklin E. Foster, JD; Bill Garcia, MICP; Mike Gray; Janet A. Head, RN, MS; Kenneth Hines; Steven Kidd; Mark A. Kirk, MD; Kevin Kraus, BS, EMT-P; Richard A. Lazar; Mark Lockhart, NREMT-P; Julie Long; Glenn H. Luedtke, NREMT-P; Mary Beth Michos, RN; Gary P. Morris; Keith Neely, EMT-P, MPA; Gregory Noll; Michael P. Peppers, PharmD; Dwight Polk, BA, NREMT-P; William Raynovich; Lou E. Romig, MD, FAAP; José V. Aalazar, BA, NREMT; Randy L. Sanders; Carol J. Shanaberger; JoAnn Shew, RN, CS, MSN; John Sinclair; Todd M. Stanford, BS, PA-C, MICP; Andrew W. Stern, NREMT-P, MPA; Mike Taigman; Vickie H. Taylor; Michael W. Turner; Patricia L. Westbrook, MS, CCC; Jason T. White; Sherrie C. Wilson, EMT-P, I/C; Monroe Yancie, NREMT-P; and Rodney C. Zerr.

Second edition reviewers: Joseph J. Acker, AHT, EMT-P; Richard Alcorta, MD, FACEP; Chandra Aubin, MD; Alan J. Azzara, Esq, BA, JD, EMT-P; Catherine A. Parvensky Barwell, RN/EMT-P, MEd; James P. Boedeker, MD; William Brandes; David H. Brisson, RN, EMCA; Lawrence R. Brown, MD, PhD; Roy Edward Cox, Jr., MEd, EMT-P; Kevin Cunningham, BS, EMT-P; John Czajkowski; Heather Micholene Davis, MS, NREMT-P; Jeff G. DeGraffenreid, MEd, Paramedic; William H. Dribben, MD; William J. Dunne, MS, NREMT-P; Lisa Susan Etzwiler, MD, FAAP; Daryl Eustace; Edward Ferguson, MD; Janet Fitts, RN, BSN, CEN, EMT-P; Ken Fowke, BSc, EMA-II; Timothy Gridley; Larry Hatfield; Shirley A. Jones, MS Ed, MHA, EMT-P; Antoinette Kanne, RN, MS; Lisa Keenly, MD; Anthony C. Kessels; J. Steven Kidd; Jeffrey Levine, MD, FACS; James Linardos, MS, EMT-I; Michael Mullins, MD; Scott Mullins; Robert E. O'Connor, MD, MPH; Nathan Piemann, MD; Denise S. Pope, RN, MSN, BSN, MSN; John Eric Powell, MS, NREMT-P; Chris Richter, MD; Becky Ridenhour, PharmD; Cleeve Robertson, MD; S. Rutherford Rose, PharmD, FAACT;

Stanley Sakabu, MD, FACS; Robert J. Schappert III; Roberta J. Secrest, PhD, PharmD; Sharon Smith, MD; Karen Snyder; Andrew W. Stern, NREMT-P, MPA, MA; Gail Stewart, BS, EMT-P, CHES; Robert Theriault, RCT (Adv), CCP (F); Eric Thompson, MD; Bryan Troop, MD, FACS, FCCM; Christina Wagner, MD; Bruce J. Walz, PhD; Roxanne Ward, RN; A. Keith Wesley, MD, FACEP; and Brian S. Zachariah, MD, MBA.

Third edition reviewers: Beth Lothrop Adams, MA, RN, NREMT-P; Patrick Black, BS, NREMT-P; Chip Boehm, RN, EMT-P/FF, EMS I/C; Kristen Borchelt, NREMT-P; Angel Clark Burba, MS, NREMT-P; Heather Micholene Davis, MS, NREMT-P; Ken Davis, NREMT-P, CCEMT-P, I/C; Bill Doss, EMT-P; Steven Dralle, BA, EMT-P; James W. Drake, MS, NREMT-P; Rudy Garrett, AS, NREMT-P, CCEMT-P; Peter Glaeser, MD; Thomas James Gottschalk, NREMT-P, I/C, CCEMT-P; Shawn Harthorn, EMT, MACS; Robert Hawkes, BA, BS, NREMT-P, CCEMT-P; Seth Collings Hawkins, MD; Attila Hertelendy, MHSM, CCEMT-P, NREMT-P, ACP; John C. Hopkins, EMT-P; Arthur Hsieh, MA, NREMT-P; I. Kevin Johnson, AS, BS, NREMT-P; Mark Lockhart, NREMT-P; Joanne McCall, RN, MA, CEN, SANE-A, CFN; Kirk E. Mittleman, AAS, BS, NREMT-P/Utah EMT-P; Taz Meyer, BS, EMT-P; Susan M. Caley Opsal, MS; David S. Pecora, MS, PA-C, NREMT-P; Eric Powell, EMT-P; Virginia K. Riedy, RN, NREMT-P; Becky Ridenhour, PharmD; Blaine Riggleman, EMT-P; Judith A. Ruple, PhD, RN, NREMT-P; Gordon M. Sachs, EFO, MPA; Gail Saxowsky, RNC, MPH; Janet L. Schulte, BS, NR-CCEMT-P; Roberta J. Secrest, PhD, PharmD, RPh; Wayne Snyder, MPA, EMT-P; Robert Swor, DO, FACEP; Rob Theriault, EMCA, RCT(Adv), CCP(F); Mike Turner; Anne Walters; Robert B. Wylie, BS, EFO, CFI

Edition Four Models: Mary Jo Adams, Dixie Allen, Noah Cutshall, Morgan Luter, Dusty Sanders, David Sanders, Mandy Sanders, and Daniel Swafford.

Preface

> Chapter Openers set the stage for learning with **Objectives** and **Key Terms** with definitions.

CHAPTER
10 Review of Human Systems

OBJECTIVES

Upon completion of this chapter, the paramedic student will be able to:

1. Discuss the importance of human anatomy as it relates to the paramedic profession.
2. Describe the anatomical position.
3. Properly interpret anatomical directional terms and body planes.
4. List the structures that compose the axial and appendicular regions of the body.
5. Define the divisions of the abdominal region.
6. List the three major body cavities.
7. Describe the contents of the three major body cavities.
8. Discuss the functions of the following cellular structures: the cytoplasmic membrane, the cytoplasm (and organelles), and the nucleus.
9. Describe the process by which human cells reproduce.
10. Differentiate and describe the following tissue types: epithelial tissue, connective tissue, muscle tissue, and nervous tissue.
11. For each of the 11 major organ systems in the human body, label a diagram of anatomical structures; list the functions of the major anatomical structures; and explain how the organs of the system interrelate to perform the specific functions of that system.
12. For the special senses, label a diagram of the anatomical structures of the special senses; list the functions of each sense; and explain how the structures of the senses interrelate to perform their specialized functions.

KEY TERMS

abdominal aorta The portion of the descending aorta that passes from the aortic hiatus of the diaphragm into the abdomen, where it divides into the two common iliac arteries.
acetabulum The large, cup-shaped articular cavity at the juncture of the ilium, the ischium, and the pubis that contains the ball-shaped head of the femur.
action potential A change in membrane potential in an excitable tissue that acts as an electrical signal and is propagated in an all-or-none fashion.
adenosine triphosphate (ATP) A nucleotide composed of adenosine, an organic base, with three phosphate groups

alveoli Minute air sacs in the lungs through which gas exchange takes place between alveolar air and pulmonary capillary blood.
amino acids Organic chemical compounds composed of one or more basic amino groups and one or more acidic carboxyl groups.
antidiuretic hormone (ADH) A hormone produced in the posterior pituitary gland that regulates the balance of water in the body by accelerating the resorption of water.
anus The distal end or outlet of the rectum.
aorta The main and largest artery in the body.
anatomical position The position of standing erect with the feet and palms facing the examiner.

---

756 PART SEVEN · Medical

Viral Pneumonia

Influenza A is the most common type of **viral pneumonia** (Box 24-7). It often occurs as epidemics in populations of small groups such as schoolchildren, army recruits, and nursing home residents. The interstitial infection caused by the virus predisposes the patient to secondary bacterial pneumonia.

Bacterial Pneumonia

Until 2000, the pneumococcus bacillus (*Streptococcus pneumoniae*) accounted for 90% of bacterial pneumonias. It affected 1 in 500 people each year. The decline in cases is related to vaccination of infants against the pneumococcus bacteria. The peak incidence is in winter and early spring. A vaccine that is now available is effective against this type of pneumonia in adults.

? DID YOU KNOW?

Pneumococcal Polysaccharide Vaccine (PPSV)
Pneumococcal disease is the leading cause of vaccine-preventable disease and death in the United States. The disease can lead to serious infections of the lungs (pneumonia), blood (bacteremia), and brain (meningitis). Pneumococcal pneumonia kills about 1 out of 20 people who contract the disease; bacteremia kills about 1 person in 5; and meningitis kills about 3 people in 10.
Pneumococcal polysaccharide vaccine (PPSV) protects against 23 types of pneumococcal bacteria, including those most likely to cause serious disease. Most healthy adults who are vaccinated develop protection to most or all of these types within 2 to 3 weeks of vaccination. Usually only one dose of PPSV is needed, but under some circumstances a second dose may be given. A second dose (given 5 years after the first dose) is recommended for:
• People 65 years and older who received their first dose when they were younger than 65 and it has been 5 or more years since the first dose
• People 2 through 64 years of age who:
  • Have a damaged spleen or no spleen
  • Have sickle cell disease
  • Have HIV infection or AIDS
  • Have cancer, leukemia, lymphoma, or multiple myeloma
  • Have nephrotic syndrome
  • Have received an organ or bone marrow transplant
  • Are taking medication that lowers immunity, such as chemotherapy or long-term steroids
People to whom the vaccine should not be given include those who are allergic to the vaccine or a component of the vaccine; those who are moderately or severely ill; and women who are pregnant. Another type of pneumococcal vaccine, pneumococcal conjugate vaccine, or PCV) is routinely recommended for children younger than 5 years of age.[15]

Bacterial pneumonia also can result from the aspiration of mucus and saliva. Therefore patients in a coma or with seizures, suppressed cough reflex, and increased secretion

BOX 24-7 Influenza

Influenza is an acute, febrile disease that affects the entire body. It is associated with viral infection of the upper and lower respiratory tracts. It usually is characterized by the abrupt onset of a severe protracted cough, fever, headache, muscle ache, and mild sore throat. Of all the viruses, the influenza and parainfluenza viruses are the most common causes of serious respiratory tract infections. Moreover, they have high morbidity and mortality rates.

Influenza viruses A, B, and C (and their many strains) are known for their potential to quickly cause respiratory tract infections after exposure. (It usually occurs within 24 to 48 hours.) The virus is inhaled in respiratory droplets from infected individuals (such as when an infected person sneezes). The droplets penetrate the surface of upper respiratory tract mucosal cells. The virus eventually spreads to the lower respiratory tract, where it causes cell inflammation and destruction of the cilia. Without the cilia, clearing the airways of infected mucus is more difficult. Consequently, a secondary bacterial infection often develops. This may result in pneumonia or acute respiratory failure. (This is particularly the case in patients with chronic lung disease.)

Influenza has the potential for widespread epidemics in high-risk populations. (These include adults and children with chronic cardiorespiratory or metabolic disorders, residents of nursing homes and other institutions, and health care workers.) Current vaccines are effective against some strains of the flu. These vaccines have minimal side effects. If uncomplicated, influenza is self-limiting. Acute symptoms last 2 to 7 days. These are followed by a convalescent period of about 1 week.
NOTE: The H1N1 outbreak of 2009 affected healthy young people and pregnant women disproportionately, compared with other influenza viruses (see Chapter 28).

---

are predisposed to developing the disease. Other predisposing risk factors that may contribute to the development of bacterial pneumonia include the following:
• Infection
  • Upper respiratory tract infection (influenza)
  • Postoperative infection
• Foreign body aspiration
• Alcohol or other drug addiction
• Cardiac failure
• Stroke
• Syncope
• Pulmonary embolism
• Chronic illness
  • Chronic respiratory disease
  • Diabetes mellitus
  • Congestive heart failure
• Prolonged immobilization
• Compromised immune status

Mycoplasmal Pneumonia

Mycoplasmal pneumonia is caused by *Mycoplasma pneumoniae*. It causes respiratory tract infection in school-age children

> **Did You Know?** boxes expand on interesting and relevant information, such as unusual facts and figures, "nice-to-know" data, and "need-to-know" material.

---

576 PART SIX · Cardiovascular

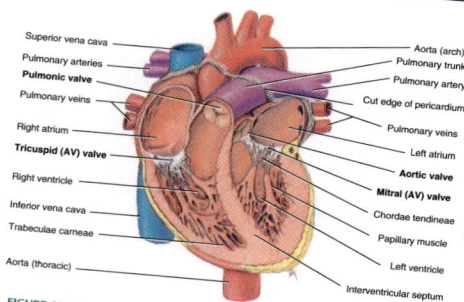

FIGURE 22-1 Internal view of the heart showing the chambers. (Applegate EM: *The anatomy and physiology learning system*, ed 3, St Louis, 2007, Saunders.)

ventricle and pulmonary trunk is the pulmonary semilunar valve. The valve between the left ventricle and the aorta is the aortic semilunar valve. When the ventricles contract, atrioventricular valves close to prevent blood from flowing back into the atria. When the ventricles relax, semilunar valves close to prevent blood from flowing back into the ventricles.

Blood Supply to the Heart

The coronary arteries are the sole suppliers of arterial blood to the heart. They deliver 200 to 250 mL of blood to the myocardium each minute during rest (Figure 22-2). The left coronary artery carries about 85% of the blood supply to the myocardium. The right coronary artery carries the rest. The coronary arteries begin just above the aortic valve where the aorta exits the heart. These arteries run along the epicardial surface. They divide into smaller vessels as they penetrate the myocardium and the endocardial (inner) surface.

The left main coronary artery supplies the left ventricle, the interventricular septum, and part of the right ventricle. Its two main branches are the left anterior descending artery and the circumflex artery. The right coronary artery supplies the right atrium and ventricle, part of the left ventricle, and the conduction system. Its two main branches are the right anterior descending branch and the marginal branch. In addition to the blood supply provided by the coronary arteries, many connections (anastomoses) exist between arterioles to provide backup (collateral) circulation. These anastomoses play a key role in providing alternative routes

of blood flow in the event one or more of the coronary vessels become blocked (Figure 22-3).

📍 CRITICAL THINKING
Why is collateral circulation important?

Coronary capillaries allow the exchange of nutrients and metabolic wastes. They merge to form coronary veins. These veins deliver most of the blood to the right atrium. The coronary sinus empties directly into the right atrium. The coronary sinus is the major vein draining the myocardium.

PHYSIOLOGY

The heart can be thought of as two pumps in one. One is a low-pressure pump (right atrium and right ventricle). This pump supplies blood to the lungs. The other is a high-pressure pump (left atrium and left ventricle). This pump supplies blood to the body. The right atrium receives blood from the systemic circulation. The right atrium receives

> Boxed **Critical Thinking** questions aid in understanding concepts and how chapter content impacts patient care.

XV

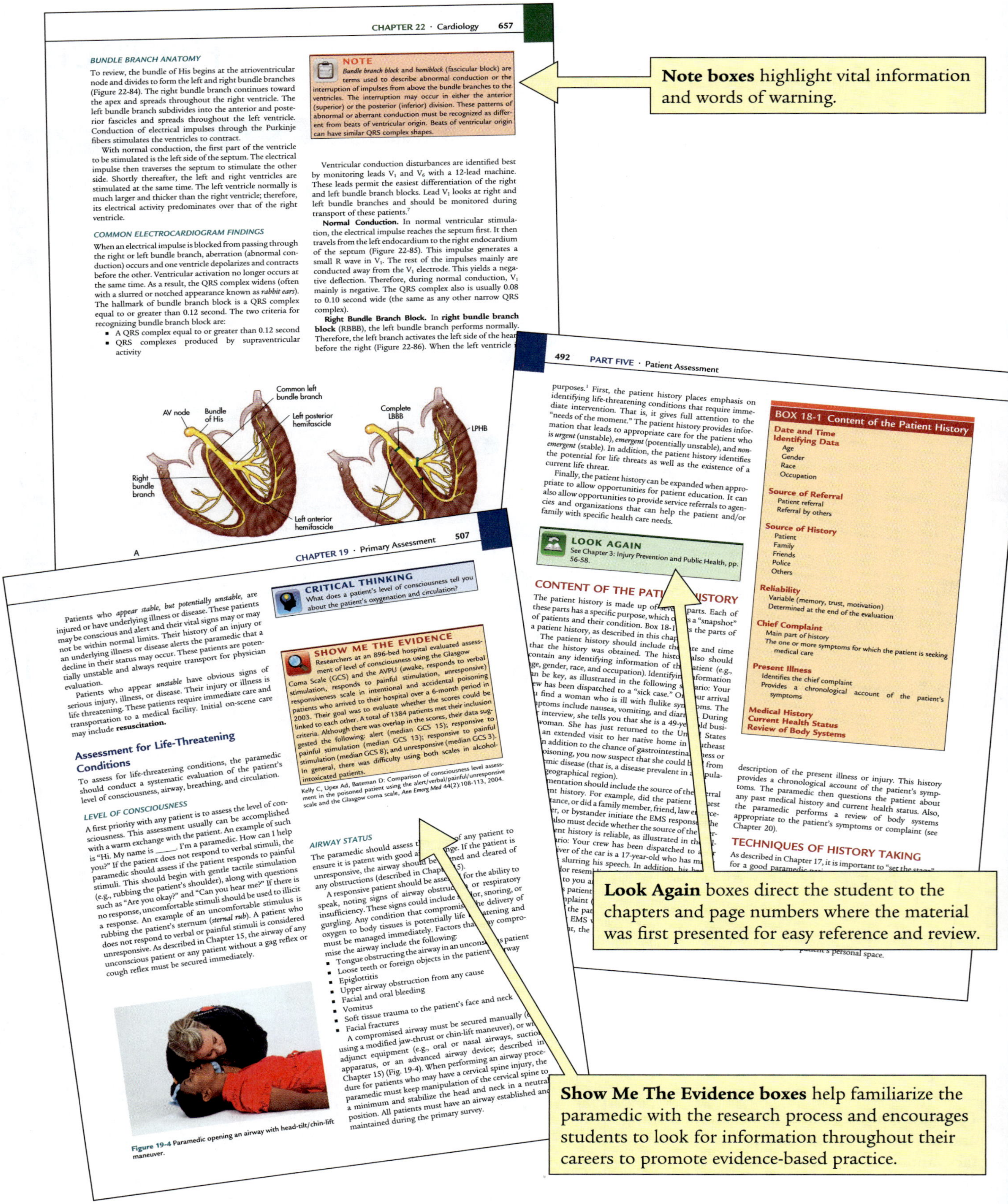

BUNDLE BRANCH ANATOMY

To review, the bundle of His begins at the atrioventricular node and divides to form the left and right bundle branches (Figure 22-84). The right bundle continues toward the apex and spreads throughout the right ventricle. The left bundle branch subdivides into the anterior and posterior fascicles and spreads throughout the left ventricle. Conduction of electrical impulses through the Purkinje fibers stimulates the ventricles to contract.

With normal conduction, the first part of the ventricle to be stimulated is the left side of the septum. The electrical impulse then traverses the septum to stimulate the other side. Shortly thereafter, the left and right ventricles are stimulated at the same time. The left ventricle normally is much larger and thicker than the right ventricle; therefore, its electrical activity predominates over that of the right ventricle.

COMMON ELECTROCARDIOGRAM FINDINGS

When an electrical impulse is blocked from passing through the right or left bundle branch, aberration (abnormal conduction) occurs and one ventricle depolarizes and contracts before the other. Ventricular activation no longer occurs at the same time. As a result, the QRS complex widens (often with a slurred or notched appearance known as *rabbit ears*). The hallmark of bundle branch block is a QRS complex equal to or greater than 0.12 second. The two criteria for recognizing bundle branch block are:

- A QRS complex equal to or greater than 0.12 second
- QRS complexes produced by supraventricular activity

NOTE
Bundle branch block and *hemiblock* (fascicular block) are terms used to describe abnormal conduction or the interruption of impulses from the bundle branches to the ventricles. The interruption may occur in either the anterior (superior) or the posterior (inferior) division. These patterns of abnormal or aberrant conduction must be recognized as different from beats of ventricular origin. Beats of ventricular origin can have similar QRS complex shapes.

Ventricular conduction disturbances are identified best by monitoring leads V_1 and V_6 with a 12-lead machine. These leads permit the easiest differentiation of the right and left bundle branch blocks. Lead V_1 looks at right and left bundle branches and should be monitored during transport of these patients.[7]

Normal Conduction. In normal ventricular stimulation, the electrical impulse reaches the septum first. It then travels from the left endocardium to the right endocardium of the septum (Figure 22-85). This impulse generates a small R wave in V_1. The rest of the impulses mainly are conducted away from the V_1 electrode. This yields a negative deflection. Therefore, during normal conduction, V_1 mainly is negative. The QRS complex also is usually 0.08 to 0.10 second wide (the same as any other narrow QRS complex).

Right Bundle Branch Block. In **right bundle branch block** (RBBB), the left bundle branch performs normally. Therefore, the left branch activates the left side of the heart before the right (Figure 22-86). When the left ventricle

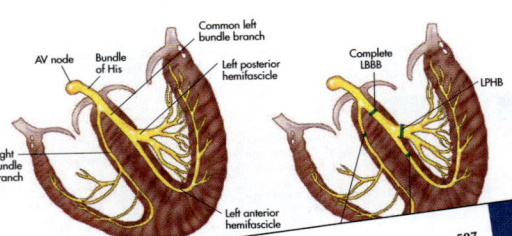

Common left bundle branch
AV node
Bundle of His
Left posterior hemifascicle
Complete LBBB
LPHB
Right bundle branch
Left anterior hemifascicle

A

Note boxes highlight vital information and words of warning.

---

purposes.[1] First, the patient history places emphasis on identifying life-threatening conditions that require immediate intervention. That is, it gives full attention to the "needs of the moment." The patient history provides information that leads to appropriate care for the patient who is *urgent* (unstable), *emergent* (potentially unstable), and *nonemergent* (stable). In addition, the patient history identifies the potential for life threats as well as the existence of a current life threat.

Finally, the patient history can be expanded when appropriate to allow opportunities for patient education. It can also allow opportunities to provide service referrals to agencies and organizations that can help the patient and/or family with specific health care needs.

LOOK AGAIN
See Chapter 3: Injury Prevention and Public Health, pp. 56-58.

CONTENT OF THE PATIENT HISTORY

The patient history is made up of several parts. Each of these parts has a specific purpose, which gives a "snapshot" of patients and their condition. Box 18-1 lists the parts of a patient history, as described in this chapter.

The patient history should include the date and time that the history was obtained. The history also should contain any identifying information of the patient (e.g., age, gender, race, and occupation). Identifying information can be key, as illustrated in the following scenario: Your crew has been dispatched to a "sick case." On your arrival you find a woman who is ill with flulike symptoms. During your interview, she tells you that she is a 49-year-old business woman. She has just returned to the United States from an extended visit to her native home in a northeast Asian country. In addition to the chance of gastrointestinal poisoning, you now suspect that she could be exposed to an endemic disease (that is, a disease prevalent in a population or geographical region).

...mentation should include the source of the ...nt history. For example, did the patient ...tance, or did a family member, friend, law e ...er, or bystander initiate the EMS response ...also must decide whether the source of the ...ient history is reliable, as illustrated in the ...rio: Your crew has been dispatched to a ...ver of the car is a 17-year-old who has m ...slurring his speech. In addition, his b ...for resem... ...to you a ...e patient ...plaint (se ...the pa ...EMS ...t, the

BOX 18-1 Content of the Patient History

Date and Time
Identifying Data
- Age
- Gender
- Race
- Occupation

Source of Referral
- Patient referral
- Referral by others

Source of History
- Patient
- Family
- Friends
- Police
- Others

Reliability
- Variable (memory, trust, motivation)
- Determined at the end of the evaluation

Chief Complaint
- Main part of history
- The one or more symptoms for which the patient is seeking medical care

Present Illness
- Identifies the chief complaint
- Provides a chronological account of the patient's symptoms

Medical History
Current Health Status
Review of Body Systems

description of the present illness or injury. This history provides a chronological account of the patient's symptoms. The paramedic then questions the patient about any past medical history and current health status. Also, the paramedic performs a review of body systems appropriate to the patient's symptoms or complaint (see Chapter 20).

TECHNIQUES OF HISTORY TAKING

As described in Chapter 17, it is important to "set the stage" for a good paramedic p...

Look Again boxes direct the student to the chapters and page numbers where the material was first presented for easy reference and review.

Patients who *appear stable, but potentially unstable,* are injured or have underlying illness or disease. These patients may be conscious and alert and their vital signs may or may not be within normal limits. Their history of an injury or an underlying illness or disease alerts the paramedic that a decline in their status may occur. These patients are potentially unstable and always require transport for physician evaluation.

Patients who appear *unstable* have obvious signs of serious injury, illness, or disease. Their injury or illness is life threatening. These patients require immediate care and transportation to a medical facility. Initial on-scene care may include **resuscitation.**

Assessment for Life-Threatening Conditions

To assess for life-threatening conditions, the paramedic should conduct a systematic evaluation of the patient's level of consciousness, airway, breathing, and circulation.

LEVEL OF CONSCIOUSNESS

A first priority with any patient is to assess the level of consciousness. This assessment usually can be accomplished with a warm exchange with the patient. An example of such is "Hi. My name is _____. I'm a paramedic. How can I help you?" If the patient does not respond to verbal stimuli, the paramedic should assess if the patient responds to painful stimuli. This should begin with gentle tactile stimulation (e.g., rubbing the patient's shoulder), along with questions such as "Are you okay?" and "Can you hear me?" If there is no response, uncomfortable stimuli should be used to elicit a response. An example of an uncomfortable stimulus is rubbing the patient's sternum (*sternal rub*). A patient who does not respond to verbal or painful stimuli is considered unresponsive. As described in Chapter 15, the airway of any unconscious patient or any patient without a gag reflex or cough reflex must be secured immediately.

CRITICAL THINKING
What does a patient's level of consciousness tell you about the patient's oxygenation and circulation?

SHOW ME THE EVIDENCE
Researchers at an 896-bed hospital evaluated assessment of level of consciousness using the Glasgow Coma Scale (GCS) and the AVPU (awake, responds to verbal stimulation, responds to painful stimulation, unresponsive) responsiveness scale in intentional and accidental poisoning patients who arrived to their hospital over a 6-month period in 2003. Their goal was to evaluate whether the scores could be linked to each other. A total of 1384 patients met their inclusion criteria. Although there was overlap in the scores, their data suggested the following: alert (median GCS 15); responsive to verbal painful stimulation (mean GCS 13); responsive to painful stimulation (median GCS 8); and unresponsive (median GCS 3). In general, there was difficulty using both scales in alcohol-intoxicated patients.

Kelly C, Upex Ad, Bateman D: Comparison of consciousness level assessment in the poisoned patient using the alert/verbal/painful/unresponsive scale and the Glasgow coma scale, *Ann Emerg Med* 44(2):108-113, 2004.

AIRWAY STATUS

The paramedic should assess the airway of any patient to ensure it is patent with good air exchange. If the patient is unresponsive, the airway should be examined and cleared of any obstructions (described in Chapter 15).

A responsive patient should be assessed for the ability to speak, noting signs of airway obstruction. Labor or respiratory insufficiency. These signs could be stridor, snoring, or gurgling. Any condition that compromises the delivery of oxygen to body tissues is potentially life threatening and must be managed immediately. Factors that may compromise the airway include the following:

- Tongue obstructing the airway in an unconscious patient
- Loose teeth or foreign objects in the patient's airway
- Epiglottitis
- Upper airway obstruction from any cause
- Facial and oral bleeding
- Vomitus
- Soft tissue trauma to the patient's face and neck
- Facial fractures

A compromised airway must be secured manually (e.g., using a modified jaw-thrust or chin-lift maneuver), or with adjunct equipment (e.g., oral or nasal airways, suction apparatus, or an advanced airway device; described in Chapter 15) (Fig. 19-4). When performing an airway procedure for patients who may have a cervical spine injury, the paramedic must keep manipulation of the cervical spine to a minimum and stabilize the head and neck in a neutral position. All patients must have an airway established and maintained during the primary survey.

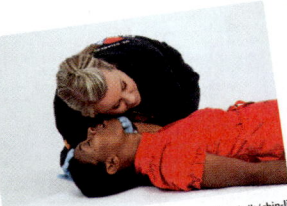

Figure 19-4 Paramedic opening an airway with head-tilt/chin-lift maneuver.

Show Me The Evidence boxes help familiarize the paramedic with the research process and encourages students to look for information throughout their careers to promote evidence-based practice.

More than 1500 photographs and illustrations–
including approximately **150 new** illustrations–support
the text content, including anatomy, physiology,
patient management guidelines, equipment, and skills.

Perfect for review, each chapter includes a bulleted
Summary and a list of **References** (most chapters
include suggested readings).

Emergency Drug Index lists 78 commonly prescribed
medications that are used in prehospital care.

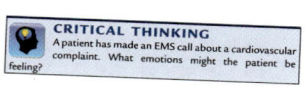

CHAPTER 22 · Cardiology   675

Anterior view   Posterior view

Midclavicular line

Left   Right

V₈ V₉

FIGURE 22-111 Lead placement for V4ᵣ and V₈ and V₉.

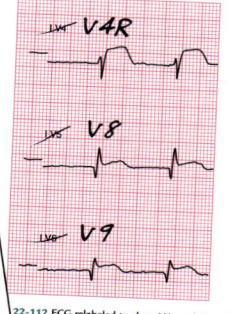

22-112 ECG relabeled to show V4ᵣ and V₈ and V₉.

CRITICAL THINKING
A patient has made an EMS call about a cardiovascular complaint. What emotions might the patient be feeling?

Chief Complaint

Cardiovascular disease may cause a variety of symptoms. Obtaining an appropriate history of each symptom is important to form a diagnostic impression of any patient with a possible coronary event. Common chief complaints include chest pain or discomfort, including shoulder, arm, neck, or jaw pain or discomfort; dyspnea; syncope; and abnormal heartbeat or palpitations.

In some patients (e.g., some women, older adults, and patients with diabetes), cardiovascular problems commonly have atypical symptoms. These include mental status changes, abdominal or gastrointestinal symptoms (including persistent heartburn), and vague complaints of feeling ill.

CHEST PAIN OR DISCOMFORT

Chest pain or discomfort is the most common chief complaint of patients with myocardial infarction. However, many causes of chest pain are not related to cardiac disease (e.g., pulmonary embolus, pleurisy, reflux esophagitis). Therefore, a history of chest pain is a key factor. The OPQRST method (or a similar method) should be used to

---

22   PART ONE · Preparatory

we are working on it. It helps us as we complete a task. Reflection in action promotes critical thinking and bridges the gap between "knowing and doing."

- **Question assumptions:** Apply critical thinking to continuously look for good ideas and new solutions. This will help to set priorities and to problem solve.
- **Reflection bias ("hindsight" bias):** Avoid the tendency to judge an experience you had. ("I knew that was going to happen.") Reflection bias is the inclination to see events that have occurred in the past as more predictable than they really were. Review the events after the fact and you

might foresee the outcome as more preventable. Replace hindsight with insight.

- **Use decision aids:** Use evidence-based decision aids and guidelines (e.g., algorithms, pocket guides) to simplify decision making and improve patient safety. Decision aids can also facilitate patients' participation in decisions about their care, when appropriate.
- **Ask for help:** You are functioning as part of a team. Don't be hesitant to ask your crew members or medical direction for help or advice, if the need arises. If you are unsure about a decision, drug dose, or procedure, remember that patient safety comes first.

SUMMARY

- The roots of prehospital emergency care may date back to the military.
- In the early twentieth century through the mid-1960s, prehospital care in the United States was provided in a few ways. Care was provided mostly by urban hospital-based systems. These systems later developed into municipal services. Care also was provided by funeral directors and volunteers who were not trained in these services.
- The operations of an effective EMS system include citizen activation, dispatch, prehospital care, hospital care, and rehabilitation.
- Each level of EMS personnel have their own distinct roles and duties. These roles include telecommunicators (dispatchers), emergency medical responders, EMTs, advanced EMTs, and paramedics. These levels combine to make an effective prehospital EMS system.
- Many professional groups and organizations help to set the standards of EMS. These groups exist at the national, state, regional, and local levels. The groups take part in development, education, and implementation. Being active in such a group helps to promote the status of the paramedic.
- Continuing education is crucial. It provides a way for all health care personnel to maintain basic technical and professional skills.

- Professionalism refers to the way in which a person conducts himself or herself. Professionalism also refers to how one follows the standards of conduct and performance established by the profession.
- The roles and duties of the paramedic can be divided into two categories: *primary* and *additional* duties.
- The two types of medical direction are online (direct) and off-line (indirect). Both are equally important. They help to ensure that the components of quality medical care are in place in an EMS system.
- A CQI program identifies and attempts to resolve problems in areas such as medical direction, financing, training, communication, prehospital management, transportation, interfacility transfer, receiving facilities, specialty care units, dispatch, public information, education, audit and quality assurance, disaster planning, and mutual aid.
- Patient safety should be a high priority during events. Errors that may cause injury or illness often handoffs, communication issues, medication airway issues, lifting or moving patients, crashes, and immobilization.

REFERENCES

1. Lyons A, Petrucelli J: *Medicine: an illustrated history*, New York, 1987, Harry N Abrams.
2. McSwain NE: Prehospital care from Napoleon to Mars: The surgeon's role, *J Am Coll Surg* 201(4):651, 2005.
3. [...] www.redcross.org/museum/registry/profile.asp?id= [...] accessed 3-15-09.
4. [...] JE: Airborne care of the ill and injured, New York, 1983, Springer-Verlag.
5. EMS: Past, Present, Future, NAEMT, www.naemt.org/ education, accessed 3-15-09.
6. National Highway Traffic Safety Administration, Health Resources and

Services Administration, Maternal and Child Health Bureau: Emergency medical services agenda [...] Washington, DC, 1999.
7. Munir GM: Access to health care in the [...] the bottom line, http://www.articlecity.com [...] and_government/article_525.shtml, accessed [...]
8. National Highway Traffic Safety [...] National EMS Scope of Practice model [...] 2005, U.S. Department of Transportation [...] Traffic Safety Administration.
9. National Highway Traffic Safety Administration, Department of Transportation: Emergency [...] leading the way, Washington, DC, [...]

Emergency Drug Index   1579

AMIODARONE (CORDARONE)

CLASS

Class III antidysrhythmic

DESCRIPTION

Amiodarone is a unique antidysrhythmic agent with multiple mechanisms of action. The drug prolongs the duration of the action potential and the effective refractory period, and when given short-term IV, probably includes noncompetitive beta-adrenergic receptor and calcium channel blocker activity.

ONSET AND DURATION

Onset: Within minutes
Duration: Variable

INDICATIONS (IV USE)

Initial treatment and prophylaxis of frequently recurring ventricular fibrillation and hemodynamically unstable ventricular tachycardia in patients unresponsive to shock delivery, CPR, and vasopressors
Recurrent hemodynamically unstable VT
Treatment of some stable atrial and ventricular dysrhythmias

CONTRAINDICATIONS

Pulmonary congestion
Cardiogenic shock
Second- or third-degree AV block if no pacemaker present
Bradycardia
Sensitivity to amiodarone or iodine

ADVERSE REACTIONS

Hypotension
Headache
Dizziness
Bradycardia
Atrioventricular conduction abnormalities
Flushing
Abnormal salivation
Pain at IV site
Liver function abnormalities
Congestive heart failure
Abnormal thyroid function

DRUG INTERACTIONS

May potentiate bradycardia and hypotension with beta blockers and calcium channel blockers.
May increase risk of atrioventricular block and hypotension with calcium channel blockers.
May increase anticoagulant effects of warfarin.
May decrease metabolism and increase serum levels of phenytoin, procainamide, quinidine, and theophyllines.
Routine use in combination with drugs that prolong the Q-T interval is not recommended.
Y-site incompatibilities with furosemide, heparin, and sodium bicarbonate

HOW SUPPLIED

50 mg/mL vials

DOSAGE AND ADMINISTRATION

Adult:
Pulseless arrest unresponsive to CPR, shock, and vasopressors: 300 mg IV/IO push. If needed, second dose of 150 mg IV/IO push
Life-threatening dysrhythmias: Max cumulative dose: 2.2 g IV/24 hr. May be given as rapid infusion 150 mg IV over first 10 min (15 mg/min) repeated every 10 min as needed. Slow infusion: 360 mg IV over 6 hr (1 mg/min). Maintenance infusion: 540 mg IV over 18 hr (0.5 mg/min)
Pediatric:
Refractory VF, pulseless VT: 5 mg/kg rapid IV/IO bolus; can be repeated to total dose of 15 mg/kg (2.2 g in adolescents) IV per 24 hr; max single dose: 300 mg
Perfusing supraventricular and ventricular dysrhythmias: Loading dose 5 mg/kg IV/IO over 20-60 min (max single dose: 300 mg); can repeat to a max of 15 mg/kg (2.2 g in adolescents) per day IV

SPECIAL CONSIDERATIONS

Pregnancy safety: Category D
Rapid infusion may cause hypotension.
Continuous electrocardiogram monitoring is required.
Slow infusion or discontinue if bradycardia or atrioventricular block occurs.
Do not give with other drugs that prolong Q-T interval (e.g., procainamide).
Maintain at room temperature and protect from excessive heat.

ASPIRIN (ASA, BAYER, ECOTRIN, ST. JOSEPH, OTHERS)

CLASS

Analgesic, antiinflammatory, antipyretic, antiplatelet

DESCRIPTION

Aspirin decreases inflammation (analgesic effect not limited to effects in CNS), dilates peripheral vessels, and decreases platelet aggregation. The use of aspirin is strongly recommended for all patients with acute coronary syndrome.

ONSET AND DURATION

Onset: 15-30 min
Duration: 4-6 hr

INDICATIONS

Mild to moderate pain or fever
Prevention of platelet aggregation in ischemia and thromboembolism
All patients [...]

Contents

PART ONE

Preparatory

1 EMS Systems: Roles, Responsibilities, and Professionalism

Upon completion of this chapter, the paramedic student will be able to:

1. Outline key historical events that influenced the development of emergency medical services (EMS) systems.
2. Identify the key elements necessary for effective EMS systems operations.
3. Outline the five components of the *EMS Education Agenda for the Future: A Systems Approach.*
4. Describe the benefits of continuing education.
5. Differentiate among the training and roles and responsibilities of the four nationally recognized levels of EMS licensure/certification: Emergency Medical Responder, Emergency Medical Technician, Advanced Emergency Medical Technician, and Paramedic.
6. List the benefits of membership in professional EMS organizations.
7. Differentiate among professionalism, professional licensure, certification, registration, and credentialing.
8. List characteristics of the professional paramedic.
9. Describe the paramedic's role in patient care situations as defined by the U.S. Department of Transportation.
10. Describe the benefits of each component of off-line (indirect) and online (direct) medical direction.
11. Outline the role and components of an effective continuous quality improvement program.
12. Recognize EMS activities that pose a high risk for patients.
13. Describe actions paramedics may take to reduce the chance of errors related to patient care.

KEY TERMS

advanced life support The provision of care that paramedics or allied health professionals render, including advanced airway management, defibrillation, intravenous therapy, and medication administration.

basic life support Care provided by persons trained in first aid, cardiopulmonary resuscitation, and other noninvasive care.

certification A process by which authority is granted to a person to take part in an activity. This person has to meet certain qualifications.

code of ethics A set of guidelines that are designed to set out acceptable behaviors for members of a particular group, association, or profession.

continuous quality improvement A management approach to customer service and organizational performance that includes constant monitoring, evaluation, decisions, and actions.

credentialing A local process that allows a paramedic to practice in a specific EMS agency (or setting).

emergency medical services A national network of services coordinated to provide aid and medical assistance from primary response to definitive care; the network involves personnel trained in rescue, stabilization, transportation, and advanced management of traumatic and medical emergencies.

extended scope of practice The expansion of health care services provided by emergency medical services personnel in the prehospital setting.

licensure A process of regulating occupations through licenses granted by a government authority.

managed care organizations Networks that provide patient care services to their members, including health maintenance organizations and preferred provider organizations.

medical oversight The ultimate responsibility and authority for the medical actions of an EMS system; usually provided by one or more physicians.

off-line (indirect) medical direction The establishment and oversight of all medical components of an EMS system, including protocols, standing orders, educational programs, and the quality and delivery of online (direct) medical direction.

online (direct) medical direction The medical direction physician or designee who directly supervises prehospital care activities via radio or phone. Online (direct) medical direction also may be responsible for the activities of the emergency department staff and others at the medical direction hospital.

paramedic A person who has completed training consistent with the National EMS Education Standards, including advanced training in clinical decision making, patient assessment, cardiac rhythm interpretation, defibrillation, drug therapy, and airway management.

patient care report A document used in the prehospital setting to record all patient care activities and circumstances related to an emergency response.

peritracheal Situated or occurring in the tissues surrounding the trachea.

registration The act of enrolling one's name in a register, or book of record.

reciprocity The practice of granting an individual licensure or certification/registration based on licensure or certification/registration by another state, agency, or association.

standing orders Specific treatment protocols used by prehospital emergency care personnel in the absence of online (direct) medical direction.

treatment protocols Guidelines that define the scope of prehospital intervention practiced by emergency services personnel.

*T*he role of the paramedic is different than that of the "ambulance driver" of the past. Today's paramedics work in sophisticated **emergency medical services** (EMS) systems. They take part in an array of professional activities. These activities enhance the paramedic's ability to provide quality service and state-of-the-art patient care in the field and in less traditional health care settings.

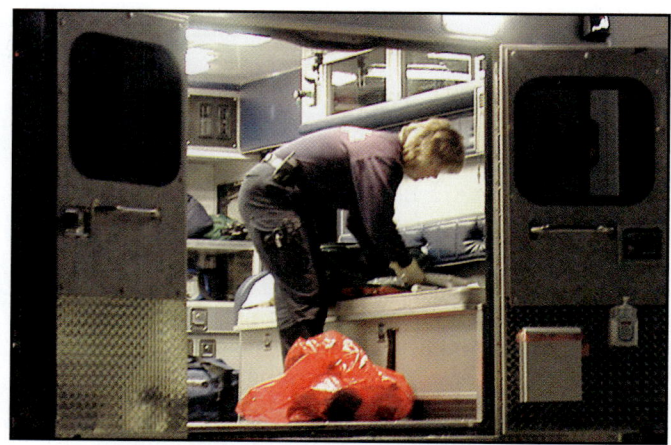

(Courtesy Ray Kemp, St. Charles, Mo.)

EMERGENCY MEDICAL SERVICES SYSTEM DEVELOPMENT

Assigning a time and place to the birth of organized prehospital emergency care is difficult. To understand EMS system development, one must first consider certain events from ancient times to the present.

Before the Twentieth Century

The ancient Egyptians used herbs and drugs as medicine. They also splinted fractured bones, and they performed some surgeries. The Edwin Smith papyrus (circa the seventeenth century BC) depicted medical practice in Egypt. This system referred to the pulsation of the heart, palpation, and abnormal motor functions associated with brain injury. Other ancient texts show that surgery was practiced by the Babylonians of Mesopotamia, an ancient region of southwest Asia, as early as 1700 BC.[1]

Organized prehospital emergency care has its roots in military history. Paintings of Roman battlefields suggest that some of the warriors cared for the injured. The first "ambulance" is thought to have been a covered cart used by one of Napoleon's surgeons, Dominique-Jean Larrey. He moved injured soldiers to treatment areas during the Napoleonic wars in the 1800s.[1] The first civilian ambulance services were established in Cincinnati and New York City in the 1860s. In the United States Civil War, there was scandal when Walt Whitman and Matthew Brady reported that

3000 wounded soldiers lay in the field for 3 days and 600 for a week during the 1862 Battle of Bull Run. In response, Surgeon General Jonathan Letterman created an ambulance service for each army corps. They evacuated 10,000 wounded soldiers within 24 hours at the Battle of Antietam in 1863.[2]

? DID YOU KNOW?
Clara Barton was an American nurse who served as a frontline volunteer during the American Civil War. She saw first-hand the value of the Red Cross during the Franco-Prussian War of 1870. These experiences encouraged her to establish a society in the United States. Under her leadership, the American Red Cross became the premier disaster relief organization in the world. Clara Barton was the founder and first president of the American Red Cross, which was established on May 21, 1881, in Washington, D.C.[3]

Twentieth Century

During World War I, medical care made rapid progress. Wounded soldiers needed urgent care for their injuries, which often were caused by machine guns and bombs. Thus the military developed battlefield ambulance corps. During World War II, the military moved wounded soldiers by airplane. Then during the Korean conflict, the military evacuated soldiers with helicopters. During the Vietnam conflict, the military improved urgent care and rapid evacuation with well-trained corpsmen. These efforts became the basis of the prehospital care of the injured today.

From the early twentieth century through the mid-1960s, prehospital care in the United States was provided in several ways. Care mostly was delivered by urban, hospital-based systems. These systems later developed into municipal services. Care also was provided by funeral directors and volunteers who had little or no training in emergency care. Most patients received minimal stabilization at the scene. Then they were transported quickly to the nearest hospital.

CRITICAL THINKING
How would you feel about moving to an area with this minimal level of emergency medical services?

Two landmarks in EMS development occurred in 1966:
1. The National Academy of Sciences–National Research Council Committee on Trauma and Shock published *Accidental Death and Disability: The Neglected Disease of Modern Society* (the "white paper"). This document lists recommendations to improve care for victims. Eleven of these recommendations are related directly to EMS (Box 1-1).
2. The U.S. Congress passed the Highway Safety Act of 1966. This act created the U.S. Department of Transportation. Congress also created the National Highway Traffic Safety Administration (NHTSA). The act provided legislative authority and funds to improve EMS and directed states to develop effective EMS programs. If the states did not develop effective EMS programs, they were subject to a loss of up to 10% of their federal highway construction funds. As a result of this act, states gave more than $142 million between 1968 and 1979 to develop EMS and early **advanced life support** (ALS) pilot programs.

Emergency medical services also emerged as a nationwide system because of death rate comparisons from World War I to Vietnam. Death rates for battlefield casualties were 8% in World War I. In World War II, they were 4.5%. In Korea, they decreased to 2.5%. Then in Vietnam, they were less than 2%. This decline was due to advances in field care for trauma patients (Box 1-2).[4] These and other factors helped formulate the blueprint for improving prehospital emergency medical care in the United States. During 1972 and 1973, federal and private sources provided $31 million to fund EMS programs in 37 states and Puerto Rico.

In 1973, Congress passed the Emergency Medical Service Systems (EMSS) Act. This act paved the way for states to benefit from federal funds. The states could obtain the

BOX 1-1 Eleven Recommendations for Emergency Medical Services Identified in the White Paper

1. Extension of basic and advanced first aid training to greater numbers of the lay public
2. Preparation of nationally acceptable texts, training aids, and courses of instruction for rescue squad personnel, police officers, firefighters, and ambulance attendants
3. Implementation of recent traffic safety legislation to ensure completely adequate standards for ambulance design and construction, ambulance equipment and supplies, and the qualifications and supervision of ambulance personnel
4. Adoption at the state level of general policies and regulations pertaining to ambulance services
5. Adoption at district, county, and municipal levels of ways and means of providing ambulance services applicable to the conditions of the locality, control and surveillance of ambulance services, and coordination of ambulance services with health departments, hospitals, traffic authorities, and communication services
6. Initiation of pilot programs to determine the efficacy of providing physician-staffed ambulances for care at the site of injury and during transportation
7. Initiation of pilot programs to evaluate automotive and helicopter ambulance services in sparsely populated areas and in regions where many communities lack hospital facilities adequate to care for seriously injured persons
8. Delineation of radio frequency channels and equipment suitable to provide voice communication between ambulances, emergency departments, and other health-related agencies at the community, regional, and national levels
9. Initiation of pilot studies across the nation for evaluation of models of radio and telephone installations to ensure effectiveness of communication facilities
10. Day-to-day use of voice communication facilities by the agencies serving emergency medical needs
11. Active exploration of the feasibility of designating a single nationwide telephone number to summon an ambulance

From National Academy of Sciences, National Research Council: *Accidental death and disability: the neglected disease of modern society*, Washington, DC, 1996, National Academy Press.

funds by forming regional EMS agencies. The act listed 15 vital parts of the EMS system (Box 1-3). Plus, the act required emergency care programs funded by the U.S. Department of Health and Human Services to plan and put into practice a regional approach for emergency response and immediate care for trauma patients. This act played a major role in creating regional EMS systems from 1974 to 1981.

CRITICAL THINKING
How does the "age" of the emergency medical services profession compare with the "age" of your parents' or grandparents' professions?

BOX 1-2 Medical Advances Made During Wartime

Civil War
- Railroads were used to evacuate casualties
- Army still used ambulances much like Napoleon's
- Death rate was very high because germs were unknown as the cause of infection; barns were used as hospitals
- U.S. Army set up the Medical Corps
- System-wide approach with ambulances on the battlefield transporting wounded to hospitals
  Aid stations
  Field hospitals
  Rear general hospitals
  This model was used until the Vietnam War

World War I
- Poor planning (no field hospitals) caused excessive evacuation times of 12-18 hours
- High mortality rates >20%
- Most died of hemorrhagic shock
- No antibiotics; sepsis was common
- Blood transfusions were just beginning to be used
- Thomas half-ring femur splint was considered the greatest advancement in trauma care at this time

World War II
- Evacuation time for wounded decreased to 4-6 hours
- Antibiotics were developed
- Plasma and blood transfusions became common
- Hospitals were located closer to the front to decrease time to surgery
- Fixed wing air transport began

Korean War
- Evacuation time averaged 2-4 hours
- Helicopter evacuation of wounded was introduced
- More use of electrolyte solutions
- Better antibiotics
- Surgical hospitals located closer to front lines

Vietnam War
- Casualties were taken directly from front lines to surgical hospitals by helicopter
- Average evacuation time was 35 minutes
- Average time to surgery was 1-2 hours
- Civilian systems have never matched these timeframes

Iraq War
- Tourniquets were reintroduced
- Hemostatic agents were developed
- Concept of CAB (circulation-airway-breathing) was developed for patients with exsanguinating hemorrhage[5]

BOX 1-3 Fifteen Required Components of the Emergency Medical Services System

1. Manpower
2. Training
3. Communications
4. Transportation
5. Facilities
6. Critical care units
7. Public safety agencies
8. Consumers
9. Access to care
10. Transfer of patients
11. Medical record keeping
12. Consumer information and education
13. Review and evaluation
14. Disaster linkage
15. Mutual aid

BOX 1-4 The 10 System Elements of the National Highway Traffic Safety Administration

1. Comprehensive emergency medical services and trauma system legislation
2. Resource management and administration
3. Professional training
4. A communication system (9-1-1, communication centers, equipment, and the ability to communicate among ambulances, hospitals, fire departments, and police)
5. A transportation system (air, ground, and water)
6. Facilities (hospitals, trauma centers, specialty centers)
7. An inclusive trauma system fully integrated with emergency medical systems
8. Physician involvement (medical oversight)
9. Public information, education, and prevention
10. Data collection, quality improvement and evaluation, and research.

From National Highway Traffic Safety Administration: *Emergency medical services: NHTSA leading the way*, Washington, DC, 1995, The Administration.

In 1981, funding for EMS development changed due to the Consolidated Omnibus Budget Reconciliation Act (COBRA). This act consolidated EMS funding into state preventive health services block grants. As a result, funding under the EMSS Act was eliminated. These block grants were paid to state health departments instead of regional EMS organizations. Because these grants could be spent on projects other than EMS, the grants fell victim to politics. Thus direct funding for EMS declined. Through cuts in funding and staff, the ability of NHTSA to support the U.S. Department of Health and Human Services effort diminished. As a result, each state had to develop and fund their EMS systems. Thus the great growth that EMS experienced in the 1960s and 1970s declined. NHTSA continues to assist EMS development.[6] In 1988 NHTSA established "10 System Elements" (the Statewide EMS Technical Assistance Program) as a recommended standard for EMS systems (Box 1-4).

In 1996 NHTSA and the Health Resources and Services Administration (HRSA) published a consensus paper that was held in high regard. This document, the *Emergency Medical Services Agenda for the Future*, was referred to as the *Agenda*. The *Agenda* was federally funded and completed by the National Association of EMS Physicians and the National Association of State EMS Directors. These organizations designed the *Agenda* to be used by government and private organizations at the national, state, and local levels. The intent of the document was to build a common vision for the future of EMS. The *Agenda* also was meant to help guide planning, decision making, and policy regarding EMS.

The *Agenda* made 14 suggestions for EMS focused on principles of public health and safety systems (Figure 1-1), including the EMS education system (described later in this chapter). The 14 attributes for EMS identified by the *Agenda* are the following:

1. Integration of health services
2. EMS research
3. Legislation and regulation
4. System finance
5. Human resources
6. Medical direction
7. Education systems
8. Public education
9. Prevention
10. Public access
11. Communication systems
12. Clinical care
13. Information systems
14. Evaluation

Box 1-5 outlines other landmarks in EMS development.

Changes in federal health care reform affect the way health care, including emergency care, is provided. Managed care and **extended scope of practice** are most relevant to EMS. *Managed care* refers to patient care services that are provided to members by **managed care organizations** (e.g., health maintenance organizations [HMOs], preferred provider organizations [PPOs], and other provider networks). These plans now cover about 60% of the U.S. population.[7] This reform affects EMS systems in the way that they provide patient care choices for their clients (e.g., emergency versus nonemergency response, resources, and personnel; transportation modes; and health care facility options).

Extended scope of practice came out of the cost-containment setting of managed care. As it relates to EMS, extended

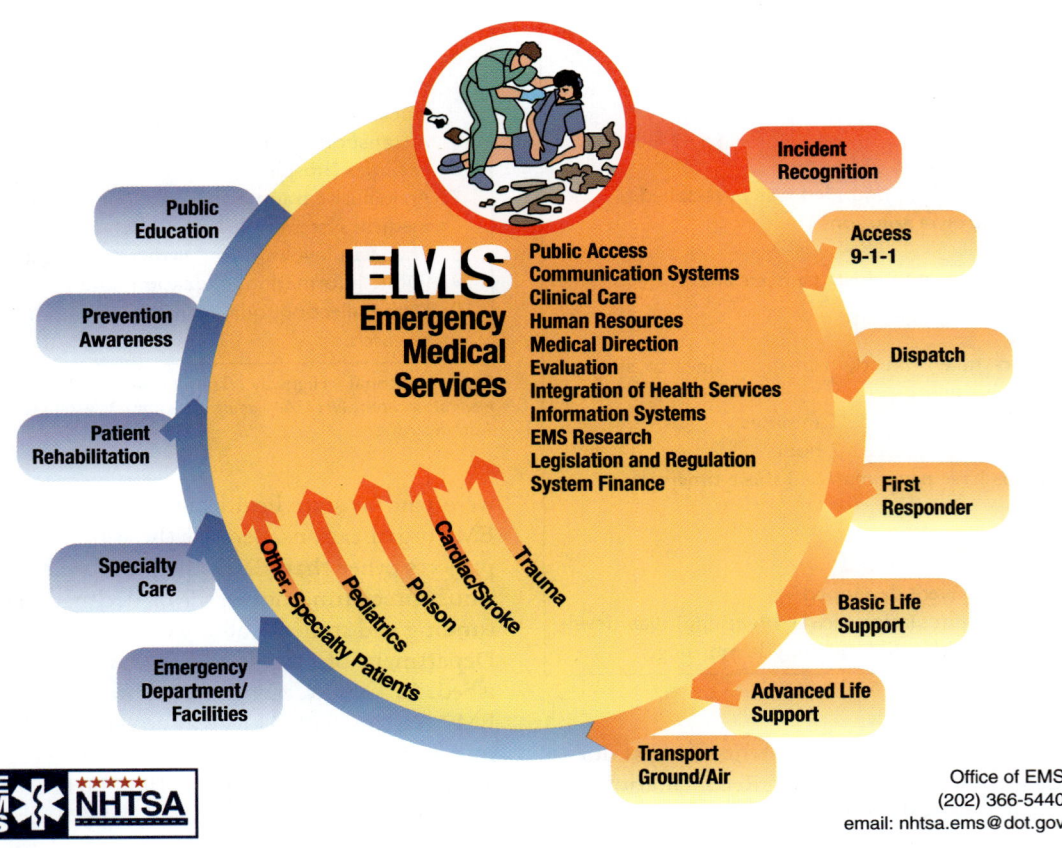

FIGURE 1-1 Emergency medical services: part of the health care system.

BOX 1-5 Other Landmarks in the Development of Emergency Medical Services

- Mid 1950s: The American College of Surgeons develops the first training programs for ambulance attendants.
- 1958: Dr. Peter Safar demonstrates the efficacy of mouth-to-mouth ventilation.
- 1960: Cardiopulmonary resuscitation is shown to be effective.
- 1967: Dr. Eugene Nagel trains Miami firefighters as paramedics at the University of Miami School of Medicine.
- 1968: The American Telephone and Telegraph Company designates 9-1-1 as the universal emergency telephone number.
- 1969: The U.S. Department of Transportation and National Highway Traffic Safety Administration (NHTSA) develop the basic training course for emergency medical technicians (EMTs).
- 1969: The Committee on Ambulance Design develops Ambulance Design Criteria, a report to the U.S. Department of Transportation and the NHTSA to complement the National Academy of Sciences–National Research Council Medical Requirements for Ambulance Design and Equipment (1968). This document recommends ambulance design standards and emergency equipment. The NHTSA agrees to issue matching federal funds to states that purchase vehicles meeting these standards.
- 1970: The National Registry of Emergency Medical Technicians is organized to standardize education, examinations, and certification of EMTs on a national level.
- 1972: President Nixon directs the U.S. Department of Health, Education, and Welfare to develop new ways to organize emergency medical services (EMS), which results in $8.5 million in contracts being awarded to develop a model EMS system.
- 1972: The University of Cincinnati establishes the first residency program to train new physicians exclusively for the practice of emergency medicine.
- 1973: The star of life is adopted as the official symbol for EMS. The six blue bars of the star of life represent the six system functions of EMS: detection, reporting, response, on-scene care, care in transit, and transfer to definitive care.
- 1974: President Gerald Ford proclaims the first National EMS Week.
- 1975: The National Association of Emergency Medical Technicians is founded.
- 1975: The American Medical Association accepts and approves the Paramedic role as an emergency health occupation.
- 1977: More than 40 EMT training agencies throughout the United States develop and test the national training standards for the paramedic for 2 years.
- 1980: The U.S. Department of Health and Human Services releases the *Position Paper on Trauma Center Designation*, which describes trauma centers within EMS systems. The paper also categorizes facilities.
- 1984: The EMS for Children program, under the Public Health Act, provides funding for enhancing the EMS system to better serve pediatric patients.
- 1986: The 1979 Public Safety Officer's Act (SB 1479) is amended to expand the $50,000 compensation to include survivors of rescue squads, ambulance crew members, and public safety department volunteers killed in the line of duty (amended in 1990).
- 1990: President George Bush signs the Trauma Care Systems Planning and Development Act (HR 1602), which provides for annual grants to states based on geographic and population size to help establish and improve trauma systems. In 1995 Congress does not reauthorize funding for this act.
- 1991: Occupational Exposure to Blood-Borne Pathogens; Final Rule (CFR 29 1910. 1030) establishes standards for workplace protection from blood-borne diseases.
- 1993: The Institute of Medicine publishes *Emergency Medical Services for Children*, which points out deficiencies in the ability of the health care system to address the emergency medical needs of pediatric patients.
- 1993: National Registry of EMTs publishes the *National EMS Education and Practice Blueprint*.
- 1995: Congress does not reauthorize funding under the Trauma Care Systems and Development Act.
- 1996: NHTSA and HRSA publish *EMS Agenda for the Future*.
- 1997: The NHTSA publishes *A Leadership Guide to Quality Improvement for Emergency Medical Services Systems*.
- 1998: The U.S. Department of Transportation revises the national standard curriculum for paramedics.
- 2000: *EMS Education Agenda for the Future* is published by NHTSA and HRSA.
- 2004: National Rural Health Association publishes *Rural and Frontier EMS Agenda for the Future*.
- 2005: NHTSA funds National EMS Core Content: The Domain of EMS Practice.
- 2007: *The National EMS Scope of Practice Model* published by NHTSA.

scope of practice refers to expanding services of EMS personnel in the prehospital setting. Examples include providing health screenings, physical examinations, and immunizations. Expanded scope for paramedics will continue to evolve. EMS agencies and managed care programs will develop other useful patient services to enhance revenues, to further injury prevention programs, and to reflect changes in how medical care is delivered. Expanded scope also helps ensure that EMS remains a vital part of the health care system.[8]

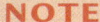

NOTE

Medicare and Medicaid are the two insurance programs of the U.S. government. Together, these insurance programs cover about 25% of the U.S. population.[7] These plans have rules that affect how patients qualify for emergency medical services transportation. The rules also decide the conditions under which reimbursement for transportation will occur. This reimbursement became standardized throughout the country in 2002. Standardization occurred through a consensus process involving national emergency medical services agencies and the Center for Medicare Services. The new Medicare fee structure caused major reductions in payment for some emergency medical services agencies but increased fees for others.

CURRENT MEDICAL SERVICES SYSTEMS

The EMS system of today is a network of coordinated services that provides medical care to the community. The coordination is defined by the NHTSA Technical Assistance Program Standards. This coordination ensures that patients are treated quickly and properly and that resources are used efficiently. Together these factors reduce health care costs (Figure 1-2). They also improve patient outcome and reduce hospital stays.[9]

State EMS systems usually are made up of local and regional agencies that manage the delivery of prehospital care. The local agencies are responsible for providing day-to-day EMS to the community. Local agencies also work with regional and state agencies to create protocols and help set standards and guidelines. Local agencies provide data collection services and coordinate mutual aid and disaster planning. Most state EMS agencies have advisory councils to help organize EMS programs and activities. These councils are made up of medical professionals, paraprofessionals, consumers, and public and private agencies with an interest in EMS. The state agency is responsible for licensing and/or certification. In addition, the state enforces state EMS regulations and develops public education programs. Moreover, the state agency acts as a liaison with national agencies. Some of these national agencies include NHTSA, the Federal Emergency Management Agency (FEMA), Homeland Security, and the Maternal Child Health Bureau of the Health Resources and Services Administration.

Emergency Medical Services System

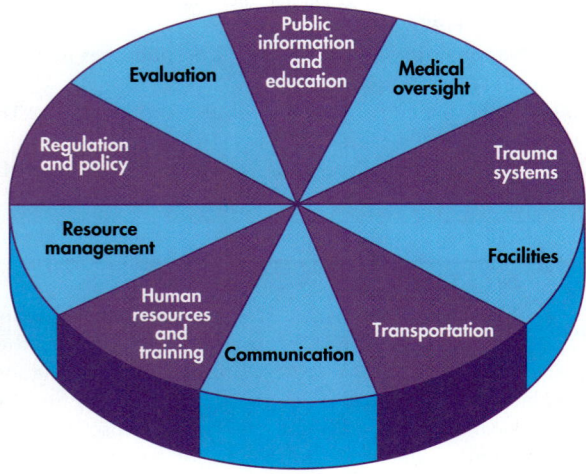

FIGURE 1-2 Ten components of the emergency medical services system. (National Highway Traffic Safety Administration, U.S. Department of Transportation: *Emergency medical services: NHTSA leading the way,* Washington, DC, 1995, The Administration; accessed at www.nhtsa.dot.gov/people/injury/ems/agenda/emsman.html#Services. Accessed April 13, 2011.)

> ### ? DID YOU KNOW?
> NEMSIS stands for the National Emergency Medical Services Information System. NEMSIS is the national repository that will be used to store EMS data from every state in the nation. Since the 1970s, the need for EMS information systems and databases has been well established, and many statewide data systems have been created. However, these EMS systems vary in their ability to collect patient and systems data and allow analysis at a local, state, and national level. For this reason, the NEMSIS project was developed to help states collect more standardized elements and eventually submit the data to a national EMS database. Such a database will be useful in:
> * Developing nationwide EMS training curricula
> * Evaluating patient and EMS system outcomes
> * Facilitating research efforts
> * Determining national fee schedules and reimbursement rates
> * Addressing resources for disaster and domestic preparedness
> * Providing valuable information on other issues or areas of need related to EMS care

Emergency Medical Services System Operations

The operations of an effective EMS system include citizen activation, dispatch, prehospital care, hospital care, and rehabilitation.

CITIZEN ACTIVATION

Emergency public safety services are highly visible in the community. However, the public is not always aware of the complex nature of these services. Citizens expect to have police and fire protection. They also expect to get a quick response with skilled personnel in a medical emergency. These expectations are due to years of available public safety service, public relations, press coverage, and national media. The public also expects such service because of public support in the form of taxes, donations, subscriptions for service, and user fees.

> ### ? DID YOU KNOW?
> In December 1971, the television show "Emergency!" made its debut to millions of viewers. The series starred Randolph Mantooth as paramedic John Gage and Kevin Tighe as his partner, paramedic Roy DeSoto. This popular TV series contributed to a change in public attitudes about fire service and prehospital emergency care. It was also during this time that many fire departments expanded their services to include EMS response.

Public involvement in EMS goes beyond funding. Citizens are often at the scene of an injury or illness. They play an important role in recognizing the need for emergency services. Citizens sometimes administer first aid, help secure the scene and gain access to the patient, and can be instrumental in managing a crisis. Educating the public is fundamental to the development of an effective EMS system. Paramedics help prepare the public to respond to a medical emergency. They also build support for EMS by helping to develop and present public health care education and prevention programs (see Chapter 3).

CRITICAL THINKING

How is the emergency medical services system funded in your community?

Once citizens recognize that an emergency exists and a call for help is made, the response is coordinated. Citizens usually contact communication centers and dispatching services by emergency phone numbers. The number 9-1-1 offers access to public safety services in most of the country. These services include fire service, law enforcement, and EMS. The availability of emergency access through 9-1-1 continues to expand across the country as areas adopt the system. In areas that do not have 9-1-1, citizens should have easy access to other emergency phone numbers. These numbers can be promoted through public awareness programs, phone stickers, and phone book covers. Other ways of engaging an emergency response include firebox pull stations, citizen band radios, voice over Internet protocol (VOIP), and cell phones. Chapter 5 covers 9-1-1 in more detail.

PREHOSPITAL CARE

Ill or injured patients may need prehospital intervention and stabilization. Interventions may involve **basic life support** (BLS) and ALS skills. Depending on the situation (e.g., entrapment, distance to the hospital, and availability of ALS), initial prehospital care may be limited. The care may consist of giving only comfort and reassurance. Care also may require spinal immobilization, airway protection, endotracheal intubation, intravenous therapy, medication administration, defibrillation, and external cardiac pacing.

HOSPITAL CARE

When the patient is brought to the emergency department, patient care resources expand. This care may include physicians, physician assistants, nurse practitioners, nurses, technicians, ancillary support staff (allied health counselors, social workers, and others), secretaries, and medical record staff. Diagnostic tests are often performed. These services may be provided by laboratory, radiology, and cardiopulmonary departments. Resources available beyond the emergency department include surgery, cardiac catheterization, intensive care, physical therapy, pharmacy, nutrition services, and many others.

REHABILITATION

After hospital delivery and definitive care, many patients receive some type of rehabilitation services. Rehabilitation often occurs before and after hospital discharge. The

services may be in the form of education and physical and occupational therapy that help the patient to recover. Rehabilitation also can help the patient to maintain maximal independence. One example of such therapy is helping patients and families adjust to required changes in lifestyle after a myocardial infarction. Another example is retraining in activities of daily living (e.g., bathing and preparing meals). Job rehabilitation also allows patients to adapt to limb impairment or loss.

EMS EDUCATION

The national standard curriculum for paramedics was last revised in 1998. That same year, EMS leaders worked with NHTSA to revise a portion of the *Agenda* (the *National Emergency Medical Services Education and Practice Blueprint* [the *Blueprint*]). This revision revealed the future of EMS education. The text was titled the *EMS Education Agenda for the Future: A Systems Approach* (the *Education Agenda*). The *Education Agenda* named core content categories for each license level. The *Education Agenda* also stressed the integration of EMS within the overall health care system. Figure 1-3 is a diagram of a model that came from the revision.[10] New to this revision was the definition of cognitive (knowledge), psychomotor (skills), and affective (attitude) objectives.

The NHTSA and HRSA also funded the *National EMS Core Content*, which was published in 2005. This document defined the entire domain of out-of-hospital practice. It also identified the universal body of knowledge and skills for EMS personnel. This project was led by the National Association of EMS Physicians and the American College of Emergency Physicians.

The *National EMS Scope of Practice Model* (*Scope of Practice*) was published in 2007. This consensus document defined the four levels of EMS personnel described in this chapter. It also defined the practices and minimum skills for each level. Each educational level assumes mastery of previous competencies for each license level. Each individual must demonstrate each skill within his or her scope of practice and for patients of all ages.

Development of the *National EMS Education Standards* (the *Standards*) was led by the National Association of EMS Educators (NAEMSE). The *Standards* replace NHTSA's national standard curricula that had been the cornerstone of EMS education since the 1960s. The *Standards* define the competencies, clinical behaviors, and judgments that must be met by entry-level EMS personnel at each licensure level. The goal was to meet practice guidelines as defined by the *National EMS Scope of Practice Model*. Content and concepts defined by the *National EMS Core Content* were also integrated within the *Standards*.[11] Box 1-6, EMS History, outlines the timeline of these publications and standards.

NOTE

Each EMS licensure level represents a *significant* difference in skills, risk, knowledge, level of supervision and autonomy, judgment, and clinical decision making.

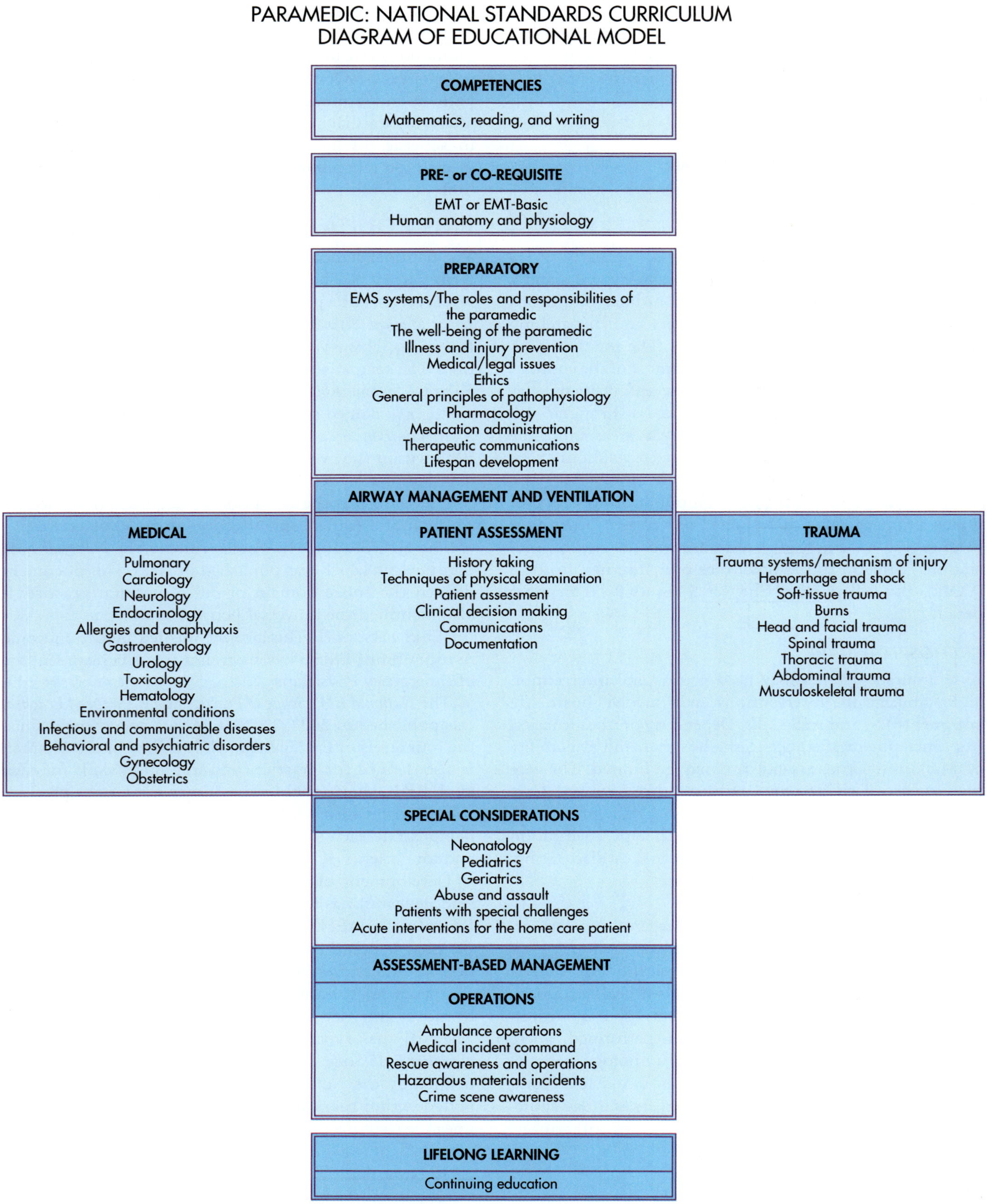

PARAMEDIC: NATIONAL STANDARDS CURRICULUM
DIAGRAM OF EDUCATIONAL MODEL

COMPETENCIES

Mathematics, reading, and writing

PRE- or CO-REQUISITE

EMT or EMT-Basic
Human anatomy and physiology

PREPARATORY

EMS systems/The roles and responsibilities of
the paramedic
The well-being of the paramedic
Illness and injury prevention
Medical/legal issues
Ethics
General principles of pathophysiology
Pharmacology
Medication administration
Therapeutic communications
Lifespan development

AIRWAY MANAGEMENT AND VENTILATION

MEDICAL	**PATIENT ASSESSMENT**	**TRAUMA**
Pulmonary	History taking	Trauma systems/mechanism of injury
Cardiology	Techniques of physical examination	Hemorrhage and shock
Neurology	Patient assessment	Soft-tissue trauma
Endocrinology	Clinical decision making	Burns
Allergies and anaphylaxis	Communications	Head and facial trauma
Gastroenterology	Documentation	Spinal trauma
Urology		Thoracic trauma
Toxicology		Abdominal trauma
Hematology		Musculoskeletal trauma
Environmental conditions		
Infectious and communicable diseases		
Behavioral and psychiatric disorders		
Gynecology		
Obstetrics		

SPECIAL CONSIDERATIONS

Neonatology
Pediatrics
Geriatrics
Abuse and assault
Patients with special challenges
Acute interventions for the home care patient

ASSESSMENT-BASED MANAGEMENT

OPERATIONS

Ambulance operations
Medical incident command
Rescue awareness and operations
Hazardous materials incidents
Crime scene awareness

LIFELONG LEARNING

Continuing education

FIGURE 1-3 Diagram of Department of Transportation education model. (U.S. Department of Health and Human Services, Health Resources and Services, Health Resources and Services Administration, Maternal and Child Health Bureau: *Emergency medical services agenda for the future,* Washington, DC, 1999, The Administration.)

NOTE

The *Education Agenda* recommends that EMS students graduate from a nationally accredited EMS educational program to be eligible for National EMS Certification (Figure 1-4). This is to ensure consistency and quality of EMS personnel. National certification is the element critical to extend **reciprocity** to EMS personnel educated in other states. In the future, EMS educational programs will likely require review by the Committee on Accreditation of Educational Programs for Emergency Medical Services Professions (CoAEMSP). The goal of this accreditation is to ensure quality of education and to ensure that appropriate educational infrastructures and resources are available for students in EMS programs. For more information, see The Commission's website at www.caahep.org.

The Five Components of the EMS Agenda: http://www.nhtsa.dot.gov/people/injury/ems/EdAgenda/final/agenda6-00.htm, accessed 2-10-09.

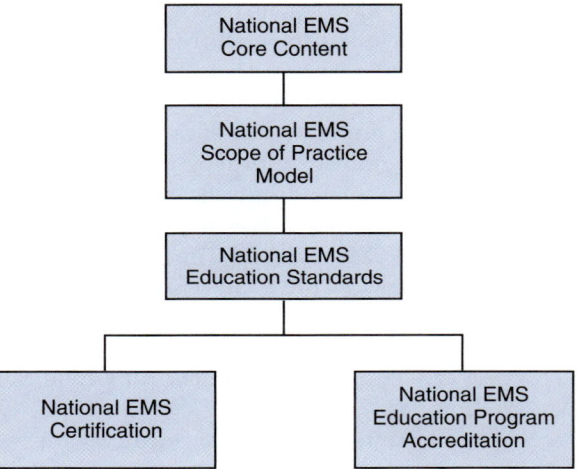

FIGURE 1-4 The five components of the EMS agenda. (National Registry of Emergency Medical Technicians; *Education Agenda for the Future, A Systems Approach*, Columbus, Ohio, 2000.)

BOX 1-6 Timeline of EMS Education Publications and Standards in the United States

- 1969: AAOS: Emergency Care and Transportation of the Sick and Injured (the "Orange Book")
- 1996: EMS Agenda for the Future
- 1971: EMT-Ambulance National Standard Curriculum
- 1998: National Standard Curriculum for EMT-Paramedic (revised)
- 2000: Education Agenda for the Future: A Systems Approach
- 2004: National EMS Practice Analysis
- 2005: National EMS Scope of Practice
- 2006: EMS at the Crossroads (Institute of Medicine [IOM]) report
- 2007: National EMS Scope of Practice
- 2009: National EMS Education Standards
- Supported by NHTSA for future implementation
  National EMS Certification
  National EMS Program Accreditation

Continuing Education

Continuing education provides a way for all health care practitioners to retain primary technical and professional skills. It also helps the paramedic move from competency (at graduation) to higher, more expert levels of practice. Continuing education aids in learning new and advanced skills and knowledge. Some skills learned during the initial course of study are not used often. New information, procedures, and resources that enhance patient care are continuously being developed to help maintain skill proficiency. Continuing education can take many forms, including the following:

- Conferences and seminars
- Lectures and workshops
- Quality improvement reviews
- Skill laboratories
- Certification and recertification programs
- Refresher training programs
- Journal studies
- Multimedia presentations
- Internet-based learning
- Case presentations
- Independent study

EMERGENCY MEDICAL SERVICES PERSONNEL LEVELS

Various levels of personnel and medical direction come together to make an effective prehospital EMS system. The levels include dispatcher, Emergency Medical Responder (EMR), Emergency Medical Technician (EMT), Advanced Emergency Medical Technician (AEMT), and Paramedic. Each EMS level described here has satisfied training based on the *National EMS Education Standards*. They function as part of a comprehensive EMS response, under **medical oversight**. (The following descriptions of EMS practitioner levels are adapted from the *National EMS Education Standards*.)[11]

Dispatcher

A dispatcher is a telecommunicator. This person serves as the primary contact with the public. The dispatcher directs the proper agencies to the scene. These agencies may include ground and air ambulances, fire departments, law enforcement, utility services, and others. The term *telecommunicator* applies to call takers, dispatchers, radio operators, data terminal operators, or any combination of such functions in a public service answering point located in a fire, police, or EMS communications center (see Chapter 5). An effective EMS dispatch communications system includes the following functions:

- *Receive and process calls for EMS assistance.* The dispatcher receives and records calls for EMS assistance and selects an appropriate course of action for each call. To do this, the dispatcher must obtain as much information as possible about the emergency event. This information includes name, call-back number, and address. The dispatcher may also have to deal with distraught callers.

- *Dispatch and coordinate EMS resources.* The dispatcher directs the proper emergency vehicles to the correct address. This person also coordinates the emergency vehicles while en route to the scene, to the medical facility, and back to the operations base (Figure 1-5).
- *Relay medical information.* The dispatch center can provide a telecommunications channel among appropriate medical facilities and EMS personnel; fire, police, and rescue workers; and private citizens. This can consist of phone, radio, or biomedical telemetry.
- *Coordinate with public safety agencies.* The dispatcher aids communications between public safety (fire, law enforcement, rescue) and the EMS system. This coordinates services such as traffic control, escort, fire suppression, and extrication. The dispatcher must know the location and status of all EMS vehicles and whether support services are available. In larger systems, computer-aided dispatching is used. This provides for one or more of the following abilities:
  - Automatic entry of 9-1-1
  - Automatic interface to vehicle location with or without map display
  - Automatic interface to mobile data terminal
  - Computer messaging among multiple radio operators, call takers, or both
  - Dispatch note taking, reminder aid, or both
  - Ability to monitor response times, response delays, and on-scene times
  - Display of call information
  - Emergency medical dispatch review
  - Manual or automatic updates of unit status
  - Manual entry of call information
  - Radio control and display of channel status
  - Standard operating procedure review
  - Telephone control and display of circuit status

Many EMS and public service agencies require specialized training for their dispatch personnel. The dispatcher then can give directions to the caller while the caller waits for EMS arrival. The training may include the USDOT training program for the emergency medical dispatcher, which is described further in Chapter 5.

> **CRITICAL THINKING**
> What type of dispatching is provided in your community? Are dispatchers trained to the level of emergency medical dispatcher?

Emergency Medical Responder (EMR)

The EMR (also known as First Responder) may be the first trained person in an EMS system to arrive on a scene. These responders may include personnel from fire departments and law enforcement agencies. They also may include designated commercial medical response teams, athletic trainers, and others. The primary focus of the EMR is to initiate immediate lifesaving care to critical patients who access the EMS system. This person has the basic knowledge and skills necessary to provide basic lifesaving interventions while awaiting additional EMS response. The EMR can also assist higher-level personnel at the scene and during transport. They perform basic interventions with minimal equipment. The EMR can do the following:

1. Recognize the seriousness of the patient's condition or extent of injuries.
2. Assess requirements for emergency medical care.
3. Administer appropriate emergency medical care for life-threatening injuries relative to airway, breathing, and circulation.

Emergency Medical Technician (EMT)

The EMT (formerly known as EMT-Basic) is trained in all phases of basic life support. This training includes the use of automated external defibrillators and the administration of some emergency medications. The primary focus of the EMT is to provide basic emergency medical care and transportation for critical and emergent patients who access the EMS system. They perform interventions with the basic equipment typically found on an ambulance. They also assist paramedics in the care of patients during transport.

Advanced Emergency Medical Technician (AEMT)

The AEMT was formerly known as EMT-Intermediate. The degree of training and skills that the AEMT practices varies between states and EMS systems. Training can include ALS procedures such as **peritracheal** airway adjuncts, intravenous therapy, defibrillation, cardiac rhythm interpretation,

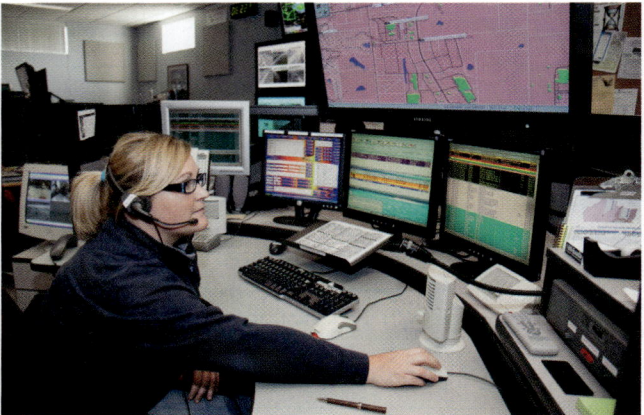

FIGURE 1-5 Computer dispatch screen.

and administration of some emergency medications. The primary focus of the AEMT is to provide basic and limited advanced emergency medical care and transportation for critical and emergent patients who access the EMS system.

Paramedic

The **paramedic** (formerly known as EMT-Paramedic) is trained in all aspects of basic and advanced life support procedures that are relevant to prehospital emergency care. The paramedic has advanced training in patient assessment, clinical decision making, cardiac rhythm interpretation, defibrillation, drug therapy, and airway management (Box 1-7). The paramedic provides emergency care based on advanced assessment skills and the formulation of a field diagnosis. The paramedic's specific roles and duties are discussed later in this chapter.

NATIONAL EMERGENCY MEDICAL SERVICES GROUP INVOLVEMENT

Many groups and organizations help to set the standards of EMS (Box 1-8). These groups exist at the national, state, regional, and local levels. They take part in development, education, implementation, lobbying, and setting standards for EMS. Membership and participation in professional organizations help promote the professional status of the paramedic. These groups expose the paramedic to trends in emergency care, continuing education, and to resource experts. The organizations also provide for national representation. They have a unified voice in other health care organizations and issues of national matters. The EMS standard-setting groups have many roles. Their primary role, however, is to set standards with input from members of the profession and the community. By doing so, they help ensure that the public is protected from individuals and agencies that do not meet professional standards for licensure and/or certification.

One such organization is the National Registry of Emergency Medical Technicians (NREMT). The National Registry helps develop professional standards in the EMS industry. This organization verifies competencies for EMTs and paramedics by preparing and conducting certification examinations. The organization also simplifies the process of state-to-state mobility and reciprocity for its members.

BOX 1-7 Description of the Paramedic Profession

The description of the paramedic profession provides the philosophy and rationale for the depth and breadth of coverage.

- Paramedics have fulfilled requirements prescribed by an accrediting agency to practice the art and science of out-of-hospital medicine under medical direction. Through performing assessments and providing medical care, their goal is to prevent and reduce mortality and morbidity caused by illness and injury. Paramedics primarily provide care to emergency patients in an out-of-hospital setting.
- Paramedics possess knowledge, skills, and attitudes consistent with the expectations of the public and the profession. Paramedics recognize that they are an essential component of the continuum of care and serve as linkages among health resources.
- Paramedics strive to maintain high-quality, reasonable-cost health care by delivering patients directly to appropriate facilities. As advocates for patients, paramedics seek to be proactive in affecting long-term health care by working with other provider agencies, networks, and organizations. The emerging roles and responsibilities of the paramedic include public education, health promotion, and participation in injury- and illness-prevention programs. As the scope of service continues to expand, the paramedic will function as a facilitator of access to care and as an initial treatment provider.
- Paramedics are responsible and accountable to medical direction, the public, and their peers. Paramedics recognize the importance of research and actively participate in the design, development, evaluation, and publication of research. Paramedics seek to take part in lifelong professional development, perform peer evaluation, and assume an active role in professional and community organizations.

From U.S. Department of Transportation, National Highway Transportation Administration: *EMT-Paramedic national standard curriculum*, Washington, DC, 1998, The Department.

BOX 1-8 Sampling of National Emergency Medical Services Organizations and Associations

American Ambulance Association
American College of Emergency Physicians
American College of Surgeons
Association of Air Medical Services
Emergency Nurses' Association
National Association of EMS Educators
National Association of EMS Physicians
National Association of Emergency Medical Technicians
International Association of Fire Chiefs
International Association of Fire Fighters
National Association of Search and Rescue
National Association of State EMS Officials
National Flight Nurses' Association
National Flight Paramedic Association
National Registry of Emergency Medical Technicians

DID YOU KNOW?
Every five years, the NREMT conducts a *National EMS Practice Analysis*. This has been done since 1994. The purpose of the study is to gather data on what EMS personnel actually do as part of their practice in providing emergency care. This helps the NREMT to revise and tailor their certification examinations. These data are also used in developing the EMS curricula that affect current practice.

The LEADS project is another important area of research conducted by the NREMT. LEADS stands for the *Longitudinal Emergency Medical Technician Attributes and Demographics Study*. The study is hosted by the NREMT and is conducted once each year. It is designed to describe the EMT population in the United States, their work activities, working conditions, and job satisfaction. The project began in August 1998. It is led by a team of researchers made up of state EMS directors, state EMS training coordinators, EMS system managers, emergency physicians, EMS educators, survey researchers, and staff of the NREMT. The NREMT is a leader in the areas of research in EMS education and practice. For more information about the Practice Analysis or LEADS study, see http://www.nremt.org.

CRITICAL THINKING
What issues do you think your national emergency medical services association should address to enhance patient care in your area?

LICENSURE, CERTIFICATION, AND REGISTRATION

Paramedics are granted permission to practice their skills by three processes: licensure, certification, and registration. The exact wording of granting this permission varies by state.

Licensure

Licensure is a process of regulating occupations. In this process a license is granted by a government authority. The license allows a person to engage in a profession or activity that otherwise would be unlawful. Some states and local authorities require that paramedics have a license.

Certification

Certification grants authority to a person to take part in an activity. The person receives a document from a government or nongovernment entity showing that the person has met the requirements to practice an activity. Some states or local authorities require that paramedics be certified.

NOTE
Some persons believe that licensed professionals have greater status than those who are certified or registered. This belief is unfounded. A certification granted by a state and conferring a right to engage in a trade or profession is in fact a license.

Registration

Registration is the act of enrolling one's name in a register, or book of record. For example, paramedics can be licensed or certified in their state and can be registered with the National Registry of Emergency Medical Technicians.

Credentialing

Credentialing is a local process that allows a paramedic to practice in a specific EMS agency (or setting). Credentialing processes are typically guided by the local medical director (Figure 1-6).

PROFESSIONALISM

Training and performance standards have helped to define EMTs and paramedics as health care professionals. The term *profession* refers to a body of knowledge or expertise. The members of such a field are often self-regulated through licensing or certification that confirms competence. In addition, most professions adhere to standards. These standards include initial and continuing education requirements. *Professionalism* refers to the way in which a person follows the standards of a profession. These standards may include conduct and performance standards. These standards also usually include adhering to a **code of ethics** approved by the profession (see Chapter 7).

Health Care Professionals

Health care professionals conform to the standards of their profession. By providing quality patient care and striving for high standards, they instill pride in the profession and earn the respect of others. EMS professionals occupy positions of public trust and are highly visible role models. As

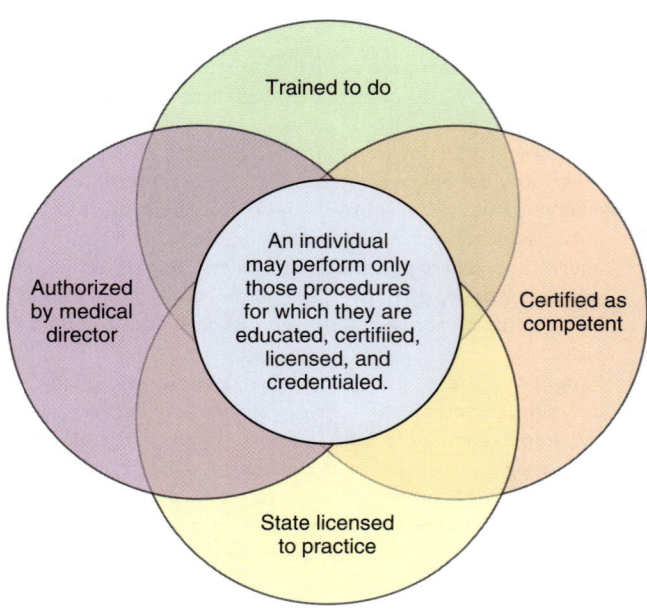

FIGURE 1-6 The relationship among education, certification, licensure, and credentialing.

such, the public has high expectations of EMTs and paramedics while they are both "on" and "off" duty. Therefore, professional conduct at all times and a commitment to excellence in daily activities complement the image of the EMS professional. Image and behavior are vital to establishing credibility and instilling confidence. The professional paramedic represents his or her employer; the EMS agency; the state, county, city, or district EMS office; and his or her peers.

Attributes of the Professional Paramedic

Many aspects of being professional can be applied to the role of the paramedic. Eleven of these attributes follow:[10]

1. *Integrity*. Integrity means being honest in all actions. Integrity may be the most important behavior for EMS professionals. The public assumes EMS professionals have integrity. Actions that show integrity include being truthful, not stealing, and providing complete and correct documentation.

2. *Empathy*. Empathy is identifying with and understanding the feelings, situations, and motives of others. EMS professionals must always show empathy to patients, families, and other health care professionals. Behavior that demonstrates empathy includes showing caring, compassion, and respect for others; understanding the feelings of the patient and family; being calm and helpful to those in need; and being supportive and reassuring of others.

3. *Self-motivation*. Self-motivation is the internal drive for merit and self-direction. Self-motivation can mean taking the lead to finish tasks, to improve behavior, and to follow through without supervision. Some marks of self-motivation are showing enthusiasm for learning, being committed to **continuous quality improvement** or CQI (described later in this chapter), and accepting constructive feedback.

4. *Appearance and personal hygiene*. Paramedics are aware of how they present themselves as representatives of their profession. They must ensure that their clothing and uniforms are clean and in good repair. They must be aware of the importance of personal hygiene and good grooming.

5. *Self-confidence*. Paramedics must trust and rely on themselves, often in difficult situations. One key task is to assess personal and professional strengths and weaknesses. The ability to trust personal judgment shows self-confidence.

6. *Communications*. An important part of the paramedic's job is communicating. Paramedics must be able to convey key information to others verbally and in writing. They must demonstrate communication skills by speaking clearly, writing legibly, and listening actively. Finally, paramedics must be able to adjust communication strategies to various situations.

7. *Time management*. Time management refers to organizing and prioritizing tasks to make the best use of time.

Examples include being punctual and completing tasks and assignments on time.

8. *Teamwork and diplomacy*. The paramedic must be able to work well with others to achieve common goals. As a member of the EMS team, the paramedic must place the success of the team above personal success. This is done by supporting and respecting other team members, being flexible and open to change, and communicating with co-workers to resolve problems. (See Chapter 5.)

9. *Respect*. Respect means having regard for others and showing consideration and appreciation. Paramedics are polite to others and avoid the use of derogatory or demeaning terms. They know that showing respect brings credit to themselves, their association, and their profession.

10. *Patient advocacy*. The paramedic must always act as the patient's advocate, even when the patient disagrees with the care. Paramedics should not attempt to impose their personal beliefs on patients or allow personal biases (religious, ethical, political, social, legal) to impact patient care. The needs of the patient are always placed above self-interests. The paramedic also must protect the patient's confidentiality.

11. *Careful delivery of service*. Paramedics deliver the highest quality of patient care. With this care comes attention to detail and proper prioritization of care. They also must evaluate their performance and attitude on every call. As part of the careful delivery of service, paramedics master and refresh their skills; perform full equipment checks; and ensure safe ambulance operations. Paramedics also follow policies, procedures, and protocols and comply with the orders of their supervisors.

CRITICAL THINKING
Which of these professional attributes represent your strengths? Which ones do you think you need to work on?

ROLES AND RESPONSIBILITIES OF THE PARAMEDIC

The paramedic may practice patient care at an emergency scene, from an emergency scene to the hospital, between health care facilities, or in other health care settings as permitted by state and local laws. The paramedic's roles and duties can be divided into two groups: primary responsibilities and additional responsibilities[10] (Box 1-9).

Primary Responsibilities

The paramedic must be prepared physically, mentally, and emotionally for the job. Preparation includes being committed to positive health practices (see Chapter 2). It also includes having the proper equipment and supplies

BOX 1-9 Roles and Responsibilities of the Paramedic

Primary Responsibilities	Additional Responsibilities
Preparation	Community involvement
Response	Support of primary care efforts
Scene assessment	Advocation of citizen involvement in emergency medical services
Patient assessment	Participation in leadership activities
Recognition of injury or illness	Personal and professional development
Patient management	
Appropriate patient disposition	
Patient transfer	
Documentation	
Returning to service	

BOX 1-10 Sampling of Specialized Care Facilities

Burn specialization center
Cardiac treatment center
Clinical laboratory service
Emergency department
Facility with acute hemodialysis capability
Facility with acute spinal cord or head injury management capability
Facility with reperfusion capability
Facility with special radiological capabilities
High-risk obstetrical facility
Hyperbaric treatment center
Intensive care unit for trauma patients
Neurology center
Operating suite
Pediatric facility
Postanesthesia recovery room or surgical intensive care unit
Psychiatric facility
Rehabilitation facility
Stroke center
Toxicology (including hazardous material or decontamination) service
Trauma center

and maintaining adequate knowledge and skills of the profession. The paramedic must respond to the scene in a safe and timely manner. Scene assessment must consider personal safety; safety of the crew, patients, and bystanders; and the mechanism of injury or probable cause of illness.

The paramedic must quickly perform patient assessment to determine the injury or illness. Integrating assessment findings with knowledge of disease or injury helps the paramedic formulate a field impression. It also helps set priorities of care and transportation. Managing an emergency often entails following protocols and interacting with medical direction as needed. The care provided by the paramedic should minimize secondary injury. After stabilizing the patient in the field, the paramedic should provide for transport to an appropriate facility. Transportation may include a ground or air ambulance. The type of transport needed for optimal patient care is based on the patient's condition, distance from the hospital, travel time, and other factors. Choosing the most appropriate facility requires knowledge of available resources, hospital designations, and categorization (Box 1-10). The hospital destination decision should be made jointly between the paramedic and the patient in cooperation with medical oversight. Knowledge of transfer agreements and local transport protocols is also helpful.

The paramedic is the patient's advocate as responsibility for care shifts to the staff at the receiving facility. The staff must be briefed about the patient's condition at the scene and during transport. The paramedic also needs to provide thorough and accurate documentation in the **patient care report** (PCR). The PCR should be completed in a timely manner so that the EMS crew can return to service. The crew should prepare the ambulance for return to service by replacing equipment and supplies (per agency protocol). The crew also should review the call openly. This can help to identify ways to improve the patient care services that were provided at the scene and during transport.

Additional Responsibilities

Other duties of the paramedic include community involvement, support of primary care efforts, advocating citizen involvement in the EMS system, participation in leadership activities, and personal and professional development.

A paramedic can be involved in the community and can be a role model for the profession in many ways. The paramedic can advocate illness and injury prevention programs (see Chapter 3) and can participate as a leader in community activities. A few ways to improve the health of the community include teaching CPR, first aid, and injury prevention. These activities help to ensure proper use of EMS resources. They can also improve the integration of EMS with other health care and public safety agencies.

Communities and their health care organizations often enlist paramedics to support primary care efforts, and prevention and wellness programs. Paramedics can help to inform the public of the best use of prehospital and other non-EMS health care resources. Examples include alternatives to ambulance transportation, nonhospital emergency department clinical providers, and freestanding emergency clinics. These programs that teach when, where, and how to use EMS and emergency departments promote the best use of health care resources.

Encouraging citizens to be involved in EMS improves the system as a whole. Citizens can help to set the needs and parameters for EMS use in the community. They can offer an objective view into quality improvement and problem solving. In addition, having involved citizens creates informed, independent advocates for the EMS system.

> **NOTE**
>
> Some EMS agencies organize community emergency response teams (CERTs). These teams help prepare citizens to respond to disaster-type emergencies. Members are trained to provide instant help to victims, organize volunteers, and support first responder efforts.

Paramedics can take part in leadership activities in their communities in many ways. One example is conducting primary injury prevention initiatives (activities and risk surveys). Another example is assisting media campaigns to promote EMS issues and other health programs. (See Chapter 3.)

Finally, a paramedic has a responsibility for personal and professional development. There are many methods to accomplish this. Examples include continuing education, student mentoring, membership in professional organizations, and joining professional teams. Other methods include becoming involved in work-related issues that affect career growth, exploring alternative career paths in the EMS profession, conducting and supporting research initiatives, and being actively involved in legislative issues related to EMS.

MEDICAL DIRECTION FOR EMERGENCY MEDICAL SERVICES

The medical direction physician is the medical leader for the EMS system. The physician serves as a resource and as a patient advocate. This relationship between medical direction and the paramedic is critical to an effective EMS system. It allows for the delivery of advanced prehospital care. The ideal medical direction physician is properly educated as an EMS medical director. The physician also is motivated to provide the following[12]:

- EMS system design and operations
- Education and training of EMS personnel
- Participation in personnel selection
- Participation in equipment selection
- Development of clinical protocols in cooperation with expert EMS personnel
- Participation in CQI and problem resolution
- Direct input into patient care
- Interface between EMS systems and other health care agencies
- Advocacy within the medical community
- Guidance as the "medical conscience" of the EMS system (advocating for quality patient care)

> **SHOW ME THE EVIDENCE**
>
> Researchers asked nationally registered EMS professionals how much contact they had with their medical director in the previous 6 months. For that period 62.5% of respondents indicated contact with the medical director during education, a call review, or on the scene. Paramedics were more likely (78.5%) than EMT-Intermediates (62.3%) or EMT-Basics (47.6%, $p < 0.001$) to have had contact with the medical director. Urban EMS professionals were more likely to have had MD contact than rural respondents (64.9% vs. 59.2%, $p < 0.001$).

From: Studnek JR, Fernandez AF, Margolis GS, O'Connor RE: Describing the amount of medical director contact among nationally registered emergency medical services professionals. Abstract published in *Prehosp Emerg Care,* 12(1): 115, 2008.

Types of Medical Direction

The two types of medical direction are **online (direct) medical direction** and **off-line (indirect) medical direction**.[13] Both types ensure the quality of medical care in an EMS system. Most prehospital care is provided through standing orders and patient care protocols (varies by state). There are times, however, when a patient care issue falls outside the scope of standing orders or an unusual situation at the scene arises. When this occurs, the paramedic may need to contact online medical direction by radio or phone to convey the patient's information and to receive orders through direct consultation with a physician or physician designee. This designee may be a registered nurse or physician assistant. The designee also may be a paramedic trained to give ALS orders in the medical direction system. Online medical direction allows for instant and specific care, telemetry, and CQI while paramedics are on the scene. As a rule, online medical direction supersedes off-line medical direction.[14]

An advisory group often is the voice behind the off-line direction, but it also can be provided by one or more medical directors. A director must have full medical direction authority. He or she also must have knowledge of how the EMS system operates. This type of direction can be *prospective* or *retrospective*. Prospective off-line direction covers the authority to set **treatment protocols** and **standing orders** (Box 1-11). Such knowledge includes training for care and triage in the prehospital arena, as well as the choice of equipment, supplies, and personnel. Retrospective off-line direction includes any actions that take place after the EMS call. An example is reviewing a patient care report and providing CQI.

On-Scene Physicians

Some of the first ambulance personnel were physicians. Yet, rarely is a medical direction physician on the scene providing direct field supervision of EMS personnel. At times, however, a physician (*physician intervenor*) may witness the injury or illness. Perhaps the patient's private physician is on the scene when EMS arrives. When this occurs, positive

BOX 1-11 Protocols

Treatment protocols are written guidelines that define the scope of prehospital care for emergency medical services (EMS) personnel. The medical director of the EMS or members of a regional EMS advisory group create them. The paramedic must adhere to these protocols. The paramedic must follow the protocols unless advised otherwise by medical direction.

Standing orders are more specific than protocols. Standing orders usually are included in a protocol when a delay in treatment would harm the patient. Most protocols and standing orders comply with national standards. They also comply with state EMS medical practice arts and regional guidelines. An example of a national standard is the American Heart Association guidelines for advanced cardiac life support. Another is the American College of Surgeons standards for advanced trauma life support. Protocols define the standard of care for paramedic crews and online physicians. The cases in which the paramedic acts strictly by standing orders usually are few. These situations may include intubation of a nonbreathing patient or first-line medication administration in cardiac arrest. Situations also may include events in which radio contact has failed and a delay could threaten the patient outcome.

BOX 1-12 Quality Assurance and Continuous Quality Improvement

Quality assurance (QA) is a system of quality management that by tradition was linked with spotting deviations from a standard (e.g., protocols). Quality assurance also altered these deviations through some type of punitive action. Continuous quality improvement (CQI) is a modified form of QA. Continuous quality improvement focuses on the system and not the individual, thus removing much of the punitive aspect associated with a QA program. Continuous quality improvement is less rigid than QA. In addition, CQI considers many factors that often apply to EMS. Continuous quality improvement includes the entire medical direction system and involves all health providers in the problem-solving process.

The EMS worker should use input from CQI activities to adapt treatment protocols and educational activities when needed. The goal of CQI is to find and fix problems in a positive manner. Continuous quality improvement also is aimed at improving the overall system. CQI activities include a review of the following:

- Outcome measures of prehospital care (e.g., scene times, procedure completion rates, and mortality reviews)
- Care while treatment is ongoing (concurrent reviews)
- Written EMS patient care paperwork (retrospective reviews)
- Random or selected radio communication tapes
- New procedures, equipment, or therapies

interaction between the on-scene physician and the EMS crew is essential.

> **NOTE**
>
> An on-scene physician may not be familiar with functions of emergency medical services or medical oversight responsibilities. The lines of authority and responsibility for these physicians vary from state to state. Each EMS agency should have a policy that defines interaction with physicians on the scene.

If a nonmedical direction physician or the patient's physician is on the scene, EMS personnel must follow protocols. If no protocols are in place, the paramedic should immediately contact online medical direction. The policies of many EMS agencies require that the physician on the scene can assume responsibility for patient care and provide medical direction.[15] Together the physicians can make choices about the patient's care. With permission of medical direction, a physician on the scene may take control of the patient's care. If a physician on the scene tries to direct care in opposition to medical direction, EMS personnel should have law enforcement intervene. This will ensure that the scene is safe and the EMS care goes uninterrupted.

IMPROVING SYSTEM QUALITY

A major goal of any EMS system is to evaluate and improve care continually. One way to meet this goal is through a modified form of quality assurance. This form of quality assurance is known as *continuous quality improvement* (CQI), which is the ongoing study and improvement of a process, system, or organization (Box 1-12).

A CQI program identifies and attempts to improve problems in certain areas. Key areas that are monitored in most EMS systems include:

- Medical direction
- Financing
- Training
- Communications
- Prehospital management and transportation
- Interfacility transportation
- Receiving facilities
- Specialty care units
- Dispatch
- Public information and education
- Audit and quality assurance
- Disaster planning and mutual aid

Continuous quality improvement is a process that involves all caregivers in the problem-solving aspect (Figure 1-7). Continuous quality improvement stresses the value of enabling frontline personnel to perform their jobs well. With this group approach, all parties can be involved in elaborating on the cause of the problem. They can work together to develop remedies and can design a course of action to correct the problem. Then they can enforce the plan and reexamine the issue to see whether the problem has been resolved.

> **CRITICAL THINKING**
>
> The number of needle-stick injuries in your agency has increased. How might the continuous quality improvement process affect this situation?

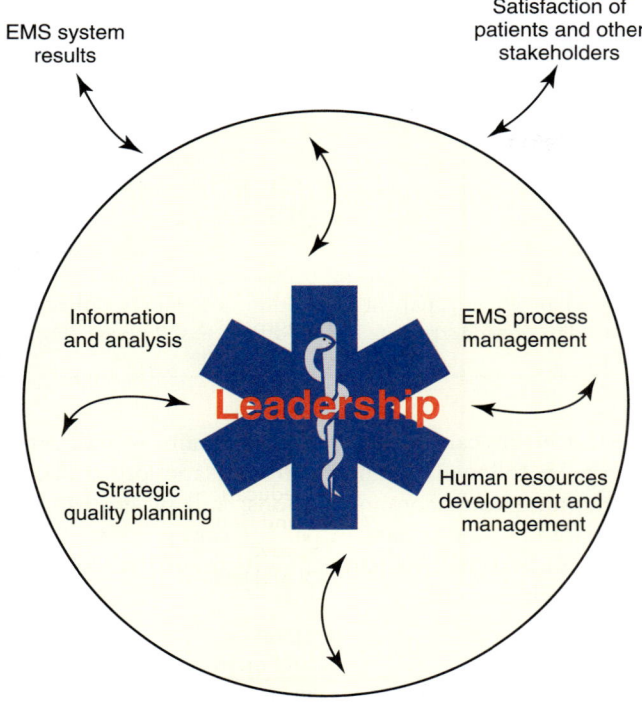

FIGURE 1-7 Leadership guide to quality improvement for EMS. (U.S. Department of Transportation, Health Resources and Services Administration, Maternal and Child Health Bureau, *A leadership guide to quality improvement,* Washington, DC, 1999, The Administration.)

Key actions or categories for EMS leaders to improve quality within their organization are as follows[9]:

1. *Leadership* involves efforts by senior leadership and management. These persons lead by example to integrate CQI into the strategic planning process and throughout the entire organization. Such integration promotes quality values and CQI techniques in work practices.

2. *Information and analysis* deal with managing and using the data needed for effective CQI. Continuous quality improvement is based on management by fact. Thus information and analyses are critical to CQI success.

3. *Strategic quality planning* has three main parts. The first is developing long- and short-term goals for structural, performance, and outcome quality standards. The second is finding ways to achieve those. The third is measuring the effectiveness of the system in meeting quality standards.

4. *Human resource development and management* refers to developing the full potential of the EMS workforce. This effort is guided by the principle that the entire EMS workforce is motivated to achieve new levels of service and value.

5. *Emergency medical services process management* concerns the creation and maintenance of high-quality services. Within the context of CQI, process management refers to the improvement of work activities. Process management also refers to improving work flow *across* functional or departmental boundaries.

6. *Emergency medical systems results* entail assessment of the quality results achieved and examining the success of the organization in achieving CQI.

7. *Satisfaction of patients and other stakeholders* involves ensuring ongoing satisfaction. Those internal and external to the EMS system must be satisfied with the services provided.

Benefits gained by applying these seven guidelines and recommendations are many. They include improvements in service and patient care delivery, economic efficiency, and profitability. They also help improve patient and community satisfaction and loyalty, and healthful outcomes.

SHOW ME THE EVIDENCE

The 2007 U.S. Metropolitan Municipalities' EMS Medical Directors' Consortium describe an evidence-based model to measure quality within suburban and urban EMS systems. They include specific key interventions and numbers-needed-to-treat that should be measured in the areas of ST-elevation myocardial infarction (STEMI), pulmonary edema, asthma, seizure, trauma, and cardiac arrest. The interventions to be evaluated in CQI are those that have been demonstrated by research to have a positive impact on patient outcome. For example, in a patient with trauma, prehospital records should be evaluated for scene time <10 minutes and transport to a trauma center.

From: Myers JB, Slovis CM, Eckstein M, et al: Evidence-based performance measures for emergency medical services systems: a model for expanded EMS benchmarking, *Prehosp Emerg Care* 12(2): 141-151, 2008.

PATIENT SAFETY

Patient safety is one of the most urgent health care challenges. In 1996, the Institute of Medicine (IOM) launched an ongoing effort to assess and improve the nation's quality of care. The report brief of this initiative is titled *To Err is Human: Building a Safer Health System.* This study found that[16]:

- Health care in the United States is not as safe as it should be—and can be.
- At least 44,000 people, and perhaps as many as 98,000 people, die in hospitals each year as a result of medical errors that could have been prevented.
- Preventable medical errors in hospitals exceed attributable deaths to such feared causes as motor-vehicle wrecks, breast cancer, and AIDS.
- High error rates with serious consequences are most likely to occur in intensive care units, operating rooms, and emergency departments.
- Most errors are caused by faulty systems, processes, and conditions (Box 1-13).

High-Risk Activities

There are many activities that can lead to medical errors in EMS. Some of the more high-risk activities include:

BOX 1-13 Types of Errors

Diagnostic
- Error or delay in diagnosis
- Failure to employ indicated tests
- Use of outmoded tests or therapy
- Failure to act on results of monitoring or testing

Treatment
- Error in the performance of an operation, procedure, or test
- Error in administering the treatment
- Error in the dose or method of using a drug
- Avoidable delay in treatment or in responding to an abnormal test
- Inappropriate (not indicated) care

Preventive
- Failure to provide prophylactic treatment
- Inadequate monitoring or follow-up of treatment

Other
- Failure of communication
- Equipment failure
- Other system failure

Types of Errors from IOM report, http://www.iom.edu/Object.File/Master/4/117/ToErr-8pager.pdf, accessed August 26, 2010.

- Ambulance crashes
- Dropping patients
- Hand-offs
- Communication issues
- Medication issues
- Poor sterile technique
- Airway issues
- Spinal immobilization

DID YOU KNOW?
Hand-offs involve the transfer of rights, duties, and obligations from one person or team to another. Hand-offs should include the continuity and safety of the patient's care. For hand-offs to be effective, a solid foundation in communications is necessary. Face-to-face communications through a standardized process is the best way to transfer patient care. This should include an opportunity to ask and respond to questions. The hand-off includes current information about the patient, such as care, treatment, condition, and recent or anticipated changes in the patient's condition. A memory aid that can be used to provide structure in handoffs is *I Pass the Baton* (Figure 1-8).[17]

Most errors can be avoided by maintaining skill proficiency; by following established rules and protocols; by maintaining team communications; and by ensuring an adequate knowledge base in patient care procedures and related EMS duties. Patient safety issues will be discussed throughout this text.

SHOW ME THE EVIDENCE
Researchers in the UK surveyed four emergency departments and one ambulance service to investigate the hand-over process from ambulance personnel to the ED staff. They found a lack of active listening skills in the ED staff led to frustration of the EMS crews. They report that ambulance staff should be prepared to repeat their report, especially for seriously ill or injured patients. Reports for critically ill patients should be delivered in two phases: with essential information reported at the time of handoff and more detailed information conveyed after initial care of the patient in the ED has begun. They recommend more ED education on this process.

From: Jenkin A, Abelson-Michell N, Cooper S: Patient handover: time for a change? *Accid Emerg Nurs* 15(3): 141-147, 2007.

I PASS the BATON

I	Introduction	Individuals involved in the handoff identify themselves, their roles and jobs
P	Patient	Name, identifiers, age, sex, location
A	Assessment	Present chief complaint, vital signs, symptoms, and diagnosis
S	Situation	Current status and circumstances, including code status, level of certainty or uncertainty, recent changes, and response to treatment
S	Safety concerns	Critical lab values and reports, socioeconomic factors, allergies and alerts, such as risk for falls
the		
B	Background	Comorbidities, previous episodes, current medications, and family history
A	Actions	Detail what actions were taken or are required and provide a brief rationale for those actions
T	Timing	Level of urgency and explicit timing, prioritization of actions
O	Ownership	Who is responsible (nurse/doctor/team), including patient and family responsibilities?
N	Next	What will happen next? Any anticipated changes? What is the plan? Any contingency plans?

FIGURE 1-8 Transferring patient care safely.

Preventing Medical Errors

Patient safety solutions have been developed by the World Health Organization (WHO), in collaboration with the Joint Commission, and The Joint Commission International. This group defined *patient safety solutions* as: "Any system design or intervention that has demonstrated the ability to prevent or mitigate patient harm stemming from the processes of health care." In 2007, the International Steering Committee approved nine solutions for patient safety (Box 1-14).[18]

BOX 1-14 Nine Patient Safety Solutions

1. **Look-Alike, Sound-Alike Medication Names:** Confusing drug names is one of the most common causes of medication errors and is a worldwide concern. With tens of thousands of drugs currently on the market, the potential for error created by confusing brand or generic drug names and packaging is significant.

2. **Patient Identification:** The widespread and continuing failures to correctly identify patients often leads to medication, transfusion, and testing errors; wrong person procedures; and the discharge of infants to the wrong families.

3. **Communication During Patient Hand-Overs:** Gaps in hand-over (or hand-off) communication between patient care units, and between and among care teams, can cause serious breakdowns in the continuity of care, inappropriate treatment, and potential harm for the patient.

4. **Performance of Correct Procedure at Correct Body Site:** Considered totally preventable, cases of wrong procedure or wrong site surgery are largely the result of miscommunication and unavailable, or incorrect, information. A major contributing factor to these types of errors is the lack of a standardized preoperative process.

5. **Control of Concentrated Electrolyte Solutions:** Although all drugs, biologics, vaccines, and contrast media have a defined risk profile, concentrated electrolyte solutions that are used for injection are especially dangerous.

6. **Assuring Medication Accuracy at Transitions in Care:** Medication errors occur most commonly at transitions. Medication reconciliation is a process designed to prevent medication errors at patient transition points.

7. **Avoiding Catheter and Tubing Misconnections:** The design of tubing, catheters, and syringes currently in use is such that it is possible to inadvertently cause patient harm through connecting the wrong syringes and tubing and then delivering medication or fluids through an unintended wrong route.

8. **Single Use of Injection Devices:** One of the biggest global concerns is the spread of human immunodeficiency virus (HIV), the hepatitis B virus (HBV), and the hepatitis C virus (HCV) because of the reuse of injection needles.

9. **Improved Hand Hygiene to Prevent Health Care-Associated Infection (HAI):** It is estimated that at any point in time more than 1.4 million people worldwide are suffering from infections acquired in hospitals. Effective hand hygiene is the primary preventive measure for avoiding this problem.

Methods to Help Prevent Medical Errors in EMS

Methods to avoid medical errors in EMS can be grouped into environmental methods and individual methods.

Environmental methods that can help prevent medical errors include having clear and established protocols for procedures; ensuring that there is sufficient lighting for patient assessment and patient care procedures; and performing patient care duties with minimal interruptions. Organizing and packaging drugs (e.g., separating adult and pediatric drugs) to avoid confusing the medications is another example of an environmental method to reduce medical errors. Another example of a safety method to reduce medical error is securing equipment in the patient compartment of the ambulance. Another is safely securing adult and pediatric patients during transport.

DID YOU KNOW?
Medication Error Survey: Paramedic Self-Reported Medication Errors

BACKGROUND: Continuing quality improvement (CQI) reviews reflect that medication administration errors occur in the prehospital setting. These include errors involving dose, medication, route, concentration, and treatment.

METHODS: A survey was given to paramedics in San Diego County. The survey tool was established on the basis of previous literature reviews and questions developed with previous CQI data.

RESULTS: A total of 352 surveys were returned, with the paramedics reporting a mean of 8.5 years of field experience. They work an average of 11.0 shifts/month with an average of 25.4 hours and 6.7 calls/shift. Thirty-two (9.1%) responding paramedics reported committing a medication error in the last 12 months. Types of errors included dose-related errors (63%), protocol errors (33%), wrong route errors (21%), and wrong medication errors (4%). Issues identified as contributing to the errors include failure to triple check, infrequent use of the medication, dosage calculation error, and incorrect dosage given. Fatigue, training, and equipment setup of the drug box were not listed as contributing factors. The majority of these errors were self-reported to the CQI representative (79.1%), with 8.3% being reported by the base hospital radio nurse, 8.3% found upon chart review, and 4.2% noted by paramedic during call but never reported.

CONCLUSIONS: Nine percent of paramedics responding to an anonymous survey report medication errors in the last 12 months, with 4% of these errors never having been reported in the CQI process. Additional safeguards must continue to be implemented to decrease the incidence of medication errors.

From: Vilke GM, Tornabene SV, Stepanski B, et al: Paramedic self-reported medication errors, *Prehosp Emerg Care* 11(1):80-84, 2007.

Individual methods include personal activities to improve patient safety. These include:

■ **Reflection in action:** Think during an event (during action) when things do not go as planned. Reflection in action allows us to reshape what we are working on *while* we are working on it. It helps us as we complete a task. Reflection in action promotes critical thinking and bridges the gap between "knowing and doing."

- **Question assumptions:** Apply critical thinking to continuously look for good ideas and new solutions. This will help to set priorities and to problem solve.
- **Reflection bias ("hindsight" bias):** Avoid the tendency to judge an event, because a bad outcome is known from a previous experience you had. (*"I knew that was going to happen."*) Reflection bias is the inclination to see events that have occurred in the past as more predictable than they really were. Review the events after the fact and you might foresee the outcome as more preventable. Replace hindsight with insight.

- **Use decision aids:** Use evidence-based decision aids and guidelines (e.g., algorithms, pocket guides) to simplify decision making and improve patient safety. Decision aids can also facilitate patients' participation in decisions about their care, when appropriate.
- **Ask for help:** You are functioning as part of a team. Don't be hesitant to ask your crew members or medical direction for help or advice, if the need arises. If you are unsure about a decision, drug dose, or procedure, remember that patient safety comes first.

SUMMARY

- The roots of prehospital emergency care may date back to the military.
- In the early twentieth century through the mid-1960s, prehospital care in the United States was provided in a few ways. Care was provided mostly by urban hospital-based systems. These systems later developed into municipal services. Care also was provided by funeral directors and volunteers who were not trained in these services.
- The operations of an effective EMS system include citizen activation, dispatch, prehospital care, hospital care, and rehabilitation.
- Each level of EMS personnel have their own distinct roles and duties. These roles include telecommunicators (dispatchers), emergency medical responders, EMTs, advanced EMTs, and paramedics. These levels combine to make an effective prehospital EMS system.
- Many professional groups and organizations help to set the standards of EMS. These groups exist at the national, state, regional, and local levels. The groups take part in development, education, and implementation. Being active in such a group helps to promote the status of the paramedic.
- Continuing education is crucial. It provides a way for all health care personnel to maintain basic technical and professional skills.

- Professionalism refers to the way in which a person conducts himself or herself. Professionalism also refers to how one follows the standards of conduct and performance established by the profession.
- The roles and duties of the paramedic can be divided into two categories: *primary* and *additional* duties.
- The two types of medical direction are online (direct) and off-line (indirect). Both are equally important. They help to ensure that the components of quality medical care are in place in an EMS system.
- A CQI program identifies and attempts to resolve problems in areas such as medical direction, financing, training, communication, prehospital management and transportation, interfacility transfer, receiving facilities, specialty care units, dispatch, public information and education, audit and quality assurance, disaster planning, and mutual aid.
- Patient safety should be a high priority during every call. Errors that may cause injury or illness often involve handoffs, communication issues, medication issues, airway issues, lifting or moving patients, ambulance crashes, and immobilization.

REFERENCES

1. Lyons A, Petrucelli J: *Medicine: an illustrated history*, New York, 1987, Harry N Abrams.
2. McSwain NE: Prehospital care from Napoleon to Mars: The surgeon's role, *J Am Coll Surg* 201(4):651, 2005.
3. http://www.redcross.org/museum/registry/profile.asp?id=33, accessed 3-15-09.
4. McNeil E: *Airborne care of the ill and injured*, New York, 1983, Springer-Verlag.
5. EMS: Past, Present, Future, NAEMT, www.naemt.or/education, accessed 3-15-09.
6. National Highway Traffic Safety Administration, U.S. Department of Health and Human Services, Health Resources and Services Administration, Maternal and Child Health Bureau: Emergency medical services agenda for the future, Washington, DC, 1999.
7. Munir GM: Access to health care in the U.S.: Problems and the bottom line, http://www.articlecity.com/articles/politics_and_government/article_525.shtml, accessed 2-10-09.
8. National Highway Traffic Safety Administration: The National EMS Scope of Practice model, Washington, DC, 2005, U.S. Department of Transportation/National Highway Traffic Safety Administration.
9. National Highway Traffic Safety Administration, U.S. Department of Transportation: Emergency medical services: NHTSA leading the way, Washington, DC, 1995.

10. National Registry of Emergency Medical Technicians: National emergency medical services education and practice blueprint, Columbus, Ohio, 1993.
11. National Highway Traffic Safety Administration. The National EMS Education Standards, Washington, DC, 2009, U.S. Department of Transportation/National Highway Traffic Safety Administration, DOT.
12. National Association of EMS Physicians, National Highway Traffic Safety Administration, Maternal and Child Health Bureau: National standard curriculum for medical direction, Washington, DC, 1998.
13. Kuehl AE (Ed): Prehospital systems and medical oversight, National Association of EMS Physicians, ed 3, Lenexa, KS, 2002, Mosby.
14. National Highway Traffic Safety Administration: A leadership guide to quality improvement for emergency medical services (EMS) systems, Washington, DC, 1997.
15. American College of Emergency Physicians: Direction of out-of-hospital care at the scene of medical emergencies, Revised and approved by the ACEP Board of Directors, April 2008.
16. Institute of Medicine: Shaping the future for health, November 1999, National Academy of Sciences, 2000, http://www.iom.edu/~/media/Files/Report%20Files/1999/To-Err-is-Human/To%20Err%20is%20Human%201999%20%20report%20brief.pdf, accessed August 4, 2010.
17. Department of Defense Patient Safety Program: Healthcare communications toolkit to improve transitions in care, Washington, D.C., 2008.
18. The Joint Commission, Joint Commission Resources, Joint Commission International: Patient Safety Solutions, 2008, http://www.ccforpatientsafety.org/Patient-Safety-Solutions, accessed 2-6-09.

SUGGESTED READINGS

Brown WE, Dickinson PD, Misselbeck WJ, Levine R: Longitudinal emergency medical technician attribute and demographic study, *Prehosp Emerg Care* 6(4):433-439, 2002.

National Registry of Emergency Medical Technicians: http://www.nremt.org, accessed 8-4-2010.

The NEMSIS Technical Assistance Center: http://www.nemsis.org/index.html, accessed 2-23-09.

Institute of Medicine of the National Academies. Future of emergency care series: Emergency medical services at the crossroads, Washington DC, 2006, National Academic Press.

Meisel ZF, Hargarte S, Vernick J: Addressing prehospital patient safety using the science of injury prevention and control, *Prehosp Emerg Care* 12(4), 411-416, 2008.

Page J: The Paramedics: an illustrated history of paramedics in their first decade, Morristown NJ, 1979, Backdraft Publications.

Page J: The Magic of 3 A.M: essays on the art and science of emergency medical services, Carlsbad, CA, 2002, JEMS Communications.

Page J: The Modern History of EMS: making a difference 2.0 (DVD), St Louis, 2004, Elsevier Mosby.

2 Well-Being of the Paramedic

OBJECTIVES

Upon completion of this chapter, the paramedic student will be able to:

1. Describe the components of wellness and associated benefits.
2. Discuss the paramedic's role in promoting wellness.
3. Outline the benefits of specific lifestyle choices that promote wellness, including proper nutrition, weight control, exercise, sleep, and smoking cessation.
4. Identify risk factors and warning signs of cancer and cardiovascular disease.
5. List measures to take to reduce the risk of infectious disease exposure.
6. Outline actions to be taken following a significant exposure to a patient's blood or other body fluids.
7. Identify preventive measures to minimize the risk of work-related illness or injury associated with exposure, lifting and moving patients, hostile environments, vehicle operations, and rescue situations.
8. List signs and symptoms of addiction and addictive behavior.
9. Describe guidelines for working effectively in a diverse workplace.
10. Distinguish between normal and abnormal anxiety and stress reactions.
11. Give examples of stress-reduction techniques.
12. Outline the 10 components of critical incident stress management.
13. Given a scenario involving death or dying, identify therapeutic actions you may take based on your knowledge of the dynamics of this process.

KEY TERMS

adaptation A cellular response to stress of any kind to escape and protect from injury; a central part of the response to changes in the physiological condition.

addiction A compulsive, uncontrollable dependence on a substance, habit, or practice to such a degree that cessation causes severe emotional, mental, or physiological reactions.

adrenaline An endogenous adrenal hormone that helps prepare the body for energetic action.

anxiety A state or feeling of apprehension, uneasiness, agitation, uncertainty, or fear resulting from the anticipation of some threat or danger.

autonomic nervous system The part of the nervous system that regulates involuntary vital functions, including the activity of cardiac muscle, smooth muscle, and glands.

circadian rhythm A pattern based on a 24-hour cycle, especially repetition of certain physiological phenomena, such as sleeping and eating.

distress Negative, debilitating, or harmful stress.

eustress Positive, performance-enhancing stress.

posttraumatic stress disorder An anxiety disorder that can occur following a traumatic event.

stress A nonspecific mental or physical strain caused by any emotional, physical, social, economic, or other factor that initiates a physiological response.

universal precautions Infection control practices in health care that are observed with every patient and procedure and that prevent exposure to blood-borne pathogens.

The paramedic has a demanding job that requires physical and mental well-being. By adopting a lifestyle that enhances personal wellness, paramedics can improve their health and prolong their careers. A healthful lifestyle also helps paramedics to serve as role models and coaches for others.

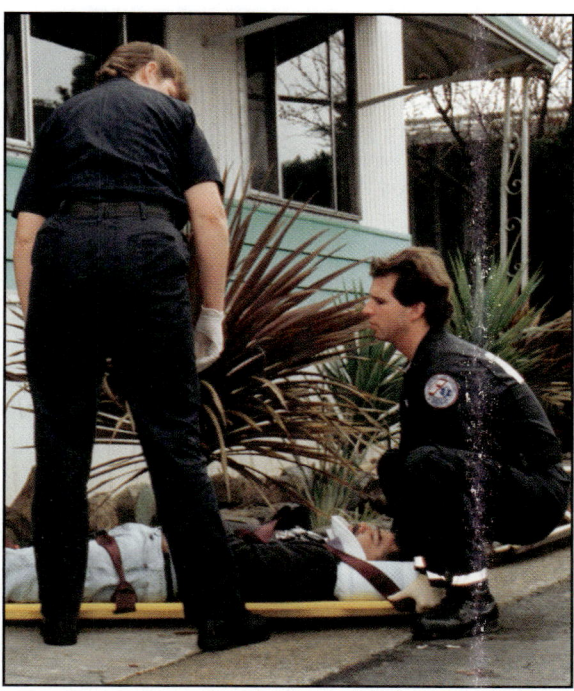

WELLNESS COMPONENTS

Wellness has two main aspects: physical well-being and mental and emotional health. Both aspects are key to the paramedic's personal health and ability to safely deliver emergency care. They are also important to manage stressful events that are inherent in the profession.

Physical Well-Being

Several factors play a major role in maintaining physical health. These factors include good nutrition, physical fitness, ample sleep, and the prevention of disease and injury.

NUTRITION

Nutrients are foods that hold the elements necessary for body function. The six categories of nutrients are carbohydrates, fats, proteins, vitamins, minerals, and water.

Carbohydrates are composed of carbon, hydrogen, and oxygen. Carbohydrates are obtained primarily from plant foods. The only important source of animal carbohydrates is lactose (milk sugar). Plants store carbohydrates as starch. Starch is made up of granules enclosed by cellulose walls that swell and burst when cooked. This feature makes cooked starchy foods easier to digest than raw, uncooked starchy foods.

All dietary fats contain a mixture of saturated and unsaturated fatty acids. Saturated fats are found mainly in meat and dairy products and in some vegetable fats. These fats raise the cholesterol levels in the blood by shutting down the process that normally removes excess cholesterol from the body. Unsaturated fats are subdivided further into polyunsaturated and monounsaturated fats. Polyunsaturated fats are found in safflower, sunflower, corn, soybean, and cottonseed oils and in some fish. These fats help rid the body of newly formed cholesterol. Omega-3 fatty acids are found mainly in cold-water fish such as tuna, salmon, and mackerel. These fats are a form of polyunsaturated fats. All polyunsaturated fats, including the omega-3 fats, are considered important to human health. Monounsaturated fats are liquid vegetable oils. Examples of these fats include canola and olive oils. Like polyunsaturated fats, these also may decrease blood cholesterol levels (Box 2-1). Trans-fats are unsaturated fatty acids formed when vegetable oils are processed and made more solid or into a more stable liquid. Trans-fats are present in a wide range of foods. These foods include those products made with partially hydrogenated oils, such as baked goods and fried foods, and some margarine products. Trans-fats also occur naturally in low amounts in meats and dairy products. Although trans-fats are unsaturated, they appear similar to saturated fats in terms of their effect on blood cholesterol levels.

> **NOTE**
>
> Cholesterol is present in all foods of animal origin and is concentrated heavily in fat and in poultry skin. Cholesterol is a white, waxy substance found in every cell. Not all cholesterol is harmful; an adequate amount of cholesterol is needed for body functions. Cholesterol is manufactured in the liver and is carried through the bloodstream. Adding cholesterol to the diet can raise blood cholesterol levels and increase the risk of heart disease and stroke.

Proteins are made of hydrogen, oxygen, carbon, and nitrogen (and most contain sulfur and phosphorus). Proteins are vital to building body tissue during growth, maintenance, and repair. When proteins are digested, they break down into amino acids (classified as *essential* or *nonessential*). Essential amino acids are needed for body growth and cellular life. They must be obtained in food because they are *not* made in the body. Nonessential amino acids are not needed for body health and growth and can be made in the body. Proteins that contain all the essential amino acids are *complete proteins* and are found in meats and dairy products. Proteins that are missing one or more essential amino acids are *incomplete proteins* (e.g., those in grains and vegetables).

BOX 2-1 A Primer on Fats and Oils

Not All Fats and Oils Are Created Equal

Fats and oils are made up of basic units called fatty acids. Each type of fat or oil is a mixture of different fatty acids.

- **Saturated Fatty Acids** are found chiefly in animal sources such as meat and poultry, whole or reduced-fat milk, and butter. Some vegetable oils like coconut, palm kernel oil, and palm oil are saturated. Saturated fats are usually solid at room temperature.
- **Monounsaturated Fatty Acids** are found mainly in vegetable oils such as canola, olive, and peanut oils. They are liquid at room temperature.
- **Polyunsaturated Fatty Acids** are found mainly in vegetable oils such as safflower, sunflower, corn, flaxseed, and canola oils. Polyunsaturated fats are also the main fats found in seafood. They are liquid or soft at room temperature. Specific polyunsaturated fatty acids, such as linoleic acid and alpha-linolenic acid, are called essential fatty acids. They are necessary for cell structure and making hormones. Essential fatty acids must be obtained from foods we choose.
- **Trans–Fatty Acids** are formed when vegetable oils are processed into margarine or shortening. Sources of trans-fats in the diet include snack foods and baked goods made with "partially hydrogenated vegetable oil" or "vegetable shortening." Trans–fatty acids also occur naturally in some animal products such as dairy products.

Cholesterol Is Different

Blood (serum) cholesterol and dietary cholesterol are two different types of cholesterol. Dietary cholesterol is found in food of animal origin such as egg yolks, organ meats, and full-fat dairy products. Blood cholesterol is a waxy substance that occurs naturally in our body. It is used to make estrogen and testosterone, and bile, which is needed for digestion. However, if the level of cholesterol in the blood is too high, cholesterol and other fats can stick to the artery walls.

Because blood cholesterol is waxy and cannot dissolve in water, it is carried through the blood in packages called lipoproteins. High-density lipoprotein (HDL) is a "good" package for cholesterol and low-density lipoprotein (LDL) is a "bad" package for cholesterol.

HDL cholesterol collects excess cholesterol in the blood and carries it to the liver. The liver reprocesses or excretes it. HDL may also help remove some of the cholesterol deposited on the artery walls.

Excess LDL cholesterol can increase the risk of heart disease because it is LDL cholesterol that accumulates on the artery walls. The type of fats and oils we eat helps control LDL levels.

Fat and Cholesterol: Know Your Limits

The guidelines for fat intake are well known: for healthy Americans, consume no more than 30% of total calories from fat. The "30 percent" guideline means:

- 7%-10% of total calories from saturated fats
- About 10%-15% of total calories from monounsaturated fats
- About 10% of total calories from polyunsaturated fats

Healthy Americans should limit their cholesterol intake to less than 300 milligrams per day.

From Duyff RL: *American Dietetic Association complete food and nutrition guide*, ed 3, Hoboken, New Jersey, 2006, John Wiley & Sons.

Proteins can be used as a source of energy but should be spared for their more important role in body health by the sufficient intake of carbohydrates.

Vitamins are organic substances that are present in minute amounts in foods. Because vitamins are crucial for metabolism and cannot be made in adequate amounts by the body, they must be gained through food or vitamin supplements. (An ample intake of vitamins through a balanced diet should make vitamin supplements unnecessary in healthy people.) Vitamins are water soluble or fat soluble. Vitamins C and B complex contain eight water-soluble vitamins. Water-soluble vitamins cannot be stored in the body. They must come from the daily diet. Fat-soluble vitamins (vitamins A, D, E, and K) can be stored in the body. Therefore a daily dietary intake of these vitamins is not required (Box 2-2).

Minerals are inorganic elements that play a key role in biochemical reactions in the body. These minerals include calcium, chromium, iron, magnesium, potassium, selenium, sodium, and zinc. Like vitamins, minerals come from the diet (Table 2-1).

Water is the most important nutrient because cellular function depends on a fluid environment. Water composes

BOX 2-2 Free Radicals and Antioxidants

Free radicals are natural by-products of chemical reactions in the body that can produce cellular injury. The buildup of these free radicals increases with age. The buildup is thought to be the cause of many diseases, including heart disease, diabetes, and some cancers. Substances that can generate free radicals can be found in fried foods, alcohol, tobacco smoke, pesticides, and air pollution. Other substances to which persons often are exposed also may create free radicals.

Antioxidants are known as free radical scavengers. They are compounds that reduce the formation of free radicals or react with and neutralize them, making them nontoxic to cells. Antioxidants occur naturally in the body. They also occur naturally in certain foods such as fruits, vegetables, and whole grains. Beta carotene (a form of vitamin A) and vitamins C and E are popular antioxidant supplements. These may benefit a person's health.

50% to 60% of the total body weight. (Infants have the greatest percentage of body water; older adults have the least.) Water is obtained through consumption of liquids and fresh fruits and vegetables. Water is also produced when food is oxidized during digestion.

TABLE 2-1 The ABCs of Nutrition

	Function	Source
Vitamins		
A	Proper eye function; keeps skin, hair, and nails healthy; helps maintain healthy gums, glands, bones, teeth; helps ward off infection; may protect against lung cancer	Liver,* dairy products,* fish, carrots, yellow squash, dark-green leafy vegetables, corn, tomatoes, papaya
B_1 (thiamine)	Helps convert carbohydrates into biological energy; promotes proper nerve function	Pork,* unrefined and enriched cereals, organ meats,* legumes, nuts*
B_2 (riboflavin)	Crucial in the production of body energy	Milk,* cheese,* yogurt,* green leafy vegetables, fruits, bread, cereals, meats*
B_3 (niacin)	Lowers cholesterol levels in blood only in very high doses; may protect against cardiovascular disease	Yeast, meats* including liver,* cereals, legumes, seeds*
B_6	Essential for protein breakdown and absorption	Beef,* poultry,* fish, pork,* bananas, nuts,* whole grains, vegetables
B_{12}	Essential for the healthy function of nerve tissue	Meats,* meat products,* shellfish, fish, poultry,* eggs*
Biotin	Needed for breakdown of glucose (a type of sugar) and formation of certain fatty acids necessary for several important body functions	Meats,* poultry,* fish, eggs,* nuts,* seeds,* legumes, vegetables
C (ascorbic acid)	Strengthens blood vessel walls; keeps gums healthy; promotes healing of cuts and wounds	Strawberries, citrus fruits, tomatoes, cabbage, cauliflower, broccoli, greens
D	Helps build and maintain teeth and bones; needed for body to absorb calcium	Egg yolks,* fish and cod liver oil,* fortified milk and butter*
E	Helps form red blood cells, muscle tissue, and other tissues; may protect against heart disease	Poultry,* seafood, seeds,* nuts,* cooked greens, wheat germ, fortified cereals, eggs*
K†	Needed for normal clotting of blood	Spinach, broccoli, brussels sprouts, kale, turnip greens
Minerals		
Calcium	Helps build strong bones and teeth; promotes proper muscle and nerve function; helps blood to clot; helps activate enzymes needed to convert food to energy; may protect against the development of fragile, porous bones	Milk,* cheese,* yogurt,* buttermilk, other dairy products,* green leafy vegetables†
Chromium	Works with insulin to maintain normal blood glucose	Whole-grain cereals, condiments (black pepper, thyme), meat products,* cheeses*
Iron	Essential to make hemoglobin, the oxygen-carrying component of red blood cells	Red meat* and liver,* shellfish and fish, legumes, dried apricots, fortified breads and cereals
Magnesium	Activates enzymes needed to release energy in body; promotes bone growth; needed to make cells and genetic material	Green leafy vegetables, beans, nuts,* fortified wholegrain cereals and breads, oysters, scallops
Potassium	With sodium, helps to regulate body's fluid balance; plays a major role in muscle contraction, nerve conduction, beating of the heart	Bananas, citrus fruits, dried fruits, deep yellow vegetables, potatoes, legumes, milk,* bran cereal
Selenium	Interacts with vitamin E to prevent breakdown of cells in body	Organ meats,* seafood, meats,* cereals and grains, egg yolks,* mushrooms, onions, garlic
Sodium	Helps maintain body fluid balance	Salt, processed foods, foods in brine, salted crackers and chips, cured meats, soy sauce (Note: sodium is so prevalent that low intake is very rare. The problem is avoiding excessive intake of sodium.)
Zinc	Boosts the immune system and helps fight disease; element in more than 100 enzymes—proteins that are essential to digestion and other functions	Red meats,* some seafoods, grains

From U.S. Department of Agriculture's Center for Nutrition Policy and Promotion, Washington, DC, accessed at www.usda.gov.
*These foods are high in fat and/or cholesterol. Use sparingly or substitute low-fat versions, where possible.
†Green leafy vegetables and other foods rich in vitamin K can contribute to blood clotting. If you take a drug that prevents blood clotting, talk to your physician before changing your diet.

DIETARY RECOMMENDATIONS

Various health care groups make recommendations for a healthful diet. These groups include the U.S. Department of Agriculture (USDA), the U.S. Department of Health and Human Services, and the Food and Drug Administration. Box 2-3 lists the nutritional recommended intake values and Table 2-2 and Box 2-4 give the dietary recommendations for the general population as recommended by the American Heart Association, the National Institutes of Health, and the USDA.

CRITICAL THINKING
Does your average diet meet these guidelines? If not, in what areas do you need to make changes?

FOOD GUIDANCE PYRAMID

In 2005, the USDA revised and simplified the original food guide pyramid, established in 1992. The food pyramid is known as MyPyramid. It was designed to educate the public and health professionals about diet and lifestyle that was consistent with the *2005 Dietary Guidelines for Americans* (revised in 2010).[1]

BOX 2-3 Nutritional Components of the TLC Diet

Nutrient	Recommended Intake
Saturated fat*	<7% of total calories
Polyunsaturated fat	Up to 10% of total calories
Monounsaturated fat	Up to 20% of total calories
Total fat	25%-35% of total calories
Carbohydrate (esp. complex carbs)	50%-60% of total calories
Fiber	20-30 g/day
Protein	~15% of total calories
Cholesterol	<200 mg/day

TABLE 2-2 Summary of Diet and Lifestyle Recommendations from the American Heart Association Nutrition Committee 2006

Population Goals	Major Guidelines
Consume an overall healthy diet	Consume a variety of fruits, vegetables, and grain products, especially whole grains; choose fat-free and low-fat dairy products, legumes, poultry, and lean meats; and eat fish, preferably oily fish, at least twice a week.
Aim for a healthy body weight BMI 18.5-24.9 kg/m²	Achieve and maintain healthy weight throughout life with increased effort aimed at helping individuals avoid inappropriate weight gain during childhood years and subsequent weight gain during adult years. Increase emphasis on prevention of weight gain in the first place.
Aim for a desirable lipid profile LDL-C <100 mg/dL optimal 100-129 mg/dL near or above optimal 130-159 mg/dL borderline high 160-189 mg/dL high ≥190 mg/dL very high TG <150 mg/dL HDL-C >40 mg/dL (men) >50 mg/dL (women)	Reduce daily intake of saturated fat (<7%), trans-fat (<1%), and cholesterol (300 mg). Avoid excess body weight. Drug therapy is often prescribed for those at moderate or high risk. Dietary changes are recommended for all individuals.
Aim for a normal BP Systolic BP <120 mm Hg Diastolic BP <80 mm Hg	Reduce salt intake; induce weight loss by caloric deficit, moderation of alcohol (among those who drink), increased potassium intake. Stress consumption of a healthy diet such as the DASH diet that emphasizes fruits and vegetables and low-fat dairy. Include whole grains, poultry, fish, and nuts. Reduce fat, red meat, sweets, and sugar-containing beverages. Replace some carbohydrates either with protein from plant sources or with monounsaturated fat.
Be physically active	All adults should accumulate ≥30 minutes of physical activity most days of the week. At least 60 minutes of physical activity most days of the week is recommended for children and those adults attempting to lose weight or maintaining weight loss.
Avoid use and exposure to tobacco products	Eliminate the use of tobacco products and minimize exposure to second-hand smoke.

From Lichtenstein AH, Appel LJ, Brands M, et al: Diet and lifestyle recommendations revision 2006: a scientific statement from the American Heart Association Nutrition Committee, *Circulation* 114:82-96, 2006.

BOX 2-4   USDA Dietary Guidelines for Americans: Key Recommendations

Balancing Calories to Manage Weight
- Prevent and/or reduce overweight and obesity through improved eating and physical activity behaviors
- Control total calorie intake to manage body weight. For people who are overweight or obese, this will mean consuming fewer calories from foods and beverages
- Increase physical activity and reduce time spent in sedentary behaviors
- Maintain appropriate calorie balance during each stage of life—childhood, adolescence, adulthood, pregnancy and breastfeeding, and older age

Foods and Food Components to Reduce
- Reduce daily sodium intake to fewer than 2300 milligrams (mg) and further reduce intake to 1500 mg among persons who are 51 and older and those of any age who are African-American or have hypertension, diabetes, or chronic kidney disease. The 1500-mg recommendation applies to about half of the U.S. population, including children, and the majority of adults
- Consume fewer than 10% of calories from saturated fatty acids by replacing them with monounsaturated and polyunsaturated fatty acids
- Consume fewer than 300 mg per day of dietary cholesterol
- Keep trans fatty acid consumption as low as possible by limiting foods that contain synthetic sources of trans fats, such as partially hydrogenated oils, and by limiting other solid fats
- Reduce the intake of calories from solid fats and added sugars
- Limit the consumption of foods that contain refined grains, especially refined grain foods that contain solid fats, added sugars, and sodium
- If alcohol is consumed, it should be consumed in moderation—up to one drink per day for women and two drinks per day for men—and only by adults of legal drinking age

Foods and Nutrients to Increase
Individuals should meet the following recommendations as part of a healthy eating pattern while staying within their calorie needs
- Increase vegetable and fruit intake
- Eat a variety of vegetables, especially dark green and red and orange vegetables and beans and peas
- Consume at least half of all grains as whole grains. Increase whole-grain intake by replacing refined grains with whole grains

- Increase intake of fat-free or low-fat milk and milk products, such as milk, yogurt, cheese, or fortified soy beverages*
- Choose a variety of protein foods, which include seafood, lean meat and poultry, eggs, beans and peas, soy products, and unsalted nuts and seeds
- Increase the amount and variety of seafood consumed by choosing seafood in place of some meat and poultry
- Replace protein foods that are higher in solid fats with choices that are lower in solid fats and calories and/or sources of oils
- Use oils to replace solid fats when possible
- Choose foods that provide more potassium, dietary fiber, calcium, and vitamin D, which are nutrients of concern in American diets. These foods include vegetables, fruits, whole grains, and milk and milk products

Recommendations for Specific Population Groups
Women Capable of Becoming Pregnant?†
- Choose foods that supply heme iron, which is more readily absorbed by the body, additional iron sources, and enhancers of iron absorption such as vitamin C-rich foods
- Consume 400 micrograms (mcg) per day of synthetic folic acid (from fortified foods and/or supplements) in addition to food forms of folate form a varied diet‡

Women Who Are Pregnant of Breastfeeding?
- Consume 8 to 12 ounces of seafood per week from a variety of seafood types
- Due to their high methyl mercury content, limit white (albacore) tuna to 6 ounces per week and do not eat the following four types of fish: tilefish, shark, swordfish, and king mackerel
- If pregnant, take an iron supplement as recommended by an obstetrician or other health care provider

Individuals Age 50 Years and Older
- Consume foods fortified with vitamin B_{12}, such as fortified cereals or dietary supplements

Building Health Eating Patterns
- Select an eating pattern that meets nutrient needs over time at an appropriate calorie level
- Account for all foods and beverages consumed and assess how they fit within a total healthy eating pattern
- Follow food safety recommendations when preparing and eating foods to reduce the risk of foodborne illnesses

*Fortified soy beverages have been marketed as *"soymilk,"* a product name consumers could see in supermarkets and consumer materials. However, the FDA's regulations do not contain provisions for the use of the term soymilk. Therefore, in this document, the term *fortified soy beverage* includes products that may be marketed as soymilk.
†Includes adolescent girls.
‡Folic acid is the synthetic form of the nutrient, whereas folate is the form found naturally in foods.

> **NOTE**
> In 2011, the MyPlate image was introduced for the consumer. MyPlate is a visual place setting that is intended to simplify eating recommendations for the general public, using five food groups: grains, vegetables, fruits, dairy, and protein.

MyPyramid has 12 sets of possible recommendations based on age, gender, and activity level. The new pyramid stresses activity and moderation along with the proper mix of food groups in a person's diet (Fig. 2-1). MyPyramid contains five food groups. They are:

1. Grains, recommending that half or more of grains be eaten as whole grains

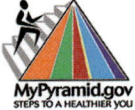

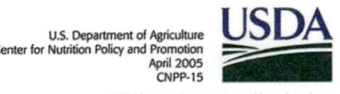

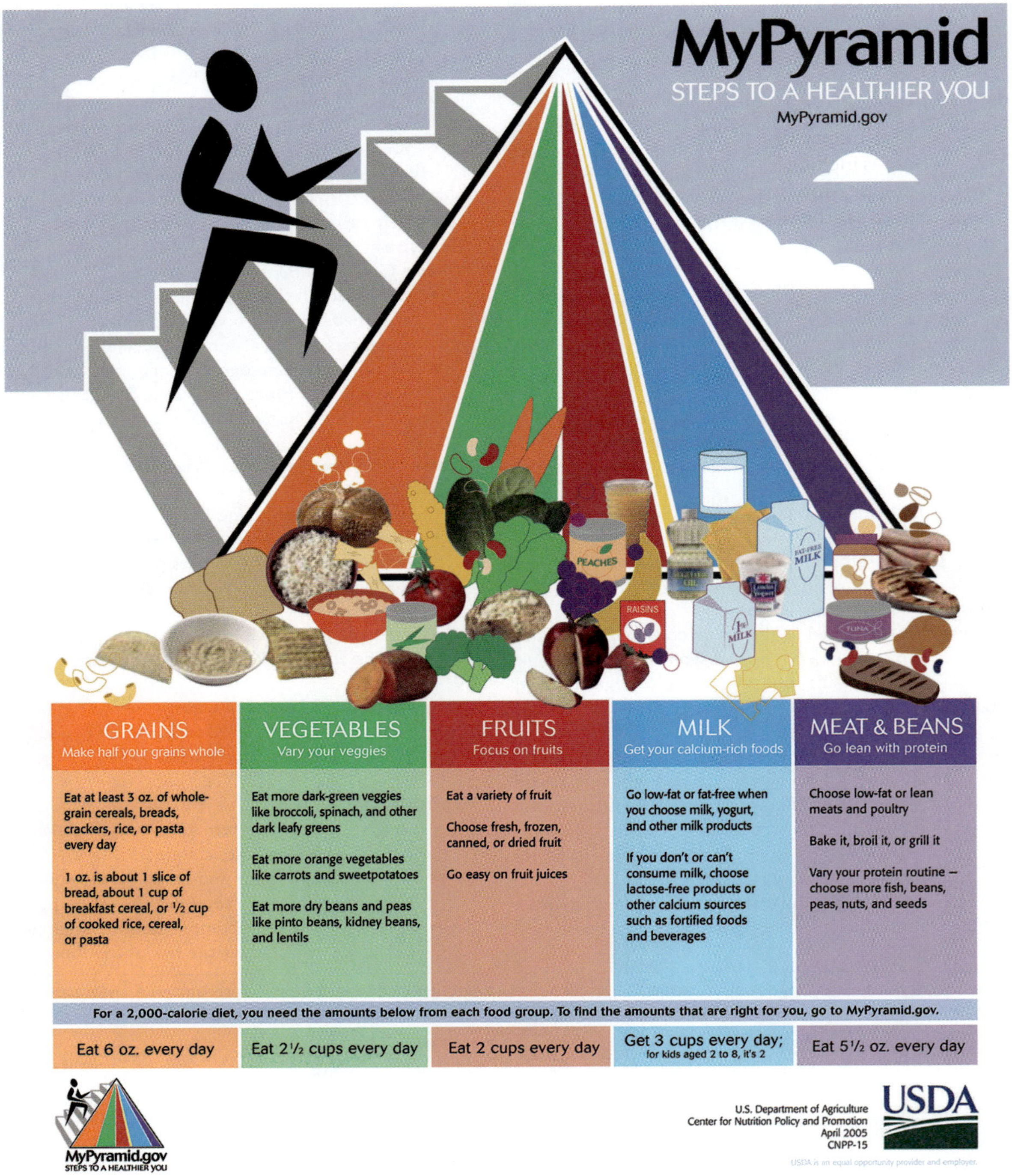

FIGURE 2-1 MyPyramid. (From Nix S: *William's basic nutrition & diet therapy,* ed 13, St Louis, 2009, Mosby.)

2. Vegetables, emphasizing dark green vegetables, orange vegetables, and dry beans and peas
3. Fruits, emphasizing variety, deemphasizing fruit juices
4. Milk, including milk-based foods
5. Meat and beans (proteins), emphasizing low-fat and lean meats as well as peas, nuts, and seeds

Two other categories of the MyPyramid are physical activity and discretionary calories. Physical activity is shown in the figure by a person climbing steps. Discretionary calories are those from candy, alcohol, and other foods. These calories are shown in the figure by the narrowed tip of each colored band. The slogan in the figure "Steps to a Healthier You" is to remind people that they can benefit from small steps to improve their diet and lifestyle.

Principles of Weight Control. Persons who are overweight tend to be at higher risk for developing certain illnesses. These illnesses include high blood pressure, diabetes mellitus, heart disease, and some cancers. The tenets of weight control are to eat the right balance of foods in moderation, limit fat consumption, and exercise regularly (Box 2-5).

Anyone committed to weight control for a healthier life should set realistic goals. For example, the general recommendation is a steady weight loss goal of 1/2 to 1 lb per week. (3500 calories is equal to 1 pound. An extra 500 calories per day results in a 1 pound gain per week; 500 fewer calories per day results in a 1 pound loss per week.) A healthful lifestyle is balanced with proper nutrition and exercise. A healthful diet includes a variety of foods that are low in fat, saturated fat, and cholesterol. A healthful diet also includes plenty of grain products, vegetables, and fruit (Box 2-6). A diet should also contain modest amounts of simple sugars, salt, and sodium. Alcoholic beverages should be avoided or consumed only in moderation. Finally, a system for checking weight control progress is essential. Adjustments and professional advice sometimes may be needed to achieve weight control goals.

BOX 2-5 Getting a Handle on Fat

Eat foods that are less than 30% fat. Try to aim for no more than 3 g of fat per 100 calories, which provides about 27% of the total calories from fat. This is important for the following reasons:

- Each gram of fat has more than double the calories of a gram of protein or carbohydrates.
- The body uses fewer calories to store the fat as excess weight.
- In complex carbohydrates, 23% of the calories are burned to make them into a usable form in the body; only 3% of fat calories are burned before they are "worn" on the hips or abdomen.
- Decreasing fat intake to less than 30% of daily calories helps reduce cholesterol, decreases risk of heart disease, helps with weight loss, and reduces risk of diabetes.

Fat Content of Various Foods

More than 90% fat: whipped cream, pork sausage, cooking oils, margarine, butter, gravy, mayonnaise

More than 80% fat: spare ribs, bologna, cream cheese, salad dressing, high-fat steaks (T-bone, porterhouse, tenderloin, filet mignon)

More than 70% fat: Half and Half dairy creamer, peanuts, hot dogs, pork chops, most cheeses and nuts, sirloin steak, bacon, lamb chops

More than 60% fat: potato and corn chips, regular ground beef, ham, eggs

More than 50% fat: round steak, pot roast, creamed soup, ice cream, sweet rolls

More than 40% fat: whole milk, cake, doughnuts, french fries

More than 30% fat: muffins, cookies, fruit pies, low-fat milk, cottage cheese, tuna, chicken, turkey

More than 20% fat: lean fish, beef liver, ice milk

More than 10% fat: bread, pretzels, whole grains, legumes

Less than 10% fat: sherbet, nonfat milk, most fruits and vegetables, baked potato

---

? DID YOU KNOW?

Food Labels 101

Understanding food labels and food content is important for a healthy diet. To help you make healthy choices in food, follow these steps when reading food labels (Figure 2-2):

Step 1: Look at the serving size and the number of servings per container or package. The sample here shows 2 servings (2 cups) in the package. If you eat the entire package of macaroni and cheese, you double your calories and other nutrients, including your percentage of daily allowance values (%DVs). A general rule for %DVs is 5% or less is low; 20% or more is high.

Step 2: Check the calories and note how many of those calories come from fat. In the figure, the fat calories per serving are 250, and 110 of those calories are from fat. If you eat the whole package, you will consume 500 calories and 220 of those will come from fat. The general rule for calories is 40 is low, 100 is moderate, 400 or more is high.

Steps 3 and 4: Look at the nutrients on the label. The ones in yellow should be limited. Eating too much fat, saturated fats, trans-fats, cholesterol, or sodium can increase your risk of certain chronic diseases. The nutrients in blue are good for you. They can improve your health and may reduce the risk of some diseases and conditions.

Step 5: Read the footnote on the bottom of the Nutrition Facts label. This tells you that the %DVs are based on a 2000 calorie diet. This is the recommended dietary advice for all Americans. It does not change from package to package.[2]

PHYSICAL FITNESS

Physical fitness can be described as a condition that helps persons look, feel, and do their best (Figure 2-3). Physical fitness is individual and varies from person to person. Physical fitness also is influenced by age, gender, heredity, personal habits, exercise, and eating habits. Being physically fit offers many benefits, which include the following:

- Decreased resting heart rate and blood pressure
- Increased oxygen-carrying capacity

BOX 2-6 Fiber

The human body requires fiber to maintain good health and to fight disease. Fiber (found only in plant foods) may be soluble or insoluble. Examples of soluble fiber include fiber obtained from peas, beans, oats, barley, and some fruits and vegetables. This type of fiber helps control the level of blood glucose. Soluble fiber also may lower the level of blood cholesterol. Insoluble fiber (found in whole grains and many vegetables) helps hold water in the colon and can reduce or prevent constipation. This type of fiber also may help prevent intestinal disease (e.g., diverticulosis, hemorrhoids, and certain cancers). Many authorities recommend a dietary intake of 20 to 35 g of fiber each day.

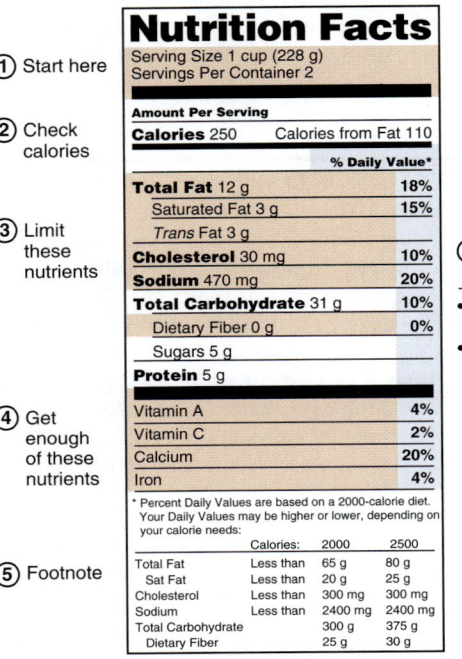

FIGURE 2-2 Food labels. (From Mahan LK, Stump S: *Krause's Food and nutrition therapy,* ed 12, St Louis, 2008, WB Saunders.)

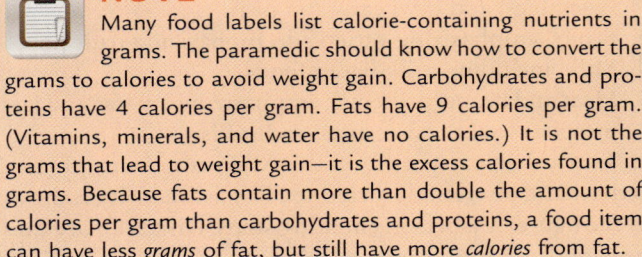

NOTE

Many food labels list calorie-containing nutrients in grams. The paramedic should know how to convert the grams to calories to avoid weight gain. Carbohydrates and proteins have 4 calories per gram. Fats have 9 calories per gram. (Vitamins, minerals, and water have no calories.) It is not the grams that lead to weight gain—it is the excess calories found in grams. Because fats contain more than double the amount of calories per gram than carbohydrates and proteins, a food item can have less *grams* of fat, but still have more *calories* from fat.

- Enhanced quality of life
- Increased muscle mass and metabolism
- Increased resistance to injury
- Improved personal appearance and self-image
- Maintenance of motor skills throughout life

Cardiovascular Endurance. A physical examination is the first step before starting a fitness program. Another step is to have a fitness assessment performed by a certified physical trainer. The purpose of these assessments is to evaluate a person's present physical condition. These exams also create baseline assessments for weight, including body mass index (Box 2-7); high blood pressure; heart disease (including family history); arthritis or other bone problems; muscular, ligament, or tendon problems; and other known or suspected diseases. These assessments help to establish a heart rate target zone as well. This is a measure used to improve cardiovascular endurance through exercise. Ideally, the heart rate target zone should be maintained during exercise for 20 minutes to increase cardiovascular endurance.

Muscle Strength. Another part of the fitness assessment tests muscular strength and endurance. Muscular strength is the ability of a muscle to exert force for a brief period. Muscle endurance is the ability of a muscle or a group of muscles to sustain repeated contractions or to continue applying force against a fixed object. Many exercises improve muscle strength and endurance.

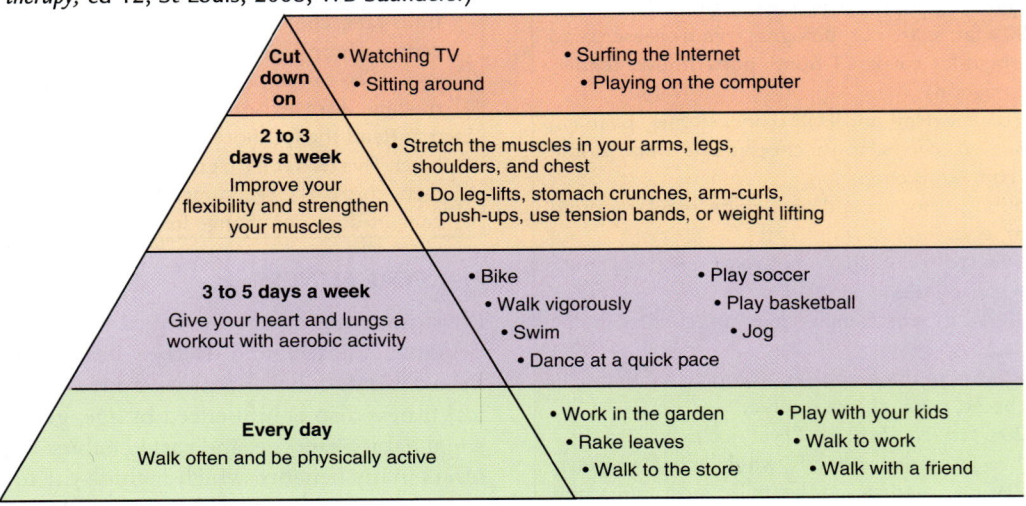

FIGURE 2-3 Exercise pyramid.

BOX 2-7 The Body Mass Index

The body mass index (BMI) is a widely used measurement of body fat that corrects for height. The BMI is the only body fat index that conveys the risk of disease or death. A healthful BMI is 19 to 25. A BMI of 25 to 29 indicates "moderately overweight." A BMI of 30 or more indicates "severely overweight." To calculate your body mass index, use the following formula:

Step 1: Multiply your weight in pounds by 0.45.

  Example: 150 pounds × 0.45 = 67.5

Step 2: Multiply your height in inches by 0.025.

  Example: 5 ft 9 in, or 69 inches × 0.025 = 1.725

Step 3: Square the answer from step 2.

  Example: 1.725 × 1.725 = 2.976

Step 4: Divide the answer in step 1 by the answer in step 3.

  Example: 67.5 ÷ 2.976 = BMI of 22.7

SHOW ME THE EVIDENCE

EMS personnel re-registering with the NREMT were surveyed to determine their body mass index (BMI). The mean BMI for study participants was 27.74 (95% CI 27.68-27.81), and 71.5% of participants were classified as having high (greater than or equal to 25) BMI. More males reported having a high BMI compared to females (79.2% vs 50.8%, respectively, $p < 0.001$). More paramedics reported the higher BMI than any of the other levels of licensure. Military EMS personnel reported the lowest prevalence of high BMI (61.7%). Fire-based EMS personnel had the highest (77.7%).

From Fernandez AR, Studnek JR: *Body mass index of emergency medical services professionals,* Poster presentation at 2008 annual meeting of the National Association of EMS Physicians, Phoenix.

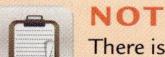

CRITICAL THINKING

Calculate your body mass index. Does it fall within the recommendations?

NOTE

There is a simple way to determine the heart rate target zone. First, multiply the established maximum heart rate of 220 minus a person's age in years. Then multiply this number by 70%.

  Example for a 25-year-old:

$$\text{Maximum heart rate} \ (220 - 25) = 195$$

$$195 \times 70\% = 136 \ \text{beats/min}$$

The tenets of training for muscle strength and endurance should consider isometric and isotonic exercises, resistance, repetitions, sets, and frequency. *Isometric* exercises are those that do not result in any movement of a joint. An example of this is a contraction performed against an immovable object such as a wall or door frame. These exercises do not significantly increase muscle bulk, but they do strengthen the muscle at the joint angle at which the contraction is performed. *Isotonic* exercises move a joint through a range of motion against resistance of a fixed weight. An example of this is lifting a barbell. These exercises add muscle bulk by creating tension within the muscle. *Resistance* refers to the amount of weight moved or lifted during isotonic exercises. A *repetition* ("rep") refers to the full execution of an exercise from start to finish. A *set* is the number of times an exercise (rep) is done from start to finish, one after another, without any rest time. *Frequency* refers to the least number of workouts that will have a positive effect on muscle strength and endurance.

Muscular Flexibility. Flexibility refers to the ability to move joints and use muscles through their full range of motion. The fitness assessment tests flexibility in several ways. A lack of normal flexibility may lead to muscle strains and other injuries.

Muscular flexibility can be improved by stretching exercises. These exercises must be done slowly, without a bouncing motion. The intensity of these exercises should be mild. A person should not strain or hold the breath and should feel no pain or discomfort. How often these exercises are done should match an individual's specific level of activity. For example, if daily work on an ambulance requires lifting patients, then regular stretching exercises specific to the paramedic's arms, back, thighs, calves, and hips would be helpful.

CRITICAL THINKING

How many minutes per week do you perform physical activities that raise your heart rate? What benefits does a paramedic gain by maintaining a high level of personal fitness?

THE IMPORTANCE OF SLEEP

Sleep plays an important role in being physically fit because it helps to rejuvenate a tired body. The average adult needs 7 to 8 hours of sleep each day. In emergency medical services (EMS), where rotating shifts and 24- and 48-hour work shifts are common, sleep deprivation may occur and interrupt the normal circadian rhythm.

Circadian is Latin for "about a day." The circadian rhythm is the physiological ebb and flow of the body as it relates to the rotation of the earth. This timing system is based roughly on the solar day as the earth rotates in its course around the sun. For example, a person gets hungry or tired, or energetic or moody, at fairly set times each day as the body systems change. The levels of melatonin and cortisol affect the periods of sleepiness and wakefulness, respectively. As will be discussed in Chapter 10, the pineal gland secretes melatonin. The adrenal glands secrete cortisol. Release of these hormones is stimulated by the dark and is suppressed by light. Thus when the line between night and day is disrupted on an ongoing basis (e.g., working rotating work shifts or responding to emergency calls in the early morning hours during a 24- or 48-hour shift), irritability, depression, and illness can result (Box 2-8).

BOX 2-8 Getting Your Z's

Working nights, 24- and 48-hour shifts, and rotating shifts can prevent you from getting enough rest. The following are some helpful tips:

- Allow some time to unwind and relax before trying to go to sleep.
- Consider exercise before sleeping as a way to reduce stress.
- Avoid stimulants (e.g., caffeine in coffee, soda, tea, and chocolate) during the last few hours of your work shift.
- Eat simple carbohydrates (e.g., cookies or candy bar) to release serotonin (a hormone that may help induce sleep).
- Keep your sleeping area cool and dark so that your body will think it is nighttime.
- Make sure your family and friends know about your work shifts and your sleeping schedule to minimize interruptions.
- Try to maintain a "normal" period of dedicated sleep time each day.
- Consult a physician about your sleep difficulties when needed.

SHOW ME THE EVIDENCE

A preliminary study published in *The Lancet Oncology*[3] provides a summary of scientific evidence of increased cancer risk in night-shift workers, as well as increased cancer risk in painters and firefighters. The study, conducted by the World Health Organization's International Agency for Research on Cancer (IARC), emphasizes the impact of night-shift work on melatonin secretion, immune function, cancer risk, and disruption of circadian rhythm. More information about this study can be found at: www.epidemiologic.org/2007/12/iarc-cancer-hazards-associated-with.html, accessed 1-28-09. IARC: Cancer hazards associated with shiftwork, painting, and firefighting.

Shift-work studies have been done by numerous agencies, including the Centers for Disease Control and Prevention and the National Institute for Occupational Safety and Health.[4] Findings in these studies suggest sleep loss:

- Makes it easier to fall asleep at inappropriate times
- Affects performance both on and off the job
- Can lead to serious injuries
- Disrupts social and family life
- Increases health risks for digestive problems and heart disease

Other studies have shown that people who have disruptions in their circadian rhythms because of extended work shifts have increased risks of motor vehicle crashes, short-term decreases in cognition and neuropsychological performance, decreased job satisfaction, and an increased likelihood for making errors that result in patient care litigation.[5,6] Research and work shift studies are still underway. The goals of these are to help shift workers and their employers modify work schedules so that changes in normal biorhythms will have the least adverse effects on employee health and productivity.

CRITICAL THINKING

Do you get enough sleep? If not, which of these strategies should you try in an attempt to increase your hours of sleep?

DISEASE PREVENTION

There are many things a paramedic can do to help prevent serious personal illness. As health care professionals, paramedics must serve as role models in helping to prevent disease.

Cardiovascular Disease. Cardiovascular disease accounts for more than 830,000 deaths each year in the United States.[7] For most persons, cardiovascular disease can be altered through living a healthful life. Boosting cardiovascular endurance can help to prevent this disease. However, other steps are also needed. These steps include the following:

- Eliminating cigarette smoking
- Controlling high blood pressure
- Maintaining a favorable body fat composition through regular exercise
- Maintaining a good total cholesterol/high-density lipoprotein ratio (Box 2-9)
- Monitoring triglyceride levels
- Controlling diabetes
- Avoiding excessive alcohol intake
- Eating healthful foods
- Reducing stress
- Obtaining risk assessments periodically

Cancer. The term *cancer* includes more than 100 diseases affecting nearly every part of the body. All these diseases are potentially life threatening. The main cause of all cancer is a change or mutation in the nucleus of a cell. Most common cancers are linked to one of three environmental risk factors: smoking, sunlight, or diet. Dietary factors are associated with some cancers of the gastrointestinal tract and may be linked to others, such as cancer of the breast, prostate, or uterus. Steps in preventing cancer include the following:

- Elimination of smoking
- Dietary changes
- Limitation of sun exposure; use of sunscreen
- Regular physical examinations
- Attention to the warning signs (Box 2-10)
- Periodic risk assessment

Infectious Disease. Most infectious diseases can be avoided by practicing good personal hygiene (including performing hand washing and following **universal precautions** and other guidelines in the workplace). These guidelines are established by the Centers for Disease Control and Prevention, the Occupational Safety and Health

BOX 2-9 Understanding the Cholesterol Numbers

Cholesterol moves through the body attached to various sizes of fat-carrying proteins. These proteins are called lipoproteins. Low-density lipoproteins (LDLs) are more common. They are thought to carry cholesterol to the cells and to promote blood vessel disease. Smaller high-density lipoproteins (HDLs) are thought to carry cholesterol to the liver. They may help prevent or slow down blood vessel disease. Very-low-density lipoproteins are made mostly of triglycerides (the main fatty substance in the fluid portion of blood) that are absorbed by the intestines and therefore are affected by fasting. (Fasting is abstaining from all or certain foods.)

Cholesterol
High blood cholesterol: 240 mg/dL or higher
Borderline high blood cholesterol: 220 to 239 mg/dL
Desirable blood cholesterol: less than 200 mg/dL

LDL Cholesterol: The "Bad or Lousy" Cholesterol
Very high LDL cholesterol: 189 mg/dL or higher
High LDL cholesterol: 160 to 189 mg/dL or higher
Borderline high LDL cholesterol: 130 to 159 mg/dL
Desirable LDL cholesterol in healthy persons: less than 100 mg/dL
Desirable LDL cholesterol in persons at risk for heart disease: less than 90 mg/dL

HDL Cholesterol: Higher Is Better
Low HDL cholesterol: less than 40 mg/dL
Desirable HDL cholesterol: greater than 60 mg/dL

Very-Low-Density Lipoproteins/Triglyceride: Lower Is Better
Should not exceed 200 to 300 mg/dL

BOX 2-10 The Seven Warning Signs of Cancer (CAUTION) as Designated by the American Cancer Society

Change in bowel or bladder habits
A sore throat that does not heal
Unusual bleeding or discharge
Thickening or lump in the breast or elsewhere
Indigestion or difficulty swallowing
Obvious change in a wart or mole
Nagging cough or hoarseness

TABLE 2-3 Personal Equipment for Protection Against Transmission of HIV and Hepatitis B Virus

Activity	Disposable Gloves	Gown	Mask	Protective Eyewear
Bleeding control (spurting blood)	Yes	Yes	Yes	Yes
Bleeding control (minimal blood)	Yes	No	No	No
Emergency childbirth	Yes	Yes	Yes*	Yes*
Intravenous therapy	Yes	No	No	No
Endotracheal intubation	Yes	No	Yes*	Yes*
Oral or nasal suctioning	Yes	No	No	No
Administration of an injection	No	No	No	No

*If splashing is likely.

DID YOU KNOW?
The Right Way to Wash Your Hands
The most important tool in your arsenal for preventing infection and protecting yourself from illness is washing your hands. Hand washing should be done whenever your hands are soiled. Hand washing should also be done between each patient contact, before eating, after using the restroom, and after coughing, sneezing, or blowing your nose. The CDC recommends vigorous scrubbing with warm soapy water for at least 15 seconds (or the time it takes to sing a short tune, such as Happy Birthday).

There are five easy steps to proper hand washing:
1. **Wet** your hands under warm running water; apply soap.
2. **Rub** your hands with soap under warm running water.
3. **Scrub** your hands for a count of at least 15 seconds. Scrub all surfaces, including the back of your hands, and wrists. Clean between your fingers and under your fingernails.
4. **Rinse** your hands under clean warm water.
5. **Dry** your hands on a paper towel or with an air dryer and use a towel to turn off the faucet.

When soap and water are not available, alcohol-based disposable hand wipes or gel sanitizers may be used. Gel sanitizers that contain at least 60% alcohol are more effective in killing bacteria and viruses than hand washing[8] and most contain ingredients that help prevent skin dryness.

Administration, the National Fire Protection Association, the Federal Emergency Management Agency, the United States Fire Administration, and others (Table 2-3). Universal precautions and other personal safety measures will be discussed throughout this text.

At a minimum, personal protective equipment to guard against the spread of infectious diseases should include the following:

■ Disposable gloves when contact with blood or other body fluids is likely
■ Masks and protective eyewear when blood splashing is likely to occur
■ Gowns to protect clothing from spurting blood (e.g., during emergency childbirth)

■ HEPA (high-efficiency particulate air) filter and N-95 respirators when tuberculosis is confirmed or suspected (see Chapters 24 and 28)

If a potential exposure to an infectious disease occurs, the paramedic should report it as soon as possible. The report should be made to the receiving hospital and to the proper designated officer in the local agency (see Chapter 28). To defend against such diseases, the Occupational Safety and Health Administration requires a periodic risk assessment be offered to staff. The risk assessment includes regular testing for diseases such as tuberculosis and monitoring of vaccinations for infectious diseases (e.g., hepatitis B).

INJURY PREVENTION

The number of injuries that occur on the job can be reduced. Knowledge of proper body mechanics during lifting and moving is helpful. Staying alert for hostile settings also is essential. A paramedic must prioritize personal safety during rescue situations. Finally, one must practice safe vehicle operations and use safety equipment and supplies.

Body Mechanics During Lifting and Moving. One in four EMS workers suffers a career-ending back injury within the first 4 years of employment, and back injury is the number one reason for leaving the EMS profession.[9] Almost one in two workers (47%) have sustained a back injury while performing EMS duties.[10]

Using proper body mechanics during lifting and moving is crucial. This helps avoid personal injury as well as injury to a partner or patient (Box 2-11). The paramedic should consider the following guidelines when lifting and moving patients or equipment:

■ Only move a victim you can handle safely; get additional help if needed.
■ Look where you are walking or crawling.
■ Move forward rather than backward when possible.
■ Take short steps, if walking.
■ Bend at the hips and knees.
■ Maintain the natural curvature of the spine when possible.
■ Lift with the legs, not the back.
■ Keep the load close to the body.
■ Keep patient's body in line when moving.

> **NOTE**
> When preparing to lift, contract the abdominals by pulling in the abdominal wall (sucking the belly button to the spine). This is the core of the body. In addition, the abdominals help stabilize the back and help produce power and strength. Lift by extending through the hips and legs, not the back. ("Think with the hips" when lifting.) The body works from the center, out. The hips are part of the "core" and more centralized than the legs. Therefore extending through the hips first adds another muscle group. It also instantly provides greater strength and power for lifting. Incorporating the hips can also help prevent knee injuries.

BOX 2-11 Prevention and Rehabilitation of Low Back Pain

The back is a complex system of ligaments, muscles, bones, nerves, and intervertebral disks. All of these parts can be injured by improper lifting techniques. Emergency medical services workers are highly vulnerable to low back pain and injury. A common cause of low back pain and injury is lordosis (an inward curvature in the lumbar spine that is normally present to some degree). Abnormal curvature in this area can result from poor posture and from being overweight with associated weak abdominal muscles. Back injury can be prevented or lessened to a significant degree by being physically fit, performing regular stretching exercises, and following some general rules of lifting:

1. Know the weight (ask the patient's weight if you can, and add the weight of the equipment). Two persons should work together to lift objects that weigh more than 60 lb.
2. Know your physical ability and limitations.
3. Keep your back positioned with a normal curvature.
4. Use your legs and abdominal muscles to support the weight; use your back muscles to maintain balance.
5. Keep the weight close to your body.
6. Communicate clearly and frequently with your partner.

If back pain or injury occurs when lifting, pushing, pulling, or stretching, tell a supervisor as soon as possible. Treatment for back pain usually begins with rest and ice or cold packs to lessen swelling. Treatment also can include pain medicine and muscle relaxants. A rehabilitation program usually will follow the injury. Rehabilitation often includes exercises to improve abdominal muscle strength. The exercises also help to improve the control of the pelvis and the flexibility of the lower back.

From *EMT: injury free*, Wilmington, Ohio, 1991, Ferno-Washington.

Hostile Environments. As part of EMS work, paramedics may sometimes find themselves in hostile situations. Such situations may include responding to violent crimes of murder, rape, robbery, domestic violence, acts of terrorism, and aggravated assault. These crimes often are linked with the use of illegal drugs. This environment may threaten one's personal safety. When these situations occur, paramedics should do the following:

■ Carefully check the scene for safety concerns and do not enter the scene until it is safe.
■ Coordinate all actions with law enforcement personnel.
■ Follow protocols for establishing medical incident command (see Chapter 54).
■ Plan entrance and escape routes.
■ Above all, stay alert and be prepared for the unexpected.

Safely managing a violent scene requires special training. The situation also calls for unity among many emergency response agencies. As members of the response team, paramedics should take part in planning, training, and practice sessions. These sessions help to ensure personal safety in hostile settings (see Chapter 58).

Rescue Situations. Many personal safety issues arise in the case of rescue. Examples include exposure to hazardous materials, bad weather, extremes in temperature, fire, toxic gases, unstable structures, heavy equipment, road hazards, and sharp edges and fragments. For every rescue response the key is to assess the scene for hazards first. One also must take personal protective measures. In addition, the scene should be monitored constantly during the operation. A safe rescue requires proper use of protective gear, special training, and safe rescue practices (see Chapter 55).

Safe Vehicle Operation. Safe operation of an emergency vehicle is important for personal safety and the safety of the crew and patient (see Chapter 53). Many factors affect safe vehicle operations, including the following:

- Safe driving of the vehicle
- Use of personal restraints for all occupants in the vehicle
- Safe and appropriate use of escorts to and from emergency scenes
- Adverse environmental conditions (e.g., inclement weather)
- Appropriate use of audible and visual warning devices
- Proceeding through intersections safely
- Parking at the emergency scene
  - Safe vehicle positioning strategies
- Maintaining due regard for the safety of all others

> **NOTE**
> Safe operations and personal safety on the roadways are of utmost importance. Emergency personnel should wear ANSII-2 reflective safety vests over turnout gear. They should also minimize the time they spend on roadways.

> **CRITICAL THINKING**
> Is there any patient situation that would call for using unsafe vehicle operations? Keep in mind that this could risk the safety of those in the ambulance or in other vehicles.

Some EMS agencies require their employees to take a specialized driver's training class. One such program is the U.S. Department of Transportation Emergency Vehicle Operation Course (EVOC). A program such as this allows EMS personnel to practice driving in a safe and controlled setting.

Safety Equipment and Supplies. Proper use of safety equipment and supplies is key to injury prevention for paramedics. Standards for protective clothing and equipment are required by the Occupational Safety and Health Administration. These and other standards (such as those set by the National Fire Protection Association) are used by many states, cities, and fire and EMS agencies to help ensure employee safety (see Chapter 54). Safety equipment and supplies include the following:

- Body substance isolation equipment
- Head protection
- Eye protection
- Hearing protection
- Respiratory protection
- Gloves
- Boots
- Coveralls
- Turnout coat and pants
- Specialty equipment
- Reflective clothing

Mental and Emotional Health

Many factors play a role in mental and emotional health. An important factor is to be aware of "warning signs" that could indicate a potential problem (e.g., signs of substance misuse and health disorders caused by **anxiety** and **stress**). Also key to maintaining good emotional health is realizing the value of having personal time; being connected with family, peers, and the community; and accepting the personal differences that make individuals unique.

SUBSTANCE MISUSE AND ABUSE CONTROL

Health care workers, emergency responders, and public service personnel are not immune to stressors that can lead to substance misuse and abuse. Studies have found that 8% to 12% of physicians were estimated to develop a substance use problem;[11] 32% of nurses reported some substance abuse;[12] and about 30% of firefighters and law enforcement officers reported problematic alcohol use.[13]

The misuse and abuse of drugs and other substances may lead to chemical dependency (**addiction**) (Box 2-12). Such dependency may have a wide range of effects on physical and mental health, including damage to vital organs, cancer, increased risk for injuries, and mental impairment (see Chapter 34). Warning signs of addiction and addictive behavior include the following:

> **BOX 2-12 Common Drugs and Substances That Are Misused or Abused**
>
> - Alcohol
> - Central nervous system stimulants (e.g., cocaine and amphetamines)
> - Cigarettes and other tobacco products
> - Hallucinogens
> - Inhalants
> - Marijuana
> - Narcotics and related drugs
> - Sedative-hypnotics
> - Tranquilizers
> - Nonprescription substances
> - Sedatives
> - Appetite suppressants
> - Laxatives
> - Cough and cold preparations
> - Nasal sprays
> - Analgesics

- Using a substance to relieve tension
- Using an increasing amount of the substance
- Lying about using the substance
- Experiencing guilt about using the substance
- Avoiding discussion about using the substance
- Experiencing interference with daily activities as a result of substance abuse

CRITICAL THINKING
Do you know anyone with these behaviors?

Methods used to manage substance abuse depend on the type of substance being misused. Substance misuse or abuse control may call for professional counseling. Physician-controlled drug therapy and support programs also may be necessary.

SMOKING CESSATION

Cigarette smoking is a major health hazard. Smoking is responsible for more than 438,000 deaths each year in the United States.[14] The health ramifications of cigarette smoking are numerous, including an increased risk of the following:

- Coronary heart disease
- Myocardial infarction
- Chronic obstructive pulmonary disease
- Sudden death
- Dying from a variety of diseases
- Miscarriage, premature birth, and birth defects

Smokers often name many reasons for continuing to smoke. These reasons may include peer pressure, relief of stress, weight control, and others. Regardless, most persons continue to smoke because of the addictive nature of nicotine. Nicotine is the stimulant in tobacco, but there are other harmful chemicals. These chemicals include hydrocarbons (tar) and carbon monoxide. Exposure to these chemicals is considered a health hazard for nonsmokers also. Nonsmokers have an increased risk of developing smoking-related illnesses through "passive smoking," or second- and third-hand smoke.

Many resources and smoking cessation programs are available to those who want to quit smoking. Support groups and quit-smoking campaigns are sponsored by the American Heart Association, the American Cancer Society, the American Red Cross, government health agencies, and local health care organizations. Other methods one may use alone or with these programs include the use of prescription and nonprescription drugs. Some examples include Chantix, Wellbutrin, dermal patches, and nicotine chewing gum. These products decrease the physical effects of smoking cessation. In a sense, they help to wean the smoker off nicotine (Box 2-13).

ANXIETY AND STRESS

Anxiety can be defined as the worry or dread about future uncertainties. *Stress* can result from the interaction

---

BOX 2-13 Body Changes When You Stop Smoking

Within 20 Minutes of Your Last Cigarette
Pulse and blood pressure drop to normal.
Body temperature of hands and feet increases to normal.

Within 8 Hours of Your Last Cigarette
Carbon monoxide level in blood drops to normal.
Oxygen level in blood increases to normal.

Within 24 Hours of Your Last Cigarette
Chance of heart attack decreases.

Within 48 Hours of Your Last Cigarette
Nerve endings begin to regenerate.
Ability to smell and taste is enhanced.

Within 72 Hours of Your Last Cigarette
Bronchial tubes relax, making breathing easier.
Lung capacity increases.

Within 2 Weeks to 3 Months After Your Last Cigarette
Circulation improves.
Walking becomes easier.
Lung function increases up to 30%.

Within 1 to 9 Months After Your Last Cigarette
Coughing, sinus congestion, fatigue, and shortness of breath decrease.
Cilia regrow in lungs, increasing the ability to handle mucus, clean the lungs, and reduce infection.

Within 5 Years of Your Last Cigarette
Lung cancer death rate for the average smoker (one pack per day) decreases.

Within 10 Years of Your Last Cigarette
Lung cancer death rate drops to 12 deaths per 100,000—almost the rate of nonsmokers.
Precancerous cells are replaced.
Risk for other cancers—such as those of the mouth, larynx, esophagus, bladder, kidney, and pancreas—decreases (20 chemicals in tobacco smoke cause cancer).
When smokers quit, the health improves over time.
    See www.cancer.org/docroot/SPC_1 when smokers_quit. asp.

---

of events that cause anxiety and the coping abilities of the person. Stress can be positive (described later in this chapter). However, stress usually is thought of as having a negative effect (e.g., fear, depression, and guilt). Recognizing and coping with anxiety and stress is important for a lasting career in the EMS profession. Signs that you may need stress management assistance include[15]:

- Disorientation or confusion and difficulty communicating thoughts
- Difficulty remembering instructions
- Difficulty maintaining balance
- Becoming easily frustrated and being uncharacteristically argumentative
- Inability to engage in problem solving and difficulty making decisions
- Unnecessary risk taking
- Tremors/headaches/nausea
- Tunnel vision/muffled hearing
- Colds or flulike symptoms
- Limited attention span and difficulty concentrating
- Loss of objectivity
- Inability to relax when off duty
- Refusal to follow orders or to leave the scene
- Increased use of drugs/alcohol
- Unusual clumsiness

PERSONAL TIME FOR MEDITATION AND CONTEMPLATION

Setting aside some personal time can boost mental and perhaps even physical health. This time can be spent meditating or contemplating. *Meditation* is a form of relaxation. To meditate, a person limits his or her awareness to a repeated or constant focus. The person may focus on something that holds some attraction (e.g., controlled breathing, a pleasant site, a fragrance, or a mantra). This quiet time provides an uninterrupted period for thoughtful introspection *(contemplation)* of important things in a person's life. Most who practice meditation do so once or twice a day for 10 to 20 minutes.

 NOTE
Spirituality is a unique quality of human existence. Spirituality should not be overlooked as a means for some to achieve mental and physical well-being.

DIVERSITY AND FREEDOM FROM PREJUDICE

The concept of **diversity** encompasses acceptance and respect of other people. It means understanding that each person is unique and recognizing our individual differences. These differences can be along the dimensions of race, ethnicity, gender, sexual orientation, socioeconomic status, age, physical abilities, religious beliefs, political beliefs, or other ideologies (Figure 2-4).

Accepting differences in people provides an opportunity to learn about others and to see variations in people in a positive light. Acceptance also affirms the value of these differences. It allows paramedics to see life from another viewpoint. Being able to work with others in a diverse workplace is also essential. Following are some general guidelines:

1. Maintain a personal attitude about others that "includes" rather than "excludes."

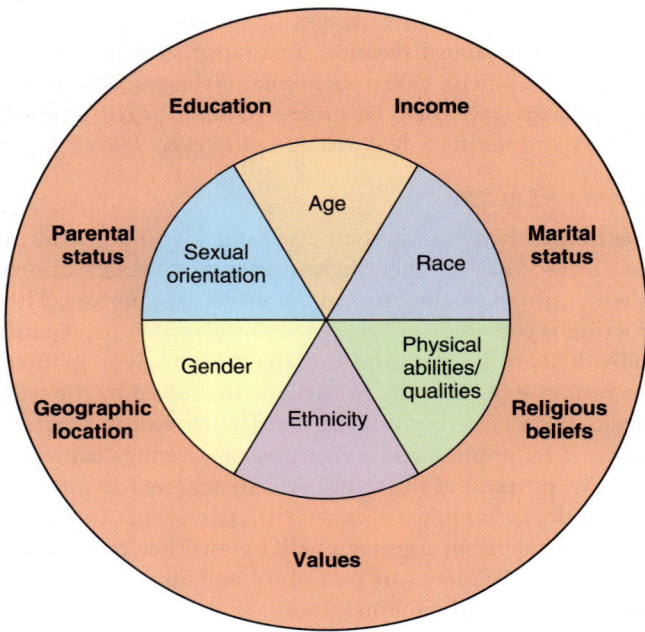

FIGURE 2-4 Dimensions of diversity.

2. Treat everyone with respect, including patients, your co-workers, those to whom you report, and those who report to you.
3. Do not assume that everyone shares your beliefs.
4. Examine your assumptions about people who are different than you.
5. Learn to listen carefully and observe those around you to be more aware of their needs, boundaries, and differences.

 NOTE
The four major ethnic minority groups in the United States are Hispanic/Latinos (Mexican-American, Puerto Rican, Cuban, Central and South American), Asians (Chinese, Korean, Japanese), Southwest Asians (Vietnamese, Laotians, Cambodians), and African Americans. Providing health care to patients of some cultures may call for special communication skills. Provision of care also may require some further education to understand the customs and beliefs of that culture (see Chapter 17).

STRESS

As previously stated, stress can be positive and negative. The responses to stress may be physical, emotional, or both. "Good" stress (**eustress**) is a positive response to stimuli. Eustress is considered protective. "Bad" stress (**distress**) is a negative response to environmental stimuli. Distress is the source of anxiety and stress-related disorders.

Phases of the Stress Response

Hans Selye was an Austrian-born professor at the University of Montreal. He coined the term *stress* in its medical usage in 1950. The three stages of the stress response he found are the alarm reaction, resistance, and exhaustion (Figure 2-5).[16] Selye called these phases the *general adaption syndrome*. He gave them this name to describe the attempt of body and mind to deal with stressful events.

ALARM REACTION

The human body can prepare itself quickly to do battle or run from danger. This "fight-or-flight" reaction occurs when a situation threatens one's safety or comfort. This reaction is considered positive (eustress) in that it prepares individuals to be alert and to defend themselves. At first, the response of the body to stress is unaffected by the type of situation. The body reacts equally to events that are pleasant or unpleasant, dangerous or exciting, happy or sad. The purpose of the response is to achieve top physical preparedness rapidly to cope with the event. Examples would be having an argument with a co-worker, performing an unfamiliar patient care procedure, and taking part in the delivery of a healthy infant.

The alarm reaction is triggered by the **autonomic nervous system** (see Chapter 10). This reaction is coordinated by the hypothalamus. The hypothalamus triggers the pituitary gland to release adrenocorticotropic hormone into the bloodstream. This stress hormone stimulates the production of glucose. The hormone also increases the concentration of nutrients in the blood that provide energy. These nutrients are needed for the response to stress. Adrenocorticotropic hormone also activates the adrenal glands for an intense sympathetic discharge of **adrenaline** and noradrenaline. These hormones cause the heart rate to increase, the blood pressure to rise, and the pupils of the eyes to dilate, which improves vision. Together these hormones relax the bronchial tree for deeper breathing, increase blood sugar (glucose) for total energy, slow the digestive process, and shift blood supply to accommodate the clotting mechanism in case the body is wounded. After these physiological events, the body is ready for an emergency (fight or flight). The body can perform feats of strength and endurance far beyond its normal capacity. The alarm reaction takes only seconds. The reaction occurs to some extent at the first exposure of the body to a stressor. When the body realizes that an event is not dangerous or does not require the alarm reaction, the response stops. The individual begins to adapt to the situation. Then bodily functions return to normal.

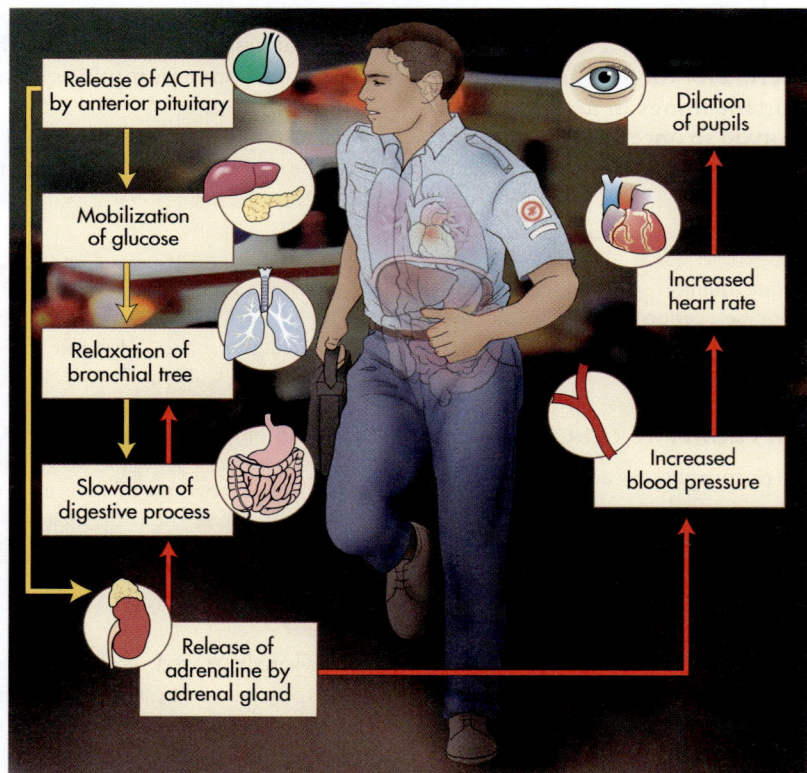

FIGURE 2-5 Physiological response to stress. During the alarm reaction, the release of adrenocorticotropic hormone (*yellow*) results in a sympathetic discharge of adrenaline (*red*). These stress hormones stimulate glucose production and cause the heart rate to increase, the blood pressure to rise, and the pupils to dilate. The bronchial tree relaxes for deep breathing, the digestive process slows, and the blood supply shifts to accommodate clotting mechanisms in case the body is wounded.

Labels in figure:
- Release of ACTH by anterior pituitary
- Mobilization of glucose
- Relaxation of bronchial tree
- Slowdown of digestive process
- Release of adrenaline by adrenal gland
- Dilation of pupils
- Increased heart rate
- Increased blood pressure

RESISTANCE

The stress response raises the level of resistance to the agent that provoked it and others like it. That is, if a particular stress persists long enough, a person's reactions change. For example, a paramedic becomes accustomed to responding to emergency scenes in an ambulance using audible and visual warning devices. Thus the alarm reaction that once occurred is no longer elicited. Therefore reactions to stressors may change over time.

EXHAUSTION

As stress continues, coping mechanisms weaken. Then resistance fails. For example, paramedics may appear to be unaffected by the stress of life-threatening emergencies. However, all of their adaptive resources have been used to reach this stage of resistance. When any reservoir of adaptive resources no longer exists, resistance to other types of stress tends to decline as well. At that point, the body may become at risk for physical and psychological illness. Rest and recovery usually are needed before a person is ready for another emergency.

Factors That Trigger the Stress Response

Each person has unique means to deal with stressful situations. Individual reactions to stress are customized based on previous exposure to a specific type of stress, perception of the stressful event, and personal coping skills. Many factors can trigger the stress response. Examples include the following:

- Loss of something that is of value
- Injury or threat of injury
- Poor health or nutrition
- Frustration
- Ineffective coping skills

PHYSIOLOGICAL AND PSYCHOLOGICAL EFFECTS OF STRESS

Anxiety is a common symptom of stress. Feeling anxious in certain situations or unusual circumstances is normal and healthy. This response provides a warning system that protects persons from being overwhelmed by a sudden stimulation. Anxiety also prepares persons for action in critical situations. This adaptive response to stress prepares the paramedic to make quick, correct decisions regarding the emergency. Anxiety also allows the paramedic to perform at maximal efficiency.

Sometimes stress is not reduced by a solution to the conflict or emergency. This may lead to an ongoing state of vigilance and alertness beyond the initial event. The paramedic then may begin to feel chronic anxiety. This kind of anxiety fails to stimulate effective coping. In addition, a person may respond to conflict or stress by anxious behavior alone. Anxiety interferes with thought processes and with relationships and work performance. A person may

develop problems concentrating, lose the ability to trust others, or become isolated or withdrawn.

Individuals who are exposed to stressful situations often or who are unable to cope with stressful events may experience a chronic state of anxiety. This state may lead to physical, emotional, cognitive, and behavioral effects (Box 2-14). Some warning signs may call for immediate evaluation and medical care. These signs include chest pain and difficulty breathing. Others call for less immediate action. The presence of one or more warning signs is an indicator of distress. However, the absence of warning signs does not preclude the chance of a stress reaction.

CAUSES OF STRESS IN EMERGENCY MEDICAL SERVICES

A variety of sources can produce stress in EMS work. Environmental stress includes noise, bad weather, confined spaces, poor lighting, spectators, rapid response to the

---

BOX 2-14 Warning Signs and Symptoms of Stress

Physical
- Cardiac rhythm disturbances
- Chest pain
- Difficulty breathing
- Nausea
- Profuse sweating
- Sleep disturbances
- Vomiting

Emotional
- Anger
- Denial
- Fear
- Feeling of being overwhelmed
- Inappropriate emotions
- Panic reactions

Cognitive
- Confusion
- Decreased level of awareness
- Difficulty making decisions
- Disorientation
- Distressing dreams
- Memory problems
- Poor concentration

Behavioral
- Changes in eating habits
- Crying spells
- Excessive silence
- Hyperactivity
- Increased alcohol consumption
- Increased smoking
- Withdrawal

scene, and life-and-death decision making. Psychosocial stress may arise from family relationships and can come from conflicts with co-workers, abusive patients, and similar sources. Personality stress relates to the way a person thinks and feels. For example, this kind of stress can include the need to be liked. Personality stress can include one's expectations and feelings of guilt and anxiety as well. Choosing a career in EMS requires developing an understanding of job-related stress and effective stress management.

REACTIONS TO STRESS

Certain types of persons may be attracted to certain types of careers. For example, some believe that EMS personnel, firefighters, police officers, and others in public safety are predisposed to stressful and demanding jobs.[17] However, no person is immune from potential conflicts in managing stress.

ADAPTATION

Adaptation is a process that involves learning successful ways to deal with stressful situations. This process usually begins with using defense mechanisms. Next, adaptation focuses on developing coping skills, followed by problem solving. Finally, adaptation concludes with mastery.

Defense mechanisms are adaptive functions of the personality (Box 2-15). They assist a person in adjusting to stressful situations and help a person to avoid dealing with problems. *Denial*, for example, is a defense mechanism. Denial might be used to separate a person from the event long enough to deal with a problem that normally would be overwhelming.

Coping is an active confronting process. Coping involves gathering information and using the information to change or adjust to a new situation. Some beneficial ways to cope include taking part in regular physical exercise and being involved in activities at work that result in financial rewards and increased productivity. Other positive ways to cope include finding humor in personal crises, and "talking through" stressful events with family, friends, and co-workers.

Persons also may use harmful or negative coping mechanisms. An individual may become withdrawn or use alcohol or other drugs. Some may have angry outbursts toward family members and co-workers. Others may become silent. These negative coping mechanisms threaten interpersonal relationships with co-workers and loved ones. They should be seen as signs that an individual is having trouble dealing with stress.

> ### NOTE
> **Burnout** can be the result of cumulative stress. The condition is defined by physical and emotional exhaustion and negative attitudes. Burnout can develop when one is exposed to chronic stress that cannot be managed with usual coping mechanisms.

Problem solving involves analyzing a problem and finding options to deal with the issue now and in the future. Problem solving allows a person to clearly identify the problem and determine a course of action. This is a healthy approach to everyday concerns.

Mastery refers to the ability to see multiple options and solutions for challenging situations. Mastery results from extensive experience and the use of effective coping mechanisms with situations that are very similar. Mastery may be difficult to achieve.

STRESS MANAGEMENT TECHNIQUES

To manage stress well, a person must recognize the early warning signs of anxiety. Some of the physical effects of anxiety an individual may notice include the following:
- Heart palpitations
- Difficult or rapid breathing
- Dry mouth
- Chest tightness or pain
- Anorexia (lack of appetite), nausea, vomiting, diarrhea, abdominal cramps, flatulence, "butterflies"
- Flushing, diaphoresis (profuse sweating), body temperature fluctuation
- Urgency and frequency in urination
- Dysmenorrhea (painful menstruation), decreased sexual drive or performance
- Aching muscles, joints

Physical effects that may not be as noticeable include the following:
- Increased blood pressure and heart rate
- Increased blood glucose levels
- Increased adrenaline production by adrenal glands
- Reduced gastrointestinal peristalsis
- Pupillary dilation

> ### CRITICAL THINKING
> Compare your reactions while on a highly stressful call in the field to those you experience when stressed about school. How are those feelings similar or different from each other?

Many warning signs appear during the emergency response or within 24 hours after the event. Some responses, however, may be delayed for some time and may not appear for months or years after the event. If signs and symptoms of stress-related illness appear, the person should seek appropriate medical or psychological help.

Intervening to relieve stress is as important as recognizing the warning signals. Methods one may use initially to manage stress include reframing, controlled breathing, progressive relaxation, and guided imagery. All of these methods require practice to perform them properly. *Reframing* involves first looking at the situation from a different emotional viewpoint and then placing it in a different "frame" that fits the facts of another situation equally well. This acts to change the meaning of the situation. *Controlled*

BOX 2-15 Common Defense Mechanisms

Repression

Repression is thought to be the mechanism underlying all other defense mechanisms. Repression is the involuntary attempt to keep certain feelings or memories from reaching conscious awareness. Traumatic events, intolerable and dangerous impulses, and other unacceptable ideas are forced out of consciousness. This defense mechanism may be seen as a result of an approach-avoidance conflict. This is a conflict between trying to recall or think about something and trying to avoid the topic because it creates fear. Once repressions form, they usually are difficult to abolish. The individual must be reassured that no danger exists in recalling the event. For example, an emergency medical services (EMS) co-worker is killed while on duty. The partner has no recall of the event from the time they arrived at the scene until after the event.

Regression

Regression is a return to earlier levels of emotional adjustment. Of all the reactions to anxiety and danger, regression may be the most dramatic and debilitating. A person returns to an earlier developmental phase of life. This phase may have been a time when tension and conflict could be avoided. For example, an EMS worker throws a temper tantrum because he was assigned driver status on a work shift when he thought he would have direct patient care duties.

Projection

Projection involves attributing one's own undesirable qualities, feelings, motives, or desires to someone else. Projection may appear as aggression toward others. However, the problem is actually self-anger. Often individuals are wrong in labeling their own motives and the motives of others. For example, a paramedic crashes an emergency vehicle en route to a call. Because of guilt, she feels that others blame her for the crash. In fact, she is blaming herself.

Rationalization

Rationalizations occur when persons feel the need to explain their behavior. This need may be a result of social training. They feel the need to explain because the true explanation would cause anxiety or guilt. A person is trying to prove that the behavior is "rational" and therefore worthy of the approval of self and others. Rationalization is a commonly used defense mechanism. For example, a paramedic performs a poor physical examination on a trauma patient. She fails to discover a femur fracture. When questioned by medical direction, she justifies her actions by saying that the police were hurrying her to clear the scene.

Compensation

Compensation is trying to cover up for a real or imagined weakness. One compensates by stressing a more positive trait or skill. This conceals frustration and anxiety by focusing attention on other behavior. For example, an EMS crew member has weak clinical skills and feels inadequate at emergency scenes. He compensates by becoming an instructor in water rescue.

Reaction Formation

Reaction formation is a defensive behavior that prevents unwanted desires from being expressed. The person exaggerates opposing attitudes and behavior, thereby expressing the opposite of the true motive. The original impulse is still present. However, the impulse is masked by actions or attitudes that do not cause anxiety or stress. For example, a paramedic is outwardly friendly to a co-worker whom she dislikes.

Sublimation

Sublimation is a form of substitution. Sublimation entails changing undesirable urges so that they are socially acceptable. Sublimation is a defense mechanism. However, the functions of sublimation are thought to extend beyond that of protection. Sublimation requires changing one's focus or energy. In this change, instinctual drives are substituted for ones that may result in a higher cultural achievement. For example, a paramedic may become angry from seeing people die in drunk-driving crashes. Thus he starts a public awareness program on the hazards of drinking and driving.

Denial

Denial is another defense mechanism. In denial the person rejects elements of reality that knowingly would be intolerable. The person gains protection from unpleasant reality by refusing to see it. The person may deny the event itself or the memory of it. For example, a person who has just lost a loved one may be unable to accept the reality of death. (Denial differs from repression. Persons who use repression as a defense mechanism seem deliberately to keep their feelings or memories at a distance from the conscious mind.)

Substitution

Substitution is a defense mechanism that switches another activity or goal for one that is desired but unreachable. Substitution may involve the redirection of an emotion from the first object to a more acceptable one. Substitution often results from frustration. For example, a co-worker is having marital problems. He feels that it is unacceptable to argue with his spouse. He substitutes and displaces his anger at work by being irritable, grouchy, and hostile toward other crew members.

Isolation

Isolation involves the separation of unacceptable impulses, acts, or ideas from their origin in memory. This defense mechanism removes the emotional charge from the event. Isolation prevents feelings from being linked to the memory. Isolation may be helpful to the paramedic who must turn off feelings until after a call. For example, a paramedic may also be a parent and may have to give care to a dying child without being overcome by emotions.

breathing is a natural stress control technique. A person concentrates on depth and rate of breathing to achieve a calming effect. Controlled breathing may begin with deep breathing, followed by less deep breathing, and finally normal breathing. *Progressive relaxation* is a stress reduction strategy in which the person systematically tightens and relaxes particular muscle groups (from head to toe or from toe to head). This "fools" the brain into initiating muscle relaxation throughout the body. *Guided imagery* is used with meditation. Another person familiar with the technique acts as a guide during a stress response. The person experiencing stress then can focus on an image that helps relieve stress. (Once guided imagery is learned, a person can use the technique without prompting.)

Other ways to fight stress include being aware of personal limitations, taking part in peer counseling, and participating in group discussions. Proper diet, exercise, sleep, and rest also help to relieve stress. In addition, pursuing positive activities outside of EMS can balance work and recreation. The responsibility for personal health and well-being belongs to the individual. However, intervention programs may be available through EMS agencies, hospitals, and other groups.

CRITICAL INCIDENT STRESS MANAGEMENT

Critical incident stress management (CISM) evolved from the early 1970s concept of critical incident stress debriefing. This program was developed to help emergency workers exposed to a major incident. CISM is based on a partnership between mental health professionals and peer group support. Although the benefits of CISM as a form of psychological first aid are debated,[18] CISM is designed to give emergency workers a chance to vent their feelings about a call or event that had a major impact (Box 2-16).

Critical incident stress management aims to help emergency workers understand their reactions. It reassures them that what they are experiencing is normal. It also reassures them that what they are feeling may be common to others involved in the incident. The process may be for one person or may include various members of the emergency team (e.g., police, EMS crew members, firefighters, and emergency department staff).

NOTE
There are many programs available to EMS personnel and their families that can help manage stress. These include employee assistance programs, counseling, spouse support programs, family life programs, pastoral services, and periodic stress evaluations. These efforts and others can be good resources to the paramedic in dealing with stress on the job (see Box 2-16).

POSTTRAUMATIC STRESS DISORDER (PTSD)

Posttraumatic stress disorder is an anxiety disorder that can occur following a traumatic event. These events can include:

- Combat or military exposure
- Child sexual or physical abuse
- Terrorist attacks
- Sexual or physical assault
- Serious incidents, such as a car crash
- Natural disasters, such as a fire, tornado, hurricane, flood, or earthquake

Recent studies have indicated that EMS personnel are more likely than the general public to suffer from PTSD.[19] The emotional difficulties that can result from dealing regularly with traumatic calls can lead to increased absenteeism from work, a troubled family life, and increased alcohol or other drug use. PTSD may also increase the risk of suicide.

There are four types of symptoms associated with PTSD. They include reexperiencing, numbing, avoidance, and arousal.[20]

1. Reexperiencing is a mental "replay" of the event. It is often accompanied by strong, emotional reactions. This can occur during waking hours or during sleep (nightmares).
2. Avoidance refers to efforts to evade activities, places, or people that remind those with the disorder of the traumatic event.
3. Numbing is typically experienced as a loss of emotion, particularly positive feelings.
4. Arousal reflects excessive psychological activation. Examples include a heightened sense of being "on guard" as well as difficulty with sleep and concentration.

The symptoms of PTSD are often managed with counseling, behavior therapy, and sometimes medication. Brief "time-out" periods from work (1 to 8 weeks) and support from co-workers and supervisors may also aid EMS personnel in their recovery (Box 2-17).[21]

BOX 2-16 Potential Situations for Critical Incident Stress Management

- Line-of-duty injury or death
- Disaster
- Emergency worker suicide
- Infant/child death
- Extreme threat to emergency worker
- Prolonged incident that ends in loss or success
- Victims known to operations' personnel
- Death/injury of civilian caused by operations
- Other significant event

BOX 2-17 Techniques for Reducing Crisis-Induced Stress

- Allow adequate rest for emergency workers.
- Provide food and fluid replacement.
- Limit exposure to the incident.
- Change assignments.
- Provide postevent defusing/debriefing.

CRITICAL THINKING
Imagine which type of call would be a critical incident for you personally.

DEALING WITH DEATH, DYING, GRIEF, AND LOSS

Death and dying always will be part of health care delivery. Medical science has given society the ability to postpone death in some instances and perhaps lessen its physical pain. However, the fight for self-preservation is still inevitably lost.

Patient and Family Needs

In the delivery of EMS, paramedics at times will give care to a dying person surrounded by loved ones. In such cases, the emotional needs of the dying patient, family, and loved ones should be of utmost importance. The patient and significant others will need to be comforted, given privacy, and treated with respect and dignity. Loved ones may need to express feelings of rage, anger, despair, and guilt. They may need the paramedic to provide control and direction for this solemn event. The paramedic's role in these cases is important and may be a determining factor in the way survivors adjust to their loss (Box 2-18).

Stages of the Grieving Process

In 1968 Elisabeth Kübler-Ross began her work on the psychological aspects of death and dying. Her studies identified five predictable stages of dying: denial, anger, bargaining, depression, and acceptance. Kübler-Ross found that patients and loved ones dealing with the death process generally experience the following five stages:[22]

1. *Denial* is characterized by the feeling "No, not me." Denial is an expected response to news of a life-threatening illness or situation. The news is so overwhelming that it must be absorbed slowly. The patient seeks other opinions, verifies the accuracy of medical reports, or simply seems to ignore what he or she has been told. Denial is a valuable defense mechanism.

Denial is troubling only when no indication exists that the patient understands the seriousness of the situation. Most patients, families, and friends deny death to some degree to continue with the daily business of living.

2. *Anger* can be viewed as the "Why me?" phase. Anger is probably the most difficult for persons who care about or are trying to help the dying person. In this phase, the person rejects all efforts to help or console. This anger is really the anger of the dying person toward all the persons who continue to live. More accurately, anger may be anger directed toward God because He does not appear to have acted fairly or justly with the dying person.

3. *Bargaining* is reflected in a "Yes, me, but ..." frame of mind. The person admits the reality of being sick and of probably dying, but the person tries to bargain for extension or quality of life. These bargains usually are secret, frequently are made with God, and rarely are kept. For example, a father promises to be a "perfect patient" if only he can live to see his son's wedding.

4. *Depression* is the "Yes, me" reaction to anticipated death. Depression involves preparing to say and saying goodbye to everything and everyone a person has known and loved. The inherent sadness of this phase is appropriate and should be respected.

5. *Acceptance,* the simple and quiet "Yes," grows out of individuals' convictions that they have done what they could to be ready to die. Personal energy and interpersonal interests decrease significantly. During this phase, relatives and friends usually need more help than the dying person. The dying person's most important wish at this point is not to die alone.

NOTE
Dying patients and their loved ones may fluctuate between these stages and may or may not experience all five stages.

SHOW ME THE EVIDENCE
Researchers surveyed families of patients in whom they terminated resuscitation of asystolic cardiac arrest in the field. They found that field resuscitation termination was accepted by the patients' families. The system had predefined termination criteria and a preplan that included a mechanism for family support (other than the EMS crew). Follow-up of these nontransported families in 3 to 6 months indicated that their grief adjustment trended more positively than that observed in families whose deceased family member was transported.

From Edwardsen EA, Chiumento S, Davis E: Family perspective of medical care and grief support after field termination by emergency medical services personnel, *Prehosp Emerg Care* 6(4):440-444, 2002.

Paramedics rarely are involved in a patient's process of coming to terms with death. However, they often see the reactions of patients and families going through the death process. For example, denial may be obvious in some family members. These people may not appear to see or

---

BOX 2-18 Hospice Programs

Hospice programs began in England in 1967. They since have become a standard service of many health care institutions in the United States. Their goal is to help the terminally ill patient, family, and loved ones cope when death is expected. The hospice philosophy supports home care for the patient. Home care provides for a more natural environment. In addition, volunteers and health care professionals provide counseling and other psychological support to the patient and family during the death process. Hospice programs are well respected in the medical community. The programs play an important role in helping patients and their families accept death as a natural event in life.

acknowledge the seriousness of a situation in which decisions about resuscitation must be made. Anger may be directed at the paramedic crew or other health care workers. Bargaining may occur in the form of a mother who says, "Please save my child, and I promise that I'll always make her wear her seat belt!" The paramedic must realize the psychological aspects of the stages of grief.

When it is necessary to give news of a sudden death to a family, the paramedic's initial contact can influence the grief response greatly. The paramedic should gather the family in a private area and advise them of the patient's death, with a brief account of the situation causing the death. The paramedic should use the words *death* or *dead* and should avoid euphemisms such as "he's passed on" or "she's no longer with us." The paramedic should be compassionate and allow time for the news to be absorbed and for questions to be asked. The family members should be allowed to see the relative if they choose. They should be told in advance if resuscitation equipment is still connected to the patient. These efforts, along with empathic interaction with the family, help relatives deal with the loss of a loved one (Box 2-19).

Common Needs of the Paramedic When Dealing With Death and Dying

Dealing with death is difficult for everyone. Thus the paramedic's feelings and emotions also must be considered. The paramedic may experience some of the same stages of grief

described earlier. These reactions are normal and a great deal of effort to disguise or suppress these emotions may be required at the scene or while rendering care. However, the paramedic should discuss these feelings as soon as possible with friends, co-workers, and family in a constructive way that will lessen the emotional burden. Like others, the paramedic will need a chance to process the incident and obtain closure. Available resources, such as employee assistance programs and counseling and pastoral services, help avoid the effects of cumulative stress.

> ### CRITICAL THINKING
> What personal experiences have you had with death? How did you or others who were close to the deceased react to the initial news of the death?

Developmental Considerations When Dealing With Death and Dying

The way persons cope with their own death or the death of a loved one depends on their age, maturity, and understanding of death. The paramedic should be sensitive to the emotional needs of all age groups during this crisis. The following guidelines may be helpful when offering advice to family members who will be helping the young or elderly cope with the death of a loved one.[23]

Children up to age 3 probably will sense that something has happened in the family. They will realize that others are sad and crying. They also may be aware of increased activity in the household. The family should be urged to watch for changes in eating or sleeping patterns and for an increase in irritability. In addition, the family should be sensitive to the child's needs and try to maintain consistency in the child's routines and with significant persons in the child's life.

Children 3 to 6 years of age do not have a concept of the finality of death. They may believe that the person will return and may ask "when" continually. This age group believes in magical thinking and may feel that they are responsible for the death. They also may believe that everyone else they love will die too. The family should watch for changes in the child's behavior patterns with friends and at school, for difficulty sleeping, and for changes in eating habits. The family should emphasize that the child is not responsible for the death. The family should reinforce the fact that crying is normal when persons are sad and should encourage children to talk about their feelings.

Children 6 to 9 years of age are beginning to understand the finality of death. They want detailed explanations for the death and can differentiate fatal illness from just "being sick." Like the 3- to 6-year-olds, these children may be afraid that other loved ones will die too. This age group may be uncomfortable with expressing their feelings and may act silly or embarrassed when talking about death. The paramedic should suggest to the family that they talk about the

BOX 2-19 Recommended Communication Strategies

A situation involving death and dying is uncomfortable. Communication with the patient and loved ones may be difficult. The following recommendations for communications and activities may help a paramedic deal with dying patients and their families:

- Answer questions honestly for the patient and family and explain all activities.
- Do not initiate the subject of dying; let it come from the patient or family.
- If the patient or family asks you whether the patient is going to die, advise that you are doing everything you possibly can but that the situation is critical. This allows a brief time for the patient and family to prepare themselves.
- Do not falsely reassure the patient or family (e.g., "everything's going to be okay").
- Use compassionate, nonverbal communication (facial expression, touching).
- Offer to contact someone if the patient is alone.
- If family is not present, assure the patient that emergency department personnel will notify them. If they are nearby, encourage the family to come to the patient immediately or to meet the patient at the emergency department.
- Allow the family to stay with the patient when appropriate.

normal feelings of anger, sadness, and guilt and that they share their own feelings about death with the child. The family members should not hesitate to cry because crying will let the child know that expression of feelings is acceptable.

Children 9 to 12 years of age are aware of the finality of death. They may want to know the details surrounding the event. They will be concerned with practical matters involving their lifestyle and may try to "act like an adult." (Most of these children, however, will show regression to an earlier stage of emotional response.) The paramedic should suggest to the family that they set aside time to talk to the child about feelings and encourage the sharing of memories to aid in the grief response.

Older adults usually show concern for other family members. In addition, they may be worried about their further loss of independence and about financial matters at hand. Family members should be sensitive and understanding about these issues because they are real for this age group.

PREVENTION OF DISEASE TRANSMISSION

Emergency workers often manage ill and injured patients. Thus prevention of disease transmission must be a priority in daily practice. Specific concerns arise for personal health and safety. One concern includes being aware of common sources of exposure. Another includes using personal protection. Finally, one must know what to do if an exposure has occurred (Box 2-20).

Common Sources of Exposure

Common sources of exposure to infectious agents in the prehospital setting include needlesticks and broken or scraped skin. Mucous membranes such as those that line the eyes, nose, and mouth also are a source for entry of infectious agents or microorganisms. As a result, the paramedic must practice universal precautions during all patient care encounters (see Chapter 14).

Paramedic Protection From Airborne and Blood-Borne Pathogens

The following list contains some general guidelines to help prevent exposure to infectious diseases (a more complete discussion of infectious disease is presented in Chapter 28).
1. Follow engineering and work practices. Maintain good personal health and hygiene habits. (Wash hands frequently and pay attention to general cleanliness.)
2. Maintain immunizations for tetanus, diphtheria, pertussis, polio, hepatitis B, MMR (measles, mumps, and rubella), and influenza.

> ### BOX 2-20 Disease Transmission Terminology
>
> Airborne and blood-borne pathogens are organisms respectively carried through air and blood (and other body fluids). These organisms create disease in the human body or host. Some pathogens (e.g., certain bacteria) can survive outside a host. Others (such as viruses) can survive only in the human cell (see Chapter 28). Exposure occurs in cases of contact with a likely infectious body fluid or other infectious agent. Certain steps are used to destroy infectious organisms that may have come in contact with equipment and instruments. These steps include cleaning, disinfection, and sterilization. Universal precautions are practices to prevent or reduce contact with body substances and other infectious agents.

3. Conduct a periodic screening for tuberculosis.
4. Practice universal precautions in all encounters with patients.
5. Properly clean, disinfect, and dispose of used materials and equipment immediately.
6. Use puncture-resistant containers to dispose of needles and other sharp objects.
7. Separate and label all soiled laundry (clothes, bed linens). Also separate and label all equipment. Do this until the items can be cleaned and disinfected properly.
8. Conduct a periodic risk assessment of health.

Documentation and Management of an Exposure

The paramedic must be familiar with laws, regulations, and national standards that address issues of infectious disease and take personal protective measures against exposure. In the event of a potential exposure to an infectious disease or a significant exposure to a patient's blood or body fluids, the paramedic should do the following:
1. Wash the area of contact with soap and water thoroughly and immediately.
2. Immediately document the situation in which the exposure occurred.
3. Describe actions taken to reduce chances of infection.
4. Comply with all required reporting responsibilities and time frames.
5. Cooperate with incident investigation.
6. Be screened for antibody titers and potential infectious diseases.
7. Obtain proper immunization boosters.
8. Obtain a full medical follow-up.

SUMMARY

- Wellness has two main aspects: physical well-being and mental and emotional health.
- As health care professionals, paramedics have a responsibility to serve as role models in disease prevention.
- Persons who are overweight tend to be at risk for developing certain illnesses. A healthful diet includes a variety of foods that are low in fat, saturated fat, and cholesterol. The calories in the diet should be regulated to prevent unwanted weight gain.
- Physical fitness can be described as a condition that helps individuals look, feel, and do their best.
- Sleep helps to rejuvenate a tired body.
- Steps to reduce cardiovascular disease include the following: improving cardiovascular endurance, eliminating cigarette smoking, controlling high blood pressure, maintaining a normal body fat composition, maintaining good total cholesterol/high-density lipoprotein ratio, monitoring triglyceride levels, controlling diabetes, avoiding excessive alcohol, eating healthy foods, reducing stress, and making a periodic risk assessment.
- Most common cancers are linked to one of three environmental risk factors: smoking, sunlight, and diet.
- The paramedic's duty is to be familiar with laws, regulations, and national standards that address issues of infectious disease. The paramedic also must take personal protective measures to guard against exposure.
- Actions to take after significant exposure include disinfection, documentation, incident investigation, screening, immunization, and medical follow-up.
- Injuries on the job can be minimized. Knowledge of body mechanics during lifting and moving is helpful. Also, being alert for hostile settings is key. Prioritization

- of personal safety during rescue situations is wise. In addition, paramedics must practice safe vehicle operation. They must use safety equipment and supplies as well.
- The misuse and abuse of drugs and other substances may lead to chemical dependency (addiction). This may have a wide range of effects on physical and mental health.
- The concept of diversity encompasses acceptance and respect of other people. It is important to realize that each person is unique and to recognize individual differences.
- "Good" stress is eustress. Eustress is a positive response to stimuli and is considered protective. "Bad" stress is distress. Distress is a negative response to environmental stimuli and is the source of anxiety and stress-related disorders.
- Adaptation is a process in which persons learn effective ways to deal with stressful situations. This dynamic process usually begins with using defense mechanisms. Next, one develops coping skills, followed by problem solving, and culminating in mastery.
- Critical incident stress management is designed to help emergency personnel understand their reactions to a call or event that had a major emotional impact. The process reassures them that what they are experiencing is normal and may be common to others involved in the incident.
- Often news of a sudden death must be given to a family. The paramedic's initial contact can influence the grief process greatly.
- The five stages of dying identified by Dr. Elisabeth Kübler-Ross are denial, anger, bargaining, depression, and acceptance.

REFERENCES

1. USDA: *Dietary Guidelines for Americans*, 2010. www.cnpp.usda.gov/dietaryguidelines. Accessed July 1, 2011.
2. U.S. Food and Drug Administration: *Protecting your health*, www.fda.gov, accessed 7-26-10.
3. Straif K, Baan R, Grosse Y, et al: *Carcinogenicity of shiftwork, painting, and fire-fighting*, Lancet Oncol 12(8):1065-1066, 2007.
4. Caruso C, Hitchcock EM, Dick RB, et al: *Overtime and extended work shifts, U.S. Department of Health and Human Services, Centers for Disease Control and Prevention, National Institutes of Occupational Safety and Health*, www.cdc.gov/niosh/docs/2004-143/pdfs/2004-143.pdf, accessed 8-4-2010.
5. Barger LK, Cade BE, Ayas NT, et al: Extended work shifts and the risk of motor vehicle crashes among interns, *N Engl J Med* 352(2):125-134, 2005.
6. Rouch I, Wild P, Ansiau D, et al: Shiftwork experience, age, and cognitive performance, *Ergonomics* 48(10):1282-1293, 2005.
7. American Heart Association: *Heart and disease stroke statistics update: a report from the American Heart Association*, Dallas, 2010, The Association.
8. Mayo Clinic: *Handwashing: an easy way to prevent infection*, www.mayoclinic.com/health/hand-washing/HQ00407, accessed 7-30-10.
9. *Facts about EMS back and musculoskeletal disorders (MSD's)*, www.mytactical.com/downloads/SAM_S_EMS_BACK_INJURY_FACTS.doc, accessed 7-30-10.
10. Dailey B: Musculoskeletal injury prevention: protect yourself from on-the-job injuries, *JEMS* 31(4):61-73, 2010.
11. Cicala RS: Substance abuse among physicians: what you need to know, *Hospital Physician* 39(7):39-46, 2007.
12. Trinkoff AM, Storr CL: Substance use among nurses: differences between specialties, *Am J Public Health* 88(4):581-585, 1998.

13. Boxer PA, Wild D: Psychological distress and alcohol use among firefighters, *Scand J Work Environ Health* 19(2):121-125, 1993.
14. Centers for Disease Control and Prevention: *Fact sheet: health effects of cigarette smoking*, 2008, www.cdc.gov/tobacco/data_statistics/fact_sheets/fast_facts/index.htm, accessed 7-30-10.
15. U.S. Department of Health and Human Services, Substance Abuse and Mental Health Services Administration, Center for Mental Health Services: *Tips for managing and preventing stress, a guide for emergency and disaster response workers*, www.samhsa.gov, accessed 7-13-10.
16. Selye H: *The stress of life*, New York, 1956, McGraw-Hill.
17. Mitchell J, Bray G: *Emergency services stress: guidelines for preserving the health and careers of emergency services personnel*, Englewood Cliffs, NJ, 1990, Brady.
18. Department of Mental Health and Substance Dependence: *Mental and social aspects of health of populations exposed to extreme stressors*, WHO/MSD/MER/03.01, Geneva, 2003, World Health Organization.
19. Medscape Psychiatry & Mental Health: *Posttraumatic stress disorder in urban EMS workers*, www.medscape.com/viewarticle/430883, accessed 7-30-10.
20. U.S. Department of Veterans Affairs: *How is PTSD measured?* http://ncptsd.va.gov/ncmain/ncdocs/fact_shts/fs_lay_assess.html, accessed 7-30-10.
21. International Medical Corp: *Coping in the aftermath of Hurricane Katrina: some brief guidance notes on stress, grief and loss for front line teams*, www.who.int/hac/techguidance/ems/IMC_Guidance_Stress_Grief_Loss.pdf, accessed 1-29-09.
22. Elisabeth Kübler-Ross, *On death and dying*, Macmillan, New York, 1969, Scribner.
23. Bassuk EL, Fox SS, Prendergast KJ: *Behavioral emergencies*, Boston, 1983, Little, Brown.

SUGGESTED READINGS

Amtmann J, Amtmann K: Fit to respond: strength training for EMS professionals, *JEMS* 31(7):53-56, 2006.
Blanchet D: Lift with your head, *EMS* 35(8), 2006.
Dickinson ET: When an exposure is not an exposure, *JEMS* 32(10):59-62, 2007.

Upon completion of this chapter, the paramedic student will be able to:

1. Identify roles of the emergency medical services community in injury prevention.
2. Describe the epidemiology of trauma in the United States.
3. Define injury.
4. Describe Haddon's matrix and the injury triangle.
5. Describe public health goals and activities.
6. Outline the aspects of the emergency medical services system that make it a desirable resource for involvement in public health activities.
7. Describe essential activities for the active participation of emergency medical services in community wellness activities.
8. List situations in which paramedics may participate in injury prevention.
9. Differentiate among primary, secondary, and tertiary health prevention activities.
10. Evaluate a situation to determine opportunities for injury prevention.
11. Identify resources necessary to conduct a community health assessment.
12. Relate how alterations in the epidemiological triangle can influence injury and disease patterns.
13. Describe strategies to implement a successful injury prevention program.

community health assessment An assessment of a target community to identify needs and resources required to provide prevention and wellness promotion activities.

epidemiology The study of the detriments of disease events in populations.

injury Intentional or unintentional damage to the person resulting from acute exposure to thermal, mechanical, electrical, or chemical energy or from the absence of essentials such as heat and oxygen

injury risk Real or potentially hazardous situations that put individuals at increased risk for sustaining an injury.

injury surveillance The ongoing systematic collection, analysis, and interpretation of injury data essential to the planning, implementation, and evaluation of public health practice.

primary injury prevention The practice of preventing an injury from occurring.

public health A field of medicine that deals with the physical and mental health of all people in a community.

secondary and tertiary prevention The care and rehabilitation activities, respectively, that are intended to prevent further problems from an event that has already occurred.

secondary injury prevention A concept that recognizes that injuries will occur and that is centered on reducing severity of the injury as it is occurring.

teachable moment The time after an injury has occurred when the patient and observers remain acutely aware of what has happened and may be more receptive to being taught ways that the event or illness could have been prevented.

years of productive life The calculation obtained by subtracting the age of teh victim's death from 65 (the average age of retirement)

A community has a duty to promote injury prevention. This prevention can occur in the form of leadership and educational activities. One goal of injury prevention is to decrease the incidence of preventable illness and injury. A final goal is to prevent persons from needing costly medical care. As a member of the health care system the paramedic can be a key resource in injury prevention programs (Box 3-1).

INJURY EPIDEMIOLOGY

Injuries that are unintentional are the leading cause of death among all persons 1 to 44 years of age. Unintentional injuries are the fifth leading cause of death among all age groups, exceeded only by heart disease, cancer, stroke, and chronic obstructive pulmonary disease.[1] In 2008, 118,000 injury-related deaths occurred in the United States.

Unintentional injuries result in more years of life lost before age 65 than any other cause of death. From a financial perspective the effect of fatal and nonfatal unintentional injuries was $652.1 billion in 2006. This equaled about $5700 per household (Figure 3-1). The quality of life lost from these injuries is valued at another $3080.1 billion. This makes the total cost $3732.2 billion in 2006[1] (Table 3-1). About 36% of all emergency department visits in the United States are related to injury. This percentage accounted for more than 41 million visits to emergency departments in 2005 (Box 3-1).

> ### NOTE
>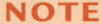
> While you make a 10-minute speech about bicycle safety to a classroom of children, at least 2 persons will be killed by unintentional injury. Another 498 will be disabled. A death caused by unintentional injury occurs in the United States every 4 minutes.[1]

OVERVIEW OF INJURY PREVENTION

Traditionally, emergency medical services (EMS) has been a reactionary medical discipline that waits until patients are injured or ill before being used. Reactionary medical care is termed *the acute care phase of injury control,* or *tertiary injury prevention.* Although EMS excels in acute care, a full system of injury control is made up of several facets, with acute care being one aspect. The injury control strategy of preventing rather than simply treating an injury is known as **primary injury prevention.**

Preventive strategies yield better outcomes than treatment strategies in terms of lives saved and money spent. Identifying prevention strategies relies heavily on data collection. Success also depends on teaching injury prevention to patients. Paramedics are respected in the community and generally are welcomed into homes and businesses. Thus paramedics have a unique opportunity to find injury patterns and intervene on behalf of persons at risk.

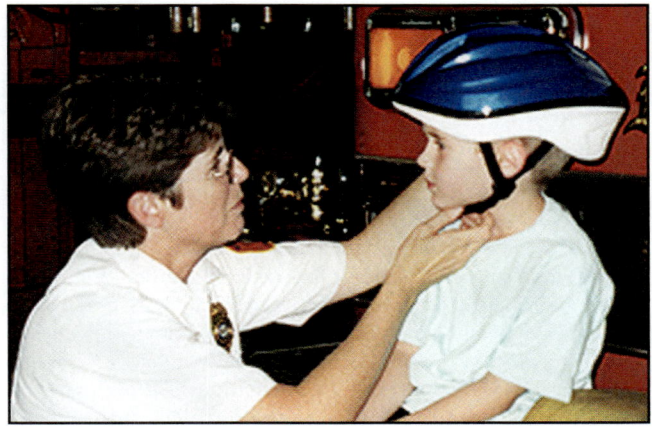

(Courtesy Kim McKenna, St. Charles, Mo.)

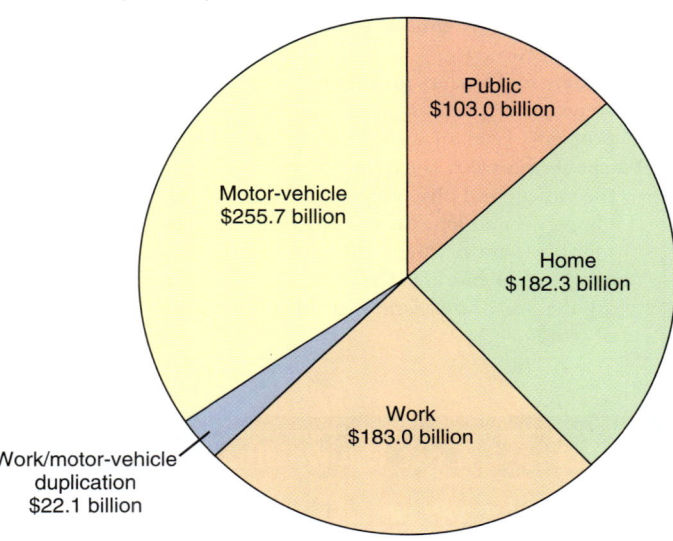

FIGURE 3-1 Cost of unintentional injuries by class in 2008. (From National Safety Council: *Injury facts,* Itasca, Ill, 2009, The Council.)

> ### DID YOU KNOW?
> **The National Health Interview Survey**
> The National Health Interview Survey is conducted annually by the National Center for Health Statistics. This survey samples U.S. households to obtain data about the health status of household members. This includes any injuries that were sustained during the 5 weeks before the survey. In 2005 the survey found that most injuries (46.6%) occurred in or around the home. This was followed by injuries at recreational or sports facilities (14.2%) and then by injuries on streets, highways, and parking lots (13.3%).[2] It is this kind of data collection performed by various government agencies and health organizations (discussed later in this chapter) that guides the focus of injury prevention initiatives in this country.

Injury Concepts
DEFINITION OF INJURY

A puzzling factor that hindered the study of injury and therefore injury prevention was the apparent unrelated nature of injuries. On the surface, no relationship seemed

BOX 3-1 Injury and Illness Prevention Terminology

Injury: Intentional or unintentional damage to the person resulting from acute exposure to thermal, mechanical, electrical, or chemical energy or from the absence of essentials such as heat and oxygen

Injury risk: Real or potentially hazardous situations that put individuals at increased risk for sustaining an injury

Injury surveillance: The ongoing collection, analysis, and interpretation of injury data essential to the planning, implementation, and evaluation of public health practice; closely integrated with the timely dissemination of these data to those who need to know, with the final link in the chain being the application of these data to prevention and control

Primary injury prevention: The practice of preventing an injury from occurring

Secondary and tertiary prevention: The care and rehabilitation activities, respectively, that are intended to prevent further problems from an event that has already occurred

Teachable moment: The time after an injury has occurred when the patient and observers remain acutely aware of what has happened and may be more receptive to being taught ways that the event or illness could be prevented

Years of productive life: The calculation obtained by subtracting the age of the victim's death from 65 (the average age of retirement)

TABLE 3-1 Cost Equivalents, 2008

The Cost of	Is Equivalent to
All injuries ($701.9 billion)	62 cents of every dollar paid in federal personal income taxes, **or**
	50 cents of every dollar spent on food in the United States
Motor vehicle crashes ($255.7 billion)	Purchasing 300 gallons of gasoline for each registered vehicle in the United States, or more than $1200 per licensed driver
Work injuries ($183 billion)	46 cents of every dollar of corporate dividend to stockholders, **or**
	11 cents of every dollar of pretax corporate profits, **or**
	Exceeds the combined profits reported by the top 22 Fortune 500 companies
Home injuries ($182.3 billion)	A $222,600 rebate on each new single-family home built, **or**
	45 cents of every dollar of property taxes paid
Public injuries ($103 billion)	A $11.2 million grant to each public library in the United States, **or**
	A $93,100 bonus for each police officer and firefighter

Courtesy National Safety Council: *Injury facts,* Itasca, Ill, 2010, The Council.

to exist between a vehicle crash and a poisoning, or between a gunshot wound and a drowning. However, it now is known that all injuries are the result of either (1) tissue damage caused by the transfer of energy to the human body (this energy may be mechanical, thermal, electrical, chemical, or radiant) or (2) tissue damage caused by the absence of needed energy elements such as heat or oxygen (see Chapter 37). So in essence, all injuries are related.

THE INJURY TRIANGLE AND HADDON'S MATRIX

Injury is also a disease process. Three factors are necessary to cause a disease: host, agent, and environment. Together these three factors are known as *the injury triangle* (Figure 3-2). In the injury triangle the host is the victim, the agent of injury is energy, and the environment provides a place for the agent and host to come together over time. The actual injury event may take only a fraction of a second, but the events that lead up to an injury and the events that occur as a result of an injury may take place over seconds, months, or even years.

NOTE

Changing one or more of the factors in the injury triangle can alter disease or injury patterns.

In the mid-1960s, William Haddon (the "father" of injury prevention) developed an analytical tool to aid in understanding the entire injury sequence. This tool is now known as *Haddon's matrix.* The three factors of the injury triangle are placed in a table on a timeline that is divided into three phases. These phases are preevent, event, and postevent. For example, the Haddon's matrix in Table 3-2 charts the events that may occur before, during, and after a car crash. The table helps one to see that injuries often result from a predictable and therefore preventable chain of events. The matrix also affirms that most injuries are linked with many causes.

The *preevent phase* is the period before the release of injury-causing energy. During this time the person's performance is greater than the task demands and energy is under control. Events in this phase tend to influence the *likelihood* that an injury will occur. Because the injury

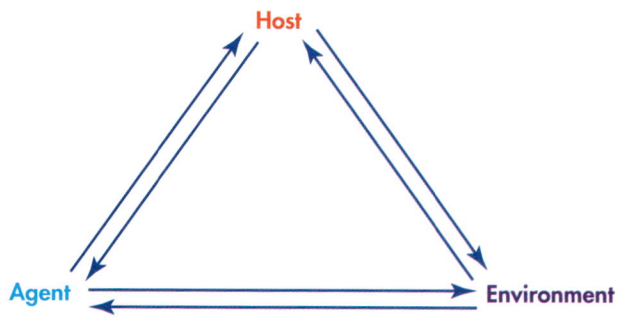

FIGURE 3-2 Epidemiological injury triangle.

TABLE 3-2 Haddon's Matrix for Automobile Crashes

Phase	FACTOR		
	Host	Agent	Environment
Preevent	Impaired capabilities, age, fatigue, alcohol/drug use, driving experience, adherence to driving laws	Defective equipment, dirty windows, improper maintenance, equipment design	Road shoulder too narrow, poor lighting, weather conditions, highway not divided, inadequate notification signs, road design, and construction
Event	Injury threshold caused by aging, chronic disease, alcohol, use of restraints, ejection	Failure of doors, impact with sharp objects in the vehicle, vehicle size	Lack of guardrails, large trees near roadside, oncoming traffic
Postevent	Type or extent of injury, knowledge of first aid, alcohol	Bursting gas tanks, entrapment	Quality of rescue, EMS, hospitals, rehabilitation

has yet to occur, primary injury prevention can take place in this phase. The time frame can be seconds to years, depending on what events come into play to cause the injury.

The *event phase* is the period during which the person's performance falls below the demands of the task. The result is the release of uncontrolled energy. The time frame usually is a fraction of a second to a few minutes. Events in this phase affect the transmission of energy. **Secondary injury prevention** recognizes that injuries are going to occur and is centered on reducing the severity of the injury as it is occurring.

The *postevent phase* is the period after the injury has occurred. This phase can last from a few seconds to years. In this time frame, tertiary injury prevention takes place and traditional EMS exists. The focus of tertiary injury prevention is to lessen the long-term adverse effects of the injury.

The Three E's of Injury Prevention

Three broad practices typically have been used to establish injury prevention programs. The first *E* of injury prevention is education. The second *E* is enforcement. The third *E* is engineering. A proactive, prevention-oriented paramedic can play a key role in all three strategies.

EDUCATION

The purpose of education is to persuade high-risk persons or groups to change risky behavior. It also is meant to teach these persons to adopt safety precautions. Education is considered an active countermeasure. This practice requires the person to do something to take advantage of knowledge learned and often requires the person to make a behavioral change. Education is the most often used approach in injury prevention. It is most effective when used with enforcement and engineering. Examples of educational programs include:

- Alcohol and other drug prevention
- Burn prevention
- Drowning prevention
- Elder safety
- Fall prevention
- Pedestrian and bicycle safety
- Poison prevention
- School safety and school-based programs
- Sports safety
- Suicide prevention
- Violence prevention

SHOW ME THE EVIDENCE

A North Carolina EMS service developed a program called "Welcome to the World." Paramedics trained in childhood injury prevention visited 110 families with newborns to provide home safety inspections. If hazards were identified they were corrected immediately or referred to another agency for correction. Paramedics also provided injury prevention education. They found that in families with one child 88% had smoke detectors, 64% had bath water <120° F, 94% had correct crib slat spacing, and 98% had a car seat. Only 38% of the homes with one child were deemed "infant-safe."

From Brice JH, Overby BA, Hawkins ER, et al: Determination of infant-safe homes in a community injury prevention program, *PEC* 10(3):397-402, 2006.

ENFORCEMENT

Enforcement occurs through force of law. It requires that persons adopt certain behaviors that reduce risk. Mandatory personal restraints (e.g., lap and shoulder restraints) and motorcycle helmet use laws are examples of this approach. Like education, enforcement is seen as an active countermeasure. It requires the person to adhere to the law to benefit from it, so the success of this approach depends on the compliance of individuals. Success also depends on the ability to enforce these laws. Even so, enforcement is more effective than education alone. Enforcement strategies that have been proven to reduce vehicle-related injury include:

- Child restraint laws
- "Click It or Ticket" programs

- Ignition interlock programs for repeat offenders
- Minimum legal drinking age laws
- Reducing legal blood alcohol concentrations
- Sobriety checkpoints and DUI enforcement
- Speed limit enforcement
- Zero tolerance for young drivers

ENGINEERING

Engineering refers to product or environmental design. This design automatically provides protection or decreases the likelihood that an injury-producing incident will occur. This approach builds safety into a product. Thus a person does not have to do anything to benefit from engineering. Engineering is a passive countermeasure. Examples include air bags in cars and sprinkler systems in buildings. Engineering has proved to be the most effective of the three *E*'s. However, engineering also is the most expensive approach to undertake. Examples of engineering used to prevent injury for paramedics include:

- Disposable equipment
- Latex gloves
- Needleless syringes and injection ports
- Nonslip footwear and nonskid surfaces
- Particulate air filters and masks
- Personal protective equipment
- Sharps containers

BASIC PRINCIPLES OF PUBLIC HEALTH

Most people know what is meant by the term *medical care*. And even though many people benefit from *public health,* they are less familiar with the term—specifically its missions and functions. Public health is different than medical care. Although there are many definitions of **public health**, the term can be defined as a field of medicine that deals with the physical and mental health of all people in a community. The focus of public health is more on prevention of disease than on treatment of disease. Important areas of public health include water supply, waste disposal, air pollution, and food safety. Other examples of public health goals and accomplishments include:

- Widespread vaccination programs
- Clean drinking water and sewage systems
- Declines in infectious disease
- Fluoridated water supplies
- Reduction in use of tobacco products
- Prenatal care services

Public Health Laws, Regulations, and Guidelines

Laws, regulations, and guidelines for public health initiatives are provided by local, state, and government agencies. Box 3-2 provides a sampling of state, federal, and international public health resources.

BOX 3-2 A Sampling of State, Federal, and International Public Health Resources

- Agency for Toxic Substances and Disease Registry (ATSDR)
- American Public Health Association (APHA)
- Association of Public Health Laboratories
- Association of Schools of Public Health (ASPH)
- Association of State and Territorial Health Officials (ASTHO)
- Centers for Disease Control and Prevention (CDC)
- Centers for Medicare & Medicaid Services (CMS)
- Food and Drug Administration (FDA)
- Health Resources and Services Administration (HRSA)
- National Academy of Sciences, Institute of Medicine (IOM)
- National Association of County and City Health Officials (NACCHO)
- National Association of Local Boards of Health (NALBOH)
- National Institutes of Health (NIH)
- National Organization of State Offices of Rural Health
- Public Health Foundation
- U.S. Department of Health and Human Services (DHHS)
- U.S. Environmental Protection Agency (EPA)
- World Health Organization (WHO)

Others involved in public health include medical professionals such as physicians, nurses, and EMS personnel. Area hospitals, clinics, public service agencies, and other government and nongovernment agencies also play important roles in providing public health services in a community.

FEASIBILITY OF EMERGENCY MEDICAL SERVICES INVOLVEMENT IN PUBLIC HEALTH

The United States has more than 840,669 EMS personnel.[3] As noted in *Emergency Medical Services: Agenda for the Future,* "People attracted to the EMS service are among society's best, and desire to contribute to their community's health. The composition of the EMS workforce reflects the diversity of the population it serves."[4] Thus it seems fitting that EMS plays a role in educating the public as a part of promoting health. EMS is a public health system and a workforce that is a valuable human resource. The following points support the feasibility of EMS interface with public health and injury prevention. EMS personnel are:

- Often the most medically educated persons in rural settings
- Role models with high profiles
- Seen as the champions of the customer
- Welcome in homes, schools, and other settings
- Seen as authorities on injury and prevention
- Often the first to note situations that pose a risk for illness or injury (e.g., unsanitary conditions and unsafe home environments)

CRITICAL THINKING

Did you ever have a class or program taught by a fire-fighter or paramedic when you were a child? How did you feel about the firefighter and paramedic?

NOTE

As managed care evolves, a demand on EMS for sup-portive care and intervention will increase. Paramedics and emergency medical services agencies must adapt to new roles in the health care delivery system.

Essential Community Leadership Activities

For paramedics and other public service personnel to play active roles in community health and injury prevention programs, the community must take the following steps to ensure successful participation among these groups (Box 3-3).

PROTECT EMERGENCY MEDICAL SERVICES PERSONNEL FROM INJURY

A basic first step for preventing injury and promoting well-ness in a community is to protect the well-being of EMS personnel. Policies should help to ensure EMS safety during an emergency response, while at the scene, and during patient transportation. Protection can be accomplished with traffic safety laws and public education. Protection also can be enhanced with the help of law enforcement, fire service personnel, and other public service agencies.

All EMS workers must have access to personal protective equipment. This equipment helps to reduce the risk of eye, back, and skin injury. Other valuable safety tactics include helmets to reduce head injury, reflective clothing to increase visibility, and steel-toed shoes to prevent foot injury. Other goals of personal protection are to reduce exposure to com-municable diseases and hazardous chemicals. Communi-ties can reduce injuries related to work through personal

safety programs. Communities also can reduce injuries by creating a wellness program for EMS workers (see Chapter 3).

PROVIDE EDUCATION TO EMERGENCY MEDICAL SERVICES PERSONNEL

Primary and continuing education programs for EMS per-sonnel should include the basics of primary injury preven-tion. Community leaders should help to create a liaison between EMS programs and public and private specialty groups. These groups may include hospitals, other public health and safety agencies, safety councils, social services, religious organizations, colleges, and universities. This link will help provide specific education and training. Coopera-tion among these groups can help locate target groups for prevention activities and encourage sharing of program establishment tasks.

SUPPORT AND PROMOTE COLLECTION AND USE OF INJURY DATA

Communities should create policies that promote injury documentation by EMS personnel. Communities should review and at times modify the tools for data collection so that prompt recording of data is both feasible and realistic. The data collected should contribute to local, state, and national surveillance programs. For instance, these programs may include head and spinal cord injury regis-tries, among others.

DID YOU KNOW?
Data Collection Registries

A registry (disease or trauma registry) is a file of uniform data. It describes persons who meet certain criteria. The registry collects medical and demographic data in an ongoing and systematic way to serve predetermined purposes.[5] These purposes include (1) facilitating and coordinating rehabilitation and other needed services, (2) gathering data for injury preven-tion and control, (3) gathering data for health care planning, and (4) evaluating services provided to injured persons.[6]

The first computerized trauma registry was introduced in 1969 at Cook County Hospital in Chicago, Illinois.[5] In 1985 the CDC began to promote the development of surveillance systems for clusters of injuries (sentinel injuries) at both the state and national levels. Since then, many states have developed statewide registries to track traumatic brain injuries, spinal cord injuries, and other classes of trauma. Federal agencies working with medical organizations and other groups help coordinate national-level standardizations of trauma registries. EMS and trauma care professionals play a major role in gathering these data. It helps in monitoring and evaluating the quality of trauma care in trauma center hospitals and trauma care systems.

OBTAIN SUPPORT AND RESOURCES FOR PRIMARY INJURY PREVENTION ACTIVITIES

The community needs to provide budgetary support for injury prevention programs. Community leaders may need to seek financial resources for fees and equipment,

BOX 3-3 Essential Community Leadership Activities

Communities have the responsibility to assist and support paramedics in the following activities:

- Protect the paramedic from injury.
- Provide primary injury prevention education to EMS personnel.
- Support and promote collection and use of injury data.
- Obtain support and resources for primary injury prevention activities.
- Empower individual paramedics to conduct primary injury prevention activities.

NOTE: Emergency medical services, through expanded scope of practice, will be performing these leadership activities for injury prevention and wellness.

publicity, and networking with other injury prevention organizations. In addition, the community needs to initiate or attend meetings of local organizations that are involved or that are requesting involvement in injury prevention. Grants can be obtained from state and national groups to help fund these initiatives. Examples of such organizations include the Centers for Disease Control and Prevention and Emergency Medical Services for Children. Grants may also be obtained from private donors, community block grants, and institutions. The funding may not always be easy to obtain. Regardless of how funding is obtained, EMS workers have a duty to provide prevention initiatives on any call where a preventable event has occurred.

EMPOWER INDIVIDUAL EMERGENCY MEDICAL SERVICES PERSONNEL TO CONDUCT PRIMARY INJURY PREVENTION ACTIVITIES

As stated previously, the community must financially support injury prevention programs. It must also promote interest and involvement in injury prevention activities from EMS personnel. This support can influence individual participation in the following ways:

- Providing rotating assignments to prevention programs
- Providing salary for off-duty injury prevention activities
- Rewarding and/or remunerating participation for on- and off-duty prevention activities

Essential Paramedic Activities

Activities that are essential for paramedics are based on education. These activities include knowing and practicing the personal injury prevention strategies. Examples of these strategies include:

- Appropriate use of audible and visual warning devices
- Availability and use of law enforcement
- Exercise and conditioning
- Practice of on-scene survival techniques
- Proper driving techniques
- Recognition of health hazards and high-profile crime areas
- Safety restraint use (self, patient, passenger)
- Secure equipment in patient care compartment
- Safe approach to parking at, and exiting, the scene
- Safe driving
- Scene safety precautions
- Stress management (personal, family, work)
- Traffic control (vehicles, bystanders)
- Use of on-scene survival resources
- Use of personal protective equipment (reflective clothing, helmets)
- Use of proper lifting and moving techniques
- Personal wellness

The paramedic also needs to know about illnesses and injuries common to various age groups and associated with different recreational activities, workplaces, and other facilities in the community (Box 3-4).

BOX 3-4 Other Essential Paramedic Activities

Other essential paramedic activities include review of illness and injuries common to the following:

Infancy (low birth weight; mortality and morbidity)
Childhood (intentional, unintentional, or alleged intentional events)
Childhood violence to self and others
Adults
Geriatric patients
Recreational activities
Workplace hazards
Day care centers (licensed and nonlicensed)
Early release from hospital
Discharge from urgent care or other outpatient facilities
Signs of emotional stress that can lead to intentional, unintentional, or alleged events
Self-medication
Dangers of noncompliance (borrowing, not taking medicines on time or finishing the regimen)
Storage of medicine
Overmedication and polypharmacy

 SHOW ME THE EVIDENCE
Nationally registered EMS personnel were asked to describe their use of seat belts while in the front seat of the ambulance. "High" seat belt users had always worn their seat belts in the past year. "Low" seat belt users had never worn their seat belts in the past year. Those who worked in an EMS system with a seat belt policy were more likely to wear seat belts. Paramedics and EMS personnel who worked in rural areas were less likely to wear seat belts.

From Studneck JR, Ferketich A: Organizational policy and other factors associated with emergency medical technician seat belt use, *J Safety Res* 38(1):1-8, 2007.

Implementation and Prevention Strategies

In addition to the primary personal injury prevention strategies just listed, there are other key strategies. The paramedic needs to use these prevention strategies both for patient care considerations and to recognize the signs and symptoms of exposure to danger and the need for outside assistance. EMS personnel must document primary care and injury data as well. Finally, on-scene education is essential.

PATIENT CARE CONSIDERATIONS

The paramedic needs to identify signs and symptoms of suspected abuse and recognize potentially abusive situations. Such recognition helps to ensure the safety of the EMS crew and the patient (see Chapter 50). Preplanning for these events helps to identify outside resources that may play an important role in injury prevention. Examples include child protective services, abuse support groups, and rape/crisis intervention programs.

RECOGNITION OF DANGEROUS SITUATIONS

A priority for the paramedic is personal safety. Thus the EMS worker must stay alert for signs of dangerous situations. This includes recognizing general and specific environmental hazards. This will help the paramedic to assess a patient's need for preventive information. They will also help the paramedic assess a patient's need for direction. Examples include the following:

- Safety hazards in the home
- Inadequate housing conditions
- Inadequate food and clothing
- Absence of protective devices (e.g., smoke detectors)
- Hazardous materials (e.g., lead-based paint and dangerous chemicals)
- Communicable disease (and potential for transmission)
- Signs of abuse or neglect

 CRITICAL THINKING
Do you know a paramedic who was injured on the job? How did the injury occur? Can you identify any measures that could have prevented it?

RECOGNITION OF THE NEED FOR OUTSIDE RESOURCES

Most communities have outside resources that can be helpful to their citizens. The providers of these resources and services are usually eager to assist with the development of injury prevention strategies. Such programs may be sponsored by municipal, community, and religious organizations. Box 3-5 provides a sampling of outside resources and services that are available in most communities.

DOCUMENTATION

Taking precise notes of patient care and primary injury data is crucial. This documentation offers a record of the events of the encounter. The notes are also helpful to others who will be taking part in the patient's care (see Chapter 4). Gathering primary injury data can be useful in designing injury prevention strategies. For example, one might study a large number of patients who received head injuries while riding a horse. This study may help one to observe that helmet use was notably absent in all seriously injured patients. Primary injury data include the following:

- Scene conditions
- Mechanism of injury
- Use of protective devices
- Absence of protective devices
- Risks at the scene
- Other factors as noted by the EMS agency

On-Scene Education

- The EMS response to an injury or near-injury may provide for a **teachable moment.** This is a moment in which the patient and the family may be open to injury prevention tips and strategies. The paramedic can use

BOX 3-5 Sampling of Outside Resources and Services

Municipal
Animal control services
Child protective services
Fire service personnel
Law enforcement personnel
Social services

Community
Abuse support groups for spouses, children, and older adults
Alternative health care services (e.g., free clinics)
Alternative means of transportation
Alternative modes of education
Assistance for food, shelter, and clothing
Day care services
Disaster services (e.g., American Red Cross)
Immunization programs
Managed care organizations
Mental health resources and counseling
Rape or crisis intervention
Rehabilitation programs
Services for the disabled
Work-study programs

Religious
Family counseling
Grief support
Pastoral services
Support groups

this opportunity to assess hazards in an environment. The paramedic also can provide on-scene, one-on-one injury prevention education. The teachable moment involves a three-step process[7]:

1. *Observe the scene*: The first step is to look for contributing factors or hazards at the scene that may have caused or could cause an injury event. Examples include floor rugs without a nonslip backing and inoperable smoke detectors.

2. *Gather information:* The next step is to gather information from individuals and observers. What did they see? Why do they think the injury occurred? Has this been a common occurrence? Patients, family members or bystanders, and first responders may have valuable insight about a situation that caused an injury event.

3. *Make assessments:* The final step is to make decisions from the information that has been gathered. The first assessment is to decide whether the situation is critical or noncritical. If the situation is critical, the focus must be on patient care. If the situation is noncritical, a teachable moment exists. This is the opportunity to conduct one-on-one injury prevention counseling that may help to prevent another injury. Another assessment uses the information gathered through observation and history taking.

The paramedic uses this step to decide whether high-risk persons, high-risk behaviors, or a high-risk setting exists. Based on the assessment of risks, the paramedic can create a remedy.

Three common on-scene remedies are *discussion, demonstration,* and *documentation.* Discussion involves talking about proper behavior or action with the person at risk. Injury prevention discussions are a 30- to 60-second process. The message must be offered in a patient-appropriate manner. This manner depends on age, education, and socioeconomic status. The message should be conveyed in a nonjudgmental, "here are the facts" tone of voice. Although discussion may not always work, the paramedic should attempt it.

It may be possible to demonstrate proper behavior as an injury prevention strategy. For example, the paramedic could replace a safety cap on a pill bottle and explain the importance of doing so. The paramedic could put a fresh battery in a smoke detector. Or the paramedic could move a throw rug on a slippery floor to a safer location. These demonstrations on the scene draw attention to likely hazards and can help prevent future injury.

The paramedic should document what was seen, heard, and done at the scene. Written histories allow for follow-up by the receiving personnel. Other injury prevention groups also can use these histories in their data-gathering efforts. Lastly, histories make it easier for review in the EMS organization to improve injury prevention.

Other Injury Prevention Roles in Emergency Medical Services

In addition to the injury prevention strategies just listed, EMS personnel can play a major role in improving public health and safety. They can do this through support of legislative change and through involvement in primary prevention programs. Box 3-6 lists a sampling of these other injury prevention roles.

CRITICAL THINKING
At some point, you probably will visit an older adult family member or friend. Can you identify any potential hazards that exist in that person's home?

PARTICIPATION IN PREVENTION PROGRAMS

Prevention programs that are effective first call for a **community health assessment.** This assessment is needed before the intervention can take place. The assessment also is required before the education can begin. A systematic approach to a health assessment and prevention programs includes the following steps (Figure 3-3):

1. Gather information and identify the problem and population.
2. Identify prevention strategies.
3. Choose the best strategy.
4. Develop the plan.
5. Implement the plan.
6. Evaluate and revise the plan as needed.

Community Health Assessment

Paramedics may likely have limited time and resources to allot to prevention and wellness promotion. To maximize available time and resources, paramedics can perform a community health assessment to identify the target for community health education (Figure 3-4).

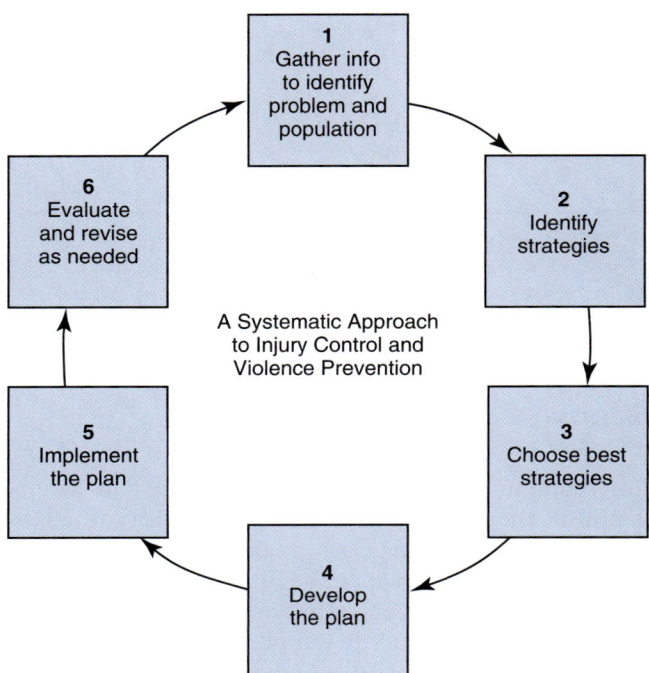

FIGURE 3-3 A systematic approach to health assessment and injury prevention programs.

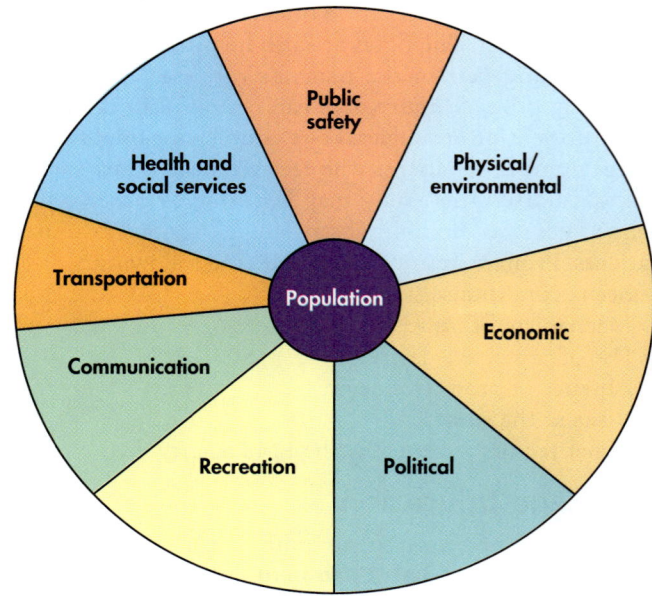

FIGURE 3-4 Community health assessment.

BOX 3-6 A Sampling of Injury Prevention Strategies*

Bicycle Safety
Bicycle helmet programs

Brain Injury
Brain injury prevention programs

Burns
Fire prevention programs
Smoke detector programs

Children
Babysitter training classes
Child abuse prevention programs
Child safety seat programs
Child safety programs
Drowning prevention programs
Emergency medical services for children (EMSC) programs
Parenting classes
Playground safety programs
Safe kids programs
Safe school programs
Swimming classes
Youth advocacy groups

Community Safety
Safe communities programs

Elderly
Programs to reduce elderly falls

Firearm Safety
Gun safety programs

Home Safety
Home assessment programs

Legal/Political
Being involved as an expert or advisor in the political process during the debate over laws dealing with the following:
- Child and adolescent safety laws
- Drunk driving laws
- Engineering regulations (building safety into a product)
- Gun legislation
- Helmet laws

Many Internet sites have information on ways to prevent medical illness. Some of this material can be passed on to the paramedic's patients. The information can be provided informally or through a program with handouts or public service activities. Sites include the following:
- Acquired immunodeficiency syndrome
- Cancer
- Cardiovascular health
- Childhood illnesses
- Influenza
- Healthful lifestyle
- Heat-related illness
- Medical conditions A to Z (Centers for Disease Control and Prevention site)
- Parenting
- Premenstrual syndrome
- Senior citizen illnesses
- Stroke

Most local physician offices have brochures that EMS personnel can hand out in cooperation with the local doctor.

Neurological Injury
Head injury prevention programs

Nutrition
Proper nutrition programs

Occupational Safety
Occupational illness and injury prevention programs

Pedestrian Safety
Pedestrian safety programs

Poisoning
National Poisoning Prevention Week

Posttraumatic Stress Syndrome
Programs for the community
Programs for EMS and other public safety personnel

Public Driving
Programs to prevent driving while intoxicated
Programs to prevent running of red lights
Programs to promote seat belt use

Rehabilitation
Rehabilitation support groups

Research
Universities throughout the United States research many illness and injury prevention strategies. These schools often welcome input from EMS personnel. This input may be in the form of volunteer work in data collection. Input also may be ride-alongs by the researchers. Input can even help in the actual writing of the research documents. Emergency medical services personnel should search for injury prevention centers, illness prevention centers, EMS research centers, and schools of public health within colleges and universities in their local area.

Smoking
Smoking cessation programs

Substance Abuse
Addiction programs
Substance abuse prevention programs
Substance abuse prevention programs for youth

Suicide
Suicide prevention programs

Trauma
National Trauma Awareness Week

Violence
Violence prevention programs
Violence survivor programs

This list is compiled from programs already in place. Some of these are national and some are local. The student should seek those programs that already exist in his or her area. If a program does not exist locally, chances are it exists somewhere in the United States. If interested, the student should search the Internet or other sources and find a comparable guide for starting a local program.

*This box should encourage the paramedic student to search for prevention programs that are of personal interest because the work likely will be voluntary and without pay.

This assessment often is a large undertaking and may be conducted more effectively through a group effort with other health agencies to evaluate the following:

- Population demographics
- Morbidity statistics
- Mortality statistics
- Crime and fire information
- Community resource allocation
- Hospital data (e.g., emergency department visits and length of stay)
- Senior citizen needs
- Education standards
- Recreational facilities
- Environmental conditions
- Other factors

> **NOTE**
>
> *Morbidity statistics* refers to the disease rate of a population or geographic region. *Mortality statistics* refer to the number of deaths per unit of population in a specific region or for a specific age group, disease, or other classification. This number is usually expressed as deaths per 1000, 10,000, or 100,000 (see Chapter 8).

This "landscape" view of the health of a community can yield data that are valuable, and sometimes unexpected, about the target population. The assessment also can identify factors that relate or contribute to certain health risks. After the assessment the paramedic should choose the target for health education carefully and then use a fitting intervention. Ideally, the paramedic should compare the data from the assessment with those of another population (Box 3-7). This population should have similar demographics. For example, a city of similar size within the state would be a good choice.

Community Health Intervention

After identifying a health risk, the paramedic must implement a plan that attempts to reduce or eradicate the risk. This plan also should attempt to help improve the health of the community. The three levels of health prevention activities are *primary, secondary,* and *tertiary.* Primary prevention prevents problems and disease development before they occur. Examples include seat belt education, laws requiring wearing of helmets while bicycling, and vaccination programs. Secondary prevention activities find issues and promote early intervention. They also prevent complications and/or progression of disease. For example, health screenings to detect hypertension is a secondary prevention activity. Tertiary prevention activities correct and prevent further deterioration of a disease or problem. An example of this is providing EMS services in a community. The three types of prevention activities often overlap. Box 3-8 provides examples of each activity.[8]

BOX 3-7 Sampling of Community Health Information Sources

American Heart Association
American Red Cross
Births and deaths (including cause)
Call types and response times
Census data (public library, Internet)
Centers for Disease Control and Prevention
Chamber of Commerce
Clustering of illnesses and injuries
Communication
Crime rate statistics
Disaster planning
Distribution of age, sex, race, ethnicity
Distribution of grant monies
Education and literacy rates
Emergency coordinating council
Emergency medical services
Employment statistics
Environmental hazards (sanitation, air quality)
Federal Emergency Management Agency (FEMA)
Federal government
Fire service
Fire-related injuries and fatalities
Form of government
Geographic distribution
Health departments (city, county, state, Internet)
Health services and school lunch programs
Hospitals
Housing and tax information
Industry and economic figures
Infectious disease statistics
Law enforcement
Local government
Location and frequency of fires
National Safety Council
Newspapers, radio, and television stations
Parks and recreation
Population demographics
Religious organizations
Response times
School board
Socioeconomic status
State trauma registry statistics

Community Health Education

A good injury prevention program must serve the entire target population in a community. This also is the mark of a successful program. The community must try to improve the education and training for EMS and other public service agencies. In that way special groups can be included in the prevention program. Examples include training emergency personnel to communicate effectively with the following:

- Various ethnic, cultural, and religious groups
- Non–English-speaking populations
- Those with learning disabilities
- Those who are physically challenged

DID YOU KNOW?
Immunization Programs

Paramedics are trained to administer medications and can play a vital role in immunization programs in a community. Numerous studies have demonstrated the feasibility of EMS agencies in administering vaccines. The programs followed CDC guidelines[9] and were performed under strict medical oversight. Citizens were recruited through public service campaigns to visit EMS stations, places of worship, retail establishments, and other public places to receive the vaccine. It was found that paramedics can safely provide immunizations and can sometimes reach populations who otherwise would not have received the medication.[10]

In the event of a pandemic disease outbreak or other disease emergency requiring large-scale vaccination, it is likely that paramedics will provide vaccines and antiviral drugs at emergency dispensing sites (EDSs) in the community.[11,12] (See Chapter 28 and Chapter 58 for more discussion.)

CRITICAL THINKING

What method of health education is most likely to change your personal behaviors? Would that same method be equally effective for a 5-year-old or a 70-year-old person?

The paramedic must consider the reading level and age of the target population. Recognizing these considerations helps the paramedic prepare educational materials and make the materials more effective. Before starting any type of large-scale educational program, the paramedic should test the program on a target audience. This test will evaluate the appeal of the materials and ensure understanding of the message. EMS personnel can provide community health education to promote wellness and injury prevention in numerous ways, including the following:

BOX 3-8 Examples of Prevention Activities

Primary Prevention Activities
Influenza/pneumococcal immunization
Smoking cessation
Preventive dental care
Car seat distribution and installation

Secondary Prevention Activities
General health screenings
Colonoscopy
Mammography
Blood pressure screenings

Tertiary Prevention Activities
Lowering cholesterol after myocardial infarction (MI)
Treating hypertension after stroke
Providing exams for eye and foot problems in diabetic patients

Verbal
- Lectures
- Informal discussions
- Informal teaching on an EMS call
- Podcasts
- Radio programs

Written/static visual
- Bulletin boards, exhibits
- Flyers, pamphlets, posters
- Models
- Slides, photographs

Dynamic visual
- Videotapes
- Television
- Internet resources (blogs, websites)

SUMMARY

- Emergency medical services personnel are members of the community health care system. They can be an important resource in injury prevention.
- Unintentional injuries are the fifth leading cause of death. This cause is exceeded only by heart disease, cancer, stroke, and chronic obstructive pulmonary disease.
- The United States has more than 800,000 EMS personnel. This valuable human resource plays a major role in public education. This component of health promotion seems only fitting.
- It is crucial that paramedics play an active role in the health of a community. Thus the community must protect the EMS worker from injury. The community also needs to provide education to paramedics. The community should supply support and promote the collection and use of injury data as well. In addition, the community must obtain resources for primary injury prevention activities. Lastly, the community needs to empower paramedics to conduct primary injury prevention.
- Paramedics must have a basic knowledge of personal injury prevention. They also should know about maladies and injuries common to various age groups and associated with different recreational activities, workplaces, and other facilities in the community.
- The paramedic needs to note the signs and symptoms of abuse and abusive situations. In addition, the paramedic should notice exposure to danger.

Continued

- Paramedics should identify and use outside community resources. Plus they should document primary injury data properly. Moreover, they should identify and properly use the teachable moment.
- The paramedic must maximize time and resources. Thus the paramedic should identify targets for community health education. The paramedic can do this by performing a community health assessment.
- To identify community education goals, the paramedic must understand several factors: (1) illness or injury is related to the extent or exposure to an agent; (2) illness or injury also is related to the strength of the agent; (3) illness or injury is linked to the susceptibility of the individual (host); and (4) illness or injury is related to the biological, social, and physical environment.
- Primary injury prevention involves preventing an injury from occurring. Secondary and tertiary prevention help to prevent further problems from an event that has already occurred.
- A good injury prevention program must serve the whole target population in a community. An effective program also takes into account reading level and age. These aspects are the mark of a successful program. The paramedic can provide community health education in diverse ways, including verbal, written/static material, and dynamic visual presentations.

REFERENCES

1. National Safety Council: *Injury facts*, Itasca, Ill, 2010, The Council.
2. Adams PF, Day AN, Vickerie JL: *Summary health statistics for the US population: National Health Interview Survey, 2005. Vital and health statistics, Series 10 (No. 233)*, Hyattsville, Md, 2007, National Center of Health Statistics.
3. Bureau of Labor Statistics, U.S. Department of Labor: Occupational outlook handbook, 2008-09 Edition, emergency medical technicians and paramedics, www.bls.gov/oco/ocos101.htm, accessed 7-15-10.
4. National Highway Traffic Safety Administration: *Emergency medical services: agenda for the future*, Washington, DC, 1996, The Administration.
5. Pollock D: *Trauma registries and public health surveillance of injuries*, www.cdc.gov/nchs/data/ice/ice95v1/C11.pdf, accessed 2-4-09.
6. Binder S, Corrigan JD, Langlois JA: The public health approach to traumatic brain injury: an overview of CDC's research and programs, *J Head Trauma Rehabil* 20(3):189-195, 2005.
7. Yancey AH II, Martinez R, Kellermann AL: Injury prevention and emergency medical services: *The "Accidents Aren't" program*, Atlanta, Ga, 2001, Emory University.
8. Breslow E, Cengage G, editors: *Disease prevention, encyclopedia of public health*, 2002, www.enotes.com/public-health-encyclopedia/disease-prevention, accessed 2-6-09.
9. Centers for Disease Control and Prevention: *Vaccine information statements (VISs)*, www.cdc.gov/vaccines/pubs/vis/default.htm, accessed 2-24-09.
10. Mosesso VN Jr, Packer CR, McMahon J, et al: *Influenza immunizations provided by EMS agencies: the MEDICVAX project*, *Prehosp Emerg Care* 7(1):74-78, 2003.
11. Massachusetts Department of Public Health: *Emergency dispensing site management and operations, to the template for local infectious disease emergency planning and response*, www.mass.gov/dph/topics/bioterrorism/idep.doc, accessed 7-31-10.
12. U.S. Department of Transportation: *EMS pandemic influenza guidelines for statewide adoption*, May 2007, www.nhtsa.gov/people/injury/ems/PandemicInfluenzaGuidelines/Task61136Web/PDFs/Task%206.1.13.6Lo.pdf, accessed 7-31-10.

SUGGESTED READINGS

American Academy of Pediatrics, Committee on Injury and Poison Prevention: *Injury prevention and control for children and youth*, ed 3, Elk Grove Village, Ill, 1997, The Academy.

Eisenberg M, Garson G: *Closing the loop: SPHERE brings EMS & public health together*, *JEMS* 31(6):56-59, 2006.

Garrison HG, Foltin GL, Becker LR, et al: The role of emergency medical services in primary injury prevention, *Ann Emerg Med* 30:80-91, July 1997.

Institute of Medicine, Division of Health Promotion and Disease Prevention, Committee on Injury Prevention and Control: *Reducing the burden of injury*, Washington, DC, 1999, National Academy Press.

Kinnane JM, Garrison HG, Coben JH, et al: Injury prevention: is there a role for out-of-hospital emergency medical services? *Acad Emerg Med* 4:306-312, 1997.

Russo T: Pandemic planning, *EMS* 35(10):51-61, 2006.

Stanhope M: *Public health nursing: population-centered health care in the community*, ed 7, St Louis, 2007, Mosby.

Williams K, White L, Plorde M, et al: Empowering the patient, *JEMS* 33(12):43-49, 2008.

OBJECTIVES

Upon completion of this chapter, the paramedic student will be able to:

1. Identify the purpose of the patient care report.
2. Describe the uses of the patient care report.
3. Outline the components of an accurate, thorough patient care report.
4. Describe the elements of a properly written emergency medical services (EMS) document.
5. Describe an effective system for documenting the narrative section of a prehospital patient care report.
6. Identify important differences in the documentation of special situations.
7. Describe the appropriate method for revising or correcting the patient care report.
8. Recognize consequences that may result from inappropriate documentation.

KEY TERMS

military time A precise method of expressing time that is used by the armed forces and is based on a 24-hour clock.

narrative The portion of the patient care report that presents a chronological description of the call.

objective information Information based on observable facts, such as clinical signs or symptoms.

patient care report A document used in the prehospital setting to record all patient care activities and circumstances related to an emergency response.

pertinent negative findings Findings that warrant no medical care or intervention but that provide evidence of the thoroughness of the patient examination and the history of the event.

pertinent oral statements Statements made by the patient and other individuals at the scene.

pertinent positive findings Signs or symptoms that help substantiate the patient's condition.

subjective information Information based on opinions expressed by patients or others.

The **patient care report** is used to document the essential elements of patient assessment, care, and transport. It is a legal document, and next to providing good patient care, it is the paramedic's best protection from liability action.

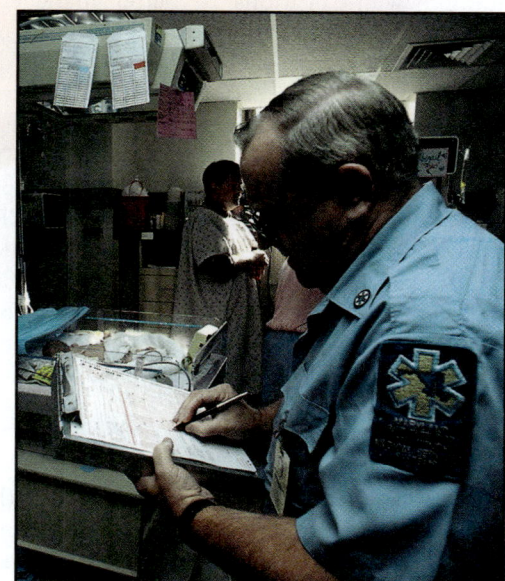

(Courtesy Maryland Institute for Emergency Medical Services Systems and Acadian Ambulance Service, Baltimore.)

IMPORTANCE OF DOCUMENTATION

Thorough written documentation is important for many reasons (Box 4-1). It provides a tangible and legal record of an incident. It often is used by physicians, nurses, and others involved in the patient's care. Hospital staff members read the patient care report (PCR) to understand the patient's initial condition and the type of care given in the field. The EMS agency and medical direction may use the PCR to monitor care in the field, evaluate an individual paramedic's performance, and conduct review conferences and other educational forums. The four main reasons for charting patient care[2] are to:

- Demonstrate the continuity of the patient care provided
- Create a legal record of the patient care provided
- Assist in financial reimbursement and cost recovery for patient care services and equipment and supplies
- Assist in quality improvement studies and EMS research

> **NOTE**
> The requirements for retaining medical records vary throughout the United States. Most medical records (including patient care reports) are maintained for at least 10 years.[1] These records are kept as a safety measure in case legal action involving a statute of limitations arises. *Thorough documentation is essential. It leads to accurate recall if litigation occurs.*

Data collection and recordkeeping are important for identifying quality improvement issues (see Chapter 1). Such issues that may be identified through the PCR, resulting in policy changes to improve patient care, include:

- Minimizing the time spent at the scene with critical trauma patients
- Adding new medications to better manage some medical emergencies
- Changing the placement of emergency vehicles during peak response times in certain demographic areas

The PCR also documents any unique scene situations that may have affected patient care. For example, traffic may have caused a long response time. A trapped patient may have required prolonged extrication. The PCR also helps track certain patient care skills of the paramedic (e.g., insertion of intravenous lines, intubation, and defibrillation). The EMS agency's training division may require tracking of these skills. In some states, documentation of advanced life support (ALS) skills may be required for relicensure or recertification.

GENERAL CONSIDERATIONS

The PCR should be legible and carefully detailed (Figure 4-1). It is a legal document and part of the patient's medical record. Therefore, slang terms and medical abbreviations that are not universally accepted should not be used. Common medical abbreviations and symbols used in EMS documentation are presented in Chapter 9.

The report should include all dates and response times, noted in **military time** (Box 4-2). In addition, any difficulties encountered en route or during patient treatment, extrication, or transport should be described. The report also should include observations at the scene, any previous medical care provided (and by whom), and the time of patient extrication, if appropriate (Box 4-3). The times of all significant occurrences and interventions are useful to the receiving physician and should be recorded. In particular, the PCR provides a legal and accurate recording of the following incident times:

- Time of the call
- Time of dispatch
- Time of arrival at the scene
- Time at patient's side
- Time of vital signs assessments

Incident Number

Grid & Page

| 1 | 8 | 3 | 0 | 3 | 2 |

Date of Run · Ambulance Service # · Vehicle License #

St. Charles County Ambulance District   Medic
Ambulance Service Name

LOCATION OF PICKUP
☐ Same as patient address

Name of Hospital, Nursing Home, Clinic, or Street, Route, Highway #

City · County

State · Zip · EMD Code · Condition Code

Explain CC

PATIENT DESTINATION

Name of Hospital, Nursing Home, Clinic, Ambulance Service, Home, etc.

City · State

Referring/Personal Physician _____

Receiving Physician _____

Driver _____ Lic #

Attendant #1 _____ Lic #

Attendant #2 _____ Lic #

Person Receiving Patient _____

Medical Control Name/Hospital _____

PATIENT INFORMATION
Date of Birth · Age in Years
Month · Day · Century · Year

Last Name · First Name · M.I.

Street, Route, etc. · Home phone

City · State · Zip

Patient's SS # · Employer

Guarantor's/Spouse's/Guardian's name (if different from patient) · Relationship

Guarantor's/Spouse's/Guardian's address · Guarantor's/Spouse's/Guardian's phone

City · State · Zip

Guarantor's/Spouse's/Guardian's SS # · Employer

Primary Insurance Company · Group · Policy Number

Primary Insurance Address

Secondary Insurance Company · Group · Policy Number

Secondary Insurance Address

Medicare # · State

Medicaid # · State

☐ Hospice
☐ Worker's Comp
☐ VA
☐ Private Pay

RACE:
☐ 1 Black
☐ 2 White
☐ 3 Hispanic
☐ 4 Other

SEX:
☐ 1 Male
☐ 2 Female

TYPE OF RUN
TO SCENE ☐ Lights/Siren
1 Emergency response required
2 Non-emergency response (routine)
FROM SCENE ☐ Lights/Siren
01 Life threatening, transported
02 Urgent, transported
03 Routine, transported
04 Treated, transferred care _____
05 Treated, transported by private vehicle
06 Treated and released ☐ Care sheet
07 No treatment required
08 Patient refused care and/or transport
09 Dead at scene, not transported
10 Cancelled / disregard
11 No patient found
12 Crank call/Unfounded
13 Stand-by
14 Citizen Assist

TREATMENT AUTHORIZATION
1 On-line A radio B telephone
2 On-scene ☐ Release
3 Protocol # _____
4 Written orders (patient specific)
5 Orders refused
6 Unknown
7 Not Applicable

PRIOR CARE BY
0 Ambulance Service 1 ALS
1 Police 2 BLS
2 Fire _____
3 Medical Facility
4 Bystander
5 Other _____
6 Family
7 Not Applicable

TIMES
Call Received
Unit Dispatched
Unit En Route
1st Unit Arrive Location/Staged
Ambulance Arrive Location
Arrive Patient
Depart Location
Arrive Destination
Unit Available
Depart Destination

ODOMETER
At Scene
At Destination

PLACE OF INCIDENT
0 Home
1 Farm
2 Mine/Quarry
3 Industrial Place
4 Recreation or Sport
5 Street or Highway
6 Public Building
7 Residential Institution (Hospital)
8 Other
9 Unspecified

PROTECTIVE EQUIPMENT
1 None
2 Unknown
3 Seat Belt
4 Child Seat
5 Air Bag
6 Belt & Bag
7 Helmet
8 Other
9 Not Applicable

DESTINATION DETERMINATION
01 Closest Facility (none below)
02 Patient/Family choice
03 Patient physician choice
04 Managed care
05 Law enforcement choice
06 Protocol
07 Specialty resource center
08 On-line medical direction
09 Diversion _____ (name hospital diverted from)
10 Other
11 Unknown
12 Not applicable

FACTORS AFFECTING EMS
01 Adverse weather
02 Adverse road conditions
03 Traffic problems
04 Unsafe scene
05 Language barrier
06 Extrication >20 minutes
07 Hazardous materials
08 Crowd control
09 Med. Control failure
10 Other _____
11 Not applicable

TRAUMA ASSESSMENT
Circle boxes that apply

	Amputation	Burn	Crush	Dislocation/FX	Blunt	Gunshot	Laceration	Puncture/Stab	Pain	Soft Tissue
Head	00	10	20	30	40	50	60	70	80	90
Face/Eye/Ear	01	11	21	31	41	51	61	71	81	91
Neck	02	12	22	32	42	52	62	72	82	92
Spine	03	13	23	33	43	53	63	73	83	93
Thorax	04	14	24	34	44	54	64	74	84	94
Abdomen/Pelvic Contents	05	15	25	35	45	55	65	75	85	95
Upper Arm/Shoulder	06	16	26	36	46	56	66	76	86	96
Lower Arm/Hand/Elbow	07	17	27	37	47	57	67	77	87	97
Upper Leg/Hip	08	18	28	38	48	58	68	78	88	98
Lower Leg/Foot/Knee	09	19	29	39	49	59	69	79	89	99

Cause of Injury

ILLNESS ASSESSMENT
01 Abdominal pain/problems
02 Airway obstruction
03 Allergic reaction
04 Altered level consciousness
05 Behavioral/psychiatric
06 Cardiac arrest
07 Cardiac rhythm disturbance
08 Chest pain/discomfort
09 Diabetic symptoms
10 Hyperthermia
11 Hypothermia
12 Hypovolemia/shock
13 Inhalation injury (toxic gas)
14 Poisoning/drug ingestion
15 Pregnancy/O.B. delivery
16 Respiratory arrest
17 Respiratory distress
18 Seizure
19 Smoke inhalation
20 Stroke/CVA
21 Syncope/fainting
22 Vaginal hemorrhage
23 Other _____
24 Unknown
25 Not applicable (trauma)

REVISED TRAUMA SCORE COMPONENTS (R.T.S.)
Systolic BP
Respiratory Rate
Glasgow Coma Score
Eye Opening **G**
Best Verbal Response **C**
Best Motor Response **S**
Total R.T.S.

PEDIATRIC TRAUMA SCORE COMPONENTS (P.T.S.)
Weight
Airway
Systolic Blood Pressure
Central Nervous System
Wounds
Fractures
TOTAL P.T.S.

☐ Patient has a DNR
☐ Patient has an Advanced Directive

PERSONAL EFFECTS (describe below)
☐ Clothing ☐ Meds ☐ Glasses ☐ Dentures
☐ Patient stated none

☐ All items left with ☐ staff / ☐ patient / ☐ family / ☐ friend at receiving facility

PCR LF-10 no highlight.doc

Revision date: 7/28/2006

FIGURE 4-1 Example of a patient care report. (Courtesy St. Charles County Ambulance District, St. Charles, Mo.)

INITIAL ASSESSMENT

Airway: [1] Clear [2] Noisy [3] Obstructed [4] OPA/NPA [5] EOA [6] ETT [7] C-Spine precautions Comments

Breathing: [1] Normal [2] Fast [3] Slow [4] Absent [5] Labored [6] Shallow [7] BVM [8] Other O₂ _____ lpm [9] cannula [10] NRB

Circulation Assessed at: [1] Radial [2] Carotid [3] Brachial [4] Femoral [5] Pedal [6] Apical Comments

Pulse: [1] Normal [2] Strong [3] Weak [4] Absent [5] Regular [6] Irregular [7] CPR Comments

Skin: [1] Pink [2] Flushed [3] Pale [4] Ashen [5] Cyanotic [6] Warm [7] Cool [8] Hot [9] Cold [10] Dry [11] Moist [12] Wet

Neuro: [1] Alert [A] Person [B] Place [C] Time [2] Verbal [3] Pain [4] Unresponsive Comments

Time	BP	Pulse	Resp.	SaO₂	Temp	Time	EMTP	Intervention/ Medication	Route	Dosage	Time	EMTP	Intervention/ Medication	Route	Dosage

EKG [1] N/A [2] 3/4 Lead [3] 12 Lead [4] Pads [5] CPFS (see below) [6] 12- Lead Faxed ☐ ALS Assessment Weight/Kg

Onset Date: Time:

PPE [1] Gown [2] Gloves [5] Turnout coat [6] Bunker pants [7] Helmet [3] Mask [4] Eye protection [8] Leather gloves [9] Other _____

Chief Complaint: **Pt Treated For:**

HEENT	☐ PERL ☐ Pink mucosa ☐ Not examined ☐ See narrative
Neck	☐ No JVD ☐ Trachea Midline ☐ Not examined ☐ See narrative
Chest	☐ CEBBS ☐ ERF ☐ Not examined ☐ See narrative
Abdomen	☐ Soft, non-tender ☐ Not examined ☐ See narrative
Pelvis	☐ Intact to press ☐ Not examined ☐ See narrative
Extremity	☐ No pedal edema ☐ Nail beds pink ☐ Not examined ☐ See narrative
Back	☐ No deformity ☐ No pain upon palp ☐ Not examined ☐ See narrative
Gen/Rec	☐ No incontinence ☐ No bleeding ☐ Not examined ☐ See narrative
Skin	☐ Normal color, warm, dry ☐ Not examined ☐ See narrative
Neuro	☐ MAE ☐ SAE ☐ Not examined ☐ See narrative
Forms	☐ CPFS ☐ ETTFS
Trauma	☐ Class I ☐ Class II ☐ Class III

Hx:

Rx Meds: ☐ See attached list ☐ List given to receiving staff – attach list if given to receiving staff

Narcotic authorization Signature: **Allergies:** _____ ☐ NKDA

AID/DIAGNOSTIC/TREATMENT Supervisor Name: _____

D	A1	A2	S		D	A1	A2	S		D	A1	A2	S		D	A1	A2	S	
01	01	01	01	Bag mask/Demand valve	17	17	17	17	Drug administered: Updraft	33	33	33	33	Glucose test _____ mg/dl	49	49	49	49	Pulse oximetry
02	02	02	02	Bleeding controlled	18	18	18	18	Drug administered: P.O.	34	34	34	34	Hemodynamic monitor	50	50	50	50	Restraints
03	03	03	03	Blood specimen drawn	19	19	19	19	Drug administered: Rectal	35	35	35	35	I.V. administered # _____	51	51	51	51	Spinal immobilization: LBB
04	04	04	04	C.P.R.	20	20	20	20	Drug administered: Sub-L	36	36	36	36	I.V. failed # _____	52	52	52	52	Spinal Immobilization: KED
05	05	05	05	Cardiac pacing # _____ mA	21	21	21	21	Oral tracheal tube	37	37	37	37	I.V. maintained	53	53	53	53	Spinal immobilization: PEDS
06	06	06	06	Cardioversion	22	22	22	22	Oral tracheal tube failed	38	38	38	38	Infusion pump	54	54	54	54	Suction airway
07	07	07	07	Cricothyrotomy	23	23	23	23	Nasal tracheal tube	39	39	39	39	Intraosseous infusion # _____	55	55	55	55	Thoracentesis
08	08	08	08	Cricothyrotomy failed	24	24	24	24	Nasotracheal tube failed	40	40	40	40	Intraosseous infusion failed	56	56	56	56	Stretcher
09	09	09	09	Defibrillation	25	25	25	25	Obturator airway	41	41	41	41	Isolette _____ FiO₂	57	57	57	57	Other _____
10	10	10	10	Defibrillation by AED	26	26	26	26	Obturator airway failed	42	42	42	42	Mechanical ventilator	58	58	58	58	V/S
11	11	11	11	Doppler	27	27	27	27	EKG monitor	43	43	43	43	N.G. tube	59	59	59	59	Physical Exam
12	12	12	12	Drug administered: IV push	28	28	28	28	End Tidal CO₂	44	44	44	44	N.G. tube failed					
13	13	13	13	Drug administered: IV drip	29	29	29	29	Extremity splint: traction	45	45	45	45	O.B. delivery					
14	14	14	14	Drug administered: IM	30	30	30	30	Extrication _ _ _ _	46	46	46	46	Oxygen by cannula _____ lpm					
15	15	15	15	Drug administered: Sub-Q	31	31	31	31	Rapid Extrication _ _ _ _	47	47	47	47	Oxygen by mask _____ lpm					
16	16	16	16	Drug administered: ETT	32	32	32	32	Extremity splint: fixation	48	48	48	48	P.C.P.D. applied					

FIGURE 4-1, cont'd

- Time (or times) of medication administration and certain medical procedures as defined by local protocol
- Time of departure from the scene
- Time of arrival at the medical facility (when a patient is transported)
- Time back in service

NOTE

The National EMS Information System (NEMSIS) has developed an EMS Dataset Schema.[3] This is a comprehensive list of all potential elements of information that would be collected about an emergency incident. It includes information that would be considered important from the perspectives of an EMS system, EMS personnel, and an EMS patient. The data elements in the EMS dataset provide documentation of the system performance and clinical care. The purpose of the Dataset Schema is to create a national EMS database that contains information from local and state EMS agencies across the nation. To date, 48 states and three territory members have agreed to participate and to support the EMS data initiatives set by NEMSIS.

SHOW ME THE EVIDENCE

In one study, researchers compared the times used to record medical information in five hospitals and three EMS systems in Indianapolis, Indiana. They compared the times of clocks in these systems to the Coordinated Universal Time (UTC) kept by an atomic clock in Boulder, Colorado. The 152 clocks included in the study showed an average difference from UTC of 1 minute and 45 seconds. The differences ranged from 12 minutes and 34 seconds slow to 7 minutes and 7 seconds fast. The researchers concluded that the time sources studied varied considerably in their ability to keep accurate time.

Cordell WH, Olinger ML, Kozak PA, Nyhuis AW: Does anybody really know what time it is? Does anybody really care? *Ann Emerg Med* 23:1032-1036, 1994.

When testimony must be given years after an incident, the PCR may be the only means by which a paramedic can recall accurately the events of an emergency call. Paramedics must include as much detail as possible in the PCR, because this level of detail is useful both for present and for future use (see Chapter 6).

CRITICAL THINKING

Documentation of specific times on the PCR is important. How can this information be useful?

THE NARRATIVE

The **narrative** section of the PCR provides a chronological account of the call. Paramedics should write the narrative concisely and clearly, using simple words. They should not use uncommon abbreviations or unnecessary terms or include duplicate information. A standard format

established by medical direction can help ensure completeness. Such a format also aids quality improvement reviews. Components of the narrative of the PCR include the following:

- Initial contact
- All patient care activities (including medications and treatments; also, care provided by others at the scene)
- Initial assessment and vital signs
- Chief complaint
- Pertinent significant medical history
- Clock time of hospital contact
- Time of physician's orders and advice (name of physician)
- Pertinent positive and negative findings
- Pertinent oral statements
- Changes in the patient's status
- Patient's response to treatment
- Vital sign reassessment
- Electrocardiogram (ECG) interpretation
- Diagnostic readings (e.g., capnography, pulse oximetry, serum glucose)
- Use of support services
- Time of delivery to health care facility and patient's condition
- Name of receiving health care worker
- Signature of paramedic

NOTE

Paramedics should never use documentation to creatively reconstruct patient care. If the paramedic did not document the care, it was not done. Conversely, if the care was not done, the paramedic should not document it.

SHOW ME THE EVIDENCE

Salt Lake City researchers compared PCRs produced after implementation of a quality improvement (QI) program that provided feedback on documentation with documentation done before the program was initiated. They found that with the QI program, documentation in the PCRs improved in 13 of the 19 parameters evaluated. These researchers concluded that a QI program can improve documentation in an EMS system.

Joyce SM, Dutkowski KL, Hynes T: Efficacy of an EMS quality improvement program in improving documentation and performance, *Prehosp Emerg Care* 1:140-144, 1997.

Pertinent findings may be classified as positive or negative. Both types should be documented in the PCR, because both can help determine the course of treatment. **Pertinent positive findings** are signs or symptoms that help substantiate the patient's condition. Examples of positive findings include difficulty breathing, numbness or paralysis, and altered mental status. **Pertinent negative findings** are findings that warrant no medical care or intervention but that show the thoroughness of the paramedic's examination of the patient and the history of the event. Examples of negative findings include the absence of diminished breath sounds, the absence of skin rashes, and the absence of abdominal tenderness. **Pertinent oral statements** are those made by the patient and other individuals on the scene. These statements should also be recorded. Statements that may have an impact on patient care or resolution of the situation include the following:

- Mechanism of injury
- Patient's behavior
- Aid given before arrival of EMS
- Safety-related information (including disposition of weapons)
- Information of interest to crime scene investigators
- Disposition of valuable personal property (e.g., jewelry and wallets)

The paramedic should enclose in quotation marks any statements made directly by patients or others that relate to possible criminal activity. In addition, an admission of suicidal intention should be recorded in quotes.

Failed skills should be documented in the PCR, such as unsuccessful attempts to start an intravenous line or to perform endotracheal intubation. The narrative also should include the use of support services and mutual aid assistance (e.g., helicopter, coroner, rescue or extrication team). As the last step, the paramedic should sign the PCR.

CRITICAL THINKING
Why should you note the previous care given by bystanders in your report?

The PCR should list everyone who took part in the patient's care before delivery to the emergency department (ED). Because a copy of the report is placed in the patient's hospital medical record, paramedics may need to leave a finished copy at the receiving hospital. This means that the report must be completed in a timely fashion at the receiving hospital so that the EMS crew can be available for another call. If possible, the report should be left with the patient at the hospital.

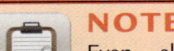

NOTE
Even electronic reports that allow automatic selections require a narrative. Details such as the patient's appearance, the individual's home or vehicle, the mechanism of injury, and specific statements made by the patient often are not included in an electronic report if a narrative is not written.

ELEMENTS OF A PROPERLY WRITTEN EMS DOCUMENT

A properly written EMS document is accurate and complete, legible, timely, unaltered, and free of nonprofessional or extraneous information.

1. *Accurate and complete.* All relevant information must be provided in the narrative and check-box sections of the report; this ensures accuracy. Completion of all areas of the report (even a section that was unused) is the sign of a precise, full document. The paramedic should make sure medical terms, abbreviations, and acronyms are used properly and spelled correctly.
2. *Legible.* All writing, especially in the narrative, must be easily read by others. Check-box markings should be clear and consistent from the top page of the report to all underlying pages.
3. *Timely.* Ideally, the documentation is completed immediately after the paramedic completes the patient care. Delays in recording can result in serious omissions, which may be interpreted as negligent patient care.
4. *Unaltered.* If an error is made during documentation, the paramedic should draw a single line through the error and then date and initial the error (Figure 4-2). Any changes to a completed report should be accompanied by a proper "revision/correction" supplement with the date and time of revision.
5. *Free of nonprofessional and extraneous information.* The PCR must be free of jargon, slang, personal bias, libelous or slanderous remarks, and irrelevant opinions or impressions.

NOTE
An EMS report should be considered confidential. Paramedics must comply with all patient privacy provisions as outlined by the policies of their agency and by the Health Insurance Portability and Accountability Act (HIPAA) (see Chapter 6).

These same five principles of documentation apply to computer-generated PCRs (Figure 4-3) and other computer-generated forms. Other, related documentation (e.g., ECG

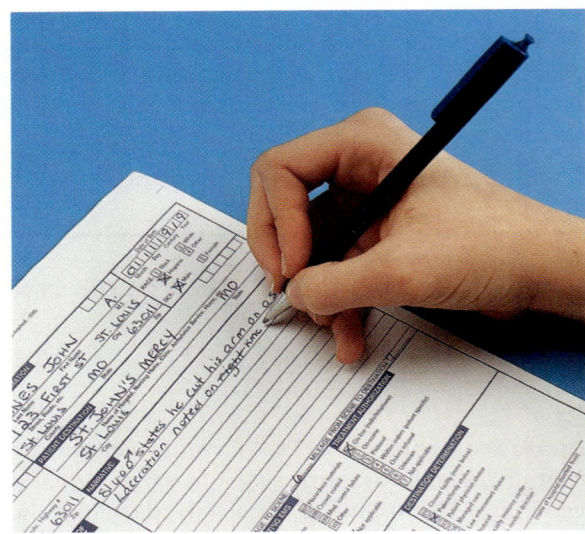

FIGURE 4-2 Correction of a patient care report.

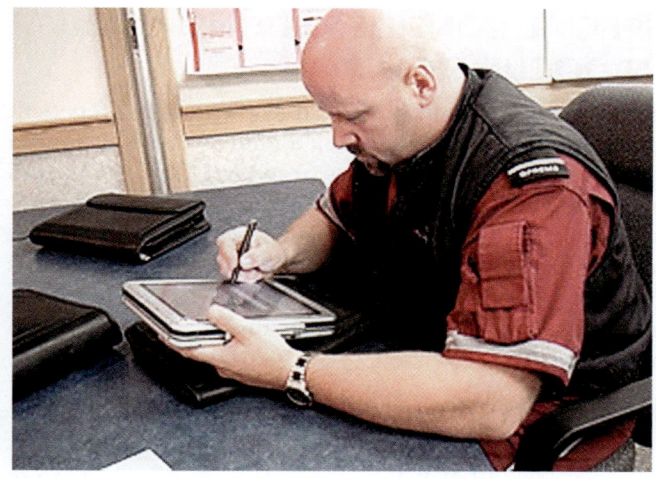

FIGURE 4-3 Paramedic completing an electronic patient care report. (Courtesy Grande Prairie Regional EMS, Alberta, Canada.)

or capnography tracings, photographs, insurance information) should be properly labeled and attached, scanned, or uploaded with the report.

SYSTEMS OF NARRATIVE WRITING

As with all other aspects of emergency care, paramedics should develop a systematic approach to writing the PCR narrative. Many approaches can be used for this purpose. However, the best practice is to adopt only *one* approach and to use it consistently; this helps prevent omissions in report writing. Regardless of the system used, the paramedic must make sure that **objective information,** rather than **subjective information,** is the focus of the report.

> **NOTE**
>
> *Objective information* is supported by facts and direct observation (e.g., an obvious fracture). *Subjective information* cannot be supported by facts (e.g., the patient appears depressed). When including subjective information in the narrative, the paramedic should enter the patient's own words, enclosed within quotation marks. Some subjective observations should be documented carefully and reported to medical direction, such as behavior by a child that may indicate physical or sexual abuse in the home.

Formats that have been established to organize the narrative include the SAMPLE history; the SOAP format; the CHART format; and the CHEATED charting method.

- The elements of the *SAMPLE history* are signs and symptoms *(S)*, allergies *(A)*, medications *(M)*, past medical history *(P)*, last meal or oral intake *(L)*, and events before the emergency *(E)*. (The patient history is presented in detail in Chapter 18.)
- The *SOAP format* can be used to organize a patient report for most patient care encounters. The elements of this format are:

- Subjective data: All of the patient's symptoms, including the chief complaint, associated symptoms, history, current medications, and allergies, in addition to information provided by the patient, bystanders, and family.
- Objective data: Pertinent physical examination information, including vital signs, level of consciousness, physical examination findings, ECG data, pulse oximetry readings, and blood glucose determinations.
- Assessment data: The paramedic's clinical impression of the patient based on subjective and objective data.
- Plan of patient management: Treatment that has been provided and any requests for additional treatment.
- The *CHART format* is an alternative to the SAMPLE and SOAP methods. It includes the following elements:
  - Chief complaint: The patient's primary complaint.
  - History: The history of the current illness; any significant medical history; the patient's current health status; and a review of systems.
  - Assessment: The paramedic's general impression; vital signs; physical examination findings; diagnostic tests; and field diagnosis.
  - Rx (treatment): Standing orders or protocols; direct orders from online medical direction.
  - Transport: Effects of interventions; mode of transportation; ongoing assessment findings.
- The *CHEATED charting method* begins with the initial patient contact and ends when the patient is delivered to the ED. The elements are:
  - Chief complaint: The reason the patient requested EMS assistance.
  - History: Past and present medical history, nature of incident, mechanism of injury.
  - Examination: The physical assessment.
  - Assessment: General impression and diagnosis.
  - Treatment: Any care rendered.
  - Evaluation: Patient's response to care provided (improvement or deterioration).
  - Disposition: The transfer of patient care to another health care professional.

Other approaches also may be used to write the narrative. These include the head-to-toe physical approach; a review of primary body systems approach; a chronological, call-incident approach; and a patient management approach.

The *head-to-toe physical approach* often is used in the PCR narrative. Paramedics may use this approach to record their findings after performing a full head-to-toe physical examination. Findings are noted in the narrative in the same order as they occurred in the examination. For example, findings from the examination of the patient's head are noted first (e.g., pupillary response). The paramedic ends by noting circulatory findings (e.g., the character of a pedal pulse or capillary refill) from the examination of the patient's extremities.

A *review of primary body systems approach* may be used when the examination is performed for a chief complaint that focuses on one body system. For example, for chest pain with suspected myocardial infarction, the paramedic would limit the findings to the cardiorespiratory system. Findings may include a description of the patient's pain, vital signs, ECG findings, associated breathing difficulties, significant medical history, allergies, and medication use.

The *chronological, call-incident approach* begins by noting the time of arrival at the patient's side and the initial examination findings, the time of vital sign assessment and reassessment, and a chronological listing of all patient care interventions performed at the scene and en route to the ED. This type of report commonly is used to document the events involving a patient with major trauma who has extended on-scene time. This format also may be used during a cardiac arrest event when numerous medications and electrical therapy are administered.

The *patient management approach* is used to organize and record the complete patient management plan. The report covers the emergency response from start to finish. This approach might describe in detail how the patient was found, what interventions were performed and why, and any important assessment findings. The patient management approach differs slightly from the others described in that it provides a more complete picture of the events at the scene, during care, and during transport of the patient.

CRITICAL THINKING

How many meanings can you think of for the word *lethargic*? Look it up in the dictionary. Should you use this word to document a patient's mental status? Why?

SPECIAL CONSIDERATIONS IN DOCUMENTATION

Several considerations in the documentation of patient care deserve special mention. Some of these include a patient's refusal of care or transport, situations and events in which transportation is not needed, interagency and interfacility transfers, mass casualty situations, and exposure or injury reporting. Other special situations (e.g., legal reporting, caring for intoxicated patients, and cases of abuse and neglect) are discussed in Chapters 6 and 51.

Patient's Refusal of Care or Transport

A patient's refusal of care or transport is a major area of potential liability for paramedics and EMS agencies (see Chapter 6). Thorough documentation of these situations is crucial and should include the following:

- The physical assessment findings
- The paramedic's advice to the patient about the benefits of treatment and the risks associated with refusing care
- The advice provided by medical direction by telephone or radio
- Clinical information that suggests the patient is able to make heath care decisions (e.g., the individual's level of consciousness)
- The signatures of any witnesses to the event, according to local protocol
- A complete narrative, including quotations or statements made by others

If the patient refuses care or transport, the paramedic should document the incident in exacting detail (Figure

---

REFUSAL OF MEDICAL CARE

I hereby voluntarily acknowledge and state that I have been advised regarding the state of my present physical condition. I have been advised of the risks/complications of my condition and the dangers of refusing medical treatment. I understand the risks, complications and/or dangers of refusing medical treatment as explained by St. Charles County Ambulance District personnel. With full knowledge of the possible consequences of my refusal of care, I hereby voluntarily refuse medical care and transportation by St. Charles County Ambulance District. Furthermore, I, for myself, my heirs, executors, administrators and assigns forever release and fully discharge St. Charles County Ambulance District, its officers, employees, medical consultants, hospitals, borrowed servants or agents from any and all liability or claims of whatever nature arising out of St. Charles County Ambulance District's effort to provide me with medical care and/or transportation and my consequent refusal, and I, therefore, agree to hold them completely and totally harmless and without fault unconditionally. *I have read and fully understand all of the above.*

I also acknowledge that I have received a copy of the St. Charles County Ambulance District Notice of Privacy Practices. A copy of this form is as valid as the original.

☐ Medical Control Contact   Talked to: _____

☐ Patient refused specific treatment (explain in narrative) _____

Date __/__/__   Signature **X** _____   Date __/__/__   Witness X _____

FIGURE 4-4 Refusal of care form. (Courtesy St. Charles County Ambulance District, St. Charles, Mo.)

4-4). The paramedic also should make it clear that the patient may call again for help despite the initial refusal. When possible, friends or family members should be encouraged to stay with the patient.

Cases in Which Care and Transport Are Not Needed

At times, care and transportation of a patient are not required, perhaps because of the patient's condition or because a request for help is canceled. After evaluating the patient or the scene, the paramedic may determine that circumstances do not warrant EMS transport (e.g., for a car crash without injuries or a patient who has left the scene). At this point, the paramedic should advise the dispatch center and document the event. If the EMS unit is canceled en route to the scene, the paramedic should make note of the canceling authority and the time of the cancellation. The canceling authority, for example, may be the dispatch center or the EMS supervisor. As with refusal of care, thorough documentation of these events can protect the paramedic from potential liability (see Chapter 6).

Interagency and Interfacility Transfers

Interagency transfers are those in which patient care duties are assigned (or "turned over") to another EMS unit. For example, a basic life support unit may intercept an ALS unit that is better able to manage the patient's needs; or, a fire rescue squad that provided initial emergency care but that does not have transport duties or capabilities may turn a patient in critical condition over to air ambulance personnel for speedier transport to a hospital. Documentation, tracking, and reporting systems should be established for these situations and followed consistently.

Interfacility (hospital to hospital) transfers occur between critical care hospitals and other facilities as approved by medical direction. They are arranged by the sending hospital to maximize the patient's safety and care. Some interfacility transfers are done for critical care patients, such as pediatric trauma patients, patients with severe burns, transplant candidates, cardiac patients, and patients with indwelling medical devices that support life (see Appendix, Advanced Practice Procedures for Critical Care Paramedics.) In some cases medical personnel from the sending hospital accompany the patient during the interfacility transfer. These personnel may include physicians, critical care nurses, respiratory therapists, or other specialty care professionals. Most sending hospitals have special interfacility transfer forms to document care en route; to provide for any standing orders; and to document the transfer of patient care at the new destination.

Some patients are transferred because of insurance requirements or to receive specialized care not available at the sending hospital. Paramedics should use a standard PCR or other form designated by their EMS agency to document these transfers.

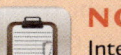

NOTE

Interfacility transfers differ from the nonemergency transfer of a patient from a private physician's office, nursing home, convalescent care center, or other facility that may not be equipped to provide acute patient care needs.

Mass Casualty Events

A major incident may result in a large number of patients, and comprehensive documentation may have to be postponed until patients have been triaged and transported for definitive care (see Chapter 54). These are difficult and unusual situations; in these circumstances, the paramedic should follow local documentation procedures.

Exposure and Injury Reporting

EMS agencies have special forms for documenting and reporting a possible unprotected exposure to infectious disease organisms, hazardous chemicals, or a job-related injury. These reports are developed by the local EMS agency and their legal advisers. They must follow state and federal guidelines, as well as those established by the Occupational Safety and Health Administration (OSHA) and the Centers for Disease Control and Prevention (CDC), if applicable. (Reporting of a possible exposure to infectious disease organisms or hazardous chemicals is discussed in detail in Chapters 28 and 57).

Paramedics who have been injured on the job or who believe that they may have been exposed to an infectious disease organism should follow agency protocol and do the following:

1. Immediately contact the EMS supervisor or designated officer.
2. Seek medical care.
3. Thoroughly document the event.

DOCUMENT REVISION AND CORRECTION

As noted previously, a PCR sometimes must be revised or corrected. Most EMS agencies provide separate report forms for this purpose. If a separate report is needed, the paramedic should do the following:

- Make the revision or correction as soon as the need for it is realized.
- Note the purpose of the revision or correction and the reason the information did not appear on the original document.
- Note the date and time the revision or correction was made.
- Make sure the revision or correction was made by the original author of the document.

Acceptable methods of making revisions or adding information to a document vary by agency. Some include making the change to the original form; such changes must be initialed, and the date and time must be noted (this method should not be used for electronic patient reports unless the program has a built-in mechanism to track the changes). Other methods include writing the corrections in the narrative; attaching a new report to the original; and providing supplemental narratives on a separate form, which is attached to the original. The paramedic should follow the policies set by the EMS agency and medical direction for revising or correcting reports.

> **CRITICAL THINKING**
> Consider this situation: Your supervisor asks you to change your documentation so that the insurance company will pay for the transport. What would you do?

CONSEQUENCES OF INAPPROPRIATE DOCUMENTATION

Incorrect or incomplete documentation can have serious consequences that have medical and legal implications. With an inaccurate, incomplete, or illegible PCR, caregivers may provide improper care to a patient. For example, a paramedic fails to mention that a patient with a possible myocardial infarction is allergic to *amiodarone.* The patient later becomes unconscious in the ED as a result of a ventricular rhythm disturbance. *Amiodarone,* an antidysrhythmic, might be administered, but in this case it

> **BOX 4-4 Documentation Responsibilities of the Paramedic**
>
> The paramedic's professional responsibilities with regard to documentation include the following:
> - View the task of documentation as one of utmost importance.
> - Assume responsibility for self-assessment of all documentation.
> - Appreciate the importance of good documentation to all health care personnel.
> - Strive to set a good example in the completion of the documentation task.
> - Respect the confidential nature of an EMS report.

could prove lethal for the patient. A thorough PCR completed in a professional manner may influence the decision of an attorney considering the merits of an impending lawsuit for negligence or malpractice. (The converse also is true if the documentation is not thorough and professional.)

Documentation should never become routine or superficial (Box 4-4). Good documentation should be completed in a timely manner and with careful attention to detail. This helps ensure that the PCR is medically and legally sound.

SUMMARY

- The patient care report is used to document the key elements of patient assessment, care, and transport.
- The four primary reasons for written documentation are that the medical community involved in the patient's care uses it; it is a legal record; it is important for reimbursement; and it is essential to data collection.
- The PCR should include dates and response times, difficulties encountered, observations at the scene, previous medical care provided, a chronological description of the call, and significant times.
- A properly written EMS document is accurate and complete, legible, timely, unaltered, and free of nonprofessional or extraneous information.

- Many approaches can be used to write the narrative. The paramedic should adopt only one approach and use it consistently to prevent omissions in report writing.
- Special documentation is necessary when a patient refuses care or transport; when care or transport is not needed; and for mass casualty events.
- Most EMS agencies have separate forms for revising or correcting the patient care report.
- Incorrect or incomplete documentation may have medical and legal implications.

REFERENCES

1. McWay D: *Legal aspects of health information management*, ed 2, Clifton Park, NY, 2003, Delmar.
2. National Highway Traffic Safety Administration: The National EMS Education Standards, Washington, DC, 2009,
U.S. Department of Transportation/National Highway Traffic Safety Administration, DOT.
3. NEMSIS Technical Assistance Center: EMS Dataset Schema. www.nemsis.org/softwaredevelopers/downloads/emsDataset. html. Accessed August 2, 2010.

SUGGESTED READINGS

Angell L, et al: *Documentation: the language of nursing*, Upper Saddle River, NJ, 2000, Prentice Hall.
Graham DH: Motivation for documentation, *EMS* 23:39-40, 2004.

Marelli T, Harper S: *Nursing documentation handbook*, St Louis, 2000, Mosby.
Milewski R, et al: *Documentation: field guide*, Boston, 2000, Jones & Bartlett.
Welsley K: Write it right: keeping your PCR clinical and factual, *JEMS* 33:42-44, 2008.

OBJECTIVES

Upon completion of this chapter, the paramedic student will be able to:

1. Outline the phases of the communications that occur during a typical emergency medical services (EMS) event.
2. Describe the role of communications in EMS.
3. Outline the basic model of communications.
4. Define common EMS communications terms.
5. Describe ways to communicate effectively using the primary modes of EMS communications.
6. Outline the elements of an EMS communications system.
7. Describe the characteristics of EMS communications operation modes.
8. Describe the role of dispatching as it applies to prehospital emergency medical care.
9. Outline techniques for relaying EMS communications clearly and effectively.
10. Describe the regulation of EMS communications.
11. Distinguish between EMS frequency ranges.
12. Outline procedures for EMS communications.

KEY TERMS

communications The process by which one individual or group transmits information to others.

decoding The process by which the intended meaning of information is interpreted.

duplex mode A communications mode in which traffic may be transmitted and received simultaneously through two different frequencies, one for transmitting and one for receiving.

EMS communications The delivery of patient and scene information (either in person, in writing, or through communications technology) to other members of the emergency response team.

encoding The process by which information is organized through a medium or channel.

Federal Communications Commission (FCC) A federal agency that has jurisdiction over interstate and international telephone and telegraph services and satellite communications.

multiplex mode A communications mode in which two or more different types of information can be transmitted simultaneously, in either or both directions, over the same frequency.

simplex mode A communications mode in which information can be transmitted or received in only one direction at a time. Simultaneous transmission cannot occur.

SOAP format A memory aid used to organize written and verbal patient reports; *SOAP* stands for *s*ubjective data, *o*bjective data, *a*ssessment data, and *p*lan of patient management.

team dynamics The unseen forces that operate in a team between different groups of people; will enable a group of people to act as one.

telemedicine Technological communications that allow the transmission of photographs, video, and other information directly from the scene to a hospital for physician evaluation and consultation.

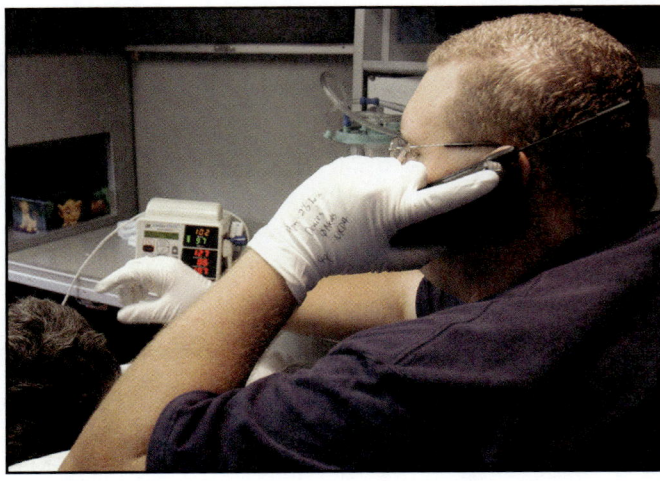

E*MS communications* refers to the delivery of information about the patient and the scene. The information may be delivered in person, in writing, or through various electronic devices to other members of the emergency response team. These members include telecommunicators, EMS personnel, emergency response workers, EMS system control and administration staff, and medical direction. This chapter addresses the complexities of communications that are vital aspects of the EMS system.

Courtesy Ray Kemp, St. Charles, Mo.

PHASES OF COMMUNICATIONS DURING A TYPICAL EMS EVENT

A typical EMS event involves five phases of communications.[1] The first phase is the occurrence of the event. The second phase is the detection of the need for emergency services. The third phase is the notification and emergency response. The fourth phase is the EMS responders' arrival, treatment of the patient, and preparation for transport. (Treatment may require consultation with medical direction.) The fifth phase is preparation of the EMS crew for the next response.

In many urban areas, the public requests help by a phone call. This call goes to a communications center or *public safety answering point* (PSAP). Communications specialists receive the call. In the most modern systems, details about the origin of the call and any history of a response to that locale are displayed automatically on a console (Figure 5-1). The call taker uses digital technology to send these details to the telecommunicator, who sends a response unit to the scene. In some PSAP systems, the caller is given prearrival instructions by emergency medical dispatchers or other qualified personnel. The communication with the caller continues until the first EMS unit arrives at the scene.

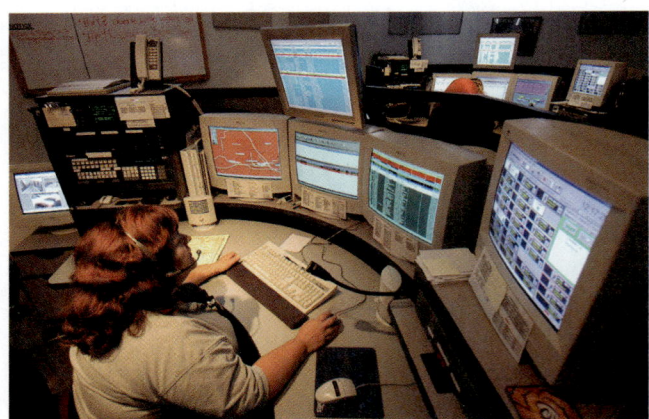

FIGURE 5-1 Communications console (dispatch).

DID YOU KNOW?
Vehicle Telemetry

Vehicle telemetry systems (e.g., OnStar, Tele-Aid, and others) are installed on some newer automobiles. They use a collection of sensors that send crash data to an adviser if the vehicle is involved in a moderate or severe front, rear, or side impact crash. Depending on the type of system, the data may include information on the severity of the crash, the direction of impact, airbag deployment, multiple impacts, and a rollover (if the system is equipped with appropriate sensors). Advisers can relay this information to emergency dispatchers, helping them quickly to determine the appropriate combination of emergency personnel, equipment, and medical facilities that may be needed. Telemetry systems also can pinpoint the location of the vehicle if it is equipped with a global positioning system (GPS). Since OnStar launched its program in 1996, the company has assisted its subscribers and others on the roadway in more than 100,000 crashes.[2]

NOTE
As described in Chapter 1, a *telecommunicator* is a person trained in public safety telecommunications. The term applies to call takers, dispatchers, radio operators, data terminal operators, or any combination of such functions in a public safety answering point located in a fire, police, or EMS communications center.

The EMS unit is dispatched to the scene. The paramedic crew advises the communications center of its response and arrival status by radio or electronically using a computer data terminal. The paramedics provide care at the scene of the emergency. They prepare ("package") the patient for transport and then deliver the individual to the receiving facility. After reporting has been done, the paramedics make the EMS vehicle ready for the next emergency call.

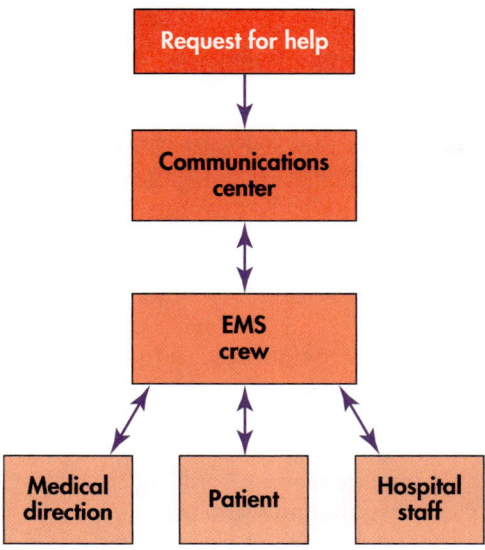

FIGURE 5-2 EMS communications.

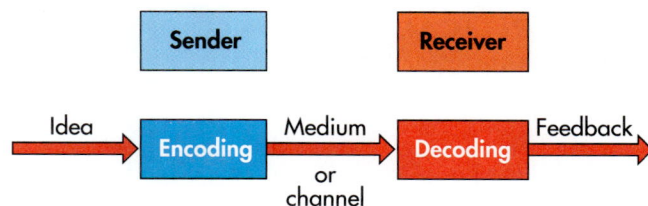

FIGURE 5-3 Basic model of communication.

ROLE OF COMMUNICATIONS IN EMERGENCY MEDICAL SERVICES

Verbal, written, and electronic communications allow the delivery of information between the person requesting help and the telecommunicator and between the telecommunicator and the paramedic. Communications occur between the paramedic, patient, hospital, and direct/online medical direction (if needed) and between the paramedic and hospital personnel who receive the patient on arrival at the emergency department (Figure 5-2). Good communication occurs only when key elements are in place. These elements make up the basic model of communications.

Basic Model of Communications

Communications can be verbal, nonverbal, or written in form. They serve a vital information function in the course of decision making. **Communications** is the process by which one individual or group transmits meaning to others. The basic model of communications describes the relationships between an idea, encoding, a sender, a medium or channel, a receiver, decoding, and feedback (Figure 5-3).

> **NOTE**
> The elements of successful communication described here apply to *all* types of communication between people. This includes communications with friends, family, co-workers, other emergency personnel, and other health care professionals. Successful communication is an important part of **team dynamics.**

The *idea* is the meaning that is intended in the communication. Conveying the idea requires two things. First, the sender must organize the intended meaning through a medium or channel; this is called **encoding.** (For example, the medium or channel may be written or verbal, facial or

body expression, or voice modulation.) Second, the communication must be interpreted by the receiver; this is called **decoding.** The receiver provides feedback that indicates the idea was received. If the communication is fully successful, the idea intended by the sender will overlap with the feedback provided by the receiver. (That is, the receiver interprets, or decodes, the idea exactly as intended by the sender.) Four common barriers can prevent successful communication.[3]

1. *Attributes of the receiver.* Different people react in different ways to the same message or idea. A variety of personal reasons may affect the interpretation of the message. These reasons may include cultural differences, language barriers, or sensory deficits. For example, a patient from one culture may find personal touch comforting, whereas a patient from another culture may be offended by touching.

2. *Selective perception.* People tend to listen to only part of an idea or message. They block out other information. They do this for a variety of reasons (e.g., values, mood, motives of the sender). They may block out an idea when new information conflicts with established values, beliefs, or expectations. For example, a paramedic supervisor may not welcome or respect the input of a newly licensed paramedic.

3. *Semantic problems.* Commonly used words may have different meanings for different people. A common issue is the use of vague or abstract words or phrases. These words invite varying interpretation. Another problem is the use of medical terms and technical language (jargon); the receiver may not be able to understand these. For example, a paramedic may refer to a patient as "comatose" during a radio report to the hospital. The hospital staff member may ask for further clarification using the *a*lert, *v*erbal, *p*ainful, *u*nresponsive (AVPU) scale (see Chapter 19).

4. *Time pressures.* Time pressures can lead to distortions in communications. A major temptation when pressed for time is to bypass or "short circuit" normal channels. In these cases the immediate demands of the situation are met. However, a number of unintended consequences can result. For example, a paramedic may not document the medications administered at the scene to a patient in cardiac arrest. This can cause confusion about the next appropriate drug to be used.

CRITICAL THINKING
What tends to happen to you when you are talking with someone who continually interrupts you?

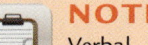
NOTE
Verbal communications can be affected by the terms used. Likewise, the effectiveness of written documentation can be impeded by the use of technical terms. Semantic jargon also can hinder the message. These types of terms often cannot be understood clearly by all parties.

Paramedics should consider this basic model of communications and the common barriers that block good communications. These elements are the key to recall when a paramedic is conveying information to or receiving information from telecommunicators, coworkers, patients, bystanders, medical direction, and hospital personnel.

Proper Verbal Communications During an EMS Event

The role of proper verbal communications during an EMS event is to exchange system and patient information with other members of the response team. Communications must be done according to local protocol and patient privacy standards and regulations (see Chapters 4 and 6).

The terms used in EMS communications should be clear and conveyed in short narrative form. Technical or semantic jargon that cannot be understood clearly by all parties should be avoided. Some EMS systems use a code to shorten radio transmissions. However, the English language usually is preferred for written and verbal messages. Paramedics should keep in mind that many radio and phone communications are recorded. These recordings may be replayed for patient care audits, media broadcasts, and disciplinary hearings and also during legal proceedings. Professional conduct is important in all communications. In many communities, members of the public use scanners to monitor emergency services. Paramedics, therefore, must take steps to preserve a patient's confidentiality. They should not speak the patient's name or use descriptive phrases over unsecured airwaves.

Proper Written Communications during an EMS Event

As described in Chapter 4, written documentation during an EMS event serves several key purposes. It provides a written and legal record of the event. It conveys key clinical information from one part of the medical chain (EMS) to the next (the emergency department). In addition, documentation is an expected component of professional work. Written documentation of patient care activities becomes part of the patient's medical record. Other important ways in which written data can be used in the EMS system include the following:

- Medical audits
- Quality improvement/quality management
- Billing
- Data collection
- Research

In addition to the patient care report (PCR), other types of documentation may be required by an EMS agency, such as:

- Personnel records documenting training and work assignments
- Call records that list or log dates, times, and other specifics of a call
- Vehicle maintenance records documenting vehicle service at regular intervals
- Vehicle and equipment cleaning records documenting procedures used to disinfect vehicle and emergency equipment
- Drug and equipment inventory records verifying daily checks of drug and fluid expiration, security measures for controlled substances as required by state and federal drug enforcement agencies; and monitor-defibrillator, radio, and telemetry checks
- Incident reports that document problem calls or unusual circumstances
- Records of significant exposures to communicable disease organisms or biological hazards
- Records of any possible hazardous substances to which the patient or paramedic may have been exposed

Technological Advances in the Collection and Exchange of Information

As technology evolves, it alters the way EMS gather and exchange information. Technology reduces the reliance on more traditional means of verbal and written communications. Examples of such advances include portable wireless voice and data devices, satellite terminals, global positioning systems (GPSs) for tracking emergency vehicles, diagnostic devices, laptop or handheld computers, and personal digital assistants (PDAs) (Figure 5-4). These and other devices can allow for real-time capture of EMS events and data. They can allow advanced notification and reduce the time to in-hospital diagnosis and therapy.

NOTE
Laptops and handheld computers can send patient information from a scene to a receiving hospital or a host computer. Then the data can be transferred electronically into a final report and patient record. This electronic information has the same legal status as a written document. The data take the place of the paper record of the incident.

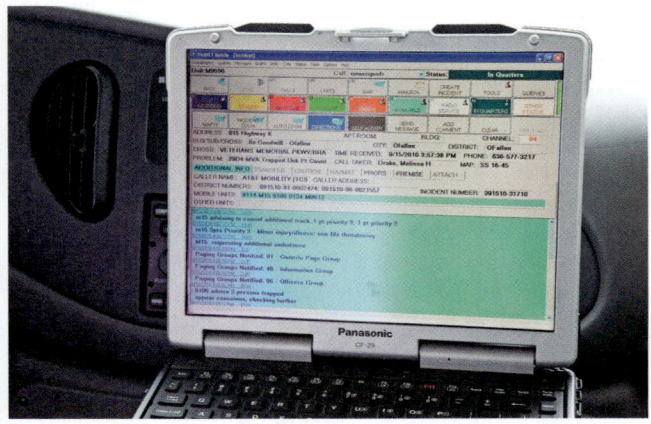

FIGURE 5-4 Rugged computer used for EMS documentation.

COMMUNICATIONS SYSTEMS

The terms used to describe emergency communications technology are specific to the industry (Box 5-1). The following sections provide an overview of the simple and complex communications systems and their requirements as established by the **Federal Communications Commission (FCC).**[4]

Simple Systems

The minimum requirements for radio equipment used by an ambulance service include a self-contained desktop transceiver with a speaker, microphone, antenna, and mobile unit, as well as a two-way radio with multiple-frequency capability in the vehicle. Most EMS agencies also use handheld portable radios (often called simply *portables*). These radios are capable of communications contact with the base station and data recording. The portable radio protects the crew and aids optimum patient care by allowing continued contact with the communications center and medical direction. The data recording part of the device is on the dispatch or hospital radio or telephone. It offers medical and legal protection for the service and can verify transmissions when contact is disrupted.

Complex Systems

More advanced radio communications systems include remote consoles, high-power transmitters, repeaters, satellite receivers, and high-power multifrequency vehicle radios. Some services also use mobile transmitter steering, vehicular repeaters, mobile encode-decode capabilities, mobile data terminals, microwave links, and other sophisticated communications devices.

BASE STATIONS

Base stations usually are located on a high spot, such as a hill, mountain, or tall building. This location ensures optimum transmission and reception. Base stations generally are connected by telephone lines to dispatch centers, where all elements of the EMS response are coordinated.

Depending on the locale, one dispatch center may be responsible for all fire, police, and EMS communications activities. Base station transmitters usually are equipped with an antenna to boost their signal.

MOBILE TRANSCEIVERS

Vehicle-mounted transmitters usually operate at lower outputs than base stations. They provide a range of 10 to 15 miles over average terrain. Transmission over flat land or water increases this range. However, transmission over mountainous terrain, dense foliage, or urban areas with tall buildings reduces the range. Transmitters with higher outputs are available. These transmitters may offer greater ranges for transmission. Multichannel units are preferred over single-channel radios because an EMS system uses many channels.

PORTABLE TRANSCEIVERS

Portable transceivers are hand-held or hand-carried devices. They are used when the paramedic is working away from the emergency vehicle. Portable transceivers usually have a limited range. Many systems boost the signal through a mobile or vehicular repeater. Portable transceivers may be single-channel or multichannel units.

REPEATERS

Repeaters act as a special type of long-range transceiver. They receive transmissions from a low-power portable or mobile radio on one frequency. At the same time, they retransmit it at a higher power on another frequency. Repeaters may be fixed or vehicle-mounted; EMS systems often use both. Repeaters are needed for large geographical areas. They are used to increase coverage between two or more portable or mobile units. Repeaters allow low-power units to receive other radio messages. They also allow two or more low-power units to communicate with each other when distances or obstructions normally would hinder such communications.

REMOTE CONSOLE

Most EMS systems use dispatch services located away from base stations. These remote centers control all base station functions. The remote center and base station are connected by dedicated telephone lines, microwave relay, or other radio means. Hospitals also often are equipped with a terminal that receives and displays telemetry transmissions. The remote console provides contact with paramedic crews in the field. Consoles for these systems include an amplifier, a speaker, a microphone, receiving capabilities, and remote control circuits.

SATELLITE RECEIVERS AND TERMINALS

Satellite receivers sometimes are used, depending on the area and the terrain. They are used to ensure that low-power units are always within coverage. The satellite receivers are strategically located and are connected to the base station or repeater by dedicated phone lines, radio, or microwave

BOX 5-1 Communications Terminology

9-1-1: A three-digit telephone number used to facilitate reporting of an emergency that requires a response by a public safety agency.

9-1-1 service area: The geographical area that has been granted authority by a state or local government body to provide 9-1-1 service.

abandoned call: A call placed to 9-1-1 in which the caller disconnects before the call can be answered by the public safety answering point (PSAP) telecommunicator.

advanced mobile phone service: The analog or digital radio interface used in wireless telephone systems.

alternate PSAP: A PSAP designated to receive calls when the primary PSAP is unable to do so.

alternate routing: A system for routing 9-1-1 calls to one or more designated alternate locations if all 9-1-1 trunks to a primary PSAP are busy or out of service. Alternate routing may be activated upon request or automatically, if detectable, when 9-1-1 equipment fails or the PSAP itself is disabled.

amplitude modulated: The encoding of a carrier wave by variation of its amplitude in accordance with an input signal.

attendant position: The customer premises equipment at which the telecommunicator answers and responds to calls.

automatic alarm and automatic alerting device: Any automated device that can access the 9-1-1 system for emergency services upon activation but that does not provide for two-way communication. Many states prohibit dialing of 9-1-1 by an automated device.

automatic call distributor: Equipment that automatically distributes incoming calls to available PSAP call takers in the order the calls are received or queues calls until a call taker becomes available.

automatic location identification: The automatic display at the PSAP of the caller's telephone number, the address or location of the telephone, and supplementary emergency services information.

automatic number identification (ANI): The telephone number associated with the access line from which a call originates.

backup PSAP: Typically, a disaster recovery answering point that serves as a backup to the primary PSAP and is not located in the same place as the primary PSAP.

basic 9-1-1: An emergency telephone system that automatically connects 9-1-1 callers to a designated answering point. Call routing is determined only by the originating central office. Basic 9-1-1 typically does not support ANI or automatic location identification.

call relay: Forwarding of pertinent information by a PSAP telecommunicator to the appropriate response agency; not to be confused with telephone relay service.

calling party hold: The capability of the PSAP to maintain control of a 9-1-1 caller's access line, even if the caller hangs up.

calling party's number: The callback number associated with a wireless telephone; similar to ANI for wireline telephones.

cell: The wireless telecommunications (cellular or PCS) antenna serving a specific geographical area.

circuit route: The physical path between two terminal locations.

computer-aided dispatch: A computer-based system that aids PSAP telecommunicators by automating selected dispatching and recordkeeping activities.

consolidated PSAP: An arrangement in which one or more public safety agencies choose to operate as a single 9-1-1 entity.

dedicated trunk: A telephone circuit used for a single purpose, such as transmission of 9-1-1 calls.

direct dispatch: The performance of 9-1-1 call answering and dispatching by personnel at the primary PSAP.

diverse routing: The practice of routing circuits along different physical paths to prevent total loss of 9-1-1 service in the event of a facility failure.

emergency call: A telephone request for public safety agency emergency services that requires immediate action to save a life, report a fire, or stop a crime; it may include other situations as determined locally.

emergency ring back: The capability of a PSAP telecommunicator to ring the telephone on a held circuit (a basic 9-1-1 feature); requires calling party hold; also known as *re-ring*.

emergency service trunks: Message trunks capable of providing ANI, connecting the serving central office of the 9-1-1 calling party and the designated enhanced 9-1-1 control office.

enhanced 9-1-1 (E9-1-1): An emergency telephone system that includes network switching, database, and customer premises equipment elements capable of providing selective routing, selective transfer, fixed transfer, ANI, and automatic location identification.

forced disconnect: The capability of a PSAP attendant to disconnect a 9-1-1 call even if the calling party remains off the hook; used to prevent overloading of 9-1-1 trunks.

global positioning system (GPS): A satellite-based technology for determining location.

highway call box: A telephone enclosed in a box and placed along a highway that allows a motorist to summon emergency and nonemergency assistance.

management information system: A program that collects, stores, and collates data into reports to allow interpretation and evaluation of information such as performance, trends, and traffic capacities.

master street address guide: A database of street names and house number ranges within their associated communities defining emergency service zones and their associated emergency service numbers to enable proper routing of 9-1-1 calls.

National Emergency Number Association: A not-for-profit corporation established in 1982 to further the goal of "One Nation—One Number." The association is a networking source that promotes research, planning, and training. It strives to educate, set standards, and provide certification programs, legislative representation, and technical assistance for implementing and managing 9-1-1 systems.

primary PSAP: A PSAP to which 9-1-1 calls are routed directly from the 9-1-1 control office.

public safety answering point (PSAP): A facility equipped and staffed to receive 9-1-1 calls. A primary PSAP receives the calls directly. If the call is relayed or transferred, the next receiving PSAP is designated a secondary PSAP.

selective routing: The routing of a 9-1-1 call to the proper PSAP based on the location of the caller. Selective routing is controlled by the emergency service number, which is derived from the customer's location.

telecommunicator: As used in 9-1-1, a person trained and employed in public safety telecommunications. The term applies to call takers, dispatchers, radio operators, data terminal operators, or any combination of such functions in a PSAP.

trunk: Typically, a communication path between central office switches or between the 9-1-1 control office and the PSAP.

Modified from National Emergency Number Association Technical Committee and PSAP Operational Standards Committee: *NENA master glossary of 911 terminology*, Arlington, Va, 1998, The Association.

relay. "Voting systems" automatically select the best audio signal. These systems pick up the signal from among multiple satellite receivers and the main base station receiver. (These also are used in other types of communications systems.)

Commonly available satellite terminals incorporate ground stations and transportable stations. They provide voice, data, and video communications. Portable satellite terminals are useful when other systems are not available. For example, they may be used during major disasters.

ENCODERS AND DECODERS

Selective call encoders look like a phone dial or the buttons of a push-button phone. When activated, the encoder transmits tone pulses or pairs of tones over the air. Receivers with decoders recognize the specific codes. This in turn opens the audio circuits of the receivers. Two-tone sequential paging alerts personnel using two pairs of specific frequency tones to address pagers and alert monitors selectively. A selective-address system usually has a code for calling all units within radio range (all call).

Hospitals in certain regions of the United States are tied together by radio systems known as Hospital Emergency Administrative Radio (HEAR [by Motorola]) or Emergency Administrative Communications (EACOM by Ericson). Radios for these systems use 1500 Hz rotary pulse dialing to transmit specific groups of rotary tone pulses to designated hospital-based receivers. Most ambulance services have access to this system.

CELLULAR TELEPHONES

Many EMS systems use cellular phones (analog and digital). Cell phones are an alternative to dedicated EMS communications systems. One benefit of cell phones is that they have more channels. In addition, a cell phone offers a fairly secure link between EMS workers and area hospitals. A cell phone also allows the online physician to speak directly with the patient. However, the use of cell phones for emergency services also has some disadvantages. For example, network usage might limit channel access. Also, high network usage might create problems in maintaining continuous communications in some areas, which would be especially problematic in a community disaster. Other issues are lack of priority access and the fact that calls could not be monitored by other members of an emergency response team. For these reasons, many EMS agencies that use cell phones have a backup option. They often have backup radio communications capabilities (Box 5-2).

DID YOU KNOW

The U.S. Congress recently mandated conversion to *all digital television* (DTV) broadcasting, because digital frequencies are more efficient than analog frequencies. In addition, ending analog broadcasts will free up those frequencies for public safety communications and emergency response networks.

BOX 5-2 Cellular Phone Technology

An analog cell phone is actually a radio that allows two people to communicate on one frequency. The analog signal fluctuates with the rise and fall of the caller's voice. This produces a wildly oscillating electrical wave (a "copy" of speech). The signal can be heard at the receiver's end. Digital cell phones use the same radio technology but different frequencies. Moreover, they compress the caller's voice into digital 1s and 0s that remain stable for the length of their travel. At the receiver's end, the digital information is converted back to voice. A digital signal generally is thought to provide better sound quality. It also is thought to provide a more secure method of transmission than analog methods. In addition, digital technology provides the platform for wireless services such as data transmission and interactive computers.

DIGITAL MODES

Digital communication modes include digital phones, telemetry, facsimile ("fax") transmissions, and digital signals used in some wireless phone, paging, and alerting systems. Telemetric communications and facsimiles are transmitted using electronic signals, which are converted into audio tones. These tones are converted back into electronic signals by the receiver decoder. The signals then can be displayed or printed. Transmission of a patient's electrocardiogram is an example of telemetry.

COMPUTER TECHNOLOGIES

Computer technology (e.g., that used with automated external defibrillators [AEDs] and other devices) is capable of "saving" (preserving a record of) every step of data entry. Computers allow for (1) documentation in near real time; (2) sorting of information in many categories; (3) creation of multiple reporting formats; and (4) quick online and retrieval system data access. Computer terminals also are used by some communications centers to dispatch units automatically to a scene. As with most technologies, computer devices are subject to human error and machine limitations. Therefore, they require regular upgrades and user education.

NOTE

Advances in EMS communications technology and **telemedicine** continue to proceed at a rapid pace. Video cameras, fax machines, cellular networks, and the Internet now allow photographs, videos (including movie-type imaging), and other information to be sent directly from the scene to a hospital for physician evaluation and consultation.

Operation Modes Used for EMS Communications

The operation modes commonly used in EMS communications are the simplex, multiplex, duplex, and trunked modes.

SIMPLEX MODE

The **simplex mode** (Figure 5-5) requires a transmitter and receiver at each end of the communications path. Both elements operate on the same frequency. However, only one end may operate at a time. This mode allows speakers to send a message without interruption, although it slows the communications process and precludes the ability to discuss an emergency event.

DUPLEX MODE

The **duplex mode** (Figure 5-6) uses two frequencies that allow both parties to communicate at the same time. The advantage of this mode is that either party can interrupt the other to facilitate discussion. However, a tendency exists for each end to interrupt the other.

MULTIPLEX MODE

The **multiplex mode** (Figure 5-7) has the advantage of transmitting telemetry and voice simultaneously from a field unit. With this mode either party can interrupt as needed, which facilitates discussion. As with the duplex mode, each party tends to interrupt the other. In addition, voice transmission may interfere with the transmission of data. Multiplex is the most common mode currently used by most EMS systems.

TRUNKED SYSTEM

Trunking refers to systems that have five or more repeaters that work as a group. Each repeater is on a different channel. The trunking system may belong to a single user (e.g., a specific EMS agency or police department), or it may be shared by a number of public service agencies. When radio transmissions originate, computerized scanning automatically finds an available repeater in the system. The computer then switches the transmission to the chosen repeater. As one fleet captures an open channel, it locks out all other users who share the system. This bars interference from other agencies. The trunked system is advantageous in major metropolitan operations in which radio frequencies are used heavily.

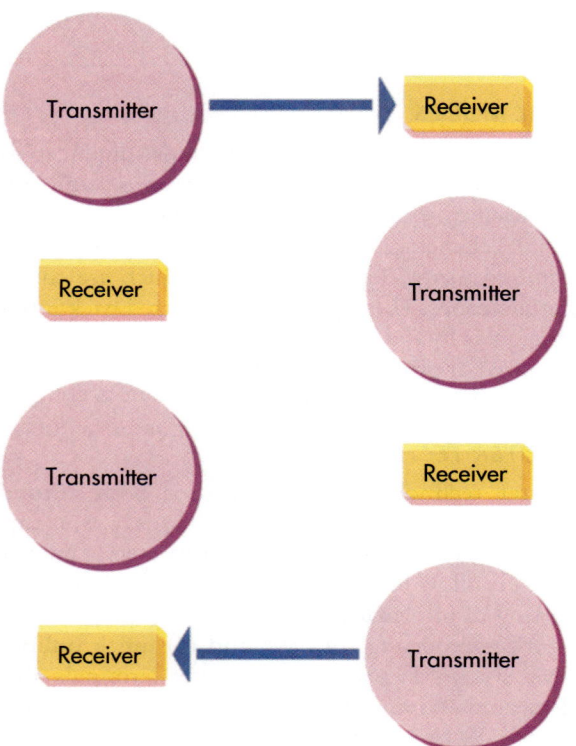

FIGURE 5-5 Simplex mode requires a transmitter and a receiver at each end of the communications path, both operating on the same frequency. In this mode, only one end may operate at a time.

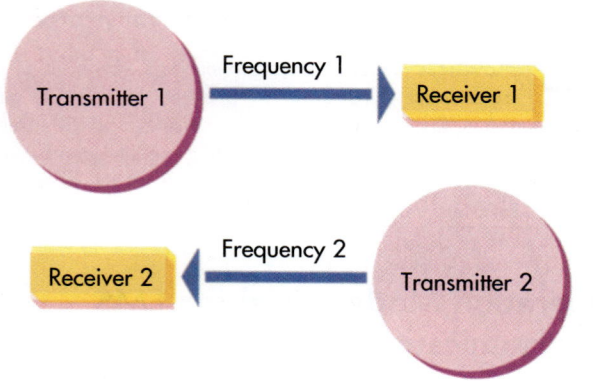

FIGURE 5-6 Duplex mode requires two frequencies so that both ends can communicate simultaneously.

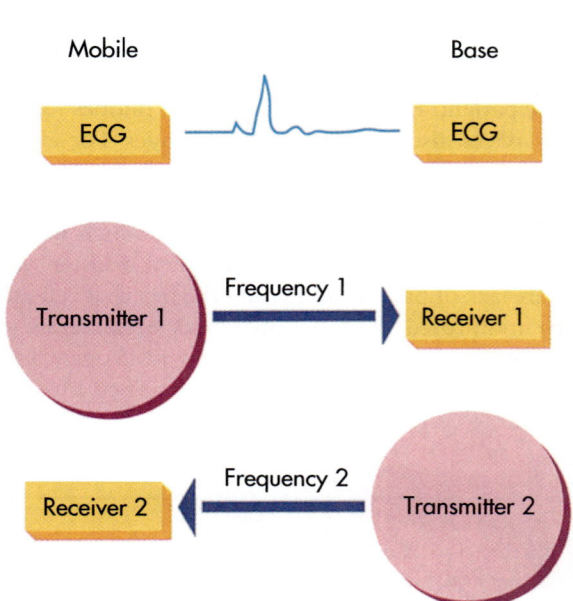

FIGURE 5-7 Multiplex mode operates similarly to duplex mode but has added capabilities, such as simultaneous electrocardiogram and voice transmission.

COMPONENTS AND FUNCTIONS OF DISPATCH COMMUNICATIONS SYSTEMS

The dispatch communications system is the public safety answering point (Box 5-3). The following are some of the functions of an effective EMS dispatch communications system.[5]

- *Receive and process calls for EMS assistance:* Calls for EMS assistance are received and recorded by the dispatcher, who selects an appropriate course of action for each call. This function involves obtaining as much information as possible about the emergency event, including the caller's name, callback number, and address; it also may involve dealing with distraught callers. In addition, emergency care instructions may be provided while the EMS crew is dispatched.
- *Dispatch and coordinate EMS resources:* The dispatcher directs the proper emergency vehicles to the correct address. In addition, the dispatcher coordinates the movements of emergency vehicles while en route to the scene, to the medical facility, and back to the operations base.
- *Relay medical information:* The dispatcher may provide a telecommunications channel between appropriate medical facilities and EMS personnel; firefighters, the police, and rescue workers; and private citizens. The channel may consist of telephone, radio, or biomedical telemetry.
- *Coordinate with public safety agencies:* The dispatcher provides for communications between public safety units (fire department, law enforcement, rescue workers) and elements of the EMS system. This facilitates the coordination of services such as traffic control, escort, fire suppression, and extrication. The dispatcher ensures an integrated, well-coordinated system. To do so, the dispatcher must know the location and status of all EMS vehicles. The dispatcher also must know the availability of support services (e.g., utility companies, coroner). In larger systems, computer-aided dispatching may be used. This advanced technology allows one or more of the following capabilities or functions:

- Automatic emergency medical dispatch
- Automatic entry of 9-1-1
- Automatic call notification/request for assistance
- Automatic interface to automatic vehicle location (AVL) with or without map display (Figure 5-8)
- Automatic interface to mobile data terminal
- Computer messaging among multiple radio operators, call takers, or both
- Dispatch note taking, reminder aid, or both
- Emergency medical dispatch review
- Manual or automatic updates of unit status
- Manual entry of call information
- Radio control and display of channel status
- Standard operating procedure review
- Telephone control and display of circuit status

SHOW ME THE EVIDENCE

EMS calls from 2 years in an emergency medical dispatch (EMD) system in a California suburb that totaled 500 or more in one dispatch category were compared to the prehospital patient care report for those same calls. The researchers wanted to see whether the dispatch code predicted prehospital use of medications and other interventions. They found that the EMD system had "only a modest ability" to predict which patients would need advanced life support (ALS) interventions. More medicines were given to patients with shortness of breath, chest pain, diabetic problems, and altered mental status.

From Sporer KA et al: Can emergency medical dispatch codes predict prehospital interventions for common 9-1-1 call types? *Prehosp Emerg Care* 12:470-478, 2008.

BOX 5-3 9-1-1, Enhanced 9-1-1, and Computer-aided Dispatch Systems

In 1988 the number 9-1-1 was designated as the universal emergency telephone number (see Chapter 1). The number was chosen by the American Telephone and Telegraph Company. The number offers the public a toll-free number for reaching a public safety answering point. (This service is still not available in all areas.) Since 1988, enhanced 9-1-1 has been created. This system, which is used in many areas of the country, allows for automatic caller location and identification. It also shows the caller's number and address on a terminal at the communications center.

The most advanced centers use a computer-aided dispatch system that monitors the available resources. The system makes an assignment based on access and routes for the ambulance closest to the map grid shown on the terminal. Global positioning systems tell the telecommunicator or system status controller which unit is closest to the origin of the call by air miles or by road miles if an intelligent map (also known as a "smart map") is used automatically to route the unit closest to the scene. That unit then is sent to the scene. The telecommunicator monitors the call from beginning to end and records status changes using digital media (e.g., tapes, CDs, or DVDs).

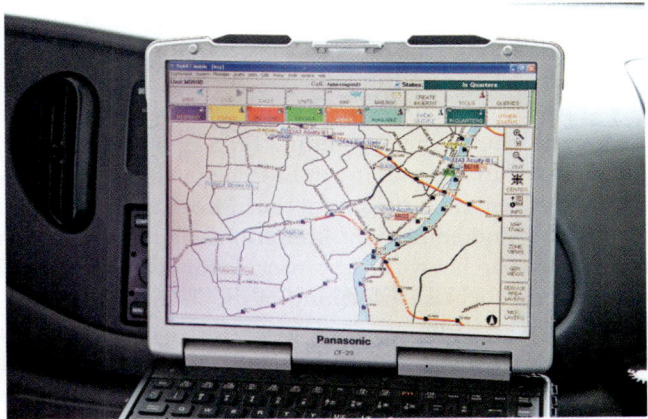

FIGURE 5-8 AVL mapping system in an ambulance cab.

DID YOU KNOW?
Enhanced 9-1-1

The rules established by the Federal Communications Commission (FCC) for wireless enhanced 9-1-1 (E9-1-1) are intended to improve the effectiveness and reliability of wireless 9-1-1 services by providing 9-1-1 dispatchers with additional information on wireless 9-1-1 calls. The wireless E9-1-1 rules apply to all wireless licensees, broadband Personal Communications Services (PCS) licensees, and certain Specialized Mobile Radio (SMR) licensees.

The FCC has divided its wireless E9-1-1 program into two parts, phase I and phase II. Under phase I, within 6 months of a valid request by a local public safety answering point (PSAP), wireless carriers must provide the PSAP with the telephone number of the originator of a wireless 9-1-1 call and the location of the cell site or base station transmitting the call.

Under phase II, within 6 months of a valid request by a PSAP, wireless carriers must begin providing more precise information to PSAPs, specifically, the caller's latitude and longitude. This information must meet FCC accuracy standards, generally to within 50 to 300 m, depending on the type of technology used. The deployment of E9-1-1 requires the development of new technologies and upgrades to local 9-1-1 PSAPs, in addition to coordination among public safety agencies, wireless carriers, technology vendors, equipment manufacturers, and local wireline carriers.

From Public Safety and Homeland Security Bureau: *Enhanced 9-1-1: wireless services.* http://www.fcc.gov/pshs/services/911-services/enhanced911/Welcome.html. Accessed August 3, 2010.

Dispatcher Training

Many EMS and public safety agencies require specialized medical training for their dispatch personnel. This training may include the Association of Public Communications Officials and Emergency Medical Dispatch Program (which is based on the National Standard Curriculum for Emergency Medical Dispatch, established by the National Highway Traffic Safety Administration). Emergency medical dispatchers are trained to do the following[6]:

- Use locally approved emergency medical dispatch guide cards (customized to local protocols and EMS response priorities)
- Quickly and properly determine the nature of the call
- Determine the priority of the call
- Dispatch the appropriate response
- Provide the caller with instructions to help treat the patient until the responding EMS unit arrives

A background of training in EMS helps the telecommunicator understand functions of the EMS system, personnel capabilities, and equipment limitations. The training also arms the dispatcher with the protocols for giving prearrival instructions, such as performing cardiopulmonary resuscitation (CPR) or administering *aspirin* to a patient with a coronary event. These protocols may mitigate the event before the EMS unit arrives.

A variety of dispatching systems and procedures are in place across the United States. Some are the simple call received–ambulance dispatched types; others are the more advanced call prioritization–prearrival instructions systems.

SHOW ME THE EVIDENCE

A prospective, experimental, before-and-after trial was conducted in a small Connecticut city with a population of 125,000 in which a first responder fire department engine company was routinely dispatched on most EMS calls. The purpose of the study was to see whether changing the emergency medical dispatch (EMD) protocol would reduce the call volume of first responder engine companies without affecting patient safety. Before the protocol was implemented, engine companies responded to 84.3% of calls. In the after phase, they were dispatched to 39.1% of EMS calls. The researchers estimated that only 0.55% of patients were undertriaged. They cautioned that these results may not be applicable to all EMS systems because of the diversity of response modes and dispatch protocols. They concluded that in their system, EMD protocols can safely limit the number of first responder runs.

From Cone D et al: Can emergency medical dispatch systems safely reduce first-responder call volume? *Prehosp Emerg Care* 12:479-485, 2008.

Call Prioritization—Prearrival Instructions Systems

In a call screening–prearrival instructions system, an emergency medical dispatcher, paramedic, or nurse determines the type of assistance needed for an emergency call. This may involve referring the caller to other services, choosing a basic life support (BLS) or an advanced life support (ALS) response, selecting a private or public EMS agency, and determining the appropriate use of audible and visual warning devices.

While dispatching the proper unit, the dispatcher can give the caller prearrival instructions. These instructions are crucial for several reasons:

- They provide the caller with instant help.
- They complement the call prioritization process.
- They allow the dispatcher to give updated information to responding units.
- They may be lifesaving in critical incidents.
- They provide emotional support for the caller, bystander, or victim.

CRITICAL THINKING
What are some possible consequences of a dispatching error?

REGULATION

As stated previously, radio communications in the United States are regulated by the FCC. This commission develops rules and regulations for the use of all radio equipment and

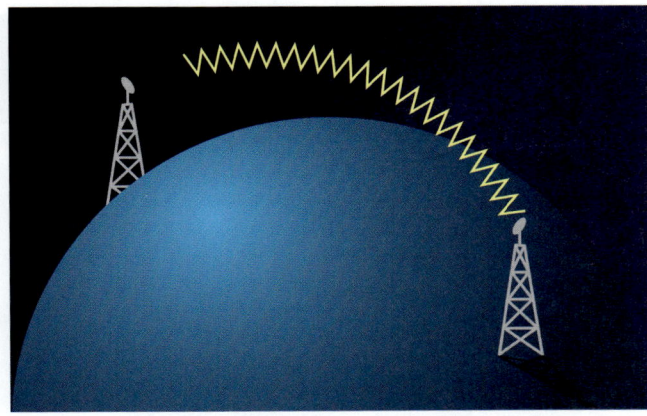

FIGURE 5-9 VHF low band.

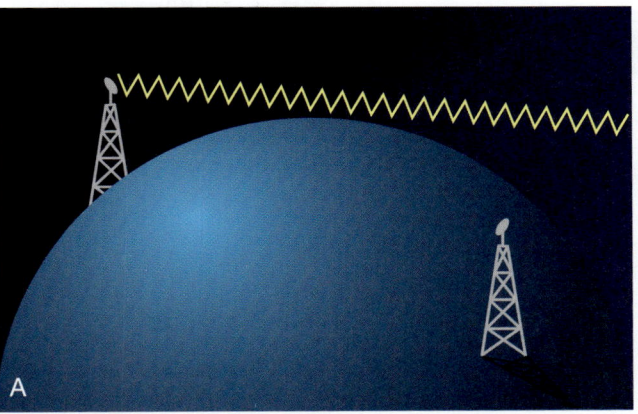

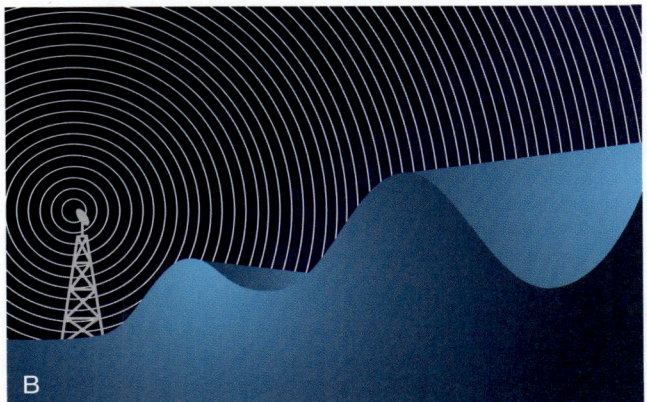

FIGURE 5-10 VHF high band.

frequencies. In addition to the FCC, state and local governments may have rules and regulations for radio operations. Paramedics must be knowledgeable about these agencies and must follow their guidelines. The primary functions of the FCC include the following:

- Licensing and frequency allocation
- Establishing technical standards for radio equipment
- Establishing and enforcing rules and regulations for equipment operation, including monitoring frequencies for appropriate usage and spot-checking for appropriate licenses and records

CRITICAL THINKING
Why are these rules and regulations needed for good EMS communications?

EMS Frequency Ranges

For public safety radio, very high frequency (VHF) may be defined as VHF low band (32 to 50 megahertz [MHz]) and VHF high band (150 to 174 MHz). A number of VHF low-band and VHF high-band frequencies are assigned strictly to two-way use or one-way paging. These frequencies normally operate in a simplex mode. UHF frequencies are used in either half-duplex, duplex, or multiplex modes.

VHF low-band signals (Figure 5-9) generally have the greatest range. They usually cover a greater distance than VHF high band or ultra high frequency (UHF) band. However, these low-band signals follow the curvature of the earth's surface; therefore, they are subject to noise interference and physical or structural interference. Consequently, although these signals have the best range, they may not provide the best coverage.

VHF high-band (Figure 5-10) signals generally have medium range. They travel in straight lines rather than following the earth's curvature. This virtual "straight line" characteristic means that high-band signals more easily reflect around buildings and other structures. These signals may provide better radio coverage in some areas.

In 1974 the FCC established a system of radio frequencies called *Special Emergency Radio Services* (SERS). These frequencies were to be used by EMS systems, hospitals, school buses, and rescue operations. Of the approximately 75 radio channels in this group, 10 UHF channels were designated for medical communications: eight for paramedic to hospital communications and two for dispatching (Table 5-1). EMS-only communications were confined to the 450 to 470 MHz UHF frequency band and five VHF frequencies.

UHF-band signals (Figure 5-11) generally have a limited range. They are more "straight line sensitive" than VHF high-band signals. However, the UHF band's ability to reflect or bounce around buildings exceeds that of the VHF high band. In metropolitan areas, UHF band may be the most effective frequency. Of the three bands, UHF is the least susceptible to noise interference. UHF also can reach into and out of structures more easily.

Public Safety 800 MHz Frequencies

Over the years, the growth of EMS systems and other public service operations has resulted in overcrowded frequencies and radio congestion. In 1987 the FCC allocated an additional band (821 to 824 MHz and 866 to 869 MHz) to SERS assignments. This helped resolve some of the communications problems. The 800 MHz signals generally

TABLE 5-1 UHF Channels Designated for Medical Communication

	Base Transmit	Base Receive	Recommended Use
Med 1	463.000	468.000	EMS to medical direction
Med 2	463.025	468.025	EMS to medical direction
Med 3	463.050	468.050	EMS to medical direction
Med 4	463.075	468.075	EMS to medical direction
Med 5	463.100	468.100	EMS to medical direction
Med 6	463.125	468.125	EMS to medical direction
Med 7	463.150	468.150	EMS to medical direction
Med 8	463.175	468.175	EMS to medical direction
Med 9	462.950	467.950	Dispatch
Med 10	462.975	467.975	Dispatch

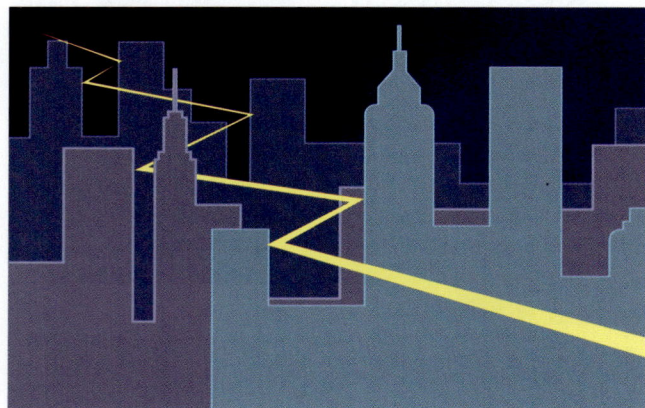

FIGURE 5-11 UHF band.

NOTE

Cellular phone companies also use the 800 MHz band. This can cause congestion and can interfere with public service communications, especially during a large-scale incident or major disaster. This type of communications gridlock occurred during the 9/11 attacks on the World Trade Center in New York in 2001. Work is underway to "reband" the 800 MHz system. This will increase the space of the frequencies to accommodate the communications needs of commercial carriers and public service agencies.

have a limited range, because they are more straight line than VHF high-band signals. With the use of repeaters, however, the 800 MHz band is able to reflect or bounce around buildings better than are the VHF high band and the UHF 400 MHz band. As such, the 800 MHz spectrum is best suited for use in urban areas.

To ensure the efficiency of the 800 MHz band, the FCC established "trunking" requirements. In the systems required, five or more repeaters (each on a different channel) work together as a group. The trunking system may belong to a single user, such as a specific EMS agency or police department. The system also may be shared by a number of public service agencies. As explained previously, when a radio transmission is originated, computerized scanning automatically finds an available repeater in the system. It then switches all radios in the fleet to the selected repeater. As one fleet captures an open channel, it locks out all other users who share the system. This prevents interference from other agencies. Several groups have helped the FCC reorganize the management of frequencies for public service operations, with the goal of improving the ability of public service agencies to communicate with each other.

In 1995 the FCC, along with the National Telecommunications and Information Administration (NTIA), established the Public Safety Wireless Advisory Committee (PSWAC) with the goal of addressing the communications needs of public service agencies through the year 2010. One of their recommendations has been the formation of a national broadband license for public safety.[7] The FCC remains committed to a policy goal of a nationwide 700 MHz broadband network for public safety. It currently is acquiring a number of frequencies in the 700 MHz band that had been used by television channels before the switch to all-digital TV in 2009.

PROCEDURES FOR EMS COMMUNICATIONS

Most EMS systems use a standard radio communications protocol. This protocol includes the desired format for message transmission and key words and phrases. This format aids professional and efficient radio communication within the system. General guidelines for radio communications include the following:

- Think before you speak (formulate the message) to ensure that the communication will be effective.
- Speak at close range (2 to 3 inches) when talking into a microphone.
- Speak slowly and clearly. Enunciate each word distinctly and avoid words that are difficult to hear.

- Speak in a normal pitch without emotion.
- Be brief and concise. Break up long messages into shorter ones.
- Avoid codes unless they are systems-approved. Avoid dialect or slang.
- Advise the receiving party when the transmission has been completed.

- Confirm that the receiving party has received the message.
- Always be professional, polite, and calm.

CRITICAL THINKING

Can you think of three reasons a concise EMS radio report is essential?

? DID YOU KNOW?

NATO Alphabet Chart

The NATO alphabet assigns code words to the letters of the English alphabet acrophonically (e.g., *alfa* for A, *bravo* for B, and so on). This system ensures uniform pronunciation of critical combinations of letters and numbers, making them more easily understood by those who transmit and receive voice messages. It also ensures the intelligibility of voice signals over radio links.

A–Alfa	**B**–Bravo	**C**–Charlie	**D**–Delta	**E**–Echo	**F**–Foxtrot
G–Golf	**H**–Hotel	**I**–India	**J**–Juliet	**K**–Kilo	**L**–Lima (*Lee-ma*)
M–Mike	**N**–November	**O**–Oscar	**P**–Papa	**Q**–Quebec	**R**–Romeo
S–Sierra	**T**–Tango	**U**–Uniform	**V**–Victor	**W**–Whiskey	**X**–Xray
Y–Yankee	**Z**–Zulu				

From North Atlantic Treaty Organization: *NATO phonetic alphabet chart.* http://74.125.95.132/search?q=cache:BFkrJ90WLsUJ:www.lindagranfield.com/ NATO_alphabet.doc+%2nato%22+Alphabet+chart%22&hl=en&ct=clnk&cd=1&gl=us&lr=lang_en. Accessed August 3, 2010.

Relaying Patient Information

A standard format of transmission may be developed as a protocol for some EMS agencies. This format allows the best use of communications systems: (1) it limits radio air time; (2) physicians can receive details quickly about the patient's condition; and (3) the chance that any critical details will be omitted is reduced (Box 5-4). (Patient assessment findings are presented in Part Five.)

Patient information can be reported to the hospital or dispatcher by radio or phone. Although the order of information delivery may vary by EMS system and scenario, the radio report should be brief and concise and should contain the following:

- Unit and personnel identification
- Description of the scene or incident
- Patient's age, gender, and approximate weight (if drug orders are needed)
- Patient's chief complaint
- Associated symptoms
- Brief pertinent history of the present illness or injury
- Pertinent medical history, medications, and allergies
- Pertinent physical examination findings, such as:
    Level of consciousness
    Vital signs
    Neurological examination
    General appearance and degree of distress
    Electrocardiogram results (if applicable)
    Diagnostic findings (e.g., serum glucose)
    Trauma index or Glasgow Coma Scale (if applicable)
    Other pertinent observations and significant findings
- Any treatment given
- Estimated time of arrival

BOX 5-4 Sample Radio Report

"This is paramedic Sanders with Medic One. We are en route to your facility with a 6 minute ETA. We have a 17-year-old female with a possible head injury. We were called to the scene for a patient who had fallen from her skateboard and struck her head. On arrival, the patient appeared drowsy and confused. Bystanders described the patient as having a seizure lasting less than 1 minute after her fall. The patient has a large hematoma on the left temporal area of her head. No other signs of trauma are noted. Pupils are equal and react to light. No medical history is available. We have the patient on 15 liters of oxygen by nonrebreather. She is immobilized with a C-collar and long spine board. I have established a 16-gauge IV in her left forearm with normal saline, TKO. She is still drowsy but rouses to voice at this time. BP 118/64, respirations are 16 and regular, pulse is 88 with normal sinus rhythm. SpO$_2$ is 99%; skin is pink, warm and dry. Lung sounds are clear. Blood sugar is 136 mg/dL. No orders requested at this time."

- Request for orders from or further questions for the medical direction physician

NOTE

The use of telemetry to transmit a patient's electrocardiogram usually is reserved for patients who require diagnosis of a 12-lead electrocardiogram (see Chapter 22). Telemetry transmission uses excessive air time. If such a transmission is warranted, 15 to 30 seconds of electrocardiogram transmission usually is adequate.

SOAP Format

Many paramedics use the **SOAP format** (see Chapter 4) or a similar method to organize their written and verbal patient reports. To review, *SOAP* is an acronym for the following:

- *Subjective data:* All patient symptoms, including the chief complaint, associated symptoms, history, current medications and allergies, and information provided by bystanders and family members.
- *Objective data:* Pertinent physical examination information, including vital signs, level of consciousness, physical examination findings, electrocardiogram results, pulse oximetry readings, and blood glucose determinations.
- *Assessment data:* The paramedic's clinical impression of the patient based on subjective and objective data.
- *Plan of patient management:* Treatment that has been provided and any requests for additional treatment.

General Procedures for the Exchange of Information

When communicating with medical direction, the paramedic should repeat all orders received from the physician. Any order that is unclear should be confirmed. The paramedic should also repeat all drug orders for confirmation.

The receiving hospital should be informed of any significant changes in the patient's status before and during transport. General procedures for the exchange of information include the following:

- Protect the patient's privacy.
- Use proper unit numbers, hospital numbers, names, and titles.
- Avoid slang and profanity.
- Use the echo procedure (repeat what was heard) when receiving directions from the dispatcher or physician.
- Obtain confirmation that the message was received.

When performing the hand-off of patient care to the receiving facility (see Chapter 6), the paramedic should make the final verbal report to the person who will be assuming responsibility for the patient. This report may be only a short update if the person receiving the patient has been following the care given in the field and en route to the emergency department. If this person is not familiar with the patient, the report should be complete. In either case, all pertinent information about the patient should be conveyed during the hand-off.

SUMMARY

- EMS communications refer to the delivery of information. The patient and scene information is delivered to other key members of the emergency response team.
- Typical EMS events have five phases: (1) the occurrence of the event; (2) detection of the need for emergency services; (3) notification and emergency response; (4) EMS arrival, treatment of the patient, and preparation of the patient for transport; and (5) EMS preparation for the next response.
- Communications is the process by which one person or group transmits meaning to others. The sender encodes a message that the receiver decodes. Four barriers to communication include the attributes of the receiver; selective perception; semantic problems; and time pressures.
- Proper verbal and written communications allows the delivery of information between the members of the emergency team, the patient, and the community. Communications should be brief, clear, and confidential.
- EMS communications involve both simple and complex systems. A simple system includes a desktop transceiver and two-way radio. Complex systems include high-power communications capabilities.

- Operation modes used in EMS communications include the *simplex mode*, which permits only one person to talk at a time; the *duplex mode*, which allows two people to converse at the same time; the *multiplex mode*, which can transmit telemetry and voice simultaneously; and *trunked systems*, which use five or more repeaters to provide communications channels in busy systems.
- The functions of an effective dispatch communications system include receiving and processing calls for EMS assistance, dispatching and coordinating EMS resources, relaying medical information, and coordinating with public safety agencies. Some emergency dispatchers provide prearrival instructions for patient care.
- In the United States, the FCC regulates communications over the radio. Paramedics must be familiar with and follow the rules and guidelines of the FCC and those of state and local regulatory agencies.
- EMS frequency ranges include VHF bands, UHF bands, and 800 MHz.
- Establishing a standard format for transmission of patient information is important. It allows the best use of communications systems: it reduces the use of radio air time; allows physicians to receive details about the patient quickly; and reduces the chance that any critical details will be omitted.

REFERENCES

1. National Highway Traffic Safety Administration: *Paramedic national standard curriculum*, Washington, DC, 1998, The Department. www.onstar.com. Accessed August 3, 2010.
2. GM continues to work to enhance U.S. and Canada's emergency response system. OnStar helps in more than 100,000 automatic crash response incidents. http://f.email.onstar.com/i/32/322163447/OnStar_100k.pdf. Accessed July 5, 2011.
3. Szilagyi A, Wallace M: *Organizational behavior and performance*, ed 5, Glenview, Ill, 1990, Addison-Wesley.
4. Federal Communications Commission: Code of regulations, Title 47. www.fcc.gov. Accessed August 4, 2010.
5. National Highway Traffic Safety Administration: *Emergency medical dispatch: national standard curriculum*, Washington, DC, 1996, US Government Printing Office.
6. APCO Institute: *Emergency medical dispatch services*, South Daytona, Fla, 2009, The Institute. www.apcointl.org/institute. Accessed 8/4/2010.
7. Public Safety Wireless Advisory Committee: Final report of the Public Safety Wireless Advisory Committee to the Federal Communications Committee, September 11, 1996. http://pswac.ntia.doc.gov/pubsafe/publications/PSWAC_AL.PDF. Accessed August 4, 2010.

SUGGESTED READINGS

Institute of Medicine, Committee on the Future of Emergency Care in the United States Health System: *Emergency medical services—at the crossroads: future of emergency care*. Washington, DC, 2007.

Stokes A: Reconciling fractured communications data: a response to the IOM report, *EMS* 36:46-55, 2007.

National Highway Traffic Safety Administration: *Emergency medical services: education agenda for the future*, Washington, DC, 1996, The Administration.

NENA Technical Standards & Documents, 03-002: Enhanced MF Signaling, E9-1-1 Tandem to PSAP, http://www.nena.org/technical/standards/w-descriptions, accessed 4-13-11.

6 Medical and Legal Issues

OBJECTIVES

Upon completion of this chapter, the paramedic student will be able to:

1. Describe the basic structure of the legal system in the United States.
2. Explain how laws affect the paramedic's practice.
3. List situations the paramedic is legally required to report in most states.
4. Describe the four elements of a claim of negligence.
5. Describe measures paramedics may take to protect themselves from claims of negligence.
6. Describe the paramedic's responsibilities regarding patient confidentiality.
7. Outline the process for obtaining expressed, informed, and implied consent.
8. Describe legal complications relating to consent.
9. Describe actions to be taken in a refusal of care situation.
10. Describe legal considerations in situations that require the use of force.
11. Describe legal considerations related to patient transportation.
12. Outline legal implications related to resuscitation and death of a patient.
13. List the paramedic's responsibilities at a crime scene.

KEY TERMS

abandonment The act of terminating medical care without legal excuse or of turning care over to personnel who do not have the training and expertise appropriate for the patient's medical needs.

administrative law Regulations developed by a government agency to provide details about the function and process of the law.

advance directive A legal document in which an individual specifies what should be done for his or her health if the person is unable to make medical decisions because of injury, illness, or lack of decisional capacity.

assault Creating apprehension; also, unauthorized handling and treatment of a patient.

battery Physical contact with a person without consent and without legal justification.

borrowed servants A legal doctrine that refers to a servant who serves two "masters" (e.g., an Emergency Medical Technician [EMT] who is employed by a municipality but who is supervised by a paramedic).

breach of duty A breach of a professional duty to act.

civil law An area of law that deals with "private" complaints brought by one person (the plaintiff) against another person (the defendant); also known as *tort law*.

common law Law that comes from societal acceptance of customs or norms of behavior over time; also known as *case law* or *judge-made law*.

compensable damages Damages awarded in a lawsuit that may include medical expenses, lost earnings, conscious pain and suffering, and wrongful death.

criminal law A type of law in which the federal, state, or local government prosecutes individuals for violating a law.

decisional capacity Patients' ability to make their own health care decisions.

defamation Saying something untrue about a person's character or reputation without legal privilege or the person's consent.

dependent practice A medical provider who provides a certain type of care that falls under the same scope of practice as a physician but that requires medical oversight.

depositions Testimonies taken under oath in places other than a courtroom.

discovery The judicial process in which documents are exchanged and depositions and interrogatives are taken.

duty to act The duty of a party to take necessary action to prevent harm to another party; this duty may be formal or contractual.

emancipation The state of being legally released from parental control and supervision.

expressed consent Verbal or written consent to treatment.

false imprisonment Intentional and unjustifiable detention of a person.

Good Samaritan laws State laws that are passed to encourage people to help others in an emergency without fear of litigation.

implied consent The presumption that an unconscious or incompetent person would consent to lifesaving care.

informed consent Consent obtained from a patient after all facts necessary for the person to make a reasonable decision have been explained.

interrogative A set of questions about a lawsuit that is answered in consultation with the party's lawyer.

invasion of privacy The release, without legal cause, of details about a patient's private life that might expose the person to ridicule, notoriety, or embarrassment.

involuntary consent Treatment granted by authority of law.

legislative law Laws made by legislative branches of government.

libel Making false statements about a person with malicious intent or reckless disregard for the falsity of the statements; includes statements made in writing or through the mass media.

malfeasance Performing a wrongful or unlawful act.

malpractice insurance Liability insurance carried by health care professionals.

mandatory reporting The requirement by law that health care professionals report certain types of cases, such as abuse and neglect.

medical malpractice Professional negligence by act or omission by health care personnel in which the care provided deviates from accepted standards of practice in the medical community and causes injury to the patient.

medical practice act A law that governs the practice of medicine.

misfeasance Performing a legal act in a manner that is harmful or injurious.

negligence Failure to use such care as reasonably prudent EMS personnel would use in similar circumstances.

nonfeasance Failure to perform a required act or duty.

protected health information (PHI) Any information about health status, provision of health care, or payment for health care that can be linked to a specific individual.

proximate cause Proof that a negligent act or lack of action caused an injury or worsened an existing injury.

punitive damages Damages awarded in a lawsuit that may be in excess of compensable damages; damages meant to punish the person at fault and to deter others from causing such harm in the future.

regulations Legal restrictions promulgated by a government authority.

scope of practice With regard to EMS personnel, the range of duties and skills paramedics are allowed and expected to perform when necessary.

settlement An agreement to accept an amount of money in exchange for a promise not to pursue a legal claim.

slander Making false verbal statements about a person.

standard of care A measure of competence of a professional.

statutes Formal written enactments of a legislative authority that governs a state, city, or county.

transcript A formal record of questions and answers that may be used during a trial.

vicarious liability A form of liability in which one person is liable for the negligent actions of another person, even though the first person was not directly responsible for the injury.

*H*istorically, only hospitals and physicians were affected by **medical malpractice**. *This is because EMS personnel were not expected to meet professional standards of patient care. However, with state and national certification, licensure, and the paramedic's role as a health care professional, medical liability for EMS personnel and their employers has become a real concern.*

LEGAL DUTIES AND ETHICAL RESPONSIBILITIES

The paramedic's legal duties are to the patient, the employer, the medical director, and the public. These duties are defined by **statutes** and **regulations** that are based on commonly accepted standards of medical care. As do other health care professionals, paramedics have ethical responsibilities in addition to legal duties. These ethical responsibilities include the following:

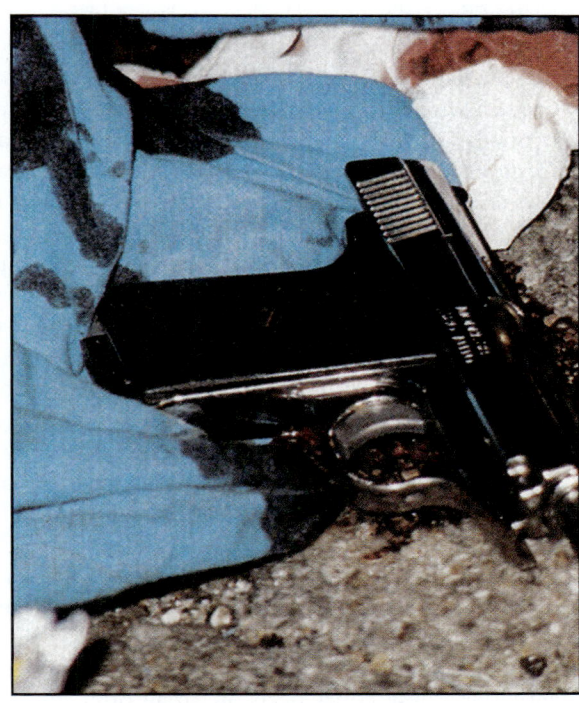

(Courtesy Ronald Olschwanger.)

- Responding with respect to the physical and emotional needs of every patient
- Maintaining mastery of skills
- Participating in continuing education and refresher training
- Critically reviewing one's own performance and taking steps to improve it
- Reporting honestly
- Respecting confidentiality
- Working cooperatively and with respect with other emergency personnel and health care professionals
- Staying current on new concepts and modalities

Failure to perform EMS duties properly can result in civil or criminal liability. As described in this chapter, the best legal protection is providing appropriate assessment and care to the patient. This care should be coupled with correct and full written documentation.

> ### NOTE
> Laws pertaining to patient care delivery vary by state. Every paramedic should be aware of the medical practice act in his or her state and other regulatory statutes that pertain to EMS. If necessary, the paramedic should consult with a private attorney experienced in EMS law or the state attorney general's office (or its equivalent) to clarify state laws and their application to EMS activities. The information in this chapter is *general* information and is not intended to be a complete guide to the legislative system, EMS laws, or regulations of any state.

THE LEGAL SYSTEM

The structure of the legal system in the United States is composed of five types of law: legislative law, administrative law, common law, criminal law, and civil law.[1]

- **Legislative law** is made by legislative branches of government. Examples of these branches are city councils, district boards, general assemblies, and Congress. The power of these bodies to make law is defined by statutes, state constitutions and, in the case of Congress, the U.S. Constitution.
- **Administrative law** refers to regulations developed by a government agency to provide details about the function and process of the law. An example is the general requirement for paramedic licensure. These regulations may address areas such as examinations, licenses, and maintenance of records. Regulatory agencies may hold disciplinary hearings on the revocation or suspension of licenses. An example of a regulatory agency is a state EMS bureau.
- **Common law** is also known as case law or judge-made law. This law is derived from societal acceptance of customs or norms of behavior over time. It is based on the decisions of judges within the state and federal judicial systems. With reference to patient care activities, these court decisions may offer guidance in defining acceptable conduct, negligence, and the

interpretation of state statutes and regulations that apply to EMS.
- **Criminal law** is a type of law in which the federal, state, or local government prosecutes individuals for violating a law. Criminal laws are enacted to protect society (a "public" complaint). Violation of criminal law may be punishable by fine or imprisonment or both.
- **Civil law** (tort law) deals with "private" complaints brought by one person (the *plaintiff*) against another person (the *defendant*). These complaints are for an illegal act or wrongdoing (*tort*) for which the plaintiff asks the court to award damages. Most EMS activities that result in litigation are civil suits.

How Laws Affect the Paramedic

As previously stated, the U.S. legal system has been active on issues relating to medical malpractice. To avoid litigation, paramedics must be knowledgeable about these issues. They also must know how these issues can affect patient care activities.

SCOPE OF PRACTICE

Scope of practice for paramedics refers to the range of duties and skills they are allowed and expected to perform when necessary. These duties are set by state law or regulation. Scope of practice defines the boundaries between the paramedic and the lay person. It also defines the boundaries between professionals (e.g., EMTs, paramedics, and physicians).[2] For example, the scope of practice for most paramedics in most states includes endotracheal intubation, administration of medications, and other basic and advanced life support procedures. If a paramedic commits a scope of practice violation, it is a criminal offense.

>
> ### CRITICAL THINKING
> Why is it necessary to define the scope of practice for a profession?

MEDICAL DIRECTION

As is explained in Chapter 1, medical direction is a required component of paramedic practice. Medical direction may be provided online (direct) or off-line (indirect), depending on state and local requirements. EMS systems also should have a policy to guide paramedics in dealing with physicians on the scene (these physicians may be known as *bystander physicians* or *physician interveners*). Some states have cards for paramedics to give to on-scene physicians. The cards officially prohibit interference with paramedics performing their duties. The use of these cards often requires legislative or regulatory support.

>
> ### LOOK AGAIN
> See Chapter 1: EMS Systems: Roles, Responsibilities, and Professionalism, pp. 17-18.

MEDICAL PRACTICE ACT

A **medical practice act** is a law that governs the practice of medicine. Medical practice acts are in place to protect the public and the health care profession. This legislation varies by state. Medical practice acts may do the following:

- Designate restricted acts that prohibit certain tasks from being performed by nonphysicians
- Authorize physicians to delegate certain tasks to non-licensed personnel
- Provide for the authorization and the withdrawal of **dependent practice;** for example, how and to what extent paramedics may perform medical acts as a function of their licensure or certification

>
> **NOTE**
> *Dependent providers* include paramedics, physician assistants, nurse practitioners, surgical assistants, certified nurse midwives, physical therapists, and other health care professionals who provide care that is within the same scope as that of physicians. Dependent providers must receive medical oversight and supervision from physicians.[3] Again, the provisions of medical practice acts vary by state.

LICENSURE AND CERTIFICATION

As is described in Chapter 1, paramedic licensure or certification (or both) may be required by state or local authorities. *Licensure* is a process of occupational regulation. In this process a government agency (e.g., a state medical board) grants permission for a person who meets established qualifications to engage in a profession. *Certification* may be granted by a governmental body (e.g., city, county, or state) or a nongovernmental certifying agency or professional association. An example of such a group is the National Registry of Emergency Medical Technicians. The terms *certification* and *licensure* often are used to refer to the same process. A certification granted by a state that confers a right to engage in a trade or profession is in fact a license.

> **CRITICAL THINKING**
> How do licensure and certification help ensure the safety of your community?

MOTOR VEHICLE LAWS

Motor vehicle laws usually define the standards for equipping and operating emergency vehicles. As do most laws, these codes vary by state. Emergency vehicle operations and motor vehicle codes are addressed further in Chapter 53.

> **NOTE**
> Criminal statutes do not always require proof of intent or intentional conduct for an action to be seen as criminal in nature. For example, an emergency vehicle crash from reckless driving may result in civil and criminal lawsuits. Excessive speed, failure to consider road and weather conditions, and improper use or nonuse of audible and visual warning devices are key areas of liability for all emergency drivers. The paramedic should be well aware of state motor vehicle codes and laws that apply to emergency vehicle operations.

MANDATORY REPORTING REQUIREMENTS

Paramedics and health care workers may be required by law to report certain cases. This is called **mandatory reporting.** Mandatory reporting usually applies to cases involving spousal abuse or abuse or neglect of children or older adults. It also include cases involving rape, sexual assault, gunshot wounds, stab wounds, animal bites, and some communicable diseases (Box 6-1). The content of the report and to whom it must be made are set by law, regulation, or policy. Local protocols set by medical direction and the EMS agency give guidance in these areas. Some states have penalties if mandatory reporting is not satisfied. Many reporting statutes provide immunity for the person reporting the situation. Immunity helps lessen the fear of legal consequences from such reporting should the report be false or unfounded. These statutes prohibit lawsuits against individuals who file reports or offer a defense in court in the event of a lawsuit.

> **CRITICAL THINKING**
> Imagine that your state requires the reporting of gunshot wounds. Your patient has a small-caliber flesh wound. The patient refuses care and begs you not to tell anyone so that her privacy will be protected. What would you do?

PROTECTION FOR THE PARAMEDIC

Some state and federal regulations provide legal protection for the paramedic. Examples include notification of exposure to infectious disease, protection provided by immunity statutes, and laws that describe special crimes against EMS personnel. These regulations vary by state and local jurisdictions.

> ### BOX 6-1 Cases Reportable under Law in Most States
>
> - Neglect or abuse of children
> - Neglect or abuse of older adults
> - Spousal abuse
> - Rape, sexual assault
> - Gunshot wounds
> - Stab wounds
> - Animal bites
> - Certain communicable diseases

Notification of Infectious Disease Exposure. The Ryan White Comprehensive AIDS Resources Emergency Act of 1990 (PL 101-381) requires that emergency responders be advised if they have been exposed to infectious diseases. These diseases include hepatitis, tuberculosis, bacterial (meningococcal) meningitis, rubella (German measles), and human immunodeficiency virus (see Chapter 28). The act also requires that employers name a designated officer to coordinate communications between the hospital and the emergency response organization in case of an exposure. The responder is to be notified within 48 hours of determination of the exposure so that postexposure management procedures can be taken.

In December, 2006, the Ryan White Treatment Modernization Act of 2006 (PL 109-415) was signed into law. The part of the law in the original act that covered notification of disease exposure to first responders was stricken from the legislation. In 2009 the language that was dropped from the bill in 2006 was reinstated.[4] In addition to the Ryan White act, many states have laws that require emergency responders to be notified if they have been exposed to an infectious disease.

> ### CRITICAL THINKING
> Reflect on the time before the Ryan White law of 1990. At that time, why would some health care facilities not report significant infectious disease exposures to EMS personnel?

Immunity Statutes. Protection of state and other government entities from litigation derives from an ancient English common law. This immunity was based on the concept that "the king can do no wrong." In modern law, this means that government agencies cannot be held liable for the negligent acts of their employees. Since the 1950s, the trend in many states has been to discard this doctrine or limit its application. In some states, for example, immunity, if exercised, may apply only to the government agency and not to the individual employee or operator of an emergency vehicle. Governmental immunity statutes vary throughout the country. Therefore, EMS personnel may or may not be protected by this statute.

All 50 states have some form of **Good Samaritan laws.** The intent of these laws is to encourage people to help others in an emergency without fear of a lawsuit. As a rule, a person who gives emergency first aid in good faith, without expecting to be paid, and in a manner that another person with similar training would, is covered by these laws. However, these laws generally do not protect health care workers from acts of gross negligence, reckless disregard, or willful or wanton misconduct. The laws also generally do not apply to paid, on-duty EMS personnel.

> ### CRITICAL THINKING
> Imagine that your state has no Good Samaritan laws. Would this affect your decision about whether to stop and aid an ill or injured person while off duty?

Special Crimes Against a Paramedic. Paramedics may become victims of *assault* or *battery* while performing their duties. To deter crimes against paramedics, some localities have enacted ordinances that provide the same level of protection for EMS personnel as for law enforcement personnel. These ordinances make it illegal to harm or threaten to harm EMS crews or to obstruct patient care. The paramedic should use good judgment and work closely with the dispatch center and police so that dangerous situations can be avoided. *Paramedics must remember that if the scene is not safe and cannot be made safe, the EMS crew should retreat from the scene and not enter the area until it has been properly secured.*

The Legal Process

An injury lawsuit against a paramedic consists of a series of specific steps (Figure 6-1). The lawsuit begins with an incident in which a person feels that he or she has been injured as a result of negligent patient care. This person is the plaintiff. The plaintiff hires an attorney who conducts a case investigation to determine the merit of the complaint. The investigation may include examining patient care reports, textbooks, journal articles, and local protocols. If the attorney believes the plaintiff's case has merit, a complaint is prepared and filed in court. The complaint outlines the negligent conduct that resulted in the alleged injury. After the complaint has been filed in court, the complaint and a summons are served on the defendant, and the litigation process is initiated. The summons usually is

Anatomy of an Injury Lawsuit

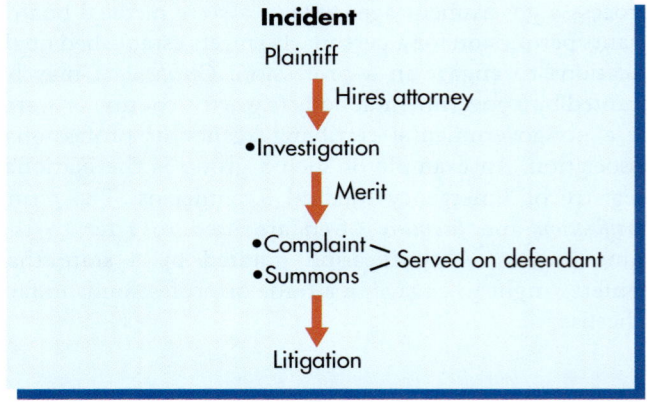

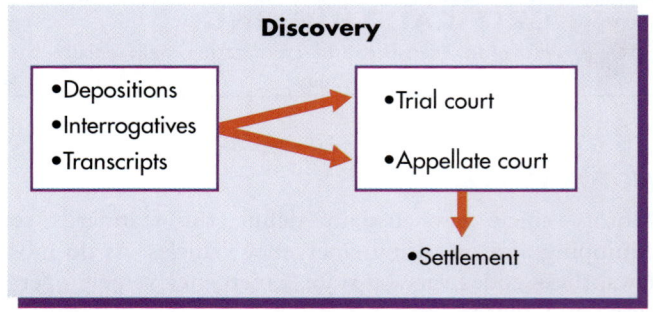

FIGURE 6-1 Anatomy of a lawsuit.

served by a sheriff or other authorized person. It requires that the defendant answer the complaint or risk automatically losing the case. At this point, the defendant and all parties involved (e.g., the paramedic, ambulance service, and hospital) usually retain an attorney to defend against the lawsuit.

The next step in the legal process is known as **discovery.** This step usually involves the exchange of documents and the taking of depositions and interrogatives. **Depositions** are testimonies taken under oath at a location other than in a courtroom. The person giving the deposition answers a list of questions from the attorney for the other side. A court reporter types the questions and answers and prepares a **transcript** that may be used during the trial. When a person gives a deposition, his or her attorney should always be present. An **interrogative** is a set of questions about the lawsuit that is answered in consultation with the party's lawyer. The interrogative then is given to the lawyer for the other side. During discovery, each side is entitled to receive all key information having to do with the lawsuit. Other documents that may be gathered during discovery are patient care reports, computer dispatch records, and recordings of radio messages related to the incident. After discovery, the case either is settled out of court or goes to trial. Quality improvement (QI) materials are "discoverable" in some states.

CRITICAL THINKING
Consider a case that occurred 5 years ago. How important would your written documentation of that case be?

During the trial, each party presents its side of the case. Based on the evidence, a judge or jury determines liability and any damages to be awarded to the plaintiff. Either side may appeal the decision of the trial court, but the appeal usually can be based only on errors in law made by the trial court.

Settlement may occur at any stage during the litigation. In settlement the plaintiff agrees to accept an amount of money in exchange for a promise not to pursue the claim. After the case is settled, it is dismissed.

NOTE
The legal process may involve both trial and appellate courts. A trial court determines the outcome of individual cases. The outcome may be determined by a judge or by a jury. The appellate court hears appeals of decisions by trial courts or other appeals courts. Decisions reached in the appellate court may set precedent for later cases of a similar nature.

LEGAL ACCOUNTABILITY OF THE PARAMEDIC

Paramedics are responsible for acting in a way that is reasonable and prudent. They should provide a level of care and transportation consistent with their education, training, and local protocol. If paramedics fail to meet these responsibilities, the result may be legal liability.

NOTE
Nearly anyone can be sued, regardless of the validity of the complaint. A lawsuit itself is not an indication of guilt or wrongdoing unless the allegations are proved.

Components of Negligence

Lawsuits involving patient care usually result from civil claims of **negligence;** that is, the failure to act as a reasonable, prudent paramedic would act in similar circumstances. In most states, four elements must be present to prove negligence: (1) a duty to act existed; (2) the actions performed were at a level that deviated from the standard of care (**breach of duty**); (3) damage to the patient or other individual (plaintiff) occurred; and (4) the breach was the proximate cause of the damage.

CRITICAL THINKING
Certain advanced life support (ALS) interventions pose a greater risk of causing harm to the patient compared with basic life support (BLS) skills. As a paramedic, what ALS interventions do you think you will perform that have this increased risk?

DUTY TO ACT

Paramedics assume a "duty" to provide emergency care when requested while working for an EMS service. This duty may be formal (contractual). The duty also may be informal (volunteer). Once a paramedic assumes the **duty to act,** the paramedic must *continue to act.* That is, the duty must not be interrupted until (1) patient care has been transferred to another health care worker whose training and experience meet the patient's needs; (2) it is abundantly clear that the patient no longer needs assistance; or (3) the patient-caregiver relationship is terminated by the patient. Among the paramedic's duties are:

- Respond and render care
- Obey laws and regulations
- Operate emergency vehicles reasonably and prudently
- Provide care and transportation to the expected standard
- Provide care and transportation consistent with the scope of practice and local medical protocols
- Continue care and transportation through to its appropriate conclusion

NOTE

The authorization of dependent practice between a physician and a paramedic may be effective only when the paramedic is on duty. Therefore, an off-duty paramedic who provides emergency care usually must act in a basic life support capacity unless the paramedic has specific authorization from medical direction to perform advanced life support procedures while off duty.

BREACH OF DUTY

As mentioned earlier, for negligence to exist, the plaintiff first must prove two of the required elements: that the paramedic had a duty to act and that the actions performed were at a level that deviated from the standard of care (breach of duty). The paramedic must exercise the degree of care, skill, and judgment that any other similarly trained paramedic would provide under similar circumstance. This **standard of care** is established by court testimony and referenced to public codes, standards, criteria, and guidelines related to the situation. Many states consider national standards when defining acceptable care. If the paramedic violated written national or state standards, the plaintiff may have a less difficult time proving breach of duty.

NOTE

The *standard of care* is a measure of competence of a professional (i.e., whether you did the right thing and did it properly). The standard of care may vary, depending on the situation; however, the scope of practice should not.[1] The standard of care differs from the *scope of practice*. The scope of practice identifies specific medical practices that are permitted by licensure, certification, or both.

Breach of duty may occur by **malfeasance** (performing a wrongful or unlawful act), **misfeasance** (performing a legal act in a manner that is harmful or injurious), or **nonfeasance** (failure to perform a required act or duty). In some cases negligence may be so obvious that it does not require extensive proof. The Latin phrase *res ipsa loquitur* means "the thing speaks for itself." This phrase implies that the facts are so clear that without a doubt the injury could have been caused only by negligence. *Negligence per se* means that negligence is shown by the fact that a statute or ordinance was violated and injury resulted.

DAMAGE TO THE PATIENT OR OTHER INDIVIDUAL (PLAINTIFF)

The third element of negligence is proof of damage; in other words, proof that the plaintiff suffered **compensable damages.** These damages may include medical expenses, lost earnings, conscious pain and suffering, and wrongful death. **Punitive damages** may be awarded in excess of compensable damages. These damages are meant to punish the person at fault and to deter others from causing such harm in the future. Punitive damages usually are not covered by

malpractice insurance (this topic is discussed later in the chapter).

PROXIMATE CAUSE

Finally, the plaintiff must prove that the negligent act or lack of action caused the injury or made an existing injury worse. This is known as **proximate cause.** The plaintiff also must prove that the injury or further harm was foreseeable by the paramedic. The element of proximate cause sometimes is difficult to establish. Proof of proximate cause often calls for expert witnesses. These witnesses address issues of duty, standard of care, and conflicting views of causation. For example, was a cervical spine injury caused by the car crash or was it the result of rescue efforts by the EMS crew? Negligent conduct is possible in areas besides direct patient care. Such areas include patient transportation to a medical facility contrary to medical direction advice, trauma center designation, or other known special patient care needs and facility capabilities. Another example is failure to maintain equipment, supplies, or vehicles. Negligent or reckless driving also is an area for potential negligent conduct.

CRITICAL THINKING

Do you think an effective quality management program can reduce the risk of negligent lawsuits? Explain your reasoning.

Defenses to Negligence Claims

Several practices provide the best protection for health care professionals against claims of negligence. They include training, competent patient care skills, and full documentation of all patient care activities. The following are other defenses to negligence and their pros and cons.

1. Good Samaritan laws
   - Generally do not protect EMS personnel from acts of gross negligence, reckless disregard, or willful or wanton misconduct.
   - Generally do not prohibit the filing of a lawsuit.
   - May provide coverage for paid or volunteer EMS personnel.
   - Vary from state to state.
2. Government immunity
   - Trend is toward limiting protection.
   - May protect only government agency, not EMS personnel.
   - Varies from state to state.
3. Statute of limitations
   - Limits the number of years after an incident during which a lawsuit can be filed.
   - Is set by law and may differ for cases involving adults and children.
   - Varies from state to state.
4. Contributory negligence
   - Plaintiff may be found to have contributed to his or her own injury.

- Damages awarded may be reduced or eliminated based on the plaintiff's contribution to the injury.

SHOW ME THE EVIDENCE

A descriptive study was performed as a retrospective review of litigation against ambulance services in England over the previous 10 years. The authors found 272 cases. The most common reason given for the lawsuit was "lack of assistance or care" followed by failure or delay in treatment or diagnosis. The authors concluded that areas on which the ambulance services should focus included obstetrical care, recognition of spinal injury, and decisions not to transport.

From Dobbe A, Cooke M: A descriptive review and discussion of litigation claims against ambulance services, *Emerg Med J* 25:455-458, 2008.

LIABILITY INSURANCE

All practicing active health care professionals should have adequate liability insurance. This is also known as **malpractice insurance.** These policies offer coverage for legal defense and potential judgments against the policyholder. Malpractice insurance falls into two groups: *primary policies* and *umbrella policies.* Primary policies are personal policies. They offer certain limits of coverage for the types of risks against which the professional is insured. For example, a policy with a $100,000 limit pays up to that amount for covered damages caused by the insured.

CRITICAL THINKING

What kind of liability insurance protects you now as an Emergency Medical Technician? What type of liability insurance protects you as a student paramedic in a clinical experience?

Umbrella policies are liability insurance policies carried by employers of paramedics. For example, an ambulance service or a hospital may carry such a policy. These policies often have additional limits of coverage. These additional limits apply to on-duty employees who perform activities within the scope of practice authorized by the employer, policy, or protocol. A $1,000,000 umbrella policy, for example, covers damages caused by the insured in excess of those limits in the underlying primary policy. The amount of coverage of such umbrella policies may vary by hospital and EMS agency. The umbrella policy may not cover the employee's liability. In such a case, a separate individual policy may be desirable. A variety of companies offer the individual insurance coverage. Group plans often are less expensive, though, and may offer better coverage than the more costly individual policies.

SPECIAL LIABILITY CONCERNS

Several liability concerns are unique to prehospital care. One issue is the liability of the medical director. Another issue is the liability for "borrowed servants." Concerns also may arise relating to civil rights.

LIABILITY OF THE PARAMEDIC MEDICAL DIRECTOR

As stated earlier, paramedics function as dependent providers under medical oversight. As a result, the medical direction physician assumes legal responsibility for the patient who receives care in the prehospital setting. This is known as **vicarious liability.** This liability may hold true for actions that are performed through online medical direction. Vicarious liability also may hold true for off-line medical direction in which care is guided by the use of physician-developed protocols and standing orders. Therefore, negligence on the part of a paramedic may become the responsibility of the medical direction physician (and the paramedic's employer) even in the absence of direct supervision.

Vicarious liability arises from the relationship between the employer and employee. It also arises by virtue of the paramedic's role as a principal agent who is authorized to perform for the benefit of another. The paramedic is not an employee of the medical direction physician per se. Still, the paramedic acts as an agent in place of the physician. For this reason, the law may regard the actions of the paramedic as a legal responsibility of the medical direction physician.

LIABILITY FOR BORROWED SERVANTS

Borrowed servants is another legal doctrine. The doctrine refers to a servant who serves two "masters." An example of this is an EMT who is employed by a municipality but supervised by a paramedic. This doctrine can create liability for the supervising paramedic. It also can create liability for the employer and the medical direction physician (through vicarious liability). The amount of liability for the supervising paramedic depends on the degree of supervision and control given to the paramedic by the employer.

The borrowed servant doctrine is based on a theory that when a person has control over someone else's employee, he or she should be responsible for that person's acts. This is the case even though no employer-employee relationship exists. Paramedics who normally have full supervisory control over EMTs must protect the patient's interests by making sure the EMTs perform patient care properly.

CIVIL RIGHTS

The first civil rights measure was enacted in 1866.[5] This law prohibited discrimination based on race. Since then, civil rights laws have been modified several times to make it illegal to discriminate by reason of race, color, gender, religion, national origin and, in the case of health care, ability to pay (Box 6-2). In the case of a municipal ambulance service, a patient could bring a claim under the civil rights act for a number of possible violations in addition to discrimination. These violations could include treatment and transport without proper consent.

Another law, the Rehabilitation Act of 1973, prohibits discrimination against handicapped people solely based on the individual's handicap. This act applies to any program

BOX 6-2   Cobra and Obra

The Consolidated Omnibus Budget Reconciliation Act (COBRA) took effect in 1986. The act now is known as the Emergency Medical Treatment and Active Labor Act (EMTALA). The act addressed the medical screening, stabilization, and transfer of patients who have emergency medical conditions or who are in active labor for Medicare-participating hospitals. The act also addressed the issue of "patient dumping," which is the transfer, diversion, or premature discharge of patients from a hospital because they are unable to pay. The act set penalties of up to $20,000 for each violation. The act was amended as the Omnibus Budget Reconciliation Act (OBRA 1989, 1990, and 1993; revised 2000 and 2003).[6] This amendment clarified and strengthened enforcement of the COBRA rules. It also raised the possible fine to $50,000 per infraction. The major provisions of OBRA include the following:

- Medical screening as it relates to the capabilities of the sending and receiving hospitals
- Stabilization of the patient at a referring hospital (legal and financial responsibility)
- Provision of appropriate transfer methods after making sure the patient's condition is stable and the person has consented to the transfer
- Definition of "appropriate transfer" as the provision of the needed level of care and resources available during the transfer
- Whistle blower protection for physician and hospital staff

or activity that receives federal funding. These programs may include EMS agencies that receive Medicare or Medicaid reimbursement. Title II of the Americans with Disabilities Act also allows for equal accessibility for public services by people with disabilities. This includes receiving appropriate patient care regardless of disease condition. For example, these conditions may include acquired immunodeficiency syndrome (AIDS), infection with the human immunodeficiency virus (HIV), tuberculosis (TB), and other communicable diseases.

Protection Against Negligence Claims

Paramedics must be aware of the ways patient care activities can pose a threat of litigation for negligence. The best protections against such claims are:

- Education, training, continuing education, and skills retention
- Appropriate quality improvement
- Appropriate medical direction, online and off-line
- Accurate, thorough documentation (see Chapter 4)
- Professional attitude and demeanor

CRITICAL THINKING

Think back to a call you took as an emergency medical technician that did not go well and in which the patient did not do well. Did that call meet any of the elements of negligence? What measures could you take to prevent the recurrence of that type of situation?

PARAMEDIC-PATIENT RELATIONSHIPS

The relationship formed between the paramedic and the patient during a patient care encounter is a legal one. Consequently, legal issues may arise from the provision of patient care. These issues include confidentiality, consent (including the occasional use of force to restrain a patient), and transportation.

Confidentiality

Paramedics have a legal and ethical duty to protect a patient's privacy. Information from a patient usually can be conveyed without the patient's consent to other health care workers involved in the patient's care. For example, such information may include a history of communicable disease. Similarly, paramedics may report to law enforcement personnel and testify in court about information obtained from a patient about an incident or crime. However, potential liability for invasion of privacy and defamation (libel or slander, discussed later) exists in some cases. For example, potential liability exists in cases in which information is released with malicious intent or reckless disregard. Potential liability also exists in cases in which **protected health information (PHI)** is released to individuals not legally entitled to the information.

HEALTH INSURANCE PORTABILITY AND ACCOUNTABILITY ACT (HIPAA)

The privacy provisions of the Health Insurance Portability and Accountability Act of 1996 (HIPAA) were published in 2003 by the Department of Health and Human Services. Compliance with the privacy rule is mandatory. The act requires all health care providers to do the following[7]:

- Protect the privacy of patients' protected health information, disclosing the minimum amount needed for treatment, billing, and operations
- Safeguard that information physically and administratively
- Grant certain rights to patients regarding that information

Compliance with HIPAA is required for all health plans (payers of health care), health care clearinghouses (facilitators of electronic data exchange between standard and nonstandard formats for payers and providers), and health care providers who conduct certain financial and administrative transactions electronically. These groups are known as *covered entities*. They must comply with certain standards regarding the protection of personal health information. They also must comply with the coding of electronic transactions. In addition, they must follow proper security measures for electronic information. EMS agencies are direct providers of health care to patients. They generate protected health records with information that identifies a person (e.g., name, Social Security number, and address). These records also contain medical information about the person (e.g., include injury or illness and treatments provided). If EMS agencies transmit or have ever transmitted this PHI electronically in connection with any of the transactions designated under HIPAA (e.g., billing or fund transfers), they are covered entities and are subject to HIPAA regulations (Box 6-3).

DEFINITION OF CONFIDENTIALITY

Information related to a patient's history, assessment findings, and any treatment rendered generally is considered confidential information. This information can be in an electronic, a written, or a verbal format. As a rule, the release of this information for purposes other than treatment, payment (e.g., filing insurance claims), or ambulance service operations requires written permission from the patient or legal guardian. Exceptions to this general rule include the following[8]:

- Federal, state, or local law that requires release of information
- Health care fraud and abuse detection
- Certain public health activities, such as reporting a birth, death, or disease, as required by law, as part of

a public health investigation; to report child or adult abuse or neglect or domestic violence; to report adverse events, such as product defects; or to notify a person about exposure to a possible communicable disease as may be required by law

- Health oversight activities, including audits or government investigations, inspection, disciplinary proceedings, and other administrative or judicial actions undertaken by the government by law to oversee the health care system
- Judicial and administrative proceedings as required by a court or an administrative order or in some cases in response to a subpoena or other legal process
- Law enforcement activities in limited situations, such as when a warrant has been issued for the request or when the information is needed to locate a suspect or stop a crime
- Military, national defense and security, and other special government functions
- To avert a serious threat to the health and safety of a person or the public at large
- Workers' compensation purposes and in compliance with workers' compensation laws
- Coroners, medical examiners, and funeral directors who need information to identify a deceased person, determine the cause of death, or to carry out their duties as authorized by law
- Organizations that handle organ procurement or organ, eye, or tissue transplantation (if the patient is an organ donor), or to an organ donation bank, as necessary to facilitate organ donation and transplantation
- Research purposes (subject to strict oversight)
- Patients who are inmates or in the custody of a law enforcement official, as needed (1) for the correctional institution to render health care; (2) to protect the patient's health or the health and safety of others; or (3) for the safety and security of the correctional institution or law enforcement

In some cases, confidential patient information may need to be released without the patient's consent. The paramedic must adhere to all reporting requirements and procedures established by state and local laws, the EMS agency, and medical direction. Even then, only the minimum necessary details should be released.

IMPROPER RELEASE OF INFORMATION

Improper release of confidential information or the release of inaccurate information can result in liability. Liability may come into play in two areas, invasion of privacy and defamation (libel and/or slander).

Invasion of Privacy. Invasion of privacy is the release, without legal justification, of details about a patient's private life that might expose the person to ridicule, notoriety, or embarrassment. For example, a paramedic is caring for a public official who was in a car crash. After the call the paramedic tells everyone at the ambulance base that the

---

BOX 6-3 Health Insurance Portability and Accountability Act (HIPAA)

The privacy provisions of the Health Insurance Portability and Accountability Act of 1996 (HIPAA) were published in 2003 by the U.S. Department of Health and Human Services. Compliance with the privacy rule is mandatory. The act requires all health care providers to do the following:

- Protect the privacy of patients' protected health information, disclosing the minimum amount needed for treatment, billing, and operations.
- Safeguard that information physically and administratively.
- Grant certain rights to patients regarding that information.

Compliance with HIPAA is required for health plans (payers of health care), health care clearinghouses (facilitators of electronic data exchange between standard and nonstandard formats for payers and providers), and health care providers who conduct certain financial and administrative transactions electronically. These groups are known as *covered entities*. They must comply with certain standards regarding the protection of personal health information. They also must comply with the coding of electronic transactions. In addition, they must keep proper security measures for electronic information.

EMS agencies are direct providers of health care to patients. They generate protected health records that have information that identifies a person (e.g., name, Social Security number, and address). These records also contain medical information about the person, such as an injury or illness and the treatments provided. If an EMS agency transmits or has ever transmitted this protected health information electronically in connection with any of the transactions designated under HIPAA (e.g., billing or fund transfers), it is a covered entity and is subject to HIPAA regulations.

Modified from National EMS Data Analysis Resource Center: *The application of HIPAA privacy to emergency medical service providers.* www.nedarc.org/HIPAA/hipaa_and_ems.htm. Accessed June 8, 2003.

official had a Nazi tattoo on his left shoulder. A custodian at the base hears the discussion and tells his wife, who works at the official's office building. The next day, a flyer is distributed with a caricature of the official in the back of an ambulance with this tattoo. Within a few days, the EMS agency is contacted by the official's attorney, who claims an invasion of privacy. (The fact that the information released is true is not a defense for invasion of privacy.)

> **NOTE**
> Invasion of privacy is different from defamation. In most cases of invasion of privacy, the information is true, but it is information a person wants to keep private. Defamation causes injury to reputation, whereas invasion of privacy causes injury to feelings.[9]

> **CRITICAL THINKING**
> Have you ever been in a situation in which you or a colleague said something about a patient that you think may have violated confidentiality? What did you do about it?

Defamation. Defamation refers to making an untrue statement about someone's character or reputation without legal privilege or the person's consent. **Libel** refers to false statements about a person made in writing or through the mass media with malicious intent or reckless disregard for the falsity of the statements. **Slander** refers to false verbal statements about a person made with malicious intent or reckless disregard for the falsity of the statements. If the paramedic in the previous example had lied about the official's tattoo, he or she and the office worker who made and distributed the flyer could be sued for libel and slander.

> **NOTE**
> In defining a defamatory statement, the courts have looked to whether the statement exposed the plaintiff to public hatred, contempt, ridicule, or degradation. Proof must exist of actual harm to the person's reputation.[8]

Consent

The rights of patients have been defined and clarified by legislation and by the judicial system through malpractice litigation. A basic concept of law and medical practice is a patient's rights. These involve the **decisional capacity** of patients and their right to choose what medical care and transport to receive.

> **CRITICAL THINKING**
> Imagine being called to care for a patient who clearly is having signs and symptoms of a heart attack but is alert and refusing care. How would you feel? What strategies would you use to try to persuade the patient to allow you to provide care and transport?

To give consent, the patient must be of legal age and must be able to make a reasoned decision about the following:

- Nature of the illness or injury
- Treatment recommended
- Risks and dangers of treatment
- Alternative treatments and associated risks
- Dangers of refusing treatment (including transport)

> **SHOW ME THE EVIDENCE**
> A study was done on whether paramedics can safely decide which patients do not need ambulance transport. Paramedics at a New Mexico EMS service were asked (before transport) to predict whether their patient could be transported by means other than ambulance. The paramedic's opinion was compared to the patient's emergency department differential diagnosis. Of the 236 calls evaluated, the paramedics thought 53% of the patients could have been transported by other means. Of that group, 24% needed ambulance transport (as defined by the study criteria). Paramedics were likely to undertriage patients in three situations; all involved abnormal vital signs, but also an unremarkable chief complaint, intoxication, or psychological problems. The authors concluded that the paramedics in the study group were not capable of making non-transport decisions safely or accurately.

From Hauswald M: Can paramedics safely decide which patients do not need ambulance transport or emergency department care? *Prehosp Emerg Care* 6:383-386, 2007.

TYPES OF CONSENT

Informed consent is patient consent that signifies the individual knows, understands, and agrees to the care rendered. This consent is given based on full disclosure of the information. Verbal or written consent to the treatment is called **expressed consent.** (Consent also can be expressed nonverbally by actions or simply by the patient allowing care to be provided.)

> **NOTE**
> Consent generally must be obtained before treatment is initiated. However, paramedics do not have to obtain the same degree of informed consent as other health care personnel. For example, in-hospital staff members must obtain a higher degree of consent. Because the paramedic is working in an emergency situation, the patient must only agree or at least must not object to the general nature of the treatment.

Implied consent presumes that an unconscious person without decisional capacity who needs emergency care would consent to lifesaving care if able to do so. Unconscious patients and victims of shock, head injury, and alcohol or other drug intoxication are examples of patients to whom emergency care should be provided in the absence of informed consent. It should be noted, however, that an adult with decisional capacity who regains consciousness can revoke consent at any time during care and transport. This commonly is seen in situations involving diabetic patients and those with seizure disorders who may choose to refuse *insulin* or anticonvulsant medicines.

Involuntary consent refers to treatment that is granted by the authority of law. An example is caring for patients who are held involuntarily for mental health evaluation. Another example is patients who may be held under arrest or who are in protective custody. The paramedic must follow established policies and procedures when providing care to these patients. (Law enforcement personnel may not order a paramedic to treat a patient who has decisional capacity and who objects to the treatment.)

SPECIAL CONSENT SITUATIONS

Situations may arise in which obtaining consent for treatment is difficult. Such cases may involve minors, adults without decisional capacity, patients in an institution, or prisoners. In such cases, consent for medical care may need to be obtained from a parent, legal guardian, representative of a state agency, or other legal authority. If a delay in obtaining consent would pose a threat to the patient's life, however, the person should be treated. EMS personnel should be familiar with state laws governing these unique circumstances and should follow agency protocols. When a situation arises with consent issues, paramedics should *always* make sure medical direction is contacted and involved in the decision-making process, and they should carefully document all events.

Minors. In most states a person is a minor until age 18. This is the case unless the person is emancipated. **Emancipation** is the legal release of an individual from parental control and supervision. Emancipation may include minors who are married, who are parents, who are in the armed forces, and who are living independently and are self-supporting. An example of the latter is college students who do not live at home or do not receive financial aid.

Unemancipated minors are those who are under parental control and supervision. These minors are not legally able to give or withhold consent (although consent should be sought before treatment). The consent of a parent, legal guardian, or court-appointed custodian usually is required. If a delay in obtaining consent would pose a threat to the minor's life, the emergency doctrine of treating and transporting the patient without consent applies. Although the courts will assume that the parents would have consented, the paramedic should thoroughly document the nature of the emergency and the reason the minor required urgent care.

Adults Without Decisional Capacity. With regard to obtaining consent, providing emergency care for adults without decisional capacity is similar to caring for minors. These patients may not be able legally to give or refuse consent. Decisional capacity may be impaired by a number of factors, such as disease, injury, anxiety, mental illness, mental retardation, and alcohol or other drug use. The patient may not be mentally or emotionally able to make sound decisions about his or her care. Therefore, the emergency doctrine of treating and transporting without consent should be applied. Emergency care should be provided without consent only when a life-threatening illness or injury exists and only when a legal guardian is not present to grant or refuse consent. The paramedic should involve medical direction in these decisions.

Prisoners or Arrestees. Incarceration or detention generally does not deny a person the right to make choices about medical treatment. However, a prisoner or arrestee may have a limb- or life-threatening injury or illness and may refuse to give consent. In these cases, the court or law enforcement agency that has the patient in custody sometimes may authorize treatment. The authority of law provides consent through the emergency doctrine. Paramedics who often provide care in prison settings should be aware of local and state laws regarding consent for this population.

Refusal of Care or Transport. An adult with decisional capacity has the right to refuse medical care. This is true even if the choice could result in death or permanent disability. Refusal of care may be based on religious beliefs, inability to pay, fear, or lack of understanding of medical procedures. Paramedics should be sensitive to these concerns; they should explain each procedure carefully and answer any questions the patient has. Documentation of this effort on the patient care report is prudent.

> **NOTE**
>
> When a patient refuses care or transport, the paramedic should try to ensure that the patient has decisional capacity. The following steps may be helpful:
>
> 1. Make a visual assessment that includes responsiveness, level of consciousness, orientation, obvious injuries, respiratory distress, and gait.
> 2. Make an initial assessment to evaluate airway, breathing, circulation, and disability.
> 3. Measure vital signs, including pulse, blood pressure, and respiratory rate and effort. Use pulse oximetry or blood glucose testing (or both) when clinically indicated.
> 4. Perform a focused examination as dictated by the patient's complaint (if any).
> 5. Make sure the patient understands the nature of his or her condition and the medical consequences of the patient's medical care decision.
> 6. Consult with medical direction and thoroughly document the event.

Involving medical direction, law officers, family members, and friends at the scene may help persuade the patient to accept care and transportation. Despite these efforts, however, some patients still refuse care. If this occurs, the paramedic should make sure before leaving that the patient understands that he or she can call again for help despite the initial refusal. In addition, family members or friends should be encouraged to stay with the patient, if possible. Cases involving refusal of care are a major cause of lawsuits against EMS agencies. The paramedic should always consult with medical direction about these cases.

When attempting to provide care to any patient who refuses care, the paramedic should thoroughly document the event. The names and addresses of others who witnessed the event should be recorded, as should all attempts to obtain consent. In addition, the paramedic should advise the patient of the medical risks of refusing care and record this advice on the patient care report (PCR). Law enforcement officers and other allied health professionals at the scene should be asked to make similar records of the event. Many EMS systems require the paramedic to obtain a "release of liability" signed by the patient and a disinterested witness. The release should note the refusal of care or of transportation, or both (Figure 6-2).

Some EMS systems require EMS crews to contact medical direction while at the scene. At that time, the paramedics review the case with the physician or physician designee. Medical direction personnel may discuss the situation with the patient while the call is recorded. This policy may be useful in suppressing legal action. However, the most critical legal document of refusal is the written PCR prepared by the paramedic.

LEGAL COMPLICATIONS RELATED TO CONSENT

Four other key legal issues are related to consent: abandonment, false imprisonment, assault, and battery. These may result in a civil or criminal violation.

Abandonment. Abandonment is the improper termination of care or the turning over of care to personnel without the training and expertise appropriate for the patient's medical needs. Abandonment may occur at the scene or when the patient is delivered to the emergency department (ED). Examples include allowing an emergency medical responder (EMR) to provide care for a patient who requires advanced life support care and placing a patient in critical condition in the care of an unlicensed ED "tech" at the receiving hospital.

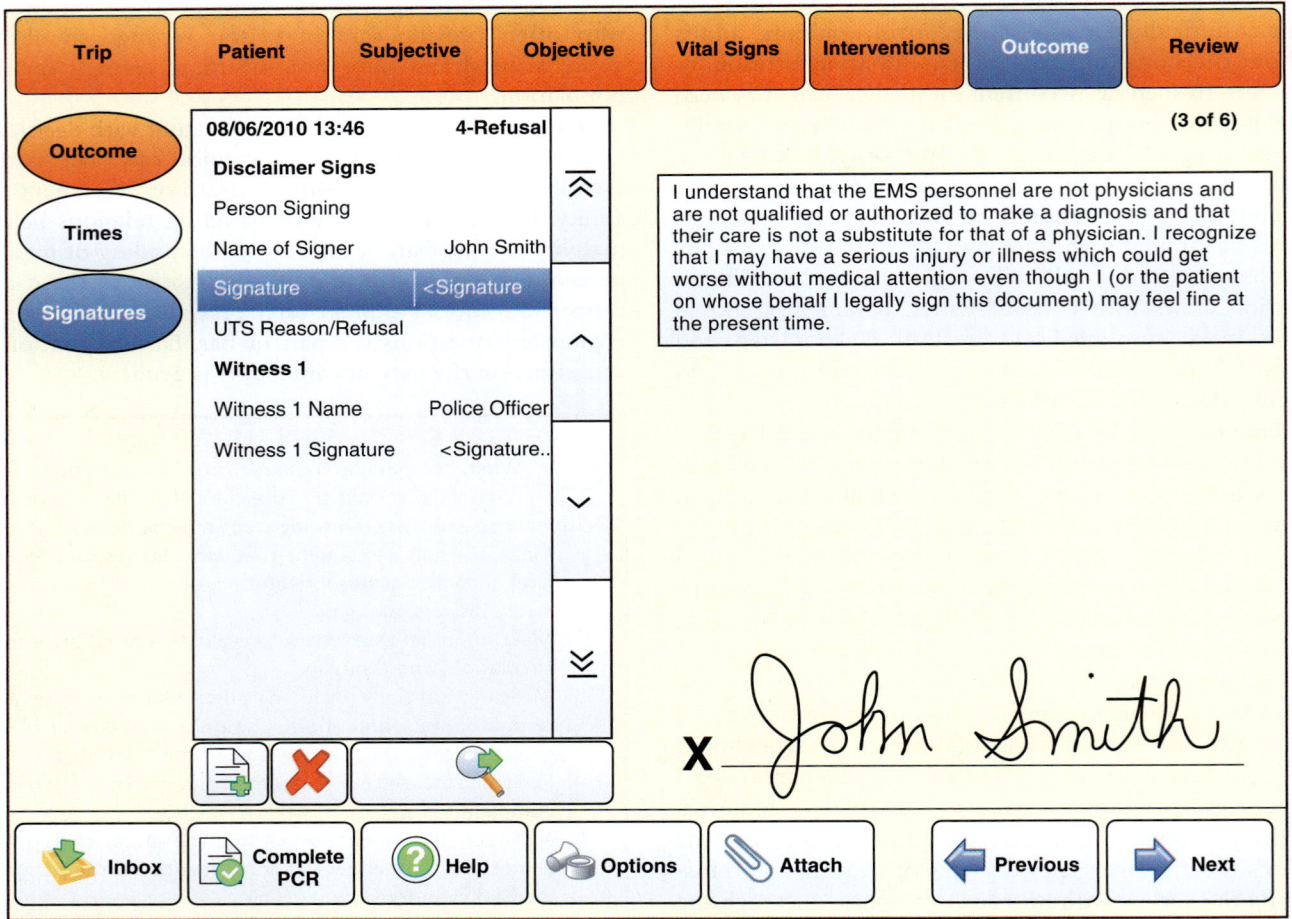

FIGURE 6-2 Electronic refusal form.

False imprisonment. **False imprisonment** is the intentional and unjustifiable detention of a person. Examples include charges brought by a patient who was transported without consent or who was restrained without proper cause or authority.

Assault. **Assault** is the creation of apprehension or the unauthorized handling and treatment of patients. An example is threatening to restrain a patient unless the patient "quiets down."

Battery. **Battery** refers to physical contact with a person without the individual's consent and without legal cause. An example is drawing a patient's blood without permission or authorization.

The paramedic can prevent problems in these other areas of liability by using good judgment. In addition, the paramedic must be sensitive to any special needs of the patient in crisis. Unusual situations or actions should be recorded on the PCR. Medical direction and law enforcement should be involved when needed.

Use of Force

Occasionally, reasonable force or restraints may be needed to deal with unruly or violent patients. These patients may be unable to make sound decisions about their care. An example is a patient with a behavioral emergency. Another example is a patient with an altered level of consciousness caused by injury, substance abuse, or illness.

Most law enforcement agencies have the authority to place a patient in protective custody, thereby permitting some patients to be treated. EMS personnel should become involved in restraining patients only when it can be done safely and there is reason to suspect that patients are a threat to themselves or others. Agency protocols should be followed when restraint of patients is necessary. Some protocols require that violent patients be put in protective custody by law enforcement personnel before paramedics become involved in patient care. The use of reasonable force to restrain a patient must always be humane and should never be punitive. (Physical restraint and the use of sedative drugs [chemical restraint] to help subdue a patient are described in Chapter 35.)

Transportation

As previously stated, once the paramedic has assumed the duty to act and has begun patient care, the paramedic must continue care until (1) the patient is transferred to another health care worker with training and expertise appropriate for the patient's medical needs; (2) the patient clearly no longer needs care; or (3) the patient ends the patient-caregiver relationship. A key aspect of this continuum of care is patient transport.

USE OF EMERGENCY VEHICLE OPERATING PRIVILEGES

In operating the emergency vehicle, the driver must conform to laws, regulations, and policies. The driver also must operate the vehicle in a manner that safeguards the patient,

crew, and public. Operators of emergency vehicles usually are given right-of-way privileges, allowing the driver to do the following:

- Travel slightly faster than the posted speed limit
- Move safely from one lane into the opposite lane of traffic
- Safely enter and pass through intersections on a red light
- Use audible and visual warning devices appropriately
- Park in unauthorized areas

> **CRITICAL THINKING**
> Your supervisor decides that exceeding the posted speed limit (even with audible and visual warning devices) is too dangerous to the community. The supervisor disallows it on all but cardiac arrest calls. What do you do?

Paramedics should be aware of the laws in their state regarding right of way and should not abuse these privileges. Excessive speed and improper use of audible and visual warning devices are examples of privileges that sometimes are abused. Most states recommend that emergency vehicles not exceed the posted limits more than 10 miles per hour during response or patient transport[10] (see Chapter 53).

CHOICE OF PATIENT DESTINATION

The choice of hospital to which the patient is taken should be based on the patient's needs and the hospital's capability. If possible, the paramedic should honor the patient's choice. Examples of limitations on hospital selection include hospitals on diversion status because of patient load and the need for specialty care that can be provided only at designated facilities (Box 6-4). Protocols for hospital selection must be established. In addition, medical direction should be involved when a patient's choice of hospital cannot be honored. For example, some EMS agencies use a "nearest hospital" rule. This may be the case even if the nearest hospital is not the facility requested by the patient.

PAYER PROTOCOLS

In some cases health care plan restrictions may affect when and where a patient can be taken for medical care. For example, Medicare, which is the largest single payer of ambulance services in the United States,[11] has complex rules about the types of services and patient transports that are eligible for reimbursement. Paramedics must have a basic understanding of these programs so that the EMS agency can be paid for its services. In addition, such knowledge helps paramedics help patients determine which services are likely to be covered by their insurance policies.

In emergencies involving a threat to life or limb, payer protocols should not be a factor in providing patient care or transportation to the closest appropriate facility. However, the paramedic must provide a full description of patient care activities on the patient care report. This is

BOX 6-4 Categorization of Hospital Resource Capabilities

The American Medical Association recommended categorization of hospital emergency services in the early 1970s. In 1990 a task force of the American College of Surgeons' Committee on Trauma published *Resources for Optimal Care of the Injured Patient* (which was revised in 1999 and amended in 2000 and 2006). The publication described three levels of trauma centers based on resources, admissions, staff, research, and education involvement.

- *Level I* institutions can provide total care for every aspect of injury. The trauma center is qualified to care for the most severely injured patient, especially in the surgical critical care setting.
- *Level II* institutions provide care that supplements treatment in level I facilities; they also serve as the primary care institutions in less populated areas.
- *Level III* institutions provide services such as assessment, resuscitation, emergency surgery, and stabilization. Patients may be transferred to higher level institutions as needed.

Note: The American College of Surgeons also has designated level IV facilities, which are primarily referral centers. Some states recognize level IV centers.

Categorization of hospital resources identifies hospitals capable of handling trauma patients. It also enables EMS personnel to transport patients rapidly to the correct medical facility. Based on the guidelines established by the American College of Surgeons, some state government agencies have designated certain institutions as trauma centers. Other specialized care facilities, such as pediatric trauma centers, burn centers, hyperbaric centers, and poison treatment centers, provide care for critically ill or injured patients with special needs.

In 1991 the Department of Health and Human Services and EMS division committees provided financial grants for states to develop comprehensive statewide trauma systems as part of the Trauma Systems Planning and Development Act of 1990. These grants were last awarded in 1994.

the agreement of family members, or approval of physicians. As a rule, patients who are pulseless should be resuscitated (unless directed otherwise by a physician), until one of the following occurs[12]:

- Restoration of effective, spontaneous circulation and ventilation
- Transfer of care to a senior emergency medical professional
- The presence of reliable criteria indicating irreversible death
- The health care provider is unable to continue because of exhaustion or dangerous environmental hazards or because continued resuscitation places the lives of others in jeopardy
- A valid DNAR order is presented
- Online authorization from the medical control physician or by prior medical protocol for termination or resuscitation

According to the American Heart Association, unwitnessed deaths in the presence of known serious, chronic, debilitating disease or in the terminal state of fatal illness may be a reliable criterion in some settings to believe that CPR is not indicated. CPR also is not indicated for traumatic arrests with extended response or transport times.[12] At some emergency scenes, the paramedic may have difficulty determining whether resuscitation should be initiated. For example, a family member may request CPR for a patient despite the existence of a No CPR order (Box 6-5). In this situation (or if the paramedic suspects that the No CPR order is invalid), the paramedic should initiate resuscitation and contact medical direction.

 CRITICAL THINKING
You are called to care for a debilitated older adult in full cardiac arrest. The family members tell you that they want nothing done and are sobbing and begging you not to resuscitate the patient. They do not have the written documentation needed by your agency to permit the do not resuscitate order. What do you do? How would you feel about your decision?

crucial; some claims are rejected for reimbursement because of poor documentation.

RESUSCITATION ISSUES

Issues involving resuscitation are complex. They often pose certain legal and ethical considerations for the patient, family, EMS crew, and medical direction. Resuscitation issues that relate directly to EMS include withholding or stopping resuscitation (termination of resuscitation [TOR]), advance directives, potential organ donation, and death in the field.

Withholding or Stopping Resuscitation

As stated previously, informed adult patients with decisional capacity have the right to refuse medical care, including cardiopulmonary resuscitation (CPR). This right does not depend on the presence or absence of terminal illness,

In most circumstances, paramedics should err on the side of providing resuscitation and life support if any issue is unclear. If evidence later indicates that resuscitation should be withheld, life support measures can be stopped.

The determination to stop resuscitation in the prehospital setting should be made by EMS authorities and medical directors, who generally should ensure the following:

- Tracheal intubation has been successfully performed.
- Intravenous access has been achieved, and rhythm-appropriate medications and countershocks for ventricular fibrillation or pulseless ventricular tachycardia have been administered according to advanced cardiac life support protocols.

BOX 6-5 Do Not Resuscitate (DNR) Orders

Orders that specify no cardiopulmonary resuscitation (CPR) attempts (i.e., do not resuscitate [DNR] and do not attempt resuscitation [DNAR]) are the result of a decision made between the patient and the physician that CPR should be withheld in the event of cardiac arrest. However, such orders do not limit other forms of treatment, such as oxygen, fluid replacement, and drug administration. Some nursing home orders specify the levels of care and support to be provided; for example, the orders may specify no intubation.

BOX 6-6 Cardiac Terminology*

Agonal: A cardiac rhythm frequently seen as the last rhythm in an unsuccessful resuscitation attempt; also called "dying heart" rhythm.

Asystole: The absence of mechanical and electrical activity in the heart.

Countershock: A high-intensity, short-duration electrical shock applied to the area of the heart.

Ventricular fibrillation/pulseless ventricular tachycardia: Pulseless rhythms of the heart.

*See Chapter 22 for a more detailed discussion of cardiac conditions.

- Persistent asystole or agonal electrocardiographic patterns are present, and no reversible causes have been identified (Box 6-6).

Advance Directives

In 1991 a federal law known as the Patient Self-Determination Act of 1990 was passed. The law required all facilities that accept Medicare or Medicaid to recognize any kind of **advance directive.** Examples of such directives are a *durable power of attorney for health care* and a *do not resuscitate order* (Figure 6-3). These legal documents are executed to inform health care personnel of a patient's wishes in the event the person becomes incapacitated and unable to convey these wishes directly. The person's wishes may include treatment or the withholding of treatment. Many states also have passed legislation regarding *living wills* and the *right to die with dignity*. These laws are for patients with a terminal illness.

The EMS service must work closely with medical direction to develop procedures and protocols that help EMS personnel contend with these laws and policies. Advance directives should not be confused with No CPR orders. Advance directives require interpretation by a physician and must be formulated into a treatment plan. This treatment plan may include No CPR orders consistent with the patient's wishes. Medical direction must establish and implement policies for dealing with advance directives.

The EMS crew may be dispatched to a dying patient who has asked not to be resuscitated. In such a case, the crew

should contact medical direction immediately so that decisions can be made about the patient's care. If medical direction determines that the patient is not to receive medical intervention to prolong life, paramedics should provide reasonable measures of comfort. Emotional support to family members and loved ones also is important during this time.

NOTE

EMS and medical direction should work closely with the families and physicians of terminally ill patients in private homes and hospice programs. This allows these individuals to make appropriate use of the EMS system and to know when to call 9-1-1. Even though resuscitation may not be indicated, EMS personnel may be needed to manage pain and to treat an acute medical illness or a traumatic injury and to provide transport to a hospital. Policies must be set and adopted by local or state EMS authorities to allow people to decline resuscitation attempts but still have access to other emergency medical care and ambulance transport.

Potential Organ Donation

Each day in the United States, about 77 people receive organ transplants. However, 19 people on the waiting list die because not enough organs are available (Box 6-7).[13] The donation of organs and tissues and the transplantation process are complex. Donation and transplantation require the effort of many health care professionals. Paramedics can play a key role in the evaluation of potential donors by identifying appropriate patients, establishing communication with medical direction, and providing emergency care to help maintain viable organs.

Identifying likely donors who are dead or near dead is a vital role for EMS agencies in organ procurement. Paramedics can identify a donor by searching for a donor card (Figure 6-4). They also can look for a notation on a driver's license that indicates the person's intent to be a donor or not to be a donor. Another method is to talk with next of kin about the patient's intent to donate tissue or organs at death (Box 6-8). Even if the patient has no donor card or other document, the family still has the right to make the decision to donate. Tissue procurement organizations provide special training for EMS personnel that can teach them how to approach the family about organ donation.

Once the patient has been identified as a potential donor, paramedics should contact medical direction. Then the proper organ procurement agencies should be notified. These agencies are staffed 24 hours a day to assist in all aspects of the donation, including gathering the proper documentation. The paramedic should carefully and thoroughly record all patient care activities, vital sign assessments, and scene events (e.g., presence of drug paraphernalia) that may affect the agency's evaluation of the potential donor.

Donations usually are separated into two groups: vital, or heartbeating, donors; and the more common donor who

OUTSIDE THE HOSPITAL DO-NOT-RESUSCITATE (OHDNR) ORDER

I, _____, authorize emergency medical services personnel to
(name)
withhold or withdraw cardiopulmonary resuscitation from me in the event I suffer cardiac or respiratory arrest. Cardiac arrest means my heart stops beating and respiratory arrest means I stop breathing.

I understand that in the event that I suffer cardiac or respiratory arrest, this OHDNR order will take effect and no medical procedure to restart breathing or heart functioning will be instituted.

I understand this decision will **not** prevent me from obtaining other emergency medical care and medical interventions, such as intravenous fluids, oxygen or therapies other than cardiopulmonary resuscitation such as those deemed necessary to provide comfort care or to alleviate pain by any health care provider (e.g. paramedics) and/or medical care directed by a physician prior to my death.

I understand I may revoke this order at any time.

I give permission for this OHDNR order to be given to outside the hospital care providers (e.g. paramedics), doctors, nurses, or other health care personnel as necessary to implement this order.

I hereby agree to the "Outside The Hospital Do-Not-Resuscitate" (OHDNR) Order.

Patient – Printed or Typed Name	Date
Patient's Signature or Patient Representative's Signature	Date

REVOCATION PROVISION

I hereby revoke the above declaration.

Patient's Signature or Patient Representative's Signature	Date

I AUTHORIZE EMERGENCY MEDICAL SERVICES PERSONNEL TO WITHHOLD OR WITHDRAW CARDIOPULMONARY RESUSCITATION FROM THE PATIENT IN THE EVENT OF CARDIAC OR RESPIRATORY ARREST.

I affirm this order is the expressed wish of the patient/patient's representative, medically appropriate and documented in the patient's permanent medical record.

Attending Physician's Signature (**Mandatory**)		Date
Attending Physician – Printed or Typed Name	Attending Physician's License No.	Attending Physician's Telephone No.
Address – Printed or Typed		Facility or Agency Name

THIS OHDNR ORDER SHALL REMAIN WITH THE PATIENT WHEN TRANSFERRED OUTSIDE THE HEALTH CARE FACILITY.

Emergency Medical Services personnel shall not comply with an outside the hospital do-not-resuscitate order when the patient or the patient's representative expresses to such personnel in any manner, before or after the onset of a cardiac or respiratory arrest, the desire to be resuscitated or if the patient is or is believed to be pregnant.

Statutory citation 190.600-190.621 RSMo
9/07

FIGURE 6-3 Advance directive.

BOX 6-7 The Wait for Organ Transplantation

Every 16 minutes, a new name is added to the national transplant waiting list. The following statistics reflect the national patient waiting list for organ transplant on July 1, 2011, as reported by the United Network for Organ Sharing (UNOS). UNOS is a private, nonprofit organization that has a contract with the federal government to manage the nation's organ transplant system.

Transplant Type	Patients Waiting
Heart	3208
Heart-lung	65
Intestine	252
Kidney	95,274
Kidney-pancreas	2255
Liver	17,060
Lung	1817
Pancreas	1387
Total	**121,318***

*UNOS policies allow patients to be listed with more than one transplant center (multiple listing); therefore the number of registrations is greater than the actual number of patients. Also, some patients are waiting for more than one organ; therefore, the total number of patients is lower than the sum of patients waiting for each organ.

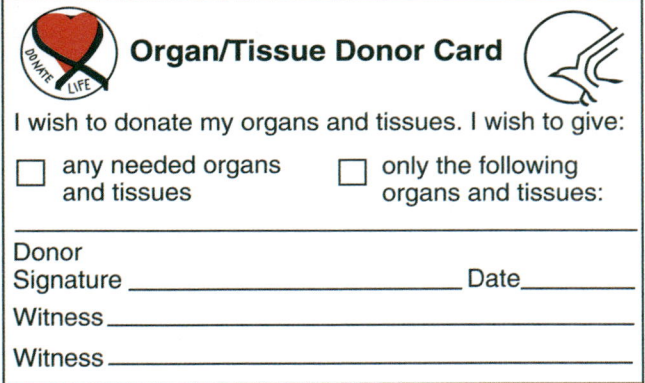

I wish to donate my organs and tissues. I wish to give:

☐ any needed organs and tissues ☐ only the following organs and tissues:

_____

Donor
Signature _____ Date_____

Witness_____

Witness_____

FIGURE 6-4 Organ donor card.

BOX 6-8 Legal Next of Kin

When a patient dies in the prehospital setting, organ and tissue donation should be offered as the final option to the surviving family members. This option should be offered regardless of the decision to transport the patient to the hospital. Obtaining consent for organ or tissue donation is a delicate subject. The paramedic should approach the issue with compassion and in a positive manner. When approaching a family for organ donation, the paramedic must obtain consent from the next of kin. This relationship is defined by law. The accepted legal order is as follows:

1. Spouse (even if separated but not divorced)
2. Adult son or daughter (over age 18)
3. Parents (for any unmarried child)
4. Siblings (in the event both parents are deceased and the donor is unmarried or divorced with no adult children)
5. Legal guardian

has no heartbeat (nonvital tissue donor). Vital donors may donate the heart, liver, kidneys, lungs, and pancreas. These donors must meet the criteria for brain death (Box 6-9). In addition, the donor's heartbeat and circulation must be maintained until the vital organs have been harvested. The nonvital (no heartbeat) tissue donor can donate corneas, skin, bones, tendons, heart valves, and saphenous veins up to 24 hours after cardiac death.

The paramedic plays a key role in helping to maintain viable organs in the prehospital setting by preserving organ function. This is accomplished by airway management and by proper fluid resuscitation to maintain blood pressure and organ perfusion (see Chapter 36). For all nontransported individuals who die at the scene, eye care should be provided using lubrication and saline solution or a commercial product (e.g., Lacri-Lube). In addition, the eyes should be taped closed so that donation of the cornea can continue to be an option for the family.

Death in the Field

Policies for determining death in the field should be established by medical direction in accordance with state and local protocols. Determination of death usually is confirmed by the following signs:

- No spontaneous electrical activity in the heart, as confirmed by an electrocardiogram in several leads
- No spontaneous respirations
- Absent cough and gag reflex
- No spontaneous movement
- No response to painful stimuli
- Fixed and midpoint pupils

Other signs also used to determine death include the presence of dependent lividity and rigor mortis (Box 6-10). When paramedics encounter an apparent death in the field, they should do the following:

- Contact medical direction and follow established state and local protocols
- Document any observations or unusual findings at the scene
- Notify appropriate authorities per protocol (e.g., the police and the coroner)
- Disturb the scene as little as possible
- Provide emotional support to surviving family members and loved ones at the scene

BOX 6-9 Criteria for Brain Death

Brain death has been defined as the state of an individual who has sustained either (1) irreversible cessation of circulatory and respiratory functions or (2) irreversible cessation of all functions of the entire brain, including the brain stem.[14] These clinical findings usually are confirmed in the hospital by electroencephalogram or a brain flow scan. In most states, brain death must be declared by two separate physicians, and neither physician can be involved in the removal or transplantation of the organs.

BOX 6-10 Physiological Changes That Occur after Death

Within minutes after death, postmortem changes begin to occur in the body. The surface of the skin becomes pale and yellowish; body temperature falls and reaches that of the environment within 24 hours; blood pressure and muscle tension decrease; and the pupils become dilated. Blood and fluids begin to drain away from the face, nose, and chin as gravity causes blood to settle in the most dependent (i.e., lowest) tissues. This drainage results in a bluish purple discoloration in the tissues known as *postmortem lividity*.

Within 6 hours after death, muscle stiffening occurs as a result of chemical changes in the body. This is known as *rigor mortis*. Smaller muscles in the face usually are affected first. Rigor mortis is followed by a stiffening of the entire body within 12 to 14 hours. Signs of tissue decay usually are obvious within 24 to 48 hours after death, depending on environmental temperatures. Rigor mortis diminishes and the body becomes flaccid within 12 to 14 hours. As the body decays, the skin loosens from the underlying tissues, and swelling and bloating become evident.

CRIME SCENE RESPONSIBILITIES

Paramedics play two important roles in the management of crime and other incident scenes. The first is to provide patient care (the primary focus). The second is to help preserve evidence at the scene when possible. Personal safety always is the first priority in any emergency response. If the scene is not safe and cannot be made safe, the EMS crew should not enter the area until it has been secured by the appropriate personnel.

CRITICAL THINKING

Consider this scenario: At the scene of a shooting, you see a patient with slow, gasping respirations; however, the police will not let you enter the crime scene. How do you think you would feel? What would you do?

When responding to a crime scene, paramedics should be in direct radio communication with law enforcement officers at the scene. This provides the paramedics with information on scene safety, the number of patients, and the need for additional resources, which may include more EMS vehicles or personnel, air medical transport, fire service or specialized rescue units, and hazardous materials teams. If the police are not on the scene or if the EMS crew is the first to respond, paramedics should maintain contact with the dispatch center so that appropriate information can be relayed to law enforcement officials. Paramedics must always keep in mind that law enforcement officers are in charge of the crime scene; paramedics are in charge of patient care. EMS crews should work closely with law enforcement officers, who also provide protection for the EMS crew.

BOX 6-11 Crime Scene Preservation

Lifesaving procedures always take precedence over forensic considerations. However, the paramedic should disturb the scene as little as possible so as to help preserve evidence. Some forensic considerations include the following:

- Park the ambulance away from skid marks, tire prints, or other evidence.
- Follow the same path to and from the ambulance and patient.
- Avoid stepping on blood stains.
- Do not touch or move weapons or other environmental clues unless absolutely necessary for patient care.
- Document the exact condition of the patient and the wound's appearance on arrival at the scene, including the environment of the patient and the body's position in relation to objects and doorways.
- If possible, cut or tear clothing along a seam to avoid altering tears made by a penetrating object. Do not cut through a hole made in the clothing by a wounding object.
- Do not shake clothing; keep all clothing in a paper bag rather than a plastic bag that may alter evidence; do not give clothing to the victim's family members.
- Save any avulsed tissue for forensic pathological examination.
- If a bullet is retrieved, place it in a padded container to prevent marring and secure the evidence until it is delivered to the authorities; obtain a receipt.
- Document any dying declarations made by patients.
- Report all actions and alterations made to the crime scene to the police.

In addition to providing patient care, the paramedic should observe and document the overall scene and make an effort to protect potential evidence (Box 6-11). Steps for ensuring scene safety include the following:

- Approach the scene only after it has been secured
- Approach the scene from a direction that appears safe and allows for easy exit
- Maintain constant radio contact with the police or dispatch
- Survey and assess the scene before approaching the patient
- Keep all unnecessary individuals away from the patient
- Initiate conversations with bystanders only when necessary

DOCUMENTATION

As described in Chapter 4, the PCR serves several functions. A particularly important function is providing a legal record of the patient care delivered in the field. The report also becomes a permanent part of the patient's hospital record.

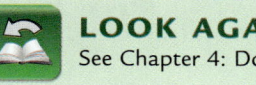

LOOK AGAIN

See Chapter 4: Documentation, pp. 63-67.

In the legal professions, the general belief is that "if it was not written down, it was not done." The paramedic's record of an emergency call is one of the first items reviewed in the case of a lawsuit for negligence or malpractice. Memory is faulty. Moreover, claims may not be filed until years after an event. As a result, EMS personnel may be expected to testify to events years after they occurred. Paramedics are allowed to refer to written reports to refresh their memory about details while testifying. Therefore, accuracy and attention to detail are crucial in documentation. The characteristics of an effective PCR include the following:

- *It is completed promptly.* The PCR is a record made "in the course of business" not long after the event. Timely completion is essential to the PCR becoming part of the hospital record.
- *It is completed thoroughly.* The PCR should cover assessment, treatment, and other relevant facts. The report should paint a complete, clear picture of the patient's condition and the care provided.
- *It is completed objectively.* The paramedic should make observations and not assumptions or conclusions. The use of emotional and value-laden words or phrases should be avoided.
- *It is completed accurately.* Descriptions should be as precise as possible; the paramedic should not use abbreviations or jargon that is not commonly understood.
- *It is written so as to maintain confidentiality.* The paramedic should follow policy for the release of patient information. When possible, the paramedic should obtain the patient's consent before the release. All records, whether paper or electronic, should be stored in a secure location with access limited by department policy.

All patient care records must be maintained in a secure location at least for the duration of the statute of limitations. This statute varies by state from 2 to 6 years for personal injury lawsuits. Patient records involving minors may have to be kept for a longer time, because the statute of limitations may not begin until the minor is 18 years of age. (This also varies from state to state.)

> **CRITICAL THINKING**
>
> Think back to the first call you were on when a patient refused medical care. Can you remember exact details of his level of consciousness, what you told him about the risks of refusing care, and what you told him to do if the problem got worse? Do you think all those facts are in the written documentation of that call in the event of litigation?

SUMMARY

- The structure of the legal system in the United States is composed of five types of law: legislative law, administrative law, common law, criminal law, and civil law. The law requires that paramedics perform within their scope of practice and follow all legal guidelines applicable to their practice.
- To safeguard against litigation, paramedics must be knowledgeable about legal issues. They also must know about the effects of these issues.
- Paramedics and health care workers may be required by law to report some cases. These include cases of abuse or neglect of children and older adults and spousal abuse. They also include cases involving rape, sexual assault, gunshot wounds, stab wounds, animal bites, and some communicable diseases.
- Some states and federal agencies require notification of EMS personnel of exposure to infectious disease. Also, some states have passed immunity statutes, as well as laws that describe special crimes against EMS personnel.
- Lawsuits related to patient care usually result from civil claims of negligence. This refers to the failure to act as a reasonable, prudent paramedic would act in such circumstances.
- Most legal authorities stress that protection against claims of negligence has three elements: the first is training; the second is competent patient care skills; and the third is full documentation of all patient care activities.
- For the most part, confidential information includes any details about a patient that are related to the patient's history. Any assessment findings also are included, as is any treatment given. As a rule, the release of these details requires written permission from the patient or legal guardian. (There are some exceptions.)
- A mentally competent adult with decisional capacity has the right to refuse medical care. This is true even if the decision could result in death or permanent disability.
- Four legal complications related to consent are abandonment, false imprisonment, assault, and battery.
- An adult patient with decisional capacity has certain rights. The patient has the right to decide what medical care (and transportation) to receive. This is a basic concept of law and medical practice.
- Legal responsibility for the patient continues until patient care is transferred to another member of the health care system or the patient clearly no longer requires care. Legal issues related to patient transport include the level of care during transportation, use of

Continued

the emergency vehicle operating privileges, choice of patient destination, and payer protocols.

- Resuscitation issues that relate directly to EMS personnel include withholding or stopping resuscitation, advance directives, potential organ donation, and death in the field.
- EMS personnel play two important roles when responding to a crime scene: focusing on patient care and preserving evidence at the scene when possible.
- In the legal field, the general belief is that "if it was not written down, it was not done." Therefore, thoroughness and attention to detail are vital in documentation.

REFERENCES

1. Burnham W: *Introduction to the law and legal system of the United States*, ed 4, St Paul, Minn, 2006, Thomson West.
2. National Highway Traffic Safety Administration: *The National EMS Scope of Practice Model*, Washington, DC, 2005, The Administration.
3. Hafter J, Fedor V: *EMS and the law*, Boston, 2003, Jones & Bartlett.
4. Ryan White Care Act Extension Success, October 2009, *EMS Insider* 36:(10), 2009.
5. Jefferies J, Karlan PS, Low PW, et al: *Civil rights actions: enforcing the Constitution*, ed 2, New York, 2007, Foundation Press.
6. *Emergency Medical Treatment and Active Labor Act.* www.emtala.com/law/index.html. Accessed August 31, 2010.
7. US Department of Health and Human Services: *Summary of the HIPAA privacy rule.* www.hhs.gov/ocr/privacy/hipaa/understanding/summary/index.html. Accessed July 17, 2010.
8. American Medical Association: *Patient confidentiality.* www.ama-assn.org/ama/pub/physician-resources/legal-topics/patient-physician-relationship-topics/patient-confidentiality.html. Accessed July 17, 2010.
9. Aiken TD: *Legal and ethical issues in health occupations*, ed 2, St Louis, 2009, Saunders.
10. National Highway Traffic Safety Administration: *Emergency vehicle operator course (ambulance): instructor guide, national standard curriculum*, Washington, DC, 1995, The Administration.
11. US Government Accountability Office (GAO): *Ambulance providers: costs and expected Medicare margins vary greatly*, Washington, DC, 2007, The GAO.
12. American Heart Association: American Heart Association guidelines for cardiopulmonary resuscitation and emergency cardiovascular care, *Circulation* 122(18 suppl):S639-S946, 2010.
13. US Department of Health and Human Services: *Organ donation*. www.organdonor.gov. Accessed August 26, 2010.
14. Guidelines for the determination of death: report of the medical consultants on the diagnosis of death to the President's Commission for the Study of Ethical Problems in Medicine and Biochemical and Behavioral Research, *JAMA* 246:2184-2186, 1981.

7   Ethics

OBJECTIVES

Upon completion of this chapter, the paramedic student will be able to:

1. Define ethics and bioethics.
2. Distinguish between professional, legal, and moral accountability.
3. Outline strategies for resolving ethical conflicts.
4. Describe the role of ethical tests in resolving ethical dilemmas in health care.
5. Discuss specific prehospital ethical issues, including the allocation of resources, decisions surrounding resuscitation, confidentiality, and consent.
6. Identify ethical dilemmas that may arise with regard to care in futile situations, the obligation to provide care, patient advocacy, and the paramedic's role as physician extender.

KEY TERMS

autonomy The principle of self-determination; that is, a person's ability to make moral decisions, including those affecting personal medical care.

beneficence A duty to confer benefits; the practice of good deeds; an obligation to benefit others or to seek their good.

bioethics The systematic study of moral dimensions, including the moral vision, decisions, conduct, and policies of the life sciences and health care.

ethics The discipline relating to right and wrong, moral duty and obligation, moral principles and values, and moral character; a standard for honorable behavior designed by a group with expected conformity.

morals Social standards or customs; dealing with what is right or wrong in a practical sense.

unethical Conduct that fails to conform to moral principles, values, or standards.

Ethical dilemmas will always be a part of prehospital care. At times paramedics must perform duties that may involve conflicts in moral judgment. Examples include issues of patient confidentiality, patient's rights, and honoring a do not resuscitate order. Such ethical issues are dynamic. The ethical dilemmas of today may be decided by law tomorrow.

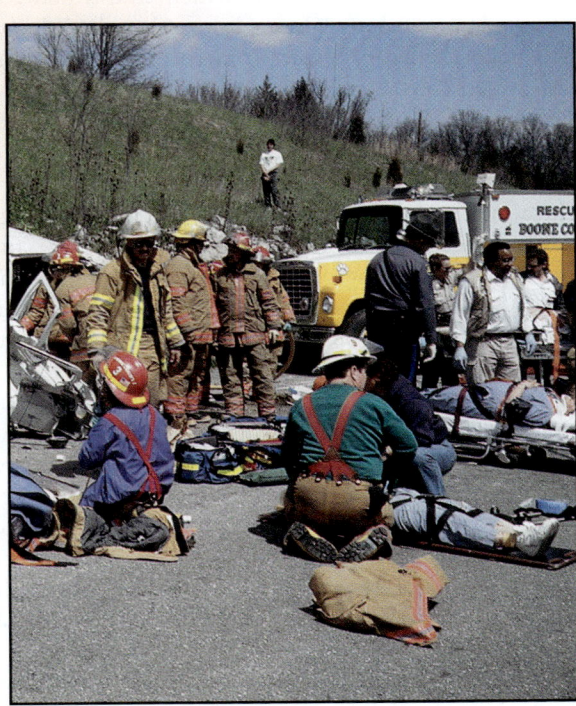

(Courtesy Ken Hines, Columbia, Mo.)

ETHICS OVERVIEW

Ethics is the field relating to right and wrong, duty and obligation, principles and values, and character.[1] Ethics is a basis for honorable actions designed by a group with expected conformity. **Morals** refer to social standards or customs, or dealing with what is right or wrong in a practical sense. The term **unethical** refers to conduct that fails to conform to these moral principles, values, or standards.[2] Ethical decisions are based on an appraisal of moral judgments—a concept that places the responsibility on individuals.

DID YOU KNOW?
The Difference Between Morals and Ethics

The difference between morals and ethics can seem confusing. The two concepts have similarities, but a basic, subtle difference exists. *Morals* define personal character. *Ethics* stresses a social system in which those morals are applied. In other words, ethics points to standards or codes of behavior expected by the group to which a person belongs. This could be the ethics of a social group, a religion, a company, a profession, or even a family. Therefore, although a person's moral code usually is unchanging, the ethics that the person practices can depend on the groups to which he or she belongs.

To help clarify the difference between morals and ethics, consider the following examples:

- *Example 1:* A defense attorney must defend a man she believes is guilty of murder. The attorney believes that murder is wrong and immoral and that this person would be a danger to society if found not guilty and released. However, the legal system and the ethics of the profession to which she belongs require that her client be defended as vigorously as possible. He also must receive a fair trial. In this case, the attorney's ethics must override her personal morals.
- *Example 2:* You teach your child that it is wrong to steal. That becomes the child's moral code. The fact that your child does not steal when given the opportunity is an example of the child's ethics.

The concept of ethics dates back to the ancient Greek philosophers, such as Hippocrates, Socrates, Plato, and Aristotle. They turned the focus toward questions of ethics and virtue (how one should live) for moral accountability and away from choice and fate, which traditionally had been guided by astrology. These philosophers laid the basis for a science of medical ethics (bioethics), the analysis of choice in medicine (Box 7-1).[3]

Bioethics is the systematic study of moral dimensions, including the moral vision, decisions, conduct, and policies of the life sciences and health care. Bioethics uses a variety of ethical methodologies in an interdisciplinary setting.

Many ethical and other value choices can be made instinctively, by drawing on longstanding personal beliefs, commitments, and habits. For example, most people believe it is wrong to steal, to be deceitful, or to commit murder. In health care, however, paramedics are faced with life issues that involve a patient. The patient may have beliefs, commitments, and habits that may be different from the paramedic's personal experience. Throughout history, guidance in these situations has been provided through a variety of professional codes. These codes represent the collective wisdom of a group. The EMT Code of Ethics and the American Medical Association's Principles of Medical Ethics are examples of professional codes (Boxes 7-2 and 7-3).

As with professional codes, an individual's personal code of ethics consists of principles of proper conduct. These values can help one make moral choices. A personal code is

BOX 7-1 The Earliest Hippocratic Oath

The Oath of Hippocrates is a brief statement of principles. It is thought to have been conceived during the fourth century BC. The oath protected the rights of the patient. It also addressed the moral character of the physician as a healer. The Hippocratic oath was modified in the tenth or eleventh century to eliminate reference to pagan gods. The oath remains an expression of ideal conduct for the physician.

I swear by Apollo the physician and Asclepius and Hygieia and Panacea and all the gods and goddesses, making them my witnesses, that I will fulfill according to my ability and judgment this oath and this covenant:

To hold him who has taught me this art as equal to my parents and to live my life in partnership with him, and if he is in need of money to give him a share of mine, and to regard his offspring as equal to my brothers in male lineage and to teach them this art—if they desire to learn it—without fee and covenant; to give a share of precepts and oral instruction and all the other learning to my sons and to the sons of him who has instructed me and to pupils who have signed the covenant and have taken an oath according to the medical law, but to no one else.

I will apply dietetic measures for the benefit of the sick according to my ability and judgment; I will keep them from harm and injustice.

I will neither give a deadly drug to anybody if asked for it, nor will I make a suggestion to this effect. Similarly I will not give to a woman an abortive remedy. In purity and holiness I will guard my life and my art.

I will not use the knife, not even on sufferers from stone, but will withdraw in favor of such men as are engaged in this work.

Whatever houses I may visit, I will come for the benefit of the sick, remaining free of all intentional injustice, of all mischief and in particular of sexual relations with both female and male persons, be they free or slaves.

What I may see or hear in the course of treatment or even outside of the treatment in regard to the life of men, which on no account one must spread abroad, I will keep to myself, holding such things shameful to be spoken about.

If I fulfill this oath and do not violate it, may it be granted to me to enjoy life and art, being honored with fame among all men for all time to come; if I transgress it and swear falsely, may the opposite of all this be my lot.

SHOW ME THE EVIDENCE

Adams and colleagues conducted a study to identify the ethical conflicts experienced by prehospital personnel. A single observer interviewed a convenience sample of 607 paramedics.*

The authors found ethical conflicts in 14.4% of the paramedics' responses. Ethical dilemmas were related to informed consent (27%); the duty of paramedics in threatening situations (19%); requests to limit resuscitation (14%); patients' decision-making capacity (17%); resource allocation (10%); confidentiality (8%); truth telling (3%); and training (1%).

*These researchers cautioned against applying their results to the broad EMS population, because their sample was not random.
Adams J, Siminoff L, Wolfson A: Ethical conflicts in the prehospital setting, *Ann Emerg Med* 21:1259-1265, 1992.

BOX 7-2 The EMT Code of Ethics

Professional status as an Emergency Medical Technician and Emergency Medical Technician–Paramedic is maintained and enriched by the willingness of the individual practitioner to accept and fulfill obligations to society, other medical professionals, and the profession of Emergency Medical Technician. As an Emergency Medical Technician at the basic level or an Emergency Medical Technician–Paramedic, I solemnly pledge myself to the following code of professional ethics:

A fundamental responsibility of the Emergency Medical Technician is to conserve life, to alleviate suffering, to promote health, to do no harm, and to encourage the quality and equal availability of emergency medical care.

The Emergency Medical Technician provides services based on human need, with respect for human dignity, unrestricted by consideration of nationality, race, creed, color, or status.

The Emergency Medical Technician does not use professional knowledge and skills in any enterprise detrimental to the public well-being.

The Emergency Medical Technician respects and holds in confidence all information of a confidential nature obtained in the course of professional work unless required by law to divulge such information.

The Emergency Medical Technician, as a citizen, understands and upholds the law and performs the duties of citizenship; as a professional, the Emergency Medical Technician has the never-ending responsibility to work with concerned citizens and other health care professionals in promoting a high standard of emergency medical care to all people.

The Emergency Medical Technician shall maintain professional competence and demonstrate concern for the competence of other members of the Emergency Medical Services health care team.

An Emergency Medical Technician assumes responsibility in defining and upholding standards of professional practice and education.

The Emergency Medical Technician assumes responsibility for individual professional actions and judgment, both in dependent and independent emergency functions, and knows and upholds the laws which affect the practice of the Emergency Medical Technician.

An Emergency Medical Technician has the responsibility to be aware of and participate in matters of legislation affecting the Emergency Medical Technician and the Emergency Medical Services System.

The Emergency Medical Technician adheres to standards of personal ethics which reflect credit upon the profession.

Emergency Medical Technicians, or groups of Emergency Medical Technicians, who advertise professional services, do so in conformity with the dignity of the profession.

The Emergency Medical Technician has an obligation to protect the public by not delegating to a person less qualified any service which requires the professional competence of an Emergency Medical Technician.

The Emergency Medical Technician will work harmoniously with, and sustain confidence in, Emergency Medical Technician associates, the nurse, the physician, and other members of the emergency medical services health care team.

The Emergency Medical Technician refuses to participate in unethical procedures and assumes the responsibility to expose incompetence or unethical conduct of others to the appropriate authority in a proper and professional manner.

Courtesy Charles Gillespie, MD
Adopted by The National Association of Emergency Medical Technicians, 1978. http://www.naemt.org/about_us/emtoath.aspx. Accessed 4-19-11

a critical reflection on one's life. For the paramedic, a personal code of ethics must take into account professional, legal, and moral responsibilities (Box 7-4).

Professional Accountability

As professionals, paramedics conform to a standard set by their level of training and regional practice. Paramedics are accountable to the patient, the medical director, and the EMS system for meeting the standard of care. Duties include commitment to high-quality patient care; continuing education; skill proficiency; and licensure or certification or both. The paramedic is accountable by law to that level of training and that standard of care. A paramedic who is accountable to the profession is more likely to provide good patient care and make decisions that are ethically acceptable.

Legal Accountability

Through patient care activities, the paramedic also assumes a role in the health care legal system (see Chapter 6). Legal issues often are intertwined with ethical issues. However,

ethics is not synonymous with law. (Ethics deals with moral actions; law deals with legal actions.) Many ethical decisions occur outside the boundaries of the law, and many legal decisions may not be ethical. An example is a patient who has a living will in a state in which the legality of advance directives has not been resolved. Another example is a terminally ill patient who requests assisted suicide in a state where the practice is illegal. The paramedic should consider the importance of legal accountability as it relates to medical ethics and abide by the law when ethical conflicts occur.

Moral Accountability

Moral accountability refers to *personal* ethics; that is, personal values and beliefs. Combining moral, legal, and professional accountability may be difficult in an emergency. At times the paramedic must draw on personal ethics to resolve conflicts among these roles and duties. Moreover, the paramedic must decide on a course of action. When dealing with ethical questions, paramedics should remember the following key points[4,5]:

BOX 7-3 American Medical Association Principles of Medical Ethics*

- A physician shall be dedicated to providing competent medical care, with compassion and respect for human dignity and rights.
- A physician shall uphold the standards of professionalism, be honest in all professional interactions, and strive to report physicians deficient in character or competence, or engaging in fraud or deception, to appropriate entities.
- A physician shall respect the law and also recognize a responsibility to seek changes in those requirements which are contrary to the best interests of the patient.
- A physician shall respect the rights of patients, colleagues, and other health professionals, and shall safeguard patient confidences and privacy within the constraints of the law.
- A physician shall continue to study, apply, and advance scientific knowledge, maintain a commitment to medical education, make relevant information available to patients, colleagues, and the public, obtain consultation, and use the talents of other health professionals when indicated.
- A physician shall, in the provision of appropriate patient care, except in emergencies, be free to choose whom to serve, with whom to associate, and the environment in which to provide medical care.
- A physician shall recognize a responsibility to participate in activities contributing to the improvement of the community and the betterment of public health.
- A physician shall, while caring for a patient, regard responsibility to the patient as paramount.
- A physician shall support access to medical care for all people.

*These principles were adopted by the American Medical Association's House of Delegates on June 17, 2001. They also have been adopted by the American College of Emergency Physicians.

BOX 7-4 Perspectives on Ethical Living

Socrates: The unexamined life is not worth living. Know thyself. Morality is the necessity of the heart. The soul is that which is.

Plato: Justice is the harmony of all virtues. Truth belongs to the mind.

Aristotle: Sense reveals only individual existence. The universal is immanent in the individual. Man finds his ethic only in his natural self-realization.

Zoroastrianism and Parsis: Good thoughts, good words, good deeds. The Reality is one, the wise by many men call it.

Buddhism: Let a man lift himself up by his own self; let him not depress himself; for he himself is his friend and he himself is his enemy.

Confucianism: Seek to be in harmony with all your neighbors.

Taoism: Being in one's inmost heart in kindly sympathy with all things.

Christianity: Love thy neighbor as thyself.

Judaism: Perform righteousness on earth that ye may find treasures in heaven.

Islam: Do what God likes, and avoid what He dislikes.

CRITICAL THINKING

Which of the perspectives on ethical living presented in Box 7-4 best speaks for your personal philosophy?

1. *Emotion may not be a reliable determinant for ethical decision making. Conscience should be monitored.* The conscience can be a reasonably good guide if one's conscience is well informed concerning right or wrong. Rational decision making relies on research and prudence to determine what is right. However, as a result of some knowledge deficit, the paramedic may come to a flawed decision.

2. *Decisions must not be based solely on the opinions of others; nor should they be based on global protocols meant to guide, not dictate (e.g., codes of the profession).* If paramedics encounter a situation with which they have not previously dealt, they are likely to make a poor or even an unethical decision. In these circumstances, paramedics should consult with medical direction, coworkers, a supervisor, or a set of guidelines or other resources. Consultation is better than limiting oneself to one's own knowledge base or principles. At times, input from patients and their loved ones can be a key source of information and can lead to a better decision.

3. *Once the ethical question has been answered, the answer becomes a "rule" to guide behavior, at least in that particular setting.* Once the rule has been identified, it should become a barrier to acting in opposition to the rule. Paramedics are expected to avoid breaking the rule without a strong reason for their actions.

DID YOU KNOW?

The Heinz Dilemma

Lawrence Kohlberg was a well-known theorist in the field of moral development. During his research, he posed a moral dilemma (called the *Heinz dilemma*) to young children and asked for a specific course of action to three scenarios. A brief description of each scenario follows.[6]

1. A woman was near death from a unique cancer. A physician had developed a drug that could cure her. The cost of the drug was $4000 per dose, but it cost the physician only $2000 to produce it. The woman's husband (Heinz) could raise only $2000. He asked the physician who developed the drug to accept the $2000 and said that he would pay the remaining $2000 at a later date. The physician refused. *Should Heinz break into the laboratory to steal the drug for his wife. Why or why not?*

2. Heinz broke into the laboratory and stole the drug. The break-in and theft were reported in newspapers the next day. A policeman (Officer Brown), a friend of Heinz, remembered seeing him the previous evening running away from the laboratory. *Should Brown report what he saw? Why or why not?*

3. Officer Brown reported what he saw. Heinz was arrested and brought to court. If convicted, he would face up to 2

years in prison. Heinz was found guilty. *Should the judge sentence Heinz to prison? Why or why not?*

Kohlberg was not interested so much in the answers to the questions in each scenario being wrong or right. He was more interested in the *reasoning* behind the participants' decisions. The responses were then classified into various stages of reasoning in his theory of moral development.

> **NOTE**
>
> With regard to answering ethical questions, no one knows all the answers. In addition, none of the tools or techniques work in every case to arrive at the "right" decision. Nonetheless, paramedics are accountable for personal and professional actions and decisions. Seeking counsel and guidance in such decisions is always prudent.

RAPID APPROACH TO ETHICAL PROBLEMS IN AN EMERGENCY

A method of ethical case analysis, or "rules of thumb" process, has been designed to serve as a way to deal rapidly with ethical problems in an emergency.[7] The steps of this process are as follows:

1. Ask yourself whether you have experienced a similar ethical problem in the past. If so, use that experience as a precedent for this problem and follow the previously established rule. (The paramedic must evaluate these rules periodically.)

2. If you have not already experienced a similar ethical problem, buy time for deliberation and for consulting with co-workers and medical direction.

3. If buying time for deliberation is not an option, use a set of three tests to help you make a decision[8] (Figure 7-1):
   - Test 1 (*impartiality test*): Would you accept the action if you were in the patient's place?
   - Test 2 (*universalizability test*): Would you feel comfortable having this action performed in all relevantly similar circumstances?
   - Test 3 (*interpersonal justifiability test*): Are you able to provide good reasons to justify and defend your actions to others?

The impartiality test is a good means of correcting partiality or personal bias. The universalizability test helps do away with moral decision difficulty. The interpersonal justifiability test requires that the paramedic define reasons for proceeding that others would approve. If all three tests can be answered in the affirmative, the paramedic has a fair probability that the action falls within the scope of being ethically acceptable. Even though disagreement may occur about a specific set of values, general agreement often exists about what constitutes wrong actions.

ETHICAL TESTS IN HEALTH CARE

The most basic question of ethical tests in health care is, "What is in the patient's best interest?" However, doing what is best, or what one thinks is best, is not enough to

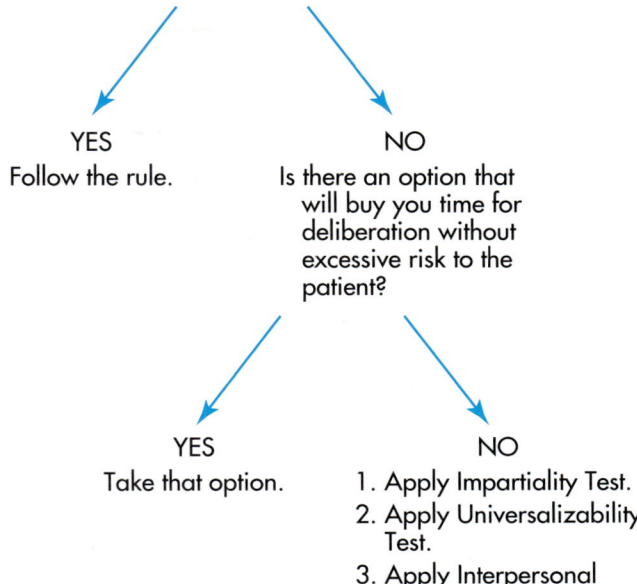

FIGURE 7-1 Rapid approach to resolving ethical problems in an emergency. (Modified from Iserson KV: *An approach to ethical problems in emergency medicine,* Baltimore, 1986, Williams & Wilkins.)

justify actions. One must determine what the patient wants. The paramedic can do this using statements by the patient (if the patient has decisional capacity) and written statements. Family input also is helpful (if the patient shows altered mental status or a lack of decisional capacity). The role of "good faith" in making ethical decisions ("Am I doing my best to help and not harm my patient?") should be balanced with the wishes of the patient and the family. The global concept of health care is providing patient benefit and avoiding harm. It recognizes and respects the patient's autonomy. The concept also recognizes the various legal issues that affect the delivery of health care (Box 7-5).

RESOLVING ETHICAL DILEMMAS

At times, ethical dilemmas can be difficult to resolve. This may be the case when global concepts of health care are in conflict. Therefore, the resolution can be guided by the health care community and by the public. The role of the health care community in resolving these conflicts is to set standards of care. The health care community also must provide research and treatment protocols. Finally, the health care community must make prospective and retrospective reviews of decisions and policies. The intent of the reviews is to educate the paramedic and improve the quality of patient care.

BOX 7-5 Global Concepts of Ethical Health Care

For an ancient Greek physician, therapeutic activity was subject to the following rules:
- Help the patient or at least to do no harm
- Refrain from interfering if the illness is incurable and inevitably mortal
- Insofar as possible, attack the cause of the disease therapeutically

Today, these global concepts of ethical health care can be stated as follows:
- Provide patient benefit.
- Do no harm.

BOX 7-6 Commonly Accepted Bioethical Values

Allocation of resources: Consistent access to quality medical services; the distribution of health-related services among various people and uses.

Autonomy: Self-determination; a person's ability to make moral decisions, including those affecting personal medical care. The three components of autonomy are *agency* (awareness of oneself as having desires and intentions and acting on them); *independence* (absence of influences that so control what a person does that it cannot be said the person wants to do it); and *rationality* (rational decision making).

Beneficence: A duty to confer benefits; the practice of good deeds; an obligation to benefit others or seek their good.

Confidentiality: The presumption that certain information will not be revealed to others without the patient's permission. Confidentiality, like privacy, is valued because it protects individual preferences and rights.

Nonmaleficence: The prevention of harm, from the Hippocratic tradition that established *primum non nocere* ("Above all, do no harm"); a prohibition against actions with foreseeable harmful effects.

Personal integrity: Adherence to a personal set of values and moral standards.

The role of the public in managing ethical conflicts in medicine includes creating laws, setting public policy, and allocating resources to protect the patient's rights. It also includes participating in the use of advance directives and other self-determination documents to make the patient's wishes known (see Chapter 6).

 LOOK AGAIN
See Chapter 6: Medical and Legal Issues, pp. 102-104.

ETHICAL ISSUES IN PARAMEDIC PRACTICE

All paramedics face ethical issues during the course of their careers. Most issues deal with the patient's right to self-determination and the paramedic's duty to provide patient care (Box 7-6). The concept of the patient's right to self-determination is known as **autonomy,** and the concept of the paramedic's duty to provide patient care is known as **beneficence.** Some of the more common issues (and sample case studies) are described in this section. For each case study, the paramedic should apply the rapid approach to emergency medical problems (described previously) and answer the following ethical questions:

1. What is in the patient's best interest?
2. What are the patient's rights?
3. Does the patient understand the issues at hand?
4. What is the paramedic's professional, legal, and moral accountability?

Allocation of Resources

Fairness in the allocation of resources and obligations is a commonly accepted bioethical value. Fairness is incorporated into society-wide health care policies. This perceived "right" to universal access to an adequate level of health care is a complex economic issue that is affected by the need to contain health care costs. Two factors affect true parity in the allocation of resources. The first is a person's access

to health insurance. This may define which medical services are covered or excluded. The second is treatment decisions made when resources are inadequate to meet patient care needs. This may occur, for example, during a disaster involving multiple casualties. When rationing of care is required, it should be based on ethically oriented criteria.[8]

The allocation of resources (*medical rationing*) is more of a policy than a clinical concept. However, allocation can pose ethical dilemmas in prehospital care, as illustrated in the following case study.

CASE STUDY 1

A paramedic crew has been dispatched to the home of a 74-year-old man. The man complains of chest pain and shortness of breath. The patient is in obvious distress and provides a significant cardiac history. He asks to be taken to the Veterans Administration hospital (30 miles away), where he had heart surgery several years ago. Based on the patient's history, the physical examination findings, and the electrocardiogram (ECG), the paramedic crew, in consultation with medical direction, elects to take the patient to a closer hospital so that his condition can be stabilized. The patient becomes anxious and complains of increasing chest pain. He tells the paramedic crew that he has no medical insurance and demands to be taken to the Veterans Administration hospital.

CASE STUDY 2

The paramedic crew has been dispatched to a restaurant where an elderly woman has collapsed. She has suffered cardiac arrest, and a waiter is performing cardiopulmonary resuscitation. The ECG monitor reveals ventricular fibrillation. Defibrillatory shocks are delivered, but the rhythm remains unchanged. As resuscitation measures are continued, the woman's husband says to the paramedics, "She said she didn't want this. Her living will is at home. Please stop what you're doing and let her go."

Confidentiality

Most people are considered to have a basic right to privacy. The principle of confidentiality refers to a person's private and personal information. This information should not be disclosed by a health care professional to other people without the patient's consent. As is described in Chapter 6, doing so is illegal and may violate laws and regulations designed to protect a patient's privacy, such as state and federal laws and the regulations established by the Health Insurance Portability and Accountability Act (HIPAA).

LOOK AGAIN
See Chapter 6: Medical and Legal Issues, pp. 96-97.

In some cases, the release of such information may be required by law. An example of such a case is the disclosure to others involved in the patient's care that a patient has tested positive for infection with the human immunodeficiency virus (HIV). However, conflict between ethics and confidentiality may arise, particularly if the public health would benefit from the disclosure of confidential information, as described in the following case study.

CASE STUDY 3

The paramedic crew has been dispatched to a motor vehicle crash. A young man struck another car head-on, killing the driver of that car. The patient is shaken but has only minor injuries. As the patient is prepared for transport, he confides to the paramedic that he had used cocaine shortly before the crash. He asks the paramedic to keep the information confidential and not to tell the police officers at the scene.

CRITICAL THINKING
Your partner uses the phone number from the patient care report to contact a former patient and ask for a date. Do you think that action violates any ethical principles? If so, which ones?

CONSENT

As is explained in Chapter 6, patients with decisional capacity have a legal right to decide on the medical care they will receive. This right is a basic element of the relationship between the patient and physician and is described in the American Medical Association's Principles of Medical Ethics. The right also can be inferred from the EMT Code

of Ethics. Cases in which patients refuse lifesaving care can produce legal and ethical conflicts, as shown in the following case study.

CASE STUDY 4

The paramedic crew has been dispatched to an office building where a 55-year-old woman collapsed at a business meeting. She is alert and oriented, complains of chest pain, and is pale and diaphoretic. The paramedics advise the patient of the possibility of a heart attack and the need for immediate care and transport for evaluation by a physician. The patient insists on waiting until after the meeting has concluded to seek medical care on her own, and she asks the EMS crew to leave.

OTHER ETHICAL PRINCIPLES FOR PATIENT CARE SITUATIONS

Other ethical principles of patient care arise in cases related to care in futile situations, legal obligations to provide care, patient advocacy and paramedic accountability, and the paramedic's role as a physician extender.

Care in Futile Situations

An action is seen as *futile* if it serves no purpose or is totally ineffective. A paramedic providing care in a case that may be futile should consult with medical direction. Consultation can help the paramedic decide on a course of action. An example of a futile situation in health care is continuing resuscitation initiated by bystanders when the patient clearly has expired. Another example is providing life support measures for a patient who has fatal injuries. The definition of *futility* may pose an ethical dilemma. This may be especially true when a dispute or lack of agreement exists about the goals of treatment. Not all futility judgments are controversial. For example, cardiopulmonary resuscitation is futile in patients with obvious signs of death, such as decapitation, rigor mortis, tissue decompensation, or extreme dependent lividity.[9]

CRITICAL THINKING
You arrive at a home where you find a 3-month-old baby who obviously has been dead for several hours. The mother is screaming, "Help her! Help her!" Your partner decides to proceed with advanced life support care even though it is clearly futile. Is this decision ethical?

Obligation to Provide Care

In the prehospital setting, the paramedic's duty to provide care is seldom an issue; the patient's request for emergency service presents a legal duty to act. In other areas of health care, though, an obligation to provide care other than emergency care may be affected by several factors. Examples include a patient's ability to pay for service, the patient's insurance, or other economic factors. As is described in

Chapter 6, some laws protect well-meaning caregivers from liability (e.g., Good Samaritan legislation). Other laws protect patients from unethical health care practices (e.g., the Emergency Medical Treatment and Active Labor Act [EMTALA]). An example of such practices is "economic triage," in which evaluation of the impact of the patient's care is based on fiscal aspects important to the hospital. Another example is "patient dumping," in which a patient in unstable condition is transferred or discharged from a hospital for financial reasons.

Patient Advocacy and Paramedic Accountability

While providing care, the paramedic serves as the patient's advocate. This advocacy may conflict at times with the paramedic's accountability to the patient, the physician medical director, and the health care system (e.g., health maintenance organization [HMO] protocols). In such a case, the paramedic should discuss all options with medical direction. *As a rule, it is prudent and ethical to err on the side of providing for the needs of the patient when conflict arises.* Examples of ways in which a paramedic can serve as the patient's advocate include the following:

- Educating patients about the delivery of health care and the role they can play to help change the nation's health care system
- Making sure health care decisions are made by patients and their physicians and are based on the patient's medical needs, not financial considerations
- Informing patients of health care reform initiatives in the federal, state, and private sectors
- Promoting patient access to reliable information about state-of-the-art medical technologies and treatments

- Promoting fairness and equality in America's health care system

Paramedic's Role as Physician Extender

As a physician extender, the paramedic generally is responsible for following the orders of the medical director or the director's designee. However, sometimes these orders may not seem appropriate. For example, the paramedic may believe that a medication order is contraindicated for the patient (e.g., giving narcotics when the patient is hypotensive). Also, a medication may be medically acceptable but may not be in the patient's best interest (e.g., an order for an intravenous [IV] drug to treat asthma before the patient's inhaler has been tried). A third example of such a case is a medication that is medically acceptable but morally wrong (e.g., an off-label use of a drug) (see Chapter 13).

The converse also can occur. For example, a paramedic might request treatment in a situation in which the field diagnosis is unsure, or the physician may lack information needed to approve the request. When a conflict occurs between medical direction and the paramedic, communication is the key to resolving short-term and long-term concerns.

> **CRITICAL THINKING**
>
> Your patient is in critical condition, and you cannot secure the airway. Medical direction tells you to divert because the hospital has no open beds in the intensive care unit. You repeat the urgency of your patient's condition and are still told to divert. You elect to override the physician's order and transport the patient to that hospital. Can you justify disobeying the physician's order?

SUMMARY

- *Ethics* is the discipline relating to right and wrong, moral duty and obligation, moral principles and values, and moral character. *Bioethics* is the science of medical ethics. *Morals* refers to social standards or customs.
- Paramedics must meet a standard established by their level of training and regional practice. They must abide by the law when ethical conflicts occur.
- A paramedic must act in a way that is seen as morally acceptable.
- The rapid approach to resolving ethical issues is a process. It involves reviewing past experiences; deliberation (if possible); and performing the impartiality test, universalizability test, and interpersonal justifiability test to reach an acceptable decision.
- Two concepts of ethical health care are to provide patient benefit and to do no harm.

- All resources must be allocated fairly. This is an accepted bioethical value.
- Advance directives, living wills, and other self-determination documents can help the paramedic make decisions about the appropriateness of resuscitation in the prehospital setting.
- A health care professional is not allowed to reveal details supplied by the patient to others without the patient's consent. This is the principle of confidentiality.
- In some cases, patients refuse lifesaving care. These cases can produce legal and ethical conflicts.
- Other areas likely to raise ethical questions in the prehospital setting include providing care in futile situations, the paramedic's obligation to provide care, patient advocacy, and the paramedic's role as physician extender.

REFERENCES

1. Sanderson B: *History of ethics to 30 BC: ancient wisdom and folly*, Santa Barbara, Calif, 2002, World Peace Communications.
2. American Medical Association, Council on Ethical and Judicial Affairs: *Code of medical ethics: current opinions with annotations*, Chicago, 2009, The Association.
3. Veatch R: *Medical ethics*, ed 2, Sudbury, Mass, 1997, Jones & Bartlett.
4. National Highway Traffic Safety Administration: *EMT-Paramedic national standard curriculum*, Washington, DC, 1998, US Department of Transportation.
5. Bourn S: Through traffic keep right, *J Emerg Med Serv JEMS* 21(5):26, 1996.
6. Rosen P, Barkin R: *Emergency medicine: concepts and clinical practice*, ed 7, St Louis, 2010, Mosby.
7. Iserson K, et al: *Ethics in emergency medicine*, ed 2, Tucson, Ariz, 1995, Galen Press.
8. American Heart Association: Guidelines 2005 for cardiopulmonary resuscitation and emergency cardiovascular care, International Consensus on Science, *Circulation* 112: (IV-211, 2005.
9. American Heart Association (2010): 2010 American Heart Association guidelines for cardiopulmonary resuscitation and emergency cardiovascular care, *Circulation* 122(18 suppl 3):S639-S946, 2010.

CHAPTER 8

Research Principles and Evidence-Based Practice

OBJECTIVES

Upon completion of this chapter, the paramedic student will be able to:

1. Explain the importance of emergency medical services (EMS) research.
2. Describe the differences between types of EMS research.
3. Outline the 10 steps in performing research that are identified in this chapter.
4. Define evidence-based practice.
5. Describe the criteria for evaluating a research paper.

KEY TERMS

alternative time sampling Sampling to prevent bias by assigning a treatment group based on the day, week, or month in which patients are encountered in a study.

blinding A research specification that dictates that parties are not made aware of the study, treatment, or outcome to be measured.

convenience sampling The process of choosing the individuals who are easiest to reach, or sampling that is easily done; the sample does not represent the entire population.

descriptive statistics Numerical facts or data that do not try to infer anything about a subject that goes beyond the data; can be qualitative or quantitative.

evidence-based practice Practice that is based on current scientific evidence.

hypothesis A statement of the relationship between two or more variables.

inferential statistics A form of statistics that enables the researcher to conclude (infer) whether the relationships seen in a sample are likely to occur in the larger population.

institution review board (IRB) A committee that performs critical oversight functions (scientific, ethical, and regulatory) for research conducted on human subjects.

level of significance The risk of committing a type I error.

mean The arithmetic average of a group being studied.

median A number that is found by first arranging the measurement according to size from smallest to largest, then by choosing the one in the middle; the midpoint of a distribution score.

mode The number that occurs more often than any other number in a set of data.

nuisance variables Variables that can make drawing accurate conclusions from a study difficult.

null hypothesis An exact statement that the results are a chance of variation (the opposite of the hypothesis).

parameter An aspect of a population that is difficult or impossible to measure.

population: A large group of people or places or objects that are the main focus of a scientific query.

qualitative analysis The nonnumerical organization and interpretation of observations.

quantitative analysis Use of the mean, median, and mode to describe the most commonly occurring values in a sample.

random sample A subset of individuals chosen from a larger set; a sample chosen randomly and entirely by chance.

sampling error Error that results from observation of a sample rather than the whole population.

selection bias A distortion of evidence or data that arises from the way the data are collected.

statistically significant A descriptive term used when the observed phenomenon represents a significant departure from what might be expected by chance alone.

statistics A summary of characteristics of numerical facts or data.

systematic sampling A statistical method that involves the selection of a population from an ordered sampling so as to ensure equal probability.

type I error Rejection of the null hypothesis when the hypothesis was true.

type II error Failure to accept the alternative hypothesis when the alternative hypothesis was true.

unblinding A research specification by which all parties are made aware of the study, treatment, and outcome to be measured.

*E*MS systems are committed to providing effective and efficient health care to acutely ill and injured patients. As the National Highway Traffic Safety Administration has said, EMS agencies face a challenge today. Practices have been based on tradition and expert opinion. They need to be transformed into practices based on guidelines and protocols that have been developed through thoughtful, systematic examination of scientific evidence and data.[1] The paramedic of today must have a basic knowledge of research principles. This knowledge is necessary for conducting research and interpreting published studies. Paramedics also must be willing to help collect research data, which provide important information for the continued development of EMS care.

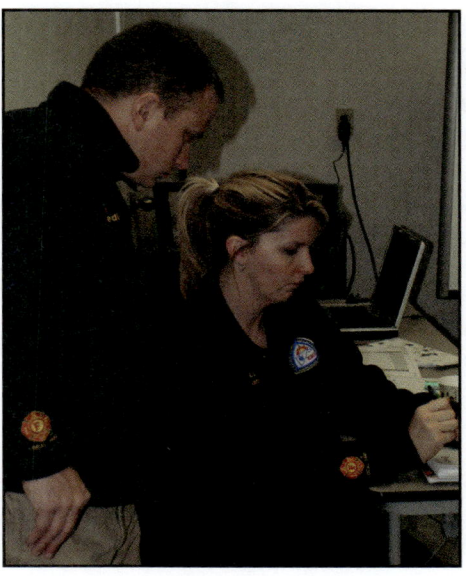

Courtesy Rick Brady

EMS RESEARCH

Research is a desirable activity for an EMS system. In fact, research is essential to the evolution of emergency medical services. Quality EMS research helps shed light on the intended effects and cost-effectiveness of EMS interventions. The National EMS Research Agenda, published in 2001, states, "Research is essential to ensure that the best possible care is provided in the prehospital setting."[2] This research is based on data and can lead to changes in professional standards, training, equipment, procedures, and improved patient care. In addition, EMS research increases respect for EMS professionals (Box 8-1).

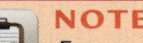

NOTE
For too long, prehospital care has been driven more by what we *think* is right than by what we *know* is right.[1] A system-wide process is needed to ensure that prehospital care is based on current and scientific evidence. This is known as **evidence-based practice**.

CRITICAL THINKING
How do you feel about research?

Types of Research

EMS research has many applications. One application involves gathering data to allow conclusions to be drawn about which procedures, techniques, and equipment are

sound. Another application involves gathering data to answer clinically valuable questions and to find results that lead to system improvements. Research is carried out through standard research methods, which include the following:

- *Descriptive (observational) method*: A research design in which events are monitored and analyzed without any attempt to manipulate or alter the outcome.
- *Experimental method*: A research design in which an intervention is introduced and the effects are monitored for an outcome.
- *Prospective method*: A research design in which the specific question, hypothesis, and data collection are defined before the study begins.
- *Retrospective method*: A research design in which the specific question, hypothesis, and data collection are defined after the data already exist.
- *Cross-sectional method*: A research design in which a group of subjects is studied during a specified (usually short) period.

BASIC PRINCIPLES OF RESEARCH

This chapter describes 10 basic steps for conducting research[3] (Figure 8-1):

1. Prepare a question.
2. Write a hypothesis.
3. Decide what to measure and the best way to measure it.
4. Define the population.
5. Identify study limitations.
6. Seek approval of the study.
7. Obtain informed consent.
8. Gather data after conducting pilot trials.
9. Analyze the data with an awareness of the pitfalls in interpreting the data.

BOX 8-1 Importance of Research in Emergency Medical Services

- Production of outcome-based research
- New procedures, medications, and treatment
- Quality assurance
- Improved patient outcomes
- Professionalism

10. Determine what to do with the research product (publish, present, perform follow-up studies).

Prepare a Question

EMS research begins with the posing of a specific problem or question. The research then is carried out using the standard research methods described previously. Examples of problems or questions specifically related to EMS might include the following:

- What factors predict success for paramedic students on the National Registry of EMTs written examination?
- Is the incidence of complications greater with prehospital peripheral vascular access than with hospital peripheral vascular access?
- Does the paramedic uniform influence a patient's satisfaction?
- What is the incidence of violence in an EMS system?

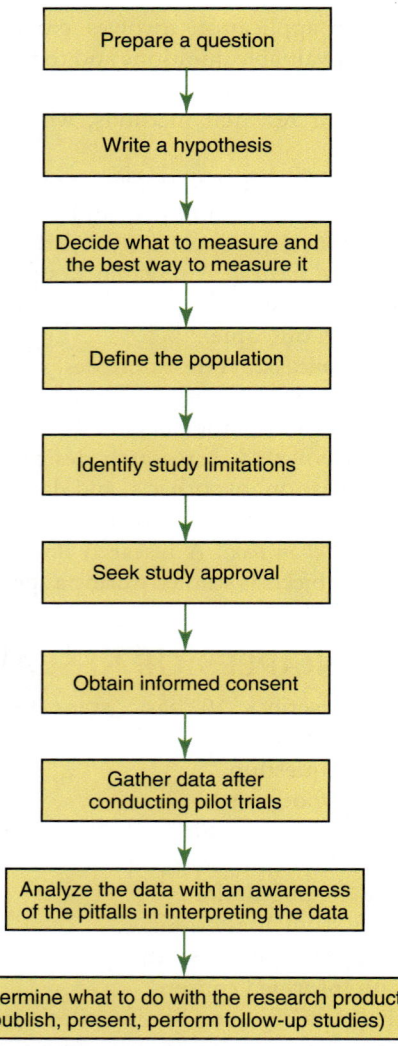

FIGURE 8-1 Ten steps for conducting research.

- Does the paramedic's shift length influence the number of medical errors?

NOTE
Paramedics should search medical literature for related research. The research should be evaluated for validity and reliability (described later in this text). Reference sources for literature review include peer-reviewed studies, government publications, and literature searches on the Internet.

Write a Hypothesis

After a problem or question to be studied has been identified, a statement to be tested by the study must be defined. This statement is called the **hypothesis.** The hypothesis states the relationship between two or more variables. A *variable* is any factor or entity that can vary in amount or type. For example, the problem might be the ability of one drug to lower a patient's blood pressure more effectively than another drug. A hypothesis for the drug study might be that drug A lowers blood pressure better and with fewer side effects than drug B. A major goal of this step is to decide what to measure and how to measure it.

Define the Population

The next step in the research process is to define the **population** for the study. The population can be any group of people (e.g., all patients with a diastolic blood pressure greater than 100 mm Hg), or any group of places or objects. If the population group is large, the researcher can use a sample (e.g., all patients over 50 years of age who have a diastolic blood pressure greater than 100 mmHg). The researcher should draw the sample randomly. That way, the patients in the study have an equal chance of being assigned to one group (drug A study) or the other (drug B study).

Identify Study Limitations

Drawing a **random sample** prevents **selection bias** (placing the best or worst patients in a study group). The researcher can ensure random sampling with computer software programs, random digits, and even with the flip a coin. Another way to limit bias is with **systematic sampling.** With this method, patients are put into groups in the order in which they are encountered in the prehospital setting. For example, the first patient seen is put into group A, the second into group B, the third into group A, and so on. The researcher also can use **alternative time sampling** to prevent bias by assigning a treatment group based on the day, week, or month in which patients are encountered in the study. **Convenience sampling** is the least preferred method. With this method, patients are assigned to groups when a particular person or crew is working. Even with carefully designed methods, a **sampling error** may occur. Errors result from the fact that even the best sample will not work perfectly to represent the population. This is because of the chance inclusion of one person in the study group rather than the chance inclusion of someone else.

In addition to the bias of the researcher, bias can occur on the part of the participants in the study. Bias may be a result of the expectations of the participants. To lessen bias, the researcher can use **blinding** (either single, double, or triple). In a *single blind* method, one party (the patient, the paramedic, or the person gathering the data) is unaware of (blinded to) the treatment at the time it is given. That party also is unaware of the effect to be measured during the study. In a *double blind* study, two parties are blinded. In a *triple blind* study, all parties are blinded. **Unblinding** refers to making all parties aware of the study, treatment, and outcome to be measured.

Seek Approval of the Study

When planning for research involving human subjects, researchers use an **institutional review board (IRB).** IRBs (also known as *independent ethics committees* [IECs] or *ethical review boards* [ERBs]) came into wide use as a result of a mandate from the U.S. Public Health Services in 1966.[4] This mandate required a review by a "committee of institutional associates" for any federally funded research that used human subjects. In the United States, regulations have empowered IRBs to approve research, require modifications in planned research before approval, or disapprove research. These regulations were developed by the U.S. Food and Drug Administration (FDA) and the Department of Health and Human Services (DHHS) (specifically the Office for Human Research Protections [OHRP]). An IRB performs critical oversight functions for research conducted on human subjects. The research is required to be scientific, ethical, and regulatory.

CRITICAL THINKING

Why do you think the development of institution review boards was needed for research?

Obtain Informed Consent

With informed consent, the subject voluntarily agrees to take part in the research project. The subject has decisional capacity and understands what is being presented. With respect to EMS research and the problems associated with obtaining informed consent in emergency situations,

DID YOU KNOW?
Institution Review Boards

Currently most IRBs involved in EMS research consist of physicians, attorneys, psychologists, ethicists, allied health professionals, and lay members of the community. In fact, many peer-reviewed EMS journals ask for a record that the research was approved by an IRB. Institution review boards seek to reduce the risk of patients unknowingly entering into research that could harm them in any way. In 1981 the U.S. Department of Health and Human Services established the following regulations for research practice (CFR title 45, part 46; revised, 2005).[5] These regulations are observed by most IRBs.

1. Risks to subjects are minimized by using procedures consistent with sound research design that do not unnecessarily expose subjects to risk and, whenever appropriate, by using procedures already being performed on the subjects for diagnostic or treatment purposes.
2. Risks to subjects are reasonable in relation to anticipated benefits, if any, to subjects, and the importance of the knowledge that may reasonably be expected to result. In evaluating risks and benefits, the IRB should consider only risks and benefits that may result from the research (as distinguished from risks and benefits of therapies subjects would receive even if not participating in the research). The IRB should not consider possible long-range effects of applying knowledge gained in the research (e.g., the possible effects of the research on public policy) as among the research risks that fall within the purview of its responsibility.
3. Selection of subjects is equitable. In making this assessment, the IRB should take into account the purposes of the research and the setting in which the research will be conducted, and should be particularly cognizant of the special problems of research involving vulnerable populations, such as children, prisoners, pregnant women, mentally disabled persons, or economically or educationally disadvantaged persons.
4. Informed consent will be sought from each prospective subject or the subject's legally authorized representative in accordance with and to the extent required by *46.116.*
5. Informed consent will be appropriately documented in accordance with and to the extent required by *46.117.*
6. When appropriate, the research plan makes adequate provision for monitoring the data collected to ensure the safety of subjects.
7. When appropriate, adequate provisions are made to protect the privacy of subjects and to maintain the confidentiality of data.
8. When some or all of the subjects are likely to be vulnerable to coercion or undue influence (e.g., children, prisoners, pregnant women, mentally disabled persons, or economically or educationally disadvantaged persons), additional safeguards are included in the study to protect the rights and welfare of these subjects.

alternatives to informed consent have been developed, including the following[3]:

■ *Consent at a distance.* The base station physician administers informed consent to the subject by radio or telephone.

- *Consent by proxy.* The paramedic administers informed consent to the subject.
- *Stepped consent.* The paramedic provides the subject with a brief overview of the experimental therapy. Full informed consent is obtained at the hospital.
- *Cohort consent.* Permission is obtained to enter into the study at some future time (e.g., during an asthma exacerbation or sickle cell crisis).
- *Deferred consent.* This type of consent is used during resuscitation; the subject's condition is stabilized and the person receives experimental therapy without permission, after which the family is approached for traditional informed consent.
- *Surrogate consent.* Lay people are presented with the experimental protocol and are asked to state whether they believe the treatment is appropriate.
- *Consent jury.* A lay panel determines certain aspects of the experimental protocol, particularly potential risks and complications that must be presented during a request for consent.

> **NOTE**
> A waiver of informed consent may be permitted in some emergency research. To be granted this waiver, the researchers must prove that they have informed the community about the research. The research team must also solicit feedback from the community about the proposed research. This is known as *community consultation and public disclosure.*

> **SHOW ME THE EVIDENCE**
> Nelson and colleagues collected a cross-sectional, standardized survey conducted by two sets of random-digit telephone surveys, paper surveys at community meetings, and Web-based surveys. Their goal was to comply with federal law that allows research to be conducted using very strict criteria without having prior consent of the patient. The surveys were done to fulfill the law's requirement for community consultation and public disclosure. The authors found that community meetings were poorly attended and that phone surveys were effective for gauging public opinion. However, they recommended targeted surveys to reach special populations.

Nelson M et al: Community consultation methods in a study using exception to informed consent, *Prehosp Emerg Care* 12:417-425, 2008.

Gather and Analyze Data

Data from the research study should be gathered and analyzed using statistical methods. The term **statistics** refers to numerical facts or data. These facts or data are classified and put into a chart to present key details about a subject. Statistics can be descriptive or inferential.

DESCRIPTIVE STATISTICS

Descriptive statistics does not try to conclude (infer) anything about a subject that goes beyond the data. This type of statistics provides a description of the sample of objects or people being studied. It does not infer anything from the data; it simply reports it. Descriptive statistics can be qualitative or quantitative.

Qualitative analysis is nonnumerical; it is the organization and interpretation of observations. The sample size in qualitative research usually is very small. Qualitative analysis is used to find key underlying dimensions and patterns in a group. For example, it would show the age and gender of a sample. Qualitative analysis uses text and few numbers to describe the research findings. The conclusions from qualitative research involve themes, trends, or theories derived from interviews, discussion, or observation of the study population.

Quantitative analysis in descriptive statistics uses the mean, median, and mode to describe the most commonly occurring values in a sample. The **mean** is the arithmetic average of the group (e.g., the average age of the people in the sample). The **median** is found first by arranging the measurement according to size from smallest to largest and then by choosing the one in the middle (or the mean of the two that are nearest to the middle). The median sometimes is referred to as the *50th percentile*. The median frequently is used to divide a sample into two halves. The **mode** is the number that occurs more often than any other number in a set of data. The following is an example of quantitative analysis:

Your sample has 13 participants. Their ages are 53, 53, 53, 54, 55, 55, 56, 57, 59, 60, 64, 71, and 79. The *mean* (average) age of the group is 59.15 years; the *median* (middle) age is 56; and the *mode* age is 53.

INFERENTIAL STATISTICS

Inferential statistics is used to infer whether the relationships seen in a sample are likely to occur in the larger population. The researcher can use these statistics to decide whether the results of the study support or contradict the initial hypothesis. To do this, one must assume the opposite of what one may want to prove. This is done by stating a **null hypothesis.** A null hypothesis is a default position, such as that a specific treatment has no effect or that the results are a chance of variation (the opposite of what you expect to prove). This is done in court, where the accused is assumed to be innocent until proved guilty beyond a reasonable doubt. The assumption that the accused is not guilty is a null hypothesis. If the assumption cannot be rejected, the accused goes free. However, this does not always mean that the accused actually is innocent. A *research hypothesis* is the opposite of the null hypothesis (e.g., the accused is guilty until proved innocent).

> **NOTE**
> The sureness with which a null hypothesis can be rejected is called *confidence.* The *confidence interval* is the range where a researcher "expects" something to be true, leaving open the possibility of being wrong. The *degree of confidence* measures the probability of that expectation to be true. It is linked with the width of the confidence interval and often is reported in research journals.

It is easy to be very confident that something will be within a very wide range, and vice versa. For example, one can be fairly confident that a classroom of children would prefer soda over water. The degree of confidence and the width of the confidence interval for this study would be quite large. However, if the question to be studied is, "Do children prefer Coke, Pepsi, or Mountain Dew?" the degree of confidence and the width of the confidence interval become narrow.

When a statistical test reveals that the probability is rare that a set of results is attributable to chance alone, this result is called **statistically significant.** *Statistically significant* means that the observed phenomenon represents a significant departure from what might be expected by chance alone.

The **level of significance** is the probability of a **type I error** that an investigator is willing to risk in rejecting a null hypothesis. Generally, the *level of significance* refers to the probability of the event occurring as a result of chance. The level of significance is the acceptable risk of sampling errors and is established through mathematical equations. The level of significance is usually 0.05 (1 chance in 200) or 0.01 (1 chance in 100) that the difference between two groups is larger than expected as a result of chance alone (too large to be reasonably attributed to chance). If the level of significance is lowered from 0.05 to 0.01, the probability of rejecting a true hypothesis is decreased and the probability of accepting a false hypothesis is increased. A **type II error** occurs when an investigator fails to accept the alternative hypothesis when in fact the alternative hypothesis was true. In other words, the null hypothesis was accepted when it was not true. Researchers must set their level of significance before they begin their research.

1. The *introduction* provides a brief historical background of the research. It also relates any previously published research. The introduction provides both a rationale for the study and the research hypothesis.
2. The *methods section* describes how the experiment was done so that it can be replicated by others. This section should define the inclusion or exclusion criteria for the study (how patients were chosen). It also should contain the statistical methods used to analyze the data.
3. The *results section* provides answers to study questions and data (e.g., tables and figures). This information supports the research findings.
4. The *discussion section* lets the author interpret the research findings. Limitations of the project usually are also given here. This section frequently offers suggestions for improving the study through follow-up research.
5. The *conclusion* provides a succinct summary of the four preceding sections (Box 8-2).

PRESENTING THE RESULTS AND FOLLOW-UP STUDIES

Presenting the results of a study can help put research into practice. Presentations can be made to peers, professional organizations, and higher education institutions. Clinical studies can lead to improvements in patient outcomes. Funding may be available for follow-up studies. These studies may be done through collaborative efforts with public agencies, corporations, and foundations. Studies also may be funded and supported through state and federal government programs that support research

NOTE
In statistics, rejection of the null hypothesis when it is true (a false alarm) is referred to as a *type I error*. Acceptance of the null hypothesis when it is false (failure to detect a real phenomenon) is a *type II error*. A type II error occurs when the phenomenon is *too* small to see.

Determine What to Do with the Results

The final step in EMS research is to determine what to do with the results of the study. Several options are available, including publishing the results, presenting the results, and performing follow-up studies.

PUBLISHING THE RESULTS

The findings from research may be published in a professional journal for peer evaluation. (Sometimes just an abstract, or summary, of the research is published. Published abstracts have not gone through the same rigorous peer-review process as a full article.) The format for writing a manuscript for scientific literature has five basic sections:

BOX 8-2 Fifteen Steps for Evaluating and Interpreting Research

1. Was the research peer reviewed?
2. What was the research hypothesis?
3. Was the study approved by an institutional review board and conducted ethically?
4. What was the population studied?
5. What were the inclusion and exclusion criteria for the study?
6. What method was used to draw a sample of patients?
7. How many patient groups participated?
8. How were patients assigned to groups?
9. What type of data was gathered?
10. Does the study appear to have had a sufficient number of patients enrolled?
11. Does the study fail to account for any potential confounding variables?
12. Were the data properly analyzed?
13. Is the author's conclusion logical and based on the data?
14. Could the results apply in local EMS systems?
15. Are the patients in the study similar to those seen in the local EMS system?

consortia. (A *consortium* is a group of individuals and/or organizations that pool resources and information to achieve a common goal.) An example of organizations that may be members of a local research consortium is area hospitals and EMS agencies that collect and share data.

EVIDENCE-BASED PRACTICE

Traditional medical practice has been based on medical knowledge, intuition, and judgment. With the emphasis moving toward evidence-based practice, many medical specialties have developed evidence-based guidelines for specific conditions, such as traumatic brain injury, spinal injury, and ST-segment elevation myocardial infarction. (These conditions are addressed by subject matter later in the text.)

> **NOTE**
> The National Guideline Clearinghouse (NGC) is a public resource for evidence-based, clinical practice guidelines and related documents. The mission of the NGC is to provide physicians and other health professionals with an accessible means of obtaining objective, detailed information on clinical practice guidelines. Another goal of the NGC is to disseminate practice guidelines for implementation and use.[6]

High-quality patient care should focus on procedures that have been proven useful in improving patient outcomes.[7] Paramedics should participate in EMS research, data collection, and the sharing of information. These efforts aid in the design of a system-wide process for prehospital care that reflects the current state of scientific evidence (Figure 8-2).

Reviewing Research

When reviewing research articles, paramedics should read the article critically to determine whether the findings are relevant to their practice. They should look carefully at the following components[8]:

1. *Population.* Is the sample adequate and is it similar to your practice? For example, a study that evaluates response times without lights and sirens conducted in a rural setting may not be relevant to an urban EMS system. Another example is a study conducted in an area that has a significantly different ethnic makeup than your practice area. This could influence results if the study subject involves disease processes that are more prevalent in some ethnic communities.

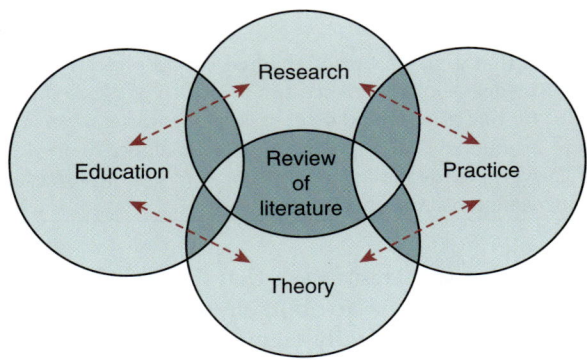

FIGURE 8-2 Relationship of the review of the literature to theory, research, education, and practice. (LoBiondo-Wood G, Haber J: *Nursing research: methods and critical appraisal for evidence-based practice,* ed 7, St Louis, 2010, Mosby.)

2. *Inclusion and exclusion criteria.* A study of patients with chest pain that did not include patients older than age 65, for example, would eliminate a key group at risk for heart disease and death.
3. *Data collection.* Is there anything that could have influenced the data collection? If the study used the experimental method, how were the groups randomized? Was the method clearly described? Could the method have varied based on the person delivering care? Were the conditions in the control group and the experimental group the same?
4. *Results.* Are the numbers presented clearly? When percentages are presented, are the underlying numbers reported? If a statistically significant difference was seen in the outcome, is it also clinically significant?
5. *Discussion and conclusion.* Is the conclusion consistent with the results reported? Did the authors properly report correlations and relationships, rather than predictions? Did they link the research to relevant literature? Were the limitations of the study pointed out clearly? Did the researchers make specific suggestions for future research? Did you identify any major flaws in the conclusion?
6. *How does this research relate to your practice?* Does the research suggest an area of improvement for your system? Does it suggest an area that should be monitored in your quality improvement program? Is there a reason to seek out more literature on the same subject to propose a change in your system?

SUMMARY

- The paramedic must be familiar with research principles. This knowledge is needed to conduct research, collect research data, and interpret published studies.
- Research is essential to improving patient care.
- Two main types of research are the descriptive method and the experimental method. Data are collected by various methods. These methods may be prospective, retrospective, or cross-sectional.
- The 10 steps of EMS research are (1) prepare a question; (2) write a hypothesis; (3) decide what to measure and how to measure it; (4) define the population; (5) identify the study limitations; (6) seek IRB approval; (7) obtain informed consent; (8) gather data after conducting pilot trials; (9) analyze the data; and (10) present the data.

- Descriptive statistics does not try to infer anything about a subject that goes beyond the data.
- Qualitative analysis provides a nonnumerical description of the population. Quantitative data analysis evaluates the data using numbers.
- Inferential statistics infers whether the relationships seen in a sample are likely to occur in the larger population. In this type of study, researchers develop a null hypothesis.
- EMS care should be evidence-based; that is, interventions and procedures should be proven to benefit the patient.
- Paramedics should read research articles critically to determine whether the article is relevant to their practice.

REFERENCES

1. National Highway Traffic Safety Administration, Office of EMS: *EMS update*, Washington, DC, Fall 2008–Winter 2009, The Administration.
2. National Highway Traffic Safety Administration and the Maternal Child Health Bureau: *National EMS research agenda*, Washington, DC, 2001, Health Resources Administration.
3. Menegazzi J: *Research: the who, what, why, when and how*, Wilmington, Ohio, 1994, Ferno-Washington.
4. Hicks S: *How the past influenced human research protection legislation*, Washington, DC, 2007, US Department of Health and Human Services.
5. US Department of Health and Human Services: *Code of federal regulations,* Title 45, Public, Part 46, Protection of human subjects, Washington, DC, revised June 23, 2005, effective June 23, 2005, The Department.
6. National Guideline Clearinghouse, Agency for Healthcare Research and Quality, US Department of Health and Human Services. www.guideline.gov. Accessed August 10, 2010.
7. National Highway Traffic Safety Administration: *The National EMS Education Standards*, Washington, DC, 2009, U.S. Department of Transportation/National Highway Traffic Safety Administration, DOT.
8. Pyrczak F: *Evaluating research in academic journals: a practical guide to realistic evaluation*, Glendale, 2008, Pyrczak Publishing.

SUGGESTED READINGS

Brown LH, et al: *An introduction to EMS research*, Upper Saddle River, NJ, 2002, Pearson Education.

Jaeger RM: *Statistics: a spectator sport*, New York, 1990, Sage Productions.

LoBiondo-Wood G, Haber J: *Nursing research: methods and critical appraisal for evidence-based practice*, ed 7, St Louis, 2010, Mosby.

PART TWO

Anatomy and Physiology

9 Medical Terminology

OBJECTIVES

Upon completion of this chapter, the paramedic student will be able to:

1. Explain the use of medical terms to describe organs and processes.
2. Explain the role of a prefix, root word, combining vowel, and suffix in a medial term.
3. Interpret selected examples of medical prefixes, root words, combining vowels, and suffixes.
4. Distinguish between singular and plural forms of medical terms.
5. Use accepted medical abbreviations appropriately.
6. Differentiate between similar medical terms and abbreviations

KEY TERMS

combining vowels Vowels often used between root words and suffixes or between two or more root words.

prefix One or more root syllables at the beginning of a word; a prefix often describes location or intensity.

root words Medical words that may be combined to describe a particular structure or condition.

suffix A word part that appears at the end of a medical word; the suffix often describes a patient's condition or diagnosis.

A necessary skill for working in the health care profession is the ability to speak and understand the language of medicine. This skill is required for conveying patient information to other members of the heath care team. In addition, medical terminology is universally understood. It provides a clear and concise way to document patient care activities.

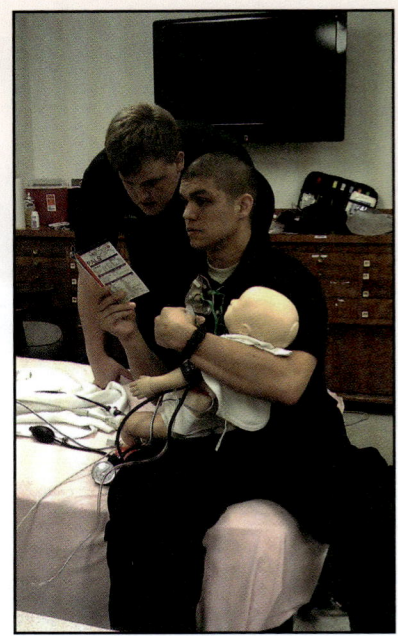

(Courtesy Kim McKenna, St. Charles, Mo.)

THE LANGUAGE OF MEDICINE

The language of medicine offers intriguing challenges both to medical historians and to linguists. The oldest written sources of Western medicine are the Hippocratic writings from the fourth and fifth centuries BC. This was the beginning of the Greek era of the language of medicine. This era lasted even after the Roman conquest. During the Renaissance (fourteenth to seventeenth centuries), the Greek language was not widely understood. Over time, Greek words were translated into Latin. As a result, most medical terms today are derived from Greek, and many have Latin roots. Medical terms that describe a disease are usually of Greek origin. Medical terms used to describe anatomy are usually of Latin origin.[1]

> **NOTE**
>
> Most major medical journals are written in English. In addition, English has become the language of choice at international medical conferences. Newer medical terms are being coined from ordinary English words. Examples include *bypass*, *shunt*, *pacemaker*, and *screening*. Non-English-speaking countries often translate these terms into their own language. These countries also accept and use English acronyms, such as AIDS (acquired immune deficiency syndrome) and CPR (cardiopulmonary resuscitation).

WORD PARTS OF MEDICAL TERMINOLOGY

Medical terms (Table 9-1) are used as descriptives for:

- Body structures and systems
- Anatomical regions and locations
- Diseases and other health problems
- Medical and surgical procedures
- Diagnostic tests
- Medical instruments

Most medical terms can be broken down into one or more word parts. For the sake of simplicity, these word parts are known as *prefixes, suffixes, root words,* and some *linking* or *combining vowels.* A knowledge of the basic word parts can help paramedics understand medical terminology and use it correctly (Figure 9-1).

Prefixes

A **prefix** is one or more root syllables at the beginning of a word. In medical terminology, a prefix often describes location and intensity. For example, the word *abnormal* begins with the prefix *ab*, which means "away from." This is followed by *normal*, which means "within a balance." Therefore, *abnormal* describes something that is not within balance. Other common prefixes are listed in Table 9-2.

Suffixes

A **suffix** appears at the end of a medical word. In medical terminology, a suffix often describes a patient's condition or diagnosis. For example, *bronchitis* begins with the root word *bronchi* (a respiratory structure). The root word, *bronchi*, is followed by the suffix *itis*, which means "inflammation." Therefore, *bronchitis* describes inflammation of the bronchi. Other common suffixes are listed in Table 9-3.

Root Words

Root words are medical words that may be combined to describe a particular structure or condition. They usually are derived from Latin or Greek nouns, verbs, or adjectives.

TABLE 9-1 Examples of Medical Terms

Body Structures and Systems
Aden/o: Gland
Cardi/o: Heart
Cyt/o: Cell
Hist/o: Tissue
Neur/o: Nerve
Viscer/o: Internal organs

Anatomical Regions and Locations
Anteroposterior: Pertaining to the front and to the back
Bilateral: Pertaining to two sides
Caudal: Pertaining to the tail
Cephalic: Pertaining to the head
Dorsal: Pertaining to the back

Diseases and Other Health Problems
Aphagia: Without swallowing (inability to swallow)
Carcinoma: Cancerous tumor (malignant)
Dyspnea: Difficulty breathing
Neoplasm: New growth (of abnormal tissue or tumor)
Sepsis: Systemic infection

Medical and Surgical Procedures
Appendectomy: Surgical removal of the appendix
Endoscopy: Visual examination of a hollow organ or body cavity
Hemodialysis: Removal of impurities from the blood
Laryngoscopy: Visual examination of the larynx
Nephrectomy: Surgical removal of a kidney

Medical Instruments
Capnometer: Used to measure carbon dioxide
Ophthalmoscope: Used to evaluate the eye
Otoscope: Used to evaluate the inner ear
Oximeter: Used to measure oxygen
Sphygmomanometer: Used to measure blood pressure

Diagnostic Tests
Arterial blood gases (ABGs): A test performed on arterial blood to determine levels of oxygen, carbon dioxide, and other gases
Computed tomography (CT) scan: Computerized imaging of body organs in sectional slices
Magnetic resonance imaging (MRI): An imaging technique in which magnetic and radio waves are used to produce images of organs and tissues in all three planes of the body
Purified protein derivative (PPD) skin test: A test performed on individuals who have been recently exposed to tuberculosis
Ultrasonography: An imaging technique in which scans are obtained through the use of high-frequency sound waves

For example, *cardiopulmonary* begins with the root word *cardio*, which means "heart"; the next root word is *pulmonary*, which means "lungs." Therefore, *cardiopulmonary* refers to the cardiac and respiratory systems. Other common root words are listed in Table 9-4.

Combining Vowels

Combining vowels are also known as *linking vowels.* Combining vowels make medical terms easier to pronounce. The vowel most often used is *o.* An example of the use of a combining vowel is shown in the preceding box for the term

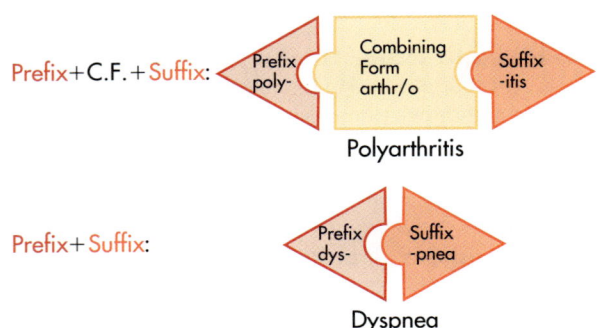

Polyarthritis

Dyspnea

FIGURE 9-1 The relationship of prefixes, suffixes, and combining words. (Leonard PC: *Quick and easy medical terminology,* ed 6, St Louis, 2011, Saunders.)

sternocleidomastoid: *stern—**o**—cleid—**o**—mastoid.* Other vowels, such as *i* and *a,* are also used. Combining vowels often are used between root words and suffixes, as well as between two or more root words. They are not used between prefixes and root words. Table 9-5 presents guidelines for the use of combining vowels.

PLURAL FORMS OF MEDICAL TERMS

As do words in any language, medical terms need both a singular form and a plural form. Because most medical terms are Greek or Latin in origin, some unusual rules must be followed to change a singular word into its plural form. These rules are presented in Table 9-6.

TABLE 9-2 Common Prefixes

Prefix	Meaning	Example
a-, an-	without, lack of	apnea (without breath)
		anemia (lack of blood)
ad-	to, toward	adhesion (something stuck to or remaining close to)
angio-	vessel	angiogram (the study of vessels)
ante-	before, forward	antenatal (occurring or formed before birth)
anti-	against, opposed to	antipyretic (against fever)
arter-	artery	arteriogram (study of arteries)
arthro-	pertaining to a joint	arthroscopy (inspection of a joint)
bi-	two	bilateral (both sides)
bio-	life	biology (the study of life)
brady-	slow	bradycardia (slow heart rate)
cardi-	pertaining to the heart	cardiography (recording the movements of the heart)
cerebr-	brain	cerebral (pertaining to the brain)
cerv-	neck	cervical (pertaining to the neck)
chole-	pertaining to bile	cholelithiasis (stones in the gallbladder)
contra-	against, opposite	contrastimulant (against stimulating)
cost-	pertaining to a rib	costal margin (margin of the lower limit of the ribs)
cyst-	pertaining to the bladder or any fluid-containing sac	cystitis (inflammation of the urinary bladder)
cyt-	cell	cytology (the study of cells)
di-	twice, double	diplopia (double vision)
dys-	with difficulty	dyspnea (difficulty breathing)
ecto-	out from	ectopic (out of place)

TABLE 9-3 Common Suffixes

Suffix	Meaning	Example
-algia	pertaining to pain	neuralgia (pain along a nerve)
-centesis	puncturing	thoracentesis (puncturing into a pleural space)
-cyte	cell	leukocyte (white cell)
-ectomy	a cutting out	tonsillectomy (surgical removal of the tonsils)
-emia	blood	anemia (a decrease in blood hemoglobin)
-esthesia	sensation	anesthesia (without sensation)
-genic	causing	carcinogenic (cancer causing)
-ology	science of	psychology (the science or study of behavior)
-ostomy	creation of an opening	gastrostomy (artificial opening into the stomach)
-osis	condition	psychosis (condition of the mind)
-paresis	weakness	hemiparesis (one-sided weakness)
-phagia	eating	polyphagia (excessive eating)
-pnea	breathing	dyspnea (difficulty breathing)
-pathy	disease	neuropathy (disease of the peripheral nerves)
-phasia	speech	aphasia (loss of the power of speech)
-plasty	repair of, tying of	angioplasty (repair of damaged vessels)
-rhythmia	rhythm	dysrhythmia (variation from a normal rhythm)
-rrhagia	bursting forth	hemorrhage (flowing of blood)
-rrhea	flowing	pyorrhea (discharge of pus)
-scopy	examination by inspection	laparoscopy (examination of the abdominal cavity with a laparoscope)
-uria	pertaining to urine	polyuria (excessive secretion of urine)

TABLE 9-4 Common Root Words

Root Word	Meaning	Root Word	Meaning
adeno-	gland	mal-	bad
arter-	artery	meningo-	meninges
arthro-	joint	myo-	muscle
asthenia-	weakness	nephro-	kidney
bio-	life	neuro-	nerve
bucc-	cheek	noct-	night
burs-	pouch or sac	oculo-	eye
carc-	cancer	orchi-	testicle
cardio-	heart	osteo-	bone
caut-	to burn	oto-	ear
cephalo-	head	ov-	egg
cerv-	neck	pariet-	wall
chole-	bile	phago-	to eat
chondro-	cartilage	pharyngo-	throat
cysto-	bladder	phlebo-	vein
cyto-	cell	photo-	light
dermo-	skin	pneumo-	air
edem-	swelling	procto-	rectum
entero-	intestine	pseud-	false
eryth-	red	psych-	mind
eti-	cause	pyo-	pus
febr-	fever	rhino-	nose
flex-	to bend	sclero-	hardness
gastro-	stomach	sept-	wall
glyco-	sugar	somat-	body
gyn-	female	stern-	chest
hemo-	blood	tact-	to touch
hepato-	liver	thoraco-	chest
hydra-	water	uro-	urinary
iod-	distinct	varic-	dilated vein
leuko-	white	vaso-	vessel

TABLE 9-5 Guidelines for Using Combining Vowels

1. When a word root and a suffix are connected, a **combining vowel** *IS USED* if the suffix *DOES NOT BEGIN* **with a vowel.**
   arthr/**o**/pathy

2. When a word root and a suffix are connected, a **combining vowel** *USUALLY IS NOT USED* **if the suffix** *BEGINS* **with a vowel.**
   hepat/ic

3. When two word roots are connected, a **combining vowel** *USUALLY IS USED* **even if vowels are present at the junctions.**
   oste/**o**/arthr/it/is

4. When a prefix and a word root are connected, a **combining vowel** *IS NOT USED.*
   sub/hepat/ic

From LaFleur Brooks M: *Exploring medical language,* ed 7, St Louis, 2009, Mosby.

MEDICAL ABBREVIATIONS, ACRONYMS, AND SYMBOLS

Many EMS systems develop agency-approved medical abbreviations. Medical abbreviations, including acronyms and symbols, promote efficient communication and documentation. Communication and documentation of medical information require thoroughness, precision, and accuracy. Medical abbreviations, acronyms, and symbols are a form of medical shorthand. They are universally understood by other members of the heath care team. Some of the more

TABLE 9-6 Guidelines for Pluralizing Medical Terms

Guideline	Singular Form	Plural Form
1. If the term ends in "a", the plural is formed by adding an "e".	bursa	bursae
2. If the term ends in "ex" or "ix", the plural is formed by changing ex/ix to "ices".	vertebra	vertebrae
	appendix	appendices
	cervix	cervices
3. If the term ends in "is", the plural is formed by changing the is to "es".	diagnosis	diagnoses
	neurosis	neuroses
	metastasis	metastases
4. If the term ends in "itis", the plural is formed by dropping the s and adding "des".	arthritis	arthritides
	meningitis	meningitides
5. If the term ends in "nx" the plural is formed by changing the x to "g" and adding "es".	phalanx	phalanges
	larynx	larynges
6. If the term ends in "on", the plural is formed by dropping the on and adding "a".	criterion	criteria
	ganglion	ganglia
7. If the term ends in "um", the plural is formed by changing um to "a".	diverticulum	diverticula
	ovum	ova
8. If the term ends in "us", the plural is formed by changing us to "i".	alveolus	alveoli
	bronchus	bronchi
	malleolus	malleoli

From National Safety Councils of Canada: *Introduction to medical terminology,* 2005.

common medical abbreviations, acronyms, and symbols used in EMS systems can be found in Box 9-1.

NOTE

Many medical abbreviations and acronyms may have common, multiple meanings. For example, the acronym **PE** may be used for *physical examination, pulmonary edema,* or *pulmonary embolism.* Therefore, it is important for every EMS agency or medical direction system to have an approved list of medical abbreviations and acronyms. This helps ensure precision in documentation. It also facilitates patient assessments and patient histories. In addition, approved lists may provide for medical-legal protection if cases are reviewed for litigation.

Do Not Use List

In May, 2005, The Joint Commission (formerly known as the Joint Commission on Accreditation of Healthcare Organizations, or JCAHO) affirmed its "Do Not Use" list of abbreviations (originally created in 2004).[2] The list, which is updated annually, is designed to eliminate the use of abbreviations, acronyms, symbols, and drug dose designations that could be confusing or dangerous and that might result in errors. Many EMS agencies and health care facilities use this list as part of their documentation protocol (Table 9-7).

SHOW ME THE EVIDENCE

Brunetti and colleagues found that nearly 5% of the errors reported to Medmarx, a national database for medication errors, were related to abbreviation use. Many of the abbreviations involved in the errors were on the official "Do Not Use" list of abbreviations established by The Joint Commission (formerly known as the Joint Commission on Accreditation of Healthcare Organizations).

From Brunetti L, Santell JP, Hicks RW: The impact of abbreviations on patient safety, *The Joint Commission Journal on Quality and Patient Safety* 33:576-583, 2007.

PRONUNCIATION OF MEDICAL TERMS

Correct spelling and pronunciation of medical terms are necessary for good communication. These skills are expected of health care professionals. A good way to learn (and remember) the spelling and pronunciation of medical terms is first to consider the way the terms are built. This is done by analyzing the root words, prefixes, and suffixes described earlier in the chapter. Understanding root words and memorizing these terms and their correct spelling, can help paramedics build a medical vocabulary.

The pronunciation of medical terms often varies, because no "rigid rules" exist. In addition, medical terms often are pronounced somewhat differently even among medical professionals. Some medical terms can be acceptably pronounced in more than one way (Table 9-8). A common

BOX 9-1 Common Medical Abbreviations Used by EMS Systems*

°C	degrees Centigrade	CPAP	continuous positive airway pressure
°F	degrees Fahrenheit	CPK	creatine phosphokinase
ABG	arterial blood gas	CPR	cardiopulmonary resuscitation
Ac	before meals	CSF	cerebrospinal fluid
ACS	acute coronary syndrome	CT	computed tomography
ad lib	freely as desired	CVA	cerebrovascular accident,
ADHD	attention deficit/hyperactivity disorder		costovertebral angle
ADL	activities of daily living	CVP	central venous pressure
AED	automated external defibrillator	D&C	dilation and curettage
Afib	atrial fibrillation	D_5W	5% dextrose in water
AICD	automatic implanted cardioverter	DB	diabetes
	defibrillator	dc	discontinue
AIDS	acquired immunodeficiency syndrome	DIC	disseminated intravascular coagulation
ALS	amyotrophic lateral sclerosis	diff	differential blood count
AM	morning	dil	dilute
A.M.A.	against medical advice	DJD	degenerative joint disease
AMI	acute myocardial infarction	dL	deciliter
amp	ampule	DM	diastolic murmur
ARC	AIDS-related complex	DNR/DNAR	do not resuscitate
ARDS	acute respiratory distress syndrome	DOE	dyspnea on exertion
AS	aortic stenosis	DVT	deep vein thrombosis
ASD	atrial septal defect	dx, DX	diagnosis
BE	barium enema	EBV	Epstein-Barr virus
bid	two times a day	ECF	extracellular fluid
BiPAP	Bilevel positive airway pressure	ECG	electrocardiogram
BLS	basic life support	ECT	electroconvulsive therapy
BM, bm	bowel movement	ED	emergency department
BNP	brain natriuretic peptide	EDC	estimated date of confinement
BMR	basal metabolic rate	EDD	estimated date of delivery
BP	blood pressure	EEG	electroencephalogram
BPH	benign prostatic hypertrophy	EKG	electrocardiogram
BPM	beats per minute	elix	elixir
BSA	body surface area	EMG	electromyogram
BUN	blood urea nitrogen	ENG	electronystagmography
BVM	bag valve mask	ER	emergency room
	with	ESR	erythrocyte sedimentation rate
c/o	complains of	ESRD	end-stage renal disease
Ca	calcium, cancer, carcinoma	EST	electroshock therapy
CAD	coronary artery disease	$etCO_2$	end-tidal carbon dioxide
cap	capsule	ETOH	ethyl alcohol
CAT	computed axial tomography	Fe	iron
cath	catheter, catheterize	FEV	forced expiratory volume
CBC	complete blood count	FHR	fetal heart rate
CBR	complete bed rest	FRC	functional residual capacity
CC	chief complaint	FUO	fever of unknown origin
CCU	coronary care unit, critical care unit	Fx, fx	fracture, fractional urine test
CDC	Centers for Disease Control and	g, gm, Gm	gram
	Prevention	GCS	Glasgow Coma Scale
CHF	congestive heart failure	GERD	gastroesophageal reflux disease
CHO	carbohydrate	GI	gastrointestinal
Cl	chlorine	Grava I, II, III, etc.	pregnancy one, two, three, etc.
cm	centimeter	gt, gtt	drop, drops
cm^3	cubic centimeter	GTT	glucose tolerance test
CNS	central nervous system	GU	genitourinary
CO	carbon monoxide	GYN, Gyn	gynecological
CO_2	carbon dioxide	H_2O	water
COPD	chronic obstructive pulmonary disease	H^+	hydrogen ion

Continued

BOX 9-1 Common Medical Abbreviations Used by EMS Systems—cont'd

h/o	history of	MCV	mean cell volume, mean corpuscular volume
H&P	history and physical examination	mg	milligram
HAV	hepatitis A virus	Mg	magnesium
Hb	hemoglobin	MG	myasthenia gravis
HBV	hepatitis B virus	MI	myocardial infarction
Hct, HCT	hematocrit	min	minute(s)
Hg	mercury	MICU	medical intensive care unit
Hgb	hemoglobin	mL	milliliter
HIV	human immunodeficiency (AIDS) virus	mm	millimeter
HSV	herpes simplex virus	mm^3	cubic millimeter
HTN	hypertension	mm Hg	millimeters of mercury
IBD	irritable bowel disease	MOI	mechanism of injury
I&O	intake and output	MRI	magnetic resonance imaging
IC	inspiratory capacity	MS	multiple sclerosis
ICP	intracranial pressure	mV	millivolt
ICU	intensive care unit	N	nitrogen
IDDM	insulin-dependent diabetes mellitus	Na	sodium
Ig	immunoglobulin	NG	nasogastric
IgA, etc.	immunoglobulin A, etc.	NICU	neonatal intensive care unit
IM	Intramuscular	NIPPV	noninvasive positive pressure ventilation
INR	International normalized ratio	NOI	nature of illness
IO	intraosseous	NPA	nasopharyngeal airway
IPPB	intermittent positive-pressure breathing	NPO	nothing by mouth
ITD	impedance threshold device	NS	normal saline
IV	intravenous	O$_2$	oxygen
IVP	intravenous push; intravenous pyelogram	OCD	obsessive compulsive disorder
IVPB	intravenous piggy back	OD	overdose
J	joules	OG	orogastric
K	potassium	OPA	oropharyngeal airway
kg	kilogram	ORIF	open reduction and internal fixation
KUB	kidney, ureters, and bladder (radiograph)	OT	occupational therapy
KVO	keep vein open	OTC	over-the-counter
L	liter	oz	ounce
L&A	light and accommodation	Paco$_2$	partial pressure of carbon dioxide (arterial blood)
LBBB	left bundle branch block	Pao$_2$	partial pressure of oxygen (arterial blood)
LE	lupus erythematosus		
LLL	left lower lobe	para I, ... II, etc	unipara, bipara, etc.
LLQ	left lower quadrant	PAT	paroxysmal atrial tachycardia
LMP	last menstrual period	pc	after meals
LNMP	last normal menstrual period	PCI	percutaneous coronary intervention
LP	lumbar puncture	Pco$_2$	partial pressure of carbon dioxide
LR	lactated Ringer's solution	PCP	pulmonary capillary pressure, phencyclidine
LUL	left upper lobe		
LUQ	left upper quadrant	PCV	packed cell volume
LV	left ventricle	PCWP	pulmonary capillary wedge pressure
LVAD	left ventricular assist device	PE	pulmonary embolism, physical examination
LVH	left ventricular hypertrophy		
M	meter	PEEP	positive-end expiratory pressure
MAP	mean arterial pressure	PEF	peak expiratory flow
min	minim	per	through, by way of
max	maximum	PERRLA	pupils equal, round, and reactive to light and accommodation
MAP	mean arterial pressure		
mcg, mg	microgram	PET	positron emission tomography
MCH	mean corpuscular hemoglobin	PG	prostaglandin
MCHC	mean corpuscular hemoglobin concentration	pH	hydrogen ion concentration (acidity and alkalinity)

BOX 9-1   Common Medical Abbreviations Used by EMS Systems—cont'd

PID	pelvic inflammatory disease	sib	sibling
PIH	pregnancy-induced hypertension	SICU	surgical intensive care unit
PKU	phenylketonuria	SIDS	sudden infant death syndrome
PM	postmortem	Sig	write on label
pm	evening	SL	sublingual
PMS	premenstrual syndrome	SLE	systemic lupus erythematosus
PND	paroxysmal nocturnal dyspnea, postnasal drip	sol	solution, dissolved
		sos	if necessary
Po_2	partial pressure of oxygen	sp gr, SG, sg	specific gravity
PO, po	orally	Sub-Q, subQ	Subcutaneous
PPD	purified protein derivative	SpCO	saturated pressure carbon monoxide
ppm	parts per million	SpMet	saturated pressure methemoglobin
prn	when required, as often as necessary	SSS	sick sinus syndrome, specific soluble substance, short-stay surgery
PSVT	paroxysmal supraventricular tachycardia	stat	immediately
PT	physical therapy; prothrombin time	STD	sexually transmitted disease
PTSD	post-traumatic stress disorder	STEMI	ST elevation myocardial infarction
PTT	partial thromboplastin time	susp	suspension
PVC	premature ventricular complex	T_3	triiodothyronine
q	every	T_4	tetraiodothyronine
q2h	every 2 hours	T&A	tonsillectomy and adenoidectomy
q3h	every 3 hours	TAH	total abdominal hysterectomy
q4h	every 4 hours	TB, TBC	tuberculosis
qh	every hour	TCP	transcutaneous pacing
QID	four times a day	TdP	torsades de pointes
qn	every night	Tdap	tetanus, diphtheria, acellular pertussis
qod	every other day	TIA	transient ischemic attack
qns	quantity not sufficient	TIBC	total iron-binding capacity
R/O	rule out	TID	three times a day
RA	rheumatoid arthritis	TKO	to keep open
RBBB	right bundle branch block	TPN	total parenteral nutrition
RDS	respiratory distress syndrome	TPR	temperature, pulse, and respirations
Rh+	positive Rh factor	UA	Unstable angina; urinalysis
Rh-	negative Rh factor	URI	upper respiratory infection
RHD	rheumatic heart disease	UTI	urinary tract infection
RLL	right lower lobe	VC	vital capacity
RLQ	right lower quadrant	VD	venereal disease
RML	right middle lobe	VDH	valvular disease of the heart
ROM	range of motion	VDRL	Venereal Disease Research Laboratory (test for syphilis)
ROS	review of systems		
ROSC	return of spontaneous circulation	VF	ventricular fibrillation
RSI	rapid sequence intubation	VS	vital signs
RSV	respiratory syncytial virus	VSD	ventricular septal defect
RUL	right upper lobe	V_T	tidal volume
RUQ	right upper quadrant	VF	ventricular fibrillation
Rx	take; treatment	VT	ventricular tachycardia
s̄	without	WBC	white blood cell, white blood count
SB	sternal border	WNL	within normal limits
sec	second(s)	WPW	Wolff-Parkinson White

*Adapted From Potter PA, Perry AG: Basic nursing: essentials for practice, ed 6, St Louis, 2007, Mosby.

TABLE 9-7 The Joint Commission's "Do Not Use" Abbreviations List

OFFICIAL "DO NOT USE" LIST*

Do Not Use	Potential Problem	Use Instead
U (unit)	Mistaken for "0" (zero), the number "4" (four) or "cc"	Write "unit"
IU (International Unit)	Mistaken for IV (intravenous) or the number 10 (ten)	Write "International Unit"
Q.D., QD, q.d., qd (daily)	Mistaken for each other	Write "daily"
Q.O.D., QOD, q.o.d., qod (every other day)	Period after the Q mistaken for "I" and the "O" mistaken for "I"	Write "every other day"
Trailing zero (X.0 mg)†	Decimal point is missed	Write X mg
Lack of leading zero (.X mg)		Write 0.X mg
MS	Can mean morphine sulfate or magnesium sulfate	Write "morphine sulfate"
MSO_4 and $MgSO_4$	Confused for one another	Write "magnesium sulfate"

ADDITIONAL ABBREVIATIONS, ACRONYMS, AND SYMBOLS
(FOR POSSIBLE FUTURE INCLUSION IN THE OFFICIAL "DO NOT USE" LIST)

Do Not Use	Potential Problem	Use Instead
> (greater than)	Misinterpreted as the number "7" (seven) or the letter "L"	Write "greater than"
< (less than)	Confused for one another	Write "less than"
Abbreviations for drug names	Misinterpreted due to similar abbreviations for multiple drugs	Write drug names in full
Apothecary units	Unfamiliar to many practitioners. Confused with metric units	Use metric units
@	Mistaken for the number "2" (two)	Write "at"
Cc	Mistaken for U (units) when poorly written	Write "mL" or "milliliters"
μg	Mistaken for mg (milligrams) resulting in 1000-fold overdose	Write "mcg" or "micrograms"

Joint Commission on Accreditation of Healthcare Organizations, 2010.http://www.jointcommission.org/assets/1/18/Official_Do%20Not%20Use_List_%206_10.pdf. Accessed 4-19-11

*Applies to all orders and all medication-related documentation that is handwritten (including free-text computer entry) or on preprinted forms.

†**Exception:** A "trailing zero" may be used only where required to demonstrate the level of precision of the value being reported, such as for laboratory results, imaging studies that report size of lesions, or catheter/tube sizes. It may not be used in medication orders or other medication-related documentation.

TABLE 9-8 Guide to Pronunciation of Medical Terms

The following is a simple guide for practicing the pronunciation of medical terms. The pronunciations are only approximate; however, they are adequate to meet the needs of the beginning student.

In respelling for pronunciation, words are minimally distorted to indicate phonetic sound.

Example:
 doctor (dok-tor)
 gastric (gas-trik)

A special mark, called the *macron* (ˉ), is used to indicate long vowel sounds.

Example:
 donate (dō-nāt)
 hepatoma (hep-a-tō-ma)
 ā as in *ate, say*
 ē as in *eat, beet, see*
 ī as in *I, mine, sky*
 ō as in *oats, so*
 ū as in *unit, mute*

Vowels with no markings have the short sound.

Continued

TABLE 9-8 Guide to Pronunciation of Medical Terms—cont'd

Example:
  discuss (dis-kus)
  medical (med-i-kal)
  a as in *at, lad*
  e as in *edge, bet*
  i as in *itch, wish*
  o as in *ox, top*
  u as in *sun, come*
An accent mark indicates the stress on a certain syllable. The primary accent is indicated by capital letters, and the secondary
  accent (which is stressed but not as strongly as the primary accent) is indicated by italics.
Example:
  altogether (*all*-tū-GETH-er)
  pancreatitis (*pan*-krē-a-TĪ-tis)

From LaFleur Brooks M: *Exploring medical language,* ed 7, St Louis, 2009, Mosby.

example is *angina* (an′ jin a) with the emphasis on the first syllable and a short i and (an jin′ a) with the emphasis on the second syllable and a long i. Some medical terms look alike and sound alike but have very different meanings.

NOTE
Paramedics who can spell a medical term accurately usually can also pronounce it correctly.

The pronunciation of medical terms is best perfected by using the word frequently and by saying the word aloud. If the paramedic is unsure of any word, the correct spelling and pronunciation should be checked in a medical dictionary.

DID YOU KNOW?
Confusing Medical Terms
Some medical terms look alike and sound alike, but have very different meanings. Some common ones that are easily confused include:
- **Arterio** means artery. **Athero** means plaque or fatty substance. **Arthro** means joint.
- **Ileum** is a part of the small intestine. **Ilium** means part of the hip bone.
- **Mucous** means resembles mucus. **Mucus** is the substance secreted from the membranes.
- **Myco** means fungus. **Myelo** means both bone marrow and spinal cord. **Myo** means muscle.
- **Palpation** is an examination technique. **Palpitation** means a pounding racing heart.
- **Pyelo** means the renal pelvis. **Pyo** means pus.
- **Viral** means a virus. **Virile** means having masculine traits.

SUMMARY

- Medical terminology is the language of medicine. It is important to know the language to interpret patient information and communicate it to other health care personnel.
- Medical terms are used to describe body structures, systems, and functions; anatomical regions and locations; diseases and other health problems; medical and surgical procedures; diagnostic tests; and medical instruments.
- Medical terms are broken down into several parts. These parts include prefixes, suffixes, root words, and some combining vowels.
- A prefix is a root syllable at the beginning of a word that describes location or intensity.
- A suffix comes at the end of a word and describes a condition or diagnosis.
- Root words describe a structure or condition. Root words may be combined with other root words, a prefix, and/or a suffix.

- Combining vowels join syllables in medical terms to make them easier to pronounce.
- Medical terms are interpreted by analyzing each word part and then combining them to determine the meaning.
- Specific rules govern the conversion of medical terms from the singular form to the plural form. For example, *vertebra* becomes *vertebrae; diagnosis* becomes *diagnoses; phalanx* becomes *phalanges;* and *alveolus* becomes *alveoli.*
- Medical abbreviations, acronyms, and symbols are a form of medical shorthand. It is important for paramedics to use the abbreviations approved within their EMS system.
- Paramedics must be able to pronounce medical terms correctly so that their intended meaning is communicated clearly.

REFERENCES

1. Wulff H: The language of medicine, *R Soc Med* 97:187-188, 2004.

2. The Joint Commission: The official "do not use" list of abbreviations. http://www.jointcommission.org/assets/1/18/Official_Do%20Not%20Use_List_%206_10.pdf. Accessed 4-19-11.

SUGGESTED READINGS

Chabner DE: *Medical terminology: a short course,* ed 5, St Louis, 2009, Saunders.

Flashcard Exchange: www.flashcardexchange.com/

Leonard PC: *Quick and easy medical terminology,* ed 5, St Louis, 2007, Saunders.

CHAPTER
10 Review of Human Systems

OBJECTIVES

Upon completion of this chapter, the paramedic student will be able to:

1. Discuss the importance of human anatomy as it relates to the paramedic profession.
2. Describe the anatomical position.
3. Properly interpret anatomical directional terms and body planes.
4. List the structures that compose the axial and appendicular regions of the body.
5. Define the divisions of the abdominal region.
6. List the three major body cavities.
7. Describe the contents of the three major body cavities.
8. Discuss the functions of the following cellular structures: the cytoplasmic membrane, the cytoplasm (and organelles), and the nucleus.
9. Describe the process by which human cells reproduce.
10. Differentiate and describe the following tissue types: epithelial tissue, connective tissue, muscle tissue, and nervous tissue.
11. For each of the 11 major organ systems in the human body, label a diagram of anatomical structures; list the functions of the major anatomical structures; and explain how the organs of the system interrelate to perform the specific functions of that system.
12. For the special senses, label a diagram of the anatomical structures of the special senses; list the functions of the anatomical structures of each sense; and explain how the structures of the senses interrelate to perform their specialized functions.

KEY TERMS

abdominal aorta The portion of the descending aorta that passes from the aortic hiatus of the diaphragm into the abdomen, where it divides into the two common iliac arteries.

acetabulum The large, cup-shaped articular cavity at the juncture of the ilium, the ischium, and the pubis that contains the ball-shaped head of the femur.

action potential A change in membrane potential in an excitable tissue that acts as an electrical signal and is propagated in an all-or-none fashion.

adenosine triphosphate (ATP) A nucleotide composed of adenosine, an organic base, with three phosphate groups attached to it; it stores energy in muscles.

adipose tissue A specialized connective tissue that stores lipids; also known as *fat tissue.*

aerobic oxidation A biochemical reaction that increases the positive charges on an atom or the loss of negative charges in the presence of oxygen.

afferent division The division of the peripheral nervous system that transmits impulses from the periphery to the central nervous system.

afferent neurons Neurons that carry action potentials from the periphery to the CNS.

aldosterone A steroid hormone produced by the adrenal cortex to regulate the sodium and potassium balance in the blood.

alveoli Minute air sacs in the lungs through which gas exchange takes place between alveolar air and pulmonary capillary blood.

amino acids Organic chemical compounds composed of one or more basic amino groups and one or more acidic carboxyl groups.

antidiuretic hormone (ADH) A hormone produced in the posterior pituitary gland that regulates the balance of water in the body by accelerating the resorption of water.

anus The distal end or outlet of the rectum.

aorta The main and largest artery in the body.

anatomical position The position of standing erect with the feet and palms facing the examiner.

anterior The front, or ventral, surface.

appendicular region The region comprised of the limbs, or extremities.

appendicular skeleton The bones of the upper and lower extremities.

aqueous humor The clear, watery fluid that circulates in the anterior and posterior chambers of the eye.

arachnoid layer The delicate, weblike, middle membrane that covers the brain.

areola The circular, pigmented area surrounding the nipple.

areolar connective tissue A loose tissue that consists of delicate webs of fibers and a variety of cells embedded in a matrix of soft, sticky gel.

arterioles Small branches of arteries.

arteriovenous anastomoses Vessels that allow blood to flow from arteries to veins without passing through capillaries; also known as *arteriovenous shunts*.

atrial natriuretic factor (ANF) A peptide released from the atria when atrial blood pressure is increased; it lowers blood pressure by increasing urine production, thus reducing blood volume.

atrioventricular node An area of specialized cardiac muscle that receives the cardiac impulse from the sinoatrial node and conducts it to the bundle of His.

atrioventricular valve A valve in the heart through which blood flows from the atria to the ventricles.

auricle The part of the external ear that protrudes from the head; also known as the *pinna*.

autonomic nervous system The division of the peripheral nervous system that acts as a control system for visceral processes; it functions largely below the level of consciousness.

autonomic reflex Any of a large number of normal reflexes governing and regulating the functions of the viscera

autophagia A condition in which the body obtains nutrition through consumption of its own tissues.

axial region The region comprised of the head, neck, thorax, and abdomen.

axial skeleton The bones of the head, neck, and torso.

bacteria Single-celled microorganisms that cause an infection characteristic of that species.

basophils White blood cells that promote inflammation; they readily stain with specific dyes.

bicuspid valve One of the two atrioventricular valves located between the left atrium and ventricle; also known as the mitral valve.

bile A bitter, yellow-green secretion of the liver that is stored in the gallbladder.

blood The fluid and its suspended, formed elements that circulate through the heart, arteries, capillaries, and veins.

bone A highly specialized form of hard, connective tissue; it consists of living cells and mineralized matrix.

bony labyrinth Part of the inner ear; it contains the membranous labyrinth.

Bowman's capsule The expanded beginning of a renal tubule.

bronchioles Small branches of the bronchi.

bulbourethral glands Small glands located just below the prostate gland that lubricate the terminal portion of the urethra and contribute to seminal fluid; also known as Cowper's glands.

bundle of His A band of fibers in the myocardium through which the cardiac impulse is transmitted from the atrioventricular node to the ventricles.

calcaneus The heel bone, the largest of the tarsal bones.

cancellous bone Lattice like tissue normally present in the interior of many bones where spaces usually are filled with marrow; also known as *spongy bone*.

capillaries Tiny vessels that connect arterioles to venules.

cardiac muscle A special striated muscle of the myocardium that contains dark, intercalated disks at the junctions of the abutting fibers; it is characterized by special contractile abilities.

cardiac output The volume of blood pumped each minute by the ventricle.

cardiac sphincter A ring of muscle fibers at the juncture of the esophagus and stomach.

carina A downward and backward projection of the lowest tracheal cartilage, forming a ridge between the openings of the right and left primary bronchi.

carpal bones The bones of the carpus, or wrist.

cartilage Firm, smooth, nonvascular connective tissue.

cartilaginous joints Joints that are slightly movable.

cecum A cul-de-sac constituting the first part of the large intestine.

cell The functional basic unit of life.

central nervous system (CNS) The system composed of the brain and spinal cord.

centrioles Usually paired organelles that lie in the centrosome.

centrosome A specialized zone of cytoplasm close to the nucleus that contains two centrioles.

cerebellum The second largest part of the brain; it plays an essential role in producing normal movements.

cerebral cortex A thin layer of gray matter, made up of neuron dendrites and cell bodies, that comprises the surface of the cerebrum.

cerebrospinal fluid (CSF) The fluid that fills the subarachnoid space in the brain and spinal cord and is found in the cerebral ventricles.

cerebrum The largest and uppermost part of the brain; it controls consciousness, memory, sensations, emotions, and voluntary movements.

cervix The lower part of the uterus.

chromatin granules The material within the cell nucleus from which chromosomes are formed.

chromosomes Organized structures of deoxyribonucleic acid (DNA) and protein that are found in cells.

chyme The semifluid mass of partly digested food passed from the stomach into the duodenum.

cilia Small, hairlike processes on the outer surfaces of some cells.

clitoris Erectile tissue in the vestibule of the vagina.

compact bone Hard, dense bone that usually is found at the surface of skeletal structures, as distinguished from cancellous bone.

conjunctiva A mucous membrane that covers the anterior surface of the eyeball and the lining of the eyelids.

connective tissue Tissue that supports and binds other body tissues and parts.

cornea The convex, transparent, anterior part of the eye.

coronary arteries The two arteries that arise from the base of the aorta and carry blood to the muscle of the heart.

costal cartilages Cartilages that connect the sternum and the ends of the ribs; they allow the chest to move in respiration.

coxae The hip joints; the head of the femur and the acetabulum of the innominate bone.

cranial vault The eight skull bones that surround and protect the brain; the brain case.

cricoid cartilage The most inferior laryngeal cartilage.

cricothyroid membrane The membrane joining the thyroid and cricoid cartilages.

cytoplasm All of the substance of a cell other than the nucleus

cytoplasmic membrane The plasma membrane.

deoxyribonucleic acid (DNA) A type of nucleic acid that comprises the genetic material of cells.

dermatome The skin surface area supplied by a single spinal nerve.

dermis Dense, irregular connective tissue that forms the deep layer of the skin.

diaphragm The dome-shaped, musculofibrous partition that separates the thoracic and abdominal cavities.

diaphysis The shaft of a long bone, consisting of a tube of compact bone that encloses the medullary cavity.

diencephalon The parts of the brain between the cerebral hemispheres and the mesencephalon

differentiation A process in which cells become specialized in one type of function or act in concert with other cells to perform a more complex task.

dorsal root A sensory component that conveys afferent nerve processes to the spinal cord.

ductus deferens A thick, smooth muscular tube that allows sperm to exit from the epididymis through the ejaculatory duct; also known as the *vas deferens*.

duodenum The first subdivision of the small intestine.

dura mater The outermost layer of the meninges.

efferent division The division of the peripheral nervous system that transmits action potentials from the central nervous system to effector organs such as muscles and glands

efferent neurons Neurons that carry impulses away from the central nervous system to the periphery.

electrolytes Cations or anions in solution that conduct an electrical current.

endocrine glands Glands that secrete hormones into the blood rather than through a duct.

endocrine system A collection of glands that produce and secrete hormones.

endoplasmic reticulum A network of connecting sacs or canals that wind through the cytoplasm of a cell, serving as a miniature circulatory system for the cell.

enzymes A protein produced by living cells that catalyzes chemical reactions in organic matter.

eosinophil A white blood cell that inhibits inflammation; it readily stains with acidic dyes.

epicardium The portion of the serous pericardium that covers the heart's surface; also known as the *visceral pericardium*.

epidermis The outer portion of the skin; it is formed of epithelial tissue that rests on or covers the dermis.

epididymis A tightly coiled tube, lying along the top of and behind the testes, where sperm matures.

epidural space The space above or on the dura.

epiglottis A lidlike cartilage that overhangs the entrance to the larynx.

epiphyseal plate The site of bone elongation; also known as the *growth plate*.

epithelial tissue The cellular covering of internal and external surfaces of the body, including the lining of vessels and other small cavities.

erection The condition of hardness, swelling, and elevation observed in the penis and to a lesser degree in the clitoris, usually caused by sexual arousal.

erythrocytes Red blood cells.

esophagus The muscular canal extending from the pharynx to the stomach.

eukaryotes Cells with a true nucleus; they are found in all higher organisms and in some microorganisms.

eustachian tube The auditory canal; it extends from the middle ear to the nasopharynx; also known as the *auditory tube*.

exocrine gland A gland that secretes chemicals and hormones into a duct.

external ear The portion of the ear that includes the auricle and external auditory meatus; it terminates at the eardrum.

extracellular matrix Nonliving chemical substances located between connective tissue cells.

extracellular Occurring outside a cell or cell tissues or in cavities or spaces between cell layers or groups of cells.

femur The thigh bone, which extends from the pelvis to the knee; the largest and strongest bone in the body.

fibrous connective tissue A connective tissue that consists mainly of bundles of strong, white collagenous fibers arranged in parallel rows.

fibrous joints Joints that are immovable.

fibula The bone of the leg, lateral to and smaller than the tibia.

flat bones Bones that have a thin, flattened shape, such as certain skull bones, the ribs, the sternum, and the scapulae.

gallbladder A pear-shaped excretory sac on the visceral surface of the right lobe of the liver; it serves as a reservoir for bile.

ganglia A group of nerve cell bodies in the peripheral nervous system.

glomerulus The mass of capillary loops at the beginning of each nephron.

glottic opening The vocal cords and the space between them.

glycoproteins A large group of conjugated proteins in which the nonprotein substance is a carbohydrate.

Golgi apparatus Specialized endoplasmic reticulum that concentrates and packages materials for secretion from the cell.

gray matter The gray tissue that makes up the inner core of the spinal column.

hemoglobin A complex protein-iron compound in the blood that carries oxygen to the cells from the lungs and carbon dioxide away from the cells to the lungs.

hematopoietic tissue Tissue related to the process of formation and development of various types of blood cells.

hepatic artery The branch of the aorta that delivers blood to the liver.

histamine An amine released by mast cells and basophils that promotes inflammation.

homeostasis A state of equilibrium in the body with respect to functions and composition of fluids and tissues.

humerus The largest bone of the upper arm, comprising a body, head, and condyle.

hymen A mucous membrane that may partly or entirely occlude the vaginal outlet.

hyoid bone The U-shaped bone between the mandible and the larynx.

hypothalamus A portion of the diencephalon of the brain that activates, controls, and integrates the peripheral autonomic nervous system, endocrine processes, and many somatic functions, such as body temperature, sleep, and appetite.

ileum The distal portion of the small intestine.

iliac crest The upper free margin of the ilium.

ilium One of the three bones that make up the innominate bone.

inferior Toward the feet; below a point of reference in the anatomical position.

inferior vena cava The vein that returns blood from the lower limbs and the greater part of the pelvic and abdominal organs to the right atrium.

inflammatory response A tissue reaction to injury or an antigen; it may include pain, swelling, itching, redness, heat, and loss of function.

inguinal canal The passage through the lower abdominal wall that transmits the spermatic cord in the male and the round ligament in the female.

inner ear The part of the ear that contains the sensory organs for hearing and balance

integumentary system The largest organ system in the body, consisting of the skin and accessory structures.

intercellular Occurring between or among cells.

interstitial fluid Fluid that occupies the space outside the blood vessels and/or outside the cells of an organ or tissue.

intracellular Occurring within cell membranes.

intraocular pressure Pressure within the eye that keeps the eye inflated.

ions Atoms or groups of atoms that carry a charge of electricity by virtue of having gained or lost one or more electrons.

iris The colored contractile membrane of the eye that can be seen through the cornea.

irregular bones Bones that are not representative of the other three categories (long, short, or flat bones).

ischium One of the three parts of the hipbone; it joins the ilium and the pubis to form the acetabulum.

jejunum One of the three portions of the small intestine.

joint capsule A well-defined structure that encloses a joint.

jugular notch The superior margin of the manubrium; it is palpated easily at the anterior base of the neck; also known as the *suprasternal notch*.

kidney One of the pair of organs that cleanse the body of the waste products continually produced by metabolism.

Krebs cycle A sequence of enzymatic reactions, involving the metabolism of carbon chains of sugar, fatty acids, and amino acids, that yield carbon dioxide, water, and high-energy phosphate bonds.

lacrimal gland The tear gland located in the superolateral corner of the orbit.

large intestine The portion of the digestive tract comprising the cecum; the appendix; the ascending, transverse, and descending colons; and the rectum.

laryngopharynx The lowest part of the pharynx.

larynx The voice box, located just below the pharynx.

lateral recumbent A position in which the patient lies on the right or left side.

left atrium One of the four chambers of the human heart; the left atrium receives oxygenated blood from the lungs and pumps it into the left ventricle.

lens The crystalline portion of the eye.

leukocytes White blood cells.

limbic system The part of the brain involved with emotions and olfaction.

lipid bilayer The central layer of the cytoplasmic membrane; it is composed of a double layer of lipid molecules.

lipoproteins Conjugated proteins in which lipids form an integral part of the molecule; lipoproteins are synthesized primarily in the liver.

liver An organ in the upper abdomen that aids in digestion and removes waste products and cellular debris from the blood; the largest solid organ in the human body.

long bones Bones that are longer than they are wide, such as the humerus, ulna, radius, femur, tibia, fibula, and phalanges.

loop of Henle The U-shaped portion of the renal tubule.

lymph nodes Encapsulated masses of lymphoid tissue found among lymph vessels.

lymph nodules Small, densely packed spherical nodes or aggregations of lymph cells embedded in the reticular meshwork of the lymphatic system; they are found mainly in the tonsils, spleen, and thymus.

lymphatic system The network of vessels, ducts, nodes, valves, and organs involved in protecting and maintaining the internal fluid environment of the body.

lymphocytes A type of white blood cell formed in lymphoid tissue.

lysosomes Membranous-walled organelles that contain enzymes, which enable the lysosome to function as an intracellular digestive system.

macrophages Phagocytic cells in the immune system.

mammary glands External accessory sex organs in females; the breasts.

medial malleolus The rounded process on the medial side of the ankle joint.

mediastinum The area of the body that includes the trachea, esophagus, thymus, heart, and great vessels.

medulla The lowest part of the brainstem, which controls vital functions; an enlarged extension of the spinal cord; also known as the *medulla oblongata*.

meninges Fluid-containing membranes surrounding the brain and spinal cord.

mesencephalon One of the three parts of the brainstem; also known as the *midbrain*.

mesentery Connective tissue that holds some of the abdominal organs to the body wall.

metabolism The culmination of all chemical processes that take place in living organisms.

metacarpals The five bones that extend from the carpus to the phalanges.

metatarsals The five bones that comprise the metatarsus.

middle ear An air-filled space in the temporal bone that contains the auditory ossicles.

mitochondria Small, spherical, rod-shaped or thin filamentous structures in the cytoplasm of cells; a site of adenosine triphosphate production.

mitosis Cell division that results in two daughter cells with exactly the same number and type of chromosomes as the mother cell.

monocytes A type of white blood cell found in the lymph nodes, spleen, bone marrow, and loose connective tissue.

mons pubis The prominence caused by a pad of fatty tissue over the symphysis pubis in the female.

motor neuron A neuron that innervates skeletal, smooth, or cardiac muscle fibers; also known as an *interneuron*.

mucus The viscous, slippery secretion of mucous membranes and glands.

mycoplasma A genus of microscopic organisms that lack rigid cell walls; mycoplasma are considered the smallest free-living organisms.

myofilaments Extremely fine, molecular, threadlike structures that help form the myofibril of muscle; thick myofibrils are formed of myosin, and thin myofilaments are formed of actin.

nephron The functional unit of the kidney.

neuroglia The supporting or nonneuronal tissue cells of the central and peripheral nervous system.

neurons The functional units of the nervous system, consisting of the nerve cell body, the dendrites, and the axon.

neutrophils Small, phagocytic white blood cells with a lobed nucleus and small granules in the cytoplasm; neutrophils stains readily with neutral dyes.

nucleoplasm The protoplasm of the nucleus, as contrasted with that of the cell.

nucleus The central controlling body within a living cell.

obturator foramen A large opening on each side of the lower portion of the hipbone, formed posteriorly by the ischium, superiorly by the ilium, and anteriorly by the pubis.

oculomotor nerve The third cranial nerve, which contains sensory and motor fibers; it provides for movement in most of the muscles of the eye, for constriction of the pupil, and for accommodation of the eye to light.

olfactory Of or pertaining to the sense of smell.

oocytes Incompletely developed ova.

optic nerve The nerve that carries visual signals from the eye to the crossing of the optic tracts.

organ A structure made up of two or more kinds of tissues organized to perform a more complex function than any one tissue alone.

organelles Various particles of living substance that are bound within most cells, such as the mitochondria, the Golgi apparatus, the endoplasmic reticulum, the lysosomes, and the centrioles.

ovarian follicles Spherical cell aggregations in the ovary that contain an oocyte.

ovaries The pair of female gonads found on each side of the lower abdomen beside the uterus.

pancreas A fish-shaped, nodular gland located across the posterior abdominal wall in the epigastric region of the body; it secretes various substances, including digestive enzymes, insulin, and glucagon.

parasympathetic nervous system The subdivision of the autonomic nervous system, usually involved in activating vegetative functions such as digestion, defecation, and urination.

parietal peritoneum The serous membrane that covers the body cavity wall.

patella A flat, triangular bone at the front of the knee joint; the kneecap.

penis The external reproductive organ of the male.

pericardial sac The sac that surrounds the heart.

perineum The pelvic floor and associated structures occupying the pelvic outlet, bounded anteriorly by the pubic symphysis, laterally by the ischial tuberosities, and posteriorly by the coccyx.

periosteum Tough connective tissue that covers the bone.

peripheral nervous system A subdivision of the nervous system consisting of nerves and ganglia.

phagocytosis The process by which cells ingest solid substances, such as other cells, bacteria, bits of necrosed tissue, and foreign particles.

phalanges Any bone of a finger or toe.

phospholipids A class of compounds, widely distributed in living cells, that contain phosphoric acid, fatty acids, and a nitrogenous base.

pia mater The innermost layer of the meninges; it directly covers the brain.

pituitary gland A small gland attached to the hypothalamus; it supplies numerous hormones that govern many vital processes.

plasma membrane The outer covering of a cell that contains the cellular cytoplasm; also known as the *cell membrane*.

platelet A fragment of a cell; it contains granules in the central part and clear protoplasm peripherally but has no definite nucleus.

pleural cavity The area of the body that surrounds the lungs.

pleural space The potential space between the visceral and parietal layers of the pleura.

polysaccharides Carbohydrates that contain three or more molecules of simple carbohydrate.

pons The part of the brainstem between the medulla and midbrain.

portal vein A vein that branches like an artery in the liver and ends in capillary-like sinusoids that convey the blood to the inferior vena cava through the hepatic veins.

posterior The back, or dorsal, surface.

precapillary sphincter The smooth muscle sphincter that regulates blood flow through a capillary.

prokaryotes Cells without a true nucleus; instead, nuclear material is scattered throughout the cytoplasm.

prone A position in which the patient lies on the stomach (face down).

prostate gland The gland that lies just below the male bladder; its secretion is one of the components of semen.

puberty The period of life when the ability to reproduce begins.

pubis One of a pair of pubic bones that, with the ischium and the ilium, form the hipbone and join the pubic bone from the opposite side at the pubic symphysis.

pulmonary surfactant Certain lipoproteins that reduce the surface tension of pulmonary fluids, allowing the exchange of gases in the alveoli of the lungs and contributing to the elasticity of pulmonary tissue.

pulmonary trunk The large elastic artery that carries blood from the right ventricle of the heart to the right and left pulmonary arteries.

pulmonary veins The veins that carry oxygenated blood from the lung to the left atrium.

pupil The opening in the center of the iris that regulates the amount of light entering the eye.

Purkinje fibers Myocardial fibers that are a continuation of the bundle of His and that extend into the muscle walls of the ventricles.

radius One of the bones of the forearm; it lies parallel to the ulna.

rectum The segment of the large intestine continuous with the descending sigmoid colon just proximal to the anal canal.

red marrow Specialized soft tissue found in many bones of infants and children; in the spongy bone of the proximal epiphyses of the humerus and femur; and in the sternum, ribs, and vertebral bodies of adults. It is essential in the manufacture of red blood cells.

renal pyramids Pyramidal masses seen on longitudinal section of the kidney; they contain part of the loop of Henle and the collecting tubules.

respiration The process of the molecular exchange of oxygen and carbon dioxide in the body's tissues.

reticular activating system A functional system in the brain that is essential for wakefulness, attention, concentration, and introspection.

reticular formation A small, thick cluster of neurons nestled in the brainstem that controls breathing, the heartbeat, blood pressure, level of consciousness, and other vital functions.

retina The nervous tunic of the eye; it is continuous with the optic nerve.

retroperitoneal Behind the peritoneum.

ribonucleic acid (RNA) A nucleic acid found in the nucleus and the cytoplasm of cells that transmits genetic instructions from the nucleus to the cytoplasm. In the cytoplasm, RNA functions in the assembly of proteins.

ribosome The "factory" of a cell, in which protein is synthesized.

right atrium One of the four chambers of the human heart; it receives deoxygenated blood from the body through the vena cava and pumps it into the right ventricle.

sarcomere The contractile unit of skeletal muscle; it contains thick and thin myofilaments.

sclera The opaque membrane covering the eyeball.

scrotum The sac of skin that contains the testes.

sebaceous glands Glands of the skin, usually associated with a hair follicle, that produce sebum.

sebum The secretion of sebaceous glands; it prevents drying and protects against some bacteria.

semen The male reproductive fluid.

seminal vesicle One of two glandular structures that empty into the ejaculatory ducts; its secretion is one of the components of semen.

septum A thin wall dividing two cavities or masses of soft tissue.

serum Blood plasma without its clotting factors.

short bones Bones that are approximately as broad as they are long, such as the carpal bones of the wrist and the tarsal bones of the ankle.

sinoatrial node An area of specialized heart tissue that generates the cardiac electrical impulse.

sinuses The cavities in the bones of the skull that connect to the nasal cavities by small channels.

skeletal muscle Muscle tissue that appears microscopically to consist of striped myofibrils; also known as *striated muscle* and *voluntary muscle*.

small intestine The longest portion of the digestive tract; it is divided into the duodenum, jejunum, and ileum.

smooth muscle One of two kinds of muscle; it is composed of elongated, spindle-shaped cells in muscles not under voluntary control, such as smooth muscle of the intestines, stomach, and other visceral organs; also known as *visceral muscle, involuntary muscle,* and *nonstriated muscle.*

somatic nervous system The part of the nervous system composed of nerve fibers that send impulses from the central nervous system to skeletal muscle.

somatomotor neurons Neurons that innervate skeletal muscles.

spermatogenesis The process of development of spermatozoa.

spermatozoa The male sex cells, which are composed of a head and a tail; sperm contains genetic information transmitted by the male.

spinal nerve One of 31 pairs of nerves formed by the joining of the dorsal and ventral routes that arise from the spinal cord.

spleen A large, highly vascular lymphatic organ situated in the upper part of the abdominal cavity between the stomach and the diaphragm; it responds to foreign substances in the blood, destroys worn-out erythrocytes, and is a storage site for red blood cells.

sternal angle The point at which the manubrium joins the body of the sternum; also known as the *angle of Louis*.

sternoclavicular joint The double gliding joint between the sternum and the clavicle.

sternomanubrial joint The point at which the manubrium joins the body of the sternum; also known as the sternal angle or angle of Lewis.

sternum The elongated, flattened bone that forms the middle portion of the thorax.

subarachnoid space The area below the arachnoid membrane but above the pia mater that contains cerebrospinal fluid.

subclavian vein The continuation of the axillary vein in the upper body; it extends from the lateral border of the first rib to the sternal end of the clavicle, where it joins the internal jugular to form the brachiocephalic vein.

subcutaneous tissue The adherent layer of adipose tissue just below the dermal layer; also known as the *hypodermis*.

subdural space The space between the dura mater and the arachnoid.

superior Situated above or higher than a point of reference in the anatomical position.

superior vena cava The vein that returns blood from the head and neck, upper limbs, and thorax to the right atrium.

supine A position in which the patient lies on the back (face up).

sweat glands Glands that produce sweat or viscous organic secretions; also known as *sudoriferous glands*.

sympathetic nervous system A subdivison of the autonomic nervous system that usually is involved in preparing the body for physical activity.

symphysis pubis The joint that connects the coxal bones of the pelvis.

synapse Functional membrane-to-membrane contact of a nerve cell with another nerve cell, muscle cell, gland cell, or sensory receptor; it serves to transmit action potentials from one cell to another.

synovial joints Joints that are freely movable.

system Interconnected functions or organs in which a stimulus or an action in one area affects all other areas.

tarsal bones The bones of the ankle.

taste buds The peripheral taste organs that are distributed over the tongue and the roof of the mouth.

testes The male gonads, which produce the male sex cells, or sperm.

thalamus Tissue located just above the hypothalamus; it helps to produce sensations, associates sensations with emotions, and plays a part in arousal.

thymus A single, unpaired gland located in the mediastinum; the primary central gland of the lymphatic system.

thyroid membrane The fibrous membrane that joins the hyoid and the thyroid cartilages.

tibia The second longest bone of the skeleton; it is located at the medial side of the leg.

tonsils Large collections of lymphatic tissue beneath the mucous membrane of the oral cavity and pharynx.

trachea A cylindrical tube in the neck composed of cartilage and membrane; it conveys air to the lungs.

tricuspid valve The valve located between the right atrium and ventricle.

tunic One of the enveloping layers of a part; one of the coats of a blood vessel; one of the coats of the eye; one of the coats of the digestive tract.

tympanic membrane The cellular membrane that separates the external ear from the middle ear; also known as the *eardrum*.

ulna One of the bones of the forearm.

ureters A pair of tubes that carry the urine from the kidneys into the bladder.

urethra A small tubular structure that drains urine from the bladder; in men, it also serves as a passageway for semen during ejaculation.

urinary bladder The muscular, membranous sac in the pelvis that stores urine for discharge through the urethra.

uterine tubes A pair of ducts that open at one end into the uterus and at the other end into the peritoneal cavity, over the ovary; also known as the *fallopian tubes*.

uterus The hollow, pear-shaped internal female organ of reproduction.

uvula The cone-shaped process hanging down from the soft palate that helps prevent food and liquid from entering the nasal cavities.

vagina The part of the female genitalia that forms a canal from the orifice through the vestibule to the uterine cervix.

vascular tunic The choroid, ciliary body, and iris.

ventral root The nerve that conveys efferent nerve processes away from the spinal cord.

ventricles Small cavities; the term usually refers to the right and left ventricles of the heart.

viruses Minute, parasitic microorganisms without independent metabolic activity that can replicate only within a cell of a living plant or animal host.

visceral peritoneum The serous membrane that covers the abdominal organs.

visceral reflex A reflex mediated by autonomic nerves and initiated in the viscera

vitreous humor The transparent, jellylike material that fills the space between the lens and the retina.

vocal cords The two folds of elastic ligaments covered by mucous membrane that stretch from the thyroid cartilage to the arytenoid cartilage; vibration of the vocal cords is responsible for voice production; also known as the *true vocal cords.*

vulva The external genitalia of the female.

xiphoid process The smallest of three parts of the sternum; it articulates caudally with the body of the sternum and laterally with the seventh rib.

yellow marrow Specialized soft tissue (mainly adipose) found in the compact bone of most adult epiphyses.

Human anatomy is the study of how the human body is organized. The paramedic must know anatomy to assess a patient by body region. This knowledge also helps the paramedic communicate well with other members of the health care team.

TERMINOLOGY

Directional terms used by medical professionals refer to the human body in the **anatomical position**. This position describes a person standing erect with the feet and palms facing the examiner. A patient in the **supine** position is lying on the back (face up). A patient in the **prone** position is lying on the stomach (face down). A patient in the **lateral recumbent** position is lying on the right or left side. Regardless of the patient's position, the paramedic should always report patient information with reference to the anatomical position (Figure 10-1).[1]

Directional terms, such as *up* or *down, front* or *back*, and *right* or *left*, also are expressed in anatomical terminology (Table 10-1). The terms always refer to the patient, not the examiner (e.g., the patient's left arm).

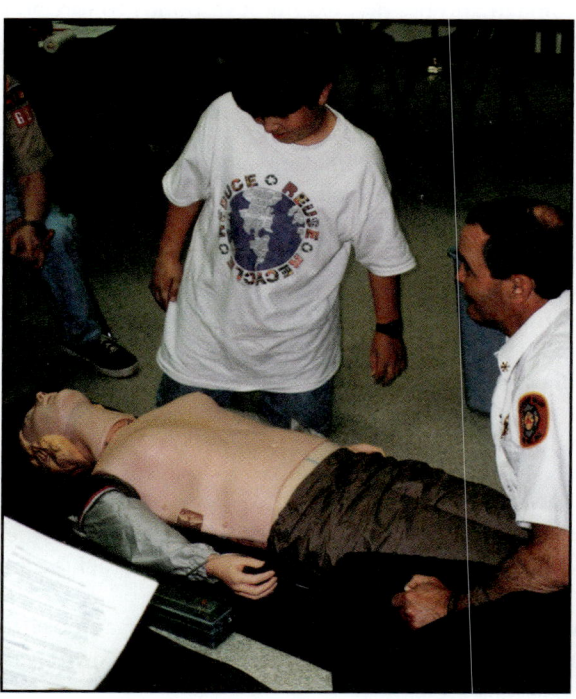

(Courtesy Florissant Valley Fire Protection District, Florissant, Mo.)

Anatomical Planes

The relationships of internal body structures are classified into anatomical planes. These planes may be viewed as imaginary straight-line divisions of the human body (Figure 10-2). The *sagittal plane* runs vertically through the middle of the body, creating right and left sections. A plane that is to one side of the midline is said to be *parasagittal*. The transverse (or horizontal) plane divides the body into top and bottom sections. These are known as **superior** and **inferior** sections. The frontal (or coronal) plane divides the body into front and back. These are known as **anterior** and **posterior** sections.

Body Regions

The human body is divided into a number of regions.[2] This division helps to organize anatomical structures. The **appendicular region** is made up of the limbs, or extremities. The **axial region** is made up of the head, neck, thorax, and abdomen. The abdomen usually is divided into four quadrants: the upper right, lower right, upper left, and

SHOW ME THE EVIDENCE
Walters and colleagues sought to develop a program that would both introduce medical students to continuing education and enhance paramedics' knowledge of anatomy. They chose anatomy because paramedics have some previous knowledge of the subject, and the researchers thought that this knowledge could help the paramedics predict injury based on external physical findings in trauma cases. Five medical students provided anatomy education to 19 paramedics using case-based instruction and cadaver laboratories. At the conclusion, all the paramedics passed the post test and reported above average satisfaction with the program. A survey was performed 3 months later, and the mean paramedic scores indicated that the paramedics believed the course had very likely or absolutely affected their patient care and understanding of injury.

Walters WA, Bailey H, Kaplan L: Can preclinical medical students be integrated into the continuing medical education process by instructing prehospital care providers? *Am J Surg* 179:229-233, 2000.

An imaginary plane divides the abdominal cavity from the pelvic cavity. The division is drawn between the symphysis pubis and the sacral promontory. The latter is the projecting portion of the pelvis at the base of the sacrum. The abdominal and pelvic cavities are lined with a thin sheet of membranous tissue. This thin sheet of tissue secretes serous fluid. The serous membrane that covers the abdominal organs is known as the **visceral peritoneum**. The serous membrane that covers the body cavity wall is known as the **parietal peritoneum**. Peritoneal organs are held in place by connective tissue called **mesentery**. The mesentery holds some of the abdominal organs to the body wall and offers a pathway for nerves and vessels to reach the organs. Abdominopelvic organs that do not have mesentery or peritoneum are said to be **retroperitoneal**. This means that they are behind the peritoneum. These organs include the kidneys, adrenal glands, pancreas, portions of the colon, and the urinary bladder. The pelvic cavity is enclosed by the bones of the pelvis. The abdominal and pelvic cavities often are referred to collectively as the *peritoneal* or *abdominopelvic cavity* (Figure 10-4).

CELL STRUCTURE

The **cell** is the basic unit of life. Cells are highly organized units composed of protoplasm, or living matter. The three main parts of all human cells are the cytoplasmic membrane **(plasma membrane)**, cytoplasm, and nucleus.

Cytoplasmic Membrane

The **cytoplasmic membrane** encloses the **cytoplasm** and forms the outer boundary of the cell. The cytoplasmic membrane is believed to have two layers of phosphate-containing fat molecules. These molecules are known as **phospholipids**. The layers form a fluid framework for the cytoplasmic membrane (Figure 10-5). Substances outside this membrane are considered **extracellular** (outside of cells) or **intercellular** (between cells). Substances inside this membrane are **intracellular**. The functions of the cytoplasmic membrane are to enclose and support the cell contents and regulate what moves into and out of the cell.

The central layer of the cytoplasmic membrane is a **lipid bilayer**. This layer is composed of a double layer of lipid molecules. The lipid bilayer has a liquid quality, and protein molecules "float" on the inner and outer surfaces. Some of these proteins have carbohydrate molecules bound to them. The protein molecules are thought to function as membrane channels, carrier molecules, receptor molecules, **enzymes**, or structural supports in the membrane (see Chapter 11).

Cytoplasm

The cytoplasm lies between the cytoplasmic membrane and the nucleus. The nucleus can be viewed as a round or spherical structure in the center of the cell. Specialized structures

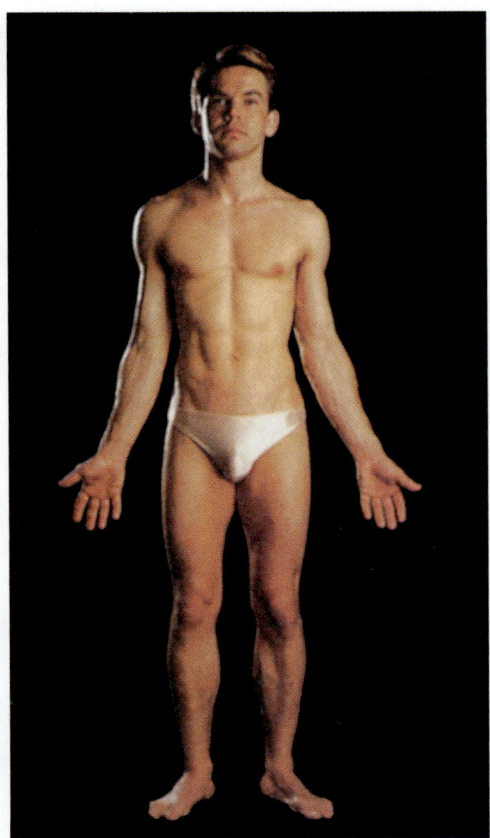

FIGURE 10-1 Anatomical position. A person in the anatomical position stands with the feet and the palms of the hands facing forward with the thumbs to the outside. (Thibodeau GA, Patton KT: *Structure and function of the body*, ed 13, St Louis, 2008, Mosby.)

lower left (Figure 10-3). The dividing lines consist of two imaginary divisions. These divisions run horizontally through the umbilicus and vertically from the **xiphoid process** through the **symphysis pubis**.

Body Cavities

The three major cavities of the human body are the thoracic cavity, the abdominal cavity, and the pelvic cavity. The thoracic cavity is divided into two portions by a midline structure known as the **mediastinum**. The mediastinum includes the trachea, esophagus, thymus, heart, and great vessels. The lungs are located on either side of this midline structure. The thoracic cavity is surrounded by the rib cage. This cavity is separated from the abdominal cavity by the diaphragm.

The thorax contains two pleural cavities (which contain the lungs) and a pericardial cavity (which contains the heart). These cavities are lined with a serous membrane. The serous membrane that comes in contact with the organ is *visceral*. The serous membrane that comes in contact with the cavity wall is *parietal*. These membranes produce a thin, lubricating film of fluid. This fluid reduces the friction that occurs during movement of organs against other organs or body cavities.

TABLE 10-1 Directional Terms

Term	Definition
Left	Toward the left side
Right	Toward the right side
Superior	Situated above another structure (usually synonymous with "cephalic")
Inferior	Situated below another structure (usually synonymous with "caudal")
Cephalic	Toward the head of the body
Caudal	Toward the distal end of the spine
Proximal	Closer than another structure to the point of attachment to the trunk
Distal	Farther than another structure from the point of attachment to the trunk
Medial	Toward the midline of the body
Lateral	Away from the midline of the body
Anterior	The front of the body (synonymous with "ventral")
Posterior	The back of the body (synonymous with "dorsal")
Ventral	Pertaining to the front
Dorsal	Pertaining to the back

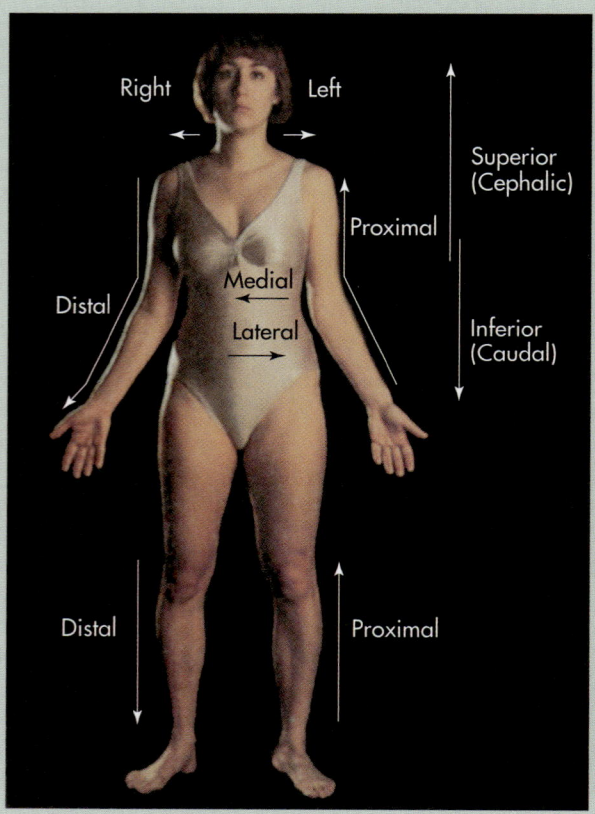

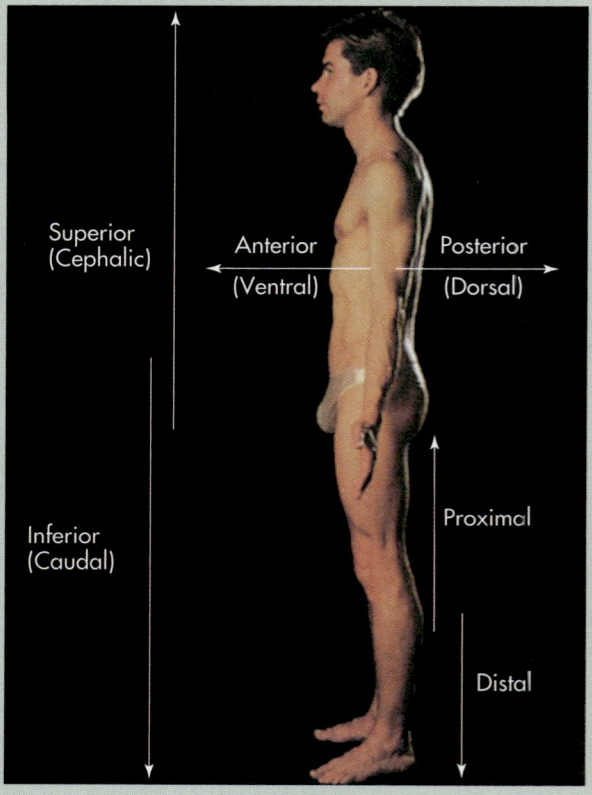

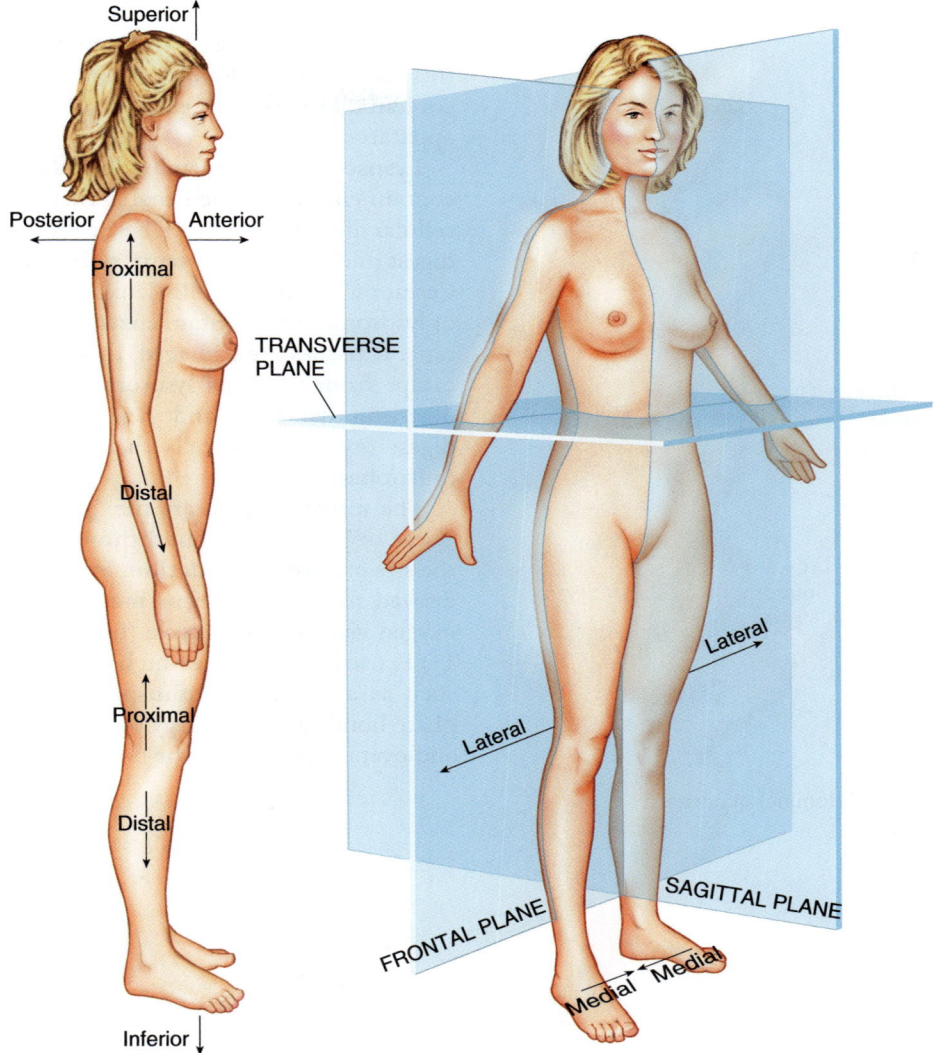

FIGURE 10-2 Body planes. (Patton KT, Thibodeau GA: *Anatomy and physiology*, ed 7, St Louis, 2007, Mosby.)

in the cell, known as **organelles**, are located in the cytoplasm. These structures perform functions important to the cell's survival (Table 10-2 and Figure 10-6).

The **endoplasmic reticulum** is a chain of connecting sacs or canals that winds through the cytoplasm of the cell. In essence, the endoplasmic reticulum serves as a tiny circulatory system for the cell. The tubular passages or canals in the endoplasmic reticulum carry proteins and other substances through the cytoplasm of the cell from one area to another. The two types of endoplasmic reticulum are *smooth endoplasmic reticulum* and *rough endoplasmic reticulum*. Smooth endoplasmic reticulum is found in cells that handle or produce fatty substances. This organelle also plays a part in detoxification processes through the chemical action of **enzymes**. Rough endoplasmic reticulum is found in cells that produce proteins to be secreted for use outside the cell.

Ribosomes are the "factories" in the cells where protein is synthesized. Ribosomes are macromolecules of protein and **ribonucleic acid (RNA)** that are composed of thousands of atoms. Ribosomes usually are bound to the endoplasmic reticulum but also are found free in cytoplasm. Ribosomes form complexes with strands of RNA, which through the genetic code provide the blueprint for the new protein. Individual **amino acids** are attached in long chains with peptide bonds to form the new proteins.

The **Golgi apparatus** concentrates and packages materials for secretion from the cell. This organelle consists of tiny sacs composed of smooth endoplasmic reticulum. These sacs are stacked one on the other near the nucleus. The Golgi apparatus concentrates and in some cases chemically modifies the proteins. It does this by synthesizing and attaching carbohydrate molecules to the proteins to form **glycoproteins** or by attaching lipids to the proteins to

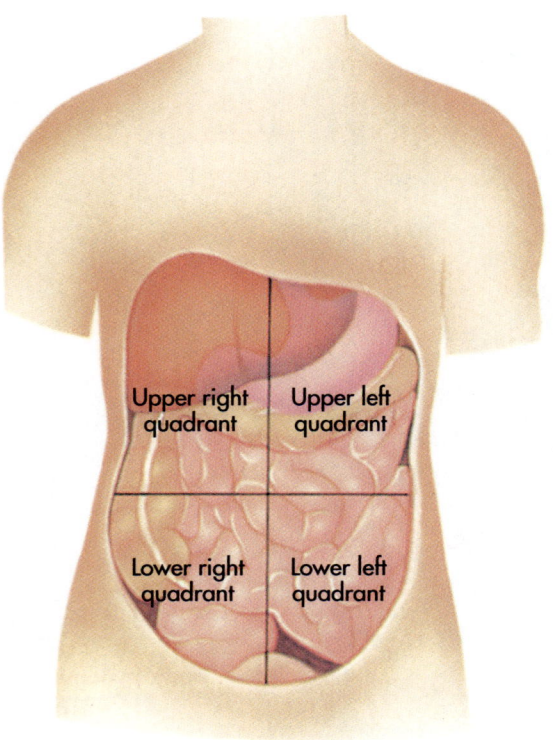

FIGURE 10-3 Abdominal quadrants.

form **lipoproteins**. These concentrated globules move slowly outward to and through the cell membrane. At this point, the globules break open and spill their contents. **Mucus** is an example of a product of the Golgi apparatus.

Lysosomes are membranous-walled organelles that contain enzymes, which enable them to function as intracellular digestive systems. These enzymes include those that digest nucleic acids, proteins, **polysaccharides**, and lipids. Certain white blood cells (leukocytes) have large numbers of lysosomes that contain enzymes to digest engulfed bacteria. If tissues are damaged, these powerful enzymes may escape from ruptured lysosome sacs into the cytoplasm, digesting damaged and healthy cells. Lysosomes also digest organelles of cells that are no longer functional **(autophagia)**.

The **mitochondria** are the "power plants" of the cell. These organelles are found throughout the cell. They are the site of **aerobic oxidation**. In the mitochondria, energy derived from the efficient **metabolism** of nutrients and oxygen via the **Krebs cycle** (further described in Chapter 11) is used to synthesize high-energy triphosphate bonds, such as **adenosine triphosphate (ATP)**. These triphosphate bonds are the energy source for the muscles, nerves, and overall function of the body.

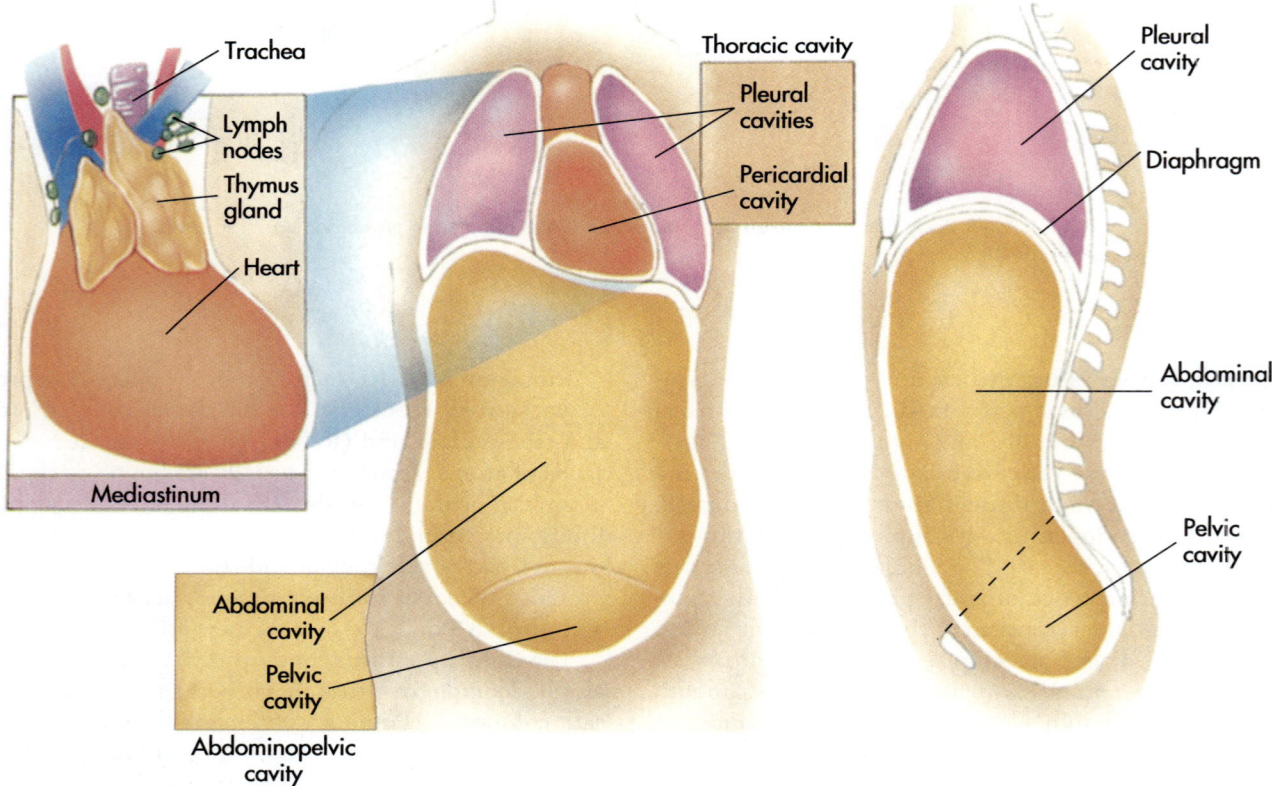

FIGURE 10-4 Body cavities. The thoracic cavity includes the two pleural cavities and the pericardial cavity. Some of the contents of the mediastinum are shown on the left. The abdominopelvic cavity contains the abdominal cavity and the pelvic cavity.

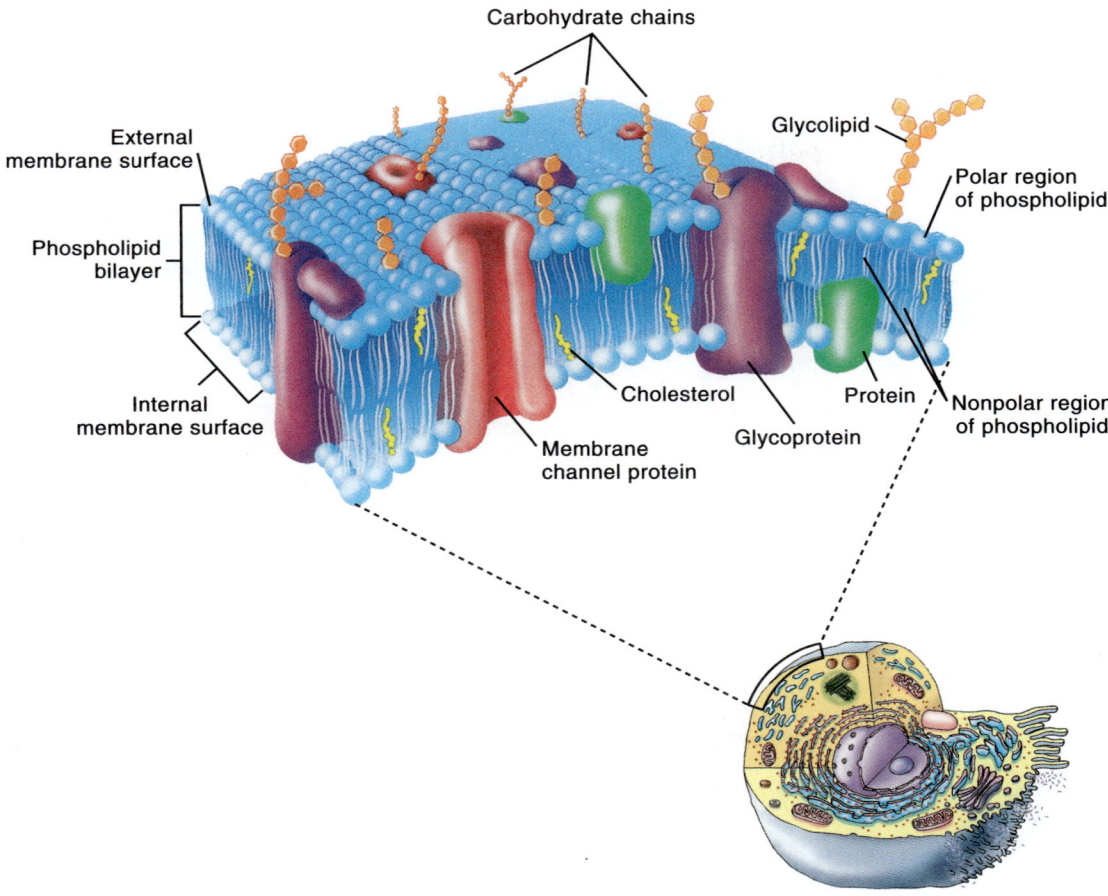

FIGURE 10-5 Fluid mosaic model of the plasma membrane. (Patton KT, Thibodeau GA: *Anatomy and physiology,* ed 7, St Louis, 2007, Mosby.)

TABLE 10-2 Some Major Cell Structures and Their Functions

Structure	Function
Centrioles	Function in cell reproduction.
Cilia	Short, hairlike extensions on the free surfaces of some cells capable of movement.
Endoplasmic reticulum	Ribosomes attached to rough endoplasmic reticulum synthesize proteins; smooth endoplasmic reticulum synthesizes lipids and certain carbohydrates.
Flagella	Single projections of cell surfaces that are much larger than cilia; the only example in human beings is the "tail" of a sperm cell.
Golgi apparatus	Synthesizes carbohydrates, combines them with proteins, and packages the product as globules of glycoproteins.
Lysosomes	The "digestive system" of the cell.
Mitochondria	Synthesize adenosine triphosphate; the "powerhouses" of the cell.
Nucleoli	Play an essential role in the formation of ribosomes.
Nucleus	Dictates protein synthesis, thereby playing an essential role in other cell activities, namely active transport, metabolism, growth, and heredity.
Plasma membrane	Serves as the boundary of the cell. Protein and carbohydrate molecules on the outer surface of the plasma membrane perform various functions; for example, they serve as markers that identify the cells of each individual or as receptor molecules for certain hormones.
Ribosomes	Synthesize proteins; the "protein factories" of the cell.

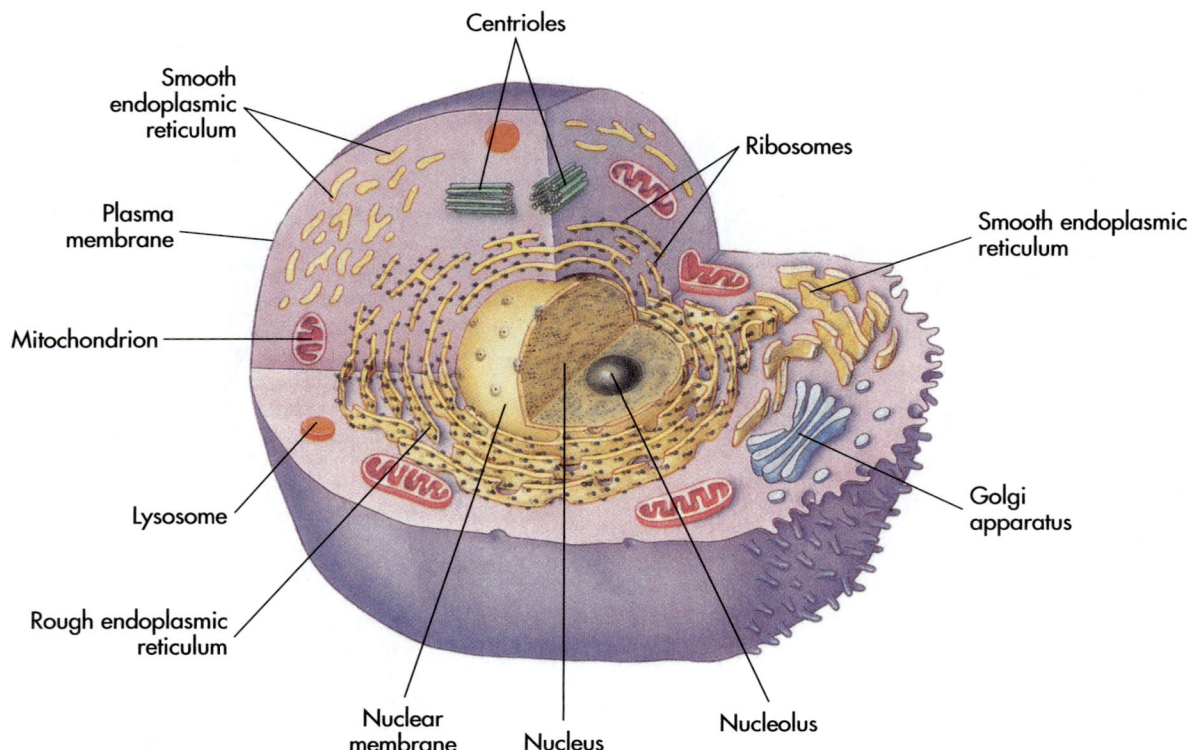

FIGURE 10-6 Artist's interpretation of cell structure. (Thibodeau GA, Patton KT: *Structure and function of the body,* ed 13, St Louis, 2008, Mosby.)

CRITICAL THINKING

Your patient has severe lung disease and poor oxygenation. What effect will this have on cellular energy production?

Centrioles are paired, rod-shaped organelles that lie at right angles to each other in a specialized zone of cytoplasm. This zone is known as the **centrosome**. Each centriole is composed of microtubules, which play an important role in the process of cell division. At some point in their existence, all human cells contain a nucleus in which the genetic material of the cell is located. The nucleus is a large, membrane-bound organelle that ultimately controls all other organelles in the cytoplasm. The nucleus may be spherical, elongated, or lobed, depending on the type of cell in which it is found. The nucleus usually is located near the center of the cell; however, some cells, such as red blood cells (erythrocytes), lose their nucleus as they develop. Other cells, such as certain bone cells, have more than one nucleus. The most significant categorizing feature of cells is the presence or absence of a nucleus.

Nucleus

The **nucleus** is a relatively large structure that is not always near the center of the cell. The cell nucleus is surrounded by a nuclear membrane. This membrane encloses a special type of protoplasm known as **nucleoplasm**. The nucleoplasm contains a number of specialized structures. Two of these are the nucleolus and the chromatin granules. The nucleolus consists of **deoxyribonucleic acid (DNA)**, which programs the formation of RNA, and protein, which makes ribosomes. These ribosomes then migrate through the nuclear membrane into the cytoplasm of the cell and produce proteins. **Chromatin granules** are threadlike structures made up of proteins and DNA. During cell division, the chromatin condenses to form the 23 pairs of **chromosomes** characteristic of human cells. The information in nuclear DNA determines most of the chemical events that occur within the cell. The basic functions of the nucleus are cell division and control of genetic information. Not all cells are capable of continuous division, and some cells (e.g., nerve cells) cannot reproduce.

DID YOU KNOW?

Human Genome Project

In 1990 the U.S. Human Genome Project was started through a coordinated effort by the U.S. Department of Energy and the National Institutes of Health. The project was completed in 2003. The goals of the project were the following:

- Identify all of the approximately 20,000 to 25,000 genes found in human deoxyribonucleic acid (DNA)
- Determine the sequences of the 3 billion chemical base pairs that make up human DNA
- Store this information in databases

- Improve tools for data analysis
- Transfer related technologies to the private sector
- Address the ethical, legal, and social issues (ELSI) that may arise from the project

A *genome* is all the DNA in an organism, including its genes. Genes carry information for making all the proteins required by all organisms. These proteins determine, among other things, how the organism looks, how well its body metabolizes food or fights infection, and sometimes even how it behaves.

Knowledge of the effects of DNA variations among individuals can lead to revolutionary new ways to diagnose, treat, and someday prevent the thousands of disorders that affect human beings. Besides providing clues to understanding human biology, learning about nonhuman DNA sequences or organisms can lead to an understanding of their natural capabilities. This knowledge can then be applied to solving challenges in health care, agriculture, energy production, environmental remediation, and carbon sequestration.

Modified from the US Department of Energy, Human Genome Management Information Systems (HGMIS): *About the Human Genome Project.* www.ornl.gov/sci/techresources/Human_Genome/project/about.shtml. Accessed September 11, 2010.

Major Classes of Cells

Free-living cells of multicellular "social" organisms are divided into two major classes. They are divided by the way genetic material is organized inside them. The two main types are **eukaryotes** ("true nucleus") and **prokaryotes** ("before nucleus").

Eukaryotes are larger than prokaryotes and have a more extensive intracellular anatomy. They have a separate membrane-bound nucleus. The nucleus holds the genetic material (chromosomes, DNA). The fluid filling of eukaryotes is divided into the nucleoplasm and the cytoplasm. The nucleoplasm is inside the nuclear membrane. The cytoplasm is outside the nuclear membrane. Nearly all human body cells are eukaryotes, as are those of all living organisms. Exceptions to this are bacteria, cyanobacteria (blue-green algae), and **mycoplasmas;** these are prokaryotes. **Bacteria** and mycoplasmas cause many diseases in human beings and other animals. **Viruses** have a close association with cells but are not classified as cells.

In the simpler, prokaryote cells, the genetic material and enzymes required for energy production, cell growth, and cell division are contained in the jellylike cytoplasm. The cytoplasm is surrounded by the plasma membrane. Unlike eukaryotes, these cells have a simple internal organization. Prokaryotes do not have a nucleus that is bound by a plasma membrane. Their DNA is attached to the plasma membrane.

Chief Cellular Functions

Cells have evolved in myriad ways to fulfill specific tasks in the human body. Through **differentiation** (maturation), cells become specialized in one type of function or act in concert with other cells to perform a more complex task. For example, red blood cells carry out only one function:

they transport respiratory gases around the body. The cells in the pancreas synthesize and secrete large amounts of the digestive enzymes required to break down foods. The seven chief cellular functions are as follows:

1. Movement (muscle cells)
2. Conductivity (nerve cells)
3. Metabolic absorption (kidney and intestinal cells)
4. Secretion (mucous gland cells)
5. Excretion (all cells)
6. Respiration (all cells)
7. Reproduction (most cells)

Cell Reproduction

All human cells, with the exception of reproductive (sex) cells, reproduce by a process known as **mitosis**. In this process, cells divide to multiply; one cell divides to form two cells. Many cell types in the body (e.g., epithelial, liver, and bone marrow cells) undergo cell division throughout an individual's life. Other cell types (e.g., nerve and skeletal muscle cells) divide until near the time of birth.

BODY TISSUES

The characteristics of cell structure and composition are used to classify tissue types. Four main types of tissue make up the many organs of the body: epithelial tissue, connective tissue, muscle tissue, and nervous tissue.

Epithelial Tissue

Epithelial tissue covers surfaces or forms structures derived from body surfaces (e.g., glands). This tissue consists almost entirely of cells that have little or no intercellular material between them. The tissue forms continuous sheets that contain no blood vessels. Epithelium covers the outside of the body. It also lines the digestive tract, the blood vessels, and many body cavities.

CRITICAL THINKING

Think about the role of each of the tissue types. Compare these roles with the types of materials used to construct a building. How does each tissue type serve as a component for building a body?

Epithelial tissues can be subdivided by the shape and arrangement of the cells found in each type. If classified according to shape, epithelial cells are *squamous* (flat and scalelike), *cuboidal* (cube-shaped), or *columnar* (more tall than wide). If classified according to arrangement, epithelial cells are *simple* (a single layer of cells of the same shape), *stratified* (multiple layers of cells of the same shape), or *transitional* (several layers of cells of differing shapes).

Connective Tissue

Connective tissue is the most abundant type of tissue in the body. Connective tissue is also the most widely distributed type. It consists of cells separated from each other by intercellular material. This material is known as the

extracellular matrix. This nonliving matrix gives most connective tissue its fundamental characteristics and is the basis for separating connective tissue into the following seven subgroups.

1. **Areolar connective tissue** is a loose tissue. It consists of delicate webs of fibers and a variety of cells embedded in a matrix of soft, sticky gel. Areolar connective tissue is the "loose packing" material of most organs and other tissues. It attaches the skin to the underlying tissues. The areolar connective tissue contains three major types of protein fibers: collagen, reticulum, and elastin.

2. **Adipose tissue** (fat tissue) is a specialized connective tissue that stores lipids. Lipids take up less space per calorie than carbohydrates or proteins. This tissue, therefore, not only acts as an insulator and protector but also as a site of energy storage.

3. **Fibrous connective tissue** is made up mainly of bundles of strong, white collagenous fibers in parallel rows. Tendons are composed of this type of connective tissue. Fibrous connective tissue is characterized by strength and inelasticity.

4. **Cartilage** is made up of cartilage cells (chondrocytes). These cells are located in tiny spaces and are distributed throughout a somewhat rigid matrix. The makeup of cartilage varies by its location and ultimate role. For example, *hyaline cartilage* is found at articulating surfaces and is firm and smooth. *Fibrocartilage* is more flexible and supple. Cartilage makes up part of the human skeleton and covers the articulating surfaces of bones. In addition, cartilage forms the major skeletal tissue of the embryo before it is replaced by bony tissue. The type of cartilage depends on the relative amounts of collagen, elastin, and ground substance. Ground substance is composed of nonfibrous protein and other organic molecules and fluid. Increased amounts of collagen or elastin allow cartilage to spring back after being compressed. Because blood vessels do not penetrate the substance of cartilage, cartilage heals slowly after injury.

5. **Bone** is a highly specialized form of hard, connective tissue. It consists of living cells and mineralized matrix. The strength and rigidity of this matrix allow bone to support and protect other tissues and organs. Bones are classified according to their shape. **Long bones**, for example, are longer than they are wide (Figure 10-7). The humerus, ulna, radius, femur, tibia, fibula, and phalanges are long bones. **Short bones** are about as broad as they are long. Examples of short bones are the carpal bones of the wrist and the tarsal bones of the ankle. **Flat bones** have a thin, flattened shape. Examples of flat bones are certain skull bones, the ribs, sternum, and scapulae. **Irregular bones** are bones that do not fit any of the other three categories. Examples of irregular bones include vertebrae and facial bones.

Each growing long bone consists of a **diaphysis** (shaft), an *epiphysis* at the end of each bone, and an **epiphyseal plate** (growth plate). The epiphyseal plate is the site of bone elongation. When bone growth stops,

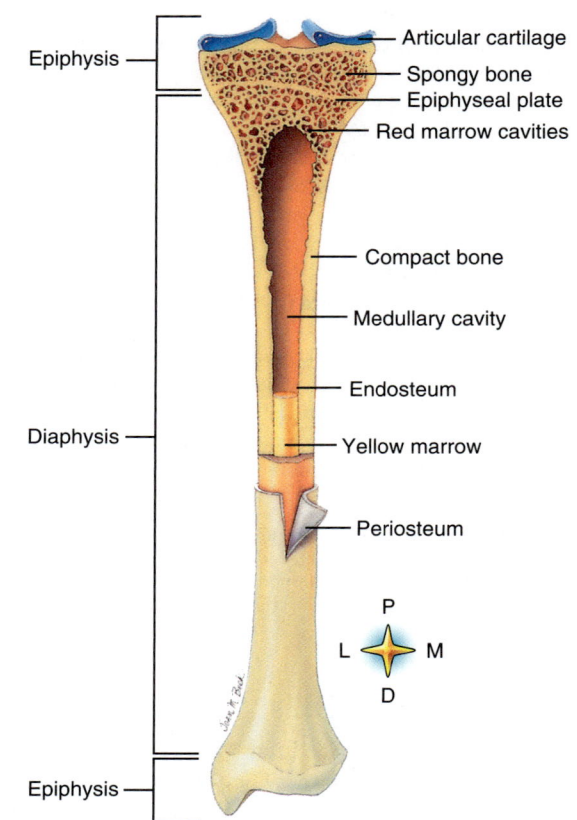

FIGURE 10-7 Long bone. (Patton KT, Thibodeau GA: *Anatomy and physiology,* ed 7, St Louis, 2007, Mosby.)

the epiphyseal plate becomes ossified. The plate then is called the *epiphyseal line*. An injury to this area can impair bone growth if it is not recognized and treated properly (see Chapter 44).

> **💡 CRITICAL THINKING**
> Intraosseous infusion is a critical intervention that can save a life. It is used to administer fluids and drugs. This infusion requires the insertion of a needle into the humerus or bone of the leg. Why could failure to identify anatomical landmarks or to place the needle correctly in the epiphysis in a child be harmful?

Bones contain large cavities and smaller cavities. An example of a large cavity is the medullary cavity in the diaphysis. Smaller cavities include the epiphyses of long bones and throughout the interior of other bones. These spaces are filled with **yellow marrow** (mainly adipose tissue) or **red marrow** (the site of blood formation). Blood supply to most bones is excellent. Therefore, some bones, such as the tibia and sternum, are suitable choices for venous access by means of intraosseous infusion (described in Chapter 14).

Bones can be classified further as cancellous or spongy bone and compact bone. **Cancellous bone** has spaces between the plates of the bone and resembles a sponge. **Compact bone** is essentially solid. Unlike cartilage, bone has a rich blood supply and can repair itself much more readily than cartilage.

6. **Blood** is a unique connective tissue because the matrix between the cells is liquid. The liquid matrix of blood allows it to flow rapidly through the body. Blood carries nutrients, oxygen, waste products, and other materials.

7. **Hematopoietic tissue** is the connective tissue in the marrow cavities of bones. This tissue also is in organs such as the spleen, tonsils, and lymph nodes. This tissue is responsible for the formation of blood cells and cells of the lymphatic system that are important in the defense against disease.

Muscle Tissue

Muscle tissue is a contractile tissue and is the force behind all body movement. It is highly specialized to contract or shorten forcefully. Muscle tissue is classified as skeletal, cardiac, and smooth (visceral) muscle, according to the anatomical location and function. When classified by appearance, muscle is *striated* or *nonstriated*. When classified by function, muscle is *voluntary* (consciously controlled) or *involuntary* (not normally consciously controlled). The three types of muscles are *striated voluntary* (skeletal) muscle, *striated involuntary* (cardiac) muscle, and *nonstriated involuntary* (smooth) muscle.

Skeletal muscle attaches to bones. It represents a large portion of the total weight of the human body. Contraction of these muscles is responsible for body movement. **Cardiac muscle** is the muscle of the heart. Contraction of the cardiac muscle pumps blood throughout the body. **Smooth muscle** is widespread throughout the body and is responsible for a variety of functions. Examples include movement in the digestive, urinary, and reproductive systems.

Nervous Tissue

Nervous tissue is characterized by its ability to conduct electrical signals, which are known as **action potentials**. Nervous tissue consists of two basic kinds of cells: neurons and neuroglia.

Neurons, or nerve cells, are the actual conducting cells of nervous tissue. They are composed of three major parts: cell body, dendrite, and axon. The cell body contains the nucleus and is the site of general cell functions. Dendrites and axons are nerve cell processes (projections of cytoplasm surrounded by membrane). Dendrites receive electrical impulses and conduct them toward the cell body. Axons usually conduct impulses away from the cell body. Neurons take many different sizes and shapes, especially in the brain and spinal cord.

Neuroglia are the support cells of the brain, spinal cord, and peripheral nerves. These cells are divided into several subgroups that nourish, protect, and insulate neurons.

ORGAN SYSTEMS

An **organ** is a structure made up of two or more kinds of tissues that are organized to perform a more complex job than any one tissue can perform. A **system** is a group of organs arranged to perform a more complex job than any one organ can perform (Figure 10-8). The human body has 11 major organ systems[3]:

1. Integumentary system
2. Skeletal system
3. Muscular system
4. Nervous system
5. Endocrine system
6. Circulatory system
7. Lymphatic system
8. Respiratory system
9. Digestive system
10. Urinary system
11. Reproductive system

Integumentary System

The **integumentary system** is the largest organ system of the body. It consists of the skin and accessory structures such as hair, nails, and a variety of glands. The functions of this system include protecting the body against injury and dehydration. The integumentary system also defends against invading microorganisms and regulates temperature.

 CRITICAL THINKING
Consider your knowledge of the functions of the skin. What signs, symptoms, or complications would you expect in a patient with burns covering half the body?

SKIN

The skin is a sheetlike organ composed of two distinct layers of tissue, the epidermis and the dermis (Figure 10-9). The **epidermis** is the outermost layer of the skin. It consists of tightly packed epithelial cells. Cells of the innermost layer of the epidermis can undergo mitosis and can repair themselves if injured. Because of this characteristic, the body can maintain an effective barrier against infection, even when subjected to injury and normal wear and tear.

The **dermis** is the deeper of the two layers of the skin. The dermis is largely made up of connective tissue. It is much thicker than the epidermis and contains collagenous and elastic fibers. The dermis also contains a specialized network of nerves and nerve endings. These nerves provide sensory information about pain, pressure, touch, and temperature. At various levels of the dermis are muscle fibers, hair follicles, sweat and sebaceous glands, and many blood vessels.

The layers of the skin are supported by a thick layer of loose connective tissue and fat. This is known as **subcutaneous tissue**. Subcutaneous tissue insulates the body from temperature extremes. It serves as a source of stored energy

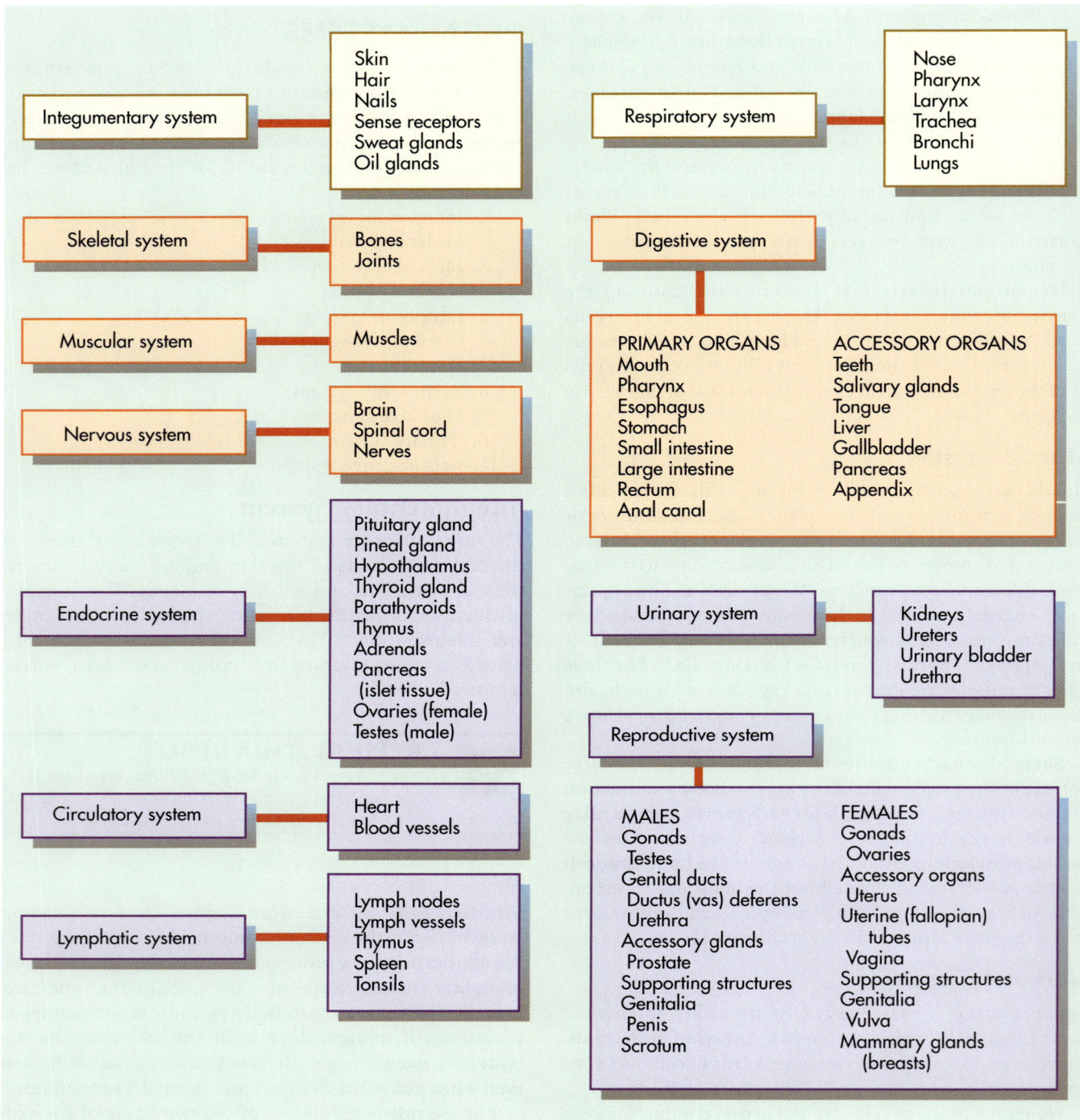

FIGURE 10-8 Body systems and their organs.

and acts as a shock absorber to protect underlying tissue from injury.

HAIR

Hair growth begins when cells of the epidermal layer of the skin grow into the dermis, forming a small tube called the *hair follicle*. Hair growth begins from a small, cap-shaped cluster of cells called the *hair papilla*. The part of the hair that lies hidden in the follicle is known as the *root,* and the visible part is called the *shaft*. Smooth muscles known as *arrector pili* are associated with each hair follicle. Movement of the hair follicle by the arrector pili produces pressure on the skin (resulting in "goose bumps") and pulls the hairs upward.

NAILS

Nails are produced by cells in the epidermis. The visible part of the nail is the *nail body*. The root of the nail lies in a

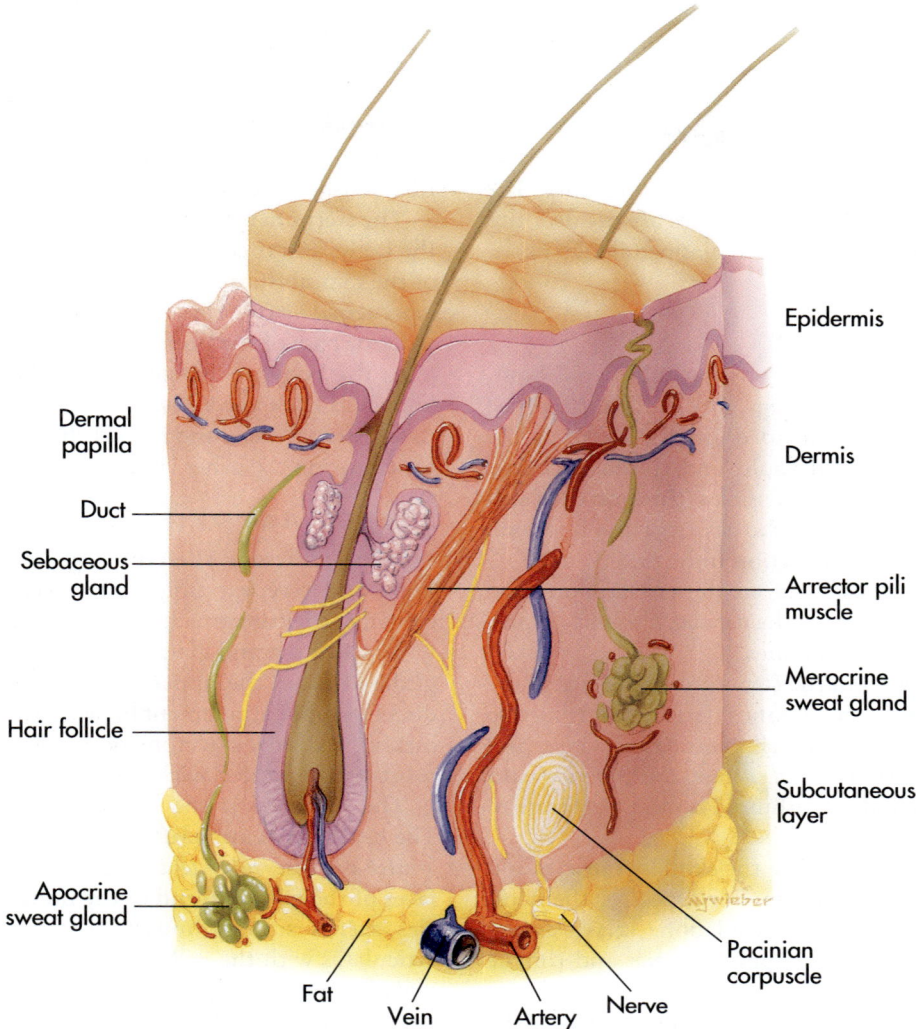

Epidermis

Dermal papilla

Duct

Sebaceous gland

Dermis

Arrector pili muscle

Merocrine sweat gland

Hair follicle

Subcutaneous layer

Apocrine sweat gland

Pacinian corpuscle

Fat

Vein

Artery

Nerve

FIGURE 10-9 Microscopic view of the skin.

groove and is hidden by a fold of skin known as the *cuticle*. The crescent-shaped white area of the nail is called the *lunula* and is most visible on the thumbnail. The nail bed that lies under the nail contains many blood vessels. In healthy individuals, this layer of epithelium appears pink through the translucent nail body.

GLANDS

The major glands of the skin are the sebaceous and sweat glands. Most **sebaceous glands** are found in the dermis and secrete oil **(sebum)** for the hair and skin. This oil prevents drying and protects against some bacteria. Sebum secretion increases during adolescence, stimulated by increased blood levels of the sex hormones. Other skin glands include the *ceruminous glands* of the external auditory meatus, which produce cerumen (earwax), and the *mammary glands*.

Sweat glands (sudoriferous glands) are the most numerous skin glands. They usually are classified as merocrine or apocrine, according to their mode of secretion. *Merocrine sweat glands* are the most common. They open directly onto the surface of the skin through sweat pores. The coiled portion of the gland produces a fluid that is mostly water but also contains some salts (mainly sodium chloride) and small amounts of ammonia, urea, uric acid, and lactic acid. As the body temperature rises, the sweat glands produce sweat. The sweat evaporates and cools the body. *Apocrine glands* usually open into hair follicles. These glands are found in the axillae and genitalia and around the anus. These glands become active at puberty through the influence of sex hormones. Apocrine glands secrete an organic substance that is odorless when released but is quickly metabolized by bacteria to cause body odor.

CRITICAL THINKING
The ability to sweat is impaired in the elderly. What implications does this have?

Skeletal System

The skeletal system consists of bones and associated connective tissues. These tissues include cartilage, tendons, and ligaments. The skeletal system offers a rigid framework for support and protection. It also provides a system of levers on which muscles act to produce body movements. The skeletal system contains 206 bones. Bones are divided into two groups, the axial skeleton and the appendicular skeleton (Figure 10-10).

AXIAL SKELETON

The **axial skeleton** is made up of the skull, hyoid bone, vertebral column, and thoracic cage. The skull is composed of 28 bones. These bones are divided into three groups: the auditory ossicles, the cranial vault, and the facial bones (Figure 10-11). The six auditory ossicles (three on each side of the head) are located inside the cavity of the temporal bone. The auditory ossicles function in hearing.

The **cranial vault** consists of six bones that surround and protect the brain. They are the *parietal, temporal, frontal, occipital, sphenoid,* and *ethmoid* bones.

The 14 facial bones form the structure of the face in the anterior skull. However, these bones do not contribute to the cranial vault. They include the *maxilla, mandible,* and *zygomatic, palatine, nasal, lacrimal, vomer,* and *inferior nasal concha* bones. The frontal and ethmoid bones contribute to the cranial vault and the face.

The **hyoid bone** is attached to the skull by muscles and ligaments and "floats" in the superior aspect of the neck, just below the mandible. The hyoid bone serves as the attachment point for several important neck and tongue muscles.

The vertebral column consists of 33 bones, which can be divided into five regions: 7 cervical vertebrae, 12 thoracic vertebrae, 5 lumbar vertebrae, 5 sacral vertebrae (fused), and 4 coccygeal vertebrae (fused) (Figure 10-12).

The weight-bearing portion of a vertebra is a bony disk called the *body*. Intervertebral disks are located between the bodies of adjacent vertebrae. The disks serve as shock absorbers for the vertebral column. They also provide additional support for the body. In addition, the disks prevent the vertebral bodies from rubbing against each other. The spinal cord is protected by the vertebral arch and the dorsal portion of the body. A *transverse process* extends laterally from each side of the arch, and a single *spinous process* is present at the point of junction. Much vertebral movement is accomplished by the contraction of skeletal muscles attached to the transverse and spinous processes.

The thoracic cage protects vital organs in the thorax. It also prevents the thorax from collapsing during respiration. The thoracic cage consists of the thoracic vertebrae, ribs with their associated **costal cartilages**, and the **sternum** (Figure 10-13).

The 12 pairs of ribs can be divided into *true ribs* or *false ribs*. The superior seven ribs (the true ribs) articulate with the thoracic vertebrae and attach directly through their costal cartilages to the sternum. The inferior five ribs (the false ribs) articulate with the thoracic vertebrae but do not attach directly to the sternum. The eighth, ninth, and tenth ribs are joined to a common cartilage, which is attached to the sternum. The eleventh and twelfth ribs are "floating" ribs that have no attachment to the sternum.

The sternum is divided into three parts: the manubrium, the body, and the xiphoid process. At the superior margin of the manubrium is the **jugular notch** (also known as the *suprasternal notch*). This notch can be easily palpated at the anterior base of the neck. The point where the manubrium joins the body of the sternum is the **sternal angle** (also known as the *angle of Louis*). The second rib is found lateral to the sternal angle and is used clinically as a starting point for counting the other ribs.

APPENDICULAR SKELETON

The **appendicular skeleton** consists of the bones of the upper and lower extremities. It also consists of their girdles, by which they are attached to the body.

The scapula and clavicle form the pectoral girdle. This girdle attaches the upper limbs to the axial skeleton. The direct point of attachment between the bones of the appendicular and axial skeletons occurs at the **sternoclavicular joint** between the clavicle and the sternum.

The **humerus** is the second longest bone in the body. The head of the humerus articulates with the scapula. The *greater and lesser tubercles* are on the lateral and anterior surfaces of the proximal end of the humerus. There the tubercles act as sites of muscle attachments. The humerus articulates with the **radius** and **ulna** at its distal end. The *capitulum* (lateral aspect of the humerus) articulates with the head of the radius. The *trochlea* (medial aspect of the humerus) articulates with the ulna. Proximal to the trochlea and capitulum are the *medial* and *lateral epicondyles,* respectively. These sites act as muscle attachments for the muscles of the forearm. Figure 10-14 illustrates the bones of the upper extremity.

The large bony process of the ulna (the *olecranon process*) can be felt at the point of the elbow. This process fits into a large depression on the posterior surface of the humerus known as the *olecranon fossa*. The structural relationship between these two processes makes movement of the joint possible. The distal end of the ulna has a small head that articulates with the radius and wrist bones. The posterior-medial side of this head has a small *styloid process* to which the ligaments of the wrist are attached. The proximal end of the radius articulates with the humerus. The medial surface of the head constitutes a smooth cylinder where the radius rotates against the radial notch of the ulna. Major anterior arm muscles (biceps brachii) are attached to the *radial tuberosity*.

The wrist is composed of eight carpal bones, which are arranged in two rows of four each. Five **metacarpals** are attached to the **carpal bones** and constitute the bony framework of the hand. Twenty-eight **phalanges** make up

Axial skeleton   **Appendicular skeleton**   **Axial skeleton**

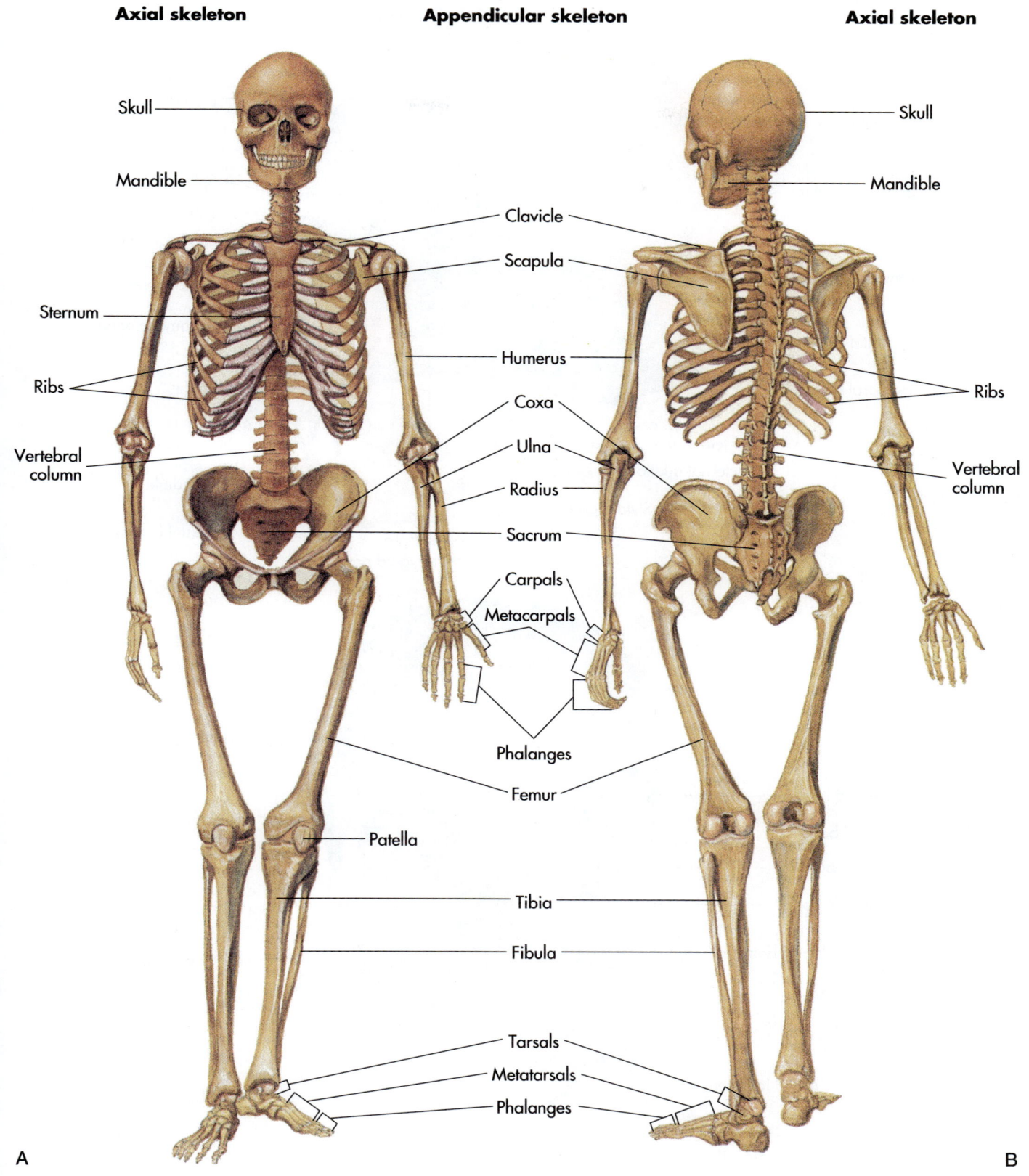

Skull

Mandible

Sternum

Ribs

Vertebral
column

Clavicle

Scapula

Humerus

Coxa

Ulna

Radius

Sacrum

Carpals

Metacarpals

Phalanges

Femur

Patella

Tibia

Fibula

Tarsals

Metatarsals

Phalanges

Skull

Mandible

Ribs

Vertebral
column

A

B

FIGURE 10-10 Anterior view **(A)** and posterior view **(B)** of the skeleton.

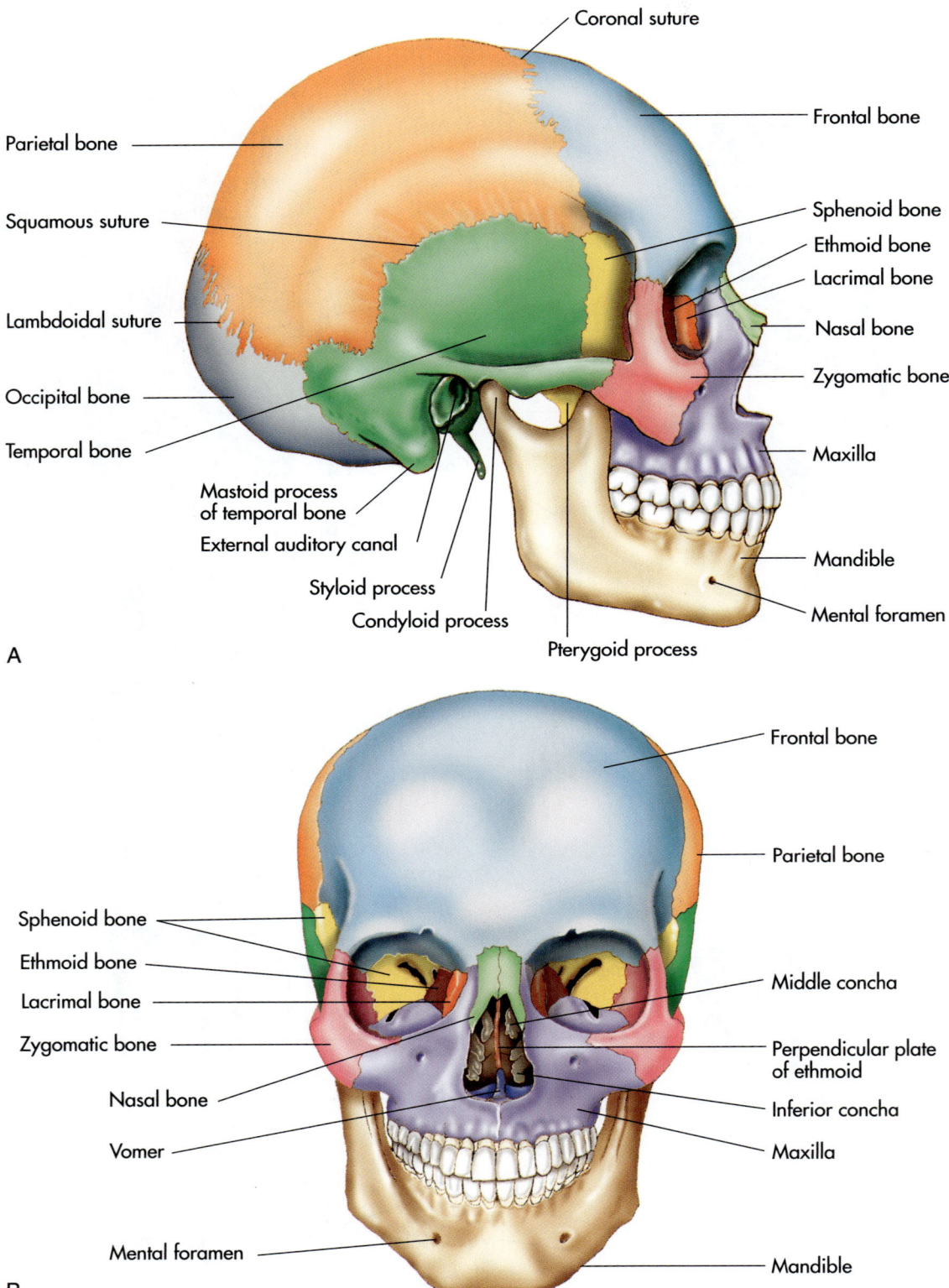

FIGURE 10-11 Skull viewed from the right side (**A**) and the front (**B**).

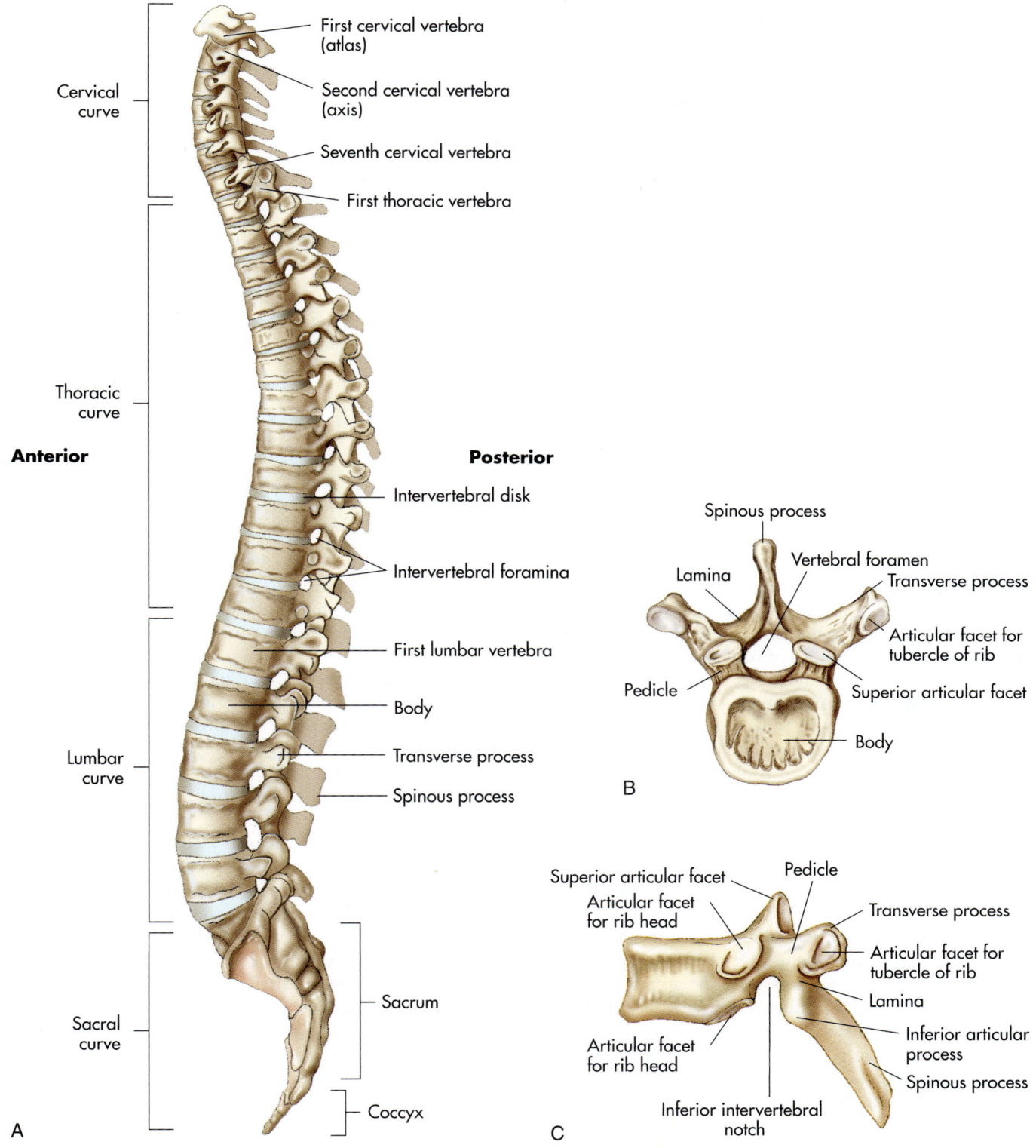

Cervical curve

First cervical vertebra (atlas)

Second cervical vertebra (axis)

Seventh cervical vertebra

First thoracic vertebra

Thoracic curve

Anterior

Posterior

Intervertebral disk

Intervertebral foramina

First lumbar vertebra

Body

Transverse process

Spinous process

Lumbar curve

Sacrum

Sacral curve

Coccyx

A

Spinous process

Lamina

Vertebral foramen

Transverse process

Articular facet for tubercle of rib

Pedicle

Superior articular facet

Body

B

Superior articular facet

Articular facet for rib head

Pedicle

Transverse process

Articular facet for tubercle of rib

Lamina

Inferior articular process

Spinous process

Articular facet for rib head

Inferior intervertebral notch

C

FIGURE 10-12 A, Vertebral column viewed from the left side. **B,** Superior view of the vertebrae. **C,** Lateral view of the vertebrae.

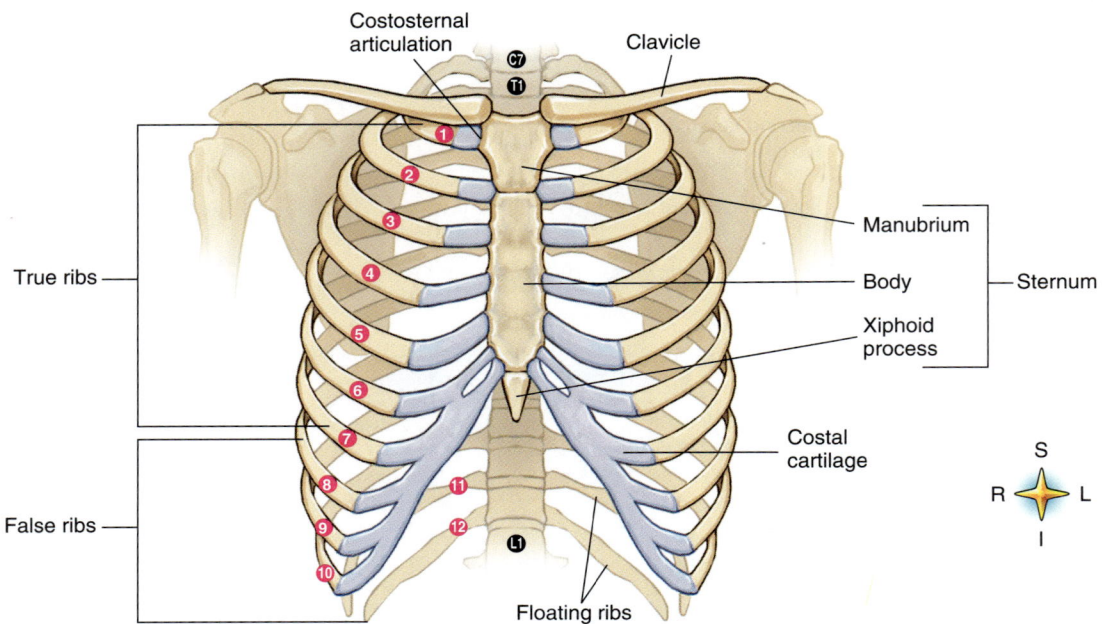

FIGURE 10-13 Thoracic cage. Note the costal cartilages and their articulations with the body of the sternum. (Patton KT, Thibodeau GA: *Anatomy and physiology,* ed 7, St Louis, 2007, Mosby.)

the 10 digits of the hands. Each thumb has two phalanges, and each finger has three phalanges.

The pelvic girdle attaches the legs to the trunk (Figure 10-15). The girdle consists of two **coxae** (hip bones). One is located on each side of the pelvis. Each coxa surrounds a large **obturator foramen**, through which muscles, nerves, and blood vessels pass to the leg. A fossa called the **acetabulum** is located on the lateral surface of each coxa. The acetabulum is the point of articulation of the lower limb with the girdle. During development, each coxa is formed by the fusion of three separate bones: the **ilium**, the **ischium**, and the **pubis**. The superior portion of the ilium is the **iliac crest**. The crest ends anteriorly as the anterior-superior iliac spine and posteriorly as the posterior-superior iliac spine.

The **femur** is the longest bone in the body. The femur has a neck that is well defined. It also has a prominent rounded head that articulates with the acetabulum. The proximal shaft has two tuberosities: a *greater trochanter,* which is lateral to the neck, and a smaller or *lesser trochanter,* which is inferior and posterior to the neck. Both trochanters are attachment sites for muscles that attach the hip to the thigh. The distal end of the femur has *medial* and *lateral condyles* that articulate with the tibia. Located laterally and proximally to the condyles are the *medial* and *lateral epicondyles*. These are sites of muscle and ligament attachment. Figure 10-16 illustrates the bones of the lower extremity.

Distally, the femur also articulates with the **patella**, which is located in a major tendon of the thigh muscle. The patella allows the tendon to turn the corner over the knee.

The two bones of the leg are the tibia and the fibula. The **tibia** is the larger of the two and supports most of the weight of the leg. A *tibial tuberosity* can be seen and palpated just inferior to the patella. The proximal end of the tibia has *flat medial* and *lateral condyles* that articulate with the condyles of the femur. The distal end of the tibia forms the **medial malleolus**, which helps to form the medial side of the ankle joint.

The **fibula** does not articulate with the femur. However, the fibula does have a small proximal head that articulates with the tibia. The distal end of the fibula forms the lateral malleolus to create the lateral aspect of the ankle joint.

The foot consists of seven **tarsal bones** (Figure 10-17). The talus articulates with the tibia and the fibula to form the ankle joint. The **calcaneus** is located inferior and just lateral to the talus, supporting the bone. The calcaneus protrudes posteriorly where the calf muscles attach to it. The calcaneus is identified easily as the heel. The foot consists of tarsals, **metatarsals**, and phalanges. These bones are arranged in a manner similar to the metacarpals and phalanges of the hand, the great toe being analogous to the thumb. The ball of the foot is the junction between the metatarsals and the phalanges. Strong ligaments and leg muscle tendons normally hold the foot bones firmly in their arched position.

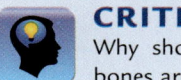 **CRITICAL THINKING**
Why should you anticipate blood loss when large bones are fractured?

BIOMECHANICS OF BODY MOVEMENT

With the exception of the hyoid bone, every bone in the body connects to at least one other bone.

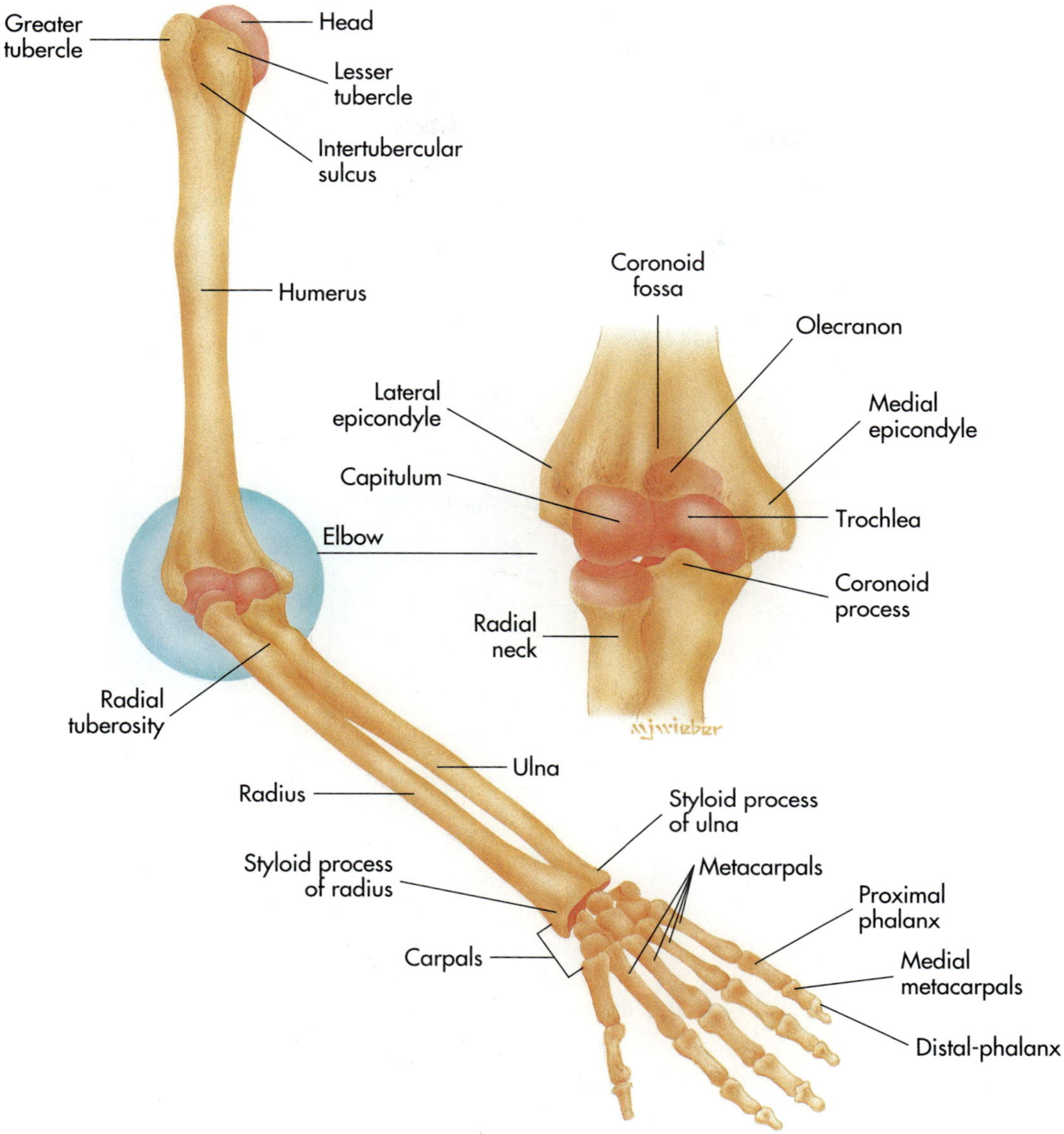

Greater tubercle

Head

Lesser tubercle

Intertubercular sulcus

Humerus

Coronoid fossa

Olecranon

Lateral epicondyle

Medial epicondyle

Capitulum

Elbow

Trochlea

Coronoid process

Radial neck

Radial tuberosity

mjwiebier

Ulna

Radius

Styloid process of ulna

Metacarpals

Styloid process of radius

Proximal phalanx

Medial metacarpals

Carpals

Distal-phalanx

FIGURE 10-14 Bones of the upper extremity.

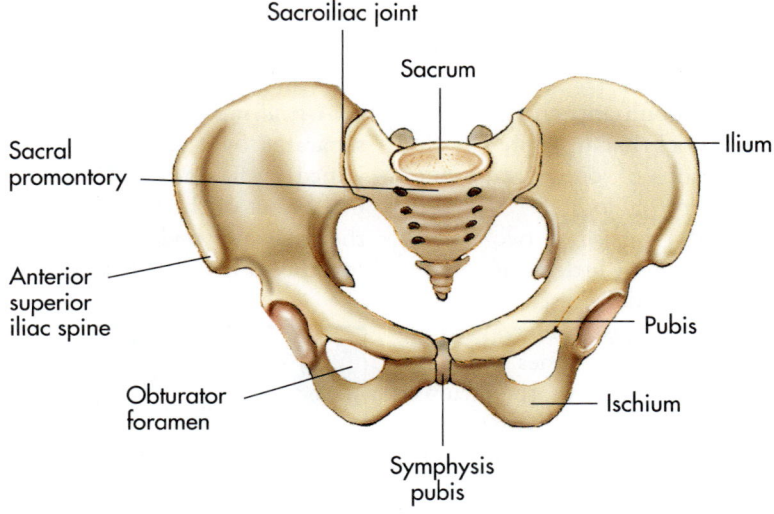

Sacroiliac joint

Sacrum

Sacral promontory

Ilium

Anterior superior iliac spine

Pubis

Obturator foramen

Ischium

Symphysis pubis

FIGURE 10-15 Complete pelvic girdle (anterior view).

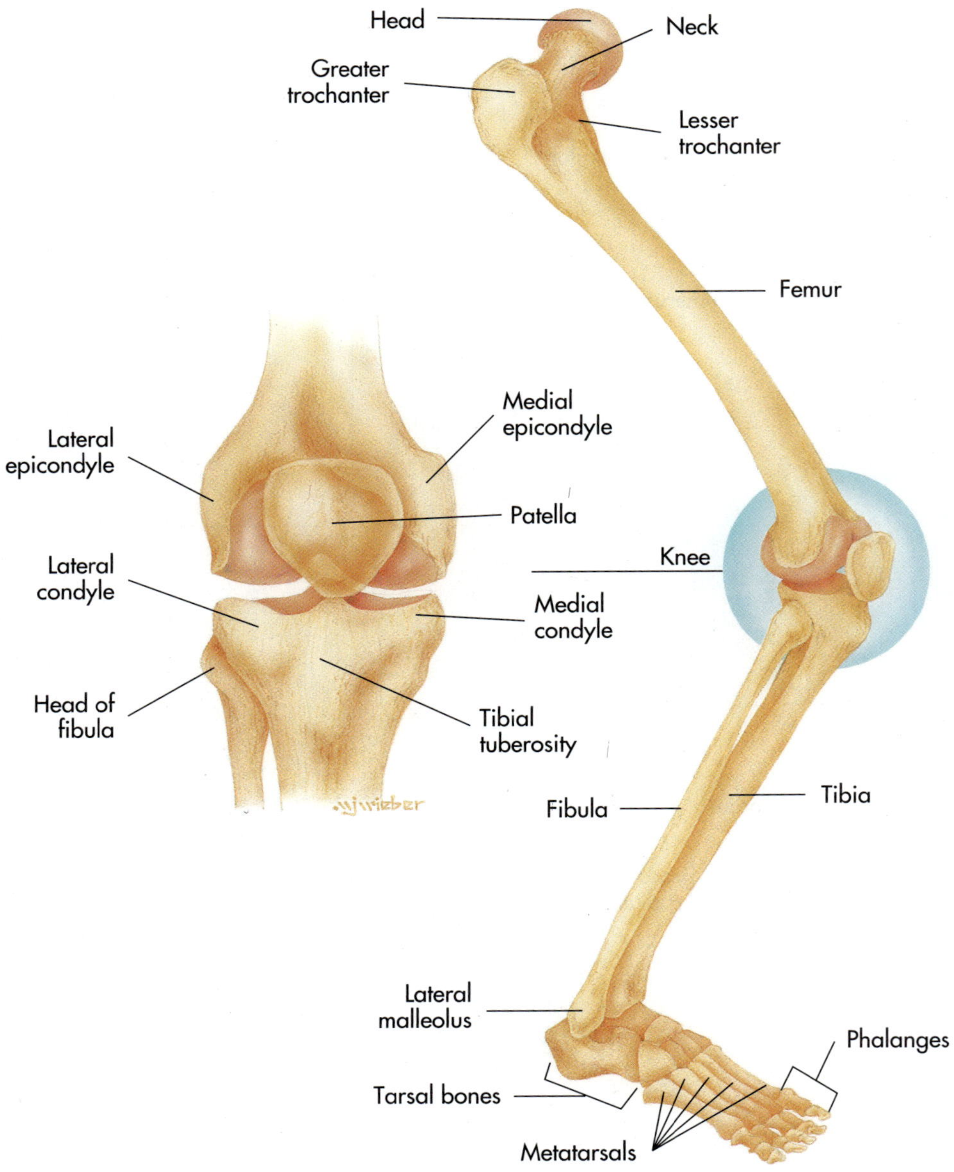

Head — Neck

Greater trochanter — Lesser trochanter

Femur

Medial epicondyle

Lateral epicondyle

Patella

Lateral condyle

Knee

Medial condyle

Head of fibula

Tibial tuberosity

Tibia

Fibula

Lateral malleolus

Phalanges

Tarsal bones

Metatarsals

FIGURE 10-16 Bones of the lower extremity.

The connections, or joints, commonly are named according to the bones or portions of bones that are united at the joint. The three major classifications of joints are fibrous joints, cartilaginous joints, and synovial joints.

Fibrous Joints. Fibrous joints consist of two bones united by fibrous tissue; these joints have little or no movement. Fibrous joints are further classified, based on structure, as sutures, syndesmoses, or gomphoses. *Sutures* (seams between flat bones) are located in the skull bones and may be completely immobile in adults. In newborns, the sutures have gaps between them, called *fontanels* (Figure 10-18); these gaps are fairly wide to allow "give" to the skull during birth and to allow growth of the head during development.

A *syndesmosis* is a fibrous joint in which the bones are separated by a greater distance than in a suture and are joined by ligaments. These ligaments may provide some movement of the joint. An example of this type of joint is the *radioulnar syndesmosis,* which binds the radius and ulna together (Figure 10-19).

CRITICAL THINKING

Why might the structure of the skull sutures be a disadvantage with head trauma in an adult?

A *gomphosis* consists of a peg that fits into a socket. The peg is held in place by fine bundles of collagenous

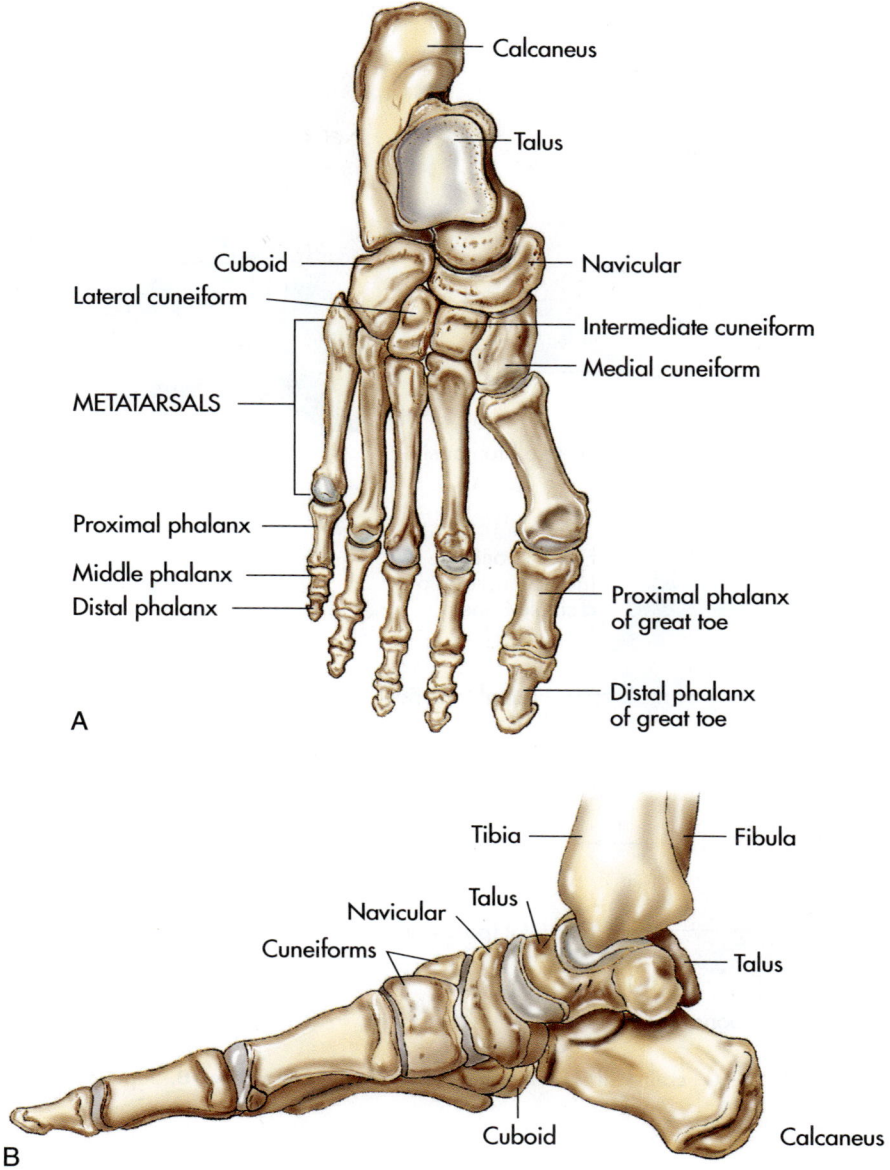

Calcaneus

Talus

Cuboid

Lateral cuneiform

Navicular

Intermediate cuneiform

Medial cuneiform

METATARSALS

Proximal phalanx

Middle phalanx

Distal phalanx

Proximal phalanx of great toe

Distal phalanx of great toe

A

Tibia

Fibula

Talus

Navicular

Cuneiforms

Talus

Cuboid

Calcaneus

B

FIGURE 10-17 Bones of the right ankle and foot. **A,** Dorsal view. **B,** Medial view.

connective tissue. The joints between the teeth and the sockets along the processes of the mandible and maxilla are examples of gomphoses.

Cartilaginous Joints. Cartilaginous joints unite two bones by means of hyaline cartilage (synchondroses) or fibrocartilage (symphyses). A synchondrosis allows only slight movement at the joint. A common example of this type of joint is the epiphyseal plate of a growing bone. Another example is the cartilage rod between most of the ribs and the sternum. Symphyseal joints are slightly movable because of the flexible nature of the fibrocartilage. Symphyses include the junction between the manubrium and the body of the sternum in adults, the symphysis pubis of the coxae, and the intervertebral disks.

Synovial Joints. Synovial joints contain synovial fluid, which is a thin lubricating film that allows considerable movement between articulating bones. Most joints that unite the bones of the appendicular skeleton are synovial. The articular surfaces of bones in synovial joints are covered with a thin layer of hyaline cartilage. This cartilage provides a smooth surface where the bones meet. The joint is enclosed by a **joint capsule**. The capsule consists of an outer fibrous capsule and an inner synovial membrane. The synovial membrane lines the joint and produces synovial fluid. Synovial joints are classified into six divisions according to the shape of the adjoining articular surfaces (Figure 10-20):

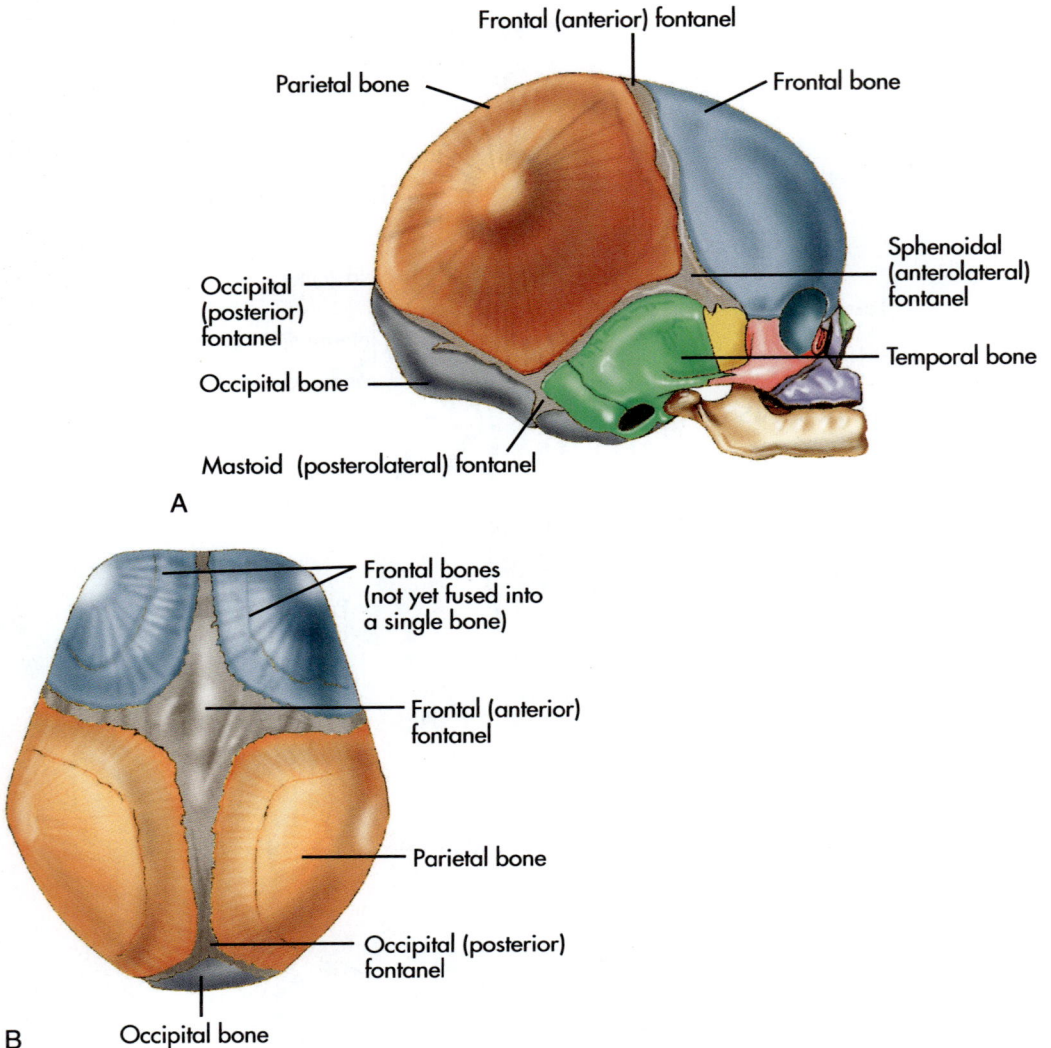

FIGURE 10-18 Fetal skull showing the fontanels. **A,** Lateral view. **B,** Superior view.

1. *Plane* or *gliding joints* consist of two opposed flat surfaces that are about equal in size. Examples of these joints are the articular processes between the vertebrae.

2. *Saddle joints* consist of two saddle-shaped articulating surfaces oriented at right angles to each other. Movement in these joints can occur in two planes. An example of a saddle joint is the carpometacarpal joint of the thumb.

3. *Hinge joints* consist of a convex cylinder in one bone applied to a corresponding concavity in another bone. These joints permit movement in one plane only. Examples of hinge joints are the joints of the elbow and knee.

4. *Pivot joints* consist of a relatively cylindrical bony process. This process rotates within a ring composed partly of bone and partly of ligament. An example of a pivot joint is the articulation of the head of the radius with the proximal end of the ulna.

5. *Ball-and-socket joints* consist of a ball (head) at the end of one bone and a socket in an adjacent bone into which a portion of the ball fits. These joints allow wide ranges of movement in almost any direction. Examples are the shoulder and hip joints.

6. *Ellipsoid joints* are modified ball-and-socket joints. The articular surfaces are ellipsoid rather than spherical. The shape of the joint limits movement, making it similar to a hinge motion, but the motion occurs in two planes. The *atlantooccipital joint* is an ellipsoid joint.

Types of Movement. Movement may be described as it relates to the position of the body.[3] In other words, movement can be described by motion away from the anatomical position or motion toward it. (Table 10-3 lists examples of each type of movement; also see Figures 10-21 to 10-25.)

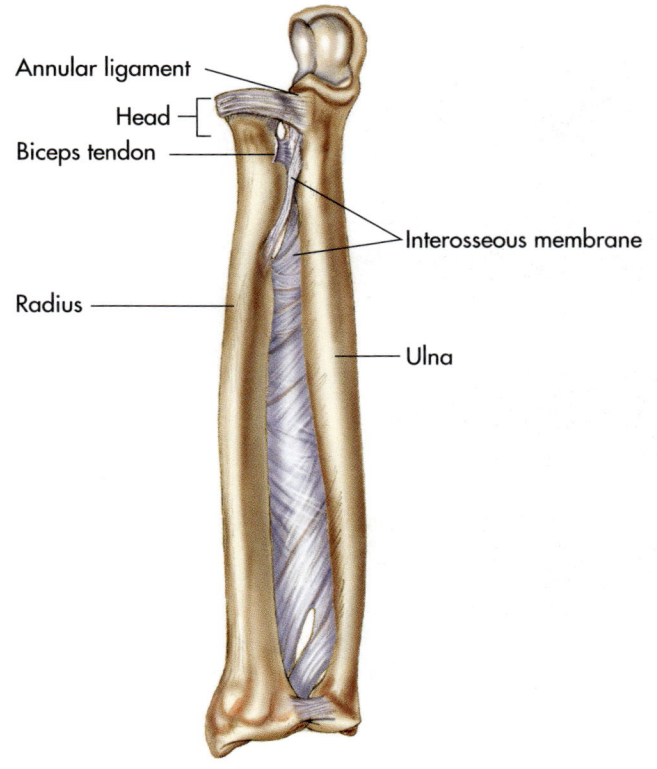

Annular ligament

Head

Biceps tendon

Interosseous membrane

Radius

Ulna

FIGURE 10-19 Radioulnar syndesmosis of the right forearm.

TABLE 10-3 Body Movement Terminology

Term	Definition
Flexion	Bending
Extension	Stretching out
Protraction	Movement in the anterior direction
Retraction	Movement in the posterior direction
Abduction	Movement away from the midline
Adduction	Movement toward the midline
Inversion	Turning inward
Eversion	Turning outward
Excursion	Movement from side to side
Rotation	Movement of a structure around its axis
Circumduction	Movement in a circular motion
Pronation	Rotation of the forearm so that the anterior surface is down
Supination	Rotation of the forearm so that the anterior surface is up
Elevation	Movement of a structure in a superior direction
Depression	Movement of a structure in an inferior direction
Opposition	Movement of the thumb and little finger toward each other
Reposition	Movement of a structure to its original position

 CRITICAL THINKING
Why would it be an asset to use movement terms in your radio report or written patient care report?

Muscular System

The three primary functions of the muscular system are movement, postural maintenance, and heat production. As previously discussed, the major types of muscles are skeletal, cardiac, and smooth muscle. Skeletal muscle is far more common than other types of muscle in the body and is the focus of this section. Cardiac and smooth muscle are presented later in this text. (Table 10-4 compares these muscle types.)

PHYSIOLOGY OF SKELETAL MUSCLE

Muscle tissue is made up of specialized contractile cells or muscle fibers. Skeletal muscle contracts in response to electrochemical stimuli. Nerve cells regulate the function of skeletal muscle fibers by controlling the series of events that results in muscle contraction.

Each skeletal muscle fiber is filled with thick and thin **myofilaments**. These are fine, threadlike structures. The *thick myofilaments* are formed from the protein *myosin*. The *thin myofilaments* are composed of the protein *actin*. The **sarcomere**, the contractile unit of skeletal muscle, contains thick and thin myofilaments. During the contraction process, energy obtained from ATP molecules enables the two types of myofilaments to slide toward each other, shortening the sarcomere and eventually the entire muscle.

A nervous impulse enters the muscle fiber through a specialized nerve known as a **motor neuron**. The point of contact between the nerve ending and the muscle fiber is the neuromuscular junction, or **synapse** (Figure 10-26). Each muscle fiber receives a branch of an axon. Each axon innervates more than a single muscle fiber. When a nerve impulse passes through this junction, specialized chemicals are released, causing the muscle to contract.

CRITICAL THINKING
Consider that exposure to a chemical nerve weapon caused too much chemical stimulation at the synapse for the muscles of the eye. What might you find in your examination of the eye?

SKELETAL MUSCLE MOVEMENT

Most muscles extend from one bone to another and cross at least one joint. Muscle contraction causes most body movements by pulling one of the bones toward the other across the movable joint. The points of attachment of each muscle are the origin and the insertion. The *origin* is the end of the muscle attached to the more stationary of the two bones. The *insertion* is the end of the muscle attached to the bone undergoing the greatest movement. Some muscles of

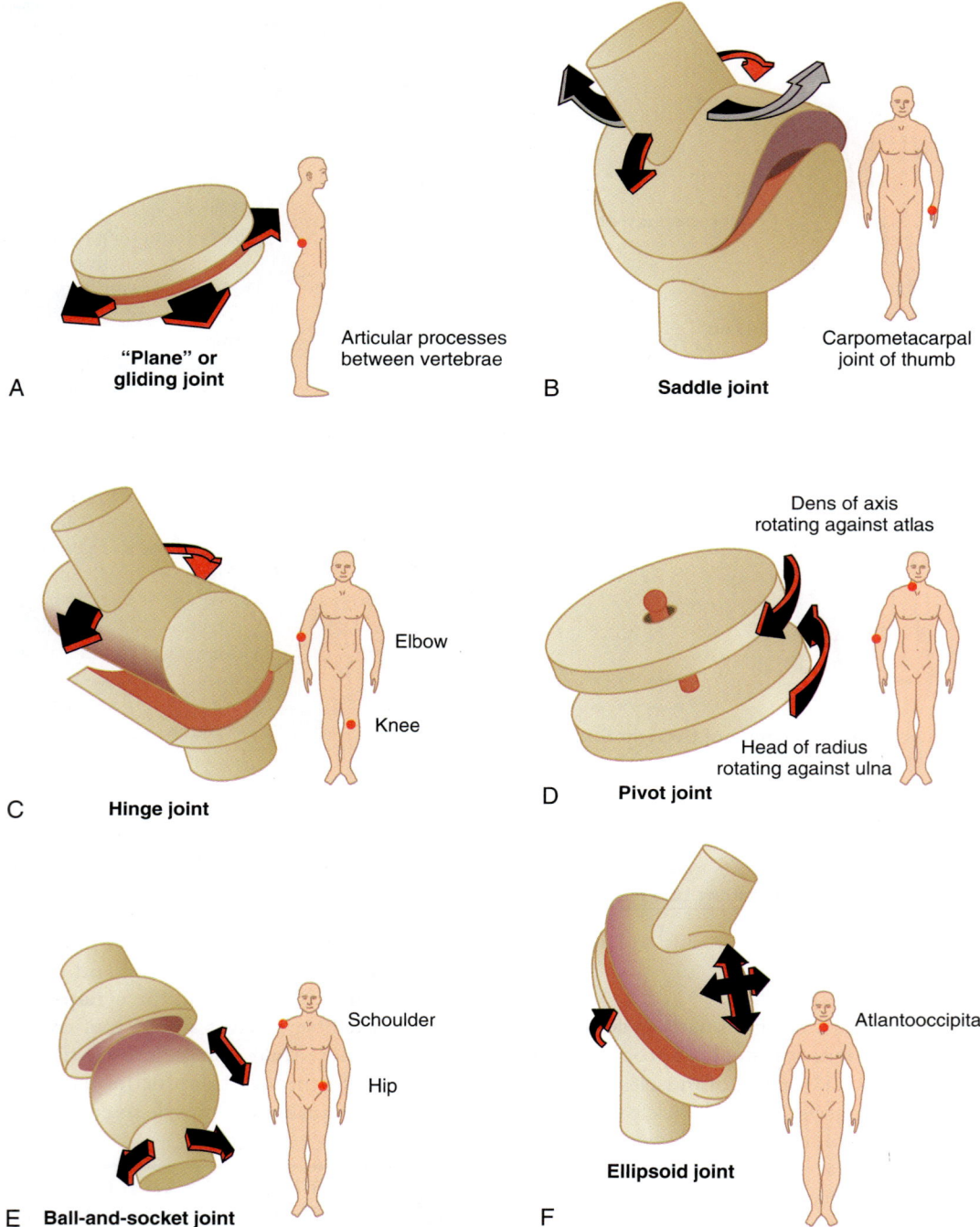

A **"Plane" or gliding joint** — Articular processes between vertebrae

B **Saddle joint** — Carpometacarpal joint of thumb

C **Hinge joint** — Elbow, Knee

D **Pivot joint** — Dens of axis rotating against atlas, Head of radius rotating against ulna

E **Ball-and-socket joint** — Schoulder, Hip

F **Ellipsoid joint** — Atlantooccipital

FIGURE 10-20 Types of synovial joints and selected examples. **A,** Plane. **B,** Saddle. **C,** Hinge. **D,** Pivot. **E,** Ball-and-socket. **F,** Ellipsoid.

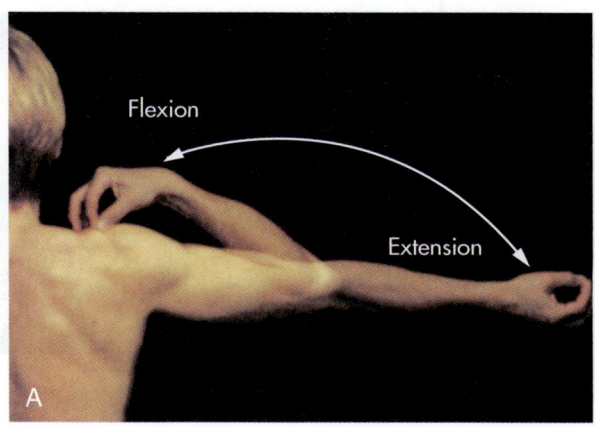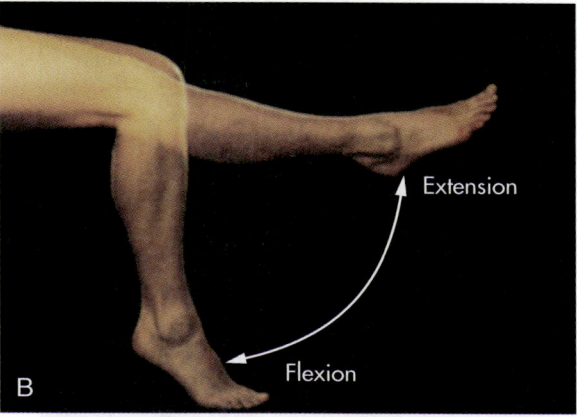

FIGURE 10-21 Flexion and extension of the elbow **(A)** and the knee **(B)**.

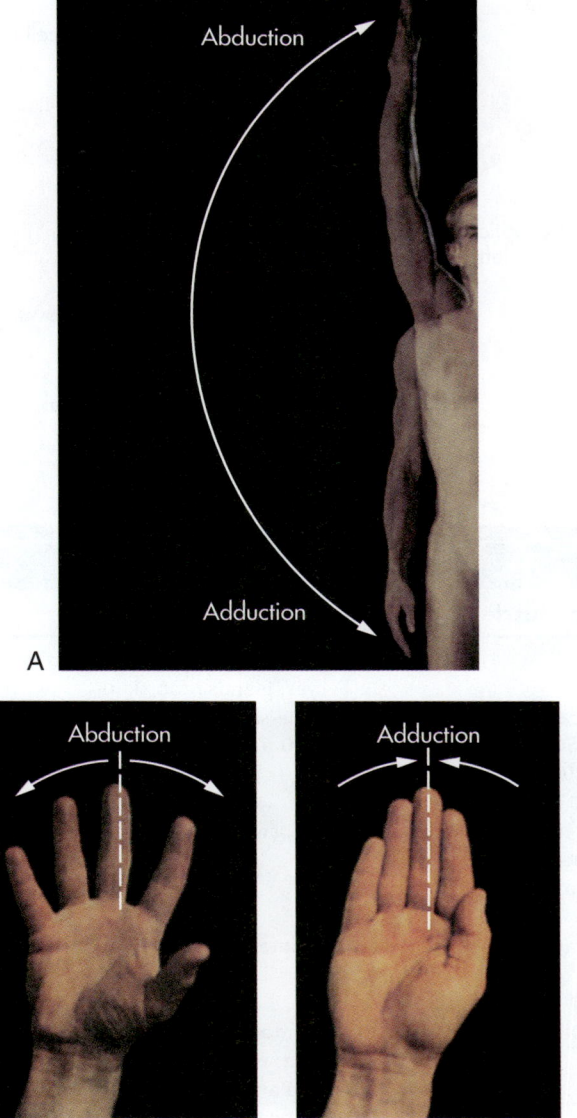

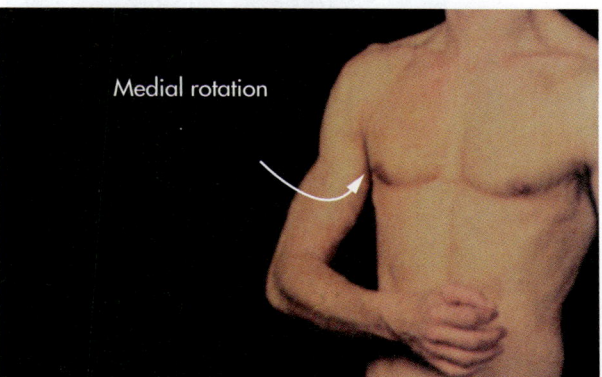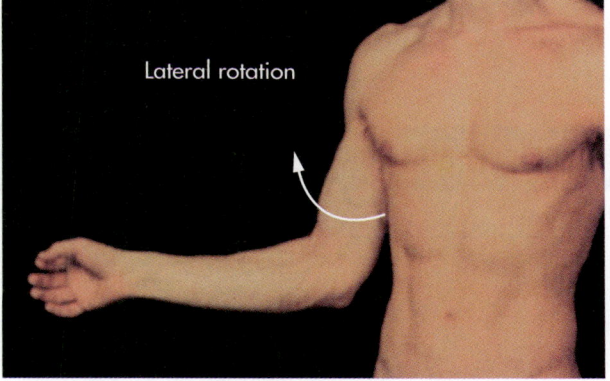

FIGURE 10-23 Medial and lateral rotation of the humerus.

FIGURE 10-22 Abduction and adduction of the upper extremity **(A)** and the fingers **(B)**.

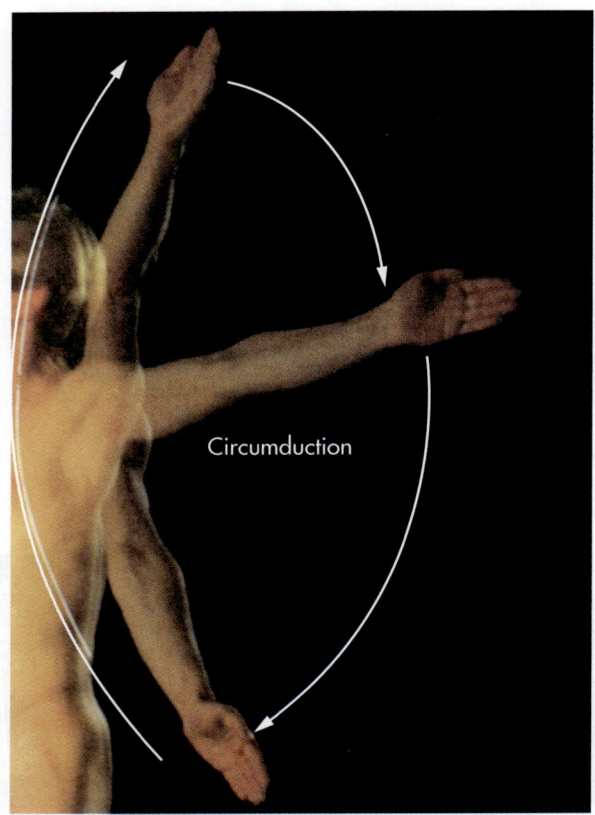

FIGURE 10-24 Circumduction of the shoulder.

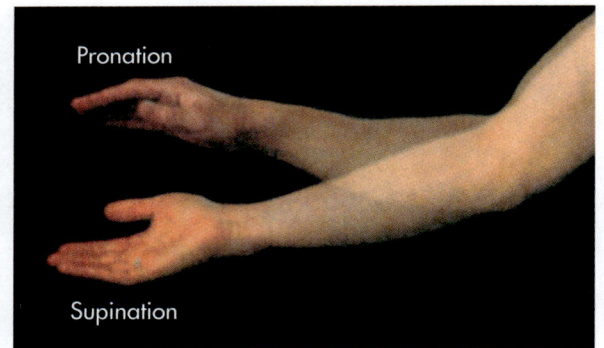

FIGURE 10-25 Pronation and supination.

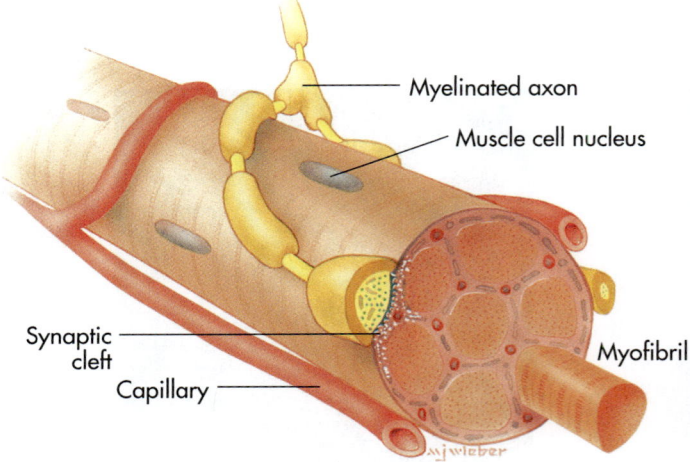

FIGURE 10-26 Neuromuscular junction.

TABLE 10-4 **Comparison of Muscle Types**			
Features	**Skeletal Muscle**	**Cardiac Muscle**	**Smooth Muscle**
Location	Attached to bones	Heart	Walls of hollow organs, blood vessels, eyes, glands, and skin
Cell shape	Long and cylindrical (1-40 mm in length; may extend the entire length of a muscle; 10-100 μm in diameter)	Cylindrical and branched (100-500 μm in length; 100-200 μm in diameter)	Spindle-shaped (15-200 μm in length, 5-10 μm in diameter)
Nucleus special features	Multiple, peripherally located	Single, centrally located Intercalated disks join the cells to each other	Single, centrally located
Striations	Yes	Yes	No
Control	Voluntary	Involuntary	Involuntary
Capable of spontaneous contraction	No	Yes	Yes
Function	Body movement	Pumps blood	Food movement through the digestive tract, emptying of the urinary bladder, regulation of blood vessel diameter, change in pupil size, contraction of many gland ducts, movement of hair, and many other functions

the face are not attached to bone at both ends; rather, they attach to the skin, which moves when muscles contract.

As some muscles contract and others relax at the same time, movement is created. Muscles that work together to cause movement are called *synergists*. A muscle that opposes another muscle (moves the structure in an opposite direction) is called an *antagonist*. The muscle that is the main cause of a movement is called the *prime mover*. For example, the biceps brachii, brachialis, and triceps brachii muscles are involved in flexion and extension of the forearm at the elbow joint. The *biceps brachii* is the prime mover during flexion. The *brachialis* is the synergistic muscle. When the biceps brachii and the brachialis muscles flex the forearm, the *triceps brachii* relaxes. The triceps is the antagonist. During extension of the forearm, the triceps brachii is the prime mover. The biceps and brachialis are the antagonistic muscles. The synergists and antagonists coordinate their activity, making movement smooth (Figure 10-27).

Types of Muscle Contraction. Muscle contractions can be labeled as *isometric* or *isotonic*. This depends on the type of contraction that predominates. In isometric contractions the length of the muscle does not change. However, the amount of tension increases during the contraction. Isometric contractions are responsible for the constant length of the postural muscles of the body. During isotonic contractions, the amount of tension created by the muscle is constant, but the length of the muscle changes. An example of isotonic contraction is the movement of the arms or fingers. Most muscle contractions are a mix of the two types of contractions.

Postural Maintenance. Postural maintenance is a result of muscle tone, the constant tension produced by muscles of the body for long periods. This tone keeps the back and legs straight, the head in an upright position, and the abdomen from bulging. These positions balance the distribution of weight. Therefore, they put less strain on muscles, tendons, ligaments, and bones.

Heat Production. The energy needed to create muscle contraction is derived from ATP. Most of the energy released in the breakdown of ATP during a muscular contraction is used to shorten the muscle fibers. Some energy, though, is lost as heat during the chemical reaction. The normal body temperature comes in large part from this metabolism in skeletal muscle. If the body temperature drops below a certain level, the nervous system induces shivering. Shivering is rapid contractions of skeletal muscle that produce shaking rather than coordinated movements. The muscle movement increases heat production up to 18 times that of resting levels. The heat made during shivering can exceed that from moderate exercise. This helps to raise the body temperature to its normal range.

CRITICAL THINKING
Children under 3 months of age cannot shiver. How will you account for that in your prehospital care for patients in this age group?

Nervous System

The nervous system and the endocrine system are the main regulatory and coordinating systems of the body. The nervous system rapidly sends out information. This occurs by means of nerve impulses conducted from one area of the body to another. The endocrine system sends out information more slowly. This takes place by means of chemicals secreted by ductless glands into the bloodstream. These chemicals and hormones then are circulated to other parts of the body. The constancy of the internal environment of the body is **homeostasis**. This constancy is sustained to a large degree by these regulatory and coordinating actions.

DIVISIONS OF THE NERVOUS SYSTEM

The human body has a single nervous system. This is the case even though some of its subdivisions are referred to as separate systems. Each subdivision has structural and functional aspects that distinguish it from the others (Figure 10-28).

The **central nervous system (CNS)** is made up of the brain and spinal cord. These organs are encased in and protected by bone. The brain and spinal cord are continuous with each other. The **peripheral nervous system (PNS)** consists of the nerves and ganglia. The **ganglia** are collections of nerve cell bodies located outside the CNS. Forty-three pairs of nerves originate from the CNS to form the PNS; 12 pairs, the cranial nerves, originate from the brain, and the remaining 31 pairs, the spinal nerves, originate from the spinal cord. The **afferent division** transmits action potentials from the sensory organs to the CNS. The **efferent division** transmits action potentials from the CNS to effector organs such as muscles and glands (Figure 10-29). The efferent division is divided further into the **somatic nervous system** and the **autonomic nervous system**. The somatic nervous system transmits impulses from the CNS to skeletal muscle. The autonomic nervous system transmits action potentials from the CNS to smooth muscle, cardiac muscle, and certain glands.

CRITICAL THINKING
How are the cranial nerves like the Supreme Court?

CENTRAL NERVOUS SYSTEM

As stated before, the CNS consists of the brain and spinal cord. The adult brain has four major regions: the brainstem (consisting of the medulla, pons, and midbrain); the diencephalon (which includes the thalamus and hypothalamus); the cerebrum; and the cerebellum (Figure 10-30). Table 10-5 describes the functions of these divisions.

Brainstem. The medulla, pons, and midbrain constitute the brainstem. The brainstem connects the spinal cord to the remainder of the brain and is responsible for many essential functions. All but two of the 12 cranial nerves enter or exit the brain through the brainstem.

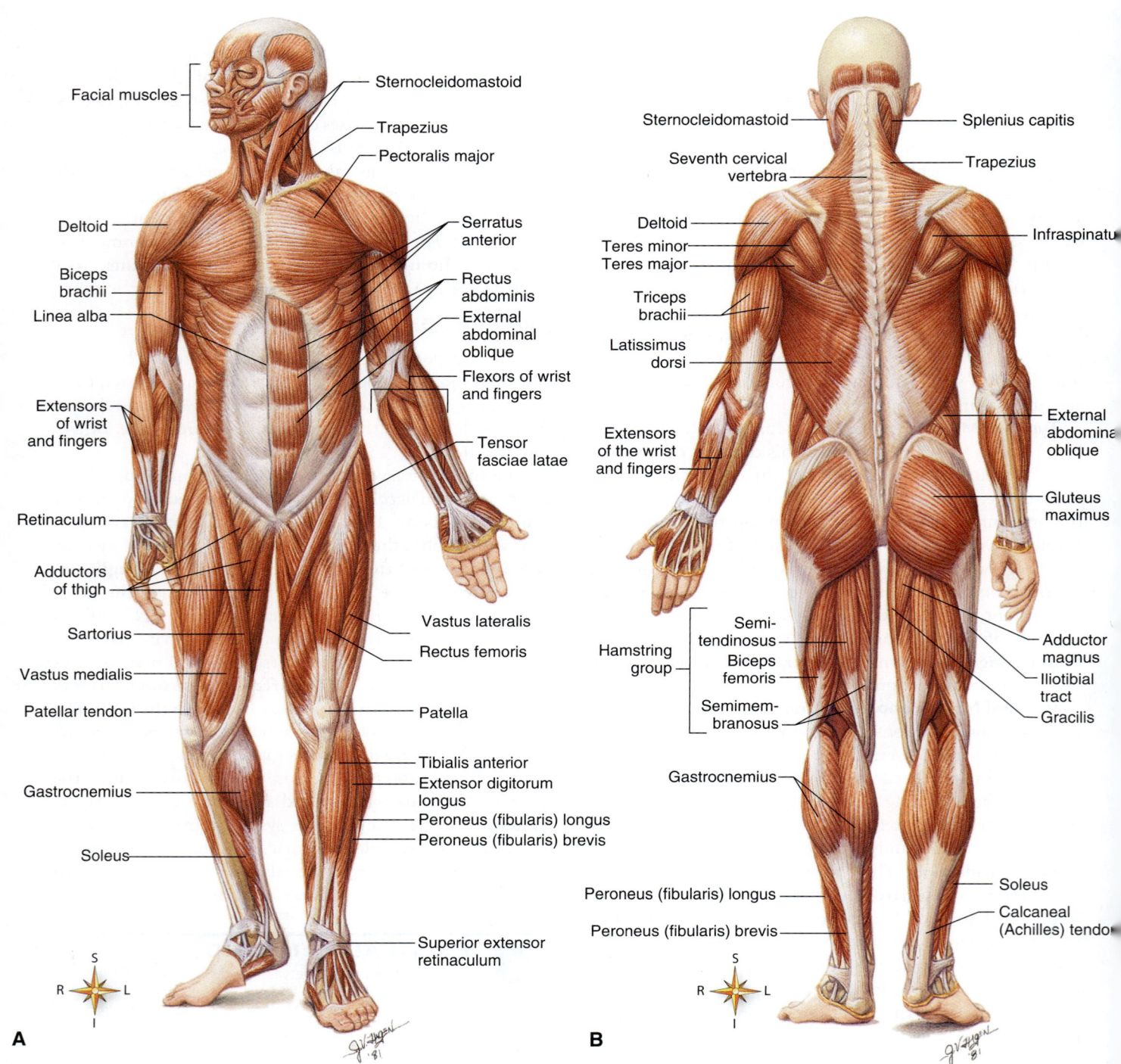

FIGURE 10-27 A, Anterior view of the body's musculature. **B,** Posterior view of the body's musculature. (Patton KT, Thibodeau GA: *Anatomy and physiology,* ed 7, St Louis, 2007, Mosby.)

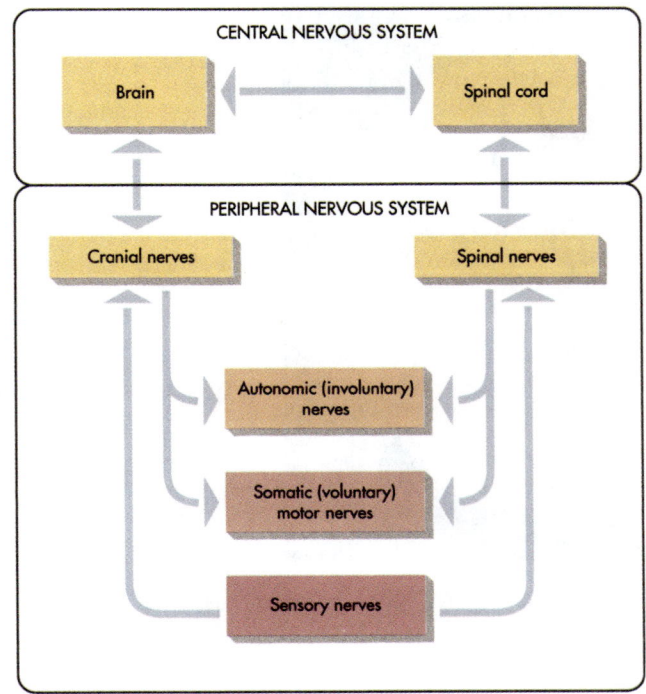

FIGURE 10-28 Divisions of the nervous system. (Thibodeau GA, Patton KT: *Structure and function of the body,* ed 13, St Louis, 2008, Mosby.)

The **medulla**, also known as the *medulla oblongata,* is the most inferior portion of the brainstem. The medulla acts as a conduction pathway for ascending and descending nerve tracts. It controls several body functions, such as regulation of the heart rate, blood vessel diameter, breathing, swallowing, vomiting, coughing, and sneezing.

> ### CRITICAL THINKING
> You have a patient with an injury that affects the medulla. What is the initial prehospital management priority? Why?

The **pons** contains ascending and descending nerve tracts. It relays information from the cerebrum to the cerebellum. In addition, the pons houses the sleep center and respiratory center that, along with the medulla, help control breathing.

The midbrain, or **mesencephalon**, is the smallest region of the brainstem. The midbrain is involved in hearing through audio pathways in the CNS. The midbrain also is involved in visual reflexes such as visual tracking of moving objects and turning of the eyes. Other parts of the midbrain help regulate the automatic functions that require no conscious thought. These functions include, for example, coordination of motor activities and muscle tone.

The **reticular formation** is a group of nuclei scattered throughout the brainstem. It receives axons from a large number of sources, especially from the nerves that

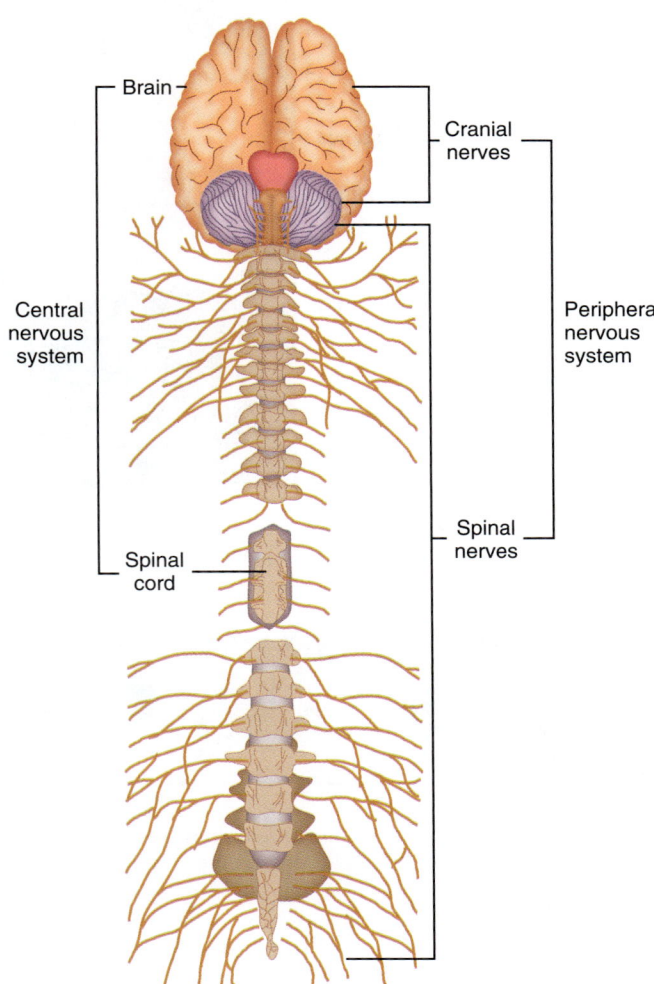

FIGURE 10-29 The central nervous system consists of the brain and spinal cord. The peripheral nervous system consists of the cranial nerves, which arise from the brain, and the spinal nerves, which arise from the spinal cord.

innervate the face. The reticular formation and its connections are known as the **reticular activating system**. This system is involved in the sleep-wake cycle. The reticular activating system also is important in arousing and maintaining consciousness. Coma after head injury results from damage to this system.

Diencephalon. The **diencephalon** is the part of the brain between the brainstem and the cerebrum. Major components of this organ include the thalamus and hypothalamus. The **thalamus** is the largest portion of the diencephalon. It receives sensory input from various sense organs of the body and relays these impulses to the **cerebral cortex**. The thalamus also has other functions, such as influencing mood and general body movements linked with strong emotions such as fear or rage.

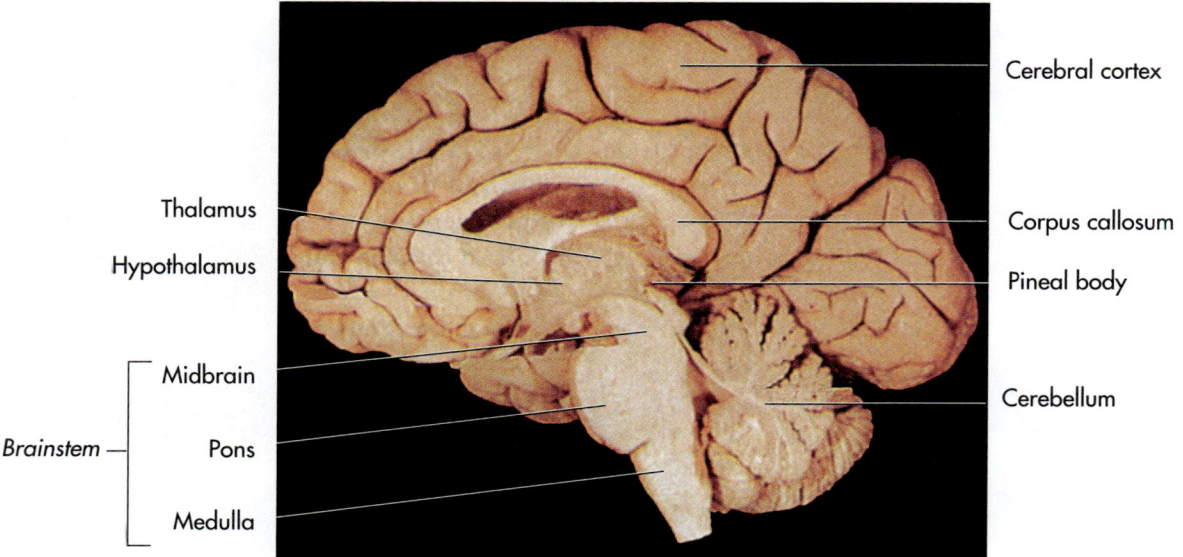

Thalamus

Hypothalamus

Cerebral cortex

Corpus callosum

Pineal body

Brainstem

Midbrain

Pons

Medulla

Cerebellum

FIGURE 10-30 Section of preserved brain. (Thibodeau GA, Patton KT: *Structure and function of the body,* ed 13, St Louis, 2008, Mosby.)

TABLE 10-5 Functions of Major Divisions of the Brain	
Brain Area	**Function**
Brainstem	
Medulla	Two-way conduction pathway between the spinal cord and higher brain centers; cardiac, respiratory, and vasomotor control centers
Pons	Two-way conduction pathway between areas of the brain and other regions of the body; influences respiration
Midbrain	Two-way conduction pathway; relay point for visual and auditory impulses
Diencephalon	
Hypothalamus	Regulation of body temperature, water balance, sleep-cycle control, appetite, and sexual arousal
Thalamus	Sensory relay station from various body areas to cerebral cortex; emotions and alerting or arousal mechanisms
Cerebellum	Muscle coordination; maintenance of equilibrium and posture
Cerebrum	Sensory perception, emotions, willed movements, consciousness, and memory

The **hypothalamus** is a major controller in the brain. It acts as a gatekeeper in determining what information is passed along to the cerebrum. The hypothalamus is an active participant in emotions, hormonal cycles, and sexuality. (Table 10-6 gives a summary of the various hypothalamic functions.)

Cerebrum. The **cerebrum** is the largest portion of the brain. It is divided into left and right hemispheres, and each hemisphere is divided into lobes named for the bones that lie over them (Figure 10-31).

The *frontal lobe* is important in voluntary motor function, motivation, aggression, and mood. The *parietal lobe* is the major center for the reception and evaluation of most sensory information, except for smell, hearing, and vision. The *occipital lobe* functions in the reception and integration of visual input. The occipital lobe is not distinctly separate from other lobes. The *temporal lobe* receives and evaluates olfactory and auditory input. The temporal lobe plays a key role in memory. A thin layer of **gray matter**, made up of neuron dendrites and cell bodies, composes the surface of the cerebrum (cerebral cortex).

The **limbic system** is made up of portions of the cerebrum and diencephalon. This system influences emotions, visceral responses to those emotions, motivation, mood, and sensations of pain and pleasure.

Cerebellum. The **cerebellum** is the second largest part of the human brain. It is involved in gross motor coordination and helps produce smooth movements. A major job of the cerebellum is to compare impulses from the motor cortex with those from moving structures (e.g., the position of the body or of body parts that innervate the joints and tendons of the structure being moved). The cerebellum compares the intended movement with the actual one. If a difference is detected, the cerebellum sends impulses to the motor cortex and the spinal cord to correct the discrepancy. Loss of cerebellar functioning results in inability to make exact movements.

Spinal Cord. The spinal cord lies within the spinal column and extends from the occipital bone to the level of the second lumbar vertebra. The spinal cord has a *central*

TABLE 10-6 Hypothalamic Functions

Function	Description
Autonomic	Helps control heart rate, urine release from the bladder, movement of food through the digestive tract, and blood vessel diameter.
Endocrine	Helps regulate pituitary gland secretions and influences metabolism, ion balance, sexual development, and sexual functions.
Muscle control	Controls muscles involved in swallowing and stimulates shivering in several muscles.
Temperature regulation	Promotes heat loss when the hypothalamic temperature increases by increasing sweat production (anterior hypothalamus) and promotes heat production when the hypothalamic temperature decreases by promoting shivering (posterior hypothalamus).
Regulation of food and water intake	Hunger center promotes eating, and satiety center inhibits eating; thirst center promotes water intake.
Emotions	Large range of emotional influences over body functions; directly involved in stress-related and psychosomatic illnesses and with feelings of fear and rage.
Regulation of the sleep-wake cycle	Coordinates responses to the sleep-wake cycle with other areas of the brain (e.g., the reticular activating system).

gray portion and a *peripheral white portion*. The white matter consists of nerve tracts, and the gray matter consists of nerve cell bodies and dendrites. The **dorsal root** conveys afferent nerve processes to the cord, and the **ventral root** conveys efferent nerve processes away from the cord. Spinal ganglia, or dorsal root ganglia, contain the cell bodies of sensory neurons (Figure 10-32).

CRITICAL THINKING

An older adult patient has a new onset of staggering gait. What area of the brain do you suspect has altered function?

The spinal cord is the main reflex center of the body. Many of these reflexes are **autonomic** or **visceral**. An example of this is an increased heart rate in response to decreased blood pressure. Another example is the stretch reflex (knee-jerk reflex). The body also has withdrawal reflexes (i.e., removing a limb or other body part from a painful stimulus). In addition to acting as a primary reflex center, the spinal cord tracts carry impulses to the brain in afferent, ascending tracts. These tracts also carry motor impulses from the brain in efferent, descending tracts. (Ascending and descending pathways are addressed further in Chapter 25.)

FIGURE 10-31 Lobes of the cerebrum. (Thibodeau GA, Patton KT: *Structure and function of the body,* ed 13, St Louis, 2008, Mosby.)

Frontal lobe
Fissure of Rolando
Parietal lobe
Fissure of Sylvius
Temporal lobe
Occipital lobe

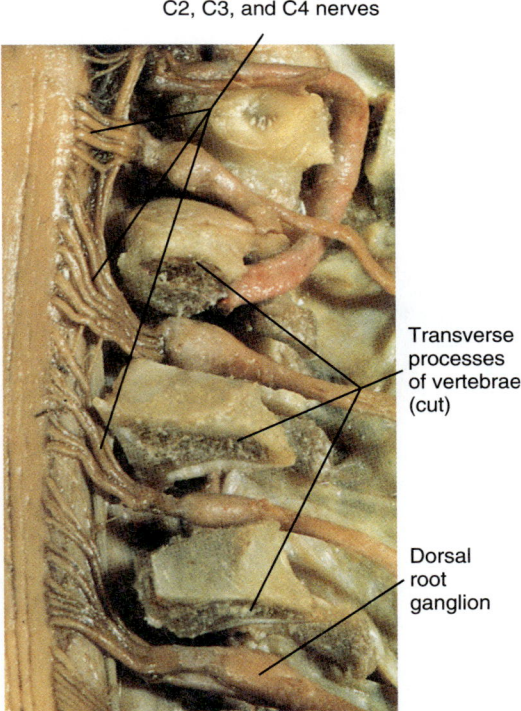

FIGURE 10-32 Dissection of the cervical segment of the spinal cord. (Thibodeau GA, Patton KT: *Structure and function of the body,* ed 13, St Louis, 2008, Mosby.)

Dorsal roots of C2, C3, and C4 nerves

Transverse processes of vertebrae (cut)

Dorsal root ganglion

The organs of the nervous system are surrounded by a tough, fluid-containing membrane. This membrane is known as the **meninges**. The meninges are surrounded by bone and have three connective tissue layers. The most superficial and thickest layer is the **dura mater**. It consists of two layers around the brain and one layer around the spinal cord. The two layers of the dura mater are fused around most of the brain but are separate in several places. The dura mater of the brain is attached tightly and is continuous with the **periosteum** of the cranial vault, whereas the dura mater of the spinal cord is separated from the periosteum of the vertebral canal by the **epidural space**.

The **arachnoid layer** is the second meningeal layer. The space between this layer and the dura mater is known as the **subdural space**, which contains a small amount of serous fluid. The third meningeal layer is the pia mater. The **pia mater** lies external to a basement membrane formed by special cells called the *glia limitans*, which completely envelops the CNS. The space between the pia mater and the arachnoid layer is the **subarachnoid space**. This space is filled with blood vessels and cerebrospinal fluid (Figure 10-33).

The **cerebrospinal fluid (CSF)** is similar to plasma and **interstitial fluid** (the fluid that occupies the space outside the blood vessels). CSF bathes the brain and spinal cord and acts as a cushion around the CNS. It is formed continually from fluid filtering out of the blood in a network of brain capillaries and cells known as the *choroid plexus*. This special fluid fills the ventricles of the brain, the subarachnoid space, and the central canal of the spinal cord.

PERIPHERAL NERVOUS SYSTEM

The PNS collects information from numerous sources inside the body and on the body surface. The PNS relays this information by way of afferent fibers to the CNS. The CNS then evaluates the information. Efferent fibers in the PNS relay information from the CNS to various parts of the body, primarily to muscles and glands.

Spinal Nerves. The **spinal nerves** arise from many rootlets along the dorsal and ventral surfaces of the spinal cord. All of the 31 pairs of spinal nerves, except for the first pair of spinal nerves and the spinal nerves in the sacrum, exit the vertebral column though adjacent vertebrae. The first pair of spinal nerves exits between the skull and the first cervical vertebrae. The spinal nerves in the sacrum exit through the bone. Eight spinal nerve pairs exit the vertebral column in the cervical region, 12 in the thoracic region, 5 in the lumbar region, 5 in the sacral region, and 1 in the coccygeal region (Figure 10-34).

Each spinal nerve except the first has a specific cutaneous sensory distribution. Detailed mapping of the skin surface reveals a close relationship between the source on the cord of each spinal nerve and the level of the body it innervates. (A grasp of this relationship is vital when the paramedic examines a patient with a spinal cord injury.) The skin surface areas supplied by a single spinal nerve are known as **dermatomes** (Figure 10-35).

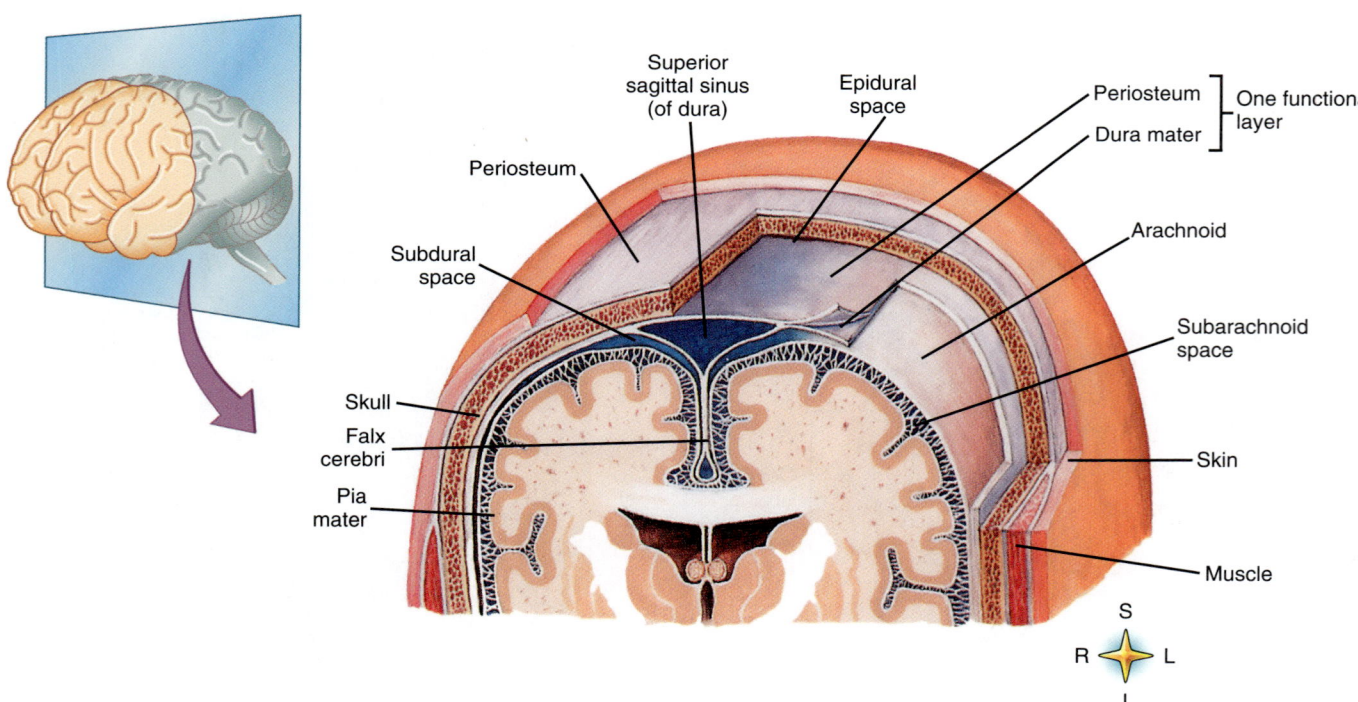

FIGURE 10-33 Meningeal coverings of the brain and spinal cord. (Patton KT, Thibodeau GA: *Anatomy and physiology*, ed 7, St Louis, 2007, Mosby.)

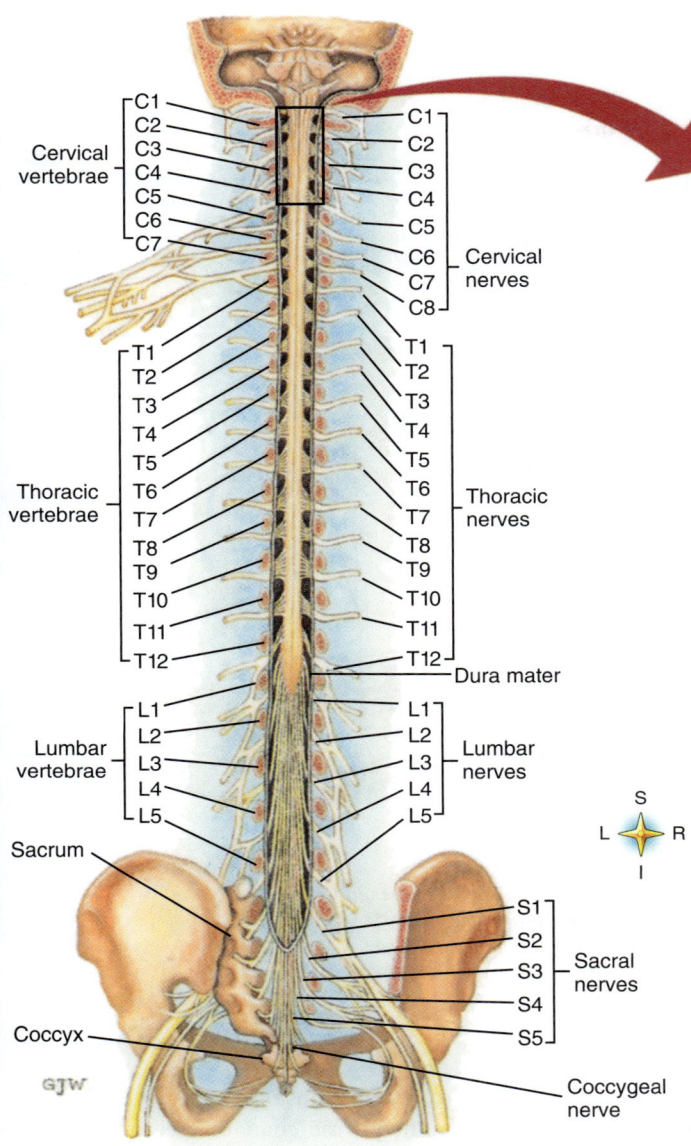

FIGURE 10-34 Spinal cord and spinal nerves. (Thibodeau GA, Patton KT: *Structure and function of the body*, ed 13, St Louis, 2008, Mosby.)

CRITICAL THINKING
Does a person with a spinal cord injury at the C5 level have movement in the hands?

Cranial Nerves. The 12 cranial nerves are divided into three general groups: sensory, somatomotor and proprioception, and parasympathetic (Figure 10-36). *Sensory functions* include the special senses, such as vision. They also include the more general senses, such as touch and pain. *Somatomotor functions* control the skeletal muscles through motor neurons. *Proprioception* provides the brain with information about the position of the body and its various parts, including joints and muscles. *Parasympathetic function*

involves the regulation of glands, smooth muscle, and cardiac muscle (functions of the autonomic nervous system). Some cranial nerves have only one of the three functions. However, other cranial nerves have more than one function (Table 10-7).

AUTONOMIC NERVOUS SYSTEM

As stated before, the PNS is made up of afferent and efferent neurons. **Afferent neurons** carry action potentials from the periphery to the CNS. **Efferent neurons** carry action potentials from the CNS to the periphery. Afferent neurons give information to the CNS. These data may stimulate somatomotor and autonomic reflexes. Therefore, afferent neurons cannot be put easily into groups by function. However, efferent neurons clearly differ structurally and functionally. They can be put into the somatomotor nervous system or the autonomic nervous system.

Somatomotor neurons innervate skeletal muscles. These neurons play a key role in locomotion, posture, and equilibrium. The movements controlled by the somatomotor nervous system usually are conscious movements. The effect of these neurons on skeletal muscle is always excitatory. Neurons of the autonomic nervous system innervate smooth muscle, cardiac muscle, and glands. These neurons usually are controlled unconsciously. The effect of autonomic neurons on their target tissue is inhibitory or excitatory.

The autonomic nervous system is made up of two divisions, the **sympathetic nervous system** and the **parasympathetic nervous system**. Both of these divisions consist of autonomic ganglia and nerves. The action potentials in sympathetic neurons generally prepare a person for physical activity. Parasympathetic stimulation, however, activates vegetative functions such as digestion, defecation, and urination.

The functions of the autonomic nervous system help to maintain homeostasis or to quickly restore homeostasis (Table 10-8). Many internal organs receive fibers from parasympathetic and sympathetic divisions (Figure 10-37). Therefore, they are continually bombarded by sympathetic and parasympathetic impulses. These impulses influence the function of these organs in opposite or antagonistic ways. For example, the heart receives sympathetic impulses that increase the heart rate. The heart also receives parasympathetic impulses that decrease the heart rate. The ratio between these two forces determines the actual heart rate.

CRITICAL THINKING
You administer a drug that blocks the action of the parasympathetic nervous system. What happens to the patient's heart rate?

Endocrine System

The **endocrine system** is made up of glands. These glands secrete hormones into the circulatory system (Figure 10-38). The endocrine and nervous systems have considerable

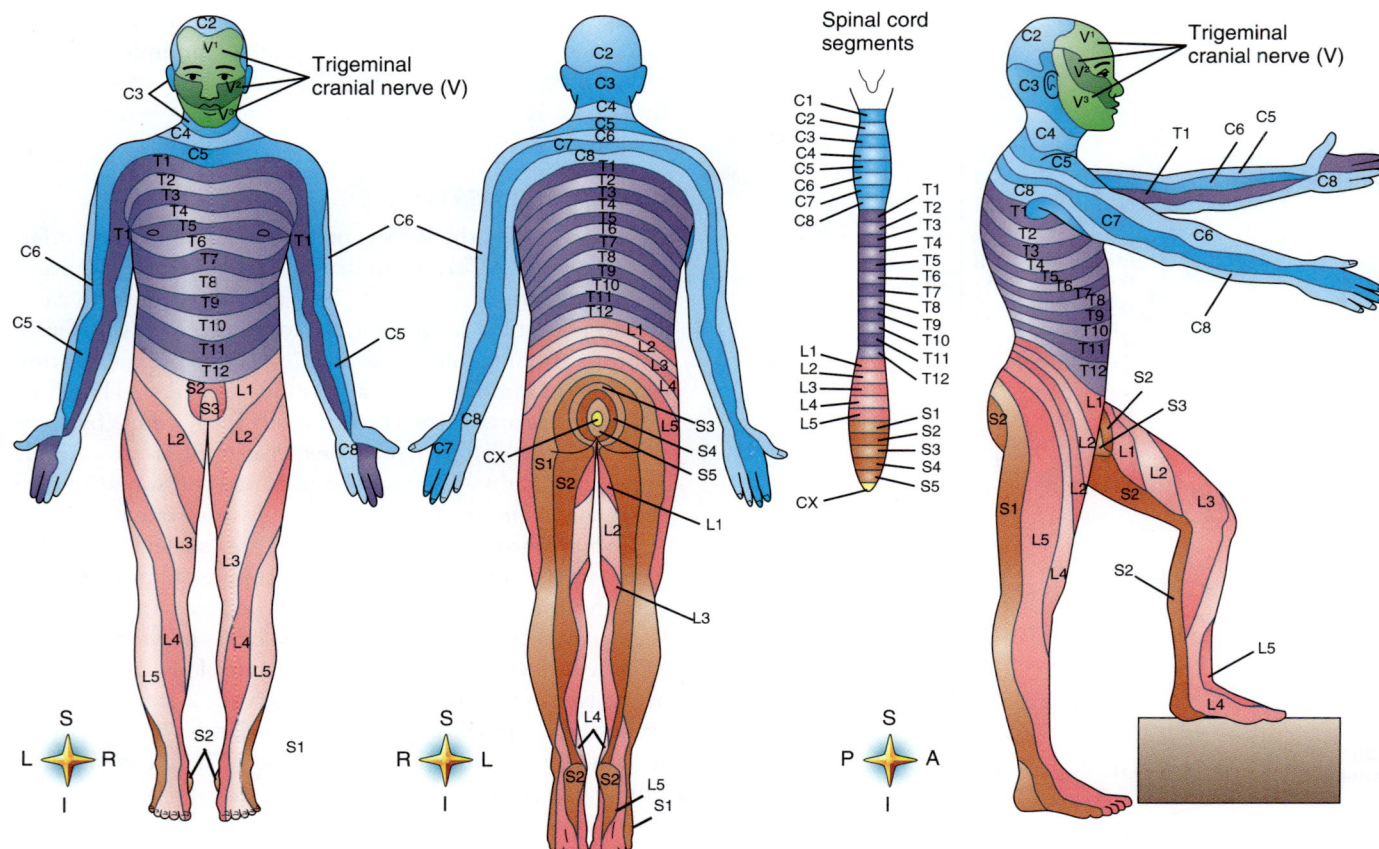

FIGURE 10-35 Dermatome map. Letters and numbers indicate the spinal nerves innervating a given region of the skin. (Patton KT, Thibodeau GA: *Anatomy and physiology,* ed 7, St Louis, 2007, Mosby.)

overlap. The overlap is functional and anatomical. Some neurons secrete regulatory chemicals that function as hormones *(neurohormones),* such as **antidiuretic hormone (ADH),** into the circulatory system. Other neurons innervate **endocrine glands** and influence their secretory activity. However, some hormones secreted by the endocrine glands affect the nervous system.

Hormones, including neurohormones, are classified as proteins, polypeptides, derivatives of amino acids, or lipids. Lipid hormones are steroids or derivatives of fatty acids. Hormones are dissolved in blood plasma and are distributed quickly throughout the body. In general, the amount of hormone that reaches the target tissue directly correlates with the concentration of the hormone in the blood. (Table 10-9 lists endocrine glands, hormones, and their functions.)

Some hormones are present in fairly constant levels in the circulatory system. Amounts of other hormones change suddenly in response to certain stimuli. Still others change in fairly constant cycles. For example, *thyroid hormones* in the blood vary within a small range of concentrations. Their concentration is maintained continuously. *Epinephrine* is

released in large amounts in response to stress or exercise. The concentration of epinephrine changes greatly. *Reproductive hormones* increase and decrease cyclically in women during their reproductive years.

Circulatory System

Blood vessels extend throughout the body. These vessels carry blood to and from all tissues. Blood performs a number of important functions: (1) it transports nutrients and oxygen to tissues; (2) it carries carbon dioxide and waste products away from tissues; (3) it carries hormones produced in the endocrine glands to their target tissues; (4) it plays a key role in temperature regulation and fluid balance; and (5) it protects the body from bacteria and foreign substances. These and other functions of blood help to maintain homeostasis.

BLOOD COMPONENTS

Blood is a special form of connective tissue. It consists of cells and cell fragments *(formed elements)* surrounded by a liquid intercellular matrix (plasma). About 95% of the volume of formed elements consists of red blood cells

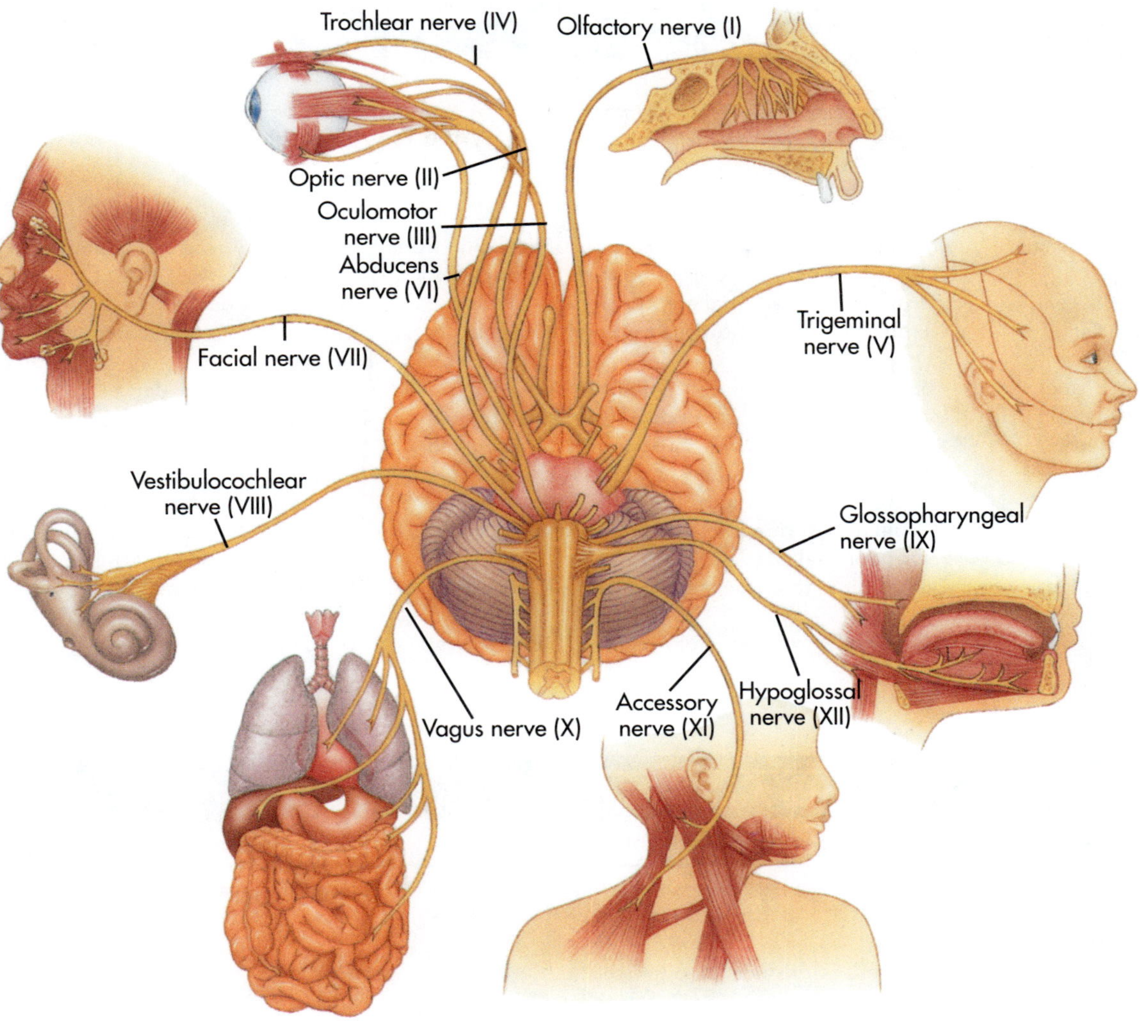

FIGURE 10-36 Origin of the cranial nerves. (McCance KL, Huether SE: *Pathophysiology: the biologic basis for disease in adults and children,* ed 5, St Louis, 2005, Mosby.)

(erythrocytes). The remaining 5% consists of white blood cells (leukocytes) and cell fragments called *platelets.*

Plasma. Plasma is a pale yellow fluid composed of about 92% water and 8% dissolved or suspended molecules. Plasma contains proteins such as *albumin, globulins,* and *fibrinogen.* When the proteins that produce clots are removed from the plasma, the remaining fluid is called **serum**.

Formed Elements. Three formed elements of blood are erythrocytes, leukocytes, and platelets or thrombocytes (cell fragments) (Table 10-10). Formed elements are produced in the embryo and fetus. They are also produced in tissues such as the liver, thymus, spleen, lymph nodes, and red bone marrow.

1. **Erythrocytes** are the most numerous of the formed elements. One drop of male blood has about 5.2 million erythrocytes; one drop of female blood has about 4.5 million erythrocytes. The major erythrocyte contents include lipids, ATP, and the enzyme *carbonic anhydrase*. The main component of erythrocytes is **hemoglobin**. This is the protein that gives blood its red color. The primary functions of erythrocytes are to transport oxygen from the lungs to the various tissues of the body and to transport carbon dioxide from the tissues to the lungs. Under normal conditions, about 2.5 million erythrocytes are destroyed and replaced by the body each second. The average erythrocyte circulates for 120 days.

CRITICAL THINKING

If the number of erythrocytes drops, a person may become short of breath during mild exertion. Why does this happen?

TABLE 10-7 Functions of the Cranial Nerves

Nerve	Name	Impulse Conduction	Functions
I	Olfactory	From nose to brain	Sense of smell
II	Optic	From eye to brain	Vision
III	Oculomotor	From brain to eye muscles	Eye movements
IV	Trochlear	From brain to external eye muscles	Eye movements
V	Trigeminal	From skin and mucous membranes of head and from teeth to brain; also from brain to chewing muscles	Sensations of face, scalp, and teeth; chewing movements
VI	Abducens	From brain to external eye muscles	Turning eyes outward
VII	Facial	From taste buds of tongue to brain; from brain to facial muscles	Sense of taste; contraction of muscles of facial expressions
VIII	Acoustic	From ear to brain	Hearing; sense of balance
IX	Glossopharyngeal	From throat and taste buds of tongue to brain; also from brain to throat muscles and salivary glands	Sensation of throat, taste, swallowing movements; secretion of saliva
X	Vagus	From throat, larynx, and organs in thoracic and abdominal cavities to brain; also from brain to muscles of throat and to organs in thoracic and abdominal cavities	Sensations of throat and larynx and of thoracic and abdominal organs; swallowing, voice production, slowing of heartbeat, acceleration of peristalsis
XI	Spinal accessory	From brain to certain shoulder and neck muscles	Shoulder movements, turning movements of head
XII	Hypoglossal	From brain to muscles of tongue	Tongue movements

TABLE 10-8 Functions of the Autonomic Nervous System

Visceral Effectors	Sympathetic Control	Parasympathetic Control
Heart muscle	Accelerates heartbeat	Slows heartbeat
Smooth Muscle		
Of most blood vessels	Constricts blood vessels	None
Of blood vessels in skeletal muscles	Dilates blood vessels	None
Of the digestive tract	Decreases peristalsis; inhibits defecation	Increases peristalsis
Of the anal sphincter	Stimulates-closes sphincter	Inhibits-opens sphincter for defecation
Of the urinary bladder	Inhibits-relaxes bladder	Stimulates-contracts bladder
Of the urinary sphincters	Stimulates-closes sphincter	Inhibits-opens sphincter for urination
Of the eye:		
Iris	Stimulates radial fibers—dilation of pupil	Stimulates circular fibers—constriction of pupil
Ciliary	Inhibits—accommodation for far vision (flattening of lens)	Stimulates—accommodation for near vision (bulging of lens)
Of hairs (pilomotor muscles)	Stimulates—goose bumps	No parasympathetic fibers
Glands		
Adrenal medulla	Increases epinephrine secretion	None
Sweat glands	Increase sweat secretion	None
Digestive glands	Decrease secretion of digestive juices	Increase secretion of digestive juices

2. **Leukocytes** are white blood cells that do not contain hemoglobin (therefore, they are clear). The several types of leukocytes are involved in guarding the body against invading microorganisms. They also remove dead cells and debris. Some leukocytes are grouped by their appearance. This is based on the presence or absence of cytoplasmic granules. The classifications include neutrophils, eosinophils, and basophils. Other types of leukocytes are nongranular. These leukocytes are named according to nuclear morphology and major site of proliferation. These include lymphocytes and monocytes.

- **Neutrophils** are the most common type of leukocyte in the blood. These cells normally remain in the circulation for 10 to 12 hours. They then move into tissue to seek out and destroy bacteria and other foreign matter **(phagocytosis)**. Neutrophils also

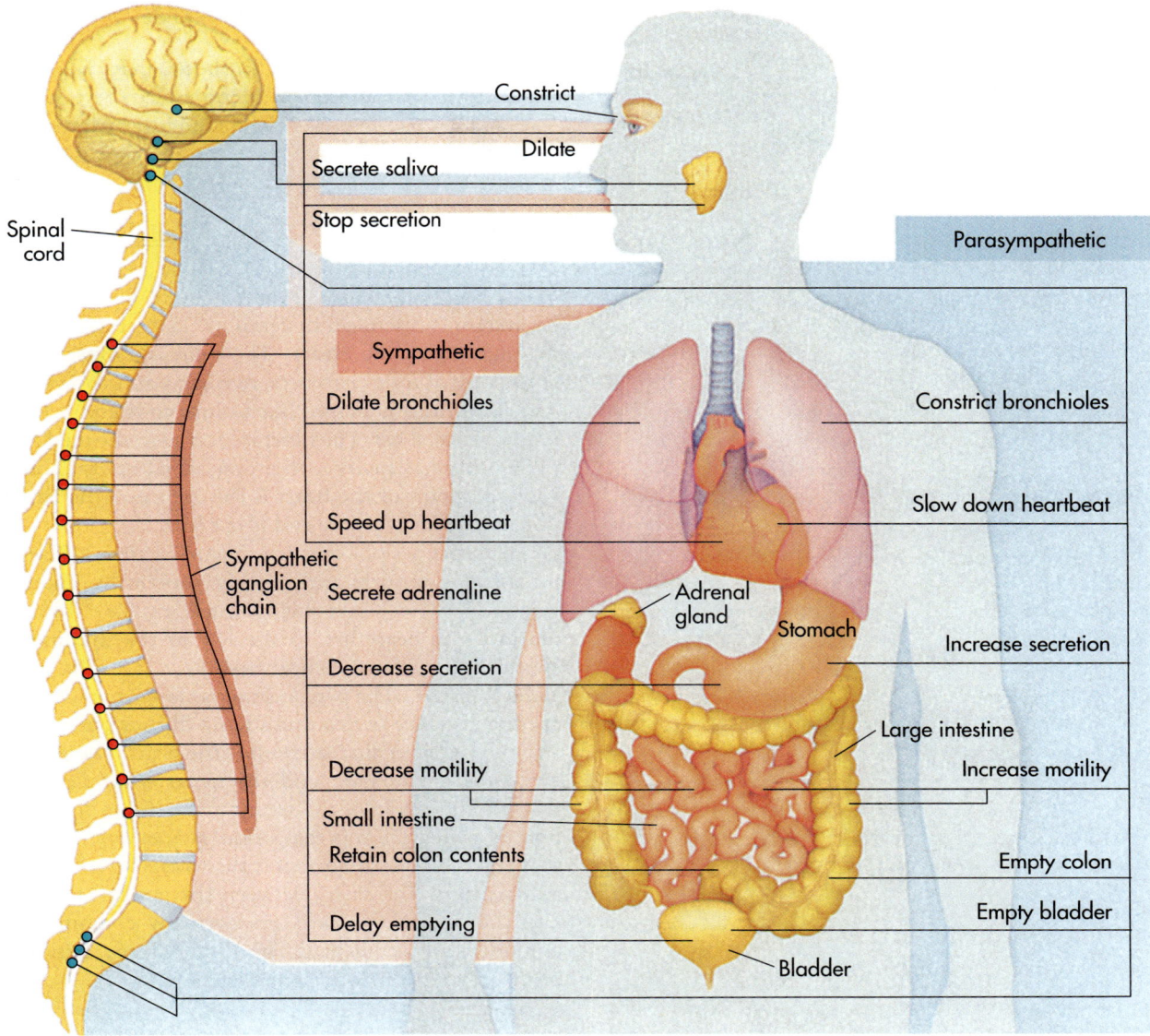

FIGURE 10-37 Innervation of major target organs by the autonomic nervous system. The sympathetic fibers are highlighted in red, and the parasympathetic fibers are highlighted in blue. (Thibodeau GA, Patton KT: *Structure and function of the body,* ed 13, St Louis, 2008, Mosby.)

secrete lysosomes that can destroy certain bacteria. Neutrophils usually survive for 1 to 2 days after leaving the circulation.

- **Eosinophils** leave the circulation to enter the tissues during an inflammatory reaction. Their numbers usually are elevated in the blood of individuals with allergies and certain parasitic infections. These cells have phagocytic properties. However, they are not thought to be as important in this function as neutrophils.

- **Basophils** are the least common of all leukocytes. They also are called mast cells when in tissues. Like eosinophils, basophils leave the circulation and migrate through tissues to play a role in allergic and inflammatory reactions. In addition, they release

heparin, which inhibits blood clotting. They also release **histamine**, which is important to the **inflammatory response** (see Chapter 2).

- **Lymphocytes** are the smallest of all leukocytes. They are capable of migrating through the cytoplasm of other cells. The many different types of lymphocytes play a major role in immunity, including antibody production. Lymphocytes originate in bone marrow. They are most abundant in lymphoid tissues; that is, the **lymph nodes**, **spleen**, **tonsils**, **lymph nodules**, and **thymus**.

- **Monocytes** are the largest of the leukocytes. They remain in the circulation for about 3 days before changing into **macrophages**. These large "eating" cells migrate through various tissues. An increase in

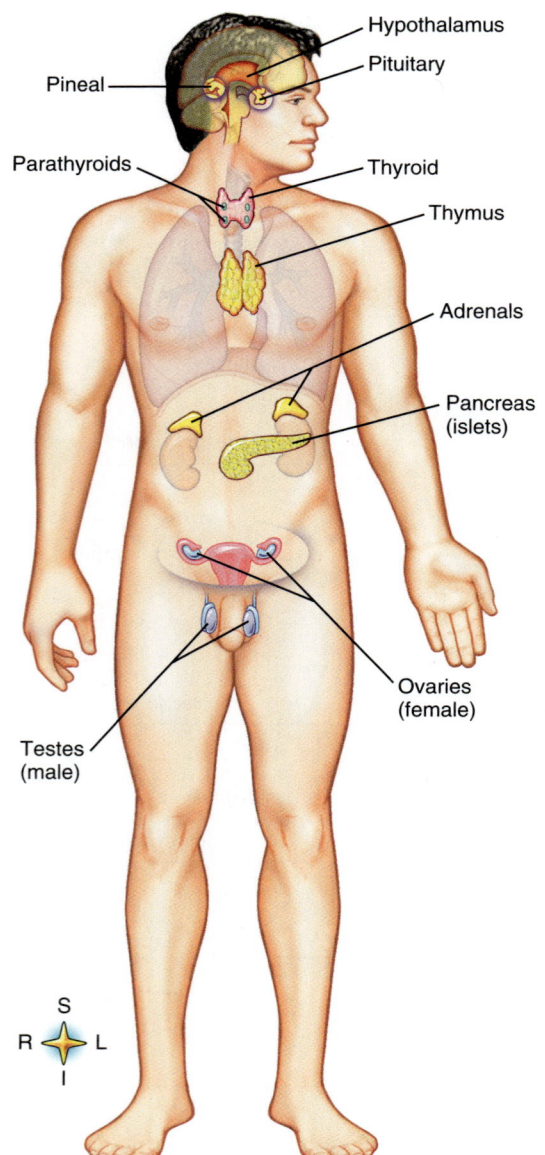

Hypothalamus
Pituitary
Pineal
Parathyroids
Thyroid
Thymus
Adrenals
Pancreas
(islets)
Ovaries
(female)
Testes
(male)

FIGURE 10-38 Locations of major endocrine glands. (Patton KT, Thibodeau GA: *Anatomy and physiology,* ed 7, St Louis, 2007, Mosby.)

the number of monocytes is common in patients with chronic infections.

3. **Platelets** are produced in bone marrow. They are 40 times as common in blood as leukocytes. Platelets play a key role in preventing blood loss by forming plugs that seal holes in small vessels and by forming clots that seal off larger wounds in the vessels.

CARDIOVASCULAR SYSTEM

The heart and cardiovascular system are responsible for circulating blood throughout the body. (The cardiovascular system is discussed in detail in Chapter 22.)

Anatomy of the Heart. The heart is a muscular pump consisting of four chambers, two **atria** and two **ventricles**. The adult heart is shaped like a blunt cone and is about the size of a closed fist. The heart is located in the mediastinum of the thoracic cavity in the pericardial cavity. The blunt, rounded point of the heart is the *apex*, and the larger, flat portion at the opposite end is the *base*.

The heart lies obliquely in the mediastinum. The base is directed posteriorly and slightly superiorly. The apex is directed anteriorly and slightly inferiorly. Two thirds of the mass of the heart lies to the left of the midline of the sternum (Figures 10-39 and 10-40).

Pericardium. The pericardium is also known as the **pericardial sac**. The pericardium has a fibrous outer layer and a thin inner layer that surrounds the heart. These layers are the *fibrous pericardium* and the *serous pericardium*, respectively. The portion of the serous pericardium that lines the fibrous pericardium is the *parietal pericardium*. The portion that covers the heart surface is the *visceral pericardium* or the **epicardium**. The cavity between the parietal pericardium and the visceral pericardium normally contains a small amount of *pericardial fluid*. This fluid reduces friction as the heart moves within the pericardial sac.

CRITICAL THINKING

Why would a sudden increase in the amount of pericardial fluid be harmful?

TABLE 10-9 Endocrine Glands, Hormones, and Their Functions	
Gland/Hormone	**Function**
Anterior Pituitary	
Thyroid-stimulating hormone	Tropic hormone; stimulates secretion of thyroid hormones
Adrenocorticotropic hormone	Tropic hormone; stimulates secretion of adrenal cortex hormones
Follicle-stimulating hormone	Tropic hormone
	Female: Stimulates development of ovarian follicles and secretion of estrogens
	Male: Stimulates seminiferous tubules of testes to grow and produce sperm
Luteinizing hormone	Tropic hormone
	Female: Stimulates maturation of ovarian follicle and ovum; stimulates secretion of estrogen; triggers ovulation; stimulates development of corpus luteum (luteinization)
	Male: Stimulates interstitial cells of the testes to secrete testosterone

TABLE 10-9 Endocrine Glands, Hormones, and Their Functions—cont'd

Gland/Hormone	Function
Melanocyte-stimulating hormone	Stimulates synthesis and dispersion of melanin pigment in the skin
Growth hormone	Stimulates growth in all organs; mobilizes food molecules, causing an increase in blood glucose concentration
Prolactin (lactogenic hormone)	Stimulates breast development during pregnancy and milk secretion after pregnancy
Posterior Pituitary*	
Antidiuretic hormone	Stimulates retention of water by the kidneys
Oxytocin	Stimulates uterine contractions at the end of pregnancy; stimulates the release of milk into the breast ducts
Hypothalamus	
Releasing hormones (several)	Stimulate the anterior pituitary to release hormones
Inhibiting hormones (several)	Inhibit secretion of hormones by the anterior pituitary
Thyroid	
Thyroxine, triiodothyronine	Stimulate the energy metabolism of all cells
Calcitonin	Inhibits the breakdown of bone; causes a decrease in blood calcium concentration
Parathyroid	
Parathyroid hormone	Stimulates the breakdown of bone; causes an increase in blood calcium concentration
Adrenal Cortex	
Mineralocorticoids: aldosterone	Regulate electrolyte and fluid homeostasis
Glucocorticoids: cortisol (hydrocortisone)	Stimulate gluconeogenesis, causing an increase in blood glucose concentration; also have antiinflammatory, antiimmunity, and antiallergy effects
Sex hormones (androgens)	Stimulate sexual drive in the female but have negligible effects in the male
Adrenal Medulla	
Epinephrine (adrenaline), norepinephrine	Prolong and intensify the sympathetic nervous response during stress
Pancreatic Islets	
Glucagon	Stimulates liver glycogenolysis, causing an increase in blood glucose concentration
Insulin	Promotes glucose entry into all cells, causing a decrease in blood glucose concentration
Ovary	
Estrogens	Promotes development and maintenance of female sexual characteristics
Progesterone	Promotes conditions required for pregnancy
Testis	
Testosterone	Promotes development and maintenance of male sexual characteristics
Thymus	
Thymosin	Promotes development of immune-system cells
Placenta	
Chorionic gonadotropin, estrogens, progesterone	Promote conditions required during early pregnancy
Pineal	
Melatonin	Inhibits tropic hormones that affect the ovaries; may be involved with the internal clock of the body
Heart (atria)	
Atrial natriuretic hormone	Regulates fluid and electrolyte homeostasis

*Posterior pituitary hormones are synthesized in the hypothalamus but are released from axon terminals in the posterior pituitary.

TABLE 10-10 Classes of Blood Cells

Cell Type	Function
Erythrocyte	Oxygen and carbon dioxide transport
Neutrophil	Immune defenses (phagocytosis)
Eosinophil	Defense against parasites
Basophil	Inflammatory response
B lymphocyte	Antibody production (precursor of plasma cells)
T lymphocyte	Cellular immune response
Monocyte	Immune defenses (phagocytosis)
Platelet	Blood clotting

Coronary Vessels. Seven large veins normally carry blood to the heart: four **pulmonary veins** carry blood from the lungs to the left atrium; the **superior vena cava** and **inferior vena cava** carry blood from the body to the right atrium; and the coronary sinus carries blood from the walls of the heart to the right atrium. Two arteries, the aorta and the pulmonary trunk, exit the heart. The **aorta** carries blood from the left ventricle to the body. The **pulmonary trunk** carries blood from the right ventricle to the lungs. The right and left **coronary arteries** exit the aorta near the point where the aorta leaves the heart. They supply the heart muscle with oxygen and nutrients (Figure 10-41).

Heart Chambers and Valves. The right and left chambers of the heart are separated by a **septum**. The *interatrial septum* separates the **right atrium** and the **left atrium**. The *interventricular septum* separates the two ventricles. The atria open into the ventricles through the *atrioventricular canals*. An **atrioventricular valve** on each atrioventricular canal is composed of cusps or flaps. These valves allow blood to flow from the atria into the ventricles. Yet they prevent blood from flowing back into the atria. The atrioventricular valve between the right atrium and right ventricle has three cusps; it is called the **tricuspid valve**. The atrioventricular valve between the left atrium and left ventricle has two cusps and is called the **bicuspid valve** (or *mitral valve*).

The aorta and pulmonary trunk possess *aortic and pulmonary semilunar valves*. These valves meet in the center of the artery to block blood flow. Blood flowing out of the ventricles pushes against each valve, forcing it open. However, when blood flows back from the aorta or pulmonary trunk toward the ventricles, the valves close.

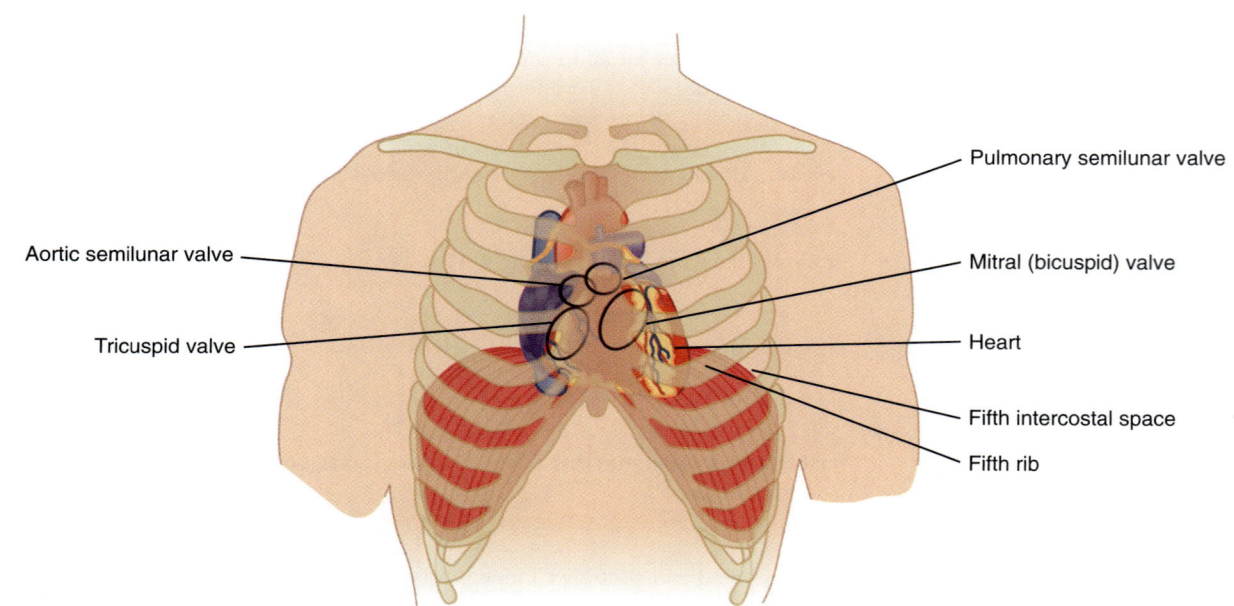

FIGURE 10-39 Location of the heart in the thorax.

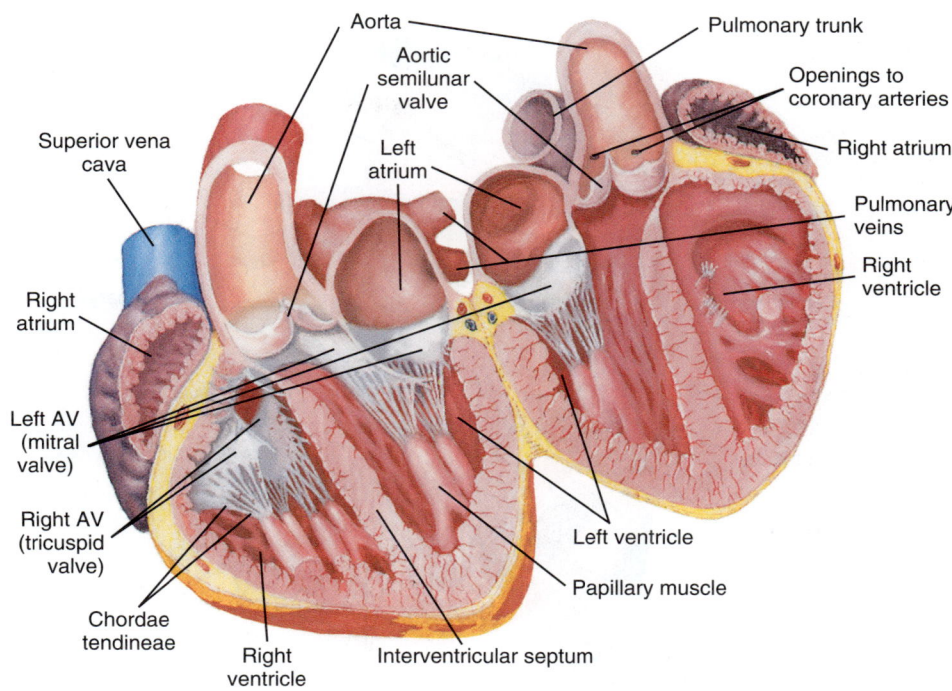

FIGURE 10-40 Internal view of the heart. (Patton KT, Thibodeau GA: *Anatomy and physiology,* ed 7, St Louis, 2007, Mosby.)

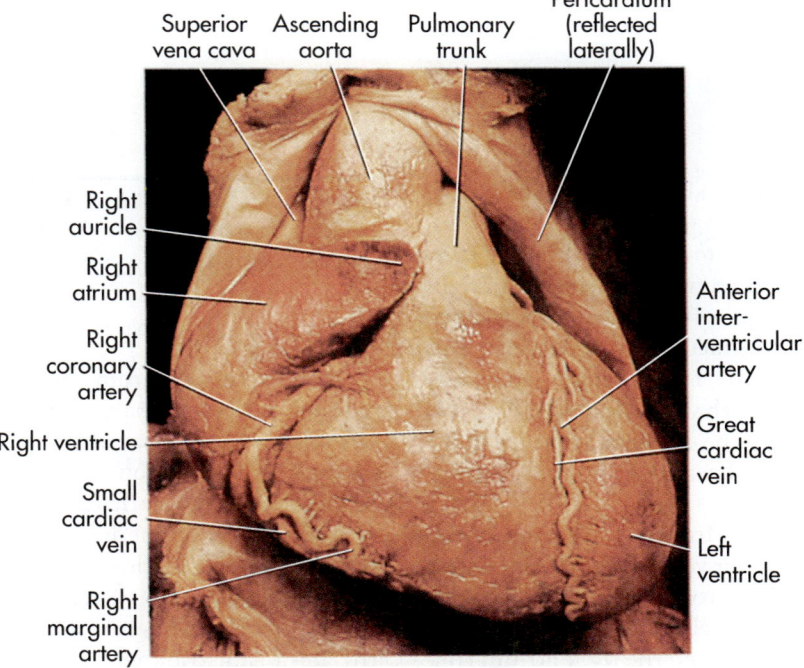

FIGURE 10-41 Anterior surface of the heart.

Conduction System of the Heart. The muscle tissue of the heart has the unique ability for spontaneous, rhythmic self-excitation. This excitation occurs by way of four structures embedded in the wall of the heart. These structures are the **sinoatrial node**, the **atrioventricular node**, the **bundle of His**, and the **Purkinje fibers** (Figure 10-42).

Impulse conduction normally begins in the sinoatrial node. From there the impulse spreads in all directions through both of the atria, causing an atrial contraction. As the electrical impulses reach the atrioventricular node, they are relayed to the ventricles through the bundle of His and the Purkinje fibers. This impulse conduction causes both

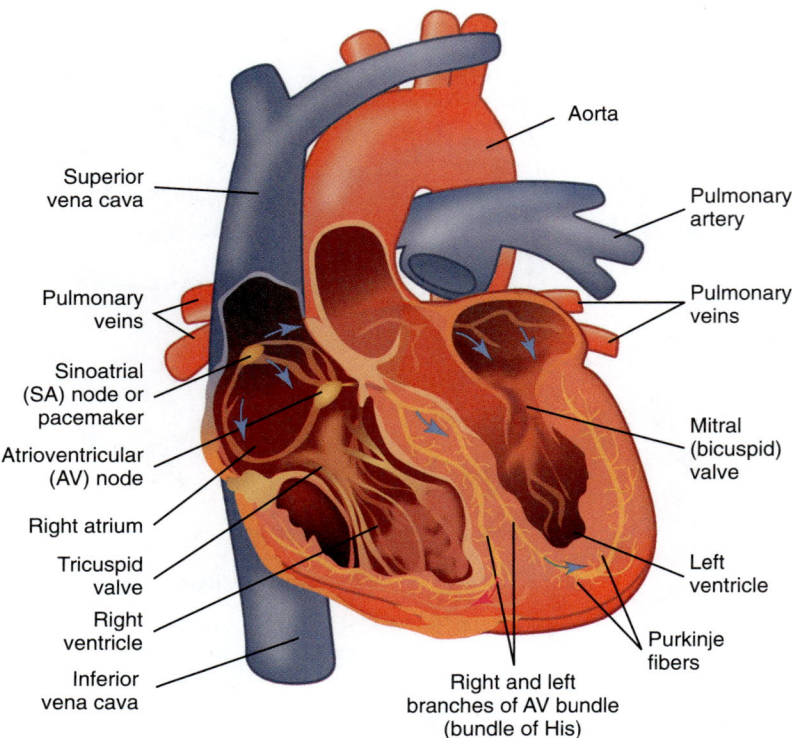

FIGURE 10-42 Conduction system of the heart.

of the ventricles to contract shortly after the atrial contraction.

Route of Blood Flow Through the Heart. This text presents blood flow through the heart with a discussion of right and left heart circulation (Figure 10-43). It is important to remember that both atria contract at the same time. This contraction is followed shortly thereafter by essentially simultaneous contraction of both ventricles.[4] Knowing this is key to understanding clearly the electrical impulses of the heart, pressure changes, and heart sounds that are discussed in other chapters.

Blood enters the right atrium from the systemic circulation via the inferior and superior venae cavae. Blood enters from the heart muscle via the coronary sinus. Most of this blood passes into the right ventricle as the ventricle relaxes after the previous contraction. When the right atrium contracts, the blood left in the atrium is pushed into the ventricle. The contraction of the right ventricle pushes blood against the tricuspid valve, forcing it closed. The contraction also pushes blood against the *pulmonary semilunar valve*, forcing the valve open. This flow allows blood to enter the pulmonary trunk. The pulmonary trunk divides into left and right pulmonary arteries that carry blood to the lungs. In the lungs the blood releases carbon dioxide and picks up oxygen.

CRITICAL THINKING
A clot forms in the right atrium of the heart. Will it be circulated to the extremities? Why?

Blood returning from the lungs enters the left atrium through four pulmonary veins. The blood passing from the left atrium to the relaxed left ventricle opens the bicuspid valve. The contraction of the left atrium completes the filling of the left ventricle.

Contraction of the left ventricle pushes blood against the bicuspid valve, closing the valve. The pressure of the blood against the aortic semilunar valve causes it to open. This allows blood to enter the aorta. Blood flowing through the aorta is distributed to all parts of the body except for the pulmonary vessels in the lungs.

PERIPHERAL CIRCULATION

Blood is pumped from the ventricles of the heart into large elastic arteries. These arteries branch repeatedly to form many gradually smaller arteries. As these vessels become smaller, the amount of elastic tissue in the arterial wall decreases. At the same time, the amount of smooth muscle increases.

Normal Blood Flow

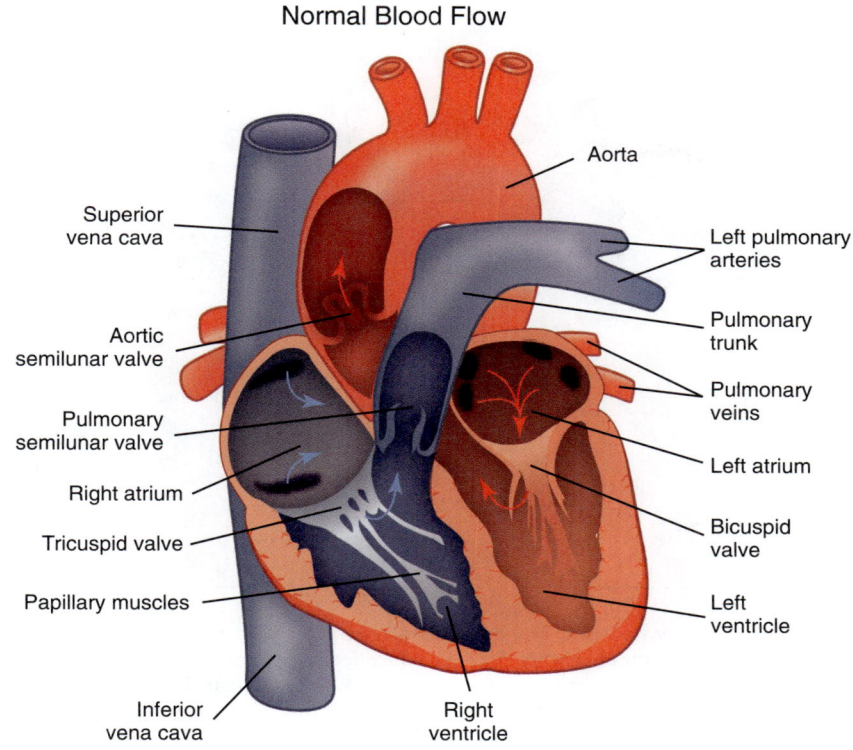

FIGURE 10-43 Frontal section of the heart showing the four chambers and the direction of blood flow through the heart.

Blood flows from the **arterioles** into **capillaries** and from capillaries into the venous system. Compared with artery walls, vein walls are thinner and contain less elastic tissue and fewer smooth muscle cells. As veins approach the heart, the walls increase in diameter and thickness.

Capillary Network. Arterioles supply blood to each capillary network (Figure 10-44). Blood flows through this network and into the venules. The ends of the capillaries closest to arterioles are *arterial capillaries*. The ends closest to venules are *venous capillaries*.

Blood flow through arterioles may continue through *metarterioles* and into a *thoroughfare channel* to a venule in a relatively constant way; or, blood may enter the *capillary circulation*. Flow in the capillaries is regulated by smooth muscle cells. These cells are known as **precapillary sphincters**. The exchange of nutrients and waste products is the major role of the capillaries.

Arteries and Veins. Blood vessel walls are made up of three layers of elastic tissue and smooth muscle. (Capillaries and venules are the exception.) These layers also are known as **tunics**. The layers are the *tunica intima* (inner layer), the *tunica media* (middle layer), and the *tunica adventitia* (outer layer). The thickness and composition of each layer vary with the type and diameter of the blood vessel.

Large elastic arteries often are called *conducting arteries*, because they are the arteries with the largest diameter.

These vessels have more elastic tissue and less smooth muscle than any other arteries. Medium and small arteries have fairly thick muscular walls. These arteries also have elastic membranes that are well developed. These vessels are called distributing arteries because the smooth muscle allows these vessels partially to regulate blood supply to various body regions. The vessels do this by constriction or dilation. Arterioles are the smallest arteries in which the three tunics can be detected. As do small arteries, arterioles can vasodilate and vasoconstrict.

Venules have only a few isolated smooth muscle cells and are similar in structure to the capillaries. Venules collect blood from the capillaries and transport it to small veins. These veins in turn transport the blood to the medium-sized veins. Nutrient exchange occurs across the walls of the venules, but as the small veins increase in thickness, the degree of nutrient exchange decreases.

As venules increase in diameter, the vessels become veins with walls that are a continuous layer of smooth muscle cells. Medium-sized and large veins collect blood from small veins and deliver it to the large venous trunks. Large veins transport blood from the medium-sized veins to the heart.

Veins with a large diameter have valves that allow blood to flow to but not from the heart. Medium-sized veins have many valves, and the veins of the lower extremities have

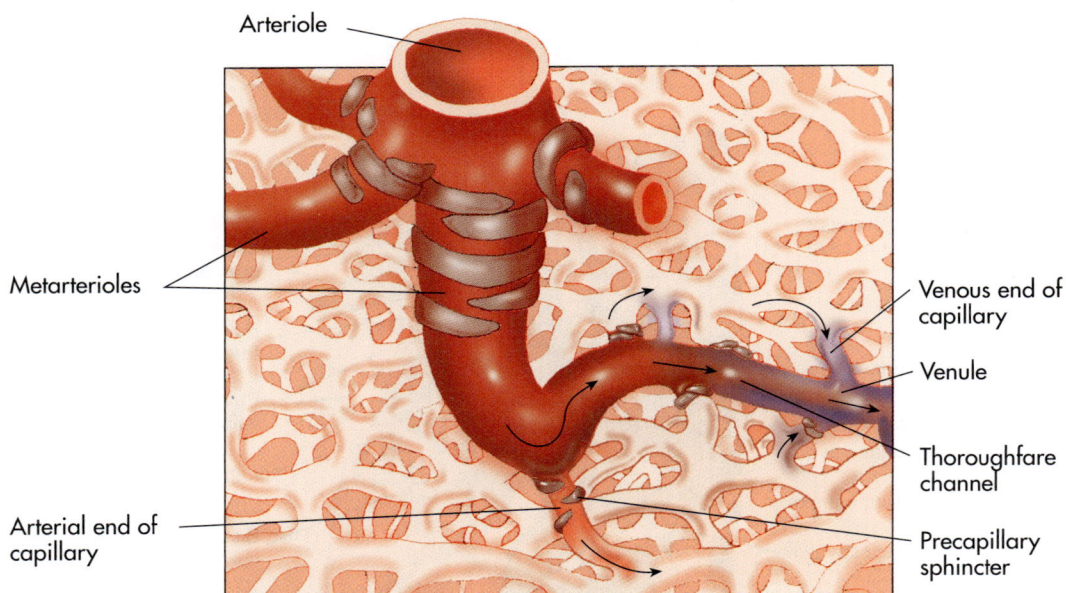

Arteriole

Metarterioles

Venous end of capillary

Venule

Arterial end of capillary

Thoroughfare channel

Precapillary sphincter

FIGURE 10-44 Capillary network. The metarteriole, giving rise to the network, feeds directly from the arteriole into the thoroughfare channel, which feeds into the venule. The network forms numerous branches that transport blood from the thoroughfare channel and may return to the thoroughfare channel.

more valves than do those of the upper extremities. These valves help prevent the backflow of blood, especially in dependent tissues.

Arteriovenous anastomoses allow blood to flow from arteries to veins without passing through capillaries. Natural *arteriovenous shunts* occur in large numbers in the soles of the feet, palms, and nail beds, where they regulate body temperature. Pathological shunts can result from injury or tumors. These shunts can cause a direct flow of blood from arteries to veins. Severe shunts may lead to "high output" heart failure from increased venous return to the heart and its resultant demand on **cardiac output** (see Chapter 22).

PULMONARY CIRCULATION

Blood from the right ventricle is pumped into the pulmonary trunk. This trunk splits into the right and left pulmonary arteries. These arteries move blood to the respective lungs, where oxygen and carbon dioxide are exchanged. Two pulmonary veins exit each lung and enter the left atrium. Pulmonary veins are the only veins in the body that carry oxygenated blood. Pulmonary arteries are the only arteries in the body that carry deoxygenated blood.

SYSTEMIC CIRCULATION

Oxygenated blood enters the heart from the pulmonary veins. The blood passes through the left atrium into the left ventricle. Then the blood passes from the left ventricle into the aorta. From the aorta, blood is distributed to all parts of the body. The arteries of systemic circulation include the aorta, coronary arteries, arteries of the head and neck, arteries of the upper and lower limbs, the thoracic aorta and its

branches, the **abdominal aorta** and its branches, and the arteries of the pelvis (Figure 10-45).

The veins of systemic circulation include coronary veins, veins of the head and neck, veins of the upper and lower limbs, veins of the thorax, veins of the abdomen and pelvis, and the *hepatic portal system*, which transports blood from the digestive tract to the liver (Figure 10-46).

Lymphatic System

The **lymphatic system** is considered part of the circulatory system because it consists of a moving fluid that comes from the body and returns to the blood. Unlike the circulatory system, the lymphatic system only carries fluid away from the tissues.

As stated before, the lymphatic system includes lymph, lymphocytes, lymph nodes, tonsils, spleen, and the thymus gland. The lymphatic system has three basic functions: (1) to help maintain fluid balance in tissues; (2) to absorb fats and other substances from the digestive tract; and (3) to act as part of the body's immune defense system.

The lymphatic system begins in the tissues as *lymph capillaries*. These capillaries differ in structure from blood capillaries. Lymph capillaries have a series of one-way valves. These valves allow fluid to enter the capillary. However, the valves prevent fluid from passing back into the interstitial spaces. Almost all body tissues have lymph capillaries; the exceptions are the CNS, bone marrow, and tissues without blood vessels (e.g., cartilage, epidermis, and cornea). Lymph capillaries join to form larger lymph capillaries that resemble small veins.

Lymph nodes are distributed along various lymph vessels. Most lymph passes through at least one node before

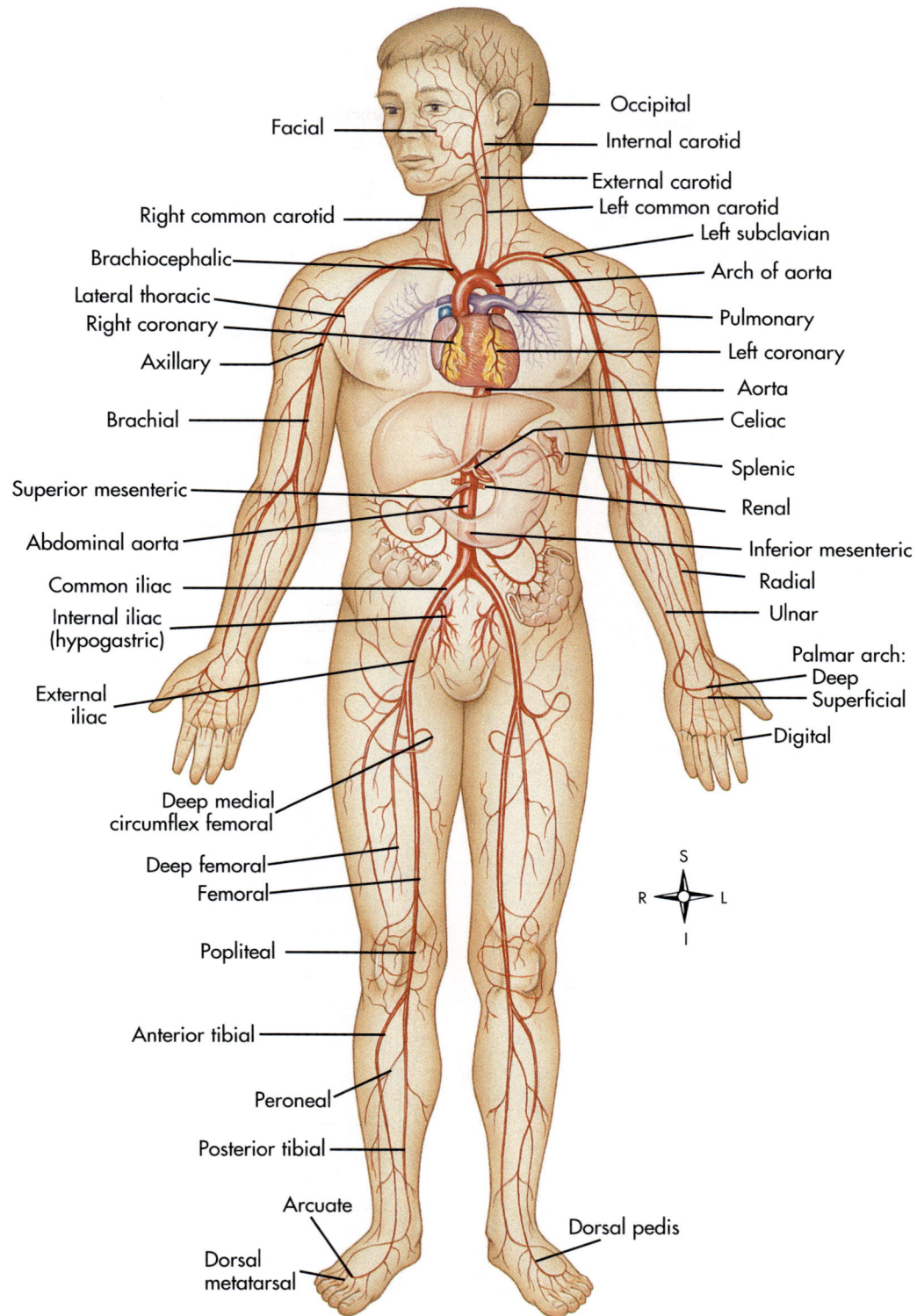

Facial

Right common carotid

Brachiocephalic
Lateral thoracic
Right coronary
Axillary

Brachial

Superior mesenteric

Abdominal aorta

Common iliac

Internal iliac
(hypogastric)

External
iliac

Deep medial
circumflex femoral

Deep femoral
Femoral

Popliteal

Anterior tibial

Peroneal

Posterior tibial

Arcuate

Dorsal
metatarsal

Occipital
Internal carotid
External carotid
Left common carotid
Left subclavian
Arch of aorta
Pulmonary
Left coronary
Aorta
Celiac
Splenic
Renal
Inferior mesenteric
Radial
Ulnar
Palmar arch:
Deep
Superficial
Digital

Dorsal pedis

S
R — L
I

FIGURE 10-45 Principal arteries of the body. (McCance KL, Huether SE: *Pathophysiology: the biologic basis for disease in adults and children,* ed 5, St Louis, 2005, Mosby.)

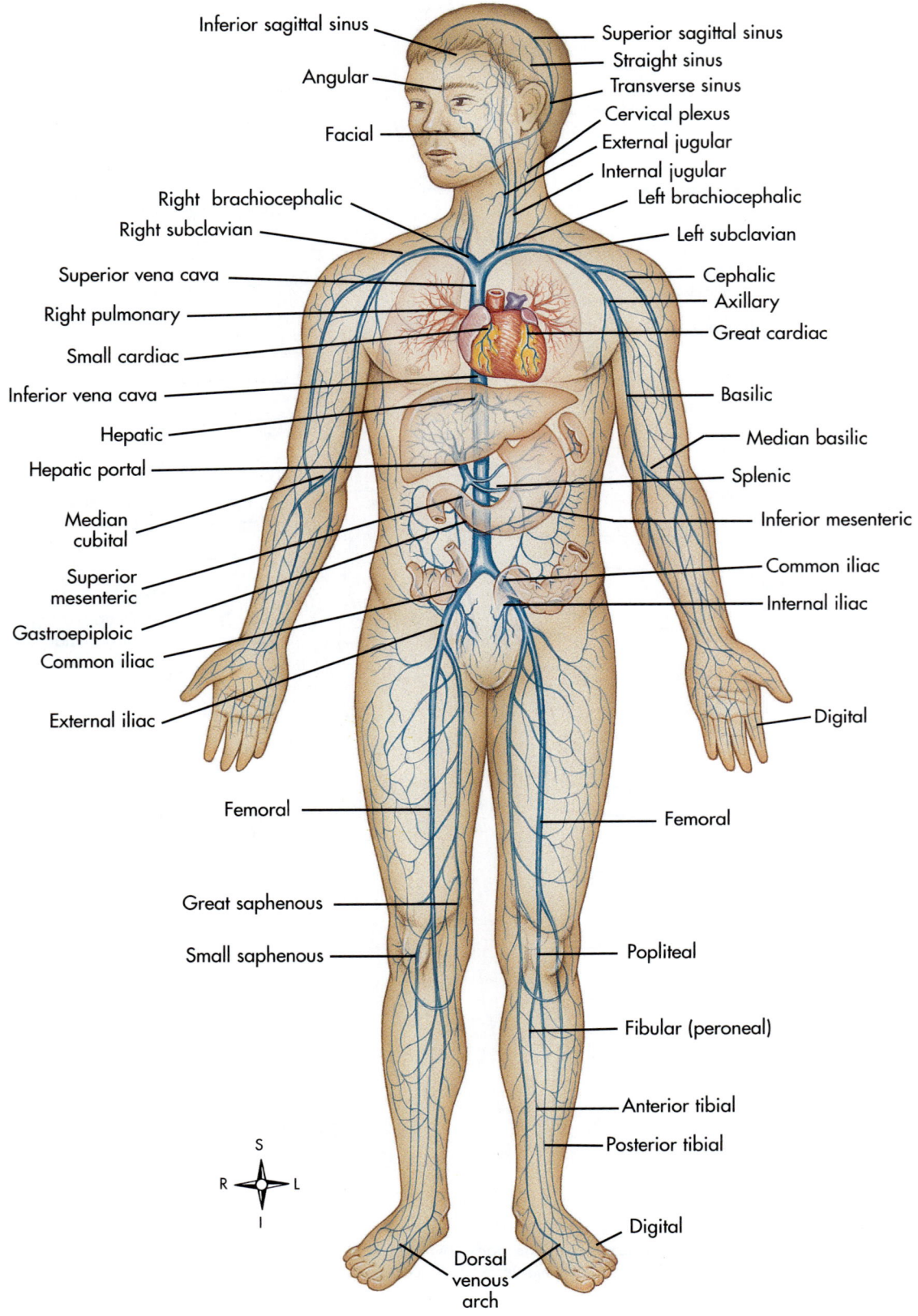

Inferior sagittal sinus
Angular
Facial
Right brachiocephalic
Right subclavian
Superior vena cava
Right pulmonary
Small cardiac
Inferior vena cava
Hepatic
Hepatic portal
Median cubital
Superior mesenteric
Gastroepiploic
Common iliac
External iliac
Femoral
Great saphenous
Small saphenous

Superior sagittal sinus
Straight sinus
Transverse sinus
Cervical plexus
External jugular
Internal jugular
Left brachiocephalic
Left subclavian
Cephalic
Axillary
Great cardiac
Basilic
Median basilic
Splenic
Inferior mesenteric
Common iliac
Internal iliac
Digital
Femoral
Popliteal
Fibular (peroneal)
Anterior tibial
Posterior tibial
Digital

Dorsal venous arch

S
R — L
I

FIGURE 10-46 Principal veins of the body. (McCance KL, Huether SE: *Pathophysiology: the biologic basis for disease in adults and children*, ed 5, St Louis, 2005, Mosby.)

entering the blood. The node filters the lymph as it passes through the node. Filtering removes microorganisms and foreign substances, preventing them from entering the general circulation. Three major collections of lymph nodes are located on each side of the body: *inguinal nodes, axillary nodes,* and *cervical nodes.* If a part of the body is inflamed or otherwise diseased, the nearby lymph nodes become swollen and tender as they limit the spread of microorganisms and foreign substances.

After passing through lymph nodes, lymph vessels converge toward the right or left **subclavian vein**. Vessels from the upper right limb and the right side of the head enter the right lymphatic duct. Lymph vessels from the rest of the body enter the larger thoracic duct. The *right lymphatic duct* drains the right thorax, right upper limb, and right side of the head and neck and opens into the right subclavian vein. The *thoracic duct* drains the left thorax, the left upper extremity, and the left side of the head and neck. The duct ends by entering the left subclavian vein. All fluid drained from the tissue spaces eventually returns to the venous circulation.

Lymph serves a unique transport role. It returns tissue fluid, proteins, fats, and other substances to the general circulation. The lymphatic system does not form a closed ring or circuit, as does the true circulatory system. Once lymph has formed, it flows only once through its system of lymphatic vessels before draining into the right and left subclavian veins.

> ### CRITICAL THINKING
> A woman has had a radical mastectomy (removal of breast and lymph tissue). Why might she have a chronically swollen arm?

Respiratory System

Oxygen is a basic element needed for normal cell metabolism. Carbon dioxide is a major waste product of this process. The organs of the respiratory system and the cardiovascular system transport oxygen to individual cells. These organs then transport carbon dioxide from the cells to the lungs. In the lungs the carbon dioxide is released into the air.

The respiratory system is a complex part of the human body. The aim of this section is to familiarize the paramedic student with the respiratory anatomy. (Further discussion of the respiratory system is presented in Chapter 15.)

AIRWAY ANATOMY

The structures of the respiratory system are divided into the upper airway and the lower airway. They are divided by their locations relative to **the glottic opening** (i.e., the vocal cords and the space between them). For the purpose of this text, all airway structures above the glottis are considered to be *upper airway.* All structures below the glottis are considered to be *lower airway* (Figure 10-47).

UPPER AIRWAY STRUCTURES

The entrance to the respiratory tract begins with the nasal cavity. This cavity includes the nasopharynx, oropharynx, laryngopharynx, and larynx.

Nasopharynx. Air passes into the nasal cavity through the nostrils, or *nares.* The right and left nasal cavities are separated by the *nasal septum,* a bony partition covered with a mucous membrane. This membrane has a rich blood supply that warms and humidifies the nasal lining and the inspired air as it passes through the nose. Inside each nostril a slight enlargement, known as the *vestibule,* is lined with coarse hairs that trap foreign substances carried into the nasal cavity by inspired air. The floor of the nasal cavity is composed of the *hard palate;* the lateral walls are formed by bony ridges coated with respiratory mucosa. These ridges are known as *conchae,* or *turbinates.*

Two patches of yellow-gray tissue lie just beneath the bridge of the nose. These patches compose the *olfactory membranes.* Located in the roof of the nasal cavity, these membranes contain the receptors for the sense of smell. The nasal cavities also connect to the middle ear cavities through the auditory (or eustachian) tubes.

> ### CRITICAL THINKING
> Why might a chronic cocaine abuser have a higher risk of sinus infection?

Sinuses are cavities in the bones of the skull that connect to the nasal cavities by small channels (Figure 10-48). The four groups of sinuses, each named for the skull bone in which it lies, are the *frontal sinuses,* above the eyebrows; *maxillary sinuses* (the largest sinuses), in the cheekbones; *ethmoid sinuses,* just behind the bridge of the nose; and *sphenoid sinuses,* in a bone that cradles the brain, slightly anterior to the **pituitary gland**. These hollow chambers are lined with mucous membranes that secrete mucus into the nasal cavities. They are thought to help add resonance to the voice and to reduce the weight of the skull.

The back of each nasal cavity opens into the nasopharynx. This is the superior part of the pharynx. The nasopharynx extends from the internal nares to the level of the **uvula**. Like the nasal cavity, the nasopharynx is lined with mucous membrane.

Oropharynx. At the level of the uvula, the nasopharynx ends and the oropharynx begins. The oropharynx extends down to the level of the **epiglottis**. Anteriorly, the oropharynx opens into the oral cavity. The oral cavity is made up of the lips, cheeks, teeth, tongue (which is attached to the mandible), hard and soft palates, and palatine tonsils. The *palatine tonsils* and the *pharyngeal tonsils* (located in the roof and posterior wall of the nasopharynx) form a partial ring of lymphoid tissue. This tissue surrounds the respiratory tract. This ring is completed by the *lingual tonsils.* The tonsils lie on the floor of the oropharyngeal passageway at the base of the tongue.

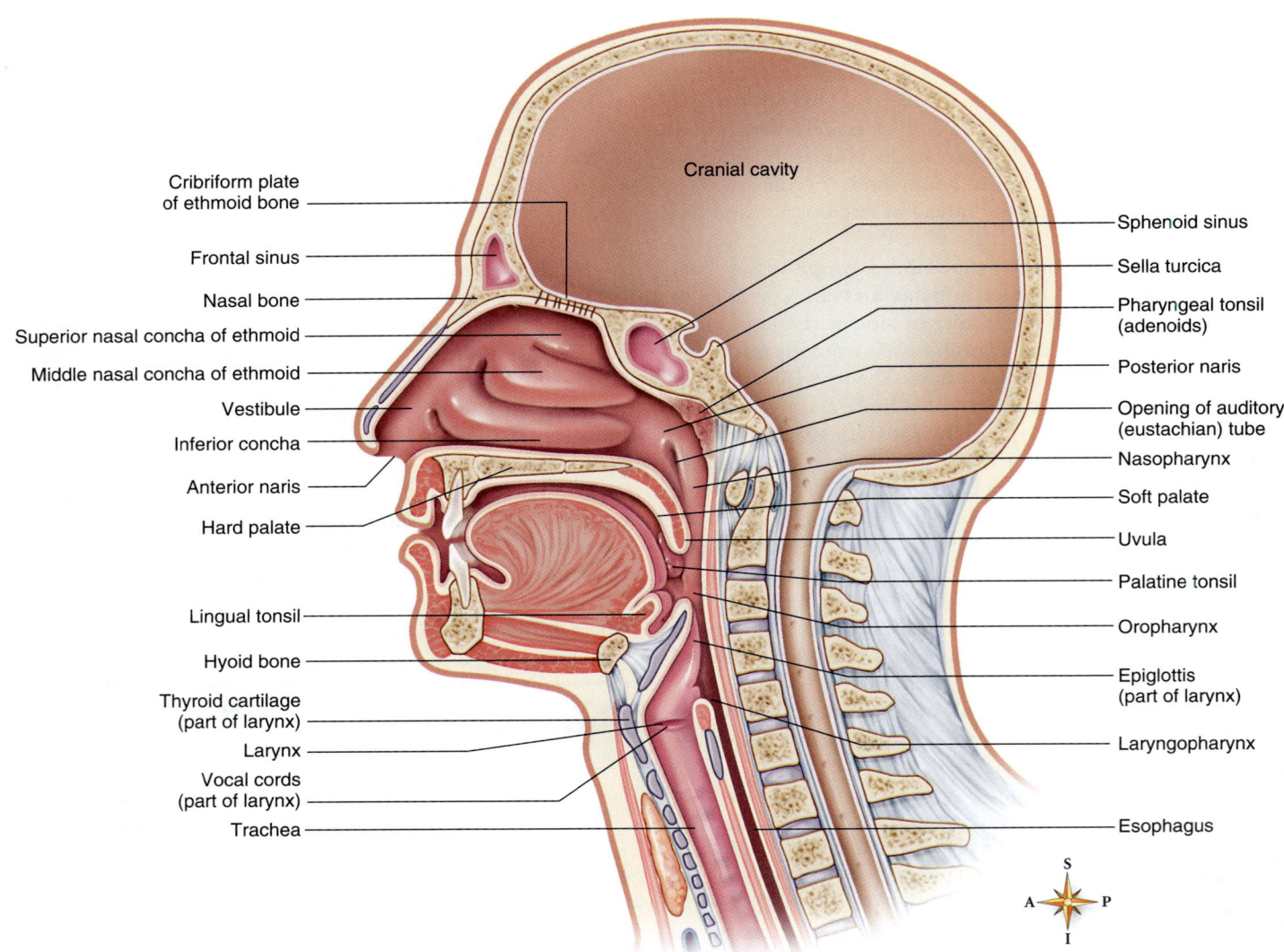

FIGURE 10-47 Airway structures. (Patton KT, Thibodeau GA: *Anatomy and physiology,* ed 7, St Louis, 2007, Mosby.)

Laryngopharynx. The **laryngopharynx** extends from the tip of the epiglottis to the glottis and the **esophagus**. It is lined with mucous membrane, which protects the internal surfaces from abrasion.

Larynx. The laryngopharynx opens into the **larynx,** which lies in the anterior neck (Figure 10-49). The larynx serves three main functions: (1) it is the air passageway between the pharynx and the lungs; (2) it is a protective sphincter that prevents solids and liquids from passing into the respiratory tree; and (3) it is involved in the production of speech.

The larynx consists of an outer casing of nine cartilages connected to each other by muscles and ligaments. Six of the nine cartilages are paired; three are unpaired. The largest, most superior of the cartilages is the unpaired thyroid cartilage, or *Adam's apple.* This prominence is hardly

visible in children or adult females but is visible in males after puberty.

The most inferior cartilage of the larynx is the unpaired **cricoid cartilage**. This is the only complete cartilaginous ring in the larynx. This cartilage forms the base of the larynx on which all other cartilages rest. The third unpaired cartilage is the epiglottis.

The six paired cartilages are stacked in two pillars between the cricoid cartilage and the thyroid cartilage. The largest inferior cartilages are ladle-shaped and are known as the *arytenoid cartilages*. The middle pair are horn-shaped and are known as *corniculate cartilages*. The smallest, most superior cartilages are wedge-shaped and are known as *cuneiform cartilages*.

The U-shaped hyoid bone is tucked beneath the mandible. As previously mentioned, the hyoid is the only bone

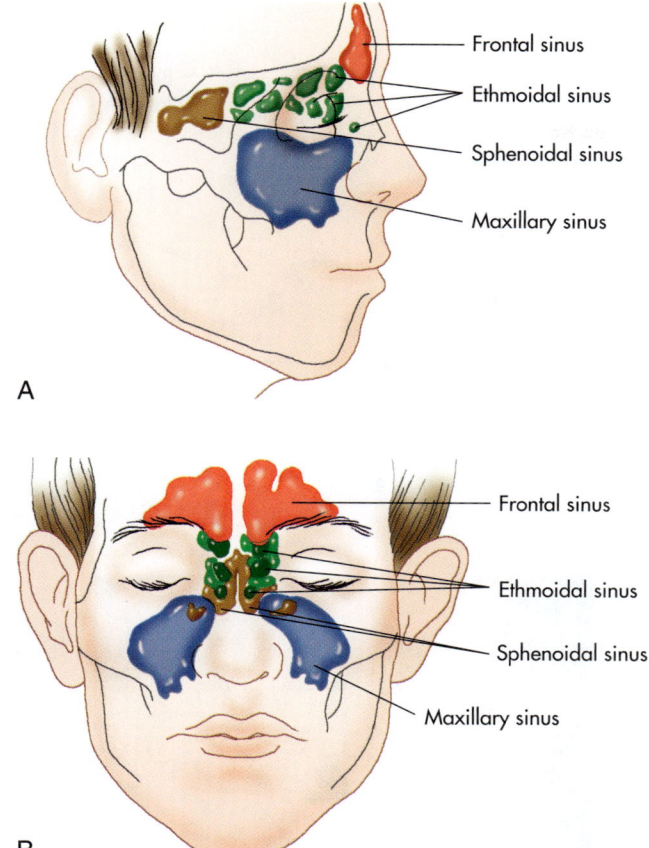

A

B

FIGURE 10-48 Paranasal sinuses. **A,** Side view. **B,** Front view.

of the human body that does not articulate with another bone. The hyoid bone helps to suspend the airway by anchoring the muscles (particularly those of the tongue) to the jaw. The fibrous membrane that joins the hyoid and the thyroid cartilage is called the **thyroid membrane**. The membrane joining the thyroid and cricoid cartilages is called the **cricothyroid membrane**.

Two pairs of ligaments extend from the anterior surface of the arytenoid to the posterior surface of the thyroid cartilage. The superior pair forms the *vestibular folds,* or false vocal cords, which are not involved directly in the production of voice sounds. The inferior pair of ligaments composes the **vocal cords**, or true vocal cords, which participate directly in the production of voice sounds. When a person talks, air expelled from the lungs rushes up the throat to the larynx. In the larynx, the air creates sound by vibrating the vocal cords. Muscles tighten the folds of the cords to produce the high-pitched tones and relax the cords to produce the deeper tones. The lips, tongue, and jaw further modify the sounds into intelligible words.

CRITICAL THINKING

Why can't a person talk when an endotracheal tube is correctly positioned in the trachea?

LOWER AIRWAY STRUCTURES

Below the glottis are the structures of the lower airway and lungs. These structures include the trachea, the bronchial tree (primary bronchi, secondary bronchi, and bronchioles), the alveoli, and the lungs (Figure 10-50).

Trachea. The **trachea** is the air passage from the larynx to the lungs. It is composed of dense connective tissue and smooth muscle reinforced with 15 to 20 C-shaped pieces of cartilage that form an incomplete ring. This ring protects the trachea and maintains an open passage for air. The adult trachea is about 1.5 cm in diameter and 9 to 15 cm long. The trachea is located anterior to the esophagus and extends from the larynx to the fifth thoracic vertebra.

The trachea is lined with *ciliated epithelium* that contains many goblet cells. These cilia protect the lower airway. They sweep mucus, bacteria, and other small particles toward the larynx. At the larynx, the mucus and its contents may be expelled through coughing, or they may enter the esophagus, where they are swallowed and digested. Constant exposure to some irritants (e.g., cigarette smoke) may produce a tracheal epithelium that lacks cilia and goblet cells. When this protective mechanism is disrupted, mucus and bacteria may contribute to disease.

 NOTE

A centimeter is equal to 0.4 inch. One inch is equal to 2.54 cm.

Bronchial Tree. The lower airway may be thought of as an inverted tree; the many subdivisions become narrower and shorter until they terminate at the alveoli. The large branches are *primary bronchi,* which divide into smaller secondary bronchi and bronchioles.

The trachea divides into the *right* and *left primary bronchi* at the level of the angle of Louis (the **sternomanubrial joint**). The point of bifurcation of the trachea into the right and left mainstem bronchi is called the **carina**. The right primary bronchus is shorter, wider, and more vertical. Like the trachea, the primary bronchi are lined with ciliated epithelium. They are supported by C-shaped cartilage rings. As the bronchi sequentially branch into smaller subdivisions, the amount of cartilage decreases. The bronchi also become more and more muscular until no cartilage is present. The primary bronchi extend from the mediastinum to the lungs.

The primary bronchi divide into the *secondary bronchi* as they enter the right and left lungs. Two secondary lobar bronchi in the left lung conduct air to its two lobes; three in the right lung conduct air to its three lobes. The secondary bronchi then divide into the *tertiary segmental bronchi,* of which there are 10 in the right lung and nine in the left. The tertiary bronchi extend to the individual segments of each lobe of the lung (lobule). The bronchial tree continues to branch several times. As the cartilage continues to decrease and the diameter is reduced to about 1 mm, the bronchi become **bronchioles**.

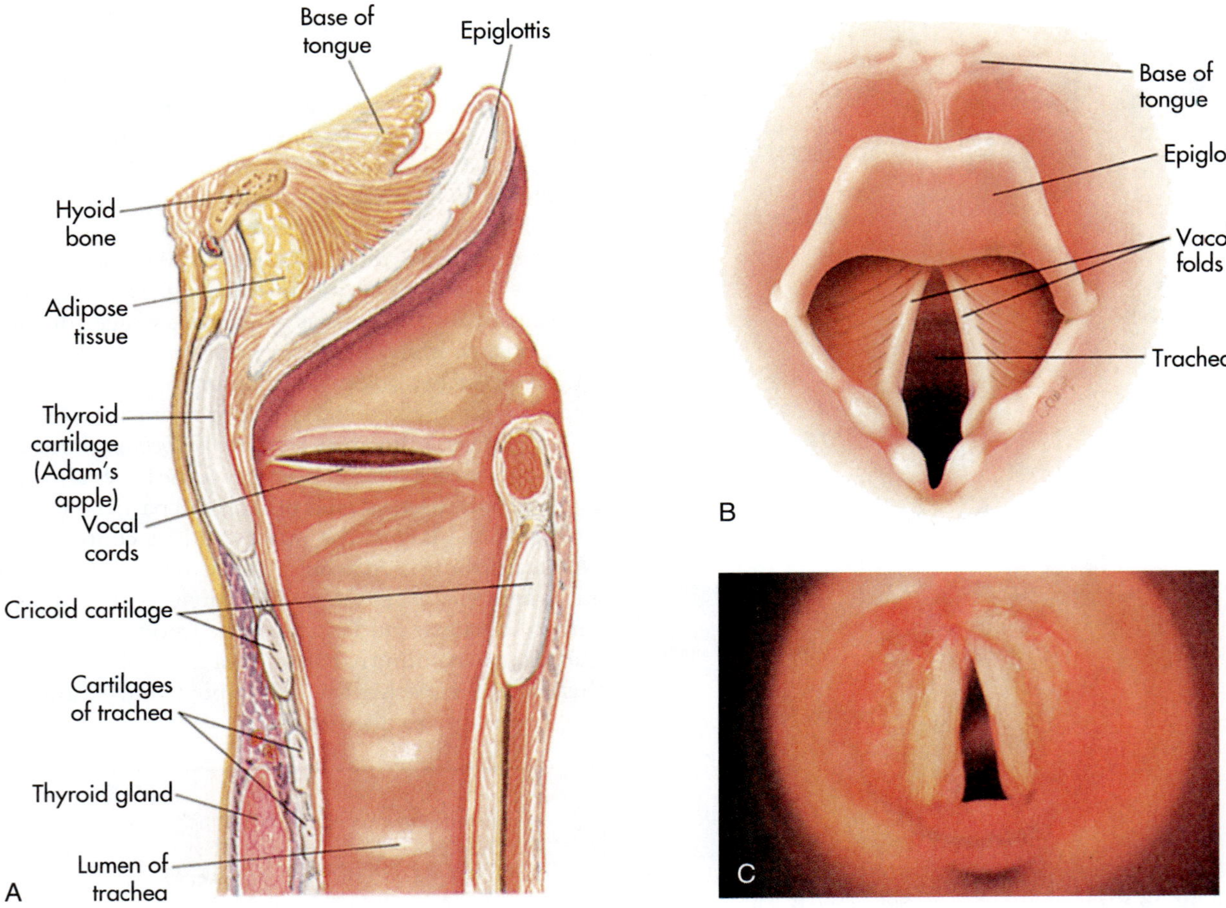

Base of tongue   Epiglottis

Hyoid bone

Adipose tissue

Thyroid cartilage (Adam's apple)

Vocal cords

Cricoid cartilage

Cartilages of trachea

Thyroid gland

Lumen of trachea

A

Base of tongue

Epiglottis

Vacol folds

Trachea

B

C

FIGURE 10-49 Larynx. **A,** Sagittal section. **B,** Superior view. **C,** Photograph taken with an endoscope. (Thibodeau GA, Patton KT: *Structure and function of the body,* ed 13, St Louis, 2008, Mosby.)

CRITICAL THINKING
What is the benefit of having many bronchiole branches?

NOTE
A millimeter is equal to 0.04 inch. One inch is equal to 25.4 mm.

The walls of the bronchioles are devoid of cartilage. Their muscles are sensitive to certain circulating hormones, such as epinephrine. Contraction and relaxation of these muscles alter resistance to air flow. The bronchioles can constrict if the smooth muscle contracts forcefully. (An example of this is an asthma exacerbation.) Bronchioles continue to divide. In time they become *terminal bronchioles.* Ultimately, they become *respiratory bronchioles.* Each respiratory bronchiole divides to form *alveolar ducts.* These ducts end as grapelike clusters of tiny, hollow air sacs. These sacs are called *alveoli.* Most respiratory gas exchange takes place in the alveoli.

Alveoli. The **alveoli** are the functional units of the respiratory system. They are the main constituent of lung tissue. The two lungs have about 300 million alveoli. The wall of an alveolus consists of a single layer of epithelial cells and elastic fibers. These fibers permit the alveolus to stretch and contract during breathing. The exchange of oxygen and carbon dioxide in the lungs takes place in the alveoli (see Chapter 15).

Each alveolus is surrounded by a fine network of blood capillaries. These capillaries are arranged so that air in the alveolus is separated by a thin respiratory membrane from the blood in the alveolar capillaries. The large surface area of the respiratory membrane may be reduced by respiratory diseases, such as *emphysema* and *lung cancer.* Such diseases restrict the exchange of oxygen and carbon dioxide.

Alveoli are coated with **pulmonary surfactant,** a thin film made by alveolar cells. This fluid keeps the alveoli from collapsing. In addition, pores in the alveolar membrane allow for a limited flow of air between alveoli. This collateral ventilation offers some protection for an alveolus that is occluded by disease.

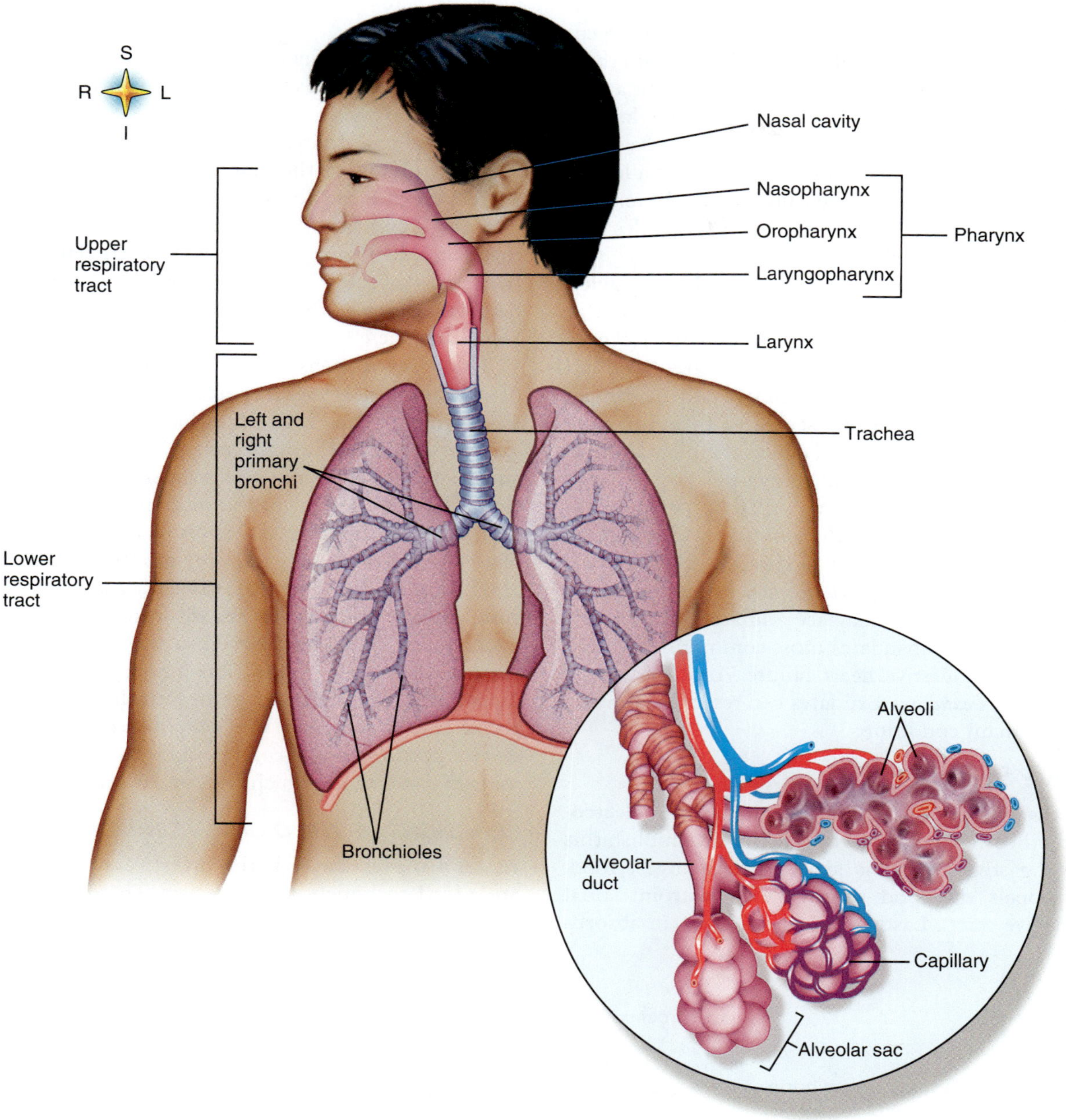

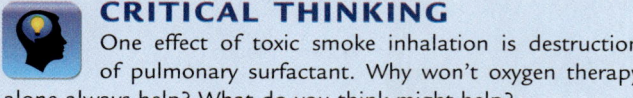

S

R L

I

Nasal cavity

Nasopharynx

Oropharynx ⎤
⎥ Pharynx
Laryngopharynx ⎦

Larynx

Upper respiratory tract

Trachea

Left and right primary bronchi

Lower respiratory tract

Bronchioles

Alveoli

Alveolar duct

Capillary

Alveolar sac

FIGURE 10-50 Structural plan of the respiratory system. The inset shows alveolar sacs; the exchange of oxygen and carbon dioxide takes place through the walls of the grapelike alveoli. (Patton KT, Thibodeau GA: *Anatomy and physiology,* ed 7, St Louis, 2007, Mosby.)

CRITICAL THINKING
One effect of toxic smoke inhalation is destruction of pulmonary surfactant. Why won't oxygen therapy alone always help? What do you think might help?

Lungs. The lungs are large, paired, spongy organs; their main function is **respiration**. Although smooth muscle is present in the bronchioles of the lungs, the lungs expand and contract during the respiratory cycle as a result of the expansion of the thoracic cavity during inspiration and the elastic recoil during expiration. The lungs are attached to the heart by the pulmonary artery and veins. The two lungs are separated by the mediastinum and its contents (the heart, blood vessels, trachea, esophagus, lymphatic tissues, and vessels). The point of entry for the bronchi, vessels, and nerves of each lung is known as the *hilum,* or root, of each lung. At birth the lungs are rose pink. However, by adulthood the lungs are slate gray with dark patches because of the particulate matter that is inhaled and deposited in the tissues. An adult lung weighs less than 2 pounds.

Each lung is conical, with the base resting on the **diaphragm** and the apex extending to a point about 2.5 cm superior to each clavicle. The right lung is divided into three lobes. The left lung is slightly smaller than the right and is divided into two lobes. Each lobe is divided into lobules separated by connective tissue. Major blood vessels and bronchi do not cross this connective tissue; this allows a diseased lobule to be removed surgically, leaving the remaining lung relatively intact. The left lung has nine lobules, and the right lung has 10 lobules.

Both lungs are surrounded by a separate **pleural cavity**. The lungs are attached to each other only at the point of entry of the bronchi, vessels, and nerves of each lung (Figure 10-51). The two layers of the pleura (the *visceral* layer and the *parietal* layer) are so close they are virtually in contact with each other. The pleurae are separated by a thin fluid that acts as a lubricant. This fluid allows the pleural membranes to slide past each other during respiration.

Between the two pleurae is a potential space known as the **pleural space**. When significant chest wall injury or pathologic pulmonary condition occurs, the pleural space may become filled with air *(pneumothorax)* or blood *(hemothorax)*. Another fluid that may accumulate in the pleural space is *transudates*. Transudates most commonly accumulate because of congestive heart failure. Another type of fluid collection is *exudates*. Exudates can result from infectious or malignant conditions.

Digestive System

The digestive system provides the body with water, **electrolytes**, and other nutrients used by cells. To accomplish this task, the digestive system is specialized to ingest food. It then propels the food through the gastrointestinal tract (digestive tract). Lastly, the digestive system absorbs nutrients across the wall of the lumen of the gastrointestinal tract.

The gastrointestinal tract is an irregularly shaped tube. Associated accessory organs (mainly glands) secrete fluid into the digestive tract. The first part of the digestive tract is the oral cavity. The *salivary glands* and tonsils are accessory organs of the oral cavity. The oral cavity opens posteriorly into the pharynx. The pharynx opens inferiorly into the esophagus. The esophagus opens inferiorly into the stomach (through the muscular **cardiac sphincter**). In the stomach small glands secrete acids and enzymes that help with digestion. The cardiac sphincter stops food from reentering the esophagus when the stomach contracts.

The stomach opens into the **duodenum**, the first section of the small intestine. Important accessory structures in this segment of the gastrointestinal tract are the **liver**, the **gallbladder**, and the **pancreas**. The **jejunum**, the major site of absorption, is the next segment of the **small intestine**. The last segment of the small intestine is the ileum. The **ileum** is similar in function to the jejunum but has fewer digestive enzymes and provides less absorption.

The last section of the digestive tract is the **large intestine;** its functions are to absorb water and salts and to concentrate undigested food into feces. The major accessory glands secrete mucus. The first segment of the large intestine is the **cecum** with its attached appendix. The cecum is followed by the *ascending, transverse, descending,* and *sigmoid* portions of the colon and the rectum. The **rectum** joins the anal canal, which ends at the **anus**.

FUNCTIONS OF THE DIGESTIVE TRACT

As food moves through the digestive system, secretions are added to liquefy and digest it. These secretions also provide lubrication. The processes of *secretion, movement,*

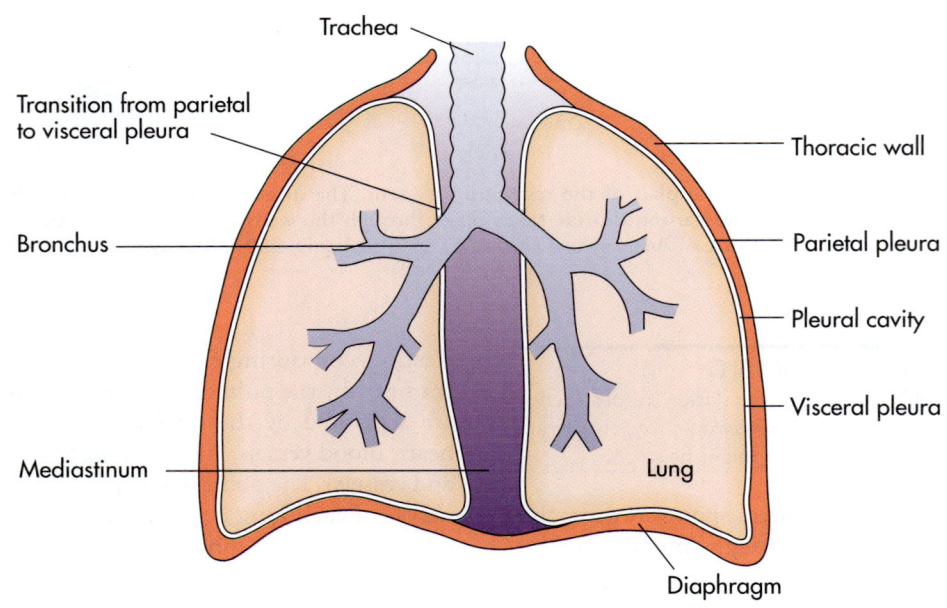

FIGURE 10-51 Lungs surrounded by the pleural cavities.

and *absorption* are regulated by nervous and hormonal mechanisms.

ORAL CAVITY

Saliva contains a digestive enzyme referred to as *salivary amylase*. This enzyme begins the chemical digestion of carbohydrates. In addition, saliva prevents bacterial infection in the mouth. It does this by washing the oral cavity with certain substances. These substances offer a weak antibacterial action. Salivary gland secretion is stimulated by the parasympathetic and sympathetic nervous systems. The parasympathetic nervous system controls salivation in the relaxed state.

The teeth chew food in the mouth to break it up, which aids swallowing and processing. Food then is swallowed by voluntary and involuntary actions. The pharynx elevates to receive the food from the mouth. As the pharyngeal muscles contract, the upper esophageal sphincter relaxes, the esophagus opens, and the food is pushed into the esophagus. During this phase of swallowing, the vocal folds are moved medially. The epiglottis is tipped posteriorly to close the entrance of the airway and prevent aspiration.

Muscular contractions in the esophagus occur in *peristaltic waves*. These waves push the food through the esophagus toward the stomach. The contractions cause the cardiac sphincter (also known as the *lower esophageal sphincter*) to relax, and they then push the food into the stomach.

STOMACH

The stomach acts primarily as a storage area and mixing chamber for ingested food. Although some digestion and absorption occur in the stomach, these are not its major functions. The stomach secretes mucus to protect the surface of the stomach wall and duodenum. The stomach is lined by mucous membranes that contain thousands of microscopic gastric glands. These gastric glands secrete *hydrochloric acid, intrinsic factor*, gastrin, and *pepsinogen*.

The stomach produces about 2 to 3 L of gastric secretions each day. Secretion is regulated by nervous and hormonal mechanisms. The ingested food is mixed well with the secretions of the stomach glands to produce a semisolid mixture called **chyme**. Movements resembling peristalsis slowly force chyme toward the *pyloric sphincter*, through the *pyloric opening*, and into the duodenum (Figures 10-52 and 10-53).

> **NOTE**
> A liter is equal to 1.06 quarts. One gallon is equal to 3.79 L.

SMALL INTESTINE

The mucosa of the small intestine produces secretions that contain mucus, electrolytes, and water. These substances lubricate the intestinal wall. They also protect the intestine from the acidic chyme and digestive enzymes. In addition, secretions of the liver and pancreas enter the small intestine to aid the digestive process.

The main functions of the small intestine are the mixing and propulsion of chyme and the absorption of fluid and nutrients. Peristaltic contractions move the chyme through the small intestine toward the *ileocecal sphincter*. At this point, the chyme enters the cecum. When the chyme causes the cecum to distend, the sphincter closes. This closure

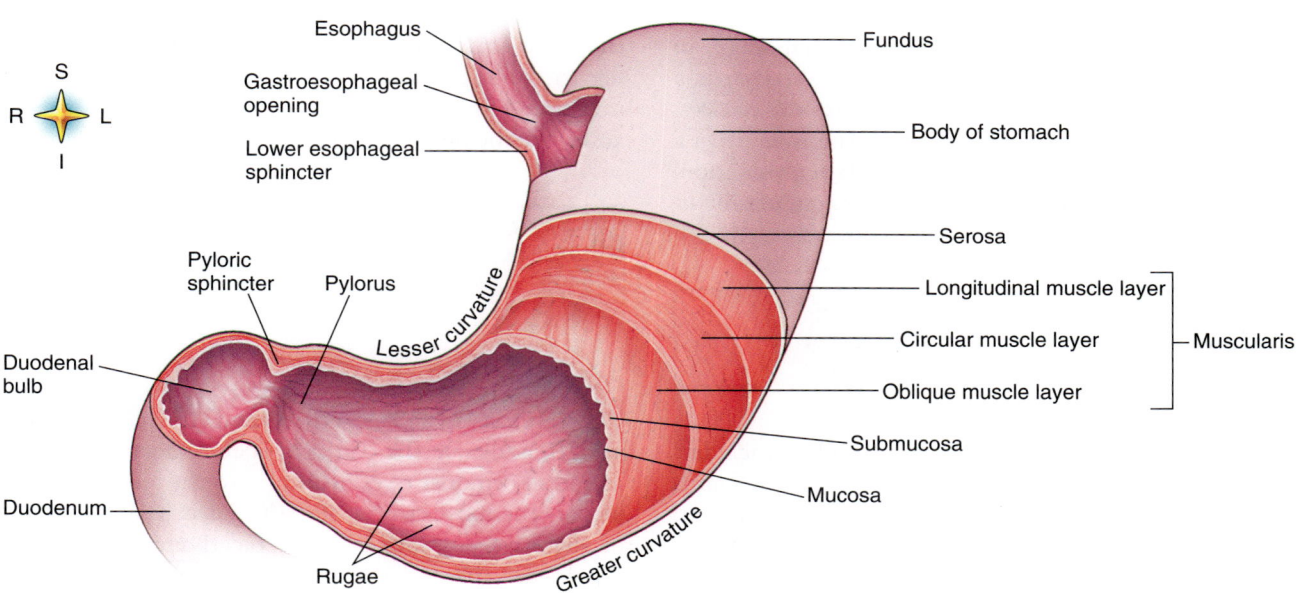

FIGURE 10-52 Muscle layers of the stomach wall. (Patton KT, Thibodeau GA: *Anatomy and physiology*, ed 7, St Louis, 2007, Mosby.)

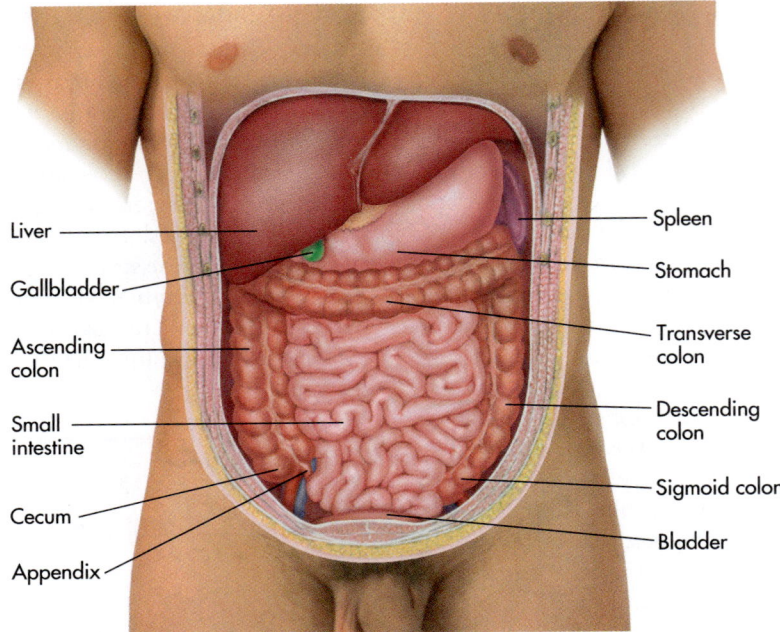

FIGURE 10-53 Digestive organs. (Patton KT, Thibodeau GA: *Anatomy and physiology,* ed 7, St Louis, 2007, Mosby.)

slows the rate of movement of chyme from the small intestine into the large intestine. Closure also prevents material from returning to the ileum from the cecum.

CRITICAL THINKING
What might happen if the excretion of protective mucus in the small bowel is impaired?

LIVER

The liver is the largest internal organ. It serves a number of biochemical functions. It lies just under the diaphragm in the upper regions of the abdominal cavity. The liver is a vascular organ that gets a blood supply from two sources, the **hepatic artery** and the **portal vein**. The liver plays a major role in iron metabolism, plasma protein production, detoxification of drugs and other substances circulating in plasma, and many other biochemical pathways.

NOTE
A milliliter is equal to 0.5 teaspoon volume. One tablespoon volume is equal to 15 mL.

The liver secretes about 600 to 1000 mL of **bile** each day. Bile contains no digestive enzymes, but it dilutes stomach acid and emulsifies fats. Most bile salts are reabsorbed in the ileum and are carried back to the liver in the blood. Other bile salts are lost through feces.

In addition to secreting bile, the liver has other functions that are needed for healthy survival. The liver plays a major role in the metabolism of certain foods. It also helps maintain a normal blood glucose concentration. The liver is a line of defense against many byproducts of metabolism that are toxic if they collect in the body. Blood proteins (e.g., *albumin, fibrinogen, globulins,* and *clotting factors*) also are made and released into the circulation by the liver.

GALLBLADDER

Bile is secreted regularly by the liver and is stored in the gallbladder. When chyme containing lipid or fat enters the duodenum, the gallbladder is stimulated by the hormones *cholecystokinin* and *secretin*. These hormones are secreted by the intestinal mucosa. The stimulation causes the gallbladder to contract, forcing concentrated bile into the small intestine. The only role of the gallbladder is to concentrate and store the bile made by the liver.

CRITICAL THINKING
When is the person who suffers from gallstones (cholelithiasis) most likely to have pain? Why?

PANCREAS

The pancreas is an **exocrine gland**. It secretes *pancreatic juice*. In addition, the pancreas is an endocrine gland that secretes hormones (e.g., insulin) into the blood. Pancreatic juice is the most critical digestive juice. The juice consists of digestive enzymes, sodium bicarbonate, and alkaline substances that neutralize the hydrochloric acid in the chyme entering the small intestine. Pancreatic juice also holds *amylase*. The amylase continues the digestion that began in the oral cavity.

LARGE INTESTINE

Chyme moves through the small intestine in 3 to 5 hours. Passage through the large intestine, however, takes 18 to 24 hours. Processes involving the absorption of water and salts, the secretion of mucus, the action of microorganisms, and the conversion of chyme produce feces. Feces remain in the colon until eliminated through defecation.

The contents of the large intestine are forced toward the anus by peristaltic contractions. These contractions occur three or four times a day. During the movement of chyme through the large intestine, bacteria act on material that escaped digestion in the small intestine. As a result of this action, more nutrients may be released and absorbed. Some of the bacteria also synthesize vitamin K. This vitamin is needed for normal blood clotting to produce the vitamin B complex. Once formed, these vitamins are absorbed from the large intestine and enter the blood.

Distention of the rectal wall by feces starts the defecation reflex. This reflex causes weak contractions and relaxations of the *internal anal sphincter*. The *external anal sphincter* (under conscious cerebral control) stops the passage of feces out of the rectum until it is relaxed. During defecation, pressure in the abdominal cavity increases. This pressure forces the contents of the colon through the anal canal and out the anus.

Urinary System

The urinary system works with other body systems to maintain homeostasis. It does this by removing waste products from the blood and by helping to maintain a constant body fluid volume and composition. The kidneys also are involved in the control of red blood cell production and metabolism of vitamin D. The urinary system is made up of two kidneys, two ureters, the urinary bladder, and the urethra.

CRITICAL THINKING
Think about patients with renal failure. Why should you anticipate anemia and decreased calcium levels?

KIDNEYS

Each **kidney** is shaped much like a kidney bean. The two kidneys lie on the posterior abdominal wall behind the peritoneum. They are on either side of the vertebral column near the lateral border of the *psoas muscles*. The superior pole of each kidney is protected by the rib cage. The right kidney is slightly lower than the left because of the superior position of the liver. A fibrous *renal capsule* surrounds each kidney, as does a dense deposit of adipose tissue that protects the kidney from injury.

The kidney is divided into an *outer cortex* and an *inner medulla*. The medulla consists of a number of triangular divisions. These divisions are called the **renal pyramids**. They extend into the cortex (Figure 10-54). The *papilla* is the innermost end of a pyramid. Several large urinary

tubes (*calyces*) extend to the renal pelvis from the kidney tissue.

The basic functional unit of the kidney is the **nephron**. The nephron is made up of a large terminal end (called a *renal corpuscle*), a proximal convoluted tubule, the **loop of Henle**, and a distal convoluted tubule. The distal convoluted tubule empties into a collecting duct. This duct carries the urine from the cortex of the kidney to the calyces. The terminal end of the nephron is enlarged to form **Bowman's capsule**. The wall of Bowman's capsule is indented to form a double-walled chamber occupied by a network of blood capillaries known as the **glomerulus**. Together, the glomerulus and Bowman's capsule form the renal corpuscle.

URETERS, URINARY BLADDER, AND URETHRA

The **ureters** extend from the renal pelvis to the urinary bladder. The triangular area of the bladder wall between the two ureters and the urethra is called the *trigone*. (Figure 10-55 depicts the male urinary bladder.) This region differs from the rest of the bladder wall in that it does not expand during bladder filling.

The **urinary bladder** is a hollow, muscular organ. It lies in the pelvic cavity just posterior to the pubic symphysis. The size of the bladder depends on the volume of urine.

CRITICAL THINKING
Why is the bladder more susceptible to injury when full than when empty?

At the junction of the urethra and the urinary bladder, smooth muscle of the bladder forms the *internal urinary sphincter*. The external urinary sphincter surrounds the urethra as the urethra extends through the pelvic floor. These sphincters control the flow of urine through the urethra. In the male, the urethra extends to the end of the penis, where it opens to the outside. The female urethra is much shorter than the male urethra. It opens into the vestibule anterior to the vaginal opening.

URINE PRODUCTION

Nephrons are the structural parts of the kidney and are the location where urine is produced. The more than 2 million nephrons form urine in a three-step process of filtration, reabsorption, and secretion.

1. The first step of urine formation is the passage of fluid from the glomerular capillaries. This fluid passes into Bowman's capsule. Blood flowing through the glomeruli exerts pressure. This pressure pushes water and small dissolved molecular substances out of the glomeruli and into the Bowman's capsule. Simply stated, glomerular blood pressure causes filtration through the glomerular capillaries. Glomerular filtration normally occurs at the rate of 125 mL/min or 180 L/day (glomerular filtration rate). Ninety percent of this filtrate is reabsorbed. Healthy individuals produce 1 to 2 L of urine a day.

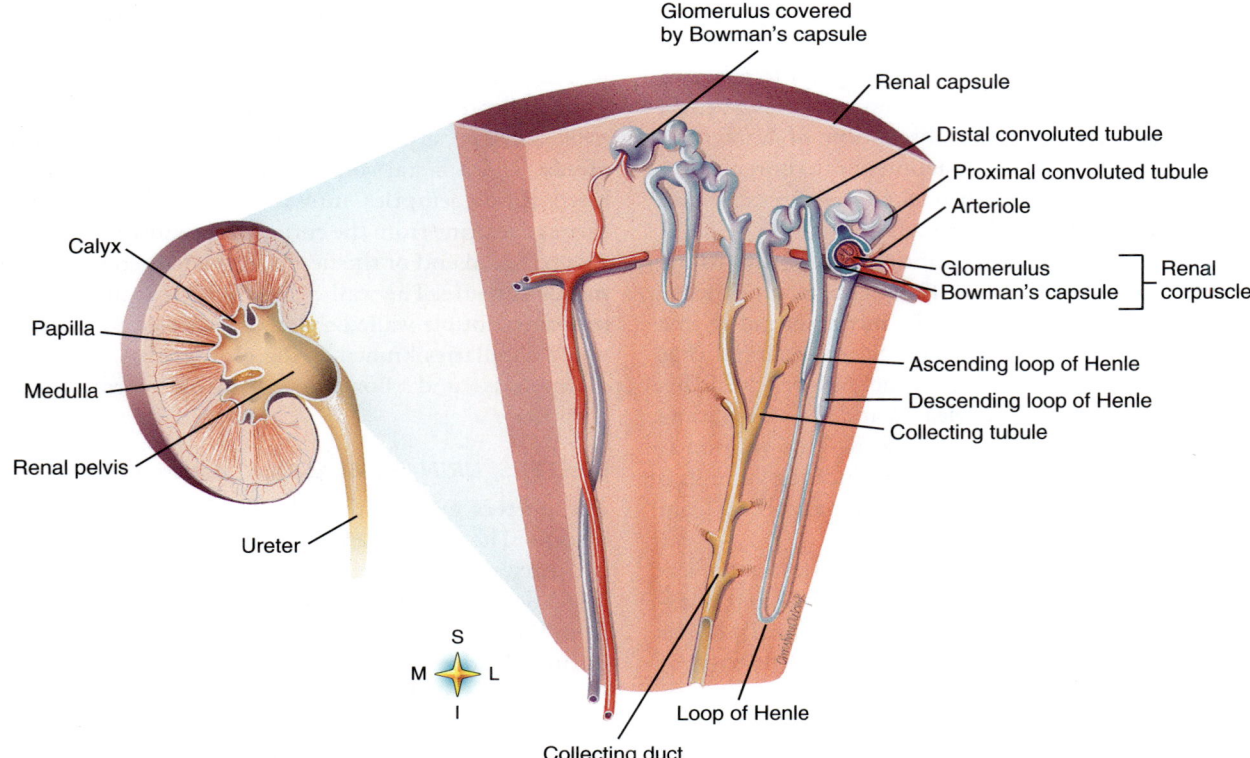

FIGURE 10-54 Magnified wedge cut from a renal pyramid. (Thibodeau GA, Patton KT: *Structure and function of the body,* ed 13, St Louis, 2008, Mosby.)

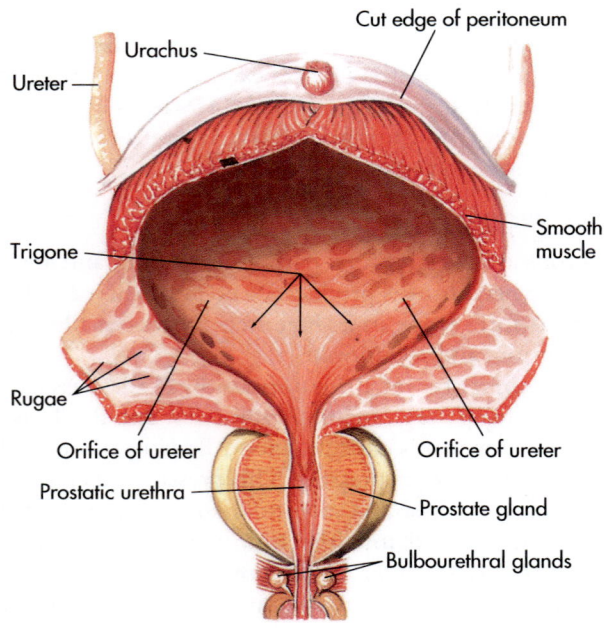

FIGURE 10-55 Male urinary bladder. (Christensen BL, Kockrow EO: *Adult health nursing,* ed 6, St Louis, 2010, Mosby.)

2. Upon leaving the renal capsule, the filtrate flows through the proximal convoluted tubule, the loop of Henle, the distal convoluted tubule, and into the collecting duct. During this process, many substances in the filtrate are reabsorbed by the blood capillaries around the tubules. These substances reenter the general circulation. Substances that are reabsorbed include water, glucose and other nutrients, and most of the sodium and other **ions**.

3. Secretion is the process by which substances move into urine in the distal convoluted tubule and collecting duct from blood in the capillaries around these structures. Reabsorption moves substances out of the urine and into the blood. Secretion, however, moves substances out of the blood and into the urine. Secreted substances include hydrogen and potassium ions, ammonia, and certain drugs. (Figure 10-56 depicts the formation of urine.)

URINE REGULATION

The body usually can control the amount and makeup of the urine it secretes. This involves hormonal mechanisms, autoregulation, and sympathetic nervous system stimulation.

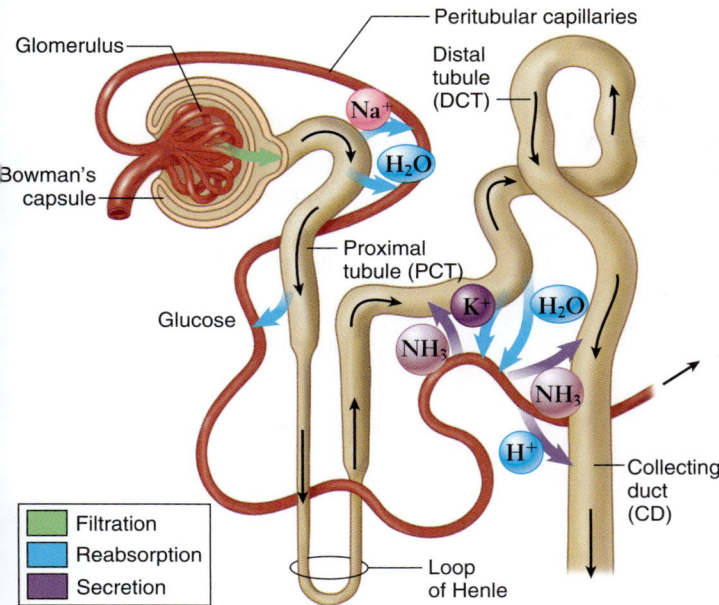

Glomerulus

Bowman's capsule

Peritubular capillaries

Distal tubule (DCT)

Proximal tubule (PCT)

Glucose

Na^+

H_2O

K^+ H_2O

NH_3

NH_3

H^+

Collecting duct (CD)

Loop of Henle

- Filtration
- Reabsorption
- Secretion

FIGURE 10-56 Formation of urine. The steps in urine formation in successive parts of a nephron are filtration, reabsorption, and secretion. (Patton KT, Thibodeau GA: *Anatomy and physiology,* ed 7, St Louis, 2007, Mosby.)

Aldosterone is a steroid hormone secreted by the adrenal gland. It passes through the circulatory system from the adrenal gland to the kidney. Aldosterone stimulates the tubules to reabsorb sodium salts and water.

Antidiuretic hormone (ADH), which is secreted by the posterior pituitary gland, tends to reduce the amount of urine produced by making distal and collecting tubules permeable to water, thus increasing water reabsorption. As a result, water is retained by the body in the presence of ADH.

Atrial natriuretic factor (ANF) is a hormone secreted from the cells in the right atrium of the heart when the pressure in the right atrium increases. This hormone inhibits ADH secretion. It also reduces the kidneys' ability to concentrate urine. As a result, the body produces a large volume of dilute urine.

Prostaglandins and *kinins* are substances formed in the kidneys that affect kidney function. These substances are believed to influence the rate of filtrate formation and sodium ion reabsorption.

Autoregulation is the ability of the kidneys to regulate a stable glomerular filtration rate over a wide range of systemic blood pressures. When small increases in glomerular capillary pressure occur, the rate of filtrate formation increases substantially. Therefore, large increases in the arterial blood pressure increase the rate of urine production. Conversely, when the arterial blood pressure decreases, urine production decreases. Through autoregulation the kidneys change the degree of constriction or dilation of the arterioles in the renal capsule to maintain glomerular

capillary pressure and urine production within normal limits over a wide range of arterial blood pressures.

Sympathetic neurons innervate the blood vessels of the kidney. The sympathetic stimulation in response to severe stress, intense exercise, or circulatory shock constricts the small arteries and the afferent arterioles. This reduces renal blood flow.

Reproductive System

Most organs and systems of the human body are the same in the male and female. However, the reproductive systems are different. The purpose of the male reproductive system is to make **spermatozoa** and to transfer the spermatozoa to the female. The purpose of the female reproductive system is to make **oocytes**. Other purposes include receiving the spermatozoa to enable fertilization, conception, gestation, and birth.

MALE REPRODUCTIVE SYSTEM

The male reproductive system consists of the testes, epididymis, ductus deferens, urethra, seminal vesicles, prostate gland, bulbourethral glands, scrotum, and penis (Figure 10-57).

The **testes** are ovoid organs in the scrotum that develop as retroperitoneal organs in the abdominopelvic cavity. The testes move from the abdominal cavity to the scrotum by way of the **inguinal canal**. This canal is common to men and women. Normally the inguinal canal is closed, but it persists as a weak spot in the abdominal wall where the testes pass through it. If the inguinal canal weakens or ruptures, an *inguinal hernia* may result.

Interstitial cells of the testes secrete the male hormone *testosterone*. Before **puberty** (12 to 14 years of age), the testes remain relatively simple and unchanged. At the time of puberty, however, the interstitial cells increase in number and size. At this time, the production of spermatozoa begins. The testes contribute about 5% of the seminal fluid **(semen)**.

The final maturation of spermatozoa occurs in the **epididymis.** This is a convoluted, comma-shaped structure on the posterior side of the testis. Infection or injury can block a single epididymis or both of them. This in turn can result in infertility.

The **ductus deferens** (also called the *vas deferens*) emerges from the tail of the epididymis. This duct ascends to the *seminal vesicle,* finally associating with the blood vessels and nerves that supply the testis. These structures and their coverings constitute the *spermatic cord.* The ductus deferens and the spermatic cord structures ascend and pass through the inguinal canal to enter the abdominal cavity. The ductus deferens crosses the lateral wall of the cavity. The duct then travels over the ureter and loops over the posterior surface of the urinary bladder to approach the prostate gland. The ductus deferens is surrounded by smooth muscle. This muscle helps propel sperm through the duct.

The **urethra** is a passageway for urine and male reproductive fluids. It can be divided into three parts: the *prostatic*

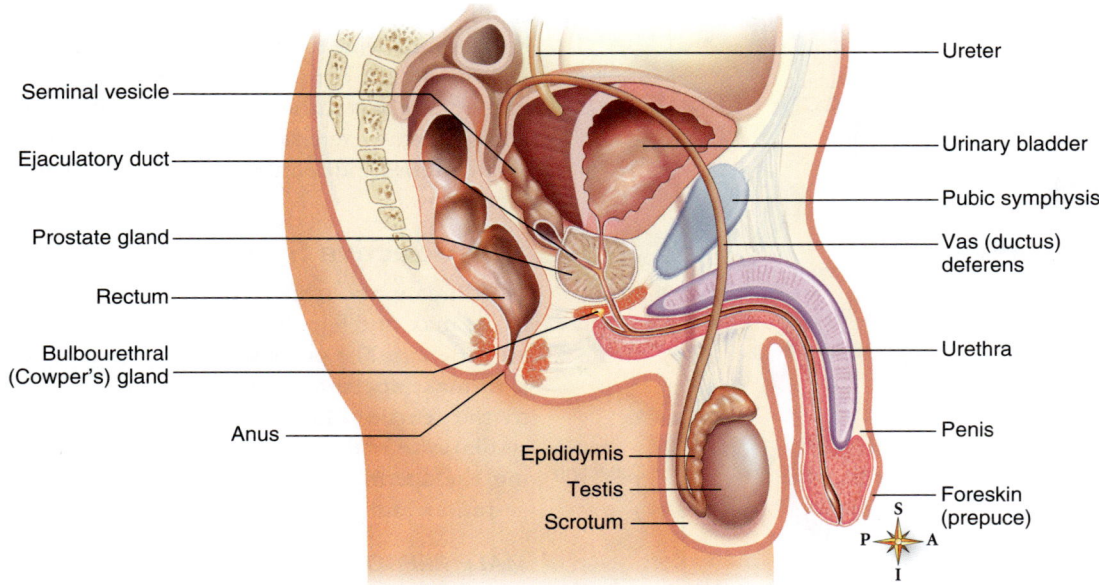

FIGURE 10-57 Sagittal section of the male pelvis. (Patton KT, Thibodeau GA: *Anatomy and physiology,* ed 7, St Louis, 2007, Mosby.)

portion (the portion that passes through the prostate gland); the *membranous portion* (which extends from the prostatic urethra through the muscular floor of the pelvis); and the *spongy portion* (which extends the length of the penis).

The **seminal vesicle** is a sac-shaped gland that lies adjacent to each ductus deferens. A short duct from the seminal vesicle joins the ductus deferens to form the *ejaculatory duct.* These ducts project into the prostate gland and end by opening into the urethra. Seminal vesicles produce about 60% of seminal fluid.

The **prostate gland** consists of glandular and muscular tissue. It is about the size and shape of a walnut. The gland is located dorsal to the symphysis pubis at the base of the bladder and surrounds the prostatic urethra and the two ejaculatory ducts. Twenty to 30 small *prostatic ducts* secrete prostatic fluid into the prostatic urethra. The prostate gland contributes about 30% of seminal fluid.

The **bulbourethral glands** are a pair of small glands located near the membranous portion of the urethra. In young adults these glands are each about the size of a pea, but they decrease in size with age. The gland is a compound mucous gland with small ducts that unite to form a single duct from each gland. The two bulbourethral glands enter the spongy urethra at the base of the penis. They add secretions to semen, contributing about 5% of seminal fluid.

The **scrotum** is divided into two internal compartments by a connective tissue septum. Beneath the skin of the scrotum is a layer of *superficial fascia* (loose connective tissue) and a layer of cutaneous muscle. This muscle is called the *dartos muscle.* The *dartos* and *cremaster muscles* of the abdomen are crucial for regulating temperature in the testes (which is required for **spermatogenesis**). They pull the testes near

the body in cold temperatures. They also allow the testes to descend away from the body in warm temperatures and during exercise.

 CRITICAL THINKING
If a patient's prostate gland is greatly enlarged by benign or malignant disease, what symptoms would you expect?

The **penis** consists of three columns of erectile tissue. Engorgement of this tissue with blood causes the penis to enlarge and become firm, producing an **erection**. The penis is the male organ of copulation and functions in the transfer of spermatozoa from the male to the female.

FEMALE REPRODUCTIVE SYSTEM

The female reproductive organs consist of the ovaries, uterine (or fallopian) tubes, uterus, vagina, external genital organs, and mammary glands. The internal reproductive organs lie within the pelvis between the urinary bladder and the rectum. These organs are held in place by a group of ligaments (Figure 10-58).

The small **ovaries** are attached to the posterior of the broad ligament called the *mesovarium.* Two other ligaments associated with the ovary are the *suspensory ligament* and the *ovarian ligament.* The ovarian arteries, veins, and nerves traverse the suspensory ligament. They enter the ovary through the mesovarium. Each ovary has a dense outer portion called the *cortex.* Each ovary also has a looser inner portion called the *medulla.* Many small vesicles, called **ovarian follicles** (each of which contains an oocyte), are distributed throughout the cortex.

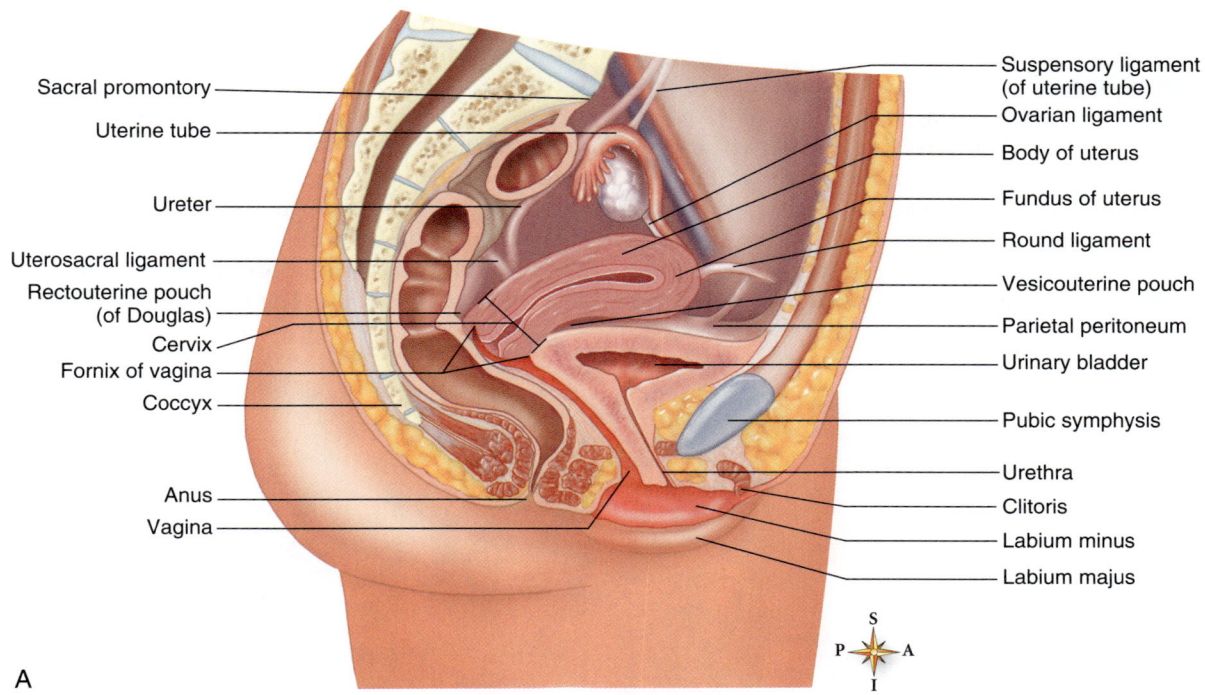

A

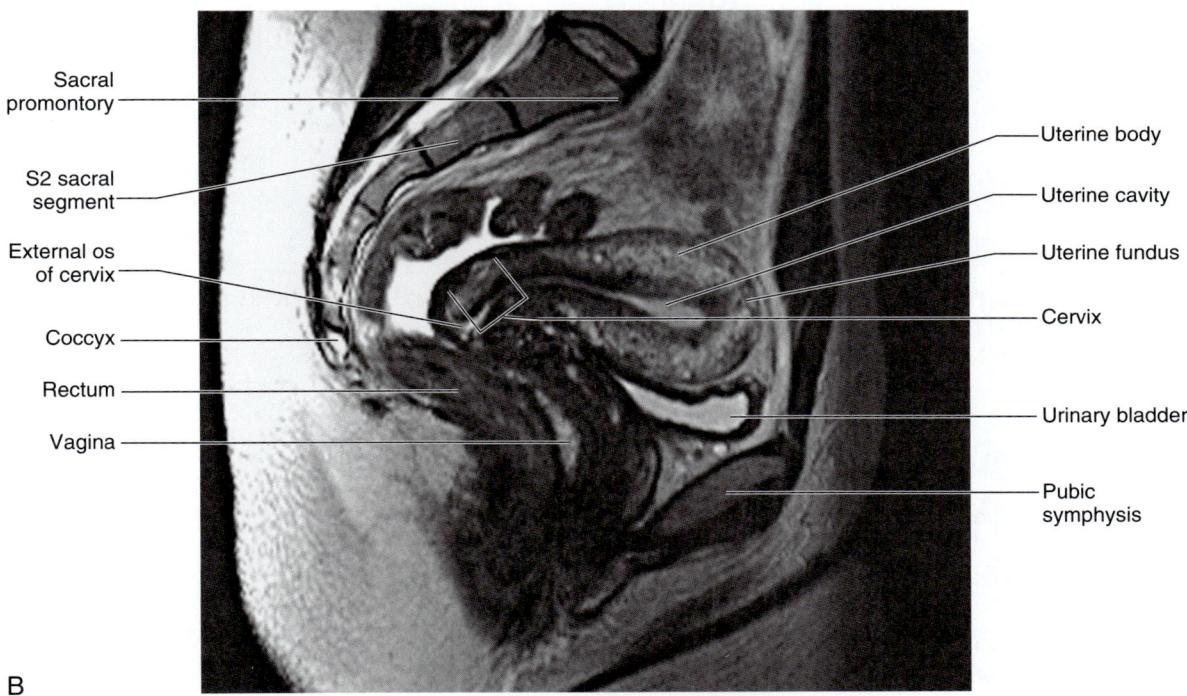

B

FIGURE 10-58 Sagittal section of the female pelvis. (Patton KT, Thibodeau GA: *Anatomy and physiology,* ed 7, St Louis, 2007, Mosby.)

The **uterine tubes** are ducts for the ovaries. Each tube is located along the superior margin of the broad ligament. Each one opens right into the peritoneal cavity to receive the oocyte. Once inside the uterine tube, the oocyte is transported by cilia and peristaltic contractions of the smooth muscle in the uterine tube.

The **uterus** is the size and shape of a medium-sized pear. It is oriented in the pelvic cavity with the larger rounded portion (the *fundus*) directed superiorly. The narrower portion, the **cervix**, is directed inferiorly. The main portion of the uterus (the *body*) is positioned between the fundus and the cervix. The major ligaments that hold the uterus in place are the *broad ligament, round ligaments,* and *uterosacral ligaments* (Figure 10-59).

The **vagina** is the female organ of copulation. It functions to receive the penis during intercourse. The vagina extends from the uterus to the outside of the body. It provides a passageway for menstrual flow and for childbirth. The smooth muscle layer of the vagina allows the organ to increase in size to accommodate the penis during intercourse and to stretch greatly during delivery. The vaginal orifice is covered by a thin mucous membrane called the

hymen. The openings in the hymen usually are enlarged during the first sexual intercourse but also may be perforated or torn during strenuous exercise.

The external genitalia is referred to as the **vulva**. The vulva consists of the vestibule and its surrounding structures (Figure 10-60). The vestibule is the space into which the vagina and urethra open. It is bordered by a pair of thin, longitudinal skin folds called the *labia minora*. A small erectile structure, called the **clitoris**, is located in the anterior margin of the vestibule. The two labia minora unite over

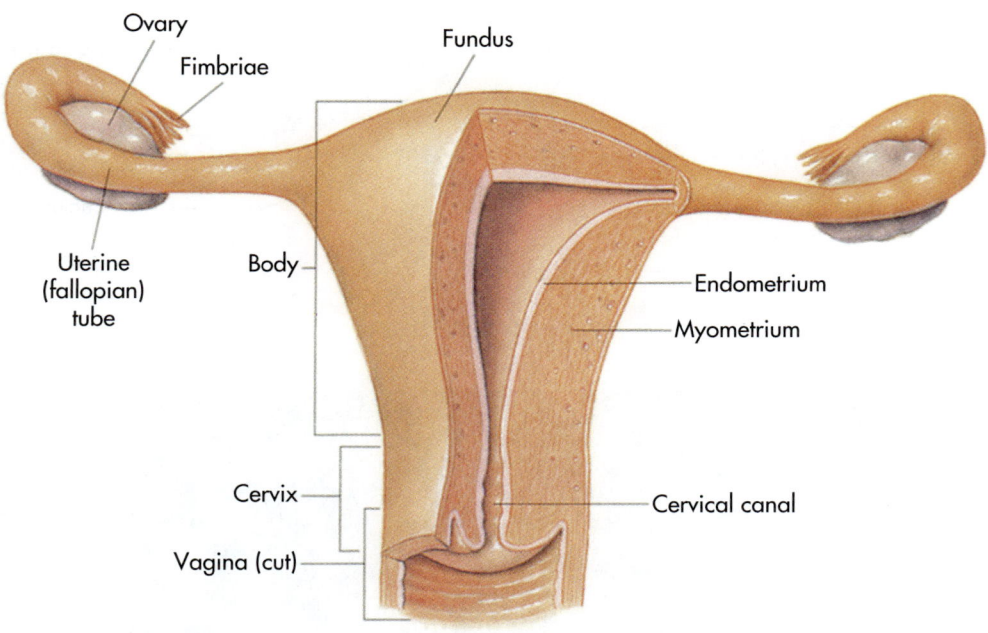

FIGURE 10-59 Internal anatomy of the female pelvis. (Thibodeau GA, Patton KT: *Structure and function of the body,* ed 13, St Louis, 2008, Mosby.)

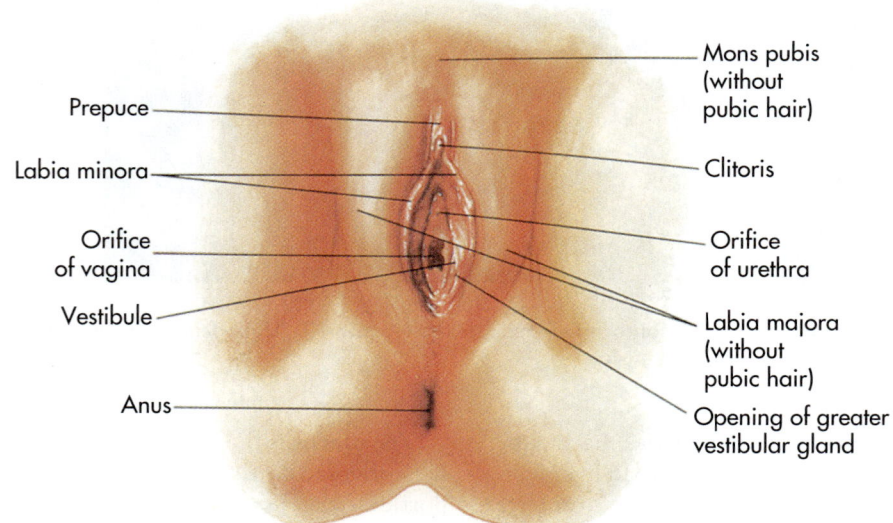

FIGURE 10-60 Female external genitalia. (Thibodeau GA, Patton KT: *Structure and function of the body,* ed 13, St Louis, 2008, Mosby.)

the clitoris to form a fold of skin known as the *prepuce*. Lateral to the labia minora are two prominent folds of skin called the *labia majora*. These folds unite anteriorly in an elevation over the pubic symphysis to form the **mons pubis**. Most of the time, the labia majora are in contact with each other. They conceal the deeper structures within the vestibule.

The **perineum** is divided into triangles by perineal muscles. The *urogenital triangle* contains the external genitalia. The posterior anal triangle contains the anal opening. The region between the vagina and the anus is called the *clinical perineum*. This area sometimes tears during childbirth.

The **mammary glands** are the organs of milk production. They are located in the breasts, or *mammae*. Externally, the breasts of males and females have a raised nipple surrounded by a circular pigmented **areola**. Nipples are sensitive to tactile stimulation. They may become erect in response to sexual arousal. The areolae normally have a slightly bumpy surface due to the presence of areolar glands just below their surface. Secretions from these glands protect the nipple and areola from chafing during nursing.

Female breasts begin to enlarge during puberty (usually between ages 12 and 13) under the effect of *estrogen* and *progesterone*. Each adult female mammary gland is made up of 15 to 20 glandular lobes covered by adipose tissue. Each lobe has a single *lactiferous duct*. This duct subdivides to form smaller ducts, each of which supplies a lobule. These ducts expand at their ends to form secretory sacs called *alveoli*. The alveoli secrete milk during nursing (Figure 10-61).

SPECIAL SENSES

Senses provide the brain with information about the outside world. Four senses are recognized as special senses: (1) *smell*, (2) *taste*, (3) *sight*, and (4) *hearing* and *balance*. (The sense of touch now is considered a general sense, which consists of several types of nerve endings scattered throughout the body and not localized to a specific area.)

Olfactory Sense Organs

The smell receptors for the fibers of the **olfactory** (first cranial) nerve lie in the mucosa of the upper part of the nasal cavity (Figure 10-62). Most of the nasal cavity is involved with respiration. Only a small part is devoted to smell.

The dendrites of olfactory neurons extend to the epithelial surface of the nasal cavity, where they form vesicles. These vesicles have long **cilia**. The cilia lie in a thin, mucous film on the epithelial surface. Olfactory cells are stimulated by molecules in the air. The resulting nerve impulses travel through the olfactory nerves in the *olfactory bulb* and *olfactory tract*. In the olfactory tract the impulses enter the thalamic and olfactory centers of the brain. In the brain the nervous impulses are interpreted as specific odors.

The exact mechanism of olfactory stimulation is not understood clearly. The range of smells is thought to be actually just a combination of seven main odors: (1) camphoraceous, (2) musky, (3) floral, (4) pepperminty, (5) ethereal, (6) pungent, and (7) putrid. Olfactory receptors are sensitive, even to slight odors. However, they also are fatigued easily. The olfactory system quickly adapts to

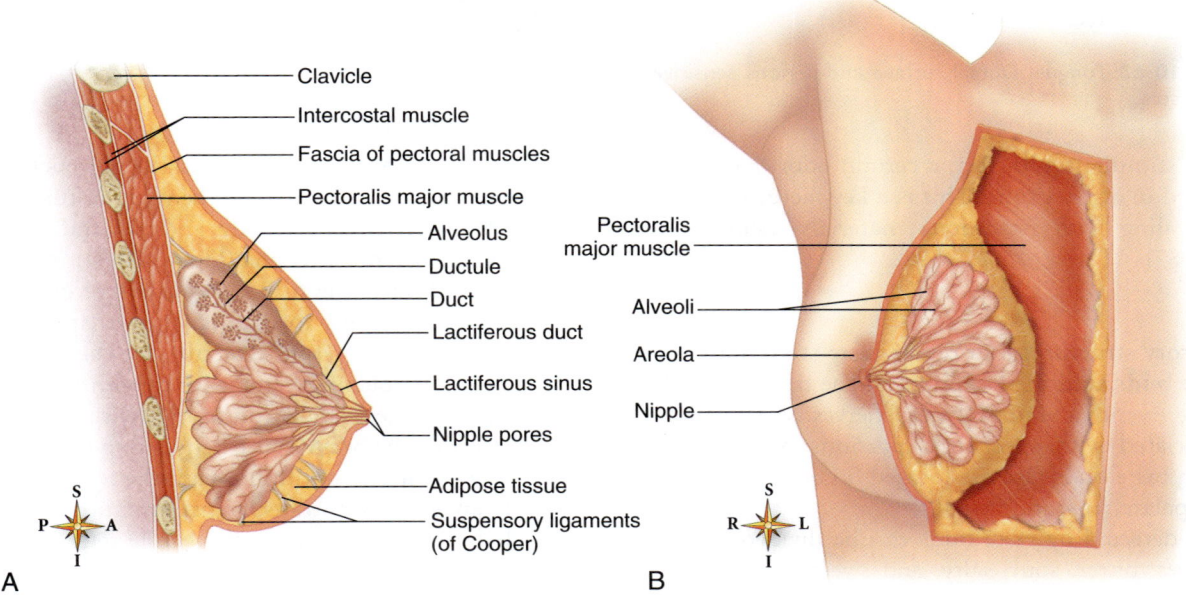

Clavicle
Intercostal muscle
Fascia of pectoral muscles
Pectoralis major muscle
Alveolus
Ductule
Duct
Lactiferous duct
Lactiferous sinus
Nipple pores
Adipose tissue
Suspensory ligaments (of Cooper)

Pectoralis major muscle
Alveoli
Areola
Nipple

A

B

FIGURE 10-61 Blood supply, mammary glands, and duct system of the right mamma. (Patton KT, Thibodeau GA: *Anatomy and physiology*, ed 7, St Louis, 2007, Mosby.)

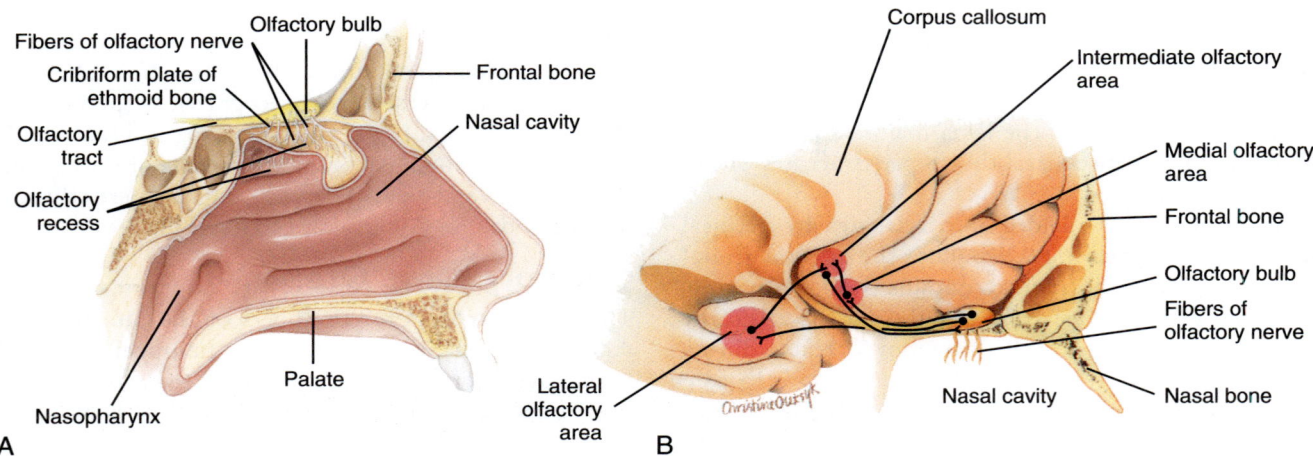

FIGURE 10-62 Olfactory structures. Gas molecules stimulate olfactory cells in the nasal epithelium. Sensory information is conducted along nerves in the olfactory bulb and olfactory tract to sensory processing centers in the brain. (McCance KL, Huether SE: *Pathophysiology: the biologic basis for disease in adults and children,* ed 5, St Louis, 2005, Mosby.)

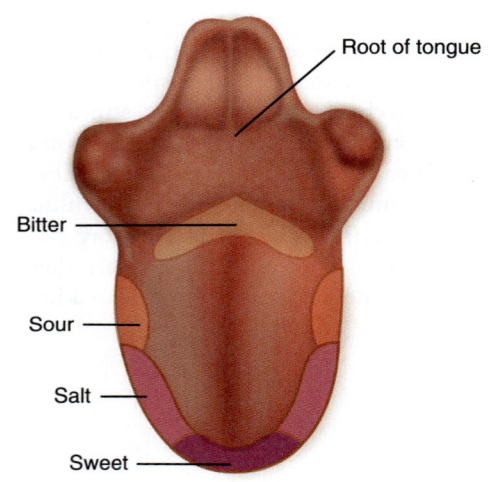

FIGURE 10-63 Tongue. Dorsal surface and regions sensitive to various tastes.

ongoing stimulation. In fact, a certain odor may cease to be noticed in a short time. This is a key factor to consider when dealing with hazardous materials incidents (see Chapter 57).

Taste

The sensory structures that detect taste stimuli are called the **taste buds**, and the receptors for the taste nerve fibers are in the seventh and ninth cranial nerves. Most taste buds are associated with specialized portions of the tongue. However, taste buds also are located on other areas of the tongue, palate, lips, and throat.

Taste detected by taste buds can be divided into four basic types: bitter, sour, salty, and sweet. The tip of the tongue reacts more strongly to sweet and salty tastes, the back of the tongue to bitter taste, and the sides of the tongue to sour taste (Figure 10-63). All the other taste sen-

sations result from a combination of taste bud and olfactory receptor stimulation.

Visual System

The visual system includes the *eyes,* the *accessory structures* (eyelids, eyebrows, eyelashes, and tear glands), and the *optic nerve, tracts,* and *pathways.* The second cranial nerve **(optic nerve)** conducts impulses from the eye to the brain. In the brain these impulses create the sensation of vision. The third cranial nerve **(oculomotor nerve)** conducts impulses from the brain to the muscles of the eye, where they cause contractions that move the eye.

> **CRITICAL THINKING**
> Why is an examination of the eyes a key part of the neurological evaluation?

ANATOMY OF THE EYE

The eye is composed of three layers: the fibrous tunic, consisting of the sclera and cornea; the vascular tunic, consisting of the choroid, ciliary body, and iris; and the nervous tunic, consisting of the retina (Figure 10-64).

1. The **sclera** is the firm, opaque, white outer layer of the eye. It helps to maintain the shape of the eye, protects the internal structures of the eye, and provides an attachment point for the muscles that move the eye. The sclera is continuous with the meningeal layers of the brain that extend along the optic nerve. The **cornea** is continuous with the sclera. The cornea is an avascular, transparent structure that permits light to enter the eye. It also bends and refracts entering light.

2. The **vascular tunic** contains most of the blood vessels of the eyeball. The part of this layer associated with the sclera is the *choroid.* Anteriorly, the vascular tunic

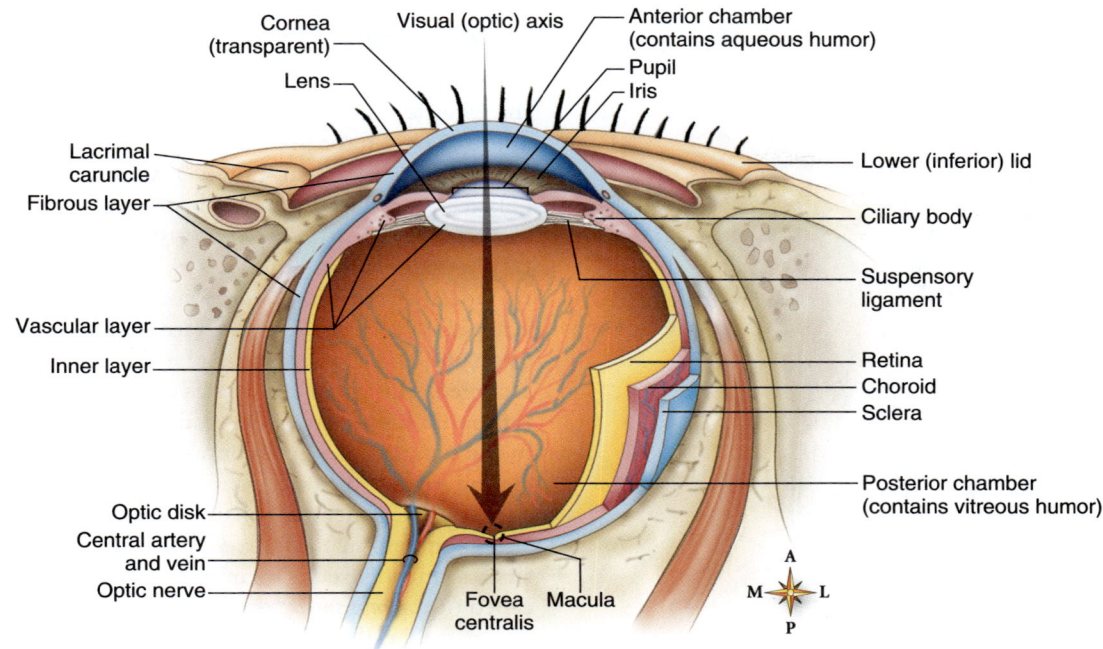

FIGURE 10-64 Horizontal section through the left eyeball. The eye is viewed from above. (Patton KT, Thibodeau GA: *Anatomy and physiology*, ed 7, St Louis, 2007, Mosby.)

consists of the *ciliary body* and the *iris*. The ciliary body consists of ciliary muscles (which can change the shape of the lens) and of complex capillaries involved in producing **aqueous humor**. The **iris** is the colored part of the eye. It consists mainly of smooth muscle that surrounds the **pupil**. Light enters through the pupil, and the iris regulates the amount of light by controlling the size of the pupil.

3. The **retina** consists of an outer pigmented retina and an inner sensory layer, which responds to light. The sensory retina contains photoreceptor cells, called *rods* and *cones,* and numerous relay neurons. Rods are the receptors for night vision. Cones are the receptors for daytime and color vision.

COMPARTMENTS OF THE EYE

The two compartments of the eye are separated by a **lens**. The lens is suspended between the two eye compartments by ligaments. These two compartments are known as the *anterior* and *posterior chambers*. The anterior chamber is filled with *aqueous humor*. This helps maintain **intraocular pressure** (pressure within the eye that keeps the eye expanded), refract light, and provide nutrition for the anterior chamber.

The posterior chamber of the eye is surrounded almost completely by the retina. The chamber is filled with a transparent, jelly-like substance called **vitreous humor**. Like aqueous humor, the vitreous humor helps maintain intraocular pressure. In addition, the fluid helps to hold the retina in place and functions in the refraction of light in the eye.

ACCESSORY STRUCTURES OF THE EYE

The accessory structures of the eye protect, lubricate, move, and aid in the function of the eye. These structures include the eyebrows, eyelids, conjunctivae, and lacrimal gland.

Eyebrows protect the eyes by providing shade from direct sunlight. They also prevent perspiration from running into the eyes.

Eyelids protect the eyes from foreign objects. Blinking, which normally occurs about 25 times per minute, helps lubricate the eyes by spreading tears over their surfaces. Eyelids also help regulate the amount of light entering the eyes.

The **conjunctiva** is a thin, transparent mucous membrane. It covers the inner surface of the eyelids and the outer surface of the sclera.

The **lacrimal gland** makes lacrimal fluid (tears) that leaves the gland through several ducts, passing over the anterior surface of the eyeball. The gland is in the superolateral corner of the orbit. The gland makes tears to moisten the surface of the eye, lubricate the eyelids, and wash away foreign objects. Tears also contain lysosomes that destroy some forms of bacteria.

Most tears evaporate from the surface of the eye. Excess fluid is collected in the medial corner of the eye by the lacrimal canals through a *punctum* (the opening of each canal). The lacrimal canals open into a *lacrimal sac.* This sac in turn continues into the *nasolacrimal duct* (Figure 10-65).

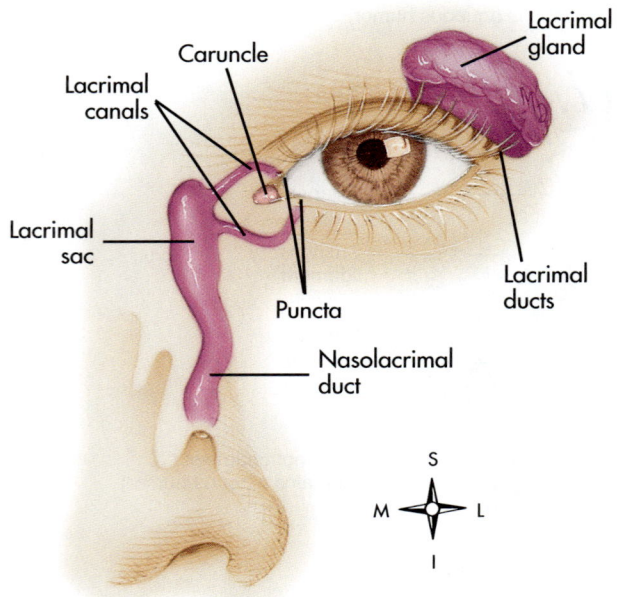

FIGURE 10-65 Lacrimal structures of the eye. (McCance KL, Huether SE: *Pathophysiology: the biologic basis for disease in adults and children,* ed 5, St Louis 2005, Mosby.)

Hearing and Balance

The organs of hearing can be divided into three portions: the external ear, the middle ear, and the inner ear (Figure 10-66). The external ear and middle ear are involved only in hearing. The inner ear, however, functions in hearing and balance. The special senses of hearing and balance are transmitted by the *vestibulocochlear nerve* (eighth cranial nerve).

The **external ear** includes the *auricle,* or *pinna.* It also includes the *external auditory meatus,* which opens into the *external auditory canal.* The external auditory canal is lined by hairs and ceruminous glands. These glands make cerumen. This canal terminates medially at the eardrum, or **tympanic membrane**. The middle ear is an air-filled space in the temporal bone. It contains the auditory ossicles.

The **inner ear** holds the sensory organs for hearing and balance. The inner ear consists of interconnecting tunnels and chambers in the *bony labyrinth.* Inside the bony labyrinth is another set of membranous tunnels and chambers called the *membranous labyrinth.* This labyrinth is filled with a clear fluid called *endolymph.* The space between the membranous and bony labyrinths is filled with a fluid called *perilymph.* These fluids are similar to cerebrospinal fluid.

The **auricle** is shaped to collect sound waves. It directs sound waves toward the external auditory meatus. From the meatus, sound waves travel through the auditory canal

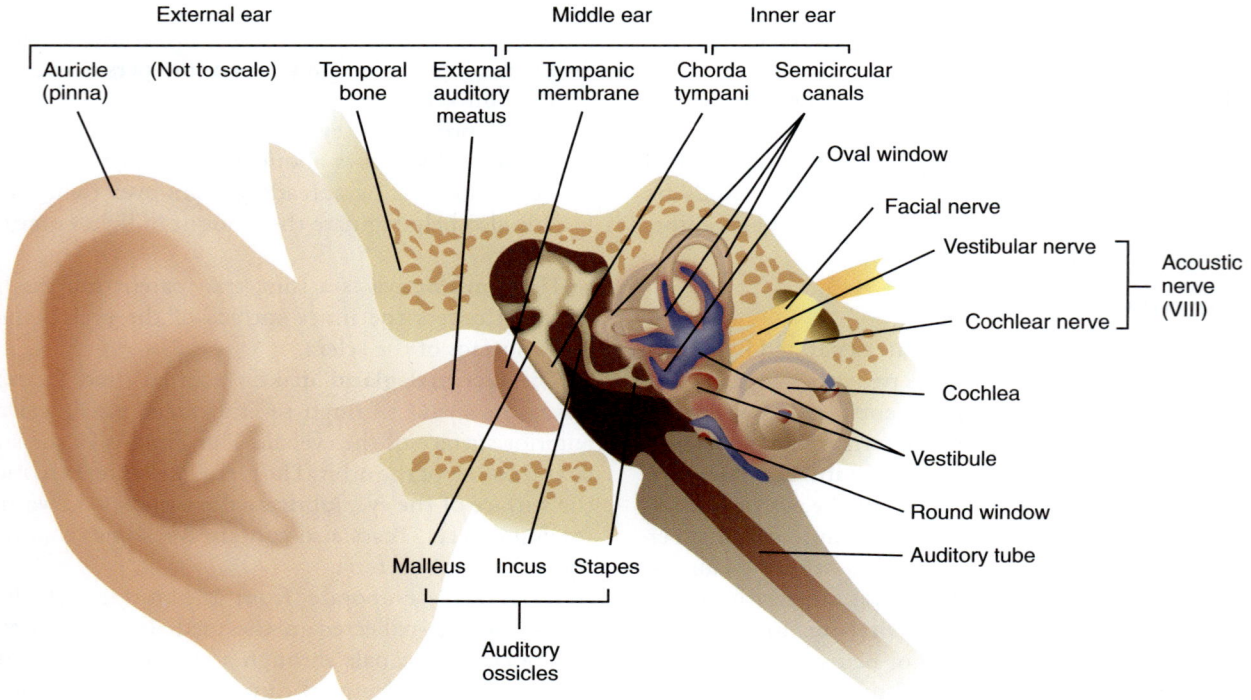

FIGURE 10-66 External, middle, and inner ear.

to the tympanic membrane, causing the membrane to vibrate.

The **middle ear** is connected to the inner ear by two membrane-covered openings. These are the *round window* and the *oval window*. Two other openings that are not covered by membranes offer a passageway for air from the middle ear. One opens into the *mastoid air cells*. The second opening, the auditory (or eustachian) tube, opens into the pharynx. The **eustachian tube** allows the equalization of air pressure between the outside air and the middle ear cavity. (Children have shorter eustachian tubes. Consequently, bacteria can travel more easily from infected areas in the throat to the middle ear. This difference between children and adults is responsible for the increased frequency of earaches and ear infections in children.) The auditory ossicles of the middle ear (called the *malleus, incus,*

and *stapes*) transmit vibrations from the tympanic membrane to the oval window.

CRITICAL THINKING

Besides pain and impaired hearing, what other symptom would you look for in a patient with an inner ear problem?

The **bony labyrinth** of the inner ear is divided into three regions. These are called the *vestibule,* the *cochlea,* and the *semicircular canals*. The vestibule and semicircular canals are involved primarily in balance. The cochlea is involved in hearing. The hearing sense organ, which lies inside the cochlea, is called the *organ of Corti*. In young, healthy individuals, the frequencies that can be detected by the ear range (over octaves) from 20 to 20,000 cycles per second.

SUMMARY

- The paramedic must understand human anatomy fully. This understanding helps the paramedic organize a patient assessment by body region. Knowledge of anatomy also helps the paramedic communicate well with medical direction and other members of the health care team.
- The anatomical position refers to a person standing erect with the feet and palms facing the examiner.
- Directional terms are expressed in anatomical terminology. Examples of these are *up* or *down* (superior or inferior) *front* or *back* (anterior or posterior), and *right* or *left*. These terms always refer to the patient, not the examiner. Internal body structure is classified into anatomical planes of the human body. These planes can be thought of as imaginary straight-line divisions.
- The appendicular region of the body includes the limbs, or extremities. The axial region consists of the head, neck, thorax, and abdomen.
- The abdomen usually is divided into four quadrants: upper right, lower right, upper left, and lower left.
- The three major cavities of the human body are the thoracic cavity, the abdominal cavity, and the pelvic cavity.
- The thoracic cavity contains the trachea, esophagus, thymus, heart, great vessels, lungs, and the cavities and membranes that surround them. The abdominopelvic cavity is surrounded by membranes and contains organs and blood vessels.
- The cytoplasmic membrane encloses the cytoplasm. The membrane forms the outer boundary of the cell.
- Cytoplasm lies between the cytoplasmic membrane and the nucleus. Specialized structures in the cell (organelles) are located in the cytoplasm. These organelles perform functions that are vital to the cell's survival. The nucleus is a large, membrane-bound organelle. It ultimately controls all other organelles in the cytoplasm.

- All human cells, except for the reproductive (sex) cells, reproduce by a process known as *mitosis*. In this process, cells divide to multiply.
- Four main types of tissue make up the many organs of the body: epithelial tissue, connective tissue, muscle tissue, and nervous tissue. Epithelial tissue covers surfaces and forms structures. Connective tissue is made of cells separated from each other by intercellular material. This material is known as the *extracellular matrix*. Muscle tissue is contractile tissue and is responsible for movement. Nervous tissue has the ability to conduct electrical signals, known as *action potentials*.
- A *system* is a group of organs arranged to perform a more complex function than any one organ can perform alone. The eleven major organ systems in the body are the integumentary, skeletal, muscular, nervous, endocrine, circulatory, lymphatic, respiratory, digestive, urinary, and reproductive systems.
- The integumentary system consists of the skin and accessory structures such as the hair, nails, and a variety of glands. The functions of the integumentary system include protecting the body against injury and dehydration, defending against infection, and regulating temperature.
- The skeletal system consists of bone and associated connective tissues, including cartilage, tendons, and ligaments. The skeletal system provides a rigid framework for support and protection. It also provides a system of levers on which muscles act to produce body movements.
- The three primary functions of the muscular system are movement, postural maintenance, and heat production.
- The nervous system and the endocrine system are the major regulatory and coordinating systems of the body. The nervous system rapidly sends information. It does

Continued

this by means of nerve impulses conducted from one area of the body to another. The endocrine system sends information more slowly. It does this by means of chemicals secreted by ductless glands into the bloodstream.

- The heart and cardiovascular system are responsible for circulating blood throughout the body. Blood performs many important functions: it transports nutrients and oxygen to tissues; it carries carbon dioxide and waste products away from tissues; it carries hormones produced in endocrine glands to their target tissues; it plays a key role in temperature regulation and fluid balance; and it protects the body from bacteria and foreign substances.
- The lymphatic system is made up of lymph, lymphocytes, lymph nodes, tonsils, spleen, and thymus gland. The lymphatic system has three basic functions: to help maintain fluid balance in tissues; to absorb fats and other substances from the digestive tract; and to play a role in the body's immune defense system.
- The organs of the respiratory system and the cardiovascular system move oxygen to cells. They move carbon dioxide from cells to the locations where it is released into the air. The entrance to the respiratory tract begins at the nasal cavity and includes the nasopharynx, oropharynx, laryngopharynx, and larynx. Below the glottis are the structures of the lower airway and lungs. These structures include the trachea, bronchial tree, alveoli, and lungs.

- The digestive system provides the body with water, electrolytes, and other nutrients used by cells. The gastrointestinal tract is an irregularly shaped tube. Associated accessory organs (mainly glands) secrete fluid into the digestive tract.
- The urinary system works with other body systems to maintain homeostasis. It does this by removing waste products from the blood. It also does this by helping to maintain a constant body fluid volume and composition. The urinary system comprises two kidneys, two ureters, the urinary bladder, and the urethra.
- The purpose of the male reproductive system is to make and transfer spermatozoa to the female. The purpose of the female reproductive system is to make oocytes and to receive the spermatozoa for fertilization, conception, gestation, and birth. The male reproductive system consists of the testes, epididymis, ductus deferens, urethra, seminal vesicles, prostate gland, bulbourethral glands, scrotum, and penis. The female reproductive organs consist of the ovaries, uterine (or fallopian) tubes, uterus, vagina, external genital organs, and mammary glands.
- Senses provide the brain with information about the outside world. Four senses are recognized as special senses: smell, taste, sight, and hearing and balance.

REFERENCES

1. Seidel HM, et al: *Mosby's guide to physical examination*, ed 6, St. Louis, 2006, Mosby.
2. Patton KT, Thibodeau GA: *Anatomy and physiology*, ed 7, St. Louis, 2010, Mosby.
3. Seeley RR, et al: *Anatomy & physiology*, ed 9, Columbus, Ohio, 2010, McGraw-Hill.
4. Snell RS, Smith MS: *Clinical anatomy of emergency medicine*, St. Louis, 1993, Mosby. 1993

SUGGESTED READINGS

Get Body Smart: www.getbodysmart.com/.

Gould B, Dyer R: Pathophysiology for the health professions, ed 4, St Louis, 2011, Mosby.

McCance K, Huether S: Pathophysiology: the biologic basis for disease in adults and children, ed 6, St Louis, 2010, Mosby.

US Cancer Institute's Surveillance, Epidemiology and End Results (SEER) Program: http://training.seer.cancer.gov/module_anatomy/unit1_1_body_structure.html#.

11 General Principles of Pathophysiology

Upon completion of this chapter, the paramedic student will be able to:

1. Describe the normal characteristics of the cellular environment and the key homeostatic mechanisms that strive to maintain an optimal fluid and electrolyte balance.
2. Outline pathophysiological alterations in water and electrolyte balance and list their effects on body functions.
3. Describe the treatment of patients with particular fluid or electrolyte imbalances.
4. Describe the mechanisms in the body that maintain normal acid-base balance.
5. Outline pathophysiological alterations in acid-base balance.
6. Describe the management of a patient with an acid-base imbalance.
7. Describe the changes in cells and tissues that occur with cellular adaptation, injury, neoplasia, aging, or death.
8. Outline the effects of cellular injury on local and systemic body functions.
9. Describe changes in body functions that can occur as a result of genetic and familial disease factors.
10. Outline the causes, adverse systemic effects, and compensatory mechanisms associated with hypoperfusion.
11. Describe the ways in which the inflammatory and immune mechanisms respond to cellular injury or antigenic stimulation.
12. Explain how changes in immune status and the presence of inflammation can adversely affect body functions.
13. Describe the impact of stress on the body's response to illness or injury.
14. Describe factors that influence disease.

KEY TERMS

acid A compound that yields hydrogen ions when dissociated in solution.

acid-base balance The body's balance between acidity and alkalinity.

acidosis A condition marked by a high concentration of hydrogen ions (i.e., a pH below 7.35).

active transport A carrier-mediated process that can move substances against a concentration gradient.

aerobic Of or pertaining to the presence of air or oxygen.

afterload The total resistance against which blood must be pumped; also known as peripheral vascular resistance.

aldosterone A steroid hormone produced by the adrenal cortex to regulate the sodium and potassium balance in the blood.

alkalosis A condition marked by a low concentration of hydrogen ions (i.e., a pH above 7.45).

allergens Substances that can produce hypersensitivity reactions in the body.

allergy A hypersensitivity reaction to intrinsically harmless antigens, most of which are environmental.

alpha-adrenergic receptor Any one of the postulated adrenergic components of receptor tissues that responds to norepinephrine and to various blocking agents.

ammonium ion The monovalent cation NH_4.

anaerobic Of or pertaining to the absence of oxygen.

anaphylaxis An exaggerated, life-threatening hypersensitivity reaction to a previously encountered antigen.

angiotensin I The inactive form of angiotensin, formulated by the stimulation of renin, which is converted to angiotensin II.

angiotensin II A potent vasoconstrictor that also acts to stimulate the secretion of antidiuretic hormone.

angiotensin-converting enzyme A circulating enzyme that participates in the body's renin-angiotensin system, which mediates extracellular volume and arterial vasoconstriction.

anion An ion with a negative charge.

antibody A substance produced by the body that destroys or inactivates a specific substance (antigen) that has entered the body.

antigens Substances (usually proteins) that cause the formation of an antibody and that react specifically with that antibody.

anuria The inability to urinate; the cessation of urine production; a diminished urinary output of less than 100 to 250 mL per day.

areflexia A neurological condition characterized by the absence of reflexes.

arteriovenous anastomosis A vessel that allows blood to flow from arteries to veins without passing through capillaries; also known as an *arteriovenous shunt*.

ascites An abnormal intraperitoneal accumulation of fluid containing large amounts of protein and electrolytes.

atherosclerosis A common arterial disorder characterized by yellowish plaques of cholesterol, lipids, and cellular debris in the inner layers of the walls of large and medium-sized arteries.

atrial natriuretic factor A peptide released from the atria when atrial blood pressure is increased; it lowers blood pressure by increasing urine production, thus reducing blood volume.

atrophy Decrease in size (shrinkage) of a cell, which adversely affects cell function.

autoimmunity An abnormal characteristic or condition in which the body reacts against constituents of its own tissues.

autolysis The spontaneous disintegration of tissues or cells by the action of their own autogenous enzymes.

B lymphocytes The lymphocytes responsible for antibody-mediated immunity.

base A chemical compound that combines with an acid to form a salt; also known as an alkali.

beta-adrenergic receptor Any of the postulated adrenergic components of receptor tissues that respond to epinephrine and various blocking agents.

bivalent cation An ion with two positive charges.

botulism An often fatal form of food poisoning caused by the bacillus *Clostridium botulinum*.

capillaries Tiny vessels that connect arterioles to venules.

capillary network A complex, interconnected structure where a single blood cell traveling from an arteriole to a venule via a capillary bed passes through capillary segments.

capsid A protein coat that encloses a virus.

carbonic acid An aqueous solution of carbon dioxide.

carbonic anhydrase The enzyme that converts carbon dioxide into carbonic acid.

cardiac output The volume of blood pumped each minute by the ventricles.

carrier molecule A protein that combines with solutes on one side of a membrane, transporting the solute to the other side; it is used in mediated transport mechanisms.

cathartic A substance that accelerates defecation.

cation An ion with a positive charge.

central nervous system ischemic response An increase in blood pressure caused by vasoconstriction that occurs when oxygen levels are too low, carbon dioxide levels are too high, or pH is too low in the medulla.

chemotactic factors Biochemical mediators that are important in activating the inflammatory response.

complement system A group of proteins that coat bacteria; the proteins then either help kill the bacteria directly or assist neutrophils (in the blood) and macrophages (in the tissues) to engulf and destroy the bacteria.

congenital Present at birth.

cortisol A steroid hormone that occurs naturally in the body.

cytochromes Proteins in the liver that play a role in drug detoxification.

dehydration An excessive loss of water from the body tissues; it may follow prolonged fever, diarrhea, vomiting, acidosis, and other conditions.

diabetes mellitus A complex disorder of carbohydrate, fat, and protein metabolism that primarily results from partial or complete lack of insulin secretion by the beta cells of the pancreas or occurs because of defects in the insulin receptors.

diffusion The process by which solid, particulate matter in a fluid moves from an area of higher concentration to an area of lower concentration, resulting in an even distribution of the particles in the fluid.

dysplasia Abnormal cellular growth.

dysrhythmia Variation from a normal rhythm.

edema The accumulation of fluid in the interstitial spaces.

endotoxin A toxin contained in the cell walls of some microorganisms, especially gram-negative bacteria.

exotoxin A toxin secreted or excreted by a living organism.

extracellular fluid The fluid found outside the cells, including that in the intravascular and interstitial compartments.

facilitated diffusion A carrier-mediated process that moves substances into or out of cells from a high to a low concentration.

glycolysis An anaerobic process during which glucose is converted to pyruvic acid.

hemodialysis A procedure in which impurities or wastes are removed from the blood; it is used in treating renal insufficiency and various toxic conditions.

hemoglobin A complex protein-iron compound in the blood that carries oxygen to the cells from the lungs and carbon dioxide away from the cells to the lungs.

hydrogen ion The acidic element in a solution.

hypercalcemia A higher than normal concentration of calcium in the blood.

hyperkalemia A higher than normal concentration of potassium in the blood.

hypermagnesemia A higher than normal concentration of magnesium in the blood.

hypernatremic A term describing a higher than normal concentration of sodium in the blood.

hypernatremic dehydration The loss of more water than sodium.

hyperphosphatemia High levels of alkaline phosphate in the blood.

hyperplasia An excessive increase in the number of cells.

hypersensitivity reaction An altered immunological response to an antigen that results in a pathological immune response upon reexposure.

hypertonic A term used to describe a solution that causes cells to shrink.

hypertrophy An increase in the size of a cell.

hypokalemia A lower than normal concentration of potassium in the blood.

hypomagnesemia A lower than normal concentration of magnesium in the blood plasma.

hyponatremic A term describing a lower than normal concentration of sodium in the blood.

hyponatremic dehydration The loss of more sodium than water.

hypoperfusion Severely inadequate circulation that results in insufficient delivery of oxygen and nutrients necessary for normal tissue and cellular function; also known as shock.

hypophosphatemia Low levels of alkaline phosphate in the blood.

hypotonic A term used to describe a solution that causes cells to swell.

hypotonicity of the muscles Decreased muscle tone or tension.

hypoxemia A lower than normal oxygen content of the blood as measured in an arterial blood sample.

immune response A defense function of the body that produces antibodies to destroy invading antigens and malignancies.

infarction Cell death.

inflammatory response A tissue reaction to injury or to an antigen; it may include pain, swelling, itching, redness, heat, and loss of function.

interstitial fluid Fluid that occupies the space outside the blood vessels and/or outside the cells of an organ or tissue.

intracellular fluid The fluid found in all body cells.

ischemia A state of insufficient perfusion of oxygenated blood to a body organ or part.

isoimmunity An immune response directed against beneficial foreign tissues.

isotonic A term used to describe a solution that causes cells neither to shrink nor to swell.

isotonic dehydration Excessive loss of sodium and water in equal amounts.

ketone bodies The normal metabolic products of lipid and pyruvate within the liver; excessive production leads to their excretion in urine.

Krebs cycle A sequence of enzymatic reactions involving the metabolism of carbon chains of sugar, fatty acids, and amino acids to yield carbon dioxide, water, and high-energy phosphate bonds.

lactate A salt of lactic acid.

lactic acidosis A disorder characterized by an accumulation of lactic acid in the blood, resulting in a lowered pH in muscle and serum.

leukocytosis An abnormal increase in the number of circulating white blood cells.

malaise A vague feeling of weakness or discomfort.

mast cells Specialized cells of the inflammatory response.

mediated transport mechanisms Mechanisms that use carrier molecules to move large, water-soluble molecules or electrically charged molecules across cell membranes.

membrane permeability A quality of cell membranes that permits the passage of solvents and solutes into and out of cells.

metaplasia A change from one cell type to another that is better able to tolerate adverse conditions; a conversion into a form that is not normal for that cell.

metarteriole One of the small peripheral blood vessels that contain scattered groups of smooth muscle fibers in their walls; they are located between the arterioles and the true capillaries.

multiple organ dysfunction syndrome The progressive failure of two or more organ systems after a severe illness or injury.

necrosis Death of a cell or group of cells as the result of disease or injury.

negative feedback mechanisms Mechanisms that tend to produce a response that balances a change in a system.

neoplasia New and abnormal development of cells, which may be benign or malignant.

nonelectrolyte A substance with no electrical charge.

oliguria A diminished capacity to form or pass urine.

osmolality The osmotic pressure of a solution.

osmosis The diffusion of solvent (water) through a membrane from a less concentrated solution to a more concentrated solution.

osmotic pressure The force required to prevent the movement of water across a selectively permeable membrane.

overhydration Water excess or water intoxication.

paresthesia A sensation of numbness, tingling, or "pins and needles."

partial pressure The pressure exerted by a single gas.

pathophysiology The abnormal functions and diseases of the human body.

peripheral vascular resistance The total resistance against which blood must be pumped; also known as afterload.

pH An inverse logarithm of the hydrogen ion concentration.

phagocytosis The process of ingestion by cells of solid substances such as other cells, bacteria, bits of necrosed tissue, and foreign particles.

pitting edema Observable indentation of body tissues that persists after applying pressure to an area swollen from fluid accumulation.

polyuria Excessive secretion of urine.

postcapillary sphincter The smooth muscle sphincter at the venous end of a capillary that regulates blood flow through the capillary.

precapillary sphincter The smooth muscle sphincter at the arterial end of a capillary that regulates blood flow through the capillary.

preload The amount of blood returning to the ventricle.

renin A proteolytic enzyme that surrounds each arteriole as it enters a glomerulus; it affects blood pressure by catalyzing the change of angiotensin I to angiotensin II.

respiratory acidosis An abnormal condition characterized by an increased arterial P_{CO_2}, excess carbonic acid, and an increased plasma hydrogen ion concentration.

respiratory alkalosis An abnormal condition characterized by decreased P_{CO_2}, decreased hydrogen ion concentration, and increased blood pH.

Rh factor An antigenic substance present in the erythrocytes of most persons; a person lacking the Rh factor is Rh negative.

semipermeable membrane A membrane that allows some fluids and substances to pass through it but not others, usually dependent on size, shape, electrical charge, or other chemical properties of the substance or fluid.

shock A condition of severely inadequate blood flow to the body's peripheral tissues that is associated with

life-threatening cellular dysfunction; also known as hypoperfusion.

solutes Substances dissolved in solution.

Starling hypothesis The concept that describes the movement of fluid across the capillary wall (net filtration).

stroke volume The volume of blood ejected from one ventricle in a single heartbeat.

T lymphocytes The lymphocytes responsible for cell-mediated immunity.

tetany The involuntary contraction of skeletal muscles.

toxic shock syndrome A severe, acute disease caused by infection with strains of *Staphylococcus aureus*.

toxoid A toxin that has been treated with chemicals or with heat to reduce its toxic effects but that retains its antigenic power.

virulence The relative strength of a pathogen.

Chapter 10 described anatomy and physiology—the structure and function of the human body. This chapter discusses pathophysiology—the abnormal functions and diseases of the human body. Paramedics need to understand the physical and biological principles of disease. This will help them to anticipate, direct, and provide appropriate care to their patients.

 NOTE
This chapter is intended to provide an introduction and overview of pathophysiology. Additional discussions of disease processes are presented throughout this textbook as indicated by subject matter.

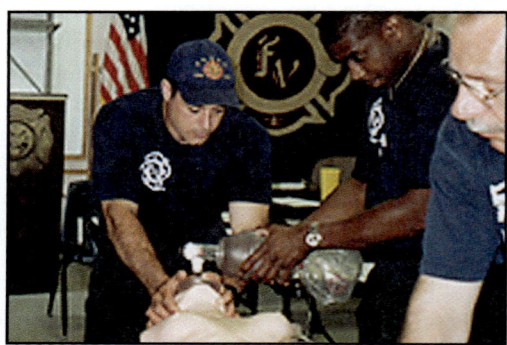

(Courtesy Kim McKenna, St. Charles, Mo.)

 LOOK AGAIN
See Chapter 10: Review of Human Systems, pp. 151-155.

SECTION ONE
Cellular Physiology

BASIC CELLULAR REVIEW

As discussed in Chapter 10, the cell is the basic unit of higher life forms. All cells have various key components and structures. These include *cell membranes,* membranes that isolate individual cells and separate each cell's internal (cellular) environment from its external environment, and *enzymes,* proteins that mediate biochemical processes. Other key components and structures are the *internal membranes* that encapsulate chemicals, and the genetic material for replication. Cells form the four basic types of tissue:

- Epithelial tissue
- Connective tissue (including hematological tissue)
- Muscle tissue
- Nervous tissue

CELLULAR ENVIRONMENT

The cells of the human body live in a fluid environment that consists mainly of water. Body water is essential for two reasons. First, it is the medium in which all metabolic reactions occur. Second, the body's health depends on precise regulation of the volume and composition of this fluid. The body has two fluid compartments: the intracellular fluid and the extracellular fluid (Figure 11-1).

Intracellular and Extracellular Fluid

Intracellular fluid (ICF) is the fluid found inside all body cells. It accounts for 40% of total body weight. **Extracellular fluid** (ECF) is the fluid found outside the cells. This includes the intravascular and interstitial compartments. ECF accounts for about 20% of total body weight, with the intravascular component (blood plasma) composing about

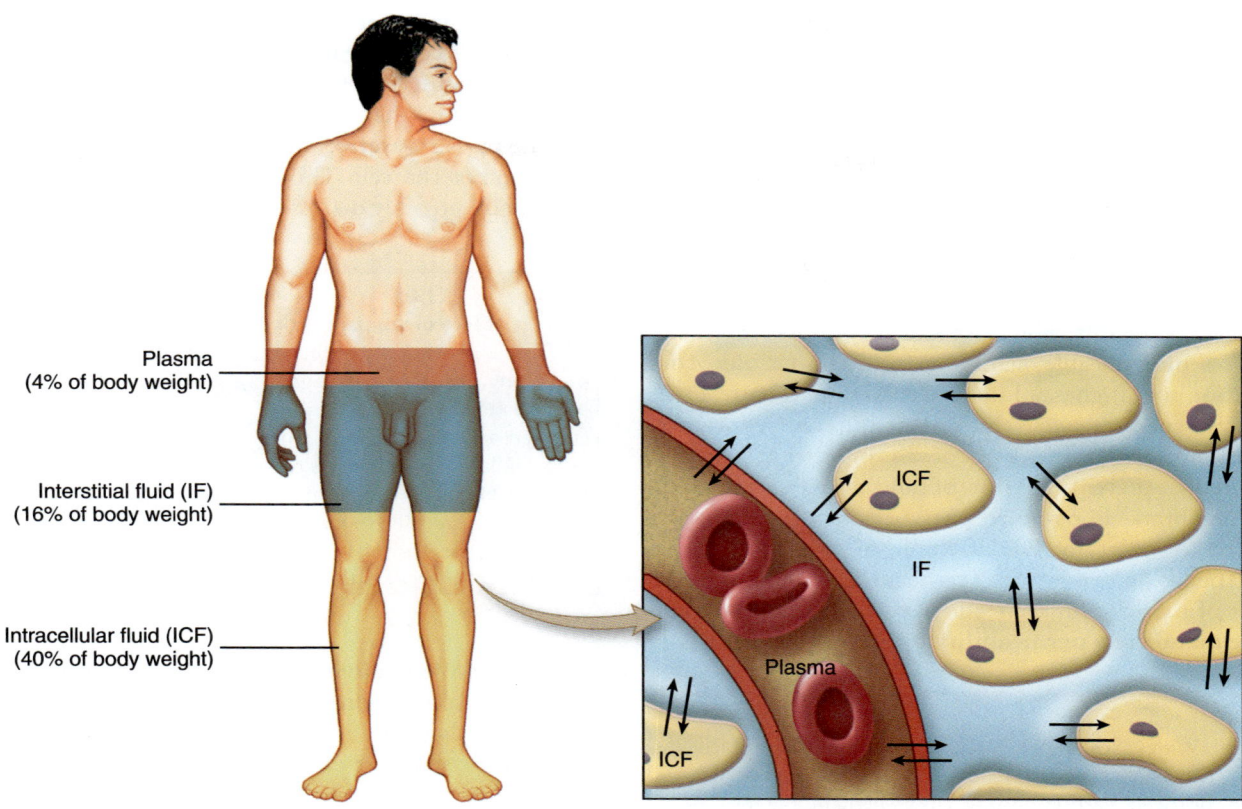

FIGURE 11-1 Fluid compartments of the body.

Plasma
(4% of body weight)

Interstitial fluid (IF)
(16% of body weight)

Intracellular fluid (ICF)
(40% of body weight)

one third. The extracellular fluid between the cells and outside the vascular bed (i.e., connective tissue, cartilage, and bone) is known as **interstitial fluid** (IF). This category also includes special fluids, such as cerebrospinal fluid and intraocular fluid. The IF accounts for about 15% to 16% of total body weight.

Aging and the Distribution of Body Fluids

Body mass consists mainly of water. In fact, water accounts for 50% to 60% of total body weight in adults. The distribution and amount of total body water (TBW) vary according to age. For example, about 80% of a newborn infant's body weight is TBW. During childhood, TBW decreases to 60% to 65% of body weight, and it declines further with age (Table 11-1). TBW in the elderly decreases to 45% to 55%, increasing the risk of dehydration and electrolyte abnormalities (see Chapter 49).

> **NOTE**
> In older adults the normal reduction in total body water (TBW) becomes a significant factor if fever or dehydration is present. With illness or injury, loss of body fluids can be severe or life-threatening.

TABLE 11-1 Total Body Water (TBW) Relative to Body Type

Body Build	Adult Male (% TBW)	Adult Female (% TBW)	Infant (% TBW)
Normal	60	50	70
Lean	70	60	80
Obese	50	42	60

From McCance KL, Huether SE: *Pathophysiology: the biologic basis for disease in adults and children,* ed 6, St Louis, 2010, Mosby.

Water Movement Between Intracellular Fluid and Extracellular Fluid

Body fluids constantly move from one compartment to another. In healthy individuals, the volume in each compartment remains about the same. To keep the volume stable, the body uses **osmosis, diffusion,** and **mediated transport mechanisms.** To understand illness and disease, the paramedic first must understand how fluids in the body move and how changes in these fluids can occur.

OSMOSIS

For the body to function well, molecules must be able to move within a cell or across cell membranes. Membranes separate fluid compartments. Most of these membranes allow water to pass freely. They also regulate the flow of **solutes** (substances dissolved in solution) on the basis of size, shape, electrical charge, or other chemical properties. These membranes are referred to as **semipermeable membranes.** *Channels* in these membranes permit the passage of solutes. The channels may be open at all times to specific solutes, or they may be closed at times, depending on the cell's composition. Because the cell membrane can regulate the flow of solutes, the cell can maintain **homeostasis** (stability in the body's internal environment).

Osmosis is the diffusion or spreading of water molecules across a semipermeable membrane from a lower solute concentration to a higher solute concentration. (Figure 11-2). Osmosis separates two solutions of different concentrations by blocking the transport of salts or other solutes. The pressure that prevents the flow of fluid across a semipermeable membrane is **osmotic pressure;** it is the pressure required to maintain cellular equilibrium. Osmotic pressure depends on two factors: (1) the number and molecular weight of particles on each side of the cell membrane and (2) the **membrane permeability** to these particles.

> **NOTE**
> With gases, the driving force of osmosis is produced by the partial pressures of the dissolved gases (such as oxygen, nitrogen, carbon dioxide) and water. In any mixture of gases, the combination of the pressures exerted by all the gases is the **total pressure.** The pressure exerted by a single gas is the **partial pressure.** The partial pressure of a gas in a mixture is denoted by the letter "P" preceding the gas (e.g., the partial pressure of oxygen [P_{O_2}] or the partial pressure of carbon dioxide [P_{CO_2}]) (see Chapter 15).

When a living cell is placed in a solution that has a higher solute concentration (and a lower water concentration) than that inside the cell, the solution is called a **hypertonic** solution. When the cell is placed in this solution, the osmotic pressure exerted on it produces a net movement of water out of the cell. This causes the cell to dehydrate, shrink, and possibly die.

> **NOTE**
> **Electrolytes** are salt substances whose molecules dissociate into charged components when in water, producing positively and negatively charged ions. An ion with a positive charge is called a **cation.** An ion with a negative charge is called an **anion.** Sodium is the most abundant cation in the extracellular fluid (ECF). It is responsible for the osmotic balance of the ECF space. Potassium is the most abundant cation in the intracellular fluid (ICF). It maintains the osmotic balance of the ICF space. The body also has **nonelectrolytes** (substances with no electrical charge), such as glucose and urea.

Likewise, when a living cell is placed in a solution that has a lower solute concentration (and a higher water concentration) than that inside the cell, the solution is called a **hypotonic** solution. Osmotic pressure draws water from the solution into the cell. The net movement of water into the cell causes it to swell and possibly burst (**lyse**).

A cell may be placed in a solution that has the same solute and water concentrations as the solution inside the cell. This solution is called **isotonic.** Isotonic solutions have no net movement of water molecules (Figure 11-3 and Box 11-1).

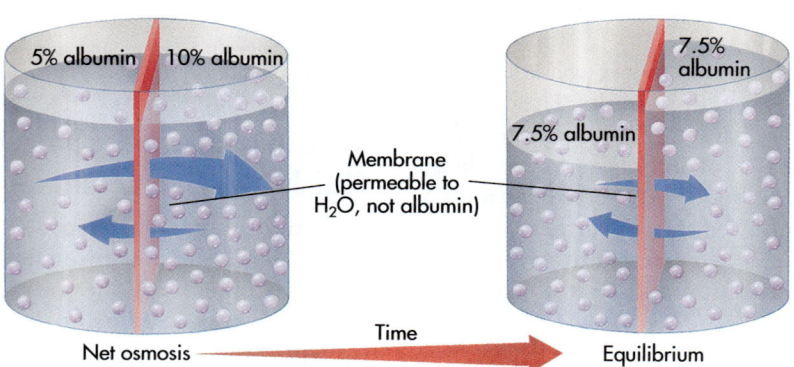

FIGURE 11-2 Osmosis. Osmosis is the diffusion of water through a selectively permeable membrane. The membrane shown in this diagram is permeable to water but not to albumin. Because there are relatively more water molecules in 5% albumin than in 10% albumin, more water molecules osmose from the more dilute into the more concentrated solution (as indicated by the *large arrow* in the diagram on the left) than osmose in the opposite direction. The overall direction of osmosis, in other words, is toward the more concentrated solution. Movement across the membrane continues until the concentrations of the solution equalize.

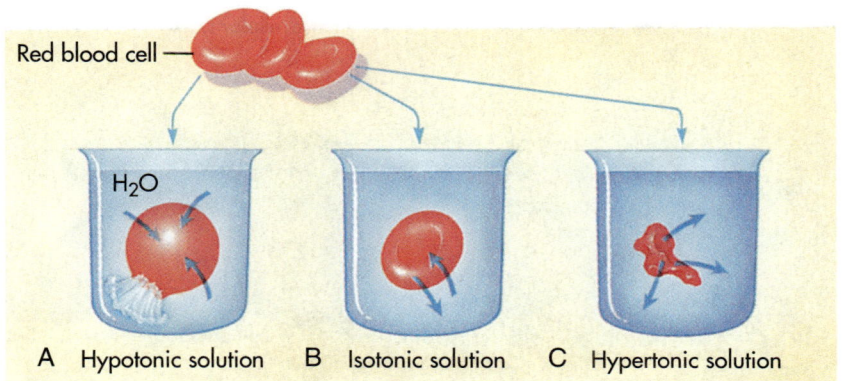

FIGURE 11-3 Effects of hypotonic, isotonic, and hypertonic solutions on red blood cells. **A,** The *hypotonic solution,* which has a low ion concentration, causes swelling and lysis of the cells. **B,** In the *isotonic solution,* which has a normal ion concentration, the cells keep their normal shape. **C,** The *hypertonic solution,* which has a high ion concentration, causes shrinkage (*crenation*) of the cells.

BOX 11-1 Fluid Replacement Therapy

Intravenous therapy is based on hypertonic, hypotonic, and isotonic properties.

Hypotonic Solutions

A *hypotonic solution* has a lower solute concentration than that of normal cells. When a hypotonic solution is infused into a normally hydrated patient, water is drawn from the solution into the cells. Hypotonic solutions supply the patient with calories. They also replenish salt and water. They are used to hydrate patients. They are used to prevent dehydration as well. An example of a hypotonic solution is 2.5% dextrose in water. Another is 0.45% normal saline ($\frac{1}{2}$NS). Although technically isotonic (see below), 5% dextrose in water (D_5W) acts physiologically as a hypotonic solution. This is because the solute (glucose) is actively transported into cells, leaving excess free water behind.

Isotonic Solutions

In an *isotonic solution,* the concentration of solute molecules is the same as that found in most normal cells. When an isotonic solution is infused into a normally hydrated patient, water is neither drawn out of the cells nor moved into them. Rather, water stays in the vascular space. Isotonic solutions are usually given to replace extracellular fluid. This fluid may have been depleted as a result of blood loss or severe vomiting. In fact, an isotonic solution may be prescribed for any patient in whom the chloride loss equals or exceeds the sodium loss. An example of an isotonic solution is 0.9% normal saline. Another is lactated Ringer's solution.

Hypertonic Solutions

A *hypertonic solution* has a higher concentration of solute molecules than that found in normal cells. When a hypertonic solution is infused into a normally hydrated patient, it draws water from the cells into the vascular space. Examples of hypertonic solutions are mannitol (Osmitrol), sodium bicarbonate, and 50% dextrose (D_{50}).

These solutions are often used to treat cerebral edema (mannitol), metabolic acidosis (bicarbonate), and profound hypoglycemia (50% dextrose). In addition, recent studies have suggested that some hypertonic solutions (e.g., Dextran, hetastarch, and sodium chloride [3%, 5%, and 7.5%, respectively]) should be used for volume restoration after trauma.[3] By drawing tissue fluid into the vascular space, hypertonic solutions may reduce both the volume of the infusion and the development of pulmonary problems after resuscitation.

DIFFUSION

Diffusion is a result of the constant motion of all the atoms, molecules, or ions in a solution. It is a passive process in which molecules or ions move from an area of higher concentration to an area of lower concentration (Figure 11-4). An area of high concentration has more solute particles than an area of low concentration. More solute particles move from the higher concentration to the lower one. Once at *equilibrium,* the movement of solutes in one direction is balanced by equal movement in the opposite direction.

The concentration of a solute may be greater at one point in the solvent than it is at another point. This means that a **concentration gradient** exists. Solutes diffuse *down* their concentration gradients from high to low concentration until equilibrium is achieved. Some nutrients enter and some waste products leave the cell by diffusion. Maintenance of the proper intracellular concentrations of certain substances depends on this process.

CRITICAL THINKING

What happens to a raisin that is put into a cup of water and left there for an hour? Why does this change occur? Is the water hypotonic, hypertonic, or isotonic relative to the inside of the raisin? Does a concentration gradient exist?

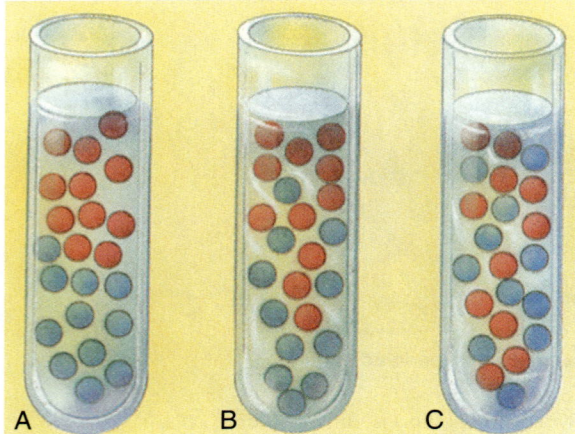

FIGURE 11-4 Diffusion. **A,** A solution (red, representing one type of molecule) is layered onto another solution (blue, representing a second type of molecule). A concentration gradient exists that favors the passage of red molecules into the blue solution, because the blue solution has no red molecules. Likewise, a concentration gradient exists that favors the passage of blue molecules into the red solution, because the red solution has no blue molecules. **B,** Red molecules move with their concentration gradient into the blue solution, and the blue molecules move with their concentration gradient into the red solution. **C,** Red and blue molecules are distributed evenly throughout the solution. Even though the red and blue molecules continue to move randomly, equilibrium exists. This means that no net movement occurs because no concentration gradient exists.

MEDIATED TRANSPORT MECHANISMS

A number of vital molecules (e.g., glucose) cannot enter most cells by diffusion. Also, a number of products (e.g., some proteins) cannot exit most cells by diffusion. *Mediated transport mechanisms* are required to move large, water-soluble molecules or electrically charged molecules across the cell membranes. These mechanisms use carrier molecules. **Carrier molecules** are proteins that combine with solute molecules on one side of a membrane. They then change shape, pass through the membrane, and release the solute molecule on the other side (Figure 11-5).

Carrier-mediated transport can be divided into two types: active transport and facilitated diffusion. **Active transport** moves substances *against* a concentration gradient, from *areas of lower concentration to areas of higher concentration*. The cell must expend energy to work against this concentration gradient. Active transport occurs at a faster rate than diffusion.

Facilitated diffusion moves substances into and out of cells from an *area of higher concentration to an area of lower concentration*. For these materials, the direction of movement is *with* the concentration gradient. As with active transport, this movement occurs more quickly than in normal diffusion. However, unlike in active transport, facilitated diffusion does not require the cell to expend energy. The moving force in facilitated diffusion is a downhill concentration gradient.

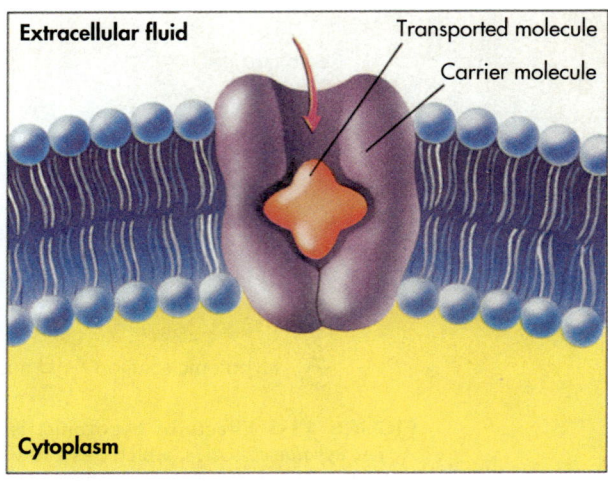

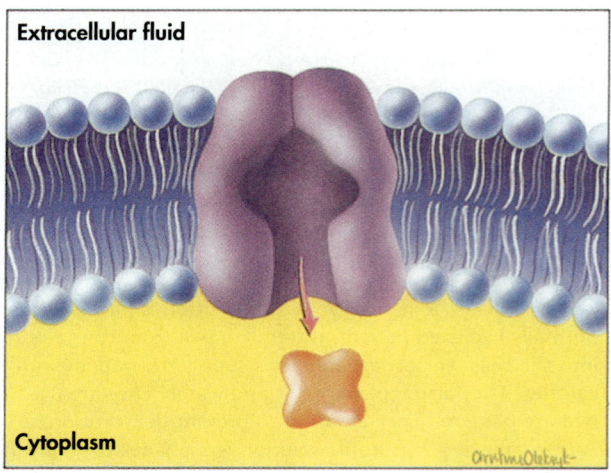

FIGURE 11-5 Mediated transport by a carrier molecule. **A,** The carrier molecule binds with a molecule on one side of the plasma membrane and changes shape. **B,** The molecule is released on the other side of the plasma membrane.

Water Movement Between Plasma and Interstitial Fluid

Fluid is transferred between the circulating blood and the interstitial fluid as a result of pressure changes. These changes occur at the arterial and venous ends of the capillary. The human body has about 10 billion capillaries. Few of the body's functional cells are farther than $5/1000$ inch (20 to 30 micrometers) from a capillary.

ANATOMY OF THE CAPILLARY NETWORK

A **capillary** is a thin-walled tube of endothelial cells. Capillaries do not have elastic or connective tissue or smooth muscle that would impede the transfer of water and solutes. Blood enters the capillary network from the arterioles. It flows through the **capillary network** and into the venules. The ends of the capillaries closest to the arterioles are *arteriolar capillaries*. The ends closest to the venules are *venous* *capillaries*. The exchange of nutrients and metabolic end products takes place at the capillary level.

The arterioles lead directly to capillaries. In some tissues the **arterioles** give rise to metarterioles. The metarterioles then give rise to capillaries. As described in Chapter 10, most tissues appear to have two distinct types of capillaries: *true capillaries* and *thoroughfare channels*. From a metarteriole, blood may flow into a thoroughfare channel that connects arterioles and venules directly, bypassing the true capillaries. Blood flow through thoroughfare channels is relatively constant. From the thoroughfare channels, fluid commonly exits and reenters the network of true capillaries.

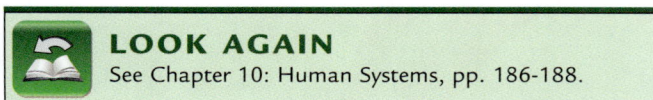

LOOK AGAIN
See Chapter 10: Human Systems, pp. 186-188.

The capillaries of some tissues have small cuffs of smooth muscle. These cuffs, which encircle the proximal and distal portions of the capillary, are known as *capillary sphincters*. The sphincter at the arterial end is known as the **precapillary sphincter.** The sphincter at the venous end is known as the **postcapillary sphincter.** These sphincters control capillary blood flow by opening and closing the entrance and exit to the capillary. Blood flow in true capillaries is not uniform. It depends on the contractile state of the arterioles and the precapillary and postcapillary sphincters (if present).

The blood flow through the capillaries that provides the exchange of gases and solutes between blood and tissue is referred to as *nutritional flow*. Blood that bypasses the capillaries in traveling from the arterial to the venous side of the circulation is known as *nonnutritional*, or *shunt flow*. True **arteriovenous anastomoses** (AV shunts) occur naturally in the sole of the foot, the palm of the hand, the terminal phalanges, and the nail bed. These shunts are important for the regulation of body temperature. Some evidence suggests the presence of AV shunts upstream from the capillary sphincters.[1]

Sympathetic fibers innervate all blood vessels of the body, except for the capillaries, the capillary sphincters, and most metarterioles. Sympathetic innervation of blood vessels includes both *vasoconstrictor* and *vasodilator* (vasomotor) fibers. However, the vasoconstrictor fibers are the most important in regulating blood flow. During normal circulation in the healthy body when arterial blood pressure is adequate, arterioles are open (though with some vasomotor tone), AV shunts are closed, and about 20% of the capillaries are open at any given time (Figure 11-6).

Diffusion Across the Capillary Wall. Tissue cells do not exchange material directly with blood. The interstitial fluid always acts as a "middle man." Nutrients must diffuse across the capillary wall into the interstitial fluid to enter cells. Metabolic end products, such as carbon dioxide and lactic acid, first must move across cell membranes into interstitial fluid to diffuse into the plasma.

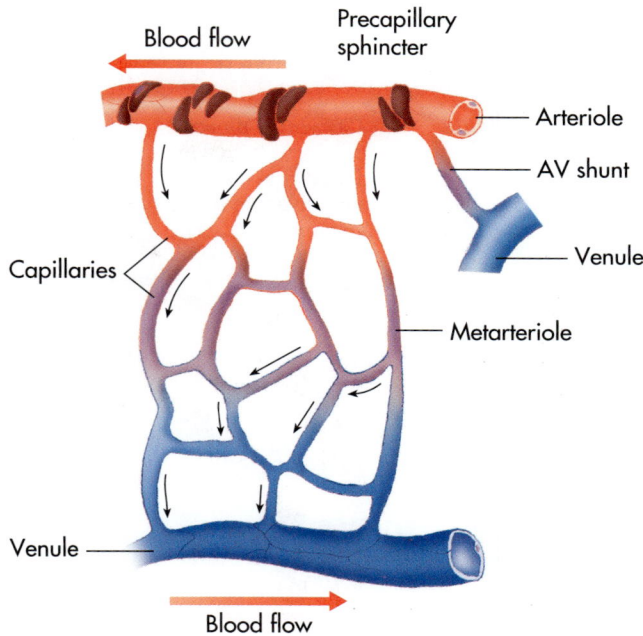

FIGURE 11-6 Microcirculation. The circular structures on the arteriole and venule represent smooth muscle fibers; branching solid lines represent sympathetic nerve fibers. The arrows indicate the direction of blood flow.

At the arteriole end of the capillary, the forces moving fluid out of the capillary are greater than the forces attracting fluid into it. At the venous end, these forces are reversed. Thus more fluid is attracted into the capillary at the venous end. Hydrostatic and osmotic pressures are the two forces responsible for this movement of fluid. The hydrostatic pressure (created with each heartbeat) forces water out of the arterial end of the capillary. The osmotic pressure results from the presence of plasma proteins (mostly albumin), which are too large to pass through the wall of the capillary; this pressure is referred to as *blood colloid osmotic pressure* or *oncotic pressure*.

At the venous end of the capillary, the hydrostatic pressure is lower. The concentration of proteins in the capillary increases slightly. This occurs because of the movement of fluid out of the arteriolar end. The result is a greater plasma protein concentration and a greater colloid osmotic pressure. Consequently, nearly all the fluid that leaves the capillary at its arteriolar end reenters the capillary at its venous end. The remaining fluid enters the lymphatic capillaries. Eventually it is returned to the general circulation. The movement of fluid across the capillary wall is called *net filtration*. It is best described by the **Starling hypothesis:**[2]

Net filtration = Forces favoring filtration −
Forces opposing filtration

The forces favoring filtration include capillary hydrostatic pressure and the interstitial oncotic pressure. The forces opposing filtration are the plasma oncotic pressure and the interstitial hydrostatic pressure.

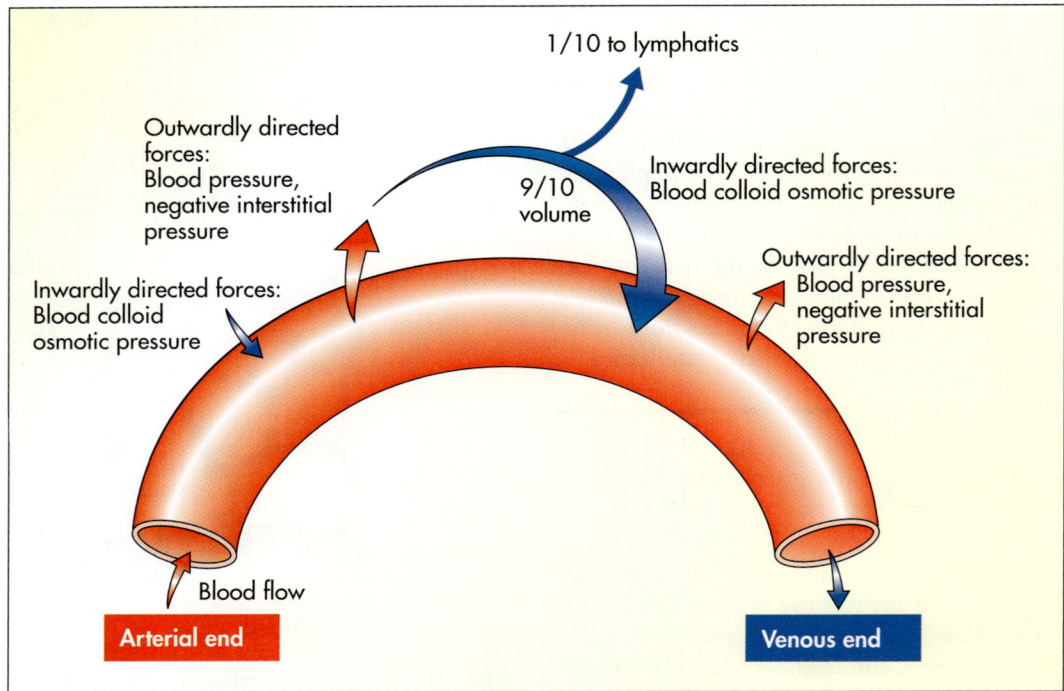

FIGURE 11-7 Total pressure differences between the inside and the outside of the capillary at its arteriolar and venous ends. At the arteriolar end, the sum of the forces causes fluid to move from the capillaries into the tissues. At the venous end, the sum of the forces attracts fluid into the capillary.

Fluid also may be exchanged across the capillary wall as a result of the cyclic dilation and constriction of the precapillary sphincter. When this sphincter dilates, the pressure rises in the capillary. This forces fluid to move into the interstitial spaces. When the precapillary sphincter constricts, the pressure in the capillary drops. Thus fluid moves into the capillary (Figure 11-7).

CAPILLARY AND MEMBRANE PERMEABILITY

A key factor in the movement of fluid across the capillary wall is the integrity of the capillary membrane. Changes in membrane permeability may allow plasma proteins to escape into the interstitial space. The resultant increase in interstitial oncotic pressure changes the relationship defined by the Starling hypothesis. It leads to osmotic movement of water into the interstitial space. This, in turn, results in tissue edema.

Alterations in Water Movement

Edema is the accumulation of fluid in the interstitial spaces. It can be caused by any condition that leads to a net movement of fluid out of capillaries and into the interstitial tissues. Edema is a problem of *fluid distribution*. It does not always indicate a *fluid excess*.

PATHOPHYSIOLOGY OF EDEMA

Normal flow of fluid through the interstitial spaces depends on the following four factors:

1. The capillary hydrostatic pressure that filters fluid from the blood through the capillary wall
2. The oncotic pressure exerted by the proteins in the blood plasma, which attracts fluid from the interstitial space back into the vascular compartment
3. The permeability of the capillaries, which determines how easily fluid can pass through the capillary wall
4. The presence of open lymphatic channels, which collect some of the fluid forced out of the capillaries by the hydrostatic pressure of the blood and return the fluid to the circulation

When any of these four factors is disturbed, changes in water movement can develop. The mechanisms most often responsible for edema are (1) an increase in the hydrostatic pressure, (2) a decrease in the plasma oncotic pressure, (3) an increase in capillary permeability, and (4) lymphatic obstruction.

Increased Capillary Hydrostatic Pressure. An increase in hydrostatic pressure can be caused by venous obstruction or sodium and water retention. With venous obstruction, the hydrostatic pressure of fluid in the capillaries can become great enough to cause fluid to escape into the interstitial spaces. Conditions that can lead to venous obstruction and edema include **thrombophlebitis** (the formation of a blood clot and inflammation in a vein), chronic venous disease, hepatic obstruction (blockage of hepatic veins or common bile duct), tight clothing around an extremity, and prolonged standing.

Sodium and water retention can cause an increase in circulating fluid volume (volume overload) and edema. *Congestive heart failure* (CHF) and *renal failure* are two conditions associated with sodium and water retention.

Decreased Plasma Oncotic Pressure. Decreases in plasma albumin concentration lead to a decrease in the plasma oncotic pressure. As a result, fluid moves into the interstitial space. This condition most often results from liver disease or protein malnutrition.

Increased Capillary Permeability. Increases in capillary permeability result in greater than normal filtration of fluid into the interstitial space. This condition usually is associated with allergic reactions. It also is linked to inflammation and the immune response triggered by trauma. (The immune response is described later in this chapter.) Examples of such trauma are burns or crushing injuries. In such cases, proteins escape from the vascular bed. As a consequence, the capillary oncotic pressure decreases, and the fluid oncotic pressure increases. The result is edema.

Lymphatic Obstruction. When lymphatic channels are blocked by infection or are surgically removed, proteins and fluid can accumulate in the interstitial space. This obstruction blocks the normal pathway by which fluid is returned from the interstitial space into the circulation. This leads to edema in the region that normally is drained by the lymphatic channels. Conditions that can cause obstruction in the channels include certain malignancies and parasitic infections, and the surgical removal of lymphatics. Surgical removal may occur after a radical mastectomy (surgical removal of an entire breast), which requires removal of the axillary lymph nodes.

CLINICAL MANIFESTATIONS OF EDEMA

Edema may be localized or generalized. *Localized edema* usually is limited to an injury site or an organ system. For example, an injury site may be a sprained ankle. An affected organ system may be the brain (*cerebral edema*) or the lungs (*pulmonary edema*). Edema of specific organs such as the brain, lungs, or larynx can threaten life.

Generalized edema is more widespread. It is most obvious in dependent parts of the body. It usually is noted first in the legs and ankles when the individual is standing or sitting. It is noted in the sacrum and buttocks when the person is lying down. Generalized edema usually causes weight gain, swelling, and puffiness. It is often linked to other symptoms caused by an underlying illness. In industrialized countries, the diseases that most often cause generalized edema are heart disease, kidney disease, and liver disease. In developing countries, the most common causes are malnutrition and parasitic disease.[3] When edematous tissue is compressed with a finger (e.g., over the ankle or tibia), the fluid is pushed aside, leaving a "pit" or indentation that gradually refills with fluid. This condition is called **pitting edema** (Box 11-2). The accumulation of fluid in the peritoneal cavity is a condition called **ascites.**

BOX 11-2 Pitting Edema Scale

+1 Minor pitting of the skin without visible deformation; depression disappears quickly.

+2 No obvious distortion of the skin; depression typically normalizes within 10 to 15 seconds.

+3 Noted deformity of the skin; depression produces a definite pit that persists longer than 1 minute.

+4 Obvious gross deformity of the skin; depression produces a very deep pit that persists longer than 2 minutes.

CRITICAL THINKING

The rest, ice, compression, and elevation (RICE) treatment is used for swelling from a sprained ankle. Why does this treatment reduce tissue edema?

Water Balance, Sodium, and Chloride

Water follows the osmotic gradient established by changes in the sodium concentration. Hence sodium and water balance are closely related.

WATER BALANCE

Water balance is mainly regulated by antidiuretic hormone (ADH) (see Chapter 10). The secretion of ADH and the perception of thirst help regulate water balance. Release of ADH is triggered by an increase in the plasma **osmolality** (the osmotic pressure of a solution). It also may be triggered by a decrease in the circulating blood volume and a decline in venous and arterial pressures. An increase in plasma osmolality stimulates hypothalamic neurons (called *osmoreceptors*). This causes the individual to feel thirsty. It also increases the release of ADH from the posterior pituitary gland.

In response to the release of ADH, water is reabsorbed into the plasma from the distal renal tubules and collecting ducts of the kidneys. This reduces the amount of water lost in the urine. Also, as the water is reabsorbed, the plasma osmolality decreases, returning to normal. Volume-sensitive receptors, as well as pressure-sensitive receptors (*baroreceptors,* which are found in the heart and great vessels), also can stimulate the release of ADH when body fluids are depleted. These fluids may be lost from conditions such as vomiting, diarrhea, or excess sweating.

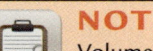

NOTE

Volume-sensitive receptors and baroreceptors are nerve endings that are sensitive to changes in volume and pressure, respectively. Volume-sensitive receptors are located in the right and left atria and the thoracic vessels. Baroreceptors are found in the aorta, pulmonary arteries, and carotid sinus.

SODIUM AND CHLORIDE BALANCE

As mentioned before, sodium is the major ECF cation. Sodium balance is regulated by **aldosterone.** (Aldosterone is a hormone secreted by the adrenal cortex.) Along with chloride and bicarbonate, sodium regulates osmotic forces. Hence, it regulates water balance. (Chloride is the major ECF anion. It provides electroneutrality in relation to sodium. Increases or decreases in chloride concentration occur in proportion to changes in sodium concentration.)

Secretion of aldosterone is triggered by a decrease in sodium levels. It also is triggered by an increase in potassium levels. Aldosterone causes the distal tubules of the kidneys to increase both the reabsorption of sodium and the secretion of potassium.

The enzyme **renin** also is secreted by the kidneys. This occurs when the circulating blood volume is reduced or the sodium-water balance is disrupted. Renin stimulates the formation of **angiotensin I.** This is then changed to **angiotensin II.** Angiotensin II is a potent vasoconstrictor. It acts to stimulate the secretion of ADH, which results in the reabsorption of sodium and water. It also results in an increase in the systemic blood pressure. (This is described later in the chapter.) This mechanism for regulating levels of sodium and water is known as the *renin-angiotensin-aldosterone system* (Figure 11-8).

Natriuretic hormone also helps to regulate sodium concentration. It does this by promoting the secretion of sodium in the urine. One result is a decrease in tubular reabsorption of sodium. Another result is a subsequent loss of sodium and water. **Atrial natriuretic factor** is a substance released from the atrial cells of the heart. (It is described in Chapter 10 and later in this chapter.) This substance also helps control the balance of sodium and water. It does this by promoting renal elimination of sodium.

ALTERATIONS IN SODIUM, CHLORIDE, AND WATER BALANCE

In the healthy body, homeostatic mechanisms maintain a constant balance between the intake and excretion of water. The water gained each day basically equals the water lost. The body gains water mainly in two ways: (1) when a person drinks fluids and eats moist foods and (2) when water is formed through the oxidation of hydrogen in food during the metabolic process. The body loses water through the kidneys as urine, through the bowel as feces, through the skin as perspiration, through exhaled air as vapor, and by the excretion of tears and saliva. Two abnormal states of body fluid balance can occur. If the water lost exceeds the water gained, a water deficit occurs. This is **dehydration.** If the water gained exceeds the water lost, a water excess occurs. This is **overhydration.**

DEHYDRATION

Dehydration may be described in three ways. **Isotonic dehydration** is excessive loss of sodium and water in equal amounts. **Hypernatremic dehydration** is the loss of more water than sodium. **Hyponatremic dehydration** is the loss of more sodium than water.

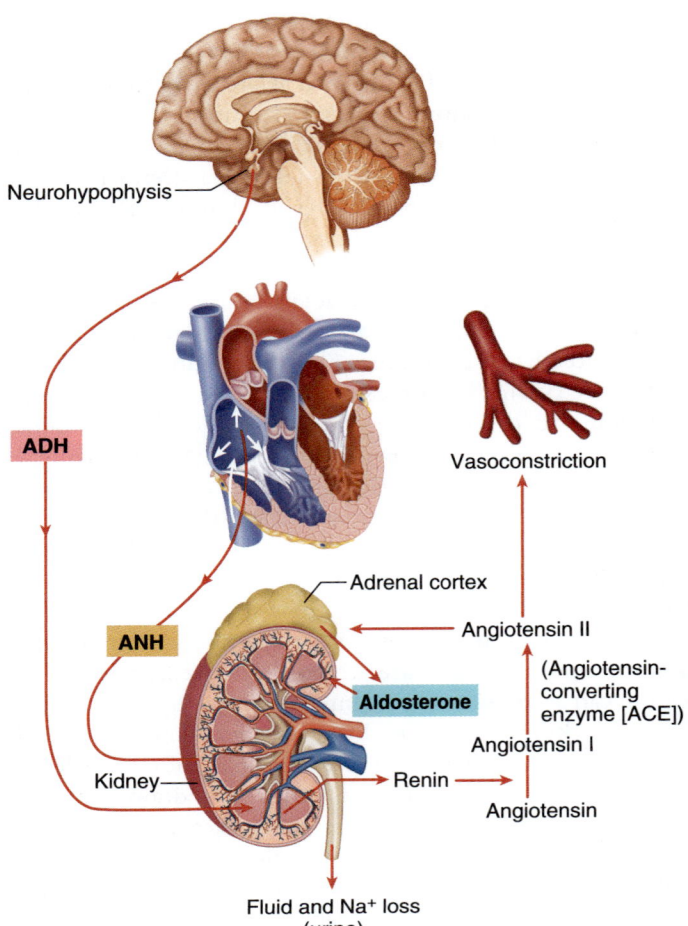

FIGURE 11-8 Three mechanisms that influence total plasma volume. The antidiuretic hormone (ADH) mechanism and renin-angiotensin-aldosterone system (RAAS) tend to increase water retention and thus increase total plasma volume. The atrial natriuretic hormone (ANH) mechanism antagonizes these mechanisms by promoting water loss and thus promoting a decrease in total plasma volume. (From Patton KT, Thibodeau GA: *Anatomy and physiology*, ed 7, St Louis, 2007, Mosby.)

> ### CRITICAL THINKING
> Consider the causes of dehydration and your knowledge of anatomy and physiology. What two age groups do you think are at highest risk for dehydration? Why?

Isotonic Dehydration

Possible Causes
   Usually severe or long-term vomiting or diarrhea
   Systemic infection
   Intestinal obstruction

Signs and Symptoms
   Dry skin and mucous membranes
   Poor skin turgor
   Longitudinal wrinkles or furrows of the tongue
   Oliguria (decreased urinary output)

Anuria (essentially no urinary output [100 mL or less in 24 hours])

Acute weight loss

Depressed or sunken fontanelles in infants

Treatment

An intravenous infusion of an isotonic solution is administered. The solution has a solute concentration equal to that of blood (0.9% sodium chloride or normal saline typically is used).

Hypernatremic Dehydration

Possible Causes

Excessive use or misuse of diuretics

Continued intake of sodium in the absence of water consumption

Excessive loss of water with little loss of sodium

Profuse, watery diarrhea

Signs and Symptoms

Dry, sticky mucous membranes

Flushed, doughy skin

Intense thirst

Oliguria or anuria

Increased body temperature

Altered mental status

Treatment

Volume replacement is administered. This usually begins with isotonic fluids, because the patient often is both salt and water depleted, with the water supply being more depleted. (Isotonic fluids are relatively hypotonic in these patients.)

Hyponatremic Dehydration

Possible Causes

Use of diuretics

Excessive perspiration (heat-related illness)

Salt-losing renal disorders

Increased water intake (e.g., excessive use of water enemas)

Signs and Symptoms

Abdominal or muscle cramps

Seizures

Rapid, thready pulse

Diaphoresis (profuse sweating)

Cyanosis

Treatment

Intravenous fluid replacement (i.e., normal saline or lactated Ringer's solution) is administered. Occasionally, hypertonic saline is given (e.g., in seizures caused by hyponatremia).

OVERHYDRATION

Because overhydration is an increase in body water, it results in a decrease in the solute concentration. (The total body amount of solute actually may be increased. However, because body water is increased more, the solute concentration is decreased.) This water excess may result from parenteral administration of excessive fluids, impaired cardiac function, impaired renal function, or some endocrine dysfunctions. Signs and symptoms of overhydration may include the following:

- Shortness of breath
- Puffy eyelids
- Edema
- **Polyuria** (voiding of a large volume of urine within a given time)
- Moist crackles (on pulmonary examination)
- Acute weight gain

Treatment for overhydration depends on the cause. Water restriction is the main treatment for excessive water administration. It also is the main treatment for certain endocrine problems. A diuretic may be indicated for patients with cardiac impairment. It also may be the treatment for patients with renal impairment. When profound hyponatremia is associated with overhydration (a low serum sodium level and associated seizures or altered consciousness), administration of saline may be indicated.

🔍 SHOW ME THE EVIDENCE
Overhydration

Researchers in California reviewed the records of 545 patients reported to have ecstasy intoxication. Their goal was to determine whether the incidence of hyponatremia differed in males and females. Of the 188 cases with a documented sodium level, 38.8% were hyponatremic. Of the patients with hyponatremia, 75.3% were women and 24.7% men. Females had increased odds of hyponatremia (odds ratio [OR] 4.0; 95% confidence interval [CI] 2.1 to 7.6). Females with hyponatremia had a higher incidence of coma.

From Rosenson J, Smollin C, Sporer K, et al: Patterns of ecstasy-associated hyponatremia in California, *Ann Emerg Med* 49(2):164-171, 2007.

ELECTROLYTE IMBALANCES

In addition to water and sodium imbalances, disturbances may occur in the balance of electrolytes other than sodium. These electrolytes include potassium, calcium, and magnesium (Table 11-2).

Potassium. Potassium is the major positively charged ion in ICF. The body must keep potassium levels within a narrow range. This allows normal function of the nerves, cardiac system, and skeletal muscle. *Obligate* potassium losses are losses that cannot be avoided. These usually are minimal. In addition, they normally can be replenished through the diet. Excess potassium usually is excreted by the kidneys. Potassium plays a key role in muscle contraction, enzyme action, nerve impulse conduction, and cell membrane function. Potassium imbalances interfere with neuromuscular function. They may cause cardiac rhythm disturbances (**dysrhythmias**). These may even include sudden cardiac death.

Hypokalemia is an abnormally *low* level of potassium in the blood. It can be caused by reduced dietary intake (rare), poor potassium absorption, increased gastrointestinal losses from vomiting or diarrhea, renal disease, infusion of solutions low in potassium, or the use of some

TABLE 11-2 Electrolyte Concentrations of Intracellular and Extracellular Fluid

Predominant Cations	Normal Adult Range
Intracellular	
Potassium (K⁺)	3.5-5.0 mEq/L
Magnesium (Mg⁺⁺)	1.5-2.0 mEq/L
Extracellular	
Sodium (Na⁺)	135-145 mEq/L

Predominant Anions	Normal Adult Range
Intracellular	
Phosphate (PO₄³⁻)	50-60 units/L
Extracellular	
Chloride (Cl⁻)	90-108 mEq/L
Bicarbonate (HCO₃⁻)	22-30 mEq/L

medications (most commonly diuretics, but steroids, theophylline, and others have also been implicated). The most common cause of hypokalemia in the United States is the use of diuretics. About 80% of patients who are receiving diuretics become hypokalemic.[4] Signs and symptoms of hypokalemia may include the following:

- Malaise
- Skeletal muscle weakness
- Cardiac dysrhythmias
- Decreased reflexes
- Weak pulse
- Faint or distant heart sounds
- Shallow respiration
- Low blood pressure
- Anorexia
- Vomiting
- Gaseous distention
- Excessive thirst (rare)

In-hospital treatment of hypokalemia involves intravenous or oral administration of potassium.

CRITICAL THINKING
What common illness mimics many of the signs and symptoms of fluid and electrolyte imbalance?

Hyperkalemia is an abnormally *high* level of potassium in the blood. This condition may be caused by acute or chronic renal failure, burns, crush injuries, severe infections or other conditions in which large amounts of potassium are released, excessive use of potassium salts, and a shift of potassium from the cells into the extracellular fluid (such as occurs in acidosis, described later in this chapter). Signs and symptoms of hyperkalemia may include the following:

- Cardiac conduction disturbances
- Irritability
- Abdominal distention
- Nausea
- Diarrhea
- Oliguria
- Weakness (an early sign) and paralysis (a late sign of severe hyperkalemia)

In-hospital treatment for hyperkalemia involves restriction of potassium. It also involves administration of a cation exchange resin, either orally or through a nasogastric tube. For severe potassium level elevation, **hemodialysis** may be indicated. In an emergency, administration of *calcium* intravenously can be lifesaving. This is especially true with cardiac dysrhythmias, which are life-threatening. Other critical efforts include intravenous administration of glucose and *insulin.* This helps to lower the serum potassium level. It forces potassium movement intracellularly along with the glucose. *Sodium bicarbonate* also causes potassium to move back into the cells. High-dose nebulized *albuterol* may also be administered to lower potassium levels. *Albuterol* does this by stimulating the release of insulin, which in turn stimulates the sodium-potassium pump, causing potassium to be shifted into the cells.[5]

Calcium. Calcium is a **bivalent cation** (an ion with two positive charges). It is essential for a variety of body functions. These include neuromuscular transmission, cell membrane permeability, hormone secretion, growth and ossification of bones, and muscle contraction (including smooth, cardiac, and skeletal muscle). Calcium intake in a balanced diet usually is sufficient for normal body needs. Calcium is excreted through urine, feces, and perspiration.

Hypocalcemia is an abnormally low level of calcium in the blood. It may result from endocrine dysfunction (mostly underactivity of the parathyroid gland). It may also result from renal insufficiency; a decreased intake or malabsorption of calcium; or **toxic shock syndrome.** Another cause of hypocalcemia is a deficiency of, malabsorption of, or inability to activate vitamin D (which is responsible for calcium absorption). Signs and symptoms of hypocalcemia may include the following:

- **Paresthesia** (numbness or tingling sensation)
- **Tetany** (muscle twitching)
- Abdominal cramps
- Muscle cramps
- Neural excitability
- Personality changes
- Abnormal behavior
- Convulsions
- Heart failure

In-hospital treatment for hypocalcemia involves intravenous administration of calcium ions. Calcium salt and vitamin D may be given orally for maintenance.

Hypercalcemia is an abnormally high level of calcium in the blood. It may be caused by various tumors. Other common causes include parathyroid overactivity, thyroid dysfunction, diuretic therapy, some cancers, and excessive administration of vitamin D (as in the treatment of *osteoporosis*). Calcium can be deposited in various body tissues, including many organ systems. Examples include the gastrointestinal system, central nervous system, renal system, neuromuscular system, and cardiovascular system. Signs and symptoms of hypercalcemia include the following:

- **Hypotonicity of the muscles** (decreased muscle tone or tension)
- Renal stones
- Altered mental status, seizures, coma
- Deep bone pain
- Cardiac dysrhythmias

The treatment of hypercalcemia is aimed at controlling the underlying disease. It may include hydration and/or drug therapy to decrease the calcium level. In-hospital therapy for severe hypercalcemia may include forced diuresis with normal saline and *furosemide.* The patient also may be given calcium-lowering drugs. Examples of these are thyrocalcitonin, steroids (glucocorticoids), and plicamycin (a cytotoxic drug that inhibits bone reabsorption of calcium). Hemodialysis may be needed in patients with heart failure or renal insufficiency.

> **NOTE**
>
> Changes in the level of phosphate in the blood also can occur. This can result in hypophosphatemia or hyperphosphatemia. **Hypophosphatemia,** an abnormally low serum phosphate level, may be caused by intestinal malabsorption or increased excretion of phosphate by the kidneys. **Hyperphosphatemia,** an abnormally high serum phosphate level, is associated with acute or chronic renal failure or diminished activity of the parathyroid gland.

Magnesium. Like calcium, magnesium is a bivalent cation. It activates many enzymes. Magnesium is distributed throughout the body approximately as follows: 50% in an insoluble state in bone; 45% as an intracellular cation; and 5% in extracellular solution. Magnesium is excreted by the kidneys. Its physiological effects on the nervous system resemble those of calcium.

Hypomagnesemia is an abnormally low level of magnesium in the blood. It may be encountered in conditions involving alcoholism, diabetes, malabsorption disorders, starvation, diarrhea, diuresis, and diseases that cause hypocalcemia and hypokalemia. The condition is characterized by increased irritability of the central nervous system. Signs and symptoms of hypomagnesemia include the following:

- Tremors
- Nausea or vomiting
- Diarrhea
- Hyperactive deep reflexes
- Confusion (including hallucinations)
- Seizures or myoclonus (muscle spasms)
- Cardiac dysrhythmias (which may lead to cardiac arrest)

Treatment for significant, symptomatic hypomagnesemia involves intravenous administration of a solution that contains magnesium. Magnesium sulfate would be given to treat **torsades de pointes** associated with hypomagnesemia. (Torsades de pointes is a type of ventricular dysrhythmia, described in Chapter 22.)

Hypermagnesemia is an abnormally high level of magnesium in the blood. It occurs mainly in patients with chronic renal insufficiency. It also can occur in patients who take large amounts of magnesium-containing compounds. Examples of such compounds are **cathartics** (e.g., magnesium citrate, magnesium sulfate) and antacids (e.g., magnesium hydroxide). Hypermagnesemia causes central nervous system depression, profound muscular weakness, and **areflexia** (absence of reflexes). It also causes cardiac rhythm disturbances, which may lead to sudden death. Signs and symptoms of hypermagnesemia include the following:

- Sedation
- Confusion
- Muscle weakness
- Respiratory paralysis

The most effective treatment for hypermagnesemia is hemodialysis. It can return blood levels to normal in about 4 hours. Calcium salts may be given parenterally as well. These act as an antagonist to magnesium. Administration of intravenous glucose and *insulin* also drives magnesium back into the cells. This treatment can be used in emergencies when respiratory depression or cardiac conduction defects are present.

Acid-Base Balance

Acids are produced by the body through normal metabolism. Two types of acids are produced: *respiratory acids* (culminating in carbon dioxide [CO_2]) and *nonrespiratory (metabolic) acids.* **Bases** are used in metabolic disturbances to return the body's plasma to normal pH. For physiological functioning, the balance between acids and bases must be kept in a narrow range. The body's main regulators of **acid-base balance** are the lungs and the kidneys. The lungs secrete respiratory acids. The kidneys secrete metabolic acids.

pH

Hydrogen ions are protons with a positive charge. In chemistry, a hydrogen ion that loses its charge is marked with a positive sign (H^+). Likewise, a hydrogen ion that gains a charge is marked with a negative sign (H^-). *Acids* are materials that release or donate hydrogen ions. *Bases* (alkaline substances) receive, or absorb, hydrogen ions. Thus they neutralize positively charged ions. The concentration of hydrogen ions is expressed as the **pH.** This indicates the *potential for hydrogen.* A small change in pH is very important: *The strength of an acid or a base changes by 10 times with **each** unit change of pH.* For example, a pH that changes by 0.3 unit (e.g., from 7.4 to 7.1) doubles the concentration of hydrogen ions (Box 11-3). The pH is neutral (6.8 to 7) when equal numbers of positive and negative ions are present. A solution increases in acidity as the pH

BOX 11-3 pH Values

A solution of pH 1 is 1 million times as acidic as a solution of pH 7.
pH 2 is 100,000 times as acidic as pH 7.
pH 3 is 10,000 times as acidic as pH 7.
pH 4 is 1000 times as acidic as pH 7.
pH 5 is 100 times as acidic as pH 7.
pH 6 is 10 times as acidic as pH 7.
pH 7 is neutral (distilled water).
pH 8 is 1/10 as acidic as pH 7, or 10 times as alkaline.
pH 9 is 1/100 as acidic as pH 7, or 100 times as alkaline.

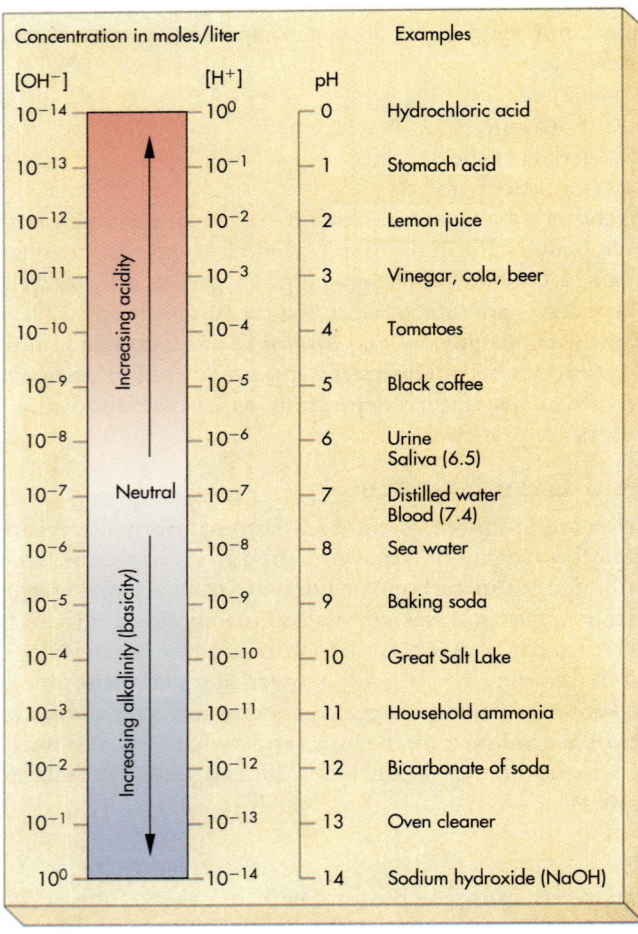

FIGURE 11-9 The pH scale. A pH of 7 is considered neutral. Values less than 7 are acidic (the lower the number, the more acidic the substance). Values greater than 7 are basic (the higher the number, the more basic the substance). Representative fluids and their approximate pH values are listed.

decreases. It increases in alkalinity (basicity) as the pH rises (Figure 11-9).

BUFFER SYSTEMS

The healthy body is sensitive to changes in the concentration of hydrogen ions. In fact, it tries to maintain the pH of extracellular fluid at 7.4. This is carried out through three related compensatory mechanisms. These are *carbonic acid–bicarbonate buffering*, *protein buffering*, and *renal buffering*. These mechanisms are stimulated by changes in the pH. They require normal organ function to be effective in maintaining acid-base balance.

Carbonic Acid–Bicarbonate Buffering. Bicarbonate, carbon dioxide, and carbonic acid are always present in a dynamic balance in the blood. **Bicarbonate** (HCO_3^-) arises from the transport of carbon dioxide in the blood. Under the influence of the enzyme **carbonic anhydrase** (found in the alveoli, walls of the lungs, and epithelial cells in the renal tubules), carbon dioxide dissolves in the water of blood. It reacts with water in red blood cells to form **carbonic acid** (H_2CO_3). Carbonic acid dissociates into hydrogen and bicarbonate ions. Because of the effects of carbonic acid or sodium bicarbonate, the buffering must occur through the lungs or kidneys. This means that the pH can be increased or decreased in one of three ways: (1) by the renal system that excretes or retains sodium bicarbonate; (2) by the respiratory system that excretes or retains carbonic acid, or its component carbon dioxide; or (3) by both systems acting together. At a physiological pH of 7.4, the normal ratio of carbonic acid to bicarbonate is 1:20 (1 part of carbonic acid to every 20 parts of sodium bicarbonate), and is summarized by the chemical equation:

$$CO_2 + H_2O \rightleftarrows H_2CO_3 \rightleftarrows H^+ + HCO_3^-$$

Bicarbonate may bind with a cation to form base bicarbonate (e.g., $NaHCO_3$). The ratio of carbonic acid to base bicarbonate determines the pH. As long as there is 1 *milliequivalent* (mEq) of carbonic acid for each 20 mEq of base bicarbonate in the extracellular fluid, the pH stays within normal limits.

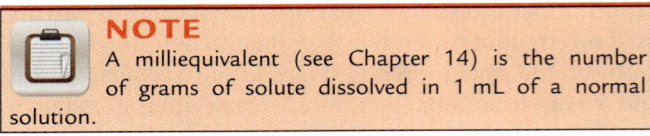

NOTE
A milliequivalent (see Chapter 14) is the number of grams of solute dissolved in 1 mL of a normal solution.

The carbonic acid–bicarbonate compensatory mechanism is triggered immediately by changes in pH. The respiratory rate helps maintain this balance (Figure 11-10). This is the most important buffering system in extracellular fluid. It can buffer up to 90% of the hydrogen ions in extracellular fluid and has little effect on the cells.[6]

Protein Buffering. Both intracellular and extracellular proteins have negative charges. Both also can serve as buffers for changes in the pH. However, most proteins are inside cells. Protein buffering, therefore, is mainly an intracellular buffer system. **Hemoglobin** (Hb) is an excellent intracellular buffer, because it can bind with hydrogen ions (forming a weak acid) and carbon dioxide.

After oxygen is released in the peripheral tissues, hemoglobin binds with carbon dioxide and hydrogen ions. As the blood reaches the lungs, these actions are reversed.

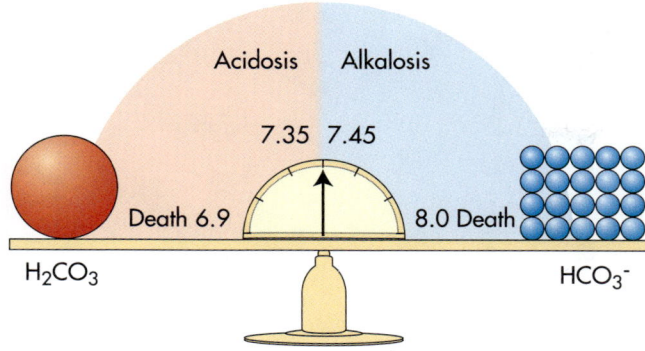

FIGURE 11-10 Bicarbonate buffer system. When body fluids are in acid-base balance, the ratio of bicarbonate (HCO_3^-) to carbonic acid (H_2CO_3) normally is 20:1, and the pH is between 7.35 and 7.45.

Hemoglobin binds with oxygen, releasing carbon dioxide and hydrogen ions. The released hydrogen ions combine with bicarbonate ions, forming carbonic acid. The carbonic acid dissociates into carbon dioxide and water. Then the lungs exhale the carbon dioxide. Therefore in normal circumstances, respirations help maintain pH. The respiratory centers are more responsive to pH changes than to changes in the oxygen level of the tissues. For this reason, the amount of carbon dioxide in the blood (and hence the pH), rather than the need for oxygen in the tissues, controls the rate of breathing in healthy individuals. Within minutes of a decrease in the pH, alveolar ventilation increases in an effort to lower the carbon dioxide concentration.

Renal Buffering. The kidneys help maintain an acid-base balance through three mechanisms. One is the recovery of bicarbonate, which is filtered into the tubules. Another is the excretion of hydrogen ions against a gradient to acidify the urine. The third is the excretion of **ammonium ions** (NH_4), each of which carries a hydrogen ion with it. The renal system compensates for acid-base imbalances slowly compared with the protein and bicarbonate buffer systems. The kidneys can take several hours to days to restore the pH to the normal physiological range.

> **NOTE**
> The concentration of carbonic acid is controlled by the lungs. (Carbonic acid is dissolved carbon dioxide.) The concentration of bicarbonate is controlled by the kidneys.

ACID-BASE IMBALANCE

As stated previously, acid-base balance is maintained mainly through two factors: a respiratory element and a metabolic element. Any condition that increases the concentration of carbonic acid or decreases the concentration of base bicarbonate causes **acidosis.** Any condition that increases the concentration of base bicarbonate or decreases the concentration of carbonic acid causes **alkalosis.** In discussing acid-base imbalance, it is important to remember that

acidosis makes the pH *more* acidic than normal. Alkalosis makes the pH *less* acidic than normal (Box 11-4). Also, a patient can have both disorders at the same time (e.g., respiratory acidosis and metabolic alkalosis, described later). When two disturbances are present, one usually dominates. The other attempts to compensate.

ACIDOSIS

The accumulation of acid and the resulting acidosis (pH below 7.35) cause the pH to be more acidic compared to the normal pH of 7.4. (A decrease in pH means an increase in acidity.) A discussion of respiratory and metabolic acidosis follows.

Respiratory Acidosis. Respiratory acidosis is caused by the retention of carbon dioxide. This leads to an increase in the partial pressure of carbon dioxide (P_{CO_2}). This state usually is caused by an imbalance in the production of carbon dioxide and its elimination through alveolar ventilation (Figure 11-11). Respiratory acidosis can be summarized by the following chemical equation:

$$\downarrow Respiration = \uparrow CO_2 + H_2O \rightarrow \uparrow H_2CO_3 \rightarrow \uparrow H^+ + HCO_3^-$$

Reductions in alveolar ventilation may occur as a result of the following:

- Respiratory depression
- Respiratory arrest
- Cardiac arrest
- Neuromuscular impairment
- Medications (e.g., sedatives, hypnotics)
- Chest wall injury (e.g., flail chest, pneumothorax)
- Pulmonary disorders (e.g., airway obstruction, chronic obstructive pulmonary disease, pulmonary edema)

> **NOTE**
> In respiratory acidosis, the primary abnormality is failure of the lungs to excrete carbon dioxide efficiently.

When the respiratory system cannot continue as a compensatory mechanism to correct the acidosis, the body's renal system must conserve bicarbonate and excrete more

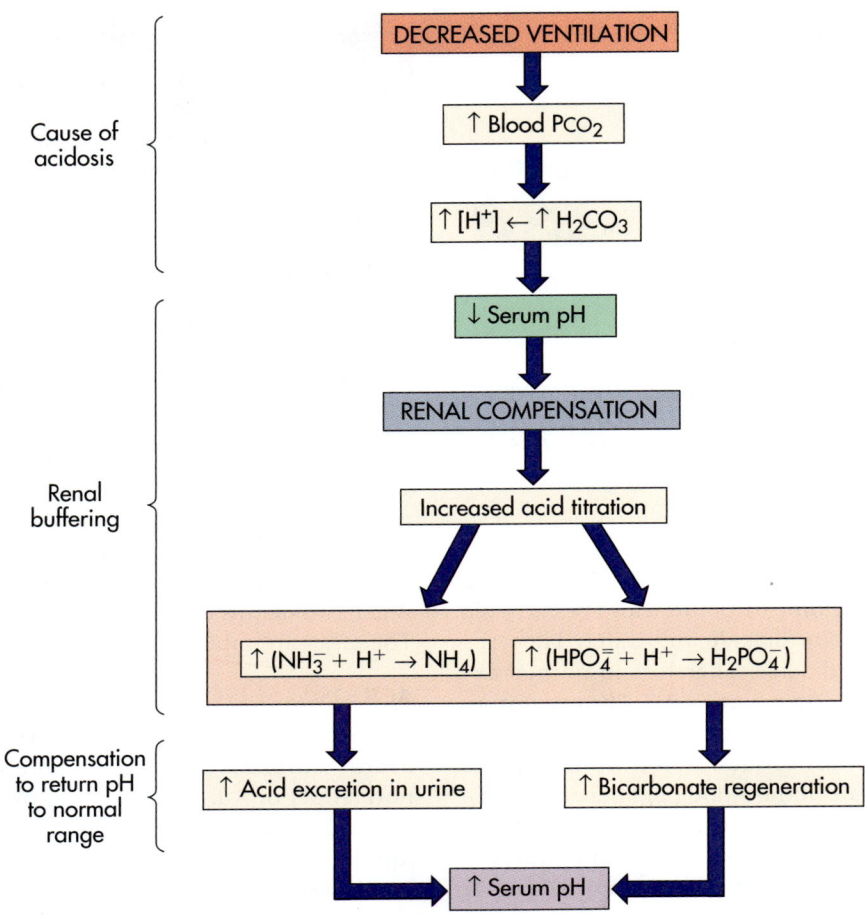

FIGURE 11-11 Respiratory acidosis. An excess of carbon dioxide in the body results in acidosis.

hydrogen ions to help bring the pH into normal limits. The kidneys take some time to restore pH. Thus the patient in respiratory acidosis should be treated by improving ventilation to quickly eliminate carbon dioxide. This may be done by assisting ventilations to decrease the P_{CO_2}. Supplemental oxygen also should be given to help correct any accompanying **hypoxemia** (which itself can lead to acidosis).

> ### CRITICAL THINKING
> What kind of acid-base imbalance exists in a patient you have just defibrillated and resuscitated from cardiac arrest? How are you going to treat that imbalance?

Metabolic Acidosis. Metabolic acidosis results from a buildup of acid or a loss of base. When excessive acid is produced by the body, the acid spills into the extracellular fluid. This, in turn, consumes some bicarbonate buffers. The result is an increase in acid and a decrease in available base (Figure 11-12). Metabolic acidosis can be summarized by the following equation:

$$\uparrow H^+ + HCO_3^- \rightarrow \uparrow H_2CO_3 \rightarrow H_2O + \uparrow CO_2$$

The increase in available hydrogen ions forces the reaction to the right. This decreases the amount of base bicarbonate.

> ### NOTE
> Metabolic acidosis occurs when the amount of acid generated by the body exceeds the body's buffering capacity.

The healthy respiratory system instantly tries to compensate for the acidosis. It does this by increasing the rate and depth of breathing to reduce carbon dioxide levels. As the carbon dioxide concentration falls, so does the concentration of carbonic acid. This moves the pH toward normal. In addition, the kidneys excrete more hydrogen ion to equilibrate the excess acid in the extracellular fluid.

The four most common forms of metabolic acidosis encountered in the prehospital setting are lactic acidosis, diabetic ketoacidosis, acidosis caused by renal failure, and acidosis caused by ingestion of toxins (poisons).

Lactic Acidosis. Lactic acid is made when a large number of cells are inadequately perfused. This results in

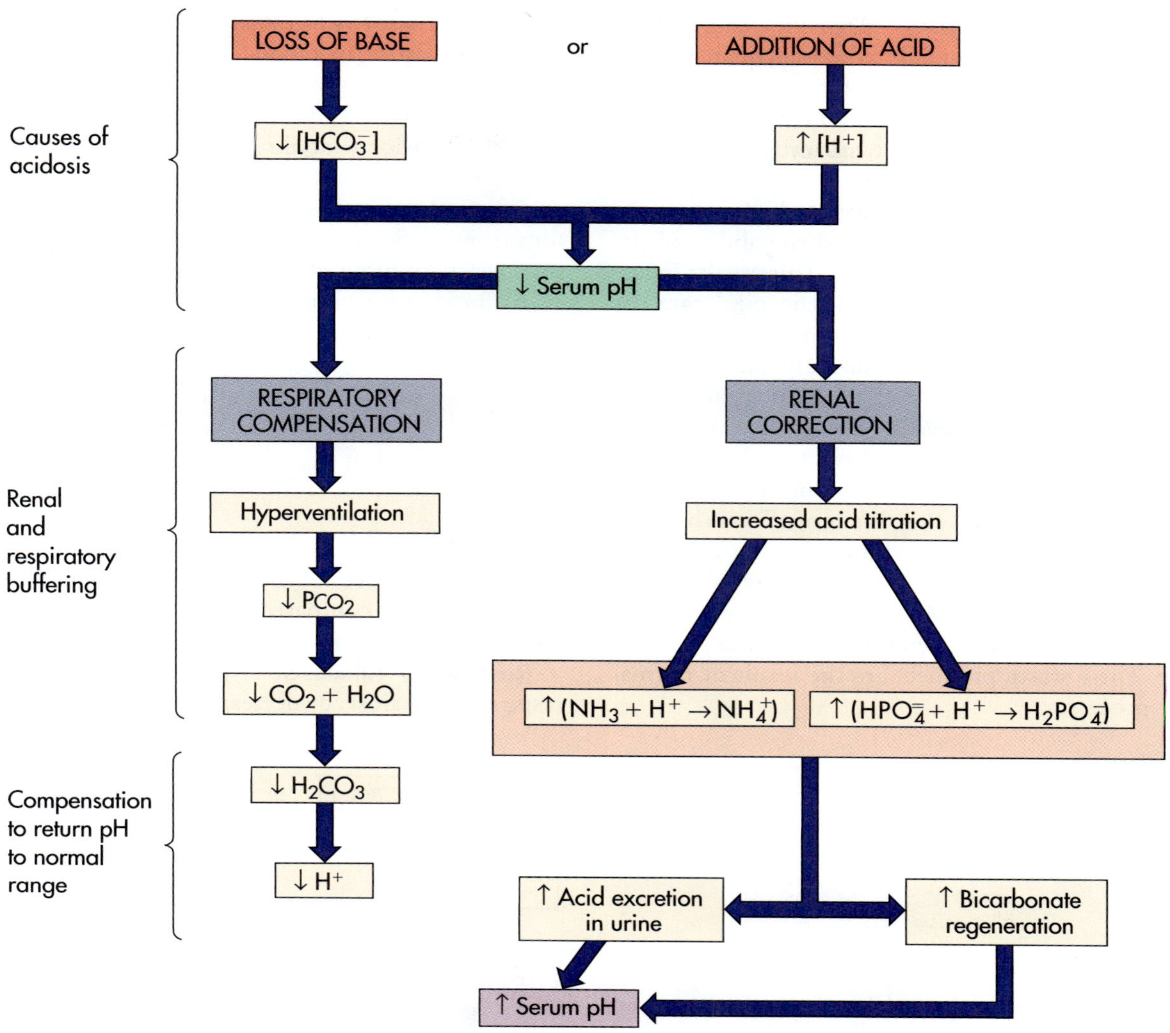

Causes of acidosis

LOSS OF BASE   or   ADDITION OF ACID

$\downarrow [HCO_3^-]$ $\uparrow [H^+]$

$\downarrow$ Serum pH

Renal and respiratory buffering

RESPIRATORY COMPENSATION   RENAL CORRECTION

Hyperventilation   Increased acid titration

$\downarrow PCO_2$

$\downarrow CO_2 + H_2O$ $\uparrow (NH_3 + H^+ \rightarrow NH_4^+)$ $\uparrow (HPO_4^- + H^+ \rightarrow H_2PO_4^-)$

Compensation to return pH to normal range

$\downarrow H_2CO_3$

$\downarrow H^+$ $\uparrow$ Acid excretion in urine $\uparrow$ Bicarbonate regeneration

$\uparrow$ Serum pH

FIGURE 11-12 Metabolic acidosis. With an excess of metabolic acids, bicarbonate is consumed and hydrogen ions are liberated, resulting in acidosis. (From McCance KL, Huether SE: *Pathophysiology: the biologic basis for disease in adults and children,* ed 5, St Louis, 2005, Mosby.)

a shift from **aerobic** (with oxygen) to **anaerobic** (without oxygen) metabolism. The end product of anaerobic metabolism is lactic acid. The lactic acid releases hydrogen ions and becomes **lactate.** This creates systemic acidosis. Normally, the liver changes lactate back into glucose, or lactate is oxidized to carbon dioxide and water. When lactic acid is produced faster than it is metabolized, **lactic acidosis** occurs. The most common causes of systemic lactic acidosis are extreme exertional states (e.g., seizures), **ischemia** (reduced blood supply) in large muscles or organs (e.g., *mesenteric ischemia*), circulatory failure, and shock. Specific complications associated with lactic acidosis are thought to include the following:

- Decreased force of cardiac contraction
- Decreased peripheral response to catecholamines
- Hypotension and shock
- Cardiac muscle that is refractory to defibrillation

CRITICAL THINKING

Think about the last time you ran so fast you had a muscle cramp. What acid-base changes were occurring inside your body? How did your body compensate for those changes?

Treatment of lactic acidosis involves reestablishing tissue perfusion and cardiac output. This allows the liver to regenerate bicarbonate by metabolizing lactate to carbon dioxide and water. Hyperventilation is sometimes advised to induce **respiratory alkalosis** in these cases. Vigorous rehydration to support circulation, and perhaps intravenous administration of *sodium bicarbonate* for immediate compensation (if the patient is in cardiac arrest), may also be indicated. Correction of lactic acidosis often depends on identification and rectification of the underlying cause.

Diabetic Ketoacidosis. Ketoacidosis usually is a complication of **diabetes mellitus.** It also may be seen in alcoholics (*alcoholic ketoacidosis*). Diabetic ketoacidosis usually results when a patient fails to take adequate **insulin.** It also may develop when the need for insulin increases. This may occur, for example, in cases of infection or trauma. Insulin is required for many cells to absorb glucose. With impaired glucose utilization, fatty acids are metabolized, producing **ketone bodies** and releasing hydrogen ions. Large amounts of ketone bodies exceed the ability of the body's buffering system to compensate. This results in acidosis and a decrease in blood pH. Prehospital care for patients with diabetic ketoacidosis involves administration of normal saline for volume repletion. (The pathophysiology of diabetes is further addressed in Chapter 26).

Acidosis Caused by Renal Failure. The kidneys help maintain acid-base balance. They do this by reabsorbing or secreting either bicarbonate or hydrogen ions as needed. This keeps the pH constant. Renal failure affects the compensatory mechanisms of the kidneys to varying degrees. Patients with moderate to severe renal failure often have mild to moderate acidosis. Acidosis results because the failing kidneys are unable to excrete the acid waste products efficiently. These waste products are the result of normal metabolic processes.

Acidosis Caused by Ingestion of Toxins. Ingestion of some toxins can cause metabolic acidosis. Examples of such toxins are ethylene glycol, methanol, and salicylate, a component of **aspirin.** These and other toxins lead to the production of toxic metabolites. They may result in acid-base disorders. These disorders are characterized by metabolic acidosis and compensatory respiratory alkalosis. Treatment for various toxic ingestions frequently includes gastrointestinal evacuation but also may require hemodialysis, diuresis, hydration to promote excretion, and specific antagonistic or antidotal therapy.

 NOTE
In a patient with renal failure, administration of intravenous (IV) fluids may rapidly lead to overhydration.

ALKALOSIS

Alkalosis (pH above 7.45) causes the blood and body fluids to be less acidic compared to the normal pH of 7.4. (An increase in pH means a decrease in acidity.)

Respiratory Alkalosis. Hyperventilation may produce respiratory alkalosis by decreasing the P_{CO_2} (Figure 11-13).

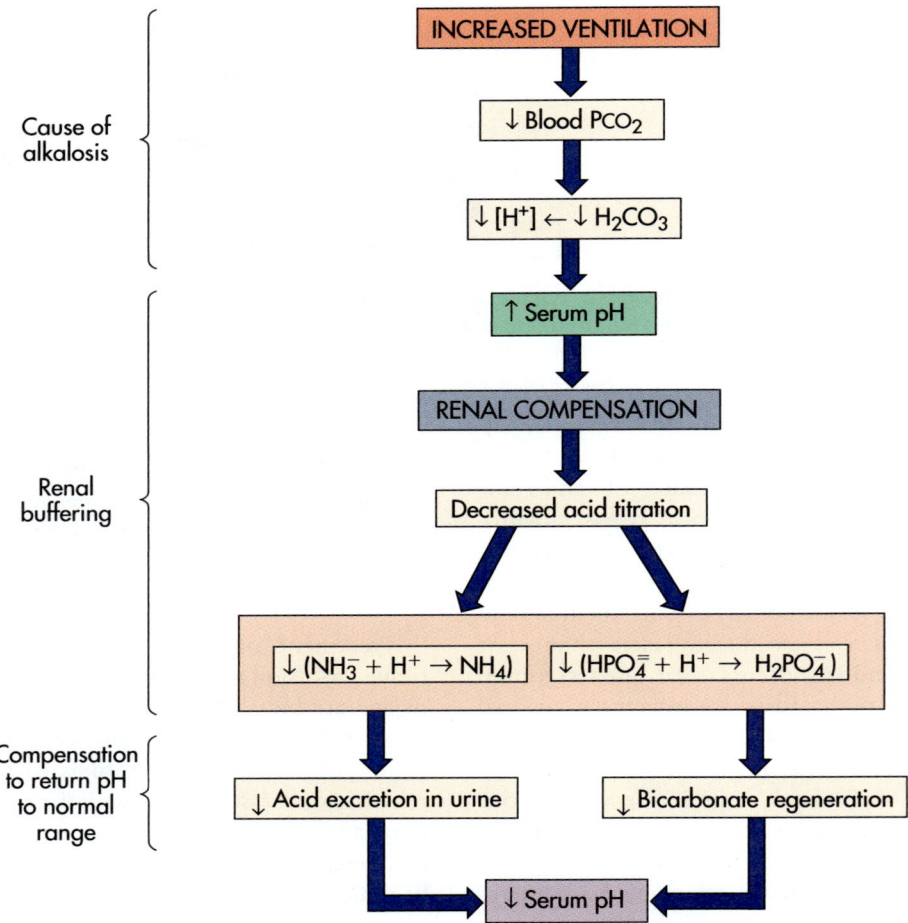

FIGURE 11-13 Respiratory alkalosis. A deficit of carbon dioxide results in respiratory alkalosis.

Hyperventilation is common in patients who are acutely ill. It is often seen in the early stages of *sepsis, peritonitis, shock,* and *respiratory ailments*. Respiratory alkalosis can be summarized by the following chemical equation:

$$\uparrow \text{Respiration} = \downarrow CO_2 + H_2O \rightarrow \downarrow H_2CO_3 \rightarrow \downarrow H^+ + HCO_3^-$$

> **NOTE**
> Respiratory alkalosis is caused by hyperventilation. This lowers the partial pressure of carbon dioxide (P_{CO_2}) in the alveoli (the air cells in the lungs) and subsequently the P_{CO_2} in the blood.

When carbonic acid is lacking because of excessive elimination of carbon dioxide, the blood pH rises. Thus the kidneys must excrete bicarbonate ions and retain hydrogen ions. They do this in an effort to return the pH to normal. Treatment of respiratory alkalosis is directed at correcting the underlying cause of the hyperventilation. An initial approach is to administer low-concentration oxygen to the patient. Another is to provide calming measures to assist the patient with slow, controlled breathing.

Metabolic Alkalosis. Metabolic alkalosis (rare) most often results from loss of hydrogen ions (primarily from the stomach), ingestion of large amounts of absorbable base sodium bicarbonate (baking soda) or calcium carbonate (Tums, other antacids), or excessive intravenous administration of alkali (e.g., intravenous injection of *sodium bicarbonate*). The use of diuretics also may be a factor (Figure 11-14). Metabolic alkalosis can be summarized by the following chemical equation:

$$\downarrow H^+ + HCO_3^- \rightarrow \downarrow H_2CO_3^- \rightarrow H_2O + \downarrow CO_2$$

The loss of hydrogen ions is the initial cause of metabolic alkalosis. This may result from vomiting (loss of hydrochloric acid), suctioning of gastric contents, or increased renal excretion of hydrogen ions in the urine. When vomiting occurs, gastric acid (i.e., hydrochloric acid) is lost, but volume also is depleted.

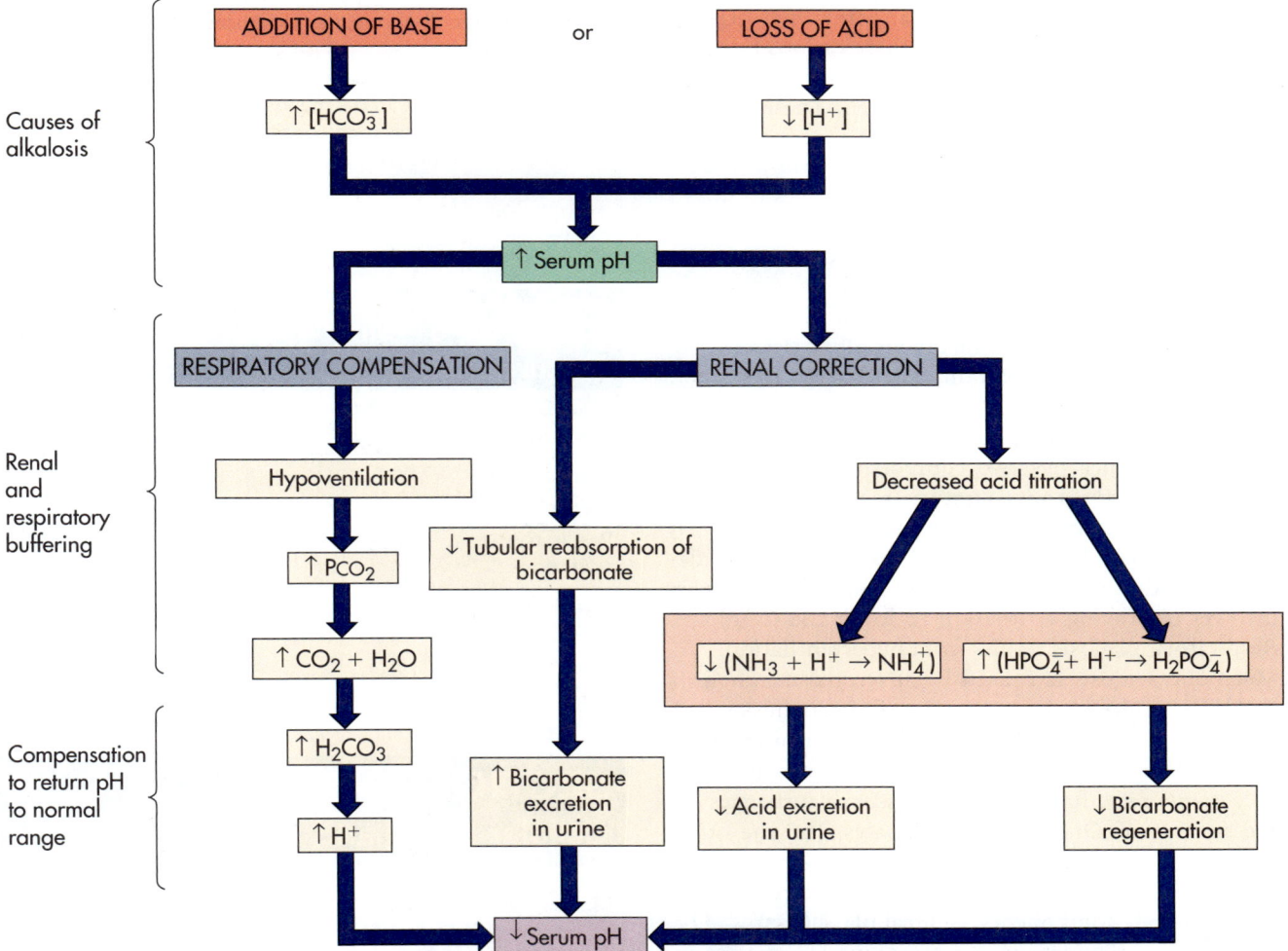

FIGURE 11-14 Metabolic alkalosis. An excess of bicarbonate results in metabolic alkalosis. (From McCance KL, Huether SE: *Pathophysiology: the biologic basis for disease in adults and children,* ed 5, St Louis, 2005, Mosby.)

Chronic use of diuretics can result in volume depletion. The loss of sodium chloride and potassium causes a relative increase in bicarbonate concentration. (The kidneys defend against volume depletion. They increase reabsorption of sodium and thus water.) When sodium is reabsorbed, either potassium or hydrogen ions must be excreted. This action helps to maintain electrical neutrality. The excretion of hydrogen ions can lead to a net increase in bicarbonate level. This, in turn, can lead to metabolic alkalosis.

At first, the respiratory system tries to compensate. It does so by retaining carbon dioxide. However, this mechanism is limited by the development of hypoxemia. (Hypoventilation causes a rise in the PCO_2 and a decrease in the partial pressure of oxygen [PO_2]. This, in turn, stimulates respiration).

Treatment of metabolic alkalosis is aimed at correcting the underlying condition. Volume depletion, if present, should be corrected. This should be done with isotonic solutions. Hypokalemia may require correction with potassium replacement.

MIXED ACID-BASE DISTURBANCES

Many conditions may cause mixed abnormalities of acid-base regulation. These conditions include various forms of shock. In patients in shock, simultaneous respiratory and metabolic alterations are commonly seen. These develop because pathophysiological changes occur in both the respiratory and the metabolic components of the acid-base system (Box 11-5; also see Table 11-3). Examples of mixed acid-base disturbances include the following:

- Combined respiratory and metabolic acidosis
- Metabolic acidosis and respiratory alkalosis
- Respiratory acidosis and metabolic alkalosis
- Combined respiratory and metabolic alkalosis

Acid-base balance can be a difficult concept to master. In providing emergency care, the paramedic should remember the following primary points:

1. Acid-base balance has two components: a respiratory (CO_2) factor and a nonrespiratory (metabolic) factor.
2. Respiratory acidosis is caused by an increase in the CO_2 level of the blood and body fluids as a result of inadequate breathing. The treatment of respiratory acidosis involves improving ventilation to lower the CO_2 level. Respiratory alkalosis results from hyperventilation.
3. Metabolic acidosis is caused by anaerobic metabolism and lactic acidosis. The treatment of metabolic acidosis involves neutralizing the acid by reestablishing tissue perfusion and cardiac output. Metabolic alkalosis is rare.
4. A patient may have two acid-base disturbances at the same time. One usually dominates, and the other attempts to compensate.
5. The patient's pH is always a product of both respiratory and metabolic components. Neutral pH is 6.8 to 7. The normal pH of blood is 7.4. A decrease in pH indicates an increase in acidity (more acid than normal); an increase in pH indicates a decrease in acidity (less acid than normal).

BOX 11-5 Acid-Base Determination and Other Laboratory Studies

Blood Gas Analysis

Blood gas values are measured for two reasons. One reason is to determine whether the patient is well oxygenated. The second reason is to determine the patient's acid-base status. Most often, blood gas values are measured in a sample of arterial blood obtained in a heparinized syringe (see Appendix A: Advanced Practice Procedures for Critical Care Paramedics). Arterial samples are used for this test more often than venous samples for a good reason. Arterial samples give more direct information about the lungs' ability to oxygenate blood and remove carbon dioxide.

Acid-Base Determination

The patient's acid-base status is assessed by measuring the partial pressure of carbon dioxide (PCO_2) and the hydrogen ion concentration (pH) of the arterial blood. The pH level indicates whether an acid or a base state is present. The PCO_2 value indicates whether a respiratory component is a factor in the acidosis or alkalosis. (For instance, it may show whether alveolar hypoventilation or hyperventilation is present.) Table 11-3 summarizes the abnormalities that occur in mixed acid-base disturbances.

Currently, paramedics are not expected to determine the pH by blood gas analysis in the prehospital setting. Pulse oximetry allows continual assessment of the arterial oxygen saturation without invasive procedures. (Under normal circumstances, a saturation of 90% correlates with a partial pressure of oxygen [PO_2] in arterial blood of 60 mm Hg.)

TABLE 11-3 Simple Acid-Base Disturbances

Acid Base Disturbance	Initial Chemical Change	Compensatory Response	pH
Respiratory acidosis	↑PCO_2	↑HCO_3^-	↓
Respiratory alkalosis	↓PCO_2	↓HCO_3^-	↑
Metabolic acidosis	↓HCO_3^-	↓PCO_2	↓
Metabolic alkalosis	↑HCO_3^-	↑PCO_2	↑

SECTION TWO
Cellular Injury and Disease

ALTERATIONS IN CELLS AND TISSUES

Certain concepts are crucial to an understanding of the disease process. One of these concepts is the way that cells and tissues react to injury, both structurally and functionally. Changes in the structure and function of cells and tissues can result from cellular adaptation, injury, neoplasia (actual formation of a tumor), aging, and death.

Cellular Adaptation

Cells adapt to their environment (Figure 11-15). They do so to escape and to protect themselves from injury. (An adapted cell is neither normal nor injured.) Adaptations are common. They are a central part of the response to changes in the physiological condition. In many instances the adaptation allows the cell to function more efficiently. For this reason, it can be difficult to distinguish between a pathological response and an extreme adaptation to changing conditions. The following is a list of the five most significant adaptive changes in cells:

1. Atrophy (a decrease in cell size)
2. Hypertrophy (an increase in cell size)
3. Hyperplasia (an excessive increase in the number of cells)
4. Metaplasia (a change from one cell type to another that is better able to tolerate adverse conditions; a conversion into a form that is not normal for that cell)
5. Dysplasia (abnormal changes in mature cells)

Atrophy is a decrease in cellular size that adversely affects cell function. It can affect any organ. However, it is seen most often in skeletal muscle, the heart, the secondary sex organs, and the brain. Causes include decreased use,

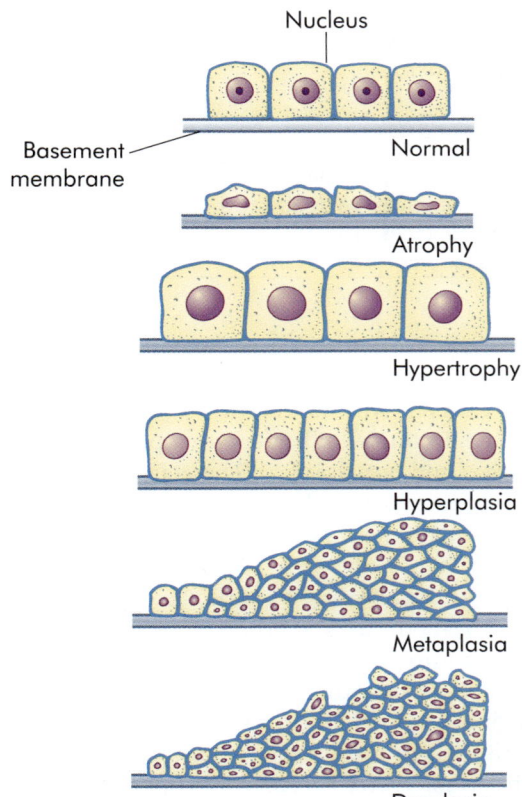

FIGURE 11-15 Adaptive changes in cells. (From Huether SE, McCance KL: *Understanding pathophysiology,* ed 4, St Louis, 2008, Mosby.)

chronic inflammation, poor nutrition or starvation, inadequate hormonal or nervous stimulation, and reduced blood supply. An example of atrophy is a skeletal muscle that is reduced in size because of prolonged wearing of a cast. Atrophy may be reversed (in some cases) when normal function is restored.

Hypertrophy is an increase in the size of cells. (This occurs without an increase in the number of that type of cell.) Along with the increase in the size of the cells comes an increase in the size of the affected organ. Hypertrophy results when cells are required to do more work to achieve a task. Examples of "normal" or physiological hypertrophy are a weight lifter's large muscles, increased growth of the uterus during pregnancy, and the development of sexual organs in adolescence (initiated by sex hormones). Examples of pathological hypertrophy are enlargement of the heart (myocardial hypertrophy) and of the kidneys (which also can be physiological).

 CRITICAL THINKING

What happens to muscle strength when the muscle cells are affected by each of these conditions: atrophy, hypertrophy, and hyperplasia?

Hyperplasia is an excessive increase in the number of cells. This results in an increase in the size of a tissue or an organ. Hyperplasia occurs in response to increased demand. It may be a pathological event. It also may be a normal adaptive mechanism that allows certain organs to regenerate (*compensatory hyperplasia*). The formation of a callus is an example of compensatory hyperplasia. Another example is the increased formation of red blood cells that occurs at high altitudes. An example of pathological hyperplasia is *endometrial hyperplasia*. This condition can cause excessive menstrual bleeding. Hyperplasia and hypertrophy often occur together.

Metaplasia is a change into a form that is not normal for that cell. It also can be seen as the reversible replacement of normal tissue cells by other cells that may be better able to tolerate poor environmental conditions. An example of metaplasia is the change that occurs in the bronchial lining as a result of smoking. The normal ciliated epithelial cells are replaced by nonciliated squamous epithelial cells. The latter cells are more resistant to irritation. (*Bronchial metaplasia* can be reversed if the individual quits smoking.) Chronic inflammation of the cervix also can result in metaplasia.

Dysplasia is the development of abnormal changes in mature cells. The cells vary in size, shape, and color, and their relationship to one another also is abnormal. Dysplastic changes frequently are seen as precancerous. They occur most often in epithelial tissue. These changes often result from chronic irritation or inflammation. They frequently are found in cells near cancerous cells. Dysplasia is not considered a true cellular adaptation. Rather, it is seen as an atypical hyperplasia.

Cellular Injury

Many processes can injure a cell. The mechanisms involved in cellular injury are complex. The specific site of injury often is characteristic of a certain pathological process. As a rule, cellular injury occurs if the cell is unable to maintain homeostasis as a result of the following factors:

1. Hypoxic injury
2. Chemical injury
3. Infectious injury (e.g., bacteria, viruses)
4. Immunological and inflammatory injury
5. Genetic factors
6. Nutritional imbalances
7. Physical agents

HYPOXIC INJURY

Hypoxic injury is the most common cause of damage to a cell. It may result from a decrease in the amount of oxygen in the air, loss of hemoglobin or altered hemoglobin function, a decrease in the number of red blood cells, diseases of the respiratory or cardiovascular system, external compression (e.g., in trauma), or poisoning and loss of **cytochromes** (proteins in the liver that play a role in drug detoxification). Hypoxic injury commonly is a result of **atherosclerosis** (narrowing of the arteries) and **thrombosis** (complete blockage of an artery or a vein by a blood clot). Prolonged ischemia leads to **infarction,** or cell death (see Chapter 22). Atherosclerosis and thrombosis are leading causes of *myocardial infarction* and *stroke.*[7]

> **NOTE**
> Cells need an adequate supply of oxygen. Without oxygen they cannot generate enough energy to maintain the mechanisms (ion pumps) that move some substances across the cell membrane. Lack of oxygen also causes cellular swelling.

CHEMICAL INJURY

Many chemical agents can damage a cell. Examples include heavy metals (e.g., lead), carbon monoxide, ethanol, drugs, and complex toxins. Some of these chemicals injure cells directly (e.g., *curare* and *cyanide*). Others, when metabolized, produce a toxin that affects the cells (e.g., *carbon tetrachloride* [CCl_4]).

The injury begins with a biochemical interaction. The interaction occurs between a toxic substance and an integral part of the cell's structure. Some drugs and toxins (e.g., salicylate, certain venoms) affect the cellular membrane. This interaction can damage the plasma membrane. It can lead to increased permeability, cellular swelling, and irreversible cellular injury (see Chapter 32). Other toxins, such as carbon monoxide, mainly affect the cytochrome system found in the mitochondria. This leads to a halt in oxidative metabolism. Still other toxins affect the genetic material (a primary target for chemotherapeutic drugs).

INFECTIOUS INJURY

The **virulence** of microorganisms such as bacteria and viruses depends on their ability to survive and reproduce in the human body. The disease-producing potential of microorganisms depends on their ability to do the following:

- Invade and destroy cells
- Overcome the organism's defense system
- Produce toxins
- Produce hypersensitivity reactions

Bacteria. The survival and growth of bacteria are determined by the success of the body's defenses. They also depend on the bacteria's ability to resist these mechanisms (see Chapter 28). Many bacteria that survive and multiply in the body produce toxins. These can injure or destroy cells and tissues. The toxins take two forms: **exotoxins** (toxins secreted or excreted by a living organism) and **endotoxins** (toxins contained in the cell walls of some living organisms).

Bacteria make exotoxins when they have been identified by viruslike particles called *bacteriophages*. These particles carry the genetic material needed to make the toxin. Exotoxins are produced by a microorganism. Then they are excreted into the medium surrounding the microorganism. Exotoxins have highly specific effects. These effects are produced by the release of exotoxins as metabolic products during bacterial growth. Several of the *streptococci* (bacteria that cause sore throats and rheumatic fever) produce an exotoxin. The bacterium *Clostridium botulinum*, which causes the severe food poisoning known as **botulism,** also produces an exotoxin.

> **NOTE**
> **Toxoids** are modified (harmless) toxins. They are used as vaccines so that the body can develop specific **antibodies** to them. The best-known toxoid is *tetanus toxoid,* which is made from tetanus toxin.

Endotoxins are complex molecules. They are contained in the cell walls of some bacteria. Endotoxins are released during treatment with antibiotics or when the cell walls disintegrate. Examples of bacteria that produce endotoxins are *gonococci* and *meningococci*. (These are the bacteria that respectively cause gonorrhea and meningitis.) Endotoxins do not stimulate the production of strong antibodies. For this reason, it has not been possible to develop vaccines against endotoxin-bearing bacteria. Instead, to fight these bacteria, the body uses a group of proteins collectively called the **complement system.** These proteins coat the bacteria and then either help kill the microorganisms directly or aid neutrophils (in the blood) or macrophages (in the tissues) in the process of microorganism destruction. The *reticuloendothelial system* (composed of cells in the spleen, lymph nodes, liver, bone marrow, lungs, and intestines) works with the lymphatic system to dispose of the debris produced by the immune system's attack on invading organisms.

Bacteria that make endotoxins are also called *pyrogenic bacteria*. They are called this because they activate the inflammatory process. They also produce fever directly through the release of cell membrane toxins. As part of the inflammatory process, white blood cells are released from the bone marrow. This is the cause of the increased white blood cell count that is commonly found with infection. Inflammation also increases capillary permeability. This allows substances that destroy bacteria to migrate from the capillaries to the site of infection (see Chapter 28). Fever is caused by the release of *endogenous pyrogens* (proteins that act on the thermoregulatory centers of the hypothalamus). These proteins are released by macrophages or by circulating white blood cells that are attracted to the injury site.

CRITICAL THINKING
Will treating a fever with antipyretic drugs cause the body to rid itself of the toxin that caused the fever?

A **hypersensitivity reaction** is a life-threatening pathogenic mechanism of bacterial toxins. Few toxins are capable of producing this type of reaction. An immunological response occurs with the first exposure to the toxin. *Hypersensitivity* develops the next time the individual is exposed to the toxin. The result is an inflammatory response. At times, the response is so extreme that the person is killed instead of the bacteria. For example, the complement system can activate blood clotting and can cause white blood cells to aggregate and form "clumps," which block blood vessels.

The net effect of overactivation of the complement system by endotoxins is the blockage of small blood vessels in the lungs (with the clumps) and the formation of tiny blood clots in small arteries elsewhere in the body. Luckily, this life-threatening reaction is rare. Moreover, the complement system normally acts as an efficient defense against most bacterial toxins without causing any damage. (Hypersensitivity reactions are further described later in this chapter and in Chapter 27).

NOTE
When the body's defenses fail and microorganisms multiply in the blood, **bacteremia** develops. This may lead to *septicemia*, a severe systemic infection in which pathogens are present in the bloodstream. The endotoxins (along with a number of proteins involved in the inflammatory response) cause vasodilation. This reduces blood pressure and oxygen delivery. The result is shock. Other signs of an inflammatory response to bacteremia may include chills, fever, and an altered level of consciousness. Rashes or red streaks also may be associated with bacteremia. (The red streaks are called *lymphangitis*.)

CRITICAL THINKING
In septic shock, toxins damage the cell membrane, making it more permeable. This allows fluids to leak out of the blood vessels more freely. How could that affect cardiac output?

Viruses. Viruses cause many human diseases. These include the *common cold, influenza, chickenpox, smallpox, hepatitis, herpes,* and *acquired immunodeficiency syndrome* (AIDS). Viruses are intracellular parasites that work very differently from bacteria (Figure 11-16). Viruses lack much of the machinery that allows bacterial cells and other types of cells to grow rapidly and multiply. They can reproduce only by infecting the living cells of host tissue. (They often destroy the host cell.) Viruses usually consist of a protein coat (**capsid**) that encloses a core of nucleic acid. They have no organelles and therefore have no metabolism. They do not produce endotoxins or exotoxins.

Viruses need nucleic acid (either deoxyribonucleic acid [DNA] or ribonucleic acid [RNA]) to replicate. (Unlike all other cellular forms of life, viruses never have both DNA and RNA.) Cells are thought to engulf the virus particles by surrounding them with part of the cell membrane. Once inside the cell, the virus loses the capsid and begins to replicate the viral nucleic acids. Some viruses cause the cell to burst. Others replicate without destroying the cell.

The capsid enables the virus particle to resist **phagocytosis,** even though viruses often trigger a very strong immune response. Viruses can rapidly cause permanent and lethal injury in hosts, regardless of the host's state of immunosuppression. Rabies, smallpox, and influenza are examples of viral diseases that are highly infectious and that have high rates of illness (morbidity) and death (mortality).

NOTE
Phagocytosis is the process of ingestion of solid substances by cells. Substances ingested may include other cells, bacteria, pieces of necrosed (dead) tissue, and foreign particles.

Viral infections are easier to prevent than to treat. Vaccines have proven to be the best guard against viral disease (Box 11-6). Viral infections usually cause active illness. The

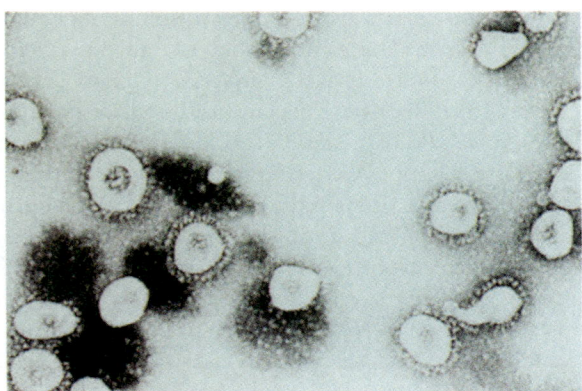

FIGURE 11-16 Coronavirus particles. (From U.S. Department of Health Education and Welfare, Public Health Service, Centers for Disease Control and Prevention, Atlanta, Ga.)

BOX 11-6 Influenza Vaccines

Influenza viruses are categorized into three major types: A, B, and C.

Type A mutates every 2 to 3 years. (Type A influenza viruses have caused worldwide epidemics, killing tens of thousands of people.) Type B mutates every 3 to 6 years. Type C apparently does not mutate. The mutations allow the virus to escape containment by the immune system. This is true even if a person had a previous influenza infection. Each year, virologists and epidemiologists analyze cultures from the southern hemisphere (where the flu season occurs during the northern hemisphere's summer). They try to determine which strains are likely to appear in the upcoming flu season and use this information to prepare effective vaccines. If the expected strain strikes, the vaccine can protect about 75% of those who have been vaccinated. It takes about 2 weeks after the vaccination to build antibodies (see Chapter 28).

signs and symptoms are based on the type and location of the cells infected. For this reason, certain viruses tend to cause respiratory illness (e.g., influenza). Others cause gastroenteritis (*enteroviruses*), central nervous system disease (e.g., *St. Louis B encephalitis, rabies*), or liver disease (*hepatitis*).

IMMUNOLOGICAL AND INFLAMMATORY INJURY

Cellular membranes are damaged by direct contact with cellular and chemical components of the immune and inflammatory responses. These components include phagocytic cells (*monocytes, neutrophils,* and *macrophages*) and substances such as *antibodies, lymphokines, complements,* and *proteases* (see Chapters 28 and 32). If the cell membrane is injured or if the transport mechanism (which moves potassium into the cell and sodium out of it) begins to fail, intracellular water level increases. This causes the cell to swell. If the swelling continues, the cell eventually may rupture.

INJURIOUS GENETIC FACTORS

Genetic disease results from a chromosomal abnormality or a defective gene. These genetic defects may be inherited. (An example of such a disease is *sickle cell anemia*.) They also may result from spontaneous mutations. (An example is *Down syndrome*.) Some genetic disorders can alter the cell's structure and function. Genetic disorders can cause changes in the structural or metabolic component of the specific target cells. *Huntington's disease* and *muscular dystrophy* are examples of conditions caused by such disorders (see Chapter 32).

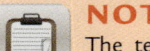

NOTE

The term **congenital** refers to any abnormality that is present at birth. This is the case even though the abnormality may not be detected until much later.

INJURIOUS NUTRITIONAL IMBALANCES

Cells need adequate amounts of essential nutrients to function normally. If the needed nutrients are not obtained through the diet and transported to the cells, pathophysiological effects on the cells can occur. Damaging effects also can occur if excessive amounts of nutrients are consumed and transported to the cells. Examples of conditions caused by injurious nutritional imbalances include *protein-calorie malnutrition, obesity, hyperglycemia, scurvy,* and *rickets.*

INJURIOUS PHYSICAL AGENTS

Many physical agents can damage cells and tissues. Examples of physical agents (including environmental agents) that can cause cellular or tissue injury include the following:

- Temperature extremes (e.g., hypothermic and hyperthermic injury)
- Changes in atmospheric pressure (e.g., blast injury, decompression sickness)
- Ionizing radiation (e.g., radiation injury)
- Nonionizing radiation (e.g., radio waves, microwaves)
- Illumination (light injury [e.g., vision injury, skin cancer])
- Mechanical stresses (e.g., noise-induced hearing loss, overuse syndromes)

Manifestations of Cellular Injury

An injured cell may show various types of abnormalities in its form and structure. These are known as *morphological abnormalities*. The two most common abnormalities of this type are *cellular swelling* and *fatty change*. Cellular injury is indicated by both local and systemic signs.

CELLULAR MANIFESTATIONS

In injured cells (and in some healthy cells), several substances accumulate. They include fluids and electrolytes, triglycerides (lipids), glucose, calcium, uric acid, protein, melanin, and bilirubin. These substances normally are present in certain cells of the body. However, abnormal intracellular accumulation may lead to cellular damage. Also, injured cells may be unable to rid themselves of excessive amounts of water, sodium, or calcium. This leads to increased injury. If water, sodium, or calcium continues to accumulate, the cells become permanently damaged.

Macrophages ingest debris from injured cells. Some macrophages circulate throughout the body. Others remain fixed in tissues (e.g., the liver and the spleen). Phagocytes migrate to injured tissue. They engulf dying cells and abnormal extracellular substances. As more phagocytes migrate to injured tissue to engulf the metabolites, the affected tissue begins to swell. Phagocytosis by the fixed macrophages of the reticuloendothelial system causes enlargement of the liver (*hepatomegaly*) or the spleen (*splenomegaly*). This is seen with many diseases that are associated with abnormal accumulation of various metabolic products (*amyloidosis*) or abnormal cells (*hemolytic disease*).

Cellular Swelling. As described previously, the swelling in injured cells results from membrane changes that allow potassium to leak rapidly out of the cell and sodium and water to enter the cell. The increase in intracellular sodium concentration increases the osmotic pressure. This draws more water into the cell. If the swelling affects all cells in an organ, the organ increases in weight and becomes distended. Cellular swelling usually is reversible.

> **NOTE**
> Inflammation is associated with cellular swelling. This is true whether the cause is infection, trauma, or an autoimmune reaction. Inflammation is often accompanied by fever.

Fatty Change. Fatty change occurs when the enzyme systems that metabolize fat are impaired or overwhelmed. When this happens, lipids accumulate inside the cell. This is common in liver cells (*fatty liver*), because these cells are actively involved in the metabolism of fat. Hepatic metabolism and secretion of lipids are crucial to proper body function. For this reason, deficiencies in these processes lead to major pathological changes. Alcohol abuse is a common cause of fatty liver. It usually is a precursor to cirrhosis.

Systemic Manifestations. Cellular injury produces many systemic manifestations. These include fever, malaise, loss of well-being, change in appetite, altered heart rate, an abnormal rise in WBCs (**leukocytosis**), and pain. In addition, testing of extracellular fluid may reveal the presence of cellular enzymes released by injured cells or tissue.

Cellular Death and Necrosis

A cell dies if it has been irreparably damaged. Shortly after cell death, structural changes begin to occur in the nucleus and cytoplasm. The *lysosome* (a membranous sac of digestive enzymes found in many cells) begins to undergo membrane breakdown. This releases the lysosomal enzymes, which begin to digest the cell. The nucleus shrinks and dissolves or breaks into fragments (Box 11-7).

BOX 11-7 Normal Cellular Aging and Death

Cellular aging and death are common processes. They are natural functions of the cell cycle. As the cell ages, it becomes less efficient in executing its functions. It also is more at risk of damage from harmful environmental agents. With progressive damage, cells lose their ability to repair themselves. In time, they begin to malfunction. Changes in immunological cells slowly lead to decreased immunity and an increased risk of infectious disease. Malignancies increase with age as a result of decreased immunity. This also is due to an increased incidence of malignant transformation of various in cells. Other examples of the manifestations of aging in cells include gray hair, reduced muscle mass, menopause, arteriosclerosis, memory and vision impairment, and arthritis.

Necrosis is the death of cells or tissues caused by injury or disease. It also can occur by cellular self-destruction (**autolysis**). Different types of necrosis tend to occur in different organs or tissues. The type may indicate the cause of cellular injury. Necrotic changes take several hours to develop. They are easy to recognize on histological examination by their structure and staining characteristics.

HYPOPERFUSION

The term **hypoperfusion** is used to describe decreased circulation of blood and nutrients to tissues and organs. If this condition is prolonged, hypoperfusion can result in permanent cellular dysfunction and death. Hypoperfusion can be caused by a number of medical and traumatic conditions.

Pathogenesis

Hypoperfusion often is the result of a decrease in cardiac output. Decreased cardiac output, if prolonged, leads to **shock** (a continued state of hypoperfusion), *multiple organ dysfunction syndrome,* and other disease states associated with impaired cellular metabolism.

DECREASED CARDIAC OUTPUT

Cardiac output (also known as the *cardiac minute volume*) is the total amount of blood pumped by the ventricles each minute. It is usually expressed in liters per minute (L/min). Cardiac output is a crucial determinant of organ perfusion. It depends on several factors. These include the strength of contraction, the rate of contraction, and the amount of available blood returning through the veins (*venous return*) to the ventricles (**preload**).

> **NOTE**
> Cardiac output is determined by multiplying the heart rate by the stroke volume (i.e., the volume of blood ejected by the ventricles during each heartbeat). For example, if the ventricles contract 64 times per minute and eject 70 mL of blood with each contraction, the cardiac output would be 64 beats per minute multiplied by 70 mL per beat, or 4.48 L/min.

COMPENSATORY MECHANISMS

The body uses compensatory mechanisms to manage blood pressure and cardiac output. These include a number of **negative feedback mechanisms.** A negative feedback mechanism is any mechanism that tends to balance a change in a system. A number of negative feedback mechanisms are crucial to the process of maintaining cardiac output and tissue perfusion. These include baroreceptor reflexes, chemoreceptor reflexes, the central nervous system ischemic response, hormonal mechanisms, reabsorption of tissue fluids, and splenic discharge of stored blood (seen in animals but minimal in humans).

Baroreceptor Reflexes. As mentioned earlier, baroreceptors (Figure 11-17, *A*) are pressure-sensitive nerve endings found in the heart and great vessels. They keep blood pressure and cardiac output within a normal range.

Normal blood pressure produces a constant, low-level stimulation of the baroreceptors. When the blood pressure moves out of the normal range, either up or down, stimulation of the baroreceptors increases (Box 11-8). The baroreceptor reflexes then act to correct the condition. If the arterial blood pressure increases, the baroreceptor reflexes act to lower blood pressure. Likewise, if the arterial blood pressure decreases, the baroreceptor reflexes act to increase blood pressure (see Figure 11-17, *A*).[8] When baroreceptor stimulation ceases because of a fall in arterial pressure, the negative feedback mechanism evokes several cardiovascular responses (see Box 11-8). Vagal (parasympathetic) stimulation is reduced, and sympathetic response is increased. The increase in sympathetic impulses results in increased **peripheral vascular resistance** (PVR). It also results in an increase in the heart rate and stroke volume. Sympathetic responses also cause generalized arteriolar vasoconstriction. This reduces the size of the vascular compartment. As the veins constrict, blood is shifted into the central circulation. This, coupled with the constriction of blood vessels in the skin, muscles, and viscera, helps maintain perfusion of the central organs. The vasoconstriction in these peripheral vascular beds results in the characteristic pale, cool skin seen in patients suffering from *hypovolemic shock.*

> **NOTE**
> Peripheral vascular resistance is the resistance to blood flow in the systemic circulation (small arteries, arterioles, venules, veins). **Afterload** is the systemic vascular resistance on the left side of the heart. It is the pressure against which the left ventricle must contract to eject its contents.

BOX 11-8 Baroreceptor Responses to Changes in Blood Pressure: Sympathetic Nervous System

Baroreceptors (see Figure 11-17, *A*) help maintain blood pressure and cardiac output in two ways. Both of these are negative feedback mechanisms. Baroreceptors lower blood pressure in response to increased arterial pressure. They also increase blood pressure in response to decreased arterial pressure. Normal blood pressure partially stretches the arterial walls so that the baroreceptors produce a constant, low level frequency stimulation. This stimulation increases progressively from a lower pressure limit of 60 mm Hg to a maximum at 180 to 200 mm Hg. Impulses from the baroreceptors travel through the vagus and the Hering nerve to the glossopharyngeal nerve. There, they inhibit the vasoconstrictor center of the medulla. They also excite the vagal center. These impulses result in vasodilation in the peripheral circulatory system. They also cause a decrease in the heart rate and strength of contraction. The combined effect is a decrease in arterial pressure.

When low blood pressure stimulates a response in the baroreceptors, the effects on the heart include increases in the strength and rate of contraction. Peripheral effects include arteriolar constriction, decreased blood vessel size, and increased peripheral vascular resistance.

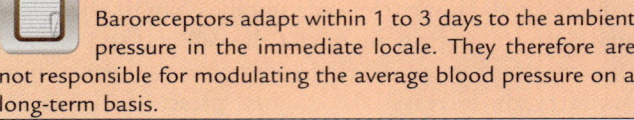

> **NOTE**
> Baroreceptors adapt within 1 to 3 days to the ambient pressure in the immediate locale. They therefore are not responsible for modulating the average blood pressure on a long-term basis.

Chemoreceptor Reflexes. When low arterial pressure leads to hypoxemia, acidosis, or both, peripheral chemoreceptor cells are stimulated. These are found in the carotid and aortic bodies. Because of the location of these bodies, the chemoreceptor cells have a vast blood supply. When the PO_2 or pH decreases, chemoreceptor cells stimulate the vasomotor center of the medulla. At the same time, the rate and depth of ventilation are increased. This helps to eliminate excess carbon dioxide. It also helps to maintain acid-base balance. Chemoreceptors (see Figure 11-17, *B*) are more involved in the regulation of respiration than in the regulation of the cardiovascular rate and rhythm or blood pressure. However, during profound hypotension or acidosis, chemoreceptors will produce vasoconstriction. This vasomotor stimulation results in enhanced peripheral vasoconstriction, which is initiated by the baroreceptors.

Central Nervous System Ischemic Response. Blood flow to the vasomotor center of the medulla can be reduced enough to cause ischemia. When this occurs, the neurons in the vasomotor center become excited. This raises the arterial blood pressure. This effect is known as the **central nervous system ischemic response.** The degree of sympathetic vasoconstriction can be intense. It can be so intense that it elevates the arterial pressure for as long as 10 minutes, sometimes to more than 200 mm Hg. If the ischemia lasts longer than a few minutes, the vagal centers are activated. This results in vasodilation in the periphery and *bradycardia* (a slowed heart rate). Like the chemoreceptor reflex, the central nervous system ischemic response functions only in emergency situations. Moreover, it does not become active until the arterial blood pressure falls below 50 mm Hg.

Hormonal Mechanisms. Several hormonal mechanisms also help to control arterial pressure through negative feedback. These include the adrenal medullary mechanism, the renin-angiotensin-aldosterone mechanism, and the vasopressin mechanism.

Adrenal Medullary Mechanism. When sympathetic stimulation of the heart and blood vessels increases, stimulation of the adrenal medulla also increases. The hormones secreted by the adrenal medulla are *epinephrine* and *norepinephrine.* The effect of these hormones on the cardiovascular system is very similar to that produced by the sympathetic nervous system. As a result, the heart rate, the stroke volume, and vasoconstriction increase.

Renin-Angiotensin-Aldosterone Mechanism. As described before, *renin* is an enzyme. It is released by the kidneys into the circulatory system. Renin changes the structure

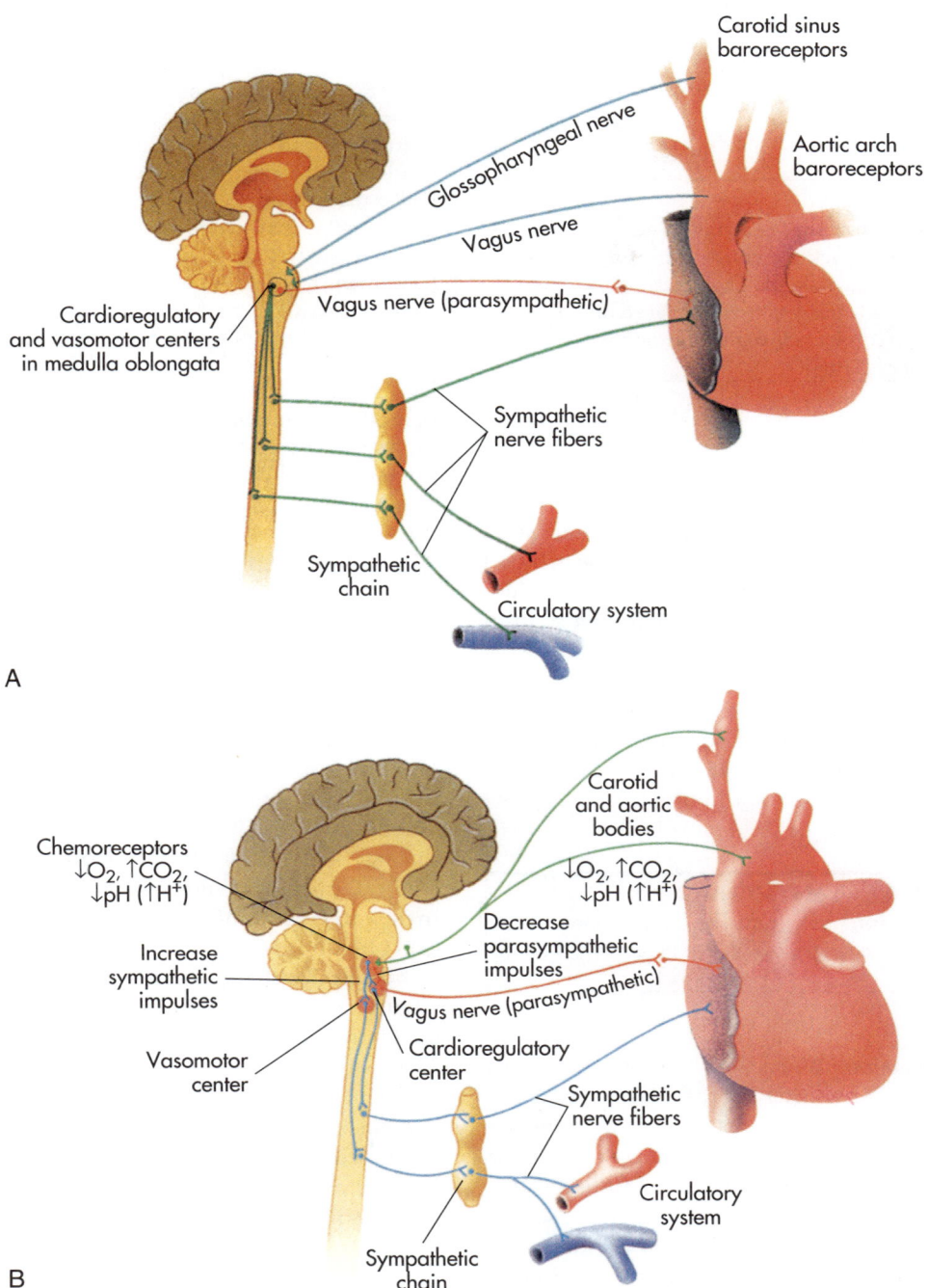

FIGURE 11-17 A, Baroreceptor reflexes. Baroreceptors in the carotid sinuses and the aortic arch detect changes in blood pressure. Impulses are conducted to the cardioregulatory and vasomotor centers. The heart rate can be decreased by the parasympathetic system; the heart rate and stroke volume can be increased by the sympathetic system. The sympathetic system can also constrict or dilate blood vessels. **B,** Chemoreceptor reflexes. Chemoreceptors in the medulla and carotid and aortic bodies detect changes in blood oxygen, carbon dioxide, or pH levels. Impulses are conducted to the medulla. In response, the vasomotor center can cause constriction or dilation of blood vessels through the sympathetic system, and the cardioregulatory center can cause changes in the pumping activity of the heart through the parasympathetic and sympathetic systems during emergency situations. Moreover, it does not become active until the blood pressure falls below 50 mm Hg.

of the plasma protein angiotensinogen, thereby producing angiotensin I. This, in turn, is converted by **angiotensin-converting enzyme** (mostly in the lungs), creating angiotensin II (active angiotensin).

> **NOTE**
> Angiotensin-converting enzyme (ACE) inhibitors are drugs that block the conversion of the precursor angiotensin I to the active molecule angiotensin II. As a result, blood pressure is lowered, and less stress is placed on the heart. Examples of ACE inhibitors include *captopril* (Capoten), *enalapril* (Vasotec), and *lisinopril* (Prinivil).

Angiotensin II causes vasoconstriction in the arterioles and to a lesser degree in the veins. This vasoconstriction results in increased peripheral vascular resistance, increased venous return to the heart, and a resultant increase in blood pressure. Angiotensin II also stimulates the release of aldosterone. Aldosterone acts on the kidneys to conserve sodium and water.

The renin-angiotensin-aldosterone mechanism is an important regulatory loop for increasing the blood pressure in circulatory shock. It takes about 20 minutes to become effective in hypovolemia caused by hemorrhagic shock. It remains active for about 1 hour.

> **CRITICAL THINKING**
> You are assessing your patient's radial pulse. What compensatory changes can you evaluate while doing this?

Vasopressin Mechanism. When the blood pressure drops or the concentration of solutes in the plasma increases (*increased serum osmolality*), the hypothalamic neurons are stimulated. This causes the anterior pituitary to increase secretion of vasopressin, or antidiuretic hormone (ADH). ADH acts directly on the blood vessels. It causes vasoconstriction within minutes after a rapid fall in the blood pressure. ADH also reduces the rate of urine production by enhancing reabsorption of water. This helps to maintain blood volume and blood pressure.

> **NOTE**
> *Atrial natriuretic factor* (ANF) also helps to control arterial pressure through a negative feedback mechanism. Its release is triggered by a rise in atrial pressure. (This is usually a sign of volume overload.) ANF increases the rate of urine production. Loss of water through the urine decreases blood volume. The result is a decrease in the atrial pressure. This is the only hormonal system actively used to decrease volume and pressure.

> **SHOW ME THE EVIDENCE**
> The brain natriuretic peptide (BNP) blood test is used to diagnose left ventricular failure (LVF). In 2001 researchers in Paris, France, conducted a prospective study to determine if this test could be used when treating prehospital patients complaining of difficulty breathing. A total of 52 adults older than 50 years who exhibited dyspnea were included (with some exclusions). During patient care, prehospital physicians categorized the cause of dyspnea as cardiac, respiratory, or uncertain. The BNP values did not affect treatment. BNP values were compared to the clinical diagnoses made by the physicians. All cardiac diagnoses were confirmed by BNP values. The BNP value established or corrected the original diagnosis in 33% of the cases, most frequently the uncertain patients. The authors concluded that BNP is a reliable indicator of LVF and that it appears to be a beneficial factor to enhance prehospital care. They cautioned that more studies are needed.

From Teboul A, Gaffinel A, Meune C, et al: Management of acute dyspnoea: use and feasibility of brain natriuretic peptide (BNP) assay in the prehospital setting, *Resuscitation* 61(1):91-96, 2004; doi: 10.1016/j.resuscitation.2003.12.005.

Reabsorption of Tissue Fluids. Arterial hypotension, arteriolar constriction, and reduced venous pressure during hypovolemia lower the blood pressure in the capillaries (*hydrostatic pressure*). This decrease promotes reabsorption of interstitial fluid into the vascular compartment. Large amounts of fluid may be drawn into the circulation during hemorrhage. It has been estimated that about 0.25 mL/min/kg of body weight, or 1 L/hr in the adult male, can be autoinfused from the interstitial spaces after acute blood loss.

Splenic Discharge of Blood. Some of the blood that circulates through the spleen continues through the microcirculation. It is stored in an area called the *venous sinuses*. The venous sinuses can store more than 300 mL of blood. Sudden reductions in blood pressure cause the sympathetic nervous system to stimulate constriction of these sinuses. Constriction can expel as much as 200 mL of this blood into the venous circulation to help restore blood volume or pressure in the circulation.

> **NOTE**
> An increase in preload or afterload or a decrease in stroke volume can lead to volume overload and pulmonary edema. This, in turn, can reduce tissue perfusion and impair cellular metabolism (see Chapter 22).

Types of Shock

Shock is classified according to the primary cause (Box 11-9). Although these classifications are separate and distinct, two or more types may be combined. Brief descriptions of the five types of shock are given here. A more detailed discussion of shock is presented in Chapter 36.

BOX 11-9 Common Etiological Classifications of Shock

Hypovolemic shock
Cardiogenic shock
Neurogenic shock
Anaphylactic shock
Septic shock

- *Hypovolemic shock* is most often caused by hemorrhage. It also may be caused by severe dehydration. In either case, circulating volume is lost.
- *Cardiogenic shock* results when the heart's pumping action cannot deliver adequate circulation for tissue perfusion.
- *Neurogenic shock* results most often from spinal cord injury that is accompanied by loss of sympathetic vasomotor tone.
- *Anaphylactic shock* occurs when the body is exposed to a substance that produces a severe allergic reaction.
- *Septic shock* most often results from a serious systemic bacterial infection.

Regardless of the classification, the underlying defect in shock is inadequate tissue perfusion.

Multiple Organ Dysfunction Syndrome

Multiple organ dysfunction syndrome (MODS) is the progressive failure of two or more organ systems. This occurs after a very severe illness or injury. Sepsis and septic shock are common causes of MODS. However, it may follow any period of prolonged shock, regardless of the cause (see Chapter 36).

> **NOTE**
> Multiple organ dysfunction syndrome (MODS) was first described in 1975. The death rate is 60% to 90%. The rate nears 100% if three or more organs are involved, if sepsis is present, and if the patient is older than 65 years.[9]

PATHOPHYSIOLOGY

Any process that triggers the body's inflammatory response may initiate MODS. (This includes traumatic, septic, and burn injury.) The syndrome begins with vascular endothelial damage. This damage is caused by the release of endotoxins and inflammatory mediators into the circulation. When the vascular endothelium is damaged, it becomes permeable. It allows fluid and cells to leak into the interstitial spaces. This, in turn, contributes to hypotension and hypoperfusion. The release of mediators activates three major plasma enzyme cascades, or processes: *complement, coagulation,* and *kallikrein/kinin.*

The plasma protein cascade systems are responsible for mediating the inflammatory response. Each system consists of a series of inactive enzymes (*proenzymes*). These are

BOX 11-10 Clinical Manifestations of Multiple Organ Dysfunction Syndrome

After resuscitation (within 24 hours), a patient with multiple organ dysfunction syndrome (MODS) develops a low-grade fever, tachycardia, dyspnea, and altered mental status (confusion, altered level of consciousness). The lungs also begin to fail. This results in acute respiratory distress syndrome (ARDS). After 7 to 10 days, bacteremia commonly develops. Signs of kidney and liver failure appear as well. During days 14 to 21, renal and liver failure become severe, and the gastrointestinal (GI) and immune systems fail, followed by cardiovascular collapse. If the patient does not improve by the end of the third week, survival is unlikely. Death usually occurs between day 21 and day 28.

converted to active enzymes. This, in turn, initiates a cascade in which the *substrate* (a substance changed by an enzyme in a chemical reaction) of the activated enzyme is the next component of the system.

Complement activates phagocytes and induces further inflammation and damage to the endothelium. As a result of the endothelial damage, coagulation becomes uncontrolled. This results in the formation of microvascular thrombi and tissue ischemia. Activation of the kallikrein/kinin system releases *bradykinin* (a potent vasodilator), which contributes to low systemic vascular resistance. The overall effect of these three systems is a hyperinflammatory and hypercoagulable state that leads to edema formation, cardiovascular instability (hypotension), and clotting abnormalities. These inflammatory processes alter the normal pathways both of systemic blood flow and of blood flow in the individual organs. The result is a hyperdynamic circulation where the cardiovascular system responds to a decrease in PVR by an elevation in cardiac output that is above normal. It is also marked by an increase in the amount of blood returning to the heart through the veins. Blood is shunted past some regional capillary beds. Changes in capillary permeability allow the formation of interstitial edema. As a result, the delivery of oxygen to the tissues is decreased. In addition, the capillaries become blocked by tiny blood clots and by clumps of inflammatory cells. The resultant ischemia contributes to MODS.

The same hormonal responses that help conserve volume in shock cause the body to enter into a hypermetabolic (*catabolic*) state, altering carbohydrate, fat, and lipid metabolism to meet the increased demand for energy. In time, the sympathetic drive and the hyperdynamic circulation place great demands on the heart. The net result is depletion of oxygen and fuel supplies. The decrease in oxygen delivery to the cells, the hypermetabolism, and the associated myocardial depression create an imbalance in oxygen supply and demand. This is soon followed by tissue hypoxia with cellular acidosis and impaired cellular function. Finally, multiple organ failure begins (Box 11-10 and Figure 11-18).

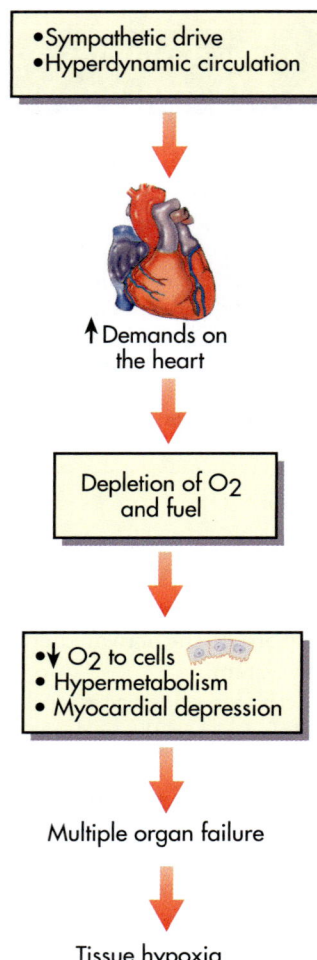

FIGURE 11-18 Multiple organ dysfunction syndrome.

Glucose is a key fuel for the production of energy. It is really the only fuel that can be used anaerobically under conditions of cellular hypoxia (as occurs in a state of shock). Under these conditions, glucose is metabolized to *lactate* and *pyruvate*. This produces a net sum of 2 ATP molecules. If oxygen is present (aerobic metabolism), pyruvate enters the **Krebs cycle.** This is a sequence of reactions that breaks down a molecule of pyruvic acid into molecules of carbon dioxide and water (Figure 11-19). The Krebs cycle is 18 times more efficient at producing ATP than is glycolysis. (Glycolysis is the breakdown of glucose to lactate.) The Krebs cycle cannot occur in the absence of oxygen. Anaerobic production of ATP is inefficient. Thus, with anaerobic metabolism, the rate of **glycolysis** must be greatly increased to meet the body's energy demands. This leads to an increase in the production of lactic acid and resultant metabolic acidosis.

As tissue metabolites (and hydrogen ions) continue to accumulate, they stimulate vasodilation. This vasodilation opposes the previously described hormonally regulated constriction of the precapillary sphincters, thereby reducing the body's ability to continue vital tissue perfusion by maintaining the proper size of the vascular compartment. (The *postcapillary sphincters* are more resistant to the vasodilating effects of tissue metabolites. They stay constricted long after the *precapillary sphincters* dilate.) This in turn increases the capillary hydrostatic pressure. The result is fluid loss from the vascular space into the interstitial space. In addition, the insufficient energy production of anaerobic metabolism affects the cell's ability to maintain a normal sodium-potassium differential across the cell membrane. Intracellular potassium leaks out of the cell; sodium leaks into the cell. This creates cellular swelling and a decreased transmembrane potential. Energy production is further impaired. Finally, the cells are irreversibly damaged.

SELF-DEFENSE MECHANISMS

The body's first lines of defense against illness and injury are the external barriers. These include the skin and the mucous membranes of the digestive, respiratory, and genitourinary tracts. These structures form a barrier between the internal organs and the environment (see Chapter 28). When they are breached, chemicals, foreign bodies, or microorganisms are allowed to enter cells and tissues. The second and third lines of defense then are activated. These are the **inflammatory response** and the **immune response,** respectively.

Inflammatory Response

Inflammation is a local reaction to cellular injury. The response may be triggered by physical, thermal, or chemical damage. It also may be caused by microbial infection. When a microbial invasion occurs, this line of defense is activated. It prevents further invasion of the pathogen by isolating, destroying, or neutralizing the microorganism. As a rule, the response is protective and is considered beneficial. However, if the response is sustained or directed toward the host's own **antigens,** healthy tissue may be destroyed.

No specific therapy exists for MODS. However, early detection is critical, because it allows supportive measures to be started at once.

Impairment of Cellular Metabolism

Energy is required for nearly all of the cellular activities that support life. The active transport pumps in the cell membrane consume a large portion of the cell's energy. They use this energy to maintain a normal fluid and electrolyte composition inside the cell. Adenosine triphosphate (ATP) and other high-energy phosphate molecules provide the fuel for all the energy-related functions of the cell. In the healthy body, most cellular metabolism is aerobic metabolism. Anaerobic metabolism occurs when the metabolic need for energy exceeds the oxygen supply. However, anaerobic metabolism can supply only a small fraction of the energy produced by aerobic metabolism. (Anaerobic metabolism generates 2 ATP molecules for every molecule of glucose. Aerobic metabolism generates 36 ATP molecules for every molecule of glucose.) By itself, anaerobic metabolism cannot meet the body's energy needs.

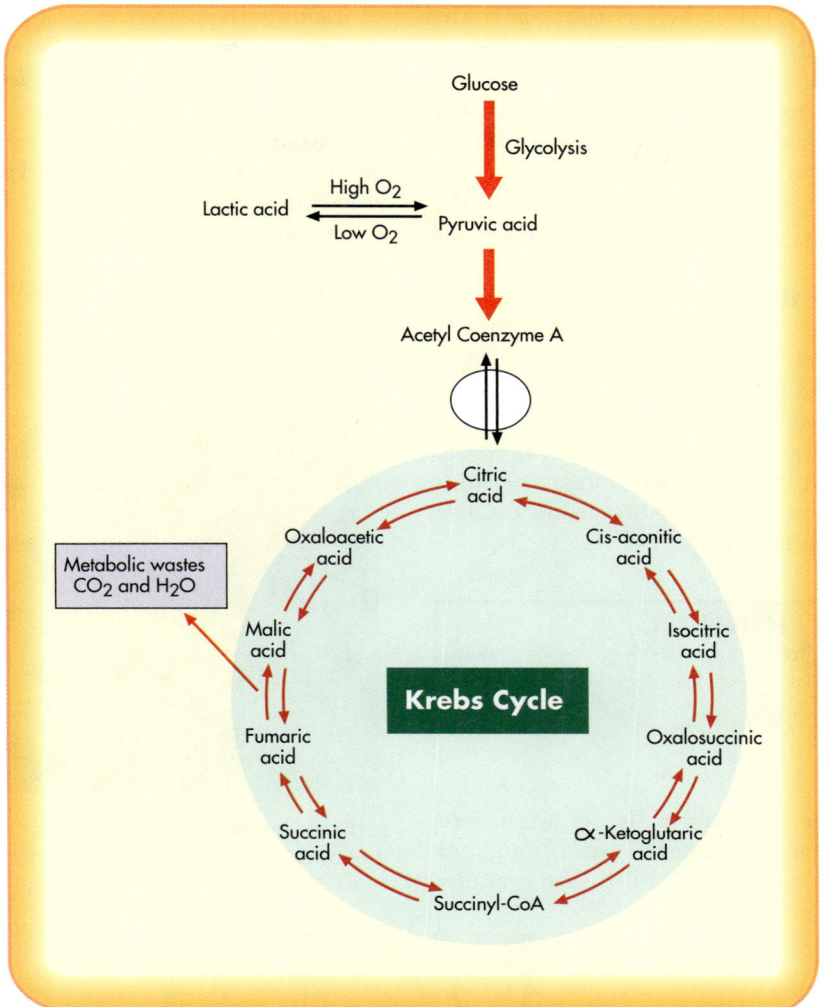

FIGURE 11-19 Krebs cycle.

STAGES OF THE INFLAMMATORY RESPONSE

The inflammatory response may be divided into three separate stages. These are the *cellular response to injury,* the *vascular response to injury,* and *phagocytosis.*

Cellular Response to Injury. Metabolic changes occur with any type of cellular injury. The most common primary effect of cellular injury is damage to the cell's aerobic metabolism and ATP-generating process (*oxidative phosphorylation*). This leads to a decrease in energy reserves. When the energy sources are depleted, the sodium-potassium pump can no longer work effectively. The cell begins to swell as sodium ions accumulate. The organelles in the cell also swell. This swelling, along with increasing acidosis, leads to further impairment of enzyme function. It also leads to further deterioration of the cell's membranes. In time, the membranes of the cellular organelles begin to leak. The release of hydrolytic enzymes by the lysosomes contributes further to cellular destruction and autolysis. As the cellular contents are dissolved by enzymes, the inflammatory response is stimulated in surrounding tissues.

Vascular Response to Injury. After cellular injury, localized **hyperemia** (an increase in organ blood flow) develops as the surrounding arterioles, venules, and capillaries dilate. The associated increase in filtration pressure and capillary permeability causes fluid to leak from the vessels. It leaks into the interstitial space. This creates edema. Leukocytes (particularly neutrophils and monocytes) begin to collect along the vascular endothelium. As a result of the release of **chemotactic factors** (chemicals that attract white blood cells to the site of inflammation), they soon migrate to the injured tissue.

Phagocytosis. As described earlier, *phagocytosis* is the process by which leukocytes engulf, digest, and destroy pathogens. The circulating macrophages are also responsible for clearing the injured area of dead cells and other debris. *Intracellular phagocytosis* is the ingestion of bacteria and dead cell fragments. It occurs at the site of tissue invasion. It may extend into the general circulation if the infection becomes systemic. Intracellular phagocytosis stimulates the release of chemicals that induce lysis of the leukocytes. These leukocytes combine with dead organisms, proteins, and fluid to form an inflammatory exudate (commonly known as *pus*). This exudate is a by-product of the inflammatory process associated with bacterial infection. Exudate may be watery (serous exudate), as is seen with blisters; thick and clotted (*fibrinous exudate*), as is seen with lobar pneumonia; or pus filled (*purulent exudate*), as is seen with cysts or abscesses. If bleeding occurs, the exudate is described as *hemorrhagic exudate*.

> ### CRITICAL THINKING
> Consider these signs or symptoms: heat, redness, pain, and swelling. What pathophysiological inflammatory response causes each of these?

MAST CELLS

As described in Chapter 10, **mast cells** are specialized cells (Figure 11-20). They are widely distributed throughout connective tissues. Their cytoplasm is filled with granules

containing *vasoactive amines* (histamine, serotonin) and chemotactic factors. When tissue is injured, the mast cells discharge their granules (*degranulation*) as part of the inflammatory response. Mast cell degranulation is stimulated by physical injury (e.g., thermal or mechanical trauma), chemical agents (e.g., toxins, snake and bee venoms), or hypersensitivity reactions. It also may be a direct result of the activity of complement components.

LOCAL AND SYSTEMIC RESPONSE TO ACUTE INFLAMMATION

Acute inflammation may be characterized by both local and systemic effects (Figure 11-21). Local responses

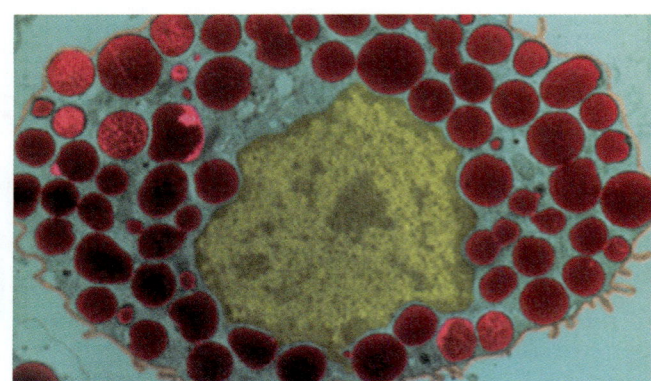

FIGURE 11-20 Mast cell in bone marrow. (From Patton KT, Thibodeau GA: *Anatomy and physiology,* ed 7, St Louis, 2007, Mosby.)

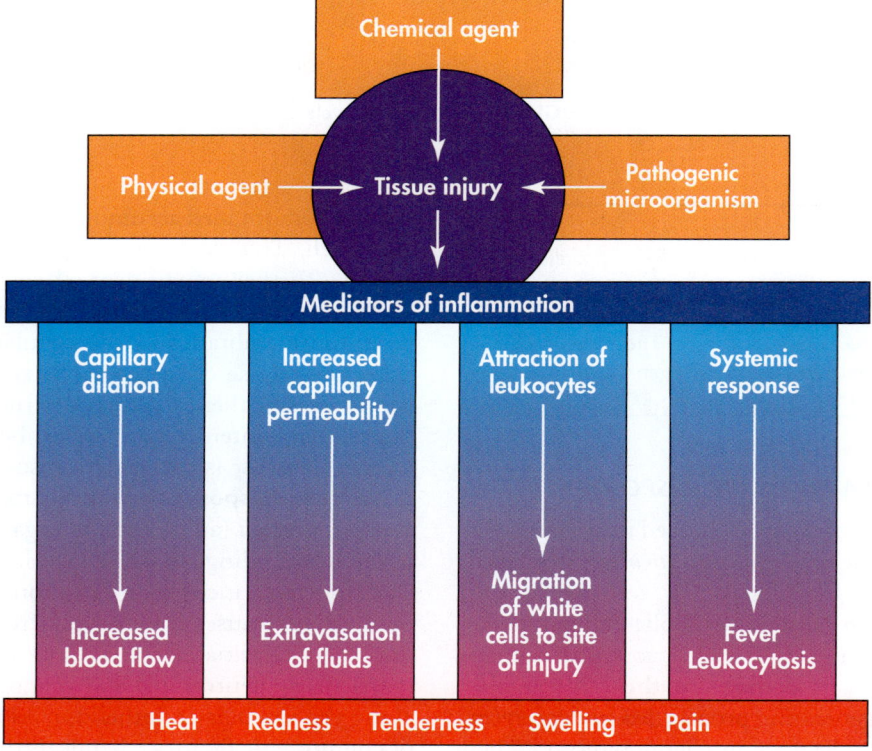

FIGURE 11-21 Inflammation. (Modified from Crowley L: *Introduction to human disease,* ed 3, Boston, 1992, Jones & Bartlett.)

include vascular changes (vasodilation and increased vascular permeability) and the formation of exudate. Systemic responses include fever, leukocytosis, and an increase in the level of circulating plasma proteins. The characteristic signs of localized inflammation are heat, redness, tenderness, swelling, and pain.

RESPONSES TO CHRONIC INFLAMMATION

Chronic inflammation lasts 2 weeks or longer. It can result from a persistent acute inflammatory response. This type of response may be caused by bacterial contamination by a foreign body (e.g., wood splinter, glass), persistent infection, or continued exposure to an antigen. If the inflammatory process is severe or prolonged, the body attempts to repair or replace tissue that has been damaged. The body produces connective tissue fibers and new blood vessels for use in the repair process. If the area of tissue destruction is large, scar tissue forms.

Immune Response

The skin and the inflammatory response are the first two defense mechanisms the body uses to protect itself from injurious agents (see Chapter 27). They respond to every agent using the identical nonspecific mechanism. The immune response, however, is specific to each individual pathogen. Immunity may be natural, present at birth, or acquired. *Acquired immunity* develops through exposure to a specific antigenic agent or pathogen. It can be induced through vaccination (immunization) against certain infectious diseases. An example of such a disease is measles.

Acquired immunity is further classified as humoral immunity and cell-mediated immunity. *Humoral immunity* is associated with the production of antibodies that combine with and eliminate foreign material. *Cell-mediated immunity* is characterized by the formation of a group of lymphocytes that attack and destroy foreign material (see Chapter 28). Cell-mediated immunity is the body's best defense against viruses, fungi, parasites, and some bacteria. It also is the mechanism the body uses to reject transplanted organs.

> ### 💡 CRITICAL THINKING
> Consider hepatitis, feline leukemia, and chickenpox. What kind of immunity protects you from each of these infections?

> ### 📋 NOTE
> The immune response is affected by age. Most infants are born with enough natural immunity to protect themselves from disease until they have made their own antibodies. However, the cells of the immune system become less efficient with age. Older people become more susceptible to disease. The aging immune system also becomes less able to eliminate abnormal cells that may develop.

INDUCTION OF THE IMMUNE RESPONSE

As defined previously, an *antigen* is a substance that reacts with preformed components of the immune system. For example, it may react with lymphocytes and antibodies. An antigen may be a molecule or a molecular complex. An *immunogen* is a specific type of antigen, one that also can bring about, or induce, the formation of antibodies. (Some antigens, therefore, are not immunogens because they are unable to induce the immune response.) To be immunogenic, the antigenic molecule must be:
- Sufficiently foreign to the host
- Sufficiently large
- Sufficiently complex
- Present in sufficient amounts

The immune response is triggered after foreign materials have been cleared from the area of inflammation. After phagocytes digest the pathogens, antigenic material appears on their surface. The antigen is recognized by receptors on lymphocytes as foreign, or "non-self." Then, a chain of events is set in motion to destroy or neutralize the antigen. Briefly, this involves two primary changes that occur among the lymphocytes. Some mature into plasma cells (derived from **B lymphocytes**), which produce antibody. Others mature into sensitized lymphocytes (**T lymphocytes**). These are capable of interacting directly with the foreign antigen to neutralize or destroy it. (The immune response is presented in more detail in Chapters 27 and 28.)

BLOOD GROUP ANTIGENS

In the early 1900s researchers discovered that human blood had individual variations. A donor's blood was separated into plasma and red blood cell components and mixed with separated blood samples from another donor. Two reactions were noted. When combined with foreign plasma, the red cells either clumped together (*agglutinated*) or showed no change. Scientists also found that two distinct *agglutinins* (substances on red blood cells that act as antigens) were responsible for the clumping. Based on possible combinations of these antigens, four types of human blood were identified: A, B, AB, and O (Figure 11-22).

Type A blood has anti-B antibodies in the plasma. It therefore clumps type B blood. Type B blood has anti-A antibodies. It therefore clumps type A blood. Type AB blood has neither antibody. Therefore people with this blood type can be given any of the four types of blood (*universal recipient*). Type O blood has both anti-A and anti-B antibodies but no antigens. It can therefore be given to patients with any blood type. Type O blood has become known as the *universal donor*.

> ### 📋 NOTE
> *Immune tolerance* refers to the immune system's ability to allow self-antigens (versus non–self-antigens) to exist by preventing their recognition by lymphocytes and antibodies.

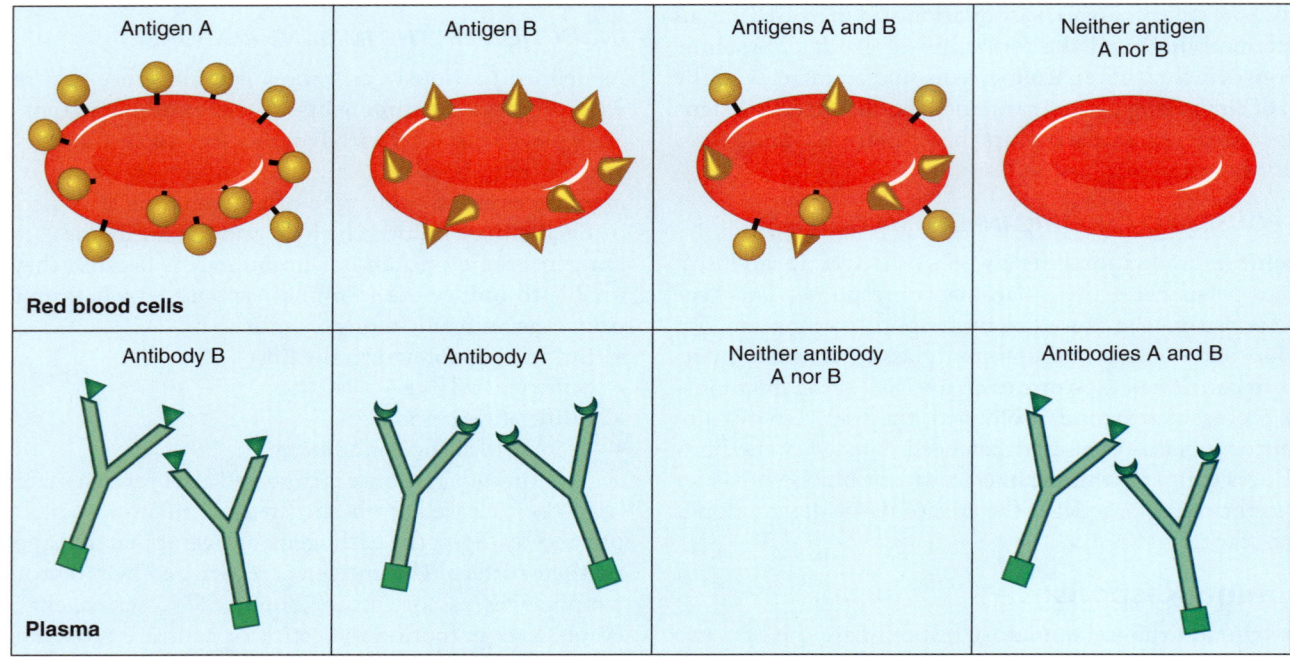

FIGURE 11-22 ABO blood groups. In type A blood, the red blood cells have type A surface antigens and the plasma has type B antibodies. In type B blood, the red cells have type B surface antigens and the plasma has type A antibodies. In type AB blood, the red cells have both type A and type B surface antigens but no plasma antibodies. In type O blood, the red cells have no ABO surface antigens but the plasma has A and B antibodies.

SHOW ME THE EVIDENCE

This group investigated the use of a hemoglobin-based oxygen carrier for prehospital resuscitation of trauma patients. A total of 714 injured patients with a systolic BP of ≤90 mm Hg were randomly given either PolyHeme or crystalloid fluid for resuscitation. They found no statistically significant difference in death rates at 30 days between the two groups. There were more adverse effects in the PolyHeme group. The researchers propose that PolyHeme may be considered as a substitute when blood is not available.

From Moore EE, Moore FA, Fabian TC, PolyHeme Study Group, et al: Human polymerized hemoglobin for the treatment of hemorrhagic shock when blood is unavailable: the USA multicenter trial, *J Am Coll Surg* 208(1):1-13, 2009.

Rh FACTOR

In the late 1940s another determinant in human blood was discovered: the **Rh factor.** (The acronym Rh was taken from the word rhesus, the species of monkey used in the research.) Researchers found that when the blood of a rhesus monkey was injected into a rabbit, the rabbit's immune system developed antibodies. When a sample of the rabbit's plasma was mixed with a sample of human red blood cells, the human cells usually agglutinated (*Rh positive*). About 85% of Americans have Rh-positive blood. Incompatibility between Rh-positive and Rh-negative blood can cause a harmful immune response (e.g., through

transfusion or during childbirth). The percentages of ABO and Rh blood groups in the general population are as follows:

O positive	38.4%
O negative	7.7%
A positive	32.3%
A negative	6.5%
B positive	9.4%
B negative	1.7%
AB positive	3.2%
AB negative	0.7%

VARIANCES IN IMMUNITY AND INFLAMMATION

The immune responses usually are protective. They help to protect the body from harmful microorganisms and other injurious agents. At times, however, these responses may be inappropriate. They may even have undesirable effects.

Hypersensitivity: Allergy, Autoimmunity, and Isoimmunity

Hypersensitivity is an altered immunological reactivity to an antigen. It results in a pathological immune response upon reexposure. These abnormal responses include allergy, autoimmunity, and isoimmunity. **Allergy** refers to an exaggerated immune response that is provoked by environmental allergens. **Autoimmunity** is an immune response against the host's own cells. (These are *self-antigens*.) **Isoimmunity** is an immune response directed against beneficial foreign tissues. (Examples of these are blood transfusions and transplanted organs.) Of these three responses, allergy is the most common. It also is the least life-threatening (see Chapter 27).

Autoimmunity and isoimmunity are responsible for some diseases, including the following:

- Graves' disease
- Rheumatoid arthritis
- Myasthenia gravis
- Immune thrombocytopenic purpura
- Isoimmune neutropenia
- Systemic lupus erythematosus (SLE)
- Rh and ABO isoimmunization
- Multiple sclerosis (MS)

MECHANISMS OF HYPERSENSITIVITY

Hypersensitivity reactions may be immediate or delayed. With *immediate hypersensitivity*, antibodies present in the serum trigger an antigen-antibody reaction upon reexposure. Mild reactions of this type include itching and hives. Severe reactions may include life-threatening respiratory distress and **anaphylaxis** (see Chapter 27).

Delayed hypersensitivity reactions are a product of cell-mediated immunity. In these reactions, the body develops hypersensitivity after exposure to a foreign antigen from bacteria, parasites, or other microorganisms. The reaction may take from several hours to 2 days to appear and may reach maximal severity several days later. An example of a delayed hypersensitivity reaction is the response against grafted tissue. The results of a brush with poison ivy are a more common example.

IgE Reactions. Antibodies, or *immunoglobulins (Ig)*, are produced by plasma cells in response to antigenic stimulation. Five distinct classes of immunoglobulins are produced in humans (Box 11-11). IgE accounts for less than 1% of the antibodies in normal serum. It is responsible for immediate (type I) hypersensitivity reactions. With type I reactions, the response is mediated through IgE, which is bound to mast cells or basophils. When an antigen reacts with an IgE molecule bound to a mast cell or circulating basophil, these cells promptly release a host of chemical mediators into the extracellular space. The target organs and the manifestations of the reaction vary, ranging from hives to hay fever to asthma to life-threatening anaphylaxis (see Chapter 27).

NOTE

Hypersensitivity reactions are divided into four distinct types: *type I* (IgE-mediated allergic reactions), *type II* (tissue-specific reactions), *type III* (immune complex–mediated reactions), and *type IV* (cell-mediated reactions). These types are further described in Chapters 13 and 27.

BOX 11-11 Classes of Immunoglobulins

IgG Immunoglobulins

IgG immunoglobulins account for 70% to 75% of the antibodies in normal serum. IgG is most abundant in blood. However, it also is found in lymph, cerebrospinal, synovial, and peritoneal fluid and breast milk. It is the main antibody involved in secondary immune responses. IgG is the only immunoglobulin that crosses the placenta. It provides temporary immunity in neonates.

IgM Immunoglobulins

IgM immunoglobulins account for about 5% to 10% of the antibodies in normal serum. Most anti-A or anti-B antibodies are of the IgM class. IgM triggers the increased production of IgG in acute infections and the complement fixation required for an effective antibody response.

IgA Immunoglobulins

IgA immunoglobulins account for about 15% of the antibodies in normal serum. This immunoglobulin is found in blood, secretions such as tears and saliva, and the respiratory tract, stomach, and accessory organs. IgA combines with a protein in the mucosa and defends body surfaces against invading microorganisms.

IgE Immunoglobulins

IgE immunoglobulins account for less than 1% of the antibodies in normal serum. IgE is found in some tissues and on the surface membranes of basophils and mast cells. IgE is responsible for immediate hypersensitivity reactions.

IgD Immunoglobulins

IgD immunoglobulins account for less than 1% of the antibodies in normal serum. The precise biological function of IgD is unknown.

Immunity and Inflammation Deficiencies

Immunity and inflammation deficiencies describe the failure of these mechanisms of self-defense to function at normal capacity. The source of the deficiency may be *congenital* (present at birth) or *acquired*. Acquired immune deficiencies may be caused by infection. Examples include the human immunodeficiency virus (HIV), cancer (in particular the leukemias), immunosuppressive drugs, and aging. Whether the source is congenital or acquired, the deficiency usually is caused by a disruption in the function of the lymphocytes, although neutrophil dysfunction also has been described. Research is underway to find replacement therapies for immune deficiencies (Box 11-12).

ACQUIRED DEFICIENCIES

Acquired immune deficiencies are far more common than congenital forms (Box 11-13). They may be classified into the following groups:

- Nutritional deficiencies (e.g., severe deficits in calorie or protein intake)

BOX 11-12 Replacement Therapies for Immune Deficiencies

Intravenous replacement of infection-fighting antibodies
Transplantation of tissue
Blood transfusions
Gene therapy (technology still in infancy)

BOX 11-13 Acquired Immune Deficiencies

The following are associated with acquired immune deficiencies:

- Pregnancy
- Infancy
- Infection (e.g., maternal rubella during pregnancy [congenital], maternal cytomegalovirus infection [during pregnancy], measles, leprosy, tuberculosis)
- Down syndrome
- Malignancies (e.g., Hodgkin's disease, leukemia, myeloma)
- Stress caused by surgery or emotional trauma
- Malnutrition
- Aging
- Diabetes
- Alcoholic cirrhosis
- Sickle cell anemia
- Immunosuppressive treatment
- Anesthesia

From McCance K, Huether S: *Pathophysiology: the biologic basis for disease in adults and children,* ed 6, St Louis, 2010, Mosby.

- Iatrogenic deficiencies (deficiencies caused by some form of medical treatment)
- Deficiencies caused by trauma (e.g., bacterial infection, burns)
- Deficiencies caused by stress (depressed immune function)
- Acquired immunodeficiency syndrome (AIDS)

NOTE

Acquired immunodeficiency syndrome (AIDS) currently is the best-known example of acquired dysfunction of the immune system. The human immunodeficiency virus (HIV) causes AIDS. It results in a debilitating illness that is manifested by various opportunistic infections and malignancies. Until recently, these were almost always fatal. The disease was first identified in 1981. Since then it has become a global health problem. It affects an estimated 33 million people worldwide[10] (see Chapter 28).

CRITICAL THINKING

Think about a time when you or someone close to you became ill because of an acquired immune deficiency. What kind of deficiency caused it? Was it preventable?

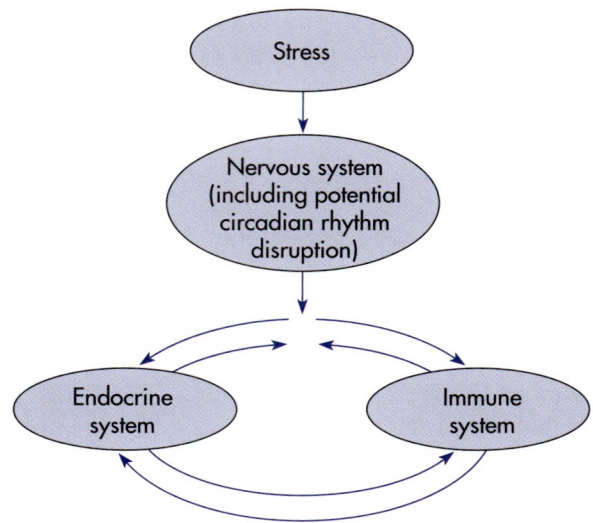

FIGURE 11-23 Interaction of the emotional state, the central nervous system, and the body's defense against infection and abnormal cell division.

STRESS AND DISEASE

Prolonged emotional or psychological stress can result in physical illness. This type of illness can produce disturbances in three important areas: cognition, emotion, and behavior. The growing evidence of the link between stress and disease has created a field of science called psychoneuroimmunology. *Psychoneuroimmunology* is the study of the three-way interaction of the emotional state, the central nervous system, and the body's defense against external infection and abnormal cell division (Figure 11-23).

Neuroendocrine Regulation of Stress

As described in Chapter 2: Well-Being of the Paramedic, the sympathetic nervous system is activated during the stress response. Stress causes the adrenal glands to release catecholamines (epinephrine, norepinephrine, and dopamine) into the bloodstream (Table 11-4). At the same time, the hypothalamus stimulates the pituitary gland to release the hormones ADH, prolactin, growth hormone, and adrenocorticotropic hormone (ACTH). ACTH, in turn, stimulates the cortex of the adrenal gland to release cortisol (Table 11-5).

CATECHOLAMINES

Catecholamines act by stimulating two major classes of receptors. These are **alpha-adrenergic receptors** and **beta-adrenergic receptors.** These two classes are further subcategorized into *alpha-1 receptors, alpha-2 receptors, beta-1 receptors,* and *beta-2 receptors.*

- Alpha-1 receptors are postsynaptic. They are located on the effector organs (e.g., blood vessels, skeletal muscle). The main role of the alpha-1 receptors is to stimulate the contraction of smooth muscle. The alpha-2 receptors are found on the presynaptic nerve endings. Stimulation of

TABLE 11-4 Physiological Effects of Catecholamines*

Organ	Process or Result
Brain	Increased blood flow
	Increased glucose metabolism
Cardiovascular system	Increased rate and force of contraction
	Peripheral vasoconstriction
Pulmonary system	Increased oxygen supply
	Bronchodilation
	Increased ventilation
Muscle	Increased glycogenolysis
	Increased contraction
	Increased dilation of skeletal muscle vasculature
Liver	Increased glucose production
	Increased gluconeogenesis
	Increased glycogenolysis
	Decreased glycogen synthesis
Adipose tissue	Increased lipolysis
	Increased fatty acids and glycerol
Skin	Decreased blood flow
Skeleton	Decreased glucose uptake and utilization (decreases insulin release)
Gastrointestinal and genitourinary tracts	Decreased protein synthesis
Lymphoid tissue	Increased protein breakdown (lymphoid tissue shrinks)

From McCance K, Huether S: *Pathophysiology: the biologic basis for disease in adults and children,* ed 6, St Louis, 2010, Mosby.
*Some of these responses require the presence of glucocorticoids (e.g., cortisol) for maximal activity.

the alpha-2 receptors serves as a negative feedback mechanism by inhibiting further release of norepinephrine.

- The beta-1 receptors are located mainly in the heart. Beta-2 receptors are located primarily in the bronchiolar and arterial smooth muscle. The beta receptors perform a number of functions. They stimulate the heart; dilate bronchioles and blood vessels in skeletal muscle, brain, and heart; and aid in glycogenolysis. Epinephrine activates both the alpha and the beta receptors (Table 11-6); norepinephrine mainly excites the alpha receptors. (Alpha and beta receptors are discussed in more detail in Chapter 13.)

CORTISOL

Cortisol (hydrocortisone) circulates in the plasma. It mobilizes substances that are needed for cellular metabolism. The main metabolic effect of cortisol is the stimulation of gluconeogenesis. It also enhances the elevation of blood glucose level. It does this by reducing glucose utilization. Cortisol also acts as an *immunosuppressant;* it reduces the reproduction of lymphocytes, particularly among the T

lymphocytes. This, in turn, leads to a decrease in cellular immunity.

Cortisol also reduces the migration of macrophages into an inflamed area. It reduces phagocytosis, partly by stabilizing the lysosomal membranes. This decrease in immune cell activity may be beneficial, because it prevents immune-mediated tissue damage. Two factors determine whether cortisol's effects are adaptive or destructive. These factors are the type of stress event and the length of exposure to the stressor.

Role of the Immune System

Many immunological conditions and diseases seem to be triggered by stress (Table 11-7). However, the exact mechanisms that link stress to these diseases and conditions have not yet been clearly defined. It is believed that the immune, nervous, and endocrine systems communicate through complex pathways. Also, they may be affected by factors involved in the stress reaction.

Interrelationship of Stress, Coping, and Illness

As noted earlier in this chapter and in Chapter 2, the damage caused by stress is determined by the nature, intensity, and duration of the stressors. It also is affected by the way in which a person perceives the stressors and how well the individual is able to cope with them. The ability to notice the signs and symptoms of stress and to use stress management tactics is crucial to good health. Stress-reduction techniques include meditation, exercise, and guided imagery. In healthy individuals, such methods can help prevent harmful physiological and psychological illness arising from stress.

GENETICS AND FAMILIAL DISEASES

People are born with a genetic predisposition to the development of certain diseases. The genetics of some diseases, like *hemophilia* or *sickle cell anemia,* are well understood (see Chapter 32). Patients either have no genetic predisposition, are carriers of the disease, or have the disease. Other disease processes (like *arthritis, diabetes,* and *hypertension*) certainly are linked to genetics, but are strongly associated with environmental factors as well. Medical researchers attempt to reduce the incidence or severity of these inherited medical conditions through environmental manipulation.

Factors Causing Disease

Factors that cause disease may be simplistically classified as *genetic* or *environmental.* However, there is a strong interaction between the two (Box 11-14). For example, genes cannot exert their effects without an environment in which to operate, and environmental factors act differently on different people. Conversely, the environment may be the same, but people have unique genetic makeups. Therefore the interaction between genetics and environment is very complex.

TABLE 11-5   Physiological Effects of Cortisol

Function	Effects
Carbohydrate and lipid metabolism	Diminishes peripheral uptake and utilization of glucose; promotes gluconeogenesis in liver cells; enhances gluconeogenic response to other hormones; promotes lipolysis in adipose tissue
Protein metabolism	Increases protein synthesis in liver and depresses protein synthesis (including immunoglobulin synthesis) in muscle, lymphoid tissue, adipose tissue, skin, and bone; increases plasma level of amino acids; stimulates deamination (an oxidative reaction) in liver
Inflammatory function	Decreases circulating eosinophils, lymphocytes, and monocytes; increases release of polymorphonuclear leukocytes from bone marrow; decreases accumulation of leukocytes at site of inflammation; delays healing; permissive for vasoconstrictive action of norepinephrine
Lipid metabolism	Promotes lipolysis in extremities and lipogenesis in face and trunk
Immune reserve	Decreases tissue mass of all lymphoid tissues (e.g., decreases protein synthesis); promotes rapid decrease in circulating lymphocytes, eosinophils, basophils, and macrophages; inhibits production of interleukin-1 and interleukin-2 and consequently blocks cell-mediated immunity and generation of fever
Digestive function	Promotes gastric secretion
Urinary function	Enhances urinary excretion
Connective tissue	Decreases proliferation of fibroblasts in connective tissue (thereby delaying healing)
Muscle	Maintains normal contractility and maximal work output for skeletal and cardiac muscle
Bone	Decreases bone formation
Vascular system and myocardial function	Maintains normal blood pressure; increases responsiveness of arterioles to constrictive action of adrenergic stimulation; optimizes myocardial performance
Central nervous system	Modulates perceptual and emotional functioning (although mechanism for this is unknown), which are essential for normal arousal and initiation of daytime activity

Modified from McCance KL, Huether SE: *Pathophysiology: the biologic basis for disease in adults and children,* ed 6, St Louis, 2010, Mosby.

TABLE 11-6   Physiological Actions of Alpha and Beta Receptors

Receptor	Physiological Actions
Alpha-1 receptor	Increased glycogenolysis; smooth muscle contraction (blood vessels, genitourinary tract)
Alpha-2 receptor	Smooth muscle relaxation (gastrointestinal tract); smooth muscle contraction (some vascular beds); inhibition of lipolysis, renin release, platelet aggregation, and insulin secretion
Beta-1 receptor	Stimulation of lipolysis, myocardial contraction (increased rate, increased force of contraction)
Beta-2 receptor	Increased hepatic gluconeogenesis; increased hepatic glycogenolysis; increased muscle glycogenolysis; increased release of insulin, glucagon, and renin; smooth muscle relaxation (bronchi, blood vessels, genitourinary tract, gastrointestinal tract)

Modified from McCance KL, Huether SE: *Pathophysiology: the biologic basis for disease in adults and children,* ed 6, St Louis, 2010, Mosby.

GENETIC FACTORS

Heredity is governed by the laws of chance and probability. This exists because each pair of chromosomes is sorted at random when packaged into eggs and sperm. More than 100,000 genes are involved in a person's genetic makeup. Thus the range of variation is huge. Different types of genetic diseases can arise. These can occur because of individual genetic changes or because of abnormalities involving an entire chromosome.

Sometimes mistakes occur when chromosomes are packaged. This results in rearrangement of the chromosomes. Entire chromosomal abnormalities lead to diseases such as *Down syndrome* or *Turner's syndrome*. More often, only a single gene on the chromosome is passed on, resulting in an abnormal protein. This is the type of genetic defect responsible for sickle cell anemia and hemophilia. Some conditions may involve more than one gene (i.e., they are *polygenic*) and a number of factors, but they still may have a strong inherited component. These diseases include *coronary artery disease* (CAD), hypertension, and cancer.

NOTE
Genes are not unchangeable units of inheritance. Under some circumstances, they can be affected by environmental influences (see Box 11-14).

TABLE 11-7 Examples of Stress-Related Diseases and Conditions

Target Organ or System	Disease or Condition
Cardiovascular system	Coronary artery disease
	Hypertension
	Stroke
	Disturbances of heart rhythm
Muscles	Tension headaches
	Muscle contraction backache
Connective tissues	Rheumatoid arthritis (autoimmune disease)
	Related inflammatory diseases of connective tissue
Pulmonary system	Asthma (hypersensitivity reaction)
	Hay fever (hypersensitivity reaction)
Immune system	Immunosuppression or deficiency
	Autoimmune diseases
Gastrointestinal system	Ulcer
	Irritable bowel syndrome
	Diarrhea
	Nausea and vomiting
	Ulcerative colitis
Genitourinary system	Diuresis
	Impotence
	Frigidity
Skin	Eczema
	Neurodermatitis
	Acne
Endocrine system	Diabetes mellitus
	Amenorrhea
Central nervous system	Fatigue and lethargy
	Type A behavior (impatience, competitive/aggressive attitude)
	Overeating
	Depression
	Insomnia

From McCance KL, Huether SE: *Pathophysiology: the biologic basis for disease in adults and children,* ed 4, St Louis, 2002, Mosby.

BOX 11-14 Example of Environmental Influence in Genetic Selection

The gene that causes sickle cell anemia was recognized to be much more common in environments in which malaria was prevalent. People with sickle cell disease have sickle-shaped red blood corpuscles, which clog the capillaries. This condition often proves fatal. However, in people who are carriers of the sickle cell trait, fewer than 1% of the red corpuscles are abnormal. These individuals do not die of sickle cell anemia, and they are more resistant to malaria than those who do not carry the sickle cell trait. Thus the trait proved protective, and its prevalence increased as a result of natural selection.

ENVIRONMENTAL FACTORS

Many common chronic diseases may occur because of a mismatch between genetic and environmental factors (Tables 11-8 and 11-9). Important environmental factors include the following:

- Microorganisms and immunological exposure
- Personal habits and lifestyle
- Chemical substances
- Physical environment
- Psychosocial environment

The goal in preventing disease is to find the genetic and environmental influences that lead to major diseases. This knowledge will help individuals who have specific susceptibilities. They will be able to change certain environmental factors. This, in turn, may lessen their risk of developing the illness.

AGE AND GENDER

Age and gender also seem to play a role in the incidence of *familial* (hereditary) diseases. This is especially true for diseases that are not caused by a single genetic defect. In the

TABLE 11-8 Environmental Factors That Affect the Occurrence of Disease

Factors	Examples
Microorganisms and immunological exposure	Bacteria
	Viruses
	Fungi
	Protozoa
	Vectors (e.g., insects and animals)
	Allergens
Personal habits and lifestyle	Smoking
	Physical exercise
	Dietary intake
Chemical substances	Toxins
	Pollutants
	Medications
	Solvents, fumes
	Contaminants
Physical environment	Climate
	Radiation
	Physical trauma
	Geographic location (e.g., sun exposure, altitude)
	Community (e.g., water and food supplies)
Psychosocial milieu	Family status (e.g., bereavement, loss, status change)
	Stress
	Coping skills
	Social isolation
	Ethnic and racial customs
	Religious customs

TABLE 11-9 Populations with Shared Disease Tendencies*

Disease	Rate Among Populations	Suggested Environmental Factors	Shared Gene Pool
Early coronary artery disease	Very high in Finland (very low in Japan)	Animal fat intake	Genes for high blood cholesterol
Colon cancer	Low in developing countries (e.g., Africa); high in "westernized" countries (e.g., United States, Europe)	Dietary fiber and fat intake	None
Thalassemia (a type of anemia)	High in individuals of Mediterranean descent; low in other areas	None	Major dominant gene for thalassemia
Malaria (and many other infectious diseases)	High in some parts of Africa and Asia; low in United States and Europe	Trypanosomes, mosquitoes, disease control measures	None
Early non–insulin-dependent diabetes and obesity	Native Americans	Change from scarce food supply to plenty	Apparent shared gene pool among various Native American tribes
Lung cancer	Low in Mormons and Seventh Day Adventists	Health code forbids use of tobacco	None
Skin cancers	Higher among Caucasians than African Americans; higher in "Sun Belt"	Ultraviolet light	Inherited level of skin pigmentation

From McCance KL, Huether SE: *Pathophysiology: the biologic basis for disease in adults and children,* ed 6, St Louis, 2010, Mosby.
*These tendencies are the result of shared environmental factors, a common gene pool, or both.

polygenic disorders, the combined effects of genes and environment over time play a role. These combined influences may result in diseases linked to age-related changes in metabolism. This may explain why heart disease, hypertension, and cancer are seen more often in people older than age 40.

Gender is associated with sex-specific diseases that arise from hormonal and anatomical differences. Two examples are breast cancer in women and testicular cancer in men. Lifestyle and environmental differences in gender-related activities also may play a role. These differences may be responsible for the predisposition to some diseases. Examples of gender, lifestyle, and environmental combinations include the higher rate of lung cancer and coronary artery disease in men who smoke cigarettes.

Analyzing the Risk of Disease

Epidemiologists are researchers who study disease "rates" and analyze risk factors. Disease rates help to describe the occurrence of disease. Risk factors are indicators of a person's predisposition to development of a disease.

DISEASE RATES

Three statistics are commonly used to assess the impact of a disease on a society. These are the incidence rate, the prevalence rate, and the mortality rate. The *incidence rate* refers to the number of new cases detected during a given period per the number of people in the population surveyed. The period is usually 1 year. The *prevalence rate* refers to the number of people *living* with the disease per the

number of people in the population surveyed. The *mortality rate* refers to the number of people who died from the disease during a given period per the number of people in the population surveyed. The given period, again, is often 1 year.

RISK FACTOR ANALYSIS

The presence of certain risk factors in any group of people is linked to an increased disease rate in that group. Diseases may have *causal* and *noncausal* risk factors. With causal risk factors, removal or elimination of the risk factors delays or prevents the disease. Noncausal risk factors can help predict a person's chances of developing the disease, but they have no direct effect on the underlying cause (Figure 11-24). Risk factors cannot precisely predict whether a person will develop a disease. However, they can provide clues about the individual's likelihood of developing the disease.

Combined Effects and Interaction of Risk Factors

When one or more risk factors interact, the individual effects of risk factors may be greatly magnified. For example, some risk factors alone may pose little or no danger of disease. However, if another risk factor is added, the danger increases substantially.

FAMILIAL DISEASE TENDENCY

In some cases the members of a family (brothers and sisters, parents with children, spouse pairs, twins) are more prone

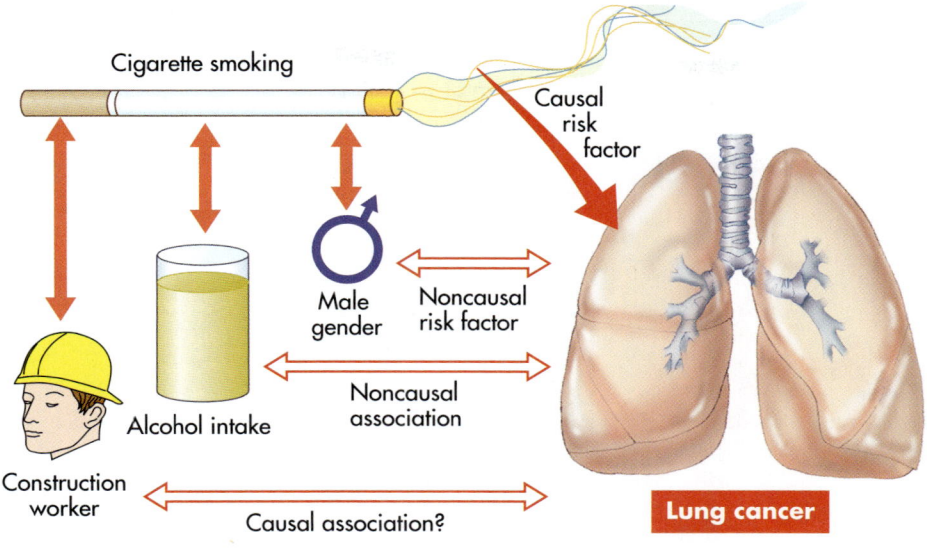

FIGURE 11-24 Causal and noncausal risk factors and associations.

to some diseases than are the people of the general population. Often the familial risk factors are genetic or shared factors in the environment. Examples include illnesses such as heart disease and pulmonary disease. These result from decisions such as choosing to smoke or consuming a diet high in fat.

> ### CRITICAL THINKING
> Think about how many risk factors you have for heart disease. Which of these factors are genetic and which ones could you eliminate by modifying your habits or environment?

AGING AND AGE-RELATED DISORDERS

Advanced age is a risk factor for many diseases, such as heart attack, stroke, and cancer. This likely represents the cumulative effects of genetics and environmental factors. Disorders related to age occur throughout life (Table 11-10). Some disorders, such as dental cavities and "strep throat," are more common in younger age groups. The degenerative disorders (e.g., arthritis) are more common in older age groups.

Common Familial Diseases and Associated Risk Factors

Individuals who are high risk can take steps to avoid many familial diseases (Table 11-11). Examples of such diseases include coronary artery disease and colorectal cancer. These conditions are described in detail throughout this text.

TABLE 11-10 Age-Related Disorders

Age	Disorders
Birth to 14 years	Congenital disorders Allergy Infection Cancer (leukemia, Wilms' tumor, medulloblastoma, retinoblastoma) Trauma or injury Diabetes (early onset)
15 to 30 years	Allergy (asthma) Endocrine disorders Trauma or injury (suicide) Venereal disease
31 to 40 years	Ulcer Hypertension Breast cancer Homicide Suicide Complications of pregnancy Alcoholism
41 to 60 years	Heart disease (hypertension, rheumatic disorder, infarction) Kidney disease (glomerular nephritis) Liver disease (cirrhosis) Cancer (lung, colon, breast, ovary)
61 to 80 years	Cardiovascular disease Cancer (lung, colon, prostate)
81 to 100 years	Cancer (leukemia, lymphoma, prostate cancer) Dementia (Alzheimer's disease, Parkinson's disease) Osteoporosis Infection Cardiovascular disease Trauma or injury (fracture)

Modified from King DW, Fenoglio CM, Lefkowitch JH: *General pathology: principles and dynamics,* Philadelphia, 1988, Lea & Febiger.

TABLE 11-11 Common Familial Diseases and Associated Environmental Risk Factors

Disease	Environmental Risk Factors
Immunological Disorders	
Asthma and other allergies	Fur, dust, pollen, mold (other allergens)
Rheumatic fever	Group A *Streptococcus* bacterial infection
Cancer	
Breast cancer	Obesity, high dietary fat intake, alcohol ingestion, hormones
Colorectal cancer	Inadequate fiber intake, high dietary fat intake
Lung cancer	Cigarette smoke, environmental pollutants
Endocrine Disorders	
Diabetes mellitus type 1 (insulin-dependent)	Viral infection, longstanding difficulty (years) controlling blood glucose level
Diabetes mellitus type 2 (non–insulin-dependent)	Obesity; high-sugar, low-fiber dietary intake; longstanding difficulty (years) controlling blood glucose level
Hypertension	Diet, obesity, inadequate exercise (sedentary lifestyle)
Hematological Disorders	
Drug-induced hemolytic anemia	Aspirin, antibiotics, infection
Sickle cell anemia	Precipitated by cold weather, infection
Hemochromatosis	Ingestions (iron), transfusions
Cardiovascular Disorders	
Coronary artery disease	Exercise, alcohol ingestion, diet high in fat and salt, smoking, obesity, stress
Cardiomyopathies	Infection, ingestion of alcohol or use of other drugs
Mitral valve prolapse	Infection
Hypertension and stroke	Diet high in fat and salt, obesity
Renal Disorders	
Gout	Poor diet, injury, stress
Kidney stones	Decreased water intake
Gastrointestinal Disorders	
Malabsorption Disorders	
Lactose intolerance	Ingestion of milk products
Ulcerative colitis	Stress, consumption of trigger foods
Crohn's disease	Stress, consumption of trigger foods
Peptic ulcers	Stress, diet that causes gastric irritation, infection
Gallstones	High dietary fat intake, obesity
Obesity	Diet high in fat, sugar, and total calories; stress that affects appetite; cultural perceptions
Neuromuscular Disorders	
Multiple sclerosis	Virus, warm environment (heat-producing exercise, warm ambient temperature), stress
Alzheimer's disease	Decreased mental stimulation later in life
Psychiatric Disorders	
Schizophrenia	Uncertain influence; dramatic success with drug treatment
Manic depression	Uncertain influence; dramatic success with drug treatment

SUMMARY

- Two facts illustrate the importance of body water. First, body water is the medium in which all metabolic reactions occur. Second, the precise regulation of the volume and composition of body fluids is essential to health. Water follows osmotic gradients established by changes in sodium concentrations. Thus sodium balance and water balance are closely related.

- Two abnormal states of body fluid balance can occur. If the water gained exceeds the water lost, a state of water excess, or overhydration, exists. If the water lost exceeds the water gained, a state of water deficit, or dehydration, exists.

- In addition to fluid imbalances, disturbances in the balance of electrolytes (other than sodium) may occur. These electrolytes include potassium, calcium, and magnesium. Imbalances of these electrolytes can interfere with neuromuscular function. They may even cause cardiac rhythm disturbances.

- The treatment of isotonic dehydration may include volume replacement with isotonic or occasionally hypotonic solutions. The treatment of hypotonic dehydration may involve intravenous replacement with normal saline or lactated Ringer's solution. Occasionally hypertonic saline (e.g., in seizures caused by hyponatremia) is used. Interventions for overhydration depend on the cause. These interventions may include water restriction, administration of a diuretic, or, if hyponatremia is present, administration of saline.

- In-hospital treatment of hypokalemia involves intravenous or oral potassium replacement. Management of hyperkalemia may involve potassium restriction, enteral administration of a cation exchange resin, or intravenous administration of glucose and insulin, sodium bicarbonate, or calcium.

- Treatment of hypocalcemia involves intravenous administration of calcium ions. The management of hypercalcemia may include controlling the underlying disease, hydration, and, occasionally, drug therapy such as with furosemide and other calcium-lowering drugs.

- Hypomagnesemia typically is corrected by the administration of intravenous magnesium sulfate. The most effective treatment for hypermagnesemia is hemodialysis. Calcium salts that antagonize magnesium may also be given.

- The healthy body is sensitive to changes in the concentration of hydrogen ions (pH). It tries to maintain the pH of extracellular fluid at 7.4. This is accomplished through three interrelated compensatory mechanisms: carbonic acid–bicarbonate buffering, protein buffering, and renal buffering.

- Metabolic acidosis occurs when the amount of acid generated exceeds the body's buffering capacity. The four most common forms of metabolic acidosis encountered in the prehospital setting are lactic acidosis, diabetic ketoacidosis, acidosis resulting from renal failure, and acidosis caused by ingestion of toxins. Treatment for metabolic acidosis is aimed at correcting the underlying cause.

- Loss of hydrogen is the initial cause of metabolic alkalosis. This may be caused by vomiting (hydrochloric acid loss), suctioning of gastric contents, or increased renal excretion of hydrogen ion in the urine. Treatment is directed at correcting the underlying condition. Volume depletion, if present, should be corrected with isotonic solutions.

- Respiratory acidosis is caused by the retention of carbon dioxide. This leads to an increase in the PCO_2. This condition usually is caused by an imbalance in the production of carbon dioxide and its elimination through alveolar ventilation. Treatment for respiratory acidosis involves improving ventilation quickly to eliminate carbon dioxide.

- Hyperventilation may produce respiratory alkalosis by decreasing the PCO_2. Treatment of respiratory alkalosis is directed at correcting the underlying cause of the hyperventilation. An initial approach is to administer low-concentration oxygen to the patient. Another is to provide calming measures to assist the patient with slow, controlled breathing.

- An understanding of the processes of disease is crucial. This requires a knowledge of the structural and functional reactions of cells and tissues to injurious agents. Changes in cells and tissues can be caused by adaptation, injury, neoplasia, aging, or death.

- An injured cell may have an abnormal physical shape or size. Cell injury has both cellular and systemic indications.

- Certain factors cause disease. For the most part, these factors may be classified as genetic or environmental. However, a strong interaction occurs between the two.

- The term hypoperfusion is used to describe inadequate tissue circulation. Hypoperfusion may result from decreased cardiac output. Decreased cardiac output can lead to shock, multiple organ dysfunction syndrome, and other disease states associated with impaired cellular metabolism. Negative feedback mechanisms important in maintaining cardiac output and tissue perfusion are baroreceptor reflexes, chemoreceptor reflexes, the central nervous system ischemia response, hormonal mechanisms, reabsorption of tissue fluids, and splenic discharge of stored blood.

- The external barriers are the body's first line of defense against illness and injury. These barriers include the skin and the mucous membranes of the digestive, respiratory, and genitourinary tracts. When these barriers are breached, chemicals, foreign bodies, or microorganisms are allowed to penetrate cells and tissues. Then the second and third lines of defense are activated. These

Continued

are the inflammatory response (second) and the immune response (third). Both the external barriers and the inflammatory response respond to all organisms using the identical nonspecific mechanism. The immune response is specific to individual pathogens.

- Immune responses usually are protective. They help to protect the body from harmful microorganisms and other injurious agents. At times these responses may be inappropriate. They may even have undesirable effects. Examples of inappropriate responses include hypersensitivity and immunity or inflammation deficiencies.

- Many immune-related conditions and diseases are associated with stress. However, the exact mechanisms causing these illnesses have not yet been clearly defined. It is believed that the immune, nervous, and endocrine systems communicate through complex pathways and that they may be affected by factions involved in the stress reaction.

- Factors that cause disease are complex. They may involve genetic or environmental factors or a combination of both. Age and gender also influence illness.

REFERENCES

1. Snell RS, Smith MS: *Clinical anatomy of emergency medicine*, St Louis, 1993, Mosby.
2. McCance KL, Brashers VL: *Pathophysiology*, ed 6, Maryland Heights, Mo, 2010, Mosby.
3. Muller O, Krawinkel M: Malnutrition and health in developing countries, *CMAJ* 173(3), 2005.
4. Garth D: *Hypokalemia*, http://emedicine.medscape.com/article/767448-overview, accessed 8-10-10.
5. Parham W, Mehdirad AA, Biermann KM, et al: Hyperkalemia revisited, *Tex Heart Inst J* 33(1):40-47, 2006.
6. Infusion Nurses Society: *Infusion therapy in clinical practice*, ed 2, Philadelphia, 2001, Saunders.
7. American Heart Association: *Heart disease and stoke statistics: 2010 update at-a-glance*, Dallas, 2010, The Association.
8. Seeley RR, Stephens T, Tate P: *Anatomy and physiology*, ed 6, New York, 2006, McGraw Hill.
9. McCance K, Huether S: *Pathophysiology: the biologic basis for disease in adults and children*, ed 5, St Louis, 2006, Elsevier.
10. World Health Organization: *HIV burden*, Dec 1, 2008, Regional Office of South-East Asia.

SUGGESTED READINGS

Alberts B, et al: *Molecular biology of the cell*, ed 4, New York, 2001, Garland.

Berne RM, Levy MN, editors: *Physiology*, ed 4, St Louis, 1998, Mosby.

Halperin ML, Goldstein MB: *Fluid, electrolyte, and acid-base physiology*, ed 3, Philadelphia, 1999, WB Saunders.

Vander AJ, et al: *Human physiology: the mechanisms of body function*, ed 6, New York, 1994, McGraw-Hill.

CHAPTER
12 Life Span Development

OBJECTIVES

Upon completion of this chapter, the paramedic student will be able to:

1. Describe the normal vital signs and body system characteristics of the newborn, neonate, infant, toddler, preschooler, school-aged child, adolescent, young adult, middle-aged adult, and older adult.
2. Identify key psychosocial features of the infant, toddler, preschooler, school-aged child, adolescent, young adult, middle-aged adult, and older adult.
3. Explain the effect of parenting styles, sibling rivalry, peer relationships, and other factors on a child's psychosocial development.
4. Discuss the physical and emotional challenges faced by the older adult.

KEY TERMS

adolescent A person 13 to 18 years of age.

attachments Physical and emotional bonds that develop between infants and their family members or caregivers.

Babinski reflex A reflex movement in which the great toe bends upward when the outer edge of the sole is stroked.

cognitive development The construction of thought processes, including remembering, problem solving, and decision making, from childhood through adolescence to adulthood.

early adulthood People 20 to 40 years of age.

family function The ways a family deals with daily problems and conflicts and whether this is done in a respectful, productive, and nonaggressive way.

infant A child 28 days to 1 year of age.

late adulthood People 61 years of age or older.

masturbation Sexual stimulation, especially of one's own genitals, often to the point of orgasm.

menarche The first menstruation and the commencement of the cyclic menstrual function.

menopause The cessation of menses.

middle adulthood People 41 to 60 years of age.

Moro reflex A normal infant response elicited by a sudden loud noise. The infant flexes the legs, makes an embracing gesture with the arms, and usually gives a brief cry.

neonate An infant in the first 28 days of life.

newborn An infant within the first few hours of life.

passive immunity Immunity acquired by transmission of antibodies from the mother, through placental transfer, to the fetus; a form of acquired immunity in which antibodies against disease are acquired naturally.

periodontal disease Disease that affects tissues that surround or support the teeth.

preschooler A child 3 to 5 years of age.

palmar grasp The curling of an infant's fingers in response to a touch on the palm of the hand; it is a normal infant response.

puberty The period of life when the ability to reproduce begins.

reciprocal socialization A term that refers to a child's temperament and the responses it elicits from adults and family members. This interaction forms the basis for early social interactions with others and with the child's environment.

reproductive maturity The time at which a person has attained the ability to reproduce.

rooting reflex A normal infant response elicited by touching or stroking the side of the cheek or mouth; this causes the infant to turn the head toward that side and to begin to suck.

school age The age group comprising children 6 to 12 years.

self-concept The accumulation of knowledge about one's self; including beliefs regarding personality traits, physical characteristics, abilities, values, goals, and roles.

self-esteem A person's overall evaluation or appraisal of his or her own worth.

separation anxiety A normal period during development in which a child experiences anxiety when separated from the primary caregiver.

sibling rivalry Jealousy or competitiveness between brothers and sisters.

sucking reflex A normal infant response in which touching the infant's lips with the nipple of a breast or bottle causes involuntary sucking movements.

temperament A person's style of behavior; the way the person interacts with the environment. It is the basis on which children develop relationships.

terminal drop A theory that a decline in intelligence in older adulthood may be caused by the person's conscious or unconscious perception of coming death.

toddler A child 1 to 3 years of age.

Paramedics provide care to patients from all age groups. Often a patient's complaints are directly related to the growth and developmental characteristics common for that person's age group. Therefore, it is important that paramedics study and understand the physiological and psychosocial development of human beings at different stages in life.

> **NOTE**
> Age groups and developmental characteristics are defined in the *EMS Education Standards.*[1] These are general descriptions of development across the life span. They may differ slightly from other references in this and other textbooks. The age groups presented in this chapter are infants (birth to 1 year of age); toddlers (1 to 3 years of age); preschoolers (3 to 5 years of age); school-age children (6 to 12 years of age); adolescents (13 to 18 years of age); early adulthood (20 to 40 years of age); middle adulthood (41 to 60 years of age); and late adulthood (61 years of age or older).

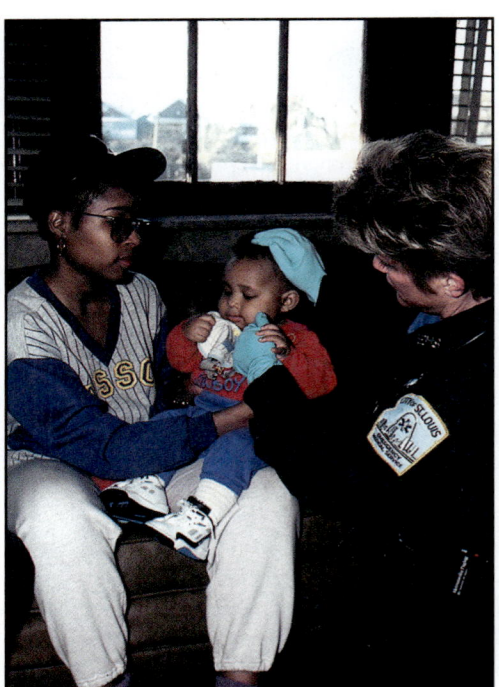

(Courtesy Monroe Yancie, St Louis, Mo.)

NEWBORN

The term **newborn** is used for infants in the first few hours of life (Figure 12-1). A child younger than 28 days is known as a **neonate.** The term **infant** is used for a child 28 days to 1 year of age.

Vital Signs

During the first 30 minutes of life, the newborn's heart rate is 100 to 200 beats per minute (bpm). By 1 year of age, the heart rate averages 120 bpm. At birth, the respiratory rate usually is 40 to 60 breaths/minute. This rate drops to 30 to 40 breaths/minute within a few minutes after delivery. By 1 year of age, a rate of 25 breaths/minute is considered normal. The average systolic blood pressure increases from 70 mm Hg at birth to 90 mm Hg at 1 year. Body temperature during infancy ranges from 98° to 100° F (36.7° to 37.8° C).

> **CRITICAL THINKING**
> Why are newborn, infant, and neonate considered distinct stages?

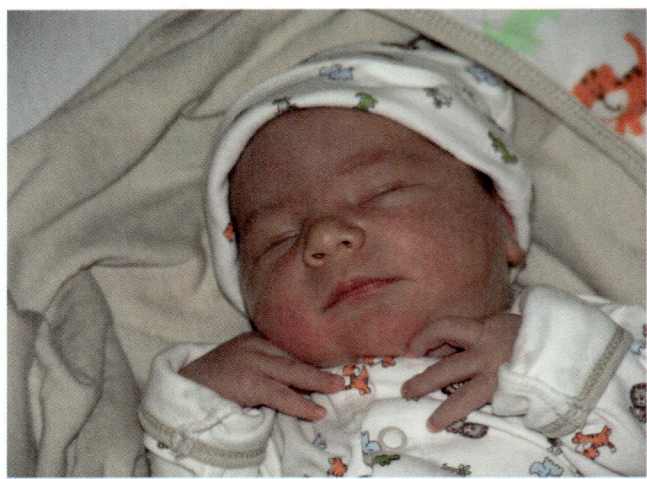

FIGURE 12-1 Newborn. (Courtesy Ben Sanders, O'Fallon, Mo.)

Weight

A full-term newborn normally weighs 3 to 3.5 kg (7 to 8 pounds). The baby's head accounts for about 25% of the total body weight; its circumference is equal to that of the baby's chest. For the first few days of life, the total body weight may decrease 5% to 10% as a result of excretion of *extracellular fluid* (fluid outside the cells). By the second week of life, the birth weight has been regained, and the child's weight exceeds the newborn weight. Although some babies gain weight faster than others, most gain an average of 140 to 168 g (5 to 6 ounces) per week. The increase in an infant's body weight should follow a steady upward curve at about 30 g (1 ounce) per day during the first month of life (this will double the birth weight within 4 to 6 months and triple it within 9 to 12 months). Monitoring the infant's weight every few weeks is a good way to keep track of development.

> **NOTE**
> One kilogram (kg) is equal to 2.2 pounds (lb). One gram (g) is equal to $\frac{1}{480}$ ounce (oz). These and other equivalents are described in Chapter 14.

> **CRITICAL THINKING**
> What considerations for patient care are necessary based on the size of the infant's head?

Cardiovascular System

A newborn's body must make some physiological changes to survive outside the womb. For example, the cardiovascular system must begin to work apart from the maternal circulation. Shortly after birth, the *ductus venosus, ductus arteriosus,* and *foramen ovale* constrict; these structures are unique to the fetal circulation. They close permanently within the first year of life. This results in an increase in systemic vascular resistance. It also results in an increase in aortic, left ventricular, and left atrial pressures. In addition, pulmonary vascular resistance decreases. This occurs because the lungs expand as the baby begins to breathe, which reduces the pulmonary arterial, right ventricular, and right atrial pressures (see Chapters 46 and 47). The left ventricle of the newborn's heart becomes stronger during the first year of life.

Respiratory System

Fetal lungs are filled with fluid. During delivery, the thorax is compressed, and the lung fluid is drained as the newborn gasps for air. Once the newborn gasps, the lung fluid that is left is absorbed through the lymphatic and pulmonary circulations. These strong first breaths open the alveoli and allow subsequent respirations to occur more easily. The principal support for the chest wall comes from muscles rather than bones. These accessory muscles are immature and tire easily. The normal practice of using these muscles for breathing increases the infant's susceptibility to the accumulation of lactic acid in the blood (*lactic acidosis*). In addition, collateral ventilation between the alveoli and bronchioles is decreased because newborns have fewer alveoli.

> **NOTE**
> Infants and small children are "belly breathers." They require full diaphragmatic excursion to produce normal respirations. The use of abdominal muscles to breathe continues until about age 7, when children become more "chest breathers."

A baby's short, narrow airways are less stable than those of adults. Breathing occurs primarily through the nose during the first month of life. With infection or stress, the baby breathes more rapidly and may quickly lose body heat and fluids.

Nervous System

A healthy newborn can respond to a wide variety of stimuli and has a range of *reflexes* (Table 12-1). A number of these reflexes are essential for life outside the womb. These include the reflexes associated with breathing and eating. Other important reflexes are those that result from stress or discomfort. For example, obstruction of the airways may trigger a sneeze or cough. Facial stimulation causes the baby to make sucking movements with the lips **(sucking reflex)** and to turn the head and move the lips toward the touch **(rooting reflex).** Crying may indicate hunger, pain, or discomfort from heat or cold. Some reflexes appear to have no useful purpose and gradually disappear during the first few months of life. These include the **Babinski reflex, the Moro reflex,** and the **palmar grasp.**

> **NOTE**
> The Babinski reflex is a normal response in infants and young children. However, in an older child or adult, it may indicate damage to the spinal cord (see Chapter 41).

Sleep is thought to be important to normal functioning of the brain. Newborns sleep an average of 16 to 18 hours a day. Sleep and wakefulness are evenly distributed over 24 hours. This sleep pattern gradually decreases to 14 to 16 hours a day with a 9- to 10-hour concentration of sleep at night. By 4 months of age, an infant generally sleeps through the night but can be easily roused.

During the first year of life, a baby makes major advances in physical and mental skills. The brain and nervous system gradually mature during this period. To make room for brain growth, the *posterior fontanelle* (unclosed joint between the bones of the skull) remains open until about 3 months of age. The *anterior fontanelle* remains open for 9 to 18 months after birth. The anterior fontanelle usually is level

TABLE 12-1	Reflexes Associated with Infancy	
Reflex	**Test**	**Normal Finding**
Babinski	The examiner gently strokes the sole of the infant's foot.	The toes spread outward and upward.
	The examiner presses on the palms of an infant who is lying on the back (supine).	The mouth opens, and the eyes close.
Moro	A loud or startling noise is made near the infant.	The infant stretches the arms and legs, spreads the fingers, and then hugs self.
Palmar grasp	The examiner puts an object or a finger in the infant's palm.	The fingers curl around the object or finger.
Rooting	The examiner gently touches the infant's cheek or an area near the lips.	The infant's head turns toward the stimulation, and the mouth puckers.
Stepping	The examiner holds the infant upright with the feet touching a solid surface.	The infant makes stepping movements that resemble walking.
Sucking	The infant's mouth comes in contact with the nipple of a breast or bottle.	The infant's lips begin to pucker and suck.
Tonic neck	The infant is placed in the supine position.	The infant turns the head and then extends the arm and leg on the side of the body toward which the head is turned.

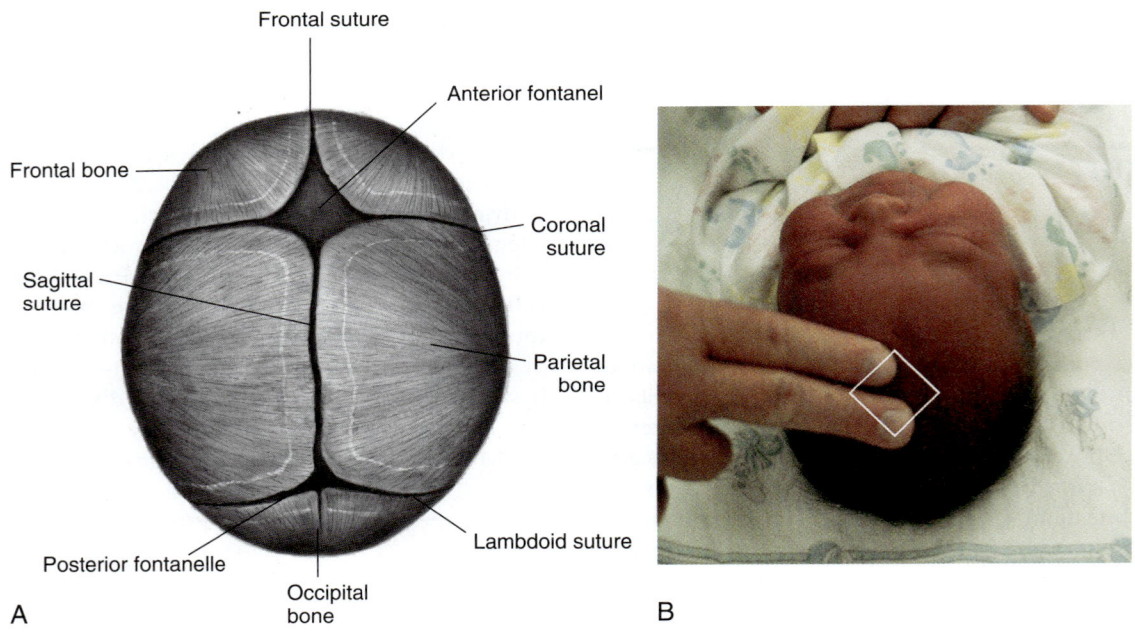

FIGURE 12-2 A, Location of the sutures and fontanelles. **B,** Palpation of the anterior fontanelle. (Price DL, Gwin JF: *Pediatric nursing: an introductory text,* ed 10, St Louis, 2008, Saunders.)

with or slightly below the surface of the skull. It is a good indicator of adequate hydration (with dehydration, the anterior fontanelle may fall below the level of the skull and appear sunken) (Figure 12-2). By the end of the first year, the development of mature nerves is virtually complete. The muscles have matured to the point that many infants can stand and walk with little or no assistance (Figure 12-3).

Musculoskeletal System

At birth the only hard bones are in the fingers. As long bones mature, hormones act on the cartilage in the epiphyses of growing bones. This results in the deposition of calcium salts and the replacement of soft cartilage with hard bone. The *epiphyseal plate* lengthens, and bones thicken as new layers of bone are deposited on existing bone. Factors that influence bone growth include genetics, the production of growth hormone and thyroid hormone, nutrition, and the child's general health status. In infants, muscle weight accounts for about 25% of the entire musculoskeletal system. Motor control in the infant moves from head to toe and from the core to the periphery of the body. Therefore, infants should be able to lift the head before they are able to sit; also, they can crawl before they are able to walk.[2] The arms and legs are proportionately smaller in the infant. These proportions change throughout the life span (Figure 12-4).

Immune System

Babies are born with enough natural immunity from disease to protect them until they can make their own antibodies. This is known as **passive immunity.** Passive immunity arises from the mother's antibodies, which are passed through the blood to the fetus. If the baby is breast-fed, they also are passed through the mother's milk. Passive immunity lasts only about 6 months after birth. After that interval, childhood immunizations against disease (e.g., *pertussis*, *diphtheria*, and *tetanus*) usually are recommended (see Chapter 48).

Metabolism

An infant's metabolic rate is much higher than that of older children or adults. Infants consume more fluids, calories, minerals, and vitamins per pound. They also lose more fluid from the respiratory and integumentary systems than do older children. This predisposes them to dehydration. It also increases the risk of heat- and cold-related illnesses in this age group.[2]

Other Developmental Milestones

Development during infancy depends on the interaction of *heredity* and the *environment*. Growth and development should be compared with standard growth charts showing norms. Box 12-1 lists some developmental milestones from birth to 12 months of age.

Psychosocial Development

The relationship with the caregiver (usually the mother) is a major factor in a baby's psychosocial development. This person is the baby's main source of comfort. The caregiver also represents the baby's main means of coping with stresses in the environment. Such stresses can include fear, pain, and anxiety. Erik Erikson,[3] a proponent of the psychosocial theory, saw human development as the interaction between a person's genes and the environment. He

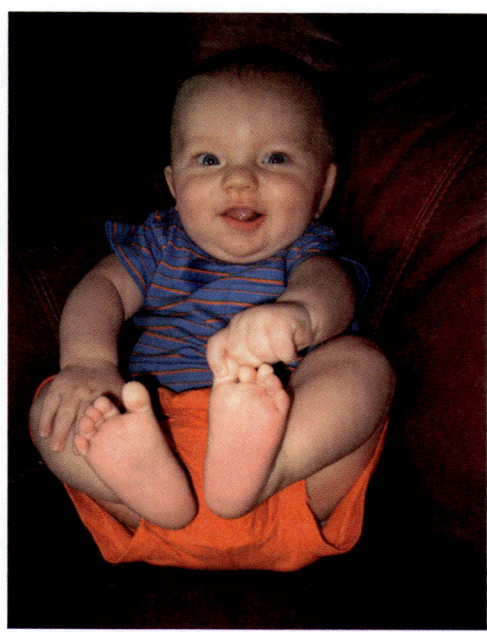

FIGURE 12-3 Infant. (Courtesy Dustin Sanders, O'Fallon, Mo.)

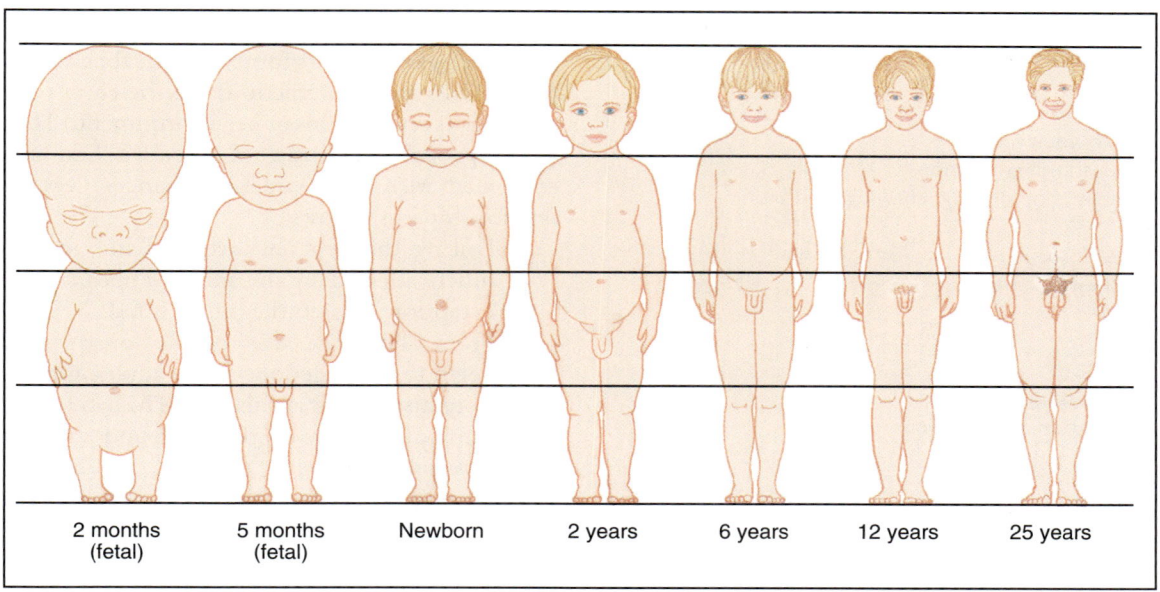

FIGURE 12-4 Changes in body proportions with growth. (McKinney ES et al: *Maternal child nursing,* ed 3, St Louis, 2009, Saunders.)

BOX 12-1 Developmental Milestones (Birth Through 12 Months)

Growth and development should be compared with standard growth charts showing established norms. It is important to remember that infants move through these stages at different rates.

1 Month
- Brings hands within range of eyes and mouth
- Keeps hands in tight fists
- Recognizes some sounds

2 Months
- Tracks objects with eyes
- Recognizes familiar faces

3 Months
- Moves objects to mouth with hands

4 Months
- Drools without swallowing
- Reaches out to people

5 Months
- Sleeps through the night without food
- Gains weight to twice birth weight
- Eruption of teeth may begin

6 Months
- Sits upright in high chair
- Makes one-syllable sounds (ma, mu, da, di)

7 Months
- Fears strangers
- Quickly changes from crying to laughing

8 Months
- Responds to "No"
- Sits without assistance

9 Months
- Responds to adult anger
- Pulls self to standing position
- Explores objects by sucking, chewing, and biting

10 Months
- Recognizes own name
- Crawls well

11 Months
- Attempts to walk unaided
- Shows frustration at restrictions

12 Months
- Walks with assistance
- Gains weight to three times birth weight

theorized that life moves through a series of overlapping stages. Each stage is marked by a crisis that must be resolved. According to Erikson, the most critical stage, which occurs in infancy (up to 1½ years of age), is the trust versus mistrust stage.[3] This stage is based on the infant's knowledge of two things: (1) that the surroundings are safe and predictable and (2) that causes and effects can be anticipated. For example, parental care is warm and loving, but punishment may result from not following rules. Consistency, or lack of it, in this type of care is the basis for trust versus mistrust issues.

TEMPERAMENT

Temperament is a person's style of behavior. It also is the way a person interacts with the environment. Moreover, it is the basis on which children form relationships. Behavioral traits seen in children by 2 to 3 months of age can be used to define three general types of temperament.[4] About 35% of children do not fit any of these categories, but rather demonstrate blends of these characteristics.

- *Easy children.* Easy children are characterized by regularity of bodily functions and low or moderate intensity of reaction. They accept new situations rather than withdraw from them. About 40% of children are easy children.
- *Difficult children.* Difficult children are characterized by irregularity in bodily functions and intense reactions. They withdraw from new situations. Children in this profile have a high activity level and an increased injury risk. About 10% of children are difficult children.
- *Slow-to-warm-up children.* Slow to warm up children are characterized by a low intensity of reaction and a somewhat negative mood. They adjust slowly to new situations. About 15% of children fall into this category.

A child's temperament and the responses this temperament elicits from adults form the basis for *early social interactions*. (Early social interactions are the child's interactions with others and with his or her environment.) This is known as **reciprocal socialization.** A baby's first interactions, combined with developmental changes, lead to specific relationships, as follows[5]:

- During the first few weeks of life, infants are not much affected by an adult's appearance. The only exception is when the infant is fed.
- From about the start of the fourth week, infants begin to direct actions at the adults. Emotional reactions also appear at this time. The baby shows obvious signs of pleasure at the sight and sound of adults, especially females.
- During the second month, more complex and sensitive reactions emerge. These include smiling and vocal sounds aimed at the mother. Animated behavior is shown during interactions.
- By 3 months of age, the infant has formed a need for social interactions. That need continues to grow and

is nourished by adults until the end of the second or the beginning of the third year. At that time, a need for peer interaction develops.

As the infant grows, his or her interactions become more complex. Bonding develops between the infant and family members. These bonds are considered **attachments.** For example, at 4 months of age, an infant shows *perceptual discrimination*. This means the child visually tracks the mother. At 9 months of age, an infant cries when the mother leaves. This is known as **separation anxiety** or *stranger anxiety*.

Separation from true attachments (e.g., separation from a parent) may result in a series of behaviors. The first is *protest* (loud crying, extreme restlessness, and rejection of all adults). Second is *despair* (nonstop crying, inactivity, and withdrawal). Third is *detachment* (a renewed but distant interest in surroundings, even if the mother comes back). Some psychologists believe that attachments continue through a person's life span. When possible, the parent should be allowed to hold the child during the assessment. This accomplishes two goals: first, the child and parent will be less anxious; second, the assessment will be easier to perform if the child is calm and not crying.

TODDLER AND PRESCHOOL YEARS

A child 1 to 3 years of age generally is considered a **toddler.** A child 3 to 5 years of age is considered a **preschooler** (Figure 12-5).

Vital Signs

A toddler's heart rate usually is 80 to 130 bpm. In preschoolers the heart rate is 80 to 100 bpm. Respirations for toddlers and preschoolers average 20 to 30 breaths/minute. A normal systolic blood pressure for toddlers is 70 to 100 mm Hg. For preschoolers it is 80 to 100 mm Hg. The normal body temperature for both age groups is 96.8° to 99.6° F (36° to 37.6° C).

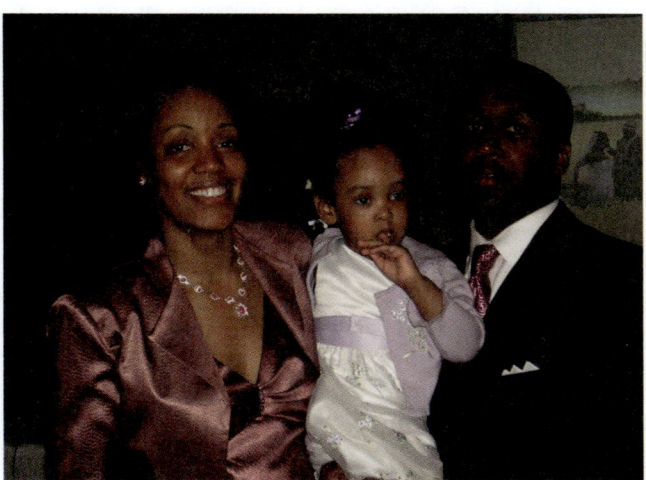

FIGURE 12-5 Preschooler. (Courtesy Kim Robinson, University City, Mo.)

Review of Body Systems

As children enter the toddler and preschool age groups, changes occur in some body systems.

Cardiovascular System. The capillary beds become better developed. They therefore are better able to assist in the body's thermoregulation. Hemoglobin approaches adult levels.

Respiratory System. The ear, nose, and throat structures in toddlers and preschoolers are similar to those in infants. Infants are at greatest risk for serious respiratory illness. Nevertheless, toddlers and preschoolers may acquire such infections in nursery school or preschool. Repeated upper respiratory tract infections may occur. However, they are rarely an indication of underlying disease in toddlers and preschoolers. The use of respiratory muscles changes from primarily abdominal to chest as the child nears school age.

Nervous System. *Myelination* (the maturation of nerve cells) begins in the third trimester and continues for about 10 to 12 years. This eventually provides for a smooth flow of neural impulses throughout the brain, increasing **cognitive development.** Even so, by age 2 much of the nervous system is completely developed. The brain weight is about 90% that of the adult brain. Visual acuity averages 20/30. Hearing essentially is mature by 3 to 4 years of age.

Musculoskeletal System. Muscle mass and bone density increase. Most children walk well with a normal gait by 2 years of age. Fine motor skills (e.g., scribbling with a pencil, stacking building blocks) become evident in toddlers and preschoolers.

Immune System. Passive immunity no longer protects toddlers and preschoolers. They become more susceptible to minor respiratory and gastrointestinal infections.

Endocrine System. The endocrine organs mature and increase production of growth hormone, insulin, and corticosteroid. Children in the toddler and preschool age groups gain an average of 2.9 kg (6½ pounds) a year.

Renal System. The kidneys are well developed by age 2. At this time, many children begin to gain control of bladder and bowel functions. *Specific gravity* is a measure of the concentrating ability of the kidneys. This value and other measurements of urinary function are similar to those in adults (see Chapter 30).

Psychosocial Development

By 2 years of age, children have developed unique personality traits and moods, as well as specific likes and dislikes. Basic language skills are mastered by age 3. Refinement of these skills continues through childhood. Toddlers and preschoolers also begin to recognize the difference between men and women. They begin to model themselves after people of their own gender. Box 12-2 lists other social milestones in the development of toddlers and preschoolers.

BOX 12-2 Social Milestones in Children 1 to 5 Years of Age

1 to 3 Years
- Can combine two different words
- Can complete some word phrases
- Follows directions
- Can point to a named part of the body
- Shows symbolic play when playing with toys
- Can remove some clothing

3 to 5 Years
- Can give first and last name
- Recognizes colors
- Speech is understandable to strangers.
- Completes short sentences and questions
- Can state name of a friend
- Begins to accept temporary absence of primary caregiver
- Plays independently in the presence of other children
- Shows increased level of confidence
- Shows sympathy at appropriate times (e.g., when another child is injured)
- Likes to hear and tell stories

TABLE 12-2 Parenting Styles and Associated Traits in Children

Authoritarian Style	Authoritative Style	Permissive Style
Low motivation to achieve	High motivation to achieve	Low motivation to achieve
Low self-esteem	Self-assertiveness	Low self-esteem
Shyness (girls)	Self-reliance	Lack of responsibility
Hostility (boys)	Friendliness, cooperativeness	Aggressiveness

> **NOTE**
>
> Toddlers are active and have a brief attention span. At this age they are at risk for falls, choking, pedestrian/motor vehicle collisions, and burn injuries. Just as with infants, many toddlers do not verbalize feelings of pain or fear directly.[2] Toddlers often have a comfort item, such as a blanket or special toy. When possible, allow the child to hold this during assessment and transport.

> **CRITICAL THINKING**
>
> Reassuring and nonthreatening language should be used when treating toddlers and preschoolers. Consider how a 3-year-old child might interpret statements such as, "I'm going to give you a shot" or "You'll feel a stick in your arm."

PATTERNS OF PARENTING

Patterns of parenting begin to have an effect on children in the toddler and preschool years (Table 12-2). Most parenting styles fall into one of three categories[6]:

- *Authoritarian*: Authoritarian parents see obedience as a virtue. Conflicts with parents result in the child being punished. Children of authoritarian parents are not given much freedom or independence. Traits seen in these children may include low motivation to achieve, shyness, and hostility. These children also may have low **self-esteem.**
- *Authoritative*: Like authoritarian parents, authoritative parents think that rules must be followed. In this style of parenting, however, the child is given reasons for the rules. The child also is allowed to express a

viewpoint, even though the parent has the final say. Authoritative parenting encourages a child to be independent. This style of parenting produces the most successful children. They tend to be responsible, assertive, self-reliant, and have high self-esteem.
- *Permissive*: Permissive parents give their children a lot of freedom. They are tolerant and accepting of the child's behavior, including both aggressive and sexual urges. These parents demand very little from their children. In fact, they tend to view their role as one of helping or serving the child. This style is the opposite of the other two parenting patterns. Traits seen in children raised by permissive parents are similar to those seen in children raised by authoritarian parents. These children are not especially independent, cooperative, or assertive. They often are discontented, distrustful, self-centered, and have low self-esteem.

SIBLING RIVALRY

First-born children often have a special relationship with their parents. They usually are expected to show self-control and responsibility when interacting with younger children. Parents are likely to be stricter with their first-born child, more demanding, and less consistent. They often spend more time with that child than with children who are born later. Because of these and other factors, **sibling rivalry** often becomes evident in the toddler and preschool age groups.

The characteristics of each child are one factor that influences how sibling conflicts occur. For example, a child may be fussy or easily bored or frustrated. A second factor is **family function;** this is the way the family deals with daily problems and conflicts and whether it is done respectfully, productively, and nonaggressively. Sibling rivalry also can be useful in child development. For example, disputes with brothers and sisters can promote crucial skills. These can include learning to value another person's point of view, learning to compromise and negotiate, and learning to control aggressive impulses.

PEER RELATIONSHIPS

Peer relationships offer a source of information about the child's world outside the family. They also expose the child to other types of families. In the toddler and preschool age groups, peer bonds are formed with others near the same age and maturity. These relationships often begin during play. Play may involve exploring a new toy, acting out fantasies, or using the imagination for new situations. Play also allows children to develop the ability to play simple games and competitive games with rules. This can lead to *problem-solving skills* and cognitive development. Play that involves others fosters interpersonal relationships. Toward the end of the preschool period, children begin to form lasting friendships. The importance of peer bonds and peer-group functions increases throughout childhood.

OTHER FACTORS THAT CAN AFFECT PSYCHOSOCIAL DEVELOPMENT

Two other key factors can have a significant impact on psychosocial development in the toddler and preschool age groups. These factors are *divorce* and *exposure to aggression or violence.*

About half of first marriages in the United States end in divorce.[7] Several factors determine the effect divorce has on toddlers and preschoolers. These include the child's age, cognition, and social competencies, and the child's sense of dependence on or independence from the parents. Children of divorced parents tend to have a higher rate of behavior problems as a result of family conflicts and stress than do children who live in a two-parent home.[8] These problems may arise from a number of factors, including (1) social, economic, and emotional turmoil (including loyalty conflicts); (2) the child's reaction to the loss of the parent who leaves; (3) a change in the custodial parent's behavior toward the child; and (4) the type of day care the child attends as a result of the divorce. Common reactions to divorce in young children include depression, withdrawal, a fear of abandonment, and fear that their parents no longer love them. The parents' ability to recognize and respond to the child's needs is important for helping the child deal with the effects of divorce.

Exposure to violence may increase a child's acceptance of this type of behavior. For example, some children may regularly watch television shows or video games with aggressive overtones. These children may model their behavior on these activities. It is particularly important that parents screen shows and play activities for children in the toddler and preschool age groups.

> **NOTE**
> Exposure to alcohol or other drugs also can be a negative factor in a child's behavior. Drug or alcohol abuse in the home environment increases the risk for child abuse. Child abuse is not limited to abuse by parents, but parents account for 80% of offenders.[2] Abuse can be inflicted by babysitters, relatives, domestic partners, or casual acquaintances. Abuse occurs at every socioeconomic level and often is precipitated by a stressful situation in the family (e.g., unemployment, marital problems, chronic illness, poverty).

SCHOOL-AGE YEARS

Children are considered **school age** from 6 to 12 years of age. The heart rate in this age group is 70 to 110 bpm, the respiratory rate is 20 to 30 breaths/minute, the systolic blood pressure is 80 to 120 mm Hg, and the body temperature averages 98.6° F (37° C) (Figure 12-6).

> **NOTE**
> School-age children are more independent. Often children of this age begin to play sports. Injuries in school-age children may be related to bicycle or other wheeled activities and to other sports. Failure to wear proper protective equipment often accounts for some of these injuries.

Review of Body Systems

The growth of children in the school-age years is slower and steadier than during infancy and the toddler and preschool years. School-age children gain an average 6.6 cm (2½ inches) in height per year (2.54 centimeters [cm] is equal to 1 inch.) Most bodily functions reach adult levels in this age group. Box 12-3 presents several important developmental milestones for school-age children.

Nervous System. About 95% of the skull's growth is complete by age 10. In addition, children's skills and abilities become more varied as their nervous and musculoskeletal systems develop. Brain function increases in both hemispheres. The child's ability to concentrate and learn develops rapidly in this age group.

Reproductive System. The reproductive system becomes active when a child reaches **puberty.** Puberty is brought about by increasing levels of sex hormones in the body. For

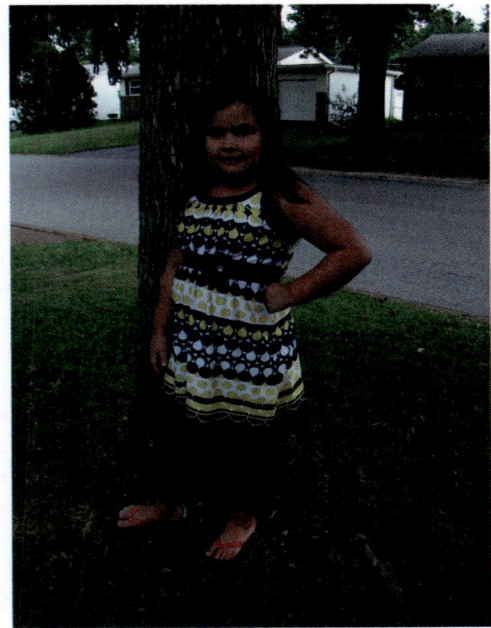

FIGURE 12-6 School-age child. (Courtesy Laura Lamadrid, Hazelwood, Mo.)

BOX 12-3 Developmental Milestones in School-Age Children (6 to 12 Years)

Physical Development
- Weight gain begins to consist more of muscle than fat; physical strength increases.
- Psychomotor skills (e.g., throwing, jumping, running) improve.
- Boys experience a "growth spurt" around age 12.
- Body changes indicate approaching puberty.
- Proportions of face and body become closer to those of adults.
- Eyes reach maturity in size and function.
- Permanent teeth begin to develop.
- Right- or left-handedness becomes well established.

Cognitive, Social, and Emotional Development
- Child is permitted more self-regulation with less supervision in the family setting.
- Parents usually spend less time with the child.
- Child's moral reasoning capabilities develop.
- Child gradually gains an understanding of the concept of death.
- Sexual interest grows rapidly with onset of puberty.
- Friendships become based on loyalty and mutual support.
- Social skills of giving, receiving, and sharing are learned.

day. In addition, school-age children begin to face the normal challenges of daily life. Fear of new situations (e.g., attending school) and peer pressure are predictable stressors for this age group.

Moral development occurs over time through experience. For school-age children, control of behavior begins to shift from external sources (e.g., what parents believe is right or wrong) to more internal self-control. With this internal control, these children justify the morality of their choices.

Many theories attempt to explain moral development. Kohlberg's theory proposes six stages, extending from about 4 years of age through adulthood. The stages occur at three age-related levels of development: preconventional reasoning, conventional reasoning, and postconventional reasoning[9] (Box 12-4). Most experts agree that loving, caring, and positive bonds play key roles in moral education.

SHOW ME THE EVIDENCE
Researchers in England weighed children between the ages of 1 and 10 years to test the accuracy of a shortcut for evaluating weight in children [i.e., $2(Age + 4) = Weight (kg)$]. According to the study, this weight formula underestimated the weight of children by a mean of 18.8% (confidence interval, 95%). The authors found that the most accurate formula for their population of children was $3(Age + 7) = Weight (kg)$.

Luscombe M, Owens B: Weight estimation in resuscitation: Is the current formula still valid? *Arch Dis Child* 92:412-415, 2007.

both genders, these hormone levels begin increasing before any external signs appear. The timing of puberty varies greatly. On average, it starts 2 years earlier in girls (between ages 8 and 13) than in boys (between ages 13 and 15).

Lymphatic System. The lymphatic system plays a key role in fighting disease and infection. This system undergoes many changes throughout a child's growth until puberty, when growth slows. Until that time, the lymphatic tissues in school-age children are proportionally larger than in adults.

Psychosocial Development

Between the ages of 6 and 12, the child's world expands outward from the family. At this time, relationships are formed with friends, teachers, coaches, caregivers, and others. As interactions with others increase, the school-age child begins to compare himself or herself with others, thus developing a **self-concept.** Some situations can create stress and affect self-esteem. Self-esteem is often based on external factors (e.g., popularity with peers, experience of rejection, emotional support from family and friends). It seems to be higher in the early years of school age. Low self-esteem can have damaging effects in later development.

Psychosocial development varies by individual. Some children seem very *mature.* Others seem very *immature.* During this stage, behavior may depend on the child's mood and experience with various types of people. It may even be determined simply by what happened on a certain

ADOLESCENCE

An individual 13 to 19 years of age is an **adolescent** (Figure 12-7). Normal vital signs for this age group are a heart rate of 55 to 105 bpm, respirations of 12 to 20 breaths/minute, a systolic blood pressure of 100 to 120 mm Hg, and a body temperature of 98.6° F (37° C). Adolescence is the final phase of change in growth and development. Organs rapidly increase in size, including the heart, kidneys, spleen, and liver. Blood chemistry values are nearly the same as those in adults (see Chapter 32). Activity of the sebaceous glands causes the skin to toughen. Growth of bone and muscle mass is nearly completed during the 2- to 3-year adolescent growth spurt.

During adolescence an individual reaches **reproductive maturity.** In girls, the first external sign of puberty is a change in one or both nipples. The nipples change into what is known as a *breast bud.* A few months later, pubic hair and underarm hair begin to grow, and the breasts enlarge. Within about 2 years after the appearance of the breast bud and after body fat reaches 18% to 20% of body weight, **menarche** (first menstruation) usually occurs. Changes in the endocrine system cause the release of *gonadotropin, luteinizing hormone,* and *follicle-stimulating hormone.* These hormonal substances promote estrogen and

BOX 12-4   Kohlberg's Stages of Moral Development

Preconventional Reasoning (About 4 to 10 Years)

From 4 to 10 years of age, children respond to cultural control mainly to avoid punishment and attain satisfaction. The first two stages occur at this level:

- Stage 1—Punishment and obedience: Children obey rules and orders to avoid punishment; the child has no concern about moral rectitude.
- Stage 2—Naïve instrumental behaviorism: Children obey rules but only out of pure self-interest. They are vaguely aware of fairness to others but only for their own satisfaction. The concept of *reciprocity* comes into play (i.e., "You scratch my back, I'll scratch yours.")

Conventional Reasoning (About 10 to 13 Years)

From 10 to 13 years of age, children desire approval both from individuals and society. They not only conform, they actively seek to support society's standards. The next two stages occur at this level:

- Stage 3—Good boy/good girl mentality: Children seek the approval of others. They begin to judge behavior by intention (e.g., "She meant to do well.")
- Stage 4—Law and order mentality: Children are concerned with authority and with maintaining the social order. Correct behavior is "doing one's duty."

Postconventional Reasoning (13 Years and Older)

If true morality (an internal moral code) is to develop, it appears during these years. The person does not appeal to other people for moral decisions. Such decisions are made by an "enlightened conscience." The final two stages occur at this level:

- Stage 5—The person makes moral decisions legalistically or contractually: This means that the best values are those supported by law, because they have been accepted by society as a whole. If a conflict arises between human need and the law, people work to change the law.
- Stage 6—An informed conscience defines what is right: An individual's actions are not based on fear, a need for approval, or legal demands, but on the person's own internalized standards of right and wrong.

Modified from Kohlberg L: A cognitive-developmental analysis of children's sex-role concepts and attitudes. In MacCoby E, editor: *The development of sex differences,* Stanford, Calif, 1996, Stanford University Press.

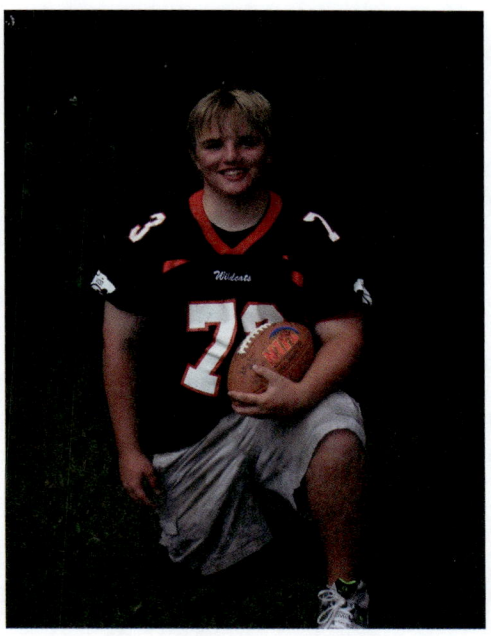

FIGURE 12-7 Adolescent. (Courtesy Laura Lamadrid, Hazelwood, Mo.)

> **NOTE**
> Teen pregnancy is also known as adolescent pregnancy. Although most teenagers do not plan to become pregnant, some do. Teen pregnancies carry extra health risks for the mother and the baby. Teenagers often do not receive timely prenatal care, and they have a higher risk for pregnancy-related high blood pressure and its complications. Risks for the baby include premature birth and a low birth weight.[10]

In boys, gonadotropin promotes testosterone production. Testosterone is a hormone produced by the testes. It causes the development of the male secondary sex characteristics. These include color and texture changes in the scrotum and an increase in the size of the testes. With these changes, the penis begins to enlarge and assume an adult shape, and pubic hair grows. At about age 14, a boy's first ejaculation of semen occurs during **masturbation** or sleep. Other male secondary sex characteristics that occur during late adolescence and early adulthood include deepening of the voice, facial hair, underarm hair, and sometimes the growth of chest hair.

The development of secondary sex characteristics in both genders coincides with the last period of rapid growth in adolescence. Rapid growth usually is preceded by an increase in body fat. This body fat decreases during the period of growth and increases again in later years. Girls retain more fat than boys in the subcutaneous tissue in the areas of the breasts, thighs, and buttocks. Boys gain an average of 20 cm (8 inches) in height before age 21, when growth usually stops. Growth in girls is less dramatic. It usually is complete by age 18. During the period of rapid growth in adolescence, the hands and feet grow first. The arms and legs then begin to lengthen, and the shoulders

progesterone production. Progesterone affects breast development and the menstrual cycle. Estrogen causes the development of the female secondary sex characteristics, such as disposition of subcutaneous fat in the breast, thighs, and buttocks and the development of axial and pubic hair. Estrogen also promotes the buildup of endometrium in the uterus.

become broader. Finally, the trunk of the body grows. The bones of the upper and lower jaw also grow. As a result, the face can change dramatically in appearance within a short time, especially in boys.

Psychosocial Development

In addition to physical changes, adolescence usually involves some emotional turmoil (Box 12-5). Adolescents may "try on" identities. These young people also begin to develop their adult personality. Conflicts with parents over school, manners, dress, hygiene, curfews, and other topics are common, because the adolescent has begun to express independence. As a result of these conflicts, most adolescents draw away from their parents. At the same time, they may emotionally move more toward their peers.

Friendships with others who are also trying on various identities may result in the use of alcohol and other drugs, sexual experimentation, and extreme forms of behavior or dress. Antisocial behavior tends to peak at about the eighth- or ninth-grade level.

In the teenage years, both boys and girls are very concerned about their appearance. Comparisons continually are made among peers. Concerns about body image are common in this age group. These include weight issues, body odor, acne, and dandruff. All these conditions can arise from the hormonal changes associated with adolescence. During adolescence many teenagers, especially girls, become obsessed with weight loss. They may try fad diets to control their figures. Eating disorders are common in this age group. Obsession with weight loss may lead to bulimia, anorexia nervosa, and severe depression. In fact, depression and suicide are more common among adolescents than in any other age group.[1]

CRITICAL THINKING
It may be best to interview the adolescent and the parents separately. Why might this be important?

NOTE
Learning to drive an automobile occurs during adolescence. Motor vehicle collisions represent the top cause of death in children of this age. Homicide is now the second-leading cause of death in adolescents in the United States, and suicide is third. According to the Centers for Disease Control and Prevention (CDC), most of these homicides and about one half of the suicides involve a firearm.[11]

EARLY ADULTHOOD

Early adulthood spans the period from 20 to 40 years of age (Figure 12-8). Average vital signs for this age group are a heart rate of 70 bpm, respirations of 16 to 20 breaths/minute, a blood pressure of 120/80 mm Hg, and a body temperature of 98.6° F (37° C). At the onset of early adulthood, individuals are reaching their physical peak. This is achieved between 19 and 26 years of age. Lifelong habits and routines develop. Body systems are at their optimum performance. This also is the age group in which pregnancy is most likely to occur. However, the aging process has begun. Some of the effects of aging (e.g., slowed reaction times, hearing loss, vision deficiencies) gradually become evident during this stage of life. Good health in early adulthood tends to be centered on lifestyle and physical fitness. Unintentional injury is the leading cause of death in this age group.

Psychosocial Development

The ability to love usually is well developed by early adulthood. This includes both romantic and affectionate love. Also, newly formed families bring on new challenges and

---

BOX 12-5 Psychosocial Development of Adolescents (13 to 18 Years)

Some variations from the following descriptions are to be expected. Also, some characteristics and traits may be affected by other developmental issues.

13 to 14 Years
- Struggles with identity issues
- Displays moodiness
- Develops close friendships
- Pays less attention to parents
- Interests and clothing styles are influenced by peer groups.
- Shows ability to work
- Has same-sex friends
- Develops need for privacy
- Experiments with body (masturbation)
- May experiment with cigarettes, alcohol, and marijuana
- Has capacity for abstract thought

14 to 17 Years
- Becomes self-involved
- Shows extreme concern with body image and sexual attractiveness
- Examines personal and inner experiences
- Channels sexual and aggressive energies into creative activities (e.g., poetry, writing, music)
- Develops feelings of sexual love and passion
- Selects role models
- Shows greater capacity for setting goals

17 to 18 Years
- Develops secure personal identity
- Shows greater emotional stability
- Has heightened sense of humor
- Shows pride in work
- Shows stable interests and concern for others
- Has higher level of concern for the future
- Develops clear sexual identity and ability for sensual love
- Shows gradual interest in adult behavior
- Accepts social norms and cultural traditions
- Can set goals and follow through with plans

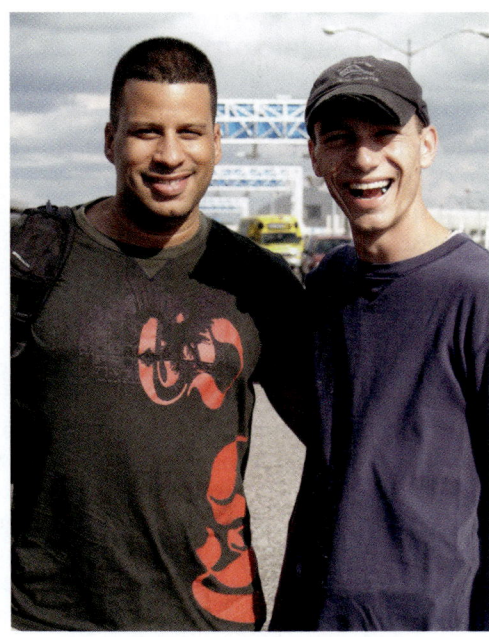

FIGURE 12-8 Early adulthood. (Courtesy Chad Sanders, Wentzville, Mo.)

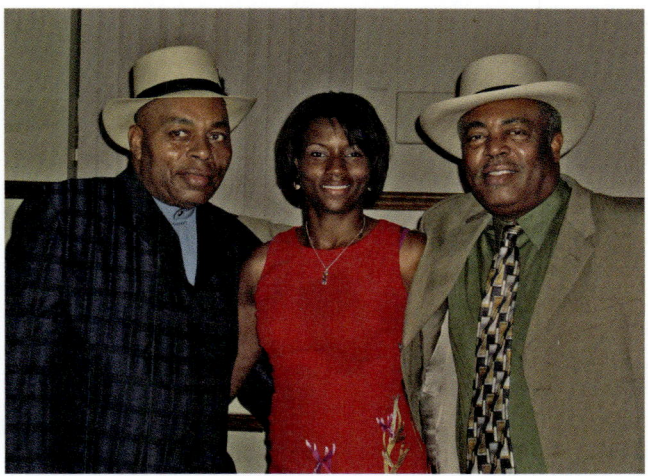

FIGURE 12-9 Middle adulthood. (Courtesy Norma Boozer, Florissant, Mo.)

stresses during this period. The highest levels of job stress are felt in this age group. Even so, fewer psychological issues related to well-being arise during early adulthood than during any other phase of life. Most individuals in this age group focus their attention on career and family as part of their psychosocial development. Their pursuits include the following:

- Selecting a mate
- Learning to live with a marriage partner
- Raising children
- Managing a home
- Finding a congenial social group
- Developing adult leisure time activities
- Selecting a secure and stable occupation
- Establishing and maintaining an economic standard of living

MIDDLE ADULTHOOD

Middle adulthood extends from 41 to 60 years of age (Figure 12-9). The average vital signs are the same as for early adulthood. Also, body systems continue to work at a high level. However, the physiological aspects of aging may become more obvious during this stage. For example, cardiovascular health becomes a concern. Hearing and vision changes occur. **Periodontal disease** may develop. Weight control becomes more difficult. Cancer tends to strike often. For women, **menopause** normally occurs between age 45 and 55. This marks the end of reproductive capacity.

Psychosocial Development

Middle adulthood generally is a productive time for social and professional recognition. It often is a period of financial security. However, because of the physical changes just described, the person in middle adulthood often becomes concerned with the "social clock." The individual may feel a sense of time pressure to meet lifelong goals. Common causes of stress in this age group include financial commitments and responsibility for the care of elderly parents. Another stress is concern for young adult children who have moved out and are on their own. As the last child leaves home, a depression or sense of loss is not unusual for many parents *(empty nest syndrome)*. Others feel a sense of freedom and enjoy a greater chance for self-fulfillment.

Some adults in middle age experience a "midlife crisis." They may make sudden and sometimes irrational changes in their life (similar to the identity issues seen in the teenage years). This may occur because of health worries, a change in physical appearance as a result of aging, or a change in the level of sexual activity with a spouse. However, most middle-aged adults tend to approach problems in their lives more as challenges than as threats. Important goals, for example, often are (1) to help their children to be responsible and happy adults; (2) to accept and adjust to aging parents; and (3) to accept the physiological changes of middle age.

LATE ADULTHOOD

People reach **late adulthood** at 61 years of age (Figure 12-10). Vital signs in this age group depend on the individual's health status. Moreover, they are affected by the physiological changes in body systems that normally occur during this stage of life. A person's life span is determined by health, genetics, and other factors. The theoretical maximum life span for human beings is 120 years.[1]

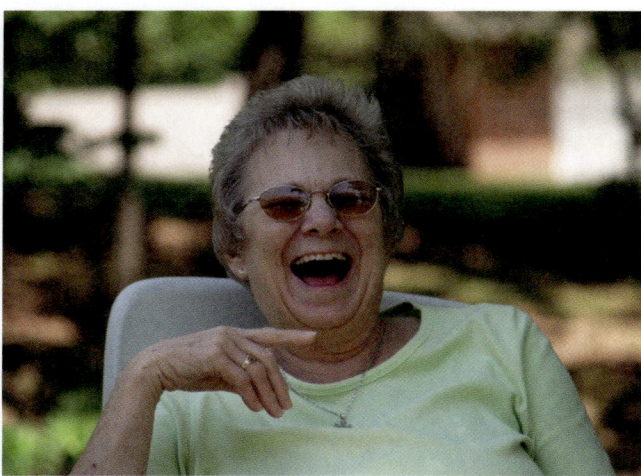

FIGURE 12-10 Late adulthood. (Courtesy Shirley Bohnert, St. Charles, Mo.)

? DID YOU KNOW?

According to *The State of Aging and Health in America 2004*, 70 million Americans—1 in 5—will be 65 or older by 2030. The fastest growing segment of the older population is elders age 85 or older. This segment is expected to double, from 5 million in 2003 to 10 million by 2030, and then to double again to 20 million by 2050.[12]

Review of Body Systems

Body system changes associated with late adulthood vary from person to person (Figure 12-11 and Box 12-6). They also vary from organ to organ and from function to function (see Chapter 49). Some occur dramatically. Others occur gradually. Some functions even remain constant well into old age. This variation can be seen in a number of systems. For example, a decrease in cardiac output and the ability to metabolize carbohydrates becomes evident early on. Changes in skin texture and hair color occur throughout late adulthood. The speed of nerve conduction and the manufacture of red blood cells do not decline until late old age.

🔍 SHOW ME THE EVIDENCE

Jacobs and colleagues reviewed current trauma literature to try to discover the reasons older adults have higher mortality and poorer outcomes after injury. Although they did not identify any clear cause for this poor prognosis, they noted that elderly patients who received prompt treatment at a trauma center had better outcomes. They also pointed out that undertriage of injured patients in this age group was a problem. The authors noted the need for more well-designed prospective research in this area.

From Jacobs D: Special considerations in geriatric injury, *Curr Opin Crit Care* 9:535-539, 2003.

Psychosocial Development

Society's attitude toward age can either enhance or detract from an older person's sense of self-worth. Some cultures credit wisdom to age; others consider the elderly to be more of a burden. For those who enjoy good health and retirement, late adulthood is a time of happiness and personal fulfillment. For others, this period is marked by financial burdens and physical and emotional challenges.

FINANCIAL BURDENS

Most people in late age begin to accept and adjust to retirement. They also adjust to having a reduced income. However, they face new issues. For example, some must pay for health care, and they may need to establish new living arrangements. About 95% of older adults live in their homes. These individuals choose not to reside in home care facilities such as nursing homes and assisted care communities. The financial requirements for either type of living arrangement can be a burden for the older adult and the family. For example, an older person living at home may require in-home health and home care services to assist with tasks of daily living. An older person who lives in a home care facility may need constant nursing care and other types of supervision. These situations, plus the cost of health insurance, prescription medicines, and other health care needs, can create financial burdens, even for those who plan well for their retirement. In 2007, about 3.6 million older adults in the United States were living below the poverty level, and more than 2 million were considered to be near-poor.[13]

CRITICAL THINKING

In an older patient's home, what clues may indicate that the person is under a financial strain or burden?

PHYSICAL AND EMOTIONAL CHALLENGES

In addition to the physical challenges linked to aging and the related health consequences, older adults face emotional challenges. Two emotional dilemmas are commonly faced in advancing years. One is accepting a decline in cognition. The other is dealing with the dying or death of a companion.

Aging does not always produce a decline in brain function. However, some conditions can cause a loss of mental faculties. Such conditions include circulatory disorders and some diseases common in older adults (e.g., *Parkinson's disease*). Problems with short-term memory, learning, attention, and judgment may develop. This decline in mental capability is an important concern and a cause of depression in older adults.

Terminal drop refers to the theory that a decline in intelligence in later years may be caused by a person's

THE MOST TYPICAL AGING CHARACTERISTICS
OF A PERSON AGED 75 YEARS

Hearing less acute

Taste and smell diminished

Loss of height on average
approximately 3 inches,
and possibly a stoop

Joints and bones become troublesome.
Thinning of bones causes them to
become lighter and more brittle.

Graying of hair

Reduced ability of
the eyes to focus

Limit for hard work lowered

Loss of tissue elasticity causes
skin to wrinkle and sag

Steady exercise delays
muscle fiber loss
and maintains strength

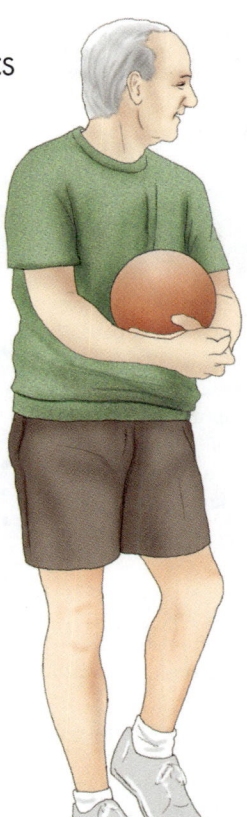

Neurons are lost and neurotransmitters diminish in number

Lung function decreases
and lung capacity diminishes

Blood pressure rises

Gut shrinks — food processing
becomes more difficult

Osteoarthritis often develops

By 80 years of age, vessel
elasticity declines by about 50%

Balance becomes less accurate

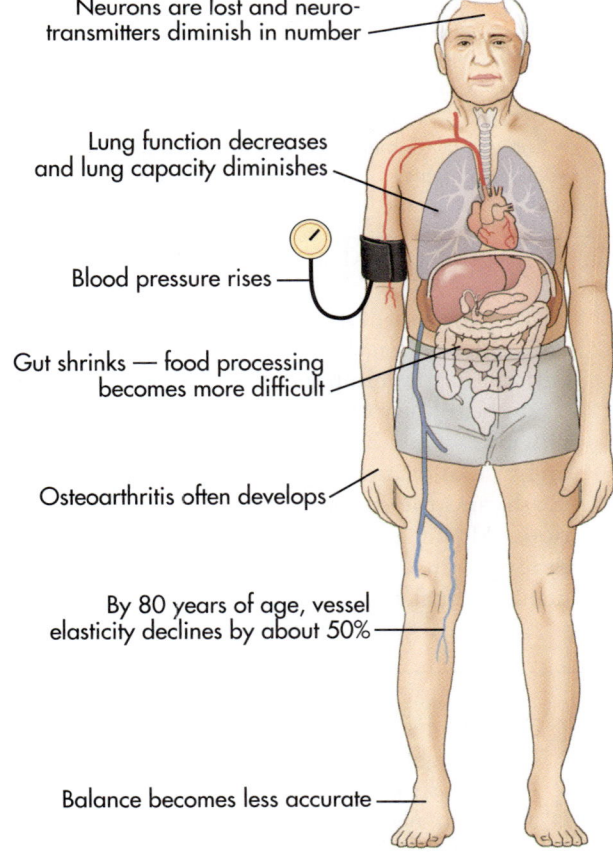

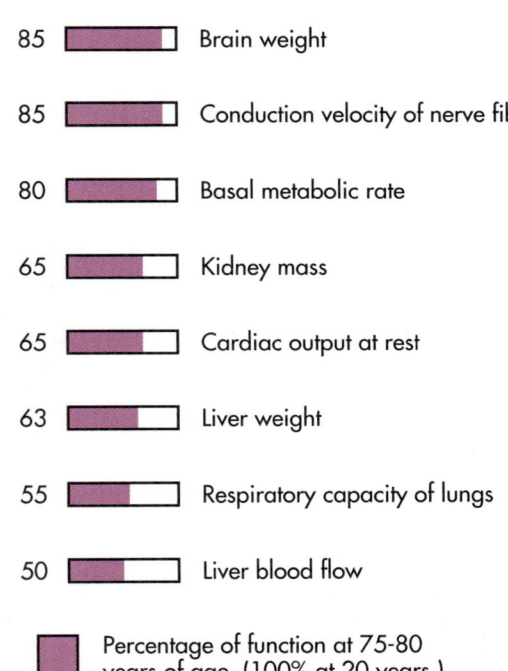

85	Brain weight
85	Conduction velocity of nerve fiber
80	Basal metabolic rate
65	Kidney mass
65	Cardiac output at rest
63	Liver weight
55	Respiratory capacity of lungs
50	Liver blood flow

Percentage of function at 75-80
years of age. (100% at 20 years.)

FIGURE 12-11 Body changes that occur in late adulthood.

BOX 12-6 Physiological Changes Associated With Late Adulthood

Cardiovascular System
- Functional changes occur as blood vessels thicken and peripheral resistance increases.
- By 80 years of age, vessel elasticity declines by about 50%.
- Blood flow to organs decreases.
- Baroreceptor sensitivity is reduced, and blood pressure tends to rise.
- Increased workload of the heart causes cardiomegaly, changes in the mitral and aortic valves, and decreased myocardial elasticity.
- The heart becomes less able to respond to exercise.
- The number of pacemaker cells in the heart diminishes, resulting in dysrhythmias (tachycardias are not well tolerated).
- The functional blood volume and platelet count decrease.
- The number of red blood cells decreases in late old age.
- Iron levels are poor.

Respiratory System
- Functional changes occur in the mouth, nose, and lungs.
- Lung function decreases, and lung capacity diminishes.
- The elasticity of the diaphragm declines, and the chest wall weakens.
- Diffusion through the alveoli diminishes from lifelong exposure to pollutants.
- Less oxygen becomes available for uptake by the blood.
- Coughing becomes ineffective because of weakened chest wall function and bone structure.

Nervous System
- Neurons are lost, and neurotransmitters diminish in number.
- Some taste buds are lost, and the olfactory sense diminishes.
- Pain perception decreases.
- The kinesthetic sense (sense of body movement) is lessened.
- Visual acuity diminishes.
- Reaction time declines.
- Hearing changes occur.
- The sleep-wake cycle is disrupted.

Musculoskeletal System
- Muscle mass is replaced by fibrous tissue.
- Progressive bone loss occurs, and changes in bones and joints become troublesome.
- Balance becomes less accurate.
- Osteoarthritis often develops.
- Shrinking of vertebral disks leads to loss of height and stooping posture.

Gastrointestinal System
- Secretion of saliva and gastric juices is reduced.
- Peristalsis and gastrointestinal secretions decrease.
- The esophageal sphincter becomes less effective, and internal intestinal sphincters lose tone.
- Vitamin and mineral deficiencies occur.
- Changes in the liver affect the metabolism of some drugs and foods.

Endocrine System
- Glucose metabolism and the production of insulin decrease.
- Production of triiodothyronine (T_3) by the thyroid gland declines.
- Production of cortisol decreases by about 25%.
- The pituitary gland becomes about 20% less effective.
- Women's reproductive glands begin to atrophy.

Renal System
- About 50% of the nephrons in the kidneys are lost.
- The filtration surface in the kidneys is reduced.
- Salt and water balance is compromised.
- Abnormal glomeruli become more common.
- The frequency of urination and the amount of urine eliminated decrease.

---

conscious or unconscious perception of coming death.[8] (This decline is measured by a change in IQ test results.) Such a perception may cause the person to begin withdrawing from the world anywhere from a few weeks up to 5 years before death. Terminal drop may become evident by changes in mood or mental functioning or by the way the body responds. It also may be linked to the presence of a disease (e.g., cancer). According to the terminal drop theory, the higher a person's IQ in old age, the longer the person is likely to live after the IQ test.

The dying or death of a partner can be one of the most stressful events in life. The ways in which a person deals with the death or imminent death of a partner are based on a number of factors. These include the person's cultural or religious views, the cause and timing of death, the length and type of relationship, the person's quality of life before death, and the support of friends, family, and organizations. Most people experience a variety of emotions in dealing with death and dying. These range from initial denial to final acceptance (see Chapter 2).

SUMMARY

- A newborn is a baby in the first hours of life. A neonate is a baby younger than 28 days. An infant is a child 28 days to 1 year of age.
- The newborn normally weighs 3 to 3.5 kg (7 to 8 pounds). This weight typically triples in 9 to 12 months.

The infant's head accounts for about 25% of the total body weight.
- At birth, structures unique to fetal circulation constrict and normally close within the first year of life. Fluid is expelled from the lungs during the first few breaths.

- Respiratory muscles and alveoli are not fully developed.
- Infants are born with protective reflexes related to breathing, eating, and stress or discomfort.
- At birth the anterior and posterior fontanels are open. Bone growth occurs at the epiphysis of the bones.
- Some passive immunity is conferred at birth and through the mother's breast milk.
- The caregiver is the major factor in the infant's psychosocial development.
- Temperament is a person's behavioral style. It is the way the person interacts with the environment.
- Toddlers are children 1 to 3 years of age. Preschoolers are children 3 to 5 years of age.
- The hemoglobin level in toddlers and preschoolers approaches that of adults. The brain in this age group is about 90% of the adult brain weight. Muscle mass and bone density increase. Walking occurs by age 2, and fine motor skills develop. Control of bowel and bladder are achieved.
- Parenting styles can be described as authoritarian, authoritative, or permissive.
- Sibling rivalry, peer relationships, divorce, and exposure to aggression and violence affect a child's development.
- School-age children range from 6 to 12 years of age. Physical growth slows, but brain function and the ability to learn quickly develop in this age group. Many children reach puberty during this time. Self-esteem and moral development are critical at this age.
- Adolescents are 13 to 19 years of age. The growth of bone and muscle mass is nearly complete in this age group. Reproductive maturity has been reached. Adolescence often involves some emotional turmoil, and antisocial behavior may be seen.
- Early adulthood spans the period from 20 to 40 years of age. Lifelong habits and routines develop. Body systems are at their optimal performance.
- Middle adulthood extends from 41 to 60 years of age. The physiological aspects of aging become more apparent in this age group. Menopause in women occurs during this stage.
- People reach late adulthood at 61 years of age. Body system changes vary widely from person to person, but the systemic changes of aging become apparent. Some adults in this age group face financial, physical, and emotional challenges.

REFERENCES

1. National Highway Traffic Safety Administration: *National EMS education standards and instructional guidelines*, Washington, DC, 2008, US Department of Transportation.
2. Price DL: *Pediatric nursing: an introductory text*, ed 10, Philadelphia, 2007, Saunders.
3. Erikson E: *Childhood and society*, ed 2, New York, 1963, WW Norton.
4. Dacey J, Travers J: *Human development: across the lifespan*, ed 5, New York, 2004, McGraw-Hill.
5. Hartup WW: Peer relations. In Mussen PH, Hetherington EM, editors: Handbook of child psychology, vol 4, *Socialization, personality, and social development*, ed 4, New York, 1983, Wiley.
6. Baumrind D: *Early socialization and the discipline controversy*, Morristown, NJ, 1975, General Learning Press.
7. Divorcerate.org: *Divorce rate*. www.divorcerate.org/. Accessed July 28, 2010.
8. Divorce-support-and-care.com: *Are children of divorced parents more likely to suffer negative effects?* www.divorce-support-and-care.com/children-of-divorced-parents-more-likely.html. Accessed March 10, 2009.
9. Kohlberg L: A cognitive-developmental analysis of children's sex-role concepts and attitudes. In MacCoby E, editor: *The development of sex differences*, Stanford, Calif, 1996, Stanford University Press.
10. Medline Plus: *Teenage pregnancy*. www.nlm.nih.gov/medlineplus/teenagepregnancy.html. Accessed August 10, 2010.
11. Centers for Disease Control and Prevention: *Injury: a risk at any stage of life—2006*. www.cdc.gov/ncipc/fact_book/factbook.htm. Accessed May 19, 2009.
12. Gordon C: *Live well, live long: health promotion and disease prevention for older adults*. http://74.125.95.132/search?q=cache:aLZFq4zxEREJ:www.asaging.org/cdc/issue_briefs/Issue_Brief_1.pdf+%22population+reports%22+%22older+adults%22&hl=en&ct=clnk&cd=10&gl=us&lr=lang_en. Accessed August 10, 2010.
13. US Census Bureau: *Income, poverty, and health insurance coverage in the United States: 2007*, Washington, DC, 2008, US Government Printing Office.

SUGGESTED READING

Northington W, Yates A: Caring for the aged: the pathophysiology of aging and its significant implications for prehospital care, *JEMS* 30:70-79, 81, 83-5; quiz 88-89, 2005.

PART THREE

Pharmacology

13 Principles of Pharmacology and Emergency Medications

OBJECTIVES

Upon completion of this chapter, the paramedic student will be able to:

1. Define the term "drug."
2. Identify the four types of drug names.
3. Outline drug standards and legislation and the enforcement agencies pertinent to the paramedic profession.
4. Distinguish between characteristics of routes of drug administration.
5. Discuss factors that influence drug absorption, distribution, and elimination.
6. Describe how drugs react with receptors to produce their desired effects.
7. List variables that can influence drug interactions.
8. Distinguish among drug forms.
9. Describe the paramedic's responsibilities to understand drug profiles.
10. Identify special considerations for administering pharmacological agents to pregnant patients, pediatric patients, and older patients.
11. Outline drug actions and care considerations for a patient who is given drugs that affect the nervous, cardiovascular, respiratory, endocrine, and gastrointestinal systems.
12. Explain the meaning of drug terms that are necessary to interpret information in drug references safely.

KEY TERMS

absorption The process by which drug molecules are moved from the site of entry into the body into the general circulation.

acetylcholine A neurotransmitter, widely distributed in body tissues, with the primary function of mediating the synaptic activity of the nervous system.

adrenergic Of or pertaining to the sympathetic nerve fibers of the autonomic nervous system, which use epinephrine or epinephrine-like substances as neurotransmitters.

agonists Drugs that combine with receptors and initiate the expected response.

alpha-adrenergic receptor Any one of the postulated adrenergic components of receptor tissues that responds to norepinephrine and to various blocking agents.

antagonists Agents designed to inhibit or counteract the effects of other drugs or undesired effects caused by normal or hyperactive physiological mechanisms.

anticholinergic Of or pertaining to the blocking of acetylcholine receptors, resulting in inhibition of transmission of parasympathetic nerve impulses.

beta-adrenergic receptor Any of the postulated adrenergic components of receptor tissues that respond to epinephrine and various blocking agents.

biological half-life The time required to metabolize or eliminate half the total amount of a drug in the body.

biotransformation The process by which a drug is converted chemically to a metabolite.

blood-brain barrier An anatomical-physiological feature of the brain thought to consist of walls of capillaries in the central nervous system and surrounding glial membranes; its function is to prevent or slow the passage of chemical compounds from the blood into the central nervous system.

blood coagulation A process that results in the formation of a stable fibrin clot that entraps platelets, blood cells, and plasma.

chemical name The exact designation of a chemical structure as determined by the rules of chemical nomenclature.

cholinergic Of or pertaining to the effects produced by the parasympathetic nervous system or drugs that stimulate or antagonize the parasympathetic nervous system.

contraindications Medical or physiological factors that make it harmful to administer a medication that would otherwise have a therapeutic effect.

controlled substance Any drug defined in the categories of the Comprehensive Drug Abuse Prevention and Control Act (also known as the Controlled Substances Act) of 1970.

cumulative action The effect that occurs when several doses of a drug are administered or when absorption occurs more quickly than removal by excretion or metabolism or both.

distribution The transport of a drug through the bloodstream to various tissues of the body and ultimately to its site of action.

drug Any substance taken by mouth; injected into a muscle, blood vessel, or cavity of the body; or applied topically to treat or prevent a disease or condition.

drug interaction Modification of the effects of one drug by the previous or concurrent administration of another drug, thereby increasing or diminishing the pharmacological or physiological action of one or both drugs.

drug-protein complex A complex formed by the attachment of a drug to proteins, mainly albumin.

drug receptors Parts of a cell (usually an enzyme or large protein molecule) with which a drug molecule interacts to trigger its desired response or effect.

dystonia A condition characterized by local or diffuse changes in muscle tone, resulting in painful muscle spasms, unusually fixed postures, and strange movement patterns.

effective dose 50 (ED$_{50}$) The amount of drug that produces a therapeutic response in 50% of those who take it.

effector organ A muscle or gland that responds to nerve impulses from the central nervous system.

endorphin Any of several peptides secreted in the brain that have a pain-relieving effect like morphine.

excretion The elimination of toxic or inactive metabolites, primarily by the kidneys; the intestines, lungs, and mammary, sweat, and salivary glands also may be involved.

first-pass metabolism The initial biotransformation of a drug during passage through the liver from the portal vein that occurs before the drug reaches the general circulation.

generic name The official, established name assigned to a drug.

idiopathic Arising from an obscure or unknown cause.

idiosyncrasy An abnormal or peculiar response to a drug.

loading dose A large quantity of drug that temporarily exceeds the capacity of the body to excrete the drug.

maintenance dose The amount of a drug required to keep a desired steady state of drug concentration in tissues.

neurotransmitter A chemical that is released from one neuron at the presynaptic nerve fiber.

nonselective beta-blocking agents Agents that block beta$_1$- and beta$_2$-receptor sites.

official name The name of a drug that is followed by the initials USP (*United States Pharmacopeia*) or NF (*National Formulary*), denoting its listing in one of the official publications; usually the same as the generic name.

orphan drug A medication that has been developed specifically to treat a rare medical condition.

parenteral Of or pertaining to any medication route other than the alimentary canal.

partial reabsorption The reabsorption from the renal tubule by passive diffusion.

pharmaceutics The science of dispensing drugs.

pharmacodynamics The study of how a drug acts on a living organism.

pharmacokinetics The study of how the body handles a drug over a period of time, including the processes of absorption, distribution, biotransformation, and excretion.

placebo An inactive substance or a less than effective dose of a harmless substance; it is used in experimental drug studies to compare the effects of the inactive substance with those of the experimental drug.

placental barrier A protective biological membrane that separates the blood vessels of the mother and the fetus.

potentiation Enhancement of the effect of a drug, caused by concurrent administration of two drugs in which one drug increases the effect of the other.

selective beta-blocking agents Agents block beta$_1$ or beta$_2$ receptors.

summation The combined effects of two drugs that equal the sum of the individual effects of each agent.

synergism The combined action of two drugs that is greater than the sum of each agent acting independently.

tardive dyskinesia A potentially irreversible neurological disorder characterized by involuntary repetitious movements of the muscles of the face, limbs, and trunk.

therapeutic action The desired, intended action of a drug.

therapeutic index A measurement of the relative safety of a drug.

therapeutic range The range of plasma concentrations that is most likely to produce the desired drug effect with the least likelihood of toxicity; the range between minimal effective concentration and toxic level.

tolerance A physiological response that requires that a drug dosage be increased to produce the same effect formerly produced by a smaller dose.

trade name The trademark name of a drug, designated by the drug company that sells the medication.

untoward effects Side effects that prove harmful to the patient.

*P*harmacology *can be defined as the science of drugs used to prevent, diagnose, and treat disease. Pharmacology deals with the interactions between living systems and chemical molecules. The paramedic must have a thorough understanding of a drug and its actions before it is administered. This understanding will help to ensure maximum effectiveness and will reduce the potential for harm.*

> **NOTE**
>
> This chapter introduces the paramedic to general principles of pharmacology and emergency medications commonly used in the prehospital setting. A more complete description of the emergency drugs discussed in this chapter can be found in the Emergency Drug Index. Medications described in this text that are included in the index are denoted by boldface italic type
>
> The drug information presented in this section conforms to current medical literature, to manufacturers' monographs, and to the clinical practice of the general medical community at the time of publication. Although every effort has been made to ensure accuracy and completeness, the authors, editors, medical advisers, and publisher disclaim liability for any discrepancies, incongruities, undetected errors, omissions in content, or reader misunderstanding. Local protocol for drug administration may vary from the information presented in this chapter. The paramedic should follow the guidelines established by medical direction.

SECTION ONE
Drug Information

HISTORICAL TRENDS IN PHARMACOLOGY

The science of pharmacology may date back as early as 10,000 to 7000 BC.[1] Medicinal herbs are thought to have been among the plants grown by human beings in the Neolithic period. Yet whether the herbs were thought to have healing properties is not known. A number of medicines are mentioned in the Bible. Some of these include gums, spices, oils, and maybe even narcotics. Drugs derived from plants were used heavily throughout the Middle Ages. They were used as digestives, laxatives, and diuretics (Figure 13-1).

The concept of "chemical medicine" was born in the seventeenth century. Some preparations introduced during the seventeenth and eighteenth centuries are still in use today. Opium *(morphine)* is a good example of one drug still in use. Accurate studies of drug dosage in the nineteenth century led to the development of manufacturing facilities to produce drugs. In addition, knowledge of the expected actions of these drugs became more exact. Important drug discoveries in the twentieth and twenty-first

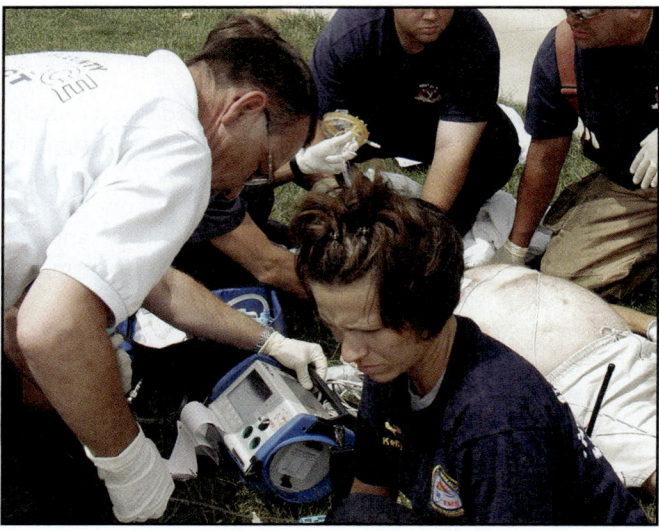

(Courtesy Ray Kemp. St. Charles, Mo.)

centuries (e.g., *insulin*, antibiotics, and fibrinolytics) have had major effects on common illnesses such as diabetes, bacterial infections, and cardiovascular disease.

Modern health care and **pharmaceutics** are undergoing many changes due in large part to consumer awareness of disease prevention. Changes also come from the consumers' drive to take responsibility for their health and wellness. The health care and pharmaceutical industries actively seek to develop new drugs, treatments, cures, or other methods to prevent diseases that affect aging, everyday living, or life span. The federal government also provides incentives to pharmaceutical companies to research and develop less profitable drugs. These drugs are called **orphan drugs.** They treat rare, chronic diseases such as hemophilia, leprosy, Cushing's syndrome, and Tourette's syndrome.

> **NOTE**
>
> The term orphan drug refers to a medication that has been developed specifically to treat a rare medical condition (an *orphan disease*). The assignment of orphan status to a disease and to any drugs developed to treat it is a matter of public policy in many countries. Medical breakthroughs have resulted from these assignments. Some of these medical advancements would not have otherwise been achieved because of the economics of drug research and development.
>
> Investigational drugs are drugs that are under study and not yet approved by the U.S. Food and Drug Administration for sale in the United States. The most common way patients receive these drugs is by taking part in clinical trials. Specific criteria must be met to receive an investigational drug outside a clinical trial. In general, these drugs are provided free of charge.

Drug Names

A **drug** may be defined as "any substance taken by mouth, injected into a muscle, blood vessel, or cavity of the body, or applied topically to treat or prevent a disease or

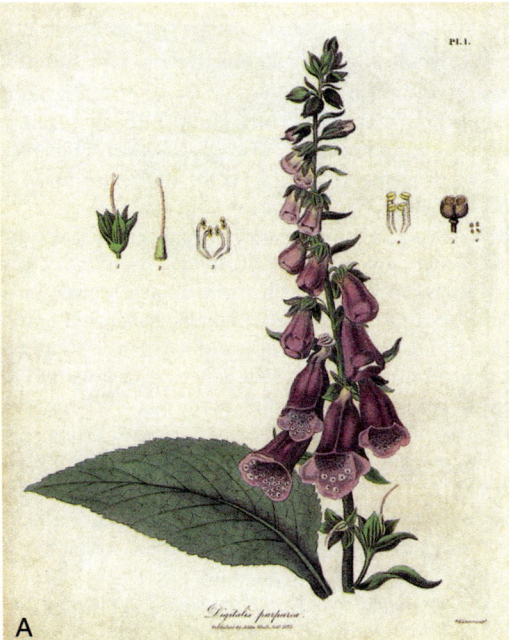

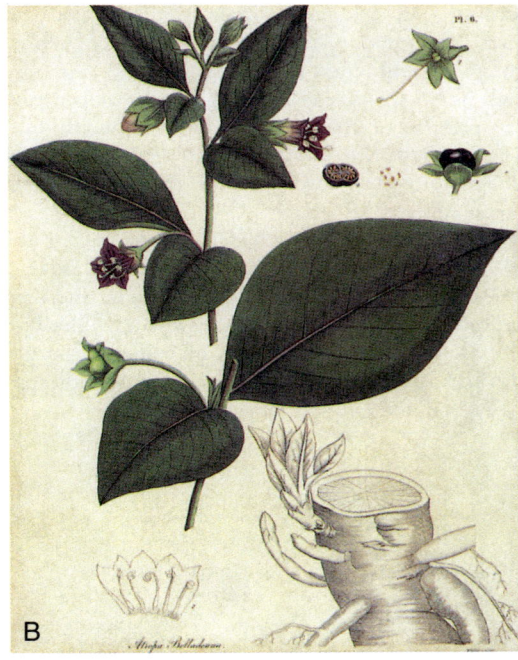

FIGURE 13-1 A, Foxglove. **B,** Deadly nightshade. These are the plant sources of digoxin and atropine, respectively. (From Page CP et al: *Integrated pharmacology*, ed 3, St Louis, 2006, Mosby.)

condition."[2] Drugs have been identified or derived from five major sources. These sources are plants (alkaloids, glycosides, gums, and oils), animals and human beings, minerals or mineral products, microorganisms, and chemical substances made in the laboratory (Box 13-1).

Drugs can be identified by the following four types of names:

BOX 13-1 Examples of Drugs and Their Sources

Plant Sources
Digoxin
Morphine sulfate
Atropine sulfate

Animal and Human Sources
Epinephrine
Insulin
Adrenocorticotropic hormone

Mineral or Mineral Product
Calcium chloride
Iodine
Iron
Sodium bicarbonate

Microorganism Sources
Penicillin
Streptomycin

Laboratory-Produced Chemicals
Diazepam (Valium)
Lidocaine (Xylocaine)
Midazolam (Versed)

1. **Chemical name:** The chemical name is an exact description. It describes the chemical composition of the drug. It also describes its molecular structure.
2. **Generic name** (nonproprietary name): This name often is an abbreviated form of the chemical name. The generic name is used more commonly than the chemical name. Generic drugs usually have the same therapeutic efficacy as nongeneric drugs. However, they generally are less expensive. This is the official name approved by the U.S. Food and Drug Administration (FDA).

DID YOU KNOW?

FDA approval is the final step in the process of drug development. The first step is for the new drug to be tested in the laboratory. If the results are promising, the drug company or sponsor must apply for FDA approval to test the drug in people. This is called an Investigational New Drug (IND) Application. Once the IND is approved, clinical trials can begin. Clinical trials are research studies to determine the safety and to measure the effectiveness of the drug in people. Once clinical trials are completed, the sponsor submits the study results in a New Drug Application (NDA) or Biologics License Application (BLA) to the FDA. This application is carefully reviewed; if the drug is found to be reasonably safe and effective, it is approved.[3]

3. **Trade name** (brand or proprietary name): The trade name is a trademark name designated by the drug company that sells the medication. Trade names are proper nouns, and the first letter is capitalized. This text

shows the trade name in parentheses after the generic name of the drug. The trade name usually is suggested by the first manufacturer of the drug.

4. **Official name:** The official name of a drug is followed by the initials *USP* (*United States Pharmacopeia*) or *NF* (*National Formulary*). These initials denote the listing of the drug in one of the official publications. In most cases the official name is the same as the generic name.

An example of the four names for a drug would be as follows:

Chemical name:	(−)-17-allyl-4-5α-epoxy-3,14-dihydroxymorphinan-6-one-hydrochloride
Generic name:	naloxone hydrochloride
Trade name:	Narcan
Official name:	naloxone hydrochloride USP

Sources of Drug Information

Several publications offer information on various drugs, their preparation, and recommended administration. These references include the *American Medical Association Drug Evaluation,* the *American Hospital Formulary Service Drug Information,* medication package inserts, the *Physicians' Desk Reference,* and the *Nursing Drug Reference* (Box 13-2). Paramedics should be familiar with these and with other emergency pharmacology manuals as well. This is crucial particularly regarding drugs that often are administered in the prehospital setting. Reliable Internet sources and computer application software (e.g., Epocrates) for hand-held devices (e.g., PDAs, Smartphones) also can be a good source of information about pharmacotherapeutics. In addition, the findings of current research can be found on the Internet. This research provides details about certain drug studies and treatments.

Drug Standards and Legislation

Before 1906 little control was exercised over the use of medications. Drugs often were sold or distributed by traveling medicine men, drugstores, mail order companies, and legitimate and self-proclaimed physicians. The ingredients of drugs were not required to be listed. In fact, many drug products contained opium, heroin, and alcohol, which could be potentially harmful to the user.

In 1906 Congress passed the Pure Food and Drug Act. This act was meant to protect the public from mislabeled or adulterated drugs. The act prohibited the use of false and misleading claims for drugs. The act also restricted the sale of drugs with a potential for abuse (Table 13-1). The act designated the *United States Pharmacopeia* and the *National Formulary* as official standards and empowered the federal government to enforce these standards. In 1980 the United States Pharmacopeial Convention purchased the *National Formulary.* This made the *United States*

BOX 13-2 Drug References

American Medical Association Drug Evaluation: The *Drug Evaluation* provides information on drug groups, dosages, prescribing information, and usage. It also covers valid clinical applications of drug use that differ from those approved by the Food and Drug Administration thus far.

Hospital Formulary: The *Hospital Formulary,* a manual published by the American Society of Hospital Pharmacists, provides an overview in monograph form of nearly every available (approved and unapproved) drug in the United States. The formulary is updated regularly and is available in all hospital pharmacies and in many emergency departments. The *Hospital Formulary* is considered by many to be the most reliable source of information on medications and drugs.

Medication package inserts: Most medications are packaged with written literature describing product use. These inserts provide valuable information as new drugs are introduced, and the health care professional should consult them to become familiar with the product.

Physicians' Desk Reference: The *Physicians' Desk Reference,* published yearly by the Medical Economics Company, is a concise compilation of drug information, including FDA-approved indications, contraindications, and adverse effects. In addition to providing product information through several cross-referenced indexes, the textbook serves as an identification guide by showing actual-size, color pictures of commonly prescribed medications. The *Physicians' Desk Reference* also lists emergency telephone numbers for poison control centers throughout the United States.

Nursing Drug Reference: The *Nursing Drug Reference* is published yearly and includes nursing considerations, side effects, adverse reactions, precautions, interactions, and contraindications for drug and intravenous therapy. The textbook contains an alphabetical listing of commonly prescribed drugs and detailed monographs for drugs recently approved by the Food and Drug Administration.

Pharmacopeia the only official book of drug standards in the United States. In addition to the *United States Pharmacopeia,* other drug standards and legislation are listed in Box 13-3.

Standardization of drugs is necessary because drugs made by different manufacturers (brand name versus generic) may vary significantly in strength and activity. The strength, purity, or effectiveness of a drug can be measured through chemical analysis in a lab. This process is known as *assay.* A concentration of a drug can be determined by comparing its effect on an organism, animal, or isolated tissue to that of a drug that produces a known effect. This process is known as *bioassay* (biological assay). Bioassay is used to measure the bioequivalence, or relative therapeutic effectiveness, of two chemically equivalent drugs.

TABLE 13-1 Controlled Substances

Characteristics	Dispensing Restrictions	Examples
Schedule I Has high abuse potential Has no accepted medical use; for research, analysis, or instruction only May lead to severe dependence	Approved protocol is required.	Heroin, marijuana (cannabis), tetrahydrocannabinols, lysergic acid diethylamide (LSD), mescaline, peyote, psilocybin, methaqualone, MDMA (ecstasy)
Schedule II Has high abuse potential Has accepted medical uses May lead to severe physical or psychological dependence or both	Written prescription is necessary (signed by the practitioner); only emergency dispensing is permitted without written prescription (only required amount may be prescribed for emergency period). No prescription refills are allowed. Container must have warning label.*	Opium, morphine sulfate, hydromorphone, meperidine, codeine, oxycodone, methadone, secobarbital, pentobarbital, amphetamine, fentanyl, methylphenidate, cocaine, and others
Schedule III Has less abuse potential than drugs in schedules I and II Has accepted medical uses May lead to moderate to low physical dependence or high psychological dependence	Written or oral prescription is required. Prescription expires in 6 months. No more than five refills are allowed in a 6-month period. Container must have warning label.*	Preparations containing limited quantities of or combined with one or more active ingredients that are noncontrolled substances (codeine, hydrocodone, morphine sulfate, dihydrocodeine, or ethylmorphine) and nonnarcotic drugs such as derivatives of barbituric acid, except those that are listed in another schedule, glutethimide, methyprylon, chlorphentermine, paregoric, and others
Schedule IV Has lower abuse potential compared with schedule III drugs Has accepted medical uses May lead to limited physical or psychological dependence	Written or oral prescription is required. Prescription expires in 6 months, with no more than five refills allowed. Container must have warning label.*	Barbital, phenobarbital, chloral hydrate, meprobamate, fenfluramine, chlordiazepoxide, diazepam, oxazepam, clorazepate, flurazepam, lorazepam, dextropropoxyphene, pentazocine, mazindol, alprazolam, and others
Schedule V Has low abuse potential compared with schedule IV drugs Has accepted medical uses May lead to limited physical or psychological dependence	Drug may require written prescription or may be sold without prescription (check state law).	Medications (generally for relief of coughs or diarrhea) that contain limited amounts of certain opioid controlled substances

*The warning must read "Caution: Federal law prohibits the transfer of this drug to any person other than the patient for whom it was prescribed."

> **NOTE**
>
> The Controlled Substances Act was passed in 1970. A controlled substance is any drug that is defined in the categories of the Act. These categories include opium and its derivatives, hallucinogens, depressants, and stimulants. It is illegal for any person to possess a controlled substance, unless the substance was obtained by a valid prescription or physician's order. A person may also possess a controlled substance if the possession of the drug is pursuant to actions in the course of professional practice. The authority for use of controlled substances and other prescription drugs is a function of state agencies. These agencies operate under restrictions of the federal government. The restrictions are provided by the federal Drug Enforcement Agency. Paramedics and other allied health workers who administer drugs should be familiar with state laws governing the administration and storage of drugs. They also should be familiar with the record-keeping requirements. Violations of the act are punishable by fine or imprisonment, or both.

BOX 13-3 History of Drug Standards and Legislation

1912: Congress passed the Sherley Amendment prohibiting fraudulent therapeutic claims.

1914: The Harrison Narcotic Act was passed to control the sale of narcotics and to help curb drug addiction or dependence. This was the first narcotic act to be passed by any nation, and it established the word narcotic as a legal term.

1938: Prompted by more than 100 deaths in 1937 from ingestion of a diethylene glycol solution of sulfanilamide, the federal Food, Drug, and Cosmetic Act was passed. This act contained a provision to prevent marketing of a new drug before it was tested properly. In addition, the act required that the label list all ingredients used in preparing the drug and the directions for drug use.

1952: The Durham-Humphrey Amendment changed the 1938 drug act, restricting the dispensing of legend (prescription) drugs. Legend drugs must bear the legend "Caution: Federal law prohibits dispensing without prescription."

1962: The Kefauver-Harris Amendment required that the safety and efficacy of a new drug be proved before the drug could be approved for use.

1970: The Comprehensive Drug Abuse Prevention and Control Act (also known as the Controlled Substances Act) superseded the Harrison Narcotic Act of 1914. The Controlled Substances Act classifies a controlled substance by its use and abuse potential. Drugs are classified into numbered schedules from schedule I (drugs with highest abuse potential) to schedule V (drugs with lowest abuse potential) (see Table 13-1).

Drug Regulatory Agencies

In July 1973 the Drug Enforcement Agency, an agency of the Department of Justice, became the sole legal drug enforcement body in the United States. Other regulatory bodies or services include the following:

CRITICAL THINKING

News stories often feature miracle drugs. These drugs are used in other countries but are not yet available in the United States. They are not available because they lack Food and Drug Administration approval. Why would the Food and Drug Administration not automatically approve drugs already known to be helpful in the international market?

- Food and Drug Administration: The FDA is responsible for enforcing the federal Food, Drug, and Cosmetic Act of 1937. The FDA may seize offending goods and criminally prosecute individuals involved.
- Public Health Service: The Public Health Service is an agency of the U.S. Department of Health and Human Services. One of the duties of the Public Health Service is to regulate biological products, which include viruses, therapeutic serums, antitoxins, or analogous products applicable in the prevention or cure of human diseases

or injuries. The agency examines and licenses these products and inspects and licenses the establishments that produce them.

- Federal Trade Commission: The Federal Trade Commission is an agency of the federal government directly responsible to the President of the United States. Its principal action with respect to drugs lies in its power to suppress false or misleading advertising aimed at the public.
- Canadian drug control: In Canada the Health Protection Branch of the Department of National Health and Welfare is responsible for administering and enforcing the Food and Drugs Act, the Proprietary or Patent Medicine Act, and the Narcotics Control Act.
- International drug control: International control of drugs began in 1912 when the first "Opium Conference" was held at The Hague. Various international treaties were adopted, obligating governments to control narcotic substances. These treaties were consolidated in 1961 into one document, known as the *Single Convention on Narcotic Drugs*, which became effective in 1964. Later the International Narcotics Control Board was established to enforce this law.

CRITICAL THINKING

Your patient is acutely ill. She reports taking only an herbal medicine, which is not found in standard drug reference materials. Where can you or the medical staff find information about these alternative therapies?

SECTION TWO
Mechanisms of Drug Action

GENERAL PROPERTIES OF DRUGS

Drugs may act in the body in many ways. Some of these actions are desirable (a *therapeutic effect*). Others are considered undesirable or even harmful (a *side effect*). Drugs also may interact with other drugs. Interaction may produce uncommon and frequently unpredictable effects. (Allergic reactions to drugs are discussed in Chapter 27.) In addition, drugs generally exert several effects rather than a single one.

NOTE

It is critical for the paramedic to perform a thorough patient assessment. The paramedic also must obtain a pertinent medical (and drug) history from the patient. Being able to recognize and understand the reasons why certain drugs are prescribed for certain conditions or diseases is important. This knowledge can help establish a field diagnosis for the patient based on the assessment and physical findings. By having a thorough understanding of drug actions/interactions, the paramedic should be able to use the right drug to manage the illness, disease, or condition.

One should note that *drugs do not confer any new functions on a tissue or organ; they only modify existing functions.* As is described later in this chapter, the actions of a drug are achieved by a biochemical interaction between the drug and certain tissue components in the body (usually receptors). A drug that interacts with a receptor to stimulate a response is known as an **agonist.** A drug that attaches to a receptor but does not stimulate a response is called an **antagonist.** Box 13-4 contains other pharmacological terms and their definitions.

To produce the desired effect, a drug first must enter the body. Then the drug must reach appropriate concentrations at its site of action. This process is influenced by three phases of drug activity: the *pharmaceutical phase,* the *pharmacokinetic phase,* and the *pharmacodynamic phase.*

Pharmaceutical Phase

Pharmaceutics is the science of dispensing drugs. One aspect of this field is the study of the ways in which the forms of drugs (solid or liquid) influence pharmacokinetic and pharmacodynamic activities (described in the following sections). All drugs must be in solution to cross the cell membranes to achieve absorption. The term *dissolution* refers to the rate at which a solid drug goes into solution after ingestion. The faster the rate of dissolution, the more quickly the drug is absorbed.

Pharmacokinetic Phase

Pharmacokinetics is the study of how the body handles a drug over a period of time. This includes the processes of absorption, distribution, biotransformation, and excretion. These factors affect a patient's response to drug therapy.

DRUG ABSORPTION

Absorption involves the movement of drug molecules from the entry site to the general circulation. The degree to which drugs attain pharmacological activity depends partly on the rate and extent to which they are absorbed. The rate and extent in turn depend on the ability of the drug to cross the cell membrane. The drug crosses the membrane through the processes of passive diffusion and active transport (described in Chapter 11). Most drugs enter the cell by passive diffusion. Yet some drugs require a carrier-mediated mechanism to assist them across the membrane.

LOOK AGAIN

See Chapter 11: General Principles of Pathophysiology, pp. 218-220.

BOX 13-4 Pharmacological Terminology

Antagonism: The opposition of effects between two or more medications that occurs when the combined (conjoint) effect of two drugs is less than the sum of the drugs acting separately

Contraindications: Medical or physiological factors that make it harmful to administer a medication that would otherwise have therapeutic value

Cumulative action: The tendency for repeated doses of a drug to accumulate in the blood and organs, causing increased and sometimes toxic effects; it occurs when several doses are administered or when absorption occurs more quickly than removal by excretion or metabolism

Depressant: A substance that decreases a body function or activity

Drug allergy: A systemic reaction to a drug resulting from previous sensitizing exposure and the development of an immunological mechanism

Drug dependence: A state in which withdrawal of a drug produces intense physical or emotional disturbance; previously known as habituation

Drug interaction: Beneficial or detrimental modification of the effects of one drug by the prior or concurrent administration of another drug that increases or decreases the pharmacological or physiological action of one or both drugs

Idiosyncrasy: Abnormal or peculiar responses to a drug (accounting for 25% to 30% of all drug reactions) thought to result from genetic enzymatic deficiencies or other unique physiological variables and leading to abnormal mechanisms of drug metabolism or altered physiological effects of the drug

Potentiation: The enhancement of effect caused by the concurrent administration of two drugs in which one drug increases the effect of the other drug

Side effect: Undesirable and often unavoidable effect of using therapeutic doses of a drug; action or effect other than those for which the drug was originally given

Stimulant: A drug that enhances or increases body function or activity

Summation: The combined effect of two drugs such that the total effect equals the sum of the individual effects of each agent (1 + 1 = 2)

Synergism: The combined action of two drugs such that the total effect exceeds the sum of the individual effects of each agent (1 + 1 = 3 or more)

Therapeutic action: The desired, intended action of a drug

Tolerance: Decreased physiological response to the repeated administration of a drug or chemically related substance, possibly necessitating an increase in dosage to maintain a therapeutic effect (tachyphylaxis)

Untoward effect: A side effect that proves harmful to the patient

---

Absorption begins at the site of administration. The rate and extent of absorption depend on the following factors[4]:

1. *The nature of the absorbing surface (cell membrane) the drug must traverse:* If a drug must pass through a single layer of cells such as the intestinal epithelium, transport is faster than if the drug must pass through several layers of cells (e.g., the skin). In addition, the greater the surface area of the absorbing site, the greater the absorption and the quicker the drug takes effect. For example, the small intestine offers a large absorption area, whereas the stomach has a relatively small absorption surface area.

2. *Blood flow to the site of administration:* A rich blood supply enhances absorption, and a poor blood supply delays it. For example, a patient with diminished blood flow may

not respond to intramuscular administration of a drug because diminished circulation reduces absorption. In contrast, intravenous administration of a drug immediately places the drug in the circulatory system, where it is absorbed completely and delivered to its target tissue.

3. *The solubility of the drug:* The more soluble the drug, the more rapidly it is absorbed. For example, drugs that are prepared in oily solutions are absorbed more slowly than drugs dissolved in water or in isotonic sodium chloride.

4. *The pH of the drug environment:* In solution, many drugs exist in an ionized (electrically charged) and nonionized (uncharged) form. A nonionized drug is lipid (fat) soluble and readily diffuses across the cell membrane. An ionized drug is lipid insoluble and generally does not cross the cell membrane. Most drugs do not ionize fully following administration. Rather, they reach an equilibrium between their ionized and nonionized forms, allowing for the nonionized form to be absorbed. Both the mechanism and the extent of ionization depend on whether the drug is an acid or a base. An acidic drug such as *aspirin* is relatively nonionized and does not dissociate well in an acidic environment such as the stomach; therefore it is absorbed easily in the stomach. A drug that is basic in the same acidic environment tends to ionize and is not absorbed easily through the gastric membrane. The reverse occurs when the drug is in an alkaline medium.

5. *The drug concentration:* Drugs administered in high concentrations tend to be absorbed more rapidly than those administered in low concentrations. In some situations, administration of a **loading dose** (large dose) first that temporarily exceeds the capacity for excretion of the drug is necessary. This rapidly establishes a therapeutic drug level at the receptor site. A **maintenance dose** (smaller dose) then can be administered to replace the amount of drug excreted. Thus loading doses are based more on the volume of distribution (of which body size is an important component) and less on capacity for excretion (e.g., renal failure). Maintenance doses are exactly the opposite.

6. *The form of the drug dosage:* Drug absorption can be manipulated by pharmaceutical processing. An example is a combination of an active drug with another substance that is slowly released or a drug that resists digestive action (e.g., those with enteric coatings).

CRITICAL THINKING

Consider a common condition seen in the prehospital setting. This condition requires that drugs be given at higher than usual doses to achieve therapeutic levels. What is the condition?

ROUTES OF DRUG ADMINISTRATION

The mode of drug administration affects the rate at which onset of action occurs. Route of administration also may affect the therapeutic response that results. The routes of drug administration are categorized as follows:

- Enteral (administration along any portion of the gastrointestinal tract)
- Parenteral (administration by any route other than the gastrointestinal tract)
- Pulmonary (administration by inhalation or through an endotracheal tube)
- Topical (administration by application to the skin and mucous membranes)

The route of administration greatly influences drug absorption (Table 13-2). Chapter 14: describes the methods used to administer drugs by various routes.

Enteral Route. Drugs administered along any portion of the gastrointestinal tract are said to use the enteral route (Box 13-5). Administration may be orally, rectally, or through a gastric tube. The enteral method of giving drugs is the safest, most convenient route. This route also is the most economical route of administration. Yet the enteral route is the least reliable and slowest of the common routes because of the frequent changes in the gastrointestinal environment (e.g., with food contents, emotional state, and physical activity). This route allows four types of absorption: oral absorption, gastric absorption, absorption from the small intestine, and rectal absorption.

Oral Absorption. The oral cavity has a rich blood supply. However, little absorption normally occurs in the mouth. Certain drugs, such as *nitroglycerin* (Nitrostat) tablets and some hormones, are prepared to be absorbed orally. When administered by sublingual or buccal routes, these drugs rapidly dissolve in the salivary secretions and are absorbed by the oral mucosa. Drugs that are absorbed in the upper gastrointestinal tract enter the systemic circulation. They

TABLE 13-2 Comparison of Drug Absorption Rates by Common Routes of Administration

Route	Rate of Absorption
Enteral	Slow
Sublingual	Rapid
Subcutaneous	Slow
Intramuscular	Moderate
Intravenous	Immediate (no absorption required)
Endotracheal	Rapid
Intraosseous	Immediate
Pulmonary	Rapid
Topical	Moderate

BOX 13-5 Some Emergency Drugs Administered via the Enteral Route

Activated charcoal
Aspirin

initially bypass gastrointestinal fluids and the liver. Drugs absorbed in the stomach and intestines pass through the portal vein system of the liver. They are subject to **first-pass metabolism** in the liver. (*First-pass metabolism refers to the concentration of a drug being reduced before it reaches the systemic circulation. It will be described in full later in this chapter.*) In the sublingual route the drug is placed under the tongue. The tablet or spray dissolves in the salivary secretions. The effects of sublingual medication usually are clear within a few minutes. With buccal administration the drug is placed between the teeth and mucous membrane of the cheek. As in the sublingual route, absorption by buccal administration usually is rapid.

CRITICAL THINKING

Nitroglycerin spray may be more effective in geriatric patients than the tablet form. Why do you think this is the case?

Gastric Absorption. The stomach also has a rich blood supply but is not considered an important site of drug absorption. The length of time a medication remains in the stomach varies, depending on the pH of the environment and gastric motility. As previously described, weakly acidic drugs tend to remain nonionized. These drugs are absorbed readily into the circulation. In comparison, basic drugs ionize in the stomach and are absorbed poorly. Altering the gastric emptying rate may alter the rate and extent of drug absorption. Many drugs are administered on an empty stomach with sufficient water (8 oz) to ensure rapid passage into the small intestine. Other drugs cause gastric irritation and usually are given with food.

Absorption From the Small Intestine. The small intestine has a rich blood supply. Thus it has a larger absorption area than the stomach. Most drug absorption occurs in the upper part of the small intestine. The pH of intestinal fluid is alkaline, which increases the rate of absorption of basic drugs. Prolonged exposure allows more time for drug absorption. An increase in intestinal motility (e.g., diarrhea) decreases exposure to the intestinal membrane and diminishes absorption.

Rectal Absorption. The surface area of the rectum is not large. However, the rectum is vascular and capable of drug absorption. Drugs administered rectally are subject to erratic absorption because of rectal contents, local drug irritation, and the uncertainty of drug retention. Fifty percent of a drug that has been administered rectally is estimated to bypass the liver after absorption. This makes first-pass metabolism by the liver less than that of an orally given dose.

CRITICAL THINKING

The drugs given rectally in emergencies usually are anticonvulsants. Why do you think this route would be chosen over the oral or intravenous route?

BOX 13-6 Examples of Emergency Drugs Administered via the Parenteral Route

Adenosine (Adenocard)
Amiodarone (Cordarone)
Atropine
Dextrose 50%
Diazepam (Valium)
Diphenhydramine (Benadryl)
Dopamine (Intropin)
Epinephrine (Adrenalin)
Fentanyl (Sublimaze)
Lidocaine (Xylocaine)
Lorazepam (Ativan)
Midazolam (Versed)
Morphine
Naloxone (Narcan)
Oxytocin (Pitocin)
Vasopressin (Pitressin)
Verapamil (Isoptin)

Parenteral Route. Drugs administered by injection are said to use the parenteral route (Box 13-6). The commonly used parenteral routes for administering medications include the following:

1. *Subcutaneous route:* A subcutaneous injection is given beneath the skin into the connective tissue or fat immediately beneath the dermis. This route is used only for small volumes of drugs (0.5 mL or less) that do not irritate tissue. The rate of absorption usually is slow and can provide a sustained effect.

2. *Intramuscular route:* An intramuscular injection is given into the skeletal muscle. Absorption generally occurs more rapidly than with a subcutaneous injection because of greater tissue blood flow.

3. *Intravenous route:* An intravenous injection is given directly into the bloodstream, bypassing the absorption process. This route produces an almost immediate pharmacological effect. Most intravenous drugs should be administered slowly to help prevent adverse reactions.

4. *Intradermal route:* An intradermal injection is made just below the epidermis. This route primarily is used for allergy testing and to administer local anesthetics. Drugs given by this route are not absorbed into the general circulation.

5. *Intraosseous route:* An intraosseous injection is given directly into the bone marrow cavity of pediatric and adult patients through an established intraosseous infusion system. Agents infused by this method are thought to circulate via the medullary cavity of the bone. Through the numerous venous channels of long bones, fluids or drugs rapidly enter the central circulation. The length of time from injection to entry into the systemic circulation is thought to equal that of the intravenous route.[5] Emergency medications known to be effective when administered via the intraosseous route are ***amiodarone***

(Cordarone), *epinephrine* (Adrenalin), *atropine, sodium bicarbonate, dopamine* (Intropin), *dobutamine* (Dobutrex), and *lidocaine* (Xylocaine).

> ### NOTE
> Although all resuscitation drugs can be given by the intraosseous (IO) route, administration of ceftriaxone, chloramphenicol, phenytoin, tobramycin, and vancomycin may result in lower peak serum concentrations.[6]

6. *Endotracheal route*: Access to the endotracheal route generally is through an endotracheal tube, which allows drug delivery into the alveoli and systemic absorption via the capillaries of the lungs. Administration of drugs via an endotracheal tube usually is reserved for situations in which an intravenous or intraosseous line cannot be established. Medications that can be administered by the endotracheal tube include *naloxone* (Narcan), *atropine, vasopressin* (Pitressin), *epinephrine* (Adrenalin), and *lidocaine* (Xylocaine). Administration of 2 to $2\frac{1}{2}$ times the recommended intravenous dose (diluted in 10 mL of normal saline) is recommended when medication is given by this route.[7]

> ### NOTE
> A mnemonic for the five medications that may be administered via the pulmonary route through an endotracheal tube is *N-A-V-E-L*, which stands for *naloxone, atropine, vasopressin, epinephrine,* and *lidocaine.*

Pulmonary Route. Medication can be administered by inhalation in the form of gas or fine mist (aerosol). The most commonly used inhalation medications are bronchodilators (Box 13-7). However, the pulmonary circulation can absorb a number of other medications if necessary, such as drugs for endotracheal administration.

Because of the large surface area and the rich capillary network of the alveoli, drug absorption into the bloodstream is rapid. Bronchodilators and steroids can be given by inhalation devices, such as a nebulizer (described in Chapter 14). A nebulizer propels the drug into alveolar sacs. Drugs that are given by a nebulizer device produce mainly local effects. Occasionally, nebulized drugs can produce

unwanted systemic effects. An example of these effects is an elevated heart rate (tachycardia).

Topical Route—Skin. In most cases, drugs applied topically to the skin and mucous membranes are absorbed rapidly (Box 13-8). Only lipid-soluble compounds are absorbed through the skin. The skin acts as a barrier to most water-soluble compounds. To prevent adverse systemic effects, intact skin surfaces should be used as an administration site. Massaging the skin helps to promote drug absorption because it dilates capillaries and increases local blood flow.

Topical Route—Nasal. As described in Chapter 10, the nasal mucosa is highly vascular. The delivery of medication via the intranasal route results in rapid absorption of the medication into the bloodstream and cerebrospinal fluid. This results in therapeutic drug levels that are effective in the management of seizures, pain, hypoglycemia, opiate overdose, and other medical conditions (Box 13-9). Using the intranasal route greatly reduces the risk of needle-stick injury. Some vaccines are also administered by the intranasal route in select patient groups. Examples of these include live attenuated influenza vaccine (LAIV) and influenza virus vaccine live (Intranasal FluMist) (see Chapter 14).

DRUG DISTRIBUTION

Distribution is the transport of a drug through the bloodstream. The drug is transported to various tissues of the body and ultimately to its site of action. After a drug has entered the circulatory system, it is distributed rapidly throughout the body. The rate at which distribution occurs depends on the permeability of capillaries to the drug molecules.

To review, lipid-soluble drugs readily cross capillary membranes to enter most tissues and fluid compartments. Lipid-insoluble drugs require more time to arrive at their point of action. Cardiac output and regional blood flow

> ### BOX 13-8 Emergency Drugs Administered via the Topical Route
>
> Lidocaine (lidocaine gel)
> Nitropaste (Nitro-Bid ointment)

> ### BOX 13-7 Emergency Drugs Administered via the Pulmonary Route
>
> Albuterol (Proventil, Ventolin)
> Amyl nitrite
> Epinephrine racemic (microNefrin)
> Levalbuterol (Xopenex)
> Metaproterenol (Alupent)
> Nitrous oxide/oxygen (Nitronox)
> Oxygen

> ### BOX 13-9 Emergency Drugs Administered via the Nasal Route
>
> Diazepam (Valium)
> Fentanyl (Sublimaze)
> Glucagon
> Haloperidol (Haldol)
> Lidocaine (Xylocaine)
> Lorazepam (Ativan)
> Midazolam (Versed)
> Naloxone (Narcan)

also affect the rate and extent of distribution into body tissues. Generally, a drug is distributed first to organs that have a rich blood supply. These organs include the heart, liver, kidneys, and brain. Then, depending on its composition, the drug enters tissue with a lesser blood supply, such as muscle and fat.

Drug Reservoirs. Drugs may accumulate at certain locations that act as storage sites. At these sites the drugs form reservoirs by binding to specific tissues. As serum levels decline, tissue-bound drug is released from its storage site into the bloodstream. The released drug maintains the serum drug levels and may permit sustained release of the drug over time. This allows continued pharmacological effect at the receptor site. The two general processes that create drug reservoirs are *plasma protein binding* and *tissue binding.*

As drugs enter the circulatory system, they may attach to plasma proteins (mainly albumin), forming a **drug-protein complex.** The extent to which this binding occurs affects the intensity and duration of the effect of the drug. The albumin molecule is too large to diffuse through the membrane of the blood vessel. Thus albumin traps the *bound drug* in the bloodstream. A drug bound to plasma protein is pharmacologically inactive. The protein becomes a circulating drug reservoir. The *free drug* (non–protein-bound drug) exists in proportion to the protein-bound fraction and is the only portion of the drug that is biologically active. As the free drug is eliminated from the body, the drug-protein complex dissociates, and more drug is released to replace the free drug that was metabolized or excreted. This process is summarized in the following equation:

$$Free\ drug + Protein \Rightarrow Drug\text{-}protein\ complex$$

Albumin and other plasma proteins provide a number of binding sites. Yet two drugs can compete for the same site and displace each other. Certain combinations of drugs may be given at the same time. As a result, this competition can have serious consequences. For example, a patient taking the anticoagulant drug warfarin (Coumadin) may be given quinidine (e.g., Quinaglute Dura Tabs). The quinidine may displace some of the protein-bound warfarin. This may cause warfarin toxicity and in turn can lead to severe hemorrhage.

Other factors that influence the binding ability of a drug include the concentration of plasma proteins (especially albumin), the number of binding sites on the protein, the *affinity* (attraction) of the drug for the protein, and the acid-base balance of the patient. Various disease states, such as liver disease, alter the ability of the body to handle many medications. These alterations result from a decrease in serum albumin levels (albumin is manufactured by the liver) and a decrease in hepatic metabolism. These and other factors may result in more free drug being available for distribution to tissue sites (increased free drug fraction and enhanced pharmacological response).

A second type of "drug pooling" occurs in fat tissue and bone. Lipid-soluble drugs have a high affinity for adipose tissue, where these drugs are stored. Because fat tissue has low blood flow, it serves as a stable reservoir for drugs. Some lipid-soluble drugs can remain in body fat for as long as 3 hours after administration. Other drugs (e.g., tetracycline) have an unusual affinity for bone. These drugs accumulate in bone after being absorbed onto the bone crystal surface.

> **CRITICAL THINKING**
> Tetracycline typically is not given to pregnant women because of the harmful effects it has on the development of the baby's teeth. Why would it affect the teeth?

Barriers to Drug Distribution. The blood-brain barrier and the placental barrier are protective membranes. These membranes prevent the passage of certain drugs into these body sites. The **blood-brain barrier** consists of a single layer of capillary endothelial cells. These cells line the blood vessels entering the central nervous system. The cells are tightly joined at common borders by continuous intercellular junctions. This special arrangement permits only lipid-soluble drugs to be distributed into the brain and cerebrospinal fluid. Examples of such drugs are general anesthetics and barbiturates. Drugs that are poorly soluble in fat (e.g., many antibiotics) have trouble passing this barrier. Thus they cannot enter the brain.

The **placental barrier** is made up of membrane layers. These layers separate the blood vessels of the mother and the fetus. Like the blood-brain barrier, the placental barrier is not permeable to many lipid-insoluble drugs. Thus the placenta offers some protection to the fetus. However, the placenta does allow the passage of certain non–lipid-soluble drugs. Examples of these are steroids, narcotics, anesthetics, and some antibiotics. If these drugs are given to the pregnant mother, they may affect the developing embryo or fetus or the neonate. (Pregnancy Category ratings for drugs are described later in this chapter.)

BIOTRANSFORMATION

After absorption and distribution, the body eliminates most drugs, first by biotransformation and then by excretion. **Biotransformation** (metabolism) is a process in which drugs are chemically converted to *metabolites* (smaller components). The purpose of biotransformation usually is to "detoxify" a drug and render it less active. The liver is the primary site of drug metabolism. However, other tissues also can be involved. Some of these include the plasma, kidneys, lungs, and the intestinal mucosa.

Orally administered drugs that are absorbed through the gastrointestinal tract normally travel to the liver before entering the general circulation. When this occurs, a large amount of the drug may be metabolized before reaching the systemic circulation. This is known as *first-pass metabolism.* This reduces the amount of drug that is available for distribution in the body. Medications affected by this initial

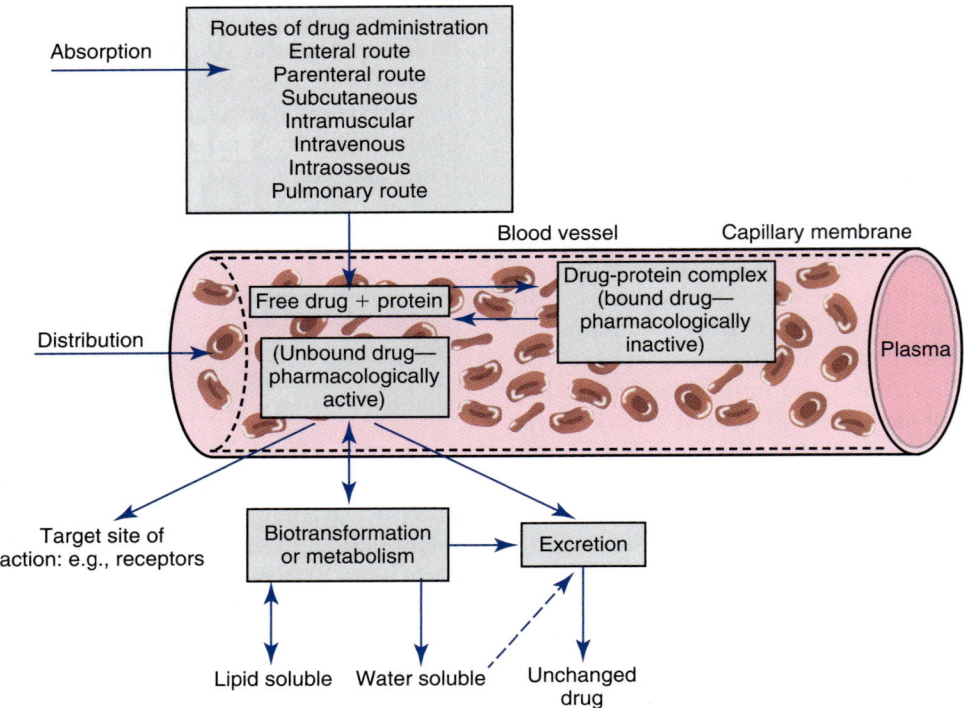

FIGURE 13-2 Pharmacokinetic phase of drug action, showing absorption, distribution, biotransformation, and excretion of drugs. Only free drug is capable of movement for absorption, distribution to the target site of action, biotransformation, and excretion. The drug-protein complex represents bound drugs; because the molecule is large, it is trapped in the blood vessel and serves as a storage site for the drug.

biotransformation in the liver may be given in higher dosages or administered parenterally (intravenously or intramuscularly) to bypass the liver.

Individuals metabolize drugs at variable rates. For example, patients with liver, renal, or cardiovascular disease are expected to have prolonged drug metabolism. Infants with immature metabolic capacity and older adults with degenerative metabolic function experience depressed biotransformation. If drug metabolism is delayed, drug accumulation and cumulative drug effects may occur. Therefore the paramedic may need to consider dosage reductions (particularly maintenance doses) for patients in these categories (Figure 13-2).

EXCRETION

Excretion is the elimination of toxic or inactive metabolites. The kidney is the primary organ for excretion. However, the intestine, the lungs, and the mammary, sweat, and salivary glands also may be involved.

Excretion by the Kidneys. A drug can be excreted in the urine unchanged. Or a drug can be excreted as a chemical metabolite of its previous form. Renal excretion consists of three mechanisms: passive glomerular filtration, active tubular secretion, and partial reabsorption (Figure 13-3).

Passive glomerular filtration is a simple filtration process. Filtration can be measured as the *glomerular filtration rate* (GFR) (described in Chapter 10). The GFR is the

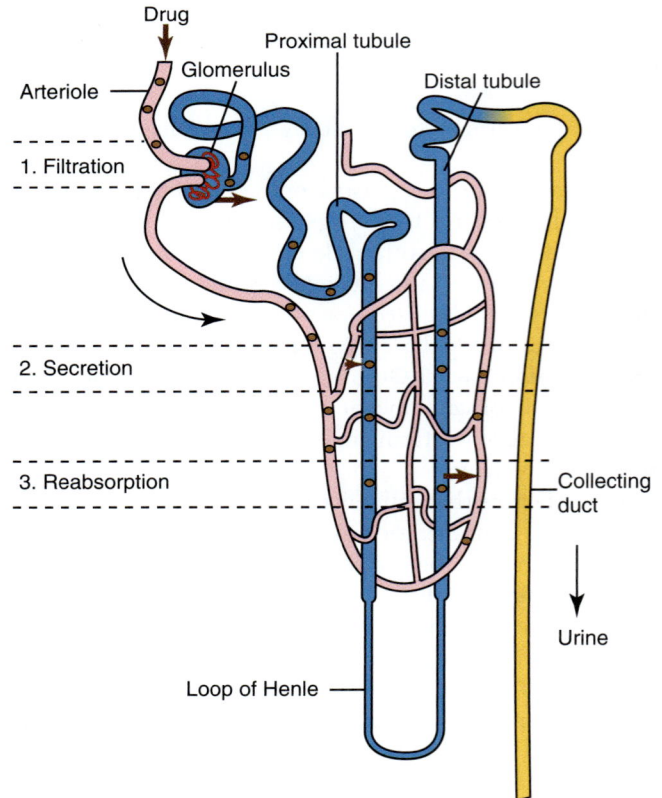

FIGURE 13-3 Drug excretion process.

total quantity of glomerular filtrate formed each minute in all nephrons of both kidneys. (This measure is usually expressed in milliliters.) The availability of a drug for glomerular filtration depends on its free concentration in plasma. Unbound drugs and water-soluble metabolites are filtered by the glomeruli. Drugs highly bound to protein do not pass through this structure.

LOOK AGAIN
See Chapter 10: Review of Human Systems, pp. 199-201.

After filtration, lipid-soluble compounds are reabsorbed by the renal tubules. Thus they reenter the systemic circulation. Water-soluble compounds are not reabsorbed. Therefore they are eliminated from the body. Because of the proportional relationship between free and bound drug, as free drug is filtered from the blood, bound drug is released from its binding sites into the plasma. The rate of excretion and the **biological half-life** of the drug (described later in this chapter) depend on how quickly bound drug is released.

CRITICAL THINKING
You pick up your patient at the renal dialysis center. How will you know which medicines you can administer safely?

Active tubular secretion occurs in the renal tubules, where free drug can be transported or secreted from the blood across the structure called the proximal tubule and from there deposited in the urine. Drugs actively secreted by the renal tubules can compete with other drugs for the same active transport process. *Amiodarone* (Cordarone) and *digoxin* (Lanoxin) is an example of a competitive drug interaction, in which the first drug reduces the removal or clearance of the second drug. (The term *clearance* refers to the complete removal of a drug by the kidneys.) The result of this competition for removal is an increase in the plasma concentration of the second drug.

Partial reabsorption is the reabsorption from the renal tubule by passive diffusion. Such reabsorption can be influenced greatly by the pH of the tubular urine. Weak acids are excreted more readily in alkaline urine. They are secreted more slowly in acidic urine. This is because they are ionized in alkaline urine but nonionized in acidic urine. The reverse is true for weak bases. For example, an increase in urinary pH decreases the reabsorption and increases the clearance of weak acids such as *furosemide* (Lasix) and *aspirin.* However, a decrease in urinary pH increases the clearance of weak bases such as amphetamine and tricyclic antidepressants.

As a rule, substances that are completely or almost completely excreted by the normal kidney can be removed by an artificial process that resembles glomerular filtration. This process is *hemodialysis* (see Chapter 29). Hemodialysis can be used to remove a wide variety of substances. It is not very effective for drugs that are highly tissue- or protein-bound. Moreover, hemodialysis is of limited benefit for the removal of rapidly acting toxins.

Excretion by the Intestine. Drugs are eliminated through the intestine by biliary excretion. After liver metabolism the metabolites are carried in bile and passed into the duodenum. The metabolites then are eliminated with the feces. Some drugs are reabsorbed by the bloodstream. They are returned to the liver and then later excreted by the kidneys.

Excretion by the Lungs. Some drugs can be eliminated by the lungs. Examples are general anesthetics, volatile alcohols, and inhaled bronchodilators. Certain factors can alter drug elimination via the lungs. These factors include the rate and depth of respiration and cardiac output. Deep breathing and an increase in cardiac output (which increases pulmonary blood flow) promote excretion. However, respiratory compromise and decreased cardiac output may occur during illness or injury. This can prolong the period required to eliminate drugs through the lungs.

Excretion by the Sweat and Salivary Glands. Sweat is an unimportant means of drug excretion. However, this method can cause various skin reactions and can discolor the sweat. Drugs excreted in saliva usually are swallowed and are eliminated in the same manner as other orally administered medicines. Certain substances given intravenously can be excreted into saliva. This may cause the person to complain about the "taste of the drug" even though it was given intravenously. Examples include *adenosine* (Adenocard) and calcium chloride.[8]

Excretion by the Mammary Glands. Many drugs or their metabolites are excreted through the mammary glands in breast milk. Nursing mothers are advised not to take any medicine except under the supervision of a physician. Mothers usually are advised to take prescribed medicines immediately after breastfeeding. This diminishes any risk to the infant.

FACTORS THAT INFLUENCE THE ACTION OF DRUGS

Many factors can alter the response to drug therapy, including age, body mass, gender, pathological state, genetic factors, psychological factors, environment, and time of administration. The paramedic should recognize these factors and should consider individual responses. The paramedic also must consider complications that may result from drug therapy.

Age. For the most part, pediatric and geriatric patients are known to be highly sensitive to drugs. In a child, this sensitivity results in part from the immature hepatic and renal systems. In an older adult, sensitivity results from the natural decline of these systems. These aspects of body function can reduce the efficiency of excretory and metabolic mechanisms. The older patient also may have underlying disease processes. This can create unexpected responses to drug therapy. Medication doses for children usually are modified based on body weight or surface area (see Chapter 48).

Body Mass. Many drugs are given according to body mass (kilograms). An indirect relationship exists between body mass and the final concentration of drug in a patient for any given dosage (i.e., the larger the patient, the lower the concentration for any given dose of drug). The average adult drug dose is calculated on the basis of drug quantity needed to produce a particular effect when administered to 50% of the population. This population includes only persons between the ages of 18 and 65 who weigh about 150 lb (68 kg). Therefore the appropriate drug doses for children who weigh less than 150 lb and are less than 18 years old are always based on body mass.

Gender. Drug effects differ in men and women. These differences result partly from size differences. Women usually are smaller in body mass than men are. Thus they may have higher concentrations of a drug when the standard dose is administered without consideration of size. Differences in the relative proportions of fat and water in the bodies of men and women also can cause variations in drug distribution.

Environment. Drugs that affect mood and behavior may be susceptible to the individual's environment and the personality of the user. For example, sensory deprivation and sensory overload may affect a person's response to a drug. The physical environment also can affect the actions of some drugs for some persons. For example, temperature extremes and changes in altitude may increase sensitivity to some drugs.

> ### CRITICAL THINKING
> You can alter the environment in the ambulance. How might you do this to promote the action of pain-relieving drugs that you have given your patient?

Time of Administration. As previously described, the presence or absence of food in the gastrointestinal tract affects the manner in which drugs are tolerated and absorbed. Other factors that may influence drug activity and reactions to drug therapy include a person's biological rhythms (e.g., sleep-wake cycles and circadian rhythms, described in Chapter 2).

Pathological State. Illness or injury and the severity of symptoms also can play a role in a person's sensitivity to drugs. Illness or injury can affect the type and amount of drug needed to achieve a desired effect. In addition, underlying disease processes such as circulatory, hepatic, or renal dysfunction can interfere with the physiological actions of the drug and drug elimination.

Genetic Factors. Genetics can alter the response of some persons to a number of drugs. For example, this can occur through inherited diseases or enzyme deficiencies or altered receptor site sensitivities. The results of genetic abnormalities may manifest as idiosyncrasies (peculiar responses to a drug) or may be mistaken for drug allergies.

Psychological Factors. A patient's belief in the effects of a drug may strongly influence and potentiate drug effects. For example, a **placebo** (e.g., a sugar pill) can have the same result as a pharmacological agent if the patient thinks it will have the desired effect. In contrast, patient hostility and mistrust can lessen the perceived effects of a drug. The paramedic can enhance the action of a drug by telling the patient that the drug is going to work and when it will take effect.

Pharmacodynamic Phase

Pharmacodynamics is the study of how a drug acts on a living organism. This includes the pharmacological response observed relative to the concentration of the drug at an active site in the organism. As stated earlier, drugs do not confer any new function on a tissue or organ of the body; rather, they modify existing functions. Most drug actions are thought to result from a chemical interaction between the drug and various receptors throughout the body. The most common form of drug action is the **drug-receptor interaction.**

DRUG-RECEPTOR INTERACTION

It is generally believed that most drugs bind to **drug receptors** to produce their desired effect (Box 13-10). According to this theory, a specific portion of the drug molecule (the active site) selectively combines or interacts with some molecular structure (the reactive site on the cell surface or within the cell). This interaction produces a biological effect. These reactive cellular sites are known as *receptors*.

The relationship of a drug to its receptor may be thought of as a key fitting into a lock (Figure 13-4). The drug represents the key. The receptor represents the lock. The drug molecule with the best fit to a receptor produces the best

> ### BOX 13-10   Drug-Receptor Interaction Terms
>
> *Affinity:* The propensity of a drug to bind or attach itself to a given receptor site
> *Agonist:* A drug that combines with receptors and initiates the expected response
> *Antagonist:* An agent that inhibits or counteracts effects produced by other drugs or undesired effects caused by normal or hyperactive physiological mechanisms
> *Efficacy (intrinsic activity):* The ability of a drug to initiate biological activity as a result of binding to a receptor site
> *Noncompetitive antagonist:* An agent that combines with different parts of the receptor mechanism and inactivates the receptor so that the agonist cannot be effective regardless of its concentration (Noncompetitive antagonist effects are considered to be irreversible or nearly so.)
> *Partial antagonist:* An agent that binds to a receptor and stimulates some of its effects but may antagonize the action of other drugs with greater efficacy. (Antagonists frequently share some structural similarities with their agonists.)

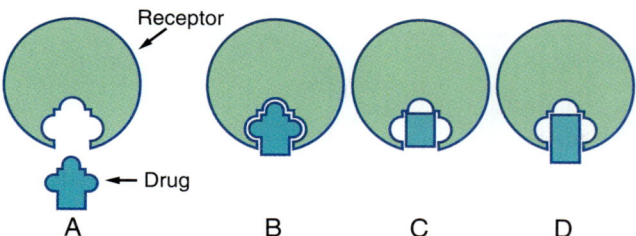

FIGURE 13-4 Lock and key fit between a drug and the receptors through which it acts. The site on the receptor that interacts with a drug has a definite shape. A drug that conforms to that shape can bind and produce a biological response. In this example, only the shape along the lower surface of the drug molecule is important in determining whether the drug binds to the receptor. (From Clayton BD, Stock YN, Harroun RD: *Basic pharmacology for nurses,* ed 14, St Louis, 2007, Mosby.)

response. Following absorption a drug is believed to gain access to a receptor after it leaves the bloodstream and is distributed to tissues that contain receptor sites. To review, drugs that bind to a receptor and cause an expected physiological response are referred to as *agonists.* Conversely, drugs that bind to a receptor and prevent a physiological response or other drugs from binding are referred to as *antagonists.*

DRUG-RESPONSE ASSESSMENT

In the prehospital setting the response to drug therapy often can be assessed by observing the effect of the drug on specific physical findings. Examples include monitoring blood pressure after administration of an antihypertensive medication and assessing pain relief after administration of an analgesic.

Each drug has its own characteristic rate of absorption, distribution, biotransformation, and excretion. Thus the effectiveness of some drugs cannot be monitored solely by the patient's response. For example, medications such as theophylline, **digoxin** (Lanoxin), and **phenytoin** (Dilantin) must reach a certain concentration at the target site to achieve the desired effect. Tissue concentrations often are proportional to and can be estimated from drug levels in the blood determined by laboratory analysis. Therapeutic drug levels in the blood, or serum, generally indicate ranges in tissue drug concentration that produce the desired therapeutic response.

Plasma-level profiles (Box 13-11) demonstrate the relationship between the concentration of drug in the plasma and the effectiveness of the drug over time (Figure 13-5). These profiles depend on the rate of absorption, distribution, biotransformation, and excretion after drug administration.

The **therapeutic range** for most drugs is based on the concentration that provides the highest probability of response with the least risk of toxicity. The dosage (loading and maintenance) required to achieve a therapeutic concentration varies because of the previously described factors that influence the actions of drugs: age, body mass, gender,

> ### BOX 13-11 Plasma-Level Profile Terms
>
> *Duration of action:* The period from onset of drug action to the time when a drug effect is no longer seen
>
> *Loading dose:* A bolus of a drug given initially to attain a therapeutic plasma concentration rapidly
>
> *Maintenance dose:* The amount of drug necessary to maintain a steady therapeutic plasma concentration
>
> *Minimum effective concentration:* The lowest plasma concentration that produces the desired drug effect
>
> *Onset of action or latent period:* The interval between the time a drug is administered and the first sign of its effect
>
> *Peak plasma level:* The highest plasma concentration attained from a dose
>
> *Termination of action:* The point at which the effect of a drug is no longer seen
>
> *Therapeutic range:* The range of plasma concentrations most likely to produce the desired drug effect with the least likelihood of toxicity (the range between minimum effective concentration and toxic level)
>
> *Toxic level:* The plasma concentration at which a drug is likely to produce serious adverse effects

pathological state, and genetic and psychological factors. In most patients, doses in the therapeutic range have a high probability of producing the desired effect and a low probability of toxicity. However, some patients fail to respond to doses in the therapeutic range. Still others may develop drug toxicity.

BIOLOGICAL HALF-LIFE

The rate of biotransformation and excretion of a drug determines its biological half-life. The *biological half-life* is defined as the time it takes to metabolize or eliminate 50% of a drug in the body. For example, a 100-mg injection of a drug is given. Its half-life is 4 hours. Thus 50 mg will be eliminated in the first 4 hours, 25 mg (half of the remaining 50 mg) will be eliminated in the second 4 hours, and so on. A drug is considered to be eliminated from the body after five half-lives have passed.

> **CRITICAL THINKING**
>
> Adenosine (Adenocard) is an intravenous antidysrhythmic medicine. Adenosine has a half-life of only 1 to 3 seconds. How will this brief half-life influence the speed and frequency of administration of this drug?

The half-life of a drug is crucial when determining the frequency of administration. A drug that has a short half-life (e.g., 2 to 3 hours) must be administered more often to maintain a therapeutic range than a drug with a long half-life, such as 12 hours. The half-life of a drug may be lengthened considerably in persons with liver dysfunction or renal disorders. These and other disease processes may require a reduction in drug dosage, or the interval between doses may have to be lengthened.

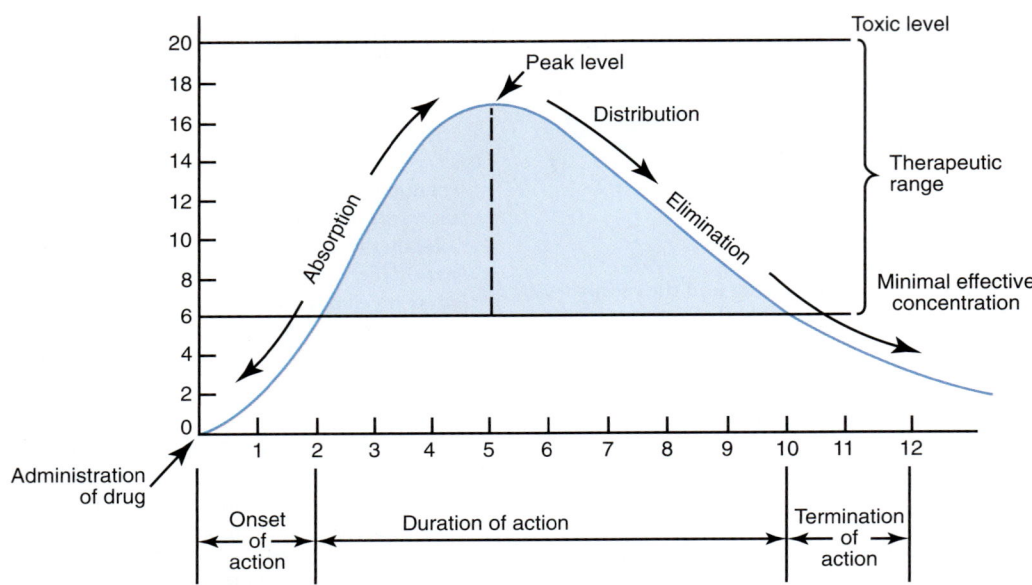

FIGURE 13-5 Plasma-level profile of a drug. (From McKenry LM, Tessier E, Hogan MA: *Mosby's pharmacology in nursing*, ed 22, St Louis, 2006, Mosby.)

THERAPEUTIC INDEX

The **therapeutic index** (TI) is a measurement of the relative safety of a drug. The index represents the ratio between two factors. The first factor is **lethal dose 50** (LD_{50}). This is the dose of a drug that is lethal in 50% of laboratory animals tested. The second factor is **effective dose 50** (ED_{50}). This is the dose that produces a therapeutic effect in 50% of a similar population. The therapeutic index is calculated as follows:

$$TI = \frac{LD_{50}}{ED_{50}}$$

A *wide* TI range indicates a drug is fairly safe. A *narrow* TI means the concentration range between effective levels of the drug and lethal levels of the drug is small. Therefore there is little room for error and it is easy to administer a toxic dose. The closer the ratio is to 1, the narrower the therapeutic index, and the greater the danger in administering the drug. In certain drugs, such as *digoxin* (Lanoxin), the difference between the effective dose and the lethal dose is small. In contrast, drugs such as *naloxone* (Narcan) have a wide margin between the effective dose (Figure 13-6).

DRUG INTERACTIONS

Many variables can influence drug interactions, including intestinal absorption, competition for plasma protein binding, biotransformation, action at the receptor site, renal excretion, and alteration of electrolyte balance. Not all drug interactions are dangerous; some may even be beneficial.

Some drug-drug interactions are clinically significant and can be dangerous. The paramedic should be aware of common drug-drug interactions. In addition, the paramedic should seek medical direction before giving drugs concurrently. (See the Emergency Drug Index.) The following drugs are associated with clinically significant drug-drug interactions:

- Blood thinners
- Tricyclic antidepressants (TCAs)
- Monoamine oxidase (MAO) inhibitors
- Amphetamines
- Digitalis glycosides
- Diuretics
- Antihypertensives

Other factors that can influence drug interactions include the following:

- Drug-induced malabsorption of food and nutrients
- Food-induced malabsorption of drugs
- Enzyme alterations that affect the metabolism of food or drugs
- Alcohol consumption
- Cigarette smoking that affects drug metabolism or excretion
- Food-initiated alteration of drug excretion

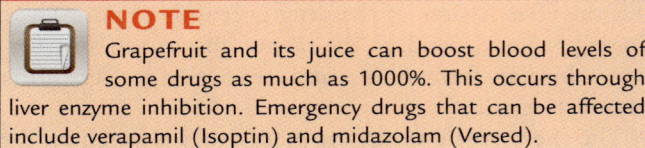

NOTE
Grapefruit and its juice can boost blood levels of some drugs as much as 1000%. This occurs through liver enzyme inhibition. Emergency drugs that can be affected include verapamil (Isoptin) and midazolam (Versed).

Finally, some drugs are incompatible with each other. For example, *calcium chloride* will precipitate (or crystallize) when mixed with *sodium bicarbonate*.

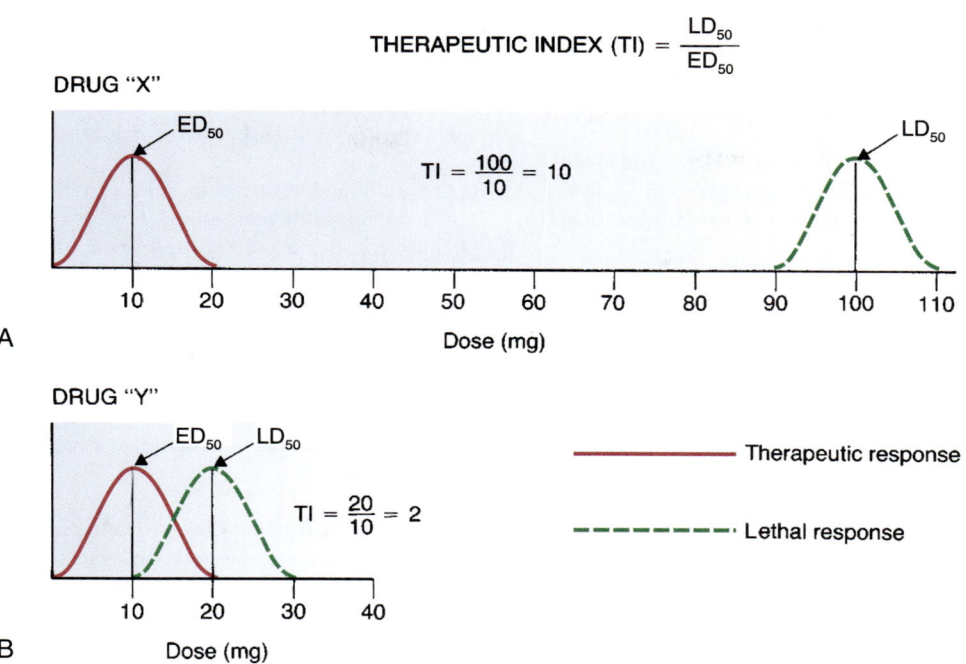

FIGURE 13-6 Plasma-level profile of a drug. (From Lehne R: *Pharmacology for nursing care,* ed 7, St Louis, 2009, Elsevier.)

DRUG FORMS, PREPARATIONS, AND STORAGE

Drugs and drug preparations are available in many forms (Box 13-12). Each one has specific indications, advantages, and disadvantages. These preparations are explained throughout the chapter and in the Emergency Drug Index.

Certain rules should guide the manner in which drugs are secured, stored, distributed, and justified. The paramedic should follow agency protocol and also local and state regulations. EMS personnel must be aware that temperature, light, moisture, and shelf life can affect drug potency and effectiveness.

DRUG PROFILES AND SPECIAL CONSIDERATIONS IN DRUG THERAPY

A paramedic should be familiar with the drug profiles of any drug he or she administers. Not all aspects of drug profiles can be committed to memory. Thus the paramedic should make regular use of pharmacology references (e.g., handbooks and pocket guides) and seek medical direction as needed. Paramedics are legally, morally, and ethically responsible for safe and effective drug administration (see Chapter 14). As part of the professional practice of patient management, paramedics must do the following:

- Use correct precautions and techniques when administering medications.
- Observe and document the effects of drugs.
- Be current in their knowledge base regarding changes in trends in pharmacology.
- Establish and maintain professional relationships with other members of the health care team.
- Understand pharmacodynamics of the drugs they administer.
- Carefully evaluate patients to identify drug indications and contraindications.
- Take a drug history from patients that includes the following information:

  Prescribed medications (name, strength, daily dosage)
  Over-the-counter medications
  Vitamins
  Alternative drug therapies (e.g., homeopathic medicines and herbal medicines)
  Any drug allergies or adverse drug reactions
- Strictly adhere to standing orders or protocols for drug administration or consult with online medical direction.

The components of a drug profile include the following:

Drug names: Usually the generic and trade names; may include chemical names

Classification: The group to which the drug belongs

Mechanism of action: The pharmacodynamic properties of a drug; the way in which a drug causes its effects

Indications: Conditions for which the drug is administered as approved by the FDA

BOX 13-12 Various Forms of Drug Preparations

Preparations for Oral Use

Liquids

Aqueous solution: substance dissolved in water and syrups

Aqueous suspension: solid particles suspended in liquid

Emulsion: fat or oil suspended in liquid with an emulsifier

Spirits: alcohol solution

Elixir: aromatic, sweetened alcohol and water solution

Tincture: alcohol extract of plant or vegetable substance

Fluid extract: concentrated alcoholic liquid extract of plant or vegetables

Extract: syrup or dried form of pharmacologically active drug, usually prepared by evaporating a solution

Solids

Capsule: soluble case (usually gelatin) that contains liquid, dry, or beaded drug particles

Tablet: compressed, powdered drugs in the form of a small disk

Troche or lozenge: medicated tablets that dissolve slowly in the mouth

Powder or granules: loose or molded drug substance for administration with or without liquids

Preparations for Parenteral Use

Ampule: sealed glass container for liquid injectable medication

Vial: glass container with rubber stopper for liquid or powdered medication

Cartridge or Tubex: single-dose unit of parenteral medication to be used with a specific injecting device

Intravenous Infusions (Suspended on Hanger at Bedside)

Flexible collapsible plastic bags (25 to 250 mL): used for continuous infusion of fluid replacement with or without medications

Intermittent intravenous infusions: usually secondary intravenous setup of a small plastic bag (25 to 250 mL) to which medication is added. The infusion runs as a "piggyback," hung separately from the primary intravenous infusion via a secondary administration tubing set usually for 20 to 120 minutes. The primary intravenous solution is run between medication doses or may be co-infused if the solutions are compatible

Heparin or saline lock: a port site for direct administration of intermittent intravenous medications without the need for primary intravenous solution

Preparations for Topical Use

Liniment: liquid suspension for lubrication that is applied by rubbing

Lotion: liquid suspension that can be protective, emollient, cooling, astringent, antipruritic, or cleansing

Ointment: semisolid medicine in a base for local protective, soothing, astringent, or transdermal application for systemic effects (nitroglycerin, scopolamine, estrogen)

Paste: thick ointment primarily used for skin protection

Plasters: solid preparations that are adhesive, protective, or soothing

Cream: emulsion that contains aqueous and oily bases

Aerosol: fine powder or solution in a volatile liquid that contains a propellant

Preparations for Use on Mucous Membranes

Drops for eyes, ears, or nose: aqueous solutions with or without gelling agent to increase retention time in the eye

Topical instillation of aqueous solution of medications: usually for topical action but occasionally for systemic effects (enema, douche, mouthwash, throat spray, gargle)

Aerosol sprays, nebulizers, and inhalers: aqueous solutions of medication delivered in droplet form to the target membrane, such as the bronchial tree (bronchodilators)

Nasal drugs: an alternative route for drugs with poor bioavailability and high-molecular-weight compounds such as peptides, steroids, and vaccines

Foam: powder or solution of medication in volatile liquid with propellant (vaginal foams for contraception)

Suppositories: usually medicinal substances mixed in a form but malleable base (cocoa butter to facilitate insertion into a body cavity [rectum or vagina])

Miscellaneous Drug Delivery Systems

Intradermal implants: pellets that contain a small deposit of medication and are inserted into a dermal pocket; they are designed to allow medication to leach slowly into tissue and usually are used to administer hormones such as testosterone or estradiol

Micropump system: small, external pump attached by belt or implanted that delivers medication via a needle in a continuous steady dose (insulin, anticancer chemotherapy, opioids)

Membrane delivery systems: drug-laden membranes are instilled into the eye to deliver a steady flow of medication (pilocarpine or corticosteroids)

Pharmacokinetics: How the body handles the drug over time; includes absorption, distribution, biotransformation, excretion, and onset and duration

Side/adverse effects: Untoward or undesired effects that may be caused by the drug

Dosages: The amount of drug to be administered

Routes of administration: How the drug is given

Contraindications: Conditions in which it may be harmful to administer the drug

Special considerations: How the drug may affect pediatric patients, geriatric patients, pregnant patients, and other special groups (described next)

Storage requirements: How the drug should be stored

Special Considerations in Drug Therapy

Special considerations in drug therapy must be taken into account when one is caring for pregnant patients, pediatric patients, and older adult patients. These considerations are described next. They also are described throughout this text by subject matter and in the Emergency Drug Index.

SHOW ME THE EVIDENCE

This descriptive paper reviews 21,298 adverse drug events (ADEs) seen in emergency departments in 2004 and 2005. They found patients 65 years of age or older were more likely to experience ADEs and to need subsequent hospitalization as a result of the ADE. Drugs that were involved in ADEs most often included insulin, warfarin, antibiotics, and digoxin. On the whole, drugs that required frequent outpatient monitoring were implicated most often.

From Budnitz D, Pollock D, Weidenbach K et al: Emergency department surveillance for adverse drug events, *JAMA* 296(15):1858-1866, 2006.

PREGNANT PATIENTS

Before administering any drug to a pregnant patient, the paramedic should consider the expected benefits and the possible risks to the fetus. Drugs given to a pregnant patient may cross the placental barrier and harm the fetus or may be communicated to a newborn during breastfeeding. The FDA has established a scale to indicate drugs that may be harmful to a fetus during pregnancy (Box 13-13).

PEDIATRIC PATIENTS

Special considerations for administration of drugs to pediatric patients are presented here and throughout the text. Following is a summary of the pharmacokinetics that influence dosing principles in the neonate, infant, and pediatric populations.

Age. The effects of drugs are unpredictable among infants because of the variation in the development and maturation of the different organ systems.

CRITICAL THINKING

Drug doses vary for pediatric and neonatal patients. They are almost always related to weight. How can you ensure accuracy of dosing for these patients in critical situations when seconds count, even though you know the wrong dose calculation could be lethal?

Absorption. Drug absorption in infants and children follows the same basic principles as it does in adults. A factor that influences drug absorption is blood flow at the site of intramuscular or subcutaneous administration. Blood flow usually is determined by the patient's cardiovascular function. Certain physiological conditions might reduce blood flow to the muscle and subcutaneous tissue. These conditions include shock, vasoconstriction, and heart failure. The smaller muscle mass of the infant further complicates drug absorption because of diminished peripheral perfusion to these areas. For orally administered drugs, underlying gastrointestinal function may influence drug absorption.

BOX 13-13 Pregnancy Category Ratings for Drugs

Drugs have been categorized by the Food and Drug Administration according to the level of risk to the fetus. These categories are listed for each drug herein under Pregnancy Safety and are interpreted as follows[1]:

Category A: Controlled studies in women fail to demonstrate a risk to the fetus in the first trimester, and there is no evidence of risk in later trimesters; the possibility of fetal harm appears to be remote.

Category B: Either (1) animal reproductive studies have not demonstrated a fetal risk but there are no controlled studies in pregnant women or (2) animal reproductive studies have shown an adverse effect (other than decreased fertility) that was not confirmed in controlled studies on women in the first trimester, and there is no evidence of risk in later trimesters.

Category C: Either (1) studies in animals have revealed adverse effects on the fetus and there are no controlled studies in women or (2) studies in women and animals are not available. Drugs in this category should be given only if the potential benefit justifies the risk to the fetus.

Category D: There is positive evidence of human fetal risk, but the benefits for pregnant women may be acceptable despite the risk, as in life-threatening diseases for which safer drugs cannot be used or are ineffective. An appropriate statement must appear in the "Warnings" section of the labeling of drugs in this category.

Category X: Studies in animals or human beings have demonstrated fetal abnormalities, there is evidence of fetal risk based on human experience, or both; the risk of using the drug in pregnant women clearly outweighs any possible benefit. The drug is contraindicated in women who are or may become pregnant. An appropriate statement must appear in the "Contraindications" section of the labeling of drugs in this category.

Liquids and suspensions disperse quickly in gastrointestinal fluids. Thus they are more readily absorbed than tablet or capsule forms. Increases in peristalsis (e.g., diarrheal conditions) and lowered gastrointestinal enzyme activities tend to decrease overall absorption of orally or rectally administered medications.

Distribution. Most drugs are distributed in body water. Thus increases in total body water and extracellular volume can increase the volume of the distribution. Compared with adults, infants have proportionately higher volumes of total body water (70% to 75% compared with 50% to 60%). Infants also have a higher ratio of extracellular to intracellular fluid (40% compared with 30%); higher dosages of water-soluble drugs may be needed to have effective blood levels in the newborn.

Another key factor that affects drug distribution is drug binding to plasma proteins. In general, protein binding of drugs is reduced in the infant; therefore the concentration of free drug in plasma is increased. This can result in a greater drug effect or toxicity. Regarding central nervous system effects, the blood-brain barrier in the infant is much less effective than in adults. This allows drugs greater access to this area.

Biotransformation. Various liver enzyme systems for metabolism generally mature unevenly. The infant therefore has a decreased ability to metabolize drugs. This predisposes the infant to developing toxicity from drugs metabolized by the liver. In addition, many drugs given to infants have slower renal clearance times and longer half-lives in the body. Thus the paramedic must adjust dosages based on age and weight.

Elimination. The glomerular filtration rate is much lower in newborns than in older infants, children, and adults. Therefore drugs eliminated through renal function are cleared from the body slowly in the first few weeks of life. Renal excretory mechanisms progress to maturity after 1 year of age. Before that age, excretion of some substances through the renal system may be delayed because of immaturity. This may result in higher serum levels and a longer duration of action than intended.

OLDER ADULT PATIENTS

Key changes in drug responses occur with age in most individuals. Factors associated with aging that significantly affect pharmacokinetics include the likelihood of multiple diseases requiring the use of several drugs (also referred to as *polydrug usage*). In addition, nutritional problems, decreased ability to metabolize drugs, and the possibility of decreased drug dosing compliance for a variety of reasons can influence the effects of drugs. This summary is meant to serve as a review of the pharmacokinetics that influence dosing principles in the older adult.

Age. Declines in the functional capacity of most major organ systems begin in young adulthood. These changes continue throughout life. Older adults do not lose specific function at a quicker rate than young and middle-aged adults; rather, they have less physiological reserves. Decreases in physiological function (glomerular filtration rate, cardiac function, maximal breathing capacity) generally are accepted as beginning by age 45. Decreased renal function has the greatest impact on medication administration and drug clearance.

Absorption. Little evidence exists of major changes in drug absorption with age. Yet conditions associated with age may alter the rate at which some drugs are absorbed. Examples of these conditions include altered nutritional habits, greater consumption of nonprescription drugs (e.g., antacids and laxatives), and changes in gastric emptying. The reduced production of gastric acid and slowed gastric motility may have an impact and may result in unpredictable rates of dissolution and absorption of weakly acidic drugs.

Distribution. Changes in body composition have been noted in the older adult. Such changes include reduced lean body mass, reduced total body water, and increased fat as a percentage of body mass. Levels of serum albumin—which binds many drugs, especially weak acids—also usually decline. This affects drug distribution; it decreases protein binding of drugs. This results in an increase in the amount of free drug in the circulation. Thus the ratio of bound to free drug in these patients may be significantly altered.

Biotransformation. The ability of the liver to metabolize drugs does not appear to decline consistently with age for all drugs. But disorders common with aging can impair liver function. One such example is congestive heart failure. Hepatic recovery from injury, such as that caused by alcohol or viral hepatitis, declines as well.

Certain drugs generally are believed to be metabolized more slowly in older adults. This is thought to be the case because of decreased liver blood flow. This decrease may lead to drug accumulation and toxicity. The paramedic must use caution when administering repeated doses of a medication that is metabolized primarily in the liver (e.g., *lidocaine* [Xylocaine]) to a patient with a history of liver disease. Older patients with severe nutritional deficiencies also may have impaired hepatic function.

Elimination. Renal function is the most critical factor for clearance of most drugs from the body. A natural reduction in renal function occurs with aging and usually is caused by loss of functioning nephrons and a decrease in blood flow. Both of these result in a decreased GFR. A decrease in renal function caused by decreases in renal blood flow also may occur because of congestive heart failure. The practical result of renal impairment is a prolongation of the half-life of many drugs and the possibility of accumulation to toxic levels. Other reversible conditions (e.g., dehydration) can cause further reduction in renal clearance of drugs.

Drug Administration Problems. Older adults commonly do not comply with their drug therapy. Noncompliance may be intentional or unintentional on their part but rarely affects the administration of emergency drugs. Still, the paramedic must be familiar with the most common factors that contribute to drug administration problems in older adults. This is crucial because noncompliance or errors may be a factor in the patient's condition. Following are some common causes of noncompliance and medication errors:

- The expense of drugs may lead to noncompliance in patients with fixed incomes. Older patients may not take prescribed medications routinely or may be unwilling to receive medications in emergency situations.
- Noncompliance in taking prescribed medications may result from forgetfulness or confusion, especially if the patient has several prescriptions and different dosing intervals.
- Older patients may forget instructions on the need to complete medication because symptoms have disappeared. Disappearance of symptoms often is regarded by the patient as the best reason to stop the therapy.
- Errors in self-administered medications may result from physical disabilities such as arthritis or visual impairment.

- Noncompliance may be deliberate. A patient may be opposed to taking a drug because of past experiences. A careful drug history is especially important when caring for older adults. The paramedic should remember that a patient has the right to refuse medication.

SECTION THREE
Drugs That Affect the Nervous System

REVIEW OF ANATOMY AND PHYSIOLOGY

The actions of many drugs depend on which branch of the autonomic nervous system they affect and whether the branch is stimulated or inhibited by drug therapy. The following is a discussion of the anatomy and physiology of the nervous system as they pertain to pharmacology (Box 13-14).

As described in Chapter 10, the *central nervous system* (CNS) consists of the brain and spinal cord. The CNS serves as the collection point for nerve impulses (Figure 13-7). The *peripheral nervous system* consists of cranial and spinal nerves and all their branches (those nerves outside the CNS). The peripheral nervous system connects all parts of the body to the CNS. The *somatic nervous system* controls functions that are under conscious, voluntary control such as skeletal muscles and sensory neurons of the skin. The *autonomic nervous system,* comprised mostly of motor nerves, controls functions of involuntary smooth muscles, cardiac muscles, and glands. Four types of nerve fibers are found in most nerves:

LOOK AGAIN

See Chapter 10: Review of Human Systems, pp. 171-177.

1. *Visceral afferent* (sensory) *fibers,* which convey impulses from the internal organs to the CNS
2. *Visceral efferent* (motor) *fibers,* which convey impulses from the CNS to the internal organs, glands, and the smooth and cardiac (involuntary) muscles
3. *Somatic afferent* (sensory) *fibers,* which convey impulses from the head, body wall, and extremities to the CNS
4. *Somatic efferent* (motor) *fibers,* which convey impulses from the CNS to the striated (voluntary) muscles

Simply put, the peripheral (sensory) nervous system receives stimuli from the body. The CNS interprets these

BOX 13-14 Emergency Drugs: Nervous System

Atropine
Diazepam (Valium)
Dopamine (Intropin)
Epinephrine (Adrenalin)
Etomidate (Amidate)
Fentanyl (Sublimaze)
Hydromorphone (Dilaudid)
Lorazepam (Ativan)
Magnesium sulfate
Midazolam (Versed)
Morphine (Astramorph/PF)
Naloxone (Narcan)
Succinylcholine (Anectine)

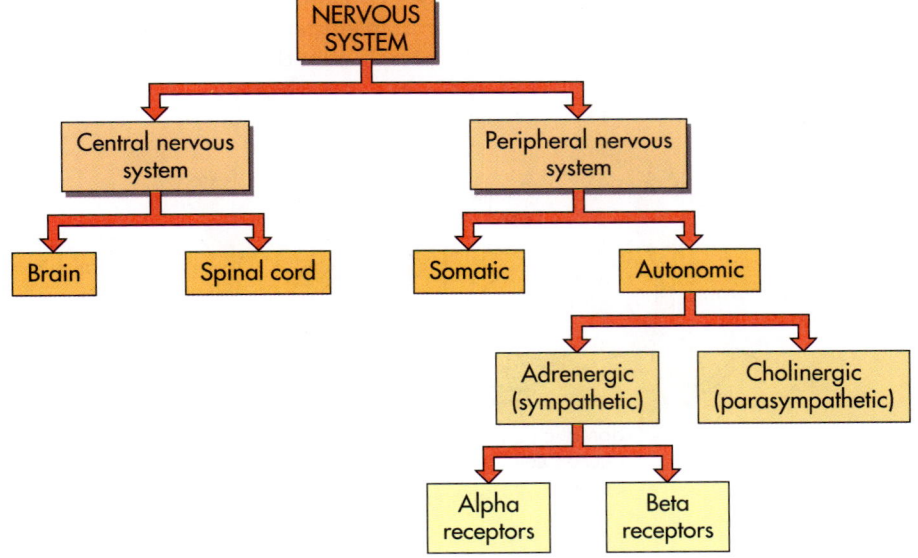

FIGURE 13-7 Overview of the nervous system. (From Lehne RA: *Pharmacology for nursing care,* ed 7, St Louis, 2010, Saunders.)

stimuli. The peripheral (motor) nervous system initiates responses to the stimuli. Together the visceral afferent and visceral efferent nerve fibers form the autonomic nervous system. In contrast, the somatic afferent and somatic efferent nerve fibers form the somatic nervous system. Thus the autonomic nervous system and the somatic nervous system can be regarded as subdivisions of the peripheral nervous system (Box 13-15).

Autonomic Division of the Peripheral Nervous System

The autonomic division of the peripheral nervous system provides almost every organ with a double set of nerve fibers: *sympathetic* (also known as **adrenergic**) and *parasympathetic* (also known as **cholinergic**). The cell bodies of the neurons in these two divisions are located in different areas of the CNS. They also exit the spinal cord at different levels. The sympathetic fibers exit from the thoracic and lumbar regions of the spinal cord. The parasympathetic fibers exit from the cranial and sacral portions of the spinal cord.

The sympathetic and parasympathetic systems generally work as *physiological antagonists* on **effector organs.** That is,

BOX 13-15 Organization of the Nervous System	
Central Nervous System	**Peripheral Nervous System**
Brain	Cranial nerves
Spinal cord	Visceral afferent nerve fibers
	Visceral efferent nerve fibers
	Somatic afferent nerve fibers
	Somatic efferent nerve fibers
Spinal nerves	Visceral afferent nerve fibers
	Visceral efferent nerve fibers
	Somatic afferent nerve fibers
	Somatic efferent nerve fibers

one division carries impulses that inhibit a certain function. The other division usually carries impulses that augment that function. As a rule, the sympathetic system prepares the body for vigorous muscular activity, stress, and emergencies (fight or flight). The sympathetic nervous system tends to affect widespread areas of the body for sustained periods of time. In contrast, the parasympathetic system lowers muscular activity, operates during nonemergency situations, conserves energy, and produces selective and localized responses of short duration. The sympathetic and parasympathetic systems operate at the same time. Yet one usually has more dominant effects at any given time.

Autonomic innervation by the sympathetic and parasympathetic nervous systems may be viewed as involving a two-neuron chain. This chain exists in a series between the CNS and the effector organs. This two-neuron chain is composed of a *preganglionic neuron,* located in the CNS, and a *postganglionic neuron,* located in the periphery (Figure 13-8). The area that serves as a functional junction between these two neurons is known as a *synapse.* The preganglionic fibers pass between the CNS and the nerve cell bodies in the peripheral nervous system (ganglia). The postganglionic fibers pass between the ganglia and the effector organ. Many of the sympathetic ganglia lie close to the spinal cord. Others lie about midway between the spinal cord and the effector organ. The parasympathetic ganglia lie close or within the walls of the effector organ. The difference in location of the ganglia in these two divisions is the anatomical reason for the widespread responses caused by the sympathetic division versus the localized responses caused by the parasympathetic division.

Neurochemical Transmission

Most neurons are separated electrically from each other. Because of this separation, the fibers communicate by way of **neurotransmitters.** These are chemicals that are released from one neuron at the presynaptic nerve fiber. These neurotransmitters then cross the synapse where they may be accepted by the next neuron at a specialized site called a

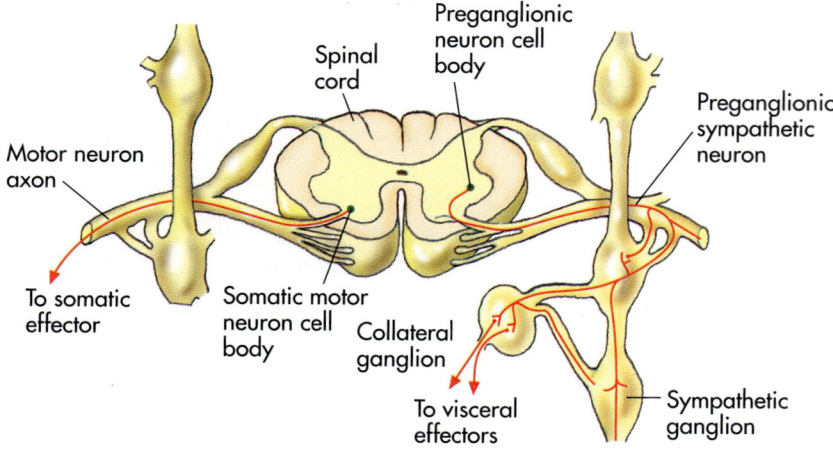

FIGURE 13-8 Autonomic conduction pathways.

receptor. (Neurotransmitters bind only to specific receptors on the postsynaptic membranes that recognize them.) The neurotransmitter then is deactivated or taken up into the presynaptic neuron.

In the sympathetic and parasympathetic divisions, the neurotransmitter for the preganglionic fiber at the junction between the preganglionic fiber and the synapse is **acetylcholine.** The neurotransmitter at the junction between the parasympathetic postganglionic fiber and the effector cell is also acetylcholine. Fibers that release acetylcholine are known as *cholinergic fibers.* All preganglionic neurons of the autonomic division and all postganglionic neurons of the parasympathetic division are cholinergic.

>
> **NOTE**
> All preganglionic nerves use the same neurotransmitter: acetylcholine.

The neurotransmitter between the sympathetic postganglionic fiber and the effector cell is **norepinephrine.** This chemical is a member of the catecholamine family. Fibers that release norepinephrine are known as *adrenergic fibers.* (This is a term derived from *noradrenaline,* the British name for norepinephrine.) Most postganglionic neurons of the sympathetic division are adrenergic; that is, they release norepinephrine. However, a few are cholinergic. The actions of the autonomic nervous system depend on the interaction between the neurotransmitter released by the ganglionic cells and the receptor effector cells. For example, stimulation of the sympathetic nerves causes excitatory effects in some organs and inhibitory effects in others. Likewise, parasympathetic stimulation causes excitation in some organs but inhibition in others.

> **NOTE**
> Two different neurotransmitters exist for postganglionic neurons. All parasympathetic postganglionic neurons release acetylcholine onto their target tissue. Most sympathetic postganglionic neurons release norepinephrine onto their target tissue.

The parasympathetic and sympathetic systems function continuously. They innervate many of the same organs at the same time. Thus the opposing actions of the two systems balance one another. (Most organs, however, are controlled predominantly by one or the other of the two systems.) As previously stated, the sympathetic system usually dominates during stressful events. The parasympathetic system is most active during periods of emotional and physical calmness.

Transmission of Nerve Impulses in the Autonomic Nervous System

Both branches of the autonomic nervous system have multiple receptors. The variety among neurotransmitters and receptors accounts for the differences in response to stimulation of sympathetic and parasympathetic nerves (excitatory or inhibitory).

The parasympathetic nervous system has nicotinic and muscarinic receptors (Figure 13-9). **Nicotinic receptors** (stimulated by nicotine) are found at the neuromuscular junctions of skeletal muscles. They also are found on the postganglionic neurons of the parasympathetic nervous system. **Muscarinic receptors** (stimulated by the mushroom poison muscarine) are found at the neuromuscular junction of cardiac and smooth muscle. They also are found on glands and on the postganglionic neurons of the sympathetic nervous system. Drugs that can activate nicotinic receptors typically do not activate muscarinic receptors. The difference between nicotinic and muscarinic receptors is crucial in drug therapy. For example, when acetylcholine binds to nicotinic receptors, an excitatory response occurs. When acetylcholine binds to muscarinic receptors, it results in excitation or inhibition. This depends on the target tissue in which the receptors are found (Table 13-3). When acetylcholine binds to muscarinic receptors in cardiac muscle, the heart rate slows. When it binds to muscarinic receptors in smooth muscle cells of the gastrointestinal tract, the rate and amplitude of contraction increase. *Atropine* blocks muscarinic but not nicotinic receptor sites. (Thus *atropine* affects the heart rate but does not cause paralysis.) A drug such as curare (a nicotinic receptor blocker), however, causes paralysis.

> **NOTE**
> The two types of cholinergic receptors are nicotinic receptors and muscarinic receptors. Nicotinic responses are of *fast onset and short duration* and are excitatory. Nicotinic receptors are associated with preganglionic neurons of both branches of the autonomic nervous system. Muscarinic receptors are of *slow onset and long duration* and may be excitatory or inhibitory. These receptors are associated with the neuromuscular junction.

> **CRITICAL THINKING**
> Imagine that your patient has eaten some poisonous mushrooms containing muscarine. What signs or symptoms related to pulse rate would you expect? What signs or symptoms related to gastrointestinal tract activity should be evident? Lastly, what signs or symptoms related to pupil diameter should be present?

For the sympathetic (adrenergic) nervous system, the major receptor types belong to two structural categories. These are the **alpha-adrenergic receptors** and the **beta-adrenergic receptors** (and their subgroups, described in the following text). Norepinephrine binds to and activates both types of receptor molecules. Yet norepinephrine has more affinity for alpha receptors. The hormone epinephrine is produced by the adrenal medulla and is classified as an adrenergic substance. Epinephrine has nearly equal

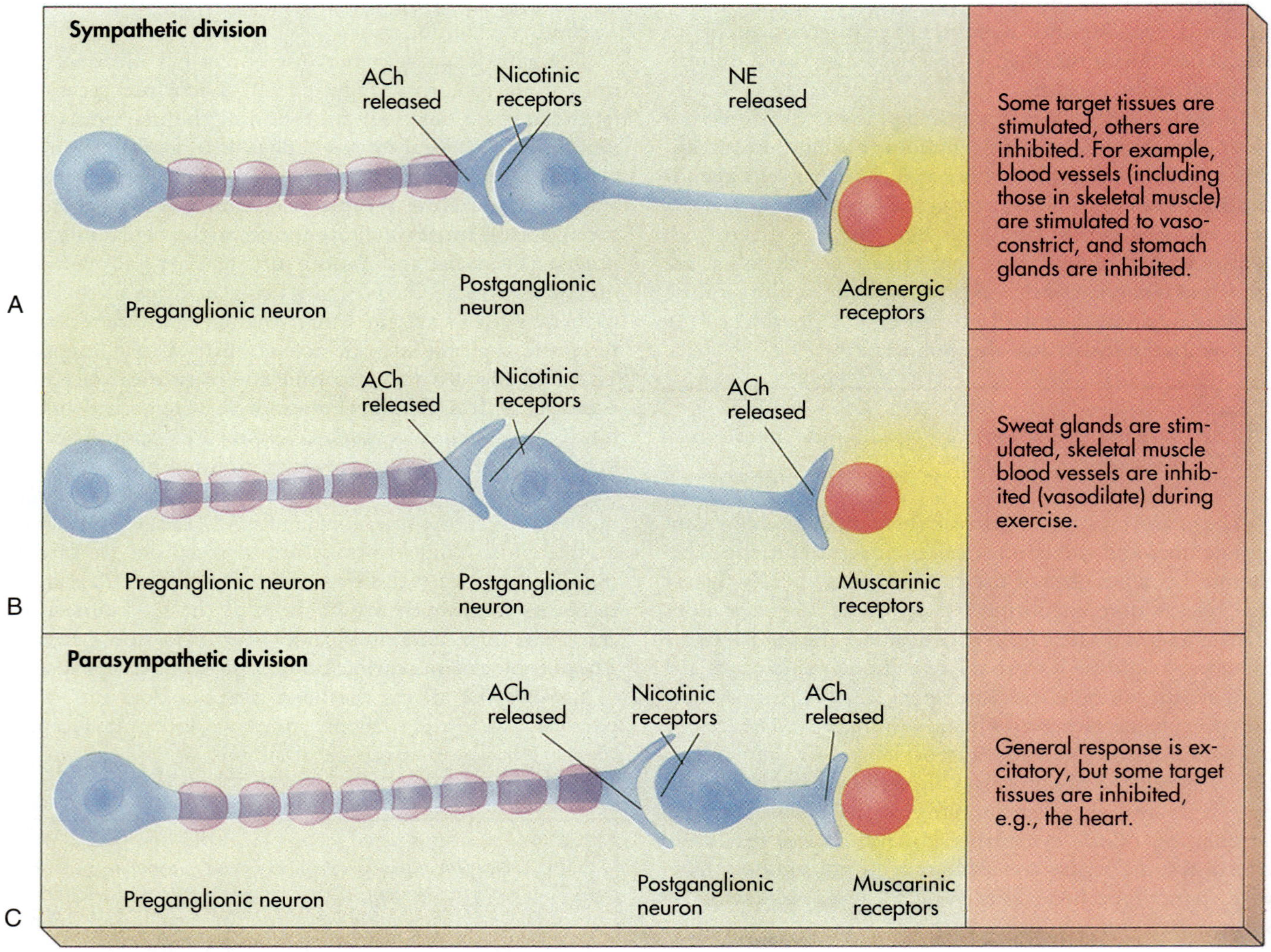

Sympathetic division

A Preganglionic neuron — ACh released — Nicotinic receptors — Postganglionic neuron — NE released — Adrenergic receptors	Some target tissues are stimulated, others are inhibited. For example, blood vessels (including those in skeletal muscle) are stimulated to vaso-constrict, and stomach glands are inhibited.
B Preganglionic neuron — ACh released — Nicotinic receptors — Postganglionic neuron — ACh released — Muscarinic receptors	Sweat glands are stim-ulated, skeletal muscle blood vessels are inhib-ited (vasodilate) during exercise.

Parasympathetic division

C Preganglionic neuron — ACh released — Nicotinic receptors — Postganglionic neuron — ACh released — Muscarinic receptors	General response is ex-citatory, but some target tissues are inhibited, e.g., the heart.

FIGURE 13-9 Location of the nicotinic, muscarinic, and adrenergic receptors in the autonomic nervous system. Nicotinic receptors are found on the cell bodies of sympathetic and parasympathetic postganglionic cells in the autonomic ganglia. **A,** Adrenergic receptors are found in most target tissues innervated by the sympathetic division. **B,** Some sympathetic target tissues have muscarinic receptors. **C,** All parasympathetic target tissues have muscarinic receptors. *ACh,* Acetylcholine; *NE,* norepinephrine.

affinity for both receptors. In tissues containing alpha- and beta-receptor cells, one type is more abundant. As a result, that type has a predominant effect. Both receptors can be excitatory or inhibitory. For example, beta receptors are stimulatory in cardiac muscle. Yet they are inhibitory in intestinal smooth muscle (Table 13-4).

> **NOTE**
> The two major types of adrenergic receptors are alpha and beta. Both receptors can be excitatory or inhibitory.

Drugs That Affect the Autonomic Nervous System

The nervous and endocrine systems are responsible for controlling and coordinating body functions. These two systems share three characteristics: a high level of integration in the brain, the ability to influence functions in distant regions of the body, and the extensive use of *negative feedback mechanisms* (described in Chapter 11). One main difference between the two systems is the mode of transmission of information.

TABLE 13-3 Sites for Muscarinic and Nicotinic Actions of Acetylcholine

Site	Muscarinic Actions*	Nicotinic Actions
Cardiovascular		
Blood vessels	Dilation	Constriction
Heart rate	Slowed	Increased
Blood pressure	Decreased	Increased
Gastrointestinal		
Tone	Increased	Increased
Motility	Increased	Increased
Sphincters	Relaxed	—
Glandular secretions	Increased salivary, lacrimal, intestinal, and sweat secretion	Initial stimulation and then inhibition of salivary and bronchial secretions
Other		
Skeletal muscle	—	Stimulation
Autonomic ganglia	—	Stimulation
Eye	Pupil constriction Decreased accommodation	— —
Blocking agent	Atropine	Tubocurarine
Remarks	Above effects increase as dosage increases	Increased dosage inhibits effects and causes receptor blockade

*Usual sites for therapeutic effects.

LOOK AGAIN
Chapter 11: General Principles of Pathophysiology, pp. 238-240.

The endocrine system transmission is chiefly chemical. The information moves via blood-borne hormones. The hormones are not targeted for a specific organ. Instead, they diffusely affect many cells and organs at the same time. In contrast, the nervous system mainly relies on rapid electrical transmission of information over nerve fibers. Chemical impulses carry signals only between nerve cells and their effector cells in a localized manner, perhaps affecting only a few cells. (Drugs that affect the endocrine system are presented later in this chapter.)

CLASSIFICATIONS

The autonomic drugs mimic or block the effects of the sympathetic and parasympathetic divisions of the autonomic nervous system (Box 13-16). These drugs can be classified into four groups:

1. Cholinergic (*parasympathomimetic*) drugs, which mimic the actions of the parasympathetic nervous system
2. Cholinergic blocking (*parasympatholytic*) drugs, which block the actions of the parasympathetic nervous system
3. Adrenergic (*sympathomimetic*) drugs, which mimic the actions of the sympathetic nervous system or the adrenal medulla
4. Adrenergic blocking (*sympatholytic*) drugs, which block the actions of the sympathetic nervous system or adrenal medulla

Cholinergic Drugs. As described earlier, acetylcholine plays a key role in the parasympathetic and sympathetic

BOX 13-16 Anatomical and Functional Terms for the Autonomic Nervous System

The anatomical names and functional terms for the autonomic nervous system often are used interchangeably: sympathetic or adrenergic, and parasympathetic or cholinergic. The terms *parasympathomimetic* and *sympathomimetic* mean to mimic or to produce an effect similar to activation of either system. The words *parasympatholytic* and *sympatholytic* mean to block the normal effects seen with activation of either system. The term *anticholinergic* is synonymous with *parasympatholytic*.

Anatomical Name	Functional Term	Primary Neurotransmitter
Sympathetic	Adrenergic	Norepinephrine
Parasympathetic	Cholinergic	Acetylcholine

divisions of the nervous system. Acetylcholine has two major effects in the nervous system: (1) a stimulant effect on the ganglia, adrenal medulla, and skeletal muscle (the nicotinic effect) and (2) stimulant effects at postganglionic nerve endings in cardiac muscle, smooth muscle, and glands (the muscarinic effect). Drugs that affect nicotinic or cholinergic receptor sites on autonomic ganglia are ganglionic-stimulating drugs (e.g., nicotine and nicotine gum) and ganglionic-blocking drugs (e.g., **mecamylamine**).

Cholinergic drugs (choline esters) act directly with cholinergic receptors on postsynaptic membranes, or they act indirectly by inhibiting the enzyme that normally destroys acetylcholine. This inhibition results in an accumulation of acetylcholine. This in turn causes a longer and more intense

TABLE 13-4 Autonomic Innervation of Target Tissues

Organ	Effect of Sympathetic Stimulation*	Effect of Parasympathetic Stimulation*
Heart		
Muscle	Increased rate and force (b)	Slowed rate (c)
Coronary arteries	Dilation (b),† constriction (a)†	Dilation (c)
Systemic blood vessels		
Abdomen	Constriction (a)	None
Skin	Constriction (a)	None
Muscle	Dilation (b, c), constriction (a)	None
Lungs		
Bronchi	Dilation (b)	Constriction (c)
Liver	Release of glucose into blood (b)	None
Skeletal muscles	Breakdown of glycogen to glucose (b)	None
Metabolism	Increase of up to 100% (a, b)	None
Glands		
Adrenal glands	Release of epinephrine and norepinephrine (c)	None
Salivary glands	Constriction of blood vessels and slight production of thick, viscous secretion (a)	Dilation of blood vessels and thin, copious secretion (c)
Gastric glands	Inhibition (a)	Stimulation (c)
Pancreas	Inhibition (a)	Stimulation (c)
Lacrimal glands	None	Secretion (c)
Sweat glands		
Merocrine glands	Copious, watery secretion (c)	None
Apocrine glands	Thick, organic secretion (c)	None
Gut		
Wall	Decreased tone (b)	Increased motility (c)
Sphincter	Increased tone (a)	Decreased tone (c)
Gallbladder and bile ducts	Relaxation (b)	Contraction (c)
Urinary bladder		
Wall	Relaxation (b)	Contraction (c)
Sphincter	Contraction (a)	Relaxation (c)
Eye		
Ciliary muscle	Relaxation for far vision (b)	Contraction for near vision (c)
Pupil	Dilation	Constriction (c)
Erector pili muscles	Contraction (a)	None
Blood	Increased coagulation (a)	None
Sex organs	Ejaculation (a)	Erection (c)

*(a), Mediated by alpha receptors; (b), mediated by beta receptors; (c), mediated by cholinergic receptors.
†Normally blood flow through coronary arteries increases as a result of sympathetic stimulation of the heart because of increased demand by cardiac tissue for oxygen. In experiments that isolate the coronary arteries, however, sympathetic nerve stimulation, acting through alpha receptors, causes vasoconstriction. The beta receptors are relatively insensitive to sympathetic nerve stimulation but can be activated by drugs.

response at various effector sites. Cholinergic drugs have little therapeutic value. For the most part, they are not thought of as emergency drugs. The main exception to this is *physostigmine* (Antilirium), which is an indirect-acting cholinergic drug. *Physostigmine* (Antilirium) may be used to manage extreme cases of poisoning resulting from atropine-type drugs (see Chapter 34). Indirect-acting cholinergic drugs are used to treat myasthenia gravis, a condition characterized by weakness of the skeletal muscles (described in Chapter 33). These drugs work to elevate the concentration of acetylcholine at myoneural junctions. This in turn increases muscle strength and function.

Cholinergic blocking (**anticholinergic**) agents have many uses in emergency medicine. These drugs work by blocking the muscarinic effects of acetylcholine. Thus they decrease the action of acetylcholine on its effector organ.

The best known cholinergic blocking drug used in emergency care is *atropine.* Atropine is a belladonna alkaloid that acts as a competitive antagonist. Atropine works by occupying muscarinic receptor sites. This action prevents or reduces the muscarinic response to acetylcholine. Large doses dilate the pupils, inhibit accommodation of the eyes, and increase the heart rate by blocking the cholinergic effects of the heart. Synthetic substitutes for *atropine* have been created to obtain only the antispasmodic effects of the drug. (For example, they may be used to treat gastric and duodenal ulcers.) These synthetic drugs include dicyclomine (Bentyl) and glycopyrrolate (Robinul).

Adrenergic Drugs. Adrenergic drugs are designed to produce activities like those of neurotransmitters. The three types of adrenergic agents are *direct acting*, *indirect acting*, and *dual acting* (direct and indirect).

Direct-Acting Drugs. Three naturally occurring catecholamines are present in the body: epinephrine, norepinephrine, and dopamine. Epinephrine acts mainly as an emergency hormone. Epinephrine is released by the adrenal medulla. Norepinephrine acts as a critical neurotransmitter of nerve impulses. Dopamine is a precursor of epinephrine and norepinephrine. Dopamine has a neurotransmitter role of its own in certain parts of the CNS. Examples of synthetic catecholamine drugs and the three endogenous catecholamines are *epinephrine* (Adrenalin), *norepinephrine* (Levophed), *dopamine* (Intropin), and *dobutamine* (Dobutrex).

Catecholamines depend on their ability to act directly with alpha and beta receptors. Two subgroups of **alpha receptors** have been identified. These are alpha₁ and alpha₂. *Alpha₁* **receptors** are postsynaptic receptors. They are located on the effector organs. The chief role of the alpha₁ receptor is to stimulate contraction of smooth muscle. In the vasculature, this results in an increase in blood pressure. *Alpha₂ receptors* are found on presynaptic and postsynaptic nerve endings. When stimulated, presynaptic receptors inhibit the further release of norepinephrine. Like alpha₁ receptors, alpha₂ postsynaptic receptors produce vasoconstriction to increase resistance in blood vessels and thus increase blood pressure.

Beta receptors are subdivided into beta₁ and beta₂ receptors based on their response to drugs. However, the division also follows anatomical distinctions. *Beta₁ receptors* are located mainly in the heart. *Beta₂ receptors* are located mainly in the bronchiolar and arterial smooth muscle. Beta receptors stimulate the heart; dilate bronchioles; dilate blood vessels in the skeletal muscle, brain, and heart; and aid in glycogenolysis (the breakdown of glycogen to glucose) (Table 13-5).

> **NOTE**
> Use of a memory aid to differentiate the physiological effects of beta receptors may be helpful: A person has one heart (beta₁ effects) and two lungs (beta₂ effects).

Norepinephrine acts mainly on alpha receptors. It causes almost pure vasoconstriction of the blood vessels. Epinephrine acts on alpha and beta receptors. It produces a mixture of vasodilation and vasoconstriction. This effect depends on the number of alpha and beta receptors present in the target tissue. The following are the most important alpha and beta activities in human beings:

1. Alpha activities
   - Vasoconstriction of arterioles in the skin and splanchnic area, resulting in a rise in blood pressure and peripheral shunting of blood to the heart and brain from the shifting of blood volume
   - Pupil dilation
   - Relaxation of the gut
2. Beta activities
   - Cardiac acceleration and increased contractility
   - Vasodilation of arterioles supplying the skeletal muscle
   - Bronchial relaxation
   - Uterine relaxation

Indirect-Acting and Dual-Acting Drugs. Indirect-acting adrenergic drugs act indirectly on receptors. They do this by triggering the release of the catecholamines norepinephrine and epinephrine. These chemicals then activate the alpha and beta receptors. Dual-acting adrenergic drugs have indirect and direct effects. An example of a drug in this group is ephedrine (ephedrine sulfate).

Adrenergic blocking agents may be classified into alpha- and beta-blocking drugs. Alpha-blocking drugs block the vasoconstricting effect of catecholamines. They are used in certain cases of hypertension. They also are used to help prevent necrosis when *norepinephrine* (Levophed) or *dopamine* (Intropin) has leaked, or extravasated, into the tissues. They have limited clinical application in the prehospital setting.

> **NOTE**
> All drugs with alpha effects should be administered through a secure intravenous line. This line should be well positioned in a large vein because of the possibility of extravasation and tissue necrosis.

Beta-blocking agents have greater clinical application. They often are used in emergency care. These drugs block beta receptors. They inhibit the action of beta receptors at the effector site. Beta-blocking agents are grouped into **selective beta-blocking agents** and **nonselective beta-blocking agents.** The selective blocking agents block beta₁ or beta₂ receptors. The nonselective beta-blocking agents block beta₁- and beta₂-receptor sites. Selective beta₁-blocking agents also are known as *cardioselective blockers* because they block the beta₁ receptors in the heart with minimal beta₂ activities in the lungs. Examples of important selective beta₁-blocking agents are *metoprolol* (Lopressor, Toprol-XL) and *atenolol* (Tenormin). These drugs are antihypertensives and antidysrhythmics. They are used in managing hypertension. They also are used in select patients with suspected myocardial infarction and high-risk unstable angina.

Nonselective beta-blocking agents inhibit beta receptors in the smooth muscle both of the bronchioles and of the blood vessels. Examples include the antianginal antihypertensives **nadolol** (Corgard) and *propranolol* (Inderal), and the antihypertensive *labetalol* (Normodyne, Trandate). (*Labetalol* also has some alpha-blocking activity.)

TABLE 13-5 Actions of Autonomic Nervous System Neuroreceptors

Effector Organ or Tissue	Receptor	Adrenergic Effect	Cholinergic Effect
Eye, iris			
Radial muscle	α_1	Contraction (mydriasis)	—
Sphincter muscle		—	Contraction (miosis)
Eye, ciliary muscle	β_2	Relaxation for far vision	Contraction for near vision
Lacrimal glands	—	—	Secretion
Nasopharyngeal glands	—	—	Secretion
Salivary glands	α_1	Secretion of potassium and water	Secretion of potassium and water
	β	Secretion of amylase	—
Heart			
SA node	β_1	Increased heart rate	Decreased heart rate; vagus arrest
Atrial	β_1	Increased contractility and conduction velocity	Decreased contractility; shortened action potential duration
AV junction	β_1	Increased automaticity and propagation velocity	Decreased automaticity and propagation velocity
Purkinje system	β_1	Increased automaticity and propagation velocity	—
Ventricles	β_1	Increased contractility	—
Arterioles			
Coronary	α_1, β_2	Constriction, dilation	Dilation
Skin and mucosa	α_1, α_2	Constriction	Dilation
Skeletal muscle	α, β_2	Constriction, dilation	Dilation
Cerebral	α_1	Constriction (slight)	—
Pulmonary	α_1, β_2	Constriction, dilation	—
Mesenteric	α_1	Constriction	—
Renal	α_1, β_1, β_2,	Constriction, dilation	—
Salivary glands	α_1, α_2	Constriction	Dilation
Veins, systemic	α_1, β_2	Constriction, dilation	—
Lung			
Bronchial muscle	β_2	Relaxation	Contraction
Bronchial glands	α_1, β_2	Decreased secretion; increased secretion	Stimulation
Stomach			
Motility	α_1, β_2	Decreased (usually)	Increased
Sphincters	α_1	Contraction (usually)	Relaxation (usually)
Secretion	—	Inhibition (?)	Stimulation
Liver	α, β_2	Glycogenolysis and gluconeogenesis	Glycogen synthesis
Gallbladder and ducts	—	Relaxation	Contraction
Pancreas			
Acini	α	Decreased secretion	Secretion
Islet cells	α_2, β_2	Decreased secretion; increased secretion	—
Intestine			
Motility and tone	α_1, β_1, β_2	Decreased	Increased
Sphincters	α_1	Contraction (usually)	Relaxation (usually)
Secretion	α_2	Inhibition (?)	Stimulation
Adrenal medulla	—	—	Secretion of epinephrine and norepinephrine (nicotinic effect)
Kidney			
Renin secretion	α_1, β_1	Decreased; increased	—
Ureter			
Motility and tone	α_1	Increased	Increased
Urinary bladder			
Detrusor muscle	β_2	Relaxation (usually)	Contraction
Trigone and sphincter	α_1	Contraction	Relaxation
Sex organs, male	α_1	Ejaculation	Erection
Skin			
Pilomotor muscles	α_1	Contraction	—
Sweat glands	α_1	Localized secretion	Generalized secretion
Fat cells	α_2; $\beta_1(\beta_3)$	Inhibition of lipolysis; stimulation of lipolysis	—
Pineal gland	β	Melatonin synthesis	—

CRITICAL THINKING
Physicians usually will not prescribe a nonselective beta blocker such as propranolol (Inderal) for patients with a history of asthma. Explain why this is true.

Narcotic Analgesics and Antagonists

Narcotic analgesics relieve pain. Narcotic antagonists reverse the effects of some narcotic analgesics. Pain has two components. The first is the sensation of pain. This involves the nerve pathways and the brain. The second is the emotional response to pain. This may be a result of the individual's anxiety level, previous pain experience, age, gender, and culture. Box 13-17 lists and defines classifications of pain.

Opiates are drugs that contain or are extracted from opium. The term *opioid* refers to synthetic drugs. These drugs have pharmacological properties that are similar to those of opium or *morphine.* Morphine is the chief alkaloid of opium. Opioids work by binding with opioid receptors in the brain and other body organs. This alters the patient's perception of pain and the emotional response to a pain-causing stimulus. Opioid analgesics include *morphine,* codeine (methylmorphine), hydromorphone (Dilaudid), *meperidine* (Demerol), *fentanyl* (Duragesic, Sublimaze), methadone (Dolophine, Methadose), oxycodone (Oxy-Contin, Percodan, Tylox, Percocet), hydrocodone (Lortab, Vicodin), and propoxyphene (Darvon, Dolene).

NOTE
Endorphins serve as the body's own supply of "opiates." Endorphins are produced by the pituitary gland and the hypothalamus during strenuous exercise, excitement, pain, and orgasm. They resemble the opiates in their abilities to produce analgesia by binding to opiate receptors, thereby blocking pain. They also produce a sense of well-being. Endorphins work as "natural pain relievers," whose effects may be enhanced by other medications.

BOX 13-17 Classifications of Pain

Acute pain: Pain sudden in onset that usually subsides with treatment (e.g., pain associated with acute myocardial infarction, acute appendicitis, renal colic, or traumatic injuries)
Chronic pain: Persistent or recurrent pain that is difficult to treat (e.g., pain that accompanies cancer and rheumatoid arthritis)
Referred pain: Visceral pain felt at a site distant from its origin (e.g., pain from a myocardial infarction felt in the arm)
Somatic pain: Pain arising from skeletal muscles, ligaments, vessels, or joints
Superficial pain: Pain arising from the skin or mucous membrane
Visceral pain: "Deep" pain arising from smooth musculature or organ systems that may be difficult to localize and is often described as dull or aching

Opioid analgesics may produce undesirable effects such as nausea and vomiting, constipation, urinary retention, orthostatic hypotension, respiratory depression, and CNS depression. Most of these effects can be overcome by careful administration and close patient monitoring.

Opioid antagonists block the effects of opioid analgesics by displacing the analgesics from their receptor sites. (Examples of such effects are opioid-induced respiratory depression and sedation.) *Naloxone* (Narcan), naltrexone (Trexan), and *nalmefene* (Revex) are opioid antagonists.

Opioid agonist-antagonist agents have analgesic and antagonist effects. They are thought to have pharmacokinetic and adverse effects similar to those of *morphine.* They may antagonize some opioid receptors competitively. Yet they may have varying degrees of agonist effect at other opioid receptor sites. Examples of these drugs include pentazocine (Talwin) and nalbuphine (Nubain). These drugs generally have a lower potential for creating dependency than opioid analgesics. In addition, withdrawal symptoms are not as severe as those of the opioid agonist drugs. They may initiate withdrawal symptoms in addicts.

Nonnarcotic Analgesics

Nonnarcotic analgesics act by a peripheral mechanism that interferes with local mediators released when tissue is damaged. These mediators stimulate nerve endings and they cause pain. When nonnarcotic analgesics are used, the nerve endings in damaged tissues are stimulated less often. This differs from the mechanism of narcotic analgesics that act at the level of the CNS. An example of a nonnarcotic analgesic is *ketorolac* (Toradol), a nonsteroidal antiinflammatory drug (NSAID) that exhibits analgesic activity. Another is tramadol (Ultram). Other nonnarcotic analgesics include cyclooxygenase (COX) inhibitors and oral NSAIDs such as ibuprofen (Advil), naproxen (Aleve), and acetaminophen (described later in this chapter).

CRITICAL THINKING
A nonnarcotic analgesic may be selected instead of a narcotic for a paramedic returning to work on the ambulance. Why?

Anesthetics

Anesthetic drugs are CNS depressants. They have a reversible action on nervous tissue. The three major types of anesthesia are general, regional, and local. *General anesthesia* is achieved by intravenous or inhalation routes and is the most common type of anesthesia used during surgery to induce unconsciousness. *Regional anesthesia* is obtained by injecting a local anesthetic drug. The drug is injected near a nerve trunk or at specific sites in a large region of the body (e.g., spinal block). *Local anesthesia* is achieved topically to produce a loss of sensation. Local anesthesia also can be achieved by injection to block an area surrounding an operative field, making it insensitive to pain (e.g., minor wound repair) (Box 13-18).

BOX 13-18 Examples of Anesthetics

Inhalation Anesthetics

Gases
Cyclopropane
Nitrous oxide; oxygen (Nitronox)

Volatile Liquids
Halothane (Fluothane)
Methoxyflurane (Penthrane)
Enflurane (Ethrane)
Isoflurane (Forane)
Sevoflurane (Ultane)
Desflurane (Suprane)

Intravenous Anesthetics

Ultrashort-Acting Barbiturates
Thiopental sodium (Pentothal)
Thiamylal sodium (Surital)
Methohexital sodium (Brevital Sodium)

Nonbarbiturates
Etomidate (Amidate)
Fentanyl (Sublimaze)
Sufentanil (Sufenta)
Alfentanil (Alfenta)
Propofol (Diprivan)

Dissociative Anesthetics
Ketamine (Ketalar)

Neuroleptic Anesthetics
Droperidol-fentanyl (Innovar injection)

Local Anesthetics

Topical
Benzocaine (Anbesol)
Ethyl chloride cocaine
Lidocaine (Xylocaine)
Tetracaine (Pontocaine)

Injectable
Lidocaine (Xylocaine)
Procaine (Novocain)

BOX 13-19 The Physiology of Sleep

Sleep can be viewed as a series of rhythms. Each has its own brain wave patterns. These rhythms can be divided into two major categories: rapid eye movement (REM) and non–rapid eye movement (non-REM). During sleep, a person moves through REM sleep. Then the person moves through four stages of non-REM sleep. Rapid eye movement, or active, sleep is the time of irregular body activity, vivid dreaming, and rapid eye movements. During REM sleep, the eyes move back and forth under the closed lids as they follow the action of a dream. The heart rate, blood pressure, and respirations may become irregular. During non-REM sleep, the person drifts out of wakeful awareness. The muscles relax, and the blood pressure, heartbeat, and breathing begin to decline. The brain sends signals to the arms, legs, and other large muscles to stop moving. At that point, "sleep paralysis" occurs. The first REM period lasts nearly 10 minutes. The whole cycle repeats itself usually four to five times each night. Each cycle lasts an average of 90 minutes. As the night continues, REM periods lengthen and non-REM periods shorten. The final REM period of the night may last as long as 1 hour.

may be a sedative or a hypnotic, depending on the dose used.

As stated before, alcohol has actions that are characteristic of sedative-hypnotic or antianxiety drugs. Alcohol is a major source of drug abuse and dependency.

Scattered throughout the brainstem is a group of nuclei, collectively called the *reticular formation*. The reticular formation and its neural pathways compose a system known as the *reticular activating system* (described in Chapter 10). This system is involved with the sleep-wake cycle. Through these pathways, the reticular activating system collects incoming signals from the senses and viscera. The system then processes and passes these signals to the higher brain centers. The reticular activating system determines the level of awareness to the environment. Thus the reticular activating system also governs actions and responses to the environment. Antianxiety and sedative-hypnotic agents and alcohol act by depressing this system.

 LOOK AGAIN
See Chapter 10: Review of Human Systems, pp. 171-173.

CLASSIFICATIONS

Two prototypical groups of drugs are used to treat anxiety and to induce sleep. These are the benzodiazepines and barbiturates, respectively. Benzodiazepines make up the drug class most often used today to treat anxiety and insomnia. Barbiturates compose an older drug class with many uses. These uses range from sedation to anesthesia.

Benzodiazepines. Benzodiazepines were introduced in the 1960s as antianxiety drugs. At present, they are among the most widely prescribed drugs in clinical medicine. This

Antianxiety and Sedative-Hypnotic Agents and Alcohol

Antianxiety and sedative-hypnotic agents and alcohol are presented together because of their similarities in pharmacological action. Antianxiety agents are used to reduce feelings of apprehension, nervousness, worry, or fearfulness.

Sedatives and hypnotics are drugs that depress the CNS, produce a calming effect, and help induce sleep (Box 13-19). The major difference between a sedative and a hypnotic is the degree of CNS depression induced by the agent. For example, a small dose of an agent administered to calm a patient is called a *sedative;* a larger dose of the same agent sufficient to induce sleep is called a *hypnotic*. Thus an agent is partly because of their wide therapeutic index. Mortality and morbidity from an oral overdose is rare, unless taken with other CNS depressants, such as alcohol.[9] Benzodiazepines are thought to work by binding to specific receptors in the cerebral cortex and limbic system. (These systems together govern emotional behavior.) These drugs are highly lipid soluble and are distributed widely in the body tissues. They also are highly bound to plasma protein, usually more than 80%. Benzodiazepines have four actions: anxiety reducing, sedative-hypnotic, muscle relaxing, and anticonvulsant. All benzodiazepines are schedule IV drugs because of their potential for abuse. Commonly prescribed benzodiazepines are alprazolam (Xanax), clonazepam (Klonopin), *diazepam* (Valium), flurazepam (Dalmane), *midazolam* (Versed), *lorazepam* (Ativan), and temazepam (Restoril).

> ### CRITICAL THINKING
> Consider that you are preparing to reduce a dislocated shoulder. Why would a benzodiazepine be preferred over a narcotic?

> ### NOTE
> Flumazenil (Romazicon) is a specific benzodiazepine receptor antagonist. Flumazenil has been shown to be effective in reversing benzodiazepine-induced sedation and coma[10] (see Chapter 34 and the Emergency Drug Index).

Barbiturates. Barbiturates were once the most commonly prescribed class of medications for sedative-hypnotic effects. However, they virtually have been replaced by the benzodiazepines. Barbiturates are divided into four classes according to their duration of action: *ultrashort acting, short acting, intermediate acting,* and *long acting.* The differences in onset and duration of action depend on their lipid solubility and protein-binding properties. Ultrashort-acting barbiturates commonly are used as intravenous anesthetics. These drugs act rapidly and can produce a state of anesthesia in a few seconds. An example of an ultrashort-acting barbiturate is thiopental sodium (Pentothal).

Short-acting barbiturates produce an effect in a short time (10 to 15 minutes). They also peak over a short period (3 to 4 hours). This class of drugs rarely is used to treat insomnia; it more often is used for preanesthesia sedation and in combination with other drugs for psychosomatic disorders. Examples include pentobarbital (Nembutal) and secobarbital (Seconal).

Intermediate-acting barbiturates have an onset of 45 to 60 minutes. They peak in 6 to 8 hours. Short-acting and intermediate-acting barbiturates produce similar patient responses. Examples of intermediate-acting barbiturates include amobarbital (Amytal) and butabarbital (Butisol).

Long-acting barbiturates require more than 60 minutes for onset. They peak over 10 to 12 hours. These agents are used to treat epilepsy and other chronic neurological disorders (see Chapter 25). They also are used to sedate patients with severe anxiety. Examples of long-acting barbiturates include mephobarbital (Mebaral) and phenobarbital (Luminal).

Miscellaneous Sedative-Hypnotic Drugs. The previously discussed drug classes do not include all of the antianxiety and sedative-hypnotic drugs. In fact, a number of other antianxiety and sedative-hypnotic drugs do not fall into these classes. These agents are more similar to barbiturates than benzodiazepines because they are generally shorter acting. Examples of miscellaneous drugs with antianxiety and sedative-hypnotic effects are chloral hydrate (Noctec), eszopiclone (Lunesta), and zolpidem (Ambien). In addition to these drugs, antihistamines such as hydroxyzine (Vistaril, Atarax) have pronounced sedative effects. Etomidate (Amidate) is another nonbarbiturate, hypnotic anesthetic used for premedication for tracheal intubation and cardioversion.

Alcohol Intake and Behavioral Effects

Alcohol is a general CNS depressant that can produce sedation, sleep, and anesthesia. In addition, alcohol enhances the sedative-hypnotic effects of other drug classes, including all general CNS depressants, antihistamines, phenothiazines, narcotic analgesics, and tricyclic antidepressants. If alcohol is taken with other drugs, this enhancement could result in coma or death. Blood alcohol is measured in milligrams per deciliter (mg/dL). Characteristic behavioral effects can be predicted based on the amount of alcohol consumed and blood alcohol levels. Behavioral effects associated with alcohol intake are described further in Chapter 34.

Anticonvulsants

Anticonvulsant drugs are used to treat seizure disorders. The most notable of these disorders is epilepsy. Epilepsy is a neurological disorder characterized by a recurrent pattern of abnormal neuronal discharges within the brain. These discharges result in a sudden loss or disturbance of consciousness, sometimes associated with motor activity, sensory phenomena, or inappropriate behavior. Epilepsy is estimated to occur in 0.5% to 1% of the population. In 50% of these cases, the cause is unknown (primary or idiopathic epilepsy). Secondary epilepsy is epilepsy that can be traced to trauma, infection, a cerebrovascular disorder, or some other illness. (Epilepsy is discussed further in Chapter 25.)

Anticonvulsant drugs work by depressing the excitability of neurons that fire to initiate the seizure. These drugs also suppress the neurons responsible for the spread of the seizure discharge. Anticonvulsants are presumed to modify the ionic movements of sodium, potassium, or calcium across the nerve membrane. Thus they reduce the response to incoming electrical or chemical stimulation. Benzodiazepines also stimulate major inhibitory neurotransmitters in the CNS. Many patients need drug therapy throughout their lives to control seizure disorders.

Several drugs are available for the control of seizure disorders. The choice of drug depends on the type of seizure disorder (*generalized, partial,* or *status;* described in Chapter 25). The choice of drug also depends on the patient's tolerance and response to the prescribed medication. Box 13-20 presents classes of anticonvulsant drugs.

Central Nervous System Stimulants

Central nervous system stimulants are classified by where they exert their major effects in the nervous system: on the cerebrum, on the medulla and brainstem, or in the hypothalamic limbic regions. All CNS stimulants work to increase excitability by blocking activity of inhibitory neurons or their respective neurotransmitters or by enhancing the production of the excitatory neurotransmitters. Some of the more common CNS stimulant drugs are anorexiants and amphetamines.

ANOREXIANTS

Anorexiants are appetite suppressants. They are used to treat obesity. They work by producing a direct stimulant effect on the hypothalamic and limbic regions. They perhaps have this effect on other areas of the nervous system as well. Examples of anorexiants include phendimetrazine (Plegine) and mazindol (Mazanor, Sanorex).

A new class of drugs (gastrointestinal lipase inhibitors, or fat blockers) block the absorption of about 30% of dietary fat. These drugs sometimes are used to manage obesity along with a reduced-calorie diet. An example of a gastrointestinal lipase inhibitor is orlistat (Xenical).

> **DID YOU KNOW?**
> At one time, a two-drug combination of fenfluramine and phentermine (Fen-Phen) was used to manage obesity. The combination was withdrawn from the market in 1997. It was found to have serious complications. These included potentially fatal primary pulmonary hypertension and valvular heart disease.

AMPHETAMINES

Amphetamines stimulate the cerebral cortex and reticular activating system. This stimulation increases alertness and responsiveness to environmental surroundings. Amphetamines mainly are used to treat *attention deficit hyperactivity disorder* (ADHD), *attention deficit disorder* (ADD), and *narcolepsy.* For the most part, ADHD is seen in children and adolescents and is characterized by a short attention span and impulsive behavior. (ADHD and ADD are described further in Chapter 35.)

Individuals with narcolepsy experience excessive drowsiness, sudden sleep attacks during daytime hours, and sometimes sleep paralysis. Medications used to treat these disorders include methamphetamine (Desoxyn), amphetamine-mixed salts (Adderall), and dextroamphetamine tablets and elixir. Nonamphetamine CNS stimulants used to treat ADHD and ADD include methylphenidate (Ritalin, Concerta), atomoxetine (Strattera), and pemoline (Cylert). Paradoxically, amphetamines and other stimulants have a calming effect on persons with ADHD. Likely, the drugs achieve this effect by increasing neurotransmitter levels of dopamine.

Psychotherapeutic Drugs

Psychotherapeutic drugs include antipsychotic agents, antidepressants, and lithium. These drugs are used to treat psychoses and affective disorders, especially schizophrenia, depression, and mania (see Chapter 35).

CENTRAL NERVOUS SYSTEM AND EMOTIONS

The neurotransmitters acetylcholine, norepinephrine, dopamine, serotonin, and monoamine oxidase have a major effect on emotion (Figure 13-10). Alterations in the levels of these chemicals are linked to changes in mood and behavior. Drug therapy alleviates symptoms by temporarily modifying unwanted behavior.

> **NOTE**
> Acetylcholine is released from central neural tissue into the cerebrospinal fluid during activity. Norepinephrine and dopamine have widespread inhibitory effects. They influence functions such as sleep and arousal, affect, and memory. Serotonin levels affect mood and behavior. Monoamine oxidase is an enzyme that inactivates dopamine and serotonin, both of which are produced during intense emotional states.

BOX 13-20 Classes of Anticonvulsant Drugs

Barbiturates
Phenobarbital (Luminal)

Benzodiazepines
Clonazepam (Klonopin)
Diazepam (Valium)
Lorazepam (Ativan)

Hydantoins
Fosphenytoin (Cerebyx)
Phenytoin (Dilantin)

Succinimides
Ethosuximide (Zarontin)
Zonisamide (Zonegran)

Other
Carbamazepine (Tegretol)
Divalproex (Depakote)
Gabapentin (Neurontin)
Lamotrigine (Lamictal)
Magnesium sulfate
Topiramate (Topamax)
Valproic acid (Depakene)
Levetiracetam (Keppra)

From McKenry L, Leda M: *Mosby's pharmacology in nursing,* ed 22, St Louis, 2005, Mosby.

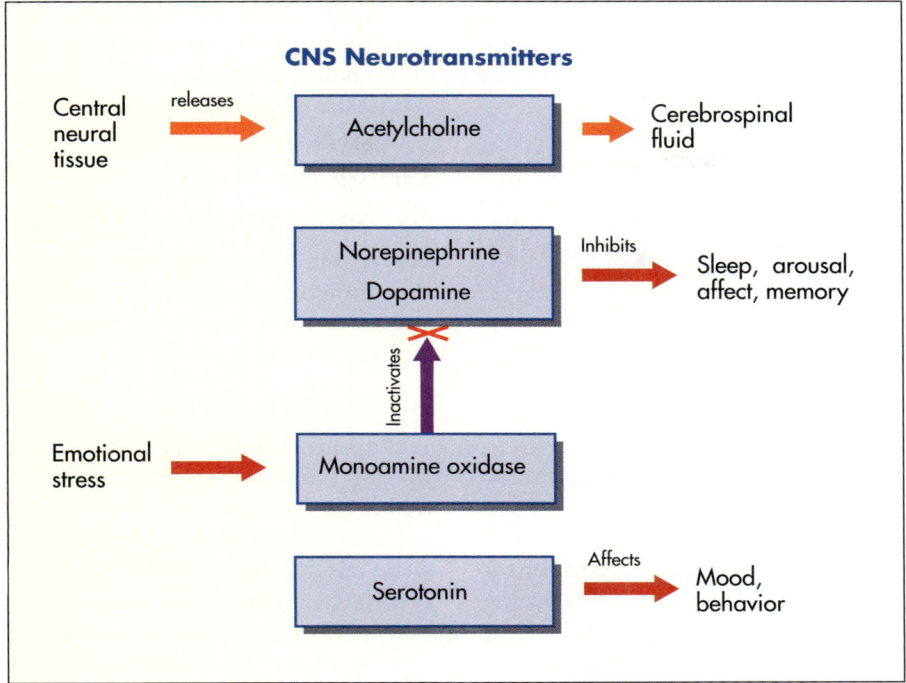

FIGURE 13-10 Neurotransmitters in the brain and their effects on emotion.

ANTIPSYCHOTIC AGENTS

The main use of antipsychotic drugs is to treat *schizophrenia*. This class of drugs is the only clearly effective treatment for this condition. There are other psychiatric indications for the use of antipsychotic drugs. These drugs are used to treat Tourette's syndrome. They also are used to control disturbing behavior in patients with senile dementia associated with Alzheimer's disease. Effective antipsychotic (neuroleptic) drugs block dopamine receptors in specific areas of the CNS. These drugs can be classified into the following groups:
- Phenothiazine derivatives
  Chlorpromazine (Thorazine)
  Thioridazine (Mellaril)
  Fluphenazine (Prolixin)
- Butyrophenone derivatives
  Haloperidol (Haldol)
- Dihydroindolone derivatives
  Molindone (Moban)
- Dibenzoxazepine derivatives
  Loxapine (Loxitane)
- Thienbenzodiazepine derivatives
  Olanzapine (Zyprexa)
- Atypical agents
  Clozapine (Clozaril)
  Risperidone (Risperdal)

With continued use of certain antipsychotics, some patients develop supersensitivity of dopamine receptors. This can lead to tardive dyskinesia or dystonia. **Tardive dyskinesia** is a potentially irreversible neurological disorder characterized by involuntary repetitious movements of the muscles of the face, limbs, and trunk. Other identifying features include excessive blinking of the eyelids, lip smacking, tongue protrusion, foot tapping, and rocking side-to-side. **Dystonia** is characterized by local or diffuse changes in muscle tone. This condition can result in painful muscle spasms, unusually fixed postures, and strange movement patterns.

ANTIDEPRESSANTS

Antidepressants are used to treat affective disorders (mood disturbances) including depression, mania, and elation. Tricyclic antidepressants, selective serotonin reuptake inhibitors, and MAO inhibitors are prescribed for depression; lithium (an antimanic drug) is the preferred treatment for mania (see Chapter 35).

> **NOTE**
>
> Depression may be exogenous or endogenous. *Exogenous depression* results from a person's response to a loss or disappointment (e.g., "the blues"). This type of depression is considered normal. It is usually temporary and remits without the use of drug therapy. *Endogenous depression,* however, lasts 6 months or longer. This type of depression is characterized by the absence of external causes; it may be the result of genetic or biochemical alterations. Antidepressants often are needed to treat this disorder. Depression is discussed further in Chapter 35.

Tricyclic Antidepressants. Tricyclic antidepressants (TCAs) are thought to treat depression by increasing levels (blocking the reuptake) of the neurotransmitters norepinephrine and serotonin. Examples include nortriptyline

(Pamelor) and amitriptyline (Elavil). Excessive doses of these drugs (e.g., TCA overdose) have the potential for cardiac dysrhythmias and cardiovascular collapse (see Chapter 34).

Selective Serotonin Reuptake Inhibitors. Selective serotonin reuptake inhibitors work to block the reabsorption or reuptake of serotonin. This makes more of the chemical available to the brain. These drugs do have some side effects; for example, insomnia, headache, and diarrhea are common complaints. However, these drugs often treat depression without the adverse effects of other antidepressants, such as the dry mouth caused by tricyclic antidepressants or the dietary restrictions mandated by MAO inhibitors. Examples of selective serotonin reuptake inhibitors are fluoxetine (Prozac), sertraline (Zoloft), paroxetine (Paxil), escitalopram (Lexapro), fluvoxamine (Luvox), and citalopram (Celexa).

Monoamine Oxidase Inhibitor Antidepressants. Central-acting monoamines, especially norepinephrine and serotonin, are thought to cause depression and mania. Monoamine oxidase is an enzyme found in nerve cells. It is thought to be produced during tense emotional states. The enzyme is responsible for metabolizing norepinephrine within the nerve. Monoamine oxidase inhibitors block this enzyme. This leads to increased levels of norepinephrine. Examples of MAO inhibitors used to treat depression include isocarboxazid (Marplan), phenelzine (Nardil), and tranylcypromine (Parnate). Monoamine oxidase inhibitors also are used as antihypertensive agents (described later in this chapter).

NOTE

The monoamine oxidase inhibitors used in psychiatric practice are irreversible inhibitors of both forms (A and B) of brain monoamine oxidase. These drugs are rarely used today because of their potentially dangerous interactions with dietary tyramine and other agents that have sympathomimetic or serotoninergic properties.[11]

Lithium. Lithium is a cation that is closely related to sodium. Both cations are transported actively across cell membranes. However, lithium cannot be pumped as effectively out of the cell as sodium. Lithium therefore accumulates in the cells. This results in a decrease in intracellular sodium concentration and perhaps an improvement in the symptoms of a manic state. In addition, lithium appears to enhance some of the actions of serotonin. Lithium may decrease levels of norepinephrine and dopamine. It also appears to block the development of dopamine receptor

supersensitivity that may accompany long-term therapy with antipsychotic agents. Lithium carbonate is used to treat manic disorders, such as bipolar disorders. Lithium has a narrow therapeutic range, so toxicity is common.

Drugs for Specific Central Nervous System–Peripheral Dysfunction

Several movement disorders result from an imbalance of dopamine and acetylcholine. Two of the most common are Parkinson's disease (including parkinsonism syndromes) and Huntington's disease.

PARKINSON'S DISEASE

Parkinson's disease is a chronic disabling disease characterized by rigidity of voluntary muscles. Parkinson's disease also is characterized by tremor of the fingers and extremities. The disease most often affects persons over age 60, although it may occur in younger persons. Parkinson's disease may occur especially after acute encephalitis or cases of carbon monoxide or metallic poisoning or from the use of some illicit drugs. The disease is thought to result from an abnormally low concentration of dopamine. *Parkinsonism syndromes* mimic the symptoms of Parkinson's disease. They usually are of an unknown cause (**idiopathic**) but may result from treatment with antipsychotic drugs (*drug-induced parkinsonism*) that block dopaminergic receptors (e.g., **haloperidol** [Haldol], metoclopramide [Clopra, Emex], and phenothiazines [e.g., Thorazine, Mellaril]). Symptoms of Parkinson's disease include the following:

- Immobile facial expression (parkinsonism facies)
- Bobbing of the head
- Resting tremor
- Pill-rolling of the fingers
- Shuffling gait
- Forward flexion of the trunk
- Loss of postural reflexes

HUNTINGTON'S DISEASE

Huntington's disease is an inherited disorder characterized by progressive dementia and involuntary muscle twitching (chorea). Like Parkinson's disease, Huntington's disease is thought to be related to an imbalance of dopamine, acetylcholine, and perhaps other neurotransmitters.

Drugs With Central Anticholinergic Activity

Drugs that inhibit or block acetylcholine are referred to as *anticholinergic*. They work by restoring the normal dopamine-acetylcholine balance in the brain. Common anticholinergic agents include benztropine (tablets and injections), ethopropazine hydrochloride, and **ipratropium** (Atrovent). Another commonly prescribed anticholinergic is donepezil (Aricept) that is used to treat dementia in patients with mild-to-moderate Alzheimer's disease.

Drugs That Affect Dopamine in the Brain

Three classifications of drugs affect dopamine in the brain: those that release dopamine, those that increase brain levels of dopamine, and dopaminergic agonists (Box 13-21). Levodopa (L-dopa) is a drug that increases brain levels of dopamine. Levodopa is the current drug of choice in the treatment of movement disorders associated with dopamine-acetylcholine imbalance.

MONOAMINE OXIDASE INHIBITORS

Two types of MAO inhibitors have been identified. The first one is *monoamine oxidase A,* which metabolizes norepinephrine and serotonin. The second one is *monoamine oxidase B,* which metabolizes dopamine. Selegiline (Deprenyl) is a selective inhibitor of monoamine oxidase B. It retards the breakdown of dopamine. Selegiline often is used along with levodopa because it enhances and prolongs the antiparkinsonism effects of levodopa. (Selegiline allows the dose of levodopa to be reduced.)

Skeletal Muscle Relaxants

Skeletal muscle contraction is evoked by a nicotinic cholinergic transmission process. Just as the autonomic ganglionic transmission can be modified by drugs, so too can skeletal muscle contractions. Skeletal muscle relaxants can be classified as central-acting, direct-acting, and neuromuscular blockers.

CENTRAL-ACTING MUSCLE RELAXANTS

Central-acting drugs are used to treat muscle spasms. They are thought to work by producing CNS depression in the brain and spinal cord. Antispastic agents include carisoprodol (Soma), cyclobenzaprine (Flexeril), and *diazepam* (Valium).

DIRECT-ACTING MUSCLE RELAXANTS

Direct-acting muscle relaxants directly affect skeletal muscles to produce muscle relaxation. This results in a decrease in muscle contraction. Dantrolene (Dantrium) is an example of a direct-acting muscle relaxant.

NEUROMUSCULAR BLOCKERS

Neuromuscular blocking drugs produce complete muscle relaxation and paralysis. They do this by binding to the nicotinic receptor for acetylcholine at the neuromuscular junction. Neuromuscular nerve transmission is thus blocked. Nerve transmission remains blocked for a variable period depending on the type and amount of neuromuscular blocker used.

Neuromuscular blockers sometimes are used to achieve total paralysis before endotracheal intubation (described in Chapter 15), to relieve muscle spasms of the larynx, to suppress tetany, to treat depression resulting from electroconvulsive therapy, and to allow for breathing control by a respirator. These blocking agents can produce complete paralysis. Thus a patient's breathing must be supported. The effectiveness of ventilation and oxygenation must be monitored closely. (These muscle relaxants do not inhibit pain or seizure activity.) Examples of neuromuscular blockers include *pancuronium* (Pavulon), *vecuronium* (Norcuron), and *succinylcholine* (Anectine).

NOTE

The two types of neuromuscular blocking drugs are *depolarizing agents* and *nondepolarizing agents.* Depolarizing agents (e.g., *succinylcholine*) substitute themselves into the neuromuscular junction. They bind to receptors for acetylcholine (ACh) and have a rapid onset and brief duration of action. This makes them the drug of choice for endotracheal intubation. Nondepolarizing agents bind to the receptors for ACh at the neuromuscular junction. They do this without initiating depolarization of the muscle membrane. Nondepolarizing agents (e.g., *pancuronium*) have a longer onset and duration than depolarizing agents.

SECTION FOUR
Drugs That Affect the Cardiovascular System

REVIEW OF ANATOMY AND PHYSIOLOGY

The heart consists of many interconnected branching fibers or cells that form the walls of the two atria and two ventricles (see Chapter 10). Some of these cells are specialized to conduct electrical impulses. Others have contraction as their main role. All of these cells are nourished through a profuse network of blood vessels (coronary vasculature). Cardiac drugs are classified by their effects on these tissues. Boxes 13-22 and 13-23 list cardiac drugs and pharmacological terms that describe their actions.

BOX 13-21 Drugs That Affect Dopamine in the Brain

Amantadine (Symmetrel)
Bromocriptine (Parlodel)
Carbidopa-levodopa (Sinemet)
Levodopa (Larodopa)
Pergolide (Permax)

LOOK AGAIN

See Chapter 10: Review of Human Systems, pp. 182-186.

BOX 13-22 Emergency Drugs: Cardiovascular System

Drugs Used to Treat Dysrhythmias

Adenosine (Adenocard)
Amiodarone (Cordarone)
Atropine

Beta-Adrenergic Blockers
Atenolol (Tenormin)
Metoprolol (Lopressor, Toprol-XL)

Calcium Channel Blockers
Diltiazem (Cardizem)
Verapamil (Isoptin)

Dopamine (Intropin)
Isoproterenol (Isuprel)
Lidocaine (Xylocaine)
Magnesium
Procainamide (Pronestyl)

Drugs Used to Optimize Cardiac Output and Blood Pressure

Calcium chloride
Digoxin (Lanoxin)
Dobutamine (Dobutrex)
Dopamine (Intropin)
Epinephrine (Adrenalin)
Nitroglycerin (Nitrostat, Tridil)
Norepinephrine (Levophed)
Vasopressin (Pitressin)

BOX 13-23 Pharmacological Terms to Describe Actions of Cardiovascular Drugs

Chronotropic: Chronotropic drugs affect heart rate. If the drug accelerates the heart rate (e.g., isoproterenol [Isuprel]), it is said to have a positive chronotropic effect. A drug that decreases the heart rate (e.g., verapamil [Isoptin]) is said to have a negative chronotropic effect.

Dromotropic: Dromotropic drugs affect conduction velocity through the conducting tissues of the heart. If a drug accelerates conduction, it is said to have a positive dromotropic effect. Examples of drugs with positive dromotropic effects include isoproterenol (Isuprel) and phenytoin (Dilantin). Drugs with negative dromotropic effects delay conduction (e.g., verapamil [Isoptin] and adenosine [Adenocard]).

Inotropic: Inotropic drugs strengthen or increase the force of cardiac contraction (a positive inotropic effect). Some examples include digoxin (Lanoxin), dobutamine (Dobutrex), epinephrine (Adrenalin), and isoproterenol (Isuprel). A drug that weakens or decreases the force of cardiac contraction has a negative inotropic effect. An example of such a drug is propranolol (Inderal).

Cardiac Glycosides

Cardiac glycosides are naturally occurring plant substances. They have characteristic effects on the heart. These compounds contain a carbohydrate molecule (sugar). When combined with water, the molecule is converted into a sugar plus one or more active substances. Glycosides may work by blocking certain ionic pumps in the cellular membrane. This indirectly increases the calcium concentration to the contractile proteins. A key cardiac glycoside is **digoxin** (Lanoxin). **Digoxin** is used to treat heart failure and to manage certain tachycardias (see Chapter 22).

Digitalis glycosides affect the heart in two distinct ways. First, they increase the strength of contraction. This is a **positive inotropic effect.** Second, they have a dual effect on the electrophysiological properties of the heart. They have a modest negative chronotropic effect. (This causes slight slowing of the heart rate.) They also have a profound negative dromotropic effect, decreasing conduction velocity of impulses in the heart.

Many patients who take cardiac glycosides develop side effects at one time or another because of the narrow therapeutic index of the drugs. The symptoms may be neurological, visual, gastrointestinal, cardiac, or psychiatric. These symptoms often are vague and the patient can easily attribute them to a viral illness. A high index of suspicion in patients taking cardiac glycosides who report experiencing flulike symptoms is important. The most common side effects of cardiac glycosides are anorexia, nausea or vomiting, visual disturbances (flashing lights, altered color vision), and **dysrhythmias** (cardiac rhythm disturbances), usually slowing of the heart rate with varying degrees of blocked conduction (see Chapter 22).

> **NOTE**
> **Proarrhythmias** are serious dysrhythmias that are generated by antidysrhythmic agents. All antidysrhythmic drugs have some degree of proarrhythmic effects. The sequential use of two or more antidysrhythmic drugs compounds these effects. As a rule, it is best not to use more than one agent to manage dysrhythmias (unless absolutely necessary).

The toxic effects of cardiac glycosides are dose related. These effects may be increased by the presence of other drugs, such as diuretics. These other drugs may predispose the patient to cardiac rhythm disturbances. Dysrhythmias may include bradycardias, tachycardias, and even ventricular fibrillation. For these reasons, patients taking these drugs require close monitoring. Treatment for digitalis toxicity may include correction of electrolyte imbalances, neutralization of the free drug, and use of antidysrhythmics. A patient with a low potassium level is much more likely to develop digoxin toxicity.

Antidysrhythmics

Antidysrhythmic drugs are used to treat and prevent disorders of cardiac rhythm. The pharmacological agents that suppress dysrhythmias may do so by direct action on the cardiac cell membrane (*vasopressin* [Pitressin]), by indirect action that affects the cells (*propranolol* [Inderal]), or both.

Cardiac rhythm disturbances may be caused by a number of factors. These include ischemia, hypoxia, acidosis or alkalosis, electrolyte abnormalities, excessive catecholamine exposure, autonomic influences, drug toxicity, or scarred and diseased tissue. Dysrhythmias result from disturbances in impulse formation, disturbances in impulse conduction, or both.

CLASSIFICATIONS

Antidysrhythmic drugs have been classified into categories based on their fundamental mode of action on cardiac muscle. Drugs that belong to the same class do not always produce identical actions. However, all antidysrhythmic drugs have some ability to suppress *automaticity*.

> **NOTE**
> Local protocols and standing orders assist and guide EMS personnel. These orders often are established to allow paramedics to use certain drugs in certain cases. With these orders in place, paramedics can act without seeking medical direction. One such example is antidysrhythmic drugs for a patient with specific cardiac conduction disturbances. Another is first-line cardiac life support drugs for a patient in cardiac arrest.

Class I. Class I drugs are sodium channel blockers. These work to slow conduction. They are divided further into subclasses (Ia, Ib, and Ic) based on the extent of sodium channel blockade. Examples of Class Ia drugs include quinidine (Quinaglute, Duraquin), disopyramide (Norpace), and *procainamide* (Pronestyl). Class Ib drugs decrease or have no effect on conduction velocity. Examples include *lidocaine* (Xylocaine) and *phenytoin* (Dilantin). Class Ic drugs profoundly slow conduction and are indicated only for control of life-threatening ventricular dysrhythmias. An example of a Class Ic drug is flecainide (Tambocor).

> **CRITICAL THINKING**
> How might the signs of shock in a patient taking digoxin (Lanoxin) or propranolol (Inderal) vary from what might be expected normally?

Class II. Class II drugs are beta-blocking agents. These drugs reduce adrenergic stimulation of the heart. An example is *metoprolol* (Lopressor).

Class III. Class III drugs produce potassium channel blockade. This increases the contractility. Unlike other antidysrhythmic agents, drugs in this class do not suppress automaticity. They also have no effect on conduction velocity. These drugs are thought to cease dysrhythmias that result from the reentry of blocked impulses. An example of such a drug is *amiodarone* (Cordarone).

Class IV. Class IV drugs are also known as *calcium channel blockers*. These drugs are thought to work by blocking the inflow of calcium through the cell membranes of the cardiac and smooth muscle cells. This action depresses the myocardial and smooth muscle contraction, decreases automaticity, and in some cases decreases conduction velocity. Examples of calcium channel blockers include *verapamil* (Isoptin) and *diltiazem* (Cardizem).

Antihypertensives

High blood pressure affects as many as 50 million adults and children in the United States[9] and has been related directly to an increased incidence of stroke, cerebral hemorrhage, heart and renal failure, and coronary heart disease. The exact mechanism of action of many antihypertensive drugs is unknown. The ideal antihypertensive drug should accomplish the following:

- Maintain blood pressure within normal limits for various body positions
- Maintain or improve blood flow without compromising tissue perfusion or blood supply to the brain
- Reduce the workload of the heart
- Have no undesirable side effects
- Permit long-term administration without intolerance

CLASSIFICATIONS

Certain drugs are used to reduce blood pressure in patients with chronic hypertension. These drugs usually are given in low-dose combinations and are *titrated* (gradually adjusted) to effect. These drugs include diuretics, sympathetic blocking agents (sympatholytic drugs), vasodilators, angiotensin-converting enzyme (ACE) inhibitors, calcium channel blockers, and the newer class, angiotensin II receptor antagonists.

Diuretics. Diuretics are the drugs of choice in managing hypertension. They often are used with other antihypertensive agents. Diuretics cause a loss of excess salt and water from the body by the kidneys. The decrease in plasma and extracellular fluid volume decreases preload and stroke volume. The decrease in fluid volume has a direct effect on the size of the arterioles, resulting in lowered blood pressure. This response causes an initial decline of cardiac output. That is followed by a decrease in peripheral vascular resistance. These responses result in a lowering of the blood pressure.

Thiazides are diuretics that work well to lower blood pressure. Many antihypertensive agents cause retention of sodium and water. Yet thiazides may be given concomitantly (along with other drugs) to help prevent this side effect. An example of a thiazide diuretic is hydrochlorothiazide (HCTZ).

Loop diuretics are strong, short-acting agents. They inhibit sodium and chloride reabsorption in the loop of

Henle. These drugs cause excessive loss of potassium. They also cause an increase in the excretion of sodium and water. Loop diuretics have fewer side effects than most other antihypertensives. However, hypokalemia and profound dehydration can be a result of their use. These agents are prescribed to patients who have renal insufficiency. They also may be given to patients who cannot take other diuretics. An example of a loop diuretic is *furosemide* (Lasix).

> **NOTE**
>
> Many drugs are excreted by the kidneys. Thus patients with renal system dysfunction (acute or chronic renal failure) may accumulate drugs in their systems. These patients often require modifications in drug doses and dosing intervals. These changes are in addition to diet modification and fluid restriction.

Potassium-sparing agents can be effective as an antihypertensive when they are used in combination with other diuretics. They promote sodium and water loss without a loss of potassium. These agents are used to treat hypertensive patients who become hypokalemic from other diuretics. They also can be used by patients who are apparently resistant to the antihypertensive effects of other diuretics. Potassium-sparing agents are also used to treat some edematous states. (An example of such is cirrhosis of the liver with ascites.) An example of a potassium-sparing agent is spironolactone (Aldactone).

Sympathetic Blocking Agents. Sympathetic blocking agents may be classified as *beta-blocking agents* and *adrenergic-inhibiting agents*. Beta-blocking agents are used to treat cardiovascular disorders, including patients with suspected myocardial infarction, high-risk unstable angina, and hypertension. These drugs work by decreasing cardiac output and inhibiting renin secretion from the kidneys. Both actions result in lower blood pressure. Beta-blocking drugs compete with epinephrine for available beta-receptor sites as well. This inhibits tissue and organ response to beta stimulation. Examples of beta-blocking agents include the following:

- Beta$_1$-blocking agents (cardioselective)
  Acebutolol (Sectral)
  Atenolol (Tenormin)
  Metoprolol (Lopressor, Toprol-XL)
- Beta$_1$- and beta$_2$-blocking agents (nonselective)
  Labetalol (Normodyne, Trandate) (also has alpha$_1$-blocking properties)
  Nadolol (Corgard)
  Propranolol (Inderal)

Adrenergic-inhibiting agents work by modifying the actions of the sympathetic nervous system. They are effective antihypertensive drugs. Arterial pressure is influenced through various mechanisms of the heart, blood vessels, and kidneys. Sympathetic stimulation increases the heart rate and force of myocardial contraction, constricts arterioles and venules, and causes the release of renin from the

kidneys. Blocking this sympathetic stimulation can reduce blood pressure.

Adrenergic-inhibiting agents are classified as *centrally acting adrenergic inhibitors* or *peripheral adrenergic inhibitors*. The mechanism by which many of these agents work is unknown. Generally, most of these agents are believed to have multiple sites of action. Examples include the following drugs:

- Centrally acting adrenergic inhibitors
  Clonidine hydrochloride (Catapres)
  Methyldopa (Aldomet)
  Prazosin hydrochloride (Minipress)
- Peripheral adrenergic inhibitors
  Doxazosin (Cardura)
  Guanethidine sulfate (Ismelin)
  Reserpine (Sandril, Serpasil)
  Phentolamine (Regitine)
  Phenoxybenzamine (Dibenzyline)
  Terazosin (Hytrin)

Vasodilator Drugs. Vasodilator drugs act directly on the smooth muscle walls of the arterioles, veins, or both. They lower peripheral resistance. Thus they lower blood pressure. This stimulates the sympathetic nervous system and also activates the baroreceptor reflexes. In turn this leads to an increase in heart rate, cardiac output, and renin release. Medications that inhibit the sympathetic response usually are given with vasodilator drugs.

In addition to their use as antihypertensives, some vasodilator drugs work to treat angina pectoris (ischemic chest pain). For example, nitrates dilate veins and arteries. Their dilating effects on veins lead to venous pooling of blood. They also reduce the amount of blood return to the heart. Thus these effects reduce *left ventricular end-diastolic pressure and volume* (the volume of blood in the left ventricle at the end of filling) (see Chapter 22). The subsequent decrease in wall tension helps to reduce myocardial oxygen demand and also relieves the chest pain of myocardial ischemia. Vasodilator drugs are classified as *arteriolar dilators* and *arteriolar and venous dilators*. Examples of each include the following:

- Arteriolar dilator drugs
  Hydralazine (Apresoline)
  Minoxidil (Loniten)
- Arteriolar and venous dilator drugs
  Sodium nitroprusside (Nipride, Nitropress)
  Nitrates and nitrites
  Amyl nitrite inhalant
  Isosorbide dinitrate (Isordil, Sorbitrate)
  Nitroglycerin sublingual tablet (Nitrostat)
  Nitropaste (Nitro-Bid ointment, Nitrostat, Nitrol)
  Intravenous *nitroglycerin* (Tridil)

Angiotensin-Converting Enzyme (ACE) Inhibitor Drugs. As described in Chapter 11, the renin-angiotensin-aldosterone system plays a key role in maintaining blood pressure. This system also plays a key role in sodium and fluid balance. A disturbance in this system can result in hypertension, edema, and congestive heart failure.

In addition, kidney damage can result in an inability to regulate the release of renin through normal feedback mechanisms. This causes elevated blood pressure in some patients.

LOOK AGAIN
See Chapter 11: General Principles of Pathophysiology, pp. 239-240.

Angiotensin II is a strong vasoconstrictor that raises blood pressure and also causes the release of aldosterone. Aldosterone contributes to sodium and water retention. By inhibiting conversion of the precursor angiotensin I to the active molecule angiotensin II (a process triggered by ACE), the renin-angiotensin-aldosterone system is suppressed and blood pressure is lowered. Examples of ACE inhibitors include *captopril* (Capoten), *enalapril* (Vasotec), benazepril (Lotensin), fosinopril (Monopril), *lisinopril* (Prinivil, Zestril), and quinapril (Accupril).

Calcium Channel Blockers. Calcium channel blocking agents such as *verapamil* (Isoptin), amlodipine (Norvasc), felodipine (Plendil), and *diltiazem* (Cardizem, Tiazac) reduce peripheral vascular resistance by inhibiting the contractility of vascular smooth muscle. They dilate coronary vessels through the same mechanism. The effects of these drugs are important in treating hypertension, decreasing the oxygen requirements of the heart (through decreased afterload), and increasing oxygen supply (by abolishing coronary artery spasm), thus relieving the causes of angina pectoris. The various drugs in this class differ in degree of selectivity for coronary (and peripheral) vasodilation or decreased cardiac contractility.

Angiotensin II Receptor Antagonists

Angiotensin II receptor antagonists are a newer class of antihypertensive agent. They block the renin-angiotensin-aldosterone system more completely than ACE inhibitors. They lower blood pressure by selectively inhibiting the actions of angiotensin II receptors, which include vasoconstriction, renal tubular sodium reabsorption, aldosterone release, and stimulation of central and peripheral sympathetic activity. These drugs are used to manage hypertension in those who cannot cope with the adverse effects of ACE inhibitors (e.g., dry cough). The drugs appear to be equally effective in lowering systolic and diastolic pressure. They also are being studied for their effectiveness in treating congestive heart failure, diabetic nephropathy, and vascular diseases such as atherosclerosis. Drugs in this classification include candesartan (Atacand), irbesartan (Avapro), losartan (Cozaar, Hyzaar), telmisartan (Micardis), and valsartan (Diovan) (Figure 13-11).

Antihemorrheologic Agents

Antihemorrheologic agents are used to treat peripheral vascular disorders caused by pathological or physiological obstruction (e.g., arteriosclerosis). These drugs improve blood flow and the delivery of oxygen to ischemic tissues. They do this by restoring red blood cell flexibility to traverse narrow vessels, and by lowering blood viscosity. An example of an antihemorrheologic agent is pentoxifylline (Trental).

SECTION FIVE
Drugs That Affect the Blood

ANTICOAGULANTS, FIBRINOLYTICS, AND BLOOD COMPONENTS

Bleeding and thrombosis are altered states of hemostasis. An understanding of the drugs that affect blood coagulation and the use of fibrinolytic agents and blood components is crucial. In the prehospital arena, these concepts will assist in the management of patients.

Anticoagulants

As described in Chapter 10, platelets are small cell fragments in the blood. They provide the initial step in normal repair of blood vessels. **Blood coagulation** is a process that results in the formation of a stable fibrin clot that entraps platelets, blood cells, and plasma. The end result of this process is called a blood clot or thrombus. Abnormal thrombus formation is the major cause of myocardial infarction (from coronary thrombosis) and stroke (from cerebral vascular thrombosis) (see Chapter 22).

LOOK AGAIN
See Chapter 10: Review of Human Systems, pp. 178-182.

Thrombus formation can occur in both the venous and arterial systems. An example of thrombosis in the venous system is pulmonary embolus and deep vein thrombosis. The three major risk factors for various thromboses are *stasis, localized trauma,* and *hypercoagulable states.* Stasis (reduced blood flow) results from immobilization or venous insufficiency. Stasis is responsible for the increased incidence of *deep vein thrombosis* (DVT) in many bedridden patients. Localized trauma may initiate the clotting cascade and may cause arterial and venous thrombosis. *Hypercoagulability* is the increased likelihood of blood to become abnormally thick and thus increase the formation of fibrin complexes in the blood vessels. It is the cause of the increased incidence of deep vein thrombosis in women who take birth control pills. Hypercoagulability is also a factor in clotting problems for many of the familial thrombotic disorders (see Chapter 22).

Arterial thrombi commonly are associated with atherosclerotic plaques, hypertension, and turbulent blood flow that damages the endothelial lining of blood vessels. Damage to the endothelium causes platelets to stick and *aggregate* (clump) in the arterial system. Arterial thrombi are

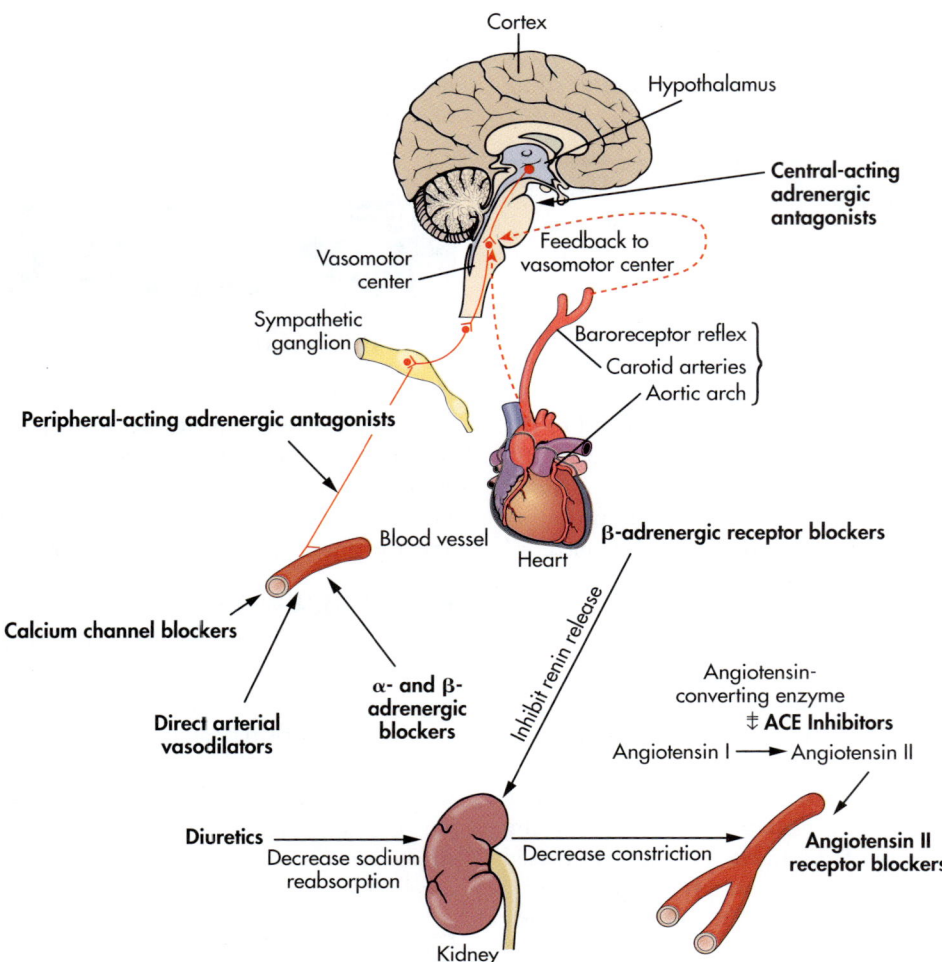

FIGURE 13-11 Sites of action of antihypertensive agents.

composed mostly of platelets, but they also involve the chemical substances that contribute to the coagulation process (in particular, fibrinogen and fibrin). Myocardial infarctions and strokes are often the result of arterial thrombi.

AGENTS THAT AFFECT BLOOD COAGULATION

Drugs that affect blood coagulation may be classified as *antiplatelet, anticoagulant,* and *fibrinolytic agents.* They each act at a different phase in the clotting process.

Antiplatelet Agents. Drugs that interfere with platelet aggregation are known as *antiplatelet* drugs. These drugs sometimes are prescribed prophylactically (as a precaution) for patients at risk of developing arterial clots. They also are prescribed for those who have suffered myocardial infarction or stroke. Antiplatelet agents also are given to patients with certain valvular heart diseases, valvular prostheses (replacement valves), and various intracardiac shunts

(a passage that allows blood to flow from one part of the heart to another). Among the most common oral antiplatelet drugs are ***aspirin,*** dipyridamole (Persantine), clopidogrel (Plavix), and ticlopidine (Ticlid).

> **NOTE**
>
> Platelet adhesion, activation, and aggregation that result in the formation of an arterial thrombus are pivotal in the pathogenesis of acute coronary syndromes (acute myocardial infarctions). Studies indicate that the administration of a glycoprotein IIb/IIIa receptor antagonist may reduce ischemic complications after plaque fissure or rupture. (These drugs inhibit glycoprotein receptors in the membrane of platelets and help prevent platelet aggregation.) These drugs may be included along with aspirin, heparin, and beta blockers during in-hospital reperfusion therapy for select patients. Examples of glycoprotein IIb/IIIa inhibitors include ***abciximab*** (ReoPro), ***eptifibatide*** (Integrilin), and ***tirofiban*** (Aggrastat).

Anticoagulant Agents. Anticoagulant drug therapy is used to prevent intravascular thrombosis. The therapy works by decreasing blood coagulability. Such therapy commonly is used to prevent postoperative thromboembolism. Anticoagulant agents also are used during hemodialysis and in reperfusion therapy for some patients with acute coronary syndromes (see Chapter 22). Anticoagulant therapy is a preventive measure against future clot formation. The therapy has no direct effect on a blood clot that has formed already or on ischemic tissue injured by inadequate blood supply as a result of a thrombus. The major side effect of anticoagulant therapy is hemorrhage and bleeding complications. Examples of anticoagulant agents include warfarin (Coumadin) and *heparin.*

> **NOTE**
> Natural (unfractionated) heparin and its derivative, low-molecular-weight heparin (LMWH), are effective and indicated for the prevention of venous thromboembolism. Heparin also is indicated for the treatment of venous thrombosis, pulmonary embolism, and acute myocardial infarction. In addition, heparin is administered to patients who undergo cardiac surgery using cardiac bypass, vascular surgery, and coronary angioplasty; in patients with coronary stents; and in selected patients with coagulation disorders.[12]
> Natural heparin is usually administered in the hospital. It is given intravenously (IV) and requires laboratory monitoring. LMWH (e.g., enoxaparin [Lovenox, Clexane]) may be given IV or subcutaneously in weight-adjusted doses. LMWH does not require laboratory monitoring and therefore may be given in the out-of-hospital or home setting. LMWH is given in the prehospital setting to some patients with ischemic chest pain and myocardial infarction (see Chapter 22).

Fibrinolytic Agents. Fibrinolytic drugs dissolve clots after their formation. They do so by promoting the digestion of fibrin. Fibrinolytic therapy has become the treatment of choice for treating acute myocardial infarction in certain groups of patients. Fibrinolytic therapy also has become the treatment of choice in managing some stroke patients. The goal is to reestablish blood flow and prevent ischemia and tissue death. Fibrinolytic therapy also has been used in acute pulmonary embolism, deep vein thrombosis, and peripheral arterial occlusion. Fibrinolytics are used in the prehospital setting in some areas of the United States. These drugs include anistreplase (APSAC, Eminase), *alteplase* (t-PA), *reteplase* (Retavase), *streptokinase* (Streptase), and tenecteplase (TNKase) (see Chapter 22 and Emergency Drug Index).

> **CRITICAL THINKING**
> Fibrinolytics have the potential to dissolve clots. This in turn may reverse the serious effects of myocardial infarction and stroke. So why are fibrinolytics not given to everyone who is suspected of having these conditions?

Antihemophilic Agents

Hemophilia (further described in Chapter 32) is a group of hereditary bleeding disorders in which the affected individual lacks one of the factors needed for the coagulation of blood. These disorders are characterized by persistent and uncontrollable bleeding that can occur after even a minor injury. Bleeding may occur into joints, the urinary tract, and at times the CNS. *Hemophilia A* is the classic form of hemophilia and is caused by a deficiency of factor VIII. *Hemophilia B* results from a deficiency in factor IX complex. Replacement therapy of the missing clotting factor can be effective in managing hemophilia. These include factor VIII (Factorate), factor IX (Konyne), and antiinhibitor coagulant complex (Autoplex).

> **NOTE**
> Coagulation factors refer to the 13 proteins contained in blood plasma. These proteins interact to produce a blood clot.

Hemostatic Agents

Hemostatic agents hasten clot formation. The formation of clots in turn reduces bleeding. Systemic hemostatic agents (e.g., Amicar and Cyklokapron) generally are used to control rapid blood loss after surgery by inhibiting fibrinolysis. Topical hemostatic agents (e.g., Gelfoam and Novacell) are used to control capillary bleeding during surgical and dental procedures.

Hemostatic agents are now being used in the prehospital setting and in combat medical care. Celox, WoundStat, and QuickClot work by absorbing plasma from blood, thereby reducing clotting times. Chitosan, a substance derived from shrimp shells, is another hemostatic agent that adheres to and seals wounds[13] (see Chapter 38).

Blood and Blood Components

The healthy body maintains a normal balance of blood and its components. However, illness and injury such as hemorrhage, burns, and dehydration may affect this balance. These conditions may impair this balance and require replacement therapy (see Appendix: Advanced Care Procedures for Critical Care Paramedics).

Knowledge of how to manage an imbalance of blood or blood components is crucial. The usual treatment of choice is to replace the sole blood component that is deficient. Replacement therapy may include transfusing the following:

- Whole blood (red blood cells and plasma; rarely used)
- Packed red blood cells (red blood cells without plasma)
- Fresh-frozen plasma (plasma without red blood cells or platelets)
- Plasma expanders (dextran)
- Platelets
- Cryoprecipitate (multiple clotting factors)

BOX 13-24 Examples of Antihyperlipidemic Drugs

Atorvastatin (Lipitor)
Fenofibrate (Tricor)
Fluvastatin (Lescol)
Gemfibrozil (Lopid)
Pravastatin (Pravachol)
Simvastatin (Zocor)
Nicotinic acid (Niacin)
Rosuvastatin (Crestor)

BOX 13-25 Emergency Drugs: Respiratory System

Albuterol (Proventil, Ventolin)
Levalbuterol (Xopenex)
Epinephrine (Adrenalin) 1:1000
Racemic epinephrine (microNephrin)

- Fibrinogen (found in fresh frozen plasma [FFP] and cryoprecipitate)
- Albumin
- Gamma globulins (antibodies)

Antihyperlipidemic Drugs

Hyperlipidemia refers to an excess of lipids in the plasma. Several types of hyperlipidemia occur; all are associated with elevated levels of cholesterol and triglycerides (described in Chapter 2). This condition is thought to play a role in the development of atherosclerosis. Thus antihyperlipidemic drugs sometimes are used along with diet and exercise to control serum lipid levels (Box 13-24).

LOOK AGAIN
See Chapter 2: Well Being of the Paramedic, pp. 25-28.

SECTION SIX
Drugs That Affect the Respiratory System

REVIEW OF ANATOMY AND PHYSIOLOGY

The respiratory system includes all structures that are involved in the exchange of oxygen and carbon dioxide. Serious narrowing of any portion of the respiratory tract may be an indication for drug therapy (Box 13-25). Emergencies involving the respiratory system usually are caused by reversible conditions such as asthma, emphysema with infection, and foreign body airway obstruction (see Chapter 15).

LOOK AGAIN
See Chapter 10: Review of Human Systems, pp. 191-196.

Smooth muscle fibers line the tracheobronchial tree. They directly influence the diameter of the airways. The bronchial smooth muscle tone is maintained by impulses from the autonomic nervous system. Parasympathetic fibers from the vagus nerve stimulate bronchial smooth muscle through the release of acetylcholine. This neurotransmitter interacts with the muscarinic receptors on the membranes of the cell, producing bronchoconstriction.

Sympathetic fibers mainly affect beta$_2$ receptors in the lungs through the release of epinephrine from the adrenal medulla and the release of norepinephrine from the peripheral sympathetic nerves. The epinephrine reaches the lungs via the circulatory system. Epinephrine interacts with beta$_2$ receptors to produce smooth muscle relaxation and bronchodilation. Thus the beta$_2$ receptor plays the dominant role in bronchial muscle tone. (Although beta$_1$ receptors also are found on bronchial smooth muscle, their ratio to beta$_2$ receptors is 1:3.)

Bronchodilators

Bronchodilator drugs are the primary treatment for obstructive pulmonary disease such as asthma, chronic bronchitis, and emphysema. These drugs are classified as sympathomimetic drugs or xanthine derivatives. Many of these drugs are administered by inhalation via a nebulizer or pressure cartridge (see Chapter 24).

SYMPATHOMIMETIC DRUGS

Sympathomimetic drugs are grouped according to their effects on receptors. Nonselective adrenergic drugs have alpha, beta$_1$ (cardiac), and beta$_2$ (respiratory) activity. Nonselective beta-adrenergic drugs have beta$_1$ and beta$_2$ effects. Selective beta$_2$-receptor drugs act primarily on beta$_2$ receptors in the lungs (bronchial smooth muscle). Box 13-26 summarizes the alpha, beta$_1$, and beta$_2$ activities of the adrenergic drugs used as bronchodilators.

Nonselective adrenergic drugs stimulate alpha and beta receptors. The alpha activity lessens vasoconstriction to reduce mucosal edema. Beta$_2$ activity produces bronchodilation and vasodilation. Undesirable beta$_1$ effects include an increase in heart rate and force of contraction. Undesirable beta$_2$ effects include muscle tremors and CNS stimulation. Examples of nonselective adrenergic drugs include nonprescription epinephrine inhalation aerosol (Bronkaid Mist, Primatene Mist) and epinephrine inhalation solution

BOX 13-26 Alpha, Beta₁, and Beta₂ Activities of Adrenergic Drugs Used as Bronchodilators

Alpha Effects (Vasoconstriction)
Vasoconstriction
Increased blood pressure
Decreased bronchial congestion
Increased duration of action for coadministered beta₂ drugs

Beta₁ Effects
Cardiac stimulation
Increased heart rate
Increased force of contraction
Possible palpitations and dysrhythmias
Relaxation of gastrointestinal tract
Some bronchodilation and increased heart rate
Fewer effects than with subcutaneous administration

Beta₂ Effects
Bronchiole dilation
Stimulation of skeletal muscles (tremors)
Vasodilation (mainly in blood vessels supplying muscle)
Glycogenolysis

Central Nervous System Effects
Anxiety
Dizziness
Insomnia
Irritability
Nervousness
Sweating
Lower incidence of systemic effects than with subcutaneous administration

(Adrenalin). **Racemic epinephrine** inhalation solution (microNephrin) is another nonselective adrenergic drug. It is used mainly to manage upper airway swelling associated with *croup* (see Chapter 24).

Nonselective beta-adrenergic drugs are not selective for beta₂ receptors. Thus they have a wide range of effects (described earlier in this chapter). This class of drug is no longer recommended for the management of asthma.[14] Examples of nonselective beta-adrenergic drugs include **epinephrine** (Adrenalin, Asmolin, and others), ephedrine (Ephed II), and ethylnorepinephrine (Bronkephrine), each of which has some alpha activity; isoproterenol inhalation solution (Aerolone, Vapo-Iso, Isuprel); and isoproterenol inhalation aerosol (Isuprel Mistometer, Norisodrine Aerotrol).

The action of beta₂-selective drugs lessens the incidence of unwanted cardiac effects caused by beta₁-adrenergic agents. Patients with hypertension, cardiac disease, or diabetes can better tolerate this group of bronchodilators. Examples of selective beta₂-receptor drugs include **albuterol** (Proventil, Ventolin), **levalbuterol** (Xopenex), pirbuterol (Maxair), bitolterol (Tornalate), salmeterol (Serevent),

formoterol (Foradil aerolizer), and isoetharine (Bronkosol, others).

NOTE
Some bronchodilators act rapidly ("rescue inhalers") whereas others provide slow relief. If a patient claims to have used his or her inhaler, it is important to ask the patient which inhaler was used.

XANTHINE DERIVATIVES

The xanthine group of drugs includes caffeine, theophylline, and theobromine. These drugs relax smooth muscle (particularly bronchial smooth muscle), stimulate cardiac muscle and the CNS, increase diaphragmatic contractility, and promote diuresis through increased renal perfusion. The action of various theophylline compounds depends on the concentration of theophylline, which is the active ingredient. Theophylline products vary in their rate of absorption and therapeutic effects. Aminophylline (Amoline, Somophyllin, Theo-Dur, Aminophyllin), dyphylline (Dilor, Droxine, Lufyllin), and theophylline (Bronkodyl, Elixophyllin, Somophyllin-T, others) are some of the many theophylline-containing preparations. Theophylline preparations generally are not considered a first-line drug in the treatment of acute reactive airway disease such as asthma. This is because of their high side effect profile and slow onset of action.

Other Respiratory Drugs

A number of other drugs can be used to treat asthma and other obstructive pulmonary diseases. These drugs include prophylactic asthmatic agents such as cromolyn sodium (Intal, sodium cromoglycate); aerosol corticosteroid agents such as beclomethasone dipropionate (Vanceril inhaler, Beclovent); **dexamethasone** (Decadron); antileukotrienes such as montelukast (Singulair) and zafirlukast (Accolate); and muscarinic antagonists (anticholinergics) such as **ipratropium** (Atrovent) and glycopyrrolate (Robinul). These drugs reduce the allergic or inflammatory response to a variety of stimuli. They also have an effect on bronchial smooth muscle. In the acute care setting, intravenously administered steroids (e.g., **methylprednisolone** [Solu-Medrol]) may be given in an attempt to decrease the inflammatory response and improve airflow.

Mucokinetic Drugs

Mucokinetic drugs are used to move respiratory secretions along the tracheobronchial tree. These agents work by altering the consistency of these secretions. Thus the secretions can be removed from the body more easily. Persons with chronic pulmonary disease often use mucokinetic drugs. These drugs help to clear their respiratory passages. They also improve ciliary activity in the airways. Mucokinetic drugs include diluents (water, saline solution), aerosols, and mucolytic drugs or expectorants (Mucomyst).

> **NOTE**
> *Mucus* is a normal secretion produced by the surface cells in the mucous membranes. *Sputum* is an abnormal viscous secretion. Sputum consists mainly of mucus. Sputum originates in the lower respiratory tract.

Oxygen and Miscellaneous Respiratory Agents

Oxygen is mainly used to treat hypoxia and hypoxemia. Oxygen is a colorless, odorless, and tasteless gas. It is essential for sustaining life. (Oxygen and oxygen delivery are described in detail in Chapter 15.)

DIRECT RESPIRATORY STIMULANTS

Direct respiratory stimulants are known as *analeptics*. These act directly on the medullary center of the brain to increase the rate and depth of respirations. These drugs are considered inferior to mechanical ventilatory measures to treat respiratory depression and to counteract drug-induced respiratory depression caused by anesthetics. An example of a direct respiratory stimulant is doxapram (Dopram).

REFLEX RESPIRATORY STIMULANTS

Spirits of ammonia is given by inhalation and acts as a reflex respiratory stimulant. The noxious vapor is used sometimes in cases of fainting. The vapor works by irritating sensory nerve receptors in the throat and stomach. These nerve receptors send afferent messages to the control centers of the brain to stimulate respiration.

RESPIRATORY DEPRESSANTS

Respiratory depressants include opiates and barbiturate drugs previously described. Respiratory depression is a common side effect of these drugs. However, they seldom are given to intentionally inhibit rate and depth of respiration.

COUGH SUPPRESSANTS

The cough is a protective reflex to expel harmful irritants. It may be *productive* when removing irritants or secretions from the airway, or *nonproductive* (dry and irritating). When the cough is prolonged or secondary to an underlying disorder, treatment with antitussive drugs may be indicated. Box 13-27 presents a few narcotic and nonnarcotic antitussive agents.

BOX 13-27 Examples of Narcotic and Nonnarcotic Antitussive Agents

Narcotic Agent
Codeine

Nonnarcotic Agents
Benzonatate (Tessalon)
Dextromethorphan (Sucrets, Robitussin DM)

ANTIHISTAMINES

Histamine is a chemical mediator found in almost all body tissues. The concentration is highest in the skin, lungs, and gastrointestinal tract. The body releases histamine when exposed to an antigen, such as pollen or insect stings. This results in increased localized blood flow, increased capillary permeability, and swelling of the tissues. In addition, histamine produces contractile action on bronchial smooth muscle.

Allergic responses involving histamines and other chemical mediators include local effects such as angioedema, eczema, rhinitis (runny nose), urticaria (hives), and asthma. Systemic effects from the release of histamine and certain other mediators may result in anaphylaxis (see Chapter 27).

Antihistamines compete with histamine for receptor sites. Thus they prevent the physiological action of histamine. Two types of histamine receptors are H_1 *receptors* (these act mainly on the blood vessels and the bronchioles) and H_2 *receptors* (these act mainly on the gastrointestinal tract). In addition to blocking some actions of histamine, antihistamines also have anticholinergic or atropine-like action. This may result in tachycardia, constipation, drowsiness, sedation, and inhibition of secretions. Most antihistamines have a local anesthetic effect as well. This effect may soothe the skin irritation caused by an allergic reaction. The chief clinical use of antihistamines is for allergic reactions. However, they also sometimes are prescribed to control motion sickness or as a sedative or antiemetic. Examples of antihistamines are dimenhydrinate (Dramamine), **diphenhydramine** (Benadryl), **hydroxyzine** (Vistaril), **promethazine** (Phenergan, others), and the newer H_1-receptor antagonists, for example, loratadine (Claritin), cetirizine (Zyrtec), and fexofenadine (Allegra).

SEROTONIN

Serotonin is a naturally occurring vasoconstrictor material found in platelets and in the cells of the brain and intestine. It has several pharmacological actions, which are exerted on various smooth muscles and nerves. Serotonin is not administered as a drug, but has a major influence on other drugs and some disease states. It is helpful in repairing damaged blood vessels, stimulates smooth muscle contraction, and acts as a neurotransmitter in the CNS, where it has an effect on sleep, pain perception, and some mental illnesses.

ANTISEROTONINS

Antiserotonins are serotonin antagonists. They work to inhibit responses to serotonin and its influence on other drugs and disease states. Specific antiserotonins block smooth muscle contraction and vasoconstriction and inhibit the action of serotonin in the brain. Some antiserotonins are used to treat vascular headaches and allergic disorders. Examples of these drugs include cyproheptadine (Periactin), lysergic acid diethylamide (LSD), and methysergide maleate (Sansert).

SECTION SEVEN
Drugs That Affect the Gastrointestinal System

REVIEW OF ANATOMY AND PHYSIOLOGY

As described in Chapter 10, the gastrointestinal system is composed of the digestive tract, the biliary system, and the pancreas. The primary function of the gastrointestinal system is to provide the body with water, electrolytes, and other nutrients used by cells. Drug therapy for the gastrointestinal system can be divided into two groups: drugs that affect the stomach and drugs that affect the lower gastrointestinal tract. In emergency care, conditions of the stomach or gastrointestinal tract that may require drug therapy usually are limited to nausea and vomiting (Box 13-28.)

LOOK AGAIN

See Chapter 10: Review of Human Systems, pp. 196-199.

Drugs That Affect the Stomach

Conditions of the stomach that may require drug therapy include hyperacidity, hypoacidity, ulcer disease, nausea, vomiting, and hypermotility.

ANTACIDS

Antacids buffer or neutralize hydrochloric acid in the stomach. They are prescribed for the relief of symptoms associated with hyperacidity. These conditions include peptic ulcer, gastritis, esophagitis, heartburn, and hiatal hernia. Common over-the-counter antacids include Alka-Seltzer, Gaviscon, and Rolaids.

ANTIFLATULENTS

Antiflatulents prevent the formation of gas in the gastrointestinal tract. Gas retention is a common condition with diverticulitis, ulcer disease, and spastic or irritable colon (see Chapter 29). These drugs sometimes are used along with antacids. Simethicone (Mylicon) is an example of an antiflatulent.

DIGESTANTS

Digestant drugs promote digestion in the gastrointestinal tract. They work by releasing small amounts of digestive enzymes in the small intestine. Examples of digestants include pancreatin (Creon) and pancrelipase (Pancrease).

EMETICS AND ANTIEMETICS

Vomiting is usually an involuntary action that is coordinated by the emetic center of the medulla. Vomiting may be initiated through the CNS as a secondary reaction to emotion, pain, or disequilibrium (motion sickness); through irritation of the mucosa of the gastrointestinal tract or bowel; or through stimulation from the chemoreceptor trigger zone of the medulla by circulating drugs and toxins (e.g., opiates or digitalis).

Emetics. Emetics induce vomiting. They rarely are administered today as part of the treatment for drug overdoses and poisonings. These drugs include apomorphine and syrup of ipecac. The treatment of drug overdoses and poisoning is addressed further in Chapter 34.

Antiemetics. Drugs used to treat nausea and vomiting include antagonists of histamine, acetylcholine, and dopamine as well as other drugs. These drugs work best when they are given before rather than after nausea and vomiting have begun. For example, drugs used to treat motion sickness or vertigo should be taken 30 minutes before traveling. Common antiemetics include scopolamine (Transderm-Scōp), dimenhydrinate (Dramamine), *diphenhydramine* (Benadryl), *hydroxyzine* (Vistaril), meclizine (Antivert), *promethazine* (Phenergan), prochlorperazine (Compazine), and *ondansetron* (Zofran).

NOTE

Cannabinoids are drugs that are derived from hemp plants. They have been used experimentally to prevent vomiting in patients who receive cancer chemotherapy. Examples of these drugs include dronabinol (Marinol) and nabilone (Cesamet). These drugs use a synthetic derivative of the active ingredient in marijuana.

BOX 13-28 Emergency Drugs: Gastrointestinal System

Activated charcoal
Diphenhydramine (Benadryl)
Hydroxyzine (Vistaril)
Metoclopramide (Reglan)
Ondansetron (Zofran)
Prochlorperazine (Compazine)
Promethazine (Phenergan)

SHOW ME THE EVIDENCE

Researchers in Oregon investigated the effect of ondansetron (Zofran). In the 6 months of data collection, they evaluated the effect of administration of this drug to 952 EMS patients who had nausea and vomiting. They found no adverse effects. Vomiting decreased significantly in 462 patients (from 60% to 30%). They concluded that ondansetron was moderately effective. The researchers recommended further studies to compare this drug to other antiemetics.

From Warden CR, Moreno R, Daya M: Prospective evaluation of ondansetron for undifferentiated nausea and vomiting in the prehospital setting, *PEC* 12(1):87-91, 2008.

CYTOPROTECTIVE AGENTS

Cytoprotective agents are drugs that protect cells from damage. They are used along with other drugs to treat peptic ulcer disease by protecting the gastric mucosa. Examples of these drugs include sucralfate (Carafate) and misoprostol (Cytotec).

H₂-RECEPTOR ANTAGONISTS

As described previously, the action of histamine is mediated through H_2 receptors. Histamine has been associated with gastric acid secretion. H_2-receptor antagonists block the H_2 receptors. They reduce the volume of gastric acid secretion and its acid content. Examples of H_2-receptor antagonists include cimetidine (Tagamet), ranitidine (Zantac), and famotidine (Pepcid).

PROTON PUMP INHIBITORS

Proton pump inhibitors are used for treatment of symptomatic gastroesophageal reflux disease, short-term treatment of erosive esophagitis, and maintenance of erosive esophagitis healing. Some agents also are approved for use with antibiotics to treat *Helicobacter pylori* infection (associated with duodenal ulcers). The proton pump (potassium adenosine triphosphate enzyme system) is the final pathway for secretion of hydrochloric acid by the parietal cells of the stomach. Proton pump inhibitors decrease hydrochloric acid secretion by inhibiting the actions of the parietal cells. In addition, the gastric pH of the stomach is altered. Examples of proton pump inhibitors include esomeprazole (Nexium), lansoprazole (Prevacid), omeprazole (Prilosec), pantoprazole (Protonix), and rabeprazole (AcipHex).

Drugs That Affect the Lower Gastrointestinal Tract

Constipation and diarrhea are two common conditions of the lower gastrointestinal tract. Both conditions may require drug therapy. Drugs used to manage these conditions include laxatives and antidiarrheals.

LAXATIVES

Laxatives produce defecation. They are used to evacuate the bowel and to soften hardened stool for easier passage. Situations that may indicate the need for laxative use include the following:

- Constipation
- Neurological diseases (e.g., multiple sclerosis or Parkinson's disease)
- Pregnancy
- Rectal disorders
- Drug poisoning
- Surgery and endoscopic examination

Numerous types of laxatives are available. Many can be purchased without a prescription. Examples include saline laxatives (Epsom salt, Milk of Magnesia), stimulant laxatives (Dulcolax, castor oil, Ex-Lax), bulk-forming laxatives (Mitrolan, Metamucil), lubricant laxatives (mineral oil), fecal moistening agents (Colace, glycerin suppositories), and those used for bowel evacuation (GoLYTELY, Chronulac). Regular or excessive use of laxatives is common in older adults and in those with eating disorders. Laxative abuse may result in permanent bowel damage and electrolyte imbalance.

ANTIDIARRHEAL DRUGS

Antidiarrheal drugs are used to reduce an abnormal frequency of bowel evacuation. Common causes of acute and chronic diarrhea include bacterial or viral invasion, drugs, diet, and numerous disease states (e.g., diabetes insipidus and inflammatory bowel syndromes). Drugs used to treat diarrhea include the following:

- Adsorbents
  Bismuth subsalicylate (Pepto-Bismol)
- Anticholinergics
  Donnatal
- Opiates
  Paregoric
  Codeine
- Other agents
  Diphenoxylate (Lomotil)
  Loperamide (Imodium)

SECTION EIGHT
Drugs That Affect the Eye and Ear

TREATMENT OF EYE DISORDERS

Drugs That Affect the Eye

Drugs used to treat eye disorders include antiglaucoma agents, mydriatics and cycloplegics, antiinfective/antiinflammatory agents, and topical anesthetics.

ANTIGLAUCOMA AGENTS

Glaucoma is an eye disease in which the pressure of the fluid in the eye is abnormally high (see Chapter 23). The pressure is so high that it causes compression or obstruction of the small internal blood vessels of the eye, the fibers of the optic nerve, or both. The result is nerve fiber destruction and partial or complete loss of vision. Glaucoma is a common eye disorder in persons over age 60 and is responsible for 15% of blindness in adults in the United States.[11] Agents used to reduce the pressure in chronic glaucoma include cholinergic and anticholinesterase drugs. Some of these drugs (e.g., pilocarpine) dilate the pupil of the eye, and some constrict the pupil; others (e.g., acetazolamide) slow the secretion of aqueous fluid. If these drug therapies fail, surgery may be indicated. If glaucoma is diagnosed early, drugs can control it for a lifetime. Most physicians recommend testing for glaucoma every 2 years after age 35.

MYDRIATIC AND CYCLOPLEGIC AGENTS

Mydriatic and cycloplegic agents are applied topically. They cause dilation of the pupils and paralysis of accommodation to light. They are used to treat inflammation and to relieve ocular pain by helping the eye to rest. These drugs are used during routine eye examinations and in ocular surgery as well. Examples of these drugs include atropine ophthalmic solution, cyclopentolate hydrochloride ophthalmic solution (Cyclogyl), homatropine ophthalmic solution (Isopto Homatropine), epinephrine, and oxymetazoline (OcuClear).

> ### CRITICAL THINKING
> You are caring for an older adult patient. This patient had mydriatic eye drops instilled by an ophthalmologist. If you did not know this history, what might you consider after your physical examination of this patient?

ANTIINFECTIVE/ANTIINFLAMMATORY AGENTS

Antiinfective and antiinflammatory agents are used to treat eye conditions such as conjunctivitis, stye, and keratitis (corneal inflammation caused by bacterial infection). Examples of these drugs include bacitracin (Baciguent), chloramphenicol (Chloroptic), erythromycin (Ilotycin), and natamycin (Natacyn).

TOPICAL ANESTHETIC AGENTS

Local anesthetics are used to prevent pain in surgical procedures and eye examinations. They also are used in the treatment of some eye injuries (e.g., a corneal abrasion). These drugs usually have a rapid onset (within 20 seconds) and last 15 to 20 minutes. Examples of these drugs include proparacaine (Ophthaine, Alcaine) and *tetracaine* (Ak-T-Caine, Pontocaine). Other eye medications include artificial tear solutions and lubricants to provide additional moisture, irrigation solutions, and antiallergic agents to relieve symptoms of itching, tearing, and redness. Many of these drugs and solutions are available without a prescription.

Drugs That Affect the Ear

Drugs used to treat disorders of the external ear canal include antibiotics, steroid/antibiotic combinations, and miscellaneous preparations. These drugs include the following:
- Antibiotics used to treat infections
  Chloramphenicol (Chloromycetin Otic)
  Gentamicin sulfate (Garamycin)
- Steroid/antibiotic combinations used to treat superficial bacterial infections
  Neomycin sulfate/polymyxin B sulfate/hydrocortisone (Cortisporin Otic)
  Neomycin/colistin/hydrocortisone (Coly-Mycin S Otic)
- Miscellaneous preparations used to treat earwax accumulation, inflammation, pain, fungal infections, and other minor conditions

Boric acid in isopropyl alcohol (Aurocaine 2)
Triethanolamine with chlorobutanol in propylene glycol (Cerumenex)

Persons with inner ear infections or serious illness associated with hearing impairment may require antibiotics with systemic effects, following physician evaluation. These actions will help to prevent complications (see Chapter 23).

> # SECTION NINE
> Drugs That Affect the Endocrine System

REVIEW OF ANATOMY AND PHYSIOLOGY

The endocrine system works to control and integrate body functions. (Box 13-29 presents emergency drugs that affect the endocrine system.) Information from various parts of the body is carried via blood-borne hormones to distant sites. Hormones are natural chemical substances. They act after they have been secreted into the bloodstream from endocrine glands (ductless glands that secrete internally). These glands include the anterior and posterior pituitary, thyroid, parathyroid, and adrenal glands and the thymus, pancreas, testes, and ovaries. Hormones from the various endocrine glands work together to regulate vital processes, including the following:
- Secretory and motor activities of the digestive tract
- Energy production
- Composition and volume of extracellular fluid
- Adaptation (e.g., acclimatization and immunity)
- Growth and development
- Reproduction and lactation

> ### LOOK AGAIN
>
> See Chapter 10: Review of Human Systems, pp. 177-178.

Drugs That Affect the Pituitary Gland

As described in Chapter 10, the hormones of the anterior and posterior pituitary gland are important for regulating the secretion of other hormones in the body. Box 13-30 lists

> ### BOX 13-29 Emergency Drugs: Endocrine System
>
> Dexamethasone (Decadron)
> Dextrose 50%
> Glucagon
> Insulin
> Methylprednisolone (Solu-Medrol)
> Oxytocin (Pitocin, Syntocinon)

BOX 13-30 Drugs That Affect the Anterior and Posterior Pituitary Gland

Anterior Pituitary Gland Drugs
Used to treat growth failure in children caused by growth hormone deficiency:
Somatrem (Protropin)
Somatropin (Humatrope)

Posterior Pituitary Gland Drugs
Used to treat the symptoms of diabetes insipidus resulting from antidiuretic hormone deficiency:
Vasopressin (Pitressin)

BOX 13-31 Drugs That Affect the Thyroid and Parathyroid Glands

Thyroid Drugs
Used to treat hypothyroidism and to prevent goiters:
Thyroxine
Iodine products
Levothyroxine (Synthroid, Levoxyl)

Parathyroid Drugs
Used to treat hyperparathyroidism:
Vitamin D
Calcium supplements

BOX 13-32 Drugs That Affect the Adrenal Cortex

Glucocorticoids
Betamethasone (Celestone)
Dexamethasone (Decadron)
Methylprednisolone (Solu-Medrol)
Triamcinolone (Aristocort)

Mineralocorticoids
Desoxycorticosterone acetate (DOCA)
Fludrocortisone (Florinef)

Adrenal Steroid Inhibitors
Aminoglutethimide (Cytadren)
Metyrapone (Metopirone)

---

drugs that affect the anterior and posterior pituitary. (Disorders of the endocrine glands are described further in Chapter 26.)

Drugs That Affect the Thyroid and Parathyroid Glands

The thyroid hormone controls the rate of metabolic processes and is required for normal growth and development. Parathyroid hormone regulates the level of ionized calcium in the blood. Parathyroid hormone does this through the release of calcium from bone, the absorption of calcium from the intestine, and the regulation of calcium excretion by the kidneys.

Disorders of the thyroid gland include goiter (enlargement of the thyroid gland), hypothyroidism (thyroid hormone deficiency), and hyperthyroidism (thyroid hormone excess). Disorders of the parathyroid include hypoparathyroidism and hyperparathyroidism. Box 13-31 lists the drugs used to treat these disorders (see Chapter 26).

Drugs That Affect the Adrenal Cortex

The adrenal cortex secretes three major classes of steroid hormones: glucocorticoids (cortisol), mineralocorticoids (primarily aldosterone), and sex hormones. Glucocorticoids raise blood glucose level, deplete tissue proteins, and suppress the inflammatory reaction. Mineralocorticoids regulate electrolyte and water balance. Sex hormones are estrogen, progesterone, and testosterone and are produced in small amounts by men and women. The sex hormones have little physiological effect under normal circumstances. Box 13-32 lists drugs that affect the adrenal cortex. Two disorders of the adrenal cortex are Addison's disease (adrenal cortical hypofunction) and Cushing's disease (adrenal cortical hyperfunction) (see Chapter 26).

Drugs That Affect the Pancreas

As described in Chapter 10, the pancreas is an exocrine gland and an endocrine gland. The exocrine portion secretes hormones into ducts, providing digestive juices to the small intestine. The endocrine portion of the pancreas consists of pancreatic islets (islets of Langerhans). These cells produce the hormones that directly enter the circulatory system.

Hormones of the Pancreas

The pancreatic hormones play a key role in regulating the concentration of certain nutrients in the circulatory system. The pancreas secretes two major hormones: insulin and glucagon.

Insulin is the primary hormone that regulates glucose metabolism. In general, insulin increases the ability of the liver, adipose tissue, and muscle to take up and use glucose. Glucose not immediately needed for energy is stored in the skeletal muscle, liver, and other tissues. This stored form of glucose is called *glycogen*.

Glucagon mainly influences the liver, although it has some effect on skeletal muscle and adipose tissue. In general, glucagon stimulates the liver to break down glycogen so that glucose is released into the blood. Glucagon also inhibits the uptake of glucose by muscle and fat cells. The balancing action of these two hormones protects the body from hyperglycemia (high blood sugar) and hypoglycemia (low blood sugar).

This balance of hormonal actions is important when one considers the metabolic problems that can occur in

BOX 13-33 Drugs That Affect the Pancreas

Insulin Preparations

Rapid Acting
Insulin lispro (Humalog)
Insulin aspart (NovoLog)

Short Acting
Regular (Humulin R, Novolin R)

Intermediate Acting
NPH (Humulin N, Novolin N)
Lente (Humulin L, Novolin N)

Long Acting
Insulin Detemir (Levemir)
Insulin Glargine (Lantus)

Oral Hypoglycemic Agents

Glimepiride (Amaryl)
Glipizide (Glucotrol)
Glyburide (Micronase, Diabeta)
Metformin (Glucophage)
Pioglitazone (Actos)

Combination Drugs
Glyburide/metformin (Glucovance)
Glipizide/metformin (Metaglip)
Rosiglitazone/metformin (Avandamet)

Hyperglycemic Agents

Dextrose
Diazoxide (Proglycem)
Glucagon
Oral glucose (Glutose, Insta-Glucose)

diabetes mellitus. The relationship of glucagon and insulin to other hormones and substances such as **dextrose 50%** (D50) and **thiamine** (vitamin B$_1$) is addressed in Chapter 26. Box 13-33 lists drugs that affect the pancreas.

SECTION TEN
Drugs That Affect the Reproductive System

TREATMENT OF DISORDERS OF THE REPRODUCTIVE SYSTEM

Drugs That Affect the Female Reproductive System

Drugs that affect the female reproductive system include synthetic and natural substances such as hormones, oral contraceptives, ovulatory stimulants, and drugs used to treat infertility.

LOOK AGAIN
See Chapter 10: Review of Human Systems, pp. 202-205.

FEMALE SEX HORMONES

Two main types of hormones are secreted by the ovary: estrogen and progesterone. Supplemental estrogen is indicated for estrogen deficiency or replacement, treatment of breast cancer, and as prophylaxis for osteoporosis in postmenopausal women (controversial). Progesterone (and synthetic progestins) may be used to treat hormonal imbalance, endometriosis, and specific cancers and to prevent pregnancy when used properly.

ORAL CONTRACEPTIVES

Oral contraception is the most effective form of birth control and is known as "the pill." Oral contraception is a combination of estrogen and progesterone. This combination results in the suppression of ovulation (see Chapter 31). Several types of oral contraceptives and drug combinations are available. All are nearly 100% effective in preventing pregnancy, when taken properly.

DID YOU KNOW?
Emergency contraception is a method of preventing pregnancy to be used after a contraceptive fails or after unprotected sex. It is not for routine use.[15] Emergency contraceptives (Previn and Plan B™) are also known as post-coital pills, or morning-after pills. They contain the hormones estrogen and progestin (levonorgestrel), either separately or in combination. Emergency contraceptives can reduce the chance of pregnancy when taken as directed up to 72 hours (3 days) after unprotected sex. These drugs have recently been approved by the FDA for women 17 years of age and older. They are available without prescription and do not require parental consent.

OVULATORY STIMULANTS AND INFERTILITY DRUGS

The absence of ovulation in women is *anovulation*. The condition may be pathological in women with abnormal bleeding or infertility. The condition sometimes is treated with gonadotropins, thyroid preparations, estrogen, and synthetic agents. One example of a drug used to induce ovulation and increase fertility is clomiphene citrate (Clomid).

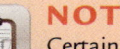

NOTE
Certain drugs are used during labor and delivery. These drugs help to increase (oxytocin [Pitocin]) or decrease (ritodrine [Yutopar]) uterine contractility. In prehospital care, oxytocin is used to control hemorrhages that occur after the delivery of the infant and placenta (see Chapter 46).

Drugs That Affect the Male Reproductive System

The male sex hormone is testosterone. Adequate amounts of this hormone are needed for normal development and for the maintenance of male sex characteristics.

>
> **LOOK AGAIN**
> See Chapter 10: Review of Human Systems, pp. 201-202.

Testosterone therapy is indicated for the treatment of hormone deficiency (e.g., testicular failure), impotence, delayed puberty, female breast cancer, and anemia. The choice of dosage and length of therapy depend on the diagnosis, age of the patient, and intensity of side effects/adverse reactions. An example of an oral testosterone drug is methyltestosterone (Metandren).

>
> **NOTE**
> *Impotence* is the inability of a man to achieve or maintain an erection. This can lead to decreased sexual function. The condition afflicts as many as 30 million men in the United States.[16]

Drugs That Affect Sexual Behavior

Sexual drive (libido) can be affected by psychological, social, and physiological factors or by a combination of these. Negative effects of these factors can result in a lack of interest in sexual activity in men and women and impotence in men.

DRUGS THAT IMPAIR LIBIDO AND SEXUAL GRATIFICATION

Some drugs interfere with sympathetic nervous stimulation. At times they may cause sexual dysfunction. Drugs may interfere with the nervous system mechanisms (directly and indirectly) that are responsible for sexual arousal. Some of these drugs include antihypertensives, antihistamines, antispasmodics, sedatives and tranquilizers, antidepressants, alcohol, and barbiturates.

DRUGS THAT ENHANCE LIBIDO AND SEXUAL GRATIFICATION

A patient may change medicines (under physician supervision) to avoid drug-induced sexual dysfunction. In addition, a patient may be prescribed drugs to enhance libido and sexual gratification. Drugs that enhance sexual function include levodopa (L-dopa), tadalafil (Cialis), vardenifil (Levitra), and sildenafil citrate (Viagra).

>
> **NOTE**
> The administration of nitroglycerin (Nitrostat) or nitrate/nitrite medications is contraindicated in patients who have taken Cialis, Levitra, or Viagra within the previous 24 to 48 hours because the combination can cause a lethal drop in blood pressure. Other drugs that may produce untoward effects in patients taking drugs to enhance sexual gratification include some antibiotics, cimetidine, and some antihypertensive medications.[17] The paramedic should question the patient about the use of sexual enhancement drugs before administering any of these medications.

SECTION ELEVEN
Drugs Used in Neoplastic Diseases

ANTINEOPLASTIC AGENTS

Antineoplastic agents are used in cancer chemotherapy. They are used to prevent the increase of malignant cells (Box 13-34). These drugs do not directly kill tumor cells. Rather they interfere with cell reproduction or replication through various mechanisms.

>
> **NOTE**
> Any person who handles antineoplastic agents should be trained properly in the safety procedures. These drugs are considered cytotoxic (toxic to human cells).

Antineoplastic agents are nonselective. They are injurious to all cells in the body. Side effects from these drugs may include infection, hemorrhage, nausea and vomiting, and changes in bowel habits. Short-term toxicity from these agents may affect the pulmonary, cardiovascular, renal, and integumentary systems. Prehospital care for these patients mainly is supportive and is aimed at providing comfort measures and emotional support.

BOX 13-34 Examples of Antineoplastic Agents*

Doxorubicin (Adriamycin)
5-Fluorouracil (Adrucil)
Mechlorethamine (Mustargen)
Methotrexate (Amethopterin, MTX)
Streptozocin (Zanosar)
Cistiplatin (Platinol-AQ)
Carmustine (BCNU)
Chlorambucil (Leukeran)
Cyclophosphamide (Cytoxan)
Melphalan (Alkera)
Tamoxifen (Nolvadex)
Interferon

*Varies greatly, depending on the type of cancer

TREATMENT OF INFECTIOUS DISEASE AND INFLAMMATION

Antibiotics

Antibiotics are used to treat local or systemic infection. Antibiotics kill or suppress the growth of microorganisms. They do this by disrupting the bacterial cell wall, by disturbing the functions of the cell membrane, or by interfering with the metabolic functions of the cell. This group of drugs includes penicillins, cephalosporins, and related products; macrolide antibiotics; tetracyclines; fluoroquinolones; and miscellaneous antibiotic agents (e.g., metronidazole [Flagyl] and spectinomycin [Trobicin]). Antibiotics are much more toxic to bacteria than they are to a patient. Some antibiotics, though, may produce hypersensitivity. This can lead to a fatal reaction if the drug is given to a sensitized patient (see Chapter 27).

> **NOTE**
> In time, some bacteria that are at first sensitive to antibiotics may become resistant to them. The bacteria develop ways to evade the effect of a drug. Widespread use and misuse of antibiotics lead to the development of resistant strains of bacteria. Bacterial resistance may even complicate treatment when a person is infected with an antibiotic-resistant organism.

PENICILLINS

Penicillins are active against gram-positive and some gram-negative bacteria (Box 13-35). Penicillins are used to treat many infections, including tonsillitis, pharyngitis, bronchitis, and pneumonia. Examples of penicillins include amoxicillin (Amoxil), ampicillin (Amcill), dicloxacillin (Dynapen), and penicillin V potassium (Pen Vee K). Penicillin can produce severe anaphylactic reactions.

CEPHALOSPORINS

Cephalosporins (and related products) resemble penicillins. Yet they are active against gram-positive and gram-negative bacteria. Cephalosporins are used widely to treat

> **BOX 13-35 Gram's Stain**
>
> Gram's stain is an iodine-based stain used to differentiate various types of bacteria. Examples of gram-positive bacteria are staphylococci, streptococci, and pneumococci. Examples of gram-negative bacteria are gonococci and meningococci.

ear, throat, and respiratory tract infections. They also are useful for treating urinary tract infections. Urinary tract infections often are caused by bacteria that are resistant to penicillin-type antibiotics. Examples of cephalosporins and related products include cefazolin (Ancef), cephalothin (Keflin), cephalexin (Keflex), and cefotaxime (Claforan). About 6% to 10% of those who are allergic to penicillins are also allergic to cephalosporins.

MACROLIDE ANTIBIOTICS

Macrolides (erythromycins) are used to treat infections of the skin, chest, throat, and ears. Macrolides are useful for treating pertussis (whooping cough), legionnaires' disease, and pneumonia (see Chapter 28). Examples of erythromycin drugs include Eryc, EMycin, E.E.S, and Erythrocin. Other antibacterial agents include azithromycin (Zithromax) and clarithromycin (Biaxin).

TETRACYCLINES

Tetracyclines are active against many gram-negative and gram-positive organisms (*broad-spectrum*). Tetracyclines commonly are used to treat conditions such as acne, bronchitis, syphilis, gonorrhea, and certain types of pneumonia. Examples of tetracyclines include demeclocycline (Declomycin), doxycycline (Vibramycin), and tetracycline (Achromycin). Tetracyclines may discolor developing teeth. Thus they usually are not prescribed for children under the age of 12 or for pregnant women.

> **CRITICAL THINKING**
> Explain how antibiotics and infectious organisms work like a lock and key.

FLUOROQUINOLONES

Fluoroquinolone antibiotics are the treatment of choice for some human gastrointestinal infections, particularly severe food-borne illness caused by *Campylobacter* or *Salmonella* bacteria. They are also used to treat urinary tract infections, bone and joint infections, some types of pneumonia, and other human illness. Examples of fluoroquinolones include ciprofloxacin (Cipro), gatifloxacin (Tequin), and levofloxacin (Levaquin).

Antifungal and Antiviral Drugs

As discussed, persons can be infected by bacterial organisms; in addition, they can be infected by fungi and viral diseases.

ANTIFUNGAL DRUGS

Some fungi are harmlessly present at all times in areas of the body such as the mouth, skin, intestines, and vagina. These fungi are prevented from multiplying through competition from bacteria. The actions of the immune system also prevent them from multiplying. Fungal infections are more common and serious in persons taking antibiotics long term (antibiotics destroy the bacterial competition), in those who are immunosuppressed as a complication of illness (e.g., infection with the human immunodeficiency virus), and in those who are taking corticosteroids or immunosuppressant drugs (described later in this chapter). Fungal infections can be classified broadly into superficial infections, subcutaneous infections, and deep infections (Box 13-36). Examples of antifungal drugs include tolnaftate (Tinactin), fluconazole (Diflucan), and nystatin (Mycostatin). About 50 species of fungi can cause illness and sometimes fatal disease in human beings.

> **NOTE**
>
> A few drugs may shorten the duration of symptoms from the influenza viruses, if taken early in the illness. These drugs include oseltamivir (Tamiflu) and zanamivir (Relenza). These drugs are effective against some A and B influenza viruses. Others include amantadine (Symmetrel) and rimantadine (Flumadine). These drugs are effective against influenza virus A (see Chapter 28).

ANTIVIRAL DRUGS

To date, few effective drugs exist to treat minor viral infections such as colds. In fact, few drugs exist for use in any viral infections. This is due partly to the relative delay in the onset of symptoms that occurs in viral diseases. This delay in turn makes drug therapy difficult once the disease is established. Some viral infections are trivial and harmless (e.g., warts). Yet others are serious diseases such as influenza, rabies, acquired immunodeficiency syndrome, and probably some types of cancers (Table 13-6).

Many agents have been tested as antiviral drugs. However, few have been proved to work against specific virus-infected cells without toxic effects to uninfected cells. Examples of specific antiviral drugs include acyclovir (Zovirax) and valacyclovir (Valtrex), which is effective against herpes infection. Others are zidovudine (Retrovir, AZT, ZDV), lamivudine (Epivir), and the combination drug lamivudine/zidovudine (Combivir). At present, these drugs are used to treat human immunodeficiency infection.

PROTEASE INHIBITORS

The complete mechanism of action of protease inhibitors is not understood clearly. Yet they appear to inhibit the replication of retroviruses (e.g., HIV) in acute and chronically infected cells. (A retrovirus is a virus that travels and tries to enter host cells with an RNA genome.) Side effects and adverse reactions of these drugs include nausea and vomiting, headache, malaise, fever, and flulike symptoms. Examples of protease inhibitors include indinavir (Crixivan), ritonavir (Norvir), and saquinavir (Invirase).

> **NOTE**
>
> The administration of antiviral drugs and protease inhibitors to a health care worker who has been exposed to body fluids that may contain human immunodeficiency virus or another virus known or suspected to be resistant to antiviral drugs is important and is a postexposure prophylaxis recommendation by the Centers for Disease Control and Prevention.[18]

Other Antimicrobial Drugs and Antiparasitic Drugs

Various drugs are used to treat atypical microbial infection (e.g., *Mycobacterium tuberculosis* and *M. leprae*) and infection and disease caused by parasite and insect vector (e.g., trichomoniasis and malaria). Box 13-37 lists examples of these drugs and their classifications.

BOX 13-36 Categories of Fungal Infections

Examples of Superficial Infections

Candidiasis (thrush): Affects the genitals or inside of the mouth and vaginal and intertriginous areas
Tinea (including ring worm, athlete's foot, jock itch): Affects external areas of the body

Examples of Subcutaneous Infections (Rare)

Mycetoma (Madura foot): Occurs in tropical countries
     Sporotrichosis: May follow inoculation of spores through a puncture or scratch

Examples of Deep Infections

Aspergillosis
Blastomycosis
Candidiasis (that spreads from its usual site to the esophagus, urinary tract, or other internal sites)
Cryptococcosis
Histoplasmosis

TABLE 13-6 Common Viruses and Viral Diseases or Conditions

Viral Family	Diseases or Conditions
Papovavirus	Warts
Adenovirus	Cold sores, genital herpes, chickenpox, herpes zoster (shingles), congenital abnormalities (cytomegalovirus)
Picornavirus	Poliomyelitis, viral hepatitis A and B, respiratory tract infections, myocarditis, rhinovirus (common cold)
Togavirus	Yellow fever, encephalitis
Orthomyxovirus	Influenza
Paramyxovirus	Mumps, measles, rubella
Coronavirus	Common cold
Rhabdovirus	Rabies
Retrovirus	Acquired immunodeficiency syndrome, degenerative brain disease, possibly cancer

BOX 13-37 Examples of Antimicrobial and Antiparasitic Drugs

Antimalarial Agents
Chloroquine phosphate (Aralen and generics)
Hydroxychloroquine (Plaquenil and generics)
Atovaquone plus proguanil (Malarone)
Quinine (Quinamm) (plus doxycycline, tetracycline, or clindamycin)
Mefloquine (Lariam)

Antitubercular Agents
Isoniazid (Isozid, INH)
Rifampin (Rifadin)
Rifabutin
Rifapentine
Ethambutol
Pyrazinamide

Antiamebic Agents
Emetine
Iodoquinol (Yodoxin)
Paromomycin (Humatin)

Antihelminthic Agents
Diethylcarbamazine (Hetrazan)
Mebendazole (Vermox)

Antiprotozoal Agents
Metronidazole (Flagyl)

Leprostatic Agents
Clofazimine (Lamprene)
Dapsone (DDS)

Cephalosporins
Cephalexin (Keflex)
Cefazolin (Ancef)
Cefaclor (Ceclor)
Cefprozil (Cefzil)
Cefuroxime (Ceftin)
Ceftriaxone (Rocephin)
Cefdinir (Omnicef)
Cefepime (Maxipime)

Fluoroquinolones
Ciprofloxacin (Cipro)
Levofloxacin (Levaquin)
Moxifloxacin (Avelox)

Penicillins
Amoxicillin (Amoxil)
Ampicillin (Polycillin)
Dicloxacillin (Dynapen)
Penicillin G
Penicillin V

NOTE
Malaria is still a prevalent disease in tropical areas and may be carried into the United States by refugees, immigrants, and travelers. Tuberculosis is on the rise in individuals with acquired immunodeficiency syndrome. Tuberculosis also is increasing in persons who are homeless, persons who abuse drugs, and those taking immunosuppressant drugs.

Antiinflammatory and Nonsteroidal Antiinflammatory Drugs

INFLAMMATION

Inflammation is a defense mechanism of body tissues in response to physical trauma, foreign biological and chemical substances, surgery, radiation, and electricity. Regardless of the event producing inflammation, the response is similar. For example, if bacterial infection or an injury to the tissues occurs, chemical mediators are released or activated. These mediators cause vasodilation and increased blood flow (localized warmth and redness at the site). This process brings phagocytes and other leukocytes to the area. The process prevents the spread of infection by limiting the infected site. Finally, phagocytes clean the area. The damaged tissues are repaired.

LOOK AGAIN
See Chapter 11: General Principles of Pathophysiology, pp. 242-245.

Inflammation can be localized or systemic. Local inflammation is confined to a specific area of the body. Symptoms include redness, heat, swelling, pain, and loss of function. Systemic inflammation occurs in many parts of the body. In addition to local symptoms at the inflammation site, red bone marrow produces and releases large numbers of neutrophils that promote phagocytosis, pyrogens stimulate fever production, and increased vascular permeability in severe cases may result in decreased blood volume. Drugs used to treat inflammation or its symptoms may be classified as analgesic-antipyretic drugs and nonsteroidal antiinflammatory drugs (NSAIDs). A number of medications have both properties.

ANALGESIC-ANTIPYRETIC DRUGS

An antipyretic drug is one that reduces fever. The temperature-regulating mechanism of the body is located in the anterior hypothalamus. (This is known as the thermostat of the body.) Normally, the set point of this hypothalamic center is about 98.6° F (37° C). When an inflammatory response occurs in the body, endogenous pyrogens are released by the phagocytic leukocytes. This produces fever. Analgesic-antipyretic drugs work by reversing the effect of the pyrogen on the hypothalamus. Thus the set point of the hypothalamus is returned to normal. The analgesic effects of these drugs act on peripheral pain receptors to block activation. Examples of these drugs include the following:

- Acetaminophen (Datril, Tylenol, Panadol, and others)
- *Aspirin*/acetylsalicylic acid (A.S.A, Aspergum, Bayer Aspirin, and others)
- *Aspirin* (buffered) (Aluprin, Bufferin, Alka-Seltzer, and others)

NONSTEROIDAL ANTIINFLAMMATORY DRUGS

Aspirin is the prototype of the nonsteroidal antiinflammatory drug. New drugs also have been developed, and like *aspirin* they are analgesic, antipyretic, and antiinflammatory. These drugs often are prescribed for patients with various inflammatory conditions. (One such condition is rheumatoid arthritis.) The new drugs also often are prescribed for those who cannot tolerate *aspirin.* In addition, these drugs may be used to treat painful joint disorders (with or without inflammation) such as osteoarthritis, low back pain, and gout. One should note that like *aspirin,* the other nonsteroidal antiinflammatory agents may decrease platelet activity. This could result in gastrointestinal bleeding. Long-term use of some NSAIDs has been linked to an increased risk for heart attack and stroke[19] (see Chapter 33).

> **NOTE**
> Gout is a metabolic disease associated with high levels of uric acid in the blood (hyperuricemia). Gout is characterized by attacks of acute pain, swelling, and tenderness of joints. The condition is treated with uricosuric drugs, colchicine, and nonsteroidal antiinflammatory drugs.

Nonsteroidal antiinflammatory drugs are thought to act by inhibiting specific enzymes so that prostaglandins (substances that promote inflammation and pain) are not formed. Examples of these drugs include the following:

- *Aspirin* (Bayer Timed-Release, Bufferin, and others)
- Diflunisal (Dolobid)
- Ibuprofen (Advil, Motrin, Nuprin, and others)
- Indomethacin (Indocin and others)
- Naproxen (Anaprox, Aleve, Naprosyn)
- Sulindac (Clinoril)
- *Ketorolac* (Toradol)
- Cyclooxygenase-2 inhibitors (COX-2 inhibitors)
  Celecoxib (Celebrex)
  Valdecoxib (Bextra)

SECTION THIRTEEN
Drugs That Affect the Immunological System

REVIEW OF ANATOMY AND PHYSIOLOGY

As described earlier in this chapter and in Chapter 11, the immunological system is composed of cells and organs. These cells and organs defend the body against invasion by foreign substances. Organs and tissues of the immune system include the spleen, tonsils, lymph nodes, and thymus (Figure 13-12).

> **LOOK AGAIN**
> See Chapter 10: Review of Human Systems, pp. 242-247.

Drugs Used to Treat the Immune System

IMMUNOSUPPRESSANTS

Immunosuppressant drugs reduce the activity of the immune system. They do this by suppressing the production and activity of lymphocytes. These drugs are given after transplant surgery to help prevent the rejection of foreign tissues. They also are administered to halt the progress of autoimmune disorders when other treatments are ineffective. Examples of immunosuppressant drugs include antirejection drugs (used in organ transplantation), anticancer drugs, and corticosteroids.

> **CRITICAL THINKING**
> It would be important to know that a patient with altered level of consciousness is taking an immunosuppressant drug. Why is this?

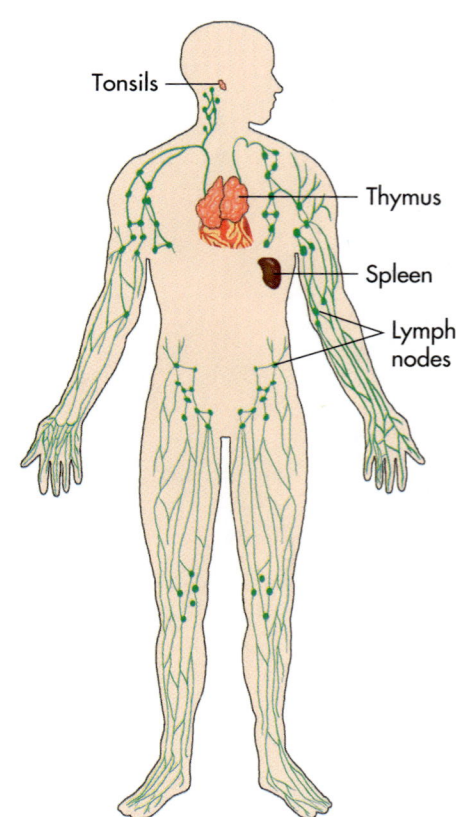

FIGURE 13-12 Organs and tissues of the immune system. (From Clayton BD, Stock YN, Harroun RD: *Basic pharmacology for nurses,* ed 14, St Louis, 2007, Mosby.)

IMMUNOMODULATING AGENTS

Immunomodulating agents are drugs that increase the efficiency of the immune system. These agents activate the immune defenses or modify a biological response to an unwanted stimulus. These drugs include vaccines that protect against specific infectious agents. One group of drugs belonging to this group is the interferons. (They are used to treat viral infections such as hepatitis C and certain types of cancer.) Another drug in this group is zidovudine (AZT, Retrovir). (Zidovudine is used to treat acquired immunodeficiency syndrome.) Some immunomodulating agents enhance the ability of a vaccine to stimulate the immune system. Thus they are added to the vaccine for this reason (see Chapter 28).

SERUMS AND VACCINES

Serum is the clear fluid that separates from blood when blood clots. Serum contains salts, glucose, and proteins. Serum also includes antibodies formed by the immune system. Antibodies are formed to fight against infection. Serum from the blood of a person (or in rare cases an animal) infected with a microorganism usually contains antibodies. Therefore that serum may protect against that microorganism if the serum is injected into someone else. This relationship forms the basis for passive immunization (see Chapter 28).

> **NOTE**
>
> The two main types of immunization are *passive* and *active*. In passive immunization, antibodies are injected into a person. The antibodies provide instant but short-lived protection against specific disease-causing bacteria, viruses, or toxins. Active immunization stimulates the body to make its own antibodies. These antibodies fight against such microorganisms and confer longer-lasting immunity.

Vaccines contain killed or modified microorganisms (live attenuated organisms) that usually do not cause the disease. The vaccines are given to a person to produce specific immunity. This immunity may be for a disease-causing bacterial toxin, virus, or bacterium (active immunization). The infectious agent may invade the body at a later time. At that time, the sensitized immune system quickly produces antibodies to destroy the agent or the toxin it produces. Examples of live attenuated vaccines are those given to protect against measles, mumps, rubella, yellow fever, and polio. Diphtheria and tetanus vaccines contain inactivated bacterial toxins. Cholera, typhoid fever, pertussis, rabies, viral hepatitis B, influenza, and Salk injected polio vaccines contain killed organisms. (In the case of hepatitis B the vaccine contains only part of the hepatitis B virus. See Chapter 28.)

> **? DID YOU KNOW?**
> **Immune Globulin**
>
> Immune globulin (IG) is a sterilized solution obtained from pooled human blood plasma that contains the immunoglobulins (or antibodies) required for protection against infectious agents that cause various diseases. Antibodies are substances in the blood plasma that fight infections. Our bodies create antibodies (or immunity) against disease-causing agents when infections occur. These antibodies can protect us from becoming ill if we are exposed to the same infectious agents sometime in the future. When someone is given IG, that person is using other people's antibodies to help fight or prevent an illness from occurring. This protection is temporary and should not be confused with getting an immunization, which provides longer-term protection.
>
> Special IG formulations are produced from donors with high levels of antibodies against hepatitis B (hepatitis B immune globulin, HBIG), rabies (rabies immune globulin, RIG), tetanus (tetanus immune globulin, TIG), and varicella (chickenpox) (varicella-zoster immune globulin, VZIG). Immune globulins are sometimes called gamma globulins or immune serum globulins. IG administered by injection persists in the body for several months. The protective effect of the injection disappears after approximately 3 months. If risk of exposure to disease continues, individuals may require additional IG.

From Public Health Department, Seattle and King County: *Important information about immune globulins (IG) for the prevention of communicable disease,* available at http://depts.washington.edu/druginfo/Vaccine/HealthDept/ImmuneGlobulin.html, accessed 5-13-09.

SUMMARY

- A drug is any substance taken by mouth; injected into a muscle, blood vessel, or cavity of the body; or applied topically to treat or prevent a disease or condition.
- Drugs can be identified by four types of names. These include the chemical name; generic or nonproprietary name; trade, brand, or proprietary name; and official name.
- The Drug Enforcement Agency is the sole legal drug enforcement body in the United States. Other regulatory bodies or services include the FDA; the Public Health Service; the Federal Trade Commission; in Canada, the Health Protection Branch of the Department of National Health and Welfare; and for international drug control, the International Narcotics Control Board.
- Drugs do not confer any new functions to a tissue or organ; they only modify existing functions. A drug that interacts with a receptor to stimulate a response is known as an agonist. A drug that attaches to a receptor but does not stimulate a response is called an antagonist.

Continued

- Pharmacokinetics is the study of how the body handles a drug over a period of time.
- The degree to which drugs attain pharmacological activity depends partly on the rate and extent to which they are absorbed. Absorption in turn depends on the ability of the drug to cross the cell membrane. The rate and extent of absorption depend on the nature of the cell membrane the drug must cross, blood flow to the site of administration, solubility of the drug, pH of the drug environment, drug concentration, and drug dosage form.
- The route of drug administration influences drug absorption. These routes can be classified as enteral, parenteral, pulmonary, and topical.
- Distribution is the transport of a drug through the bloodstream to various tissues of the body and ultimately to its site of action. After absorption and distribution, the body eliminates most drugs. The body first biotransforms the drug and then excretes the drug. The kidney is the primary organ for excretion; however, the intestine, lungs, and mammary, sweat, and salivary glands also may be involved.
- The blood-brain barrier and the placenta are barriers to distribution of some drugs.
- Many factors can alter the response to drug therapy, including age, body mass, gender, pathological state, time of administration, genetic factors, and psychological factors.
- Most drug actions are thought to result from a chemical interaction. This interaction is between the drug and various receptors throughout the body. The most common form of drug action is the drug-receptor interaction.
- Many variables can influence drug interactions, including intestinal absorption, competition for plasma protein binding, biotransformation, action at the receptor site, renal excretion, and alteration of electrolyte balance.
- Paramedics are held responsible for the safe and effective administration of drugs. In fact, they are responsible for each drug they provide to a patient. They are legally, morally, and ethically responsible.
- Elements of the drug profile the paramedic should know include the following: drug names, classification, mechanism of action, indications, pharmacokinetics, side/adverse effects, dose, route of administration, contraindications, special considerations, and storage requirements.
- Alterations in drug administration may be needed when caring for children, pregnant patients, or older adults.
- Autonomic drugs mimic or block the effects of the sympathetic and parasympathetic divisions of the autonomic nervous system. These drugs are classified into four groups: cholinergic (parasympathomimetic) drugs, cholinergic blocking (parasympatholytic) drugs, adrenergic (sympathomimetic) drugs, and adrenergic blocking (sympatholytic) drugs.
- Narcotic analgesics relieve pain. Narcotic antagonists reverse the narcotic effects of some analgesics. Nonnarcotic analgesics interfere with local mediators released when tissue is damaged in the periphery of the body. These mediators stimulate nerve endings and cause pain.
- Anesthetic drugs are CNS depressants that have a reversible effect on nervous tissue. Antianxiety agents are used to reduce feelings of apprehension, nervousness, worry, or fearfulness. Sedatives and hypnotics are drugs that depress the CNS. They produce a calming effect. They also help induce sleep. Alcohol is a general CNS depressant that can produce sedation, sleep, and anesthesia.
- Antianxiety agents are used to reduce feelings of apprehension, nervousness, worry, or fearfulness. Sedatives and hypnotics are drugs that depress the CNS, produce a calming effect, and help induce sleep. Alcohol has characteristics of both of these drug groups.
- Anticonvulsant drugs are used to treat seizure disorders. Most notably they treat epilepsy.
- All CNS stimulants work to increase excitability. They do this by blocking the activity of inhibitory neurons or their respective neurotransmitters or by enhancing the production of the excitatory neurotransmitters.
- Psychotherapeutic drugs include antipsychotic agents, antidepressants, and lithium. These drugs are used to treat psychoses and affective disorders, especially schizophrenia, depression, and mania.
- Movement disorders such as Parkinson's disease can result from an imbalance of dopamine and acetylcholine. Drugs that inhibit or block acetylcholine are referred to as anticholinergic. Three classes of drugs affect brain dopamine levels: those that release dopamine, those that increase brain levels of dopamine, and dopaminergic agonists.
- Skeletal muscle relaxants can be classified as central acting, direct acting, and neuromuscular blockers.
- Cardiac drugs are classified by their effects on specialized cardiac tissues. Cardiac glycosides are used to treat congestive heart failure and certain tachycardias. Antidysrhythmic drugs are used to treat and prevent disorders of cardiac rhythm. The pharmacological agents that suppress dysrhythmias may do so by direct action on the cardiac cell membrane (lidocaine), by indirect action that affects the cell (propranolol), or both. The four classes of antidysrhythmic drugs are sodium channel blockers, beta blockers, potassium channel blockers, and calcium channel blockers.
- Antihypertensive drugs used to reduce blood pressure are classified into six major categories: diuretics, sympathetic blocking agents (sympatholytic drugs), vasodilators, calcium channel blockers, angiotensin-converting

enzyme (ACE) inhibitors, and angiotensin II receptor antagonists.

- Antihemorrheologic agents are used to treat peripheral vascular disorders. These disorders are caused by pathological or physiological obstruction (e.g., arteriosclerosis). These agents improve blood flow to ischemic tissues.

- Drugs that affect blood coagulation may be classified as antiplatelet, anticoagulant, or fibrinolytic agents. Drugs that interfere with platelet aggregation are known as antiplatelet or antithrombic drugs. Anticoagulant drug therapy is designed to prevent intravascular thrombosis. The therapy decreases blood coagulability. Fibrinolytic drugs dissolve clots after their formation. These drugs work by promoting the breakdown of fibrin.

- Hemophilia is a group of hereditary bleeding disorders. These disorders involve a deficiency of one of the factors needed for the coagulation of blood. Replacing the missing clotting factor can help manage hemophilia.

- Hemostatic agents accelerate clot formation, thus reducing bleeding. Systemic hemostatic agents are used to control blood loss after surgery. They work by inhibiting the breakdown of fibrin. Topical hemostatic agents are used to control capillary bleeding. They are used during surgical and dental procedures.

- The treatment of choice in managing a loss of blood or blood components is to replace the blood component that is deficient. Replacement therapy may include transfusing whole blood (rare), packed red blood cells, fresh-frozen plasma, plasma expanders, platelets, cryoprecipitate, fibrinogen, albumin, or gamma globulins.

- Antihyperlipidemic drugs sometimes are used along with diet and exercise to control serum lipid levels, which may include high levels of cholesterol and triglycerides.

- Bronchodilator drugs are the primary form of treatment for obstructive pulmonary disease such as asthma, chronic bronchitis, and emphysema. These drugs may be classified as sympathomimetic drugs and xanthine derivatives.

- Mucokinetic drugs are used to move respiratory secretions, excessive mucus, and sputum along the tracheobronchial tree.

- Oxygen is used chiefly to treat hypoxia and hypoxemia.

- Direct respiratory stimulant drugs act directly on the medullary center of the brain. These drugs are analeptics. They increase the rate and depth of respiration.

- A cough may be prolonged or result from an underlying disorder. In such a case, treatment with antitussive drugs may be indicated.

- The main clinical use of antihistamines is for allergic reactions. They also are used to control motion sickness or as a sedative or antiemetic.

- Drug therapy for the gastrointestinal system can be divided into drugs that affect the stomach and drugs that affect the lower gastrointestinal tract. Antacids buffer or neutralize hydrochloric acid in the stomach. Antiflatulents prevent the formation of gas in the gastrointestinal tract. Digestant drugs promote digestion in the gastrointestinal tract. They do this by releasing small amounts of hydrochloric acid in the stomach. Drugs used to treat nausea and vomiting include antagonists of histamine, acetylcholine, and dopamine as well as other drugs, the actions of which are not understood clearly.

- Cytoprotective agents and other drugs are used to treat peptic ulcer disease by protecting the gastric mucosa. H_2-receptor antagonists block the H_2 receptors. They also reduce the volume of gastric acid secretion and its acid content. Proton pump inhibitors decrease hydrochloric acid secretion by inhibiting the actions of the parietal cells.

- Two common conditions of the lower gastrointestinal tract may require drug therapy: constipation and diarrhea. Drugs used to manage these conditions include laxatives and antidiarrheals.

- Drugs used to treat eye disorders include antiglaucoma agents, mydriatics, cycloplegics, antiinfective/antiinflammatory agents, and topical anesthetics.

- Drugs used to treat disorders of the ear include antibiotics, steroid/antibiotic combinations, and miscellaneous preparations.

- The endocrine system works to control and integrate body functions. A number of drugs are used to treat disorders of the anterior and posterior pituitary, the thyroid and parathyroid glands, and the adrenal cortex.

- The pancreatic hormones play a key role in regulating the amount of certain nutrients in the circulatory system. The two main hormones secreted by the pancreas are insulin and glucagon. Imbalances in either of these may necessitate drug therapy. This therapy is meant to correct metabolic derangements. Oral hypoglycemic agents help lower blood glucose level by a variety of mechanisms.

- Drugs that affect the female reproductive system include synthetic and natural substances such as hormones (estrogen and progesterone), oral contraceptives, ovulation stimulants, and drugs used to treat infertility.

- The male sex hormone is testosterone. Adequate amounts of this hormone are needed for normal development and maintenance of male sex characteristics.

- Erectile dysfunction drugs are used to enhance sexual function.

- Antineoplastic agents are used in cancer chemotherapy to prevent the increase of malignant cells.

- Antibiotics are used to treat local or systemic infection. This group includes penicillin, cephalosporins, and related products; macrolide antibiotics; tetracyclines; fluoroquinolones; and miscellaneous antibiotic agents.

- Persons can be infected by bacterial organisms, fungi, and viruses. Examples of antifungal drugs include

Continued

tolnaftate (Tinactin), fluconazole (Diflucan), and nystatin (Mycostatin).

- Few drugs exist for use in any viral infections. One antiviral drug is acyclovir (Zovirax). This drug is effective against herpes infection. Another one is zidovudine (Retrovir, AZT), which currently is used to treat human immunodeficiency virus infection.
- Drugs used to treat inflammation or its symptoms may be classified as analgesic-antipyretic drugs and nonsteroidal antiinflammatory drugs. A number of medications have both properties.
- Immunosuppressant drugs reduce the activity of the immune system. They do this by suppressing the production and activity of lymphocytes. These drugs are prescribed after transplant surgery. They can help to prevent the rejection of foreign tissues. They also are sometimes given to halt the progress of autoimmune disorders.
- Immunomodulating agents are drugs that help the immune system to be more efficient. They do this by activating the immune defenses and by modifying a biological response to an unwanted stimulus.
- Serum contains agents of immunity. These are antibodies. The antibodies can protect against an organism if the serum is injected into someone else. This forms the basis for passive immunization. Vaccines are composed of killed or altered microorganisms. These are administered to a person to produce specific immunity to a disease-causing bacterial toxin, virus, or bacterium (active immunization).

REFERENCES

1. Lyons A, Petrucelli R: *Medicine: an illustrated history*, New York, 1987, Abradale Press.
2. Glanze W, editor: *Mosby's medical, nursing, and allied health dictionary*, ed 7, St Louis, 2006, Mosby.
3. *National cancer information factsheet*, www.cancer.gov/cancertopics/factsheet/therapy/investigational-drug-access, accessed 4-20-09.
4. McKenry L, Salerno E: *Mosby's pharmacology in nursing*, ed 22, St Louis, 2005, Mosby.
5. Buck M: Intraosseous administration of drugs in infants and children, *Pediatr Pharm* 12(12), 2006.
6. Buck ML, Wiggins BS, Sesler JM: Intraosseous drug administration in children and adults during cardiopulmonary resuscitation, *Ann Pharmacother* 41(10):1679-1686, 2007.
7. American Heart Association: *Guidelines 2000 for cardiopulmonary resuscitation and emergency cardiovascular care*, International Consensus on Science, Dallas, 2000, The Association.
8. Gahart B, Nazareno AR: *2010 Intravenous medications: a handbook for nurses and health professionals*, ed 26, St Louis, 2010, Mosby.
9. Bronstein AC, Spyker DA, Cantilena LR Jr, et al: 2008 Annual Report of the American Association of Poison Control Centers' National Poison Data System (NPDS): 26th Annual Report, *Clin Toxicol (Philadelphia)* 47(10):911-1084, 2009.
10. Rosen P, Barkin R: *Emergency medicine: concepts and clinical practice*, ed 6, St Louis, 2006, Mosby.
11. Goldman L: *Cecil medicine*, ed 23, Philadelphia, 2007, Saunders.
12. Hirsh J, Warkentin TE, Shaughnessy SG, et al: Heparin and low-molecular-weight heparin mechanisms of action, pharmacokinetics, dosing, monitoring, efficacy, and safety, *Chest* 119:64S-94S, 2001.
13. Perkins T: Keeping it under control, *EMS Magazine,* July 2008.
14. National Heart Lung and Blood Institute: *Guidelines for the diagnosis and management of asthma (EPR-3)*, www.nhlbi.nih.gov/guidelines/asthma/, accessed 5-13-09.
15. Food and Drug Administration: *FDA's decision regarding plan B: questions and answers*, www.fda.gov/CDER/DRUG/infopage/planB/planBQandA.htm, accessed 4-27-09.
16. National Kidney and Urologic Diseases Clearinghouse, National Institutes of Health: *Erectile dysfunction*, http://kidney.niddk.nih.gov/kudiseases/pubs/ED/index.htm, accessed 7-30-09.
17. Hazinski MF, et al: *2010 handbook of emergency cardiovascular care for healthcare providers*, Dallas, 2010, American Heart Association.
18. U.S. Department of Health and Human Services, Centers for Disease Control and Prevention: Public Health Service guidelines for the management of health care worker exposures to HIV and recommendations for postexposure prophylaxis, *MMWR* 47(No. RR-7):1-46, 1998.
19. Food and Drug Administration: *Medication guide for nonsteroidal anti-inflammatory drugs (NSAIDs)*, www.fda.gov/cder/Offices/ODS/MG/Cataflam.pdf, accessed 4-27-2009.

Herbal Products

The use of herbs and herbal products is common in the United States; it is estimated that nearly half of all Americans use herbs on a regular basis.[1,2] Unlike prescription drugs and over-the-counter medications, herbal products used as supplements are not regulated by the Food and Drug Administration (FDA). Proof of product purity and accuracy in the amount of active ingredient in each pill is not required, and there are no standards on the accuracy and amount of information that must be provided on the label of herbal products. Some herbal products have been shown to be effective, whereas others have been shown to be ineffective. In addition, some herbs when taken internally can interact with prescription medications, producing untoward effects. Therefore all persons should advise their physician and pharmacist if they are using herbal supplements. Although there are hundreds of herbal ingredients and thousands of herbal products that can be purchased without a prescription, the following section provides information about common herbal supplements used in the United States.

Herbal Supplements

Bilberry

(Airelle, Bleaberry, Burren, Dyeberry, Huckleberry, Hurtleberry, Myrtle, Trackleberry, Whortleberry)

COMMON USES

Diarrhea; improving vision; mouth/throat inflammation.

CONTRAINDICATIONS/INTERACTIONS

May inhibit platelet aggregation; should not be used before surgery or near maternal delivery; should not be used with other drugs or herbs that might affect clotting, including aspirin, nonsteroidal antiinflammatory agents, heparin, or warfarin.

Black Cohosh

(*Actaea racemosa, Cimicifuga racemosa,* Black Snakeroot, Bugbane, Rattletop)

COMMON USES

Hot flashes and other menopausal symptoms.

CONTRAINDICATIONS/INTERACTIONS

Women with breast cancer may want to avoid black cohosh until its effects on breast tissue are understood. Individuals with liver disorders or who develop abdominal pain, dark urine, or jaundice should avoid or discontinue use. No known interactions with other drugs.

Cranberry

(Arandano, Moosebeere, Mossberry)

COMMON USES

Urinary tract disorders; susceptibility to kidney stones.

CONTRAINDICATIONS/INTERACTIONS

None noted.

Echinacea

(Black Sampson, Hedgehog, Kansas Snakeroot, Red Sunflower, Purple Cone Flower)

COMMON USES

Preventing and treating infection (especially the cold or flu); low immune status.

CONTRAINDICATIONS/INTERACTIONS

May boost certain areas of the immune system and exacerbate a person's systemic disease. Not recommended in patients with autoimmune diseases, multiple sclerosis, AIDS, HIV infection, or tuberculosis, or in transplant patients or persons taking immunosuppressive drugs (e.g., anti-HIV drugs).

Ephedra

(Ma-Huang, Desert Herb, Ephedrine)

COMMON USES

Bronchodilator; nasal decongestant; weight loss; stimulant.

CONTRAINDICATIONS/INTERACTIONS

May enhance side effects of beta blockers and MAO inhibitors. Overuse may cause hypertension. May increase blood pressure in hypertensive patients.

Evening Primrose

(Fever Plant, King's Cureall, Night Willow-Herb, Scabish, SunDrop)

COMMON USES

Premenstrual syndrome; hot flashes; inflammatory disorders; migraine headache.

CONTRAINDICATIONS/INTERACTIONS

May cause uterine contraction in pregnant women; may lower seizure threshold (increasing drug dosage requirements) in patients with seizure disorders and in those taking phenothiazine (e.g., patients with schizophrenia).

Feverfew

(Bachelors Buttons, Featherfew)

COMMON USES

Fevers, headaches (including migraine headaches), stomach aches, toothaches, insect bites, infertility, and problems with menstruation and with labor during childbirth; psoriasis, allergies, asthma, tinnitus, rheumatoid arthritis, dizziness, nausea, and vomiting.

CONTRAINDICATIONS/INTERACTIONS

Should be avoided during pregnancy (may cause uterus to contract). No serious side effects or interactions have been noted.

Garlic

(Camphor of the Poor, Nectar of the Gods, Rust Treacle, Stinking Rose)

COMMON USES

Improving circulation; lowering blood lipid levels; hypertension; inflammatory disorders; menstrual disorders; childhood earaches; diarrhea; colds and flu symptoms; and numerous other ailments.

CONTRAINDICATIONS/INTERACTIONS

May augment anticoagulant effect and may increase bleeding time; should not be used with other drugs or herbs that might affect clotting, including aspirin, nonsteroidal antiinflammatory agents, heparin, or warfarin; should not be used before surgery or near maternal delivery.

Ginger

COMMON USES

Nausea; motion sickness; morning sickness; inflammation; indigestion.

CONTRAINDICATIONS/INTERACTIONS

May inhibit platelet aggregation (in large doses); should not be used with other drugs or herbs that might affect clotting, including aspirin, nonsteroidal antiinflammatory agents, heparin, or warfarin; should not be used before surgery or near maternal delivery.

Ginkgo Biloba

(Duck Foot, Kew, Madenhair, Silver Apricot)

COMMON USES

Memory improvement; altitude sickness; poor circulation; inflammatory disorders; impotence.

CONTRAINDICATIONS/INTERACTIONS

Augments anticoagulant effect and may increase bleeding time; should not be used with other drugs or herbs that might affect clotting, including aspirin, nonsteroidal antiinflammatory agents, heparin, or warfarin; should not be used before surgery or near maternal delivery; may lower seizure threshold in patients with seizure disorders.

Ginseng

COMMON USES

Physical and mental exhaustion; stress; viral infection; diabetes; headache.

CONTRAINDICATIONS/INTERACTIONS

May lower blood glucose levels; should not be used by persons with diabetes; may alter bleeding or clotting times; should not be used with other drugs or herbs that might affect clotting, including aspirin, nonsteroidal antiinflammatory agents, heparin, or warfarin; should not be used before surgery or near maternal delivery; may contain cardiac glycosides and should not be used by persons taking digoxin.

Grape Seed

(Activin, Oligomeric Proanthocyanidins [OPCs], Red Wine Extract)

COMMON USES

Antioxidant; chronic disease prevention; leg cramps; inflammation.

CONTRAINDICATIONS/INTERACTIONS

None noted.

Kava Kava

(Ava Pepper, Awa, Intoxicating Pepper, Kawa, Kew, Sakau, Tonga)

COMMON USES

Nervous anxiety; insomnia; stress.

CONTRAINDICATIONS/INTERACTIONS

May enhance the effects of alcohol or other sedating substances; should be avoided in persons taking antidepressants, pain medications, tranquilizers, antihistamines, and anticholinergic drugs; may antagonize the effect of dopamine and should be avoided in persons with Parkinson's disease; may increase the effects of anesthesia and should be avoided before surgery; extended use may cause discoloration of the skin, nails, and hair; chronic use may produce neurological symptoms; should be avoided in pregnant women and nursing mothers.

Milk Thistle

(Holy Thistle, Lady's Thistle, Marian Thistle, St. Mary Thistle, Silymarin)

COMMON USES

Liver disorders (alcohol or drug induced, hepatitis B, hepatitis C); breast and prostate cancer.

CONTRAINDICATIONS/INTERACTIONS

Should be avoided in persons who have allergies to ragweed, marigolds, daisies, or chrysanthemums; safety during pregnancy has not been established.

Saw Palmetto

(American Dwarf Palm, Cabbage Palm, Sabal, Shrub Palmetto)

COMMON USES

Benign prostatic hypertrophy (BPH); urinary problems.

CONTRAINDICATIONS/INTERACTIONS

May have antihormone effects; should be avoided in persons with hormone-dependent cancers and during pregnancy.

St. John's Wort

(Demon Chaser, Goatweed, Hypericum, Klamath Weed, Finasteride)

COMMON USES

Anxiety; depression; sleep disorders; viral infection.

CONTRAINDICATIONS/INTERACTIONS

May potentiate the effects of MAO inhibitors, selective serotonin reuptake inhibitors (SSRIs), and tricyclics; should not be used in persons with serious depression or suicidal tendencies; may increase levels of dopamine and norepinephrine and should be avoided in persons with hypertension; may decrease serum levels of digoxin, theophylline, reserpine, and some HIV drugs; inhibits iron absorption; may cause stomach upset, sleep disturbance; photosensitivity.

Valerian Root

(All-Heal, Amantilla, Baldrian, Capon's Tail, Heliotrope, Setwall, Vandal Root)

COMMON USES

Anxiety; stress; depression; insomnia.

CONTRAINDICATIONS/INTERACTIONS

May enhance the effects of alcohol or other sedating substances; should be avoided in persons taking antidepressants, pain medications, tranquilizers, antihistamines, anticholinergic drugs, and the herb Kava Kava; may increase the effects of anesthesia and should be avoided before surgery.

14 Venous Access and Medication Administration

OBJECTIVES

Upon completion of this chapter, the paramedic student will be able to:

1. Convert selected units of measurement into the household, apothecary, and metric systems.
2. Identify the steps in the calculation of drug dosages.
3. Calculate the correct volume of drug to be administered in a given situation.
4. Compute the correct rate for an infusion of drugs or intravenous fluids.
5. List measures for ensuring the safe administration of medications.
6. Describe actions paramedics should take if a medication error occurs.
7. List measures for preserving asepsis during parenteral administration of a drug.
8. Explain drug administration techniques for the enteral and parenteral routes.
9. Describe the steps for safely initiating an intravenous infusion.
10. Identify complications and adverse effects associated with intravenous access.
11. List the steps for safely initiating intravenous access.
12. Describe the steps for safely initiating an intraosseous infusion.
13. Explain drug administration techniques for percutaneous routes.
14. Identify special considerations in the administration of pharmacological agents to pediatric patients.
15. Explain the technique for obtaining a venous blood sample.
16. Describe the safe disposal of contaminated items and sharps.

KEY TERMS

air embolism The presence of air bubbles in the bloodstream.

apothecary system A system of graduated liquid volumes arranged in order of heaviness; it is based on the grain.

catheter fragment embolism The shearing or detachment of an intravenous (IV) catheter, allowing the embolus to travel in the bloodstream.

cellulitis An inflammation of the skin characterized most commonly by local heat, redness, pain, swelling, and occasionally by fever, malaise, chills, and headache.

centimeter A metric unit of length equal to $\frac{1}{100}$ of a meter, or 0.3937 inches.

deciliter A metric unit of volume equal to $\frac{1}{10}$ of a liter.

embolus A blockage or free-moving thrombus in a blood vessel.

extravasation The passage or escape of blood, serum, or lymph into the tissues.

grain The smallest unit of mass in apothecaries' weights, equal to about 65 mg.

gram A metric unit of mass equal to $\frac{1}{1000}$ of a kilogram.

hematoma formation The collection of blood or fluids at the site of injection or cannulation.

household system A common system of measurement that includes the *glass, cup, tablespoon, teaspoon, drop, quart,* and *pint.*

infiltration The process by which a fluid passes into tissues.

kilogram A metric unit of mass equal to 1000 grams, or 2.2046 pounds.

liter A metric unit of capacity equal to 1 cubic decimeter, 61.025 cubic inches, or 1.0567 liquid quarts.

medical asepsis The removal or destruction of disease-causing organisms or infected material.

meter A metric unit of length equal to 1000 millimeters.

metric system A system of measurement that includes the *meter, liter,* and *gram.*

microgram A metric unit of mass equal to $\frac{1}{1,000,000}$ of a gram.

milligram A metric unit of mass equal to $\frac{1}{1000}$ of a gram.

milliliter A metric unit of capacity equal to $\frac{1}{1000}$ of a liter.

millimeter A metric unit of length equal to 1/1,000 of a meter

necrosis The death of tissue.

phlebitis Inflammation of a vein, often accompanied by the formation of a clot; also known as thrombophlebitis.

pulmonary embolism The blockage of a pulmonary artery by foreign matter, such as fat, air, tumor tissue, or a thrombus that usually arises from a peripheral vein.

sepsis Infection.

thromboembolism A condition in which a blood vessel is blocked by an embolus carried in the bloodstream from the site of formation of the clot.

thrombosis The formation of a blood clot (thrombus) in a blood vessel.

sloughing The separation of tissue.

universal precautions Infection control practices in health care, observed for every patient and procedure, that prevent exposure to blood-borne pathogens.

*T*he ability to gain venous access safely and to administer prescribed medications are key elements of professional paramedic practice. This chapter addresses techniques for drug administration. It also emphasizes the paramedic's patient care responsibilities with regard to medication therapy.

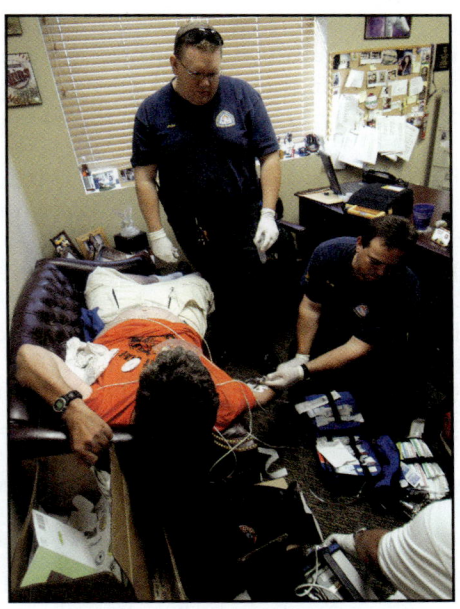

(Courtesy Ray Kemp, St. Charles, Mo.)

> **NOTE**
> Mathematical skills are important in the administration of drugs. These skills include multiplication and division, figuring percentages, and working with Roman numerals, fractions, decimal fractions, and proportions. Paramedics must have a good working knowledge of these principles and must be adept at calculations.

MATHEMATICAL EQUIVALENTS USED IN PHARMACOLOGY

Three systems for measuring drug dosages are in common use today. These are the **metric system,** the **apothecary system,** and the common **household system** (Box 14-1). Each system deals with units of mass and volume. A physician may use any of these three systems in ordering drugs.

Metric System

The French developed the metric system of weights and measures in the latter part of the eighteenth century. Congress declared it to be the official measurement system in the United States in 1866.[1] Use of the metric system is not required in the United States. However, it has been adopted by the medical sciences and pharmacies. It is used to weigh currency at the federal mints. The military also uses it. About 92% of the countries of the world use the metric system. The International System of Units is the modern form of the metric system. It is often abbreviated as SI, from the French *Le Système International d'Unités.*

The basic metric units of measurement are the meter, the liter, and the gram. The **meter** is the unit for linear measurement. The **liter** is the unit for capacity or volume. The **gram** is the unit for weight. A meter is slightly longer than a yard. A liter is slightly more than a quart. A gram is slightly more than the weight of a metal paper clip.

BOX 14-1 Systems of Equivalents

Metric System
1 g = 0.001 kg
1 g = 1000 mg
1 L = 1000 mL

Apothecary System
1 grain (gr) = $\frac{1}{60}$ dram (dr) or $\frac{1}{480}$ oz
60 gr = 1 dr
8 dr = 1 oz (or K)
1 minim (m) = $\frac{1}{60}$ fluid drams (f dr) or $\frac{1}{480}$ fluid ounces (f oz)
60 m = 1 f dr (or f l)
8 f dr = 1 f oz (or f K)

Household System
1 lb = 16 oz
1 pt = $\frac{1}{2}$ quart (qt) = $\frac{1}{8}$ gallon (gal)
1 pt = 16 f oz = 32 tablespoons (T)
1 T = 3 teaspoons (t)
1 t = 5 mL
1 T = 15 mL
1 pt = 480 mL
1 qt = 960 mL
1.0 gal = 3.84 L

The basic units of the metric system can be divided or multiplied by 10, 100, or 1000 parts to form secondary units. These secondary units differ from each other by 10 or some multiple of 10. Subdivisions of these basic units are made when the decimal is moved to the left. Multiples of the basic units are made when the decimal is moved to the right. The names of the secondary units are formed by putting a Greek or Latin prefix on the primary unit (Table 14-1).

The meter (m) is the unit of length from which the other metric units of length are derived (Figure 14-1). The **centimeter** (cm) and the **millimeter** (mm) are the primary linear measurements used in medicine. For example, they are used to measure the size of body organs and to measure blood pressure.

The liter (L) is the unit of capacity or volume (Figure 14-2). A fractional part of a liter is expressed in milliliters (mL) or cubic centimeters (cc). The liter is equal to 1000 mL (1000 cc). A **milliliter,** therefore, is $\frac{1}{1000}$ of a liter. A **deciliter** is $\frac{1}{10}$ of a liter. The National Bureau of Standards recommends that the units of measure *ml* or *mL* and *dl* or *dL* be used to express fractional parts of a liter.

The gram (g) is the metric unit used to weigh drugs and various pharmaceutical preparations (Figure 14-3). The gram equals the weight of 1 mL of distilled water at 4° C. A **kilogram** (kg) is equal to 1000 grams, or 2.2 pounds. A **milligram** (mg) is equal to $\frac{1}{1000}$ of a gram. A **microgram** (mcg) is equal to $\frac{1}{1,000,000}$ of a gram.

METRIC STYLE OF NOTATION

The National Bureau of Standards recommends the following style of metric notation except when it conflicts with the proper use of English[2]:

- Units are not capitalized (gram, not Gram).
- Unit abbreviations are not followed by a period (mL, not m.L. or mL.).

TABLE 14-1 Common Metric Prefixes	
Prefix	**Meaning**
kilo-	1000 times greater
deci-	10 times less
centi-	100 times less
milli-	1000 times less
micro-	1 million times less

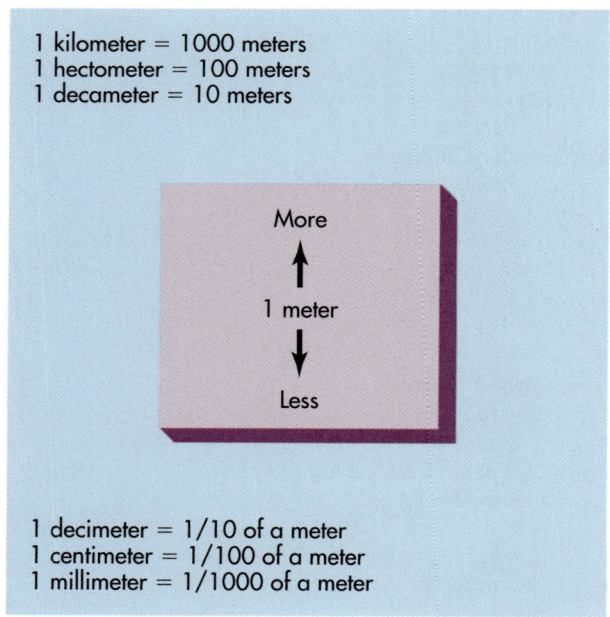

1 kilometer = 1000 meters
1 hectometer = 100 meters
1 decameter = 10 meters

More
1 meter
Less

1 decimeter = 1/10 of a meter
1 centimeter = 1/100 of a meter
1 millimeter = 1/1000 of a meter

FIGURE 14-1 The *meter* measures length.

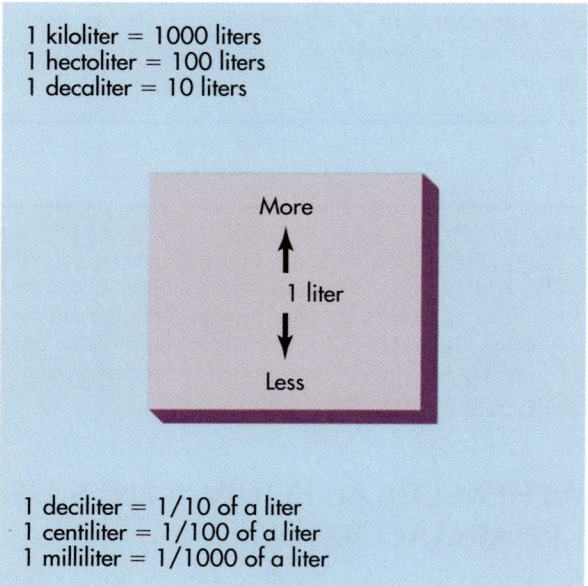

1 kiloliter = 1000 liters
1 hectoliter = 100 liters
1 decaliter = 10 liters

More
1 liter
Less

1 deciliter = 1/10 of a liter
1 centiliter = 1/100 of a liter
1 milliliter = 1/1000 of a liter

FIGURE 14-2 The *liter* measures capacity.

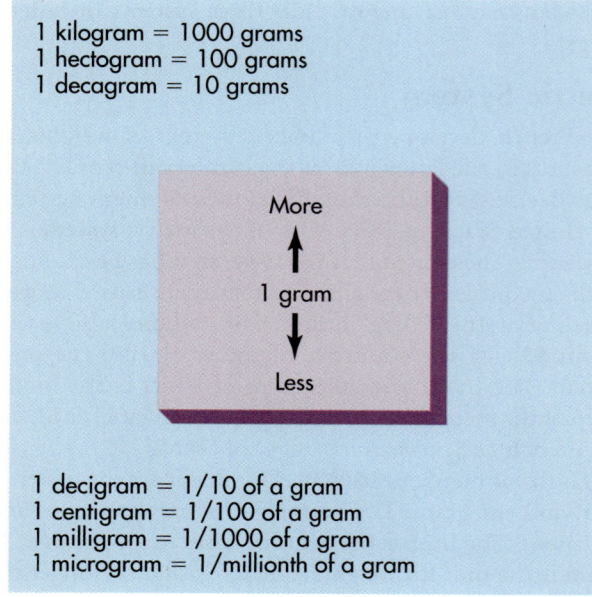

1 kilogram = 1000 grams
1 hectogram = 100 grams
1 decagram = 10 grams

More
1 gram
Less

1 decigram = 1/10 of a gram
1 centigram = 1/100 of a gram
1 milligram = 1/1000 of a gram
1 microgram = 1/millionth of a gram

FIGURE 14-3 The *gram* measures weight.

- A single space is left between the quantity and the symbol (24 kg, not 24kg).
- Unit abbreviations are not pluralized (kg, not kgs).
- As a rule, fractions are not used, only decimal notation (0.25 kg, not ¼ kg).
- For numerical quantities less than 1, a 0 is placed to the left of the decimal point (0.75 mg, not .75 mg).
- Trailing zeros should not be used after a decimal point (2 mg, not 2.0 mg).

CRITICAL THINKING
Placing a 0 to the left of the decimal point reduces the likelihood of a drug dosing error. Why?

Apothecary System

The apothecary system is less precise and less convenient than the more widely adopted metric system. This system is seldom used in the medical sciences. Only a few medications are now available in units of the apothecary system. *Aspirin* and *nitroglycerin* are two examples.

The primary unit of mass in the apothecary system is the **grain** (gr). The grain was derived from the age-old standard of the weight of a single grain of wheat (about 60 to 65 mg). *Aspirin* (5 gr) contains 325 milligrams of medication (5 grain × 65 mg = 325 mg). *Nitroglycerin* generally is labeled with both milligrams (0.3 to 0.4 mg) and grains (1/150 or 1/200 gr). Other units of mass used in the apothecary system are the *dram* (dr), *ounce* (oz), and *pound* (lb). Sixty grains equals 1 dram, and 8 drams equals 1 ounce.

The primary unit of volume in the apothecary system is the *minim* (m). The minim equals the volume of water that would weigh 1 gr (about 0.005 or 0.006 mL). The equivalent of 60 m is 1 fluid dram (f dr), and 8 f dr equals 1 fluid ounce (f oz).

In written prescriptions, the apothecary system puts the abbreviation before the numeral. Whole numerical amounts usually are set in lower case Roman numerals. For example, 10 grains would be grains x. Fractional amounts usually are given in Arabic numerals rather than decimal form. For example, ¼ grain would be grain ¼, not 0.25 grain.

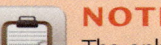

NOTE
The only apothecary conversion needed in emergency drug therapy is pounds to kilograms: 1 kilogram = 2.2 pounds. When the weight of an adult patient is converted from pounds to kilograms, the whole number can be rounded up when the number to the right of the decimal point is 5 or greater. For example, 70.9 kg could be rounded up to 71 kg.

Household System

Household measures include the *glass, cup, tablespoon, teaspoon, drop, quart,* and *pint.* Standard measures of the household system are not available in most homes. For example, the average coffee cup may hold 5 to 9 ounces or more. The average household teaspoon may hold 4 to 6 mL of liquid. Household measurements are only approximations.

Temperature Conversions

The *Fahrenheit* and *Celsius* (centigrade) temperature scales are used to measure temperature. These measurements are compared by their freezing points and their boiling points. On the Fahrenheit scale, water freezes at 32° and boils at 212°. On the Celsius scale, water freezes at 0 degree and boils at 100°. Throughout most of the world, the Celsius scale is the preferred temperature scale used in scientific and engineering fields. Most of the general population in the United States is more accustomed to the Fahrenheit scale. This is probably because the Fahrenheit scale is used by the U.S. media in weather forecasts.

Normal body temperature is 98.6° Fahrenheit, or 37° Celsius (centigrade). A simple formula can be used to convert temperatures. To convert a Celsius reading to Fahrenheit, multiply the Celsius reading by 9/5 or 1.8. Then add 32. To convert a Fahrenheit reading to Celsius, subtract 32 from the Fahrenheit reading. Then multiply by 5/9 or 0.555. (Figure 14-4).

NOTE
Remember these temperature conversion formulas:
Celsius to Fahrenheit: (° C 9/5) + 32
Fahrenheit to Celsius: (° F − 32) (5/9)

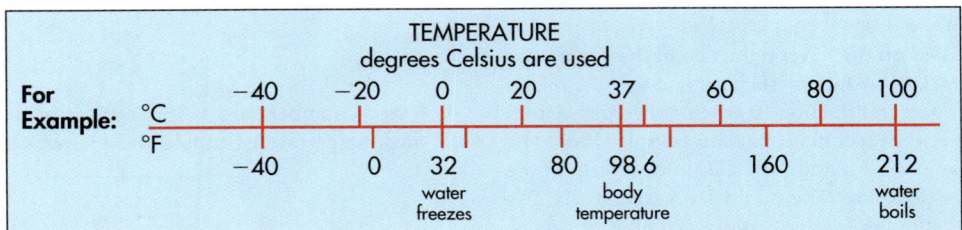

FIGURE 14-4 Temperature conversions.

DRUG CALCULATIONS

While providing emergency care, the paramedic must calculate adult and pediatric drug dosages and infusion rates, as well as the strength of drug solutions and diluted solutions. These tasks involve the use of basic math skills in a logical order. This requires a working knowledge of decimals, fractions, ratios, and proportions. This text offers common equations used for drug calculations. These equations are accepted in the medical community. Other drug calculation methods may work as well (Box 14-2).

Calculation Methods

Calculation methods must be precise and reliable. To perform drug calculations, paramedics should:

- Convert all units of measure to the same unit and system
- Check the computed dosage to determine whether it is reasonable
- Use one dosage calculation method consistently

CONVERSION OF UNITS OF MEASURE

Most emergency drug preparations do not require conversion. This is because most drugs are packaged in milligrams and administered in milligrams. However, some drugs, such as *dopamine,* are packaged in milligrams but administered in micrograms (mcg). These drugs must be converted to like units. When conversion to like units is required, the conversion must be completed before the drug dose is calculated.

Example

You are to administer ***dopamine*** at a rate of 800 mcg per minute. You have 200 mg of the drug in 250 mL of solution. Convert 800 mcg to 0.8 mg so that both measures of weight are in the same units:

$$800\,\text{mcg} \div 1000 = 0.8\,\text{mg}$$

CRITICAL THINKING
Imagine that you failed to convert the 800 mcg of dopamine to 0.8 mg in this example. Would you overdose or underdose your patient?

NOTE
Math tip: Move the decimal point to the right when multiplying (converting the measurement to smaller units). Move it to the left when dividing (converting the measurement to larger units).

When the dose is given per unit of weight (kg), the patient's weight must be converted from pounds to kilograms. This should be done before the total dose to be given is calculated.

BOX 14-2 "T" Method of Calculating Conversions, Drug Doses, and Intravenous Flow Rates

The "T" method for calculating conversions, drug doses, and intravenous (IV) flow rates does not require advanced mathematical skills. The following are guidelines for using this method to calculate a drug dose.

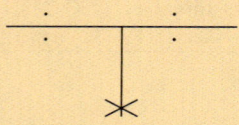

1. One T is required for every step in the calculation. To use the T method, you must know two things: (1) the prescribed dose, and (2) the gram or milligram or microgram per mL concentration of the drug.
2. The number entered on the lower right side of the T is always a "given in 1" (a known factor, such as known in 1 mL or known in 1 kg), or a multiple of 10 when converting within the metric system, that will never have to be solved for. The answer solved for in the equation will always be on top of the T or in the lower left side. The number on top of the T is always the larger number (either a known number or one to be solved for). The number in the lower left side is always the

smaller number (either a known number or one to be solved for).

| Larger Number ||
| Smaller Number | Given in 1 |

3. If a number is placed on top of the T, it will always be divided by the other number in the T to find the answer.

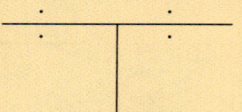

4. If both numbers are in the bottom of the T, multiplication must be performed to find the answer.

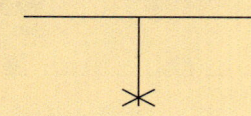

BOX 14-2 "T" Method of Calculating Conversions, Drug Doses, and Intravenous Flow Rates—cont'd

Example 1:

You are to administer meperidine 25 mg IM. You have 50 mg of the drug in 1 mL of solution. How many milliliters will you give?

Step 1:

Place the "given" (50 mg/in 1 mL) in the lower right corner of the T:

$$\frac{\quad\quad\quad}{\quad\begin{array}{c}50 \text{ mg}\\ \text{in}\\ 1 \text{ mL}\end{array}}$$

Step 2:

Place the larger number (the desired dose of 25 mg) on top of the T:

$$\frac{25 \text{ mg}}{\quad\begin{array}{c}50 \text{ mg}\\ \text{in}\\ 1 \text{ mL}\end{array}} \cdot$$

Step 3:

Divide 25 by 50 (basic formula) to obtain the smaller number (the required dose of 0.5 mL):

$$\frac{25 \text{ mg}}{\boxed{0.5 \text{ mL}} \quad 50 \text{ mg}} \cdot$$

Example 2:

You are to administer lidocaine 1 mg/kg IV to a 177-pound man. You have 100 mg in 5 mL of solution. How many milliliters will you give? This calculation requires four steps (four Ts).

Step 1:

Convert the patient's weight to kilograms:

$$\frac{177 \text{ lb}}{\boxed{80 \text{ kg}} \quad \begin{array}{c}2.2 \text{ lb}\\ \text{in}\\ 1 \text{ kg}\end{array}} \cdot$$

Step 2:

Calculate the prescribed dose in milligrams:

$$\frac{80 \text{ mg}}{1 \text{ mg} \times 80 \text{ kg}} \cdot$$

Step 3:

Determine the mg/mL concentration of the drug (remember, this example uses 5 mL of solution, not 1 mL):

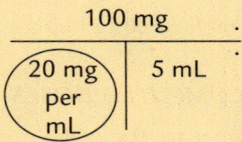

Step 4:

Use the basic formula to calculate the dose:

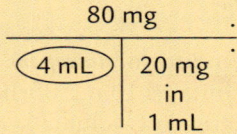

Example 3:

You are to administer atropine 0.02 mg/kg IV to a pediatric patient who weighs 30 pounds. You have 1 mg of the drug in 10 mL of solution. How many milliliters will you give? This calculation requires four steps (four Ts).

Step 1:

Convert the patient's weight to kilograms:

$$\frac{30 \text{ lb}}{\boxed{13.6 \text{ kg}} \quad \begin{array}{c}2.2 \text{ lb}\\ \text{in}\\ 1 \text{ kg}\end{array}} \cdot$$

Step 2:

Calculate the prescribed dose in milligrams:

$$\frac{0.27 \text{ mg}}{0.02 \text{ mg} \times 13.6 \text{ kg}}$$

Step 3:

Determine the mg/mL concentration of the drug:

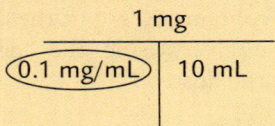

Step 4:

Use the basic formula to calculate the dose:

$$\frac{0.27 \text{ mg}}{\boxed{2.7 \text{ mL}} \quad \begin{array}{c}0.1 \text{ mg/}\\ \text{in 1 mL}\end{array}}$$

Example

You are to give 1 mg/kg of *lidocaine* to a patient who weighs 132 lb. Divide 132 by 2.2 to convert pounds to kilograms (132 lb = 60 kg). The total dose equals 1 mg/kg multiplied by 60 kg. This equals 60 mg.

$$132\,\text{lb} \div 2.2 = 60\,\text{kg}$$

$$1\,\text{mg/kg} \times 60\,\text{kg} = 60\,\text{mg}$$

ASSESSMENT OF COMPUTED DOSES

Many emergency drugs are packaged in units that contain enough drug for a normal adult dose. After computations are performed, the paramedic should decide whether the answer is reasonable.

Example

You are to administer 8 mg of *diazepam.* It is supplied in a 2 mL ampule that contains 10 mg of the drug. Therefore, a reasonable calculation of volume would be less than 2 mL.

METHODS OF CALCULATION

Many drug calculations can be performed almost intuitively. This is because many drugs are packaged to supply one adult dose. However, a paramedic should never rely on intuitive calculations, no matter how simple the drug dose may seem. The three methods of calculation discussed below are in common use.

METHOD 1: BASIC FORMULA ("DESIRE OVER HAVE")

For method 1, information must be substituted in the following formula:

$$\frac{D}{H} \times Q = X$$

In this formula, D is the desired dose to be given. H is the known dose on hand. Q is the unit of measure or volume on hand. X is the unit of measure to be given. Many consider "desire over have" to be the easiest formula to use. It works for nearly all emergency drug calculations.

Example

You are to administer 25 mg of *diphenhydramine.* You have a 10 mL vial that contains 50 mg of the drug. How many milliliters will you give? Using the "desire over have" formula, calculate the dose.

$$\frac{25\,\text{mg}}{50\,\text{mg}} \times 10\,\text{mL} = X$$

$$\frac{25}{5} \times 1\,\text{mL} = X$$

$$5 \times 1\,\text{mL} = X$$

$$X = 5\,\text{mL}$$

 NOTE
Math tip: When using the basic formula, always divide the bottom number into the top number.

METHOD 2: RATIOS AND PROPORTIONS

Method 2 uses ratios and proportions to calculate the drug dosage. A *ratio* compares two numbers and is the same as a fraction. When used to calculate drug doses, a ratio refers to the weight or quantity of a drug in solution. For example, the ratio of 10 mg of *morphine* in 1 mL of solution is 10 mg to 1 mL. A *proportion* is an equation made up of two ratios; it states that the two ratios are equal. For example, ⅔ is equal to ⁴⁄₆ (2 : 3 :: 4 : 6); therefore the ratios are equivalent and the proportions are true.

To use method 2, the equation must be set up to ensure that the same units of measure are stated in the same sequence (e.g., mg : mL = mg : x mL). x is the quantity (e.g., mL) to be solved. The formula can be expressed as

Dose on Hand : Volume on Hand :: Desired Dose : Desired Volume

Example

You are to administer 40 mg of *furosemide.* You have 100 mg of the drug in 10 mL of solution. How many milliliters will you give? Calculate the dose using ratios and proportions:

$$100\,\text{mg} : 10\,\text{mL} :: 40\,\text{mg} : x\,\text{mL}$$

Multiply inside numbers *(means)* and outside numbers *(extremes).* Drop the unit of measurement terms.

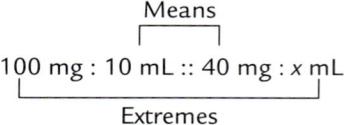

 NOTE
Math tip: Remember the phrases *middle for means* and *end for extremes.* In a proportion, the product of the means is always equal to the product of the extremes.

Solve the proportion by dividing both sides of the equation by the number before × (100).

$$\frac{100x}{100} \times \frac{400}{100} = 4\,\text{mL}$$

To check your answer, multiply the means and then multiply the extremes. The sum product will be equal if the proportion is true.

$$\left.\begin{array}{l} 100 \times 4 = 400 \\ 10 \times 40 = 400 \end{array}\right\} \text{Sum parts are equal}$$

METHOD 3: DIMENSIONAL ANALYSIS

Dimensional analysis works well for complex drug calculations. These may call for several conversions of a similar basic dimensional unit so that all units of measure are changed to like units (e.g., milligrams). Dimensional analysis is based on the same tenet as the basic formula. However, it does not require memorization of the "desire over have" equation. All conversion factors are set up in one equation. They are separated by multiplication signs.

NOTE

Math tip: When using dimensional analysis, convert all units to the easiest math operation. This reduces the chance of error.

Example

You are to administer 0.8 mg of **naloxone**. The drug is packaged in 1 mL of solution containing 0.4 mg of the drug.

Step 1: Set up the equation, placing the desired unit of measure in the answer to the left of the equal sign. Place the first factor to the right of the equal sign. Make sure it is the same unit as the answer.

$$mL = \frac{1\,mL}{0.4\,mg} \times \frac{0.8\,mg}{1}$$

Step 2: Cancel like units of measure in the numerator and denominator, and reduce the fraction, if needed:

$$mL = \frac{1\,mL}{0.4\,\cancel{mg}} \times \frac{0.8\,\cancel{mg}}{1}$$

NOTE

Math tip: The only unit remaining after canceling the like units should be the unit of the answer. If this is not the case, the equation is set up incorrectly.

Step 3: Multiply the numerators and then the denominators.

$$mL = \frac{1\,mL}{0.4} \times \frac{0.8}{1}$$

Step 4: Divide the numerator by the denominator to solve the equation.

$$mL = \frac{0.8\,mL}{0.4} = 2\,mL$$

Calculating Intravenous Flow Rates

To calculate intravenous (IV) flow rates, paramedics must know three factors: (1) the volume to be infused; (2) the period of time, in minutes, over which the fluid is to be infused; and (3) the number of drops (gtt) per milliliter the infusion set delivers *(drop factor)*. The flow rate can then be calculated using the following equation:

$$gtt/min = \frac{Volume\ to\ be\ infused \times Drop\ factor}{Duration\ of\ infusion\ (minutes)}$$

Example

You are to give 250 mL of normal saline over 90 minutes. Your infusion set delivers 10 gtt/mL. Calculate the drops per minute using the above formula.

$$gtt/min = \frac{250\,\cancel{mL} \times 10\,gtt/\cancel{mL}}{90\,minutes} = \frac{2500\,gtt}{90\,min} = 27.7\ or\ 28\ gtt/min$$

NOTE

The two intravenous (IV) infusion sets most often used in emergency care are microdrip tubing and macrodrip tubing. Microdrip tubing delivers 60 gtt/mL. Macrodrip tubing delivers 10, 15, or 20 gtt/mL. *Math tip:* When a drop factor of 60 is used, the gtt/min always equals the mL/hour infusion.

CRITICAL THINKING

When is it best to use microdrip tubing? When is it better to use macrodrip tubing?

Calculating Infusion Rates

Paramedics may need to administer medications by continuous IV infusion. Calculating the correct drip rate is crucial (Boxes 14-3 and 14-4). This helps prevent overdosing or underdosing of the patient. To properly calculate and give a prescribed drug by continuous infusion, paramedics must know three things: (1) the prescribed dose; (2) the concentration of the drug in 1 mL of solution; and (3) the drop factor of the IV infusion set. The calculation then is made using the following IV drip formula:

$$gtt/min = \frac{Prescribed\ dose \times Drop\ factor}{Concentration\ of\ drug\ in\ 1\,mL}$$

Example

You are to administer a **procainamide** infusion at 3 mg/min. You have 1 g of the drug in 250 mL of 5% dextrose in water (D_5W). The infusion set delivers 60 gtt/mL. How many drops per minute will you deliver?

Convert all units to like measurements and calculate the concentration of the drug in 1 mL.

$$1\,g \times 1000 = 1000\,mg$$

$$1000\,mg \div 250\,mL = 4\,mg/mL$$

Calculate the drops per minute using the IV drip formula:

$$gtt/min = \frac{3\,mg/min \times 60\,gtt/mL}{4\,mg\ in\ 1\,mL} = \frac{180}{4} = 45\ gtt/min$$

Calculating Drug Dosages for Infants and Children

The doses of some medications for infants and children are administered in the same proportion to body weight as the doses for adults. Others are given in very reduced doses.

BOX 14-3 "Clock" Method of Calculating Flow Rates

Visualizing a clock can help paramedics calculate the flow rate for an intravenous (IV) medication. For example, if the concentration of a drug in solution is 4 mg/mL and microdrip tubing is used that delivers 1 mL in 60 drops, and 60 drops are delivered in 1 minute, then 4 mg will be delivered with every 60 drops of solution. Picturing a clock where 4 mg and 60 drops are at the 12 position, you can calculate that 15 drops/minute will deliver 1 mg/minute; 30 drops will deliver 2 mg/min; and 45 drops will deliver 3 mg/min. You can use this same method with any drug in solution when microdrip is used.

Lidocaine Infusion Clock

- Mix 2 g of lidocaine in 500 mL D$_5$W or NS (or 1 g in 250 mL) = 4 mg/mL
- Infusion dose range = 2-4 mg/min
- When administered with a minidrip (60 gtt/mL) IV administration set, lidocaine drip rates resemble a seconds "clock"

60 gtt/min = 4 mg/min

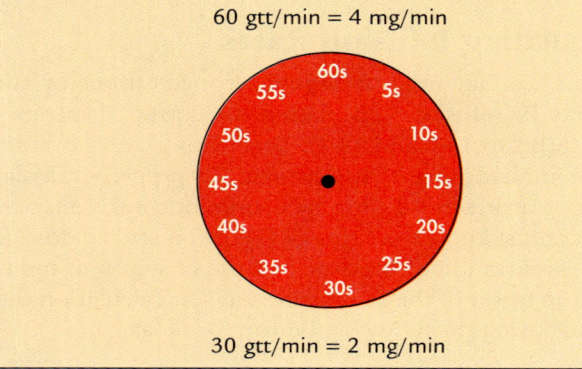

30 gtt/min = 2 mg/min

BOX 14-4 Shortcut for Calculating Dopamine Drips

Dopamine is a very strong drug. Calculating the correct dose can daunt the best mathematician. The following is a shortcut for calculating dopamine infusions using 60 drops/minute intravenous (IV) tubing and a standard mixture of drug in solution (e.g., 400 mg in 250 mL; 800 mg in 500 mL).

Formula:

$$\frac{\text{Dose} \times \text{Weight (kg)} \times 60 \text{ gtt/mL}}{1600} = \text{Drops per minute}$$

Example:

You are to administer 5 mcg/kg of dopamine per minute to a 75 kg patient.

$$\frac{5\,\mu g \times 75\,kg \times 60 \text{ gtt/mL}}{1600} = 14 \text{ Drops per minute}$$

DRUG ADMINISTRATION

During the administration of any drug, safety should always be a high priority.

Safety Considerations and Procedures

Paramedics should follow these guidelines when administering drugs to patients.

- Focus on the procedure and avoid distractions (including when preparing the medicines).
- In the prehospital setting, carefully follow all standing orders and protocols for drug therapy. Make sure that any medication orders received from medical direction are fully understood. Repeat all orders back to medical direction for confirmation. Before administering any drug, state the *name* of the drug, the *dose*, and the *route* by which it is to be given. If the order is unclear or if there is reason to question the order, ask medical direction to repeat it. In the emergency department or other patient care areas, make sure you have a written or electronic order for every medication you administer. Verify the patient's name on the person's armband or identification tag and scan the tag (per protocol for electronic recordkeeping). Also, verify that the patient is not allergic to the medication. Strictly follow these *five patient rights* of drug administration: Make sure the *right* patient receives the *right* dose of the *right* drug via the *right* route at the *right* time. Also make sure to document the drug administration accurately and thoroughly.
- Make a habit of reading the drug label and comparing it to the medication order at least three times before administration:
  - First—when removing the drug from the drug kit or supply area

This is due to differences in the child's ability to metabolize the drug. In general, the total dose administered to a child rarely exceeds a normal adult dose (see Chapter 13). Paramedics often calculate pediatric drug doses in the prehospital setting by using memory aids or with the advice of medical direction. Some of the memory aids are charts, tapes, pocket guides, and dosage wheels (Figure 14-5). Personal electronic devices (e.g., personal digital assistants [PDAs]) with drug calculation software also are available (Figure 14-6). The most precise way to calculate a pediatric drug dose is based on the child's body surface area. (Body surface area as a function of weight is discussed in Chapter 48.) The wisest course is to have someone double-check the dose before a medication is administered to a child.

NOTE

Paramedics who administer a medication do so by the authority provided by medical direction. The paramedic has both a professional and a legal responsibility to follow all patient management protocols, policies, and procedures. These policies specify the regulations of drug administration. This includes policies on the stocking and supply of drugs.

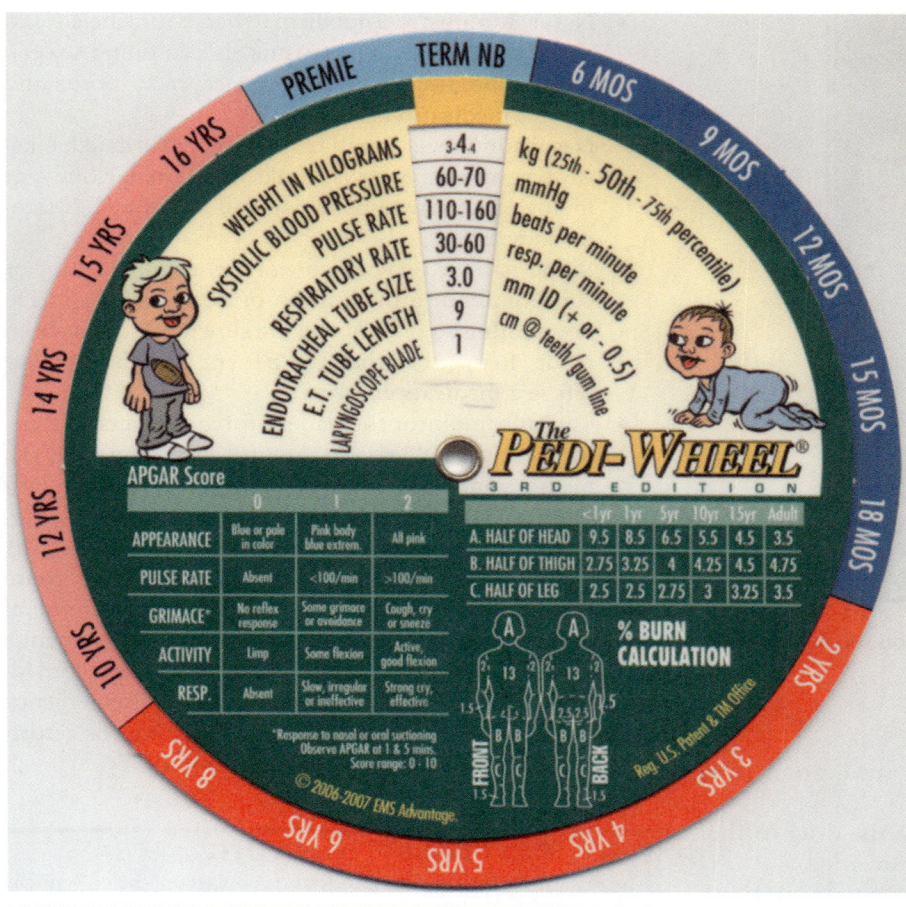

FIGURE 14-5 Pedi Wheel. (Courtesy Harley Don and 2010 EMS Advantage.)

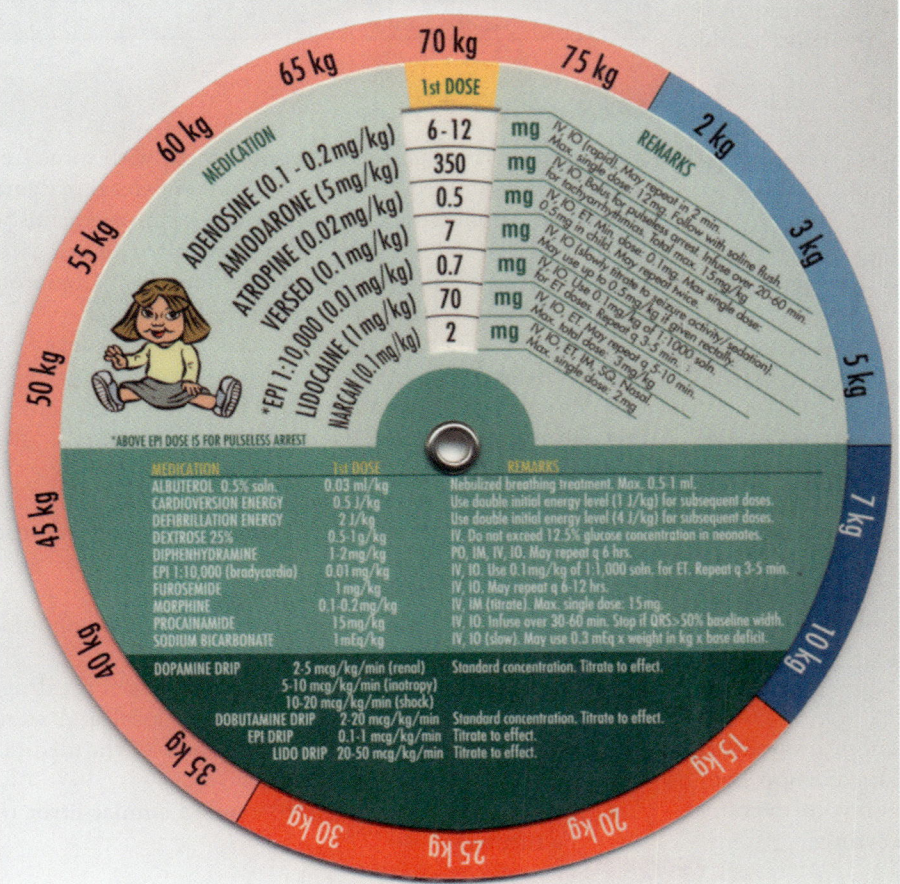

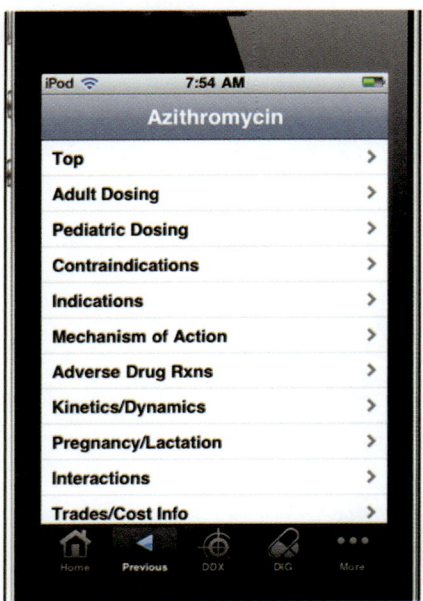

FIGURE 14-6 Drug references are available on wireless devices. (Courtesy PEPID, Rocklin, Calif.)

- Second—when preparing the medication for administration
- Third—just before administering the drug to the patient (before the container is discarded)
- Always check the correct route of administration. Some medications can be prepared for administration by several routes. For instance, the route could be intramuscular or intravenous.
- Make sure the information on the label matches the prescriber's order.
- Never give a medicine from an unlabeled container. Also, never give a medicine from a container on which the label is not legible.
- If you are unsure of your drug calculation, have a coworker check it. You also can contact medical direction for verification.
- Handle multidose vials carefully and with aseptic technique. This prevents drugs from being wasted or contaminated.

> **NOTE**
>
> As a rule, a multidose vial should be discarded after a single patient use. Also, the safest course is to restrict each medication vial to a single patient, even if it is a multidose vial. Proper aseptic technique should always be followed.

- When preparing more than one injection, always label the syringe immediately. Keep the medication container with the syringe. Do not rely on your memory to recall which solution is in which syringe.

- Never administer a medicine that is unlabeled and that was prepared by someone else. In doing so, you accept the responsibility for accuracy, dose, and correct medication.
- Never administer a medication that is outdated. Likewise, never give one that looks discolored, cloudy, or in any other way unusual, or as if someone has tampered with it.
- If the patient or your co-workers express doubt or concern about a medication or dose, recheck it. Do not administer it until you are sure no error has been made. Remember that the patient has the right to refuse a medication.
- Carefully monitor the patient for any adverse effects. Monitor for at least 5 minutes after you give the medication. (Intramuscular and oral medicines may require longer monitoring.)
- Document all medications given. This includes the name of the drug, the dosage, and the time and route of administration. When documenting parenteral medications, note the site of injection. The patient's response, adverse as well as intended, also is recorded.
- Follow government guidelines and local emergency medical services (EMS) policies regarding the return and disposal of any unused medication.

> **CRITICAL THINKING**
>
> Your clinical preceptor hands you an unlabeled syringe of medication and tells you to give it by intramuscular injection. What do you do?

Medication Errors

Medication errors *(adverse drug events)* occur with some frequency. An estimated 1.5 million people (hospital patients and nursing home residents) receive the wrong medicine or the incorrect dose of medicine in the United States each year. Of these, about 7000 people die annually.[3] Common causes of medication errors include the following:

- The prescriber ordered the wrong dose of medication.
- Drug calculations were incorrect.
- Drugs were administered by the wrong route.
- The drug was given to the wrong patient.
- The wrong drug was given to the patient.

If a medication error occurs, paramedics should do the following:

- Accept responsibility for the error.
- Immediately advise medical direction or the prescriber.
- Assess and monitor the patient for effects of the drug.
- Document the error as required by local and state drug administration policies and those of the medical direction institution.
- Modify personal practice to avoid a similar error in the future.

- Follow EMS agency procedures for documentation and quality improvement activities.

NOTE

Most injectable medications are given as their mass concentration (mg/mL or mcg/mL). For only a few drugs (e.g., epinephrine) is the concentration expressed as a ratio or percentage. These expressions are error prone because (1) practitioners may not recognize or understand the difference between dose concentrations (e.g., 1:1000 or 1 mg/mL and 1:10,000 or 0.1 mg/mL); and (2) numbers in the thousands are easily confused, because they have so many zeros (e.g., at a quick glance, 1,000 may be mistaken for 10,000). Paramedics should be especially careful when administering epinephrine. They should always have a co-worker double-check the dose and route of administration. This can help prevent a life-threatening drug error.

LOOK AGAIN

See Chapter 4: Documentation, pp. 71-72.

SHOW ME THE EVIDENCE

Vilke and colleagues surveyed paramedics in San Diego County to determine their experience with drug errors. According to the 352 surveys returned, 9.1% of paramedics reported committing a drug error within the last 12 months. Most of the errors reported were dose related (63%). Other errors were related to: protocol (33%); wrong route (21%); and wrong medication (4%). Of the errors noted in the survey, 4.2% had been noted during the call but had not been previously reported by the paramedic. The authors noted the need for additional safeguards to reduce the incidence of medication errors.

From Vilke G et al: Paramedic self-reported medication errors, *Prehosp Emerg Care* 10:457-462, 2006.

MEDICAL ASEPSIS

Medical asepsis is the removal or destruction of disease-causing organisms or infected material. Medical asepsis is performed by using "clean" technique (rather than sterile technique). *Clean technique* includes hygienic measures, cleaning agents, antiseptics, disinfectants, and barrier fields.

NOTE

Sterile technique means using sterile equipment and sterile fields that are free of all forms and types of life. This is also known as *surgical asepsis*. *Clean technique* focuses on destroying or inhibiting only pathogens (not all forms and types of life).

Antiseptics and Disinfectants

Antiseptics and disinfectants are chemical agents. They are used to kill specific groups of microorganisms. They generally are not very effective against spores of bacteria and fungi, many viruses, and some resistant bacterial strains. Disinfectants are used only on nonliving objects and are toxic to living tissue. Antiseptics are applied only to living tissue and are more dilute, to prevent cell damage. Some chemical agents have both antiseptic and disinfectant properties. Examples of these are alcohol and some chlorine compounds (Box 14-5 and Table 14-2).

NOTE

New disinfection methods are under consideration by the Environmental Protection Agency (EPA) and the Food and Drug Administration (FDA). These include a persistent antimicrobial drug coating that can be applied to inanimate and animate objects (Surfacine); a high-level disinfectant with reduced exposure time (orthophthalaldehyde); and an antimicrobial drug that can be applied to animate and inanimate objects (superoxidized water).[4]

UNIVERSAL PRECAUTIONS IN MEDICATION ADMINISTRATION

As described in Chapter 2, **universal precautions** are infection control practices in health care that are observed with every patient and procedure and that prevent exposure to blood-borne pathogens. (Personal protective measures are described in the appendix for this chapter and in Chapter 28.) When administering drugs, paramedics should follow hand washing procedures. They also should follow gloving procedures if indicated. Face shields should be used during administration of endotracheal drugs and whenever splashing of blood or body fluids is likely.

NOTE

Many consider hand washing the most crucial step in reducing the risk of transmission of organisms from one person to another or from one site to another on the same patient.[4] Hand washing protects both the paramedic and the patient. If soap and water are not available, a sanitizing gel, foam, or wipe should be used.

BOX 14-5 Examples of Antiseptics and Disinfectants

Antiseptics	Disinfectants
• Hexachlorophene	• Cresol
• Silver nitrate	• Carbolic acid
• Benzoyl peroxide	• Lysol

TABLE 14-2 Sterilization and Disinfection Methods for Equipment Used by Paramedics*

Organisms Destroyed	Methods	Uses
Sterilization All forms of microbial life, including high numbers of bacterial spores	Steam under pressure (autoclave), gas (ethylene oxide), dry heat, or immersion in an Environmental Protection Agency (EPA)-approved chemical sterilant for a prolonged period (e.g., 6 to 10 hours or according to the manufacturer's instructions). *Note*: Liquid chemical sterilants should be used only on instruments that cannot be sterilized or disinfected with heat.	Instruments or devices that penetrate the skin or come into contact with normally sterile areas of the body (e.g., scalpels, needles). Use of disposable invasive equipment eliminates the need to reprocess these items. When indicated, however, arrangements should be made with a health care facility for reprocessing of reusable invasive instruments.
High-Level Disinfection All forms of microbial life except high numbers of bacterial spores	Hot water pasteurization (176° to 212° F [80° to 100° C] for 30 minutes), or exposure to an EPA-registered chemical sterilant, except for a short exposure time (10 to 45 minutes or as directed by the manufacturer).	Reusable instruments or devices that come into contact with mucous membranes (e.g., laryngoscope blades, endotracheal tubes).
Intermediate-Level Disinfection *Mycobacterium tuberculosis*, vegetative bacteria, most viruses, and most fungi but not bacterial spores	EPA-registered hospital disinfectant chemical germicides with a label claim of tuberculocidal activity; commercially available hard surface germicides; or solutions with at least 500 parts per million (ppm) free available chlorine (a 1:100 dilution of common household bleach—approximately 1 cup of bleach per 1 gallon of tap water).	Instruments and equipment that come into contact only with intact skin (e.g., stethoscopes, blood pressure cuffs, splints) and that have been visibly contaminated with blood or bloody body fluids. Surfaces must be cleaned of visible material before the germicide is applied.
Low-Level Disinfection Most bacteria, some viruses, some fungi, but not *Mycobacterium tuberculosis* or bacterial spores	EPA-registered hospital disinfectants (no label claim for tuberculocidal activity).	Routine housekeeping or removal of soiling in the absence of visible blood contamination.
Environmental Disinfection	Any cleaner or disinfectant agent intended for environmental use.	Environmental surfaces that have become soiled and that should be cleaned and disinfected (e.g., floors, woodwork, ambulance seats, countertops).

*To ensure the effectiveness of any sterilization or disinfection process, equipment and instruments first must be thoroughly cleaned of all visible soiling.

ENTERAL ADMINISTRATION OF MEDICATIONS

Enteral medications are drugs that are administered and absorbed through the gastrointestinal tract. Enteral drugs are administered by the oral, gastric, or rectal route.

LOOK AGAIN
See Chapter 13: Principles of Pharmacology and Emergency Medications, pp. 283-286.

Oral Route

The oral route is the most frequently used method of drug administration. The patient should be in an upright or sitting position. The pill, tablet, or capsule should be placed in the patient's mouth and swallowed with enough fluid (4 to 8 ounces) to make sure the drug reaches the stomach. Some oral drugs, such as **ondansetron,** are placed on the tongue and allowed to dissolve without water. Medication should not be administered orally if the patient cannot swallow or does not have an effective gag reflex.

BOX 14-6 Forms of Solid and Liquid Oral Medications

- Caplets
- Capsules
- Time-released capsules
- Lozenges
- Pills
- Tablets
- Elixirs
- Emulsions
- Suspensions
- Syrups

CRITICAL THINKING

Think of some clinical situations in which oral administration of a drug would not be the best technique. Why is this so?

Many oral drugs are manufactured in solid and liquid forms (Box 14-6). If the medication is in a liquid suspension, the stock bottle or unit dose should be shaken thoroughly before the drug is poured for administration. A drug not packaged as a unit dose should be measured in a medicine cup or a medicine dropper or by syringe.

Administration of Medications by Gastric Tube

Most drugs that can be given orally can also be given via a gastric tube. Orogastric tubes are placed through the mouth and into the esophagus and stomach. Nasogastric tubes are placed through the nose and esophagus and into the stomach. Before giving a drug by this route, the paramedic must make sure the tube has been inserted correctly (see Chapter 29). This can be done by injecting 30 to 50 mL of air into the tube and auscultating the epigastric region for the sound of air movement. Once correct insertion has been verified, the drug is administered through the tube, followed by a small amount of water (about 30 mL). The water flushes the drug and helps to maintain the patency of the tube. An emergency drug that is given by gastric tube is *activated charcoal.*

NOTE

The traditional method of auscultating the epigastric area to confirm correct tube placement may not always be reliable.[5] Other ways to confirm correct placement include asking the patient to speak (if the tube is in the trachea, the patient will be unable to talk); visually inspecting the posterior pharynx for the presence of a coiled tube; aspirating gently on the syringe to obtain gastric fluid; and measuring the pH of the aspirate.[6] These methods require special training. The paramedic should follow protocols approved by medical direction.

BOX 14-7 Procedure for Administering Rectal Drugs*

1. Carefully restrain the child. If possible, place the child in a knee-chest or lateral recumbent position with the legs flexed at the hips and the knees.
2. Draw the drug dose into a syringe and remove the needle. (A slightly higher dose may be required because absorption is incomplete. Consult medical direction.)
3. Insert the lubricated syringe just beyond the external sphincter (aiming just above the junction of the skin and mucous membranes and toward the rectal wall).
4. Inject the solution into the rectum.
5. Aid drug retention by squeezing the buttocks together with manual pressure.

*Although the procedure is described for a child, it also is appropriate for adults.

Rectal Administration of Medications

Some drugs, such as suppositories, are made for rectal administration (Box 14-7). Other drugs can be given by the rectal route when vascular access cannot be established. Emergency drugs that can be given rectally include *diazepam* and *lorazepam* (Figure 14-7).

PARENTERAL ADMINISTRATION OF MEDICATIONS

Parenteral drugs are administered outside the gastrointestinal tract. This term usually refers to injections. Drugs are administered parenterally by the intradermal, subcutaneous, intramuscular, intravenous, and intraosseous routes. (Percutaneous medications also are discussed in this section.) Blood collection procedures (phlebotomy procedures) are discussed later in this chapter.

NOTE

Parenteral administration of drugs can be very hazardous. This is because drugs given by injection are usually thought to be irretrievable. Also, a slight risk of infection exists, because the skin is broken. Other possible hazards associated with parenteral administration include pain with drug administration, cellulitis or abscess formation, necrosis, skin sloughing, nerve injury, prolonged pain, and periostitis (inflammation of connective tissue covering bones). The use of aseptic technique, ensuring an accurate drug dosage, finding the proper site for the injection, and administering the injection at the proper rate are essential to minimizing the risk of harm.

Equipment Used for Injections

SYRINGES AND NEEDLES

The choice of syringe and needle depends on three factors: (1) the route of administration, (2) the characteristics of the fluid (e.g., aqueous or oil based), and (3) the volume of

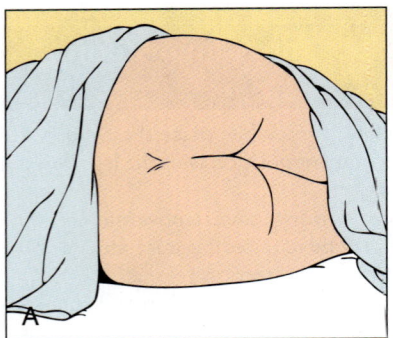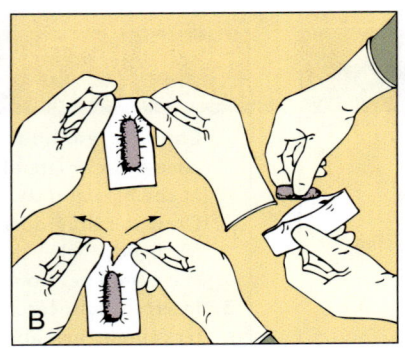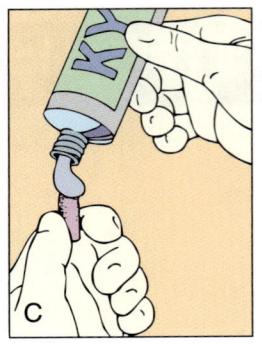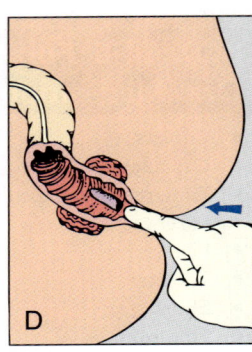

FIGURE 14-7 Rectal drug administration. **A,** Position the patient in the lateral recumbent position and drape. **B,** Unwrap the suppository and remove it from the package. **C,** Apply a water-soluble lubricant. **D,** Gently insert the suppository about 1 inch past the internal sphincter. (Clayton BD, Stock YN, Harroun RD: *Basic pharmacology for nurses,* ed 14, St Louis, 2007, Mosby.)

medication. Syringes in common use today are made of disposable plastic. Sizes range from 1 mL tuberculin and insulin syringes to 60 mL irrigation syringes.

Tuberculin syringes are marked in 0.01 mL gradients. They should be used when the volume to be given is small. Insulin syringes are available in 0.5 and 1 mL volumes. They are marked in 1-unit increments. When used with the specified strength of insulin, this syringe allows the patient to draw up the correct dose easily without doing any calculations. Tuberculin and insulin syringes should not be substituted for each other. Figure 14-8 shows syringes used to measure varying amounts of liquids and liquid medications accurately.

Needles vary in length and gauge. Length ranges from ⅜ inch to 3 inches or longer. Gauge ranges from 12 gauge (large lumen) to 30 gauge (small lumen). Smaller lumen (larger gauge) needles usually are used for intradermal injections. Subcutaneous injections usually are given with a ⅝-inch, 23- or 25-gauge needle. Intramuscular injections usually are given with a 1- to 2-inch, 19- or 21-gauge needle; occasionally a 16- or 18-gauge needle is used.

In 2000 Congress passed the Healthcare Worker Needlestick Prevention Act. The following year, the Occupational Safety and Health Administration (OSHA) amended its Bloodborne Pathogens Standard to recommend needleless systems or "needle safe" devices (sharps with engineered sharps protection). These devices collect body fluids or deliver medications without the use of a needle, which helps prevent blood exposure and needlestick injuries (Box 14-8). Examples of these devices include self-sheathing hypodermic syringes, retractable needles for injections, self-blunting phlebotomy needles, retracting lancets, filter straws, vial access cannulas, and disposable retracting scalpels.

CONTAINERS USED FOR PARENTERAL MEDICATIONS

Medications given by injection usually are supplied in three forms. They come in *single-dose ampules, multidose vials,* or *prefilled syringes.* Single-dose ampules are glass containers that hold one dose of a medication for injection. After use,

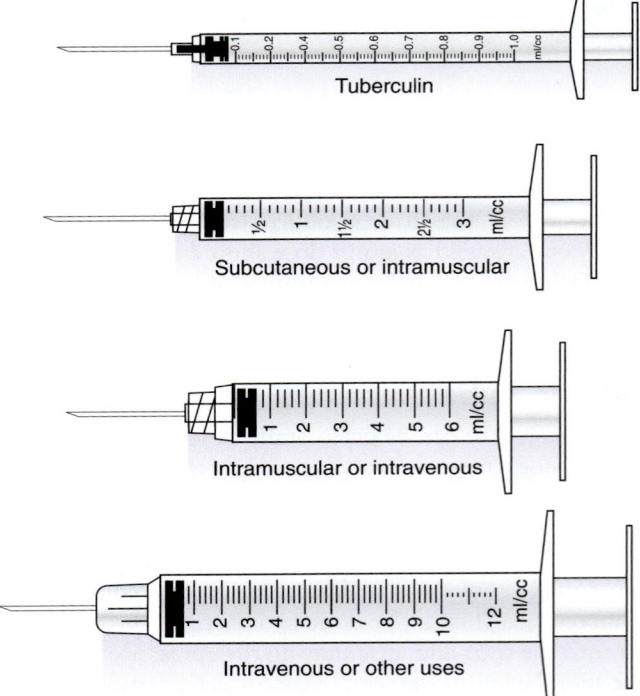

FIGURE 14-8 Types of syringes.

the ampule is discarded into a sharps container. Multidose vials are glass containers that come with rubber stoppers. These permit several medication doses to be withdrawn for injection. In general, these are intended for single-patient use.

To prepare a prescribed medication for injection, the paramedic should choose the appropriate needle and syringe. The size of the syringe must be in proportion to the volume of solution to be given. To withdraw medication from an ampule or vial, the paramedic should follow these steps:
1. Assemble the equipment (alcohol swab or gauze, syringe, 18-gauge filter needle or filter straw to withdraw

medication if using an ampule, and appropriate-gauge needle for injection).

2. Compute the volume of medication to be given.
3. If using a vial (Figure 14-9):
   (a) Clean the rubber stopper with alcohol.
   (b) Inject a volume of air into the vial equivalent to the amount of solution to be withdrawn. (This prevents the formation of a vacuum in the vial. A vacuum can make the solution difficult to withdraw.) Withdraw the volume required and remove the syringe from the vial.
   (c) Gently push in the plunger of the syringe to expel air from the solution.
4. If using an ampule (Figure 14-10):
   (a) Lightly tap or shake the ampule to dislodge any solution from the neck of the container.
   (b) Wrap the neck of the glass ampule with an alcohol swab or gauze dressing to protect the fingers.
   (c) Grasp the ampule, snap off the top, and discard the top in an appropriate medication disposal container. (The ampule is designed to break easily when pressure is exerted at the neck.)
   (d) Carefully insert an 18-gauge filter needle or filter straw into the solution, without allowing it to touch the edges of the ampule, and draw the solution into the syringe.
   (e) Carefully remove the 18-gauge needle or filter screw and discard it in the appropriate container. Attach the needle to be used for injection.
   (f) Gently push in the plunger of the syringe to expel air.

Mixing Medications. Two compatible drugs can be mixed into one injection if the total volume of the dosage is within accepted limits. For example, this technique can be used with **butorphanol** and **hydroxyzine.** When mixing medications, it is crucial not to contaminate one with the other and to maintain aseptic technique. Any doubt about compatibility should be discussed with medical direction. It also can be verified by consulting a proper reference, such as a drug compatibility chart. To mix medications, the paramedic should take the following steps.

BOX 14-8 Prevention of Needle and Sharps Injuries

Each year, health care workers suffer 600,000 to 1 million injuries from conventional needles and sharps.[15] Infection with the hepatitis C virus (HCV) is the most common infection caused by needle-stick and sharps injury.[16] However, transmission of other diseases also is possible. These diseases include human immunodeficiency virus (HIV) infection, hepatitis B, syphilis, herpes simplex, herpes zoster, Rocky Mountain spotted fever, and tuberculosis. The following precautions can help prevent exposure to these pathogens.

- Paramedics should get help when administering infusion therapy or injections to uncooperative patients.
- Needles should not be recapped, purposely bent or broken by hand, removed from disposable syringes, or otherwise manipulated by hand. If a needle must be recapped or removed because there is no alternative or because a specific medical procedure requires it, the paramedic should use a mechanical device or a one-handed technique. Needleless products should be used when available.
- Disposable syringes and needles, scalpel blades, and other sharp items should be placed in puncture-resistant containers for disposal.

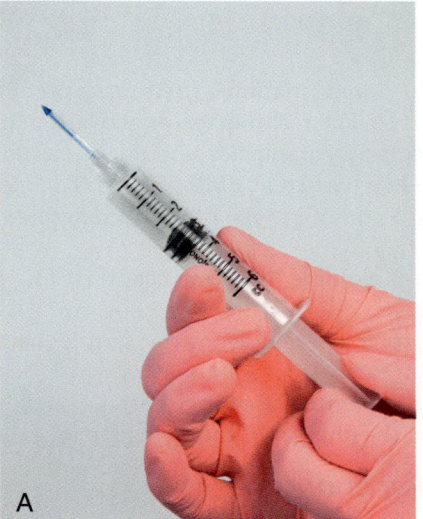
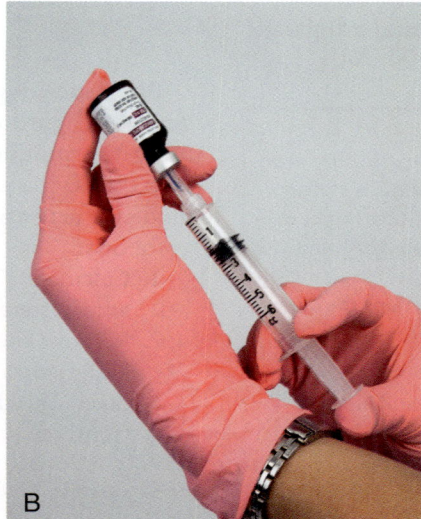
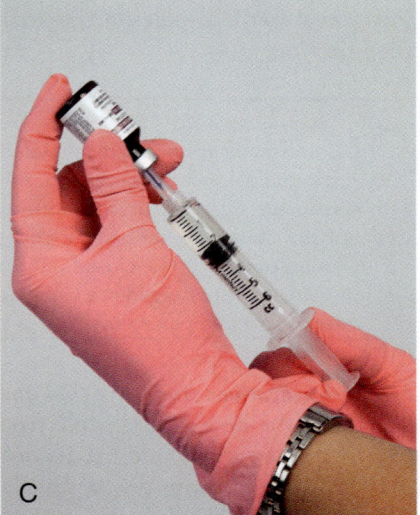

FIGURE 14-9 Withdrawing medication from a vial. **A,** Draw into the syringe an amount of air equal to the volume to be given. **B,** Inject air into the drug vial. **C,** Draw the drug into the syringe.

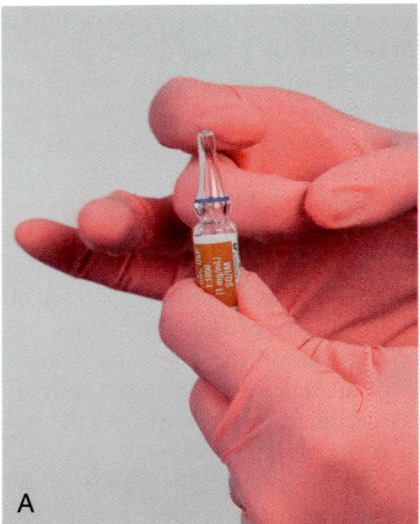 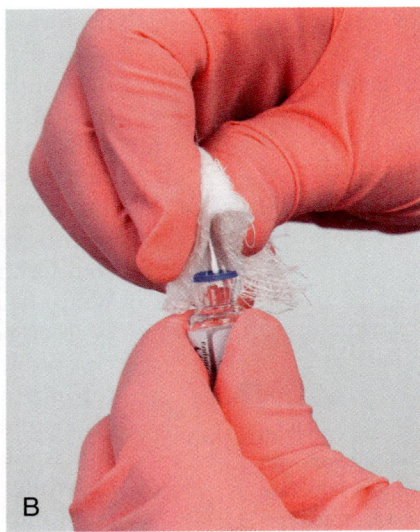 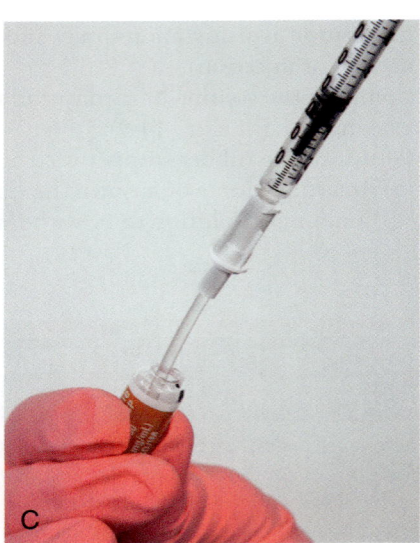

FIGURE 14-10 Withdrawing medication from an ampule. **A,** Tap the ampule to remove drug from the neck. **B,** Break off the top of the ampule with a gauze pad. **C,** Use a filter straw to withdraw the medication from the ampule.

Mixing Medications from Two Vials

1. Use only one syringe to mix the drugs.
2. Aspirate a volume of air equivalent to the dose of the first drug. Inject the air into vial A, making sure the needle or vial access cannula does not touch the solution. Withdraw the needle or vial access cannula.
3. Aspirate a volume of air equivalent to the dose of the second drug. Inject the air into vial B. Withdraw the required medication from vial B.
4. Put a new sterile needle or vial access cannula on the syringe and insert it into vial A. Be careful not to push in the plunger or expel the drug from the syringe into the vial. This would pose a risk of infection and result in mixing of the drugs.
5. Withdraw the desired amount of the drug from vial A into the syringe.
6. Put a new sterile needle on the syringe and administer the injection.

> **NOTE**
> Some medications are dry powders that must be reconstituted before administration. An example is glucagon. Carefully read the manufacturer's information. Use the correct amount of the diluent prescribed for this purpose. Always mix the diluent and powder in the closed vial before withdrawing the dose. Some drugs are packaged in a vial that contains the diluent and powder in two compartments (Mix-o-Vial).

Mixing Medications from One Vial and One Ampule

1. Withdraw the desired drug dose from the vial first.
2. Use the same syringe and needle or filter straw to withdraw medication from the ampule.
3. Put a new sterile needle on the syringe (if the medication is to be given by the intramuscular or subcutaneous route) and administer the injection.

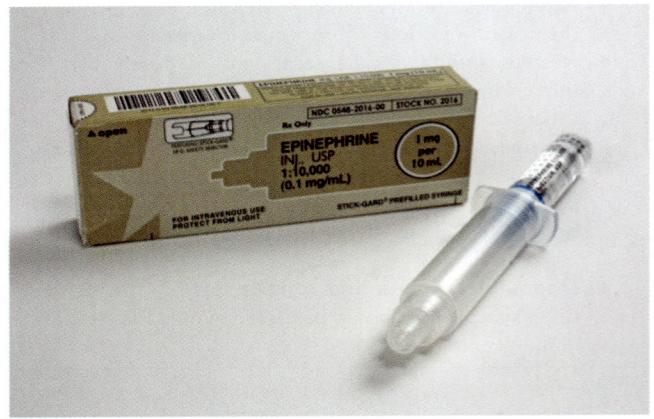

FIGURE 14-11 Prefilled medication syringe.

Prefilled Syringes. Several manufacturers make prefilled syringes (Figure 14-11). The techniques for activating and using the products vary. Paramedics should be familiar with the devices used by particular EMS systems. The technique for activating a common type of prefilled syringe is as follows:

1. Calculate the volume of medication to be administered.
2. Remove the protective caps from the syringe barrel and medication cartridge.
3. Screw the cartridge into the syringe barrel.
4. Gently push in the plunger of the syringe to expel air.

PREPARING THE INJECTION SITE

The injection site is prepared by cleansing the area using aseptic technique. The Guidelines for Prevention of Intravascular Catheter-Related Infections, published by the

Centers for Disease Control and Prevention (CDC), state that "although 2% chlorhexidine-based preparation is preferred, tincture of iodine, an iodophor, or 70% alcohol can be used."[7]

The steps in preparing the injection site are as follows:

1. Thoroughly scrub the site with the appropriate cleanser to remove dirt, dead skin, and other surface contaminants.
2. If using a chlorhexidine-based preparation, scrub the area up and down and then side to side. If using other products, clean the site with overlapping, concentric circles and moving outward from the site.
3. Allow the site to dry.

Intradermal Injections

An intradermal injection is made just below the *epidermis,* or outer layer of skin (Figures 14-12 and 14-13). This site is commonly used for allergy testing and for administration of local anesthetics. A tuberculin syringe usually is used for intradermal injections. The volume injected usually is less than 0.5 mL. Common sites for intradermal injections are the medial surface of the forearm and the back. The steps for administering an intradermal injection are as follows:

1. Choose the injection site and cleanse the skin surface.
2. Hold the skin taut with one hand.
3. With the other hand, hold the syringe (with the needle bevel up) at a 10- to 15-degree angle to the injection site.
4. Gently puncture the skin. Insert the needle until the bevel is completely under the skin surface. Inject the medication. (Intradermal injections usually produce a raised wheal that resembles a mosquito bite.)
5. Withdraw the needle and dispose of the equipment appropriately.

Subcutaneous Injections

Subcutaneous injections are given to place medication below the skin into the subcutaneous layer (Figure 14-14). The volume of such an injection usually is less than 0.5 mL. It is administered through a ½- or ⅝-inch, 23- or 25-gauge needle. In the prehospital setting, the drug most often given by this route is **epinephrine.** The steps for subcutaneous injections are as follows (Figure 14-15):

1. Choose the injection site and cleanse the area.
2. Elevate the subcutaneous tissue by gently pinching the injection site.

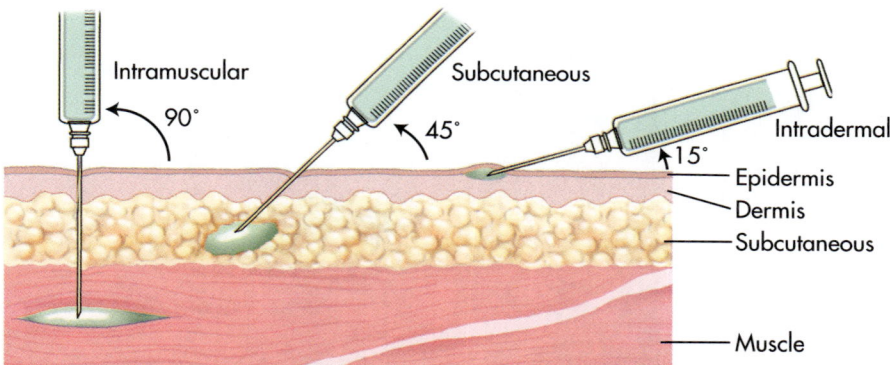

FIGURE 14-12 Comparison of angle of injection and deposition of medication for intramuscular, subcutaneous, and intradermal injections.

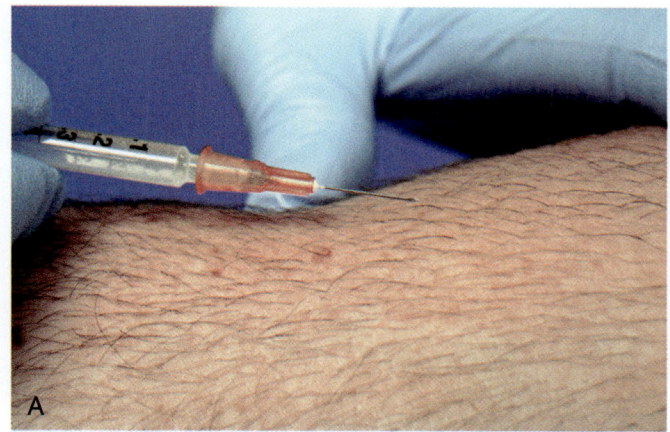
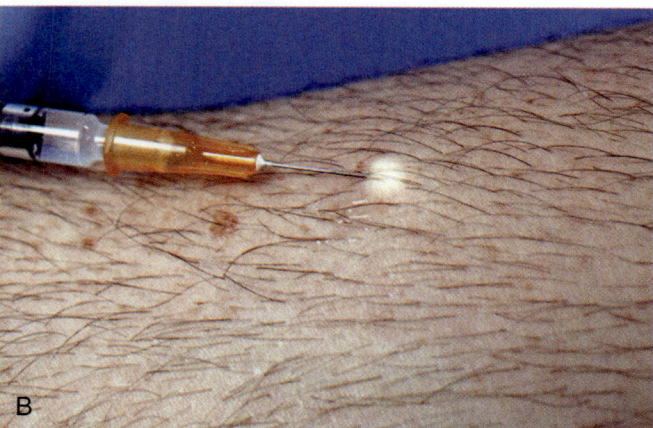

FIGURE 14-13 Intradermal injection. Choose the site and cleanse the skin. **A,** Then, with the bevel up, insert the needle at a 15-degree angle. **B,** Wheal produced by the injection.

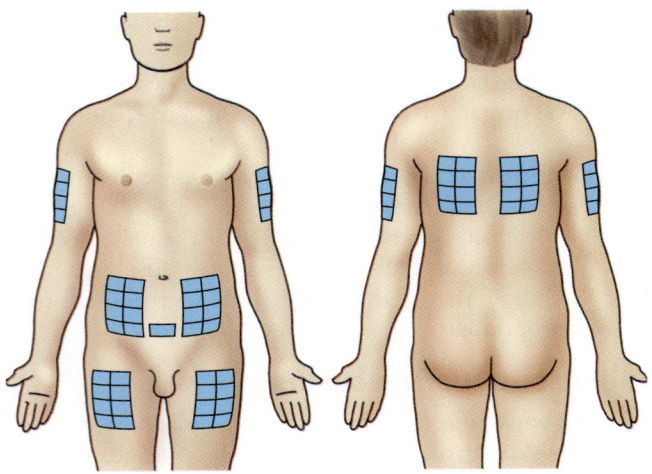

3. With the needle bevel up, insert the needle at a 45-degree angle in one quick motion.

4. Pull back slightly on the plunger (aspirate) to ensure needle placement. If no blood is aspirated, gently but smoothly inject the medication. If blood is present on aspiration, it indicates inadvertent vascular injection. When this occurs, withdraw the needle, discard the medication and equipment, and begin again.

5. After the injection, withdraw the needle at the same angle at which it was inserted. Use an alcohol swab to massage the site. This helps distribute medication and promote absorption by dilating blood vessels in the area and increasing blood flow.

FIGURE 14-14 Sites commonly used for subcutaneous injections.

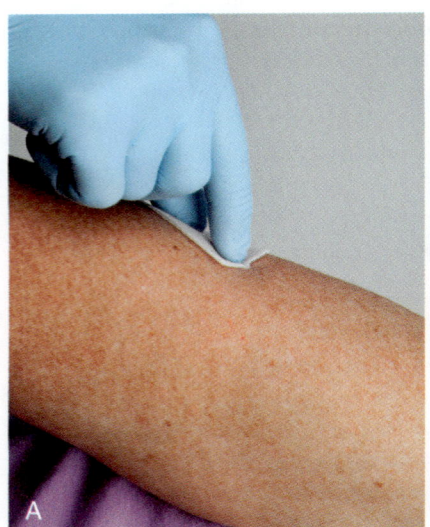

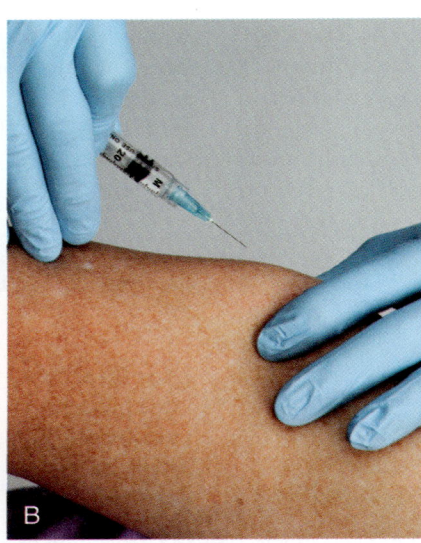

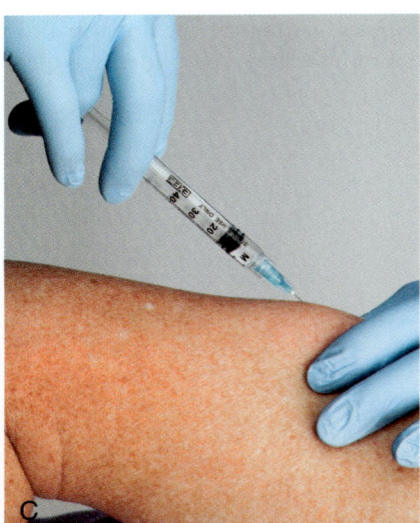

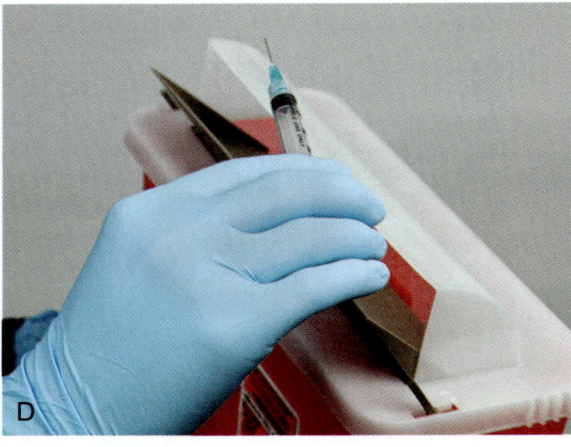

FIGURE 14-15 Subcutaneous injection. **A,** Cleanse the skin. **B,** Grasp the skin to maximize the amount of subcutaneous tissue available and insert the needle. Aspirate unless contraindicated. **C,** Slowly push the plunger to administer the medication. **D,** Discard the needle and syringe in an appropriate sharps container.

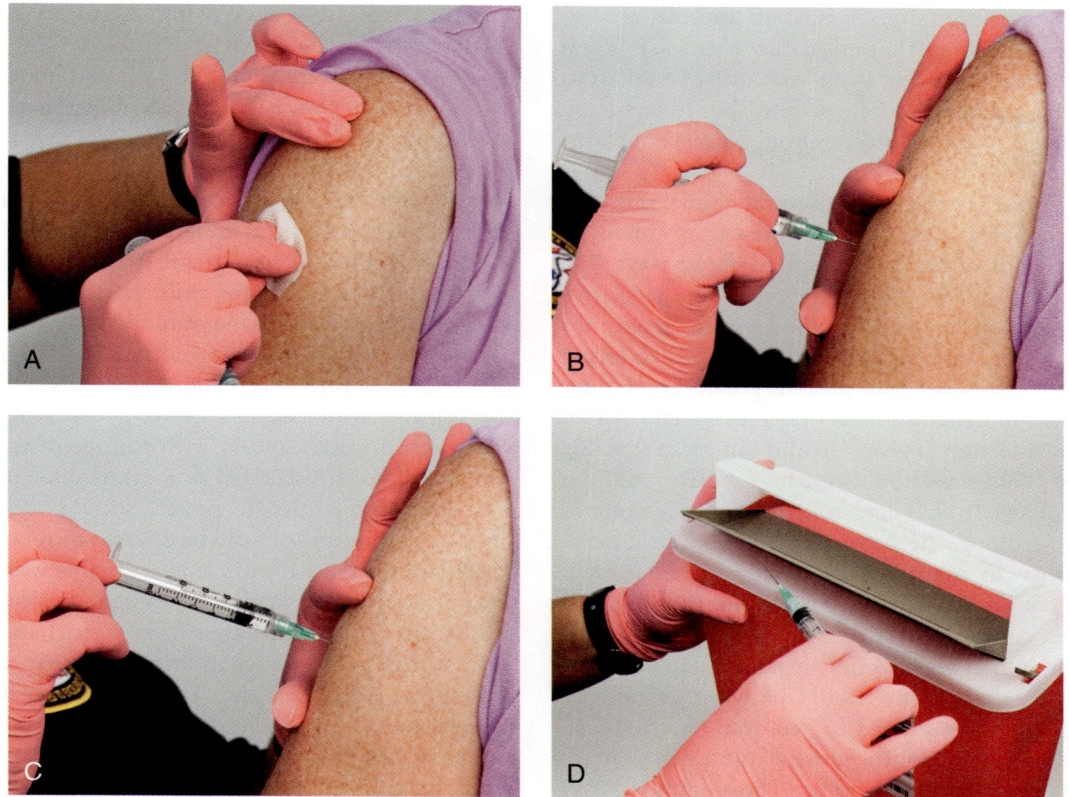

FIGURE 14-16 Intramuscular injection. A, Choose the site and cleanse the skin. B, Pull the skin tight and insert the needle. C, Aspirate and then slowly push the plunger to inject the medication. D, Discard the needle and syringe in an appropriate sharps container.

Intramuscular Injections

Deeper injections are made into muscle tissue. These pass through the skin and subcutaneous tissue. They are given when a drug is too irritating to be injected subcutaneously or when a greater volume or faster absorption is desired. (Irritation still may occur with administration by this route.) A maximum volume of 5 mL may be given by intramuscular injection in a large muscle mass (e.g., gluteal muscle).

The type of needle used depends on four factors: (1) the site of the injection; (2) the condition of the tissue; (3) the size of the patient; and (4) the type of drug to be injected (i.e., small-lumen needles are used for thin solutions, and larger lumen needles are used for suspensions and oils). Because the muscle layer is below the subcutaneous layer, a longer needle generally is used (usually 1½ inches and 19 or 21 gauge). The procedures for intramuscular injections are the same as those described before (Figure 14-16). However, the needle is inserted at a 90-degree angle. Also, the skin is held taut, not pinched.

Several muscles are commonly used for intramuscular injections. These are the deltoid muscle, several gluteal muscles (dorsogluteal site), the vastus lateralis muscle, the rectus femoris muscle, and the ventrogluteal muscle. The deltoid muscle is located in the upper arm. It forms a

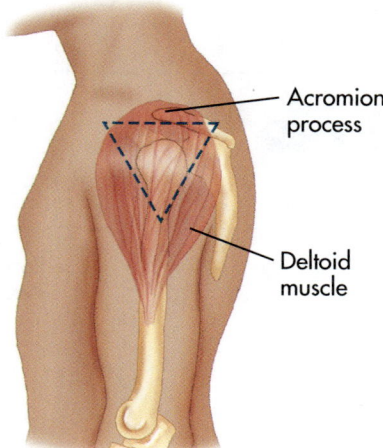

FIGURE 14-17 The injection site for the deltoid muscle roughly forms an inverted triangle, with the acromion process as the base. The muscle may be visible in well-developed patients.

triangular shape, with the base of the triangle along the acromion process and the peak of the triangle ending approximately one third of the way down the lateral aspect of the upper arm (Figure 14-17). This muscle is used primarily for vaccinations involving only a small volume of drug. This is because the muscle is small and can accommodate only small doses of injection (1 mL or less). When injections are made in this location, care must be taken to avoid hitting the radial nerve. The patient should be sitting upright or lying flat and should be told to relax the arm muscles.

The dorsogluteal site consists of several gluteal muscles. The gluteus medius muscle is most often used for injections. The dorsogluteal site can be defined in two ways. The first method is to divide the buttocks on one side into imaginary quadrants; the medication is administered into the upper outer quadrant. The second method is to locate the posterior-superior iliac spine and the greater trochanter of the femur. An imaginary line is drawn between the two landmarks; the injection is given up and out from this line (Figure 14-18). This site should not be used for children under 3 years of age. In that age group, the muscles are not yet well developed and the proximity of the sciatic nerve (the largest nerve in the body) poses a risk. Large, well-developed muscles can accommodate an injection of up to 5 mL. However, volumes over 3 mL may be uncomfortable for the patient. When an injection is administered at the dorsogluteal site, the patient should be lying prone. The toes should be pointing inward to promote muscle relaxation. Another complication of gluteal injections is inadvertent injection into the hip joint. The paramedic can minimize this risk by paying attention to anatomical landmarks.

The vastus lateralis and the rectus femoris muscles lie side by side in the thigh. To identify the necessary landmarks, the paramedic should place one hand on the patient's upper thigh and one hand on the lower thigh. The area between the hands is the middle third of the thigh and the middle third of the underlying muscle (Figure 14-19). The vastus lateralis lies lateral to the midline and is the preferred injection site for children. It is well developed in all patients and has few major blood vessels and nerves that can be injured. The rectus femoris is located in the midline of the middle third of the thigh. This site is most often used for self-injection because of its accessibility. Acceptable volumes for injection vary with the age of the patient and the size of the muscle. Up to 5 mL may be injected into a well-developed adult. The patient should be sitting upright or lying supine and should be advised to relax the muscles.

The ventrogluteal muscle is accessible when the patient lies in a supine or lateral recumbent position. The paramedic should palpate the greater trochanter using the palm, with the index finger pointing to the anterior-superior iliac spine. The paramedic's remaining three fingers should extend toward the iliac crest. The injection is made into the center of the V formed by the fingers (Figure 14-20). This injection site may be used for all patients. It is a desirable site because it has no large nerves or fat tissue. In the adult, this muscle may accommodate up to 5 mL of drug.

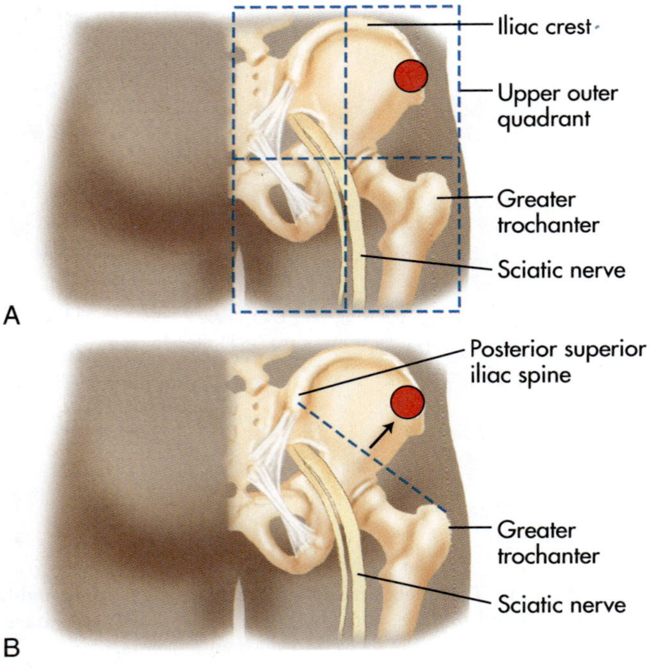

> **NOTE**
> Some intramuscular medications (e.g., promethazine) should be administered into a large muscle. In such cases, use one of the leg or hip injection sites.

FIGURE 14-18 The injection area for the dorsogluteal site can be defined in two ways. **A,** Divide the buttocks on one side into imaginary quadrants. Use the center of the upper outer quadrant as the injection site. **B,** Locate the posterior-superior iliac spine and the greater trochanter by palpation. Draw an imaginary line between the two. The injection site should be above and out from that line.

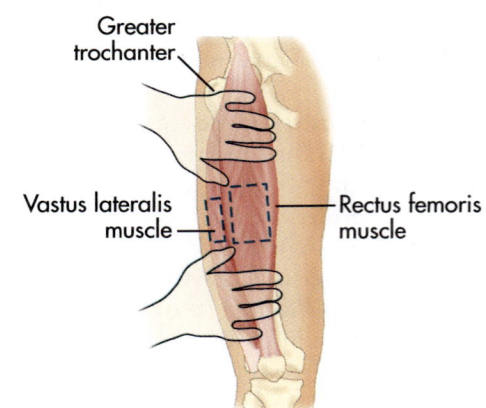

FIGURE 14-19 The injection sites for the vastus lateralis muscle and the rectus femoris muscle can be defined through landmarks. Place one hand below the greater trochanter. Place the other hand above the knee. The space between the two hands defines the middle third of the underlying muscle. The rectus femoris is on the anterior thigh. The vastus lateralis is on the lateral side.

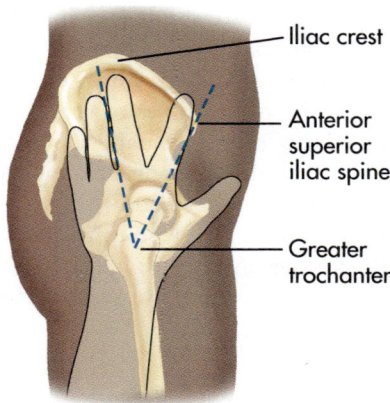

FIGURE 14-20 The injection site for the ventrogluteal muscle is defined by placing the palm of one hand on the trochanter of the femur. A V is then made with the fingers of that hand. One side runs from the greater trochanter to the anterior-superior iliac spine. The other side runs from the greater trochanter to the iliac crest. The injection is made into the center of the V.

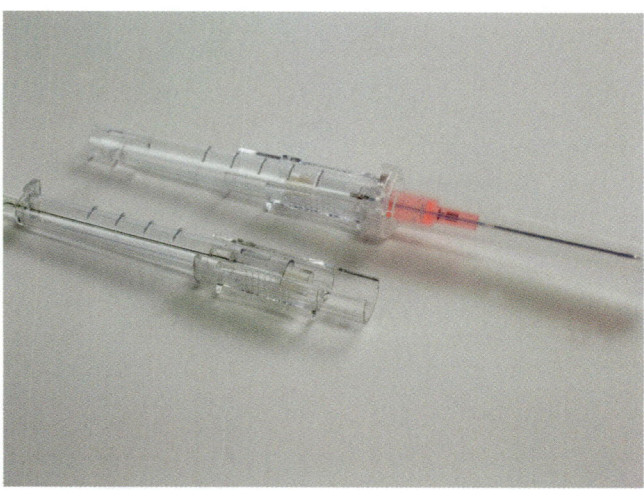

FIGURE 14-21 Various types of intravenous (IV) catheters.

Intravenous Therapy

Intravenous cannulation is used to gain access to the body's circulation. It is indicated for three reasons: (1) to administer fluids; (2) to administer drugs; and (3) to obtain specimens for laboratory testing. The intravenous route puts the drug directly into the bloodstream. This bypasses all barriers to drug absorption.

CRITICAL THINKING
What are the benefits of choosing the upper extremity for intravenous access in an adult?

Intravenous Fluid Administration

In the prehospital setting, the route of choice for fluid therapy is through a peripheral vein in an extremity. If the arms have no major injury, upper extremity veins should be used. (Some EMS agencies advise against using upper extremity sites if a major injury to the neck or upper thorax has occurred on that side.) If upper extremity sites are not available, lower extremity sites may be used. IV fluids often used in the prehospital setting include normal saline, lactated Ringer solution, and mixtures of glucose and water. For the most part, normal saline and lactated Ringer solution are used for fluid replacement. They also are used as a means of administering a drug.

TYPES OF INTRAVENOUS CATHETERS

The three main types of intravenous catheters are (1) the hollow needle (butterfly) type; (2) the indwelling plastic catheter *over* a hollow needle (e.g., Protective Cath, Autoguard, Accuvance Safety) (Figure 14-21); and (3) the

indwelling plastic catheter inserted *through* a hollow needle (e.g., Intracath; this type is seldom used in the prehospital setting).

Hollow needles are not advised for IV fluid replacement in the prehospital setting, because stabilizing the needle is very difficult. In some cases a butterfly catheter may be used for a pediatric patient if it can be stabilized adequately. This sometimes can be achieved by using armboards or other immobilization devices. In the prehospital setting, use of the over-the-needle catheter is preferred. This type of catheter is easily secured. Also, it is more comfortable for the patient.

PERIPHERAL INTRAVENOUS INSERTION

An area commonly used for peripheral intravenous therapy is the hands. Another is the arms. This includes the antecubital fossae (AC space). Other sites are the long saphenous veins in the leg and the external jugular veins in the neck. However, the incidences of embolism (described later) and infection are higher at the latter two sites. Figures 14-22 through 14-24 show sites and techniques for peripheral cannulation.

Another factor in the selection of a puncture site for intravenous therapy is the patient's clinical status. Injuries or diseases involving an extremity interfere with the use of veins in that extremity for venipuncture or venous cannulation. Examples of such conditions include trauma, infection at the site, dialysis fistula, and a history of mastectomy.

The following are the steps involved in peripheral venous insertion of a cannula.

1. If the patient is conscious, explain the procedure. Give the reason intravenous therapy is necessary and describe the procedure.
2. Assemble the equipment (Figure 14-25).
   (a) Inspect the prescribed fluid for contamination, appearance, and expiration date. Never use fluids

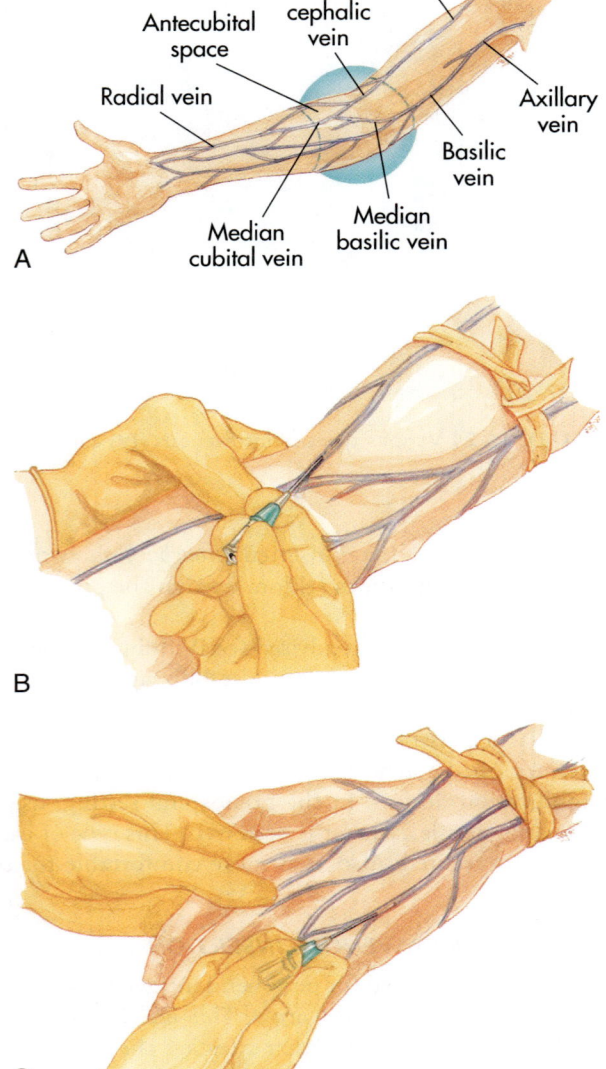

A

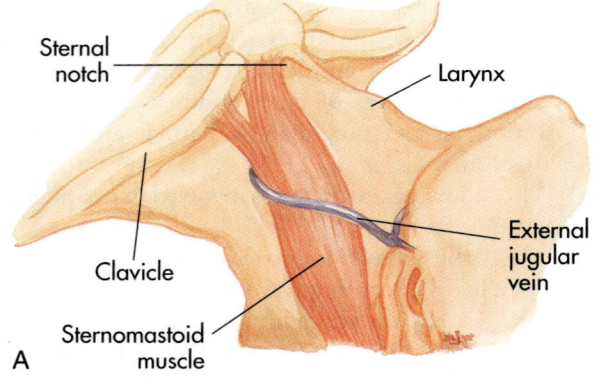

B

C

that are cloudy, outdated, or in any way suspect for contamination.

(b) Prepare the microdrip or macrodrip infusion set. Attach the infusion set to the bag of solution. (Microdrip tubing usually is used for precise drug infusions; macrodrip tubing usually is used for fluid administration.)

3. Clamp the tubing and squeeze the reservoir on the infusion set until it fills halfway. Then open the clamp and flush the air from the tubing. Close the clamp.

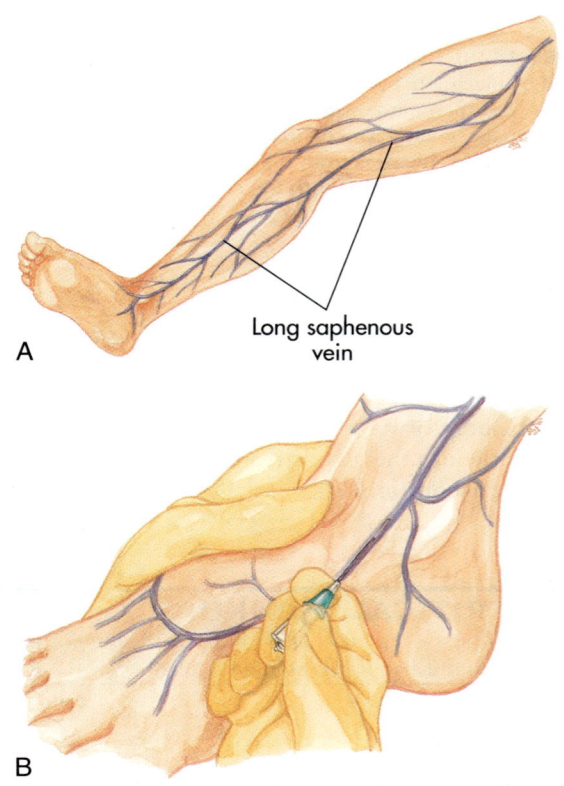

A

B

FIGURE 14-22 A, Veins of the upper extremity. **B,** Antecubital venipuncture. **C,** Dorsal hand venipuncture.

FIGURE 14-23 A, Long saphenous vein. **B,** Venipuncture of the long saphenous vein.

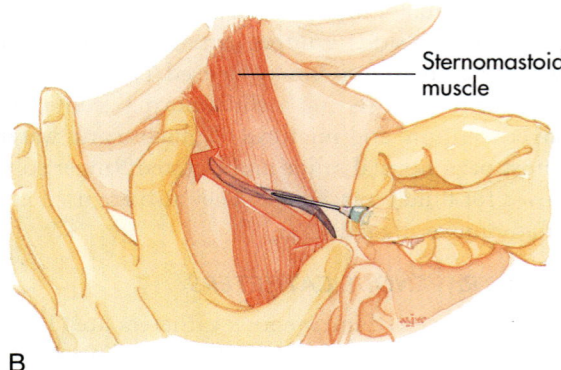

A

B

FIGURE 14-24 A, Anatomy of the external jugular vein. **B,** External jugular venipuncture.

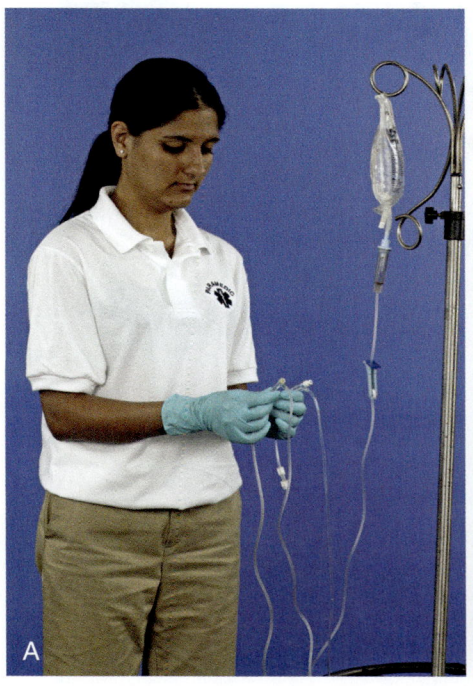
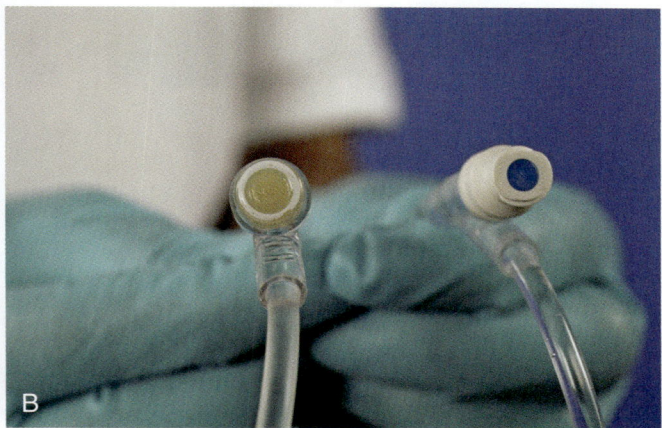

FIGURE 14-25 **A**, Intravenous infusion setup. **B**, Needle and needleless ports.

4. Select the catheter. A large-bore catheter (14 to 16 gauge) should be used for fluid replacement. A smaller bore catheter (18 to 20 gauge) should be used for "keep open" lines. Keep open lines are used to maintain hydration and to establish a channel for IV medication if needed.

5. Prepare other equipment:
   - Antiseptic to cleanse the skin
   - Sterile dressings or 4 × 4 gauze pads
   - Adhesive tape, torn or cut into several strips
   - Syringes and Vacutainers for blood samples
   - Tourniquet (rubber drain tubing or blood pressure cuff may be used)

6. Put on gloves for personal and patient protection.

7. Select the puncture site (Figure 14-26, *A*). If using an upper extremity, allow the patient's arm to hang dependent and apply the tourniquet several inches above the antecubital space. (The tourniquet should be just tight enough to tamponade venous vessels but not occlude arterial flow.) When selecting a suitable vein, begin by looking at the dorsum of the hand and forearm. Choose a vein that is fairly straight and easily accessible. The forearm is better than the hand because it allows hand movement and is more easily secured after cannulation. If a second puncture attempt is necessary, the second puncture should always be *proximal* to the first puncture. Therefore the vein selected for initial cannulation should be the most suitable distal vein. Avoid veins near joints, where immobilization is difficult, and veins near injured areas. If the long saphenous vein is chosen,

begin site selection near the medial malleolus of the foot. To locate the external jugular vein, place the patient in a supine head-down position and turn the patient's head toward the opposite side.

8. Prepare the puncture site and cleanse the area (Figure 14-26, *B*):
   (a) Thoroughly clean the site with an antiseptic to remove dirt, dead skin, blood, and other surface contaminants. Allow the area to dry.
   (b) Clean the site using overlapping, concentric circles and moving outward.

9. Stabilize the vein by applying distal pressure and tension to the point of entry. With the bevel up, pass the needle through the skin and into the vein at a 15- to 20-degree angle from the side or directly on top (Figure 14-26, *C*). (Using a "bevel down" technique in infants and children may facilitate entry into constricted peripheral veins.[8]) Advance the needle and catheter about 2 mm beyond the point where blood return in the hub of the needle was first encountered. Slide the catheter over the needle and into the vein (Figure 14-26, *D*). (Avoid touching the catheter with the fingers.) While stabilizing the catheter, withdraw the needle. Apply pressure on the proximal end of the catheter to stop escaping blood. Obtain blood samples, if needed, with a syringe or Vacutainer.

10. Release the tourniquet and attach the IV tubing (Figure 14-26, *E*). Open the tubing clamp and allow the fluid infusion to begin at the prescribed flow rate (Figure 14-26, *F*).

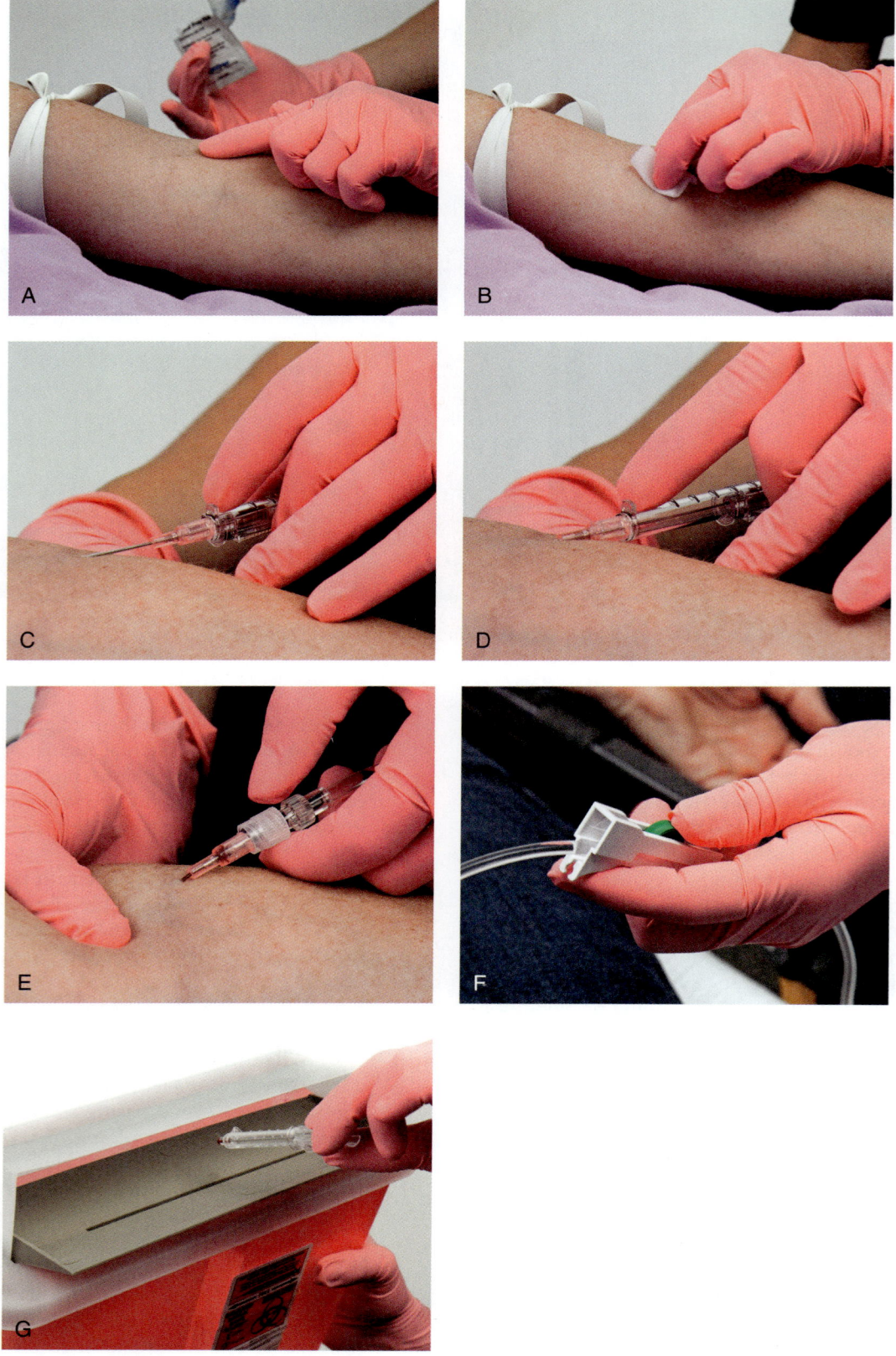

FIGURE 14-26 Intravenous (IV) catheterization technique. **A,** Apply a tourniquet above the desired site and identify the vein. **B,** Cleanse the site. **C,** Stabilize the vein and pass the needle into the vein from the side or directly on top. **D,** Slide the catheter over the needle and into the vein. While stabilizing the catheter, withdraw the needle into the protective sheath. **E,** Release the tourniquet and attach the IV tubing. **F,** Open the tubing clamp. Adjust the infusion to begin at the prescribed flow rate. **G,** Apply a dressing and secure it. Make sure the needle has been discarded in an appropriate container.

11. Cover the puncture site with an occlusive dressing to ensure asepsis and to secure the line (Figure 14-26, *G*). Anchor the tubing and secure the catheter. Catheter movement can increase the risk of phlebitis and cause migration of pathogens along the cannula into the vein.

12. Document the infusion procedure. Also, make sure the needle has been discarded in an appropriate container (Figure 14-26, *H*).

? DID YOU KNOW?

Troubleshooting an Intravenous Infusion

If intravenous (IV) fluids are not flowing well or have completely stopped flowing, the paramedic should attempt to correct the problem before abandoning the IV site. Troubleshooting of an IV infusion should begin at the patient and proceed to the IV bag. The following are some common problems and solutions to consider for IV flow problems.

1. Make sure the tourniquet has been removed. If it is still in place, remove it.
2. The patient's joint above the insertion site may be flexed. Reposition the extremity or splint the extremity with a board.
3. The patient may be lying on the IV tubing, or the tubing may be kinked, restricting flow. Reposition the patient. Secure the tubing using a loop to prevent kinking.
4. Make sure the flow clamp and any other clamps are open. Adjust the clamp as needed and recalculate the drop rate.
5. The catheter tip may be lodged against the wall of the vein. Gently reposition the catheter.
6. The securing tape or device may be too tight, restricting flow. Reapply it if necessary.
7. Gravity may prevent fluid flow when the IV tubing is too far below the insertion site. Lift and reposition the IV tubing.
8. The IV bag may not be high enough above the insertion site. Raise the bag at least 3 feet above the insertion site.

If these attempts do not resolve the fluid flow problem, the IV line should be removed and another IV site should be chosen in the opposite extremity, if possible. If the insertion site is swollen or is leaking fluid into surrounding tissues (infiltration), the catheter should be removed.

Complications of Intravenous Techniques

About 25 million Americans have IV catheters placed each year.[9] Intravenous therapy is a very important part of medical treatment for acute illnesses, cancer, surgery, anesthesia, and trauma. However, it can have complications. Possible complications include local complications, systemic complications, infiltration, and air embolism.

📋 NOTE

More than 85% of hospitalized patients receive some type of IV therapy, and many of the IV lines are established in the prehospital setting. Most lawsuits related to IV therapy involve infiltration or phlebitis.[10] To protect against litigation, it is important for paramedics to document the following:

- Type, length, and gauge of the catheter inserted
- Date and time of insertion
- Number and location of attempts
- Any complications with placement of the IV
- Name of the vein
- Type of dressing applied to the site
- How the patient tolerated the procedure
- Any comments the patient made about the insertion procedure
- Name of the person inserting the device

LOCAL COMPLICATIONS

Local complications may involve hematoma formation, thrombosis, cellulitis, phlebitis, and sloughing and necrosis of tissue.

- **Hematoma formation** is the collection of blood or fluids at the site of injection or cannulation. The hematoma usually is small enough that it resolves spontaneously. It rarely requires surgical treatment, drainage, or other interventions.
- **Thrombosis** is the formation of a blood clot (thrombus) inside a blood vessel. It occurs when the blood vessel is injured. A clot that remains in place can become a **thromboembolism** and enter the circulatory system.
- **Cellulitis** is a potentially serious bacterial infection of connective tissue. It is associated with severe inflammation of dermal and subcutaneous skin. Cellulitis can be caused by the introduction of normal skin flora after an injection or cannulation. Cellulitis appears as a swollen, red area of skin that feels hot and tender. It can spread to any part of the body. Cellulitis usually is treated with antibiotics.
- **Phlebitis** is inflammation of a vein. It is common after insertion of an IV catheter. It can result if a catheter is too large for the vein or has been left in place longer than 48 hours. Phlebitis causes localized redness and warmth at the IV site. It may extend a short distance along the course of the cannulized vein. Phlebitis increases the risk of clot formation in a vein. It is treated with antiinflammatory medicines.
- **Sloughing** and **necrosis** of tissue can occur from infiltration of some IV medicines (e.g., *dextrose 50%, sodium bicarbonate, promethazine*). Sloughing (the separation of tissue) and necrosis (tissue death) can be prevented by taking care to choose a stable vein of adequate size for drug administration. Frequent

monitoring of the IV site for position and patency before, during, and after drug administration also is important.

SYSTEMIC COMPLICATIONS

Systemic complications include sepsis, pulmonary embolism, catheter fragment embolism, and arterial puncture.

- **Sepsis** is a bacterial infection in the bloodstream. It can be caused by the use of contaminated equipment, poor aseptic technique, and prolonged IV therapy. Signs and symptoms of sepsis include a body temperature of 100.4° F (greater than 38° C) or 96.8° F (less than 36° C), profuse sweating, nausea and vomiting, diarrhea, abdominal pain, tachycardia, hypotension, an increased white blood cell count, and altered mental status. Treatment includes the use of broad-spectrum antibiotics (see Chapter 32).
- **Pulmonary embolism** is the sudden blocking of an artery in the lung. It is caused by the collection of solid material (**embolus**) brought through the bloodstream. It also may occur as a result of air bubbles introduced through an IV catheter (*air embolism*, described later). Signs and symptoms include a sudden onset of chest pain, shortness of breath, tachycardia, and hypotension. The patient should be placed on high-concentration oxygen and a cardiac monitor and should be transported for evaluation and treatment by a physician. (Pulmonary embolism is further described in Chapter 24.)
- **Catheter fragment embolism** can occur during the insertion of an IV catheter. It can result if part of the catheter is sheared off (detached), allowing the embolus to travel in the bloodstream. It also can occur when there is motion at the cannula and the hub. An example is a catheter that is poorly secured or placed at areas of flexion. Reinsertion of a needle through the catheter during intravenous insertion can also produce a fragment embolism. Signs and symptoms include sharp pain at the insertion site, chest pain, and tachycardia. If a catheter fragment embolism is suspected, the IV should be stopped; the vein should be palpated for the catheter tip; and a venous tourniquet should be applied above the tip to prevent further movement of the fragment.

> **NOTE**
> A needle should never be reinserted through a catheter. If IV insertion fails, the catheter should be removed, and a new IV catheter should be placed. When IV therapy is discontinued, the catheter should be examined to verify that it is intact and has not been sheared.

- Most arteries lie deep within the tissues. However, some may lie close to the surface. Inadvertent arterial puncture during IV therapy is noted by the presence of pulsating and bright red blood in the catheter hub. Arteries are not suited for drug administration. In addition, arterial puncture can cause diminished blood supply to areas nourished by the affected artery. If arterial puncture occurs, the catheter should be removed and direct pressure applied to the site for at least 5 minutes. (Apply direct pressure for at least 10 minutes if the patient is on anticoagulant therapy.) A new IV should be placed. The incident should be well documented on the patient care report.

> **NOTE**
> Nerves, tendons, and ligaments can be injured during IV therapy. These injuries may be caused by improper technique or lack of knowledge of anatomy. The patient may complain of intense pain, numbness, and an electric shock–type pain if a nerve is damaged. Injuries to nerves, tendons, and ligaments may be temporary or permanent. Patient management includes removing the IV catheter; inserting a new IV line; and providing careful documentation.

INFILTRATION

Infiltration may occur when the needle or catheter has been displaced or when blood or fluid leaks from around the catheter and escapes into the tissues (**extravasation**). It also can occur if a vein is punctured more than once during initiation of IV access. Signs and symptoms include:

- Coolness of the skin at the puncture site
- Swelling at the puncture site, with or without pain
- Sluggish or absent flow rate

If infiltration is suspected, the paramedic should lower the fluid reservoir to a dependent position to check for the backflow of blood into the tubing. (The absence of backflow suggests infiltration.) If any of the signs and symptoms are present, the intravenous flow should be discontinued (Box 14-9). The needle or catheter should be removed immediately. Moreover, a pressure dressing should be applied to the site. An alternative puncture site should be chosen and the infusion restarted with new equipment. In

---

BOX 14-9 Discontinuation of an Intravenous Infusion

To discontinue an intravenous (IV) infusion and remove the IV catheter, follow these steps:

1. Put on gloves.
2. Carefully remove any securing tape and dressings.
3. Close the drip chamber to stop the flow of fluid.
4. Place sterile gauze over the insertion site and apply gentle pressure with one hand. With the other hand, quickly withdraw the catheter, pulling straight back from the angle of insertion. Check that the catheter is intact.
5. Apply firm pressure to the insertion site for 2 to 5 minutes to prevent bleeding or bruising.
6. Cover the insertion site with a bandage.
7. Appropriately dispose of all equipment.

addition, the incident should be documented. Medication should not be injected into an IV line if there is a possibility it has infiltrated.

AIR EMBOLISM

Air embolism is uncommon. However, it can be fatal. The volume of air the human bloodstream can tolerate has not been firmly established. However, fatalities have been reported after 100 mL of air entered the cardiovascular system.[11] A total of 10 mL of air can be fatal in a critically ill patient.

The embolism is caused by air entering the bloodstream via the catheter tubing. The risk of air embolism is greatest when a catheter is passed into the central circulation, where negative pressure may actually pull in air (see Appendix A). Air can enter the circulation either on insertion of the catheter or when the tubing is disconnected to replace solutions or add new extension tubing (Box 14-10). With subsequent pumping, blood foaming occurs in the heart. If enough air enters the heart chamber, it can impede the flow of blood. This, in turn, can lead to shock. Signs and symptoms of air embolism include hypotension, cyanosis, weak, rapid pulse, and loss of consciousness. If air embolism is suspected, the following steps should be taken:

1. Close the tubing.
2. Turn the patient on the left side with the head down. (If air has entered the heart chambers, this position may keep the air in the right side of the heart and away from the cardiac valves. The pulmonary artery may absorb small air bubbles.)
3. Check tubing for leaks.
4. Administer high-concentration oxygen.
5. Notify medical direction.

Accidental disconnection of the IV tubing can cause an air embolism. This may occur during patient movement. The chance of an air embolism can be minimized by making sure all tubing connections are secure. Also, fluid containers should be changed before they are empty.

Intravenous Medications

Medications can be given directly into the vascular system via the venous route by injection or infusion. An intravenous injection can be administered through a previously established IV infusion line, heparin or saline lock, or implantable port (e.g., Port-A-Cath, Hickman catheter). It also can be administered directly into the vein with a sterile needle or butterfly device. An IV infusion is given by adding a drug to an infusing intravenous solution. (An example of such a solution is normal saline.) Another method is to dilute the drug in a larger volume of fluid and administer the medication IV push, or through a volume control, in-line device (e.g., burette, Volutrol, infusion pump) (Figure 14-27). Sometimes the medication is given by intermittent infusion through an existing infusion site (*intravenous piggyback* or *secondary set*).

Intravenous injections normally involve a small amount of medication. These are called *intravenous push* or *intravenous bolus* medications. To give such an injection (Figure 14-28), the paramedic should clean the injection port or needleless port of the IV line with antiseptic. The medication is then injected slowly (usually over 1 to 3 minutes). The rate of injection depends on the type of medication and the patient's response. Most intravenous tubing has one-way valves to prevent the backflow of medication. If such a valve is not present or cannot be identified, the tubing above the injection site should be clamped during drug administration. After the injection, the infusion of fluids is continued.

Intravenous infusions for drug administration can take several forms. To add a medication to the fluid reservoir of an established IV line, the paramedic should follow these steps (Figure 14-29):

BOX 14-10 Replacement of Intravenous Solutions

At times a bag of intravenous (IV) fluids must be replaced during an infusion. To do this, prepare all equipment in advance and follow these steps:

1. Hold the infusing bag upside down in one hand and remove the spike chamber. Discard the old bag.
2. Quickly insert the spike chamber into the new bag and squeeze the chamber.
3. Insert an 18-gauge needle into an injection port in the IV tubing to allow air to be expelled from the tubing before it reaches the patient.
4. After the air has been expelled, remove the needle and adjust the flow rate of the infusion.
5. Document the time the IV fluids were replaced.

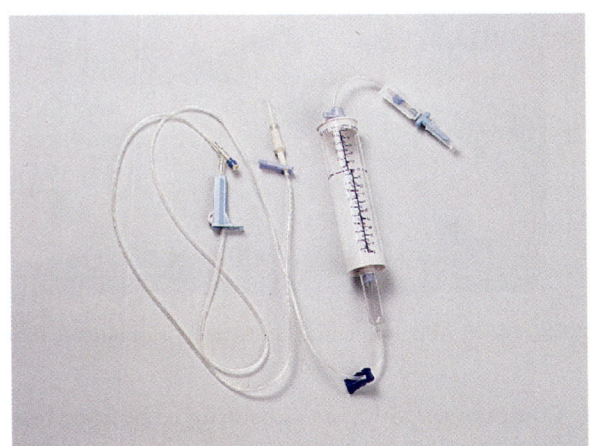

FIGURE 14-27 Buretrol, a volume control device. (Shade BR: *Mosby's EMT-intermediate textbook for the 1985 National Standard Curriculum,* revised edition, St Louis, 2007, Mosby.)

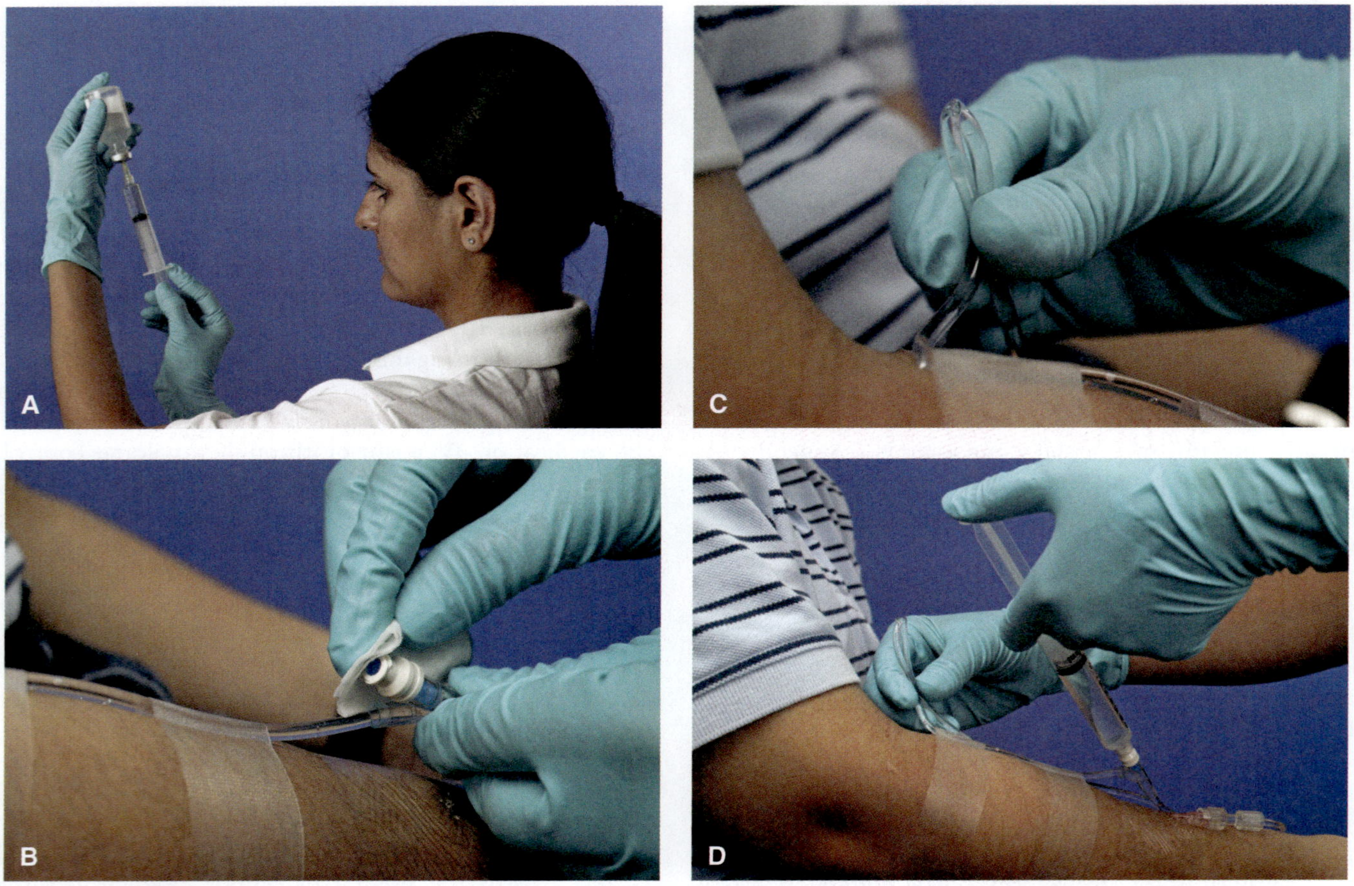

FIGURE 14-28 Administration of a drug by the intravenous (IV) route. **A,** Prepare the correct volume of the drug. **B,** Cleanse the injection port. **C,** If the tubing does not have a one-way valve, pinch the line to clamp it. **D,** Inject the drug at the recommended rate. Resume IV flow (with a small flush if indicated) and monitor the patient.

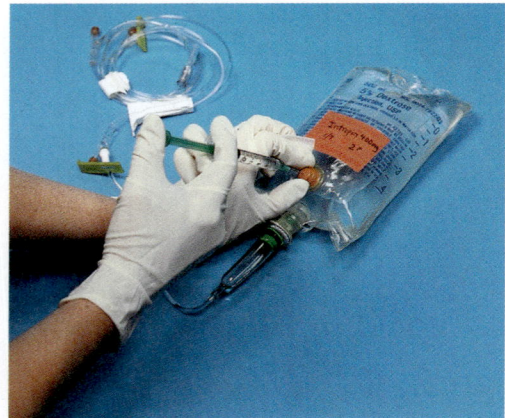

FIGURE 14-29 Adding medication to an intravenous reservoir.

1. Compute the volume of the drug to be added to the fluid reservoir.
2. Draw up the prescribed dose into a syringe. If prefilled syringes are used, note the volume of medication in the syringe and the dose to be used.

3. Cleanse the rubber sleeve of the fluid reservoir with an antiseptic.
4. Puncture the rubber sleeve (if a needle is used) and inject the prescribed medication into the fluid reservoir.
5. Withdraw the needle (if a needleless system is not used) and discard the needle and syringe. Gently mix the medication with the fluid by agitating the reservoir.
6. Label the fluid reservoir with (1) the name of the medication added, (2) the amount of the medication added, (3) the resultant concentration of the medication in the reservoir, (4) the date and time the infusion was prepared, and (5) the name of the paramedic who prepared the infusion.
7. Calculate the rate of administration in drops per minute as prescribed.

A number of in-line volume control devices allow more accurate delivery of medication diluted in precise amounts of fluids than can be achieved by simply setting the drip rate manually. These devices often are used to give intravenous medications to children and adults who need precise

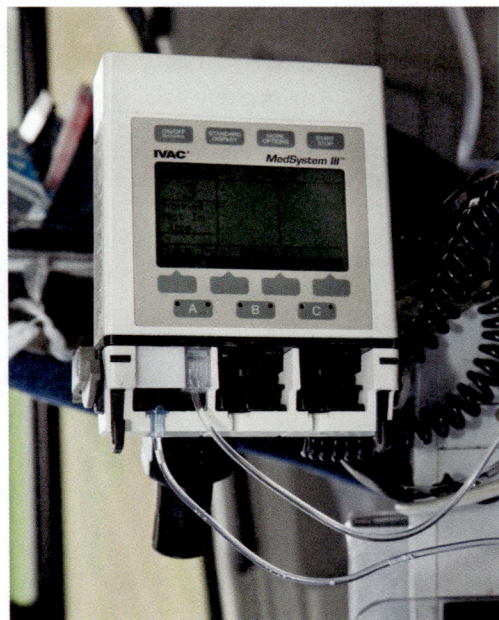

FIGURE 14-30 Intravenous infusion pump.

doses. Medications that can readily cause toxicity when given too rapidly (e.g., antidysrhythmics, vasopressors) are well suited to this delivery method. In-line devices include electronic flow rate regulators that regulate fluid passage by means of a magnetically activated metal ball valve. They also include infusion pumps that exert pressure on tubing or fluid by pumping against pressure gradients. Paramedics should follow the instructions of the equipment's manufacturer. They also should become familiar with these devices before using them (Figure 14-30). Other mechanical (nonelectric) devices are available (e.g., Dial-A-Flow). These devices are used by some EMS agencies to closely regulate the flow rate.

Intermittent infusions are given via a setup that is secondary to the primary IV infusion. The piggyback medication is hung in tandem and connected to the primary setup (Figure 14-31). Most intermittent diluted drug infusions (except **lidocaine** and **dopamine**) are meant to have a total infusion time of 20 or 30 minutes to 1 hour. The time depends on the drug and the patient's response. To prepare an intermittent infusion, the paramedic should follow these steps:

1. Prepare the prescribed medication. Add it to the secondary fluid as described here.
2. Bleed the air out of the secondary administration set. Attach a 1-inch, 18-gauge needle if a needleless system is not available.
3. Cleanse the medication port of the primary infusion tubing. Insert the needle or insert the tubing from the piggyback medication.
4. Tape the needle (if present) or carefully secure the tubing to the medication port.

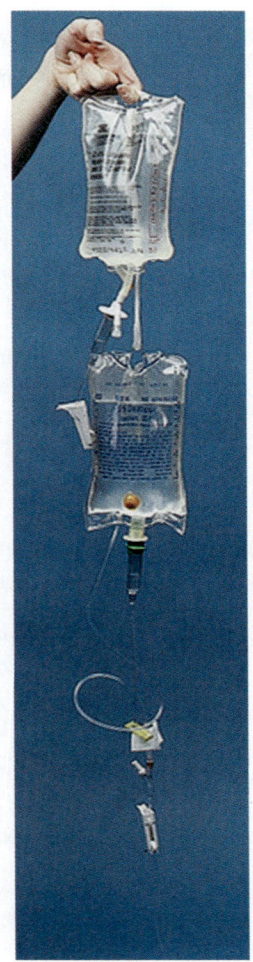

FIGURE 14-31 Intravenous piggyback setup.

5. Calculate the flow rate of the secondary infusion in drops per minute.
6. Lower the primary infusion reservoir so that its center of gravity is lower than the secondary infusion reservoir.
7. Clamp the tubing of the primary infusion to allow the piggyback medication to infuse. Open the piggyback line flow clamp. Adjust the flow rate to the desired dose. After administration of the piggyback medication, restart the primary infusion. Discard the piggyback equipment.
8. Always label the bag with the medication.
9. Document the effect on the patient.

Another device used to administer a drug intravenously is a drug pump. Drug pumps are used by patients who need a slow injection of medication in the home. Examples may be patients who are undergoing cancer chemotherapy, patient-controlled analgesia, and insulin pumps. These devices may consist of a syringe with a battery attachment, a pager device, or a large pump that regulates the injection of medication. Drug pumps are used to give medication subcutaneously, intravenously, or in some cases, into the epidural space. They also can be attached to indwelling

BOX 14-11 Indwelling Vascular Devices

Heparin or Saline Lock

A heparin or saline lock is a peripheral intravenous (IV) cannula. It has no attached IV tubing (Figure 14-32). These devices allow ready access to peripheral veins. They are used for brief administration of medications. They also are used for IV therapy that is administered frequently on an outpatient basis (e.g., chemotherapy). The cannula is filled with 0.5 to 1 mL of a heparin or saline solution. This prevents clotting when the device is not in use.

To gain access to the peripheral vein, draw 4 mL of normal saline into a syringe. Use aseptic technique. Flush 2 mL of the normal saline through the heparin lock reservoir before and after infusion of the prescribed medication or IV fluid. After IV therapy, inject 0.5 to 1 mL of heparin or 3 mL of 0.9% normal saline into the reservoir. This keeps the lock patent.

Central Venous Access Devices (CVADs)

There are four types of CVADs: nontunneled catheters, tunneled catheters, peripherally inserted central catheters (PICCs), and implanted ports (Figure 14-33). The tip of the CVAD rests in the superior vena cava (the tip of a femoral CVAD is in the inferior vena cava). If the tip moves into the atria, complications can occur. Nontunneled CVADs are inserted through the skin into the subclavian vein. They can be inserted in an emergency. Tunneled CVADs are silicone catheters inserted into the subclavian vein in the operating room or radiographic procedure room. They are designed to stay in place for years. Examples of tunneled CVADs include Hickman, Broviac, Groshong, Hohn, and Leonard catheters. Peripherally inserted central catheters usually are introduced through a vein in the antecubital fossa. They are designed for short-term treatment (up to 6 months). Because they are longer than the other CVADs, drawing blood or infusing fluids quickly through these lines sometimes is more difficult.

Most CVADs have a volume of 1 to 3 mL. Be careful not to introduce air when drawing blood, administering drugs, or initiating IV fluids, because an air embolus could result. Follow these steps to access a tunneled, nontunneled, or peripherally inserted CVAD:

1. Prepare the equipment (use only 10 mL or larger syringes; smaller syringes can create high pressure and damage the catheter).
2. Draw up 3 to 5 mL of normal saline (at least twice the volume of the catheter).

3. Put on gloves. Use aseptic technique.
4. Explain the procedure to the patient.
5. Clamp the catheter with the attached clamp or padded smooth shunt clamp (Groshong catheters have a built-in valve and should not be clamped).
6. Wipe the site with povidone-iodine and allow it to dry.
7. Connect the syringe and unclamp the catheter. Withdraw 5 mL blood **(if blood cannot be withdrawn, do not use the catheter).**
8. Replace the clamp.
9. Attach the syringe of normal saline to the catheter. Remove the clamp and flush (do not use excessive pressure).
10. Replace the clamp and remove the syringe.
11. Connect the IV tubing to the catheter. Make sure the tubing is free of air.
12. Remove the clamp and begin the infusion.
13. Tape the connection site between the tubing and catheter. Administer fluids and drugs.

Implantable Ports

An implantable port is a CVAD that is surgically inserted in a pocket under the skin (Figure 14-34). It has a self-sealing septum over a small chamber or reservoir. Each time the port is used, the skin must be punctured by a needle. A regular needle could damage the port, requiring immediate surgery. A special, noncoring Huber needle should be used. Implantable ports should not be accessed in the ambulance if the patient is stable. If the septum is punctured or the port becomes infected, a surgical technique is needed to replace it. The steps for accessing the port are as follows:

1. Palpate the skin and locate the port.
2. Use sterile technique to clean the area with alcohol and then povidone-iodine.
3. Feel for the edge of the port housing and stabilize the port with one hand.
4. Insert the Huber needle through the skin and port septum until contact is made with the back of the port.
5. Confirm correct placement by aspirating blood.
6. Flush with saline and connect the IV tubing (make sure it is free of air).
7. Cover the Huber needle with a transparent dressing. Start the infusion.

NOTE

To prevent damage to central venous catheters, paramedics should:

- Use a clamp on the clamping sleeve provided on silicone catheters
- Avoid using scissors or other sharp objects around the device
- Use only small-gauge needles (22 to 25 gauge) with a needle length of 1 inch or less when accessing the injection port
- Administer fluids or medications gently (never force them)

vascular devices such as the Port-A-Cath or Hickman catheter (Box 14-11).

Intraosseous Medications

Studies have shown that intraosseous (IO) infusion is relatively safe and effective in both children and adults.[8] Fluids and drugs infused through IO access pass quickly from the marrow cavities of long bones into the sinusoids. Then they pass to large venous channels and emissary veins. Next, they pass into the systemic circulation. Normal saline, lactated

Ringer solution, D₅W, plasma, blood, and most advanced life support (ALS) medications may be infused quickly by this route (Figure 14-35). Drugs administered by the IO route should be followed by a saline flush of at least 5 mL. This ensures that the drug is delivered into the central circulation.

IO infusion is indicated in ill or injured patients who require vascular access for drugs or fluids when peripheral cannulation is difficult or unobtainable.[12] Examples include cardiopulmonary arrest and peripheral vascular collapse (as in shock, major trauma, or burns). The procedure also may be indicated in patients in whom vascular access is impaired by obesity or edema and in patients with life-threatening status asthmaticus. Status asthmaticus is an acute exacerbation of asthma that does not respond to standard treatments (see Chapter 24).

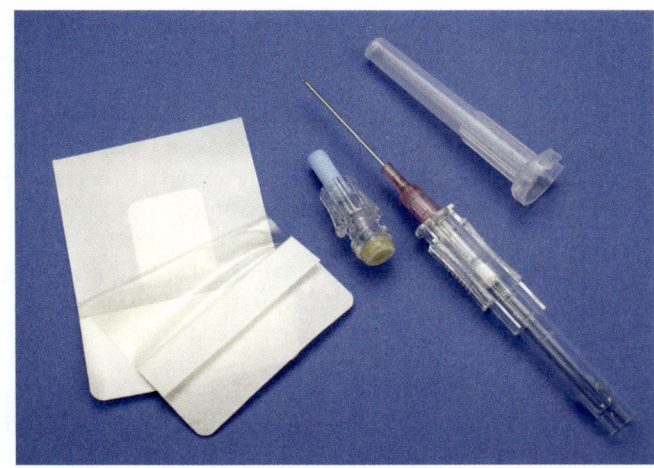

FIGURE 14-32 Saline lock.

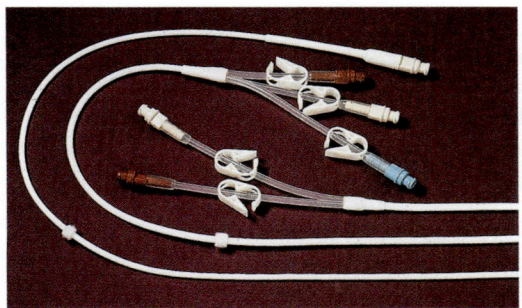

FIGURE 14-33 Single-lumen, dual-lumen, and triple-lumen central venous access device (CVAD) catheters.

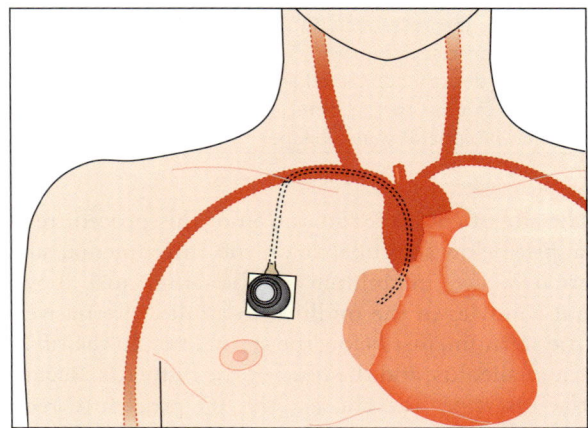

FIGURE 14-34 Port-A-Cath.

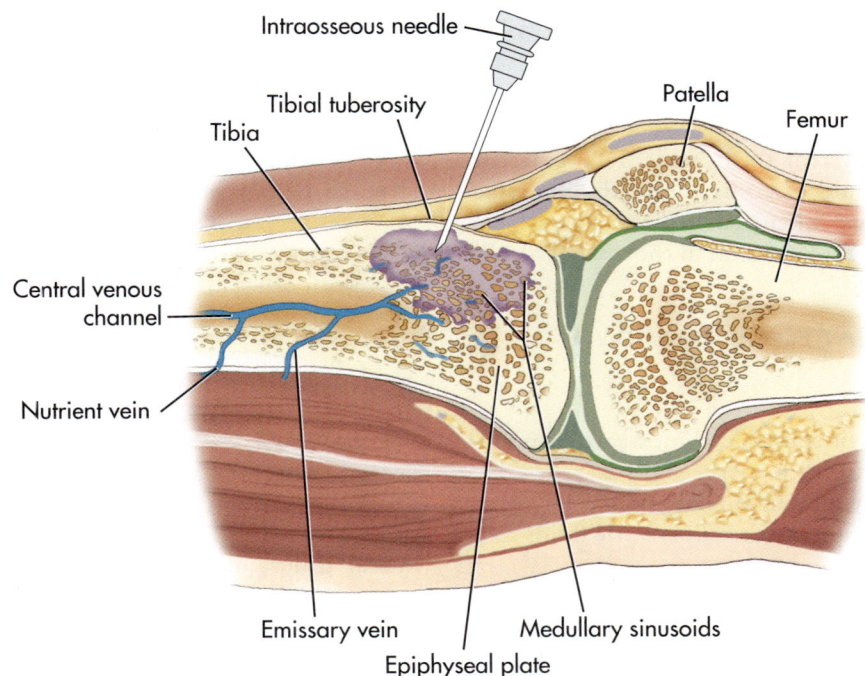

Intraosseous needle

Tibial tuberosity

Patella

Femur

Tibia

Central venous channel

Nutrient vein

Emissary vein

Epiphyseal plate

Medullary sinusoids

FIGURE 14-35 Obtaining intraosseous access.

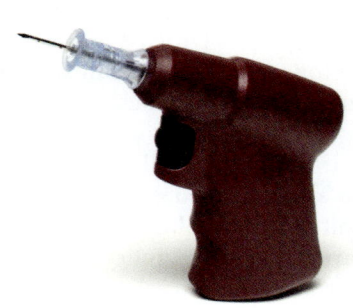

FIGURE 14-36 EZ-IO access. (Courtesy Vidacare Corp., San Antonio, Texas.)

> **NOTE**
>
> The intraosseous (IO) space can be thought of as a "noncollapsible vein." This space is surrounded by bone and is directly connected to the central circulation. In the absence of trauma to the bone, the IO space remains patent, even when peripheral veins collapse.

The site of choice for initiation of this procedure is the tibia, just below the tubercle on the anteromedial surface. Alternative sites in children are the femur, just above the lateral condyles in the midline. In adults, alternative sites are the sternum, just below the sternal notch; the tibia; the medial malleolus; and the head of the humerus. Regardless of the insertion site chosen, the IO procedure requires special IO devices. This is especially true in adults, whose bones are more difficult to penetrate than the bones of children. These devices are designed to insert the IO needle safely through the cortex into the marrow of long bones. A number of commercial IO devices are available. These include the Bone Injection Gun (BIG), Cook Disposable IO Infusion Needle (Sur-Fast Needle), EZ-IO infusion system (Figure 14-36), First Access for Shock and Trauma (F.A.S.T.1) IO infusion system, the Jamshidi IO needle, and others. Paramedics should carefully follow the manufacturer's recommendations when using these devices. The procedures for initiating IO infusion in the tibia of a child are shown in Figure 14-37.

NECESSARY EQUIPMENT FOR IO INFUSION

- Antiseptic
- Tape
- Bone marrow needle or commercial intraosseous needle
- IV tubing (pediatric infusion set)
- IV fluids (specified by medical direction): normal saline, lactated Ringer solution, or special pediatric fluids
- Pressure infusion bag or pump

INSERTION TECHNIQUE (FIGURE 14-37)

1. Put on gloves for personal and patient protection.
2. Cleanse the site as previously described for peripheral cannulation.

3. Prepare the needle for insertion. Insert the needle pointing away from the epiphyseal plate. Advance it to the periosteum.
4. Using a boring or screwing motion (or the device-specific technique), advance the needle until it penetrates the bone marrow (usually noted by decreased resistance and a slight popping sound).
5. Remove the stylet.
6. Aspirate bone marrow into a saline-filled syringe. (Bone marrow may not always be aspirated.)
7. Infuse saline by syringe to ensure placement of the needle and to clear clots.
8. Secure the needle with tape and a securing screw if so equipped (although the needle usually is well stabilized by the bone).
9. Attach standard IV tubing and fluids to infuse under gravity or pressure as prescribed by medical direction.
10. Apply a dressing to the site.
11. Document the procedure.

CONTRAINDICATIONS

- Fracture of the site or proximal to the site
- Traumatized extremity
- Cellulitis
- Burns that may be infected by the technique
- Congenital bone disease

POTENTIAL COMPLICATIONS

Technical Complications
- Subperiosteal infusion from improper placement
- Penetration of posterior wall of medullary cavity, resulting in soft tissue infusion
- Slow infusion from clotting of marrow

Systemic Complications. IO devices are short-term emergency devices. They usually are removed within 24 hours of insertion to prevent systemic complications.
- Osteomyelitis (occurs in fewer than 0.6% of cases, usually with prolonged infusion)
- Fat embolism (rare)
- Slight periostitis at the injection site (usually clears within 2 to 3 weeks)
- Infection (acceptably low rate, comparable to that with other infusion techniques)
- Fracture

ADMINISTRATION OF PERCUTANEOUS MEDICATIONS

Percutaneous drug administration is the administration of drugs that are absorbed through the mucous membranes or skin. These include topical drugs, sublingual drugs, buccal drugs, inhaled drugs, endotracheal drugs, nasal drugs, and drugs for the eye and ear.

Topical Drugs

In addition to the various emollients and antibiotic ointments, the most commonly used transdermal emergency

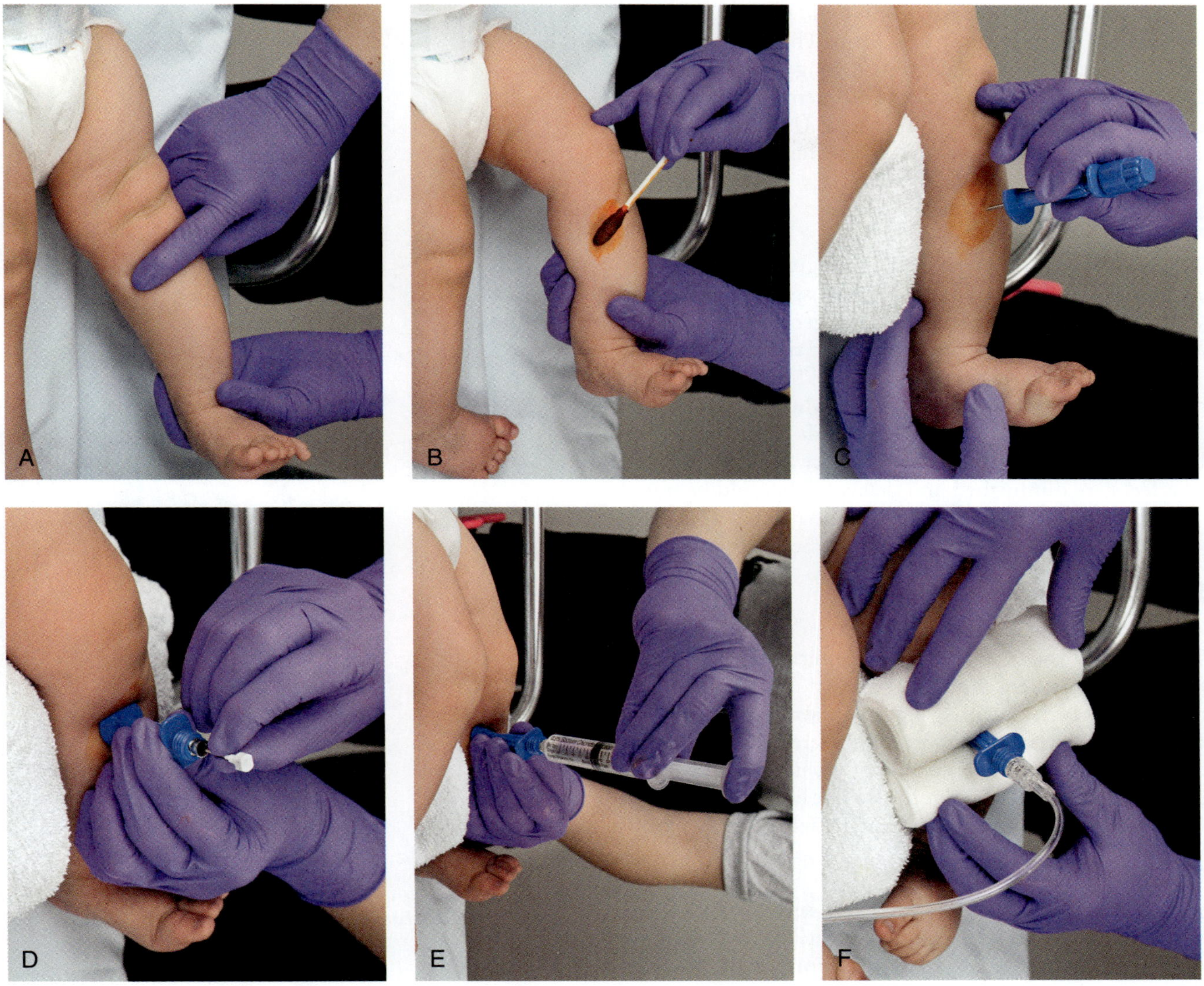

FIGURE 14-37 Intraosseous infusion. **A,** Assess the site, **B,** Cleanse the site. **C,** Using a screwing motion, insert the bone marrow needle away from the epiphyseal plate. Advance the needle until a pop is felt (this occurs when the needle penetrates the marrow). **C,** Remove the stylet. **D,** Aspirate for marrow and then flush with saline. **E, F,** Attach the intravenous tubing and adjust the infusion to the prescribed flow rate. Check for signs of infiltration.

medication is **nitroglycerin.** Two types of topical nitroglycerin preparations are available: **nitropaste** and transdermal **nitroglycerin** delivery patches. These can be applied to any clean, dry area of the upper arm or hair-free portion of the chest. **Nitropaste** has a lanolin-petrolatum base. It is applied in ½-inch increments with special papers to measure the dose. Transdermal **nitroglycerin** patches have an adhesive back (Figure 14-38). They are available in a solid or semi-solid form, depending on the manufacturer. Paramedics should always wear gloves when applying or removing these medications to prevent inadvertent self-absorption of the drug. (More information is available in the *Emergency Drug Index.*) The onset of drug action for transdermal medications is slower and the duration is longer.

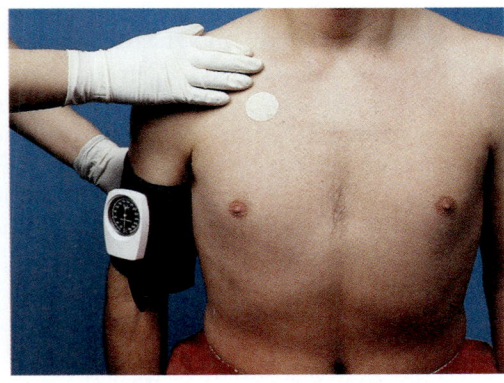

FIGURE 14-38 Application of a nitroglycerin patch.

Drugs such as *fentanyl,* scopolamine, clonidine, and estrogen are also used in patch form. These drug patches can affect the patient unfavorably during illness. Paramedics should be able to recognize the different types of patches and should remove them if indicated. Usual sites for the patches are behind the ear and on the chest, back, hip, and upper arms.

Sublingual Drugs

The most frequently prescribed sublingual (SL) drugs are nitrates (e.g., *nitroglycerin*), which are used to treat angina pectoris. Other SL drugs used in emergency care are *lorazepam,* which is used to treat anxiety, and *captopril,* which is used to manage congestive heart failure. Sublingual tablets should be placed under the tongue, where they dissolve. The patient should not drink fluids while the drug is being absorbed. If the patient inadvertently swallows the tablet, the effects are diminished and delayed. It should be noted that older adults have decreased saliva. Therefore, absorption can be slow and unpredictable in these patients.

Buccal Drugs

Buccal drugs are held between the patient's cheek and gum. They dissolve to achieve their desired effects. As with sublingual drugs, the patient should not drink fluids while the drug is being absorbed. Glucose gel preparations are an example of an emergency medication administered via the buccal route. This route should not be used for patients with altered level of consciousness. It should also not be used in patients who cannot swallow or who have an ineffective gag reflex.

Inhaled Drugs

In addition to oxygen and *nitrous oxide,* several other drugs may be administered by means of inhalation. These include bronchodilators, corticosteroids, antibiotics, and mucokinetic agents delivered through aerosolization.

Aerosols are liquid or solid particles of a substance dispersed in gas or solution. The effectiveness of aerosolization therapy depends on the number of droplets that can be suspended in the gas or solution, the rate of oxygen or gas flow, the particle size (diameter in microns), output (cc/min), and the rate and depth of the patient's breathing. Rapid, shallow breathing reduces the number and retention of droplets that reach the deep bronchioles of the lungs. The delivery of drugs by this method has certain advantages over other routes. Specifically, these are rapid onset of the drug's effect and fewer or less intense systemic side effects.

Aerosols are made by devices called *nebulizers.* Intermittent positive pressure breathing (IPPB) devices are designed for in-hospital use. Out-of-hospital devices include metered-dose inhalers (pressure cartridges) and handheld nebulizers. Handheld nebulizers operate by means of a compressed air or oxygen source regulated by a flowmeter.

METERED-DOSE INHALER

The metered-dose inhaler (MDI) is now the most commonly used device in aerosol therapy (Figure 14-39). It is

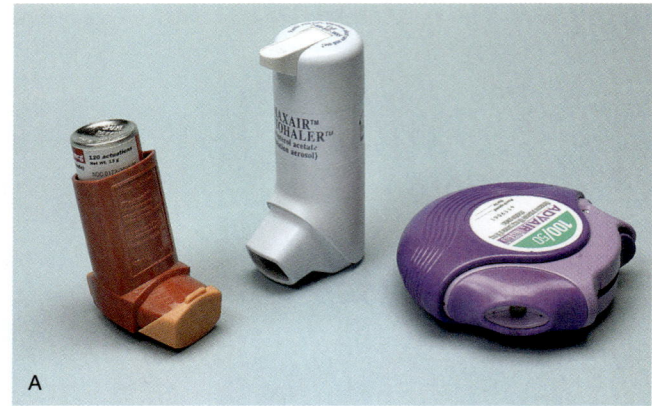

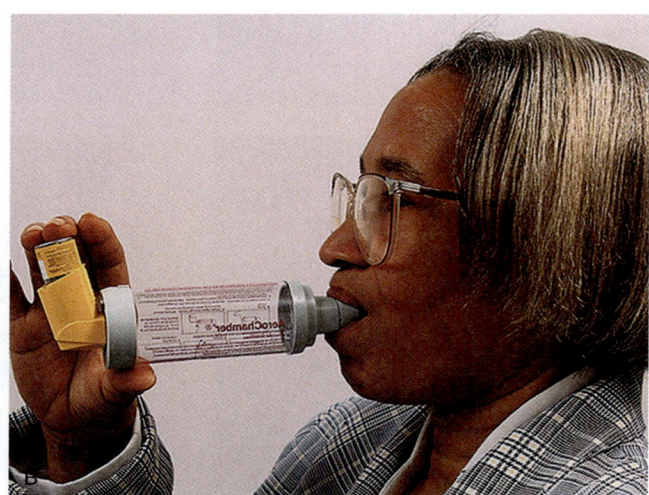

FIGURE 14-39 A, Metered-dose inhalers (MDIs). **B,** Metered-dose inhaler with an extender or spacer. (Clayton BD, Stock YN, Cooper S: *Basic pharmacology for nurses,* ed 15, St Louis, 2010, Mosby.)

convenient and delivers a measured dose with each push of the cartridge. MDIs usually are prescribed for self-treatment of asthma. Other medications prepared in MDIs are *ipratropium,* and *albuterol.* Paramedics should follow these steps to administer a drug by this method:

1. Remove the mouthpiece and protective cap from the canister (the drug container).
2. Carefully snap off the cap and turn the mouthpiece sideways.
3. Insert the canister stem into the hole inside the mouthpiece.
4. Shake the canister and mouthpiece well.
5. Invert the MDI and hold it close to the patient's mouth. Instruct the patient to exhale, pushing as much air from the lungs as possible.
6. Place the mouthpiece in the patient's mouth. Instruct the patient to close the lips loosely around it, with the tongue underneath the mouthpiece. As the patient inhales deeply over 5 seconds, press down on the canister quickly and then release it.

7. Instruct the patient to hold his or her breath 5 to 10 seconds before exhaling.

8. Repeat the procedure in 5 to 10 minutes to take advantage of possibly deeper penetration by a second round of therapy (if required). Most MDI medications are administered using aerochambers (spacers). These are beneficial devices for children and for patients with problematic conditions. For example, some patients might need additional time to inhale the medication. Others may lack coordination. Still others may be hampered by a high level of anxiety or by a diminished ability to inhale for 5 seconds. Aerochambers allow the patient to receive the maximum benefit of the drug and do not require exact synchronization.

CRITICAL THINKING

What happens to the medication if the patient does not use the metered-dose inhaler (MDI) properly?

HANDHELD NEBULIZERS

Handheld nebulizers are another means of administering some medications via inhalation in the prehospital setting. Various manufacturers make disposable nebulizer kits. The kits usually include a mouthpiece or aerosol mask, oxygen tubing, and reservoir tubing (Figure 14-40). These devices are attached to a nonhumidified portable or on-board oxygen source. They use the Bernoulli principle to create an aerosol mist (sometimes referred to as a *jet* or *pneumatic nebulizer*). Medications appropriate for nebulization therapy include **albuterol, atropine, ipratropium, levalbuterol,** and **metaproterenol**.

The specific procedure may vary slightly. It may depend on the patient's ability to tolerate the treatment by mouthpiece or mask. A tight seal around the mouthpiece is required. The patient therefore must be able to cooperate

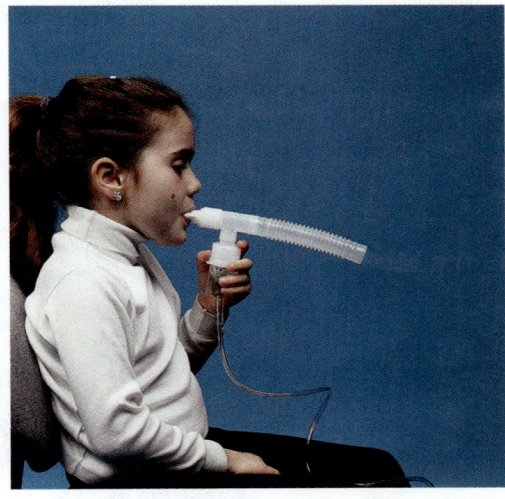

FIGURE 14-40 Administration of medication with a handheld nebulizer.

during treatment. Both mouthpiece and mask methods have advantages. With treatment by mouthpiece, less of the drug is wasted. However, patients with severe dyspnea who are mouth breathers tolerate mask administration much better.

To administer a medication with a handheld nebulizer, paramedics should follow these steps:

1. Using aseptic technique, mix the prescribed drug with a specified amount of normal saline. Then instill it into the nebulizer. Some medications come in a packaged unit dose and have a fixed amount of diluent (usually 0.9% normal saline).

2. Attach the nebulizer to a T-piece and mouthpiece and connect it with tubing to the unit delivering nonhumidified oxygen (for the hypoxic patient) or compressed air. (If the patient cannot use the mouthpiece, a simple face mask may be used in its place.)

3. Adjust the oxygen flowmeter to a rate of 4 to 6 L/min to create a steady, visible mist. (This rate usually offers a steady mist without too much wastage of medication. The higher the flow rate, the greater the medication use.) If an aerosol mask is used, the oxygen flow rate should be kept at 6 to 8 L/min. This prevents the buildup of exhaled carbon dioxide in the mask.

4. When the mist is visible, begin treatment. Instruct the patient to inhale slowly and deeply by mouth. Have the person hold a breath for 3 to 5 seconds before exhaling. This results in topical deposition of the aerosol particles deep within the tracheobronchial tree. Inhalation and exhalation should be continued until the aerosol canister is depleted of the medication. Repeat treatments usually are not given more often than every 15 to 20 minutes (usually to a maximum of three). Treatment of severe asthma, however, may include continuous administration of nebulized beta agonists, tailored to the patient's response.

The patient must be cooperative to undergo nebulization therapy. The individual must be able to follow instructions to breathe deeply so that the drug can be absorbed. This therapy would be ineffective if the patient is unable to inhale the drug sufficiently or if bronchospasm is too severe. In such cases, administration via another route should be considered. Nebulizer treatments may be administered to a patient who is artificially ventilated by placing it into the ventilation circuit of the bag-valve-mask (BVM) or ventilator.

Notable changes in the heart rate or dysrhythmias may occur during nebulization therapy. If these occur, treatment should be stopped and medical direction should be contacted for further orders. Paramedics and ambulance crews should avoid the medication vapor stream during nebulization therapy.

Endotracheal Drugs

The endotracheal (ET) route is an alternative route of drug administration. It may be used when IV or IO access cannot be established. (Absorption through the ET route is unpredictable and less effective than the IV or IO routes; therefore, the ET drug dose must be increased.) Emergency drugs that may be administered by this route are **naloxone, atropine, vasopressin, epinephrine,** and **lidocaine.** (Memory aid: N-A-V-E-L) When giving medication by this route, paramedics should follow these steps (Figure 14-41):

1. Make sure the ET tube is in the correct position. This can be checked by direct visualization and by auscultation (see Chapter 15).
2. Make sure oxygenation and ventilation of the patient's lungs are adequate.
3. Prepare the medication so that it is 2 to 2½ times the intravenous dose. Dilute the dose to 10 mL with normal saline (or prepare a 10 mL normal saline flush, per protocol).
4. Remove the air source from the ET tube. Inject the medication through a catheter deep into the tube or inject it directly into the tube and follow with a normal saline flush (per protocol). (Some ET tubes have a drug port; with these tubes, the air source need not be removed for drug administration.)
5. Resume ventilations with one to two full ventilations. This helps ensure that the medication penetrates as deeply as possible into the pulmonary tree (which enhances absorption).
6. Monitor the patient for the desired therapeutic effect and for any side effects.

Drugs for the Eye, Nose, and Ear

Eye medications usually are supplied in the form of drops or ointments. To administer these drugs, the paramedic should have the patient lie down or sit with the head tilted back. Stabilizing the patient's head with one hand, the paramedic uses the thumb or fingers of the other hand to pull down the lower lid gently. The medication should be applied into the conjunctival sac of the lower lid, never onto the eyeball (Figure 14-42).

Nose drops are best administered with the patient lying down with the head over the edge of a bed in a midline position. The drops are instilled into each nostril. The patient should be instructed not to blow the nose for several minutes to allow absorption of the drug. To administer a drug via the nasal route, the paramedic should instruct the patient to hold the head upright or tilted back and to block one nostril. The patient then inhales through the open nostril while squeezing the spray applicator to release the atomized drug (Figure 14-43).

> **NOTE**
> Giving atomized nasal drugs has some advantages. For example, because the nasal route is needleless, the risk of needle-stick injury is eliminated. Also, nasal drugs can be administered safely in a moving ambulance or rescue vehicle. The nasal route may be preferred with combative patients and small children and when IV access is difficult to obtain.
> Many emergency medications have been approved for nasal administration. Examples include diazepam (Valium), fentanyl (Sublimaze) glucagon, haloperidol (Haldol), lidocaine (Xylocaine), lorazepam (Ativan), midazolam (Versed), and naloxone (Narcan). *Any drug that can cause hypotension should not be administered intranasally without an established IV line.*

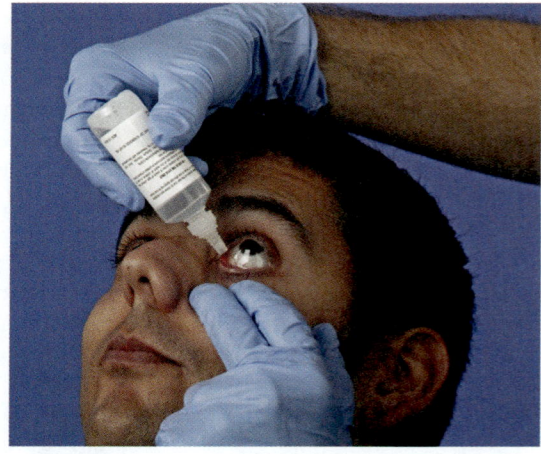

FIGURE 14-42 Administration of eye medication.

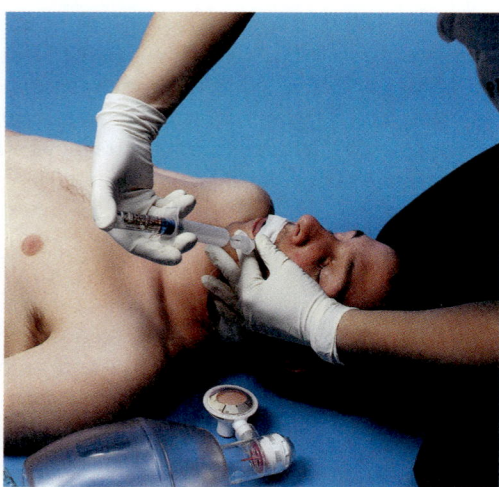

FIGURE 14-41 Administration of a drug through an endotracheal (ET) tube.

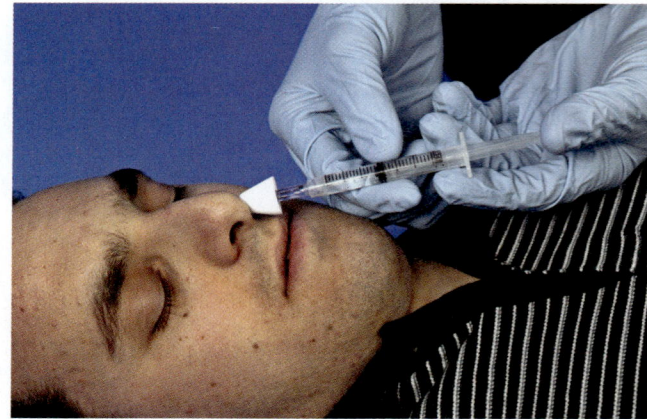

FIGURE 14-43 Nasal administration of naloxone.

Ear medications usually are provided in the form of drops. The patient should lie down with the affected ear up. With adults or children over age 3, the paramedic should gently pull the top of the ear up and back to straighten the ear canal. The prescribed number of drops is then instilled. In children under age 3, the ear is pulled down and straight back. The patient should remain in the ear-up position for about 10 minutes to allow the medicine to disperse. To prevent contamination of the drops, the paramedic should not allow the tip of the dropper to come into contact with the ear canal. Placing a cotton ball in the ear canal after administration of the drug may reduce seepage of the drops onto the face.

> **SHOW ME THE EVIDENCE**
> Barton and coworkers prospectively studied the effectiveness of administering intranasal (IN) naloxone to unconscious prehospital patients in Denver. Of the 30 patients studied, 11 responded either to intravenous (IV) or to IN naloxone. Ten responded to IN naloxone alone, with an average response time of 3.4 minutes. Seven of these patients did not require IV therapy. The authors conclude that the intranasal route should be considered for treatment of suspected overdose in the prehospital setting. Use of this route avoids the use of needles and may reduce the risk of exposure to blood-borne pathogens.

From Barton E et al: Intranasal administration of naloxone by paramedics, *Prehosp Emerg Care* 6:54-58, 2002.

SPECIAL CONSIDERATIONS FOR PEDIATRIC PATIENTS

Administering drugs to infants and children can be quite difficult. This is especially true in emergency situations. The following guidelines may be helpful for this process.

- Try to establish a positive relationship with the child. Accept fearful or anxious behavior as a natural response.
- Be honest with the child when explaining a medication or procedure that will be unpleasant or painful.
- If appropriate, allow the child to help administer the medication (e.g., by holding the medicine cup or by placing a pill in the mouth).
- When administering oral liquid drugs to infants or small children, hold the child (or have the parent hold the child) in a semireclined position. Place the oral medication syringe or administration device alongside the tongue. Slowly inject the medication, allowing the child to swallow small amounts at a time.
- Use mild physical restraint only if it is required. Explain to the child why it is needed.
- Enlist the assistance of parents or other caregivers when possible.
- When parenteral medications are required, stabilize the injection site well and give the injection quickly. Two or more individuals should be available to hold a child over 4 years of age, even if the child promises to "be still."
- Remember when administering medications that the younger and smaller the child, the smaller the margin for error.

> **SHOW ME THE EVIDENCE**
> Pediatric medication doses are calculated according to the patient's weight. Bernius and colleagues recognized that this increases the risk of drug dose errors. They evaluated whether the use of a protocol-specific pediatric code card resulted in more accurate drug dose and volume calculation by prehospital care providers. They evaluated drug dose calculation in 523 advanced life support (ALS) providers during training in Maryland and the District of Columbia. For the 246 who used the code card, the mean correct response rate was 94%; for the 277 who did not use the card, the rate was 65%.

From Bernius M et al: Prevention of pediatric drug calculation errors by prehospital care providers, *Prehosp Emerg Care* 12:486-494, 2008.

OBTAINING A BLOOD SAMPLE

Venous blood samples often are obtained in the prehospital setting for glucose testing and for laboratory determinations performed in the hospital. If possible, these samples should be obtained when an IV line is established and always before any fluids are infused. When obtaining a blood sample from an IV site, the paramedic should follow these steps:

1. Prepare all equipment in advance.
2. After removing the needle from the IV catheter, exert manual pressure above the IV site to prevent the free flow of blood from the catheter.
3. While stabilizing the site, insert the Vacutainer into the hub of the IV catheter.
4. Push blood collection vacuum tubes (Table 14-3) into the barrel of the Vacutainer to draw blood from the IV catheter.
5. After obtaining the required specimens, attach the IV tubing and begin infusion.
6. Label the sample with the patient's name and the time and date it was obtained.

> **CRITICAL THINKING**
> Why should a venous blood sample never be drawn above an IV infusion site?

If no IV line is to be used, the paramedic must obtain the blood sample using a Vacutainer (Figure 14-44) or a needle and syringe and then transfer the sample to an evacuation tube. The steps for obtaining a blood sample using a needle and syringe are as follows:

1. Apply a tourniquet above the selected site.
2. Cleanse the site as previously described for venipuncture.
3. Using an 18- or 20-gauge needle attached to a 10- or 12-mL syringe, enter the vein.

TABLE 14-3 Types of Blood Sample Tubes and Order of Blood Draws

To prevent contamination of tubes with additives from other tubes, it is important to draw the tubes in a *specific* order. This called the *order of the draw*. The following is the collection sequence for evacuated tubes when multiple tubes must be drawn[13]:

1. Yellow top or bottles: Sterile/blood cultures
2. Royal blue: Red label for trace metal analysis
3. Light blue coagulation tube (If only coagulation tests are ordered *and* a butterfly catheter is used, draw a discard tube to collect the air in the tubing. If this is not done, a short draw (insufficient amount of blood for the sample) results, which will be rejected by the laboratory.)
4. Red: Nonadditive
5. Red Gel separator tube (speckled or "tiger" top)
6. Green (heparin)
7. Green/gray mottled plasma separator tube (PST) with heparin
8. Lavender/purple top and/or pink (ethylenediamine tetraacetic acid [EDTA])
9. Gray top (oxalate/fluoride tube)

Stopper Color	Additive/ Preservative	Tests Done on Blood Sample	Comments
Green	Heparin	Electrolytes, glucose; cardiac enzymes	Invert tube several times. Heparin prevents blood from clotting without killing cells.
Gray	Oxalate/fluoride	Blood alcohol Lactate levels Fasting glucose assays	
Lavender	EDTA anticoagulant	Blood cell count, hemoglobin (Hb), hematocrit (Hct), erythrocyte sedimentation rate (ESR) Glycohemoglobin A1C T8 for human immunodeficiency virus (HIV)	Invert tube several times to prevent clotting (do not shake). EDTA tubes are used to collect samples for whole-blood hematology testing.
Light blue	Sodium citrate	Prothrombin time (PT), activated partial thrombin time (aPTT), fibrinogen levels D-dimer	Tube must be filled completely. Invert tube several times to prevent clotting. Sodium citrate tubes are used to collect samples primarily for coagulation studies. Such tests often are needed for patients with bleeding problems (e.g., in the abdomen, brain, or elsewhere).
Red	None	Serum electrolytes, liver and other enzymes, therapeutic drug levels, blood bank procedures	The tube need not be inverted, because the objective is to produce a clot. Some companies make tubes with clot activators, which hasten clotting to speed testing.
Yellow	Glass particles to speed up clotting process	All immunology tests	Tubes with clot activators

Primary Source: Becton, Dickinson: *BD Vacutainer venous blood collection: tube guide.* www.bd.com/vacutainer. Accessed August 1, 2010.

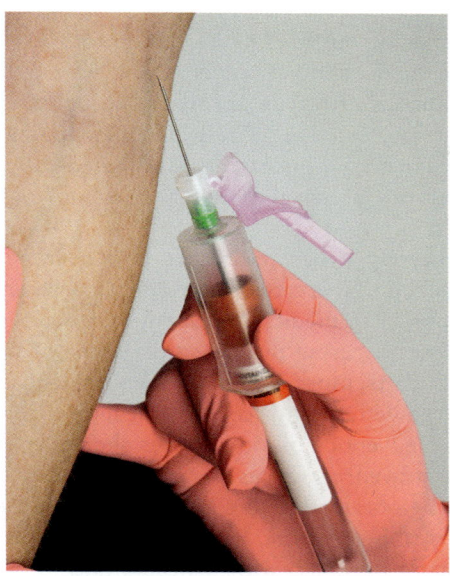

FIGURE 14-44 Obtaining a blood sample with a Vacutainer.

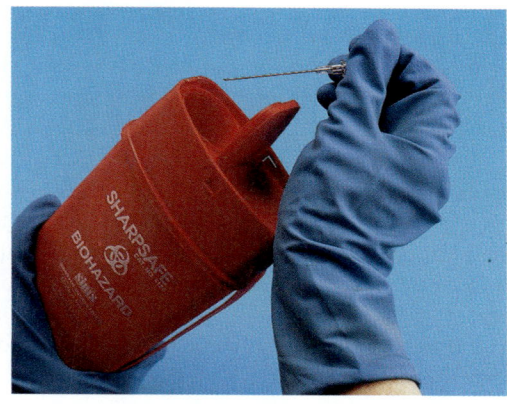

FIGURE 14-45 Disposal of a needle in a sharps container.

7. Label the sample with the patient's name and the time and date it was obtained.

4. With an even, steady motion, draw back on the plunger to obtain the sample.
5. After the sample has been obtained, release the tourniquet, withdraw the needle, and apply manual pressure to the site.
6. Immediately transfer the sample to the appropriate evacuation tube. Do not force additional blood into the tube; each tube has the correct amount of vacuum for the amount of blood required in the vial. Forcing blood into a vacuum tube can cause expulsion of contents and can lead to unnecessary injury or exposure to contents.

DISPOSAL OF CONTAMINATED ITEMS AND SHARPS

Needles and other sharp objects can injure the patient, the paramedic, coworkers, and others. They also can be a source of infection with hepatitis or the human immunodeficiency virus (HIV). The CDC recommends that needles not be capped, bent, or broken before disposal. Rather, they should be discarded with the syringe intact in a special container (i.e., sharps container) that is clearly marked (Figure 14-45). These containers should be puncture proof and leak proof. When full (as indicated by the "Full line," which usually is no more than three fourths of the space), the container should be discarded according to established policies for disposition of contaminated items and sharps.

SUMMARY

- Three systems for measuring drug dosage are in use today. These are the metric system, the apothecary system (no longer recommended), and the common household system. Each system deals with units of mass and volume. Any of these three systems may be used by a physician when ordering drugs.
- Paramedics should choose a drug calculation method that is precise. It also should be reliable. Paramedics should
  (1) Convert all units of measure to the same size and system
  (2) Assess the computed dosage to determine whether it is reasonable
  (3) Use one method of dose calculation consistently
- Many drug calculations can be performed almost intuitively. Nevertheless, paramedics should never rely on intuitive calculations. Methods of calculation include the basic formula (desire over have), ratios and proportions, and dimensional analysis.

- Intravenous flow rates can be calculated using the following formula:

$$\text{Drops/min} = \frac{\text{Volume to be infused} \times \text{Drops/mL of infusion set}}{\text{Total time of infusion (min)}}$$

- Safety procedures should be a high priority during the administration of any medication. The paramedic must make sure the *right* patient receives the *right* dose of the *right* drug via the *right* route at the *right* time.
- A medication error may occur. In such a case, paramedics should take responsibility for their actions. They should quickly advise medical direction. They also should assess and monitor the patient for effects of the drug. They must document the error as required by local, state, and medical direction policies. In addition, they must change their personal practice to prevent a similar error in the future.

Continued

- Medical asepsis is accomplished by using clean technique, which involves hygienic measures, cleaning agents, antiseptics, disinfectants, and barrier fields.
- Enteral drugs are administered and absorbed through the gastrointestinal tract. They are given by the oral, gastric, and rectal routes. Parenteral drugs are administered outside the intestine. They are usually injected. Parenteral drugs are given by the intradermal, subcutaneous, intramuscular, intravenous, and intraosseous routes.
- In the prehospital setting, the route of choice for fluid replacement is through a peripheral vein in an extremity. The over-the-needle catheter generally is preferred in this setting.
- Several possible complications are associated with all intravenous techniques. These include local complications, systemic complications, infiltration, and air embolism.
- Fluids and drugs that are infused by the intraosseous route pass from the marrow cavities into the sinusoids. Next, they pass into large venous channels and emissary veins. Then they pass into the systemic circulation. The site of choice for IO infusions in children is the tibia, one to two fingerbreadths below the tubercle on the anteromedial surface. Other sites for IO infusions include the distal tibia, humerus, and sternum (adults).
- Percutaneous drugs are absorbed through the mucous membranes or skin. These include topical drugs, sublingual drugs, buccal drugs, inhaled drugs, endotracheal drugs, nasal drugs and drugs for the eye and ear.
- Administering drugs to infants and children can be quite difficult. This often is especially true in emergency situations. Paramedics frequently calculate pediatric drug doses by using memory aids. Some of these aids include charts, tapes, and dosage books. Doses also are calculated with the advice of medical direction.
- If possible, venous blood samples should be obtained when intravenous access is established. They also should be obtained before any fluids are infused. If no IV line is to be used and a blood sample is still needed, it must be obtained with a needle and syringe (or a special vacuum needle and sleeve).
- The CDC recommends that needles not be capped, bent, or broken before disposal. Rather, they should be left on the syringe and discarded in an appropriate, clearly marked container that is puncture proof and leak proof.

REFERENCES

1. Moseley R: *Everything you always wanted to know about metrics*, Valdese, NC, 1978, R&R Enterprises.
2. Salerno E: *Pharmacology for health professionals*, St Louis, 2007, Mosby.
3. Institute of Medicine: *Preventing medication errors*, Washington DC, 2006, National Academies Press.
4. Centers for Disease Control and Prevention: *New disinfection and sterilization methods.* www.cdc.gov/ncidod/eid/vol7no2/rutala.htm. Accessed August 11, 2010.
5. Dobranowski J, Fitzgerald J, et al. Incorrect positioning of nasogastric feeding tubes and the development of pneumothorax, *Can Assoc Radiol J* 43:35, 1992.
6. Potter PA, Perry AG: *Basic nursing: essentials for practice*, ed 6, St Louis, 2002, Mosby.
7. Centers for Disease Control and Prevention: Guidelines for prevention of intravascular catheter-related infections, *MMWR Morb Mortal Wkly Report* 51(No RR-10):1-36, 2002.
8. American Heart Association: *Pediatric advanced life support*, Dallas, 2006, The Association.
9. Campbell J: Intravenous drug therapy, *Prof Nurse* 11:437-442, 1996.
10. Iyer PW, Levin BJ, editors: *Nursing malpractice*, ed 3, Tucson, Ariz., 2007, Lawyer & Judges Publishing.
11. Abbott Laboratories: *Needle and cannula technique*, Chicago, 1977, Abbott.
12. Fowler R, Gallagher JV, Isaacs SM, et al: The role of intraosseous vascular access in the out-of-hospital environment (resource document to the NAEMSP position statement), *Prehosp Emerg Care* 11:63-66, 2007.
13. University of Michigan Health System, Department of Pathology: *Blood bank: FAQs.* www.pathology.med.umich.edu/bloodbank/faqs.html. Accessed August 11, 2010.
14. Centers for Disease Control and Prevention: *2007 guideline for isolation precautions: preventing transmission of infectious agents in healthcare settings.* www.cdc.gov/hicpac/2007IP/2007isolation Precautions.html. Accessed August 11, 2010.
15. Centers for Disease Control and Prevention: Evaluation of safety devices for preventing percutaneous injuries among healthcare workers during phlebotomy procedures, *MMWR Morb Mortal Wkly Rep* 46:21-25, 1997.
16. Centers for Disease Control and Prevention: Recommendations for prevention and control of hepatitis C virus (HCV) infection and HCV-related chronic disease, *MMWR Morb Mortal Wkly Rep* 47(RR-19):1-39, 1998.
17. Centers for Disease Control and Prevention: Precautions to prevent transmission of HIV: universal precautions—recommendations for prevention of HIV transmission in health care settings, C virus (HCV) infection and HCV-related chronic disease, *MMWR* 36(Suppl 2S):1-18S, 1987.

SUGGESTED READINGS

Brown M, Mulholland J: *Drug calculations: process and problems for clinical practice*, ed 8, St Louis, 2008, Mosby/Elsevier.

Gorrell M: IO you one, *JEMS* 31:16, 2006.

Hohenhaus S: Giving liquid medications to pediatric patients, *J Emerg Nurs* 32:69-70, 2006.

Paparella S: IO needles: they're not just for kids anymore, *J Emerg Nurs* 34:318-319, 2008.

Thomas D: Lesson learned: basic evidence–based advice for preventing medication errors in children, *J Emerg Nurs* 31:490-493, 2005.

Wolfe T, Barton E: Nasal drug delivery in EMS: reducing needle-stick risk, *JEMS* 28:52-63, 2003.

Universal Precautions and Standard Precautions: Measures to Prevent Disease Transmission[17]

Universal precautions (i.e., universal blood and body fluid precautions) were developed by the Centers for Disease Control and Prevention (CDC) in 1987. They are the minimum standard of practice recommended by the Occupational Safety and Health Act of 1991 and by all health care agencies.

Universal precautions should be used in the care of all patients. However, they are especially important for paramedics and others who work in emergency care. These health care professionals face a higher risk of exposure to blood. Also, the patient's infection status usually is unknown at this point. The following are the procedures for universal precautions.[14]

1. All health care workers should routinely use appropriate barrier precautions to prevent skin and mucous membrane exposure when contact with blood or other body fluids of any patient is anticipated. Gloves should be worn for touching blood and body fluids, mucous membranes, or nonintact skin of all patients; for handling items or surfaces soiled with blood or body fluids; and for performing venipuncture and other vascular access procedures. Gloves should be changed after contact with each patient. Masks and protective eyewear or face shields should be worn during procedures that are likely to generate droplets of blood or other body fluids, to prevent exposure of mucous membranes of the mouth, nose, and eyes. Gowns or aprons should be worn during procedures that are likely to generate splashes or a spray of blood or other body fluids.

2. The hands and other skin surfaces should be washed immediately and thoroughly if they become contaminated with blood or other body fluids. The hands should be washed immediately after removing gloves.

3. All health care workers should take precautions to prevent injuries caused by needles, scalpels, and other sharp instruments or devices during procedures, when cleaning used instruments, during disposal of used needles, and when handling sharp instruments after procedures. Needles should not be recapped, purposely bent or broken by hand, removed from disposable syringes, or otherwise manipulated by hand. After use, disposable syringes and needles, scalpel blades, and other sharp items should be placed in puncture-resistant containers for disposal. The containers should be located as close as practical to the area where these items are used. Large-bore reusable needles should be placed in a puncture-resistant container for transport to the processing area.

4. Saliva has not been implicated in the transmission of the human immunodeficiency virus (HIV). However, to minimize the need for emergency mouth-to-mouth resuscitation, mouthpieces, resuscitation bags, or other ventilation devices should be available for use in areas where the need for resuscitation is predictable.

5. Health care workers with exudative lesions or weeping dermatitis should refrain from all direct patient care and from handling patient care equipment until the condition resolves.

6. Pregnant health care workers are not known to be at greater risk of contracting HIV infection than health care workers who are not pregnant. However, if a health care worker becomes infected with HIV during pregnancy, the infant is at risk of infection as a result of perinatal transmission. Because of this risk, pregnant health care workers should be especially familiar with and strictly follow precautions for minimizing the risk of HIV transmission.

Implementation of universal precautions for all patients eliminates the need for the isolation category of blood and body fluid precautions, which previously was recommended by the CDC for patients known to be or suspected of being infected with blood-borne pathogens. Isolation precautions (e.g., against enteric, acid-fast bacillus [AFB]) should be used as necessary if associated conditions such as infectious diarrhea or tuberculosis are diagnosed or suspected.

Standard precautions should not be confused with universal precautions. Standard precautions combine the major features of universal precautions (UP) and body substance isolation (BSI) and are based on the principle that all blood, body fluids, secretions, excretions except sweat, nonintact skin, and mucous membranes may contain transmissible infectious agents.

Standard precautions include a group of infection prevention practices that apply to all patients, regardless of suspected or confirmed infection status, in any setting in which health care is delivered. These include hand hygiene; use of gloves, gown, mask, eye protection, or face shield, depending on the anticipated exposure; and safe injection practices. Also, equipment or items in the patient's environment likely to have been contaminated with infectious body fluids must be handled in a manner to prevent transmission of infectious agents (e.g., wear gloves for direct contact, contain heavily soiled equipment, properly clean and disinfect or sterilize reusable equipment before use on another patient).

The application of standard precautions during patient care is determined by the nature of the health care worker–patient interaction and the extent of anticipated exposure to blood, body fluids, or pathogens. For some interactions (e.g., performing venipuncture), only gloves may be needed; during other interactions (e.g., intubation), use of gloves, gown, and face shield or mask and goggles is necessary. Education and training in the principles and rationale for recommended practices are critical elements of standard precautions, because they facilitate appropriate decision making and promote adherence when the health care worker is faced with new circumstances. An example of the importance of the use of standard precautions is intubation, especially under emergency circumstances in which infectious agents may not be suspected but later are identified (e.g., severe acute respiratory syndrome coronavirus [SARS-CoV], *Neisseria meningitidis*). Standard precautions also are intended to protect patients by ensuring that health care personnel do not carry infectious agents to patients on their hands or on equipment used during patient care.

PART FOUR

Airway

Chapter 15: Airway Management, Respiration, and Artificial Ventilation

CHAPTER
15 Airway Management, Respiration, and Artificial Ventilation

KEY TERMS

accessory muscles Muscles that sometimes assist in breathing; they include the scalenes and the sternocleidomastoid (deep muscles of the neck and thorax), posterior neck and back muscles, and abdominal muscles.

alveoli Small outpouchings of walls of alveolar space through which gas exchange takes place between alveolar air and pulmonary capillary blood.

anatomical dead space The volume of the conducting airways from the external environment down to the terminal bronchioles.

apneustic center A group of neurons in the pons that has a stimulatory effect on the inspiratory center.

atelectasis An abnormal condition characterized by the collapse of lung tissue; it prevents respiratory exchange of oxygen and carbon dioxide.

atmospheric pressure The pressure of the gas around us, which varies with differences in altitude. At sea level, it is 760 mm Hg.

biphasic positive airway pressure (BiPAP) Airway support that combines partial ventilatory support and continuous positive airway pressure; it allows the pressure to vary during each breath cycle.

Bohr effect The property of hemoglobin by which an increasing concentration of protons and/or carbon dioxide reduces the oxygen affinity for hemoglobin.

Boyle's law The principle of gas activity that states that gas flows from an area of higher pressure or concentration to an area of lower pressure or concentration; also known as the general gas law.

capnography The measurement of carbon dioxide concentrations in exhaled air; sometimes referred to as etCO$_2$ and PetCO$_2$.

carina of the trachea A downward and backward projection of the lowest tracheal cartilage; it forms a ridge between the openings of the right and left primary bronchi.

compliance The ease with which the lungs and thorax expand during pressure changes. The greater the compliance, the easier the expansion.

continuous positive airway pressure (CPAP) Airway support that transmits positive pressure into the airways of a spontaneously breathing patient throughout the respiratory cycle.

diaphragm The dome-shaped, musculofibrous partition that separates the thoracic and abdominal cavities.

diffusion The process by which solid, particulate matter in a fluid moves from an area of higher concentration to an area of lower concentration, resulting in an even distribution of the particles in the fluid.

expiratory reserve volume The amount of gas that can be forcefully exhaled after expiration of the normal tidal volume.

expiration Breathing out (exhalation), normally a passive process.

external respiration The transfer (diffusion) of oxygen and carbon dioxide between the inspired air and pulmonary capillaries.

extubation Removal of an endotracheal tube.

Fick principle The assumption that the amount of oxygen delivered to an organ is equal to the amount of oxygen consumed by that organ plus the amount of oxygen carried away from that organ. This principle is used to determine cardiac output.

gag reflex A normal neural response triggered by touching the soft palate or posterior pharynx.

Hering-Breuer reflex A reflex in which afferent impulses from stretch receptors in the lungs arrest inspiration; expiration then occurs; inflation and deflation reflexes are triggered to prevent overinflation of the lungs.

hypocarbia A state of diminished carbon dioxide in the blood; also called *hypocapnia.*

hypoxemia A state of decreased oxygen content of arterial blood.

hypoxia A state of decreased oxygen content at the tissue level.

hypoxic drive The low arterial oxygen pressure stimulus to respiration that is mediated through the carotid bodies.

inadvertent hyperventilation Excessive ventilation that is thought to result in increased intrathoracic pressure and decreased coronary perfusion pressure; also known as rescuer hyperventilation.

inspiration The act of drawing air into the lungs.

inspiratory reserve volume The maximum volume of air that can be inspired after a normal inspiration.

intercostal muscles Internal and external muscles between the ribs that contract to raise the ribs, thereby increasing the front-to-back (anterior-posterior) and side-to-side dimensions of the chest cavity.

internal respiration The transfer (diffusion) of oxygen and carbon dioxide between the capillary red blood cells and the tissue cells.

intrapulmonic pressure The pressure of the gas in the alveoli.

intrathoracic pressure The pressure in the pleural space; also known as the *intrapleural pressure.*

jugular notch The superior margin of the manubrium palpated easily at the anterior base of the neck; also known as the *suprasternal notch.*

left mainstem bronchus One of two main bronchi that branch from the trachea at the level of the carina.

lobules Small lobes or subdivisions of a lobe.

lower airway Airway structures below the glottis.

mediastinum A portion of the thoracic cavity in the middle of the thorax between the pleural sacs containing the two lungs; it extends from the sternum to the vertebral column and contains all the thoracic viscera except the lungs.

minute volume The amount of gas inhaled or exhaled in 1 minute. It is found by multiplying the tidal volume by the respiratory rate.

oxyhemoglobin Oxygenated hemoglobin.

partial pressure The pressure exerted by a single gas.

phrenic nerve A nerve composed mostly of motor nerve fibers that produce contractions of the diaphragm; also provides sensory innervation for many components of the mediastinum and pleura.

physiological dead space The sum of the anatomical dead space plus the volume of any nonfunctional alveoli.

pneumotaxic center A group of neurons in the pons that have an inhibitory effect on the inspiratory center.

positive end-expiratory pressure (PEEP) Airway support that maintains a degree of positive pressure at the end of exhalation.

pressure gradient The force produced by differences between atmospheric pressure, intrapulmonic pressure, and intrathoracic pressure.

pulmonary surfactant Certain lipoproteins that reduce the surface tension of pulmonary fluids, allowing the exchange of gases in the alveoli of the lungs and contributing to the elasticity of pulmonary tissue.

pulmonary ventilation The movement of air into and out of the lungs. This process brings oxygen into the lungs and removes carbon dioxide.

pulsus paradoxus An abnormal decrease in systolic blood pressure in which it drops more than 10 to 15 mm Hg during inspiration compared with expiration.

residual volume The volume of air remaining in the lungs after a maximum expiratory effort.

respiration The exchange of oxygen and carbon dioxide between an organism and the environment.

respiratory membrane The membrane in the lungs across which gas exchange with the blood occurs.

right mainstem bronchus One of two main bronchi that branch from the trachea at the level of the carina.

secondary bronchi Branches from a primary bronchus that conduct air to each lobe of the lungs.

surfactant Lipoproteins that reduce the surface tension of pulmonary fluids.

terminal bronchioles The ends of the conducting airways.

tidal volume The volume of air inspired or expired in a single, resting breath.

torr A measurement in millimeters of mercury.

total pressure The combination of pressures exerted by all the gases in any mixture of gas.

upper airway Airway structures above the glottis.

sternal angle The point at which the manubrium joins the body of the sternum; also known as the angle of Louis.

vallecula A furrow between the glossoepiglottic folds on each side of the posterior oropharynx.

ventilation The mechanical movement of air into and out of the lungs that makes respiration possible.

vocal cords The two folds of elastic ligaments covered by mucous membrane that stretch from the thyroid cartilage to the arytenoid cartilage; vibration of the vocal cords is responsible for voice production; also known as the true vocal cords.

An inadequate airway coupled with ineffective ventilation is a major cause of preventable death and cardiopulmonary complications in both medical and trauma patients. A thorough understanding of the respiratory system and mastery of airway management and ventilation are essential aspects of prehospital emergency care.

SECTION ONE
The Airway

AIRWAY ANATOMY

Successful management of the airway requires an understanding of the upper and lower airway structures and functions. For the purpose of this text, all airway structures above the glottis are considered the **upper airway**. All structures below the glottis are considered the **lower airway** (Box 15-1 and Figure 15-1). Airway anatomy was presented in Chapter 10; the following discussion serves as a review.

 LOOK AGAIN
See Chapter 10: Review of Human Systems, pp. 191-196.

BOX 15-1 Structures of the Upper and Lower Airways

Upper Airway Structures
Nasopharynx
Frontal, maxillary, ethmoid, sphenoid sinuses
Oropharynx
Laryngopharynx
Larynx

Lower Airway Structures
Trachea
Bronchial tree
Alveoli
Lungs

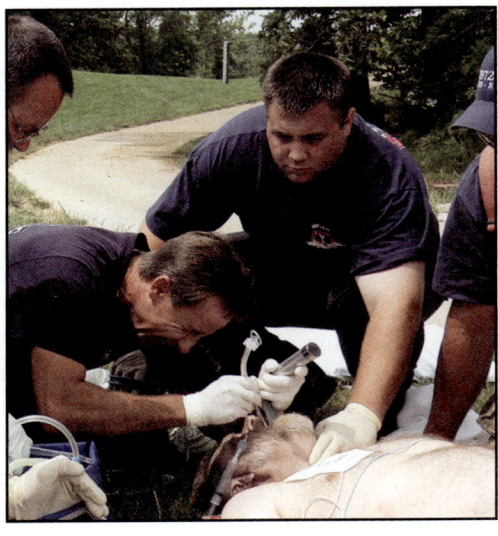

(Courtesy Ray Kemp, St. Charles, Mo.)

Upper Airway

The human airway has two openings, the nose and the mouth. Air passes through the nose into the nasopharynx. This is the superior part of the pharynx. Air passes through the mouth into the oropharynx. The nasopharynx ends and the oropharynx begins at the level of the uvula. The oropharynx extends to the level of the epiglottis. The laryngopharynx (also known as the *hypopharynx*) extends from the tip of the epiglottis to the glottis and esophagus. The laryngopharynx opens into the larynx, which lies in the anterior neck (Figure 15-2).

 NOTE
An important anatomical landmark in the laryngopharynx is the vallecula. The **vallecula** is a depression just behind the root of the tongue and between the folds of the throat. This area identifies where the curved blade of the laryngoscope is placed during endotracheal intubation to facilitate direct visualization of the glottis. (Endotracheal intubation is described later in this section.)

 NOTE
When visualizing a patient's airway, remember that the floor of the nose is the roof of the mouth.

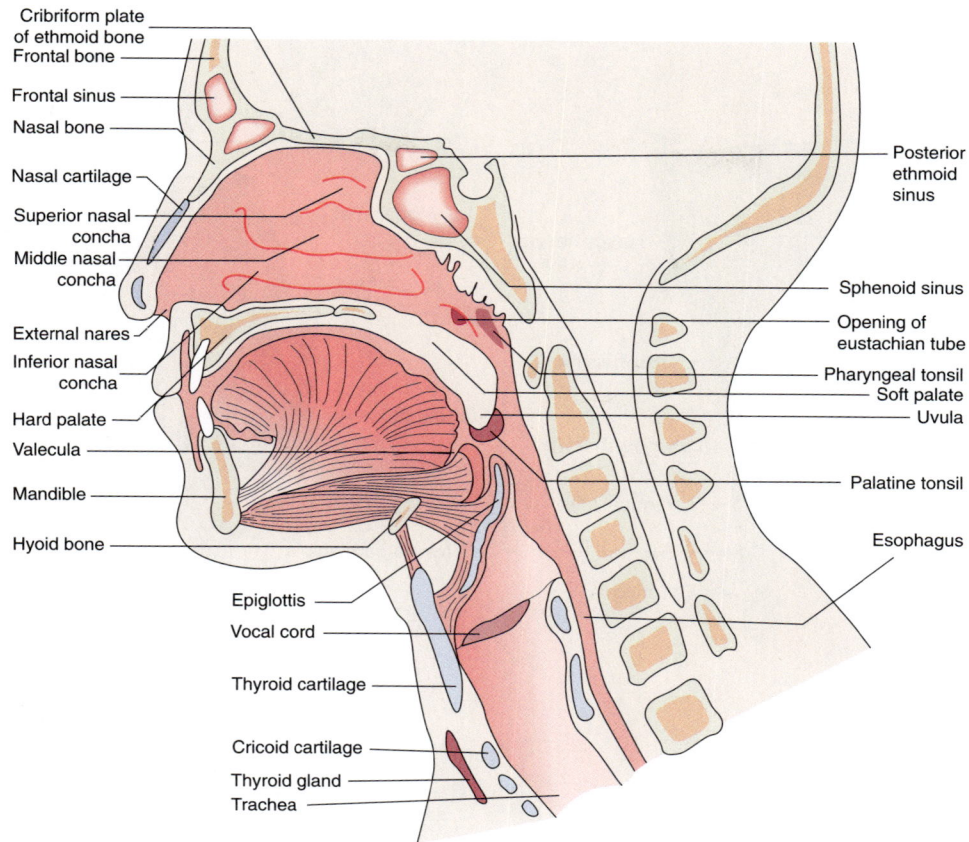

FIGURE 15-1 Midsagittal section through the upper airway. (From Wilkins RL, et al: *Egan's fundamentals of respiratory care,* ed 9, St Louis, 2009, Mosby.)

The larynx consists of an outer casing of nine cartilages. These cartilages are connected to each other by muscles and ligaments. Six of the nine cartilages are paired; three are unpaired. The unpaired thyroid cartilage is the largest, most superior of the cartilages. This structure is also known as the *Adam's apple*. The most inferior cartilage of the larynx is the unpaired cricoid cartilage. This cartilage is the only complete cartilage ring in the larynx. The third unpaired cartilage is the epiglottis. The six paired cartilages are stacked in two pillars between the cricoid cartilage and the thyroid cartilage. They are the *arytenoid cartilages,* the *corniculate cartilages,* and the *cuneiform cartilages.* The U-shaped hyoid bone is located beneath the mandible. The hyoid bone helps support the airway by anchoring muscles to the jaw. The thyroid membrane joins the hyoid bone and the thyroid cartilage. This fibrinous membrane is known as the *cricothyroid membrane.* The larynx also contains the true and false vocal cords. As described in Chapter 10, the **vocal cords** (Figure 15-3) regulate the flow of air to and from the lungs for the production of voice sounds. The endotracheal (ET) tube is passed through the open vocal cords of the larynx during endotracheal intubation. The larynx extends from the lower part of the pharynx to the trachea. On either side of the larynx is a recess called the *piriform sinus.* Foreign

materials that are swallowed may become lodged in these areas.

Lower Airway

The trachea lies anterior to the esophagus. It is the air passage from the larynx to the lungs. The trachea begins at the border of the cricoid cartilage and ends where it bifurcates into the right and left main bronchi; this bifurcation is at the level of the **jugular notch**. The trachea is composed of 16 to 20 incomplete cartilaginous rings. These rings open posteriorly to prevent the trachea from collapsing.

The **carina of the trachea** is a downward and backward projection of the last tracheal cartilage. It forms a ridge that separates the opening of the **right mainstem bronchus** and the **left mainstem bronchus**. The carina occurs at the **sternal angle** (also known as the *angle of Louis*).

> **NOTE**
> The right main bronchus is wider, shorter, and more vertical than the left one. Because of this, the right main bronchus is the more common site of foreign body obstruction.

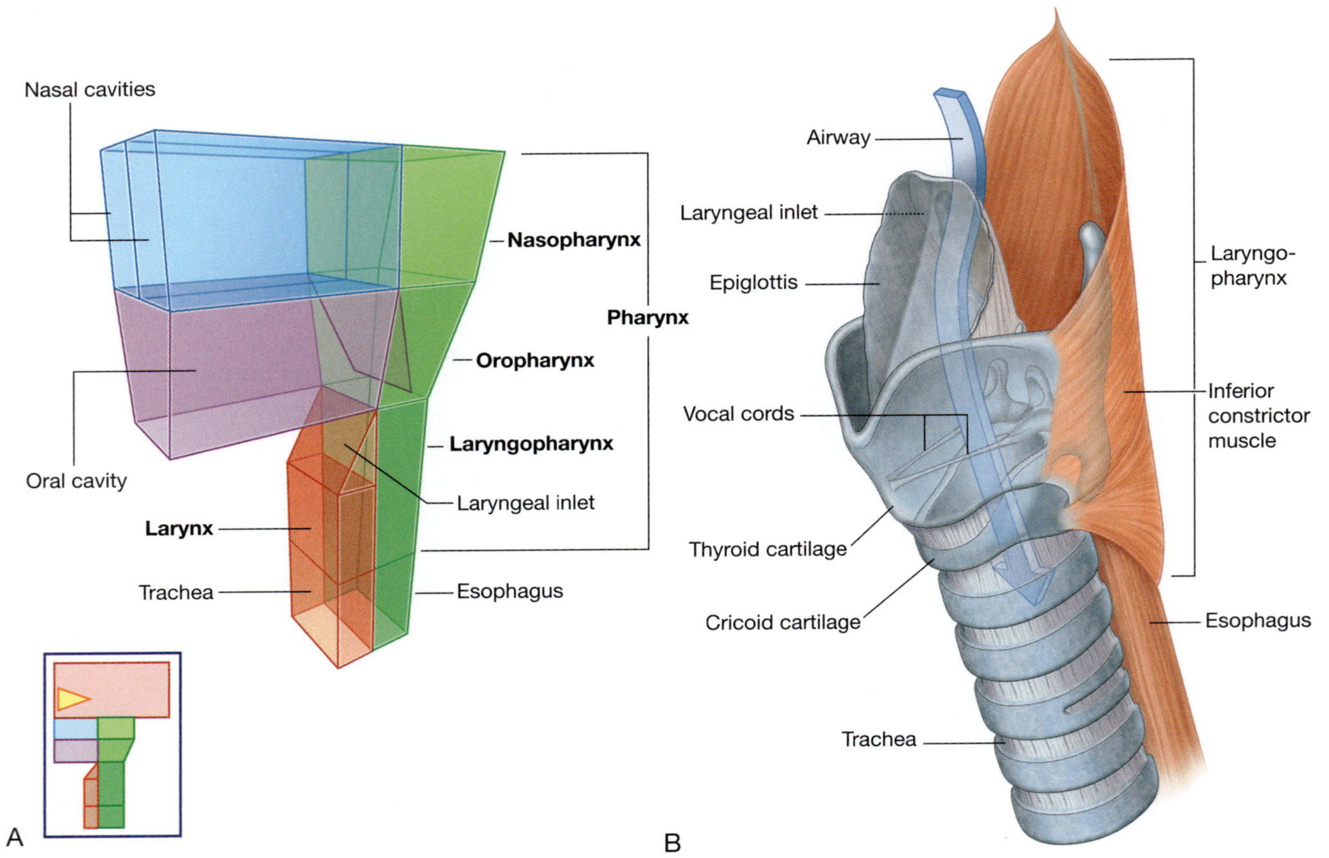

Nasal cavities

Nasopharynx

Pharynx

Oropharynx

Laryngopharynx

Laryngeal inlet

Oral cavity

Larynx

Trachea

Esophagus

A

Airway

Laryngeal inlet

Epiglottis

Vocal cords

Thyroid cartilage

Cricoid cartilage

Trachea

Laryngo-pharynx

Inferior constrictor muscle

Esophagus

B

FIGURE 15-2 Specialized structures of the neck. **A,** Conceptual view. **B,** Anatomical view. (From Drake R: *Gray's anatomy for students,* ed 2, Philadelphia, 2010, Churchill Livingstone.)

The right and left main bronchi pass from the bifurcation of the trachea to the lungs to form the bronchial tree. The right and left main bronchi further branch into **secondary bronchi.** They divide again into tertiary segmental bronchi and finally **terminal bronchioles**. The terminal bronchioles are the smallest airways without alveoli. The terminal bronchioles divide into respiratory bronchioles and then alveolar ducts (Figure 15-4).

> **NOTE**
> Like the trachea, the bronchi are supported by cartilaginous rings. As the bronchi branch into smaller subdivisions, the amount of cartilage decreases and the bronchi become increasingly muscular. This continues until no cartilage is present. Bronchial smooth muscle has beta$_2$ adrenergic receptors. Therefore, the muscles are sensitive to certain hormones (e.g., epinephrine). The muscles also are sensitive to beta$_2$ receptor drugs such as albuterol. Stimulation of the beta$_2$ adrenergic receptors causes the bronchial smooth muscles to relax.

The **alveoli** are the functional units of the respiratory system. They make up most of the lung tissue. The alveoli also are where most of the respiratory gas exchange takes place. Together the two lungs have about 300 million

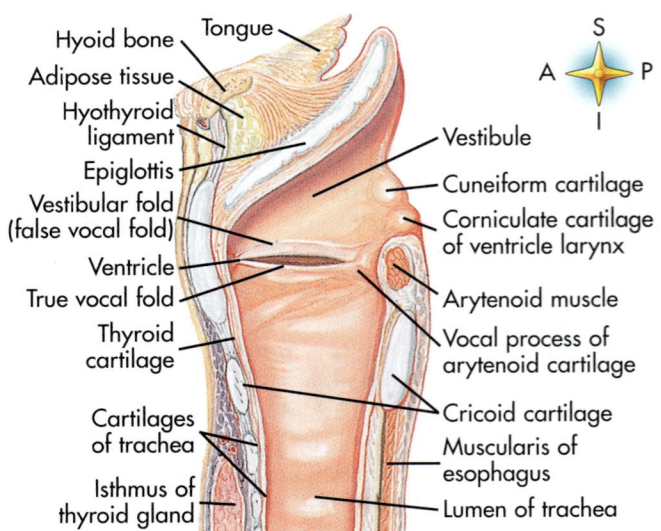

Hyoid bone

Tongue

Adipose tissue

Hyothyroid ligament

Epiglottis

Vestibular fold (false vocal fold)

Ventricle

True vocal fold

Thyroid cartilage

Cartilages of trachea

Isthmus of thyroid gland

Vestibule

Cuneiform cartilage

Corniculate cartilage of ventricle larynx

Arytenoid muscle

Vocal process of arytenoid cartilage

Cricoid cartilage

Muscularis of esophagus

Lumen of trachea

S   A   P   I

FIGURE 15-3 Vocal cords.

alveoli.[1] Each alveolus is surrounded by a fine network of blood capillaries. The capillaries are arranged so that air in the alveolus is separated from the blood by a thin **respiratory membrane.** The alveoli are coated with **pulmonary surfactant.** The surfactant is a thin film produced

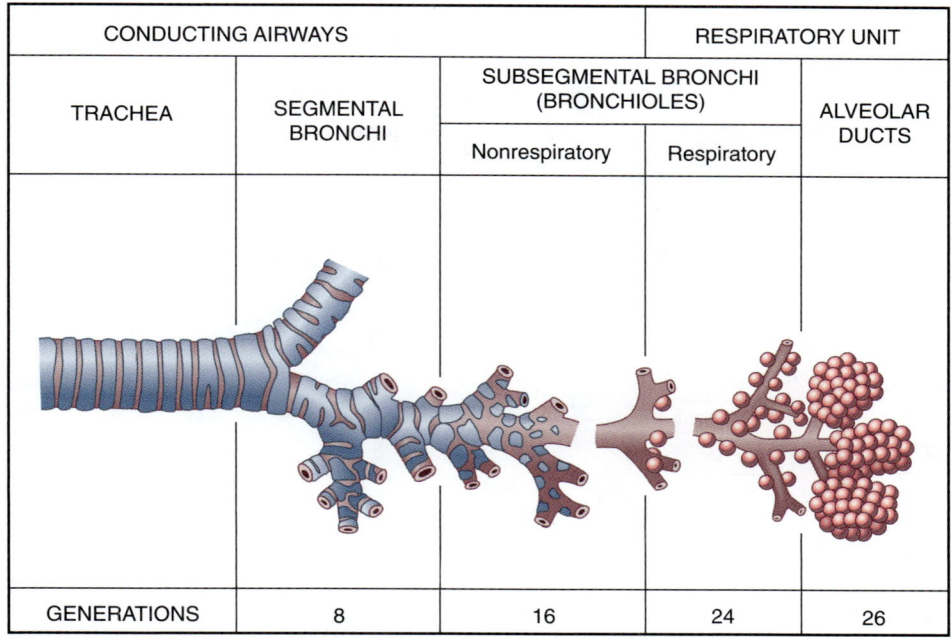

CONDUCTING AIRWAYS				RESPIRATORY UNIT
TRACHEA	SEGMENTAL BRONCHI	SUBSEGMENTAL BRONCHI (BRONCHIOLES)		ALVEOLAR DUCTS
		Nonrespiratory	Respiratory	
GENERATIONS	8	16	24	26

FIGURE 15-4 Structures of the lower airway (From McCance KL, Huether SE: *Pathophysiology: the biologic basis for disease in adults and children,* ed 6, St Louis, 2009, Mosby.)

by the alveolar cells that prevents the alveoli from collapsing.

The lungs are large, paired, spongy organs. They are attached to the heart by pulmonary arteries and veins. The two lungs are separated by the **mediastinum.** The contents of the mediastinum include the heart, blood vessels, trachea, esophagus, lymphatic tissue, and vessels. Each lung is shaped like a cone, with its base resting on the diaphragm. The left lung is smaller than the right and is divided into two lobes. The right lung has three lobes. Each lobe is divided into **lobules**. The left lung has nine lobules, and the right lung has 10 lobules. Both lungs are surrounded by a separate pleural cavity. The two layers of pleura are visceral and parietal. They are separated by a serous fluid. This fluid acts as a lubricant to allow the pleural membranes to slide past each other during breathing. The primary function of the lungs is **respiration** (the exchange of oxygen and carbon dioxide between an organism and the environment) (Figure 15-5).

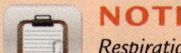 **NOTE**

Respiration should not be confused with *ventilation*. **Ventilation** is the mechanical movement of air into and out of the lungs. Ventilation makes respiration possible.

SUPPORT STRUCTURES OF THE AIRWAY

The support structures of the airway include the thoracic cage, the phrenic nerve, and the mediastinum.

As described in Chapter 10, the thoracic cage protects vital organs. It also prevents collapse of the thorax during ventilation. The thoracic cage consists of the thoracic vertebrae, ribs and their associated costal cartilages, and the sternum (Figure 15-6). Muscles involved in ventilation include the **intercostal muscles** and the **diaphragm.** The intercostal muscles and accessory muscles (described later in this chapter) are used only during exercise, exertion, or distress. They are not used during quiet breathing. The diaphragm is the most important muscle for ventilation. When the diaphragm contracts, the abdominal contents are pushed downward and the intercostal muscles move the ribs upward and outward. This movement increases the volume and decreases the pressure in the thoracic cavity.

 LOOK AGAIN

See Chapter 10: Review of Human Systems, pp. 158-162.

The **phrenic nerve** is composed mostly of motor nerve fibers. These motor nerve fibers produce contractions of the diaphragm. The phrenic nerve also provides sensory innervation for many components of the mediastinum and pleura. This is also true for the upper abdomen, especially the liver, and the gallbladder. The *right phrenic nerve* passes over the brachiocephalic artery, posterior to the subclavian vein, and then crosses the root of the right lung anteriorly. It leaves the thorax by passing through an opening in the diaphragm. The right phrenic nerve passes over the right atrium. The *left phrenic nerve* passes over the pericardium of the left ventricle and enters the diaphragm separately.

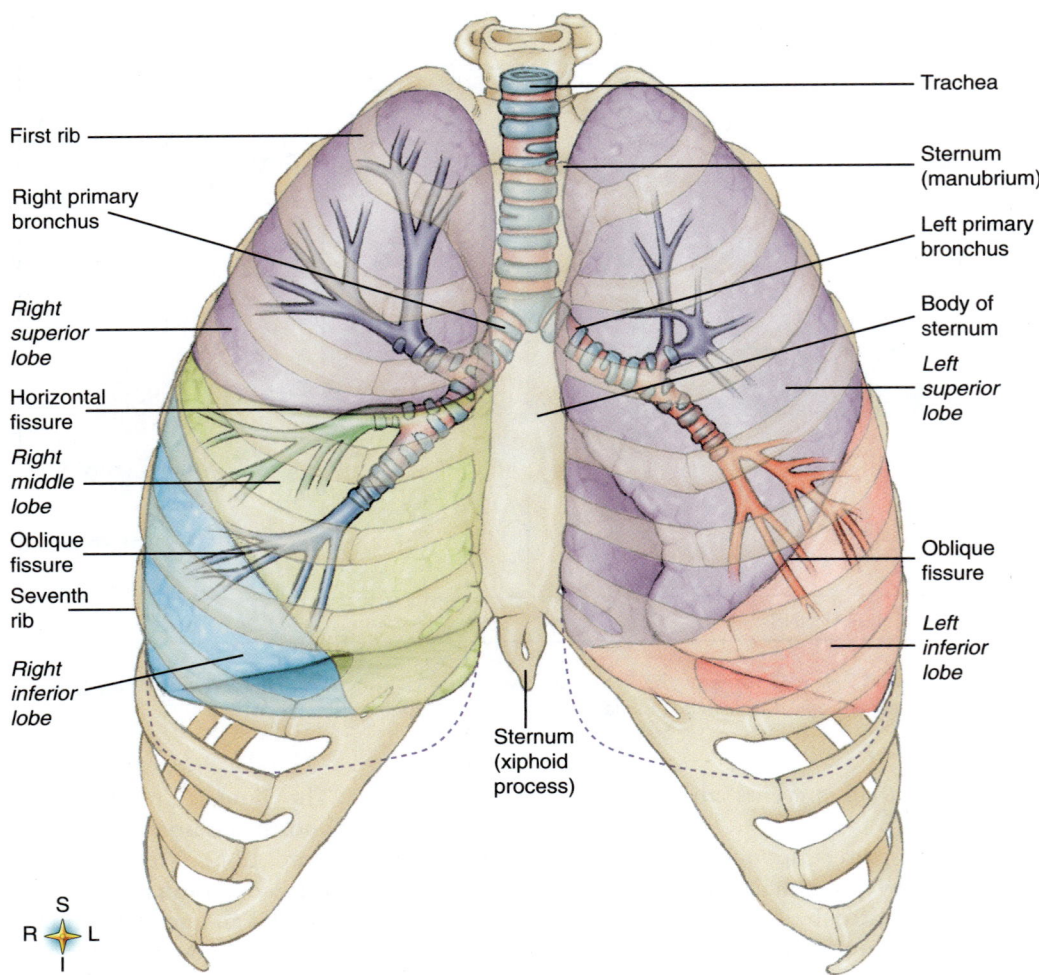

First rib

Right primary
bronchus

*Right
superior
lobe*

Horizontal
fissure

*Right
middle
lobe*

Oblique
fissure

Seventh
rib

*Right
inferior
lobe*

Trachea

Sternum
(manubrium)

Left primary
bronchus

Body of
sternum

*Left
superior
lobe*

Oblique
fissure

*Left
inferior
lobe*

Sternum
(xiphoid
process)

FIGURE 15-5 Lungs. The trachea is an airway that branches to form an inverted tree of bronchi
and bronchioles. Note that the right lung has three lobes and the left lung has two lobes. (From
Thibodeau GA, Patton KT: *Structure and function of the body,* ed 13, St Louis, 2008, Mosby.)

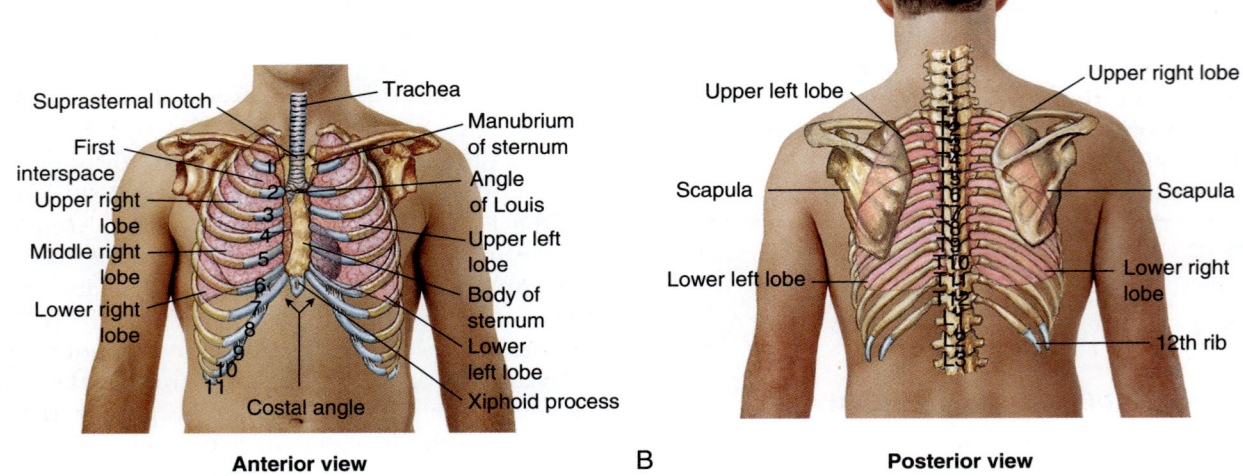

Suprasternal notch

First
interspace

Upper right
lobe

Middle right
lobe

Lower right
lobe

Costal angle

Trachea

Manubrium
of sternum

Angle
of Louis

Upper left
lobe

Body of
sternum

Lower
left lobe

Xiphoid process

Upper left lobe

Scapula

Lower left lobe

Upper right lobe

Scapula

Lower right
lobe

12th rib

A   **Anterior view**

B   **Posterior view**

FIGURE 15-6 Thorax and underlying structures. **A,** Anterior view. **B,** Posterior view. (From
Wilson SF, Giddens JF: *Health assessment for nursing practice,* ed 4, St Louis, 2009, Mosby.)

> **NOTE**
> The phrenic nerve originates from the spinal cord between cervical nerves C3 and C5. Injury to the spinal cord or brainstem may damage the nerve cells that stimulate the phrenic nerve, which facilitates contraction of the diaphragm (see Chapter 41).

As stated earlier, the contents of the mediastinum include the heart, blood vessels, trachea, esophagus, lymphatic tissue, and vessels. The mediastinum is the central compartment of the thoracic cavity and therefore is a supporting structure of the respiratory system. It lies between the right and left pleura in and near the median sagittal plane of the chest. It extends from the sternum in front to the vertebral column behind. It is continuous with the loose connective tissue of the neck, and extends inferiorly onto the diaphragm. The mediastinum contains all the thoracic viscera except the lungs (Figure 15-7).

SECTION TWO
Respiratory Physiology

MECHANICS OF RESPIRATION

As described previously, *respiration* is the exchange of oxygen and carbon dioxide between an organism and the environment. Oxygen is an essential nutrient for a living organism to produce energy. Carbon dioxide is a byproduct of energy production that must be removed from the body. For this gas exchange to occur, air must move freely into and out of the lungs. This brings oxygen into the lungs and removes carbon dioxide. This *mechanical process* is known as **pulmonary ventilation.**

The two phases of respiration are external respiration and internal respiration. **External respiration** is the transfer (diffusion) of oxygen and carbon dioxide between the inspired air and pulmonary capillaries. **Internal**

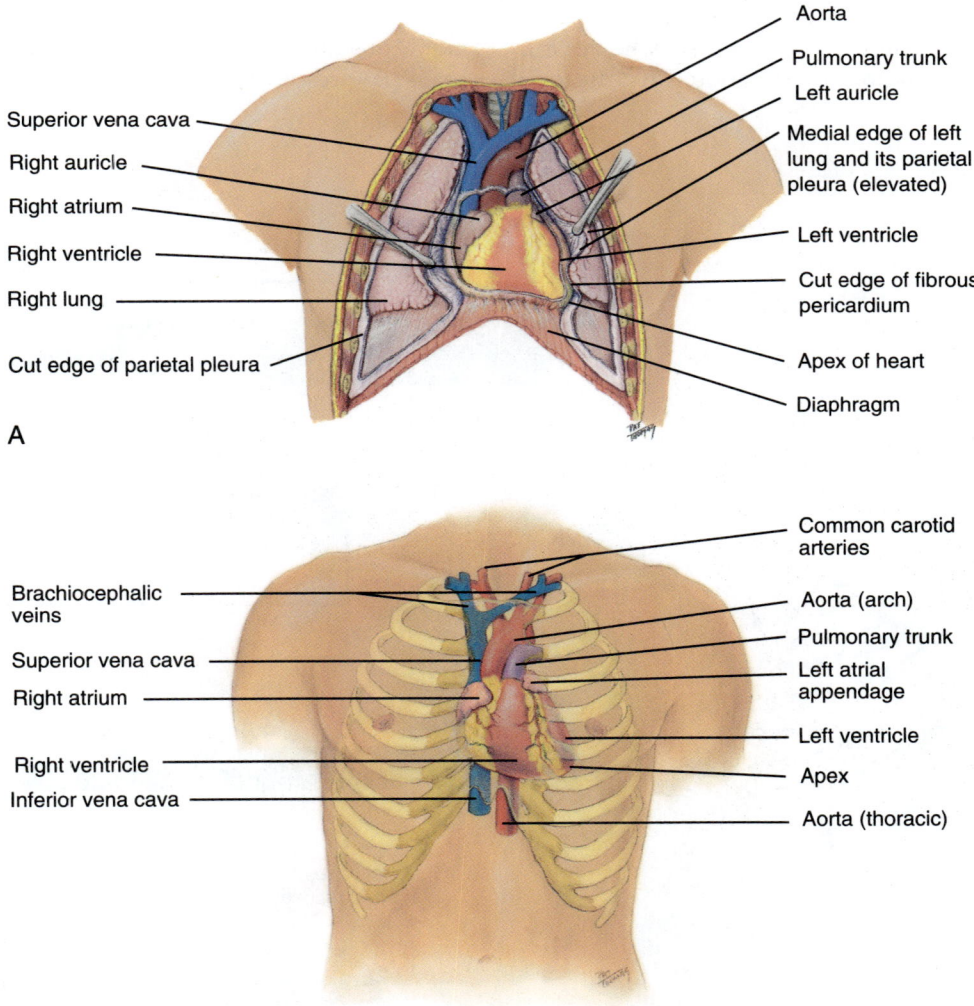

FIGURE 15-7 A, Frontal view of the mediastinum, showing the position of the heart **(B).** (Appelgate EM: *The anatomy and physiology learning system,* ed 3, St Louis, 2007, Saunders.)

respiration is the transfer (diffusion) of oxygen and carbon dioxide between the capillary red blood cells and the tissue cells.

Pressure Changes and Ventilation

Gas flows from an area of higher pressure or concentration to an area of lower pressure or concentration. For gas to flow into the lungs, a **pressure gradient** is required. This pressure gradient is produced by differences between atmospheric pressure, intrapulmonic pressure, and intrathoracic pressure (also known as *intrapleural pressure*).

> ### CRITICAL THINKING
> Think of two medical conditions that could impair (1) external respiration and (2) internal respiration.

Atmospheric pressure is the pressure of the gas around us. It varies with differences in altitude. At sea level, it is 760 mm Hg. **Intrapulmonic pressure** is the pressure of the gas in the alveoli. Depending on the size of the thorax, this pressure varies a little above and below 760 mm Hg. The intrapulmonic pressure also depends on whether it is measured during inspiration or expiration. **Intrathoracic**

pressure is the pressure in the pleural space. It normally is less than the atmospheric pressure (usually 751 to 754 mm Hg). However, it may exceed the atmospheric pressure during coughing or straining during bowel movements.

During **inspiration** the chest wall expands. This increases the size of the thoracic cavity and expands the lungs. The expansion results from muscle movement and negative pressure in the pleural space. As the thorax expands, the lung space increases. This causes a drop in the intrapulmonic pressure of about 1 mm Hg below atmospheric pressure. The pressure gradient results in gas flow into the lungs. At end inspiration the thorax and alveoli stop expanding. The intrapulmonic pressure becomes equal to the atmospheric pressure, and gas no longer moves into the lungs (Figure 15-8).

As the chest wall relaxes during **expiration,** the muscles of ventilation are at rest. The process of inspiration reverses. Elastic recoil causes the thorax and lung space to decrease in size. This increases the intrapulmonic pressure. The pressure gradient created in the thoracic cavity produces a decrease in alveolar volume and increases the intrapulmonic pressure about 1 mm Hg over the atmospheric pressure. The pressure gradient results in gas flow out of the

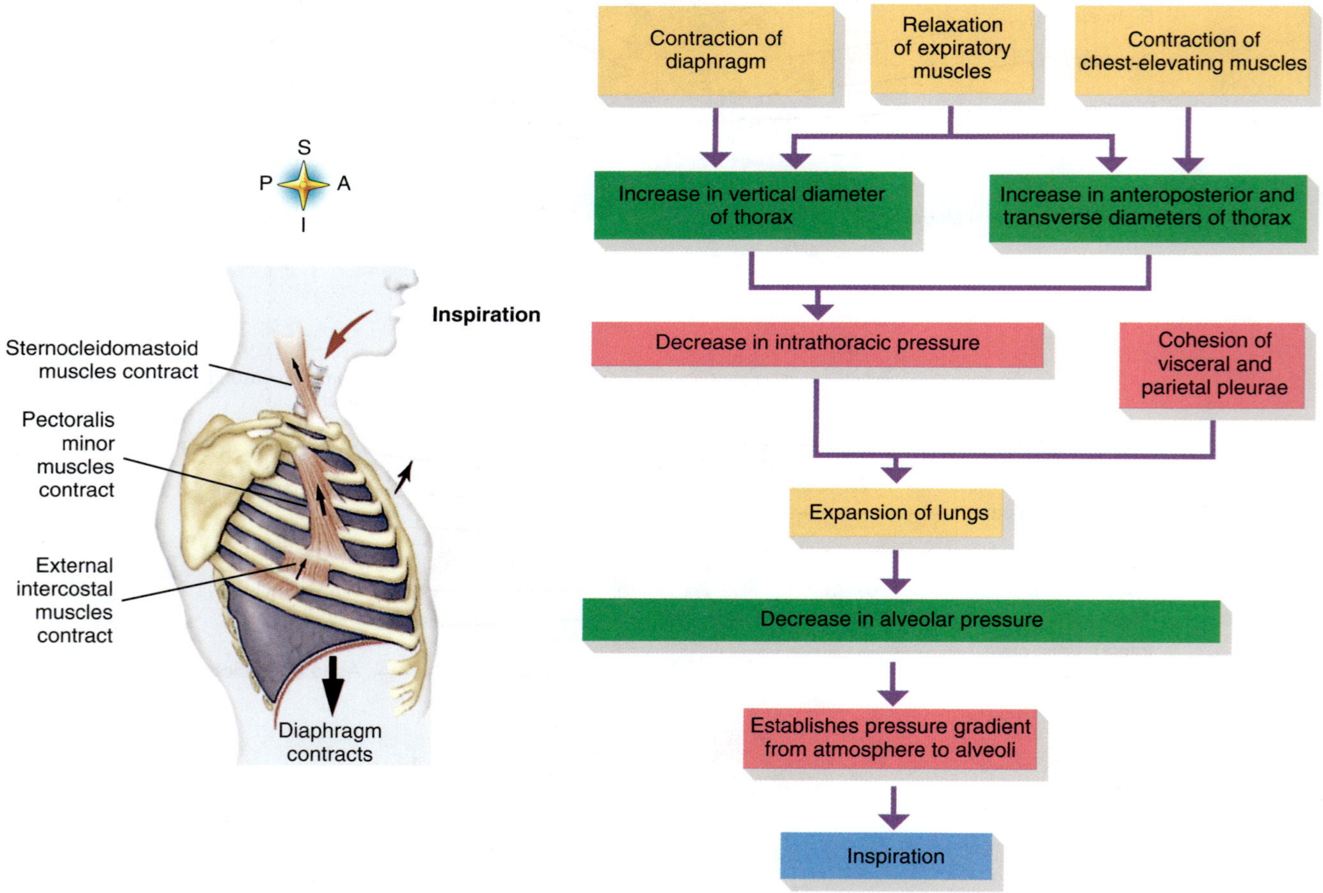

FIGURE 15-8 Mechanics of inspiration. (From Patton KT, Thibodeau GA: *Anatomy and physiology,* ed 7, St Louis, 2007, Mosby.)

lungs. At the end of expiration the opposing forces and pressures become equal. The thoracic volume no longer decreases. The intrapulmonic pressure becomes equal to the atmospheric pressure, and gas movement out of the lungs stops (Figure 15-9).

> **NOTE**
>
> **Boyle's law** states that as a pressure of a gas decreases, its volume expands. Conversely, as a pressure of a gas increases, its volume decreases. (Pressure is inversely proportional to volume.) Simply put, during inspiration, when the thorax contracts, the volume in the chest increases, negative pressure occurs, and air enters the lungs. This process is reversed during expiration.

Muscles of Ventilation

Expansion of the lungs and thorax is caused by the movement of the diaphragm and the internal and external intercostal muscles (Figure 15-10). On inspiration, the diaphragm contracts and the dome of the diaphragm flattens. This increases the superior-inferior dimension of the chest cavity. The internal and external intercostal muscles also contract. This raises the ribs. It also increases the front-to-back (anterior-posterior) and side-to-side dimensions of the chest cavity.

> **CRITICAL THINKING**
>
> How does interruption of the chest wall from a stab wound change the mechanics of breathing?

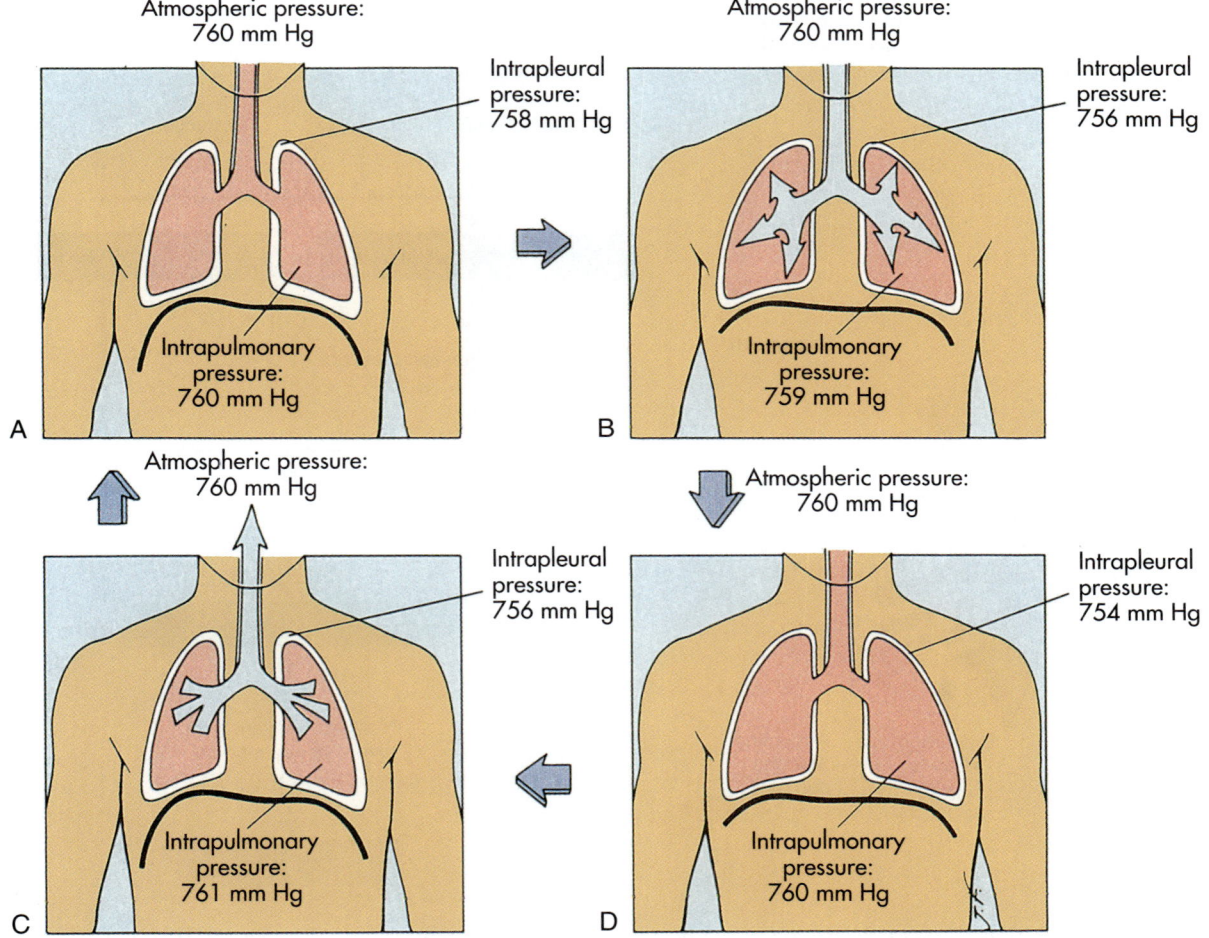

FIGURE 15-9 Pressure changes during inspiration and expiration. **A,** At the end of expiration, intrapulmonary pressure equals atmospheric pressure, and no movement of air occurs. **B,** During inspiration, the volume of the pleural space increases, causing the pressure in the intrapulmonary spaces (alveoli) to decrease. Air then flows from the outside of the body, where the pressure is greater (760 mm Hg), into the alveoli, where it is lower (759 mm Hg). **C,** At the end of inspiration, intrapulmonary pressure again equals atmospheric pressure, and no movement of air occurs. **D,** During expiration, the volume of the pleural spaces decreases, causing the intrapulmonary pressure to increase. Because the intrapulmonary pressure exceeds the atmospheric pressure, air flows out of the lungs.

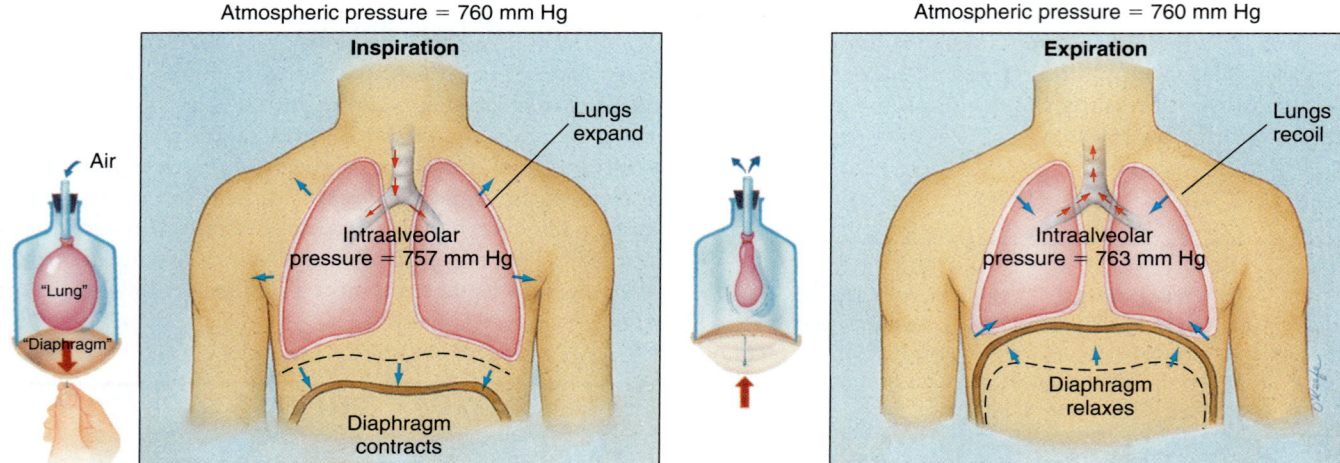

FIGURE 15-10 During inhalation, the diaphragm contracts, increasing the volume of the thoracic cavity. The increase in volume results in a decrease in pressure, which causes air to rush into the lungs. During expiration, the diaphragm returns to an upward position, reducing the volume of the thoracic cavity. Air pressure increases and forces air out of the lungs. (Patton KT, Thibodeau GA: *Anatomy and physiology,* ed 7, St Louis, 2007, Mosby.)

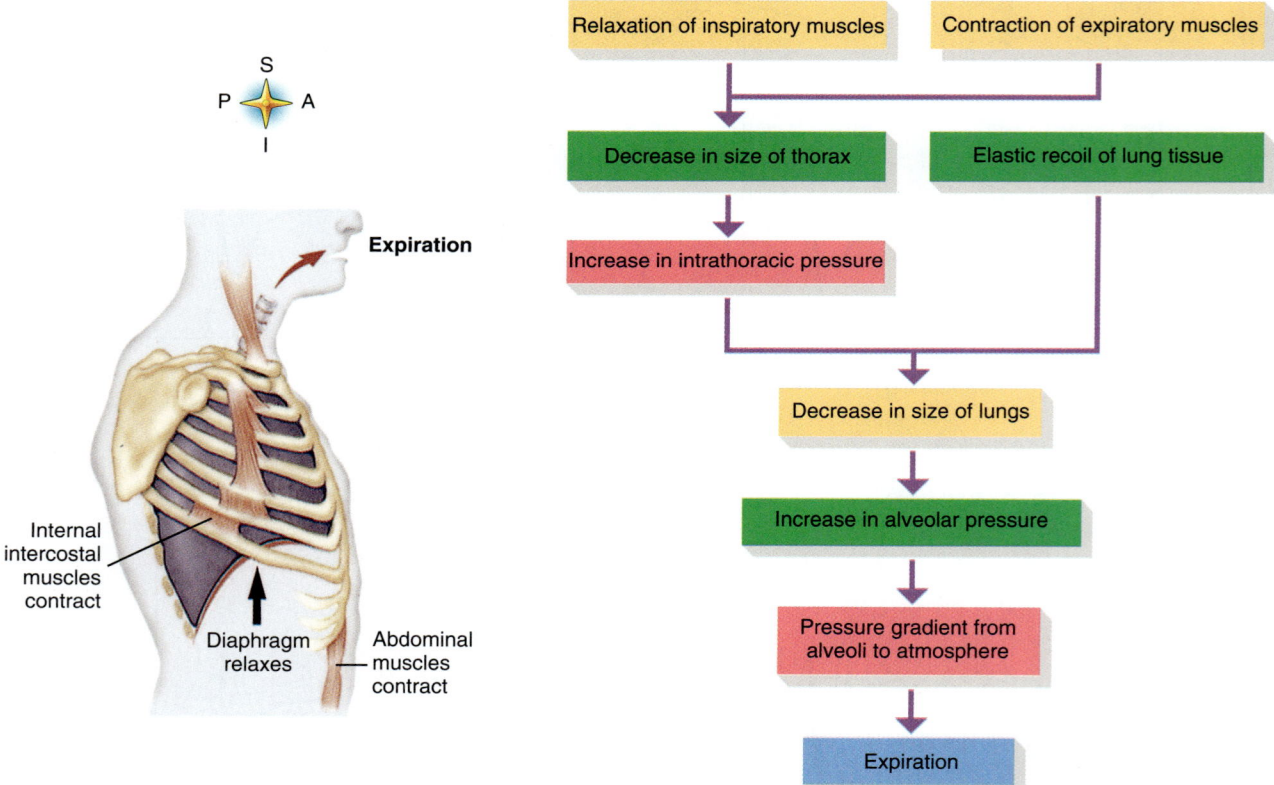

FIGURE 15-11 Relaxation of the diaphragm and contraction of the chest-depressing muscles (the internal intercostal muscles) reduce the thoracic volume. This increases pressure in the lungs, pushing air out. (Patton KT, Thibodeau GA: *Anatomy and physiology,* ed 7, St Louis, 2007, Mosby.)

Expiration is a passive motion. During expiration, relaxation of the diaphragm and internal intercostal muscles allows the elastic recoil properties of the lungs to reduce the size (or volume) of the thoracic cavity (Figure 15-11). The ease with which the lungs and thorax expand during pressure changes is known as **compliance.** The greater the compliance, the easier the expansion. Diseases that reduce compliance increase the energy required for breathing. Examples of such diseases are asthma, bronchitis, and pulmonary edema. Other diseases, such as emphysema, increase lung compliance by breaking down the elastic fibers that surround lung tissue. This may be the result of overstretching of the fibers from chronic coughing.[2,3] These patients have no problem inflating the lungs but have extreme difficulty exhaling air (see Chapter 24).

Work of Breathing

In people who are healthy, the energy needed for normal, quiet breathing is about 3% of the total body expenditure.[4] Factors that increase the amount of energy needed for ventilation include loss of pulmonary surfactant (e.g., from smoke inhalation), an increase in airway resistance (e.g., from asthma), or a decrease in pulmonary compliance (e.g., from cystic fibrosis). These factors can increase the energy requirement to as much as one third of the total body expenditure.[5]

The pulmonary alveoli have a tendency to collapse. This is the result of recoil caused by the elastic fibers and the surface tension of the alveolar walls. The surface tension is created because water molecules are attracted to each other in the alveolar membrane. Pulmonary surfactant lowers the surface tension. It does this by intermingling with the water molecules to reduce the cohesive force. This helps prevent collapse of the alveolus at the end of expiration.

> **NOTE**
>
> **Atelectasis** is the collapse (diminished volume) of all or part of the lung. This condition can be caused by obstruction, such as from a foreign body, tumor, or mucous plugging. It also may be caused by compression (e.g., pneumothorax). A deficiency in surfactant (e.g., decreased production or inactivation of surfactant) is another cause. Continuous positive airway pressure (CPAP), biphasic positive airway pressure (BiPAP), and positive end-expiratory pressure (PEEP) can prevent the collapse of alveoli. These airway therapies increase the amount of gas that remains in the lungs at the end of expiration. This prevents the collapse of alveoli and improves the ease and work of breathing in patients who have respiratory distress. (CPAP and PEEP are described later in this chapter and in Chapter 24.)

Surfactant is composed of lipoproteins that reduce the surface tension of pulmonary fluids. Surfactant is constantly being replenished by certain alveolar cells. Its production is thought to be stimulated by normal ventilation. If this production decreases, as occurs in pneumonia, very high ventilation pressures may be needed to produce lung expansion.

The elastic forces of the lung oppose lung expansion. Viscous and frictional forces often play the central role in impeding airflow into and out of the lungs. Much of the resistance to airflow is provided by the upper airways of the respiratory tract. The nasal passages cause about 50% of the total airway resistance during nose breathing. The mouth, pharynx, larynx, and trachea account for approximately 20% to 30% of airway resistance during quiet

mouth breathing. This may increase to about 50% during times of increased ventilation (e.g., during vigorous exercise).[5]

Airway resistance falls greatly as the bronchial tree continues to branch toward the alveoli. Still, the presence of airway secretions or bronchiolar constriction can lead to increased airway resistance. These factors may occur separately. More often, they occur at the same time (e.g., as in asthma). When resistance to airflow increases, the usual pressure gradient needed for ventilation is inadequate. Therefore, muscular effort is needed to create a larger pressure gradient.

Structural changes in the lungs or thorax as a result of trauma or disease also may increase the amount of work needed for effective ventilation. This increased work usually is obvious from the use of **accessory muscles** during labored breathing. The accessory muscles include the scalenes and the sternocleidomastoid (deep muscles of the neck and thorax), posterior neck and back muscles, and the abdominal muscles (Figure 15-12).

Lung Volumes and Capacities

At rest, the average adult breathes about 12 to 24 times a minute. One fifth of this inspired air never reaches the alveoli for gas exchange. Instead, it fills the upper respiratory tract and lower nonrespiratory bronchioles.[6] This area is referred to as **anatomical dead space.** The term **physiological dead space** refers to the anatomical dead space plus the volume of any nonfunctional alveoli. Usually the anatomical and physiological dead spaces are nearly identical. However, this is not always the case. In patients with respiratory diseases, such as emphysema, the alveolar walls begin to degenerate. The destruction of these walls can increase the size of the physiological dead space up to 10 times that of the anatomical dead space (Figure 15-13).

The lungs can hold about eight times the amount of air brought in by a normal resting inhalation. From the first breath of life, the lungs are never fully emptied. Even after forced expiration, a "residual volume" of air remains in the alveoli. This residual volume is replenished slowly. At least 16 breaths, and at times more, are needed to renew the residual volume of air in the lungs.[7]

The **tidal volume** is the volume of gas inhaled or exhaled during a normal breath. The tidal volume of the average adult is about 500 to 600 mL. Of this, 150 mL remains in the anatomical dead space (the bronchi, bronchioles, and other prealveolar structures) until it is exhaled during the next respiratory cycle. Therefore, 150 mL of the atmospheric gas inhaled during each inspiration never reaches the alveoli. It is merely moved into and out of the airways. A paramedic observing the rise and fall of a patient's chest is indirectly observing tidal volume.

The **inspiratory reserve volume** is the amount of gas that can be forcefully inhaled after inspiration of the normal tidal volume. This amount is usually 2000 to 3000 mL. The **expiratory reserve volume** is the amount of

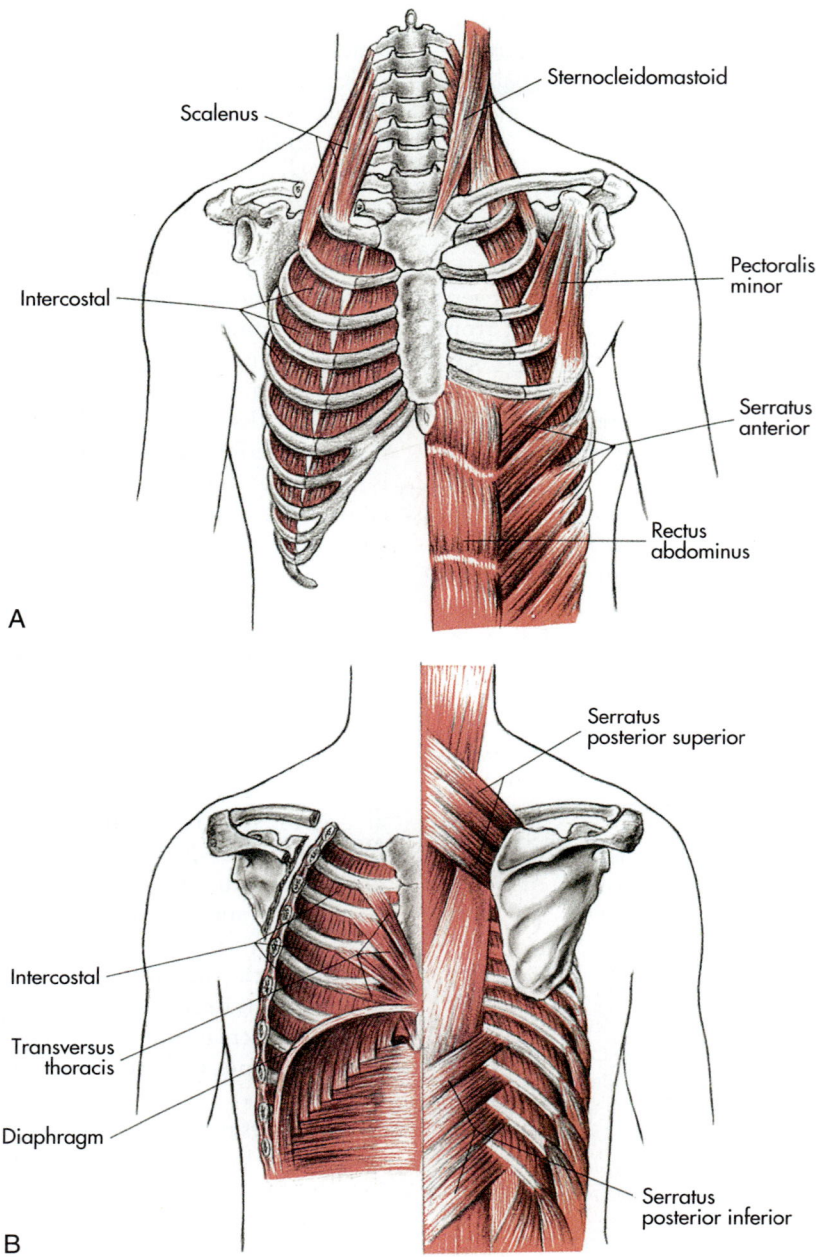

FIGURE 15-12 Muscles of ventilation. **A,** Anterior view. **B,** Posterior view. (From Seidel H et al: *Mosby's guide to physical examination,* ed 6, St Louis, 2007, Mosby.)

gas that can be forcefully exhaled after expiration of the normal tidal volume. This volume usually is less than the inspiratory reserve volume (about 1200 mL). The **residual volume** is the gas that remains in the respiratory system after forced expiration. The normal residual volume is 1000 to 1200 mL.

The combined measurements of tidal volume, inspiratory reserve volume, expiratory reserve volume, and residual volume constitute the maximum volume to which the lungs can be expanded.

Pulmonary capacities are the sum of two or more pulmonary volumes. The more common pulmonary capacities are as follows (Figure 15-14):

- *Inspiratory capacity*: Inspiratory capacity is the tidal volume plus the inspiratory reserve volume. This capacity reflects the amount of gas a person can inspire maximally after a normal expiration (about 3500 mL).
- *Functional residual capacity*: Functional residual capacity is the expiratory reserve volume plus the residual

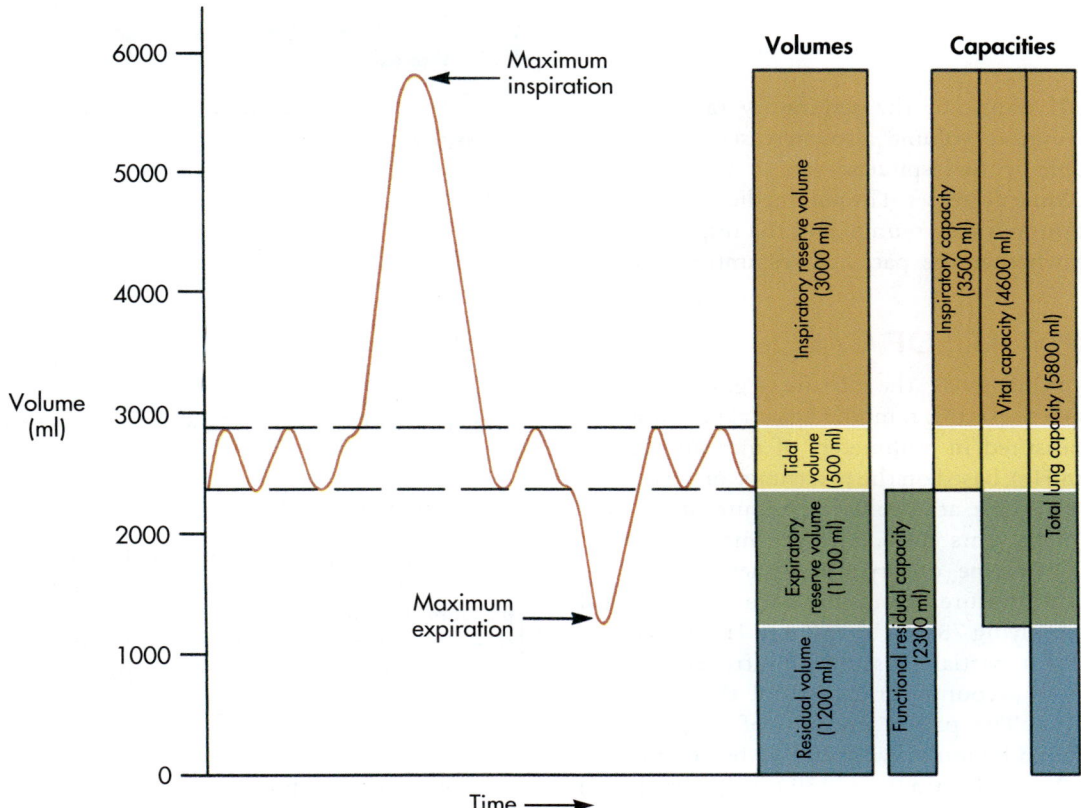

FIGURE 15-13 Lung volumes and capacities. Tidal volume during resting conditions. (From Seeley R: *Anatomy and physiology,* ed 2, St Louis, 1992, Mosby.)

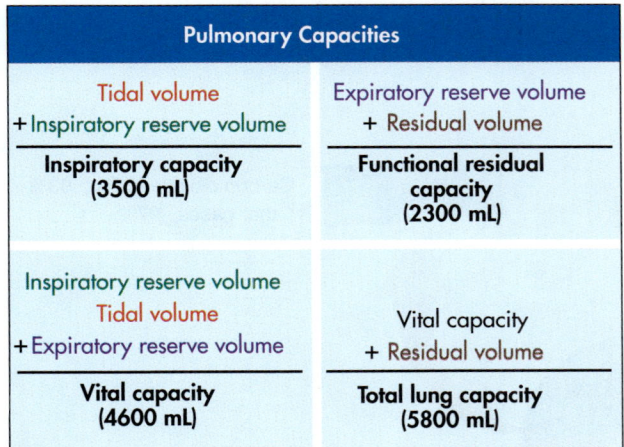

FIGURE 15-14 Pulmonary capacities.

volume. This capacity reflects the amount of gas remaining in the lungs at the end of a normal expiration (about 2300 mL).

- *Vital capacity*: Vital capacity is the volume of gas that can move on deepest inspiration and expiration or the sum of the inspiratory reserve volume, the tidal volume, and the expiratory reserve volume. This capacity is about 4600 mL.

- *Total lung capacity*: Total lung capacity is the sum of the vital capacity and the residual volume (about 5800 mL).

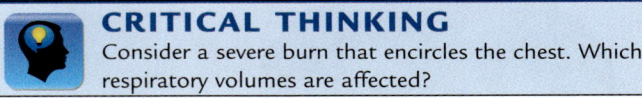

CRITICAL THINKING

Consider a severe burn that encircles the chest. Which respiratory volumes are affected?

Minute Volume and Minute Alveolar Ventilation

The **minute volume** is the amount of gas inhaled or exhaled in 1 minute. It is found by multiplying the tidal volume by the respiratory rate. For example, a patient's respiratory rate may be 10 breaths per minute, and the resting tidal volume may be 500 mL. Thus the average minute volume is 5 L/min.

Much of the gas that is inspired during breathing fills the anatomical dead space before reaching the alveoli. That air therefore is unavailable for gas exchange. The amount of inspired gas available for gas exchange during 1 minute is referred to as the *minute alveolar ventilation*. The minute alveolar ventilation is calculated by subtracting the amount of dead space from the tidal volume and then multiplying the result by the respiratory rate:

Minute alveolar ventilation = (Tidal volume − Dead space) ×
Respiratory rate

If the tidal volume or the respiratory rate, or both, increase, the minute volume also increases. Likewise, if the tidal volume or the respiratory rate, or both, decrease, the minute volume decreases. The paramedic must note the depth of breathing (tidal volume) and the respiratory rate to determine whether the patient's respiratory status is adequate.

MEASUREMENT OF GASES

As described in Chapter 11, the mixture of gases that make up the atmosphere exerts a combined partial pressure. This pressure is measured in millimeters of mercury, or **torr** (1 torr = 1 mm Hg), based on the percentage of a particular gas (Table 15-1). The atmospheric pressure at sea level (760 mm Hg) represents 100%. Nitrogen makes up about 78.62% of the volume of dry atmospheric gas at sea level. The partial pressure that results from nitrogen is calculated by multiplying 78.62% by 760 mm Hg. This equals 597 mm Hg, or a partial pressure of nitrogen (PN_2) of 597 torr. Oxygen accounts for 20.84% of the volume of atmospheric gas. The partial pressure of oxygen (PO_2), therefore, is found by multiplying 20.84% by 760 mm Hg. This equals 159 mm Hg, or a PO_2 of 159 torr (Figure 15-15).

LOOK AGAIN
See Chapter 11: General Principles of Pathophysiology, p. 216.

TABLE 15-1 Concentration of Gases

Gas	Concentration
Atmospheric Gases	
Nitrogen	597 torr (78.62%)
Oxygen	159 torr (20.84%)
Carbon dioxide	0.3 torr (0.50%)
Water (vapor)	3.7 torr (6.2%)
Alveolar Gases	
Nitrogen	569 torr (74.9%)
Oxygen	104 torr (13.7%)
Carbon dioxide	40 torr (5.2%)
Water (vapor)	47 torr (6.2%)

NOTE
To review: In any mixture of gases, the combination of the pressure exerted by all the gases is the **total pressure**. The pressure exerted by a single gas is the **partial pressure**. The partial pressure of a gas in a mixture is denoted by a *P* preceding the gas. For example, the partial pressure of oxygen is PO_2. The partial pressure of carbon dioxide is PCO_2.

Another partial pressure can be measured when gas comes into contact with water. The water molecules convert into a gas, evaporate, and exert a partial pressure. This partial pressure is known as *water vapor pressure* (PH_2O).

The compositions of alveolar gas and dry atmospheric gas are not the same. This is a result of several factors:

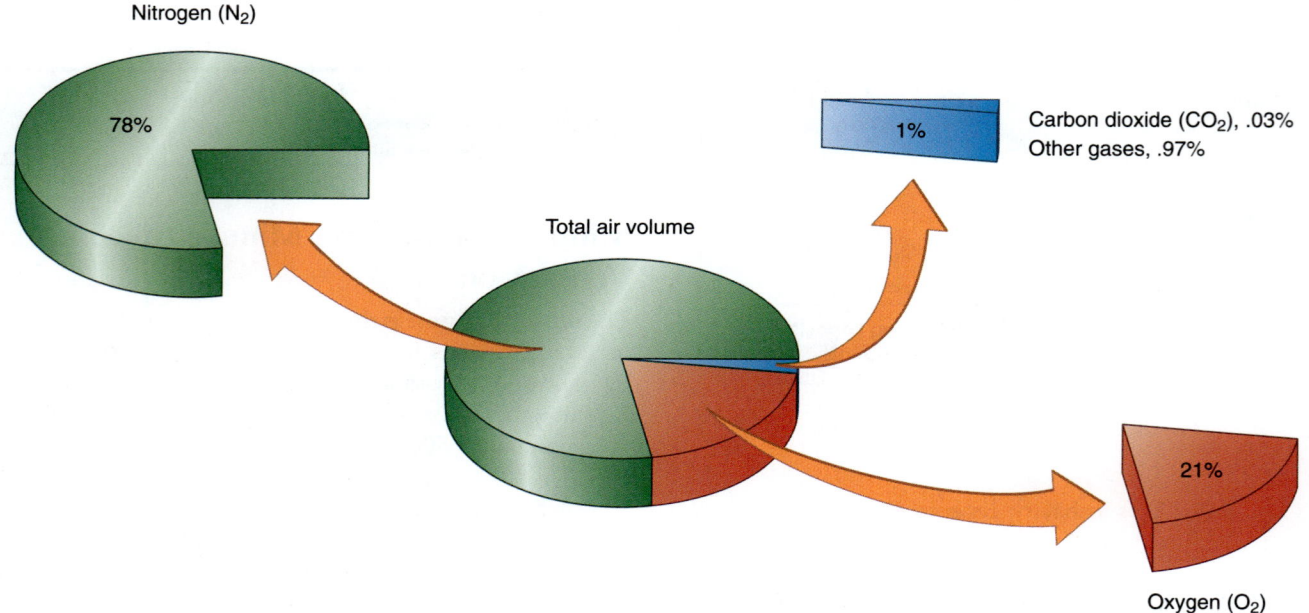

FIGURE 15-15 Partial pressure of gases in atmospheric air. (Patton KT, Thibodeau GA: *Anatomy and physiology*, ed 7, St Louis, 2007, Mosby.)

humidification of the air entering the respiratory system by the body, the exchange of oxygen and carbon dioxide between the alveoli and the blood, and incomplete emptying of the alveoli with expiration.

PULMONARY CIRCULATION

The process of gas exchange in the lungs is the opposite of that which occurs in the tissues throughout the rest of the body. As inspired gas enters the lungs, the respiratory system brings oxygen to the blood and removes carbon dioxide. Blood that is low in oxygen returns to the heart from all parts of the body. Passing through the right side of the heart, the blood flows into either lung through the pulmonary artery. From there it flows into the smaller pulmonary arterioles. Then it flows into capillaries that surround each of the hundreds of millions of alveoli inside the lungs (Figure 15-16).

The alveoli are now filled with a high concentration of oxygen molecules and a low concentration of carbon dioxide molecules as a result of the inhaled air. They have the pressure gradient required for gas exchange. Oxygen molecules move into the surrounding capillaries at the same time that carbon dioxide molecules move into the alveoli to be exhaled. The blood is now rich in oxygen. It flows through the pulmonary venules into the pulmonary veins. From there it flows into the left atrium and then into the left ventricle. Next, it flows back out through the aorta to the body's tissues. To supply enough oxygen to the body tissues, an alveolus fills and empties more than 15,000 times in a day of normal breathing.[8]

Exchange and Transport of Gases in the Body

The volume of oxygen taken up in the lungs can be measured. It can be calculated from the difference in the amount of oxygen in inspired and expired air. The volume of carbon dioxide that is eliminated can be determined in a similar way.

As noted in Chapter 10, *metabolism* is defined as all the chemical changes that occur in the body. In a healthy body with a constant metabolism, the relationship between tissue carbon dioxide production and oxygen consumption is fixed. In general, the amount of oxygen taken up by the

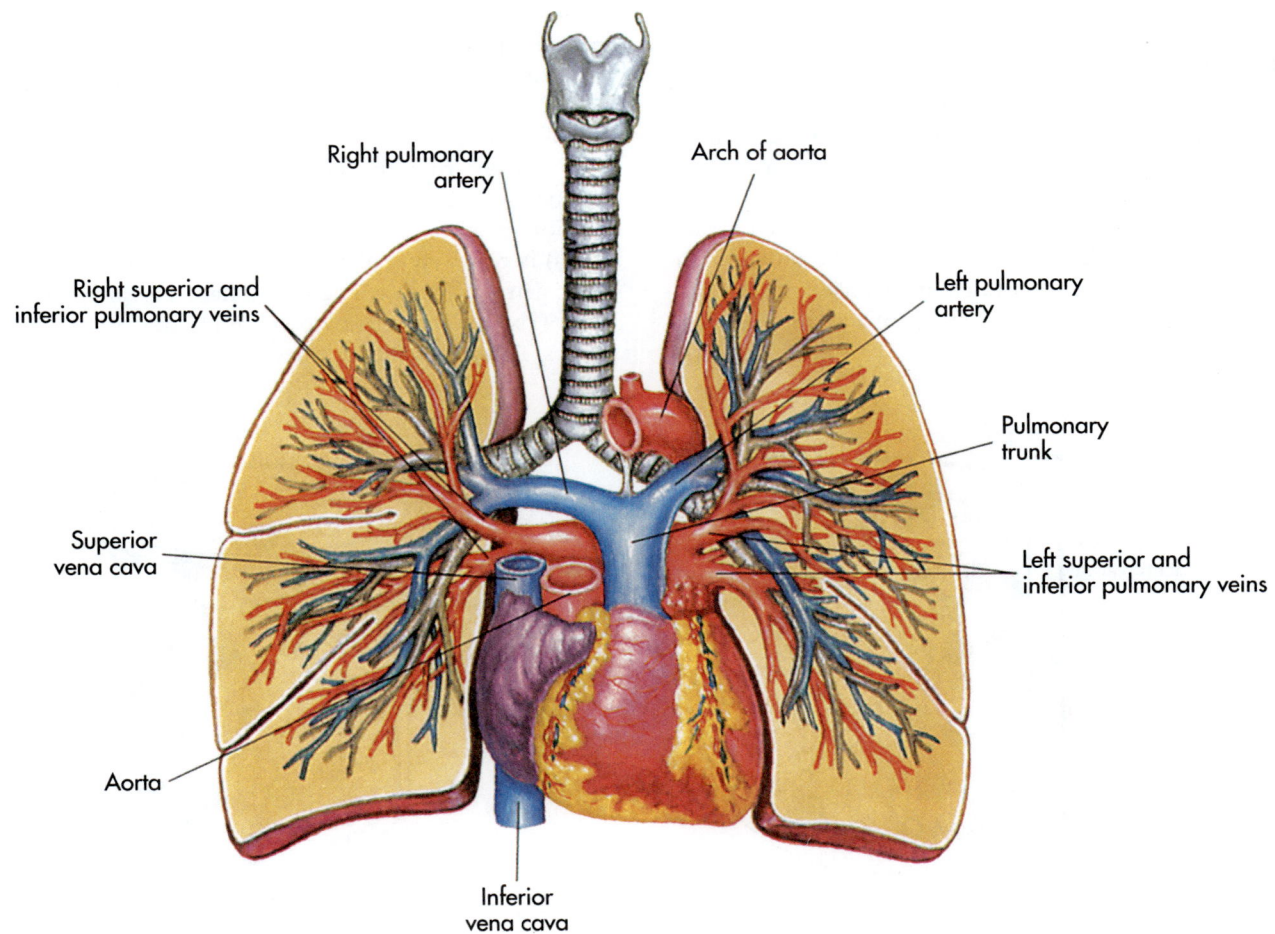

Right pulmonary artery

Right superior and inferior pulmonary veins

Superior vena cava

Aorta

Inferior vena cava

Arch of aorta

Left pulmonary artery

Pulmonary trunk

Left superior and inferior pulmonary veins

FIGURE 15-16 Pulmonary circulation. (Wilson S: *Respiratory disorders,* St Louis, 1990, Mosby.)

capillary blood is greater than the amount of carbon dioxide released by the blood to the alveolar gas. Thus the expired volume is slightly less than the inspired volume.

At rest, the combined consumption of all the body cells is about 200 mL of oxygen per minute. About the same amount of carbon dioxide is produced by the cells. Because about 20% of atmospheric gas is oxygen, the total oxygen inspired is 20% multiplied by 5 L, or about 1 L of oxygen per minute. Of this, 200 mL crosses the alveoli into the pulmonary capillaries. The remaining 800 mL is exhaled. The 200 mL of oxygen is added to the quantity of oxygen already in the pulmonary capillaries. It is then transported to body tissues by the circulatory system. After the body cells use the necessary oxygen, the oxygen remaining in the blood returns to the heart and lungs. This exchange of oxygen and carbon dioxide is carried out by the passive process of diffusion. As described in Chapter 11, **diffusion** is the tendency for molecules in solution to move from an area of higher concentration to an area of lower concentration.

LOOK AGAIN
See Chapter 11: General Principles of Pathophysiology, pp. 217-218

Diffusion

Molecules of gases are in constant, random motion. This motion is fueled by collisions with other molecules. If the blood is divided by a permeable barrier, such as a capillary wall or cell membrane, many gas molecules come in contact with and cross the barrier. The likelihood is much greater that highly concentrated molecules will strike and cross the membrane than less concentrated molecules. Thus the concentration of molecules on either side of a permeable membrane tends to equilibrate (Figure 15-17).

The diffusion of gases through liquid is determined by the pressure of the gases. It also is determined by the solubility of the gases in liquid (Figure 15-18). When a free gas comes into contact with liquid, the number of gas molecules that dissolve in the liquid is directly proportional to the pressure of the gas. When the free gas pressure is higher than the pressure of the gas in the liquid, enough molecules dissolve in the liquid to allow the free gas pressure to equal the dissolved gas pressure.

On the other hand, if a liquid containing a dissolved gas at a high pressure is exposed to a free gas at a lower pressure, gas molecules leave the liquid and enter the free gas until the pressures become equal (the *general gas law*). This is the underlying theme of the exchange of gases between the cells and the capillary blood throughout the body. The partial pressure of the free gas (PO_2) in the lungs is greater than the partial pressure of the dissolved oxygen in the bloodstream. Thus oxygen diffuses from the lungs to the blood. The partial pressure of oxygen in the blood is higher than that in the peripheral tissues. Thus oxygen diffuses from the blood into the tissues.

In addition to its pressure, the solubility of a gas also is a factor. The solubility of gases in a liquid affects the behavior of the gases. The ease with which gases dissolve determines the absolute number of gas molecules that diffuse through the liquid at a given pressure. For example, a liquid may be exposed to two different gases at the same pressure. The number of molecules of each gas that diffuse may not be the same because of the differing solubilities of the two gases.

Blood entering the pulmonary capillaries is systemic venous blood that has been circulated to the lungs via the pulmonary arteries. The partial pressure of carbon dioxide (PCO_2) is relatively high in this blood; the partial pressure of oxygen (PO_2) is low. The alveoli have a greater concentration of oxygen than the blood entering the pulmonary capillaries. Thus oxygen molecules diffuse from the alveoli into

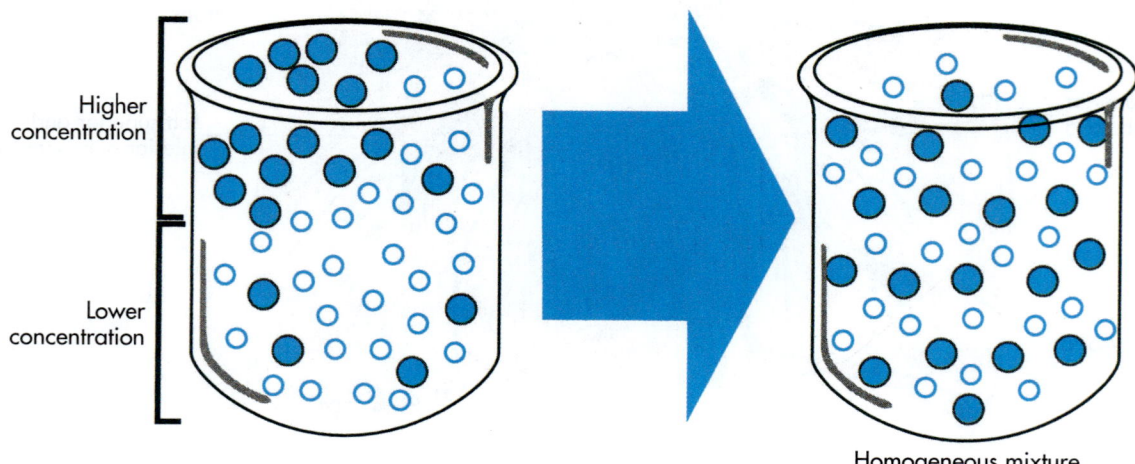

Higher concentration

Lower concentration

Homogeneous mixture

FIGURE 15-17 Random movement of gas proceeds from a higher concentration to a lower concentration until a homogeneous mixture of gases is achieved.

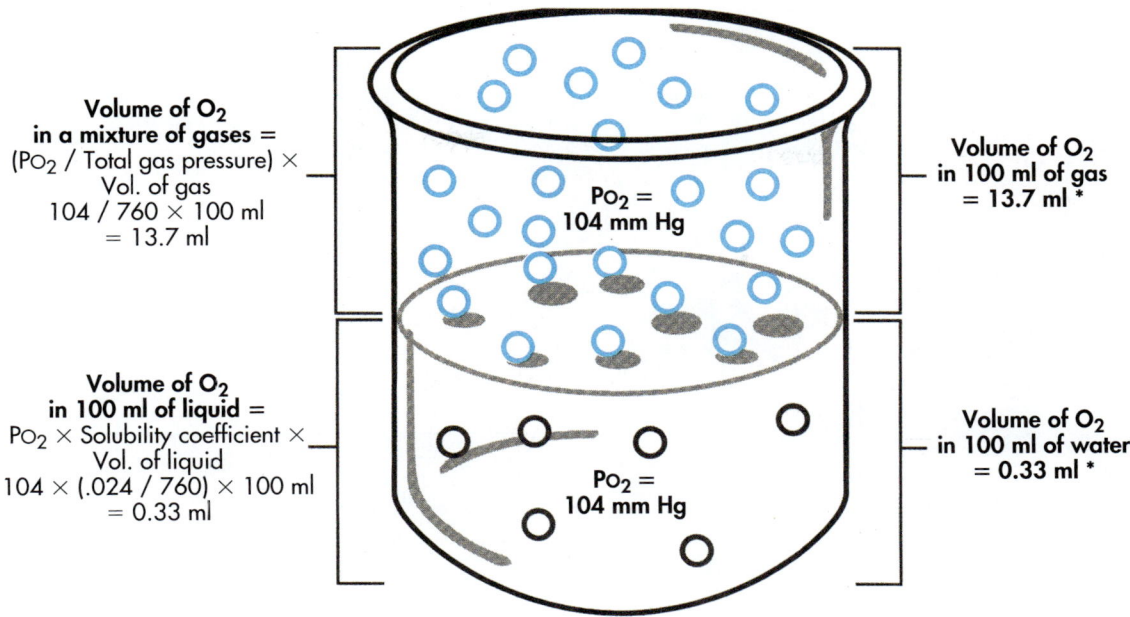

Volume of O_2
in a mixture of gases =
(PO_2 / Total gas pressure) ×
Vol. of gas
104 / 760 × 100 ml
= 13.7 ml

PO_2 =
104 mm Hg

Volume of O_2
in 100 ml of gas
= 13.7 ml *

Volume of O_2
in 100 ml of liquid =
PO_2 × Solubility coefficient ×
Vol. of liquid
104 × (.024 / 760) × 100 ml
= 0.33 ml

PO_2 =
104 mm Hg

Volume of O_2
in 100 ml of water
= 0.33 ml *

FIGURE 15-18 At equilibrium, the concentration of a gas in a liquid is determined by the partial pressure of the gas and by the solubility of the gas in the liquid at atmospheric pressure (760 mm Hg) and 98.6° F (37° C).

the blood. Carbon dioxide moves from the blood, where it is more concentrated, into the alveoli, where it is less concentrated (Figure 15-19).

> **NOTE**
> Oxygen and carbon dioxide do not readily dissolve in blood plasma. Transport molecules are required. These include hemoglobin for oxygen, and bicarbonate and hemoglobin for carbon dioxide.

The blood flowing through the pulmonary capillaries is separated from the alveolar air by a thin layer of tissue. This layer is known as the *respiratory membrane*. The membrane is composed of the alveolar wall (surfactant, epithelial cells, and basement membrane), interstitial fluid, and the wall of the pulmonary capillary (basement membrane and endothelial cells). The differences in the partial pressures of oxygen and carbon dioxide on the two sides of the membrane result in diffusion. Oxygen moves into the blood and carbon dioxide into the alveoli. With this diffusion, the capillary blood PO_2 level rises. The capillary blood PCO_2 level falls. Diffusion of these gases stops when alveolar and capillary partial pressures equalize. In healthy people this gas exchange occurs so quickly that the blood leaving the lungs to be pumped through the arteries has nearly the same PO_2 (80 to 100 mm Hg) and PCO_2 (35 to 40 mm Hg) as alveolar air.

The diffusion of gases at the capillary-alveolar level can be affected in a number of ways. Some respiratory diseases (e.g., emphysema) destroy and collapse the alveolar walls.

This results in the formation of fewer but larger alveoli. The degenerative process reduces the total area available for diffusion. In some diseases the alveolar-capillary membrane becomes thick or less permeable. This forces gas molecules to travel farther. Thus it reduces the rate of diffusion. An example of such a disease is pulmonary edema. With this condition, fluid collects in the alveoli and pulmonary interstitial space. This forces gases to diffuse through a thicker than normal layer of fluid and tissue.

Oxygen Content of Blood

Oxygen is present in the blood in two forms: (1) physically dissolved in the blood and (2) chemically bound to hemoglobin (Hb) molecules. Compared with carbon dioxide and nitrogen, oxygen is relatively insoluble in water. Only 0.3 mL of oxygen can be dissolved in 100 mL of blood at the normal alveolar and arterial PO_2 of 100 mm Hg. In contrast, 197 mL of oxygen (about 98%) is carried in red blood cells. In red blood cells, it is chemically bound to hemoglobin **(oxyhemoglobin)** (Figure 15-20).

> **NOTE**
> *Hematocrit* is a blood test that measures the proportion of blood volume occupied by red blood cells. Normal values are about 46% for men and about 38% for women.

Hemoglobin can unload carbon dioxide and absorb oxygen 60 times faster than blood plasma.[4] When fully converted to oxyhemoglobin (HbO_2), each hemoglobin

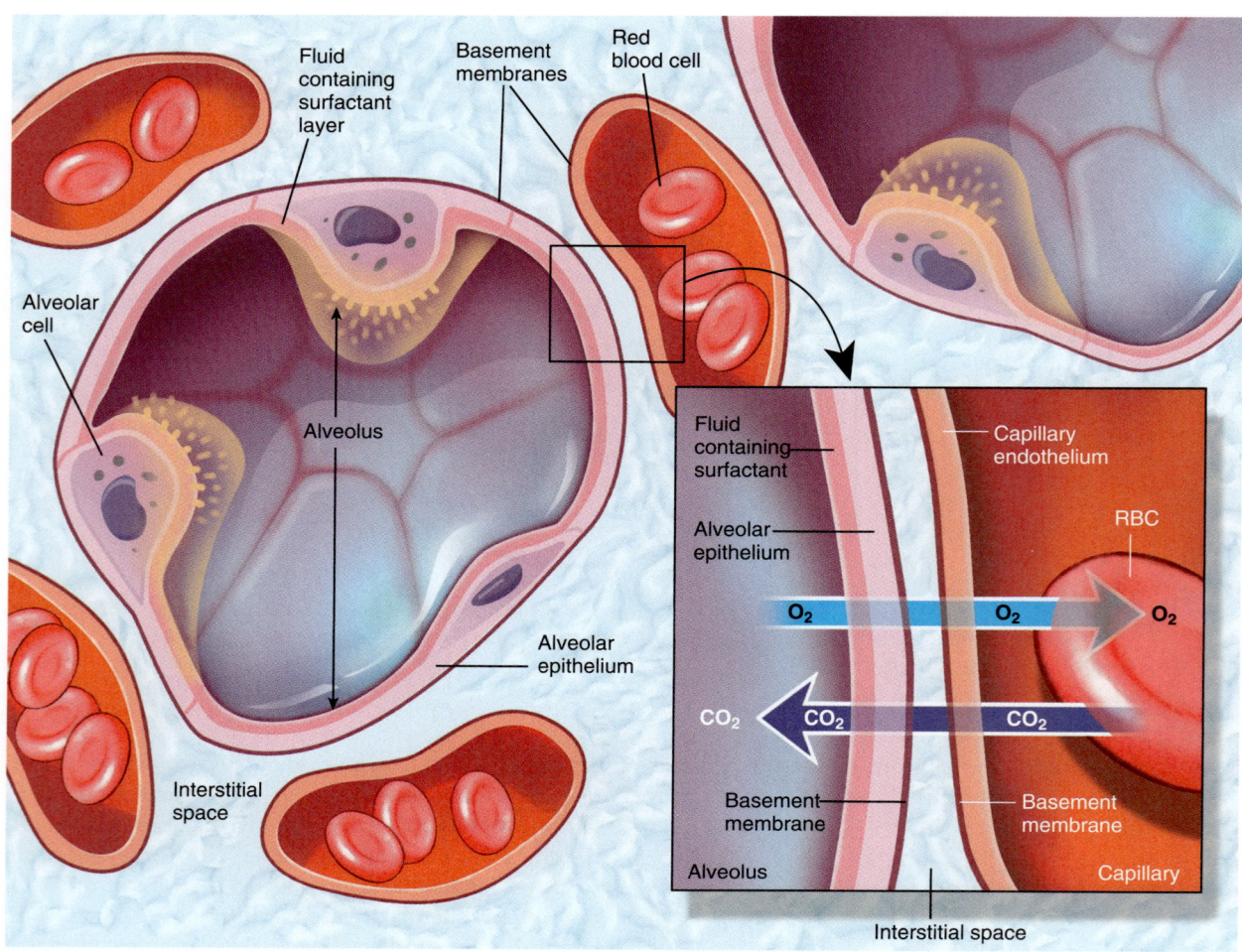

FIGURE 15-19 Gas exchange structure of the lung. Each alveolus is continually ventilated with fresh air. The inset shows a magnified view of the respiratory membrane composed of the alveolar wall (fluid coating, epithelial cells, and basement membrane), interstitial fluid, and the wall of a pulmonary capillary (basement membrane and endothelial cells). The gases, carbon dioxide (CO_2) and oxygen (O_2), diffuse across the respiratory membrane. (Patton KT, Thibodeau GA: *Anatomy and physiology*, ed 7, St Louis, 2007, Mosby.)

molecule can carry four molecules of oxygen. At this point, the Hb molecule is said to be *fully saturated*. Hemoglobin nears full saturation at a P_{O_2} of 80 to 100 mm Hg.

The degree to which hemoglobin combines with oxygen increases rapidly when the P_{O_2} is 10 to 60 mm Hg. This is because about 90% of total hemoglobin is combined with oxygen when the P_{O_2} is 60 mm Hg. Further increases in P_{O_2} produce only small increases in the amount of oxygen bound to hemoglobin. If the P_{O_2} falls slightly, the amount of oxyhemoglobin decreases only slightly. It still provides adequate oxygenation to tissues. The body adapts to higher P_{O_2} values (Figure 15-21).

NOTE

The concept of the body adapting to higher partial pressure of oxygen (P_{O_2}) values is important when dealing with patient situations involving high altitudes, excessive exercise, or cardiac and pulmonary disease. The P_{O_2} in the blood plasma is the most important factor in determining the extent to which oxygen combines with hemoglobin. Oxyhemoglobin, however, does not contribute to the P_{O_2} of the blood. Only the physically dissolved oxygen molecules can create gas pressure. This oxygen uptake by hemoglobin molecules removes dissolved oxygen from blood plasma. It also maintains a low P_{O_2}, allowing diffusion to continue (see Figure 15-21). (Laws that affect gas pressures [e.g., Boyle's law, Dalton's law, and Henry's law] are further described in Chapter 45.)

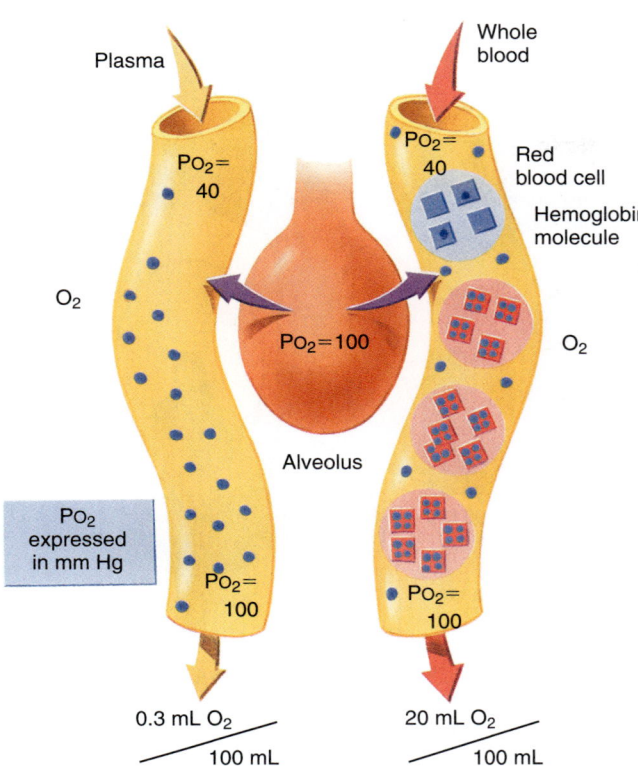

Plasma

Whole blood

$PO_2= 40$

Red blood cell

$PO_2= 40$

Hemoglobin molecule

O_2

$PO_2=100$

O_2

Alveolus

PO_2 expressed in mm Hg

$PO_2= 100$

$PO_2= 100$

0.3 mL O_2 / 100 mL

20 mL O_2 / 100 mL

FIGURE 15-20 Oxygen-carrying capacity of the blood. If blood consisted only of plasma, the maximum amount of oxygen that could be transported would be only about 0.3 mL per 100 mL of blood. However, because the red blood cells contain hemoglobin molecules, which act as "oxygen sponges," the blood can actually carry up to 20 mL of dissolved O_2 per 100 mL of blood. (Patton KT, Thibodeau GA: *Anatomy and physiology*, ed 7, St Louis, 2007, Mosby.)

> **NOTE**
> Diagnostic tests that can be used in the field to monitor the oxygen content of blood and the effectiveness of ventilation include pulse oximetry monitoring, peak expiratory flow testing, end-tidal carbon dioxide monitoring, and esophageal detection device monitoring. (These techniques are described later in this chapter and in Chapter 24.)

Carbon Dioxide Content of Blood

As described in Chapter 11, the amount of carbon dioxide produced by the body is fairly constant. It is determined by the body's rate and type of metabolism. If the metabolic rate increases, more carbon dioxide is produced. For instance, this may occur during exercise. In contrast, as the metabolic rate decreases, less carbon dioxide is produced. This may occur during sleep. Certain types of metabolic processes also result in increased carbon dioxide production. An example is anaerobic metabolism that occurs in the absence of oxygen. Another example is the body's production of ketoacids when metabolism occurs in the absence of insulin.

> **LOOK AGAIN**
> See Chapter 11: General Principles of Pathophysiology, pp. 227-230.

Carbon dioxide is transported in the blood in three major forms: plasma, blood proteins, and bicarbonate ions. As with oxygen, the solubility of carbon dioxide in water is minimal. It accounts for 8% of the carbon dioxide carried in plasma. About 20% of the carbon dioxide is present in blood proteins (including hemoglobin). About 72% is in the form of bicarbonate ions. When arterial blood flows through tissue capillaries, oxyhemoglobin gives up oxygen to the tissues. At the same time, carbon dioxide diffuses from the tissues into the blood. As a result, a small amount of the carbon dioxide dissolves in the plasma.

> **NOTE**
> It should be noted that if the SaO_2 is 100% the PaO_2 can range from 80-500 mmHg. This explains the recommendation that SaO_2 be maintained at 94% in patients who have chest pain, stroke, or a return of spontaneous circulation. *More oxygen is not always better.*

> **NOTE**
> The way in which a patient's lungs are ventilated can change the pH of blood. It also may enhance or hinder oxygenation at the tissue level. For example, carbon dioxide levels may be high (resulting in a drop in pH in capillary blood). As a result, the oxygen affinity for hemoglobin is reduced. On the other hand, if carbon dioxide levels are low (resulting in a rise in pH in capillary blood), the oxygen affinity for hemoglobin is increased. The response of hemoglobin to changes in pH is called the **Bohr effect** (Figure 15-22; also see Figure 15-23).

Venous blood entering the lungs has a PO_2 of 40 mm Hg and a hemoglobin saturation of 75%. Oxygen diffuses from the alveoli (because of its higher PO_2 of 100 mm Hg) into the plasma. This diffusion raises the plasma PO_2. This produces an increase in the uptake of oxygen by the hemoglobin molecules. In the tissue capillaries, this process is reversed. As the blood enters the capillaries, the plasma PO_2 is greater than the PO_2 in the fluid surrounding the capillaries. This causes diffusion across the capillary membranes to the cells of the tissues.

As described in Chapter 11, oxygen-free hemoglobin binds more readily to carbon dioxide than hemoglobin binds with oxygen. Thus some of the carbon dioxide that

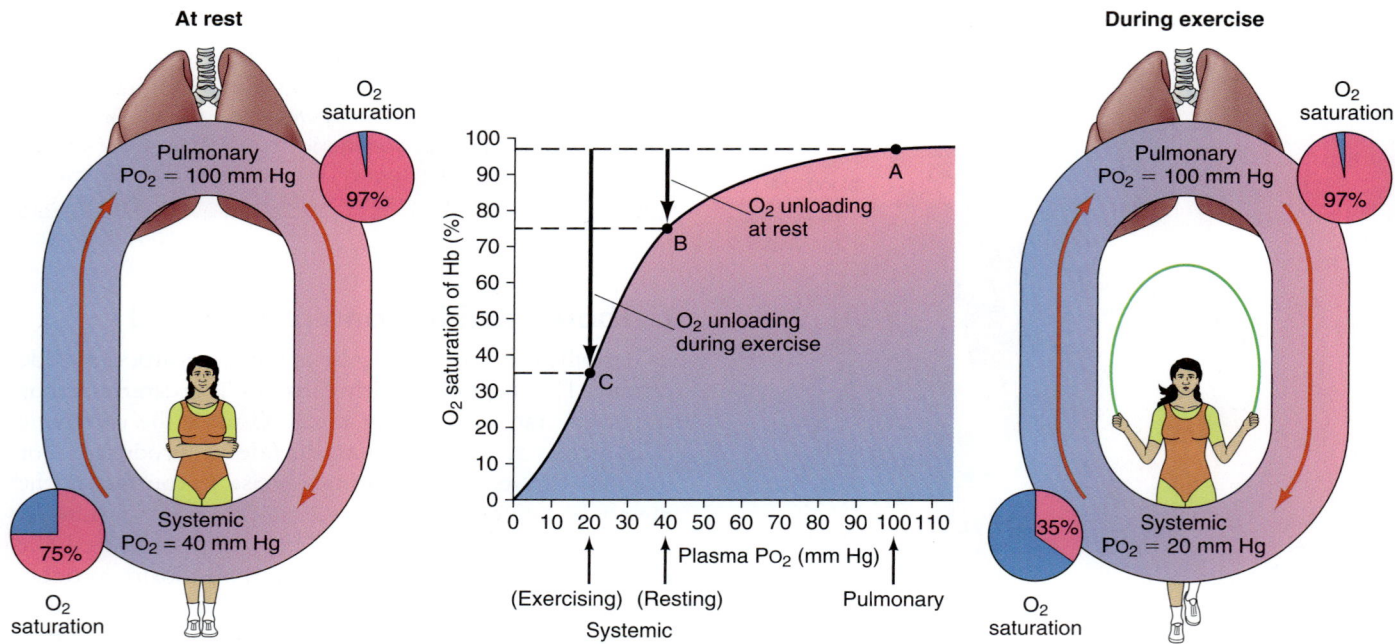

FIGURE 15-21 Oxygen (O_2) unloading at rest and during exercise. At rest, fully saturated hemoglobin (Hb) unloads almost 25% of its O_2 when it reaches the low partial pressure of oxygen (PO_2) environment (40 mm Hg) in systemic tissues *(left inset)*. During exercise, the tissue PO_2 is even lower (20 mm Hg). Consequently, fully saturated Hb unloads about 70% of its O_2 *(right inset)*. As the graph shows, a slight drop in the tissue PO_2 (from *B* to *C*) greatly increases O_2 unloading. (Patton KT, Thibodeau GA: *Anatomy and physiology,* ed 7, St Louis, 2007, Mosby.)

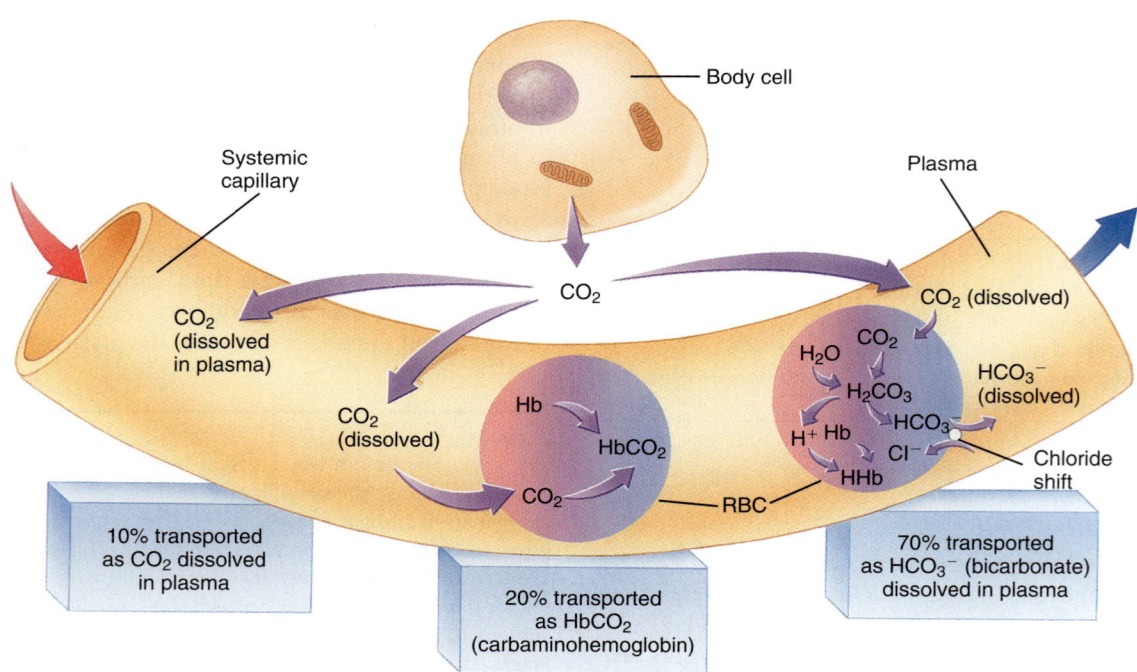

FIGURE 15-22 Interaction of the partial pressure of oxygen (PO_2) and the partial pressure of carbon dioxide (PCO_2) on gas transport by the blood. An increase in the PCO_2 in systemic tissues decreases the affinity between hemoglobin (Hb) and oxygen (O_2). This appears as a right shift of the oxygen-hemoglobin dissociation curve. The phenomenon is known as the *Bohr effect*. A right shift can also be caused by a decrease in the plasma pH. (Patton KT, Thibodeau GA: *Anatomy and physiology,* ed 7, St Louis, 2007, Mosby.)

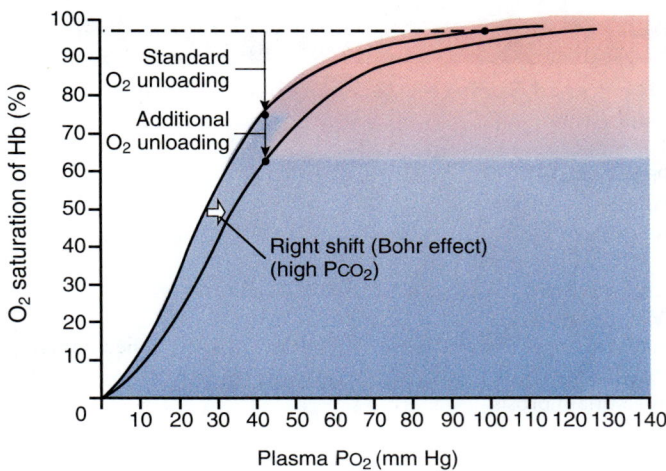

FIGURE 15-23 Carbon dioxide transport in the blood. Carbon dioxide (CO_2) dissolves in the plasma. Some of the dissolved CO_2 enters red blood cells (RBCs) and combines with hemoglobin (Hb) to form carbaminohemoglobin ($HbCO_2$). Some of the CO_2 enters RBCs and combines with water (H_2O) to form carbonic acid (H_2CO_3); this process is facilitated by an enzyme (carbonic anhydrase) present inside each cell. Carbonic acid then dissociates to form hydrogen ion (H+) and bicarbonate (HCO_3^-). The H+ combines with the hemoglobin. The HCO_3^- diffuses down its concentration gradient into the plasma. As HCO_3^- leaves each red blood cell, chloride (Cl^-) enters. This phenomenon is known as the *chloride shift*. It prevents an imbalance in charge. (Patton KT, Thibodeau GA: *Anatomy and physiology,* ed 7, St Louis, 2007, Mosby.)

diffuses into red blood cells binds to hemoglobin to form carbaminohemoglobin (HbNHCOOH). The remainder of the carbon dioxide reacts with water to form carbonic acid. Bicarbonate, in contrast to carbon dioxide, is very soluble in water. Venous blood rich in carbon dioxide is returned to the lungs. Because the blood PCO_2 is greater than that in the alveoli, carbon dioxide from the blood diffuses into the alveoli. From there it is exhaled and eliminated from the body (Figure 15-23).

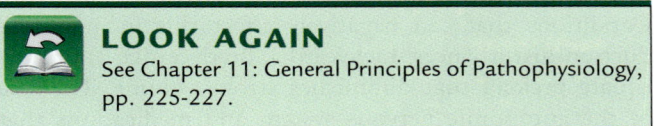

LOOK AGAIN
See Chapter 11: General Principles of Pathophysiology, pp. 225-227.

Factors That Influence Blood Oxygenation

In healthy people, the process of breathing fully oxygenates the blood at the alveolar-capillary level. It also allows carbon dioxide to be eliminated. The movement and utilization of oxygen in the body to perfuse tissues can be described by the Fick principle. (This is a method also used to measure cardiac output.) According to the **Fick principle,** the amount of oxygen the lungs deliver to the blood is directly related to the amount of oxygen the body consumes. The

movement and utilization of oxygen are based on the following conditions[9]:

1. An adequate amount of oxygen must be available to saturate the hemoglobin on red blood cells as they pass by alveolar membranes in the lungs. This requires adequate ventilation of the lungs through the patient's airway, a high partial pressure of oxygen in inspired air (FiO_2), and minimal obstruction to the diffusion of oxygen across the alveolar-capillary membrane.

2. The red blood cells must be circulated to the tissue cells. This requires adequate cardiac function, an adequate volume of blood flow, and proper routing of blood through the vascular channels.

3. The red blood cells must be able to load oxygen in the pulmonary capillaries. They also must be able to unload the oxygen at the site of peripheral tissue cells. This requires normal hemoglobin levels, circulation of the oxygenated red blood cells to the tissues in need, close approximation of the cells to the capillaries to allow for diffusion of oxygen, and ideal conditions of pH, temperature, and other factors.

NOTE
In medical care, FiO_2 is the fraction of inspired oxygen in a gas mixture. It is expressed as a number from 0 (0%) to 1 (100%). For example, the FiO_2 of normal room air is 0.21 (21%). The FiO_2 can be manipulated with airway devices that provide supplemental oxygen.

Hypoxemia is a state of decreased oxygen content of the arterial blood. It may lead to **hypoxia** (decreased oxygen content at the tissue level). Some abnormal conditions can result in inadequate blood oxygenation (Box 15-2). These conditions are described later in this chapter and throughout this text by subject matter.

DID YOU KNOW?
Ventilation/Perfusion Ratio
In respiratory physiology, the ventilation/perfusion ratio (V/Q ratio) is a measurement used to assess the efficiency and adequacy of the matching of two variables: alveolar ventilation and pulmonary perfusion.[10]
    V (ventilation)—the air that reaches the lungs
    Q (perfusion)—the blood that reaches the lungs
These two variables constitute the main determinants of the blood oxygen concentration. The matching of these two variables is vital to life. The V/Q ratio can be affected by circulation disturbances in blood volume that may result from cardiorespiratory disease, trauma, and systemic illness.
The V/Q ratio is measured by using a ventilation/perfusion scan. This imaging test gauges the circulation of air and blood in a patient's lungs. The ventilation part of the test evaluates the ability of air to reach all parts of the lungs. The perfusion part

BOX 15-2 Abnormal Conditions That Can Affect Blood Oxygenation

Depressed Respiratory Drive
Head injury
Central nervous system depressants (anesthetics, narcotics, sedatives)

Paralysis of Respiratory Muscles
Spinal injury
Inhalation injury
Neuromuscular disease

Increased Resistance in the Respiratory Airways
Asthma
Bronchitis
Emphysema
Congestion

Decreased Compliance of the Lungs and Thoracic Wall
Interstitial lung disease as a result of inhalation of toxic substances
Infection (pneumonia, tuberculosis)
Lung cancer
Connective tissue diseases
Chronic pulmonary hypertension

Chest Wall Abnormalities
Chest wall injury (flail chest)
Scoliosis
Eschar (full-thickness burn contractions)

Decreased Surface Area for Gas Exchange
Emphysema
Tuberculosis
Pneumonia
Pulmonary edema
Atelectasis

Increased Thickness of the Respiratory Membrane
Pulmonary edema (caused by heart failure, pneumonia, infections)
Interstitial fibrosis

Ventilation-Perfusion Mismatching*
Asthma
Pneumonia
Pulmonary embolus
Pulmonary edema
Myocardial infarction
Respiratory distress syndrome
Shock

Reduced Capacity of the Blood to Transport Oxygen
Anemias
Hemoglobin alterations
Carbon monoxide poisoning
Methemoglobinemia

*Ventilated alveoli that are not perfused or perfused alveoli that are not ventilated.

of the test evaluates how well the blood circulates within the lungs. Normally, alveolar ventilation is about 4 L/minute, and pulmonary capillary blood flow (perfusion) is about 5 L/minute. Therefore, the normal V/Q ratio is 4:5, or 0.8. An area with no ventilation (V/Q = 0) is called a *shunt*. An area with no perfusion (V/Q of infinity) is called *dead space*. An increased V/Q ratio is seen with disorders in which ventilation is greater than perfusion (increased partial pressure of arterial oxygen [PaO_2], decreased partial pressure of arterial carbon dioxide [$PaCO_2$]). Examples of such disorders include pulmonary embolism and pneumothorax. A decreased V/Q ratio is seen with disorders in which perfusion is greater than ventilation and there is an increased shunting of blood. Examples of these disorders include obstructive lung diseases that cause alveolar hypoventilation.

Although the V/Q ratio is not a prehospital evaluation tool, it is important that paramedics understand the relationship between alveolar ventilation and pulmonary perfusion. It also is important that they understand the way ventilation/perfusion mismatching (ventilated alveoli that are not perfused or perfused alveoli that are not ventilated) can affect patients with respiratory compromise.

Blood Volume Circulation Disturbances

Disturbances in the effective circulation of blood can affect the body's ability to nourish the tissues and maintain adequate cellular oxygenation. These circulation disturbances can result from cardiac disease, trauma, and problems with systemic vascular resistance[11]: The heart rate must be capable of circulating blood through the vascular system for adequate tissue perfusion (Box 15-3). Conditions that can negatively affect this include conduction disturbances, tachycardia, bradycardia, and inadequate preload that diminishes stroke volume. The role of the autonomic nervous system and medications that affect alpha and beta stimulation of the heart also are important for adequate cardiac function.

Finally, vascular resistance in the systemic circulation (*total peripheral resistance*) must be adequate to maintain blood pressure and cardiac output. One factor that affects total peripheral resistance is the capacitance of blood vessels (functioning precapillary arterioles). Another is the smooth muscle effects initiated by alpha and beta cholinergic receptors. As described in Chapter 11, total peripheral resistance can be affected by hypoxia, acidosis and the effectiveness of the buffer systems, temperature changes, neural factors, and catecholamines.

BOX 15-3 Blood Volume Circulation Disturbances

Blood volume circulation disturbances can occur as a result of conditions that affect vascular resistance, cardiac disease that affects cardiac output, injury, and systemic illness.[11]

Changes in Vascular Resistance
Orthostatic hypotension
Oncotic fluid pressure
Hydrostatic fluid pressure
Capacitance of the venules and veins

Cardiac Disease Affecting Cardiac Output
Heart rate (tachycardia, bradycardia)
Stroke volume (preload, afterload)
Alpha and beta stimulation of the heart
Conduction disturbances
Congestive heart failure

Injury
Head, chest, and spinal trauma
Blood loss
Shock

Systemic Illness
Acid-base disturbances
Anemia
Infection
Renal disease
Respiratory disease

LOOK AGAIN
See Chapter 11: General Principles of Pathophysiology, pp. 238-240.

REGULATION OF RESPIRATION

Respiration is controlled by a number of factors. When paramedics evaluate a patient, key elements they must consider include the various mechanisms responsible for rhythmic ventilation. The rate and depth of breathing are also crucial factors.

Voluntary Control of Respiration

Breathing is mainly an involuntary process. Within limits, however, the pattern of respiration can be consciously altered. For example, voluntary hyperventilation can lead to a decrease in the blood PCO_2, vasodilation of the peripheral blood vessels, a decrease in blood pressure, or a combination of these effects. Hyperventilation causes excessive loss of exhaled carbon dioxide, which produces **hypocarbia,** resulting in cerebral vascular constriction, reduced cerebral perfusion, paresthesia (tingling sensation), dizziness, or even feelings of euphoria.

Breathing also can be affected by voluntary apnea. An example of this is when children hold their breath. In such cases the arterial blood PCO_2 increases, whereas the PO_2 decreases. As the apneic period continues, the abnormal levels of PCO_2 and PO_2 trigger the respiratory centers. These changes in the levels override the child's conscious control of breathing. If loss of consciousness occurs, the respiratory center resumes normal function.

CRITICAL THINKING
If a prolonged, deep breath is held, what vagal effects might the patient experience?

Nervous Control of Respiration

The inspiratory muscles are the diaphragm and intercostal muscles. These are composed of skeletal muscle. They cannot contract unless they are stimulated by nerve impulses. The two phrenic nerves responsible for moving the diaphragm originate from the third, fourth, and fifth cervical spinal nerves. The 11 pairs of intercostal nerves originate from the first through the eleventh thoracic spinal nerves. The nerve impulses that control these respiratory muscles originate in neurons of the medulla. This inspiratory and expiratory center is influenced by the pons, hypothalamus, the reticular activating system (RAS), and the cerebral cortex. The center is innervated by afferent activity in the vagus, glossopharyngeal, and somatic nerves (Figure 15-24).

NOTE
The respiratory center in the medulla is bilateral. Each lateral area is made up of two groups of neurons: the *dorsal respiratory group (DRG)* and the *ventral respiratory group (VRG)*. The DRG is involved in the generation of respiratory rhythm. This group is primarily responsible for inspiration. The VRG has both inspiratory and expiratory neurons. This group plays a secondary role in inspiratory activity, after the DRG. The neurons in the VRG remain almost inactive during normal quiet respiration. When the respiratory drive for increased pulmonary ventilation becomes greater than normal, respiratory signals spill over into the VRG from the DRG area. The VRG then contributes to the respiratory drive. The VRG is responsible for motor control of inspiratory and expiratory muscles during exercise. Together, these two groups of neurons are responsible for the basic rhythm of ventilation.

The inspiratory center neurons are spontaneously active. They exhibit a pattern of activity followed by fatigue and then activity again. When active, they send impulses along the spinal cord to the phrenic and intercostal nerves. This stimulates the muscles of inspiration. (Head and spinal trauma, stroke, and some diseases can interrupt nervous control.)

The expiratory center is inactive during quiet respiration. The exact nervous system mechanisms that control the activity of this center are unknown. However, the

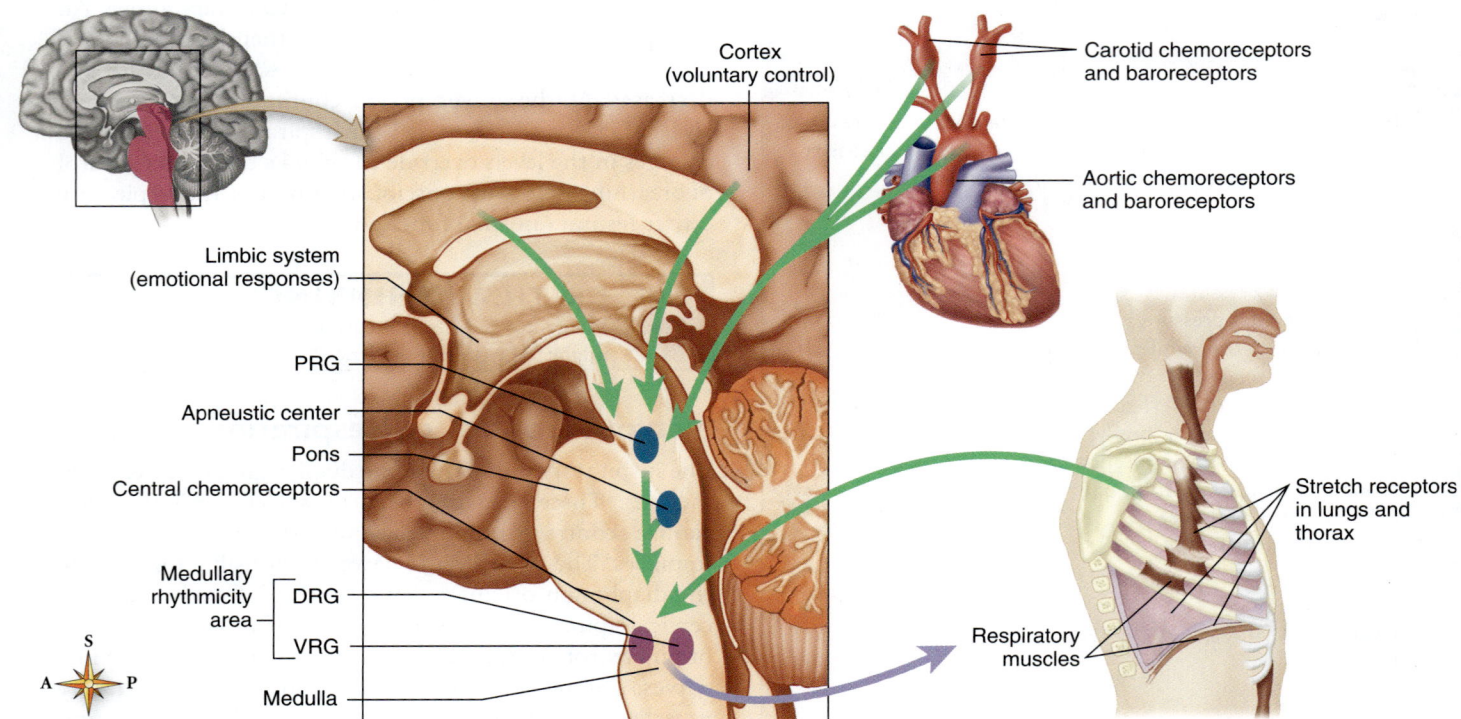

FIGURE 15-24 Regulation of breathing. The dorsal respiratory group (DRG) and ventral respiratory group (VRG) of the medulla represent the medullary rhythmicity area. The pontine respiratory group (PRG, or pneumotaxic center) and apneustic center of the pons influence the basic respiratory rhythm by means of neural input to the medullary rhythmicity area. The brainstem also receives input from other parts of the body; information from chemoreceptors, baroreceptors, and stretch receptors can alter the basic breathing pattern, as can emotional (limbic) and sensory input. Despite these subconscious reflexes, the cerebral cortex can override the "automatic" control of breathing to some extent to allow such activities as singing or blowing up a balloon. Green arrows show flow of information to the respiratory control centers. The purple arrow shows the flow of information from the control centers to the respiratory muscles that drive breathing. (Patton KT, Thibodeau GA: *Anatomy and physiology,* ed 7, St Louis, 2007, Mosby.)

expiratory center appears to be stimulated when the activity of the inspiratory center increases. (For example, this may occur during heavy or labored breathing.) When activated, the expiratory center counters the inspiratory center, responding to a forceful inspiration with a forceful expiration.

Two distinct neural mechanisms are responsible for the basic respiratory rhythm established by the inspiratory and expiratory centers: the **Hering-Breuer reflex** and the pneumotaxic center. The vagus nerve conveys sensory information from the thoracic and abdominal organs. Some of the vagus nerve fibers end in stretch or inflation receptors in the walls of the bronchi, bronchioles, and lungs. When the stretch receptors are stimulated by expansion of the lungs, information is communicated by the vagus nerve to the medulla. The medulla produces discharges of inhibitory impulses. This, in turn, causes inspiration to stop *(inflation reflex)*. The cessation of inspiration is followed by expiration or deflation of the lungs. As expiration continues, the

stretch receptors are no longer stimulated. This allows the inspiratory center to become active again *(deflation reflex)*. Thus the Hering-Breuer reflexes limit inspiration and prevent overinflation of the lungs.

The **pneumotaxic center** is located in the pons above the respiratory center in the medulla. It has an inhibitory effect on the inspiratory center. When the activity of the inspiratory center stops, inhibitory impulses from the pneumotaxic center stop. When this occurs, the inspiratory center is free to send impulses to initiate inspiration again. The pneumotaxic center appears to be active only in labored breathing. In quiet breathing the stretch receptors are the main control mechanisms for rhythmic breathing.

The **apneustic center** is located in the lower portion of the pons. Nerve impulses from this area stimulate the inspiratory center. The apneustic center neurons are constantly active during normal respiratory rates. However, they are overridden by the pneumotaxic center when the demand for increased ventilation arises.

CRITICAL THINKING
What change in breathing would you expect in a patient who has an injury affecting the pons?

Chemical Control of Respiration

The activities of the respiratory centers are determined by changes in oxygen and carbon dioxide concentrations. They also are determined by the hydrogen ion concentration (pH) of body fluids. (An example of such a fluid is cerebrospinal fluid.) The partial pressure of carbon dioxide is the major factor that controls respiration.[12]

The chemoreceptive area in the medulla has neurons that are sensitive to changes in carbon dioxide and pH. An increase or decrease in the plasma PCO_2 is accompanied by changes in pH. An increase in the PCO_2 and the resulting decrease in pH adversely affect cellular metabolism. Excess carbon dioxide must be eliminated to return the pH to normal. For example, the body responds to an increase in PCO_2 of 5 mm Hg with an increase in ventilation of 100%. On the other hand, a decrease in PCO_2 inhibits ventilation. The carbon dioxide created by normal metabolism is allowed to accumulate and return the PCO_2 to normal. Through these adaptive measures, the PCO_2 is kept within a normal range of 35 to 45 mm Hg (Figure 15-25).

Compared with the body's sensitivity to pH and carbon dioxide levels, oxygen plays a fairly small part in regulating respiration. However, if the PO_2 levels in the arterial blood fall and the pH and PCO_2 are held constant, ventilation increases.

Chemoreceptors monitor the arterial PO_2. They are located in the medulla and peripherally at the bifurcation of the common carotid arteries and in the arch of the aorta. These peripheral receptors are known as the **carotid and aortic bodies.** The carotid and aortic bodies are in intimate contact with the arterial blood of the great vessels. Thus their blood supply is greater than their use of oxygen. Moreover, the PO_2 of their tissues is very close to that of arterial blood. The nerve fibers from these bodies enter the brainstem. There they synapse with the neurons of the medulla and initiate a respiratory response.

Carbon dioxide and hydrogen ion concentrations are the major regulators of respiration. However, a reduced PO_2 in the arterial blood can play a part in regulating respiration. When a patient is hypotensive (e.g., in shock), the PO_2 in the arterial blood may fall to low levels. This stimulates the sensory receptors in the carotid and aortic bodies. This, in turn, leads to an increased rate and depth of ventilation. This can occur without a significant change in the blood PCO_2. However, it usually is accompanied by metabolic acidosis, which occurs secondary to anaerobic metabolism[12] (as described in Chapter 11).

LOOK AGAIN
See Chapter 11: General Principles of Pathophysiology, pp. 228-230.

PO_2 plays a role in respiratory regulation at high altitudes. At these altitudes, the barometric pressure is low. This causes the PO_2 in the arterial blood to drop. The low PO_2 levels stimulate the carotid and aortic bodies. Lowered barometric pressure does not affect the body's ability to eliminate carbon dioxide. The increase in ventilation (triggered by the lowered arterial PO_2) results in a drop in the carbon dioxide levels in the blood.

Patients with severe emphysema or chronic bronchitis have chronically elevated PCO_2 levels. These patients may rely on the low PO_2 as the stimulus for ventilation **(hypoxic drive).** In diseases with chronic elevation of PCO_2, the chemoreceptors become less sensitive to a high carbon dioxide level. They fail to be stimulated by it. Over time, hypoxia becomes the only remaining respiratory drive.

Control of Respiration by Other Factors

A number of other factors may play a role in the control of respiration. These include body temperature, drugs and medications, pain, emotion, and sleep.

An increase in body temperature can affect the respiratory center neurons. Such an increase may be caused by a febrile illness or an increase in physical activity. The increase can cause an increase in ventilation. On the other hand, major decreases in body temperature can lower the ventilation rate. An extreme example of this can occur during severe hypothermia. With this, patients can appear almost apneic (see Chapter 45).

Some drugs, such as *epinephrine,* stimulate ventilation. They do this by promoting cellular metabolism during stressful events and vigorous exercise. However, drugs such as *diazepam* and *morphine* may reduce ventilations. A person who takes an overdose of narcotics or barbiturates can become apneic.

Pain anywhere in the body may produce a reflex stimulation of ventilation. Examples include performing a sternal rub on a patient or stepping into a cold shower. Also, certain emotions, such as laughing or crying, require an increase in the movement of air into and out of the lungs. Situations involving fear and anger cause rapid breathing.

As the body's activity and metabolism slow, so does the formation of impulses to stimulate the respiratory centers. During times of decreased activity, ventilation also decreases.

Modified Forms of Respiration

The cough reflex and the sneeze reflex are protective mechanisms. The function of each is to dislodge foreign matter or irritants from the respiratory passages. Coughing generally is preceded by an inspiration of greater than normal force (about 2.5 L of gas). The glottis then closes, and the muscles of the thorax contract forcibly. This causes an increase in intrapulmonic pressure. The pressure change in the lungs increases to about 100 mm Hg.[13] When this pressure is reached, the vocal cords part, and air escapes from the lungs at high velocity. This air carries foreign materials and particles of mucus out of the lungs.

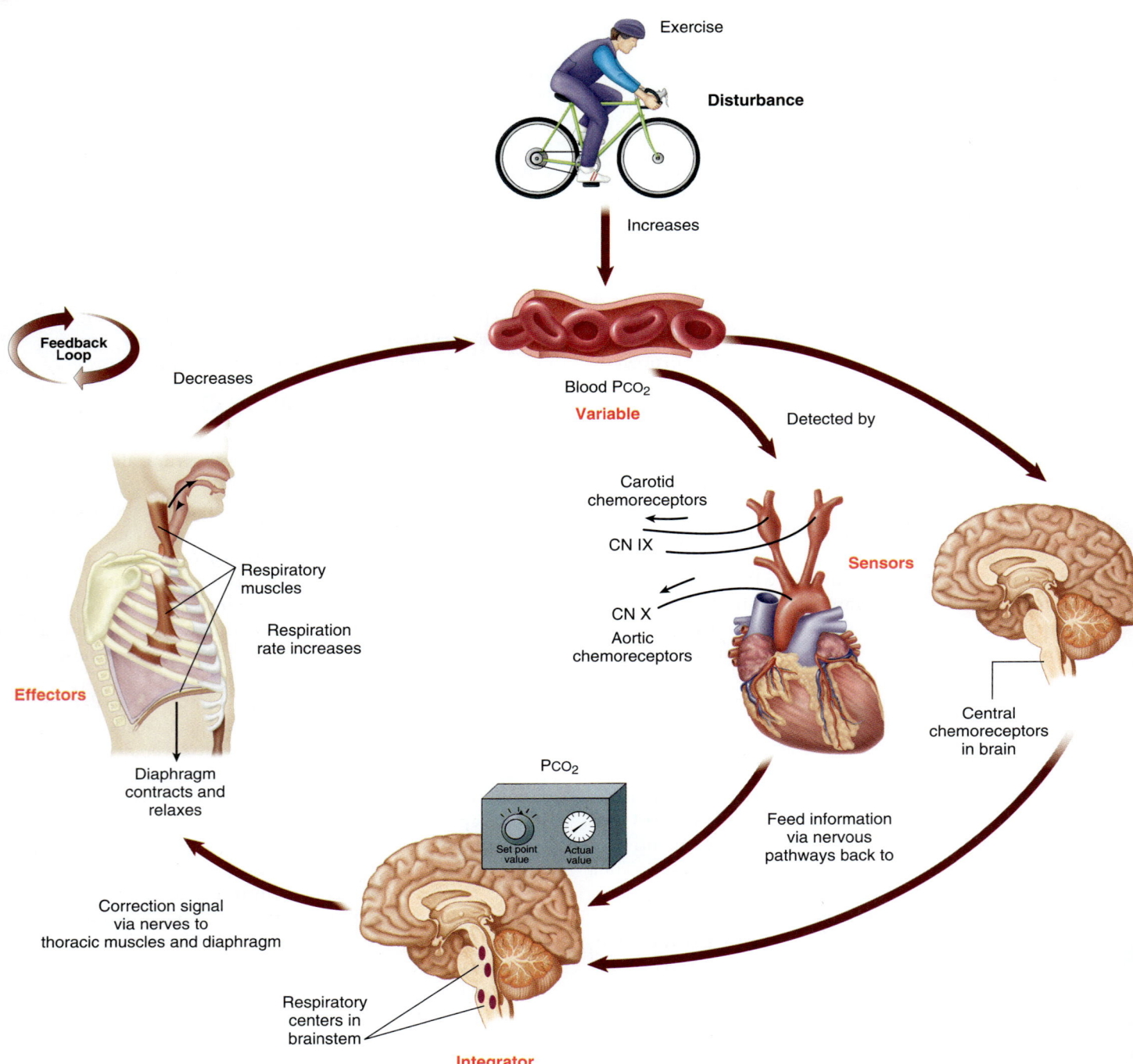

FIGURE 15-25 Negative feedback control of respiration. The diagram summarizes the feedback loop by which the respiratory rate is increased in response to a high plasma partial pressure of carbon dioxide (P_{CO_2}). Increased cellular respiration during exercise causes a rise in the plasma P_{CO_2}. This is detected by central chemoreceptors in the brain and perhaps by peripheral chemoreceptors in the carotid sinus and aorta. Feedback information is relayed to integrators in the brainstem. These respond to the increase in P_{CO_2} above the set point by sending nervous correction signals to the respiratory muscles, which act as effectors. The effector muscles increase their alternating contraction and relaxation, thereby increasing the rate of respiration. As the respiration rate increases, the rate of CO_2 loss from the body increases and the P_{CO_2} drops accordingly. This brings the plasma P_{CO_2} back to its set point value. (Patton KT, Thibodeau GA: *Anatomy and physiology,* ed 7, St Louis, 2007, Mosby.)

Sneezing is a violent expulsion of gas. The gas is forced or directed through the nasal cavity. It may occur as a result of nasal irritants, stimulation of the fifth cranial nerve (trigeminal nerve) in the nose, or exposure to bright lights. During the sneeze reflex, the uvula and the soft palate are depressed to direct air through both the nasal passages and the oral cavity.

Other forms of modified respiration include the sigh and the hiccough (in rare cases, these are chronic disorders). Sighing is a slow, deep inspiration followed by a prolonged expiration. This modified respiratory effort is thought to be a protective reflex to hyperinflate the lungs and to reexpand alveoli that might have been collapsed (atelectasis).

The hiccough results from a spasmodic contraction of the diaphragm with the sudden inspiration cut short by the closure of the glottis. Hiccoughs serve no known useful physiological purpose. They usually stop with time. However, they may indicate a pathological condition.

Special Considerations in Older Patients

Respiratory disorders create distinctive problems for the older patient. As a result of aging, the respiratory function of older patients may be compromised. Pulmonary changes that occur as a result of aging reduce vital capacity (Figure 15-26). They also increase the physiological dead space.

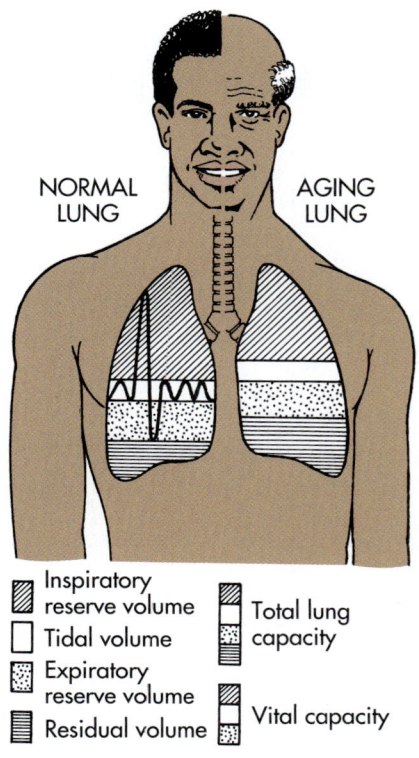

FIGURE 15-26 Changes in lung volumes with aging. Note particularly the decrease in vital capacity and the increase in residual volume that occur with aging. (McCance KL, Huether SE: *Pathophysiology: the biologic basis for disease in adults and children,* ed 6, St Louis, 2009, Mosby.)

Ventilation/perfusion mismatching also tends to increase. This leads to a gradually lowered PO_2. The changes in pulmonary physiology include the following[14]:

1. Alterations in lung and chest wall compliance
   - Increased thoracic rigidity
   - Decreased elastic recoil (total lung capacity remains unchanged because of opposing loss of chest wall compliance and weakened respiratory muscles)
2. Enlarged alveolar ducts and sacs
   - Fewer alveoli
   - Less alveolar surface for gas exchange

The aging process also changes the body's ventilatory control mechanisms. As a person grows older, for example, the body's arterial PO_2 falls. Yet no significant change in arterial PCO_2 occurs. Several methods have been developed to calculate the expected PO_2 in older people. One method is to keep in mind that a person who is 70 years old is expected to have a PO_2 of 70 mm Hg. Using this value as a baseline, the expected change is a 1 mm Hg decrease in PO_2 for every year over 70 or a 1 mm Hg increase in PO_2 for every year under 70. For example, a person who is 75 years old would be expected to have a PO_2 of 65 mm Hg. A person who is 65 years old would be expected to have a PO_2 of 75 mm Hg.[15]

The functioning of the body's chemoreceptors also declines with age. This results in a diminished ventilatory response to hypoxia, hypercapnia, and similar conditions. It also may predispose the older individual to respiratory failure. It is important that older patients with respiratory compromise from any cause receive immediate intervention, oxygenation, and ventilatory support.

SECTION THREE
Respiratory Pathophysiology

Many conditions can cause respiratory compromise and hypoxia (Table 15-2). Some of these conditions are described in this chapter and throughout the text by subject matter.[11]

UPPER AIRWAY OBSTRUCTION

A common cause of poor ventilation is upper airway obstruction. In patients who are conscious, this type of obstruction typically is caused by inhalation of food, a foreign body, or fluid (vomitus, saliva, blood, neutral liquids). In any patient who has poor ventilation from any cause, the most critical lifesaving maneuvers a paramedic can perform are establishing and maintaining a clear airway. This should always be a first-order priority of patient care. Early detection, early intervention, and education of the general public in basic life support measures are major factors in preventing unnecessary deaths from airway compromise.

TABLE 15-2 Conditions That Can Cause Respiratory Compromise

Interruption of Nervous Control
Drugs
Trauma
Muscular dystrophy
Poliomyelitis
Neuromuscular junction blocking agent

Structural Damage to the Thorax
Chest trauma

Bronchoconstriction
Respiratory diseases

Disruption of Airway Patency
Infection
Trauma/burns
Foreign body obstruction
Allergic reaction
Unconsciousness (loss of airway tone)

Oxygen Deprivation
Suffocation
Strangulation
Oxygen-deficient atmosphere

External Respiration (Environmental Factors)
Altitude
Closed environment
Toxic or poisonous environment

Internal Respiration (Pathology Related to Changes in Alveolar-Capillary Gas Exchange)
Emphysema
Pulmonary edema
Pneumonia
Environmental/occupational exposure
Drowning

Ventilation Deficiencies
Tachypnea
Mechanical ventilation with noncompliant lungs
Breathing against an elevated diaphragm

Decreases in Lung Compliance
Pneumonia
Cystic fibrosis
Trauma

Ventilation/Perfusion Mismatch
Ventilation Defects
Pulmonary edema
Pneumonia
Atelectasis
Obstruction caused by mucous plugs
Increased dead space ventilation as a result of emphysema

Perfusion Defects
Pulmonary emboli
Disruption of normal chest architecture

Disruption in Oxygen Transport with Diminished Oxygen-Carrying Capacity
Anemia
Blood loss

Disruption in Effective Circulation
Shock
Blood loss
Diminished peripheral resistance
Cardiac failure
Emboli
Increased capillary permeability

Disruptions at the Cellular Level
Acid-base disturbances
Poisons/toxins
Blood sugar changes
Hormone effects
Drugs
Hypoxia

NOTE
Brain damage may occur 4 to 6 minutes after interruption of breathing and circulation. After 6 minutes of circulatory arrest, brain damage almost always occurs. After 10 minutes of circulatory arrest, some portions of the brain have been irreversibly damaged to the point of death.[2]

Foreign Body Airway Obstruction

About 3000 deaths each year result from foreign body obstruction of the airway.[16] Immediate removal of the obstruction might have prevented the resulting hypoxemia, unconsciousness, or cardiopulmonary arrest that caused these deaths. The management of foreign body airway obstruction by health care professionals, as recommended by the American Heart Association, is summarized in Table 15-3.

NOTE
Methods for relieving foreign body airway obstruction (FBAO) in an unconscious victim of any age have been simplified for lay rescuers. Lay rescuers should begin standard cardiopulmonary resuscitation (CPR) when an unrelieved, responsive choking victim becomes unresponsive or when an unresponsive person suspected of having an FBAO is encountered, evaluated, and treated. The only difference from regular CPR is that the lay rescuer should open the airway widely whenever ventilations are attempted. This is done to look for a foreign object and remove it if seen. Blind finger sweeps are not to be used by lay rescuers for victims of any age.

TABLE 15-3 Management of Foreign Body Airway Obstruction

Infant (<1 yr)	Objectives	Adult (>12 to 14 yr)	Child (1-12 to 14 yr)
Conscious victim	1. Assessment: Check for signs of severe airway obstruction. 2. Act to relieve obstruction.	Ask, "Are you choking?" Determine whether victim can cough or speak. Perform subdiaphragmatic abdominal thrusts until object is expelled or patient loses consciousness.	Observe for breathing difficulty. Give five back blows. Give five chest thrusts until the object is expelled or the baby becomes unresponsive.
	3. Be persistent. 4. Position victim.		
Victim who loses consciousness		Turn on back as unit, supporting head and neck; position face up, arms by sides.	
	5. Check for foreign body. 6. Give rescue breaths.	Open airway with head-tilt chin-lift maneuver. Check for foreign body. Attempt rescue breathing (slow ventilations [1 sec]). If first ventilation attempt is unsuccessful, reposition head and reattempt ventilation.	
	7. Act to relieve obstruction.	Begin cardiopulmonary resuscitation (CPR). Check for foreign body each time airway is opened. Repeat steps 6 through 7 until obstruction is relieved or until advanced procedures become possible (i.e., use of Kelly clamp or Magill forceps, or cricothyrotomy).	
Unconscious victim	1. Assessment: Determine unresponsiveness.	Tap or gently shake shoulder. Shout, "Are you okay?" Send someone to activate EMS.	Tap or gently shake shoulder.
	2. Position victim.	Turn on back as unit, supporting head and neck; position face up, arms by sides.	
	3. Open airway.	Open airway with head-tilt chin-lift maneuver.	Open airway with head-tilt chin-lift maneuver without hyperextension.
	4. Assessment: Determine breathlessness. 5. Give rescue breaths.	Maintain an open airway. Place ear over mouth; observe chest. Look, listen, and feel for breathing (no longer than 10 seconds). Seal mouth to mouth with barrier device or bag-valve device.	Seal mouth to nose/mouth with barrier device.
		Attempt rescue breathing (give 2 ventilations 1 sec each). If first ventilation is unsuccessful, reposition head and reattempt ventilation.	
	6. Act to relieve obstruction. 7. Check for foreign body.	Begin CPR. Check for foreign object each time you open the airway.	
	8. Provide rescue breathing. 9. Be persistent.	Check for foreign object each time you open the airway until advanced procedures become possible (i.e., use of Kelly clamp or Magill forceps, or cricothyrotomy).	

Modified from American Heart Association: *Basic life support for healthcare providers,* Dallas, 2010, The Association.

AIRWAY OBSTRUCTION IN A CONSCIOUS PATIENT

Meat is the most common cause of foreign body airway obstruction in conscious adults. (However, a variety of other foods and foreign objects is responsible for obstruction in children and in some adults.) Factors associated with choking include large, poorly chewed pieces of food, an elevated blood alcohol level, and poorly fitting dentures. The patient often is middle-aged or older.

CRITICAL THINKING
How can you relieve a foreign body airway obstruction using only your hands?

Foreign bodies may cause partial or complete airway obstruction. A patient with a partly obstructed airway usually can speak. The person usually can cough forcefully in an effort to expel the object. If air exchange is adequate, the rescuer should not intervene.[17] A patient with a partial obstruction should be monitored closely. The person should be encouraged to persist with spontaneous coughing and breathing efforts. If the obstruction persists or air exchange becomes severely compromised (evidenced by a silent cough, also wheezing, increased respiratory difficulty, decreased air movement, and cyanosis), the patient should be managed as though a complete airway obstruction existed.

Patients with complete airway obstruction cannot speak (aphonia), exchange air, or cough. They often grasp the neck between the thumb and fingers. (This is a universal sign of choking.) These patients need immediate rescuer intervention. Complete airway obstruction causes hypoxemia. It can lead to an acute myocardial infarction in patients with atherosclerotic cardiovascular disease. Airway obstruction inevitably leads to cardiac arrest in all patients if not corrected within minutes.

AIRWAY OBSTRUCTION IN AN UNCONSCIOUS PATIENT

Although upper airway obstruction may lead to loss of consciousness and cardiopulmonary arrest, more often the obstruction is caused by unconsciousness and cardiopulmonary arrest.[17] The primary source of upper airway obstruction in an unconscious patient is the tongue.

The tongue is attached to the mandible by the muscles that form the floor of the mouth. The normal tone of these muscles allows for air exchange by keeping the posterior pharynx open. If a patient is unconscious or has neuromuscular dysfunction, relaxation of these muscles may cause the airway to be blocked by the tongue. Airway obstruction by the tongue is common in the following situations:

- Cardiac arrest
- Trauma
- Stroke
- Intoxication with alcohol, barbiturates, or psychotropic drugs
- Paralysis caused by muscle relaxants
- Myasthenia gravis
- Fractured facial and nasal bones

SHOW ME THE EVIDENCE

Soroudi and colleagues performed a retrospective review of prehospital records for a 17-month period (2003 to 2005). They evaluated calls involving adult foreign body airway obstruction that were received by a California EMS service with a call volume of 250,000 per year. Of the 513 calls identified, 17 patients died. The mean patient age was 65 years. Meat and medications were the most common cause of obstruction. Performance of the Heimlich maneuver improved the patient's condition in 86.5% of cases. Direct laryngoscopy with use of Magill forceps was successful in three patients.

Soroudi A, Shipp H, Stepanski B, et al: Adult foreign body airway obstruction in the prehospital setting, *Prehosp Emerg Care* 11:25-29, 2007.

Laryngeal Spasm and Edema

Spasmodic closure of the vocal cords often is caused by an aggressive intubation technique. (Endotracheal intubation is discussed later in this chapter.) It also may occur during **extubation** (removal of the ET tube). This may be the case especially if the patient is semiconscious. Laryngeal spasm is best managed with aggressive ventilation and a forceful upward pull on the jaw. At times it may require the use of muscle relaxants. Maintaining steady pressure against the cords with the ET tube sometimes overcomes the spasmodic closure.

Swelling of the glottic and subglottic tissues of the airway can close off the larynx. The formation of edema may result from inflammatory or mechanical causes such as epiglottitis, croup, allergic reaction, thermal injuries, strangulation, blunt trauma, or drowning. Associated swelling may partly or completely obstruct the airway. Aggressive airway management (including the consideration for cricothyrotomy) is required for the patient's survival when this occurs.

Fractured Larynx

The most common cause of external trauma to the larynx is a motor vehicle crash. If a trauma patient has localized laryngeal pain on palpation or swallowing, stridor, hoarseness, difficulty with speech (dysphonia), or hemoptysis (coughing up blood), a fracture of the larynx should be suspected. Laryngeal injury can result in a lack of support for the vocal cords. This may cause them to collapse into the tracheal-laryngeal opening, obstructing the airway. Subcutaneous emphysema, dysphagia (difficult swallowing), and throat discomfort that increases with coughing or swallowing indicate the possibility of an impending airway obstruction as a result of a fracture. The paramedic should remain alert to the possibility of laryngeal fracture. This is important because laryngeal edema can rapidly close off the airway.

Certain types of injury may cause laryngeal fracture. Examples include a clothesline injury and blunt trauma to the neck. A laryngeal fracture requires rapid intervention. Cricothyrotomy may be required. The paramedic must secure an open airway before laryngeal edema and hemorrhage cause complete closure.

Tracheal Trauma

Trauma to the trachea is rare but serious. The most common site of tracheal injury is the area bordered by the cricoid cartilage and the third tracheal ring. This injury seldom occurs as an isolated event. More often it is associated with injuries to the surrounding esophagus and cervical spine. Central nervous system (CNS) injuries and abdominal and thoracic trauma also usually accompany tracheal injury. (Tracheal trauma is described in more detail in Chapter 40.)

ASPIRATION BY INHALATION

Aspiration is the active inhalation of food, a foreign body, or fluid (e.g., vomitus, saliva, blood, neutral liquids) into the airway. Depending on the type and degree of aspiration, the syndrome may cause spasm, mucus production, atelectasis, a change in pH (if the substance is acidic), or coughing. Prevention of aspiration is far superior to any known treatment. Aspiration is prevented mainly by controlling and maintaining the airway. Paramedics should always be prepared for the chance of aspiration in patients with a diminished level of consciousness.

About 80% of the approximately 3000 deaths each year from foreign body aspiration occur in children.[16] Running with food or other objects in the mouth, seizures, and forced feeding are among the risk factors in this age group. Hot dogs and peanuts are foods children commonly aspirate. In adults, obstruction may be caused by dental or nasal surgery, loss of consciousness, swallowing of poorly chewed food, and alcohol intoxication.

Large food particles and other foreign bodies can block the airway. This may cause hypoventilation of lower lung segments. The size of the particle determines which airway is obstructed and to what extent.

Approximately 60% of foreign bodies are found in the right mainstem bronchus, 19% in the left, and 21% at the larynx or vocal cords.[18] (The left mainstem bronchus branches from the trachea at a 45- to 60-degree angle. Thus foreign body occlusion of this bronchus is less likely than of the right mainstem bronchus, which is shorter, wider, and more vertical.) When the larynx or trachea is completely obstructed, the victim can die of asphyxiation within minutes.

The average adult stomach has a capacity of 1.4 L. It manufactures an additional 1.4 L of gastric juices in each 24-hour period. Hydrochloric acid is manufactured by special cells in the gastric mucosa. With the assistance of a protein-dissolving enzyme (pepsin), this acid helps break down large pieces of food into smaller ones.

Vomitus contains not only partly digested food particles but also acidic gastric fluid. Saliva is a watery, slightly acidic fluid. It is secreted in the mouth by the major salivary glands and the smaller salivary glands in the mucous membranes that line the mouth. Saliva contains the digestive enzyme amylase. This enzyme helps break down carbohydrates. Saliva also contains a number of other substances. These include minerals (e.g., sodium, calcium, and chloride), proteins, mucin (the principal constituent of mucus), urea, white blood cells, debris from the lining of the mouth, and bacteria.

The consequences of aspiration of neutral liquids (liquids that are neither acidic nor basic) are easier to reverse with supportive therapy than the consequences of aspiration of acids or bases. Nonetheless, aspiration of a large volume of neutral liquids also is associated with a high mortality rate.

Pathophysiology of Aspiration

Two conditions are associated with a high risk of aspiration: (1) a diminished level of consciousness and (2) mechanical disturbances of the airway and gastrointestinal (GI) tract.

A diminished level of consciousness may be caused by trauma, alcohol or other drug intoxication, a seizure disorder, cardiopulmonary arrest, a stroke, or a CNS dysfunction. The common element of these conditions is depression or loss of the gag reflex, with or without a full stomach. The **gag reflex** is a normal neural reflex triggered by touching the soft palate or posterior pharynx.

Iatrogenic obstructions (i.e., those caused by medical procedures) are a common type of mechanical obstruction. This type of obstruction results from the use of various devices to control upper airway problems. Examples include removal of certain airway devices (risk of vomiting on removal), placement of a nasogastric tube (the artificial opening through the esophageal sphincter increases the risk of regurgitation and aspiration), and intubation, which requires an adequate seal at the tracheal orifice to prevent aspiration. These mechanical airway devices are discussed later in this chapter.

Other mechanical or structural problems that may lead to a high risk of aspiration include tracheostomy and esophageal motility disorders, such as hiatal hernia and esophageal reflux. Other individuals at risk include those with intestinal obstructions and those fed by gastric tube.

The chance of aspiration increases whenever vomiting occurs. Vomiting follows stimulation of the vomiting center of the medulla. This stimulation can result from irritation anywhere along the GI tract, from information passed to the medulla from the frontal lobes of the brain, or from disturbances in the balance mechanism (vestibular system) of the inner ear. Once this center is stimulated, the following seven events occur:

1. A deep breath is taken.
2. The hyoid bone and larynx are elevated. This opens the preesophageal sphincter.
3. The opening of the larynx closes.
4. The soft palate is elevated, closing the posterior nares.
5. The diaphragm and the abdominal muscles contract forcefully. This compresses the stomach and increases the intragastric pressure.
6. The lower esophageal sphincter relaxes. The stomach contents are propelled into the lower esophagus.
7. If the patient is unconscious or unable to protect the airway, pulmonary aspiration may occur.

Effects of Pulmonary Aspiration

The severity of pulmonary aspiration depends on the pH of the aspirated material, the volume of the aspirate, and whether particulate matter (e.g., food) and bacterial contamination are present in the aspirate. It generally is accepted that severe pulmonary damage occurs when the pH of an aspirated material is 2.5 or lower. When the pH is below 1.5, the patient usually dies. The mortality rate among patients who aspirate grossly contaminated material (as occurs in bowel obstruction) approaches 100%.

The toxic effects on the lungs of gastric acid (which has a pH below 2.5) can be equated with those of chemical burns. These are severe injuries that produce pulmonary changes such as destruction of surfactant-producing alveolar cells, alveolar collapse and destruction, and destruction of pulmonary capillaries. The permeability of the capillaries increases with massive flooding of the alveoli and bronchi with fluid. The resulting pulmonary edema creates areas of hypoventilation, shunting, and severe hypoxemia. The massive fluid shift from the intravascular area to the lungs also may produce hypovolemia severe enough to require volume replacement.

> **NOTE**
> The risk of pulmonary aspiration can be minimized by continuously monitoring the patient's mental status, properly positioning the patient to allow for drainage of secretions, limiting ventilatory pressures to prevent gastric distention, and using suction devices and esophageal or endotracheal (ET) intubation. Airway protection should be provided if the risk of aspiration exists. It also should be provided promptly after an occurrence of aspiration.

SECTION FOUR
Ventilation

ESSENTIAL PARAMETERS OF AIRWAY EVALUATION

Evaluation of the respiratory system is presented in depth in Chapter 20. This discussion is limited to essentials of airway evaluation that are used to identify immediate signs of life-threatening airway compromise. The essential parameters of airway evaluation are rate, regularity, and effort, in addition to recognition of airway problems that might indicate respiratory distress.

> **NOTE**
> This section serves as a review of techniques of airway assessment and airway management used by emergency medical responders (EMRs), emergency medical technicians (EMTs), and advanced emergency medical technicians (AEMTs). It also addresses advanced procedures used by paramedics.

Rate, Regularity, and Effort

The normal respiratory rate in a resting adult is 12 to 24 breaths/minute. Regularity is defined as a steady inspiratory and expiratory pattern. Breathing at rest should be effortless. It also should be marked by only subtle changes in rate or regularity.

Patients in respiratory distress often compensate for their inability to breathe easily by sitting upright with the head tilted back (*upright sniffing position*), by leaning forward on the arms (*tripod position*), or by lying down with the head and thorax slightly elevated (*semi-Fowler's position*). These patients frequently avoid lying flat, or supine.

> **CRITICAL THINKING**
> Why would lying flat on the back (i.e., in the supine position) most likely worsen respiratory distress?

Recognition of Airway Problems

Respiratory distress may be caused by upper or lower airway obstruction, inadequate ventilation, impairment of the respiratory muscles, ventilation/perfusion mismatching, diffusion abnormalities, or impairment of the nervous system. Dyspnea often is associated with hypoxia.

> **NOTE**
> Recognition and management of respiratory failure are crucial to the patient's survival. The brain can survive only a few minutes of anoxia. All therapies will fail if the airway is not adequate.

OBSERVATION TECHNIQUES

Visual clues can aid the recognition of airway problems. Paramedics should note the patient's preferred position to facilitate breathing. They also should assess the rise and fall of the patient's chest. Other visual clues to respiratory distress include the following:

- Gasping for air
- Cyanosis
- Nasal flaring
- Pursed-lip breathing
- Retraction of the intercostal or subcostal muscles, suprasternal notch, and supraclavicular fossa during respirations (Figure 15-27)

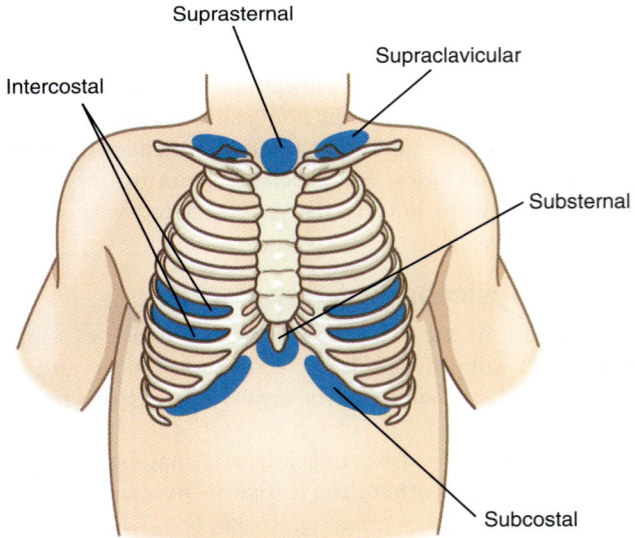

FIGURE 15-27 Areas of chest muscle retraction. (McCance KL, Huether SE: *Pathophysiology: the biologic basis for disease in adults and children,* ed 6, St Louis, 2009, Mosby.)

> **NOTE**
>
> **Pulsus paradoxus** is an exaggeration of the normal blood pressure variation that occurs with breathing. It is defined as a fall in systolic pressure of 10 mm Hg or more on spontaneous inspiration. At times it is associated with a change in the quality of the pulse. The condition occasionally is observed in patients with asthma or chronic obstructive pulmonary disease (COPD) and in victims of blunt or penetrating chest trauma (see Chapter 42). Pulsus paradoxus is difficult to measure. The paramedic should rely on more obvious signs and symptoms of respiratory distress.

AUSCULTATION, PALPATION, AND PERCUSSION TECHNIQUES

Air movement can be evaluated by listening to respirations without using a stethoscope (Figure 15-28) or by using a stethoscope to assess bilateral lung fields. Palpation of the

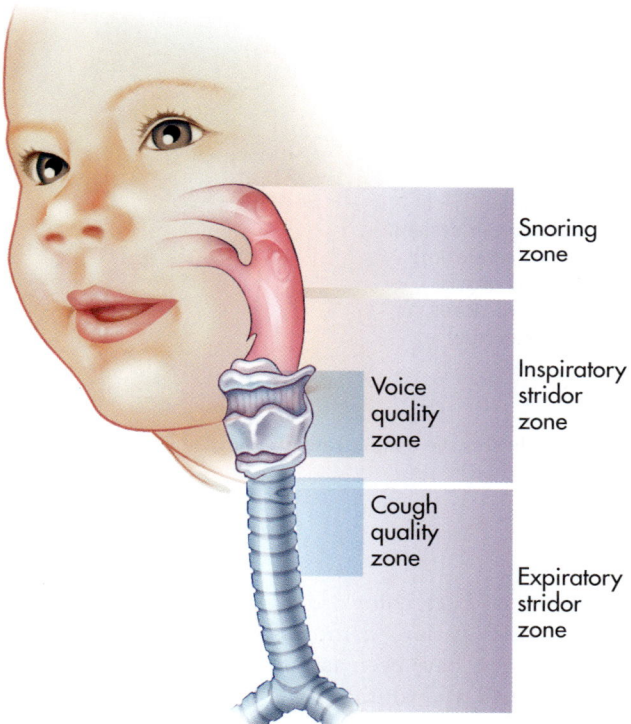

Snoring zone

Voice quality zone

Inspiratory stridor zone

Cough quality zone

Expiratory stridor zone

FIGURE 15-28 A loud, gasping snore suggests enlarged tonsils or adenoids. With inspiratory stridor, the airway is compromised at the level of the supraglottic larynx, vocal cords, subglottic region, or upper trachea. Expiratory stridor, or central wheeze, results from narrowing or collapse of the lower trachea or bronchi. Airway noise during both inspiration and expiration often represents a fixed obstruction of the vocal cords or subglottic space. Hoarseness or a weak cry is a byproduct of obstruction of the vocal cords. If a cough is croupy or low pitched, a tracheal disorder should be suspected. (McCance KL, Huether SE: *Pathophysiology: the biologic basis for disease in adults and children,* ed 6, St Louis, 2009, Mosby.)

chest wall helps determine the presence or absence of paradoxical (contrary) motion of the chest wall, inspiration, expiration, and any retraction of accessory muscles. Percussion may be helpful in some circumstances. This technique can be used to help determine the presence of air or blood in the chest cavity when diminished breath sounds or unequal chest wall movement is present (see Chapter 20).

OTHER SIGNS OF RESPIRATORY DISTRESS

Other signs that indicate possible causes of respiratory distress include resistance or changing compliance when assisting or delivering respirations with a bag-valve-mask (seen in asthma, chronic obstructive pulmonary disease [COPD], and tension pneumothorax), and the presence of pulsus paradoxus.

History

Obtaining a history to determine the progression and duration of the dyspneic event also helps guide the direction of patient care. For example, the paramedic should ask whether the event was sudden in onset or occurred over time. If it occurred over time, the length of that period should be determined. The paramedic also should ask whether any known causes or triggers initiated the difficulty breathing and if the respiratory distress is continuous or recurring. Other questions that should be asked in obtaining a patient's history include the following:

- What makes it better?
- What makes it worse?
- Do any other symptoms occur at the same time (e.g., cough, chest pain, fever)?
- Has any treatment with drugs been attempted?
- Has the patient taken all medications and treatments as prescribed?

It also is crucial to determine whether the patient has been previously evaluated or hospitalized for this condition and whether the person has ever been intubated because of respiratory problems.

Changes in the Respiratory Pattern

As previously stated, the breathing process should be comfortable, regular, and performed without distress. Abnormal respiratory patterns are commonly seen in ill or injured patients (Figure 15-29 and Box 15-4). Recognizing these patterns may help paramedics determine the proper patient care.

Inadequate Respiration

Inadequate respiration can occur when the body cannot compensate for increased oxygen demand or cannot maintain a normal range of oxygen/carbon dioxide balance. Numerous factors can cause inadequate ventilation and respiration, including infection, trauma, brainstem injury, and a noxious or hypoxic atmosphere. A patient with respiratory compromise may have a number of symptoms and various respiratory rates and breathing patterns. Some medical experts distinguish between inadequate ventilation

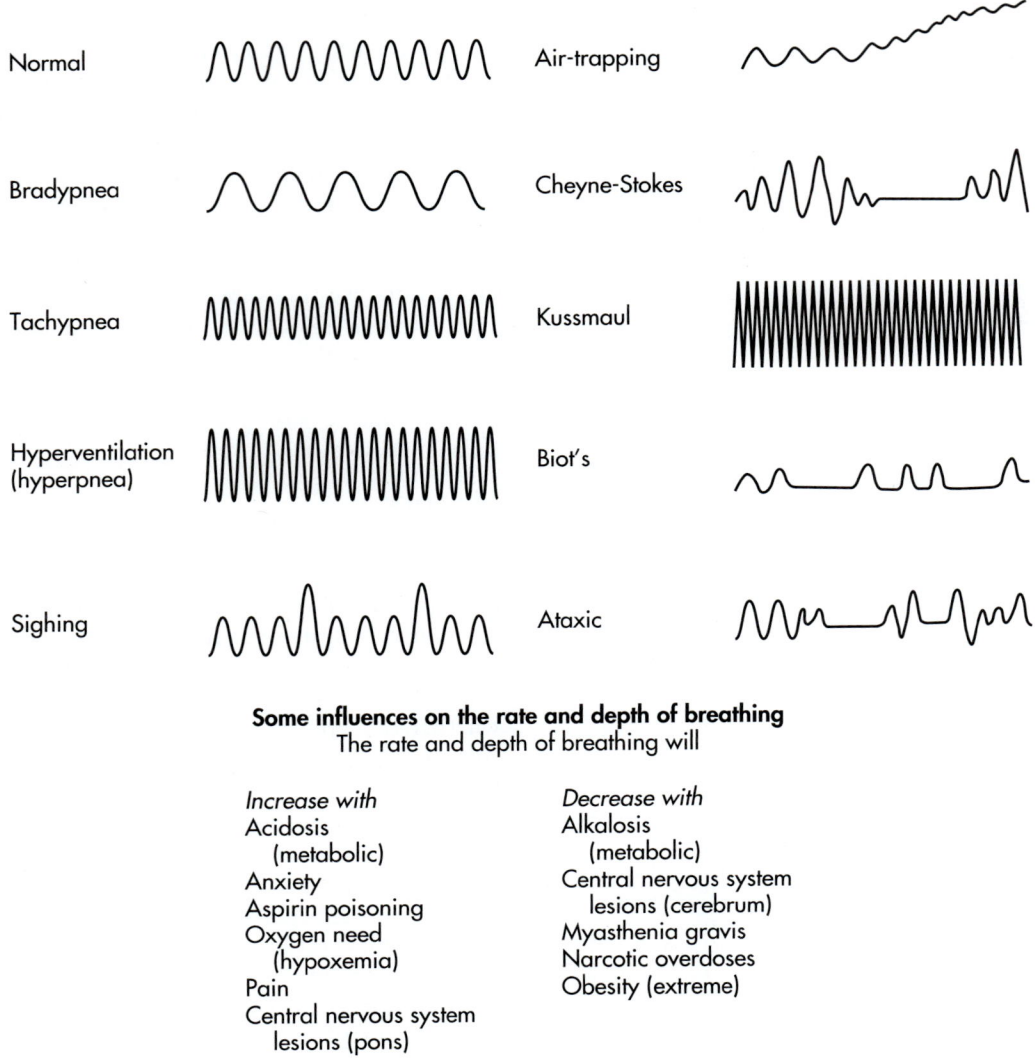

Some influences on the rate and depth of breathing
The rate and depth of breathing will

Increase with
Acidosis
　(metabolic)
Anxiety
Aspirin poisoning
Oxygen need
　(hypoxemia)
Pain
Central nervous system
　lesions (pons)

Decrease with
Alkalosis
　(metabolic)
Central nervous system
　lesions (cerebrum)
Myasthenia gravis
Narcotic overdoses
Obesity (extreme)

FIGURE 15-29 Patterns of respiration. The horizontal axis indicates the relative rate; the vertical swings indicate the relative depth.

caused by a problem in the mechanics of breathing (usually defined by the P_{CO_2}) and inadequate oxygenation but normal ventilation, as seen in pulmonary embolus and often pneumonia.

SUPPLEMENTAL OXYGEN THERAPY

Supplemental oxygen therapy may be provided for two reasons: (1) enriched oxygen in the atmosphere increases the oxygen content in pulmonary capillary blood; and (2) increasing the available oxygen allows the patient to compensate without increasing the work of breathing.

Oxygen Sources

The most common form of oxygen used in the prehospital setting is pure oxygen gas, delivered in liters per minute (LPM). This gas is stored under pressure in stainless steel or lightweight alloy cylinders (Figure 15-30). These cylinders have been color coded by the U.S. Pharmacopeia to distinguish various compressed gases. Steel green and white cylinders have been assigned to all grades of oxygen. Stainless steel and aluminum cylinders are not painted. Common sizes of oxygen cylinders (and their factors) used in emergency care include the following (Box 15-5):

Cylinder	Factor
D cylinder (425 L of oxygen)	0.16
Jumbo D cylinder (640 L of oxygen)	0.28
E cylinder (680 L of oxygen)	0.28
M cylinder (3450 L of oxygen)	1.56

Oxygen cylinders are filled under a pressure of 2000 to 2200 pounds per square inch (psi). Therefore, safety is critical when this equipment is handled. The paramedic should make sure the correct regulator is firmly attached before moving an oxygen cylinder. Also, a cylinder should never be

BOX 15-4 Abnormal Respiratory Patterns

Agonal respiration: A type of breathing that usually follows a pattern of gasping succeeded by apnea. It generally indicates the onset of respiratory arrest or the breathing pattern of a dying person.

Ataxic pattern: A type of cluster or irregular breathing pattern characterized by a series of inspirations and expirations. Ataxic respiration usually is associated with a structural or compressive lesion in the medullary respiratory centers.

Biot pattern: A respiratory pattern involving irregular respirations varying in depth and interrupted by intervals of apnea (absence of breathing). Although similar to Cheyne-Stokes respiration, this pattern lacks the repetitiveness of that type and often is irregular. Biot respiration usually is seen in patients with head injuries who have increased intracranial pressure. Unlike Cheyne-Stokes respiration, the Biot ataxic pattern frequently produces ventilatory failure and may lead to apnea.

Bradypnea: A persistent respiratory rate slower than 12 breaths/minute. This abnormal rate may be a result of the patient guarding against respiratory discomfort caused by chest wall injury, respiratory failure, cerebrovascular accident (CVA), pulmonary infection, or narcotic poisoning. However, bradypnea is more commonly caused by respiratory drive depression that occurs secondary to neurological disturbances.

Central neurogenic hyperventilation: A pattern of breathing marked by rapid and regular ventilations at a rate of about 25 breaths/minute. Increasing regularity, rather than rate, is an important diagnostic sign, because it indicates an increasing depth of coma.

Cheyne-Stokes respiration: A regular, periodic pattern of breathing with equal intervals of apnea followed by a crescendo-decrescendo sequence of respirations. Cheyne-Stokes respirations are thought to represent a level of cortical dysfunction of the brain. Although some children and older adults breathe in this pattern during sleep, it is usually seen in patients who are seriously ill or injured.

Eupnea: Normal breathing.

Hyperventilation: A persistent, rapid, deep respiration that often results in hyperpnea. Compared with tachypnea, hyperpnea usually is slower and much deeper. Its causes include exercise, anxiety, metabolic disturbances (e.g., diabetic ketoacidosis), and central nervous system illness.

Kussmaul respiration: An abnormally deep, very rapid sighing respiratory pattern characteristic of diabetic ketoacidosis or other metabolic acidosis.

Tachypnea: A persistent respiratory rate that exceeds 20 breaths/minute. It may be common in patients who are in pain, frightened, or anxious. The many other causes of tachypnea include fractured ribs, pneumonia, pneumothorax, pulmonary embolus, and pleurisy.

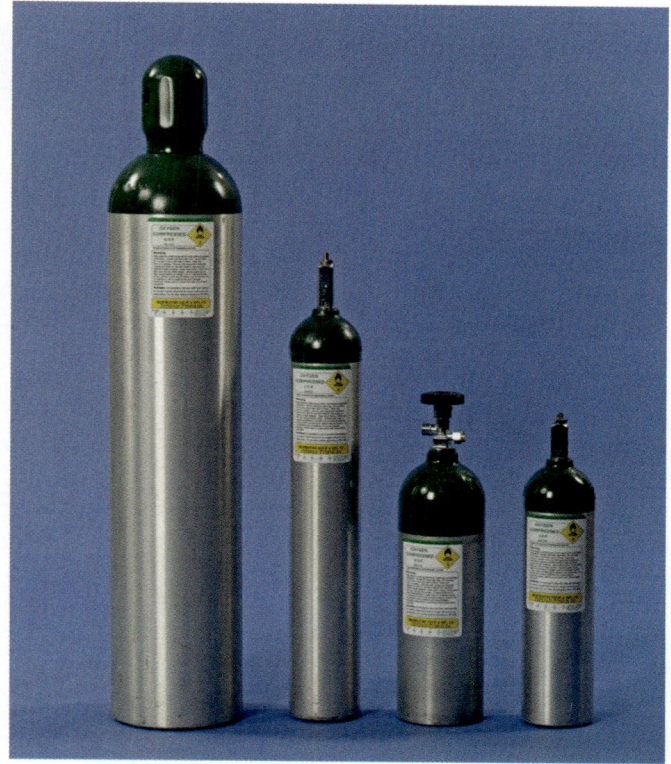

FIGURE 15-30 Oxygen cylinders: M, E, jumbo D, and D.

BOX 15-5 Calculating Oxygen Tank Life

This method can be used to estimate the amount of oxygen available in an oxygen cylinder. First, subtract the safe residual pressure (200 psi) from the tank pressure. Second, multiply the result by the tank's factor (cylinder constant). This equals the volume of gas. Third, divide the volume of gas by the liters per minute (LPM) delivery. This equals the tank life in minutes.

Example

The tank pressure in an E cylinder is 650 psi. You are delivering 6 L/minute of oxygen to the patient.

Step **1**. Subtract the safe residual pressure from the tank's psi:

$$650 - 200 = 450$$

Step **2**. Multiply the result by the E cylinder factor to obtain the volume of gas:

$$450 \times 0.28 = 126$$

Step **3**. Divide the volume of gas by the LPM delivery to determine the tank life in minutes:

$$126 \div 6 = 21 \text{ minutes}$$

handled by the neck assembly alone. Most oxygen cylinders are considered "empty" at 200 psi. (This is the safe residual pressure.) As a rule, tanks with less than 500 psi are too low to keep in service.

LIQUID OXYGEN

Liquid oxygen (LOX) has been cooled to its aqueous state. However, it converts to a gaseous state when warmed. The liquid form is used by some air medical services and by other EMS agencies when the weight and space that a standard oxygen system occupies must be considered. The main advantage of liquid oxygen is that a much larger volume of gaseous oxygen can be stored in an aqueous state. One disadvantage of liquid oxygen is the cost. (LOX is more expensive than pressurized oxygen.) Another is the fact that the units generally require upright storage. Finally, special requirements are necessary for large-volume storage and cylinder transfer.

REGULATORS

High-pressure regulators are used to transfer cylinder gas from tank to tank. They are attached to cylinder stems and allow cylinder gas to be delivered under high pressure. *Therapy regulators* are used to deliver a safe pressure of oxygen to patients (Figure 15-31). They are attached to the cylinder stem. Therapy regulators work through a regulator mechanism whereby 50 psi escape pressure is reduced ("stepped down") to 30 psi for safe delivery to the patient.

> **NOTE**
> Therapy regulators (used for delivery of oxygen to patients) are attached to smaller oxygen cylinders by a yoke assembly with a pin index safety system. This system prevents the paramedic from using a regulator with the wrong type of gas. It requires that the yoke pins match the corresponding holes in the valve assembly for oxygen to be delivered. Larger oxygen cylinders have valve assemblies with a threaded outlet specific to medical oxygen.

FLOWMETERS

Flowmeters control the amount of oxygen delivered to the patient (Figure 15-32). These devices are connected to the pressure regulator. They are adjusted to deliver oxygen at a set number of liters per minute. Some EMS agencies attach disposable humidifiers to the flowmeter. This provides moisture to the dry oxygen coming from the supply cylinder. Humidified oxygen is desirable for long-term oxygen administration and for patients with croup, epiglottitis, or bronchiolitis (see Chapter 24).

Oxygen Delivery Devices

Patients who have spontaneous respirations can receive supplemental oxygen through several different oxygen delivery devices. These include a nasal cannula, simple face mask, partial rebreather mask, nonrebreather mask, and Venturi mask (Table 15-4). Each of these devices has advantages and disadvantages.

NASAL CANNULA

The nasal cannula (Figure 15-33) delivers low-concentration oxygen through two small plastic prongs placed into the nostrils. Nasal cannulas should not be used in patients with poor respiratory effort, severe hypoxia, or apnea. They also should not be used in patients who breathe primarily through the mouth. As a rule, the nasal cannula is well

TABLE 15-4 Oxygen Delivery Devices

Device	Flow Rate (L/min)	Oxygen (O_2)% Delivered
Nasal cannula	1-6	24-44
Simple face mask	6-10	35-60
Partial rebreather mask	6-10	35-60
Nonrebreather mask	10-15	80-95
Venturi mask	4-8	24-50

L/min, Liters per minute.

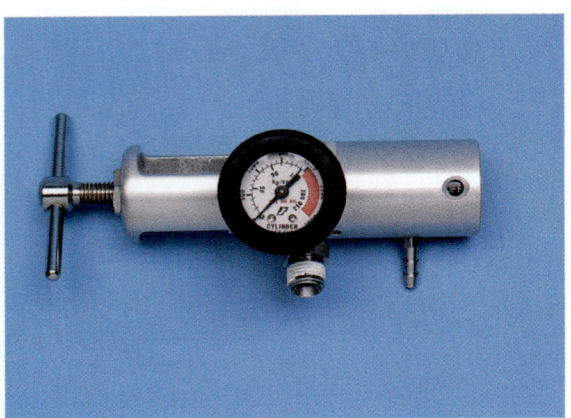

FIGURE 15-31 Therapy regulator.

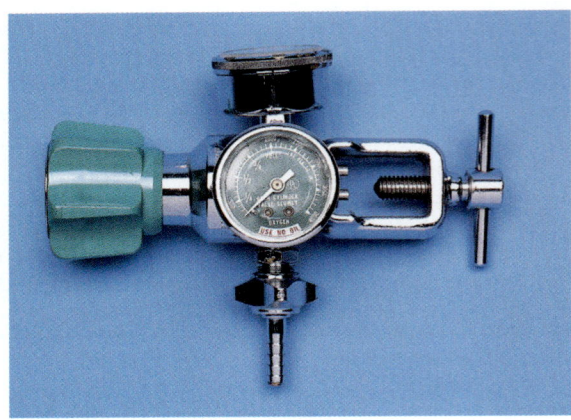

FIGURE 15-32 Flowmeter.

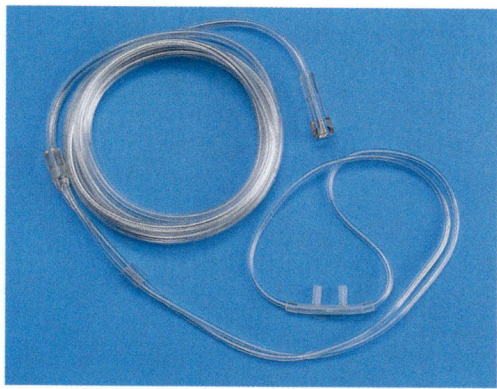

FIGURE 15-33 Nasal cannula.

TABLE 15-5 Approximate Oxygen Concentration for Liters Per Minute Flow	
Liters Per Minute	**Oxygen Concentration**
1	24%
2	28%
3	32%
4	36%
5	40%
6	44%

tolerated. However, it does not deliver high-volume/high-concentration oxygen. The relationship of approximate oxygen concentrations to liter per minute flow is listed in Table 15-5.

Obtaining oxygen concentrations greater than 30% to 35% is difficult with a nasal cannula. This is because the patient continues to breathe through the mouth during oxygen administration. The mouth breathing reduces the concentration of oxygen inspired through the nose. The device also is ineffective if the patient's nose is blocked by blood or mucus. For these reasons, use of the nasal cannula is limited to patients who would benefit from low-concentration oxygen delivery. This may include some patients with chest pain and patients with chronic pulmonary disease. The maximum oxygen flow rate for a nasal cannula is 6 L/min.

SIMPLE FACE MASK

The simple face mask (Figure 15-34) is a soft, clear plastic mask that conforms to the patient's face. Small perforations in the mask allow atmospheric gas to be mixed with oxygen during inhalation. They also permit the patient's exhaled air to escape. Oxygen concentrations of 35% to 60% can be delivered through this device with a flow rate of 6 to 10 L/min. A flow rate of less than 6 L/minute can produce an accumulation of carbon dioxide in the mask; therefore, oxygen delivery through any face mask should always exceed this minimum. Flow rates above 10 L/minute do not enhance oxygen concentration. All masks must be well

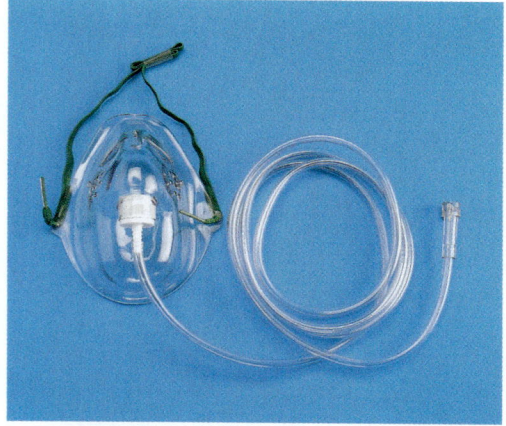

FIGURE 15-34 Simple face mask.

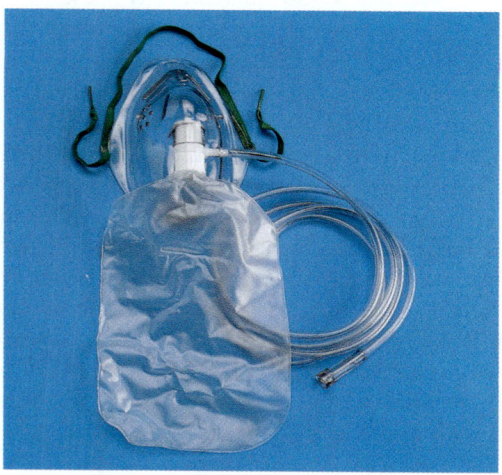

FIGURE 15-35 Partial rebreather mask.

fitted to the patient's face for optimal benefit. Leaks reduce the oxygen concentration.

PARTIAL REBREATHER MASK

The partial rebreather mask (Figure 15-35) has an attached oxygen reservoir bag. The bag should be filled before the patient uses the mask. This device has vent ports covered by one-way disks. These allow a portion of the patient's exhaled gas to enter the reservoir bag and be reused. The remainder of the carbon dioxide–loaded gas escapes into the atmosphere. Oxygen concentrations of 35% to 60% can be delivered with a flow rate that prevents the reservoir bag from collapsing completely on inspiration. Partial rebreather masks should not be used in patients with apnea or poor respiratory effort. As with the simple face mask, delivery of volumes above 10 L/minute with this device does not enhance oxygen concentration.

NONREBREATHER MASK

The nonrebreather mask (Figure 15-36) is similar in design to the partial nonrebreather mask. However, a flutter valve assembly in the mask piece stops the patient's exhaled air

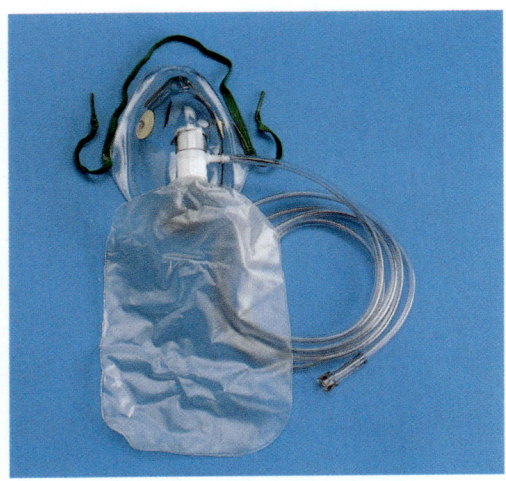

FIGURE 15-36 Nonrebreather mask.

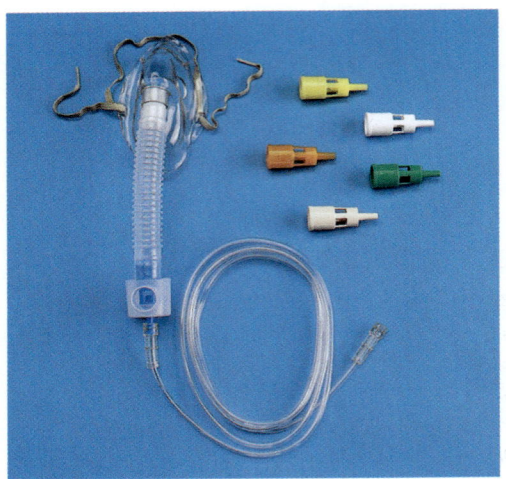

FIGURE 15-37 Venturi mask.

from returning to the reservoir bag. This device delivers oxygen concentrations up to and above 95%. The flow rate must be adequate to keep the reservoir bag partly inflated during inspiration. (Patients with severe respiratory distress may need up to 20 L/minute to maintain inflation of the reservoir bag.) Paramedics should make sure the mask is seated firmly over the patient's mouth and nose. They also should make sure the reservoir bag is never less than two-thirds full. This device most often is used in patients who need high-concentration oxygen delivery (10 to 15 L/minute). As with other masks, it should not be used in patients with apnea or poor respiratory effort.

CRITICAL THINKING
What could happen if the oxygen source is disconnected from a nonrebreather mask?

VENTURI MASK

The Venturi mask (Figure 15-37) is a high-airflow oxygen entrainment delivery device. It delivers a precise fraction of inspired oxygen (FiO_2) at typically low concentrations. The device originally was designed to deliver 30% to 40% concentrations. However, it since has been adapted to deliver higher oxygen percentages. The Venturi mask uses "jet mixing" of atmospheric gas and oxygen to achieve the desired mixture.

Color-coded adapters in various sizes are attached to the mask to control the oxygen flow rate. (Standard-size adapters are 3, 4, and 6 L/minute.) The color codes and adapters state the exact liter flow to use to obtain the precise FiO_2. Choosing a different liter flow greatly alters the FiO_2 delivered. The various Venturi masks deliver 24% to 50% oxygen. They are advised for patients who rely on a hypoxic respiratory drive. This includes, for example, patients with COPD. The main benefit of the Venturi mask is that it allows precise regulation of the FiO_2. It also permits the paramedic

to titrate oxygen for the patient with COPD so as not to exceed the patient's hypoxic drive while allowing enrichment of supplemental oxygen. Care must be taken to match the proper FiO_2 to the correct flow rate. Otherwise, the Venturi mask does not deliver the indicated FiO_2.

AUGMENTING PATIENT VENTILATIONS

Some patients who have spontaneous breathing but who also have dyspnea or respiratory compromise need assistance to improve airflow and oxygenation. Methods to improve a patient's arterial oxygenation include continuous positive airway pressure (CPAP) and biphasic positive airway pressure (BiPAP). CPAP and BiPAP can improve oxygenation through positive pressure during spontaneous breathing, reduce the work of breathing, prevent atelectasis, and allow for drug administration. These methods also may prevent the need for intubation and the risks and complications associated with invasive airway procedures. Indications and contraindications for CPAP and BiPAP are presented in Box 15-6.

Continuous Positive Airway Pressure

Continuous positive airway pressure (CPAP) transmits positive pressure into the airways of a spontaneously breathing patient throughout the respiratory cycle. The increase in airway pressure allows for better diffusion of gases and reexpansion of collapsed alveoli. This results in improvement of gas exchange and a reduction in the work of breathing. CPAP can be applied invasively in a patient with spontaneous breathing (through an ET tube). It also can be applied noninvasively through a face or nose mask. Mask CPAP is provided through a tight-fitting face mask that is connected to a battery-operated or oxygen-driven breathing circuit. This breathing circuit may have a fixed or an adjustable FiO_2 and a fixed or an adjustable pressure valve that delivers pressures of 5 to 10 cm H_2O or more

BOX 15-6 Indications and Contraindications for CPAP and BiPAP

Indications

Acute respiratory distress syndrome (ARDS)
Asthma
Chronic obstructive pulmonary disease (COPD)
Congestive heart failure (CHF)
Pneumonia
Pulmonary edema
Submersion (near-drowning) incidents

Contraindications

Patients who are unconscious
Children under 14 years of age
Upper airway trauma
Hypotension or shock
Facial/chest trauma
Pneumothorax
Barotrauma
Inability to breathe spontaneously
Inability to maintain mask seal
Stoma or tracheotomy
Serious dysrhythmias
Nausea or vomiting
Gastrointestinal (GI) bleeding or recent GI surgery

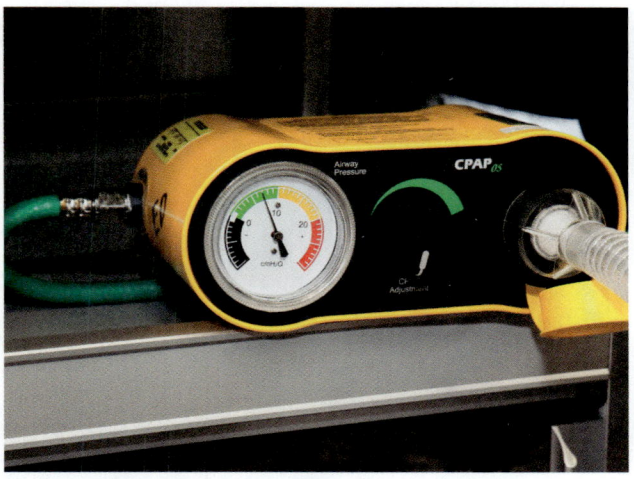

FIGURE 15-38 CPAP machine.

extensive coaching and reassurance from the paramedic. Use of CPAP with standard drug therapy to treat pulmonary edema has been shown to reduce the need for intubation.[21] (Early hospital notification allows for CPAP to be available on arrival at the emergency department [ED].)

(Figure 15-38). (A normal protocol for most EM services is 7 to 10 cm H_2O.)

NOTE

Continuous positive airway pressure (CPAP) is generally well tolerated by patients. However, CPAP may have adverse effects on the circulation or pulmonary system, especially at higher pressures. Such effects include decreased venous return, decreased cardiac output, and pulmonary barotrauma. All patients should be closely monitored for signs and symptoms of adverse effects. If CPAP is used, start with low pressures (5 to 7.5 cm H_2O) and increase in increments of 2 cm H_2O as tolerated by the patient. Respiratory goals may include an exhaled tidal volume greater than 7 mL/kg, a respiratory rate of less than 25, oxygen saturation greater than 90%, and perhaps most important, patient comfort.[19]

CPAP lowers the mean airway pressure. In addition to its use in patients with pulmonary edema, CPAP also may benefit patients with obstructive airway disease.[3] (Nasal CPAP is used in the home for patients with a history of sleep apnea.) Patients who receive CPAP usually are quite anxious. About 5 minutes after the mask is applied, the patient should be observed for signs and symptoms of improvement. These include reduced effort of breathing, increased ease in speaking, slowing respiratory and heart rate, and increased PaO_2. The patient is likely to require

SHOW ME THE EVIDENCE

From 2002 to 2006, Thompson and coworkers compared the outcomes for 71 patients in severe respiratory distress who had no chest pain. Two groups were randomized for treatment, either with standard care or with standard care and continuous positive airway pressure (CPAP). The researchers found that patients treated with CPAP were less likely to require endotracheal intubation and less likely to die.

Thompson J et al: Out-of-hospital continuous positive airway pressure ventilation versus usual care in acute respiratory failure: a randomized controlled trial, *Ann Emerg Med* 52:232-241, 2008.

BIPHASIC POSITIVE AIRWAY PRESSURE

Biphasic positive airway pressure (BiPAP), also known as *bi-level positive airway pressure,* combines partial ventilatory support and CPAP. This allows the pressure to vary during each breath cycle. When the patient inhales, the pressure is similar to CPAP. When the patient exhales, the pressure drops, making it easier to breathe. BiPAP is applied by face mask or nose mask through a noninvasive ventilator device with two settings (Figure 15-39). The device provides a 5 cm H_2O pressure difference between *inspiratory positive airway pressure (IPAP)* and *expiratory positive airway pressure (EPAP)*. BiPAP is a leak-tolerant system; that is, the unit can respond and adjust to leaks. CPAP is not a leak-tolerant system. It allows IPAP and EPAP settings to be titrated (adjusted) to reach a desired range of positive end-expiratory pressure (described later). In selected patients with

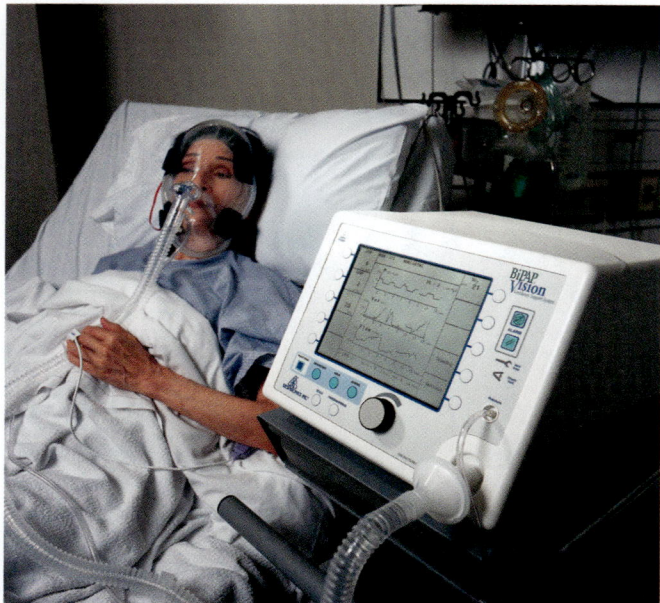

FIGURE 15-39 BiPAP machine. (Shade BR et al: *Mosby's EMT-Intermediate textbook for the 1999 National Standard Curriculum,* ed 3, St Louis, 2007, Mosby.)

respiratory distress caused by COPD, pulmonary edema, pneumonia, or asthma, BiPAP may eliminate the need for endotracheal intubation.

> **NOTE**
>
> With biphasic positive airway pressure (BiPAP), the inspiratory positive airway pressure (IPAP) setting may range from 4 to 24 cm H_2O, and the expiratory positive airway pressure (EPAP) setting may vary from 2 to 20 cm H_2O. Typical initial settings for BiPAP are 8 to 10 cm H_2O IPAP and 2 to 4 cm H_2O EPAP. These settings presume that the lower pressures allow patient tolerance and training. When using BiPAP, the paramedic should remember that the inspiratory pressure must be maintained higher than the expiratory pressure at all times to ensure biphasic flow. In addition, the flow must be synchronized with the patient's respiratory efforts.[22]

PROCEDURE FOR ADMINISTERING CONTINUOUS POSITIVE AIRWAY PRESSURE

Methods for delivering continuous positive airway pressure vary by device and by the manufacturer's guidelines. The following are general guidelines.

1. Treat the patient's underlying conditions as needed.
2. Assess for indications and contraindications.
3. Place the patient in a sitting position or similar position of comfort.
4. Assess vital signs and lung sounds before and during therapy. (The systolic pressure should be above 90 mm Hg.) Vital signs should be assessed every 5 minutes.
5. Attach an electrocardiograph (ECG) and pulse oximeter.

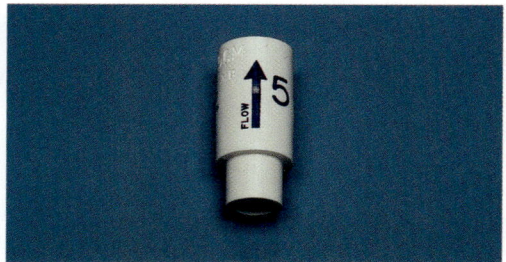

FIGURE 15-40 PEEP valve.

6. Explain the procedure to the patient.
7. Anticipate and control anxiety (consider sedation with benzodiazepines, per protocol).
8. Provide coaching as needed.
9. Connect CPAP to oxygen source; begin CPAP pressure at 5 to 7.5 cm H_2O.
10. Apply the mask and check for air leaks. Use head straps if needed and if tolerated by the patient.
11. Administer nebulized medications as indicated.
12. Treatment should be given continuously throughout transport to the ED. (CPAP therapy should be continued until arrival in the ED.) CPAP may be stopped if the patient cannot tolerate the mask; if the airway requires suctioning or intervention; if respiratory distress worsens; or if a pneumothorax is suspected.

Note: Intermittent positive pressure ventilation and/or intubation should be considered if the patient is removed from CPAP therapy in the prehospital setting. Some patients require intubation in the prehospital setting even with CPAP therapy. Intubation should be considered with:

- Deterioration of mental status
- Increase in $EtCO_2$
- Decrease in SpO_2
- Progressive fatigue
- Ineffective tidal volume
- Respiratory or cardiac arrest

POSITIVE END-EXPIRATORY PRESSURE

As do CPAP and BiPAP, **positive end-expiratory pressure (PEEP)** maintains a degree of positive pressure at the end of exhalation. PEEP is given to patients who have been intubated and who are receiving mechanical ventilation. (PEEP is considered an invasive procedure.) Positive pressure at the end of exhalation keeps the alveoli open and pushes fluid from the alveoli back into the interstitium or capillaries.

In the prehospital setting, ventilatory support with PEEP can be provided through a PEEP valve. These valves are hollow cylinders that have a weight in the lumen (e.g., a Boehringer valve or other special PEEP delivery device) (Figure 15-40). The PEEP device is connected to the expiratory port of a bag-valve device. The valve is available in pressures of 5, 10, and 15 cm H_2O. It creates PEEP by forcing the patient to exhale against the weight of the metal ball. Some transport ventilators have built-in PEEP controls.

RESCUE BREATHING AND MECHANICAL VENTILATION

Ventilation of a patient can be provided by several methods in the prehospital setting. These include rescue breathing (mouth to mouth, mouth to nose, mouth to stoma), mouth-to-mask breathing, bag-mask devices, and automatic transport ventilators. The following discussion of ventilation methods follows the recommendations of the American Heart Association.[23]

>
> **NOTE**
> Providing ventilations with barrier protection should always be a priority when performing rescue breathing. Even so, mouth-to-mouth, mouth-to-nose, and mouth-to-stoma ventilations are presented here for a complete discussion.

Rescue Breathing

As discussed previously, inspired air has an oxygen concentration of about 21%. Of this 21%, about 4% is used by the body. The remaining 17% is exhaled. Ventilation by rescue breathing can provide adequate oxygenation to a patient with respiratory insufficiency.

Rescue breathing has some advantages: no equipment is needed, and it is immediately available. However, it also has disadvantages. One disadvantage is the limitation of the vital capacity of the rescuer. (About 500 to 600 mL is needed to ventilate an adult.) Another drawback is the low amount of oxygen delivered in expired air compared with other methods of ventilation with supplemental oxygen. Also, a rescuer may have difficulty forcing air past any obstructions in the airway. Transmission of a disease through direct body fluid contact is a risk. Another risk is the transmission of an unknown communicable disease at the time of the event. Complications common to all rescue breathing techniques include the following:

- Hyperinflation of the patient's lungs
- Gastric distention
- Blood/body fluid contact concerns
- Rescuer hyperventilation

>
> **NOTE**
> Rescuer hyperventilation is also known as **inadvertent hyperventilation.** This commonly occurs during the delivery of cardiopulmonary resuscitation (CPR) when a patient in cardiac arrest is ventilated excessively. Excessive ventilation is thought to result in increased intrathoracic pressure that causes decreased venous return and decreased coronary perfusion pressure. Rescuer hyperventilation is believed to have a negative effect on survival rates for patients who have suffered cardiac arrest[24] (see Chapter 22). Impedance threshold devices (ITDs) with pressure-sensitive valves are available to limit the influx of air during chest wall compressions. The ITD also lowers intracranial pressure during the decompression phase of CPR. This, combined with increased cardiac output, may result in greater cerebral perfusion.[25] Studies, however, have yet to determine the relative contribution of the ITD to improved outcome.[23]

>
> **CRITICAL THINKING**
> What are two harmful effects of gastric distention during artificial ventilation?

MOUTH-TO-MOUTH METHOD

Paramedics should use the following guidelines in delivering ventilations mouth to mouth:

1. If no spinal injury is suspected, position the patient with optimum head tilt and chin lift. (If a spinal injury is suspected, maintain in-line stabilization and keep the airway open through the jaw-thrust maneuver without the head-tilt technique [described later in this chapter].) If this technique does not open the airway, use the head-tilt chin-lift maneuver. If necessary, clear the airway of vomitus, body fluids, and foreign objects.
2. Pinch the patient's nostrils closed.
3. Inhale a normal breath.
4. Seal your mouth over the patient's mouth, which should be slightly open.
5. Exhale into the patient's mouth over 1 second, until the chest rises visibly.
   Each adult ventilation is about 500 to 600 mL of air.
6. Break contact with patient's mouth and inhale another normal breath.
7. Deliver another breath (as described in step 5).
8. Continue rescue breathing at a rate of 10 to 12 breaths/minute (1 breath every 5 to 6 seconds) as needed. If an advanced airway is placed, reduce the rate to 8 to 10 breaths/minute (1 breath every 6 to 8 seconds).

Mouth-to-mouth breathing usually results in the exchange of saliva between the victim and the rescuer. Transmission of the hepatitis B virus (HBV) and the human immunodeficiency virus (HIV) during rescue breathing has not been documented. However, rare instances of herpes transmission during cardiopulmonary resuscitation (CPR) have been reported.[17] When possible, personal barrier protection devices should be used.

MOUTH-TO-NOSE METHOD

Mouth-to-nose ventilation is very similar to the technique described for mouth-to-mouth rescue breathing. The differences in the mouth-to-nose method are as follows:

- If no spinal injury is suspected, the rescuer must keep one hand on the patient's forehead to maintain an open airway while using the other hand to close the patient's mouth. (If a spinal injury is suspected, the jaw-thrust without head-tilt technique should be used. The rescuer's cheek is used to seal the patient's mouth.)
- The patient's nose is left open.
- The rescuer's mouth is placed over the patient's nose with as tight a seal as possible.
- During passive exhalation by the patient, the rescuer's mouth is removed from the patient's nose and the

patient's mouth is opened for exhalation. The head-tilt or jaw-thrust position must be maintained to ensure an open airway.

Mouth-to-nose ventilation may be appropriate for patients who have injuries to the mouth and lower jaw and for patients with missing teeth or dentures (which makes a tight seal around the mouth difficult). It also may overcome psychological barriers in having mouth-to-mouth contact with a patient.

VENTILATION OF INFANTS AND CHILDREN

To provide ventilations to infants and children, the paramedic should use the mouth-to-mouth-and-nose technique:

1. Position the patient with a *slight* head tilt and chin lift sufficient to open the airway. Hyperextension of a pediatric patient's neck may block the airway. (Use spinal precautions as needed [see Chapter 41]).
2. During ventilation, the rescuer's mouth should cover both the mouth and nose of the infant or small child up to 1 year of age.
3. Exhale into the patient's mouth until the chest rises.
4. When allowing for passive exhalation, break contact with the patient's mouth and nose.
5. Provide ventilations at a rate of 12 to 20 breaths/minute (1 breath every 3 to 5 seconds). When an advanced airway has been placed, reduce the rate to 8 to 10 breaths/minute (1 breath every 6 to 8 seconds).
6. Deliver each breath over 1 second.
7. Make sure the chest rises.

MOUTH-TO-STOMA METHOD

A *stoma* is a temporary or permanent surgical opening in the neck of a patient who has had a laryngectomy or tracheostomy (Figure 15-41). The airway of such a patient has been surgically interrupted. The larynx is no longer connected to the trachea (Box 15-7).

The stoma created by a laryngectomy is large and round; the edge of the tracheal lining can be seen attached to the skin. The stoma in tracheostomy patients usually is no more than several millimeters in diameter. It usually contains one or two concentric tubes (one fitting inside the other) made of plastic or metal. The method of ventilating these patients is the same, regardless of the type of stoma.

Stomas and breathing tubes may become clogged with secretions, encrusted mucus, and foreign matter, leading to inadequate ventilation. If cleaning is needed, wipe the neck opening with gauze. If the breathing tubes are clogged, they can be removed or suctioned. The tracheostomy tube or stoma is suctioned by passing a sterile suction catheter through the external opening into the trachea. *Do not insert the catheter more than 7 to 12 cm (3 to 5 inches) into the trachea.* Once the airway is partly open, begin ventilations by the mouth-to-stoma method (mouth-to-stoma ventilation is bacteriologically cleaner than the mouth-to-mouth method) by using a pediatric-size pocket mask over the top

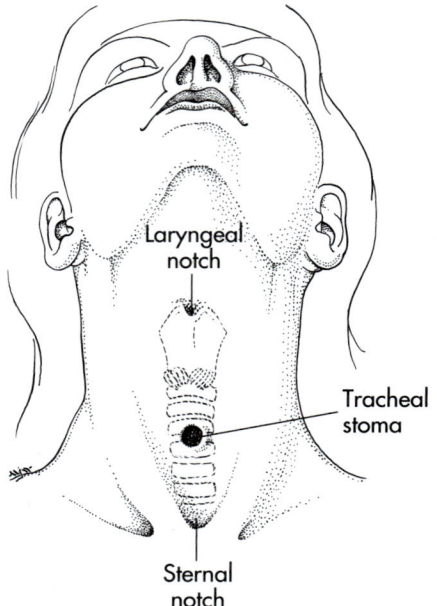

FIGURE 15-41 Stoma.

BOX 15-7 Special Considerations for Patients Who Have Had a Laryngectomy

When providing care for a patient who has had a laryngectomy, paramedics sometimes may need to suction the tracheostomy tube or remove, clean, and replace a tube that has become obstructed by mucus. (Patients who have had a laryngectomy have a less effective cough. As a result, mucous plugs often obstruct breathing tubes.)

The steps for suctioning a breathing tube are as follows:

1. Preoxygenate the patient.
2. Inject 3 mL of sterile saline down the trachea.
3. Step 2 usually results in coughing. If it does not, instruct the patient to exhale.
4. Insert the suction catheter into the trachea until resistance is met (without negative pressure).
5. Step 4 usually results in coughing. If it does not, instruct the patient to cough or exhale.
6. Suction while withdrawing the catheter.

If the breathing tube cannot be cleared and requires replacement, follow these steps:

1. Lubricate a same-size tracheostomy tube or endotracheal (ET) tube (5 mm or larger).
2. Instruct the patient to exhale.
3. Gently insert the tube 1 to 2 cm (about ½ to ¾ inch) beyond the balloon cuff.
4. Inflate the cuff.
5. Confirm the patient's comfort and verify the patency and proper placement of the tube.

Stenosis (spontaneous narrowing of a stoma) may be life-threatening. It also makes replacing a tracheostomy tube difficult or impossible. When stenosis is a factor, an ET tube must be placed before total obstruction occurs.

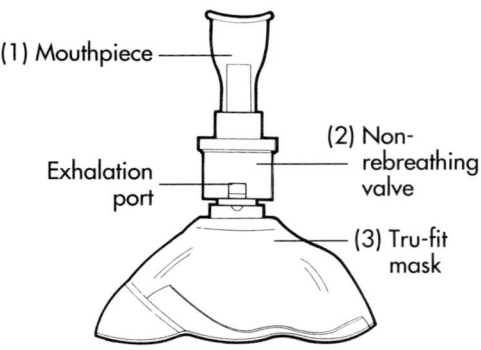

(1) Mouthpiece

(2) Non-rebreathing valve

Exhalation port

(3) Tru-fit mask

FIGURE 15-42 Mouth-to-mask device.

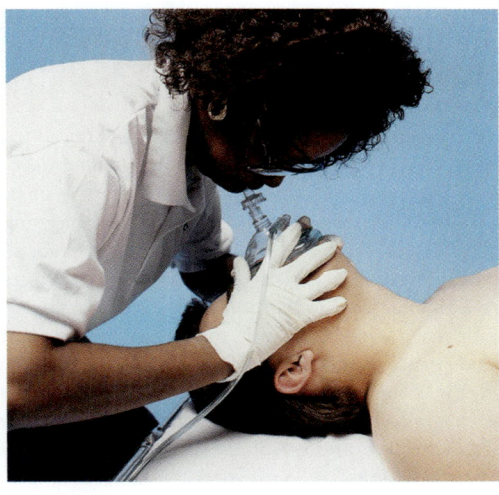

FIGURE 15-43 Mouth-to-mask ventilation technique (cephalic technique).

of the stoma or by securing the airway with an ET tube placed through the stoma.

The technique for stoma ventilation is basically the same as that for other methods of artificial ventilation. However, the patient's head should be kept straight (rather than tilted back), with the shoulders slightly elevated. This position allows more effective ventilation. If the patient's chest does not rise or if air is heard to escape through the patient's upper airway, the patient may be a "partial neck breather." These patients are able to inhale and exhale some air through their nose and mouth. If this occurs, the patient's nostrils must be pinched closed and the mouth sealed with the palm of one hand during ventilation.

Mouth-to-Mask Devices

Mouth-to-mask devices have become popular. They are used as an alternative to mouth-to-mouth methods of ventilation. These masks are constructed of a clear, flexible material. They are available with one-way valves, bacterial filters, and ports for supplemental oxygen delivery (Figure 15-42). They are made by a number of manufacturers and are available in a variety of sizes. The mouth-to-mask technique offers several advantages:

- It eliminates direct contact with the patient's mouth and nose.
- It provides more effective ventilation than the mouth-to-mouth method or a bag-valve-mask device.
- It reduces the risk of disease transmission.
- It allows delivery of supplemental oxygen.
- The one-way valve eliminates exposure to exhaled gases and sputum.
- The mask is easy to apply.

TECHNIQUE

The mask device can be used in patients with or without spontaneous respirations (Figure 15-43). To apply the mask, the paramedic should follow these steps:

1. If no spinal injury is suspected, position the patient with optimum head tilt and chin lift. Use an oropharyngeal or a nasopharyngeal airway if the patient is unconscious. (If a spinal injury is suspected, spinal precautions should be followed.)

2. Connect the one-way valve to the mask. Oxygen tubing should be connected to the inlet port with an oxygen flow rate of 10 to 12 L/minute. Using supplemental oxygen provides a higher concentration of oxygen in the inspired air. An oxygen flow rate of 10 L/minute, combined with rescuer ventilations, can supply an oxygen concentration of 50%.

3. Position yourself at the patient's head (cephalic technique) or side (lateral technique). Clear the airway of secretions, vomitus, and foreign objects. Place the mask on the patient's face and create an airtight seal. Using the thumb side of the palm with both hands, apply pressure to the sides of the mask. If using the cephalic technique, apply upward pressure to the mandible just in front of the earlobes, using the index, middle, and ring fingers of both hands while maintaining head tilt. If using the lateral technique, seal the mask by placing the index finger and thumb of the hand closer to the top of the patient's head along the border of the mask and place the thumb of the other hand along the lower margin of the mask. Place the remaining fingers of the hand closer to the patient's feet and lift the jaw while performing a head-tilt chin-lift.

4. Blow into the opening of the mask, observing chest rise and fall. If available, a second rescuer may apply cricoid pressure (Box 15-8). Cricoid pressure may help prevent gastric inflation during positive pressure ventilation and reduce the chance of regurgitation and aspiration.

5. Remove the mask from the patient's face to allow for passive exhalation.

If oxygen is not available, the tidal volumes and inspiratory times for mouth-to-mask ventilation should be the same as for mouth-to-mouth breathing, assuring visible chest rise. If supplemental oxygen is used with the face mask, provide a minimum flow rate of 10 to 12 L/minute.

BOX 15-8 Application of Cricoid Pressure

Applying pressure to the solid ring of the cricoid cartilage (Sellick maneuver) can occlude the esophagus and may reduce the risk of regurgitation and aspiration. This type of pressure also can help minimize gastric distention during bag-mask ventilation, and may improve visualization of the vocal cords during intubation. Studies suggest that cricoid pressure can interfere with effective ventilation. It is no longer recommended for routine use during ventilation during adult cardiac arrest.[23]

Cricoid pressure should be used with caution if a cervical spine injury is suspected, because it may cause additional damage to the spine. Complications include laryngeal trauma with excessive force and esophageal rupture from unrelieved high gastric pressures.

NOTE

All paramedics should be proficient in delivering effective oxygenation and ventilation with a bag-mask device to adults, children, and infants. This is the preferred method of ventilatory support, particularly if the transport time is short.[23]

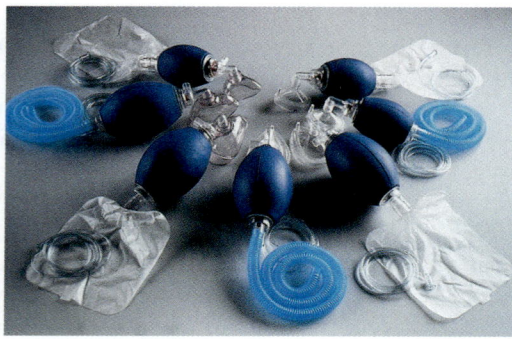

FIGURE 15-44 Disposable and reusable adult and pediatric bag-mask devices.

Bag-Mask Devices

Bag-mask devices consist of a self-inflating bag and a nonrebreathing valve (Figure 15-44). They can be used with a mask, an ET tube, or another invasive airway device. An adequate bag-valve unit should have the following components:

1. A self-refilling bag that is disposable or easily cleaned or sterilized
2. A nonjam valve system that allows a minimum oxygen inlet flow of 15 L/minute
3. A non-pop-off valve
4. Standard 15 and 22 mm fittings
5. A system for delivering high-concentration oxygen through an inlet port at the back of the bag or by an oxygen reservoir
6. A nonrebreathing valve.[26]

The device also should perform in all common environmental conditions and under extremes of temperature. It should be available in both adult and pediatric sizes. The mask should be clear to detect vomiting early.

When the bag-mask device is compressed, air is delivered to the patient through a one-way valve. The air inlet to the bag is closed during delivery. When the bag is released, the patient's expired gas passes through an exhalation valve into the atmosphere. This prevents the patient's exhaled air from reentering the bag-mask device. As the patient exhales, atmospheric air and supplemental oxygen from the reservoir refill the bag.

Use of the bag-mask device with a mask is difficult because of the problem of creating an effective seal between the mask and the patient's face while maintaining an open airway. For this reason, it has been recommended that two rescuers use the device. One should hold the mask and maintain the airway while the other compresses the bag with two hands. If three rescuers are available, one rescuer can be solely responsible for maintaining the mask seal while providing spinal precautions as indicated.

When properly used, the bag-mask device has many benefits. The rescuer can provide a wide range of inspiratory pressures and volumes to adequately ventilate patients of varying sizes and underlying pathological conditions. It can be used to assist patients with shallow respirations. It performs adequately in extremes of environmental temperatures. Oxygen concentrations ranging from 21% (room air concentration) to nearly 100% (using supplemental oxygen and a reservoir) can be achieved. In addition, manual compression of the bag can give the rescuer a sense of the patient's lung compliance, which is an advantage over mechanical methods of ventilation.

TECHNIQUE

Ventilation with the bag-mask device is best accomplished when the patient has been intubated with an ET tube or a supraglottic device (e.g., the esophageal-tracheal Combitube, King LT-D airway, or laryngeal mask airway, which are described later in this chapter). If the patient has not been intubated, the bag-mask device may be used with a mask. The following technique is recommended for use with the bag-mask device.

1. The rescuer is positioned at the top of the patient's head.
2. If no spinal injury is suspected, place the patient in the optimum head-tilt chin-lift position, with the patient's head elevated in extension. (If a spinal injury is suspected, spinal precautions should be used.) If the jaw-thrust maneuver does not produce an open airway, use the head-tilt chin-lift maneuver.

3. Clear the airway of secretions, vomitus, and foreign objects. If the patient is unconscious, insert an oropharyngeal or a nasopharyngeal airway. The patient's mouth should remain open under the mask.

4. Connect an oxygen source. Then flush the reservoir with high-concentration oxygen.

5. Place the mask on the patient's face, making a tight seal. This can be accomplished by placing the thumb on the nose area and an index finger on the chin and then spreading the remaining fingers along the mandible. The anterior displacement of the mandible must be maintained. To compress the bag, the rescuer's other hand presses the bag against his or her body (e.g., the thigh), or another rescuer compresses the bag with two hands as recommended by the American Heart Association (AHA). The bag should be compressed smoothly, delivering approximately 500 to 600 mL over 1 second (for the average adult) to produce visible chest rise.

PEDIATRIC CONSIDERATIONS

Smaller bag-mask devices are needed for infants and children. This helps to reduce the chances of overinflation and barotrauma. Bag-mask devices are used mainly for pediatric patients who are in respiratory arrest. Bag-mask devices are equipped with a fish mouth– or leaf flap–operated outlet valve should not be used to provide supplemental oxygen to an infant or a child breathing spontaneously. If the valve fails to open during inspiration, the child receives only the exhaled gases from within the mask itself. For this reason, bag devices for ventilation of full-term neonates, infants, and children should have a minimum volume of 450 to 500 mL.[20] An adult (1000 mL) bag may be needed to adequately ventilate older children. At least 10 to 15 L/minute of oxygen flow is needed to maintain an adequate oxygen volume in the reservoir of a pediatric bag (Figure 15-45). Adjust the flow rate to 15 L/min when using an adult bag.

> **NOTE**
> A child's flat nasal bridge makes achieving a mask seal difficult. In addition, compressing the mask against the face may result in obstruction. The mask seal is best achieved with jaw displacement using two rescuers to provide bag-mask ventilation.

Technique. The following procedure is used to artificially ventilate a pediatric patient with a bag-mask device:

1. Make sure the mask fits properly by using a length-based resuscitation tape or by measuring from the bridge of the nose to the cleft of the chin.

2. Make sure the mask is properly positioned and sealed. Place the mask over the mouth and nose (do not compress the eyes). With one hand, place a thumb on the mask at the apex and place the index finger on the mouth at the chin (like a C clamp). With gentle pressure, push down on the mask to establish an adequate seal. Maintain the airway by lifting the bony prominence on the chin, with the remaining fingers placed on the mandible, forming an E. Avoid putting pressure on the soft area under the chin.

3. Provide ventilations at a rate of 12 to 20 breaths/minute.

4. Deliver each breath over 1 second; both rescuers should make sure it produces visible chest rise.

5. Assess bag-mask ventilation by observing adequate rise and fall of the chest, by listening for lung sounds at the third intercostal space and midaxillary line, and by checking for improvement in skin color or heart rate, or both (see Chapter 19).

> **CRITICAL THINKING**
> What should you do if you find that ventilating a nonintubated patient suddenly has become more difficult?

Automatic Transport Ventilators

Several types of time-cycled, gas-powered, automatic transport ventilators (ATVs) are available. One commonly used in prehospital emergency care is the Autovent (Figure 15-46). Other, more sophisticated ATVs are used for intrahospital transport of patients who require ventilatory support (see Appendix A, Advanced Practice Procedures for the Critical Care Paramedic.) Most ATVs consist of a plastic control module. This module is connected by tubing to any 50 psi gas source (e.g., air or different concentrations of oxygen, including 100% oxygen). Depending on the model, the exit valve of the control module is connected by one or two tubes to the patient valve assembly to deliver selected tidal volumes (400 to 1200 mL for adults, 200 to 600 mL for children). Another control selects respiratory rates of 8 to 22 breaths/minute for adults and 8 to 30 breaths/minute

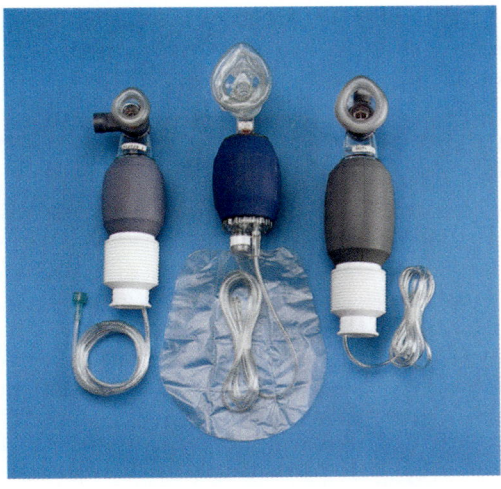

FIGURE 15-45 Pediatric bag-mask device.

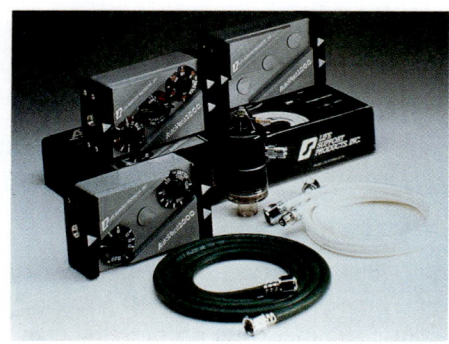

FIGURE 15-46 Autovent 1000, 2000, and 3000.

for children. (Most ATVs are not to be used in children under 5 years of age.) Most units provide a 40 L/minute flow of oxygen. This flow remains constant despite changes in the patient's airway or lung compliance.

> **NOTE**
> Automatic transport ventilators (ATVs) should have a default rate of 10 breaths/minute for adults and 20 breaths/minute for children. The paramedic should be able to adjust the rate once the patient has been intubated with a tracheal tube or alternative airway.[23]

The volume of gas delivered by the automatic ventilator is determined by the length of time the manual trigger is depressed or by the inspiratory effort of the spontaneously breathing patient. Most units are designed to limit the inspiratory pressure to 60 to 80 cm H_2O. When this pressure is reached, an alarm sounds and excess gas flow is vented off, preventing possible lung damage. On a nonintubated patient, ATVs allow the paramedic to use both hands to obtain a tight face-to-mask seal. On an intubated patient, ATVs allow the paramedic to perform other tasks. Most ATVs should not be used in patients who are awake, who have an obstructed airway, and/or who have increased airway resistance (e.g., pneumothorax, asthma, pulmonary edema).

> **NOTE**
> As described earlier, spontaneous breathing produces negative intrathoracic pressure during inspiration. It also plays an important role in maintaining cardiac output. It does this by enhancing venous return to the heart. Ventilations that are assisted with positive pressure ventilation using automatic transport ventilators (ATVs) or bag-mask devices produce positive intrathoracic pressure during inspiration. This reduces venous return and cardiac output. That is, cardiac output decreases as air pressure increases. The paramedic should remember that assisted ventilations can impair cardiac output, even in patients with healthy hearts. This effect is exaggerated when the patient is ventilated at an excessive rate or tidal volume. The use of an impedance threshold device to limit the influx of air in the lungs should be considered.[27]

AIRWAY MANAGEMENT

Science and technology have produced many devices for providing airway management. However, the paramedic must not neglect basic airway management procedures. *A basic procedure that secures a safe and functional airway is better than a more technically difficult procedure.* Airway management should progress rapidly from the least to the most invasive procedures and devices (Figure 15-47). Paramedics also should make sure they are always equipped with the appropriate personal protective equipment for these procedures (Box 15-9).

> **NOTE**
> Unconscious patients lack the muscular tone and control to maintain a patent airway. For this reason, an airway must be established and maintained in the initial assessment of all unconscious patients. Most injuries severe enough to cause loss of consciousness are severe enough to cause spinal injury. Spinal precautions should be considered in trauma patients who need airway management or ventilatory support until an x-ray film of the spine has been made.

Manual Techniques for Airway Management

Manual techniques for airway management have been described by the AHA. These include the head-tilt chin-lift method, the jaw-thrust method, and the jaw-thrust without head-tilt method. The paramedic should not use manual maneuvers to open the airway in patients who are responsive or when attempts to open the patient's mouth are met with resistance. All such maneuvers are hazardous if spinal injury is a factor. In addition, none of these maneuvers protects against aspiration.

The head-tilt chin-lift maneuver (Figure 15-48) is preferred for opening the airway when a spinal injury is not suspected. The head tilt is performed by placing one hand on the victim's forehead and applying firm backward pressure with the palm to tilt the head back. The fingers of the other hand then are placed under the bony part of the lower jaw (near the chin) and lifted to bring the chin forward. These fingers support the jaw and help maintain the head-tilt position.

BOX 15-9 Personal Protective Equipment

The Centers for Disease Control and Prevention (CDC) recommend that health care workers, in addition to taking the normal precautions for personal protection from communicable diseases, use masks, eyewear (e.g., safety glasses and face shields), and gowns when splashing of blood or other body fluids is likely. During airway management, certain patient reactions may occur. These may include vomiting and coughing. Exposure to blood and other body fluids also is possible. Because of these possibilities, the paramedic should observe barrier precautions.

ADVANCED AIRWAY MANAGEMENT

Note: Indications of emergency endotracheal intubation are (1) the inability of the rescuer to adequately ventilate the unconscious patient with a bag and mask, and (2) the absence of protective reflexes (coma or cardiac arrest).

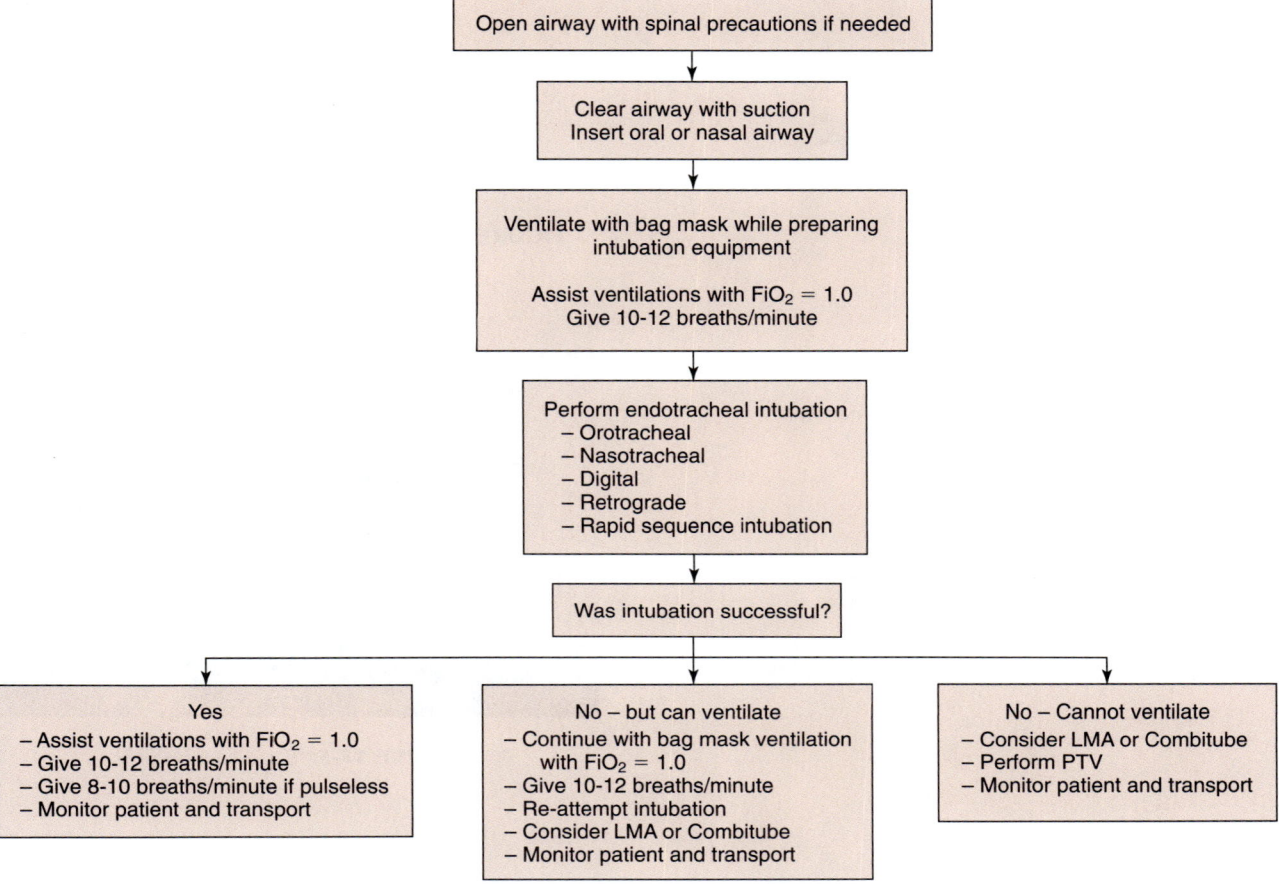

Note:
*If more than one intubation attempt is required, there should be a period of adequate ventilations between attempts.
 Correct tube placement should be verified with primary and secondary confirmation methods.

FIGURE 15-47 Advanced airway management.

The jaw-thrust maneuver (Figure 15-49) may be used to gain additional forward displacement of the mandible if no spinal injury is suspected. This is achieved by grasping the angles of the patient's lower jaw and lifting with both hands, one on each side. This displaces the mandible forward while tilting the head back. However, if the paramedic is unable to open the airway with the jaw thrust maneuver, the head-tilt chin-lift maneuver should be performed. An open airway remains the highest priority, even for an unresponsive trauma victim.

If a spinal injury is suspected, the jaw-thrust without head-tilt maneuver (Figure 15-50) should be used to open the airway. During this maneuver, the patient's head should be stabilized. Also, the cervical spine should be immobilized

with neutral, in-line stabilization. The jaw-thrust maneuver should then proceed without extension of the neck.

SUCTION

Suction can be used to remove vomitus, saliva, blood, food, and other foreign objects that might block the airway or increase the likelihood of pulmonary aspiration by inhalation. Many factors can predispose a person to aspiration. For this reason, every patient should be considered a possible aspiration victim.

Suction Devices

Fixed and portable mechanical suction devices are available through a number of manufacturers. Fixed suction devices

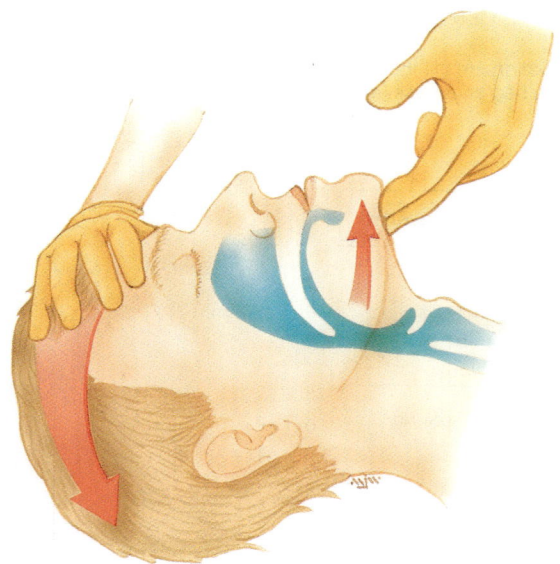

FIGURE 15-48 Head-tilt chin-lift maneuver.

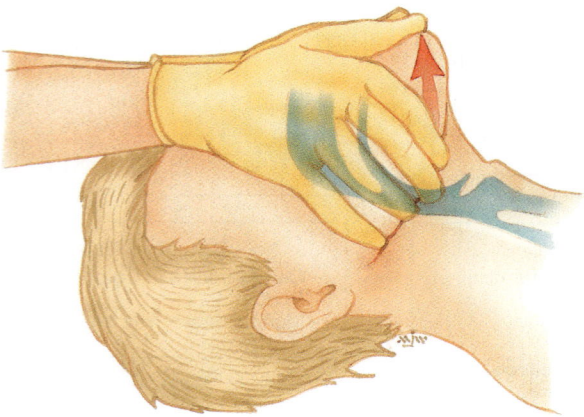

FIGURE 15-49 Jaw-thrust maneuver.

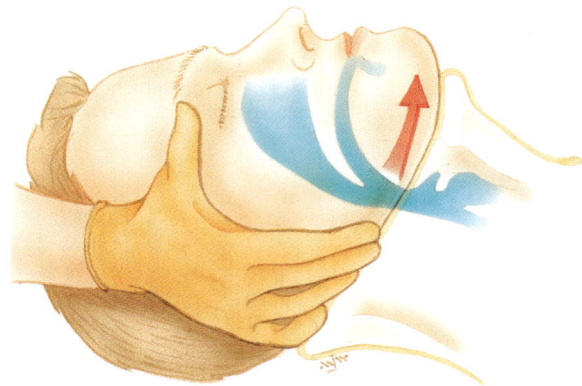

FIGURE 15-50 Jaw-thrust without head-tilt maneuver.

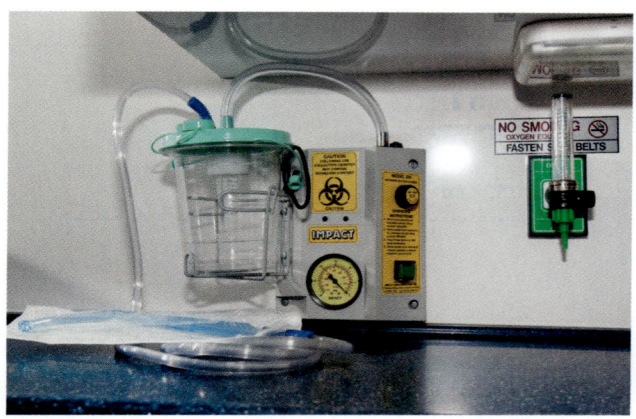

FIGURE 15-51 Fixed suction unit.

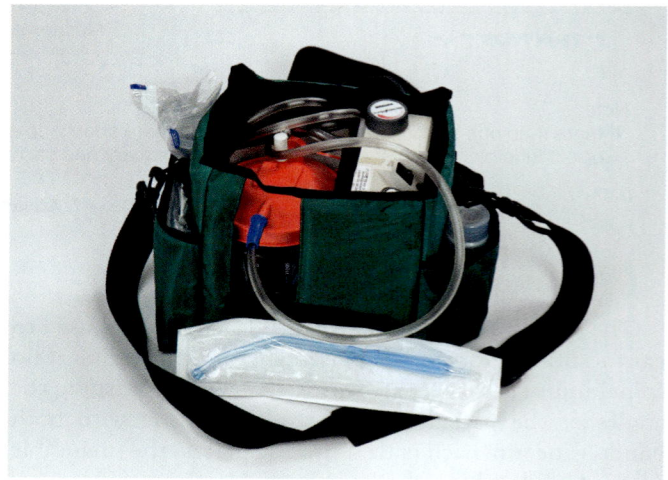

FIGURE 15-52 Portable suction unit.

(Figure 15-51) are mounted in patient care areas of hospitals and nursing homes. They also are used in many emergency vehicles. These systems are electrically operated by vacuum pumps or powered by the vacuum produced by a vehicle engine manifold. Fixed suction devices furnish an air intake of at least 40 L/minute. They provide a vacuum of more than 300 mm Hg when the tube is clamped.

Portable suction devices may be oxygen or air powered, electrically powered, or manually powered (Figure 15-52). To operate effectively, these devices should furnish an air intake of no less than 20 L/minute.

Suction Catheters

Suction catheters are used to clear secretions and debris from the oral cavity and airway passages. The two broad classifications of catheters are whistle-tip suction catheters and tonsil-tip suction catheters.

The whistle-tip catheter is a narrow, flexible tube. It is used primarily for tracheobronchial suctioning to clear

secretions through either an ET tube or the nasopharynx (Figure 15-53). This catheter is designed with molded ends and side holes to cause minimal trauma to the mucosa. It should be lubricated before insertion. A side opening in the proximal end is covered with the thumb to produce suction.

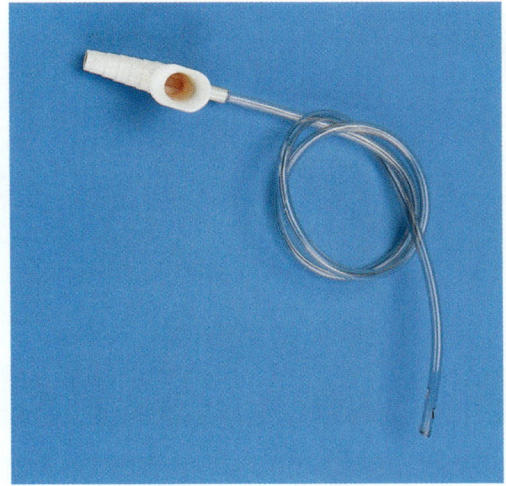

FIGURE 15-53 Soft (whistletip) suction catheter.

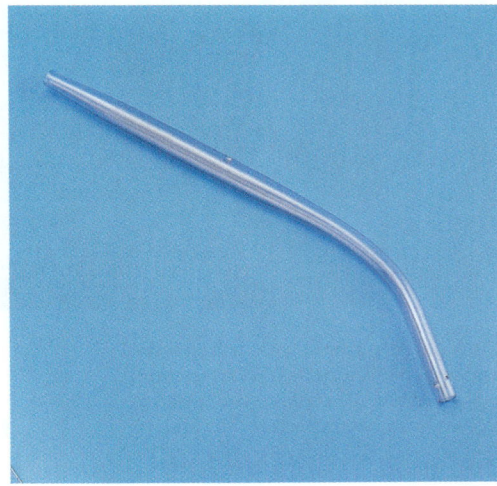

FIGURE 15-54 Rigid (tonsil tip, or Yankauer) suction catheter.

Using sterile technique, the paramedic advances the catheter to the desired location. Suction is applied intermittently as the catheter is withdrawn.

The tonsil-tip (Yankauer) suction catheter is a rigid pharyngeal catheter. It is used to clear secretions, blood clots, and other foreign material from the mouth and pharynx (Figure 15-54). The device is carefully inserted into the oral cavity under direct visualization. It then is slowly withdrawn while suction is activated.

Before any suctioning is begun, all equipment should be checked. Also, the suction should be set between −80 and −120 mm Hg. (Higher suction is needed for tracheobronchial suctioning.) If possible, the patient's lungs should be oxygenated with 100% oxygen for at least 2 minutes before suction is initiated. *Suction should never be applied for longer than 10 seconds in adult patients. It should never be applied for longer than 5 seconds in pediatric patients.* If more suctioning is needed, the patient's lungs should be reoxygenated first. Possible complications from suctioning include the following:

- Sudden hypoxemia that occurs secondary to decreased lung volume during the application of suction
- Severe hypoxemia that may lead to cardiac rhythm disturbances and cardiac arrest
- Airway stimulation that may increase arterial pressure and cardiac rhythm disturbances
- Coughing that may result in increased intracranial pressure with reduced blood flow to the brain and increased risk of herniation in patients with head injury
- Soft tissue damage to the respiratory tract

TRACHEOBRONCHIAL SUCTIONING

Before tracheobronchial suctioning is performed through an ET tube (Figure 15-55), the patient must be oxygenated with 100% oxygen for 5 minutes.[7] For tracheal suctioning, a Y- or T-piece or a lateral opening should lie between the suction tube and the source of the on-off suction control. Using sterile technique, the paramedic advances the catheter to the desired location (about the level of the carina.) Suction is applied intermittently by closing the side opening as the catheter is withdrawn in a rotating motion. The patient's cardiac rhythm should be monitored throughout the procedure. If dysrhythmias or bradycardia develops, suctioning should stop. The patient then should be manually ventilated and oxygenated. Before suctioning is resumed, the patient should be ventilated with 100% oxygen for about 30 seconds.

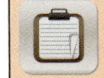

> **NOTE**
> It may be necessary to instill 3 to 5 mL of sterile saline down the endotracheal (ET) tube to loosen secretions before suctioning.

GASTRIC DISTENTION

Gastric distention results from the trapping of air in the stomach. As the stomach enlarges, it pushes against the diaphragm and interferes with lung expansion. The abdomen becomes more and more distended (especially in small children). Resistance may be felt to bag-mask ventilation.

Management. Management of gastric distention begins by slightly increasing the bag-mask ventilation inspiratory time. (Large-volume suction should be readily available.) If possible, the patient should be placed in a left lateral recumbent position. Gastric distention that cannot be managed with these techniques may require insertion of a gastric tube (Figure 15-56).

GASTRIC TUBES

Gastric distention is very common in patients who are ventilated but have not been intubated. Gastric decompression for gastric distention or vomiting control can be achieved through nasogastric (NG) or orogastric emptying or

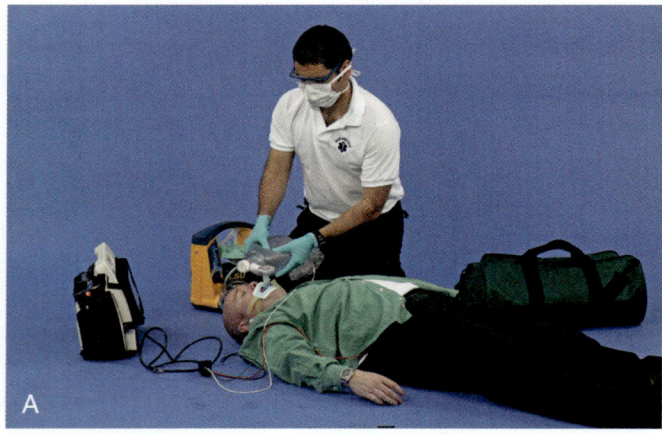
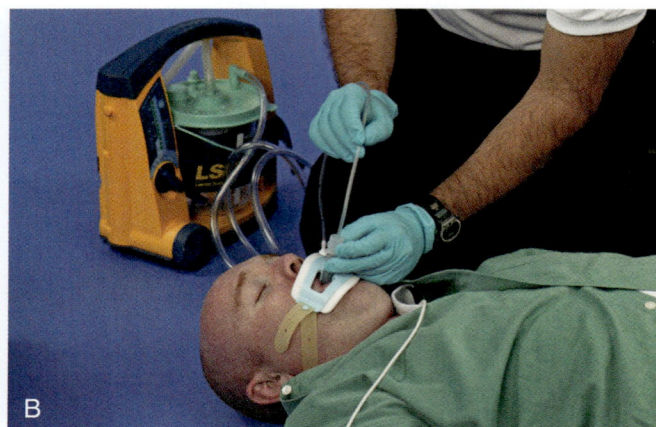
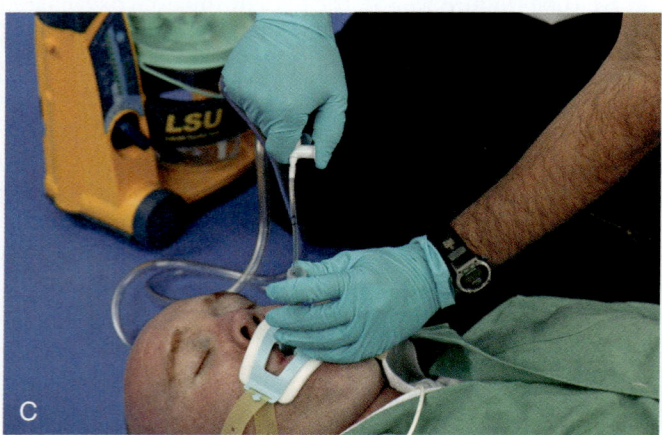
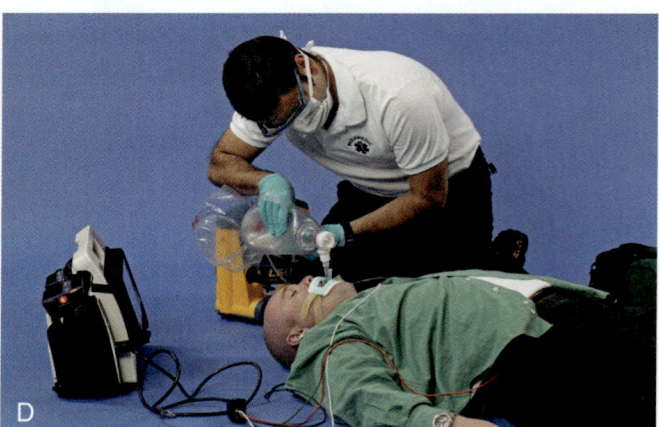

FIGURE 15-55 Tracheobronchial suctioning. **A,** Bag the intubated patient with a bag-valve device. **B,** Introduce the suction catheter through the endotracheal tube without suction. **C,** Withdraw the catheter with suction intermittently applied while observing the electrocardiographic (ECG) rhythm. **D,** Ventilate the patient and reevaluate the respiratory status.

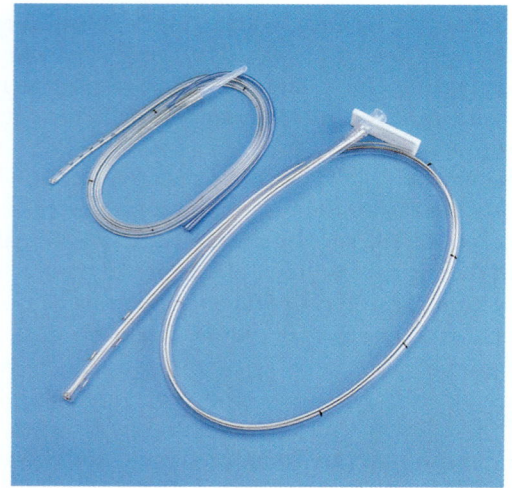

FIGURE 15-56 *Top,* Nasogastric/orogastric tube. *Bottom,* Oral gastric lavage tube.

decompression of the stomach. Gastric decompression is done with extreme caution in patients who have esophageal trauma or esophageal disease. Gastric decompression should not be performed if an esophageal obstruction is present. NG decompression should not be attempted in a patient with facial trauma or esophageal varices (large, swollen veins in the esophagus that are susceptible to hemorrhage).

Nasogastric Decompression

1. Prepare the patient.
   (a) Place the head in a neutral position.
   (b) Preoxygenate.
   (c) Instill a topical anesthetic per protocol (check for allergies).
   (d) Locate the larger nostril.
2. Measure the NG tube from the patient's nose to the ear and from the ear to the xiphoid to determine the correct insertion length. Lubricate the tube with viscous

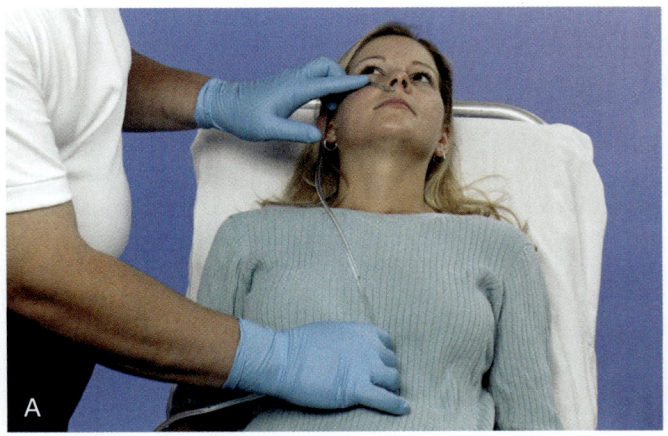
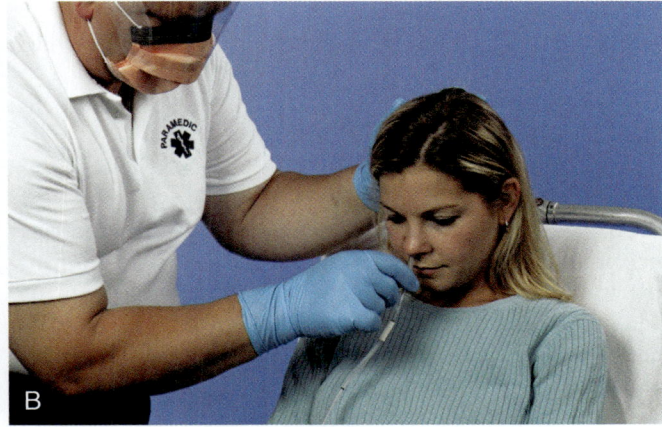
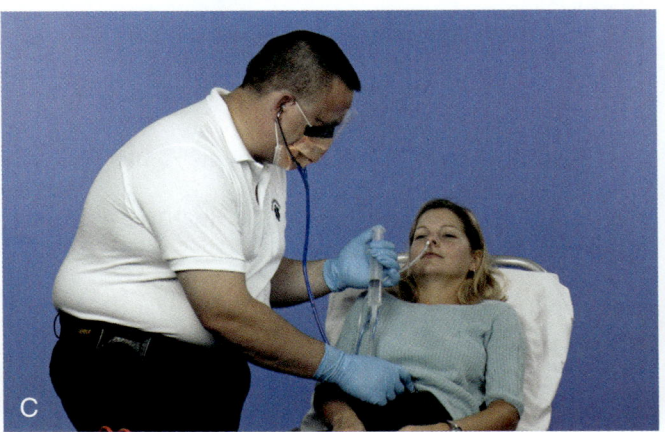
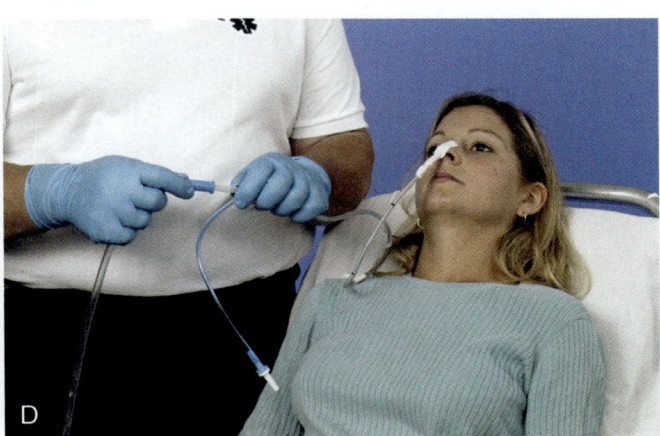

FIGURE 15-57 Insertion of a nasogastric tube. **A,** Position the patient. Measure the tube from the nose to the ear and from the ear to the xiphoid process. **B,** Lubricate the tube and insert it into the larger nostril. Advance the tube to the proper length. **C,** Verify correct placement of the tube by injecting 30 to 50 mL of air while auscultating over the epigastric area. **D,** Secure the tube and attach the suction unit.

lidocaine or water-soluble lubricant per protocol (Figure 15-57).

3. Advance the tube gently along the nasal floor and into the stomach. (Having the patient swallow during insertion may help advance the tube into the esophagus and prevent tracheal insertion.) If the patient is conscious and starts to cough vigorously, ask him or her to speak. If the patient is unable to do so, the tube likely has passed through the vocal cords.

4. Confirm placement per agency protocol.
   (a) Auscultate the epigastric region while injecting 30 to 50 mL of air.
   (b) Note gastric contents in the NG tube.
   (c) Make sure no reflux appears around the NG tube.

5. Secure the NG tube in place and attach to suction if indicated.

> ### DID YOU KNOW?
> Many clinical sites no longer use auscultation as a method to verify nasogastric (NG) tube placement. pH testing and radiographic verification are used instead. Aspiration of gastric contents provides a means of measuring fluid pH and of verifying placement of the tube tip in the gastrointestinal tract. The aspirate is obtained by attaching a catheter-tipped syringe to the end of the tube and pulling back gently on the syringe. (The aspirate usually is cloudy and green, off-white, tan, bloody, or brown.) The pH of the aspirate is measured with color-coded pH paper (Gastroccult), which is graded in whole numbers from 1 to 11. Gastric secretions usually are highly acidic (preferably a 4 or lower), compared with intestinal aspirates (usually greater than 4), or respiratory secretions (usually greater than 5.5).[28]

Orogastric Decompression

1. Prepare the patient and tube as described for NG insertion.
2. Introduce the orogastric tube down the midline of the oropharynx and into the stomach.
3. Confirm placement. Secure the orogastric tube as described for NG insertion.

Complications of Gastric Decompression. Whatever the method chosen, gastric decompression is uncomfortable for the patient. It may induce nausea and vomiting even when the gag reflex is suppressed. In addition, gastric tubes interfere with mask seals. They also interfere with visualization of airway structures during intubation. Complications of the procedures include nasal, esophageal, or gastric trauma; tracheal placement; and gastric tube obstruction.

MECHANICAL ADJUNCTS IN AIRWAY MANAGEMENT

The use of mechanical devices for airway management should never delay manual opening of the airway. These devices should be used only after efforts have been made to open the airway manually.

Nasopharyngeal Airway (Nasal Airway)

Nasal airways (Figure 15-58) are used to maintain an open airway passage in unconscious patients or in patients who are responsive but not alert enough to control their own airway. Insertion of a nasal airway may be useful as a temporary airway maintenance maneuver. It may be used to control the airway in patients with seizures or possible cervical spine injury. It also may be used before nasotracheal intubation (described later in this chapter). In addition, it can serve as a guide for insertion of an NG tube.

CRITICAL THINKING
Think about two or three specific patient conditions that would warrant the use of a nasal airway.

DESCRIPTION

Nasal airways are soft and pliable. They have a gentle curve, and the outer end is flared. Nasal airways are available in a variety of sizes to accommodate infants and adults. They range in length from 17 to 20 cm (about 7 to 8 inches) and in size from 12 to 36 French. (As with most other catheters, the French scale system is used to indicate internal diameter. Each unit of the scale equals about $\frac{1}{3}$ mm. A 21 French catheter, for example, is 7 mm [about $\frac{1}{3}$ inch] in diameter.)

To determine the correct size, the paramedic should choose an airway with a tube length equal to the distance from the tip of the patient's nose to the earlobe (Figure 15-59).

The following are recommended sizes of nasopharyngeal airways:

- Large adult: 8 to 9 mm (0.3 to 0.35 inch) internal diameter (24 to 27 French)
- Medium adult: 7 to 8 mm (about $\frac{1}{3}$ inch) internal diameter (21 to 24 French)
- Small adult: 6 to 7 mm (about $\frac{1}{4}$ inch) internal diameter (18 to 21 French)

INSERTION

The nasal airway should be lubricated with a water-soluble lubricant. This helps ease the airway through the nasal cavity. The device is placed in the nostril with the beveled tip (designed to protect nasal structures) directed toward the nasal septum. The airway is gently passed close to the midline, along the floor of the nostril, following the natural curve of the nasal passage. The airway should not be forced. If resistance is encountered, rotating the tube slightly may help, or insertion can be attempted through the other nostril (Figure 15-60).

After insertion, the nasal airway rests in the posterior pharynx behind the tongue. If the patient begins to gag, the

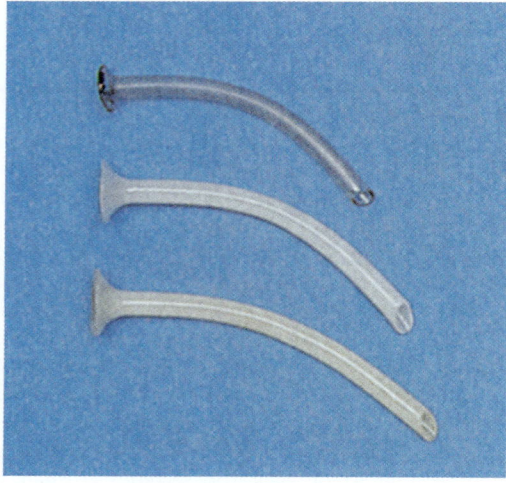
FIGURE 15-58 Nasal airways.

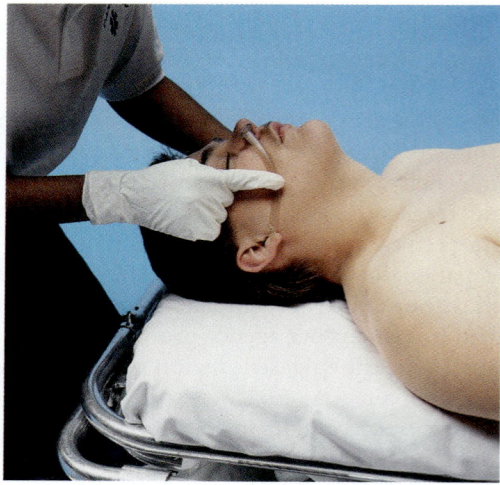
FIGURE 15-59 Measuring a nasal airway.

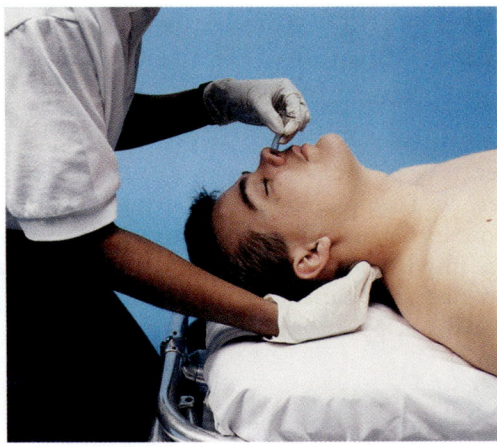

FIGURE 15-60 Insertion of a nasal airway.

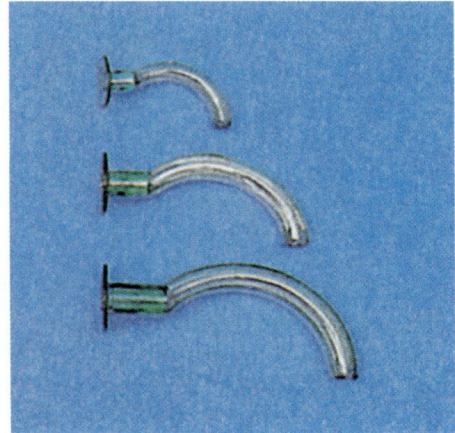

FIGURE 15-61 Oral airways.

tube may be stimulating the posterior pharynx. It may be necessary to remove the airway or withdraw it 0.5 to 1 cm (¼ to ½ inch) and reinsert it. The paramedic should maintain displacement of the mandible with either the head-tilt chin-lift or the jaw-thrust without head-tilt maneuver when using this airway.

> **NOTE**
> The cuffed oropharyngeal airway (COPA) is a modified oral airway. It has a distal inflatable cuff and proximal standard 15 mm connector. This allows attachment of a bag-mask device to the airway. The COPA may be a useful adjunct in airway management during resuscitation.

ADVANTAGES

- A nasal airway is well tolerated by conscious and semi-conscious patients with an intact gag reflex.
- Insertion is a quick procedure.
- A nasal airway may be used when insertion of an oropharyngeal airway is contraindicated or difficult because of oral trauma or soft tissue injury.

POSSIBLE COMPLICATIONS

- Long nasal airways may enter the esophagus.
- The airway may precipitate laryngospasm and vomiting in patients with a gag reflex.
- The airway may injure the nasal mucosa, causing bleeding and possibly airway obstruction.
- Small-diameter airways may become obstructed by mucus, blood, vomitus, and the soft tissues of the pharynx.
- A nasal airway does not protect the lower airway from aspiration.
- Suctioning through a nasal airway is difficult.

Oropharyngeal Airway (Oral Airway)

Oral airways are designed to prevent the tongue from obstructing the glottis. They are indicated in unconscious or semiconscious patients who have no gag reflex, and in intubated patients who are trying to bite the ET tube.

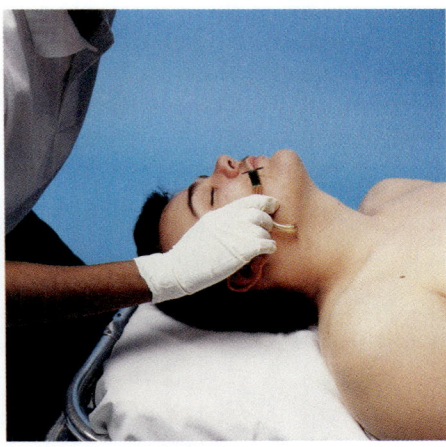

FIGURE 15-62 Measuring an oral airway.

DESCRIPTION

The oral airway is a semicircular device designed to hold the tongue away from the posterior wall of the pharynx. Most oropharyngeal airways are made of disposable plastic. The two types of airways most often used are the Guedel airway and the Berman airway. The Guedel airway is distinguished by its tubular design. The Berman airway is distinguished by the airway channels along each side of the device (Figure 15-61).

Like nasopharyngeal airways, oral airways are available in a variety of sizes ranging from infant to adult. The size is based on the distance in millimeters from the flange to the distal tip. The proper size for the patient may be determined by placing the airway next to the face so that the flange is at the level of the patient's central incisors and the bite block segment is parallel to the patient's hard palate. The airway should extend from the corner of the mouth to the tip of the earlobe or the angle of the jaw (Figure 15-62). The following sizes are recommended[20]:

- Large adult: 100 mm (about 4 inches) (Guedel size 5)
- Medium adult: 90 mm (about 3.5 inches) (Guedel size 4)
- Small adult: 80 mm (about 3.1 inches) (Guedel size 3)

INSERTION

Before an oral airway is inserted, the mouth and pharynx should be cleared of all secretions, blood, or vomitus. In an adult or older child, the oral airway may be inserted upside down or at a 90-degree angle (Figure 15-63, *A*). This helps the paramedic avoid catching the tongue during insertion. As the oral airway passes the crest of the tongue, it is rotated into the proper position. It should be situated against the posterior wall of the oropharynx. Another method of insertion is recommended for pediatric patients (Figure 15-63, *B*). (It also can be used in adults.) A tongue blade is used to displace the tongue inferiorly and anteriorly. The airway then is inserted and moved posteriorly toward the back of the oropharynx, following the normal curve of the oral cavity. Regardless of the method of insertion, care must be taken to prevent trauma to the face and oral cavity. In addition, the paramedic should make sure the patient's lips and tongue are not caught between the teeth and the airway.

CRITICAL THINKING

Why is the alternative method of oral airway insertion used for infants and young children?

Proper placement of the airway is confirmed by observable chest wall expansion. It also is confirmed by good breath sounds on auscultation of the lungs during ventilation. It is important to remember that even with an oral airway in place, the patient's head must be kept in proper position. This helps ensure a patent airway.

ADVANTAGES

- An oral airway secures the tongue forward and down, away from the posterior pharynx.
- It provides easy access for airway suction.
- It serves as a bite block to protect an ET tube and the airway in the event of seizures.

POSSIBLE COMPLICATIONS

- Oral airways that are too small may fall back into the oral cavity, resulting in blockage of the airway.
- Long airways may press the epiglottis against the entrance of the trachea, producing a complete airway obstruction.
- The airway may stimulate vomiting and laryngospasm in a patient with a gag reflex.
- The airway does not protect the lower airway from aspiration.
- Improper insertion may push the tongue back, causing it to obstruct the airway.

ADVANCED AIRWAY PROCEDURES

Advanced airway procedures described in this text include subglottic and supraglottic procedures (Box 15-10). The subglottic procedures are endotracheal intubation, digital or blind intubation, and nasotracheal intubation. The supraglottic procedures include the laryngeal mask airway (LMA), the esophageal-tracheal Combitube (ETC), and the King LT-D airway. All these procedures require special training. Before performing advanced airway procedures, the paramedic must either receive authorization from medical direction or must be operating under written protocols. These written protocols are developed by medical

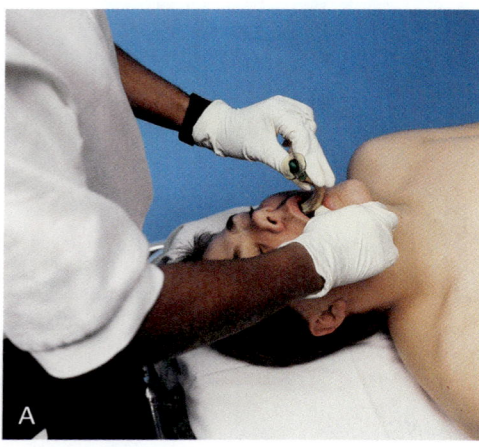

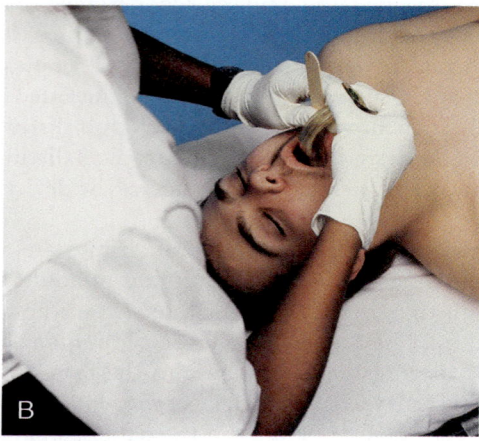

FIGURE 15-63 **A,** Inserting an oral airway upside down. **B,** Recommended method of inserting an oral airway in pediatric patients.

BOX 15-10 Advanced Airway Procedures

Subglottic Procedures
Endotracheal intubation
Digital or blind intubation
Nasotracheal intubation

Supraglottic Procedures
Laryngeal mask airway
Esophageal-tracheal Combitube
King LT-D airway

direction and the EMS agency. The paramedic also should be aware that long-term complications may result from these procedures. This may be true even when the procedures are performed properly. Such complications include aspiration, tracheal stenosis, transient dysphagia, and voice changes.

> **NOTE**
> Some EMS medical directors prefer the use of supraglottic procedures over subglottic procedures to initially secure a patient's airway. Paramedics should follow protocols and standing orders when providing advanced airway care.

Endotracheal Intubation

Tracheal intubation is the preferred technique for controlling the airway in patients who are unable to maintain an open airway. Indications for tracheal intubation include the following situations:

- The rescuer is unable to ventilate an unconscious patient with conventional methods (mouth-to-mask method, bag-mask device).
- The patient cannot protect his or her own airway (coma, respiratory and cardiac arrest).
- Prolonged artificial ventilation is needed.

The advantages of tracheal intubation are:

- The airway is isolated, which prevents aspiration of material into the lower airway.
- Ventilation and oxygenation are easier.
- Suctioning of the trachea and bronchi is easier.
- Wasted ventilation and gastric insufflation are prevented during positive pressure ventilation.
- A route is provided for administration of some medications (e.g., **naloxone, atropine, vasopressin, epinephrine,** and **lidocaine** [N-A-V-E-L]).

> **SHOW ME THE EVIDENCE**
> Cudnick and colleagues prospectively reviewed the records of patients transported by ground or air for two level I trauma centers in the state trauma registry (Oregon) from 2000 to 2003. Patients younger than 15 years and those whose out-of-hospital (OOH) time was longer than 100 minutes were excluded. Of the remaining 8707 patients, 570 (6.5%) underwent an intubation attempt in the field. The researchers found that the OOH time was 10.7 minutes longer for patients intubated with rapid sequence intubation (RSI) (95%; confidence interval [CI], 7.7 to 13.8) and 5.2 minutes longer for patients intubated without RSI (95%; CI, 2.2 to 8.1).
>
> Cudnick M, Newgard C, Wang H, Bangs C, & Herrington R, IV: Endotracheal intubation increases out-of-hospital time in trauma patients, *Prehosp Emerg Care* 11:224-229, 2007.

DESCRIPTION

The common ET tube is a flexible tube open at both ends (Figure 15-64). The proximal end has a standard 15 mm (about 0.6 inch) adapter. This adapter connects to various

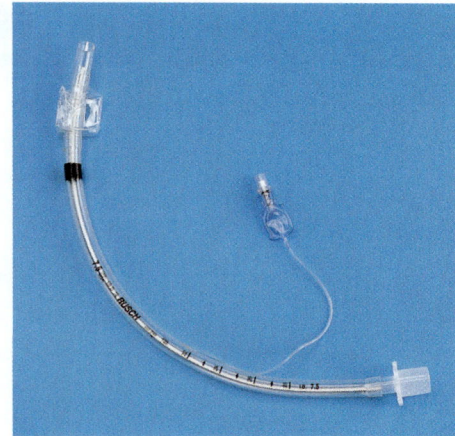

FIGURE 15-64 Endotracheal (ET) tube.

oxygen delivery devices for positive pressure ventilation. The end of the tube that is inserted into the trachea is beveled to aid placement between the vocal cords. The adult tube size (5 or larger) has a balloon cuff that closes off the remainder of the tracheal opening. This cuff prevents aspiration of fluids around the tube. It also minimizes air leakage during ventilation. The cuff is attached to a small tube. This tube has a one-way inflating valve with a port designed to fit a standard syringe. A properly positioned ET tube with the cuff inflated allows administration of high concentrations of oxygen at controlled pressures.

- In addition to the common ET tube, specialized variations are available. An example is a tube with medication ports for ET drug administration.

ENDOTRACHEAL TUBE SIZES

The markings on the ET tube indicate the internal diameter of the tube in millimeters. (The tubes are available in graduated sizes from 2.5 to 10 mm.) The length of the tube from the distal end is indicated in centimeters at several levels. Recommended ET tube sizes are 7 to 8 mm (about ⅓ inch) internal diameter for men and 7 mm (about ¼ inch) internal diameter for women.[23] Tube sizes are expressed simply as "size 6" or "size 7," without the millimeter designation.

Infant and pediatric ET tubes are available with and without balloon cuffs. Children under 8 to 10 years of age have a circular narrowing at the level of the cricoid cartilages. This narrowing serves as a functional cuff. It minimizes air leakage at the cricoid ring. Accordingly, uncuffed ET tubes are sometimes used for this age group (see Chapter 24).

Various methods can be used to determine the correct ET tube size for infants and children. Tracheal tube size for children older than 1 year may be estimated using one of the following equations[20]:

Uncuffed tube:

$$\text{Tracheal tube size (mm)} = \frac{\text{Age (yr)}}{4} + 4$$

TABLE 15-6   Tracheal Tube and Suction Catheter Sizes*

Approximate Age/Size (Weight)	Internal Diameter of Tracheal Tube (mm)	Suction Catheter Size (F)
Premature infant (<1 kg)	2.5	5
Premature infant (1-2 kg)	3.0	5 or 6
Premature infant (2-3 kg)	3-3.5	6 or 8
Infant (6-9 kg)	3.0 cuffed	8
	3.5 uncuffed	
Toddler (10-11 kg)	3.5 cuffed	10
	4.0 uncuffed	
Small child (12-14 kg)	4.0 cuffed	10
	4.5 uncuffed	
Child (15-18 kg)	4.5 cuffed	10
	5.0 uncuffed	
Child (19-23 kg)	5.0 cuffed	10
	5.5 uncuffed	
Large child (24-29 kg)	6 cuffed	10
Adolescent/Small adult (30-36 kg)	6.5 cuffed	12
Adult female	7 cuffed	12 or 14
Adult male	7 or 8 cuffed	14

*These sizes are approximations and should be adjusted on the basis of clinical experience. Tracheal tube selection for a child should be based on the child's size or age. One size larger and one size smaller should be allowed for individual variation. Color coding based on length or on the size of the child may facilitate approximation of correct tracheal tube size.

Cuffed tube:

$$\text{Tracheal tube size (mm)} = \frac{\text{Age (yr)}}{4} + 3.5$$

A more reliable method for selecting the correct ET tube size is to use length-based resuscitation tapes (for children up to 35 kg) (see Chapter 48). Suggested sizes for ET tubes and suction catheters for adult and pediatric patients are listed in Table 15-6.[9]

NECESSARY EQUIPMENT

A laryngoscope is required for visualization of the glottis during tracheal intubation. Although various makes are available, all have a number of features in common. The standard laryngoscope includes a handle made of plastic or stainless steel. The handle contains the batteries for the light source and attaches to a plastic or stainless steel blade with a bulb placed in the distal third. The electrical contact between the blade and the handle is made at a connection point called the *fitting*. The indentation of the blade is attached to the bar of the handle. When the blade is elevated to a right angle with the laryngoscope handle, the blade snaps into place and the bulb lights (Figure 15-65). (Failure of the bulb to light may be the result of a loose connection between the bulb and the bulb socket, a damaged bulb, or faulty batteries.) Other necessary equipment includes a 10 mL syringe for cuff inflation, water-soluble lubricant, and suction equipment.

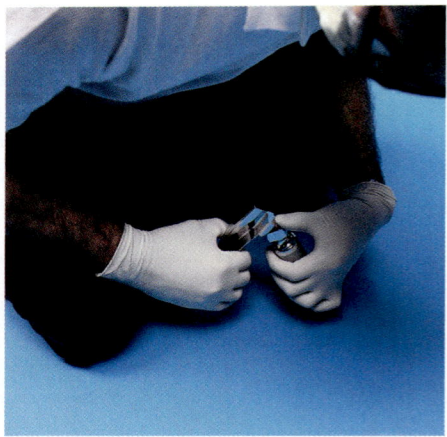

FIGURE 15-65 Attaching a blade to the handle of a laryngoscope.

Two types of blades (available in various sizes) are used with the laryngoscope: a straight blade, such as the Miller, Wisconsin, or Flagg blade (Figure 15-66), and a curved blade, such as a MacIntosh blade (Figure 15-67). The tip of a straight blade is applied directly to the epiglottis to expose the vocal cords. Advocates of the straight blade claim it provides more exposure of the glottis and less need for a stylet. A straight blade usually is recommended for infant intubation. This is because it provides greater displacement of the tongue into the floor of the mouth and better visualization of the glottic structures.

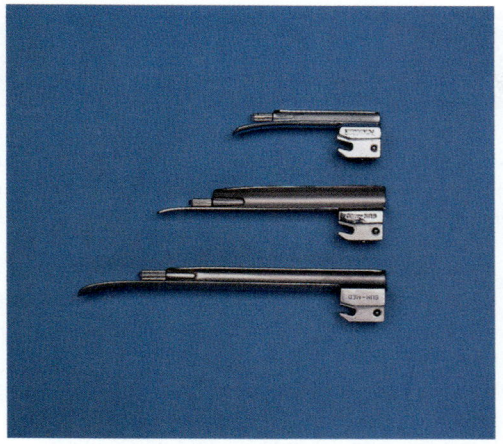

FIGURE 15-66 Types of straight laryngoscopic blades.

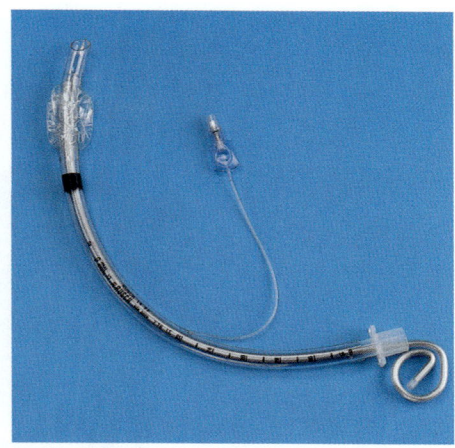

FIGURE 15-68 ET tube with malleable stylet.

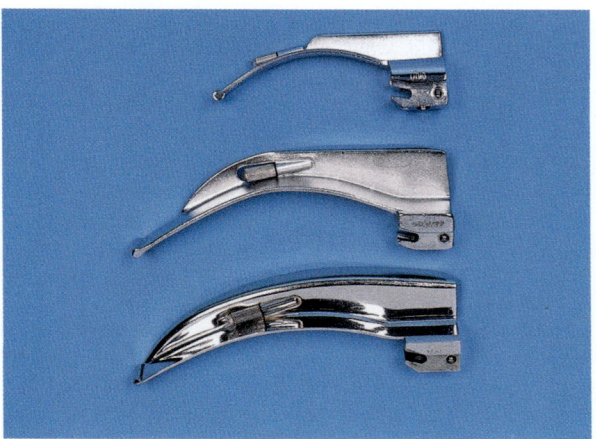

FIGURE 15-67 Types of curved laryngoscopic blades.

and may facilitate proper placement of the ET tube. If used, the stylet must be recessed 2.5 to 5 cm (1 to 2 inches) from the distal end of the ET tube to prevent injury to the patient. Recession of the stylet tip is maintained by bending the proximal end of the stylet over the proximal rim of the adapter so that it does not advance through the lumen with manipulation of the ET tube. If the stylet is allowed to extend beyond the distal end of the tube, the mucosal surface of the larynx or trachea or the vocal cords may be damaged. A gum elastic bougie (Figure 15-69) or tube introducer can be used to assist with ET tube placement. This large flexible device is placed in the trachea under direct visualization using a laryngoscope. The tracheal tube then is passed over the bougie and into position in the trachea.

> ## CRITICAL THINKING
> Ask several paramedics and anesthesiologists which laryngoscope blade they prefer and why.

The curved blade design is intended to be inserted into the vallecula. Placement of the blade displaces the tongue to the left to elevate the epiglottis without touching it. Advocates of the curved blade claim it reduces the chance of dental trauma. They also claim it provides more room for passage of the ET tube. The choice of blade is a matter of personal preference and the patient's anatomy. Paramedics should acquire expertise in using both curved and straight blades; some patients can be intubated more easily with one type than the other. Occasions also may arise when only one type of blade is available. Versatility with both curved and straight blades may improve the patient's chances of survival.

A malleable stylet (preferably plastic coated) may be inserted through the ET tube before intubation (Figure 15-68). The stylet conforms to any desired configuration

> ### NOTE
> Lighted stylets, or "light wands," are available to assist in intubation (they are useful only in low-light environments and are intended only for adult patients). These devices have a high-intensity light at the distal end. The light is powered by a small battery housing at the operator end (Figure 15-70). This device aids placement of the endotracheal (ET) tube, because the paramedic can see the light from the end of the ET tube passing through the soft tissues of the neck.
>
> Lighted stylets also can be used to help verify placement after intubation by other methods. Once the cuff has been inflated and lung sounds auscultated, the stylet is advanced through the ET tube. A bright light below the thyroid cartilage indicates proper placement. If the illumination creates a dim, indistinct light, the esophagus probably has been intubated.

Some EMS agencies also use Magill forceps (Figure 15-71), a scissors-style clamp with circular tips. It may be used to help direct the tip of the ET tube into the larynx during intubation and to remove some foreign bodies (Box 15-11).

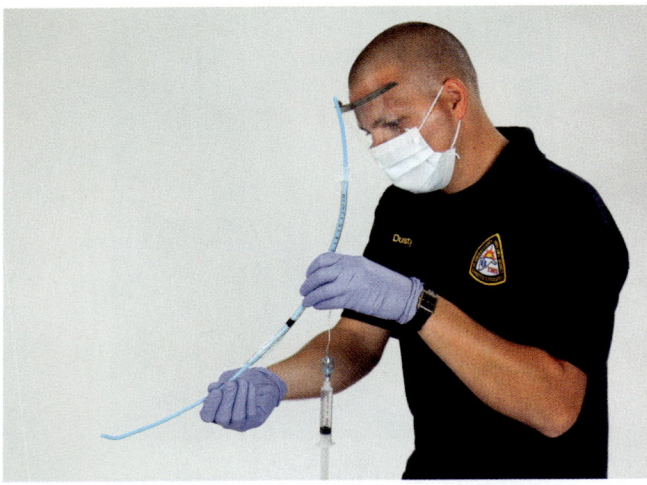

FIGURE 15-69 Gum elastic bougie (tube introducer).

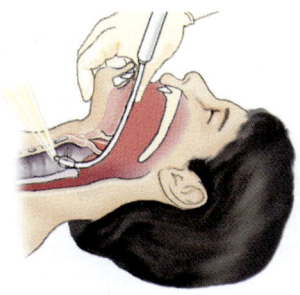

FIGURE 15-70 Fiberoptic intubation. The endotracheal tube is inserted with the aid of a lighted stylet.

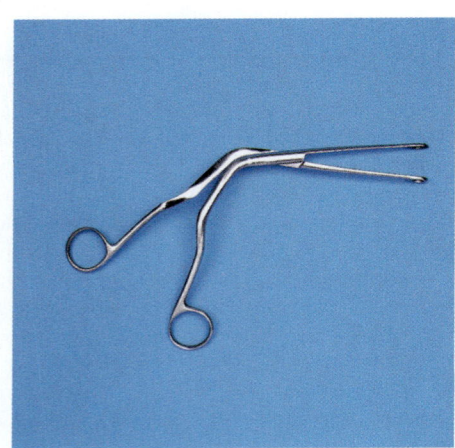

FIGURE 15-71 Magill forceps.

PREPARING FOR INTUBATION

The patient should be ventilated by other standard procedures before intubation (e.g., mouth-to-mask method, bag-mask device). The paramedic should assess the adequacy of ventilation by observing the chest rise and fall during

---

ventilation, by auscultating for breath sounds, and by noting the patient's skin color. Before intubation, the patient should be ventilated with 100% oxygen. In a pulseless patient, the goal is to avoid interrupting chest compressions for longer than 10 seconds. Interruptions for intubations should be minimized by preparing equipment beforehand. Chest compressions should be interrupted only for the placement of the tube. Chest compressions should resume immediately after the tube is distal to the vocal cords. When more than one attempt is required, the patient should receive adequate ventilation, oxygenation, and chest compressions before each attempt. The patient's lungs should then be well ventilated and oxygenated for 15 to 30 seconds by other means before intubation is attempted again. Pulse oximetry and the electrocardiogram (ECG) should be monitored continuously during intubation attempts.

Before intubation, all equipment should be examined and tested for defects. The paramedic should check the integrity of the cuff of the ET tube by inflating the balloon with 5 to 8 mL of air and checking for leaks in the cuff or inlet port. The blade of the laryngoscope should be snapped into place to examine the light bulb. The bulb should be secured in its socket and checked for brightness ("light, bright, and tight").

ANATOMICAL CONSIDERATIONS

The ET tube may be passed into the trachea through the mouth (orotracheal method) or through the nose (nasotracheal method). The orotracheal method is used most often. It is performed under direct visualization of the glottic opening. The nasotracheal route basically is a "blind" (nonvisualized) technique. The following anatomical structures are key landmarks during intubation:

- The trachea is in the midline of the neck with the superior entry at the level of the glottic opening. With orotracheal intubation, the vocal cords should be visualized while the tube is passed to ensure entry into the trachea.
- The uvula is suspended from the midline of the soft palate. It is used as a guide for correct placement of the laryngoscope.
- The epiglottis is attached to the base of the tongue. It should be visualized and elevated to expose the glottis and vocal cords. Pressure on the solid ring of the cricoid can block the esophagus, reducing the risk of regurgitation during the intubation attempt. It also may help the paramedic better visualize the entrance of the trachea by pushing it slightly posterior.

The trachea extends to the level of the second intercostal space anteriorly, at which point it divides into the left and right mainstem bronchi. The right main bronchus branches off at a very slight angle to the trachea, whereas the left branches at a 45- to 60-degree angle.

> **NOTE**
>
> An endotracheal (ET) tube that has been advanced too far most often enters the right main bronchus, bypassing and occluding the origin of the left main bronchus. If this occurs, atelectasis and pulmonary insufficiency of the left lung may result. Therefore, evaluation of ET tube placement by auscultation of both lungs is crucial. With proper ET tube placement, breath sounds should be of almost equal intensity over the two lung fields. Certain pathological conditions (e.g., pneumothorax, hemothorax, surgical removal of a lung) may result in unequal breath sounds even when an ET tube is in the proper position.

Orotracheal Intubation

In preparation for orotracheal intubation, a patient who is not a trauma victim should be placed in the sniffing position (Figure 15-72). In this position, the neck is flexed at the fifth and sixth cervical vertebrae. The head is extended at the first and second cervical vertebrae. This aligns the

three axes of the mouth, pharynx, and trachea (the oropharyngolaryngeal axis), allowing direct visualization of the larynx (Figure 15-73). (When trauma is not a factor, placing a few layers of towels under the patient's head to elevate it may be helpful.)

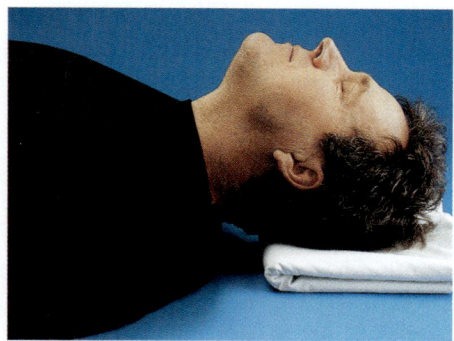

FIGURE 15-72 Sniffing position.

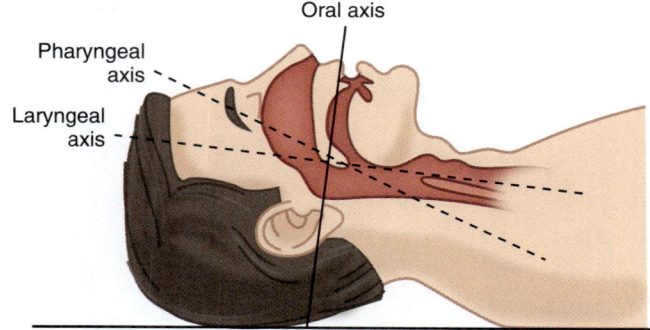

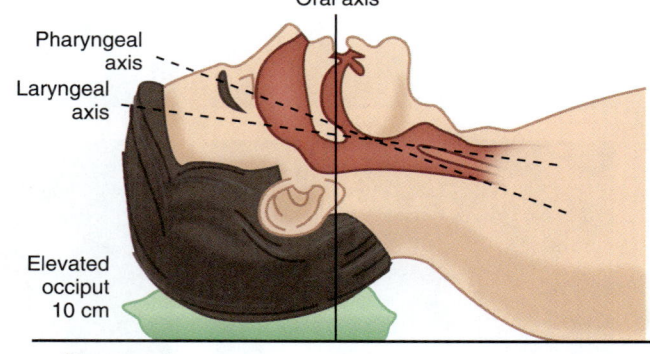

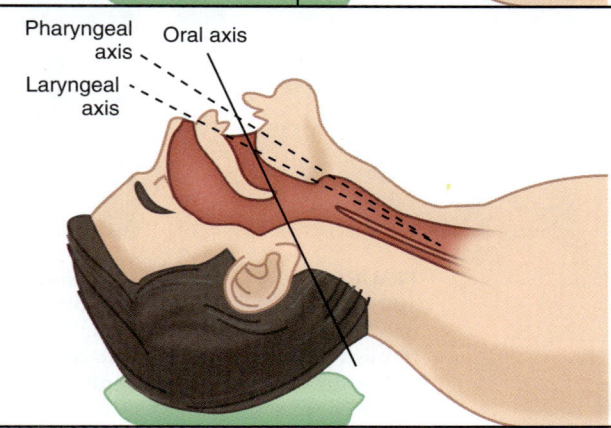

FIGURE 15-73 Oropharyngolaryngeal axis.

The orotracheal tube should be lubricated. Also, a stethoscope, stylet, and suction equipment (with large-bore catheters) should be readily available. As for all advanced airway procedures, the patient's lungs should be ventilated with 100% oxygen before intubation. The orotracheal intubation procedure is as follows (Figure 15-74):

1. Position yourself at the patient's head.
2. Inspect the oral cavity for secretions and foreign material. Suction the mouth and pharynx if needed.
3. Open the patient's mouth with the fingers of the right hand. Retract the patient's lips on the teeth or gums to avoid pinching them in the blade. The "crossed-finger technique" also may be useful in opening the patient's mouth. To perform this procedure, cross the right thumb and index finger to form an X. Place the thumb on the patient's lower incisors and the index finger on the patient's upper incisors; apply crossed-finger pressure to open the patient's mouth.

4. Grasp the lower jaw with the right hand and draw it forward and upward. Remove any dentures.
5. Holding the laryngoscope in the left hand, insert the blade into the right side of the mouth, displacing the tongue to the left. Move the blade toward the midline and the base of the tongue and identify the uvula. It is essential to work gently and avoid pressure on the lips and teeth.
6. When using a curved blade, advance the tip of the blade into the vallecula, the space between the base of the tongue and the pharyngeal surface of the epiglottis (Figure 15-75). When using a straight blade, insert the tip under the epiglottis (Figure 15-76). The glottic opening is exposed by exerting upward traction on the handle. Never use a prying motion with the handle and do not use the teeth as a fulcrum.
7. Advance the ET tube through the right corner of the mouth and, under direct vision, through the vocal

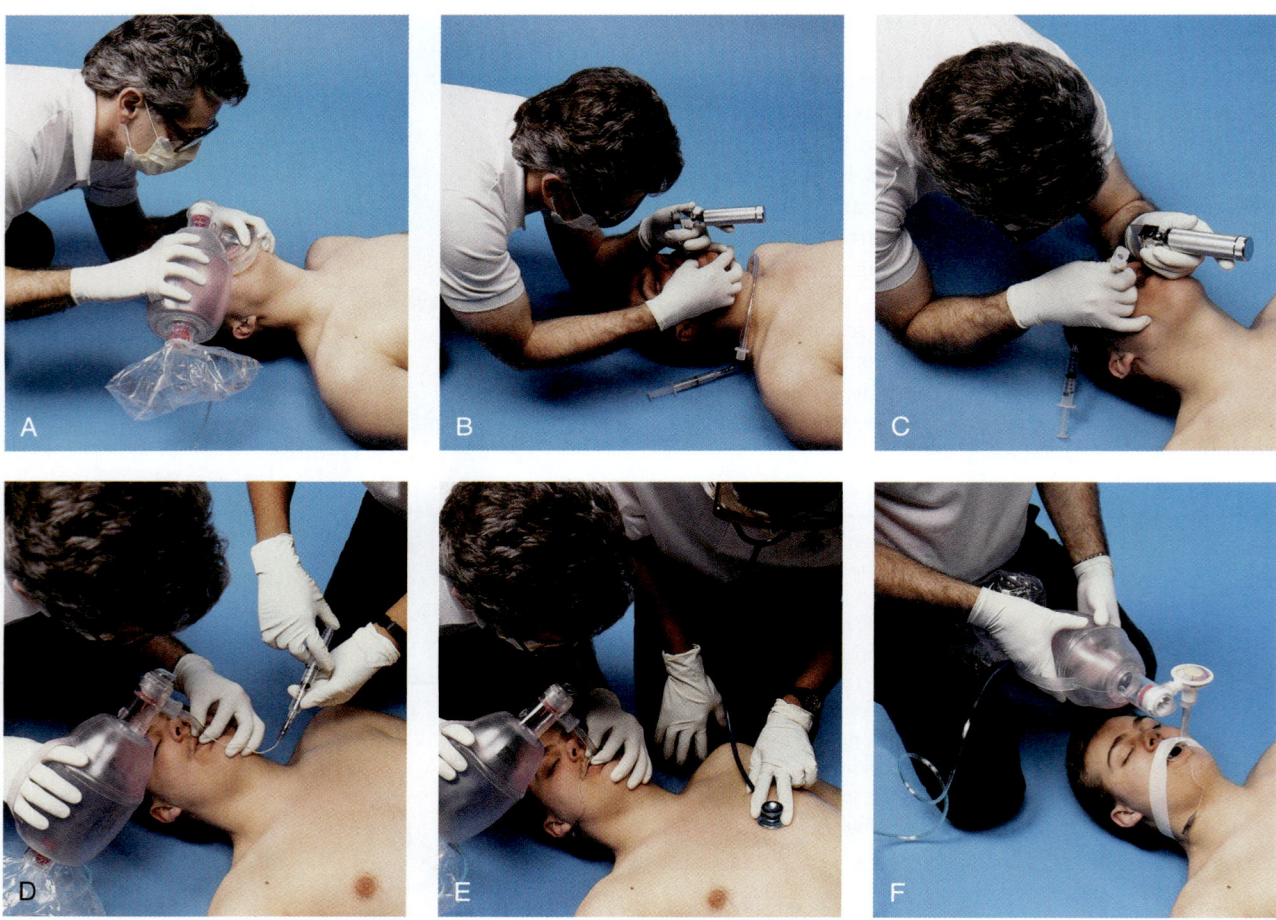

FIGURE 15-74 Orotracheal intubation. **A,** Before intubation, ventilate the patient's lungs with 100% oxygen. **B,** Hold the laryngoscope in the left hand and insert the blade into the right side of the patient's mouth, displacing the tongue to the left. **C,** Advance the endotracheal (ET) tube through the right corner of the mouth and, under direct vision, through the vocal cords. **D,** Inflate the cuff with about 10 mL of air. Ventilate the patient's lungs with a mechanical airway device. **E,** Confirm correct placement of the ET tube by primary and secondary confirmation methods. **F,** Secure the ET tube in place and provide ventilatory support with supplemental oxygen.

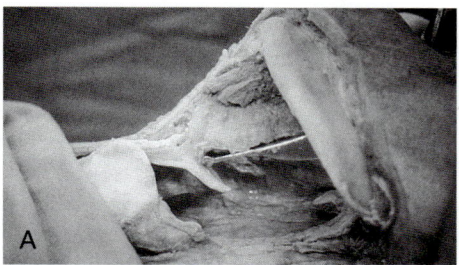

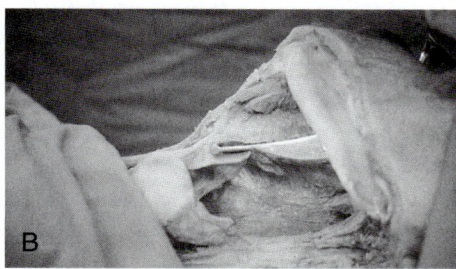

FIGURE 15-75 A, When a curved laryngoscopic blade is used, the tip of the blade is inserted into the vallecula. **B,** Direct pressure is exerted on the blade upward and toward the feet, and a lifting motion is used to expose the vocal cords.

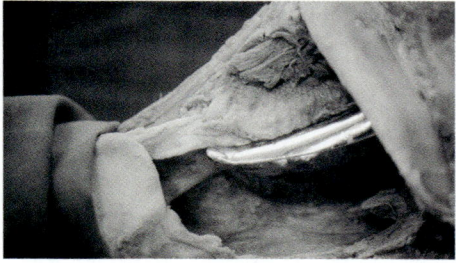

FIGURE 15-76 A straight laryngoscopic blade is used to lift the epiglottis, directly exposing the vocal cords.

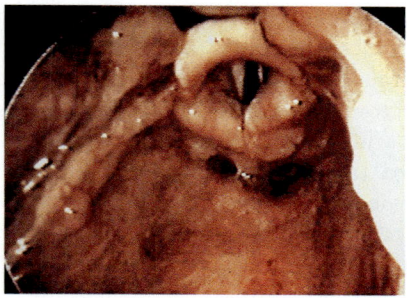

FIGURE 15-77 View of the vocal cords.

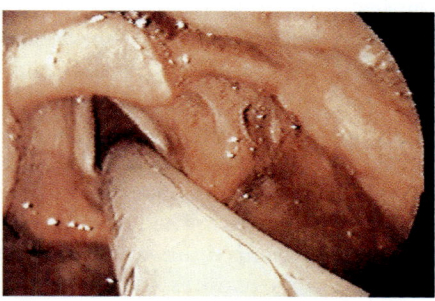

FIGURE 15-78 Endotracheal tube passing through the vocal cords.

9. Inflate the cuff with about 10 mL of air to prevent any air leaks around the tracheal cuff seal.[5]
10. Attach the tube to a mechanical airway device and ventilate the patient's lungs.
11. During ventilation, confirm accurate tube placement using primary and secondary confirmation methods.[23]

Primary Confirmation Methods. Initially confirm proper tube placement by auscultating over the epigastrium, the midaxillary region, and the anterior chest line on the right and left sides of the chest. If stomach gurgling is present or chest expansion is absent, immediately deflate the cuff and remove the tracheal tube. Reattempt intubation after oxygenating the patient's lungs with 100% oxygen for 15 to 30 seconds. When appropriate tube placement has been confirmed, reconfirm and note the tube mark at the front of the patient's teeth. Secure the tube to the patient's head and face with tape or a commercially available device. Then reevaluate lung sounds to ensure that the tube was not inadvertently repositioned. Finally, insert an oral airway or bite block. This prevents the patient from biting down and blocking the airway.

cords (Figure 15-77). If a stylet has been used, it should be removed from the tube after the tube passes through the cords into the trachea.

8. After viewing the vocal cords, make sure the proximal end of the cuffed tube has advanced past the cords about 1 to 2.5 cm ($\frac{1}{2}$ to 1 inch) (Figure 15-78). The tip of the tube should then be halfway between the vocal cords and the carina. This position allows some displacement of the tube tip during flexion or extension of the patient's neck without extubation or movement of the tip into the mainstem bronchus. (In the average adult, the distance from teeth to carina is 27 cm (about 11 inches). The paramedic should check the depth markings on the ET tube during intubation. In the average adult, the tube is properly positioned when the patient's teeth are between the 19 and 23 cm marks on the tube. This places the tip of the tube 2 to 3 cm ($\frac{3}{4}$ to 1$\frac{1}{2}$ inches) above the carina. The average tube depth in men is 22 cm (about 9 inches) ("teeth and tube at 22"). The average tube depth in women is 21 cm (about 8$\frac{1}{2}$ inches).

> **NOTE**
>
> If breath sounds are decreased or absent in the left lung, the orotracheal tube may have passed into the right mainstem bronchus, effectively bypassing the origin of the left main bronchus. If this is the case, the cuff should be deflated and the tube withdrawn 1 to 2 cm (about $\frac{1}{2}$ to $\frac{3}{4}$ inch). The cuff then should be reinflated, and tube placement should be verified as explained previously.

Secondary Confirmation Methods. A second method of determining correct tube placement requires the use of mechanical devices. These include end-tidal carbon dioxide detectors, esophageal detectors, and pulse oximetry for patients who have a perfusing rhythm. These devices are described later in this chapter. Tube confirmation should include both clinical and mechanical methods. Do not rely on a single method. Confirm correct placement immediately after intubation and each time a patient is moved.

Enhanced Optical Intubation

Enhanced optical intubation devices are available and in use by some EMS systems and are appropriate for both oral and nasal intubation procedures. Visualization of the glottis is improved in these laryngoscopes by optical or video magnification. These devices include the AirTraQ, C-MAC, GlideScope, McGrath, Shikani, Storz, and others. Using an enhanced optical laryngoscope, the glottis can be visualized and intubation performed while viewing a video monitor. Like other advanced airway techniques, intubation using these devices requires special training that is manufacturer specific, as well as authorization from medical direction. Any patient who meets the criteria for intubation (described earlier) can be intubated with an optical, video or fiberoptic device[29] (Figure 15-79).

Video-assisted intubation involves inserting a video laryngoscope into the patient's mouth and then into the pharynx. Upon visual confirmation of the glottic opening, the ET tube is advanced through a specially-designed channel or alongside the laryngoscope. The tube is placed in the trachea under direct vision, using the video monitor.

Digital (Blind) Intubation

Before the advent of laryngoscopes, intubation was performed by the intubator inserting his or her fingers into the patient's mouth. The fingers were used to guide the ET tube into the trachea. This is not a common prehospital procedure. However, digital intubation may be necessary in cases of patient entrapment, in patients whose airway is blocked from view by large amounts of blood or other secretions, or if equipment fails. Digital intubation also may be used in certain disaster or tactical situations in which victims are widespread and equipment is in short supply. The procedure for digital (blind) intubation is as follows:

1. Position yourself at the patient's left side. If a spinal injury is suspected, have a second rescuer maintain in-line spinal immobilization.
2. Ventilate the patient with 100% oxygen before intubation.
3. Use a bite stick or other device to hold the patient's mouth open. This helps protect the rescuer's fingers.
4. Bend the tube and stylet combination into a J or hockey stick configuration.
5. Insert your gloved left middle and index fingers into the patient's mouth. Alternating fingers, "walk" down

the patient's tongue, pulling the tongue and epiglottis away from the glottic opening.

6. When you feel a flap of cartilage covered by mucous membrane with your middle finger, you have reached the epiglottis (Figure 15-80, *A*). Maintain contact and advance the ET tube with your right hand. Use the index finger of your left hand as a guide (Figure 15-80, *B*). The index finger maintains the tube position against the middle finger, leading the tip of the tube into the glottic opening. It may be helpful for a second rescuer to perform the Sellick maneuver to close off the esophagus and help prevent aspiration.
7. Once the cuff of the ET tube passes the tips of the paramedic's fingers, inflate the cuff, remove the stylet, and verify placement in the usual manner.
8. Secure the tube as previously described.

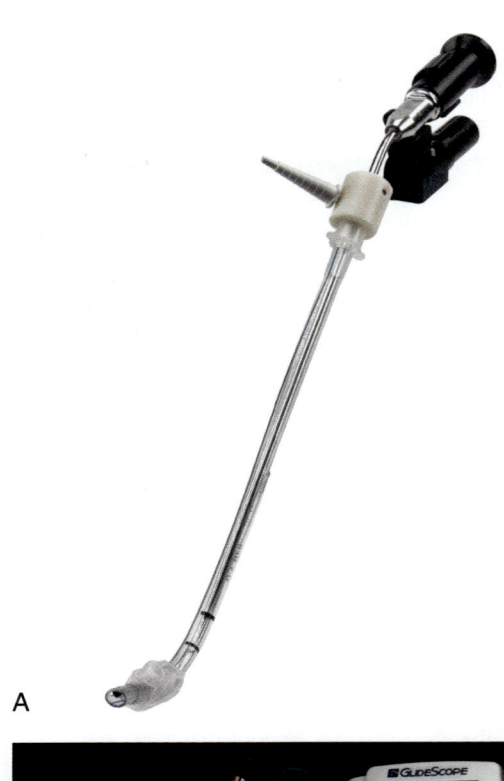

A

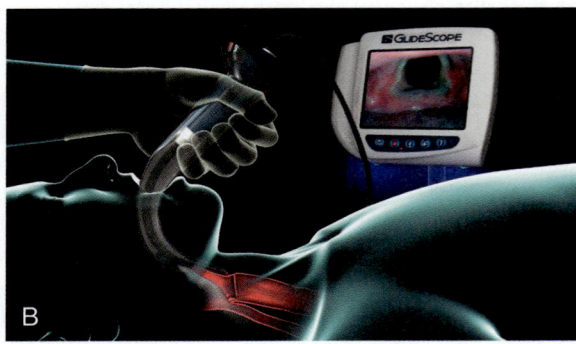

FIGURE 15-79 A, Shikani Seeing Optical Stylet. **B,** GlideScope. **(A** courtesy Clarus Medical, Minneapolis, Minn; **B** courtesy Verathon, Bothell, Wash.)

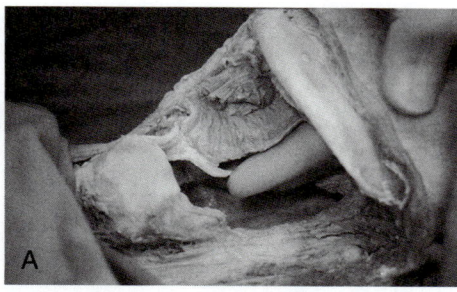

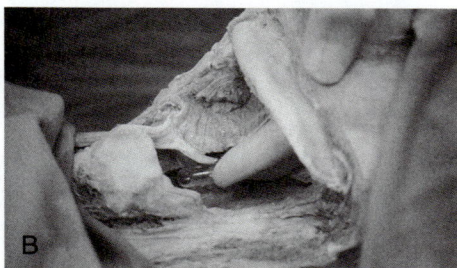

FIGURE 15-80 A, Locate the epiglottis with the tips of the fingers of one hand. **B,** Using the palpated epiglottis as a landmark, guide the endotracheal (ET) tube into the larynx.

Correct ET tube placement should be confirmed often. At a minimum, reconfirm placement each time a patient is moved or has a sudden change in condition.

Potential Complications from Intubation Procedures

- Accidental intubation of the esophagus
- Accidental intubation of a bronchus
- Lacerated lips or tongue (oral)
- Dental trauma from the laryngoscope (oral)
- Lacerated pharyngeal or tracheal mucosa
- Tracheal rupture
- Avulsion of an arytenoid cartilage
- Vocal cord injury
- Vomiting and aspiration of stomach contents
- Significant release of epinephrine and norepinephrine, leading to hypertension, tachycardia, or cardiac rhythm disturbances
- Vagal stimulation (particularly in infants and children), resulting in bradycardia and hypotension
- Increased intracranial pressure in patients with a head injury
- Hypoxia related to prolonged intubation attempts
- Displacement when the patient moves or is moved

In addition, rupture of the cuff, inflation port malfunction, or severance or kinking of the inflation tube may cause cuff malfunction and air leakage.

Nasotracheal Intubation

At times nasotracheal intubation may be the airway procedure of choice. This may be the case in patients who have spontaneous respirations, when laryngoscopy is difficult, or when the motion of the cervical spine must be limited. Examples of such conditions include the following:

- Medication overdose
- Asthma or anaphylaxis
- Chronic obstructive pulmonary disease
- Stroke
- Seizure (status epilepticus with constant seizure activity)
- Altered mental status

These and other situations may make aligning the oropharyngolaryngeal axis difficult. This rules out successful orotracheal intubation. It should be noted that nasotracheal intubation is a blind procedure. It carries a high risk of improper tube placement, because the paramedic cannot visualize the vocal cords.

In general, conscious patients tolerate a nasotracheal tube better than an orotracheal tube. Also, a nasotracheal tube often causes less trauma to the tracheal mucosa. This is because the tube moves less inside the trachea with head motion than does an orotracheal tube. If time allows, the paramedic should prepare the patient using a vasoconstrictor spray and topical anesthetic. (Examples of these are phenylephrine spray and lidocaine jelly.) These measures may make the patient more comfortable. They also reduce the risk of nasal hemorrhage, which may occur secondary to the procedure. If time allows, placement of a soft nasopharyngeal airway before the procedure may show which nostril is more passable. This also may compress the mucosa, allowing less traumatic placement of the ET tube (Figure 15-81).

 NOTE
Nasotracheal intubation is not recommended in patients who are apneic, who have midfacial fractures or nasal fractures, or who are suspected of having a basilar skull fracture.

INSERTION

The procedure for inserting a nasotracheal tube is as follows:

1. Choose a cuffed ET tube that is 1 mm smaller than optimal for oral intubation. (Most ET tubes are designed for both orotracheal and nasotracheal intubation. Some longer ET tubes are designed specifically for this procedure. A ringed ET tube [Endotrol] also is available that controls the tip of the ET tube, aiding entry into the trachea.) Prepare and check all needed equipment (balloon cuff, syringe, suction, stethoscope). Stylets are not used in nasotracheal intubation. This is because the stylet reduces flexibility and increases the risk of injury during blind insertion.

2. Ventilate the patient with 100% oxygen before intubation.

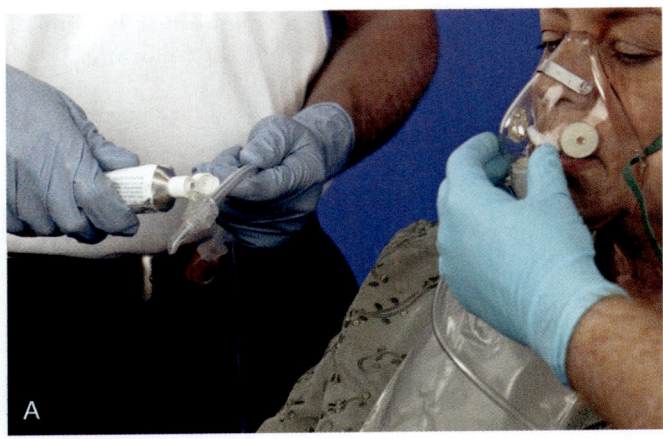

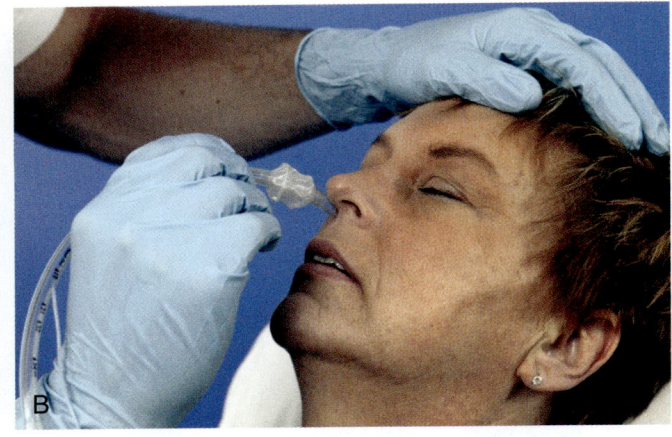

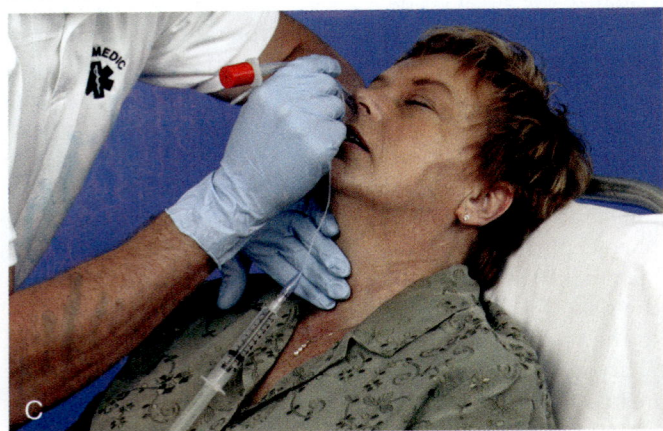

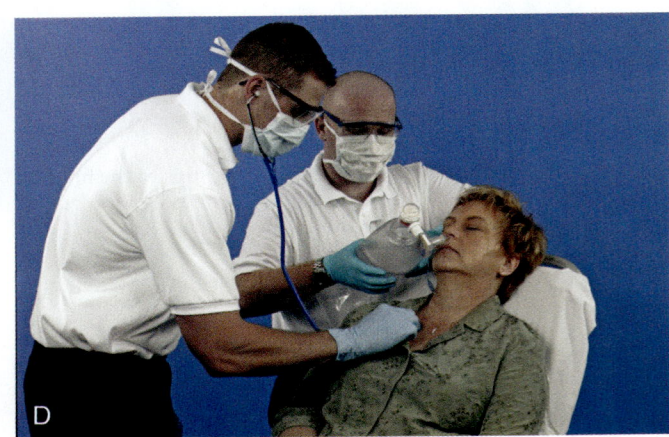

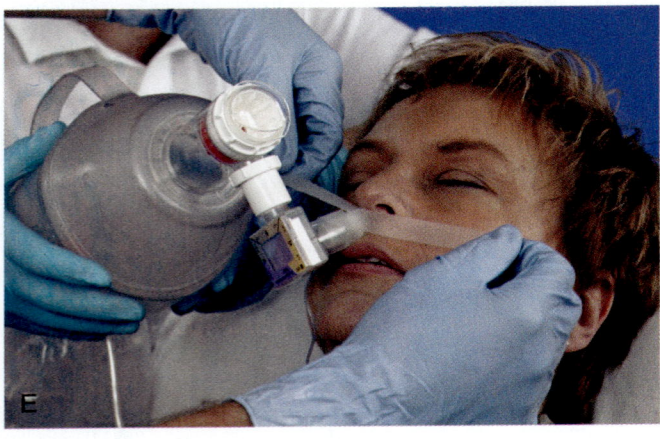

FIGURE 15-81 Nasotracheal intubation. **A,** Oxygenate the patient while the nasotracheal tube is prepared and lubricated. **B,** Insert the tube into the larger nostril. **C,** Palpate the larynx while listening for airflow over the tube as it is advanced. **D,** Ventilate the patient and confirm correct placement of the tube. **E,** Secure the tube and monitor the patient.

3. Lubricate the ET tube with a water-soluble or lidocaine jelly.

4. Insert the tube with the flange facing the nasal septum. Advance the tube along the nasal floor of the nostril that is clearer and more direct. If both nostrils appear open, advance through the larger nostril first. If the chosen nostril is impassable, try the other nostril before selecting an ET tube that is 0.5 mm smaller in diameter.

5. Stand beside the patient with one hand on the tube and the thumb and index finger of the other hand palpating the larynx. The curve of the tube should follow the natural curve of the airway. Gently advance the tube while rotating it medially 15 to 30 degrees until maximal airflow is heard through the tube. (Airflow sounds can be amplified by placing a simple device called the Beck airway airflow monitor [BAAM] whistle on the end of the endotracheal tube.) Gently

and swiftly advance the tube during early inspiration. Voluntary tongue extrusion in cooperative patients is helpful. Otherwise, the tongue can be wrapped with gauze and pulled forward. Flexion of the neck (if no spinal instability is suspected) and posterior pressure on the thyroid cartilage may help position the larynx.

6. Externally observe the advancement of the tube toward the carina. Misting or condensation on the tube should be evident as the tube approaches tracheal placement. This occurs because the patient's exhaled breath has a high concentration of water vapor. The water vapor promptly condenses on exposure to cooler room air. However, tube misting is not always a reliable indicator of proper tube position.

7. On completion of intubation, verify proper tube placement as described before. Inflate the cuff with about 10 mL of air and secure the tube in place. Ventilations may then be assisted with supplemental oxygen, or the patient's lungs can be ventilated by mechanical means.

8. If intubation fails, withdraw the tube and redirect it after ventilating and oxygenating the patient. It may be possible to recognize tube misplacement by inspecting and palpating the neck for bulges.

> **NOTE**
> Another device used to aid placement of the nasotracheal tube is the airway whistle, or Beck Airway Airflow Monitor (BAAM). The whistle, which is attached to the standard 15 mm endotracheal connector, amplifies the patient's breathing as the tube is advanced through the posterior nasopharynx. As the tube is advanced farther, the sound increases in intensity. Deviation from the airflow tract results in a decrease in or loss of the whistle sound, indicating a need for tube redirection. Once intubation is complete, the airway whistle is removed.

POSSIBLE COMPLICATIONS

- Epistaxis (nosebleed)
- Vagal stimulation
- Injury to the nasal septum or turbinates
- Retropharyngeal laceration
- Vocal cord injury
- Avulsion of an arytenoid cartilage
- Esophageal intubation
- Intracranial tube placement if the patient has a basilar skull fracture

Intubation with Spinal Precautions

Nasal or oral intubation may be performed in patients suspected of having a spinal injury. The procedure is as follows:

1. Auscultate for bilateral breath sounds while manual or mechanical ventilations are in progress. This provides a baseline.

2. One rescuer should apply manual in-line stabilization from the patient's side. The rescuer places the hands over the patient's ears. The little fingers should be under the occipital skull. The thumbs should be on the face over the maxillary sinuses. Stabilization (without distraction) should be maintained in a neutral position throughout the procedure. Thin padding under the patient's head may be necessary to maintain neutral, in-line positioning.

> **NOTE**
> Intubation of patients suspected of having a spinal injury is controversial[30] and should be authorized by medical direction. Any type of airway manipulation may be dangerous. If the paramedic and medical direction elect to intubate the trachea of a patient suspected of having a spinal injury, in-line stabilization must be maintained. Two trained rescuers are required. Video-assisted devices may be helpful in these situations.

3. In one method of intubation, the primary paramedic is positioned at the patient's head. The legs straddle the patient's shoulders and arms, and the patient's head is secured between the paramedic's thighs. The grip of the primary rescuer in this position and of the other rescuer (from the side) prevents the head from moving during the intubation. In this position, the primary paramedic may need to lean back to visualize the vocal cords (Figure 15-82). With another method, the primary paramedic lies prone at the patient's head, and the other rescuer (at the patient's side) maintains the in-line position alone (Figure 15-83).

FACE-TO-FACE OROTRACHEAL INTUBATION

Face-to-face orotracheal intubation (Figure 15-84) may be used when the paramedic cannot take a position above the patient's head (e.g., the patient is in a sitting position). In

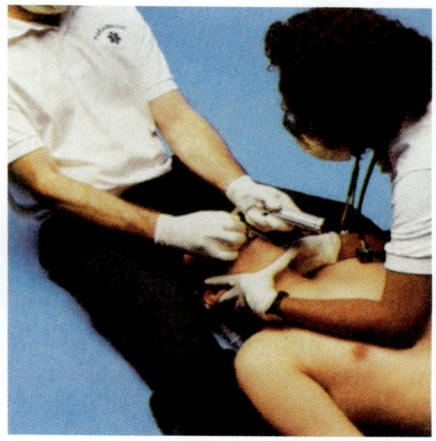

FIGURE 15-82 Intubation in a sitting position.

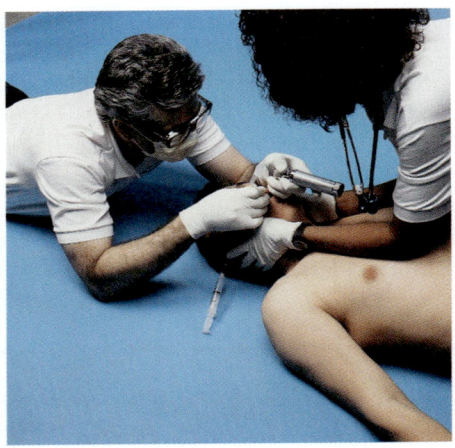

FIGURE 15-83 Intubation in a prone position.

this method of intubation, a second rescuer maintains in-line immobilization of the patient's neck and head from behind the patient. The primary rescuer takes a position facing the patient. The patient's mouth is opened with the left hand. The laryngoscope is held in the right hand, and the blade is inserted into the patient's mouth, following the normal curve of the tongue. After visualizing the vocal cords from a position above the patient's mouth, the primary rescuer passes an ET tube between the cords with the left hand. The cuff is inflated and the syringe removed. The patient then is ventilated with a bag-mask device. After proper placement has been confirmed as previously described, the ET tube is secured in place. Video laryngoscopy devices can be helpful when spinal motion needs to be restricted and in face-to-face situations.

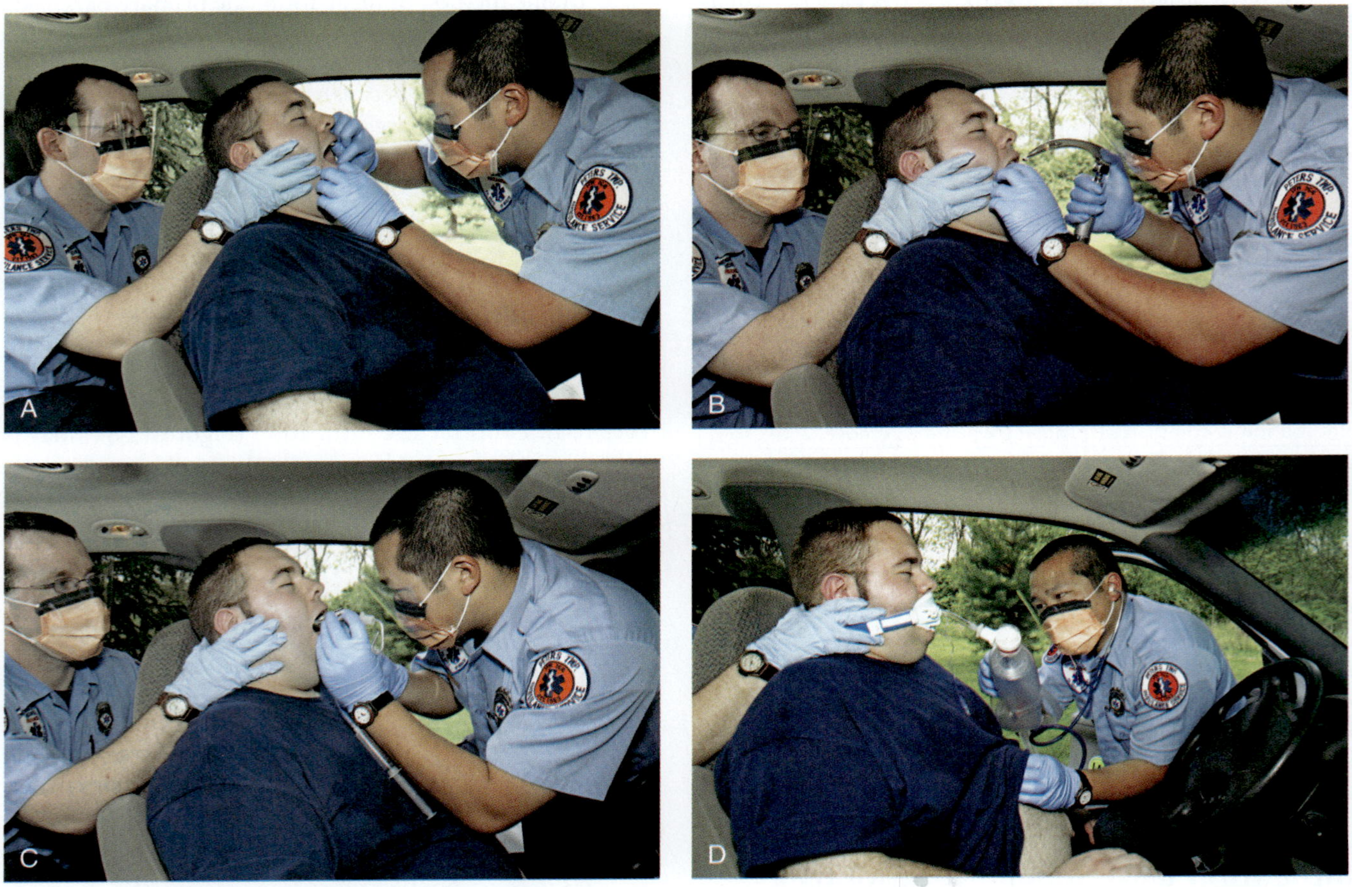

FIGURE 15-84 Face-to-face orotracheal intubation. **A**, One rescuer maintains in-line immobilization. The primary rescuer takes a position facing the patient and opens the person's mouth. The primary rescuer then should follow these steps: **B**, Hold the laryngoscope in the right hand and insert it into the patient's mouth. **C**, With the left hand, pass the endotracheal (ET) tube into the mouth and through the vocal cords. **D**, Inflate the cuff. Ventilate the patient and confirm correct placement of the tube. Secure the tube in place.

EXTUBATION

The ET tube is not usually removed in the prehospital setting. However, the patient may develop intolerance to the tube. Also, sedating the patient to improve tolerance may not be possible. In such cases medical direction may advise extubation. If time allows, the patient's lungs first should be ventilated with 100% oxygen. To remove the ET tube, the paramedic should tilt the patient or backboard to one side and proceed as follows:

1. Have suction available. (The oral cavity and the area above the cuff should be suctioned before the ET tube is removed.)
2. Deflate the cuff completely.
3. Swiftly withdraw the tube on cough or expiration.
4. Assess the patient's respiratory status.
5. Provide high-concentration oxygen; assist ventilations as needed.

NOTE
Patients who are awake are at high risk of laryngospasm immediately after extubation. Also, they may be difficult to reintubate should respiratory distress or failure recur.

Advantages of Endotracheal Intubation

- It provides complete airway control.
- It helps prevent aspiration.
- It prevents gastric distention.
- It may provide a route for administration of some drugs.
- Positive pressure ventilation can be delivered.
- It allows tracheal suctioning.
- High concentrations of oxygen and large volumes of ventilation can be delivered.

Special Considerations for Pediatric Intubations

In addition to the differences in airway and ventilation procedures for pediatric patients, the anatomical differences of the pediatric airway must be considered.[23] These anatomical differences include the following:

1. The infant's upper airway is relatively small; the tongue is disproportionately large. Therefore posterior displacement of the tongue easily obstructs the airway. In addition, the larger tongue of the pediatric patient tends to make laryngoscopy more difficult. Have another rescuer pull on a corner of the mouth to increase visualization.
2. The epiglottis is shaped like the Greek letter omega (Ω). It is narrower and longer in children than in adults. Because of this, the epiglottis is more difficult to control with a laryngoscopic blade. The larynx lies more anteriorly in relation to the base of the tongue than in the adult. It also is elevated under the base of

the tongue, making visualization more difficult. The glottic opening is at the third cervical vertebra in premature neonates, the third to fourth cervical vertebrae in term neonates, and the fourth to fifth cervical vertebrae in adults.

3. During the first few months of life, the infant's vocal cords slope from back to front. As a result, the ET tube frequently gets hung up in the angle formed by the cords. This problem can be minimized by rotating the ET tube or by having a second rescuer perform the Sellick maneuver during intubation.
4. The cricoid cartilage is the narrowest part of the airway in the infant and young child. As the child reaches 8 to 10 years of age, the vocal cords become the narrowest part. This remains the case into adulthood.
5. The distance from the vocal cords to the carina varies and can be correlated with the patient's height. This distance is about 4 to 5 cm (2 to 2½ inches) at birth and 6 to 7 cm (3 to 3½ inches) by 6 years of age. During placement of the ET tube, the tube should be advanced until breath sounds are lost unilaterally (usually on the left side). It should then be withdrawn slowly until breath sounds return, indicating that the tube tip is at the carina. After the return of breath sounds, the tube should be withdrawn 2 to 3 cm (¾ to 1½ inches) farther, placing it at a safe distance above the carina and below the cords. The tube then should be secured with tape or a commercial device.

NOTE
The correct depth of insertion for an endotracheal (ET) tube in children over age 2 can be approximated by adding one half the patient's age to 12.

$$\text{Depth of insertion (cm)} = \frac{\text{Patient's age}}{2} + 12$$

Alternatively, the depth of insertion can be estimated by multiplying the internal diameter of the tube by 3.[20]

Depth of insertion (cm) = ET tube internal diameter × 3

6. Children use the diaphragm as the major muscle for ventilation. They require full diaphragmatic excursion to breathe. Gastric distention caused by swallowing air or artificial ventilation can inhibit the child's respiratory efforts. Infants are nose breathers until 3 to 5 months of age.
7. Deciduous teeth begin to develop at about 6 months. These are lost between 6 and 8 years. They may become dislodged during airway procedures such as intubation and oral airway insertion and by the child biting on the airway.

During any airway procedure, the paramedic should remember that the airway structures of children are very fragile and easily damaged. Therefore, great care must be taken not to injure these patients.

Adjuncts to Aid Confirmation of Endotracheal Tube Placement

Several adjuncts often can help the paramedic determine correct ET tube placement. These include end-tidal carbon dioxide detectors, bulb- or syringe-type esophageal detection devices, and pulse oximeters. As stated previously, confirmation of tube placement requires more than one method of assessment.

END-TIDAL CARBON DIOXIDE DETECTORS

Capnography is the measurement of carbon dioxide concentrations in exhaled air. This measurement is made possible by end-tidal carbon dioxide ($EtCO_2$) detectors. $EtCO_2$ detectors are designed to help verify placement of the ET tube. They also are designed to reveal inadvertent esophageal intubation. These devices provide a noninvasive estimate of alveolar ventilation, carbon dioxide production, and arterial carbon dioxide content. Their use as an adjunct to assessment of ET tube placement is strongly encouraged.[20,23]

> **NOTE**
> The color indicators of colorimetric carbon dioxide (CO_2) detectors can be affected by vomitus. They also can be affected if the patient recently drank a carbonated beverage (if the endotracheal tube is placed in the esophagus).

Three types of carbon dioxide detectors are available: disposable colorimetric devices and electronic capnometry and capnography devices. Colorimetric devices contain a chemical indicator that is sensitive to carbon dioxide. When the detector is attached to the ET tube, the color of the indicator changes with elevated carbon dioxide. These elevations would be expected in the trachea but not in the esophagus. A memory aid for colorimetric devices is as follows: *yellow* (yes, the ET tube is correctly placed in the trachea); *tan* (think about it; the ET tube may not be in the trachea); and *purple* (problem; the ET tube is not in the trachea). Colorimetric devices provide limited information and can be used only for short periods. Exposure to secretions may render them ineffective (Figure 15-85).

> **NOTE**
> Cardiac output is very low during cardiopulmonary resuscitation. Consequently, colorimetric devices may show no color change even when the endotracheal (ET) tube is in the trachea. In such cases, a second method of confirming tube placement should be used, such as an esophageal detector device.

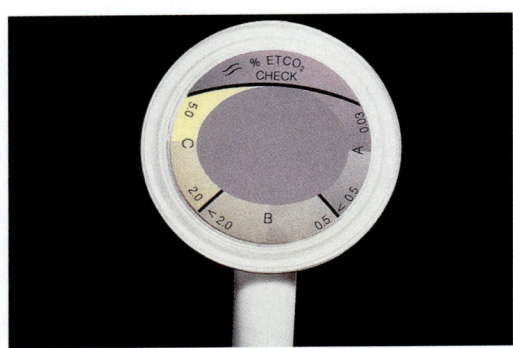

FIGURE 15-85 Colorimetric end-tidal carbon dioxide (CO_2) detector.

A capnometer is an electronic device for measuring the $EtCO_2$. The monitor probe or sampling tubing is connected between the ET tube and the bag-valve device. Because capnometers display a numerical end-tidal CO_2 value, changes can be measured over time.

Capnography is a method of measuring carbon dioxide that displays and records both a numerical value for the $EtCO_2$ and a dynamic wave form. This provides a visual display of the rate, depth, and effectiveness of the patient's ventilation. It does not measure oxygenation. Because carbon dioxide is a waste product of metabolism, capnography also provides an indirect measure of perfusion. This is important during cardiopulmonary resuscitation. A decline in $EtCO_2$ values may indicate that chest compressions are not fast enough or deep enough. Capnographic wave forms also can provide information about bronchoconstriction. When the terminal bronchioles are constricted, the upslope of the capnographic waveform resembles a shark's fin. This is related to uneven emptying of air from the narrowed airways. Paramedics can monitor the capnographic waveform to evaluate the effectiveness of bronchodilator treatment (see Chapter 24).

> **SHOW ME THE EVIDENCE**
> Wirtz and colleagues sought prospectively to find the incidence of unrecognized prehospital endotracheal tube misplacement in patients arriving at two emergency departments (ED) in New York City from 17 EMS agencies from February, 2003 to June, 2004. Only one agency used end-tidal carbon dioxide (CO_2) detectors. Paramedics intubated 132 patients during the study period. Eleven endotracheal tubes were placed in the esophagus, and one was placed in the hypopharynx. In addition, 15% of patients had right mainstem intubation on arrival at the ED. Eleven of the 12 patients with unrecognized esophageal intubation died.
>
> Wirtz D, Ortiz C, Newman D, Zhitomirsky I: Unrecognized placement of endotracheal tubes by ground prehospital providers, *Prehosp Emerg Care* 11:213-218, 2007.

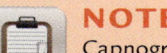

NOTE

Capnography provides a breath-by-breath measurement of a patient's ventilation. It therefore can quickly reveal a trend in a patient's condition and provide early warning of a decline in a patient's respiratory status. Capnography is useful for monitoring patients with asthma, congestive heart failure, diabetes, shock, pulmonary embolus, acidosis, and other conditions. A high end-tidal carbon dioxide (EtCO$_2$) reading in a patient with altered mental status or severe dyspnea may indicate hypoventilation and the need for tracheal intubation.

SHOW ME THE EVIDENCE

Silvestri and coworkers performed a prospective observational study for 10 months in 2002 on all adult and pediatric patients who had out-of-hospital endotracheal intubation and were taken to a level I trauma center. Use of continuous end-tidal carbon dioxide (EtCO$_2$) monitoring was available but not required by all of the participating EMS services. During this period, 153 patients who arrived at the trauma center had been intubated and met the study criteria. Continuous EtCO$_2$ monitoring was used for 93 (61%) patients; none of these patients had unrecognized misplaced intubation. In the group in which continuous EtCO$_2$ monitoring was not used, 13 patients had esophageal intubation and one patient had hypopharyngeal placement. This constituted a 23% misplacement rate.

Silvestri S, Ralls G, Krauss B, et al: The effectiveness of out-of-hospital use of continuous end-tidal carbon dioxide monitoring on the rate of unrecognized misplaced intubation within a regional emergency medical services system, *Ann Emerg Med* 45:497-502, 2005.

Electronic devices can confirm successful tracheal tube placement within seconds of an intubation attempt. They also can detect subsequent tracheal dislodgement.[23] An infrared analyzer measures the percentage of carbon dioxide gas at each phase of respiration (Figure 15-86). Capnometers provide a numerical reading of exhaled CO$_2$ levels. The information also may be displayed in a digital waveform using a capnograph with printout capability (similar to an ECG tracing) (Figure 15-87 and Box 15-12). Both colorimetric and electronic devices may be useful as indicators of circulation during some cardiac arrest situations, because an increase in the EtCO$_2$ concentration seems to be related to effective perfusion during external chest compression.[31] Some capnometers can be used in patients who have not been intubated (i.e., using a device that resembles a nasal cannula). They are helpful in determining the effectiveness of EMS treatments.

NOTE

Capnography also can be used as an early indication of return of spontaneous circulation (ROSC). Studies have shown that when a patient experiences ROSC, the first indication often is a sudden rise in the end-tidal carbon dioxide (EtCO$_2$) level. This rise occurs as the rush of circulation washes untransported CO$_2$ from the tissues. Likewise, a sudden drop in the EtCO$_2$ may indicate the patient has lost pulses and cardiopulmonary resuscitation (CPR) may need to be initiated.[32]

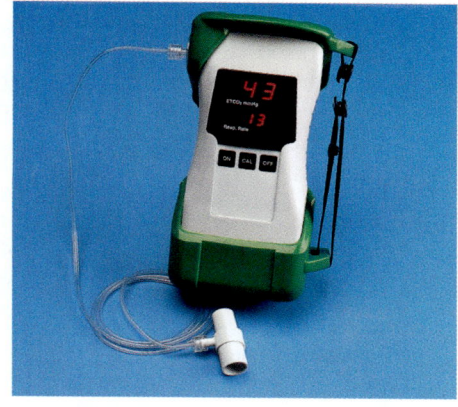

FIGURE 15-86 Digital (or electronic) end-tidal carbon dioxide (CO$_2$) detector.

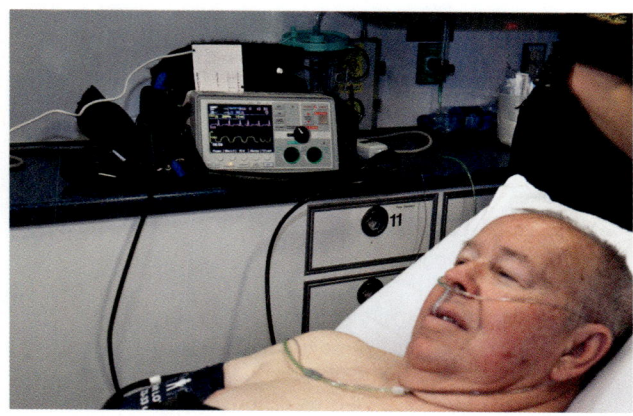

FIGURE 15-87 Monitor displaying continuous capnographic waveform.

CRITICAL THINKING

Your patient is in full arrest. Consequently, the measurements from your end-tidal carbon dioxide (EtCO$_2$) detector are inconclusive. Also, you can't get the oxygen saturation monitor to work. You are not sure whether you hear breath sounds clearly. What should you do?

BULB- AND SYRINGE-TYPE ESOPHAGEAL DETECTORS

Esophageal detection devices (e.g., the Toomey syringe) are attached to the end of the ET tube (Figure 15-88). They operate on the principle that the esophagus is a collapsible tube. As such, a vacuum is created when air is removed from the esophagus. This occurs with the bulb device after it is compressed or when air is withdrawn by the syringe device if the ET tube is in the esophagus. If the ET tube has been correctly placed in the trachea, the bulb device easily refills with air or the syringe device is easily aspirated when the plunger is pulled back. Esophageal detection devices also can be used to verify correct placement of multilumen

BOX 15-12 Capnographic Waveforms

Capnography waveforms on the monitor screen are condensed to provide assessment information in a 4-second view. Printouts of waveforms provide the same information in "real time" and may differ in duration from that of the monitor screen. The following are example waveforms for both intubated and nonintubated patients.*

Normal Ranges

Arterial partial pressure of carbon dioxide ($PaCO_2$): 35-45 mm Hg
Capnography end-tidal carbon dioxide ($EtCO_2$): 35-45 mm Hg
   (4-6 vol%)

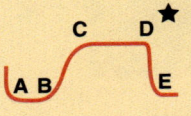

A–B	Respiratory baseline
B–C	Expiratory upslope
	Exhaled CO_2 mixes with airway dead space gases
C–D	Expiratory plateau
D	End-tidal value—peak CO_2 concentration—normally at the end of exhalation
D–E	Inspiratory downstroke

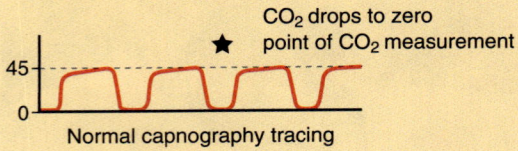

★ CO_2 drops to zero point of CO_2 measurement

Normal capnography tracing

Intubated Patients

In an intubated patient, capnography may be used to:

- Verify endotracheal (ET) tube placement
- Monitor or detect ET tube dislodgement
- Monitor loss of circulatory function
- Assess the adequacy of cardiopulmonary resuscitation (CPR) compressions
- Confirm return of spontaneous circulation

Examples

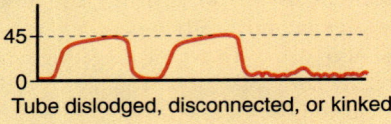

Tube dislodged, disconnected, or kinked

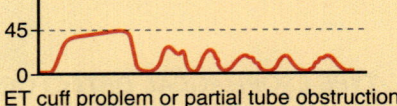

ET cuff problem or partial tube obstruction

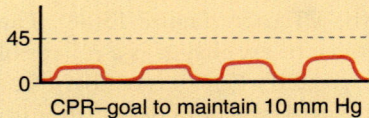

CPR—goal to maintain 10 mm Hg

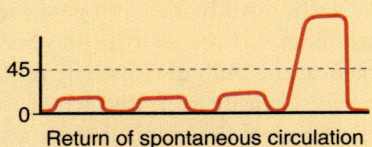

Return of spontaneous circulation

Nonintubated Patients

In a nonintubated patient, capnography may be used to:

- Assess asthma and chronic obstructive pulmonary disease (COPD)
- Document and monitor procedural sedation
- Detect apnea or inadequate breathing
- Measure hypoventilation
- Evaluate hyperventilation

Examples

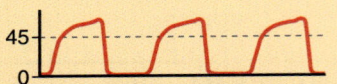

Waveform has a "shark fin" appearance during bronchospasm

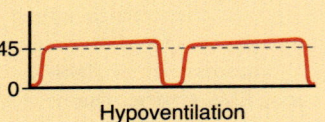

Hypoventilation

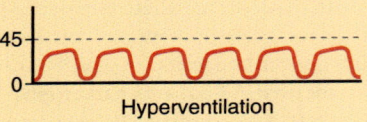

Hyperventilation

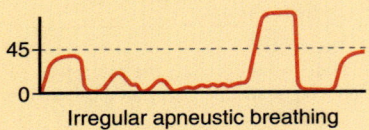

Irregular apneustic breathing

Causes of Elevated $EtCO_2$

- Decreased ventilation secondary to:
  - Head trauma
  - Overdose
  - Respiratory failure (severe asthma, COPD)
  - Sedation
  - Stroke
- Increased CO_2 production
  - Fever
  - Shivering

Causes of Low $EtCO_2$

- Ventilation problem
  - Esophageal intubation
  - Airway obstruction
- Inadequate blood flow
  - Cardiac arrest (lower if poor compressions; lower values predict poor outcome)
  - Tension pneumothorax
  - Pericardial tamponade
  - Reduced cardiac output
- Ventilation/perfusion (V/Q) mismatch
  - Pulmonary embolism
- Decreased production of carbon dioxide
  - Hypothermia
- Sampling error
  - Inadequate tidal volume delivery
  - CO_2 sampling tubing blocked

Modified from Ornato JP, Peberdy MA: Prehospital end-tidal carbon dioxide monitoring—it's not all hot air, *JEMS*, March, 1993.
*The level of sedation and severity of conditions may affect the respiratory rate and $EtCO_2$ level.

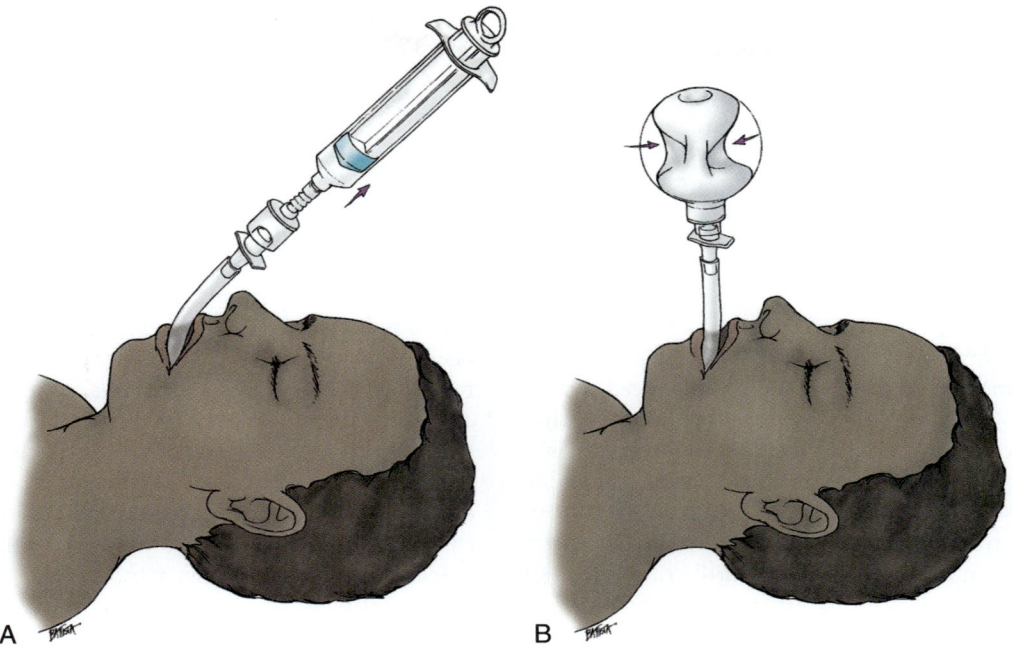

FIGURE 15-88 Esophageal intubation detector. **A,** Syringe. **B,** Bulb.

airways (described later in this chapter), provided the device is applied before the first breath is delivered after intubation.

PULSE OXIMETRY

Pulse oximeters (Figure 15-89) help determine how well the patient is being oxygenated. They measure the transmission of red and near-infrared light through arterial beds. Hemoglobin absorbs red and infrared light waves differently when it is bound with oxygen (oxyhemoglobin) from when it is not (reduced hemoglobin). Oxyhemoglobin absorbs more infrared than red light. Reduced hemoglobin absorbs more red than infrared light. Pulse oximetry reveals the arterial saturation (SpO_2) by measuring this difference.

The oximeter probe is placed on an area of thin tissue, such as a finger, toe, or earlobe. One side of the probe sends wavelengths of light through the arterial bed. The other side detects the presence of red or infrared light. Using this balance of red and infrared colors, the oximeter calculates the oxygen saturation of the blood and displays it on the monitor screen.

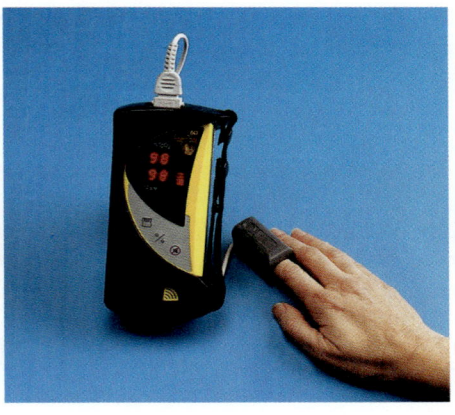

FIGURE 15-89 Pulse oximeter. (Shade BR et al: *Mosby's EMT-Intermediate textbook for the 1999 National Standard Curriculum,* ed 3, St Louis, 2007, Mosby.)

The percentage of hemoglobin saturated with oxygen is denoted as the SaO_2. It depends on a number of factors. These include the PCO_2, pH, temperature, and whether the hemoglobin is normal or altered. The lower range of normal for the SpO_2 is 93% to 95%. The upper range is 99% to 100%. Once the SpO_2 falls below 90% (corresponding to a PO_2 of 60 mm Hg), further decreases are associated with a marked decline in oxygen content (Box 15-13).

Difficulties and inaccuracies may result from the use of pulse oximeters. Therefore, paramedics should consider them only as another tool to assist the monitoring of a patient's oxygenation levels. Circumstances that may produce false readings include the following[33]:

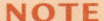

> **NOTE**
> Comprehensive assessment of a patent's ventilation and perfusion status requires blood gas analysis (an in-hospital procedure). As described in Chapter 11, blood gas analysis is used to assess pH, the partial pressure of arterial carbon dioxide ($PaCO_2$), bicarbonate, and base deficit. (Methods used to obtain arterial blood gas samples are presented in the Appendix: Advanced Practice for the Critical Care Paramedic.

- Dyshemoglobinemia (hemoglobin saturation with compounds other than oxygen (e.g., carbon monoxide, methemoglobinemia)
- Excessive ambient light (sunlight, fluorescent lights) on the oximeter's sensor probe
- Patient movement
- Hypotension
- Hypothermia/vasoconstriction
- Patient use of vasoconstrictive drugs
- Jaundice

Laryngeal Mask Airway

The laryngeal mask airway (LMA) is an advanced airway control device. It may be used in the prehospital setting when conventional endotracheal intubation is unsuccessful, when access to the patient is limited, when an unstable neck injury may be present, or when appropriate positioning of the patient for tracheal intubation is impossible.[23] Some LMAs also allow endotracheal intubation through the device. This allows easier placement of the tube.

> **NOTE**
> The laryngeal mask airway (LMA) does not offer full protection against aspiration. However, aspiration is uncommon with this device. A small number of patients cannot be ventilated adequately with the LMA. Also, it is contraindicated in conscious patients and in those with an intact gag reflex.

BOX 15-13 Oxygen Saturation and Partial Pressure (PO_2)

With 90% saturation: PO_2 drops to 60 mm Hg
With 75% saturation: PO_2 drops to 40 mm Hg
With 50% saturation: PO_2 drops to 27 mm Hg

DESCRIPTION

The LMA is available in several sizes (ranging from size 1 for neonates to size 5 for adults.) It consists of a proximal tube with standard adapters for connecting ventilatory devices. The tube is connected to a distal mask that is inflated by means of a pilot tube and balloon (Figure 15-90).

INSERTION

The LMA is inserted through the mouth into the pharynx. It is advanced until resistance is felt as the distal portion of the tube locates in the hypopharynx. When the device has been properly inserted, the black line marked on the LMA rests midline against the patient's upper lip. Inflating the cuff seals the larynx and leaves the distal opening of the tube just above the glottis, providing a clear, secure airway. After the pilot cuff has been inflated, proper placement is confirmed by observing equal rise and fall of the chest, by ensuring bilateral breath sounds, and with end-tidal CO_2 detectors and pulse oximetry monitoring (in a patient who has a perfusing rhythm) (Figure 15-91). Use of the LMA requires special training and authorization from medical direction. The LMA may be difficult to maintain during patient movement, which can make it difficult to use during patient transport.

NECESSARY EQUIPMENT

- Water-soluble lubricant
- Syringes
- Bag-valve device
- Oxygen source and connecting tubing
- Suction equipment
- Stethoscope
- One or more confirmation devices

COMMON ADVANTAGES

- Less skilled training or maintenance is required than for endotracheal intubation.

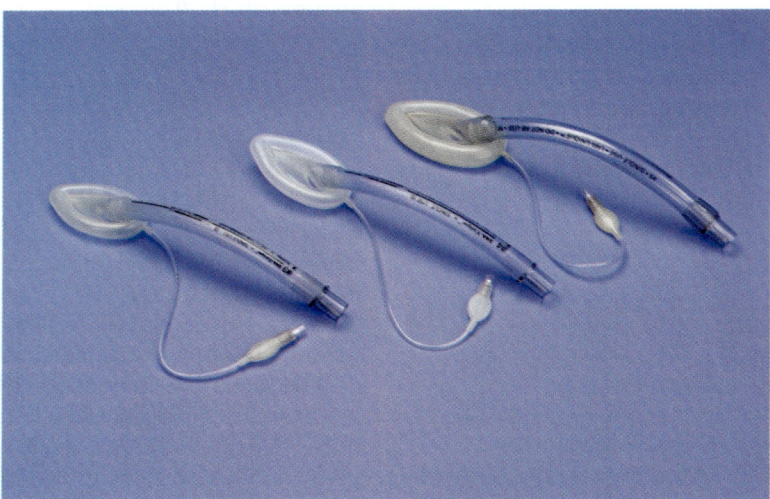

FIGURE 15-90 Laryngeal mask airways.

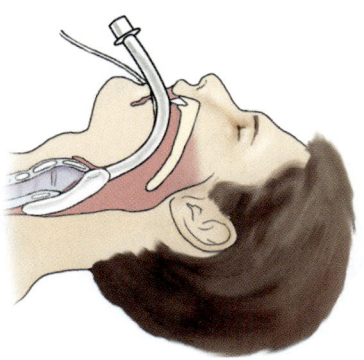

FIGURE 15-91 A patient with a laryngeal mask airway (LMA).

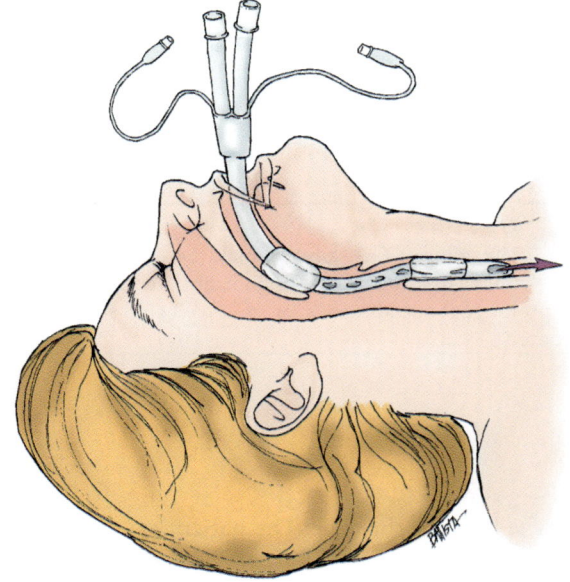

FIGURE 15-92 Placement of the esophageal-tracheal Combitube airway.

- Laryngoscopy and visualization of the vocal cords are not required.
- Minimal spinal movement is required for insertion.
- Endotracheal intubation can be achieved through some LMAs.

COMMON DISADVANTAGES

- The patient must be unresponsive and have no gag reflex.
- Not all patients can be adequately ventilated with the LMA.
- The airway must be removed when the patient becomes responsive or agitated.
- The airway does not provide as much protection from aspiration as the ET tube.

COMMON CONTRAINDICATIONS

- Presence of a gag reflex
- Caustic ingestion
- Esophageal trauma or disease

Esophageal-Tracheal Combitube

The esophageal-tracheal Combitube (ETC, Combitube) allows for either esophageal or tracheal insertion. It is a plastic tube with twin lumens that are separated by a partition wall. One tube resembles an ET tube and has an open distal end. The other tube is blocked by an obturator at the distal end. Both tubes use low-pressure balloons that provide a seal for either the trachea or the esophagus, depending on placement. There are also holes on one side of the tube between the balloons that allow for ventilation through tube 1. When inflated, the large pharyngeal balloon fills the space between the base of the tongue and the soft palate, anchoring the tube in position. The Combitube usually finds its way into the esophagus because of the stiffness and curve of the tube and the shape and the structure of the pharynx.

The Combitube is another option for airway control when endotracheal intubation is indicated but is unsuccessful or unavailable. The LMA and Combitube provide superior ventilation compared with face masks in cardiac arrest.[23] The Combitube reduces but does not eliminate the risk of aspiration. Some EMS agencies prefer the Combitube as a rescue device for endotracheal intubation because the device can be easily and quickly inserted.

INSERTION

The Combitube is inserted by gently guiding the device into the esophagus or trachea (Figure 15-92). The tube should be inserted into the midline and to a depth that puts the printed ring at the level of the teeth. (This insertion is achieved without hyperextension or flexion of the patient's head. It also is done without visualization of the glottic opening.) The pharyngeal and distal balloons then are inflated. This isolates the oropharynx above the upper balloon and the esophagus (or trachea) below the lower balloon. Ventilation is at first provided through the esophageal lumen. (This is due to the significant chance of esophageal placement with blind insertion.) In this position, air passes into the pharynx and beyond the glottis into the trachea. The placement is confirmed by the primary and secondary confirmation methods described previously.

If breath sounds and chest movement are absent with ventilation through the esophageal lumen (tube 1), ventilation should be performed through the tracheal lumen (tube 2) without changing the position of the airway. Air passes through this lumen directly into the trachea. Placement is confirmed in the usual manner.

NECESSARY EQUIPMENT

- Water-soluble lubricant
- Syringes
- Bag-mask device
- Oxygen source and connecting tubing
- Suction equipment
- Stethoscope

The various kinds of balloon-system devices share advantages, disadvantages, and contraindications.

ADVANTAGES

- Airways cannot be placed improperly.
- Less skill training or skill maintenance is needed than for endotracheal intubation.
- Minimal spinal movement is required for insertion.
- Suctioning is easily done.

DISADVANTAGES

- The patient must be unresponsive and without a gag reflex.
- The airway must be removed when the patient becomes responsive or agitated.
- Proper identification of the tube's location may be difficult, leading to ventilation through the wrong lumen.
- The trachea cannot be suctioned when the tube is in the esophagus.
- The airway should be replaced with an ET tube as soon as possible.

CONTRAINDICATIONS

- Patient height less than 5 feet or age under 14 years
- Caustic ingestion
- Esophageal trauma or disease
- Presence of a gag reflex

King LT-D Airway

The King LT-D airway is a disposable supraglottic device designed for positive pressure ventilation as well as for patients who are breathing spontaneously. It is an alternative to mask ventilation and tracheal intubation.

The King LT-D airway has a single tube that is placed only into the esophagus. (The tube's large size and short length virtually eliminates the possibility of placement into the trachea.) The tube is curved and has a proximal and distal cuff. As with the ETC, a large balloon is inflated in the oropharynx. At the same time, a smaller cuff is inflated in the esophagus by the same port that inflates the large cuff. Ventilations are delivered by attaching a bag-mask device to the proximal end of the tube. With each ventilation, the air escapes through holes in the tube between the cuffs. Some LT King-D airways also provide for passage of tubes for gastric decompression. The King LT-D is available in multiple sizes, based on a patient's height (Figure 15-93).

Use of the King LT-D airway is indicated when tracheal intubation cannot be established in two attempts *and* when a patient is unable to adequately maintain his or her airway, has an altered mental status (Glasgow Coma Score of 8 or lower), or has respiratory compromise. Contraindications to use of the airway include patients who are less than 4 feet tall, patients who have an intact gag reflex, patients who have ingested caustic substances, and patients with known esophageal disease.

Before the airway is inserted, the cuff should be tested for integrity and then deflated (Figure 15-94). Lubricant is applied to the back side of the airway, with care taken not

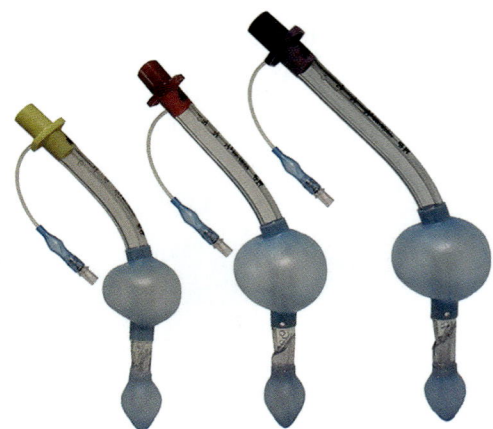

FIGURE 15-93 King LT-D airways. (Henry MC, Stapleton ER: *EMT prehospital care,* ed 4, St Louis, 2009, Mosby.)

 NOTE
The King LT-D airway may be considered *before* tracheal intubation if significant access issues exist (e.g., prolonged entrapment) or if a difficult intubation is anticipated.

to clog the holes in the tube. The patient's head should be placed in a neutral position, observing spinal precautions if indicated. Before insertion, the patient's lungs are preoxygenated with 100% oxygen. The patient's mouth should be opened, using a head-tilt or chin-lift maneuver. The tube is advanced gently behind the base of the patient's tongue while the tube is rotated back to the midline. The tube's blue orientation line should face the patient's chin. The tube then is gently advanced until the base of the connector is aligned with the patient's teeth or gums. The airway is inflated with the appropriate volume of air.

The bag-mask device is connected to the adaptor on the tube, and ventilations are provided. While providing ventilations, the paramedic gently withdraws the tube until ventilation compliance becomes easy and free flowing. Cuff inflation may be adjusted if necessary to maintain a seal of the airway at the peak ventilatory pressure used. Correct placement is confirmed by listening for breath sounds, observing chest rise and fall, the presence of $EtCO_2$, and a stable or rising SpO_2. Equal and bilateral breath sounds should be confirmed. The device is secured, and placement of a bite block should be considered.

The position of the King LT-D airway should be rechecked after each patient movement, on transfer of care to another provider, and after an ascent or a descent of more than 1000 feet.

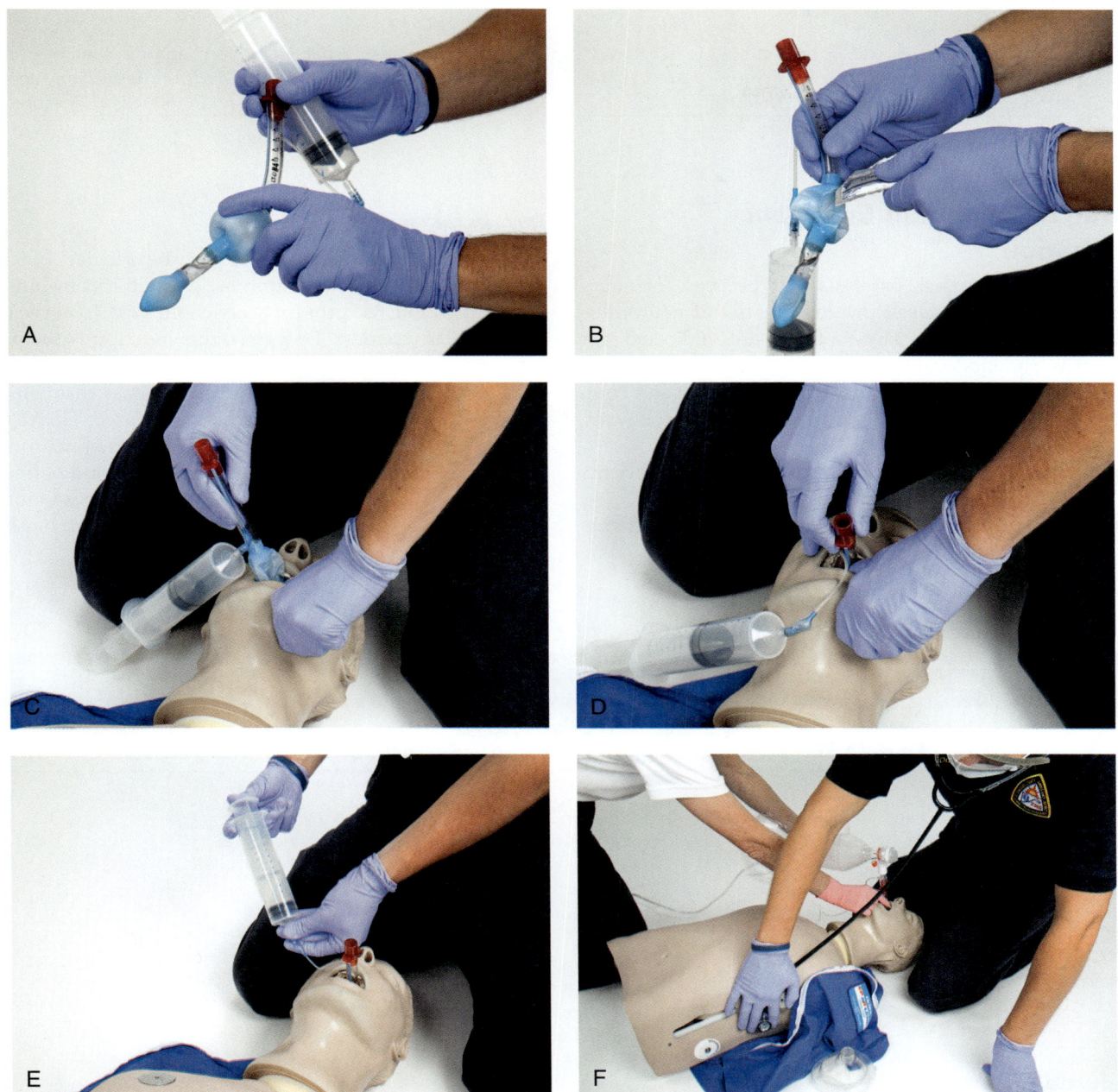

FIGURE 15-94 King LT-D airway insertion. **A,** Assemble the necessary equipment and inflate and then deflate the cuffs. **B,** Apply a water-soluble lubricant. **C,** Insert the airway behind the base of the tongue while rotating back to the midline. **D,** Align the base of the connector with the teeth or gums. **E,** Inflate the cuffs with the appropriate volume of air. **F,** Verify proper placement.

PHARMACOLOGICAL ADJUNCTS TO AIRWAY MANAGEMENT AND VENTILATION

Sedation sometimes is used in airway management and ventilation to reduce anxiety, induce amnesia, and decrease the gag reflex. Possible indications for sedation include combative patients, patients who require aggres-sive airway management but who are too alert to tolerate intubation, and agitated trauma patients. The classes of drugs commonly used for sedation in these situations are tranquilizers, barbiturates, benzo-diazepines, and narcotics. Two medications commonly used for drug-assisted intubation are *midazolam* (a short-acting benzodiazepine) and *etomidate* (a nonbarbiturate hypnotic).

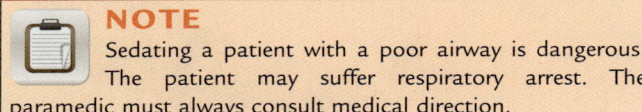

NOTE
Sedating a patient with a poor airway is dangerous. The patient may suffer respiratory arrest. The paramedic must always consult medical direction.

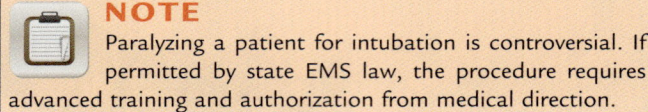

NOTE
Paralyzing a patient for intubation is controversial. If permitted by state EMS law, the procedure requires advanced training and authorization from medical direction.

Paralytic Agents in Emergency Intubation

Although controversial, paralysis may be used for emergency intubation. Paralysis involves the use of neuromuscular blocking drugs. These drugs are indicated for combative patients who need to be intubated. For instance, a patient suffering a head injury may be agitated and combative. These drugs should not be used in the following situations:

- Patients who will be difficult to ventilate (e.g., patients with facial hair)
- Patients who will be difficult to intubate (e.g., patients with short necks, obstructions)

PHARMACOLOGY

As described in Chapter 13, neuromuscular blockers produce skeletal muscle paralysis. They do this by binding to the nicotinic receptor for acetylcholine (ACh) at the neuromuscular junction. To review, this junction is the point of contact between the nerve ending and the muscle fiber (see Chapter 10). When nerve impulses pass through this junction, ACh and other chemicals are released. This release causes the muscle to contract. The two types of neuromuscular blocking drugs are depolarizing agents and nondepolarizing agents. Neuromuscular blockers should not be administered to patients until sufficient sedation has been achieved.

TABLE 15-7 Drugs Commonly Used for Pharmacologically Assisted Intubation

Drug	Dose (Adult) IV/IO	Dose (Pediatric) IV/IO	Indications	Complications/Side Effects
Pretreatment				
Oxygen	High flow Assist ventilation as needed to achieve oxygen saturation of 100% if possible	High flow Assist ventilation as needed to achieve oxygen saturation of 100% if possible	All patients undergoing pharmacologically assisted intubation	—
Lidocaine	1-2 mg/kg	1-2 mg/kg	Brain injury	Seizure
Atropine	—	0.01-0.02 mg/kg **(minimum dose, 0.1 mg; maximum dose, 0.5 mg)**	Pediatric intubation, prevention of bradycardia and excess secretions	Tachycardia
Induction of Sedation				
Midazolam (Versed)	0.1-0.3 mg/kg (maximum single dose, 10 mg)	0.1-0.3 mg/kg (maximum single dose, 10 mg)	Sedation	Respiratory depression/apnea, hypotension
Fentanyl (Sublimaze)	2-5 mcg/kg	2-5 mcg/kg	Sedation	Respiratory depression/apnea, hypotension, bradycardia
Etomidate	0.2-0.4 mg/kg (limit 1 dose; consider cortisone stress doses for a patient in shock)	0.2-0.4 mg/kg	Sedation, induced anesthesia	Apnea, hypotension, vomiting
Chemical Paralysis				
Succinylcholine	1-1.5 mg/kg	1-1.5 mg/kg	Muscle relaxation and paralysis (short duration)	Hyperkalemia, muscle fasciculations

From: 2010 Handbook of Emergency Cardiovascular Care for Healthcare Providers, American Heart Association, 2010, Dallas, Tex
IV, Intravenous; *IO,* Intraosseous.

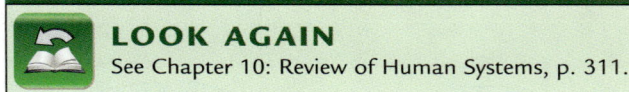

LOOK AGAIN
See Chapter 10: Review of Human Systems, p. 311.

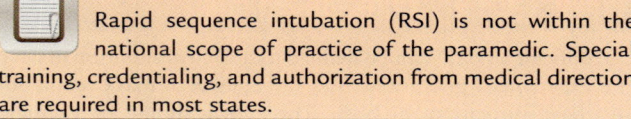

NOTE
Rapid sequence intubation (RSI) is not within the national scope of practice of the paramedic. Special training, credentialing, and authorization from medical direction are required in most states.

Depolarizing agents invade the neuromuscular junction and bind to the receptors for ACh. These drugs produce depolarization of the muscular membrane. Thus they often lead to fasciculations (uncontrollable muscle twitching). These drugs also may lead to some muscular contractions. An example of a depolarizing agent is *succinylcholine.* Succinylcholine has a rapid onset of action. Yet it has the briefest duration of action of all the neuromuscular blocking drugs. This makes it the drug of choice for emergency endotracheal intubation.

Nondepolarizing agents also bind to the receptors for ACh. However, they block the uptake of ACh at the neuromuscular junction without initiating depolarization of the muscle membrane. Examples of nondepolarizing drugs include *vecuronium* and *rocuronium.* These drugs have a longer onset and duration than depolarizing agents.

Neuromuscular blocking agents produce complete paralysis. Consequently, ventilatory support must be provided. Ventilation and oxygenation must be closely monitored to ensure that they are adequate. If the patient is conscious, the paramedic should explain the effects of the medication before administering it. Administration of *atropine* should be strongly considered, particularly in children, before a neuromuscular blocking agent is administered. *Lidocaine* given before administration of a neuromuscular blocking agent may blunt any increase in intracranial pressure associated with intubation. Finally, *diazepam, etomidate, midazolam,* or another sedative approved by medical direction should be used in any conscious patient to whom a blocking agent is administered; neuromuscular blocking agents do not inhibit pain or seizure activity (Table 15-7).

Rapid Sequence Intubation

Rapid sequence intubation (RSI) involves the administration of a potent sedative and a neuromuscular blocking agent at the same time to achieve optimal intubation conditions in less than 1 minute.[34] The blocking agent most often used is *succinylcholine* (see the Emergency Drug Index (EDI)). In addition to providing optimal intubation conditions, RSI also minimizes the risk of aspiration of gastric contents. RSI is indicated in the following situations[35]:

- Emergency intubation is warranted.
- The patient has a "full" stomach.
- Intubation is predicted to be successful (i.e., the patient does not have a difficult airway) (Box 15-14).
- If intubation fails, ventilation is predicted to be successful.

RSI is not indicated for patients in cardiac arrest or for deeply comatose patients when immediate intubation is required. Relative contraindications include concern that intubation or mask ventilation would be unsuccessful; significant facial or laryngeal edema, trauma, or distortion; or a spontaneously breathing patient who requires upper airway muscle tone and positioning (e.g., upper airway obstruction, epiglottitis).[23]

RSI is an organized approach to endotracheal intubation. It involves specific steps and actions that lead to rapid sedation and paralysis without positive pressure ventilation once the procedure begins. The purpose of RSI is to achieve optimum and rapid tracheal intubation in patients at risk for aspiration. The procedure is intended to take the patient from a conscious, breathing state to a state of unconsciousness. This is accomplished with complete neuromuscular paralysis. Intubation is performed without interposed mechanical ventilation. The six steps of RSI (the six *P*s) are preparation, preoxygenation, pretreatment, paralysis (with sedation), placement of the tube, and postintubation management (Boxes 15-15 and 15-16).

TECHNIQUE

1. **Preparation**
   - Assess the patient for difficulty of intubation (e.g., using the Mallampati score [see Box 15-14]).
   - Prepare all drugs and equipment.
   - Make sure the patient has one or more patent IV lines.
   - Explain the procedure to the patient.
2. **Preoxygenation (done simultaneously with preparation)**
   - Preoxygenate the patient with 100% oxygen for 5 minutes (an essential step of the "no bagging" approach of RSI).
   - Consider using a pulse oximeter.
3. **Pretreatment (done 3 minutes before intubation)**
   - Consider giving *lidocaine* to protect against a rise in intracranial pressure and to prevent laryngospasm.
   - Consider giving beta blockers or opioids to reduce a sympathoadrenal response (e.g., a drop in blood pressure) to intubation.
4. **Paralysis (with sedation)**
   - Administer a sedative (per protocol) to produce unconsciousness. This should be immediately followed by a rapid push of the neuromuscular blocker (see the EDI).
   - Apply cricoid pressure as the patient loses consciousness to prevent vomiting. (Once neuromuscular blockade has been established, active vomiting cannot occur.)
   - Do not initiate ventilations unless the patient's oxygen saturation falls below 90%.

BOX 15-14   Difficult Airway

A "difficult airway" can be defined as a clinical situation in which an experienced practitioner has difficulty with mask ventilation, tracheal intubation, or both. The airway should be examined before airway management in all patients. This is done to identify physical characteristics that may indicate the presence of or potential for a difficult airway. Paramedics should assess the following airway features.[36]

Feature	Sign of Difficult Airway
Length of upper incisors	Relatively long
Relation of maxillary and mandibular incisors with normal jaw closure	Prominent overbite
Visibility of uvula	Not visible when tongue is protruded (e.g., > Mallampati class II)
Shape of palate	Highly arched or very narrow
Length of neck	Short
Thickness of neck	Thick
Range of motion of head and neck	Patient cannot touch tip of chin to chest or extend neck.

Mallampati Signs as Indicators of Difficult Intubation

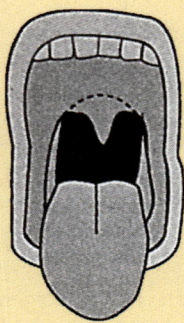 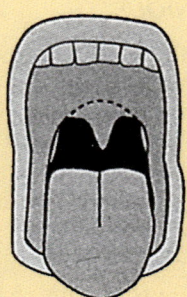

Class I: soft palate, uvula, fauces, pillars visible

No difficulty

Class II: soft palate, uvula, fauces visible

No difficulty

Class III: soft palate, base of uvula visible

Moderate difficulty

Class IV: hard palate only visible

Severe difficulty

Mallampati Signs as Indicators of Difficult Intubation

Class I (soft palate, uvula, fauces, pillars visible)—No difficulty
Class II (soft palate, uvula, fauces visible)—No difficulty
Class III (soft palate, base of uvula visible)—Moderate difficulty
Class IV (hard palate only visible)—Severe difficulty
   The following also may be indicators of a potentially difficult Airway:

- An immobilized trauma patient
- Morbidly obese patient
- Children
- Limited jaw opening
- Upper airway conditions (e.g., burns, neck injury, epiglottitis)
- Facial trauma
- Laryngeal trauma

If a difficult airway is evident, advanced airway management is required, as presented in the algorithm in Figure 15-95.

CRITICAL THINKING

How would you decide whether a patient needs more sedation after a paralytic has been given?

BOX 15-15 Six *P*s of Rapid Sequence Intubation

1. Preparation
2. Preoxygenation
3. Pretreatment
4. Paralysis (with sedation)
5. Placement of the tube
6. Postintubation management

- Within 45 seconds of administration of *succinylcholine*, the patient will be relaxed enough for intubation.

5. **Placement**
   - Perform orotracheal intubation and confirm proper placement of the tube.

6. **Postintubation management**
   - Secure the tube in place.
   - Begin mechanical ventilation.
   - Monitor the patient continuously.

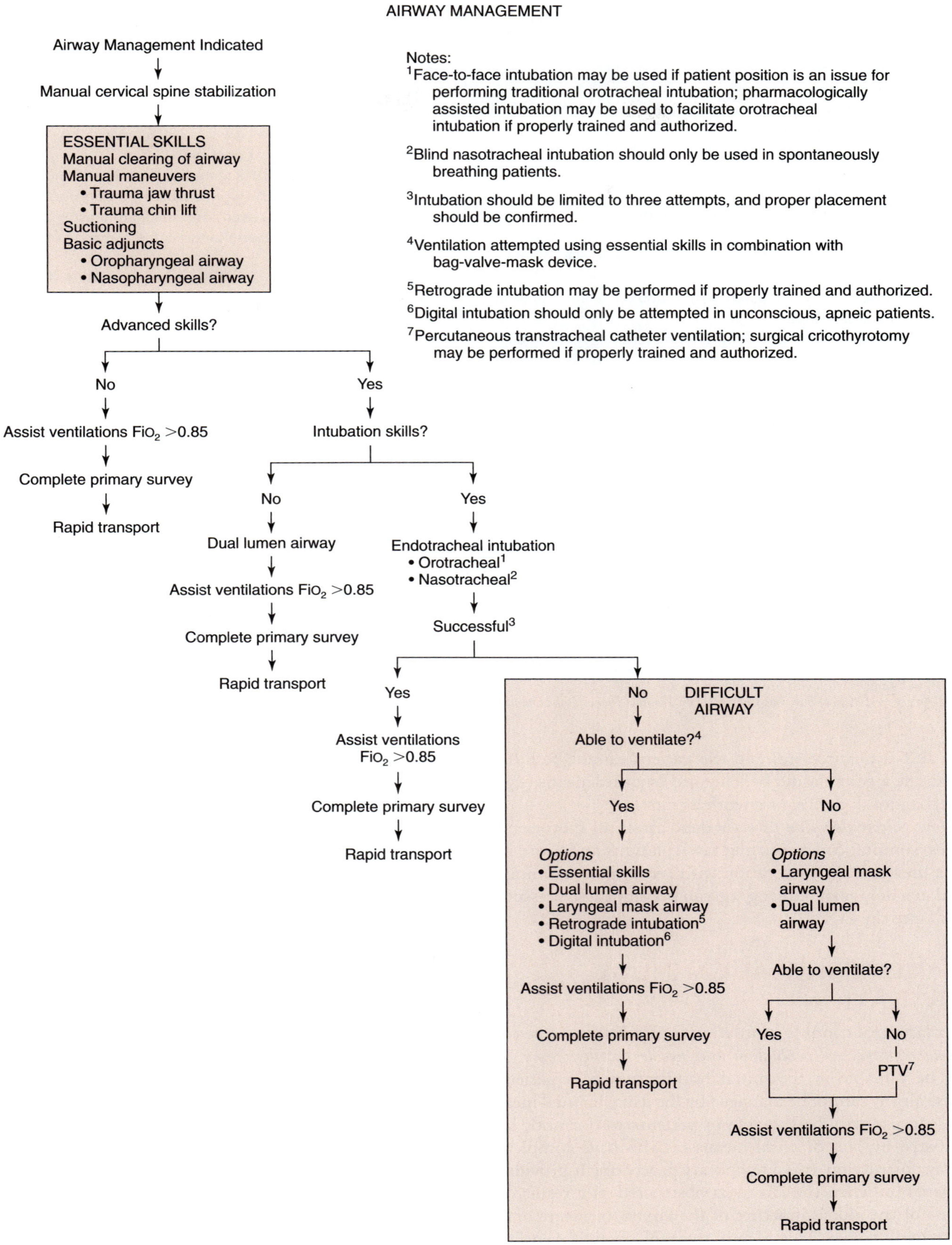

AIRWAY MANAGEMENT

Airway Management Indicated

↓

Manual cervical spine stabilization

↓

ESSENTIAL SKILLS
Manual clearing of airway
Manual maneuvers
 • Trauma jaw thrust
 • Trauma chin lift
Suctioning
Basic adjuncts
 • Oropharyngeal airway
 • Nasopharyngeal airway

↓

Advanced skills?

No

↓

Assist ventilations FiO_2 >0.85

↓

Complete primary survey

↓

Rapid transport

Yes

↓

Intubation skills?

No

↓

Dual lumen airway

↓

Assist ventilations FiO_2 >0.85

↓

Complete primary survey

↓

Rapid transport

Yes

↓

Endotracheal intubation
 • Orotracheal[1]
 • Nasotracheal[2]

↓

Successful[3]

Yes

↓

Assist ventilations
FiO_2 >0.85

↓

Complete primary survey

↓

Rapid transport

No   **DIFFICULT AIRWAY**

↓

Able to ventilate?[4]

Yes

↓

Options
 • Essential skills
 • Dual lumen airway
 • Laryngeal mask airway
 • Retrograde intubation[5]
 • Digital intubation[6]

↓

Assist ventilations FiO_2 >0.85

↓

Complete primary survey

↓

Rapid transport

No

↓

Options
 • Laryngeal mask airway
 • Dual lumen airway

↓

Able to ventilate?

Yes   **No**
              PTV[7]

↓

Assist ventilations FiO_2 >0.85

↓

Complete primary survey

↓

Rapid transport

Notes:
[1]Face-to-face intubation may be used if patient position is an issue for performing traditional orotracheal intubation; pharmacologically assisted intubation may be used to facilitate orotracheal intubation if properly trained and authorized.

[2]Blind nasotracheal intubation should only be used in spontaneously breathing patients.

[3]Intubation should be limited to three attempts, and proper placement should be confirmed.

[4]Ventilation attempted using essential skills in combination with bag-valve-mask device.

[5]Retrograde intubation may be performed if properly trained and authorized.

[6]Digital intubation should only be attempted in unconscious, apneic patients.

[7]Percutaneous transtracheal catheter ventilation; surgical cricothyrotomy may be performed if properly trained and authorized.

FIGURE 15-95 Difficult airway algorithm. (NAEMT: *Prehospital trauma life support*, ed 7, St Louis, 2011, Mosby.)

BOX 15-16 Sample Protocol for Rapid Sequence Intubation (RSI)

1. Make sure the required equipment is available.
   - Oxygen supply
   - Bag-mask of appropriate size and type
   - Nonrebreathing mask
   - Laryngoscope with blades
   - Endotracheal (ET) tubes
   - Gum elastic bougie
   - Surgical and alternative airway equipment
   - RSI medications
   - Materials or devices to secure ET tube after placement
   - Suction equipment
2. Make sure at least one patent intravenous (IV) line is present (two are preferable).
3. Preoxygenate the patient using a nonrebreathing mask or bag-mask with 100% oxygen. Preoxygenation for 3 to 4 minutes is preferred.
4. Apply cardiac and pulse oximetry monitors.
5. If the patient is conscious, strongly consider the use of sedative agents.
6. Consider administration of sedative agents and lidocaine if potential or confirmed traumatic brain injury (TBI) is a factor.
7. After administration of paralytic agents, use the Sellick maneuver (cricoid pressure) to reduce the potential for aspiration.
8. Confirm tube placement immediately after intubation. Continuous cardiac and pulse oximeter monitoring is required during and after RSI. Reconfirm tube placement periodically throughout transport and each time the patient is moved.
9. Use repeat doses of sedative and paralytic agents as needed.

Procedure

1. Assemble the required equipment.
2. Make sure the IV lines are patent.
3. Preoxygenate the patient with 100% oxygen for approximately 3 to 4 minutes if possible.
4. Place the patient on cardiac and pulse oximeter monitors.
5. Administer a sedative (e.g., midazolam) if appropriate.
6. If TBI is possible or has been confirmed, administer lidocaine (1.5 mg/kg) 2 to 3 minutes before administration of a paralytic agent.
7. For pediatric patients, administer atropine (0.01-0.02 mg/kg) 1 to 3 minutes before paralytic administration to minimize the vagal response to intubation.
8. Administer a short-acting paralytic agent (e.g., succinylcholine) intravenously. Paralysis and relaxation should occur within 30 seconds. Using the Sellick maneuver may also be helpful.
   - Adult dosage: 1 to 2 mg/kg
   - Pediatric dosage: 1 to 2 mg/kg
9. Insert an ET tube. If initial attempts are unsuccessful, precede repeat attempts with preoxygenation.
10. Confirm ET tube placement.
11. If repeated attempts to achieve endotracheal intubation fail, consider placement of an alternative or surgical airway.
12. Use a long-acting paralytic agent (e.g., vecuronium) to continue paralysis.
    - Initial dose: 0.1 mg/kg IV push
    - Subsequent doses: 0.01 mg/kg every 30 to 45 minutes
13. Repeat doses of sedative medications also may be needed.

Note: Requirements vary with individual patients.

From: *American College of Surgeons Committee on Trauma, Prehospital Trauma Life Support,* ed 7, St. Louis, 2011, Elsevier.

If RSI is unsuccessful and the patient cannot be intubated, the airway should be managed by other means (e.g., ETC, bag-mask device, or cricothyrotomy).

Note: **Succinylcholine** directly depolarizes all motor end plates, simultaneously causing fasciculations and a rise in these pressures. Premedication with **vecuronium,** administered in a dosage of 0.01 mg/kg, can prevent these pressure rises[34] (see the EDI).

TRANSLARYNGEAL CANNULA VENTILATION

Translaryngeal cannula ventilation is also known as *percutaneous transtracheal ventilation* and *needle cricothyrotomy*. It may be valuable in the initial stabilization of a patient whose airway cannot be managed by the usual manual measures. It also may be valuable in patients who cannot be intubated by oral or nasal means or who have complete airway obstruction. It is a temporary procedure. It provides oxygenation when the airway is obstructed as a result of edema of the glottis, fracture of the larynx, or severe oropharyngeal hemorrhage. Translaryngeal cannula ventilation requires special training and authorization from medical direction.

Description

Translaryngeal cannula ventilation provides high-volume, high-pressure oxygenation of the lungs. This occurs through cannulation of the trachea below the glottis. The procedure delivers a large volume of oxygen through a small port at high pressure to the lungs. This oxygen delivery (50 psi) is much greater than can be achieved with other methods (e.g., 1 psi with a therapy regulator).

Necessary Equipment

- A 12- or 14-gauge over-the-needle catheter with a 5 or 10 mL syringe
- Alcohol or povidone-iodine swabs
- Adhesive tape or appropriate ties
- Pressure-regulating valve and pressure gauge attached to a high-pressure (30 to 60 psi) oxygen supply. (Most oxygen tanks and regulators can provide 50 psi at 15 L/minute or when opened to flush.)
- High-pressure tubing connecting the high-pressure regulating valve to a hand-operated release valve (5-foot tubing is recommended).
- A release valve connected by tubing to the catheter (this may be provided via a Y- or T-connector, through a

three-way stopcock directly attached to the high-pressure tubing, or by cutting a hole in the oxygen line to provide a "whistle stop" effect).

Technique

The steps in translaryngeal cannula ventilation are as follows (Figure 15-96):

1. Make sure the patient is supine. Also make sure the cricothyroid membrane has been identified. (If a spinal injury is suspected, in-line stabilization may be provided as for nasal and tracheal intubation.)
2. Stabilize the larynx using the thumb and middle finger of one hand. With the other hand, palpate the small depression below the thyroid cartilage (the Adam's apple). Slide the index finger down to locate the cricothyroid membrane.
3. Insert the needle of the syringe downward through the midline of the membrane at a 45- to 60-degree angle toward the patient's carina. Apply negative pressure to the syringe during insertion. The entrance of air into the syringe indicates that the needle is in the trachea (Figure 15-97, A).

4. Advance the catheter over the needle toward the carina and remove the needle and syringe (Figure 15-97, B). Take care not to kink the catheter when removing the needle and syringe.
5. Hold the hub of the catheter to prevent accidental dislodgement while providing ventilation. Remove the end of the oxygen tubing from the hub of the cannula and connect it to the oxygen regulator. Provide for a release valve as described previously.

> ### CRITICAL THINKING
> What conditions could make it difficult to locate the anatomical landmarks for translaryngeal cannulation or cricothyrotomy?

When the release valve is closed, oxygen under pressure is introduced into the trachea. The pressure is adjusted to a level that allows adequate lung expansion. The patient's chest must be observed closely. The release valve must be opened to allow for exhalation. The correct ratio of inflation to deflation varies, depending on whether upper airway obstruction is present. For an open upper airway, an

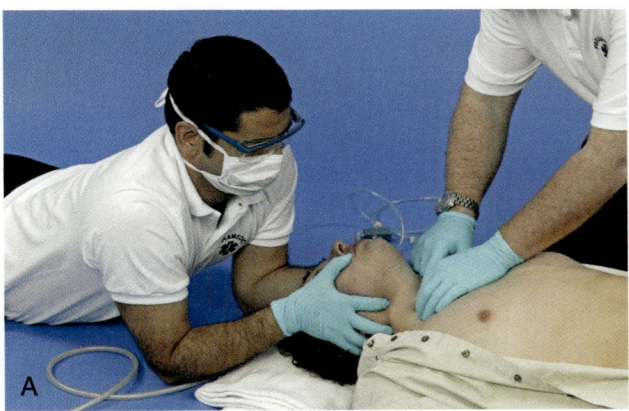
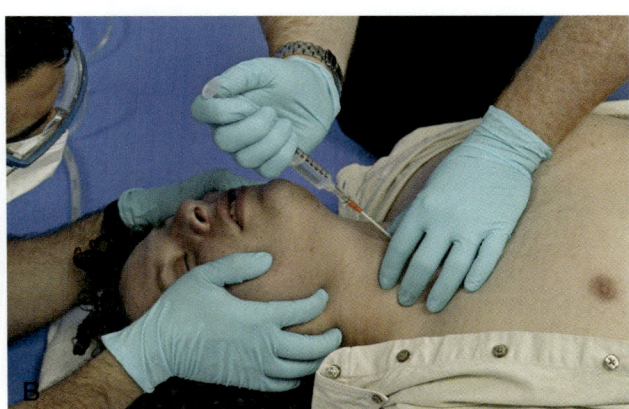
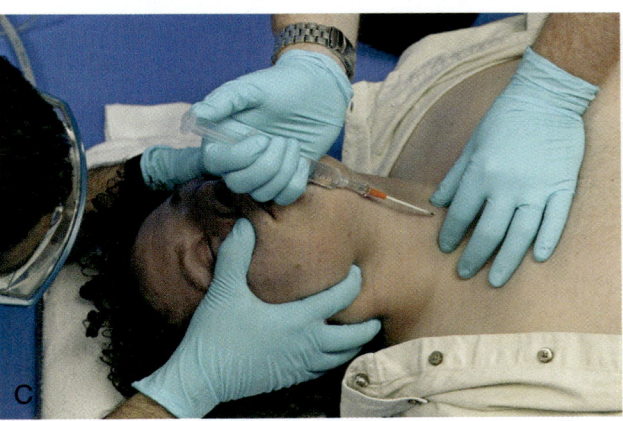
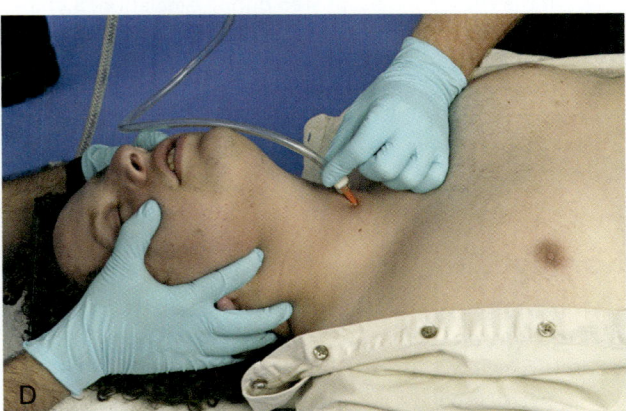

FIGURE 15-96 Translaryngeal cannula ventilation. **A,** Stabilize the larynx and identify the cricothyroid membrane. **B,** Insert the needle of the syringe downward through the midline of the membrane toward the carina. **C,** While inserting the needle, draw back on the plunger of the syringe. If air enters the syringe, the needle is in the trachea. **D,** After removing the needle and syringe, stabilize the catheter and connect the end of the oxygen tubing from the hub of the cannula to the oxygen regulator. Provide for a release valve.

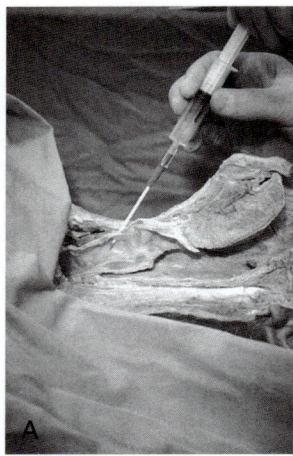

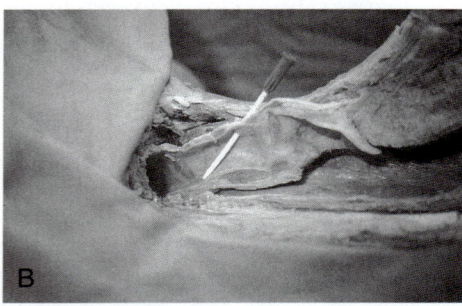

FIGURE 15-97 A, Insert a large-bore catheter through the crico-thyroid membrane, directing it toward the feet. While inserting the catheter, draw back on the plunger of the syringe; when air enters the syringe, the needle is in the airway. **B,** Slide the catheter off the stylet into the larynx.

inspiratory to expiratory ratio of 1 to 4 seconds is adequate. A ratio of about 1 to 8 seconds is needed to prevent baro-trauma (injuries caused by excessive pressures [e.g., pneu-mothorax]) when the upper airway is obstructed.[37]

> **NOTE**
> If the chest remains inflated during exhalation, a com-plete upper airway obstruction may be present. In such cases a longer expiratory time should be allowed. If this does not produce adequate deflation, a second large-bore catheter may be inserted through the cricothyroid membrane next to the first one. If the chest remains distended, a cricothyrotomy should be performed.

Advantages

- Translaryngeal cannula ventilation is the least invasive of surgical procedures.
- It can be initiated quickly.
- When performed by a trained paramedic, it is simple, inexpensive, and effective.
- Minimal spinal movement is needed for insertion.

Disadvantages

- The technique is an invasive procedure.
- Constant monitoring is required.

- Jet ventilation is required
- The airway is not protected.
- The procedure does not allow for efficient elimination of carbon dioxide.
- The patient's lungs can be ventilated adequately only for 30 to 45 minutes.

Possible Complications

- High pressure during ventilation and air entrapment may cause pneumothorax.
- Hemorrhage may occur at the insertion site. The thyroid and esophagus also may be perforated if the needle is advanced too far.
- Direct suctioning of secretions is impossible.
- Subcutaneous emphysema may occur.

Removal

Translaryngeal cannula ventilation is a temporary emer-gency procedure. It provides time for the use of other airway management techniques. The catheter should be removed only after successful orotracheal or nasotracheal intubation or after a cricothyrotomy or a tracheostomy has been per-formed. Removal involves withdrawing the catheter and dressing the wound.

CRICOTHYROTOMY

Cricothyrotomy is a surgical procedure. It allows rapid entrance to the airway through the cricothyroid membrane. The procedure can be performed quickly. It is much faster and easier than a tracheostomy. In addition, it does not require manipulation of the cervical spine.

Description

Cricothyrotomy can provide ventilation and oxygenation when airway control is not possible by other means. It should not be performed on patients who can be orally or nasally intubated. Few situations require this surgical pro-cedure. Relative indications for cricothyrotomy include severe facial or nasal injuries that preclude oral or nasal intubation, massive midfacial trauma, possible spinal trauma preventing adequate ventilation, anaphylaxis, and chemical inhalation injuries. Like translaryngeal cannula ventilation, cricothyrotomy requires special training and authorization from medical direction.

> **NOTE**
> Remember: Cricothyrotomy should be considered *only when you cannot intubate AND cannot ventilate.* If you cannot intubate but you *can* ventilate—do not cut the neck.

Necessary Equipment

Commercially prepared cricothyrotomy kits are available through a number of manufacturers (Figure 15-98). If such a kit is not available, the following equipment is required:
- Scalpel blade
- Size 6 (preferred) or size 7 ET tube or tracheostomy tube

- Antiseptic solution
- Oxygen source
- Suction device
- Bag-valve device

Technique

In patients suspected of having a spinal injury, in-line stabilization should be maintained throughout the procedure. If possible, the neck should be cleaned with alcohol or another antiseptic solution. The steps in the surgical procedure are as follows (Figure 15-99):

1. Locate the anatomical landmarks of the neck. Identify the cricothyroid membrane.
2. Make a 2 cm (¾ inch) horizontal incision with the scalpel at the level of the cricothyroid membrane. (Some physicians may recommend a vertical skin incision instead of a horizontal one.)
3. Open the incision in the cricothyroid membrane by inserting the scalpel handle. Rotate it 90 degrees. This allows placement of a size 6 or size 7 ET tube or tracheostomy tube, which will not damage the larynx. The cuff should be inflated and the tube tied securely.
4. Provide ventilation by a bag-mask device with the highest available oxygen concentration.
5. Determine the adequacy of ventilation. This can be done through bilateral auscultation and observation of rise and fall of the chest.
6. Use a secondary confirmation method such as end-tidal CO_2.

>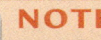
> ### NOTE
> Use of a smaller diameter endotracheal (ET) tube may aid successful placement. Once the tube is in the airway, the paramedic should be careful not to advance it more than a few centimeters. This helps prevent mainstem intubation.

Possible Complications

- Prolonged procedure time
- Hemorrhage

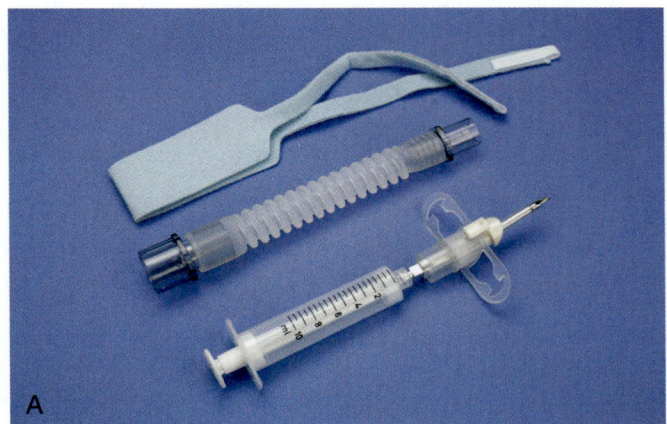

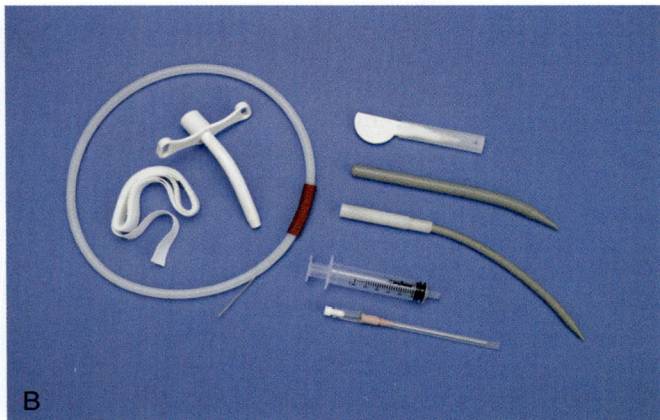

FIGURE 15-98 Commercial cricothyrotomy kits.

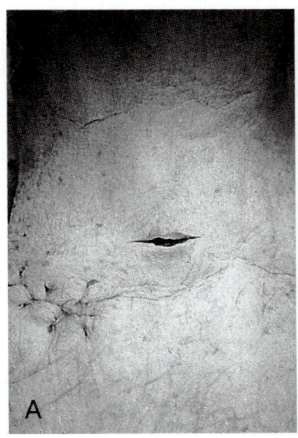
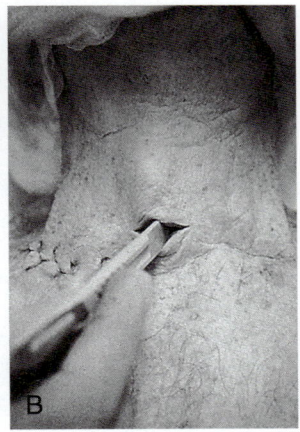
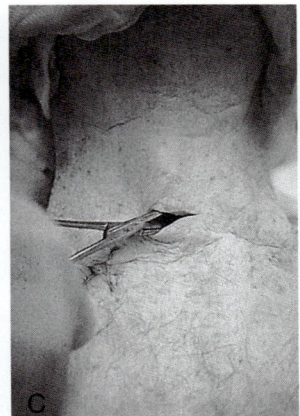
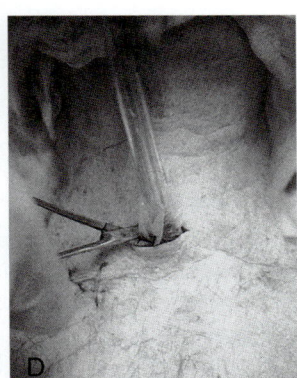

FIGURE 15-99 Surgical cricothyrotomy. **A,** Make an incision through the cricothyroid membrane. **B,** Open the hole by twisting the handle of a scalpel in it, *or* **C,** Open the hole with a clamp. **D,** Insert the endotracheal (ET) tube.

- Aspiration
- Possible misplacement
- False passage
- Perforation of the esophagus
- Injury to the vocal cords and carotid and jugular vessels lateral to the incision (the patient must be immobilized)
- Subcutaneous emphysema

Contraindications

- Inability to identify anatomical landmarks
- Underlying anatomical abnormality (e.g., tumor, subglottic stenosis)

- Tracheal transection
- Acute laryngeal disease caused by trauma or infection
- Small child under 10 years of age (in these patients, insertion of a 12- to 14-gauge catheter over the needle may be safer than a cricothyrotomy)

Removal

In the prehospital setting, no attempt should be made to remove ET tubes used during an emergency cricothyrotomy.

SUMMARY

- The upper airway opens at the nose and mouth and extends to the glottic opening.
- Structures of the lower airway include the trachea, right and left bronchus, bronchi, bronchioles, and the functional units of the lungs, the alveoli.
- The base of the lungs rests on the diaphragm. The right lung has three lobes and the left has two.
- The primary muscles of ventilation are the diaphragm and the intercostal muscles.
- The phrenic nerve enervates the diaphragm.
- *Respiration* is the exchange of oxygen and carbon dioxide between an organism and the environment. *Pulmonary ventilation* involves the movement of gas into and out of the lungs.
- *External respiration* is the transfer of gases between the inspired air and pulmonary capillaries. *Internal respiration* is the transfer of gases between the blood and tissue cells.
- During inspiration, the size of the thoracic cavity increases. This creates negative pressure inside the chest relative to atmospheric pressure, so air rushes into the lungs.
- During exhalation the chest muscles relax passively, and air is forced out of the lungs.
- The work of breathing increases if surfactant is lost, airway resistance increases, or pulmonary compliance decreases.
- The normal adult respiratory rate is 12 to 24 breaths/minute.
- No gas exchange occurs in the anatomical dead space. The physiological dead space includes the anatomical dead space plus any nonfunctioning alveoli.
- *Tidal volume* is the amount of gas inhaled or exhaled with each normal breath.
- The respiratory rate multiplied by the tidal volume equals the minute volume.
- Atmospheric gas contains approximately 79% nitrogen, 21% oxygen, and less than 1% carbon dioxide.

- As the pulmonary capillaries pass the alveoli, carbon dioxide diffuses into the alveoli and oxygen diffuses into the pulmonary capillaries.
- Oxygen is carried in the blood on hemoglobin. A small amount is also dissolved in the plasma. The amount of oxygen dissolved in the blood influences the extent to which oxygen binds with hemoglobin. The normal partial pressure of arterial blood oxygen (PaO_2) is 80 to 100 mm Hg. Venous PO_2 in the lungs is only 40 mm Hg; as a result, oxygen diffuses easily from the alveoli into the pulmonary capillaries.
- The respiratory centers normally are controlled by the pH of body fluids, which is influenced by carbon dioxide levels. Oxygen plays a role in the regulation of breathing in abnormal situations.
- Body temperature, medications, pain, emotion, and sleep also influence breathing.
- Modified forms of respiration are protective and include coughing, sneezing, and sighing.
- Older adults experience changes in ventilation and respiration that lead to a gradual decline in PO_2.
- Respiratory compromise and hypoxia can be caused by interruption of nervous control, structural damage to the thorax, bronchoconstriction, disruption of airway patency, oxygen deprivation, environmental factors, changes in alveolar-capillary gas exchange, ventilation deficiencies, decreases in lung compliance, ventilation/perfusion mismatching, disrupted oxygen transport, disrupted circulation, or cellular disruptions.
- Upper airway obstruction can rapidly cause death if not corrected.
- *Aspiration* is the inhalation of food, fluid, or foreign bodies into the lungs. This can cause airway obstruction and chemical damage with collapse of alveoli.
- The paramedic must assess the rate, regularity and rhythm of breathing. Also note the patient's position,

color, and heart rate. A thorough patient history should be obtained.

- Respiratory distress may be caused by upper or lower airway obstruction, inadequate ventilation, impairment of the respiratory muscles, ventilation/perfusion mismatching, diffusion abnormalities, or impairment of the nervous system.
- Supplemental oxygen is administered to increase the oxygen content in pulmonary capillaries and to help the patient compensate.
- Oxygen gas is administered by a variety of devices that regulate the concentration of oxygen delivered to the patient.
- Patient ventilation is provided by several methods, including rescue breathing (mouth to mouth, mouth to nose, mouth to stoma), mouth-to-mask breathing, bag-mask devices, and automatic transport ventilators.
- Airway management should progress from the least to most invasive methods. Airway management begins with manual maneuvers.
- Oropharyngeal or tracheal suction is used to remove liquids and foreign objects from the airway.
- Gastric distention can impair ventilation, and it increases the risk of aspiration. Orogastric or nasogastric tubes are inserted to reduce gastric distention.
- After manual airway maneuvers have been performed, mechanical adjuncts can be used to maintain the airway. Nasopharyngeal airways are used to maintain the airway in patients with a gag reflex. An oropharyngeal airway is inserted in patients with no gag reflex.
- Advanced airways include those that intubate the trachea and peritracheal airways, such as the laryngeal mask airway (LMA), King LT-D airway, and esophageal-tracheal Combitube (ETC) airway.

- Endotracheal intubation permits direct ventilation of the trachea, protection against aspiration, and a route for administering some medications. The ET tube may be inserted orally or nasally (in breathing patients). Adjuncts to assist with intubation include the stylet, tube introducer (bougie), and Magill forceps.
- It is essential to confirm proper placement of the ET tube. Methods of confirmation include auscultation of breath sounds; absence of gastric sounds; use of an esophageal detector device, and measurement of the end-tidal carbon dioxide and oxygen saturation.
- The laryngeal mask airway is inserted blindly into the hypopharynx in unresponsive patients with no gag reflex.
- An esophageal-tracheal Combitube is a twin-lumen airway placed blindly in unconscious patients with no gag reflex. In most cases the distal lumen is positioned in the esophagus, and inflation of balloons in the hypopharynx permits ventilation through tube 1. In rare cases, when the distal lumen is positioned in the trachea, the patient is ventilated through tube 2.
- Sedation sometimes is used in airway management and ventilation to reduce anxiety, induce amnesia, and decrease the gag reflex.
- In some EMS systems, neuromuscular blocking agents are used with sedation to permit endotracheal intubation.
- When an airway cannot be introduced through the nose or mouth and the patient cannot be ventilated, translaryngeal cannula ventilation or cricothyrotomy may be performed to access the airway by creating an opening in the cricothyroid membrane in the neck.

REFERENCES

1. Thibodeau GA, Patton KT: *Anatomy and physiology*, ed 7, St Louis, 2010, Mosby.
2. Emphysema.org: *About emphysema*. www.emphysema.org. Accessed August 6, 2010.
3. Pilbeam SP: *Mechanical ventilation: physiological and clinical applications*, ed 4, St Louis, 2006, Mosby.
4. Sherwood L: *Human physiology: from cells to systems*, ed 7, Belmont, Calif, 2007, Brooks/Cole.
5. Sukker MY, Ardawi MSM, El Munshid HA: *Concise human physiology*, ed 2, Oxford, England, 2000, Blackwell Sciences.
6. Springhouse: *Professional guide to diseases*, ed 9, Philadelphia, 2009, Lippincott Williams & Wilkins.
7. Beamis J, Mathur P, Mehta AC, editors: *Interventional pulmonary medicine*, ed 2, Bethesda, Md, 2010, Informa Health Care.
8. Bagdanov K: *Biology in physics: Is life matter?* Orlando, Fla, 2002, Academic Press.
9. Martin H: *Physiologic basis of respiratory disease*, Hamilton, Ontario, 2005, BC Decker.
10. Stockley R, Rennard S, Rabe K, et al, editors: *Chronic obstructive pulmonary disease*, Malden, Mass, 2007, Blackwell Publishing.
11. National Highway Traffic Safety Administration. *The National EMS Education Standards*. Washington, DC, 2009, U.S. Department of Transportation/National Highway Traffic Safety Administration, DOT.
12. McCance KL, Huether SE: *Pathophysiology: the biologic basis for disease in adults and children*, ed 6, St Louis, 2009, Mosby.
13. Casha A, Yang L, Cooper GJ: Measurement of chest wall forces on coughing with the use of human cadavers, *J Thorac Cardiovasc Surg* 118:1157-1158, 1999.
14. Sorenson H, Thorson JA: *Geriatric respiratory care*, Florence, Ky, 1998, Delmar.
15. Bosker G, Schwartz GR, Jones JS, et al: *Geriatric emergency medicine*, St Louis, 1990, Mosby.
16. National Safety Council: *Injury facts*, Chicago, 2010, The Council.
17. American Heart Association: *Basic life support for healthcare providers*, Dallas, 2010, The Association.

18. Tintinalli J, et al: *Emergency medicine: a comprehensive study guide*, ed 6, New York, 2003, McGraw-Hill.

19. Caples SM, Gay PC: Noninvasive positive pressure ventilation in the intensive care unit: a concise review, *Crit Care Med* 33:2651, 2005.

20. American Heart Association: *Pediatric advanced life support*, Dallas, 2006, The Association.

21. American Heart Association: Guidelines 2000 for cardiopulmonary resuscitation and emergency cardiovascular care, International Consensus on Science, *Circulation* 2000.

22. Ferrer M, Valencia M, Nicolas JM, et al: Early noninvasive ventilation averts extubation failure in patients at risk: a randomized trial, *Am J Respir Crit Care Med* 173:164-170, 2006.

23. American Heart Association. (2010). *2010 American Heart Association Guidelines for Cardiopulmonary Resuscitation and Emergency Cardiovascular Care. Circulation* 122(18 Supplement 3), S639-S946, 2010.

24. American Heart Association: *Clinical investigation and reports: hyperventilation-induced hypotension during cardiopulmonary resuscitation*. http://circ.ahajournals.org/cgi/content/full/109/16/1960?ck=nck. Accessed August 5, 2009.

25. Wigginton J: *The inspiratory impedance threshold device for treatment of patients in cardiac arrest: business briefing—emergency medicine review*. September 2005. www.touchbrieFigurescom. Accessed August 9, 2010.

26. American Heart Association: *ACLS provider manual*, Dallas, 2010, The Association.

27. Paradis NA, Halperin HR, Kern KB, et al, editors: *Cardiac arrest: the science and practice of resuscitation medicine*, ed 2, New York, 2007, Cambridge University Press.

28. Clayton BD, Stock Y, Harroun R: *Basic pharmacology for nurses*, ed 14, St Louis, 2007, Mosby.

29. Pott LM, Murray WB: Review of video laryngoscopy and rigid fiberoptic laryngoscopy, *Curr Opin Anaesthesiol* 21:750-758, 2008.

30. American College of Surgeons: *Upper airway management: advanced trauma life support*, Chicago, 2004, The College.

31. Garnet R, Ornato JP, Gonzalez ER et al: End-tidal carbon dioxide monitoring during cardiopulmonary resuscitation, *JAMA* 257:1379, 1987.

32. Gravenstein J, editor: *Capnography: clinical aspects, carbon dioxide over time and volume*, New York, 2004, Cambridge University Press.

33. Mackreth B: Assessing pulse oximetry in the field, *JEMS* 15:56, 1990.

34. Hamilton GC, Sanders AB, Strange G: *Emergency medicine: an approach to clinical problem-solving*, ed 2, Philadelphia, 2002, Saunders.

35. Marx JA et al: *Emergency medicine: concepts and clinical practice*, ed 5, St Louis, 2002, Mosby.

36. American Society of Anesthesiologists: *Practice guidelines for management of the difficult airway*. http://74.125.95.132/search?q=cache:zeAW_2T-r0QJ:www.asahq.org/publicationsAndServices/Difficult%2520Airway.pdf+difficult+airway,+defined&cd=1&hl=en&ct=clnk&gl=us&lr=lang_en. Accessed August 14, 2010.

37. Stothert J et al: High pressure transtracheal ventilation: the use of large-gauge intravenous-type catheters in the totally obstructed airway, *Am J Emerg Med* 8:184, 1990.

SUGGESTED READINGS

American College of Emergency Physicians: Verification of endotracheal tube placement: policy statement, *Ann Emerg Med* 54:141-142, 2009.

Guyette F, Greenwood M, Neubecker D et al: Alternate airways in the prehospital setting (resource document to NAEMSP position statement), *Prehosp Emerg Care* 11:56-61, 2007.

National Association of EMS Physicians: Alternate airways in the out-of-hospital setting: position statement of the National Association of EMS Physicians, *Prehosp Emerg Care* 11:248-250, 2007.

National Association of EMS Physicians: Verification of endotracheal tube placement following intubation: position statement, *Prehosp Emerg Care*, 11:248-250, 1999 (reaffirmed January, 2007).

PART FIVE

Patient Assessment

16 Scene Size-Up

Upon completion of this chapter, the paramedic student will be able to:

1. Describe the purpose of scene size-up.
2. Outline the components of scene size-up.
3. Recognize factors that may contribute to an unsafe scene.
4. Describe scene evaluation techniques.
5. Identify steps in scene management.
6. Outline measures to lower the risks associated with illness or injury at an unsafe scene.
7. Identify additional resources that may be needed to manage multiple patient incidents.

KEY TERMS

mechanism of injury The nature of the force that produced physical injury.

nature of the illness The principal characteristics and causes of an illness.

personal protective equipment Clothing or specialized equipment that provides some protection to the wearer.

safe holding area An area away from the emergency scene that provides for safety.

scene size-up An assessment of the scene to ensure scene safety for the paramedic crew, patient(s), and bystanders; a quick assessment to determine the resources needed to manage the scene adequately

*S**cene safety is always a priority in any EMS response.[1] This chapter provides a basic overview of scene safety. It also emphasizes the importance of personal safety for both the paramedic and the patient.* From Rick Brady

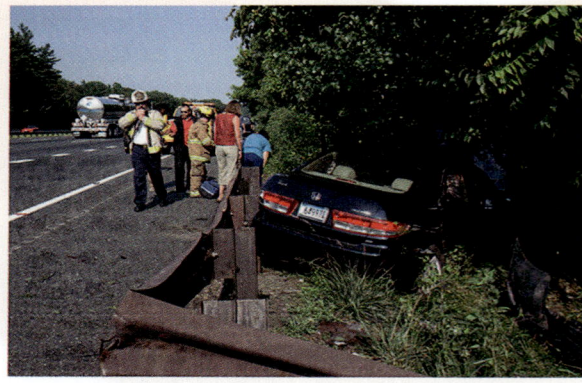

SCENE SIZE-UP

Scene size-up refers to a quick assessment of an emergency scene. The purpose of the assessment is to determine what resources are needed to safely manage the event. Scene size-up is a continuous evaluation of the scene that begins when the call is received. It requires quickly gathering facts about the situation, analyzing the problems and potential problems, and determining the appropriate response.

> 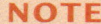 **NOTE**
> The paramedic must be constantly alert to situations that may change the needs of a particular incident. Scene size-up continues until the incident has been successfully managed and completed.

When a call is received for an emergency response, the paramedic should obtain as much information from the dispatcher as possible. Information from the dispatch center that will help in scene size-up includes:

- Exact location
- Type of occupancy (e.g., manufacturing, roadway, residence)
- Number of patients
- Type of situation (e.g., medical, trauma, vehicle collision)

- Hazards on the scene
- Unique issues (e.g., key boxes, known medical or access problems)

Obtaining this information and regular updates from the dispatch center will help the paramedic determine the need for additional resources. These resources may include additional ambulances, fire-rescue services, mutual aid, utility services (e.g., electrical power lines and gas lines), law enforcement, air medical services, and hazardous materials (Hazmat) teams, just to name a few (Box 16-1).

CRITICAL THINKING

What type of information might you obtain during dispatch that would make you concerned that a hazardous materials incident exists?

SCENE SAFETY

There are many factors that can affect scene safety in an emergency response. Examples include environmental hazards, the presence of hazardous substances, violence, and rescue-related hazards (Box 16-2) (see Part 11: EMS Operations).

Environmental Hazards

Dealing with the environment is a unique aspect of prehospital care (see Chapter 45). Hot weather conditions can expose the patient to thermal injury. An example is thermal burns from placing a patient on a spine board that is left uncovered on hot asphalt. Likewise, heat-related illness (hyperthermia) can quickly escalate if the EMS crew does not take immediate measures to remove the patient from the hot environment. All patients who are at risk for hyperthermia should be moved to a cooler environment to begin care.

Cold weather poses many challenges as well. An ill or injured patient is less able to regulate body temperature, allowing hypothermia to develop quickly. Patients who are at risk for hypothermia should be immediately sheltered from the wind and moved to a warm environment. Wet clothing should be quickly removed and the patient should be covered with warm, dry blankets. Warming measures may need to be initiated.

Caring for patients in a thunderstorm can be dangerous to everyone on the scene. Patients should be quickly moved to a location that is protected from lightning and other storm hazards. The paramedic should assume that wires downed from high winds are charged and dangerous until trained personnel verify their safety.

Many environmental hazards will warrant specialized rescue teams and additional resources. An example is rescue of a patient in water or on ice. Low light conditions can make patient assessment difficult and can easily contribute to personal injury. Portable light should be available to properly assess for hazards. Large rescue scenes should be properly lighted by requesting additional resources.

Hazardous Substances

Chemical, biological, radiological, and explosive hazards may be encountered from industrial accidents or terrorist incidents. Paramedics should be alert to dispatch information that indicates the potential for any of these hazards. Reports of large numbers of patients with similar signs or symptoms should signal the potential for one of these incidents. Assessment of a scene with a possible hazardous materials spill should be carefully planned. Scene assessment should begin at a distance using binoculars to look for the presence of indicators of hazardous materials. Indicators include container shape, smoke or vapor clouds, and identifying Hazmat placards. These scenes should not be entered until they have been secured and made safe by specialized teams, which may include law enforcement personnel, hazardous materials teams, or public health specialists. Specific information related to this type of response will be presented in Chapters 57 and 58.

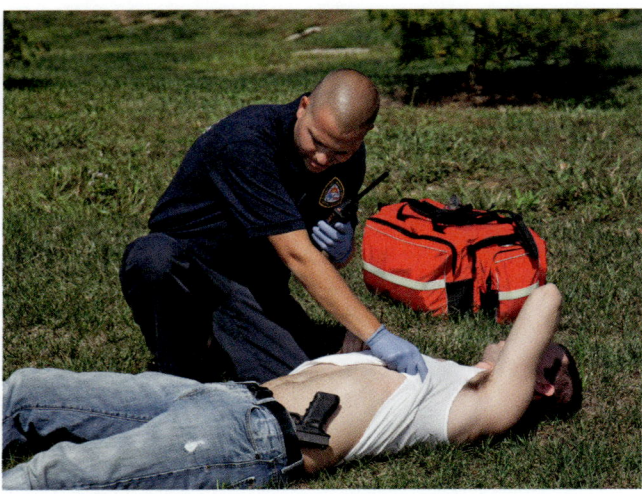

FIGURE 16-1 Patient with a concealed weapon.

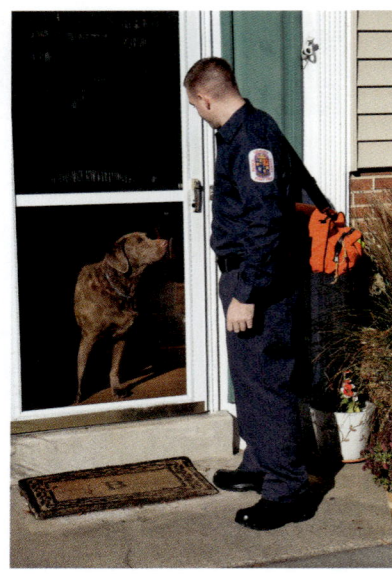

FIGURE 16-2 Paramedics preparing to enter a home with a large dog.

Violence

Many factors can contribute to a violent scene. An example is verbal aggression toward the EMS crew out of concern for the safety and well-being of a loved one. Drugs or behavioral illness can also alter a patient's behavior and create a dangerous situation. When patients or others on the scene display aggressive or violent behavior, the EMS crew should retreat from the scene until it has been secured by law enforcement personnel.

Paramedics should be alert for the presence of weapons at any scene. Traditional weapons include knives or guns. Other objects within reach of the patient also can be used as a weapon. Examples include tools, kitchen appliances, and household chemicals. In some states, concealed weapons are legal. All patients should be asked if they are carrying a knife, gun, or other weapon. If so, safely removing and securing the weapon during transport should be dictated by department policy (Figure 16-1).

Dogs or other pets can be a hazard to rescuers, particularly if they perceive their owner may be harmed. If dangerous animals are unsecured, the patient or a family member should be asked to contain them. If that is not possible, local animal control specialists should be summoned (Figure 16-2).

When responding to a known violent crime scene, the EMS crew should remain at a safe distance. This staging position should be maintained until law enforcement personnel have secured the area. Many crime scenes are not completely safe, even when law enforcement personnel are present. The paramedic should stay alert for clues that a dangerous situation can ensue or escalate.

> **NOTE**
> Paramedics should always keep in mind that a scene that appears safe can quickly become unsafe. All public service agencies play an important role in ensuring the safety of emergency response personnel.

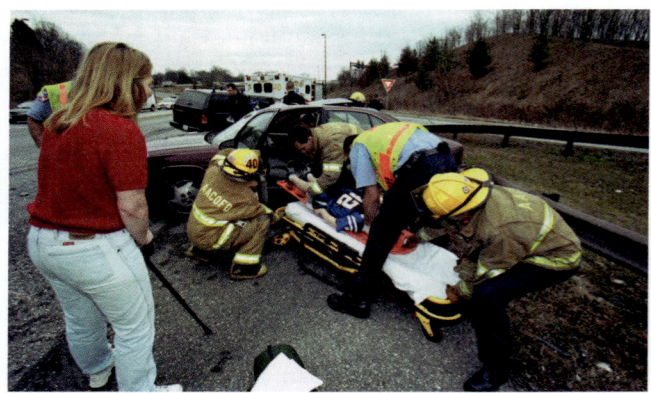

FIGURE 16-3 Extrication in progress.

Rescue-Related Hazards

Scenes involving rescue can be very dangerous. Common motor vehicle collisions often involve patient extrication, sharp metal, broken glass, unstable vehicles, and leaking fluids that increase the risk of fire. If it is safe to approach a vehicle involved in a collision, the paramedic should put the patient's vehicle in park and turn off the ignition before beginning patient care. The extrication itself may create additional hazards related to the powerful cutting and spreading tools; a shifting vehicle; or the possibility that an air bag will violently deploy (see Chapter 55). Paramedics should not remain in the vehicle during extrication unless properly trained and wearing appropriate protective equipment (Figure 16-3).

Each time a paramedic enters a roadway to provide care, there is a risk of being struck by oncoming traffic. Measures to reduce this risk should be taken on all roadway calls, regardless of the roadway speed limit. The ambulance should be positioned in a safe location. Other emergency vehicles and response personnel should park their units in a manner that shields the ambulance and the affected vehicles from oncoming traffic. Appropriate ANSI Class II vests (traffic vests) and other protective gear should be worn as outlined in departmental policies. A safety officer should monitor the scene at all times. Egress from the roadway should be made as quickly as possible. Safe roadway operations will be further addressed in Chapter 53.

IS THE SCENE SAFE?

YES — Don't accept significant risk — Stabilize the scene — Establish patient contact

NO — Do not enter until safe — Minimize hazards — Request specialized resources

FIGURE 16-4 Scene safety algorithm.

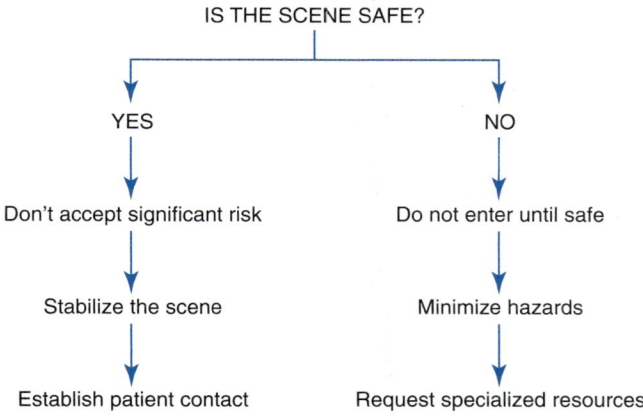

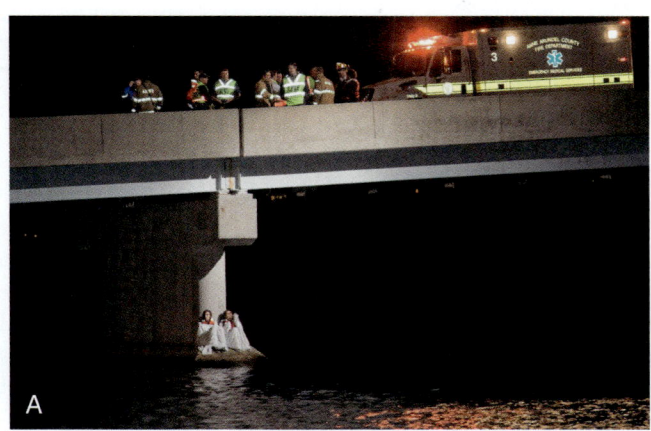

FIGURE 16-5 Water rescue.

Specialized rescues require advanced training and equipment. Examples include scenes that involve high- and low-angle rescue, trench rescue, confined space rescue, water rescue, and unstable structure rescue. Each specialized rescue event can pose a variety of hazards. Paramedics should not assist with the rescue or enter the scene until it has been made safe for entry (Figure 16-4) (see Chapter 55).

EVALUATION OF THE SCENE

When evaluating the scene, the paramedic must always ask *"Is the scene safe?"* If the scene is not safe and cannot be made safe, the scene should not be entered. Rather, the EMS crew should remain in a **safe holding area** and request additional resources. Only when the scene has been secured should the area be entered by EMS personnel. If no safety hazards exist, the paramedic should establish patient contact and proceed with patient assessment (Figure 16-5).

Sometimes it may be possible to quickly make a scene safe to enter. For example, if the incident is on a busy roadway, emergency vehicles can be quickly positioned to provide protection for emergency personnel. Another way to make a scene safer to enter is to wear reflective vests and clothing to improve rescuer visibility (Figure 16-6). However, it must be stressed that making a scene safe to enter should only be considered when it can be done without accepting significant risk to the paramedic or the patient.

SCENE MANAGEMENT

Successful management of an emergency scene requires many considerations. Specific considerations to be discussed in this chapter include:

- Impact of the environment on patient care
- Addressing scene hazards
- Violent scenes
- Need for additional/specialized resources
- Standard precautions
- Multiple patient situations

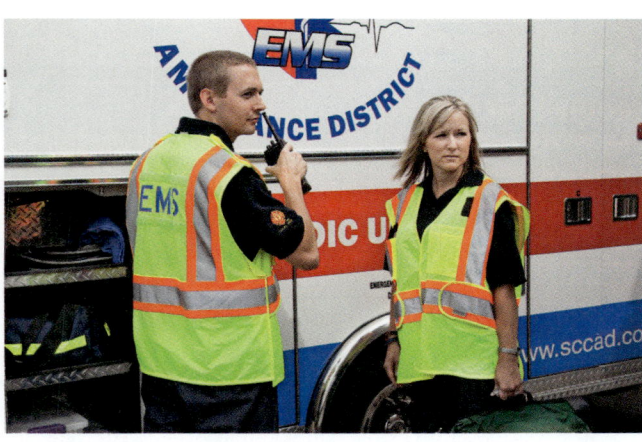

FIGURE 16-6 Reflective ANSI Class 2 vests.

Impact of the Environment on Patient Care

A quick, visual survey of the scene should be made on all emergency calls. For medical calls, the paramedic should first determine the **nature of the illness.** This includes being observant of the patient's surroundings for possible clues to the nature of the emergency. For example, are there empty pill bottles or drug paraphernalia nearby? Is the patient wearing a medical alert necklace or bracelet? Are there any unusual odors? Are there any hazards at the scene that could suddenly make the scene unsafe?

For trauma calls, it is important to quickly determine the **mechanism of injury** (see Chapter 37). Visual clues can be significant in directing patient care and in anticipating patient care that may be needed while at the scene and during transport. For example, was a steering wheel, dashboard, or windshield damaged in a motor vehicle collision? Were the occupants in the car wearing personal restraints? Was the patient wearing a helmet when she crashed her motorcycle? What is the length of the knife that was used to stab the victim? Are there any hazards at the scene that could suddenly make the scene unsafe?

CASE STUDY 1

You respond to a residence for an "accidental injury." When you arrive you find a tearful pregnant woman and her boyfriend. She is quiet and appears fearful. Her boyfriend says she fell down the stairs. You note bruising around her abdomen and other injuries not consistent with that story.

CRITICAL THINKING

Case Study 1. How can you make this scene safer for both you and your patient?

Addressing Hazards

As stated previously, all emergency scenes should be assessed for any environmental conditions or hazards. To ensure scene safety, any hazard must be addressed. Environmental conditions and hazards that could affect patient care or the safety of patients, bystanders, or emergency personnel include:

- Weather or extreme temperatures
- Toxins and gases
- Secondary collapses and falls
- Unstable conditions

After making the scene safe for the paramedic, the safety of the patient becomes the next priority. The paramedic should attempt to correct any hazards that might threaten the health or safety of the patient. If a hazard cannot be alleviated, the patient should be moved to a safer environment. Likewise, any condition that poses a threat to bystanders should be minimized. They too should be moved to a safer area.

CASE STUDY 2

You are dispatched for multiple patients with headache and vomiting at a residence. The power is out because of severe storms. When you arrive on the scene you hear the sound of a generator running in the house.

CRITICAL THINKING

Case Study 2. What actions can you take as you arrive on the scene to treat these patients in a manner that is safe for both you and your patients?

Additional and specialized resources may be needed to address hazards at the scene. These resources should be requested as soon as possible. The need for additional resources should be anticipated quickly when the scene is initially scanned for mechanism of injury or nature of illness. For example, if there are multiple patients, additional ambulances will be needed. Fire service will be needed if there are fire or electrical hazards, chemical spills, biological threats, unsafe structures, and rescue or extrication requirements. Utility services may be required to manage downed power lines or to secure natural gas lines. Law enforcement personnel may be needed to control traffic, to manage bystanders, and to contain any violence at the scene (see Chapter 55).

NOTE

Paramedics should never enter a scene or approach a patient if the threat of violence exists. The EMS crew should retreat from the scene and remain in a safe area until the scene has been secured by law enforcement personnel. *If the scene is not safe and cannot be made safe, do not enter.*

Standard Precautions

As described in Chapter 14, the use of standard precautions should be part of any EMS response. To review, standard precautions are based on the principle that all blood, body fluids, secretions, excretions (except sweat), nonintact skin, and mucous membranes may contain transmissible infectious agents.

> **LOOK AGAIN**
> See Chapter 14: Venous Access and Medication Administration, pp. 380-381.

Standard precautions include a group of infection prevention strategies. These strategies apply to all patients, regardless of suspected or confirmed infection status. They also apply to any health care delivery setting where patient care activities take place. The extent of precautions used is determined by the anticipated likelihood of exposure to blood, body fluids, or pathogens. Standard precautions are implemented by thorough hand washing and by wearing:

- Gloves
- Protective eyewear
- Masks
- Gowns

> **NOTE**
> *Universal precautions* is the practice of avoiding contact with a patient's body fluids by wearing personal protective equipment. These precautions were developed for protection of health care personnel. *Standard precautions* combine major features of universal precautions and body substance isolation. These precautions focus on the protection of patients.

> **CASE STUDY 3**
> You are dispatched for a woman with abdominal pain. As you enter the patient's bedroom, you note that she is squatting and screaming "the baby is coming, the baby is coming!"

> **CRITICAL THINKING**
> Case Study 3. How can you minimize your risk of exposure to blood or bloody body fluids on this call?

PERSONAL PROTECTIVE EQUIPMENT

Personal protective equipment (PPE) includes any clothing or specialized equipment that provides some protection to the wearer (Figure 16-7). PPE protects the paramedic and other emergency personnel from substances that may pose a health or safety risk. PPE should be appropriate for the potential hazard. (PPE will be further addressed in Part 11: EMS Operations.) Examples of PPE include:

- Steel-toe boots
- Helmets
- Turnout gear
- Heat-resistant outerwear
- Reflective clothing
- Bullet-proof vests in high crime areas
- Safety glasses
- Hearing protection
- Self-contained breathing apparatus (SCBA)
- Leather gloves

Multiple Patient Situations

When responding to an incident where there are multiple patients, the paramedic should anticipate the need for additional support. Often times, the dispatch center has made this determination and requested assistance before EMS arrives at the scene. As stated earlier in this chapter, additional and specialized resources that may be needed are based on the nature of the incident. These may include additional ambulances and/or air medical service, additional manpower to sort and care for the injured, additional medical supplies, special equipment for extrication and fire suppression, specialized rescue teams, utility services, Hazmat decontamination, and traffic and crowd control, to name a few.

The goals of managing an event with multiple patients are to ensure scene safety, protect the patients, and protect the bystanders. Bystanders will need to be removed from the patient care area and isolated from the scene. Barricades may sometimes need to be erected and manned by law enforcement personnel to ensure the goals of managing the event. Large-scale scenes or major incidents will likely require a command structure to safely manage the scene. These command structures are known as *Incident Command System* (ICS) or *Incident Management System* (IMS). These systems organize interagency functions and responsibilities of emergency personnel and public service agencies at the

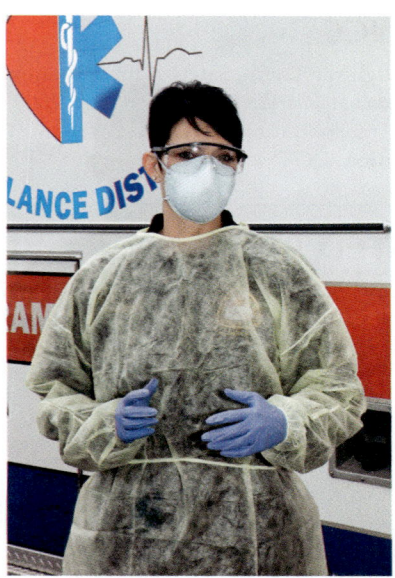

FIGURE 16-7 Example of personal protective equipment (PPE).

scene. Command structures play a vital role in scene management whenever available resources are insufficient to manage the number of casualties or the type of emergency. (Command systems will be described in detail in Chapter 54.) Examples of major incidents are listed below and in Box 16-2.

- Highway crashes
- Air crashes
- Major fires
- Train derailments
- Building collapse
- Acts of violence or terrorism
- Search and rescue operations
- Hazardous materials releases
- Natural disasters

CASE STUDY 4

Your unit is first to arrive at the scene of the call dispatched as a "motor vehicle collision." You find a school bus that left the roadway and rolled. You see multiple injured children. There is major damage to the bus and smoke is rising from the engine compartment. As you begin triage, your partner calls dispatch to establish command, to provide a brief size-up of the situation, and to request fire, rescue, and additional ambulances. Several parents in their cars have arrived at the scene.

 CRITICAL THINKING
Case Study 4. What challenges will you face in managing this scene?

SUMMARY

- Scene size-up is a quick assessment of an emergency scene. It is designed to determine resources needed to manage the scene safely and effectively.
- Dispatch information that assists with scene size-up includes location, type of location, type of situation, possible hazards, and unique issues.
- Special rescue, transport, fire, or other public safety resources may need to be dispatched to help manage the scene.
- Many factors can contribute to an unsafe scene. These may include environmental hazards, hazardous substances, violence, and rescue-related hazards.
- Scene assessment should always begin by asking, "Is the scene safe?" If it is not, identify measures that eliminate or reduce the risk to permit safe entry.

- Perform an initial scene survey. On medical calls attempt to determine the nature of the illness. On trauma calls gather information related to the mechanism of injury.
- If hazards cannot be corrected, remove the patient from the scene as quickly as safely possible.
- Standard precautions should be used for all patients to minimize the risk of exposure to blood or bloody body fluids.
- Other specialized personal protective equipment may be needed based on the nature of the hazard and the training and role of the paramedic on the scene.
- Multiple patient situations require many resources. Priorities should always be scene safety with protection of the patient and bystanders. Incident command should be established.

REFERENCE

1. National Highway Traffic Safety Administration: *The National EMS Education Standards*. Washington, DC, 2009, U.S. Department of Transportation/National Highway Traffic Safety Administration, DOT.

SUGGESTED READING

Wesley K: *Psychiatric patient assaults*, *JEMS.com*, 2007, www.jems.com/news_and_articles/columns/Wesley/PsychiatricPatient Assaults.html, accessed 10/10/09.

17 Therapeutic Communications

OBJECTIVES

Upon completion of this chapter, the paramedic student will be able to:

1. Define therapeutic communications.
2. List the elements of effective therapeutic communications.
3. Identify internal factors that influence effective communications.
4. Identify external factors that influence effective communications.
5. Explain the elements of an effective patient interview.
6. Summarize strategies for gathering appropriate patient information.
7. Discuss methods of assessing the individual's mental status during the patient interview.
8. Describe ways the paramedic can improve communication with a variety of patients. Such patients include (1) those who are unmotivated to talk; (2) hostile patients; (3) children; (4) older adults; (5) hearing-impaired patients; (6) blind patients; (7) patients under the influence of drugs or alcohol; (8) sexually aggressive patients; and (9) patients whose cultural traditions are different from those of the paramedic.
9. Describe methods to communicate in a culturally sensitive manner.

KEY TERMS

closed-ended questions Questions that are restrictive in form and can be answered with a "yes" or "no."

cultural imposition Forcing one's beliefs, values, and patterns of behavior on people from another culture.

decoding The act of interpreting symbols and format.

empathy The ability to see a situation from the viewpoint of the person experiencing it.

encoding The act of placing a message in an understandable format (either written or verbal).

ethnocentrism Seeing one's own life as the most acceptable or best; acting in a superior manner toward another culture's way of life.

open-ended questions Questions asked in a narrative form that cannot be answered with a "yes" or "no."

private space A comfortable distance from the patient's body; usually about 4 to 5 feet or twice the patient's arm length away (also known as *personal space*).

sympathy The expression of one's feelings about another person's problem.

therapeutic communications A planned, deliberate, professional act that involves the use of communication techniques to achieve two purposes: (1) a positive relationship with the patient and (2) a shared understanding of information between the patient and the paramedic. These two factors aid in the attainment of the desired patient care goals.

Therapeutic communications *can have several important effects. It can improve the paramedic's interaction with the patient, ensure better patient care, defuse potentially violent situations or prevent them from escalating, and reduce the risk of lawsuits.*

COMMUNICATION

Communication is the basic element of human interaction. It involves both verbal and nonverbal behavior. Moreover, it includes all the symbols and clues people use to convey

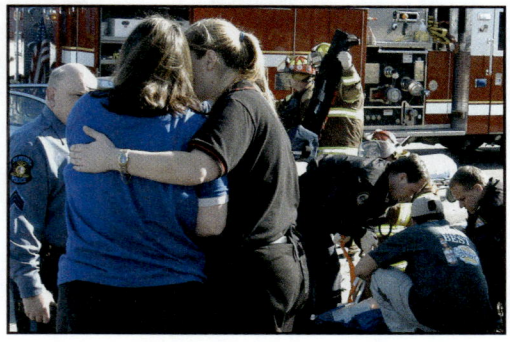

(Courtesy Ray Kemp. St. Charles, Mo.)

and receive meaning.[1] The process of communication has several elements. The paramedic must be aware of each element to interact effectively with a patient. Each element is crucial, and information and meaning can be gained or lost if any one element is changed (Figure 17-1). To achieve good communication, all participants must take equal responsibility for their part in the process. Communication is successful only when each person clearly understands the message.

> **NOTE**
> This chapter deals with communication between paramedics and their patients. However, these suggestions and techniques also can be used to improve communication between crew members, nurses, physicians, dispatchers, and other emergency personnel.

Elements of the Communication Process

Communication is a dynamic process. It has six elements: the source, encoding, the message, decoding, the receiver, and feedback.

SOURCE

Verbal communication uses spoken or written words (common symbols) to express ideas or feelings. (This is the *source* of the communication.) These common symbols should be simple, short, and direct to avoid confusion. Box 17-1 lists methods that can be used to achieve clarity in verbal communications.

> **CRITICAL THINKING**
> Think about the last time you had a misunderstanding with someone. Would any of the techniques listed in Box 17-1 have improved the situation?

FIGURE 17-1 The process of communication.

ENCODING

Encoding is the act of placing a message in a format that, when translated, is understood by both the sender and the receiver. The format may be either written or verbal. Encoding is the responsibility of the sender (*encoder*), because the sender defines the content and emotional tone of the message. In the process of communication, the sender role may pass from one person to another as information is exchanged. For example, the paramedic may initially be the sender of the message by asking a patient for information. When the patient responds, that person assumes the role of the sender.

MESSAGE

The *message* is the information that is sent or expressed by the sender. It should be clear and organized. It should be communicated in a manner familiar to the person receiving it. The message may include verbal and nonverbal symbols (e.g., spoken words, facial expressions, gestures). As a rule, the more ways (or formats) in which a message is communicated, the more likely the receiver is to understand it. For example, combining soothing words and a reassuring touch for a patient in pain communicates the message of compassion better than spoken words alone.

Not all symbols have universal meaning. For example, a reassuring touch might be welcome to persons of certain cultures, whereas those of other cultures may find it offensive. Paramedics must take into account the cultural differences of people in their service area. They should also consider how they will deal with a language barrier before attempting to send a message.

> **NOTE**
> It is estimated that at least 17.9% of the U.S. population (47 million people) speak a language other than English at home.[2]

DECODING

Decoding is the interpretation of symbols and formats. It prompts the receiver to respond to the sender's message. The decoding process can fail if symbols or words sent in

---

BOX 17-1 Techniques for Verbal Communication

- Use fewer words to avoid confusion.
- Use words that express an idea simply.
- Do not use vague phrases.
- Use examples (including demonstrations) if they will make the message easier to understand.
- Repeat the important parts of a message.
- Do not use technical jargon.
- Speak at an appropriate speed or pace.
- Do not pause for long periods or quickly change the subject.

the message are unfamiliar to both parties. It also can fail if interpretation of the message is based on different understandings of symbols or format. For example, the word *pain* may mean horrific discomfort to one person. However, it may mean a mild annoyance to another. Therefore, when communicating with a patient, the paramedic must carefully select words that cannot easily be misinterpreted.

> **NOTE**
>
> Some medical conditions, such as a stroke, can make it more difficult for a person to encode or decode a message.

RECEIVER

The receiver is essentially the *decoder*. This is the person intended to understand the message. As with the role of sender, the role of receiver switches back and forth between participants during the communication process.

> **CRITICAL THINKING**
>
> Have you ever attended a class in which nothing made sense? Contemplate the reason you did not understand the content. Was it an encoding problem or a decoding problem?

FEEDBACK

Feedback is the receiver's response to the sender's message. The quality of the feedback reveals whether the intended meaning of the message was received. If the intended meaning was not received, the sender must clarify the message by modifying its content and reassessing the new feedback. Like the message, feedback may be verbal or nonverbal.

INTERNAL FACTORS IN EFFECTIVE COMMUNICATION

To communicate well with patients, paramedics must genuinely like people. They must be able to empathize with others. They also must have the ability to listen (Box 17-2). Each of these internal factors plays an important role in therapeutic communications.

Liking Others

As a "helping profession," health care depends on the relationships forged between patients and health care personnel. These relationships are based on trust and caring. In fact, they cannot be achieved without a genuine concern for others and an understanding of human strengths and weaknesses. Patients must trust and believe that a paramedic *wants* to care for their needs. Paramedics can convey this trust to patients by accepting them as individuals.

Empathy

Empathy is the ability to see a situation from the viewpoint of the person experiencing it. It is widely accepted as a clinical aspect of a helping profession. **Sympathy,** on the other

---

BOX 17-2 Active Listening Attitudes and Guidelines

1. Listen to understand, not to ready yourself to reply, contradict, or argue back. This attitude is extremely important.
2. Remember that *understanding* involves more than simply knowing the dictionary meaning of the words used. It involves paying attention to the patient's tone of voice, facial expressions, and overall behavior.
3. Look for clues to what the individual is trying to say. As best you can, put yourself in the patient's shoes. Try to see the world as the patient sees it. Accept the patient's feelings as facts that must be taken into account, whether you share them or not.
4. Put aside your own views and opinions for the time being. Realize that you cannot listen to yourself inwardly and at the same time truly listen to the patient.
5. Control your impatience. Listening is faster than talking. The average person speaks about 120 words a minute. People can listen to about 400 words a minute. Do not jump ahead of the patient. Give the person time to tell the story. A patient does not always say what the paramedic expects to hear.
6. Do not prepare an answer while you listen. Get the whole message before deciding what to say. The patient's last sentence may put a whole new slant on what was said before.
7. Show the patient that you are alert and interested. This encourages the patient and improves communication.
8. Do not interrupt. Ask questions only to obtain more information. Do not try to trap the patient or force the individual into a corner.
9. Expect the patient's use of words to differ from yours. Do not quibble about terms—try to determine what was meant.
10. Your purpose is the opposite of a debater's goal. Look for areas of agreement, not for weak spots to attack with a barrage of counterarguments.
11. Before giving an answer in a particularly difficult discussion, summarize what you understand the patient to have said. If the patient disagrees with this version, clear up the contested points before giving your own views.
12. Let patients describe themselves and their interests, position, and opinions.

Adapted with permission from Legal Advocates for Abused Women, St Louis.

---

hand, is the expression of one's feelings about another person's problem. Unlike sympathy, empathy uses sensitive and objective communication. This helps patients explain and explore their feelings so that problem solving can occur (Box 17-3).

Ability to Listen

Listening is an active process. It requires complete attention and practice. To be an effective listener, the paramedic should[3]:

BOX 17-3 Empathy versus Sympathy

The case below shows the difference between empathy and sympathy. It also shows how empathy can help the paramedic soothe the patient and gain his trust.

Your emergency medical services (EMS) crew is sent to the home of a 60-year-old man with substernal chest pain. When you arrive, the patient is sitting on the living room sofa with his wife. They are upset and afraid that he might die. Your crew begins standard procedures for a possible heart attack and prepares to transport the patient to the emergency department. On the way to the hospital, the paramedic and the patient, who is accompanied by his wife, have the following conversation:

Paramedic: Even though you're feeling better, I can tell you're worried and afraid.

Patient: Yes, I am. I'm afraid I'm going to die.

Paramedic: Would you like me to explain to you and your wife what will happen after we arrive in the emergency department? I can also explain what the doctors and nurses will do to make sure you get the best possible care.

Patient: Yes, we would like that very much.

The use of empathy, shown in this conversation, allows the paramedic to accomplish three things: (1) calm the patient and his wife; (2) provide the couple with useful information; and (3) partly address their concerns. If the paramedic had used sympathy alone (e.g., "I understand how you feel, but don't worry, everything will be okay"), the patient's fears would have been ignored. Also, the problem of the couple's agitation would not have been solved.

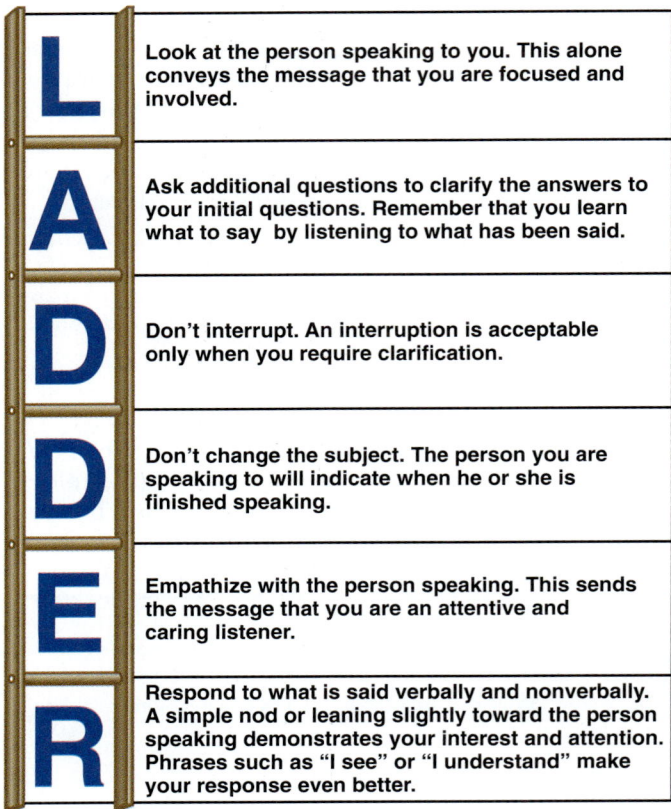

L	Look at the person speaking to you. This alone conveys the message that you are focused and involved.
A	Ask additional questions to clarify the answers to your initial questions. Remember that you learn what to say by listening to what has been said.
D	Don't interrupt. An interruption is acceptable only when you require clarification.
D	Don't change the subject. The person you are speaking to will indicate when he or she is finished speaking.
E	Empathize with the person speaking. This sends the message that you are an attentive and caring listener.
R	Respond to what is said verbally and nonverbally. A simple nod or leaning slightly toward the person speaking demonstrates your interest and attention. Phrases such as "I see" or "I understand" make your response even better.

FIGURE 17-2 The ladder of listening.

1. Face patients while speaking.
2. Maintain natural eye contact to show a willingness to listen.
3. Assume an attentive posture (avoid crossing the legs and arms, because this may convey a defensive attitude).
4. Avoid distracting body movements (e.g., wringing the hands, tapping the feet, or fidgeting with an object).
5. Nod in acknowledgment when patients talk about important points or look for feedback.
6. Lean toward the speaker to communicate involvement.

One device for remembering ways to improve communication is the listening ladder (Figure 17-2). This device has six steps to listening. They can easily be remembered from the acronym LADDER.[4]

EXTERNAL FACTORS IN EFFECTIVE COMMUNICATION

Effective communication requires a suitable setting. The paramedic has control over a number of the external factors that affect the setting. Some of these are privacy, interruptions, eye contact, and personal dress. Control of these factors results in a better interaction between the paramedic and the patient.

Privacy, Interruptions, and the Physical Environment

When possible, the paramedic should ensure privacy during the encounter. This helps to eliminate distractions and to reduce any inhibitions the patient may feel. Interruptions should be kept to a minimum. When possible, the lighting should be adequate. Noise and interference should be minimized. In addition, the patient interview should be initiated away from distracting equipment.

The paramedic should be aware of the patient's **private space.** This is a comfortable distance from the patient's body. It is about 4 to 5 feet[5] or twice the patient's arm length away. Private space (also known as *personal space*) is a form of subconscious personal protection that varies by individual and by culture. Some patients may become defensive if this space is invaded. Entering this space usually causes the patient to back away.

Eye Contact

The paramedic should maintain eye contact with the patient as much as possible, even when taking notes. Eye contact is a type of nonverbal communication. It can help express gentleness, sincerity, and authority and can help make the patient feel safe and secure. If possible, the paramedic should be positioned at eye level (equal seating) with the patient.

Personal Dress

Communication with a patient begins with first impressions. Paramedics' appearance should be professional. Their clothing should be clean and should meet professional standards (e.g., uniforms provided by the EMS agency). These standards help the patient instantly identify the paramedic. They also help to set the tone of the paramedic-patient encounter.

PATIENT INTERVIEW

The ability to conduct a successful patient interview may be as important as physical assessment skills. The information gathered often helps to decide the direction of the physical examination. The patient interview should be initiated early and should continue throughout the patient encounter.

Because of the emergency nature of their work, paramedics often think in terms of specific illnesses and injuries. They often must categorize patients into general groups, such as trauma or medical cases. However, good emergency care requires the paramedic to view each patient as an individual. Moreover, it requires paramedics to attend to a patient's needs in a caring, concerned, and receptive manner.

Communication Techniques

The paramedic should approach the conscious patient and make a personal introduction by name and title: "Hello. My name is [name], and I am a paramedic with [name of EMS agency]. What's your name?" A verbal exchange with the patient will provide information about a person's level of consciousness and sensorium. It also may provide information on any hearing or speech impediments and language barriers. During the introduction, the paramedic should maintain eye contact with the patient.

Nonverbal communication can send a message of negative feelings. It also can convey the insecurities of both the patient and the paramedic. Voice inflection, facial expression, and body position are examples of these nonverbal cues. They may reflect anger, fear, or impatience. Similarly, performing patient care procedures with trembling, sweaty hands may make the patient question the paramedic's skills. Nonverbal cues should be used to gain the patient's trust and cooperation. These can help the paramedic provide the best care for the patient.

Touch is a form of communication. It shows compassion and reassurance. Small gestures can help comfort a person in distress. A few examples are holding a patient's hand, squeezing a shoulder, or wiping tears from a patient's eyes. Experience and familiarity with patient care activities help determine the appropriateness of these gestures.

In talking with patients, the paramedic must listen to what is said and interpret what is said. Patients may say they feel fine. Yet their appearance and tone of voice may indicate that they are ill and afraid. If paramedics are unsure of the message in a patient's response, they should ask additional questions that will help them better understand what the patient is trying to communicate.

Most patients do not understand medical terminology. In addition, many have only a vague understanding of the way their bodies work. For these reasons, common words and phrases that are easy to understand should be used. The paramedic should guide and direct the patient interview without manipulating the patient's response. In other words, the paramedic should avoid asking **leading questions** (questions that can be answered with only "Yes" or "No"). **Open-ended questions** encourage a free-form response. For example, the paramedic should ask, "When did this pain begin?" rather than "Did the pain begin this morning?"

DID YOU KNOW?
Open-Ended vs. Closed-Ended Questions
Open-ended questions are asked in a narrative form. They cannot be answered with a "yes" or "no." They encourage the patient to talk.

Closed-ended questions can be answered with a "yes" or "no." They are restrictive and may not provide much information.

Open-Ended Questions	Closed-Ended Questions
How can I help you?	Can I help you?
Where is the pain in your chest?	Do you have chest pain?
How are you feeling today?	Do you feel better today than yesterday?
When was your last meal?	Did you eat today?
What medicines do you take?	Do you take any medicines?
What examples can you give me?	Can you give me an example?
Where else do you hurt?	Is this the only place that hurts you?
Can you tell me how this happened?	Has this happened before?
Can you describe your pain?	Does your pain feel sharp?
What else would you like to ask me?	Does this answer your question?

The paramedic should ask only one question at a time. The patient should be given ample time to answer the question before another question is asked. If the patient's response does not seem relevant to the question, the response should be clarified. Paramedics should be flexible. They should not discount the patient's experiences or information.

If possible, all questions asked by the patient should be answered. However, this does not mean that paramedics must provide a full explanation for each inquiry. Rather, a sensitive response that addresses the question is adequate. Paramedics should choose an answer carefully and should try to ensure the answer does not increase the patient's anxiety.

SHOW ME THE EVIDENCE

Researchers in Chicago evaluated characteristics of how physicians communicated with patients during the patient history and physical exam and during discharge instructions in 93 emergency department visits. Emergency medicine residents introduced themselves in only two thirds of cases and almost never (8%) indicated their training status. Sixty-three percent of the physicians began the history with an open-ended question; however, in only 20% of cases were patients permitted to complete their answer without interruption. Patients were interrupted in an average of 12 seconds. Discharge instructions lasted an average of 76 seconds and only 16% of patients were asked if they had questions. The researchers conclude that more provider education is needed.

From Rhodes K, Vieth T, Miller A et al: Resuscitating the physician-patient relationship, *Ann Emerg Med* 44(3):262-267, 2004.

Responses

There are many different tactics and responses that can be used to conduct a successful patient interview (Box 17-4). For example, the paramedic may use silence. This gives a patient more time to gather his or her thoughts. The paramedic also may *echo* (paraphrase) a patient's words. Echoing allows the paramedic to clarify or expand on the information provided. It also lets the patient know that the paramedic is listening. Empathy can be used to encourage a patient to talk more openly. Other tactics include asking a patient to clarify confusing statements and forcing the patient to focus on one factor of the interview (confrontation). At times the paramedic may need to interpret information by linking events, making associations, or inferring a cause based on what can be seen or concluded. Additional information (explanation) also can be given to a patient. This can persuade the person to share facts or objective information. Finally, paramedics can summarize information by asking the patient open-ended questions that can be used to review and to clarify important details.

Traps in Interviewing

Paramedics must be aware of some traps that can be damaging to the patient interview. These include the following:

BOX 17-4 Helpful Techniques for the Patient Interview

- Silence—Gives patients more time to gather their thoughts.
- Reflection—Echoing (i.e., paraphrasing) patients' words allows them to clarify or expand on the information provided.
- Empathy—Encourages patients to talk more openly.
- Clarification—Lets patients rephrase a word or thought that is confusing to the paramedic.
- Confrontation—Focuses patients' attention on one specific factor of the interview.
- Interpretation—Links events; makes associations or implies a cause; is based on observation or conclusion.
- Explanation—Provides information to patients; encourages sharing of facts or objective information.
- Summary—Provides a review of the interview; the paramedic can ask open-ended questions that allow patients to clarify details.

- Providing false reassurance
- Offering poor or unwanted advice
- Showing approval or disapproval
- Giving an opinion that takes away the patient's part in decision making
- Changing the subject inappropriately
- Stereotyping the patient or complaint
- Using professional jargon
- Talking too much
- Asking leading or biased questions
- Interrupting the patient
- Asking the patient "Why" questions (these can be viewed as accusations)
- Being defensive in response to criticism

Developing a Good Rapport With the Patient

Skill in developing good rapport with a patient requires experience and practice. In most patient encounters, paramedics can follow some general guidelines to help establish good rapport:

1. Put patients at ease by letting them know you are "on their side"; that is, that you respect their comments, and you are there to help them.
2. Be alert for and respond to visual clues that a patient needs help.
3. Show compassion.
4. Assess the patient's level of understanding and insight. Use words and explanations at their level.
5. Show expertise.

 CRITICAL THINKING

A suicidal patient keeps telling you that you do not care about him. What communication techniques could you use to persuade this patient that you are concerned about him?

STRATEGIES FOR OBTAINING INFORMATION

Patients generally communicate with health care personnel in three ways. The first is by pouring out the information in the form of complaints. The second is by revealing some problems while hiding others they think are embarrassing. The third is by hiding the most embarrassing parts of their problem from the paramedic (and personally denying the issue). The best way to obtain information from the patient is to use techniques for open-ended and closed (direct) questions. These techniques include resistance, shifting focus, recognizing defense mechanisms, and distraction.

> **NOTE**
> Closed-ended questions allow the paramedic to obtain specific information that focuses on a certain aspect of the patient's condition. "What part of your back hurts?" and "When was your last meal?" are two examples of closed-ended questions.

Resistance

Often a patient is reluctant to give information for one of two reasons. First, the patient may want to maintain a personal image and is afraid of losing that image. Second, the patient may fear that the paramedic will respond with rejection and ridicule. Paramedics, therefore, should be nonjudgmental. This helps them to obtain information from patients (Box 17-5). To develop a trusting relationship, the paramedic must be willing to talk to the patient about *any* condition in a professional manner.

Shifting Focus

A patient may be hesitant to discuss an obvious problem. In this situation, the paramedic may have to shift the focus of the questions away from that problem. For example, a man with groin pain at first may describe the pain (especially to a female paramedic) as being in his "lower back." By shifting the focus of questioning to low back pain, the paramedic can use another group of questions that focus on the presence or absence of radiating pain. This new angle of questioning can make patients feel more comfortable when describing their condition.

Defense Mechanisms

As described in Chapter 2: Well-Being of the Paramedic, paramedics should recognize common defense mechanisms. If possible, they should try to anticipate them. For example, a distraught parent with a seriously ill child may show regression or denial. The parent may be unable to provide needed information at the emergency scene. Confrontation may be required in these and similar situations to force the parent to deal with key issues. Confrontation can clarify roles. It also can help others identify problems and goals. However, this technique should be used only to obtain information critical for medical care. Confrontation must be performed in a professional way. This allows the patient to become aware of inconsistencies in interfering behavior or thoughts.

> **LOOK AGAIN**
> See Chapter 2: Well-Being of the Paramedic, pp. 42-44.

Distraction

Paramedics may use distraction to help patients recognize irrational thoughts or behavior. This type of behavior may be seen in hostile situations in which patients "act out." In such cases, paramedics need to point out the unacceptable behavior. They also need to let patients know the self-defeating nature of the behavior. Often, this distraction prompts patients to let the paramedic control the situation until they can gain self-control. When dealing with an angry or hostile patient, paramedics should:

- Avoid raising their voices to match the angry person's tone
- Have the person identify and describe the cause of anger
- Restate the cause of the anger
- Offer a solution (if possible) or empathize and acknowledge the person's feelings

METHODS OF ASSESSING MENTAL STATUS DURING THE INTERVIEW

Three methods can be used to assess a patient's mental status: observation, conversation, and exploration. (Assessment of the level of consciousness is discussed in more detail in other chapters.)

Observation

The first step in assessing mental status is to observe the patient. Paramedics should note the patient's appearance, level of consciousness, and normal or abnormal body movements. Physical characteristics, dress, and grooming can provide clues to the patient's well-being, social status,

---

BOX 17-5 Approaching Sensitive Issues

Discussing sensitive issues can be awkward for both the patient and the paramedic. Such issues might include alcohol use, sexual subjects, and suicide risk. Still, these issues must not be avoided when the information is needed to ensure good patient care. The paramedic should use the following guidelines when sensitive issues are discussed with patients:

- Make sure privacy is maintained.
- Be confident, direct, and firm with your questions.
- Do not apologize for asking a sensitive question.
- Do not be judgmental.
- Use words that are understandable, but do not be patronizing.
- Be patient and proceed slowly.

religion, culture, and self-concept. Conscious patients generically are alert and able to speak intelligently. Body movements (e.g., gestures, facial expressions) should be appropriate for the situation. Abnormal body movements may indicate an unstable situation. Such movements may include unusual posture or gait, or clenched fists.

Conversation

Conversation with patients should reveal whether they know who they are, where they are, and the day or date (i.e., whether they are oriented to person, place, and time). If the patient knows these things, the remote, recent, and intermediate facets of memory probably are intact. The patient should be able to speak at a normal pace and with even flow. Responses should not have long pauses or rapid shifts. (However, such nuances vary by geographical location.) During normal conversation, the patient should be able to demonstrate clear thinking, a normal attention span, and the ability to concentrate on and understand the discussion.

> **NOTE**
> Evaluating a patient's orientation to person, place, and date (*oriented × 3*) also can include other parameters. Some health care professionals use time or event (e.g., most recent holiday) as a fourth component in the assessment (*oriented × 4*).

A patient's responses to the environment (*affect*) should be appropriate for the situation. Normal reactions to stress may include autonomic responses. Some of these are sweating and trembling and odd facial movements (e.g., muscle twitching around the mouth, nose, and eyes). Reactive movements, such as not holding eye contact during conversation, should be noted. Other actions may indicate that a patient is uncomfortable or anxious. These include grooming movements, such as fixing the hair and straightening the clothes.

Exploration

Exploration offers a way to assess the patient's emotions. For example, by observing that the patient's mood is anxious, excited, or depressed and by noting the individual's energy level, the paramedic can gauge the mental status. Exploration can be done simply by interacting with the patient. This allows the paramedic to observe the appropriateness of behaviors and ideas. An objective assessment must consider the patient's culture and educational background. It also must take into account the person's values, beliefs, and previous experiences.

Because time is often a consideration when providing emergency care, the following "basic" questions can be used during exploration with patients of various cultures.[6]
1. What do you think caused your problem?
2. Why do you think it started when it did?
3. What does your sickness do to you? How does it work?

4. How severe is your sickness? How long do you expect it to last?
5. What problems has your sickness caused you?
6. What do you fear about your sickness?
7. What kind of treatment do you think you should receive?
8. What are the most important results you hope to receive from this treatment?

>
> **CRITICAL THINKING**
> The mental status examination is critical, both for medical reasons and for legal reasons. Why do you think this is so?

SPECIAL INTERVIEW SITUATIONS

At times paramedics may have to use special skills to interact successfully with a patient who is uncooperative or frightened or who has a disability (also see Chapter 18: History Taking).

Patients Who Do Not Talk

Although most patients are more than willing to talk, some need more time and varying techniques to participate in a successful interview. Difficult interviews generally stem from four sources[5]:
1. The patient's condition may affect the ability to speak.
2. The patient may fear talking because of psychological disorders, cultural differences, or age.
3. The patient may have a cognitive impairment.
4. The patient may want to deceive the paramedic.

HELPFUL TECHNIQUES

The following techniques may be useful for communicating with a patient who is unmotivated to talk:
- Start the interview in the normal way. If the patient does not talk, review the nature of the call as received from the dispatch center. Take time to develop a rapport with the patient.
- Use open-ended questions to get a response. If this is unsuccessful, try direct questions.
- Provide positive feedback to appropriate responses from the patient.
- Make sure the patient understands the question. (Consider whether a language barrier or a hearing difficulty is a factor.)
- Continue asking questions to obtain critical information needed to provide treatment. (Nonessential information may be difficult to obtain.)
- Question family members or others at the scene. If the patient has been uncommunicative for a long period, try to rule out a disease or disorder as the reason.
- Use summary and interpretation of events or conditions. Also, ask the patient if your summary and interpretation are correct.

- Ask the patient questions about your care, equipment, or profession in an attempt to create conversation. If the patient responds, answer all questions fully (not with one-word answers).
- Realize that all the information needed may not be obtained.
- Observe the patient's affect and record what you see. This sets a mental status baseline for later evaluations.
- Consider asking questions for which answers are known. This helps to gauge the patient's credibility.

> **NOTE**
>
> Patients who are unconscious or unresponsive may be able to receive stimuli. Hearing is thought to be the last sensation lost with unconsciousness. It also is thought to be the first regained with consciousness.[4] The paramedic must not say anything near an unconscious patient that would not be said if the patient were fully conscious.

Hostile Patients

Paramedics should be alert for signs that a situation may turn violent. This is part of ensuring personal safety. Such signs may include clenched fists, a rising voice level, a threatening facial expression, or a history of violence toward others. If such a situation exists or is expected, the EMS crew should retreat from the scene and request the help of law enforcement officers. If safe retreat is not an option, the paramedics should stay far enough away from the patient to ensure their personal safety (see Chapter 35). Some guidelines that can be used in interviewing a hostile patient are:

- Try to use normal interviewing techniques.
- Never leave the patient alone without adequate assistance.
- Set limits and establish boundaries with the patient.
- Explain the advantages of cooperation to the patient.
- Follow local protocol for dealing with hostile patients, including the use of physical and chemical restraints.

Patients With Age-Related Factors

Communicating with children and older adults should not be difficult or a challenge. It works best when the paramedic takes into account the common developmental characteristics of a particular age group (see Chapter 12).

COMMUNICATING WITH CHILDREN

When communicating with children, the paramedic often must establish rapport with two people—the child and the parent. With children 1 to 6 years old, most conversation should be directed first to the parent. (Offering a toy may distract the child while the parent is interviewed.) The paramedic should be aware that information from the parent is that person's point of view, and the parent might be feeling defensive. Paramedics should not be judgmental if the parents had not provided proper care or safety for the child before EMS arrival. (Be observant but not confrontational.)

The paramedic should gradually begin to make contact with the child during the parent interview. This can be done by moving to eye level to speak with the child and by using a quiet, calm voice. It should be remembered that children are especially responsive to nonverbal cues. Box 17-6 lists special considerations for communicating with children of various ages. (Assessing pediatric patients will be further discussed in Chapter 48.)

COMMUNICATING WITH OLDER ADULTS

Many older adults are dealing with age-related diseases and the inevitability of death. Interviewing older adults may take longer than interviewing younger persons. Older patients may tire easily. They also may have physical disabilities that distort speech. Touch is generally important to most older adults. When interviewing an older person, the paramedic should always use the individual's last name and Mr., Mrs., or Ms. unless the patient requests otherwise. In addition, the patient should be able to see the paramedic's face easily. Eye contact should be maintained, and speech should be clear and slow. Additional time may be needed to gather patient information. Using short, open-ended questions and talking with family members usually are the best approaches for the patient interview. (Assessing the older adult will be further addressed in Chapter 49.)

Hearing-Impaired Patients

When dealing with a patient with a hearing impairment, the paramedic should determine the patient's preferred method of communicating. It may be lip-reading, signing, or writing. Writing often is the best out-of-hospital method for communicating with a deaf patient. If the patient prefers lip-reading, the paramedic should (1) face the patient squarely, (2) ensure lighting is adequate, (3) speak slowly using short words and phrases, and (4) enunciate clearly. Because many deaf patients lip-read, paramedics must speak clearly in full view of these patients. It is

> ## BOX 17-6 Tips for Communicating With Children of Various Ages
>
> - Infants respond best to firm, gentle handling and a quiet, calm voice. Older infants may have stranger anxiety. If possible, the parent should remain in view of the child.
> - Preschoolers see the world only from their perspective and base everything on past experience. Use short sentences and give concrete explanations (e.g., "You will need to hold still so that I can splint your arm and make you feel better").
> - Adolescents want to be adults. Treat them with respect and use age-appropriate words. Do not talk to or treat them as if they were small children.

important to note that some deaf patients may nod "Yes" even if they do not understand the question.

If a patient is thought to be hearing-impaired or deaf, the paramedic should try to gain the person's attention. This can be done by a gentle touch or by slowly waving the hands in front of the patient. The paramedic also may try speaking a little louder or speaking into the patient's ear if the person is not wearing a hearing aid. If a hearing-impaired patient needs to be transported to a medical facility, the paramedic should inform the emergency department staff as soon as possible about the impairment. This allows arrangements to be made for personnel to aid in communications with the patient. (This is also a good practice with patients who do not speak English.) Finger-spelling and simple sign language are easily learned and can assist the paramedic in communicating with deaf patients in the prehospital setting.

Blind Patients

When communicating with a blind patient, it should be ascertained whether the patient also has a hearing impairment. (However, it is unusual for sightless people also to be deaf.) Paramedics should identify themselves in a normal voice. All questions about the emergency scene and the surroundings should be answered. In addition, all examination and treatment procedures should be explained in detail before touching the patient.

Most patients who have disabilities are very independent. They may resent unsolicited help. If a sightless person has a guide dog and the situation permits, the two should not be separated. If the dog was injured during the emergency event, the dispatch center should be quickly advised. This will allow for special arrangements to be made to care for the dog.

Patients Under the Influence of Street Drugs or Alcohol

If street drugs or alcohol play a part in an emergency, paramedics should ensure their personal safety. They should also be prepared for unpredictable patient behavior. (The help of law enforcement officers may be needed to ensure scene safety.) During the patient interview, simple and direct questions should be asked. Any action that might be viewed by the patient as a threat or confrontation should be avoided (see Chapters 34 and 35).

Sexually Aggressive Patients

Paramedics should confront male or female patients who make improper sexual advances. This ensures that the patient is aware of the professional role of the paramedic. Unusual incidents and observations of witnesses to inappropriate actions should be documented. If possible, sexually aggressive patients should receive care from paramedics of the same gender. It also is best to have a chaperone or witness present during the care and transportation of the patient. Some EMS services use audio devices during transport to record all interactions with sexually aggressive patients. (The use of these devices may require the patient's legal consent.)

Transcultural Considerations

When speaking with a patient from another culture, paramedics should introduce themselves and then ask the patient to do the same. Paramedics must be aware that they may be viewed as a cultural stereotype to the patient and family. For this reason, the roles of everyone involved in providing care (paramedics, patient, and family members) must be clearly understood. Box 17-7 outlines pitfalls to avoid when caring for patients of other cultures.

Two pitfalls that paramedics must avoid when speaking with patients of a different culture are ethnocentrism and cultural imposition. **Ethnocentrism** is seeing one's own life as the most acceptable or best. It includes acting in a superior manner toward another culture's way of life. **Cultural imposition** is forcing one's beliefs, values, and patterns of behavior on people from another culture. Paramedics do not fall into these pitfalls on purpose. Yet they must be sensitive to how their actions and words may be seen by those of another culture. Other factors to consider in communicating with patients of another culture are:

- Some cultures expect health care workers to have all the answers to their illness.
- Different cultures accept illness or injury in different ways.

BOX 17-7 General Guidelines for Working With an Interpreter

As a paramedic, you sometimes will be asked to assist a patient who does not speak English. Often someone in the home or at the scene can help you communicate with the person. When working with an interpreter, use the following guidelines:

1. Explain to the interpreter the key information you are trying to get before you begin the interview.
2. Ask a child to interpret only if no adult interpreter is available.
3. Speak directly to the patient or to a family member when asking questions. This establishes the primary relationship with that individual (not the interpreter). It also allows you to observe nonverbal clues.
4. Ask questions that require one response at a time. For example, ask, "Do you have pain?" rather than "Do you have any pain, trouble breathing, or nausea?"
5. Try not to interrupt the patient, family member, or interpreter when that person is speaking.
6. Do not make comments about the patient or family to the interpreter; the patient or family may know some English.
7. Use simple language. Do not use medical terms for which other languages may have no similar words.
8. After the interview, if time permits, ask for the interpreter's impressions and observations of the interview.

Modified from Wong D: *Whaley and Wong's nursing care of infants and children,* ed 5, St Louis, 1995, Mosby.

- Nonverbal cues (e.g., handshaking and touching) are perceived differently in different cultures.
- Some cultures consider direct eye contact impolite or aggressive; patients may avert their eyes during an interview.
- Paramedics should not use touch as a means of reassurance with members of different cultural groups because touch may be easily misunderstood.
- Language barriers may present communication difficulties (Box 17-8).

- Personal space is often defined by culture. It also varies by individual (Box 17-9).

CRITICAL THINKING

Do you know anyone whose personal space requirements are much greater or much less than those listed in Box 17-9? How would this affect your interview with that person?

BOX 17-8 10 Tips for Improving the Caregiver-Patient Relationship Across Cultures

1. Do not treat the patient in the same manner you would want to be treated. Culture determines the roles for polite, caring behavior and will formulate the patient's concept of a satisfactory relationship.
2. Begin by being more formal with patients who were born in another culture. In most countries, a greater distance between caregiver and patient is maintained through the relationship. Except when treating children or very young adults, it is best to use the patient's last name when addressing him or her.
3. Do not be insulted if the patient fails to look you in the eye or ask questions about treatment. In many cultures, it is disrespectful to look directly at another person (especially one in authority) or to make someone "lose face" by asking him or her questions.
4. Do not make any assumptions about the patient's ideas about the ways to maintain health, the cause of illness, or the means to prevent or cure it. Adopt a line of questioning that will help determine some of the patient's central beliefs about health/illness/illness prevention.
5. Allow the patient to be open and honest. Do not discount beliefs that are not held by Western biomedicine. Often, patients are afraid to tell Western caregivers that they are visiting a folk healer or are taking an alternative medicine concurrently with Western treatment because in the past they have experienced ridicule.
6. Do not discount the possible effects of beliefs in the supernatural on the patient's health. If the patient believes that

the illness has been caused by *embrujado* (bewitchment), the evil eye, or punishment, the patient is not likely to take any responsibility for his or her cure. Belief in the supernatural may result in his or her failure to either follow medical advice or comply with the treatment plan.

7. Inquire indirectly about the patient's belief in the supernatural or use of nontraditional cures. Say something like, "Many of my patients from ___ believe, do, or visit___. Do you?"
8. Try to ascertain the value of involving the entire family in the treatment. In many cultures, medical decisions are made by the immediate family or the extended family. If the family can be involved in the decision-making process and the treatment plan, there is a greater likelihood of gaining the patient's compliance with the course of treatment.
9. Be restrained in relating bad news or explaining in detail complications that may result from a particular course of treatment. "The need to know" is a unique American trait. In many cultures, placing oneself in the physician's hands represents an act of trust and a desire to transfer the responsibility for treatment to the physician. Watch for and respect signs that the patient has learned as much as he or she is able to handle.
10. Whenever possible, incorporate into the treatment plan the patient's folk medication and folk beliefs that are not specifically contradicted. This will encourage the patient to develop trust in the treatment and will help ensure that the treatment plan is followed.[7]

BOX 17-9 General Guidelines on Personal Space*

Intimate Zone
- 0 to 1½ feet
- Visual distortion occurs
- Best for assessing breath and other body odors

Personal Distance
- 1½ to 4 feet
- Perceived as an extension of self
- Speaker's voice is moderate
- Body odors are not apparent
- Much of the physical assessment occurs at this distance

Social Distance
- 4 to 12 feet
- Used for impersonal business transactions
- Perceptual information is much less detailed
- Much of the patient interview occurs at this distance

Public Distance
- 12 feet or farther
- Interaction with others is impersonal
- Speaker's voice must be projected
- Subtle facial expressions are imperceptible

*These are only general guidelines. Some cultures are more comfortable at a variety of distances when communicating.

SUMMARY

- Therapeutic communications is a planned act. It is also a professional act. The paramedic, working with the patient, obtains information that is used to meet patient care goals.
- Communication is a dynamic process. It has six elements: the source, encoding, the message, decoding, the receiver, and feedback.
- To effectively communicate with patients, paramedics must genuinely like people. They must be able to empathize with others. They also must have the ability to listen.
- Good communication requires a favorable physical environment. Factors such as privacy, interruption, eye contact, and personal dress are external influences. These factors can be controlled. This allows the paramedic to better communicate with the patient.
- The patient interview often decides the direction of the physical examination. Good care means that the paramedic sees each patient as an individual. It also means that the patient's needs are met in a caring, concerned, and receptive way.

- Open-ended and closed-ended (direct) questions can be used to get information from the patient. Techniques include resistance, shifting focus, recognizing defense mechanisms, and distraction.
- The first step with any patient is to assess mental status. This can be done by observing the patient's appearance and level of consciousness. The paramedic also can look for normal or abnormal body movements. During normal conversation, the patient should be able to show clear thinking, a normal attention span, and the ability to concentrate on and understand the discussion. The patient's responses to the environment (i.e., affect) should be appropriate to the situation.
- Difficult interviews generally arise from four situations: (1) the patient's condition may affect the ability to speak; (2) the patient may fear talking because of psychological disorders, cultural differences, or age; (3) a cognitive impairment may be present; or (4) the patient may want to deceive the paramedic.
- Paramedics should avoid ethnocentrism and cultural imposition when caring for patients from other cultures.

REFERENCES

1. Satir V: *The new peoplemaking*, Palo Alto, Calif, 1988, Science & Behavior Books.
2. U.S. Census Bureau: *Language use and English-speaking ability: 2000*, www.census.gov/prod/2003pubs/c2kbr-29.pdf, accessed 8-13-10.
3. Potter PA, Perry AG: *Fundamentals of nursing: concepts, process, and practice*, ed 5, St Louis, 2001, Mosby.
4. Moore M: *Embracing the mystery*, Madison, Wis, 1999, MJM Publishing.
5. Rathus SA: *Psychology: concepts and connections*, ed 9, New York, 2008, Wadsworth Publishing.
6. Kleinman A: *Patients and healers in the context of culture*, Berkeley, Calif, 1980, University of California Press.
7. Salimbene S, Graczykowski JW: *10 tips for improving the caregiver/patient relationship across cultures*, Amherst, Mass, 1995, Inter-Face International, Amherst Educational Publishing, pp. 23-25.

SUGGESTED READINGS

Knox H: Pain assessment and ethnicity, *Ann Emerg Med* 27(4):421-423, 1996.

Millard W: Ignoring it isn't an option: racial bias in emergency medicine, *Ann Emerg Med* 53(5):A19-A23, 2009.

University of Virginia School of Medicine: *Monograph on cultural competency*, 2009, www.med-ed.virginia.edu/courses/culture/, accessed 10/17/09.

18 History Taking

OBJECTIVES

Upon completion of this chapter, the paramedic student will be able to:

1. Describe the purpose of effective history taking in prehospital patient care.
2. List components of the patient history as defined by the National EMS Education Standards.
3. Outline effective patient interviewing techniques to facilitate history taking.
4. Describe how the paramedic uses clinical reasoning.
5. Outline the process to determine differential diagnoses.
6. Identify strategies to manage special challenges in obtaining a patient history.

KEY TERMS

chief complaint A patient's primary complaint.

clinical reasoning Use of the results of questions to think about associated problems and body system changes related to the patient's complaint.

current health status A focus on the patient's current state of health, environmental conditions, and personal habits.

differential diagnosis The process of weighing the probability of one disease versus that of other diseases possibly accounting for a patient's illness.

family history Illness or disease in a patient's family or family's background that may be relevant to the patient complaint.

history taking Information gathered during the patient interview.

opening questions Questions that determine why the patient is seeking medical care or advice.

past medical history A patient's medical background that may offer insight into the patient's current problem.

present illness Identification of the chief complaint and a full, clear, chronological account of the symptoms.

History taking *refers to details that are gathered during an interview with a patient. History taking provides an account of medical and social events in a patient's life. The history also indicates environmental factors that may have an impact on the patient's condition. Obtaining a patient history gives structure to patient assessment. History taking often is crucial to establish priorities in patient care.*

COMPONENTS OF THE PATIENT HISTORY

The patient history that is obtained in the prehospital setting is focused on the patient's problem or the reason EMS was summoned (*a problem-based history*). It has several

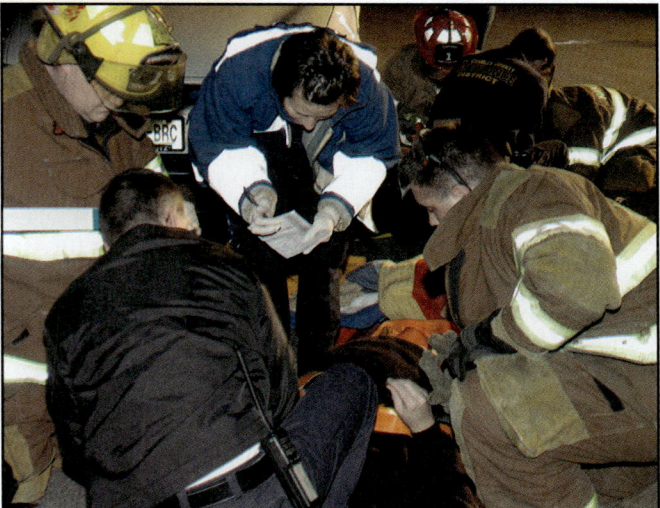

(Courtesy Ray Kemp, St. Charles, Mo.)

purposes.[1] First, the patient history places emphasis on identifying life-threatening conditions that require immediate intervention. That is, it gives full attention to the "needs of the moment." The patient history provides information that leads to appropriate care for the patient who is *urgent* (unstable), *emergent* (potentially unstable), and *non-emergent* (stable). In addition, the patient history identifies the potential for life threats as well as the existence of a current life threat.

Finally, the patient history can be expanded when appropriate to allow opportunities for patient education. It can also allow opportunities to provide service referrals to agencies and organizations that can help the patient and/or family with specific health care needs.

LOOK AGAIN
See Chapter 3: Injury Prevention and Public Health, pp. 56-58.

CONTENT OF THE PATIENT HISTORY

The patient history is made up of several parts. Each of these parts has a specific purpose, which offers a "snapshot" of patients and their condition. Box 18-1 lists the parts of a patient history, as described in this chapter.

The patient history should include the date and time that the history was obtained. The history also should contain any identifying information of the patient (e.g., age, gender, race, and occupation). Identifying information can be key, as illustrated in the following scenario: Your crew has been dispatched to a "sick case." On your arrival you find a woman who is ill with flulike symptoms. The symptoms include nausea, vomiting, and diarrhea. During your interview, she tells you that she is a 49-year-old businesswoman. She has just returned to the United States from an extended visit to her native home in Southeast Asia. In addition to the chance of gastrointestinal illness or food poisoning, you now suspect that she could be ill from an endemic disease (that is, a disease prevalent in a population or geographical region).

Documentation should include the source of the referral and patient history. For example, did the patient request EMS assistance, or did a family member, friend, law enforcement officer, or bystander initiate the EMS response? The paramedic also must decide whether the source of the referral and patient history is reliable, as illustrated in the following scenario: Your crew has been dispatched to a car crash. The driver of the car is a 17-year-old who has minor injuries. He is slurring his speech. In addition, his breath smells of an odor resembling alcohol. He denies alcohol or other drug use to you and the law enforcement officers at the scene. Is this patient history reliable?

The chief complaint (explained later in this chapter) is the main part of the patient history. The chief complaint is the reason why EMS was summoned. After identifying the chief complaint, the paramedic obtains a history and

---

BOX 18-1   Content of the Patient History

Date and Time
Identifying Data
Age
Gender
Race
Occupation

Source of Referral
Patient referral
Referral by others

Source of History
Patient
Family
Friends
Police
Others

Reliability
Variable (memory, trust, motivation)
Determined at the end of the evaluation

Chief Complaint
Main part of history
The one or more symptoms for which the patient is seeking medical care

Present Illness
Identifies the chief complaint
Provides a chronological account of the patient's symptoms

Medical History
Current Health Status
Review of Body Systems

---

description of the present illness or injury. This history provides a chronological account of the patient's symptoms. The paramedic then questions the patient about any past medical history and current health status. Also, the paramedic performs a review of body systems appropriate to the patient's symptoms or complaint (see Chapter 20).

TECHNIQUES OF HISTORY TAKING

As described in Chapter 17, it is important to "set the stage" for a good paramedic-patient encounter. This is done by establishing a good first impression and by making the environment conducive to free-flowing communication. The paramedic should do the following:

- Establish a professional demeanor with the patient.
- Ensure patient comfort and provide a safe environment.
- Greet the patient by name or surname and avoid demeaning terms (e.g., "Granny," "Pop," or "Hon").
- Avoid entering the patient's personal space.

- Inquire about the patient's feelings.
- Be sensitive to the patient's feelings and experiences.
- Watch for signs of uneasiness.
- Use language that is appropriate and easily understood.
- Ask open-ended questions and direct questions (if needed).

> **LOOK AGAIN**
> See Chapter 17: Therapeutic Communications, pp. 483-485.

> **NOTE**
> Remember that your demeanor and appearance are very important in "setting the stage." Just as you are watching the patient, the patient will be watching you.

Opening questions are questions that determine why the patient is seeking medical care or advice. Opening questions may incorporate facilitation, reflection, clarification, empathetic responses, confrontation, interpretation, and asking patients about their feelings.

Facilitation: Use your posture and positive actions or words to encourage the patient to say more. Maintain eye contact and use phrases such as "go on" and "I'm listening." These phrases encourage the patient to continue talking.

Reflection: Repeat or "echo" what the patient tells you. This encourages additional responses. Reflection usually will not bias the patient's story or interrupt the patient's train of thought.

Clarification: Ask questions to better grasp vague statements or words.

Empathy: Ask about the patient's feelings and show empathy to interpret the patient's feelings. This will help to gain your patient's trust.

Confrontation: Some issues may necessitate confronting patients about their feelings. For example, one may ask a patient who is severely depressed, "Have you ever thought about killing yourself?"

Interpretation: When appropriate, go beyond confrontation and make an inference from the patient's response. For example, draw an inference from the patient who says, "I think I'm going to die." One may infer that the patient may be gravely ill.

Ask patients about their feelings: Use therapeutic techniques described in Chapter 17 to encourage patients to explain how they feel.

Chief Complaint

As previously stated, the **chief complaint** is the patient's primary complaint, and is usually the reason for the EMS response. The complaint may be verbal (e.g., complaint of chest pain) or nonverbal (e.g., pain or distress expressed by a facial grimace). Most chief complaints are characterized by pain, abnormal function, a change in the patient's

normal state, or an unusual observation made by the patient (e.g., heart palpitations).

> **NOTE**
> When exploring the chief complaint, it is important to ask every patient:
> "What do you think is wrong with you?"
> "What are your specific concerns about your condition?"
> "What do you think caused your problem?"
> The patient's answers to these questions may be very relevant.

The paramedic should be aware that a chief complaint may be misleading. Also, a problem may be more serious than the complaint indicates. For example, the patient who has fallen down a flight of steps may complain of an injured ankle. However, physical examination may reveal possible internal injuries. Or, the patient may have fallen because of sudden paralysis on one side of the body related to a stroke. In addition, patients often modify or substitute their chief complaint. They may do this to hide a problem they find embarrassing or difficult to discuss. For example, a chief complaint of vaginal bleeding may be modified as "a heavy period." Actually, the bleeding was an abrupt hemorrhage that occurred during intercourse. Likewise, a chief complaint of "frequent headaches" may be substituted for feelings of depression with suicidal thoughts. Thus determining the *true* reason for the patient's concern is one of the skills of history taking. After identifying the patient's chief complaint (and managing any life-threatening situations), the paramedic should obtain a history of the present illness and any relevant medical history.

> **NOTE**
> Remember that the true needs of the patient may not be the stated chief complaint.

> **CRITICAL THINKING**
> What illnesses or injuries could cause a chief complaint of confusion?

History of Present Illness

The **present illness** identifies the chief complaint and provides a full, clear, and chronological account of the patient's symptoms. Obtaining a full history of the present illness takes skill. It takes skill in asking proper questions related to the chief complaint and in interpreting the patient's response. For example, a patient's complaint of low back pain suggests a muscle strain. During direct questioning in the interview, however, the patient reveals a history of a burning sensation with urination and a low-grade fever for the past several days. This information suggests a urinary tract infection or renal stones. Thus the history of the present illness may be more crucial than the obvious chief complaint. The mnemonic *OPQRST* helps define the patient's complaint by focusing on essential elements of

---

BOX 18-2 OPQRST Mnemonic

O (onset/origin): What were you doing when the pain started? Do you have a history of this problem?

P (provokes): What provokes the symptoms? What makes the symptoms better? What makes them worse?

Q (quality): What does the pain feel like? Is it sharp, dull, burning, or tearing?

R (region): Where is the symptom? Where does it go? Is it in one or more areas?

S (severity): On a scale of 1 to 10, with 1 being the least and 10 being the worst, what number would you give your pain or discomfort?

T (time): How long have you had this symptom? When did it start? When did it end? How long did it last?

BOX 18-3 SOCRATES Survey

S: Site
O: Onset (e.g., sudden, gradual)
C: Character (e.g., dull, sharp, stabbing)
R: Radiation
A: Associated symptoms (e.g., what else did you notice?)
T: Time, course, duration
E: Exacerbating and relieving factors
S: Severity (using a scale of 1 to 10)

---

assessment (Box 18-2). Use of this or another memory device (e.g., *SOCRATES* survey) will help lead the paramedic through a thorough series of questions to better understand the chief complaint (Box 18-3). The paramedic should take notes while obtaining the health history. Most patients realize that it is difficult to remember all details and accept note taking.

ONSET/ORIGIN

Onset and origin identify what the patient was doing when the pain began. The paramedic also notes whether there is any history of a similar episode. Questions to ask to obtain this information may include the following:
- "Did the pain or discomfort begin suddenly, or did it occur gradually over time?"
- "When did you last feel well?"
- "What were you doing when the pain started?"
- "Did the pain begin during a period of activity or while at rest?"
- "Have you ever had this type of pain or discomfort before? If so, is it the same or is it different than what you're experiencing now?"

PROVOKE/PALLIATION

Provoke and palliation refer to precipitating factors associated with the patient's complaints. Questions to ask to identify precipitating factors may include the following:
- "What makes your pain or discomfort better?"
- "What makes your pain or discomfort worse?"
- "Does the pain increase or decrease when you take a breath?"
- "Does lying down or sitting up affect your level of discomfort?"
- "Have you taken any medications for your symptoms? If so, did the medications make you feel better?"

QUALITY

Quality refers to how the patient perceives the pain or discomfort. Questions to ask to determine quality of the pain include the following:

- "What does the pain feel like?"
- "Can you describe the pain to me?"
- "Is the pain sharp or dull?"
- "Is the pain constant, or does it come and go?"

REGION/RADIATION

Region and radiation refer to the location of the pain and whether it is localized or associated with pain elsewhere in the body. Questions to ask to identify region and radiation include the following:
- "Where is the pain?"
- "Can you point with one finger to the exact location of the pain?"
- "Does the pain stay in the same place or does it move?"
- "If the pain moves, where does it go? Does the pain go to more than one area?"

SEVERITY

Severity refers to how the patient rates the level of the pain or discomfort. Severity also provides a baseline for future evaluation of the patient's pain. Questions to ask the patient include the following:
- "On a scale of 1 to 10, with 1 being the least and 10 being the worst, how would you rate your pain or discomfort?"
- "How bad is the pain?"
- "Does the intensity of the pain vary or does it stay the same?"
- "Have you had this type of pain before? If so, how is this pain different, or is it exactly the same?" (Figure 18-1)

 SHOW ME THE EVIDENCE

These researchers performed a retrospective study of 1227 ambulance run sheets to evaluate the feasibility of using pain scales for measuring prehospital pain level and for determining the severity of pain in prehospital patients older than age 13. This was conducted after implementation of a pain assessment protocol. Pain was assessed in 84% of conscious patients using either a verbal rating scale (VRS) or a numerical rating scale (NRS). A total of 31% of patients in their sample reported moderate to severe pain. These findings confirmed that use of the VRS and NRS to assess pain was possible in the field.

McLean S, Domeier R, DeVore H, et al: The feasibility of pain assessment in the prehospital setting, *PEC* 8 (2):155-161, 2004.

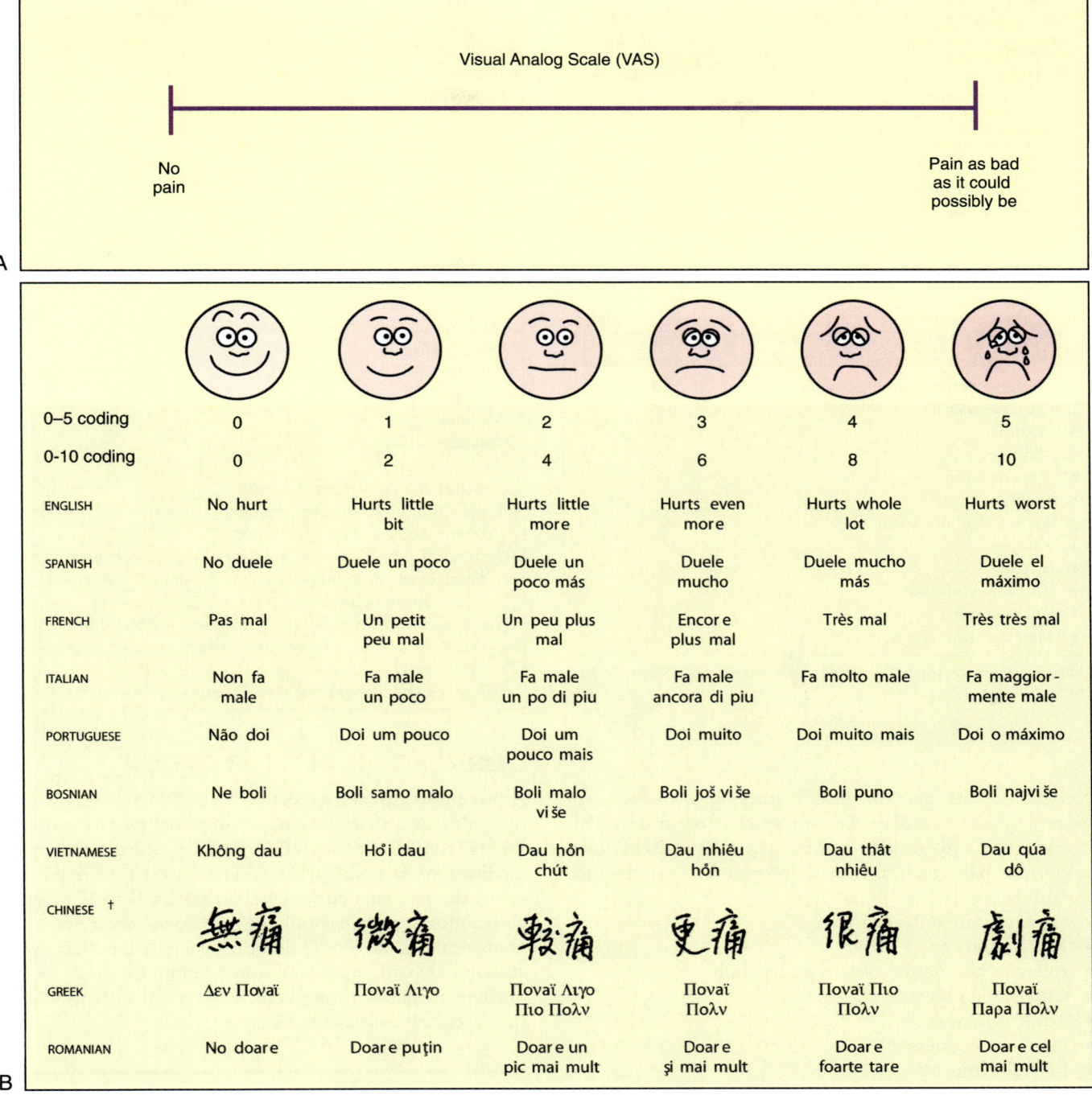

FIGURE 18-1 A, Visual analog pain scale. B, Wong FACES pain rating scale. (From Wold GH: *Basic geriatric nursing,* ed 4, St Louis, 2008, Mosby.)

TIME

Time refers to the duration of the pain or discomfort. Questions to ask to clarify the duration of the patient's pain or discomfort include the following:
- "How long have you been feeling this way?"
- "Have you had this same type of pain before, and if so, how long did it last?"
- "When did the pain or discomfort start?"

- "How long did the pain or discomfort last?"
- "When did the pain or discomfort end?"

Past Medical History

An important element of history taking is obtaining the patient's **past medical history.** This step can occur after the paramedic gains a good grasp of the patient's chief

BOX 18-4 Elements of the SAMPLE Survey

S: Signs and symptoms
A: Allergies
M: Medications
P: Past medical history
L: Last meal or oral intake
E: Events before the emergency

BOX 18-5 Complex Medical Histories

Adult patients with complex medical histories should be asked if they have ever had:
- Asthma
- Diabetes
- Hypertension
- Jaundice
- Myocardial infarction
- Seizures
- Stroke
- Thromboembolism
- Tuberculosis
- Hospital admissions

Nonsensical memory tool: All Day Helps Jack Make Sticks & Stones To Take Home.

BOX 18-6 Personal Habits and Environmental Conditions

Personal Habits
Tobacco use
Alcohol, other drugs, and related substances
Diet
Screening tests
Immunizations
Sleep patterns
Exercise and leisure activities
Use of safety measures
Home situation, spouse, or significant other
Physical abuse or violence
Sexual history
Daily life
Important experiences
Religious beliefs
Patient outlook

Environmental Conditions
Home conditions: housing; cleanliness; temperature; economic condition; pets and their health
Occupation: description of past and present work; exposure to heat, cold, and industrial toxins; similar complaints of illness among co-workers
Travel: exposure to contagious diseases; residence in tropics; water and milk supply; and other possible sources of infection
Military record: geographical areas; exposure to chemicals

complaint. The past medical history may include, for example, diabetes, and cardiac or respiratory disorders. This history may add insight into the patient's current state. Important past medical history information may include the following:
- General state of health
- Medications
- Allergies and nature of allergic reactions
- Childhood illnesses
- Adult illnesses
- Psychiatric illnesses
- Previous injuries
- Physical disability attributable to previous illness or injury
- Surgeries
- Hospitalizations

A variety of memory devices are used to recall key questions for gathering medical history. One example is the *SAMPLE Survey* (Box 18-4). Regardless of the patient's past medical history, there are important, direct questions that should be asked of every patient (Box 18-5). The answers to these specific questions can be significant in the development of a field impression. Pertinent positives and pertinent negatives can help build a complete picture of the patient's medical history.

CURRENT HEALTH STATUS

A **current health status** focuses on a patient's current state of health. It also considers personal habits and environmental conditions (Box 18-6). Details regarding allergies, medications, last oral intake, and family history can be critical to the patient's current health status. Female patients with abdominal pain should be questioned about their last menstrual period (if of child-bearing age). All patients with abdominal pain should be asked about their last bowel movement. Finally, the paramedic should identify events that occurred before the emergency.

? DID YOU KNOW?
Family History/Social History
A family history can give clues to possible predisposition to medical illness. It is known that certain diseases and health conditions tend to run in families. Examples include heart disease, cancer, hypertension, and stroke. Family history can also provide insight into why a patient may be anxious about contracting a particular disease. For example, a patient whose sister and aunt developed schizophrenia in their late twenties might be overly concerned that his son's irrational behavior is a sign of the same disease. When obtaining a medical history of family members or blood relatives, the paramedic should ask about family member health, ages, and causes of death for parents, siblings, spouse, and children.

A patient's social history can also be important. Questions should be focused on aspects of a patient's social history that may be affected by or connected to illness risk factors. Topics that may be appropriate to discuss include:

- Family (marriage, children)
- Dynamics in the home
- Dynamics in the workplace
- Financial circumstances
- Activities (work and leisure)

Other elements of a social history that may affect risk factors for illness include smoking, drinking, and drug use (past or present); sexual habits; current and previous occupation(s); and any recent travel abroad. Family pets and exposure to animals or birds can also be important and should be part of the patient's social history.

NOTE
Many persons have a life-threatening allergy to latex. Latex is a common substance found in emergency medical services care equipment.

MEDICATIONS

The paramedic should ask whether the patient takes any medications on a regular basis and, if so, for what reasons. In addition to information about prescribed medicines, information about the use of over-the-counter medicines is important. The paramedic also should ask about the use of herbs, naturopathic, and homeopathic medicines. This line of questioning should include the reason and frequency of use. If possible, the paramedic should determine whether the patient adheres to a medication regimen. The medication history may offer clues to the chief complaint. For example, a diabetic patient may have taken insulin but may have eaten at odd intervals. Other examples include a patient with chest pain who takes various cardiac drugs, an irrational patient who takes prescribed sedatives, and a trauma patient who takes blood-thinning drugs. In some cases it is helpful to examine the prescription fill date to determine whether the patient has been taking the medications as prescribed. Older adults with dementia may neglect to take medications or take them more often than prescribed.

CRITICAL THINKING
What would you do if you could not recognize the names or indications for the patient's home medicines?

The patient's medication history may not always be relevant to the problem at hand. However, the history can point to potential problems that may be seen during the patient care episode. There may be times when it is wise to directly ask a patient if he or she has taken specific drugs.

For example, before giving **nitroglycerin** it is important to ask the patient if he has taken any drugs for erectile dysfunction such as Cialis, Levitra, or Viagra. Administration of **nitroglycerin** to patients who have recently taken these drugs can cause life-threatening hypotension.

NOTE
Patients should also be questioned about alcohol use and illicit drug use. A direct line of questions is best. For example, "Mr. Jones, it is policy to ask all patients these questions, so please don't be offended. Have you used alcohol today? Have you taken any tablets or inhaled any drugs today that were not prescribed for you? Have you injected any drugs?"

LAST ORAL INTAKE

The time of the last meal or fluid intake is important when considering potential airway problems in a patient who loses consciousness or whose condition begins to deteriorate. Determining the patient's last oral intake also may help rule out some problems such as food poisoning and food allergies. For example, symptoms of certain types of food poisoning do not usually appear for several hours. In contrast, patients who are sensitive to certain foods would develop an allergic reaction immediately after eating the foods. Some of these foods are peanut oil and shellfish. Oral intake can also point to some illnesses. For example an undiagnosed or uncontrolled patient with diabetes may report excessive hunger or thirst. In the case of some older adults, they may have inadequate food intake related to inability to procure or prepare food.

NOTE
The time of the patient's last oral intake is crucial. The time can help to determine the appropriateness of surgery. Generally, if a patient has consumed any food or drink within the previous 6 to 8 hours, surgery is delayed if possible. The delay is to prevent the patient from aspirating the stomach contents. This may occur during the induction of anesthesia. However, immediate surgery may be indicated after recent oral intake. If so, a nasogastric tube is inserted to evacuate the stomach.

FAMILY HISTORY

A **family history** of illness or disease may be relevant to the chief complaint. The paramedic should establish whether a family history of heart disease, high blood pressure, cancer, tuberculosis, stroke, diabetes, kidney disease, current contagious illness, or other ailments exists. The paramedic also should note the presence or absence of hereditary diseases during the interview. Examples of these diseases include hemophilia or sickle cell anemia. Through experience, the paramedic will develop a "personal line" of questioning to further analyze a patient's particular symptoms.

LAST MENSTRUAL PERIOD

The paramedic should obtain a menstrual history when interviewing female patients between the ages of 12 and 55 years who have abdominal pain. The patient should be asked when her last period was and if it was normal for her. This questioning may prompt the patient to discuss other significant symptoms. These symptoms may include vaginal discharge, bleeding, and pregnancy history. The patient's response should determine the need to pursue additional questions regarding contraceptive use, venereal disease, urinary tract infections, and ectopic pregnancy (see Chapter 31).

LAST BOWEL MOVEMENT

The paramedic should ask a patient about his or her bowel habits to determine whether they have been normal or abnormal. A patient with abdominal pain may describe a recent history of diarrhea, constipation, or bloody bowel movements. This information will be helpful to the receiving physician to assess the patient for bowel obstruction, dehydration, or lower gastrointestinal bleeding. At this time, the paramedic also should ask the patient about any symptoms of abnormal urinary function. These symptoms may include blood in the urine, urethral discharge, pain or burning with urination, frequent urination, or the inability to void (see Chapter 30).

EVENTS BEFORE THE EMERGENCY

The paramedic should ask the patient and bystanders about events or actions that occurred before the emergency. For example, was a fainting episode preceded by exertion or straining? Did a loss of consciousness occur before or after a fall? An attempt should be made to correlate any event with the progression of an illness or injury.

GETTING MORE INFORMATION

With experience, paramedics learn to communicate with more skill. They learn to obtain a more complete picture of a patient's illness or injury. They are able to obtain more information about a symptom or complaint. Thus they are able to use clinical reasoning to evaluate associated problems and possible effects on body systems. Defining the attributes of a symptom may require the paramedic to ask direct questions. It may also involve obtaining a history on sensitive topics. Such topics may include alcohol or other drug use, physical abuse or violence, and sexual issues. When questioning a patient about sensitive issues, the paramedic should follow these guidelines:

1. Remember that privacy is essential with all patients, regardless of age or gender.
2. Be direct and firm and do not apologize for asking a question.
3. Avoid confrontation.
4. Be nonjudgmental.
5. Use language that is easily understood but not patronizing.
6. Encourage the patient to ask any relevant questions.
7. Document carefully and use the patient's words (noted by quotation marks) when possible.

CLINICAL REASONING

The depth and focus of the patient interview are based on the case at hand. However, the paramedic should gather as much information as possible at the scene and during transport to the hospital. Questions to the patient should be selected based on the patient's chief complaint and present problem. The paramedic uses the answers to think about associated problems and body system changes related to the patient's complaint. This is known as **clinical reasoning.**

Clinical reasoning requires integrating the patient's history with the physical assessment findings. It also requires knowledge of anatomy, physiology, and pathophysiology to direct appropriate questions to the patient. The answers to the questions are analyzed by the paramedic as they are received. As such, the paramedic must be prepared to change the direction of questioning based on careful evaluation of the answers.

The Process of Clinical Reasoning

Clinical reasoning should begin with the broad possibility of systems that could contribute to the patient's complaint. In addition, it requires the paramedic to consider the patient's current symptoms, past medical history, and abnormal symptoms and physical findings. These findings are then analyzed by anatomical location. This must consider all systems found in that location that may cause or contribute to the patient's problem. The findings are then interpreted in terms of a pathological process (Table 18-1).

During clinical reasoning, the possible body systems involved must be narrowed down or ruled out. Doing so allows the paramedic to develop a working hypothesis of the nature of the problem. This is known as differential diagnosis: the process of weighing the probability of one disease versus that of other diseases possibly accounting for a patient's illness. The differential diagnosis is then tested with questions and assessments relating to systems with similar types of signs and symptoms. Finally, the competing possibilities are considered and the paramedic selects the most likely problem to treat. Careful attention must be

NOTE
Before completing the patient history, the paramedic should ask every patient these three questions:
1. Is there anything else you would like to tell me that I haven't asked you about?
2. Is there anything you are worried about that we have not discussed?
3. Do you have any questions for me?

TABLE 18-1   Assessment by Body Systems

General symptoms	Fever, chills, malaise, fatigue, night sweats, weight changes
Skin, hair, and nails	Rashes, itching, swelling
Musculoskeletal	Joint pain, loss of motion, swelling, redness, warmth, deformity
Head and neck	
General	Headache, loss of consciousness
Eyes	Visual acuity, blurring, diplopia, photophobia, pain, vision changes, flashing
Ears	Hearing loss, pain, discharge, tinnitus, vertigo
Nose	Sense of smell, rhinorrhea, obstruction, epistaxis, postnasal discharge, sinus pain
Throat and mouth	Sore throat, bleeding, pain, dental issues, ulcers, changes in taste
Endocrine system	Thyroid enlargement, temperature intolerance, skin changes, swelling of hands and feet, weight changes, polyuria, polydipsia, polyphagia, changes in body and facial hair
Male	Erectile dysfunction, penile discharge, testicular pain
Female	Menstrual regularity, last menstrual period, dysmenorrhea, vaginal discharge, bleeding, pregnancy, contraception use
Chest and lungs	Dyspnea, cough (productivity/description), wheezing, hemoptysis, TB* status
Heart and blood vessels	Chest pain (onset, duration, quality, provocation, palliation), palpations, orthopnea, edema, past cardiac evaluation and tests
Hematologic system	Anemia, bruising, fatigue
Lymph system	Enlarged or tender lymph nodes
Gastrointestinal system	Appetite, digestion, food allergies or intolerance, heartburn, nausea, vomiting (frequency, color, texture, contents), diarrhea, hematemesis, bowel regularity, stool changes (frequency, color, texture, odor), flatulence, jaundice, past GI evaluation and tests
Genitourinary system	Dysuria, pain (flank, suprapubic), frequency, urgency, nocturia, hematuria, polyuria, STDs
Neurologic system	Seizures, syncope, loss of sensation, weakness, paralysis, loss of coordination or memory, twitches, tremors
Psychiatric	Depression, mood changes, difficulty concentrating, anxiety, suicidal or homicidal ideation, irritability, sleep disturbances, fatigue on waking

*GI, Gastrointestinal; STD, sexually transmitted disease; TB, tuberculosis.

paid to the signs and symptoms that do not fit with the working diagnosis (Figure 18-2).

SPECIAL CHALLENGES

History taking often presents special challenges. Each patient is unique. Thus each patient encounter is slightly different from all others. The paramedic must be able to adapt quickly to the special requirements of each encounter. That way the paramedic can obtain the needed information quickly. Some challenges that commonly affect history taking follow.

Silence

Silence is often uncomfortable and has many meanings and uses. For example, patients may use silence to collect thoughts, recall details, or decide whether they trust the paramedic. Silence also can defuse an emotionally tense event effectively. The paramedic should stay alert for nonverbal clues of distress or anxiety. These clues may include a worried expression or loss of eye contact, which often precede a silent period during the patient encounter. As a rule, when patients are ready to talk again, they will express feelings more clearly. A patient's silence also may result from a paramedic's lack of sensitivity, understanding, or compassion. An appropriate and caring "bedside manner" is key to good patient care.

Overly Talkative Patients

Interviewing talkative patients can be frustrating when there is limited time to obtain a health history. Although there are no perfect solutions in these situations, the following techniques may be helpful:

- Accept a less comprehensive history.
- Let the patient speak freely for the first several minutes.
- Ask questions that invite brief "yes" or "no" answers when appropriate.
- Summarize the patient's comments frequently.
- Refocus the discussion as needed.

Patients With Multiple Symptoms

Some patients (especially older patients) have a longer medical history because of age, chronic illness, and medication use. In addition, many older patients are likely to suffer from more than one illness. The paramedic should expect a longer interview and should use the techniques presented in Chapter 17. These techniques will help patients with multiple symptoms focus on the most relevant aspects of the chief complaint.

 LOOK AGAIN
See Chapter 17: Therapeutic Communications, pp. 487-488.

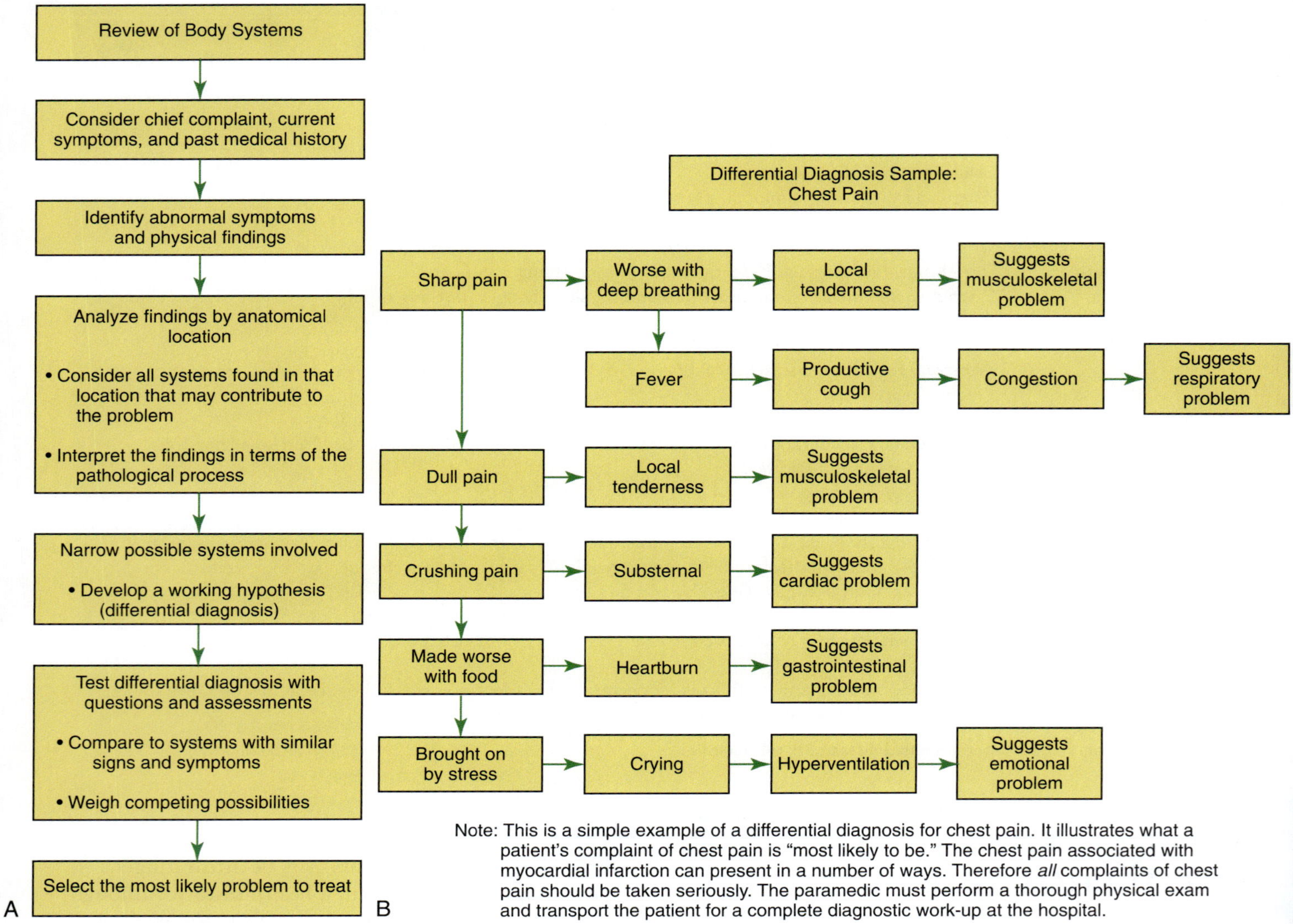

```
┌─────────────────────────────┐
│   Review of Body Systems    │
└─────────────────────────────┘
              │
              ▼
┌─────────────────────────────┐
│ Consider chief complaint,   │
│ current symptoms, and past  │
│ medical history             │
└─────────────────────────────┘
              │
              ▼
┌─────────────────────────────┐
│ Identify abnormal symptoms  │
│ and physical findings       │
└─────────────────────────────┘
              │
              ▼
┌─────────────────────────────┐
│ Analyze findings by         │
│ anatomical location         │
│ • Consider all systems      │
│   found in that location    │
│   that may contribute to    │
│   the problem               │
│ • Interpret the findings    │
│   in terms of the           │
│   pathological process      │
└─────────────────────────────┘
              │
              ▼
┌─────────────────────────────┐
│ Narrow possible systems     │
│ involved                    │
│ • Develop a working         │
│   hypothesis                │
│   (differential diagnosis)  │
└─────────────────────────────┘
              │
              ▼
┌─────────────────────────────┐
│ Test differential diagnosis │
│ with questions and          │
│ assessments                 │
│ • Compare to systems with   │
│   similar signs and         │
│   symptoms                  │
│ • Weigh competing           │
│   possibilities             │
└─────────────────────────────┘
              │
              ▼
┌─────────────────────────────┐
│ Select the most likely      │
│ problem to treat            │
└─────────────────────────────┘
A
```

Differential Diagnosis Sample: Chest Pain

```
Sharp pain ─► Worse with ─► Local ─► Suggests
              deep breathing  tenderness  musculoskeletal problem
                  │
                  ▼
              Fever ─► Productive ─► Congestion ─► Suggests
                       cough                       respiratory problem

Dull pain ─► Local ─► Suggests
             tenderness  musculoskeletal problem

Crushing pain ─► Substernal ─► Suggests cardiac problem

Made worse ─► Heartburn ─► Suggests
with food                   gastrointestinal problem

Brought on ─► Crying ─► Hyperventilation ─► Suggests
by stress                                   emotional problem
B
```

Note: This is a simple example of a differential diagnosis for chest pain. It illustrates what a patient's complaint of chest pain is "most likely to be." The chest pain associated with myocardial infarction can present in a number of ways. Therefore *all* complaints of chest pain should be taken seriously. The paramedic must perform a thorough physical exam and transport the patient for a complete diagnostic work-up at the hospital.

FIGURE 18-2 A, Review of body systems. **B,** Differential diagnosis sample—chest pain.

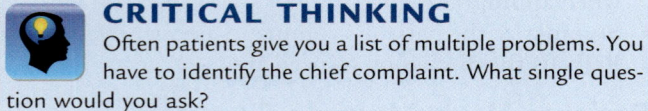

> ### CRITICAL THINKING
> Often patients give you a list of multiple problems. You have to identify the chief complaint. What single question would you ask?

Anxious Patients

It is normal for the patient, family, and bystanders to be anxious in an emergency situation. The paramedic must be sensitive to the nonverbal clues of anxiety and be supportive in a calm and confident way. The professional and caring attitude of the paramedic often helps to reduce the patient's anxiety. The paramedic should be aware that the anxiety may not be related directly to the illness or injury. For example, an older patient on a fixed income may worry about the cost of a hospital stay. A victim of a car crash may worry about liability and losing car insurance.

False Reassurance

The paramedic may be tempted to provide false reassurance in certain cases. Examples of this are saying "it's all right" or "everything's going to be okay." Although these false reassurances may comfort an ill or injured patient, they should be avoided until they can be given with confidence. False reassurance or over-reassurance may block open dialogue between the paramedic and the patient. The paramedic should reassure the patient that the patient's medical condition is understood and that good patient care is available. Patients also will be comforted to know that the outcome is hopeful (if appropriate) and that they will be treated with dignity and respect during their care. These verbal reassurances generally work well in most patient care situations.

Anger and Hostility

Anger and hostility are not very different from anxious behavior. They are similar in that they are natural responses in some emergency situations. The paramedic should expect these reactions at times to be displaced toward the EMS crew. The paramedic must always ensure personal and scene safety. However, anger and hostility toward the patient is never appropriate. A much more effective approach includes maintaining a calm, confident manner and setting limits on acceptable behavior.

Intoxication

Patients who are intoxicated with alcohol or other drugs should be managed with caution. Their behavior may be difficult to predict. Intoxicated patients should not be challenged or aggravated. Similar to managing patients who are angry or hostile, scene safety must be ensured and limits of acceptable behavior must be set. To ensure scene safety, the paramedic should call for assistance from law enforcement personnel when needed.

Crying

Crying can reduce tension and may help reestablish the patient's emotional stability during an emergency. If crying is excessive or uncontrollable, the paramedic should be patient. Compassion should be shown using direct eye contact to help control the crying. Reducing exhaustive crying conserves energy and promotes comfort.

Depression

Communicating with a depressed patient can be difficult. The types and causes of depression are many (see Chapter 35). The depression seen in an emergency often is due to moderate to high anxiety. Depression also may be enhanced by alcohol or substance use. The paramedic should use the communication techniques described previously for anxious patients. If possible, the paramedic should identify the seriousness of the patient's state. A physician's evaluation is encouraged.

Sexually Attractive or Seductive Patients

Paramedics and patients may be sexually attracted to each other. The paramedic should accept these feelings as normal. However, the feelings should not affect the paramedic's behavior. If a patient becomes seductive or makes sexual advances, the paramedic should firmly set limits of what is acceptable. It should be made clear that the relationship is a professional one. As discussed in Chapter 17, providing same-gender care often is the best practice. If this is not possible, an extra caregiver (or a chaperone) should stay with the patient.

Confusing Behavior or Histories

Emergency situations are often intense. In these situations, emotions can run high. Thus the paramedic should expect to find confusing histories and inappropriate or abnormal behavior. Factors that may contribute to these situations include mental illness, delirium, dementia, drug use, illness, and injury. Identifying a pattern of patient behavior may be difficult. Still the paramedic should try to identify one (e.g., signs and symptoms consistent with a certain disorder). In addition, the paramedic should attempt to lead the patient in an appropriate line of questioning.

Developmental Disabilities

The paramedic should not overlook the aptitude of patients with intellectual disabilities to provide adequate information. Patients with developmental disabilities should be interviewed just like other patients, using easily understood words and phrases. An obvious omission in the patient's answers reveals the need for more questioning. Questions may need to be stated more clearly. If the patient has severe mental retardation, the paramedic should try to obtain information from family or friends (see Chapter 51).

Communication Barriers

As discussed in Chapter 17, barriers to communication may result from social or cultural differences. These barriers also may occur because of sight, speech, or hearing impairments. The paramedic should seek assistance if possible. Family members, translators, and those with special training in communicating with the blind or the deaf may be helpful in these situations.

LOOK AGAIN
See Chapter 17: Therapeutic Communications, pp. 487-489.

Talking With Family and Friends

Friends and family are often at the scene of an emergency. Therefore the paramedic should consider them a good source of information. This is especially the case when the patient cannot provide all of the necessary information because of illness or injury. Sometimes family or friends are unavailable and more patient information is needed. In these cases, the paramedic should try to locate a third party (e.g., a neighbor) who can help supply the missing details.

SUMMARY

- Obtaining a patient history offers structure to the patient assessment. The history often identifies life threats and sets priorities in patient care.
- Content of the patient history includes date and time, identifying data, source of referral, history, reliability, chief complaint, present illness, past medical history, current health status, and review of body systems.
- The paramedic should ensure patient comfort. Several methods are available to accomplish this. The paramedic should avoid entering the patient's personal space. Sensitivity to the patient's feelings and watching for signs of uneasiness also are important. The paramedic should use appropriate language and ask open-ended and direct questions. The paramedic should use therapeutic communication techniques as well.
- Clinical reasoning requires integrating the patient's history with the physical assessment findings. It also requires knowledge of anatomy, physiology, and pathophysiology to direct appropriate questions to the patient.
- Differential diagnosis is the process of weighing the probability of one disease versus other diseases as accounting for a patient's illness.
- Many challenges can affect history taking. One of these challenges is silent or talkative patients. Another is patients with multiple symptoms. Then there are anxious, angry, or hostile patients. The paramedic also may see intoxication, crying, depression, and sexually attractive or seductive patients. False reassurance is a major issue to consider. Patients may present confusing behaviors and histories. Two other issues are developmental disabilities and communication barriers. In these last two cases, the issue of talking with family and friends can be complex as well.

REFERENCE

1. National Highway Traffic Safety Administration: *The National EMS Education Standards*. Washington, DC, 2009, U.S. Department of Transportation/National Highway Traffic Safety Administration, DOT.

SUGGESTED READINGS

Carpenito L, Editor: *Nursing diagnosis: application to clinical practice*, ed 12, Philadelphia, 2008, Lippincott Williams & Wilkins.

Edgerly D: *EMS assessments and differential diagnosis*, 2009, www.jems.com/news_and_articles/columns/Edgerly/ems_assessments_and_differential_diagnosis.html, accessed 10/22/10.Monahan F, Neighbors M: *Nursing care of adults*, Philadelphia, 1994, WB Saunders.

Potter PA, Perry AG: *Fundamentals of nursing*, ed 6, St Louis, 2007, Mosby.

Quinn K: *The ins and outs of patient meds: knowing about common mediations leads to improved patient care*, 2008, www.jems.com/news_and_articles/articles/jems/3304/the_ins_and_outs_of_patient_meds.html, accessed 10/22/10.

Seidel H, Ball JW, Dains JE, et al: *Mosby's guide to physical examination*, ed 6, St Louis, 2006, Mosby.

19 Primary Assessment

OBJECTIVES

Upon completion of this chapter, the paramedic student will be able to:

1. Identify the components of the scene size-up.
2. Identify the priorities in each component of patient assessment.
3. Outline the critical steps in primary patient assessment.
4. Describe findings in the primary assessment that may indicate a life-threatening condition.
5. Discuss interventions for life-threatening conditions that are identified in the primary assessment.
6. Distinguish priorities in the care of the medical versus trauma patient.

KEY TERMS

general impression An immediate assessment of the environment and the patient's chief complaint used to determine whether the patient is ill or injured and the nature of the illness or the mechanism of injury.

primary survey A component of the patient assessment to recognize and manage all immediate life-threatening conditions.

priority patients Patients who need immediate care and transport.

*T*he prehospital setting usually lacks emergency physicians on the scene and diagnostic services. Because of this, priorities of care must be set based on patient assessment. These priorities include scene safety, recognition and management of life-threatening conditions, and identification of patients who require rapid stabilization and transport for definitive care. This chapter provides an overview of patient assessment with an emphasis on the primary survey. More in-depth assessment strategies are presented in Chapter 20: Secondary Assessment and throughout this text by subject matter.

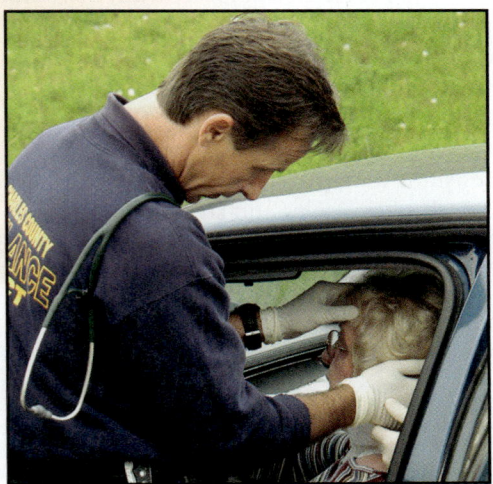

Courtesy Ray Kemp, St. Charles, Mo.

SCENE SIZE-UP AND PERSONAL SAFETY

Scene size-up and personal safety are the first steps taken during every EMS response. These steps ensure scene safety for the paramedic crew, patient(s), and bystanders. The assessment of the scene and surroundings offers key information to the paramedic. As described in Chapter 16: Scene Size-Up, the priorities in scene size-up include the following:

- Determine the nature of the incident.
- Determine the maximum potential number of persons already ill or injured and needing care.
- Assess for hazards at the scene.

- Initiate a mass casualty plan if indicated (see Chapter 54).
- Notify the dispatch center to request more resources (e.g., law enforcement, fire, rescue, utility companies) and to alert area hospitals (as needed).
- Determine the best access routes and staging areas for responders.
- Secure the area as rapidly as possible, clearing unneeded persons from the scene.
- Begin triage (if needed).

Even scenes that seem safe may be dangerous. Paramedics should never enter a potentially unsafe scene until they know it is safe to approach the patient. Examples of unsafe scenes include crash-and-rescue scenes, areas with toxic substances and low oxygen, crime scenes where violence is likely, and scenes that have unstable surfaces (e.g., slope, ice, or water). Personal safety is the paramedic's first priority.

> ### CRITICAL THINKING
> Do you know a paramedic who has been injured on a scene? What caused the injury? Could the injury have been prevented?

Protective Clothing

The National Fire Protection Association[1] and Occupational Safety and Health Administration[2,3] standards for protective clothing and personal protective equipment have been adopted by many emergency response agencies. At a minimum, paramedics should have access to the following personal protective equipment, although not all will be required on every call (Figure 19-1):

- Impact-resistant protective helmet with ear protection and chinstrap
- Safety goggles with vents to prevent fogging
- Lightweight, puncture-resistant turnout coat
- Slip-resistant waterproof gloves
- Boots with steel insoles and steel toe protection

Personal Protection From Blood-Borne Pathogens

As described in Chapter 14, The Occupational Safety and Health Act of 1991 adopted the recommendations established by the Centers for Disease Control and Prevention for personal protection from blood-borne pathogens. These universal precautions have been adopted by most states and public service entities. Now universal precautions are the minimum standard of practice recommended by the Occupational Safety and Health Administration (OSHA 29 CFR Part 1910.120). These precautions are intended to be used in the case of *all* patients in which there is a risk of exposure to blood or body fluids. They also are intended to be used when the infection status of the patient is unknown. The paramedic should wash his or her hands before and after patient contact to reduce the risk of communicable disease infection. In addition, items of personal protection from blood-borne pathogens should include disposable gloves and masks, eye protection, and gowns when necessary. Table 19-1 summarizes the patient care activities and the recommended level of protection for these activities.

> ### LOOK AGAIN
> See Chapter 14: Venous Access and Medication Administration, pp. 380-381.

PATIENT ASSESSMENT PRIORITIES

After ensuring scene safety and that needed resources are available or have been requested (Figure 19-2), patient assessment can begin (Figure 19-3). Patient assessment involves the following priorities[4]:
1. Primary survey/primary assessment
2. Integration of treatment/procedures to preserve life
3. Evaluation of the priority of patient care and transport

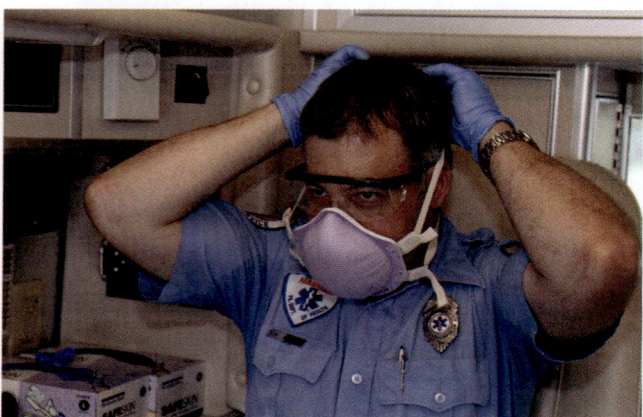

FIGURE 19-1 Personal protective equipment.

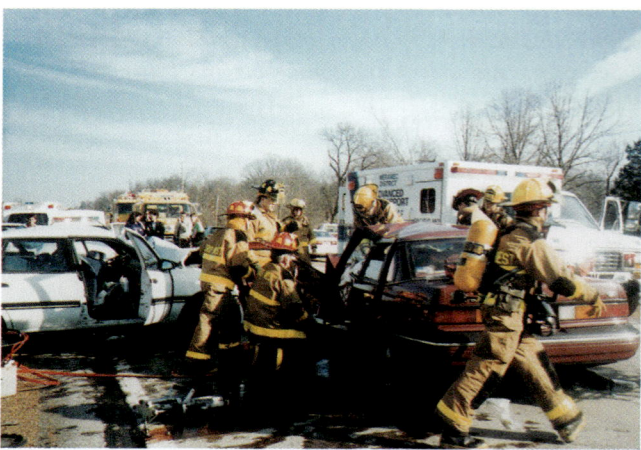

FIGURE 19-2 Many resources may be needed at an emergency scene. (Courtesy O'Fallon Fire Protection District, O'Fallon, Mo.)

TABLE 19-1 Examples of Recommended Personal Protective Equipment for Worker Protection Against HIV and HBV Transmission* in Prehospital† Settings

Task or Activity	Gloves	Gown	Protective Mask‡	Eyewear
Bleeding control with spurting blood	Yes	Yes	Yes	Yes
Bleeding control with minimal bleeding	Yes	No	No	No
Emergency childbirth	Yes	Yes	Yes, if splashing is likely	Yes, if splashing is likely
Blood drawing	Yes	No	No	No
Starting an intravenous line	Yes	No	No	No
Endotracheal intubation, esophageal obturator use	Yes	No	No, unless splashing is likely	No, unless splashing is likely
Oral/nasal suctioning, manually cleaning airway	Yes§	No	No, unless splashing is likely	No, unless splashing is likely
Handling and cleaning of instruments	Yes	No, unless soiling is likely	No	No, unless microbial contamination is likely
Measuring blood pressure	No	No	No	No
Measuring temperature	No	No	No	No
Giving an injection	No	No	No	No

HBV, Hepatitis B virus; *HIV*, human immunodeficiency virus.

*The examples provided in this table are based on application of universal precautions. Universal precautions are intended to supplement rather than replace recommendations for routine infection control, such as hand washing and using gloves to prevent gross microbial contamination of hands (e.g., contact with urine or feces).

†Defined as setting where delivery of emergency health care takes place away from a hospital or other health care facility.

‡Refers to protective masks to prevent exposure of mucous membranes to blood or other potentially contaminated body fluids.

§Although not clearly necessary to prevent HIV or HBV transmission unless blood is present, gloves are recommended to prevent transmission of other agents (e.g., herpes simplex virus).

Primary Survey/Primary Assessment

A **primary survey** is performed on all patients to establish priorities of care. The purpose of the primary survey is to recognize and manage all immediately life-threatening conditions. This assessment establishes priorities of care, which may include **resuscitation** (Box 19-1). The primary survey consists of the paramedic's general impression of the patient. This general impression is initially based on the patient's age and appropriate appearance.

General Impression of the Patient

The **general impression** is the paramedic's immediate assessment of the setting and the patient's chief complaint. The paramedic uses the general impression to determine whether the patient:

- Appears stable
- Appears stable, but potentially unstable
- Appears unstable

The general impression of a patient is formed based on both the patient and the environment in which you find the patient. It involves a visual assessment of the patient as he or she is approached (before being close enough to begin a physical assessment). As the scene is entered, the general setting should be observed for any clues of illness, injury, or mechanism of injury. Factors that help the paramedic form a general impression are based on:

- *Position.* Is the patient upright? Prone? Contorted in an unusual position? Tripod position?

BOX 19-1 Resuscitation

Resuscitation may be called for during the initial assessment. The paramedic begins resuscitative measures such as airway maintenance, ventilatory assistance, and cardiopulmonary resuscitation immediately as needed after recognizing a life-threatening condition. Several emergency care procedures generally are required in situations involving seriously ill or injured patients. Nearly all medical and trauma patients need some form of supplemental oxygen. Other resuscitation procedures for medical and trauma patients are as follows:

Resuscitation Procedures for Medical Patients
- Oxygen and airway control
- Insertion of an intravenous line to administer drugs or volume-expanding fluid
- Administration of resuscitation medications
- Administration of electrical therapy (e.g., defibrillation, cardioversion, external pacing)

Resuscitation Procedures for Trauma Patients
- Oxygen and airway control
- Cervical spine immobilization
- Insertion of intravenous lines for volume-expanding fluid
- Administration of resuscitation medications
- Application of a pneumatic antishock garment if appropriate

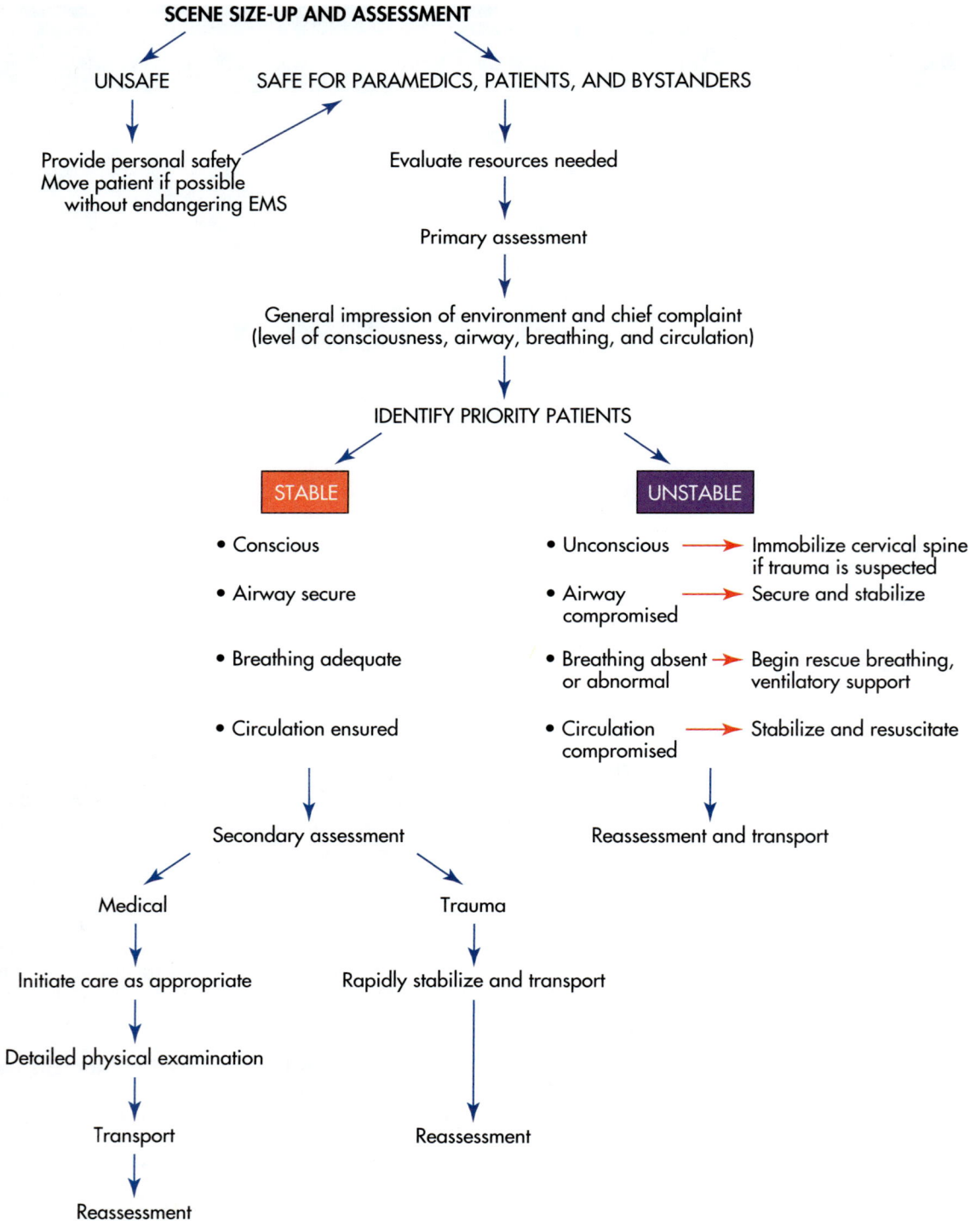

FIGURE 19-3 Components of patient assessment.

- *Work of breathing.* Is the patient breathing quietly or struggling to breathe?
- *Apparent attentiveness.* Are the patient's eyes closed or open? Does the patient turn to look at you as you enter? Is he or she staring blankly?
- *Skin color.* Is the patient pale, pink, or cyanotic?
- *Any obvious wounds noted.* Is there any bleeding or gross deformity evident?

- *Any body fluids noted.* Is there any visible blood, vomit, urine, or feces?

Patients who *appear stable* usually require only minimal care at the scene. These patients do not have life-threatening illness or injury. They are conscious and alert and their vital signs are within normal limits. Some stable patients will not require transport for physician evaluation.

Patients who *appear stable, but potentially unstable,* are injured or have underlying illness or disease. These patients may be conscious and alert and their vital signs may or may not be within normal limits. Their history of an injury or an underlying illness or disease alerts the paramedic that a decline in their status may occur. These patients are potentially unstable and always require transport for physician evaluation.

Patients who appear *unstable* have obvious signs of serious injury, illness, or disease. Their injury or illness is life threatening. These patients require immediate care and transportation to a medical facility. Initial on-scene care may include **resuscitation.**

Assessment for Life-Threatening Conditions

To assess for life-threatening conditions, the paramedic should conduct a systematic evaluation of the patient's level of consciousness, airway, breathing, and circulation.

LEVEL OF CONSCIOUSNESS

A first priority with any patient is to assess the level of consciousness. This assessment usually can be accomplished with a warm exchange with the patient. An example of such is "Hi. My name is _____. I'm a paramedic. How can I help you?" If the patient does not respond to verbal stimuli, the paramedic should assess if the patient responds to painful stimuli. This should begin with gentle tactile stimulation (e.g., rubbing the patient's shoulder), along with questions such as "Are you okay?" and "Can you hear me?" If there is no response, uncomfortable stimuli should be used to elicit a response. An example of an uncomfortable stimulus is rubbing the patient's sternum (*sternal rub*). A patient who does not respond to verbal or painful stimuli is considered unresponsive. As described in Chapter 15, the airway of any unconscious patient or any patient without a gag reflex or cough reflex must be secured immediately.

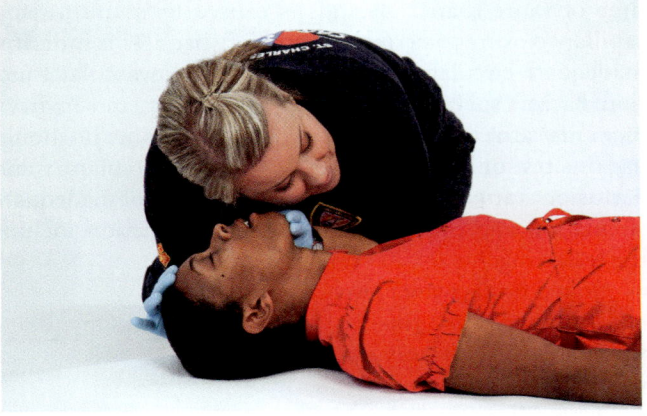

Figure 19-4 Paramedic opening an airway with head-tilt/chin-lift maneuver.

CRITICAL THINKING
What does a patient's level of consciousness tell you about the patient's oxygenation and circulation?

SHOW ME THE EVIDENCE
Researchers at an 896-bed hospital evaluated assessment of level of consciousness using the Glasgow Coma Scale (GCS) and the AVPU (*a*wake, responds to *v*erbal stimulation, responds to *p*ainful stimulation, *u*nresponsive) responsiveness scale in intentional and accidental poisoning patients who arrived to their hospital over a 6-month period in 2003. Their goal was to evaluate whether the scores could be linked to each other. A total of 1384 patients met their inclusion criteria. Although there was overlap in the scores, their data suggested the following: alert (median GCS 15); responsive to painful stimulation (median GCS 13); responsive to painful stimulation (median GCS 8); and unresponsive (median GCS 3). In general, there was difficulty using both scales in alcohol-intoxicated patients.

From Kelly C, Upex AD, Bateman D: Comparison of consciousness level assessment in the poisoned patient using the alert/verbal/painful/unresponsive scale and the Glasgow Coma Scale, *Ann Emerg Med* 44(2):108-113, 2004.

AIRWAY STATUS

The paramedic should assess the airway of any patient to ensure it is patent with good air exchange. If the patient is unresponsive, the airway should be opened and cleared of any obstructions (described in Chapter 15).

A responsive patient should be assessed for the ability to speak, noting signs of airway obstruction or respiratory insufficiency. These signs could include stridor, snoring, or gurgling. Any condition that compromises the delivery of oxygen to body tissues is potentially life threatening and must be managed immediately. Factors that may compromise the airway include the following:

- Tongue obstructing the airway in an unconscious patient
- Loose teeth or foreign objects in the patient's airway
- Epiglottitis
- Upper airway obstruction from any cause
- Facial and oral bleeding
- Vomitus
- Soft tissue trauma to the patient's face and neck
- Facial fractures

A compromised airway must be secured manually (e.g., using a modified jaw-thrust or chin-lift maneuver), or with adjunct equipment (e.g., oral or nasal airways, suction apparatus, or an advanced airway device; described in Chapter 15) (Figure 19-4). When performing an airway procedure for patients who may have a cervical spine injury, the paramedic must keep manipulation of the cervical spine to a minimum and stabilize the head and neck in a neutral position. All patients must have an airway established and maintained during the primary survey.

NOTE
The American Heart Association now recommends that patients who are in obvious cardiac arrest should be treated first with chest compressions. This is then followed by an assessment of airway and breathing (C-A-B).[7] See Chapter 22.

CRITICAL THINKING
Securing a patent airway should always receive priority over spinal immobilization. However, both are crucial tasks in the primary survey.

The patient whose airway is obstructed by a foreign object should be managed using the guidelines currently recommended by the American Heart Association and the American Red Cross. If these maneuvers fail, medical direction may recommend direct laryngoscopy or cricothyrotomy (see Chapter 15).

BREATHING STATUS

The breathing of a responsive patient can be assessed as (1) adequate rate and quality; (2) too fast (greater than 24 breaths/min); too slow (less than 8 breaths/min); or absent (e.g., choking from airway obstruction). The breathing of an unresponsive patient can be assessed as (1) adequate rate and quality; (2) inadequate; or (3) absent.

Breathing can be assessed by evaluating the rate, depth (tidal volume), and symmetry of chest movement. The patient's chest wall should be exposed and palpated for structural integrity, tenderness, and crepitus. Use of muscles of respiration (accessory muscles) in the neck, chest, and abdomen should be observed and noted. The paramedic should auscultate the lungs for the presence of bilateral breath sounds and should listen to the patient's speech. A patient who has difficulty speaking without pain or who cannot talk without gasping for air may need ventilatory support. Respiratory abnormalities discovered during the primary survey that may indicate a potentially life-threatening condition include the following:

- Cyanosis
- Respiratory distress with dyspnea or hypoxia
- Asymmetrical chest wall movement
- Chest injury (e.g., tension pneumothorax, flail segment, open chest wound)
- Tracheal deviation
- Distended neck veins

Ill or injured patients with ineffective respirations need oxygen and ventilatory support. These patients require supplemental high-concentration oxygen. If the respiratory rate of a critically ill or injured patient is less than 8 or more than 24 respirations per minute, ventilatory assistance may be needed.[4] The paramedic may coordinate assisted ventilation with the patient's respiratory efforts. Or the paramedic may intersperse assisted ventilation between the patient's own respiratory efforts as needed to maintain adequate oxygenation.

CRITICAL THINKING
Some patients with respirations between 8 and 24 breaths/min may require assisted ventilation. Can you think of any such situations?

If respirations are absent, the paramedic should initiate rescue breathing with a pocket mask. Positive-pressure ventilation, which can be provided via a bag-valve device with supplemental oxygen, should follow. Endotracheal intubation or other advanced airway devices may be indicated. The paramedic also should consider spinal precautions and barrier protection with all airway procedures (see Chapter 15).

CIRCULATORY STATUS

The patient's circulatory status should be evaluated after assessing airway and breathing. For trauma patients, this assessment includes a quick head-to-toe survey to identify and control severe bleeding. The paramedic should assess the patient's skin color, moisture, and temperature quickly. The pulse should be evaluated for quality, rate, and regularity.

Pulse. A quick evaluation of the patient's radial or carotid pulse may reveal any of the following: a normal rate of 60 to 100 beats/min, tachycardia (a fast rate, greater than 100 beats/min), bradycardia (a slow rate, less than 60 beats/min), an absent rate (asystole), or an irregular heart rate. The site of an obtainable pulse also may offer critical details about a patient's systolic blood pressure and tissue perfusion.[5] For example, if a radial pulse is not palpable in an uninjured extremity, the patient may be in a decompensated state of shock (hypoperfusion). A patient will lack a palpable femoral or carotid pulse when in cardiac arrest.

Capillary Refill Time. The capillary filling time may offer crucial details about the patient's cardiovascular status. The capillary refill test is thought to be most reliable in children younger than 12 years of age. The paramedic performs this test by blanching the patient's nail bed or the fleshy eminence at the base of the thumb, and then measuring the time it takes for normal color to return. A filling time of more than 2 seconds is caused by shunting and capillary closure to peripheral capillary beds. This indicates inadequate circulation and impaired cardiovascular function. Factors such as the patient's age, gender, and environment may affect the filling time. Thus the paramedic should use this test only as a possible indicator of circulatory and perfusion status.[6] Other signs and symptoms of inadequate circulation and impaired cardiovascular function include the following:

- Altered or decreased level of consciousness
- Distended neck veins
- Increased respiratory rate
- Pale, cool, diaphoretic skin
- Distant heart sounds
- Restlessness
- Thirst

NOTE

When an unconscious patient lacks a palpable femoral or carotid pulse, chest compressions should be initiated and cardiac arrest protocols should be followed[7] (see Chapter 22). In cases of severe external hemorrhage, bleeding should be controlled using direct pressure and elevation. If arterial bleeding is not controlled with direct pressure, a tourniquet should be applied (see Chapter 38). In most cases, these procedures to control bleeding also are effective during transport. Regardless of the cause, all patients with circulatory compromise need rapid stabilization. This may include intravenous administration of fluids and medications and rapid transportation to an appropriate medical facility.

Disability—Brief Neurological Evaluation

If time permits, a brief neurological (neuro) evaluation should be performed on all patients during the primary survey. The brief neuro exam includes level of consciousness, pupil size and reactivity, speech, and motor function. The purpose of this brief neuro exam is to gather information about any level of altered consciousness. (The neurological examination will be described in detail in Chapter 20.)

- *Level of consciousness:* The initial assessment of level of consciousness performed early in the primary survey classifies a patient as responsive or unresponsive. The brief neuro exam goes further by establishing that a patient is alert; is oriented to person, place, and date; and is aware of his or her surroundings. A patient who does not "pass" this test is assumed to be disoriented. Any deviations to a "normal" test should be recorded and reported to personnel at the receiving hospital. Other assessments, such as the Glasgow Coma Scale and stroke assessments, also may be indicated when evaluating the patient's level of consciousness (see Chapter 20).
- *Pupil size and reactivity.* As a rule, healthy people have pupils that are equal in size and react in concert to light. That is, both pupils should constrict at the same time when exposed to light and should dilate at the same time when exposed to darkness. Causes of unequal pupils and impaired reactivity include ocular prostheses, eye trauma, head trauma, stroke, and conditions that may impair oxygenation.
- *Speech.* A healthy person's speech should be clear and easy to understand. Slurred speech, difficulties with speech, or nonsensical speech can result from stroke, seizure, head or facial injury, medical conditions that cause speech impairment, and alcohol or other drug use.
- *Motor function.* An uninjured patient should be able to move all extremities on command and without difficulty. The patient's walk and gait should be smooth and

fluid. Conditions that may affect motor function and movement include extremity injury, stroke, head injury, alcohol or other drug use, and medical conditions such as multiple sclerosis and arthritis.

NOTE

A primary purpose of the brief neuro exam is to form a baseline assessment for future evaluations. This base line can then be compared to assessments performed by hospital staff after the patient has been delivered to the emergency department. Baseline assessments help identify negative and positive trends that may occur during the course of a patient's care.

Exposure

Some trauma patients require only minimal care and do not need to have their bodies fully exposed at the scene. Examples include stable patients with minor injuries that are isolated to a specific body part. Other patients with significant injury and those patients who are potentially unstable should be completely undressed as part of the primary survey. Exposure of the body may reveal other injuries that are not easily visible when the patient is clothed. Examples include bullet wounds, stab wounds, hidden fractures, and large areas of bruising or hematoma formation. When full-body exposure is indicated, every effort should be made to ensure the patient's privacy. Ideally, a paramedic of the same gender should remove the patient's clothing, make a visual inspection, and then appropriately cover the patient for privacy and warmth.

Assessment of Vital Functions

The paramedic should obtain a baseline set of vital signs for every patient. Vital functions to be assessed include pulse rate, respiratory rate, and blood pressure. Other assessments may be indicated as well. These include monitoring the patient's oxygen saturation using pulse oximetry, and electrocardiogram (ECG) monitoring. Like the brief neuro exam, baseline measurements of vital functions help to identify positive and negative trends in the course of the patient's care. They also help to identify priority patients. As a rule, vital signs should be measured and recorded every 15 minutes for stable patients, and at least every 5 minutes for patients who are unstable or potentially unstable.

IDENTIFYING PATIENTS WHO NEED PRIORITY CARE AND TRANSPORT

The paramedic uses the findings from the primary survey to identify life threats and priority patients. These are unstable patients or potentially unstable patients who need stabilization and rapid transport to an emergency facility. Examples of priority patients include those who have the following:

- Poor general impression
- Decreased level of consciousness (depressed or absent gag or cough reflex)
- No response to commands (unresponsiveness)
- Difficulty breathing
- Shock (hypoperfusion)
- Complicated childbirth
- Chest pain with a systolic pressure less than 100 mm Hg
- Uncontrolled bleeding
- Severe pain anywhere
- Multiple injuries

Integration of Treatment/Procedures Needed to Preserve Life

In some cases, definitive care for medical patients can be initiated in the prehospital setting. For example, patients who have altered consciousness related to hypoglycemia or narcotic overdose should receive immediate interventions that may completely reverse their life-threatening signs and symptoms. In the case of severe respiratory emergencies, prehospital care can relieve severe hypoxic signs and symptoms before arrival at the hospital. Because of this, the time spent on-scene with medical patients may be slightly longer.

NOTE

For patients with stroke or myocardial infarction, life-saving care can begin at the scene, but simultaneous and rapid transport is also needed. The combination of initial on-scene care and rapid transport allows for time-sensitive and definitive treatment to be delivered at the hospital.

In contrast, most seriously injured trauma patients require short scene times and rapid transport. These patients should be taken to an appropriate trauma center or other medical facility for definitive care. Patients with internal bleeding, major fractures, head injury, and multiple-system trauma need life-saving care. This care can be provided only by specially trained physicians and support staff. Minimal time should be spent at the scene with these patients. Most trauma life-support training programs (e.g., basic trauma life support, prehospital trauma life support, and advanced trauma life support) recommend that patients needing immediate transport be stabilized and prepared for transport ("packaged") within 10 minutes after arrival of EMS.[5] Field management should be limited to airway control and ventilatory support, spinal immobilization, and major fracture stabilization. Intravenous fluid therapy should be initiated en route to the hospital. (Trauma management is addressed further in Part 9: Trauma.)

SUMMARY

- Sizing-up the scene consists of the initial steps performed on every emergency medical services response. These steps help to ensure scene safety. They also provide valuable information to the paramedic.
- Paramedics should ensure they have access to and wear appropriate personal protective equipment to protect against injury or illness related to an unsafe scene or infectious diseases.
- The primary assessment includes the paramedic's general impression of the patient, the assessment for life-threatening conditions, and the identification of priority patients requiring immediate care and transport.

- Assessment of life-threatening conditions entails a systematic evaluation of the patient's level of consciousness, airway, breathing, circulation, and disability. The patient should also be appropriately exposed during the primary assessment to detect life threats.
- Information from the primary survey is used to identify life threats and prioritize patients.
- The paramedic begins resuscitative measures such as airway maintenance, ventilatory assistance, and cardiopulmonary resuscitation immediately after recognizing the life-threatening condition that necessitates each respective maneuver.

REFERENCES

1. National Fire Protection Association: *Standards on protective clothing for structural fire fighting; NFPA 1999*, Quincy, Mass, 2008 edition, The Association.
2. Occupational Safety and Health Administration: *Fire brigade regulation*, 29 CFR 1910.156, Washington, DC, 1980, The Administration.
3. Occupational Safety and Health Administration: *Hazardous waste operations and emergency response (HAZWOPER)*, Standard 1910.120, Washington, DC, 1990, The Administration.
4. National Highway Traffic Safety Administration: *The National EMS Education Standards*. Washington, DC, 2009, U.S. Department of Transportation/National Highway Traffic Safety Administration, DOT.

5. National Association of Emergency Medical Technicians: *PHTLS: Prehospital Trauma Life Support*, ed 7, St. Louis, 2011, Mosby.

6. Baraff LJ: Capillary refill: is it a useful clinical sign? *Pediatrics* 92(5):723-724, 1993.

7. American Heart Association: 2010 American Heart Association Guidelines for Cardiopulmonary Resuscitation and Emergency Cardiovascular Care, *Circulation* 122(18 Supplement 3):S639-S946, 2010.

SUGGESTED READING

Edgerly D: Assessing your assessment, 2008, JEMS www.jems.com:80/news_and_articles/columns/Edgerly/Assessing_Your_Assessment.html Accessed 10/16/10.

20 Secondary Assessment

OBJECTIVES

Upon completion of this chapter, the paramedic student will be able to:

1. Define the purpose of the secondary assessment.
2. Describe physical examination techniques commonly used in the prehospital setting.
3. Describe the examination equipment commonly used in the prehospital setting.
4. Describe the general approach to physical examination.
5. Outline the steps of a comprehensive physical examination.
6. Detail the components of the mental status examination.
7. Distinguish between normal and abnormal findings in the mental status examination.
8. Outline the steps in the general patient survey.
9. Distinguish between normal and abnormal findings in the general patient survey.
10. Describe physical examination techniques used for assessment of specific body regions.
11. Distinguish between normal and abnormal findings when assessing specific body regions.
12. Outline the process of patient reassessment.
13. State modifications to the physical examination that are necessary when assessing children.
14. State modifications to the physical examination that are necessary when assessing the older adult.

KEY TERMS

anisocoria Normal or congenital unequal pupil size.

aphasia Loss of the power of speech.

apical impulse A pulsation of the left ventricle of the heart, palpable and sometimes visible at the fifth intercostal space to the left of the midline.

ataxia Failure of muscle coordination.

auscultation A technique that requires the use of a stethoscope and is used to assess body sounds produced by the movement of various fluids or gases in organs or tissues.

bronchial breath sounds Breath sounds heard only over the trachea and are the highest in pitch.

bronchovesicular breath sounds Normal breath sounds heard over the major bronchi and over the upper right posterior lung field.

bruit An abnormal sound or murmur heard while auscultating an artery, organ, or gland.

crackle A fine, bubbling sound heard on auscultation of the lung; it is produced by air entering distal airways and alveoli that contain serous secretions.

crepitus A grating sound associated with rubbing of bone fragments.

deep tendon reflexes Reflexes elicited by sensory afferents from muscle rather than bone.

diastolic blood pressure The minimum level of blood pressure measured between contractions of the heart.

dysconjugate gaze Deviation of the eyes to opposite sides.

dysarthria Difficult and poorly articulated speech resulting from poor control over the muscles of speech.

dysphonia An abnormality in the speaking voice, such as hoarseness.

epistaxis Bleeding from the nose.

heart murmur An abnormal heart sound caused by altered blood flow into a chamber or through a valve.

inspection A visual assessment of the patient and surroundings.

nystagmus Involuntary jerking movements of the eyes.

palpation A technique in which an examiner uses the hands and fingers to gather information from a patient by touch.

percussion A technique used to evaluate the presence of air or fluid in body tissues.

pericardial friction rub A dry, grating sound heard with a stethoscope during auscultation; suggestive of pericarditis.

PERRL Acronym for pupils that are equal, round, and react to light.

physical examination An assessment of a patient that includes examination techniques, measurement of vital signs, an assessment of height and weight, and the skillful use of examination equipment.

pleural friction rub A rubbing or grating sound that occurs as one layer of the pleural membrane slides over the other during breathing.

pronator drift test A test to evaluate balance and upper extremity weakness; performed by having the patient close the eyes and hold both arms out from the body.

pulse deficit A condition that exists when the radial pulse is less than the ventricular rate; it indicates a lack of peripheral perfusion.

reassessment The ongoing assessment that follows the paramedic's initial evaluation of the patient.

rhonchi Abnormal sounds heard on auscultation of a respiratory airway obstructed by thick secretions, muscular spasm, neoplasm, or external pressure.

Romberg's test A test to evaluate stance and balance; performed by having the patient stand erect with the feet together and arms at the sides.

secondary assessment Consists of physical examination techniques, measurement of vital signs, an assessment of body systems, and the skillful use of examination equipment.

six cardinal fields of gaze A test to evaluate extraocular muscle function; performed by having the patient visually track an object in six visual fields in an H pattern.

stridor An abnormal, high-pitched musical sound caused by obstruction in the trachea or larynx.

subcutaneous emphysema The presence of air in the subcutaneous tissues.

superficial reflexes Reflexes elicited by sensory afferents from skin.

systolic blood pressure The blood pressure measured during the period of ventricular contraction.

temporomandibular joint dysfunction Acute or chronic inflammation in the temporomandibular joint.

thrill A fine vibration felt by an examiner's hands over the site of an aneurysm or on the pericardium.

tidal volume The volume of gas inhaled or exhaled during a normal breath.

tympany A hollow drum-like sound produced when a gas-containing cavity is percussed.

vesicular breath sounds Breath sounds heard over most of the lung fields; the major normal breath sound.

wheeze A form of rhonchus characterized by a high-pitched, musical quality; it is caused by high-velocity airflow through narrowed airways.

The paramedic must have a wide range of knowledge and skills to perform a comprehensive physical examination and to make effective clinical care decisions. This chapter presents the techniques of the basic physical examination. Some of the techniques presented will have application to examinations more likely to be performed in the expanded scope of practice activities. The goal of this chapter is to prepare the paramedic with the tools and skills needed to perform a thorough physical examination in any patient care setting.

NOTE

Chapter 19 addressed the components of the primary survey. That chapter focused on recognizing and managing life-threatening conditions in the initial patient care encounter. This chapter is devoted to the techniques of the detailed physical examination—the examination performed in the secondary assessment. Like the primary survey, the secondary assessment integrates patient assessment findings with knowledge of pathophysiology. This helps to form a final impression and to identify an appropriate treatment plan.

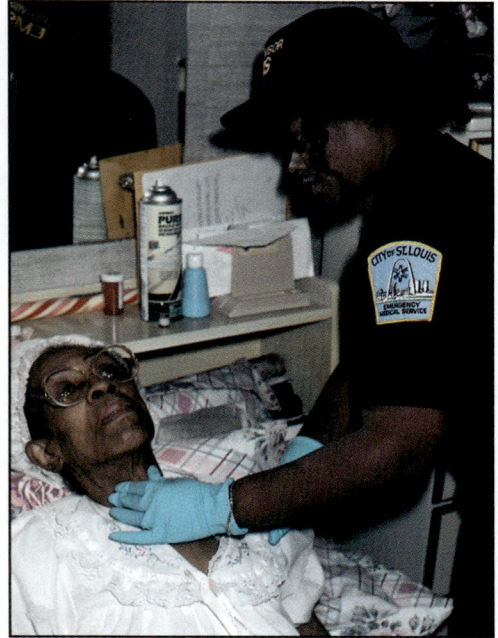

(Courtesy Monroe Yancie, St. Louis, Mo.)

SECONDARY ASSESSMENT: APPROACH AND OVERVIEW

The **secondary assessment** consists of physical examination techniques, measurement of vital signs, an assessment of body systems, and the skillful use of examination equipment (Box 20-1). Physical examination techniques will vary by patient, depending on the chief complaint, present illness, and history. The appropriate assessment of the patient depends on:

- The stability of the patient
- The complaint and history

- The patient's ability to communicate
- The potential for unrecognized illness

NOTE

Some aspects of the physical assessment may not be appropriate for all patients. For example, if the patient has a life-threatening injury or illness, a primary survey and rapid transport may be all that is provided in the prehospital phase of care. If the patient is stable, however, and has a significant history, a more thorough secondary assessment may be indicated. The order of care for this group of patients is:

1. Scene size-up
2. Primary survey
3. Secondary assessment
4. Reassessment

Examination Techniques

Four techniques commonly are used in the physical examination. These are inspection, palpation, percussion, and auscultation. These terms are referred to often in this text because they relate to the evaluation of specific body systems. Depending on the situation, these techniques may be the sole method for evaluating a patient. For example, this may be the case with an unconscious trauma patient. In other cases, these techniques may be integrated with history taking and other care procedures. If time permits, the paramedic should explain each technique that requires touch to the patient before performing it.

CRITICAL THINKING

You arrive at the scene of a motor vehicle crash. What will you look for during your initial patient inspection?

INSPECTION

Inspection is the visual assessment of the patient and the surroundings. This technique can alert the paramedic to the patient's mental status. Inspection also can alert the paramedic to possible injury or underlying illness. Patient hygiene, clothing, eye gaze, body language and position, skin color, and odor are significant inspection findings. The EMS response may be to the patient's home. In this case, the paramedic should make a visual inspection for cleanliness, prescription medicines, illegal drug paraphernalia, weapons, and signs of alcohol use. These and other items seen by EMS personnel can play a key role in determining patient care activities.

PALPATION

Palpation is a technique in which the paramedic uses the hands and fingers to gather information by touch. Generally, the paramedic uses the palmar surface of the fingers

BOX 20-1 Components of the Physical Examination

Examination Techniques

Inspection
Palpation
Percussion
Auscultation

Measurement of Vital Signs

Pulse
Respirations
Blood pressure
Temperature (especially in children)

Assessment of Height and Weight Equipment

Blood pressure cuff
Ophthalmoscope
Otoscope
Stethoscope

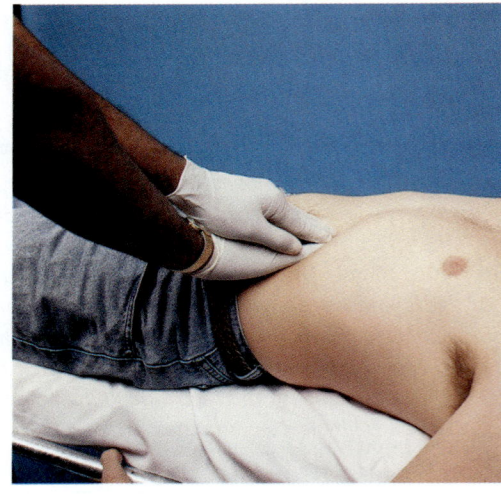

FIGURE 20-1 Deep bimanual palpation.

and the finger pads to palpate for texture, masses, fluid, and **crepitus** and to assess skin temperature (Figure 20-1). The dorsal and ulnar hand surfaces may also be used. Palpation may be either superficial or deep; *the applications for each are addressed throughout this chapter.* Examining a patient by palpation is a form of invasion of the patient's body. Therefore the approach should be gentle and should be initiated with respect.

PERCUSSION

Percussion is used to evaluate the presence of air or fluid in body tissues. This technique is performed by the paramedic striking one finger against another to produce vibrations and sound waves of underlying tissue. Sound waves are heard as percussion tones (resonance). They are determined by the density of the tissue being examined. The denser the body area, the lower the pitch of the percussion tone. To percuss, the paramedic places the first joint of the middle finger of the nondominant hand on the patient, keeping the rest of the hand poised above the skin. The fingers of the other hand should be flexed and the wrist action loose. The paramedic then snaps the wrist of the dominant hand downward with the tip of the middle finger tapping the joint of the finger that is on the body surface. The tap should be sharp and rigid, percussing the same area several times to interpret the tone (Figure 20-2). Box 20-2 describes percussion tones and examples of each. As with any other examination technique, percussion requires practice to obtain the skill needed for the physical examination.

AUSCULTATION

Auscultation calls for the use of a stethoscope. This technique is used to assess body sounds made by the movement of various fluids or gases in the patient's organs or tissues. Auscultation is best performed in a quiet environment to focus on each body sound being assessed. The paramedic should isolate a particular area to note characteristics of intensity, pitch, duration, and quality. In the prehospital setting, auscultation most often is used to assess blood pressure and to evaluate breath sounds, heart sounds, and bowel sounds. To auscultate, the paramedic should place the diaphragm of the stethoscope firmly against the patient's skin for stabilization (Figure 20-3). If a bell end piece is used, it should be positioned lightly on the body surface. This prevents the damping of vibrations.

> **NOTE**
> The bell and diaphragm end pieces of a stethoscope selectively emphasize sounds of different frequencies. The bell is central for listening to low-pitched sounds (e.g., certain heart sounds). In contrast, the diaphragm filters out low-pitched sounds and therefore emphasizes high-pitched ones. Examples of high-pitched sounds include breath sounds and bowel sounds.

Examination Equipment

Basic equipment used during the comprehensive physical examination includes the stethoscope, ophthalmoscope, otoscope, and blood pressure cuff. The ophthalmoscope and otoscope are nontraditional EMS tools. They are being introduced to the paramedic with expanded scope of practice. These devices will not be used routinely with patients in the prehospital setting.

> **NOTE**
> Monitoring devices such as capnography, electrocardiography, and devices used to test blood chemistry are also frequently used in the prehospital setting. These devices will be described throughout this text by subject matter.

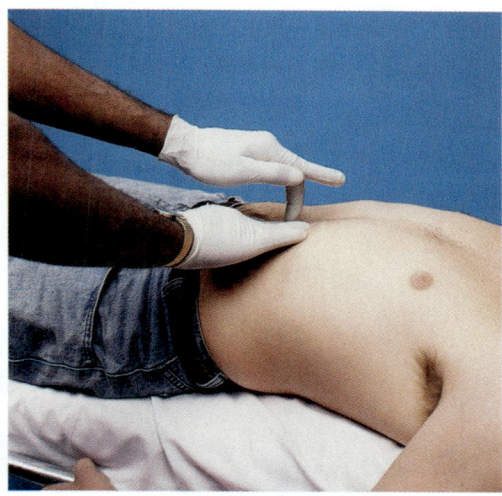

FIGURE 20-2 Percussion technique.

BOX 20-2 Percussion Tones and Examples

Percussion Tone	Example
Tympany (the loudest)	Gastric bubble
Hyperresonance	Air-filled lungs (e.g., chronic obstructive pulmonary disease and pneumothorax)
Resonance	Healthy lungs
Dullness	Liver
Flat (the quietest)	Muscle

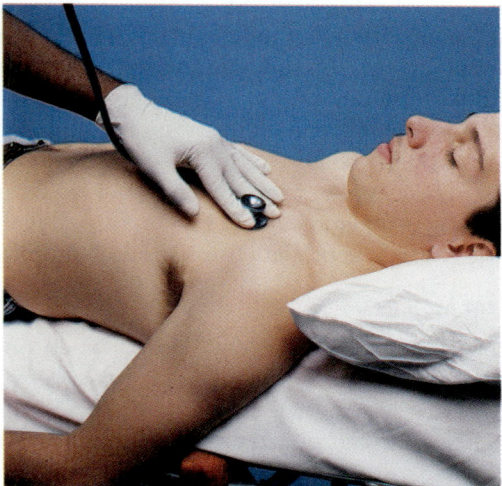

FIGURE 20-3 Position of the stethoscope between the index and middle fingers.

STETHOSCOPE

The stethoscope is used to evaluate sounds created by the cardiovascular, respiratory, and gastrointestinal systems. The three major types of stethoscopes are acoustic stethoscopes, magnetic stethoscopes, and electronic stethoscopes (Figure 20-4).

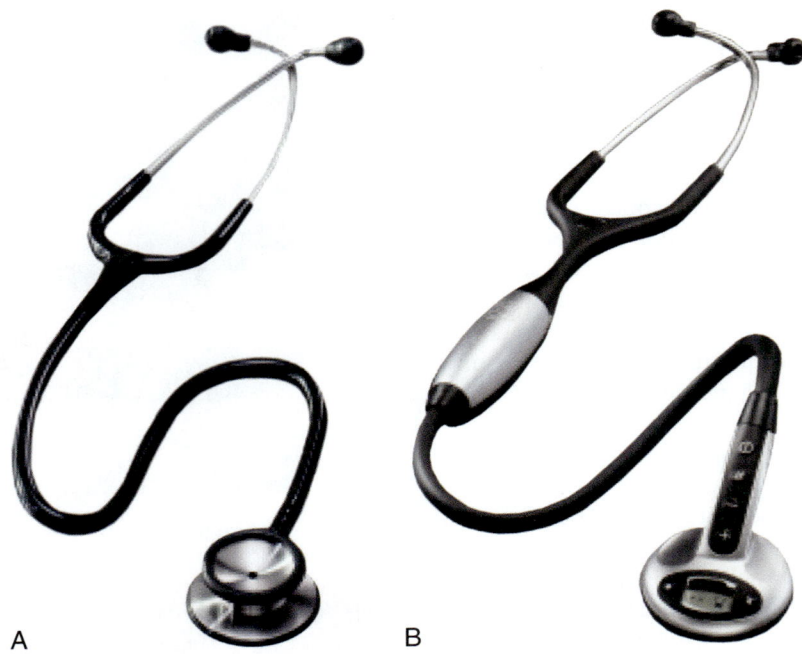

FIGURE 20-4 Stethoscope types. **A,** Acoustic. **B,** Electronic. (Courtesy 3M Healthcare, St Paul, Minn.)

Acoustic stethoscopes transmit sound waves from the source to the paramedic's ears. Most have a rigid diaphragm. This diaphragm transmits high-pitched sounds. The bell end piece transmits low-pitched sounds.

Magnetic stethoscopes have a single diaphragm end piece. The end piece contains an iron disk and a permanent magnet. The air column of the diaphragm is activated as magnetic attraction is established between the iron disk and the magnet. A frequency dial adjusts for high-, low-, and full-frequency sounds.

Electronic stethoscopes convert sound vibrations into electrical impulses that are amplified. The impulses are transmitted to a speaker where they are converted to sound. These devices can compensate for environmental noise. Thus they may be beneficial for use in the prehospital setting.

OPHTHALMOSCOPE

The ophthalmoscope is used to inspect structures of the eye, including the retina, choroid, optic nerve disk, macula (an oval, yellow spot at the center of the retina), and retinal vessels. This device has a battery light source, two dials, and a viewer (Figure 20-5). The dial at the top of the battery changes the light image. The dial at the top of the viewer allows for the selection of lenses. (Five lenses are available, but the large white light generally is used.)

OTOSCOPE

The otoscope is used to examine deep structures of the external and middle ear. This device is basically an ophthalmoscope with a special ear speculum attached to the battery tube (Figure 20-6). Ear specula are available in a number of sizes to conform to various ear canals. (The paramedic

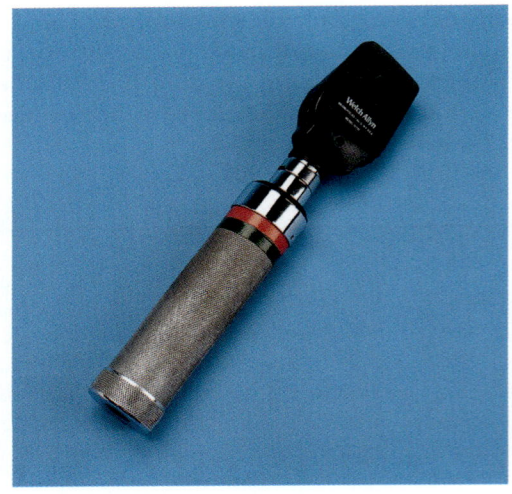

FIGURE 20-5 Ophthalmoscope.

should choose the largest one that fits comfortably in the patient's ear.) The light from the otoscope allows one to visualize the tympanic membrane.

BLOOD PRESSURE CUFF

The blood pressure cuff (sphygmomanometer) most commonly is used along with the stethoscope to measure systolic and diastolic blood pressure. The common blood pressure cuff used in the prehospital setting consists of a pressure gauge that registers millimeter calibrations, a synthetic cuff with Velcro closures that encloses an inflatable rubber bladder, and a pressure bulb with a release valve. Blood pressure cuffs are available in a number of sizes.

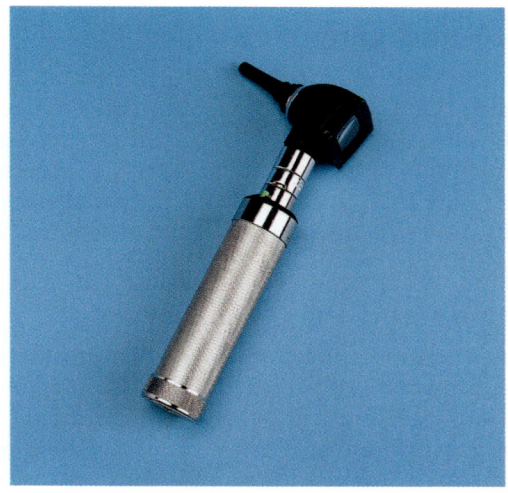

FIGURE 20-6 Otoscope.

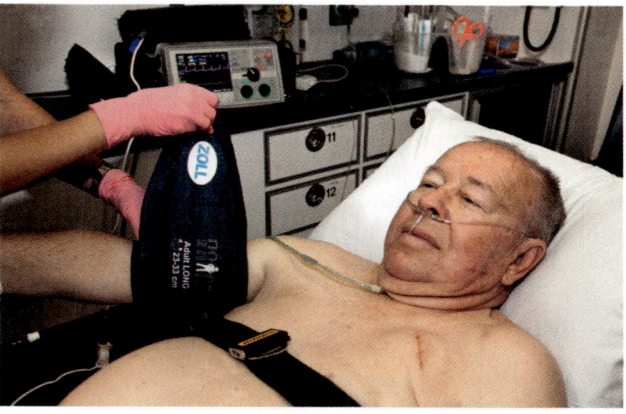

FIGURE 20-7 Electronic blood pressure device.

Adult widths should be one third to one half the circumference of the limb. For children, the width should cover about two thirds of the upper arm or thigh. (Blood pressure cuffs that are too large give a falsely low reading; cuffs that are too small give a falsely high reading.)

Electronic devices that automatically measure a patient's vital signs are used by hospitals and EMS agencies to monitor the patient's blood pressure, pulse rate, body temperature, end-tidal carbon dioxide concentration, and oxygen saturation level at regular intervals (Figure 20-7).

General Approach to the Physical Examination

The physical examination is performed as a step-by-step process. Special emphasis is placed on the patient's present illness and chief complaint. The paramedic should know that most patients view a physical exam with some anxiety. They often feel vulnerable and exposed. Therefore it is important to establish a professional trust early in the encounter. In addition, ensuring the patient's privacy and comfort when possible is very important.

Overview of a Comprehensive Physical Examination

The physical examination is a systematic assessment of the body that includes the following components:
- Mental status
- General survey
- Vital signs
- Skin
- Head, eyes, ears, nose, and throat
- Chest
- Abdomen
- Posterior body
- Extremities (peripheral vascular and musculoskeletal)
- Neurological exam

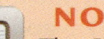

> **NOTE**
> The Centers for Disease Control and Prevention and the Occupational Safety and Health Administration have recommended that health care workers wear gloves "when handling blood-soiled items, body fluids, excretions and secretions, as well as surfaces, materials, and objects exposed to them."[1] This text assumes that all paramedics are appropriately gloved for patient care procedures. Personal protective measures are addressed in Chapter 14 and 28.

MENTAL STATUS

The first step in any encounter with a patient is to note the patient's appearance and behavior. With this step, one also should assess for level of consciousness. A healthy patient is expected to be alert and responsive to touch, verbal instruction, and painful stimuli.

Appearance and Behavior

As mentioned before, a visual assessment of the patient can yield key information. Abnormal findings may include drowsiness or the inability to respond to unpleasant or painful stimuli. Terms that are sometimes used to describe abnormal findings include *obtundation, stupor,* or *coma.* A patient who is obtunded has a decreased level of consciousness usually produced by anesthetics or analgesics. Stupor is a state of lethargy and unresponsiveness. Stuporous patients usually are unaware of their surroundings. Coma is a state of profound unconsciousness. A patient in coma has no spontaneous eye movements. These patients do not respond to verbal or painful stimuli and cannot be aroused.

> **NOTE**
> Most medical direction agencies discourage the use of these terms to describe a patient's mental status. Because these terms are vague, they may be open to interpretation. Therefore it is best to describe the patient's reactions and verbal and motor responses with indexes such as the AVPU scale or Glasgow Coma Scale (described in Chapter 19 and Chapter 40). These measurements often are considered better patient information.

POSTURE, GAIT, AND MOTOR ACTIVITY

The paramedic should observe the patient's posture, gait, and motor activity. This involves assessing pace, range, character, and appropriateness of movement. For example, most patients without physical disabilities can walk with good balance and without a limp, discomfort, or fear of falling. Abnormal findings may include **ataxia** (uncoordinated movement), paralysis, restlessness, agitation, bizarre body posture, immobility, and involuntary movements.

DRESS, GROOMING, PERSONAL HYGIENE, AND BREATH OR BODY ODORS

Dress, grooming, and personal hygiene should be appropriate for the patient's age, lifestyle, and occupation. A person's dress should be appropriate for environmental temperature and weather conditions. (Older adults and children who are improperly dressed for temperatures or who have poor hygiene may be victims of neglect.) Medical jewelry (e.g., copper bracelets for arthritis, medical insignias) should be noted. Hair, fingernails, and cosmetics may reflect the patient's lifestyle, mood, and personality. These findings can point to a decreased interest in appearance (e.g., grown-out hair or faded nail polish). This may help to estimate the length of an illness.

Breath or body odors can point to underlying conditions or illness. Examples of breath odors include alcohol, acetone (seen with some diabetic conditions), feces (seen with bowel obstruction), and halitosis from throat infections and poor dental and oral hygiene. Renal and liver disease and poor hygiene also may result in body odor.

FACIAL EXPRESSION

Facial expressions may reveal anxiety, depression, elation, anger, or withdrawal. They may also show fear, sadness, or pain. The paramedic should be alert to changes in facial expression while the patient is at rest, during conversation, during the examination, and when asking questions. Facial expressions should be appropriate to the situation.

MOOD, AFFECT, AND RELATION TO PERSONS AND THINGS

Like facial expression, the patient's mood and affect also should be appropriate to the event. Mood and affect describe the patient's emotional state and the outward display of feelings and emotions; they are expressed verbally and nonverbally. Examples of abnormal findings include an unusual happiness in the presence of major illness, indifference, thoughts of suicide, responses to imaginary persons or objects, and unpredictable mood swings.

CRITICAL THINKING
What physical clues do you look for in your friends or your partner that tell you about their mood?

Speech and Language

The patient's speech should be understandable and of a moderate pace. The paramedic should assess the quantity, rate, loudness, and fluency of the patient's speech patterns. Abnormal findings include **aphasia** (loss of speech), **dysphonia** (abnormal speaking voice), **dysarthria** (poorly articulated speech), and speech and language that changes with mood.

Thoughts and Perceptions

A healthy person's thoughts and perceptions are logical, relevant, organized, and coherent. Patients should have an insight into their illness or injury. They also should be able to show a level of judgment in making decisions or plans about their situation and their care. Although accurately assessing a person's thoughts and perceptions is difficult, the following usually are considered abnormal findings:

- Abnormal thought processes
  Flight of ideas
  Incoherence
  Confabulation
  Blocking
  Transference
- Abnormal thought content
  Obsessions
  Compulsions
  Delusions
  Suicidal ideations
  Homicidal thoughts
  Feelings of unreality
- Abnormal perceptions
  Illusions
  Visual/auditory hallucinations

Memory and Attention

Healthy persons normally are oriented to person, place, and date ("oriented times 3"). They also are usually aware of the event that initiated the EMS response ("oriented × 4"). The paramedic can use several other methods to assess a patient's memory and attention. One method is to ask the patient to count from 1 to 10 using only even or odd numbers (digit span). Another is to multiply by sevens (serial sevens). A third method is to spell simple words backward (e.g., "world"). The paramedic also should assess the patient's remote memory (e.g., birthdays) and recent memory (e.g., events of the day), and the patient's new learning ability. New learning ability can be evaluated by giving the patient new information (e.g., your name; the year and model of the ambulance). Later the paramedic would ask the patient to recall that information.

GENERAL SURVEY

After assessing a patient's level of consciousness and mental status, the paramedic performs a general survey of the patient. In addition to the assessments described previously, the patient should be evaluated for signs of distress, apparent state of health, skin color and obvious lesions, height and build, sexual development, and weight. Vital signs also are assessed during the general survey.

Signs of Distress

Obvious signs of distress include those that result from cardiorespiratory insufficiency, pain, and anxiety. Examples of these signs and symptoms are as follows:

- Cardiorespiratory insufficiency
  Labored breathing
  Wheezing
  Cough
- Pain
  Wincing
  Sweating
  Protectiveness of a painful body part or area
- Anxiety
  Restlessness
  Anxious expression
  Fidgety movement
  Cold, moist palms

CRITICAL THINKING
Combine one symptom from each of the groups of distress, and imagine how a patient with these symptoms might look and act.

Apparent State of Health

A patient's apparent state of health can be assessed by observation. The paramedic should note the patient's basic appearance as being acutely or chronically ill, frail, feeble, robust, or vigorous. Although these are subjective assessments, *frail* usually means impaired mental judgment with a dependence on others; *feeble* usually means weakness or a lack of strength; *robust* means strong and healthy; and *vigorous* means full of energy.

Skin Color and Obvious Lesions

Skin color can vary by body part and from person to person. A patient's normal skin color depends of course on race and can range from pink or ivory to deep brown, yellow, or olive. Skin color is best assessed by evaluating skin that usually is not exposed to the sun (e.g., the palms) or skin that has

less pigmentation (e.g., lips and nail beds). Box 20-3 describes abnormal skin colors and their possible causes. Obvious skin lesions that can indicate illness or injury include rashes, bruises, scars, and discoloration (Figure 20-8; Tables 20-1 and 20-2).

NOTE
Skin color, texture, and appearance can be affected by a person's age. For example, the skin color of a pediatric patient with light skin may be milky white and rose, to a deep hue of pink. A child with dark skin may have various brown, yellow, or olive-green or bluish tones. In addition, the skin of a child is usually smooth, slightly dry, and not oily or clammy. By comparison, the skin of a geriatric patient is often dry, wrinkly, with uneven pigmentation. The older patient often has thinning of the epidermal skin layers and decreased collagen production and may have various proliferative lesions associated with aging.

Height and Build

Patients generally can be described as average, tall, or short; with a slender, lanky, muscular, or stocky build. All of these factors can reflect overall health. For example, a patient can be excessively thin (as seen with some eating disorders) or trim and muscular. Age and lifestyle also may affect height and body build.

Sexual Development

Sexual characteristics should be appropriate for the patient's age and sex. Normal changes associated with puberty include facial hair and deepening of the voice in men, increased breast size in women, and hair growth in the axillary and groin areas in both sexes. As a rule, healthy men are taller, heavier, and more muscular than healthy women.

Weight

Ideally a patient's body weight should be proportionate to height and sex (Figure 20-9). Weight conditions that are easily observed in the general survey include patients who are emaciated (extremely lean from lack of nutrition), plump, or obese (body weight that is 20% greater than desirable body weight for a person's age, sex, height, and body build). A recent gain or loss is a key finding and may be clinically important. Like body height and build, body weight can reflect the patient's health, age, and lifestyle.

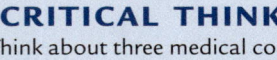
CRITICAL THINKING
Think about three medical conditions that might result in significant weight loss. Now, think about three that might cause a significant weight gain.

Vital Signs

Vital signs are a baseline measurement of function. They are used to assess respiration, pulse (circulation), and blood pressure (perfusion). The following is a brief overview of vital signs. assessment.

Text continued on p. 526

BOX 20-3 Abnormal Skin Color and Possible Causes

Color	Possible Causes
Pallor (decrease in color)	Shock, dehydration, fright
Cyanosis (bluish color)	Cardiorespiratory insufficiency, cold environment
Jaundice (yellow-orange color)	Liver disease, red blood cell destruction
Red	Fever, inflammation, carbon monoxide poisoning

Purpura—red-purple nonblanchable discoloration greater than 0.5 cm diameter.
Cause: Intravascular defects, infection

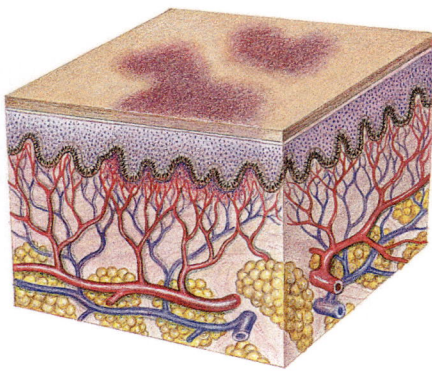

Spider angioma—red central body with radiating spiderlike legs that blanch with pressure to the central body
Cause: Liver disease, vitamin B deficiency, idiopathic

Petechiae—red-purple nonblanchable discoloration less than 0.5 cm diameter
Cause: Intravascular defects, infection

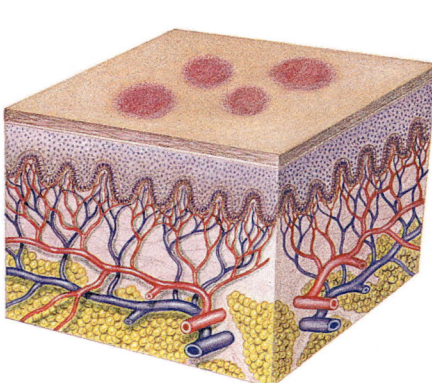

Venous star—bluish spider, linear or irregularly shaped; does not blanch with pressure
Cause: Increased pressure in superficial veins

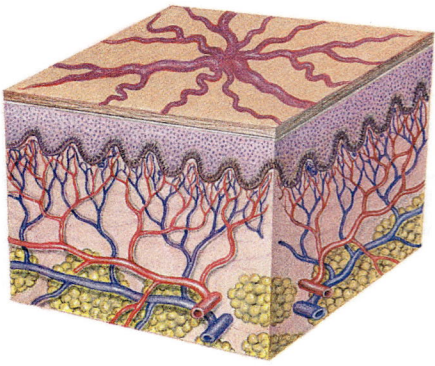

Telangiectasia—fine, irregular red line
Cause: Dilation of capillaries

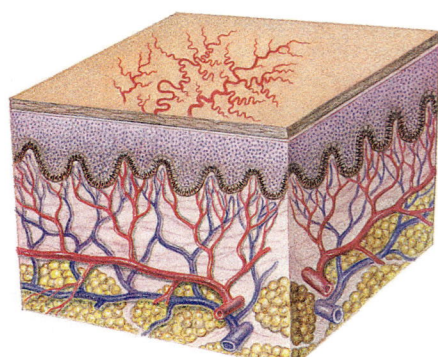

Ecchymoses—red-purple nonblanchable discoloration of variable size
Cause: Vascular wall destruction, trauma, vasculitis

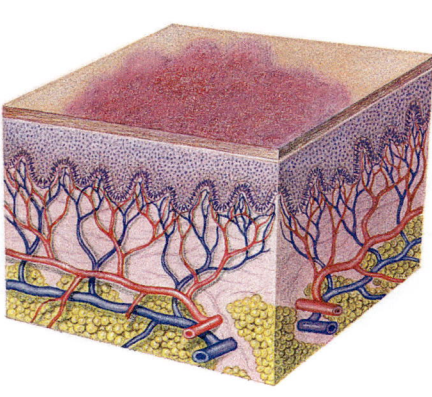

Capillary hemangioma (nevus flammeus)—red irregular macular patches
Cause: Dilation of dermal capillaries

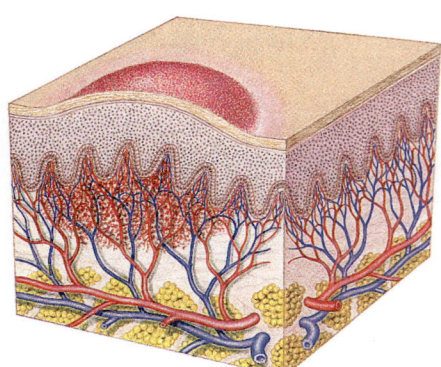

FIGURE 20-8 Characteristics and causes of vascular skin lesions. (From Seidel H, et al: *Mosby's guide to physical examination,* ed 6, St Louis, 2007, Mosby.)

TABLE 20-1 Primary Skin Lesions

Description	Examples

Macule

A flat, circumscribed area that is a change in color of the skin; less than 1 cm in diameter

Freckles, flat moles (nevi), petechiae, measles, scarlet fever

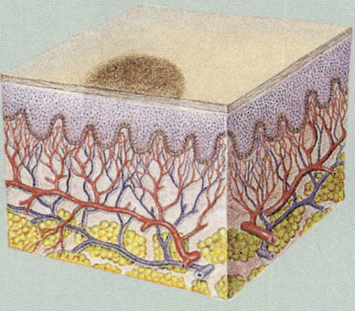

Freckles (Marks and Miller, 2006)

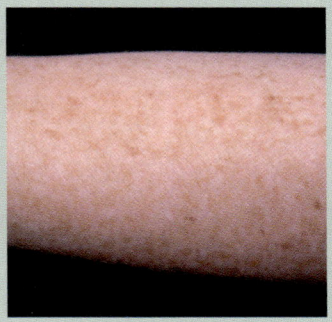

Papule

An elevated, firm, circumscribed area; less than 1 cm in diameter

Wart (verruca), elevated moles, lichen planus

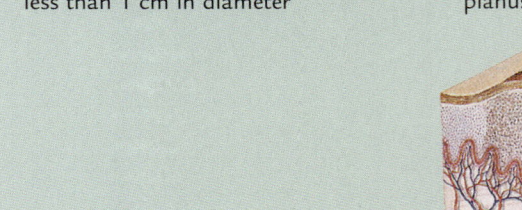

Lichen planus (Weston, Lane, and Morelli, 2007)

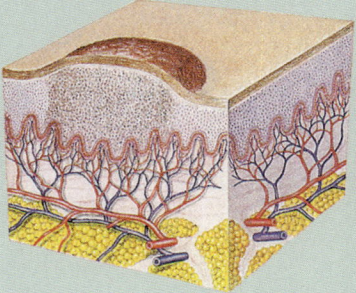

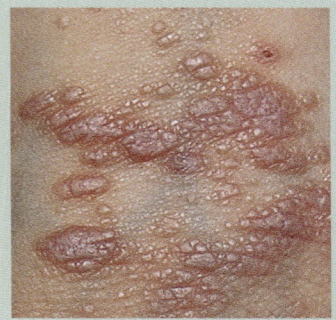

Patch

A flat, nonpalpable, irregular-shaped macule greater than 1 cm in diameter

Vitiligo, port-wine stains, Mongolian spots, café au lait patch

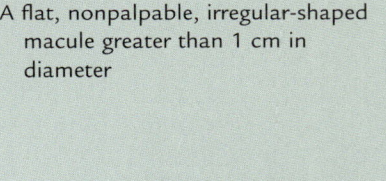

Vitiligo (White and Cox, 2006)

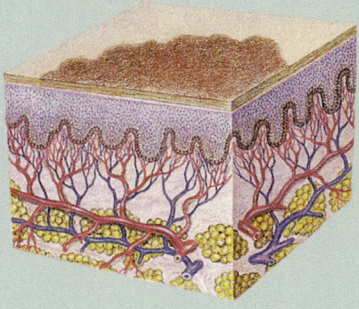

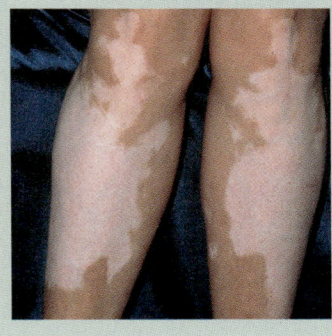

Plaque

Elevated, firm, and rough lesion with flat top surface greater than 1 cm in diameter

Psoriasis, seborrheic and actinic keratoses

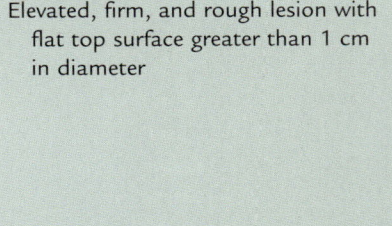

Plaque (Weston, Lane, and Morelli, 2007)

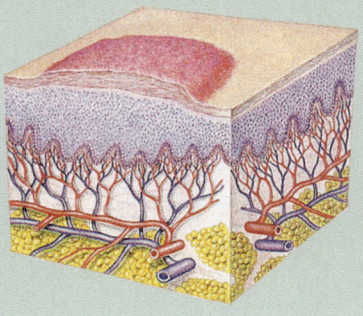

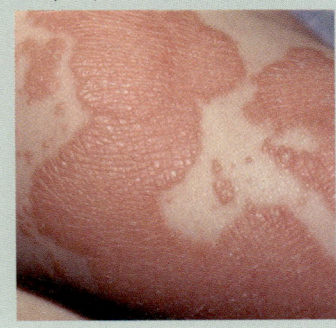

Continued

TABLE 20-1 Primary Skin Lesions—cont'd

Description	Examples

Wheal

Elevated, irregular-shaped area of cutaneous edema; solid, transient, variable diameter

Insect bites, urticaria, allergic reaction

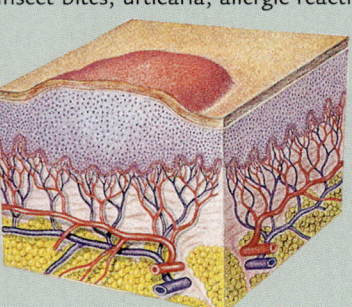

Wheal (Weston, Lane, and Morelli, 2007)

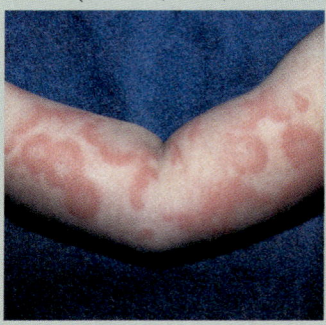

Nodule

Elevated, firm, circumscribed lesion; deeper in dermis than a papule; 1 to 2 cm in diameter

Erythema nodosum, lipomas

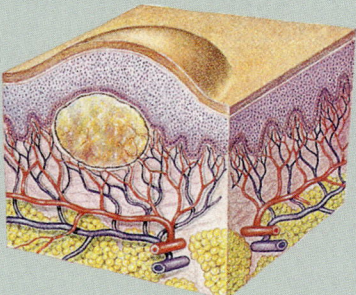

Nodule (Marks and Miller, 2006)

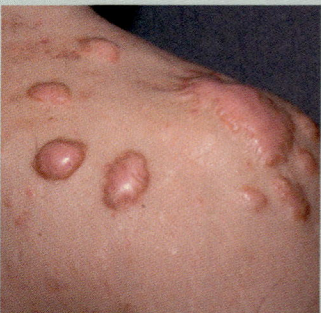

Tumor

Elevated and solid lesion; may or may not be clearly demarcated; deeper in dermis; greater than 2 cm in diameter

Neoplasms, benign tumor, lipoma, hemangioma

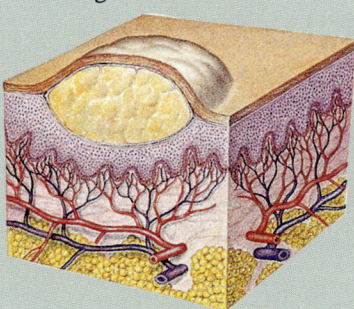

Hemangioma (Marks and Miller, 2006)

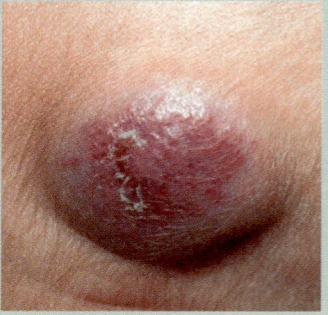

Vesicle

Elevated, circumscribed, superficial, not into dermis; filled with serous fluid; less than 1 cm in diameter

Varicella (chickenpox), herpes zoster (shingles)

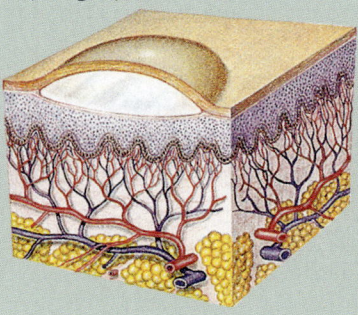

Vesicles caused by zoster (Weston, Lane, and Morelli, 2007)

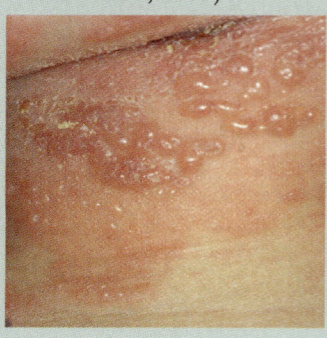

TABLE 20-1 Primary Skin Lesions—cont'd

Description	Examples	
Bulla Vesicle greater than 1 cm in diameter	Blister, pemphigus vulgaris 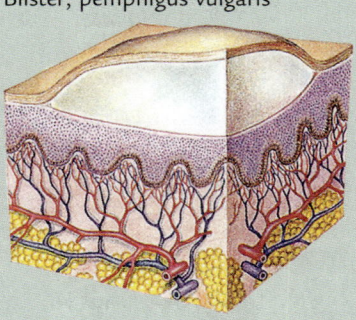	Bullous pemphigoid (White and Cox, 2006) 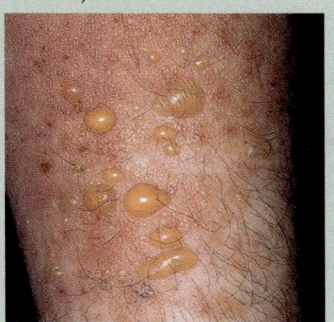
Pustule Elevated, superficial lesion; similar to a vesicle but filled with purulent fluid	Impetigo, acne 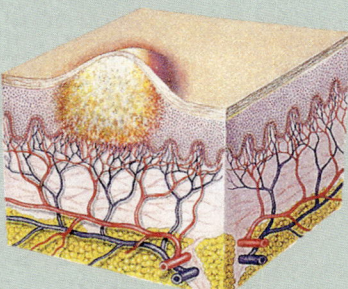	Acne (Weston, Lane, and Morelli, 2007) 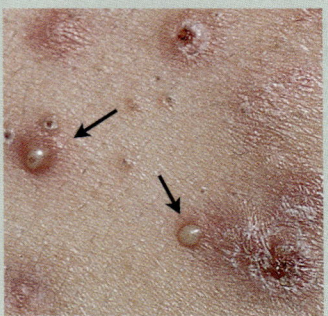
Cyst Elevated, circumscribed, encapsulated lesion; in dermis or subcutaneous layer; filled with liquid or semi-solid material	Sebaceous cyst, cystic acne 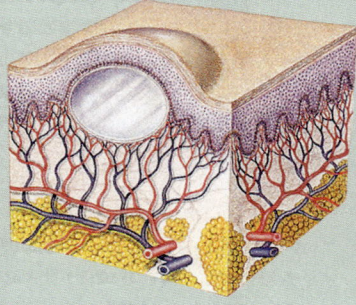	Sebaceous cyst (Weston, Lane, and Morelli, 2007) 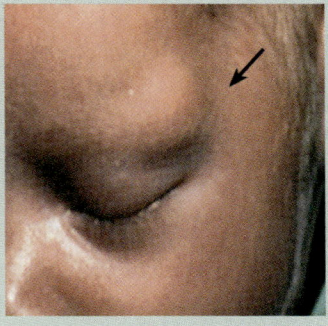
Telangiectasia Fine, irregular, red lines produced by capillary dilation	Telangiectasia in rosacea 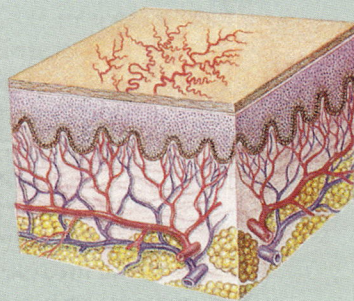	Telangiectasia (White and Cox, 2006) 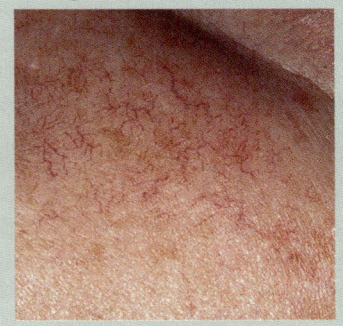

From Seidel H et al: *Mosby's guide to physical examination*, ed 6, St Louis, 2006, Mosby. Modified from Thompson JM, Wilson SF: *Health assessment for nursing practice*, ed 2, H, St Louis, 2001, Mosby.

TABLE 20-2 Secondary Skin Lesions

Description	Examples	

Scale

Heaped-up, keratinized cells, flaky skin; irregular; thick or thin; dry or oily; variation in size

Flaking of skin with seborrheic dermatitis following scarlet fever, or flaking of skin following a drug reaction; dry skin

Scale (Marks and Miller, 2006)

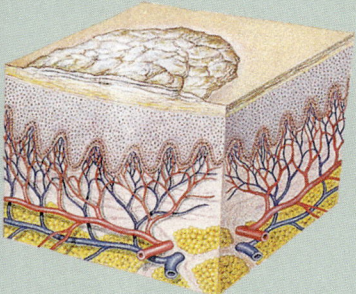
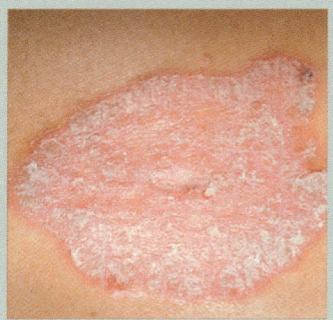

Lichenification

Rough, thickened epidermis secondary to persistent rubbing, itching, or skin irritation; often involves flexor surface of extremity

Chronic dermatitis

Atopic dermatitis (Marks and Miller, 2006)

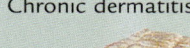
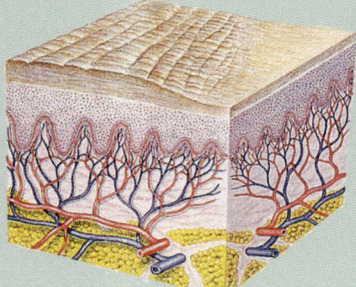
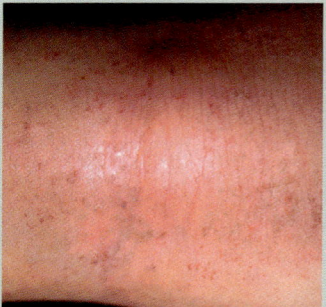

Keloid

Irregular-shaped, elevated, progressively enlarging scar; grows beyond boundaries of wound; caused by excessive collagen formation during healing

Keloid formation following surgery

Keloid (Weston, Lane, and Morelli, 2007)

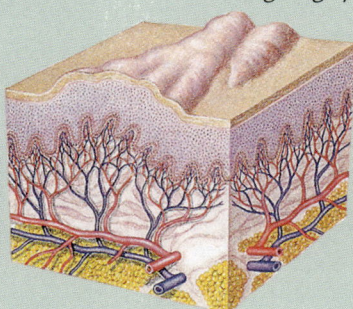
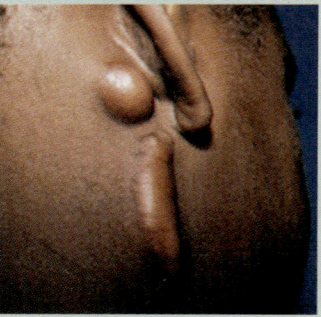

Scar

Thin to thick fibrous tissue that replaces normal skin following injury or laceration to dermis

Healed wound or surgical incision

Hypertrophic scar (White and Cox, 2006)

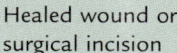
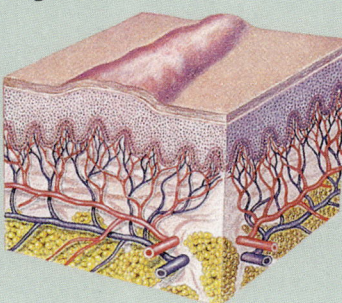
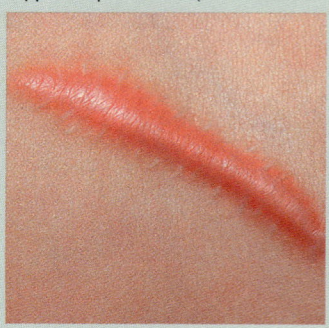

TABLE 20-2 Secondary Skin Lesions—cont'd

Description	Examples

Excoriation

Loss of epidermis; linear hollowed-out, crusted area

Abrasion or scratch, scabies

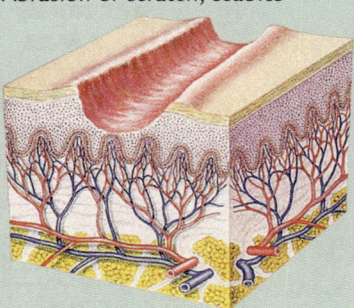

Scabies (Weston, Lane, and Morelli, 2007)

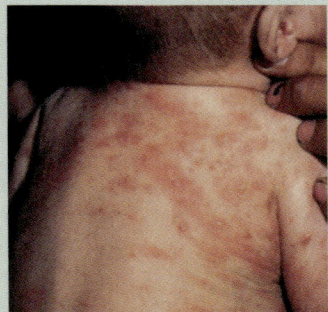

Fissure

Linear crack or break from epidermis to dermis; may be moist or dry

Athlete's foot, cracks at corner of mouth

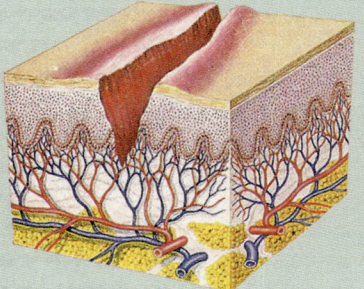

Fissure (Weston, Lane, and Morelli, 2007)

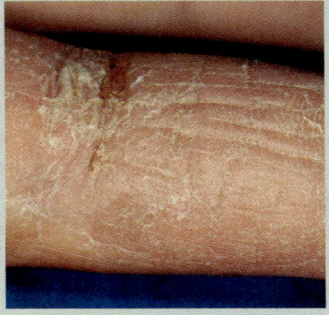

Erosion

Loss of part of epidermis; depressed, moist, glistening; follows rupture of vesicle or bulla

Varicella, variola after rupture

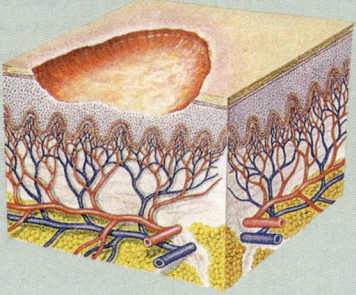

Erosion (Marks and Miller, 2007)

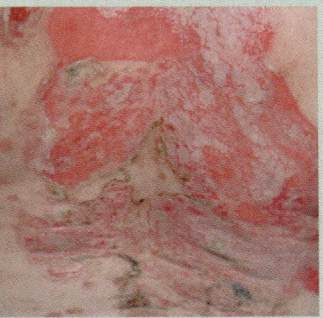

Ulcer

Loss of epidermis and dermis; concave; varies in size

Decubiti, stasis ulcers

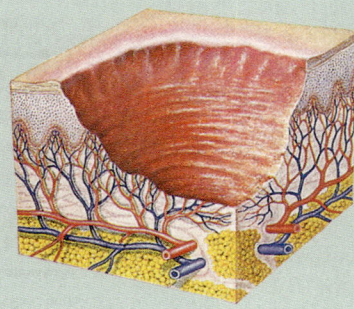

Stasis ulcer (Marks and Miller, 2007)

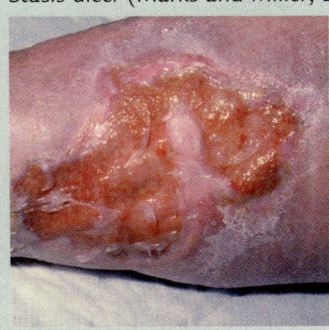

Continued

TABLE 20-2 Secondary Skin Lesions—cont'd

Description	Examples	
Crust		
Dried serum, blood, or purulent exudates; slightly elevated; size varies; brown, red, tan, or straw-colored	Scab on abrasion, eczema	Scab (Seidel et al, 2006)
Atrophy		
Thinning of skin surface and loss of skin markings; skin translucent and paper-like	Striae; aged skin	Striae (Seidel et al, 2006/courtesy Dr. Antoinette Hood, Department of Dermatology, University of Indiana, Department of Medicine)

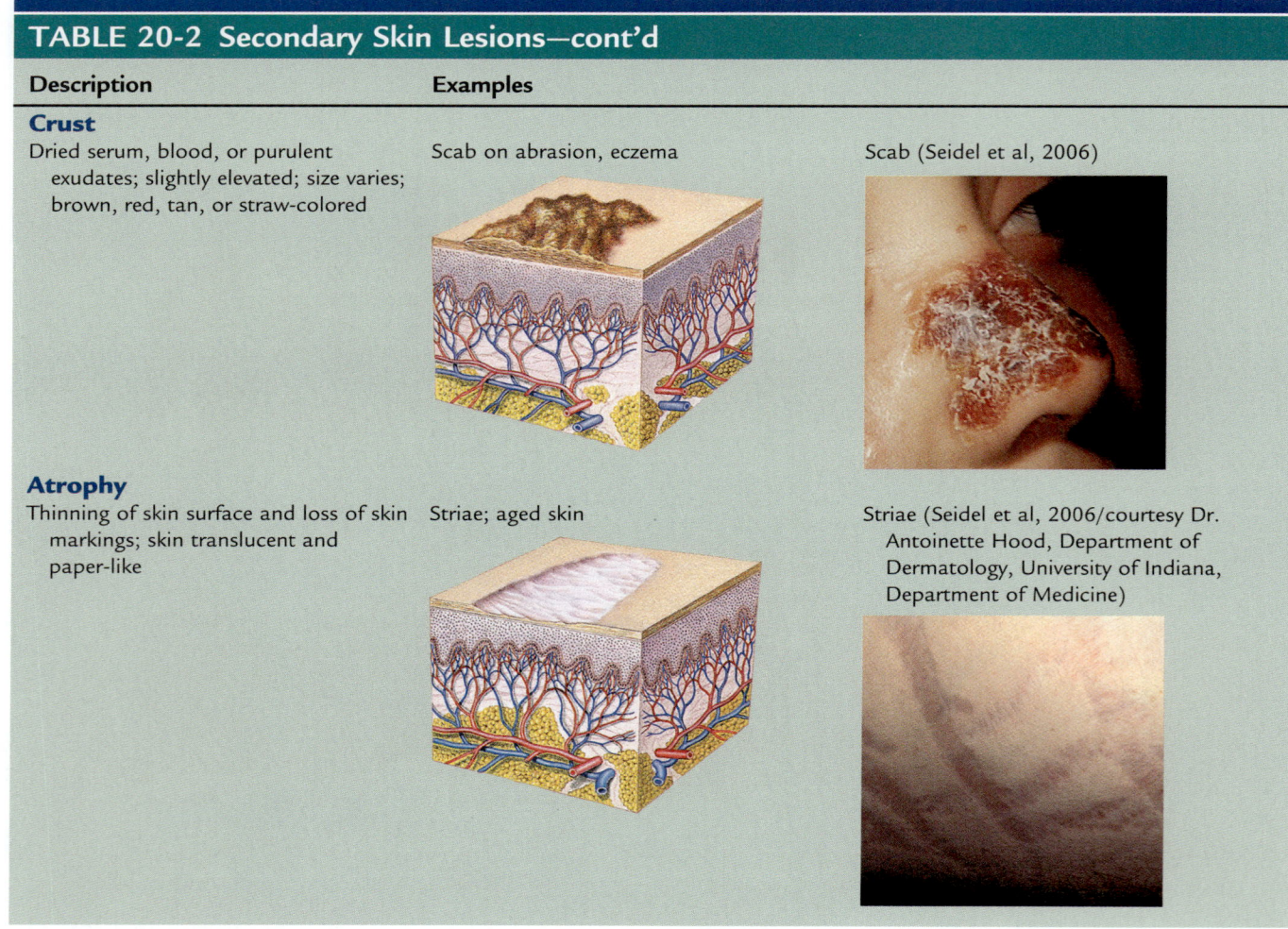

From Seidel H et al: *Mosby's guide to physical examination,* ed 6, St Louis, 2006, Mosby. Modified from Thompson JM, Wilson SF: *Health assessment for nursing practice,* ed 2, St Louis, 2001, Mosby.

RESPIRATION

The normal respiratory rate for adults is between 12 and 24 breaths per minute.[2] The respiratory rate is assessed by watching the patient breathe, by feeling for chest movement, or by auscultating the lungs. The paramedic counts the respirations for 30 seconds, and then multiplies by 2 to measure breaths per minute. Rhythm and depth of respirations are assessed by visualization and auscultation of the thorax. Abnormal findings include shallow, rapid, noisy, or deep breathing; asymmetrical chest wall movement; use of accessory muscles of respiration; or congested, unequal, or diminished breath sounds.

PULSE

A normal resting pulse rate for an adult is usually between 60 and 100 beats per minute; it may be affected by the patient's age and physical condition (Table 20-3). For example, a child's pulse rate may be 80 to 100 beats per minute. A well-trained athlete's pulse rate may be 50 to 60 beats per minute. Factors such as pregnancy, anxiety, and

fear also may produce a higher-than-normal pulse rate in healthy individuals.

Pulse rates may be obtained at the carotid artery in the neck or at any site where the artery lies close to the skin. To evaluate the radial pulse, the paramedic places the pads of the index and middle fingers at the distal end of the patient's wrist, just medial to the radial styloid. If pulsations are

TABLE 20-3 Average Vital Signs by Age

Age	Pulse (beats/min)	Respirations (breaths/min)	Blood Pressure (mm Hg)
Newborn	120-160	40-60	80/40
1 year	80-140	30-40	82/44
3 years	80-120	25-30	86/50
5 years	70-115	20-25	90/52
7 years	70-115	20-25	94/54
10 years	70-115	15-20	100/60
15 years	70-90	15-20	110/64
Adult	60-100	12-24	120/80

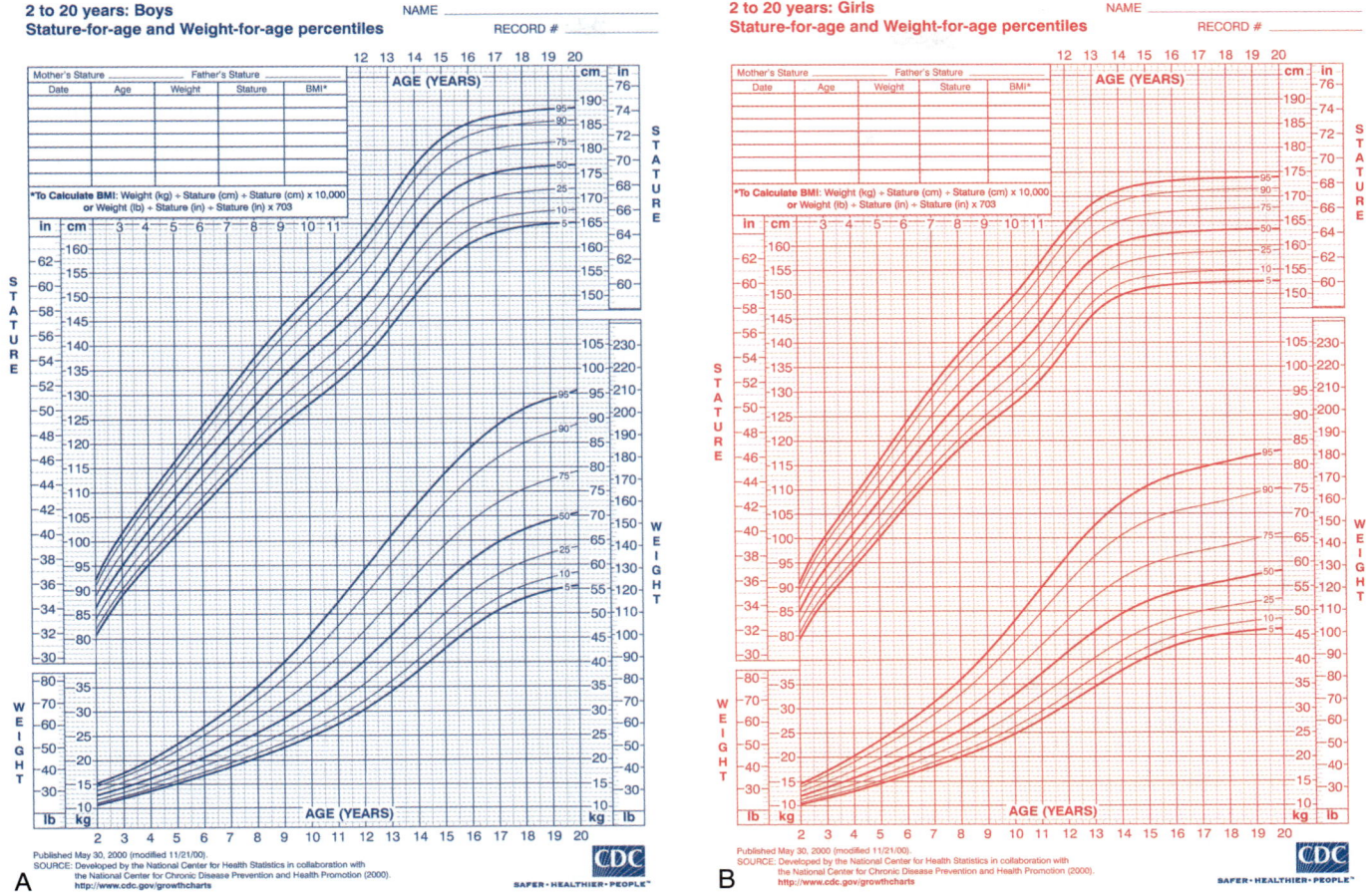

FIGURE 20-9 Physical growth curves and National Center for Health Statistics percentiles for children, age 2 through 18 years, for height and weight. **A,** Boys. **B,** Girls. (Developed by the National Council for Health Statistics in collaboration with the National Center for Chronic Disease Prevention and Health Promotion 2000.)

regular, the paramedic should count for 15 seconds and multiply that number by 4 to determine the number of beats per minute. In addition to the number of times the heart beats per minute, the regularity and strength of the pulse also are important. For example, the pulse can be regular or irregular, weak or strong. Application of an electrocardiogram monitor also is useful in evaluating cardiovascular status after initial assessment of the pulse.

BLOOD PRESSURE

The **systolic blood pressure** is the pressure exerted against the arterial walls when the heart contracts. The **diastolic blood pressure** is the pressure exerted against the arterial walls when the heart relaxes. For all age groups,[3] systolic blood pressure ideally should be less than 120 mm Hg; diastolic pressure should be less than 80 mm Hg.

Blood pressure is best measured by auscultation or by an electronic device. The blood pressure cuff is placed on the patient's arm with the lower end of the cuff positioned 1 to 2 inches (2 to 5 cm) above the antecubital (AC) space. If measured manually, the cuff is inflated to a point about 30 mm Hg above where the brachial pulse can no longer be

palpated. The stethoscope is placed over the brachial artery, and the cuff is slowly deflated at a rate of 2 to 3 mm Hg per second. As the pressure falls, the paramedic should observe the gauge and note where the first sound or pulsation is heard. This is the patient's systolic pressure. The point at which the sounds change in quality or become muffled is noted as the patient's diastolic pressure.

> **NOTE**
>
> At times, determining the correct diastolic pressure is difficult. The difference between the point of muffled tones and the complete disappearance of pulsations varies by person. In some persons, the difference is a few millimeters of mercury; however, in some persons, pulsations never totally disappear. The ability to measure accurate diastolic pressures comes from experience and requires careful listening in a quiet setting.

Blood pressure may be estimated by palpation when vascular sounds are difficult to hear with a stethoscope because of environmental noise. However, this method is less accurate than auscultation and can only estimate systolic pressure. To estimate blood pressure by palpation, the paramedic should locate the brachial or radial pulse and apply the blood pressure cuff as described before. Finger contact should be maintained at the pulse site as the cuff slowly deflates. When the pulse becomes palpable, the gauge reading denotes the systolic pressure. Like pulse rates, a patient's blood pressure may be unusually high because of fear or anxiety. Other factors, such as a patient's age and normal level of physical activity, may be the cause of unusual blood pressure readings.

Alternate sites may be used to assess blood pressure when use of the patient's upper arm is not possible. Blood pressure readings in these alternate sites vary from those taken in the arm (Figure 20-10). Other methods used to assess oxygenation and perfusion include oxygen saturation, capnography (described in Chapter 15), and capillary refill (described in Chapter 19).

LOOK AGAIN
See Chapter 15: Airway, pp. 451-455.

EXAMINATION OF THE SKIN

The skin can reveal a great deal about a patient's status. Assessment includes skin color, temperature, and moisture. As discussed before, a patient's skin color and the presence of bruises, lesions, or rashes may indicate serious illness or injury.

Skin temperature may be normal (warm), hot, or cold. Evaluations of temperature may have specific applications in some patient situations. Examples of such situations are febrile seizures and hyperthermic and hypothermic emergencies. Skin that is hot to the touch indicates a possible fever or heat-related illness or injury. Cold skin may indicate decreased tissue perfusion and cold-related illness or injury. The dorsal surface of the hand is more sensitive than the palmar surface and should be used to estimate body temperature. Normal body temperature is 37° C (98.6° F). Oral, axillary, tympanic, or rectal temperatures can be measured using electronic, digital, temporal (artery), digital dot, or tympanic-membrane thermometers (Figure 20-11). The temperature probe should be covered by a disposable sheath. The sheath helps to prevent cross-contamination.

Oral Measurement. Oral temperature usually is measured in patients over the age of 6. The readings may be affected by crying, eating, drinking, smoking, oxygen administration by mask, or nebulizer treatments, and by the position of the thermometer in the patient's mouth. When using electronic devices, a brief tone will alert the paramedic when the measurement is complete. Children can be told to hold the thermometer in a "kiss" position and not to bite on the probe.

Axillary Measurement. The axillary site often is used to take the temperature in children. The axilla frequently is used in children less than 6 years of age. The axilla also is used in children who are uncooperative or have diseases that suppress the immune system and in patients who have an altered level of consciousness. Axillary temperature is measured by placing the electronic probe firmly in the center of the patient's axillary space. The patient's arm should be held against the side of the chest. A tone will

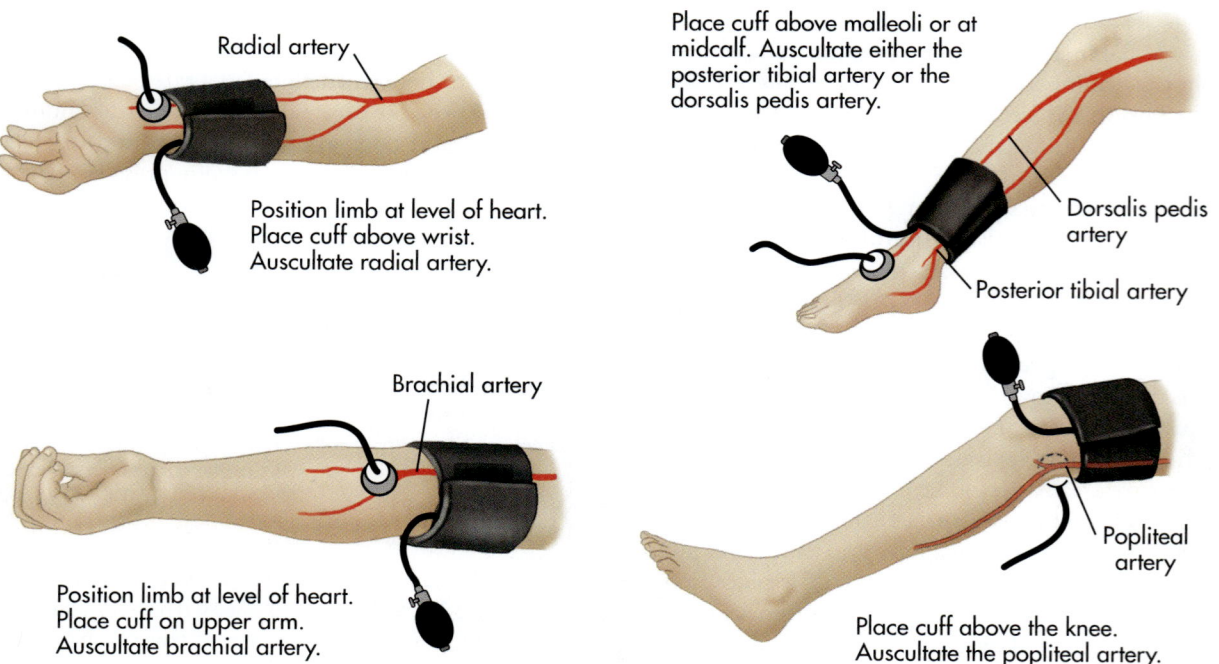

FIGURE 20-10 Blood pressure measurement sites.

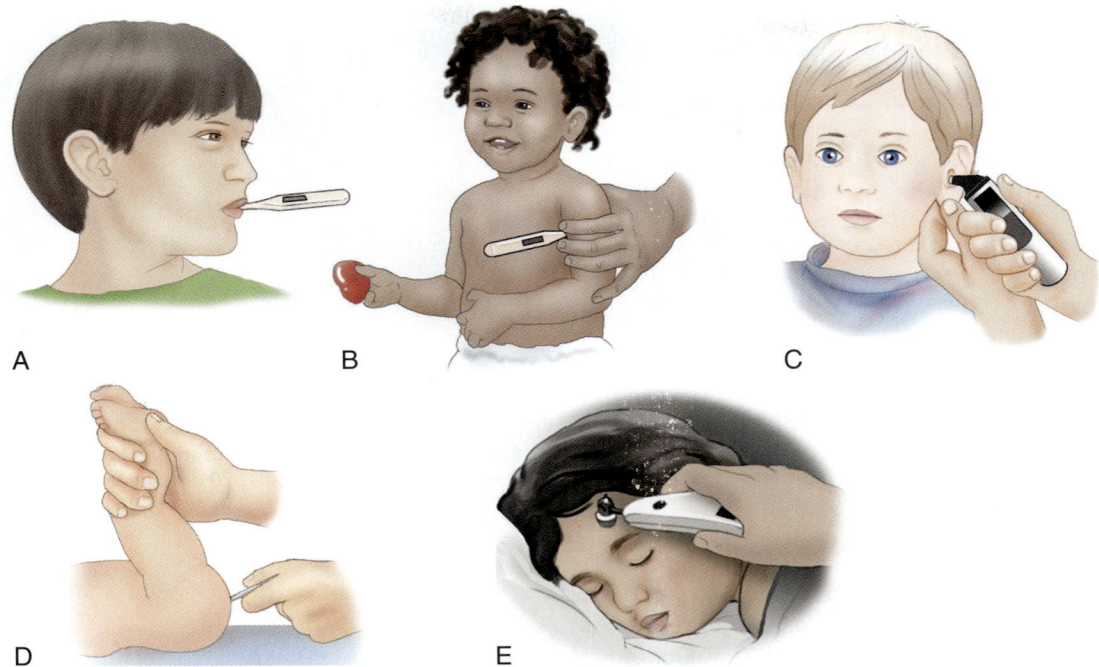

FIGURE 20-11 Temperature assessment. **A,** Oral temperature measurement. **B,** Axillary temperature measurement. **C,** Tympanic temperature measurement. **D,** Rectal temperature measurement. **E,** Temporal temperature assessment.

sound when the measurement is complete. The temperature assessed at this site is usually 1° F (0.6° C) lower than the core temperature of the body.

Tympanic Measurement. The tympanic membrane is close to the hypothalamus. This position makes the tympanic membrane an ideal place to measure core temperature. The paramedic takes this measurement by placing the tip of the probe into the patient's ear canal. To obtain the most accurate reading, the ear canal should be straightened by gently pulling the pinna of the ear down and back in children less than 3 years of age or up and back in patients 3 years of age or older. When the thermometer is in the correct position and is activated per the manufacturer's instructions, a temperature reading is obtained within seconds. Tympanic measurement is associated with significant variability in measurements. Readings can be inaccurate in patients who have had ear surgery; have otitis media or excessive earwax; have recently exercised; are in situations with extremes of temperature (incubators, wind or fans); and in children less than 3 years of age.[4]

Rectal Measurement. Measuring a patient's temperature by the rectal route poses a risk of perforation. In addition, the method can be distressing for the patient. This route generally is reserved for young children and patients who have an altered level of consciousness. When measuring rectal temperature, the paramedic should place the patient in the supine position (infants). The patient also can be placed in the left lateral recumbent position with the legs raised. This position exposes the anus. The paramedic inserts a lubricated probe no more than 2.5 cm (½ to 1 inch) into the rectum. The probe should be held securely in place until the electronic device sounds the alert. Rectal readings provide the most accurate assessment. However, they generally are impractical for prehospital use. Special hypothermic thermometers may be used to measure the rectal temperature of patients with hypothermia (see Chapter 45).

Skin moisture usually is classified as dry or wet. Dry skin is normal. Wet skin is clammy or diaphoretic. Diaphoretic skin may indicate a volume problem such as hypovolemia. It may also indicate other illness or injury that results in decreased tissue perfusion or increased sweat gland activity. Examples are cardiovascular and heat-related emergencies, respectively.

PUPILS

Examining the pupils for response to light may yield information on the neurological status of some patients. Unequal pupils (**anisocoria**) may be a normal finding in some patients. However, the pupils usually are equal and constrict when exposed to light. (The acronym **PERRL** indicates that the *p*upils are *e*qual, *r*ound, and *r*eact to *l*ight.) When testing the pupils for light response, the paramedic shines a penlight directly into one eye. The normal reaction is for the pupil exposed to the light to constrict. This occurs with a consensual constriction of the opposite eye. Table 20-4 lists abnormal pupillary reactions and possible causes.

TABLE 20-4	Abnormal Pupil Reactions
Pupil Size	**Possible Causes**
Equal	
Dilated or unresponsive	Cardiac arrest, central nervous system injury, hypoxia or anoxia, drug use (LSD [lysergic acid diethylamide], atropine, amphetamines)
Constricted or unresponsive	Central nervous system injury or disease, narcotic drug use (heroin, morphine), eye medications
Unequal	
One dilated or unresponsive	Cerebrovascular accident, head injury, direct trauma to eye, eye medications

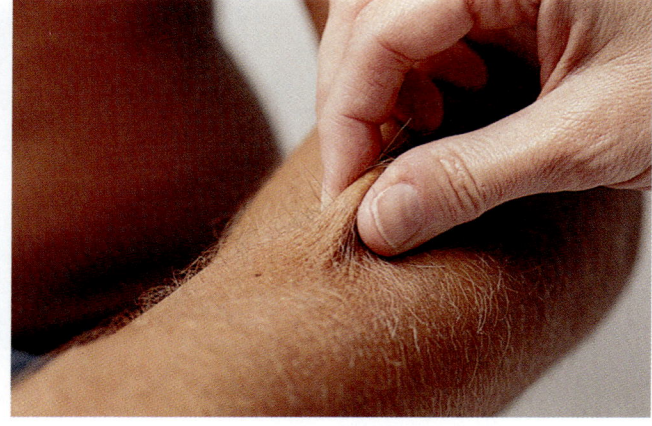

FIGURE 20-12 Assessing skin turgor. (From Potter PA, Perry AG: *Basic nursing,* ed 7, St Louis, 2011, Mosby.)

ANATOMICAL REGIONS

The remainder of this chapter discusses techniques of the physical examination as they relate to anatomical regions of the body. The paramedic should recall that anatomical and physiological aspects of the human body are age-related. They vary by person as well. An examination of the anatomical regions should be guided by a patient's chief complaint. A full examination of all regions often is not necessary in the emergency setting, but will be described here for a complete discussion. Chapter 10 serves as a review of anatomical regions of the body.

> **LOOK AGAIN**
> See Chapter 10: Review of Human Systems, pp. 146-150.

Skin

The general assessment of the skin was described previously. In addition, the comprehensive physical examination should include an evaluation of the texture and turgor of the skin, hair, and nails.[2] (All of these are part of the integumentary system.)

TEXTURE AND TURGOR

The texture of the skin normally is smooth, soft, and flexible. In older adults, though, the skin may be wrinkled and leathery from decreased amounts of collagen and subcutaneous fat as well as reduced secretion from sweat glands. Abnormal skin texture may result from lesions, rashes, tumors, and localized trauma.

Turgor refers to the elasticity of the skin (which normally decreases with age). To test skin turgor, the paramedic should pinch ("tent") a fold of skin and assess the ease and speed at which the skin returns to its normal position. (Skin on the back of the patient's hand or over the sternum are good areas to test for turgor.) Tented skin that does not quickly return to its normal position may indicate dehydration (Figure 20-12).

HAIR

As part of the examination, the paramedic should inspect and palpate the patient's hair. The paramedic should note quantity, distribution, and texture. Key findings include a recent change in the growth or loss of hair. These may result from chemotherapy or hormone and endocrine disorders (e.g., menopause and diabetes). Thinning hair is common in older men and women.

FINGERNAILS AND TOENAILS

The paramedic should note the color and shape of the patient's fingernails and toenails and also assess for the presence or absence of lesions. Uncolored nails usually are transparent. Healthy nails are smooth and firm on palpation. Box 20-4 describes abnormal findings in the nails. With age, nails often develop longitudinal striations and may have a yellow tint because of insufficient calcium.

Head, Ears, Eyes, Nose, and Throat

An examination of the structures of the head and neck involves inspection, palpation, and auscultation.

HEAD AND FACE

To examine the head, the paramedic should inspect the skull for shape and symmetry, keeping in mind that hair can hide abnormalities. The hair should be parted in several places to assess for scaliness, lumps, or other lesions. The assessment should use a systematic palpation, moving from front to back, noting any swelling, tenderness, indentations, or depressions. The scalp should move freely over the skull, and the patient should be free of pain or discomfort during the examination.

The face should be inspected for symmetry, expression, and contour, noting any asymmetry, involuntary movements, masses, or edema. The paramedic should evaluate facial skin for color, pigmentation, texture, thickness, hair distribution, and any lesions.

BOX 20-4 Abnormal Nail Findings

Beau's lines: Transverse depressions in the nail that inhibit nail growth; associated with systemic illness, severe infection, and nail injury.

Clubbing: A change in the angle between the nail and nail base that approaches or exceeds 180 degrees; associated with flattening and often enlargement of the fingertips; may indicate chronic cardiac or respiratory disease.

Onycholysis: The separation of a nail from its bed; associated with psoriasis, dermatitis, fungal infection, and other conditions.

Paronychia: Inflammation of the skin at the base of the nail; may result from local infection or trauma.

Psoriasis: Pitting, discoloration, and subungual thickening of the nail plate; may lead to splinter hemorrhages.

Splinter hemorrhages: Red or brown linear streaks in the nail bed; associated with minor nail trauma, bacterial endocarditis, and trichinosis.

Terry's nails: The presence of transverse white bands that cover the nail except for a narrow zone at the distal tip; associated with cirrhosis.

Transverse white lines: Longitudinal white streaks in the nail plate; may indicate a systemic disorder.

White spots: The presence of white spots that appear in the nail plate; usually result from minor injury or cuticle manipulation.

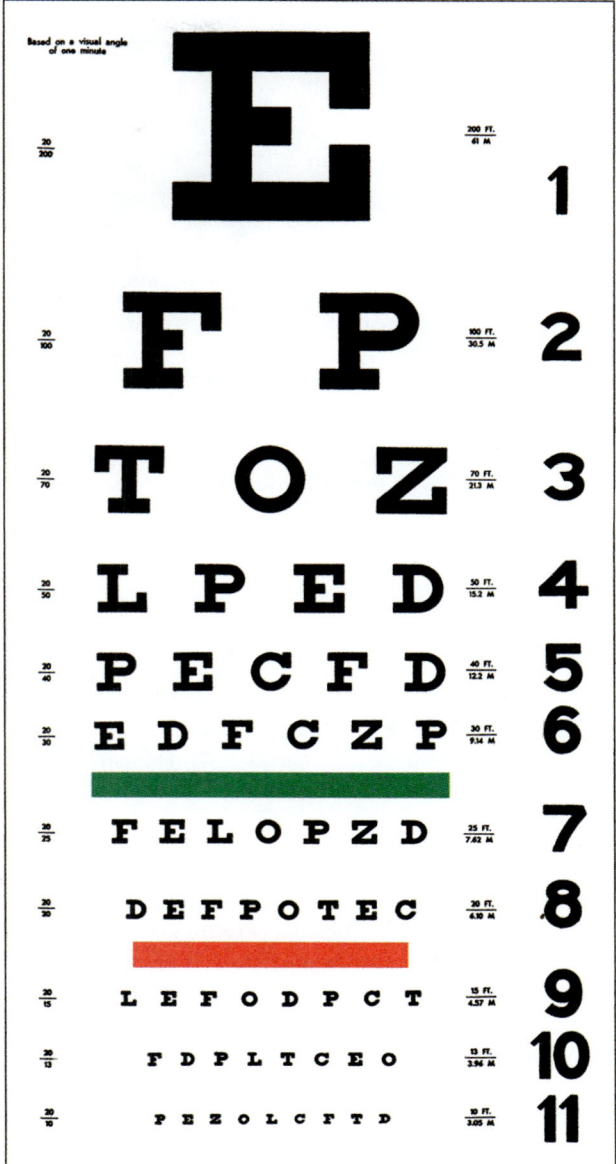

FIGURE 20-13 Snellen chart. (From Seidel H et al: *Mosby's guide to physical examination,* ed 6, St Louis, 2007, Mosby.)

EYES

The paramedic should verify that both eyes can see. Basic information is gathered during the patient history and by asking the patient about any visual disturbances. **Visual acuity** can be assessed by asking the patient to read printed material or count fingers at a distance, and by demonstrating the ability to distinguish light from dark through the use of various eye charts (e.g., a *Snellen chart*) (Figure 20-13).

Both eyes should move equally well in the **six cardinal fields of gaze** (Figure 20-14). To evaluate a patient's gaze, the paramedic should hold the patient's chin. The patient's eyes should be observed as they track a penlight or finger (or a toy, in the case of a child) when it moves through the six visual fields in an H pattern. Any **nystagmus** (involuntary jerking movements of the eyes) or **disconjugate gaze** (deviation of the eyes to opposite sides) should be noted. Another method to check visual fields is to ask the patient to look at his or her nose. The paramedic then extends his or her arms with elbows at right angles and wiggles both index fingers at the same time to test peripheral vision. Asking the patient to identify finger movements and to track a moving object can demonstrate if visual fields are grossly normal. This test should be performed in four quadrants (up, down, right, and left). The eyes should also be assessed for normal position and alignment.

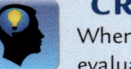

CRITICAL THINKING
When you perform an examination of the eyes, you are evaluating components of at least four body systems. What are they?

The patient's orbital area should be assessed for edema and puffiness. The eyebrows should be free of scaliness. Inspection of the eyelids consists of noting the width of *palpebral fissures* (the elliptical opening between the upper and lower lids), edema, color, lesions, condition and direction of the eyelashes, adequacy of lid closure, and drainage. The paramedic also briefly should inspect the regions of the lacrimal gland and lacrimal sac for swelling. Excessive

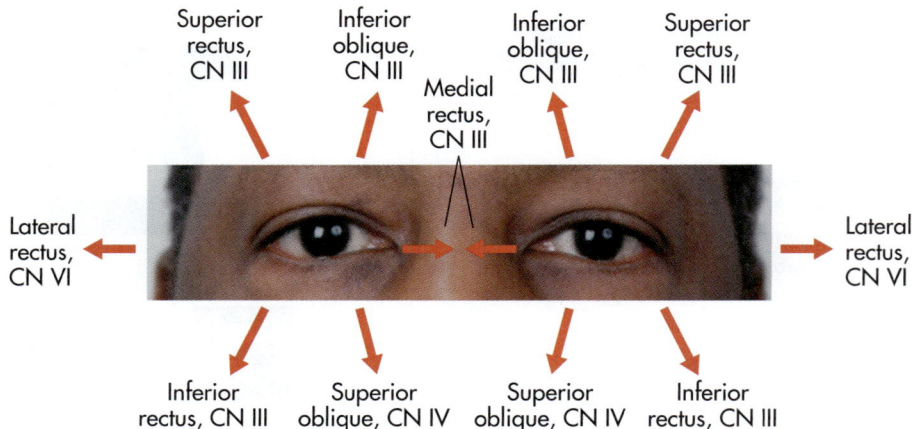

FIGURE 20-14 Six cardinal fields of gaze. Cranial nerves and extraocular muscles associated with the six cardinal fields of gaze. (From Seidel H et al: *Mosby's guide to physical examination,* ed 6, St Louis, 2007, Mosby.)

tearing or dryness of the eye should be noted (see Chapter 10).

 LOOK AGAIN
See Chapter 10: Review of Human Systems, pp. 206-208.

The patient's conjunctiva and sclera are examined by asking the patient to look up while the paramedic depresses both lower lids with the thumbs (Figure 20-15). The sclera should be white; the cornea and the iris should be clearly visible; and the pupils should be of equal size, round, and reactive to light. Palpating the patient's lower orbital rim determines structural integrity. The paramedic should be alert to the presence of contact lenses and ocular prostheses when examining a patient's eyes.

Ophthalmoscope Examination. The ophthalmoscope is used to assess the cornea for foreign bodies, lacerations, abrasions, and infection; the anterior chamber for the presence of blood or pus; and under the eyelid for the presence of foreign bodies. In addition, the retinal vessels, the optic nerve, and the retina of the fundus can be examined along with the vitreous. Ophthalmoscopic examinations should be performed in a darkened room so that the pupils are dilated. Contact lenses do not need to be removed.

To perform an examination with an ophthalmoscope, the paramedic should follow these steps for each eye:
1. Ask the patient to fixate on a distant object.
2. Sit facing the patient at the same seat height.
3. Turn on the ophthalmoscope light and select the 0 lens setting.
4. Use the right hand and eye to examine the patient's right eye and the left hand and eye to examine the patient's left eye.
5. Direct the patient to look over your shoulder, keeping both eyes open.

6. Hold the scope against your face and shine the light on the patient's pupil at a distance of about 10 inches from the face and at a 45-degree angle. A bright orange glow in the pupil ("red reflex") normally is visible (Figure 20-16).
7. Move the light slowly toward the pupil to see the structures of the fundus. Rotate the lens to improve focus as needed.
8. Inspect the size, color, and clarity of the disk and the integrity of vessels; assess for retinal lesions and the appearance of the macula. A normal examination will reveal the following[5] (Figure 20-17):

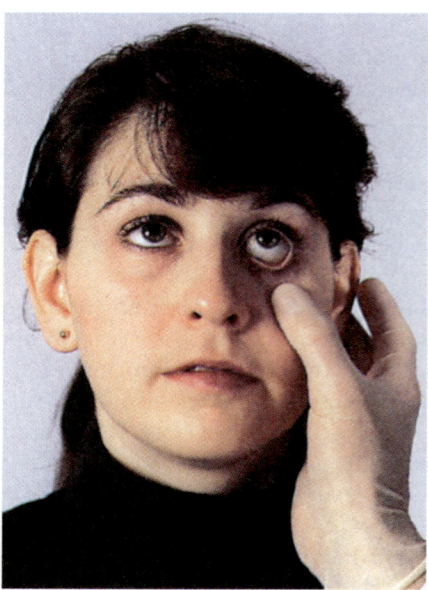

FIGURE 20-15 Examining the cornea and sclera. (From Seidel H et al: *Mosby's guide to physical examination,* ed 6, St Louis, 2007, Mosby.)

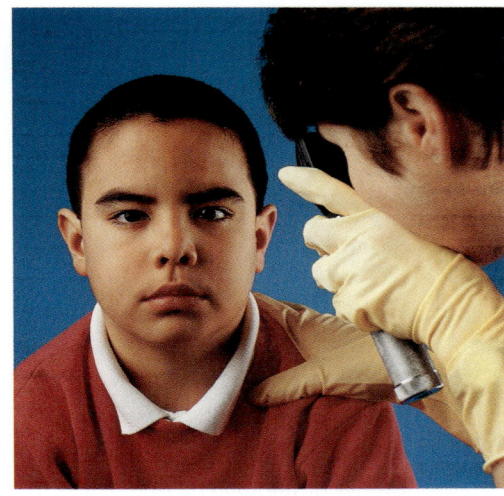

FIGURE 20-16 Paramedic using an ophthalmoscope.

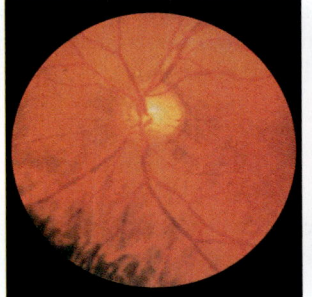 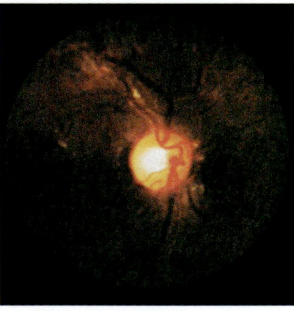

FIGURE 20-17 Normal fundus examination. (From Potter PA, Perry AG: *Basic nursing*, ed 7, St Louis, 2011, Mosby.)

- A clear, yellow optic nerve disk
- Yellow to creamy-pink retina (depending on patient's race)
- Light red arteries and dark red veins
- A 3:2 vein-to-artery ratio in size proportion
- The avascular macula

EARS

The paramedic should inspect the external ear and surrounding tissues for signs of bruising, deformity, or discoloration. No discharge should be present in either ear canal. Pulling gently on the earlobes should not produce pain or discomfort. The patient's skull and facial bones surrounding the ear should be palpated. The mastoid area should be inspected for tenderness or discoloration. A patient who is alert and able to hear and who speaks the same language as the paramedic should be able to respond to questions without many requests for repetition. Hearing aids should be noted. An assessment of gross auditory keenness can be made by covering one ear at a time and asking the patient to repeat short test words spoken in soft and loud tones.

Otoscopic Examination. An otoscope is used to evaluate the inner ear for discharge and foreign bodies and to assess the eardrum. The paramedic performs an otoscopic exam using the following steps for each ear (Figure 20-18):
1. Select the appropriate size of speculum.
2. Check the ear for foreign bodies before inserting the speculum.
3. Instruct the patient not to move during the examination to avoid injury to the canal and tympanic membrane. (Infants and young children may need to be restrained.)
4. Turn on the otoscope and insert the speculum into the ear canal, slightly down and forward. To ease insertion, pull the auricle up and backward in adults; back and downward in infants.
5. Identify cerumen and look for foreign bodies, lesions, or discharge.

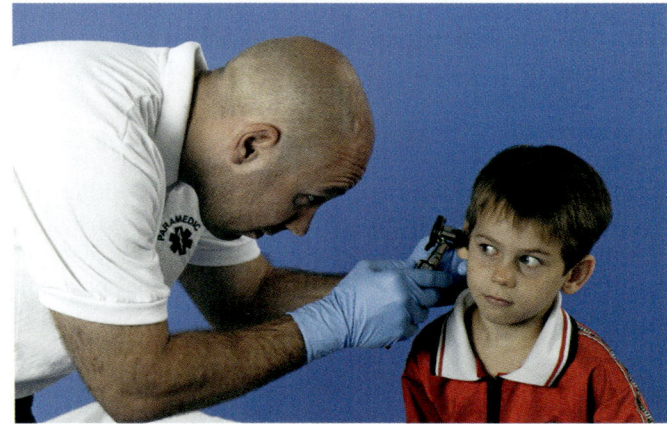

FIGURE 20-18 Paramedic performing an otoscopic exam.

6. Visualize and inspect the tympanic membrane for tears or breaks. A normal examination will reveal the following:
   - Cerumen will be dry (tan or light yellow) or moist (dark yellow or brown).
   - The ear canal should not be inflamed (a sign of infection).
   - The tympanic membrane should be translucent or pearly gray (pink or red indicates inflammation).

NOSE

The patient's nose should be inspected for shape, size, color, and stability. The column of the nose should be midline with the face and the nares positioned symmetrically. (Slight asymmetry of nares is considered normal.) The paramedic should palpate the column of the nose and surrounding soft tissues for pain, tenderness, or deformity. The frontal and maxillary sinuses may be inspected for the presence of swelling. They may also be palpated for tenderness along the bony brow on each side of the nose and the zygomatic processes.

Discharge from the nose can have a number of causes. For example, cerebrospinal fluid may be present as a result of head trauma; a bloody discharge (**epistaxis**) may result from trauma or from mucosal erosions involving blood vessels, hypertension, or bleeding disorders. A mucous discharge commonly results from allergy, upper respiratory tract infection, sinusitis, or cold exposure.

MOUTH AND PHARYNX

The paramedic should inspect the lips for symmetry, color, edema, and skin surface irregularities. The lips should be pink. Pallor of the lips is associated with anemia; cyanosis is associated with cardiorespiratory insufficiency; red lips sometimes are a late finding in carbon monoxide poisoning (see Chapter 34). The lips should show no swelling, deformity, or pain on palpation.

Healthy gums in the oral cavity are pink and free of lesions and swelling. Patchy areas of pigmentation in the mouths of African Americans are not uncommon. Enlarged gums may indicate pregnancy, leukemia, poor oral hygiene, puberty, or use of some medications (e.g., **phenytoin**). The mouth should be free of loose or broken teeth. Dental appliances may be present.

The patient's tongue should be inspected for size and color. The tongue should be positioned in the midline of the oral cavity and appear nonswollen, dull red, moist, and glistening. To inspect the oropharynx, a tongue blade is used to depress the patient's tongue. The normal palate is white or pink. If the oral cavity is inflamed or covered with exudate, an infection may be present. (Specific breath odors may indicate alcohol or other drug consumption or illness.) The tonsils normally are pink and smooth without edema, ulceration, or inflammation. A patient with a typical sore throat often has a reddened and edematous uvula and tonsillar pillars. A yellow exudate sometimes is present.

NECK

The paramedic should inspect the neck in the patient's normal anatomical position. If trauma is suspected, spinal precautions should be used. The trachea should be midline. No use of accessory muscles or tracheal tugging should occur during respiration. To palpate the neck, the paramedic places both thumbs along the sides of the distal trachea and systematically moves the hands toward the head (Figure 20-19). Care should be taken not to apply bilateral pressure to the carotid arteries, as syncope or bradycardia may result.

The lymph nodes should not be tender. (Tender or swollen lymph nodes usually are the result of inflammation.) The thyroid and cricoid cartilages should be free of pain and should move when the patient swallows. Bubbling or crackling sensations that can be palpated in the soft tissues of the neck may indicate the presence of **subcutaneous emphysema** (the presence of air in the subcutaneous tissues). The paramedic should note distended neck veins or prominent carotid arteries (see Chapter 22).

HEAD AND CERVICAL SPINE

The temporomandibular joint connects the mandible of the jaw to the temporal bone of the skull. The joint sometimes can become painful or dislocated. Normally the

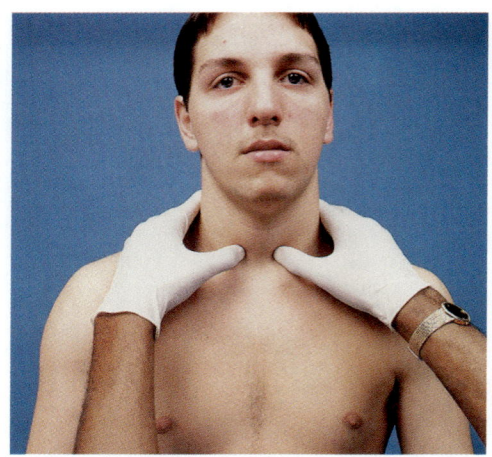

FIGURE 20-19 Position of the thumbs to evaluate the midline position of the trachea.

patient should be able to open and close the mouth without pain or limitation in movement. **Temporomandibular joint dysfunction** is a common complaint.

For the patient who has not undergone trauma, the paramedic should inspect the cervical spine by palpating for tenderness or deformities. Range of motion can be tested in the following manner:
- Flexion: touching the chin to the chest
- Rotation: touching the chin to each shoulder
- Lateral bending: touching each ear to each shoulder
- Extension: tilting the head backward

The neck of a trauma patient may need to be moved for a general or neurological examination. Any such movement must be accompanied by the application of continuous manual protection and stabilization techniques for suspected cervical spine injury (see Chapter 41).

Chest

A thorough knowledge of the structure of the thoracic cage is needed to perform an adequate respiratory and cardiac assessment. The ribs protect the vital organs within the thorax. They also offer support for respiratory movements of the diaphragm and intercostal muscles (see Chapter 10). Damage to the actual bony structure of the thoracic cavity, such as a flail chest, can prevent or limit respiratory function. The ribs of the thorax also are used as anatomical landmarks in locating specific areas for examination. Figure 20-20 shows the landmarks of the chest. The thorax can be evaluated by using imaginary lines to note examination findings (Figure 20-21). The thorax is assessed through inspection, palpation, percussion, and auscultation.

INSPECTION

The patient's chest wall should be inspected for symmetry on the anterior and posterior surfaces. The thorax is not completely symmetrical. However, a visual inspection of one side should offer a reasonable comparison to the other. Chest wall diameter often is increased in patients with

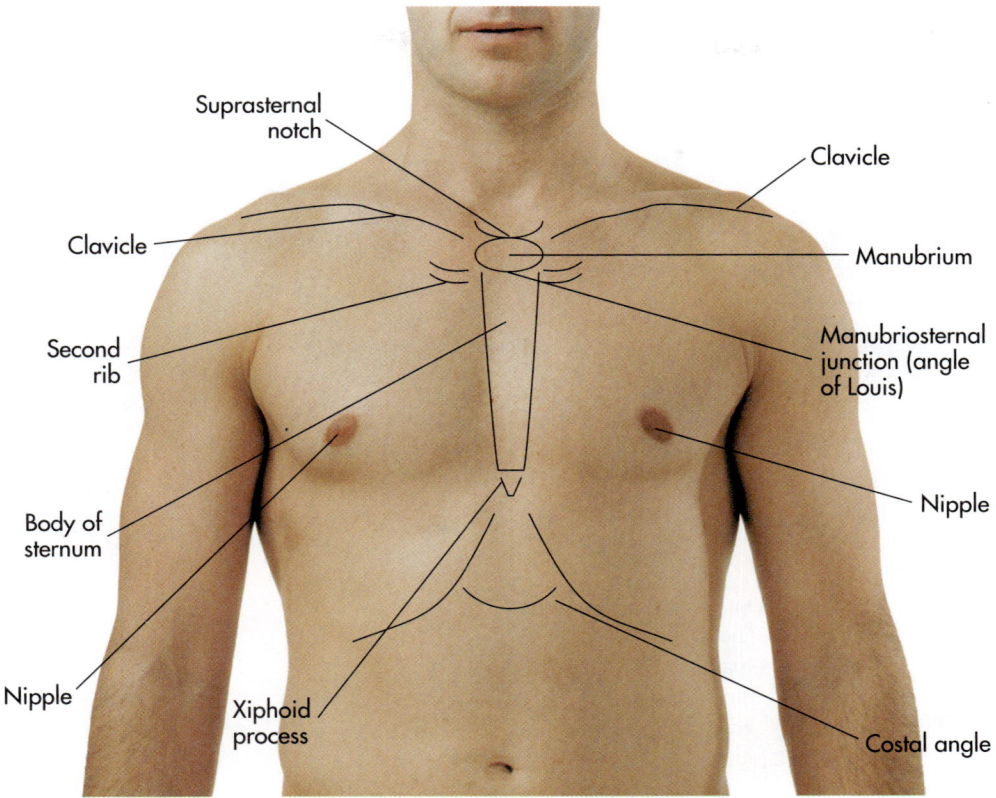

FIGURE 20-20 Topographical landmarks of the chest. (From Seidel H et al: *Mosby's guide to physical examination,* ed 6, St Louis, 2007, Mosby.)

obstructive pulmonary disease. This results in a barrel-shaped appearance of the thorax. Other causes for chest wall deformities or asymmetry include a *funnel chest* (an indentation of the lower sternum above the xiphoid process), *pigeon chest* (a prominent sternal protrusion), *thoracic kyphosis* (a posterior deviation of the spine that results in increased convexity of the chest), and *scoliosis* (a lateral deviation of the spine that results in an abnormal curvature) (Figure 20-22).

> ### CRITICAL THINKING
> Evaluate breathing in a supine patient or friend while standing to the person's side, then at the head, and finally at the feet. Which position provides the best view of the symmetry of the thorax?

The paramedic should inspect the skin and nipples for cyanosis and pallor. The presence of suture lines from chest wall surgery, skin pockets enclosing implanted pacemaker devices, implanted central venous lines or ports, and dermal medication patches (e.g., *nitroglycerin, fentanyl,* and contraceptives) should be noted. The pattern or rhythm of the patient's respirations should be assessed, noting any use of accessory respiratory muscles (e.g., intercostal or supraclavicular retractions or both). In addition, observing the rise

and fall of the patient's chest during breathing provides a rough measurement of tidal volume (see Chapter 15).

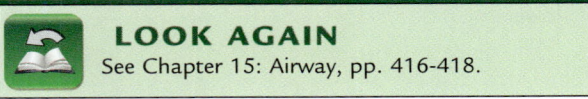

> ### LOOK AGAIN
> See Chapter 15: Airway, pp. 416-418.

PALPATION

The paramedic should palpate the thorax for pulsations, tenderness, bulges, depressions, crepitus, subcutaneous emphysema, and unusual movement and position. The examination begins by noting the position of the patient's trachea, which should be midline and directly above the sternal notch. Starting with the patient's clavicles, both sides of the patient's chest wall are firmly palpated at the same time, front to back and right side to left side. The examination should proceed systematically without pain or discomfort.

To evaluate the anterior chest wall for equal expansion during inspiration, the paramedic places both thumbs along the patient's costal margin and the xiphoid process. The palms should be lying flat on the chest wall. Equal movement should occur as the patient inhales and exhales. The posterior chest wall should be examined for

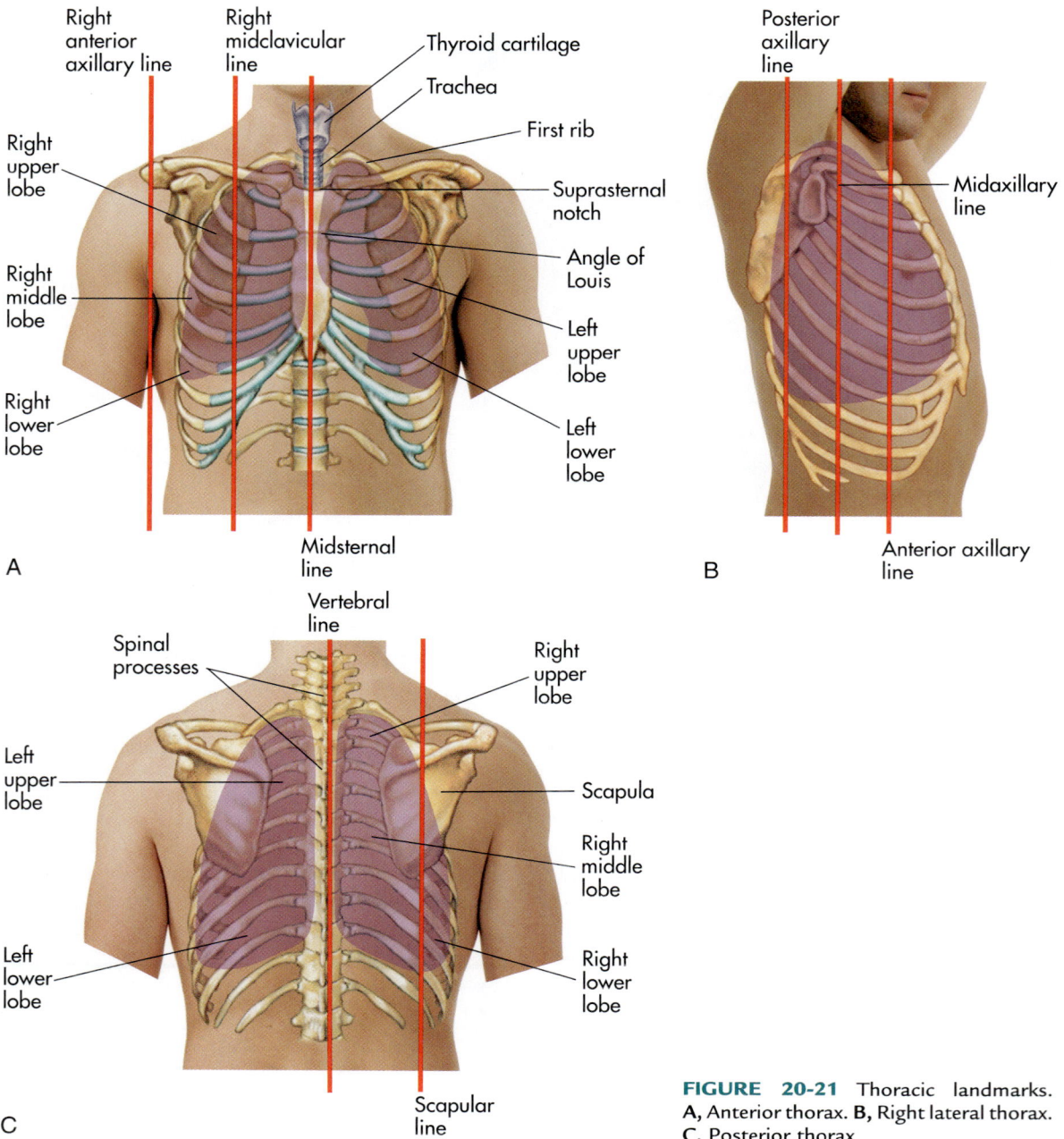

Right anterior axillary line
Right midclavicular line
Thyroid cartilage
Trachea
First rib
Suprasternal notch
Angle of Louis
Right upper lobe
Right middle lobe
Right lower lobe
Left upper lobe
Left lower lobe
Midsternal line

A

Posterior axillary line
Midaxillary line
Anterior axillary line

B

Vertebral line
Spinal processes
Left upper lobe
Left lower lobe
Right upper lobe
Scapula
Right middle lobe
Right lower lobe
Scapular line

C

FIGURE 20-21 Thoracic landmarks. **A,** Anterior thorax. **B,** Right lateral thorax. **C,** Posterior thorax.

symmetrical respiratory movement by placing the thumbs along the spinous processes at the level of the tenth rib (Figure 20-23).

PERCUSSION

The paramedic should perform percussion in symmetrical locations from side to side to compare the percussion note (Figure 20-24). *Resonance* usually is heard over all areas of healthy lungs. *Hyperresonance* is associated with overinflation, or hyperinflation, of the lungs. Hyperresonance may indicate pulmonary disease, pneumothorax, or asthma. *Dullness* or *flatness* suggests the presence of fluid or pulmonary congestion. The level and movement of the diaphragm

during breathing may be limited by disease or pain. Examples of such disease may be emphysema or tumor. An example of pain is from rib fracture.

AUSCULTATION

The thorax is best auscultated with the patient sitting upright (if possible). The patient should breathe deeply and slowly through an open mouth during the examination. The paramedic should be alert to the chance of resulting hyperventilation and fatigue that may occur in ill and older patients.

The diaphragm of the stethoscope is used to auscultate the high-pitched sounds of the patient's lungs. The

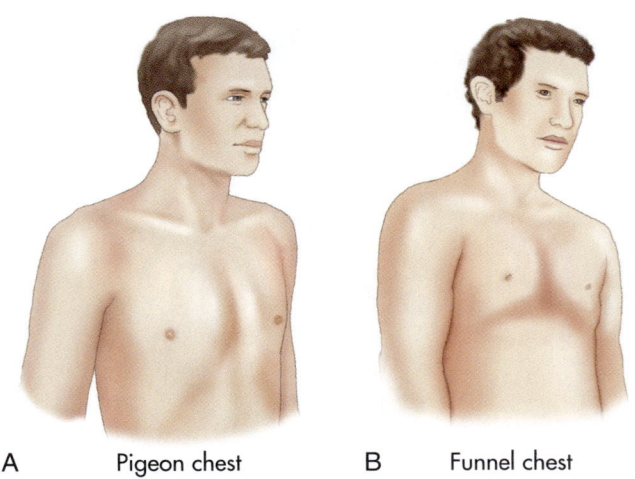

A   Pigeon chest   B   Funnel chest

FIGURE 20-22 Chest wall deformities. **A,** Pigeon chest. **B,** Funnel chest.

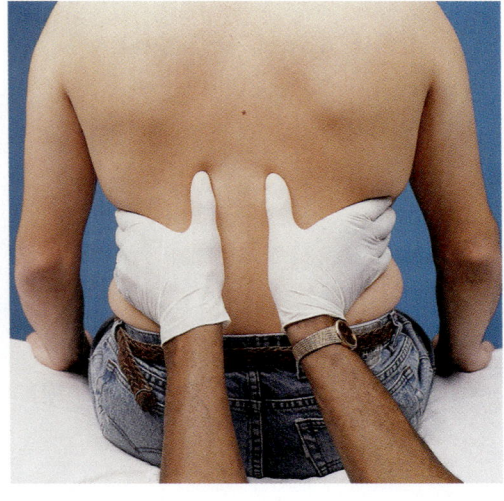

FIGURE 20-23 Palpating the thoracic expansion. The thumbs are at the level of the tenth ribs.

stethoscope is held firmly on the patient's skin and the paramedic listens carefully as the patient breathes. The chest auscultation should be systematic and thorough. Auscultation should allow evaluation of the anterior and the posterior lung fields.

Breath Sounds. Air movement creates turbulence as it passes through the respiratory tract and produces breath sounds during inhalation and exhalation. During inhalation, air moves first into the trachea and major bronchi. Then air moves into progressively smaller airways. Next, air moves to its final destination, the alveoli. During exhalation, the air flows from small airways to larger ones. This creates less turbulence. Therefore normal breath sounds generally are louder during inspiration.

Normal Breath Sounds. Normal breath sounds are classified as *vesicular, bronchovesicular,* and *bronchial* (Figure 20-25). Vesicular breath sounds are heard over most of the lung fields and are the major normal breath sound. Lungs considered "clear" make normal vesicular breath sounds. These sounds are low pitched and soft and have a long inspiratory phase and a shorter expiratory phase.

Vesicular breath sounds are classified further as *harsh* or *diminished*. Harsh vesicular sounds may result from vigorous exercise. With vigorous exercise, ventilations are rapid and deep. These harsh sounds also occur in children who have thin and elastic chest walls in which breath sounds are more easily audible. Vesicular breath sounds may be diminished in older persons who have less ventilation volume. Vesicular breath sounds also may be diminished in obese or muscular persons, whose additional overlying tissue muffles the sound.

Bronchovesicular breath sounds are heard over the major bronchi and over the upper right posterior lung field. These sounds are louder and harsher than vesicular breath sounds. Bronchovesicular breath sounds are considered to be of medium pitch. Bronchovesicular breath sounds have

equal inspiration and expiration phases. They are heard throughout respiration.

Bronchial breath sounds are heard only over the trachea and are the highest in pitch. They are coarse, harsh, loud sounds with a short inspiratory phase and a long expiration. A bronchial sound heard anywhere but over the trachea is considered an abnormal breath sound.

Abnormal Breath Sounds. Abnormal breath sounds are classified as *absent, diminished,* and *incorrectly located bronchial sounds* and as *adventitious breath sounds.* Absent breath sounds may indicate total cessation of the breathing process (e.g., complete airway obstruction). Breath sounds also may be absent only in a specific area. Causes of localized absent breath sounds include endotracheal tube misplacement, pneumothorax, and hemothorax.

Diminished breath sounds may result from any condition that lessens the airflow. Examples include endotracheal tube misplacement, pneumothorax, partial airway obstruction, and pulmonary disease. Although some airflow is present, diminished breath sounds usually indicate that some portion of the alveolar tissue is not being ventilated.

Bronchial breath sounds auscultated in the peripheral lung field indicate the presence of fluid or exudate in the alveoli. Either of these conditions may block airflow. Diseases that contribute to this condition are tumors, pneumonia, and pulmonary edema.

Adventitious Breath Sounds. Adventitious breath sounds are abnormal sounds. They are heard in addition to normal breath sounds. They may be divided into two categories: *discontinuous* and *continuous.* Adventitious breath sounds result from obstruction of the large or small airways. Adventitious breath sounds are most commonly heard during inspiration. They are classified as *crackles* (formerly known as *rales*), wheezes, and rhonchi (Figure 20-26).

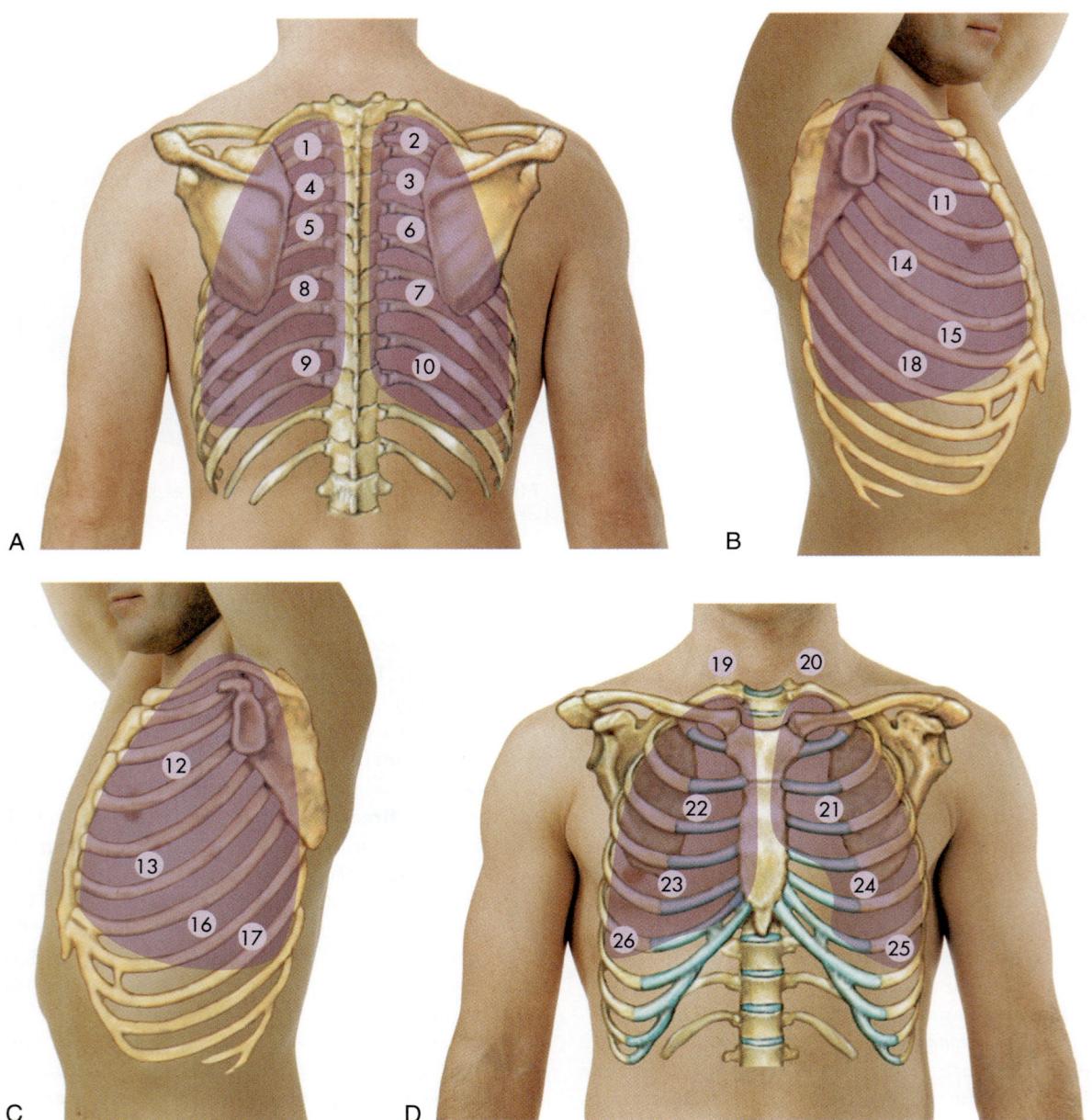

FIGURE 20-24 Suggested sequence for systematic percussion and auscultation of the thorax. **A,** Posterior thorax. **B,** Right lateral thorax. **C,** Left lateral thorax. **D,** Anterior thorax. (From Seidel H et al: *Mosby's guide to physical examination,* ed 6, St Louis, 2007, Mosby.)

Discontinuous Breath Sounds. **Crackles** are the high-pitched, discontinuous sounds that usually are heard during the end of inspiration. The sound is similar to the sound of hair being rubbed between the fingers. Crackles are caused by the disruptive passage of air in the small airways or alveoli, or both, and may be heard anywhere in the peripheral lung field.

The most typical causes of crackles are pulmonary edema and pneumonia in its early stages. Because gravity draws fluid downward, crackles often start in the bases of the lungs. Crackles may be classified further as *coarse crackles* (wet, low-pitched sounds) and *fine crackles* (dry,

high-pitched sounds). Crackles are discrete and sometimes difficult to hear and may be overridden by louder respiratory sounds. If the paramedic suspects crackles when auscultating the chest, the patient should be asked to cough. A cough may clear secretions and make crackles more audible.

Continuous Breath Sounds. **Wheezes** are also known as *sibilant wheezes.* They are high-pitched musical noises that usually are louder during expiration. Wheezes are caused by high-velocity air traveling through narrowed airways. They may occur because of asthma and other constrictive diseases and congestive heart failure. When wheezing occurs

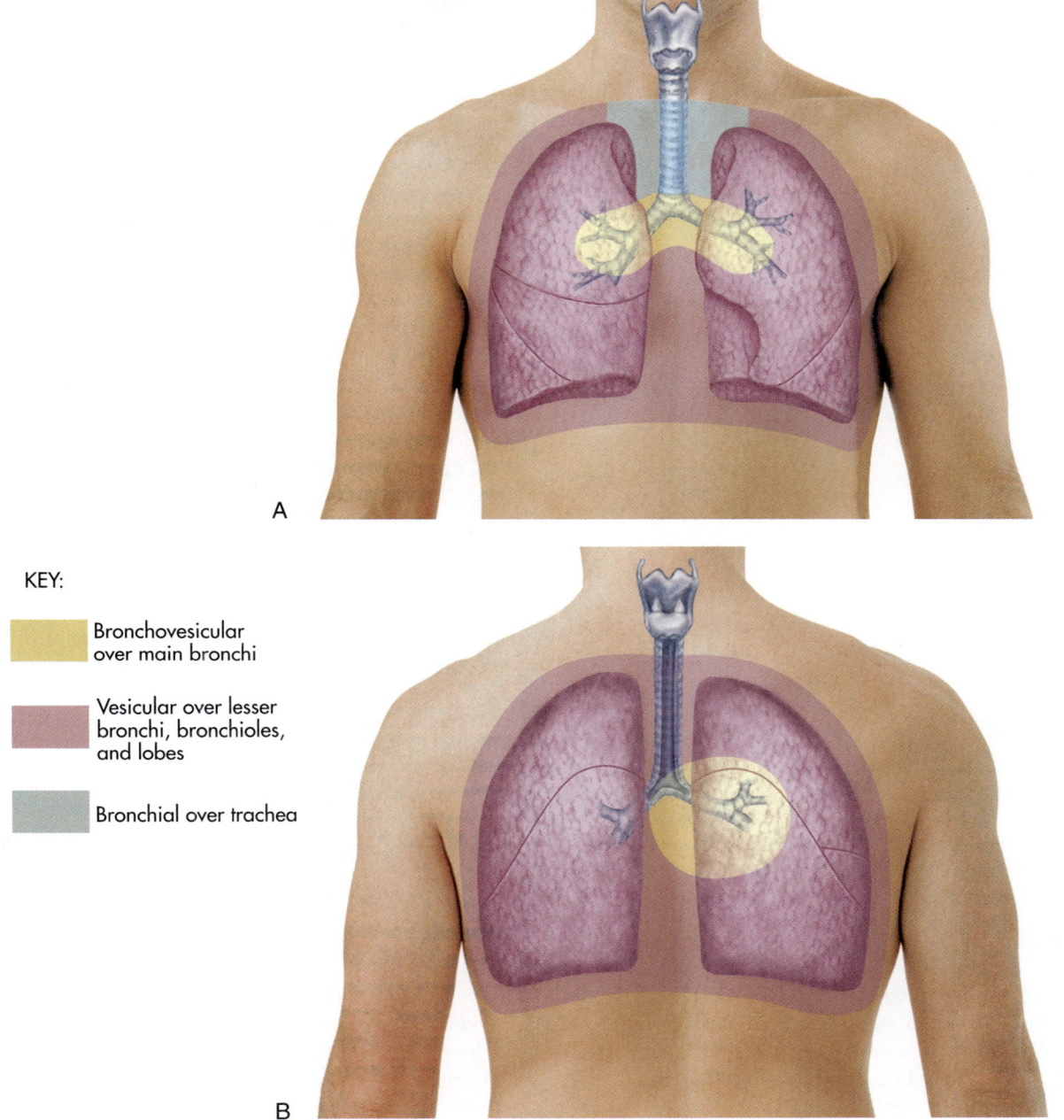

KEY:

- Bronchovesicular over main bronchi
- Vesicular over lesser bronchi, bronchioles, and lobes
- Bronchial over trachea

A

B

FIGURE 20-25 Expected auscultatory sounds. **A,** Anterior view. **B,** Posterior view. (From Seidel H et al: *Mosby's guide to physical examination,* ed 6, St Louis, 2007, Mosby.)

in a localized area, the paramedic should suspect a foreign body obstruction, tumor, or mucous plug. Wheezes are classified as mild, moderate, and severe. They should be described as occurring on inspiration or expiration or both.

> ### CRITICAL THINKING
> Breathe in and out through an open mouth. Gradually purse your lips until only a small opening is present while you continue to inhale and exhale. How do the sounds change? As you narrow the opening, is the noise louder on inspiration or expiration?

Rhonchi are also known as *sonorous wheezes*. They are continuous, low-pitched, rumbling sounds usually heard on expiration. Although rhonchi sound similar to wheezes, they do not involve the small airways. Rhonchi are less discrete than crackles and are auscultated easily. Rhonchi are caused by the passage of air through an airway obstructed by thick secretions, muscular spasm, new tissue growth, or external pressure collapsing the airway lumen. These breath sounds may result from any condition that increases secretions. Examples are pneumonia and drug overdose.

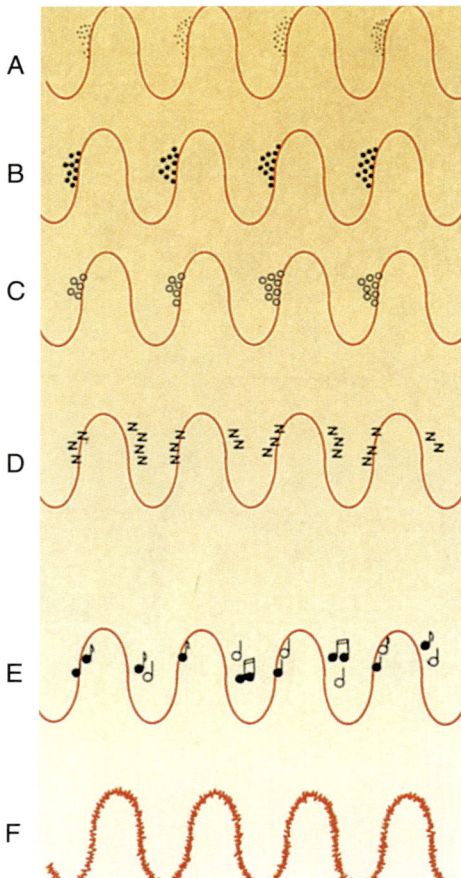

FIGURE 20-26 Adventitious breath sounds. **A,** Fine crackles. **B,** Medium crackles. **C,** Coarse crackles. **D,** Rhonchi. **E,** Wheeze. **F,** Pleural friction rub. (From Seidel H et al: *Mosby's guide to physical examination,* ed 6, St Louis, 2007, Mosby.)

SHOW ME THE EVIDENCE

In this study, researchers compared the ability of paramedics and physicians to interpret tape-recorded breath sounds. Each participant listened to a tape with crackles, rhonchi, stridor, wheezing, and normal lung sounds. The first time they listened, no patient history was provided. On a subsequent test history, age and presence or absence of dyspnea was available. On the third attempt more history was provided. Physicians' median score was 5 for each attempt; experienced paramedics' median score was 3 for trials 1 and 2 and a median score of 4 for trial 3. Scores for new paramedics were similar to those for experienced paramedics. Although significant, this study was limited by the small number of participants and the use of recorded versus real patient breath sounds.

From Wigder HN et al: Assessment of lung auscultation by paramedics, *Ann Emerg Med* 28(3):309-312, 1996.

VOCAL RESONANCE

As part of the respiratory examination, vocal sounds heard on auscultation (vocal resonance) should be assessed to evaluate the presence of lung consolidation. This consolidation usually indicates pneumonia or pleural effusion. Any change in the character of the spoken voice that is higher pitched and less muffled than normal during auscultation should be noted. Normally, the sound of the patient's voice becomes less distinct as the auscultation moves peripherally. Vocal sounds may remain loud at the periphery of the lungs or sound louder than usual over a distinct area when consolidation is present. The following tests can be used to assess vocal resonance:

Bronchophony. In this test the patient is asked to whisper "toy boat" or "blue balloons" while the lungs are auscultated. Vocal sounds will be louder where the consolidation is present.

Egophony. In this test the patient is asked to say the letter "e-e-e." If the vocal sounds more closely resemble the letter "a," lung consolidation may be present.

Whispered Pectoriloquy. The patient is asked to whisper as the posterior lungs are auscultated. If vocal sounds are transmitted clearly or there is an increased loudness of whispering during auscultation, it is often a sign of lung consolidation.

Heart

In the prehospital setting the heart must be examined indirectly. In spite of this, a skilled assessment can collect information about the size and effectiveness of the heart's pumping action. This assessment includes palpation and auscultation.

PALPATION

The **apical impulse** is a visible and palpable force. It is produced by the contraction of the left ventricle. Palpation of this impulse may be useful to compare the relationship of peripheral pulses with the pulse produced by ventricular contraction. The hearts of some patients with

Stridor usually is an inspiratory, crowing-type sound that can be heard without the aid of a stethoscope. It indicates significant narrowing or obstruction of the larynx or trachea, and may be caused by epiglottitis, viral croup, anaphylaxis, foreign body aspiration, or more than one of these factors. Stridor is heard best over the site of origin, usually the larynx or trachea. This breath sound often indicates airway compromise that may be life-threatening, especially in children. Its presence calls for careful observation for ventilatory failure and hypoxia.

Pleural Friction Rub. Although occurring outside the respiratory tree, a pleural friction rub also may be considered an adventitious breath sound. **Pleural friction rub** is a low-pitched, dry, rubbing or grating sound. It is caused by the movement of inflamed pleural surfaces as they slide on one another during breathing. The friction rub may be auscultated on inspiration and expiration and usually is loudest over the lower lateral anterior surface of the chest wall. Presence of a pleural friction rub may indicate pleurisy, viral infection, tuberculosis, or pulmonary embolism (see Chapter 24). Figure 20-27 shows a schema of breath sounds in ill and well patients.

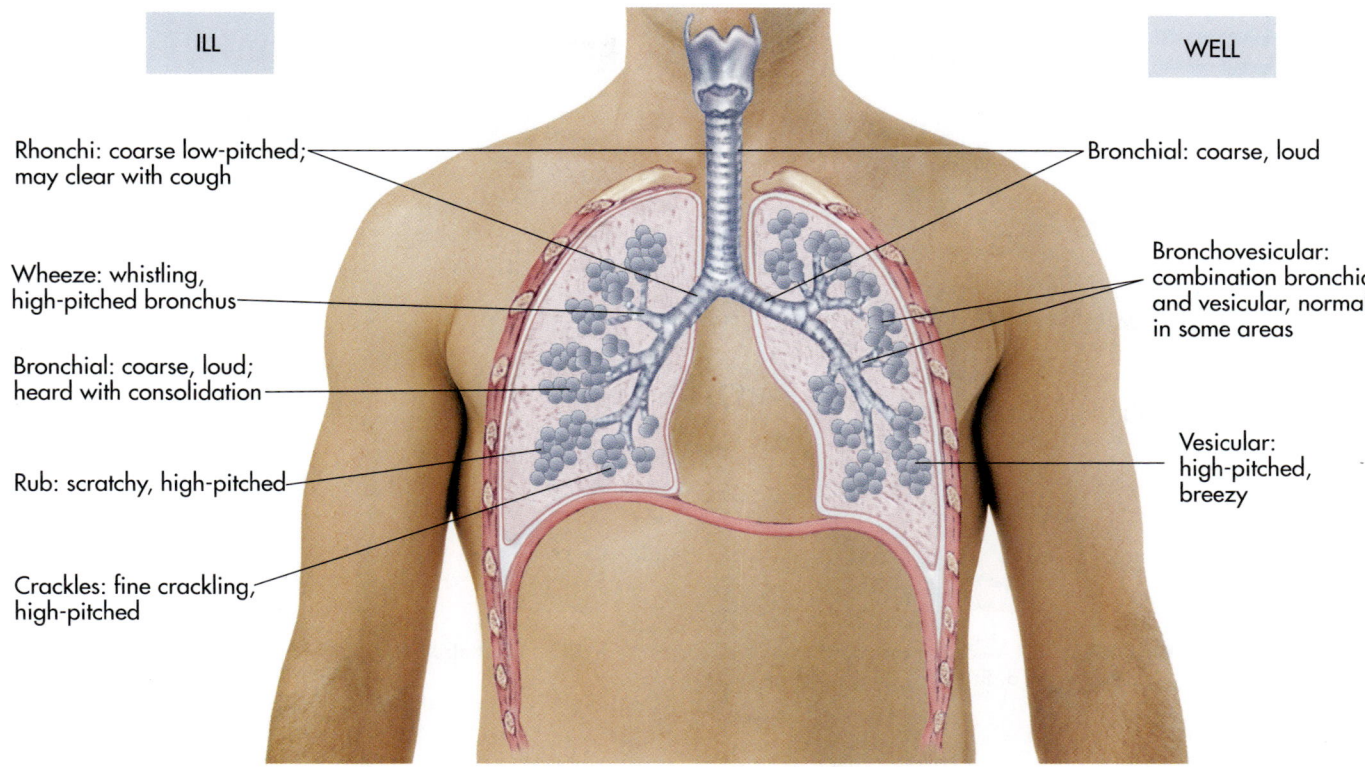

ILL

WELL

Rhonchi: coarse low-pitched; may clear with cough

Wheeze: whistling, high-pitched bronchus

Bronchial: coarse, loud; heard with consolidation

Rub: scratchy, high-pitched

Crackles: fine crackling, high-pitched

Bronchial: coarse, loud

Bronchovesicular: combination bronchial and vesicular, normal in some areas

Vesicular: high-pitched, breezy

FIGURE 20-27 Schema of breath sounds in ill and well patients (From Seidel H, et al: *Mosby's guide to physical examination,* ed 6, St Louis, 2007, Mosby.)

cardiac irregularities, for example, do not always produce a peripheral pulse with every ventricular contraction. By palpating or auscultating the apical impulse and the carotid pulse at the same time, the paramedic can note these **pulse deficits** (Figure 20-28). Factors such as obesity, large breasts, and muscularity may make this landmark hard to see or palpate.

AUSCULTATION

Heart sounds may be auscultated for frequency (pitch), intensity (loudness), duration, and timing in the cardiac cycle (Figure 20-29). A full evaluation of heart sounds calls for a high level of skill and experience, a quiet environment, and ample time to listen closely. However, the paramedic may assess two basic heart sounds quickly. These sounds may help to improve understanding of the patient's condition. The basic heart sounds S_1 and S_2 are normal sounds that occur when the heart contracts. They are best heard toward the apex of the heart at the fifth intercostal space. For evaluation of heart sounds, the patient should be sitting up and leaning slightly forward (Figure 20-30, *A*), supine (Figure 20-30, *B*), or in a left lateral recumbent position (Figure 20-30, *C*). These positions bring the heart closer to the left anterior chest wall. To listen for S_1, the paramedic should ask the patient to breathe normally and hold the breath in expiration. To listen for S_2, the paramedic should ask the patient to breathe normally again and hold the breath in inspiration.

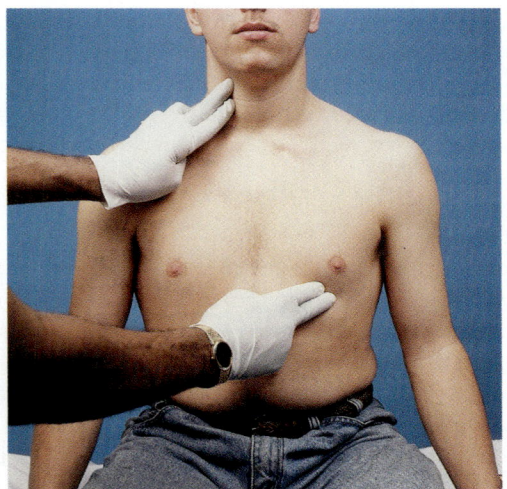

FIGURE 20-28 Simultaneous palpation of the carotid artery and apical impulse.

Heart sounds may be muffled or diminished by obesity or obstructive lung disease. Muffling also may occur as a result of the presence of fluid in the pericardial sac surrounding the heart muscle. The accumulation of fluid usually is the result of penetrating or severe blunt chest trauma, cardiac tamponade, or cardiac rupture and is considered a true emergency. Other causes of muffled or diminished heart sounds include infectious uremic pericarditis

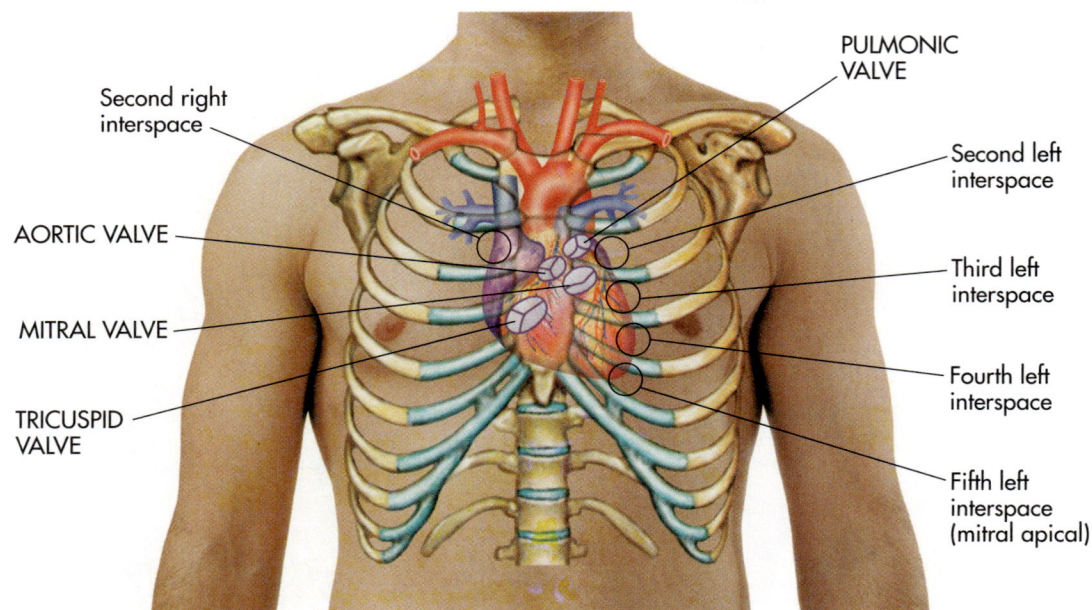

FIGURE 20-29 Areas for auscultation of the heart. (From Seidel H, et al: *Mosby's guide to physical examination,* ed 6, St Louis, 2007, Mosby.)

and malignancy. (See Chapter 22 for further discussion of abnormal heart sounds.)

Inflammation of the pericardial sac may cause a rubbing sound that is audible with a stethoscope. This is a **pericardial friction rub.** The rub may result from infectious pericarditis, myocardial infarction, uremia, trauma, and autoimmune pericarditis. These rubs have a scratching, grating, or squeaking quality. They tend to be louder on inspiration. They can be differentiated from pleural friction rubs by their continued presence when the patient holds the breath.

EXTRA SOUNDS

Extra sounds that sometimes can be heard during auscultation or can be felt by palpation include heart murmurs, bruits, and thrills. **Heart murmurs** are prolonged sounds caused by a disruption in the flow of blood into, through, or out of the heart. Most murmurs are caused by valvular defects. Some heart murmurs are serious. Others (e.g., some that occur in children and adolescents), though, are benign and have no apparent cause. Heart murmurs can be detected during auscultation of the heart.

A **bruit** is an abnormal sound or murmur that may be heard during auscultation of the carotid artery or another organ or gland. A bruit may indicate local obstruction. Bruits usually are low pitched and difficult to hear. To assess blood flow in the carotid artery, the paramedic should place the bell of the stethoscope over the carotid artery at the medial end of the clavicle. The patient is then asked to hold his or her breath (Figure 20-31).

Thrills are similar to bruits but are described as fine vibrations or tremors that may indicate blood flow obstruction. Thrills may be palpable over the site of an aneurysm or on the precordium (the area of the chest wall that overlays the heart and epigastrium). Like murmurs and bruits, thrills may be serious or benign.

Abdomen

The abdomen is divided by two imaginary lines. These lines separate the abdominal region into four quadrants. The quadrants are the upper right, lower right, upper left, and lower left (Figure 20-32). These quadrants and their contents provide the basis for inspection, auscultation, percussion, and palpation (Box 20-5).

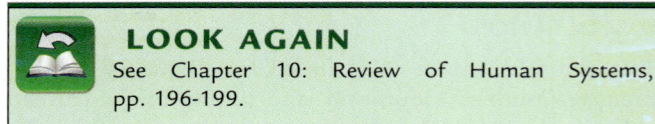

LOOK AGAIN
See Chapter 10: Review of Human Systems, pp. 196-199.

When examining a patient's abdomen, the paramedic should ensure that the patient is comfortable (with an empty bladder, if possible), and in a supine position. The paramedic's hands and stethoscope should be warm. The patient should be approached slowly and respectfully. Any painful area should be examined last to avoid "patient guarding" when the painful area is examined first. Discoloration found in the flank (*Grey Turner's sign*) or around the umbilicus (*Cullen's sign*) may indicate possible injury or disease (see Chapter 29).

INSPECTION

The paramedic should inspect the abdomen visually for signs of cyanosis, pallor, jaundice, bruising, discoloration, swelling (ascites), masses, and aortic pulsations. Surgical

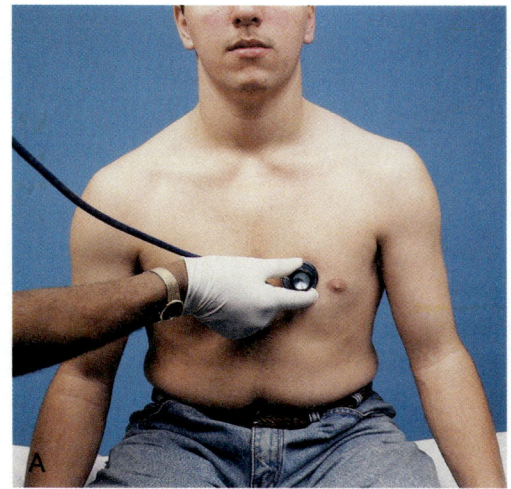

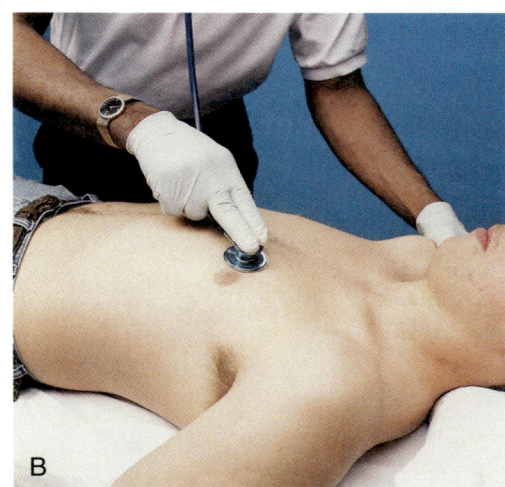

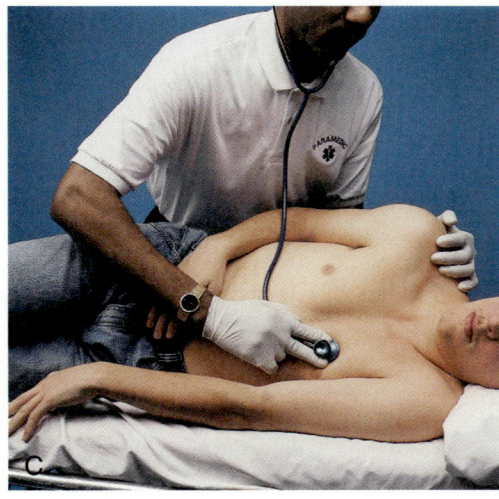

FIGURE 20-30 Patient positions for auscultation. **A,** Sitting up, leaning slightly forward. **B,** Supine. **C,** Left lateral recumbent.

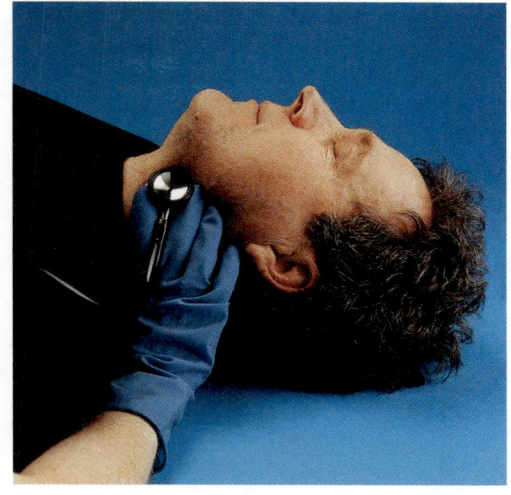

FIGURE 20-31 Evaluation of carotid bruit.

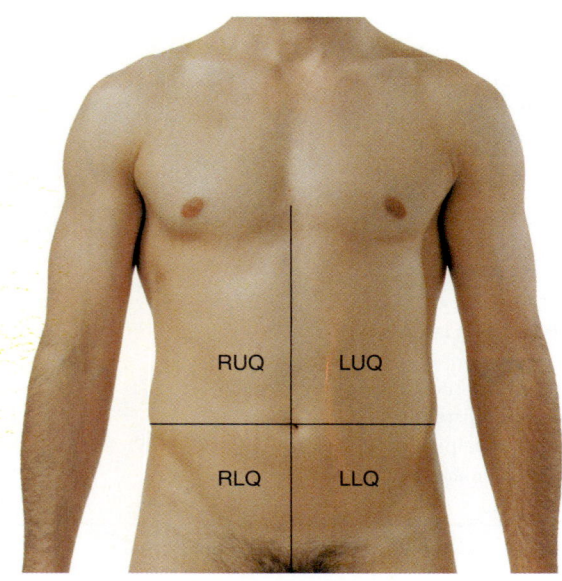

FIGURE 20-32 Four quadrants of the abdomen. *RUQ,* Right upper quadrant; *LUQ,* left upper quadrant; *RLQ,* right lower quadrant; *LLQ,* left lower quadrant.

scars and implanted medical devices should also be noted (see Chapter 22). The abdomen should be evenly round and symmetrical (Figure 20-33). Symmetrical distention of the abdomen may result from obesity, enlarged organs, fluid, or gas. Asymmetrical distention may result from hernias, tumor, bowel obstruction, or enlarged abdominal organs. A flat abdomen is common in adults who are athletic. Convex abdomens are common in children and in adults who have poor exercise habits. The umbilicus should be free of swelling, bulges, and signs of inflammation. The normal umbilicus usually is inverted, or it may protrude slightly.

BOX 20-5 Abdominal Quadrants

Right Upper Quadrant
Liver and gallbladder
Pylorus
Duodenum
Head of pancreas
Right adrenal gland
Portion of right kidney
Hepatic flexure of colon
Portions of ascending and transverse colon

Left Upper Quadrant
Left lobe of liver
Spleen
Stomach
Body of pancreas
Left adrenal gland
Portion of left kidney
Splenic flexure of colon
Portions of transverse and descending colon

Right Lower Quadrant
Lower pole of right kidney
Cecum and appendix
Portion of ascending colon
Appendix
Bladder (if distended)
Ovary and salpinx
Uterus (if enlarged)
Right ureter

Left Lower Quadrant
Lower pole of left kidney
Sigmoid colon
Portion of descending colon
Bladder (if distended)
Ovary and salpinx
Uterus (if enlarged)
Left ureter

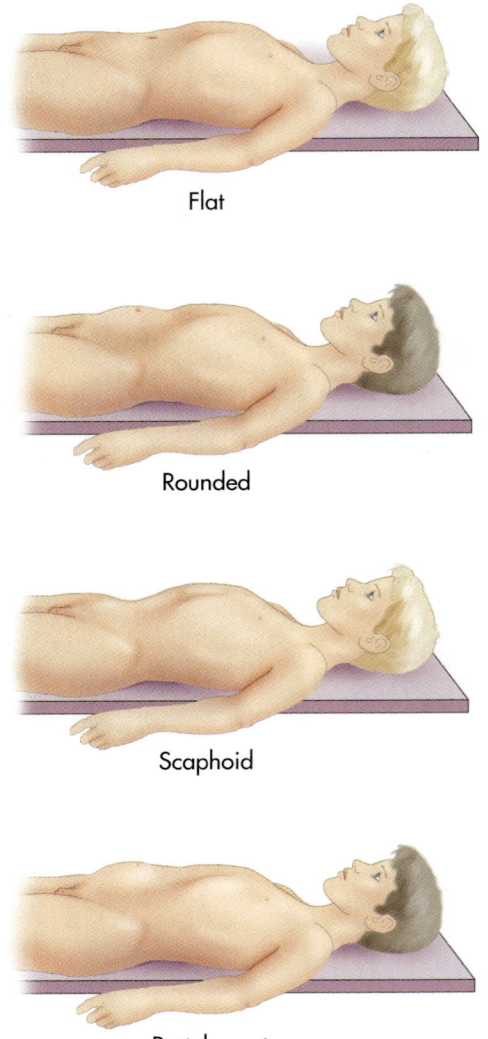

Flat

Rounded

Scaphoid

Protuberant

FIGURE 20-33 Shape of the abdomen.

Abdominal movement during respiration should be smooth and even. As a rule, males have more abdominal involvement than females during respiration, so limited abdominal movement in the male patient with symptoms may indicate a pathological abdominal condition. Visible pulsations produced by blood flow through the aorta in the upper abdomen may be normal in thin adults. However, marked pulsations may indicate an abdominal aortic aneurysm (see Chapter 22).

AUSCULTATION

Noting the presence or absence of bowel sounds to assess motility and to discover vascular sounds has limited value in the prehospital setting. Such findings do not affect or determine the approach to patient care. Moreover, the time needed for complete bowel sound assessment (about 5 minutes per quadrant) far exceeds the justifiable scene time for most patients. If auscultation is to be performed, though, it should always precede palpation. (Palpation may alter the intensity of bowel sounds.)

To auscultate bowel sounds, the paramedic holds the diaphragm of the stethoscope on the abdomen with light pressure. If bowel sounds are present, they usually are heard as rumblings or gurgles. These sounds should occur irregularly and may range in frequency from 5 to 35 per minute. Auscultation should be performed in all four quadrants. A minimum of 5 minutes per quadrant is needed to determine that normal bowel sounds are absent. Increased bowel sounds may indicate gastroenteritis or intestinal obstruction. Decreased or absent bowel sounds may indicate peritonitis (inflammation of the lining of the abdominal cavity) or ileus (inactive peristaltic activity resulting from one of several causes) (see Chapter 30).

PERCUSSION AND PALPATION

Percussion and palpation of the abdomen may help to detect the presence of fluid, air, and solid masses. The paramedic should use a systematic approach, moving from side to side or clockwise. Any rigidity, tenderness, or abnormal skin temperature or color should be noted. The patient's face should be observed for signs of pain or discomfort. If the patient is complaining of abdominal pain, the painful quadrant should be examined last so that the patient will not unnecessarily tighten or guard the abdominal area. The abdominal assessment should begin with a light palpation, using an even pressing motion. As stated before, the paramedic's hands should be warm, and sharp and quick jabs should be avoided. Palpation may be done simultaneously with percussion.

Percussion begins by evaluating all four quadrants of the abdomen in turn for tympany and dullness. (**Tympany** is the major sound that should be noted during percussion because of the normal presence of air in the stomach and intestines [gastric bubble]. Dullness should be heard over organs and solid masses.) When percussing the abdomen, proceeding from an area of tympany to an area of dullness is best. That way, the change in sound is easier to detect. Individual assessments of the liver and spleen (described in the following paragraphs) may be performed if indicated by patient complaint or mechanism of injury. Patients who may require surgery for abdominal illness or injury are best served by rapid assessment, stabilization, and transport to an appropriate medical facility.

Percussion and Palpation of the Liver. The paramedic percusses the liver by starting just above the umbilicus in the right midclavicular line in an area of tympany. Percussion should continue in an upward direction until the change from tympany to dullness occurs. This change usually occurs slightly below the costal margin. It indicates the lower border of the liver. To determine the upper border of the liver, the percussion should begin in the same midclavicular line at the midsternal level, proceeding downward until the tympany from the lung area changes to dullness (usually between the fifth and seventh intercostal spaces). Liver size and span (usually 6 to 12 cm; 2 to 5 inches) are related to age and sex. The liver usually is proportionately larger in adults than in children. The liver also is larger in males than in females.

For palpation of the liver, the patient should be supine and comfortable and should have a relaxed abdomen. The paramedic should perform the examination from the patient's right side and should begin by placing the left hand under the patient in the area of the eleventh and twelfth ribs (Figure 20-34). The right hand should be placed on the abdomen, with the fingers pointing toward the patient's head and extended, resting just below the edge of the costal margin. The conscious patient should be instructed to breathe deeply through the mouth. During exhalation, the paramedic presses upward with the hand under the patient and gently pushes in and up with the right hand. If the liver is felt, it should be firm and nontender. (A healthy liver usually cannot be palpated unless the patient is thin.)

Percussion and Palpation of the Spleen. For percussion of the spleen, the patient must be lying supine or in a right lateral recumbent position. Percussion should begin at the area of lung tympany, just posterior to the midaxillary line on the left side. When percussing downward, a change from tympany to dullness should be audible between the sixth and tenth ribs. Large areas of dullness suggest an enlarged spleen. Stomach contents and air-filled or feces-filled intestines make splenic assessment by percussion difficult. These and other factors may affect percussion tones of dullness and tympany.

Palpation is a more useful assessment technique for evaluating the spleen. The patient should be lying supine with the paramedic positioned at the patient's left side. The paramedic places the left hand under the patient, supporting the lower left rib cage. The paramedic places the right hand just below the patient's lower left costal margin (Figure 20-35). The area should be gently palpated by lifting

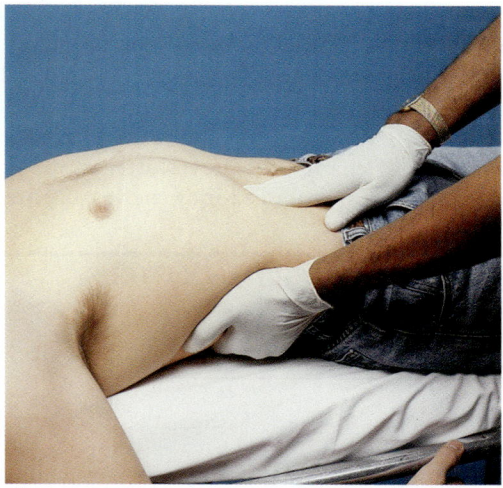

FIGURE 20-34 Palpation of the liver.

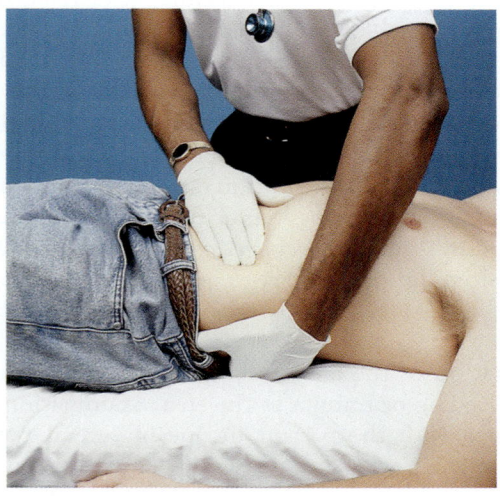

FIGURE 20-35 Palpation of the spleen.

up the left hand and pressing down with the right hand. (A normal spleen usually cannot be palpated in an adult. A palpable spleen is probably enlarged 3 times its normal size.) Palpation of the spleen can produce rupture of the organ. Palpation should be performed with caution.

Female Genitalia

Examination of the genitalia of either sex of patient can be awkward. The patient and the paramedic may feel uncomfortable. When possible, paramedics of the same sex as the patient should perform these exams. If that is not possible, a second person who acts as a chaperone should be present during the examination.

> **NOTE**
> Examination of the genitalia of both men and women should only be performed in the prehospital setting if indicated by patient complaint, pregnancy in women, or mechanism of injury.

The external genitalia should be inspected visually to note any swelling, redness, discharge, bleeding, or evidence of trauma. Discoloration or tenderness of the genital tissue may be the result of traumatic bruising. Ulcers, vesicles, and discharges (with or without pain) indicate sexually transmitted disease. If touching the anal area is necessary, the paramedic should change the gloves afterward to prevent bacteria from being introduced into the vaginal area.

> **CRITICAL THINKING**
> Examination of a patient's genitalia in the presence of another care provider is advisable. Why might this be important?

MALE GENITALIA

When examining the male genitalia, the paramedic should inspect the area visually. Bleeding or signs of trauma should be noted. The shaft of the penis should be nontender and flaccid. Rarely, patients with leukemia, sickle cell disease, or spinal injury may have a persistent painful erection (priapism). The urethral opening should be free of blood (a possible result of pelvic trauma). The opening also should be free of discharge (a sign of sexually transmitted disease). The scrotum should be nontender and slightly asymmetrical. A swollen or painful scrotum may result from infection, herniation, testicular torsion, or trauma. Discoloration of the genitals is called *Coopernail's sign* and may indicate peritoneal bleeding.

ANUS

Examination of the anus is indicated in the presence of rectal bleeding or trauma to the area. Examination can be performed with the patient in one of several positions. Most patients will find the side-lying position to be most comfortable. (The paramedic should protect the patient's privacy and use proper drapes.) Inspection of the sacrococcygeal and perineal areas should consider abnormal findings, which may include lumps, ulcers, inflammation, rashes, and excoriations (surface injuries caused by scratching or abrasions). Inflamed external hemorrhoids are common in adults and pregnant women.

EXTREMITIES

When examining the upper and lower extremities, a paramedic should pay attention to function and structure (see Chapter 10). The patient's general appearance, body proportions, and ease of movement are key. In particular, any limitation in the range of motion or an unusual increase in the mobility of a joint should be noted. Abnormal findings include the following:

- Signs of inflammation
  Swelling
  Tenderness
  Increased heat
  Redness
  Decreased function
- Asymmetry
- Crepitus
- Deformities
- Decreased muscular strength
- Atrophy

EXAMINING UPPER AND LOWER EXTREMITIES

A full assessment of the upper and lower extremities includes an evaluation of the skin and tissue overlying the muscles, cartilage, and bones. It also includes an examination of the joints. Each extremity should be assessed for soft tissue injury, discoloration, swelling, and masses. The upper and lower extremities should be symmetrical in structure and muscularity. The paramedic should assess the circulatory status of each extremity by determining skin color, temperature, sensation, and the presence of distal pulses. The bones, joints, and surrounding tissues of the extremities are assessed for structural integrity and continuity. Muscle tone should be firm and nontender. Joints are assessed for function by moving each joint through its full range of motion (described in Chapter 10). A normal range of motion occurs without pain, deformity, limitation, or instability.

> **LOOK AGAIN**
> See Chapter 10: Review of Human Systems, pp. 167-171.

Hands and Wrists. The paramedic should inspect both hands and wrists for contour and positional alignment (Figure 20-36). The wrists, hands, and joints of each finger should be palpated for tenderness, swelling, or deformity. To determine range of motion, the patient should be asked to flex and extend the wrists, make a fist, and touch the thumb to each fingertip. All movements should be performed without pain or discomfort.

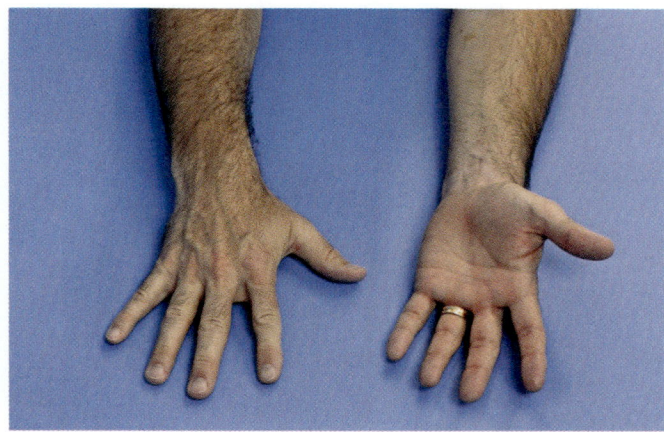

FIGURE 20-36 Hands and wrists.

Elbows. The patient's elbows should be inspected and palpated in the flexed and extended positions (Figure 20-37). To determine the range of motion of the elbow, the patient should be asked to rotate the hands from palm up to palm down. The paramedic should inspect the grooves between the epicondyle and olecranon by palpation. Pain and tenderness should not be present when pressing on the lateral or medial epicondyle.

Shoulders and Related Structures. The patient's shoulders should be inspected and palpated for symmetry and integrity of the clavicles, scapulae, and humeri. Pain, tenderness, or asymmetrical contour may indicate a fracture or dislocation. The paramedic should ask the patient to shrug shoulders and raise and extend both arms. These movements should be made without pain or discomfort. The following regions should be palpated, noting any tenderness or swelling (Figure 20-38):

- Sternoclavicular joint
- Acromioclavicular joint
- Subacromial area
- Bicipital groove

Ankles and Feet. The paramedic should inspect the patient's feet and ankles for contour, position, and size. Tenderness, swelling, and deformity are abnormal findings on palpation. The toes should be straight and aligned with each other. Range of motion can be determined by asking the patient to bend the toes, point the toes, and rotate the feet inward and outward from the ankle (Figure 20-39). These movements should be possible without pain or discomfort. The paramedic should inspect all surfaces of the ankles and feet for deformities, nodules, swelling, calluses, corns, and skin integrity.

Pelvis, Hips, and Knees. The structural integrity of the pelvis should be verified. To palpate the iliac crest and the symphysis pubis, the paramedic places both hands on each anterior iliac crest and presses downward and outward (Figure 20-40). To determine stability, the heel of the hand should be placed on the patient's symphysis pubis, pressing downward. Deformity and point tenderness of the pelvis

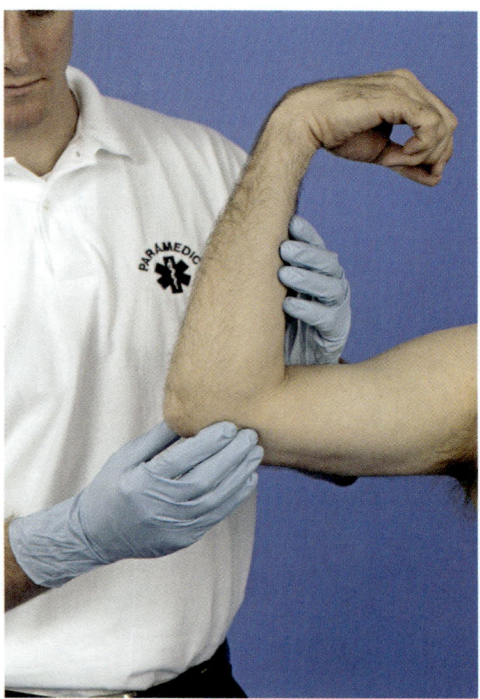

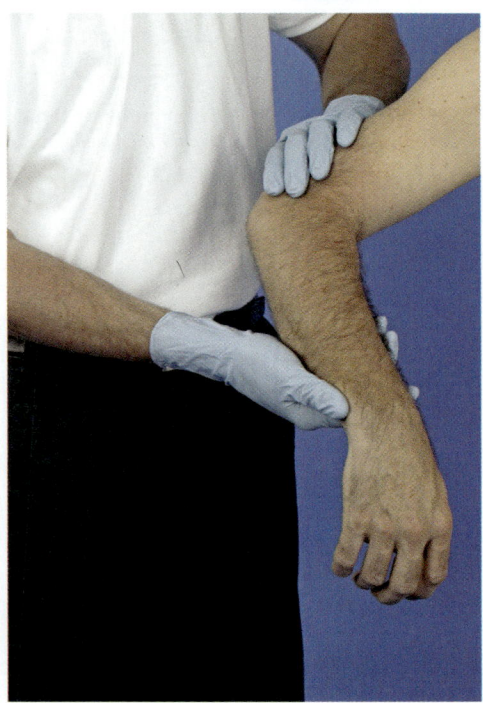

FIGURE 20-37 Palpation of the lateral and medial epicondyles.

may be signs of fracture. These signs may mask major structural and vascular injury.

The hips should be inspected for instability, tenderness, and crepitus. The paramedic can examine the supine or unconscious patient by assessing the structural integrity of the iliac crest. A mobile patient should be able to walk without discomfort. A supine patient should be able to

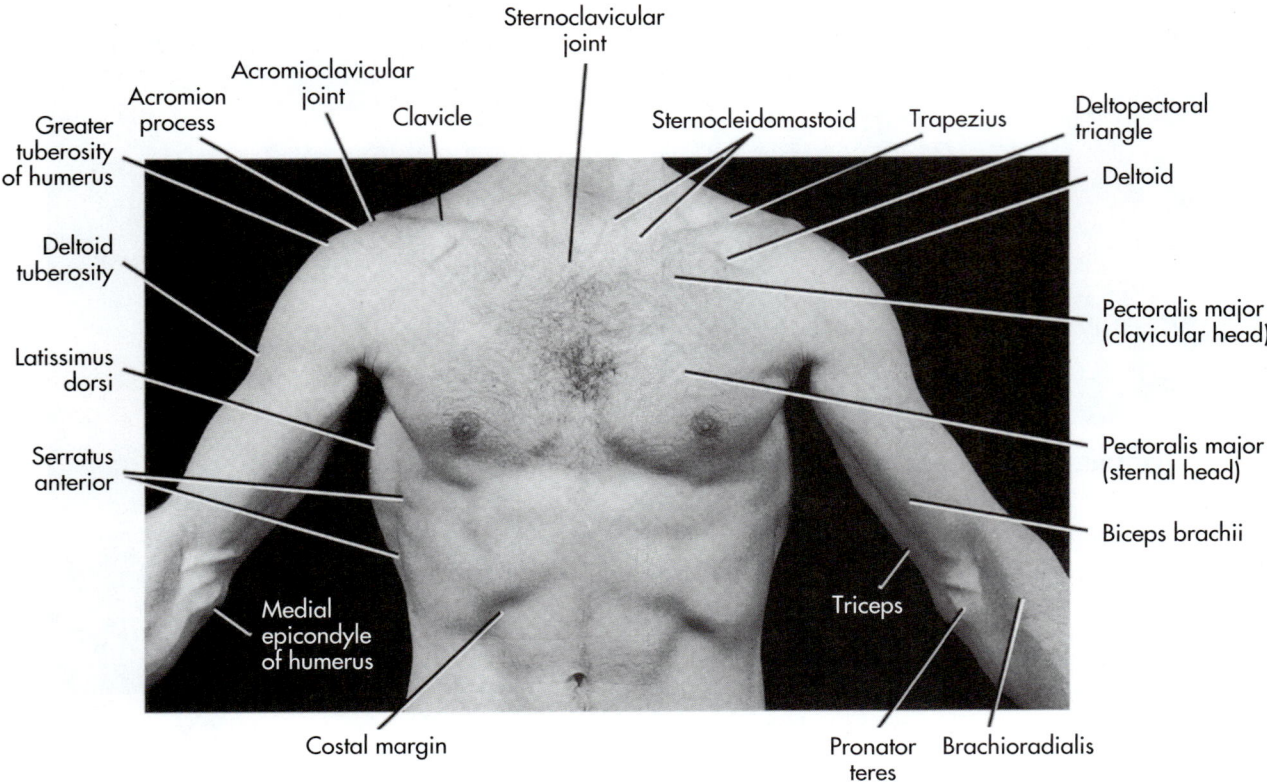

FIGURE 20-38 Evaluation of shoulder and related structures. (From Snell RS, Smith MS: *Clinical anatomy for emergency medicine,* St Louis, 1993, Mosby.)

raise the legs and knees and rotate the legs inward and outward.

The knees should be inspected and palpated for swelling and tenderness. The patella should be smooth, firm, non-tender, and midline in position. The patient should be able to bend and straighten each knee without pain.

PERIPHERAL VASCULAR SYSTEM

The peripheral vascular system includes arteries, veins, and the lymphatic system and lymph nodes. It also includes the fluids exchanged in the capillary bed. These can be evaluated during the physical examination of the upper and lower extremities.

Arms. When evaluating the arms, the paramedic should inspect from fingertips to shoulders, noting size, symmetry, swelling, venous pattern, color of the skin and nail beds, and texture of the skin. If arterial insufficiency is noted because of a weak radial pulse, the brachial pulse should be palpated. Epitrochlear nodes and brachial nodes should be nonswollen and nontender (Figure 20-41). A fine venous network on upper and lower extremities often is visible. The paramedic should be alert for enlargement of superficial veins during the exam.

Legs. During examination of the lower extremities, the patient should be supine and draped for privacy. (Shoes, socks, and hosiery should be removed for a full

examination.) The paramedic should inspect visually from the groin and buttocks to the feet, noting the following:
- Size and symmetry
- Swelling
- Venous pattern and venous enlargement
- Pigmentation
- Rashes, scars, or ulcers
- Color and texture of the skin
- Presence or absence of hair growth (indicating compromised arterial circulation)

The superficial inguinal nodes in the groin should be palpated to assess for swelling and tenderness. The paramedic should assess all lower extremity pulse sites for circulation, strength, and regularity. These sites include the femoral pulse, the popliteal pulse, the dorsalis pedis pulse, and the posterior tibial pulse (see Chapter 10). The temperature of the feet and legs should be warm, indicating adequate circulation. The paramedic can evaluate for pitting edema over the dorsum of each foot, behind each medial malleolus, and over the shins. This can be done by pressing firmly on the skin with the thumb for at least 5 seconds. Edema is said to be "pitting" when depression of the tissue remains after removal of pressure.

Abnormal Findings. Findings that are considered abnormal during a peripheral vascular assessment include the following:

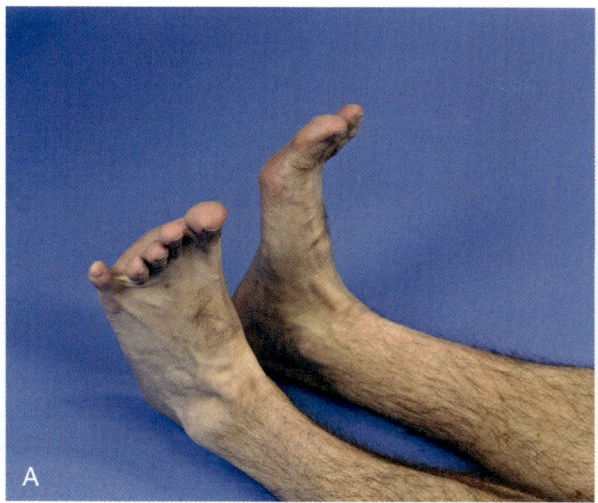

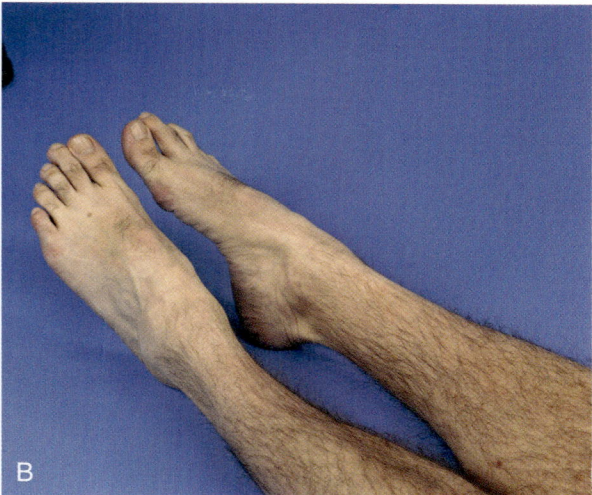

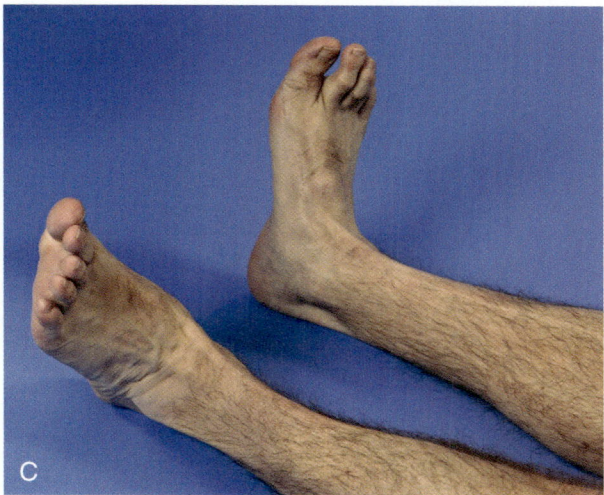

FIGURE 20-39 Motor function of the foot and ankle. **A,** Bend toes. **B,** Point toes. **C,** Rotate feet in and out.

- Swollen or asymmetrical extremities
- Pale or cyanotic skin
- Weak or diminished pulses
- Skin that is cold to the touch
- Absence of hair growth
- Pitting edema

Spine

A full physical examination includes an assessment of the spine. This begins with a visual assessment of the cervical, thoracic, and lumbar curves. From the patient's side, any curvature of the spine, including curvature associated with abnormal lordosis, kyphosis, and scoliosis should be noted (Figure 20-42). In addition, the paramedic should look for any differences in the height of the shoulders or iliac crests (hips) that may result from abnormal spinal curvature.

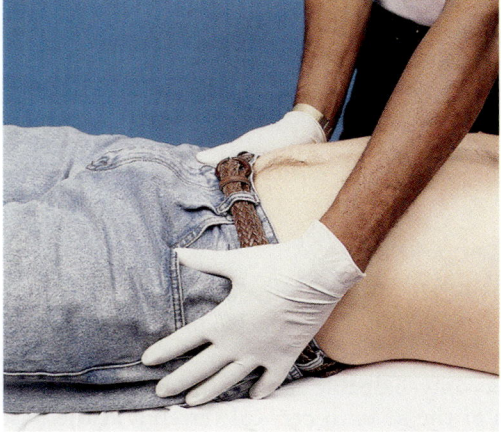

FIGURE 20-40 · Palpating the pelvis for stability.

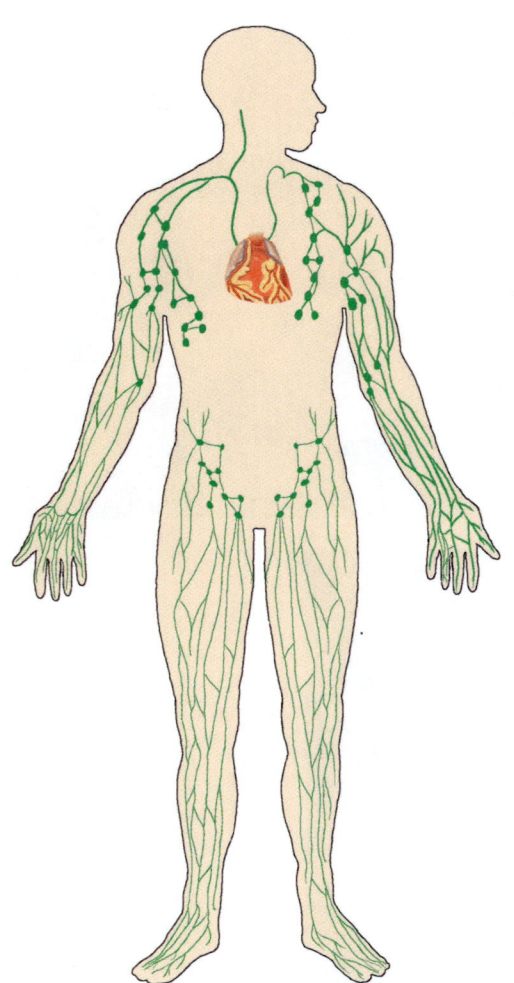

FIGURE 20-41 Nodes of upper and lower extremities.

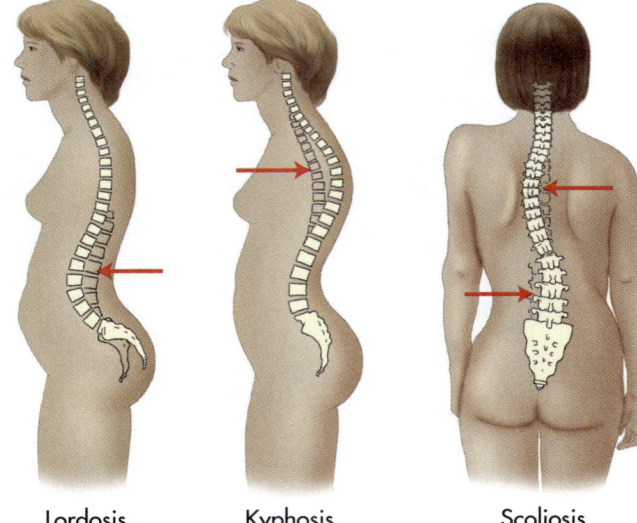

Lordosis Kyphosis Scoliosis

FIGURE 20-42 Abnormal spinal curvatures. Lordosis, kyphosis, scoliosis.

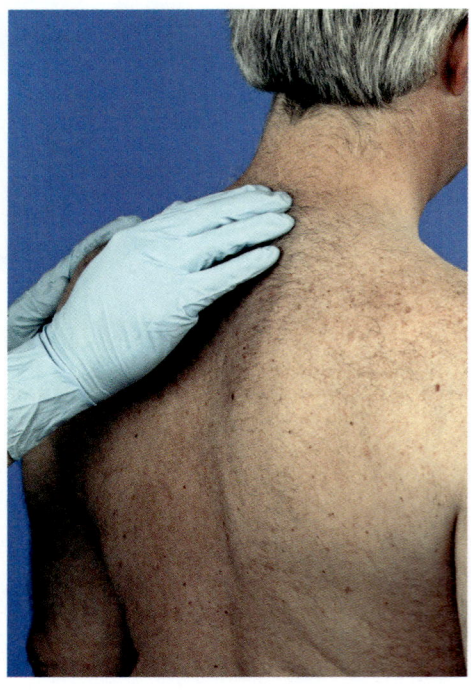

FIGURE 20-43 Palpation of the seventh cervical spinous process.

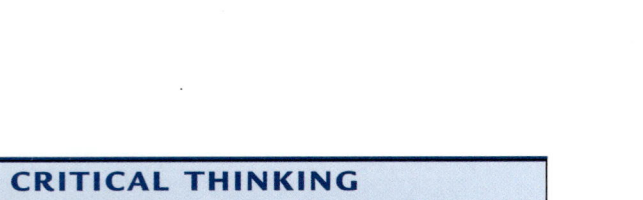

CRITICAL THINKING
Consider a case in which no deformity of the spine is found during an examination. Can spine fracture or dislocation be ruled out?

CERVICAL SPINE

The patient's neck should be in a midline position. If the patient is alert and denies neck pain, the paramedic should palpate the posterior aspect for point tenderness and swelling. The only palpable landmark should be the spinous process of the seventh cervical vertebra at the base of the neck (Figure 20-43). In the absence of suspected injury, the paramedic tests range of motion by directing the patient to

NOTE
The paramedic will need to test range of motion. However, the paramedic should never attempt to move the neck of a person who is unconscious. The paramedic also should never attempt this with a person who is unable or unwilling to do so on his or her own. Spontaneous cervical muscle spasm frequently is associated with significant cervical spine injury in the trauma victim.

bend the head forward, backward, and from side to side. These movements should not cause pain or discomfort.

THORACIC AND LUMBAR SPINE

The thoracic and lumbar areas should be inspected for signs of injury, swelling, and discoloration. Palpation should begin at the first thoracic vertebra and move downward to the sacrum. Under normal conditions, the spine is nontender to palpation. The paramedic can evaluate range of motion by asking the patient to bend at the waist forward and backward and to each side and also to rotate the upper trunk from side to side in a circular motion.

Nervous System

The details of an appropriate neurological examination vary greatly. The exam usually depends on the origin of the patient's complaint. For example, the exam may depend on whether the complaint refers to the peripheral nervous system or the central nervous system. The assessment and examination of the nervous system may be performed separately. However, neurological assessment often is completed during other assessments. A neurological examination may be organized into five categories:

- Mental status and speech
- Cranial nerves
- Motor system
- Sensory system
- Reflexes

MENTAL STATUS AND SPEECH

As discussed before, a healthy patient should be oriented to person, place, and date. Patients also should be able to organize their thoughts and converse freely (provided they have no hearing or speech impediments). Abnormal findings include unconsciousness, confusion, slurred speech, aphasia, dysphonia, and dysarthria.

CRANIAL NERVES

The 12 cranial nerves can be categorized as sensory, somato-motor and proprioceptive, and parasympathetic (see Chapter 10). The following methods can be used to assess each of the cranial nerves:

Nerve	Nerve Function and Test
Cranial nerve I	*Olfactory*: Test sense of smell with aromatic substance (Jarvis).
Cranial nerve II	*Optic*: Test for visual acuity (previously described).
Cranial nerves II and III	*Optic and oculomotor*: Inspect the size and shape of the pupils; test the pupil response to light.
Cranial nerves III, IV, and VI	*Oculomotor, trochlear, abducens*: Test extraocular movements by asking the patient to look up and down, to the left and right, and diagonally up and down to the left and right (the six cardinal directions of gaze).
Cranial nerve V	*Trigeminal*: Test motor movement by asking the patient to clench the teeth while you palpate the temporal and masseter muscles. Test sensation by touching the forehead, cheeks, and jaw on each side.
Cranial nerve VII	*Facial*: Inspect the face at rest and during conversation, noting symmetry, involuntary muscle movements (tics), or abnormal movements. Ask the patient to raise the eyebrows, frown, show upper and lower teeth, smile, and puff out both cheeks. The paramedic can assess strength of the facial muscles by asking the patient to close eyes tightly so they cannot be opened and gently attempting to raise the eyelids. Observe for weakness or asymmetry.
Cranial nerve VIII	*Acoustic*: Assess hearing acuity (previously described).
Cranial nerves IX and X	*Glossopharyngeal and vagus*: Assess the patient's ability to swallow with ease; to produce saliva; and to produce normal voice sounds. Instruct the patient to hold the breath, and assess for normal slowing of the heart rate. Testing for the gag reflex also will test the cranial nerves.
Cranial nerve XI	*Spinal accessory*: Ask the patient to raise and lower the shoulders and to turn the head.
Cranial nerve XII	*Hypoglossal*: Ask the patient to stick out the tongue and to move it in several directions.

CRITICAL THINKING

Why should abnormal findings in examination of one or more of the cranial nerves concern you?

MOTOR SYSTEM

An evaluation of a patient's motor system includes observing the patient during movement and at rest. The paramedic should evaluate abnormal involuntary movements for quality, rate, rhythm, and fullness of range. Other body movement assessments include posture, level of activity, fatigue, and emotion.

Muscle Strength. Muscle strength should be bilaterally symmetrical. In addition, the patient should be able to provide reasonable resistance to opposition. One way to evaluate muscle strength in the upper extremities is to ask the patient to extend the elbow. Then the paramedic instructs the patient to pull the arm toward the chest against opposing resistance (Figure 20-44, *A*). Muscle strength in the lower extremities is assessed by asking the

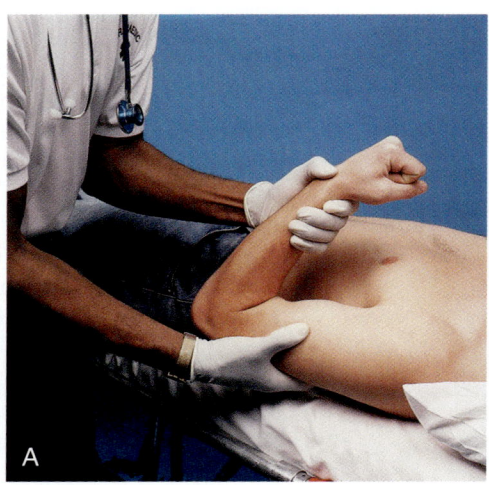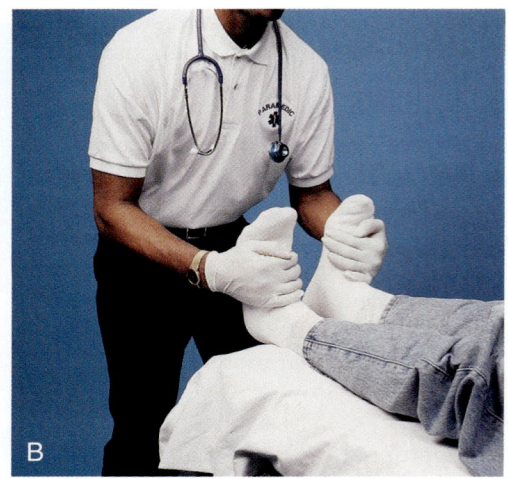

FIGURE 20-44 Evaluating muscle strength of the upper (**A**) and lower (**B**) extremities.

patient to push the soles of the feet against the paramedic's palms. Next, the paramedic directs the patient to pull the toes toward the head while the paramedic provides opposing resistance (Figure 20-44, *B*). The patient should be able to perform both of these actions easily without evident fatigue. Other methods to evaluate muscle strength and agility (illustrated in Chapter 10) include testing for flexion, extension, and abduction of the upper and lower extremities.

Coordination. To evaluate a patient's coordination, the paramedic should assess the patient's ability to perform rapid alternating movements. These include point-to-point movements, gait, and stance.

One point-to-point movement that the patient can perform easily is to touch the finger to the nose, alternating hands. Another test is to ask the patient to touch each heel to the opposite shin. Both movements should be done numerous times and quickly to assess coordination, which should be smooth, rapid, and accurate.

Gait can be evaluated in many ways. A healthy patient should be able to perform each of the following tasks without discomfort or losing balance:

- Walk heel to toe
- Walk on the toes
- Walk on the heels
- Hop in place
- Do a shallow knee bend
- Rise from a sitting position without assistance

Stance and balance can be evaluated by using **Romberg's test** and the **pronator drift test.** To perform Romberg's test, the paramedic asks the patient to stand erect with the feet together and arms at the sides (Figure 20-45). The patient's eyes initially should be open and then closed. Although slight swaying is normal, a loss of balance is abnormal (a positive Romberg's sign). A patient should be able to stand in this position with one foot raised for 5 seconds without losing balance.

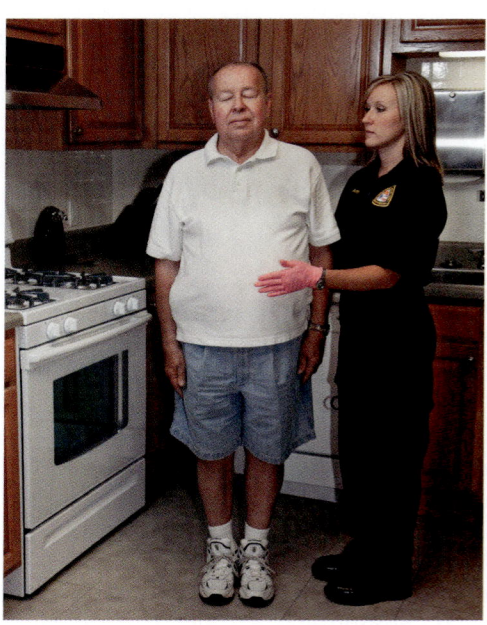

FIGURE 20-45 Romberg's test.

> **NOTE**
> The paramedic should stay close to the patient being tested for gait, stance, and balance. That way, the paramedic can help to prevent injury from a fall or loss of balance. The paramedic also should consider the patient's age and physical condition in deciding the appropriateness of these examinations.

The pronator drift test (also known as an *arm drift test*) is performed by having the patient close the eyes and hold both arms out from the body (Figure 20-46). A normal test will reveal that both arms move the same or both arms do not move at all. Abnormal findings include one arm that does not move in concert with the other or one arm that drifts down compared with the other.

SENSORY SYSTEM

The sensory pathways of the nervous system conduct sensations of pain, temperature, position, vibration, and touch. A healthy patient is expected to be responsive to each of these stimuli. Common assessments of the sensory system include evaluating the patient's response to pain and light touch. Each of the responses should be considered in relation to dermatomes (see Chapter 10).

LOOK AGAIN
See Chapter 10: Review of Human Systems, pp. 176-178.

In conscious patients the paramedic should perform a sensory examination with light touch on each hand and each foot. If the patient cannot feel light touch or is unconscious, the sensation may be evaluated by gently pricking the hands and soles of the feet with a sharp object. The paramedic should ensure the object will not penetrate the skin (e.g., a paper clip or cotton swab). The sensory examination should proceed from head to toe. The exam should compare symmetrical areas on each side of the body and the distal and proximal areas of the body. A lack of sensory response may indicate spinal cord damage (see Chapter 41).

REFLEXES

Testing a patient's reflexes can evaluate the function of certain areas of the nervous system as they relate to sensory impulses and motor neurons. Reflexes may be categorized as superficial reflexes and deep tendon reflexes (Table 20-5). Both types of reflexes should be tested as part of a thorough neurological examination.

SUPERFICIAL REFLEXES

Superficial reflexes are elicited by sensory afferents from skin. These include the upper abdominal, lower abdominal, cremasteric (for males), and plantar reflexes. All superficial reflexes are tested using the edge of a tongue blade (or similar object) or the end of a reflex hammer. An absent reflex may indicate an upper or lower motor neuron disorder.

- *Upper and lower abdominal reflex:* Place the patient supine. Gently stroke each quadrant of the abdomen with the tongue blade. A normal reflex is a slight movement of the umbilicus toward each area that is stroked.
- *Cremasteric reflex:* Place the patient supine. Gently stroke the inner thigh (proximal to distal). The testicle and scrotum should rise on the side that is stroked.
- *Plantar reflex:* Place the patient with legs extended. Gently stroke the lateral side of the foot from heel to the ball

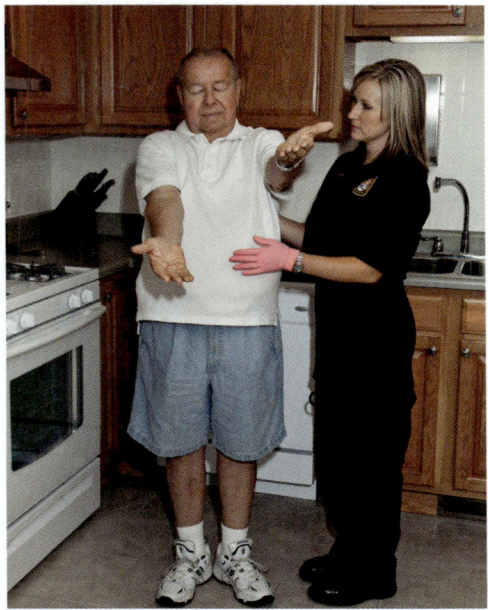
FIGURE 20-46 Pronator drift test.

TABLE 20-5 Superficial and Deep Tendon Reflexes

Reflex	Spinal Level Evaluated
Superficial	
Upper abdominal	T7, T8, and T9
Lower abdominal	T10 and T11
Cremasteric	T12, L1, and L2
Plantar	L4, L5, S1, and S2
Deep Tendon	
Biceps	C5 and C6
Brachioradial	C5 and C6
Triceps	C6, C7, and C8
Patellar	L2, L3, and L4
Achilles	S1 and S2

Modified from Rudy EB: *Advanced neurological and neurosurgical nursing,* St. Louis, 1984, Mosby.

and then across the foot to the medial side. Fanning of all the toes should occur with the direction of the stroke (Figure 20-47). The Babinski sign is present when there is dorsiflexion of the great toe with or without fanning of the other toes. It should be noted that the Babinski sign is an abnormal finding in older children and adults, but a normal response in children less than 2 years of age. Other normal reflexes for infants and children were described in Chapter 12.

LOOK AGAIN
See Chapter 12: Life Span Development, pp. 259-260.

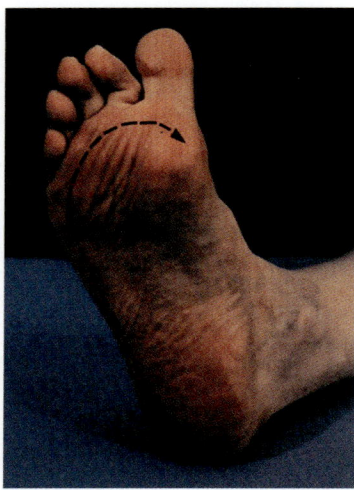

FIGURE 20-47 Plantar reflex indicating the direction of the stroke and the Babinski sign—dorsiflexion of the great toe with or without fanning of the toes.

TABLE 20-6 Scoring Deep Tendon Reflexes

Grade	Deep Tendon Reflex Response
0	No response
1+	Sluggish or diminished
2+	Active or expected response
3+	More brisk than expected, slightly hyperactive
4+	Brisk, hyperactive, with intermittent or transient clonus

DEEP TENDON REFLEXES

Deep tendon reflexes are elicited by sensory afferents from muscle rather than bone. They include the biceps reflex, brachioradial reflex, triceps reflex, patellar reflex, and the Achilles reflex. These reflexes should be tested on each extremity with a reflex hammer and a comparison made for visible and palpable responses. Deep tendon reflexes are graded using the scoring system in Table 20-6 and are recorded on a stick figure. Diminished or absent reflexes may indicate damage to lower motor neurons or the spinal cord. Hyperactive reflexes may suggest a motor neuron disorder. All reflexes are tested with the patient in a sitting position in the following manner (Figure 20-48):

- *Biceps reflex:* Flex the patient's arm to 45 degrees at the elbow. Palpate the biceps tendon in the antecubital fossa. Place your thumb over the tendon and your fingers under the elbow. Strike your thumb with the reflex hammer. Contraction of the biceps muscle should cause visible or palpable flexion of the elbow.
- *Brachioradial reflex:* Flex the patient's arm up to 45 degrees. Rest the patient's forearm on your arm with the hand slightly pronated. Strike the brachioradial tendon (about 1 to 2 inches above the wrist) with the reflex hammer. Pronation of the forearm and flexion of the elbow should occur.

- *Triceps reflex:* Flex the patient's arm at the elbow up to 90 degrees and rest the patient's hand against the side of the body. Palpate the triceps tendon and strike it with the reflex hammer, just above the elbow. Contraction of the triceps muscle should cause visible or palpable extension of the elbow.
- *Patellar reflex:* Flex the patient's knee to 90 degrees, allowing the lower leg to hang loosely. Support the leg with your hand. Strike the patellar tendon just below the patella. Contraction of the quadriceps muscle should cause extension of the lower leg.
- *Achilles reflex:* Flex the patient's knee to 90 degrees. Keep the ankle in a neutral position and hold the heel of the patient's foot in your hand. Strike the Achilles tendon at the level of the ankle malleoli. Contraction of the gastrocnemius muscle should cause plantar flexion of the foot.

REASSESSMENT

Reassessment refers to the ongoing assessment that follows the paramedic's initial evaluation of the patient. The purpose of reassessment is twofold: (1) It "re-focuses" the primary assessment to ensure that the patient continues to be stable and that initial interventions continue to be successful; (2) it also allows the paramedic to "trend" the patient's condition. That is, is the patient's condition improving or is it deteriorating while at the scene and during transport? Reassessment includes a second look at the following:

- The patient's level of consciousness
- The patient's vital signs
- The patient's response to initial care and treatment
- Positive or negative trends in the patient's condition
- Care interventions that may need to be changed or altered

Other examples of reassessment include reevaluating pulse and sensation in an extremity that has been splinted, verifying lung sounds before and after moving a patient who has been intubated, monitoring the electrocardiogram (ECG) after administering drugs, and monitoring pulse oximetry readings in a patient receiving airway support.

Reassessment also allows the paramedic to verify that nothing was missed or overlooked in the primary or secondary assessments, where the focus of patient care was on identifying and managing life-threatening conditions. Reassessment is an important aspect of providing good patient care.

SHOW ME THE EVIDENCE

Army researchers evaluated the value of vital sign trends in trauma patients. They retrospectively assessed vital signs of patients being transported to a level I trauma center in two time periods: 0-7 and 14-21 minutes. They concluded that vital sign trends over 21 minutes or less are unlikely to be diagnostically useful. Higher acuity patients' vital signs were much more variable and had periodic episodes of instability rather than a steady decline.

From Liangyou C et al: Exploration of prehospital vital sign trends for the prediction of trauma outcomes, *PEC* 13(3):286-294, 2009.

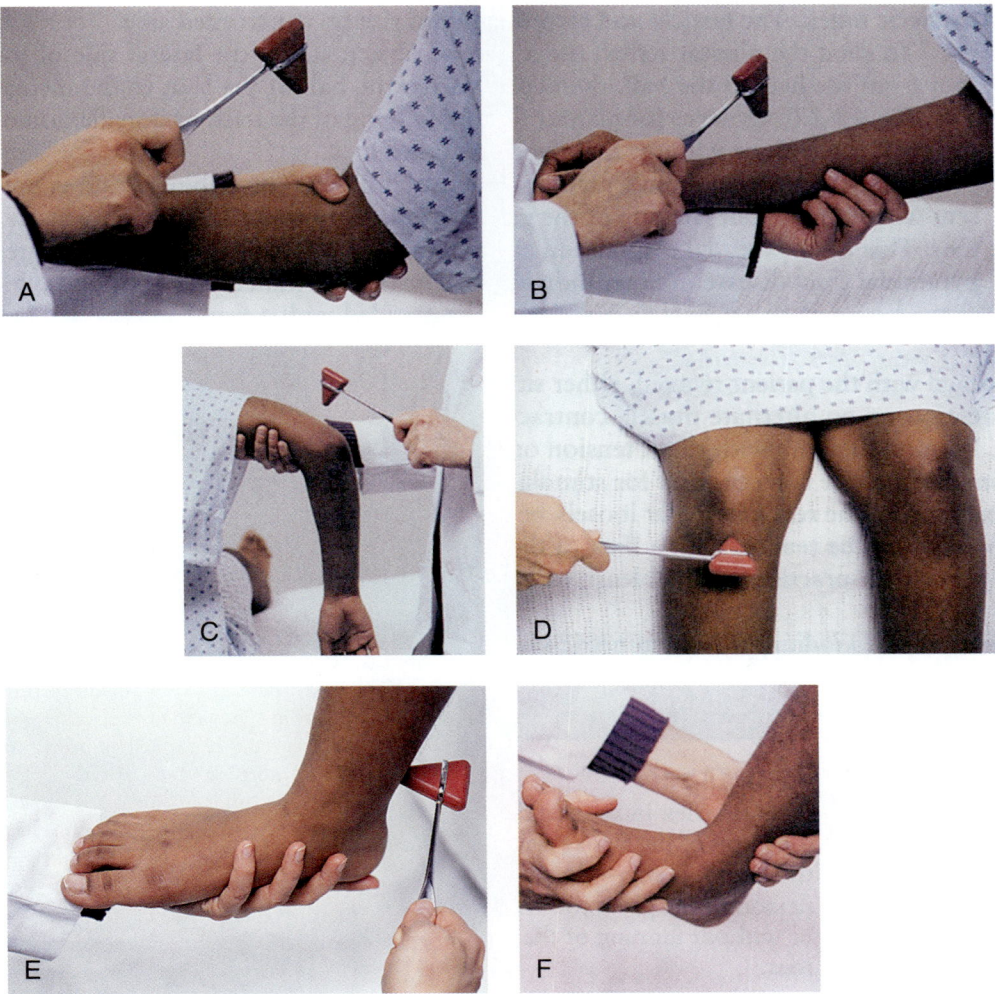

FIGURE 20-48 Location of tendons for evaluation of deep tendon reflexes. **A,** Biceps. **B,** Brachioradial. **C,** Triceps. **D,** Patellar. **E,** Achilles. **F,** Evaluation of ankle clonus.

PHYSICAL EXAMINATION OF INFANTS AND CHILDREN

Examining the ill or injured child requires special assessment skills. Children differ physiologically, psychologically, and anatomically from adults. Thus a pediatric patient assessment must take age and development into account.

Approaching the Pediatric Patient

The assessment and management objectives in caring for critically ill or injured children are similar to those for any other patient. The approach to the pediatric patient must differ, though. The initial encounter with the sick or injured child sets the tone for the entire patient care episode. Thus the paramedic must consider the patient's age. The paramedic also must be sensitive to how the child perceives the emergency environment. The following six guidelines should be considered when approaching the pediatric patient[6]:

1. Remain calm and confident. The parent's anxiety is infectious. Stay under control and take charge of the situation in a gentle but firm manner.
2. Do not separate the child from the parent unless absolutely necessary. In fact, once parents are reassured, encourage them to touch, hold, or cuddle the child when such actions are practical. This comforts the parents and the child.
3. Establish rapport with the parents and the child. Much of a child's fear and anxiety reflects the parent's behavior. When the family is calm, the child is reassured and is less fearful.
4. Be honest with the child and parent. In simple, direct, nonmedical language, explain to the parent and the child what is happening as it occurs. When a procedure is going to hurt, inform the child. Never lie. Do not give the impression that there are options when none exist. For example, do not say, "Would you like to go for a ride in the ambulance?" The child may answer "No."

5. Whenever possible, assign one paramedic to stay with the child. This person should obtain the history and be the primary person to initiate therapy. Even in a few moments, one person who remains on the child's level can establish a trusting relationship.

6. Observe the patient before the physical examination. If possible, the paramedic should at first assess the alert child with no touching. After the physical examination begins, the child's behavior may change radically. This may make it difficult to assess whether the behavior is a reaction to a physical state or to the perceived intrusion. The paramedic usually can assess the patient's general appearance, skin signs, level of consciousness, respiratory rate, and behavior easily before approaching the patient. During this observation, the paramedic also should note any area of the body that looks painful and avoid manipulating this area until the end of the examination. The paramedic should inform the child that he or she will give warning before touching the area.

CRITICAL THINKING

The next time you are in a room with an infant or small child, try this "across the room" assessment technique.

What can you tell about the level of distress and cardiopulmonary function by doing this?

General Appearance

A child's general appearance is assessed best at a distance. While the patient is in safe, familiar surroundings (e.g., a parent's arms), the paramedic visually should assess the child's level of consciousness, spontaneous movement, respiratory effort, and skin color. The child's body position also can offer helpful information. For example, the child may be lying limp or sitting upright to aid breathing. Other clues may help determine the child's willingness to cooperate during the examination. These clues may include crying, eye contact, concentration, and distractibility.

A visual inspection of the child's general appearance can be helpful. Appearance is a fairly reliable indicator of the patient's need for emergency care. Children who are seriously ill or injured usually do not attempt to hide their state. Their actions generally reflect the severity of the situation. Thus the patient's appearance is a valuable tool for the paramedic. Table 20-7 provides the key aspects of general appearance in initial assessment of the pediatric patient.

Physical Examination

A physical examination is best conducted with knowledge of the development of children and changes that occur within age groups (see Chapter 12). The guidelines that follow vary according to the child's development. However, these guidelines may be used as a reference during the exam. Parents and family members also may be a source of information. The paramedic may direct questions regarding "normal" behavior and activity levels to the parents.

TABLE 20-7 Components of General Appearance for Assessment

Assessment Finding	Evaluation Considerations
Alertness	How perceptive is the child, and how responsive is the child to the presence of a stranger or to other aspects of the environment?
Distractibility	How readily does a person, object, or sound draw the child's attention? For example, drawing a child's attention to a toy when the child initially appeared disinterested in the surroundings is a positive sign
Consolability	Can a distressed child be comforted? For example, stopping a child from crying by speaking softly or offering a pacifier or a toy is an encouraging sign.
Speech or cry	Is the speech or cry strong and spontaneous? Weak and muffled? Hoarse? Absent unless stimulated? Absent altogether?
Spontaneous activity	Does the child appear flaccid? Do the extremities move only in response to stimuli, or are movements spontaneous?
Color	Is there pallor, a flushed appearance, cyanosis, or mottling? Does the skin coloring of the trunk differ from that of the extremities?
Respiratory efforts	Are there intercostal, supraclavicular, or suprasternal retractions in the resting state? Nasal flaring also indicates respiratory difficulty.
Eye contact	Does the child appear to gaze aimlessly, or does the child maintain eye contact with objects or persons? Even small infants, when well, preferentially fix their gaze on a face rather than other objects.

BIRTH TO 6 MONTHS

Children under 6 months of age typically are not frightened by the approach of a stranger. Thus the physical examination is fairly easy. During the examination, the paramedic should maintain the child's body temperature.

Healthy and alert infants usually are in constant motion. They may have a lusty cry. If the patient is under 3 months of age, poor head control is normal. Infants are "abdominal breathers." This causes the stomach to protrude and the infant's chest wall to retract during inspiration. This diaphragmatic involvement may give the impression of labored breathing. Skin color, nasal flaring, and intercostal muscle retraction are the best indicators of respiratory insufficiency.

In the infant, assessing the fontanelles is particularly important (Figure 20-49). These sutures between the flat bones of the skull are fairly wide to allow a "give" in the skull during the birth process. (The anterior fontanelle, known as the *soft spot*, usually is present up to the age of 18 months.) The anterior fontanelle should be level with the

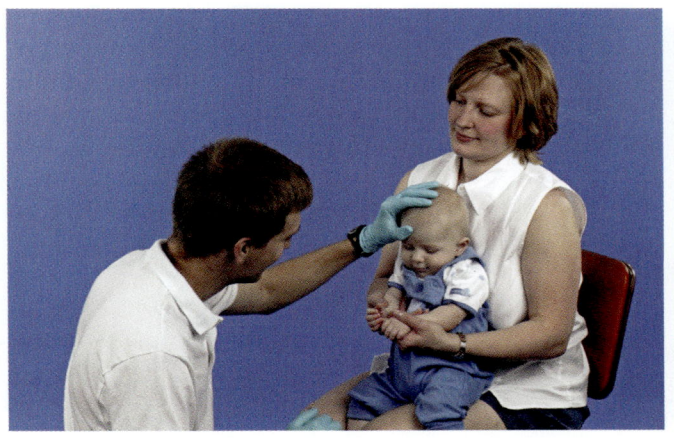

FIGURE 20-49 Palpation of the anterior fontanelle.

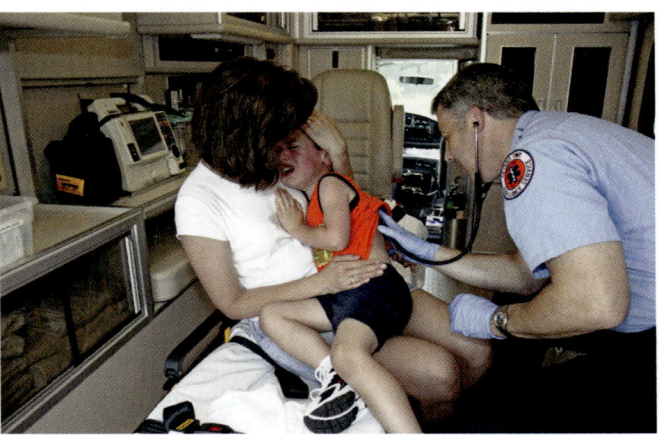

FIGURE 20-50 Examining a child.

skull or slightly depressed and soft. The fontanelle usually bulges during crying and may feel firm if the child is lying down. In the absence of injury, the fontanelle is best examined with the child in an upright position. A sunken fontanelle may indicate dehydration, and a bulging fontanelle in the noncrying upright infant may indicate an increase in intracranial pressure.

7 MONTHS TO 3 YEARS

Patients from 7 months to 3 years of age often are difficult to evaluate. They have little capacity to understand the emergency event. In addition, they are likely to experience emotional problems as a result of illness, injury, or hospitalization. Children of this age fear strangers and may show separation anxiety. If possible, parents should be present and should be allowed to hold the child during the examination (Figure 20-50). The paramedic should approach the child with a quiet, reassuring voice. If time permits, the paramedic should allow the patient to become accustomed to the examination environment.

During the physical assessment, each activity should be explained in short, simple sentences. The paramedic should give this explanation even though it may not improve cooperation. The best approach is to be gentle and firm and to complete the examination as quickly as possible. If physical restraint is necessary and if patient care activities will not be hindered, the paramedic should restrain the child with hands rather than mechanical devices (e.g., backboards).

4 TO 10 YEARS

Children in the 4- to 10-year age group are developing a capacity for rational thought. They may be cooperative during the physical examination. Depending on the child's age and the emergency scenario, the child may be able to provide a limited history of the event. These children also may experience separation anxiety and may view their illness or injury as punishment. Therefore the paramedic should approach the child slowly and speak in quiet and reassuring tones. Questions should be simple and direct.

During the examination, the paramedic should allow the child to take part by holding the stethoscope, penlight, or other pieces of equipment. This "helping" activity may lessen the child's fear. Helping also may improve the paramedic-patient relationship. Children of this age group have a limited understanding of their bodies. They also are reluctant to allow the paramedic to see or touch their "private parts" (seldom necessary in the prehospital setting). The paramedic should explain all examination procedures simply and completely. The paramedic should advise the child of any expected pain or discomfort.

ADOLESCENTS (11 TO 18 YEARS OF AGE)

Adolescents generally understand what is happening. They usually are calm, mature, and helpful. These patients are more adult than child and should be treated as such. Adolescents are preoccupied with their bodies. Usually they are concerned about modesty, disfigurement, pain, disability, and death. If appropriate, reassurance should be provided about these concerns during the examination.

During the patient interview, the paramedic should respect the patient's need for privacy. Some adolescents may hesitate to reveal relevant history in the presence of family and friends. If the adolescent gives vague answers or seems uncomfortable, the parents and patient should be interviewed privately. The possibility of alcohol or other drug use should be considered, as well as the possibility of pregnancy (for postpubescent girls).

PHYSICAL EXAMINATION OF OLDER ADULTS

As with pediatric patients, age-related physiological and psychological variations may create special challenges in patient assessment of older adults. The paramedic should not assume that all older adults are victims of age-related disorders. Individual differences in knowledge, mental reasoning, experience, and personality influence how these patients respond to examination.

Communicating With the Older Adult

Some older adults have sensory losses. This may make communications more difficult. Hearing and visual impairments, for example, are not uncommon. In addition, some older adults experience some memory loss and may become easily confused. Extra time may be needed to communicate effectively with these patients.

The paramedic should remain close to the patient during the interview. The older adult generally perceives a reassuring voice and gentle touch as comforting. Short and simple questions are best. Speaking more loudly than usual may be necessary and questions may need to be repeated. The paramedic must be patient and careful not to patronize or offend patients by assuming that they have a hearing impairment or cannot understand a particular line of questioning.

Patient History

Older patients often have multiple health problems present at the same time. Patients may be vague and nonspecific when describing their chief complaint, making it difficult to isolate a nonapparent injury or illness. Moreover, normal signs and symptoms of illness or injury may be absent because of decreased sensory function in some older adult patients.

Older patients with many health problems often take several medications. These medications increase the risk of illness from use and misuse. The paramedic should try to gather a full medication history and must be alert to the relationship among drug interactions, disease, and the aging process (see Chapter 49).

As part of the history, the paramedic should assess the patient's functional abilities and any recent changes in *instrumental activities of daily living* (IADL). Many older adults attribute these changes to age. They may not mention them unless asked. These details may help indicate patient conditions that are not readily observable. They may also reveal the need for other pertinent lines of questioning. Examples of functional abilities and instrumental activities to be discussed with the patient include the following:

- Walking
- Getting out of bed
- Dressing
- Driving a car
- Using public transportation
- Preparing meals
- Taking medications
- Sleeping habits
- Bathroom habits

Physical Examination

During examination, the paramedic should ensure comfort for the older adult patient. All exam procedures should be explained clearly. All questions should be answered sensitively. Many older patients with chronic illness may have lived with pain or discomfort for a long time. Thus their perception of what is painful may be different from that of other patients. The paramedic should observe for signs such as grimacing or wincing during the examination. These signs may indicate pain or a possible injury site. If the situation permits, the paramedic should perform the examination slowly and gently with consideration to the patient's feelings and needs.

Many older adults believe they will die in a hospital. If transportation is needed, patients may become fearful and anxious. The paramedic should be sensitive to these concerns. If appropriate, the patient should be reassured that his or her condition is not serious. The paramedic should attempt to calm these patients and advise them that they will be well treated in the hospital. All examination findings should be carefully recorded (see Chapter 4).

SUMMARY

- The secondary assessment integrates patient assessment findings with knowledge of epidemiology and pathophysiology to form a field impression and to identify an appropriate treatment plan.
- The examination techniques commonly used in the physical examination are inspection, palpation, percussion, and auscultation.
- Equipment used during the comprehensive physical examination includes the stethoscope, ophthalmoscope, otoscope, and blood pressure cuff.
- The physical examination is performed in a systematic manner. The exam is a step-by-step process. Emphasis is placed on the patient's present illness and chief complaint.

- The physical examination is a systematic assessment of the body that includes mental status, general survey, vital signs, skin, head, eyes, ears, nose and throat, chest, abdomen, posterior body, extremities, and neurological examination.
- The first step in any patient care encounter is to note the patient's appearance and behavior. This includes assessing for level of consciousness. This may include assessment of posture, gait, and motor activity; dress, grooming, hygiene, and breath or body odors; facial expression; mood, affect, and relation to person and things; speech and language; thought and perceptions; and memory and attention.

- During the general survey, the paramedic should evaluate the patient for signs of distress, apparent state of health, skin color and obvious lesions, height and build, sexual development, and weight. The paramedic also should assess vital signs.
- The comprehensive physical examination should include an evaluation of the texture and turgor of the skin, hair, and fingernails and toenails.
- Examination of the structures of the head and neck involves inspection, palpation, and auscultation.
- A full knowledge of the structure of the thoracic cage is needed. This knowledge aids in performing a good respiratory and cardiac assessment. Air movement creates turbulence as it passes through the respiratory tree. Air movement produces breath sounds during inhalation and exhalation. In the prehospital setting the paramedic must examine the heart indirectly. However, the paramedic can obtain details about the size and effectiveness of pumping action through a skilled assessment that includes palpation and auscultation.
- The four quadrants of the abdomen and their contents provide the basis for inspection, auscultation, percussion, and palpation of this body region.
- An examination of the genitalia of either sex can be awkward for the patient and the paramedic. The paramedic should inspect the genitalia for bleeding and signs of trauma (if indicated).
- Examination of the anus is indicated in the presence of rectal bleeding or trauma to the area.

- When examining the upper and lower extremities, the paramedic should direct his or her attention to function. The paramedic also should pay attention to structure.
- Assessment of the spine begins with a visual assessment of the cervical, thoracic, and lumbar curves. The assessment continues with a region-by-region examination for pain, swelling, and range of motion.
- A neurological examination may be organized into five categories: mental status and speech, cranial nerves, motor system, sensory system, and reflexes.
- Reassessment is the ongoing assessment of the patient to determine changes in condition and response to treatment.
- When approaching the pediatric patient, the paramedic should remain calm and confident. The paramedic should observe the child before beginning the physical examination. The paramedic also should make sure to avoid separation of the child and parent. Moreover, the paramedic must establish a rapport with parents and child and must be honest. One caregiver should be assigned to the child.
- The paramedic should not assume that all older adults are victims of disorders related to aging. Individual differences in knowledge, mental reasoning, experience, and personality influence how these patients respond to examination.

REFERENCES

1. Centers for Disease Control and Prevention: *Curriculum guide for public-safety and emergency-response workers: prevention of transmission of human immunodeficiency virus and hepatitis B virus,* Atlanta, 1989, U.S. Government Printing Office.
2. National Highway Traffic Safety Administration. *The National EMS Education Standards.* Washington, DC, 2009, U.S. Department of Transportation/National Highway Traffic Safety Administration, DOT.
3. U.S. Department of Health and Human Services, National Institutes of Health, National Heart, Lung, and Blood Institute: *The Seventh Report of the Joint National Committee on Prevention, Detection, Evaluation, and Treatment of High Blood Pressure,* NIH Pub. No. 03-5233, Washington, DC, 2003, National Institutes of Health.
4. Potter PA, Perry AG: *Basic nursing: essentials for practice,* ed 5, St Louis, 2007, Mosby.
5. Potter P, Perry A: *Fundamentals of nursing: concepts, process, and practice,* ed 5, St Louis, 2001, Mosby.
6. Seidel J, Henderson D, editors: *Prehospital care of pediatric patients,* California EMSC Project, Los Angeles, 1987, American Academy of Pediatrics.

SUGGESTED READINGS

Epistein O, Perkin GD, Cookson JC, et al: *Clinical examination,* London, 1992, Gower.

Seidel H, Ball JW, Dains JE, et al: *Mosby's guide to physical examination,* ed 6, St Louis, 2006, Mosby.

Snell R, Smith M: *Clinical anatomy for emergency medicine,* St Louis, 1993, Mosby.

Rock M: What about the physical exam? *JEMS* 31:5, 2006.

Clinical Decision Making

Upon completion of this chapter, the paramedic student will be able to:

1. List the key elements of paramedic practice.
2. Discuss the limitations of protocols, standing orders, and patient care algorithms.
3. Outline the key components of the critical thinking process for paramedics.
4. Identify elements necessary for an effective critical thinking process.
5. Describe situations that may necessitate the use of the critical thinking process while delivering prehospital patient care.
6. Describe the six elements required for effective clinical decision making in the prehospital setting.

KEY TERMS

application of principle A component of critical thinking in which the examiner makes patient care decisions based on conceptual understanding of the situation and interpretation of data gathered from the patient.

concept formation A component of critical thinking that refers to all elements that are gathered to form a general impression of the patient.

data interpretation A component of critical thinking in which the examiner gathers the necessary data to form a field impression and working diagnosis.

evaluation A component of critical thinking in which the examiner assesses the patient's response to care.

patient management plan A plan of care that is based on principles and applications of findings in the patient assessment.

reflection on action A component of critical thinking (usually performed after the event) in which the examiner evaluates a patient care episode for possible improvement in similar future responses.

Unique to the EMS profession is the uncertainty of the prehospital environment. The uncertainty is influenced heavily by factors that do not exist in other medical settings. Paramedics must be able to gather, evaluate, and synthesize information. They also must be able to develop and apply appropriate **patient management plans.** Finally, they must apply judgment, exercise independent decision making, and work effectively under pressure. These are the cornerstones of effective paramedic practice.

❓ DID YOU KNOW?
The Critical Thinker
The first step in critical thinking is to be aware of your assumptions. The second step is to beware of your assumptions. The final steps are to debate alternatives and look for proof. A critical thinker[1]:

- Asks pertinent questions.
- Assesses statements and arguments.
- Is able to admit a lack of understanding or information.

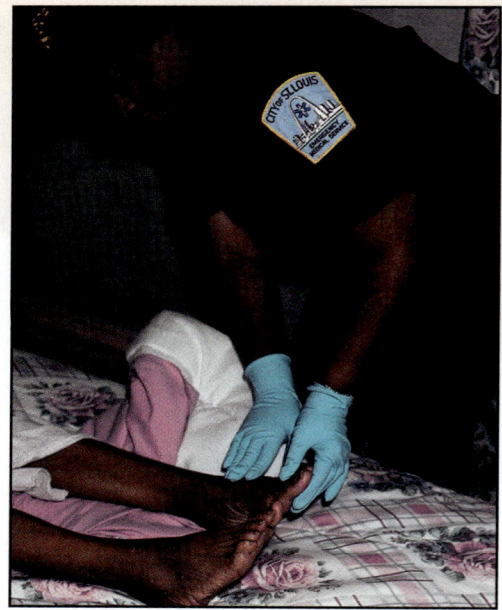

(Courtesy Monroe Yancie, St. Louis, Mo.)

- Has a sense of curiosity and creativity.
- Is interested in finding new solutions.
- Is able to clearly define a set of criteria for analyzing ideas.
- Is willing to examine beliefs, assumptions, and opinions and weigh them against facts.
- Listens carefully to others and is able to give feedback.
- Suspends judgment until all facts have been gathered and considered.
- Looks for evidence to support assumption and beliefs.
- Is able to adjust opinions when new facts are found.
- Looks for proof.
- Examines problems closely.
- Is able to reject information that is incorrect or irrelevant.

THE SPECTRUM OF PREHOSPITAL CARE

As described in Chapter 19 and Chapter 20, the paramedic must have a wide base of knowledge and skills to make good patient care decisions in the prehospital setting. On any given workday, the paramedic may be exposed to obvious critical life threats, potential life threats, and non–life-threatening situations (Box 21-1). On each call the paramedic also is expected to provide proper care and treatment.

Protocols, standing orders, and patient care algorithms help to promote a standardized approach to patient care for "classic" presentations. These presentations clearly define and outline performance parameters. However, these standards have some limitations. First, they may not apply to nonspecific patient complaints that do not fit the "model." Second, these standards do not address multiple disease etiologies or multiple treatment modalities. Third, they promote linear thinking, such as standardized care is appropriate for all patients ("cookbook medicine"). The paramedic must develop critical thinking skills to assist in unique patient care situations.

DID YOU KNOW?
Clinical Decision Rules

A key element in clinical decision making is to determine risk. Risk is the "probability that a particular adverse event occurs ..."[2] Increasingly, the medical community is devising clinical decision rules and tools that help assign the risk or probability that a patient has a particular injury or illness. These rules are based on key examination findings. *The Nexus low-risk clinical screening criteria for cervical spine injury* is an example of a clinical decision-making tool. Patients who have blunt trauma are considered low risk for cervical spine injury if they do not have tenderness over the spine, altered alertness, distracting injury, intoxication, or focal neurological changes. This tool has a sensitivity of 99% for cervical spine injury and almost 100% for clinically significant cervical spine injury. In other words, there is little chance that patients who are examined using this criterion will have a clinically significant cervical spine injury. On the other hand, the test is not very specific. A significant number of patients who have one or more positive findings also will not have cervical spine injury.[3]

Researchers are continually searching for evidence-based reliable decision-making tools—tools to help guide clinical practice and evaluate patient risk in emergency care. Areas of focus have been chest pain, syncope, triage, extremity injuries, and others. Each EMS system should evaluate the applicability of a given decision rule to their patient population before it is adopted.

CRITICAL THINKING PROCESS FOR PARAMEDICS

Specific aspects, stages, and sequences are linked with the critical thinking process. These include concept formation, data interpretation, application of principles, evaluation, and reflection on action[4] (Figure 21-1).

BOX 21-1 Spectrum of Prehospital Care

Obvious Critical Life Threats
Major multisystem trauma
Devastating single-system trauma
End-stage disease presentations
Acute presentations of chronic conditions

Potential Life Threats
Non–major multisystem trauma
Multiple disease etiologies

Non–Life-Threatening Presentations
Minor illness or injury
Emergency medical services system misuse

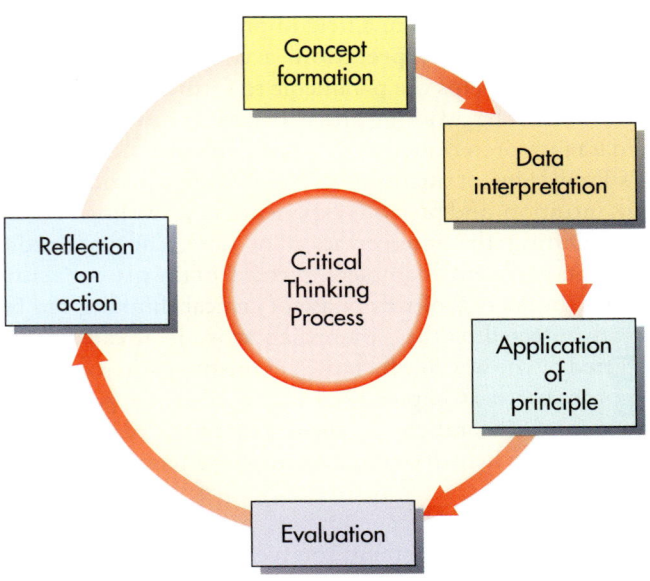

FIGURE 21-1 Critical thinking process.

Concept Formation

Concept formation refers to all elements gathered to form a general impression of the patient. Concept formation is the "what" of the patient story. These elements are described in Chapter 19 and Chapter 20 and include the following:

- Scene assessment (mechanism of injury, social setting)
- Chief complaint
- Patient history
- Patient affect
- Initial assessment and physical examination
- Diagnostic tests

SCENARIO PART ONE

Your crew has been dispatched to a local park for a person with "difficulty breathing." On your arrival at the scene, you find an 18-year-old female sitting on a park bench surrounded by her friends. The scene is safe. She is crying and tells you that she cannot catch her breath. You attempt to calm the patient and provide her with supplemental oxygen. You obtain a history from the patient and her friends that she and her boyfriend had quarreled recently and that she became emotional during the argument. Her lung sounds are clear. She has no allergies and no significant medical history other than a recent sinus infection. She denies any injury or pain. Aside from her increased respiratory rate, her vital signs are within normal range. Consider your concept formation for this patient.

> ### CRITICAL THINKING
> What effect would wrong or incomplete concept formation have on your critical thinking process during patient care? How can you enhance your concept formation skills while in your paramedic program?

Data Interpretation

Following concept formation, the paramedic must gather the needed data to form a field impression. This process is known as **data interpretation**: a component of critical thinking that helps the paramedic to form a working diagnosis. This is the "working phase" of patient care. The quality of data interpretation rests on a few elements: the paramedic's knowledge of anatomy and physiology, pathophysiology, intuition, and previous experience in providing patient care. During the interpretation of data, the paramedic attempts to obtain a complete "picture" of the patient's situation. The success of this phase of critical thinking can be greatly affected by the paramedic's attitude. It can also be affected by the way in which the paramedic-patient encounter proceeds (see Chapter 17). In some cases, the paramedic must condense and convey these data to the online physician, who can help determine appropriate actions.

SCENARIO PART TWO

While assessing this patient, you recall a similar emergency response. In that response, you provided care to a young male with difficulty breathing. He had just lost a big tennis match. At first you assumed that the patient was having breathing difficulty because of emotions that resulted from his loss. Like the female patient you are caring for now, this male patient had no allergies and no significant medical history and denied any recent injury. His vital signs were within normal range. However, lung sounds were diminished slightly on the patient's left side. The patient also complained of mild pain on inspiration. You administered supplemental oxygen. Then you rapidly transported the patient to the emergency department. After obtaining a chest x-ray film, the emergency physician confirmed your suspicion of a spontaneous pneumothorax (which resolved during the patient's hospitalization). Compare this interpretation of data to that of the female patient you are caring for now.

Application of Principles

The next step in the critical thinking process is the **application of principles** of proper patient care. These principles are based on the paramedic's conceptual understanding of the situation. They also are based on the interpretation of the data gathered from the patient. Once the paramedic establishes the field impression and working diagnosis, treatment can often be initiated through protocols and standing orders. If necessary, consultation can be made with direct/online medical direction.

SCENARIO PART THREE

Based on your experience, your knowledge of patient care, and your interpretation of the data gathered from your patient, you decide that she is hyperventilating. You initiate proper treatment with calming measures and encourage her to slow her respiratory rate. Although the female patient you are caring for presented much like the male patient you recall, your working diagnosis is different. You reach this conclusion because the female patient had clear, bilateral lung sounds. She also denied any pain on respiration.

Evaluation

The **evaluation** component of critical thinking requires an ongoing assessment of the patient's response to the care provided. Evaluation includes the following:

- Reassessment of the patient (ongoing assessment)
- Reflection of action (effectiveness of the intervention)
- Revision of field impression (a change in the working diagnosis)
- Review of the appropriateness of the protocol, standing orders, or direct orders for the patient
- Revision of the treatment or intervention as needed

SCENARIO PART FOUR

After you have provided calming measures and oxygen to your patient, she has slowed her breathing. She also appears to be more relaxed. You reassess the patient. You find that her vital signs remain normal and her lung sounds remain clear. Based on these findings, you know that your field impression of hyperventilation was correct and that there is no need to change your working diagnosis or to revise your treatment. After consulting with medical direction, the decision is made that the patient's condition does not warrant transportation for physician evaluation.

Reflection on Action

Reflection on action happens "after the event." It usually occurs through a run critique whereby the call is evaluated for improvement in similar future responses. Reflection on action provides paramedics with an avenue to add to or alter their experience base.

> ### ? DID YOU KNOW?
> **Avoiding Errors in Clinical Judgment**
> Assessing and managing patients in the prehospital environment is a difficult task. Errors in decision making are possible. To avoid errors consider using the following strategies:
> 1. Consciously think about your thinking and question your decision making.[5] Ask yourself, "Is this the right decision?" or "Does this make sense?" If the answer is no, reexamine your data, consult medical direction, or gather more information.
> 2. Recognize error-prone situations and use extra caution in those instances. For example, it is known that a significant number of patients who refuse care will seek emergency care soon after the refusal.[6] Be especially careful in those situations. Always ensure the patient knows that he or she can call again for help, even after refusing care.
> 3. Recognize your biases and use extreme caution when making decisions in situations that involve those biases. For example, you may be frustrated when caring for a patient who is intoxicated with alcohol. This may create a tendency for you to immediately attribute the patient's signs and symptoms to the intoxication. A personal bias such as this could lead you to overlook a serious head injury or other medical problem that might be the cause of the patient's presentation. Bias is a known cause of cognitive errors in medicine.[7]

> ### 🔍 SHOW ME THE EVIDENCE
> These authors evaluated 72 blunt trauma patients to compare 3 measures of intoxication in an attempt to find the best sobriety measure: blood alcohol level (BAL); a clinical sobriety assessment tool (CSAT); and physician judgment. The CSAT is a clinical sobriety tool developed by law enforcement personnel and the World Health Organization.
> The researchers found the CSAT had greater sensitivity to assess sobriety than physician judgment. There was poor agreement between CSAT and BAL data. The authors felt that chronic alcohol abusers sometimes appear sober with BAL above the designated level of intoxication.
>
> From Pattani S, Mahler S: Use of a clinical sobriety assessment tool in blunt trauma patients is more sensitive than physician judgment in determining sobriety, *Ann Emerg Med* 50(3, suppl):S64-S65, 2007.

SCENARIO PART FIVE

En route back to quarters, you discuss the call with a paramedic student. This student has just begun her field internship. Like you, she instantly thought that the patient was hyperventilating because of the fight that she had with her boyfriend. The student admitted that she had read about a spontaneous pneumothorax in her initial EMT training. However, she had never seen a patient who had one. Moreover, she would not have considered this possibility when caring for this patient. You discuss the pathology of a tension pneumothorax with her and the importance of assessing bilateral lung sounds in a patient who is having difficulty breathing. This reflection on action reinforces your data interpretation skills. It also adds to the student's experience base.

FUNDAMENTAL ELEMENTS OF CRITICAL THINKING FOR PARAMEDICS

For an effective critical thinking process, some basic elements must be present. These elements include adequate knowledge and the ability to do the following:

- Focus on specific and multiple elements of data at the same time.
- Gather and organize data and form concepts.
- Identify and deal with medical ambiguity (patients who do not "fit" the model).
- Differentiate between relevant and irrelevant data.
- Analyze and compare similar situations from past experience.
- Recall cases in which the working diagnosis was wrong.
- Articulate decision-making reasoning and construct arguments to support or discount the decision.

All of these elements were present in the previous scenario. At the scene, the paramedic dealt with the patient's symptoms and the input of friends. In addition, he focused on assessment and history findings. At the same time, he offered initial emergency care. The paramedic did this all within moments of arriving at the patient's side. He gathered and organized the data. He then concluded that the patient fit the model for hyperventilation syndrome. The paramedic also decided that the patient's sinus infection was not likely related to her present respiratory distress. He recalled a previous case where his initial working diagnosis of hyperventilation syndrome was wrong. Even so, the paramedic used clinical decision making to support the diagnosis of hyperventilation syndrome for this patient. His decision making was based on his experience and on his assessment findings.

FIELD APPLICATION OF ASSESSMENT-BASED PATIENT MANAGEMENT

Assessment-based patient management places huge responsibility on the paramedic. The paramedic must have a systematic means of analyzing a patient's problems, determining how to solve them, carrying out a plan of action, and evaluating effectiveness of the treatment. The success of assessment-based patient management in the prehospital setting depends on an integration of interpersonal skills, scientific knowledge, and physical activities (skills).

The Patient Crisis Severity Spectrum

EMS is set into action daily for many reasons. Yet few prehospital calls present true threats to life.[8] Minor medical and trauma events require little critical thinking. They result in fairly easy decision making for the paramedic. Likewise, patients with clear life threats pose limited critical thinking challenges because they often fit the "model" for standardized treatment (e.g., cardiac arrest). However, some patients fall in the spectrum between minor and life-threatening events. These patients pose the most critical thinking challenges for the paramedic. An example is a patient with mild to moderate respiratory distress. Another is a patient with diffuse abdominal pain. Either of these situations could be minor or could have life-threatening consequences.

Thinking Under Pressure

Hormonal influences from the fight-or-flight response (described in Chapter 2) can have positive and negative effects on critical decision making. The response may offer greater visual acuity and auditory keenness and improved reflexes and muscle strength. These can be positive when critical decisions must be made and action must be taken. The negative aspects of the response may include reduced critical thinking skills. This can result from a decrease in concentration and assessment ability. The key to strong performance under pressure is mental conditioning. This results in "instinctive performance" and "automatic responses" for technical procedures.

Mental Checklist for Thinking Under Pressure

Mental conditioning takes a good deal of practice. A checklist for thinking under pressure may help the paramedic to concentrate during stressful events. The mental checklist the paramedic should use is as follows:

- Stop and think.
- Scan the situation.
- Decide and act.
- Maintain clear and effective control.
- Regularly and continually reevaluate the patient.

CRITICAL THINKING

Do you think you can improve your performance under pressure by practicing imaginary critical situations in your head? Why or why not?

Practicing this checklist when under pressure will result in behaviors that improve clinical decision making. One

of these positive behaviors is staying calm (not panicking). Another is assuming a plan for the worst case (erring on the side of the patient). A third is maintaining a systematic assessment pattern. In addition, the paramedic can learn to balance the various styles of situation analysis, data processing, and decision making. Applying the styles of situational analysis (reflective versus impulsive), data processing (divergent versus convergent), and decision making (anticipatory versus reactive) allows the paramedic to provide the best possible care in most situations. In time, paramedics are able to apply all of these approaches with skill.

SITUATIONAL ANALYSIS: REFLECTIVE VERSUS IMPULSIVE

In most patient care situations, paramedics should avoid quickly stopping the pursuit of new data. One may do this to try to reach a correct working diagnosis. For example, consider a patient who has abdominal pain in his lower right quadrant. This patient should not be assigned automatically a working diagnosis of appendicitis. (This is an impulsive decision because the patient fits the model.) Rather, the paramedic should take time to reflect on other conditions, such as food poisoning, that could be the cause of the patient's pain. In other situations (e.g., a patient with foreign body airway obstruction), the impulsive decision to clear the patient's airway with chest thrusts and back blows would be the most prudent course of action to follow.

Reflective Example

When choosing an intravenous (IV) catheter for an elderly patient with small and fragile veins, the paramedic chooses a smaller gauge catheter that she knows will provide venous access, versus a larger bore catheter that might "blow the vein."

Impulsive Example

The paramedic immediately attempts IV access with a large-bore catheter because it is the gauge she "always uses."

DATA PROCESSING: DIVERGENT VERSUS CONVERGENT

Paramedics should avoid the trap of gathering only partial data that may lead them down the wrong diagnostic or therapeutic path. This is similar to impulsive situational analysis, and is known as convergent data processing. The convergent approach may be best in some cases (e.g., giving a standard drug dose to a patient in cardiac arrest). However, the convergent approach can hinder care in complex cases (e.g., an older patient with multiple complaints). A divergent approach in data processing looks at all sides of a case. The paramedic does this before arriving at a solution (e.g., multiple illnesses and polydrug use in the elderly patient).

Divergent Data Processing Example

An EMS training coordinator researches drug references and consults with medical direction for dosing suggestions for a new asthma drug being carried on the ambulance.

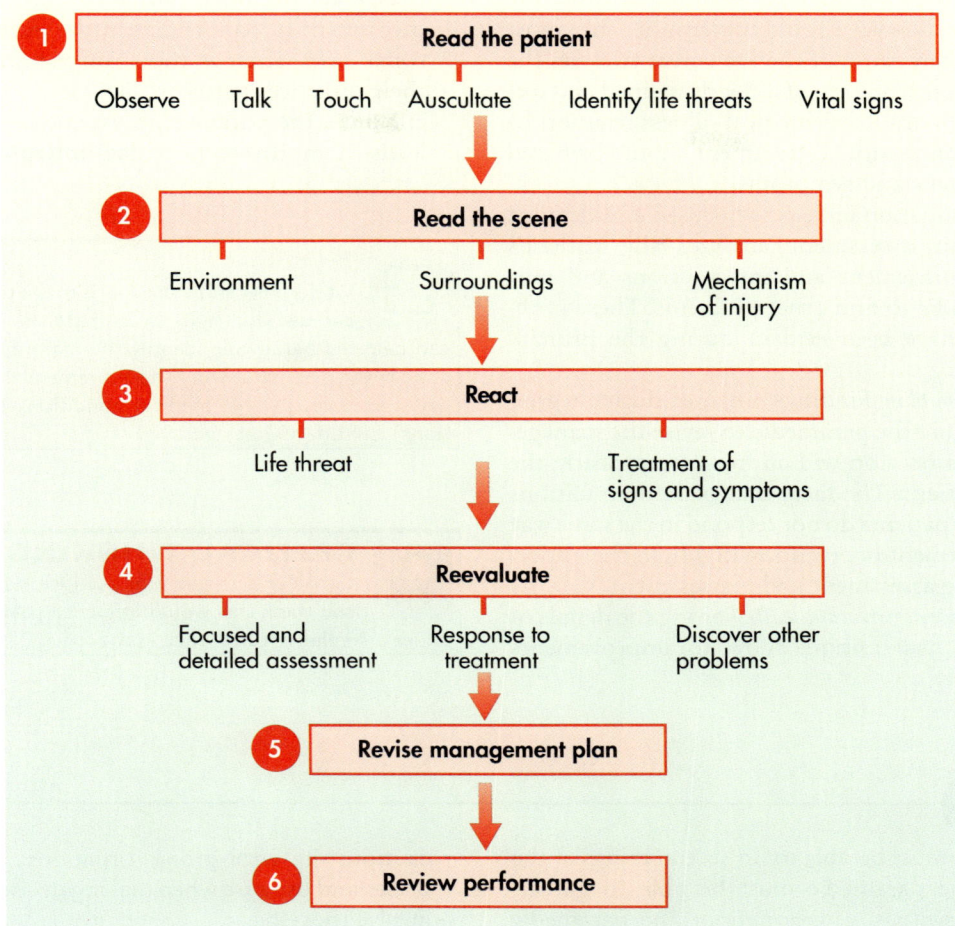

FIGURE 21-2 The six R's.

Convergent Data Processing Example

At an in-house training session, the paramedics are told "the package insert says to give this amount ..."

DECISION MAKING: ANTICIPATORY VERSUS REACTIVE

A paramedic's decision making can be seen as anticipatory or reactive. Anticipatory decision making is the process used by most health care professionals. It is based on continuing data collection and evolution of the patient's condition. With reactive decision making, decisions are made only after a problem occurs. This type of decision making can have negative effects on patient care.

Anticipatory Decision Making Example

A patient with large second-degree burns is being transported to a burn center that is 30 miles away. The paramedic requests orders for IV *morphine* before leaving the scene.

Reactive Decision Making Example

A paramedic caring for the same patient waits until the patient complains of pain before requesting the *morphine* order.

PUTTING IT ALL TOGETHER: THE SIX R'S

To put all components required for effective clinical decision making into action, the paramedic can think in terms of the six R's listed next (Figure 21-2):

1. *Read the patient*. The paramedic should observe the patient's level of consciousness and skin color. Position of the patient should be noted along with any obvious deformity or asymmetry. Talking to the patient will determine the chief complaint. This will also identify the presence of a worsening or preexisting condition. Skin temperature and moisture should be evaluated. Pulses should be assessed for rate, strength, and regularity. Auscultation of the lungs will reveal upper or lower airway problems. The paramedic should identify all life threats and obtain an accurate set of vital signs.

2. *Read the scene*. As a part of scene size-up, the paramedic should assess general environmental conditions. The paramedic should evaluate the immediate surroundings and attempt to identify any mechanism of injury or clinical clues of illness.

3. *React*. All life threats should be managed when they are found. The paramedic should determine the most common and likely cause of the life threat that fits the patient's initial presentation. If a clearly defined and recognizable presentation of medical illness cannot be defined in a priority patient, treatment should be based on presenting signs and symptoms.

4. *Reevaluate*. Reevaluation includes a focused and detailed assessment. This assessment analyzes the patient's response to management and interventions and may lead the paramedic to find other problems. These problems may not have been evident during the primary assessment.

5. *Revise management plan*. Findings obtained during reevaluation may require the paramedic to revise the management plan. This revision will address more clearly the needs of the patient. The facts that patient conditions change and that patients do not respond in the same way to identical treatment intervention highlight the importance of ongoing assessment and reassessment.

6. *Review performance at run critique*. Reviewing the details of the call through a run critique allows for improvements to be made to similar calls in the future. The interest and investment of paramedics in the outcome of their personal cases often is the strongest stimulus to change their practice patterns favorably. This process also enhances the paramedic's experience base and in turn leads to improvement of data interpretation skills.

NOTE

Vital signs can be used as a triage tool. The paramedic can use vital signs to estimate severity. Vital signs also can help the paramedic identify the majority of life-threatening conditions. The paramedic should remember that the patient's age and physical and medical conditions (including medications) can affect vital signs.

CRITICAL THINKING

Consider a negative or punitive run critique. How do you think this would influence your ability to perform under a similar circumstance in the future?

SUMMARY

- The paramedic must be able to do several things at the same time. The paramedic must be able to gather, evaluate, and synthesize information. The paramedic also must be able to develop and implement appropriate patient management plans. The paramedic must apply judgment and exercise independent decision making as well. Lastly, the paramedic must be able to think and work effectively under pressure.

- Protocols, standing orders, and patient care algorithms have several limitations. They may not apply to nonspecific patient complaints that do not fit the model. They also do not address multiple disease etiologies or multiple treatment plans. Moreover, they may promote linear thinking. Clinical decision rules may help determine risk when evaluating patients.

- The critical thinking process includes concept formation, data interpretation, application of principles, evaluation, and reflection on action.

- To reduce the risk of errors in decision making, consciously ask yourself "Is this the right decision?" Be cautious in error-prone situations. Recognize your biases and use care when making decisions in cases that involve those biases.

- For effective critical thinking, a paramedic must have a solid knowledge base. The paramedic must be able to cope with a large amount of data all at once as well. The paramedic must be able to organize these data, deal with ambiguity, and relate the situation to similar past experience. The paramedic also must be able to reason and construct arguments to support or discount the decision.

- When using assessment-based patient management, the paramedic must analyze a patient's problems, determine how to solve them, carry out a plan of action, and evaluate its effectiveness.

- Effective clinical decision making requires the paramedic to read the patient and the scene. The paramedic also must be able to react, reevaluate, and revise the management plan. Then the paramedic must be able to review performance at a run critique.

REFERENCES

1. Ferrett S: *Peak performance: success in college and beyond*, ed 7, New York, 2009, McGraw-Hill.

2. Thompson C, Dowding D: *Clinical decision and judgment in nursing*, Edinburgh, 2002, Churchill Livingstone.

3. Panacek EA, Mower WR, Holmes JF, et al: Test performance of the individual NEXUS low-risk clinical screening criteria for cervical spine injury, *Ann Emerg Med* 38(1):22-25, 2001.

4. U.S. Department of Transportation, National Highway Traffic Safety Administration: *EMT-Paramedic national standard curriculum*, Washington, DC, 1998, Author.

5. Gallagher EJ: The intrinsic fallibility clinical judgment, *Ann Emerg Med* 42(3):403-404, 2003.
6. Dawson BG, Brewer JGK: *EMS* "No Transports": an evaluation of emergency department presentation and admission rates following patient initiated "No transports," *Ann Emerg Med* 52(4, suppl):S71, 2008.
7. Croskerry P: Cognitive forcing strategies in clinical decision making, *Ann Emerg Med* 41(1):110-120, 2003.
8. National Highway Traffic Safety Administration. *The National EMS Education Standards*. Washington, DC, 2009, U.S. Department of Transportation/National Highway Traffic Safety Administration, DOT.

SUGGESTED READINGS

Alfaro-Lefevre R: *Critical thinking in nursing: a practical approach to outcome-focused thinking*, ed 4, St Louis, 2009, Saunders Elsevier.

Benner P, et al: *Clinical wisdom and interventions in critical care: a thinking-in-action approach*, Philadelphia, 1999, WB Saunders.

Croskerry P: Achieving quality in clinical decision making: cognitive strategies and detection of bias, *Acad Emerg Med* 9(11):1184-1204, 2002.

Croskerry P: Cognitive forcing strategies in clinical decision making, *Ann Emerg Med* 41(1):110-120, 2003.

Maggiore WA: How to minimize the influence of bias in patient assessment, *JEMS* 33(11), 2008.

Pesut D, Herman J: *Clinical reasoning: the art and science of critical and creative thinking*, Albany, NY, 1999, Delmar Learning.

Thompson C, Dowding D: *Clinical decision making and judgement in nursing*, London, 2002, Churchill Livingstone.

PART SIX

Cardiovascular

Chapter 22: Cardiology

OBJECTIVES

Upon completion of this chapter, the paramedic student will be able to:

1. Identify risk factors and prevention strategies associated with cardiovascular disease.
2. Describe the normal anatomy and physiology of the heart.
3. Discuss electrophysiology as it relates to the normal electrical and mechanical events in the cardiac cycle.
4. Outline the activity of each component of the electrical conduction system of the heart.
5. Describe basic monitoring techniques that permit interpretation of an electrocardiogram (ECG).
6. Explain the relationship of the ECG tracing to the electrical activity of the heart.
7. Describe in sequence the steps in ECG interpretation.
8. Identify the characteristics of normal sinus rhythm.
9. When shown an ECG tracing, identify the rhythm, site of origin, possible causes, and clinical significance and the prehospital management indicated.
10. Outline the appropriate assessment of a patient who may be experiencing a cardiovascular disorder.
11. Describe prehospital assessment and management of patients with selected cardiovascular disorders based on knowledge of the pathophysiology of the illness.
12. Describe the cause and nature of selected congenital cardiovascular defects.
13. List indications, contraindications, and prehospital considerations when using selected cardiac interventions, including basic life support, monitor-defibrillators, defibrillation, implantable cardioverter-defibrillators, synchronized cardioversion, and transcutaneous cardiac pacing.
14. List indications, contraindications, dose, and mechanism of action for pharmacological agents used to manage cardiovascular disorders.
15. Identify appropriate actions to terminate resuscitation in the prehospital setting.

KEY TERMS

abdominal aortic aneurysm A localized dilation of the wall of the abdominal aorta.

aberration Refers to the abnormal conduction of impulses through cardiac conduction pathways.

absolute refractory period The portion of the action potential during which the membrane is insensitive to all stimuli regardless of strength.

accelerated junctional rhythm A dysrhythmia that results from increased automaticity of the atrioventricular junction

acute arterial occlusion A sudden blockage of arterial flow, most commonly is caused by trauma, embolus, or thrombosis.

acute coronary syndrome (ACS) A spectrum of clinical disease that includes acute myocardial infarction and unstable angina.

acute deep vein thrombosis Occlusion of a vessel by a thrombus in any portion of the deep venous system.

acute dissecting aortic aneurysm Separation of the arterial wall of the aorta.

acute myocardial infarction (AMI) The sudden interruption of blood supply to the heart, resulting in death of cardiac tissue.

afterload The total resistance against which blood must be pumped. Also known as *peripheral vascular resistance*.

algorithms Lists used to summarize information, such as prehospital and in-hospital management recommendations.

amyloidosis A condition that results from deposits of abnormal protein in heart tissue.

aneurysm A localized dilation of a wall of a blood vessel.

angina pectoris Ischemic chest pain most often caused by myocardial anoxia as a result of atherosclerosis of the coronary arteries.

angioplasty Repair of damaged vessels.

anterior hemiblock Failure in conduction of the cardiac impulse in the anterior division of the left bundle branch.

artifact A deflection on the electrocardiogram display or tracing produced by factors other than the electrical activity of the heart.

artificial pacemaker A rhythm that is generated by regular electrical stimulation of the heart through an electrode implanted in the heart.

asystole A life-threatening cardiac condition characterized by the absence of electrical and mechanical activity of the heart.

atherosclerosis A common arterial disorder characterized by yellowish plaques of cholesterol, lipids, and cellular debris in the inner layers of the walls of large and medium-sized arteries.

atrial fibrillation A dysrhythmia that results from multiple areas of reentry within the atria or from an ectopic atrial pacemaker.

atrial flutter A dysrhythmia that usually results from rapid atrial reentry of electrical impulses.

atrial kick The priming force contributed by atrial contraction immediately before ventricular systole that acts to increase the efficiency of ventricular ejection due to acutely increased preload.

atrial tachycardia A rhythm disturbance that arises from an irritable site in the atria, producing tachycardia.

atrioventricular dissociation A conduction disturbance in which atrial and ventricular contractions occur rhythmically but are unrelated to each other.

atrioventricular node An area of specialized cardiac muscle that receives the cardiac impulse from the sinoatrial node and conducts it to the bundle of His.

atrioventricular junction An area formed by the AV node and the bundle of His; serves as the only electrical link between the atria and ventricles in a normal heart.

augmented limb leads Unipolar leads that record the difference in electrical potential in cardiac muscle.

automaticity A property of specialized excitable tissue that allows self-activation through spontaneous development of an action potential.

AV nodal reentry tachycardia A type of reentry supraventricular tachycardia, usually caused by a premature atrial contraction.

AV reentry tachycardia A type of reentry supraventricular tachycardia; results from a reentry circuit in the AV node by way of congenital accessory pathways in the heart muscle.

axis The imaginary straight line that joins the positive and negative electrodes of each ECG lead.

bifascicular block Refers to the blockage of two of three pathways (fascicles) for ventricular conduction.

bipolar lead A lead composed of two electrodes of opposite polarity.

bradycardia A heart rate of less than 60 beats per minute.

bruit An abnormal sound or murmur heard while auscultating an artery, organ, or gland.

bundle of His A band of fibers in the myocardium through which the cardiac impulse is transmitted from the atrioventricular node to the ventricles.

bundle of Kent Fibers that connect atrial muscle to ventricular muscle, bypassing the AV node; also known as *Kent fibers*.

cannon A waves Waves of pulse pressure that are visible in the jugular veins of a patient in ventricular tachycardia.

cardiac ejection fraction The percentage of ventricular blood volume released during a contraction.

cardiogenic shock Shock that results when cardiac action is unable to deliver sufficient circulating blood volume for tissue perfusion.

cardiomyopathy Any disease that affects the myocardium.

coarse ventricular fibrillation Fibrillatory waves that are greater than 3 mm in amplitude.

compensatory pause A pause following a premature beat; confirmed by measuring the interval between the R wave before the premature ventricular complex and the R wave after it.

congestive heart failure An abnormal condition that reflects impaired cardiac pumping, usually a result of myocardial infarction, ischemic heart disease, or cardiomyopathy.

contiguous leads Two or more ECG leads that are anatomically close together and that cover the same general area of the heart; specifically, the walls of the left ventricle.

delta wave A slurring or notching of the onset of the QRS complex that is a diagnostic finding in Wolff-Parkinson-White syndrome.

defibrillation The delivery of electrical current through the chest wall; used to terminate ventricular fibrillation and pulseless ventricular tachycardia.

depolarization A change in electrical charge difference across the cell membrane that causes the difference to be smaller or closer to 0 mV; a phase of the action potential in which the membrane potential moves toward zero or becomes positive.

diastole Relaxation of the atria and ventricles.

dyspnea Difficulty breathing.

dysrhythmia Variation from a normal rhythm.

ectopic focus An excitable group of cells that causes a premature heart beat outside the normally functioning sinus node of the heart.

ejection The forceful expulsion of blood from the ventricle of the heart.

electrical capture A large QRS complex produced by an artifical pacemaker which indicates ventricular contraction.

electrocardiogram (ECG) A graphic representation of the electrical activity of the heart.

end-diastolic volume The volume of blood returning to each ventricle.

endocarditis An infection of the endocardium (inner layer of the heart).

enhanced automaticity The cause of dysrhythmias in Purkinje fibers and other myocardial cells with a high resting membrane potential; it results from an acceleration of phase 4 depolarization commonly caused by abnormally high leakage of sodium ions into the cells, which causes the cells to reach threshold prematurely.

fine ventricular fibrillation Fibrillatory waves less than 3 mm in amplitude.

first-degree atrioventricular block A dysrhythmia in which there is a delay in conduction, usually at the level of the atrioventricular node.

fusion beat   A premature ventricular contraction that occurs at approximately the same time that an electrical impulse of the underlying rhythm is activating the ventricles, thereby causing ventricular depolarization to occur simultaneously in two directions; it results in a QRS complex that has the characteristics of the premature ventricular contraction and the QRS complex of the underlying rhythm.

hexaxial reference system   The system of intersecting lines of the standard limb leads and three other intersecting lines of reference: aV_R, aV_L, and aV_F leads.

high-grade atrioventricular block   Occurs when at least two consecutive atrioventricular impulses (atrial P waves) fail to be conducted to the ventricles.

high-output heart failure   A classification of heart failure where cardiac output remains high but is unable to meet the metabolic needs of the body.

hypertension   A disorder characterized by elevated blood pressure, which persistently exceeds 140/90 mm Hg.

hypertensive encephalopathy   A set of symptoms—including headache, convulsions, and coma—that result solely from elevated blood pressure.

interventricular septum   The tissue that separates the right and left ventricles of the heart.

joule   A measurement of electrical energy; one joule is the product of 1 V (potential) multiplied by 1 A (current) multiplied by 1 second.

jugular vein distention   Engorgement of jugular veins caused by an increase in central venous pressure; it is estimated by positioning the head of a supine patient at a 45-degree angle and observing the neck veins.

junctional escape beat   One or more that occurs when the rate of the SA node falls below that of the AV junction.

junctional tachycardia   A type of supraventricular tachycardia caused by a reentry mechanism in the junction of the atrioventricular node.

left axis deviation   A pattern of electrical activity that occurs in the heart there is a deviation of the axis to the left within the quadrant of 0 degrees and –90 degrees.

left bundle branch   A division in the bundle of His that provides pathways for impulse conduction.

left bundle branch block   A conduction disturbance in the left bundle branch that alters normal septal activation and sends it in the opposite direction.

left ventricular assist device (LVAD)   A battery-operated device that assumes the pumping action of the left ventricle.

left ventricular failure   A condition that occurs when the left ventricle fails to work as an effective forward pump, causing a back pressure of blood into the pulmonary circulation.

low-output heart failure   A type of heart failure where cardiac output is decreased, leading to impaired peripheral circulation and vasoconstriction.

mechanical capture   Occurs when an associated pulse is generated with the electrical capture of an artificial pacemaker.

modified chest leads   Placement of the standard limb leads of an ECG that are altered to mimic the precordial leads.

monomorphic ventricular tachycardia   Ventricular tachycardia where the QRS complex has the same morphology or fixed shape.

multifocal atrial tachycardia   A dysrhythmia that resembles wandering pacemaker but is associated with rates often in the 120 to 150 beats/minute range.

multifocal premature ventricular complex   A premature ventricular complex that originates from multiple sites in the ventricles.

myocardial contractility   The intrinsic ability of the heart to contract independent of preload and afterload.

myocarditis   Inflammation of the heart muscle.

non-STEMI   A myocardial infarction in which there is no ST-segment elevation.

P wave   The first complex of the electrocardiogram, representing depolarization of the atria.

palpitations   Irregular or forceful beating of the heart.

paroxysmal atrial tachycardia   Atrial tachycardia that begins and ends abruptly.

paroxysmal nocturnal dyspnea   An abnormal condition of the respiratory system characterized by sudden attacks of shortness of breath, profuse sweating, tachycardia, and wheezing that awaken a person from sleep; it often is associated with left ventricular failure and pulmonary edema.

paroxysmal supraventricular tachycardia   An ectopic rhythm in excess of 100 beats per minute and usually faster than 170 beats per minute that begins abruptly with a premature atrial or junctional beat and is supported by an atrioventricular nodal reentry mechanism or by an atrioventricular reentry involving an accessory pathway.

P-R interval   The time that elapses between the beginning of the P wave and the beginning of the QRS complex in the electrocardiogram.

pericarditis   Inflammation of the pericardium.

peripheral vascular resistance   The total resistance against which blood must be pumped; also known as *afterload*.

point of maximum impulse   The location or area where the apical pulse is palpated the strongest, often in the fifth intercostal space of the thorax just medial to the left midclavicular line.

polymorphic ventricular tachycardia   Ventricular tachycardia where the QRS complex has varying morphology or shape.

posterior hemiblock   Failure in conduction of the cardiac impulse in the posterior division of the left bundle branch.

potassium ion channels   Protein-lined channels in the cell membrane that prevent sodium from passing into the cell.

precordial leads   Unipolar chest leads used in 12-lead ECG monitoring that record the electrical activity of the heart in the horizontal plane.

precordial thump   A technique to restore circulation in monitored unstable ventricular tachycardia.

preexcitation syndrome   Anomalous or accelerated atrioventricular conduction associated with an abnormal conduction pathway between the atria and ventricles.

preload The volume of blood returning to the heart.

premature atrial complex A cardiac dysrhythmia characterized by an atrial beat occurring before the expected excitation and indicated on the electrocardiogram as an early P wave.

premature junctional complex A cardiac dysrhythmia that occurs during sinus rhythm earlier than the next expected sinus beat is caused by premature discharge of an ectopic focus in the atrioventricular junctional tissue.

premature ventricular complex A cardiac dysrhythmia characterized by a ventricular beat preceding the expected electrical impulse and indicated on the electrocardiogram as an early, wide QRS complex without a preceding related P wave.

proarrhythmia A new or worsened rhythm disturbance seemingly generated by antidysrhythmic therapy.

pulmonary edema The accumulation of extravascular fluid in lung tissues and alveoli.

pulse deficit A condition that exists when the radial pulse is less than the ventricular rate; it indicates a lack of peripheral perfusion.

pulseless electrical activity (PEA) The absence of a detectable pulse and the presence of some type of electrical activity other than ventricular tachycardia or ventricular fibrillation; also known as *electromechanical dissociation.*

Purkinje fibers Myocardial fibers that are a continuation of the bundle of His and that extend into the muscle walls of the ventricles.

QRS complex The principal deflection in the electrocardiogram, representing ventricular depolarization.

Q-T interval The time elapsing from the beginning of the QRS complex to the end of the T wave, representing the total duration of electrical activity of the ventricles.

R-on-T phenomenon The occurrence of a ventricular depolarization during a vulnerable period of relative refractoriness.

reentry The reactivation of tissue by a returning impulse; the sustaining mechanism in some cases of ventricular bigeminy or trigeminy, ventricular tachycardia, and paroxysmal supraventricular tachycardia.

refractory period The period after effective stimulation during which excitable tissue fails to respond to a stimulus of threshold intensity.

relative refractory period The portion of the action potential after the absolute refractory period during which another action potential can be produced with a greater than threshold stimulus strength.

repolarization The phase of the action potential in which the membrane potential moves from its maximum degree of depolarization toward the value of the resting membrane potential.

resting membrane potential The electrical charge difference inside a cell membrane measured relative to just outside the cell membrane.

return of spontaneous circulation (ROSC) Restoration of spontaneous circulation that provides evidence of more than an occasional gasp, occasional fleeting palpable pulse, or arterial waveform; the patient may or may not survive.

right axis deviation A pattern of electrical activity that occurs in the heart where there is a deviation of the axis to the right within the quadrant of +90 degrees and ±180 degrees.

right bundle branch A division in the bundle of His that provides pathways for impulse conduction.

right bundle branch block A conduction abnormality that occurs when transmission of the electrical impulse is delayed or not conducted along the right bundle branch.

right ventricular failure Failure of the right ventricle to serve as an effective forward pump; often results from left ventricular failure that produces elevated pressure in the pulmonary vascular system.

sinoatrial node An area of specialized heart tissue that generates the cardiac electrical impulse.

sinus arrest The failure of the sinus node causes short periods of cardiac standstill.

sinus bradycardia Decreased heart rate that results from slowing of the pacemaker rate of the SA node.

sinus dysrhythmia A cardiac rhythm disturbance that often is related to the respiratory cycle and to changes in intrathoracic pressure.

sinus tachycardia Increased heart rate that results from increase in the rate of the sinus node discharge.

sodium ion channels Protein-lined channels in the cell membrane that allow sodium to enter the cell during rapid depolarization.

ST segment The early part of repolarization in the electrocardiogram of the right and left ventricles.

standard limb leads Bipolar ECG leads that record the difference in electrical potential between the left arm (+), the right arm (−), and the left leg (−) electrodes.

Starling's law of the heart A rule that the force of the heartbeat is determined by the length of the fibers making up the myocardial walls.

STEMI A myocardial infarction in which there is ST-segment elevation.

stroke volume The volume of blood ejected from one ventricle in a single heartbeat.

sudden death A death that occurs within the first 2 hours after the onset of illness or injury.

supraventricular tachycardia A complex group of dysrhythmias that can be broadly defined as any tachycardia that directly or indirectly involves the atria or atrioventricular node (above the bundle of His).

syncope A brief lapse in consciousness caused by transient cerebral hypoxia.

synchronized cardioversion An electrical countershock used to terminate dysrhythmias other than ventricular fibrillation and pulseless ventricular tachycardia given after the peak of the R wave of the cardiac cycle.

systole Contraction of the atria and ventricles.

T wave A deflection in the electrocardiogram after the QRS complex, representing ventricular repolarization.

tachycardia A heart rate that exceeds 99 beats per minute.

third-degree atrioventricular block A condition that results from complete electrical block at or below the atrioventricular node; also known as *complete heart block*.

threshold potential The value of the membrane potential at which an action potential is produced as a result of depolarization in response to a stimulus.

torsades de pointes An unusual bidirectional ventricular tachycardia.

transcutaneous cardiac pacing (TCP) The delivery of repetitive electrical currents to the heart through an external artificial pacemaker; also known as *external cardiac pacing*.

Type I second-degree atrioventricular block A type of second-degree atrioventricular block that usually occurs at the level of the atrioventricular node; also known as *Wenckebach*.

Type II second-degree atrioventricular block A type of second-degree atrioventricular block that occurs when atrial impulses are not conducted to the ventricles.

U wave The gradual deviation from the T wave in the electrocardiogram, thought to represent the final stage of repolarization of the ventricles.

unifocal premature ventricular complex A premature ventricular complex that originates from a single ectopic pacemaker site.

unipolar leads Augmented limb leads that record the difference in electrical potential, using one electrode for a positive pole, but having no distinct negative pole.

unstable angina (UA) An acute coronary syndrome associated with a pattern of ischemic chest pain that has changed in its ease of onset, frequency, intensity, duration, or quality; also known as *preinfarction angina*.

unsynchronized cardioversion An electrical countershock used to terminate ventricular fibrillation and pulseless ventricular tachycardia, given without regard to where the shock occurs in the cardiac cycle.

Valsalva maneuver A vagal maneuver used to slow the heart and decrease the force of atrial contraction by stimulating postganglionic parasympathetic nerve fibers in the wall of the atria and specialized tissues of the sinoatrial and atrioventricular nodes via the vagus nerve.

valvular heart disease Any disease process that affects one or more valves of the heart: the mitral, aortic, tricuspid, or pulmonary valves.

vasovagal syncope A brief loss of consciousness that results from stimulation of the vagus nerve.

ventricular asystole Refers to the absence of all ventricular activity (cardiac standstill); may be the cause of cardiac arrest.

ventricular bigeminy A cardiac rhythm disturbance characterized by two ventricular beats in rapid succession followed by a longer interval.

ventricular escape complex A dysrhythmia that results when impulses from higher pacemakers fail to fire or to reach the ventricles; also known as *idioventricular rhythm*.

ventricular fibrillation (VF) A cardiac dysrhythmia marked by rapid, disorganized depolarization of the ventricular myocardium.

ventricular tachycardia (VT) A tachycardia that usually originates in the Purkinje fibers.

ventricular trigeminy A cardiac dysrhythmia characterized by three ventricular beats in rapid succession followed by a longer interval.

wandering pacemaker The passive transfer of pacemaker sites from the sinus node to other latent pacemaker sites in the atria and atrioventricular junction.

Wolff-Parkinson-White syndrome A syndrome of preexcitation of the ventricles of the heart; caused by an accessory pathway (bundle of Kent) that permits abnormal electrical communication from the atria to the ventricles.

Cardiovascular disease accounts for more than 500,000 deaths in the United States each year. About one half of the cases of sudden death from coronary disease take place outside the hospital and usually occur within 4 hours after onset of symptoms.[1] A large number of these deaths can be prevented by rapid entry into the EMS system, prompt provision of cardiopulmonary resuscitation, and early defibrillation.

CRITICAL THINKING
How many of your friends or family have had a heart attack or stroke? How has that illness affected their lives?

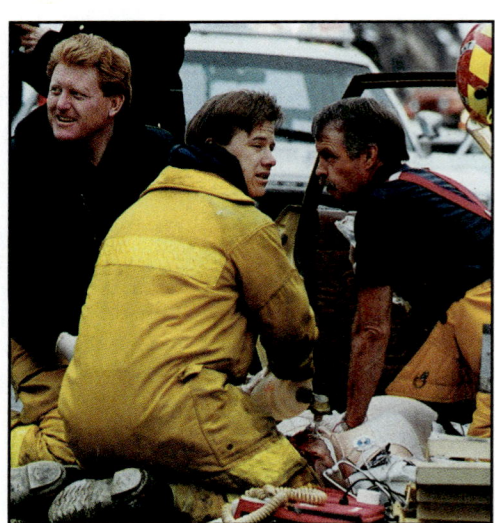

(Courtesy Thomas Cooper, Henderson, Nevada.)

RISK FACTORS AND PREVENTION STRATEGIES FOR CARDIOVASCULAR DISEASE

Although death rates from myocardial infarction have declined over the past several decades, coronary artery disease with resultant sudden death is still a major cause of morbidity and mortality and the most prominent medical emergency in the United States today.[1] The decline in death rates is due largely to heightened public awareness, the increased availability of automated external defibrillators (AEDs), improved cardiovascular diagnosis and therapy, the use of cardiovascular drugs by individuals at high risk, improved revascularization techniques, and improved and more aggressive risk factor modification.

Risk Factors and Risk Factor Modifications

Factors that pose a high risk for cardiovascular disease include advanced age, male gender, diabetes, hypertension, hypercholesterolemia, hyperlipidemia, a family history of premature cardiovascular disease, and known coronary artery disease. The risk can be increased considerably if the person has additional risk factors, such as obesity, cigarette smoking, and a sedentary lifestyle (Box 22-1). Clearly, some risk factors cannot be changed. Other risk factors, however, can be changed or modified through the following:

- Cessation of smoking
- Medical management and control of blood pressure, diabetes, cholesterol, and lipid disorders
- Exercise
- Weight loss
- Diet
- Stress reduction

Modifying cardiovascular risk factors can slow the rate of development of arterial disease. It also can reduce the incidence of acute myocardial infarction, sudden death, renal failure, and stroke.

Prevention Strategies

Paramedics and other health care professionals can support and practice activities that help prevent the development of cardiovascular disease. These strategies include community educational programs about nutrition, cessation of smoking (smoking prevention for children), early recognition and management of hypertension and cardiac symptoms, and prompt intervention (including cardiopulmonary resuscitation [CPR] and early use of an AED). These and other prevention strategies may help reduce risk factors at a young age. They also may have the greatest impact on risk factor modification (see Chapter 3).

SECTION ONE
Anatomy and Physiology of the Heart

ANATOMY REVIEW

The anatomy of the heart is described and illustrated in Chapter 10. The following is a brief review.

> **LOOK AGAIN**
> See Chapter 10: Review of Human Systems, pp. 182-188.

The human heart is a muscular organ with four chambers (Figure 22-1). It is cone shaped and about the size of a man's closed fist. It lies just to the left of the midline in the thorax. The heart is enclosed in a pericardial sac. This sac is lined with three parietal layers of serous membrane that form the wall of the heart. These three layers of tissue are the outer layer (epicardium); the middle layer (myocardium); and the inner layer (endocardium). The four chambers of the heart are the right atrium, right ventricle, left atrium, and left ventricle. The right atrium receives deoxygenated blood from the systemic veins. The left atrium receives oxygenated blood from the pulmonary veins. The heart has two types of valves that keep the blood flowing in the right direction. The valves between the atria and ventricles are the atrioventricular valves (also called *cuspid valves*); the valves at the bases of the large vessels leaving the ventricles are the semilunar valves. The right atrioventricular valve is the tricuspid valve. The left atrioventricular valve is the bicuspid (or mitral) valve. The valve between the right

---

BOX 22-1 Risk Factors for Cardiovascular Disease

Risk Factors
Age
Carbohydrate intolerance
Cigarette smoking
Cocaine use
Diabetes
Family history
Hypercholesterolemia
Hyperlipidemia
Hypertension
Previous myocardial infarction

Possible Contributing Risk Factors
Obesity
Oral contraceptive use
Personality type
Poor diet
Psychosocial tensions
Sedentary lifestyle
Stress
Excess alcohol consumption

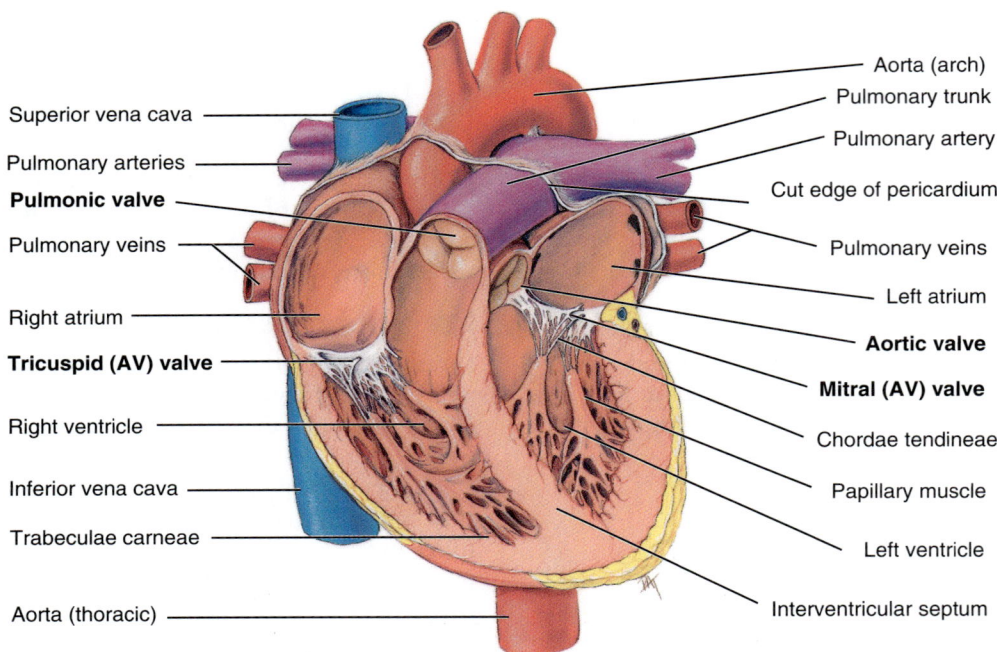

Aorta (arch)
Pulmonary trunk
Pulmonary artery
Cut edge of pericardium
Pulmonary veins
Left atrium
Aortic valve
Mitral (AV) valve
Chordae tendineae
Papillary muscle
Left ventricle
Interventricular septum

Superior vena cava
Pulmonary arteries
Pulmonic valve
Pulmonary veins
Right atrium
Tricuspid (AV) valve
Right ventricle
Inferior vena cava
Trabeculae carneae
Aorta (thoracic)

FIGURE 22-1 Internal view of the heart showing the four valves. (Applegate EM: *The anatomy and physiology learning system,* ed 3, St Louis, 2007, Saunders.)

ventricle and pulmonary trunk is the pulmonary semilunar valve. The valve between the left ventricle and the aorta is the aortic semilunar valve. When the ventricles contract, atrioventricular valves close to prevent blood from flowing back into the atria. When the ventricles relax, semilunar valves close to prevent blood from flowing back into the ventricles.

Blood Supply to the Heart

The coronary arteries are the sole suppliers of arterial blood to the heart. They deliver 200 to 250 mL of blood to the myocardium each minute during rest (Figure 22-2). The left coronary artery carries about 85% of the blood supply to the myocardium. The right coronary artery carries the rest. The coronary arteries begin just above the aortic valve where the aorta exits the heart. These arteries run along the epicardial surface. They divide into smaller vessels as they penetrate the myocardium and the endocardial (inner) surface.

The left main coronary artery supplies the left ventricle, the interventricular septum, and part of the right ventricle. Its two main branches are the left anterior descending artery and the circumflex artery. The right coronary artery supplies the right atrium and ventricle, part of the left ventricle, and the conduction system. Its two major branches are the right anterior descending branch and the marginal branch. In addition to the blood supply provided by these arteries, many connections (anastomoses) exist between arterioles to provide backup (collateral) circulation. These anastomoses play a key role in providing alternative routes

of blood flow in the event one or more of the coronary vessels become blocked (Figure 22-3).

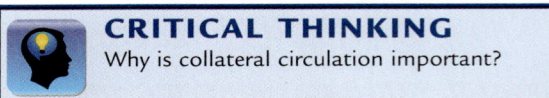

CRITICAL THINKING
Why is collateral circulation important?

Coronary capillaries allow for the exchange of nutrients and metabolic wastes. The capillaries merge to form coronary veins. These veins deliver most of the blood to the coronary sinus. The coronary sinus empties directly into the right atrium. The coronary sinus is the major vein draining the myocardium.

PHYSIOLOGY

The heart can be thought of as two pumps in one. One is a low-pressure pump (right atrium and right ventricle). This pump supplies blood to the lungs. The other is a high-pressure pump (left atrium and left ventricle). This pump supplies blood to the body. The right atrium receives venous blood from the systemic circulation and from the coronary veins. Most of this deoxygenated blood in the right atrium then passes to the right ventricle as the ventricle relaxes from the previous contraction. Once the right ventricle has received about 70% of its volume, the right atrium contracts. The blood remaining in the atrium is pushed into the ventricle. Contraction of the right ventricle pushes blood against the tricuspid valve (forcing it closed) and

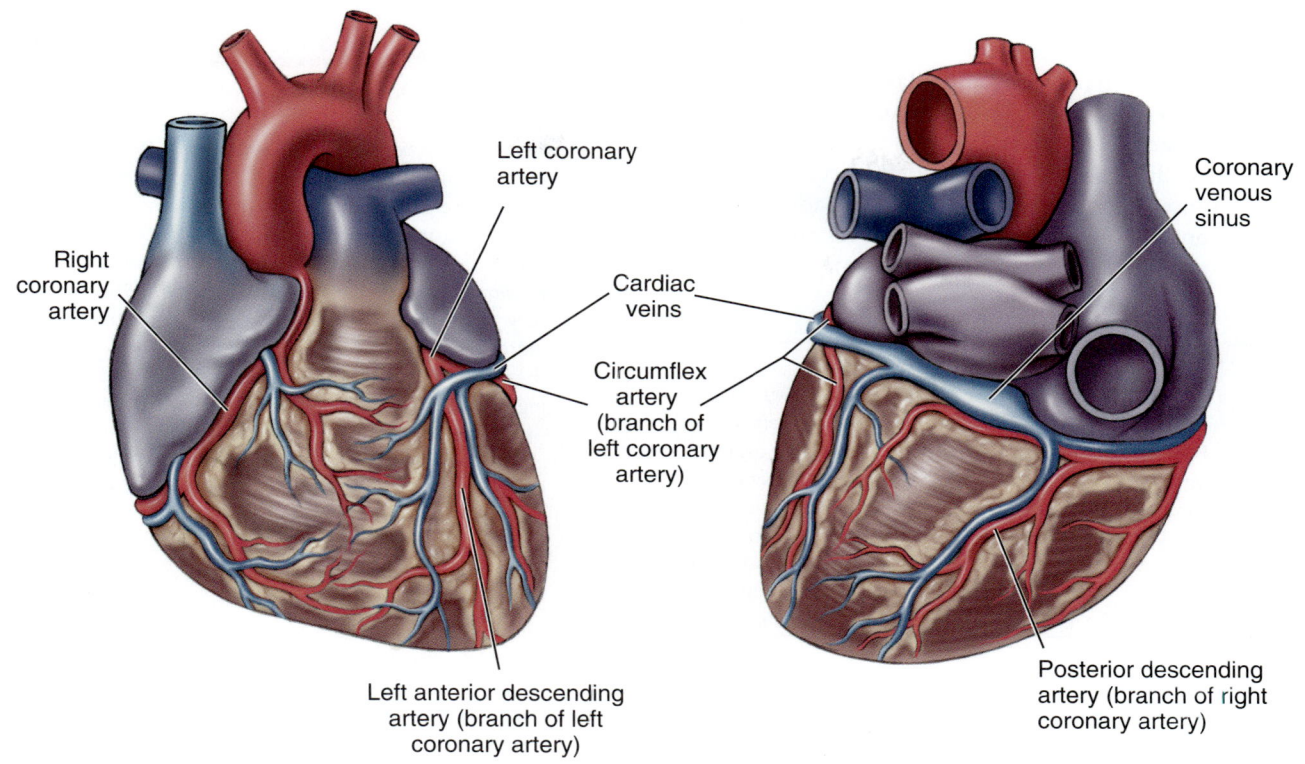

Right coronary artery

Left coronary artery

Cardiac veins

Circumflex artery (branch of left coronary artery)

Coronary venous sinus

Left anterior descending artery (branch of left coronary artery)

Posterior descending artery (branch of right coronary artery)

FIGURE 22-2 Blood supply to the myocardium: coronary blood vessels. (Herlihy B: *The human body in health and illness,* ed 3, St Louis, 2007, Saunders.)

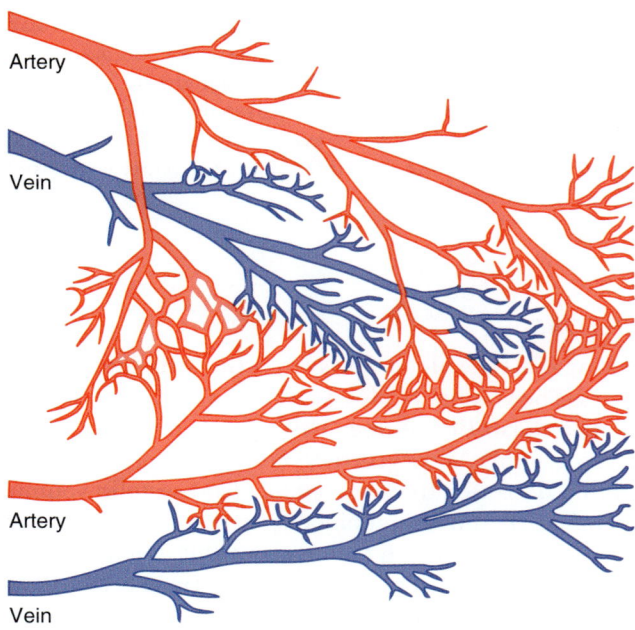

Artery

Vein

Artery

Vein

FIGURE 22-3 Minute anastomoses in the normal coronary arterial system. (Guyton AC, Hall JE: *Textbook of medical physiology,* ed 11, St Louis, 2007, Saunders.)

through the pulmonic valve (forcing it open). This allows the blood to enter the lungs via the pulmonary arteries. From the pulmonary arteries, the deoxygenated blood enters the capillaries in the lungs, where gas exchange takes place.

From the lungs the blood travels through four pulmonary veins back to the left atrium. The mitral valve opens, and blood flows to the left ventricle. Once the left ventricle has received about 70% of its volume, the left atrium contracts. The remaining blood 20% to 30% of the blood is pushed into the ventricles during atrial contraction (this is known as the **atrial kick**). The blood passing from the left atrium to the left ventricle opens the bicuspid valve when the ventricle relaxes to complete left ventricular filling. As the left ventricle contracts, blood is pushed against the bicuspid valve (closing it) and against the aortic valve (opening it). This allows blood to enter the aorta. From the aorta, blood is distributed first to the heart itself and then throughout the systemic arterial circulation.

NOTE

The atria work mainly as "primer pumps." Under most conditions, the ventricles can pump enough blood to maintain adequate blood flow to the body without the extra 30% of blood squeezed in by the atria. However, under stress, the heart may pump 300% to 400% more blood than during rest. In such conditions, the priming action of the atria becomes a key factor in maintaining pumping efficiency.

Cardiac Cycle

The pumping action of the heart is a product of rhythmic, alternate contraction (**systole**) and relaxation (**diastole**) of the atria and ventricles. (When *systole* and *diastole* are used without reference to specific chambers, they mean *ventricular* systole or diastole.) These heartbeats occur about 70 times a minute (every 0.8 second) in resting adults. These rhythmic contractions of the heart chambers are responsible for the movement of blood (Figure 22-4).

> ### NOTE
> The cardiac cycle has three phases: phase 1, ventricular filling (middle to late diastole); phase 2, ventricular systole; and phase 3, *isovolumetric relaxation* (early diastole).[2] In phase 2, ventricular systole, the atria relax and the ventricles begin contracting. Their walls close in on the blood in their chambers and ventricular pressure rises, closing the atrioventricular (AV) valve. Because, for a split second, the ventricles are completely closed chambers and blood volume in the chambers remains constant, this is called the *isovolumetric contraction* phase.

VENTRICULAR SYSTOLE AND DIASTOLE

As the ventricles begin to contract, ventricular pressure exceeds atrial pressure. This causes the atrioventricular valves to close. As the contraction proceeds, ventricular pressure continues to rise. Pressure rises until it exceeds that in the pulmonary artery on the right side of the heart and in the aorta on the left side. At that time, the pulmonary and aortic valves open. Blood then flows from the ventricles into those arteries (**ejection**).

After ventricular contraction, ventricular relaxation begins. Ventricular pressure falls rapidly. When the pressure falls below the pressure in the aorta or the pulmonary trunk, blood is forced back toward the ventricles. This closes the pulmonic and aortic valves. As the ventricular pressure drops below the atrial pressure, the tricuspid and mitral valves open. Blood then flows from the atria into the ventricles. Atrial systole occurs during ventricular diastole.

> ### CRITICAL THINKING
> What would happen if the valves were scarred and became stiff?

Stroke Volume

The **stroke volume** is the amount of blood ejected from the heart with each ventricular contraction. The stroke volume depends on three factors: **preload** (the volume of blood returning to the heart) (Box 22-2), **afterload** (the resistance against which the heart muscle must pump), and **myocardial contractility** (the performance of cardiac muscle).

BOX 22-2 Venous Return

Venous return is influenced by several factors, including the following[3]:

1. *Muscle contraction (skeletal muscle pump).* Rhythmical contraction of limb muscles, such as occurs during normal exercise (e.g., walking, running, swimming), promotes venous return by compressing and decompressing the veins.
2. *Respiratory cycle (thoracicoabdominal pump).* During respiratory inspiration, the negative pressure in the chest increases. This increase in pressure reduces right atrial pressure and increases venous return. Therefore, increasing the rate and depth of respiration increases cardiac output. Conversely, when negative pressure in the chest is reduced (e.g., from positive pressure ventilation, intermittent positive pressure breathing [IPPB], positive end-expiratory pressure [PEEP], continuous positive airway pressure [CPAP], and biphasic positive airway pressure [BiPAP]), venous return and cardiac output decrease.
3. *Decreased venous compliance.* Sympathetic activation of veins decreases venous compliance. This increases central venous pressure. It also promotes venous return by augmenting cardiac output through Starling's law of the heart. The result is an increase in the total blood flow through the circulatory system.
4. *Vena cava compression.* An increase in the resistance of the vena cava, such as occurs when the thoracic vena cava becomes compressed during a Valsalva maneuver or during late pregnancy, reduces return.
5. *Gravity.* The effects of gravity can reduce venous return. When a person stands from a supine position, cardiac output and arterial pressure decrease, because right atrial pressure falls. The flow through the entire systemic circulation falls, because the arterial pressure falls more than the right atrial pressure. Therefore, the pressure gradient driving flow throughout the entire circulatory system is decreased.

PRELOAD

During diastole, blood flows from the atria into the ventricles. The volume of blood returning to each ventricle is the **end-diastolic volume.** This volume normally reaches 120 to 130 mL. As the ventricles empty during systole, their volume decreases to 50 to 60 mL (end-systolic volume). Therefore, the amount of blood ejected during each cardiac cycle (stroke volume) in the average adult is about 70 mL.

In a patient with a healthy heart, the capacity to increase the stroke volume is great. The strong contraction of a heart during exercise, for example, can reduce the volume returning to each ventricle to as little as 10 to 30 mL. If large amounts of blood flow into the ventricles during diastole, their end-diastolic volume can be as much as 200 to 250 mL. In this way, the stroke volume can increase to more than double the normal amount. The ability of the heart to pump more strongly when it has a larger preload is explained by **Starling's law of the heart**.

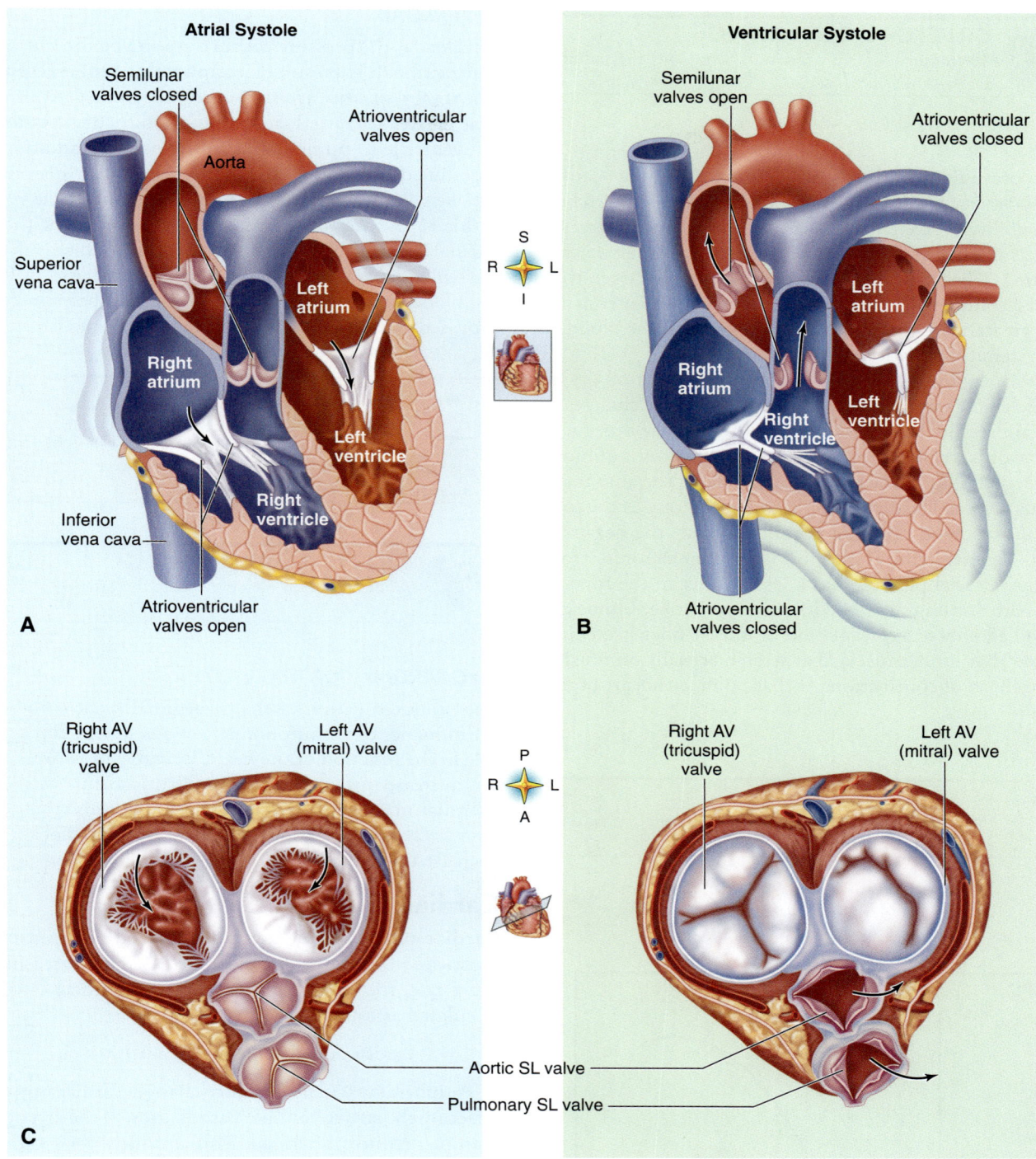

FIGURE 22-4 Heart action. **A,** During atrial systole (contraction), cardiac muscle in the atrial wall contracts, forcing blood through the atrioventricular valves and into the ventricles. **B,** During the ventricular systole that follows, the atrioventricular valves close and blood is forced out of the ventricles through the semilunar valves into the arteries. **C,** The pulmonary semilunar valves as seen from above (superior). (Thibodeau GA, Patton KT: *Structure and function of the body,* ed 13, St Louis, 2008, Mosby.)

CRITICAL THINKING
When you blow up a balloon, why does the balloon act like the heart muscle?

According to Starling's law (Figure 22-5), myocardial fibers contract more forcefully when they are stretched. (This ability of stretched muscle to contract with increased force is a quality of all striated muscle, not just cardiac muscle.) When the ventricles are filled with larger than normal volumes of blood (increased preload), they contract with greater than normal force to deliver all the blood to the systemic circulation.

The most important feature of the heart's ability to handle changes in venous blood return is that changes in arterial pressure have minimal effect on cardiac output. In other words, the heart can pump a small amount of blood or a large amount. The amount depends on the amount of venous return. The heart simply adapts, as long as the total amount of blood does not exceed the limit the heart can pump. Venous return is the most important factor in stroke volume; arterial pressure has a lesser effect in the form of afterload. Starling's law and its effect on stroke volume can be applied only to a certain limit of muscle fiber stretching. Beyond that limit, muscle fiber stretch actually diminishes the strength of contraction. At that point, the heart begins to fail.

NOTE
Preload is more important in determining cardiac output than afterload.

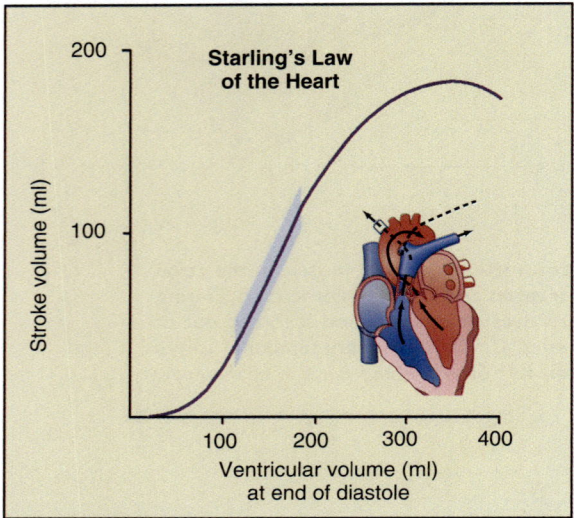

FIGURE 22-5 Starling's law of the heart. (Patton KT, Thibodeau GA: *Anatomy and physiology,* ed 7, St Louis, 2007, Mosby.)

AFTERLOAD

Afterload is the pressure within the aorta before ventricular contraction. It is a result of **peripheral vascular resistance** (the total resistance against which blood must be pumped). The greater the afterload, the more difficult it is for the left ventricle to pump blood to the body. In addition, the amount of blood ejected with ventricular contraction (stroke volume) is reduced. (The decrease in stroke volume is due to the increased pressure in the aorta that the ventricular muscle must overcome to open the aortic valve and push blood through.) As afterload is reduced (e.g., by lowering blood pressure, vasodilators), stroke volume increases, provided there is enough blood in the system.

NOTE
Although the term *afterload* generally is used to refer to the left ventricle, it also can refer to the right ventricle. For example, pulmonary hypertension increases afterload and can cause right ventricular failure.

CRITICAL THINKING
What condition would increase the afterload?

MYOCARDIAL CONTRACTILITY

The unique function of the myocardial muscle fibers and the influence of the autonomic nervous system play a major role in the function of the heart. Ischemia or various drugs can decrease myocardial contractility. Ischemia can reduce the total number of working myocardial cells (this occurs in myocardial infarction). Hypoxia or beta blockers can decrease the ability of the myocardial cells to contract.

Cardiac Output

Cardiac output is the amount of blood pumped by the ventricles in 1 minute. It can be increased by increasing the heart rate, the stroke volume, or both. Cardiac output is calculated as follows:

$$\text{Cardiac output} = \text{Stroke volume} \times \text{Heart rate}$$

Peripheral vascular resistance changes cardiac output by affecting the stroke volume. Vasodilation of the arteries, for example, reduces afterload. This produces an increase in cardiac output. In contrast, vasoconstriction increases afterload. In turn, this tends to reduce cardiac output. However, the body responds to the decrease by constricting the venous circulation. This increases the amount of blood returning to the heart and causes the heart to contract more forcefully (Starling's law). These actions help maintain or increase cardiac output.

Nervous System Control of the Heart

In addition to the heart itself, the autonomic nervous system controls the behavior of the heart (described in Chapter 10). It greatly influences the heart rate, conductivity, and contractility. The autonomic nervous system innervates the atria and ventricles. The atria are well supplied with large numbers of sympathetic and parasympathetic nerve fibers. The ventricles mainly are supplied by sympathetic nerves.

> **LOOK AGAIN**
>
> See Chapter 10: Review of Human Systems, pp. 171-177.

The parasympathetic nervous system is concerned mainly with vegetative functions (e.g., digestion and bowel and bladder function). In contrast, the sympathetic nervous system helps prepare the body to respond to stress. These sympathetic and parasympathetic control systems work in a checks-and-balance manner. They stimulate the heart to increase or decrease cardiac output according to the metabolic demands of the body.

> **CRITICAL THINKING**
>
> Consider how you regulate the hot and cold taps in a shower. How is the behavior of the autonomic nervous system similar?

PARASYMPATHETIC CONTROL

Parasympathetic control of the heart is accomplished through the vagus nerve. Control by these nerve fibers has a continuous restraining influence on the heart, primarily by reducing the heart rate and, to a lesser extent, contractility. The vagus nerve may be stimulated in several ways, such as the Valsalva maneuver, carotid sinus massage (described later in this chapter), pain, and distention of the urinary bladder. Acetylcholine is the chemical mediator of the parasympathetic nervous system.

Strong parasympathetic stimulation can decrease the heart rate to 20 or 30 beats/minute. Yet such stimulation generally has little effect on stroke volume. In fact, stroke volume may increase with a decreased heart rate. This occurs because the longer interval between heartbeats allows the heart to fill with a larger amount of blood and thus contract more forcefully (Starling's law).

SYMPATHETIC CONTROL

Sympathetic nerve fibers originate in the thoracic region of the spinal cord. They form groups of nerve fibers called *ganglia*. Their postganglionic fibers release the chemical norepinephrine. This chemical stimulates an increase in the heart rate (*positive chronotropic effect*). Norepinephrine also stimulates an increase in the force of muscle contraction (*positive inotropic effect*). Sympathetic stimulation of the heart causes the coronary arteries to dilate. It also causes constriction of peripheral vessels. These two effects, dilation and constriction, help increase the blood and oxygen

supply to the heart. The cardiac effects of norepinephrine result from stimulation of alpha- and beta-adrenergic receptors.

> **LOOK AGAIN**
>
> See Chapter 13: Principles of Pharmacology and Emergency Medications, pp. 300-304.

> **NOTE**
>
> As described in Chapter 13, the term *inotropic* refers to the force of energy of muscular contractions; *chronotropic* refers to the regularity and rate of the heartbeat; and *dromotropic* refers to conduction velocity. The effects are classified as positive or negative. For example, a positive inotropic effect would increase the strength of contraction. However, a negative dromotropic effect would decrease the speed of conduction.

Strong sympathetic stimulation of the heart may increase the heart rate notably. When rates are significantly high (greater than 150 beats/minute), the time available for the heart to fill is decreased. This produces a decrease in stroke volume.

Hormonal Regulation of the Heart

Impulses from the sympathetic nerves are sent to the adrenal medulla at the same time they are sent to all blood vessels. In response, the adrenal medulla secretes the hormones epinephrine and norepinephrine into the circulating blood in response to increased physical activity, emotional excitement, or stress.

Epinephrine has basically the same effect on cardiac muscles as norepinephrine. Epinephrine increases the rate and force of contraction. In addition, it causes blood vessels to constrict in the skin, kidneys, gastrointestinal tract, and other organs (viscera). Epinephrine also causes dilation of skeletal and coronary blood vessels. Epinephrine from the adrenal glands takes longer to act on the heart than direct sympathetic innervation does. Yet the effect lasts longer. Norepinephrine causes constriction of peripheral blood vessels in most areas of the body and also stimulates cardiac muscle.

Role of Electrolytes

As are all other cells of the human body, myocardial cells are bathed in an electrolyte solution. The major electrolytes that affect cardiac function (described in the next section) are calcium, potassium, and sodium. Magnesium is a major intracellular cation that also plays an important role. Changes in electrolytes can affect depolarization, repolarization, and myocardial contractility.

> **CRITICAL THINKING**
>
> What drugs can alter the normal balance of electrolytes in the body?

SECTION TWO
Electrophysiology of the Heart

To provide appropriate care for patients with cardiac disease, the paramedic must understand the mechanical and electrical functions of the heart. Understanding why and how the electrical conduction system can malfunction is crucial. The paramedic also must understand the effect that lack of oxygen to the cells (myocardial ischemia) has on cardiac rhythms. Two basic groups of cells in the myocardium are vital for cardiac function. One group is the specialized cells of the electrical conduction system. These cells are responsible for the formation and conduction of electrical current. The second group is the working myocardial cells. These cells have the property of contractility. They do the actual pumping of blood.

ELECTRICAL ACTIVITY OF CARDIAC CELLS AND MEMBRANE POTENTIALS

As described in Chapter 11, ions are charged particles. These particles are positive or negative. The charge depends on the ability of the ion to accept or donate electrons. In solutions containing electrolytes, particles with unlike (opposite) charges attract each other, and the particles with like charges push away from each other. This results in a tendency to produce ion pairs. These ion pairs help keep the solution neutral.

> ### 🔄 LOOK AGAIN
> See Chapter 11: General Principles of Pathophysiology, pp. 215-217.

Electrically charged particles may be thought of as small magnets. They require energy to pull them apart if they have opposite charges. They also require energy to push them together if they have like electrical charges. Therefore, separated particles with opposite charges have an electrical magnetic–like force of attraction. This gives them *potential energy* (Figure 22-6). The electrical charge creates a membrane potential between the inside and the outside of the cell. The electrical charge *(potential difference)* between the inside and outside of cells is expressed in millivolts (1 mV equals 0.001 volt). This potential energy is released when the cell membrane separating the ions becomes permeable.

Resting Membrane Potential

When the cell is in its resting state, the electrical charge difference is the **resting membrane potential**. The term *potential* is used in the electrical sense as a synonym for voltage. The inside of the cell is negative compared with the outside of the cell membrane. Also, the resting membrane potential is recorded from the inside of the cell. Therefore,

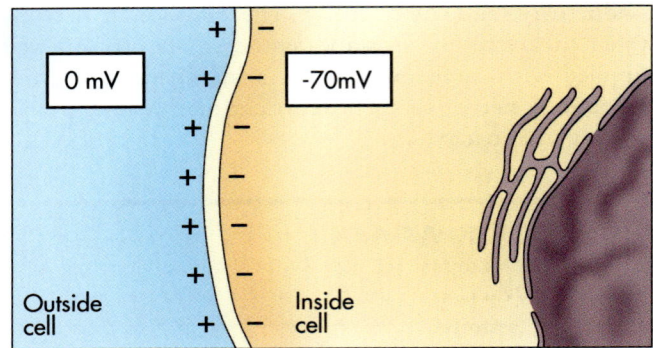

FIGURE 22-6 Electrical activity of cardiac cells and membrane potentials.

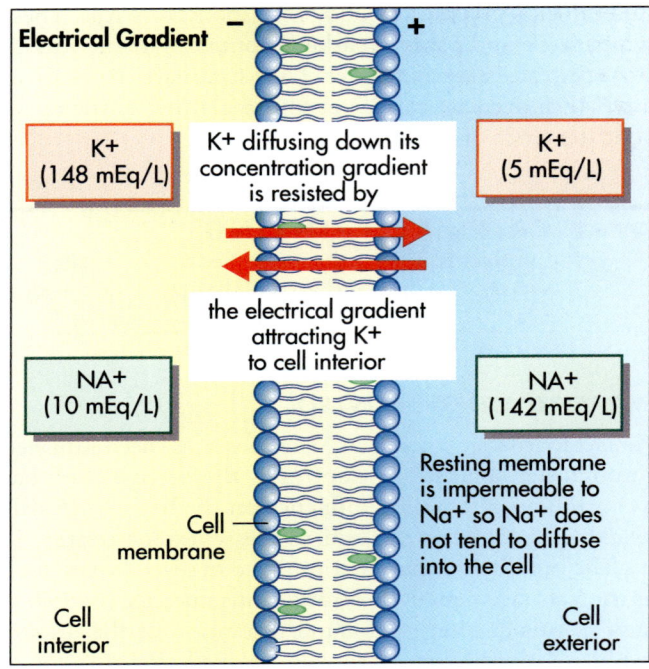

FIGURE 22-7 At equilibrium (resting conditions), the tendency for potassium ions to diffuse out of the cell is opposed by the potential difference (electrical gradient) across the cell membrane. Because the resting membrane is not permeable to sodium ions, sodium ions do not tend to diffuse into the cell.

the resting membrane potential is reported as a negative number (about –70 to –90 mV).

The resting membrane potential is a result of the balance between two opposing forces. One of these forces is the concentration gradient of ions (mainly potassium) across a permeable cell membrane. The other is the electrical forces produced by the separation of positively charged ions from their negative ion pair. The resting membrane potential mainly is established by the difference between the intracellular potassium ion level and the extracellular potassium ion level. The ratio of 148:5 produces a large chemical gradient for potassium ions to leave the cell. Yet the negative intracellular charge relative to the extracellular charge tends to keep potassium ions in the cell (Figure 22-7).

Sodium ions are positively charged ions on the outside of the cell. These ions have a chemical and electrical gradient. The gradients tend to cause sodium ions to move intracellularly, making the cell more positive on the inside compared with the outside.

Diffusion Through Ion Channels

The cell membrane is relatively permeable to potassium, somewhat less permeable to calcium chloride, and minimally permeable to sodium. The cell membrane appears to have individual protein-lined channels: **potassium ion channels** and **sodium ion channels.** These channels allow passage of a specific ion or group of ions. Permeability is influenced by electrical charge, size, and the proteins that open and close the channels *(gating proteins)*.

Potassium ion channels are smaller than sodium ion channels. They therefore prevent sodium from passing into the cell. Potassium ions are small enough to pass through sodium ion channels, but the cell favors sodium ions entering the cell during rapid depolarization. Rapid depolarization (the rapid entry of sodium ions into cells) creates a local area of current known as the *action potential*. After one patch of membrane is depolarized, the electrical charge spreads along the cell surface. This opens more channels (Figure 22-8).

> **NOTE**
> **Depolarization** occurs when the resting membrane potential changes from being more negatively charged on the inside of the cell to being more positively charged on the inside of the cell.

The contribution of unpaired ions to the resting membrane potential depends on two factors. The first factor is the diffusion of ions through the membrane by way of the ion channels. This creates an imbalance of charges. The second factor is the active transport of ions through the membrane by way of the sodium-potassium exchange pump. This also creates an imbalance of charges.

> **CRITICAL THINKING**
>
> Which of these processes of electrolyte transfer requires energy to occur?

Sodium-Potassium Exchange Pump

The specialized sodium-potassium exchange pump actively pumps sodium ions out of the cell and potassium ions into the cell. Thus this pump separates the ions across the membrane against their concentration gradients. Potassium ions are transported into the cell. This increases their concentration in the cell. Sodium ions are transported out of

the cell. This increases their concentration outside the cell (Figure 22-9).

The sodium-potassium exchange pump normally transports three sodium ions out for every two potassium ions taken in. Therefore, more positively charged ions are transferred outward than inward. This repolarizes the cell and returns it to its resting state. In the cell's resting state, the number of negative charges inside the cell is equal to the number of positive charges outside the cell.

> **NOTE**
> **Repolarization** occurs when charges inside the cell return to normal (become more negatively charged on the inside), allowing the cell to return to its normal resting state.

Pharmacological Actions

In cardiac muscle, sodium and calcium ions can enter the cell through two separate channel systems in the cell membrane. These are the fast channels and the slow channels. Fast channels are sensitive to small changes in membrane potential. As the cell drifts toward threshold level (the point at which a cell depolarizes), fast sodium channels open. This results in a rush of sodium ions into the cell and rapid depolarization. The slow channel has selective permeability to calcium and to a lesser extent to sodium. Calcium plays an electrical role by contributing to the number of positive charges in the cell. Calcium also plays a contractile role. Calcium is the ion required for contraction of cardiac muscle.

An understanding of ion channels can help paramedics understand how the heart rate and contractility respond to drugs. For example, calcium channel blockers selectively block the slow channel. Examples of such drugs are *verapamil* and *diltiazem.* These drugs limit the movement of calcium ions into the cell without altering its voltage. Other examples, such as *amiodarone* (a type III antidysrhythmic), owe much of their antidysrhythmic effects to their ability to block the fast inward sodium channel.

CELL EXCITABILITY

Nerve and muscle cells are capable of producing action potentials. This is known as *excitability.* When these cells are stimulated, a series of changes in the resting membrane potential normally causes depolarization of a small region of the cell membrane. The stimulus may be strong enough to depolarize a cell membrane to a level called the **threshold potential**. If this is the case, an explosive series of permeability changes takes place. This causes an action potential to spread over the entire cell membrane.

Propagation of Action Potential

An action potential at any point on the cell membrane acts as a stimulus to adjacent regions of the cell membrane. Thus the excitation process, once started, is spread along

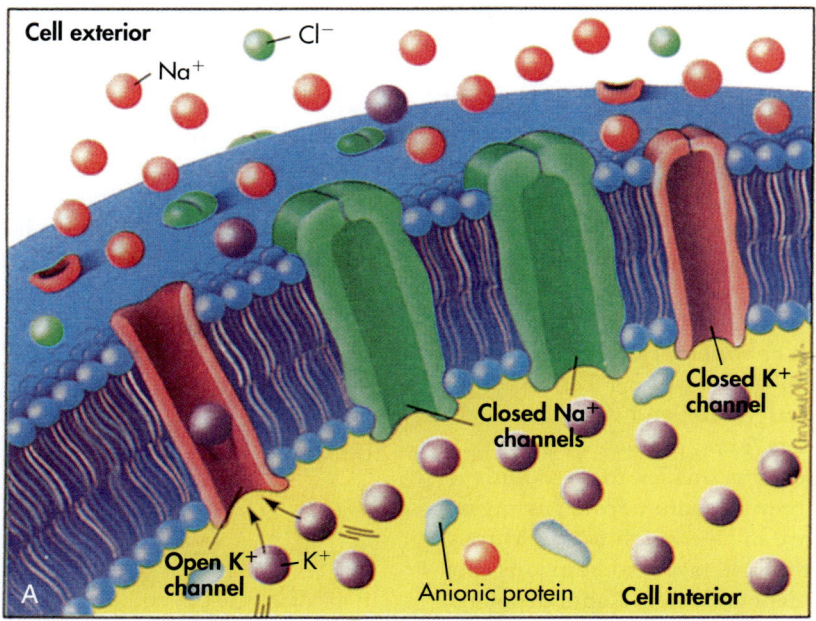

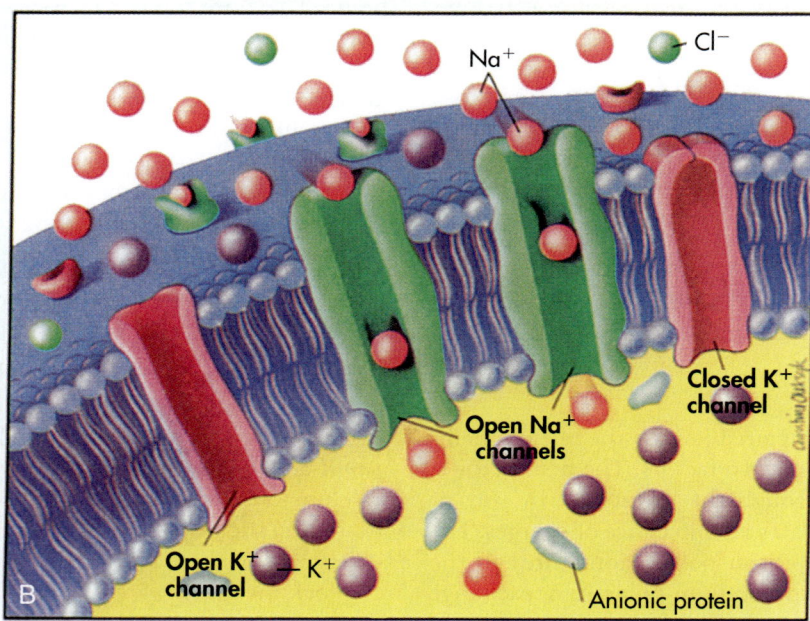

FIGURE 22-8 Effect of a stimulus that causes a voltage change across the cell membrane on the permeability of the cell membrane. **A,** Sodium channels remain closed in a resting (unstimulated) cell membrane. **B,** Depolarization of the cell membrane causes sodium channels to open. Sodium ions then diffuse down their concentration gradient into the cell, causing depolarization of the cell membrane.

the length of the cell and onto the next cell and so on. A stimulus strong enough to cause a cell to reach threshold and depolarize spreads quickly from one cell to another (this is the *all or none principle*). The cardiac action potential can be divided into five phases (phases 0 to 4) (Figure 22-10).

PHASE 0

Phase 0 is the rapid depolarization phase. It represents the rapid upstroke of the action potential. This occurs when the cell membrane reaches threshold potential. During this phase, the fast sodium channels open momentarily. In this moment, the sodium channels permit rapid entry of sodium

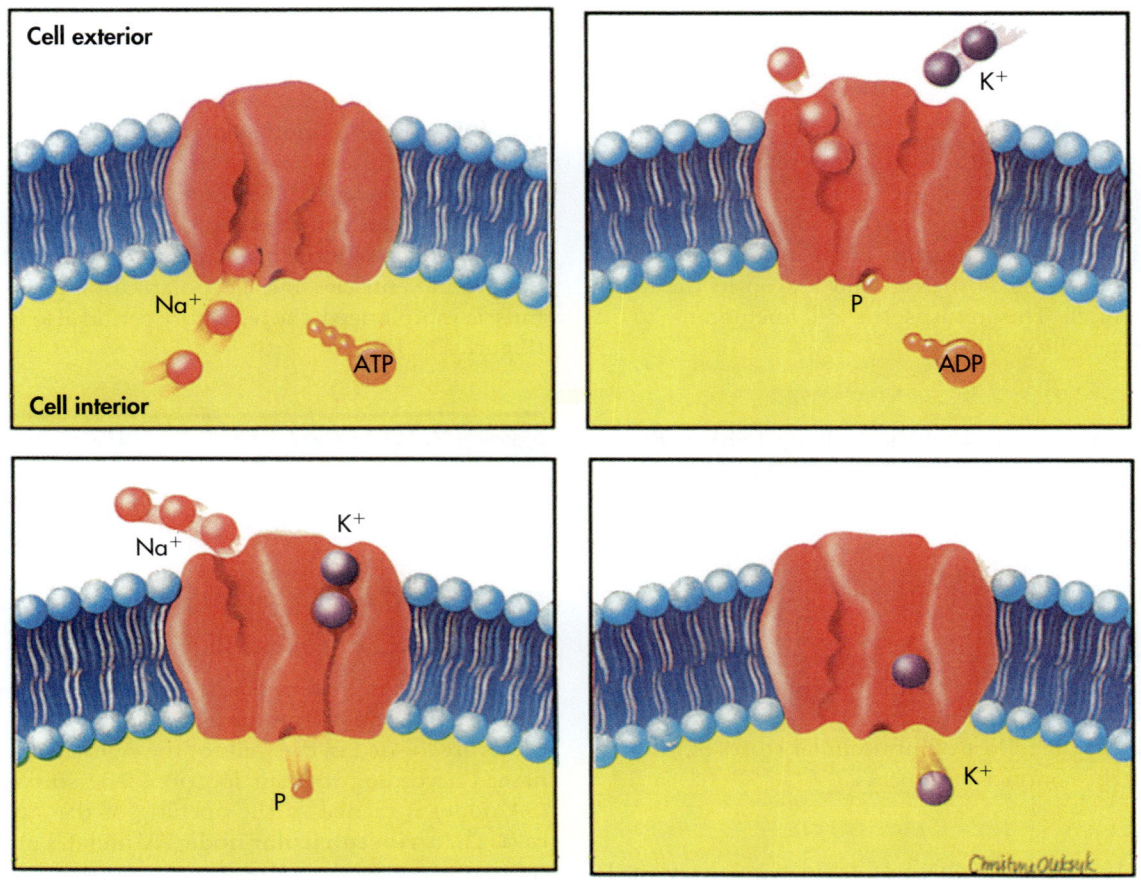

FIGURE 22-9 The sodium-potassium exchange pump actively transports sodium ions out of the cell across the cell membrane and potassium ions into the cell across the cell membrane. Adenosine triphosphate is used as the energy source. The pump can transport up to three sodium ions for every two potassium ions transported.

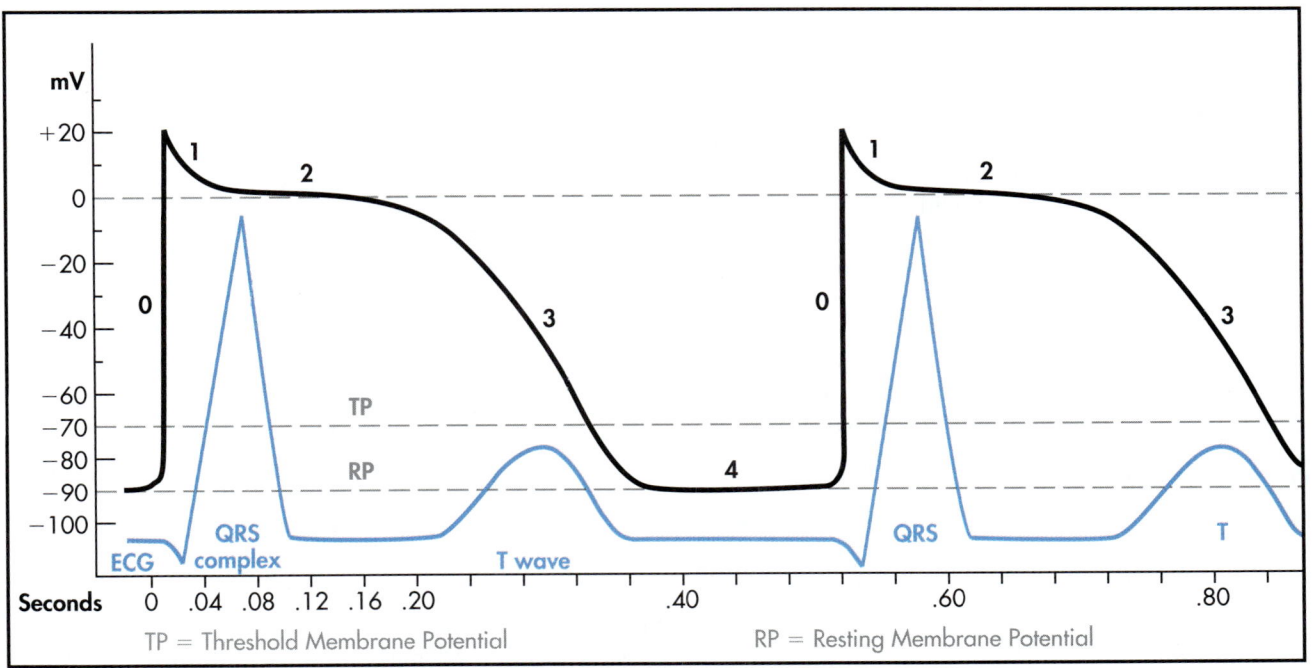

TP = Threshold Membrane Potential   RP = Resting Membrane Potential

FIGURE 22-10 Cardiac action potential of myocardial cells.

into the cell. As the positively charged ions flow into the cell, the inside of the cell becomes positively charged compared with the outside, leading to muscular contraction.

PHASE 1

Phase 1 is the early rapid repolarization phase. During this phase, the fast sodium channels close, the flow of sodium into the cell stops, and potassium continues to be lost from the cell. This results in a decrease in the number of positive electrical charges inside the cell and a drop in the membrane potential. This returns the cell membrane to its resting permeability state.

PHASE 2

Phase 2 (the plateau phase) is the prolonged phase of repolarization of the action potential. During this phase, calcium enters the myocardial cells. This triggers a large secondary release of calcium from intracellular storage sites and initiates contraction. Calcium slowly enters the cell through the slow calcium channels. At the same time, potassium continues to leave the cell. The inward calcium current maintains the cell in a prolonged depolarization state. This allows time for completion of one muscle contraction before another depolarization begins. This phase also stimulates the release of intracellular stores of calcium and aids in the contraction process.

PHASE 3

Phase 3 is the terminal phase of rapid repolarization. It results in the inside of the cell becoming negatively charged. The membrane potential also returns to its resting state. This phase is initiated by closing of the slow calcium channels and by an increase in permeability with an outflow of potassium. Repolarization is completed by the end of this phase.

PHASE 4

Phase 4 represents the period between action potentials, when the membrane has returned to its resting membrane potential. During this phase, the inside of the cell is negatively charged with respect to the outside. However, the cell still has an excess of sodium inside and an excess of potassium outside. This activates the sodium-potassium exchange pump. The excess sodium is transported out of the cell, and the potassium is transported back into the cell. During phase 4, pacemaker cells have a slow depolarization from their most negative membrane potential to a level at which threshold is reached, and phase 0 begins all over again.

Refractory Period of Cardiac Muscle

As does all excitable tissue, cardiac muscle has a **refractory period,** or resting period, in which cells are incapable of repeating a particular action. The refractory period can be further defined in two ways:

- The **absolute refractory period,** in which the cardiac muscle cell cannot respond to any stimulation, regardless of how long the stimulus is applied

- The **relative refractory period,** in which the cardiac muscle cell is more difficult than normal to excite, but the cell still can be stimulated

The refractory period ensures that the cardiac muscle is fully relaxed before another contraction begins. The refractory period of the ventricles lasts about as long as that of the action potential. The refractory period of the atrial muscle is much shorter than that of the ventricles. This allows the rate of atrial contraction to be much faster than that of the ventricles. If the depolarization phase of cardiac muscle is prolonged, the refractory period also is prolonged (Figure 22-11).

CRITICAL THINKING
How are the relative and absolute refractory periods of the heart similar to the flushing mechanism of your toilet?

ELECTRICAL CONDUCTION SYSTEM OF THE HEART

The conduction system of the heart is composed of two nodes and a conducting branch (Figure 22-12). The two nodes are located in the walls of the right atrium. They are named according to their location. The **sinoatrial node** (SA node) is medial to the opening of the superior vena cava. The **atrioventricular node** (AV node) is medial to the right atrioventricular valve. The AV node and the **bundle of His** form the **atrioventricular junction.** The AV junction serves as the only electrical link between the atria and ventricles in a normal heart. The bundle of His passes

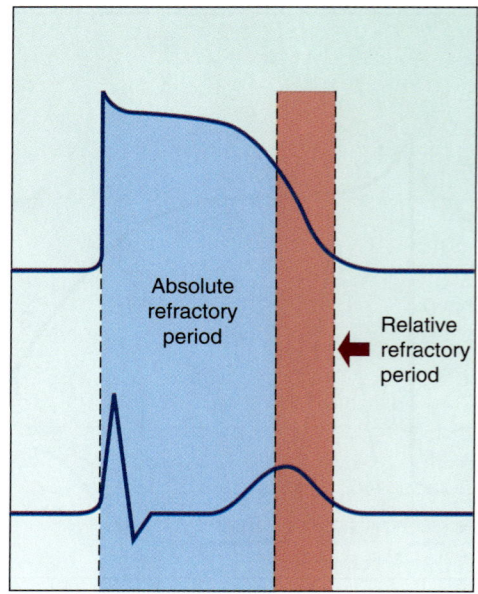

FIGURE 22-11 Absolute and relative refractory periods correlated with the cardiac muscle's action potential and with an ECG tracing. (Urden LD, Stacy KM, Lough ME: *Critical care nursing: diagnosis and management,* ed 6, St Louis, 2009, Mosby.)

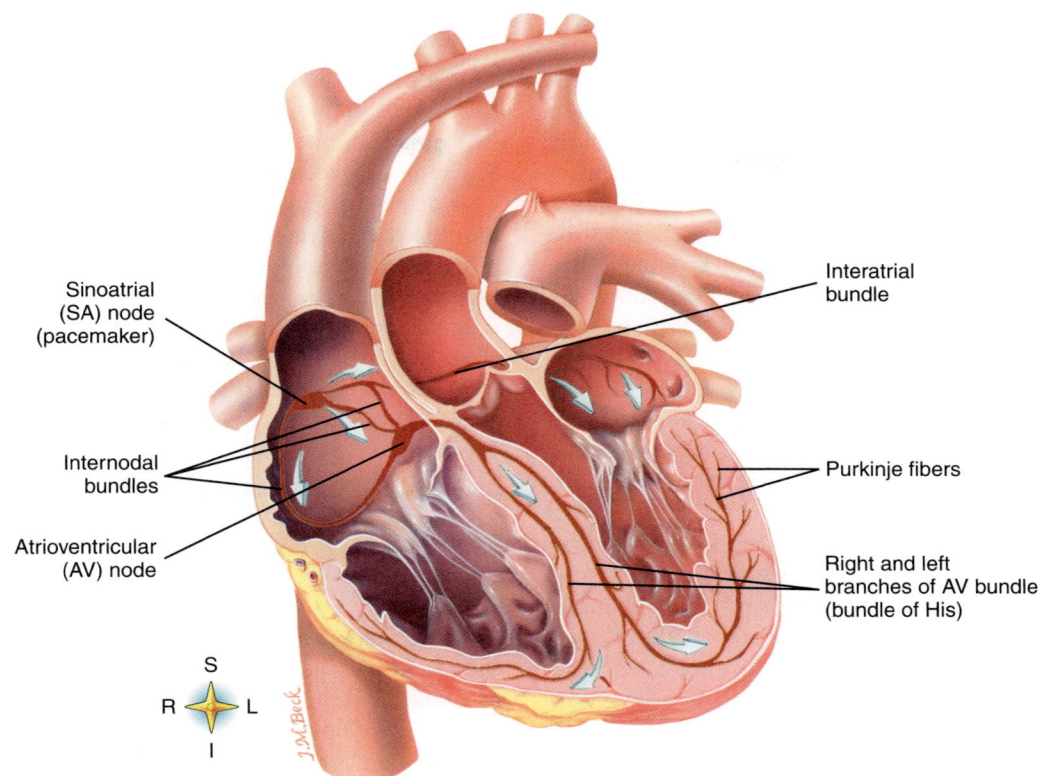

FIGURE 22-12 Conduction system of the heart. Impulses *(arrows)* travel across the wall of the right atrium from the sinoatrial node to the atrioventricular node. The atrioventricular bundle extends from the atrioventricular node through the fibrous skeleton and into the intervertebral septum, where it divides into right and left bundle branches. The bundle branches descend to the apex of the ventricle and then branch repeatedly for distribution throughout the ventricular walls.

through a small opening in the heart and reaches the **interventricular septum.** There the bundle of His divides into the **right bundle branch** and the **left bundle branch.** The left bundle branch then subdivides into the anterior-superior and posterior-inferior fascicles. These structures provide pathways for impulse conduction. A third fascicle of the left bundle branch also innervates the interventricular septum and the base of the heart.

The right and left bundle branches extend beneath the endocardium on either side of the septum to the apical portions of the right and left ventricles. The bundle branches subdivide into smaller branches. The smallest branches are called **Purkinje fibers.** The terminal Purkinje fibers spread electrical impulses from cell to cell through the myocardial fibers. This results in contraction of the heart muscle. The rapid conduction along these fibers causes depolarization of all right and left ventricular cells. These cells contract at more or less the same time, ensuring a single, coordinated contraction.

Pacemaker Activity

In skeletal and most smooth muscle, the individual cells contract only in response to hormones or nerve impulses from the central nervous system. However, unlike most other muscle cells, cardiac fibers have specialized cells known as *pacemaker cells*. These cells can generate electrical impulses spontaneously (**automaticity**). Pacemaker cells can depolarize in a repetitive manner. This rhythmic activity occurs because these tissues do not have a stable resting membrane potential (RMP). Instead, the RMP gradually decreases from its maximum repolarization potential. This continues until the RMP reaches a critical threshold, leading to depolarization. Sometimes the SA node may fail to generate an electrical impulse. If this occurs, other pacemaker cells take over. These pacemaker cells are capable of spontaneous depolarization and subsequent spread of an action potential. However, their rate is usually slower.

Sequence of Excitation in Cardiac Muscle

Under normal conditions, the chief pacemaker of the heart is the SA node. This is because the SA node reaches its threshold for depolarization more quickly than other pacemaker cells. The rapid rate of the SA node normally prevents the discharge of slower pacemakers from becoming dominant. If impulses from the SA node do not develop normally, however, the next pacemaker to reach its threshold level would take over the pacemaker duties.

Because of automaticity, cardiac cells can act as a "failsafe" means of initiating electrical impulses. The backup cells *(intrinsic pacemakers)* are arranged in cascade fashion: the farther from the SA node, the slower the intrinsic firing rate. In order, the location of cells with pacemaker capabilities and the rates of spontaneous discharge are the SA node (60 to 100 discharges/minute); AV junctional tissue (40 to 60 discharges/minute); and the ventricles, including the bundle branches and Purkinje fibers (20 to 40 discharges/minute) (Figure 22-13).

From the SA node the excitation spreads throughout the right atrium. This is made possible through four conduction tracks that make up the atrial conduction system: the AV node, *Bachmann's bundle* (in the left atrium), *Wenckebach's tract* (in the middle internodal tract), and *Thorel's tract* (in the posterior internodal tract). Through these tracts, impulses travel directly from the right to the left atrium and to the base of the right atrium. This results in virtually simultaneous contraction of the two atria. About 0.04 second is required for the impulse of the SA node to spread to the AV node. From there, propagation of the action potentials in the AV node is slow compared with the rate in the rest of the conducting system. As a result, a delay of 0.11 second occurs from the time the action potentials reach the AV node until they pass to the AV bundle. The total delay of 0.15 second allows atrial contraction to be completed before ventricular contraction begins.

After leaving the AV node, the impulse picks up speed. It travels rapidly through the bundle of His and the left and right bundle branches. The action potential passes quickly through the individual Purkinje fibers. The impulse ends in near simultaneous stimulation and contraction of the left and right ventricles. Ventricular contraction begins at the apex. Once stimulated, the special arrangement of muscle layers in the wall of the heart produces a wringing action that proceeds toward the base of the heart.

Autonomic Nervous System Effects on Pacemaker Cells

The effects of autonomic nervous system stimulation on the heart rate are mediated by acetylcholine and norepinephrine. Acetylcholine causes the cell membrane of the SA node to become more permeable to potassium ions. This delays the pacemaker in reaching threshold and thus reduces the heart rate. Parasympathetic effects also may result from stimulation of the cardiac branch of the vagus nerve, causing the heart rate to slow. An example of vagal stimulation is carotid sinus massage, described later in this chapter. Excessive vagal stimulation may result in **asystole** (the absence of electrical and mechanical activity in the heart). This is why asystole sometimes is referred to as the "ultimate bradycardia."

> **CRITICAL THINKING**
> What else can cause vagal stimulation?

Norepinephrine increases the heart rate by increasing the rate of depolarization. The result is an increase in the pacemaker discharge rate in the SA node. Norepinephrine increases the flow of potassium and calcium ions into the cell during depolarization of the action potential. As a result, sympathetic stimulation leads to an increase in the heart rate. The force of cardiac contractions also increases.

Mechanisms of Ectopic Electrical Impulse Formation

When the heart contracts as a result of stimulation by cells other than those in the SA node, the contraction is known as an ectopic beat. These isolated events sometimes are called *premature beats* because they occur early in the cycle, before the SA node normally would discharge. The new pacemaker is called an **ectopic focus**. Depending on the location of the ectopic focus, these premature complexes or contractions may be of atrial origin (premature atrial contractions [PACs]), junctional origin (**premature junctional complexes [PJCs]**), or ventricular origin (premature ventricular contractions [PVCs]). The ectopic focus may be intermittent or may be sustained and may assume the pacemaker duties of the heart (i.e., the pacemaker site that fires the fastest controls the heart).

The two basic ways ectopic impulses are generated are by enhanced automaticity and reentry.

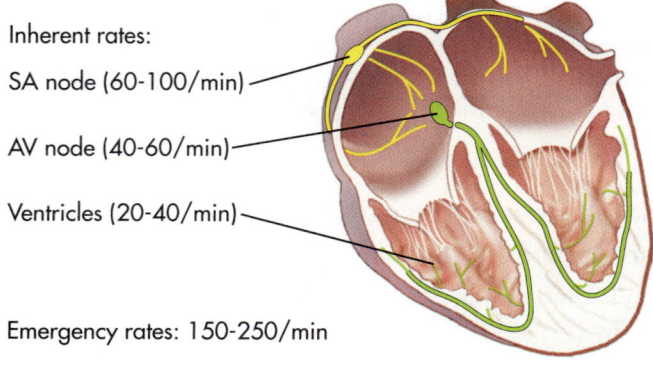

Inherent rates:

SA node (60-100/min)

AV node (40-60/min)

Ventricles (20-40/min)

Emergency rates: 150-250/min

FIGURE 22-13 Intrinsic pacemakers in the atria, atrioventricular node, and ventricles can discharge at their own inherent rate when normal pacemaking fails.

> **NOTE**
> An *ectopic beat* should not be confused with *aberrant conduction* (aberrancy). An ectopic beat is one that originates in the wrong part of the heart (away from normal). Aberrancy is abnormal conduction; that is, cardiac conduction through pathways that do not normally conduct impulses (particularly through ventricular tissue). **Aberration** can result from a number of causes, including premature atrial complexes, blocks in the bundle branches, and electrolyte abnormalities.

ENHANCED AUTOMATICITY

Enhanced automaticity is caused by an acceleration in depolarization. This commonly results from an abnormally high leakage of sodium ions into the cells, causing the cells to reach threshold prematurely. As a result, the rate of electrical impulse formation in potential pacemakers increases beyond their inherent rate.

Enhanced automaticity is responsible for **dysrhythmias** (abnormal rhythms) in Purkinje fibers and other myocardial cells. This condition may occur after the release of excess catecholamines (i.e., norepinephrine and epinephrine) or as result of digitalis toxicity, hypoxia, hypercapnia, myocardial ischemia or infarction, increased venous return (preload), hypokalemia or other electrolyte abnormalities, or *atropine* administration.

REENTRY

Reentry is the reactivation of myocardial tissue for the second or subsequent time by the same impulse (Figure 22-14). Reentry occurs when the progression of an electrical impulse is delayed or blocked (or both) in one or more segments of the electrical conduction system of the heart. A delayed or blocked impulse can enter cardiac cells that have just become repolarized. Reentry may produce single or repetitive ectopic beats. Reentry dysrhythmias can occur in the SA node, atria, AV junction, bundle branches, or Purkinje fibers. Reentry is the most common mechanism for producing ectopic beats, including cases of PVCs, ventricular tachycardia, ventricular fibrillation, atrial fibrillation, atrial flutter, and paroxysmal supraventricular tachycardia. These and other dysrhythmias are described later in the chapter.

The reentry mechanism requires that at some point, conduction through the heart must take parallel pathways. Each pathway has different conduction speeds and refractory characteristics. A premature impulse, for example, may find one branch of a conducting pathway still refractory from the passage of the last normal impulse. If this occurs, the impulse may pass (somewhat slowly) along a parallel conducting pathway. By the time the impulse reaches the previously blocked pathway, the blocked pathway may have had time to recover its ability to conduct. If the two parallel paths connect at an area of excitable myocardial tissue, the depolarization process from the slower path may enter the now repolarized tissue. This can give rise to a new impulse spawned from the original impulse. Common causes of delayed or blocked electrical impulses include myocardial ischemia, certain drugs, and hyperkalemia.

SECTION THREE
Electrocardiogram Monitoring

An **electrocardiogram** (ECG) is a graphic representation of the electrical activity of the heart. It is produced by the electrical events in the atria and ventricles and is an important diagnostic tool. This graphic reading can help identify a number of cardiac abnormalities. These include abnormal heart rates and rhythms, abnormal conduction pathways, hypertrophy or atrophy of portions of the heart, and the approximate location of ischemic or infarcted cardiac muscle.

Evaluation of the ECG requires a systematic approach. The paramedic analyzes the electrocardiogram and then relates it to the clinical assessment of the patient. The ECG tracing is only a reflection of the electrical activity of the heart. It does not provide information on mechanical events such as force of contraction or blood pressure.

> **CRITICAL THINKING**
> Aside from blood pressure, how do you evaluate the mechanical activity of the heart?

BASIC CONCEPTS OF ELECTROCARDIOGRAM MONITORING

The summation of all the action potentials transmitted through the heart during the cardiac cycle can be measured on the surface of the body. This measurement is obtained by applying electrodes connected to an ECG machine to the patient's skin. The voltage changes are fed to the machine, amplified, and displayed visually on the oscilloscope screen, graphically on ECG paper, or both. The voltage may be positive (seen as an upward deflection on the ECG tracing);

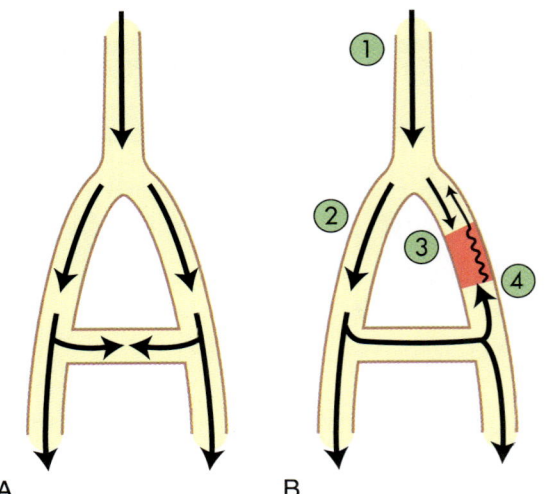

FIGURE 22-14 Reentry in terminal Purkinje fibers. **A,** Conduction through normal Purkinje fibers. The conduction velocity is uniform. **B,** Conduction through a severely depressed segment of terminal Purkinje fibers. The impulse *(1)* travels normally through normal tissue *(2)* and is blocked at the severely depressed tissue *(3)* but returns, with delay, through this tissue from the opposite direction *(4)*.

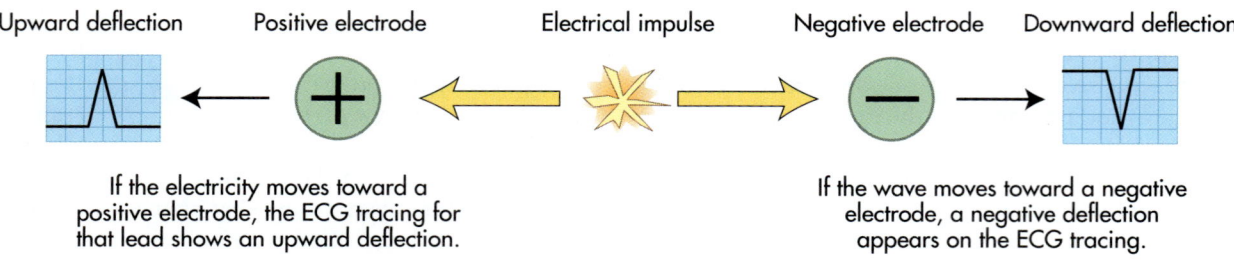

Upward deflection   **Positive electrode**   **Electrical impulse**   **Negative electrode**   **Downward deflection**

If the electricity moves toward a positive electrode, the ECG tracing for that lead shows an upward deflection.

If the wave moves toward a negative electrode, a negative deflection appears on the ECG tracing.

FIGURE 22-15 Rule of electrical flow.

negative (seen as a downward deflection on the ECG tracing); or isoelectric, when no electrical current is detected (seen as a straight baseline on the ECG tracing) (Figure 22-15).

Electrocardiograph Leads

Electrocardiograph machines offer many views of the electrical activity of the heart. They do this by monitoring voltage changes between the electrodes *(leads)* applied to the body. A modern ECG views the electrical activity of the heart from 12 leads: three standard limb leads; three augmented limb leads, and six precordial (chest) leads. The standard limb leads are I, II, III. The augmented limb leads are aV_R, aV_L, and aV_F. The precordial leads are V_1 through V_6. Each lead assesses the electrical activity of the heart from a slightly different view and produces different ECG tracings (Table 22-1).

> **NOTE**
>
> *The various views of electrical activity of the heart provided by the ECG are always from the perspective of the positive electrode.* If the net force of electrical activity moves toward the positive electrode, the waveform seen on the ECG is "up." If the net force of electrical activity moves away from the positive electrode, the waveform seen on the ECG is "down."

STANDARD LIMB LEADS

Standard limb leads are **bipolar leads.** That means they use two electrodes of opposite polarity (one pole is positive, the other, negative) to form the lead. Standard limb leads record the difference in electrical potential between the left arm (+), the right arm (−), and the left leg (−) electrodes. Lead I records the difference in electrical potential between the left arm (+) and right arm (−) electrodes. Lead II records the difference in electrical potential between the left leg (+) and right arm (−) electrodes. Lead III records the difference in electrical potential between the left leg (+) and left arm (−) electrodes. Imaginary lines *(axes)* join the positive and negative electrodes of each lead, forming a straight line between the positive and negative poles. These lines form an equilateral triangle with the heart at the center *(Einthoven's triangle)* (Figure 22-16).

The electrodes of the standard bipolar leads are placed on the following areas of the body:

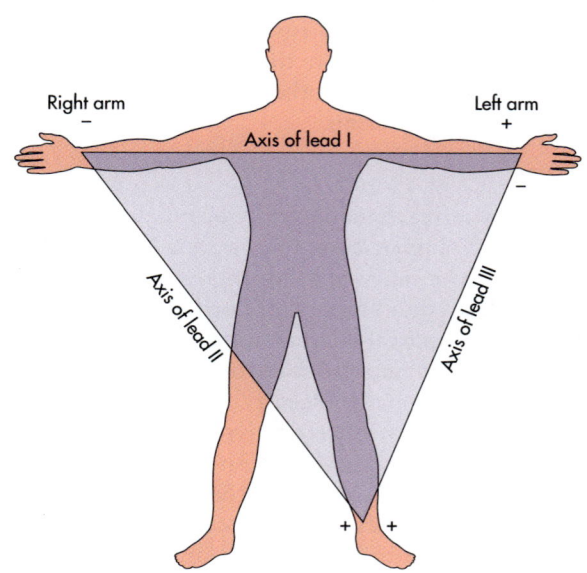

FIGURE 22-16 Leads I, II, and III make up the standard limb leads. An imaginary line joining the positive and negative electrodes of a lead is called the *axis* of the lead. The axes of these three limb leads form an equilateral triangle with the heart at the center (Einthoven's triangle).

TABLE 22-1 Comparison of Various Leads

Leads	Type	Polarity
I, II, III	Limb leads	Bipolar
aV_R, aV_L, aV_F	Limb leads	Unipolar
V_1-V_6	Chest leads	Unipolar

From Phalen T: *The 12-lead ECG in acute myocardial infarction,* St Louis, 1996, Mosby.

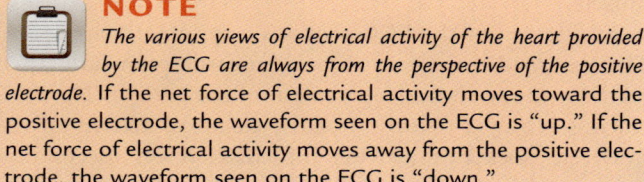

Lead	Positive electrode	Negative electrode
I	Left arm	Right arm
II	Left leg	Right arm
III	Left leg	Left arm

AUGMENTED LIMB LEADS

As do standard limb leads, **augmented limb leads** record the difference in electrical potential. However, unlike the standard limb leads, which are bipolar leads, the augmented limb leads are **unipolar leads.** This means that they have one electrode for a positive pole, but they have no distinct negative pole. The negative pole of the augmented limb leads is made by combining two of the negative electrodes. (Augmented limb leads use three electrodes to provide their view of the heart.) Augmented limb leads "augment," or magnify, the voltage of the positive lead (which usually is small). This increases the size of the complexes seen on the ECG. Augmented limb leads use the same set of electrodes as the standard limb leads and are placed on the following areas of the body:

Lead	Positive electrode	Negative electrode
aV$_L$	Left arm	Right arm, left leg
aV$_R$	Right arm	Left arm, left leg
aV$_F$	Left leg	Right arm, left arm

The aV$_R$, aV$_L$, and aV$_F$ leads intersect at angles different from those of the standard limb leads and produce three other intersecting lines of reference. When these lines of reference are combined with the lines of reference of standard limb leads, they form six lines of reference known as the **hexaxial reference system** (Figure 22-17). The hexaxial reference system is important for advanced ECG interpretation, described later in this chapter.

CRITICAL THINKING
Why is aV$_R$ seldom used in ECG analysis? What view of the heart does it provide?

PRECORDIAL LEADS

The six **precordial leads,** or *chest leads,* are unipolar leads that record the electrical activity of the heart in the horizontal plane. These leads, which are used in 12-lead ECG monitoring, measure the amplitude of the heart's electrical current. The precordial leads are projected through the anterior chest wall (through the AV node) toward the patient's back. The projection of the leads separates the body into upper and lower halves, providing the transverse or horizontal plane (Figure 22-18). The electrodes on the patient's chest are considered positive, but they are considered negative posteriorly (i.e., the patient's chest is positive; the patient's back is negative). The chest leads are numbered V$_1$ to V$_6$.

When properly positioned on the chest, the chest leads surround the heart from the right to left side (Figure 22-19). Leads V$_1$ and V$_2$ are positioned over the right side of the heart and look at the septum; V$_5$ and V$_6$ over the left side of the heart and look at the lateral wall of the

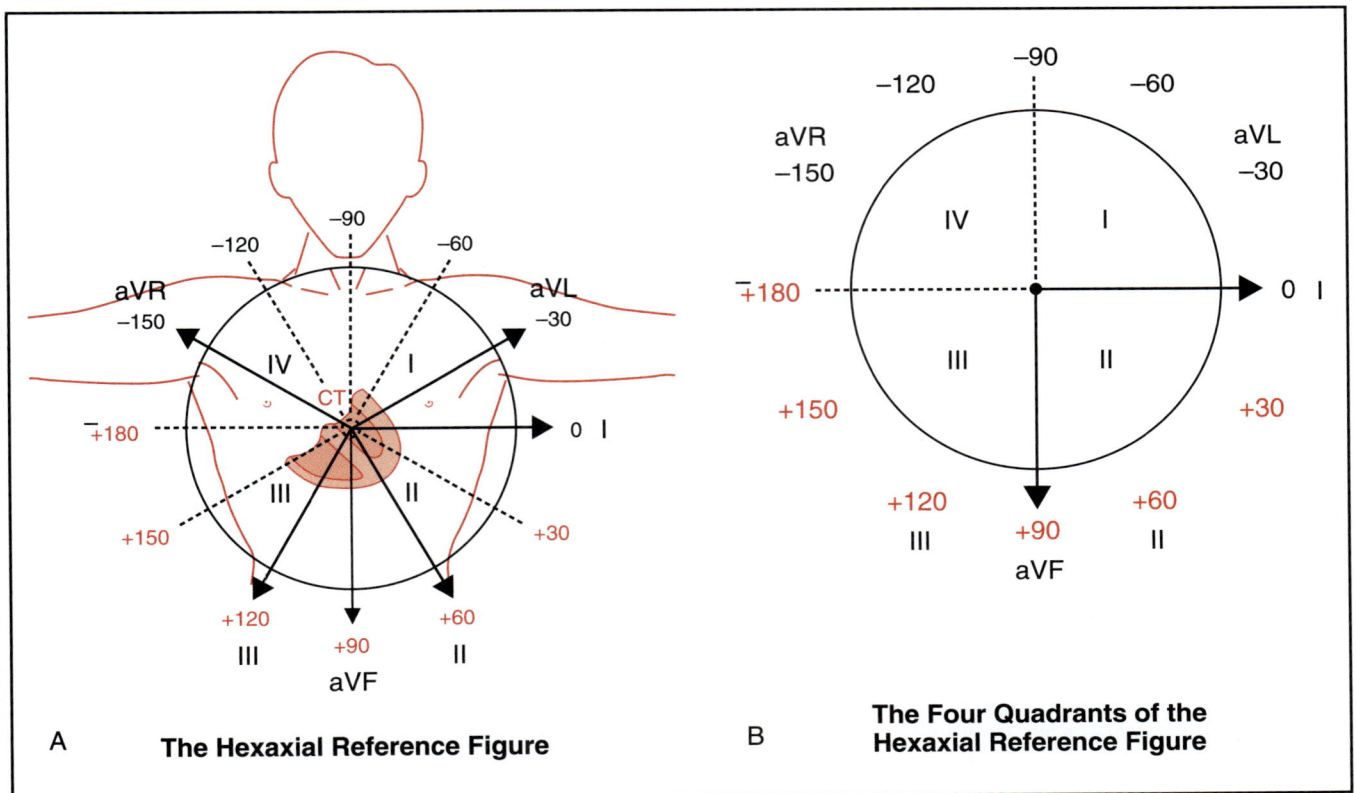

FIGURE 22-17 A, The hexaxial reference figure. **B,** The four quadrants of the hexaxial reference figure. (Wesley K: *Huszar's basic dysrhythmias and acute coronary syndromes: interpretation and management,* ed 4, St Louis, 2010, Mosby.)

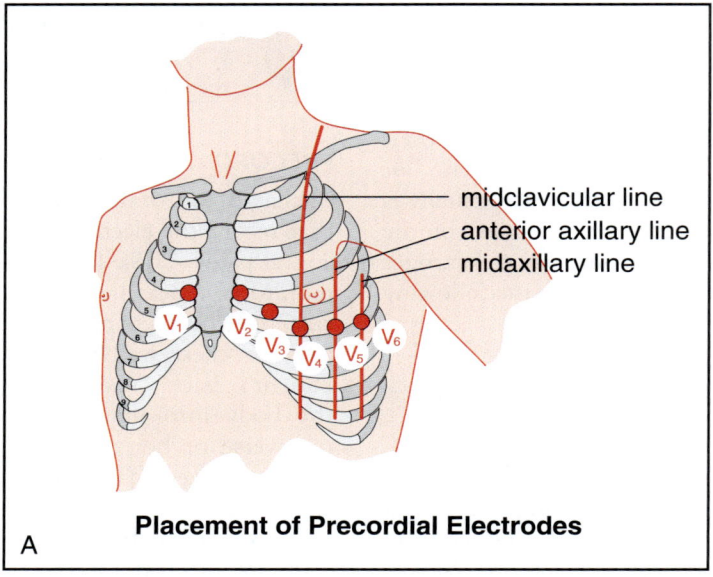

Placement of Precordial Electrodes

A

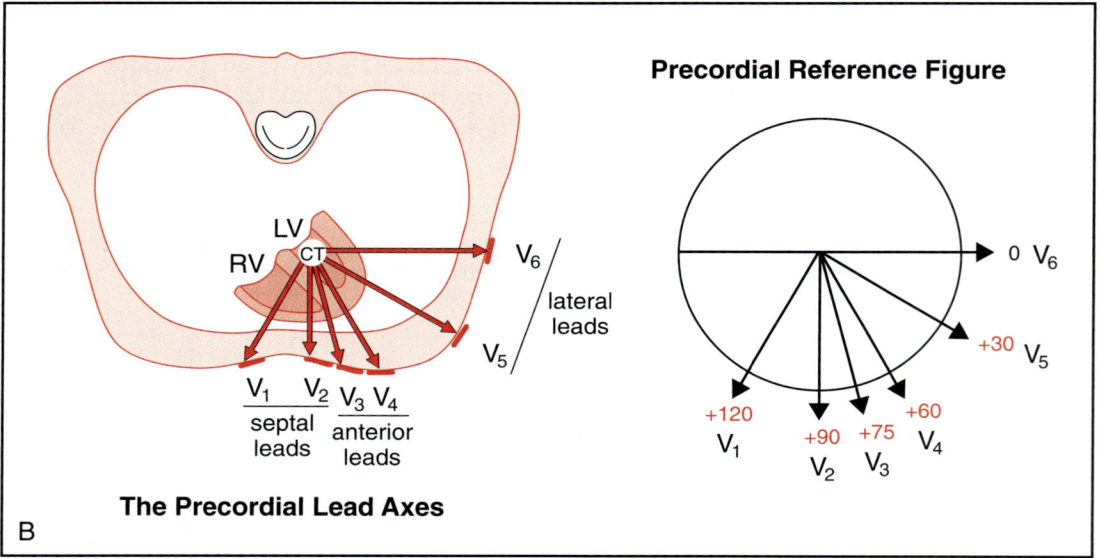

The Precordial Lead Axes

B

FIGURE 22-18 A, Placement of the precordial electrodes. **B,** Precordial lead axes and reference figure. (Wesley K: *Huszar's basic dysrhythmias and acute coronary syndromes: interpretation and management,* ed 4, St Louis, 2010, Mosby.)

left ventricle; and V_3 and V_4 over the interventricular septum (right and left ventricle, AV bundle, and right and left bundle branches). These leads look at the anterior wall of the left ventricle.

The precordial leads are placed on the chest in reference to the thoracic landmarks. Proper placement of the chest leads at specific intercostal spaces is essential for an accurate reading. The following is one method of locating the appropriate intercostal spaces[4] (Figure 22-19):

1. Locate the jugular notch and move downward until the sternal angle is found.
2. Follow the articulation to the right sternal border to locate the second rib. Just below the second rib is the second intercostal space.

3. Move down two intercostal spaces and position the V_1 electrode in the fourth intercostal space, just to the right of the patient's sternum.
4. Move across the sternum to the corresponding intercostal space and position V_2 to the left of the patient's sternum.
5. From V_2, palpate down one intercostal space and follow the fifth intercostal space to the midclavicular line to place the V_4 electrode.
6. Place lead V_3 midway between V_2 and V_4.
7. Place V_5 in the anterior axillary line in a straight line with V_4 (where the arm joins the chest).
8. Place V_6 in the midaxillary line, level with V_4 and V_5. (It may be more convenient to place V_6 first and then

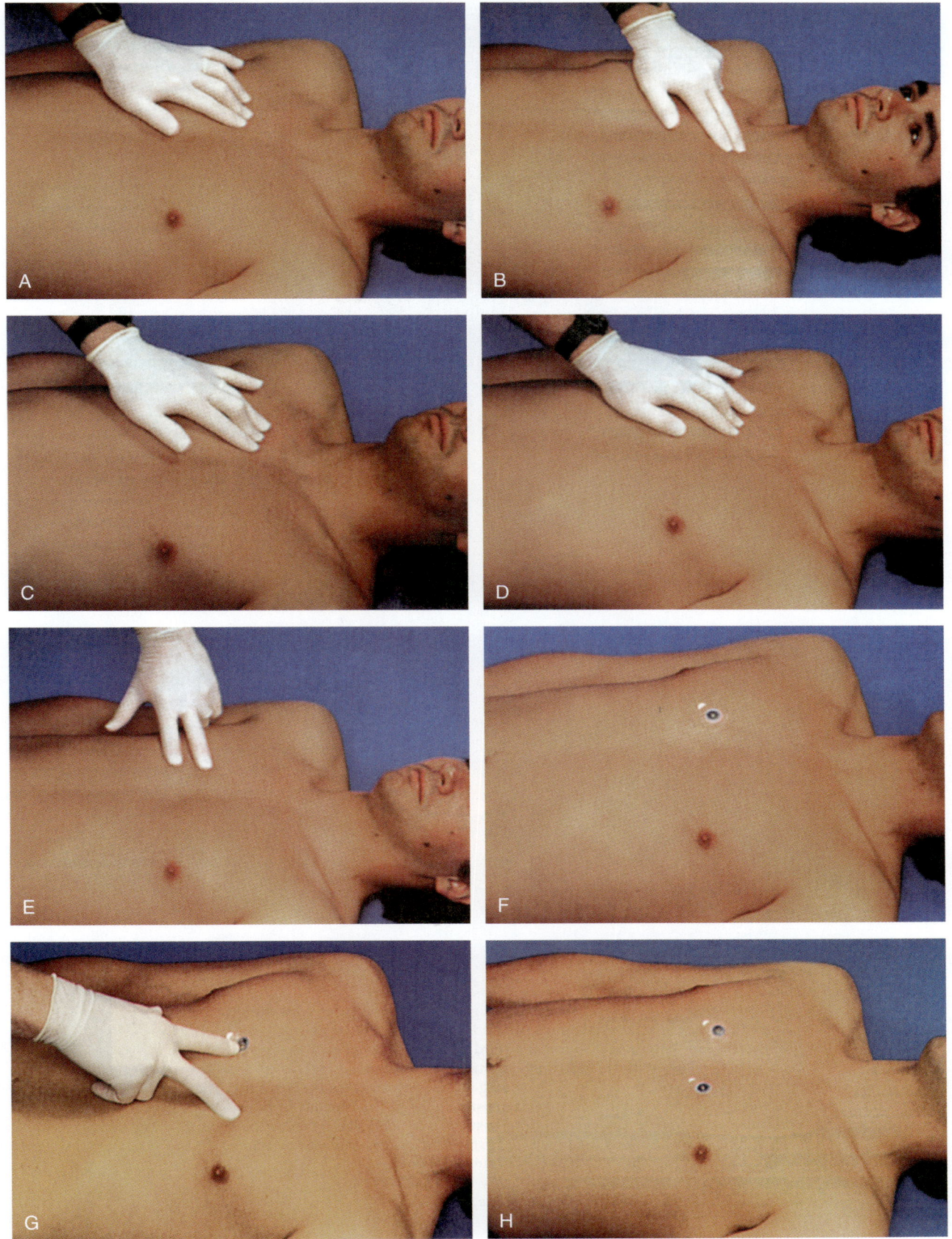

Continued on next page

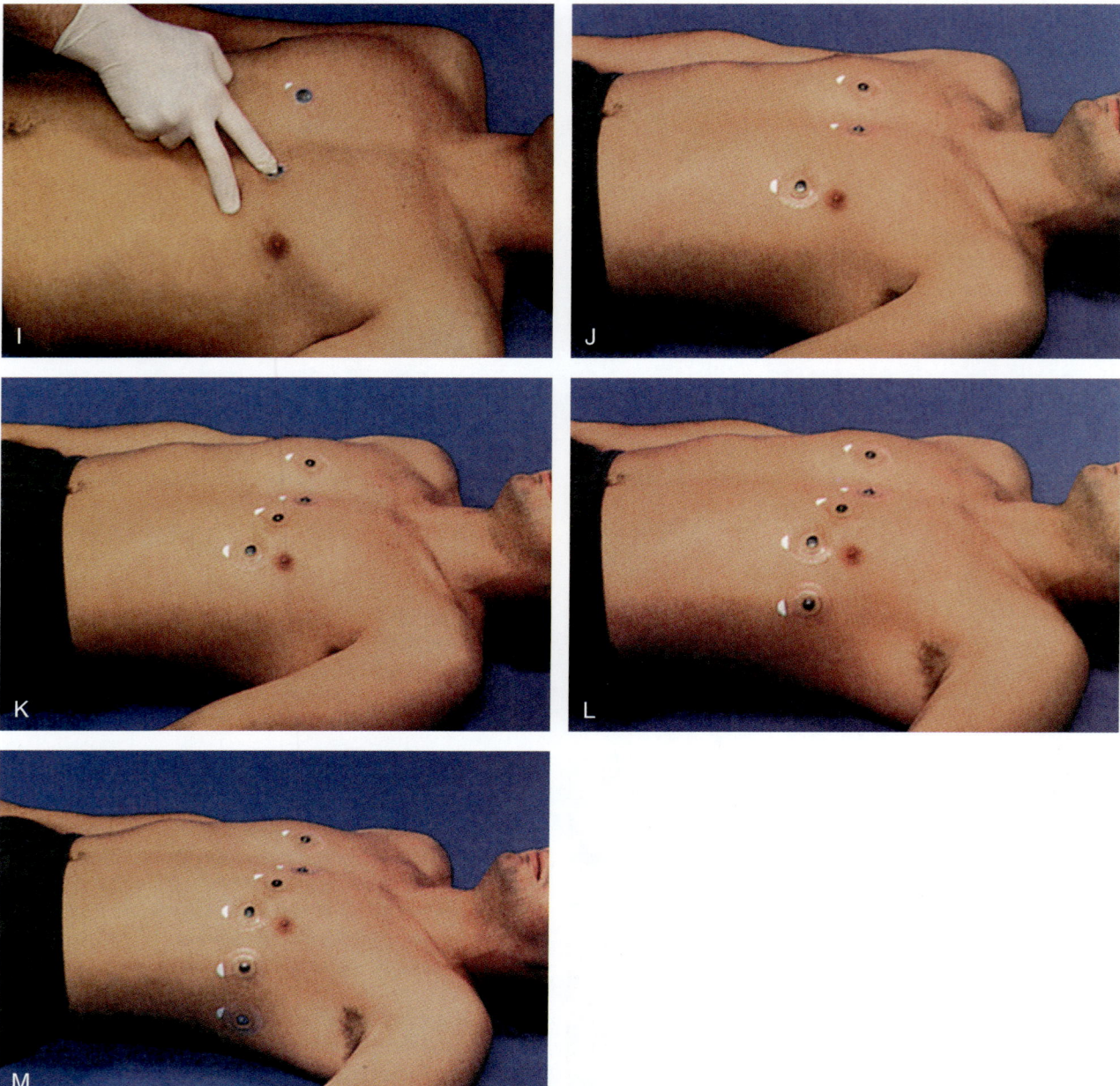

FIGURE 22-19 Proper chest lead placement.
A ▪ Locate the jugular notch.
B ▪ Palpate for the angle of Louis.
C ▪ Follow the angle of Louis to the patient's right until it articulates with the second rib.
D ▪ Locate the second intercostal space (immediately below the second rib).
E ▪ From the second intercostal space, the third and fourth intercostal spaces can be found.
F ▪ Lead V_1 is positioned in the fourth intercostal space just to the right of the sternum.
G ▪ From the V_1 position, find the corresponding intercostal space on the left side of the sternum.
H ▪ Place the V_2 electrode in the fourth intercostal space just to the left of the sternum.
I ▪ From the V_2 position, locate the fifth intercostal space and follow it to the midclavicular line.
J ▪ Position the V_4 electrode in the fifth intercostal space in the midclavicular line.
K ▪ Lead V_3 is positioned halfway between V_2 and V_4.
L ▪ Lead V_5 is positioned in the anterior axillary line, level with V_4.
M ▪ Lead V_6 is positioned in the midaxillary line, level with V_4.

V_5.) For women, place the V_4 to V_6 electrodes under the left breast to avoid any errors in the ECG tracing that may occur from breast tissue. Lift the breast away using the back of the hand (Figure 22-19).

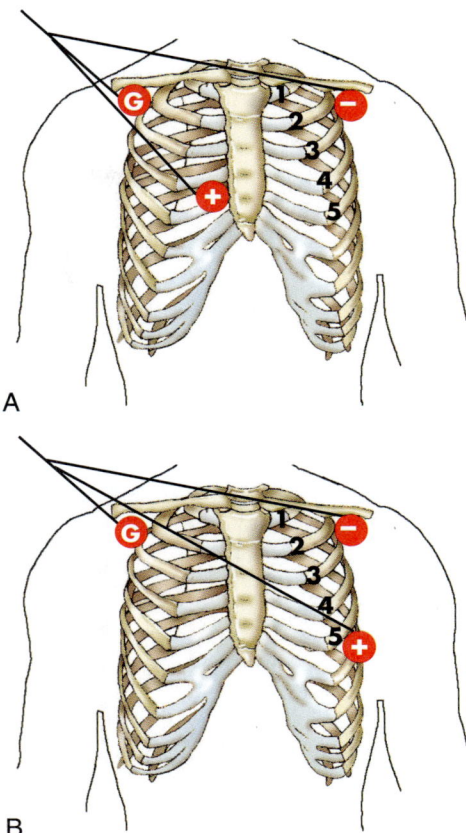

A

B

FIGURE 22-20 Monitor lead placement for MCL_1 **(A)** and MCL_6 **(B).** (Goldberger A: *Treatment of cardiac emergencies,* ed 5, St Louis, 1990, Mosby.)

> **CRITICAL THINKING**
> Consider that your patient is female. You are performing a 12-lead ECG tracing. What measures can you take to reduce her potential discomfort or embarrassment?

> **DID YOU KNOW?**
> **Modified Lead Recording**
> Placement of the limb leads can be altered to mimic the precordial leads (V_1 to V_6). These leads are referred to as **modified chest leads** and become MCL_1 to MCL_6. Modified chest leads are useful for monitoring cardiac activity in the prehospital setting when 12-lead machines are not available (e.g., equipment failure, mass disasters). These leads may help distinguish between supraventricular tachycardia and ventricular tachycardia. They also can help detect conduction blocks in the bundle branches (described later in this chapter).
> When MCL_1 is viewed, the positive electrode is placed in the V_1 position. (This is the fourth intercostal space, just to the right of the patient's sternum.) The negative electrode is placed anteriorly, just below the lateral end of the left clavicle. Electrical activity in MCL_6 is observed by placing the positive electrode on the left midaxillary line at the level of the fifth intercostal space (as for lead V_6). The negative electrode is placed anteriorly, just below the left shoulder (see Figure 22-20).

Routine Electrocardiogram Monitoring

Routine monitoring of cardiac rhythm in the prehospital setting, emergency department (ED), or coronary care unit usually is obtained in lead II or MCL_1. These are the best leads to monitor for dysrhythmias because of their ability to display P waves (atrial depolarization) on the ECG tracing. A good deal of information can be gathered from a single monitoring lead, and in many cases cardiac monitoring by a single lead is sufficient. For example, monitoring a single lead can determine how fast the heart is beating and how regular the heartbeat is. The paramedic also can determine how long conduction lasts in different parts of the heart. Single-lead monitoring does have limitations and may fail to reveal various cardiac abnormalities. In most EMS systems that provide advanced life support, the 12-lead ECG is the standard for monitoring patients with chest pain of cardiac origin.

> **CRITICAL THINKING**
> What effect does improper lead placement have on the view of the heart and the analysis of the ECG tracing?

Application of Monitoring Electrodes

The most commonly used electrodes for continuous ECG monitoring are pregelled, stick-on disks. These disks can be applied easily to the chest wall. The paramedic should observe the following guidelines to minimize artifacts in the signal and to make effective contact between the electrode and the skin:

> **CRITICAL THINKING**
> Why should alcohol or benzoin not be used under defibrillator pads?

1. Choose an appropriate area of skin, avoiding large muscle masses and large amounts of hair, which may prevent the electrode from lying flat against the skin.
2. Cleanse the area with alcohol to remove dirt and body oil. When attaching electrodes to the extremities, use the inner surfaces of the arms and legs. If necessary, trim excess body hair before placing the electrodes. If the patient is extremely diaphoretic, use tincture of benzoin to help secure application or use diaphoretic electrodes.

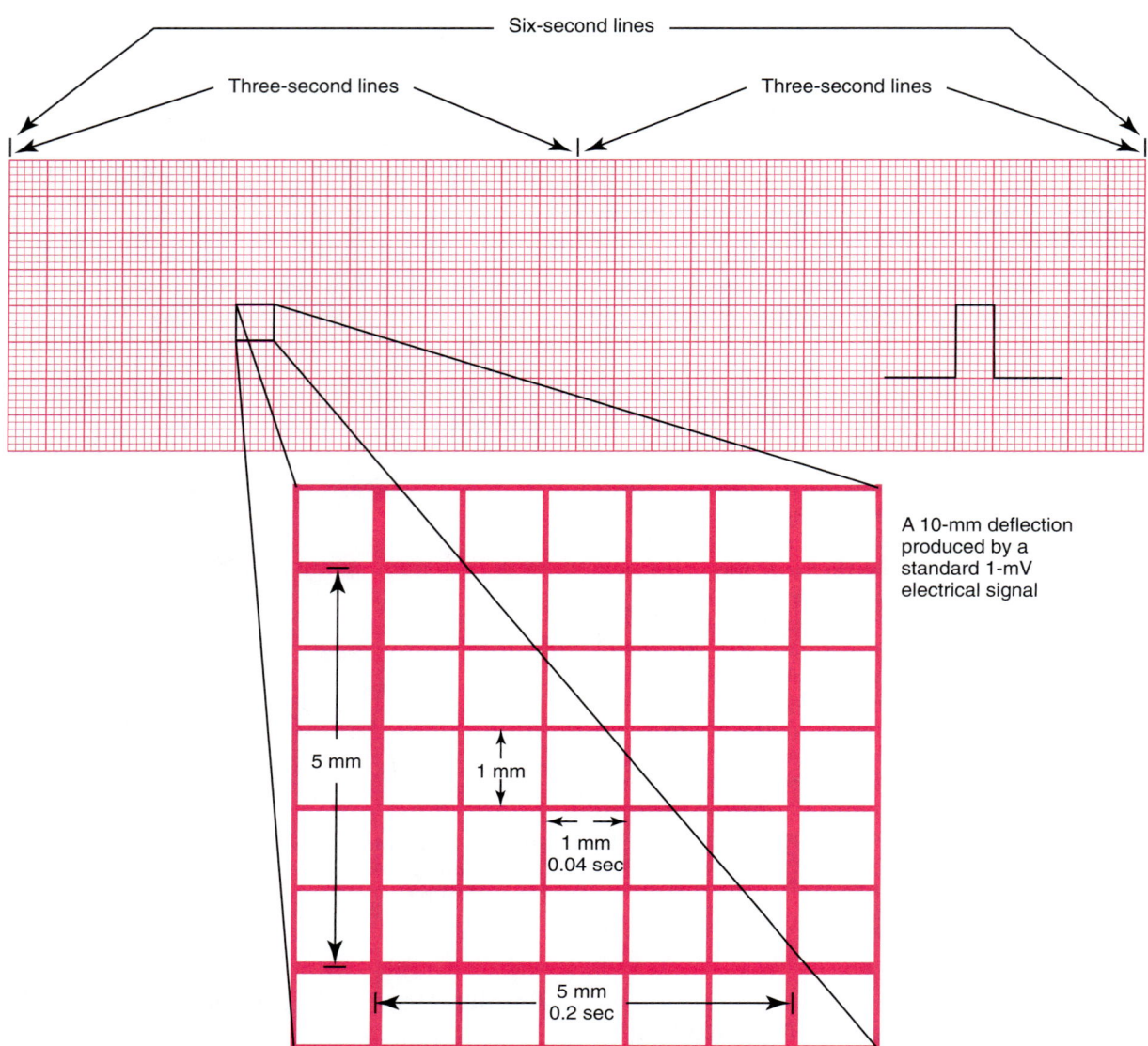

Six-second lines

Three-second lines

Three-second lines

A 10-mm deflection produced by a standard 1-mV electrical signal

5 mm

1 mm

1 mm
0.04 sec

5 mm
0.2 sec

FIGURE 22-21 Electrocardiogram graph paper.

3. Attach the electrodes to the prepared site.
4. Attach the ECG cables to the electrodes. Most cables are marked for right arm, left arm, and left leg application.
5. Turn on the ECG monitor and obtain a baseline tracing.

If the signal is poor, the paramedic should recheck the cable connections and the effectiveness of the patient's skin contact with the electrodes. Other common causes of a poor signal include body hair, dried conductive gel, poor electrode placement, and diaphoresis.

Electrocardiogram Graph Paper

The paper used in recording electrocardiograms is standardized to allow comparative analysis of an ECG wave. The graph paper is divided into squares 1 mm in height and width. The paper is divided further by darker lines every fifth square vertically and horizontally. Each large square is 5 mm high and 5 mm wide (Figure 22-21).

As the graph paper moves past the needle or pen of the ECG machine, it measures time and amplitude. Time is measured on the horizontal plane (side to side). When the ECG is recorded at the standard paper speed of 25 mm/second, each small square is equal to 1 mm (0.04 second) and each large square (the dark vertical lines) is equal to 5 mm (0.20 second). These squares measure the time it takes an electrical impulse to pass through a specific part of the heart.

Amplitude is measured on the vertical axis (top to bottom) of the graph paper. Each small square of the graph paper is equal to 0.1 mV. Each large square (five small squares) is equal to 0.5 mV. The sensitivity of the 12-lead ECG machine is standardized. When properly calibrated, a 1 mV electrical signal produces a 10 mm deflection (two large squares) on the ECG tracing. ECG machines equipped with calibration buttons should have a calibration curve placed at the beginning of the first tracing (generally a 1 mV burst, represented by a 10 mm "block" wave).

Time-interval markings are denoted by short vertical lines and usually are located on the top of the ECG graph paper. When the ECG is recorded at the standard paper speed of 25 mm/second, the distance between each short vertical line is 75 mm (3 seconds). Each 3-second interval contains 15 large squares (0.2 second multiplied by 15 squares equals 3 seconds). These markings are used as a method of heart rate calculation (i.e., counting the number of QRS complexes in 6 seconds and multiplying by 10).

RELATIONSHIP OF THE ELECTROCARDIOGRAM TO ELECTRICAL ACTIVITY

Each waveform seen on the oscilloscope or recorded on the ECG graph paper represents the conduction of an electrical impulse through a certain part of the heart. All waveforms begin and end at the isoelectric line. This line represents the absence of electrical activity in cardiac tissue. A deflection above the baseline is positive. It indicates an electrical flow toward the positive electrode. A deflection below the baseline is negative. It indicates an electrical flow away from the positive electrode.

The normal electrocardiogram consists of a P wave, QRS complex, and T wave. A U wave sometimes may be seen after the T wave. The **U wave** is thought to represent repolarization of the Purkinje fibers. It may also be associated with electrolyte abnormalities. If present, the U wave usually is a positive deflection. Other key parts of the ECG that should be evaluated include the P-R interval, ST segment, and Q-T interval. The combination of these waves represents a single heartbeat, or one complete cardiac cycle (Figure 22-22). The electrical events of the cardiac cycle are followed by their mechanical counterparts. The descriptions of ECG waveform components refer to those that would be seen in lead II monitoring (Box 22-3).

> **NOTE**
>
> A *segment* on an ECG is the region between two waves. For example, the PR segment begins at the end of the P wave and ends at the onset of the QRS complex (see Figure 22-23). An *interval* on an ECG includes one segment and one or more waves. For example, the P-R interval starts at the beginning of the P wave and ends at the onset of the QRS complex (see Figure 22-24).

P Wave

The **P wave** is the first positive (upward) deflection on the ECG. It represents atrial depolarization. It usually is rounded and precedes the QRS complex. The P wave begins with the first positive deflection from the baseline and ends at the point where the wave returns to the baseline. The duration of the P wave normally is 0.10 second or less, and its amplitude is 0.5 to 2.5 mm. The P wave usually is followed by a QRS complex. However, if conduction disturbances are present, a QRS complex does not always follow each P wave.

BOX 22-3 ECG Waves and Mechanical Counterparts

P wave: Atrial depolarization
QRS complex: Ventricular depolarization
T wave: Ventricular repolarization

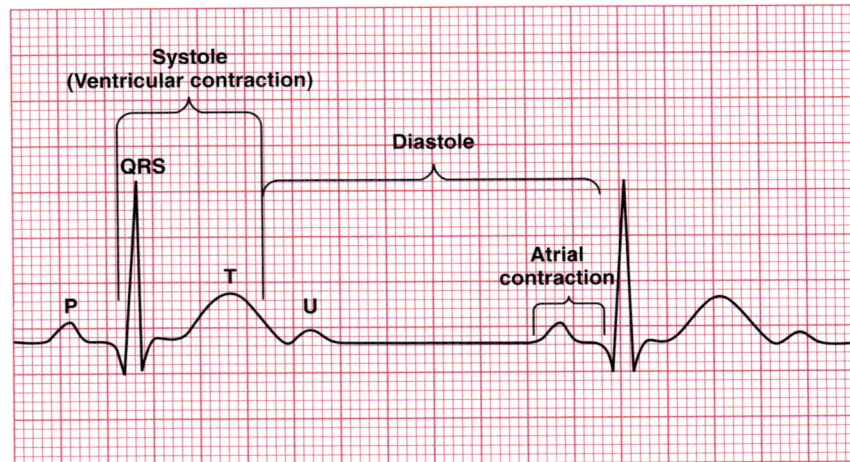

FIGURE 22-22 Summary of the electrical basis of the electrocardiogram.

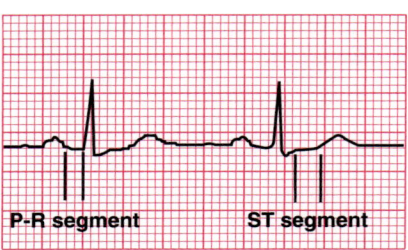

FIGURE 22-23 P-R segment and ST segment.

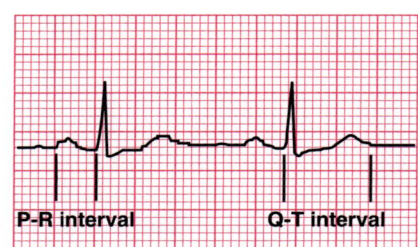

FIGURE 22-24 P-R interval and Q-T interval.

P-R Interval

The **P-R interval** is the time required for an electrical impulse to be conducted through the atria and the AV node up to the instant of ventricular depolarization. The P-R interval is measured from the beginning of the P wave to the beginning of the next deflection on the baseline (the onset of the QRS complex). The normal P-R interval is 0.12 to 0.20 second (three to five small squares on the graph paper). The P-R interval depends on the heart rate and the conduction characteristics of the AV node. When the heart rate is fast, the P-R interval normally is shorter than when the heart rate is slow. A normal P-R interval indicates that the electrical impulse has been conducted through the atria, AV node, and bundle of His normally and without delay.

QRS Complex

The **QRS complex** generally is composed of three individual waves: the Q, R, and S waves. The QRS complex begins at the point where the first wave of the complex deviates from the baseline. It ends where the last wave of the complex begins to flatten at, above, or below the baseline. The direction of the Q wave may be predominantly positive (upright), predominantly negative (inverted), or biphasic (partly positive, partly negative). A normal QRS complex is narrow and sharply pointed (when conduction is normal). Its duration generally is 0.08 to 0.10 second (two to two-and-a-half small squares on the graph paper) or less, and its amplitude normally varies from less than 5 mm to more than 15 mm.

The Q wave is the first negative (downward) deflection of the QRS complex on the ECG. However, it may not be present in all leads. The Q wave represents depolarization

of the interventricular septum or a pathological change. The R wave is the first positive deflection after the P wave. Subsequent positive deflections in the QRS complex that extend above the baseline and that are taller than the first R wave are called *R prime (R′)*, *R double prime (R″)*, and so on. The S wave is the negative deflection that follows the R wave. Subsequent negative deflections are called *S prime (S′)*, *S double prime (S″)*, and so on. Although only one Q wave may be seen in the QRS complex, more than one R wave and more than one S wave may be present. The R and S waves represent the sum of electrical forces resulting from depolarization of the right and left ventricles (Figure 22-25).

> ### CRITICAL THINKING
> What is the importance of a QRS complex duration of 0.12 second?

The QRS complex follows the P wave. The QRS complex marks the approximate beginning of mechanical contraction of the ventricles, which continues through the onset of the T wave. The QRS complex represents ventricular depolarization. This includes the conduction of an electrical impulse from the AV node through the bundle of His, Purkinje fibers, and the right and left bundle branches. This impulse results in ventricular depolarization.

ST Segment

The **ST segment** represents the early phase of repolarization of the right and left ventricles. It immediately follows the QRS complex and ends with the onset of the T wave. The point at which it takes off from the QRS complex is called the *J point*. In a normal ECG, the ST segment begins at baseline and has a slight upward slope.

The position of the ST segment commonly is judged as normal or abnormal using the baseline of the P-R or T-P interval as a reference. Deviations above this baseline are referred to as *ST segment elevation*. Deviations below baseline are referred to as *ST segment depression* (Figure 22-26). Certain conditions can cause depression or elevation of the P-R interval, affecting the reference for ST segment abnormalities. Usually the baseline from the end of the T wave to the beginning of the P wave maintains its isoelectric position and can be used as a reference. Abnormal ST segments may be seen in infarction, ischemia, and pericarditis; after digitalis administration; and in other disease states.

T Wave

The **T wave** represents repolarization of the ventricular myocardial cells. The wave occurs during the last part of ventricular contraction. The T wave is identified as the first deviation from the ST segment and ends where the T wave returns to the baseline (Figure 22-27). This wave may be above or below the isoelectric line. The T wave usually is slightly rounded and slightly asymmetrical. Deep and symmetrically inverted T waves may indicate cardiac ischemia.

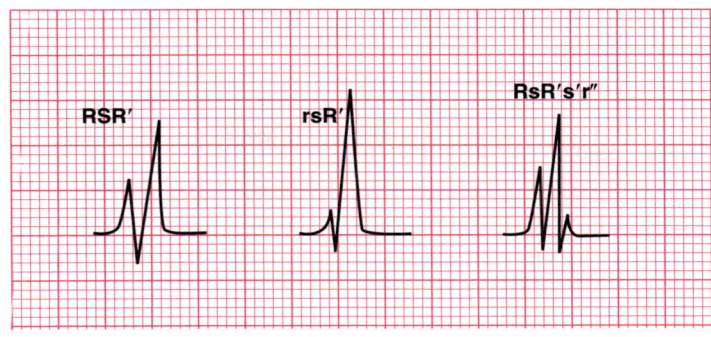

FIGURE 22-25 QRS complexes with more than one positive or negative deflection.

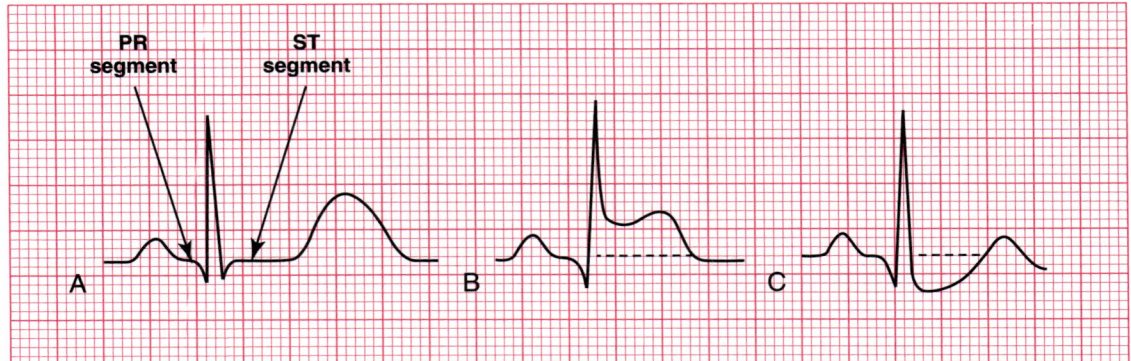

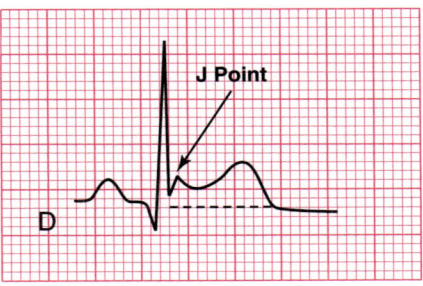

FIGURE 22-26 ST segment deviations. **A,** Use of the P-R segment as a baseline. **B,** The ST segment is elevated with respect to the P-R baseline. **C,** The ST segment is elevated with respect to the P-R baseline. **D,** J point (ST segment elevation). A prominent notch marks the takeoff of the ST segment.

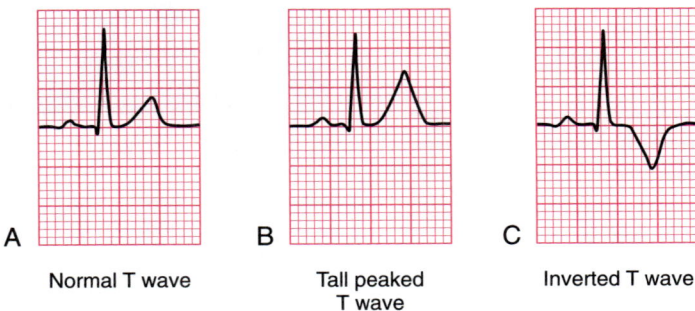

Normal T wave   Tall peaked   Inverted T wave
                         T wave

FIGURE 22-27 T waves. (Modified from Wesley K: *Huszar's basic dysrhythmias and acute coronary syndromes,* ed 4, St Louis, 2010, Mosby.)

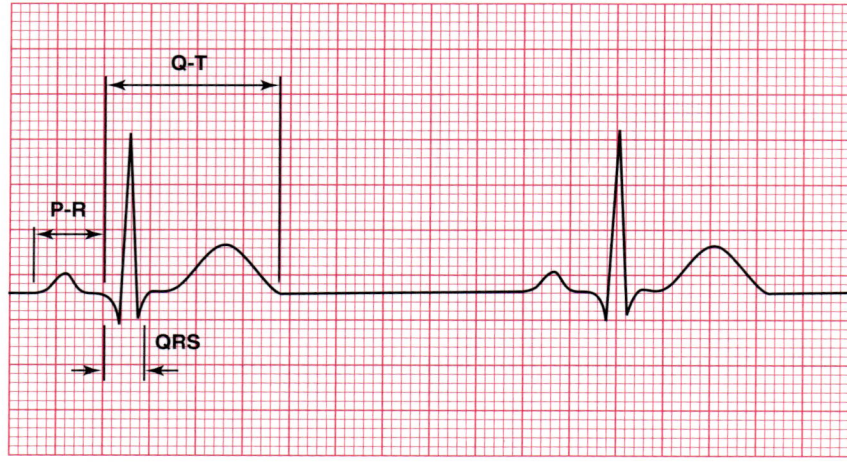

FIGURE 22-28 P-R, Q-T, and QRS intervals.

A T wave elevated more than half the height of the QRS complex *(peaked T wave)* may indicate new onset of ischemia of the myocardium or hyperkalemia.

Q-T Interval

The **Q-T interval** is measured from the beginning of the QRS complex to the end of the T wave (Figure 22-28). It represents the time from the beginning of ventricular depolarization until the end of ventricular repolarization. During the initial phase of the Q-T interval, the heart is completely unable to respond to electrical stimuli. (This is the absolute refractory period described earlier.) During the latter portion of this interval (from the peak of the T wave onward), the heart may be able to respond to premature stimuli (the relative refractory period). During this period, premature impulses may depolarize the heart. Commonly prescribed medications that may prolong the Q-T interval include quinidine, *procainamide, amiodarone,* and disopyramide. These antidysrhythmics, by virtue of their effect on the Q-T interval, may lead to potentially lethal dysrhythmias, including ventricular tachycardia, ventricular fibrillation, and an unusual bidirectional ventricular dysrhythmia called *torsades de pointes* (described later in this chapter).

> **NOTE**
> The duration of the Q-T interval depends on the heart rate. This interval usually is somewhat less than half of the preceding R-R interval. In general, a Q-T interval less than half the R-R interval is normal; one that is greater than half is abnormal; and one that is about half is considered borderline. Regardless of the heart rate, a Q-T interval greater than 0.45 second is considered abnormal.[5]

ARTIFACTS

Artifacts are marks on the ECG display or tracing caused by activities other than the electrical activity of the heart (Figure 22-29). Common causes of artifacts are improper grounding of the ECG machine, patient movement, loss of electrode contact with the patient's skin, patient shivering or tremors, and external chest compression. Two types of artifacts deserve special mention. One is alternating current interference *(60-cycle interference)*. The other one is *biotelemetry-related interference.*

Alternating current interference may occur in a poorly grounded ECG machine. Interference also may occur when an ECG is obtained near high-tension wires, transformers, and some household appliances. This results in a thick baseline made up of 60-cycle waves. The P waves may not be discernible because of the interference, but the QRS complex usually is visible. Alternating current interference also may result if the patient or the lead cable touches a metal object, such as a bed rail. Placing a blanket between the metal object and the patient may correct the interference.

Biotelemetry-related interference may occur when biotelemetry ECG signals are poorly received. This may result from weak batteries or from ECG transmission in areas with poor signaling conditions. Interference also may result if the transmitter is located a distance away from a base station receiver. Biotelemetry-related interference may produce sharp spikes and waves with a jagged appearance.

SECTION FOUR
Electrocardiogram Interpretation

STEPS IN RHYTHM ANALYSIS

Evaluation of an ECG requires a systematic approach to analyzing a given rhythm. Numerous methods can be used for rhythm interpretation. This text uses a method that first looks at the QRS complex (the most important observation in life-threatening dysrhythmias); then the P waves and the relationship between the P waves and the QRS complex; the rate; the rhythm; and finally the P-R interval. Regardless of

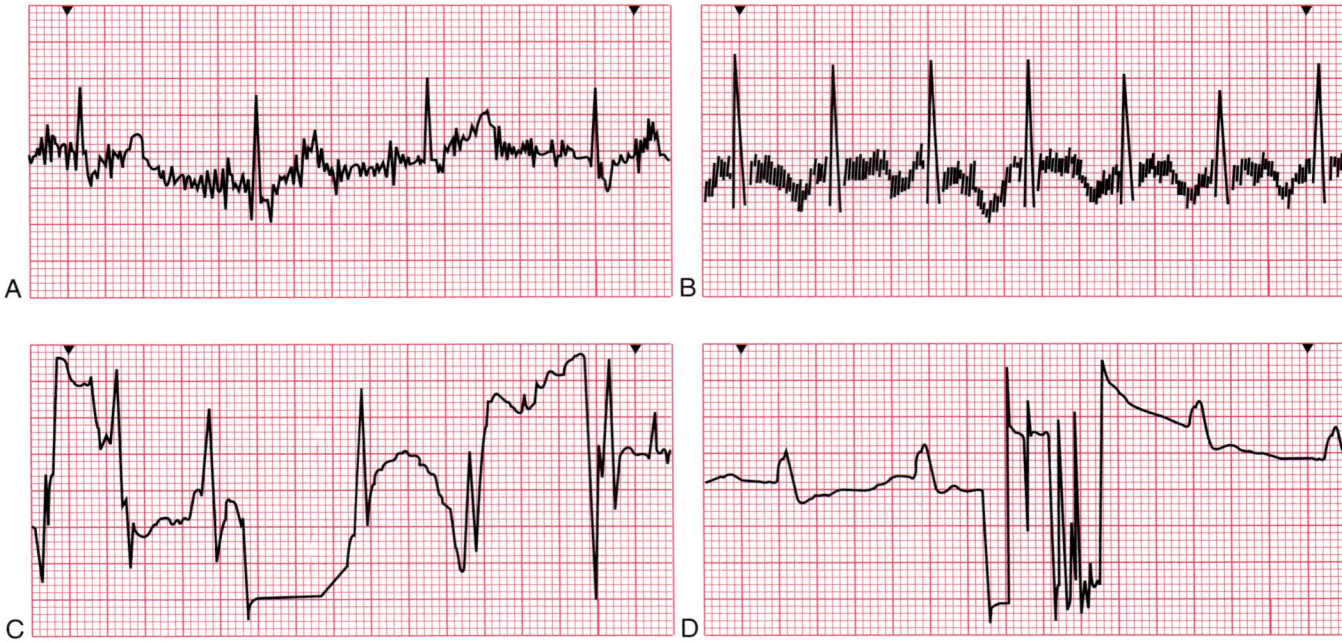

FIGURE 22-29 Artifacts. **A,** Muscle tremors. **B,** Alternating current (60 cycle) interference. **C,** Loose electrodes. **D,** Biotelemetry.

the method chosen to analyze a given rhythm, the paramedic should use a consistent format. This section of the text discusses rhythm interpretation as it pertains to standard three-lead ECG monitoring. Evaluation of 12-lead ECG monitoring is presented later in this chapter.

Five questions the paramedic must ask in any rhythm analysis to detect the presence of or potential for life-threatening rhythm disturbances are as follows:

1. Is the patient sick?
2. What is the heart rate?
3. Are there normal-looking QRS complexes?
4. Are there normal-looking P waves?
5. What is the relationship between the P waves and the QRS complexes?

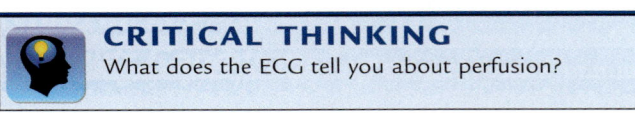

CRITICAL THINKING
What does the ECG tell you about perfusion?

Step 1: Analyze the QRS Complex

The paramedic should analyze the QRS complex for regularity and width. QRS complexes less than or equal to 0.10 second wide (less than three small squares) are supraventricular in origin. These complexes are normal. Complexes equal to or greater than 0.12 second wide may indicate a conduction abnormality in the ventricles. They also may

indicate that the focus originates in the ventricles and is abnormal (Figure 22-30). When evaluating an abnormal QRS width, the paramedic should identify the lead with the widest QRS complex, because a portion of the QRS complex may be hidden or difficult to see in some leads.

Step 2: Analyze the P Waves

The normal P wave in lead II is positive. It is smoothly rounded and usually precedes each QRS complex, indicating that the pacemaker originates in the SA node (Figure 22-31). Therefore, the paramedic should observe the following five components when evaluating P waves:

1. Are P waves present?
2. Are the P waves occurring at regular intervals?
3. Is there one P wave for each QRS complex, and is there a QRS complex after each P wave?
4. Are the P waves upright or inverted?
5. Do they all look alike? (P waves that look alike and are regular are likely from the same pacemaker.)

Step 3: Analyze the Rate

The heart rate can be analyzed in a number of ways. The methods for calculating the heart rate presented in this text are heart rate calculator rulers, the triplicate method, the R-R method, and the 6-second count method. The heart rate is determined by analyzing the ventricular rate (the QRS complex). The normal adult heart rate is 60 to 99 beats/minute. A ventricular rate less than 60 beats/minute is considered **bradycardia;** a rate equal to or greater than 100 beats/minute is considered **tachycardia.**

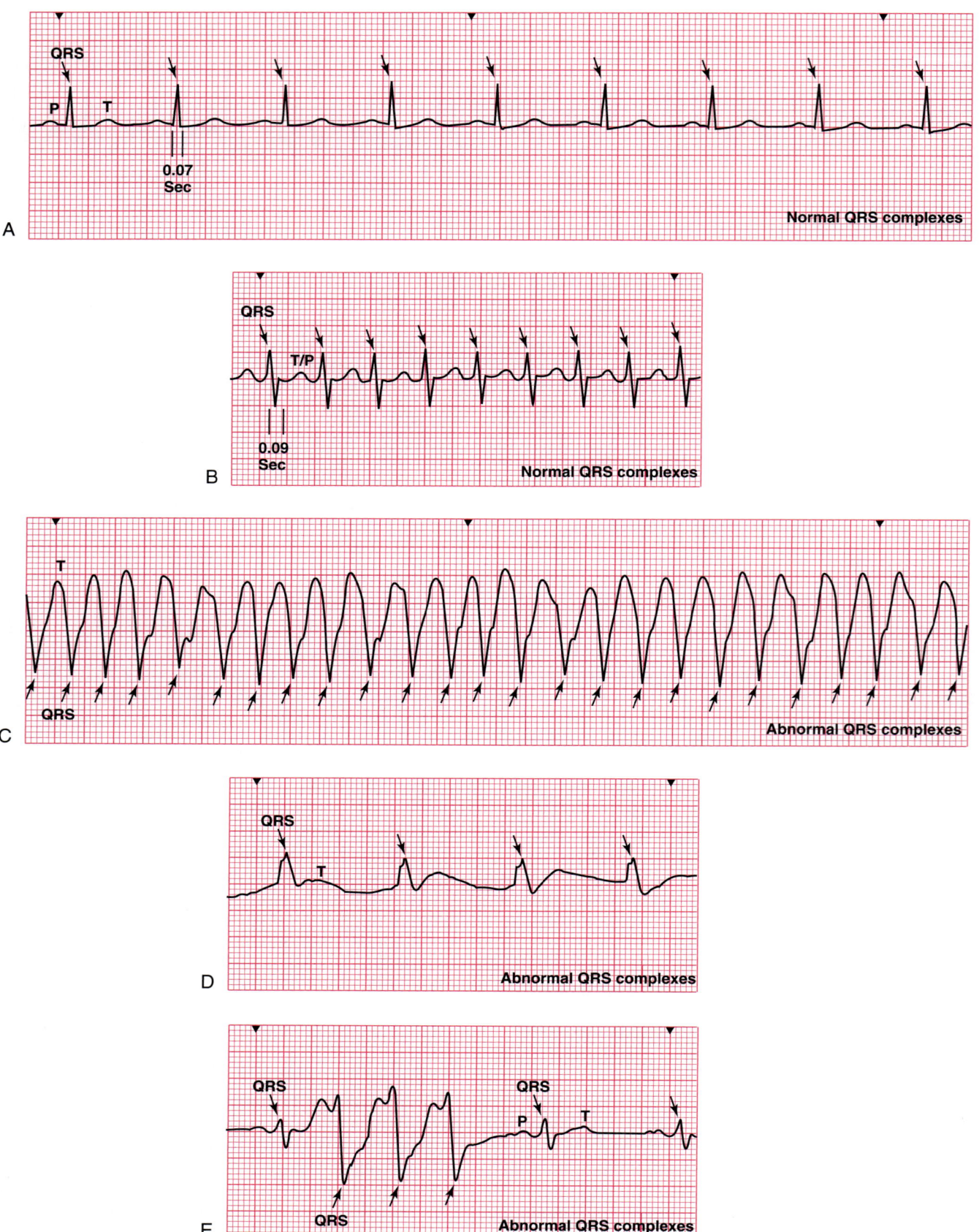

FIGURE 22-30 A and **B,** Normal QRS complexes. **C** to **E,** Abnormal QRS complexes.

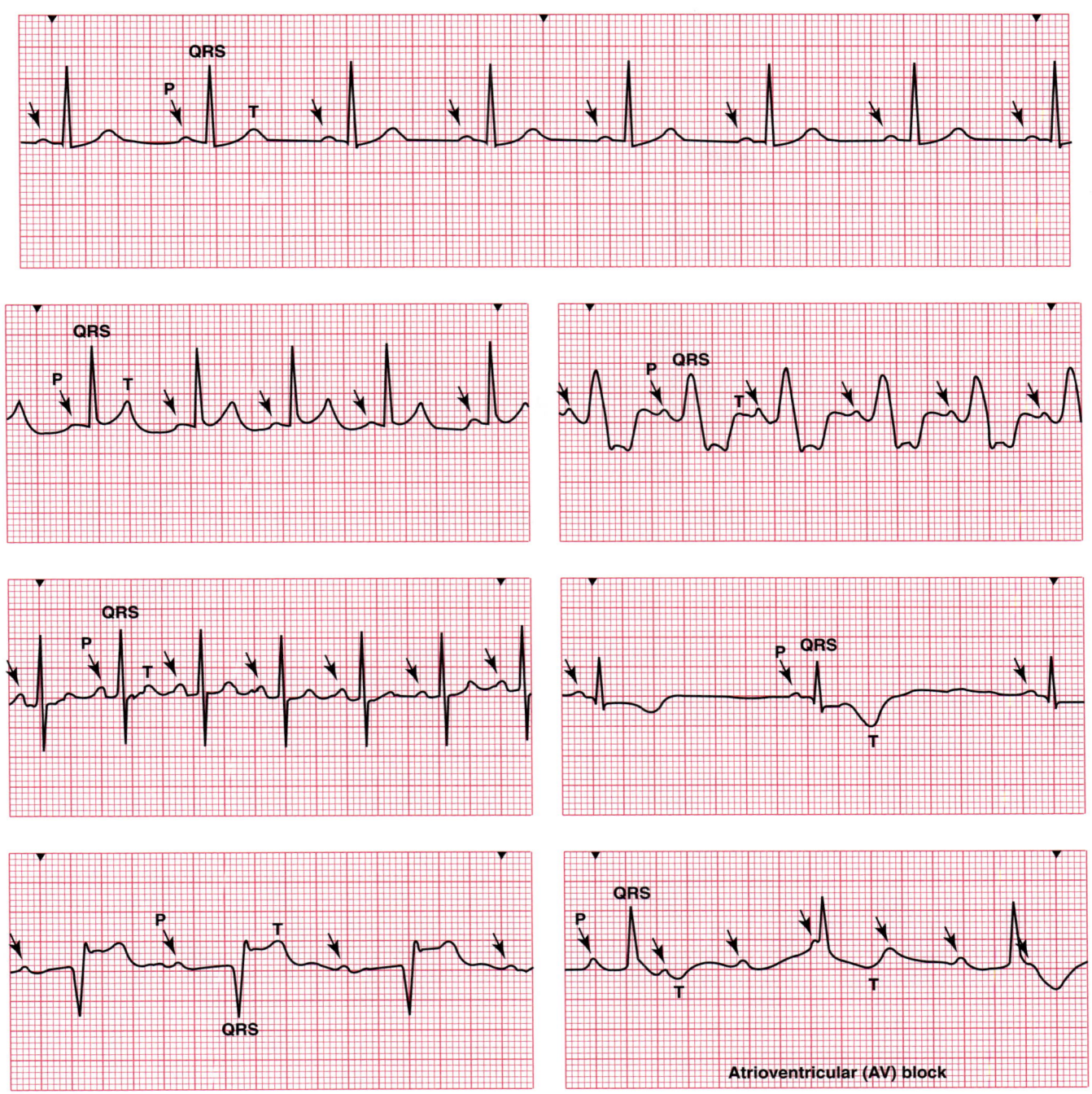

FIGURE 22-31 Normal P waves.

> **NOTE**
>
> In patients with healthy hearts, the atrial and ventricular rates are the same. This is because of the near simultaneous depolarization of the four chambers. If the atrial and ventricular rates are different (as may occur in certain dysrhythmias), the rates should be calculated separately.

HEART RATE CALCULATOR RULERS

Heart rate calculator rulers (Figure 22-32) are available from a number of manufacturers. The paramedic should follow the directions that come with the ruler. Heart rate calculator rulers are reasonably accurate if the rhythm is regular. However, the paramedic should not rely solely on a mechanical device or tool to determine the heart rate. Sometimes, a device or tool is not readily available.

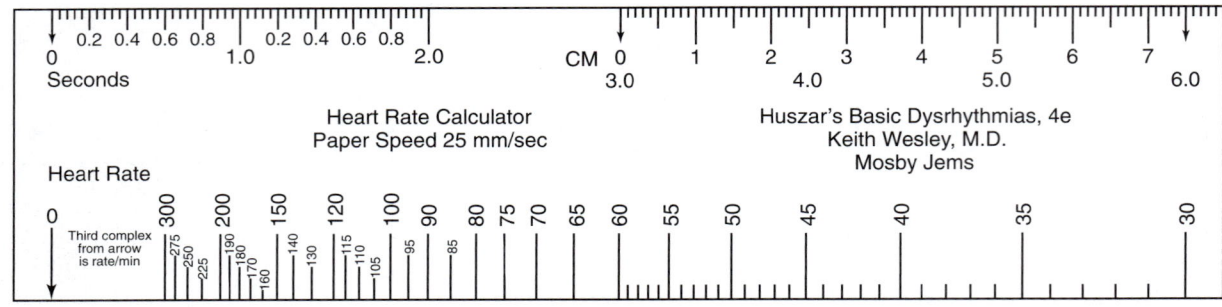

FIGURE 22-32 Heart rate calculator ruler.

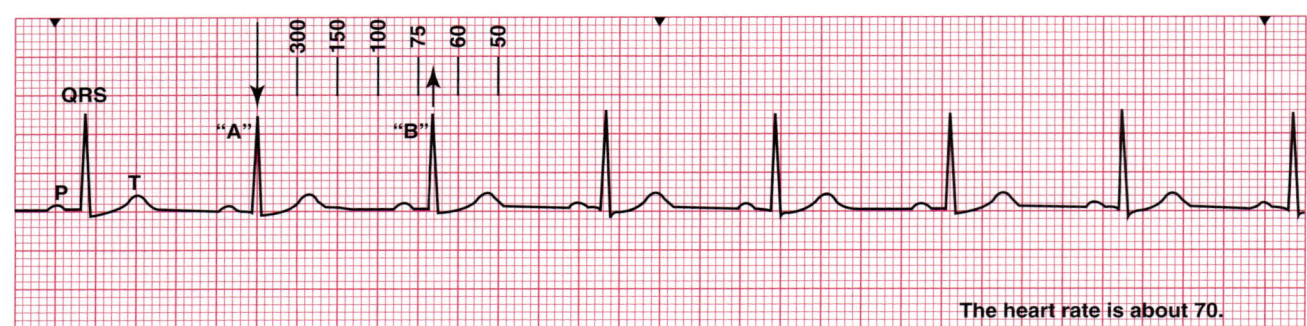

FIGURE 22-33 Triplicate method.

TRIPLICATE METHOD

The triplicate method of determining the heart rate (Figure 22-33) is accurate only under two circumstances: when the rhythm is regular and the heart rate is greater than 50 beats/minute. To use this method, the paramedic must memorize two sets of numbers: 300-150-100 and 75-60-50. These numbers are derived from the distance between the heavy black lines (each representing $\frac{1}{300}$ of a minute). Therefore, two $\frac{1}{300}$ minute units are equal to $\frac{2}{300}$ minute, which is equal to $\frac{1}{150}$ minute, or a heart rate of 150 beats/minute; three $\frac{1}{300}$ minute units are equal to $\frac{3}{300}$ minute, which is equal to $\frac{1}{100}$ minute, or a heart rate of 100 beats/minute. Using these triplicates, the paramedic can calculate heart rate as follows:

1. Select an R wave that lines up with a dark vertical line.
2. Number the next six dark vertical lines consecutively from left to right as 300-150-100 and 75-60-50.
3. Identify where the next R wave falls with reference to the six dark vertical lines. If the R wave falls on 75, the heart rate is 75 beats/minute. If the R wave falls halfway between 100 and 150, the heart rate is about 125 beats/minute.

R-R METHOD

The R-R method may be used several different ways to calculate the heart rate. As with the triplicate method, the rhythm must be regular to obtain an accurate reading.

However, the R-R method works equally well for slow rates. The three methods are as follows:

Method 1. Measure the distance in seconds between the peaks of two consecutive R waves. Then divide this number into 60 to obtain the heart rate (Figure 22-34).

Method 2. Count the large squares between the peaks of two consecutive R waves. Divide this number into 300 to obtain the heart rate (Figure 22-35).

Method 3. Count the small squares between the peaks of two consecutive R waves. Divide this number into 1500 to obtain the heart rate (Figure 22-36).

SIX-SECOND COUNT METHOD

The 6-second count method (Figure 22-37) is the least accurate method of determining the heart rate. However, it is useful for quickly obtaining an approximate rate in regular and irregular rhythms.

As previously stated, the short vertical lines at the top of most ECG graph paper are divided into 3-second intervals when run at a standard speed of 25 mm/second. Two of these intervals are equal to 6 seconds. The heart rate is calculated by counting the number of QRS complexes in a 6-second interval. This number is multiplied by 10.

 CRITICAL THINKING
Which of these rate calculation methods is fastest? Which is most accurate?

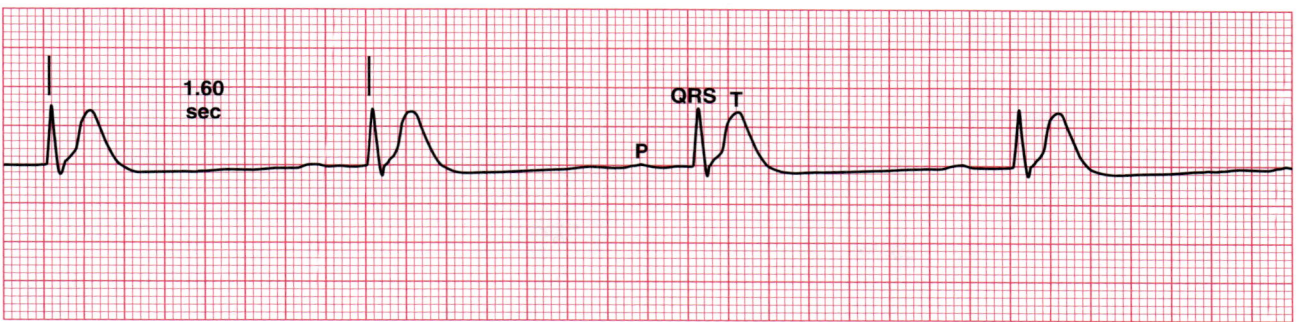

The heart rate = $\dfrac{60}{1.60\ \text{sec}}$ = 37.5 or, rounded off, 38.

FIGURE 22-34 R-R interval, method 1.

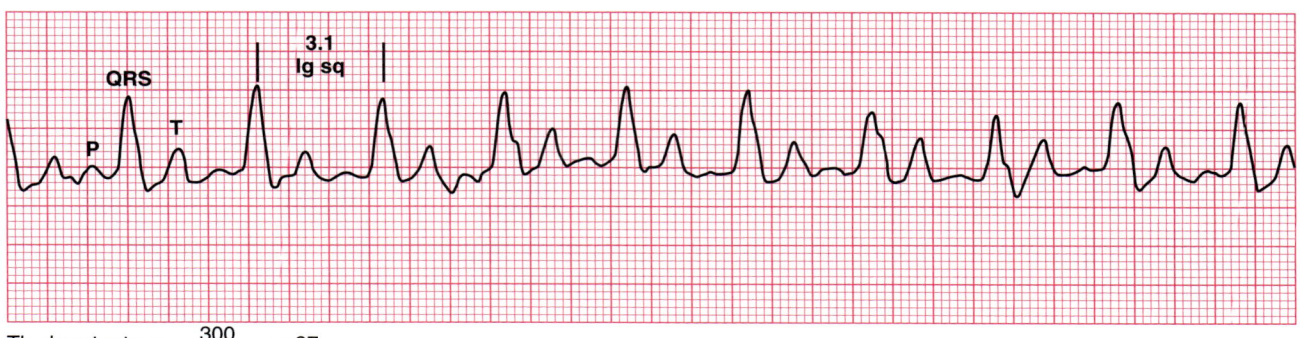

The heart rate = $\dfrac{300}{3.1\ \text{lg sq}}$ = 97.

FIGURE 22-35 R-R interval, method 2.

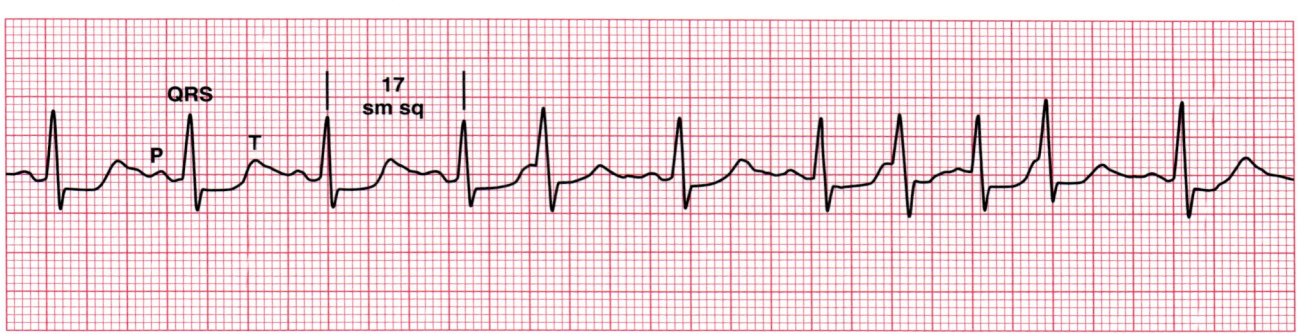

The heart rate = $\dfrac{1,500}{17\ \text{sm sq}}$ = 88.

FIGURE 22-36 R-R interval, method 3.

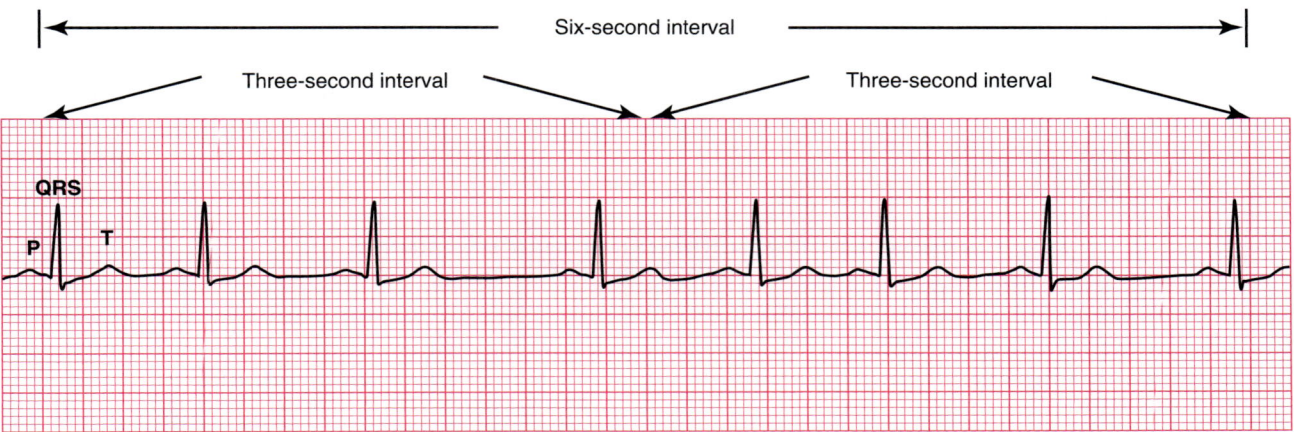

The heart rate is about 80.   (Actual heart rate is 72.)

FIGURE 22-37 Six-second count method.

Step 4: Analyze the Rhythm

To analyze the ventricular rhythm, the paramedic should compare the R-R intervals on the ECG tracing in a systematic way from left to right. This measurement may be taken using ECG calipers or pen and paper. Using calipers, the paramedic should place one tip of the caliper on the peak of one R wave and adjust the other tip so that it rests on the peak of the adjacent R wave. The paramedic then uses the caliper to map the distance of the R-R interval to evaluate evenness and regularity. (P waves may be mapped for regularity in this same way.)

In the absence of calipers, the paramedic may use a similar method of evaluating the R-R interval by using pen and paper. The paramedic places the straight edge of the paper near the peaks of the R waves and marks off the distance between the two other consecutive R waves. The paramedic then compares this R-R interval with the other R-R intervals in the ECG tracing (Figure 22-38).

If the distances between the R waves are equal or vary by less than 0.16 second (four small squares), the rhythm is

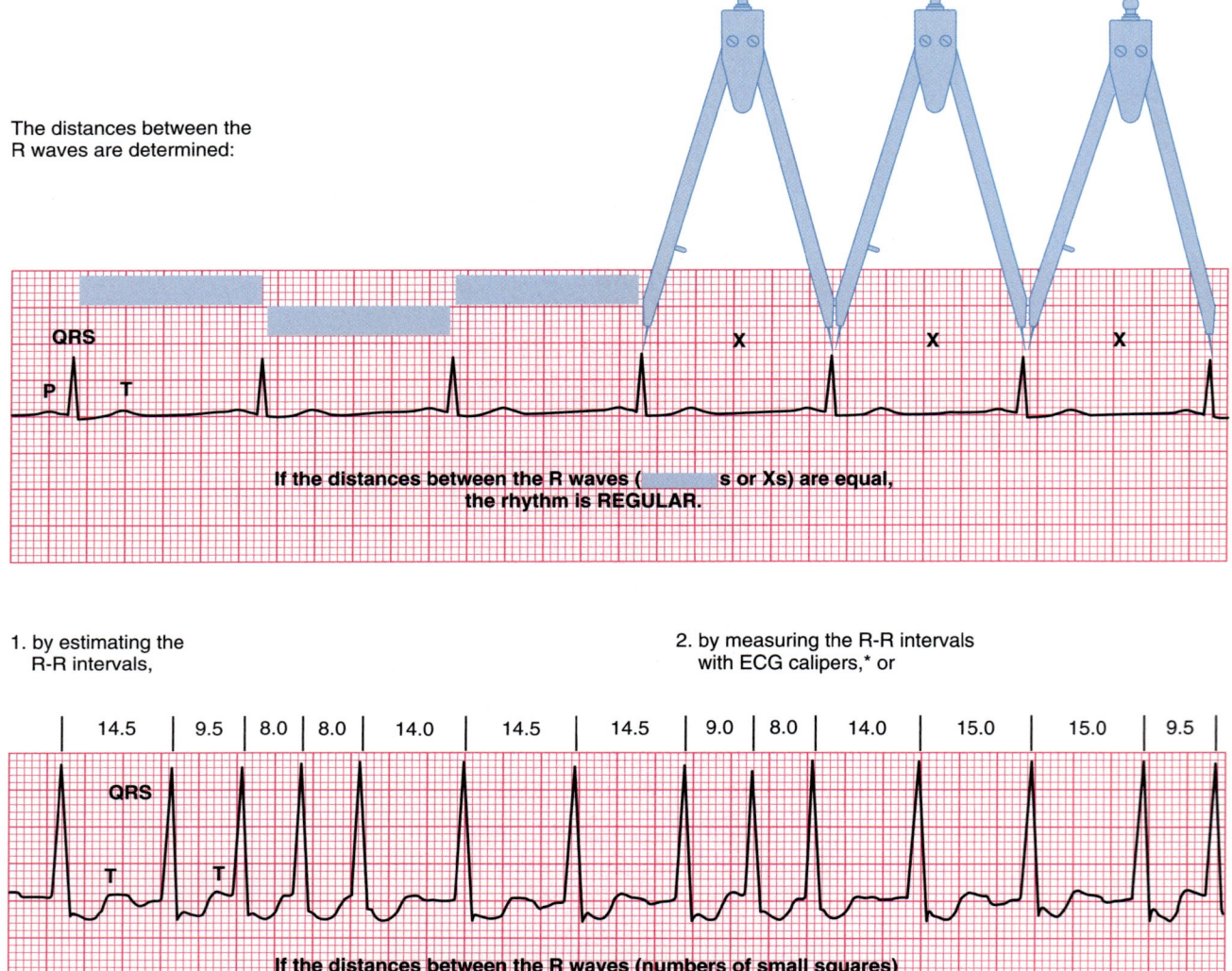

FIGURE 22-38 Determining the rhythm.

regular. If the shortest and longest R-R intervals vary by more than 0.16 second, the rhythm is irregular. Irregular rhythms may be classified further. They may be classified as *regularly irregular*. In this case, the irregularity has a pattern; it is also called "group beating." Irregular rhythms also may be *occasionally irregular*. In this case, only one or two R-R intervals are unequal. Finally, irregular rhythms may be *irregularly irregular*. In this case, the rhythm is totally irregular. No relationship is seen between the R-R intervals (Figure 22-39).

Step 5: Analyze the P-R Interval

The P-R interval indicates the time required for an electrical impulse to be conducted through the atria and AV node. The interval should be constant across the ECG tracing. A prolonged P-R interval (greater than 0.20 second) indicates a delay in the conduction of the impulse through the AV node or bundle of His. The delay is called an *atrioventricular (AV) block*. A short P-R interval (less than 0.12 second) indicates that the impulse progressed from the atria to the ventricles through pathways other than the AV node

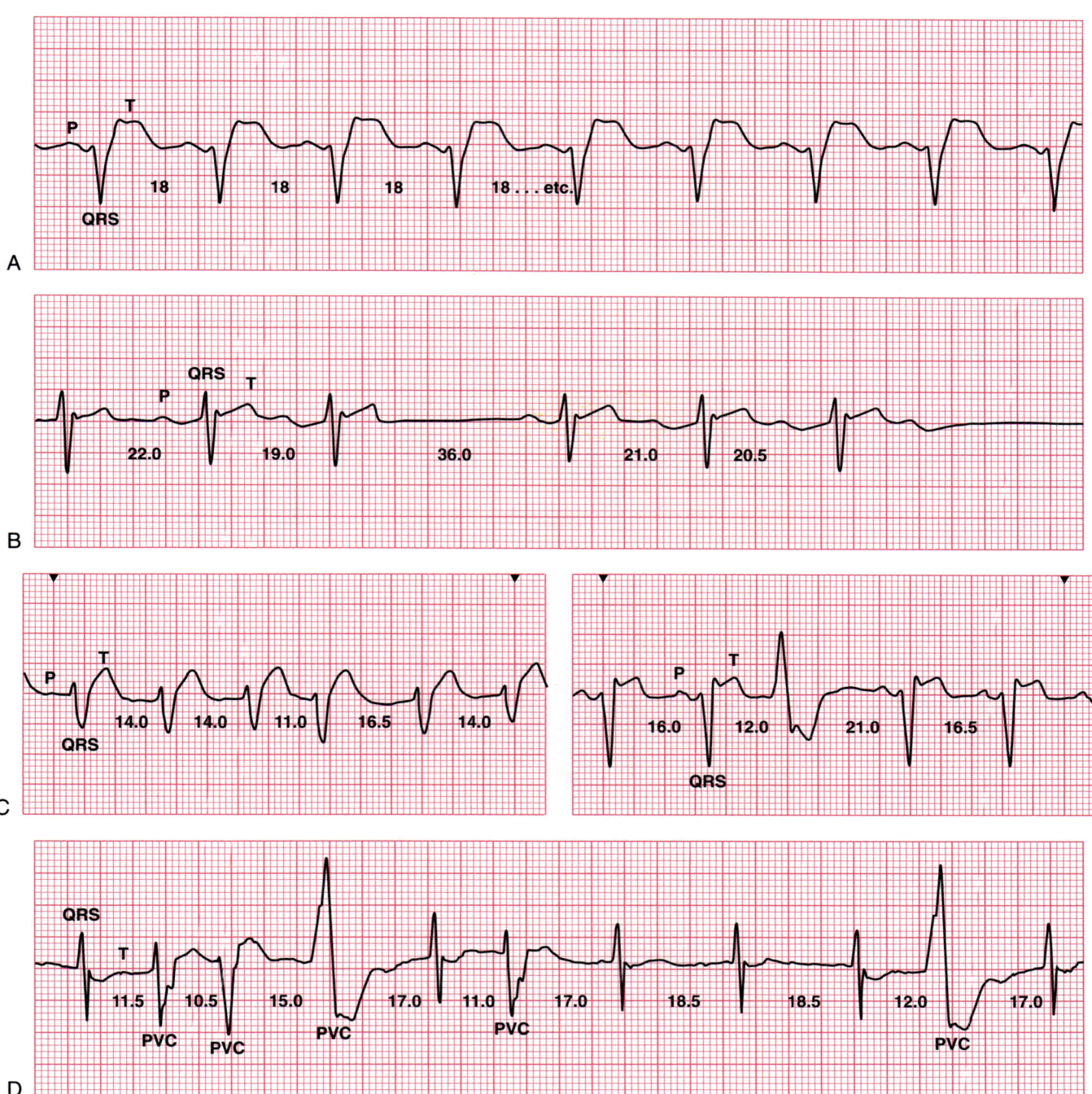

FIGURE 22-39 A, Regular rhythm. **B,** Regularly irregular rhythm. **C,** Occasionally irregular rhythm. **D,** Irregularly irregular rhythm.

(Figure 22-40). This is known as an *accessory pathway syndrome,* the most common of which is Wolff-Parkinson-White (WPW) syndrome.

> **NOTE**
> Wolff-Parkinson-White (WPW) syndrome is a genetic heart abnormality associated with early activation of the ventricles. In the presence of tachycardia, this preexcitation syndrome can be life threatening. (The syndrome is described later in this chapter.)

Analyzing a Rhythm Using the Five Steps

To review, the normal sequence of atrial and ventricular activation as it relates to the ECG tracing is as follows: Each P wave (atrial depolarization) is followed by a normal QRS complex (ventricular depolarization) and T wave (ventricular repolarization); all QRS complexes are preceded by P waves; the P-R interval is within normal limits, and the R-R interval is regular. The five steps in ECG rhythm interpretation can be applied to the rhythm in Figure 22-41.

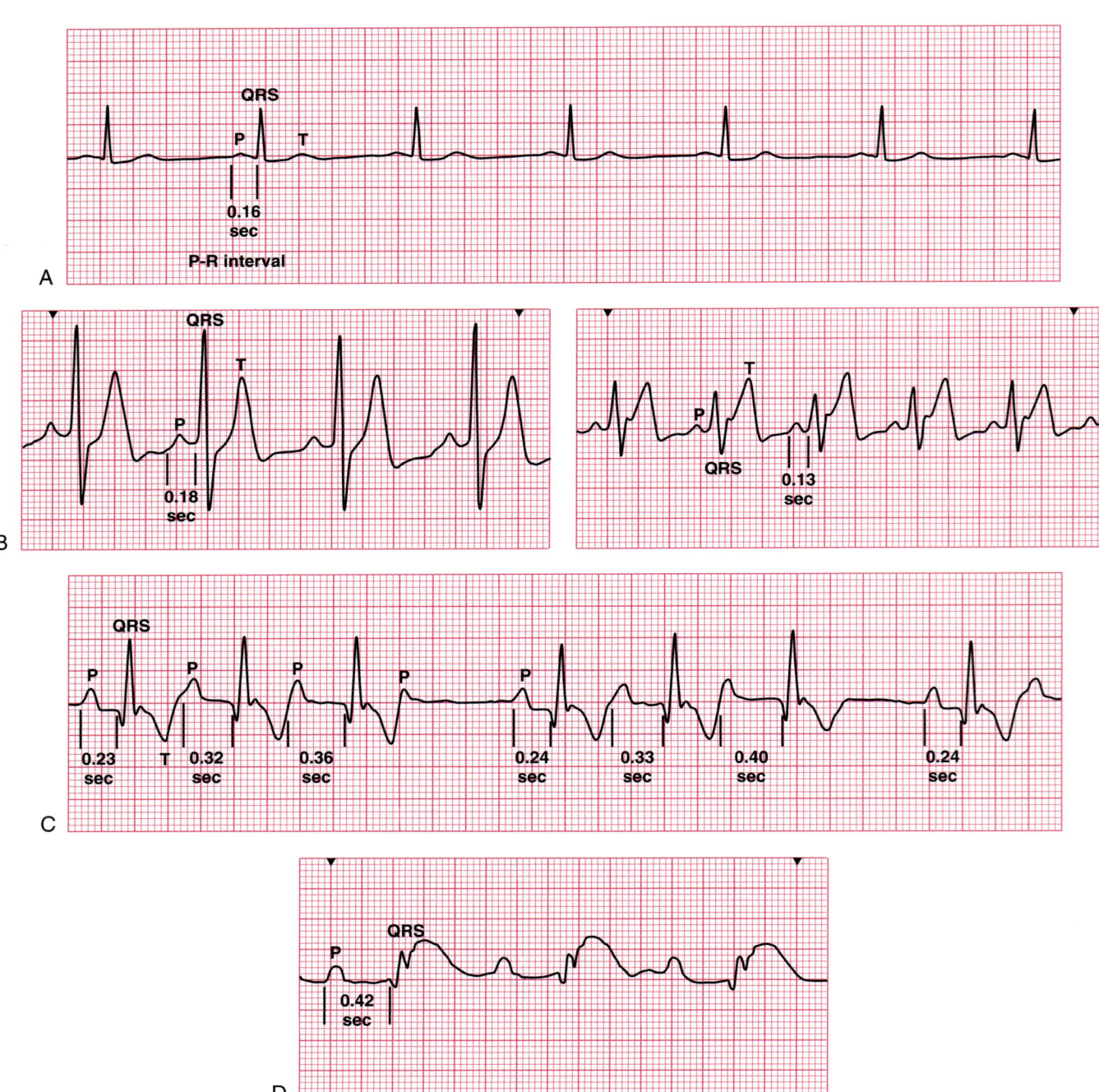

FIGURE 22-40 A and **B,** Normal P-R intervals. **C** and **D,** Abnormal P-R intervals.

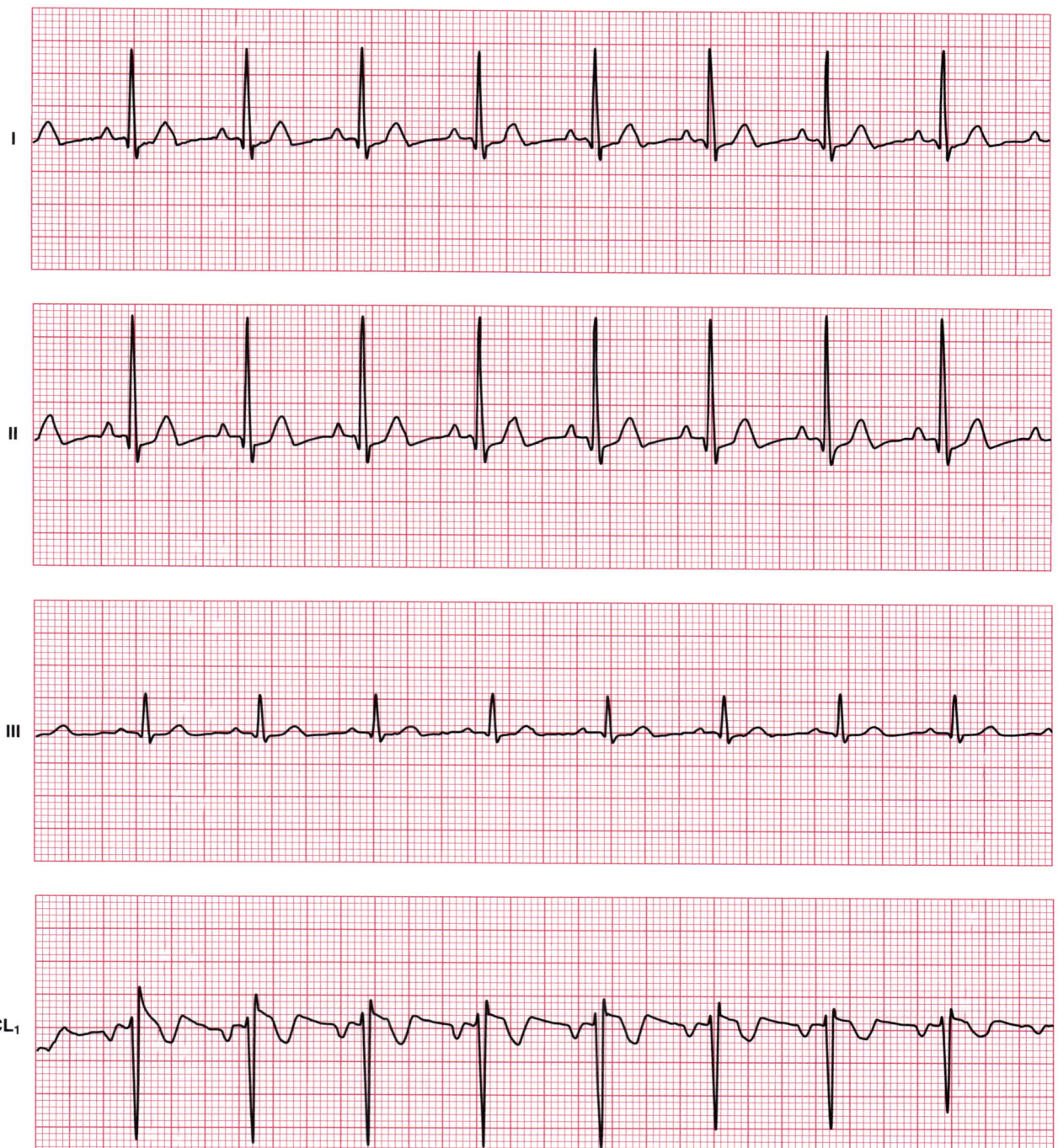

FIGURE 22-41 Normal sinus rhythm.

SECTION FIVE
Introduction to Dysrhythmias

Cardiac dysrhythmias can result from a number of physiological, pharmacological, and disease processes, including the following:

- Myocardial ischemia or necrosis
- Autonomic nervous system imbalance
- Distention of heart chambers
- Acid-base abnormalities
- Hypoxemia
- Electrolyte imbalance
- Drug effects or toxicity
- Electrical injury
- Hypothermia
- Central nervous system injury

In addition to these potential causes of dysrhythmias, some cardiac rhythm disturbances are normal, even in patients who have healthy hearts. (For example, a patient may have sinus tachycardia from stress or anxiety.) *Regardless of the cause or type of dysrhythmia, management should focus on the patient and the underlying cause. Management should not focus merely on the dysrhythmia.*

> **NOTE**
> Special considerations regarding cardiac rhythm disturbances and resuscitation in infant and pediatric patients are addressed in Chapters 47 and 48.

CLASSIFICATION OF DYSRHYTHMIAS

Classification by Rate and Pacemaker Site

The classification of dysrhythmias can be based on a number of factors. These include changes in automaticity versus disturbances in conduction, cardiac arrest (lethal) rhythms and noncardiac arrest (nonlethal) rhythms, and site of origin. For learning purposes, this text classifies rhythms by rate and pacemaker site (e.g., ventricular tachycardia and sinus bradycardia) and includes the following five groups:

1. Dysrhythmias originating in the sinoatrial node
   a. Sinus bradycardia
   b. Sinus tachycardia
   c. Sinus dysrhythmia
   d. Sinus arrest
2. Dysrhythmias originating in the atria
   a. Wandering pacemaker
   b. Multifocal atrial tachycardia
   c. Premature atrial complex
   d. Paroxysmal supraventricular tachycardia
   e. Atrial flutter
   f. Atrial fibrillation
3. Dysrhythmias originating in the atrioventricular node and surrounding tissues
   a. Premature junctional complex
   b. Junctional escape complexes or rhythms
   c. Accelerated junctional rhythm
4. Dysrhythmias originating in the ventricles
   a. Ventricular escape complexes or rhythms
   b. Premature ventricular complex
   c. Ventricular tachycardia
   d. Ventricular fibrillation
   e. Asystole
   f. Artificial pacemaker rhythms
5. Dysrhythmias that are disorders of conduction
   a. Atrioventricular blocks
      (1) First-degree atrioventricular block
      (2) Second-degree atrioventricular block type I (or Wenckebach)
      (3) Second-degree atrioventricular block type II
      (4) Third-degree atrioventricular block

b. Disturbances of ventricular conduction
c. Pulseless electrical activity
d. Preexcitation syndrome (WPW syndrome and Lown-Ganong-Levine syndrome)

> **NOTE**
> Broadly speaking, there are only four cardiac arrest rhythms: ventricular fibrillation, pulseless ventricular tachycardia, asystole, and assorted pulseless electrical activity rhythms. The two noncardiac arrest rhythms (precollapse or precardiac arrest rhythms) that are important to consider in prehospital care are those that are too slow (fewer than 60 beats/minute) and those that are too fast (more than 160 beats/minute).[1]

The text presents each dysrhythmia in lead II. For comparison, the same dysrhythmia also is shown as it would appear in leads I, III, and MCL$_1$. The text discusses how to recognize the dysrhythmia and the emergency treatment of patients with each dysrhythmia. All treatments in this chapter follow the recommendations of the American Heart Association (AHA). All treatments are referenced to the American Heart Association algorithms.

Use of Algorithms for Classification

Algorithms are lists used to summarize information. Some algorithms contain prehospital and in-hospital management recommendations. The following guidelines apply to the use of all algorithms:

1. First, manage the patient, not the monitor.
2. Algorithms for cardiac arrest presume that the condition under discussion continually persists; that the patient remains in cardiac arrest; and that cardiopulmonary resuscitation is always performed.
3. Apply different interventions when appropriate indications exist.
4. The algorithms are designed to outline the most common assessments and actions performed for the majority of patients, but they are not designed to be all-inclusive or restrictive.[6] The flow diagrams present treatments mostly in sequential order of priority. Next to a treatment or pharmacological agent may be a class recommendation (Box 22-4). The footnotes to the algorithm contain additional important information related to assessment, treatment, and evaluation.
5. Adequate airway, ventilation, oxygenation, chest compression, and defibrillation are more important than administration of medications. These measures take precedence over initiating an intravenous (IV) line or injecting pharmacological agents.
6. In the unlikely event that IV or intraosseous (IO) access is not available, some medications (naloxone, atropine, *vasopressin, epinephrine,* and *lidocaine* [N-A-V-E-L]), can be administered via an endotracheal (ET)

BOX 22-4 Classification of Recommendations for Cardiopulmonary Resuscitation and Emergency Cardiovascular Care

Class I	Benefit significantly outweighs any possible harm.
	High-level prospective studies support the treatment.
	Treatment should be performed/administered.
Class IIa	Benefit outweighs risk.
	Weight of evidence supports the treatment.
	Treatment is considered acceptable and useful.
Class IIb	Benefit equals or is greater than the risk.
	Evidence documented only short-term benefit, or lower level evidence supported its use.
	Therapy may be considered.
Class III	Risk is greater than benefit.
	Therapy is not indicated.
	Not proven to be helpful.
	May harm the patient.

Modified from the American Heart Association: 2010 American Heart Association guidelines for cardiopulmonary resuscitation and emergency cardiovascular care, *Circulation*. 112 (24)(Suppl):IV1-203, updated 2010.

---

tube. For adults, the endotracheal dose is 2 to 2½ times the IV dose. The ET tube route is the least preferred method of drug administration.

7. As a rule, intravenous medications are administered rapidly, by the bolus method in cases of cardiac arrest.

8. After each intravenous medication, a 20 to 30 mL bolus of IV fluid should be given. Also, the extremity should be elevated immediately. This enhances the delivery of drugs to the central circulation. This delivery may take 1 to 2 minutes.

9. Last, manage the patient, not the monitor.

DYSRHYTHMIAS ORIGINATING IN THE SINOATRIAL NODE

Most sinus dysrhythmias result from increases or decreases in vagal tone (parasympathetic nervous system). The SA node generally receives sufficient inhibitory parasympathetic impulses from the vagus nerve to keep the SA node in the normal rate of 60 to 100 beats/minute. However, if vagus nerve activity increases, the heart rate slows and sinus bradycardia results. If the vagus nerve is slowed or blocked, the heart rate increases and sinus tachycardia results. Dysrhythmias that originate in the SA node include sinus bradycardia, sinus tachycardia, sinus dysrhythmia, and sinus arrest. ECG features common to all SA node dysrhythmias include the following:

- Normal duration of QRS complex (in the absence of bundle branch block)
- Upright P waves in lead II
- Similar appearance of all P waves
- Normal duration of P-R interval (in the absence of atrioventricular block)

Sinus Bradycardia

DESCRIPTION

Sinus bradycardia results from slowing of the pacemaker rate of the SA node (Figure 22-42).

ETIOLOGY

Possible causes of sinus bradycardia include the following:

- Intrinsic sinus node disease
- Increased parasympathetic vagal tone
- Hypothermia
- Hypoxia
- Drug effects (e.g., digitalis, beta blockers, and calcium channel blockers)
- Myocardial infarction

RULES FOR INTERPRETATION (LEAD II MONITORING)

Sinus bradycardia has the following characteristics on the ECG:

QRS complex: Less than 0.12 second, provided no ventricular conduction disturbance is present

P waves: Normal and upright; one P wave before each QRS complex

Rate: Less than 60 beats/minute

Rhythm: Regular

P-R interval: 0.12 to 0.20 second and constant (normal), provided no atrioventricular block is present

CLINICAL SIGNIFICANCE

A decreased rate may compromise cardiac output. It may result in hypotension or other signs of shock, angina pectoris, or central nervous system symptoms (e.g.,

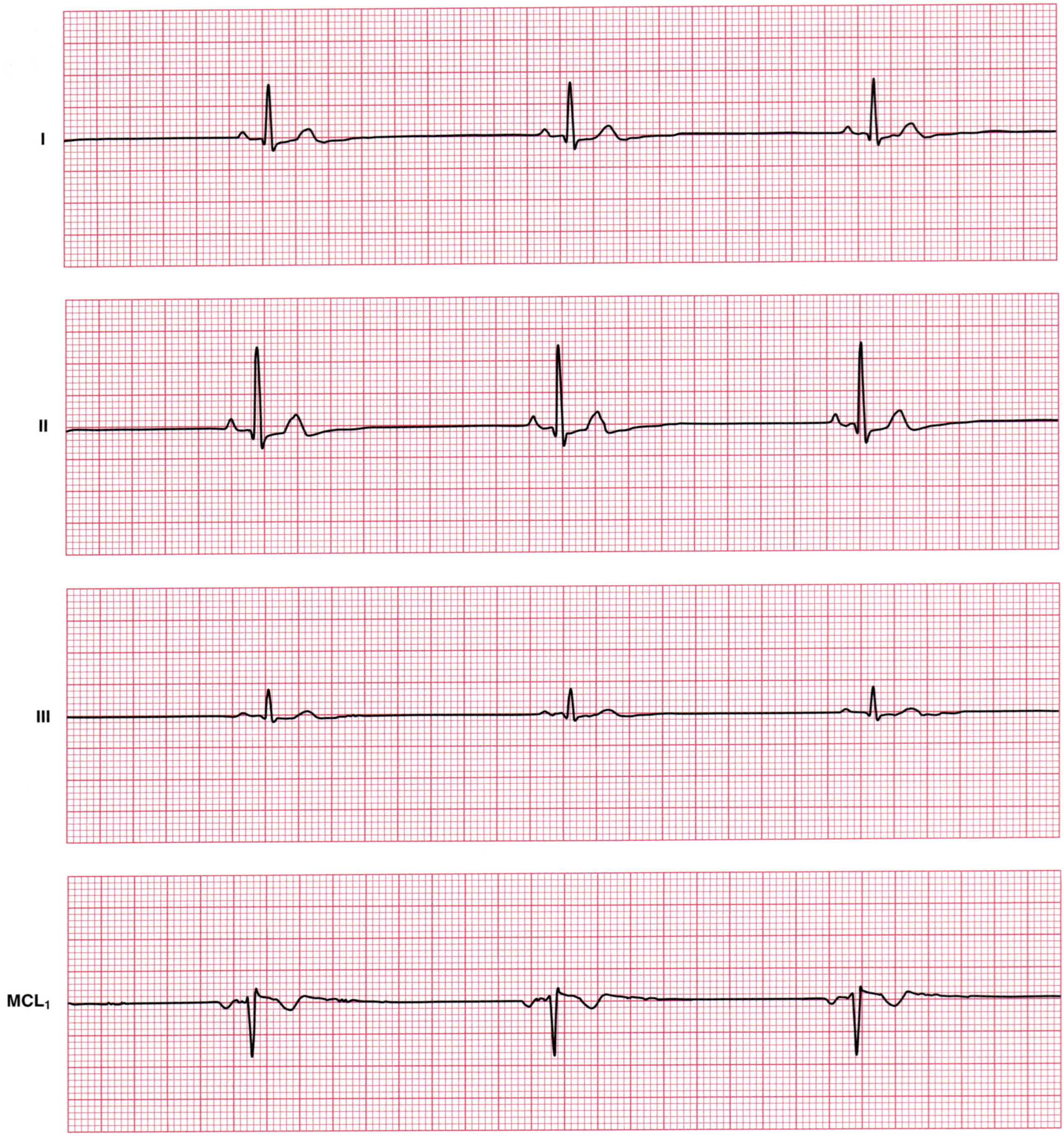

I

II

III

MCL₁

FIGURE 22-42 Sinus bradycardia.

lightheadedness, vertigo, and syncope). Sinus bradycardia can result from nausea and vomiting. The dysrhythmia is associated with overstimulation of the vagus nerve that can result in fainting (vasovagal syncope). However, sinus bradycardia may be beneficial. It may reduce myocardial oxygen consumption during myocardial infarction, provided the patient is well perfused. Sinus bradycardia also may occur after the application of carotid sinus pressure (carotid sinus massage, described later in this chapter). This dysrhythmia is common during sleep and in well-conditioned athletes.

CRITICAL THINKING
Take a poll of your classmates. How many have a resting heart rate of 60 beats/minute?

MANAGEMENT

Prehospital intervention usually is unnecessary unless hypotension, altered mental status caused by inadequate perfusion, acute heart failure, or ventricular irritability is present. (These are more common with rates below 50 beats/minute.) Management of symptomatic bradycardia is aimed at increasing the heart rate to improve cardiac output. Inotropic support also may be required (Figure 22-43). Treatment options for symptomatic bradycardia include oxygen, ventilation if indicated, *atropine,* transcutaneous pacing (the use of an external artificial pacemaker, described later in this chapter), a *dopamine* infusion, or an *epinephrine* infusion. Transcutaneous pacing is considered a class IIa intervention for symptomatic bradycardias unresponsive to atropine. Immediate pacing might be considered in unstable patients with high-degree AV block when IV access is not available.[1] Pacing is indicated for symptomatic bradycardias related to a conduction delay or block at or below the His-Purkinje level (infranodal).

> **NOTE**
> Blocks in electrical conduction may be classified as *nodal* or *infranodal*. A nodal block is one that occurs in the AV node. An infranodal block is one that occurs below the AV node. A *complete heart block* is one in which all electrical signals are blocked from the upper to lower chambers. (See conduction disorders later in this chapter.)

Atropine is administered intravenously for symptomatic bradycardia,. Administration may be repeated every 3 to 5 minutes as needed. The frequency of *atropine* administration is based on the patient's condition. *Atropine* should be administered at shorter intervals (every 3 minutes) for severely unstable patients.

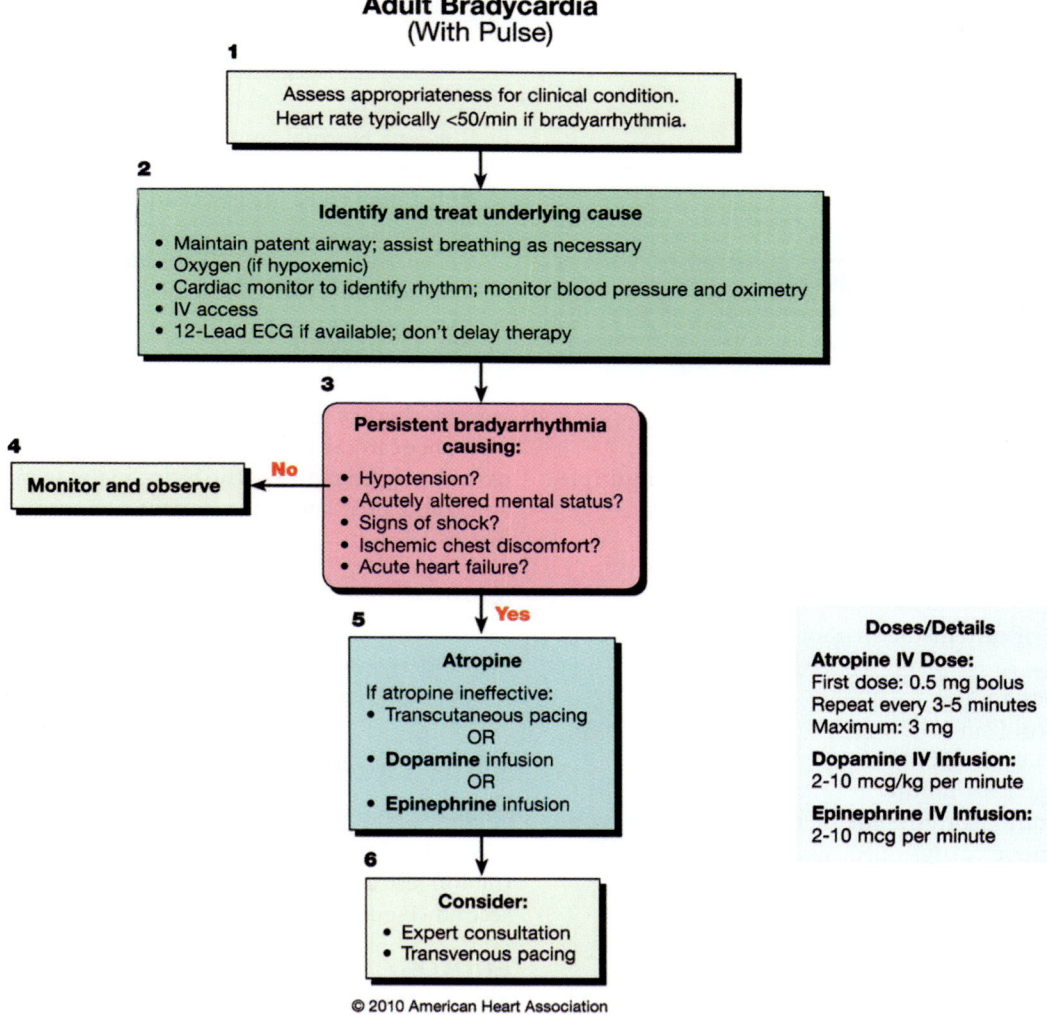

FIGURE 22-43 Bradycardia algorithm. (Reprinted with permission, American Heart Association Guidelines For CPR and ECC, *Circulation 122* [suppl 3]:S685-S919, American Heart Association, Inc, 2010.)

> **NOTE**
>
> **Atropine** should be used with caution in a patient with an acute myocardial infarction. The drug can increase the heart rate, increasing myocardial oxygen demand. This in turn can worsen ischemia or increase the size of the infarction. **Atropine** may be beneficial for the treatment of nodal blocks. The drug should be avoided for infranodal blocks and complete heart block with a wide QRS complex, because it may worsen the rhythm.

If symptoms persist after **atropine** administration, a pressor infusion such as **dopamine** or epinephrine may be needed (Box 22-5). Evaluate the need for fluid bolus infusion in hypotensive bradycardic patients before pressor infusion begins.[1]

An **epinephrine** infusion can be used for symptomatic bradycardia (Box 22-6). Generally, this is given after **atropine** and transcutaneous pacing fail to improve the patient's condition. However, an **epinephrine** infusion may be administered earlier if the patient displays severe symptoms and is deteriorating quickly.

Sinus Tachycardia

DESCRIPTION

Sinus tachycardia results from an increase in the rate of sinus node discharge (Figure 22-44).

> **CRITICAL THINKING**
>
> What effect does the excitement and commotion of the arrival of your ambulance likely have on the heart rate and blood pressure of a conscious, alert patient?

ETIOLOGY

Sinus tachycardia is common and may result from multiple factors, including the following:

- Exercise
- Fever
- Anxiety
- Ingestion of caffeine or alcohol
- Smoking
- Hypovolemia
- Hyperthyroidism
- Anemia
- Congestive heart failure
- Administration of **atropine** or any vagolytic or sympathomimetic drug (e.g., cocaine, phencyclidine, **epinephrine**)

RULES FOR INTERPRETATION (LEAD II MONITORING)

Sinus tachycardia has the following characteristics on the ECG:

QRS complex: Less than 0.12 second, provided no ventricular conduction disturbance is present

> **BOX 22-5 Dopamine Infusion**
>
> - Low-dose dopamine: 1 to 5 mcg/kg/minute. A low dose of dopamine produces a dopaminergic effect that increases renal, mesenteric, and cerebrovascular vessel dilation. The benefit of low-dose dopamine is controversial.
> - Moderate-dose dopamine: 5 to 10 mcg/kg/minute. At moderate doses, dopamine improves contractility, cardiac output, and blood pressure through alpha$_1$- and beta$_1$-receptor stimulation.
> - High-dose dopamine: 10 to 20 mcg/kg/minute. Higher doses of dopamine have an alpha-adrenergic effect producing peripheral arterial and venous vasoconstriction. (See Chapter 14 for the calculation of dopamine infusions.)

> **BOX 22-6 Epinephrine Infusion**
>
> Epinephrine infusions are used for critically unstable patients with bradycardia who have not responded to atropine or pacing. An epinephrine infusion is prepared by mixing 1 mg of epinephrine 1:1000 into 500 mL of 5% dextrose in water or 0.9% normal saline. The concentration is 2 mcg/mL. The recommended rate of infusion is 2 to 10 mcg/minute.

P waves: Normal and upright; one before each QRS complex

Rate: Equal to or greater than 100 beats/minute

Rhythm: Regular

P-R interval: 0.12 to 0.20 second (normal), provided no atrioventricular conduction block is present

CLINICAL SIGNIFICANCE

Sinus tachycardia in healthy individuals generally is a benign rhythm disturbance. If tachycardia is associated with myocardial infarction, however, it may increase the oxygen requirements of the heart, increase myocardial ischemia, and predispose the patient to more serious rhythm disturbances.

MANAGEMENT

Sinus tachycardia usually does not require treatment. When the underlying cause is removed, the tachycardia usually resolves gradually and spontaneously.

Sinus Dysrhythmia

DESCRIPTION

Sinus dysrhythmia is present when the difference between the longest and shortest R-R intervals is greater than 0.16 second (Figure 22-45).

ETIOLOGY

Sinus dysrhythmia usually is normal. It often is related to the respiratory cycle and to changes in intrathoracic pressure. These changes cause the heart rate to increase during inspiration and to decrease during expiration.

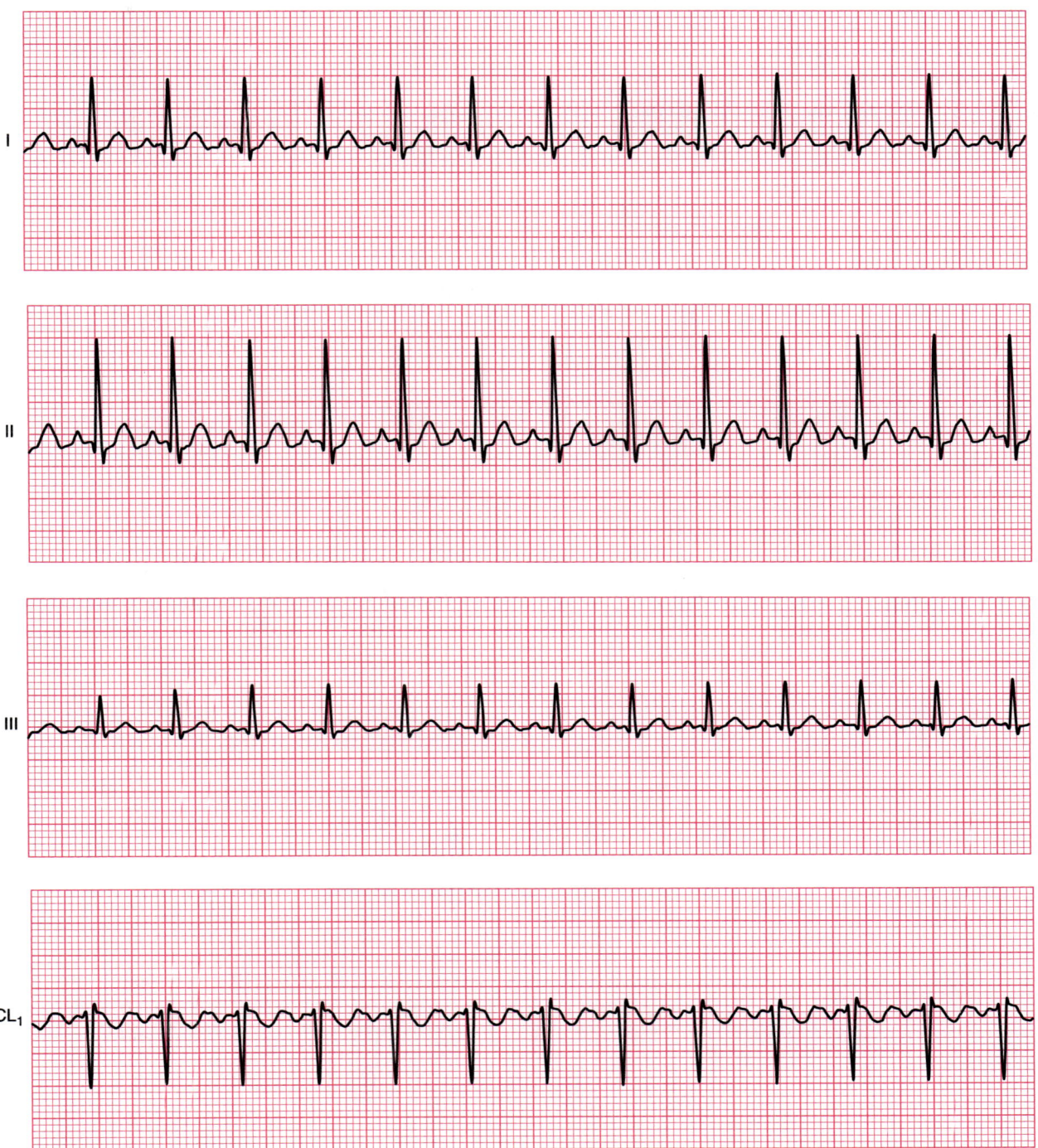

FIGURE 22-44 Sinus tachycardia.

Although sinus dysrhythmia sometimes occurs normally in healthy people, it is more common in patients with heart disease or myocardial infarction. It also is more common in patients receiving certain drugs, such as **digoxin** and **morphine.**

RULES FOR INTERPRETATION (LEAD II MONITORING)

Sinus dysrhythmia has the following characteristics on the ECG:

QRS complex: Less than 0.12 second, provided no ventricular conduction disturbance is present

P waves: Normal and upright; one P wave before each QRS complex

Rate: Usually 60 to 99 beats/minute (varies with respiration)

Rhythm: Irregular (changes occur in cycles and usually follow the patient's respiratory pattern)

P-R interval: 0.12 to 0.20 second and constant (normal)

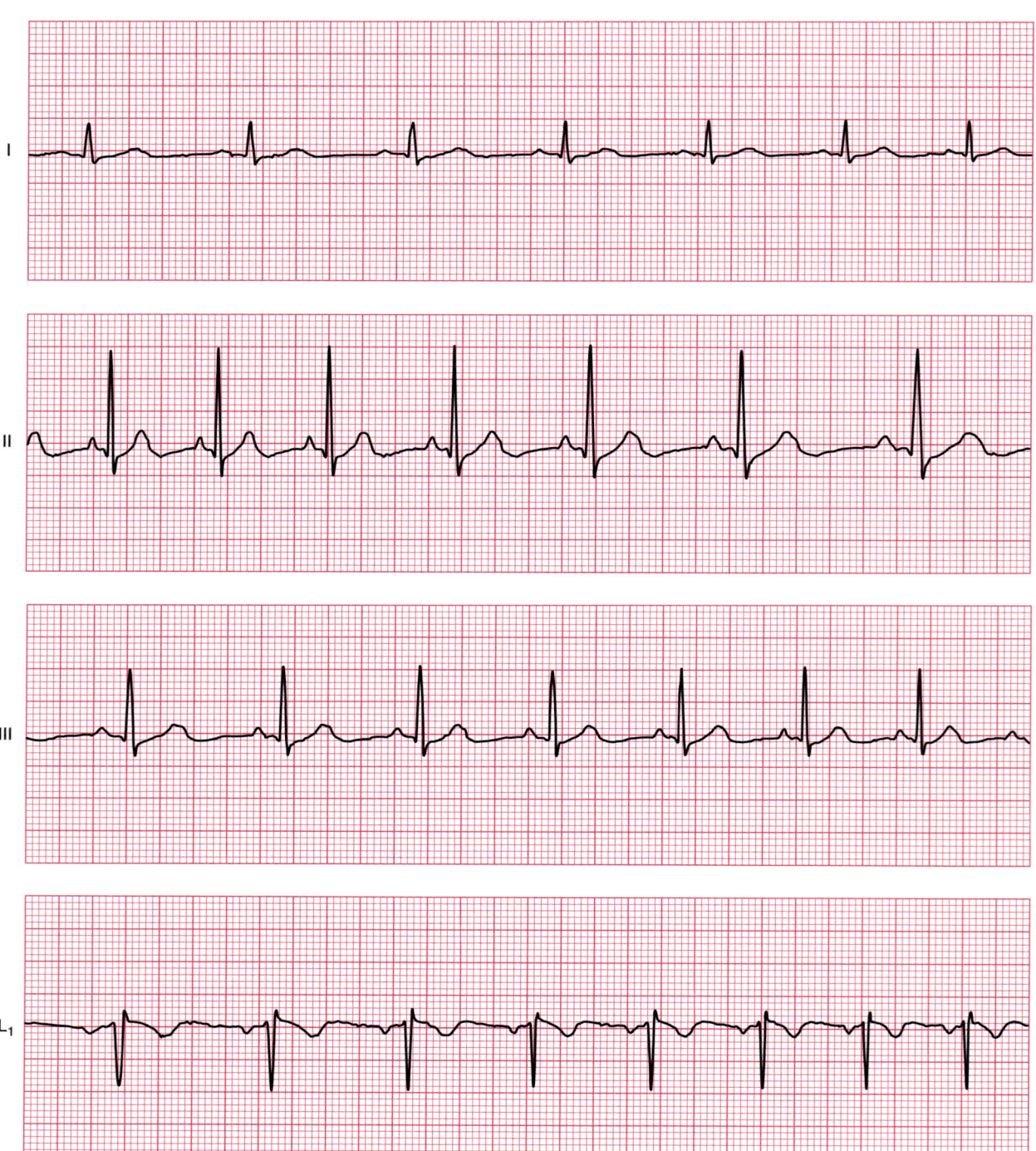

FIGURE 22-45 Sinus dysrhythmia.

CLINICAL SIGNIFICANCE

Sinus dysrhythmia is common in people of all ages. It may be associated with palpitations, dizziness, and syncope (rare).

MANAGEMENT

Sinus dysrhythmia usually is not a serious dysrhythmia. It seldom requires treatment.

Sinus Arrest

DESCRIPTION

Sinus arrest results from a depression in automaticity of the SA node (Figure 22-46). The failure of the sinus node causes short periods of cardiac standstill. This occurs until lower level pacemakers discharge (escape beats) or the sinus node resumes its normal function.

ETIOLOGY

Sinus arrest may be precipitated by an increase in parasympathetic tone on the SA node, hypoxia or ischemia, excessive administration of digitalis or *propranolol,* hyperkalemia, or damage to the SA node (acute myocardial infarction, degenerative fibrotic disease that affects the heart).

RULES FOR INTERPRETATION (LEAD II MONITORING)

Sinus arrest has the following characteristics on the ECG:

QRS complex: Less than 0.12 second, provided no bundle branch conduction disturbance is present

P waves: Normal and upright. If the electrical impulse is not generated by the SA node or blocked from entering the atria, atrial depolarization does not occur and the P wave is dropped.

Rate: Normal to slow, depending on the frequency and duration of sinus arrest

Rhythm: Irregular when sinus arrest is present

P-R interval: P-R intervals (when the P wave is present) of the underlying rhythm are normal (0.12 to 0.20 second) in the absence of atrioventricular block. Junctional escape beats may occur with no P waves.

CLINICAL SIGNIFICANCE

Frequent or prolonged episodes of sinus arrest may reduce cardiac output. The overall heart rate slows, and the atria do not contract; consequently, ventricular filling is reduced. If an escape pacemaker does not take over, ventricular asystole may result. This would cause lightheadedness followed by syncope. With this dysrhythmia, the danger exists that sinus node activity will stop completely. Another danger is that an escape pacemaker may not take over pacing. These developments would result in asystole.

MANAGEMENT

If the patient is asymptomatic, close observation is all that is required. In patients with bradycardia that produces symptoms, management may include the administration of *atropine* or transcutaneous cardiac pacing (see Figure 22-43).

DYSRHYTHMIAS ORIGINATING IN THE ATRIA

Atrial dysrhythmias may begin in the tissues of the atria or in the AV junction. Common causes of atrial dysrhythmias are ischemia, hypoxia, and atrial dilation caused by congestive heart failure, mitral valve abnormalities, or increased pulmonary artery pressures. Atrial dysrhythmias include wandering pacemaker, premature atrial complexes, paroxysmal supraventricular tachycardia, atrial flutter, and atrial fibrillation. ECG features common to all atrial dysrhythmias (provided no ventricular conduction disturbance is present) include the following:

- Normal QRS complexes
- P waves (if present) that differ in appearance from sinus P waves
- Abnormal, shortened, or prolonged P-R intervals

Wandering Pacemaker

DESCRIPTION

Wandering pacemaker (or wandering atrial pacemaker) occurs when the pacemaker shifts from the sinus node to another pacemaker site in the atria or the AV junction (Figure 22-47). The shift in the site usually is transient, back and forth along the sinoatrial node, atria, and atrioventricular junction.

ETIOLOGY

Wandering pacemaker is a type of sinus dysrhythmia. It may be normal in the very young, in older adults, and in well-conditioned athletes. The dysrhythmia generally is caused by the inhibitory vagal effect on the SA node and AV junction (often related to respiration). Vagal stimulation can cause pacemaker rates to slow. Other causes include associated underlying heart disease and the administration of digitalis.

> **NOTE**
>
> Another type of wandering atrial pacemaker is **multifocal atrial tachycardia (MAT)** (Figure 22-48). MAT resembles wandering pacemaker but is associated with rates often in the 120 to 150 beats/minute range. MAT is always considered pathological. This atrial tachycardia most often is found in patients with severe chronic obstructive pulmonary disease and may respond to management of the underlying disease. MAT often is mistaken for atrial fibrillation with rapid ventricular response (described later in this chapter).

RULES FOR INTERPRETATION (LEAD II MONITORING)

Wandering pacemaker has the following characteristics on the ECG:

QRS complex: Usually less than 0.12 second, provided no conduction block is present in the bundle branches

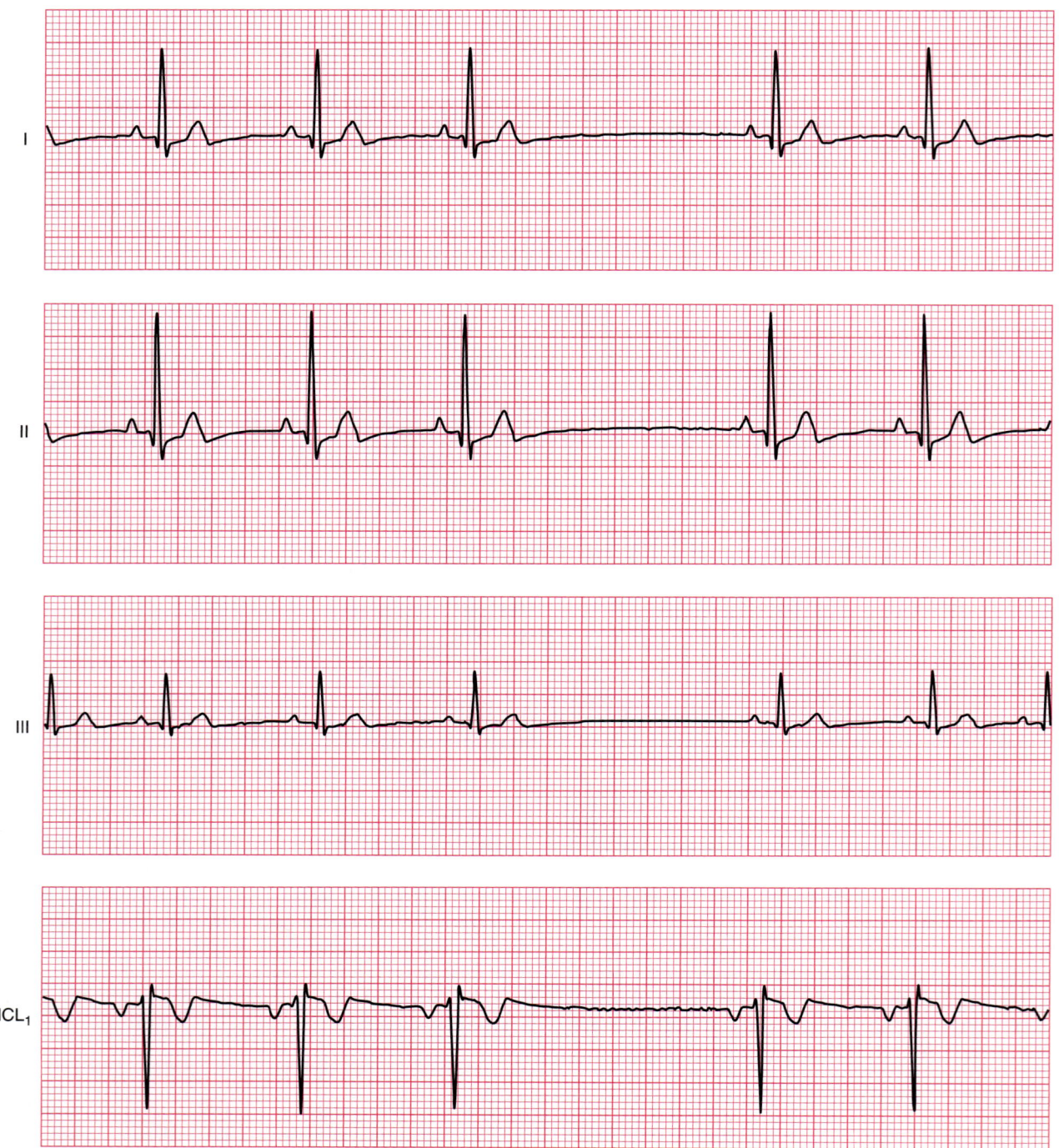

I

II

III

MCL₁

FIGURE 22-46 Sinus arrest.

P waves: Change in P-wave morphology from beat to beat. In lead II, the P waves may be upright, rounded, notched, inverted, biphasic, or buried in the QRS complex.

Rate: Usually 60 to 99 beats/minute. The rate may slow gradually when the pacemaker site shifts from the SA node to the atria or AV junction and may increase when the pacemaker site shifts back to the SA node.

Rhythm: Irregular P-R

P-R interval: Varies

CLINICAL SIGNIFICANCE

A wandering pacemaker usually does not produce serious signs and symptoms. Other atrial dysrhythmias (e.g., atrial fibrillation) occasionally are associated with this dysrhythmia.

MANAGEMENT

Sometimes a wandering pacemaker is a benign rhythm. In those instances, no management is required. Multifocal atrial tachycardia (MAT), however, may be precipitated by

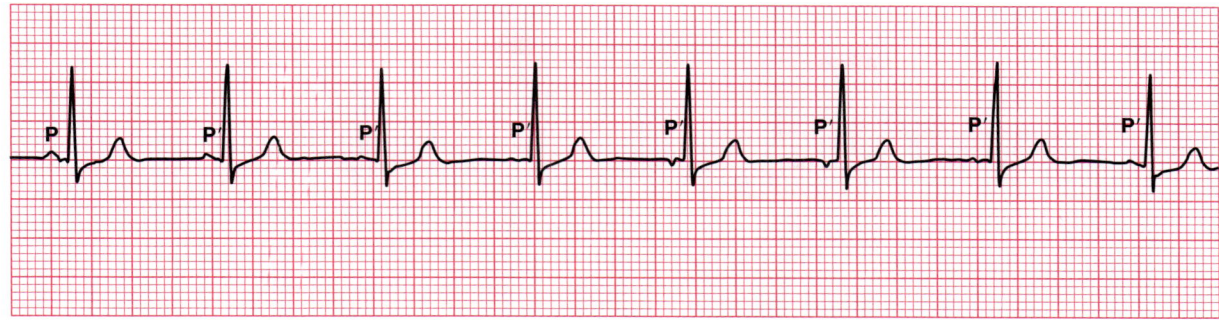

FIGURE 22-47 Wandering atrial pacemaker.

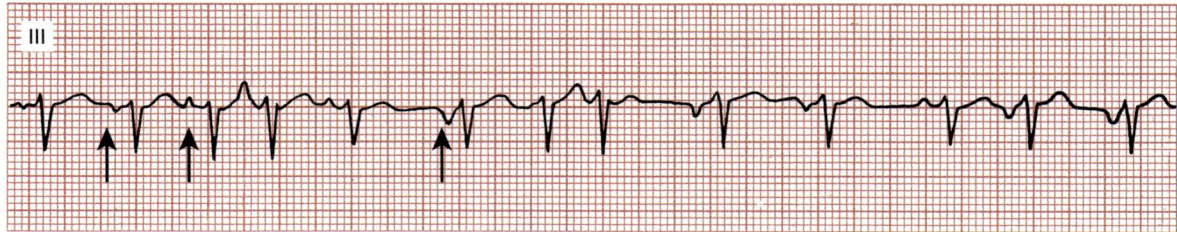

FIGURE 22-48. Multifocal atrial tachycardia. (Sole ML et al: *Introduction to critical care nursing,* ed 5, St Louis, 2009, Saunders.)

acute exacerbation of emphysema, congestive heart failure, or acute mitral valve regurgitation. Management is aimed at the underlying cause. Oxygen administration is usually the initial treatment of choice for MAT.

Premature Atrial Complex

DESCRIPTION

A **premature atrial complex (PAC)** is a single electrical impulse originating in the atria, outside the sinus node (Figure 22-49). The impulse creates a premature atrial complex (P wave). If conducted through the AV node, the impulse also causes a QRS complex before the next expected sinus beat. Because the PAC usually depolarizes the SA node prematurely, the timing of the SA node is reset. The next expected P wave of the underlying rhythm appears earlier than it would have if the SA node had not been disturbed. PACs may originate from a single ectopic pacemaker site or from multiple sites in the atria. PACs are thought to result from enhanced automaticity or a reentry mechanism (described later in this chapter).

CRITICAL THINKING

What do you feel when you palpate the pulse of a patient with premature atrial complexes?

ETIOLOGY

Premature atrial complexes may result from the following:

- Increase in catecholamines and sympathetic tone
- Use of caffeine, tobacco, or alcohol
- Use of sympathomimetic drugs *(epinephrine, albuterol, norepinephrine)*
- Electrolyte imbalance
- Hypoxia
- Digitalis toxicity
- Cardiovascular disease
- In some cases, no apparent cause

RULES FOR INTERPRETATION (LEAD II MONITORING)

Premature atrial complexes have the following characteristics on the ECG:

QRS complex: Usually less than 0.12 second. The QRS complex may be greater than 0.12 second and appear bizarre if the PAC is conducted abnormally. The QRS complex may be absent as a result of a temporary complete AV block (nonconducted PAC) that occurs during the refractory period of the AV node or ventricles.

P waves: The P wave of a PAC differs in shape from a sinus P wave. It occurs earlier than the next expected sinus P wave and may be so early that it is

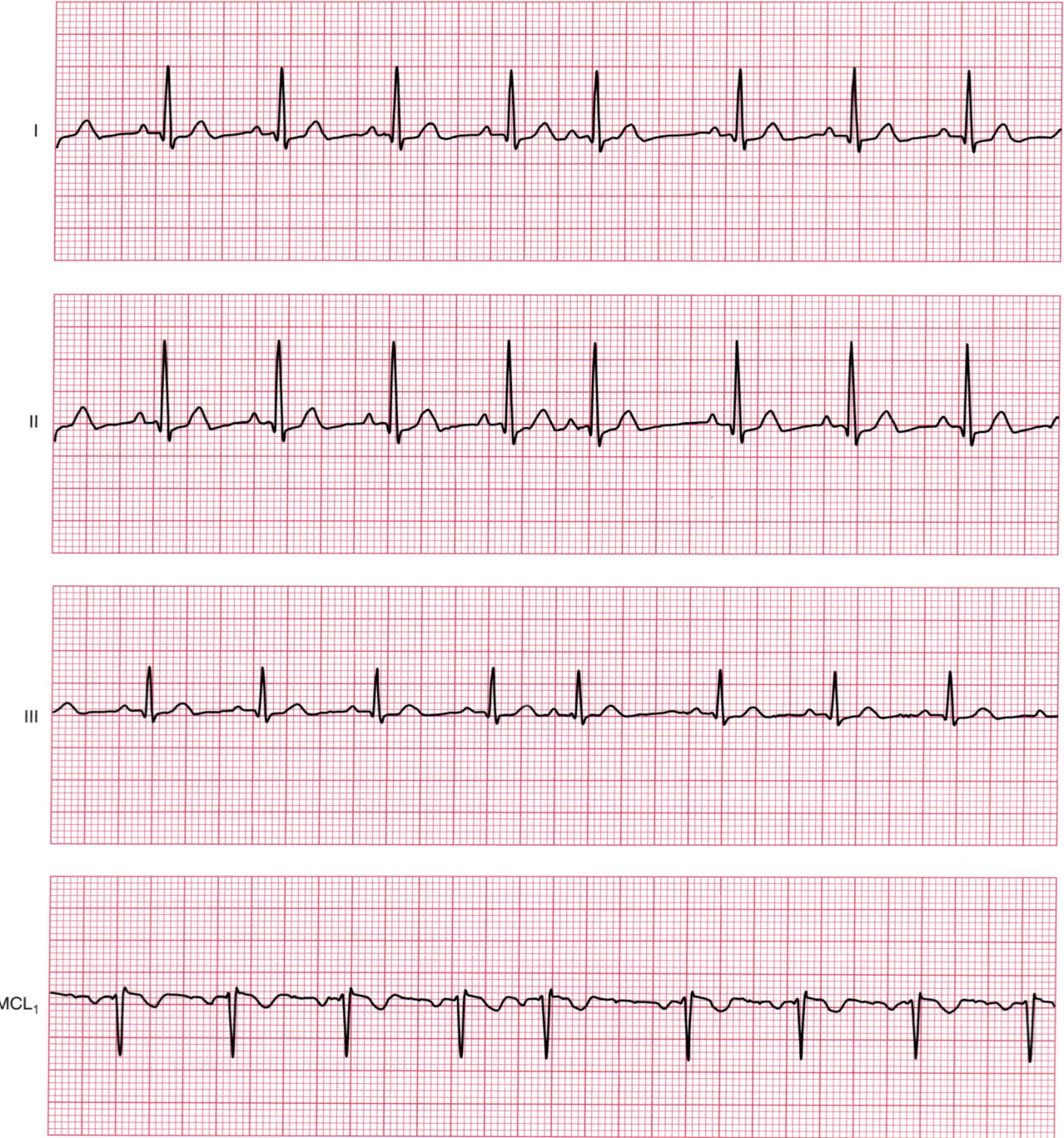

FIGURE 22-49 Premature atrial complex.

superimposed or hidden in the preceding T wave. The paramedic should evaluate the preceding T wave to see whether its shape is altered by the presence of a P wave.

Rate: Depends on the underlying rhythm

Rhythm: Usually the underlying rhythm is sinus and regular with irregular premature beats when the PACs occur.

P-R interval: Usually in the normal range but differs from those of the underlying rhythm. The P-R interval of a

PAC varies from 0.20 second when the pacemaker site is near the SA node to 0.12 second when the pacemaker site is near the AV junction.

> **NOTE**
>
> A premature atrial complex (PAC) that looks different from other PACs *(PAC with aberrancy)* on the ECG may resemble a premature ventricular complex (a more serious complex). Distinguishing between these two types of dysrhythmias is important to determining the appropriate patient care.

CLINICAL SIGNIFICANCE

Isolated PACs in healthy patients are not significant. Frequent PACs that occur in patients with heart disease may lead to serious supraventricular dysrhythmias such as multifocal atrial tachycardia, atrial tachycardia, atrial flutter, atrial fibrillation, or paroxysmal supraventricular tachycardia.

MANAGEMENT

Prehospital care usually requires only observation. PACs that are frequent or that do not produce ventricular contraction *(nonconducted PACs)* may cause symptomatic bradycardia. In these rare cases, transcutaneous cardiac pacing or *atropine* may be indicated (see Figure 22-43).

Supraventricular Tachycardias

DESCRIPTION

Supraventricular tachycardia (SVT) is a complex group of dysrhythmias. SVT can be broadly defined as any tachycardia that directly or indirectly involves the atria or AV node (above the bundle of His). SVTs described in this section include AV nodal reentry tachycardia (AVNRT), AV reentry tachycardia (AVRT), and atrial tachycardia (AT). SVTs result from rapid atrial or junctional depolarization that overrides the rate of the SA node. (Atrial fibrillation and atrial flutter are also supraventricular tachycardias and are discussed later in this chapter.)

AV nodal reentry tachycardia (AVNRT) is the most common type of reentry SVT. AVNRT usually is caused by a PAC. When the dysrhythmia begins and ends abruptly, it is known as **paroxysmal supraventricular tachycardia** (PSVT) (Figure 22-50). Most SVTs are thought to result from a reentry mechanism that involves abnormal pathways in the AV node. In patients prone to reentry SVTs, the AV node is functionally divided into two pathways: a slow (alpha) pathway with a longer refractory period and a fast (beta) pathway with a shorter refractory period (Figure 22-51). These pathways permit impulses to be conducted from the atrium to the ventricle *(antegrade conduction),* or from the ventricle to the atrium *(retrograde conduction).* Reentry SVTs occur when a premature impulse becomes blocked in the fast pathway and then travels the slow pathway. During this process, the fast pathway recovers while the slow pathway is firing. This produces a reentry tachycardia in which the electrical impulses are caught in a cycle that continuously circulates around the AV node (Figure 22-52). The cycle and the tachycardia continue until the reentry pathway is interrupted. Most SVTs are characterized by repeated episodes *(paroxysms)* of atrial tachycardia. These episodes often have a sudden onset (lasting minutes to hours) and an abrupt termination.

AV reentry tachycardia (AVRT) is the second most common type of reentry SVT. As in AVNRT, a reentry circuit is involved in the AV node. In addition, patients who have AVRT are born with a conducting tissue *(accessory pathway)* in the heart muscle. This accessory pathway bridges the atrium and ventricles outside of the AV node (Figure 22-53). The two pathways of the reentry circuit can be composed of one accessory pathway and the AV node, or it can be made up of two accessory pathways without the participation of the AV node. The accessory pathways can conduct impulses either antegrade, retrograde, or in both directions. This abnormal conduction results in preexcitation of the ventricles. (Preexcitation syndromes are discussed later in this chapter.)

Atrial tachycardia (AT) is a rhythm disturbance that arises from an irritable site in the atria. The ectopic focus overrides the SA node, producing tachycardia. AT does not require the AV junction, accessory pathways, or ventricular tissue to sustain the fast rate. The dysrhythmia presents very similar to sinus tachycardia; however, the P waves differ some in shape. The morphology of the P wave in AT depends on the location in the atrium that is responsible for the fast rate. AT that begins and ends abruptly is known as **paroxysmal atrial tachycardia** (PAT).

ETIOLOGY

SVTs may occur at any age. These dysrhythmias are common in young adults and are more common in women than in men. SVTs are not commonly associated with underlying heart disease and are rare in patients with myocardial infarction. (However, SVTs can precipitate angina pectoris or myocardial infarction in patients with heart disease.) Precipitating factors include stress, overexertion, tobacco use, caffeine consumption, and illicit drug use (e.g., cocaine). SVT is common in patients with Wolff-Parkinson-White syndrome (described later in this chapter).

RULES FOR INTERPRETATION (LEAD II MONITORING)

SVT has the following characteristics on the ECG:

QRS complex: Less than 0.12 second, provided no ventricular conduction disturbance is present

P waves: The ectopic P waves differ from the normal sinus P waves. In lead II, the P waves may be normal and upright if the pacemaker site is near the sinoatrial node but inverted if they originate near the atrioventricular junction. The P waves frequently are buried in preceding T or U waves or QRS complexes and therefore cannot be identified.

Rate: 150 to 250 beats/minute

Rhythm: Regular except at onset and termination

P-R interval: If P waves are discernible, the P-R interval often is shortened but may be normal or, rarely, prolonged.

CLINICAL SIGNIFICANCE

Supraventricular tachycardia may occur in patients with healthy hearts. Patients may tolerate it well for short periods. Often the dysrhythmia is accompanied by

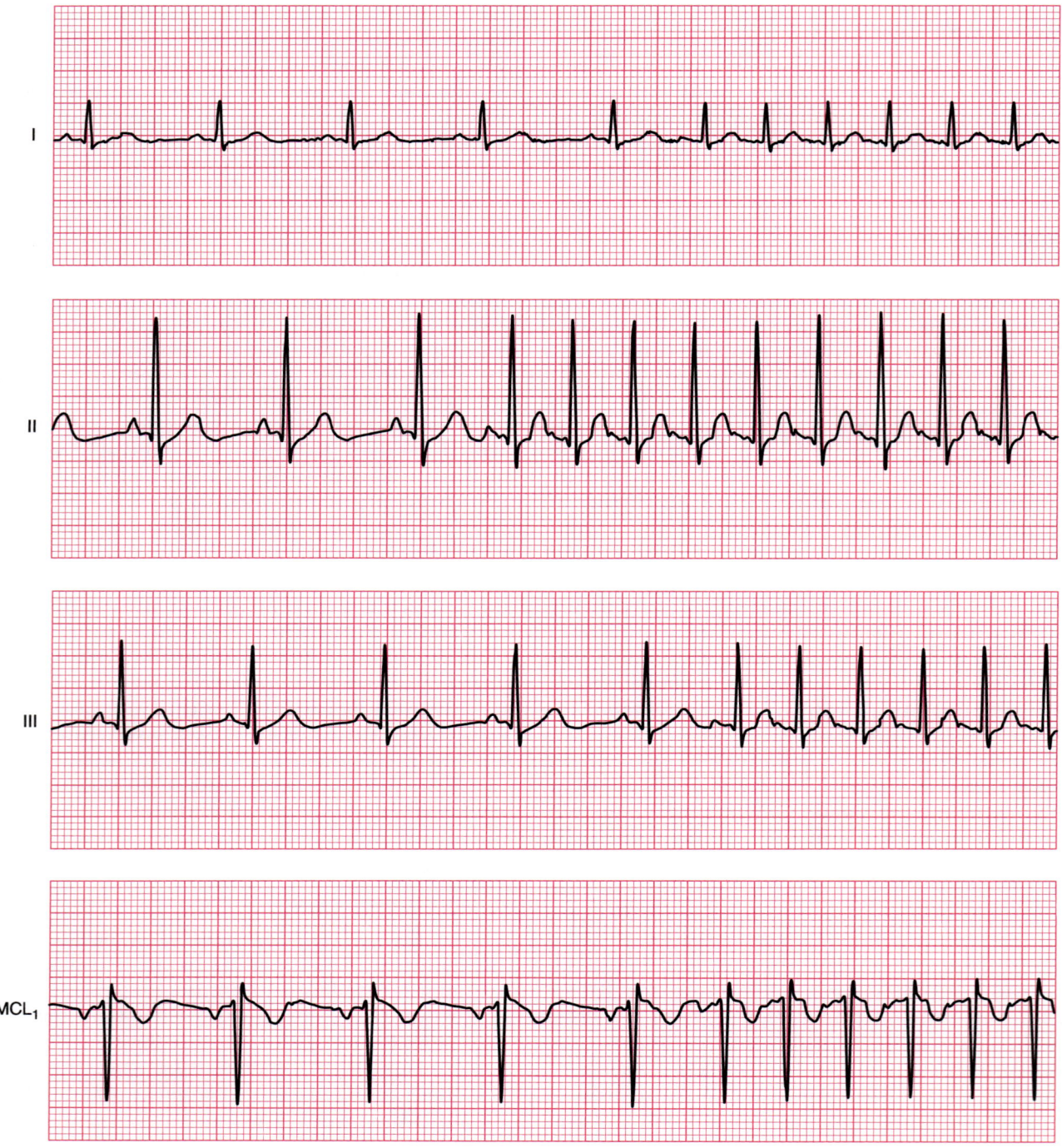

FIGURE 22-50 Paroxysmal supraventricular tachycardia.

palpitations, nervousness, and anxiety. (The patient often complains of a "racing heart.") A rapid ventricular rate may prevent the ventricles from filling fully. Therefore, SVT can compromise cardiac output in patients with existing heart disease. Decreased perfusion may cause confusion, vertigo, lightheadedness, and syncope and may precipitate angina pectoris, hypotension, or congestive heart failure. In addition, SVT increases the oxygen requirement of the heart. This may increase myocardial ischemia and the frequency and severity of the patient's chest pain.

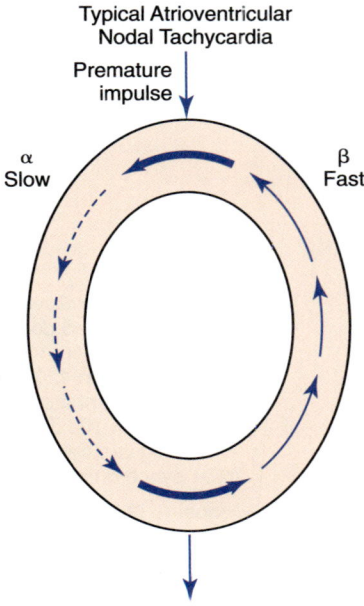

FIGURE 22-51 Atrioventricular nodal reentrant tachycardia (AVNRT) pathway.

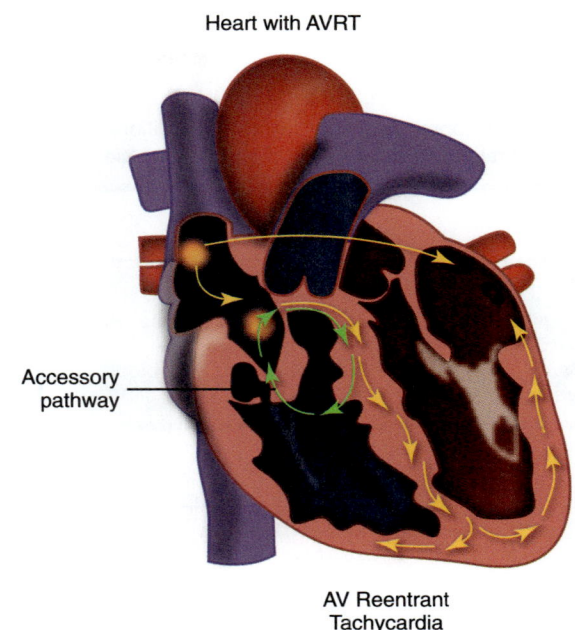

FIGURE 22-53 Atrioventricular nodal tachycardia (AVNT).

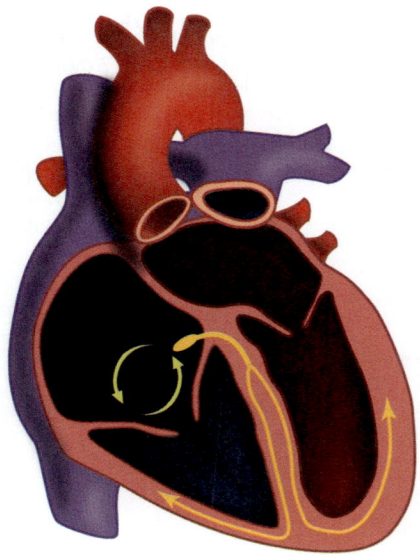

FIGURE 22-52 Atrioventricular nodal reentrant tachycardia (AVNRT).

> **NOTE**
>
> The distinctions among the various supraventricular tachycardias and ventricular tachycardia (a lethal rhythm) may be difficult to make. However, they are crucial. Two critical points to remember are these. First, if the patient has serious signs and symptoms (particularly if the ventricular rate is greater than 150 beats/minute), the paramedic should prepare for immediate cardioversion. Second, if the tachycardia complex appears wide, the paramedic should manage the rhythm as ventricular tachycardia. These two clinical rules should help manage the most difficult tachydysrhythmias. Use of modified chest leads may help identify these rhythms.

MANAGEMENT

The paramedic should manage symptomatic supraventricular tachycardia promptly. This helps reverse the consequences of the reduced cardiac output and increased workload of the heart. If the patient is stable (conscious with normal blood pressure and without chest pain, congestive heart failure, or pulmonary edema), the paramedic should attempt the following techniques to terminate the supraventricular tachycardia (Figure 22-54).

Vagal Maneuvers. Vagal maneuvers can slow the heart and reduce the force of atrial contraction. These maneuvers stimulate the parasympathetic nerve fibers in the wall of the atria and in specialized tissues of the SA and AV nodes. They can interrupt and terminate some supraventricular tachycardias. Vagal maneuvers should be attempted only under medical direction. Furthermore, the patient must be stable (conscious, normotensive, and without chest pain, congestive heart failure, or pulmonary edema). Continuous ECG monitoring and an intravenous line must be in place before beginning these procedures. **Atropine** and airway equipment should be readily available. Vagal maneuvers include the **Valsalva maneuver,** the ice pack maneuver in children, and unilateral carotid sinus pressure.

Valsalva Maneuver. The paramedic should place the patient in a sitting or semi-sitting position with the head tilted down. The patient should be instructed to take in a deep breath and to bear down as if to have a bowel movement. (Children can be instructed to blow through a straw.) The forced expiration against a closed glottis stimulates the vagus nerve and may terminate the tachycardia. The procedure may be repeated if unsuccessful.

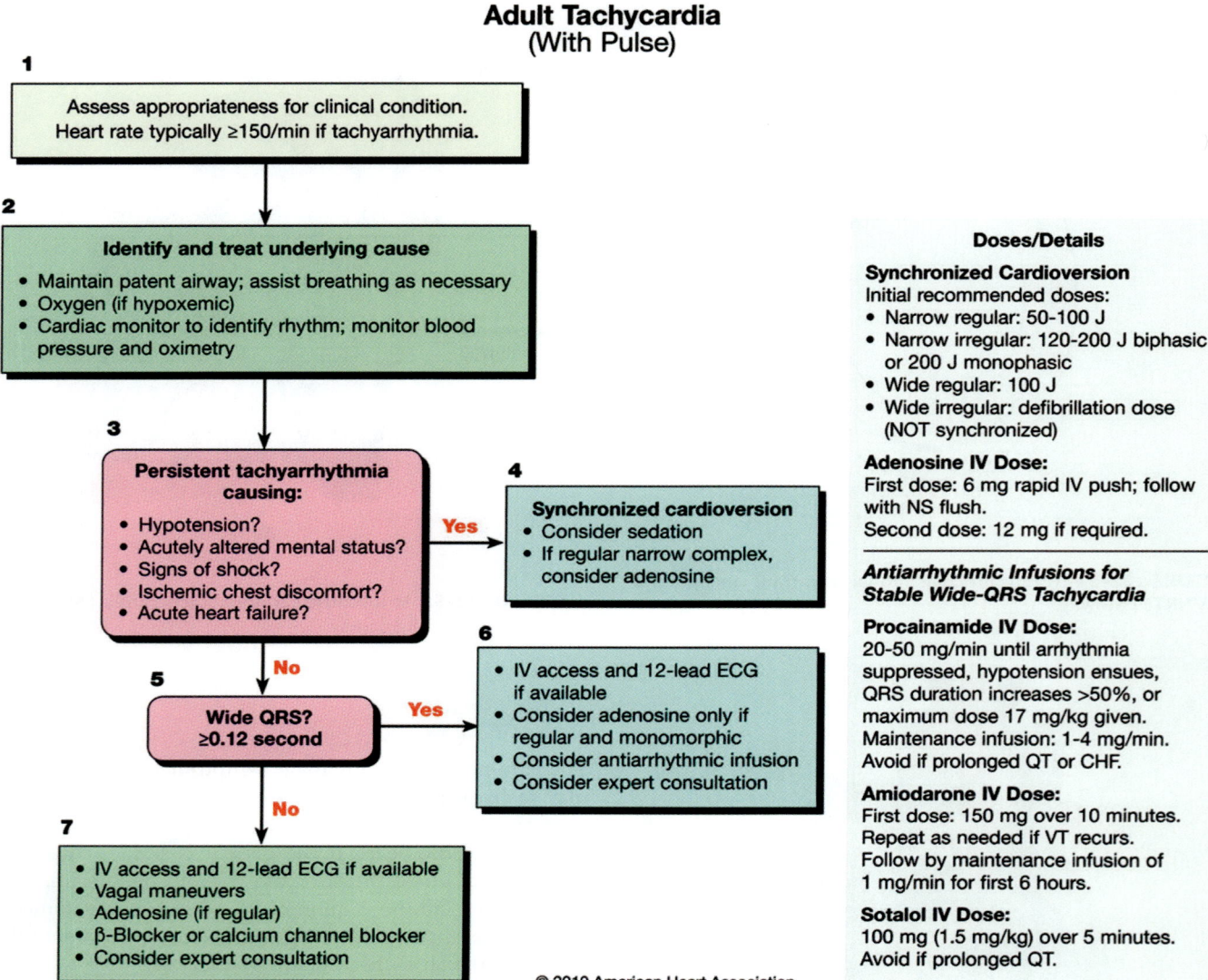

FIGURE 22-54 Tachycardia algorithm. (Reprinted with permission, American Heart Association Guidelines For CPR and ECC, *Circulation 122* [suppl 3]:S685-S919, American Heart Association, Inc, 2010.)

Ice Pack Maneuver. Placing an ice pack on the anterior neck of an infant or young child may stimulate the vagus nerve because of the *mammalian diving reflex* (see Chapter 45). (In the pediatric patient, this technique is performed with a washcloth soaked in ice water. The washcloth is placed across the patient's face, about to nostril level.) The paramedic should not attempt the ice pack maneuver if ischemic heart disease is present or suspected. The procedure may be repeated (per medical direction) if unsuccessful.

Unilateral Carotid Sinus Pressure. Carotid sinus pressure (carotid sinus massage) stimulates the carotid bodies located in the carotid arteries. The body interprets this localized pressure as an increase in blood pressure. This activates the autonomic nervous system and stimulates the vagus nerve. The heart rate slows in an attempt to lower blood pressure. The paramedic should auscultate the carotid arteries for the presence of a bruit (described in Chapter 20) before applying carotid sinus pressure. This vagal maneuver should not be used if bruits are present, if the patient is an older adult, or if the patient is known to have carotid artery disease or cerebral vascular disease. Possible complications from the procedure include cerebral emboli, stroke, syncope, sinus arrest, asystole, and an increased degree of atrioventricular block.[1] The procedure for applying unilateral carotid sinus pressure is as follows (Figure 22-55):

LOOK AGAIN
See Chapter 20: Secondary Assessment, pp. 542-543.

1. Position yourself behind the patient, who is lying supine with the neck extended and the head turned away from the side of the applied pressure.

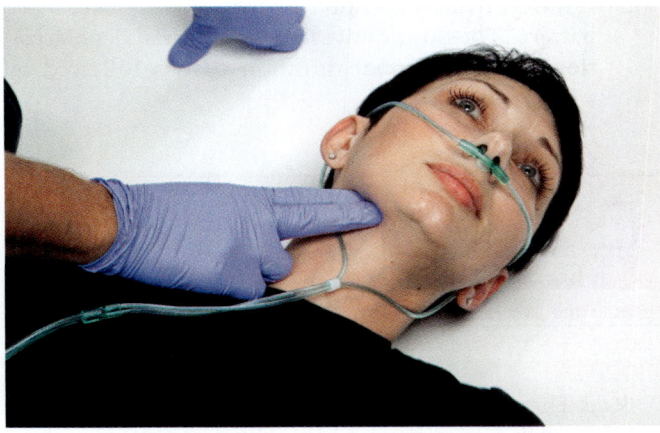

FIGURE 22-55 Carotid sinus massage.

2. Gently palpate each carotid artery to confirm the presence of equal pulses. If pulses are unequal or if one is absent, do not apply carotid sinus pressure.
3. While the patient holds his or her breath for 4 to 5 seconds, auscultate for the presence of bruits.
4. To apply carotid sinus pressure, place the index and middle fingers over the artery on the neck just below the angle of the jaw. Compress the artery firmly against the vertebral column while massaging the area. (Inform the patient that he or she may experience some pain or discomfort.) Maintain pressure no longer than 5 to 10 seconds. Discontinue the massage immediately if bradycardia or signs of heart block develop or if the tachycardia breaks. *Apply pressure to only one carotid sinus at a time. Applying bilateral carotid sinus pressure may interfere with cerebral circulation.*
5. Observe the ECG monitor and run a strip during the procedure and obtain a tracing. Repeat the procedure in 2 to 3 minutes if it is ineffective.

CRITICAL THINKING
You perform carotid sinus massage on a patient with bruits or known carotid artery disease. What might occur?

Pharmacological Therapy. If vagal maneuvers fail or are contraindicated and the patient remains stable, administration of **adenosine** (the initial drug of choice), **verapamil, diltiazem,** beta blockers **(metoprolol),** or other antidysrhythmics may end symptomatic SVT.

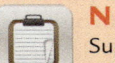

NOTE
Supraventricular tachycardia (SVT) may be the result of an underlying rhythm (e.g., atrial fibrillation with a rapid ventricular response). The prudent course is to monitor the ECG continuously and run a strip while administering **adenosine.** This allows the underlying rhythm to be captured once the heart rate slows. Other medications may be needed to treat the underlying rhythm (e.g., **diltiazem or verapamil**). It is not uncommon for the underlying rhythm to revert to SVT, requiring additional drug therapy.

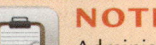

NOTE
Administration of *diltiazem or verapamil* to a patient with ventricular tachycardia can be lethal. The paramedic must carefully evaluate the patient's ECG to distinguish between SVT with aberrant conduction and ventricular tachycardia. If the complexes are wide and ventricular tachycardia is suspected, the paramedic should manage the rhythm in the same way as ventricular tachycardia.

CRITICAL THINKING
What are some of the side effects of verapamil?

Drug treatment recommended by the American Heart Association for stable narrow-complex supraventricular tachycardias is based on rhythm interpretation and the stability of the patient .People with heart disease may experience a rapid heart rate, yet remain clinically stable. These patients often are chronically ill with heart disease and have adjusted to a reduced level of cardiac function. Based on the patient history and physical examination, the paramedic should be able to distinguish between acute and chronic or stable congestive heart failure. A *sudden* onset of signs and symptoms of congestive heart failure with impaired cardiac function (e.g., jugular vein distention, dyspnea, tachycardia, chest pain, or decreased level of consciousness) indicates that the patient is unstable.

Junctional tachycardia in adults is rare; it is not paroxysmal. Ectopic atrial tachycardia is also not paroxysmal. It often continues after drug treatment to block conduction through the AV node. Unlike reentry dysrhythmias, ectopic atrial tachycardia, multifocal atrial tachycardia, and sinus tachycardia are not responsive to electrical cardioversion.

For simplicity, in symptomatic narrow complex SVT, vagal maneuvers and *adenosine* should be used first to end the tachydysrhythmia. If *adenosine* is not effective and if the patient is hemodynamically stable and has no evidence of congestive heart failure, secondary drug treatment options include calcium channel blockers and beta blockers. These agents most likely will be used after diagnosis and evaluation by a physician.

Consecutive use of calcium channel blockers, beta blockers, and primary antidysrhythmics is discouraged. The general rule is to use only one antidysrhythmic agent; using several can result in more dysrhythmias and a drop in blood pressure. Furthermore, the paramedic should avoid negative inotropic drugs (*verapamil,* beta blockers, flecainide, *procainamide,* propafenone, and sotalol) in hemodynamically unstable patients.

Several drug treatments are available for narrow-complex tachycardias (ventricular rate equal to or greater than 150 beats/minute). However, when serious signs and symptoms point to poor perfusion and clinical instability, synchronized electrical cardioversion is the treatment of choice to terminate the rhythm. (Cardioversion is presented later in this chapter.) Cardioversion should begin with a synchronized shock of 50 J or equivalent biphasic energy. (Atrial fibrillation should first be managed with a shock of 100 to 120 J biphasic.[1] If this fails, the energy may be increased in a stepwise manner per manufacturer's recommendation. Sedation should be considered before cardioversion if time permits.

> 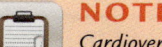 **NOTE**
> *Cardioversion* encompasses vagal, pharmacological, and electrical therapy. However, the term commonly is used to refer to electrical cardioversion.

> **CRITICAL THINKING**
> Why is the drug midazolam an ideal sedative to administer before cardioversion?

Atrial Flutter

DESCRIPTION

Atrial flutter is almost always a result of a rapid atrial reentry focus (Figure 22-56). Atrial flutter that is not slowed by preexisting atrioventricular block usually manifests a 2:1 atrioventricular conduction ratio and may look like SVT. (A 2:1 AV conduction ratio means that 50% of the atrial impulses are conducted through the ventricles.) However, 3:1, 4:1, and greater conduction ratios are not uncommon. These ratios produce a discrepancy between atrial and ventricular rates. The conduction ratios may be constant or variable. Atrial flutter may be seen with atrial fibrillation *(atrial fib-flutter).* In rare cases, atrial flutter may conduct 1:1. This results in extremely fast ventricular rates with rapid hemodynamic deterioration.

ETIOLOGY

Atrial flutter usually is seen in middle-aged or older patients who have heart disease. At times, atrial flutter also occurs in patients with healthy hearts. The dysrhythmia commonly is associated with the following:

- Cardiomyopathy
- Cardiac hypertrophy
- Digitalis toxicity (rare)
- Hypoxia
- Congestive heart failure
- Pericarditis
- Myocarditis

RULES FOR INTERPRETATION (LEAD II MONITORING)

Atrial flutter has the following characteristics on the ECG:
> *QRS complex*: Less than 0.12 second, unless ventricular conduction disturbance (aberrancy) is present
> *P waves*: Normal P waves are absent. The flutter waves (f waves) usually resemble a sawtooth or picket fence pattern. The flutter waves represent atrial depolarization in an abnormal direction that is followed by atrial repolarization.

> **NOTE**
> Flutter waves may be difficult to identify with a 2:1 ratio of atrial to ventricular complexes. The paramedic should suspect 2:1 flutter when the rhythm is regular and the ventricular rate is 150 beats/minute.

> *Rate*: The atrial rate is 250 to 300 beats/minute; the ventricular rate is regular but often less than the atrial rate.

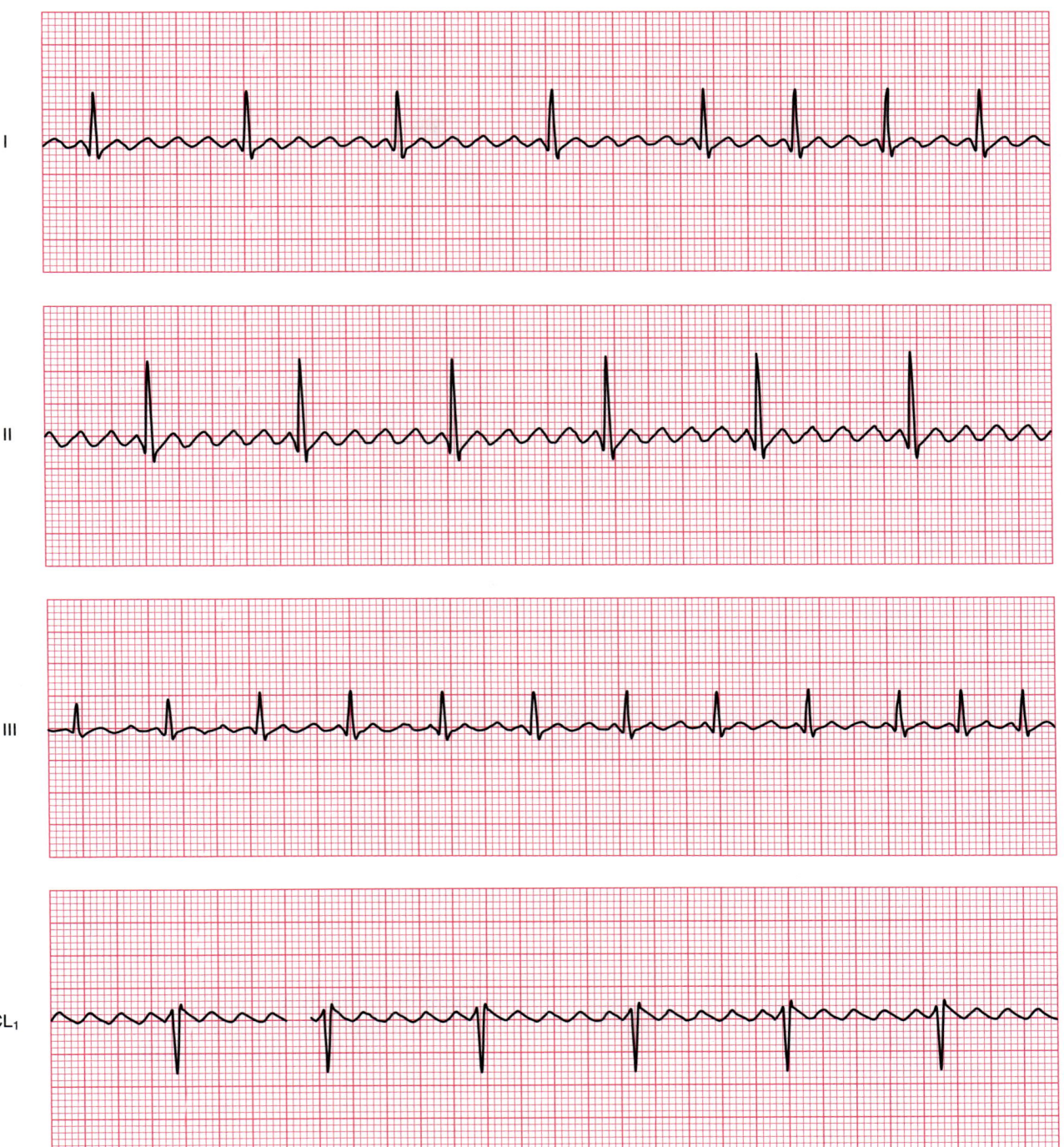

FIGURE 22-56 Atrial flutter.

Rhythm: The atrial rhythm is regular; the ventricular rate is usually regular. However, the ventricular rate may be irregular if the AV conduction ratio varies.

P-R interval: Usually constant but may vary

CLINICAL SIGNIFICANCE

With a normal ventricular rate, atrial flutter usually is well tolerated by the patient. A rapid ventricular rate produces the same signs and symptoms of decreased cardiac output that are seen in patients with SVT. In addition, in some flutter rhythms (particularly a 2:1 atrial flutter), the atria do not contract regularly and empty before each ventricular contraction. The loss of the "atrial kick" results in incomplete filling of the ventricles. This may further reduce cardiac output.

MANAGEMENT

See Management of Atrial Fibrillation and Atrial Flutter.

> **NOTE**
> The pulse rate of a patient with this dysrhythmia (and other tachycardias) might not reflect the true heart rate. This is because not all heart contractions produce enough output of blood to create a palpable pulse.

Rhythm: Irregularly irregular
P-R interval: None

> **NOTE**
> Irregularly irregular rhythms are most likely to be atrial fibrillation.

Atrial Fibrillation

DESCRIPTION

Atrial fibrillation results from multiple areas of reentry within the atria (Figure 22-57). It also can result from ectopic atrial pacemakers. (The activity of the SA node is suppressed completely by atrial fibrillation.) Atrial fibrillation produces chaotic impulses too numerous for all to be conducted by the AV node through the ventricles. AV conduction is random. This results in an irregular but usually rapid ventricular response. Medications such as digoxin, beta blockers, or calcium channel blockers often are prescribed to slow the ventricular rate.

ETIOLOGY

Sudden onset (paroxysmal) atrial fibrillation may occur in young adults after heavy alcohol ingestion ("holiday heart" syndrome) or acute stress. In these cases, the fibrillation usually is self-limited and resolves without treatment. Chronic atrial fibrillation may be intermittent. It often is associated with rheumatic heart disease, congestive heart failure, and coronary heart disease. Chronic atrial fibrillation usually requires drug therapy with digitalis (or a calcium channel blocker or beta blocker). This slows the ventricular rate to 80 to 100 beats/minute. Atrial fibrillation may be a stable rhythm that does not require management. Less commonly, it may occur in cardiomyopathy, acute myocarditis and pericarditis, and chest trauma. It rarely is caused by digitalis toxicity. However, a slow, regular ventricular response with atrial fibrillation could be the result of digitalis toxicity.

RULES FOR INTERPRETATION (LEAD II MONITORING)

Atrial fibrillation has the following characteristics on the ECG:

QRS complex: Less than 0.12 second, provided no ventricular conduction disturbance is present

P waves: P waves and organized atrial contractions are absent. Fibrillation waves (f waves) may be fine (less than 1 mm) or coarse (greater than 1 mm). Fine f waves may be so small that they appear as a wavy or flat (isoelectric) line or are absent. The f waves are irregularly shaped, rounded (or pointed), and dissimilar.

Rate: The atrial rate is 350 to 700 beats/minute (cannot be counted); the ventricular rate varies greatly, depending on conduction through the AV node (average 150 to 180 beats/minute if uncontrolled).

CLINICAL SIGNIFICANCE

The atrial kick is lost in atrial fibrillation. This loss can reduce cardiac output by as much as 15%. This, coupled with a rapid ventricular response, may cause cardiovascular decompensation (angina pectoris, myocardial infarction, congestive heart failure, or cardiogenic shock).

MANAGEMENT OF ATRIAL FIBRILLATION AND ATRIAL FLUTTER

A risk of emboli formation exists when atrial fibrillation or atrial flutter has been present for longer than 48 hours. Formation of emboli in the heart increases the risk of "throwing a clot" or systemic embolization. This most often occurs when the atrial fibrillation is converted suddenly to a sinus rhythm. The algorithm cautions against converting atrial fibrillation or atrial flutter without first giving the patient drugs that prevent blood clotting. Electrical cardioversion and the use of antidysrhythmic agents that may convert the rhythm should be avoided unless the patient is unstable or hemodynamically compromised.[6]

Using drugs to control the heart rate is the recommended initial treatment for stable, rapid atrial fibrillation or atrial flutter regardless of how long the patient has had it. Specific drug treatment depends on the patient's condition and how stable the patient is. Using several different drugs can cause a dysrhythmia to develop (a **proarrhythmia**). The paramedic should use only one drug from the list of suggested drug treatments.

In patients with a rapid atrial fibrillation or flutter with a rapid ventricular response, the rate may be controlled with **diltiazem** or beta blockers. **Amiodarone** has a potential for rhythm conversion. Thus **amiodarone** should be reserved for use within the first 48 hours of dysrhythmia onset when other medications for rate control have failed. The use of calcium channel blocking agents and beta-blocking agents warrants caution in the presence of congestive heart failure because of their negative inotropic properties. Beta-blocking agents also should be used with caution in patients with asthma and chronic obstructive pulmonary disease. Another drug that may be effective for converting the rhythm is digoxin. Digoxin should be used only if the patient developed atrial fibrillation within 48 hours or less.

If the patient reports a history of Wolff-Parkinson-White syndrome or if the paramedic forms that impression in the field before the patient developed atrial fibrillation, alternative treatment is indicated.

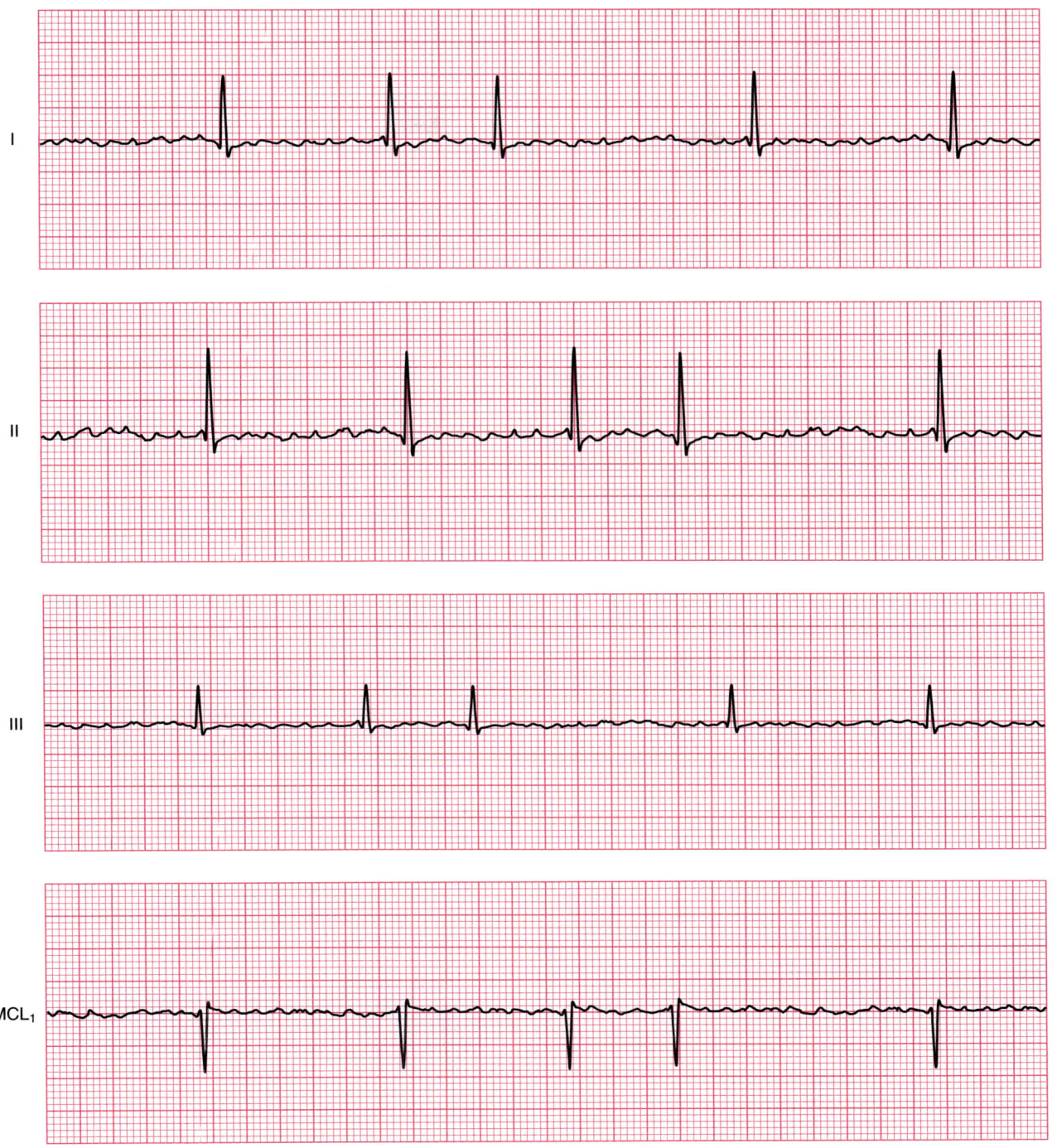

FIGURE 22-57 Atrial fibrillation.

If the patient has WPW syndrome, paramedics should not give **adenosine, diltiazem, verapamil, digoxin** or, in most cases, beta blockers. These drugs may cause a dangerous increase in the heart rate. If the patient has had the dysrhythmia for longer than 48 hours, the paramedic should avoid elective cardioversion except when the patient is unstable unless anticoagulation drugs have been given. However, when serious signs or symptoms occur, such as chest pain, shortness of breath, pulmonary congestion, a decreased level of consciousness, or hypotension, the paramedic should cardiovert the patient immediately. The initial attempt at cardioversion for atrial flutter should consist of a synchronized shock of 50 to 100 J.[1] If needed, the energy may be increased in a stepwise manner according to manufacturer's recommendations. Because atrial fibrillation is a more difficult rhythm to convert and lower joule settings have been known to cause asystole, recommendations are initially to use a synchronized shock of 100 to 120 J biphasic (200 J monophasic), followed by stepwise increases as recommended by the manufacturer if necessary (Box 22-7).[1]

BOX 22-7 Atrial Fibrillation/Flutter

With or without congestive heart failure:

Rate control   Diltiazem
Rhythm conversion   Nonemergency chemical or direct
current cardioversion should be
avoided, if possible; when indicated,
it should be performed only by an
experienced health care provider
after careful evaluation and initiation
of thromboembolic precautions.

DID YOU KNOW?
Catheter Ablation Therapy
Catheter ablation is an in-hospital procedure performed in an electrophysiology (EP) laboratory. During the procedure (which lasts several hours), three to five catheters are inserted into the heart through an artery or vein (or both) in the groin, neck, or arm. A transducer is inserted through one of the catheters so that intracardiac ultrasonography can be performed during the procedure. The ablation catheter is moved from spot to spot (mapping) to identify the origin of a dysrhythmia. A pacemaker-like device then is used to send electrical impulses to the heart to induce tachycardia. Once the area of the heart responsible for the dysrhythmia has been identified, an electrical impulse is delivered to the area through the catheter. The goal is to "disconnect" the pathway of the abnormal rhythm. Catheter ablation can be used to treat the following conditions:
- AV node reentrant tachycardia
- Accessory pathway disturbances
- Atrial fibrillation and atrial flutter
- Ventricular tachycardia

CRITICAL THINKING
What signs or symptoms would make you think these patients are unstable?

DYSRHYTHMIAS SUSTAINED OR ORIGINATING IN THE ATRIOVENTRICULAR JUNCTION

When the SA node and the atria cannot generate the electrical impulses needed to begin depolarization because of factors such as hypoxia, ischemia, myocardial infarction, and drug toxicity, the AV node or the area surrounding the AV node may assume the role of the secondary pacemaker. Rhythms that start in the AV node or AV junctional area are *junctional rhythms*. This type of rhythm usually is a benign dysrhythmia. Yet the paramedic must assess the rhythm to determine the patient's tolerance of the rhythm disturbance. Dysrhythmias that originate in the AV junction include premature junctional complexes, junctional

escape complexes or junctional escape rhythms, and accelerated junctional rhythm.

In junctional rhythms, electrical impulses travel in a normal pathway from the AV junction through the bundle of His and bundle branches to the Purkinje fibers. The pathway ends in the ventricular muscle. Conduction through the ventricles proceeds normally. The QRS complex, therefore, usually is within normal limits (0.04 to 0.10 second). However, the impulse that depolarizes the atria travels in a backward or retrograde motion. The retrograde depolarization of the atria results in one of three P wave characteristics: (1) inverted P waves in lead II with a short P-R interval; (2) absent P waves; or (3) P waves after the QRS complex.

Premature Junctional Complex
DESCRIPTION

A **premature junctional complex** (PJC) results from a single electrical impulse from the AV junction (Figure 22-58). The impulse occurs before the next expected sinus impulse.

ETIOLOGY

Isolated PJCs may occur in a healthy person without apparent cause. Yet they more often are a result of heart disease or drug toxicity. Usually PJCs result from enhanced automaticity or a reentry mechanism. Premature junctional complexes have several causes:
- Digitalis toxicity
- Other cardiac medications (quinidine, **procainamide**)
- Increased vagal tone on the SA node
- Sympathomimetic drugs (e.g., cocaine, methamphetamines)
- Hypoxia
- Congestive heart failure
- Damage to the AV junction

CRITICAL THINKING
Would the P wave be visible if it occurred during the QRS wave?

RULES FOR INTERPRETATION (LEAD II MONITORING)

Premature junctional complexes have the following characteristics on the ECG:

QRS complex: Usually less than 0.12 second, provided no ventricular conduction disturbance is present
P waves: May be associated with premature junctional complexes. P waves may occur before, during, or after the QRS complex or may be absent. If present, P waves are abnormal, differing in size, shape, and direction from normal P waves.
Rate: The heart rate is that of the underlying rhythm.
Rhythm: Usually regular, except when premature junctional complexes are present

P-R interval: Usually less than 0.12 second if the P wave precedes the QRS complex

CLINICAL SIGNIFICANCE

Occasional premature junctional complexes usually are not significant.

MANAGEMENT

No management is required.

Junctional Escape Complexes or Rhythms

DESCRIPTION

A **junctional escape beat** or rhythm (series of beats) occurs when the rate of the SA node falls below that of the AV junction (Figure 22-59). The dysrhythmia also may occur when the electrical impulses from the SA node or atria fail to reach the AV junction because of sinoatrial or

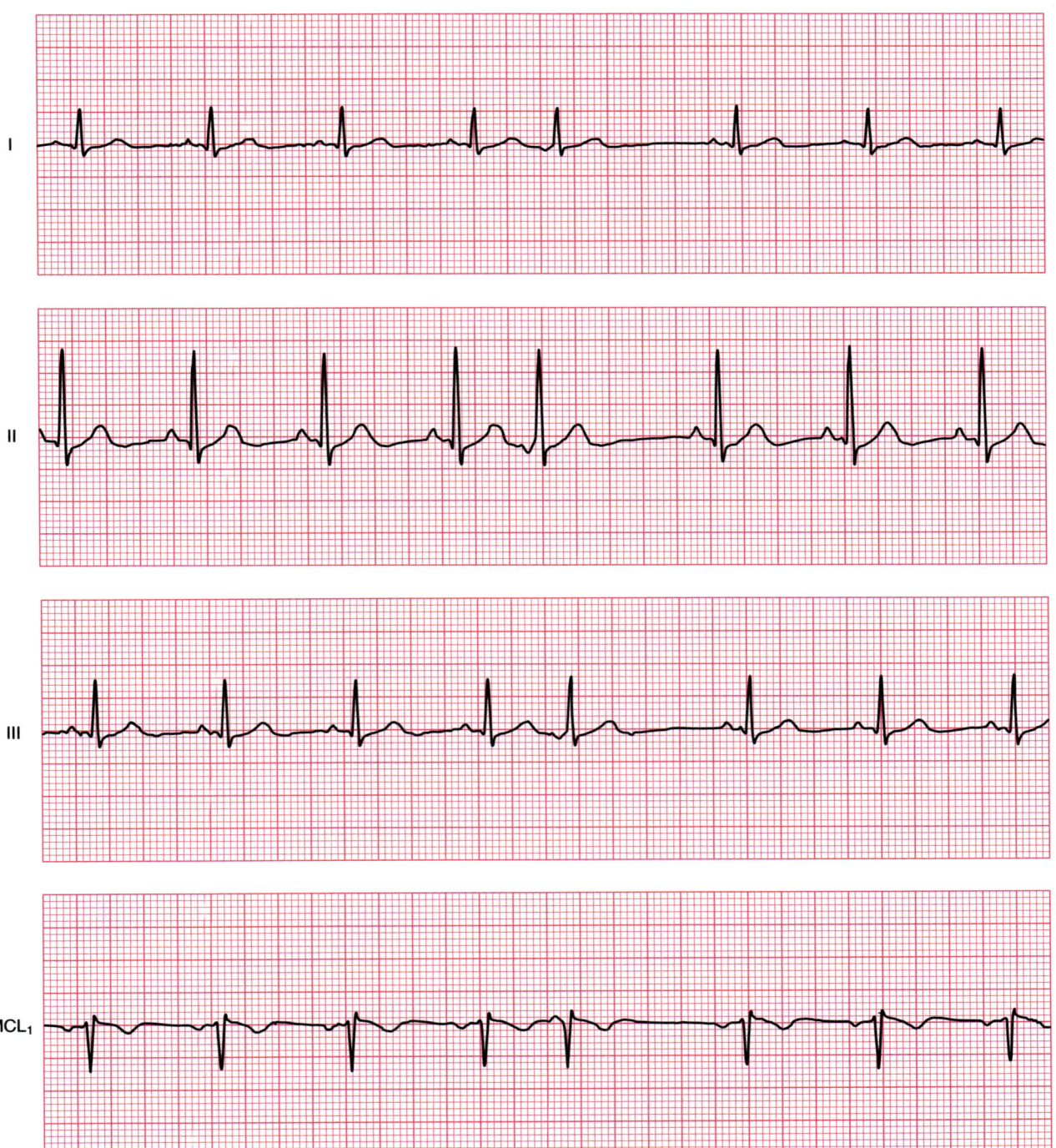

FIGURE 22-58 Premature junctional complexes.

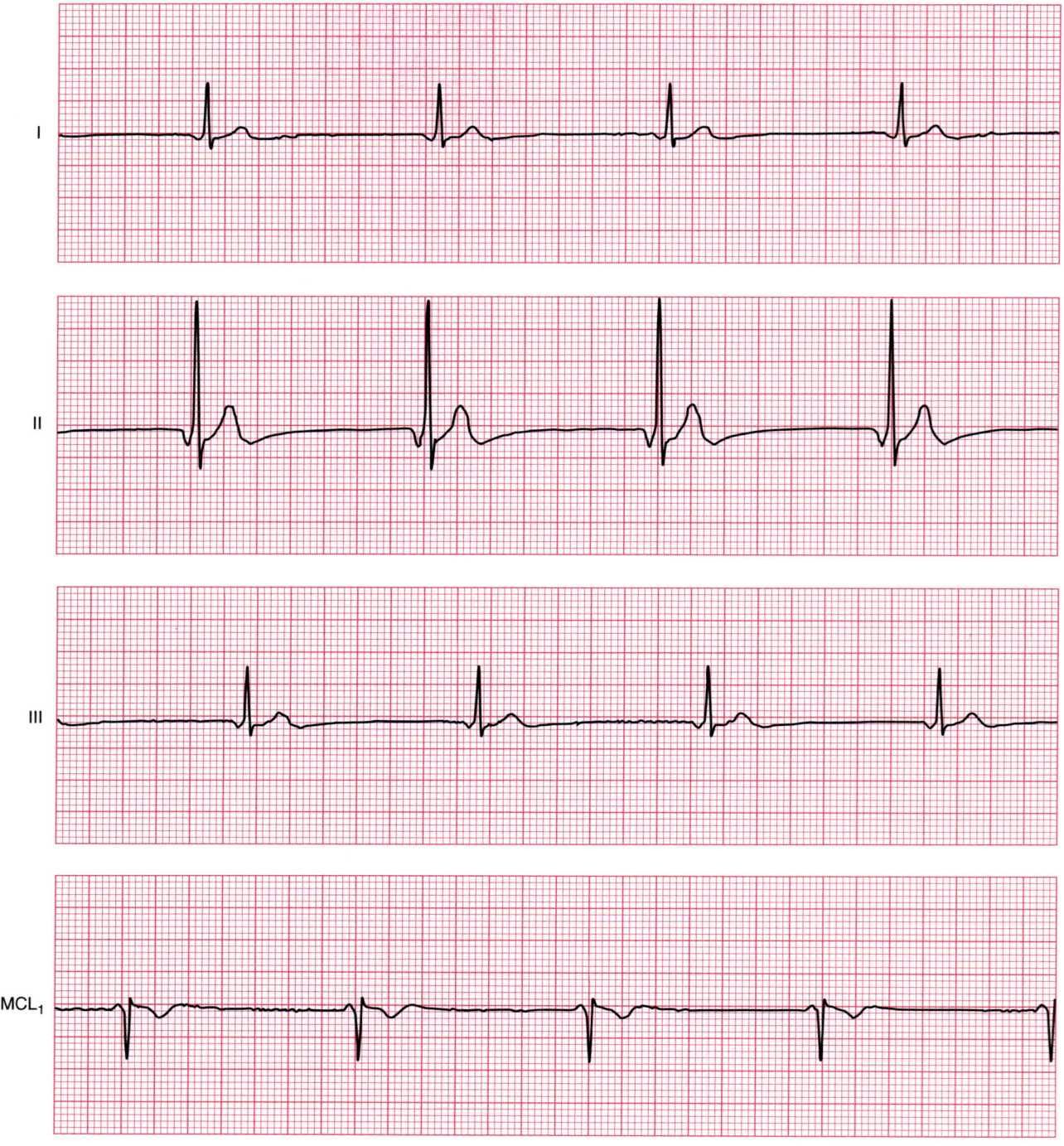

FIGURE 22-59 Junctional escape complex or rhythm.

atrioventricular block. The escape complex or rhythm provided by the AV junction serves as a safety mechanism. This mechanism prevents cardiac standstill. The AV junction begins firing at an inherent rate of 40 to 60 beats/minute within about 1 to 1.5 seconds of not receiving an impulse from the SA node.

ETIOLOGY

A junctional escape complex (isolated impulse) or a junctional escape rhythm (series of impulses) is a normal response. It may result from increased vagal tone on the sinoatrial node, a pathological slowing of the sinoatrial discharge, or complete atrioventricular block.

RULES FOR INTERPRETATION (LEAD II MONITORING)

Junctional escape complexes or rhythms have the following characteristics on the ECG:

QRS complex: Usually less than 0.12 second, provided no preexisting bundle branch block is present

P waves: May be present (with or without relationship to QRS complex) or absent. If P waves are present, they may occur before, after, or during the QRS complex. Depending on the pacemaker site, P waves may differ from normal P waves in size, shape, and direction and may be upright or inverted.

Rate: Usually 40 to 60 beats/minute but may be less

Rhythm: The ventricular rhythm usually is regular in junctional escape rhythm; it may be irregular if an isolated junctional escape complex is present.

P-R interval: If P waves precede the QRS complex, the P-R interval commonly is shortened (less than 0.12 second) and constant.

CLINICAL SIGNIFICANCE

Junctional bradycardias can cause decreased cardiac output. Therefore, patients can have signs and symptoms similar to those of other bradycardias (e.g., the signs may include lightheadedness, hypotension, and syncope). As a rule, patients tolerate junctional rhythms of 50 beats/minute or greater.

MANAGEMENT

Patients who are stable do not need to be treated. If the patient is symptomatic or if ventricular irritability is present, drug therapy (beginning with **atropine**) may be indicated. In severe cases and in patients unresponsive to **atropine,** external pacing may be necessary. If the sinoatrial node is diseased or damaged, the patient may need a permanent pacemaker (see Figure 22-43).

Accelerated Junctional Rhythm

DESCRIPTION

Accelerated junctional rhythm results from increased automaticity of the atrioventricular junction (Figure 22-60). This increase causes it to discharge faster than its intrinsic rate. (The intrinsic rate is 40 to 60 beats/minute.) This rate in turn overrides the main (sinoatrial node) pacemaker. The rate of this dysrhythmia (usually 60 to 99 beats/minute) does not truly constitute a tachycardia. Therefore, the dysrhythmia is called *accelerated junctional rhythm*. In this text, rapid junctional rhythms equal to or greater than 100 beats/minute (junctional tachycardia caused by a reentry mechanism) are discussed with other supraventricular tachycardias.

ETIOLOGY

An accelerated junctional rhythm commonly is a result of digitalis toxicity. Other causes of this rhythm include excessive catecholamine administration, damage to the atrioventricular junction, inferior wall myocardial infarction (described later in this chapter), and rheumatic fever.

RULES FOR INTERPRETATION (LEAD II MONITORING)

Accelerated junctional rhythm has the following characteristics on the ECG:

QRS complex: Usually less than 0.12 second, provided no preexisting bundle branch block is present

P waves: May be present (with or without relationship to the QRS complex), absent (retrograde atrioventricular block), or buried in the QRS complex. If present, P waves usually are inverted and appear before or after the QRS complex.

Rate: Usually 60 to 99 beats/minute

Rhythm: Regular

P-R interval: If the P wave occurs before the QRS complex, the P-R interval will be less than 0.12 second. If the P wave follows the QRS complex, it technically is an R-P interval and usually is less than 0.20 second.

CLINICAL SIGNIFICANCE

Accelerated junctional rhythm usually is well tolerated by the patient. However, heart disease and lack of oxygen to the heart muscle may cause more serious dysrhythmias.

MANAGEMENT

Accelerated junctional rhythm generally requires no immediate treatment.

 CRITICAL THINKING
Because no drug therapy is indicated, do you need to start an intravenous line on these patients?

DYSRHYTHMIAS ORIGINATING IN THE VENTRICLES

Ventricular dysrhythmias usually are considered a threat to life. Ventricular rhythm disturbances generally result from failure of the atria, atrioventricular junction, or both to initiate an electrical impulse. Such disturbances also can result from enhanced automaticity or reentry pathways in the ventricles. Enhanced automaticity and reentry can lead to premature ventricular complexes, ventricular tachycardia, and even ventricular fibrillation. Ventricular dysrhythmias often are associated with myocardial ischemia or infarction.

The ventricle is the least efficient pacemaker of the heart. It usually generates only 20 to 40 impulses per minute. However, it may discharge at rates up to 99 impulses per minute (accelerated idioventricular rhythm) or even faster (ventricular tachycardia) because of increased automaticity. Dysrhythmias originating in the ventricles include ventricular escape complexes or rhythms, premature ventricular complexes, ventricular tachycardia, ventricular fibrillation, asystole, and artificial pacemaker rhythm.

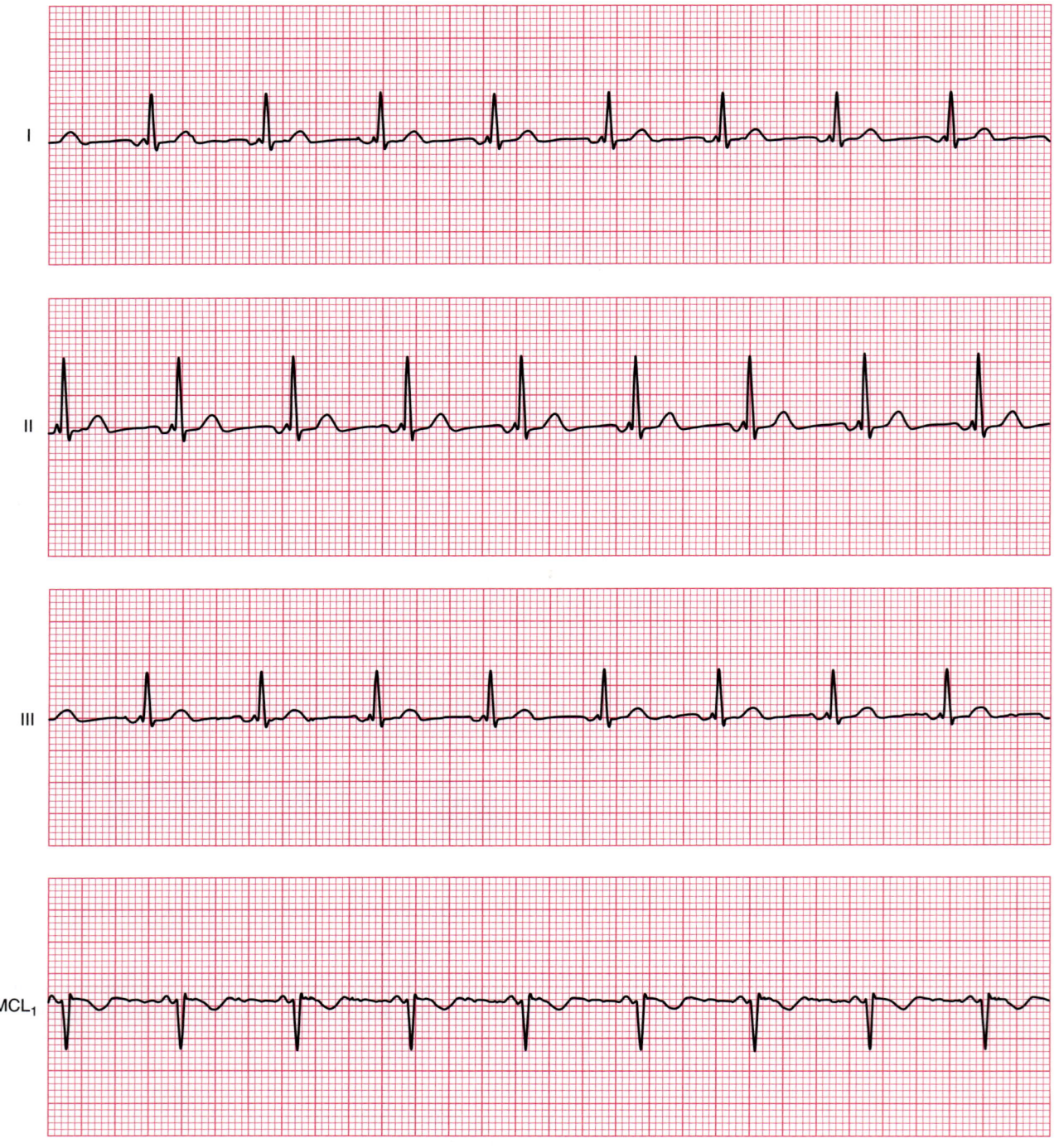

FIGURE 22-60 Accelerated junctional rhythm.

Because electrical impulses of ventricular origin start in the lower portion of the heart (the ventricular muscle, bundle branches, or Purkinje fibers), the electrical impulse must travel in a retrograde conduction pathway to depolarize the atria. The impulse may travel in an antegrade direction to depolarize the ventricles, depending on the site of initiation of the impulse. Regardless of the direction of depolarization, the normal, rapid conducting pathways are bypassed, producing three ECG features:

- QRS complexes are wide and bizarre in appearance. They are 0.12 second or greater in duration.
- P waves may be hidden in the QRS complex (this is because the atria are depolarized at about the same time as the ventricles), Alternatively, they may be superimposed on every second or third QRS complex when ventricular tachycardia with **atrioventricular dissociation** (P waves that have no set relation to the QRS complexes) is present.

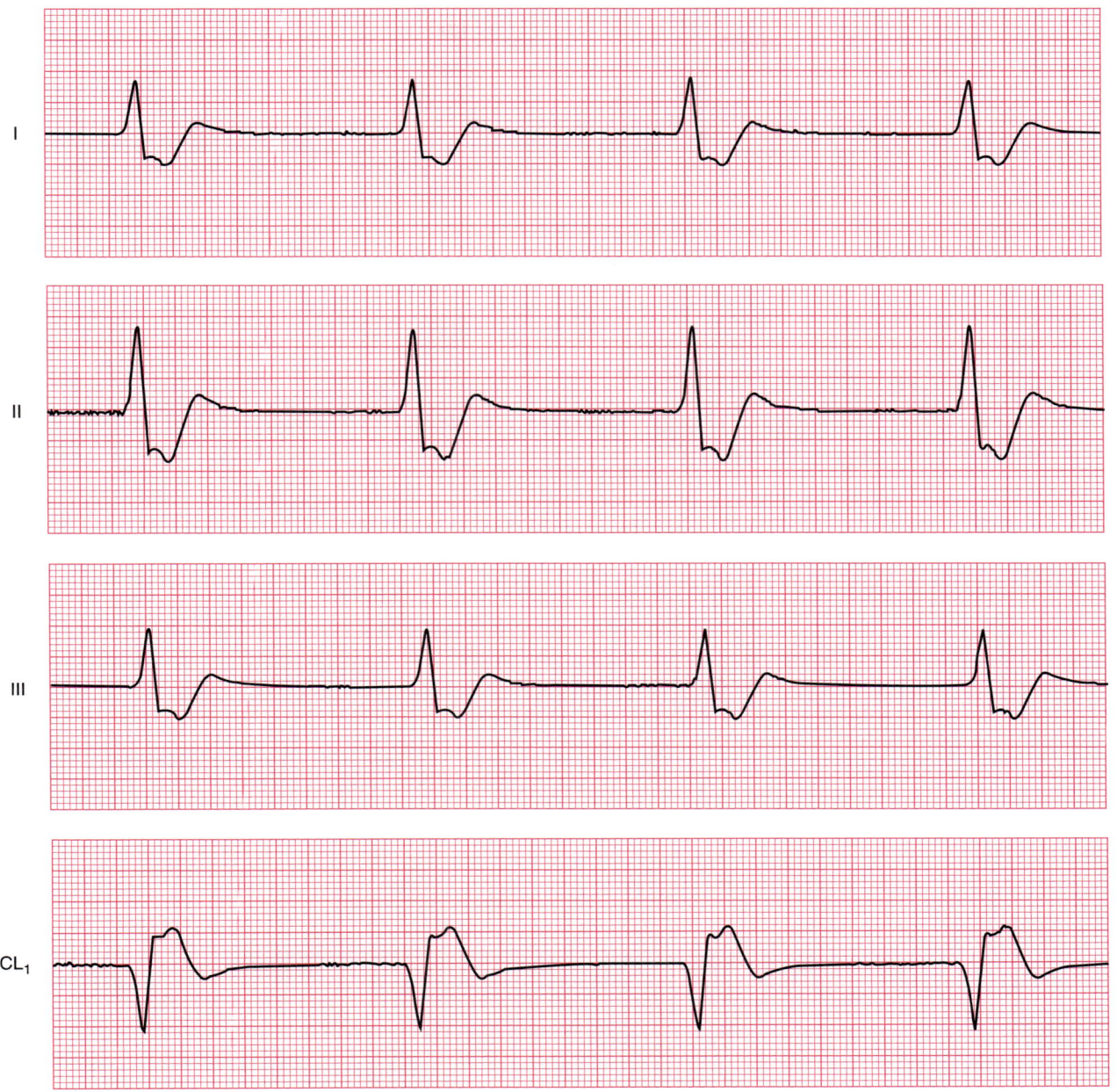

FIGURE 22-61 Ventricular escape rhythm.

- ST segments usually deviate from baseline. T waves frequently are sloped off in the opposite direction from the QRS complex.

Ventricular Escape Complexes or Rhythms

DESCRIPTION

A **ventricular escape complex** or rhythm is also known as *idioventricular rhythm* (Figures 22-61 and 22-62). The dysrhythmia results when impulses from higher pacemakers fail to fire or to reach the ventricles. It also results when the rate of discharge of higher pacemaker sites falls to less than that of the ventricles. Like the junctional escape complex or rhythm, this dysrhythmia serves as a compensatory mechanism to prevent cardiac standstill.

ETIOLOGY

Ventricular escape rhythms occur in two ways. First, the rate of impulse formation of the dominant pacemaker (usually the sinoatrial node) can fall below that of the ventricles. Second, the escape pacemaker in the atrioventricular junction can fail or fall below that of the pacemaker in the ventricles. This dysrhythmia often is seen as the first rhythm after defibrillation.

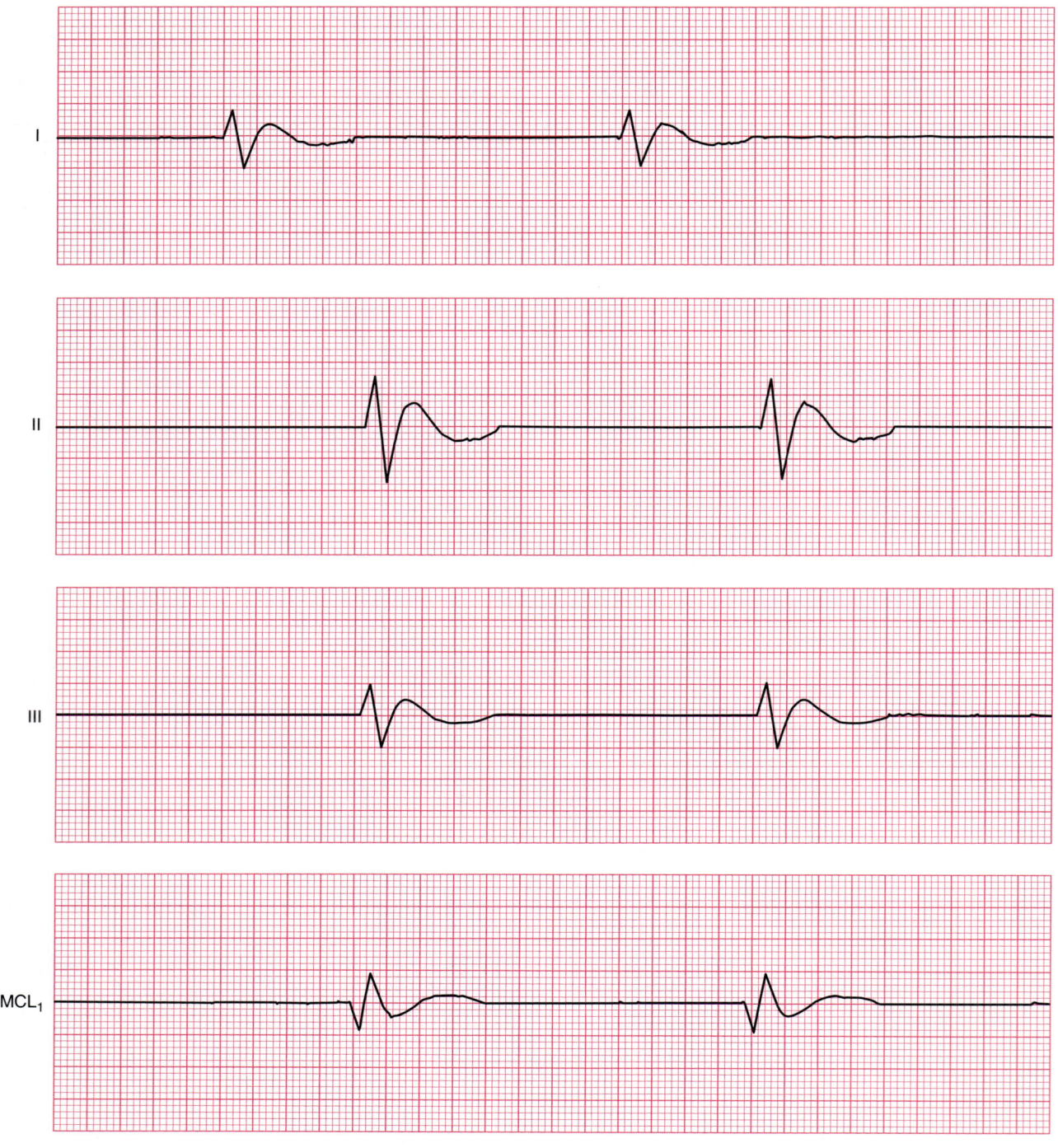

FIGURE 22-62 "Dying heart" (agonal) rhythm.

RULES FOR INTERPRETATION (LEAD II MONITORING)

Ventricular escape complexes or rhythms have the following characteristics on the ECG:

QRS complex: Generally exceeds 0.12 second and is bizarre in appearance. The shape of the QRS complex may vary in any given lead.

P waves: May be absent. If they are present and have no set relationship to the QRS complex, a third-degree atrioventricular block should be suspected.

Rate: Usually 20 to 40 beats/minute; may be lower

Rhythm: The ventricular rhythm usually is regular but may be irregular.

P-R interval: If P waves are present, the P-R interval is variable and irregular.

CLINICAL SIGNIFICANCE

A ventricular escape rhythm generally produces symptoms. This dysrhythmia is manifested by hypotension, decreased cardiac output, and decreased perfusion of the brain and other vital organs, often resulting in syncope and shock. Patient assessment is essential, because the escape rhythm may be perfusing or nonperfusing (pulseless electrical activity).

MANAGEMENT

If the rhythm is perfusing, management must be directed at increasing the heart rate by administering oxygen, transcutaneous cardiac pacing, and/or *dopamine*. Managing the escape rhythm with *lidocaine* likely would be lethal and therefore is contraindicated. If the rhythm is nonperfusing, basic life support measures should be initiated and the treatment guidelines for pulseless arrest should be followed (Figure 22-63).

CRITICAL THINKING
Why might *lidocaine* be harmful in this situation?

Premature Ventricular Complex

DESCRIPTION

A **premature ventricular complex (PVC)** is a single ectopic impulse arising from an irritable focus in either ventricle (bundle branches, Purkinje fibers, or ventricular muscle) that occurs earlier than the next expected sinus beat (Figure 22-64). This dysrhythmia is common and can occur with any underlying cardiac rhythm. The dysrhythmia results from enhanced automaticity or a reentry mechanism.

When the ventricles initiate a premature ventricular complex, the atria may or may not respond and depolarize. If atrial depolarization does not occur, a P wave is seen on the ECG. If atrial depolarization does occur, the P wave occurs but often is hidden in the QRS complex. This happens because the timing and large electrical force of ventricular depolarization block out the electrical activity from the atrial depolarization. The altered sequence of ventricular depolarization results in a wide, bizarre QRS complex. Depolarization may be deflected in the opposite direction from the QRS complex in the underlying rhythm, or it may be deflected in the same direction (this depends on the location of the focus and the lead selected). The T wave that immediately follows the premature ventricular complex usually is deflected in the opposite direction from the QRS complex of the premature ventricular complex because of the altered sequence of repolarization.

CRITICAL THINKING
Why is the QRS deflection opposite the underlying rhythm?

A premature ventricular complex usually does not depolarize the sinoatrial node or interrupt its rhythm. (For instance, the P wave of the underlying rhythm that follows the premature ventricular complex occurs at its expected time but is obstructed by the premature ventricular complex and finds the ventricles refractory.) Therefore, the ectopic impulse usually is followed by a full **compensatory pause.** Compensatory pauses are confirmed by measuring the interval between the R wave before the premature ventricular complex and the R wave after it. If the pause is compensatory, the distance is at least two times the R-R interval of the underlying rhythm. At times, a premature ventricular complex falls between two sinus beats without interrupting the rhythm; this is called an *interpolated premature ventricular complex* (Figure 22-65).

Premature ventricular complexes may originate from a single ectopic pacemaker site (unifocal premature ventricular complexes) or from multiple sites in the ventricles (multifocal premature ventricular complexes) (Figure 22-66). **Unifocal premature ventricular complexes** look alike. **Multifocal premature ventricular complexes** have varying shapes and sizes.

Multifocal premature ventricular complexes are considered more dangerous than unifocal premature ventricular complexes. In general, this is because they result from increased myocardial irritability. A premature ventricular complex that occurs about the same time as ventricular activation by a normal impulse can cause ventricular depolarization at the same time. This **fusion beat** results in a QRS complex with the characteristics of a premature ventricular complex and the QRS complex of the underlying rhythm (Figure 22-67). Fusion beats confirm that the ectopic impulse is located in the ventricle rather than the atria.

Frequently, premature ventricular complexes occur in patterns of grouped beating. **Ventricular bigeminy** occurs when every other complex is a premature ventricular complex. **Ventricular trigeminy** occurs when every third complex is a premature ventricular complex (Figure 22-68). Quadrigeminy occurs when every fourth complex is a premature ventricular complex. Consecutive premature ventricular complexes that are not separated by a complex of the underlying rhythm also can occur on the ECG: *couplets* are two premature ventricular complexes in a row; *triplets* are three premature ventricular complexes in a row (a definition for ventricular tachycardia); *salvos* are three or more ventricular complexes in a row. These terms also may be used to describe patterns of premature atrial complexes and premature junctional complexes.

As do multifocal premature ventricular complexes, frequently occurring premature ventricular complexes usually indicate that the ventricles are highly irritable. These types of premature ventricular complexes can trigger life-threatening dysrhythmias, such as ventricular tachycardia and ventricular fibrillation. This is especially the case if they

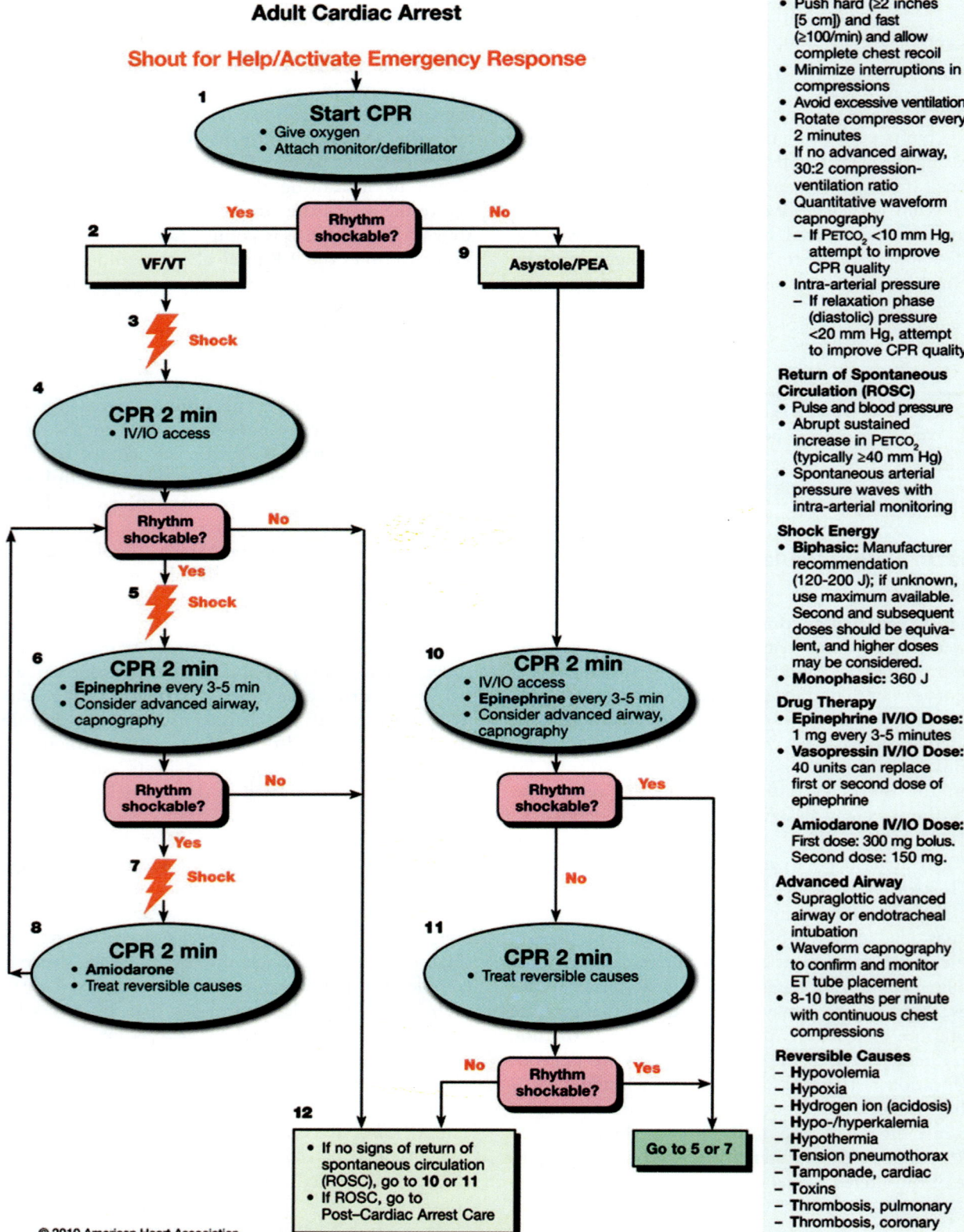

Adult Cardiac Arrest

Shout for Help/Activate Emergency Response

1 Start CPR
- Give oxygen
- Attach monitor/defibrillator

Rhythm shockable? Yes / No

2 VF/VT

9 Asystole/PEA

3 Shock

4 CPR 2 min
- IV/IO access

Rhythm shockable? No

5 Shock Yes

6 CPR 2 min
- **Epinephrine** every 3-5 min
- Consider advanced airway, capnography

Rhythm shockable? No

7 Shock Yes

8 CPR 2 min
- Amiodarone
- Treat reversible causes

10 CPR 2 min
- IV/IO access
- **Epinephrine** every 3-5 min
- Consider advanced airway, capnography

Rhythm shockable? Yes / No

11 CPR 2 min
- Treat reversible causes

Rhythm shockable? No / Yes

12
- If no signs of return of spontaneous circulation (ROSC), go to **10 or 11**
- If ROSC, go to Post–Cardiac Arrest Care

Go to 5 or 7

© 2010 American Heart Association

CPR Quality
- Push hard (≥2 inches [5 cm]) and fast (≥100/min) and allow complete chest recoil
- Minimize interruptions in compressions
- Avoid excessive ventilation
- Rotate compressor every 2 minutes
- If no advanced airway, 30:2 compression-ventilation ratio
- Quantitative waveform capnography
  - If P_{ETCO_2} <10 mm Hg, attempt to improve CPR quality
- Intra-arterial pressure
  - If relaxation phase (diastolic) pressure <20 mm Hg, attempt to improve CPR quality

Return of Spontaneous Circulation (ROSC)
- Pulse and blood pressure
- Abrupt sustained increase in P_{ETCO_2} (typically ≥40 mm Hg)
- Spontaneous arterial pressure waves with intra-arterial monitoring

Shock Energy
- **Biphasic:** Manufacturer recommendation (120-200 J); if unknown, use maximum available. Second and subsequent doses should be equivalent, and higher doses may be considered.
- **Monophasic:** 360 J

Drug Therapy
- **Epinephrine IV/IO Dose:** 1 mg every 3-5 minutes
- **Vasopressin IV/IO Dose:** 40 units can replace first or second dose of epinephrine
- **Amiodarone IV/IO Dose:** First dose: 300 mg bolus. Second dose: 150 mg.

Advanced Airway
- Supraglottic advanced airway or endotracheal intubation
- Waveform capnography to confirm and monitor ET tube placement
- 8-10 breaths per minute with continuous chest compressions

Reversible Causes
- Hypovolemia
- Hypoxia
- Hydrogen ion (acidosis)
- Hypo-/hyperkalemia
- Hypothermia
- Tension pneumothorax
- Tamponade, cardiac
- Toxins
- Thrombosis, pulmonary
- Thrombosis, coronary

FIGURE 22-63 Advanced cardiac life support (ACLS) pulseless arrest algorithm. (Reprinted with permission, American Heart Association Guidelines For CPR and ECC, *Circulation 122* [suppl 3]:S685-S919, American Heart Association, Inc, 2010.)

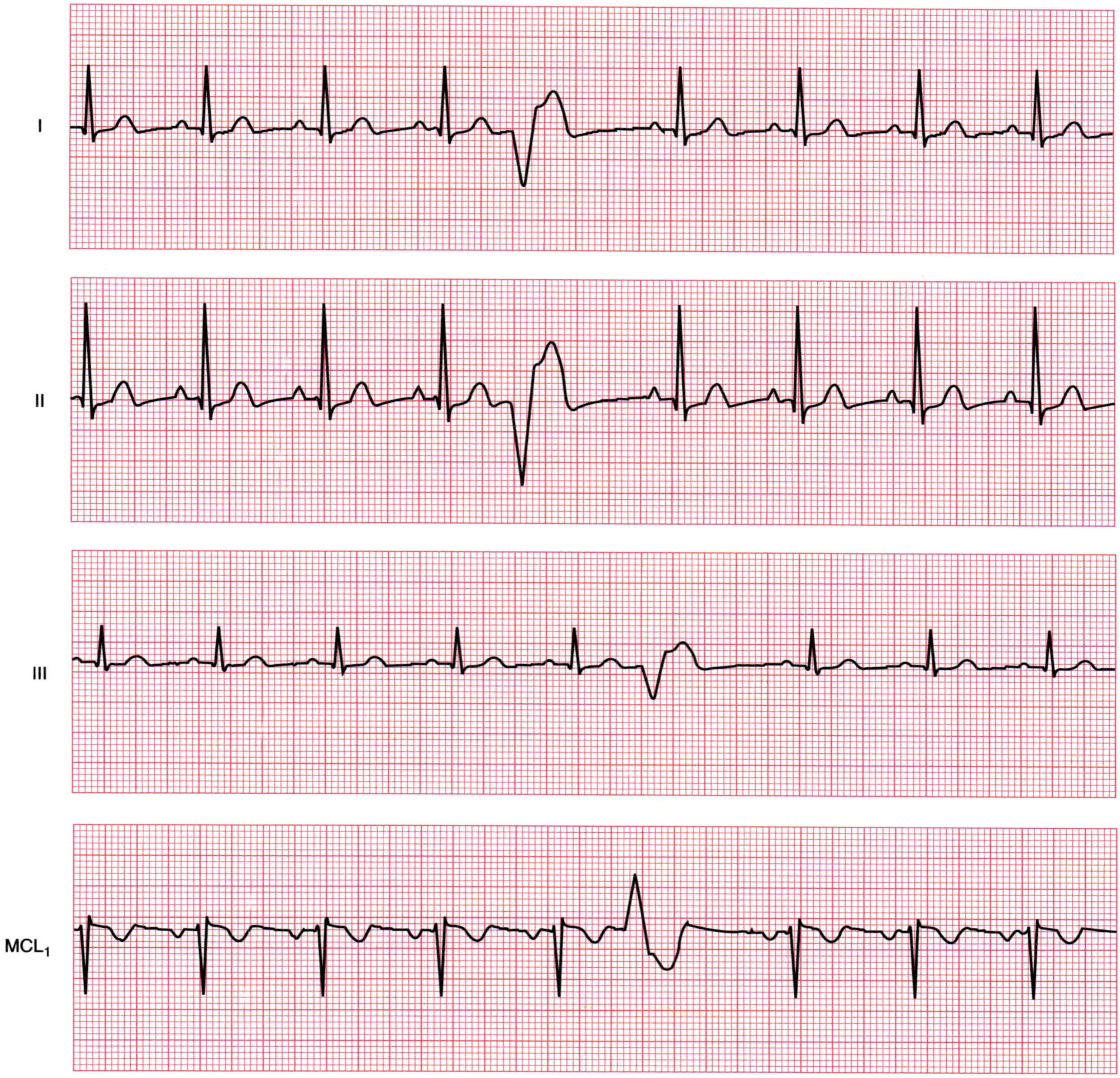

I

II

III

MCL$_1$

FIGURE 22-64 Premature ventricular complex.

occur during the T wave (relative refractory phase) of the cardiac cycle.

During this period, the heart muscle is at its greatest electrical instability. This is because in the relative refractory period, some of the ventricular muscle fibers may be partly repolarized; others may be completely repolarized; and still others may be completely refractory. Stimulation of the ventricles in the vulnerable period by an electrical impulse such as a premature ventricular complex, cardiac pacemaker, or cardioversion may cause ventricular fibrillation or ventricular tachycardia. The occurrence of a

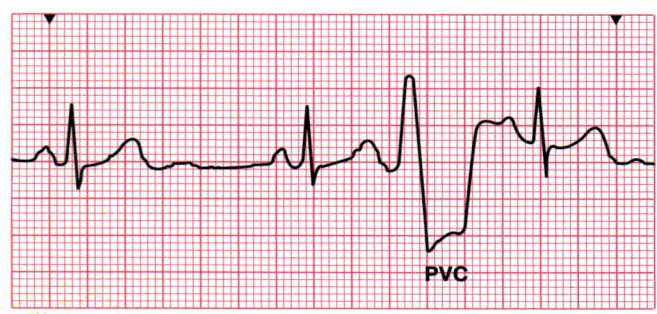

PVC

FIGURE 22-65 Interpolated premature ventricular complex.

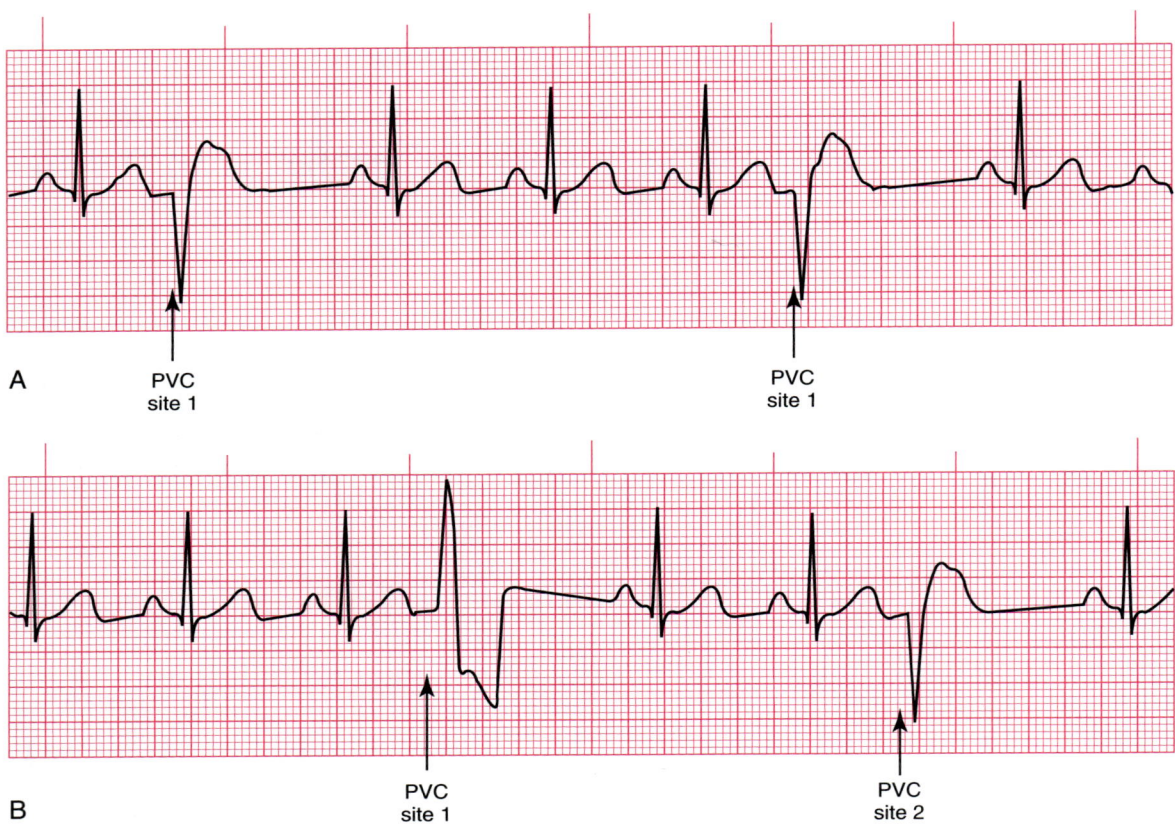

FIGURE 22-66 A, Unifocal premature ventricular complexes. **B,** Multifocal premature ventricular complexes.

ventricular depolarization during the relative refractory period is known as the **R-on-T phenomenon** (Figure 22-69).

ETIOLOGY

Isolated premature ventricular complexes do occur in healthy people without apparent cause. They usually have no significance. Pathological premature ventricular complexes usually are a result of one or more of the following:

- Myocardial ischemia
- Hypoxia
- Acid-base and electrolyte imbalance
- Hypokalemia
- Congestive heart failure
- Increased catecholamine and sympathetic tone (as in emotional stress)
- Ingestion of stimulants (alcohol, caffeine, tobacco)
- Drug toxicity
- Sympathomimetic drugs (cocaine; stimulants such as phencyclidine, *epinephrine,* and methamphetamine)

RULES FOR INTERPRETATION (LEAD II MONITORING)

Premature ventricular complexes have the following characteristics on the ECG:

QRS complex: Equal to or greater than 0.12 second. Frequently distorted and bizarre P waves may be present

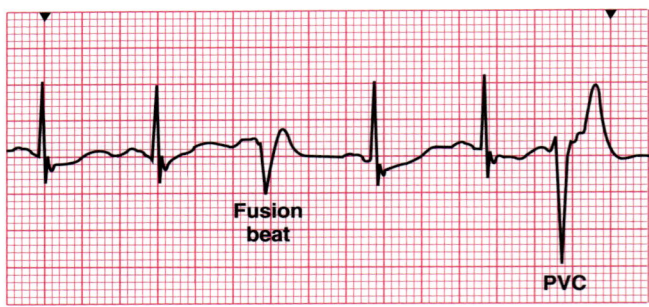

FIGURE 22-67 Fusion beat with premature ventricular complex.

or absent. If present, they usually are of the underlying rhythm and have no relationship to the premature ventricular complex.

Rate: Depends on the underlying rhythm and the number of premature ventricular complexes

Rhythm: Premature ventricular complexes interrupt the regularity of the underlying rhythm.

P-R interval: None

CLINICAL SIGNIFICANCE

Premature ventricular complexes that occur in patients without heart disease usually do not produce serious signs and symptoms, although these patients may complain of

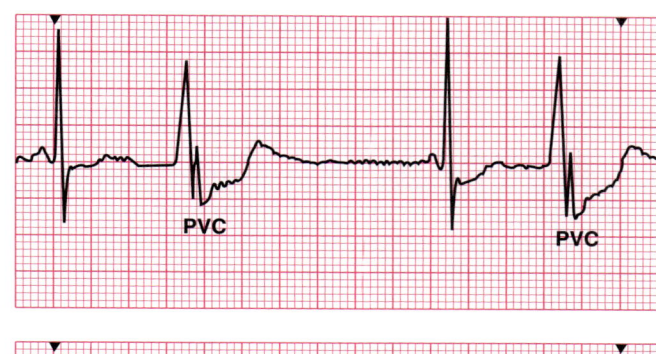

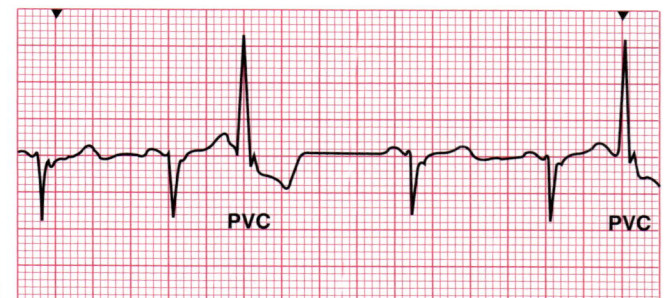

FIGURE 22-68 **A**, Bigeminy (unifocal premature ventricular complexes). **B**, Trigeminy (unifocal premature ventricular complexes).

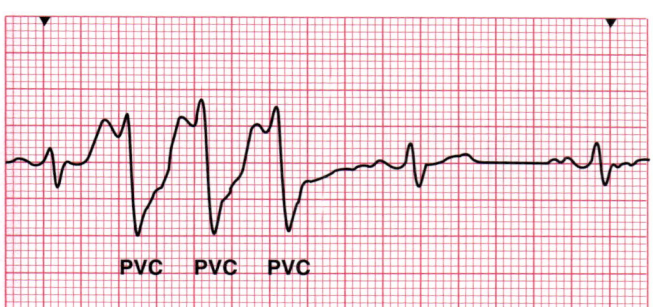

FIGURE 22-69 R-on-T phenomenon (unifocal premature ventricular complexes).

"skipped beats." Premature ventricular complexes that occur with heart disease (myocardial ischemia) may result from enhanced automaticity, a reentry mechanism, or both. These premature ventricular complexes may trigger lethal ventricular dysrhythmias. Premature ventricular complexes do not permit complete ventricular filling. Also, they may produce a diminished or nonpalpable pulse (nonperfusing premature ventricular complex). If the premature ventricular complexes occur often enough and early enough in the cardiac cycle, cardiac output drops.

Warning signs of serious ventricular dysrhythmias in patients with myocardial ischemia include frequent premature ventricular complexes, multifocal premature ventricular complexes, early premature ventricular complexes (R-on-T phenomenon), and patterns of grouped beating.

MANAGEMENT

Premature ventricular complexes that occur in patients without symptoms and without known heart disease seldom require treatment. In patients with myocardial ischemia, frequent premature ventricular complexes must be treated promptly with oxygen and antidysrhythmic drugs (e.g., beta blockers). At the hospital, the serum potassium level should be checked immediately. Hypokalemia, if present, should be treated promptly.

> **CRITICAL THINKING**
> A lidocaine drip is not regulated properly and infuses too rapidly. What signs and symptoms might the patient develop?

Ventricular Tachycardia
DESCRIPTION

Ventricular tachycardia (VT) is a dysrhythmia defined by three or more consecutive ventricular complexes that occur at a rate of more than 100 beats/minute (Figure 22-70). This dysrhythmia overrides the primary pacemaker. It starts suddenly and is triggered by a premature ventricular complex. During ventricular tachycardia, the atria and ventricles are not beating in step with each other. If ventricular tachycardia continues, the patient's condition may become unstable. Ventricular tachycardia can produce unconsciousness. Occasionally it can even lead to loss of a perfusing pulse. However, some patients in ventricular tachycardia may be able to walk and talk. The misconception that ventricular tachycardia cannot be associated with a reasonable blood pressure may result in inappropriate patient management. The origin of ventricular tachycardia is enhanced automaticity or reentry.

ETIOLOGY

Like premature ventricular complexes, ventricular tachycardia usually occurs in the presence of myocardial ischemia or significant cardiac disease. Other causes of ventricular tachycardia include the following:

- Acid-base and electrolyte imbalance
- Hypokalemia
- Congestive heart failure
- Increased catecholamine and sympathetic tone (as in emotional stress)
- Ingestion of stimulants (alcohol, caffeine, tobacco)
- Drug toxicity (digitalis, tricyclic antidepressants)
- Sympathomimetic drugs (cocaine, methamphetamines)
- Prolonged Q-T interval (may be caused by drugs or metabolic problems or may be congenital)

> **NOTE**
> Patients who have had a previous myocardial infarction with subsequent tachycardias and who are now experiencing a wide-complex tachycardia very likely are in ventricular tachycardia.

RULES FOR INTERPRETATION (LEAD II MONITORING)

Ventricular tachycardia has the following characteristics on the ECG:

QRS complex: Equal to or greater than 0.12 second and usually distorted and bizarre. The QRS complexes generally are identical, but if fusion beats are present, one or more QRS complexes may differ in size, shape, and direction.

P waves: May be absent. If present, P waves have no set relation to the QRS complex (atrioventricular dissociation). P waves occur at a slower rate than the ventricular focus and are superimposed on the QRS complexes.

Rate: Usually between 100 and 250 beats/minute

Rhythm: Usually regular (unless drug induced) but may be slightly irregular

P-R interval: If P waves are present, the P-R interval varies widely.

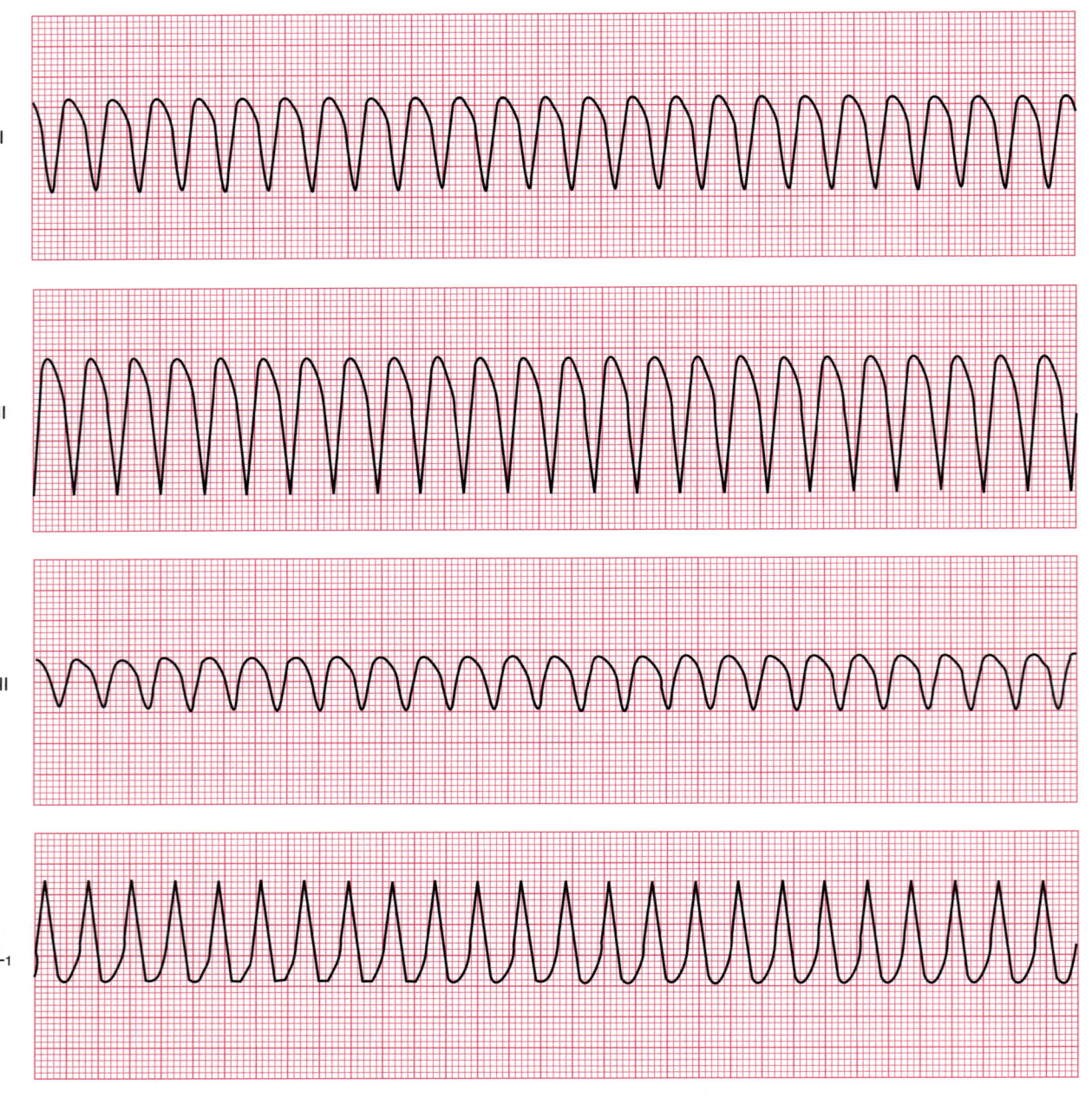

FIGURE 22-70 Ventricular tachycardia.

> **NOTE**
>
> Atrioventricular dissociation may precipitate **cannon A waves**. These are waves of pulse pressure that are visible in the jugular veins of a patient in ventricular tachycardia. Cannon A waves result when the right atrium pumps against a closed tricuspid valve; the waves of pressure consequently are directed into the jugular veins. Atrioventricular dissociation is diagnostic of ventricular tachycardia.

CLINICAL SIGNIFICANCE

Ventricular tachycardia usually indicates significant heart disease. The rapid rate and the loss of atrial kick cause a drop in cardiac output and decreased coronary artery and cerebral perfusion. The severity of symptoms varies with the rate of the ventricular tachycardia and how much heart disease is present. Ventricular tachycardia may be perfusing or nonperfusing; that is, it may produce a pulse or it may not. Ventricular tachycardia also may lead to ventricular fibrillation.

MANAGEMENT

The treatment of patients with ventricular tachycardia is based on their signs and symptoms and whether torsades de pointes is present. **Torsades de pointes** (Figure 22-71) is a type of polymorphic ventricular tachycardia. As with other supraventricular tachycardias, the paramedic should obtain a history and identify the rhythm (see Figure 22-54). If the patient is stable, a 12-lead ECG should be obtained.

Treatment of ventricular tachycardia depends on whether the QRS complex is *monomorphic* (having the same morphology or fixed shape) or *polymorphic* (having varying morphology). The paramedic should remember, however, that any wide-complex tachycardia that occurs with serious signs and symptoms (e.g., chest pain, dyspnea, decreased level of consciousness, or hypotension or other signs of shock) requires immediate cardioversion. In addition, patients who have ventricular tachycardia without a pulse should be treated as if the rhythm were ventricular fibrillation.

Treatment guidelines for **monomorphic ventricular tachycardia** are based on heart function (the cardiac ejection fraction). Signs and symptoms of failing heart function are pulmonary congestion and a decreased level of consciousness. Monomorphic ventricular tachycardia in a stable patient is managed with *procainamide.* *Adenosine* may be administered first if the nature of a regular wide-complex rhythm is uncertain.[1] Alternative drugs are *amiodarone,* and sotalol. Unstable patients with monomorphic ventricular tachycardia should receive immediate synchronized cardioversion. This should begin with an initial shock of 100 J. If no response to the first shock is seen, the dose should be increased (in stepwise fashion) according to manufacturer recommendations.[1] When unstable ventricular tachycardia is witnessed, a **precordial thump** may be performed if cardioversion is not immediately available.

PRECORDIAL THUMP

Monitored adult patients whose rhythm is observed to be unstable ventricular tachycardia may be treated with a single precordial thump, provided that a defibrillator is readily available. (A precordial thump may cause ventricular tachycardia to deteriorate to asystole, ventricular fibrillation, or pulseless electrical activity.) A precordial thump may terminate a dysrhythmia by causing ventricular depolarization and the resumption of an organized rhythm. To deliver a precordial thump, the paramedic's arm and wrist should be parallel to the long axis of the sternum to avoid rib fractures and other injury. The thump is delivered to the midsternum with the heel of the fist from 10 to 12 inches. A conscious patient should be advised of the procedure.

> **DID YOU KNOW?**
> **Cardiac Ejection Fraction**
> The **cardiac ejection fraction** is the percentage of ventricular blood volume released during a contraction. This measurement most often refers to the left ventricle (left ventricular ejection fraction [LVEF]). The LVEF is obtained through echocardiography, cardiac catheterization, or heart scans with magnetic resonance imaging, computed tomography, and nuclear medicine (nuclear stress test).
>
> A normal LVEF ranges from 50% to 70%. The LVEF may be lower if the heart muscle has been damaged by a heart attack, heart muscle disease (cardiomyopathy), or other causes. An LVEF of 35% to 40% may confirm a diagnosis of heart failure. An LVEF below 35% increases the risk of life-threatening dysrhythmias that can cause sudden cardiac arrest and sudden cardiac death. An implantable cardioverter-defibrillator (ICD) often is recommended for these patients.

Polymorphic ventricular tachycardia can degenerate into ventricular fibrillation quickly and therefore requires immediate intervention. If the patient has polymorphic ventricular tachycardia and is unstable (as is often the case), the rhythm should be treated as ventricular fibrillation with high-energy unsynchronized shocks. (Synchronization is not usually possible with irregular wave forms, such as polymorphic ventricular tachycardia.) If the rhythm is torsades de pointes, it may be the result of a prolonged

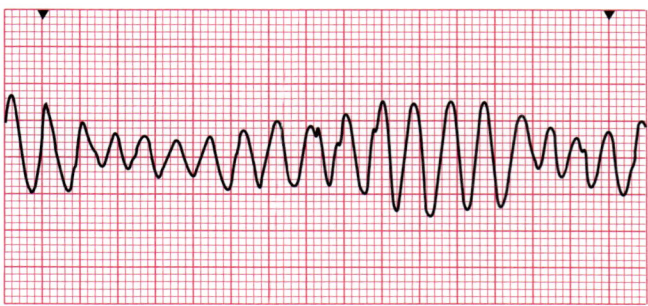

FIGURE 22-71 Torsades de pointes.

Q-T interval. Medications that prolong the Q-T interval should be discontinued. Electrolyte imbalances should be corrected, and **magnesium sulfate** should be given intravenously.

> ### NOTE
> Drugs given to treat dysrhythmias also can cause dysrhythmias *(proarrhythmic)*. Sequential use of two or more antidysrhythmic drugs increases the incidence of bradycardias, hypotension, and torsades de pointes. Avoiding the use of more than one antidysrhythmic agent in treating narrow or wide QRS complex tachydysrhythmias is strongly recommended. In most cases, if an adequate dose of a single drug is unsuccessful in ending the dysrhythmia, synchronized cardioversion is the next treatment.

Ventricular Fibrillation

DESCRIPTION

Ventricular fibrillation (VF) is a chaotic ventricular rhythm that results in pulselessness (Figure 22-72). The cause of VF is multifocal reentry in the ventricles. The electrical impulses initiated by the multiple ectopic ventricular sites do not allow the heart to fully depolarize and repolarize. As a result, organized ventricular contraction does not occur. Ventricular fibrillation is the most common initial rhythm disturbance in sudden cardiac arrest.

ETIOLOGY

Ventricular fibrillation most commonly is associated with significant heart disease. The dysrhythmias also may be precipitated by premature ventricular complexes, R-on-T phenomenon (in rare cases), or a sustained ventricular tachycardia. Other causes include the following:

- Myocardial ischemia
- Acute myocardial infarction
- Third-degree atrioventricular block with a slow ventricular escape rhythm
- Cardiomyopathy
- Digitalis toxicity
- Hypoxia
- Acidosis
- Electrolyte imbalance (hypokalemia, hyperkalemia, submersion)
- Electrical injury
- Drug overdose or toxicity (cocaine, tricyclic antidepressants)

RULES FOR INTERPRETATION (ALL LEADS)

Ventricular fibrillation has the following characteristics on the ECG:

QRS complex: Absent
P waves: Absent

Rate: No coordinated ventricular contractions are present. The unsynchronized ventricular impulses occur at rates of 300 to 500 beats/minute.
Rhythm: Irregularly irregular
P-R interval: Absent

Because organized depolarizations of the atria and ventricles are absent, P waves, QRS complexes, ST segments, and T waves are absent. Ventricular fibrillatory waves are seen on the oscilloscope as bizarre, rounded, or pointed. They also appear considerably different in shape. They also vary at random from positive to negative. These waves represent twitching of small individual groups of muscle fibers. Fibrillatory waves less than 3 mm in amplitude are called **fine ventricular fibrillation.** Those greater than 3 mm are called **coarse ventricular fibrillation** (Figure 22-73). The fibrillatory waves may be so fine they appear as a flat line, resembling ventricular asystole.

> ### NOTE
> Coarse ventricular fibrillation usually indicates the recent onset of ventricular fibrillation. It can be readily converted by prompt defibrillation. The presence of fine ventricular fibrillation that approaches asystole often means that a considerable delay has occurred since collapse. Successful defibrillation is more difficult in these cases.[2]

CLINICAL SIGNIFICANCE

Ventricular fibrillation causes all life functions to cease because of a lack of circulating blood flow. The dysrhythmia initially may result in lightheadedness. Ventricular fibrillation usually is followed within seconds by loss of consciousness, apnea, and, if left untreated, death.

MANAGEMENT

For adult resuscitation, management of ventricular fibrillation and pulseless ventricular tachycardia is the most important sequence because most adult cardiac arrests result from these two rhythm disturbances. Also, the vast majority of successful resuscitations result from the appropriate management of these two dysrhythmias (see Figure 22-63).[1] Ventricular fibrillation and nonperfusing ventricular tachycardia are managed alike: basic life support (if a defibrillator is not immediately available), defibrillation, IV/IO access, and pharmacological therapy (**epinephrine** [or **vasopressin** to replace the first or second dose] and **amiodarone** (**lidocaine** if **amiodarone** is not available). Advanced airway with capnographic monitoring should be considered after initial CPR, defibrillation, and drug administration.[1] Other interventions may be performed to treat any identified underlying cause of arrest.

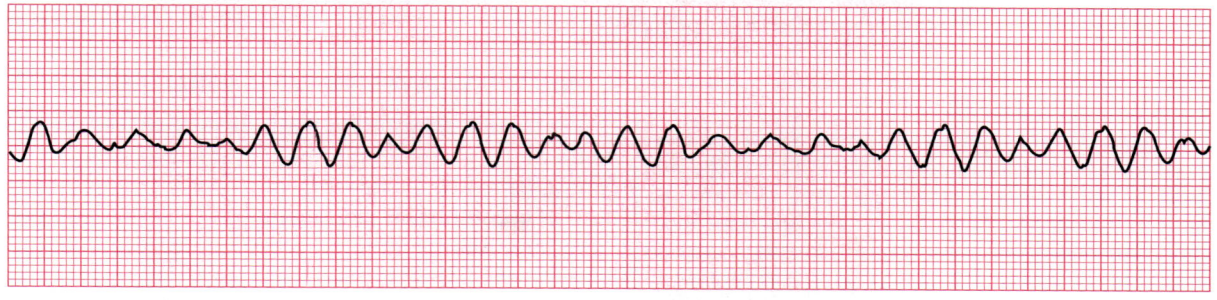

FIGURE 22-72 Ventricular fibrillation.

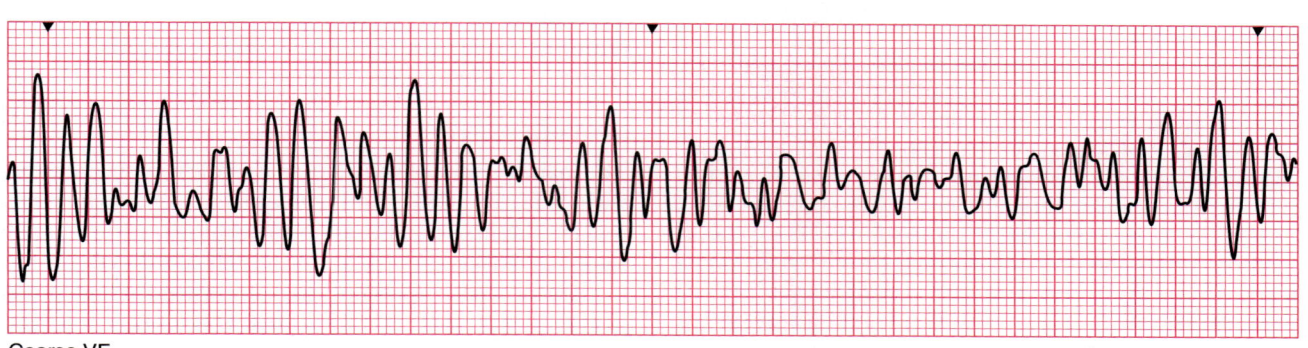

Coarse VF

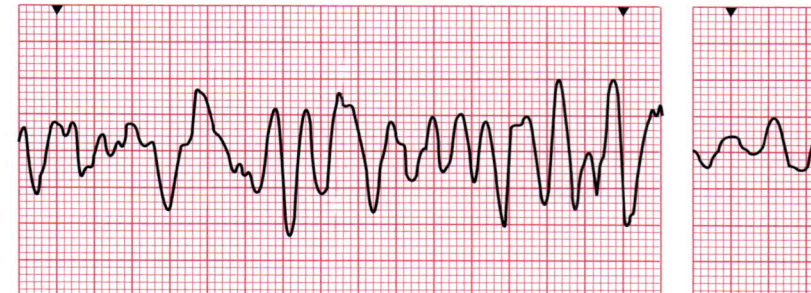

Coarse VF

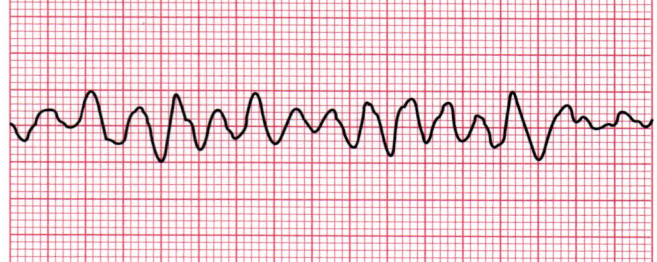

Coarse VF

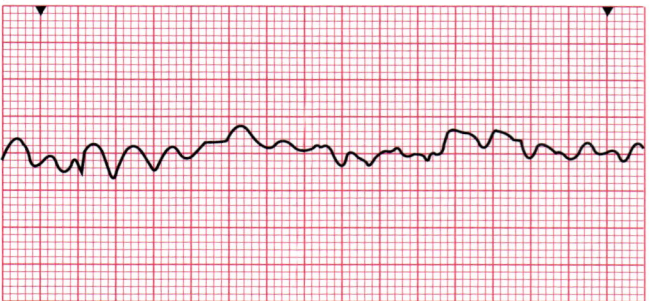

Coarse VF

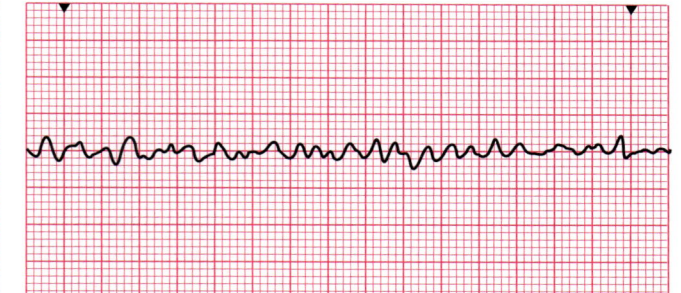

Coarse VF

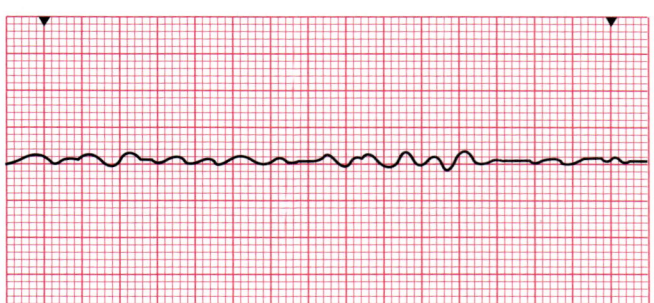

Fine VF

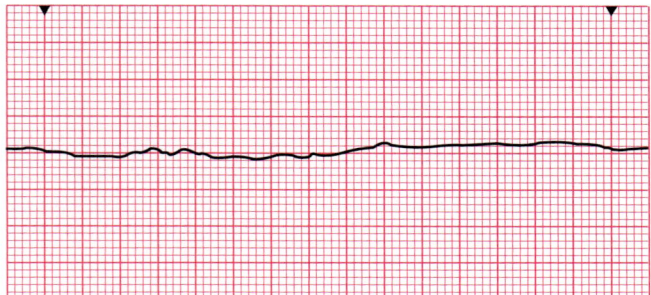

Fine VF

FIGURE 22-73 Coarse and fine ventricular fibrillation.

> ### NOTE
> With cardiac arrest, blood flow stops. Chest compressions create a small amount of blood flow to the vital organs, such as the brain and heart. The better the compressions, the more blood flow they produce. The American Heart Association recommends that chest compressions be "hard and fast" and at a rate of at least 100/minute (except in newborns). The association also recommends that chest compressions not be stopped to deliver ventilations after an advanced airway is in place when two or more rescuers are present. (When chest compressions are interrupted, blood flow stops and coronary perfusion pressure is reduced.[1])
>
> This same train of thought applies to defibrillation: minimize interruptions in chest compressions. If an EMS provider does not witness the arrest in the out-of-hospital setting, the EMS crew may perform CPR while preparing for defibrillation. If the rhythm is shockable, one shock should be delivered, and then CPR should be resumed immediately, beginning with chest compressions. CPR should be continued for another five cycles (or about 2 minutes), before the rhythm is checked again. Theory holds that even when a shock eliminates ventricular fibrillation, several minutes are required for a normal rhythm to return and for the heart to create more blood flow. A brief period of chest compressions can deliver oxygen and sources of energy to the heart. This increases the likelihood that the heart will be able to pump blood effectively after the defibrillatory shock.[6] In addition, chest compressions should not be interrupted to charge a defibrillator or to "clear" the patient for shock delivery while the defibrillator is charging. (The patient should be cleared immediately before the shock is delivered, with no time wasted in between.)
>
> Rhythm checks should be brief, and pulse checks should be performed only if an organized rhythm is observed (see Figure 22-63).

Ventricular Asystole

DESCRIPTION

Ventricular asystole (cardiac standstill) refers to the absence of all ventricular activity (Figure 22-74).

ETIOLOGY

Ventricular asystole may be the cause of cardiac arrest. It also may occur in complete heart block when there is no escape pacemaker. The dysrhythmia usually is associated with extensive heart disease. It often occurs after ventricular tachycardia, ventricular fibrillation, pulseless electrical activity, or an agonal escape rhythm in the dying heart.

RULES FOR INTERPRETATION (ALL LEADS)

Ventricular asystole has the following characteristics on the ECG:

QRS complexes: Absent
P waves: Absent or present
Rate: Absent
Rhythm: Absent
P-R interval: Absent

CLINICAL SIGNIFICANCE

Ventricular asystole produces no cardiac output and is an ominous dysrhythmia. Asystole often confirms death. The chance for resuscitation is small.

MANAGEMENT

The management of ventricular asystole is basic life support with effective CPR, and *epinephrine* (or *vasopressin* to replace the first or second dose) administration) Establish an advanced airway with an endotracheal tube or supraglottic airway with capnographic monitoring when possible (see Figure 22-63). If fine ventricular fibrillation is suspected, defibrillation is indicated. However, defibrillating asystole "just in case" is not recommended. Termination of resuscitation efforts in the prehospital setting, after meeting medical protocol (described later in this chapter), is indicated in this situation. Potential reversible causes of asystole should be considered before cessation of resuscitative efforts. These include hypoxia, hypovolemia, hyperkalemia, hypokalemia, hypothermia, tension pneumothorax, cardiac tamponade, STEMI, pulmonary edema, drug overdose, and acidosis.[1]

> ### CRITICAL THINKING
> What is the benefit to the community and to the patient's family if resuscitation is halted in the field after all appropriate guidelines have been followed?

Artificial Pacemaker Rhythms

DESCRIPTION

Artificial pacemakers generate a rhythm by regular electrical stimulation of the heart through an electrode implanted in the heart (Figure 22-75). The electrode is connected to a

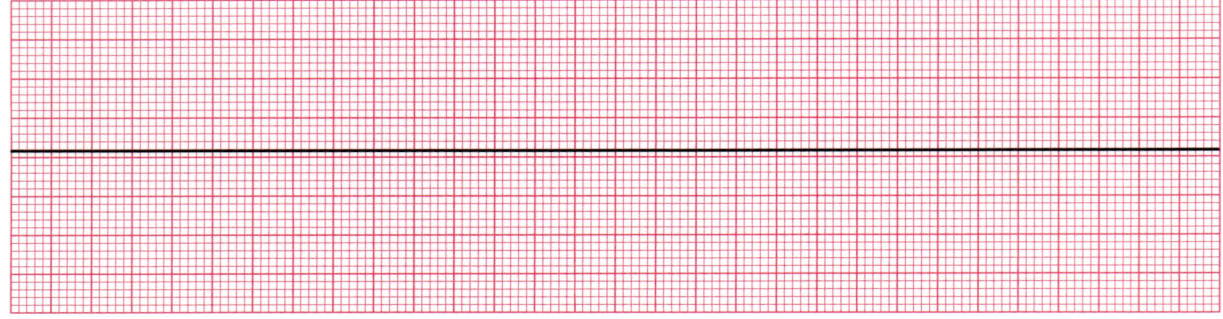

FIGURE 22-74 Ventricular asystole.

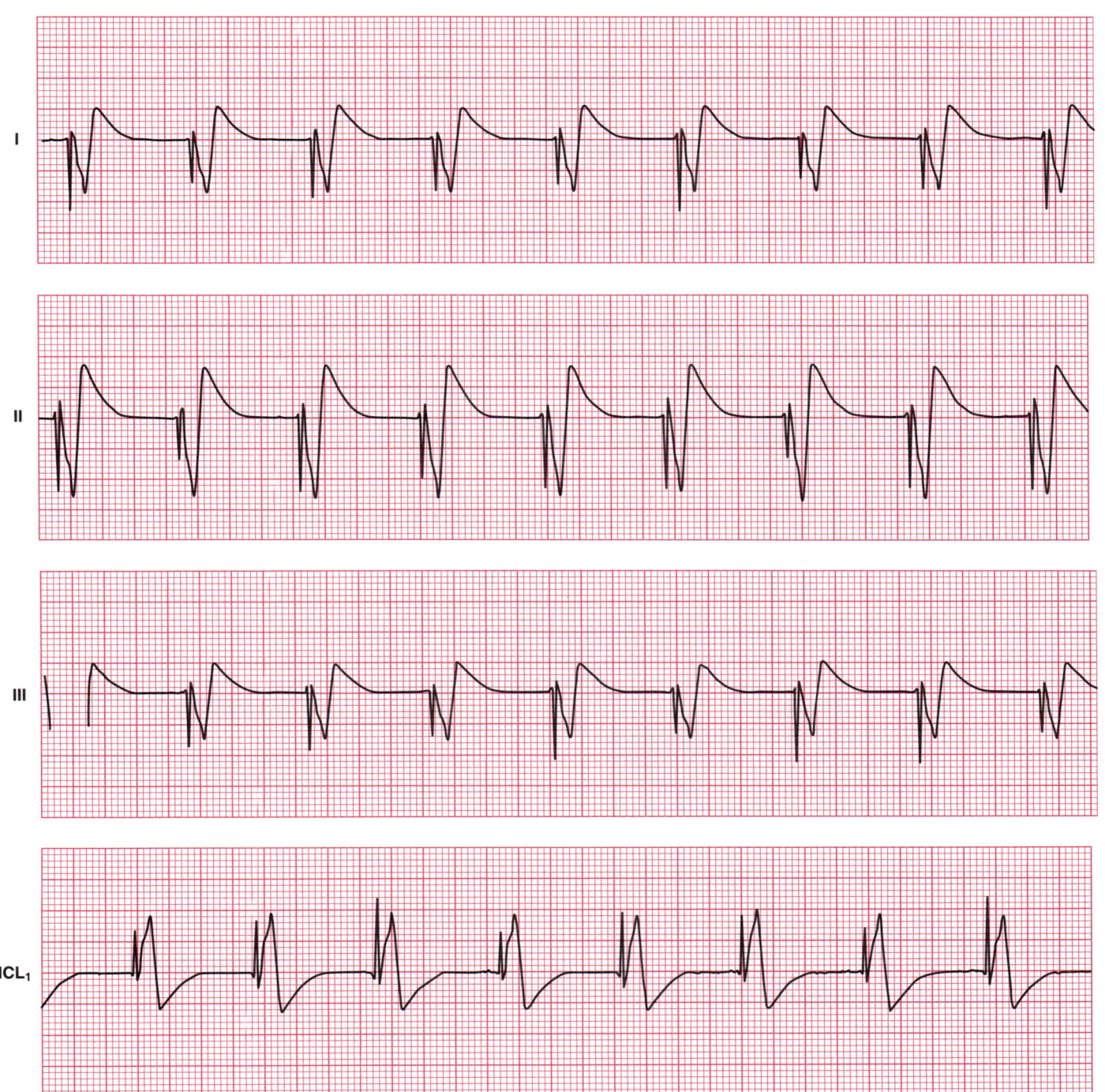

FIGURE 22-75 Artificial pacemaker rhythms.

power source (a battery cell implanted subcutaneously, typically in the right or left side of the chest). The tip of the pacemaker wire is at the apex of the right ventricle (ventricular pacemaker), in the right atrium (atrial pacemaker), or in both locations (dual-chamber pacemaker). These devices are placed in patients with complete heart block. They also are used by patients who have episodes of severe symptomatic bradycardia.

Some pacemakers fire continuously at a preset rate regardless of the patient's own electrical activity. These are known as *fixed-rate* or *asynchronous pacemakers*. They are rarely used today. Other pacemakers fire only if the patient's own rate drops below the preset rate of the pacemaker (they thereby act as an escape rhythm). These are known as *demand pacemakers*. Atrial and ventricular demand pacemakers pace the atria and ventricles when the intrinsic rate of the paced chamber drops dangerously low. *Atrial synchronous ventricular pacemakers* are synchronized with the patient's atrial rhythm. This type of pacemaker paces the ventricle after the patient's atria contract. This pacemaker is useful in patients with normal sinus node activity but various degrees of atrioventricular block. *Atrioventricular sequential pacemakers* pace the atria first and then the ventricles when normal impulses are absent or slowed in either or both chambers. If regular atrial activity is too slow, for example, the two chambers are paced sequentially to maintain the atrial kick. If the atrial rate is adequate, the atrial pacer does not fire. The ventricular pacemaker still fires if the ventricular rate is below a preset rate. This pacemaker is ideal for sick sinus syndrome and sinus arrest.

Rate-responsive pacemakers are a newer class of pacemakers. They can adjust their pacing rates to a patient's needs. They do this by sensing when cardiac output should be increased. Several methods of sensing metabolic activity are used. However, the most popular rate-responsive pacers detect patient movement to determine the best firing rate. These devices can increase both cardiac output and tolerance of physical activity. At times they may increase the patient's pacing rate inappropriately, such as if they sense muscle movement that is not caused by increased patient activity. Because the pacemaker spikes are difficult to visualize in all leads, fast pacemaker rates can easily be misinterpreted as ventricular tachycardia. Perform a 12-lead ECG if time permits.

RULES FOR INTERPRETATION (LEAD II MONITORING)

Artificial pacemaker rhythms have the following characteristics on the ECG:

QRS complex: If pacemaker induced, QRS complexes are 0.12 second or greater. Their appearance usually is bizarre, resembling a premature ventricular complex. The pacemaker is said to have electrical capture if each pacemaker spike elicits a QRS complex. If only the atria are paced, the QRS complexes usually are normal, provided no bundle branch block is present. With demand pacemakers, some of the patient's own

QRS complexes may be present. These normal QRS complexes occur without pacemaker spikes.

P waves: May be present or absent, normal or abnormal. The relationship of the P waves to the pacemaker (QRS) complex varies by type of artificial pacemaker. Pacemaker spikes precede QRS complexes induced by ventricular pacemakers, whereas dual-chambered pacemakers also produce an atrial spike followed by a P wave. The pacemaker spike is a narrow deflection on the oscilloscope and represents the electrical discharge of the pacemaker. Pacemaker spikes indicate only that a pacemaker is discharging. They provide no information about ventricular contraction or perfusion.

> ## CRITICAL THINKING
> If a pacemaker fails, what rhythms might you see on the monitor?

Rate: Varies according to the preset rate of the pacemaker. Typically the rate is 60 to 80 beats/minute.

Rhythm: Regular if pacing is constant; irregular if pacing occurs only on demand

P-R interval: The presence and duration of P-R intervals depend on the underlying rhythm and vary by the type of artificial pacemaker.

CLINICAL SIGNIFICANCE

Pacemaker spikes indicate that the patient's heart rate is regulated by an artificial pacemaker. Pacemaker spikes followed by QRS complexes indicate electrical capture. If spikes do not elicit a QRS complex, the pacemaker is not capturing the ventricle electrically. Therefore, no ventricular contraction occurs. A large percentage of pacemaker failures occur within the first month after implantation (Box 22-8).

MANAGEMENT

Pacemaker failure is a true emergency. It requires immediate recognition and rapid transport for definitive care (this may include battery replacement or temporary pacemaker insertion). Paramedics should not delay transport to attempt to stabilize these patients. Five principles apply to the treatment of patients with pacemakers:

1. When examining an unconscious patient, be alert for battery packs implanted under the skin. Also be alert for any medical alert information.
2. Manage all dysrhythmias following the appropriate algorithm.
3. Manage ventricular irritability with appropriate drug therapy without fear of suppressing ventricular response to a pacemaker rhythm, as long as pacemaker failure is not a factor.
4. For patients with artificial pacemakers, defibrillate in the usual manner. However, do not deliver the charge directly over the implanted battery pack.

BOX 22-8 Four Possible Causes of Pacemaker Malfunction

1. *Battery failure:* Currently most implanted pacemakers use a lithium-iodine cell power source. This source provides stable voltage output for about 80% to 90% of the life of the battery. (The battery life is 5 to 10 years or longer.) Battery failure usually slows the pacemaker rate. It also usually reduces the spike amplitude. If the battery fails, the patient may have bradycardia or asystole.

2. *Runaway pacemaker:* This is a pacemaker that develops rapid discharge rates, which may reach 300 beats/minute. The problem occurs as the batteries reduce their voltage output. This type of failure rarely is seen in pacemakers used today, because the newer power sources provide a gradual increase in rate as the batteries run low.

3. *Failure of the sensing device in demand pacemakers:* Demand pacemakers may fail to shut off when patients have an adequate rate of their own. When this occurs, a competition develops between the natural and artificial pacemakers of the heart. The pacemaker may discharge during the vulnerable period of the cardiac cycle. This may result in dysrhythmias.

4. *Failure to capture:* Failure of the pacemaker to capture may have a variety of causes. These may include battery failure, loose or broken catheter electrode wires, inoperable electrodes, and a shift in the location of the catheter tip. In such cases, pacemaker spikes usually are present. However, they are not followed by P waves or QRS complexes.

5. Transcutaneous cardiac pacing, if indicated, may be used in the usual manner.

Besides pacemakers, implantable cardioverter-defibrillators also are common. The battery packs of these devices are located in the subcutaneous tissues of the abdominal wall. Emergency cardiac care can be given as usual. These devices present no danger to rescuers. However, paramedics should wear gloves to help avoid unpleasant sensations when the device discharges. (Implantable cardioverter-defibrillators are described further later in this chapter.)

DYSRHYTHMIAS THAT ARE DISORDERS OF CONDUCTION

Delay or blockage of the electrical impulse conduction in the heart is called a *heart block*. Heart blocks can occur anywhere in the atria between the sinoatrial node and the atrioventricular node or in the ventricles between the atrioventricular node and the Purkinje fibers. These conduction defects can be caused by diseased tissue in the conduction system or by a physiological block, such as occurs in atrial fibrillation or atrial flutter. Causes of heart blocks include atrioventricular junctional ischemia, atrioventricular junctional necrosis, degenerative disease of the conduction system, electrolyte imbalances (e.g., hyperkalemia), and drug toxicity, especially with digitalis.

Classifications

Conduction blocks may be classified based on several characteristics: the site of the block (e.g., left bundle branch block), the degree of block (e.g., second-degree atrioventricular block), or the category of atrioventricular conduction disturbance (e.g., type I). This text presents the dysrhythmias by degree and location. However, the term *degree* does not reflect directly the gradients of severity when applied to the classification of heart blocks. Any evaluation of heart block must consider the specific rates of the atria and ventricles, the patient's clinical presentation, and the findings of a complete history and physical examination before the clinical severity of AV conduction disturbances can be determined. The dysrhythmias discussed in this section include first-degree atrioventricular block; second-degree atrioventricular block type I (or *Wenckebach*); second-degree atrioventricular block type II; third-degree atrioventricular block (complete heart block); and ventricular conduction disturbances, including bundle branch blocks and hemiblocks.

Atrioventricular Blocks

The discussion of conduction disturbances of the heart begins with the atrioventricular blocks.

FIRST-DEGREE ATRIOVENTRICULAR BLOCK

Description. **First-degree atrioventricular block** is not a true block (Figure 22-76). Rather, the disturbance is a delay in conduction, usually at the level of the atrioventricular node. First-degree atrioventricular block is not considered a rhythm in itself, because it usually is superimposed on another rhythm. Therefore, the paramedic also must identify the underlying rhythm (e.g., sinus bradycardia with first-degree atrioventricular block).

Etiology. First-degree atrioventricular block may occur for no apparent reason. The dysrhythmia sometimes is associated with myocardial ischemia, acute myocardial infarction, increased vagal (parasympathetic) tone, or digitalis toxicity.

Rules for Interpretation (Lead II Monitoring). First-degree atrioventricular block has the following characteristics on the ECG:

QRS complex: Typically normal (less than 0.12 second), with an atrioventricular conduction ratio of 1:1 (a QRS complex follows each P wave)

P waves: Present; identical waves precede each QRS complex.

Rate: The rate is that of the underlying sinus or atrial rhythm.

Rhythm: The rhythm is that of the underlying rhythm.

P-R interval: A prolonged (greater than 0.20 second), constant P-R interval is the hallmark of first-degree atrioventricular block and often is the only alteration in the ECG.

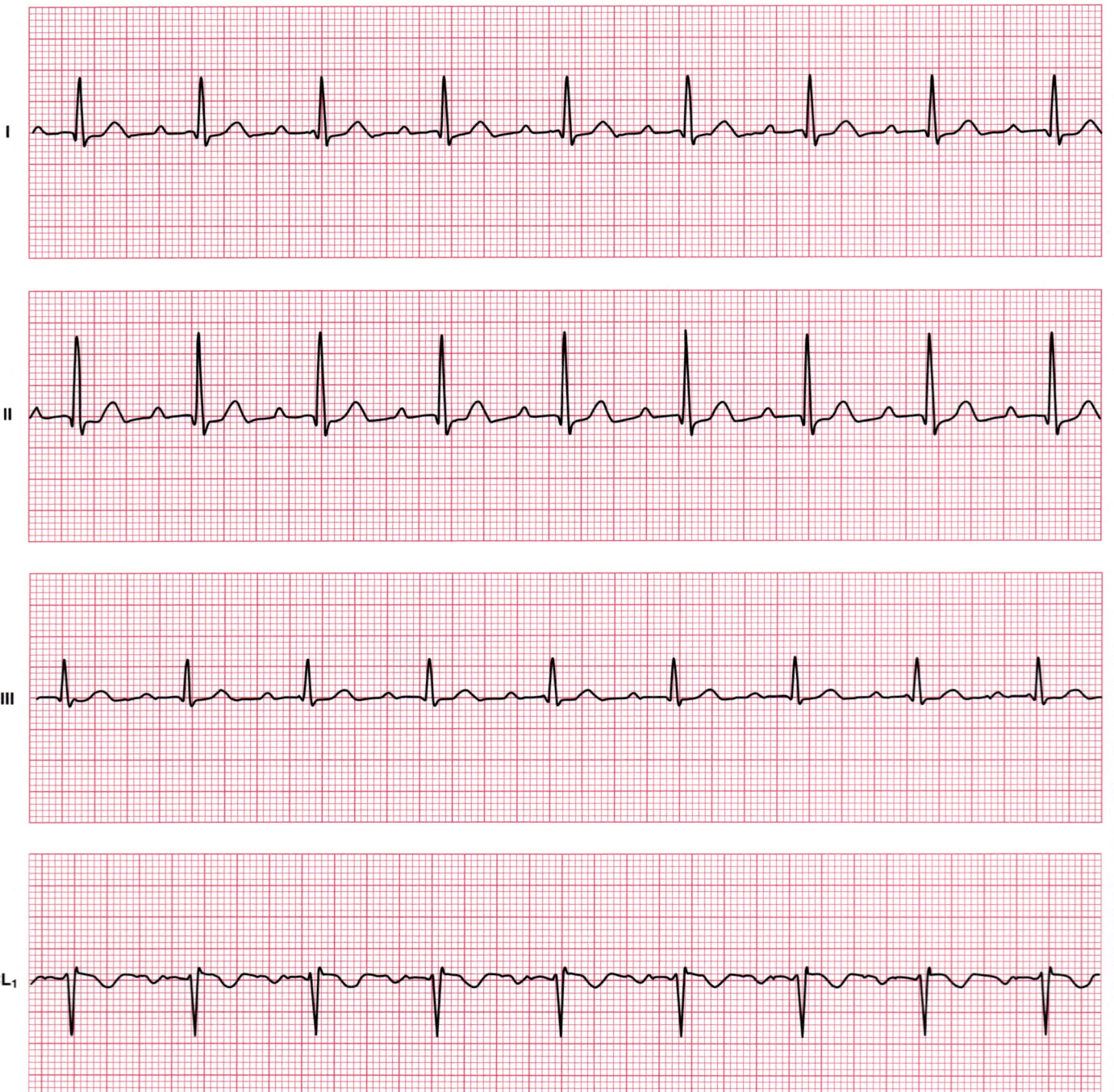

FIGURE 22-76 First-degree atrioventricular block.

Clinical Significance. As a general rule, first-degree atrioventricular block has little or no clinical significance, because all the impulses are conducted to the ventricles. In rare cases, however, a newly developed first-degree atrioventricular block progresses to a more serious atrioventricular block. The presence of first-degree AV block with a bundle branch block can signal the risk of complete heart block.[5]

Management. This dysrhythmia usually does not require treatment.

SECOND-DEGREE ATRIOVENTRICULAR BLOCK TYPE I (WENCKEBACH)

Description. **Second-degree atrioventricular block type I** is an intermittent block (Figure 22-77). It usually occurs at the level of the atrioventricular node. The conduction delay progressively increases from beat to beat until conduction to the ventricle is blocked. This dysrhythmia produces a characteristic cyclical pattern in which the P-R intervals get progressively longer until a P wave occurs that

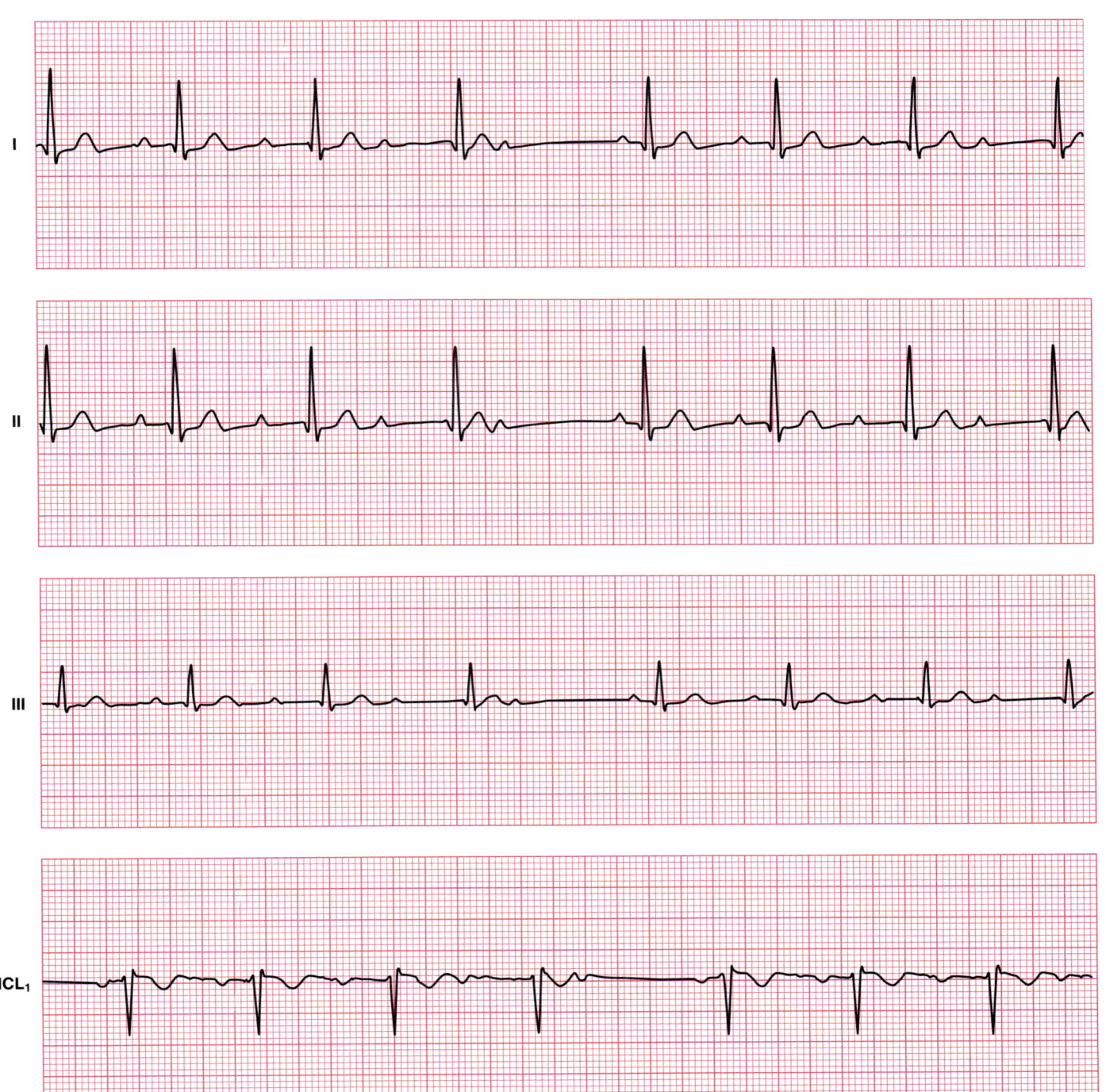

FIGURE 22-77 Second-degree atrioventricular block type I.

is not followed by a QRS complex. By the time the sinoatrial node fires again, atrioventricular conduction has had time to recover. The sequence then starts over.

Etiology. Second-degree atrioventricular block type I often occurs in acute myocardial infarction or acute myocarditis. Other causes include increased vagal tone, ischemia, drug toxicity (digitalis, propranolol, *verapamil*), head injury, and electrolyte imbalance.

Rules for Interpretation (Lead II Monitoring). Second-degree atrioventricular block type I has the following characteristics on the ECG:

QRS complex: Usually less than 0.12 second. Commonly, the atrioventricular conduction ratio (P waves to QRS complexes) is 5:4, 4:3, 3:2, or 2:1; the pattern may be constant or variable. A constant 2:1 block makes distinguishing between type I and type II blocks difficult. As a general rule, if the QRS complex is narrow, the block is probably a type I, 2:1 block. If the QRS complex is wide, the block is probably a type II, 2:1 block.[5]

P waves: Upright, uniform, and preceding the QRS complex when the QRS complex occurs

Rate: The atrial rate is that of the underlying sinus or atrial rhythm. The ventricular rate may be normal or slow but always is slightly less than the atrial rate.

Rhythm: The atrial rhythm is regular; the ventricular rhythm is irregular (characteristic group beating).

P-R interval: Progressively lengthens before the nonconducted P wave. The P-P interval is constant, but the R-R interval decreases until the dropped beat (producing grouping of QRS complexes).

Clinical Significance. Second-degree atrioventricular block type I usually is a transient and reversible phenomenon. However, it can progress to a more serious atrioventricular block. If dropped beats occur often, the patient may show signs and symptoms of decreased cardiac output.

Management. No management is required if the patient is asymptomatic. If the dropped beats compromise the heart rate and cardiac output, administration of *atropine,* transcutaneous cardiac pacing, or both may be indicated (see Figure 22-43).

SECOND-DEGREE ATRIOVENTRICULAR BLOCK TYPE II

Description. Second-degree atrioventricular block type II is an intermittent block (Figure 22-78). This dysrhythmia occurs when atrial impulses are not conducted to the ventricles. Unlike type I, this block is characterized by consecutive P waves that are conducted with a constant P-R interval before a dropped beat. This variation of atrioventricular block usually occurs in a regular sequence with the conduction ratios (P waves to QRS complexes), such as 2:1, 3:2, and 4:3 (Figure 22-79). Second-degree atrioventricular block type II usually occurs below the bundle of His.

When at least two consecutive P waves fail to be conducted to the ventricles, the atrioventricular block is referred to as a **high-grade atrioventricular block** (Figure 22-80). Clinically, serious high-grade atrioventricular blocks and those that are less serious are distinguished by the atrial and ventricular rates. A 2:1 block might be considered high grade (and certainly is clinically significant) when the patient's underlying atrial rate is 60 beats/minute. However, such a block is much less of concern if the patient's atrial rate is 120 beats/minute.

A type II 2:1 atrioventricular block sometimes may be difficult to distinguish from a type I 2:1 atrioventricular block. When assessing a patient who has two atrial complexes for each QRS complex, the paramedic should evaluate the normal cycle. If the normally conducted cycle has a prolonged P-R interval (greater than 0.20 second), a narrow QRS complex (less than 0.12 second, indicating the absence of bundle branch block), and an adequate escape rate, the patient probably has a type I 2:1 atrioventricular block. As stated previously, if the conducted QRS complex has a normal P-R interval, a wide QRS complex (greater than 0.12 second, which indicates the presence of a bundle branch block), and an adequate escape rate, a type II 2:1 atrioventricular block is most likely (Figure 22-81).

Etiology. Second-degree atrioventricular block type II usually is associated with an acute myocardial infarction that occurs in the septum. Unlike second-degree atrioventricular block type I, type II normally does not result solely from increased parasympathetic tone or drug toxicity.

Rules for Interpretation (Lead II Monitoring). Second-degree atrioventricular block type II has the following characteristics on the ECG:

QRS complex: May be abnormal (equal to or greater than 0.12 second) because of bundle branch block

P waves: Upright and uniform. Some P waves are not followed by QRS complexes.

Rate: The atrial rate is unaffected and is that of the underlying sinus, atrial, or junctional rhythm. The ventricular rate is less than that of the atrial rate and often is bradycardic.

Rhythm: Regular or irregular, depending on whether the conduction ratio is constant or variable

P-R interval: Usually constant for conducted beats and may be greater than 0.20 second

Clinical Significance. Second-degree atrioventricular block type II is a serious dysrhythmia. It usually is considered malignant in the emergency setting (unlike type I atrioventricular blocks, which usually are considered benign). Slow ventricular rates may result in signs and symptoms of hypoperfusion. This dysrhythmia may progress to a more severe heart block or even to ventricular asystole.

Management. Regardless of the patient's initial condition, treatment involves insertion of a pacemaker. Prehospital care for symptomatic patients may consist of transcutaneous cardiac pacing and possibly the administration of beta-adrenergic drugs[1] (see Figure 22-43).

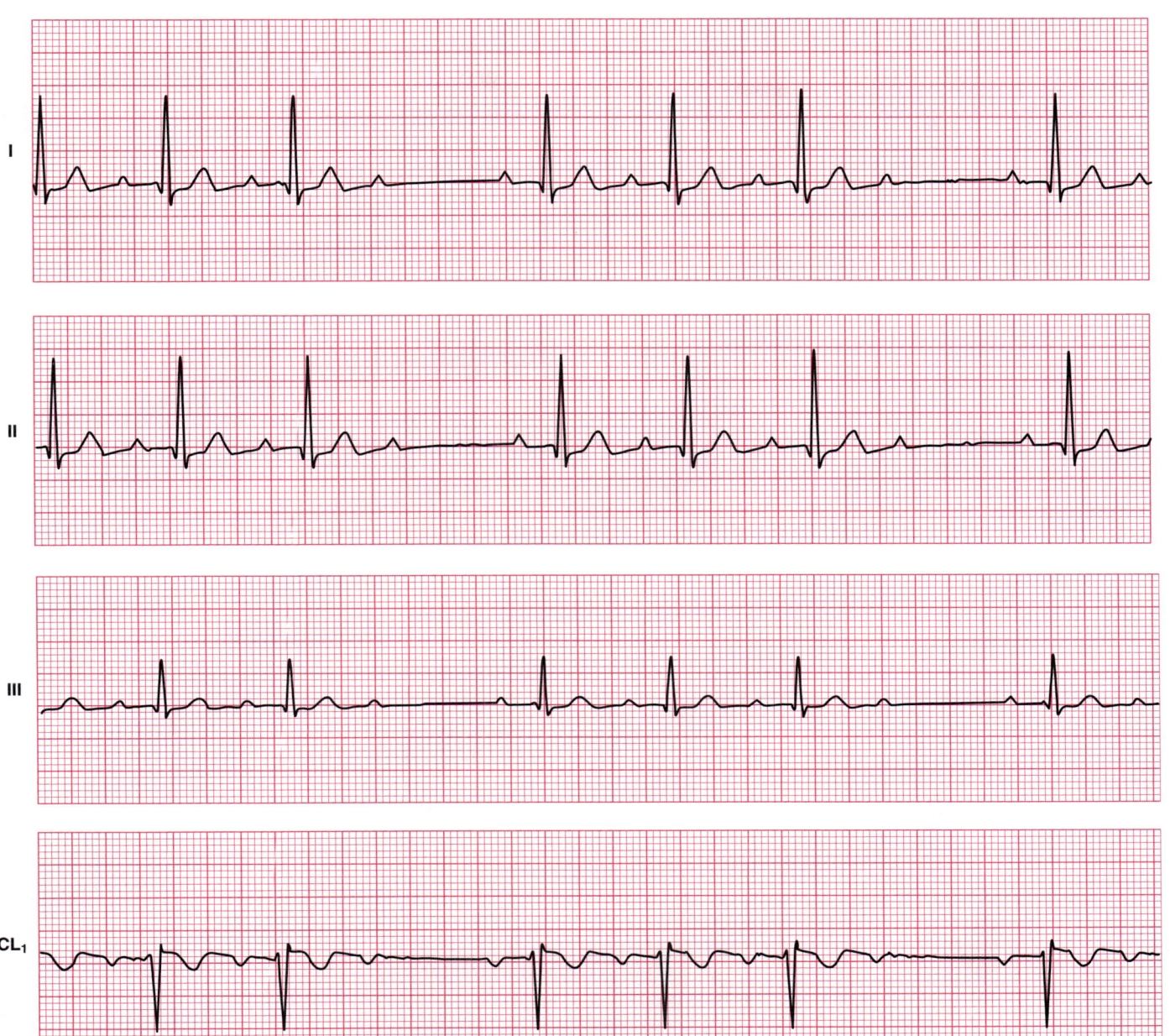

FIGURE 22-78 Second-degree atrioventricular block type II.

THIRD-DEGREE HEART BLOCK

Description. **Third-degree atrioventricular block** is also known as *complete heart block*. It results from complete electrical block at or below the atrioventricular node (infranodal) (Figure 22-82). The dysrhythmia is said to be present when the opportunity for conduction between the atria and the ventricles is present but conduction does not occur. In this condition the sinoatrial node serves as the pacemaker for the atria. An ectopic focus serves as a pacemaker in the ventricles. The result is P waves and QRS complexes that occur rhythmically, yet the rhythms are unrelated to each other (atrioventricular dissociation). The only electrical link between the atria and the ventricles is the atrioventricular node and bundle of His.

> **NOTE**
>
> *Atropine* should be used with caution in patients with complete heart block and wide-complex ventricular escape beats and also in patients with type II second-degree heart block.[1] (*Atropine* may increase the degree of block or cause third-degree atrioventricular block.) Many patients with heart block cannot be managed effectively with only medication. Immediate transport to an emergency department is indicated.

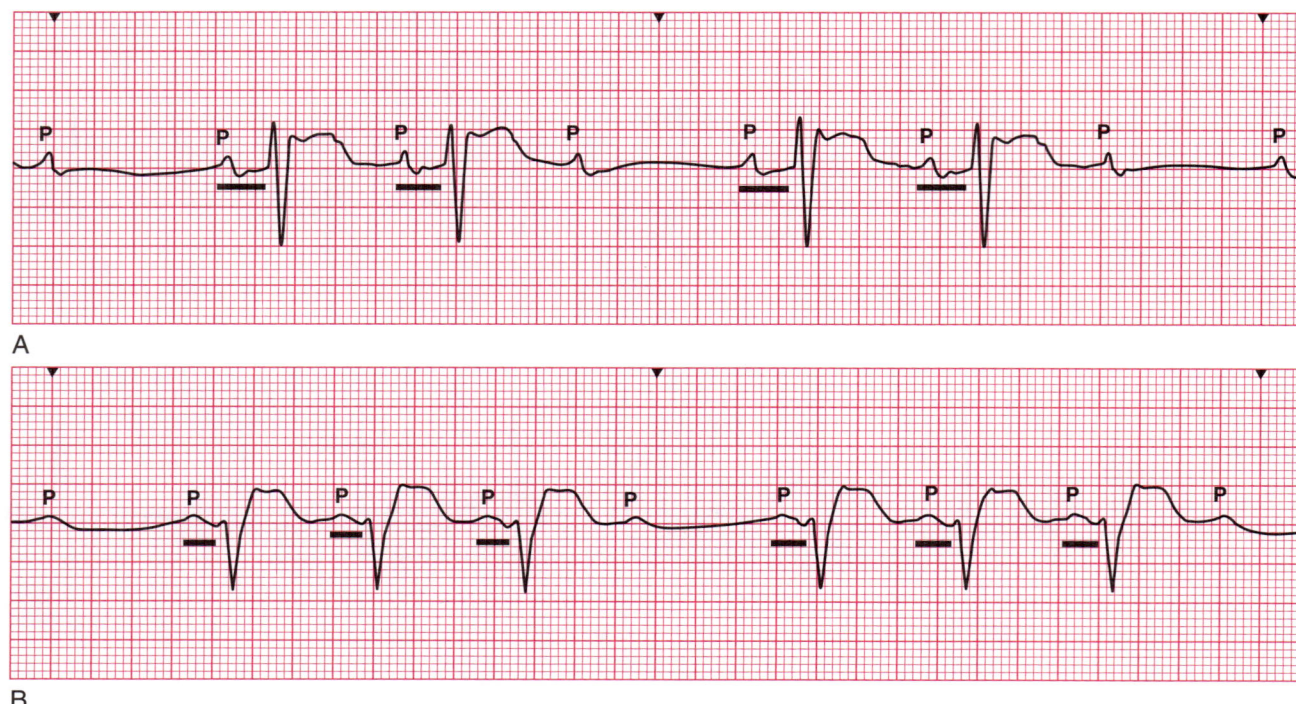

FIGURE 22-79 A, A 3 : 2 atrioventricular block. **B**, A 4 : 3 atrioventricular block.

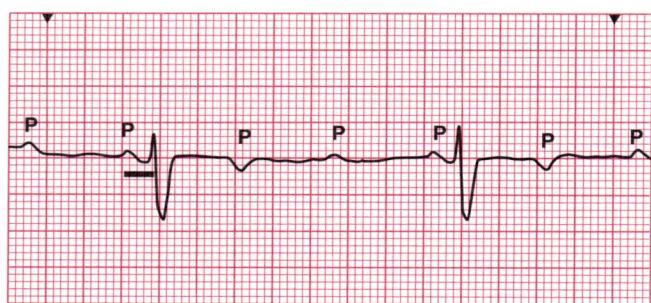

FIGURE 22-80 A 3 : 1 high-grade atrioventricular block.

Etiology. Common causes of third-degree atrioventricular block include increased vagal tone (which may produce a transient atrioventricular dissociation), septal necrosis, acute myocarditis, digitalis, beta-blocker, or calcium channel blocker toxicity, and electrolyte imbalance. The dysrhythmia also may occur in older adults as a result of chronic degenerative changes in the conduction system.

> ### CRITICAL THINKING
> When P waves and QRS complexes do not appear to be related to each other on the ECG, the paramedic should look at the shape of QRS-T waves. QRS-T waves altered by superimposed P waves suggest atrioventricular dissociation. Atrioventricular dissociation suggests third-degree atrioventricular block.

Rules for Interpretation (Lead II Monitoring). Third-degree heart block has the following characteristics on the ECG:

QRS complex: May be less than 0.12 second if the escape focus is below the atrioventricular node and above the bifurcation of the bundle branches or 0.12 second or greater if the escape focus is ventricular. A narrow QRS complex in third-degree heart block is less common than a wide QRS complex.

P waves: Present but with no relationship to the QRS complexes. In cases of atrial flutter or fibrillation, complete heart block is manifested by a slow, regular ventricular response.

Rate: The atrial rate is that of the underlying sinus or atrial rhythm. The ventricular rate typically is 40 to 60 beats/minute if the escape focus is junctional and less than 40 beats/minute if the escape focus is in the ventricles.

Rhythm: The atrial and ventricular rhythms usually are regular. The rhythms are independent of each other.

P-R interval: No relation exists between atrial and ventricular activity (Figure 22-83).

Clinical Significance. The patient may have signs and symptoms of severe bradycardia and decreased cardiac output. These are the result of the slow ventricular rate and asynchronous action of the atria and ventricles. Third-degree atrioventricular block associated with wide QRS complexes is an ominous sign. The dysrhythmia potentially is lethal. Patients with this rhythm often present as unstable.

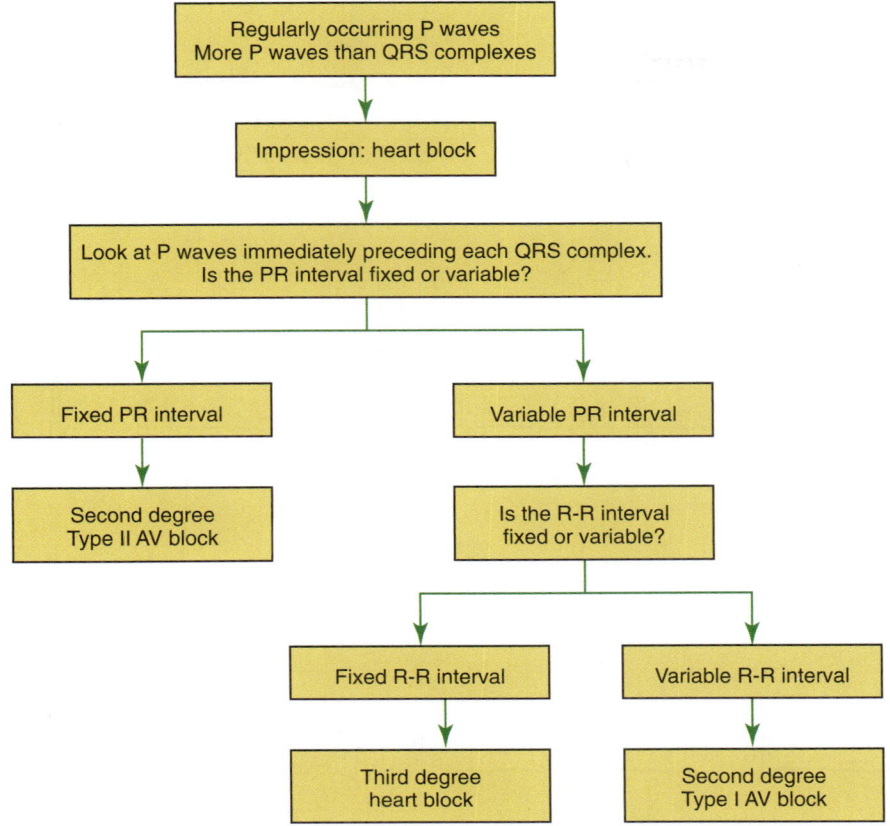

FIGURE 22-81 Identifying heart blocks.

NOTE

Complete atrioventricular block in the presence of atrial fibrillation often is caused by drug toxicity (usually *digitalis*). Almost always some atrioventricular block occurs with atrial fibrillation or flutter. Yet complete atrioventricular block is recognized by a slow, regular ventricular response. (The response usually is slower than 60 beats/minute.) The QRS complex may be normal if the escape focus is from above the bifurcation of the bundle branches.

Management. Insertion of a pacemaker is the definitive treatment for symptomatic third-degree atrioventricular block and for asymptomatic third-degree heart block with bundle branch block. Initial prehospital care includes transcutaneous cardiac pacing or administration of a *dopamine* infusion to increase the ventricular rate, if needed, and administration of an *epinephrine* infusion.

Transcutaneous cardiac pacing is a class IIb intervention for symptomatic bradycardias that do not improve after atropine administration (see Figure 22-43). *Atropine* is unlikely to help patients with complete heart block and a wide QRS complex. The vagus nerve innervates the atria and AV node, and the focus controlling the heart in a third-degree block most often is in the ventricles.

CRITICAL THINKING

What should you tell the patient before starting transcutaneous cardiac pacing?

Ventricular Conduction Disturbances

Ventricular conduction disturbances (bundle branch blocks and hemiblocks) are delays or interruptions in the transmission of electrical impulses. These disturbances occur below the level of bifurcation of the bundle of His. Detection of these blocks is important. It helps to identify the patient at increased risk of severe bradycardia and third-degree heart block. This is especially true when the patient has other forms of atrioventricular block. Common causes of bundle branch block include the following:

- Acute heart failure
- Acute myocardial infarction
- Aortic stenosis
- Cardiomyopathy
- Hyperkalemia
- Infection (e.g., carditis)
- Ischemic heart disease
- Trauma

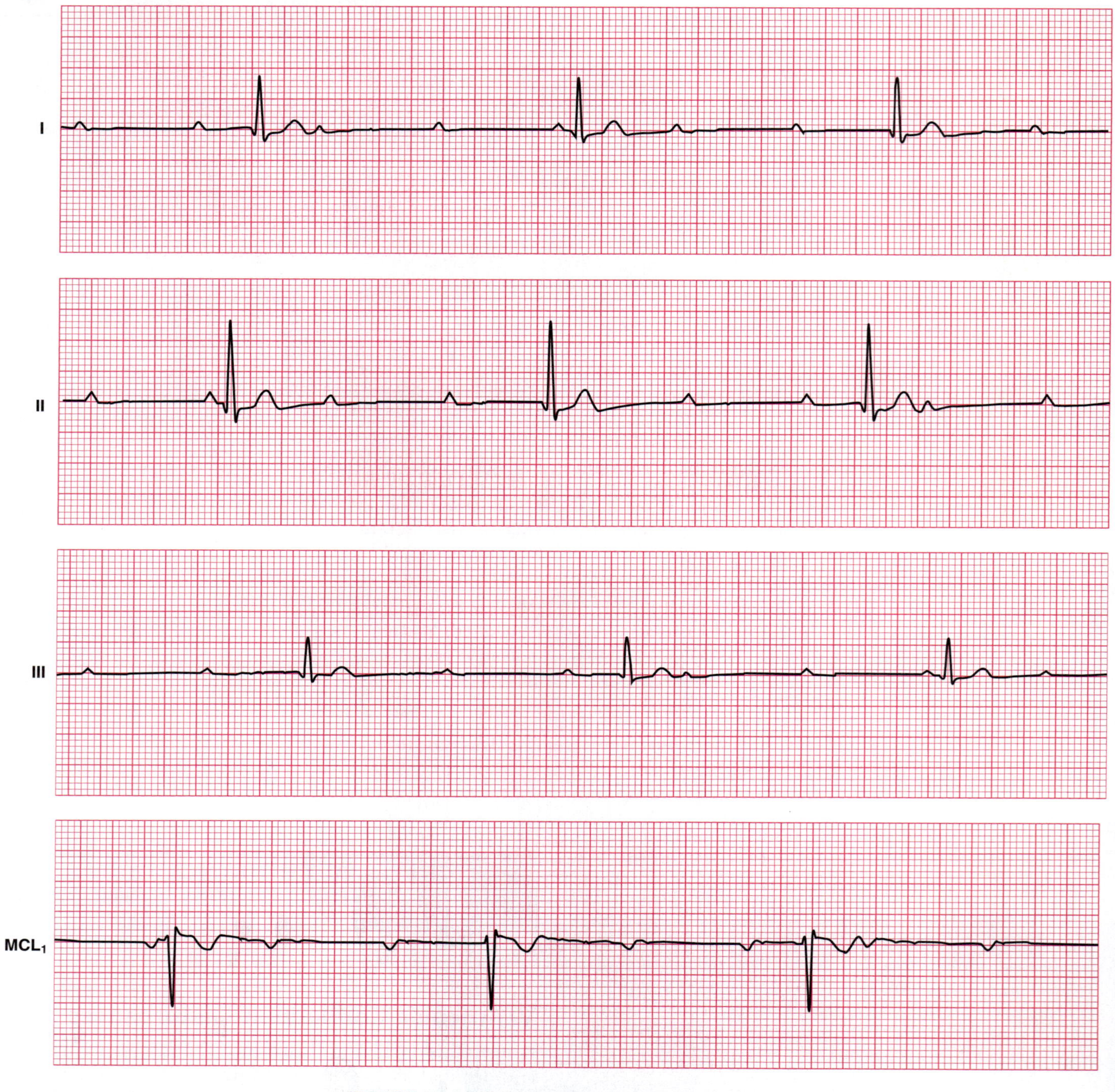

I

II

III

MCL₁

FIGURE 22-82 Third-degree atrioventricular block.

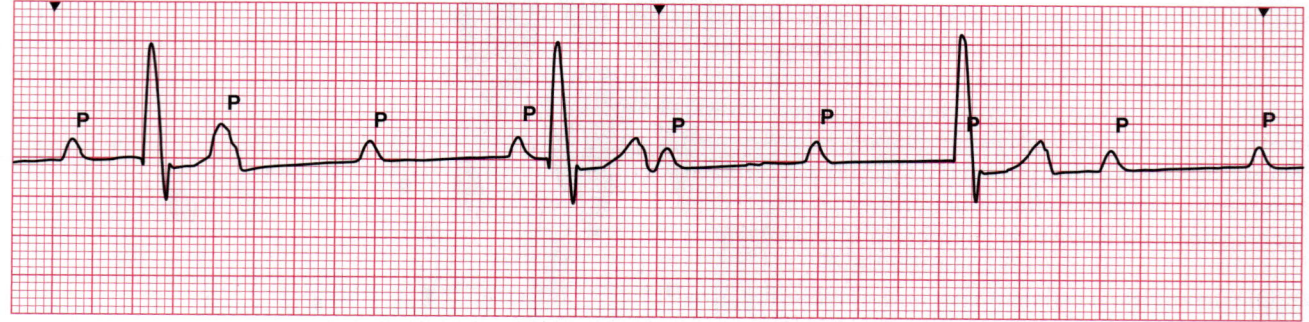

FIGURE 22-83 Third-degree block demonstrating P waves superimposed on the QRS complex.

BUNDLE BRANCH ANATOMY

To review, the bundle of His begins at the atrioventricular node and divides to form the left and right bundle branches (Figure 22-84). The right bundle branch continues toward the apex and spreads throughout the right ventricle. The left bundle branch subdivides into the anterior and posterior fascicles and spreads throughout the left ventricle. Conduction of electrical impulses through the Purkinje fibers stimulates the ventricles to contract.

With normal conduction, the first part of the ventricle to be stimulated is the left side of the septum. The electrical impulse then traverses the septum to stimulate the other side. Shortly thereafter, the left and right ventricles are stimulated at the same time. The left ventricle normally is much larger and thicker than the right ventricle; therefore, its electrical activity predominates over that of the right ventricle.

COMMON ELECTROCARDIOGRAM FINDINGS

When an electrical impulse is blocked from passing through the right or left bundle branch, aberration (abnormal conduction) occurs and one ventricle depolarizes and contracts before the other. Ventricular activation no longer occurs at the same time. As a result, the QRS complex widens (often with a slurred or notched appearance known as *rabbit ears*). The hallmark of bundle branch block is a QRS complex equal to or greater than 0.12 second. The two criteria for recognizing bundle branch block are:

- A QRS complex equal to or greater than 0.12 second
- QRS complexes produced by supraventricular activity

>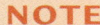
> **NOTE**
> *Bundle branch block* and *hemiblock* (fascicular block) are terms used to describe abnormal conduction or the interruption of impulses from above the bundle branches to the ventricles. The interruption may occur in either the anterior (superior) or the posterior (inferior) division. These patterns of abnormal or aberrant conduction must be recognized as different from beats of ventricular origin. Beats of ventricular origin can have similar QRS complex shapes.

Ventricular conduction disturbances are identified best by monitoring leads V_1 and V_6 with a 12-lead machine. These leads permit the easiest differentiation of the right and left bundle branch blocks. Lead V_1 looks at right and left bundle branches and should be monitored during transport of these patients.[7]

Normal Conduction. In normal ventricular stimulation, the electrical impulse reaches the septum first. It then travels from the left endocardium to the right endocardium of the septum (Figure 22-85). This impulse generates a small R wave in V_1. The rest of the impulses mainly are conducted away from the V_1 electrode. This yields a negative deflection. Therefore, during normal conduction, V_1 mainly is negative. The QRS complex also is usually 0.08 to 0.10 second wide (the same as any other narrow QRS complex).

Right Bundle Branch Block. In **right bundle branch block** (RBBB), the left bundle branch performs normally. Therefore, the left branch activates the left side of the heart before the right (Figure 22-86). When the left ventricle is

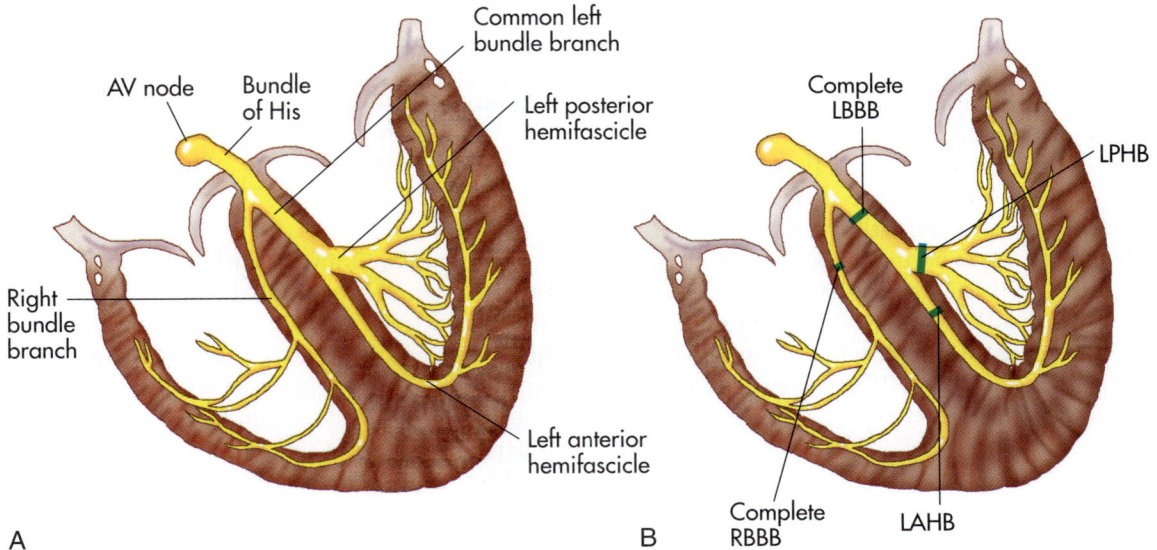

FIGURE 22-84 A, Simplified illustration of the major divisions of the ventricular conduction system. After passing through the atrioventricular node and the bundle of His, the electrical impulse is carried to the right and common left bundle branches. The latter structure divides into the left anterior and posterior hemifascicles. **B,** Possible sites of block and the conduction deficits that may be produced.

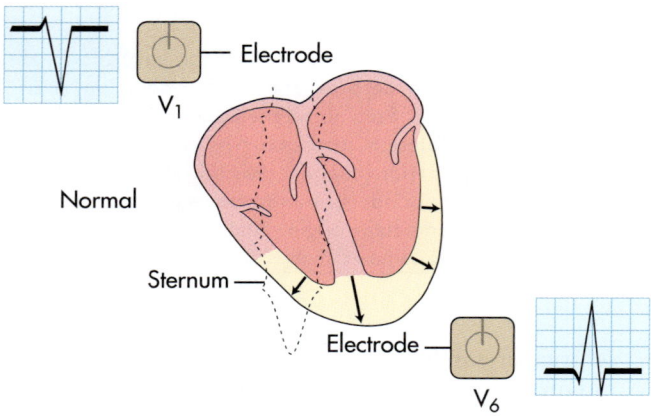

FIGURE 22-85 Normal ventricular conduction.

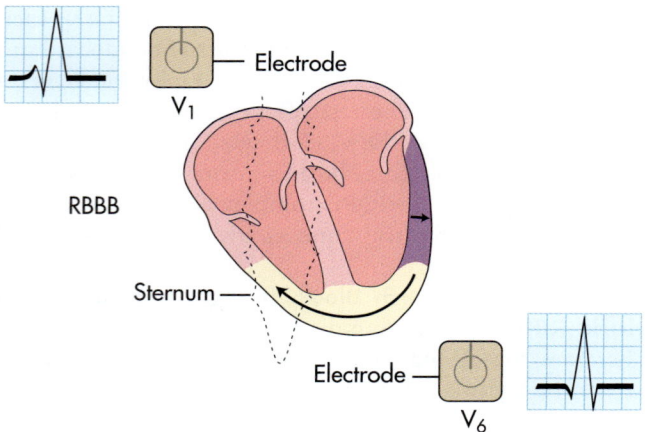

FIGURE 22-86 Right bundle branch block.

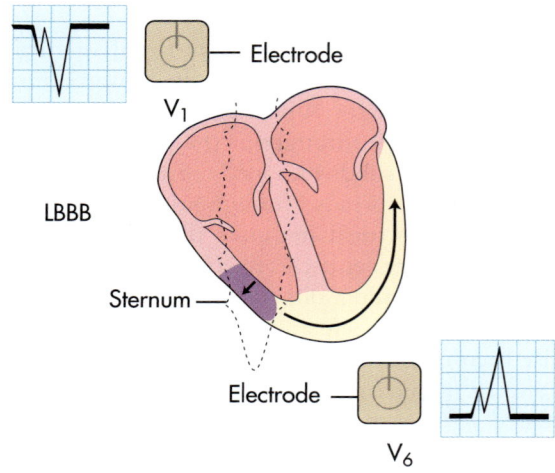

FIGURE 22-87 Left bundle branch block.

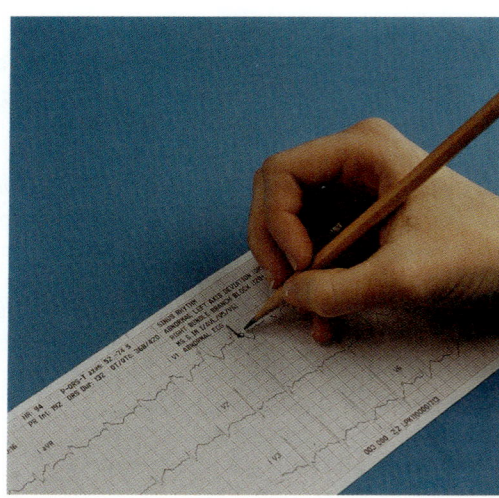

FIGURE 22-88 To distinguish left from right bundle branch blocks, find the J point of the QRS complex, draw a line backward into the QRS complex, and fill in the triangle created by this line and the last portion of the QRS complex. The direction the triangle points distinguishes the two types of blocks.

activated initially, the impulse travels away from the V₁ electrode. This yields a negative deflection (S wave). The electrical impulse then travels across the interventricular septum and activates the right ventricle. Because the impulse is coming back toward the V₁ electrode, a large positive deflection (R wave) occurs. This results in the RSR′ pattern seen in V₁ in patients with right bundle branch block. The QRS (or in this case, RSR) complex is at least 0.12 second. Whenever the two criteria for bundle branch block are met and V₁ displays an RSR′ pattern, right bundle branch block should be suspected.

NOTE

In right bundle branch block (RBBB), the left ventricle receives the electrical impulse first. In left bundle branch block (LBBB), the opposite occurs. Because one ventricle contracts slightly later than the other, two QRS complexes are produced that often appear joined.

Left Bundle Branch Block. In the more serious **left bundle branch block** (LBBB), the fibers that usually stimulate the interventricular septum are blocked. This blockage alters normal septal activation and sends it in the opposite direction (Figure 22-87). The septum is depolarized by the right bundle branch, and the right ventricle then is activated. Because the impulse is leading away from V₁, the lead shows a deep, wide S wave (QS pattern). As with right bundle branch block, the activation takes at least 0.12 second. Whenever the two criteria for bundle branch block are met and a QS pattern is seen in V₁, a left bundle branch block should be suspected. Patients with new or presumed new left bundle branch block have lost a lot of myocardium; left ventricular failure may develop and may lead to death.

BOX 22-9 Turn Signal Method of Determining Right or Left Bundle Branch Block

As a shortcut for identifying right or left bundle branch block, the paramedic should envision the turn signal mechanism in a vehicle. The turn signal is pushed "up" to turn *right* and pushed "down" to turn *left*.

When lead V_1 is monitored, the bundle branch block may be determined by the following procedure (Figure 22-88):

1. Find a QRS complex that is at least 0.12 second wide.
2. Count backward three small boxes from the beginning of the QRS complex and move straight up to see the J point.
3. Draw a line backward from the J point into the QRS complex.
4. Fill in the triangle created by this line and the last portion of the QRS complex.
5. If the triangle points up, it is a right bundle branch block.
6. If the triangle points down, it is a left bundle branch block.

The turn signal method (Box 22-9) is a means of differentiating right and left bundle branch block.

NOTE

A clear RSR′ or QS pattern in V_1 cannot always be identified. The turn signal method is another means of determining which bundle is blocked. Using this method to evaluate the ECG can help the paramedic identify which ventricle was depolarized last.

MANAGEMENT OF BUNDLE BRANCH BLOCKS AND HEMIBLOCKS

No specific treatment is necessary for persistent bundle branch blocks or hemiblocks. (New onset LBBB with chest pain may be acute coronary syndrome.) In these cases, the LBBB should be treated as ST-segment elevation myocardial infarction (STEMI). However, if other conditions (e.g., hypoxia, ischemia, electrolyte imbalance, or drug toxicity) are causing a block, these conditions should be treated. Some emergency medication administered to patients with cardiac disease (e.g., ***procainamide, digoxin,*** and ***verapamil*** or ***diltiazem***) can slow electrical impulse conduction through the atrioventricular node. To administer these medicines safely, the paramedic must make sure the patient is not at a high risk of developing complete heart block. Those at such risk include the following:

- Any patient with type II atrioventricular block
- Any patient with evidence of disease in both bundle branches
- Any patient with two or more blocks of any kind (e.g., prolonged P-R interval and anterior hemiblock, right

bundle branch block and anterior hemiblock, type I atrioventricular block, and left bundle branch block)

Prehospital care for these patients should include management of any accompanying signs and symptoms, transport, constant ECG monitoring, and anticipation of the possible need for external pacing. Emergency pacing has been recommended for the following four indications[1]:

1. Hemodynamically compromising bradycardias
2. Bradycardias with malignant escape rhythms unresponsive to pharmacological therapy
3. Overdrive pacing of refractory supraventricular or ventricular tachycardia unresponsive to pharmacological therapy or cardioversion
4. Bradyasystolic cardiac arrest (in rare situations)

The American Heart Association also recommends pacing readiness in the setting of acute myocardial infarction for patients with symptomatic sinus node dysfunction; second-degree atrioventricular block type II; third-degree heart block; or newly acquired left, right, or alternating bundle branch block or bifascicular block.[1]

Pulseless Electrical Activity

The term **pulseless electrical activity** (also known as *electromechanical dissociation*) (Figure 22-89) is defined as the absence of a detectable pulse and the presence of some type of electrical activity other than ventricular tachycardia or ventricular fibrillation.[1] The outcome of pulseless electrical activity almost always is poor unless an underlying cause can be identified and corrected. The paramedic must maintain circulation for the patient with basic and advanced life support techniques while searching for a correctable cause.

CRITICAL THINKING

What rhythms might you see on the monitor when a patient is in pulseless electrical activity?

Correctable causes of pulseless electrical activity are cardiac tamponade, tension pneumothorax, pulmonary embolism, myocardial infarction, hypoxemia, acidosis, hypokalemia, hyperkalemia, hypothermia, and overdoses (e.g., narcotics, cyclic antidepressants, beta blockers, and digitalis). Other, less correctable causes include massive myocardial damage from infarction, prolonged ischemia during resuscitation, profound hypovolemia, and massive pulmonary embolism. Patients in profound shock of any type (including anaphylactic, septic, neurogenic, and hypovolemic shock) may have pulseless electrical activity.

The paramedic should manage tension pneumothorax with needle decompression. If the patient is hypoxic, the paramedic should manage the patient by improving oxygenation and ventilation. If acute hypovolemia is present (because of hemorrhage), the paramedic should begin fluid resuscitation with volume expanders. The paramedic

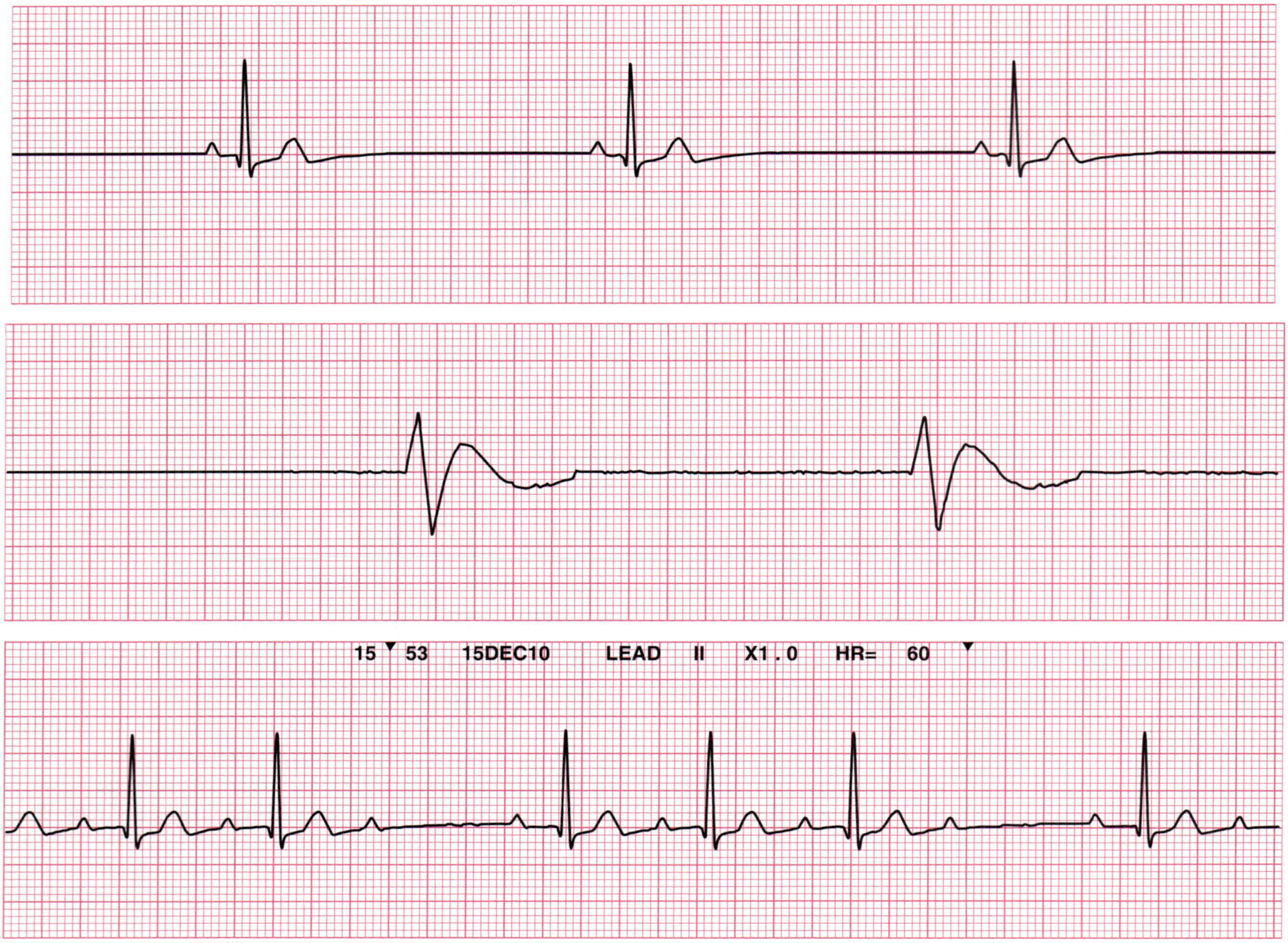

FIGURE 22-89 Various pulseless electrical activity rhythms as seen in lead II.

should manage acidosis by ensuring adequate cardiopulmonary resuscitation and hyperventilation. If preexisting acidosis (e.g., diabetic ketoacidosis), cyclic antidepressant overdose, or hyperkalemia is suspected (e.g., a patient on home dialysis), use of *sodium bicarbonate* may be indicated. *Calcium* is a specific therapy for hyperkalemia and calcium channel blocker toxicity. Both of these conditions can produce pulseless electrical activity. Besides calcium channel blockers, other drugs taken in toxic amounts can produce wide-complex pulseless electrical activity. These overdoses can be managed with specific therapy. The therapy may be effective in reestablishing a perfusing rhythm (see Figure 22-63).

> ### CRITICAL THINKING
> What patient care measures should you take in this case?

Preexcitation Syndromes

Preexcitation syndrome (anomalous or accelerated atrioventricular conduction) is associated with an abnormal conduction pathway between the atria and ventricles. This pathway bypasses the atrioventricular node or the bundle of His or both. This allows the electrical impulses to initiate depolarization of the ventricles earlier than usual. The most common preexcitation syndrome is **Wolff-Parkinson-White syndrome.**

WOLFF-PARKINSON-WHITE SYNDROME

Description. In some hearts an accessory muscle bundle (the **bundle of Kent** or *Kent fibers*) connects the lateral wall of the atrium and the ventricle, bypassing the atrioventricular node. This produces an early activation of the ventricle (Wolff-Parkinson-White syndrome).[7] WPW syndrome is thought to be of minor clinical significance unless a tachycardia is present. In that case, the syndrome can become life threatening.

Etiology. Wolff-Parkinson-White syndrome may occur in young, healthy individuals (mainly men) without apparent cause. It also may occur in multiple members of a family. It may be present in successive generations.

Rules for Interpretation (Lead II Monitoring). Wolff-Parkinson-White syndrome has the following characteristics on the ECG:

QRS complex: May be normal or wide (depending on whether conduction is retrograde or anterograde along the bundle of Kent). Conduction that occurs normally down the atrioventricular node and simultaneously in an anterograde fashion along the accessory pathway results in a meeting of the two waves of depolarization that forms a fusion (delta wave). A **delta wave** is evidenced by slurring or notching of the onset of the QRS complex and is a diagnostic finding in WPW syndrome. (Not all leads show the delta wave.) Paramedics should keep in mind that QRS widening may simulate right or left bundle branch block.

P waves: Normal

Rate: Normal unless associated with rapid supraventricular tachycardia

Rhythm: Regular

P-R interval: Usually less than 0.12 second, because the normal delay at the atrioventricular node does not occur

The three characteristic ECG findings in Wolff-Parkinson-White syndrome are a short P-R interval, a delta wave, and QRS widening (Figure 22-90).

Clinical Significance. Patients with WPW syndrome are highly susceptible to bouts of paroxysmal supraventricular tachycardias. The reason is that the accessory pathway provides a ready-made reentry circuit. This allows continued transmission of the impulse from the atria to the ventricles. Most tachydysrhythmias seen in Wolff-Parkinson-White syndrome occur with the wave of depolarization progressing from the atrioventricular node to the bundle of His to the accessory pathway. In the accessory pathway the impulse is conducted in a retrograde direction to the atria. Therefore, most tachydysrhythmias seen in WPW syndrome are narrow complexes. Patients with Wolff-Parkinson-White

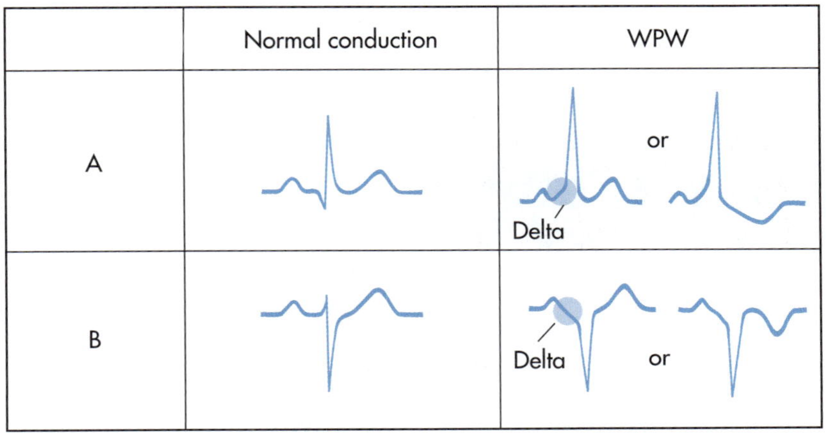

	Normal conduction	WPW
A		or Delta
B		Delta or

FIGURE 22-90 Characteristic findings in Wolff-Parkinson-White (WPW) syndrome (short P-R interval, QRS widening, and delta wave) compared with normal conduction. **A,** Usual appearance of WPW syndrome in leads where the QRS complex is predominantly upright. **B,** Appearance of WPW syndrome; the RS complex is predominantly negative.

syndrome may have attacks of paroxysmal tachydysrhythmias for many years. However, these attacks are not always benign. The atrioventricular node may be bypassed. Conduction rates also can greatly exceed those in patients whose atrioventricular node is part of the reentry circuit. This leads to rapid tachycardias. These can precipitate congestive heart failure and even death from ventricular fibrillation.

Management. Recognition of Wolff-Parkinson-White syndrome is crucial. Differentiation of the syndrome from ventricular tachycardia and uncomplicated supraventricular tachycardia also is a key factor. Many emergency drugs used to manage other reentry tachycardias are contraindicated in Wolff-Parkinson-White syndrome. AV nodal blocking agents (e.g., **adenosine,** calcium channel blockers, **digoxin,** and possibly beta blockers) should not be administered. These drugs can cause a paradoxical increase in the ventricular response to the rapid atrial impulses of atrial fibrillation. Management must be based on the patient's signs and symptoms. If the patient's heart rate is normal, no emergency care is required. If the patient has a rapid tachycardia, emergency treatment to restore normal rhythm is needed. The treatment is aimed at blocking conduction through the accessory pathways from the atria to the ventricle.

Prehospital care may include pharmacological therapy for specific dysrhythmias, vagal maneuvers, and cardioversion for severe clinical deterioration. **Verapamil** and **diltiazem** are contraindicated in wide QRS complex tachycardia because these drugs can speed conduction down the accessory pathway (greater than 280 beats/minute). This increase in conduction may lead to ventricular fibrillation and sudden death. Therefore, in patients with wide QRS complex tachycardia, the drug treatment depends on the patient's signs and symptoms and their severity.

To review, **amiodarone** is the drug of choice for presumed supraventricular tachycardia and supraventricular tachycardia with aberrant conduction. (**Procainamide** is an alternative drug that may be used.) The paramedic should perform cardioversion without delay in patients with rapid ventricular rates (greater than 150 beats/minute) who are unstable.

SECTION SIX
The 12-Lead Electrocardiogram

12-LEAD MONITORING

As stated earlier, the 12-lead ECG has become standard in many EMS systems that provide advanced life support. 12-Lead acquisition and interpretation now is recognized as a key skill for paramedics.[9] The ability to interpret a 12-lead ECG can affect transport decisions and medication and treatment selections. In addition, this skill can help paramedics predict the likelihood that a patient will become unstable. 12-Lead ECG monitoring can be used to:

- Determine the presence and location of bundle branch blocks
- Determine the electrical axis and the presence of fascicular blocks
- Identify ST-segment and T-wave changes relative to myocardial ischemia, injury, and infarction
- Identify ventricular tachycardia in wide-complex tachycardia

Lead Review

As explained earlier, ECG machines provide many views of the electrical activity of the heart by monitoring voltage changes between electrodes applied to the body. To review, the modern ECG uses 12 leads: three standard limb leads; three augmented limb leads, and six precordial (chest) leads. The standard limb leads are I, II, and III. The augmented limb leads are aV_R, aV_L, and aV_F. The precordial leads are V_1 through V_6.

NOTE

Leads should not be confused with *electrodes*. The 12-lead ECG uses only 10 electrodes. However, the machine interprets 12 leads, or "views," of the heart using computerized calculations.

The imaginary lines join the positive and negative electrodes of each lead, forming a straight line between the positive and negative poles. This straight line is known as the *axis* of the ECG lead. The axes of the standard limb leads represent the average direction of the electrical activity of the heart. If these axes are moved so that they cross a common midpoint without changing their orientation, they form a triaxial reference system (three intersecting lines of reference). Lead I is a lateral (leftward) lead. It assesses the electrical activity of the heart from a vantage point that is defined as 0 degrees on a circle. This circle is divided into an upper negative 180 degrees and a lower positive 180 degrees. Leads II and III are inferior leads. They assess the electrical activity of the heart from vantage points of +60 degrees and +120 degrees, respectively.

The augmented limb leads (Figure 22-91) record the difference in electrical potential between the positive electrode of an extremity lead and a vantage point. The vantage point of zero electrical potential is at the center of the electrical field of the heart. As a result, the axis of each lead is formed by the line from the electrode site (on the right arm, left arm, or left leg) to the center of the heart. The aV_R, aV_L, and aV_F leads intersect at angles different from the standard limb leads and produce three other intersecting lines of reference. When these six lines of reference are combined (one every 30 degrees), they form the hexaxial reference system (Figure 22-92). Lead aV_L acts as a lateral (leftward) lead. It records the electrical activity of the heart from a vantage point that looks down from the left arm. Lead aV_F

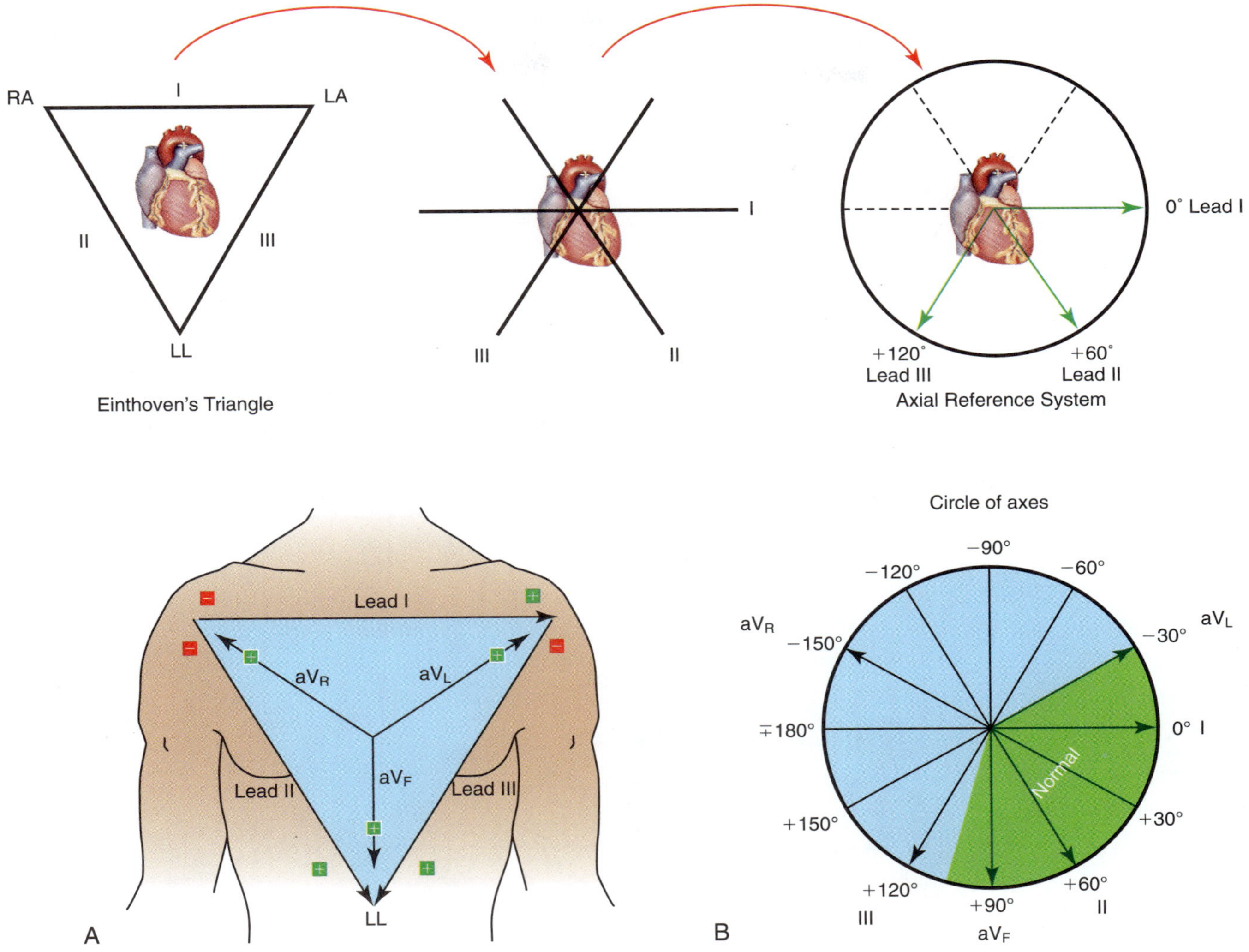

RA   I   LA

II   III

LL

Einthoven's Triangle

III   II

I

0° Lead I

+120°   +60°
Lead III   Lead II
Axial Reference System

Lead I

aV$_R$ aV$_L$

aV$_F$

Lead II   Lead III

LL

A

Circle of axes

−90°

−120°   −60°

aV$_R$ aV$_L$
−150°   −30°

∓180°   0° I

+150°   +30°

Normal

+120°   +60°
III   II
+90°
aV$_F$

B

FIGURE 22-91 Augmented limb leads.

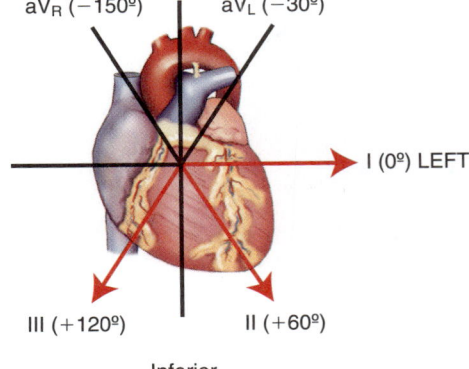

aV$_R$ (−150º)   aV$_L$ (−30º)

I (0º) LEFT

III (+120º)   II (+60º)

Inferior

FIGURE 22-92 Hexaxial reference system.

acts as an inferior lead. It records the electrical activity of the heart from a vantage point that looks up from the left lower extremity. Lead aV$_R$ is a distant recording electrode. It looks down at the heart from the right arm. Based on these lead descriptions, the lateral, or left-sided, limb leads are I and aV$_L$. The inferior leads are II, III, and aV$_F$.

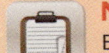

NOTE

Each of the six limb leads (three standard limb leads and three augmented limb leads) records the same cardiac activity from a different angle.

The six precordial leads (Figure 22-93) are projected through the AV node toward the patient's back. In this view, the anterior chest wall is considered positive, and the patient's back is considered negative. This horizontal plane separates the body into top and bottom halves. The chest

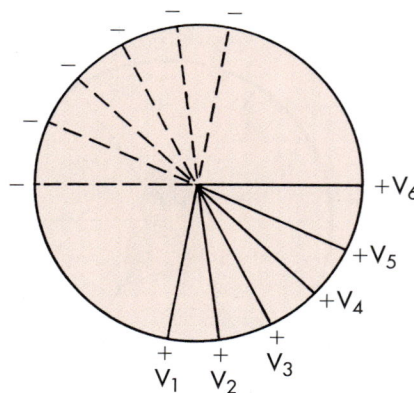

FIGURE 22-93 The precordial leads. The positive poles of the chest leads point anteriorly and the negative poles *(dashed lines)* point posteriorly. (Sole ML et al: *Introduction to critical care nursing,* ed 5, St Louis, 2009, Saunders.)

leads monitor electrical current in successive steps from the patient's right to left side. Leads V_1 and V_2 are right chest leads that view the septum of the heart (septal leads). Leads V_3 and V_4 view the anterior wall of the left ventricle (anterior leads). Leads V_5 and V_6 view the lateral wall of the left ventricle (lateral leads) (Figure 22-94).

Table 22-2 shows the area of the heart viewed by each of the 12 leads.

> **NOTE**
> Lead aV_R is the only limb lead on the right side of the body. It does not view a specific area of the heart. The aV_R lead may be useful in evaluating ST segment elevation in some coronary syndromes, in patients with acute pericarditis, in tricyclic antidepressant (TCA) poisoning, and in WPW syndrome.[10]

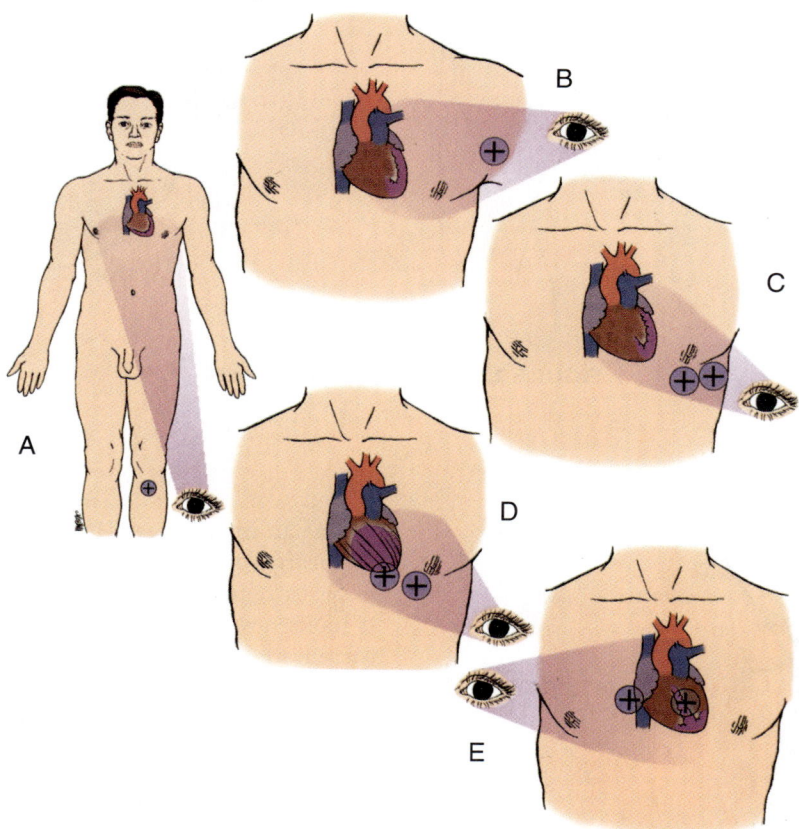

FIGURE 22-94 A, Leads II, III, and aV_F each has a positive electrode positioned on the left leg. From the perspective of the left leg, each of these leads "sees" the inferior wall of the left ventricle. **B,** From their vantage point on the left arm, leads I and aV_L "look" in at the lateral wall of the left ventricle. **C,** Leads V_5 and V_6 also view the lateral wall, because they are positioned on the axillary area of the left chest. **D,** Leads V_3 and V_4 are positioned in the area of the anterior chest. From this perspective, these leads "see" the anterior wall of the left ventricle. **E,** The septal wall is "seen" by leads V_1 and V_2, which are positioned next to the sternum. (Phalen T, Aehlert BJ: *The 12-lead ECG in acute coronary syndromes,* ed 3, St Louis, 2010, Mosby.)

TABLE 22-2 Lead Views of the Heart

Lead	Area of the Heart
II, III, aV$_F$	Inferior wall of the left ventricle
V$_1$, V$_2$	Septum
V$_3$, V$_4$	Anterior wall of the left ventricle
I, V$_5$, V$_6$, aV$_L$	Lateral wall of the left ventricle

TABLE 22-3 Lead Deflections in a Normal 12-Lead ECG

Upward (Positive)	Downward (Negative)
I, II, III, aV$_F$, aV$_L$	aV$_R$
V$_2$ through V$_6$	V$_1$

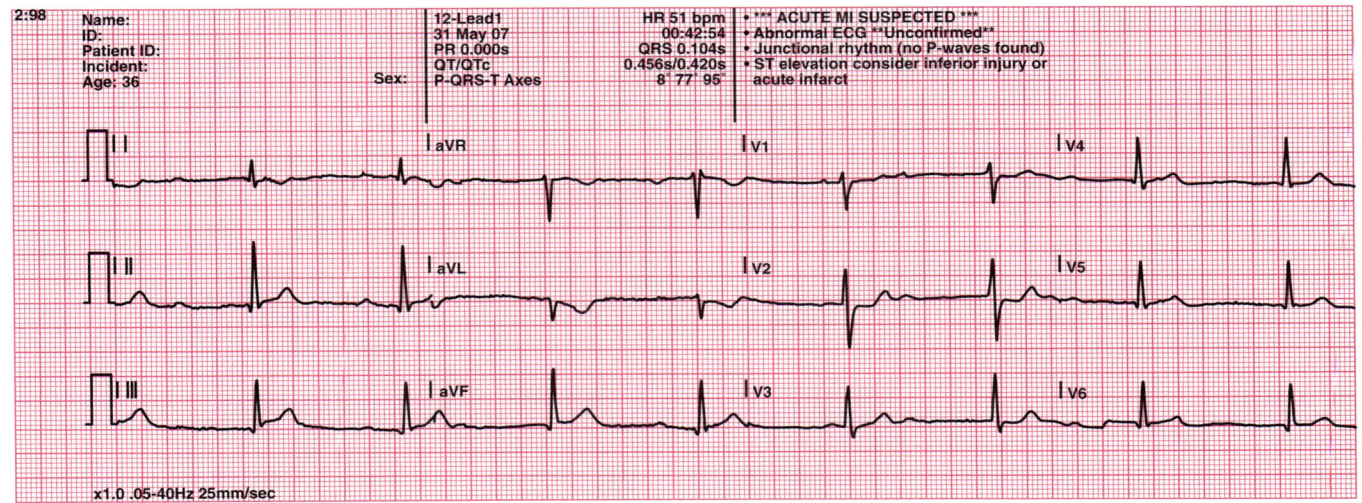

FIGURE 22-95 A 12-lead ECG strip. (Modified from Wesley K: *Huszar's basic dysrhythmias and acute coronary syndromes: interpretation and management,* ed 4, St Louis, 2010, Mosby.)

Normal 12-Lead ECG

The 12-lead ECG is recorded electronically on ECG paper in four separate columns. Column one records leads I, II, and III. Column two records aV$_R$, aV$_L$, and aV$_F$. Column three records V$_1$, V$_2$, and V$_3$. Column four records V$_4$, V$_5$, and V$_6$ (Figure 22-95). When viewing any ECG, it is important to remember that if the electrical current moves toward a positive electrode, the ECG complex will have a positive (upward) deflection from the baseline. Likewise, if the electrical current moves away from the positive electrode, the ECG complex will have a negative (downward) deflection from the baseline.

In a normal 12-lead ECG, limb leads I, II, III, aV$_F$, and aV$_L$ have a positive R wave. This is because the positive wave of depolarization in the heart cells moves toward positive electrodes (aV$_R$ is the only limb lead that has a negative complex). Chest leads are also always positive. However, leads V$_1$ through V$_6$ display the progressive nature of ventricular depolarization. As such, chest lead V$_1$ normally is negative (at or below baseline); V$_2$ is more positive; V$_3$ is progressively upright; and V$_4$ through V$_6$ are directly upright. This is called the *normal R wave progression* (Table 22-3).

12-LEAD ECG AND BUNDLE BRANCH BLOCKS

As stated earlier, heart blocks can occur in any of three areas: the SA node, the AV node, or the bundle branches. These blocks interrupt the normal passage of electrical stimulation in the heart. The sudden appearance of an AV block or bundle branch block may indicate impending myocardial infarction.

NOTE

The paramedic should always measure the P-R interval and the QRS complex of any ECG. A prolonged P-R interval indicates AV node block. A wide QRS complex indicates either ventricular tachycardia or a block in the bundle branches. Most commonly, preexisting bundle branch block is continuously present (fixed bundle branch block). The patient shows a wide QRS independent of the heart rate. However, as the heart rate increases, the QRS shape may change as a result of changes in the pattern of ventricular activation. This can lead to misdiagnosis of ventricular tachycardia in these patients.[11] Thorough evaluation of the patient, the ECG, and the electrical axis (described later) is important to correctly manage these patients.

To review, in left bundle branch block, the left ventricle depolarizes late. In right bundle branch block, the right ventricle depolarizes late. This delay results in a wide QRS complex greater than 0.12 second. With LBBB, the block often yields a QS pattern in V_1. With RBBB, the delay yields a negative S wave and a large positive R wave. This results in an RSR′ pattern. When bundle branch block is suspected, the paramedic should look at chest leads V_1 and V_2 (right chest) and leads V_5 and V_6 (left chest). If the QRS complex is wide with an RSR′ pattern in V_1 or V_2, RBBB may be present. If the wide QRS complex has a QS pattern in V_5 or V_6, LBBB may be present (Figure 22-96).

DETERMINATION OF THE AXIS

As stated previously, the electrical **axis** is the direction of electrical impulse flow in the heart that stimulates contraction. This general direction of ventricular depolarization is known as the *mean QRS vector*. Generally, the current travels down from the AV node and to the left side of the heart. Therefore, the mean QRS vector points downward and toward the patient's left side. The position of the QRS vector can be visualized in a circle that lies on top of the patient's chest. The circle is divided into degrees with the AV node at the center. The normal QRS vector is 0 to +90 degrees (Figure 22-97).

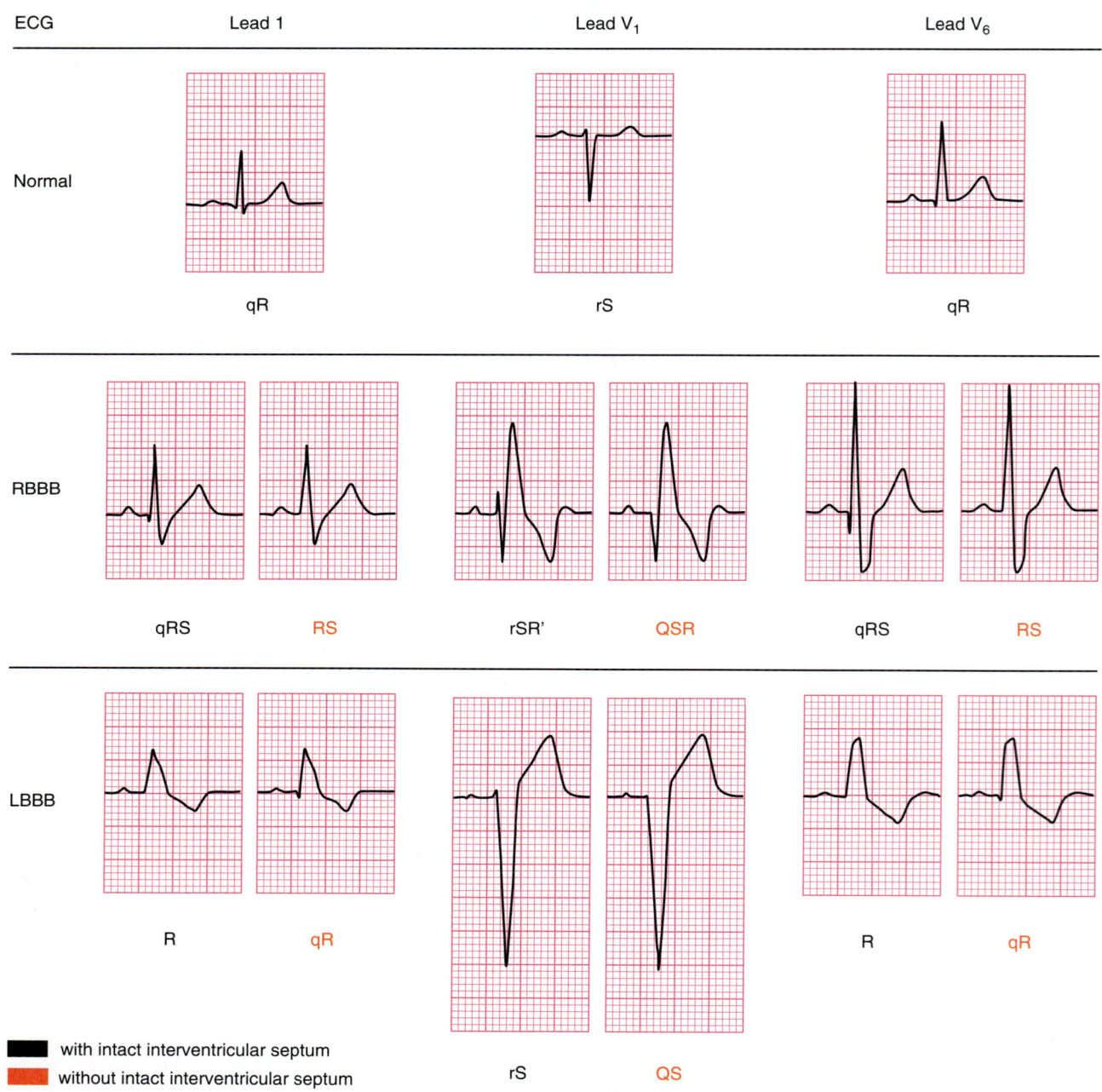

FIGURE 22-96 Comparison of leads I, V_1, and V_6 with normal conduction, right bundle branch block, and left bundle branch block.

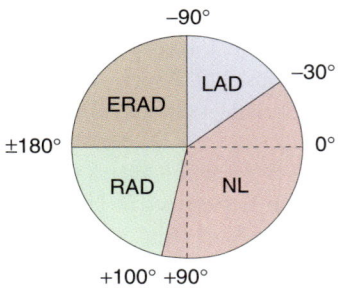

FIGURE 22-97 Frontal plane axes. Normal (NL) = −30 to +100 degrees; left axis deviation (LAD) = −30 to −90 degrees; right axis deviation (RAD) = +100 to +180 degrees; extreme right axis deviation (ERAD) = −90 to ±180 degrees. Mild RAD is considered normal in children, adolescents, and young adults. (Goldman L et al: *Cecil medicine,* ed 23, Philadelphia, 2007, Saunders.)

The QRS vector flows slightly to the left of the ventricular septum. This is because the left ventricle has more and larger cardiac cells. Generally, each person has a unique QRS vector that remains constant throughout life. However, if a person's cardiac status changes, the electrical axis and position of the heart can deviate from normal to right to left of its normal position. Box 22-10 lists common causes of axis deviation.

> **NOTE**
> The QRS vector is a representation of the electrical properties of the heart. A 12-lead ECG views the vector from 12 different angles. If the heart is displaced, the QRS vector is displaced in the same direction (right or left of normal). For example, if a patient's left ventricle is enlarged as a result of heart failure, the heart and the QRS vector are pulled to the left.

Axis is calculated automatically by modern 12-lead ECG machines (Figure 22-98). The paramedic then interprets the degree of axis by memorization or by referring to an axis chart. If the ECG machine cannot calculate axis, it can be determined by quadrant or by assessing leads I, II, and III.

Determining Axis by Quadrant

Axis can be approximated quickly by quadrant (Figure 22-99). The two key leads that can be used for approximating axis are leads I and aV$_F$. Recall that lead I is located at 0 degrees and that lead aV$_F$ is located +90 degrees from lead I. A normal axis lies within the quadrant of 0 degrees and +90 degrees. A deviation of the axis to the left **(left axis deviation)** lies within the quadrant of 0 degrees and −90 degrees. A deviation of the axis to the right **(right axis deviation)** lies within the quadrant of +90 degrees and ±180 degrees. An indeterminate axis exists when the axis lies within the quadrant of −90 degrees and ±180 degrees. By looking at the net deflection of the mean QRS vector in leads I and aV$_F$, the paramedic can make an approximate determination of axis (Table 22-4).

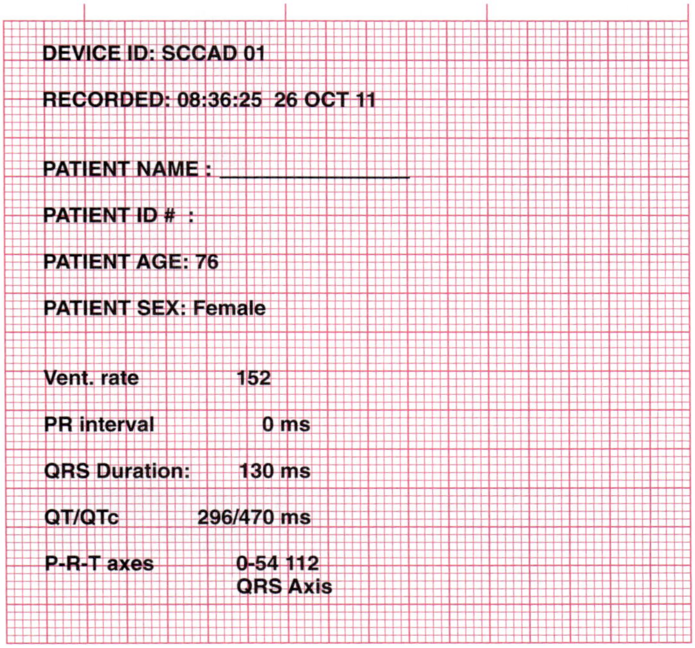

```
DEVICE ID: SCCAD 01

RECORDED: 08:36:25  26 OCT 11

PATIENT NAME : _____

PATIENT ID # :

PATIENT AGE: 76

PATIENT SEX: Female


Vent. rate            152

PR interval              0 ms

QRS Duration:        130 ms

QT/QTc           296/470 ms

P-R-T axes           0-54 112
                     QRS Axis
```

FIGURE 22-98 Axis display on ECG printout.

BOX 22-10 Common Causes of Axis Deviation

Right Axis Deviation
Anterolateral myocardial infarction
Chronic lung disease
Left posterior hemiblock
Left-sided tension pneumothorax
Pulmonary embolism
Right ventricular hypertrophy
Wolff-Parkinson-White syndrome
(May be a normal finding in children and tall, thin adults)

Left Axis Deviation
Aortic stenosis
Hypertension
Left anterior hemiblock
Mitral regurgitation
Inferior myocardial infarction
Right-sided tension pneumothorax
Ventricular pacemaker
Ventricular tachycardia
Wolf-Parkinson-White syndrome

> **NOTE**
> If the QRS complex in lead I is upright, then the vector is flowing right to left. If the QRS complex in lead aV$_F$ is upright, the vector is directed top to bottom. If the QRS complex is upright in both lead I and aV$_F$, the electrical axis must fall into the lower left or normal quadrant (see Table 22-4).

TABLE 22-4 Axis Deviation

	NET QRS DEFLECTION		
Axis	Lead I	aV$_F$	Axis Degrees
Normal	Positive	Positive	0 to +90
RAD	Negative	Positive	+90 to ±180
LAD	Positive	Negative	0 to –90
Indeterminate	Negative	Negative	–90 to ±180

LAD, Left axis deviation; *RAD,* right axis deviation.

Determining Axis by Leads I, II, and III

Axis can be evaluated by looking at the QRS complexes in leads I, II, and III (Table 22-5):

- *Normal:* QRS deflection is positive (upright) in all bipolar leads
- *Physiological left* (may be normal in some patients): QRS deflection is positive in leads I and II but negative (inverted) in lead III
- *Pathological left:* QRS deflection is positive in lead I and negative in leads II and III (indicating an anterior hemiblock)
- *Right axis:* QRS deflection is negative in lead I, negative or positive in lead II, and positive in lead III (this is

TABLE 22-5 Identifying the Axis by the QRS Complex

	QRS COMPLEX			
Axis	Lead I	Lead II	Lead III	Indications
Normal	Upright	Upright	Upright	May be normal
Physiological left	Upright	Upright	Inverted	May be normal
Pathological left	Upright	Inverted	Inverted	Anterior hemiblock
Right axis	Inverted	Inverted or upright	Upright	Posterior hemiblock*
Extreme right	Inverted	Inverted	Inverted	Ventricular in origin

*Chronic obstructive pulmonary disease (COPD) and right ventricular hypertrophy must first be ruled out.

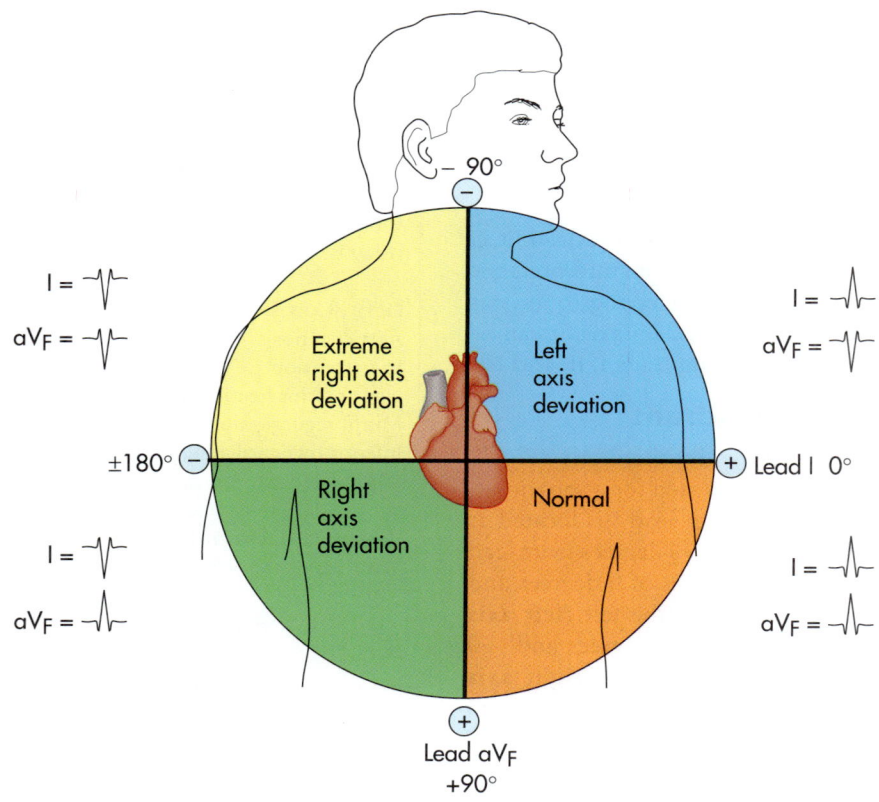

FIGURE 22-99 Approximating axis by quadrant. (Beachey W: *Respiratory care anatomy and physiology,* ed 2, St Louis, 2007, Mosby.)

pathological in any adult and may indicate a posterior hemiblock)

- *Extreme right* ("no man's land"): QRS deflection is negative in all three leads (indicating that the rhythm is ventricular in origin)

AXIS AND HEMIBLOCKS

As described earlier, a hemiblock is a failure in conduction of the cardiac impulse in either of two main divisions of the left bundle branch of the bundle of His. The interruption may occur in either the anterior (superior) or the posterior (inferior) division. Identifying the axis can be useful in determining the presence of hemiblocks.

Anterior Hemiblock

Anterior hemiblock occurs more often than **posterior hemiblock.** The anterior fascicle of the left bundle branch is a longer and thinner structure. Its blood supply comes mainly from the left anterior descending coronary artery. Anterior hemiblock is characterized by left axis deviation in a patient who has a supraventricular rhythm (Figure 22-100). Other ECG findings associated with an anterior hemiblock include a normal QRS complex (less than 0.12 second) or a right bundle branch block, a small Q wave followed by a tall R wave in lead I, and a small R wave followed by a deep S wave in lead III. In a patient who has an anterior hemiblock with a right bundle branch block, impulses can be conducted only through the ventricles by way of the posterior fascicle of the left bundle branch. These patients are at high risk of developing complete heart block.

CRITICAL THINKING
What rhythms are produced by supraventricular activity?

Posterior Hemiblock

The posterior fascicle of the left bundle branch is not blocked as easily as the anterior fascicle. This is because the bundle is much thicker and has a double blood supply (left and right coronary arteries). As a result, posterior hemiblock occurs less often. This conduction disturbance is not commonly seen alone, but rather is more often associated with right bundle branch block. For practical purposes, posterior hemiblock can be assumed in patients with right axis deviation and a QRS complex of normal width or with a right bundle branch block (Figure 22-101). Other ECG findings that indicate the presence of a posterior hemiblock include a small R wave followed by a deep S wave in lead I and a small Q wave followed by a tall R wave in lead III.

Bifascicular Block

Bifascicular block refers to the blockage of two of three pathways (fascicles) for ventricular conduction. This condition generally refers to RBBB with block of either the anterior or posterior division of the left bundle branch. (This is because anterior hemiblock combined with posterior hemiblock is difficult to distinguish from LBBB.) Bifascicular block reduces myocardial contractility and cardiac output. Patients with this condition may develop complete heart block suddenly and without warning. As a rule, the more branches with impaired conduction, the greater the chance the patient will develop complete atrioventricular block (especially in patients with acute myocardial infarction).

12-LEAD STRATEGIES FOR WIDE-COMPLEX TACHYCARDIAS

If an unstable patient's QRS complex is wide (greater than 0.12 second) and fast (greater than 150 beats/minute), immediate cardioversion may be indicated. If the patient is stable, however, the following steps in 12-lead assessment

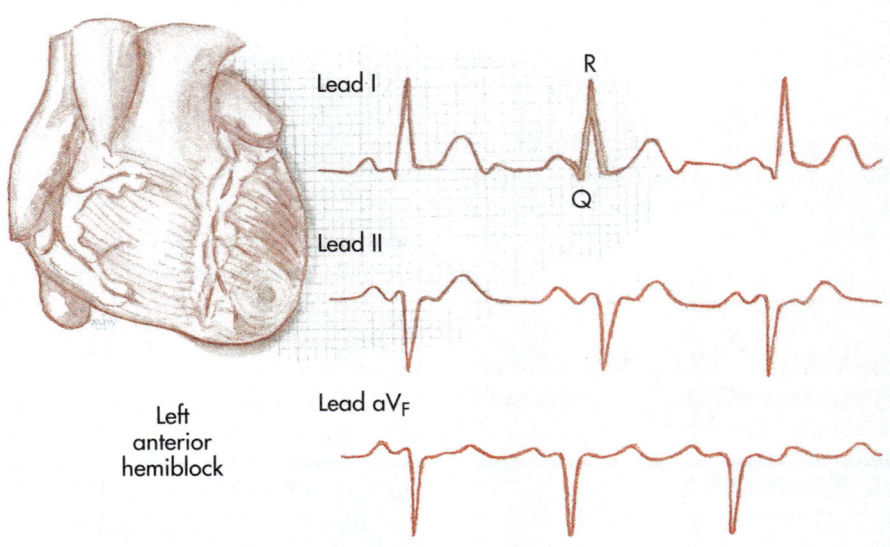

FIGURE 22-100 Anterior hemiblock.

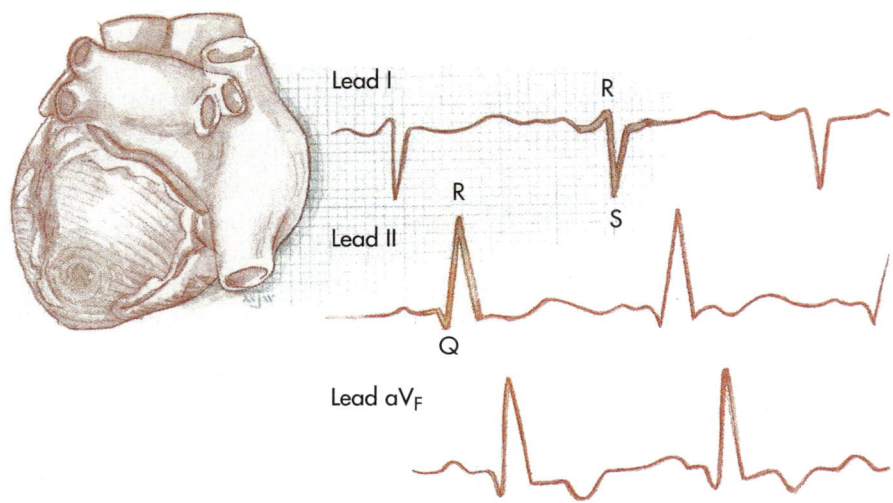

FIGURE 22-101 Left posterior hemiblock.

may help distinguish between ventricular tachycardia and other wide-complex tachycardias[12]:

1. Assess leads I, II, III, V_1, and V_6. If the QRS complex is negative in leads I, II, and III and positive in V_1, the rhythm indicates ventricular tachycardia (Figure 22-102). If these criteria are not met, proceed to step 2.

2. Assess the QRS deflection in V_1 and V_6. Regardless of the QRS deflection in leads I, II, and III, positive QRS deflections with a single peak, a taller left "rabbit ear," or an RS complex with a fat R wave or slurred S wave in V_1 indicates ventricular tachycardia. A negative QS complex, a negative RS complex, or any wide Q wave in V_6 also indicates ventricular tachycardia (Figure 22-103).

3. A negative QRS complex in lead I, a positive QRS complex in leads II and III, and a negative QRS complex in V_1 or MCL_1 indicates ventricular tachycardia (Figure 22-104).

4. If all precordial leads (V leads) are positive or negative *(precordial concordance)*, the rhythm indicates ventricular tachycardia (Figure 22-105).

5. If the R-S interval is greater than 0.10 second in any V lead (increased ventricular activation time), the rhythm indicates ventricular tachycardia (Figure 22-106).

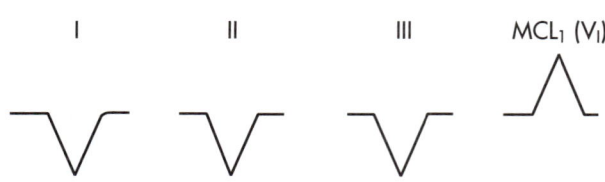

FIGURE 22-102 Criteria for ventricular tachycardia.

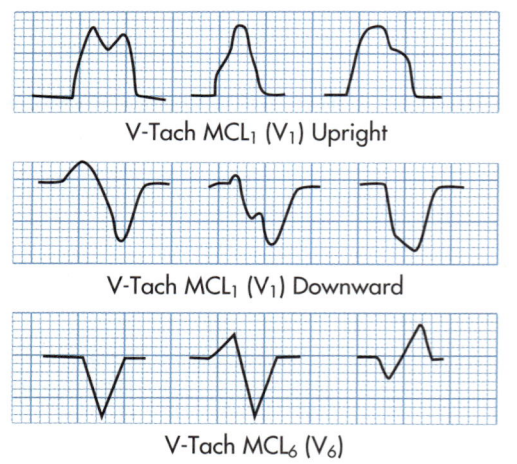

FIGURE 22-103 Step 1: A QRS complex that is negative in leads I, II, and III and positive in MCL_1 (V_1) indicates ventricular tachycardia. Step 2: Assess the QRS complex in MCL_1 (V_1) and MCL_6 (V_6). Step 3: Assess the QRS complex in leads I, II, III, and MCL_1 (V_1). (Courtesy Bob Page, Springfield, Mo.)

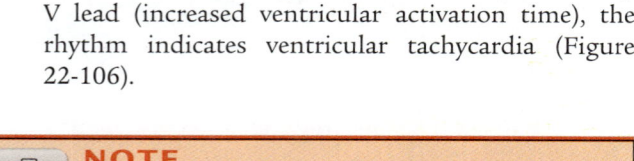

NOTE
Nonventricular tachycardia precordial concordance may occur in patients who have Wolff-Parkinson-White syndrome and associated left bundle branch block.

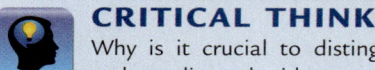

CRITICAL THINKING
Why is it crucial to distinguish between ventricular tachycardia and wide-complex tachycardias in stable patients?

CRITICAL THINKING
How would you manage a patient with ventricular tachycardia, chest pain, or difficulty breathing if you could not establish an IV line?

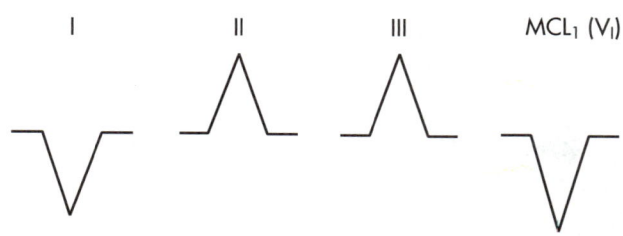

FIGURE 22-104 Right axis deviation with a downward MCL₁ indicates ventricular tachycardia.

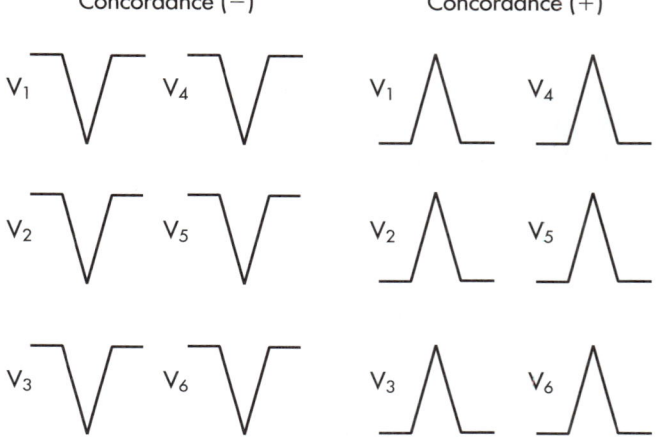

FIGURE 22-105 Ventricular tachycardia concordance.

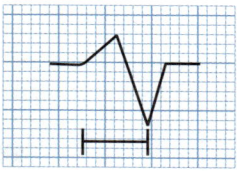

FIGURE 22-106 Ventricular tachycardia (R-S interval is .16 sec).

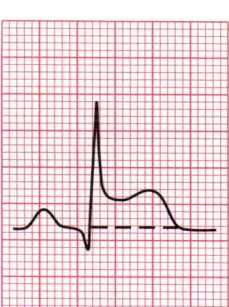

FIGURE 22-107 ST-segment elevation likely to present with acute injury.

BOX 22-11 Contiguous Leads

Contiguous leads are leads that are anatomically close together and that cover the same general area of the heart (specifically, the walls of the left ventricle). Lead aV$_R$ is the only lead that is not considered contiguous with another lead.

I	Lateral	aV$_R$	---------	V$_1$	Septal	V$_4$	Anterior
II	Inferior	aV$_L$	Lateral	V$_2$	Septal	V$_5$	Lateral
III	Inferior	aV$_F$	Inferior	V$_3$	Anterior	V$_6$	Lateral

ST-SEGMENT AND T-WAVE CHANGES

When the heart muscle is damaged, the damaged area is unable to contract effectively. The area remains in a constant depolarized state. The flow of current between the pathologically depolarized and normally repolarized areas can produce ST-segment elevation (Figure 22-107), ischemic ST-segment depression, or normal or nondiagnostic changes in the ST segment or T waves. Using these ECG findings, the paramedic can classify the patient into one of three groups[6]:

1. *ST-segment elevation myocardial infarction (STEMI):* ST-segment elevation is characterized by ST-segment elevation greater than 1 mm (0.1 mV) in two or more adjacent limb leads or any two contiguous chest leads (Box 22-11 and Figure 22-108). STEMI also occurs with presumed new LBBB.

NOTE

Numerous methods have been proposed for measuring ST-segment elevation. Some begin the measurement at the J point. Others begin the measurement at one small box (0.04 second) after the J point. More than 1 mm of ST-segment elevation in a standard limb lead or chest lead is an abnormal finding that indicates injury.

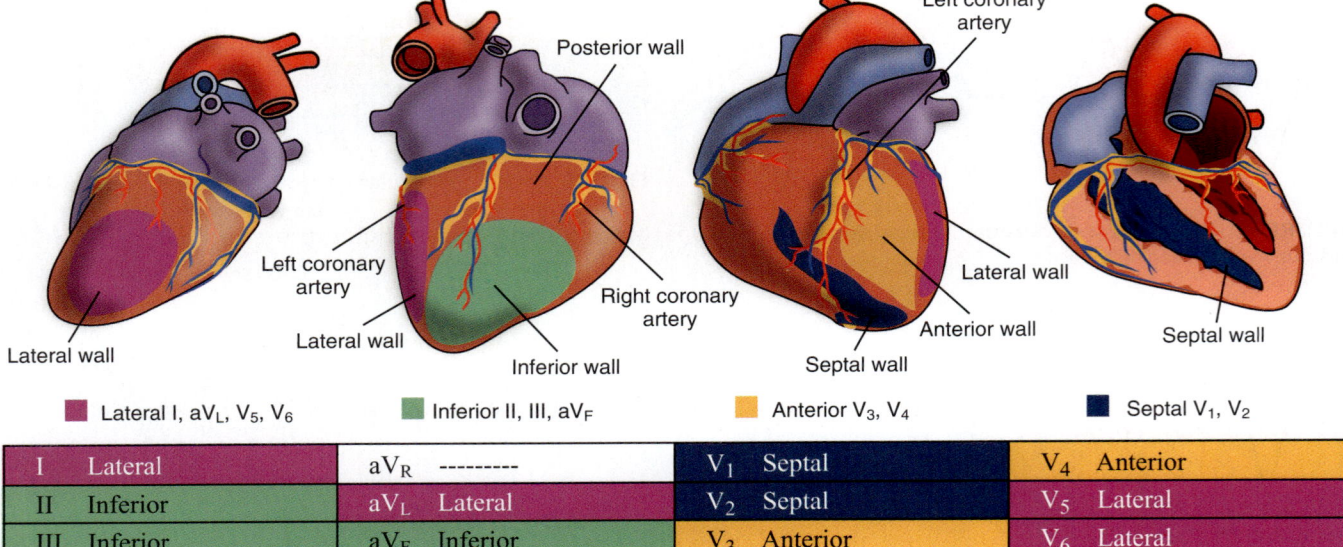

I	Lateral	aV$_R$	---------	V$_1$	Septal	V$_4$	Anterior
II	Inferior	aV$_L$	Lateral	V$_2$	Septal	V$_5$	Lateral
III	Inferior	aV$_F$	Inferior	V$_3$	Anterior	V$_6$	Lateral

FIGURE 22-108 Localizing ECG changes by lead with corresponding affected areas of the heart.

2. *High-risk non–ST-elevation myocardial infarction (non-STEMI)*: Ischemic ST-segment depression equal to or greater than 0.5 mm (0.05 mV) or dynamic T-wave inversion with pain or discomfort. Nonpersistent or transient ST-segment elevation equal to or greater than 0.5 mm (0.05 mV) for longer than 20 minutes is included in this category.

3. *Normal or nondiagnostic changes in ST segment or T wave*: These findings are inconclusive. This classification includes patients with normal ECG findings and those with ST-segment deviation of less than 0.5 mm (0.05 mV) or T-wave inversion less than or equal to 0.2 mV. Special cardiac studies and testing are needed for these patients.

> **NOTE**
> ST-segment elevation is best measured by drawing a baseline from the end of the T wave to the start of the P wave using either of the methods described previously. The ST segment then is compared with the isoelectric baseline. However, ST-segment elevation is not always present on an initial ECG tracing. This is true even when a patient is experiencing a myocardial infarction. When ST-segment elevation is present in a symptomatic patient, the paramedic should notify medical direction and transmit an ECG for evaluation (per protocol). Even if infarction is present, ST-segment elevation is a poor indicator of the type or cause of infarction (STEMI or non-STEMI). In addition, ST-segment elevation can be caused by conditions other than acute myocardial infarction, including the following:
> - Left bundle branch block
> - Some ventricular rhythms
> - Left ventricular hypertrophy
> - Pericarditis
> - Ventricular aneurysm
> - Early repolarization

USE OF A 12-LEAD ECG TO ASSESS INFARCTS

Early recognition and management of acute myocardial infarction sometimes can salvage a damaged myocardium ("time is muscle"). Paramedics can play an important role in identifying these patients by using the following five-step analysis for infarct recognition[4]:

Step 1: Identify the rate and rhythm. Manage any life-threatening dysrhythmias.

> **NOTE**
> LBBB that impairs repolarization may "look like" STEMI. If LBBB is present, ST-segment elevation measurements will not be diagnostic for infarction.

Step 2: Identify the area of infarct. ST-segment elevation is the most reliable indicator during the first hours of infarction. ST-segment elevation can be present before permanent tissue damage has occurred. If ST-segment elevation is present in a patient with chest pain, the paramedic should identify the degree of elevation and visualize the cardiac anatomy to predict which coronary artery is occluded (Figure 22-109). The paramedic should use a systematic approach for 12-lead assessment. One method is to begin by assessing the inferior leads (II, III, aV$_F$), followed by the septal leads (V$_1$, V$_2$), anterior leads (V$_3$, V$_4$), and lateral leads (V$_5$, V$_6$, I, aV$_L$). The paramedic evaluates each lead for ST-segment elevation (the most important sign of injury), deep symmetrically inverted T waves (a sign of ischemia), ST-segment depression (a reciprocal change to ST elevation), and pathological Q waves (Tables 22-6 and 22-7 and Figure 22-110).

TABLE 22-6 ST-Segment Elevation and Location of Infarct

Lead	Location of Infarct	Coronary Artery Involved
II, III, aV$_F$	Inferior wall (most common)	Right
V$_1$, V$_2$	Septal wall	Left
V$_3$, V$_4$	Anterior wall (most lethal)	Left
I, aV$_L$, V$_5$, V$_6$	Lateral wall	Left
V$_{4R}$-V$_{6R}$	Right ventricle	Right

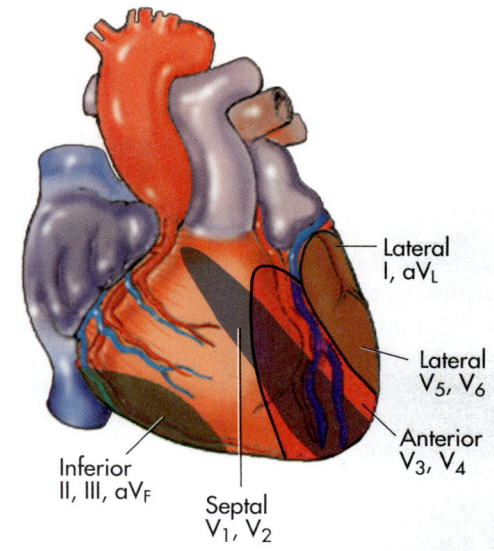

FIGURE 22-109 Multilead assessment of the heart.

TABLE 22-7 Reciprocal Changes Seen With ST-Segment Elevation Myocardial Infarction (STEMI)

Injury Site	ST Elevation	Reciprocal ST Depression
Septal	V$_1$, V$_2$	None
Anterior	V$_3$, V$_4$	None
Anteroseptal	V$_1$, V$_2$, V$_3$, V$_4$	None
Lateral	I, aV$_L$, V$_5$, V$_6$	II, III, aV$_F$
Anterolateral	I, aV$_L$, V$_3$, V$_4$, V$_5$, V$_6$	II, III, aV$_F$
Inferior	II, II, aV$_F$	I, aV$_L$
Posterior	None	V$_1$, V$_2$, V$_3$, V$_4$

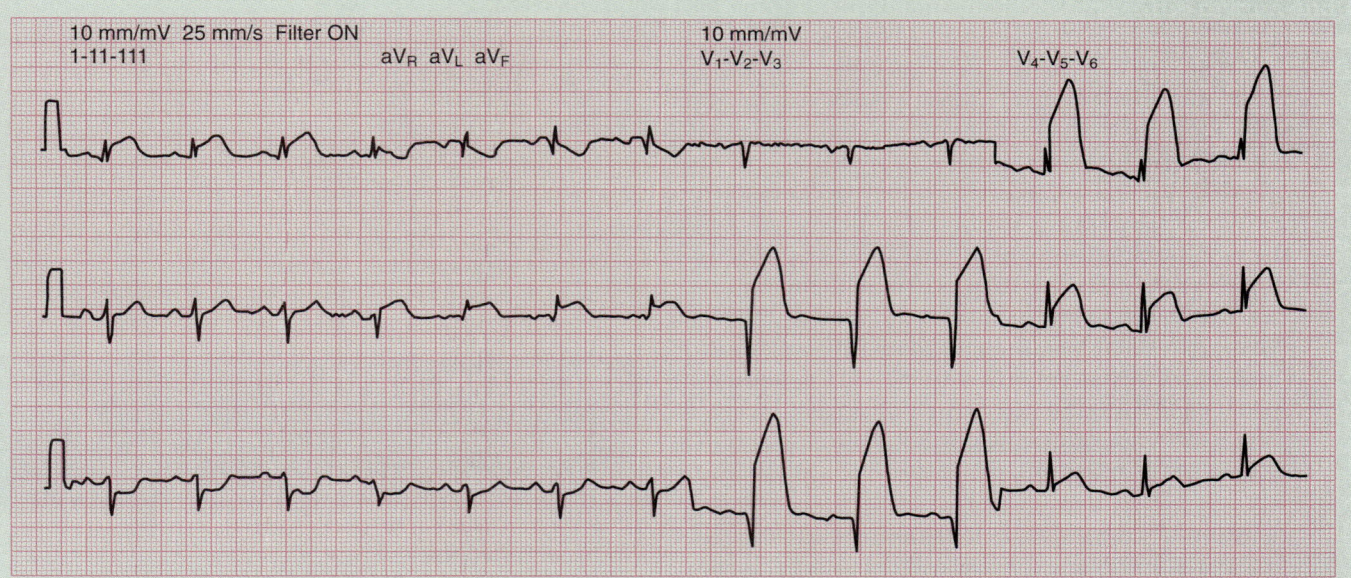

FIGURE 22-110 12-lead ECG showing STEMI and reciprocal ST-segment depression. (Andreoli TE: *Cecil essentials of medicine,* ed 7, Philadelphia, 2008, Saunders.)

In an acute STEMI, reciprocal changes may be seen between leads that face the acute injury and leads that face the lateral boundary of the injury (between ischemic and healthy tissue). Leads that face the injury often show ST-segment elevation. Leads that face the boundary often show ST-segment depression.[13] Reciprocal changes are not always visible on the 12-lead ECG during acute STEMI. However, if they are visible, this confirms the diagnosis.

At times, the extent of the infarction can be gauged by the number of leads showing ST-segment elevation. The degree of ST-segment elevation also is important. For example, large infarcts often show an ST elevation of 7 mm or more in inferior leads and 12 mm or more in anterior leads. ST-segment elevation or new or presumably new left bundle branch block is suspicious for injury.

Step 3: Consider other conditions that could be responsible for ST-segment changes (as described previously). These "infarct impostors" also may be present in a patient experiencing acute myocardial infarction. With the exception of left bundle branch block (which makes the interpretation of myocardial infarction difficult), left ventricular hypertrophy looks less like an infarction. Ventricular rhythms often produce Q waves *and* ST-segment elevation. Ventricular rhythms also do not have reciprocal ST depression. ECG changes with pericarditis are subtle. In addition, early repolarization produces no clinical symptoms.

Step 4: Assess the patient's clinical presentation. This is just as crucial as the ECG findings. Therefore, the findings of a thorough patient history and a physical examination should be incorporated into the ECG interpretation. Not all patients with acute myocardial infarction have classic signs and symptoms. Therefore, the paramedic should maintain a high degree of suspicion in the absence of pain. (This should be the case especially with diabetic patients, older adults, and postmenopausal women.) As many as 50% of patients with acute myocardial infarction have no early ECG changes. The clinical picture therefore is important.

Step 5: Recognize the infarction and initiate care. When all indications point to acute myocardial infarction, the paramedic must take steps to speed the process of data collection, physician evaluation, and definitive care (angioplasty and stent; thrombolysis when appropriate). This helps reduce the time from infarct to treatment. Clinical presentation and ECG findings that suggest an acute myocardial infarction must be confirmed by medical direction to determine appropriate care.

SHOW ME THE EVIDENCE

Eckstein and colleagues compared 234 STEMI patients who arrived at four Los Angeles hospitals where percutaneous coronary angioplasty could be performed. The authors sought to determine whether a difference existed in treatment time based on arrival by private vehicle versus arrival by ambulance with a prehospital 12-lead ECG. Although no statistically significant difference in door-to-balloon time was seen between the two groups, the time from confirmation of STEMI to balloon inflation was significantly shorter in the prehospital group.

From Eckstein M, et al: Impact of paramedic with prehospital 12-lead ECG on door-to-balloon times for patients with ST-segment elevation myocardial infarction, *Prehosp Emerg Care* 32:203-206, 2009.

15- AND 18-LEAD DIAGNOSTICS

The wall of the right ventricle and the posterior wall of the left ventricle are areas of the heart that are difficult to evaluate with the six precordial leads. ECG monitoring that includes 12 leads plus V_{4R}, V_8, and V_9 leads (a 15-lead ECG) increases sensitivity for myocardial infarctions that occur in these areas (e.g., isolated posterior myocardial infarction). For 15-lead ECG monitoring, the V_{4R} lead is placed at the fifth intercostal space in the right anterior midclavicular line. The V_8 lead is placed at the posterior fifth intercostal space in the right midscapular line. The V_9 lead is placed between the V_8 lead and the spinal column at the posterior fifth intercostal space. The 18-lead ECG monitoring (not routinely performed in the prehospital setting) uses the 15-lead ECG along with V_{5R}, V_{6R}, and V_7. These leads are placed in the same horizontal line as V_4 to V_6. V_7 is placed at the posterior axillary line. V_8 is placed at the posterior scapular line (Figure 22-111).

When a 15-lead ECG is obtained, the new 12-lead ECG printout must be labeled to identify the three leads that have been moved. A notation should be made at the top of the ECG printout, "Posterior Chest Leads." Lead V_4 should be relabeled V_{4R}; V_5 should be relabeled V_8; and V_6 should be relabeled V_9 (Figure 22-112). The more leads that reveal acute changes in the heart, the larger the area of infarct is presumed to be.

NOTE

Right ventricular (RV) infarction or ischemia may occur in up to 50% of patients with inferior wall MI. RV infarction should be suspected in patients with inferior wall infarction, hypotension, and clear lung fields. In these cases, a 15-lead ECG should be obtained to confirm the field impression. ST-segment elevation (greater than 1 mm) in lead V_{4R} is sensitive for RV infarction (sensitivity, 88%; specificity, 78%; diagnostic accuracy, 83%). These findings also are a strong predictor of increased in-hospital complications and mortality.[6]

SECTION SEVEN
Assessment of the Patient with Cardiac Disease

ASSESSMENT

A focused evaluation of any patient should identify a chief complaint. It also should cover the history of the event and any significant medical history, and it should include a

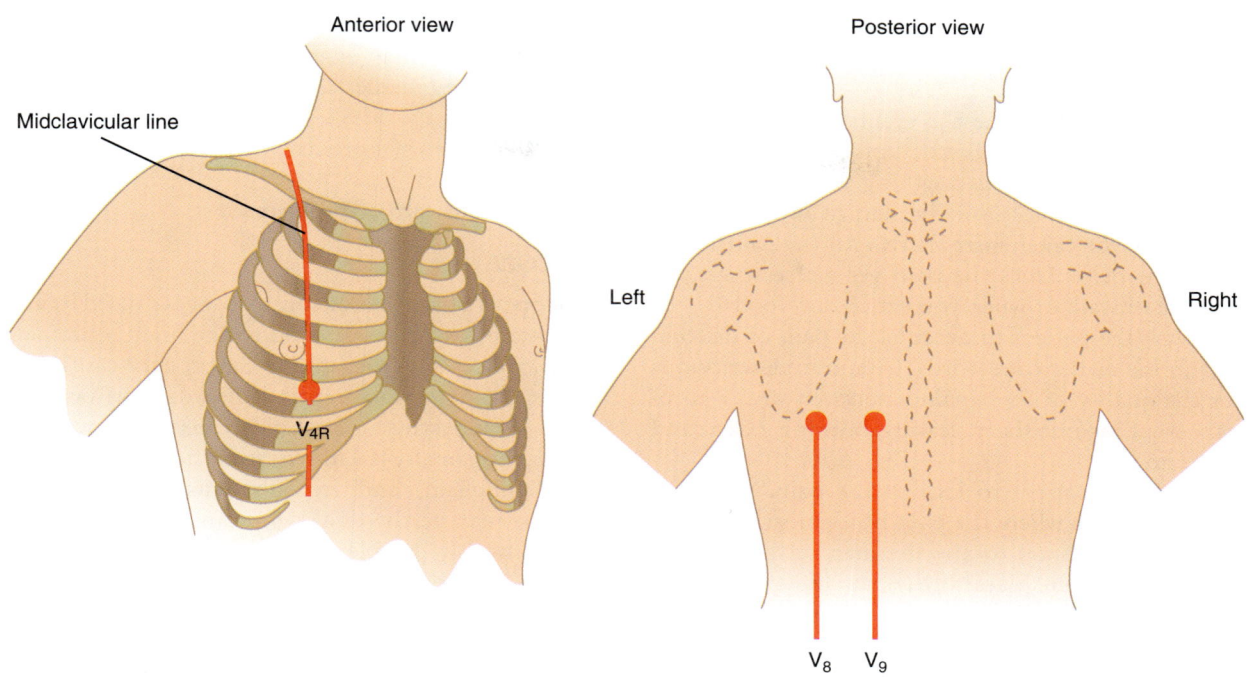

Anterior view

Posterior view

Midclavicular line

V₄R

Left

Right

V₈   V₉

FIGURE 22-111 Lead placement for V₄R and V₈ and V₉.

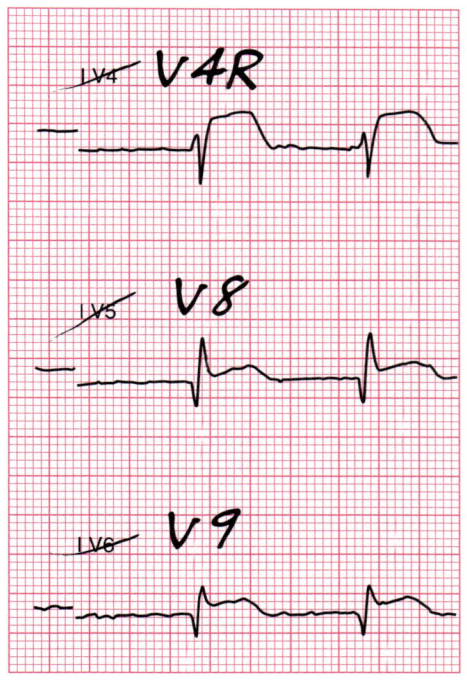

V4R

V8

V9

FIGURE 22-112 ECG relabeled to show V₄R and V₈ and V₉.

CRITICAL THINKING
A patient has made an EMS call about a cardiovascular complaint. What emotions might the patient be feeling?

Chief Complaint

Cardiovascular disease may cause a variety of symptoms. Obtaining an appropriate history of each symptom is important to form a diagnostic impression of any patient with a possible coronary event. Common chief complaints include chest pain or discomfort, including shoulder, arm, neck, or jaw pain or discomfort; dyspnea; syncope; and abnormal heartbeat or palpitations.

In some patients (e.g., some women, older adults, and patients with diabetes), cardiovascular problems commonly have atypical symptoms. These include mental status changes, abdominal or gastrointestinal symptoms (including persistent heartburn), and vague complaints of feeling ill.

CHEST PAIN OR DISCOMFORT

Chest pain or discomfort is the most common chief complaint of patients with myocardial infarction. However, many causes of chest pain are not related to cardiac disease (e.g., pulmonary embolus, pleurisy, reflux esophagitis). Therefore, a history of chest pain is a key factor. The OPQRST method (or a similar method) should be used to obtain the following information when possible:

Onset/origin: Ask the patient to describe the pain or discomfort. What does it feel like? What were you doing

physical examination. These elements are crucial in determining the cause of the emergency. They also help paramedics determine the initial patient care and anticipate potential problems during transport to a medical facility. The following discussion of patient assessment explains the approach to the patient with a cardiovascular emergency.

when the pain began? Have you ever had this type of pain before? Is it the same as or different from the last time?

Provokes: Try to determine the events surrounding the patient's symptoms. What do you think might have caused this pain? Does anything you do make the pain better or worse? Does the pain go away when you rest? Have you taken **nitroglycerin** for the pain, and if so, did it help? Does the pain get worse when you exercise or walk or when you eat certain foods?

Quality: Ask the patient to describe the pain or discomfort in his or her own words. Common descriptions for the quality of chest pain associated with a coronary event include sharp, tearing, burning, heavy, and squeezing.

Region: Ask the patient to localize the pain. With one finger, point to where the pain hurts most. Does the pain move (radiate) to another area of the body or does it stay in one place? If the pain moves, to where does it move? (Cardiac chest pain often radiates to the arms, neck, jaw, and back.)

Severity: Ask the patient to rate the pain or discomfort to establish a baseline. On a scale of 0 to 10, with 10 being the worst pain you have ever had, what number would you use to describe this pain? If you have had pain like this before, is this pain worse than the last time or not as bad as the last time?

Time: Try to determine the duration of the pain episode and document it. How long have you had this pain? Is the pain better or worse than it was when you called for help? Is the pain constant or does it come and go?

> ### CRITICAL THINKING
> What factors may influence a person's perception and description of pain?

> ### NOTE
> Chest pain is a common complaint of cocaine users. Cocaine can cause serious cardiac toxicity because of the effect of the drug on the heart. It also stimulates the central nervous system, and that also stimulates the cardiovascular system. Although rare, acute myocardial infarction can occur in these patients, even in the absence of risk factors for ischemic heart disease.[1]

DYSPNEA

Dyspnea (difficulty breathing) often is associated with myocardial infarction. It is a main symptom of pulmonary congestion caused by heart failure. Other common causes of dyspnea that may be unrelated to heart disease include chronic obstructive pulmonary disease, respiratory infection, pulmonary embolus, and asthma. Historical factors important in differentiating breathing difficulties include the following:

- Duration and circumstances of onset of dyspnea
- Anything that aggravates or relieves the dyspnea, including medications
- Previous episodes
- Associated symptoms
- Orthopnea
- Previous cardiac problems

SYNCOPE

Syncope is a brief loss of consciousness caused by a sudden decrease in oxygenated blood to the brain. Cardiac causes of syncope result from events that reduce cardiac output. The most common cardiac disorders associated with syncope are dysrhythmias. Other causes of syncope include stroke, drug or alcohol intoxication, aortic stenosis, pulmonary embolism, and hypoglycemia. In older patients, syncope may be the only symptom of a cardiac problem. Young, healthy people may have a syncopal episode. This episode may result from stimulation of the vagus nerve **(vasovagal syncope),** which can produce hypotension and bradycardia. The history of a syncopal event should include the following:

- Presyncope aura (nausea, weakness, lightheadedness)
- Circumstances of occurrence (e.g., patient's position before the event, severe pain, or emotional stress)
- Duration of syncopal episode
- Symptoms before syncopal episode (palpitation, seizure, incontinence)
- Other associated symptoms
- Previous episodes of syncope

>
> ### NOTE
> Cardiac syncope often occurs without warning. By comparison, vasovagal syncope often is preceded by a minute or two of nausea and weakness before the loss of consciousness.

>
> ### CRITICAL THINKING
> Syncopal events often occur in public places, such as a church. How can you ease the feelings of embarrassment the patient may have in this situation?

ABNORMAL HEARTBEAT AND PALPITATIONS

Many patients are aware of their own heartbeat, particularly if it is irregular (skipping beats) or rapid (fluttering). Abnormal heartbeats or **palpitations** (irregular or forceful beating of the heart) sometimes are a normal occurrence. However, they also may indicate a serious dysrhythmia. Important information to obtain with these patients includes the following:

- Pulse rate
- Regular versus irregular rhythm
- Circumstances of occurrence

- Duration
- Associated symptoms (chest pain, diaphoresis, syncope, confusion, dyspnea)
- Previous episodes and frequency
- Medication (drug stimulant) or alcohol use

Significant Medical History

The medical history is a vital part of any patient assessment. If possible, the paramedic should determine the following information.

1. *Is the patient taking prescription medications, particularly cardiac medications?* Common medications that should alert the paramedic to a possible coronary event include **nitroglycerin, atenolol, metoprolol,** and other beta blockers; **digoxin; furosemide** and other diuretics; antihypertensives; and antihyperlipidemic agents. The paramedic also should ask the patient about his or her compliance in taking medications. The use of any nonprescription drugs, such as over-the-counter (OTC) medications, **aspirin,** and herbal supplements, should also be ascertained. Alcohol use or illicit drug use may be a contributing factor in the patient's chief complaint. (For example, this may include the use of cocaine or methamphetamines.)

2. *Is the patient being treated for any other illness?* A medical history that includes angina pectoris, previous myocardial infarction, coronary artery bypass (Box 22-12), or **angioplasty** (described later) increases the likelihood of a significant coronary event. Chronic illness such as heart failure, valvular disease, renal disease, hypertension, aneurysms, diabetes, inflammatory cardiac disease (e.g., endocarditis, myocarditis), and lung disease also are indicators that heart disease may be present.

3. *Does the patient have any allergies?* Medication allergies (e.g., an allergy to **aspirin** or radiographic dye) may be important in the course of the patient's care. The paramedic should document these allergies and report them to medical direction.

4. *Does the patient have risk factors for a heart attack?* Examples of risk factors include older age, tobacco use, diabetes, a family history of heart disease, obesity, an increased serum cholesterol level (hypercholesterolemia), and illicit drug use.

5. *Does the patient have an implanted pacemaker or implantable cardioverter-defibrillator?* The presence of these devices (described later in the chapter) indicates a significant coronary history.

Physical Examination

The classic presentation of myocardial infarction is pain or discomfort beneath the sternum that lasts longer than 30 minutes. The pain often is described as crushing, pressure, squeezing, or burning. Associated signs and symptoms may include apprehension, diaphoresis, dyspnea, nausea and vomiting, and a sense of impending doom (e.g., patients feel that they are going to die). However, at times the

BOX 22-12 Coronary Bypass Surgery

Coronary bypass surgery is a commonly performed heart surgery in which blood vessels from another part of the body are used to "bypass" diseased coronary arteries. This improves blood flow in the heart. The goal of improved blood flow is to reduce chest pain and to reduce the risk of myocardial infarction. This surgical procedure is sometimes referred to as *coronary artery bypass grafting* (CABG or cabbage). A patient may have one, two, three, or more bypass grafts, depending on how many coronary arteries are blocked. Three-way and four-way coronary bypass surgery is common.

Coronary bypass surgery may be performed with or without a heart-lung machine ("on-pump" or "off-pump" surgery). During surgery, an artery is removed from the patient's chest wall or arm (internal mammary artery or radial artery) and is sewn to the coronary artery below the site of the blockage. If a vein is used (usually the saphenous vein, taken from the patient's leg), it is attached to the aorta and then grafted to the coronary artery below the blocked area. In either case, the surgery allows blood to flow more freely through the grafts to nourish the heart muscle. Grafts normally remain open and function well for 10 to 15 years, after which bypass surgery may be needed again.

Several alternatives to CABG are available, which may be appropriate for some patients. Two alternatives are specific drug therapy (e.g., thrombolytics) and atherectomy (plaque removal). Another is balloon angioplasty. In this procedure, a balloon catheter is placed over a guide wire. The catheter is used to insert a meshlike stent into a narrowed section of a coronary artery. Once positioned, the balloon is inflated. This opens the stent and pushes it against the arterial wall. The balloon then is deflated and removed, leaving the stent permanently in place to keep the artery open. Some stents are coated with a medication (drug-eluting stents) that prevents the growth of cells around the stent. This reduces the chance of the artery closing again (restenosis). Stents also may be placed without angioplasty.

presentation is atypical. The paramedic's skill in gathering a relevant medical history and performing a focused physical examination directs the patient care. For example, patients with myocardial ischemia may deny that they have chest pain. They may need to be asked specifically about tightness or squeezing in the chest.

 CRITICAL THINKING
Think of a way to ask a patient a question about chest pain that cannot be answered with a simple yes or no.

When caring for a patient who has chest pain caused by heart problems, the paramedic should understand that the patient is frightened. Chest pain is associated with life-threatening consequences. These patients should be calmed and reassured to reduce their anxiety.

PRIMARY SURVEY

In most medical emergencies involving conscious patients, the main elements of the primary survey (level of consciousness, airway, breathing, and circulation) can be evaluated during the initial paramedic-patient encounter. For example, an appropriate verbal exchange between the paramedic and the conscious patient establishes that the patient is alert, oriented, and has adequate cardiorespiratory function. However, the primary survey for a patient with a possible coronary event should include a more in-depth evaluation of the patient's level of consciousness, respirations, pulse, and blood pressure.

A change in the patient's level of consciousness (e.g., lightheadedness or confusion) may indicate decreased cerebral perfusion caused by poor cardiac output. If possible, the paramedic should determine the patient's normal level of functioning by interviewing the patient, family members, or others who are familiar with the patient (e.g., neighbors and nursing staff). In addition, the paramedic should evaluate the patient's vital signs and include a respiratory assessment, an assessment of the patient's pulse for rate and regularity, and an initial measurement of the patient's blood pressure. These findings give the paramedic a baseline. They also are important during reassessment to identify trending and to guide patient care.

PHYSICAL EXAMINATION

The physical examination of a patient with cardiac disease should be organized and complete. The paramedic should use the following look-listen-feel approach. (Chapter 20 presents a more detailed discussion of this approach.)

LOOK AGAIN
See Chapter 20: Secondary Assessment, pp. 540-542.

Look

- *Skin:* Pale and diaphoretic skin may indicate peripheral vasoconstriction and sympathetic stimulation. Cyanosis is an indicator of poor oxygenation. The paramedic should use pulse oximetry to measure hemoglobin oxygenation.
- *Jugular veins:* An increase in central venous pressure from heart failure and cardiac tamponade can produce distention of internal jugular veins. **Jugular vein distention** is best evaluated with the patient's head elevated at 45 degrees. Distention may be difficult to assess in obese patients.
- *Peripheral and presacral edema:* Edema can result from chronic back pressure in the systemic venous circulation. It may be related to right heart failure. Edema is most obvious in dependent areas. (These areas may include the ankles and the sacral region in bedridden patients.) Edema can be classified as *nonpitting* (minimal or no

depression of tissue after removal of finger pressure) or *pitting* (depression of tissue remains after removal of finger pressure).

- *Additional indicators of cardiac disease:* More subtle signs of cardiac disease that may be found on a visual inspection include a midsternal scar from coronary surgery (Figure 22-113), a **nitroglycerin** patch on the skin, an implanted pacemaker or implantable cardioverter-defibrillator in the left upper chest or abdominal wall, and medical alert identification necklaces or bracelets.

Listen

- *Lung sounds:* The paramedic should assess the patient's chest visually for accessory muscle use in breathing before listening to lung sounds. Lung sounds should be clear and equal bilaterally. As described in Chapter 20, crackles may indicate pulmonary congestion or edema.

LOOK AGAIN
See Chapter 20: Secondary Assessment, pp. 536-540.

CRITICAL THINKING
What breath sounds might you hear if the patient has congestive heart failure or pulmonary edema?

- *Heart sounds:* Abnormal heart sounds may indicate congestive heart failure in adult patients (Box 22-13). Heart sounds are best heard at the **point of maximum impulse.** The point of maximum impulse is the location where the apical impulse is most readily visible or palpable. This often is in the fifth intercostal space, just medial to the left midclavicular line. Although abnormal heart sounds are difficult to detect in the prehospital setting, they can be useful for confirming the paramedic's field impression. Even so, abnormal heart sounds do not alter prehospital care. This evaluation should never delay other patient care measures or transportation.

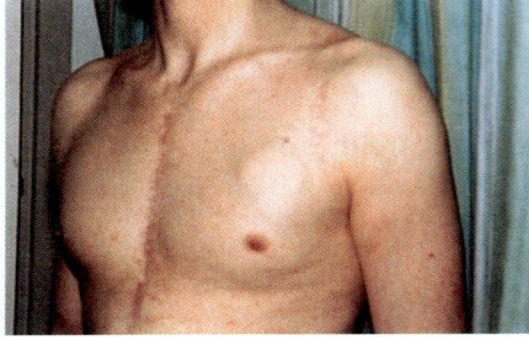

FIGURE 22-113 Midsternal scar and implanted cardiac device.

BOX 22-13 Heart Sounds

Heart sounds typically can be auscultated with a stethoscope during ventricular systole and diastole. When the ventricles contract, both atrioventricular valves close at nearly the same time. This closure causes a vibration of the valves and surrounding fluid. Vibration results in a low-pitched sound (often described as a "lubb"). Closing of the aortic and pulmonary semilunar valves at the end of ventricular systole produces a higher pitched sound (described as "dub"). These normal heart sounds are referred to as S_1 and S_2, respectively.

In rare cases a third heart sound can be heard near the end of the first third of diastole (S_3). The third heart sound is caused by turbulent blood flow into the ventricles. It may be normal, but it also may be an indicator of congestive heart failure. A fourth heart sound (S_4) may be heard during the end of diastole. This sound is thought to result from turbulence and chamber stretching caused by the atrial contraction during this part of the cardiac cycle. S_4 often is a sign of congestive heart failure in adults. S_3 and S_4 contribute to "gallop" rhythms, which are useful clinical indicators of congestive heart failure. Although heart sounds can help define the clinical picture, evaluation of these sounds should never delay emergency care or transport. To summarize:

S_1: First heart sound, which occurs with closure of the atrioventricular valves during ventricular systole.

S_2: Second heart sound, which occurs with closure of the aortic and pulmonic valves. It signifies the beginning of ventricular diastole.

S_3: Extra heart sound heard after S_2 (although it is not always present). It may be a normal finding in some patients, or it may indicate heart failure.

S_4: Extra heart sound heard in late diastole (just before S_1) It is associated with atrial contractions and often is heard in patients with congestive heart failure.

- *Carotid artery bruit:* **Bruits** are murmurs that indicate turbulent blood flow through a vessel. (This is most commonly caused by atherosclerosis.) The presence of a bruit in a patient with cardiac disease is evaluated at the carotid artery with a stethoscope and should always be assessed before carotid sinus massage (described later in this chapter) is performed. If a carotid artery bruit is present, carotid sinus massage is contraindicated. The procedure may dislodge plaque in the artery and cause a stroke.

Feel

- *Skin:* The paramedic should assess the patient's skin with the back of the hand for diaphoresis or fever. Normal skin is warm and dry.
- *Pulse:* The paramedic should assess the pulse for rate, regularity, and equality. A **pulse deficit** is a radial pulse that is less than the ventricular rate. A pulse deficit in peripheral and apical pulse sites may indicate a rhythm disturbance or vascular disease. The paramedic should note any pulse deficit and report it to medical direction.

- *Thorax and abdomen:* The paramedic should check the thorax and abdomen of a patient with cardiac disease for chest wall tenderness and pulsating masses. Chest wall tenderness is not uncommon in patients with acute myocardial infarction. A pulsating mass or distention in the abdomen or epigastric area may indicate an abdominal aneurysm (described later in this chapter).

SECTION EIGHT
Specific Cardiovascular Diseases

PATHOPHYSIOLOGY AND MANAGEMENT OF CARDIOVASCULAR DISEASE

Many true medical emergencies are cardiovascular in nature. Cardiovascular emergencies often result from atherosclerosis of the coronary arteries or peripheral arteries. The following specific medical conditions are discussed in this section:

- Acute coronary syndromes
- Atherosclerosis
- Angina pectoris
- Myocardial infarction
- Left ventricular failure and pulmonary edema
- Right ventricular failure
- Cardiogenic shock
- Cardiac tamponade
- Thoracic and abdominal aortic aneurysm
- Acute arterial occlusion
- Noncritical peripheral vascular disorders
- Hypertension

ACUTE CORONARY SYNDROMES

Acute myocardial infarction (AMI) and unstable angina (UA) are part of a spectrum of clinical disease, collectively known as **acute coronary syndromes** (ACS). ACS is the most common cause of sudden cardiac death. The pathophysiology of both AMI and UA is a ruptured or eroded atheromatous plaque. ECG findings common to ACS include ST-segment elevation, ST-segment depression, and T-wave abnormalities. As with other life-threatening conditions, time is of the essence in managing these patients. Rapid transport is indicated for any patient with chest pain of cardiac origin. Other indications for rapid transport include a sense of urgency for reperfusion; no relief of pain with medications; hypotension or hypoperfusion with central nervous system (CNS) involvement; and significant changes in the patient's ECG.[14]

The primary goals of therapy for patients with ACS include the following[1]:

- Reducing the amount of myocardial necrosis that occurs in patients with myocardial infarction, preserving left ventricular function, and preventing heart failure

- Preventing major adverse cardiac events (death, non-fatal myocardial infarction, and the need for urgent revascularization)
- Treating acute, life-threatening complications of ACS (e.g., ventricular fibrillation, pulseless ventricular tachycardia, symptomatic bradycardias, and unstable tachycardias)

Atherosclerosis

Atherosclerosis is a disease process characterized by progressive narrowing of the lumen of medium and large arteries (e.g., the aorta and its branches, cerebral arteries, and coronary arteries). The process results in the development of thick, hard atherosclerotic plaque. This plaque is referred to as *atheromata* or *atheromatous lesions*. These lesions most often are found in areas of turbulent blood flow. Such areas include vessel bifurcations or occur in vessels with a decreased lumen diameter.

Atherosclerosis is thought to result from damage to the endothelial cell from mechanical or chemical injury and perhaps inflammation (Box 22-14). This response includes platelet adhesion and clotting. Smooth muscle cells may move from the middle muscle layer into the lining of the artery. In the lining, the muscle cells form an atheroma. Over time, the atheromata become fibrous and hardened. In time, they partly or fully obstruct the opening of the arteries. In most cases, some collateral circulation develops to make up for the narrowed vessels.

MAJOR RISK FACTORS

Atherosclerosis occurs to some extent in all middle-aged and older people. The disease also occurs in some young people. Atherosclerosis is thought to be inherited. It usually is seen at a younger age in men than in women. Associated risk factors include age, a family history of heart disease, and diabetes. Some other risk factors can be reduced or eliminated. These include cigarette smoking, obesity, hypertension, and hypercholesterolemia. Some research has shown that plaque formation is not only preventable but also reversible.[1]

EFFECTS

Atherosclerosis has two major effects on blood vessels. First, it disrupts the innermost lining of the vessels. This causes loss of vessel elasticity and an increase in the formation of clots. Second, the atheroma reduces the diameter of the vessel lumen. This reduces the blood supply to tissues. Both effects result in an insufficient supply of nutrients to the tissue. This is especially true under conditions of increased tissue demand for nutrients and oxygen.

The severity of this insufficiency is related to the extent of narrowing (stenosis) of the blocked artery. The severity also depends on how long the atheroma took to develop, and the patient's ability to develop collateral circulation around the obstruction. For example, a patient who gradually develops an atherosclerotic occlusion in an artery of a lower extremity may compensate well through collateral circulation. The patient may experience only mild, intermittent pain during periods of exercise. In contrast, sudden-onset occlusion in a coronary artery (after an acute thrombus) almost always results in ischemia, injury, and necrosis to the area of the myocardium supplied by the affected artery.

Angina Pectoris

Angina pectoris is a symptom of myocardial ischemia; the term literally means "choking pain in the chest." Angina is caused by an imbalance between myocardial oxygen supply and demand. The result is a buildup of lactic acid and carbon dioxide in ischemic tissues of the myocardium. These metabolites irritate nerve endings that produce anginal pain. The most common cause of angina pectoris is atherosclerotic disease of the coronary arteries. A temporary occlusion caused by spasm of a coronary artery with or without atherosclerosis *(Prinzmetal's angina)* also can cause angina pectoris (Box 22-15). Emotional stress and any activity that increases myocardial oxygen demand may cause anginal pain, particularly in patients with atherosclerosis. Myocardial ischemia in turn puts the patient at risk for cardiac dysrhythmias.

BOX 22-14 Role of Inflammation in Heart Attack

Studies have suggested that painless inflammation deep in the body plays an important role in triggering heart attacks.[15] The inflammation may arise from such sources as chronic gum disease, lingering urinary tract infections, and others. Inflammation may weaken the walls of the blood vessels, allowing fatty buildups to burst. Inflammation can be assessed in those at risk for heart disease by testing the blood for an elevated white blood cell count and by measuring the C-reactive protein level. C-reactive protein is a chemical in the blood that is necessary for fighting injury and infection. It can be lowered with cholesterol-lowering drugs, aspirin, and other medications and through diet and exercise.

NOTE

A number of conditions can mimic the signs and symptoms of heart disease and angina pectoris (see Box 22-15). These include cholecystitis, peptic ulcer disease, aneurysm, hiatal hernia, pulmonary embolism, pancreatitis, pleural irritation, respiratory infection, and others. These conditions should be considered as part of the differential diagnosis when a patient presents with signs and symptoms of an acute coronary syndrome.

STABLE ANGINA

Angina pectoris generally is classified as *stable* or *unstable*. Stable angina usually is precipitated by physical exertion or emotional stress. The pain usually lasts 1 to 5 minutes but

BOX 22-15 Conditions That May Mimic Acute Coronary Syndrome

Acromioclavicular disease
Chest wall syndrome
Chest wall trauma
Chest wall tumors
Cholecystitis
Costochondritis
Dyspepsia
Esophageal disease
Gastric reflux
Herpes zoster
Hiatal hernia
Pancreatitis
Peptic ulcer disease
Pericarditis
Pleural irritation
Pneumothorax
Pulmonary embolism
Respiratory infection
Thoracic aortic dissection

MANAGEMENT

All patients with chest pain and signs and symptoms of myocardial ischemia should be managed as though an acute myocardial infarction were evolving (Table 22-8). The goal of management is to increase the coronary blood supply, reduce the myocardial oxygen demand, or both.

Management guidelines include the following:
1. Place the patient at rest physically and emotionally.
2. Administer oxygen if the patient is dyspneic, has signs of CHF or has an SaO_2 <94%.[1]
3. Administer *aspirin* (per protocol).
4. Initiate intravenous therapy.
5. If pain is present on paramedics' arrival, use pharmacological therapy. This may include sublingual *nitroglycerin* followed by *morphine* (IIa).
6. Monitor the ECG for dysrhythmias. Monitor a 3-lead ECG continuously and record serial 12-lead ECGs during transport. Also measure, record, and communicate any ST-segment changes. (Measurable ST-segment changes are most reliable when viewed in 12-lead mode.)
7. Transport the patient to an appropriate hospital for evaluation by a physician.

Myocardial Infarction

Acute myocardial infarction occurs with a sudden and total blockage or near blockage of blood flowing through an affected coronary artery to an area of heart muscle. This blockage results in ischemia, injury, and necrosis to the area of the myocardium distal to the occlusion. Acute myocardial infarction most often is associated with atherosclerotic heart disease.

PRECIPITATING EVENTS

The process of myocardial infarction is complex. It generally begins with the formation of an atherosclerotic plaque involving the intimal layer of a coronary artery. The plaque disrupts the smooth arterial lining and results in an uneven surface. This creates turbulent blood flow. The plaque may rupture. If rupture occurs, the injured tissue is exposed to circulating platelets. This results in the formation of a thrombus that occludes the artery. As the thrombus enlarges, it further reduces blood flow in the coronary vessel.

Acute thrombotic occlusion generally is accepted as the cause of most myocardial infarctions. Other factors that may lead to acute myocardial infarction include coronary spasm, coronary embolism, severe hypoxia, hemorrhage into a diseased arterial wall, and reduced blood flow after any form of shock. All of these may result in an inadequate amount of blood reaching the myocardium.

TYPES AND LOCATIONS OF INFARCTS

The myocardial cells beyond the occluded artery die (infarct) from lack of oxygen. The size of the infarct is determined by the needs of the tissue supplied by the occluded vessel, by the presence of collateral circulation, and by the time

may last as long as 15 minutes. Angina is relieved by rest, *nitroglycerin,* or oxygen. Stable angina attacks usually are similar and are always relieved by the same mode of therapy.

UNSTABLE ANGINA

Unstable angina *(preinfarction angina)* denotes an anginal pattern that has changed in its ease of onset, frequency, intensity, duration, or quality. (This includes any new-onset anginal chest pain.) Unstable angina may occur during periods of light exercise or at rest. The pain usually lasts 10 minutes or longer. The pain is relieved less promptly by cessation of activity or *nitroglycerin* than in stable angina. Unstable angina mimics acute myocardial infarction. The two sometimes are difficult to differentiate in the prehospital setting. Patients with unstable angina are at increased risk of acute myocardial infarction and sudden death.

The pain of angina usually is described by the patient as a pressure, squeezing, heaviness, or tightness in the chest. Although 30% of patients with angina feel pain only in the chest, others describe the pain as radiating to the shoulders, arms, neck, and jaw and through the chest to the back. Associated signs and symptoms include anxiety, shortness of breath, nausea or vomiting, and diaphoresis. The patient history often reveals previous attacks of angina. Often the patient will have taken *nitroglycerin* before paramedics arrive. If so, the paramedic should determine the age of the nitroglycerin prescription (*nitroglycerin* is unstable and quickly loses its strength), the amount of *nitroglycerin* taken, and its effect. If the pain is not relieved by rest and medication, the paramedic should suspect a myocardial infarction.

TABLE 22-8 Likelihood of Ischemic Origin of Chest Pain and Short-Term Risk

Part I. Patient With Chest Pain Without ST-Segment Elevation: Likelihood of Ischemic Origin

	A. High Likelihood	B. Indeterminate Likelihood	C. Low Likelihood
	High likelihood that chest pain has ischemic origin if patient has *any* of the findings in the column below:	Indeterminate likelihood that chest pain has ischemic origin if patient has NO findings in column A and *any* of the findings in the column below:	Low likelihood that chest pain has ischemic origin if patient has NO findings in column A or B. Patients may have any of the findings in the column below:
History	• Chief symptom is chest or left arm pain or discomfort *plus* current pain that reproduces pain of previous documented angina *and* known CAD, including MI	• Chief symptom is chest or left arm pain or discomfort • Age >70, male	• Probably ischemic symptoms • Recent cocaine use
Physical exam	• Transient mitral regurgitation • Hypotension • Diaphoresis • Pulmonary edema or rales	• Diabetes mellitus • Extracardiac vascular disease	• Age >70 years • Male gender • Chest discomfort reproduced by palpation
ECG	• New (or presumed new) transient ST deviation (≥0.5 mm) or T-wave inversion (≥2 mm) with symptoms	• Fixed Q waves • Normal ECG *or* T-wave flattening *or* T-wave inversion in leads with dominant R waves	• Abnormal ST segments *or* T waves that are not new
Cardiac markers	• Elevated troponin I or T • High (A) or indeterminate (B) likelihood of ischemia	*Any finding in column B above PLUS* • Elevated CK-MB	• Normal

Part II. Risk of Death or Nonfatal MI Over the Short Term in Patients With Chest Pain With High or Indeterminate Likelihood of Ischemia (Columns A and B in Part I)

	High Risk	Indeterminate Risk	Low Risk
	Risk is high if patient has *any* of the following findings:	Risk is indeterminate if patient has any of the following findings:	Risk is low if patient has NO high- or indeterminate-risk features; may have any of the following:
History	• Accelerating tempo of ischemic symptoms over previous 48 hours	• Previous MI *or* • Cerebrovascular disease *or* • CABG, previous aspirin use	• Peripheral-artery disease *or*
Character of pain	• Prolonged, continuing rest pain (>20 min)	• Prolonged rest angina (>20 min) now resolved (moderate to high likelihood of CAD) • Rest angina (<20 min) or pain relieved by rest or sublingual nitrates	• New-onset functional angina (class III or IV) in past 2 weeks without prolonged rest pain (but with moderate or high likelihood of CAD)
Physical exam	• Pulmonary edema secondary to ischemia • New or worse mitral regurgitation murmur • Hypotension, bradycardia, tachycardia • S₃ gallop or new or worsening rales • Age >75 years	• Age >70 years	
ECG	• Transient ST-segment deviation (≥0.5 mm) with rest angina • New or presumably new bundle branch block • Sustained VT	• T-wave inversion ≥2 mm • Pathologic Q waves or T waves that are not new	• Normal or unchanged ECG during an episode of chest discomfort
Cardiac markers	• Elevated cardiac troponin I or T	*Any of the above findings PLUS* • Elevated CK-MB	• Normal

Modified from Braunwald E, et al: ACC/AHA guideline update for the management of patients with unstable angina and non-ST segment elevation myocardial infarction-2002: Summary Article: A report of the American College of Cardiology/American Heart Association Task Force on Practice Guidelines (Committee on the Management of Patients with Unstable Angina). *Circulation* 106:1893-1900, 2002.

CABG, Coronary artery bypass grafting; *CAD,* coronary artery disease; *CK-MB,* creatine kinase, myocardial bound; *MI,* myocardial infarction.

required to reestablish blood flow. Therefore emergency care is directed at the following:

- Increasing the oxygen supply by administering supplemental oxygen
- Decreasing the metabolic needs and providing collateral circulation
- Reestablishing perfusion to the ischemic myocardium as quickly as possible after the onset of symptoms

Most acute myocardial infarctions involve the left ventricle or interventricular septum. These areas are supplied by either of the two major coronary arteries. (However, some patients sustain damage to the right ventricle.) If the occlusion is in the left coronary artery, the result is an anterior, lateral, or septal wall infarction. Inferior wall infarction (of the inferior-posterior wall of the left ventricle) usually is a result of right coronary artery occlusion.

Infarction also can be classified into one of three ischemic syndromes based on the rupture of an unstable plaque in an epicardial artery: **unstable angina, non-STEMI,** and **STEMI.**[1] These three acute coronary syndromes share common risk factors, and their management overlaps a good deal. Sudden cardiac death may occur with any of these syndromes.

- In *unstable angina,* the early thrombus has not obstructed coronary blood flow completely. This partial occlusion produces symptoms of ischemia. The blockage eventually may result in complete occlusion and produce a non-STEMI. Fibrinolytic therapy (described later in this chapter) is not effective in unstable angina. In fact, such therapy may accelerate the occlusion. Therapy with antiplatelet agents is most effective at this time because the thrombus is rich in platelets.
- *Non-STEMI* occurs as microemboli from the thrombus become lodged in the coronary arteries. This produces minimal damage to the myocardium. However, these patients are at highest risk for progression to myocardial infarction. Non-STEMIs are evident only with ST-segment depression or T-wave abnormalities.
- *STEMI* occurs when the thrombus occludes the coronary vessel for a prolonged period. The infarct is diagnosed by the development of elevated ST segments in two or more contiguous (adjacent) leads. (Figure 22-114). The clot is rich in thrombin; therefore, early management with fibrinolytics may help limit the size of the infarct.

DEATH OF MYOCARDIUM

When blood flow to the myocardium stops, a series of events begins. Cells switch from aerobic to anaerobic metabolism. This results in the release of lactic acid and an increase in tissue carbon dioxide levels. These changes contribute to ischemic pain (angina). As cells lose their ability to maintain their electrochemical gradients, they begin to swell and depolarize. These initial changes are reversible.

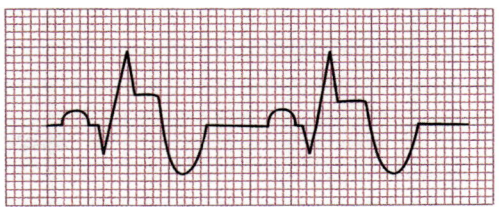

FIGURE 22-114 ST elevation and pathological Q waves. (Aehlert B: *ACLS quick review study guide,* ed 3, St Louis, 2006, Mosby.)

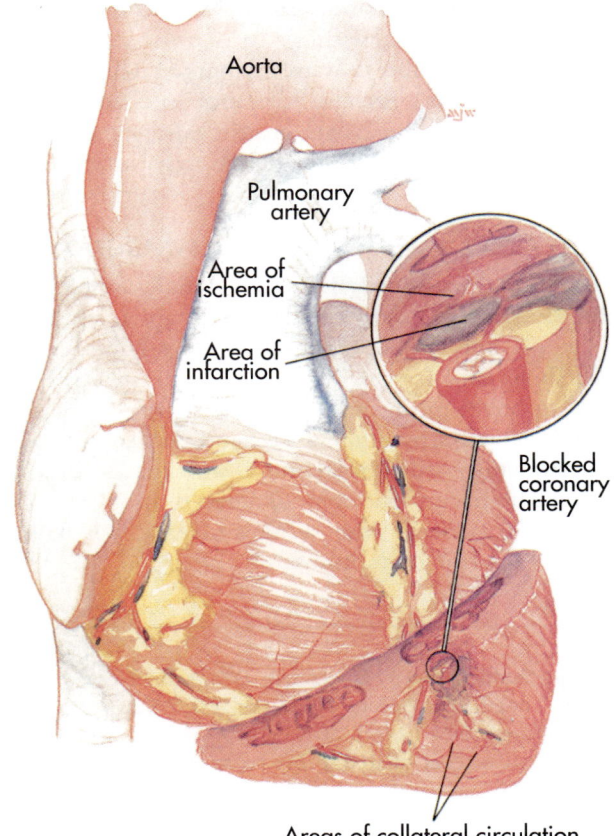

FIGURE 22-115 Areas of infarct.

However, within a few hours, if collateral flow and reperfusion are inadequate, much of the muscle distal to the occlusion dies. The area surrounding the necrotic tissue may survive because of collateral circulation. However, surviving tissue may become the origin of dysrhythmias (Figure 22-115).

Scar tissue replaces the infarcted area in a process that takes about 8 weeks. The process starts with deposits of connective tissue on about the twelfth day. Scar tissue is durable. However, it lacks elasticity, does not contract, and conducts electrical impulses poorly in the damaged area of the myocardium. The left ventricle can lose as much as 25% of its muscle and still function as an effective pump. Areas with poor perfusion after a large myocardial infarction may not develop strong scar tissue. This may result in an aneurysm. Such an aneurysm can greatly reduce the effective ventricular contractility. An aneurysm also may lead to the development of serious dysrhythmias.

The damaged myocardium is most susceptible to rupture during the first 1 to 2 weeks after a myocardial infarction, because the scar tissue has not reached adequate strength. For this reason, patient activity is limited. Prevention of hypertension and excitement during this period also is usually necessary. Even so, the hospital stay of patients with uncomplicated myocardial infarctions has been shortened. Today, most patients resume activity within 2 to 3 days, and most leave the hospital within 7 to 10 days. Many patients have a stress test before they are discharged. This test determines the patient's exercise tolerance level and whether ischemia or dysrhythmias are present during exercise. The result of this test helps determine the activities the patient may resume after discharge.

DEATH FOLLOWING MYOCARDIAL INFARCTION

Death after myocardial infarction usually results from lethal dysrhythmias (ventricular tachycardia, ventricular fibrillation, and cardiac standstill), pump failure (cardiogenic shock and congestive heart failure), or myocardial tissue rupture (rupture of the ventricle, septum, or papillary muscle). Fatal dysrhythmias are the most common cause of death from myocardial infarction. Deaths that occur within the first 2 hours after the onset of illness or injury are *sudden deaths*. Most patients who suffer sudden death have no immediate warning symptoms.

> **NOTE**
> **Sudden death** is defined as a sudden dysrhythmic death that occurs within the first 2 hours of cardiac ischemic symptoms.[6] More than 50% of cardiac deaths occur with no evidence of infarction on autopsy when resuscitation attempts fail. Sudden death without infarction is a main reason for the widespread availability of automated external defibrillators. (Another reason is that the most common death-producing dysrhythmia is ventricular fibrillation.)

SIGNS AND SYMPTOMS

Some patients with acute myocardial infarction—particularly diabetic patients, some women, and those in the older age groups—may have only symptoms of dyspnea, syncope, or confusion. However, substernal chest pain is present in 70% to 90% of patients with acute myocardial infarction. The pain generally has the same characteristics and locations as anginal pain. The pain also may radiate to the arms, neck, jaw, or back. The following signs and symptoms may accompany the pain and occasionally are present even in the absence of pain *(silent myocardial infarction)*:

- Agitation
- Anxiety
- Cyanosis
- Diaphoresis
- Dyspnea
- Nausea and vomiting
- Palpitations
- Sense of impending doom
- Weakness

>
> **CRITICAL THINKING**
> How can prehospital recognition of an acute myocardial infarction affect the care of the patient at the hospital?

The chest pain associated with acute myocardial infarction often is constant. Also, the pain often is not altered or alleviated by ***nitroglycerin*** or other cardiac medications, rest, changes in body position, or breathing patterns. With angina pectoris, the onset often occurs during periods of activity. In contrast, the onset of pain in more than half of all patients with acute myocardial infarction occurs during rest. Most patients have had warning anginal pains (preinfarction angina) hours or days before the attack. Many patients deny the possibility of an evolving myocardial infarction. They may blame the chest pain or discomfort on unrelated causes, such as fatigue or indigestion. Denial delays the request for EMS assistance during the most critical phase of the illness. According to the American Heart Association, more than 50% of deaths from ischemic heart disease occur outside the hospital within the first 4 hours after the onset of pain.[1]

>
> **CRITICAL THINKING**
> Why do you think patients deny that their signs and symptoms may be due to a heart attack?

Vital signs vary with an acute myocardial infarction. They depend on the extent of damage to the heart muscle and conduction system. They also depend on the degree and type of autonomic nervous system response. (Inferior myocardial infarctions often show a mainly parasympathetic response. In contrast, anterior myocardial infarctions commonly show a mainly sympathetic response.) For example, the patient's blood pressure may be normal, elevated (sympathetic discharge), or low (parasympathetic discharge or pump failure). The pulse rate depends on the presence or absence of dysrhythmias. The pulse rate may be normal, tachycardic, bradycardic, regular, or irregular. Respirations may be normal or increased.

> **NOTE**
> Sulfonylurea drugs (drugs for treating diabetes), such as glyburide or glipizide, may lessen the magnitude of ST-segment elevation in the presence of an infarct. Therefore, it is crucial that paramedics obtain a diabetes history for all patients with a cardiac event. Research has shown that diabetes drugs can mask the severity of a heart attack.[17]

MANAGEMENT OF AN UNCOMPLICATED ACUTE MYOCARDIAL INFARCTION

All patients with anginal chest pain are assumed to have an acute myocardial infarction until it is proved otherwise (Figure 22-116). Any patient with chest pain should be transported to a medical facility for evaluation by a physician, regardless of the apparent severity on the arrival of EMS providers, the patient's age, gender, or associated complaints. The primary goals of prehospital care are to identify a patient with possible myocardial infarction; to relieve pain and apprehension; to prevent the development of serious dysrhythmias; and to limit the size of the infarct. The paramedic should obtain a full patient history while performing the physical examination and during initial patient care. Because time is of the essence, the following aspects of patient care are a high priority:

1. Place the patient at rest or in a comfortable position. This helps reduce anxiety and the heart rate and thus oxygen demand.
2. Monitor pulse oximetry.
3. Administer low-concentration oxygen (4 L/minute) via the nasal cannula if SaO$_2$ is <94%. Patients with respiratory compromise need a higher oxygen concentration.
4. Initiate transport quickly. (If the patient is stable, do not use audible or visual warning devices, to help reduce the patient's anxiety.)
5. Administer *aspirin* (per protocol).
6. Establish an IV line with normal saline or lactated Ringer solution to keep the vein open or to supply fluid boluses (if needed).
7. Obtain baseline vital signs. Repeat the assessment often. Vital sign assessment should include auscultation of the lungs for heart failure indicators (e.g., presence of crackles).
8. Attach ECG electrodes, obtain a 12-lead ECG, document the initial rhythm, and monitor for dysrhythmias (repeat if possible during transport).
9. Administer medications (per protocol) to relieve pain and manage dysrhythmias:
   a. Medications that may be used for analgesia and to reduce preload and afterload include *nitroglycerin* followed by *morphine.*
   b. Medications that may be used to manage the various dysrhythmias include *procainamide, atropine,* diltiazem, *verapamil, adenosine, magnesium, metoprolol, amiodarone,* and others. (Refer to the appropriate treatment algorithm.)

NOTE

Nitroglycerin is a vasodilating agent that has beneficial hemodynamic effects. These include dilation of arterioles and veins in the periphery (thereby reducing preload) and dilation of the coronary arteries. This reduces the workload of the heart, lowers myocardial oxygen demand, and may relieve ischemic chest pain. Because of these hemodynamic effects, *nitroglycerin* should not be used in patients with the following conditions[4]:

- Hypotension (systolic blood pressure lower than 90 mm Hg or more than 30 mm Hg below baseline)
- Extreme bradycardia (heart rate slower than 50 beats/minute)
- Tachycardia (heart rate faster than 100 beats/minute) unless the patient has heart failure[1]

Nitroglycerin also should be given with extreme caution (if at all) to patients with suspected inferior wall myocardial infarction with possible right ventricular involvement (patients who require adequate right ventricular preload). In these patients, nitroglycerin can cause profound hypotension. *Nitroglycerin* also is contraindicated in patients who have taken medication for erectile dysfunction within the previous 24 hours (longer for some preparations).

FIBRINOLYTIC THERAPY

Studies have shown that an acute intracoronary thrombus can be dissolved (thereby restoring blood flow to the ischemic area) with salvage of ischemic myocardium if a fibrinolytic agent is administered within 12 hours after the onset of symptoms when percutaneous angioplasty (PCA) is not available within 90 minutes of first medical patient contact.[1] Some emergency medical services are authorized by medical direction to administer these agents in the prehospital setting. The American Heart Association recommends that prehospital systems focus on early diagnosis and the field administration of fibrinolytics as soon as possible after the onset of ischemic-type chest discomfort in patients with confirmed STEMI or new or presumably new left bundle branch block.[1] The AHA strongly recommends the following for EMS systems that administer fibrinolytics in the prehospital setting[1]:

- Protocols using fibrinolytic checklists
- 12-lead ECG acquisition and interpretation
- Experience in advanced life support
- Communication with the receiving institution
- Medical director with training and experience in STEMI management
- Continuous quality improvement

Common fibrinolytic agents include *streptokinase, tissue plasminogen activator,* tenecteplase, anistreplase, and *reteplase.* All these agents work through activation of the plasma protein plasminogen to dissolve the coronary thrombus. Plasminogen is converted to plasmin (the active form). Plasmin degrades fibrin, the basic component of a clot (thrombus). *Aspirin* and *heparin* are part of the "fibrinolytic package."

A fibrinolytic agent can dissolve both beneficial and pathological thrombi. Therefore, the drug is administered selectively. Most EMS systems that use fibrinolytic agents establish inclusion-exclusion criteria similar to those in Box 22-16.[6]

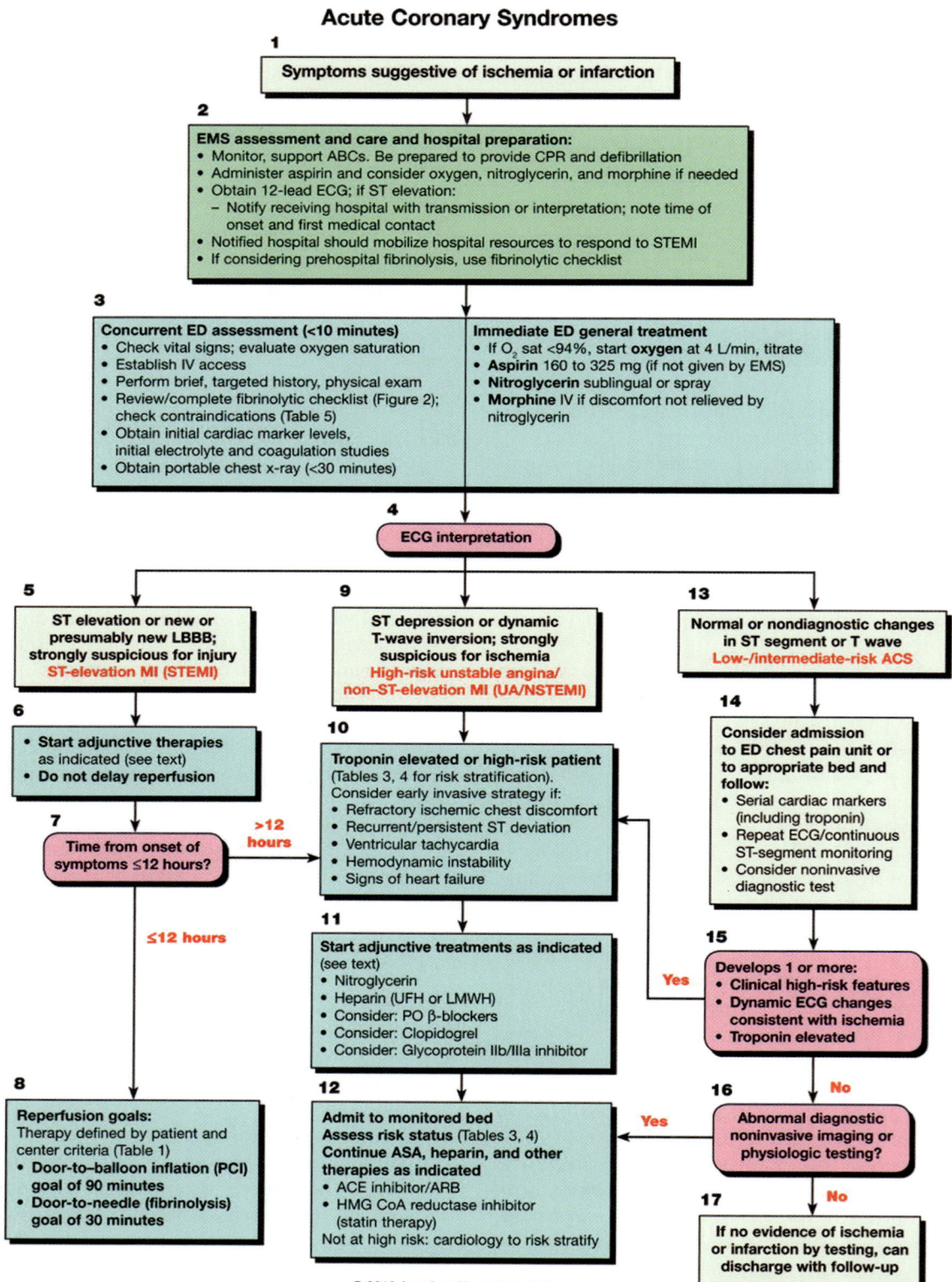

FIGURE 22-116 Acute coronary syndrome algorithm. (Reprinted with permission, American Heart Association Guidelines For CPR and ECC, *Circulation 122* [suppl 3]:S685-S919, American Heart Association, Inc, 2010.)

BOX 22-16 Possible Contraindications to Fibrinolytic Therapy

- Systolic BP >180-200 mm Hg OR diastolic BP >100-110 mm Hg
- Right vs. left arm systolic BP difference >15 mm Hg
- History of structural central nervous system disease
- Significant closed head/facial trauma within the previous 3 weeks
- Stroke >3 hours OR <3 months
- Recent (within 2 to 4 weeks) major trauma, surgery (including laser eye surgery), GI/GU bleed
- Any history of intracranial hemorrhage
- Bleeding, clotting problem, or blood thinners
- Pregnant female
- Serious systemic disease (e.g., advanced cancer, severe liver or kidney disease)

From American Heart Association. 2010 American Heart Association Guidelines for Cardiopulmonary Resuscitation and Emergency Cardiovascular Care. *Circulation*, 122(18 Supplement 3), S639-S946, 2010.

Congestive Heart Failure

Congestive heart failure is a condition in which the heart is unable to pump blood at a rate that meets the metabolic needs of the tissues. The condition affects about 5 million Americans and is responsible for 7000 to 10,000 hospital admissions each year.[17] Congestive heart failure most often is caused by volume overload, pressure overload, loss of myocardial tissue, and impaired contractility. All of these can impair left ventricular function. Precipitating causes of heart failure include myocardial infarction, pulmonary embolism, and enlarged heart *(cardiomegaly)*. This text discusses congestive heart failure in terms of left ventricular failure and pulmonary edema and also right ventricular failure (Box 22-17).

LEFT VENTRICULAR FAILURE AND PULMONARY EDEMA

Left ventricular failure occurs when the left ventricle fails to work as an effective forward pump. This causes a back pressure of blood into the pulmonary circulation. This condition may be caused by a number of forms of heart disease, such as ischemic, valvular, and hypertensive heart disease. If left unmanaged, significant left ventricular failure results in pulmonary edema.

In left ventricular failure, blood is delivered to the left ventricle, but the blood is not fully ejected from the ventricle. The increase in end-diastolic blood volume increases left ventricular end-diastolic pressure. This pressure is transmitted to the left atrium. Pressure then is transmitted to the pulmonary veins and capillaries. As pulmonary capillary hydrostatic pressure increases, the plasma portion of blood is forced into the alveoli. There plasma mixes with air. This results in the typical finding in pulmonary edema: foamy, blood-tinged sputum. If left unmanaged, the

BOX 22-17 Classification of Heart Failure

Heart failure can be classified as high-output failure or low-output failure. With **low-output heart failure,** cardiac output is decreased. This is the most common type of heart failure seen with most forms of heart disease. Low-output failure leads to manifestations of impaired peripheral circulation and vasoconstriction. With **high-output heart failure,** cardiac output remains high but is unable to meet the metabolic needs of the body. This type of heart failure is associated with hyperthyroidism, anemia, pregnancy, Paget's disease, arteriovenous fistulas, beriberi, and sepsis. In practice, differentiating between low-output and high-output heart failure sometimes is difficult and does not affect prehospital care.

Heart failure can also be classified as chronic or acute. *Chronic heart failure* typically is observed in patients with dilated cardiomyopathy or multivalvular heart disease that develops or progresses slowly. In chronic heart failure, arterial pressure tends to be well maintained until very late in the course, but peripheral edema often accumulates (these patients often have multiple events of failure). *Acute heart failure* is associated with a sudden reduction in cardiac output that often results in systemic hypotension without peripheral edema. Patients with acute heart failure usually have been entirely well but then suddenly develop a large myocardial infarction or valvular rupture in the heart (this often is a first-time event).

progressive fluid buildup can result in death from hypoxia. Myocardial infarction is a common cause of left ventricular failure. Therefore, in all patients with pulmonary edema (particularly those with an abrupt onset), an acute myocardial infarction also should be suspected.

> **NOTE**
> **Paroxysmal nocturnal dyspnea** is an abnormal condition of the respiratory system. It is characterized by sudden attacks of shortness of breath, profuse sweating, tachycardia, and wheezing that awaken a person from sleep. The condition often is associated with left ventricular failure and pulmonary edema.

Left ventricular failure results in a reduction of stroke volume. This in turn initiates several compensatory mechanisms that restore cardiac output and organ perfusion (tachycardia, vasoconstriction, and activation of the renin-angiotensin-aldosterone system). However, these mechanisms often increase myocardial oxygen demand. They therefore further decrease the myocardium's ability to contract. Box 22-18 lists the signs and symptoms of left ventricular failure and pulmonary edema.

Management. **Pulmonary edema** is an acute and critical emergency (Figure 22-117). It may lead to death unless it is treated rapidly. Emergency management is directed at reducing the venous return to the heart, improving

BOX 22-18 Signs and Symptoms of Left Ventricular Failure

- Severe respiratory distress
  - Orthopnea
  - Spasmodic cough that may produce foamy, blood-tinged sputum
  - History of paroxysmal nocturnal dyspnea (a sudden episode of dyspnea that occurs after lying down)
- Severe apprehension, agitation, confusion
- Cyanosis (if severe)
- Diaphoresis
- Adventitious lung sounds
  - Bilateral crackles that do not clear with coughing (usually present at the base of the lungs and up to the level of the scapulae)
  - Rhonchi (fluid in the upper airways)
  - Wheezes (reflex airway spasm, sometimes referred to as *cardiac asthma*)
- Jugular vein distention (indicative of back pressure through the right heart and into the venous system)
- Abnormal vital signs
  - Blood pressure: Possibly elevated
  - Pulse rate: Rapid to compensate for low stroke volume; possibly irregular if dysrhythmias are present
- Regular alterations of weak and strong beats without changes in the length of the cycle (pulsus alternans); rapid, labored respirations
- Altered level of consciousness (patient may be anxious, agitated, uncooperative, or obtunded because of poor cerebral perfusion or hypoxia)
- Chest pain
  - Presence or absence of pain
  - May be masked by respiratory distress

myocardial contractility, decreasing myocardial oxygen demand, improving ventilation and oxygenation, and rapidly transporting the patient to a medical facility.

Emergency care entails patient positioning, oxygenation, continuous positive airway pressure (CPAP), ventilatory support as needed, and pharmacological therapy. As in any other true emergency, the paramedic should perform a full but focused patient history and examination while initiating treatment. No characteristic ECG changes are associated with pulmonary edema. However, the paramedic should obtain an initial tracing. The paramedic also should monitor the patient's rhythm continuously for evidence of myocardial irritability and dysrhythmias.

The paramedic should place the patient in a sitting position with the legs dependent. This position increases lung volume and vital capacity. It also diminishes the work of respiration and reduces venous return to the heart.

The paramedic should administer high-concentration oxygen using a well-fitted face mask. Preferably the mask should be a nonrebreathing mask to optimize the amount of inspired oxygen. Some patients may require (and will

tolerate) positive pressure assistance (including CPAP or biphasic positive airway pressure [BiPAP]). Positive pressure assistance is one of the highest priorities in caring for these patients, and it reduces the need for high levels of inspired oxygen. A pulse oximeter should be used to ensure an arterial oxygen saturation of at least 90%. If this cannot be achieved with 100% oxygen or if signs of cerebral hypoxia or progressive hypercapnia are seen, tracheal intubation and assisted ventilations may be indicated.

Nitroglycerin and *morphine* may be used to reduce venous return, enhance contractile function of the myocardium, and reduce dyspnea. It should be noted that both of these drugs can lower blood pressure. Therefore, care must be taken in patients with pulmonary edema and hypotension (a systolic blood pressure less than 100 mm Hg).

In some cases of pulmonary edema, the patient will have fluid overload. In these situations, medical direction may recommend administration of furosemide[18,19].

NOTE

Some medical authorities do not recommend the administration of morphine in patients with decompensated heart failure. Studies have suggested that the use of morphine may be associated with increased adverse events in these patients. These events include a greater frequency of mechanical ventilation, prolonged hospitalization, more intensive care unit (ICU) admissions, and higher mortality.[20] The use of loop and thiazide diuretics in this patient group as part of initial stabilization also is under review.[21] The paramedic should follow local protocol established by medical direction.

The effects of *nitroglycerin* and *morphine* are:
1. Nitroglycerin
   a. Induction of peripheral vasodilation
   b. Possible reduction of preload and afterload, thereby reducing the myocardial workload and improving cardiac function
2. Morphine
   a. Decrease of venous return by dilation of the capacitance vessels of the peripheral venous bed (reduces preload)
   b. Reduction of myocardial work
   c. Reduction of anxiety

NOTE

Furosemide may be indicated in some patients with pulmonary edema who also have fluid overload. *Furosemide* has a direct relaxant (dilating) effect on the venous system and a diuretic effect that reduces intravascular volume. In these patients, *furosemide* can reduce venous return and improve breathing.

CRITICAL THINKING

What happens to the diffusion of oxygen and carbon dioxide in the lungs during this process?

Management of Acute Pulmonary Edema

Perform Primary ABCD Survey (Basic Life Support)
(Correct critical problems IMMEDIATELY as they are identified)
- Assess responsiveness, **A**irway, **B**reathing, **C**irculation, ensure availability of monitor/**D**efibrillator

Perform Secondary ABCD Survey (Advanced Life Support)
(Obtain arterial blood gas before oxygen administration if possible)
- Administer oxygen, establish IV access, attach cardiac monitor (O_2, IV, monitor)
- Assess vital signs, attach pulse oximeter, & monitor blood pressure
- Obtain & review 12-lead ECG
- Perform a focused history and physical exam

If feasible and BP permits, place patient in sitting position with feet dependent
- Increases lung volume and vital capacity
- Decreases work of respiration
- Decreases venous return, decreases preload

If systolic BP > 100 mm Hg:
- Sublingual nitroglycerin–1 tablet or 2 sprays every 5 minutes (max 3 tablets) until IV nitroglycerin or nitroprusside can take effect
- Furosemide IV 0.5 to 1.0 mg/kg (typically 20 to 80 mg) can repeat in 30 minutes if symptoms persist and BP stable
- Consider morphine IV 2-4 mg
- Consider continuous positive airway pressure (CPAP)

Consider additional preload/afterload reduction–nitroglycerin or nitroprusside IV, ACE inhibitors
- Nitroglycerin IV–start at 5 mcg/min and increase gradually until mean systolic pressure falls by 10% to 15%, avoid hypotension (SBP <90 mm hg)" **OR**
- Nitroprusside IV (If SBP > 100 mm Hg)–0.1 to 5 mcg/kg/min

Evaluate early for:
- Readily reversible cause and institute appropriate intervention (e.g., cardiac dysrhythmias, tamponade)
- Myocardial ischemia/infarction (Institute appropriate intervention–candidate for fibrinolytic therapy? PTCA?

If patient is refractory to above therapies, hypotensive, or in cardiogenic shock:
- Consider fluid or IV inotropic and/or vasopressor agents (e.g., dobutamine, dopamine, norepinephrine)

In-hospital therapy
- Consider pulmonary and systemic arterial catheterization
- Obtain echocardiogram to assist in diagnosis, evaluation, and reparability of culprit lesion or condition
- Consider need for mechanical circulatory assistance (balloon pump)

FIGURE 22-117 Acute pulmonary edema/hypotension/shock algorithm. (Aehlert B: *ACLS quick review study guide,* ed 3, St Louis, 2006, Mosby.)

Continued

RIGHT VENTRICULAR FAILURE

Right ventricular failure most often results from left ventricular failure that produces elevated pressure in the pulmonary vascular system. This pressure causes resistance to pulmonary blood flow. It also increases the workload of the right side of the heart to overcome the resistance. Over time, the right ventricle fails as an effective forward pump. This causes back pressure of blood into the systemic venous circulation. When the pressure in the systemic venous circulation becomes too high, the plasma portion of the blood is forced out into the interstitial tissues of the body. This results in edema, particularly in the dependent areas of the body. (For example, edema occurs in the lower extremities and sacrum of bedridden patients.) Right ventricular failure can result from several diseases. These include chronic hypertension (in which left ventricular failure usually precedes right ventricular failure), chronic obstructive pulmonary disease, pulmonary embolism, valvular heart disease, and infarction of the right ventricle.

Box 22-19 lists the signs and symptoms of right ventricular failure. When left and right ventricular failure occur at the same time, the signs and symptoms of each may be present. Table 22-9 can help the paramedic differentiate between the two.

Management. Right ventricular failure often is a chronic condition. It usually is not a medical emergency in itself.

Management of Hypotension/Shock–Suspected Pump Problem

Perform Primary ABCD Survey (Basic Life Support)

(Correct critical problems IMMEDIATELY as they are identified)
- Assess responsiveness, **A**irway, **B**reathing, **C**irculation, ensure availability of monitor/**D**efibrillator

Perform Secondary ABCD Survey (Advanced Life Support)

- Administer oxygen, establish IV access, attach cardiac monitor, administer fluids as needed (O₂, IV, monitor, fluids)
- Assess vital signs, attach pulse oximeter, and monitor blood pressure
- Obtain and review 12-lead ECG, portable chest x-ray,
- Perform a focused history and physical exam

Hypotension–suspected pump problem

If breath sounds are clear, consider fluid challenge of 250 to 500 -mL NS to ensure adequate ventricular filling pressure before vasopressor administration

Marked hypotension (systolic BP < 70 mm Hg)/cardiogenic shock

Pharmacologic management:
- Norepinephrine infusion (0.5 to 1 mcg/min titrated to effect) until SBP 80 mm Hg
- Then attempt to change to dopamine 2-20 mcg/kg/min until SBP 90 mm Hg
- IV dobutamine (2 to 20 mcg/kg/min) can be given simultaneously in an attempt to reduce magnitude of dopamine infusion

In-hospital therapy

Consider balloon pump left ventricular assist device or patient transfer to a cardiac interventional facility

Moderate hypotension (systolic BP 70 to 90 mm Hg)

- Dopamine 5 to 15 mcg/kg/min
- If BP remains low despite dopamine doses > 20 mcg/kg/min, may substitute norepinephrine in doses of 0.5 to 30 mcg/min
- Once SBP ≥ 90 with dopamine, add dobutamine 2 to 20 mcg/kg/min and attempt to taper off dopamine

Systolic BP 90 mm Hg

- Dobutamine 2 to 20 mcg/kg/min

Dosing:

Norepinephrine IV	0.5 to 30 mcg/min
Dopamine IV	5 to 15 mcg/kg/min
Dobutamine IV	2 to 20 mcg/kg/min

FIGURE 22-117, cont'd

BOX 22-19 Signs and Symptoms of Right Ventricular Failure

- Tachycardia
- Venous congestion
  - Engorged liver or spleen or both
  - Venous distention: Distention and pulsation of the neck veins
- Peripheral edema
  - Lower extremities or entire body (anasarca)
  - Sacral region in bedridden patients
  - Pitting edema
- Fluid accumulation in serous cavities
  - Abdominal cavity (ascites)
  - Pericardium (pericardial effusion)
  Note: Patients often can tolerate large amounts of effusion without compromise when the effusion develops over an extended period.
- History
  - Often previous myocardial infarction in patients with chronic congestive failure
  - Frequent medication history of digitalis and diuretics to control heart failure

Management of Hypotension/Shock–Suspected Volume Problem

Perform Primary ABCD Survey (Basic Life Support)

(Correct critical problems IMMEDIATELY as they are identified)
- Assess responsiveness, **A**irway, **B**reathing, **C**irculation, ensure availability of monitor/**D**efibrillator

Perform Secondary ABCD Survey (Advanced Life Support)

- Administer oxygen, establish IV access, attach cardiac monitor, administer fluids as needed (O_2, IV, monitor, fluids)
- Assess vital signs, attach pulse oximeter, and monitor blood pressure
- Obtain and review 12-lead ECG, portable chest x-ray,
- Perform a focused history and physical exam

Hypotension–suspected volume (or vascular resistance) problem

Volume replacement

- Fluid challenge (250 to 500-mL IV boluses–reassess)
- Blood transfusion (if appropriate)
- If cause known, institute appropriate intervention (e.g., septic shock, anaphylaxis)
- Consider vasopressors, if indicated, to improve vascular tone if no response to fluid challenge(s)

Note: Aggressive fluid resuscitation is not required for trauma patients with no evidence of hemodynamic compromise. Volume resuscitation in patients with hypovolemic shock should be guided by the type of trauma (penetrating vs. blunt) and by the setting (urban vs. rural). Regardless of the setting, IVs should be established while en route to the emergency department or trauma center. There should be no delay at the scene to establish IV access.

Management of Hypotension/Shock–Suspected Volume Problem

Perform Primary ABCD Survey (Basic Life Support)

(Correct critical problems IMMEDIATELY as they are identified)
- Assess responsiveness, **A**irway, **B**reathing, **C**irculation, ensure availability of monitor/**D**efibrillator

Perform Secondary ABCD Survey (Advanced Life Support)

- Administer oxygen, establish IV access, attach cardiac monitor, administer fluids as needed (O_2, IV, monitor, fluids)
- Assess vital signs, attach pulse oximeter, and monitor blood pressure
- Obtain and review 12-lead ECG, portable chest x-ray,
- Perform a focused history and physical exam

If rate too slow, use bradycardia algorithm

If rate too fast, use appropriate tachycardia algorithm

FIGURE 22-117, cont'd

TABLE 22-9 Symptoms and Signs of Chronic Heart Failure

RIGHT VENTRICULAR DYSFUNCTION		LEFT VENTRICULAR DYSFUNCTION		NONSPECIFIC FINDINGS	
Symptoms	Signs	Symptoms	Signs	Symptoms	Signs
Abdominal pain	Peripheral edema	Dyspnea on exertion	Bibasilar crackles	Exercise intolerance	Tachycardia
Anorexia	Jugular venous distention	Paroxysmal nocturnal dyspnea	Pulmonary edema	Fatigue	Pallor
Nausea	Engorged liver	Orthopnea	S_3 gallop	Weakness	Cyanosis of digits
Bloating	Engorged spleen	Tachypnea	Pleural effusion	Nocturia	Cardiomegaly
Constipation	—	Cough	Chest pain	Central nervous system symptoms	Agitation
Ascites	—	Hemoptysis	Diaphoresis		

However, if right ventricular failure is associated with pulmonary edema or hypotension, it may be a medical emergency. The paramedic should be prepared to manage the patient for either of these situations. Patient management for right ventricular failure includes the following:

1. Placing the patient at rest in a sitting or semi-Fowler position (head elevated)
2. Administering high-concentration oxygen
3. Obtaining baseline vital signs and an ECG tracing
4. Initiating an IV line to keep the vein open or to manage hypotension
5. Monitoring the ECG and oxygen saturation
6. Managing symptoms of left ventricular failure if present

> **NOTE**
> Hypotension caused by right ventricular failure (often seen in right ventricular infarction) can mimic cardiogenic shock. In this case, fluid administration helps normalize left ventricular filling. Administration of fluids is crucial and helps restore a normal blood pressure. (This is just the opposite of the hypotension associated with cardiogenic shock, in which administration of fluids worsens the condition.) Management may include 250 mL IV boluses of normal saline over 5 to 10 minutes. This helps increase myocardial strength (Starling's law). Fluid administration also improves contractility. Close observation of the patient and the vital signs is crucial.

Cardiogenic Shock

Cardiogenic shock is the most extreme form of pump failure. It occurs when left ventricular function is so compromised that the heart cannot meet the metabolic needs of the body. The result is a significant decrease in stroke volume (resulting from ineffective myocardial contraction), cardiac output, and blood pressure. All of these result in an inadequate supply of blood to the organs. Cardiogenic shock occurs in 5% to 10% of patients with acute myocardial infarction. It may be the result of acute left- or right-sided heart failure.

By definition, cardiogenic shock is present when shock persists after correction of existing dysrhythmias, volume deficit, or decreased vascular tone. Cardiogenic shock usually is caused by extensive myocardial infarction (often involving more than 40% of the left ventricle) or by diffuse ischemia. Even with aggressive therapy, cardiogenic shock has a mortality rate of 70% or higher.[22]

In addition to the signs and symptoms of myocardial infarction, patients in cardiogenic shock show clinical evidence of hypoperfusion to vital organs and significant systemic hypotension similar to that found in other forms of shock. (This makes it difficult to determine the exact cause of shock.) This evidence includes the following:

- Acidosis
- Altered level of consciousness
- Cool, clammy, cyanotic, or ashen skin
- Hypoxemia

- Profound hypotension (systolic blood pressure usually less than 80 mm Hg)
- Pulmonary congestion (crackles)
- Sinus tachycardia or other dysrhythmias
- Tachypnea

In the early stages of cardiogenic shock, the patient's heart tries to compensate. The heart rate increases. If possible, the heart also increases contractility and cardiac output. If the condition is managed inadequately, the heart progresses toward hypodynamic failure with depressed contractility, reduced stroke volume, and subsequent hypoperfusion (see Chapter 37).

MANAGEMENT

Patients in cardiogenic shock are ill (see Figure 22-117). These patients need rapid transport to a medical facility. Transport should not be delayed by attempting field treatment. Prehospital care should include airway management and ventilatory support with high-concentration oxygen, placement of the patient in a supine position (or semi-Fowler position, if the patient is dyspneic), insertion of an IV line with normal saline or lactated Ringer solution to keep the vein open, ECG monitoring, correction of dysrhythmias, and frequent evaluation of vital signs (including auscultation of the lungs and observation for jugular venous distention). A patient in respiratory failure may require intubation and ventilatory support.

> **CRITICAL THINKING**
> You have an unstable patient with signs and symptoms indicating cardiogenic shock. How should you respond when the patient asks, "Am I going to die?"

Drug therapy may include drugs that strengthen the force of contraction (inotropic agents) to improve cardiac output. Such agents include **dopamine** or **dobutamine.** The use of vasodilator drugs to reduce afterload generally is reserved for in-hospital coronary care. In such settings, the blood pressure can be evaluated more accurately. If left-sided heart failure and pulmonary edema also are present, they should be treated at the same time.

> **CRITICAL THINKING**
> What dose of each of these drugs should be given for this condition?

Cardiac Tamponade

Cardiac tamponade (described in Chapter 42) is defined as impaired diastolic filling of the heart caused by increased intrapericardial pressure and volume.[20] As the pressure of the buildup in pericardial fluid compresses the atria and ventricles, they are unable to fill adequately. This results in a decrease in ventricular filling, and stroke volume is decreased. The condition may have a gradual onset. This may result from a cancerous growth or infection, or the condition may be acute, resulting from trauma to the chest, including cardiopulmonary resuscitation. Cardiac tamponade also may result from renal disease or hypothyroidism. Signs and symptoms of cardiac tamponade include the following:

- Chest pain
- Decreased systolic pressure (a late sign)
- Ectopy
- ECG changes (usually inconclusive)
- Elevated venous pressure (an early sign) with associated jugular vein distention
- Faint or muffled heart sounds
- Shortness of breath
- Low-voltage QRS complexes and T waves
- Alternating amplitude and vector of P waves, QRS complexes, and T waves (*electrical alternans*)
- Pulsus paradoxus
- ST-segment elevation or nonspecific T-wave changes
- Tachycardia

As described in Chapter 42, the most important reliable signs of cardiac tamponade are elevated venous pressure, hypotension, and distant heart sounds (Beck's triad).

CRITICAL THINKING

Why would fluid resuscitation with large amounts of fluid not be indicated in this situation?

MANAGEMENT

First, the paramedic must obtain a thorough history to attempt to identify the cause of the cardiac tamponade. Then the paramedic should perform a physical examination. Prehospital care is directed at ensuring an adequate airway and ventilatory support and providing rapid transport for evaluation by a physician and possible drainage of the pericardial sac (pericardiocentesis). A fluid bolus may help support the circulatory system temporarily if the patient becomes hypotensive. However, definitive management requires drainage of the pericardial sac. Cardiac tamponade may result in death if the condition is not relieved.

CRITICAL THINKING

Why is drainage of the pericardial sac not done routinely in the prehospital setting?

Thoracic and Abdominal Aortic Aneurysms

Aneurysm is a nonspecific term that means "dilation of a vessel." An aneurysm may result from atherosclerotic disease (most common), infectious disease (primarily syphilis), traumatic injury, or certain genetic disorders (e.g., Marfan syndrome). Figure 22-118 shows the branches of the aorta. Abdominal aortic aneurysm and dissecting aneurysm of the aorta are presented here.

Most aneurysms develop at a weak point in the wall of an artery. This weak point results from degenerative changes in the medial layer. Weakening of the supportive elements of the vessel wall allows dilation. This causes turbulence and increasing lateral pressure. The aneurysm tends to enlarge over time as the lateral pressure increases in the dilated segment. Eventually the aneurysm may rupture. This, in turn, may produce life-threatening hemorrhage.

ABDOMINAL AORTIC ANEURYSM

Abdominal aortic aneurysm affects about 2% of the population.[22] The most common site for an abdominal aortic aneurysm is below the renal arteries and above the branching of the common iliac arteries. Abdominal aortic aneurysms are 10 times more common in men. They also are most prevalent between the ages of 60 and 70 years. An abdominal aneurysm usually is asymptomatic as long as it is stable. However, if the aneurysm begins to expand or leak, symptoms indicate impending rupture (Box 22-20).

Rupture of an abdominal aortic aneurysm may begin with a small tear in the intima. This small tear allows blood to leak into the wall of the aorta. As the process continues with increasing pressure, the tear may extend through the outer layer of the vessel. The tear then may cause bleeding into the retroperitoneal space. If bleeding is tamponaded by the retroperitoneal tissues, the patient may be normotensive on the arrival of emergency medical services. If the rupture opens into the peritoneal cavity, however, massive fatal hemorrhage may follow. In either case, major blood loss results, and hypovolemic shock ensues.

Often a patient with a rupturing aneurysm has syncope followed by hypotension with bradycardia despite the loss of a large amount of blood. The reason for bradycardia is stimulation of the vagus nerve. Fibers of the vagus nerve wrap around the aorta. When the aorta tears, the tear stretches these fibers, causing bradycardia. The bradycardia is present despite the hemorrhagic shock condition, which usually causes hypotension and tachycardia in the patient.

Management. Patients with a leaking or ruptured abdominal aneurysm appear ill. They usually need immediate surgery to repair the vessel. In 20% of patients with a leaking abdominal aortic aneurysm, the aneurysm ruptures before the patient reaches the hospital, and 80% of these patients die.[23] Therefore early recognition and rapid transport can prevent the death of these patients.

In most cases prehospital care should be limited to gentle handling, oxygen administration, cardiac monitoring (myocardial infarctions may be associated with advanced aneurysms), initiation of volume-expanding IV fluids en route to the receiving hospital, and alerting the receiving facility to prepare for imminent surgery.

Pulsatile masses (if present) are fragile and in most cases are membrane thin. The paramedic should avoid aggressive examination or deep palpation of the mass. Palpation may cause the mass to rupture. Examination, if needed, can be

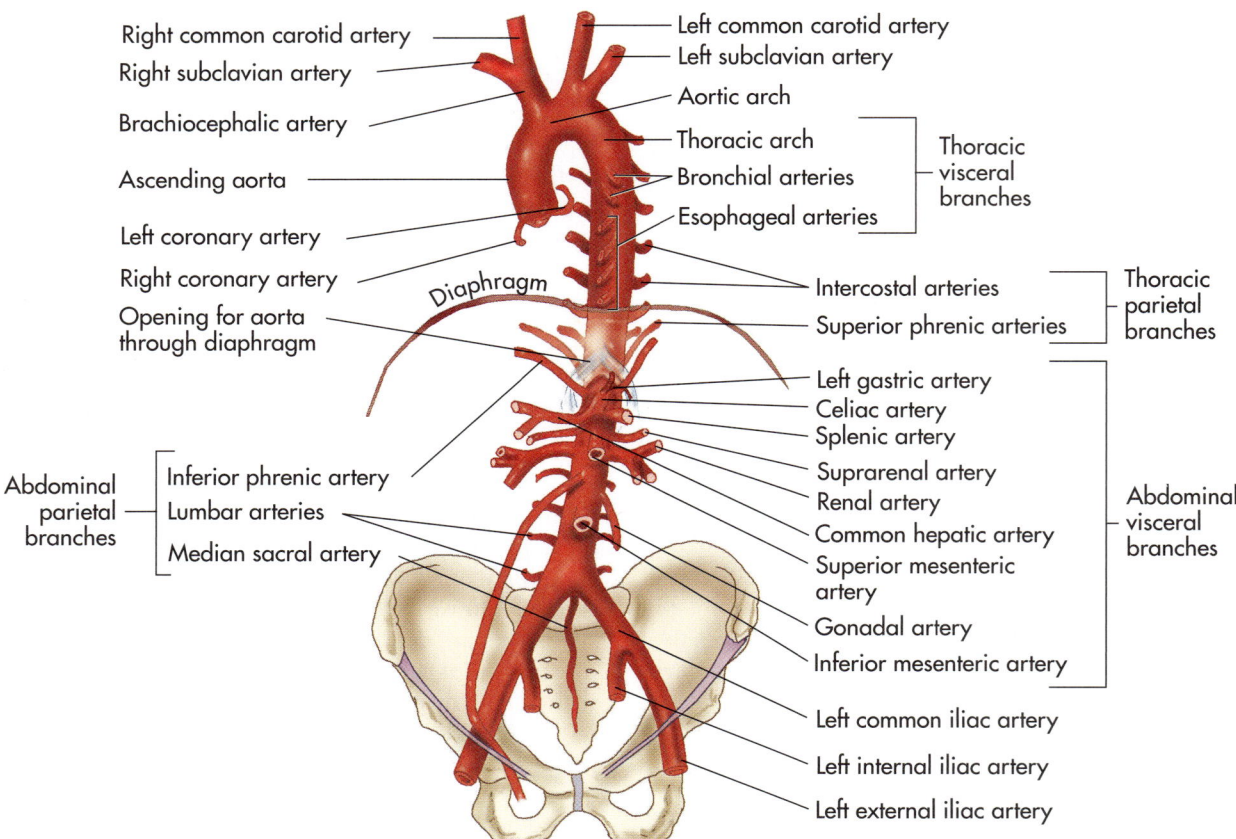

Right common carotid artery
Right subclavian artery
Brachiocephalic artery
Ascending aorta
Left coronary artery
Right coronary artery
Opening for aorta through diaphragm

Left common carotid artery
Left subclavian artery
Aortic arch
Thoracic arch
Bronchial arteries
Esophageal arteries
} Thoracic visceral branches

Diaphragm

Intercostal arteries
Superior phrenic arteries
} Thoracic parietal branches

Abdominal parietal branches {
Inferior phrenic artery
Lumbar arteries
Median sacral artery

Left gastric artery
Celiac artery
Splenic artery
Suprarenal artery
Renal artery
Common hepatic artery
Superior mesenteric artery
Gonadal artery
Inferior mesenteric artery
} Abdominal visceral branches

Left common iliac artery
Left internal iliac artery
Left external iliac artery

FIGURE 22-118 Branches of the aorta. Aortic arch, thoracic aorta, abdominal aorta, and their branches.

BOX 22-20 Signs and Symptoms of a Leaking or Ruptured Abdominal Aortic Aneurysm

- Unexplained hypotension (resulting from hemorrhage or a compensatory vasovagal response mechanism)
- Unexplained syncope (as the aneurysm ruptures, blood pressure drops transiently to zero, producing sudden cerebral hypoperfusion and syncope)
- Sudden onset of abdominal or back pain (described as "tearing" or "ripping") from the physical trauma itself or from inflammation
- Low back or flank pain (radiating to the thigh, groin, testicle, or perineum) that is unrelieved by rest or changes in position
- Signs of peritoneal irritation
- Urge to defecate (caused by retroperitoneal leakage of blood)
- Pulsatile, tender mass (may be palpated when greater than 5 cm), usually located above the umbilicus, left of the midline
- Presence or absence of distal pulses (femoral artery and below), depending on the patient's blood pressure, the occurrence of a dissection, and the degree of peripheral vascular disease
- Possible presentation as bleeding in the gastrointestinal tract if the aneurysm erodes into it

made by auscultation. This may reveal a sound similar to that of a systolic murmur or bruit.

The management of hypotension varies and depends on whether the aneurysm is leaking or ruptured. A patient suspected of having a leaking aneurysm can be maintained with mildly hypotensive blood pressure to try to prevent rupture during transport. (The hypotension associated with small leaks is thought to result from a compensatory vasovagal mechanism.) In these patients, fluid resuscitation should be minimal and less aggressive than in patients who have a ruptured aneurysm.

If rupture has occurred, hypotension, tachycardia, and loss of the pulsating mass may develop suddenly. The patient also may become unresponsive. This often is followed by full cardiac and respiratory arrest. These patients require rapid and aggressive resuscitation (intubation, ventilation, fluid replacement) and rapid transport for surgery.

ACUTE DISSECTING AORTIC ANEURYSM

Acute dissecting aortic aneurysm (separation of the arterial wall) is the most common aortic catastrophe. It affects 5 to 10 people per 1 million population each year (three times as many as a ruptured abdominal aortic aneurysm).[24] Factors that can lead to the development of dissecting aneurysm are systemic hypertension, atherosclerosis, congenital abnormalities that affect connective tissue (*Marfan* *syndrome),* degenerative changes in the connective tissue of the aortic media *(cystic medial necrosis),* trauma, and pregnancy. The syndrome affects men twice as often as women. It also is more common in African Americans.

A dissecting aneurysm of the aorta results from a small tear in the intimal layer of the vessel wall (Figure 22-119). After the tear, the process of dissection begins. The tear in the inner wall allows blood to move between the inner and outer layers. This creates a false passage between the layers of the vessel wall. Blood that enters the false passage results in the formation of a hematoma. As a result, this can rupture through the outer wall (adventitia) at any time, usually into the pericardial or pleural cavity.

Any area of the aorta may be involved. However, in most cases the dissecting aneurysm occurs in the ascending

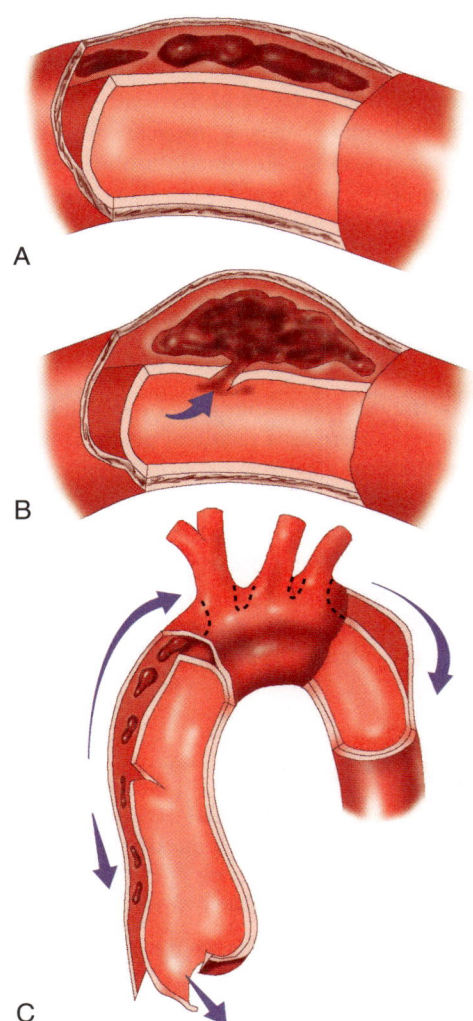

FIGURE 22-119 Pathogenesis of a dissecting aneurysm. **A,** Medial and intimal degeneration of the aortic wall sets the stage. **B,** Hemodynamic forces acting on the aortic wall produce an intimal tear, directing the bloodstream into the middle layer of the wall of the aorta. **C,** The resulting dissecting hematoma is propagated in both directions by a pulse wave produced by each myocardial contraction.

aorta. Once begun, the aneurysm may extend distally or proximally to involve all of the thoracic and abdominal aorta and tributaries, the coronary arteries, the aortic valve, and the carotid and subclavian vessels. Blood flow is reduced in any vessels bypassed by the dissection, including the carotid and other aortic arch vessels. As a result, aortic dissection may cause the following:

- Syncope
- Stroke
- Absent or reduced pulses
- Unequal blood pressure readings (right side compared to left side)
- Heart failure resulting from sudden aortic valve regurgitation
- Pericardial tamponade
- Acute myocardial infarction

Signs and Symptoms. The signs and symptoms of a dissecting aortic aneurysm depend on the site of the intimal tear (ascending or descending aorta). They also depend on the extent of dissection. More than 70% of patients with acute dissecting aneurysm of the aorta complain of severe pain in the back, epigastrium, abdomen, or extremities. They often describe this pain as the most intense pain they have ever experienced. The pain usually is sudden in onset. It may be characterized by the patient as "ripping," "tearing," or "sharp and cutting, like a knife." Pain often originates in the back (between the scapulae). The pain possibly extends down into the legs. A patient with acute dissection may appear "shocky" and have pallor, sweating, and peripheral cyanosis (from impaired perfusion), even when the blood pressure is normal or elevated. If the patient is hypotensive, the paramedic should suspect cardiac tamponade or aortic rupture.

CRITICAL THINKING
What condition has signs and symptoms similar to those of an abdominal aortic aneurysm?

Differentiating the pain of aortic dissection from that of myocardial infarction or pulmonary embolism can be difficult in the prehospital setting. The following distinctive features may help:

1. The severity of the pain is maximal from the onset (compared with the crescendo pain characteristic of acute myocardial infarction).
2. The pain may migrate from the anterior portion of the chest or interscapular area downward as dissection progresses.
3. Significant differences in blood pressure occur between the left and right arm or between the arms and the legs.
4. The peripheral pulses are unequal.
5. Neurological deficits result from occlusion of a cerebral vessel.

NOTE
Blood pressure may differ significantly in the two arms if the dissection occludes either subclavian artery, leading to a decreased blood pressure in the affected upper extremity.

Management. The goals of managing suspected aortic dissection in the prehospital setting are relieving pain and rapid transport to a medical facility. (Transport should not be delayed; analgesics should be administered en route to the hospital.) The EMS crew should be ready to initiate intubation. They also should be ready to assist ventilation in case the patient begins to decompensate. Other prehospital care measures include the following:

- Handling the patient gently
- Reducing anxiety
- Administering high-concentration oxygen
- Beginning a large-bore IV line of crystalloid solution (fluids should be kept to a minimum unless severe hypotension is present)
- Giving analgesia (e.g., *morphine* or *fentanyl*) per medical direction if the diagnosis is strongly suspected

Definitive in-hospital care generally includes reducing the myocardial contractile force to stop progressive dissection (with antihypertensives and beta blockers), monitoring of intraarterial pressure, and possibly surgical repair.

Acute Arterial Occlusion

Acute arterial occlusion is a sudden blockage of arterial flow. It most commonly is caused by trauma, embolus, or thrombosis. The severity of the ischemic episode depends on the site of occlusion and the extent of collateral circulation around the blockage. Vascular occlusion caused by thrombosis is a complication of atherosclerosis. Occlusions caused by emboli may indicate an abnormal cardiac rhythm, particularly atrial fibrillation.

CRITICAL THINKING
Why does atrial fibrillation put the patient at increased risk for emboli?

Arterial occlusion may follow blunt or penetrating trauma; it often is associated with long-bone fractures. These injuries vary from injuries to the lining of a vessel to complete severing of a vessel. The occlusion usually is evident because no signs of circulation are seen in the tissue or limb.

An embolism occurs when a blood clot breaks away and enters the arterial system. The clot travels until it reaches a narrow point in a vessel. This often is at a branching site of an artery. Ninety percent of peripheral emboli originate in the heart. Therefore, a history of cardiac disease (e.g.,

dysrhythmia, myocardial infarction, or valvular heart disease) favors a diagnosis of embolic occlusion, particularly if the patient has an asymptomatic opposite extremity with normal pulses. The most common sites of embolic occlusion are the abdominal aorta, common femoral artery, popliteal artery, carotid artery, brachial artery, and mesenteric artery (Figure 22-120).

Thrombosis usually results from atherosclerotic disease and usually occurs at a site of severe narrowing of a vessel. Unlike an embolus, a thrombus usually develops over time. As the thrombus enlarges, the collateral blood supply also can become occluded, causing progressive ischemia. The location of the ischemic pain often is related to the site of occlusion:

- Terminal portion of the abdominal aorta: Pain in both hips or lower limbs
- Iliac artery: Pain in the buttocks or hip on the involved side
- Femoral artery: Claudication (cramplike pain) in the calf of the involved leg
- Mesenteric artery: Severe abdominal pain

If severe ischemia persists, muscle necrosis occurs. Thrombotic occlusion is seen most often in men, smokers, and those over 60 years of age. Common sites of atherosclerotic (thrombotic) occlusion are depicted in Figure 22-121.

SIGNS AND SYMPTOMS

Regardless of the origin of the occlusion, the signs and symptoms of ischemia are the same and include the following:

- Pain in the extremity that may be severe and sudden in onset or absent as a result of paresthesia
- Pallor (the skin also may be mottled or cyanotic)
- Lowered skin temperature distal to the occlusion
- Changes in sensory and motor function
- Diminished or absent pulse distal to the injury
- Bruit over the affected vessel
- Slow capillary filling
- Sometimes shock (particularly with mesenteric occlusion)

NOTE
Some patients with vascular occlusion have unequal blood pressure readings in the arms. Systolic readings in the arms that differ by 15 mm Hg or more suggest vascular disease. (Normally, the difference between the arms is 5 to 10 mm Hg.)

MANAGEMENT

Acute arterial occlusion in an extremity is serious and painful. The occlusion may be limb-threatening if blood flow is not reestablished within 4 to 8 hours. The affected limb should be immobilized and protected. In addition, the patient should be transported for evaluation by a physician. Patients with mesenteric occlusion should be managed for

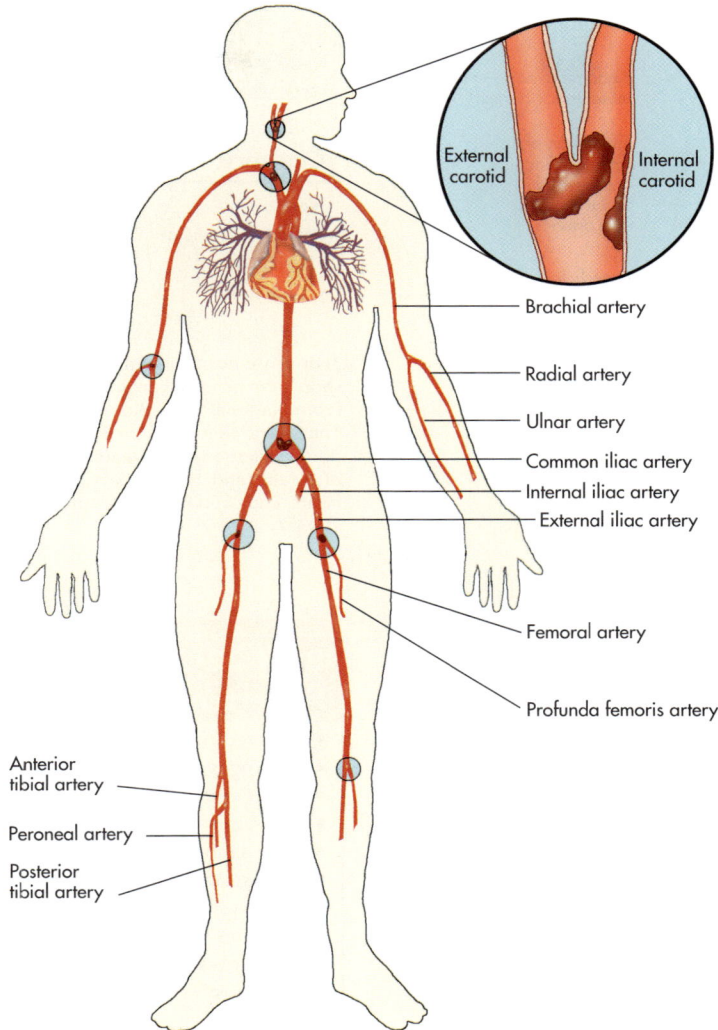

FIGURE 22-120 Common sites of embolic arterial occlusion.

shock with oxygen and IV fluids. Analgesics also may be prescribed by medical direction to relieve pain. In-hospital, definitive care may include anticoagulant or fibrinolytic therapy, transluminal arterial dilation using a balloon catheter, embolectomy, or vascular reconstruction.

Noncritical Peripheral Vascular Conditions

Noncritical peripheral vascular conditions include varicose veins, superficial thrombophlebitis (described in Chapter 11), and acute deep vein thrombosis. Of these conditions, deep vein thrombosis is the only one that can cause life-threatening pulmonary embolus. Predisposing factors to venous thrombosis include the following:

- Birth control pills
- Coagulopathies
- History of trauma
- Malignancy
- Obesity
- Pregnancy
- Recent immobilization (e.g., leg fracture)
- Sepsis
- Smoking
- Stasis or inactivity (e.g., bedridden patient or long air flights)
- Varicose veins (usually a benign condition)

ACUTE DEEP VEIN THROMBOSIS

Acute deep vein thrombosis (DVT) is a serious, common problem. Occlusion may involve any portion of the deep venous system. However, occlusion is much more common in the lower extremities. Risk factors for deep vein thrombosis include recent lower extremity trauma, recent surgery, advanced age, recent myocardial infarction, inactivity, confinement to bed, congestive heart failure, cancer, previous thrombosis, oral contraceptive therapy, sickle cell disease, and obesity. Signs and symptoms of acute deep vein thrombosis include the following:

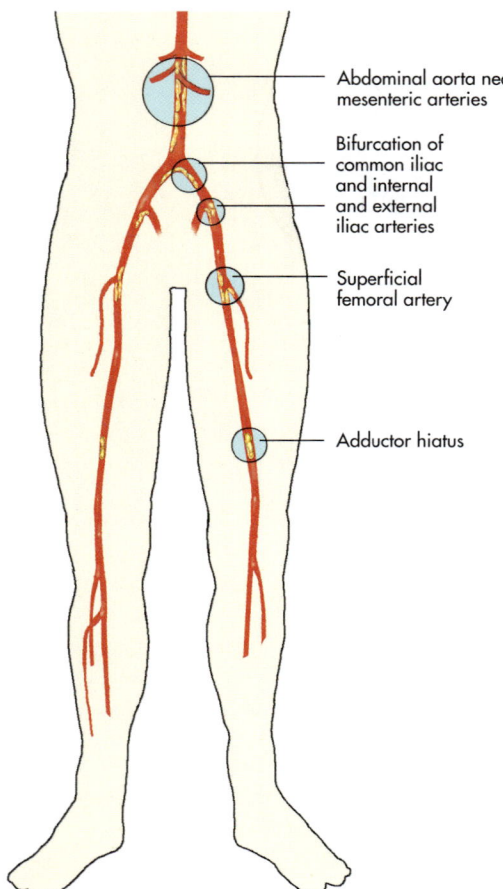

FIGURE 22-121 Common sites of atherosclerotic occlusive disease.

Abdominal aorta near mesenteric arteries

Bifurcation of common iliac and internal and external iliac arteries

Superficial femoral artery

Adductor hiatus

- Pain
- Edema
- Warmth
- Erythema or bluish discoloration
- Tenderness

MANAGEMENT

Patients with acute deep vein thrombosis require hospitalization. Prehospital care usually is limited to immobilization and elevation of the extremity and transport for evaluation by a physician. Deep vein thrombosis in the calf of the leg usually is much less serious than deep vein thrombosis of the thigh. The latter has a higher incidence of associated pulmonary embolus. Definitive care includes bed rest, administration of anticoagulants or, occasionally, fibrinolytic agents, and in rare cases, thrombectomy.

Hypertension

Hypertension is a common disorder. It afflicts about 23% of the U.S. population and is directly responsible for about 23,000 deaths a year.[25] Hypertension often is defined by a resting blood pressure consistently greater than 140/90 mm

TABLE 22-10 Blood Pressure Categories for Adults (18 Years or Older)*

Category	BLOOD PRESSURE (mm Hg) Systolic		Diastolic
Normal	<120	and	<80
Prehypertension	120-139	or	80-89
Hypertension			
Stage 1	140-159	or	90-99
Stage 2	>160		>100

*For those not taking medicine for high blood pressure and not having a short-term serious illness.
From National High Blood Pressure Education Program, JNC 7 Express, The Seventh Report of the Joint National Committee on Prevention, Detection, Evaluation, and Treatment of High Blood Pressure, U.S. Department of Health and Human Services, National Institutes of Health, National Heart, Lung and Blood Institute, NIH Publication No. 03-5233, December 2003.

BOX 22-21 Signs and Symptoms of Hypertensive Emergencies

- Altered mental status
- Changes in visual acuity
- ECG changes
- Epistaxis
- Headache
- Nausea and vomiting
- Paroxysmal nocturnal dyspnea
- Seizures
- Shortness of breath
- Tinnitus
- Vertigo

Hg (stage 1 hypertension).[26] The several categories of hypertension are based on the level of blood pressure, symptomatology, and urgency of need for intervention (Table 22-10 and Box 22-21). For the purpose of this textbook, two general categories are presented: chronic hypertension and hypertensive emergencies. (These emergencies include **hypertensive encephalopathy**.) A common cause of hypertension is discontinuing medication or other therapy prescribed by the physician.

CRITICAL THINKING
Why do patients fail to take medicines prescribed for hypertension?

CHRONIC HYPERTENSION

Chronic hypertension has an adverse effect on the function of the heart and blood vessels. It requires the heart to perform more work than normal. This leads to hypertrophy of the cardiac muscle and left ventricular failure. Chronic hypertension increases the rate at which atherosclerosis develops. This in turn increases the probability of cardiovascular, cerebrovascular, and peripheral vascular disease and the risk of aneurysm formation. Along with congestive heart failure (CHF), conditions commonly associated with chronic, uncontrolled hypertension are cerebral hemorrhage and stroke, myocardial infarction, renal failure (caused by vascular changes in the kidney), and development of thoracic or abdominal aortic aneurysm.

Many people with established hypertension have elevated peripheral resistance and elevated cardiac output (a function of Starling's law), the result of an increase in the heart rate and stroke volume.[22] The heart responds to the increased workload that results from high peripheral resistance by becoming enlarged. An enlarged heart may be able to work fine for many years. In time, though, it is no longer able to maintain adequate blood flow. The patient then develops symptoms of pump failure.

Any hypertension-related illness, such as pulmonary edema, dissecting aortic aneurysm, toxemia of pregnancy (described in Chapter 46), or stroke, requires stabilization and prompt, appropriate management. The hypertension associated with these situations often is a result of a primary problem. Managing the primary problem (e.g., toxemia) often makes controlling the patient's blood pressure easier. However, the primary cause may not be easily correctable. In situations such as dissecting aortic aneurysm, controlling the blood pressure also is a key to managing the primary problem. A life-threatening condition that develops from unmanaged or partially managed hypertension may lead to a hypertensive emergency.

HYPERTENSIVE EMERGENCIES

Hypertensive emergencies are conditions in which an increase in blood pressure leads to significant, irreversible damage to organs. This damage can occur within hours if the hypertension is not treated. The organs most likely to be at risk are the brain, heart, and kidneys. This now uncommon condition is experienced by 1% of all hypertensive patients whose illness is poorly controlled or unmanaged. As a rule, the diagnosis is based on loss of organ function. The diagnosis also is based on the rate of the rise in blood pressure, not the level of blood pressure (although the diastolic blood pressure usually is greater than 100 mm Hg). All hypertensive emergencies (except hypertension in ischemic stroke) require a 5% to 20% reduction in blood pressure within a few hours of discovery to prevent permanent organ damage. In hypertensive emergencies, blood pressure readings ranging from 220/120 mm Hg to 240/140 mm Hg are not uncommon.

Hypertensive emergencies include the following clinical conditions: (1) myocardial ischemia with hypertension, (2) aortic dissection with hypertension, (3) pulmonary edema with hypertension, (4) hypertensive intracranial hemorrhage, (5) toxemia, and (6) hypertensive encephalopathy. Hypertension per se may not be the cause of the first five

conditions. However, they all can be worsened by untreated hypertension. Hypertensive encephalopathy results solely from elevated blood pressure and a concurrently elevated intracranial pressure.

Persistent hypertension causes brain damage (hypertensive encephalopathy). It results in a decrease in blood and oxygen to the brain (cerebral hypoperfusion). It also damages the tissues that make up the blood-brain barrier. This results in fluid exudation into the brain tissue. Hypertensive encephalopathy may progress over several hours from initial symptoms of severe headache, nausea, vomiting, aphasia, and transient blindness to seizures, stupor, coma, and death. The condition is a true emergency. It requires immediate transport to a medical facility for definitive care. The goal of therapy is controlled but rapid lowering of the blood pressure to normalize cerebral blood flow. If the blood pressure is lowered too quickly, infarction of end organs (heart, kidney, brain) may occur.

NOTE
Lateralizing neurologic signs, such as hemiparesis or hemiplegia, are uncommon in hypertensive emergencies. Their presence is suggestive of stroke.[27]

CRITICAL THINKING
How does fluid leakage into the brain affect the intracranial pressure and cerebral perfusion pressure?

Prehospital management of patients with a hypertensive emergency includes the following:

- Supportive care
- Calming the patient
- Oxygen therapy
- IV line to keep the vein open
- ECG monitoring
- Rapid transport

In most cases, drug therapy for hypertensive emergencies is not initiated in the prehospital setting. However, in severe cases of hypertensive encephalopathy or if transport is delayed, medical direction may recommend the administration of antihypertensives such as **nitroglycerin** or **labetalol**. These drugs induce arteriolar vasodilation and may lower the blood pressure.

SPECIFIC HEART DISEASES

In addition to atherosclerosis that results in coronary artery disease, numerous other diseases affect the heart. These include valvular heart disease, infectious heart disease, and congenital heart disease (see Chapter 47).

Valvular Heart Disease

Valvular heart disease refers to any disease process that affects one or more valves of the heart: the mitral, aortic, tricuspid, or pulmonary valves. To review, the mitral and tricuspid valves control the flow of blood between the atria and the ventricles (the upper and lower chambers of the heart). The pulmonary valve controls the flow of blood from the heart to the lungs, and the aortic valve governs blood flow between the heart and the aorta and thereby the blood vessels to the rest of the body. (The mitral and aortic valves are the valves most frequently affected by valvular heart disease.) When one or more of these valves become narrowed, hardened, or thickened (stenotic), the valves do not open or close completely. As a result, blood does not flow with proper force or direction. A stenotic valve forces blood back up into the adjacent chamber of the heart. A valve that is unable to close properly allows blood to "leak" back (regurgitate) into the previous chamber (Figure 22-122). The defects in the pumping action of the valves can cause the heart to enlarge and thicken. This can result in a loss of elasticity and an increased risk of pulmonary embolism or stroke.

> **NOTE**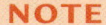
> Valve leaflets normally are very thin and flexible. However, they can become thickened, rigid, or dysfunctional in response to a disease process, such as coronary artery disease or cardiac hypertrophy. Stenosis often is accompanied by calcification and atherosclerosis-type lesions (valvular lesion).

Valvular heart disease can be congenital (described later in this chapter). It also can develop slowly, or it may be acute. Depending on the course of the disease, signs and symptoms may be similar to those seen in congestive heart failure. These may include palpitations with or without chest pain, fatigue, dizziness or syncope, and weight gain. If the cause of the valvular heart disease is a bacterial infection (e.g., endocarditis, described later), fever may be present. After evaluation by a physician, treatment may include antibiotics to manage infection, anticoagulants to prevent clot formation, balloon dilation to widen a stenotic valve, clip insertion (MitraClip, not yet approved in the United States), and sometimes surgical valve replacement. Prehospital care is primarily supportive and may include oxygen administration, ECG monitoring, IV fluids, and transport for evaluation by a physician.

Infectious Heart Disease

Infectious heart disease is caused by intravascular contamination by pathogens. The infections can damage the muscles and valves of the heart. Infections also may lead to the formation of emboli, which can travel to the brain, kidneys, lungs, or abdomen. Three common forms of infectious heart disease are endocarditis, pericarditis, and myocarditis. Most patients with infectious heart disease also have underlying heart disease or problems with the heart valves. Prehospital care for infectious heart disease is primarily supportive.

A. NORMAL VALVE

Blood flows freely forward   No backflow of blood

B. STENOSIS

Less blood flows through   No backflow of blood
narrowed opening

C. INCOMPETENT VALVE

Blood flows freely forward   Blood regurgitates
                                 backward through
                                 "leaky" valve

D. EFFECT OF AORTIC STENOSIS

4. Incomplete atrial emptying

3. Decreased cardiac output

1. Narrowing of aortic valve limits blood leaving the ventricle

2. Left ventricular hypertrophy

FIGURE 22-122 Effects of heart valve defects. (Gould BE, Dyer R: *Pathophysiology for health professions*, ed 4, St Louis, 2010, Saunders.)

> **NOTE**
> Rheumatic fever can lead to inflammation of the heart (carditis) and damage to the heart valves (rheumatic heart disease). Rheumatic fever follows infection by group A *Streptococcus* (GAS) bacteria, such as strep throat or scarlet fever. Proper diagnosis and adequate antibiotic treatment of GAS infections can prevent acute rheumatic fever in most cases. Most patients with a GAS infection respond well to antibiotic therapy.[28]

ENDOCARDITIS

Endocarditis is an infection of the endocardium (inner layer of the heart). Endocarditis usually results from a bacterium that enters the bloodstream (bacterial or infective endocarditis). Risk factors for developing endocarditis include injection drug use, permanent central venous access lines, previous valve surgery, recent dental surgery, and weakened heart valves. Patients with a history of valvular heart disease or rheumatic fever also are at higher risk for endocarditis. Complications of the disease include atrial fibrillation, blood clots, brain abscess, CNS changes, congestive heart failure, glomerulonephritis, jaundice, severe heart valve damage, and stroke.

> **NOTE**
>
> *Streptococcus viridans*, a bacterium commonly found in the mouth, is responsible for about 50% of all cases of bacterial endocarditis.[29] For this reason, prophylactic antibiotics often are prescribed for high-risk patients undergoing dental procedures or surgery involving the respiratory, urinary, or intestinal tract.

Endocarditis may develop slowly or may be sudden in onset. Signs and symptoms include:

- Abnormal urine color
- Chills (common)
- Excessive sweating (common)
- Fatigue
- Fever (common)
- Joint pain
- Muscle aches and pains
- Night sweats
- Nail abnormalities (splinter hemorrhages under the nails)
- Paleness
- Red, painless skin spots on the palms and soles *(Janeway lesions)*
- Red, painful nodes in the pads of the fingers and toes *(Osler's nodes)*
- Shortness of breath with activity
- Swelling of the feet, legs, abdomen
- Weakness
- Weight loss

Treatment consists of blood cultures to identify the bacterium causing the disease, short-term IV antibiotics, and several weeks of oral antibiotic therapy. Valve replacement surgery may be indicated in some cases.

PERICARDITIS

Pericarditis is inflammation of the pericardium (the fibrous sac surrounding the heart). It usually is a complication of viral infection, most commonly echovirus, adenovirus, or Coxsackie virus. Less frequently, it is caused by the influenza virus or infection with the human immunodeficiency virus (HIV). Pericarditis is most common in men 20 to 50 years of age and in children after a respiratory infection. Pericarditis can be associated with diseases such as autoimmune disorders, cancer (including leukemia), acquired immunodeficiency syndrome (AIDS),

hypothyroidism, kidney failure, rheumatic fever, and tuberculosis. Although the cause of the pericarditis often is unknown *(idiopathic pericarditis)*, possible causes include myocardial infarction *(post-MI pericarditis)*; injury, including surgery or trauma to the chest, esophagus, or heart; medications that suppress the immune system; myocarditis; and radiation therapy to the chest.[30] Signs and symptoms include the following:

- Swelling of the ankles, feet, and legs (occasionally)
- Anxiety
- Difficulty breathing when lying down
  - Crackles
  - Decreased breath sounds
- Chest pain caused by the inflamed pericardium rubbing against the heart
  - May radiate to the neck, shoulder, back, or abdomen
  - Often increases with deep breathing and lying flat; may increase with coughing and swallowing
  - Pleuritic chest pain (often relieved by sitting up and leaning forward)
- Pericardial friction rub
- Dry cough
- Fatigue
- Fever
- 12-lead ECG changes
  - Diffuse ST elevation
  - PR segment depression
  - Notched J point

> **NOTE**
>
> These 12-lead ECG changes are one of the "MI imposters." Pericarditis often can be distinguished from AMI in the prehospital setting by obtaining a good patient history and by noting ST elevation in all leads.[31]

Pericarditis is assessed with diagnostic imaging (chest radiograph, magnetic resonance imaging [MRI], computed tomography [CT]), blood and fluid cultures, and other laboratory tests. An ECG and echocardiogram also may be useful for ruling out myocardial infarction and enlargement of the heart. Pericarditis is managed with analgesics, antibiotics, nonsteroidal antiinflammatory drugs (NSAIDs), corticosteroids, and diuretics. With decreased cardiac function or cardiac tamponade, pericardiocentesis may be needed. Most patients recover completely within 2 to 3 months. However, the condition may recur.

MYOCARDITIS

Myocarditis is inflammation of the heart muscle. It is an uncommon disorder caused by a viral, bacterial, or fungal infection that reaches the heart. (Myocarditis also can be caused by chemical exposure, allergic reactions, or an inflammatory disease, such as rheumatoid arthritis or sarcoidosis.) The immune response associated with myocarditis can damage the heart muscle. This can cause the heart to become thick, swollen, and weak, leading to symptoms of heart failure. Some patients with myocarditis are asymptomatic. In other patients, signs and symptoms that may occur with the disease include the following:

- Abnormal heartbeat, sometimes leading to syncope
- Chest pain that may be severe
- Fever and other signs of infection (headache, muscle aches, sore throat, diarrhea, rashes)
- Joint pain or swelling
- Leg swelling
- Shortness of breath
- Decreased urine output

Myocarditis is diagnosed and managed similarly to pericarditis (described previously). If the heart muscle has been damaged, the patient may need to be treated for heart failure. Dysrhythmias may need to be managed with antidysrhythmics and insertion of a pacemaker or an implantable cardioverter-defibrillator. If a blood clot has formed in the heart chamber, anticoagulants may be prescribed. Depending on the severity of the damage to the heart, the patient may recover completely or may have permanent heart failure.

CARDIOMYOPATHY

Cardiomyopathy is a weakening of the heart muscle or a change in heart muscle structure. It often is associated with inadequate heart pumping or other heart function problems. Common causes of the disease are alcoholism and cocaine use, chemotherapy drugs, pregnancy, genetic defects, amyloidosis, end-stage kidney disease, viral infection, long-term hypertension, nutritional deficiencies, and lupus. Cardiomyopathy can be classified into three main types[32]:

- *Dilated cardiomyopathy* (the most common type) is a condition in which the heart becomes weakened and enlarged. It cannot pump blood efficiently. Many different medical problems can cause this type of cardiomyopathy, including coronary artery disease, rheumatoid arthritis, muscular dystrophy, and HIV infection.
- *Restrictive cardiomyopathy* refers to a group of disorders in which the heart chambers are unable to properly fill with blood because of stiffness of the heart. The most common causes of restrictive cardiomyopathy are **amyloidosis** (deposits of abnormal protein in heart tissue) and scarring of the heart muscle. This type of cardiomyopathy frequently occurs after a heart transplant.
- *Hypertrophic cardiomyopathy (HCM)* is a condition in which parts of the heart muscle become thicker than other parts. This thickening makes it more difficult for blood to leave the heart and forces the heart to work harder to pump blood. This type of cardiomyopathy is inherited. The first symptom of the disease among many young patients is sudden collapse, and possibly death, caused by dysrhythmias.

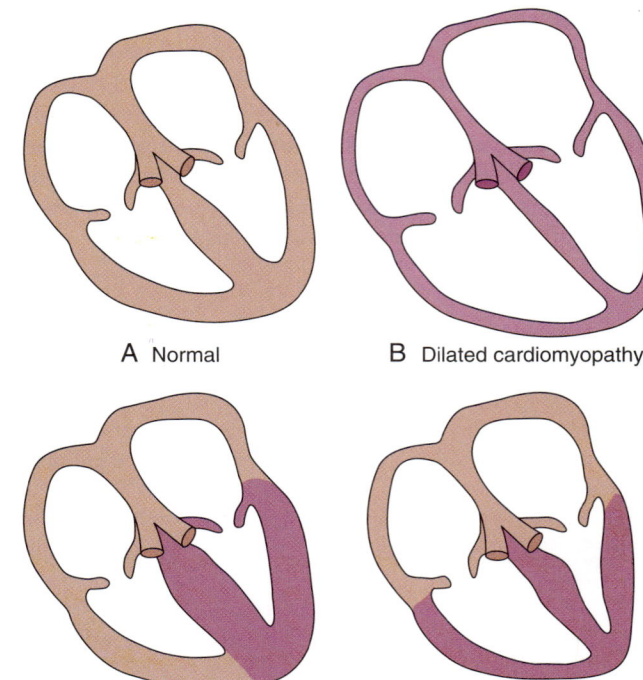

A Normal   B Dilated cardiomyopathy

C Hypertrophic cardiomyopathy   D Restrictive cardiomyopathy

FIGURE 22-123 The three types of cardiomyopathy. **A,** Normal heart. **B,** Dilated cardiomyopathy demonstrating enlargement of all four chambers. **C,** Hypertrophic cardiomyopathy showing a thickened left ventricle. **D,** Restrictive cardiomyopathy characterized by a small left ventricular volume. (Copstead-Kirkhorn LE, Banasik JL: *Pathophysiology,* ed 4, St Louis, 2010, Saunders.)

Hypertrophic cardiomyopathy is a major cause of death in young athletes who seem completely healthy but who die during heavy exercise (Figure 22-123).[33]

Signs and Symptoms

Some patients with cardiomyopathy have no signs and symptoms in the early stage of the disease. However, as the disease progresses, signs and symptoms usually appear. These may include:

- Breathlessness with exertion or even at rest
- Swelling of the legs, ankles, and feet
- Bloating (distention) of the abdomen with fluid
- Fatigue
- Irregular heartbeats that feel rapid, pounding, or fluttering
- Dizziness, lightheadedness, and fainting

The treatment of cardiomyopathy is based on the patient's age and general health and the specific type and severity of the disease. Drugs often are prescribed to improve heart function and to prevent clot formation and fluid retention. These drugs include vasodilators, digitalis, angiotensin-converting enzyme (ACE) inhibitors, anticoagulants, and diuretics. Dilated cardiomyopathies usually respond well to medication, at least initially. Treatment of some cardiomyopathies that result from viral infections may not be effective. Therapy for those with restrictive cardiomyopathy may be particularly limited. If end-stage heart failure develops, a heart transplant may be necessary.

This section addresses the various procedures, techniques, and types of equipment used to manage cardiac emergencies. These include basic life support, mechanical cardiopulmonary resuscitation devices, monitor-defibrillators (manual, fully automated, and semiautomated), defibrillation, automatic implantable cardioverter-defibrillators, synchronized cardioversion, and transcutaneous cardiac pacing. This section also offers an overview of the management of a cardiac arrest as it applies to working within an advanced cardiac life support system. The reader is encouraged to review the dysrhythmias and drug therapy presented previously in this text.

BASIC CARDIAC LIFE SUPPORT

Basic cardiac life support (BCLS) provides circulation and respiration for a victim of cardiac arrest until advanced cardiac life support (ACLS) is available. The American Heart Association has stated:

> The highest hospital discharge rate—a measure of resuscitation success—is achieved in patients for whom CPR is initiated within 4 minutes of the time of the arrest and who, in addition, are provided with ACLS management within 8 minutes of their arrest. The victim whose heart and breathing have stopped for less than 4 minutes has an excellent chance for recovery if CPR is administered immediately. After 4 to 6 minutes without circulation, brain damage may occur; after 6 minutes brain damage will almost always occur.[34]

Cardiac arrest most often is associated with cardiovascular disease and is precipitated by ventricular fibrillation or ventricular asystole. Cardiac arrest also may result from noncardiac causes, such as poisoning, drug overdose, toxic inhalation, trauma, and foreign body airway obstruction.

Physiology of Circulation Provided by External Chest Compression

Two mechanisms are thought to be responsible for blood flow during cardiopulmonary resuscitation (CPR). The first is direct compression of the heart between the sternum and the spine. This increases pressure within the ventricles enough to provide blood flow to the lungs and other organs. The second mechanism (which is thought to play a more important role than direct compression of the heart) is the generalized increase in intrathoracic pressure that occurs during CPR. This increase in intrathoracic pressure allows the left heart to act as a conduit for the passage of blood. Other mechanisms not currently known may be involved

as well. Artificial circulation generates only about 20% to 30% of the normal output of the heart.[31]

Research has been conducted for many years on ways to improve cardiopulmonary resuscitation. These methods include simultaneous chest compressions and ventilation, abdominal compression with synchronized ventilation, cardiopulmonary resuscitation augmented by pneumatic antishock garments, interposed abdominal compression, continuous abdominal binding, and plunger mechanisms for chest compression that cause active compression and active expansion. However, no alternative method has been shown to improve survival or circulation unequivocally.[1] Figure 22-124 presents the standards of cardiopulmonary resuscitation as recommended by the American Heart Association.

Mechanical Cardiopulmonary Resuscitation Devices

A number of mechanical devices (e.g., vest-type devices, plunger devices) have been designed to produce external chest compressions. Most operate to reduce intrathoracic pressure during decompression of the chest, thereby improving venous return to the heart (Box 22-22). Some devices provide chest compression and synchronized ventilation in the patient with cardiac arrest (Figure 22-125). These devices may help standardize the CPR technique, minimize the need to interrupt chest compressions, eliminate rescuer fatigue, free other rescuers to participate in advanced cardiac life support procedures, and ensure adequate compression during patient transport. In addition, they allow acceptable ECG recordings during compressions and defibrillation without interruption of CPR. There is currently no strong evidence for or against the use of these devices.[1] If used, the devices should be limited to adult patients. The use of mechanical cardiopulmonary resuscitation devices requires special training and authorization from medical direction. EMS personnel should follow the directions supplied with the equipment.

Monitor-Defibrillators

Cardiac monitor-defibrillators are classified as manual or automated external defibrillators. The latter may be semiautomated or fully automated. The paramedic should be familiar with the monitor-defibrillators used in the local EMS system or community settings.

MANUAL MONITOR-DEFIBRILLATORS

Monitor-defibrillators are available from a number of equipment manufacturers in a variety of designs and capabilities. All consist of the following:

- Patch electrodes
- Defibrillator controls
- Synchronizer switch
- Oscilloscope
- Patient cable and lead wires
- Controls for monitoring

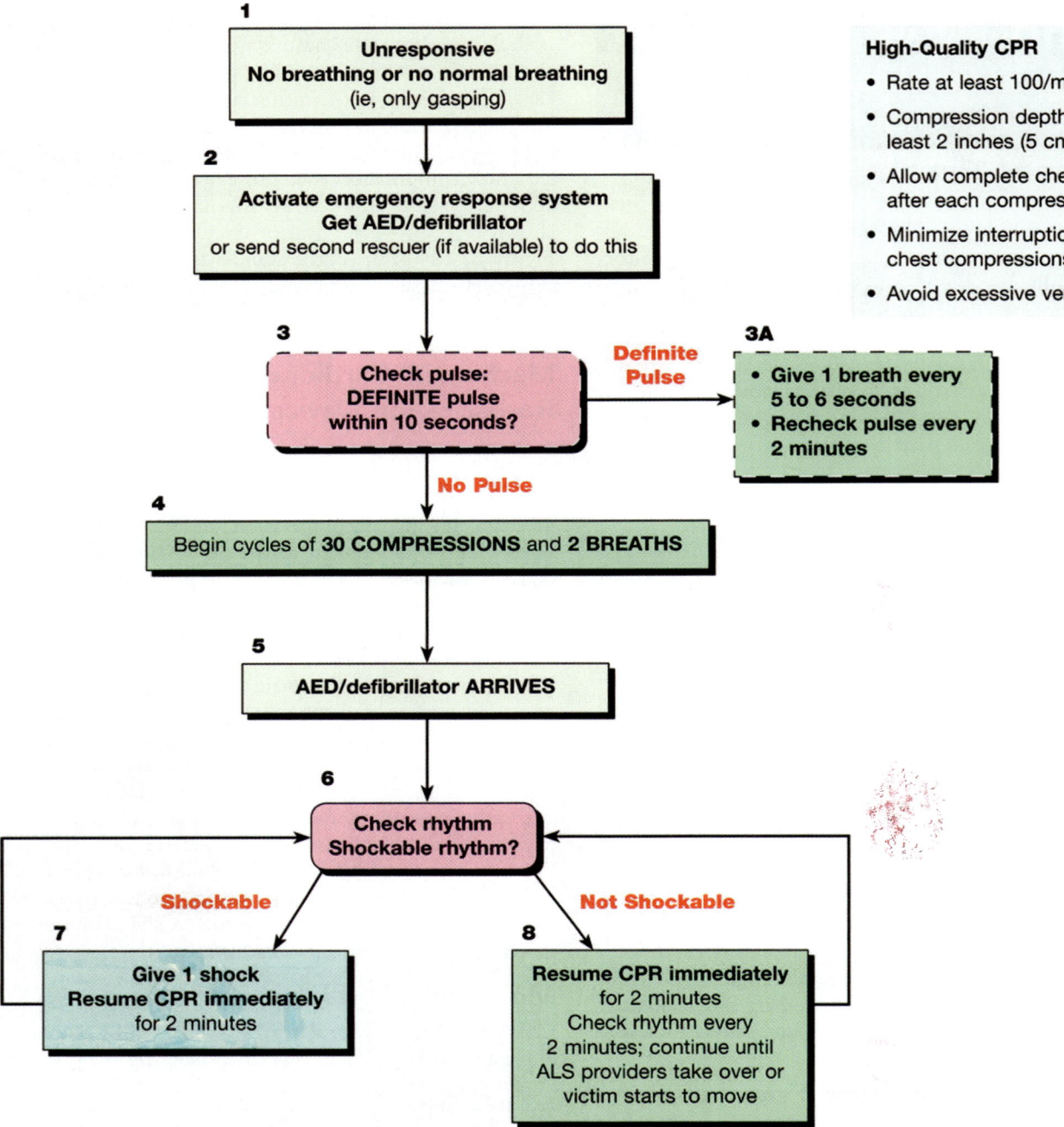

Adult BLS Healthcare Providers

1
Unresponsive
No breathing or no normal breathing
(ie, only gasping)

2
Activate emergency response system
Get AED/defibrillator
or send second rescuer (if available) to do this

High-Quality CPR
- Rate at least 100/min
- Compression depth at least 2 inches (5 cm)
- Allow complete chest recoil after each compression
- Minimize interruptions in chest compressions
- Avoid excessive ventilation

3
Check pulse:
DEFINITE pulse
within 10 seconds?

Definite Pulse →

3A
- Give 1 breath every 5 to 6 seconds
- Recheck pulse every 2 minutes

No Pulse

4
Begin cycles of **30 COMPRESSIONS** and **2 BREATHS**

5
AED/defibrillator ARRIVES

6
Check rhythm
Shockable rhythm?

Shockable

7
Give 1 shock
Resume CPR immediately
for 2 minutes

Not Shockable

8
Resume CPR immediately
for 2 minutes
Check rhythm every
2 minutes; continue until
ALS providers take over or
victim starts to move

Note: The boxes bordered with dashed lines are performed by healthcare providers and not by lay rescuers

© 2010 American Heart Association

FIGURE 22-124 Health care provider algorithm for adult basic life support. (Reprinted with permission, American Heart Association Guidelines For CPR and ECC, *Circulation 122* [suppl 3]:S685-S919, American Heart Association, Inc, 2010.)

Impedance threshold devices (ITDs) have a valve that limits the amount of air that enters the chest during the upstroke (recoil) during chest compressions. This enhances negative pressure inside the chest. The net effects of an ITD are:

- Blood flow to the heart is increased.
- Blood flow to the brain is enhanced.
- Systolic blood pressure doubles.
- Survival to the hospital may be increased.
- Chance of successful defibrillation may be increased.

The American Heart Association has classified ITDs as a class IIb intervention

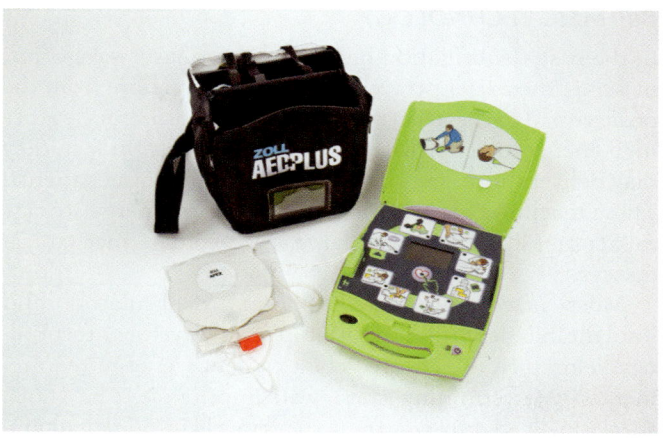

FIGURE 22-126 Automated external defibrillator.

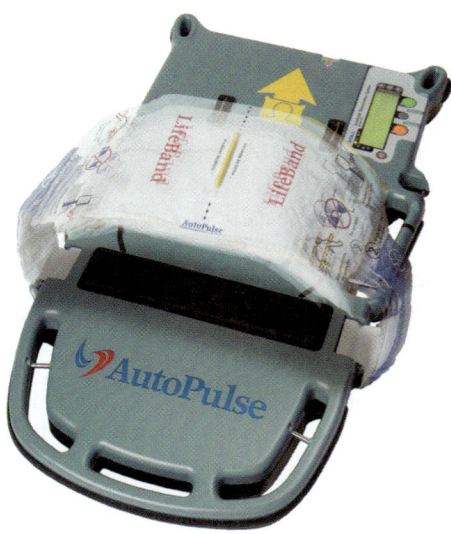

FIGURE 22-125 Mechanical cardiopulmonary resuscitation devices. Vest type.

In addition, some manual monitor-defibrillators have special features, such as data recorders, transcutaneous cardiac pacing capabilities, and 12-lead monitoring and transmission.

AUTOMATED EXTERNAL DEFIBRILLATORS

Automated external defibrillators (Figure 22-126) analyze the ECG signal. They evaluate the frequency, amplitude, and shape of the ECG waves. They are designed to be used by people with little training. They increase the number of individuals who are able to use a defibrillator in a cardiac arrest emergency. Automated external defibrillators are available for adult and pediatric patients (see Chapter 48).

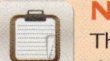

NOTE

There are many community-based first-responder defibrillation programs using automated external defibrillators. These programs and others (e.g., automated external defibrillators located in airports, businesses, schools, and on public airlines) are supported by the American Heart Association and other groups. The Food and Drug Administration (FDA) approved nonprescription sales of some automated external defibrillators for home use.

All automated external defibrillators are attached to the patient by two adhesive monitor-defibrillator pads (electrodes) and connecting cables. Automated external defibrillators are available from a number of manufacturers. They have a variety of features and controls. Most units provide programmable modules, data recorders, and voice messages to the operator. All users should become familiar with the automated external defibrillator device used in their system. Moreover, they should follow the recommendations of the manufacturer.

A fully automated defibrillator requires only that the operator attach the defibrillation pads and turn on the device. The rhythm is analyzed in the internal circuitry of the automated external defibrillator. If a shockable rhythm is detected, the automated external defibrillator charges capacitors and delivers a shock.

A semiautomated defibrillator requires the operator to press an "analyze" button to interpret the rhythm and a "shock" button to deliver the shock. The operator presses the shock control only when the automated external defibrillator identifies a shockable rhythm and "advises" the operator to press the shock button.

CRITICAL THINKING

What safety measure is still the duty of the person who operates the automated external defibrillator?

Automated external defibrillators have four safety features:

1. They can analyze ECG waves.
2. They have built-in filters that check for QRS-like signals, radio transmission waves, 60-cycle interference, and loose or poor electrode contact.
3. Most are programmed to detect spontaneous patient movements, continued heartbeat and blood flow, and movement of the patient by others.
4. They make multiple evaluations of the rhythm before making a shock advisory or delivering a shock.

BIPHASIC TECHNOLOGY

In the past, defibrillation has used monophasic waveforms, in which the current travels in only one direction, from the positive pad to the negative pad. These defibrillators require high energy to defibrillate a patient effectively. In fact, they may deliver more energy than is needed for some patients. These machines also require large batteries, energy storage capacitors, inductors, and large, high-voltage mechanical devices.

Most newer automated external defibrillators and implantable defibrillators use biphasic waveform technology. This technology predicts a patient's energy requirements by determining chest wall impedance. The shock then is delivered by a current that travels in one direction, is stopped, and then is reversed to travel in the opposite direction. This technology allows for effective defibrillation to occur with lower energy for most patients.[35] (Biphasic defibrillation of 115 and 130 J appears to be as effective as 200 and 360 J delivered with monophasic shocks.[36]) Biphasic waveforms are more effective at lower energy than monophasic waveforms. As a result, automated external defibrillators (using smaller batteries) have become smaller, lighter, more durable. They also have become less expensive to manufacture.

DEFIBRILLATION

Defibrillation is the delivery of electrical current through the chest wall. The purpose is to terminate ventricular fibrillation and pulseless ventricular tachycardia. The shock depolarizes a large mass of myocardial cells at once. If about 75% of these cells are in the resting state (depolarized) after the shock is delivered, a normal pacemaker may resume discharging. Early defibrillation is supported by the following rationales[1]:

- The most frequent initial rhythm in sudden cardiac arrest is ventricular fibrillation.
- The most effective management for ventricular fibrillation is electrical defibrillation.
- The probability of successful defibrillation decreases rapidly over time.
- Ventricular fibrillation tends to convert to asystole within a few minutes.

The modern defibrillator is designed to deliver an electrical shock via patches or pads to the patient's chest. The defibrillator accepts the electrical charge from the battery source. It stores the charge in the capacitor and then releases the current into the patient in a short, controlled burst (within 5 to 30 msec).

> **NOTE**
>
> Older defibrillators used "quick look" paddles instead of the modern pads or patches. If paddles are used, they should be coated with electrode paste or gel to reduce resistance and should be held firmly on the patient's chest with about 20 to 25 pounds of pressure.

> **SHOW ME THE EVIDENCE**
>
> Menegazzi and coworkers combined existing cardiac arrest data from four cities and analyzed it to determine which factors predicted failure of the first defibrillation. They found that first defibrillation failure increased in cases of unwitnessed arrest, if the response time was longer than 6 minutes, and if no bystander-provided CPR was performed. Menegazzi J, Hsieh M, Niemann J: Derivation of clinical predictors of failed rescue shock during out-of-hospital ventricular fibrillation, *Prehosp Emerg Care* 12:347-351, 2008.

Patch Electrodes

The electrode patches of the defibrillator (Figure 22-127) should be placed so that the heart (mainly the ventricles) is in the path of the current and the distance between the electrodes and the heart is minimized. This helps ensure adequate delivery of current through the heart. Bone is not a good conductor. For that reason, the patches should not be placed over the sternum. As recommended by the American Heart Association, one patch should be placed to the right of the upper sternum below the right clavicle and the other patch should be placed to the left of the nipple in the midaxillary line.[1] (The anterior-posterior anterolateral, anterior-left infrascapular, and anterior-right infrascapular positions also are acceptable.) Most manufacturers have adult and pediatric patches available. Adult patches usually are 8 to 12 cm in diameter. Pediatric patches are 4.5 cm in diameter. They are used for children under 1 year of age.

The resistance to current by the chest wall is called *impedance*. Impedance is determined by body size, bone structure, skin properties, underlying health conditions, and other variables. The greater the resistance, the less current delivered. Dry, unprepared skin has high impedance. To reduce resistance, the electrode patches are gelled. Care must be taken to prevent contact (bridging) between the two conductive areas on the chest wall. If contact between the two areas is made, superficial burns of the skin may result. The effective current also may bypass the heart. Even with proper technique and equipment, minor skin damage may still occur.

Stored and Delivered Energy

Electrical energy is commonly measured in **joules** (watt seconds). One joule of electrical energy is the product of 1 V (potential) multiplied by 1 A (current) multiplied by 1 second. Delivered energy is about 80% of stored energy because of losses within the circuitry of the defibrillator and resistance to the flow of current across the chest wall. As a rule, 80% of stored energy approximates the number of joules delivered to the patient. The American Heart Association currently recommends that one initial defibrillation be attempted at 120 to 200 J biphasic (follow manufacturer's instructions) or 360 J monophasic. (Box 22-23).[1] Second and subsequent shocks may be the same or higher. Initial defibrillation in pediatric patients generally is 2 J/kg. This is followed by 4 J/kg if needed.

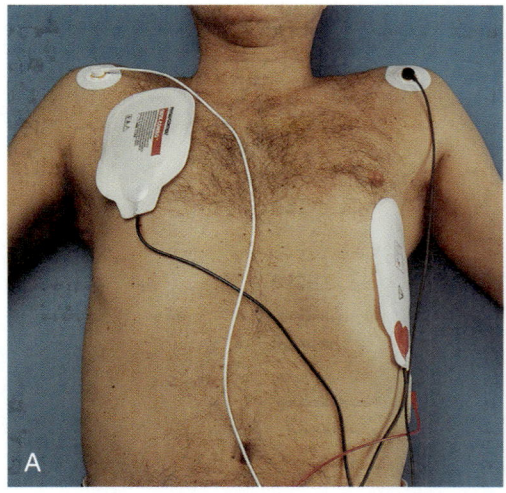 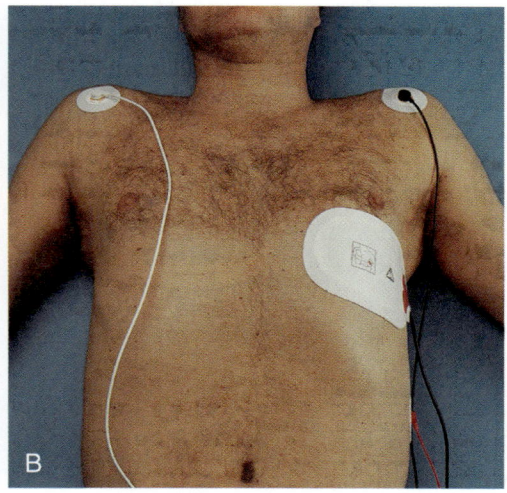

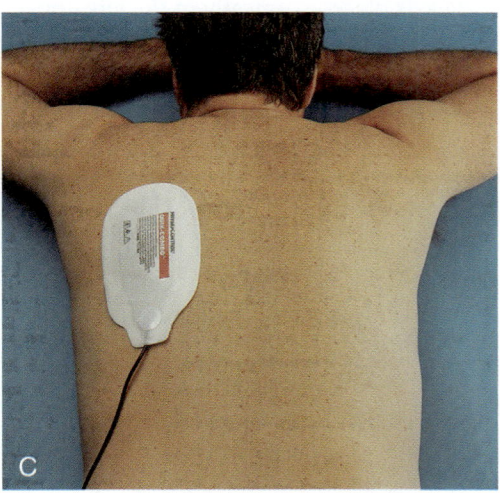

FIGURE 22-127 Proper electrode placement for defibrillation.

BOX 22-23 Current-Based Defibrillation

Current-based defibrillation has been studied as an alternative to traditional defibrillation. With current-based defibrillation, the defibrillator operator selects electrical current (amperes) versus energy (joules). This method avoids the problem of low-energy selection in the presence of high impedance (resulting in a current flow that is too low and thus failure to defibrillate). It also avoids the problem of high-energy selection in the presence of low impedance (resulting in excessive current flow, myocardial damage, and failure to defibrillate). The optimum current for ventricular defibrillation appears to be 30 to 40 A.[4]

Procedure for Defibrillation

The following is the procedure for defibrillation recommended by the American Heart Association.

1. Turn on the defibrillator.
2. Select the energy level at 120 to 200 J biphasic (based on manufacturer's recommendation) or 360 J for monophasic defibrillators.
3. Set lead I, II, or III if monitor leads are used.
4. Position electrode patches on the patient's chest (sternum-apex).
5. Visually check the monitor display and assess the rhythm. (Subsequent steps assume that ventricular tachycardia/ventricular fibrillation is present.)
6. Announce to the team members, "Charging the defibrillator."
7. Press the "charge" button on the defibrillator controls.
8. Continue CPR while the defibrillator is charging.
9. When the defibrillator is fully charged, state quickly, in a forceful voice, the following chant (or some suitable equivalent) before each shock.
   - *"I am going to shock on three. One, I'm clear."* (Check to make sure you are clear of contact with the patient, the stretcher, and the equipment.)
   - *"Two, you're clear."* (Make a visual check to ensure that no one continues to touch the patient or stretcher. In particular, do not forget about the person providing ventilations. That person's

hands should not be touching the ventilatory adjuncts, including the tracheal tube. Turn off oxygen or direct the flow away from the patient's chest.)

- *"Three, everybody's clear."* (Check yourself one more time before pressing the "shock" button.)

10. Perform five cycles of CPR.
11. Check the monitor. If ventricular fibrillation/ventricular tachycardia remains, recharge the defibrillator at once.
12. Shock at the same or higher biphasic energy (per manufacturer) or 360 J for monophasic defibrillators, repeating the verbal statements in step 9.

Operator and Personnel Safety

The following six guidelines are designed to ensure safe use of a defibrillator.[37]

1. Make sure all personnel are clear of the patient, the bed, and the defibrillator before making a defibrillation attempt.
2. Do not make contact with the patient during discharge.
3. Do not discharge current over a pacemaker or implantable cardioverter-defibrillator generator or **nitroglycerin** paste. Remove **nitroglycerin** patches before defibrillation.
4. Do not "open air" discharge the defibrillator to cancel an unwanted charge. Turn the defibrillator off to "dump" the charge. (In most models, changing the energy setting dumps the charge.)
5. Treat equipment with respect. It is safe when used properly.
6. Routinely check the defibrillator (including the batteries) to make sure the equipment is functioning properly. Follow the manufacturer's recommendations.

Defibrillator Use in Special Environments

On occasion a patient requires defibrillation in a special environment (e.g., inclement weather). The guidelines in operator and personnel safety always apply. However, additional precautions are taken in special situations.

A patient can be defibrillated in wet conditions, such as near water, in rain, or in snowy weather. The patient's chest should be kept dry between the defibrillator electrode sites. The operator's hands should be kept as dry as possible. In a rainstorm, the safest course is to find shelter.

Depending on the defibrillator and its equipment specifications, the device may not be guaranteed to work properly in nonpressurized aircraft. In addition, some electrical interference may occur between the radio equipment in the aircraft and the monitor-defibrillator or vice versa. This is affected by the distance and angle between the defibrillator and the radio equipment. Studies have demonstrated that defibrillation with current equipment would be expected to be safe in all types of rotary aircraft used for emergency

medical transport.[38] Nonetheless, the medical crew should always inform the pilot when electrical therapy is being used. In addition, the paramedic should consult with the pilot to make sure the flight instruments are well shielded from electromagnetic interference.

IMPLANTABLE CARDIOVERTER-DEFIBRILLATORS

Implantable cardioverter-defibrillators (ICDs) commonly are used in patients at risk for recurrent, sustained ventricular tachycardia or fibrillation (Figure 22-128). During implantation, the various leads of the ICD are fed through a vessel (usually the subclavian vein) into the right ventricle or placed on the epicardium. The leads are tunneled to a pulse generator in the biphasic defibrillator device. The device is placed surgically in the left upper quadrant of the abdomen. (An outline of the generator usually can be felt or seen under the patient's skin.) The leads are used to deliver shocks, monitor cardiac rhythm, and sometimes pace the heart as needed if bradycardia occurs.

 CRITICAL THINKING
These devices are used by what type of patients?

The implantable cardioverter-defibrillator works by monitoring the patient's cardiac rhythm, rate, and QRS complex morphology. When a monitored ventricular rate exceeds the preprogrammed rate, the implantable

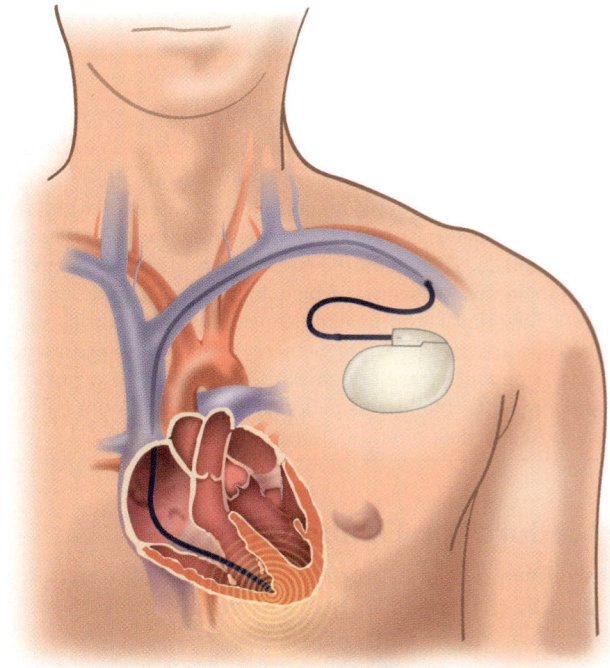

FIGURE 22-128 Implantable cardioverter-defibrillator.

cardioverter-defibrillator delivers a shock of about 6 to 30 J through the patches to restore a normal sinus rhythm. The device requires 10 to 30 seconds to sense ventricular tachycardia or ventricular fibrillation and to charge the capacitor before delivering the shock. If defibrillation does not restore a normal sinus rhythm, the implantable cardioverter-defibrillator charges again. It then delivers up to four shocks. A complete sequence of five shocks, if required, may take up to 2 minutes. If the tachycardia or fibrillation persists after five shocks, no further shocks are delivered. Once a slower rhythm (i.e., sinus or idioventricular rhythm) has been restored for at least 35 seconds, the device can deliver another series of up to five shocks if ventricular tachycardia or ventricular fibrillation recurs.

> ### 💡 CRITICAL THINKING
> A conscious patient has a device that is firing repeatedly in response to the presence of a ventricular rhythm. How can you lessen the patient's discomfort and anxiety?

The paramedic must manage patients with implantable cardioverter-defibrillators as if they did not have a device. The paramedic should follow standard ACLS protocols if the patient is in cardiac arrest or in any other way medically unstable. The American Heart Association recommends the following four guidelines for caring for a patient with an implantable cardioverter-defibrillator[1]:

1. If the implantable cardioverter-defibrillator discharges while the rescuer is touching the victim, the rescuer may feel the shock. However, the shock will not be dangerous. Personnel shocked by implantable cardioverter-defibrillators report sensations similar to contact with an electrical current.
2. Implantable cardioverter-defibrillators are protected against damage from traditional transchest defibrillation shocks. However, they require an implantable cardioverter-defibrillator readiness check after external defibrillation.
3. If ventricular fibrillation or ventricular tachycardia is present despite an implantable cardioverter-defibrillator, an external shock should be given immediately, because the implantable cardioverter-defibrillator likely has failed to defibrillate the heart. After an initial series of shocks, the implantable cardioverter-defibrillator becomes operative again only if a period of nonfibrillatory rhythm occurs to reset the unit.
4. Older implantable cardioverter-defibrillator units use patch electrodes instead of leads. These electrodes cover a portion of the epicardial surface. They may reduce the amount of current delivered to the heart from transthoracic shocks. Therefore, if transthoracic shocks of up to 360 J fail to defibrillate a patient with an implantable cardioverter-defibrillator, the chest electrode positions should be changed immediately (e.g., anterior-apex to anteroposterior). The transthoracic shocks should be repeated. The different electrode positions could increase transthoracic current flow. This in turn may facilitate defibrillation.

Because the implantable cardioverter-defibrillator can be deactivated and activated with a magnet, patients with implantable cardioverter-defibrillators should be kept away from strong magnets. This prevents accidental deactivation or reactivation of the device. The ability to use a magnet to deactivate and reactivate many of these devices can be useful when the unit is not working properly. However, use of a handheld magnet to turn the unit off or back on should be considered only with the advice and under the direction of a physician.

LEFT VENTRICULAR ASSIST DEVICE

A **left ventricular assist device** (LVAD) is a battery-operated pump that sometimes is implanted during heart surgery in a person waiting for a heart transplant ("bridge to transplant"). (The devices also are used in some patients to allow a weakened heart to recover.) The common LVAD is implanted in the patient's abdomen. A catheter in the pump pulls blood from the weakened left ventricle and then directs the blood into the aorta. (This takes stress off the left ventricle.) A second catheter is brought out of the abdominal wall to the outside of the body, where it can be attached to the pump's battery and control system.

Modern LVADs are portable, and they often are used for weeks to months while the patient waits for a donor heart to become available (Figure 22-129). LVADs also are prescribed for patients who are terminally ill and ineligible for a heart transplant. In these patients, the LVAD can improve the quality of life ("destination therapy"). Possible complications from the device include infection, internal bleeding, heart failure, and mechanical malfunction (see Chapter 52).

Special Care Considerations

Because the LVAD assumes the pumping function of the left ventricle, the patient may have no palpable pulse or measurable blood pressure. (This depends on the pulsatility of the specific device. A Doppler probe may be required for blood pressure readings.) The patient and family usually are quite knowledgeable about the LVAD and often are a valuable resource. In addition, many patients with LVADs advise emergency service agencies so that personnel can be made aware of their special equipment needs.

Because of the location of the LVAD and the tubing connecting it to the heart, the device can be dislodged during CPR, causing severe bleeding. Therefore, chest compressions to manage cardiac arrest are contraindicated in some of these patients. In addition, the procedure for defibrillation and cardioversion is specific to the LVAD and the manufacturer's recommendations.

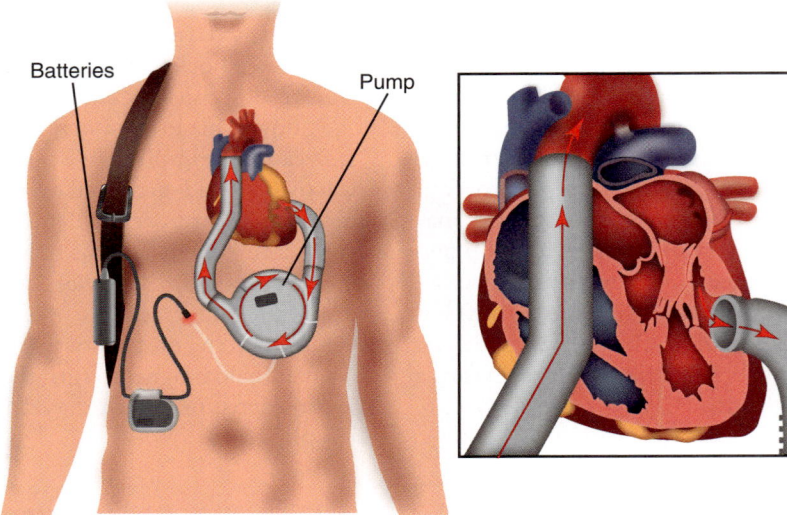

FIGURE 22-129 Left ventricular assist device.

SYNCHRONIZED CARDIOVERSION

Synchronized cardioversion (or countershock) is used to terminate dysrhythmias other than ventricular fibrillation and pulseless ventricular tachycardia. Defibrillation (**unsynchronized cardioversion**) delivers the shock on the operator's command and with no regard to where the shock occurs in the cardiac cycle. In contrast, synchronized cardioversion is designed to deliver the shock about 10 msec after the peak of the R wave of the cardiac cycle. This avoids the vulnerable relative refractory period of the ventricles. Synchronization may reduce the energy required to end the dysrhythmia. It also may decrease the chance of causing ventricular fibrillation.

When the defibrillator is placed in the synchronized mode, the ECG displayed on the oscilloscope shows a marker denoting where in the cardiac cycle the energy will be discharged. This marker should appear on the R wave; if it does not, the paramedic should select another lead. Adjustment of the ECG size may be needed if the marker does not appear. The procedure for synchronized cardioversion is as follows:

1. Consider sedation.
2. Turn on the defibrillator (monophasic or biphasic).
3. Attach monitor leads to the patient ("white to right, red to ribs, what's left over to the left shoulder") and ensure proper display of the patient's rhythm.
4. Engage the synchronization mode by pressing the "sync" control button.
5. Look for markers on R waves indicating the sync mode.
6. If necessary, adjust the monitor gain until the sync markers occur with each R wave.
7. Select the appropriate energy level.
8. Position the electrode patches on the patient (sternum-apex).

9. Announce to the team members: "Charging defibrillator."
10. Press the "charge" button on defibrillator.
11. When the defibrillator is charged, begin the final clearing chant. State firmly, in a forceful voice, the following chant before each shock:
    - *"I am going to shock on three. One, I'm clear."* (Check to make sure you are clear of contact with the patient, the stretcher, and the equipment.)
    - *"Two, you're clear."* (Make a visual check to ensure that no one continues to touch the patient or stretcher. In particular, do not forget about the person providing ventilations. That person's hands should not be touching the ventilatory adjuncts, including the tracheal tube. Turn off oxygen or direct the flow away from the patient's chest.)
    - *"Three, everybody's clear."* (Check yourself one more time before pressing the "shock" button.)
12. Press the "discharge" button.
13. Check the monitor. If tachycardia persists, increase the joules according to the electrical cardioversion algorithm.
14. Reset the sync mode after each synchronized cardioversion, because most defibrillators default back to the unsynchronized mode. This default allows an immediate shock if the cardioversion produces ventricular fibrillation.

TRANSCUTANEOUS CARDIAC PACING

Transcutaneous cardiac pacing (TCP), also known as *external cardiac pacing*, is an effective emergency therapy for bradycardia, complete heart block, and suppression of some malignant ventricular tachydysrhythmias. TCP devices have been recognized by the American Heart Association. They are used to treat bradycardia.

Artificial Pacing

Artificial pacemakers deliver repetitive electrical currents to the heart (Figure 22-130). They can act as a substitute for a natural pacemaker. The natural pacemaker may have become blocked or dysfunctional. A patient with severe sinus bradycardia, heart block, or idioventricular rhythm who can generate a pulse with cardiac contractions may respond to an external pacing device and produce a perfusing pulse. Sinus bradycardia also may be paced. Generally, though, sinus bradycardia responds well to *atropine.*

The two modes of TCP are nondemand (asynchronous) pacing and demand pacing. Most devices provide both modes. An asynchronous pacemaker delivers timed electrical stimuli at a selected rate. This occurs regardless of the patient's own cardiac activity. These pacing devices are used less often than demand pacers. This is because they may discharge during the vulnerable period of the cardiac cycle (producing the R-on-T phenomenon). The asynchronous mode generally is used only as a last resort, usually in asystole. This mode also can be used when artifact on the ECG interferes with the machine's ability to sense the patient's own heartbeat. Asynchronous pacing also can be used to override the high heart rates of tachydysrhythmias (e.g., torsades de pointes). This should be attempted only if other means of controlling the dysrhythmia have failed; it may be limited by the design of the machine.

Demand pacing senses the patient's QRS complex. The pacemaker delivers electrical stimuli only when needed. Demand pacing is much safer to apply than the nondemand mode. When the pacemaker senses an intrinsic beat, it is inhibited. If no beats are sensed, the pacemaker delivers

pacing stimuli at a selected rate. The device usually is set to discharge at a rate of 70 to 80 beats/minute beginning with 50 mA. The charge then is increased in increments, beginning at 0 mA of electricity, until electrical and mechanical capture is achieved. Generally, the patient's clinical condition (blood pressure, level of consciousness, skin color, and temperature) improves at this point.

> **NOTE**
> **Electrical capture** means that every pacer stimulus is followed by a large QRS complex, which indicates ventricular contraction. **Mechanical capture** occurs when an associated pulse is generated with the electrical capture.

The paramedic should make sure each pacemaker spike on the oscilloscope is followed by a QRS complex. If not, the current should be increased gradually until consistent capture is achieved. Unfortunately, motion artifact often makes ECG confirmation of electrical capture difficult. The only accurate method of monitoring mechanical function of the heart produced by the pacing device is the presence of a pulse with each QRS complex. Therefore, the paramedic must monitor the patient's pulse constantly. The paramedic should assess the patient's pulse rate and blood pressure on the patient's right side. This helps minimize interference from muscle artifact.

Procedure for Transcutaneous Pacing

The procedure for transcutaneous pacing is as follows:
1. Consider sedation.
2. Gather the required equipment.
3. Explain the procedure to the patient.
4. Connect the patient to a cardiac monitor and obtain a rhythm strip.
5. Obtain baseline vital signs.
6. Attach the limb leads and apply the pacing electrodes. Often the defibrillation position is used when the same pads can be used for defibrillation and pacing. The pads can also be placed in the anterior-posterior position (left of the lower sternum and just below the left scapula).
7. Select the pacing mode.
8. Select the pacing rate (usually 80 beats/minute); set the current (begin with 0 mA and then increase the current until ventricular capture is obtained).
9. Activate the pacemaker, observing the patient and the ECG.
10. Obtain rhythm strips as appropriate.
11. Continue monitoring the patient and anticipate further therapy.

> **NOTE**
> As with synchronized cardioversion, selecting the "pacing mode" should result in the appearance of light markers on intrinsic beats. Paramedics should make sure this happens so that they know the demand mode is activated and working properly.

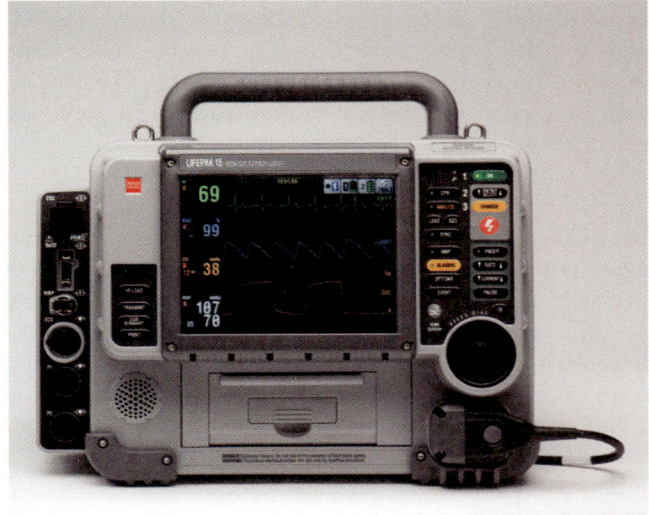

FIGURE 22-130 LifePak 15 defibrillator monitor pacer. (Courtesy Physio-Control, Redmond, Wash.)

Indications and Contraindications

The primary indications for transcutaneous cardiac pacing in the prehospital setting are symptomatic bradycardia, heart block associated with reduced cardiac output that is unresponsive to *atropine,* and pacemaker failure. As stated previously, cardiac pacing rarely is effective in cardiac arrest. It also is ineffective in pulseless electrical activity unless the underlying cause of the pulseless electrical activity is corrected. Cardiac pacing is not advised for patients with open wounds or chest burns or for patients in a wet environment.

CRITICAL THINKING
Why should patient movement be minimized during transcutaneous cardiac pacing?

Electrode Placement

Proper placement of the electrodes is one of the keys to effective external pacing. As stated previously, the defibrillation position often is used when the same pads can be used for defibrillation and pacing. Alternatively, the paramedic can apply the negative (anterior) electrode to the left of the sternum. The electrode should be centered as close as possible to the point of maximum cardiac impulse. The positive (posterior) electrode is placed directly behind the anterior electrode, just below the left scapula. In rare cases posterior placement cannot be used. In such cases the positive electrode can be placed in line with the patient's left nipple at the midaxillary line. (Anterior-anterior placement may produce pronounced chest muscle twitching.) The electrodes should be applied to clean, dry skin free of localized trauma or infection.

A conscious patient most likely will experience some pain and discomfort during transcutaneous cardiac pacing. This is related directly to the intensity of muscle contractions and the amount of applied current. Ideally, analgesia or sedation of the patient should be provided.

CARDIAC ARREST AND SUDDEN DEATH

It is becoming increasingly evident that patients who cannot be resuscitated in the prehospital setting rarely survive. This is the case even if the patient is resuscitated temporarily in the ED (Box 22-24). The patient's best chance for survival is rapid recognition and, appropriate treatment in the field. The priorities in cardiac arrest are effective CPR and rapid defibrillation (if indicated). Vascular access and advanced airway management are of secondary importance to the initial priorities and should never delay them. Prolonged field resuscitation in the face of difficulties with IV/IO access and intubation almost always is destined to fail.

BOX 22-24   Resuscitation Terminology

Resuscitation: The technique of providing efforts to return spontaneous pulse and breathing to a patient in full cardiac arrest.

Survival: Resuscitation of a patient who survives to hospital discharge.

Return of spontaneous circulation: Restoration of spontaneous circulation that provides evidence of more than an occasional gasp, occasional fleeting palpable pulse, or arterial waveform; the patient may or may not survive.

Adapted from the Utstein registry template.

Much research is under way in the area of emergency cardiac care. Some of the research deals with various drugs to improve cardiac and neurological outcomes after resuscitation. A fairly large number of patients regain cardiac function but never regain consciousness. Therefore, a good deal of interest has arisen in how to improve cerebral perfusion after cardiac arrest. This research may lead to a variety of new drugs that paramedics may use during resuscitation in the future.

Care of the Patient after Return of Spontaneous Circulation

Some patients survive cardiac arrest and have a return of spontaneous circulation (ROSC). In these situations, the principal objective of postresuscitation care is reestablishment of effective perfusion of organs and tissues.[6] Ideally, the patient is alert and awake. Patients also may be comatose, yet still have full potential for recovery with a good neurological outcome. Research is under way to improve the survival rate of patients with ROSC who remain comatose after resuscitation. Some of these methods include therapeutic hypothermia, hemodynamic and ventilation optimization, immediate coronary reperfusion with PCI, glycemic control, and neurological care and prognostication.[1]

THERAPEUTIC HYPOTHERMIA

The 2010 American Heart Association guidelines recommend inducing mild hypothermia in comatose survivors of cardiac arrest When a patient is resuscitated, reperfusion sets off a series of chemical reactions that can continue for up to 24 hours, possibly causing significant inflammation in the brain. Inducing mild hypothermia reduces the intracranial pressure, the cerebral metabolic rate, and the brain's demand for oxygen consumption. In addition, it is thought to suppress many of the chemical reactions associated with reperfusion injury, including free radical production, excitatory amino acid release, and calcium shifts.[39]

Some EMS agencies induce hypothermia in an unconscious patient after ROSC from ventricular fibrillation.[40]

(For example, cooling to induce mild hypothermia can be initiated in the prehospital setting by the application of iced IV bags or through the infusion of cold saline.) In the ED it is initiated by means of internal and external cooling methods. When a core body temperature of 91° to 92° F (28° to 32° C) has been established, the patient is transferred to intensive care. After 12 to 24 hours, the patient is slowly rewarmed to normal core body temperature.

Therapeutic hypothermia should be induced in a comatose patient within 30 to 60 minutes after resuscitation from cardiac arrest if the initial rhythm was ventricular fibrillation or out-of-hospital cardiac arrest with an initial rhythm of PEA or asystole. Therapeutic hypothermia is associated with an improved functional recovery and a better neurological outcome.[41] The technique is under study in other types of patients who may benefit from induced hypothermia, such as victims of severe stroke and adults with head injuries.[42]

HEMODYNAMIC AND VENTILATION OPTIMIZATION

The administration of 100% oxygen should be given during initial resuscitation measures. Following the return of spontaneous circulation, however, inspired oxygen should be titrated during the post-cardiac arrest phase to the lowest level required to achieve and maintain an arterial oxygen saturation of ≥94%. Doing so helps to avoid any complications associated with oxygen toxicity. In addition, excessive ventilation should be avoided. As described in Chapter 15, excessive ventilation can cause adverse hemodynamic effects from an increase in intrathoracic pressures and a potential decrease in cerebral blood flow. The American Heart Association recommends that ventilations begin at 10 to 12 breaths per minute, titrated to achieve a $PETCO_2$ of 35 to 40 mm Hg or a $PaCO_2$ of 40 to 45 mm Hg.

IV fluids and vasoactive and inotropic drugs should be titrated to optimize blood pressure, cardiac output, and systemic perfusion. Although an optimal post-cardiac arrest blood pressure remains unknown, a mean arterial pressure ≥65 mm Hg is suggested as a reasonable goal.

IMMEDIATE CORONARY REPERFUSION WITH PCI

As described earlier, all patients with ROSC should be transported to an appropriate facility that can provide effective postresuscitation care. These therapies include immediate coronary reperfusion (e.g., PCI), therapeutic hypothermia, and other treatment modalities to improve post-cardiac arrest survival.

GLYCEMIC CONTROL

The American Heart Association recommends that serum glucose levels be maintained at 144 to 180 mg/dL in adult patients with ROSC following cardiac arrest. This range prevents any increased risk for hypoglycemia. Attempts to alter serum glucose concentrations below this level should be avoided.

NEUROLOGICAL CARE AND PROGNOSTICIAN

Neurological recovery is an important component of post-resuscitation care. The goal is to restore a level of functioning that the patient had before the cardiac arrest. An accurate prognosis of neurological recovery helps in making decisions to limit or withdraw life-sustaining care.

TERMINATION OF RESUSCITATION

As described in Chapter 6, health care professionals are expected to provide basic life support and advanced cardiac life support as part of their professional duty to respond, with the following exceptions:

- When a person lies dead and has obvious clinical signs of irreversible death
- When attempts to perform CPR would place the rescuer at risk of physical injury
- When the patient or surrogate has indicated that resuscitation is not desired

The termination of resuscitative efforts in the prehospital setting should follow rules established by the local EMS system and medical direction. The rules should include consideration for advance directives and orders specifying no CPR. If at any time paramedics are presented with an advance directive (e.g., a written directive, living will, or durable power of attorney) that indicates a patient should not be resuscitated, they should follow established protocol or immediately consult with medical direction (see Chapter 6).

In some adult cases resuscitation can be appropriately terminated in the prehospital setting. For example, the National Association of EMS Physicians (NAEMSP) suggests that resuscitation can be terminated in patients who do not respond to at least 20 minutes of ALS care.[43]

The American Heart Association recommends considering terminating resuscitation when ALL of the following criteria apply[1]:

1. Arrest was not witnessed
2. No bystander CPR was provided
3. No ROSC after full ALS care in the field
4. No AED shocks were delivered

Finally, unusual clinical features (e.g., drowning, profound hypothermia, young age, toxins, electrolyte abnormalities, drug overdose) may be indicators that continued resuscitation is appropriate. Termination of resuscitation in the prehospital setting should be guided by medical direction.

SHOW ME THE EVIDENCE
Using focus groups, Grudzen and colleagues[41] interviewed EMTs and paramedics about their attitude toward a policy change that permitted cessation of resuscitation in the field for nontraumatic cardiac arrest. Overall the groups had a very positive response; they believed that except in select circumstances, this approach was beneficial to patients, families, EMS agencies, and the public. Grudzen C, et al: Paramedic and emergency medical technicians views on opportunities and challenges when forgoing and halting resuscitation in the field, *Acad Emerg Med* 16:532-538, 2009.

Procedure for Termination of Resuscitation

The process for terminating resuscitation in the field varies by protocol. The paramedic must follow the guidelines set by medical direction. When termination is considered appropriate, the paramedic should contact medical direction to convey the following information:

- Patient's medical condition
- Known causes of the arrest
- Any treatment provided
- Family's appraisal of the situation and any resistance or uncertainty

While gathering and giving this information to medical direction, the paramedic should maintain ongoing documentation of the event. (This should include continuous ECG monitoring.) Documentation aids the review of the call. The review usually is performed for quality assurance in most EMS systems.

CRITICAL THINKING
You have just terminated resuscitation in the home. What resources can you contact to help the family?

Special Considerations

In addition to attending to the needs of the patient, paramedics must consider grief support for the family.

DID YOU KNOW?
Helping a Grieving Person
Conveying the news of a death to family members, friends, and loved ones at the scene is difficult. In addition to ensuring the family's privacy, the following guidelines may be helpful in this situation.

What to Say
- Acknowledge the situation (e.g., "I'm sorry to say that [patient's name] has died").
- Express your concern (e.g., "I'm sorry this has happened to you").
- Offer your support (e.g., "Tell me what I can do to help you").

What Not to Say
"I know how you feel."
"Look at what you have to be thankful for."
"It's part of God's plan."
"He's in a better place now."
"It's over, and it's all behind you now."

Listen with Compassion
- Accept and acknowledge the feelings of the bereaved.
- Be willing to sit in silence.
- Let the bereaved talk about how their loved one died.
- Offer comfort without minimizing the loss.

Offer Practical Assistance
- Contact a neighbor or other family member.
- Make sure the bereaved has a means of transportation if needed.

Modified from *Supporting a grieving person: helping others through grief, loss, and bereavement.* http://helpguide.org/mental/helping_grieving.htm. Accessed May 26, 2010.

Support services vary by agency. Often a paramedic (or other EMS personnel) is assigned to stay with the family for a time. At times a community agency referral is arranged.

Law enforcement officers may have additional duties at the scene as part of their professional role. These duties may include an on-scene determination that the patient be assigned to a medical examiner. This may occur when the death or event is suspicious or when a patient's private physician refuses or hesitates to sign the death certificate. The paramedic must be familiar with local and state laws regarding reporting an out-of-hospital death and the disposition of the patient's remains under such circumstances.

SUMMARY

- Individuals at high risk for cardiovascular disease include males, older adults, and those with diabetes, hypertension, a family history of premature cardiovascular disease, and prior myocardial infarction. Prevention strategies include community educational programs in nutrition, cessation of smoking (smoking prevention for children), and screening for hypertension and high cholesterol.
- The left coronary artery carries about 85% of the blood supply to the myocardium. The right coronary artery carries the rest. The pumping action of the heart is a product of rhythmic, alternate contraction and relaxation of the atria and ventricles. The stroke volume is the amount of blood ejected from each ventricle with

one contraction. The stroke volume depends on the preload, afterload, and myocardial contractility. Cardiac output is the amount of blood pumped by each ventricle per minute.

- In addition to the intrinsic control of the body in regulating the heart, extrinsic control by the parasympathetic and sympathetic nerves of the autonomic nervous system is a major factor influencing the heart rate, conductivity, and contractility. Sympathetic impulses cause the adrenal medulla to secrete epinephrine and norepinephrine into the blood.
- The major electrolytes that influence cardiac function are calcium, potassium, sodium, and magnesium. The electrical charge (potential difference) between the

- inside and outside of cells is expressed in millivolts. When the cell is in a resting state, the electrical charge difference is referred to as a *resting membrane potential*. The specialized sodium-potassium exchange pump actively pumps sodium ions out of the cell. It also pumps potassium ions into the cell. The cell membrane appears to have individual protein-lined channels. These channels allow for passage of a specific ion or group of ions.

- Nerve and muscle cells are capable of producing action potentials. This property is known as *excitability*. An action potential at any point on the cell membrane stimulates an excitation process. This process is spread down the length of the cell and is conducted across synapses from cell to cell.

- The contraction of cardiac and skeletal muscle is believed to be activated by calcium ions. This results in binding between myosin and actin myofilaments.

- The conduction system of the heart is composed of two nodes and a conducting bundle. One of the nodes is the sinoatrial node. The other is the atrioventricular node.

- Parasympathetic stimulation by the vagus nerve affects primarily the SA node and the AV node, causing the heart to slow. Sympathetic stimulation increases the heart rate and contractility.

- The ECG represents the electrical activity of the heart. It is generated by depolarization and repolarization of the atria and ventricles.

- Routine monitoring of cardiac rhythm in the prehospital setting usually is obtained in lead II or V_1. These are the best leads to monitor for dysrhythmias, because they allow visualization of P waves. The paper used to record ECGs is standardized. This allows comparative analysis of an ECG wave.

- A normal ECG consists of a P wave, QRS complex, and T wave. The P wave is the first positive deflection on the ECG. The P wave represents atrial depolarization. The P-R interval is the time required for an electrical impulse to be conducted through the atria and the AV node up to the instant of ventricular depolarization. The QRS complex represents ventricular depolarization. The ST segment represents the early part of repolarization of the right and left ventricles. The T wave represents repolarization of the ventricular myocardial cells. Repolarization occurs during the last part of ventricular systole. The Q-T interval is the period from the beginning of ventricular depolarization (onset of the QRS complex) until the end of ventricular repolarization or the end of the T wave.

- The steps in ECG analysis include analyzing the QRS complex, P waves, rate, rhythm, and P-R interval.

- Dysrhythmias originating in the SA node include sinus bradycardia, sinus tachycardia, sinus dysrhythmia, and sinus arrest. Most sinus dysrhythmias are the result of increases or decreases in vagal tone.

- Dysrhythmias originating in the atria include wandering pacemaker, premature atrial complexes, paroxysmal supraventricular tachycardia, atrial flutter, and atrial fibrillation. Common causes of atrial dysrhythmias are ischemia, hypoxia, and atrial dilation caused by congestive heart failure or mitral valve abnormalities.

- When the SA node and the atria cannot generate the electrical impulses needed to begin depolarization because of factors such as hypoxia, ischemia, myocardial infarction, and drug toxicity, the AV node or the area surrounding it may assume the role of the secondary pacemaker. Dysrhythmias originating in the atrioventricular junction include premature junctional complexes, junctional escape complexes or rhythms, and accelerated junctional rhythm.

- Ventricular dysrhythmias pose a threat to life. Ventricular rhythm disturbances generally result from failure of the atria, atrioventricular junction, or both to initiate an electrical impulse. They also may result from enhanced automaticity or reentry phenomena in the ventricles. Dysrhythmias originating in the ventricles include ventricular escape complexes or rhythms, premature ventricular complexes, ventricular tachycardia, ventricular fibrillation, asystole, and artificial pacemaker rhythm.

- A 12-lead ECG can be used to help identify changes relative to myocardial ischemia, injury, and infarction; distinguish ventricular tachycardia from supraventricular tachycardia; determine the electrical axis and the presence of fascicular blocks; and determine the presence of bundle branch blocks.

- Partial delays or full interruptions in cardiac electrical conduction are called *heart blocks*. Causes of heart blocks include atrioventricular junctional ischemia, atrioventricular junctional necrosis, degenerative disease of the conduction system, and drug toxicity. Dysrhythmias that are disorders of conduction are first-degree atrioventricular block, second-degree atrioventricular block type I (Wenckebach), second-degree atrioventricular block type II, third-degree atrioventricular block, disturbances of ventricular conduction, pulseless electrical activity, and preexcitation (Wolff-Parkinson-White syndrome).

- Common chief complaints of the patient with cardiovascular disease include chest pain or discomfort, including shoulder, arm, neck, or jaw pain or discomfort; dyspnea; syncope; and abnormal heartbeat or palpitations. Paramedics should ask patients suspected of having a cardiovascular disorder whether they take prescription medications, especially cardiac drugs. Paramedics also should ask whether patients are being treated for any serious illness. They should ask whether patients have a history of myocardial infarction, angina, heart failure, hypertension, diabetes, or chronic lung disease. In addition, paramedics should ask whether patients have any allergies or other risk factors for heart disease.

Continued

- After performing the initial assessment of the patient with cardiovascular disease, the paramedic should look for skin color, jugular venous distention, and the presence of edema or other signs of heart disease. The paramedic should listen for lung sounds, heart sounds, and carotid artery bruit. The paramedic should feel for edema, pulses, skin temperature, and moisture.

- Atherosclerosis is a disease process characterized by progressive narrowing of the lumen of medium and large arteries. It has two major effects on blood vessels. First, it disrupts the intimal surface. This causes a loss of vessel elasticity and an increase in thrombogenesis. Second, the atheroma reduces the diameter of the vessel lumen. This reduces the blood supply to tissues.

- Angina pectoris is a symptom of myocardial ischemia. Angina is caused by an imbalance between myocardial oxygen supply and demand. Prehospital management includes placing the patient at rest, administering oxygen if SaO_2 <94%, initiating IV therapy, administering nitroglycerin and possibly morphine, monitoring the patient for dysrhythmias, and transporting the patient for evaluation by a physician.

- Acute myocardial infarction occurs when a coronary artery is blocked and blood does not reach an area of heart muscle. This results in ischemia, injury, and necrosis to the area of myocardium supplied by the affected artery. Death caused by myocardial infarction usually results from lethal dysrhythmias (ventricular tachycardia, ventricular fibrillation, and cardiac standstill), pump failure (cardiogenic shock and congestive heart failure), or myocardial tissue rupture (rupture of the ventricle, septum, or papillary muscle). Some patients with acute myocardial infarction, particularly those in the older age groups, have only symptoms of dyspnea, syncope, or confusion. However, substernal chest pain is usually present in patients with acute myocardial infarction (70% to 90% of patients). ST-segment elevation greater than or equal to 1 mV in at least two side-by-side ECG leads indicates an acute myocardial infarction. However, some patients infarct without ST-segment elevation. Other conditions also can produce ST-segment elevation. Prehospital management of the patient with a suspected myocardial infarction should include placing the patient at rest; administering oxygen if SaO_2 <94%; frequently assessing vital signs and breath sounds; initiating an IV line with normal saline or lactated Ringer solution to keep the vein open; monitoring for dysrhythmias; administering medications such as nitroglycerin, morphine, and aspirin; and screening for risk factors for fibrinolytic therapy; transport to an appropriate hospital.

- Left ventricular failure occurs when the left ventricle fails to function as an effective forward pump. This causes a back pressure of blood into the pulmonary circulation. This in turn may lead to pulmonary edema. Emergency management is directed at reducing the venous return to the heart, improving myocardial contractility, decreasing myocardial oxygen demand, improving ventilation and oxygenation, and rapidly transporting the patient to a medical facility.

- Right ventricular failure occurs when the right ventricle fails as a pump. This causes back pressure of blood into the systemic venous circulation. Right ventricular failure is not usually a medical emergency in itself unless it is associated with pulmonary edema or hypotension.

- Cardiogenic shock is the most extreme form of pump failure. It usually is caused by extensive myocardial infarction. Even with aggressive therapy, cardiogenic shock has a mortality rate of 70% or higher. Patients in cardiogenic shock require rapid transport to a medical facility.

- Cardiac tamponade is defined as impaired filling of the heart caused by increased pressure in the pericardial sac.

- Abdominal aortic aneurysms usually are asymptomatic. However, signs and symptoms signal impending or active rupture. If the vessel tears, bleeding initially may be stopped by the retroperitoneal tissues. The patient may be normotensive on the arrival of EMS. If the rupture opens into the peritoneal cavity, however, massive fatal hemorrhage may follow.

- Acute dissection is the most common aortic catastrophe. Any area of the aorta may be involved. However, in 60% to 70% of cases, the site of a dissecting aneurysm is in the ascending aorta, just beyond the takeoff of the left subclavian artery. The signs and symptoms depend on the site of the intimal tear. They also depend on the extent of dissection. The goals of managing suspected aortic dissection in the prehospital setting are relief of pain and immediate transport to a medical facility.

- Acute arterial occlusion is a sudden blockage of arterial flow. Occlusion most commonly is caused by trauma, an embolus, or thrombosis. The most common sites of embolic occlusion are the abdominal aorta, common femoral artery, popliteal artery, carotid artery, brachial artery, and mesenteric artery. The location of ischemic pain is related to the site of occlusion.

- Noncritical peripheral vascular conditions include varicose veins, superficial thrombophlebitis, and acute deep vein thrombosis. Of these conditions, deep vein thrombosis is the only one that can cause a life-threatening problem: pulmonary embolus.

- Hypertension often is defined by a resting blood pressure that is consistently greater than 140/90 mm Hg. Chronic hypertension has an adverse effect on the heart and blood vessels. It requires the heart to perform more work than normal. This leads to hypertrophy of the cardiac muscle and left ventricular failure. Conditions associated with chronic, uncontrolled hypertension are cerebral hemorrhage and stroke, myocardial infarction, and renal failure.

- Hypertensive emergencies are conditions in which a blood pressure increase leads to significant, irreversible end-organ damage within hours if not treated. The organs most likely to be at risk are the brain, heart, and kidneys. As a rule, the diagnosis is based on altered end-organ function and the rate of the rise in blood pressure, not the blood pressure level.
- Valvular heart disease may occur as a result of infection, or it may be related to heart disease. When one or more of these valves become narrowed, hardened, or thickened (stenotic), the valves do not open or close completely. As a result, blood does not flow with proper force or direction.
- Infectious heart disease includes endocarditis, pericarditis, and myocarditis. Complications can be severe and may include heart failure.
- Cardiomyopathy is an alteration in or weakness of the heart muscle. It can cause heart failure or sudden death. Basic cardiac life support helps maintain the circulation and respiration of a victim of cardiac arrest. Basic life support is continued until advanced cardiac life support is available. Two mechanisms are thought to be responsible for blood flow during cardiopulmonary resuscitation. One is direct compression of the heart between the sternum and the spine. This increases pressure within the ventricles to provide a small but critical amount of blood flow to the lungs and body organs. The second mechanism is increased intrathoracic pressure transmitted to all intrathoracic vascular structures. This creates an intrathoracic-to-extrathoracic pressure gradient. This gradient causes blood to flow out of the thorax. A number of mechanical devices provide external chest compression. Others provide chest compression with ventilation in a cardiac arrest patient.
- Cardiac monitor-defibrillators are classified as manual or automated external defibrillators. Defibrillation is the delivery of electrical current through the chest wall. Its purpose is to terminate ventricular fibrillation and certain other nonperfusing rhythms.
- Implantable cardioverter-defibrillators monitor the patient's cardiac rhythm. When a monitored ventricular rate exceeds the preprogrammed rate, the implantable cardioverter-defibrillator delivers a shock of about 6 to 30 J through patches. This is an attempt to restore a normal sinus rhythm.
- Synchronized cardioversion is designed to deliver a shock about 10 msec after the peak of the R wave of the cardiac cycle. (Therefore. the device avoids the relative refractory period.) Synchronization may reduce the amount of energy needed to end the dysrhythmia. It also may decrease the chances of causing another dysrhythmia.
- Transcutaneous cardiac pacing is an effective emergency therapy for bradycardia, complete heart block, and suppression of some malignant ventricular dysrhythmias. Proper electrode placement is important for effective external pacing.
- It is becoming increasingly evident that patients who cannot be resuscitated in the prehospital setting rarely survive. This is the case even if they are resuscitated temporarily in the emergency department. Cessation of resuscitative efforts in the prehospital setting should follow system-specific criteria established by medical direction.

REFERENCES

1. American Heart Association: 2010 American Heart Association guidelines for cardiopulmonary resuscitation and emergency cardiovascular care, *Circulation* 122:18(Suppl 3): S639-S946, 2010.
2. Marieb E, Hoehn K: *Human anatomy and physiology*, ed 8, San Francisco, 2009, Benjamin Cummings/Pearson Education.
3. Klabunde R: *Cardiovascular physiology concepts*, Philadelphia, 2005, Lippincott Williams & Wilkins.
4. Phalen T, Aehlert B: *The 12-lead ECG in acute myocardial infarction*, St Louis, 2006, Mosby.
5. Huszar RJ: *Basic dysrhythmias: interpretation and management*, ed 3, St Louis, 2006, Mosby.
6. American Heart Association: 2005 American Heart Association guidelines for cardiopulmonary resuscitation and emergency cardiovascular care, *Circulation* 112:(24)(Suppl):IV1-203, 2005.
7. Taigman M, Cannon S: Reading bundle branch blocks, *JEMS* 15:41, 1990.
8. Beyerbach D: *Lown-Ganong-Levine syndrome*. http://emedicine.medscape.com/article/160097-overview. Accessed February 16, 2010.
9. National Highway Traffic Safety Administration: *National EMS Education Standards*. (DOT HS 811 077A). Washington, 2009, Department of Transportation.
10. Williamson K, et al: Electrocardiographic applications of lead aVR, *Am J Emerg Med* 2006. www.ncbi.nlm.nih.gov/pubmed/17098112. Accessed February 13, 2010.
11. Wellens HJ, Conover M: *The ECG in emergency decision making*, ed 2, St Louis, 2006, Saunders.
12. Page B: *12-lead ECG interpretation workshop*, St Louis, 1998, Multi-lead Medics.
13. Hopenfeld B, Stinstra J, MacLeod R: A mechanism for ST depression associated with contiguous subendocardial ischemia, *J Cardiovasc Electrophys* 15:1200-1206, 2004.
14. ACC/AHA 2007 Guidelines for the management of patients with unstable angina/non–ST-elevation myocardial infarction, *J Am Coll Cardiol* 50:1-157, 2007.
15. American Heart Association/Centers for Disease Control and Prevention Scientific Statement: Markers of inflammation and cardiovascular disease: application to clinical and public health practice, *Circulation* 107:499-511, 2003.
16. Garratt K, Brady P, et al: Sulfonylurea drugs increase early mortality in patients with diabetes mellitus after direct

angioplasty for acute myocardial infarction, *J Am Coll Cardiol* 42(6):1017-1021, September 17, 2003.

17. ACC/AHA guidelines for the evaluation and management of chronic heart failure in the adult: executive summary, *Circulation* 104:2926-3007, 2001.

18. Ezekowitz JA, Hernandez A, Starling R, Yancy CW, Massie B, Hill JA, et al: Standardizing care for acute decompensated heart failure in a large megatrial: The approach for the Acute Studies of Clinical Effectiveness of Nesiritide in Subjects with Decompensated Heart Failure (ASCEND-HF), *American Heart Journal* 157(2):219-228, 2009.

19. Weintraub NL, Collins SP, Pange PS, Levy PD, Anderson AS, Arslanian-Engoren C, et al: Acute heart failure syndromes: emergency department presentation, treatment, and disposition: current approaches and future aims, *Circulation* 1-22, 2010. doi: 10.1161/CIR.0b013e3181f9a22310.1016/j.ahj.2008.10.002>

20. Peacock W, et al: Morphine and outcomes in acute decompensated heart failure: an ADHERE analysis, *Emerg Med J* 25:205-209, 2008.

21. Ezekowitz J, et al: Standardizing care for acute decompensating heart failure in large megatrial: the approach of the Acute Studies of Clinical Effectiveness of Nesiritide in Subjects with Decompensated Heart Failure (ASCEND-HF), *Am Heart J* 157:219-228, 2009.

22. Rosen P, Barkin R: *Emergency medicine: concepts and clinical practice*, ed 6, St Louis, 2005, Mosby

23. Grubbs T: *The ultimate emergency: managing aortic aneurysms*, *JEMS* 16:56, 1991.

24. Little R, Little W: *Physiology of the heart*, ed 4, St Louis, 1989, Mosby.

25. *Department of Health and Human Services, Centers for Disease Control and Prevention*, Washington, DC. National Vital Statistics Reports, vol 50, No 15, 2000.

26. National Joint Committee on Hypertension: *The seventh report of the Joint National Committee on Prevention, Detection, Evaluation, and Treatment of High Blood Pressure*, Washington, DC, 2004, National Institutes of Health, National Heart Lung and Blood Institute.

27. Sharma S, et al: Management of hypertensive urgency in an urgent care setting. *J Urgent Care Med.* http://jucm.net/2009-apr/clinical.shtml. Accessed February 19, 2010.

28. Armstrong C: *Practice guidelines: AHA guidelines on prevention of rheumatic fever and diagnosis and treatment of acute streptococcal pharyngitis.* www.aafp.org/afp/2010/0201/p346.html. Accessed February 20, 2010.

29. *Infectious endocarditis.* Medline Plus. www.nlm.nih.gov/medlineplus/ency/article/000681.htm. Accessed December 19, 2010.

30. *Pericarditis.* Medline Plus. www.nlm.nih.gov/medlineplus/ency/article/000182.htm. Accessed December 20, 2010.

31. Phalen T, Aehlert B: *12-Lead ECG in Acute Coronary Syndromes*, rev ed 2, St. Louis, 2006, Mosby.

32. *Cardiomyopathy.* Medline Plus. www.nlm.nih.gov/medlineplus/ency/article/001105.htm. Accessed February 10, 2010.

33. Nicholson C: *Heart failure: a clinical nursing handbook*, West Sussex, England, 2007, Wiley & Sons.

34. American Heart Association: *BLS for healthcare providers*, Dallas, 2005, The Association.

35. *The forerunner biphasic waveform technical note*, Seattle, 1997, Heartstream.

36. Brady G, et al: Multicenter comparison of truncated biphasic shocks and standard damped sine wave monophasic shocks for transthoracic ventricular defibrillation, *Pacing Clin Electrophysiol* 19:678, 1996.

37. Higgins S: *Defibrillation: what you should know*, Redmond, Texas, 1978, Physio-Control.

38. Dedrick D, et al: Defibrillation safety in emergency helicopter transport, *Ann Emerg Med* 18:69, 1989.

39. American Heart Association: *American Heart Association outlines "chilling" plan to prevent brain damage after cardiac arrest.* 2003. www.americanheart.org/presenter.jhtml?identifier=3013397. Accessed January 31, 2005.

40. Kim F, Olsufka M, et al: The use of prehospital mild hypothermia after resuscitation from out-of-hospital cardiac arrest, *J Neurotrauma* 26(3):359–363, 2009 March.

41. American Heart Association: Therapeutic hypothermia after cardiac arrest: an advisory statement by the Advanced Life Support Task Force of the International Liaison Committee on Resuscitation (ILCOR), *Circulation* 108:118, 2003.

42. Bernard SA: Treatment of comatose survivors of out-of-hospital cardiac arrest with induced hypothermia, *N Engl J Med* 346:557, 2002.

43. Bailey ED, et al: Termination of resuscitation in the prehospital setting for adult patients suffering nontraumatic cardiac arrest. National Association of EMS Physicians Standards and Clinical Practice Committee, *Prehosp Emerg Care* 4:190-195, 2000.

PART SEVEN

Medical

OBJECTIVES

Upon completion of this chapter, the paramedic student will be able to:

1. Label a diagram of the eye.
2. Describe the pathophysiology, signs and symptoms, and specific management techniques for each of the following disorders of the eye: conjunctivitis, corneal abrasion, foreign body, inflammation (chalazion and hordeolum), glaucoma, iritis, papilledema, retinal detachment, central retinal artery occlusion, and orbital cellulitis.
3. Label a diagram of the ear.
4. Describe the pathophysiology, signs and symptoms, and specific management techniques for each of the following conditions that affect the ear: foreign body, impacted cerumen, labyrinthitis, Meniere's disease, otitis media, perforated tympanic membrane.
5. Label a diagram of the nose.
6. Describe the pathophysiology, signs and symptoms, and specific management techniques for each of the following conditions that affect the nose: epistaxis, foreign body, rhinitis, and sinusitis.
7. Label a diagram of the oropharynx.
8. Describe the pathophysiology, signs and symptoms, and specific management techniques for each of the following conditions that affect the oropharynx and throat: toothache and dental abscess, Ludwig's angina, epiglottitis, laryngitis, tracheitis, oral candidiasis, peritonsillar abscess, pharyngitis/tonsillitis, and temporomandibular joint disorders.

KEY TERMS

angle-closure glaucoma A form of glaucoma associated with a physically obstructed anterior chamber angle; may be chronic or, rarely, acute.

central retinal artery occlusion The blockage of blood supply to the arteries of the retina.

cerumen A yellowish or brownish waxy secretion produced in the external ear canal; also known as earwax.

chalazion A small bump in the eyelid, caused by the blockage of a tiny oil gland in the upper or lower eyelid.

conjunctivitis Inflammation of the conjunctiva, caused by bacterial or viral infection, allergy, or environmental factors.

corneal abrasion The rubbing off of the outer layers of the cornea.

dental abscess A bacterial infection in the center of the tooth.

dentalgia The medical term for toothache.

epiglottitis Inflammation of the epiglottis; a severe form of the condition that affects primarily children is characterized by fever, sore throat, stridor, croupy cough, and an erythematous epiglottis.

epistaxis Bleeding from the nose.

glaucoma A condition in which intraocular pressure increases and causes damage to the optic nerve.

hordeolum An acute infection of the oil gland; commonly known as a stye.

iritis Inflammation of the iris of the eye.

labyrinthitis An ear disorder that involves irritation and swelling of the inner ear structure called the labyrinth.

laryngitis Inflammation of the larynx.

Ludwig's angina A type of cellulitis that involves inflammation of the tissues of the floor of the mouth, under the tongue.

Meniere's disease An abnormality of the inner ear that causes vertigo and tinnitus; associated with fluctuations in hearing loss and a sensation of pressure or pain in the affected ear.

mononucleosis A viral infection causing fever, sore throat, and swollen lymph glands, especially in the neck.

open-angle glaucoma The most common type of glaucoma; structures of the eye appear normal but fluid in the eye does not flow properly through the trabecular meshwork; also called wide-angle glaucoma.

oral candidiasis An infection of yeast fungi of the genus *Candida* on the mucous membranes of the mouth; also known as thrush.

orbital cellulitis An acute inflammation in the tissues immediately surrounding the eye, including the eyelids, eyebrow, and cheek.

otitis media Infection or inflammation of the middle ear.

papilledema Swelling of the head of the optic disc, caused by a rise in intracranial pressure (ICP).

perforated tympanic membrane A hole or rupture in the eardrum, usually from trauma or infection.

peritonsillar abscess A collection of pus in and around one or both tonsils; often caused by tonsillitis.

pharyngitis Inflammation or infection of the pharynx.

retinal detachment A separation of the light-sensitive retina from its supporting layers.

rhinitis Inflammation of the mucous membranes of the nose.

sinusitis Inflammation of one or more paranasal sinuses.

strep throat An infection of the throat caused by streptococcal bacteria.

temporomandibular joint dysfunction Acute or chronic inflammation in the temporomandibular joint.

tinnitus A ringing sound in the ears.

tonsillitis Inflammation of the tonsils.

tracheitis A bacterial infection of the upper airway and subglottic trachea.

trismus Muscle spasms of the jaw.

vertigo A sensation of faintness or an inability to maintain normal balance in a standing or seated position.

M*edical conditions that affect the ears, eyes, nose, and throat are a common occurrence in the prehospital setting.*[1] *This chapter will review the anatomy of these structures and discuss the specific findings, symptoms, and management considerations for common diseases.*

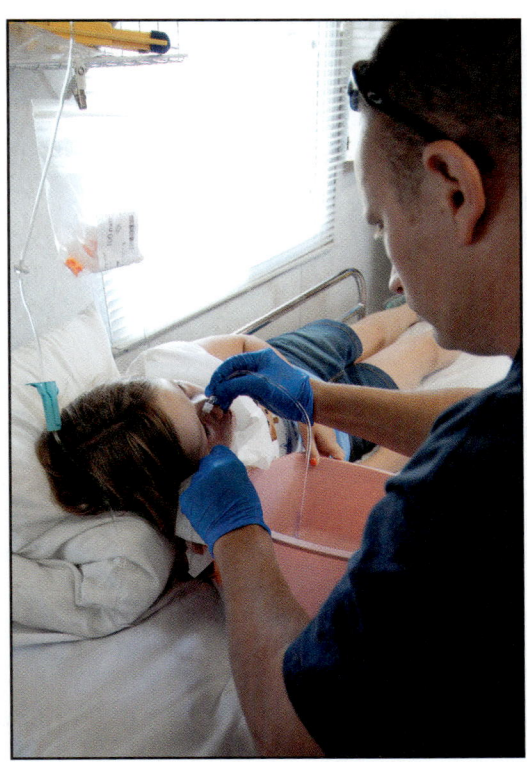

CONDITIONS OF THE EYE

As described in Chapter 10, the eye is composed of three layers: the fibrous tunic, consisting of the sclera and cornea; the vascular tunic, consisting of the choroid, ciliary body, and the iris; and the nervous tunic, consisting of the retina (Figure 23-1). In addition, there are accessory structures that protect, lubricate, move, and aid in the function of the eye. These structures include the eyebrows, eyelids, conjunctiva, and lacrimal gland. Box 23-1 lists conditions of the eyes described in this chapter.

LOOK AGAIN
See Chapter 10: Review of Human Systems, pp. 206-208.

BOX 23-1 Medical Conditions That Affect the Eye

Conjunctivitis
Corneal abrasion
Foreign body
Inflammation (chalazion and hordeolum)
Glaucoma
Iritis
Papilledema
Retinal detachment
Central retinal artery occlusion
Orbital cellulitis

NOTE
As described in Chapter 20: Secondary Assessment, eye movement is controlled by cranial nerves III, IV, and VI. The paramedic should remember that visual disturbances of the eyes may be an early indication of stroke, tumor, or other nervous system disease. These possibilities must always be considered when caring for a patient with an eye movement disorder.

CRITICAL THINKING
Which assessment will you perform on an unconscious patient to determine if there is pressure on cranial nerve III?

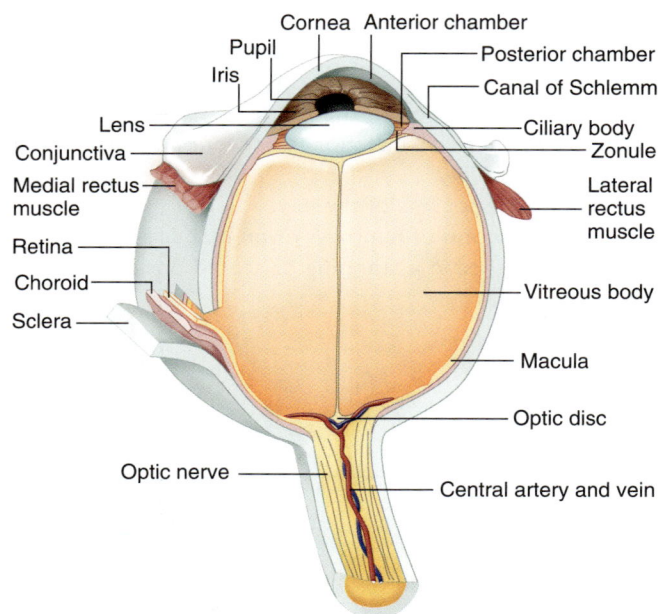

FIGURE 23-1 Anatomy of the eye. (From Goldman L: *Cecil medicine,* ed 23, Philadelphia, 2008, Saunders.)

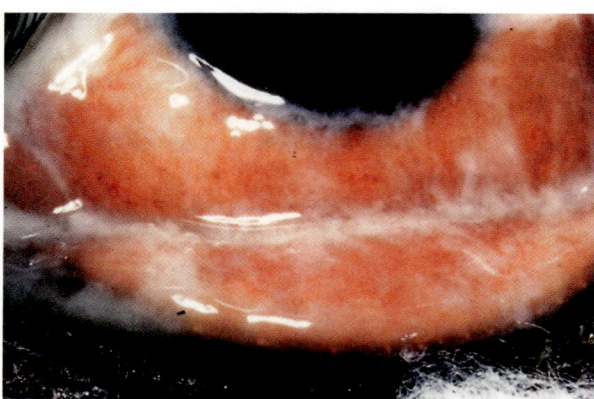

FIGURE 23-2 Gonococcal conjunctivitis showing redness and copious discharge in the eye caused by *Neisseria gonorrhoeae.* (From Mahon CR, Manuselis G: *Textbook of diagnostic microbiology,* ed 2, Philadelphia, 2000, Saunders.)

Conjunctivitis

Conjunctivitis refers to inflammation or infection of the conjunctiva (the membrane lining of the eyes). The condition is commonly called "pink eye," or "Madras eye." Two common causes of conjunctivitis are bacterial or viral infection and an allergic reaction (Figure 23-2). In newborns, conjunctivitis can result from an incompletely opened tear duct.

> **NOTE**
> Conjunctivitis can also be caused by agents that irritate the eye. Examples include an accidental exposure to chemicals and a foreign body in the eye (see Chapter 39 and Chapter 40).

Conjunctivitis caused by viral or bacterial infection is very contagious. Therefore, early diagnosis and treatment can prevent spread of the disease. This type of conjunctivitis can affect both eyes and is often associated with a cold. If the cause is viral, there may be a watery, mucous discharge. If the cause is bacterial, the discharge may be thick and yellow-green. Most bacterial infections are associated with a respiratory tract infection or sore throat. Bacterial conjunctivitis is more common in children than adults. To help prevent the spread of infectious conjunctivitis, patients who have the disease should be cautioned not to touch their eyes with their hands and to practice the following precautions:

- Wash hands thoroughly and frequently.
- Change towels and washcloths daily, and do not share them with others.
- Change pillowcase often.
- Discard eye cosmetics, particularly mascara.
- Avoid using another person's eye cosmetics or personal eyecare items.
- Follow instructions from eye physician about proper contact lens care.

Conjunctivitis can be caused by allergies. An example is exposure to an allergen such as pollen (see Chapter 27). This type of inflammation is often associated with eyes that water and itch, and sometimes with sneezing and a nasal discharge ("runny nose").

MANAGEMENT CONSIDERATIONS

Although conjunctivitis is irritating to the eye, it rarely affects vision. Bacterial causes of the condition are usually managed with antibiotic eye drops or eye ointment.[2] Symptoms generally improve within 1 to 2 days. Viral and allergic forms of conjunctivitis are usually managed with over-the-counter medicines (e.g., antihistamines and decongestants) to relieve symptoms. If severe, drugs such as steroids and antiinflammatories may be prescribed. The symptoms of viral and allergic conjunctivitis may take several days to a week or more to subside.

Corneal Abrasion

As the name implies, a **corneal abrasion** is a painful scrape or scratch on the cornea of the eye. It most often occurs from trauma, such as being struck in the eye by a tree branch or limb. It is also frequently caused by foreign bodies in the eye that lodge under the upper lid (e.g., dust, paint chips, wind debris). Corneal abrasions can also be caused by wearing contact lenses longer than recommended, or by allowing the contact lens, fingers, or nails to scratch the eye during insertion or removal of contact lenses. Signs and symptoms of a corneal abrasion include:[3]

- Pain (which can be severe)
- A sensation of a foreign body in the eye
- Tearing and redness
- Blurred vision
- Spasms of the muscles around the eye, causing the patient to squint

MANAGEMENT CONSIDERATIONS

Prehospital care for a patient with a corneal abrasion is usually limited to supportive measures to relieve pain and prevent further injury. Care may include applying a topical ophthalmic anesthetic, such as *tetracaine,* and covering the affected eye. Patients with corneal abrasion should be seen by a physician.

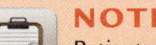

NOTE
Patients who are given *tetracaine* should be cautioned not to rub or manipulate the eye or eyelid. Doing so to an eye that has been anesthetized can worsen the injury.

Foreign Body

As stated earlier in this chapter, small foreign bodies in the eye are not uncommon. They are often irritating to the patient, but seldom affect vision. Common complaints are pain, tearing, and a sensation of fullness in the eye.

MANAGEMENT CONSIDERATIONS

Small foreign bodies can be washed or irrigated from the eye using eye cups or saline solution attached to intravenous (IV) tubing. The patient should be instructed not to rub the lid of the affected eye, which could lead to a corneal abrasion. Large or penetrating foreign bodies in the eye are serious in nature and should be managed as described in Chapter 40.

Inflammation of the Eyelid

Inflammation of the eyelid usually results from blockage of a gland or from bacterial infection. Two common conditions are chalazion and hordeolum.

Chalazion is a small bump in the eyelid, caused by the blockage of a tiny oil gland in the upper or lower eyelid. These oil glands normally secrete oil into tears (Figure 23-3). The lump appears as localized and hard, and may increase in size over days to weeks. Symptoms include tenderness, tearing, painful swelling, and sensitivity to light (*photophobia*).[4]

DID YOU KNOW?
There are about 40 oil glands (*meibomian glands*) within each upper and lower eyelid. The glands secret oil into tears, through a tiny opening located just behind the eyelashes.

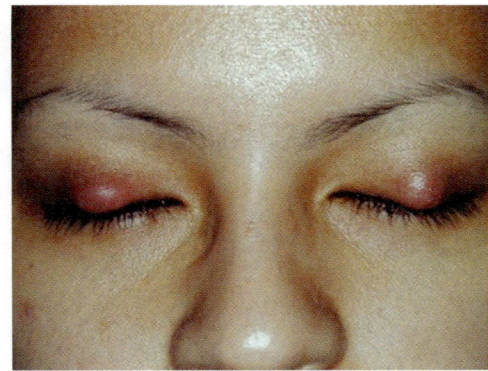

FIGURE 23-3 Bilateral chalazion in the upper eyelids. (From Goldman L: *Cecil medicine,* ed 23, Philadelphia, 2008, Saunders.)

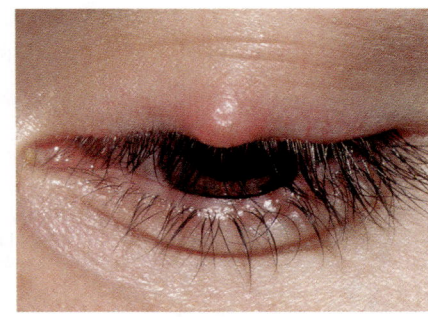

FIGURE 23-4 Acute hordeolum of upper eyelid. (From Krachmer JH, Palay DA: *Cornea color atlas*, St. Louis, 1997, Mosby.)

A **hordeolum** is commonly known as a **stye.** It represents an acute infection of the oil gland. A stye is usually more painful than a chalazion caused by inflammation, and may look infected (Figure 23-4). The pain of a stye can cause redness around the eye, the eyelid, and cheek tissue. A stye can be limited to one eyelid or can occur on both eyelids simultaneously.

MANAGEMENT CONSIDERATIONS

Inflammation of the eyelids from either of these conditions usually subsides without treatment within 5 to 7 days.[5] Home care may include applying warm compresses 3 to 4 times a day, and gentle scrubbing of the affected eyelid with warm water and a mild soap or shampoo. Patients should be advised not to squeeze or puncture the inflamed area because it can result in serious infection. Eye makeup and eye lotions and creams should be avoided until the inflammation clears. If fever or headache develops, the patient should seek physician evaluation.

Glaucoma

Glaucoma refers to a group of diseases that affect the optic nerve (Box 23-2). It develops when too much aqueous humor accumulates in the anterior chamber of the eye, between the cornea and the iris. This fluid normally flows

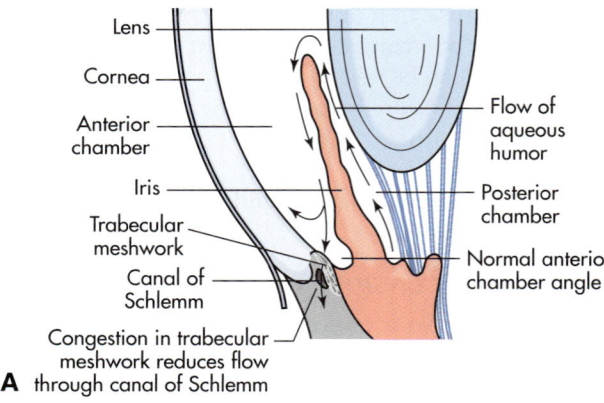

Slowly rising intraocular pressure

A, Congestion in trabecular meshwork reduces flow through canal of Schlemm

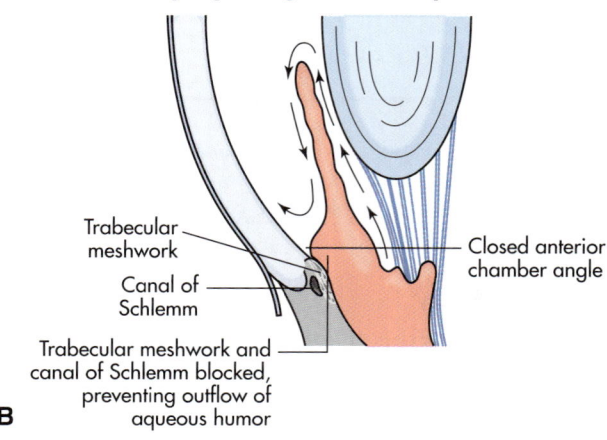

Rapidly rising intraocular pressure

B, Trabecular meshwork and canal of Schlemm blocked, preventing outflow of aqueous humor

FIGURE 23-6 A, Primary open-angle glaucoma. Congestion in the trabecular meshwork reduces the outflow of aqueous humor. **B,** Primary closed-angle glaucoma (acute). The angle between the iris and the anterior chamber narrows, obstructing the outflow of aqueous humor. (From Christensen BL, et al: *Adult health nursing,* ed 6, St Louis, 2010, Mosby.)

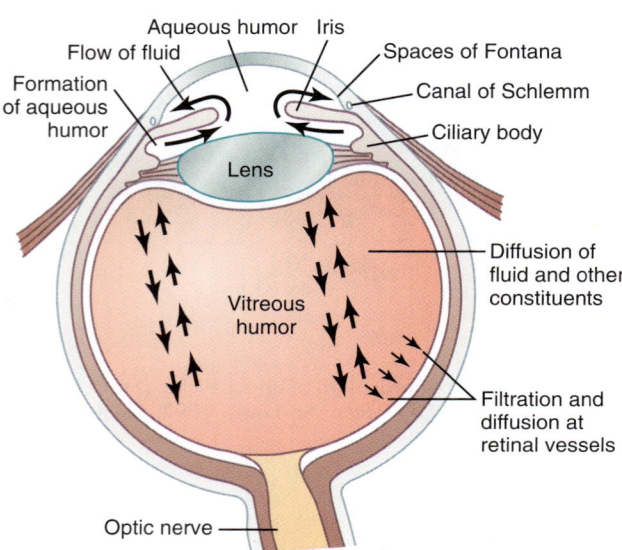

FIGURE 23-5 Formation and flow of fluid in the eye. (From Hall J: *Guyton and Hall textbook of medical physiology,* ed 12, Philadelphia, 2011, Saunders.)

out of the eye through a mesh-like channel (trabecular channel) (Figure 23-5). If this channel becomes blocked, the increase in intraocular pressure damages the optic nerve and can lead to a loss of vision. Without treatment, the condition can lead to permanent blindness. The disease usually occurs in both eyes, but affects one more than the other. The direct cause of the blockage is unknown, but seems to have a heritable **component.**[6] Other risk factors for developing the disease include:

- African-American, Hispanic, Inuit, Irish, Japanese, Russian, or Scandinavian heritage
- More than 40 years old
- Poor vision
- Diabetes
- Use of systemic corticosteroid drugs (e.g., prednisone)

Glaucoma can occur at any age (including children and infants), but occurs most often after age 40 (see Chapter 49). There may be no symptoms of the disease (early

screening every 1 to 2 years is important). The first sign of glaucoma is usually a loss of peripheral vision, which can remain unnoticed until the disease has progressed. If the rise in intraocular pressure is severe, the patient may have sudden eye pain, headache, vomiting, and blurred vision. The patient may also complain of seeing halos around lights caused by swelling of the cornea.

CRITICAL THINKING

If a patient presents with these signs and symptoms, what other conditions should you consider in your differential diagnosis?

MANAGEMENT CONSIDERATIONS

Prehospital care for patients with glaucoma is primarily supportive. If symptoms are sudden in onset, rapid transport for physician evaluation is indicated. Physician care to treat glaucoma may include eye drops to reduce the formation of fluid in the eye, laser surgery to increase the outflow of fluid in the eye, or microsurgery to create a new channel to drain the fluid from the eye. In some cases, a combination of these therapies will be needed to prevent blindness.

Iritis

Iritis (*anterior uveitis*) is inflammation of the iris of the eye. It is a serious disease that can cause blindness if not treated (Figure 23-7). Causes of iritis include eye trauma, inflammatory and autoimmune disorders, infection, and cancer. Examples of medical causes of the inflammation include rheumatoid arthritis, lupus, Crohn's disease, Lyme disease, herpes, syphilis, tuberculosis, and **leukemia.**[7] Iritis can be classified as acute or chronic. The acute form of the disease develops suddenly and usually heals within a few weeks with treatment. Chronic iritis can exist for months or years, and is associated with a higher risk of vision impairment or blindness. Iritis can affect one or both eyes. Signs and symptoms of iritis include a reddened eye, ocular or periorbital pain, photophobia, and blurred or cloudy vision.

MANAGEMENT CONSIDERATIONS

Prehospital care is primarily supportive. Physician care may include a variety of steroidal antiinflammatory eye drops, pressure-reducing eye drops, and oral and injectable steroids to reduce inflammation.

Papilledema

Papilledema is swelling of the head of the optic disc, caused by a rise in intracranial pressure (ICP). There are numerous causes of elevated ICP, including cerebral edema, bleeding within the skull, tumors, encephalitis, and increased production of cerebral spinal fluid (CSF), among others (see Chapter 25 and Chapter 40). The swelling of the optic disc is usually bilateral and may be more severe in one eye than the other. The condition is diagnosed using an ophthalmoscope (described in Chapter 20), where visible signs may include (Figure 23-8):

- Venous engorgement (usually the first sign)
- Loss of venous pulsation
- Hemorrhages over and/or adjacent to the optic disc
- Blurring of optic margins
- Elevation of optic disc
- *Paton's lines* (radial retinal lines cascading from the optic disc)

Patient complaints may include a headache that is usually worse on awakening and made worse by coughing, holding the breath, or straining. Other complaints may include nausea and vomiting and vision disturbances (double vision and vision that temporarily flickers or grays).

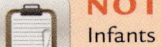

NOTE

Infants who are victims of *shaken baby syndrome* may be unconscious with papilledema. Therefore, shaken baby syndrome should be suspected with this presentation. External signs of abuse may or may not be present (see Chapter 50).

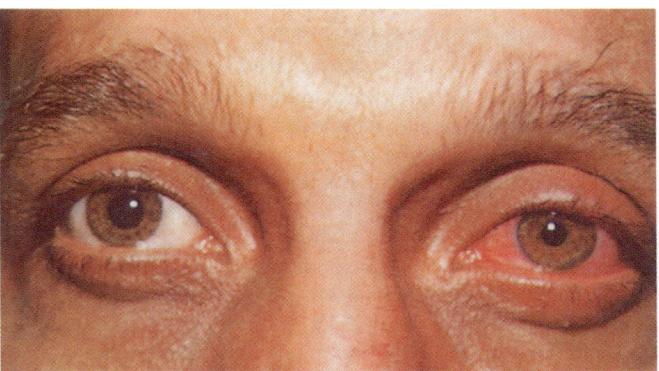

FIGURE 23-7 Iritis. (From Jarvis C: *Physical examination and health assessment,* ed 5, St Louis, 2008, Saunders.)

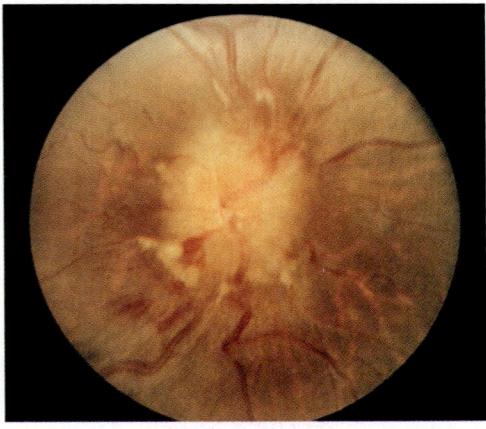

FIGURE 23-8 Severe papilledema. (Courtesy John W. Payne, MD, The Wilmer Ophthalmological Institute, The Johns Hopkins University and Hospital, Baltimore, Md.)

MANAGEMENT CONSIDERATIONS

Prehospital care is primarily supportive. Physician care will depend on the cause of the disease. After the underlying cause is determined and treated, medical care may include diuretics to reduce increased CSF and corticosteroids to reduce inflammation. If papilledema is diagnosed and managed early, permanent vision damage can often be prevented.

Retinal Detachment

As described in Chapter 10, the retina is the light-sensitive tissue that lines the inside of the eye. It also sends visual messages from the optic nerve to the brain. If the retina detaches, it is lifted or pulled from its normal position. Small areas of the retina can also be torn. These retinal *tears, breaks,* or *defects* can lead to retinal detachment. Box 23-3 describes the three different types of retinal detachment.

BOX 23-3 Types of Retinal Detachment

Rhegmatogenous—A tear or break in the retina allows fluid to get under the retina and separate it from the retinal pigment epithelium (RPE), the pigmented cell layer that nourishes the retina. These types of retinal detachments are the most common.

Tractional—In this type of detachment, scar tissue on the retina's surface contracts and causes the retina to separate from the RPE. This type of detachment is less common.

Exudative—Frequently caused by retinal diseases, including inflammatory disorders and injury/trauma to the eye. In this type, fluid leaks into the area underneath the retina, but there are no tears or breaks in the retina.[8]

Retinal detachment is a true emergency and can lead to permanent vision loss. The condition can occur at any age, but is more likely to occur in people who[8]:

- Are extremely nearsighted
- Have had a retinal detachment in the other eye
- Have a family history of retinal detachment
- Have had cataract surgery
- Have other eye diseases or disorders
- Have had an eye injury
- Have diabetes
- Have sickle cell disease

Signs and symptoms of retinal detachment include a sudden or gradual increase in either the number of floaters, which are little "cobwebs" or specks that float in your field of vision, and/or the number of light flashes in the eye. Another symptom is the appearance of a curtain over the field of vision.

CRITICAL THINKING

How would your life change if you were to lose your sight next week?

MANAGEMENT CONSIDERATIONS

Like most eye conditions, prehospital care for a patient with retinal detachment is primarily supportive. Because the condition is a true emergency, rapid transport for physician evaluation is key. Small tears in the retina may be repaired with laser surgery or a freeze treatment (*cryopexy*) to reattach the retina. Full retinal detachment requires advanced surgery and usually hospitalization. About 90% of patients can be successfully treated if managed early, with varying degrees of visual outcome. Visual results are best if the retinal detachment is repaired before the macula (the center region of the retina responsible for fine, detailed vision) detaches.[9]

Central Retinal Artery Occlusion

Central retinal artery occlusion (CRO) is the blockage of blood supply to the arteries of the retina. CRO produces sudden, painless blindness and is usually limited to one eye. This is a true ocular emergency. Retinal circulation must be reestablished within 60 to 90 minutes to prevent permanent loss of vision. Occasionally, before total occlusion occurs, the patient may experience transient episodes of blindness called *amaurosis fugax*. This can be equated to a transient ischemia attack of the retinal artery. Patients usually describe the episode as a shade coming down over the eye. Causes of CRO include embolus (carotid and cardiac), thrombosis, hypertension, or simple angiospasm (rare) associated with a migraine or atrial fibrillation. Hence, the patient will need to be thoroughly evaluated to rule out other systemic problems.

MANAGEMENT CONSIDERATIONS

Prehospital care is primarily supportive. The patient requires rapid transport to an appropriate facility. To prevent permanent damage, retinal perfusion needs to be reestablished as rapidly as possible. In-hospital care may include vasodilation techniques, ocular massage, and administration of *intraocular pressure–lowering drugs,* none of which have been shown to be extremely beneficial.[10]

Orbital Cellulitis

Orbital cellulitis is an acute infection of the tissues that surround the eye. These areas include the eyelids, eyebrow, and cheek (Figure 23-9). Orbital cellulitis is a dangerous infection that can have serious consequences if not treated. It can quickly lead to blindness, especially in children. Other complications of the disease include hearing loss, septicemia, sinus thrombosis, and meningitis.

Orbital cellulitis can be caused from bacteria (often *Haemophilus influenzae*) from a sinus infection. (This form is especially common in children less than 6 years of age, but

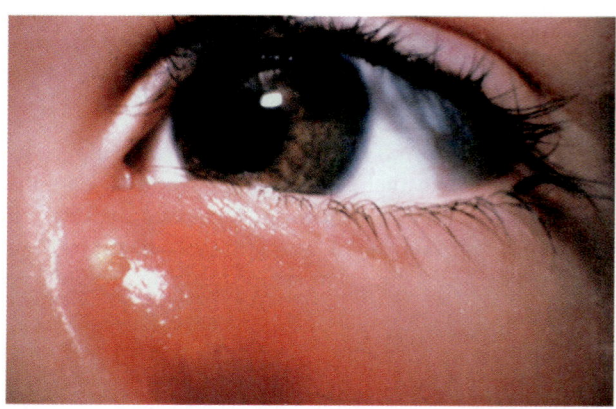

FIGURE 23-9 Orbital cellulitis. (From Marx J, et al: *Rosen's emergency medicine: concepts and clinical practice,* ed 6, St Louis, 2006, Mosby.)

the rate has decreased steadily with the HiB vaccine.[11]) The bacteria *Staphylococcus aureus, Streptococcus pneumoniae,* and beta-hemolytic streptococci may also cause orbital cellulitis. Other causes of orbital cellulitis include stye and eyelid injury with inflammation. Signs and symptoms of the disease include:

- Fever, with temperature generally >102° F (38.9° C)
- Painful swelling of upper and lower eyelids
- Shiny, red or purple eyelid
- Eye pain
- Decreased vision
- Bulging eyes
- General malaise
- Painful or difficult eye movements

MANAGEMENT CONSIDERATIONS

Prehospital care is focused on recognition of the signs and symptoms and rapid transport for physician evaluation. Patients will usually be hospitalized for diagnostic tests. Physician care may include IV antibiotics and sometimes surgery to drain any abscess associated with the illness. With prompt treatment, most patients will make a full recovery.

> ### CRITICAL THINKING
> If a patient with orbital cellulitis has developed sepsis, what additional signs and symptoms should you anticipate?

CONDITIONS OF THE EAR

As described in Chapter 10, the ear can be divided into three portions: external, middle, and inner ear. The external ear and middle ear are involved in hearing only. The inner ear functions in both hearing and balance (Figure 23-10). Common medical conditions that affect the ear are listed in Box 23-4.

>
> ### LOOK AGAIN
> See Chapter 10: Review of Human Systems, pp. 208-209.

Foreign Body

A foreign body in the ear is a fairly common occurrence, especially in toddlers. Most foreign bodies are lodged in the ear canal. Common objects found in the ears of young children include food material and toys that are usually

> **BOX 23-4 Medical Conditions That Affect the Ear**
>
> Foreign body
> Impacted cerumen
> Labyrinthitis
> Meniere's disease
> Otitis media
> Perforated tympanic membrane

FIGURE 23-10 Anatomy of the ear. (From Jarvis C: *Physical examination and health assessment,* ed 5, St. Louis, 2008, Saunders.)

inserted voluntarily. Children and adults are also subject to insects that enter the ear canal during sleep. Foreign bodies in the ear are often easily detected by complaints of pressure, discomfort, and decreased hearing in the affected ear. (If the foreign body stays undetected, serious infection can result.) Bleeding from the ear can also occur if the foreign body is sharp or is manipulated during attempts to remove it.

> ### NOTE
> It is not uncommon for young children to have multiple foreign bodies inserted in both ears and the nose. The paramedic should be alert for this possibility. All children should be reminded not to put anything "smaller than an elbow" in the ear or nose.

Foreign bodies in the ear are seldom a serious medical condition that requires emergency care. Most objects can be easily removed at a physician's office or clinic. Some foreign bodies do require immediate removal in the emergency department. These include button-type batteries than can cause chemical burns, and food and plant material that can swell when moistened. If the patient complains of significant pain or discomfort, immediate evaluation by a physician is also indicated.

MANAGEMENT CONSIDERATIONS

Prehospital care for foreign bodies in the ear is limited to gentle examination of the external auditory canal. This can be done by gently pulling back on the ear's pinna (changing the shape of the ear canal), and viewing the canal with a penlight or ear speculum. Objects that are visible may sometimes be easily removed with alligator forceps. Care should be taken not to push the object deeper into the canal. This can make the object more difficult to retrieve and may also damage the eardrum. Patients who require physician evaluation should be advised not to eat or drink before their exam, because sedation may be needed to safely remove the foreign body. In-hospital care may include diagnostic imaging, irrigation of the ear canal, suction, surgical removal of the foreign body, and prescribed antibiotics.

> ### CRITICAL THINKING
> What additional signs and symptoms might your patient experience if there is a live insect in his or her ear?

Impacted Cerumen

As described in Chapter 10, **cerumen** (earwax) is produced normally by the ceruminous glands that are located in the external auditory canal. Cerumen protects and lubricates the skin of the ear canal. It also provides some protection from bacteria, fungi, insects, and water. Cerumen is a yellowish-waxy substance that has the consistency of toothpaste. Excess cerumen can become impacted, pressing up against the eardrum and creating a foreign body in the ear. Excessive cerumen can impede the passage of sound in the ear canal, causing hearing loss. Signs and symptoms of impacted cerumen include:

- Earache, fullness in the ear, or a sensation the ear is plugged
- Partial hearing loss, which may be progressive
- Tinnitus, ringing, or noises in the ear
- Itching, odor, or discharge
- Coughing

Many patients regularly clean their ears of excess cerumen with cotton-tipped swabs. This is a dangerous practice that can push the cerumen deeper into the ear. It is recommended that cerumen not be removed from the ear canal, unless the cerumen is impacted.[12] Most forms of ear blockage respond well to home treatments to soften the wax. These treatments include irrigation and syringing with warm water or saline and wax-dissolving drops (e.g., mineral oil, baby oil, glycerin, and other commercial drops).

> ### NOTE
> Ears should not be irrigated if a person has diabetes, a perforated eardrum, a tube in the eardrum, or a weakened immune system.[12]

MANAGEMENT CONSIDERATIONS

Prehospital care for a patient with impacted cerumen is primarily supportive. Patients should be encouraged to see a physician for wax removal. This is most often performed by an otolaryngologist using special equipment and techniques.

Labyrinthitis

Labyrinthitis is an ear disorder that involves irritation and swelling of the inner ear structure called the *labyrinth* (described in Chapter 10). Inflammation of this balance-control area in the ear can cause sudden **vertigo.** It may also cause a temporary hearing loss and a ringing sound in the ears **(tinnitus).** Labyrinthitis can result from a viral infection or, more rarely, a bacterial infection. Common triggers are an upper respiratory tract infection and middle ear infection.

> ### NOTE
> Vertigo (dizziness) is an uncomfortable feeling when there is no actual movement. It is commonly described as spinning or whirling. It may also include the sensations of falling or tilting. Vertigo may cause nausea and vomiting, and may impair the patient's ability to walk or stand. Vertigo and ataxia (failure of muscle coordination) also can signal stroke (see Chapter 26).

MANAGEMENT CONSIDERATIONS

Prehospital care for patients with labyrinthitis is primarily supportive. Patients should be advised to be careful of falling and to have assistance when walking. Most cases of labyrinthitis resolve without treatment. If infection is to blame, antibiotics may be prescribed. Antiemetics may also be prescribed for symptoms of nausea and vomiting.

Meniere's Disease

Meniere's disease is an abnormality of the inner ear. Like labyrinthitis, this disease causes vertigo and tinnitus. It is also associated with fluctuations in hearing loss and a sensation of pressure or pain in the affected ear. The symptoms of Meniere's disease are associated with a change in fluid volume in the labyrinth. Causes of the disease may include environmental factors, such as noise pollution, viral infection, and biological factors. It is estimated that about 615,000 Americans have been diagnosed with the disease and that 45,500 new cases are diagnosed each year.[13]

The classic presentation of Meniere's disease is a combination of vertigo, tinnitus, and hearing loss that lasts several hours. The symptoms occur suddenly. Episodes can be as frequent as once a day or as infrequent as once per year. The vertigo is often debilitating and can lead to severe nausea and vomiting. Other symptoms of the disease may include headache, abdominal discomfort, and diarrhea.

MANAGEMENT CONSIDERATIONS

Like most other conditions that affect the ear, prehospital care for a patient with Meniere's disease is primarily supportive. There is no cure for the illness. Physician care may include medications and diet restrictions to reduce fluid retention. Drug therapy to improve blood circulation in the inner ear may also be prescribed. Eliminating tobacco use and reducing stress may help with the severity of the symptoms.

CRITICAL THINKING
What other conditions in addition to labyrinthitis and Meniere's disease can cause vertigo?

Otitis Media

Otitis media is infection or inflammation of the middle ear. (*Otitis externa* is inflammation of the outer ear and ear canal. It is commonly known as "swimmer's ear.")

Otitis media occurs between the eardrum and inner ear and involves the eustachian tube (Figure 23-11). Otitis often begins with viral or bacterial infections that cause sore throats, colds, or other respiratory problems that spread to the middle ear. Otitis media can be acute or chronic. It most commonly affects infants and young children, but can also occur in adults. Signs and symptoms of otitis media include:

- Chills
- Diarrhea
- Drainage from the ear

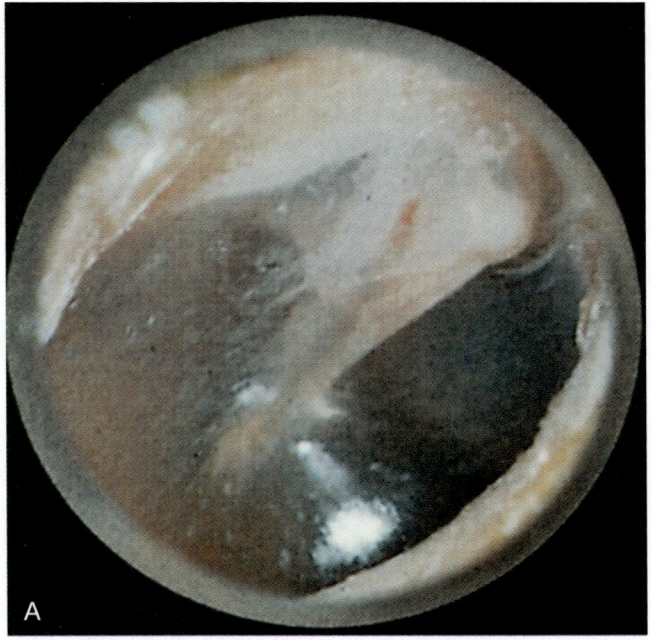

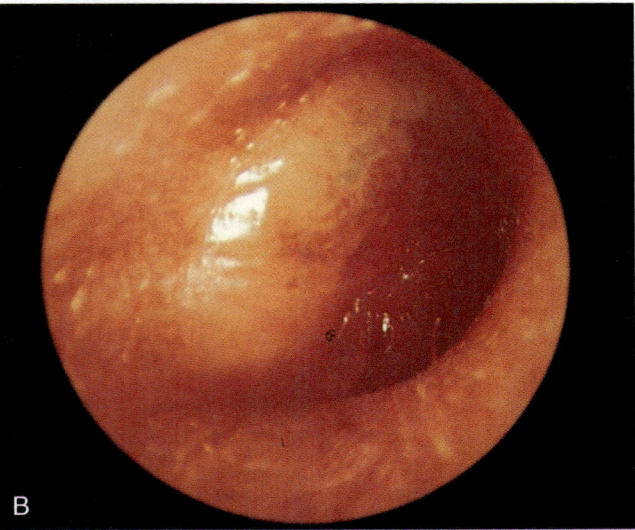

FIGURE 23-11 A, Normal tympanic membrane. **B,** Tympanic membrane with otitis media. (**A,** Courtesy Richard A. Buckingham, Clinical Professor, Otolaryngology, Abraham Lincoln School of Medicine, University of Illinois, Chicago, from Seidel HM, Ball JW, Dains JE, et al: *Mosby's guide to physical examination,* ed 5, St Louis, 2003, Mosby. **B,** Courtesy Michael Hawke, MD, from Zitelli BJ, Davis HD: *Atlas of pediatric physical diagnosis,* ed 4, St Louis, 2002, Mosby.)

- Earache
- Ear noise or buzzing
- Fever
- Hearing loss
- Discomfort in the ear or ear canal
- Irritability
- General malaise
- Nausea
- Vomiting

Otitis media causes severe pain and can have serious consequences. If untreated, the infection can travel from the middle ear to the brain and may lead to permanent hearing loss. Because the illness often strikes small children with limited speech and communications skills, the paramedic should be keen to subtle signs and symptoms such as irritability, tugging at the ear, fever, and drainage from the ear. Parents or other caregivers may notice a loss of balance, sleeplessness, and signs of hearing difficulty.

MANAGEMENT CONSIDERATIONS

Children with otitis media need to be evaluated by a physician. Until such time, the child should avoid contact with other children who are sick; the child should not be exposed to environmental smoke, which may aggravate the condition. Physician assessment will include an otoscope examination of the outer ear and eardrum. Various tests may also be used to assess middle ear fluid, eardrum movement, and hearing. Prescribed medications may include antibiotics for a bacterial infection, and agents to reduce pain and fever. Once the infection is eradicated, fluid may remain in the middle ear for several months. Follow-up with a physician is required. Other treatments may include surgical removal of the adenoids and the placement of tubes in the affected ears (myringotomy) to ventilate the middle ear. These procedures often are done at the same time.

Perforated Tympanic Membrane

Perforated tympanic membrane is a hole or rupture in the eardrum. Causes of perforation are usually from trauma or infection. Examples of traumatic causes of perforated tympanic membrane include blunt trauma to the ear, barotrauma, skull fracture, explosion or blast injury, and foreign bodies in the ear (see Part 9: Trauma). Otitis media is an example of an infection that can cause a perforated tympanic membrane (*otitis media with perforation*). Signs and symptoms of perforation caused by infection are those of middle ear infections (described previously), and include decreased hearing and an occasional bloody discharge. Pain is usually not persistent with perforation.

MANAGEMENT CONSIDERATIONS

Perforations of the tympanic membrane often cause a patient to be anxious, especially if it is related to trauma. However, prehospital care is primarily supportive. Most perforations of the eardrum heal without treatment within weeks of the rupture. Some perforations may take several months to heal. During the healing process, the affected ear should be protected from water and trauma. Perforations that do not heal on their own require advanced technologies and/or surgical intervention to close the tympanic membrane. These techniques often will restore or improve hearing.

The amount of hearing loss associated with perforations is related to the size and location of the hole in the tympanic membrane. A large hole that is close to inner ear structures will cause a greater hearing loss. The hearing loss may be severe. Chronic infection that results from perforation may also lead to progressive loss of hearing. Patients must be evaluated by a physician to determine the underlying cause.

CONDITIONS OF THE NOSE

As described in Chapter 10, the nose is the organ of smell (Figure 23-12). The nose is located in the middle of the face and is composed of several components:

- External meatus—the triangular-shaped projection in the center of the face
- External nostrils—two chambers divided by the septum
- Septum—composed primarily of cartilage and bone and covered by mucous membranes
- Nasal passages—passages that are lined with mucous membranes and cilia
- Sinuses—four pairs of air-filled cavities, also lined with mucous membranes

Common conditions that affect the nose are listed in Box 23-5.

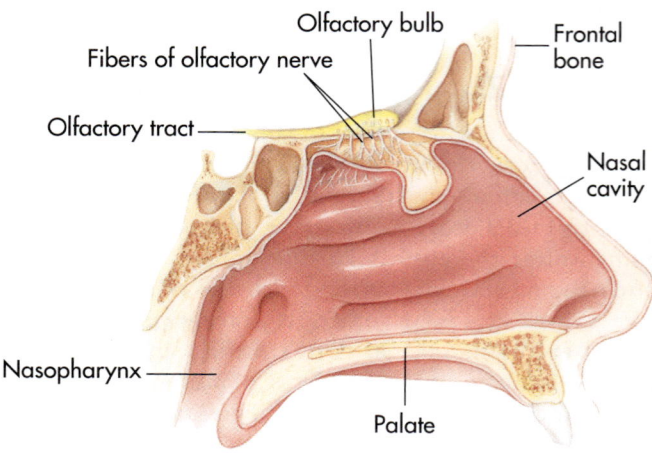

FIGURE 23-12 Anatomy of the nasal cavity. (From Shade BR: *Mosby's EMT-intermediate for the 1999 national standard curriculum,* ed 3, St Louis, 2007, Mosby.)

BOX 23-5 Conditions That Affect the Nose

Epistaxis
Foreign body
Rhinitis
Sinusitis

LOOK AGAIN
See Chapter 10: Review of Human Systems, pp. 205-206.

Epistaxis

Epistaxis is acute hemorrhage from the nostril, nasal cavity, or nasopharynx. It is a fairly common occurrence and a frequent complaint in emergency departments. Bleeding from epistaxis is most commonly *anterior*, originating from the nasal septum. Less common is *posterior* bleeding, originating from the posterior nasal cavity or nasopharynx. Local trauma (nose picking) is the most common cause of epistaxis. This is followed by facial trauma, foreign bodies, nasal or sinus infection, and prolonged breathing of dry air. Other less common causes of epistaxis include:[15]

- Nasogastric and nasotracheal intubation
- Topical nasal drugs
- Upper respiratory tract infection (especially in children)
- Oral anticoagulants
- Medical conditions that affect coagulation, such as splenomegaly, thrombocytopenia, hemophilia, platelet disorders, liver disease, renal failure, chronic alcohol use, or acquired immunodeficiency syndrome (AIDS) related conditions
- Dry climates
- Vascular abnormalities (e.g., sclerosis, neoplasm, aneurysm, endometriosis)
- Use of cocaine or other drugs that are inhaled (Figure 23-13)

NOTE
Nosebleeds can occur at any age, but are most common in children ages 2 to 10 years and in adults ages 50 to 80 years. For unknown reasons, nosebleeds most commonly occur in the morning hours.

SHOW ME THE EVIDENCE
Researchers in the United Kingdom evaluated the relative risk of epistaxis in patients taking low-dose aspirin or clopidogrel compared to patients who took none of these drugs. There was an increased risk of epistaxis in both drug groups, but little difference in risk between groups taking clopidogrel versus those taking low-dose aspirin.

Rainsbury JW, Molony NC: Clopidogrel versus low-dose aspirin as risk factors for epistaxis, *Clin Otolaryngol* 34(3):232-235, 2009.

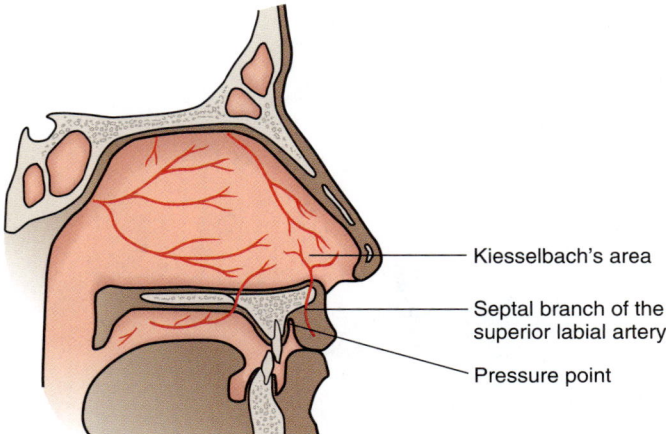

FIGURE 23-13 Epistaxis. (From Kulig K: Epistaxis. In Rosen P, et al: *Emergency medicine: concepts and clinical practice*, St Louis, 1983, Mosby.)

Kiesselbach's area
Septal branch of the superior labial artery
Pressure point

MANAGEMENT CONSIDERATIONS

Most nosebleeds can be visualized in the anterior portion of the nasal cavity. If not, the source of bleeding is likely posterior. This is especially true if the bleeding is coming from both nares, or if blood is draining into the posterior pharynx. If time permits, the patient should be questioned about previous nosebleeds, medication use that may cause or worsen epistaxis (e.g., aspirin, nonsteroidal antiinflammatory drugs [NSAIDs], Coumadin), hypertension, family history, and preexisting disease.

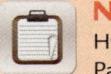

NOTE
Hypertension is rarely a direct cause of epistaxis. Patients with epistaxis usually have an elevated blood pressure because of their anxiety. However, nosebleeds in hypertensive patients are more often caused by long-standing disease and not the hypertension. Management should focus on controlling hemorrhage and reducing anxiety as the primary means of blood pressure reduction.

Prehospital care for epistaxis consists of controlling the hemorrhage and calming the patient. To control bleeding, the conscious patient should be positioned upright and leaning forward. (An unconscious patient should be positioned on the side, if not complicated by injury.) Direct pressure should be applied midway on the nose for about 5 minutes or until bleeding subsides. An emesis basin should be nearby to catch any blood or drainage. Packing the nose to control bleeding should not be attempted in the prehospital setting. If bleeding is severe or prolonged, the patient should be treated for shock and transported for physician evaluation (Figure 23-14).

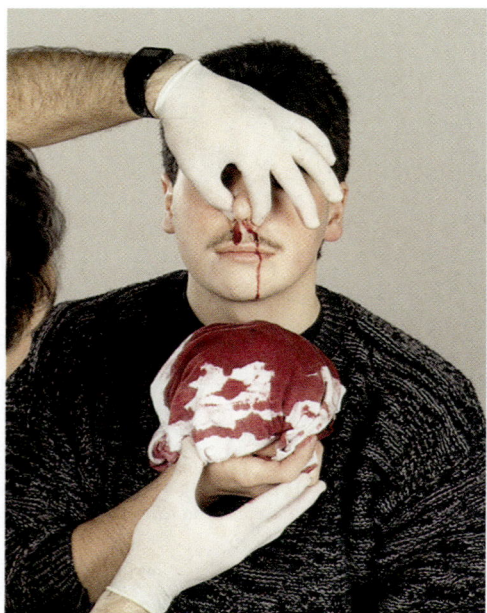

FIGURE 23-14 Epistaxis. (From Henry MC, Stapleton ER: *EMT prehospital care*, ed 4, St Louis, 2009, Mosby.)

Foreign Body

As described previously, a foreign body placed in the ear or nose is a common occurrence. Beans or other foodstuffs, beads, paper wads, and eraser tips are frequently found in the noses of young children. The foreign bodies usually lodge on the floor of the anterior or middle third of the nasal cavity. Most cases are not serious, and most foreign bodies can be easily removed by a physician. Signs and symptoms of a foreign body in the nose include obstruction to airflow in the affected nostril, nasal discomfort, tearing, and unilateral nasal discharge (sometimes foul smelling).

> **NOTE**
> If a child has inserted a foreign body in the nose, suspect that more than one object has been placed. The ears of the child should also be inspected for foreign bodies.

MANAGEMENT CONSIDERATIONS

Prehospital care for foreign bodies in the nose is limited to gentle examination of the nares. A cooperative patient may be coached to blow his or her nose to try to expel the foreign body. Foreign bodies that are easily visible may be removed with alligator forceps. The patient must be cooperative, and special care must be taken not to push the object deeper into the nasal cavity. Most likely, the patient will require physician evaluation and topical anesthesia. Small children may need to be restrained or sedated for the examination. Methods to remove foreign bodies in the nose include removal by forceps and irrigation or by use of Foley catheters: after the catheter is passed beyond the foreign body,

the balloon is inflated and the object is pulled out through the nose.

Rhinitis

Rhinitis is commonly known as a "runny nose." The term is used to describe irritation and inflammation of the mucous membranes of the nose, often caused by a virus, bacteria, or allergens (*allergic rhinitis*). A foreign body in the nose can also cause rhinitis. The hallmark feature of rhinitis is nasal drip, caused by an increase in histamine production. The increase in the amount of histamine increases the production of mucus. Other symptoms of rhinitis include nasal congestion and itchy eyes and nose.

MANAGEMENT CONSIDERATIONS

Prehospital care for a patient with rhinitis is primarily supportive. Emergency care or transport is seldom needed. Patients should be advised to follow up with their private physician if symptoms persist. Treatment for rhinitis usually consists of use of antihistamines, avoidance of exposure to suspected allergens or irritants, and sometimes administration of antibiotics if the cause is bacterial.

Sinusitis

Sinusitis (sinus infection) is inflammation of the sinuses and nasal passages. The condition can be caused by a viral, bacterial, or fungal infection. Symptoms of sinusitis include headache, and pressure in the eyes, nose, or cheek area. Often the discomfort is limited to one side of the head. Sinusitis may also be associated with a cough, fever, bad breath (halitosis), and nasal congestion. The nasal congestion can produce thick nasal secretions. Sinusitis affects 37 million people each year, making it a common health condition in the United States.[16]

As described in Chapter 10, the paranasal sinuses are four pairs of air-filled sacs that connect the space between the nostrils and the nasal passages. These include the frontal sinuses (in the forehead), the maxillary sinuses (behind the cheek bones), the ethmoid sinuses (between the eyes), and the sphenoid sinuses (behind the eyes). Normally, mucus that collects in the sinuses drains into the nasal passages and is eliminated from the body. When a patient has a cold or allergy, the sinuses can become inflamed and unable to drain, leading to congestion and infection. Sinusitis can be acute or chronic (lasting 3 months or more). Chronic sinusitis can damage the sinuses and cheekbones, and can sometimes require surgical intervention.

> **LOOK AGAIN**
> See Chapter 10: Review of Human Systems, pp. 191-193.

MANAGEMENT CONSIDERATIONS

Prehospital care for patients with sinusitis is primarily supportive. Because the signs and symptoms are easily confused with those of a cold or allergy, the chart in Box 23-6

BOX 23-6 Signs and Symptoms of Sinusitis, Allergy, and Cold

What are the symptoms of sinusitis versus a cold or allergy?

Sign/Symptom	Sinusitis	Allergy	Cold
Facial pressure/pain	Yes	Sometimes	Sometimes
Duration of illness	More than 10-14 days	Varies	Less than 10 days
Nasal discharge	Whitish or colored	Clear, thin, watery	Thick, whitish, or thin
Fever	Sometimes	No	Sometimes
Headache	Sometimes	Sometimes	Sometimes
Pain in upper teeth	Sometimes	No	No
Bad breath	Sometimes	No	No
Coughing	Sometimes	Sometimes	Yes
Nasal congestion	Yes	Sometimes	Yes
Sneezing	No	Sometimes	Yes

From Sinusitis, American Academy of Otolaryngology-Head and Neck Surgery, http://www.entnet.org/HealthInformation/Sinusitis.cfm, accessed 8-18-10.

can aid in a differential diagnosis. Patients should be encouraged to follow up with their private physician, where treatment may include antibiotics for bacterial infection, antihistamines, and decongestants.

CONDITIONS OF THE OROPHARYNX AND THROAT

As described in Chapter 10, the oropharynx begins at the level of the uvula and extends down to the level of the epiglottis. The oropharynx opens into the oral cavity. This cavity contains the lips, cheeks, teeth, tongue, the hard and soft palates, and the palantine tonsils. The throat is the anterior portion of the neck, located in front of the vertebral column. The throat consists of the pharynx and larynx. It also contains the epiglottis, which separates the esophagus from the trachea (Figure 23-15). Box 23-7 lists common conditions that affect these structures.

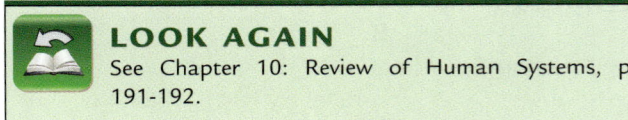

LOOK AGAIN
See Chapter 10: Review of Human Systems, pp. 191-192.

Toothache and Dental Abscess

The medical term for toothache is **dentalgia.** Toothache usually refers to pain around the teeth or jaws. Common causes of toothache include dental cavities, **dental abscess** (a bacterial infection in the center of the tooth), a cracked tooth, an exposed tooth root, and gum disease. The most common cause of toothache is a dental cavity; the second most common cause is gum disease.

The normal adult mouth has 32 teeth. Each tooth consists of two sections: the *crown* and the *root.* The crown projects above the oral mucosa around the tooth. The root fits into the bony socket of the maxilla or mandible. There

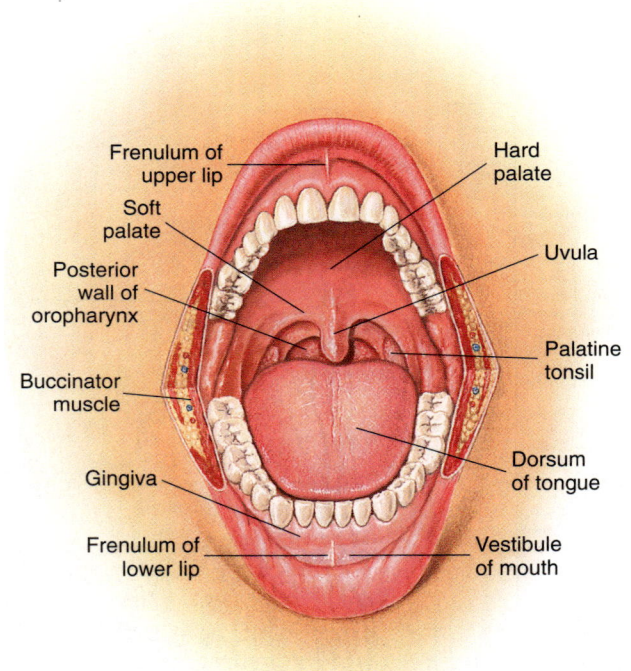

FIGURE 23-15 Anatomic structures of the oral cavity. (From Seidel H, et al: *Mosby's guide to physical examination,* ed 7, St Louis, 2011, Mosby.)

are three layers that comprise the hard tissues of the teeth. They are the *enamel,* the *dentin* (ivory), and the *cementum.* The soft tissues of the teeth include the *pulp* and *periodontal membrane* (Figure 23-16). Symptoms of toothache include:
- Sharp, throbbing, or constant pain in the tooth
- Swelling around the tooth
- Fever or headache
- Foul-tasting drainage from infection of the tooth

MANAGEMENT CONSIDERATIONS

Prehospital care for a patient with a toothache is primarily supportive. Follow-up with a private dentist or oral surgeon should be recommended. Dental care will vary by nature of the problem and may include cavity fill, tooth extraction, root canal, x-ray, phototherapy to reduce pain, and antibiotics to treat bacterial infection. Proper identification and treatment of dental infections is important. Infection that is not treated can spread to other parts of the face and skull, and may even enter the bloodstream (sepsis). Prehospital care for the patient who has suffered dental trauma will be addressed in Chapter 40.

BOX 23-7 Conditions That Affect the Oropharynx and Throat

Toothache and dental abscess
Ludwig's angina
Foreign body*
Epiglottitis
Laryngitis
Tracheitis
Oral candidiasis
Peritonsillar abscess
Pharyngitis/tonsillitis
Temporomandibular joint disorders

*Foreign body airway obstruction was described in Chapter 15.

CRITICAL THINKING
What serious medical condition should be ruled out in high-risk patients who complain of tooth or jaw pain?

Ludwig's Angina

Ludwig's angina is a type of cellulitis that involves inflammation of the tissues of the floor of the mouth, under the tongue. It can occur following dental abscess or mouth injury. Ludwig's angina is most common in adults. The disease can cause swelling of the tissues that can occur rapidly. The swelling may block the airway or prevent

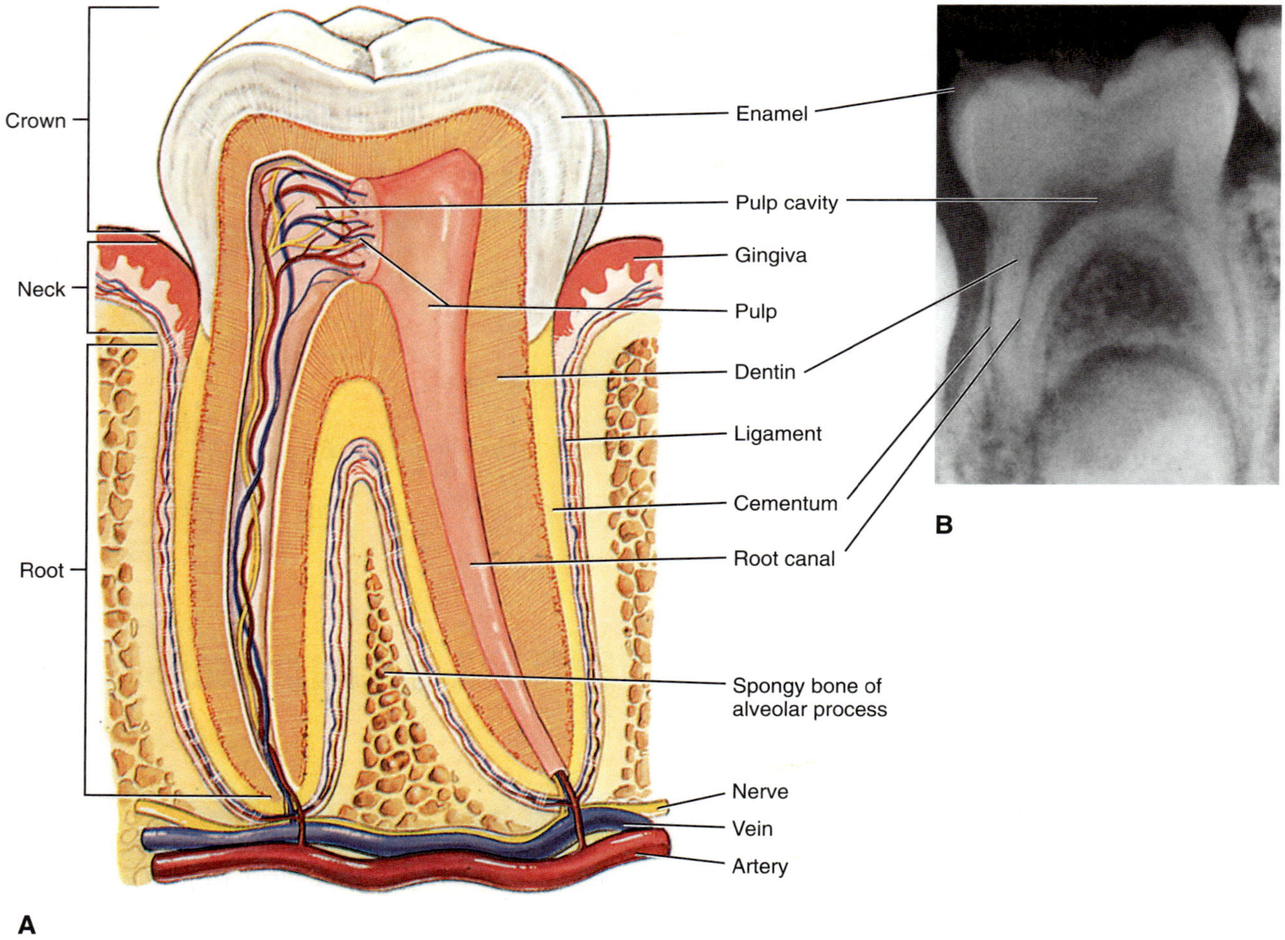

Crown

Enamel

Pulp cavity

Gingiva

Neck

Pulp

Dentin

Ligament

Cementum

Root

Root canal

Spongy bone of alveolar process

Nerve

Vein

Artery

A

B

FIGURE 23-16 Tooth anatomy. **A,** Sagittal section of a lower molar. **B,** X-ray of a healthy tooth. (From Solomon EP: *Introduction to human anatomy and physiology,* Philadelphia, 2009, Saunders.)

swallowing of saliva. Signs and symptoms of Ludwig's angina may include:

- Breathing difficulty
- Confusion or other mental changes
- Fever
- Neck pain
- Neck swelling
- Redness of the neck
- Weakness, fatigue, excessive tiredness
- Drooling
- Earache

MANAGEMENT CONSIDERATIONS

Ludwig's angina is a medical emergency that can be life threatening. Prehospital care may include airway and ventilatory support. Rapid transport to an emergency department is indicated. Physician care may include airway maintenance, computed tomography (CT) scan, blood cultures to identify the bacteria, IV/oral antibiotics, and surgery to drain fluids that are causing the swelling. Although Ludwig's angina can be successfully treated, possible complications include complete airway obstruction, sepsis, and septic shock.

Epiglottitis

As the name implies, **epiglottitis** is inflammation of the epiglottis. The disease is caused by a bacterial infection that can lead to life-threatening airway obstruction. It can occur at any age. The bacterial infection causes edema and swelling of the epiglottis and supraglottic structures. The disease usually begins suddenly in children. It frequently occurs after a child goes to bed. Signs and symptoms include sore throat, pain on swallowing, drooling, fever, and a muffled voice. Classic signs of respiratory distress usually are present.

> **NOTE**
> The HiB vaccine has greatly reduced the number of cases of epiglottitis in children.[17]

MANAGEMENT CONSIDERATIONS

Epiglottitis is a true emergency that requires prompt recognition and immediate transport for definitive care (see Chapter 48). Airway occlusion can occur suddenly. This can be precipitated by minor irritation of the throat, aggravation, and anxiety. It is therefore important that these patients be handled gently. Patients with suspected epiglottitis should not lie down. They should be transported in a position of comfort that helps them breathe and facilitate drainage of oral fluids. IV access should not be attempted in the field to avoid creating anxiety and agitation in the child. High-concentration oxygen should be applied by mask, unless it provokes anxiety. If respiratory arrest occurs before emergency department (ED) arrival, the patient

should be intubated by the most experienced paramedic (intubation will likely be difficult). In-hospital care may include airway and circulatory support, placement of a surgical airway, and IV antibiotic therapy.

Laryngitis

Laryngitis is swelling and irritation of the larynx that inflames the vocal cords. It is usually associated with hoarseness or loss of voice, and swollen glands and lymph nodes in the neck. The most common form of laryngitis is caused by a virus, and often occurs along with an upper respiratory tract infection. Other causes include allergies, bacterial infection, bronchitis, pneumonia, influenza, and exposure to irritants or chemicals.

MANAGEMENT CONSIDERATIONS

Laryngitis is usually not a serious condition and typically improves without treatment. (Only rarely does respiratory distress develop.) Prehospital care is primarily supportive. Patients should be encouraged to follow up with their private physician if symptoms persist. Recommendations may include resting the voice and humidifying the air at home. Drug therapy may include analgesics, decongestants, and antibiotics if the infection is bacterial. Young children with laryngitis may need to be seen by a specialist for further evaluation.

Tracheitis

Tracheitis is a bacterial infection of the upper airway and subglottic trachea. The major site of the disease is at the level of the cricoid cartilage, the narrowest part of the trachea. The disease generally occurs in infants and toddlers (1 to 5 years of age) but can also occur in older children. It frequently follows a viral upper respiratory tract infection (see Chapter 48). Signs and symptoms are those of respiratory distress or respiratory failure (depending on severity). These include agitation, high-grade fever, inspiratory and expiratory stridor, productive cough, hoarseness, and throat pain.

> **NOTE**
> Tracheitis is an uncommon infectious cause of upper airway obstruction, but is more prevalent than acute epiglottitis.[18]

MANAGEMENT CONSIDERATIONS

Emergency care is focused on providing airway, ventilatory, and circulatory support, and rapid transport to an appropriate medical facility. If respiratory failure or arrest develops in the field, tracheal intubation and tracheal suction are indicated. (High-pressure bag-mask ventilation may be needed because of airway swelling and accumulation of mucus or pus.) In-hospital care will include IV antibiotics after the child's airway has been stabilized.

Oral Candidiasis

Oral candidiasis (also known as *thrush*) is an infection of yeast fungi of the genus *Candida*. It affects the mucous membranes of the mouth. The infection usually appears as thick or white cream-colored deposits on the mucosal membranes (Figure 23-17). The area may appear inflamed and can be painful. Bleeding can occur from irritation of the area. Oral candidiasis most commonly affects infants and toddlers, and those with impaired immune function. The disease is contagious, but is seldom passed from person-to-person if immune systems are healthy. Persons at risk for oral candidiasis include:

- Newborns
- Those with diabetes
- Those taking antibiotics or inhaled corticosteroids
- Those with immune deficiencies (human immunodeficiency virus [HIV], AIDS, cancer)
- Those with oral piercings
- Denture wearers

MANAGEMENT CONSIDERATIONS

Emergency care is seldom required for patients with oral candidiasis. Physician care generally includes the use of topical or oral antifungal drugs. In severe cases, IV antifungal drugs may be needed.

Peritonsillar Abscess

Peritonsillar abscess (also called PTA or *quinsy*) is a collection of pus in and around one or both tonsils. The abscesses form in the area between the palatine tonsil and its capsule. It is a complication of **tonsillitis** (infection of the tonsils) and is the most common deep infection of the head and neck in adults. It is most common in persons 20 to 40 years of age who have chronic tonsillitis.[19] Presenting symptoms include fever, throat pain, and **trismus** (muscle spasms of the jaw).

MANAGEMENT CONSIDERATIONS

Prehospital care for the patient with peritonsillar abscess is primarily supportive. Physician care may include ultrasound, antibiotics, and procedures to remove the abscess

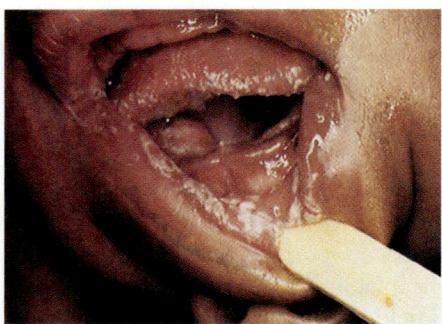

FIGURE 23-17 White, curdlike plaques of thrush (oral candidiasis, oral moniliasis), a common fungal infection in infants. (From McKinney ES, et al: *Maternal-child nursing*, ed 3, St Louis, 2009, Saunders.)

material. These procedures may include needle aspiration or incision and drainage. Tonsillectomy also may be indicated.

Pharyngitis/Tonsillitis

Pharyngitis and tonsillitis are infections in the throat that cause inflammation. If the tonsils are primarily affected, it is called tonsillitis. If the throat is primarily affected, it is called pharyngitis. Inflammation of the throat usually is associated with an underlying illness. The most common cause of inflammation is a virus, but the inflammation may also be caused by bacteria (especially streptococci), resulting in **strep throat.** Signs and symptoms that accompany pharyngitis and tonsillitis depend on underlying illness, such as the common cold, influenza, and **mononucleosis:**[20]

Sore throat with common cold:

- Sneezing
- Cough
- Low-grade fever (temperature less than 102° F) (38.9° C)
- Mild headache

Sore throat with flu:

- Fatigue
- Body aches
- Chills
- Fever (temperature higher than 102° F) (38.9° C)

Sore throat with mononucleosis:

- Enlarged lymph nodes in neck and armpits
- Swollen tonsils
- Headache
- Loss of appetite
- Swollen spleen
- Liver inflammation

> **NOTE**
>
> Tonsillitis may be caused by a bacterial or a viral infection. The condition may be acute, recurrent, or chronic. Nearly all children in the United States have at least one episode of tonsillitis. Complications associated with the disease are rare. The herpes simplex virus, *Streptococcus pyogenes* (GABHS) and Epstein-Barr virus (EBV), cytomegalovirus, adenovirus, and the measles virus cause most cases of acute pharyngitis and acute tonsillitis.[21]

MANAGEMENT CONSIDERATIONS

Prehospital care for a patient with pharyngitis or tonsillitis is primarily supportive. Emergency care is seldom needed. Physician care may include antihistamines, cough suppressants, and antipyretics. Throat cultures and blood analyses may be needed if a bacterial infection requiring antibiotics or mononucleosis is suspected. Severe or recurrent tonsillitis may require tonsillectomy.

> **CRITICAL THINKING**
>
> What complications may occur if a patient's pharyngitis is related to strep throat and is not treated?

Temporomandibular Joint Disorders

The **temporomandibular joint** (TM joint; TMJ) is the joint on each side of the head in front of the ears where the mandible meets the temporal bones (Figure 23-18). TM joint disorders are a set of conditions that cause pain in the area of the joint. They may also involve associated muscles and can cause problems using the jaw. One or both of the TM joints may be affected. The disorders can influence a person's ability to speak, eat, chew, swallow, and make facial expressions. In severe cases, TM joint disorders can affect a person's ability to breathe. TM joint disorders affect about 35 million people in the United States. Most who seek treatment are women in their child-bearing years.[22]

Some of the causes of TM joint disorders are not clearly understood. Risk factors for developing the disorders include jaw injury, arthritis, dental procedures, infection, autoimmune disease, endotracheal intubation where the jaw is stretched to visualize the airway, and clenching or grinding of the teeth. TM joint disorders may also be a symptom of other diseases such as sinus or ear infection, periodontal disease, headaches, and facial neuralgia. Poor diet, stress, and lack of sleep may also contribute to the disease. Common complaints associated with TM joint disorders include:

- Pain in the neck and shoulders
- Headache
- Jaw muscle stiffness
- Limited movement or locking of the jaw
- Painful clicking, popping, or grating in the jaw joint when opening or closing the mouth
- A change in the way the upper and lower teeth fit together or a bite that feels "off"
- Ringing in the ears
- Ear pain

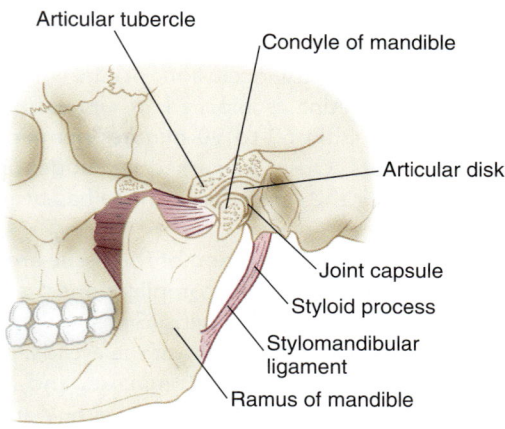

FIGURE 23-18 Structures of the temporomandibular joint. (From Seidel H, et al: *Mosby's guide to physical examination,* ed 7, St Louis, 2011, Mosby.)

- Decreased hearing
- Dizziness and vision problems.

MANAGEMENT CONSIDERATIONS

The symptoms of TM joint disorders are usually temporary, but may be painful. In addition, patients experiencing discomfort will often be anxious. Prehospital care should be focused on calming the patient and providing comfort measures. Physician care may include diagnostic tests of the head, neck, face, and jaw. A complete medical history will also be obtained to rule out other possible causes for the disorder. Health care professionals who may be involved in the patient's treatment and recovery include dentists; sleep specialists; ear, nose, and throat specialists; neurologists; endocrinologists; rheumatologists; and pain specialists.

SUMMARY

- The eye is composed of both primary vision structures and accessory structures, which protect, lubricate, move, and aid in the function of the visual structures. Cranial nerves control vision, pupil constriction, and movement of the eyes. Consider nervous system disease if these functions are impaired.
- Conjunctivitis is inflammation or infection of the eye and is sometimes called pink eye. Infectious conjunctivitis is contagious.
- A corneal abrasion is a scrape or scratch of the cornea. It is very painful and may cause tearing, redness, and blurred vision. Patch the eye and administer a topical ophthalmic anesthetic if permitted by protocol.
- Foreign bodies in the eye are very painful and cause pain and tearing. Irrigation of the eye may be indicated to remove small foreign bodies.

- Two types of eyelid inflammation are chalazion (obstructed oil gland) and hordeolum (stye).
- Glaucoma is caused by an increase in intraocular pressure related to excess aqueous humor. This results in pressure on the optic nerve and can lead to blindness if untreated. Signs and symptoms include loss of peripheral vision, pain, headache, vomiting, or blurred vision.
- Iritis is inflammation of the iris. It can cause blindness if untreated.
- Papilledema is swelling of the optic disc caused by an increase in intracranial pressure (ICP). The increased ICP may be related to illness or injury.
- The retina is the eye structure central to vision. Tears, breaks, or defects in the retina cause retinal detachment. Without treatment, retinal detachment leads to blindness. Signs and symptoms include an increase in

Continued

floaters, light flashes in the eye, or the appearance of a curtain over the field of vision.

- Central retinal artery occlusion occurs when blood supply to the retina is blocked. If circulation is not reestablished within 60 to 90 minutes permanent loss of vision occurs. Onset is marked by sudden, painless loss of vision or the sense that a shade has been pulled down over the eye.
- Orbital cellulitis is an infection of the tissue around the eye that can lead to serious complications that include blindness, sepsis, and meningitis. Signs and symptoms include fever, pain and swelling of the eyelids, eye pain, decreased vision, bulging eyes, malaise, and impaired eye movement. Immediate treatment with IV antibiotics is essential.
- When excess earwax (cerumen) accumulates in the ear it can cause earache, hearing loss, tinnitus, itching, odor, or discharge. Removal of the wax usually resolves the symptoms.
- Swelling of the inner ear causes labyrinthitis. This results in vertigo and tinnitus.
- Meniere's disease causes vertigo, tinnitus, and hearing loss. This can lead to nausea and vomiting. Stroke can cause similar symptoms and should be ruled out.
- Otitis media is an infection or inflammation of the middle ear. In addition to earache, it can produce a number of signs and symptoms.
- Infection or trauma can cause perforation of the tympanic membrane. This can result in brief pain, hearing loss, and drainage from the affected ear.
- Epistaxis is bleeding from the structures of the nose or nasopharynx. Attempt to control epistaxis by positioning the patient upright, leaning forward. Apply direct pressure on the nose until bleeding is controlled. Treat for shock if indicated.
- It is common for children to place foreign bodies in their nose. Transport for physician examination and removal.
- Rhinitis is a runny nose. Common causes are infection, allergy, or foreign body in the nose.
- Sinusitis is inflammation of sinuses and nasal passages. Signs and symptoms include cough, fever, halitosis, nasal congestion, headache, and pressure sensation over the eyes, nose or cheek.
- Toothache is frequently caused by tooth decay, abscess, cracked tooth, exposed root, or gum disease. Transport for definitive care and pain management.
- Ludwig's angina is cellulitis of the tissues under the tongue. It can cause rapid tissue swelling and airway obstruction. Signs and symptoms include dyspnea, confusion, fever, neck pain, redness or swelling, and weakness or drooling. Urgent transport is needed.
- Epiglottitis is inflammation of the epiglottis caused by bacterial infection. It can lead to airway obstruction. Signs and symptoms include sore throat, high fever, drooling, and muffled voice. Airway obstruction is possible. Perform minimal interventions unless airway obstruction occurs.
- Laryngitis is a hoarse voice and swollen lymph nodes associated with inflamed vocal cords.
- Tracheitis is a bacterial infection of the upper airway and subglottic trachea. It can cause respiratory failure and arrest. Be prepared to manage the airway and assist with ventilation if needed.
- Oral candidiasis is a yeast fungal infection of the mouth. It covers the tongue and mucous membranes with a thick cream-colored coating.

REFERENCES

1. EMS Standards.National Highway Traffic Safety Administration: *The National EMS Education Standards*, Washington, DC, 2009, U.S. Department of Transportation/National Highway Traffic Safety Administration, DOT.
2. Chisari G, Sanfilippo M, Reibaldi M: Treatment of bacterial conjunctivitis with topical ciprofloxacin and norfloxacin: a comparative study, *Infez Med* 11(1):25-30, 2003.
3. Ragge NK, Easty DL: *Immediate eye care*, St Louis, 1990, Mosby.
4. MedlinePlus: *Chalazion*, www.nlm.nih.gov/medlineplus/ency/article/001006.htm, accessed 8-18-10.
5. American Optometric Association: *Chalazion*, www.aoa.org/x9762.xml, accessed 10-19-09.
6. Ragge N: *Immediate eye care*, London, 1990, Wolfe.
7. Iritis Organization: *About iritis*. www.iritis.org/index.php, accessed 8-18-10.
8. National Eye Institute: *Retinal detachment*, www.nei.nih.gov/health/retinaldetach, accessed 8-18-10.
9. Mayo Clinic: *Retinal detachment*, www.mayoclinic.com/health/retinal-detachment/DS00254, accessed 8-18-10.
10. Emergency Nurses Association: *Sheehy's emergency nursing: principles and practice*, ed 6, St Louis, 2010, Mosby.
11. Ghosh C: Periorbital and orbital cellulitis after *H. influenza* B vaccination, *Ophthalmology* 108(9):1514-1515, 2001.
12. American Academy of Otolaryngology—Head and Neck Surgery: *Earwax*, www.entnet.org/HealthInformation/earwax.cfm, accessed 8-18-10.
13. National Institute on Deafness and Other Communication Disorders: *Meniere's disease*, www.nidcd.nih.gov/health/balance/meniere.asp, accessed 8-18-10.
14. National Institute on Deafness and Other Communication Disorders: *Ear infections in children*, www.nidcd.nih.gov/health/hearing/otitism.asp, accessed 8-18-10.
15. Bamimore O: *Epistaxis*, http://emedicine.medscape.com/article/764719-overview, 2009, accessed 8-18-10.
16. American Academy of Otolaryngology—Head and Neck Surgery: *Sinusitis*, www.entnet.org/HealthInformation/Sinusitis.cfm, accessed 8-18-10.
17. Mayo Clinic: *Epiglottitis*, www.mayoclinic.com/health/epiglottitis/DS00529, accessed 8-18-10.

18. Sujatha R: *Bacterial tracheitis*, http://emedicine.medscape.com/article/961647-overview, accessed 8-18-10.

19. Petruzzelli GJ, Johnson JT: *Peritonsillar abscess. Why aggressive management is appropriate*, Postgrad Med 88:99-100, 103-105, 108, 1999.

20. University of Maryland Medical Center: *Pharyngitis*, www.umm.edu/altmed/articles/pharyngitis-000129.htm, accessed 8-18-10.

21. American Academy of Otolaryngology—Head and Neck Surgery: *Tonsillitis, fact sheet*, www.entnet.org/HealthInformation/tonsillitis.cfm, accessed 8-18-10.

22. TMJ Association: *TMJD basics*. www.tmj.org, accessed 8-18-10.

24 Respiratory

OBJECTIVES

Upon completion of this chapter, the paramedic student will be able to:

1. Distinguish the pathophysiology of respiratory emergencies related to ventilation, diffusion, and perfusion.
2. Outline the assessment process for the patient who has a respiratory emergency.
3. Describe the causes, complications, signs and symptoms, and prehospital management of patients

diagnosed with obstructive airway disease, pneumonia, adult respiratory distress syndrome, pulmonary thromboembolism, upper respiratory tract infection, spontaneous pneumothorax, hyperventilation syndrome, and lung cancer.

KEY TERMS

acute respiratory distress syndrome A fulminant form of respiratory failure characterized by acute lung inflammation and diffuse alveolar-capillary injury.

aspiration pneumonia Inflammation of the lung tissue from foreign material entering the tracheobronchial tree.

asthma A respiratory disorder characterized by recurring episodes of paroxysmal dyspnea, wheezing on expiration caused by constriction of the bronchi, coughing, and viscous mucoid bronchial secretions.

bacterial pneumonia A type of pneumonia associated with a bacterial infection.

biphasic positive airway pressure Airway support that combines partial ventilatory support and continuous positive airway pressure; allows the pressure to vary during each breath cycle.

bleb An accumulation of fluid under the skin.

bronchiectasis An abnormal dilation of the bronchi caused by a pus-producing infection of the bronchial wall.

bullae Thin-walled blisters of the skin or mucous membranes that contain clear, serous fluid.

chronic bronchitis Obstructive airway disease of the trachea and bronchi.

continuous positive airway pressure Airway support that transmits positive pressure into the airways of a spontaneously breathing patient throughout the respiratory cycle.

deficient ambient oxygen An oxygen concentration that is less than 21%.

diffusion The process in which solid, particulate matter in a fluid moves from an area of higher concentration to an area of lower concentration, resulting in an even distribution of the particles in the fluid.

emphysema An abnormal condition of the pulmonary system characterized by overinflation and destructive changes in the alveolar walls, resulting in a loss of lung elasticity and a decrease in gases.

glottic opening The vocal cords and the space between them.

hemoptysis Coughing up of blood from the respiratory tract.

hyperventilation syndrome Abnormally deep or rapid breathing that leads to excessive loss of carbon dioxide, resulting in respiratory alkalosis.

lung cancer A disease of uncontrolled cell growth in tissues of the lung.

metastasis The movement or spreading of cancer cells from one organ or tissue to distant locations in the body.

mycoplasmal pneumonia A type of atypical pneumonia. It is caused by the bacterium *Mycoplasma pneumoniae*.

near-fatal asthma Acute asthma associated with respiratory arrest, a drop in blood pressure, and reduced cardiac output.

peak expiratory flow rate A measurement of how fast a person can exhale air.

perfusion The circulation of blood to the tissues.

pneumonia An acute inflammation of the lungs, usually caused by inhaled pneumococci of the species *Streptococcus pneumoniae*.

positive end-expiratory pressure Airway support that maintains a degree of positive pressure at the end of exhalation.

pulmonary embolism The blockage of a pulmonary artery by foreign matter such as fat, air, tumor tissue, or a thrombus that usually arises from a peripheral vein.

pulmonary respiration The exchange of gases between the cells of the body and the outside environment.

spontaneous pneumothorax A condition that results when a subpleural bleb ruptures, allowing air to enter the pleural space from within the lung.

status asthmaticus A severe, prolonged asthma attack that has not been broken with repeated doses of bronchodilators.

upper respiratory tract infection Infection of the upper airway, affecting the nose, throat, sinuses, and larynx.

ventilation The mechanical movement of air into and out of the lungs; makes respiration possible.

viral pneumonia An inflammation of the lungs caused by viral infection.

*R*espiratory emergencies are common in the prehospital setting. They account for 28% of the chief complaints in all EMS calls.[1] Each year more than 400,000 people die as a result of respiratory emergencies in the United States.[2] Therefore, patients with respiratory emergencies require the highest priority of care. The paramedic must be able to quickly assess a patient with respiratory distress, identify the cause, initiate management, and provide appropriate care en route to the hospital.

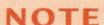

> **NOTE**
> Age-related variations in disease and methods of patient assessment are described throughout this textbook by subject matter. Respiratory diseases specific to children will be addressed in Chapter 48; those unique to older adults will be presented in Chapter 49; those associated with infectious disease (e.g., tuberculosis) will be presented in Chapter 28. Respiratory emergencies related to trauma will be presented in Part 9: Trauma.

ANATOMY AND PHYSIOLOGY REVIEW

As described in Chapter 10, the structures of the respiratory system are divided into upper and lower airways. Their location is assigned in relation to the **glottic opening** (the vocal cords and the space between them). For the purpose of this chapter, upper airway structures are those located above the glottis. Lower airway structures are those located below the glottis. The upper and lower airway structures include (Figure 24-1):

Upper Airway Structures
Nasopharynx
Oropharynx
Laryngopharynx
Larynx
Lower Airway Structures
Trachea
Bronchial tree
Alveoli
Lungs

> **LOOK AGAIN**
> See Chapter 10: Review of Human Systems, pp. 191-196.

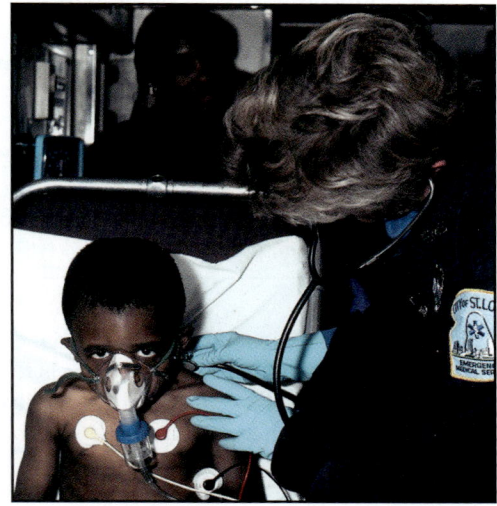

(Courtesy Monroe Yancey, St. Louis, Mo.)

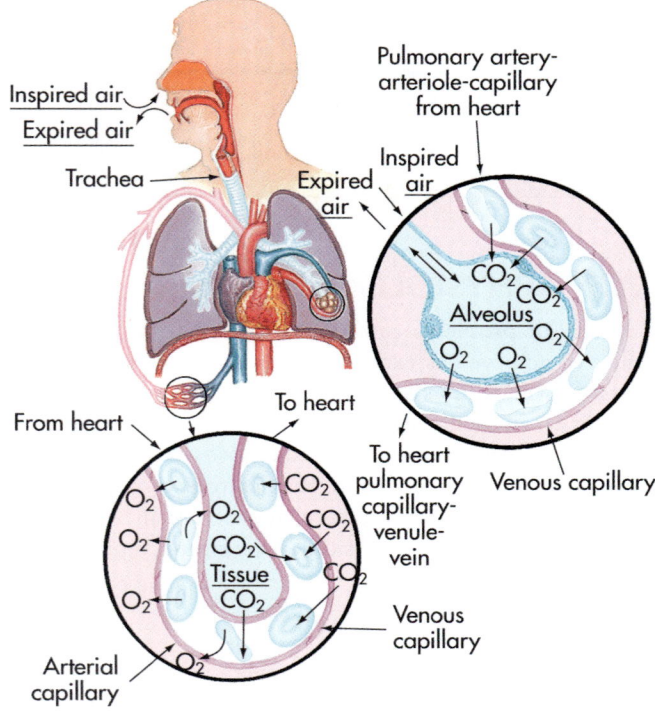

FIGURE 24-1 Structures of the pulmonary system. The circles denote the alveoli. (Modified from Wilson SF, Thompson JM: *Mosby's clinical nursing series: respiratory disorders,* St Louis, 1990, Mosby.)

Physiology

The exchange of gases between the cells of the body and the outside environment is the essence of respiratory physiology. As described in Chapter 15, for gas exchange to occur, air must move freely in and out of the lungs. This process, known as pulmonary respiration, brings oxygen to the lungs and removes carbon dioxide. This is made possible by:

- *External respiration:* the transfer of oxygen and carbon dioxide between inspired air and pulmonary capillaries
- *Internal respiration:* the transfer of oxygen and carbon dioxide between the capillary red blood cells and the tissue cells

LOOK AGAIN

See Chapter 15: Airway Management, Respiration, and Artificial Ventilation, pp. 391-411.

There are many other factors that are essential elements of pulmonary respiration. One of these factors is the structure and function of the chest wall (diaphragm, ribs, intercostal muscles, accessory muscles). Another factor is the control of respirations by the central nervous system (medulla, phrenic nerve innervation of the diaphragm, spinal nerves that innervate intercostal muscles, and reflexes that prevent overinflation). Acid-base balance mediated by the buffer systems also plays an important role in respiration (see Chapter 11).

LOOK AGAIN

See Chapter 11: General Principles of Pathophysiology, pp. 226-227.

PATHOPHYSIOLOGY

A variety of problems can affect the pulmonary system's ability to achieve gas exchange. Gas exchange must occur to provide for cellular needs and the excretion of wastes (see Chapter 10 and Chapter 15). Specific disorders responsible for respiratory emergencies include those related to ventilation, diffusion, and perfusion. Risk factors associated with the development of respiratory disease are listed in Box 24-1. The following discussion of pulmonary physiology serves as a review.

Ventilation

Ventilation is the process of air movement into and out of the lungs. For ventilation to occur, the following must be intact:

- Neurological control (to initiate ventilation)
- Nerves between the brainstem and the muscles of respiration

BOX 24-1   Risk Factors Associated With the Development of Respiratory Disease

Intrinsic Factors

Genetic predisposition may influence the development of these conditions:

- Asthma
- Obstructive lung disease
- Cancer

Cardiac or circulatory disorders may influence the development of these conditions:

- Pulmonary edema
- Pulmonary emboli

Stress may increase the following:

- Severity of respiratory complaints
- Frequency of attacks of asthma and chronic obstructive pulmonary disease (COPD)

Extrinsic Factors

Smoking increases the following:

- Prevalence of COPD and cancer
- Severity of virtually all respiratory disorders

Environmental pollutants increase the following:

- Prevalence of COPD
- Severity of all obstructive airway disorders

- Functional diaphragm and intercostal muscles
- Patent upper airway
- Functional lower airway
- Alveoli that are functional and have not collapsed

Specific pathophysiologies associated with ventilation include upper and lower airway obstruction, chest wall impairment, and problems in neurological control. Emergency treatments for ventilation problems include ensuring the upper and lower airways are open and clear and providing assisted ventilations (Box 24-2).

Diffusion

Diffusion is the process of gas exchange. This gas exchange occurs between the air-filled alveoli and the pulmonary capillary bed. Gas exchange is driven by simple diffusion in which gases move from areas of high concentration to areas of low concentration. (This occurs until the concentrations are equal.) For diffusion to occur, the following must be intact:

- Alveolar and capillary walls that are not thickened
- Interstitial space between the alveoli and capillary wall that is not enlarged or filled with fluid

Specific pathophysiologies associated with diffusion include inadequate oxygen concentration in ambient air, alveolar disorders, interstitial space disorders, and capillary bed disorders (Box 24-3). Emergency treatment for diffusion problems includes providing high-concentration oxygen. Treatment is also directed at reducing inflammation in the interstitial space.

BOX 24-2 Causes of Ventilation Problems

Upper Airway Obstruction
- Trauma
- Epiglottitis
- Laryngotracheobronchitis
- Abscess
- Foreign body obstruction
- Inflammation of the tonsils

Lower Airway Obstruction
- Trauma
- Obstructive/restrictive lung disease
- Emphysema
- Chronic bronchitis
- Mucus accumulation
- Reactive airway disease
- Smooth muscle spasm, including asthma
- Airway edema

Chest Wall Impairment
- Spontaneous pneumothorax
- Pleural inflammation
- Pleural effusion
- Neuromuscular diseases
- Muscular sclerosis
- Muscular dystrophy

BOX 24-3 Causes of Diffusion Problems

Inadequate oxygen concentration in ambient air
Alveolar pathology
Asbestosis; other environmental lung diseases
Blebs/bullae associated with COPD
Inhalation injuries
Interstitial space pathology
Pulmonary edema
Acute respiratory distress syndrome
Submersion/drowning
Acute lung syndrome (ALS)

Perfusion

Perfusion is the process of circulation of the blood through the lung tissues (capillary bed). For perfusion to occur, the following must be intact:

- Adequate blood volume
- Adequate hemoglobin in the blood
- Pulmonary capillaries that are not occluded
- Efficient pumping by the heart that provides a smooth flow of blood through the pulmonary capillary bed

Specific pathophysiologies associated with perfusion include inadequate blood volume, impaired circulatory blood flow, and capillary wall disorders (Box 24-4). Emergency treatment for perfusion problems includes ensuring an adequate circulating blood volume and hemoglobin levels. Treatment also may be needed to optimize left-sided heart function (see Chapter 22).

BOX 24-4 Causes of Perfusion Problems

Inadequate blood volume/hemoglobin levels
Hypovolemia
Anemia
Impaired circulatory blood flow
Pulmonary embolus

Unknown Pulmonary Diagnosis

If the patient's diagnosis is unknown, paramedics should try to determine whether it is primarily related to ventilation, diffusion, or perfusion, or to a combination of defects. Care for a patient with an unknown pulmonary diagnosis should be focused on the specific disorder responsible for the respiratory emergency. That is, is the problem a disorder of ventilation, diffusion, or perfusion? Ventilation disorders are managed by assisting the patient's airway using mechanical means (e.g., opening the airway, relieving airway obstructions, clearing the airway of secretions, the use of airway adjuncts). Diffusion disorders are treated to improve gas exchange between the alveoli and the pulmonary capillary bed (e.g., medications to improve breathing and reduce inflammation in the airways, continuous positive airway pressure [CPAP]). Perfusion disorders are managed by improving the circulation of blood through the lung tissues (e.g., intravenous [IV] fluids, medications to improve cardiac function). Regardless of the specific disorder, all patients with respiratory compromise should receive high-concentration oxygen and ventilatory support as needed.

> **NOTE**
> Pulmonary complaints may be associated with exposure to environments that have deficient ambient oxygen. Examples include scenes with poisonous or toxic gases. During the scene size-up, it is critical to ensure a safe environment for all EMS personnel before initiating patient contact. Rescue personnel with special training and equipment should be utilized as needed to ensure scene safety. **Deficient ambient oxygen** is defined as oxygen concentration that is less than 21%. (An oxygen concentration less than 16% is immediately dangerous.) Oxygen can be consumed or displaced by toxic or inert gas (e.g., carbon monoxide, methane gas), and is usually associated with confined or enclosed spaces. Poison gases are hazardous because they can harm lower airways, cause bronchospasm, or interfere with the blood's ability to carry oxygen or the cell's ability to use oxygen (e.g., exposure to hydrogen cyanide) (see Chapter 34).

ASSESSMENT FINDINGS

Primary Survey

A general impression of the patient can be made in the primary survey. As described in Chapter 19, the major focus of the primary survey is to detect and manage any life-threatening conditions that affect airway, breathing, and circulation. This and initiating resuscitation measures take priority over a detailed assessment. Signs of life-threatening respiratory distress in adults include the following[3]:

- Alterations in mental status
- Severe cyanosis
- Audible stridor
- Inability to speak one or two words without dyspnea
- Tachycardia (>130 beats/min)
- Pallor and diaphoresis
- Retractions and/or the use of accessory muscles to assist breathing

A quick assessment of lung sounds may be indicated in the primary survey for a patient in respiratory distress. As described in Chapter 20, abnormal breath sounds include absent or diminished breath sounds, crackles, wheezes, and rhonchi.

LOOK AGAIN
see Chapter 20: Secondary Assessment, pp. 536-540.

Focused History

The paramedic should ascertain the patient's chief complaint. A chief complaint may include dyspnea, chest pain, productive or nonproductive cough, **hemoptysis** (coughing up blood from the respiratory tract), wheezing, and signs of respiratory tract infection (e.g., fever, increased sputum production). The history should focus on the patient's previous experiences with similar or identical symptoms. The patient's objective description of severity often is an accurate indicator of the severity of the current episode if the condition is chronic.

Asking the patient, "What happened the last time you had an attack this severe?" is very useful for predicting what will happen with this episode. The following is a sample of questions that might be asked in order to obtain a focused history for a patient with respiratory distress. This format uses the acronym OPQRST (onset, provocation, quality, region/radiation, severity, and time):

Onset: "What were you doing when the breathing difficulty began? Do you think anything might have triggered it? Did your breathing difficulty begin gradually or was it sudden in onset? Did you experience any pain when the breathing difficulty began?"

Provocation: "Does lying down or sitting up make your breathing better or worse? Do you have any pain when you breathe? If so, does the pain increase when you take a deep breath or does it stay the same?"

Quality: "Is it more difficult to breathe when you inhale or exhale? If you have pain when you breathe, would you describe it as sharp or dull?"

Region/radiation: "What area of the chest has the most discomfort? Can you point with your finger to the specific area that hurts? Does the pain move anywhere or does it stay in the same place?"

Severity: "On a scale of 0 to 10 (with 10 being the worst), how would you rate the difficulty of your breathing?"

Time: "What time did the breathing difficulty start? Has it been constant since it began? If you've had this type of difficulty before, how long did it last?"

NOTE
It is important to ask patients if intubation was ever required to manage their respiratory disease. A history of previous intubation indicates severe pulmonary disease. It also suggests that intubation may be required again.

After obtaining a history of the present illness, a medication history should be obtained. A medication history includes current medications, medication allergies, cardiac medications, and pulmonary medications (e.g., in-home oxygen therapy; inhaled, oral, or parenteral sympathomimetics; inhaled or oral corticosteroids; cromolyn sodium; methylxanthines; leukotriene inhibitors, antibiotics). Obtaining a medication history (as well as when and why the patient takes these medications) may help the paramedic determine the nature of the respiratory emergency.

Secondary Assessment

The secondary assessment should be guided by the paramedic's general impression of the patient and by the patient's chief complaint. As part of the secondary assessment, the paramedic should note the patient's position, mental status, ability to speak, respiratory effort, and skin color (see Chapter 20: Secondary Assessment). Vital signs should be assessed, with the following considerations[3]:

- *Pulse rate:* Tachycardia may be a sign of hypoxemia. Bradycardia caused by respiratory problems is a warning sign of severe hypoxemia and imminent cardiac arrest.
- *Blood pressure:* Hypertension may result from the use of medications the patient takes to manage cardiac and respiratory disorders. (Patients with congestive heart failure [CHF] often are hypertensive.) Hypertension also may result from the patient's fear and anxiety. Like hypertension, hypotension can be caused by medication therapy. It may also result from fluid loss and dehydration in some respiratory illnesses. (Patients with pneumonia often are dehydrated.)
- *Respiratory rate:* The respiratory rate is not an accurate sign of respiratory status unless it is very slow. Trends are essential in evaluating a patient with chronic respiratory disease. A slowing rate in a patient who is not improving suggests exhaustion and impending respiratory insufficiency. As described in Chapter 15, abnormal patterns that may be seen in patients with severe illness or injury include tachypnea, Cheyne-Stokes respirations,

central neurogenic hyperventilation, Kussmaul respirations, ataxic respirations, apneustic respirations, and apnea.

LOOK AGAIN
See Chapter 15: Airway Management, Respiration, and Artificial Ventilation, pp. 417-419.

The patient's face and neck should be assessed for pursed-lip breathing, grunting, nasal flaring, and use of accessory muscles. (Visible head bobbing in infants indicates they are using accessory muscles to breathe.) Pursed-lip breathing and grunting helps maintain pressure in the airways (even during exhalation). This pressure helps to support bronchial walls internally that have lost their external support as a result of disease. The use of accessory muscles can quickly result in respiratory fatigue. The patient should be questioned about sputum production. An increasing amount of sputum suggests infection. Thick green or brown sputum may indicate pneumonia; yellow or pale gray sputum may be related to allergic or inflammatory causes; pink, frothy sputum is associated with severe and late stages of pulmonary edema (described in Chapter 22 and in Chapter 45). The patient's neck should be evaluated for jugular vein distention. Jugular vein distention may be a sign of right-sided heart failure resulting from severe pulmonary congestion.

The patient's chest should be inspected for injury, if indicated by history. It also should be inspected for any indicators of chronic disease. (An example is a barrel chest from long-standing chronic obstructive pulmonary disease.)

Other components of the chest examination include noting accessory muscle use or retractions to facilitate breathing, evaluating chest wall symmetry, and auscultating the patient's lungs for normal and abnormal breath sounds.

The patient's extremities should be assessed for peripheral cyanosis, pitting edema, clubbing of the fingers, and carpopedal spasm. Peripheral cyanosis is caused when a large amount of the hemoglobin in the blood is not carrying oxygen. Pitting edema is an indication of heart failure. Clubbing is an abnormal enlargement of the ends of the fingers (Figure 24-2). It indicates long-standing chronic hypoxemia. Carpopedal spasms are spasms of the hands, thumbs, feet, or toes. They often are associated with hypocapnia that results from hyperventilation.

Physical findings in a patient with respiratory disease should be documented on the patient care report. They also should be communicated to medical direction.

DIAGNOSTIC TESTING

Diagnostic testing that may be appropriate for some patients with respiratory disease includes pulse oximetry, capnometry, and the use of peak flow meters. As described in Chapter 15, pulse oximeters measure oxygen saturation. Capnography monitors end-tidal carbon dioxide level. Peak flow meters provide a baseline assessment of airflow for patients with obstructive lung disease.

NOTE
New diagnostic devices are available and are in use by some EMS and fire service agencies. These devices (e.g., Rad57) measure levels of carboxyhemoglobin (SpCO), hemoglobin (SpHB), and methemoglobin (SpMet) as well as oxygen content (SpOC).

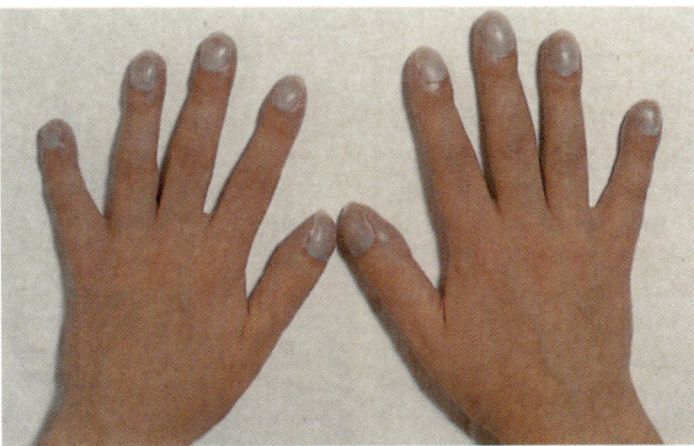

FIGURE 24-2 Severe finger clubbing in a patient with cyanotic congenital heart disease. (From Forbes CD, Jackson WD: *Color atlas and text of clinical medicine,* ed 3, London, 2003, Mosby, with permission.)

Pulse Oximetry

To review, pulse oximetry helps determine how well the patient is being oxygenated. The device does this by measuring the transmission of red and near-infrared light through arterial beds using a probe placed on a finger, toe, or earlobe. Hemoglobin that is bound with oxygen (oxyhemoglobin) absorbs more infrared than red light; reduced hemoglobin absorbs more red than infrared light. The pulse oximeter measures this difference and calculates the oxygen saturation of the blood (SaO_2). The low range of normal SaO_2 is 93% to 95%. The upper range is 99% to 100%. An SaO_2 reading below 90% indicates a PaO_2 (partial pressure of arterial oxygen) of 60 mm Hg or less. An SaO_2 of 75% indicates a PaO_2 of 40 mm Hg. An SaO_2 of 50% indicates a PaO_2 of 27 mm Hg.

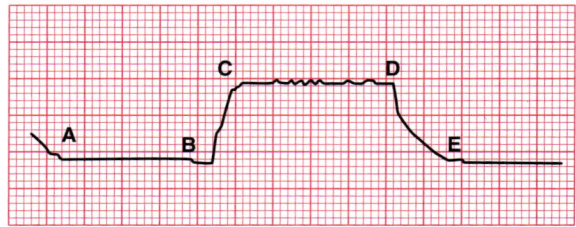

FIGURE 24-3 Capnography waveform.

LOOK AGAIN
See Chapter 15: Airway Management, Respiration, and Artificial Ventilation, pp. 451-455.

Capnography

As described in Chapter 15, capnography is a noninvasive monitoring technique that is primarily used in the prehospital setting to confirm correct tracheal tube placement. When used in conjunction with pulse oximetry and electrocardiogram (ECG) monitoring, capnography also can provide insight into ventilation, circulation, and metabolism. It is a useful indicator of efficient cardiopulmonary resuscitation and also can help confirm the diagnosis of pulmonary embolism. In patients with hemorrhage, capnography can provide continuous hemodynamic monitoring, information about tissue perfusion, and fluid resuscitation strategies for patients in shock[4] (see Chapter 36).

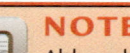

NOTE
Although capnography is a direct measurement of ventilation in the lungs, it also indirectly measures metabolism and circulation. For example, an increased metabolism will increase the production of carbon dioxide. This leads to an increase in the $EtCO_2$. A decrease in cardiac output will reduce the delivery of carbon dioxide to the lungs. This decreases the $EtCO_2$.

USE OF CAPNOGRAPHY IN MEDICAL PATIENTS WITH SPONTANEOUS RESPIRATIONS

Capnography is the graphical representation of carbon dioxide concentration exhaled through the breath. The measurements are taken by a capnography filter attached to a face mask or nasal cannula or endotracheal tube. The graphic representation is displayed as a waveform (measured in millimeters of mercury) on a *capnogram* throughout the respiratory cycle. (A *capnometer* displays only the numerical value of $PaCO_2$, not the waveform.) Each waveform on the capnogram consists of four phases (Figure 24-3). Phase 1 (*A-B*) represents air that is exhaled from the conducting airways with a low level of CO_2. Phase 2 (*B-C*) represents the mixture of air from the anatomical dead space and alveolar gas. It is here that CO_2 concentration begins to rise. Phase 3 (*C-D*) represents a plateau as alveolar gas is exhaled (*alveolar plateau*). Phase 4 (*D-E*) represents inspiration (*inspiration washout*) where *D* is the end-tidal volume (the peak concentration) and *E* is the sharp decline in CO_2 concentration. Box 24-5 shows three primary waveforms that are important in monitoring medical patients in the prehospital setting.

The waveform helps to detect any rebreathing of CO_2 and is useful in diagnosing problems associated with increased dead space.[5] For example, patients with obstructive lung disease or a pulmonary embolism often have a decreased angle for phase 2, and the slope of the curve during phase 3 often will not reach the alveolar plateau. This is associated with unequal flow rates (ventilation-perfusion mismatch) and the uneven emptying of obstructed alveoli. Ventilation-perfusion mismatch can be caused by blood shunting, as seen with atelectasis. It also can be caused by dead space in the lungs, such as occurs with pulmonary embolism. All of these conditions result in a continuous increase in CO_2 concentration. A waveform that plateaus late in the expiration phase can indicate heart failure, chronic obstructive pulmonary disease (COPD), and pulmonary embolus (Figure 24-4).

Peak Flow Meters

Peak flow meters (Figure 24-5) are used in pulmonary function tests to measure a patient's **peak expiratory flow rate** (PEFR). PEFR is a measurement of how fast a person can exhale air. These tests most often are used to help determine the severity of an asthma attack. They also can help assess the effectiveness of treatment of respiratory disease in the prehospital setting. Use of peak flow meters requires a cooperative patient who can make a maximal respiratory effort. It also requires coaching by the paramedic.

To determine baseline airflow (before drug administration), the paramedic should instruct the patient to inflate

BOX 24-5 Three Important Waveforms for Monitoring Medical Patients

1. Hyperventilation—Decreased CO_2

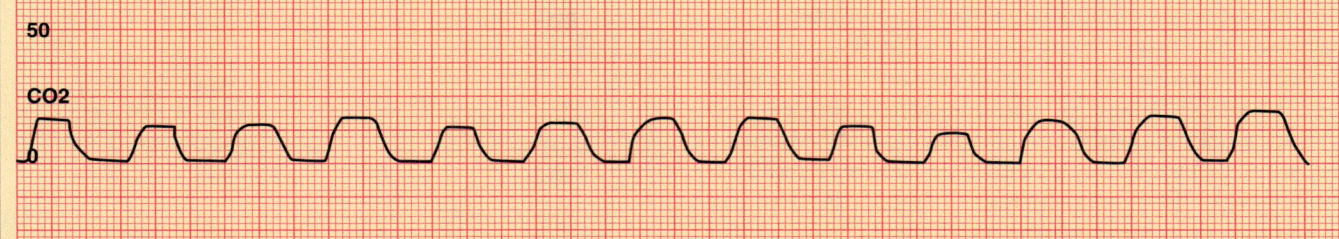

Possible causes: Anxiety, bronchospasm, pulmonary embolus, decreased cardiac output, hypotension, pulmonary edema

2. Hypoventilation—Increased CO_2

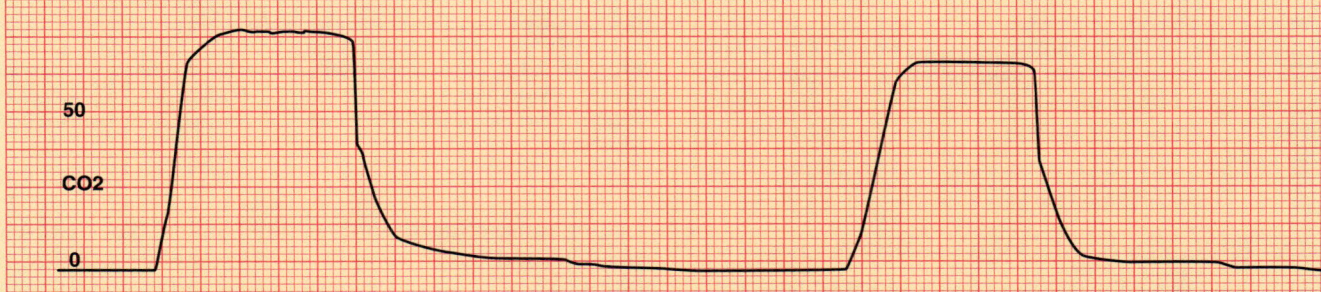

Possible causes: Sedation, overdose, dyspnea, chronic hypercapnia

3. Asthma, COPD, CHF—"Shark-fin" wave

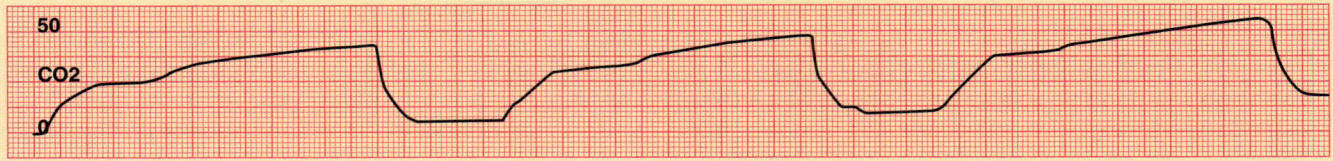

Possible causes: Bronchospasm, uneven emptying of the alveoli, breath struggle

EtCO$_2$ Values
Normal: 35 to 45 mm Hg
Hypoventilation/hypercapnia: Greater than 45 mm Hg
Hyperventilation/hypocapnia: Less than 46 mm Hg

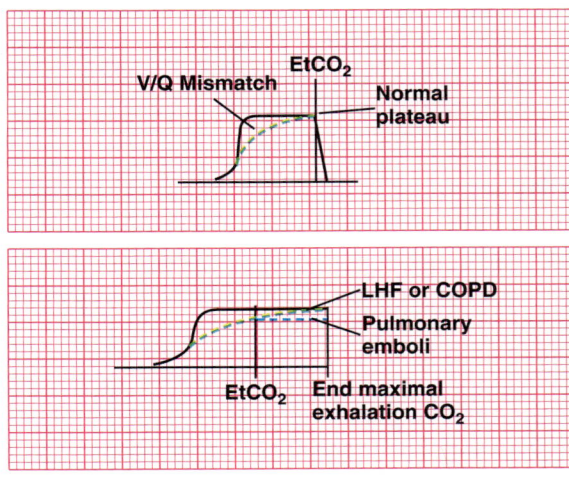

FIGURE 24-4 Abnormal EtCO$_2$ waveform.

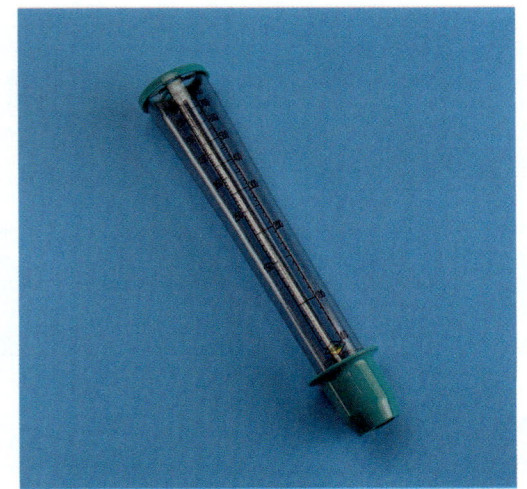

FIGURE 24-5 Peak flow meter.

the lungs fully and forcefully exhale as quickly as possible into the flow meter. (Children should be reminded to breathe out as if they were blowing out candles or blowing up a balloon.) The reading is recorded in liters per minute. This measurement should be taken two more times. The highest of the three readings is chosen as the peak value flow. This measurement is then compared with standard tables based on height, gender, and race (Table 24-1). A PEFR measurement with variability less than 20% is considered mild; 20% to 30% is moderate; and more than 30% is severe.[6] Peak flow measurements should be repeated throughout the course of management to evaluate the patient's response to drug therapy.

> **NOTE**
> Most children younger than 5 years of age cannot adequately perform peak expiratory flow rate (PEFR) tests. Also, this test should not be used with a patient in severe respiratory distress. Drug therapy to reverse the bronchospasm is the priority.

OBSTRUCTIVE AIRWAY DISEASE

Obstructive airway disease is a major health problem in the United States. It affects nearly 32 million people in the United States.[7] Predisposing factors that contribute to some forms of obstructive pulmonary disease include smoking, environmental pollution, industrial exposures, and various pulmonary infectious processes. Obstructive airway disease is a triad of distinct diseases that often coexist. They are chronic bronchitis and emphysema (together referred to as chronic obstructive pulmonary disease [COPD]) and asthma. These diseases are presented separately in this chapter. However, different degrees of each frequently are present in the same patient.

> **NOTE**
> Pulmonary function tests are used by many physicians and other health care professionals to diagnose COPD. The tests also allow them to stage the severity of the illness. The mantra advocated by many respiratory support groups is "test your lungs and know your numbers"; it provides a way for patients with COPD to assess how well they are responding to treatment and if their disease is progressing.

> **CRITICAL THINKING**
> Will patients with chronic obstructive pulmonary disease (COPD) always be able to "name" their disease when you ask about their history?

Chronic Bronchitis

Chronic bronchitis is a condition involving inflammatory changes and excessive mucus production in the bronchial tree (Figure 24-6). Although preventable, it is the fourth

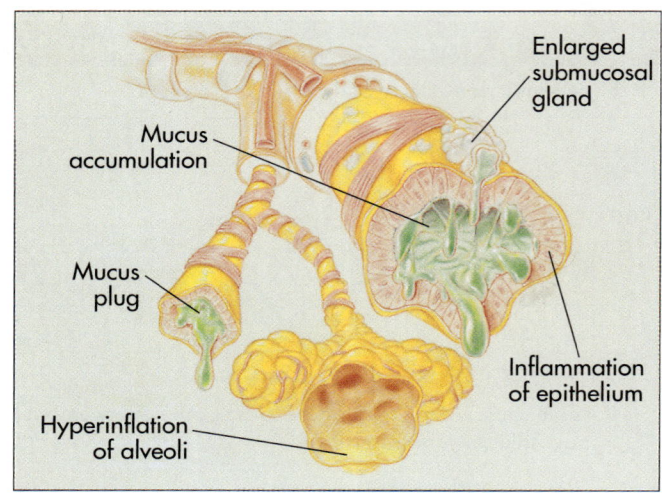

FIGURE 24-6 Chronic bronchitis. Bronchi are filled with excess mucus. (Modified from Desjardins T, Burton GG: *Clinical manifestations and assessment of respiratory disease*, ed 3, St Louis, 2006, Mosby.)

leading cause of death in the United States.[8] The disease is characterized by an increase in the number and size of mucus-producing glands. This results from prolonged exposure to irritants. (Most often the irritant is cigarette smoke.) The condition is diagnosed clinically by the presence of cough with sputum production that is present half of the time for at least 2 consecutive years.[9] The alveoli are not seriously affected and diffusion remains relatively normal.

Patients with severe chronic bronchitis have a low oxygen pressure (PO_2) because of changes in the ventilation-perfusion relationships in the lung and hypoventilation. (These patients sometimes are called "blue bloaters" because of their hypoxia and fluid retention.) The hypoventilation leads to hypercapnia (high levels of carbon dioxide [CO_2]), hypoxemia (low levels of oxygen [O_2]), and increases in arterial carbon dioxide pressure (PCO_2). Patients with chronic bronchitis have frequent respiratory tract infections. These eventually cause scarring of lung tissue. In time, irreversible changes occur in the lung. These changes may lead to emphysema or bronchiectasis. **Bronchiectasis** is an abnormal dilation of the bronchi. It is caused by a pus-producing infection of the bronchial wall.

Emphysema

Emphysema results from pathological changes in the lung. It is the end stage of a process that progresses slowly for many years. The disease is characterized by permanent abnormal enlargement of the air spaces beyond the terminal bronchioles and by destruction and collapse of the alveoli (Figure 24-7). The disease reduces the number of alveoli available for gas exchange. It also reduces the elasticity of the remaining alveoli. This loss of elasticity leads to trapping of air in the alveoli. Thus residual volume increases, whereas vital capacity remains relatively normal.

TABLE 24-1 Predicted Average Peak Expiratory Flow Rates

Predicted Average Peak Expiratory Flow Rates for Normal Children and Adolescents (L/min)

Height (Inches)	Males and Females	Height (Inches)	Males and Females
43	147	56	320
44	160	57	334
45	173	58	347
46	187	59	360
47	200	60	373
48	214	61	387
49	227	62	400
50	240	63	413
51	254	64	427
52	267	65	440
53	280	66	454
54	293	67	467
55	307		

Modified from Polger G, Promedhat V: *Pulmonary function testing in children: techniques and standards,* Philadelphia, 1971, WB Saunders.

Predicted Average Peak Expiratory Flow Rates for Normal Males (L/min)

	Height (Inches)				
Age	60	65	70	75	80
20	554	602	649	693	740
25	543	590	636	679	725
30	532	577	622	664	710
35	521	565	609	651	695
40	509	552	596	636	680
45	498	540	583	622	665
50	486	527	569	607	649
55	475	515	556	593	634
60	463	502	542	578	618
65	452	490	529	564	603
70	440	447	515	550	587

Modified from Leiner GC, et al: Expiratory peak flow rate: standard values for normal subjects use as a clinical test of ventilatory function, *Am Resp Dis* 88:644, 1963.

Predicted Average Peak Expiratory Flow Rates for Normal Females (L/min)

	Height (Inches)				
Age	55	60	65	70	75
20	390	423	460	496	529
25	385	418	454	490	523
30	380	413	448	483	516
35	375	408	442	476	509
40	370	402	436	470	502
45	365	397	430	464	495
50	360	391	424	457	488
55	355	386	418	451	482
60	350	380	412	445	475
65	345	375	406	439	468
70	340	369	400	432	461

Modified from Leiner GC, et al: Expiratory peak flow rate: standard values for normal subjects use as a clinical test of ventilatory function, *Am Resp Dis* 88:644, 1963.

NOTE: These charts are for informational purposes only. Spirometry should be used for diagnosis and staging. "Personal best" measures should be used for the asthma treatment plan.

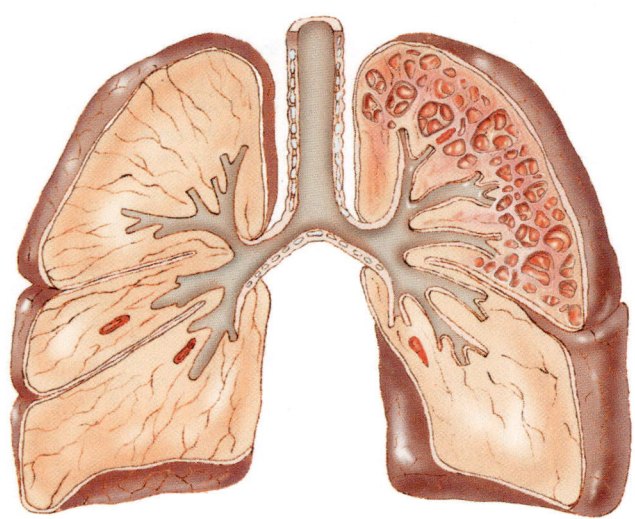

FIGURE 24-7 Cystic changes of lobar emphysema resulting from destruction of alveoli. (From Wilson SF, Thompson JM: *Mosby's clinical nursing series: respiratory disorders,* St Louis, 1990, Mosby.)

The associated reduction in arterial PO_2 leads to increased production of red blood cells and polycythemia (an elevated hematocrit value.) The elevation in hematocrit level is much more common in the patient with chronic bronchitis than in the patient who has primary emphysema. This is because the patient with chronic bronchitis is more often chronically hypoxemic. Decreases in alveolar membrane surface area and in the number of pulmonary capillaries in the lung reduce the area for gas exchange. These factors are also responsible for an increased resistance to pulmonary blood flow.

Patients with emphysema have some resistance to airflow into and out of the lungs. Yet most of the hyperexpansion is caused by air trapping secondary to loss of elastic recoil (Figure 24-8). Patients with chronic bronchitis have increased airway resistance during inspiration and expiration. In contrast, patients with emphysema have increased airway resistance only on expiration. Normally a passive, involuntary act, expiration becomes a muscular act in patients with COPD. (These patients are sometimes called "pink puffers" because of the red face they make during forced exhalation.) Over time, the chest becomes barrel-shaped from the trapping of air. Then, the patient must use accessory muscles of the neck, chest, and abdomen to move air into and out of the lungs. Full deflation of the lungs becomes more and more difficult. Finally, it becomes impossible. Often the patient with emphysema is thin because of poor dietary intake and increased caloric consumption required by the work of breathing (Table 24-2). Patients with emphysema often develop **bullae** (thin-walled cystic lesions in the lung) from the destruction of alveolar walls. **Blebs** (the collection of air within the visceral pleura) also may develop. When bullae collapse or blebs rupture, they increase the diffusion defect seen in these patients. They also can lead to pneumothorax.

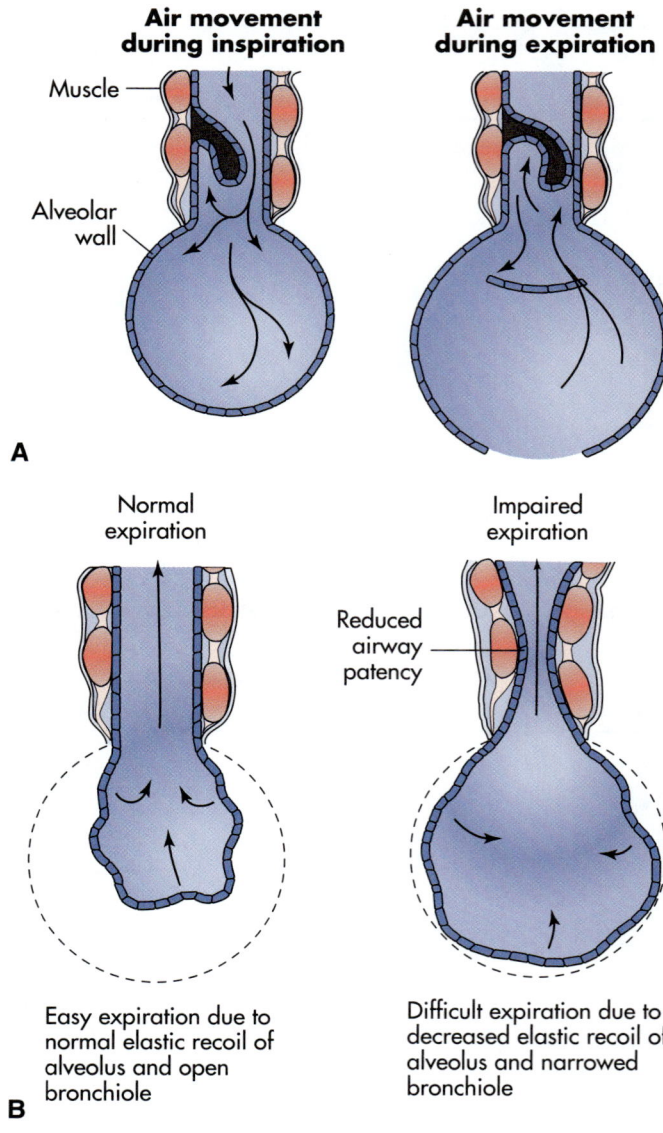

FIGURE 24-8 A, Mechanisms of air trapping in chronic obstructive pulmonary disease (COPD): Mucus plugs and narrowed airways cause air trapping and hyperinflation on expiration. During inspiration, the airways enlarge, allowing gas to flow past the obstruction. This mechanism of air trapping occurs in asthma and chronic bronchitis. **B,** Mechanism of air trapping in emphysema: Damaged or destroyed alveolar walls no longer support and hold open the airways, and alveoli lose their property of elastic recoil. Both these factors contribute to airway collapse during expiration. (Modified from Desjardins T, Burton GG: *Clinical manifestations and assessment of respiratory disease,* ed 3, St Louis, 2006, Mosby.)

CRITICAL THINKING

What effect might application of a cervical collar, use of a short spine board or vest, and immobilization supine on a long backboard have on a patient with chronic obstructive pulmonary disease (COPD) who has sustained trauma?

TABLE 24-2 Comparison of Signs and Symptoms of Emphysema and Chronic Bronchitis

Emphysema	Chronic Bronchitis
Thin, barrel-chest appearance	Typically overweight
Nonproductive cough	Productive cough with
Wheezing and rhonchi	sputum
Pink complexion	Coarse rhonchi
Extreme dyspnea on exertion	Chronic cyanosis
Prolonged inspiration	Mild, chronic dyspnea
(pursed-lip breathing)	Resistance on inspiration
	and expiration

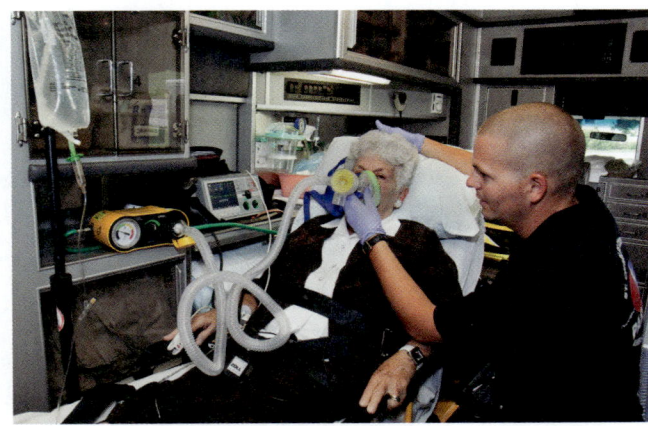

FIGURE 24-9 Patient being treated with continuous positive airway pressure. (Courtesy Rick Brady, Baltimore, Md.)

ASSESSMENT OF COPD

Patients with COPD usually are aware of and have adapted to their illness. A request for emergency care indicates that a significant change has occurred in the patient's condition. The patient with COPD usually has an acute episode of worsening dyspnea that is manifested even at rest, an increase or change in sputum production, or an increase in the malaise that accompanies the disease. Other common complaints include inability to sleep and recurrent headaches.

On EMS arrival, the patient with COPD will likely be in respiratory distress. Often the patient is sitting upright and leaning forward to aid in breathing. The patient frequently is using pursed-lip breathing to maintain positive airway pressures, in addition to using accessory muscles. Increased hypoxemia and hypercarbia may be indicated by tachypnea, diaphoresis, cyanosis, confusion, irritability, and drowsiness.

Other physical findings include wheezes, rhonchi, and crackles (see Chapter 20). Breath sounds and heart sounds also may be diminished. This is due to reduced air exchange and the increased diameter of the thoracic cavity. In late stages of decompensation, the patient may have peripheral cyanosis, clubbing of the fingers, and signs of right-sided heart failure. As described in Chapter 22, the patient's electrocardiogram may reveal cardiac dysrhythmias or signs of right atrial enlargement; these include tall, peaked P waves in leads II, III, and aV_F.

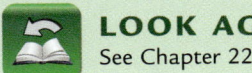 **LOOK AGAIN**
See Chapter 22: Cardiology, pp. 689-692.

MANAGEMENT

The primary goal of prehospital care for these patients is the correction of hypoxemia through improved airflow. This can be achieved through administration of oxygen and drug therapy. Drug therapy may cause serious side effects and complications, especially if the patient has used medication before EMS arrival. Therefore it is crucial for paramedics to obtain a thorough medical history regarding medication use, home oxygen use, and drug allergies.

An intravenous (IV) line should be established in all patients in respiratory distress. A cardiac monitor also should be applied. If the patient has a productive cough, coughing should be encouraged. Any sputum should be collected and delivered with the patient for laboratory analysis.

Some patients with COPD rely on a hypoxic drive for ventilatory effort. However, *the paramedic should never withhold oxygen because of fear of decreasing hypoxic drive while providing emergency care in the prehospital setting.* High-concentration oxygen should be administered with a non-rebreather mask if indicated. Pulse oximetry to measure oxygen saturation is indicated. Some of these patients will require ventilatory assistance. In addition, their breathing may require augmentation with *continuous positive airway pressure* (CPAP) or *biphasic positive airway pressure* (BiPAP) (Figure 24-9). As described in Chapter 15, CPAP improves oxygenation, reduces the work of breathing, prevents atelectasis, and allows for drug administration. Positive-pressure ventilation also may prevent the need for intubation and the risks and complications associated with invasive airway procedures.

 LOOK AGAIN
See Chapter 15: Airway Management, Respiration, and Artificial Ventilation, pp. 422-424.

The medications used in the prehospital setting to relieve bronchospasm and reduce constricted airways are the beta agonists (e.g., *levalbuterol* and *albuterol*). Other drugs that may be given after evaluation by a physician include steroids (*methylprednisolone*) and nebulized anti-cholinergics (e.g., *ipratropium*). These drugs are given for bronchodilation and stimulation of the respiratory drive. (See the Emergency Drug Index for specific drug therapy.)

Asthma

Asthma, or reactive airway disease, is a common disorder that affects nearly 23 million Americans, including 7 million children. It is responsible for 4000 to 5000 deaths each year.[8] Asthma is most common in children and young adults. Yet it can occur in any decade of life. Exacerbating factors tend to be extrinsic (external) in children. In contrast, they tend to be intrinsic (internal) in adults (Figure 24-10). Childhood asthma often improves or resolves with age. Adult asthma usually is persistent.

SHOW ME THE EVIDENCE

An abstract by Lamba et al. examines how initial prehospital $EtCO_2$ values in 299 adult asthma patients relate to patient severity. Patients with $EtCO_2$ values between 14-28 and 50-82 mm Hg were more likely to be intubated, admitted to the intensive care unit, or die than patients with $EtCO_2$ values between 29 and 49 mm Hg.

Lamba S et al: Initial out-of-hospital end-tidal carbon dioxide measurements in adult asthma patients, *Ann Emerg Med* 54(3, suppl):S51, 2009.

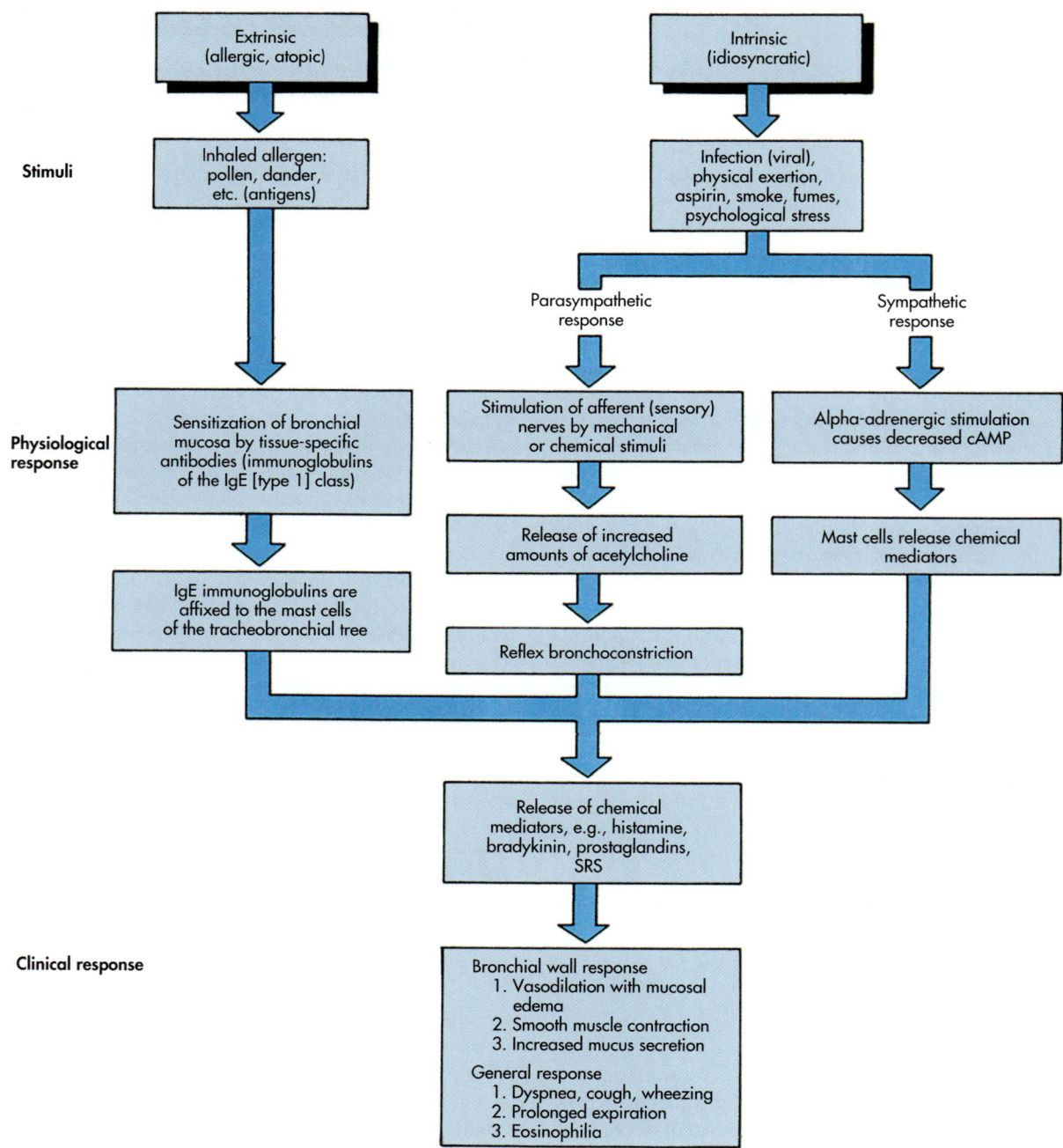

FIGURE 24-10 Extrinsic and intrinsic bronchial asthma. (From Wilson SF, Thompson JM: *Mosby's clinical nursing series: respiratory disorders,* St Louis, 1990, Mosby.)

PATHOPHYSIOLOGY OF AN ASTHMA ATTACK

Asthma generally occurs in acute episodes of variable duration. Between these episodes, the patient is relatively free of symptoms. The attack is characterized by reversible airflow obstruction caused by bronchial smooth muscle contraction; hypersecretion of mucus, resulting in bronchial plugging; and inflammatory changes in the bronchial walls. The increased resistance to airflow leads to alveolar hypoventilation, marked ventilation-perfusion mismatching (leading to hypoxemia), and carbon dioxide retention (stimulating hyperventilation) (Figure 24-11). The obstruction of inspiration and the marked obstruction of expiration cause pressure to remain high in the airways, as a result of air trapping in the lungs.

During an acute asthma attack, the combination of increased airway resistance, increased respiratory drive, and air trapping creates excessive demand on the muscles of respiration. This leads to greater use of accessory muscles and increases the chance of respiratory fatigue. If labored breathing continues, high pressures in the thorax can reduce the amount of blood returning to the left ventricle (left ventricular preload). The result is a drop in cardiac output and systolic blood pressure (**near-fatal asthma**). Pulsus paradoxus also may be seen. If the episode continues, hypoxemia and changes in blood flow and blood pressure may lead to death. Most asthma-related deaths occur outside the hospital. In the prehospital setting, cardiac arrest in patients with severe asthma has been linked to the following factors[10]:

- Severe bronchospasm and mucus plugging, which leads to asphyxia (the most common cause of asthma-related deaths)

- Cardiac dysrhythmias caused by hypoxia
- Tension pneumothorax (often bilateral)

Other conditions that may be present in patients with near-fatal asthma include cardiac disease, pulmonary disease, acute allergic bronchospasm or anaphylaxis, drug use or misuse (beta blockers, cocaine, and opiates), and recent discontinuation of long-term corticosteroid therapy (associated with adrenal insufficiency).

ASSESSMENT

When paramedics arrive, the asthmatic patient usually is sitting upright. The person may be leaning forward with hands on knees (tripod position) and using accessory muscles to aid breathing. The typical asthmatic patient is in obvious respiratory distress. Respirations are rapid and loud, and audible wheezing may be present.

> **NOTE**
> The severity of wheezing does not correlate with the degree of airway obstruction. The absence of wheezing may indicate critical airway obstruction, whereas increased wheezing may indicate a positive response to bronchodilator therapy.

The patient's mental status should be noted and monitored carefully. Lethargy, exhaustion, agitation, and confusion are serious signs of impending respiratory failure. An initial history must be obtained quickly. Questions about the onset of the current episode, its relative severity, the precipitating cause, medication use, and allergies should be specific and to the point. It is crucial to find out whether the patient has needed intubation to manage his or her previous asthma.

On auscultation, a prolonged expiratory phase may be noted. Usually wheezing is heard from the movement of air through the narrowed airways. Inspiratory wheezing (unlike inspiratory stridor) does not indicate upper airway occlusion. It suggests that the large and middle-size muscular airways are obstructed. This indicates more obstruction than if only expiratory wheezes are heard. Inspiratory wheezes also may suggest that the large airways are filled with secretions. A silent chest (i.e., no audible wheezing or air movement) may indicate such severe obstruction that the flow of air is too low to generate breath sounds. Other signs of severe asthma include the following:

- Reduced level of consciousness
- Diaphoresis and pallor
- Retractions
- Inability to speak after only one or two words
- Poor, floppy muscle tone
- Pulse rate greater than 130 beats per minute
- Respirations greater than 30 breaths per minute
- Pulsus paradoxus greater than 20 mm Hg
- Altered mental status or severe agitation
- End-tidal CO_2 >45 mm Hg

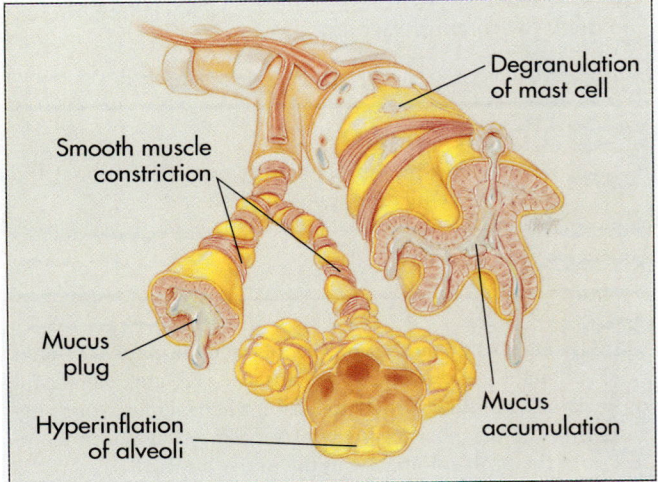

FIGURE 24-11 With bronchial asthma, thick mucus accumulation, mucosal edema, and smooth muscle spasm obstruct the small airways. Breathing becomes labored, and expiration is difficult. (Modified from Desjardins T, Burton GG: *Clinical manifestations and assessment of respiratory disease,* ed 3, St Louis, 2006, Mosby.)

Labels in figure:
Degranulation of mast cell
Smooth muscle constriction
Mucus plug
Hyperinflation of alveoli
Mucus accumulation

NOTE

Asthma attacks are true medical emergencies. Para-medics should manage these episodes aggressively. Deterioration of the patient's condition can be expected, rapid, and fatal. Therefore the paramedic must monitor the patient carefully and continuously. Initial patient management should be directed at ensuring an adequate airway, providing supplemental oxygen, and reversing the bronchospasm.

MANAGEMENT

After administration of high-concentration oxygen, drug therapy is provided (Box 24-6). Drug therapy is based on the patient's age and medication use before EMS arrival. Nebulized **albuterol** is the current cornerstone of asthma treatment in the United States. This fast-acting beta$_2$ agonist stimulates beta-adrenergic receptors and thus acts as a rapid bronchodilator. Side effects include transient tachycardia and tremor. Other nebulized drugs used to manage asthma include **levalbuterol, ipratropium,** or a combination of **albuterol** and **ipratropium.** When combined with nebulized beta-adrenergic agents and corticosteroids, IV **magnesium sulfate** can moderately improve pulmonary function in patients with asthma.[10]

If the patient is not able to tolerate nebulized medications, subcutaneous (SubQ), intramuscular (IM), or IV drug therapy will likely be indicated to treat bronchoconstriction. These drugs include **epinephrine** and **terbutaline** (see the Emergency Drug Index). CPAP or BiPAP can be beneficial in managing reactive airway disease. As described in Chapter 15, CPAP or BiPAP should only be considered if the patient is alert and has adequate spontaneous respirations.

IV fluids may be indicated for rehydration. All patients with acute asthma should be transported in a position of comfort. This helps to maximize the use of respiratory muscles. These patients should also be monitored for cardiac rhythm disturbances.

CRITICAL THINKING

Consider that the patient is unable to hold the nebulizer mouthpiece or needs to be ventilated using a bag-mask device. What can you do to promote bronchodilation?

In rare cases, advanced airway management is required for a patient having a severe asthma attack. Absolute indications for immediate intubation of the wheezing patient are apnea and coma. In addition, intubation should be considered if[11]:

- PO_2 is less than 50 mm Hg with supplemental oxygen.
- PCO_2 is greater than 50 mm Hg with acute respiratory acidosis.
- PCO_2 is increasing, despite maximal therapy.
- Patient is fatigued.
- Mental status is depressed.

If a conscious patient requires intubation and the paramedic is trained and authorized to perform rapid sequence

BOX 24-6 Asthma Medications

Nebulized Beta$_2$ Agonists
Albuterol, levalbuterol, pirbuterol, salmeterol
Inhaled anticholinergics
Ipratropium

Corticosteroids (IV)
Methylprednisolone
Hydrocortisone

Corticosteroids (Inhaled)
Triamcinolone

Leukotriene Modifiers
Montelukast, zafirlukast, zileuton
Aminophylline (IV)
Magnesium sulfate (IV)
Epinephrine or terbutaline (SubQ or IM)

IM, Intramuscular; *IV,* intravenous; *SubQ,* subcutaneous.

intubation (described in Chapter 15), consult with medical direction and consider the following critical actions[10]:

- Provide adequate sedation with **ketamine** or **etomidate.**
- Paralyze the patient with **succinylcholine** or **vecuronium** (if credentialed or authorized in your state).
- Immediately after intubation, administer 2.5 to 5 mg of **albuterol** directly into the endotracheal (ET) tube.
- Confirm ET tube placement with primary and secondary confirmation methods.
- Ventilate the patient's lungs at 6 to 10 breaths per minute and with smaller tidal volumes (6 to 8 mL/kg). Deliver breaths with a shorter inspiratory time, and prolong the expiratory time to allow for the escape of air and to avoid sudden hypotension (especially in elderly patients with emphysema).

LOOK AGAIN

See Chapter 15: Airway Management, Respiration, and Artificial Ventilation, pp. 460-464.

NOTE

Even after intubation, ventilating the patient's lungs may be difficult. The absence of any significant obstruction to airflow immediately after tracheal intubation suggests that the diagnosis of acute asthma may have been incorrect, and the problem may be in the upper airway.[10]

STATUS ASTHMATICUS

Status asthmaticus is a severe, prolonged asthma attack that has not been stopped with repeated doses of bronchodilators. It may be of sudden onset, resulting from spasm of the airways. It can also be subtle in onset, resulting from a viral respiratory tract infection or prolonged exposure to one or more allergens. Status asthmaticus is a true emergency. It calls for early recognition and immediate transport of the patient. These patients are in danger of respiratory failure.

The treatment of patients with status asthmaticus is the same as that for acute asthma attacks. Yet the urgency of rapid transport is more important. In addition, these patients usually are dehydrated. They typically require IV fluid administration. The patient's respiratory status should be monitored closely. Also, high-concentration oxygen should be administered. The need for intubation and aggressive ventilatory support should be anticipated. Continuous bronchodilator therapy with nebulized and parenteral drugs may be indicated.

 CRITICAL THINKING
When a patient treated for status asthmaticus is reassessed, would decreasing respiratory and heart rates indicate a good outcome or a bad one? Why?

Differential Considerations

Wheezing commonly is associated with asthma. However, it may be present in *all* types of diseases that cause dyspnea (Table 24-3). For example, tachypnea, wheezing, and respiratory distress may indicate heart failure, pneumonia, pulmonary edema, pulmonary embolism, pneumothorax, toxic inhalation, foreign body aspiration, and various other pathological states. Appropriate emergency care is based on the patient assessment and an accurate history.

PNEUMONIA

Pneumonia is a group of specific infections (not a single disease) that cause an acute inflammatory process of the respiratory bronchioles and the alveoli. The disease kills more than 60,000 Americans each year and is a leading cause of death in children worldwide[12] (Figure 24-12). Pneumonia can be caused by bacterial, viral, or fungal infection. Associated risk factors include cigarette smoking, alcoholism, exposure to cold, and extremes of age (the very young and very old). These diseases may be spread by respiratory droplets through contact with infected individuals. They also may be spread by inhaling bacteria from one's own nose and mouth.

Pneumonia may be classified as the viral, bacterial, mycoplasmal, or aspiration type. Pneumonia generally manifests with classic signs and symptoms (*typical pneumonia*). These include a productive cough, pleuritic chest pain, and fever that produces "shaking chills" (usually associated with the bacterial infection). It also may cause nonspecific complaints. (This particularly may be the case in older adults and debilitated patients.) Nonspecific complaints may include a nonproductive cough, headache, fatigue, and sore throat (*atypical pneumonia*).

 NOTE
Community-acquired pneumonia is an infection that is acquired from the environment. This category includes infections acquired indirectly as a result of the use of medications that change the body's ability to fight disease. The occurrence of these infections has risen in recent years. This is due to the increased percentage of the population older than age 65. It also is due to the increasing number of patients taking immunosuppressive drugs for malignancy, transplantation, or autoimmune disease.

TABLE 24-3 Diseases and Symptoms Associated With Wheezing

Disease	Symptoms
Asthma	Productive cough, tightness in chest
Bacterial pneumonia	Productive cough, pleuritic pain
Chronic bronchitis	Chronic productive cough
Emphysema	Cough
Foreign body aspiration	Cough
Heart failure	Cough, orthopnea, nocturnal dyspnea
Pneumothorax	Sudden, sharp pleuritic pain
Pulmonary disease	Tachypnea, cough, congestion
Pulmonary embolism	Sudden, sharp pleuritic pain
Toxic inhalation	Cough, pain

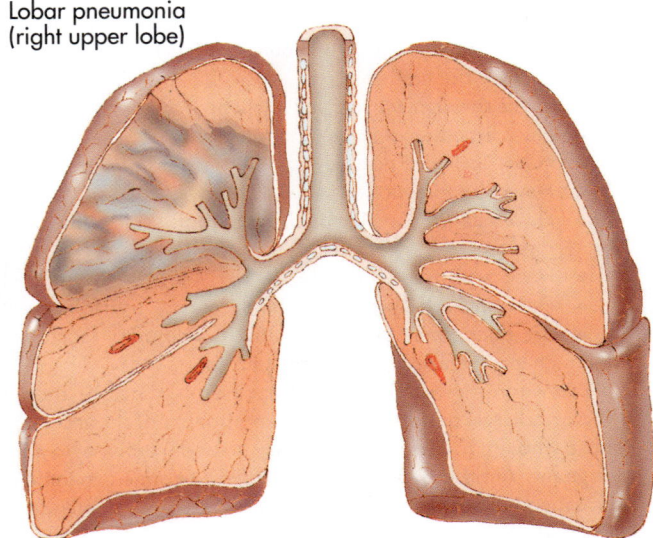

Lobar pneumonia (right upper lobe)

Pneumococcal pneumonia

FIGURE 24-12 *Pneumonia* is an inflammatory process of the respiratory bronchioles and alveoli. It is caused by infection. (From Wilson SF, Thompson JM: *Mosby's clinical nursing series: respiratory disorders,* St Louis, 1990, Mosby.)

Viral Pneumonia

Influenza A is the most common type of **viral pneumonia** (Box 24-7). It often occurs as epidemics in populations of small groups such as schoolchildren, army recruits, and nursing home residents. The interstitial infection caused by the virus predisposes the patient to secondary bacterial pneumonia.

Bacterial Pneumonia

Until 2000, the pneumococcus bacillus (*Streptococcus pneumoniae*) accounted for 90% of bacterial pneumonias. It affected 1 in 500 people each year. The decline in cases is related to vaccination of infants against the pneumococcus bacteria. The peak incidence is in winter and early spring. A vaccine that is now available is effective against this type of pneumonia in adults.

 DID YOU KNOW?

Pneumococcal Polysaccharide Vaccine (PPSV)

Pneumococcal disease is the leading cause of vaccine-preventable disease and death in the United States. The disease can lead to serious infections of the lungs (pneumonia), blood (bacteremia), and brain (meningitis). Pneumococcal pneumonia kills about 1 out of 20 people who contract the disease; bacteremia kills about 1 person in 5; and meningitis kills about 3 people in 10.

Pneumococcal polysaccharide vaccine (PPSV) protects against 23 types of pneumococcal bacteria, including those most likely to cause serious disease. Most healthy adults who are vaccinated develop protection to most or all of these types within 2 to 3 weeks of vaccination. Usually only one dose of PPSV is needed, but under some circumstances a second dose may be given. A second dose (given 5 years after the first dose) is recommended for:

- People 65 years and older who received their first dose when they were younger than 65 and it has been 5 or more years since the first dose
- People 2 through 64 years of age who:
  - Have a damaged spleen or no spleen
  - Have sickle cell disease
  - Have HIV infection or AIDS
  - Have cancer, leukemia, lymphoma, or multiple myeloma
  - Have nephrotic syndrome
  - Have received an organ or bone marrow transplant
  - Are taking medication that lowers immunity (such as chemotherapy or long-term steroids)

People to whom the vaccine should not be given include those who are allergic to the vaccine or a component of the vaccine; those who are moderately or severely ill; and women who are pregnant. Another type of pneumococcal vaccine (pneumococcal conjugate vaccine, or PCV) is routinely recommended for children younger than 5 years of age.[13]

Bacterial pneumonia also can result from the aspiration of mucus and saliva. Therefore, patients in a coma or with seizures, suppressed cough reflex, and increased secretions

---

Influenza is an acute, febrile disease that affects the entire body. It is associated with viral infection of the upper and lower respiratory tracts. It usually is characterized by the abrupt onset of a severe protracted cough, fever, headache, muscle ache, and mild sore throat. Of all the viruses, the influenza and para-influenza viruses are the most common causes of serious respiratory tract infections. Moreover, they have high morbidity and mortality rates.

Influenza viruses A, B, and C (and their many strains) are known for their potential to quickly cause respiratory tract infections after exposure. (It usually occurs within 24 to 48 hours.) The virus is inhaled in respiratory droplets from infected individuals (such as when an infected person sneezes). The droplets penetrate the surface of upper respiratory tract mucosal cells. The virus eventually spreads to the lower respiratory tract, where it causes cell inflammation and destruction of the cilia. Without the cilia, clearing the airways of infected mucus is more difficult. Consequently, a secondary bacterial infection often develops. This may result in pneumonia or acute respiratory failure. (This is particularly the case in patients with chronic lung disease.)

Influenza has the potential for widespread epidemics in high-risk populations. (These include adults and children with chronic cardiorespiratory or metabolic disorders, residents of nursing homes and other institutions, and health care workers.) Current vaccines are effective against some strains of the virus. These vaccines have minimal side effects. If uncomplicated, influenza is self-limiting. Acute symptoms last 2 to 7 days. These are followed by a convalescent period of about 1 week. *NOTE:* The H1N1 outbreak of 2009 affected healthy young people and pregnant women disproportionately, compared to other influenza viruses (see Chapter 28).

---

are predisposed to developing the disease. Other predisposing risk factors that may contribute to the development of bacterial pneumonia include the following:

- Infection
  - Upper respiratory tract infection (influenza)
  - Postoperative infection
- Foreign body aspiration
- Alcohol or other drug addiction
- Cardiac failure
- Stroke
- Syncope
- Pulmonary embolism
- Chronic illness
  - Chronic respiratory disease
  - Diabetes mellitus
  - Congestive heart failure
- Prolonged immobilization
- Compromised immune status

Mycoplasmal Pneumonia

Mycoplasmal pneumonia is caused by infection with *Mycoplasma pneumoniae*. It causes mild upper respiratory tract infection in school-age children and young adults.

Transmission is believed to occur by means of infected respiratory secretions. Therefore the condition spreads quickly among family members. This form of pneumonia can be treated effectively with antibiotics.

Aspiration Pneumonia

Aspiration pneumonia is an inflammation of the lung tissue (parenchyma). It results when foreign material enters the tracheobronchial tree. The syndrome is common in patients who have an altered level of consciousness (e.g., from head injury, seizure activity, use of alcohol or other drugs, anesthesia, infection, shock); patients who are intubated; and those who have aspirated foreign bodies. Factors common to victims of aspiration include depression of the cough or gag reflex, inability of the patient to handle secretions or gastric contents, and inability to protect the airway.

Aspiration pneumonia may be nonbacterial. (For example, it may develop after aspiration of stomach contents, toxic materials, or inert substances.) This typically is called *pneumonitis* to distinguish it from infectious pneumonia or bacterial pneumonia (as a secondary complication). Bacterial aspiration pneumonia has a poor prognosis, even with antibiotic therapy.

Management of Pneumonia

The pathophysiology of pneumonia depends on the agent that caused the disease. In viral and mycoplasmal pneumonias, the inflammatory response in the bronchi damages the cilia and the epithelium. This causes congestion. In some cases it causes hemorrhage. Signs and symptoms include chest pain, cough, fever, dyspnea, and occasionally hemoptysis. Patients usually complain of general malaise. They also complain of upper respiratory and gastrointestinal tract symptoms. Auscultation of the chest may reveal wheezing and fine crackles. In uncomplicated cases the symptoms usually resolve in 7 to 10 days.

Bacterial pneumonia begins with infection in the alveoli. In time, this infection fills the alveoli with fluid and purulent sputum. The infection spreads from alveolus to alveolus. As this occurs, large areas of the lung, even entire lobes, may become consolidated (filled with fluid and cellular debris). Consolidation reduces the available surface area of respiratory membranes. It also decreases the ventilation-perfusion ratio. Both of these effects may lead to hypoxemia. Patients with bacterial pneumonia usually have acute shaking chills, tachypnea, tachycardia, cough, and sputum production. The sputum may be rust-colored (classic for pneumococcus). More often, though, it is yellow, green, or gray. Additional symptoms include malaise, anorexia, flank or back pain, and vomiting. If the disease is uncomplicated and treated with antibiotics, the patient begins to recover within 3 to 5 days. Antibiotics usually are continued for a total of 7 to 10 days.

The physiological effects of aspiration pneumonia are based on the volume and pH of the aspirated substances. If the pH is below 2.5 (as may occur in the aspiration of

stomach contents), atelectasis, pulmonary edema, hemorrhage, and cell necrosis may occur. The alveolar-capillary membrane may be damaged as well. This, in turn, may lead to the accumulation of fluid in the alveoli. In severe cases, it may lead to adult respiratory distress syndrome (described in the next section). The patient's signs and symptoms vary with the scenario and the severity of the insult (e.g., near-drowning, foreign body aspiration, aspiration of gastric contents). Clinical features may include dyspnea, cough, bronchospasm, wheezes, rhonchi, crackles, cyanosis, and pulmonary and cardiac insufficiency. Of these patients, a good percentage develop pulmonary infection.

CRITICAL THINKING

What measures can the paramedic take to reduce a patient's risk of aspiration?

Prehospital care for patients with pneumonia includes airway support, oxygen administration, ventilatory assistance as needed, IV fluids to support blood pressure and to thin and loosen mucus, cardiac monitoring, and transport for evaluation by a physician. (Bronchodilator drugs may also be used for some patients.) In cases of aspiration, suctioning of the airway may be required. General patient management usually includes bed rest, analgesics, decongestants, expectorants, antipyretics, and antibiotic therapy. In severe cases, bronchoscopy, intubation, and mechanical ventilation may be required for some patients.

ACUTE RESPIRATORY DISTRESS SYNDROME

Acute respiratory distress syndrome (ARDS) is a fulminant form of respiratory failure. It is characterized by acute lung inflammation and diffuse alveolar-capillary injury.[14] All disorders that result in ARDS cause severe noncardiogenic pulmonary edema (described in Chapter 22). The syndrome develops as a complication of injury or illness such as trauma, gastric aspiration, cardiopulmonary bypass surgery, gram-negative sepsis, multiple blood transfusions, oxygen toxicity, toxic inhalation, drug overdose, pneumonia, and infections. Regardless of the specific cause, increased capillary permeability (high-permeability noncardiogenic pulmonary edema) results in a clinical condition in which the lungs are wet and heavy, congested, hemorrhagic, and stiff, with decreased perfusion capacity across alveolar membranes (Figure 24-13). The lungs become noncompliant. This requires the patient to increase the pressure in the airways to breathe.

The pulmonary edema associated with ARDS leads to severe hypoxemia, intrapulmonary shunting, reduced lung compliance, and, in some cases, irreversible damage to lung tissue. Unique to this syndrome is the fact that most patients who develop this condition have healthy lungs before the event that caused the disease; that is, they have

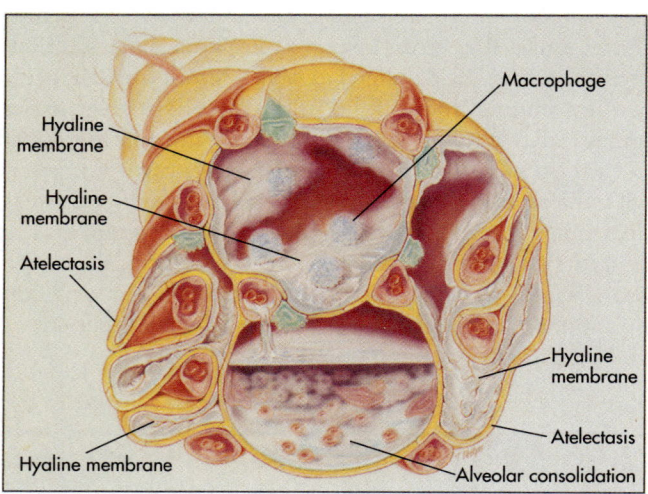

FIGURE 24-13 Cross-sectional view of alveoli in acute respiratory distress syndrome.

no history of recent respiratory illness or disease. ARDS is more common in men than in women. It affects about 190,000 people in the United States each year.[15] The death rate is greater than 65%. Complications include respiratory failure, cardiac dysrhythmias, disseminated intravascular coagulation, barotrauma, congestive heart failure, and renal failure.

Management

All patients with ARDS should be given high-concentration oxygen and ventilatory support. Depending on the underlying cause of ARDS, prehospital management may include fluid replacement to maintain cardiac output and peripheral perfusion; drug therapy to support mechanical ventilation; the use of pharmacological agents (e.g., corticosteroids) to stabilize pulmonary, capillary, and alveolar walls; and administration of diuretics.

Patients with ARDS usually have tachypnea, labored breathing, and impaired gas exchange 12 to 72 hours after the initial injury or medical crisis. The syndrome often results from another illness or injury. Therefore paramedics should consider the cause of the underlying problem. They also should provide supplemental oxygen and ventilatory support to improve arterial oxygenation (assessed by pulse oximetry). Most patients with moderate to severe respiratory distress require mechanical ventilation. This ventilation includes the use of positive end-expiratory pressure (PEEP, described in Chapter 15) or continuous positive airway pressure (CPAP). Both of these provide positive-pressure ventilation.

LOOK AGAIN

See Chapter 15: Airway Management, Respiration, and Artificial Ventilation, pp. 422-425.

PULMONARY EMBOLISM

Pulmonary embolism (PE) is a blockage of a pulmonary artery. The artery is blocked by a clot or other foreign material that has traveled there from another part of the body (Figure 24-14). Usually pulmonary embolisms originate in the lower extremities. PE is a relatively common disorder that affects about 650,000 people each year in the United States. Of this number 30% to 50% die, 10% within the first few hours after blockage.[16] In cases of severe pulmonary embolism, where shock and heart failure occur, the death rate may be greater than 50%.[17] Pulmonary embolism is responsible for 5% of all sudden deaths.[18]

PE usually begins as a venous disease. It most often is caused by migration of a thrombus from the large veins of the lower extremities, but it also can occur as a result of fat, air, sheared venous catheters, amniotic fluid, or tumor tissue. The clot or embolus dislodges and travels through the venous system to the right side of the heart. From there it migrates to the pulmonary arteries, obstructing the blood supply to a section of lung. The most common sites of thrombus formation are the deep veins of the legs and pelvis. Six factors that contribute to the development of venous thrombosis are listed in Box 24-8.

When one or more pulmonary arteries are blocked, an area does not receive blood flow; however, it continues to be ventilated. In response to the lack of blood flow, vasoconstriction occurs. If the vascular obstruction is severe (blockage of 60% or more of the pulmonary vascular supply), hypoxemia, acute pulmonary hypertension, systemic hypotension, and shock may rapidly occur, with subsequent death.

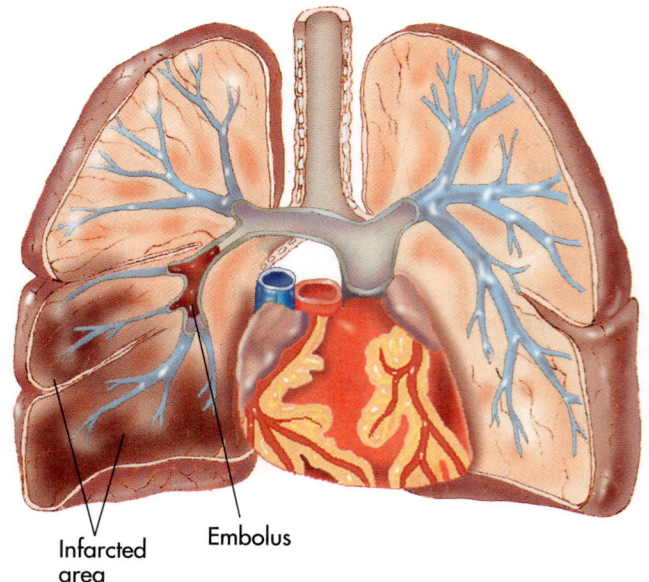

FIGURE 24-14 *Pulmonary embolism (PE) is the blockage of a pulmonary artery by foreign matter, such as a thrombus. The blockage usually arises from a peripheral vein, fat, air, or tumor tissue. The result is obstruction of the blood supply to the lung tissue. (From Wilson SF, Thompson JM: Mosby's clinical nursing series: respiratory disorders, St Louis, 1990, Mosby.)*

BOX 24-8 Contributing Factors in the Development of Venous Thrombosis

Venostasis
- Extended travel
- Prolonged bed rest
- Obesity
- Advanced age
- Burns
- Varicose veins

Venous Injury
- Surgery of the thorax, abdomen, pelvis, or legs
- Fractures of the pelvis or legs

Increased Blood Coagulability
- Malignancy
- Use of oral contraceptives
- Congenital or acquired coagulation disorders

Disease
- Chronic lung disease with polycythemia
- Congestive heart failure
- Sickle cell anemia
- Cancer
- Atrial fibrillation
- Myocardial infarction
- Previous pulmonary embolism
- Previous deep vein thrombosis
- Infection
- Diabetes mellitus

Multiple Trauma
- Long bone fracture
- Pelvic fracture

Signs and Symptoms

An embolus may be small, moderate, or massive. Thus patients with PE may have very different presentations and a wide variety of signs and symptoms. These depend on the location and size of the clot. They may include dyspnea, cough, hemoptysis (rare), pain, anxiety, syncope, hypotension, diaphoresis, tachypnea, tachycardia, fever, and distended neck veins. In addition, chest splinting, pleuritic pain, pleural friction rub, crackles, and localized wheezing may be present. If the embolism is large, sudden cardiac arrest can occur. The paramedic should consider a pulmonary embolism in any patient who has cardiorespiratory problems that cannot be otherwise explained, particularly when risk factors are present. As mentioned earlier, continuous capnometry may be useful in identifying a patient with PE.

CRITICAL THINKING
Consider that you need to distinguish a pulmonary embolism (PE) from other conditions with similar signs and symptoms. What information in the patient assessment may help?

Management

Prehospital care mainly is supportive. Supplemental high-concentration oxygen should be administered, a cardiac monitor and pulse oximeter applied, and an IV line of normal saline or lactated Ringer's solution established. The patient should be transported in a position of comfort. Definitive care requires hospitalization and in-hospital treatment with fibrinolytic or **heparin** therapy.

NOTE
The ECG may show an *S1Q3T3 pattern* in a patient with PE. This pattern is a prominent S wave in lead I, a Q wave in lead III, and a T wave in lead III. However, the ECG pattern needed for the diagnosis of pulmonary embolism is debatable. Once the diagnosis of PE has been established, however, the ECG could allow the massive forms to be distinguished. T-wave inversion in the precordial leads is the most common abnormality (68%). This represents the ECG findings that are best correlated to the severity of the PE.[19]

UPPER RESPIRATORY INFECTION

Upper respiratory infections (URIs) affect the nose, throat, sinuses, and larynx. They are among the most common of all illnesses, affecting nearly 80 million people each year.[1] These illnesses include the common cold, pharyngitis, tonsillitis, sinusitis, and laryngitis (see Chapter 23). They rarely are life-threatening. However, they often exacerbate underlying pulmonary conditions. They also may lead to significant infections in patients with suppressed immune function. A key action for preventing the spread of respiratory tract infections is hand washing. Another crucial action is covering the mouth when sneezing or coughing.

A variety of bacteria and viruses can cause URIs. Group A streptococci are responsible for 20% to 30% of cases; 50% of cases have no demonstrated bacterial or viral cause.[1] Signs and symptoms of upper respiratory tract infection include the following:

- Sore throat
- Fever
- Chills
- Headache
- Facial pain (sinusitis)
- Purulent nasal drainage
- Halitosis (bad breath)
- Cervical adenopathy (enlarged cervical lymph nodes)
- Erythematous pharynx (pharyngeal inflammation/irritation)

CRITICAL THINKING
When might an upper respiratory infection (URI) become life threatening? Give two or three examples.

Management

Most URIs are self-limiting and require little or no prehospital treatment. Prehospital care is aimed at relieving the symptoms. This is especially true for patients who have underlying lung conditions. With such conditions, oxygen administration may be indicated. Other interventions that may be indicated for patients with underlying lung conditions include administration of bronchodilators or corticosteroids. If throat cultures are obtained at the scene, the family must be notified of the results. Follow-up by a physician is also required. The paramedic should follow local protocol.

SPONTANEOUS PNEUMOTHORAX

A primary **spontaneous pneumothorax** usually results when a bleb ruptures. This allows air to enter the pleural space from within the lung. This type of pneumothorax may occur in seemingly healthy individuals who are usually between 20 and 40 years of age. Often these patients are tall, thin men with long, narrow chests. (In contrast, a secondary spontaneous pneumothorax sometimes may develop from an underlying disease, such as COPD.) In recent years the number of spontaneous pneumothoraces has increased in some populations. These groups include individuals with acquired immunodeficiency syndrome (AIDS) who have pneumonia, and drug abusers who deeply inhale free-base cocaine, marijuana, or inhalants (e.g., glue or solvents). The condition should also be considered in a patient with COPD, especially if the patient has been treated with positive-pressure ventilation.

Most primary spontaneous pneumothoraces that are well tolerated by the patient occupy less than 20% of a lung (partial pneumothorax). Signs and symptoms include shortness of breath and chest pain that often is sudden in onset, pallor, diaphoresis, and tachypnea. In severe cases in which the pneumothorax occupies more than 20% of the hemithorax, the following signs and symptoms may be present:

- Altered mental status
- Cyanosis
- Tachycardia
- Decreased breath sounds on the affected side
- Local hyperresonance to percussion
- Subcutaneous emphysema

> **NOTE**
> In severe cases a spontaneous pneumothorax may generate a *tension pneumothorax.* When this occurs, venous return to the heart is impaired. This can lead to total cardiovascular collapse. Tension pneumothorax is further described in Chapter 42.

Management

Prehospital care is based on the patient's symptoms and degree of respiratory distress. Administration of high-concentration oxygen is indicated to help resolve the pneumothorax, and airway, ventilatory, and circulatory support may be required in severe cases. These patients should be transported in a position of comfort for evaluation by a physician and possible decompression of the pleural space. Surgery may be indicated in some cases. This may be done to allow for lung reexpansion or to prevent recurrence. If signs and symptoms of tension pneumothorax develop, needle chest decompression should be performed (see Chapter 42).

HYPERVENTILATION SYNDROME

Hyperventilation syndrome is abnormally deep or rapid breathing that results in an excessive loss of carbon dioxide. (This, in turn, produces respiratory alkalosis.) As a result, the syndrome produces hypocarbia. The hypocarbia leads to cerebrovascular constriction, reduced cerebral perfusion, paresthesia, dizziness, or even feelings of euphoria. Several conditions can cause hyperventilation syndrome, including the following:

- Anxiety
- Hypoxia
- Pulmonary disease
- Cardiovascular disorders
- Metabolic disorders
- Neurological disorders
- Fever
- Infection
- Pain
- Pregnancy
- Drug use

> **CRITICAL THINKING**
> How can you distinguish between hyperventilation caused by anxiety and hyperventilation caused by a serious medical illness or toxic ingestion?

Signs and symptoms of hyperventilation syndrome include dyspnea with rapid breathing and a high minute volume, chest pain, facial tingling, and carpopedal spasm. Other assessment findings vary, based on the cause of the syndrome. A low end-tidal carbon dioxide concentration ($EtCO_2$) measurement is <35 mm Hg.

Management

If the syndrome clearly is caused by anxiety (*psychogenic dyspnea,* which is a diagnosis of exclusion), prehospital care is mainly supportive. It consists of calming measures and reassurance. Paramedics may suspect that the syndrome is a result of illness (e.g., diabetes, renal disease). They also may suspect drug ingestion. In either case care includes both oxygen administration and airway and ventilatory support. All patients who are hyperventilating should be calmed and the paramedic should coach the patient's ventilations. Attempts should not be made to slow ventilations if patients are compensating for hypoxia or metabolic acidosis. If the hyperventilation is severe or complicated by illness or drug ingestion, transport for evaluation by a physician is indicated.

LUNG CANCER

Lung cancer is an epidemic in the United States. An estimated 219,000 new cases are reported each year.[20] Most cases of lung cancer develop in individuals between 55 and 65 years of age. Of the new cases reported, most patients die of the disease within 1 year; 20% have local lung involvement, 25% have metastasis to the lymph system, and 55% have distant metastatic cancer.[21] The most common cause of lung cancer is cigarette smoking. Heavy smokers (more than 20 cigarettes a day) have a 25 times greater chance of developing lung cancer than nonsmokers.[22] Other risk factors include passive smoking (exposure to someone else's cigarette smoke) and exposure to asbestos, radon gas, dust, coal products, ionizing radiation, and other toxins.

Pathophysiology

Like other cancers, lung cancer is the uncontrolled growth of abnormal cells. At least a dozen different cell types of tumors are associated with primary lung cancer (Figure 24-15). The two major cell types of lung cancer are *small cell lung cancer* and *non–small cell lung cancer* (which is subcategorized as *squamous cell carcinoma, adenocarcinoma,* and *large cell carcinoma*). Each cell type has a different growth pattern. Each also has a different response to treatment. Most abnormal cell growth begins in the bronchi or bronchioles. The lung also is a fairly common site of **metastasis** (the spread of cancer) to other primary sites (e.g., breast cancer).

Signs and Symptoms

The signs and symptoms of early-stage disease often are nonspecific. Smokers often attribute them to the effects of smoking. These include coughing, sputum production, lower airway obstruction (noted by wheezing), and respiratory illness (e.g., bronchitis). As the disease progresses, signs and symptoms may include the following:

- Cough
- Hemoptysis (which may be severe)
- Dyspnea
- Hoarseness or voice change
- Dysphagia
- Weight loss/anorexia
- Weakness

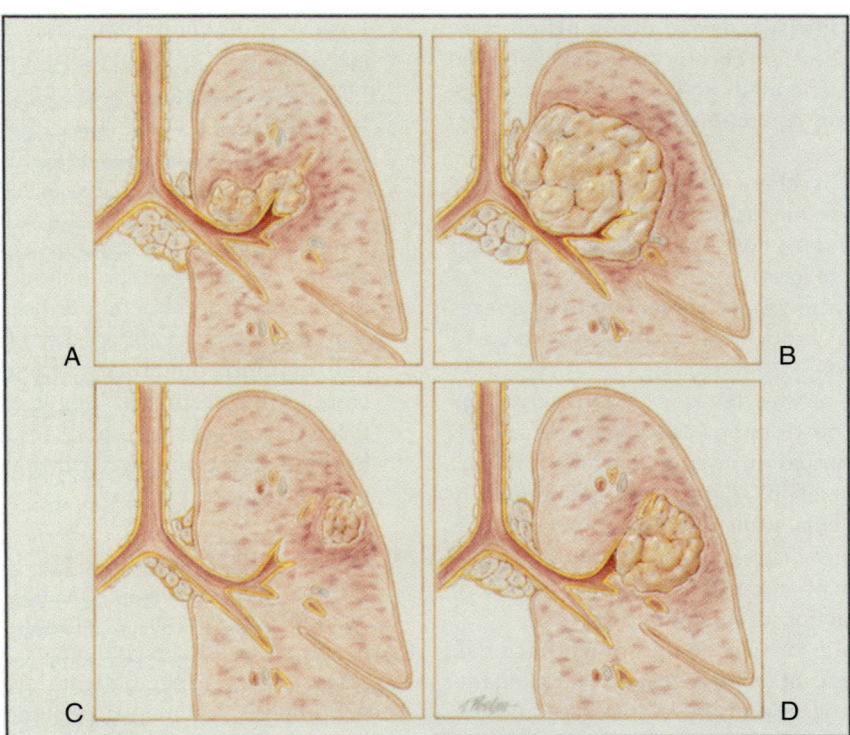

FIGURE 24-15 Cancer of the lung. **A,** Squamous cell carcinoma. **B,** Small cell (oat cell) carcinoma. **C,** Adenocarcinoma. **D,** Large cell carcinoma. (Modified from Desjardins T, Burton GG: *Clinical manifestations and assessment of respiratory disease,* ed 3, St Louis, 2006, Mosby.)

Patients with cancer may call paramedics because of complications resulting from chemotherapy or radiation therapy. Such therapy is toxic to both normal body cells and malignant cells. Associated complaints often include nausea and vomiting, fatigue, and dehydration. These patients should be offered emotional and psychological support.

> ### CRITICAL THINKING
> Should you assume that patients who have been diagnosed with lung cancer want "do not resuscitate" (DNR) status?

Management

Most patients with lung cancer are aware of their disease. Prehospital management includes airway, ventilatory, and circulatory support; oxygen administration (based on symptoms and pulse oximetry); and transport for evaluation by a physician. Depending on the severity of the patient's condition, IV fluids may be needed to improve hydration and to thin sputum. Drug therapy (e.g., bronchodilators and corticosteroids) may be needed to improve breathing. Analgesics may be required to relieve pain. End-stage patients may have advance directives or "do not resuscitate" (DNR) orders. In these cases emotional support should also be offered to the family and loved ones.

·SUMMARY

- Diseases responsible for respiratory emergencies include those related to ventilation, diffusion, and perfusion. Ventilation moves air into and out of the lungs. Diffusion is the process of gas exchange. Perfusion is circulation of blood through the tissues.
- Patients should be assessed for chief complaint, signs and symptoms of respiratory distress, and past medical history. The physical examination should determine vital signs, indicators of increased work of breathing, breath sounds, and peripheral edema or cyanosis. Capnometry, oximetry, and peak flow measurements supplement the physical examination findings.
- Obstructive airway disease is a triad of distinct diseases that often coexist. These are chronic bronchitis, emphysema, and asthma. The main goal of prehospital care for these patients is the correction of hypoxemia through improved airflow.
- Chronic bronchitis is characterized by inflammatory changes and excessive mucus production in the alveoli. These patients often have low blood oxygen levels and excess carbon dioxide levels.
- Emphysema causes abnormal enlargement of air spaces beyond the terminal bronchioles and destruction and collapse of the alveoli.
- Asthma, or reactive airway disease, is characterized by reversible airflow obstruction caused by bronchial smooth muscle contraction; hypersecretion of mucus, resulting in bronchial plugging; and inflammatory changes in the bronchial walls. The typical patient with asthma is in obvious distress. Respirations are rapid and loud. Treatment focuses on bronchodilation, hydration, and reduction of inflammation.
- Pneumonia is a group of specific infections (bacterial, viral, or fungal). These infections cause an acute inflammatory process of the respiratory bronchioles and the alveoli. Pneumonia usually manifests with classic signs and symptoms. These include a productive cough and associated fever that produces "shaking chills."

- Prehospital care of patients with pneumonia includes airway support, oxygen administration, ventilatory assistance as needed, IV fluids, cardiac monitoring, and transport.
- Adult respiratory distress syndrome is a fulminant form of respiratory failure. It is characterized by acute lung inflammation and diffuse alveolar-capillary injury. It develops as a complication of illness or injury. In ARDS, the lungs are wet and heavy, congested, hemorrhagic, and stiff, with decreased perfusion capacity across alveolar membranes. Prehospital management includes airway and ventilatory support.
- Positive end-expiratory pressure (PEEP) maintains pressure at the end of exhalation. Adding PEEP in the respiratory circuit keeps alveoli open and pushes fluid from the alveoli back in the interstitium or capillaries. Continuous positive airway pressure maintains constant airway pressure throughout the entire respiratory cycle. CPAP improves diffusion and helps reexpand collapsed alveoli. Biphasic positive airway pressure delivers variable airway pressure throughout the respiratory cycle.
- Pulmonary thromboembolism is a blockage of a pulmonary artery by a clot or other foreign material. When one or more pulmonary arteries are blocked by an embolism, a section of lung is ventilated but hypoperfused. Hypotension, shock, and death can occur. Prehospital care is mainly supportive and includes oxygen administration, IV access, and transport for definitive care.
- Upper respiratory infections affect the nose, throat, sinuses, and larynx. Signs and symptoms of a URI include sore throat, fever, chills, headache, cervical adenopathy, and an erythematous pharynx. Prehospital care is based on the patient's symptoms.
- A primary spontaneous pneumothorax usually results when a subpleural bleb ruptures. This allows air to enter the pleural space from within the lung. Signs and symptoms include shortness of breath and chest pain that

often are sudden in onset, pallor, diaphoresis, and tachypnea. Prehospital care is based on the patient's symptoms and degree of distress.

- Hyperventilation syndrome is abnormally deep or rapid breathing. This type of breathing results in an excessive loss of carbon dioxide. If the syndrome clearly is caused by anxiety, prehospital care is mainly supportive (i.e., calming measures and reassurance). The paramedic may suspect that the syndrome is a result of illness or drug ingestion. If this is the case, care may include oxygen administration and airway and ventilatory support.

- Lung cancer is an expression of the uncontrolled growth of abnormal cells. As the disease progresses, signs and symptoms may include cough, hemoptysis, dyspnea, hoarseness, and dysphagia. Prehospital management includes airway, ventilatory, and circulatory support.

REFERENCES

1. U.S. Department of Transportation, National Highway Traffic Safety Administration: *EMT-paramedic national standard curriculum*, Washington, DC, 1998, Department of Transportation (DOT).
2. Centers for Disease Control and Prevention, National Center for Health Statistics: National Vital Statistics Report 2007, www.cdc.gov/nchs/data/nvsr/nvsr57/nvsr57_12.pdf, accessed 9-17-2010.
3. National Highway Traffic Safety Administration: *The National EMS Education Standards*, Washington, DC, 2009, U.S. Department of Transportation/National Highway Traffic Safety Administration, DOT.
4. Kupnik D, Skok P: Capnometry in the prehospital setting: are we using its potential? *Emerg Med J* 24(9):614-617, 2007.
5. Gravenstein JS, Jaffe MB, Paulus DA, editors: *Capnography: clinical aspects*, Cambridge, UK, 2004, Cambridge Press.
6. Barnes PJ, Drazen JM, Rennard SI, et al: *Asthma and COPD: basic mechanisms and clinical management*, Amsterdam, 2002, Academic Press.
7. Siddiqi A, Sethi S: Optimizing antibiotic selection in treating COPD exacerbations, *Int J Chron Obstruct Pulmon Dis* 3(1): 31-44, 2008.
8. American Lung Association: Lung disease data: 2008, www.lungusa.org/assets/documents/publications/lung-disease-data/LDD_2008.pdf, accessed 9-20-2010.
9. Stein JH, Sande MA, Zvaifler NJ, et al: *Internal medicine*, ed 5, St Louis, 1998, Mosby.
10. American Heart Association: 2010 American Heart Association guidelines for cardiopulmonary resuscitation and emergency cardiovascular care, *Circulation* 122(18 suppl): S639-S946, 2010.
11. Hamilton GC, Sanders AB, Strange G, et al: *Emergency medicine: an approach to clinical problem-solving*, ed 2, Philadelphia, 2003, Saunders.
12. Centers for Disease Control and Prevention: *Pneumonia*, www.cdc.gov/nchs/FASTATS/pneumonia.htm, accessed 8-21-10.
13. Centers for Disease Control and Prevention: Pneumococcal polysaccharide vaccine (PPSV): what you need to know, www.cdc.gov/vaccines/pubs/VIS/downloads/vis-ppv.pdf, accessed 10-29-09.
14. McCance L, Huether S: *Pathophysiology: the biologic basis for disease in adults and children*, ed 5, St Louis, 2006, Mosby.
15. U.S. Department of Health and Human Services, National Institutes of Health: What is ARDS, www.nhlbi.nih.gov/health/dci/Diseases/Ards/Ards_WhatIs.html, accessed 10-29-09.
16. Tapson VF: Acute pulmonary embolism, *N Engl J Med* 358(10): 1037-1052, 2008.
17. Snow V, Qaseem A, Barry P, et al: Management of venous thromboembolism: a clinical practice guideline from the American College of Physicians and the American Academy of Family Physicians, *Ann Intern Med* 146(3):204-310, 2007.
18. Goldhaber SZ: Pulmonary thromboembolism. In Kasper DL, Braunwald E, Fauci AS, et al, editors: *Harrison's principles of internal medicine*, ed 16, New York, 2005, McGraw-Hill.
19. Ferrari E, Imbert A, Chevalier T, et al: The ECG in pulmonary embolism: predictive value of negative T waves in precordial leads, http://chestjournal.chestpubs.org/content/111/3/537.abstract, accessed 10-29-09.
20. National Cancer Institute, National Institutes of Health: Lung cancer, www.cancer.gov/cancertopics/types/lung, accessed 10-29-09.
21. Rosen P, Barkin R: *Emergency medicine: concepts and clinical practice*, ed 4, St Louis, 2006, Mosby.
22. Chiras D: *Human biology*, ed 7, Sudbury, Mass., 2012, Jones and Bartlett.

SUGGESTED READING

Pines JM: Within the inflamed lung, *JEMS.com* 32(10):64-75, 2007.

OBJECTIVES

Upon completion of this chapter, the paramedic student will be able to:

1. Describe the anatomy and physiology of the nervous system.
2. Outline pathophysiological changes in the nervous system that may alter the cerebral perfusion pressure.
3. Describe the assessment of a patient with a nervous system disorder.
4. Describe the pathophysiology, signs and symptoms, and specific management techniques for each of the following neurological disorders: coma, stroke and intracranial hemorrhage, seizure disorders, headaches, brain neoplasm and brain abscess, and degenerative neurological diseases.

KEY TERMS

absence seizures Seizures characterized by brief lapses of consciousness without loss of posture; also known as *petit mal seizures*.

acoustic neuroma A noncancerous tumor that involves the vestibular portion of the acoustic nerve (cranial nerve VIII).

action potential A change in membrane potential in an excitable tissue that acts as an electrical signal and is propagated in an all-or-none fashion.

Alzheimer's disease A disease characterized by confusion, memory failure, disorientation, speech disturbances, and inability to carry out purposeful movements.

amyotrophic lateral sclerosis (ALS) One of a group of rare disorders in which the nerves that control muscular activity degenerate in the brain and spinal cord; also called *Lou Gehrig's disease*.

arteriovenous (AV) malformation An abnormal connection between veins and arteries; it is believed to arise during fetal development or soon after birth.

atonic seizures Seizures that cause an abrupt loss of muscle tone, loss of posture, or sudden collapse ("drop attacks").

aura A sensation that may precede a migraine or seizure activity.

automatism Abnormal repetitive motor behavior (e.g., lip smacking, chewing, or swallowing), during which the patient is amnestic.

axon The main central process of a neuron that normally conducts action potentials away from the cell body of the neuron.

Babinski's sign A reflex movement in which the great toe bends upward when the outer edge of the sole is scratched; also known as *Babinski's reflex*.

Bell's palsy A paralysis of the facial muscles caused by inflammation of the facial nerve (cranial nerve VII); the condition usually is one-sided and temporary and often develops suddenly.

brain abscess An accumulation of purulent material (pus) surrounded by a capsule within the brain.

brain tumors Masses in the cranial cavity.

cell body The part of the cell that contains the nucleus and surrounding cytoplasm, exclusive of any projections or processes; it is concerned more with metabolism of the cell than with a specific function.

central nervous system (CNS) The brain and spinal cord.

cerebral aneurysm A weak or thin spot on a blood vessel in the brain that balloons and fills with blood.

cerebral blood flow (CBF) A function of the cerebral perfusion pressure and the resistance of the cerebral vascular bed.

cerebral embolism An obstruction in a cerebral artery by an embolus, usually resulting in transient or permanent impairment of cognitive, motor, or sensory function.

cerebral perfusion pressure (CPP) A measure of the amount of blood flow to the brain. It is calculated by subtracting the intracranial pressure from the mean systemic arterial blood pressure.

cerebral thrombosis The formation of a blood clot (thrombus) in an artery that supplies blood to the brain.

cerebrospinal fluid (CSF) The fluid that fills the subarachnoid space in the brain and spinal cord and in the cerebral ventricles.

cerebrovascular accident (CVA) An abnormal condition of the blood vessels of the brain characterized by occlusion by an embolus, thrombus, or cerebral hemorrhage; also called a *stroke* or "brain attack."

circle of Willis The circle of interconnected blood vessels at the base of the brain.

cluster headache A type of headache that occurs in bursts, or clusters; also known as a histamine headache.

coma An abnormally deep state of unconsciousness from which the patient cannot be aroused by external stimuli.

complex partial seizure A seizure that originates in the temporal lobe; it usually begins with an aura and is followed by repetitive motor behavior.

confabulation The invention of stories to make up for gaps in memory.

conjugate gaze Deviation of both eyes to either side at rest; the condition implies a structural lesion.

Creutzfeldt-Jakob disease (CJD) A rare, fatal brain disorder characterized by rapidly progressive dementia.

Cushing's reflex An attempt by the body to compensate for a decline in cerebral perfusion pressure by increasing the mean arterial pressure.

decerebrate rigidity A position in which a comatose patient's arms are extended and internally rotated and the legs are extended with the feet in forced plantar flexion; it usually is seen with compression of the brainstem; also known as *decerebrate posturing*.

decorticate rigidity A position in which a comatose patient's upper extremities are rigidly flexed at the elbows and at the wrists; it usually is seen with a lesion in the mesencephalic region of the brain; also known as *decorticate posturing*.

dementia A slow, progressive loss of awareness of time and place. It usually involves an inability to learn new things or recall recent events.

dendrites The branching processes of a neuron that receive stimuli and conduct potentials toward the cell body.

dysconjugate gaze Deviation of the eyes to opposite sides at rest; it implies a structural brainstem dysfunction in the pathways that traverse the brainstem from the upper midbrain to at least the level of the lower pons.

dystonia A condition characterized by local or diffuse changes in muscle tone, resulting in painful muscle spasms, unusually fixed postures, and strange movement patterns.

effector organ A muscle or gland that responds to nerve impulses from the central nervous system.

epilepsy A condition characterized by the tendency to have recurrent seizures (excluding those that arise from correctable or avoidable circumstances).

generalized seizure A seizure without an identifiable focus in the brain.

gingival hypertrophy Swelling of the gums; often associated with chronic phenytoin therapy.

Glasgow Coma Scale A standardized system for assessing the degree of impairment of consciousness in a critically ill patient and for predicting the duration and ultimate outcome of coma.

glossopharyngeal neuralgia Irritation of the glossopharyngeal nerve (cranial nerve IX).

Guillain-Barré syndrome (GBS) A rare disease associated with a viral infection or immunization that affects the peripheral nervous system, especially the spinal nerves, but also the cranial nerves.

hemifacial spasm A neuromuscular disorder characterized by frequent involuntary contractions of the muscles on one side of the face.

hemiparesis One-sided weakness.

hemorrhagic stroke A stroke caused by bleeding.

Huntington's disease (HD) A rare, hereditary disease characterized by quick, involuntary movements, speech disturbances, and mental deterioration; it is caused by degenerative changes in the cerebral cortex and basal ganglia; also known as *Huntington's chorea*.

intracranial pressure (ICP) The pressure inside the skull, brain tissue, and cerebrospinal fluid.

ischemic stroke A stroke caused by blockage of a cerebral blood vessel; also called an *occlusive stroke*.

jacksonian seizure A transitory disturbance in motor, sensory, or autonomic function resulting from abnormal neuronal discharges in a localized part of the brain; also known as a *focal seizure*.

mean arterial pressure (MAP) The arithmetic mean of the blood pressure in the arterial portion of the circulation.

migraine A severe, incapacitating headache that often is preceded by visual and/or gastrointestinal disturbances.

motor neurons Neurons are efferent neurons that innervate skeletal, smooth, or cardiac muscle fibers.

multiple sclerosis (MS) A progressive disease of the central nervous system in which scattered patches of myelin in the brain and spinal cord are destroyed.

muscular dystrophy An inherited muscle disorder of unknown cause marked by a slow but progressive degeneration of muscle fibers.

myoclonic seizures Seizures that cause brief muscle contractions, which usually occur at the same time and on both sides of the body.

neoplasm An abnormal growth; a malignant or benign tumor.

neuroglia Specialized connective tissue cells that protect and hold functioning neurons together.

neurons The functional units of the nervous system; they consist of the nerve cell body, the dendrites, and the axon.

nonepileptic seizure A seizure that stems from psychological causes rather than electrical disturbances in the brain.

nuchal rigidity Neck stiffness with flexion, which suggests meningeal irritation.

Parkinson's disease A disease caused by degeneration or damage (of unknown origin) to nerve cells in the basal ganglia in the brain.

partial seizure A seizure that originates from an identifiable cortical lesion.

peripheral nervous system (PNS) A subdivision of the nervous system consisting of nerves and ganglia.

peripheral neuropathy Diseases and disorders that affect the peripheral nervous system, including the spinal nerve roots, cranial nerves, and peripheral nerves.

Pick's disease A rare neurodegenerative disease associated with the shrinking of the frontal and temporal anterior lobes of the brain.

poliomyelitis An infectious disease caused by one of three polio viruses; asymptomatic, mild, and paralytic forms of the disease occur.

Ranvier's nodes The short intervals in the myelin sheath of a nerve fiber between adjacent Schwann cells.

reflex An automatic response to a stimulus that occurs without conscious thought; it is produced by a reflex arc.

Schwann cells Cells that form a myelin sheath around each nerve fiber of the peripheral nervous system.

seizure A temporary change in behavior or consciousness caused by abnormal electrical activity in one or more groups of neurons in the brain.

sensory neurons Neurons that transmit impulses to the spinal cord and brain from all parts of the body.

simple partial seizure A seizure that originates in the motor or sensory cortex; it usually manifests as clonic activity that is limited to one body part.

sinus headache A headache characterized by pain in the forehead, nasal area, and eyes.

spina bifida A congenital defect in which part of one or more vertebrae fails to develop completely, leaving a portion of the spinal cord exposed.

spinal cord tumors Benign or malignant tumors that originate in the cells within or next to the spinal cord.

status epilepticus Continuous seizure activity lasting 30 minutes or longer, or a recurrent seizure without an intervening period of consciousness.

subarachnoid hemorrhage Bleeding within the subarachnoid space.

synapse Functional membrane-to-membrane contact of a nerve cell with another nerve cell, muscle cell, gland cell, or sensory receptor; it transmits action potentials from one cell to another.

tension headache A headache caused by muscle contraction in the face, neck, and scalp.

tonic-clonic seizures Generalized seizures involving the entire body; also known as *grand mal seizures.*

transient ischemic attack (TIA) An acute episode of temporary neurological dysfunction resulting from focal cerebral ischemia; also called a "mini stroke."

trigeminal neuralgia Infection or disease of the trigeminal nerve (cranial nerve V); also known as *central pain syndrome.*

Acute medical disorders of the nervous system require rapid assessment and management. Paramedics must combine knowledge and skills with appropriate, aggressive intervention. These actions can help reduce mortality and morbidity. Proper recognition and treatment are the foundation for the greatest potential for rehabilitation and recovery.

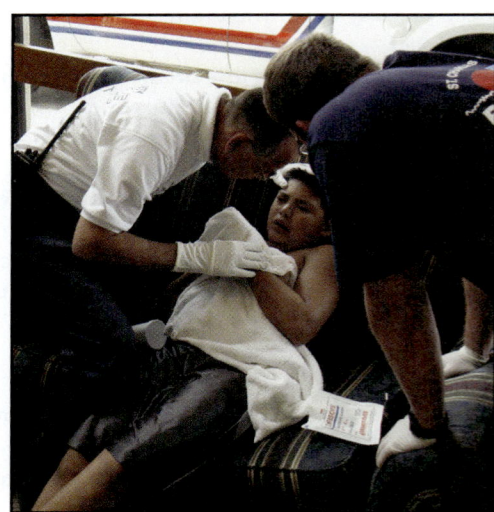

(Courtesy Ray Kemp, St. Charles, Mo.)

 LOOK AGAIN
See Chapter 10: Review of Human Systems, pp. 171-177.

ANATOMY AND PHYSIOLOGY OF THE NERVOUS SYSTEM

As described in Chapter 10, the nervous system is divided into two parts: the **central nervous system (CNS)** and the **peripheral nervous system (PNS)** (Figure 25-1). The ability of the human body to maintain a state of balance **(homeostasis)** is chiefly the result of the nervous system's ability to coordinate and regulate the body's activities. To review, the CNS consists of the brain and the spinal cord. Both of these are encased in and protected by bone. A total of 43 pairs of nerves originate from the CNS to form the PNS. Twelve pairs of cranial nerves originate from the brain. Thirty-one pairs of spinal nerves originate from the spinal cord.

Cells of the Nervous System

The cells of the nervous system include **neurons** (the basic units of the nervous system) and connective tissue cells known as **neuroglia** (specialized cells that protect and hold functioning neurons together). Each neuron has three main parts: (1) the **cell body,** which has a single, relatively

CENTRAL NERVOUS SYSTEM

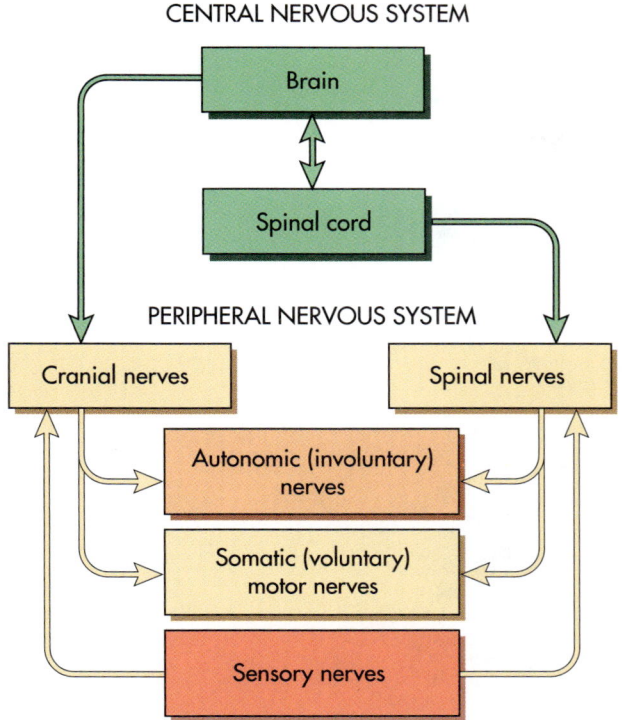

FIGURE 25-1 Divisions of the nervous system. (McSwain N: *The basic EMT: comprehensive prehospital patient care,* St Louis, 1999, Mosby.)

large nucleus with a prominent nucleolus; (2) one or more branching projections, called **dendrites;** and (3) a single, elongated projection, known as an **axon** (Figure 25-2). Dendrites transmit impulses to the cell bodies. Axons transmit impulses away from the cell bodies. Axons are surrounded by supportive and protective sheaths formed by the cytoplasmic extensions of neuroglial cells in the CNS *(unmyelinated axons)*. Axons are also surrounded by **Schwann cells** in the PNS *(myelinated axons)*.

Bundles of parallel axons with their associated sheaths are white and therefore are called *white matter*. The **action potential,** which is initiated in the neuron body, is propagated through the axons via conduction pathways or nerve tracts from one area of the CNS to another. In the PNS, bundles of axons and their sheaths are called *nerves*. Collections of nerve cells are grayer and are called *gray matter*. Gray matter is the site of integration in the nervous system. The outer surface of the cerebrum and the cerebellum consists of gray matter, which forms the cerebral cortex and the cerebellar cortex.

Types of Neurons

Neurons are classified as sensory neurons, motor neurons, or interneurons. This is based on the direction in which they transmit impulses. **Sensory neurons** transmit impulses to the spinal cord and brain from all parts of the body. **Motor neurons** transmit impulses in the opposite direction, away from the brain and spinal cord. In addition, they transmit impulses only to muscle and glandular epithelial tissue. **Interneurons** conduct impulses from sensory neurons to motor neurons. Sensory neurons also are called *afferent neurons*. Motor neurons are called *efferent neurons*. Interneurons are called *central* or *connecting neurons*.

Impulse Transmission

The transmission of nerve impulses in the nervous system is similar to the conduction of electrical impulses through the heart. In its resting state, the neuron is positively charged on the outside and negatively charged on the inside. When the neuron is stimulated by pressure, temperature, or chemical changes, the cell membrane's permeability to sodium ions increases. As a result, positively charged sodium ions rush into the interior of the neuron. This inward movement begins a wave of depolarization. The wave travels down the axon, resulting in the propagation of an action potential (Figure 25-3).

CRITICAL THINKING
Think of examples of a pressure, a temperature, and a chemical stimulus to a nerve.

In unmyelinated axons, action potentials are spread along the entire axon membrane. Myelinated axons, however, have interruptions in the myelin sheaths. These are known as **Ranvier's nodes.** These nodes allow nerve impulses to "jump" from one node to the next without spreading along the entire length of the cell *(saltatory conduction)*. Myelinated axons, therefore, conduct action potentials faster than unmyelinated axons.

Synapse

The membrane-to-membrane contact that separates the axon endings of one neuron *(presynaptic neuron)* from the dendrites of another neuron *(postsynaptic neuron)* is known as a **synapse.** The structures that compose a synapse are the presynaptic terminal, the synaptic cleft, and the plasma membrane of the postsynaptic neuron. Within each presynaptic terminal are synaptic vesicles that contain neurotransmitter chemicals (Figure 25-4).

Each action potential arriving at the presynaptic terminal initiates a series of specific events. These events result in the release of the neurotransmitter. The neurotransmitter rapidly diffuses the short distance across the synaptic cleft. It then binds to specific receptor molecules on the postsynaptic membrane. After an impulse has been generated and conducted by the postsynaptic neurons, neurotransmitter activity ends quickly. Several substances have been identified as neurotransmitters; others are thought to be neurotransmitters. Well-known neurotransmitters include acetylcholine, norepinephrine, epinephrine, and dopamine (Table 25-1).

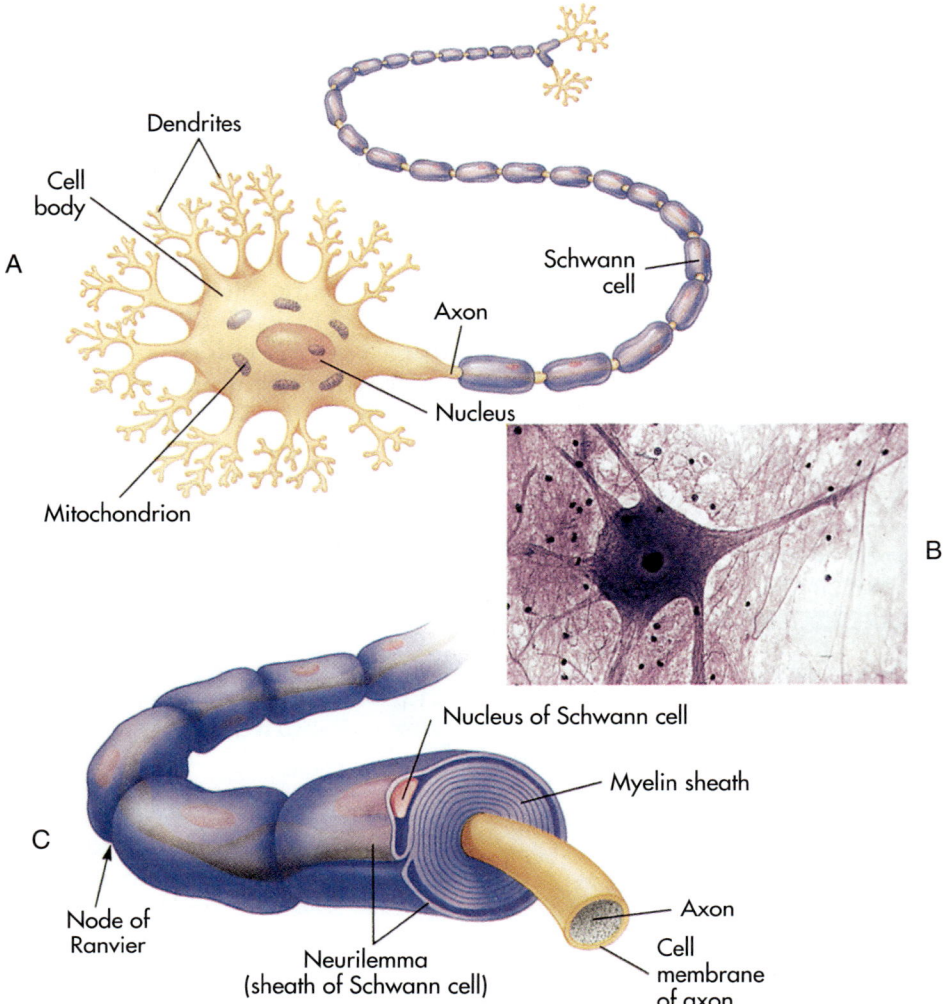

FIGURE 25-2 A, Typical neuron showing dendrites, a cell body, and an axon. **B,** Photomicrograph of a neuron. **C,** Segment of a myelinated axon cut to show details of the concentric layers of the Schwann cell filled with myelin. (Thibodeau GA, Patton KT: *Structure and function of the body,* ed 13, St Louis, 2008, Mosby.)

TABLE 25-1 Major Neurotransmitters

Neurotransmitter	Postsynaptic Effect
Acetylcholine	Excitatory
Norepinephrine	Excitatory
Epinephrine	Excitatory
Dopamine	Excitatory

Reflexes

One type of route traveled by nerve impulses is a reflex, or reflex arc. A **reflex** is the basic unit of the nervous system capable of receiving a stimulus and generating a response. Reflexes allow conduction of impulses in one direction. They have several basic components: a sensory receptor, a sensory neuron, interneurons, a motor neuron, and an effector organ. (An **effector organ** is a muscle or gland that contracts or secretes, respectively, in direct response to nerve impulses.) Individual reflexes vary in complexity. Some act to remove the body from painful stimuli. Some prevent the body from suddenly falling or moving as a result of external forces. Others are responsible for maintaining a relatively constant blood pressure, body fluid pH, blood carbon dioxide level, and water intake. All reflexes are homeostatic; that is, they function to maintain healthy survival.

Action potentials initiated in sensory receptors spread along sensory axons in the PNS to the CNS. There they synapse with interneurons. Interneurons synapse with motor neurons in the spinal cord; the motor neurons send their axons out of the spinal cord and through the PNS to muscles or glands. This causes the effector organ to respond. Figure 25-5 shows the transmission of nerve impulses that result in the patellar (knee jerk) reflex.

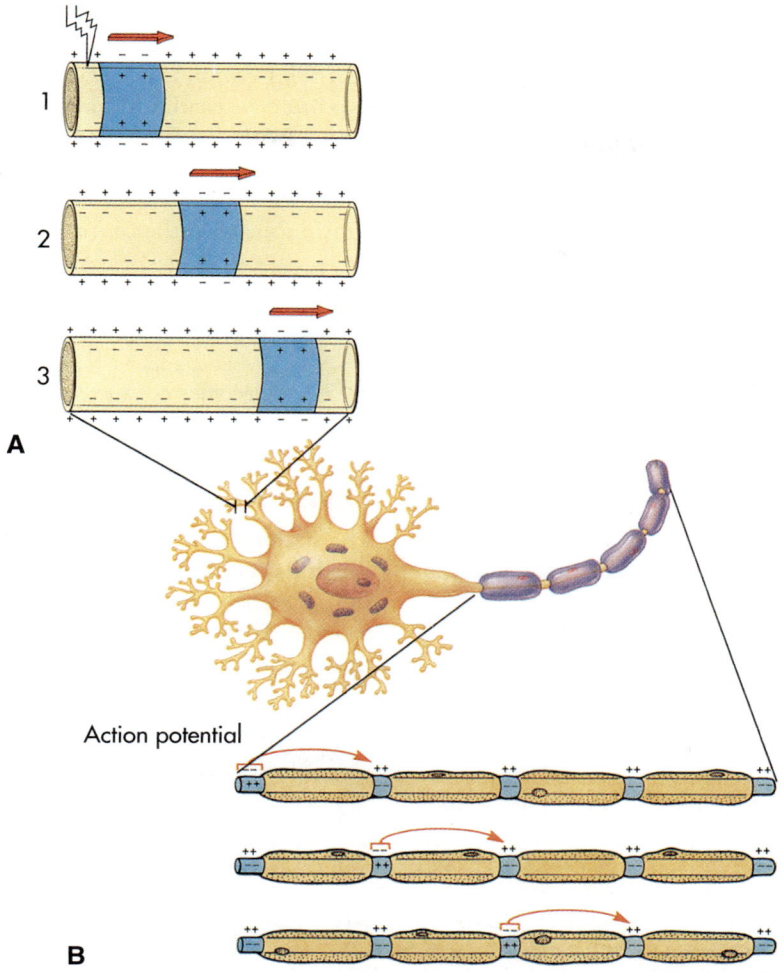

FIGURE 25-3 Conduction of nerve impulses. **A,** In unmyelinated fiber, a nerve impulse (action potential) is a self-propagating wave of electrical disturbance. **B,** In myelinated fiber, the action potential "jumps" around the insulating myelin in a rapid type of conduction called *saltatory conduction*. (Thibodeau GA, Patton KT: *Structure and function of the body,* ed 13, St Louis, 2008, Mosby.)

Blood Supply

The arterial blood supply to the brain comes from the vertebral arteries and the internal carotid arteries (Figure 25-6). The right and left vertebral arteries (supplying the cerebellum) enter the cranial vault through the foramen magnum. They unite to form the midline basilar artery. The basilar artery branches to supply the pons and the cerebellum. It divides again to form the posterior cerebral arteries. These supply the posterior portion of the cerebrum.

The internal carotid arteries enter the cranial vault through the carotid canals. These vessels give rise to the anterior cerebral arteries. The anterior cerebral arteries supply blood to the frontal lobes of the brain. They end by forming the middle cerebral arteries. These supply a large portion of the lateral cerebral cortex. A posterior communicating artery branches off each internal carotid artery and connects with the ipsilateral posterior cerebral artery. The two posterior cerebral arteries are connected at their common origin from the basilar artery. The anterior cerebral arteries are connected by an anterior communicating artery. Thus they complete a circle around the pituitary gland and the brain; this is the **circle of Willis.** The circle of Willis provides an important safeguard. It helps to ensure the supply of blood to all parts of the brain in the event of a blockage in one of the vertebral or internal carotid arteries.

The veins that drain blood from the head form the venous sinuses. (These are the spaces in the dura mater surrounding the brain.) Eventually they drain into the internal jugular veins (Figure 25-7). These veins exit the cranial vault and join with several other veins that drain the external

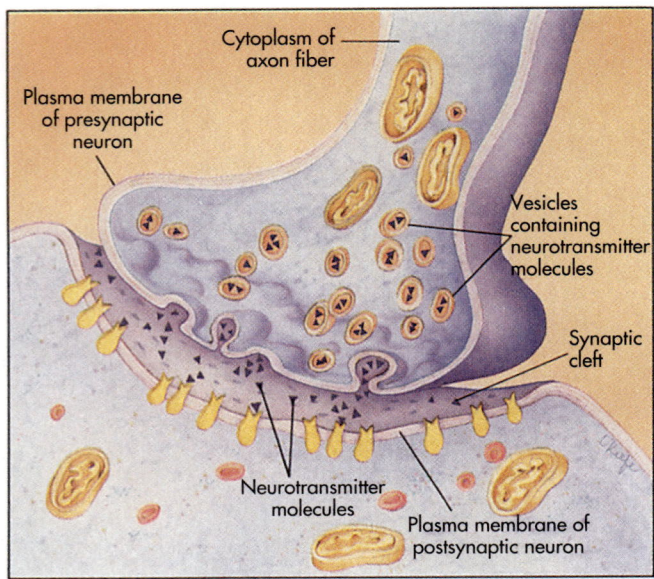

FIGURE 25-4 Components of a synapse. The diagram shows an axon terminal of a presynaptic neuron and a synaptic cleft. When an action potential arrives at the axon terminal of a presynaptic neuron, neurotransmitter molecules are released from vesicles in the axon terminal into the synaptic cleft. The combining of neurotransmitter and receptor molecules in the plasma membrane of the postsynaptic neuron initiates impulse conduction in the postsynaptic neuron. (Thibodeau GA, Patton KT: *Structure and function of the body*, ed 13, St Louis, 2008, Mosby.)

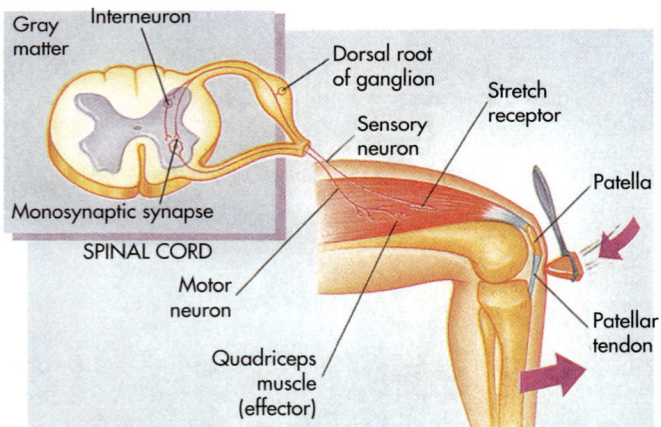

FIGURE 25-5 Neural pathway involved in the patellar (knee jerk) reflex. (Thibodeau GA, Patton KT: *Structure and function of the body*, ed 13, St Louis, 2008, Mosby.)

head and face. The internal jugular veins join the subclavian veins on each side of the body.

Ventricles

Each cerebral hemisphere contains a large space filled with **cerebrospinal fluid (CSF).** This space is known as a *lateral ventricle.* The lateral ventricles are connected posteriorly. A

third ventricle is located in the center of the diencephalon between the two halves of the thalamus. The two lateral ventricles communicate with the third ventricle through two interventricular foramina. The third ventricle communicates with the fourth ventricle (located in the superior region of the medulla) by way of a narrow canal. This canal is known as the *cerebral aqueduct.* The fourth ventricle is continuous with the central canal of the spinal cord.

> **CRITICAL THINKING**
> What happens if the flow in one of these canals becomes obstructed?

Divisions of the Brain

The major divisions of the adult brain are the brainstem (medulla, pons, midbrain, and site of the reticular formation), cerebellum, diencephalon (hypothalamus and thalamus), and cerebrum (Figure 25-8). (See Chapter 10 to review these structures.)

> **LOOK AGAIN**
> See Chapter 10: Review of Human Systems, pp. 171-174.

NEUROLOGICAL PATHOPHYSIOLOGY

Some neurological emergencies are a consequence of structural changes or damage, circulatory changes, or alterations in **intracranial pressure (ICP)** that affect **cerebral blood flow (CBF).** Three structures occupy the intracranial space: brain tissue, blood, and water. Brain tissue contains mostly water, both intracellular and extracellular. Blood is contained in the major arteries in the base of the brain; in arterial branches, arterioles, capillaries, venules, and veins in the substance of the brain; and in the cortical veins and dural sinuses. Water is located in the ventricles of the brain, in the CSF, and in extracellular and intracellular fluid. Normally the volumes of brain tissue, blood, and water are such that the pressure inside the skull is maintained within 1 mm of mercury above atmospheric pressure.

Cerebral Blood Flow

Although the brain accounts for only 2% of adult weight, 20% of total body oxygen use and 25% of total body glucose use are devoted to brain metabolism.[1] Oxygen and glucose delivery are controlled by cerebral blood flow.

Cerebral blood flow is a function of the **cerebral perfusion pressure (CPP)** and the resistance of the cerebral vascular bed. To measure the CPP, the intracranial pressure is subtracted from the **mean arterial pressure (MAP).** (The MAP is the diastolic blood pressure [DBP] plus one third of the pulse pressure [PP]: MAP = DBP + ⅓ PP). The

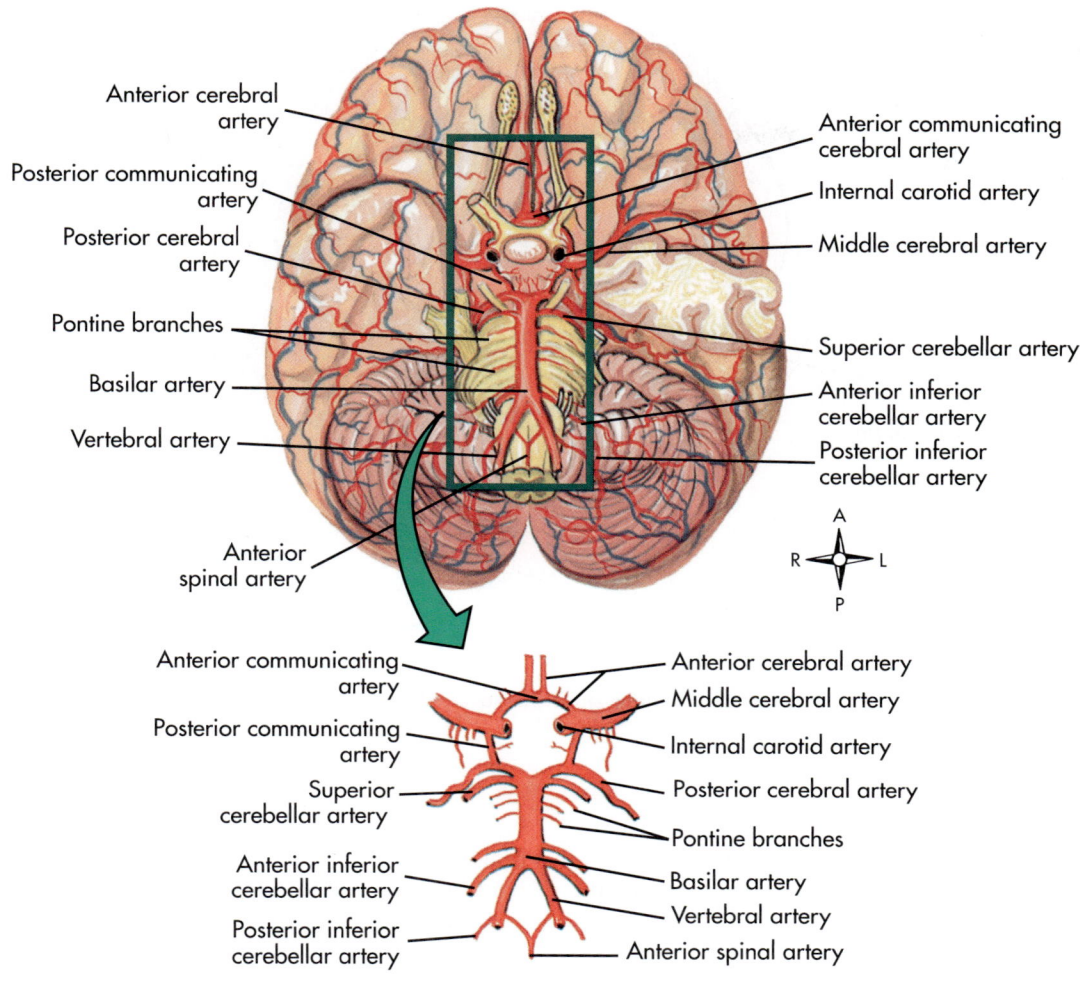

FIGURE 25-6 Inferior view of the brain showing vertebral, basilar, and internal carotid arteries and their branches. (Modified from Thibodeau GA, Patton KT: *Structure and function of the body,* ed 13, St Louis, 2008, Mosby.)

cerebral blood flow is the difference between the MAP and the ICP (CPP = MAP − ICP). The normal ICP is 10 to 15 mm Hg or less. The normal MAP ranges from 70 to 95 mm Hg. Therefore, the normal CPP is 60 to 80 mm Hg. (A CPP of 60 mm Hg is thought to be the critical minimum threshold for organ blood flow.[2]) As the ICP rises and approaches the MAP, the gradient for flow decreases and cerebral blood flow decreases; that is, when the ICP increases, the CPP decreases (Figure 25-9). As the CPP decreases, vessels in the brain dilate (cerebral vasodilation). This results in increased cerebral blood volume (increasing the ICP) and further cerebral vasodilation. In most EMS systems, the CPP is not calculated, because the MAP and ICP are not measured in the prehospital setting. Maintaining a systolic blood pressure of at least 90 mm Hg may help maintain an adequate mean arterial pressure.[3]

NOTE

Vascular tone in the normal brain is regulated by the partial pressure of arterial carbon dioxide (PCO_2), the partial pressure of arterial oxygen (PO_2), and by autonomic and neurohumoral control. The PCO_2 has the greatest effect on intracerebral vascular diameter and subsequent resistance. For example, a 40 to 80 mm Hg increase in the PCO_2 doubles the cerebral blood flow.[4] This results in increased brain blood volume and intracranial pressure.

Cerebral Perfusion Pressure

As stated previously, cerebral blood flow depends on the CPP, which is the pressure gradient across the brain. The CBF remains constant when the CPP is 50 to 160 mm Hg. If the CPP falls below 40 mm Hg, cerebral blood flow

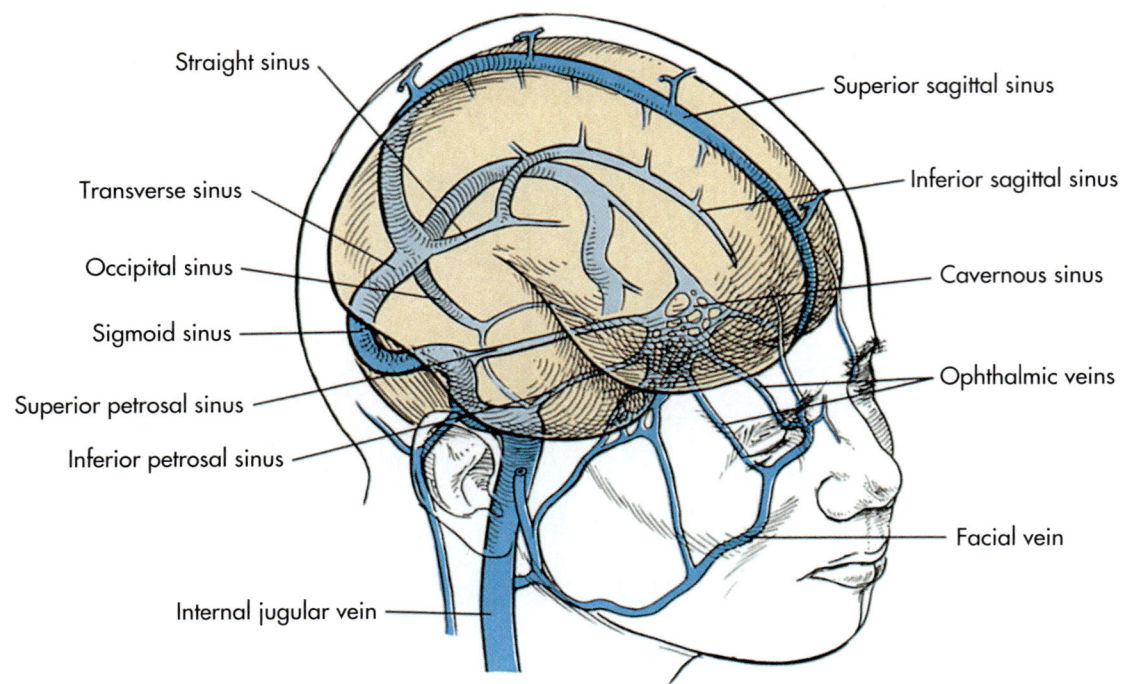

FIGURE 25-7 Venous sinuses associated with the brain.

declines. This critically affects cerebral metabolism. With mild to moderate elevation of the ICP, the MAP usually rises. The rise in the MAP causes cerebral blood vessels to constrict and prevents the increase in blood volume and CBF that normally would occur.

CRITICAL THINKING

Relate the difficulty created for cerebral blood flow by increased intracranial pressure to having a person push on a door from the outside while you try to open it from the inside. How much more difficult is it for you to open the door?

On the other hand, if the MAP falls, the cerebral arteries dilate, increasing the CBF. Therefore, with an MAP of 60 to 150 mm Hg, cerebral blood flow may be maintained in a constant state. However, when ICP elevations are marked (greater than 22 mm Hg), perfusion of brain tissue often decreases despite a rise in the systemic arterial pressure. Therefore, if a mass or cerebral edema develops, an immediate reduction in the volume of one or more of these components (brain tissue, blood, or water) must occur to prevent the ICP from rising and compressing brain tissue.

Assessment of the Nervous System

As with all patient encounters, care of a patient with a non-traumatic neurological emergency begins with the primary survey. Paramedics should have a systematic approach for examining these patients. This helps to ensure that signs and symptoms that may indicate an urgent condition are not overlooked. The goals of emergency care are (1) control

of the airway, (2) stabilization and support of the cardio-vascular system, (3) intervention to interrupt ongoing cere-bral injury, and (4) protection of the patient from further harm while at the scene and during transport to an appro-priate medical facility for definitive care.

PRIMARY SURVEY

The paramedic should begin the primary survey by deter-mining the patient's level of consciousness. An open and patent airway also must be ensured. If the patient is uncon-scious when paramedics arrive and there is reason to suspect a cervical spine injury, the patient's airway should be opened with spinal precautions and the cervical spine should be immobilized (see Chapter 41). It is important to remember that an unconscious patient is unable to maintain the airway. Therefore, airway adjuncts (including the place-ment of advanced airways) may be indicated. The patient also should be closely monitored for respiratory arrest, which may result from an increase in the ICP. The patient should be closely watched for vomiting or aspiration of stomach contents. Suction should be readily available.

NOTE

The mantra of the cardiologist is "time is muscle." Many neurologists consider that time also is brain tissue. Rapid stabilization of the patient's condition and trans-port for definitive care may be the most prudent course of action in a neurological emergency.

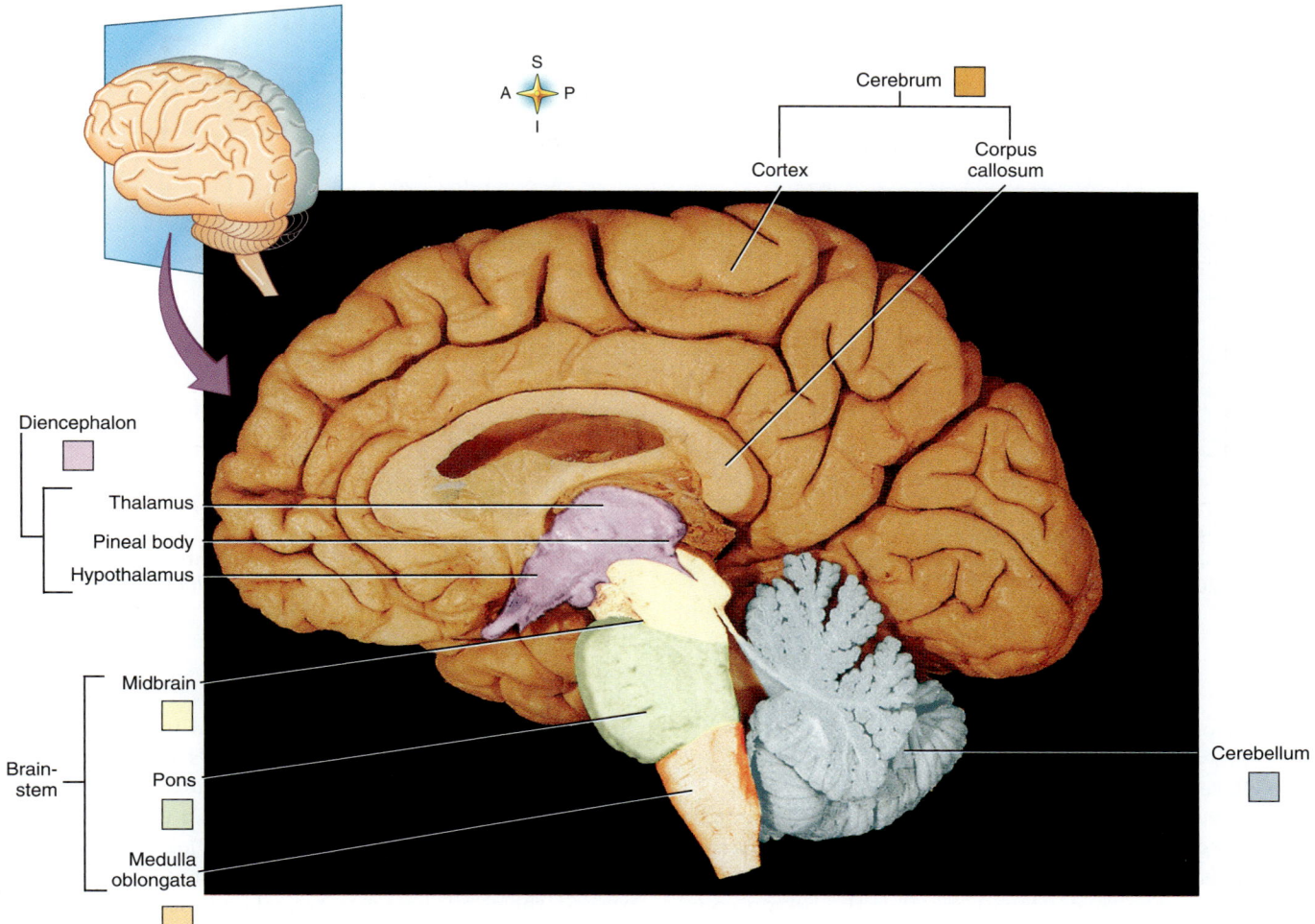

FIGURE 25-8 Divisions of the brain. A midsagittal section of the brain reveals features of its major divisions. (From Thibodeau G, Patton K: *Anatomy and physiology,* ed 18, St Louis, 2007, Elsevier.)

Support of breathing and supplemental oxygen should be provided for most patients experiencing a neurological emergency. An increase in the partial pressure of arterial carbon dioxide (Pco_2) or a decrease in the partial pressure of arterial oxygen (Po_2) results in dilation of the blood vessels. This occurs presumably because of an increase in cerebral metabolic needs. As the Pco_2 drops, blood volume and blood flow to the brain are reduced.

PHYSICAL EXAMINATION

A patient with a neurological illness may be difficult to assess. This is particularly true if the patient's mental function is impaired. Key elements of the physical examination may offer clues to the cause of the neurological emergency. These include the patient history, the history of the event, vital signs, and respiratory patterns.

History. After any life-threatening problems have been identified and managed, the paramedic should attempt to compile a thorough history. This information can be obtained from the patient (when possible) or from family members or bystanders. The following are six important elements of the patient history.

1. The patient's chief complaint
2. Details of the presenting illness
3. Pertinent underlying medical problems
   a. Cardiac disease
   b. Lung disease
   c. Neurological disease (e.g., multiple sclerosis)
   d. Previous stroke
   e. Chronic seizures
   f. Diabetes
   g. Hypertension

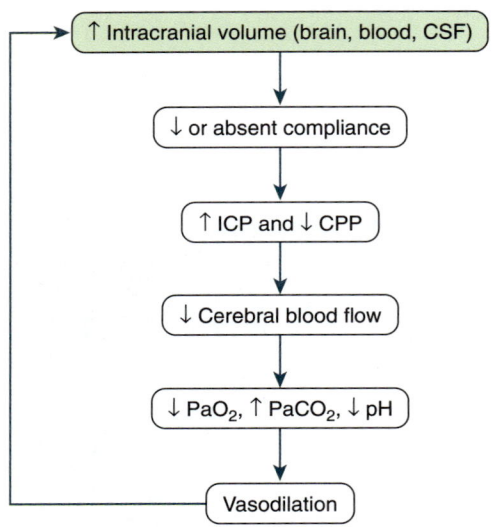

FIGURE 25-9 Pathophysiology flow diagram for increased intracranial pressure. (Sole ML: *Introduction to critical care nursing*, ed 5, St Louis, 2009, Saunders.)

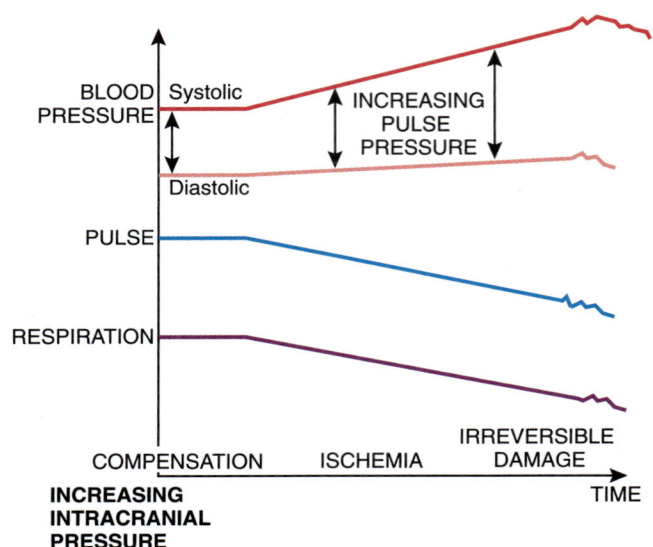

FIGURE 25-10 Vital signs with increased intracranial pressure. (Gould BE, Dyer R: *Pathophysiology or the health professional*, ed 4, St Louis, 2011, Saunders.)

4. Alcohol or other drug use
5. Previous history of similar symptoms
6. Recent injury (particularly head trauma)

If a loss of consciousness was involved, the paramedic should ascertain the events that led up to the unconscious state. This information may include the patient's position (sitting, standing, lying down), whether the person complained of a headache, and whether seizure activity or a fall occurred. At times no history is available. In such cases paramedics should assume that the onset of unconsciousness was acute. They also should assume that an intracranial hemorrhage is likely. In addition, they should be alert for any environmental clues. Examples include evidence of current prescribed medications, medical alert identification, recreational drugs, alcohol, or drug paraphernalia.

> ### CRITICAL THINKING
> How could having one of the conditions listed in the six important elements of the patient history result in a change in the patient's neurological status?

Vital Signs. The patient's vital signs should be checked and recorded often. This is important because the vital signs may change rapidly in patients with a neurological emergency. The patient's electrocardiogram (ECG) should be monitored for dysrhythmias, which are common in these situations.

When the ICP begins to rise, a conscious patient may complain of headache, nausea, and vomiting. Progressive hypertension associated with bradycardia and diminished respiratory effort is a response to lethal increases in the ICP.[5] This reflex is known as **Cushing's reflex.** The late stages of increased ICP are marked by an increase in systolic pressure, a widened pulse pressure, and a decrease in the pulse and respiratory rate (Figure 25-10). In the terminal stages, as the ICP continues to rise and brain tissue is compressed, the pupils become unequal and the body temperature usually remains elevated. The pulse rate generally decreases and the blood pressure falls, particularly after herniation occurs. Therefore, hypotension is a late and ominous sign in these patients.

Respiratory Patterns. The respiratory pattern of a patient with a neurological emergency may be normal or abnormal. In the absence of respiratory arrest caused by damage to the lower respiratory centers in the medulla, abnormalities of the respiratory rate and rhythm may occur. These abnormalities may provide clues to which area of the brain is involved. They also may indicate the severity of the neurological problem. Apnea can occur with loss of consciousness even with relatively minor head trauma. However, acute respiratory arrest usually results from involvement of the medullary respiratory center (brainstem compression or infarct). Damage to neural pathways (anywhere from the cortex down to the medulla) produces problems with the respiratory rhythm more often than respiratory arrest. Abnormal respiratory patterns (described in detail in Chapter 15) include the following:

- Cheyne-Stokes respiration
- Central neurogenic hyperventilation
- Ataxic respiration
- Apneustic respiration
- Diaphragmatic breathing

CRITICAL THINKING

Consider a patient who has ataxic or apneustic respirations. Which respiratory control center likely is affected?

NEUROLOGICAL EVALUATION

Some neurological complications are obvious (e.g., paralysis). Others may be subtle (e.g., a decreasing level of awareness). A sudden or rapidly worsening level of consciousness is the single most suggestive sign of a serious neurological condition.[6]

As described in Chapter 20, the mnemonic device AVPU (*a*lert, *v*erbal, *p*ainful, *u*nresponsive) can help determine the patient's baseline neurological status. The **Glasgow Coma Scale** (Box 25-1) should also be calculated during the initial assessment. These evaluations should be repeated and recorded often. This allows changes in the patient's mental state to be detected quickly.

When evaluating a patient's neurological status, the paramedic should report and record patient information with descriptive terms. These terms should be specific to responses to certain stimuli. (For example, "The patient has no recall of the event"; "The patient moves on command"; and "The patient does not open his eyes to painful stimuli.") Clear descriptions of the patient's response allow others involved in the patient's care to follow the progression of the condition.

Posturing, Muscle Tone, and Paralysis

Significant neurological emergencies may be associated with abnormal or unusual posturing, paralysis of a limb or several limbs, or both. Generally, disturbances of posture result from flexor spasms, extensor spasms, or flaccidity. Abnormal flexor response of one or both arms with extension of the legs is called **decorticate rigidity.** This abnormal posturing is thought to result from damage to the cortex of the brain. Abnormal extensor response of the arms with extension of the legs is called **decerebrate rigidity.** Decerebrate rigidity has a worse prognosis than decorticate rigidity. It is thought to result from damage to the

subcortical areas of the brain. Flaccidity usually is caused by brainstem or cord dysfunction. It has a dismal prognosis.

Abnormal reflexes are not uncommon with decorticate or decerebrate rigidity. Babinski's sign *(plantar reflex)* may be associated with such posturing. **Babinski's sign** is an abnormal extensor reflex in adults. (It may be normal in children in the first few years of life.) It is characterized by dorsiflexion or extension of the great toe, with or without fanning or abduction of the other toes, when the outer edge of the foot is scratched. It indicates neurological injury (Figure 25-11). A patient with a severe injury may also have relaxation of sphincter tone and may be incontinent of urine or feces or both.

NOTE

There is no "positive" or "negative" Babinski's sign. The presence of this response indicates the existence of a pathological condition.

Pupillary Reflexes

Examination of the pupils is very important in an unconscious patient. Often the diagnosis of drug use can at least be suspected based on the appearance and reaction of the pupils. If deviations from normal (in relative symmetry, size, and prompt reaction to light) are observed, it is crucial to note whether these deviations are unilateral or bilateral. If both pupils are dilated and do not react to light, the brainstem probably has been affected. This also may occur with severe cerebral anoxia.

BOX 25-1 Glasgow Coma Scale

The Glasgow Coma Scale (GCS) evaluates eye opening, verbal and motor responses, and brain stem reflex function. The scale is considered one of the best indicators of eventual clinical outcome and should be part of every examination of a patient with a medical or traumatic neurological emergency (see Table 25-1). A GCS score of 9 to 12 indicates moderate brain injury; a score of 8 or lower indicates severe brain injury.[5] (The lowest possible score is 3; the highest possible score is 15.) Hypoxemia and hypotension have been shown to cause falsely low GCS scores. Therefore, the GCS score should be measured after the primary survey and after a clear airway has been established.

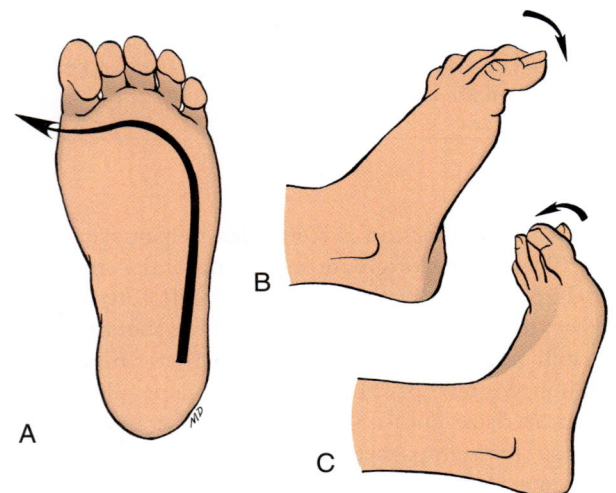

FIGURE 25-11 Babinski's reflex. **A,** Light pressure is applied with a hard object to the lateral surface of the sole, starting at the heel, going over the ball of the foot, and ending beneath the great toe. **B,** The normal response is flexion of all the toes. **C,** Babinski's reflex is seen as dorsiflexion or extension of the great toe, with or without fanning or abduction of the other toes. (Sole ML: *Introduction to critical care nursing,* ed 5, St Louis, 2009, Saunders.)

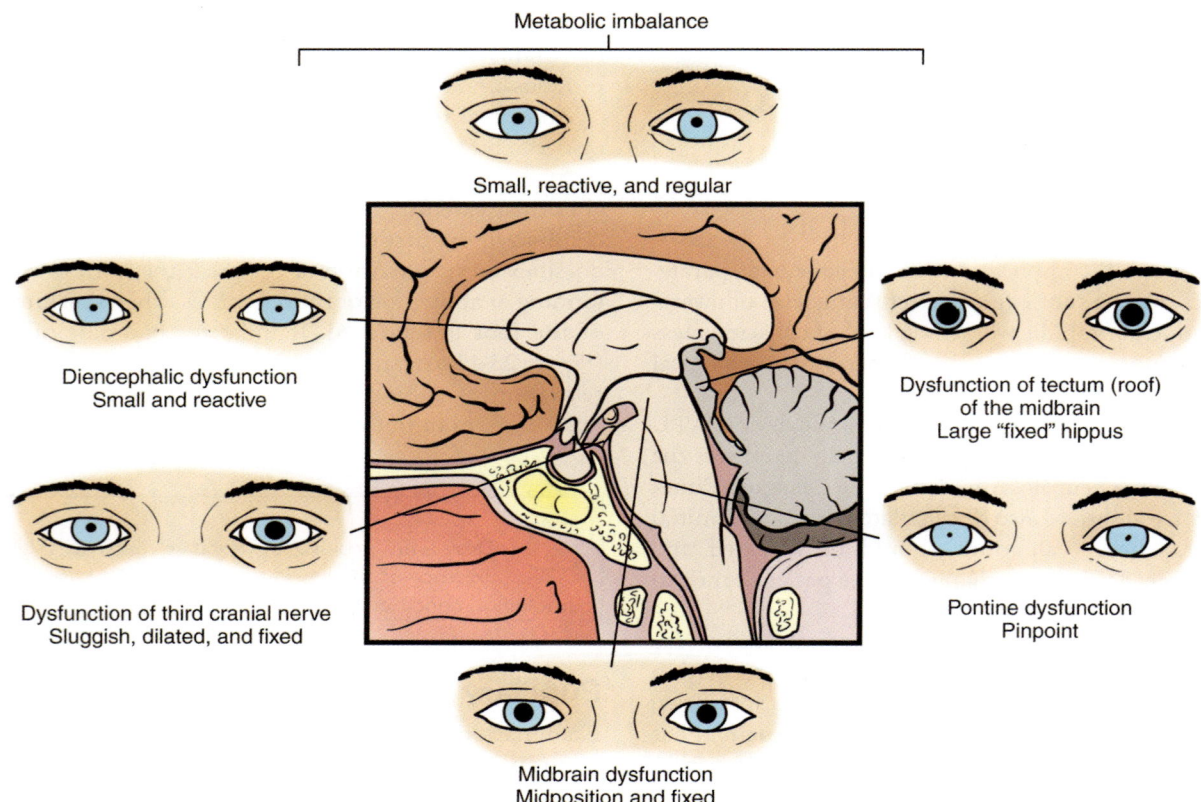

Metabolic imbalance

Small, reactive, and regular

Diencephalic dysfunction
Small and reactive

Dysfunction of tectum (roof)
of the midbrain
Large "fixed" hippus

Dysfunction of third cranial nerve
Sluggish, dilated, and fixed

Pontine dysfunction
Pinpoint

Midbrain dysfunction
Midposition and fixed

FIGURE 25-12 Pupils at different levels of consciousness.

NOTE
The response of the pupils must be considered in conjunction with the patient's mental status. Unresponsive, dilated pupils in a patient who is awake, alert, and oriented most likely are the result of topical medications used to induce pupillary dilation.

Pupillary constriction is controlled by parasympathetic fibers. These fibers originate in the midbrain and accompany the oculomotor nerve (cranial nerve III) (Figure 25-12). Pupillary dilation involves fibers that travel the entire brainstem and return in the cervical sympathetic nerves. Midbrain injury interrupts both pathways. Generally it results in fixed, midsize pupils. Compression of cranial nerve III interrupts parasympathetic nerve actions. It is manifested by a unilateral, fixed, dilated pupil. Any unconscious patient who suddenly develops a fixed, dilated pupil probably has suffered a significant neurological event.[5] This requires immediate transport to a proper medical facility. (Parasympathetic nerve roots and the functions of the cranial nerves are described in Chapter 10; methods of cranial nerve assessment are addressed in Chapter 20. Table 25-2 serves as a review of this information.)

LOOK AGAIN
See Chapter 10: Review of Human Systems, pp. 177-179.

Extraocular Movements

A conscious patient should be able to move the eyes in full directional ranges. As described in Chapter 20, paramedics can evaluate extraocular movements by asking the patient to follow the paramedic's finger movements. For this test, the paramedic moves a finger to the extreme left and then up and down and to the extreme right and then up and down. Any deviations from normal should be recorded.

LOOK AGAIN
See Chapter 20: Secondary Assessment, pp. 531-532.

CRITICAL THINKING
Which cranial nerves control eye movements?

TABLE 25-2 Cranial Nerve Assessment

Nerve	Name	Function	Test
I	Olfactory	Smell	Have patient smell a familiar odor
II	Optic	Visual acuity	Have patient identify fingers
		Visual field	Check peripheral vision
III	Oculomotor	Pupillary reaction	Shine a light in patient's eye
IV	Trochlear	Eye movement	Have patient follow finger without moving the head
V	Trigeminal	Facial sensation	Touch the face
		Motor function	Have patient hold the mouth open
VI	Abducens	Motor function	Check lateral eye movements
VII	Facial	Motor function	Have patient smile, wrinkle the face, and puff the cheeks
		Sensory	Check different tastes
VIII	Acoustic	Hearing	Snap fingers by the ear
		Balance	Perform Romberg's test
IX	Glossopharyngeal	Swallowing and voice	Have patient swallow and say "Ah"
X	Vagus	Gag reflex	Check with tongue depressor
XI	Spinal accessory	Neck motion	Have patient shrug shoulders
XII	Hypoglossal	Tongue movement and strength	Have patient stick out tongue; exert resistance with a tongue depressor

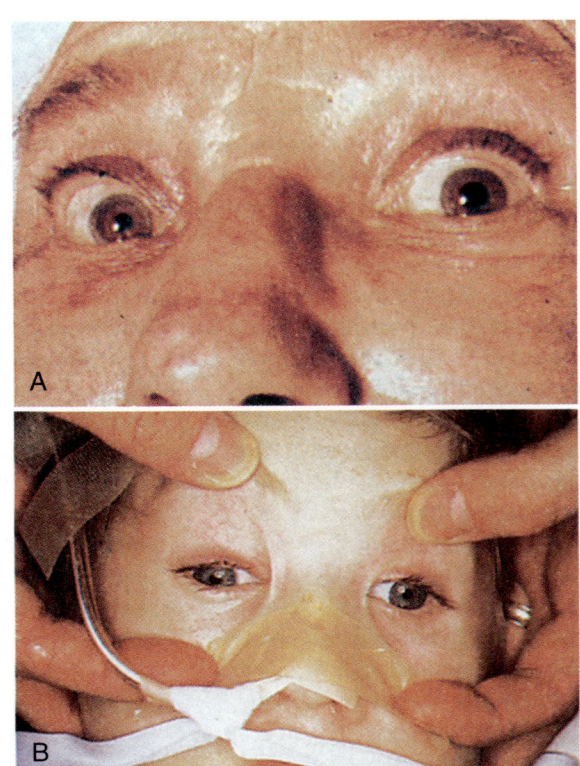

FIGURE 25-13 A, Conjugate gaze. **B,** Dysconjugate gaze. (London PS: *A colour atlas of diagnosis after recent injury,* Ipswich, England, 1990, Wolfe Medical Publications.)

Deviation of both eyes to either side **(conjugate gaze)** at rest implies damage to brain tissue (a lesion). If the lesion has an *irritative focus,* the eyes look away from the lesion. If it has a *destructive focus,* the eyes look toward the lesion.[7] Deviation of the eyes to opposite sides **(dysconjugate gaze)** at rest implies damage to the brainstem (Figure 25-13).

PATHOPHYSIOLOGY AND MANAGEMENT OF SPECIFIC CENTRAL NERVOUS SYSTEM DISORDERS

Disorders of the nervous system have many causes. Specific causes discussed in this chapter include structural and metabolic coma, stroke and intracranial hemorrhage (including transient ischemic attack), seizure disorders, headaches, and brain neoplasm and brain abscess. Several degenerative neurological diseases also are discussed.

Coma

Coma is an abnormally deep state of unconsciousness from which the patient cannot be aroused by external stimuli. In general terms, only two mechanisms produce coma: *structural lesions* and *toxic/metabolic states.* Structural lesions (e.g., a tumor or an abscess) depress consciousness by destroying or encroaching on the reticular activating system in the brainstem. Toxic/metabolic conditions involve the presence of toxins or the lack of oxygen or glucose. Either mechanism may result in depression of the cerebrum, with or without depression of the reticular activating system. Within these two primary mechanisms are six general causes of coma (Box 25-2). A mnemonic that may be helpful for remembering the common causes of coma is AEIOU-TIPS (Box 25-3).

DIFFERENTIATION OF STRUCTURAL AND TOXIC-METABOLIC CAUSES OF COMA

Structural and toxic/metabolic causes of coma differ in two primary ways. In coma of structural origin, the neurological signs often are one-sided, or asymmetrical. In toxic/metabolic coma, the neurological findings often are the same on the two sides of the body. In addition, coma of

BOX 25-2 Six General Causes of Coma

Structural Origin
- Intracranial bleeding
- Head trauma
- Brain tumor or other space-occupying lesion

Metabolic System
- Anoxia
- Hypoglycemia
- Diabetic ketoacidosis
- Thiamine deficiency
- Kidney and liver failure
- Postictal phase of seizure

Drugs
- Barbiturates
- Narcotics
- Hallucinogenics
- Depressants
- Alcohol

Cardiovascular System
- Hypertensive encephalopathy
- Shock
- Dysrhythmias
- Stroke

Respiratory System
- Chronic obstructive pulmonary disease
- Toxic inhalation (e.g., carbon monoxide poisoning)

Infection
- Meningitis
- Sepsis

BOX 25-3 Common Causes of Coma AEIOU-TIPS

A—Acidosis or alcohol
E—Epilepsy
I—Infection
O—Overdose
U—Uremia
T—Trauma
I—Insulin
P—Psychosis
S—Stroke

NOTE

Some psychiatric conditions (e.g., a *hysterical coma*) can mimic comalike states. In these conditions, the state of unconsciousness has no physical cause. Patients who appear unconscious as a result of a psychiatric condition often vigorously blink and move the eyes. They also usually respond to annoying physical or verbal stimuli. In contrast, patients with organic sources of coma are unresponsive.

Unlike toxic/metabolic coma, structural coma follows a progressive pattern of deterioration. This pattern is caused by focal pressure or compression in the brain. The syndrome often is sudden in onset, and the examination results are asymmetrical, such as muscle weakness on one side of the body **(hemiparesis).** As a rule, structural lesions damage the reticular activating system as a result of increased ICP and herniation of the brain. This type of injury requires rapid surgical correction. Knowledge of the difference between toxic/metabolic coma and structural coma can help the paramedic anticipate the course of the patient's condition.

ASSESSMENT AND MANAGEMENT

Regardless of the cause of the coma, prehospital care is directed at supporting vital functions, preventing further deterioration of the patient's condition, and administering medications, intravenous (IV) fluids, or both to manage potentially reversible causes of coma. As always, airway maintenance and ventilatory support with supplemental high-concentration oxygen are the first priorities in patient care. Rapid transport for definitive care may be indicated.

If respirations are abnormally slow or shallow, ventilations should be supported. If the patient is unconscious and has no gag reflex, the trachea should be intubated. After securing the airway, the paramedic should take the following steps to treat a patient in a coma of unknown origin.

1. Establish an IV line to keep the vein open or to manage hypotension (if present).
2. Monitor the patient's ECG.
3. Per protocol, draw a blood sample for laboratory analysis. If hypoglycemia is suspected, use a glucometer or other device to measure the serum glucose level (see Chapter 26). Administer **50% dextrose** if indicated (per protocol). If alcohol is suspected as the cause of the coma, consider administration of **thiamine** before glucose.
4. If no response is obtained with glucose administration, administer **naloxone** per protocol. This rules out or reverses narcotic depression.
5. If the patient remains comatose, transport the person in a lateral recumbent position (if not contraindicated). This aids drainage of secretions. It also minimizes the chance of aspiration of stomach contents.

toxic/metabolic origin often is slow in onset, whereas structural lesions occur acutely. Changes in pupil responses are the most important physical sign in distinguishing between structural and toxic/metabolic causes of coma. Normal pupil responses suggest that the coma has a toxic/metabolic cause. Unresponsive or asymmetrical pupils suggest a structural cause.

Closely monitor the patient's airway. Have suction readily available. Protect the patient's eyes from corneal drying by gently closing them and covering the lids with moist gauze pads.

> **NOTE**
>
> Thiamine is a B vitamin (B_1). It usually is found in adequate amounts in the normal diet. However, chronic alcoholism interferes with the intake, absorption, and utilization of thiamine. Serious neurological disease may result. The incidence of these alcohol-related neurological syndromes varies markedly in different regions of the United States. Therefore, administration of **thiamine** may be a local consideration. Paramedics should follow established protocols and consult with medical direction.

> **NOTE**
>
> Patients who are dependent on narcotics may have frank withdrawal symptoms. The paramedic should be prepared to restrain a patient who may become violent as the **naloxone** reverses the narcotic effects. Repeated doses of **naloxone** may be needed. This is because the duration of some narcotics may be longer than that of **naloxone.** Doses should be titrated to keep the patient free of respiratory depression.

Stroke and Intracranial Hemorrhage

A **cerebrovascular accident (CVA)** (also called a *stroke* or "brain attack") is a sudden interruption in blood flow to a portion of the brain, resulting in a neurological deficit. Stroke is a serious disease that affects more than 700,000 Americans each year.[8] It is associated with a 30-day mortality of 10% to 15%. It also is the third leading cause of death in the United States. A stroke frequently leaves its survivors severely disabled. According to the American Heart Association (AHA), individuals who are more likely to suffer a stroke have prior risk factors that can be classified as modifiable or nonmodifiable. Modifiable risk factors include the following:

- High blood pressure
- Cigarette smoking
- Transient ischemic attacks
- Heart disease
- Atrial fibrillation
- Diabetes mellitus
- Hypercoagulopathy
- High red blood cell count and sickle cell anemia
- Carotid stenosis

Nonmodifiable risk factors include the following:

- Age
- Gender (men are at greater risk than women)
- Race (African Americans are at greater risk than Caucasians)
- Previous stroke
- Heredity

The best way to prevent strokes is to identify individuals who are at risk and then to control as many risk factors as possible. This can be achieved with modification of poor health habits and drug therapy.

PATHOPHYSIOLOGY

As described previously, blood reaches the brain through four major vessels. These are the two carotid arteries and the two vertebral arteries. (The two carotid arteries provide about 80% of cerebral blood flow.) The two vertebral arteries combine to form the single basilar artery (supplying the remaining 20% of CBF). These two systems are interconnected at various levels. The principal level is the circle of Willis. In addition, collateral blood flow can be supplied to the brain through connections from blood vessels in the face and scalp to the dura and arachnoid coverings of the brain. The amount of collateral circulation varies from individual to individual. Beyond this, however, there is no collateral circulation in the depths of the brain.[9] Therefore, occlusion of any one of the more distal vessels may result in ischemia and infarction.

Normally, the CBF is maintained through autoregulation of cerebral vessels. These vessels constrict or dilate to preserve perfusion pressure even when the patient is hypotensive. Arterial cerebral perfusion is regulated by the level of oxygen and glucose supplied (ischemia and acidosis are profound vasodilators). Vessel occlusion or hemorrhage causes a sudden cessation of circulation to a portion of the brain. Autoregulatory mechanisms cannot readily correct this problem. The uncorrected ischemia that results within a short period leads to neuronal dysfunction and death. The onset and symptoms of the stroke depend on the area of the brain involved.

> **CRITICAL THINKING**
>
> How much oxygen and glucose can the brain store for emergency situations?

TYPES OF STROKE

Stroke is a general term that refers to the neurological manifestations of a critical decrease in blood flow to a portion of the brain, regardless of the cause. The AHA has defined two primary categories of stroke: **ischemic stroke,** also called *occlusive stroke* (stroke caused by clots); and **hemorrhagic stroke** (stroke caused by bleeding). Each of these categories is subdivided into two classes. For ischemic stroke, these are **cerebral thrombosis** and **cerebral embolism.** For hemorrhagic stroke, they are **intracerebral hemorrhage** and **subarachnoid hemorrhage** (Box 25-4).

Determining the origin of a stroke frequently is difficult and often unnecessary in the prehospital setting. (The best care for all stroke patients is support of vital functions and rapid transport for definitive care.) However, a paramedic who understands the various signs and symptoms of each

BOX 25-4 Classification of Strokes

Ischemic Strokes

Ischemic strokes are caused by blood clots. This type of stroke accounts for 85% of all strokes. This is the only type of stroke for which fibrinolytics are administered. Ischemic strokes are divided into two classes, depending on the cause:

- Cerebral thrombosis
- Cerebral embolism

Hemorrhagic Strokes

Hemorrhagic strokes are caused by ruptured blood vessels. The two classes of hemorrhagic stroke are:

- Intracerebral hemorrhage
- Subarachnoid hemorrhage

TABLE 25-3 Differentiation of Ischemic and Hemorrhagic Stroke

Ischemic Stroke	Hemorrhagic Stroke
- Most common	- Least common
- Usually the result of atherosclerosis or a tumor in the brain	- Usually the result of cerebral aneurysms, arteriovenous (AV) malformations, hypertension
- Develops slowly	- Develops abruptly
- Long history of vessel disease	- Commonly occurs during stress or exertion
- May be associated with valvular heart disease and atrial fibrillation	- May be associated with use of cocaine and other sympathomimetic amines
- History of angina, previous strokes	- May be asymptomatic before rupture

- Aphasia
- Confusion or coma
- Convulsions
- Incontinence
- Diplopia (double vision)
- Monocular blindness (painless visual loss in one eye)
- Numbness of the face
- Dysarthria (slurred speech)
- Headache
- Dizziness or vertigo
- Ataxia

A stroke caused by cerebral embolism occurs when an intracranial vessel is blocked by a foreign substance. The vessel is occluded by a fragment of a foreign substance originating outside the CNS. Common sources of cerebral emboli include atherosclerotic plaques (originating from large vessels of the head, neck, or heart). Thrombi that develop on the valves or in the chambers of the heart are very common in patients with heart valve disease and atrial fibrillation. Other, rare causes include air embolism from a chest injury and fat embolism after long-bone injury. Bacterial and fungal infections of the heart also can produce emboli. Women taking oral contraceptives and patients with sickle cell disease have an increased risk of stroke, by both thrombotic and embolic origins. Signs and symptoms of a cerebral embolus are similar to those of thrombotic stroke. However, embolic signs and symptoms develop more quickly. Also, they often are associated with an identifiable cause (e.g., atrial fibrillation).

Hemorrhagic Stroke. Cerebral hemorrhage accounts for about 15% of all strokes.[10] A hemorrhage may occur anywhere in the brain and its structures. This includes the epidural, subdural, subarachnoid, intraparenchymal, and intraventricular spaces. The most common causes are cerebral aneurysms, arteriovenous (AV) malformations, and hypertension. Cerebral aneurysms and AV malformations are congenital anomalies. They can run in families. They often are asymptomatic until they rupture. Unlike thrombotic and embolic strokes, which have relatively high survival rates, cerebral hemorrhages are fatal in 50% to 80% of cases.[11]

type of stroke is better equipped to anticipate the course of patient care (Table 25-3). Documentation of a thorough history and physical examination also helps others involved in the patient's care.

Ischemic Stroke. About 85% of strokes are the ischemic type.[10] Some of these are caused by cerebral thrombosis. The thrombosis occurs as a result of atherosclerotic plaques or pressure from a mass in the brain itself. Stroke caused by cerebral thrombosis usually is associated with a long history of blood vessel disease. Therefore, most of these patients are older. Most also have evidence of atherosclerotic disease in other areas of the body (angina pectoris, claudication, previous strokes). The signs and symptoms of thrombotic stroke usually are slower to develop than those of cerebral hemorrhage. These signs and symptoms include the following:

- Hemiparesis or hemiplegia on the side of the body opposite the lesion
- Numbness (decreased sensation) on the side of the body opposite the lesion

NOTE

A **cerebral aneurysm** is a weak or thin spot on a blood vessel in the brain that balloons and fills with blood. This bulging can put pressure on a nerve or brain tissue. The aneurysm also can rupture or leak, spilling blood into surrounding tissue. Cerebral aneurysms can occur anywhere in the brain, but most are located along a loop of arteries that run between the underside of the brain and the base of the skull.

An **arteriovenous (AV) malformation** is an abnormal connection between veins and arteries. These defects in the circulatory system are believed to arise during fetal development or soon after birth.[12] AV malformations can develop in many sites in the body. Those in the brain or spinal cord can result in hemorrhage and stroke.

Hemorrhagic strokes often occur during stress or exertion. Cocaine and other sympathomimetic-type drugs also may contribute to intracranial hemorrhage by a drug-induced rapid elevation of blood pressure. The onset of the stroke is sudden. It often begins with a headache (sometimes described as a "thunderclap headache" or the worst headache of the patient's life). The headache is accompanied by nausea, vomiting, and progressive deterioration in mental status. Some patients complain of a stiff neck. Often the patient loses consciousness or experiences a seizure at the time of the hemorrhage. As the hemorrhage expands, the ICP rises. As this occurs, the patient becomes comatose, with increasing hypertension, bradycardia, and diminished respiratory effort (*Cushing's reflex*).

CRITICAL THINKING

Why do you think mortality is higher for hemorrhagic stroke than for embolic stroke?

TRANSIENT ISCHEMIC ATTACKS

A **transient ischemic attack (TIA)** often is referred to as a "mini stroke." TIAs are episodes of cerebral dysfunction that affect a specific portion of the brain. They may last minutes to several hours. The patient returns to normal within 24 hours without permanent neurological deficit. A TIA is thought to be the most important indicator of impending stroke; about 5% of patients who have a TIA go on to have a complete stroke within 1 month if left untreated.[2] A TIA is the most important forecaster of a brain infarction.

The signs and symptoms of a TIA are the same as those that characterize stroke: weakness, paralysis, numbness of the face, and speech disturbances. All of these correspond to vascular occlusion of a specific cerebral artery. Most patients who experience a TIA are hospitalized for close observation, evaluation, and treatment of vascular disease (e.g., endarterectomy or anticoagulant or antiplatelet therapy).

Role of Paramedics in Stroke Care

In stroke care, the paramedic's role is to identify a stroke event quickly; notify medical direction; and transport the patient rapidly to a proper facility for hospital-based evaluation and treatment. Key points in the management of stroke include the eight *D*s: detection, dispatch, delivery, door, data, decision, drug, and disposition (Box 25-5). (The first three *D*s are the responsibility of the public and EMS personnel.)

BOX 25-5 Eight *D*s of Stroke Management

The first three *D*s are the responsibility of the public and emergency medical services (EMS) providers. The fourth *D* is the responsibility of EMS, and the last three *D*s are performed in the hospital.

Detection: A patient, family member, or bystander recognizes the signs and symptoms of a stroke or transient ischemic attack (TIA) and calls EMS for help.

Dispatch: EMS dispatchers prioritize the call about a suspected stroke and dispatch the appropriate EMS team with high transport priority.

Delivery: EMS providers respond rapidly, confirm the signs and symptoms of stroke, and transport the patient (delivery) to an appropriate medical facility.

Door: An appropriate medical facility is a hospital that can provide fibrinolytic therapy within 1 hour of arrival at the emergency department door.

Data: A computed tomography (CT) scan is obtained.

Decision: Candidates for fibrinolytic therapy are identified.

Drug: Eligible patients are treated with fibrinolytic therapy.

Disposition: Rapid transfer to a stroke or critical care unit.

DID YOU KNOW?

Primary Stroke Centers

The Joint Commission's Certificate of Distinction for Primary Stroke Centers recognizes centers that make exceptional efforts to foster better outcomes for stroke care. Achievement of certification signifies that the services provided have the critical elements to achieve long-term success in improving outcomes. These centers are deemed qualified to effectively provide care for the unique and specialized needs of stroke patients. The Joint Commission's Primary Stroke Center Certification program[14] was developed in collaboration with the American Stroke Association. It is based on the Brain Attack Coalition's recommendations for the establishment of primary stroke centers. As of October 1, 2009, there were more than 600 certified primary stroke centers in 49 states.

NOTE

About 85% of strokes occur at home. Public education programs focused on individuals at risk for stroke, their friends, and family members have been shown to reduce the time to arrival at the emergency department[13] (see Chapter 3). The "chain of survival" described by the American Heart Association (AHA) and the American Stroke Association (ASA) to improve stroke survival is made up of four links:

1. Rapid recognition and reaction to stroke warning signs
2. Rapid EMS dispatch
3. Rapid EMS transport and hospital prenotification
4. Rapid diagnosis and treatment in the hospital

ASSESSMENT

The primary survey of a patient who may have suffered a stroke or TIA follows the same sequence as that for any other ill or injured patient in the emergency setting. The priorities are to maintain a patent airway and to provide adequate ventilatory support with appropriate supplemental oxygen. If the patient is conscious and able to speak, a thorough history should be obtained. The following are important components of the patient history for these patients:

- Time of symptom onset
- Previous neurological symptoms (e.g., TIAs)
- Previous neurological deficits
- Initial symptoms and their progression
- Alterations in level of consciousness
- Precipitating factors
- Dizziness
- Palpitations
- Significant past medical history
  - Hypertension
  - Diabetes mellitus
  - Cigarette smoking
  - Oral contraceptive use
  - Cardiac disease
  - Sickle cell disease
  - Previous stroke

Cincinnati Prehospital Stroke Scale. In addition to the abnormal neurological signs and symptoms described previously, other methods can be used to diagnose stroke. One such method is the Cincinnati Prehospital Stroke Scale (CPSS).[15] This scale evaluates three major physical findings: facial droop, arm drift, and speech (Box 25-6). The paramedic can use this scale to help identify a patient who may be having a stroke and who needs rapid transport to a hospital. It also allows for prearrival notification of the receiving hospital. The CPSS has a sensitivity of 59% and a specificity of 89% when scored by prehospital personnel.[10]

BOX 25-6 Cincinnati Prehospital Stroke Scale*

Facial Droop (have the patient show the teeth or smile)
- Normal: The two sides of the face move equally well.
- Abnormal: One side of the face does not move as well as the other side.

Arm Drift (have the patient close the eyes and hold out both arms)
- Normal: Both arms move the same *or* both arms do not move at all (other findings, such as pronator grip, may be helpful).
- Abnormal: One arm does not move *or* one arm drifts down compared with the other.

Speech (have the patient say, "You can't teach an old dog new tricks.")
- Normal: The patient uses the correct words with no slurring.
- Abnormal: The patient slurs words, uses inappropriate words, *or* is unable to speak.

*The presence of a single abnormality on the CPSS has a sensitivity of 59% and a specificity of 89% when scored by prehospital providers.[2]

Los Angeles Prehospital Stroke Screen. The Los Angeles Prehospital Stroke Screen (LAPSS) is another means of diagnosing stroke. This screening tool requires the examiner to rule out other causes of altered level of consciousness (e.g., hypoglycemia or seizure). The examiner then must identify asymmetry (right versus left) in facial smile/grimace, grip, and arm strength (Box 25-7). Asymmetry in any category indicates a possible stroke. Like the CPSS, the LAPSS can be used quickly in the prehospital setting. The LAPSS has a specificity of 97% and a sensitivity of 93%.[10]

MANAGEMENT (FIGURE 25-14)

Once the diagnosis of stroke is suspected, *time in the field must be reduced,* because limited time is available to begin therapy. Fibrinolytics should be given less than 4 hours from the onset[2] (some centers have expanded this time frame to 6 hours or more in certain cases). Whenever possible, the paramedic should establish the time of onset of the stroke signs and symptoms. If the patient awoke with the symptoms, the time of onset should be recorded as the last time the patient was known to be normal *(last seen well).* This is important for determining whether fibrinolytics can be administered. Prehospital care is directed at managing the patient's airway, breathing, and circulation and monitoring vital signs. Besides life support, the most important care a paramedic can provide a stroke victim is quick identification of the possible stroke and rapid transport of the patient for definitive care.

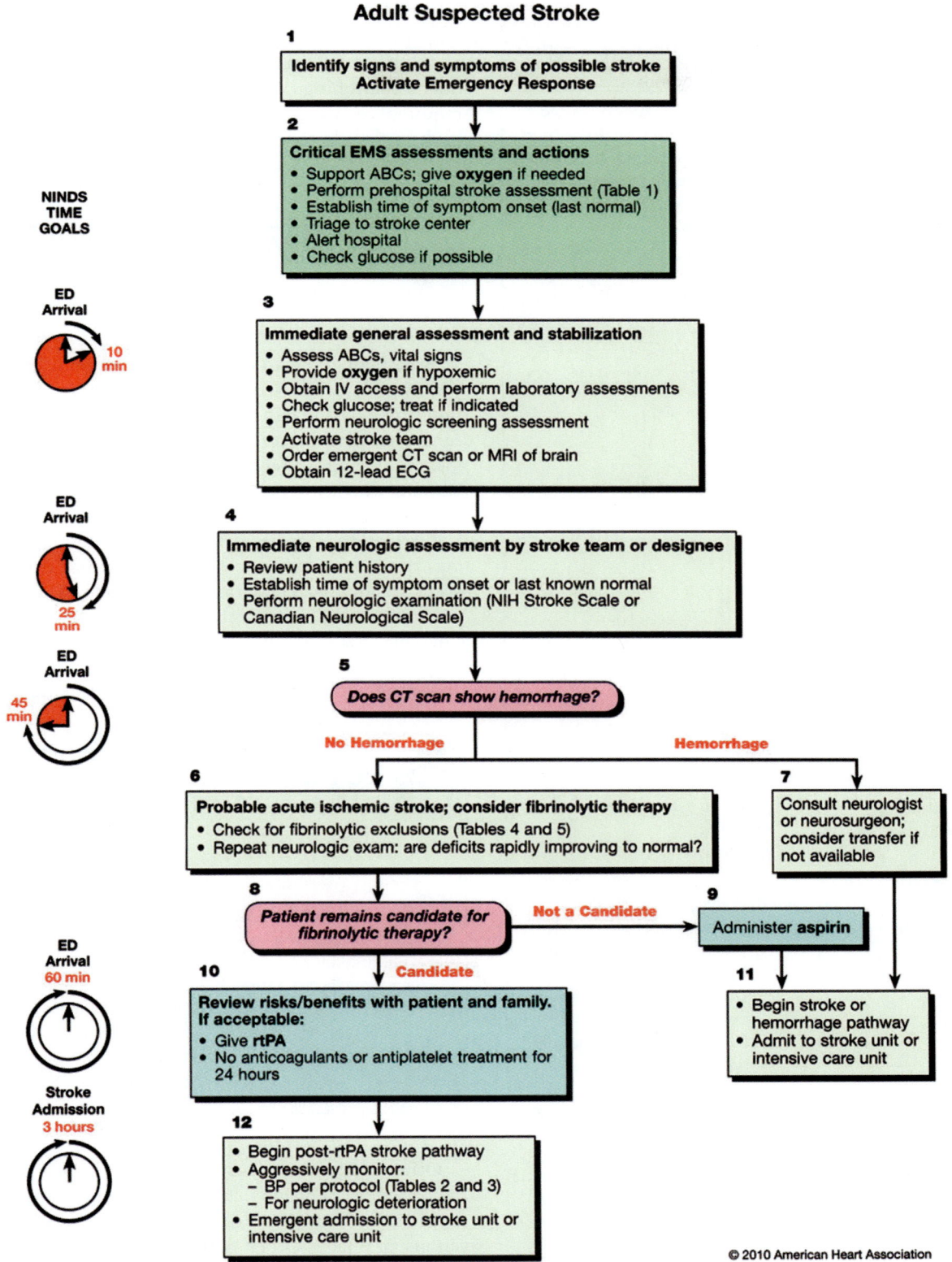

FIGURE 25-14 Goals for management of suspected cases of stroke. (American Heart Association: 2010 American Heart Association guidelines for cardiopulmonary resuscitation and emergency cardiovasular care, *Circulation* 122 (18 suppl): S639-S946, 2010.)

BOX 25-7 Los Angeles Prehospital Stroke Screen

The Los Angeles Prehospital Stroke Screen (LAPSS) is used to evaluate patients who may have an acute, noncomatose, nontraumatic neurological condition. If items 1 through 6 are **all checked Yes** (or Unknown), notify the receiving hospital before arrival of the potential stroke patient. If any are checked No, follow the appropriate treatment protocol.

Interpretation: Ninety-three percent of patients with stroke have positive findings (all items checked Yes or Unknown [sensitivity, 93%]). Of those with positive findings, 97% have a stroke (specificity, 97%). A patient may be having a stroke even if LAPSS criteria are not met.

	Yes	Unknown	No
1. Age >45	{}	{}	{}
2. History of seizures or epilepsy **absent**	{}	{}	{}
3. Symptom duration >24 hours	{}	{}	{}
4. At baseline, patient is **not** wheelchair bound or bedridden	{}	{}	{}
5. Blood glucose level is 60 to 400 mg/dL	{}	{}	{}
6. **Obvious asymmetry** (right vs. left) in **any** of the following three categories (**must be unilateral**):	{}	{}	{}

	Equal	R Weak	L Weak
Facial smile/grimace	{}	{} Droop	{} Droop
Grip	{}	{} Weak grip	{} Weak grip
	{}	{} No grip	{} No grip
Arm strength	{}	{} Drifts down	{} Drifts down
	{}	{} Falls rapidly	{} Falls rapidly

Modified from Kidwell CS, et al: Design and retrospective analysis of the Los Angeles Prehospital Stroke Screen (LAPSS), *Prehosp Emerg Care* 2:267-273, 1998.

> **NOTE**
> Some hospitals have dedicated stroke units staffed with a multidisciplinary team experienced in managing stroke. When such a facility is available within a reasonable transport interval, stroke patients who require hospitalization should be admitted there (class I).[11] The paramedic should consult with medical direction.

Airway. Paralysis of the muscles of the throat, tongue, and mouth can lead to partial or complete airway obstruction. (This is a major problem in acute stroke.) Frequent suctioning of the oropharynx and nasopharynx is required to prevent aspiration of saliva. If possible, the patient should be positioned to aid drainage of oral secretions.

> **CRITICAL THINKING**
> How can you detect paralysis of the muscles of the throat, tongue, and mouth on your physical exam?

Breathing. Inadequate ventilation should be managed with supplemental oxygen and positive-pressure ventilation. Hypoxia and hypercarbia can occur as a result of inadequate ventilation, contributing to cardiac and respiratory instability. Supplemental oxygen should be given to stroke patients who are hypoxic (oxygen saturation less than 94%) and to patients whose oxygen saturation is unknown.[11]

Circulation. Cardiac arrest is uncommon. However, it may result from a respiratory arrest. Cardiac dysrhythmias occur frequently. Therefore, the patient's ECG and blood pressure require constant monitoring. As described in Chapter 22, a difference in blood pressure readings in the upper extremities of 10 mm Hg or more may indicate aortic dissection and compromise of the brain's blood supply.

> **LOOK AGAIN**
> See Chapter 22: Cardiology, pp. 693-696.

> **NOTE**
> Many patients develop hypertension after a stroke. However, this usually does not require emergency treatment. Elevated blood pressure after a stroke is not a hypertensive emergency unless the patient has other medical indications, such as an acute myocardial infarction (AMI) or left ventricular failure. Management of hypertension in the prehospital setting is not recommended in cases of suspected stroke.[11] The paramedic should notify the receiving facility and transfer the patient to a stroke center if available.

Other Supportive Measures. If the airway is patent and the patient's condition permits, the person should be kept supine. The head should be elevated 15 degrees to aid venous drainage. Other patient care measures the paramedic can provide while en route to the receiving hospital include the following:

1. Initiate an IV line of lactated Ringer solution or normal saline (50 mL per hour).
2. Monitor ECG.
3. Perform serum glucose analysis (*50% dextrose* should be administered only if indicated).

4. If the patient cannot communicate, consider transporting a witness to confirm the time of onset. If that is not possible, obtain the most reliable information.
5. Protect paralyzed extremities.
6. Maintain normal body temperature.
7. Control seizure activity with benzodiazepines.
8. Provide comfort measures and reassurance.
9. Notify ED of possible stroke. Provide gentle transport to the appropriate receiving hospital.

Paramedics must keep in mind that a stroke patient has experienced a catastrophic event, one that may seriously affect the person's quality of life. These patients often are frightened, embarrassed, confused, and frustrated with their inability to move or communicate. They have special physical and emotional needs. As do all other patients, they deserve a compassionate, caring approach.

IN-HOSPITAL TREATMENT

On arrival at the emergency department (ED), a patient suspected of having a nonhemorrhagic stroke is evaluated as a possible candidate for fibrinolytic therapy. This evaluation includes an emergency neurological stroke assessment, which identifies the patient's level of consciousness. It also identifies the type, location, and severity of the stroke. This assessment is aided by use of the Glasgow Coma Scale and other standardized scales. These scales and other in-hospital diagnostic studies help measure neurological function. This function correlates with the severity of the stroke and the long-term outcome. These studies also help identify stroke patients who would benefit from fibrinolytic therapy. Rapid evaluation of the computed tomography (CT) scan is critical to rule out an intracranial hemorrhage. An intracranial hemorrhage is a contraindication to fibrinolytic therapy. As described in Chapter 22, fibrinolytics have potential adverse effects. Patients must be evaluated by a physician with inclusion-exclusion criteria to make sure they are candidates for fibrinolytic therapy.

LOOK AGAIN
See Chapter 22: Cardiology, pp. 685-687.

Seizure Disorders

A **seizure** is a brief alteration in behavior or consciousness. It is caused by abnormal electrical activity of one or more groups of neurons in the brain. It is estimated that 300,000 people in the United States experience a first-time seizure each year.[16] The highest incidence is among feverish children under 5 years of age. (Febrile seizures are further addressed in Chapter 48.)

CRITICAL THINKING
What feelings may parents experience after seeing their child have a febrile seizure? How should you respond to those feelings?

The underlying cause of seizures is not well understood. However, a seizure generally is believed to result from a structural lesion or problems with brain metabolism. This results in changes in the brain cell's permeability to sodium and potassium ions. When such changes occur, the neurons' ability to depolarize and emit an electrical impulse sometimes results in seizure activity. Seizures may be caused by several factors, including the following[5]:

- Stroke
- Head trauma
- Toxins (including alcohol or other drug withdrawal)
- Hypoxia
- Hypoperfusion
- Hypoglycemia
- Infection
- Metabolic abnormalities
- Brain tumor or abscess
- Vascular disorders
- Eclampsia
- Drug overdose

In the prehospital setting, determining the cause of a seizure is less important than managing the complications and recognizing whether the seizure is reversible with therapy (e.g., resulting from hypoglycemia). A tendency to have recurrent seizures is called **epilepsy** (Box 25-8). Epilepsy does not include seizures that arise from correctable or avoidable causes, such as alcohol withdrawal.

SHOW ME THE EVIDENCE
In a retrospective study in Pittsburgh, Martin-Gill and coworkers reviewed the prehospital treatment of patients whose chief complaint was seizure. The researchers' goal was to determine whether treatment followed the system's EMS seizure protocol and to evaluate patient outcomes. Of the 87 patients who met the inclusion criteria, only 11 (12.6%) had electrocardiographic (ECG) monitoring; in 55 (63.2%), attempts were made to establish an intravenous (IV) line; and 56 (64.4%) had blood glucose analysis. Twenty-eight patients (32.2%) had another seizure (17 were in the prehospital setting). Among the 17 patients who had another seizure in the field, eight had seizures that lasted longer than 1 minute. Only four of the eight patients were given diazepam. The researchers concluded that adherence to the seizure protocol was poor. They noted that individual patient differences made following one specific policy difficult.

Martin-Gill C, et al: Management of prehospital seizure patients by paramedics, *Prehosp Emerg Care* 13:179-184, 2009.

TYPES OF SEIZURES

All seizures are pathological; they are never considered normal. They may arise from almost any region of the brain and therefore have many clinical manifestations. The two most common types are generalized seizures and partial (focal) seizures.

Generalized Seizures. As the name implies, a **generalized seizure** does not have a definable origin (focus) in the

BOX 25-8 Epilepsy Statistics

- Each year, 200,000 new cases of epilepsy are diagnosed in the United States.
- The incidence is highest in infants under age 2 years and in adults over age 65.
- Each year, 45,000 children under age 15 develop epilepsy.
- Males are slightly more likely to develop epilepsy than females.
- The incidence is higher in African Americans and the socially disadvantaged.
- Trends show a decreased incidence in children and an increased incidence in the elderly.
- No cause is apparent in 70% of new cases.
- Among people with new cases of epilepsy, 50% will have generalized onset seizures.
- Generalized seizures are more common in children under age 10; after that age, more than 50% of individuals with new cases of epilepsy will have partial seizures.[16]

brain, although focal seizures may progress to generalized seizures. This class includes absence seizures and atonic, myoclonic, and tonic-clonic seizures.

Absence seizures (also known as *petit mal seizures*) occur most often in children between the ages of 4 and 12 years. They are characterized by brief lapses of consciousness without loss of posture. Often no motor activity is seen. However, some children have eye blinking, lip smacking, or isolated contraction of muscles. These seizures usually last less than 15 seconds. During this time, the patient is unaware of the surroundings. The seizures are followed by the patient's immediate return to normal. Most patients have remission by age 20 but later may develop generalized tonic-clonic (grand mal) seizures.

Atonic seizures produce an abrupt loss of muscle tone, loss of posture, or sudden collapse ("drop attacks"). These seizures can result in physical injury from falls. Children and adults with this condition sometimes wear protective headgear. These seizures tend to be resistant to drug therapy.

Myoclonic seizures cause brief muscle contractions that usually occur at the same time and on both sides of the body. (Occasionally they involve one arm or one foot.) Individuals with this disorder compare the sensation to the sudden jerk of a foot during sleep.

Tonic-clonic seizures are common and are associated with significant morbidity and mortality. They may be preceded by an **aura** (an olfactory or auditory sensation). Often the patient recognizes the aura as a warning of the imminent convulsion. The seizure itself is characterized by a sudden loss of consciousness associated with loss of organized muscle tone. The tonic phase is marked by a sequence of extensor muscle tone activity (sometimes flexion) and apnea. Tongue biting and bladder or bowel incontinence may occur. The tonic phase lasts only seconds. It is followed by a bilateral clonic phase (rigidity alternating with

relaxation). This usually lasts 1 to 3 minutes. During the clonic phase, a massive autonomic discharge occurs. This results in hyperventilation, salivation, and tachycardia. After the seizure, the patient usually experiences a period of drowsiness or unconsciousness. This resolves over minutes to hours. On regaining consciousness, the patient often is confused and fatigued. The person also may show signs of a transient neurological deficit. This part of the seizure is known as the *postictal phase*. Tonic-clonic seizures may be prolonged or may recur before the patient regains consciousness. When this occurs, the patient is said to be in status epilepticus (described later in this chapter).

CRITICAL THINKING
What could cause death after a grand mal seizure?

Partial Seizures. In contrast to generalized seizures, in which a specific seizure focus is unknown, a **partial seizure** arises from identifiable cortical lesions. Partial seizures may be classified as *simple* or *complex*. A **simple partial seizure** results mainly from seizure activity in the motor or sensory cortex. Simple motor seizures usually manifest as clonic activity that is limited to one body part. (For instance, this might be one hand, one arm or leg, or one side of the face.) *Simple sensory seizures* result in symptoms such as tingling or numbness of a body part or abnormal visual, auditory, olfactory, or taste symptoms. Patients with partial seizures generally do not lose consciousness. They usually maintain a somewhat normal mental status. However, the seizure focus may spread and lead to a generalized tonic-clonic seizure. Partial seizure activity that spreads in an orderly way to surrounding areas is known as a **jacksonian seizure.**

A **complex partial seizure** arises from focal seizures in the temporal lobe (psychomotor seizures). These manifest mainly as changes in behavior. The classic complex partial seizure is preceded by an aura. It is followed by abnormal repetitive motor behavior **(automatism),** such as lip smacking, chewing, or swallowing. During this time the patient has no memory of the event. These seizures usually are brief, lasting less than 1 minute. The patient usually regains normal mental status quickly. Like simple partial seizures, complex partial seizures also may progress to a generalized tonic-clonic seizure.

NOTE
A **nonepileptic seizure** can mimic a true seizure. However, it stems from psychological causes rather than electrical disturbances in the brain. Also, such seizures do not respond to the usual treatments. Nonepileptic seizures (*hysterical seizures* or *pseudoseizures*) sometimes can be ended by sharp commands or painful stimuli (e.g., a sternal rub). These maneuvers may help distinguish between pathological and psychogenic seizure activity. It should be noted that some nonepileptic diseases can cause life-threatening seizures. Paramedics should remember that a seizure is *never* normal. Any seizure should be taken seriously.

ASSESSMENT

The assessment process is determined by the patient's seizure state. In most cases the patient's seizure has ended before paramedics arrive. If possible, the assessment should include a thorough history and physical examination, including a neurological evaluation.

History. If the patient is in the postictal phase of the seizure, information can be gathered from family members or bystanders who witnessed the event. The following are important components of the patient history.

1. History of seizures
   a. Frequency
   b. Compliance in taking prescribed medications (e.g., ***phenytoin***, phenobarbital)
   c. Use of home medicines to control seizures (herbal medicines, vitamins)
2. Description of seizure activity
   a. Duration of seizure
   b. Typical or atypical pattern of seizure for the patient
   c. Presence of aura
   d. Generalized or focal
   e. Incontinence
   f. Tongue biting
3. Recent or past history of head trauma
4. Recent history of fever, headache, nuchal rigidity (neck stiffness with flexion, suggesting meningeal irritation)
5. Past significant medical history
   a. Diabetes
   b. Heart disease
   c. Stroke

Physical Examination. During the physical examination, maintaining a patent airway is always of prime importance. The paramedic also should be alert for signs of trauma (head and neck trauma, tongue injury, oral lacerations). These injuries may have occurred before or during the seizure. Also, the patient's mouth should be inspected for **gingival hypertrophy** (swelling of the gums). This is a sign of chronic ***phenytoin*** therapy. Other components of the physical examination include the following:

- Level of sensorium, including presence or absence of amnesia
- Cranial nerve evaluation, particularly pupillary findings
- Motor and sensory evaluation, including coordination (abnormalities may be caused by metabolic disturbances, meningitis, intracranial hemorrhage, and drug use)
- Evaluation for hypotension, hypoxia, and hypoglycemia
- Presence of urine or feces (suggesting bladder or bowel incontinence)
- Automatisms
- Cardiac dysrhythmias

CRITICAL THINKING
What are signs and symptoms of phenytoin toxicity?

NOTE

A *vagal nerve stimulator* (VNS) is used to treat some patients who have frequent partial seizures unresponsive to medication therapy. (The device also is used to manage some forms of depression.) This device usually is implanted in the left chest; lead wires are fed through the neck and tethered to the vagus nerve (cranial nerve X). The VNS sends electrical impulses regularly to the vagus nerve, causing the widespread release of gamma aminobutyric acid (GABA) and glycine in the brain. (The device also can be activated and deactivated manually by the patient.) Although the precise mode of action is unknown, a VNS is effective in controlling seizures in some patients.[17]

Differentiation of Syncope and Seizure. As described in Chapter 22, *syncope* is a complete loss of consciousness caused by a temporary reduction in cerebral blood flow. Because syncope and seizure have similar presentations, determining whether a patient has experienced a syncopal episode or a seizure can be difficult. The main difference is in the symptoms the patient experiences before and after the event. The factors listed in Table 25-4 may aid differentiation of these two conditions.

LOOK AGAIN
See Chapter 22: Cardiology, p. 676.

MANAGEMENT

The first step in the management of a patient with seizure activity is to protect the patient from injury. This is best achieved by removing obstacles in the patient's immediate area. If necessary, the patient can be moved to a safe environment, such as a carpeted or soft, grassy area. *At no time should a patient with seizure activity be restrained, nor should objects be forced between the patient's teeth to maintain an airway.* Restraining activity may harm the patient or paramedic crew. Forcing objects into the oral cavity in an effort to secure an airway or prevent the patient from biting the tongue may evoke vomiting, aspiration, or spasm of the larynx. Placement of a nasopharyngeal airway, along with end-tidal carbon dioxide ($EtCO_2$) monitoring should be considered.

Most patients with an isolated seizure can be properly managed in the postictal phase by being placed in a lateral recumbent position. This allows drainage of oral secretions

TABLE 25-4 Differentiation of Syncope and Seizure

Characteristic	Syncope	Seizure
Position	Syncope usually starts when patient is in a standing position.	Seizure may start with patient in any position.
Warning	Patient usually has a warning period of lightheadedness.	Patient has little or no warning.
Level of consciousness	Patient usually regains consciousness immediately on becoming supine; fatigue, confusion, and headache last less than 15 minutes.	Patient may remain unconscious for minutes to hours; fatigue, confusion, and headache last longer than 15 minutes.
Clonic-tonic activity	Clonic movements (if present) are of short duration.	Tonic-clonic movements occur during unconscious state.
Electrocardiographic (ECG) analysis	Bradycardia is caused by increased vagal tone associated with syncope.	Tachycardia is caused by muscular exertion associated with seizure activity.

and aids suctioning (if needed). Supplemental oxygen should be administered via a nonrebreather mask. The patient should be moved to a quiet place (away from onlookers). Patients often are embarrassed or self-conscious after a seizure. This is especially the case if incontinence has occurred. Paramedics should be sensitive to the physical and emotional needs of the patient.

All seizure patients should be encouraged to seek care. Some patients should always be transported to the ED for care and evaluation by a physician. These include patients who have a history of seizures but who experienced a seizure that is different from the usual one, and patients with a seizure that is complicated by an unusual event (e.g., trauma). All patients who have experienced a seizure for the first time should be transported to the ED for evaluation by a physician. Depending on the patient's status and seizure history, an IV line may be necessary to administer drug therapy. However, few patients who experience an isolated seizure require drug therapy in the prehospital setting.

STATUS EPILEPTICUS

Status epilepticus is ongoing seizure activity that lasts 30 minutes or longer. The term also refers to recurrent seizures without a period of consciousness between them.[5] Status epilepticus is a true emergency. Without immediate management, it can result in permanent neurological damage, respiratory failure, and death. Associated complications of status epilepticus include aspiration, brain damage, and fracture of long bones and the spine. The most common cause in adults is failure to take prescribed anticonvulsant medications.

Management. As for all patients with seizures, management priorities include securing the airway and providing ventilatory support, protecting the patient from injury and, if indicated, transporting the patient to a medical facility for evaluation by a physician. In addition, management includes stopping the seizure activity with anticonvulsant medications (e.g., *diazepam, lorazepam,* or *midazolam*).[18]

After the airway has been secured with oral or nasal adjuncts (or with intubation of the trachea during the flaccid period between seizures), high-concentration oxygen should be administered. Also, ventilation should be supported with a bag-valve device. An IV line should be established to keep the vein open and secured well with tape and roller bandage. A sample of the patient's blood should be drawn for laboratory analysis (per protocol). Medications administered in the prehospital setting may include the following:

- **50% dextrose** given by slow IV infusion (only if hypoglycemic). In some cases, hypoglycemia causes the seizure.
- **Lorazepam, diazepam,** or **midazolam** (IV route preferred) to stop the spread of the seizure focus. (If vascular access cannot be established, **lorazepam** may be given intramuscularly [IM]. It is the preferred drug choice, followed by **diazepam** and then **midazolam.**)

While administering these drugs, paramedics should closely monitor the patient's blood pressure and respiratory status. They should be prepared for respiratory arrest. If the patient's blood pressure begins to fall or if the respiratory rate or effort decreases, paramedics should stop the drug therapy and consult with medical direction.

Headache

Headaches are painful and bothersome. However, most are minor health concerns and are easily managed with analgesics. Headaches are categorized according to their underlying cause. The types of headaches are tension headache, migraine, cluster headache, and sinus headache. Therapies that may be useful in managing these headaches include prescription and over-the-counter medications, herbal remedies, meditation, acupressure, aromatherapy, and others. Headache is an extremely common medical complaint; 40% of Americans have what they consider a serious headache at some time during their lives.[19] The pain associated with headaches arises from the meninges and from the scalp and its blood vessels and muscles.

A **tension headache** is caused by muscle contractions of the face, neck, and scalp. This type of headache has a variety of causes, including stress, persistent noise, eyestrain, and poor posture. The pain of tension headaches (usually described as dull, persistent, and nonthrobbing) may last for days or weeks. The pain can cause variable degrees of discomfort. These headaches can be short-lived and infrequent or chronic. Most tension headaches can be managed effectively with analgesics such as *aspirin,* acetaminophen, or ibuprofen.

A **migraine** is a severe, incapacitating headache. These headaches often are preceded by visual or gastrointestinal (GI) disturbances or both. They usually begin with an intense, throbbing pain on one side of the head that may spread. They often are accompanied by nausea and vomiting. The symptoms of migraines are associated with constriction and dilation of blood vessels, which may be brought on by an imbalance of serotonin or hormone fluctuations. Migraines also can be triggered by excessive caffeine use, various foods, changes in altitude, and extremes of emotions. A wide range of medications are prescribed for migraines. These include beta blockers, calcium channel blockers, antidepressants, and serotonin-inhibiting drugs.

Cluster headaches are headaches that occur in bursts (clusters). They often begin several hours after a person falls asleep. The pain may be severe. It usually is located in and around one eye and generally is accompanied by nasal congestion and tearing. The painful episode often lasts 30 minutes to 2 hours. It then diminishes or disappears, recurring a day or so later. The headaches may occur every day for weeks or months before going into long periods of remission. Cluster headaches also are known as *histamine headaches.* This is because they are associated with the release of histamine from the body tissues. They are marked by symptoms of dilated carotid arteries, fluid accumulation under the eyes, tearing or lacrimation, and rhinorrhea. Cluster headaches generally are managed with antihistamines, corticosteroids, and calcium channel blockers. Cluster headaches seem to be more common in heavy smokers than in nonsmokers. Alcohol consumption and certain foods also may be implicated. These headaches are much more common in men.

A **sinus headache** is characterized by pain in the forehead, nasal area, and eyes. These headaches often produce a feeling of pressure behind the face. Allergies, inflammation, or infection of the membranes lining the sinus cavities usually is responsible for the discomfort. Sinus headaches are managed with medications such as analgesics, antihistamines, and antibiotics to treat infection.

MANAGEMENT

Many causes of headaches can be prevented. For example, triggers can be identified, such as irregular meals, prolonged travel, noisy environments, and food additives (in susceptible individuals). Headaches such as those described in the preceding paragraphs seldom require prehospital emergency care. However, a full history of the headache should be obtained. This helps identify a more serious cause of the headache, should one be present. For example, the headache may be a sign of an aneurysm or a stroke.

Important assessment findings include the following:
- The patient's general health
- Previous medical conditions
- Medications used
- Previous experience with headaches
- The time of onset

After a patient history has been obtained and a neurological examination has been performed, prehospital care for patients with tension headaches, migraines, cluster headaches, and sinus headaches is mainly supportive. Transport of the patient for evaluation by a physician may be indicated. These patients often have light sensitivity. Lights in the ambulance should be dimmed.

Central Nervous System Tumors

CNS tumors include **brain tumors** and **spinal cord tumors.** The incidence of these tumors tends to increase up to age 70 and then decrease. CNS tumors are the second most common group of tumors in children.[20]

A brain tumor, or **neoplasm,** is a mass in the cranial cavity. This mass may be either malignant or benign. Heredity may play a role in the development of brain tumors. They also are associated with several risk factors, including exposure to radiation, tobacco use, dietary habits, some viruses, and the use of some medications. The effects of the tumor depend on its size, location, and growth rate and whether any evidence of hemorrhage or edema exists. Brain tumors may cause local and generalized manifestations. Local effects are caused by the destructive action of the tumor on a particular site in the brain and by compression, which reduces cerebral blood flow (Figure 25-15). These effects are varied and may include the following[20]:
- Seizures
- Visual disturbances
- Unstable gait
- Cranial nerve dysfunction

Lesions inside the cranial vault produce pain by distending or stretching the arteries and other pain-sensitive structures of the head and neck. Headache may be present but often is a late finding in the absence of hemorrhage, which may cause a sudden onset of pain.[19] The main treatment for a cerebral tumor is surgical or radiosurgical excision. Surgical decompression may be used if total excision is not possible. Chemotherapy and radiation also may be used.

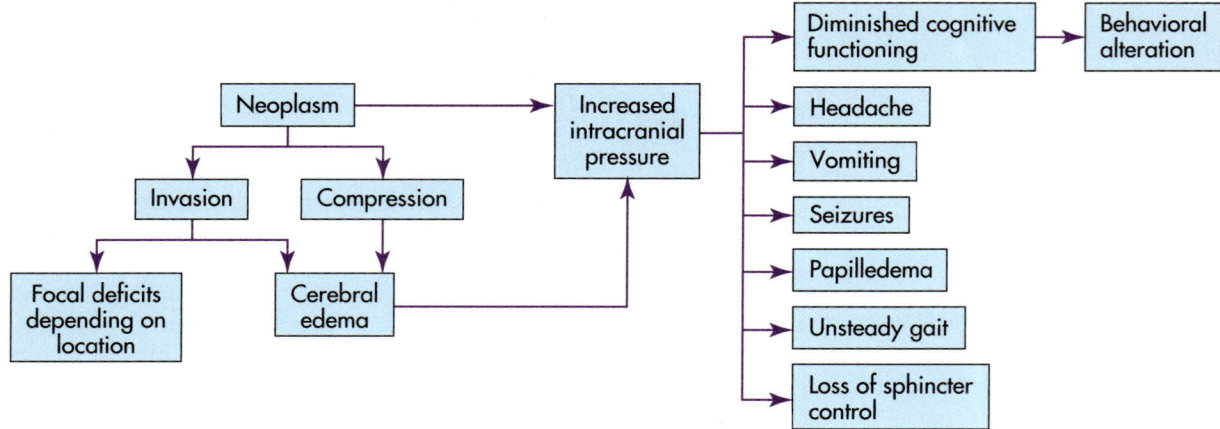

FIGURE 25-15 Origin of signs and symptoms associated with an intracranial neoplasm.

A **brain abscess** is an accumulation of purulent material (pus) surrounded by a capsule within the brain. It develops from a bacterial infection that often begins in the nasal cavity, middle ear, or mastoid cells. The condition also may develop after surgery or penetrating cranial trauma, especially when bone fragments are retained in cranial tissue. Clinical manifestations of a brain abscess are associated with intracranial infection (e.g., fever). They also are associated with an expanding intracranial mass (e.g., nausea, vomiting, seizures, and changes in mental status). Headache is the most common early symptom. Removal of fluid from the abscess or excision, accompanied by antibiotic therapy, generally is recommended to manage this disorder. The incidence of brain abscess is about 1 per 100,000 hospital admissions. The condition is twice as common in men as in women. The median age for abscess formation is 30 to 40 years.[20]

Like the brain, the spinal cord can become compressed. In the absence of trauma, compression of the spinal cord can be caused by bone, blood, abscesses, tumors, or a ruptured disk. (Compression of the spinal cord that results from trauma and associated spinal cord syndromes is discussed in Chapter 41.) Compression of the cord can disrupt normal functions, as a result of pressure on the roots of spinal nerves. Spinal cord compression can occur suddenly, causing immediate symptoms. It also may occur gradually, over weeks to months. Slight compression may cause mild symptoms, such as back pain (that may or may not radiate to the leg or foot), slight muscle weakness, and tingling in the extremities. In men, difficulty urinating and erectile dysfunction may occur. If the cause of compression is cancer, an abscess, or a hematoma, the back may be tender to the touch in the affected area. Significant compression of the cord may block nerve impulses. This can result in severe muscle weakness, numbness, retention of urine, and loss of bladder and bowel control. If all nerve impulses are blocked, paralysis and complete loss of sensation may result. Definitive care is determined by the cause of the compression. Treatment by a physician may include high doses of IV steroids to reduce inflammation, antibiotics, radiation, and other therapies. Surgery may be required to relieve the compression and prevent permanent nerve damage.

MANAGEMENT

Prehospital care of a patient with a CNS tumor may range from providing comfort and emotional support during patient transport to managing seizure activity and providing airway, ventilatory, and circulatory resuscitation. If the patient's condition permits, a focused history should be obtained and a neurological evaluation should be performed. Elements of the focused history for these patients should include the following:

- Past significant medical history (e.g., surgical removal of a tumor, radiation therapy)
- History and description of any headache
- Dizziness or loss of consciousness
- Seizure activity
- GI disturbances (vomiting, diarrhea)
- New onset of incoordination, difficulty walking or maintaining balance
- Behavioral or cognitive changes
- Weakness or paralysis
- Vision disturbances

Degenerative Neurological Diseases

There are many degenerative neurological diseases. The pathophysiology of many of these disorders is not fully understood. Some diseases may involve Schwann cells, the CSF, or axons of the CNS. Others may result from circulatory and immunological disorders and exposure to bacterial toxins and chemicals (see Chapters 28 and 57). The following specific neurological diseases are discussed in this chapter[21]:

- Dementia
- Alzheimer's disease
- Pick's disease
- Huntington's disease

- Creutzfeldt-Jakob disease
- Muscular dystrophy
- Multiple sclerosis
- Guillain-Barré syndrome
- Dystonia
- Parkinson's disease
- Cranial nerve disorders
- Bell's palsy
- Amyotrophic lateral sclerosis
- Peripheral neuropathy
- Spina bifida
- Polio

DEMENTIA

Dementia is a slow, progressive loss of awareness of time and place. It usually involves an inability to learn new things or recall recent events. Dementia often is a result of brain disease caused by strokes, genetic or viral factors, and Alzheimer's disease. Dementia generally is considered irreversible. It eventually results in full dependence on others because of progressive loss of cognitive functioning. During the course of the disease, patients often try to conceal their memory loss by **confabulation** (inventing stories to fill gaps in memory). Sudden outbursts or embarrassing conduct may be the first obvious signs of dementia. Some patients eventually regress to a "second childhood." At that point, they need full care for feeding, toileting, and physical activity. About 50% of nursing home residents have dementia. The disease affects about 20% of those over age 80 to some degree.[5] Prehospital care is primarily supportive.

> **NOTE**
>
> Any patient with altered mental status (e.g., confusion or lethargy) should be assessed for infections that may cause these symptoms. Infections that irritate and inflame the membranes of the CNS can cause neurological disorders, such as *encephalitis* and *meningitis*. These diseases are presented in Chapter 28.

ALZHEIMER'S DISEASE

Alzheimer's disease is a condition in which nerve cells in the cerebral cortex die and the brain substance shrinks. The disease is the single most common cause of dementia and is responsible for most cases in people over age 75. It is estimated that at least 5.3 million Americans are living with the disease.[22] Alzheimer's disease does not cause death directly; rather, these patients ultimately stop eating and become malnourished and immobilized. They then are prone to intercurrent infections (Box 25-9).

The cause of Alzheimer's disease is not known. Possible causes include abnormalities in glutamate metabolism, chronic infection, toxic poisoning by metals, reduction in brain chemicals (e.g., acetylcholine), and genetics. Early symptoms of Alzheimer's disease mainly are related to memory loss, especially the ability to make and recall new

> **BOX 25-9 10 Signs of Alzheimer's Disease**
>
> 1. Memory loss that disrupts daily life
> 2. Challenges in planning or solving problems
> 3. Difficulty completing familiar tasks at home, work, or leisure
> 4. Confusion with time or place
> 5. Difficulty understanding visual imagery or spatial relationships
> 6. New problems with words in speaking or writing
> 7. Misplacing things and losing the ability to retrace steps
> 8. Diminished or poor judgment
> 9. Withdrawal from work or social activities
> 10. Changes in mood or personality[22]

memories. As the disease progresses, agitation, violence, and impairment of abstract thinking occur. Judgment and cognitive disabilities begin to interfere with work and social relations. In the advanced stages of Alzheimer's disease, patients often become bedridden and totally unaware of their surroundings. Once the patient is bedridden, bed sores, feeding problems, and pneumonia shorten the person's life. Currently Alzheimer's disease has no cure. Treatment consists mainly of medications to help slow the progression of the disease and nursing and social care for the patient and relatives.

PICK'S DISEASE

Pick's disease is a rare neurodegenerative disease. It is one of the causes of frontotemporal dementia (FTD), a disease associated with the shrinking of the frontal and temporal anterior lobes of the brain. The disease is associated with changes in behavior or problems with language. These changes manifest as symptoms of behavior that can be either impulsive (disinhibited) or apathetic.[23] They include:

- Inappropriate social behavior
- Lack of social tact
- Lack of empathy
- Distractibility
- Loss of insight into the behaviors of oneself and others
- An increased interest in sex
- Changes in food preferences
- Agitation or, conversely, blunted emotions
- Neglect of personal hygiene
- Repetitive or compulsive behavior and decreased energy and motivation

Other features of the disease include symptoms of language disturbance, including difficulty making or understanding speech. Unlike Alzheimer's disease, spatial skills and memory in patients with Pick's disease remain intact. The disease has a strong genetic component; FTD often runs in families. No treatment is known to slow the progression of the disease, and the outcome is poor. Some patients are treated with behavior modification and antidepressants. Most require institutionalized care. As in other forms of dementia, prehospital care for these patients is primarily supportive.

HUNTINGTON'S DISEASE

Huntington's disease (HD) (also known as *Huntington's chorea*) results from genetically programmed degeneration of neurons in the brain. This degeneration causes uncontrolled movements, loss of intellectual faculties, and emotional disturbance. HD is a rare, inherited disease that is passed from parent to child. Early symptoms of HD are mood swings, depression, irritability, memory loss, and inability to make decisions. As the disease progresses, concentration on intellectual and personal tasks becomes increasingly difficult. Patients may become unable to feed themselves or swallow food or water. The rate of disease progression and the age of onset vary from person to person. A number of medications are used to manage the symptoms of HD, but the course of the disease cannot be altered. Prehospital care is primarily supportive.

> **NOTE**
> Each child of a parent with HD has a 50% chance of inheriting the HD gene.[24] If a child does not inherit the HD gene, he or she will not develop the disease and cannot pass it to subsequent generations. A person who inherits the HD gene will develop the disease. Genetic counseling and testing are available for people who carry the gene.

CREUTZFELDT-JAKOB DISEASE

Creutzfeldt-Jakob disease (CJD) is a rare and fatal brain disorder. Worldwide, it affects about 1 in 1 million people per year. In the United States, about 200 cases occur per year.[25] CJD usually appears in later life and runs a rapid course. Typically, the onset of symptoms occurs at about age 60, and about 90% of patients die within 1 year.

> **NOTE**
> CJD may be categorized as *classic* or *variant*. Although both forms of the disease are fatal, classic CJD, described in this chapter, is not related to *bovine spongiform encephalopathy* (BSE, or "mad cow" disease). However, strong evidence links outbreaks in Europe of the disease in cattle to the variant form of CJD in humans.[26]

CJD is characterized by rapidly progressive dementia. Initially, patients with CJD have problems with muscular coordination. They often experience personality changes, involuntary movements, impaired memory, and poor judgment. Some patients develop blindness. As the illness progresses, these patients eventually lose the ability to move

and speak; some may become comatose. Pneumonia and other infections often occur in these patients and can lead to death. No treatment exists to cure or control the disease. Prehospital care is primarily supportive.

MUSCULAR DYSTROPHY

Muscular dystrophy is an inherited muscle disorder. The disease is marked by a slow but progressive degeneration of muscle fibers. Different forms of the disease are classified by the age at which the symptoms appear, the rate at which the disease progresses, and the way in which it is inherited. *Duchenne's muscular dystrophy* is the most common type. It is caused by an absence of dystrophin, a protein that helps keep muscle cells intact. The disease affects about 1 in 3500 to 5000 male children.[27] It is inherited through a recessive sex-linked gene; therefore, only males are affected, and only females can pass on the disease.

Muscular dystrophy often is first diagnosed by the child's physician, who notices that the child is slow in learning to sit up and walk. The disease is confirmed through blood tests that reveal high levels of enzymes released from damaged muscle cells, through nerve conduction studies, and sometimes with muscle biopsy. Muscular dystrophy rarely is diagnosed before age 3. As the disease progresses, the child tends to walk with a waddle and has difficulty climbing stairs. Muscles (especially those in the calves) become bulky as wasted muscle is replaced by fat. By about age 12, affected children are no longer able to walk, and few survive their teenage years. Death usually results from pulmonary infections and heart failure.

> **CRITICAL THINKING**
> How can you determine a child's baseline level of functioning?

No effective treatment exists for muscular dystrophy. Parents or siblings of an affected child should receive genetic counseling. Some types of muscular dystrophy can be diagnosed before birth. This can be done through blood analysis and amniocentesis (testing of amniotic fluid).

MULTIPLE SCLEROSIS

Multiple sclerosis (MS) is a progressive disease of the CNS in which scattered patches of myelin in the brain and spinal cord are destroyed. The cause of MS is unknown. However, it is thought to be an autoimmune disease in which the body's defense system begins to treat the myelin in the CNS as foreign, gradually destroying it *(demyelination)*, causing scarring and nerve fiber damage.

MS is the most common acquired disease of the nervous system in young adults. To date, about 400,000 Americans have the disease. Each week, more than 200 people in the United States are diagnosed with MS.[28] The ratio of women to men affected is 3:2. The symptoms, which may be active briefly in early adult life and resume years later, vary according to the parts of the brain and spinal cord affected. Symptoms range from numbness and tingling to paralysis and incontinence and may last several weeks to several months. Damage to the white matter in the brain may lead to fatigue, vertigo, clumsiness, unsteady gait, slurred speech, blurred or double vision, and facial numbness or pain. Some patients may have mild relapses and long symptom-free periods throughout life. Others may gradually become disabled from the first attack and are bedridden and incontinent in early middle life.

The disease usually is diagnosed by ruling out other diseases. Diagnostic tests that may help identify MS include lumbar puncture, CT scanning, and magnetic resonance imaging (MRI) studies. Patients are managed with medications (e.g., corticosteroids, antidepressants, immune system medications). These help control the symptoms of an acute episode and prevent exacerbation. The disease also is managed with physical therapy to help maintain mobility and independence. Currently no cure exists.

> **CRITICAL THINKING**
> Consider the patient who has been receiving long-term steroid therapy. This person is at risk for what conditions?

GUILLAIN-BARRÉ SYNDROME

Guillain-Barré syndrome (GBS) is a rare autoimmune disorder that affects the body's peripheral nervous system. Initial symptoms of the syndrome include weakness or tingling sensations in the legs that may spread to the arms and upper body. These symptoms can increase in intensity until the muscles can no longer be used, causing total or near-total paralysis ("stocking and glove paralysis"). At this stage, the disorder is life-threatening. Patients often require mechanical ventilation to breathe. However, most patients recover from GBS, although some continue to have varying degrees of weakness.

GBS occurs a few days or weeks after the patient has had symptoms of a respiratory or GI viral infection.[29] Occasionally, surgery or vaccinations trigger the syndrome. The disorder can develop over the course of hours or days, or it may take up to 3 to 4 weeks. The syndrome is managed by supporting the patient's vital functions. Some patients are treated with plasmapheresis (the removal and replacement of plasma fluids) and high-dose immunoglobulin therapy.

DYSTONIA

The term **dystonia** refers to local or diffuse changes in muscle tone (usually abnormal muscle rigidity). These changes cause painful muscle spasms, unusually fixed postures, and strange movement patterns. Localized dystonia may result from *torticollis* (a painful neck spasm.) It also may result from *scoliosis* (an abnormal curvature of the spine). More generalized dystonia results from various neurological disorders. These include Parkinson's disease and stroke. It also may be a feature of schizophrenia or a side effect of some antipsychotic drugs (see Chapter 35). Dystonia sometimes is managed with medications such as benztropine or **diphenhydramine.** These help reverse the symptoms and prevent their recurrence.

PARKINSON'S DISEASE

Parkinson's disease is caused by degeneration of nerve cells in the basal ganglia in the brain or damage of unknown origin to those cells. The degeneration causes a lack of dopamine. This prevents the basal ganglia from modifying nerve pathways that control muscle contraction. The result is muscles that are overly tense. This causes tremor, joint rigidity, and slow movement. Parkinson's disease affects about 130 in 10,000 people, and 60,000 new cases are diagnosed in the United States each year.[30] Left untreated, the disease progresses over 10 to 15 years to severe weakness and incapacity. Parkinson's disease is the leading cause of neurological disability in people over age 60. Currently about 1 million people in the United States have the disease.

Parkinson's disease usually begins as a slight tremor in one hand, arm, or leg. In the early stages, the tremor is worse while the limb is at rest. In the later stages, the disease affects both sides of the body. It causes stiffness, weakness, and trembling of the muscles. Other symptoms include an unusual walking pattern (shuffling) that may break into uncontrollable, tiny running steps; constant trembling of the hands, sometimes accompanied by shaking of the head; a permanent rigid stoop; and an unblinking, fixed facial expression. Late in the disease, intellect may be affected. Speech becomes slow and hesitant. Depression is common.

At first Parkinson's disease is managed with counseling, exercise, and special aids in the home. As the disease progresses, management may include various combinations of drugs that either mimic or replace dopamine (e.g., levodopa). These drugs provide relief from specific symptoms. Other management measures may include brain surgery to reduce tremor and rigidity if medication therapy fails.

> **NOTE**
> *Normal pressure hydrocephalus (NPH)* is a syndrome that affects some older adults. It is caused by an abnormal increase in cerebrospinal fluid in the cavities of the brain. It may result from a subarachnoid hemorrhage, head trauma, infection, tumor, or complications of surgery. Often the cause is unknown. NPH can simulate Parkinson's disease, Alzheimer's disease, and other degenerative neurological diseases. Patients may present with a gait disorder, psychomotor slowing, incontinence, progressive dementia, and memory loss. NPH is diagnosed with a computed tomography (CT) scan or magnetic resonance imaging (MRI) studies or both. The disease is treated by surgical placement of a shunt in the brain to drain excess CSF.

CRANIAL NERVE DISORDERS

Cranial nerve disorders can affect the connections between cranial nerve centers in the brain. These disorders may lead to dysfunction of smell, vision, facial sensation or expression, taste, hearing, and balance, among others. Cranial nerve disorders discussed in this section include trigeminal neuralgia, acoustic neuroma, glossopharyngeal neuralgia, and hemifacial spasm. Because the cause of the cranial nerve disorders often is unclear, management sometimes is difficult. Treatment includes drugs to inhibit nerve impulses and sometimes surgery if the cause is a tumor or lesion. Prehospital care for patients with cranial nerve disorders is primarily supportive.

Trigeminal neuralgia (also known as central pain syndrome) refers to infection or disease of the trigeminal nerve (cranial nerve V). Patients with trigeminal neuralgia complain of paroxysmal episodes of excruciating pain (often described as recurrent bursts of an electric shock) that affect the cheek, lips, gums, or chin on one side of the face. The episode usually is very brief, lasting only a few seconds to minutes, but it may be so intense the person is unable to function during the attack. The pain of trigeminal neuralgia usually begins from a trigger point on the face. It can be brought on by touching, washing, shaving, eating, drinking, or talking. Trigeminal neuralgia is unusual in people under age 50 but may be associated with multiple sclerosis in younger people. Attacks occur in bouts that may last weeks at a time.

Acoustic neuroma is a noncancerous tumor that involves the vestibular portion of the acoustic nerve (cranial nerve VIII). Because of its position in the internal auditory canal, the tumor may also compress other cranial nerves. The tumor usually grows slowly. As it grows, it presses against the nerves that affect hearing and balance. Patients may be asymptomatic or may have mild symptoms that include loss of hearing on one side, tinnitus, and vertigo. Acoustic neuroma can be difficult to diagnose, because the symptoms are similar to those of middle ear infections.

Glossopharyngeal neuralgia is believed to be caused by irritation of the glossopharyngeal nerve (cranial nerve IX). Often the source of the irritation is never identified. Possible causes include pressure exerted by blood vessels on the glossopharyngeal nerve, lesions at the base of the skull, and tumors or infection of the throat and mouth. Symptoms include severe pain in the nose, ear, and throat. The discomfort often is triggered by coughing, chewing, laughing, or swallowing. Treatment is aimed at pain relief. Medications used to manage the disorder include analgesics, anticonvulsants, and antidepressants. In rare cases, surgery may be needed to correct the underlying cause of the pain.

Hemifacial spasm is a neuromuscular disorder characterized by frequent involuntary contractions of the muscles on one side of the face. It most often is caused by a blood vessel that presses on the facial nerve (cranial nerve VII), but it also can be caused by an injury or a tumor. The disorder occurs in both men and women, although it more frequently affects middle-aged or elderly women. The first symptom usually is an intermittent twitching of the eyelid muscle that can lead to forced closure of the eye. The spasm may then gradually spread to involve the muscles of the lower face, which may cause the mouth to be pulled to one side. Eventually the spasms involve all of the muscles on one side of the face almost continuously.

BELL'S PALSY

Bell's palsy (facial palsy) is a paralysis of the facial muscles. The paralysis is caused by inflammation of the facial nerve (cranial nerve VII) (Figure 25-16). It usually is one-sided and temporary. It often develops suddenly. Bell's palsy is the most common cause of facial paralysis; it affects 1 in 60 to 70 people in a lifetime.[31] The cause of the inflammation is unclear. However, it has been associated with many past or present infectious processes. These include Lyme disease, herpes viruses, mumps, and infection with the human immunodeficiency virus (HIV). Stroke should also be part of the paramedic's differential diagnosis.

CRITICAL THINKING
In the field, should you diagnose and release a patient who has Bell's palsy?

Bell's palsy usually causes the eyelid and corner of the mouth to droop on one side of the face. It sometimes is associated with numbness and pain. Depending on which branches of the nerve are affected, taste may be impaired, or sounds may seem oddly loud. Management may involve the use of antiviral and antiinflammatory drugs to reduce inflammation of the nerve, along with analgesics. Recovery usually is complete within 2 weeks to 2 months. A key

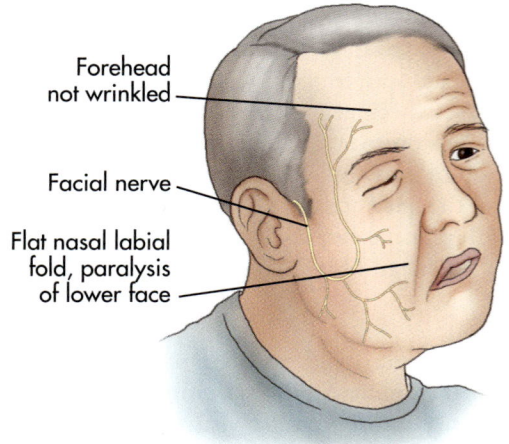

Forehead not wrinkled

Facial nerve

Flat nasal labial fold, paralysis of lower face

FIGURE 25-16 Bell's palsy. (McCance KL, Huether SE: *Pathophysiology: the biologic basis for disease in adults and children*, ed 5, St Louis, 2006, Mosby.)

component of therapy is to protect the affected eye from corneal drying and injury, which may result because the paralysis prevents the eyelid from closing. These conditions are best prevented through the use of lubricating ointments and eye patches.

AMYOTROPHIC LATERAL SCLEROSIS

Amyotrophic lateral sclerosis (ALS), also called *Lou Gehrig's disease,* is one of a group of rare disorders known as *motor neuron diseases.* In these disorders, the nerves that control muscular activity degenerate in the brain and spinal cord. ALS usually affects people over age 50. It is more common in men than in women. One or two cases of ALS are diagnosed each year per 100,000 people in the United States.[20] About 10% of ALS cases are familial.

Motor neuron diseases may involve deterioration of both upper and lower neuron tracts. When only muscles of the tongue, jaw, face, and larynx are involved, the term *progressive bulbar palsy* is used. When only corticospinal processes are affected, the term *primary lateral sclerosis* is used. When only lower motor neurons are affected, the term *progressive spinal muscular atrophy* is used. The term ALS is used for neuron signs that predominate in the extremities and trunk.

Patients with ALS often first notice weakness in the hands and arms. This is accompanied by involuntary quivering *(fasciculations).* The disease progresses to involve the muscles of all four extremities and those involved in respiration and swallowing. In the final stages of the disease, patients often are unable to speak, swallow, or move. However, awareness and intellect are maintained. Death usually occurs 2 to 4 years after the diagnosis. This is due to involvement of the respiratory muscles, aspiration pneumonia, and general inanition (starvation, failure to thrive). In some cases, life can be prolonged through the use of feeding tubes and ventilators. Care generally is aimed at providing emotional support and easing discomfort.

CRITICAL THINKING

Why is there a tendency to treat patients with amyotrophic lateral sclerosis (ALS) as if they have impaired intelligence?

PERIPHERAL NEUROPATHY

As the name implies, **peripheral neuropathy** refers to diseases and disorders that affect the peripheral nervous system. This includes the spinal nerve roots, cranial nerves, and peripheral nerves. Most neuropathies arise from damage to or irritation of either the axons or their myelin sheaths. This slows or fully blocks the passage of electrical signals. The various types of peripheral neuropathy are classified according to the site and distribution of damage. For example, damage to sensory nerve fibers may cause numbness and tingling, sensations of cold, or pain that often starts in the hands and feet and spreads toward the central body. Damage to motor nerve fibers may cause muscle weakness and muscle wasting. Damage to the nerves of the autonomic nervous system may result in blurred vision, impaired or absent sweating, fluctuations in blood pressure (and associated syncope), GI disorders, incontinence, and impotence.

Some peripheral neuropathies have no identifiable cause. Others may be related to specific causes, including the following:

- Diabetes
- Dietary deficiencies (especially of the B vitamins)
- Alcoholism
- Uremia
- Lead poisoning
- Drug intoxication
- Viral infection (e.g., Guillain-Barré syndrome)
- Rheumatoid arthritis
- Systemic lupus erythematosus
- Malignant tumors (e.g., lung cancer)
- Lymphomas
- Leukemias
- Inherited neuropathies (e.g., peroneal muscular atrophy)

When possible, management is aimed at the underlying cause (e.g., blood glucose control in a diabetic patient, improved nutrition). If management is successful and the cell bodies of the damaged nerves have not been destroyed, full recovery from the neuropathy is possible.

SPINA BIFIDA

Spina bifida is a congenital defect in which part of one or more vertebrae fails to develop completely. This leaves a portion of the spinal cord exposed. The condition can occur anywhere on the spine. However, it is most common in the lower back. Although the cause is unknown, spina bifida occurs in about 1 in 1000 births. An estimated 166,000 people in the United States are living with this birth defect.[32] It is more likely to occur with extremes of maternal age. A woman who has given birth to one child with spina bifida is 10 times more likely than the average woman to give birth to another affected child (indicating the need for genetic counseling).

Types of Spina Bifida. The severity of spina bifida depends on how much nerve tissue is exposed after the neural tube has closed. The four types of spina bifida are *spina bifida occulta, meningocele, myelomeningocele,* and *encephalocele.* Currently the condition has no cure. Treatment includes surgery, medications, and physical therapy. Most patients with spina bifida live into adulthood.

Spina bifida occulta is the most common and least serious form. There is little external evidence of the defect. Meningocele (Figure 25-17, *A*) is a type of spina bifida in which the nerve tissue of the spinal cord usually is intact and covered with a membranous sac of skin. Meningocele usually does not cause functional problems. However, it

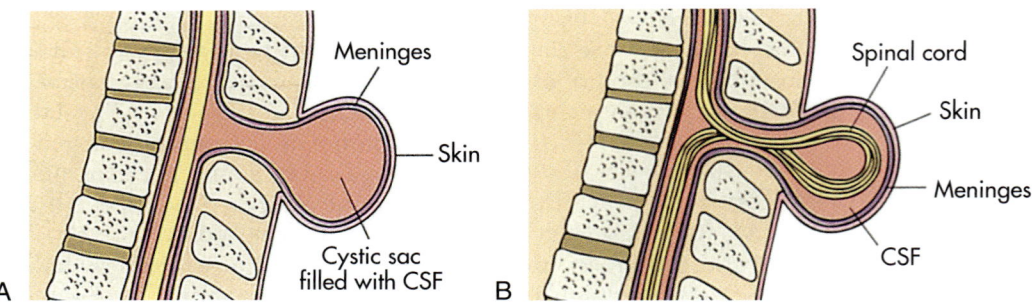

FIGURE 25-17 A, Meningocele. **B,** Myelomeningocele.

requires surgical repair early in life. Myelomeningocele (Figure 25-17, *B*) is the severest form of spina bifida. The child often is severely handicapped. This type of spina bifida is marked by a raw swelling over the spine and a malformed spinal cord that may or may not be contained in a membranous sac. The legs of these children often are deformed. Also, the condition causes partial or complete paralysis and loss of sensation in all areas below the level of the defect. Associated abnormalities of myelomeningocele include hydrocephalus (excess CSF in the skull) with brain damage, cerebral palsy, epilepsy, and developmental delay. In the fourth and very rare type of spina bifida, encephalocele, the protrusion occurs through the skull. Severe brain damage is common with this condition.

POLIO

Polio **(poliomyelitis)** is caused by the poliovirus. The virus attacks with variable severity. It may range from an infection that is not very apparent, to a febrile illness without neurological aftereffects, to aseptic meningitis, and finally to paralytic disease (including respiratory paralysis) and possibly death. The incidence of polio has declined in the United States, Canada, and Europe since the development of the Salk and Sabin vaccines in the 1950s. However, the disease may affect nonimmune adults and indigent children from other countries. It remains a serious risk for any unvaccinated individual traveling in southern Europe, Africa, or Asia. Polio vaccinations are given during infancy. In the United States, they usually are given in doses at 2, 14, and 18 months of age. An optional extra dose may be given at 6 months and a booster dose at 5 years.

CRITICAL THINKING
Ask your older friends or relatives about their memories of the polio epidemic. How did it affect their lives?

People infected with the poliovirus can pass large amounts of the virus in their feces. The virus then may be spread directly or indirectly to others by fingers-to-food transmission and by airborne transmission. Signs and symptoms of polio differ in the nonparalytic and paralytic

forms. Fever, headache, sore throat, and malaise are common to both forms. However, the paralytic form of polio also is associated with generalized pain, weakness, muscle spasms, and paralysis of limbs and other muscles. If the infection spreads to the brainstem, the person may find it difficult or may be unable to swallow or breathe. A full recovery can be made from nonparalytic polio. Of those who become paralyzed, more than half eventually make a full recovery. Some patients may develop "postpolio deterioration." They may have new weakness and pain from recovered muscles. The disease is confirmed through CSF analysis, throat culture, or testing of fecal samples.

DIFFERENTIAL DIAGNOSIS OF NEUROLOGICAL DISORDERS

The key process in differentiating among the many neurological disorders is first to consider which disorders are most likely and most dangerous. Signs and symptoms of the various disorders often overlap, making a diagnosis difficult. Also, in many cases little correlation exists between a patient's pain and the seriousness of the condition.

The differential diagnosis begins with a thorough patient history and a detailed physical examination. This assessment, combined with personal experience, can help the paramedic identify signs and symptoms of the primary illness. To review, major neurological conditions include:

- Headache disorders (e.g., migraine, cluster headache, tension headache)
- Seizure disorders
- Neurodegenerative disorders (Alzheimer's disease, Parkinson's disease, Huntington's disease, ALS [Lou Gehrig's disease])
- Cerebrovascular disease (e.g., TIA and stroke)
- Cerebral palsy
- Infections of the brain (encephalitis), brain meninges (meningitis), and spinal cord
- Infections of the peripheral nervous system
- Neoplasms and tumors of the brain and its meninges (brain tumors), spinal cord tumors, and tumors of the peripheral nerves (neuromas)

- Movement disorders (e.g., Parkinson's disease, Huntington's disease)
- Demyelinating diseases of the CNS (e.g., MS) and of the peripheral nervous system (e.g., Guillain-Barré syndrome)
- Spinal cord disorders (tumors, infection, trauma, malformations)

- Disorders of the peripheral nerves, muscle (myopathy), and neuromuscular junctions
- Traumatic injuries to the brain, spinal cord, and peripheral nerves
- Altered mental status, encephalopathy, stupor, and coma
- Speech and language disorders

SUMMARY

- The body's ability to maintain a state of balance *(homeostasis)* results from the nervous system's regulatory and coordinating activities. The vertebral arteries and the internal carotid arteries supply blood to the brain.
- Neurological emergencies may be related to structural changes or damage, circulatory changes, or alterations in intracranial pressure that affect cerebral blood flow.
- Cerebral blood flow depends on the cerebral perfusion pressure. The CPP decreases when the mean arterial pressure drops or when the intracranial pressure rises (CPP = MAP − ICP).
- The primary survey begins by determining the patient's level of consciousness and by ensuring an open and patent airway. Key elements of the physical examination that may provide clues to the nature of the neurological emergency include the patient history, the history of the event, vital signs, and respiratory patterns.
- The neurological exam may include assessment of AVPU, the Glasgow Coma Scale score, posturing or paralysis, reflexes, pupil size and response, and extraocular movements.
- *Coma* is an abnormally deep state of unconsciousness. The patient cannot be aroused from this state by external stimuli. In general, two mechanisms produce coma: structural lesions and toxic/metabolic states.
- *Stroke* is a sudden interruption in blood flow to the brain that results in a neurological deficit. Strokes can be classified as ischemic strokes or hemorrhagic strokes. A stroke scale is used to assess for the presence of stroke. Rapid transport to a stroke resource center (if available) is indicated.
- A *seizure* is a brief alteration in behavior or consciousness. It is caused by abnormal electrical activity of one or more groups of neurons in the brain. In the prehospital setting, determining the cause of a seizure is not as important as other measures. These include managing the complications and recognizing whether the seizure is reversible with therapy (e.g., it is caused by hypoglycemia).
- The four fairly common types of headaches are tension headaches, migraines, cluster headaches, and sinus headaches.

- A CNS tumor, or *neoplasm,* is a mass in the cranial cavity or spinal cord. This mass can be either malignant or benign. Heredity may play a role in the development of brain tumors. They also are associated with several risk factors. These include exposure to radiation, tobacco use, dietary habits, some viruses, and the use of some medications.
- A *brain abscess* is a buildup of purulent material (pus) surrounded by a capsule within the brain. It develops from a bacterial infection. The infection often starts in the nasal cavity, middle ear, or mastoid bone.
- Dementia is a slow, progressive loss of awareness of time and place. Alzheimer's disease is the most common cause of dementia. Pick's disease is another type of dementia. It is associated with language disturbance.
- Huntington's disease causes degeneration of neurons in the brain. This causes uncontrolled movements and intellectual and emotional impairment.
- Creutzfeldt-Jakob disease is characterized by rapid progression of dementia.
- Muscular dystrophy is an inherited muscle disorder. The cause is unknown. The disease is marked by a slow but progressive degeneration of muscle fibers.
- Damage to the white matter of the brain in multiple sclerosis may lead to fatigue, vertigo, clumsiness, unsteady gait, slurred speech, blurred or double vision, and facial numbness or pain.
- Guillain-Barré syndrome is an autoimmune disorder. It causes muscle weakness, which progresses to paralysis that includes the muscles of respiration.
- The term *dystonia* refers to local or diffuse changes in muscle tone. These may cause painful muscle spasms, unusually fixed postures, and strange movement patterns.
- Parkinson's disease usually begins as a slight tremor in one hand, arm, or leg. In the later stages, the disease affects both sides of the body, causing stiffness, weakness, and trembling of the muscles.
- The term *central pain syndrome* refers to infection or disease of the trigeminal nerve. This causes intense pain of the face.
- Acoustic neuroma is a noncancerous tumor that affects the acoustic nerve (cranial nerve VII). It impairs balance and hearing.

- Glossopharyngeal neuralgia is an irritation of the glossopharyngeal nerve (cranial nerve IX) that causes pain in the ear, nose, and throat.
- Hemifacial spasm results in involuntary contractions of muscles on one side of the face.
- *Bell's palsy* is paralysis of the facial muscles. It is caused by inflammation of the facial nerve (cranial nerve VII). The condition usually is one-sided and temporary. It often develops suddenly.
- Amyotrophic lateral sclerosis is also called *Lou Gehrig's disease.* It is one of a group of rare nervous system disorders. In these disorders, the nerves that control muscular activity degenerate in the brain and spinal cord.

- Peripheral neuropathies usually arise from damage to or irritation of either the axons or their myelin sheaths. This slows or fully blocks the passage of electrical signals.
- *Spina bifida* is a congenital defect in which part of one or more vertebrae fail to develop completely. This leaves a portion of the spinal cord exposed.
- Polio is caused by a virus. The severity of the disease can range from unapparent infection, to a febrile illness without neurological aftereffects, to aseptic meningitis, and finally to paralytic disease and possibly death.

REFERENCES

1. Magistretti P, Pellerin L, Martin J-L: *Brain energy metabolism: an integrated cellular perspective.* www.acnp.org/g4/GN401000064/CH064.HTML. Accessed August 23, 2010.
2. Bourgoing A, Leone M, Delmas A, et al: Increasing mean arterial pressure in patients with septic shock: effects on oxygen variables and renal function, *Crit Care Med* 33:780-786, 2005.
3. Gabriel E, Ghajar J, Jagoda A, et al: Guidelines for prehospital management of traumatic brain injury, Brain Trauma Foundation, *J Neurotrauma* 19:111-174, 2002.
4. Vinkin PJ, Bruyn GW, Klawans HL, et al, editors: *Handbook of clinical neurology, vascular diseases,* Part III, Amsterdam, 1989, Elsevier Science.
5. Marx JA, Hockberger R, Walls R: *Rosen's emergency medicine: concepts and clinical practice,* ed 6, Philadelphia, 2006, Mosby.
6. Menon S, Bharadwaj R, Chowdhary A, et al: Current epidemiology of intracranial abscess: a prospective 5-year study, *J Med Microbiol* 57(Part 10):1259-1268, 2008.
7. Young GB, Wijdicks E, editors: *Disorders of consciousness: handbook of clinical neurology,* Edinburgh, 2008, Elsevier.
8. American Heart Association: *Heart disease stroke statistics: 2010 update at a glance.* www.americanheart.org/downloadable/heart/1265665152970DS-3241%20Heart StrokeUpdate_2010.pdf. Accessed September 20, 2010.
9. Mohr JP, Choi D, Grotta J, et al: *Stroke: pathophysiology, diagnosis, and management,* ed 4, New York, 2004, Churchill Livingstone.
10. American Heart Association, Advanced Cardiac Life Support Provider Manual, Dallas, 2006, The Association.
11. American Heart Association: 2010 American Heart Association guidelines for cardiopulmonary resuscitation and emergency cardiovascular care, *Circulation* 122(18 suppl):S639-S946, 2010.
12. National Institute of Neurological Disorders and Stroke: *Arteriovenous malformation information page.* www.ninds.nih.gov/disorders/avms/avms.htm. Accessed September 23, 2010.
13. American Heart Association: 2010 American Heart Association Guidelines for Cardiopulmonary Resuscitation and Emergency Cardiovascular Care, *Circulation* 122(18 Supplement 3):S639-S946, 2010.
14. The Joint Commission: *Primary stroke centers: primary stroke center certification.* www.jointcommission.org/Certification Programs/PrimaryStrokeCenters. Accessed August 23, 2010.
15. Kothari R, Hall K, Brott T, et al: Early stroke recognition: developing an out-of-hospital stroke scale, *Acad Emerg Med* 4:986, 1997.
16. Epilepsy Foundation: *Epilepsy and seizure statistics.* www.epilepsyfoundation.org/about/statistics.cfm. Accessed August 23, 2010.
17. Saneto R, Sotero de Menezes MA, Ojemann JG, et al: Vagus nerve stimulation for intractable seizures in children, *Pediatr Neurol* 35:323-326, 2006.
18. American College of Emergency Physicians (ACEP) Clinical Policies Committee, Clinical Policies Subcommittee on Seizure: Clinical policy: critical issues in the evaluation of adult patients presenting to the emergency department with seizures, *Ann Emerg Med* 43:605-625, 2004.
19. Rosen P, Barkin R: *Emergency medicine: concepts and clinical practice,* ed 6, St Louis, 2006, Mosby.
20. McCance K, Huether S: *Pathophysiology: the biologic basis for disease in adults and children,* ed 6, St Louis, 2006, Mosby.
21. National Highway Traffic Safety Administration. *The National EMS Education Standards,* Washington, DC, 2009, U.S. Department of Transportation/National Highway Traffic Safety Administration, DOT.
22. Alzheimer's Association: 2010 *Alzheimer's disease facts and figures.* www.alz.org/documents_custom/report_alzfactsfigures2010.pdf. Accessed September 20, 2010.
23. National Institute of Neurological Disorders and Stroke: *Frontotemporal dementia information page.* www.ninds.nih.gov/disorders/picks/picks.htm. Accessed August 23, 2010.
24. Huntington's Disease Society of America: www.hdsa.org/. Accessed August 23, 2010.
25. National Institute of Neurological Disorders and Stroke: *Creutzfeldt-Jakob disease fact sheet.* www.ninds.nih.gov/disorders/cjd/detail_cjd.htm. Accessed August 23, 2010.
26. Centers for Disease Control and Prevention: *About CJD.* www.cdc.gov/ncidod/dvrd/cjd/. Accessed August 23, 2010.
27. Centers for Disease Control and Prevention: *Single gene disorders and disability.* www.cdc.gov/ncbddd/duchenne/who.htm. Accessed August 23, 2010.
28. National Multiple Sclerosis Society: *FAQs about MS.* www.nationalmssociety.org/about-multiple-sclerosis/what-we-know-about-ms/faqs-about-ms/index.aspx. Accessed August 23, 2010.
29. National Institute of Neurological Disorders and Stroke: *Guillain-Barré syndrome fact sheet.* www.ninds.nih.gov/disorders/gbs/gbs.htm. Accessed August 23, 2010.

30. National Parkinson Foundation: *About Parkinson's disease.* www.parkinson.org/Page.aspx?pid=225. Accessed August 23, 2010.

31. Gilden D: Clinical practice: Bell's palsy, *N Engl J Med* 351:1323-1331, 2004.

32. Spina Bifida Association: *How many people with spina bifida are there in the United States?* www.spinabifidaassociation.org/site/c.liKWL7PLLrF/b.2700311/k.13CB/How_Many_People_With_Spina_Bifida_In_The_US.htm. Accessed August 23, 2010.

SUGGESTED READINGS

National Association of EMS Physicians: NAEMSP position statement: the role of EMS in the management of acute stroke—triage, treatment, and stroke systems, *Prehosp Emerg Care* 11:312, 2007.

National Association of EMS Physicians: EMS management of acute stroke: out-of-hospital treatment and stroke system development (resource document to NAEMSP position statement), *Prehosp Emerg Care* 11:318-325, 2007.

Phrampus PE: CNS infections, *JEMS* 31:62-70, 2006.

CHAPTER
26 Endocrinology

OBJECTIVES

Upon completion of this chapter, the paramedic student will be able to:

1. Describe how hormones secreted from endocrine glands help the body maintain homeostasis.
2. Describe the anatomy and physiology of the pancreas and the ways its hormones maintain normal glucose metabolism.
3. Discuss pathophysiology as a basis for key signs and symptoms, patient assessment, and patient management for diabetes and diabetic emergencies of hypoglycemia, diabetic ketoacidosis, and hyperosmolar hyperglycemic nonketotic syndrome.

4. Discuss pathophysiology as a basis for key signs and symptoms, patient assessment, and patient management for disorders of the thyroid gland.
5. Discuss pathophysiology as a basis for key signs and symptoms, patient assessment, and management of emergencies related to Cushing's syndrome and Addison's disease.

KEY TERMS

acetate A byproduct of fatty acids in the liver.

Addison's disease A rare and potentially life-threatening disorder caused by a deficiency of the corticosteroid hormones normally produced by the adrenal cortex.

Cushing's syndrome A condition caused by an abnormally high circulating level of corticosteroid hormones produced naturally by the adrenal glands.

diabetes insipidus (DI) A metabolic disorder characterized by extreme polyuria and polydipsia that is caused by deficient production or secretion of antidiuretic hormone or inability of the kidney tubules to respond to antidiuretic hormone.

diabetes mellitus A complex disorder of carbohydrate, fat, and protein metabolism. It primarily results from a partial or complete lack of insulin secretion by the beta cells of the pancreas or from defects in the insulin receptors.

diabetic ketoacidosis An acute, life-threatening complication of uncontrolled diabetes characterized by hyperglycemia, hypovolemia, electrolyte imbalance, and a breakdown of free fatty acids, causing acidosis; also known as *diabetic coma.*

endocrine glands Glands that secrete chemicals and hormones directly into the blood rather than through a duct.

exocrine glands Glands that secrete chemicals and hormones into a duct.

gestational diabetes mellitus A disorder characterized by impaired ability to metabolize carbohydrates, usually caused by a deficiency of insulin; it occurs in pregnancy and disappears after delivery but in some cases returns years later.

glucagon A hormone produced by the alpha cells in the islets of Langerhans that stimulates the conversion of glycogen to glucose in the liver.

gluconeogenesis The formation of glycogen from fatty acids and proteins rather than carbohydrates.

glycogenolysis The breakdown of glycogen to glucose.

Graves' disease A type of excessive thyroid activity characterized by generalized enlargement of the gland (goiter) that leads to a swollen neck and often to protruding eyes (exophthalmos).

growth hormone (GH) A polypeptide hormone produced and secreted by the anterior pituitary gland; it acts as an insulin antagonist.

hormones Substances, usually a peptide or a steroid, produced by one tissue and conveyed by the bloodstream to another to effect physiological activity, such as growth or metabolism.

hormone receptors Receptors on target organs and body tissues that are able to respond to a particular hormone.

hyperglycemia A greater than normal amount of glucose in the blood.

hyperosmolar hyperglycemic nonketotic syndrome (HHNS) A diabetic state in which the level of ketone bodies is normal. It is caused by hyperosmolarity of extracellular fluid and results in dehydration of intracellular fluid.

hypoglycemia A lower than normal amount of glucose in the blood.

insulin A hormone secreted by the pancreatic islets.

ketogenesis The formation or production of ketone bodies.

ketone bodies The normal metabolic products of lipid and pyruvate within the liver; excessive production leads to their excretion in the urine.

myxedema A condition that results from a deficiency of thyroid hormone.

nonsteroid hormones Hormones synthesized chiefly from amino acids, such as insulin, parathyroid hormone, and others.

steroid hormones Hormones synthesized by endocrine cells from cholesterol; they include cortisol, aldosterone, estrogen, progesterone, and testosterone.

thyroid storm A life-threatening form of hyperthyroidism.

thyrotoxicosis Any toxic condition that results from thyroid hyperfunction.

type 1 diabetes Diabetes characterized by inadequate production of insulin by the pancreas. It may occur any time after birth and requires lifelong treatment with insulin.

type 2 diabetes Diabetes usually characterized by a decrease in the production of insulin by the pancreatic beta cells and diminished tissue sensitivity to insulin (insulin resistance).

The endocrine system and the nervous system allow the body to regulate many functions and to communicate among millions of cells. Paramedics encounter many patients with endocrine system disorders. These disorders can range from minor changes in functioning to life-threatening conditions.

ANATOMY AND PHYSIOLOGY OF THE ENDOCRINE SYSTEM

As described in Chapter 10, the endocrine system is composed of ductless glands and tissues that produce and secrete **hormones.** The major endocrine glands are the pituitary, thyroid, and parathyroid glands; the adrenal cortex and medulla; the pancreatic islets; and the ovaries and testes (Figure 26-1 and Table 26-1). Other specialized groups of cells that secrete hormones are found in the kidneys and the mucosa of the gastrointestinal (GI) tract.

LOOK AGAIN
See Chapter 10: Review of Human Systems, pp. 177-183.

Endocrine Gland Functions

Endocrine glands secrete hormones directly into the bloodstream and regulate various metabolic functions. The products of endocrine glands travel via the blood (or tissue fluids). They therefore are able to exert their effects at widespread sites, often distant from their source. The endocrine hormones are released in response to a change in the cellular environment; to maintain a normal level (i.e., homeostasis) of hormones or other substances; or to stimulate or inhibit organ functions. This integrated chemical and coordination system enables reproduction, growth and development, and the regulation of energy. Target organs and body

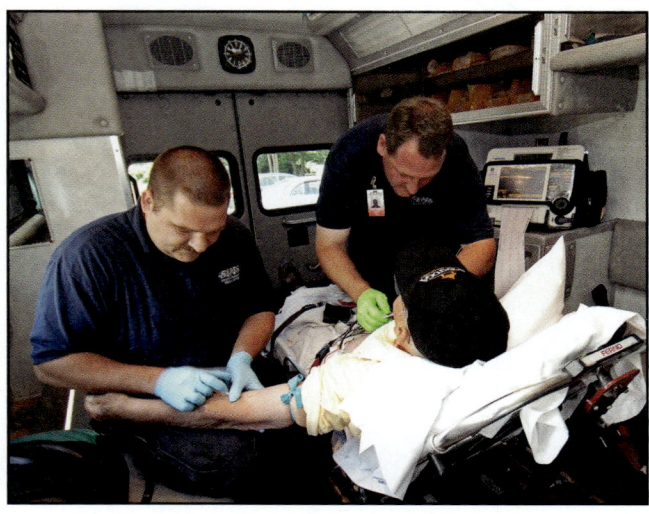

(Courtesy Ray Kemp, St. Charles, Mo.)

tissues have **hormone receptors** and are able to respond to a particular hormone.

CRITICAL THINKING
How are hormones and their target organs like a lock and key?

HORMONE RECEPTORS

Most hormones can be categorized as proteins, polypeptides, derivatives of amino acids, or lipids. As shown in Table 26-1, each hormone may affect a specific organ or tissue or can have a general effect on the entire body. Hormones also may be classified as *steroid* or *nonsteroid*. **Steroid hormones** are synthesized by endocrine cells from cholesterol. They include cortisol, aldosterone, estrogen, progesterone, and testosterone. **Nonsteroid hormones** are synthesized chiefly from amino acids. These hormones include insulin, parathyroid hormone, and others.

Hormones affect only cells with appropriate receptors. They act on these cells to initiate specific cell functions or activities. Hormone receptor sites may be on the outside of

TABLE 26-1 Review of Endocrine Glands, Hormones, and Effects of Improper Function

Endocrine Gland	Location/Description	Hormones Produced	Gland/Hormone Function	Effects of Improper Function
Hypothalamus	Lower middle of the brain	Growth hormone–releasing hormone (GHRH) Thyrotropin-releasing hormone (TRH) Corticotropin-releasing hormone (CRH) Gonadotropin-releasing hormone (GnRH) Prolactin inhibitory factor (PIF; dopamine)	Communicates with both nervous and endocrine systems Stimulates (GHRH, TRH, CRH, GnRH) or inhibits (PIF) hormone production in the pituitary	Early puberty Thyroid diseases
		Oxytocin (OT)	Uterine contraction during labor	
		Antidiuretic hormone (ADH), also called arginine vasopressin (AVP)	Water balance	Diabetes insipidus
Pituitary	Inferior to hypothalamus, posterior to sinus cavity	Prolactin (PRL)	Milk production	Hypopituitarism Galactorrhea (milk production outside of pregnancy and normal breastfeeding because of high prolactin level)
		Growth hormone (GH)	Bone growth	Acromegaly or gigantism Growth hormone deficiency
		Adrenocorticotrophic hormone (ACTH)	Stimulates cortisol	Cushing's disease
		Thyroid-stimulating hormone (TSH)	Stimulates thyroid hormone	Hyperthyroidism/hypothyroidism
		Luteinizing hormone (LH), follicle-stimulating hormone (FSH)	Regulation of testosterone and estrogen, fertility	Loss of menstrual period Loss of sex drive Infertility
Thyroid	Butterfly-shaped gland that lies flat against trachea in the anterior neck	T4 (thyroxine) T3 (triiodothyronine)	Helps regulate rate of metabolism	Thyroid diseases (including hypothyroidism and hyperthyroidism)
		Calcitonin	Helps regulate bone status, blood calcium	
Parathyroid	Four tiny glands located posterior, adjacent to, or inferior to the thyroid	Parathyroid hormone (PTH)	Regulate blood calcium	Hyperparathyroidism Hypoparathyroidism
Adrenal	Two triangular glands, each located superior to a kidney	Epinephrine (adrenaline) Norepinephrine	Blood pressure regulation, stress reaction	Pheochromocytoma (adrenal tumor results in elevated levels of epinephrine and norepinephrine)
		Aldosterone	Salt, water balance	Cushing's syndrome
		Cortisol	Stress reaction	Addison's disease
Ovaries (females only)	Two glands located in the pelvis	Estrogen Progesterone	Female sex characteristics	Polycystic ovary syndrome
Testes (males only)	Two glands located in the scrotum	Testosterone	Male sex characteristics	Hypogonadism
Pancreas	Large, gourd-shaped gland located posterior to the stomach and between the spleen and duodenum	Insulin Glucagon Somatostatin	Glucose regulation	Diabetes mellitus Zollinger-Ellison syndrome
Pineal	Inferior and posterior to the thalamus	Melatonin	Not well understood; helps control sleep patterns, affects reproduction; involved in stress response	

From http://www.endocrineweb.com/endocrinology/conditions/endocrine/endocrine_3.html. Accessed August 24, 2010.

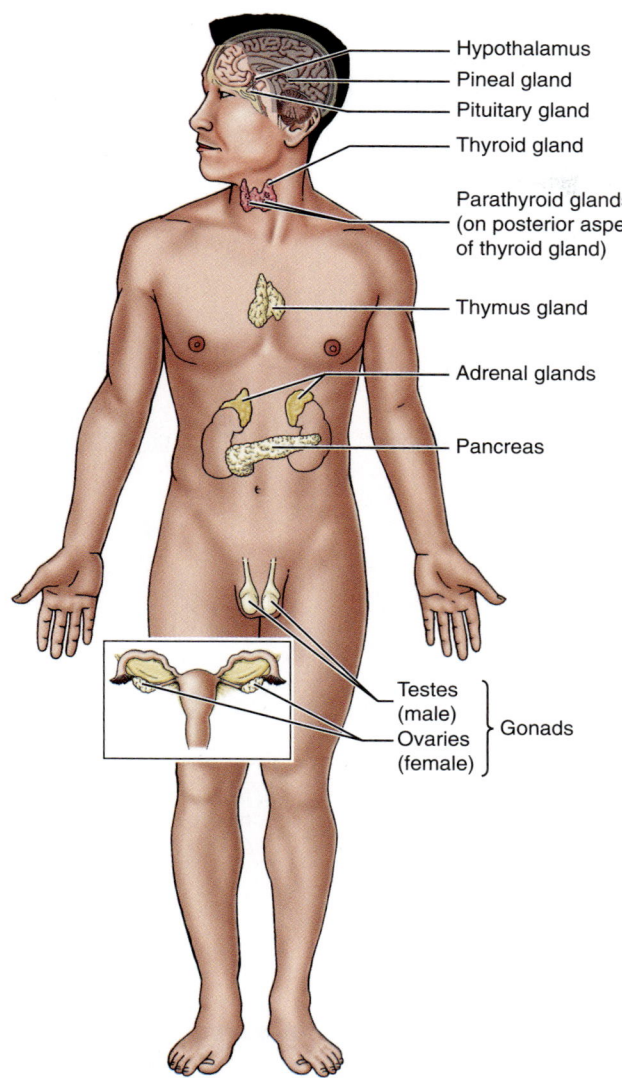

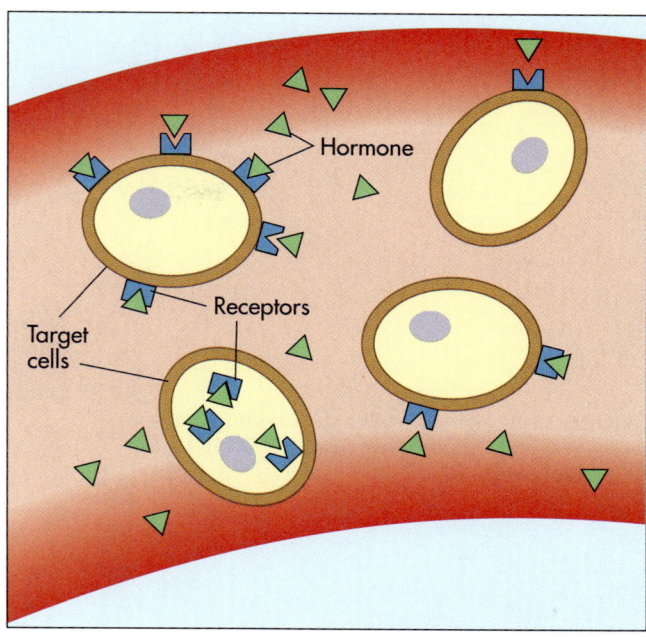

FIGURE 26-2 Target cell concept. Cells with fewer receptor sites bind with less hormone than cells with many receptor sites.

FIGURE 26-1 Major endocrine glands. (Herlihy B: *The human body in health and illness,* ed 3, St Louis, 2007, Saunders.)

the cell membrane or in the interior of the cell. Cells with fewer receptor sites bind with less hormone than cells with many receptor sites (Figure 26-2). In addition, abnormalities in the presence or absence of specific hormone receptors can result in endocrine disorders.

Regulation of Hormone Secretion

All hormones operate with feedback systems. These systems are either positive or negative. The feedback systems help maintain the optimum internal environment. An example of positive feedback can be found in childbirth. The hormone *oxytocin* stimulates and enhances labor contractions. As the baby moves toward the birth canal, pressure receptors in the cervix send messages to the brain to secrete oxytocin. Oxytocin travels to the uterus through the bloodstream. It stimulates the muscles in the uterine wall to contract more strongly. The contractions intensify and

increase until the baby is delivered. When the stimulus to the pressure receptors ends, oxytocin secretion stops. Uterine contractions also stop.

Negative feedback (Figure 26-3) is the mechanism most commonly used to maintain homeostasis. For example, after a person eats a candy bar, the following occurs:

1. Glucose from the ingested lactose or sucrose is absorbed in the intestine. Consequently, the level of glucose in the blood rises.
2. The increase in the blood glucose concentration stimulates the pancreas to release insulin. Insulin facilitates the entry of glucose into the cells. As a result, the blood glucose level falls.
3. When the blood glucose level has dropped sufficiently, the endocrine cells in the pancreas stop producing and releasing insulin.

Another example is the hypothalamus receptors that monitor blood levels of thyroid hormones. Low blood levels of thyroid-stimulating hormone (TSH) cause the release of TSH-releasing hormone from the hypothalamus. This causes the release of TSH from the anterior pituitary. TSH travels to the thyroid. There, it promotes the production of thyroid hormones, which regulate the metabolic rate and body temperature.

> **NOTE**
> Negative feedback loops can be distinguished from positive feedback loops in a relatively simple way:
> 1. Negative feedback typically attempts to bring the system/body back toward its normal state (i.e., homeostasis).
> 2. Positive feedback tends to push the system/body away from normal.

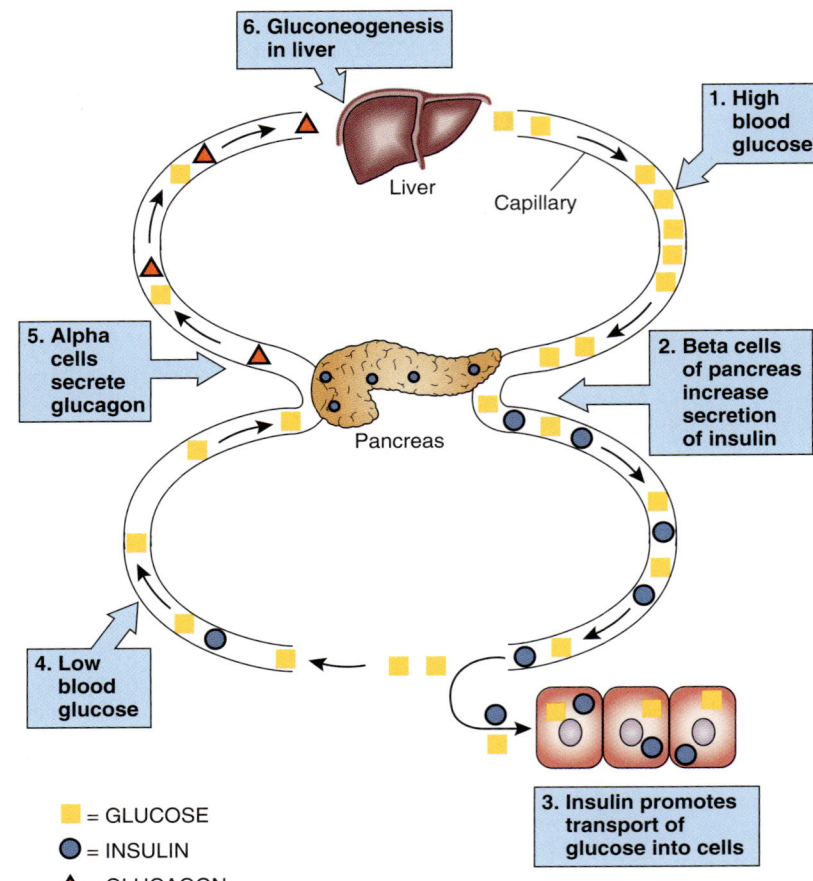

FIGURE 26-3 Negative feedback. (Gould BE: *Pathophysiology for the health professions,* ed 3, St Louis, 2006, Saunders.)

■ = GLUCOSE
● = INSULIN
▲ = GLUCAGON

SPECIFIC DISORDERS OF THE ENDOCRINE SYSTEM

Disorders of the endocrine system arise from the effects of an imbalance in the production of one or more hormones. They also arise from the effects of a change in the body's ability to use the hormones produced. The clinical effects of endocrine gland disorders are determined by the degree of dysfunction. They also are determined by the age and gender of the affected person. The specific disorders of the endocrine system presented in this chapter are presented in Table 26-2.

DISORDERS OF THE PANCREAS: DIABETES MELLITUS

Diabetes mellitus is a systemic disease of the endocrine system. It usually results from a dysfunction of the pancreas. It is a complex disorder of fat, carbohydrate, and protein metabolism that affects more than 24 million adults in the United States. It is estimated that another 57 million people have *prediabetes* (described later).[1] Diabetes mellitus is potentially lethal. It can put the patient at risk for several kinds of true medical emergencies.

TABLE 26-2 Specific Disorders of the Endocrine System

Gland	Disorder
Pancreas	Diabetes mellitus (types 1 and 2)
	Hyperosmolar hyperglycemic nonketotic syndrome (HHNS)
Thyroid	Hyperthyroidism
	Hypothyroidism
	Myxedema
	Thyroid storm
	Thyrotoxicosis
Adrenal	Addison's disease
	Cushing's syndrome

Anatomy and Physiology of the Pancreas

The pancreas is important in the absorption and use of carbohydrates, fat, and protein. It is the chief regulator of glucose levels in the blood. The pancreas is located retroperitoneally, adjacent to the duodenum on the right and extending to the spleen on the left. As described in Chapter

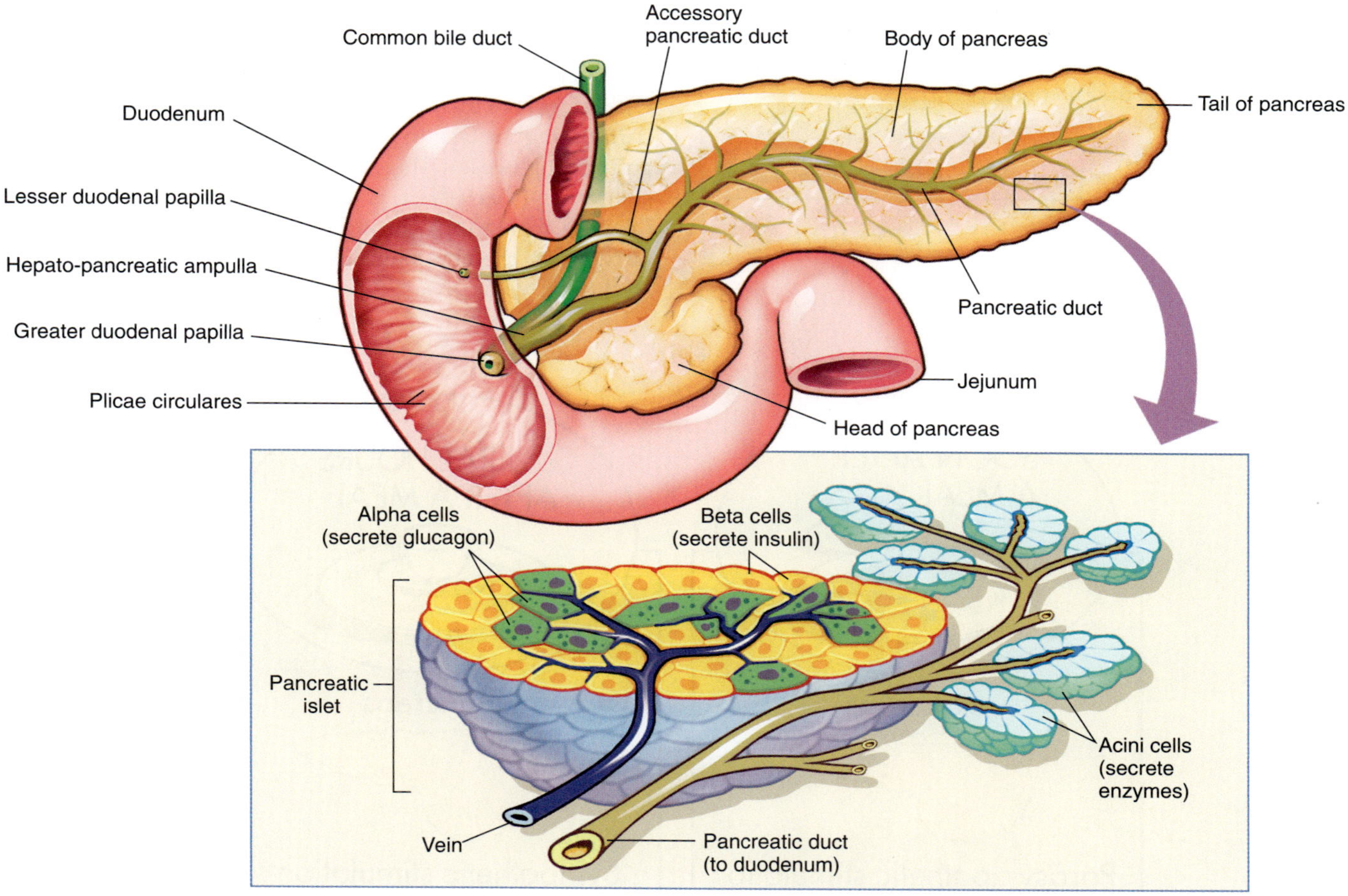

Common bile duct

Accessory pancreatic duct

Body of pancreas

Duodenum

Tail of pancreas

Lesser duodenal papilla

Hepato-pancreatic ampulla

Greater duodenal papilla

Plicae circulares

Pancreatic duct

Jejunum

Head of pancreas

Alpha cells (secrete glucagon)

Beta cells (secrete insulin)

Pancreatic islet

Acini cells (secrete enzymes)

Vein

Pancreatic duct (to duodenum)

FIGURE 26-4 Two pancreatic islets (islets of Langerhans), or hormone-producing areas, are evident among the pancreatic cells that produce the pancreatic digestive juice. (Patton KT, Thibodeau GA: *Anatomy and physiology*, ed 7, St Louis, 2010, Mosby.)

10, a healthy pancreas has exocrine and endocrine functions. To review, **exocrine glands** secrete substances through a duct onto the inner surface of an organ or the outer surface of the body. **Endocrine glands** secrete chemicals directly (not through a duct) into the bloodstream. The exocrine portion consists of *acini* (glands that produce pancreatic juice) and a duct system. The duct system carries the pancreatic fluids to the small intestine. The endocrine portion consists of pancreatic islets *(islets of Langerhans)* that produce hormones (Figure 26-4).

ISLETS OF LANGERHANS AND PANCREATIC HORMONES

About 500,000 to 1 million pancreatic islets are dispersed among the ducts and acini of the pancreas. Each islet is composed of beta cells, alpha cells, and delta cells. The beta cells produce and secrete insulin. The alpha cells produce and secrete glucagon. Delta cells produce and secrete the hormone somatostatin. This hormone inhibits the secretion of growth hormone and TSH. It also is thought to inhibit the secretion of insulin and glucagon. These

properties of somatostatin act as a buffer to prevent rapid swings in blood glucose levels. Nerves from both divisions of the autonomic nervous system innervate the pancreatic islets, and each islet is surrounded by a well-developed capillary network.

CRITICAL THINKING

Consider that part of a patient's pancreas must be removed as a result of traumatic injury. Will the patient still be able to produce insulin and glucagon?

INSULIN

Insulin is a small protein. It is released by the beta cells when blood glucose levels rise. The main functions of insulin are to increase glucose transport into cells, increase glucose metabolism by cells, increase liver glycogen levels, and decrease the blood glucose concentration toward normal (Box 26-1). Many of the functions of insulin antagonize the effects of glucagon.

BOX 26-1 Primary Functions of Insulin

- Increase glucose transport into cells
- Increase glucose metabolism by cells
- Increase liver glycogen levels
- Decrease blood glucose concentration toward normal levels

GLUCAGON

Glucagon is a protein released by the alpha cells when blood glucose levels fall. Glucagon has two major effects. One effect is to increase blood glucose levels. It does this by stimulating the liver to release glucose stores from glycogen and other glucose storage sites. (This is called **glycogenolysis.**) The other effect is to stimulate **gluconeogenesis** (glucose formation) through the breakdown of fats and fatty acids, thereby maintaining a normal blood glucose level (Figure 26-5).

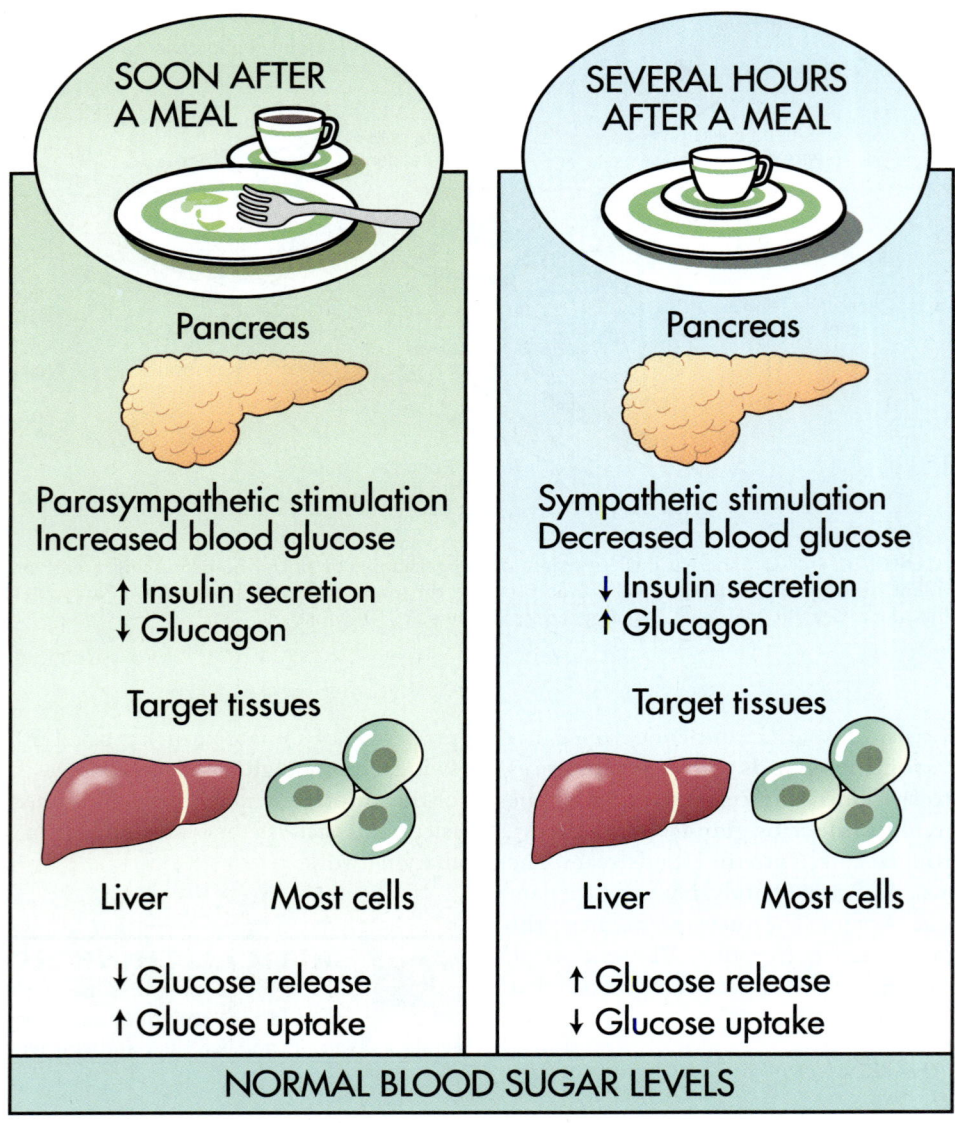

FIGURE 26-5 Regulation of insulin and glucagon secretion. Sympathetic stimulation and decreasing concentrations of glucose increase the secretion of glucagon, which acts primarily on liver cells to increase the rate of glycogen breakdown and the secretion of glucose from the liver. The release of glucose from the liver helps maintain blood glucose levels. Increasing blood glucose levels has an inhibitory effect on glucagon secretion. Increasing concentrations of glucose and amino acids stimulate the beta cells of the islets to secrete insulin. In addition, parasympathetic stimulation causes insulin secretion. Insulin acts on most tissues to increase the uptake of glucose and amino acids. As the blood levels of glucose and amino acids decrease, the rate of insulin secretion also decreases.

NOTE

Glycogenolysis and *gluconeogenesis* can be confusing terms. Glycogenolysis is the *breakdown* of glucose. Gluconeogenesis *generates* "new" glucose. (*Lysis* means to break or lyse; *neo* means new.)

GROWTH HORMONE

Growth hormone (GH) is a polypeptide hormone. It is produced and secreted by the anterior pituitary gland. GH secretion is triggered by many physiological stimuli. These include exercise, stress, sleep, and hypoglycemia. GH acts as an insulin antagonist. It decreases insulin's actions on cell membranes. This reduces the ability of muscles and adipose and liver cells to absorb glucose.

Regulation of Glucose Metabolism

Under normal conditions, the body maintains the serum glucose level in the blood at 60 to 120 mg/dL. (Normal fasting blood glucose is below 100 mg/dL.[1]) A knowledge of food intake and digestion is required to understand glucose metabolism.

DIETARY INTAKE

As described in Chapter 2, the three main organic components of food are carbohydrates, fats, and proteins. (Food also contains minerals and vitamins.) Carbohydrates are found in all sugary, starchy foods. They are a ready source of near-instant energy. They are the first food substances to enter the bloodstream after a meal is ingested. Carbohydrates yield the simple sugar glucose. If not "burned" for immediate energy, glucose is stored in the liver and muscles as glycogen for short-term energy needs, or it is stored in adipose tissue for intermediate and long-term needs.

LOOK AGAIN

See Chapter 2: Well-Being of the Paramedic, pp. 25-28.

PROCESS OF DIGESTION

Before food compounds can be used by body cells, they must be digested and absorbed into the bloodstream. Digestion begins in the mouth. It is accomplished by physical forces (chewing) and chemical (enzymatic) forces. This begins the process that reduces the food to soluble molecules and particles small enough to be absorbed. After food has been swallowed, it enters the stomach. There, various nutrients are absorbed into the circulatory system. These nutrients include glucose, salts, water, and some other substances (alcohol and certain other drugs). The remaining material (chyme) is shunted from the stomach into the intestine for further digestion.

The duodenum signals the release of hormones that mobilize the pancreas to contribute its molecule-splitting enzymes and the gallbladder to release bile salts. These enzymes and salts neutralize acids and help emulsify fats. Carbohydrates are absorbed as simple sugars. Fats are absorbed as fatty acids and glycerol. Proteins are absorbed as amino acids. These nutrients are then carried from the intestine to the liver by way of the portal vein. Water and remaining salts are absorbed from food residues in the colon. The liver synthesizes glycogen from the absorbed glucose, lipoproteins from the absorbed fatty acids, and many proteins required for health from absorbed amino acids.

Carbohydrate Metabolism. The secretion of insulin is controlled by chemical, neural, and hormonal means. An increased blood glucose concentration, parasympathetic stimulation, and GI hormones involved in the regulation of digestion cause the beta cells of the pancreas to release insulin after dietary intake of carbohydrates. Insulin travels through the blood to target tissues. There it combines with specific chemical receptors on the surface of the cell membrane to permit glucose to enter the cell (Table 26-3). This allows the cells to use glucose for energy. It also prevents the breakdown of alternative energy sources (proteins and fat cells). In addition, it promotes the uptake of glucose into the liver, where it is converted to glycogen for storage. This rapid uptake and storage of glucose normally prevents a large increase in blood glucose levels, even just after a normal meal.

CRITICAL THINKING

Why do individuals with diabetes eat carbohydrates instead of protein or fat when they sense that their glucose level is too low?

When the blood glucose level begins to fall, the liver releases glucose back into the circulating blood. Thus the liver removes excess glucose from the blood after a meal. Also, it returns it to the blood when it is needed between meals. Under normal circumstances, about 60% of the glucose in a meal is stored in the liver as glycogen and released later.

If the muscles are not exercised after a meal, much of the glucose transported into the muscle cells by insulin is stored as muscle glycogen. Muscle glycogen differs from liver glycogen. It cannot be reconverted into glucose and released into the circulation. The stored glycogen must be used by the muscle for energy.

The brain is quite different from other body tissues with regard to glucose uptake. Insulin has little or no effect on the uptake or use of glucose by the brain; the cells of the brain do not have adequate storage capacity. Also, because the brain normally uses only glucose for energy, it cannot depend on stored supplies of glycogen. Therefore, it is essential that the serum glucose be maintained at a level that provides adequate energy to these tissues. When the serum glucose level falls too low, signs and symptoms of hypoglycemia can develop quickly. These include progressive irritability, altered mental status, fainting, convulsions, and even coma.

TABLE 26-3   Effects of Insulin and Glucagon on Target Tissues

Target Tissue	Response to Insulin	Response to Glucagon
Skeletal muscle, cardiac muscle, cartilage, bone, fibroblasts, leukocytes, and mammary glands	Increased glucose uptake and glycogen synthesis; increased uptake of certain amino acids	Little effect
Liver	Increased glycogen synthesis; increased use of glucose for energy (glycolysis)	Rapid increase in the breakdown of glycogen to glucose (glycogenolysis) and release of glucose into the blood Increased formation of glucose (gluconeogenesis) from amino acids and, to some degree, from fats Increased metabolism of fatty acids, resulting in increased ketones in the blood
Adipose cells	Increased glucose uptake, glycogen synthesis, fat synthesis, and fatty acid uptake; increased glycolysis	High concentrations cause breakdown of fats (lipolysis); probably unimportant under most conditions
Nervous system	Little effect except to increase glucose uptake in the satiety center	No effect

From Seeley R: *Anatomy and physiology,* ed 2, St Louis, 1992, Mosby.

Fat Metabolism. Only a limited amount of glycogen can be stored in the liver and skeletal muscles. Therefore, one third of any glucose passing through the liver is converted to fatty acids. Under the influence of insulin, fatty acids are converted to triglycerides (storable fats.) They are stored in adipose tissue. In the absence of insulin, the stored fat is broken down. The plasma concentration of free fatty acids rapidly increases. A low level of insulin in the blood can result in high levels of triglycerides and cholesterol (in the form of lipoproteins) in the plasma. This is thought to contribute to the development of atherosclerosis in patients with serious diabetes.[1]

If needed (as in the absence of insulin), fatty acids in the liver can be metabolized and used for energy. A byproduct of the breakdown of fatty acids in the liver is **acetate.** Acetate is converted to acetoacetic acid and beta hydroxybutyric acid. These products are released into the circulating blood as **ketone bodies.** Ketone bodies may cause acidosis and coma (diabetic ketoacidosis) in a diabetic patient.

Protein Metabolism. Insulin causes the storage of proteins in addition to carbohydrates and fats. Through the actions of GH and insulin, amino acids are actively transported into the various cells of the body. Most amino acids are used as building blocks to form new proteins. (This is called *protein synthesis.*) However, some enter the metabolic cycle by being converted to glucose after initial breakdown in the liver.

In the absence of insulin, protein storage stops and protein breakdown (particularly in muscle) begins. This releases large amounts of amino acids into the circulation. The excess amino acids are used directly for energy or as substrates for gluconeogenesis. Degradation of the amino acids leads to increased excretion of urea in the urine. This "protein wasting" has serious effects in diabetes mellitus. It leads to extreme weakness and dysfunction of many organs.

GLUCAGON AND ITS FUNCTIONS

Glucagon has several functions that are the opposite of the functions of insulin. The most important is to increase the blood glucose concentration. Glucagon has two major effects on glucose metabolism. One is the breakdown of liver glycogen (glycogenolysis). The other is the generation of glucose (gluconeogenesis).

As the serum glucose level returns to normal (several hours after dietary intake), insulin secretion decreases with continued fasting. The blood sugar level then begins to drop. As a result, glucagon, cortisol, GH, and epinephrine (from sympathetic stimulation) are secreted. This initiates the release of glucose from glycogen and other glucose-storage sites. Glycogen is converted back to glucose and released into the blood. Uptake of glucose by most tissues helps maintain the blood glucose at levels necessary for normal function (Figure 26-6).

In summary, the four mechanisms for achieving adequate blood glucose regulation are as follows:

1. The liver functions as a blood glucose buffer system. It removes excess glucose from the blood and stores it as glycogen. It also returns glucose to the blood when the glucose concentration and insulin secretion decline.
2. Insulin and glucagon function as a negative feedback control system. They work to maintain normal serum

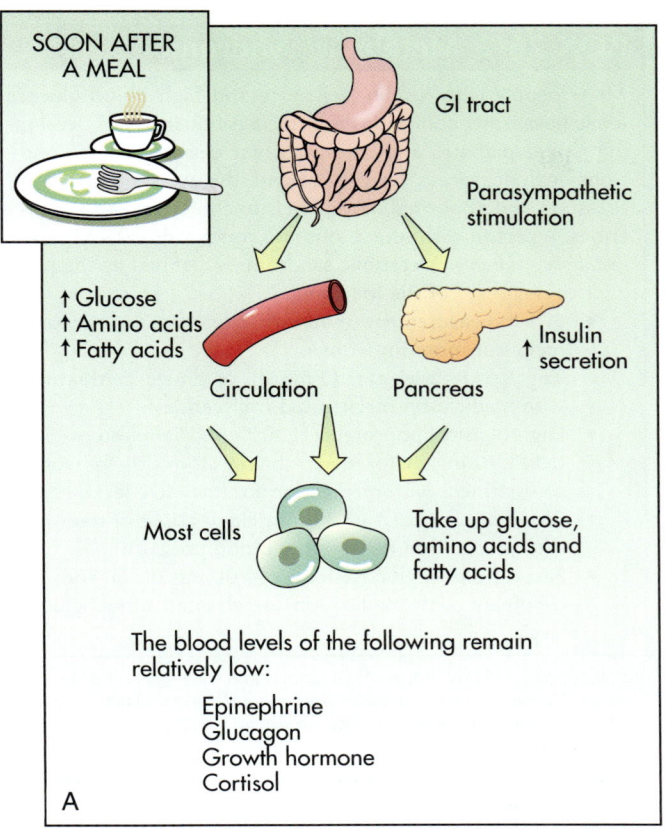

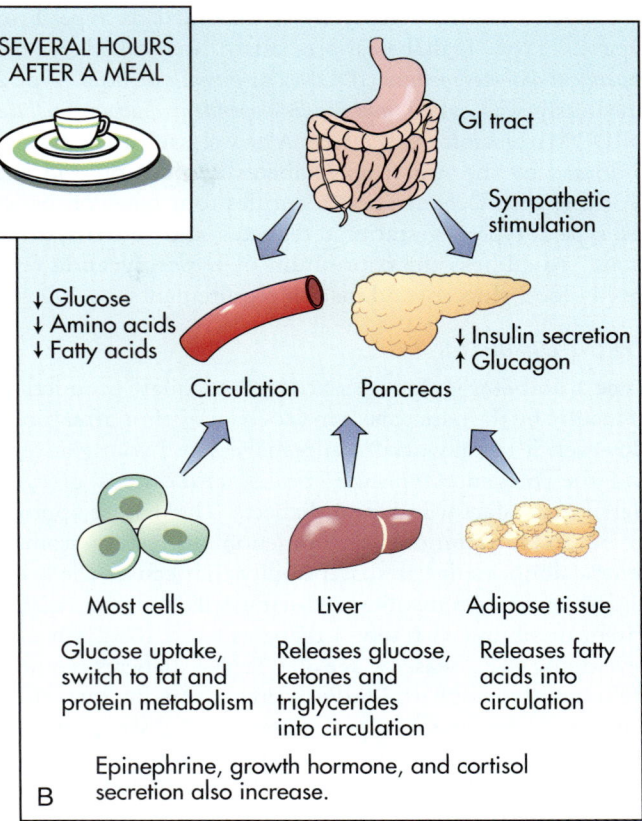

FIGURE 26-6 A, Soon after a meal, glucose, amino acids, and fatty acids enter the bloodstream from the intestinal tract. Glucose and amino acids stimulate insulin secretion. Cells take up the glucose and amino acids and use them in their metabolism. **B,** Several hours after a meal, absorption from the intestinal tract decreases, and the blood levels of glucose, amino acids, and fatty acids decrease. As a result, insulin secretion decreases, and glucagon, epinephrine, and growth hormone (GH) secretion increases. Cell uptake of glucose decreases, and the use of fats and proteins increases.

glucose concentrations. When the serum glucose level rises, insulin is secreted to lower it toward normal. On the other hand, when the serum glucose level falls, glucagon is secreted to raise the serum glucose level toward normal.

3. Low serum glucose levels stimulate the sympathetic nervous system to secrete epinephrine. Epinephrine and, to a lesser degree, norepinephrine have a glucagon-like effect that promotes liver glycogenolysis.

4. GH and cortisol play a role in less immediate regulation of serum glucose levels. They are secreted in response to more prolonged hypoglycemic episodes, such as a late overnight fast. They also increase the rate of glucose production. They tend to decrease the rate of glucose use.

CRITICAL THINKING
What signs and symptoms will a patient have in response to the release of epinephrine that occurs when the blood glucose level falls?

Pathophysiology of Diabetes Mellitus

Diabetes is the seventh leading cause of death in the United States.[2] The disease is characterized by a deficiency of insulin or by an inability of the body to respond to insulin. Diabetes often is associated with an increased intake of fluid *(polydipsia)*, excretion of large amounts of urine that contains glucose *(polyuria, glucosuria)*, and weight loss.

NOTE
Diabetes insipidus (DI) is a disorder marked by an abnormal increase in urine output, fluid intake, and often thirst. Diabetes insipidus (also called "water diabetes") is not the same as diabetes mellitus ("sugar diabetes"). The two diseases are completely unrelated, even though the symptoms of both include increased urination and thirst. DI has a variety of causes. The most common cause is a lack of vasopressin, which normally acts on the kidney to reduce urine output by increasing the concentration of the urine. Most patients with DI are aware of their disease. The paramedic should consider DI as a differential diagnosis in a patient who presents with increased urination and thirst.

Diabetes mellitus generally is classified as type 1 or type 2. Type 1 diabetes previously was called *insulin-dependent diabetes mellitus* (IDDM), or *juvenile diabetes*. Type 2 previously was called *non-insulin-dependent diabetes mellitus* (NIDDM), or *adult-onset diabetes*. A new classification system endorsed by the American Diabetes Association and the World Health Organization identifies four types of diabetes: type 1, type 2, gestational diabetes, and "other specific types," to address the continuum of **hyperglycemia** (elevated blood glucose) and insulin requirements.[1]

TYPE 1 DIABETES

Type 1 diabetes is characterized by inadequate production of insulin by the pancreas. It may occur any time after birth. However, it usually occurs in teenagers and young adults, and the incidence typically "peaks" at 12 years of age.[3] Heredity is a factor in type 1 diabetes. The disease appears to be an autoimmune phenomenon. It results from a genetic abnormality or susceptibility that causes the body to destroy its own insulin-producing cells. A person with a parent or sibling with type 1 diabetes has a 10% chance of developing the disease by age 50.[1] Type 1 diabetes requires lifelong treatment with **insulin,** exercise, and dietary regulation. The symptoms of type 1 diabetes usually appear suddenly. They include polyuria, polydipsia, dizziness, blurred vision, and rapid, unexplained weight loss. Only 5% to 10% of people with diabetes have this form of the disease.

TYPE 2 DIABETES

Type 2 diabetes usually is characterized by a decrease in the production of insulin by the pancreatic beta cells and diminished tissue sensitivity to insulin *(insulin resistance)*. People who are insulin resistant have either too few insulin receptors or faulty insulin receptors. As a result, the circulating insulin cannot be properly used. Most people with type 2 diabetes are insulin resistant. The disease occurs most often in adults over age 40, in minorities, and in overweight individuals (Box 26-2). (Obesity predisposes a person to this form of diabetes. This is because larger amounts of insulin are needed for metabolic control in obese individuals than in people of normal weight.). Type 2 diabetes accounts for 90% to 95% of all diagnosed cases of diabetes.[4] Because of the increase in childhood obesity, a growing number of children and young adults are being diagnosed with type 2 diabetes.

> **NOTE**
>
> *Prediabetes* is a condition that is becoming common in the United States. People with prediabetes have blood glucose levels that are higher than normal but not high enough for a diagnosis of diabetes. This condition increases the risk the person will develop type 2 diabetes, heart disease, and stroke. The National Institutes of Health estimate that 79 million adults age 20 and older have prediabetes. People with prediabetes are likely to develop type 2 diabetes within 10 years unless steps are taken to prevent or delay diabetes. Preventive measures include weight loss, diet modification, and exercise.

BOX 26-2　Metabolic Syndrome

Many people with insulin resistance and high blood glucose levels have other conditions that increase their risk of developing type 2 diabetes and cardiovascular disease. These conditions include excess weight around the waist, high blood pressure, and abnormal blood levels of cholesterol and triglycerides. A person with several of these conditions is said to have *metabolic syndrome*. Metabolic syndrome is defined as the presence of any three of the following:

- Waist measurement of 40 inches or more for men or 35 inches or more for women
- Triglyceride level of 150 mg/dL or above or treatment with medication for elevated triglycerides
- High-density lipoprotein (HDL; "good" cholesterol) level below 40 mg/dL for men or below 50 mg/dL for women or treatment with medication for low HDL levels
- Blood pressure of 130/85 mm Hg or above or treatment with medication for elevated blood pressure
- Fasting blood glucose level of 100 mg/dL or above or treatment with medication for elevated blood glucose levels

Modified from Grundy SM, et al: Diagnosis and management of the metabolic syndrome: an American Heart Association/National Heart, Lung, and Blood Institute scientific statement, *Circulation* 112:2735-2752, 2005.

> **CRITICAL THINKING**
> Would patients with type 1 or type 2 diabetes have an increased risk of complications related to this disease?

Most patients with type 2 diabetes require oral hypoglycemic medications, exercise, and dietary regulation to control their illness. A small number of patients require **insulin.** Warning signs, if present, develop gradually. They include all of those associated with type 1 diabetes. Fatigue, changes in appetite, and tingling, numbness, and pain in the extremities also are indicators.

GESTATIONAL DIABETES MELLITUS

Gestational diabetes mellitus develops in some women during late pregnancy. This type of diabetes usually resolves with childbirth. However, some women go on to develop type 2 diabetes within 5 to 10 years. Gestational diabetes is addressed further in Chapter 46.

OTHER SPECIFIC TYPES OF DIABETES

Although less common than type 1 and type 2 diabetes, a number of other types of diabetes exist. A person may show characteristics of more than one type. Other types of diabetes include those caused by[5]:

- Genetic defects of the pancreatic beta cells
- Genetic defects in insulin action, resulting in an inability by the body to control blood glucose levels
- Diseases of the pancreas or conditions that damage the pancreas, such as pancreatitis and cystic fibrosis
- Excess amounts of certain hormones as a result of some medical conditions that work against

the action of insulin (e.g., cortisol in Cushing's syndrome)

- Medications that reduce the action of insulin (e.g., glucocorticoids) or chemicals that destroy beta cells
- Infections, such as congenital rubella and cytomegalovirus
- Rare immune-mediated disorders
- Genetic syndromes associated with diabetes, such as Down syndrome

Effects of Diabetes

Most of the effects of diabetes can be attributed to one of the following three effects of decreased insulin levels[6]:

1. Decreased use of glucose by the body cells, which results in an increase in the serum glucose level
2. Markedly increased mobilization of fats from the fat storage areas, causing abnormal fat metabolism, which may result in the short term in ketoacidosis and in the long term in severe atherosclerosis
3. Depletion of protein in body tissues and muscle wasting

LOSS OF GLUCOSE IN THE URINE

When the amount of glucose entering the kidneys rises above the kidneys' ability to reabsorb it, a significant portion of the glucose "spills" into the urine. The loss of glucose in the urine causes diuresis. This is because the osmotic effect of glucose prevents the kidneys from reabsorbing water (osmotic diuresis). The effect is dehydration. If left untreated, dehydration can lead to hypovolemic shock.

ACIDOSIS IN DIABETES

The shift from carbohydrate to fat metabolism results in the formation of ketone bodies *(ketoacids)*. Ketone bodies are acids, and their continuous production leads to a metabolic acidosis. Often the respiratory system at least partly compensates for this acidosis (indicated by Kussmaul respirations). The kidneys' ability to clear the acid is overwhelmed by the continuous production of ketone bodies. Profound acidosis eventually occurs. This acidosis, along with the usually severe dehydration that occurs as a result of the osmotic diuresis, can lead to death. Hyperkalemia, secondary to acidosis, also leads to cardiac dysrhythmias, some of which may be lethal. Treatment of this condition can be lifesaving.

Diabetes mellitus is a systemic disease with many long-term complications, including the following[5]:

- Blindness (5000 people with diabetes lose their sight each year)
- Kidney disease (10% of patients with diabetes develop some form of kidney disease, including end-stage kidney failure, which requires dialysis or a kidney transplant)
- Peripheral neuropathy, which results in nerve damage to the hands and feet and an increased incidence of foot infections

- Autonomic neuropathy, which damages the nerves controlling voluntary and involuntary functions and may affect sexual function, bladder and bowel control, and blood pressure
- Heart disease and stroke (People with diabetes are two to four times as likely to develop heart disease as those without the disease and are two to six times as likely to have a stroke.)
- High blood glucose and blood fat levels, which contribute to atherosclerosis
- Peripheral vascular disease (also secondary to atherosclerosis), which results in the need for amputations

> **? DID YOU KNOW?**
> **Diabetic Foot**
> About 20% of patients hospitalized with diabetes have foot problems.[7] These problems result from sensory neuropathy, ischemia, and infection. The loss of sensation leads to pressure necrosis from poorly fitting footwear. In addition, small wounds on the feet frequently go unnoticed by the patient, leading to foot ulcers and infection. The most common cause of foot injury is pressure on the plantar bony prominences.
>
> Care should always be taken to assess the feet of any diabetic patient. Findings may include infected ulcerations, foreign bodies in the foot tissue, and bone abnormalities. Full-thickness ulcerations and cellulitis can be limb-threatening and can lead to sepsis. Patients with a *diabetic foot* should not be permitted to put weight or pressure on the affected area. Wounds should be dressed. Treatment by a physician may include debridement of devitalized tissue, advanced wound care, and antibiotic therapy. Some patients must be hospitalized.

Patients with diabetes also suffer from decreased immune function as a long-term complication of the disease. This places the diabetic patient at higher risk for increased morbidity and mortality from infectious diseases, such as influenza. These patients also are prone to infection-related complications from surgeries and other invasive procedures (e.g., intravenous [IV] therapy, bladder catheterization).

Management

The treatment of diabetes consists of drug therapy *(insulin* or oral hypoglycemic agents), dietary regulation, and exercise. These therapies allow patients to control their serum glucose levels. They also help restore normal metabolism. Pancreatic transplantation remains an experimental treatment for diabetes mellitus.

> **📋 NOTE**
> The A1C test is a general measure of diabetes care. It indicates the amount of glucose attached to hemoglobin A proteins. The A1C test provides a patient with an average of the person's blood glucose levels for the past 2 to 3 months. The test often is done two to four times a year. The test result is reported as a percentage. For a person without diabetes, a typical A1C level is about 5%. The American Diabetes Association (ADA) recommends an A1C target of 7% or lower. The American Association of Clinical Endocrinologists recommends a level of 6.5% or lower.[8] Many diabetic patients know their A1C number.

INSULIN

As described in Chapter 13, genetically engineered human *insulin* is available in rapid-, intermediate-, and long-acting preparations. (*Insulin* is administered by injection or nasal inhalation; it is a protein that would be digested if consumed orally.) A patient with insulin-dependent diabetes usually takes one or two doses of a long-acting *insulin* preparation each day. At meal times, these individuals also take a rapid-acting *insulin* (which lasts only a few hours).

LOOK AGAIN

See Chapter 13: Principles of Pharmacology and Emergency Medications, pp. 324-325.

An insulin infusion pump (Figure 26-7) is another means by which patients may self-administer *insulin*. The pump delivers a continuous "basal" level of *insulin*. The patient supplements the basal level with a bolus after eating. Patients calculate the amount of *insulin* to be taken based on their caloric intake. The glucose level must be monitored regularly to ensure adequate medication control. The

medication balance is delicate. The dosage of *insulin* that appears correct at one time may be too much or too little at another time. The dosage depends on various factors, such as exercise or the presence of infection.

ORAL HYPOGLYCEMIC AGENTS

Some oral hypoglycemic agents stimulate the release of insulin from the pancreas. These are effective only in patients who have functioning beta cells that produce some insulin (type 2 diabetes). Other agents help the body better utilize insulin or prevent the body from manufacturing glucose (Table 26-4). Oral hypoglycemic drugs can have important side effects. They require careful patient monitoring (e.g., periodic tests for liver and kidney function).

NOTE

Patients with type 2 diabetes who have an episode of hypoglycemia should be transported for evaluation by a physician. A patient who refuses transport should be advised of the associated risks and should be encouraged to call again for help if needed. In addition, these patients should not be left alone.

Diabetic Emergencies

Three life-threatening conditions may result from diabetes mellitus: hypoglycemia (insulin shock), hyperglycemia (diabetic ketoacidosis), and hyperosmolar hyperglycemic non-ketotic syndrome (HHNS).

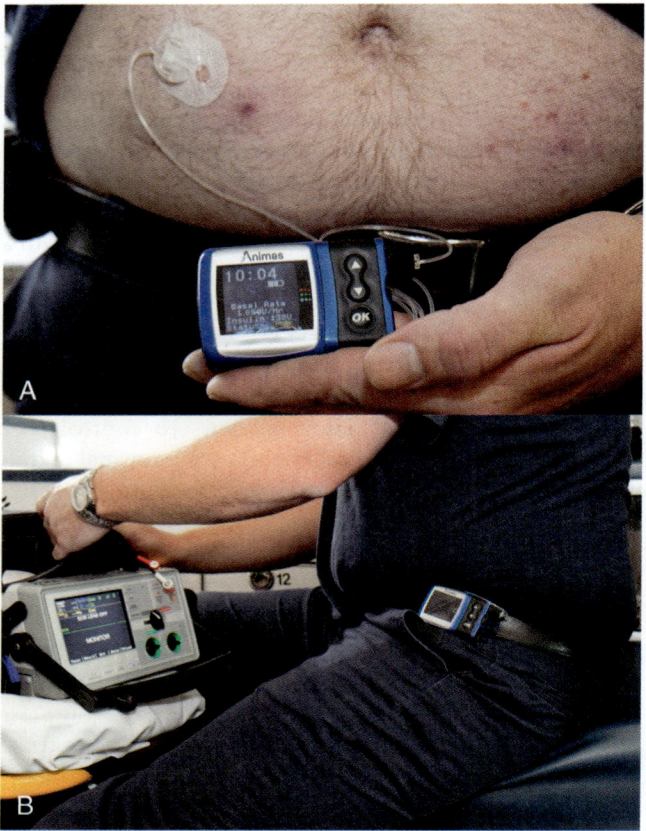

FIGURE 26-7 Insulin pump. **A,** Device and insertion site. **B,** Diabetic paramedic with an insulin pump.

TABLE 26-4 Medications Used in the Treatment of Diabetes

Generic Name	Brand Name	Effect
Biguanides		
Metformin	Glucophage	Block the liver from making sugar
Sulfonylureas (Second-Generation)		
Glimepiride	Amaryl	Raise the amount of insulin in the body
Glipizide	Glucotrol	
Glyburide	Diabeta, Glynase, PresTab, Micronase	
Meglitinides		
Repaglinide	Prandin	Raise the amount of insulin in the body
Nateglinide	Starlix	
Thiazolidinediones		
Pioglitazone	Actos	Help the body use insulin better
Rosiglitazone	Avandia	
Alpha-Glucosidase Inhibitors		
Acarbose	Precose	Slow the digestion of sugar
Miglitol	Glyset	

Agency for Health Care Research and Quality: *Pills for type 2 diabetes: a guide for adults.* http://effectivehealthcare.ahrq.gov/index.cfm/search-for-guides-reviews-and-reports/?pageaction=displayproduct&productID=28&returnpage=#45. Accessed August 24, 2010.

HYPOGLYCEMIA

Hypoglycemia is a syndrome related to blood glucose levels below 70 mg/dL.[8] Symptoms usually occur at levels below 60 mg/dL or at slightly higher blood glucose levels if the fall has been rapid. The condition also may occur in patients who are not diabetic. It usually is a result of an excessive response to glucose absorption, physical exertion, alcohol or drug effects, pregnancy and lactation, or decreased dietary intake. In patients with diabetes, hypoglycemic reactions usually are caused by the following:

- Too much ***insulin*** (or some types of oral hypoglycemic medication)
- Decreased dietary intake (a delayed or missed meal)
- Unusual or vigorous physical activity
- Administration of certain antibiotics (with oral hypoglycemic agents)

Less common causes and predisposing factors include the following:

- Chronic alcoholism (alcohol depletes liver glycogen stores)
- Adrenal gland dysfunction
- Liver disease (i.e., hepatic insufficiency or failure)
- Malnutrition
- Pancreatic tumor
- Cancer
- Hypothermia
- Sepsis
- Administration of beta blockers (e.g., ***propranolol***)
- Administration of salicylates (e.g., ***aspirin***) in ill infants or children
- Intentional overdose with ***insulin,*** oral hypoglycemic agents, or salicylates

> **NOTE**
>
> *Relative hypoglycemia* can occur when glucose levels fall rapidly below normal fasting levels for a particular person. This condition commonly is overlooked in diabetic patients who have elevated fasting levels. These patients may be symptomatic even with near-normal glucose readings. (This condition also is common in a newborn whose mother has diabetes.)

Signs and Symptoms. The signs and symptoms of hypoglycemia usually appear quickly, often within minutes. They are related to the release of epinephrine as the body tries to compensate for a drop in blood sugar. In the early stages, the patient may complain of extreme hunger. The patient may demonstrate one or more of the following signs and symptoms because of the decreased availability of glucose to the brain:

- Nervousness, trembling
- Irritability
- Psychotic (combative) behavior
- Weakness and incoordination
- Confusion

- Appearance of intoxication
- Weak, rapid pulse
- Cold, clammy skin
- Drowsiness
- Seizures
- Coma (in severe cases)
- Cardiac arrest

Hypoglycemia should be suspected in any diabetic patient who shows behavioral changes, confusion, abnormal neurological signs, or unconsciousness. This condition is a true emergency. It requires immediate administration of glucose to prevent permanent brain damage or death.

> **CRITICAL THINKING**
>
> Why might a call for a patient with diabetic ketoacidosis (DKA) be dispatched as a behavioral emergency?

DIABETIC KETOACIDOSIS

Diabetic ketoacidosis (DKA) results from an absence of or resistance to insulin (Box 26-3). The low insulin level prevents glucose from entering the cells. As a result, glucose accumulates in the blood. Consequently, the cells become starved for glucose and begin to use other sources of energy, principally fat. The metabolism of fat generates fatty acids and glycerol. The glycerol provides some energy to the cells, but the fatty acids are further metabolized to form ketoacids, resulting in acidosis.

As described in Chapter 11, acidosis increases the transport of potassium from the intracellular space into the intravascular space. The subsequent diuresis results in a high potassium concentration in the urine and a total body potassium deficit. In addition, the sodium concentration in the extracellular fluid usually decreases through osmotic dilution. The sodium is replaced by increased hydrogen ions, which adds greatly to the acidosis. As the blood sugar level rises, the patient undergoes massive osmotic diuresis. This, combined with vomiting, causes dehydration and shock. Although an overall loss of potassium occurs, the patient is still hyperkalemic. This can lead to cardiac dysrhythmias and cardiac abnormalities (e.g., peaked T waves,

> ### BOX 26-3 Common Causes of Diabetic Ketoacidosis
>
> - Inadequate insulin dose
> - Failure to take insulin
> - Infection
> - Increased stress (trauma, surgery)
> - Increased dietary intake
> - Decreased metabolic rate
> - Other, less common predisposing factors, including significant emotional stress, alcohol consumption (often associated with hypoglycemia), and pregnancy

a prolonged P-R interval, and widening of the QRS complex). Electrolyte imbalances may also cause altered neuromuscular activity, including seizures.

LOOK AGAIN
See Chapter 22: Cardiology, pp. 582-586.

NOTE
Patients may present with DKA without knowing that they are diabetic (i.e., their diabetes has not yet been diagnosed). This is especially true in children.[9]

Signs and Symptoms. The signs and symptoms of DKA usually are related to hypovolemia and acidosis. They usually are slow in onset (over 12 to 48 hours) and include the following:

- Diuresis
- Increased blood glucose level
- Warm, dry skin
- Dry mucous membranes
- Tachycardia, thready pulse
- Postural hypotension
- Weight loss
- Polyuria
- Polydipsia
- Polyphagia
- Acidosis
- Abdominal pain (usually generalized)
- Anorexia, nausea, vomiting
- Acetone breath odor (fruity odor)
- Kussmaul respirations (as the body attempts to reduce carbon dioxide levels)
- Diminished level of consciousness

Patients with DKA seldom are deeply comatose. Patients who are unresponsive should be assessed for another cause, such as head injury, stroke, or drug overdose.

NOTE
An elevation in blood glucose is common in the early phase of stroke. It is estimated that up to one third of acute stroke patients have either diagnosed or newly diagnosed diabetes. A significant proportion of these patients are likely to have *stress hyperglycemia,* mediated partly by the release of cortisol and norepinephrine. This form of hyperglycemia is associated with poor outcomes, such as a dependent state or intracerebral hemorrhage.[10] If a TIA or stroke is suspected in a patient over age 50, administration of a concentrated glucose solution may worsen cerebral damage. However, glucose should not be withheld if the patient is hypoglycemic. The paramedic should consult with medical direction.

CRITICAL THINKING
How can you distinguish Kussmaul respirations from hyperventilation?

HYPEROSMOLAR HYPERGLYCEMIC NONKETOTIC SYNDROME

Hyperosmolar hyperglycemic nonketotic syndrome (HHNS) is a condition of acute diabetic decompensation. It is a life-threatening emergency characterized by marked hyperglycemia, hyperosmolarity and dehydration, and decreased mental functioning that may lead to coma. It often occurs in older patients with type 2 diabetes or in patients with undiagnosed diabetes (Box 26-4). The syndrome is easily mistaken for DKA. It differs from DKA in that enough insulin may be present to prevent the metabolism of fats **(ketogenesis)** and the development of ketoacidosis. However, the amount of insulin may not be enough to prevent glucose use by peripheral tissues or to reduce gluconeogenesis by the liver.

HHNS develops from sustained hyperglycemia that produces a hyperosmolar state. This causes an osmotic diuresis that results in marked dehydration and electrolyte losses.[11] In HHNS, protein and fats are not used to create new supplies of glucose to the same degree as in DKA, and the ketotic cycle is either never started or does not occur until the glucose is extremely elevated.[12] These patients usually have blood glucose levels above 600 mg/dL. They also have less ketone formation. This results in less acidemia than in patients with DKA (Figure 26-8).

NOTE
HHNS can occur when a diabetic (or nondiabetic) patient is unable to drink sufficient fluids to offset urinary losses. This situation can result from stroke, Alzheimer's disease, and other diseases that can lead to dehydration. It also can occur as a result of drug use, trauma, burns, and dialysis.

HHNS tends to develop slowly, often over several days. It has a high mortality rate. Early signs and symptoms are mostly related to volume depletion. They include polyuria and polydipsia. Associated signs and symptoms may include orthostatic hypotension, dry mucous membranes, and tachycardia. CNS dysfunction may result in lethargy, confusion, and coma. Precipitating factors of HHNS include the following:

- Advanced age
- Preexisting cardiac or renal disease
- Inadequate insulin secretion or action (type 2 diabetes)
- Increased insulin requirements (stress, infection, trauma, burns, myocardial infarction)
- Medication use (thiazide and thiazide diuretics, glucocorticoids, **phenytoin,** sympathomimetics, **propranolol,** immunosuppressants)
- Supplemental parenteral and enteral feedings

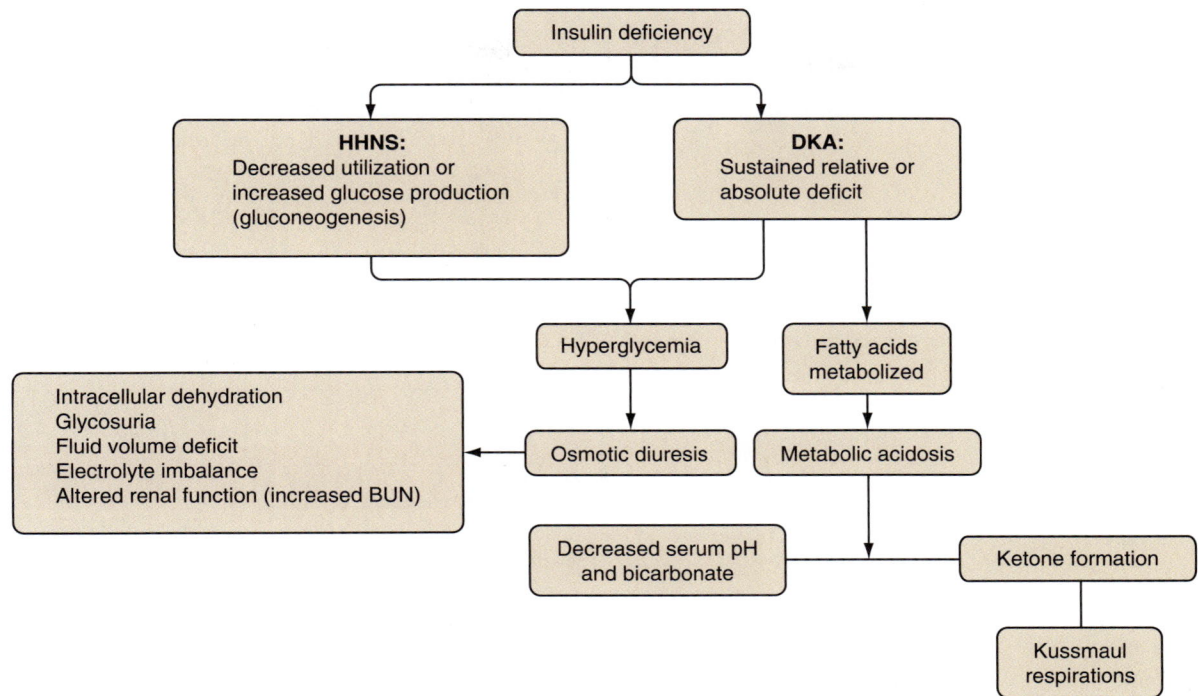

FIGURE 26-8 Pathophysiology of hyperosmolar hyperglycemic nonketotic syndrome (HHNS). (Sole ML: *Introduction to critical care nursing,* ed 5, St Louis, 2009, Saunders.)

ASSESSMENT OF THE DIABETIC PATIENT

A patient with a diabetic emergency may have a range of signs and symptoms. Many of these may mimic other, more commonly encountered conditions. Therefore, the paramedic must have a high degree of suspicion for illness related to diabetes.

In addition to the patient assessment, measures appropriate for any emergency patient encounter (primary assessment, physical examination, and treatment of life-threatening illness or injury), the paramedic should search for medical alert information, an insulin pump, insulin syringes, and diabetic medications (*insulin* often is kept in the refrigerator). Important components of the patient history in the assessment of diabetic patients include the onset of symptoms, food intake, *insulin* or oral hypoglycemic use, alcohol or other drug consumption, predisposing factors (exercise, infection, illness, stress), and any associated symptoms.

MANAGEMENT OF THE CONSCIOUS DIABETIC PATIENT

If the diabetic patient is conscious and able to talk, a pertinent history should be obtained. The paramedic should do this while assessing the patient's airway, breathing, and circulation. If appropriate, the patient should be given glucose.

Protocols may include drawing a blood sample for laboratory testing before glucose is administered. Glucose testing in the field is done with a glucometer (Figure 26-9). Patients who have a glucose reading below 70 mg/dL (varies

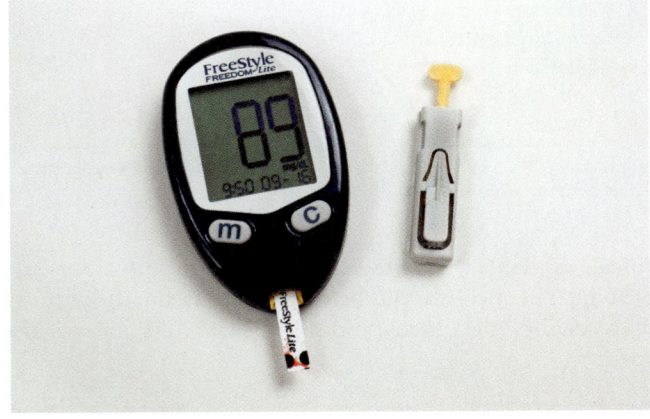

FIGURE 26-9 Glucometer for measuring serum glucose levels.

by protocol) *and* who have signs and symptoms consistent with hypoglycemia generally should be given glucose.[13] Some type I diabetic patients who have experienced a diabetic reaction may be treated at the scene and released. Others may need to be transported for evaluation by a physician. The paramedic should consult with medical direction or follow the established protocol. If a patient who received glucose refuses transport, before leaving the scene the paramedic should make sure the patient has been advised of the possibility of recurrent hypoglycemia.[14] In addition, paramedics should make sure the patient has a

BOX 26-4 Causes of Hyperglycemic Hyperosmolar Nonketotic Syndrome

External Insult
- Trauma
- Burns
- Dialysis
- Hyperalimentation

Disease Process
- Cushing's syndrome and other endocrinopathies
- Hemorrhage
- Myocardial infarction
- Renal disease
- Subdural hematoma
- Cerebrovascular accident
- Infection
- Down syndrome

Drugs
- Antimetabolites
- L-Asparaginase
- Chlorpromazine
- Chlorpropamide
- Cimetidine
- Diazoxide
- Didanosine
- Ethacrynic acid
- Furosemide
- Glucocorticoids
- Immunosuppressants
- Phenytoin
- Propranolol
- Thiazides

From Marx J, Hockberger R, Walls R: *Rosen's emergency medicine: concepts and clinical practice,* ed 6, St Louis, 2006, Mosby.

BOX 26-5 Cautions for Intravenous Administration of Glucose

- 50% Dextrose should not be administered to infants or young children or to patients with suspected stroke.
- Administration of 50% dextrose may lead to neurological complications in alcoholics and other patients with thiamine deficiency. Therefore, administration of thiamine before or during administration of dextrose should be considered for patients suspected of having a thiamine deficiency.
- IV dextrose may raise A1C levels.

BOX 26-6 Glucose Preparations

Concentrated dextrose in water is designed for intravenous administration. The preparation is available in several concentrations. High-concentration dextrose solution may infiltrate tissue, causing sloughing and necrosis of the vein.[17] Therefore, concentrated dextrose must be given through a large, stable vein. It may also be given by the intraosseous route (see the EDI). The concentrations used most often in prehospital care are:

- 50% dextrose in water (recommended for most adults)
- 25% dextrose in water (recommended for most children)
- 10% dextrose in water (recommended for most neonates)

SHOW ME THE EVIDENCE

In a randomized, controlled study, Welsh researchers evaluated the effectiveness of administering dextrose 10% in 5 g doses, compared with 50% dextrose given in 5 g doses, to treat hypoglycemia in the prehospital setting. The endpoint for treatment was a dose of 25 g or a Glasgow Coma Scale (GCS) score of 15. In both groups, patients recovered within a median time of 8 minutes. The group that received 10% dextrose required a significantly lower dose and had lower post-treatment blood glucose levels than the group that received 50% dextrose. An equal number of subjects from the two groups had a subsequent hypoglycemic event.

Moore C, Woollard M: Dextrose 10% or 50% in the treatment of hypoglycaemia out of hospital? A randomized controlled trial, *Emerg Med J* 22:512-515, 2005.

CRITICAL THINKING

What steps should you take before leaving the scene if the patient refuses transport after treatment with dextrose?

"meal" available that is high in complex carbohydrates and protein. The meal should be consumed within 30 minutes of receiving the glucose, ideally before EMS leaves the scene.[15]

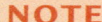

NOTE

A patient who may have taken an unintentional overdose of insulin always requires evaluation by a physician. These patients can develop delayed, profound, and protracted hypoglycemia. This is especially true with long-acting insulin preparations.[16]

The methods of glucose administration vary. If the patient is alert and able to swallow, sugar should first be administered orally. It can be given in the form of a candy bar, a glass of orange juice mixed with sugar, a nondiet soft drink, or by sublingual or buccal administration of a glucose gel preparation. An alternate method is to slowly administer **50% dextrose** (50%, 25%, or 10%) through a large, stable peripheral vein (Box 26-5). This dose may be repeated according to protocol (Box 26-6).

MANAGEMENT OF THE UNCONSCIOUS DIABETIC PATIENT

Prehospital management of any unconscious patient should be directed at airway management, administration of high-concentration oxygen, and ventilatory and circulatory support. Depending on protocol, an IV line should be established for rehydration with lactated Ringer solution or a saline solution. The flow rate should be determined by the patient's blood pressure and heart rate. Before glucose is given, a blood sample should be drawn for laboratory analysis. If alcoholism or other drug abuse is suspected, the administration of *thiamine* or *naloxone,* or both, before glucose may be indicated.

> **NOTE**
>
> Administration of one dose of **50% dextrose** only minimally worsens DKA or HNNS. The drug also is lifesaving for patients who are hypoglycemic. In the rare event the blood glucose cannot be measured rapidly, **50% dextrose** should be given.[7]

If an IV line cannot be established, **glucagon** may be given by the subcutaneous route, intramuscular route, or intranasally via mucosal atomization (per protocol). Any of these methods can help raise the serum glucose level. They do so by stimulating the breakdown of liver glycogen. However, **glucagon** is not effective in any patient with decreased liver glycogen. Examples include chronic alcoholics; those with liver disease; those who are malnourished; and those on certain diets. Definitive treatment for patients with DKA or HHNS requires administration of **insulin,** fluid replacement, electrolyte monitoring, and in-hospital observation. While at the scene and during transport, the patient should be monitored closely for serious dysrhythmias, which can lead to cardiac arrest. They result from electrolyte abnormalities (hyperkalemia) and may require drug therapy **(albuterol, calcium, sodium bicarbonate)** (see Chapter 22). In addition, a patient with HHNS may require large amounts of IV fluid (1 to 1.5 L within the first hour) for rehydration while at the scene and during transport.

DIFFERENTIAL DIAGNOSIS

The signs and symptoms of diabetic emergencies can sometimes overlap, making the exact cause of the patient's condition difficult to identify. Although blood glucose monitoring is now a standard of care, Table 26-5 may help in making a differential diagnosis in difficult cases.

DISORDERS OF THE THYROID GLAND

Common disorders of the thyroid gland include hyperthyroidism and hypothyroidism. *Hyperthyroidism* is an excess of thyroid hormones in the blood, which may result in thyrotoxicosis. *Hypothyroidism* is an insufficiency of thyroid hormones in the blood, which may result in myxedema.

Thyrotoxicosis

Thyrotoxicosis is a mild form of hyperthyroidism. **Thyroid storm** is a life-threatening form of hyperthyroidism. Thyrotoxicosis is fairly common and develops over time. Thyroid storm is a rare condition that may occur spontaneously. It may be brought on by infection, stress, or a thyroidectomy. Most cases of hyperthyroidism occur as a consequence of toxic diffuse goiter (Graves' disease).[7] **Graves' disease** is a type of excessive thyroid activity characterized by generalized enlargement of the gland (goiter), which leads to a swollen neck and, often, protruding eyes (exophthalmos) (Figure 26-10). Graves' disease most often occurs in young women. It may arise as a result of an autoimmune process in which an antibody stimulates the thyroid cells.

ANATOMY AND PHYSIOLOGY OF THE THYROID GLAND

As described in Chapter 10, the thyroid gland is situated in the front of the neck just below the larynx. It consists of two lobes, one on each side of the trachea, which are joined by a narrower portion of tissue called the *isthmus* (Figure 26-11).

> **LOOK AGAIN**
>
> See Chapter 10: Review of Human Systems, pp. 182-183.

Thyroid tissue is composed of two types of secretory cells: follicular cells and parafollicular cells (or C cells). Follicular cells make up most of the gland. They are arranged in the form of hollow, spherical follicles. They secrete the iodine-containing hormones thyroxine (T_4) and triiodothyronine (T_3). Parafollicular cells occur singly or in small groups in the spaces between the follicles. These cells secrete

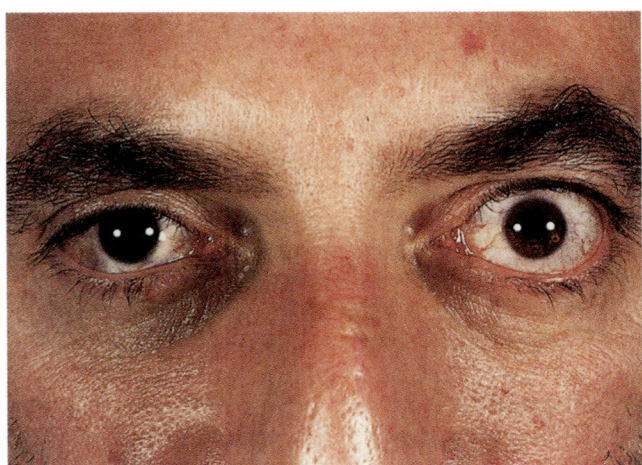

FIGURE 26-10 Protrusion of the eyes in a patient with Graves' disease. (Epstein O, et al: *Clinical examination,* ed 4, St Louis, 2008, Mosby.)

TABLE 26-5 Differential Considerations in Diabetic Emergencies

Findings	Hypoglycemia	DKA	HHNS
History			
Food intake	Insufficient	Excessive	Excessive
Insulin dosage	Excessive	Insufficient	Insufficient
Onset	Rapid	Gradual	Gradual
Infection	Uncommon	Common	Common
Gastrointestinal Tract			
Thirst	Absent	Intense	Intense
Hunger	Intense	Absent	Intense
Vomiting	Uncommon	Common	Uncommon
Respiratory System			
Breathing	Normal or rapid	Deep and rapid	Shallow/rapid
Breath odor	Normal	Acetone smell	Normal
Cardiovascular System			
Blood pressure	Normal	Low	Low
Pulse	Normal, rapid, or full	Rapid and weak	Rapid and weak
Skin	Pale and moist	Warm and dry	Warm and dry
Nervous System			
Headache	Present	Absent	Irritable
Consciousness	Irritable	Restless	Seizure or coma
	Seizure or coma	Coma (rare)	Irritable
Urine			
Glucosuria	Absent	Present	Present
Acetone	Usually absent	Usually present	Absent
Serum glucose levels	<60 mg/dL	>300 mg/dL	>600 mg/dL
Treatment response	Immediate (after glucose administration) (*Note:* If the hypoglycemic episode is prolonged or severe, response may be delayed and may require more than one dose.)	Gradual (within 6 to 12 hours after medication and fluid replacement)	Gradual (within 6 to 12 hours after medication and fluid replacement)

Modified from Clark F, et al: *Pharmacological basis of nursing,* ed 4, St Louis, 1993, Mosby.
DKA, Diabetic ketoacidosis; *HHNS,* hyperosmolar hyperglycemic nonketotic syndrome.

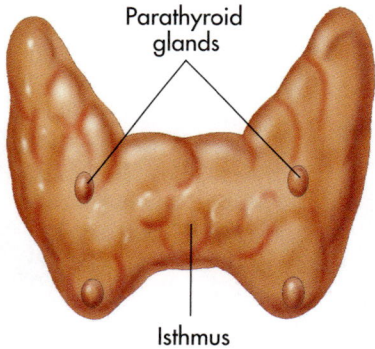

FIGURE 26-11 Thyroid gland.

the hormone calcitonin, which helps regulate the level of calcium in the body.

Thyroid hormones play a key role in controlling body metabolism. They are essential in children for normal physical growth and mental development. The secretion of T_3 and T_4 is controlled by a feedback system. This system involves the pituitary gland and the hypothalamus. (The secretion of calcitonin is regulated directly by the level of calcium in the blood, independent of the pituitary gland or hypothalamus.)

Disorders of the thyroid gland may result from defects in the gland itself or from disruption of the hypothalamic-pituitary hormonal control system (Box 26-7). The disease advances slowly. It may have nonspecific signs and symptoms over months to years. It also may culminate in an acute episode (thyroid storm). Nonspecific signs and symptoms of thyroid hyperfunction include fatigue, anxiety, palpitations, sweating, weight loss, diarrhea, and heat intolerance.

In acute episodes of thyroid storm, the signs and symptoms are those related to adrenergic hyperactivity. They may include the following:

- Severe tachycardia
- Heart failure
- Cardiac dysrhythmias
- Shock
- Hyperthermia
- Restlessness
- Agitation and paranoia

BOX 26-7 Causes of Thyroid Gland Disorders

- Congenital defects
- Genetic disorders
- Infection (thyroiditis)
- Tumors (benign or malignant)
- Autoimmune disorders
- Hormonal disorders during puberty or pregnancy
- Nutritional disorders

- Abdominal pain
- Delirium
- Coma

The paramedic should consider other causes of symptoms related to adrenergic hyperactivity, most notably hypoglycemia, use of cocaine and amphetamines, and withdrawal from alcohol and other drugs.

 CRITICAL THINKING
What medical emergencies could produce signs and symptoms similar to those of thyroid storm?

MANAGEMENT

Mild hyperthyroidism requires no emergency therapy. It is best managed with physician follow-up. Thyroid storm, however, is a true emergency that requires immediate treatment. Emergency care efforts are directed at providing airway, ventilatory, and circulatory support and rapid transport to an appropriate medical facility. In-hospital care focuses on inhibiting hormone synthesis, blocking hormone release and the peripheral effects of thyroid hormone with antithyroid drugs, and providing general support of the patient's vital functions. Beta blockers also are given to control the heart rate, tremors, and anxiety. Table 26-6 lists the signs and symptoms of hyperthyroidism and hypothyroidism.

 NOTE
All patients with disorders related to the thyroid gland should be closely monitored for cardiac dysrhythmias. Atrial fibrillation and supraventricular tachycardia are common in these patients. Efforts to control the heart rate may not be effective until the thyroid disorder has been treated.

Myxedema

Myxedema is a condition that results from hypothyroidism. It may be associated with inflammation of the thyroid gland (e.g., *Hashimoto thyroiditis*) or atrophy of the thyroid gland. It also may be a consequence of treatment for

TABLE 26-6 Signs, Symptoms, and Medications Used in Hyperthyroidism and Hypothyroidism

Hyperthyroidism	Hypothyroidism
Exophthalmos	Facial edema
Goiter	Jugular venous distention (sometimes goiter)
Warm, flushed skin	Cool skin
Sensitivity to heat	Sensitivity to cold
Fever	Hypothermia
Agitation/psychosis	Coma
Hyperactivity	Weakness
Weight loss	Weight gain
Common Medications Used in Treatment	
Iodine	Levothyroxine (Synthroid)
Methimazole (Tapazole)	Liothyronine (Cytomel)
Propylthiouracil (Propacil)	Liotrix (Euthroid)

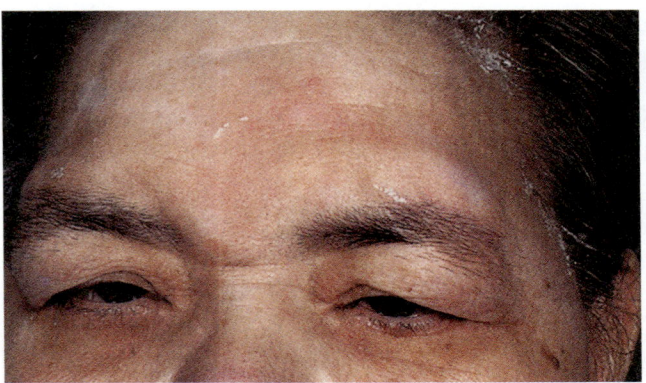

FIGURE 26-12 Myxedema. (Epstein O, et al: *Clinical examination,* ed 4, St Louis, 2008, Mosby.)

hyperthyroidism. Myxedema causes an accumulation of mucinous material in the skin. This results in thickening and coarsening of the skin and other body tissues (most notably the lips, nose, and throat) (Figure 26-12). The condition is most common in adults over age 40, especially women.

NOTE
Symptoms of hypothyroidism in children and adolescents differ from those in adults. In newborns, hypothyroidism causes *cretinism* (neonatal hypothyroidism). This condition is characterized by jaundice, poor appetite, constipation, a hoarse cry, outpouching of the navel (umbilical hernia), and slowed bone growth. If not diagnosed and treated within a few months of birth, hypothyroidism can lead to mental retardation. Hypothyroidism that begins in childhood (*juvenile hypothyroidism*) slows growth. This sometimes results in disproportionately short limbs. Tooth development also can be delayed.

Myxedema coma is a rare illness. In addition to myxedema, it is characterized by hypothermia and a reduced level of consciousness. Myxedema coma is a medical emergency that may be precipitated by the following factors:

- Exposure to cold
- Infection (usually pulmonary)
- Congestive heart failure
- Trauma
- Drugs (sedatives, hypnotics, anesthetics)
- Stroke
- Internal hemorrhage
- Hypoxia
- Hypercapnia
- Hyponatremia
- Hypoglycemia

MANAGEMENT

Prehospital care is directed at managing life-threatening conditions (airway, ventilatory, and circulatory compromise) and providing rapid transport to an appropriate medical facility for evaluation by a physician. En route, the patient's body temperature should be maintained and the ECG should be monitored closely for cardiac dysrhythmias. Once other causes of the coma have been ruled out and the patient's condition has been stabilized, treatment of myxedema can begin with oral administration of thyroxine. This treatment must be continued for life.

NOTE

The angioedema associated with thyroid disease often affects the patient's neck and throat. This may make for a difficult airway if intubation is required.

DISORDERS OF THE ADRENAL GLANDS

Two disorders of the adrenal gland are Cushing's syndrome and Addison's disease. Cushing's syndrome is caused by excessive activity of the adrenal cortex. Addison's disease is caused by inactivity of the adrenal cortex.

Anatomy and Physiology of the Adrenal Glands

As described in Chapter 10, the adrenal glands are triangular-shaped endocrine glands located on top of both kidneys (Figure 26-13). Each gland consists of a *medulla,* the center of the gland, which is surrounded by the *cortex.* The medulla is responsible for producing epinephrine and norepinephrine. The adrenal cortex produces other hormones necessary for fluid and electrolyte balance in the body (e.g., cortisone and aldosterone).

Cushing's Syndrome

Cushing's syndrome is a rare condition caused by an abnormally high circulating level of corticosteroid hormones. It mainly affects women 30 to 50 years of age. The syndrome may be produced directly by an adrenal gland tumor, which causes excessive secretion of corticosteroids. It also may be produced by administration of corticosteroid drugs, such as predinsone, dexamethasone, or methylprednisolone. These drugs are used to treat conditions such as rheumatoid arthritis, inflammatory bowel disease, and asthma. Finally, it may be produced by enlargement of both adrenal glands as a result of a pituitary tumor. The pituitary gland controls the activity of the adrenal gland by producing adrenocorticotropic hormone (ACTH). ACTH stimulates growth of the adrenal cortex.

People with Cushing's syndrome have a characteristic appearance (Figure 26-14). The face appears round ("moon face") and red (Figure 26-15). Also, the trunk tends to become obese from disturbances in fat metabolism. The limbs become wasted from muscle atrophy. Acne develops, and purple stretch marks may appear on the abdomen, thighs, and breasts. The skin often thins and bruises easily. Weakened bones are at increased risk of fracture. Other features of the disease include the following:

- Increased body and facial hair
- Hump on the back of neck ("buffalo hump")
- Supraclavicular fat pads
- Weight gain
- Hypertension
- Psychiatric disturbances (depression, paranoia)
- Insomnia
- Diabetes mellitus

CRITICAL THINKING

How do you think patients who suffer from Cushing's syndrome feel about their body image?

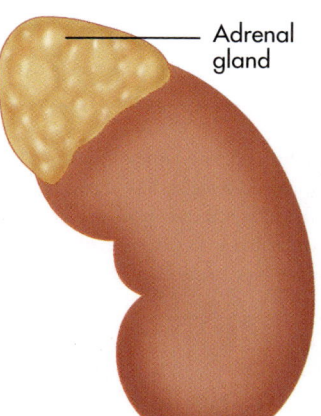

Adrenal gland

Cushing's Syndrome caused by:

- adrenal gland tumor
- corticosteroid drugs
- enlargement of adrenal glands due to pituitary tumor

FIGURE 26-13 Adrenal gland.

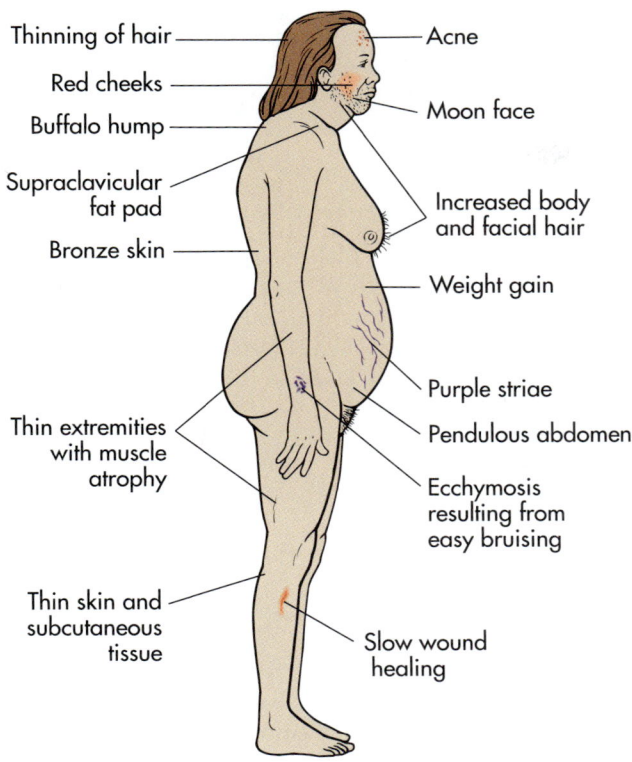

Thinning of hair

Red cheeks

Buffalo hump

Supraclavicular fat pad

Bronze skin

Thin extremities with muscle atrophy

Thin skin and subcutaneous tissue

Acne

Moon face

Increased body and facial hair

Weight gain

Purple striae

Pendulous abdomen

Ecchymosis resulting from easy bruising

Slow wound healing

FIGURE 26-14 Cushing's syndrome. (Lewis SM, Collier IC, Heitkemper MM: *Medical-surgical nursing: assessment and management of clinical problems,* ed 7, St Louis, 2007, Mosby.)

MANAGEMENT

Prehospital care for patients with Cushing's syndrome is mainly supportive. The disease is diagnosed through measurement of hormone levels in the blood and urine and by radiological imaging (e.g., computed tomography [CT] scan). If the cause of the syndrome is overtreatment with corticosteroid drugs, the condition usually is reversible when the drug dosages are adjusted. If the cause is a tumor or overgrowth of the adrenal gland, the gland may require surgical removal. If the tumor is in the pituitary gland, the usual treatment involves surgery, radiation, and medication. Treatment usually is successful. Lifelong hormone replacement therapy is required.

Addison's Disease

Addison's disease is a rare disorder that can be life threatening. It is caused by a deficiency of the corticosteroid hormones cortisol and aldosterone. These hormones normally are produced by the adrenal cortex. The disorder can be caused by any disease process that destroys the adrenal cortices. Such disease processes may include adrenal hemorrhage or infarction, infections (tuberculosis, fungi, viruses), and autoimmune diseases. However, the most common cause of Addison's disease is shrinking of the adrenal tissue. When this occurs, production of corticosteroid hormones is inadequate to meet the body's metabolic requirements. Signs and symptoms associated with this disease include the following:

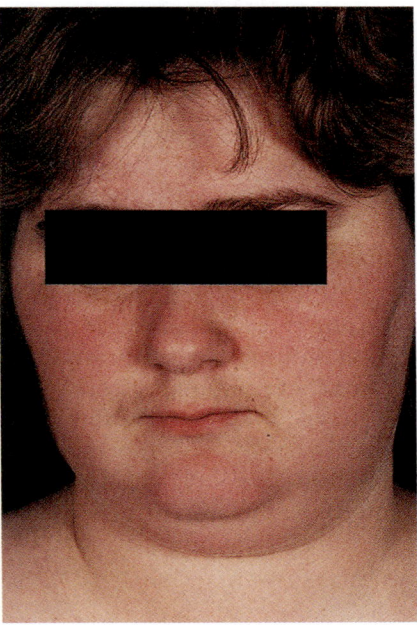

FIGURE 26-15 Moon-faced appearance in a patient with Cushing's syndrome. (Epstein O, et al: *Clinical examination,* ed 4, St Louis, 2008, Mosby.)

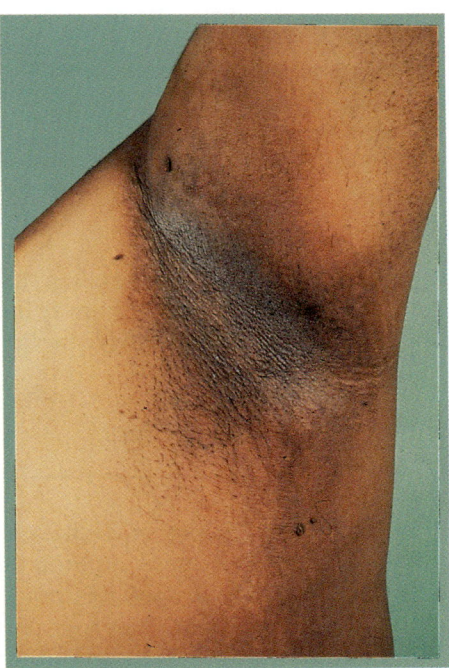

FIGURE 26-16 Hyperpigmentation in a patient with Addison's disease. (Forbes CD, Jackson WF: *Color atlas and textbook of clinical medicine,* ed 3, St Louis, 2003, Mosby.)

- Progressive weakness
- Progressive weight loss
- Progressive anorexia
- Skin hyperpigmentation (caused by increased hormone production by the pituitary gland, which stimulates melanin) (Figure 26-16)

- Hypotension
- Hyponatremia
- Hyperkalemia
- GI disturbances (nausea, vomiting, diarrhea)

Addison's disease usually has a slow onset and a chronic course. The symptoms develop gradually over months to years. However, acute episodes *(addisonian crisis)* may be brought on by emotional and physiological stress. Examples of such stressors include surgery, alcohol intoxication, hypothermia, myocardial infarction, severe illness, trauma, hypoglycemia, and infection. During these events, the adrenal glands cannot increase the production of the corticosteroid hormones to help the body cope with stress. As a result, blood glucose levels drop; the body loses the ability to regulate the content of sodium, potassium, and water in body fluids, causing dehydration and extreme muscle weakness; blood volume and blood pressure fall; and the body may not be able to maintain circulation efficiently. In these situations, airway, ventilatory, and circulatory support are required in the prehospital setting. The serum glucose level should be monitored closely. ECG findings as a result of hypokalemia may include peaked T waves, flattened P waves, and widening of the QRS complex. Some EMS services carry hydrocortisone (Solu-Cortef) to manage adrenal insufficiency.

> **NOTE**
> Many patients with Addison's disease carry injectable hydrocortisone in case of crisis. The paramedic may need to contact medical direction for an order to administer the drug to an unstable patient.

MANAGEMENT

In-hospital treatment involves maintaining the patient's vital functions and correcting the sodium deficiency and dehydration. After the life-threatening episode has been

TABLE 26-7 Signs, Symptoms and Medications Used in Adrenal Gland Disorders	
Corticosteroid Excess (Cushing's Syndrome)	**Adrenal Insufficiency (Addison's Disease)**
Weight gain	Weight loss
Weakness	Weakness
Hump on back of neck	Hypotension
Slow healing	Gastrointestinal disorders
Increased body and facial hair	Skin hyperpigmentation
Common Medications Used in Treatment	
Aminoglutethimide (Cytadren)	Dexamethasone (Decadron)
Metyrapone (Metopirone)	Fludrocortisone (Florinef Acetate)

managed, treatment consists of administration of corticosteroids. The patient often is advised to increase the dosage of these drugs during times of emotional and physiological stress.

Table 26-7 presents a comparison of the signs and symptoms of Cushing's syndrome and Addison's disease.

OTHER ENDOCRINE DISORDERS

The endocrine disorders presented in this chapter are the most common. However, there are many types of endocrine disorders and diseases. A discussion of each is beyond the scope of this textbook. The paramedic should remember that most endocrine disorders are related to hormone imbalance or nutritional deficiencies. After diagnosis, most patients require lifelong treatment.

SUMMARY

- The endocrine system consists of ductless glands and tissues. These glands and tissues produce and secrete hormones. Endocrine glands secrete their hormones directly into the bloodstream. They exert a regulatory effect on various metabolic functions. All hormones operate within feedback systems that are either positive or negative. These systems work to maintain the optimum internal environment.
- The pancreatic islets are composed of beta cells, alpha cells, and other cells. The beta cells secrete insulin. The alpha cells secrete glucagon. The function of the other cells is not completely clear. The chief functions of insulin are to increase glucose transport into cells, increase glucose metabolism by cells, increase the liver glycogen level, and decrease the blood glucose

concentration toward normal. Glucagon has two major effects: (1) it increases blood glucose levels by stimulating the liver to release glucose stores from glycogen and other glucose storage sites (glycogenosis) and (2) it stimulates gluconeogenesis through the breakdown of fats and fatty acids, thereby maintaining a normal blood glucose level.

- Diabetes mellitus is characterized by a deficiency of insulin production or an inability of the body to respond to insulin. Diabetes generally is classified as type 1 or type 2. Patients with type 1 diabetes have inadequate insulin production. Treatment consists of insulin administration, exercise, and dietary regulation. Type 2 diabetes is caused by cellular resistance to insulin and, ultimately, decreased insulin production. Most patients with type 2 diabetes require oral hypoglycemic medications, exercise, and dietary regulation to control the illness. Some require insulin administration.

- Hypoglycemia is a syndrome related to blood glucose levels below 70 mg/dL. A diabetic patient with behavioral changes or unconsciousness should be treated for hypoglycemia. This condition is a true emergency. It requires immediate administration of glucose to prevent permanent brain damage or death.

- Diabetic ketoacidosis results from an absence of or a resistance to insulin. The signs and symptoms of DKA are related to hypovolemia. They usually are slow in onset.

- Hyperosmolar hyperglycemic nonketotic syndrome is a life-threatening emergency. HHNS often occurs in older patients with type 2 diabetes. It also frequently occurs in individuals whose diabetes has not yet been diagnosed. The hyperglycemia produces a hyperosmolar state. This causes osmotic diuresis, dehydration, and electrolyte imbalances.

- Important components of the patient history in the assessment of diabetic patients include the onset of symptoms, food intake, insulin or oral hypoglycemic use, alcohol or other drug consumption, predisposing factors, and any associated symptoms.

- Any patient with a glucose reading below 70 mg/dL (varies by protocol) and signs and symptoms consistent with hypoglycemia generally should be given glucose.

- Thyrotoxicosis is any toxic condition that results from overactivity of the thyroid gland.

- Thyroid storm is a life-threatening condition resulting from an overactive thyroid gland. Thyroid hormones play a key role in controlling body metabolism. They are essential in children for normal physical growth and development.

- Myxedema is a condition that results from a thyroid hormone deficiency. Myxedema coma is a rare illness. In addition to myxedema, it is characterized by hypothermia and mental obtundation. It is a medical emergency.

- Cushing's syndrome is caused by an abnormally high circulating level of corticosteroid hormones. These are produced naturally by the adrenal glands.

- Addison's disease is a rare but life-threatening disorder. It is caused by a deficiency of the corticosteroid hormones cortisol and aldosterone. These are normally produced by the adrenal cortex.

REFERENCES

1. American Diabetes Association: *Diabetes and how it affects you.* www.diabetes.org/living-with-diabetes/planning-for-a-healthy-life/diabetes-and-how-it-affects.html. Accessed August 24, 2010.

2. National Diabetes Information Clearinghouse (NDIC): *National diabetes statistics, 2011.* http://diabetes.niddk.nih.gov/DM/PUBS/statistics/#allages. Accessed August 24, 2010.

3. McCance K, Heuther S: *Pathophysiology: the biologic basis for disease in adults and children,* ed 5, St Louis, 2006, Mosby.

4. National Diabetes Information Clearinghouse (NDIC): *National diabetes statistics, 2007.* http://diabetes.niddk.nih.gov/DM/PUBS/statistics/#allages. Accessed August 24, 2010.

5. The Facts About Diabetes: *A leading cause of death in the United States, National Diabetes Education Program, National Institutes of Health,* http://www.ndep.nih.gov/diabetes-facts/index.aspx, accessed 5-3-2011.

6. McCance K, Heuther S: *Pathophysiology: the biologic basis for disease in adults and children,* ed 6, St Louis, 2010, Mosby.

7. Marx J, Hockberger R, Walls R: *Rosen's emergency medicine: concepts and clinical practice,* ed 6, St Louis, 2006, Mosby.

8. American Diabetes Association: www.diabetes.org. Accessed August 24, 2010.

9. Agwu CJ: Screening for type 2 diabetes mellitus in children and adolescents, *Br J Diabetes Vasc Dis* 8:163-168, 2008.

10. Lindsberg P, et al: Hyperglycemia in acute stroke: advances in stroke 2003, *Stroke* 35:363, 2004.

11. Sole ML: *Introduction to critical care nursing,* ed 5, Philadelphia, 2008, Saunders.

12. Urden LD: *Priorities in critical care nursing,* ed 4, St Louis, 2004, Mosby.

13. Moghisssi E, et al: Consensus: Inpatient hyperglycemia, *Endocr Pract* 15(4):1-17, 2009.

14. Cater A, et al: Transport refusal by hypoglycemic patients after on-scene intravenous dextrose, *Acad Emerg Med* 9 (8):855-857, 2002.

15. Pollak A, editor: *Emergency care and transportation of the sick and injured,* ed 9, Sudbury, Mass, 2005, Jones & Bartlett.

16. Flomenbaum N, et al: *Goldfrank's toxicologic emergencies,* ed 8, New York, 2006, McGraw-Hill.

17. Dart R, et al: *Medical toxicology,* ed 3, Philadelphia, 2004, Lippincott Williams & Wilkins.

SUGGESTED READINGS

Becker K, et al: *Principles and practice of endocrinology and metabolism,* ed 3, Philadelphia, 2001, Lippincott Williams & Wilkins.

Gardner D, Shoback D: *Greenspan's basic and clinical endocrinology,* ed 8, New York, 2007, McGraw-Hill.

Goodman M: *Basic medical endocrinology,* ed 4, St. Louis, 2009, Elsevier.

William R, et al: *William's textbooks of endocrinology,* ed 11, Philadelphia, 2008, Saunders.

OBJECTIVES

Upon completion of this chapter, the paramedic student will be able to:

1. Outline the structure of the immune system.
2. Describe the antigen-antibody response.
3. Distinguish between natural and acquired immunity.
4. Differentiate between a normal immune response and an allergic reaction.
5. Distinguish between the four types of hypersensitivity reaction.
6. Describe the signs, symptoms, and management of local allergic reactions based on an understanding of the pathophysiology associated with this condition.
7. Identify allergens associated with anaphylaxis.
8. Describe the pathophysiology, signs and symptoms, and management of a nonsystemic allergic reaction.
9. Describe the pathophysiology, signs and symptoms, and management of anaphylaxis.
10. Define autoimmune disease.
11. Describe the pathophysiology, signs and symptoms, and prehospital considerations for patients who have collagen vascular diseases, such as systemic lupus erythematous and scleroderma.
12. Identify major complications associated with organ transplantation.
13. List infections associated with organ transplantation.
14. Outline characteristics of organ rejection.
15. Recognize side effects associated with antirejection medications.

KEY TERMS

acquired immunity Immunity that develops after exposure to specific antigens; also known as *adaptive immunity*.

allergens Substances that can produce hypersensitivity reactions in the body.

allergic reaction A hypersensitivity response to an allergen to which a person previously was exposed and to which the person has developed antibodies.

allografting The transplantation of cells, tissues, or organs between nonidentical (genetically unrelated) people.

anaphylactoid reaction An allergic reaction that is not mediated by an antigen-antibody reaction; it presents exactly like anaphylaxis but does not require previous exposure.

anaphylaxis An exaggerated, life-threatening hypersensitivity reaction to a previously encountered antigen.

angioedema A localized edematous reaction of the deep dermal or subcutaneous or submucosal tissues that appears as giant wheals.

antibodies Substances produced by the body that destroy or inactivate a specific substance (antigen) that has entered the body.

antigen-antibody reaction The binding of an antibody with an antigen of the type that stimulated the formation of the antibody; this makes the antigen more susceptible to ingestion and destruction by phagocytes or neutralization of an exotoxin.

antigens Substances (usually proteins) that cause the formation of an antibody and react specifically with that antibody.

autoimmune disease A condition that occurs when the immune system mistakenly attacks and destroys healthy body tissue.

B lymphocytes The lymphocytes responsible for antibody-mediated immunity.

basophils White blood cells that promote inflammation.

biphasic reaction An anaphylactic reaction that resolves and then recurs hours later without further exposure to the trigger.

cell-mediated immunity Immunity characterized by the formation of a population of lymphocytes that attack and destroy foreign material.

collagen vascular disease Abnormal immune system activity with inflammation in the connective tissues; it results in the accumulation of extra antibodies in the circulation.

degranulation A cellular process that releases antimicrobial substances from secretory vesicles (granules) found inside mast cells and basophils; it plays a role in allergic reactions.

eosinophils White blood cells that inhibit inflammation; they are thought to deactivate leukotrienes.

eosinophil chemotactic factor of anaphylaxis A group of active substances, including histamine and leukotrienes, that are released during an anaphylactic reaction.

erythema Redness of the skin, caused by hyperemia of the capillaries in the lower layers of the skin.

Fc receptors Proteins found on the surface of certain cells that contribute to the protective functions of the immune system. Fc receptors bind to antibodies that are attached to infected cells or invading pathogens.

histamine An amine released by mast cells and basophils that promotes inflammation.

humoral immunity One of the two forms of immunity that respond to antigens such as bacteria and foreign tissue.

IgA Immunoglobulin A; an antibody that plays a crucial role in mucosal immunity.

IgD Immunoglobulin D; an antibody present on the surface of most, but not all, B cells early in their development; IgD signals B cells to activate.

IgE Immunoglobulin E; an antibody that plays an important role in allergies; it is especially associated with type I anaphylactic reactions.

IgG Immunoglobulin G; the most abundant antibody; it is equally distributed in blood and tissue liquids.

IgM Immunoglobulin M; a basic antibody that produces B cells; the first antibody to appear in response to initial exposure to an antigen.

immune system A complex network of cells, tissues, and organs that work together to protect the body against "attacks" by foreign substances.

immunologic memory The body's ability to rapidly produce large numbers of specific immune cells after subsequent exposure to a previously encountered antigen.

immunology A broad branch of medical science that covers the study of the immune system.

immunosuppression Reduction in the activation or efficiency of the immune system; it often is caused with drugs or radiation to prevent the rejection of grafts or transplanted tissues or to control autoimmune disease.

isografting The transplantation of cells, tissues, or organs between identical twins.

leukotrienes A class of biologically active compounds that occur naturally in leukocytes and that produce allergic and inflammatory reactions.

lymphocyte A type of white blood cell formed in the lymphoid tissue.

macrophages Phagocytic cells in the immune system.

mast cells Specialized cells of the inflammatory response.

memory cells Cells that remember the same pathogen for faster antibody production with future exposures; they are produced by the division of B cells.

natural immunity Non-antigen-specific immunity that is present at birth; also known as *innate immunity* or *nonspecific immunity*.

organ transplant The replacement of a failing organ with a healthy one from a donor.

pathogen A disease-causing agent.

pathogenic microbes Microscopic pathogens that can cause infection, such as bacteria, parasites, fungi, and viruses.

phagocytosis The process of ingestion by cells of solid substances, such as other cells, bacteria, bits of necrosed tissue, and foreign particles.

pruritus A sensation that causes the desire or reflex to scratch.

Raynaud's phenomenon A condition in which cold temperatures or strong emotions cause blood vessel spasms that block blood flow to the fingers, toes, ears, and nose.

scleroderma A collagen vascular disease thought to arise when the immune system stimulates certain cells (fibroblasts) that cause increased production of collagen.

sensitization An acquired reaction in which specific antibodies develop in response to an antigen.

systemic lupus erythematosus (SLE) A chronic inflammatory disease that affects many systems of the body; it is characterized by severe vasculitis, renal involvement, and lesions of the skin and nervous system.

T lymphocytes The lymphocytes responsible for cell-mediated immunity.

thromboxanes Antagonistic prostaglandin derivatives that are synthesized and released by degranulating platelets, causing vasoconstriction and promoting the degranulation of other platelets.

urticaria A pruritic skin eruption characterized by transient wheals of various shapes and sizes that have well-defined margins and pale centers.

wheals Small areas of swelling of the skin that result from an allergic reaction.

---

*I*mmunology *is a broad branch of medical science that covers the study of the immune system. A healthy immune system is the body's best defense against disease. However, sometimes the immune system goes awry, and the body begins to attack its own tissues and organs. People with immune system disorders are susceptible to a number of diseases, some of which can be life threatening. This chapter reviews the immune system and some of the more common immune disorders that may be encountered in the prehospital setting. These include allergic reaction and anaphylaxis, collagen vascular disease, and transplant disorders.*[1]

SECTION ONE
Immune System and Allergic Reaction

OVERVIEW OF THE IMMUNE SYSTEM

As described in Chapter 11, the **immune system** is a complex network of cells, tissues, and organs. These cells, tissues, and organs work together to protect the body against "attacks" by foreign substances. Most of these substances are **pathogenic microbes,** or **pathogens.** Examples include bacteria, parasites, fungi, and viruses that can cause infection. The primary role of the immune system is to

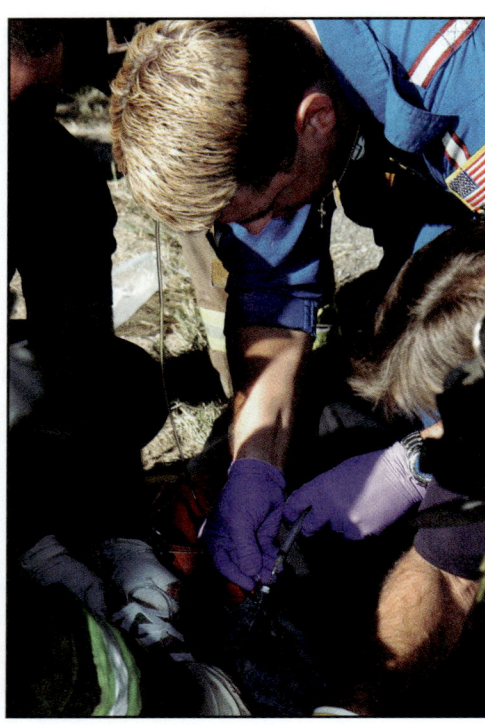

(Courtesy Ray Kemp, St. Charles, Mo.)

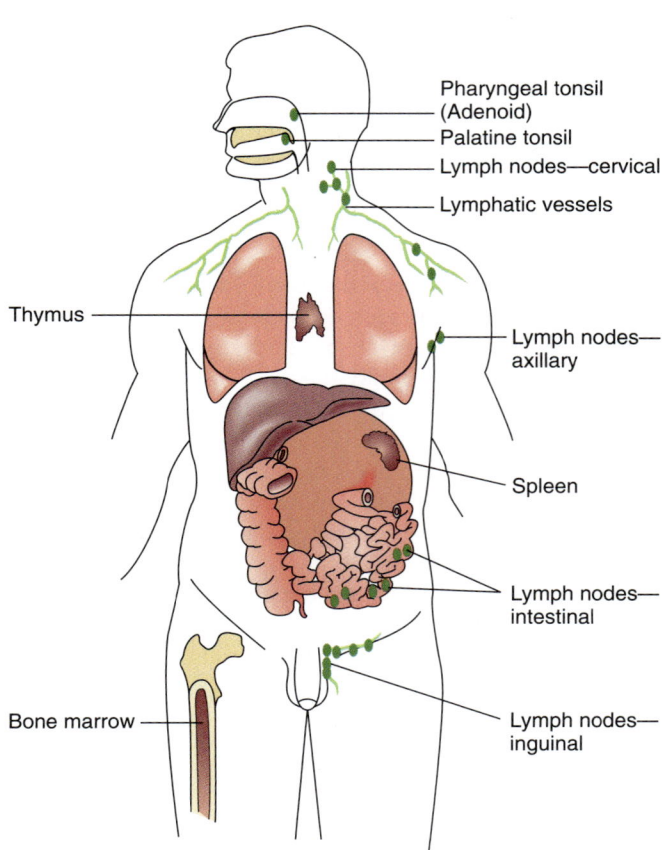

FIGURE 27-1 Structures of the immune system. (Gould BE: *Pathophysiology for the health professional*, ed 3, St Louis, 2006, Saunders.)

prevent these foreign substances from entering the body. If that fails, the immune system launches an attack so that these foreign bodies are found and destroyed.

LOOK AGAIN
See Chapter 11: Principles of Pathophysiology, pp. 242-248.

Immune System Structure

As described in Chapter 10, the organs of the immune system include the spleen, tonsils, adenoids, lymph nodes, and thymus (Figure 27-1). These organs are positioned throughout the body and are important outposts for lymphocytes, the key players in the immune system.

LYMPHOCYTES

The **lymphocyte** is the fundamental cellular unit of the immune system. About 25% of circulating white blood cells are lymphocytes. Lymphocytes are divided into two major classes: **B lymphocytes** *(B cells)* and **T lymphocytes** *(T cells)*. The roles of these two classes of lymphocytes are different and complementary.

B cells produce **antibodies.** Antibodies are proteins, not cells. In a sense, they are "magic bullets" that seek out specific invaders, or *antigens*. **Antigens** have *marker molecules* that identify them as foreign. When found, antibodies

trigger a process that destroys them. The antibodies in blood and lymph make up the humoral immunity. **Humoral immunity** is the form of immunity that responds to antigens, such as bacteria and foreign tissue.

NOTE
The process by which leukocytes destroy and digest pathogens is called phagocytosis. Circulating macro phages are specialized white cells. They are responsible for clearing the area of dead cells and debris.

T cells also respond only to specific organisms. However, instead of producing antibodies, they perform other tasks. There are three varieties of T cells: (1) *killer T cells* attack the invading organism with chemicals; (2) *helper T cells* encourage B cells to produce antibodies; and (3) *suppressor T cells* help regulate the immune response to protect the body from its own defense. The work of T cells is called **cell-mediated immunity.** Cell-mediated immunity does not involve antibodies. Rather, this form of immunity activates lymphocytes that attack and destroy foreign material.

    As discussed in Chapter 11, there are five varieties of antibodies: immunoglobulin A (IgA), immunoglobulin D (IgD), immunoglobulin E (IgE), immunoglobulin G (IgG), and immunoglobulin M (IgM). IgA is found mainly in the body's mucous membranes, where it intercepts antigens in the nose and throat. IgE binds to certain antigens to cause allergic reactions. The exact function of IgD is largely unknown. It is thought to bind to basophils and mast cells, activating the cells to produce antimicrobial factors that participate in the respiratory immune defense.[2] The largest antibody is IgM. The most common antibody is IgG. Together, these two play the major role in attacking many bacteria and other antigens.

    Each antibody consists of two chains of amino acids (the building blocks of protein). Each antibody has two long, thick amino chains that join to form a Y, and two smaller, thin chains along each branch of the Y (Figure 27-2). At the end of these four chains, the antibody binds with a specific antigen, similar to a lock and key. The *class* of immunoglobulin (e.g., IgG or IgM) enables the antibody to destroy antigens through an enzymatic chain reaction in the bloodstream.

Natural and Acquired Immunity

Once B cells and T cells have been activated by an antigen, some of these cells become **memory cells.** Many of the memory cells take up permanent residence in the lymph nodes, the gastrointestinal (GI) tract, and the spleen. Other memory cells travel through the lymphatic system and bloodstream. There they join with other lymphocytes and remain on guard for their chosen antigen. Memory cells ensure that the next time the body is exposed to the same antigen that produced the memory cell, the immune system is set into motion to destroy it. This memory is known as **immunologic memory.** The process by which this occurs is known as *immunity*. As described in Chapter 11, immunity can be either natural or acquired.

NATURAL IMMUNITY

Natural immunity is also known as *innate immunity* or *nonspecific immunity*. It is immunity that "naturally" exists. This type of immunity is not antigen-specific; it does not require previous exposure to an antigen. Natural immunity is present at birth because of antibodies the newborn receives from the mother. (The antibody IgG travels across the placenta and makes the newborn immune to the same microbes to which the mother is immune. Children who are nursed also receive IgA from breast milk to protect the infant's stomach.) Natural immunity also may have a heritable component. This type of immunity is quick to respond. It is the body's first line of defense against invading organisms.

    Natural immunity can be *passive* or *active*. The natural immunity present at birth is passive. Passive immunity also can be conveyed through serum obtained from a person who is immune to a specific infectious agent *(artificially acquired passive immunity)*. For example, gamma globulin sometimes is given to travelers who visit countries where hepatitis is widespread. Passive immunity usually provides protection for only a few weeks. It also carries the risk of causing sensitivity reactions.

    Active immunity can be triggered by infection and vaccination. For example, nondeliberate exposure to a person

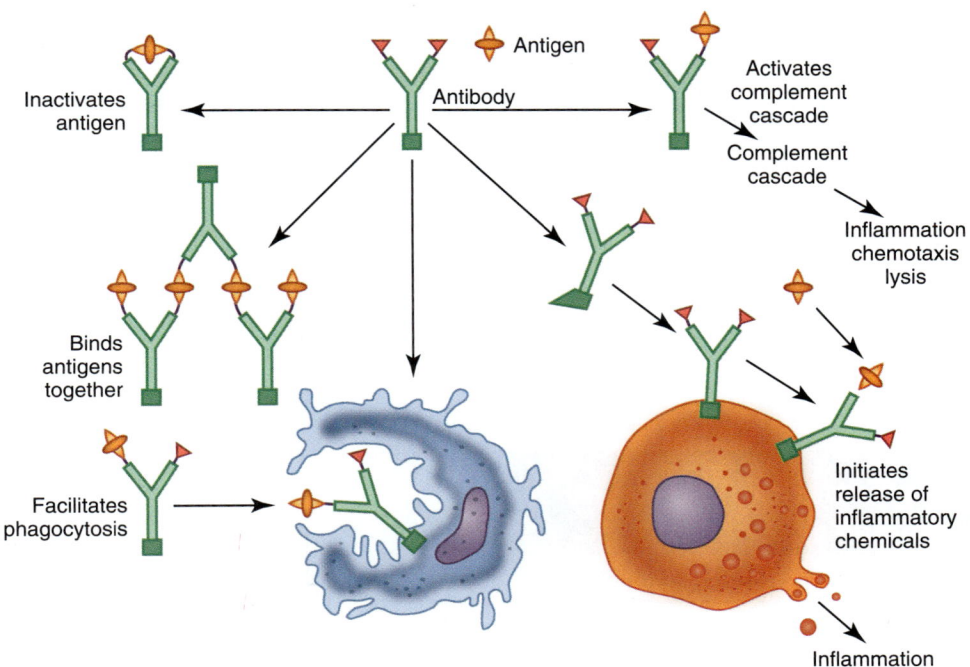

FIGURE 27-2 Antibodies act on antigens by inactivating and binding them together to facilitate phagocytosis and by initiating inflammation and activating the complement cascade.

with an illness can provide active immunity. The person exposed to the specific agent that caused the illness becomes immune to that specific disease. Vaccinations given with inactive (noninfectious) pathogens also provide active immunity. Like passive immunity, active immunity usually is short-lived.

> **NOTE**
> Natural immunity that is passive is achieved by the transfer of antibodies produced by one person *to another person*. Natural immunity that is active is the production of antibodies against a specific agent *by the immune system*. Natural immunity provides short-term protection for immediate threats. It does not change or prepare the immune system for future challenges.

ACQUIRED IMMUNITY

Acquired immunity is also known as *adaptive immunity*. It is immunity that develops after exposure to specific antigens. This type of immunity is "acquired" after the activation of B cells and T cells, which creates immunologic memory. Acquired immunity also may occur through immunization with a vaccine that contains a weak form of a specific antigen. Acquired immunity generally is a long-term immunity and often is considered permanent. It is slower to respond than natural immunity. However, immunologic memory significantly improves the rate of response to subsequent exposure to the same antigen. Acquired immunity acts as the body's second line of defense against invading organisms (Table 27-1). Like natural immunity, acquired immunity can be passive (acquired by the transfer of antibodies) or active (through immunization) (Figure 27-3).

> **NOTE**
> Acquired immunity is obtained deliberately. It changes and prepares the immune system to respond to future challenges.

IMMUNE RESPONSE

The first two lines of defense against infection (described previously) use the same mechanism to respond to all pathogens. However, the immune response is specific to

individual pathogens (see Chapter 28). The immune system that makes up the immune response has four unique characteristics:

1. It has "self-nonself" recognition; therefore, it usually responds only to foreign antigens.
2. It produces antibodies that are antigen-specific. That is, new antibodies can be produced in response to new antigens.
3. The memory cells produced by some of the antibody-producing lymphocytes allow for a more rapid response to repeat invasions by the same antigen.
4. The immune system is self-regulated. It activates only when a pathogen invades. This ability prevents healthy tissues from being destroyed. When this function goes awry, allergic reactions and autoimmune disease can occur. The immune system also may require extrinsic regulation with drugs in patients with transplanted organs or severe autoimmune diseases.

> **CRITICAL THINKING**
> What major immune disorder causes life-threatening airway, breathing, and circulation problems?

ALLERGIC REACTIONS

Antigens can enter the body exogenously (from the outside) by injection, ingestion, inhalation, or absorption (see Chapter 34). As described previously, antigens stimulate the immune system to produce antibodies. Antibodies then help neutralize the antigens and remove them from the body. This normal **antigen-antibody reaction** protects the body from disease by activating the immune response.

The immune responses normally are protective. However, they can become oversensitive. They can become directed toward harmless antigens to which people often are exposed (e.g., ragweed and pollen). When this occurs, the response is termed *allergic*. Antigens or substances that cause an allergic response are called **allergens.** Common allergens include drugs, insects, foods, latex (Box 27-1), animals, pollens, and mold. The healthy body responds to an antigen challenge through immunity.

TABLE 27-1 Characteristics of Natural and Acquired Immunity

Natural Immunity	Acquired Immunity
Non-antigen-dependent	Antigen dependent
Immediate response	Requires time between exposure and response
Results in no immunologic memory	Results in immunologic memory

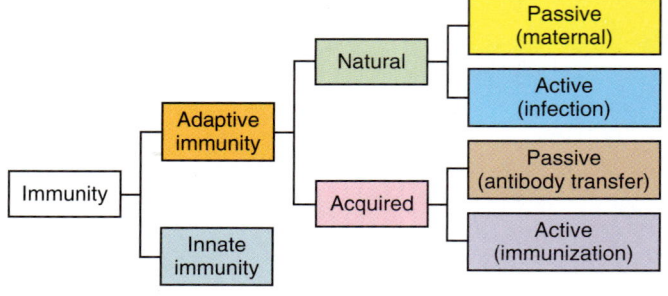

FIGURE 27-3 Passive or active immunity.

CRITICAL THINKING

Consider the list of antigens in Box 27-2. Based on this list, what are some likely locations to which you may be dispatched to care for a patient experiencing an anaphylactic reaction?

An **allergic reaction** (also known as a *hypersensitivity reaction*) is marked by an increased physiological response to an antigen after a previous exposure to the same antigen. This is known as **sensitization.** The allergic reaction starts when a circulating antibody combines with a specific foreign antigen, resulting in hypersensitivity reactions, or with antibodies bound to mast cells or basophils. To review, **mast cells** are cells found in several types of tissues. They contain granules that are rich in histamine and heparin. Mast cells are similar to **basophils,** a class of white blood cell that promotes inflammation through the release of chemical mediators (described later in the chapter). Mast cells and basophils and the release of these chemicals play an important role in allergic reactions (Figure 27-4).

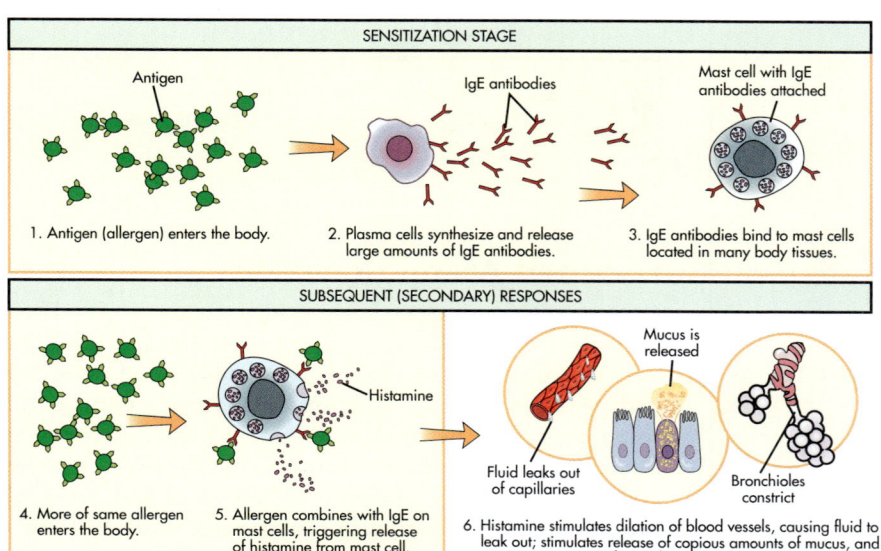

FIGURE 27-4 In an allergic reaction, antigen stimulates the production of massive amounts of immunoglobulin E, a type of antibody produced by plasma cells. IgE attaches to mast cells. This is the sensitization stage. When the antigen enters again, it binds to the IgE antibodies on the mast cells, triggering a massive release of histamine and other chemicals. Histamine in turn causes blood vessels to dilate and become leaky. This triggers the production of mucus in the respiratory tract. In some people the chemicals released by the mast cells also cause the small air-carrying ducts in the lungs to constrict, making breathing difficult.

BOX 27-1 Latex Allergies

Latex allergy is a significant concern, especially among health care workers. The first account of contact urticaria related to glove use was published in 1979. However, latex allergy was relatively unknown until after the acquired immunodeficiency syndrome (AIDS) epidemic in the mid-1980s and the resulting tremendous increase in glove use. The prevalence of sensitization to latex has been reported to range from 2.9% to 4.7% among health care workers and from 7% to 10% among operating room staff. (In addition to latex gloves, health care workers and latex-sensitive patients can be exposed to latex on medical instruments, surgical equipment, and other appliances.) Individuals considered at high risk for latex allergy include the following:

- Individuals who have had significant and early exposure to latex (e.g., patients with spina bifida or genitourinary anomalies and others who have had multiple surgeries and catheterizations)
- People with a genetic propensity to develop allergies
- Asthmatics
- Health care workers and law enforcement and fire service personnel who regularly use latex gloves
- Workers in some occupations (e.g., rubber manufacturing employees, hairdressers, food handlers, auto mechanics, tollbooth operators)

The symptoms of latex allergy can range from mild discomfort to life-threatening anaphylaxis. Most often the first manifestation of a latex allergy is urticaria, which typically is localized to the hands but may be widespread. A type I latex allergy can manifest in symptoms that include rash, lacrimation, rhinitis, wheezing, bronchospasm, laryngeal edema, hypotension, dysrhythmia and, in rare cases, respiratory or cardiac arrest.

Many health care facilities, EMS agencies, and other public service agencies have addressed this issue by developing "latex safe" environments and by using latex-free equipment for patients with latex allergy. For the health care provider, education, early recognition, prevention strategies, and implementation of safe and effective practices are essential. The National Institute for Occupational Safety and Health and many professional organizations have recommended that health care workers wear low-protein, powder-free gloves when latex gloves are necessary and synthetic gloves when the risk of exposure to blood-borne pathogens is low. Individuals not exposed to blood or body fluids (e.g., food handlers and maintenance workers) should avoid latex gloves altogether. All patients should be questioned about latex allergy; people with latex allergy should wear appropriate medical-alert identification. Sensitivity to latex should be documented on the patient care report, and this information should be conveyed to medical direction.

From Korniewicz D: Latex allergy: a current challenge. *Asepsis on the Web,* 1999. www.jnjmedical.com/asepsis/atex_allg.asp. Accessed September 22, 2004.

Allergic reactions can be mild, moderate, or severe, including anaphylaxis.[1] Mild and moderate reactions usually are localized, affecting the skin, upper and lower airways, and GI tract. They are not life threatening. Severe allergic reactions affect the same body systems but may be life threatening.

BOX 27-2 Agents That May Cause Allergies and Anaphylaxis

Drugs and Biological Agents
Antibiotics
Anticancer agents
Aspirin
Cephalosporins
Chemotherapeutics
Insulin
Local anesthetics
Muscle relaxants
Nonsteroidal antiinflammatory agents
Opiates
Vaccines

Insect Bites and Stings
Bees
Fire ants
Hornets
Wasps

Food
Cod, halibut, shellfish (e.g., shrimp)
Cottonseed
Egg white
Food additives
Mango
Milk
Peanuts, soybeans
Sesame and sunflower seeds
Strawberries
Tree-grown nuts
Wheat and buckwheat

Other
Intravenous contrast agents

TYPES OF HYPERSENSITIVITY REACTIONS

As described in Chapter 11, hypersensitivity reactions are divided into four distinct types: *type I*, anaphylactic (IgE mediated) reactions; *type II*, cytotoxic (tissue specific) reactions; *type III*, immune complex–mediated reactions; and *type IV*, delayed (cell mediated) reactions (Table 27-2). A type I (anaphylactic) reaction is the most dramatic. It may lead to life-threatening anaphylaxis (described later). Box 27-2 presents examples of antigens that may cause hypersensitivity reactions. Patients who have a known sensitivity to these or other agents should avoid exposure.

 LOOK AGAIN
See Chapter 11: Principles of Pathophysiology, pp. 246-247.

Localized Allergic Reaction

Contact with an allergen bridges adjacent antibodies. Each antibody binds with the invading organism at a different site. This changes the alignment of the antibodies on the surface of the mast cell. It causes the mast cell to burst and to release active chemical mediators into the surrounding fluid. Localized allergic reactions do not involve the entire body. In these cases, the sites of mast cell and basophil mediator release are limited. Common signs and symptoms of localized allergic reactions include the following:

- Conjunctivitis (inflammation of the conjunctiva of the eyes)
- Rhinitis (runny nose)
- Angioedema (swelling)
- Urticaria (hives)
- Pruritus (itching)

Localized allergic reactions are best managed with drugs that compete with histamine for receptor sites. This competition prevents histamine from performing its physiological actions (described later). Common antihistamines include over-the-counter oral and nasal decongestants and prescription and nonprescription *diphenhydramine.* Other

---

TABLE 27-2 Comparison of Hypersensitivity Types

Characteristics	Type I (Anaphylactic)	Type II (Cytotoxic)	Type III (Immune Complex)	Type IV (Delayed Type)
Antibody	IgE	IgG, IgM	IgG, IgM	None
Antigen	Exogenous	Cell surface	Viral (soluble)	Tissues and organs
Onset	Within minutes	Minutes to hours	3-8 hours	48-72 hours
Appearance	Wheal and flare	Lysis and necrosis	Erythema, edema, necrosis	Erythema and sclerosis
Cell type (histology)	Basophils and eosinophils	Antibody and complement	Complement and neutrophils	Monocytes and lymphocytes
Initiated by	Antibody	Antibody	Antibody	T cells
Examples	Urticaria, hay fever	Hemolytic anemia, glomerulonephritis	Lupus, serum sickness	Contact dermatitis, transplant rejection

medications that may be helpful for some local reactions include steroids and topical creams.

ANAPHYLAXIS

Anaphylaxis is an immediate, systemic, life-threatening allergic reaction. It is associated with major changes in the cardiovascular, respiratory, and cutaneous systems. Prompt recognition and appropriate drug therapy in the prehospital phase are vital to the patient's survival. *Anaphylaxis* comes from Greek terms. It means "against or opposite of protection." Anaphylaxis is the most extreme form of an allergic reaction, and it accounts for 500 to 1000 deaths a year in the United States.[3] It has a mortality rate of 3%. Rapid recognition and aggressive therapy are essential in treating this disorder.

Causative Agents

Almost any substance can cause anaphylaxis. The antigenic agents most frequently associated with anaphylaxis are penicillin (by ingestion or injection), venom from stinging insects, and food (especially nuts and shellfish). Regardless of the offending antigen, in sensitive individuals the risk of anaphylaxis increases with each exposure. To a lesser extent, the risk increases with the length of exposure or site of inoculation.

Pathophysiology of Anaphylaxis

As described previously, a person first must be exposed to a specific antigen to develop hypersensitivity. In the first exposure, the antigen enters the body by injection, ingestion, inhalation, or absorption. The antigen then activates the immune system. In susceptible individuals, large amounts of IgE antibody are produced. IgE antibodies leave the lymphatic system and bind to IgE-specific **Fc receptors** on the cell membranes of basophils that are circulating in the blood and to mast cells that are in tissues surrounding the blood vessels. The antibodies remain there and are inactive until the same antigen is introduced into the body a second time (Figure 27-5). With the next exposure to the specific antigen, the allergen cross-links at least two of the cell-bound IgE molecules. This results in **degranulation** (release of internal substances) of the mast cells and basophils and the onset of an anaphylaxis (Box 27-3).

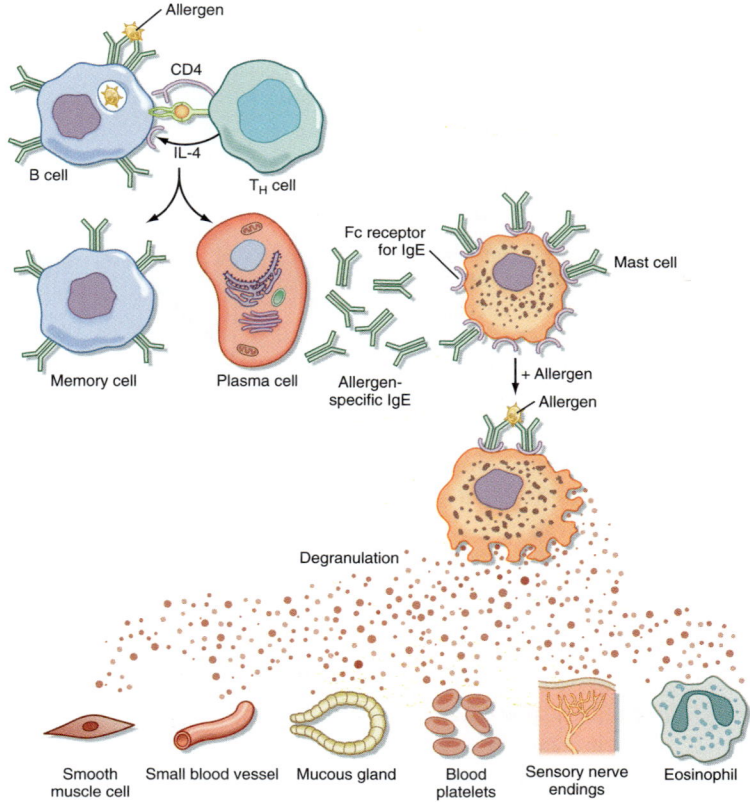

FIGURE 27-5 General mechanism underlying an allergic reaction. Exposure to an allergen activates B cells to form IgE-secreting plasma cells. The secreted IgE molecules bind to IgE-specific Fc receptors on mast cells and basophils. After a second exposure to the allergen, the bound IgE is cross-linked, which triggers the release of pharmacologically active mediators from mast cells and basophils. The mediators cause smooth muscle contraction, increased vascular permeability, and vasodilation. (Koeppen BM, Stanton BA: *Berne and Levy physiology,* ed 6, St Louis, 2010, Mosby.)

BOX 27-3 Anaphylaxis

Three conditions must be met for sensitization of an individual and generation of an anaphylactic response:

1. Antigen-induced stimulation of the immune system must occur, with specific IgE antibody formation.
2. A latent period must follow the initial antigenic exposure to allow sensitization of mast cells and basophils.
3. The person must subsequently be reexposed to the same specific antigen.

NOTE

Anaphylactoid reactions are allergic reactions that are not mediated by an antigen-antibody reaction. These reactions present exactly as does anaphylaxis, but they do not require previous exposure. For example, an anaphylactoid reaction can be caused by an IV medication that produces an excessive release of histamine in some patients. The distinction is not crucial with regard to treatment of an acute reaction; the two conditions are treated in the same way.[4]

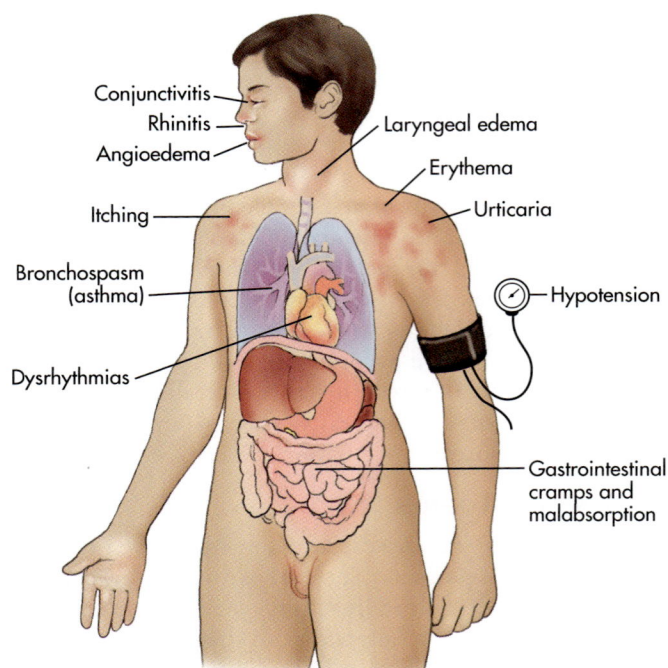

FIGURE 27-6 Manifestation of allergic reactions as a result of type I hypersensitivity includes itching, angioedema (swelling of the face, hands, feet, or genitals), edema of the larynx, urticaria (hives), bronchospasm, hypotension, dysrhythmias, and gastrointestinal cramping caused by inflammation of the gastrointestinal mucosa.

Degranulation of the target cell is associated with the release of pharmacologically active chemical mediators from inside the affected basophils and mast cells. These chemicals include histamine, leukotrienes, eosinophil chemotactic factor of anaphylaxis, neutrophils, heparin, kinins, prostaglandins, and **thromboxanes.** All of these chemicals mediate or trigger an internal systemic response.

Histamine is a protein released by mast cells and basophils. It promotes vascular permeability. It also causes dilation of capillaries and venules and contraction of smooth muscle in the GI tract and bronchial tree. An associated increase in gastric, nasal, and lacrimal secretions also occurs. This results in tearing and rhinorrhea. The increased capillary permeability allows plasma to leak into the interstitial space. This reduces the amount of intravascular volume available for the heart to pump. The profound bodywide vasodilation further reduces cardiac preload. This in turn decreases stroke volume and cardiac output. These responses lead to flushing, urticaria, angioedema, and hypotension (Figure 27-6). The onset of action of the histamine is rapid. However, the effects of histamine are short-lived, because they are quickly broken down by plasma enzymes. Figure 27-7 illustrates the pathophysiology of anaphylactic shock.

Leukotrienes are the most potent of the bronchoconstrictors, which cause wheezing. These chemical mediators also cause coronary vasoconstriction and increased vascular permeability. Leukotrienes formerly were known as *slow-reacting substances of anaphylaxis,* because their effects were delayed relative to histamine. However, the duration of action of these chemicals is much longer than that of histamine.

Eosinophil chemotactic factor of anaphylaxis is a group of active substances, including histamine and leukotrienes, that are released during an anaphylactic reaction.

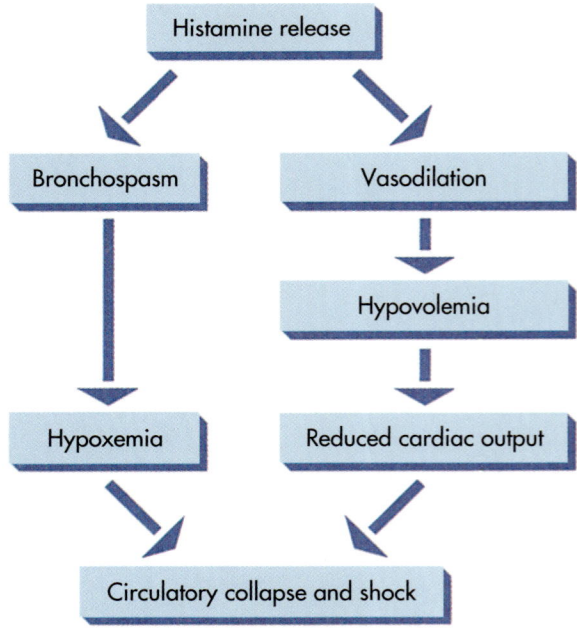

FIGURE 27-7 Pathophysiology of anaphylactic shock.

The process of anaphylaxis attracts eosinophils to the site of allergic inflammation. **Eosinophils** are thought to contain an enzyme that can deactivate leukotrienes.

The remaining chemical mediators (heparin, neutrophils, thromboxanes, prostaglandins, and kinins) exert varying effects that may include fever, chills, bronchospasm, and pulmonary vasoconstriction. These complex chemical processes rapidly can lead to upper airway obstruction and bronchospasm, dysrhythmias, cardiac ischemia, circulatory collapse, and shock.

Assessment Findings

An accurate history and physical assessment are necessary to differentiate between severe allergic reactions and other conditions that may mimic anaphylaxis (Table 27-3). A flawed prehospital assessment in this group can have life-threatening consequences. Disease entities that may present similar signs and symptoms of anaphylaxis include the following:

- Severe asthma with respiratory failure
- Upper airway obstruction
- Toxic or septic shock

- Pulmonary edema (with or without myocardial infarction)
- Drug overdose
- Dystonic reaction to antipsychotics
- Scombroid poisoning
- Angiotensin-converting enzyme (ACE) inhibitor angioedema
- Hypovolemic shock

RESPIRATORY EFFECTS

The initial signs of respiratory involvement associated with anaphylaxis may vary (Box 27-4). Signs may range from sneezing and coughing to complete airway obstruction

---

TABLE 27-3 Clinical Criteria for Diagnosing Anaphylaxis

Anaphylaxis is highly likely when any one of the following three criteria are fulfilled[5]:

1. Acute onset of an illness (minutes to several hours) with involvement of the skin, mucosal tissue, or both (e.g., generalized urticaria, pruritus or erythema, angioedema) *AND AT LEAST ONE OF THE FOLLOWING*
   a. Respiratory compromise (e.g., dyspnea, wheeze-bronchospasm, stridor, reduced peak expiratory flow [PEF], hypoxemia)
   b. Reduced blood pressure (BP) or associated symptoms of end-organ dysfunction (e.g., hypotonia [collapse], syncope, incontinence)
2. Two or more of the following that occur rapidly after exposure to *a likely allergen for that patient (minutes to several hours)*:
   a. Involvement of the skin-mucosal tissue (e.g., generalized urticaria, pruritus, erythema, angioedema)
   b. Respiratory compromise (e.g., dyspnea, wheeze-bronchospasm, stridor, reduced PEF, hypoxemia)
   c. Reduced BP or associated symptoms (e.g., hypotonia [collapse], syncope, incontinence)
   d. Persistent gastrointestinal symptoms (e.g., crampy abdominal pain, vomiting)
3. Reduced BP after exposure to *a known allergen for that patient (minutes to several hours)*:
   a. Infants and children: Low systolic BP (age-specific) or greater than 30% decrease in systolic BP*
   b. Adults: Systolic BP of less than 90 mm Hg or greater than 30% decrease from that person's baseline

*Low systolic blood pressure for children is defined as less than 70 mm Hg from 1 month to 1 year; less than (70 mm Hg + [2 × Age]) from 1 to 10 years; and less than 90 mm Hg from 11 to 17 years.

BOX 27-4 Signs and Symptoms of Anaphylaxis

Upper Airway
- Hoarseness or muffled voice
- Laryngeal or epiglottic edema
- Rhinorrhea
- Stridor

Lower Airway
- Accessory muscle use
- Bronchospasm
- Decreased breath sounds
- Increased mucus production
- Wheezing

Cardiovascular System
- Chest tightness
- Dysrhythmias
- Hypotension
- Tachycardia

Gastrointestinal System
- Abdominal cramps
- Diarrhea
- Nausea
- Vomiting

Neurological System
- Anxiety
- Coma
- Dizziness
- Headache
- Seizure
- Syncope
- Weakness

Cutaneous System
- Angioedema
- Edema
- Erythema
- Pallor
- Pruritus
- Tearing of the eyes
- Urticaria

(caused by laryngeal and epiglottic edema). The patient may complain of throat tightness and dyspnea. Stridor or voice changes also may be evident. Lower airway bronchospasm and associated hypersecretion of mucus caused by the actions of histamine, leukotrienes, and prostaglandins may produce wheezing and significant respiratory distress. Symptoms can develop with startling rapidity.

CARDIOVASCULAR EFFECTS

The cardiovascular manifestations of allergic reactions range from mild hypotension to vascular collapse and profound shock. Dysrhythmias (including severe bradycardia) are common. They may be related to the severe hypoxia and loss of circulating fluid volume that occurs. The patient may complain of chest pain if myocardial ischemia is present.

GASTROINTESTINAL EFFECTS

Nausea, vomiting, diarrhea, and severe abdominal cramping may occur in a patient having an anaphylactic reaction. The increased gastrointestinal activity is related to smooth muscle contraction, increased production of mucus, and outpouring of fluid from the gut wall into the intestinal lumen initiated by the chemical mediators.

NERVOUS SYSTEM EFFECTS

The nervous system responses are caused in large part by the impaired gas exchange and shock associated with anaphylaxis. At first the patient may be agitated and speak of a sense of impending doom. As hypoxia and shock worsen, brain functions deteriorate. This may result in confusion, weakness, headache, syncope, seizures, and coma.

CUTANEOUS EFFECTS

The most visible signs that distinguish anaphylaxis from other medical conditions relate to the skin. These signs are caused by the vasodilation induced by histamine release from the mast cells. Initially the patient may complain of warmth and **pruritus** (itching). Physical examination often reveals diffuse **erythema** (redness) and **urticaria** (hives). The hives are well-circumscribed wheals of 1 to 6 cm. Hives may be redder or more pallid than the surrounding skin. Often they are accompanied by severe pruritus (Figure 27-8). Significant swelling of the face, tongue, and deep tissues **(angioedema)** also may be present. This reflects involvement of deeper capillaries of the skin and mucous membranes. As hypoxia and shock continue, cyanosis may be evident.

> **NOTE**
> Angioedema is a localized swelling of the deep dermis or subcutaneous or submucosal tissues. It appears in the form of giant **wheals** (swelling under the skin). Patients with angioedema are at high risk for rapid deterioration.

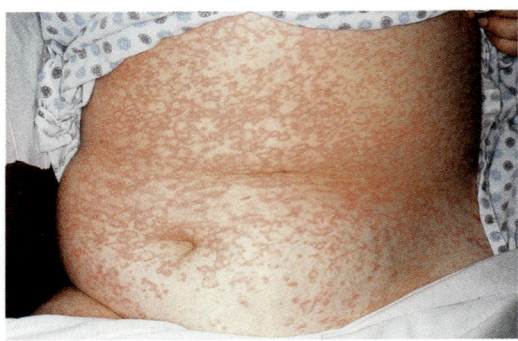

FIGURE 27-8 Urticaria as a result of an allergic reaction. (Courtesy Gary Quick, Oklahoma City, Okla.)

Primary Survey

As in any emergency, initial patient care is directed at providing adequate support for the airway, ventilation, and circulation. Drug therapy often is the definitive treatment in anaphylaxis. Therefore, drug therapy (described later) should be initiated as quickly as possible.

Airway assessment is critical, because most deaths from anaphylaxis are related directly to upper airway obstruction. A conscious patient should be evaluated for voice changes, stridor, or a barking cough. Complaints of tightness in the neck and dyspnea should alert the paramedic to impending airway obstruction. While drug therapy is underway, the airway of an unconscious patient should be assessed and secured. If air movement is blocked, an advanced airway should be placed. If laryngeal and epiglottic edema is severe, surgical or needle cricothyrotomy may be indicated to provide airway access (see Chapter 15). Early, elective intubation is indicated for patients with hoarseness, lingual edema, and posterior or oropharyngeal swelling. If respiratory function deteriorates, medical direction may recommend tracheal intubation (with sedation) without paralytic agents.[4]

The paramedic should monitor the patient closely for signs of respiratory distress, as indicated by pulse oximetry, capnography, skin color, accessory muscle use, wheezing, diminished breath sounds, and abnormal respiratory rates. Circulatory status also may deteriorate quickly. Therefore, the pulse quality, rate, and location should be assessed frequently.

History

A history may be difficult to obtain. However, ruling out other medical emergencies that may mimic anaphylaxis can be critical. The patient should be questioned about the chief complaint and the rapidity of the onset of symptoms. The signs and symptoms of anaphylaxis usually appear within 1 to 30 minutes of introduction of the antigen.[2] The onset of a reaction can be delayed if the exposure is by the oral route.

Important medical history includes previous exposure and response to the suspected antigen. In addition, the paramedic should identify the method of exposure to the antigen. Injection of an antigen often produces the most rapid and severe response. Other significant history includes chronic or concurrent illness and medication use. Preexisting cardiac disease or bronchial asthma should alert the paramedic to anticipate severe complications as a result of the allergic reaction. Certain drugs, such as beta-blocking agents, may diminish the patient's response to *epinephrine* and may necessitate the administration of other medications. The paramedic also should determine whether the patient has an emergency *epinephrine* drug kit (e.g., EpiPen [Box 27-5]) and whether the medication was administered before the paramedic crew arrived. Some patients with a history of allergic reaction may have taken an oral antihistamine (e.g., *diphenhydramine*), or they may have used aerosolized *epinephrine* (e.g., Primatene Mist or Medihaler Epi). The paramedic should try to determine whether the patient has taken these drugs, if possible. However, appropriate intervention should not be delayed.

SHOW ME THE EVIDENCE

Safdar and colleagues reviewed the literature to evaluate the use of subcutaneous epinephrine in patients with either asthma or anaphylaxis. They sought to determine its effects on older adults who did not have known cardiovascular disease. The researchers found three cases that reported adverse effects related to epinephrine administration. They noted that none of the literature included controlled studies. They concluded that insufficient evidence was available to prohibit the use of epinephrine to treat asthma or anaphylaxis in older adults with no known cardiovascular disease.

Safdar BD, Cone DC, Pham KT: Subcutaneous epinephrine in the prehospital setting, *Prehosp Emerg Care* 5:200-207, 2001.

Physical Examination

Vital signs should be assessed often. In severe reactions, most patients initially are tachycardic, tachypneic, and hypotensive if deterioration to cardiac arrest has not occurred. The paramedic should inspect the patient's face and neck for angioedema, urticaria, tearing, and rhinorrhea and should note the presence of erythema or urticaria in other body regions. Along with vital signs, the paramedic should assess airway and lung sounds often to evaluate the patient's clinical progress. Such assessment also helps the paramedic monitor the effectiveness of interventions. Cardiac monitoring should be instituted as soon as possible to aid evaluation of the patient.

Key Interventions to Prevent Arrest

Organ involvement in anaphylaxis varies. This makes a standardized approach to patient management difficult. The following key interventions commonly are used to manage anaphylaxis.[3,4]

BOX 27-5 EpiPen

EpiPen is an autoinjector prescribed for people with a history of severe allergic reactions or anaphylaxis. Each EpiPen contains a single dose of 0.3 mg of epinephrine. This dose is appropriate for people who weigh 66 pounds (29.7 kg) or more. EpiPen Junior contains 0.15 mg of epinephrine. This dose is appropriate for children who weigh 33 to 66 pounds (14.9 to 29.7 kg). The drug is administered by pushing the autoinjector into the anterior-lateral thigh and holding it in place for 10 seconds. (The EpiPen self-injects through clothing.) The EpiPen is packaged in single and 2-Pak cartons (in case a second dose of the drug is needed to manage an allergic reaction).

---

1. Place the patient in a position of comfort. Elevate the legs until replacement fluids improve the blood pressure.
2. Administer high-concentration oxygen. Early recognition of the potential for a difficult airway in anaphylaxis is paramount in patients who develop hoarseness, lingual edema, stridor, or oropharyngeal swelling. Planning for advanced airway management, including a surgical airway, is recommended.
3. Give *epinephrine* to all patients with clinical signs of shock, airway swelling, or difficulty breathing. *Epinephrine* may be given by the IM route (see the Emergency Drug Index). *IV epinephrine* should be considered immediately if life-threatening signs and symptoms are present.
4. Initiate IV therapy with normal saline solution if hypotension is present and does not respond rapidly to *epinephrine.* Repeated 1000 mL IV boluses (up to 4 L) to maintain a systolic pressure above 90 mmHg rapid infusion of 1 to 2 L (up to 4 L) may be needed initially.
5. Position the patient recumbent and elevate the legs unless precluded by vomiting or shortness of breath. Transport the patient for evaluation by a physician. Most patients are observed carefully in the hospital for up to 24 hours. Many patients do not respond promptly to therapy, and symptoms may recur in some patients **(biphasic reaction)** (Box 27-6).

NOTE

Complications of IV administration of *epinephrine* are significant and include the development of uncontrolled systolic hypertension, vomiting, seizures, dysrhythmias, and myocardial ischemia. This route should be used only in patients with a critical life-threatening condition. Intravenous administration of *epinephrine* rarely is performed in conscious patients. Intravenous administration is performed with extreme caution in rare circumstances and only with authorization from medical direction. *Epinephrine 1:1000 should never be given as an IV bolus.* The paramedic should follow the specific administration guidelines in the Emergency Drug Index.

BOX 27-6   Biphasic Reactions

As many as 25% of those who have an anaphylactic reaction experience a recurrence in the hours after the beginning of the reaction and will require further medical treatment.[6] This delayed reaction is called *biphasic,* meaning in two phases. The second phase usually occurs after an asymptomatic period of 1 to 8 hours, but a delay of up to 24 hours is possible. Epinephrine again is the treatment of choice, and the drug should be administered immediately. Post-treatment observation of these patients is necessary, and they should remain within ready access of emergency care for the next 48 hours.[7]

CRITICAL THINKING
How does *epinephrine* reverse the signs and symptoms of anaphylaxis?

OTHER DRUG THERAPY

Additional drug therapy may be helpful. However, *epinephrine* is the only drug that can reverse the life-threatening complications of anaphylaxis immediately. It is the drug of choice, because its beta stimulation produces bronchodilation; its alpha stimulation produces vasoconstriction; and it reduces the release of chemical mediators from mast cells. Pharmacological agents that may be used with *epinephrine* include antihistamine to antagonize the effects of histamine, beta agonists to improve alveolar ventilation, corticosteroids to prevent a delayed reaction, *glucagon* (for patients unresponsive to *epinephrine,* especially those taking antidysrhythmics [beta blockers]), and perhaps vasopressors to manage protracted hypotension (H2 antagonists such as cimetidine or ranitidine may be given in cases of hypotension that are unresponsive to *epinephrine*). Other drugs that may be useful in managing anaphylaxis include *albuterol* for bronchodilation, *diphenhydramine* to counter the effects of histamine, and *methylprednisolone* to reduce inflammation (Box 27-7). (See the EDI.)

NOTE
Beta blockers may increase the incidence and severity of anaphylaxis and can produce a paradoxical response to *epinephrine.*[4] For patients taking beta blockers, *glucagon* may be effective.

Key Interventions During Arrest

Cardiac arrest from anaphylaxis may be associated with profound vasodilation, intravascular collapse, tissue hypoxia, and asystole. Special considerations for resuscitation of these patients are described next.[3,4]

AIRWAY, OXYGENATION, AND VENTILATION

Swelling of the airway can make bag-mask ventilation and endotracheal intubation difficult or ineffective in patients with anaphylaxis. In addition, the landmarks for needle cricothyrotomy may not be visible because of severe

BOX 27-7   Additional Drug Therapy for Anaphylaxis

Antihistamines
Diphenhydramine
Hydroxyzine
Promethazine
Cimetidine
Ranitidine
Famotidine

Corticosteroids
Methylprednisolone
Hydrocortisone
Dexamethasone

Beta Agonists
Albuterol
Levalbuterol

Anticholinergic Bronchodilator
Ipratropium

Antiarrhythmics
Amiodarone
Lidocaine and others

Vasopressors
Dopamine
Norepinephrine
Vasopressin

Glucagon

swelling in the soft tissues of the neck. Fiberoptic intubation and digital intubation are alternative methods to consider in these situations (see Chapter 15). Smaller than normal endotracheal tubes may be needed because of associated edema.

SUPPORT OF CIRCULATION

Cardiac arrest from anaphylaxis requires rapid, aggressive volume replacement (2 to 4 L) to support circulation and the use of vasopressor drugs to support blood pressure. *Epinephrine* (including immediate use of EpiPen, if available) is the drug of choice for the treatment of vasodilation and hypotension in cardiac arrest (see the EDI). Alternative vasoactive drugs (*vasopressin*, *norepinephrine*, methoxamine, and metaraminol) may be considered in cardiac arrest secondary to anaphylaxis that does not respond to epinephrine.[3]

Asystole or pulseless electrical activity with a heart rate less than 60 beats/minute are the most common arrest rhythms in anaphylaxis (see Chapter 22). Cardiac arrest from anaphylaxis may respond to prolonged periods of cardiopulmonary resuscitation. This may be the case especially when the patient is young and has a healthy heart and cardiovascular system.

SECTION TWO
Collagen Vascular Disease

Collagen vascular disease is also known as *connective tissue disease*. Collagen is the principal structural protein of most body tissues. Many connective tissue diseases feature abnormal immune system activity with inflammation in the tissues. This is a result of an immune system that is directed against one's own body tissues **(autoimmune disease).** Collagen vascular disease may have both genetic and environmental causes. The immune system disorder results in the accumulation of extra antibodies in the circulation. Two "classic" collagen vascular diseases described in this chapter are systemic lupus and scleroderma,[1] (Other autoimmune diseases, such as rheumatoid arthritis, are discussed in Chapter 33.) Some patients have a combination of these diseases; this is known as *mixed connective tissue disease*.[9]

> **NOTE**
> Physician care for patients with collagen vascular disease often is multidisciplinary because of the nature of the disease and the affected organs and body systems. Specialists involved in this care may include rheumatologists, clinical immunologists, dermatologists, neurologists, nephrologists, cardiologists, psychologists, social workers, and others. Prehospital care is primarily supportive. When possible, these patients should be transported to their primary hospital for their specialized care.

SYSTEMIC LUPUS

Systemic lupus is a term that refers to one of many disorders of the immune system. **Systemic lupus erythematosus (SLE)** is the form of the disease most people refer to as "lupus." SLE usually first affects people between 15 and 45 years of age. However, it also can occur in childhood or later in life.

> **NOTE**
> Lupus primarily is a disease of young women, beginning mainly between the ages of 15 and 40 years. Women are six to 10 times more likely to have lupus than are men. Lupus can run in families, but the risk that a child or a brother or sister of a patient will also have lupus is still quite low. Lupus occurs in both siblings in approximately 25% to 50% of identical twins and 5% of fraternal twins.[10]

As in all autoimmune diseases, the immune system produces antibodies against the body's healthy cells and tissues. With lupus, these antibodies, called *autoantibodies*, contribute to the inflammation of various parts of the body and can damage organs and tissues. The most common type of autoantibody that develops in people with lupus is called an *antinuclear antibody* (ANA). It is so named because it reacts with parts of the cell's nucleus. Lupus can affect many parts of the body, including the joints, skin, kidneys, heart, lungs, blood vessels, and brain. These patients frequently develop inflammatory heart disease (pericarditis). They also may experience early-onset arthrosclerosis as a complication of the disease.

People with SLE can have many different symptoms (Box 27-8).[11] Some of the most common symptoms are extreme fatigue, painful or swollen joints (arthritis), unexplained fever, skin rashes, and kidney problems. A common finding in a patient with SLE is a characteristic reddish skin rash, called the *butterfly* or *malar rash*. This rash may appear across the nose and cheeks (Figure 27-9). Systemic effects of lupus may include the following[12]:

- GI ulceration or hemorrhage, abdominal pain, pancreatitis, cholecystitis, bowel infarction
- Renal failure

> **BOX 27-8 Signs and Symptoms of Lupus**
> - Painful or swollen joints and muscle pain
> - Unexplained fever
> - Red rash, most commonly on the face
> - Chest pain on deep breathing
> - Unusual loss of hair
> - Pale or purple fingers or toes from cold or stress (Raynaud's phenomenon)
> - Sensitivity to the sun
> - Swelling (edema) in legs or around eyes
> - Mouth ulcers
> - Swollen glands
> - Extreme fatigue

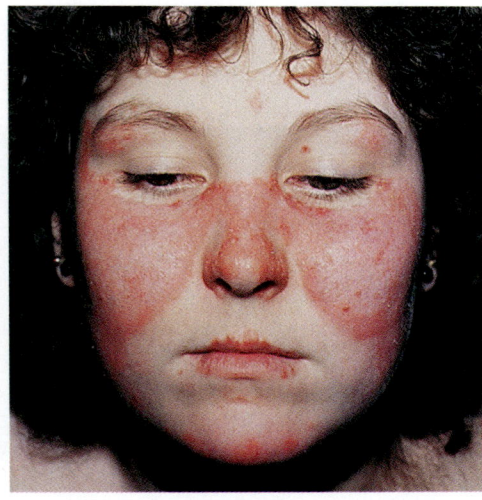

FIGURE 27-9 Systemic lupus erythematosus (SLE) flare. The classic butterfly rash occurs in 10% to 50% of patients with acute cutaneous lupus erythematosus. The rash appears over the nose and cheeks. (Christensen BL, Kockrow EO: *Adult health nursing*, ed 6, St Louis, 2010, Mosby.)

- Anemia and clotting abnormalities
- Pericarditis
- Pleurisy or pleural effusions
- Skin rash
- Behavioral changes, seizures, headaches, stroke

Management

The symptoms of SLE may be mild or serious. The goal of treatment is to prevent flareups, organ damage, and complications. Physician care may include nonsteroidal antiinflammatory drugs and corticosteroids to decrease inflammation, and antimalarials to treat fatigue, joint pain, skin rashes, and lung inflammation. Other therapies may include hormones, dietary modification, and nutritional supplements. Currently no cure is available for the disease.

SCLERODERMA

Scleroderma is derived from the Greek words *sklerosis*, meaning hardness, and *derma*, meaning skin. Scleroderma literally means hard skin. The disease is thought to result when the immune system stimulates certain cells (fibroblasts) that cause increased production of collagen. The excess collagen collects in the skin and internal organs, interfering with their function. Blood vessels and joints also can be affected. The disease is more common in women than in men. Because scleroderma can be difficult to diagnose, only rough estimates of its prevalence are available. The number of people in the United States with systemic sclerosis is estimated at 40,000 to 165,000.[13]

Scleroderma can be either localized or systemic, and both groups have subgroups. The localized forms of the disease are limited to the skin and related tissues and may involve underlying muscle. Internal organs are not affected. Localized scleroderma does not progress to systemic forms. Localized conditions often subside, but skin changes and damage from the event can be permanent (Figure 27-10). Two types of the localized condition are recognized: morphea and linear scleroderma.[14]

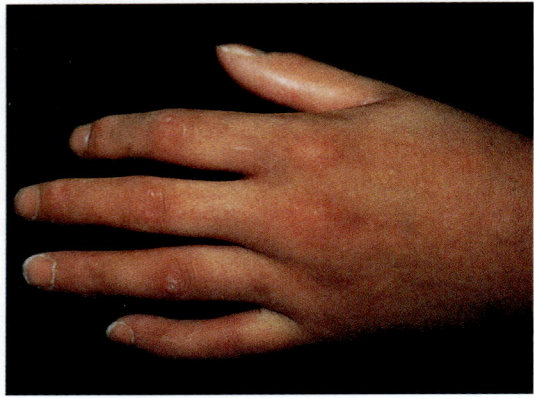

FIGURE 27-10 Scleroderma (acrosclerosis). Note the inflammation and shiny skin. (McCance KL, Huether SE: *Pathophysiology: the biologic basis for disease in adults and children,* ed 6, St Louis, 2009, Mosby.)

- *Morphea* is marked by local patches of hardened skin. Red patches of skin develop white centers with purplish borders. Lesions remain active for weeks to several years. Spontaneous softening that leaves a darkened area of skin often occurs. In localized morphea, one or a few patches are seen. In generalized morphea, the patches may grow over large areas of the body. Morphea can occur at any site. Occasionally the lesions can be extensive and gradually evolve into generalized morphea, in which the patches extend over most or all of the body surface.
- *Linear scleroderma* is characterized by a single line or band of thickened, discolored skin. The line usually runs down an arm or leg but sometimes runs down the forehead. When the band runs down the forehead, it may be called *en coup de sabre* ("sword stroke" in French).

Systemic scleroderma *(systemic sclerosis)* affects the skin, blood vessels, and major organs. Two types of systemic disease are recognized: limited and diffuse.

- ***Limited systemic sclerosis.*** In this form of scleroderma, skin thickening generally is limited to the fingers, forearms, legs, face, and neck. *Raynaud's phenomenon* may be present for years before any other symptoms develop. People with this form are less likely to develop severe organ involvement than are people with diffuse disease.
- ***Diffuse systemic sclerosis.*** In this form of scleroderma, skin thickening may occur anywhere on the body, including the trunk. Only a short period elapses between the onset of Raynaud's phenomenon and significant organ involvement. Damage typically occurs over the first 3 to 5 years, after which most patients enter a stable phase that varies in length. Organ involvement may lead to diseases and dysfunction of the esophagus, GI tract, kidneys, heart, and lungs.

NOTE

In a person with Raynaud's phenomenon, cold temperatures or emotional distress can cause the arteries feeding the hands or feet (or both) to constrict. This constriction causes the hands and feet to feel cold, turn white, and then turn blue. Once the vessels reopen (usually within 10 to 15 minutes), the hands turn red or mottled. More than 90% of individuals with scleroderma have Raynaud's phenomenon. It often is the first symptom of the disease. It also is found in patients with SLE.

CRITICAL THINKING

How might Raynaud's phenomenon affect your assessment of a patient who is hypoxic?

Management

No treatment for the complicated process that causes scleroderma has proved effective.[14] Therapies are aimed at preventing or reducing organ damage to prolong life.

Treatment decisions are made on a symptom-by-symptom and an organ-by-organ basis.

Patients with systemic scleroderma can suffer serious organ failure as a result of their disease. Thickening of vessels can lead to significant hypertension and pulmonary, cardiovascular, and renal failure. As a result, these patients can present with hypertensive crisis, renal failure, and heart failure. Drug therapy that may be needed to manage these disorders includes nitrates and calcium channel blockers to lower blood pressure, and angiotensin-converting enzyme (ACE) inhibitors to reverse renal crisis. Prehospital care may include both basic and advanced life support.

SECTION THREE
Transplant Complications

Every 10 minutes, a new name is added to the National Transplant Waiting List.[15] Many of these people are waiting for a solid organ transplant. These organs include the kidneys, liver, pancreas, heart, and lungs. In 2010, 28,663 Americans received an organ transplant.[16] Therefore, the likelihood of EMS personnel caring for a patient who has had an organ transplant is great. Common complications in patients who have received an organ transplant are related to **immunosuppression.** These include infection, rejection, and drug toxicity.[1]

> **NOTE**
>
> Two major complications associated with solid organ transplantation are infection and malignancy. These are the result of the lifelong immunosuppressive therapy that must be endured by transplant recipients to maintain function. The organisms most commonly associated with post-transplantation infection are the result of reactivation of latent infection carried by the donor organ or the recipient. They also may be due to new exposures in the community or in the hospital.[17]

INFECTION

Infection is the most common life-threatening complication of long-term immunosuppressive therapy in patients who have received an **organ transplant.**[18] Infection after transplantation of a solid organ can have many causes (Table 27-4), including:

- Community-acquired bacterial and viral diseases
- Opportunistic infections
- Infections due to *P. carinii* (also called *P. jirovecii*), *Nocardia asteroides, Aspergillus spp., Cryptococcus neoformans,* CMV, VZV, influenza, respiratory syncytial virus (RSV), *Rhodococcus equi,* and *Legionella spp.*

After a patient has been infected, the inflammatory responses associated with the invasion of microbes are impaired by immunosuppressive therapy. As a result, the signs and symptoms of infection that normally would be

TABLE 27-4 Possible Causes of Infection After Organ Transplantation

- *Month 1 (early post-transplantation):* The immune system usually is most suppressed in the first month after transplantation. Most infections during this time period are due to surgical or hospital-acquired infections. These may include infections caused by bacteria or *Candida* organisms. Infections may present as a urinary tract infection, wound infection, pneumonia, or a bloodstream infection. Herpes simplex virus (HSV) may reactivate (e.g., as cold sores). Many transplant recipients are prescribed medications to prevent the reactivation of HSV.
- *Months 2 to 6:* During this period, transplant recipients are at risk for unusual or opportunistic infections, such as *Pneumocystis carinii* pneumonia (PCP) or tuberculosis. During this phase, the transplant recipient also is at highest risk for reactivation of certain viruses, including cytomegalovirus, varicella zoster virus, Epstein-Barr virus, and the hepatitis viruses (see Chapter 28).
- Cytomegalovirus (CMV): CMV infection occurs in 44% to 85% of patients who have received a kidney, heart, or liver transplant. Symptomatic CMV disease occurs in 8% to 29% of kidney and liver transplant recipients. CMV disease can occur if a transplant recipient without a history of CMV receives an organ transplant from a donor with a history of CMV (primary infection). CMV disease also can reactivate after transplantation in a recipient who has a history of a previous CMV infection. CMV disease can present in a variety of ways, such as a flulike illness with fever, muscle aches, and fatigue, or as hepatitis. CMV is both preventable and treatable with antiviral medications such as ganciclovir, valganciclovir, and foscarnet.
- Varicella zoster virus (VZV): VZV is the virus that causes chickenpox. Ninety percent of adult transplant recipients were exposed to VZV during childhood, and they are at risk for reactivation of VZV in a form called *shingles.* Shingles is a painful, blister-like rash.
- Epstein-Barr virus (EBV): EBV is the virus that causes mononucleosis, or "mono." Transplant recipients who are not immune to EBV may get mononucleosis. Symptoms include fever, fatigue, muscle aches, and pains. EBV also may reactivate and cause post-transplantation lymphoproliferative disease (PTLD) in 1% to 2% of kidney and liver transplants, respectively. Symptoms are varied and can include fever, sore throat, abdominal pain, jaundice, or kidney and liver dysfunction. Treatment depends on the level of disease.
- Hepatitis B and hepatitis C viruses (HBV and HCV): Viral hepatitis can recur in transplant recipients who receive their transplants because of chronic hepatitis. Hepatitis B recurs in 5% to 10% of patients; hepatitis C recurs in 80% to 90% of recipients.
- *After 6 months (late post-transplantation):* Most transplant recipients do well 6 months after transplantation. They are at risk for community-acquired infections, such as urinary tract infections, influenza, and pneumococcal (bacterial) pneumonia.[19]

evident are masked. Consequently, infections often are advanced or have spread by the time of the patient complaint or clinical presentation. Established infection is difficult to treat in immunocompromised transplant recipients.[20] Significant antimicrobial toxicities are common, often as a result of diminished renal or hepatic function and drug interactions (described later).

NOTE

Paramedics should observe strict aseptic technique when caring for transplant recipients to avoid introducing infection. Vascular access should be avoided unless the need is clear.

CRITICAL THINKING

Which signs and symptoms of infection may be masked by immunosuppressive treatment?

DID YOU KNOW?
Post-Transplantation Infection
Infections in transplant recipients usually are categorized according to three phases that follow transplantation (early post-transplantation [month 1], months 2 to 6, and late post-transplantation [after 6 months]). Certain infections are more likely to occur during a specific phase.

REJECTION

Tissues or cells from another person (except an identical twin) carry nonself markers and may be recognized by the body as foreign. This is the reason some tissue transplants *(grafts)* are rejected. Most solid organ transplants are donated by nonidentical (genetically unrelated) people. This is known as **allografting.** If the transplanted tissue is donated by an identical twin, it is termed is **isografting.** Because allografts are more common than isografts, organ rejection is a major complication of solid organ transplant recipients. Rejection can be classified as *hyperacute, acute,* or *chronic* (Box 27-9).

NOTE

Rejection rates for transplant recipients have improved with advances in antirejection drugs. In the 1960s, 70% to 80% of patients experienced at least one rejection episode, and the 1-year survival rate for transplanted organs was about 65%. Newer drugs have reduced the rejection rate to 10% to 15%, and the 1-year survival rate for transplanted organs now is about 95%.[21]

Signs and symptoms of transplant rejection vary, depending on the transplanted organ and the recipient's general health. General signs and symptoms include the following:
- Pain at the site of the transplant

BOX 27-9 Classes of Rejection

Hyperacute rejection is a complement-mediated response in recipients with preexisting antibodies to the donor (e.g., ABO blood type antibodies). Hyperacute rejection occurs within minutes. The transplant must be removed immediately to prevent a severe systemic inflammatory response.
Acute rejection usually begins 1 week after transplantation. The risk of acute rejection is highest in the first 3 months after transplantation. Acute rejection occurs to some degree in all transplant recipients (except those between identical twins). This type of rejection can be successfully managed if recognized quickly.
Chronic rejection refers to cases of transplant rejection in which the rejection is due to a poorly understood chronic inflammatory and immune response against the transplanted tissue.

- General malaise
- Irritability (in children)
- Flulike symptoms
- Fever
- Weight changes
- Swelling and edema
- Change in the heart rate or blood pressure

DRUG TOXICITY

Many drugs are necessary to manage a patient who has received a solid organ transplant. Most of the medications are required for life to ensure the patient's survival and the success of the graft. The primary goals of drug therapy are to prevent organ rejection and infection. A major complication of the drug therapy is drug toxicity and adverse effects (see Chapter 13).

TYPES OF DRUGS USED IN TRANSPLANT RECIPIENTS

Oral immunosuppressant drugs commonly used in the United States include interleukin-2 (IL-2), receptor antagonist such as daclizumab (Zenapax) and basiliximab (Simulect), and OKT3 (monoclonal antibody). Other drugs include tacrolimus (Prograf), mycophenolate mofetil (CellCept), sirolimus (Rapamune), prednisone, cyclosporine (Neoral, Sandimmune, Gengraf), and azathioprine (Imuran). Medications to help prevent infections include antivirals such as acyclovir (Zovirax) or valganciclovir (Valcyte) to fight viruses, and antifungals such as fluconazole (Diflucan), nystatin (Mycostatin, Nilstat), or itraconazole (Sporanox) to fight fungal infections. Antibiotics such as sulfamethoxazole/trimethoprim (Bactrim, Septra) are used to treat bacterial infections. Three drugs commonly associated with drug toxicity and adverse drug interactions in transplant recipients are cyclosporine, azathioprine, and corticosteroids (Table 27-5).[1]

NOTE

Other medications and some foods may interact with post-transplantation medications. Complications can arise from the following:

- Some prescription medicines, such as erythromycin, clarithromycin (Biaxin), **diltiazem** (Cardizem, Tiazac), and **verapamil** (Calan, Verelan)
- Over-the-counter products, such as cimetidine (Tagamet) or herbal products or natural remedies, including St. John's wort, echinacea, black cohosh, and others.
- Eating grapefruit or drinking grapefruit juice, which can alter drug metabolism

MANAGEMENT OF PATIENTS WITH TRANSPLANT DISORDERS

Prehospital care for a patient who has received a solid organ transplant may vary from providing only comfort measures to supporting vital functions. These patients often have a long and complex medical history. Most require rapid transport for evaluation by a physician and specialty care.

TABLE 27-5 Drugs That Can Cause Toxicity in Transplant Recipients[22]

Drug	Adverse Effects
Cyclosporine	Hyperkalemia, hypomagnesemia, nausea, vomiting, diarrhea, hypertrichosis, hirsutism, gingival hyperplasia, hyperlipidemia, glucose intolerance, infection, malignancy, hyperuricemia. Multiple drug interactions are possible, primarily with agents affecting the cytochrome.
Azathioprine	Leukopenia, thrombocytopenia, gastrointestinal difficulties, hepatitis, cholestasis, alopecia. Azathioprine is compatible with cyclosporine and tacrolimus.
Corticosteroids	Cushing's disease, bone disease (osteoporosis, avascular necrosis), cataracts, glucose intolerance, infections, hyperlipidemia, growth retardation.

SUMMARY

- The immune system is designed to prevent foreign substances from entering the body. If that fails, this system should launch an attack to find and destroy these foreign substances.
- Organs of the immune system include the spleen, tonsils, adenoids, lymph nodes, and thymus.
- Lymphocytes are the primary units of the immune system. There are B lymphocytes and T lymphocytes. B lymphocytes produce antibodies. This is called *humoral immunity*. T lymphocytes provide immune protection with three types of cells. Killer T cells attack invading organisms; helper T cells encourage B-cell antibody production; and suppressor T cells regulate the immune response so that it does not attack the body. T cells provide cell-mediated immunity.
- Natural immunity is present at birth. It is not antigen-specific. Acquired immunity develops after exposure to specific antigens.
- Local allergic reactions do not produce life-threatening signs and are treated with antihistamine (e.g., diphenhydramine).
- Anaphylaxis is an immediate, systemic, and life-threatening reaction.
- Antigens are substances that trigger antibody formation.
- Antibodies bind to the antigen that produced them. Antibodies help neutralize the antigen and remove it from the body.
- An allergic reaction is an increased physiological response to an antigen after a previous exposure to the same antigen.

- Localized allergic reactions do not affect the entire body. They affect the skin, nasal passages, or eyes, not the lungs or cardiovascular system. They are treated with antihistamines (e.g., diphenhydramine).
- Anaphylaxis is a form of type I hypersensitivity reaction. It is the most extreme form of allergic reaction. Rapid recognition and aggressive therapy are needed for patient survival.
- Almost any substance can cause anaphylaxis. The risk of anaphylaxis increases with the frequency of exposure.
- Chemical substances released by basophils and mast cells cause signs and symptoms of anaphylaxis. These chemicals include histamine, leukotrienes, and other substances.
- Symptoms of anaphylaxis may include a sudden onset of hives, angioedema, and pruritus; sneezing and coughing; airway obstruction; wheezing; hypotension or vascular collapse; chest pain; nausea, vomiting, or diarrhea; and weakness, headache, syncope, seizures, or coma.
- The paramedic should determine whether the patient has used an epinephrine autoinjector or taken diphenhydramine before arrival of the paramedic crew.
- Treatment of anaphylaxis includes administration of epinephrine and, if the patient is hypotensive, 1 to 2 L of normal saline. Additional interventions may include antihistamines, inhaled beta agonists, corticosteroids, glucagon, and vasopressors.
- Autoimmune disease occurs when the body's immune system attacks normal body cells, causing harm.

Continued

- Collagen vascular disease is also called *connective tissue disease*.
- Systemic lupus erythematosus, or lupus, is a disease of young women that can damage many organs. It often causes a butterfly rash on the nose and cheeks. Severe damage to the GI organs, kidneys, lungs, and central nervous system are possible.
- Scleroderma means hard skin. It is caused by increased collagen production. Systemic scleroderma may cause Raynaud's phenomenon and dysfunction of the esophagus, GI tract, kidneys, heart, and lungs.
- Solid organ transplants include the kidneys, liver, pancreas, heart, and lungs.

- Infection, rejection, and drug toxicity are the key complications seen after organ transplant.
- Infections may include community-acquired bacterial or viral diseases, opportunistic infections, and others. Normal signs and symptoms of infection may be masked by the immunosuppressive therapy.
- When the body recognizes the transplanted tissue as "nonself," it begins to reject it. Rejection may be hyperacute (occurring within minutes), acute (occurring within 1 week), or chronic (occurring after 1 week).
- Immunosuppressive drugs have many side effects. Three drug groups known to cause many adverse effects are cyclosporines, azathioprines, and corticosteroids.

REFERENCES

1. National Highway Traffic Safety Administration: *The National EMS Education Standards*, Washington, DC, 2009, U.S. Department of Transportation/National Highway Traffic Safety Administration, DOT.
2. Chen K, Xu W, Wilson M, et al: Immunoglobulin D enhances immune surveillance by activating antimicrobial, proinflammatory and B cell-stimulating programs in basophils, *Nat Immunol* 10:889-898, 2009.
3. American Heart Association: 2010 American Heart Association Guidelines for Cardiopulmonary Resuscitation and Emergency Cardiovascular Care. *Circulation* 122(18 Supplement 3):S639-S946, 2010.
4. Marx J, Hockberger R, Walls R: *Rosen's emergency medicine*, ed 6, Philadelphia, 2006, Mosby.
5. Sampson HA, Munoz-Furlong A, Campbell RL, et al: Second Symposium on the Definition and Management of Anaphylaxis: summary report—Second National Institute of Allergy and Infectious Disease/Food Allergy and Anaphylaxis Network symposium, *Ann Emerg Med* 48:762, 2006.
6. Stark BJ, Sullivan TJ: Biphasic and protracted anaphylaxis, *J Allergy Clin Immunol* 78:76-83, 1986.
7. Ellis A, Day J: Diagnosis and management of anaphylaxis, CMAJ: *Canadian Medical Association Journal* 169:312, 2003.
8. Sampson HA, Munoz-Furlong A, Campbell RL, et al: Second symposium on the definition and management of anaphylaxis: summary report—Second National Institute of Allergy and Infectious Disease/Food Allergy and Anaphylaxis Network symposium, *Ann Emerg Med* 47:373-380, 2006.
9. Uitto J, Perejda AJ, editors: *Connective tissue disease: molecular pathology of the extracellular matrix*, New York, 1987, Marcel Dekker.
10. Arthritis Foundation: *Systemic lupus erythematous.* www.arthritis.org/disease-center.php?disease_id=29&df=whos_at_risk. Accessed August 25, 2010.
11. National Institute of Arthritis and Musculoskeletal and Skin Diseases: *Lupus.* www.niams.nih.gov/Health_Info/Lupus/default.asp#Lupus_2. Accessed November 6, 2009.
12. Christensen BL, Kockrow EO: *Adult health nursing*, St Louis, 2005, Mosby.
13. National Institute of Arthritis and Musculoskeletal and Skin Diseases: *Scleroderma.* www.niams.nih.gov/Health_Info/Scleroderma/default.asp. Accessed August 25, 2010.
14. Arthritis Foundation: *Scleroderma.* www.arthritis.org/disease-center.php?disease_id=26&df=effects. Accessed August 25, 2010.
15. United Network for Organ Sharing: *Transplant trends.* www.unos.org/. Accessed August 25, 2010.
16. Donate Life America: *Statistics*, http://donatelife.net/understanding-donation/statistics/. Accessed May 4, 2011.
17. Fishman JA, Ramos E: *Infection in renal transplant recipients in chronic kidney disease, dialysis and transplantation*, ed 2, Philadelphia, 2005, Saunders.
18. Fishman J, Rubin R: *Infection in organ-transplant recipients*, *N Engl J Med* 338:1741-1751, 1998.
19. Infectious Diseases in Solid Organ Transplant: http://www.lahey.org/Departments_and_Locations/Departments/Infectious_Diseases/Infection_Prevention/Infections_in_Solid_Organ_Transplants.aspx. Accessed May 4, 2011.
20. Bowden RA, Ljungman P, Pava CV, editors: *Transplant infections*, ed 2, Philadelphia, 2003, Lippincott Williams & Wilkins.
21. Benfield M: *Repeated transplant rejection: why does it happen?* American Association of Kidney Patients. www.aakp.org/aakp-library/Repeated-Transplant-Rejection/. Accessed August 25, 2010.
22. Pellegrino B, Schmidt RJ: *Immunosuppression.* http://emedicine.medscape.com/article/432316-overview. Accessed August 25, 2010.

SUGGESTED READINGS

Sampson HA, et al: Second symposium on the definition and management of anaphylaxis: summary report—Second National Institute of Allergy and Infectious Disease/Food Allergy and Anaphylaxis Network Symposium, *Ann Emerg Med* 47:373-380, 2006.

Venkat KK, Venkat A: Care of the renal transplant recipient in the emergency department, *Ann Emerg Med* 44:330-341, 2004.

CHAPTER
28 Infectious and Communicable Diseases

OBJECTIVES

Upon completion of this chapter, the paramedic student will be able to:

1. Identify general public health principles related to infectious disease.
2. Describe the chain of elements necessary for an infectious disease to occur.
3. Explain how internal and external barriers affect susceptibility to infection.
4. Differentiate the four stages of infectious disease: the latent period, the incubation period, the communicability period, and the disease period.
5. Describe the mode of transmission, pathophysiology, prehospital considerations, and personal protective measures to be taken for the human immunodeficiency virus (HIV), hepatitis, tuberculosis, meningococcal meningitis, and pneumonia.
6. Describe the mode of transmission, pathophysiology, signs and symptoms, and prehospital considerations for patients who have rabies or tetanus.
7. List the signs, symptoms, and possible secondary complications of selected childhood viral diseases.
8. List the signs, symptoms, and possible secondary complications of influenza, severe acute respiratory syndrome (SARS), and mononucleosis.
9. Describe the mode of transmission, pathophysiology, prehospital considerations, and personal protective measures for sexually transmitted diseases.
10. Identify the signs, symptoms, and prehospital considerations for scabies and lice.
11. Outline the reporting process for exposure to infectious or communicable diseases.
12. Discuss the paramedic's role in preventing disease transmission.

KEY TERMS

asplenia Congenital absence or surgical removal of the spleen.

bacterial endocarditis Inflammation of the endocardium and one or more heart valves; also known as *infective endocarditis*.

bacterial meningitis A life-threatening illness that results from bacterial infection of the meninges.

body lice Tiny parasites that concentrate around the waist, shoulders, axillae, and neck.

C. diff colitis Inflammation of the colon caused by the bacterium *Clostridium difficile*.

chemotactic factors Biochemical mediators that are important in activating the inflammatory response.

chickenpox An acute, highly contagious viral disease caused by a herpes virus, varicella-zoster virus; it occurs primarily in young children and is characterized by crops of pruritic vesicular eruptions on the skin; also known as *varicella*.

Chlamydia A genus of microorganisms that live as intracellular parasites; a common cause of sexually transmitted diseases and a frequent cause of sterility.

Clostridium difficile A bacterium that normally is present in small numbers in the intestines.

communicability period A stage of infection that begins when the latent period ends and continues as long as the agent is present and can spread to other hosts.

communicable disease An infectious disease that can be transmitted from one person to another.

complement system A group of proteins that coat bacteria and help to kill them directly or assist in having them taken up by neutrophils in the blood or by macrophages in the tissues.

congenital rubella syndrome A serious disease that affects about 25% of infants born to women infected with rubella during the first trimester of pregnancy; it is associated with multiple congenital anomalies, mental retardation, and an increased risk of death from congenital heart disease and sepsis during the first 6 months of life.

designated officer (DO) A person who serves as a liaison between the public safety agency and community health agencies involved in monitoring and responding to communicable diseases.

disease period A stage of infection that follows the incubation period; the duration of this stage varies with the disease.

exposure incident Any specific contact of the eyes, the mouth, other mucous membranes, or nonintact skin, or any parenteral contact, with blood, blood products, bloody body fluids, or other potentially infectious materials.

external barriers The surface of the body that is exposed to the environment. This includes the skin and the mucous membranes of the digestive, respiratory, and genitourinary (GU) tracts; the body's first line of defense against infection.

gonorrhea A sexually transmitted disease that results from contact with the causative organism *Neisseria gonorrhoeae*.

hantavirus A cause of several different forms of hemorrhagic fever with renal syndrome.

head lice Tiny parasites that concentrate around the scalp (sometimes including the eyebrows and eyelashes).

hepatitis An inflammatory condition of the liver characterized by jaundice, hepatomegaly, anorexia, abdominal and gastric discomfort, abnormal liver function, clay-colored stools, and dark urine. Viruses responsible for hepatitis are *hepatitis A virus, hepatitis B virus, hepatitis C virus, hepatitis D virus,* and *hepatitis E virus.*

hepatitis A Viral hepatitis.

hepatitis B Serum hepatitis.

hepatitis C Non-A/non-B hepatitis.

herpes simplex virus 1 An infection caused by the herpes simplex virus; it tends to occur in the facial area, particularly around the mouth and nose.

herpes simplex virus type 2 An infection caused by the herpes simplex virus; it usually is limited to the genital region.

host The human or animal exposed to an infectious agent.

host susceptibility Factors of the host that contribute to prevention or continuation of infection.

human immunodeficiency virus The viral agent responsible for acquired immunodeficiency syndrome.

incubation period The stage of infection during which an organism reproduces; it begins with invasion of the agent and ends when the disease process begins.

indigenous flora Agents found on various sites of the body that could produce disease if allowed access to the interior of the body.

infectious disease Any illness caused by a specific microorganism.

influenza A highly contagious infection of the respiratory tract transmitted by airborne droplet infection. Researchers have identified three main types of the virus (types A, B, and C).

internal barriers Protection against germs provided by the inflammatory response and the immune response; the body's second line of defense against infection.

latent period A stage of infection that begins when a pathogenic agent invades the body and ends when the agent can be shed or communicated.

latent TB infection Tuberculosis that is not symptomatic or infectious; must be treated to prevent active TB disease.

meningococcal meningitis Inflammation of the membranes that surround the spinal cord and brain; can be caused by a variety of different bacteria, viruses, and other microorganisms; also known as *spinal meningitis.*

mode of transmission The way in which diseases are transmitted; may be direct or indirect contact.

mononucleosis A viral infection causing fever, sore throat, and swollen lymph glands, especially in the neck.

mumps An acute viral disease characterized by swelling of the parotid glands.

opportunistic infections Infections that take advantage of weakness in the immune defenses.

pandemic An infectious disease outbreak that infects large numbers of people in a large geographical region and may occur worldwide.

pathogen A disease-causing agent.

pertussis An acute, highly contagious respiratory disease characterized by paroxysmal coughing that ends in a loud, whooping inspiration; also known as whooping cough.

pneumonia An acute inflammation of the lungs, usually caused by inhaled pneumococci of the species *Streptococcus pneumoniae.*

portal of entry The means by which the pathogenic agent enters a new host.

portal of exit The method by which a pathogenic agent leaves one host to invade another.

pubic lice Tiny parasites that concentrate in the pubic area.

rabies An acute, usually fatal viral disease of the central nervous system of animals; it is transmitted from animals to human beings by infected blood, tissue, or, most commonly, saliva.

resistance The immune status of the host; the ability to ward off infection.

reservoir Any person, animal, plant, soil, or substance in which an infectious agent normally lives and multiplies; typically harbors the infectious agent without injury to itself and serves as a source from which other individuals can be infected.

reticuloendothelial system Part of the immune system composed of immune cells in the spleen, lymph nodes, liver, bone marrow, lungs, and intestines; stores mature B and T cells until the immune system is activated.

rubella A contagious viral disease characterized by fever, symptoms of mild upper respiratory tract infection, lymph node enlargement, and a diffuse, fine, red maculopapular rash; it is spread by droplet infection; also known as *German measles.*

rubeola An acute, highly contagious viral disease involving the respiratory tract; it is characterized by a spreading, maculopapular, cutaneous rash and occurs primarily in young children who have not been immunized; also known as *red measles.*

scabies A contagious parasitic skin infection characterized by superficial burrows and intense pruritus; caused by the mite *Sarcoptes scabiei.*

sexually transmitted disease Refers to a group of infections that are passed from one person to another through sexual contact.

shingles An acute infection caused by reactivation of the latent varicella-zoster virus; it is characterized by painful vesicular eruptions that follow the underlying route of cranial or spinal nerves inflamed by the virus; also known as *herpes zoster*.

syphilis A sexually transmitted disease characterized by distinct stages of effects over a period of years; any organ system may be involved.

tabes dorsalis An abnormal condition characterized by the slow degeneration of all or part of the body and the progressive loss of peripheral reflexes.

TB disease Active tuberculosis.

tetanus An acute, potentially fatal infection of the central nervous system caused by the tetanus bacillus *Clostridium tetani;* characterized by muscle spasms and convulsions.

transmitted nonspecific urethritis A sexually transmitted disease characterized by inflammation or infection of the urethra in which the cause is not defined; also known as nongonococcal urethritis.

tuberculosis A chronic granulomatous infection caused by *Mycobacterium tuberculosis;* it usually affects the lungs and generally is transmitted by inhalation or ingestion of infected droplets.

universal precautions Infection control practices in health care that are observed with every patient and procedure and that prevent exposure to blood-borne pathogens.

viral meningitis A syndrome generally associated with an existing systemic viral disease (e.g., enteroviral infection, herpes virus infection, mumps, and, less commonly, influenza); also known as *aseptic meningitis*.

virulence The relative strength of a pathogen.

---

*E*mergencies that involve infectious and communicable diseases are common in the prehospital setting. They can pose a significant health risk to emergency medical services (EMS) personnel. This chapter addresses the duties of the paramedic and EMS agencies in ensuring personal protection. It also presents the causes of infectious and communicable diseases, as well as special aspects of providing care for these conditions.

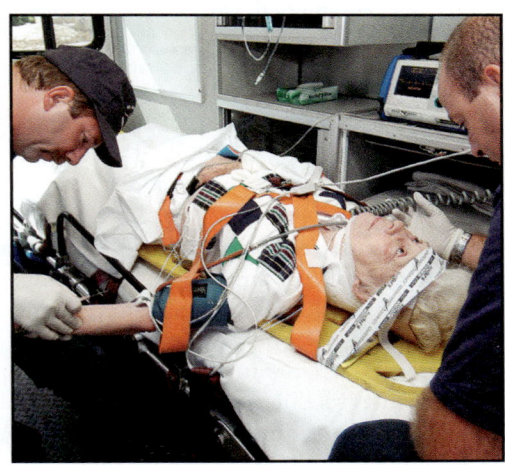

(Courtesy Ray Kemp, St. Charles, Mo.)

PUBLIC HEALTH PRINCIPLES RELATED TO INFECTIOUS DISEASES

An **infectious disease** is any illness caused by a specific germ. A **communicable disease** is an infectious disease that can be passed from one person to another. Infectious (communicable) diseases affect entire populations of people. These populations or groups of people are defined by location, age, socioeconomic status, and the relationships between the groups. Groups display varying susceptibilities to infection and varying degrees of susceptibility. In addition to demographics, other factors can affect the life cycle of an infectious agent within a population. These include:

- International travel
- Age distributions
- Population settling and migration dictated by religion
- Genetic factors
- The effectiveness of treatment once the infection has been established (Box 28-1)

When a disease outbreak occurs, local, state, private, and federal health agencies and other organizations become involved in prevention and management. Local agencies usually are the first line of defense in disease surveillance and outbreak. As described in Chapter 3, these include municipal, city, and county agencies such as health departments, fire departments, and EMS agencies.

 LOOK AGAIN
See Chapter 3: Injury Prevention and Public Health, pp. 54-57.

State agencies often are involved in the regulation and enforcement of federal guidelines. They frequently are required by statute or public law to meet or exceed federal guidelines and recommendations for prevention and management of disease outbreaks.

The private sector is composed of regional and national health care providers, local and national health

BOX 28-1 The Emergence of AIDS: An Outbreak of Disease

The presence of the human immunodeficiency virus (HIV) may have been detected as early as 1959 in Zaire. However, the virus did not become epidemic until 20 to 30 years later. The outbreak may have resulted from the migration of poor and young sexually active people from rural areas to urban centers in developing countries. This group often returned to rural areas or moved internationally because of civil wars, tourism, business travel, and the drug trade.

Acquired immunodeficiency syndrome (AIDS) was first identified in the United States in 1981. Young, previously healthy homosexual men in New York and California were found to have an unusual clustering of rare diseases (most notably Kaposi sarcoma, *Pneumocystis carinii* pneumonia, and unexplained persistent lymphadenopathy). A review of laboratory tests from that time for antibodies to HIV suggests that the virus entered the U.S. population in the late 1970s. Yet, at the end of 2008, an estimated 1,178,350 persons in the United States were living with HIV. And about 235,670 of those people do not know they are infected.[1] In 2008, an estimated 33.4 million people worldwide are living with HIV infection or AIDS. Since the epidemic began in 1981, more than 25 million people have died of AIDS.[2]

maintenance organizations, laboratories (hospital and private), infection control and disease specialists, and others. These groups influence protocols and guidelines for tracking diseases and responding to outbreaks.

Federal and national organizations include Congress, which plays an integral role in national health policy by passing public laws and drafting the federal budget; the U.S. Department of Labor's Occupational Safety and Health Administration (OSHA); and agencies under the U.S. Department of Health and Human Services, such as the Centers for Disease Control and Prevention (CDC) and the National Institute for Occupational Safety and Health (NIOSH). Other federal and national organizations involved in the prevention and management of disease outbreaks include the U.S. Department of Defense, the Federal Emergency Management Agency (FEMA), the National Fire Protection Association (NFPA), the U.S. Fire Protection Administration (USFPA), and the International Association of Firefighters (IAFF).

Local public health agencies can also play an important role during a disease outbreak in a community. These agencies can provide education to public service agencies, vaccine distribution through immunization clinics, and outbreak surveillance and tracking of infectious agents.

Agency Responsibility in Infectious Agent Exposure

National concerns regarding communicable disease and infection control have resulted in public law, guidelines, standards, and recommendations to protect health care personnel and emergency responders from infectious diseases. The components of a health care agency's exposure control plan should include the following[3]:

- Health maintenance and surveillance
- Appointment of a **designated officer (DO)** to serve as a liaison between the agency and community health agencies involved in monitoring and responding to communicable diseases
- Identification of job classifications and, in some cases, specific tasks when exposure to blood-borne pathogens is possible
- A schedule detailing when and how the provisions of blood-borne pathogen standards will be implemented
- Personal protective equipment (PPE)
- Body substance isolation (BSI)
- Procedures for evaluating exposure and postexposure counseling
- Notifying and working with local health authorities and state and federal agencies regarding exposures
- Personal, building, vehicle, and equipment disinfection and storage
- Education of employees regarding disinfection agents
- After-action analysis of the agency's response
- Correct disposal of needles and sharps in appropriate containers
- Correct handling of linens and supplies that become contaminated with body fluids during patient care
- Identification of agency and/or contracted personnel for counseling, authorization of acute medical care, and documentation

SHOW ME THE EVIDENCE

These authors reviewed existing literature to determine the incidence of blood-borne pathogens in firefighters and emergency medical technicians. Studies from St. Louis, Florida, Portland, New York City, Chicago, Baltimore, Atlanta, Fulton and Dade Counties, and Tucson were evaluated. Although there were problems with study design, they concluded that, even though the populations that EMS and firefighters encounter have a higher prevalence of HIV, HBV, and HCV than the general population, the emergency responders did not. The authors propose that this may be related to employment-related drug screening in this industry. Studies indicate that between 0% and 0.8% of first responders state they have ever injected drugs. They did find that paramedics have a higher incidence of needle-stick injury and mucous membrane and skin exposure than EMTs. Further, EMTs have a higher rate of blood-borne exposures than firefighters who are not EMTs or paramedics.

From Boal WL, Hales T, Ross C: Blood-borne pathogens among firefighters and emergency medical technicians, *PEC* 9(2):236-247, 2005.

CRITICAL THINKING

Have you had an outbreak of a communicable disease in your region? How was it controlled?

GUIDELINES, RECOMMENDATIONS, STANDARDS, AND LAWS

To protect health care workers against the spread of infection, OSHA requires that personal protective equipment be made available to all employees considered at high risk for exposure to infectious diseases. It also requires that all employees be offered preexposure prophylaxis against hepatitis B through inoculation with hepatitis vaccines.[4] The CDC and NFPA have established similar guidelines, recommendations, and standards regarding the protection of health care workers and emergency personnel from communicable disease. This includes regular testing for tuberculosis. It also includes vaccination for measles in individuals who do not have immunity (Box 28-2).

 DID YOU KNOW?
Ryan White Act
The *Ryan White Comprehensive AIDS Resources Emergency Act* (PL 101-381), passed in 1990, requires notification of emergency responders if they have been exposed to infectious diseases. It also requires that employers name a DO to direct communications between the hospital and emergency service in case of an exposure. Notification must be made within 48 hours of determination of the presence of the disease.

In December 2006, the *Ryan White Treatment Modernization Act of 2006* (PL 109-415) was signed into law. The portion of the law in the original *Act* that covered notification of disease exposure to first responders was stricken from the legislation, but was recently restored.[5] In addition, many states have laws in place that require emergency responders to be notified if they have been exposed to infectious disease.

The CDC has classified infectious disease into two types: airborne and blood-borne. An example of an airborne disease is infectious tuberculosis. Examples of blood-borne diseases spread by pathogens are the hepatitis B and C viruses and HIV. The CDC also lists less common communicable diseases. These include diphtheria, hemorrhagic fevers, meningococcal disease, plague, and rabies.

Currently, medical facilities are not required to test patients for any infectious disease. If paramedics have a significant exposure to blood or body fluids, they may submit a written notice to the DO. The DO, in turn, must submit a written request for a determination to the medical facility that treated the patient. The medical facility must try to identify the source patient and review any signs and symptoms shown by the patient that may correspond to the CDC list of infectious diseases. After determining whether a paramedic may have been exposed to an infectious disease, the medical facility must notify the DO within 48 hours of receiving the request. If it is a significant exposure and the source patient is known, the medical facility will usually ask for patient consent to test for HIV, hepatitis B virus (HBV), and hepatitis C virus (HCV) infection. In addition, the paramedic will be counseled about the need for postexposure

BOX 28-2 Recommended Immunizations for Emergency Medical Services Personnel*

Hepatitis B[†]
Diphtheria
Pertussis
Influenza
Measles
Mumps
Rubella
Tetanus
Polio

*Testing for tuberculosis (TB) may be required at the time of initial employment and annually thereafter. Additional vaccinations are recommended for EMS personnel involved in disaster services, military employment, or international work.
[†]This vaccination is required by the federal Occupational Safety and Health Administration.

prophylaxis (PEP) based on the patient's risk factors as well as the need for safe sex until follow-up results are known. If the patient refuses to be tested or the source patient is unknown, follow-up monitoring for the paramedic is arranged. Follow-up monitoring for the development of HIV, HBV, and HCV is important because PEP is most effective if started immediately.

 NOTE
Immediate testing will only reveal infection from a previous exposure—not from the exposure that prompted the immediate testing. A paramedic who tests positive for an infectious disease through an immediate test has had a previous exposure to the disease. Conversely, a paramedic who tests negative for an infectious disease through an immediate test may still have been infected from the exposure that prompted the test.

CRITICAL THINKING
What rights do you think paramedics had to obtain infectious disease information before the Ryan White law was passed?

Personal Responsibilities in Infectious Agent Exposure

Paramedics should familiarize themselves with the laws, regulations, and national standards regarding infectious disease. They should take personal protective measures against exposure to these pathogens. At times all paramedics will provide patient care to a person with an infectious disease. They must be aware of the potential consequences of the disease for public health and through contact with family members and friends. Table 28-1 and Box 28-3

TABLE 28-1 Personal Equipment for Protection Against Transmission of Human Immunodeficiency Virus (HIV) and Hepatitis B Virus

Activity	Disposable Gloves	Gown	Mask	Protective Eyewear
Bleeding control (spurting blood)	Yes	Yes	Yes	Yes
Bleeding control (minimal blood)	Yes	No	No	No
Emergency childbirth	Yes	Yes	Yes*	Yes*
Intravenous therapy	Yes	No	No	No
Endotracheal intubation	Yes	No	Yes*	Yes*
Oral or nasal suctioning	Yes	No	No	No
Administration of an injection	No	No	No	No

Modified from Centers for Disease Control and Prevention: Recommendations for preventing transmission of human immunodeficiency virus and hepatitis B virus to patients during exposure-prone invasive procedures, *MMWR* 40(RR08):1-9, 1991.
*If splashing is likely.

provide an overview of CDC guidelines. These are designed to help prevent the spread of infectious disease to public safety and emergency response workers. Paramedics should follow local protocol regarding similar or additional precautions for personal protection and should be aware of their individual responsibilities, including the following:

- A proactive attitude toward infection control
- Maintenance of personal hygiene (esthetics of patient care)
- Attention to wounds and maintenance of the skin (the external barrier to infection)
- Effective hand washing after every patient contact using warm water and antiseptic cleanser or waterless antiseptic cleanser when portable water is unavailable
- Washing or disposing of work garments before entering the home
- Handling uniforms in accordance with the agency's definition of PPE
- Proper handling and laundering of work clothes soiled with body fluids, with consideration for bathing and showering after the work shift and before returning home
- Preparing food and eating in appropriate areas
- Maintenance of general physiological and psychological health to prevent stress, which can compromise the immune system of a healthy individual
- Use of needleless or safe needle devices if available
- Proper disposal of needles and sharps in appropriate containers
- Proper disposal of body fluid–tinged linens and supplies
- Awareness and avoidance of tendencies to wipe the face and/or rub the eyes, nose, or mouth with gloved hands
- Knowledge of general classifications of exposure to determine the extent of infection control measures applied to the health care worker

UNIVERSAL PRECAUTIONS

As described in Chapter 14, the CDC published the *Recommendations for Prevention of HIV Transmission Guidelines in Health-Care Settings* (1987). This document recommended that **universal precautions** (universal blood and body fluid precautions) be used for all patients, regardless of their blood-borne infection status.[6] Since then, the U.S. Food and Drug Administration (FDA) and the CDC have worked together to further identify the body fluids to which universal precautions apply (Box 28-4).

 **LOOK AGAIN**
See Chapter 14: Venous Access and Medication Administration, pp. 380-381.

DECONTAMINATION METHODS AND PROCEDURES

Guidelines for cleaning, disinfecting, and sterilizing patient care equipment have been established by the CDC, OSHA, the Environmental Protection Agency (EPA), USFA, and other agencies and organizations. These guidelines are part of an EMS agency's protocols and standard operating procedures. The following is a brief description of these decontamination methods and procedures.[7]

Sterilization destroys all forms of microbial life. It is used for instruments that penetrate the skin or come in contact with normally sterile parts of the body (e.g., scalpels and needles). Methods that may be used for sterilization include steam under pressure (autoclave), gas (ethylene oxide), dry heat, and immersion in an EPA-approved chemical sterilant.

High-level disinfection destroys all forms of microbial life *except* high numbers of bacterial spores. It is used for reusable instruments that have contact with mucous membranes (e.g., laryngoscope blades, endotracheal tubes). Methods that may be used for high-level disinfection include hot water pressurization and exposure to an EPA-registered chemical sterilant.

Intermediate-level disinfection destroys *Mycobacterium tuberculosis,* most viruses, vegetative bacteria, and most fungi, but not bacterial spores. It is used for surfaces that come in contact with intact skin (e.g., stethoscopes, blood pressure

BOX 28-3 Guidelines for Prevention of Transmission of Human Immunodeficiency Virus (HIV) and Hepatitis B Virus to Health Care and Public Safety Workers

These general principles have been developed from existing principles of occupational safety and health. They have been developed in conjunction with data from studies of health care workers in hospitals. The basic premise is that workers must be protected from exposure to blood and other potentially infectious body fluids in the course of their work. However, data concerning the risks these worker groups face are lacking. This complicates the development of control principles. Thus the guidelines here are based on principles of prudent public health practice.

Fire and emergency medical services personnel provide medical care in the prehospital setting. The following guidelines can help rescue personnel make decisions on the use of personal protective equipment and resuscitation equipment. They also are meant to help them make decisions regarding documentation, disinfection, and disposal procedures.

Personal Protective Equipment

The proper personal protective equipment should be made available by the employer. This reduces the risk of exposure. For many situations, the rescuer's chance of being exposed to blood and other body fluids to which universal precautions apply can be determined in advance. If the chance of exposure is high, the worker should put on protective attire before beginning patient care. (Examples of high-risk situations include cardiopulmonary resuscitation, intravenous line insertion, trauma, and childbirth.) (This list is not intended to be all-inclusive.) Important pieces of protective gear include the following:

1. *Gloves.* Disposable gloves should be a standard part of emergency response equipment. All personnel should put them on before giving any care that involves exposure to blood or other body fluids to which universal precautions apply. Extra pairs should always be available. No single type or thickness of glove offers the best protection in all situations. Considerations in the choice of disposable gloves should include dexterity, durability, fit, and the task to be performed. When large amounts of blood are likely, the gloves must fit tightly at the wrist. This prevents contamination of the hands around the cuff. For care of several trauma victims, gloves should be changed between patients if the situation allows.

    More extensive personal protective measures are indicated when broken glass and sharp edges are likely to be encountered. Such a situation might include extricating a person from a motor vehicle crash. Structural firefighting gloves that meet the requirements of the federal Occupational Safety and Health Administration for firefighter gloves* should be worn in any situation in which sharp or rough surfaces are likely to be encountered.

    While wearing gloves, paramedics should avoid handling personal items (e.g., combs, pens) that could become soiled or contaminated. Gloves that have become contaminated with blood or other body fluids should be removed as soon as possible. In doing so, paramedics should take care to avoid skin contact with the exterior surface of the gloves. Contaminated gloves should be placed and transported in bags that prevent leakage. They should be disposed of properly or, in the case of reusable gloves, cleaned and disinfected as required.

2. *Mask, eyewear, and gowns.* Masks, eyewear, and gowns should be kept on all emergency vehicles that respond or may respond to medical emergencies or victim rescues. This barrier equipment should be used in accordance with the level of exposure encountered. Minor cuts or small amounts of blood do not merit the same degree of barrier use as that needed for victims with massive blood loss. Management of the patient who is not bleeding and who has no body fluids present should not routinely require the use of barrier precautions. Masks and eyewear (e.g., safety glasses) should be worn together or a face shield should be used by all personnel for any situation that is likely to involve splashes of blood or other body fluids to which universal precautions apply. Gowns or aprons should be worn to protect clothing from blood splashes. If large splashes or amounts of blood are present or anticipated, nonpermeable gowns or aprons should be worn. An extra change of work clothing should be available at all times.

3. *Resuscitation equipment.* No transmission of hepatitis B virus or HIV infection during mouth-to-mouth resuscitation has been documented. However, because of the risk of transmission of other infectious diseases through saliva, disposable airway equipment or resuscitation bags should be used. Diseases that can be spread in saliva include herpes simplex infection and *Neisseria meningitidis.* Theoretically, a risk exists of HIV and hepatitis B virus transmission during artificial ventilation of trauma victims. Disposable resuscitation equipment and devices should be used once and then discarded. If reusable, this equipment should be thoroughly cleaned and disinfected after each use according to the manufacturer's recommendations.

Mechanical respiratory assist devices (e.g., bag-valve-masks, oxygen demand-valve resuscitators) should be available on all emergency vehicles. They also should be available to all emergency response personnel who respond to medical emergencies or victim rescues.

Pocket mouth-to-mask resuscitation masks are designed to prevent personnel from coming in contact with victims' blood and blood-contaminated saliva, respiratory secretions, and vomitus. These should be provided to all personnel who provide or may provide emergency treatment.

Modified from U.S. Department of Health and Human Services, Centers for Disease Control and Prevention, National Institute of Occupational Safety and Health: *Guidelines for prevention of transmission of human immunodeficiency virus and hepatitis B virus to health-care and public-safety workers,* Washington, DC, 1989, Author.
*Standards are presented in 29 Code of Federal Register (CFR) 1910.156 and in National Fire Protection Association Standard 1973, Gloves for Structural Fire Fighters.

BOX 28-4 Clarification of Use of Universal Precautions*

Body Fluids to Which Universal Precautions Apply

- Blood and other body fluids containing visible blood
- Semen and vaginal secretions
- Human tissue
- Human fluids (cerebrospinal fluid, synovial fluid, pleural fluid, peritoneal fluid, pericardial fluid, amniotic fluid)

Body Fluids to Which Universal Precautions Do Not Apply (in the Absence of Blood)

- Feces
- Nasal secretions
- Sputum
- Sweat
- Tears
- Urine
- Vomitus

Precautions for Other Body Fluids in Special Settings

- Human breast milk in mothers infected with hepatitis B virus (HBV) (e.g., milk banking procedures)
- Saliva in some individuals infected with HBV or human immunodeficiency virus (HIV) (e.g., human bites [remote], dental procedures)

Modified from Centers for Disease Control and Prevention: Perspectives in disease prevention and health promotion update: universal precautions for prevention of transmission of human immunodeficiency virus, hepatitis B virus, and other bloodborne pathogens in health-care settings, *MMWR Morb Mortal Wkly Rep* 37(24):377, 1988.
*Established by the Centers for Disease Control and Prevention and the U.S. Food and Drug Administration.

BOX 28-5 Types of T Cells

Sensitized T cells develop into distinct groups. Each group has a specific set of functions that coordinate the activity of other components of the immune system.

- *Killer T cells* (like B cells) are sensitized and stimulated to multiply by the presence of antigens on abnormal body cells. Unlike B cells, killer T cells do not produce antibodies.
- *Helper T cells* "turn on" the activities of killer (cytotoxic) cells. They also control other aspects of the immune response.
- *Suppressor T cells* "turn off" the action of the helper and killer T cells. This prevents them from causing harmful immune reactions.
- *Inflammatory T cells* stimulate allergic reactions, anaphylaxis, and autoimmune reactions.

As described in Chapter 27, the body's immune response to an invading pathogen depends partly on the size of the pathogen. It also depends on the pathogen's ability to stimulate production of an antibody. Often, peripheral phagocytic cells encounter a pathogen first. However, circulating B and T cells also are scouting for pathogens (Box 28-5). Complex interactions occur among neutrophils, macrophages, and B and T cells. These cells assist each other in processing antigens that allow them to recognize and destroy the invading pathogens.

LOOK AGAIN
See Chapter 27: Immune System Disorders, pp. 826-828.

cuffs, splints). It also is used for surfaces that have been visibly contaminated with blood or body fluids. (Surfaces must be cleaned of visible material before disinfection.) Methods that may be used for intermediate-level disinfection include use of EPA-registered "hospital disinfectant" chemical germicides that claim to be tuberculocidal on the label, hard surface germicides, and solutions containing at least 550 parts per million (ppm) free available chlorine (1:100 dilution of common household bleach: approximately ¼ cup of bleach per 1 gallon of water).

Low-level disinfection destroys some viruses, most bacteria, and some fungi, but not *M. tuberculosis* or bacterial spores. It is used for routine housekeeping. It also is used to clean up soiling when no blood is visible. Methods that may be used for low-level disinfection include use of EPA-registered "hospital disinfectants." (The label carries no claim of tuberculocidal activity.)

Environmental disinfection cleans soiled surfaces in the environment, such as floors, ambulance seats, and counter tops. Such surfaces should be disinfected with cleaners or disinfectant agents.

The B cell's role is to produce antibody (humoral immunity). This antibody coats the pathogen and facilitates phagocytosis. Antibody can also fix *complement*. The **complement system** is a group of proteins that coat bacteria and help to kill them directly. Or the proteins can have the bacteria taken up by neutrophils in the blood or by macrophages in the tissues. T cells not only process antigen for the B cells, but also include a subpopulation of "killer cells." These cells play a major role in cell-mediated immunity (Figure 28-1).

Both the humoral and cell-mediated types of immunity take time to work. Both require previous exposure to mobilize specialized white cells. In time, these white cells differentiate between antibodies. They then organize an attack on the foreign material. By comparison, the complement system recognizes and kills invaders on first sight. It does not take time to mobilize specialized responses.

Reticuloendothelial System. The **reticuloendothelial system** (RES), described in Chapter 11, works with the lymphatic system to dispose of debris that results from the immune system attack on invading organisms. The RES is composed of immune cells in the spleen, lymph nodes,

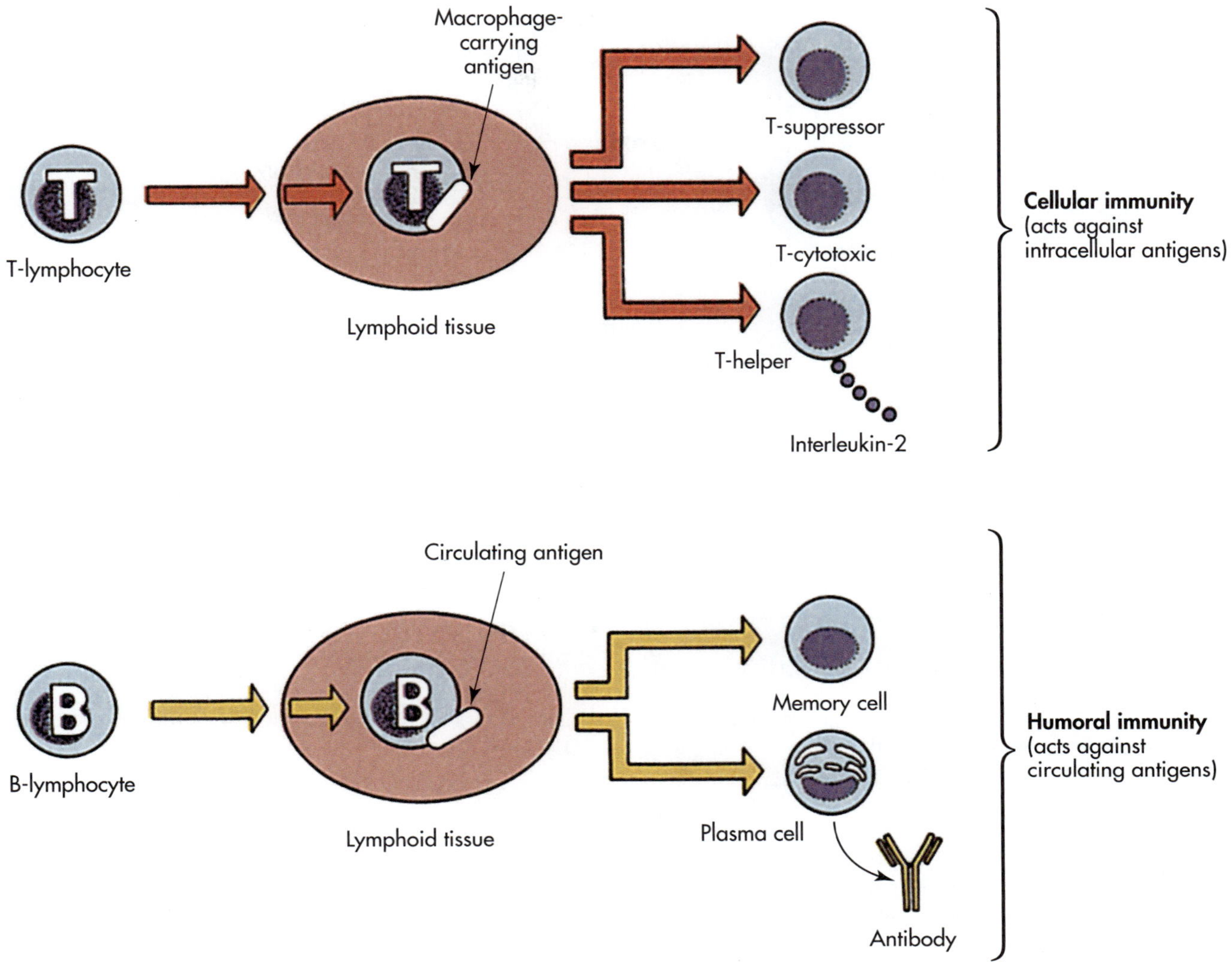

FIGURE 28-1 Cellular and humoral immunity. Cellular immunity results from activation of T cells through contact with intracellular organisms. Activated T cells differentiate and proliferate. Humoral (antibody-mediated) immunity results from the activation of B cells. (From Grimes D: *Infectious diseases,* St Louis, 1991, Mosby.)

liver, bone marrow, lungs, and intestines. These structures store mature B and T cells until the immune system is activated.

> **LOOK AGAIN**
> See Chapter 11: General Principles of Pathophysiology, pp. 234-237.

PATHOPHYSIOLOGY OF INFECTIOUS DISEASE

Infectious and communicable diseases are the second leading cause of death worldwide (after heart disease), and the third most common cause of death in the United States.[8] The development and/or manifestations of clinical disease depend on several factors, including the **virulence** (degree of pathogenicity) of the infectious agent, the number of infectious agents (dose), the **resistance** (immune status) of the **host** (the human or animal who is exposed to the infectious agent), and the correct mode of entry.[9] These factors all rely on an intact chain of elements to produce an infectious disease (Figure 28-2). The elements of the chain include the following[10]:

- The pathogenic agent
- A reservoir
- A portal of exit from the reservoir
- An environment conducive to transmission of the pathogenic agent
- A portal of entry into the new host
- Susceptibility of the new host to the infectious disease

Even if all these elements are present, exposure does not necessarily mean that a person will become infected.

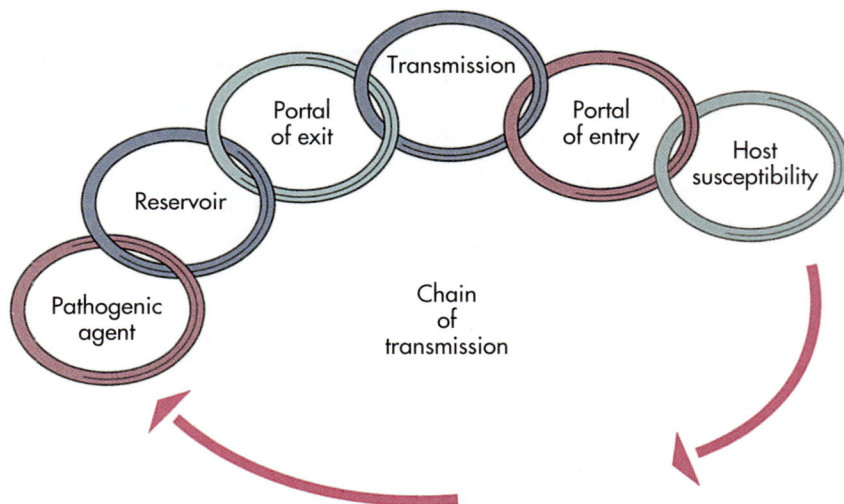

FIGURE 28-2 Chain of transmission for infection. The chain must be intact for an infection to be transmitted to another host. Transmission can be controlled by breaking any link in the chain.

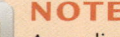

NOTE

According to the World Health Organization, five diseases cause 90% of all infectious disease deaths worldwide. In order of prevalence, they are acute respiratory tract infections (including pneumonia and influenza), AIDS, diarrheal diseases, tuberculosis, malaria, and measles.[11]

Pathogenic Agent

As described in Chapter 11, **pathogens** are organisms that can cause disease in the human host. They are classified according to shape (morphology), chemical composition, growth requirements, and viability. Pathogens rely on a host to supply their nutritional needs.

LOOK AGAIN

See Chapter 11: General Principles of Pathophysiology, pp. 242-245.

Some pathogens (e.g., certain bacteria) are metabolically equipped to survive outside a host. In contrast, others (e.g., certain viruses) can survive only in the human cell (Box 28-6). Some viruses, such as HIV and the hepatitis B virus (HBV), can survive for several hours outside a host. This is why blood products can be infectious.

Most bacteria are susceptible to certain drugs (antibiotics) (Box 28-7). These drugs either kill the bacteria or inhibit their growth. Viruses, however, are more difficult to treat because they reside in cells for most of their life cycle and become intricately enmeshed in the host cell's deoxyribonucleic acid (DNA). Factors that affect a pathogen's ability to cause disease include the following:

- The ability to invade and reproduce in a host and the mode by which it does so

- The speed of reproduction, the ability to produce a toxin, and the degree of tissue damage that results
- Potency
- The ability to induce or evade an immune response in the host

Reservoir

Pathogens may live and reproduce in humans or other animal hosts. They also may live and reproduce in an arthropod, a plant, soil, water, food, or some other organic substance, or a combination of these **reservoirs.** When infected, the human host may show signs of clinical illness. However, the host may be an *asymptomatic carrier* (i.e., a person who can pass the pathogen to others without showing signs of illness). As stated previously, the life cycle of the infectious agent depends on three factors: the demographics of the host, genetic factors, and the efficacy of therapeutic interventions once infection has been established.

Portal of Exit

The method by which a pathogenic agent leaves one host to invade another involves a **portal of exit.** The portal of exit from the human host depends on the agent. The portal may be single or multiple, involving the genitourinary (GU) tract, intestinal tract, oral cavity, respiratory tract, an open lesion, or any wound through which blood escapes. The time during which an actively infectious pathogen escapes to produce disease in another host coincides with the period of communicability (described later in this chapter). This period varies with each disease.

Mode of Transmission

The portal of exit and the portal of entry determine the **mode of transmission.** This mode may be direct or indirect. *Direct transmission* results from physical contact

BOX 28-6 Review of Infectious Agents and Their Properties

Bacteria
- Bacteria are *prokaryotic* (i.e., the nuclear material is not contained within a distinctive envelope).
- They can self-reproduce without a host cell.
- Signs and symptoms depend on the cells and tissues affected.
- Bacteria produce toxins (these are often more lethal than the bacterium itself).
- Endotoxins (chemicals, usually proteins) are integral parts of a bacterium's outer membrane and are constantly shed from living bacteria.
- Exotoxins (proteins) are released by bacteria and can cause disease symptoms by acting as neurotoxins or enterotoxins.
- Lysis of bacteria may result in the release of endotoxins.
- Bacteria can cause localized or systemic infection.

Viruses
- Viruses are living organisms without a nucleus.
- They must invade host cells to reproduce.
- Many cannot survive outside a host cell.
- Viruses may contain other microorganisms.

Fungi
- Fungi are *eukaryotic* (i.e., the nuclear material is contained within a distinct envelope).
- A protective capsule surrounds the cell wall to protect the organism from phagocytes.

Protozoa
- Protozoa are single-celled microorganisms.
- They are more complex than bacteria.

Helminths (Worms [Including Tapeworms], Roundworms)
- Helminths are pathogenic parasites.
- They are not necessarily microorganisms.

BOX 28-7 Methicillin-Resistant *Staphylococcus aureus* (MRSA)

Staphylococcus aureus (often referred to as staph) is a bacterium commonly carried on the skin and in the nose of healthy people. Sometimes staph can cause infection. Staph bacteria are one of the most common causes of skin infections in the United States.[5] Most infections are minor (e.g., pimples and boils). Most of these can be managed without antibiotics. However, some infections are serious. These include surgical wound infections, bone infections, pneumonia, septicemia, and others, which may be resistant to penicillin-related antibiotics.

MRSA is a variety of staph that is resistant to penicillin and other antibiotics. MRSA occurs more often in elderly or very sick patients in hospitals and other health care facilities; patients often have an open wound (e.g., bed sore) or an indwelling urinary catheter or are receiving intravenous (IV) therapy. Staphylococci and MRSA most often are spread by direct physical contact and not by airborne transmission. Spread may also occur through indirect contact by the touching of objects (e.g., towels, sheets, wound dressings, clothes) contaminated by the infected skin of a person with MRSA or staph bacteria. It is important for all health care providers to (1) use universal precautions, (2) practice good hand washing before and after each patient encounter, and (3) avoid contact with open wounds or material contaminated by wounds.

Staph and MRSA can also cause illness in persons outside of hospitals and health care facilities. MRSA infections that are acquired by persons who have not been recently (within the past year) hospitalized or had a medical procedure (such as dialysis, surgery, catheter insertion) are known as community-associated (CA) MRSA infections. Staph or MRSA infections in the community are usually manifested as skin infections, such as pimples and boils, and occur in otherwise healthy people. Clusters of CA-MRSA skin infections have been noted among athletes, military recruits, children, Pacific Islanders, Alaskan Natives, Native Americans, men who have sex with men, and prisoners. Factors that have been associated with the spread of MRSA skin infections include close skin-to-skin contact, openings in the skin such as cuts or abrasions, contaminated items and surfaces, crowded living conditions, and poor hygiene.[12]

---

between the source and the victim. Examples of direct transmission include oral transmission and transmission by airborne mucus droplets, fecal contamination, and sexual contact.

In *indirect transmission,* the organism survives on animate or inanimate objects for a time without a human host. Diseases can be transmitted indirectly by air, food, water, soil, or biological matter.

Portal of Entry

The **portal of entry** is the means by which the pathogenic agent enters a new host. It may be by ingestion, inhalation, percutaneous injection, crossing of a mucous membrane, or crossing of the placenta. The time it takes for the infectious process to begin in a new host varies with the disease and host susceptibility. The duration of the exposure to the

pathogen and the number of organisms required to initiate the infectious process also vary. Exposure to an infectious agent does not always produce infection.

SHOW ME THE EVIDENCE
Methicillin-Resistant *Staphylococcus aureus* (MRSA)

Researchers at a large urban ambulance service performed a cross-sectional research study to determine whether methicillin-resistant *Staphylococcus aureus* (MRSA) could be cultured from any of five locations on an ambulance. Of the 21 ambulances tested, 10 (47.6%) were positive for MRSA. Positive cultures were obtained from the steering wheel, stretcher handrail, stretcher cushion, work area beside the stretcher, and Yankauer suction tip.

From Roline CE, Crumpecker C, Dunn T: Can methicillin-resistant *Staphylococcus aureus* be found in an ambulance fleet? *PEC* 11(2):241-244, 2007.

CRITICAL THINKING
Describe a precaution or intervention that could break each of the links in the chain of disease transmission.

Host Susceptibility

Host susceptibility is influenced by a person's immune response (described in Chapters 11 and 27). It also is influenced by several other factors. Some of these factors include the following:

1. Human characteristics
   - Age
   - Gender
   - Ethnic group
   - Heredity
2. General health status
   - Nutrition
   - Hormonal balance
   - Presence of concurrent disease
   - History of previous disease
3. Immune status
   - Prior exposure to disease (conferring resistance)
   - Effective immunization against disease (conferring host immunity)
4. Geographical and environmental conditions
5. Cultural behaviors
   - Eating habits
   - Personal hygiene
   - Sexual behaviors

PHYSIOLOGY OF THE HUMAN RESPONSE TO INFECTION

The human body is regularly exposed to pathogens that can cause illness. Even so, most people do not succumb to infectious disease. This protection is provided by external and internal barriers. These barriers act as lines of defense against infection.

External Barriers

The first line of defense against infection is the surface of the body (**external barriers**), which is exposed to the environment. This includes the skin and the mucous membranes of the digestive, respiratory, and GU tracts. These areas are inhabited by **indigenous flora** (agents that could produce disease if allowed access to the interior of the body). The surface of the body forms a continuous closed barrier between the internal organs and the environment (Figure 28-3).

FLORA

Nearly the whole body surface is inhabited by normal microbial flora. The flora enhance the effectiveness of the surface barrier. They do this by interfering with the establishment of pathogenic agents in several ways. Indigenous flora compete with pathogens for space and nutrients. They

maintain a pH optimal for their own growth. This pH can be incompatible with that needed for many pathogenic agents to survive. Some flora also secrete germicidal substances and are thought to stimulate the immune system.

Normal flora play a key role in the body's defense. However, some indigenous flora can be pathogenic under certain conditions. For example, flora can cause infection when the skin or mucous membranes are interrupted. They also can cause infection when flora are displaced from their natural habitat to another area of the body. (This is a common cause of urinary tract infection after catheterization of the bladder.)

SKIN

Intact skin defends against infection. It does this in two ways. First, it prevents penetration. Second, it maintains an acidic pH level that inhibits the growth of pathogenic bacteria. In addition, microbes are sloughed from the skin's surface with dead skin cells, and oil and sweat wash microorganisms from the skin's pores.

GASTROINTESTINAL SYSTEM

The normal bacteria in the gastrointestinal (GI) system provide competition between colonies of microorganisms for nutrients and space. Normal bacteria help prevent the growth of pathogenic organisms (Box 28-8). In addition, stomach acid may destroy some microorganisms. It also may deactivate their toxic products. The digestive system eliminates pathogens through feces.

UPPER RESPIRATORY TRACT

The sticky membranes of the upper airway protect against pathogens. They do this by trapping large particles. These particles may then be swallowed or expelled by coughing or sneezing. Coarse nasal hairs and cilia also trap and filter foreign substances in inspired air. They prevent the pathogens from reaching the lower respiratory tract. In addition, the lymph tissues of the tonsils and adenoids allow a rapid local immunological response to pathogenic organisms that may enter the respiratory tract.

BOX 28-8 *Clostridium difficile*

Clostridium difficile, often called *C. difficile* or "C. diff," is a bacterium that normally is present in small numbers in the intestines. C. diff can overpopulate the colon, especially after extended antibiotic therapy. This can lead to **C. diff colitis.** The toxins attack the intestinal wall and cause ulcerations. Initially, diarrhea and cramping occur. This is followed by flulike symptoms, weakness, abdominal pain, fever, nausea, vomiting, dehydration, and bloody stools. In late stages, life-threatening inflammation of the colon can occur. This can result in sepsis and, rarely, death. Illness from C. diff most commonly affects older adults in hospitals or in long-term care facilities. The disease can be spread through the fecal-oral route. Universal precautions are indicated.

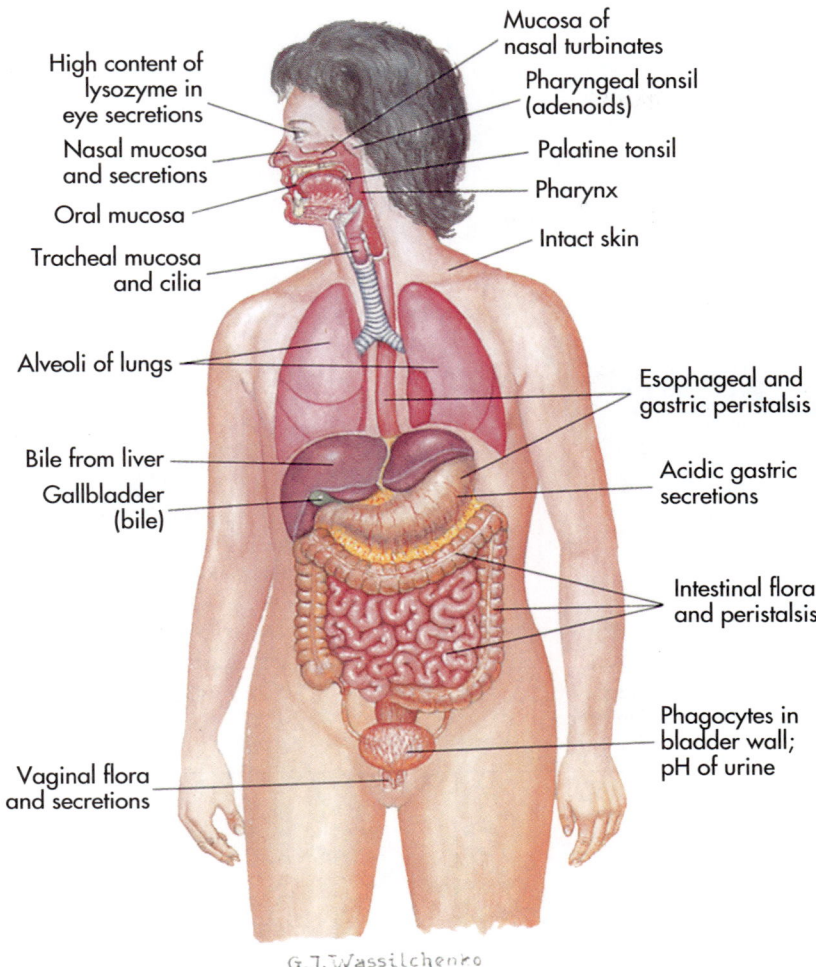

High content of lysozyme in eye secretions

Nasal mucosa and secretions

Oral mucosa

Tracheal mucosa and cilia

Alveoli of lungs

Bile from liver

Gallbladder (bile)

Vaginal flora and secretions

Mucosa of nasal turbinates

Pharyngeal tonsil (adenoids)

Palatine tonsil

Pharynx

Intact skin

Esophageal and gastric peristalsis

Acidic gastric secretions

Intestinal flora and peristalsis

Phagocytes in bladder wall; pH of urine

G.J. Wassilchenko

FIGURE 28-3 First line of defense: external barriers. (From Grimes D: *Infectious diseases,* St Louis, 1991, Mosby.)

GENITOURINARY TRACT

The natural process of urination and urine's ability to kill bacteria help prevent infections in the GU tract. Antibacterial substances in prostatic fluid and the vagina also help prevent infection in the GU system.

> **NOTE**
> Enterococci are bacteria that are normally present in the human intestines and in the female genital tract and are often found in the environment. These bacteria can sometimes cause infections. Vancomycin is an antibiotic that is often used to treat infections caused by enterococci. In some instances, enterococci have become resistant to this drug and thus are called *vancomycin-resistant enterococci* (VRE). Most VRE infections occur in hospitals. Enterococci also may become resistant to most or all other standard drug therapies (*multidrug-resistant enterococci*).

Internal Barriers

Internal barriers protect against germs when the external lines of defense cannot. Internal barriers include the inflammatory response and the immune response. These share many of the same processes and cellular components.

INFLAMMATORY RESPONSE

Inflammation (described in Chapters 11 and 27) is a local reaction to cellular injury. It occurs in response to a microbial infection. When invasion occurs, this line of defense is activated. It works to prevent further invasion of the pathogen by isolating, destroying, or neutralizing the microorganism (Figure 28-4).

The inflammatory response usually is protective and beneficial. However, it may initiate destruction of the body's own tissue. It may be destructive if the response is sustained or directed against the host's own antigens. To review, the

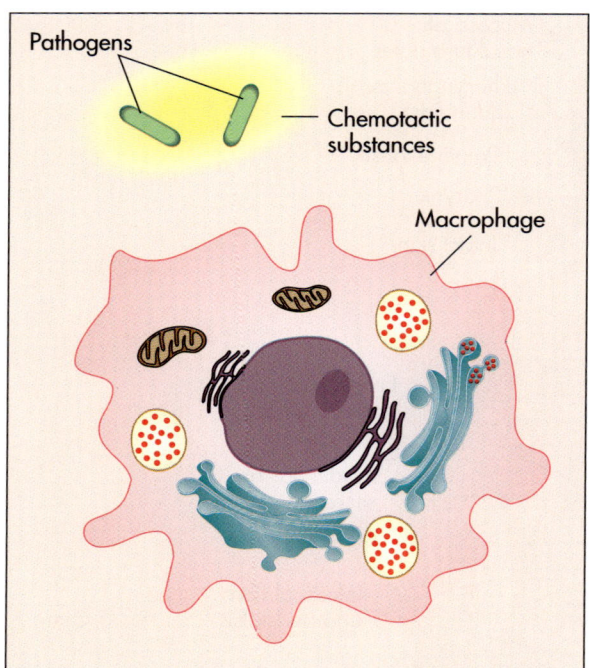

1. Injured area produces chemotactic exudate that attracts macrophages in area.

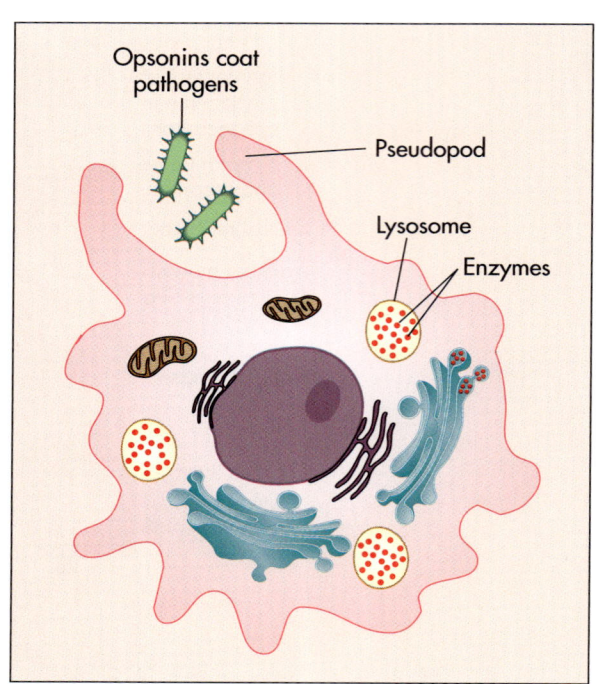

2. Opsonins facilitate phagocytosis.

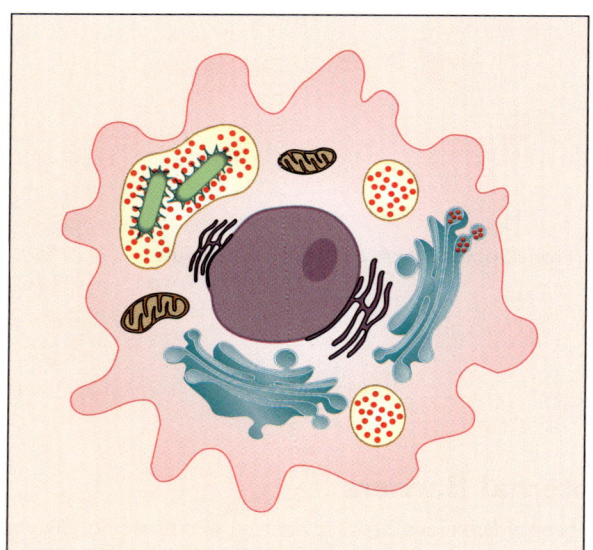

3. The engulfed pathogen becomes digested by enzymes in the lysosomes.

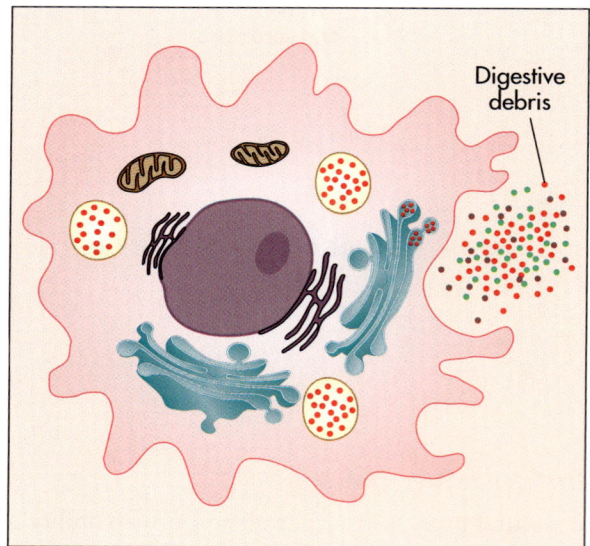

4. The macrophage expels debris after digestion is complete, including prostaglandins, interferon, and complement components. These elements continue the immune response.

FIGURE 28-4 Second line of defense: inflammatory response. (From Grimes D: *Infectious diseases,* St Louis, 1991, Mosby.)

inflammatory response may be divided into three separate stages: first, cellular response to injury; second, vascular response to injury; and third, phagocytosis.

Cellular Response to Injury. The body mounts various types of cellular response to injury. The processes responsible for the cellular injury also are complex. Some cells are the targets of specific inflammatory mediators (e.g., leukotrienes, histamine). When these cells are injured, the cell's metabolism is damaged. This leads to decreasing energy reserves in the cell. When the energy reserves are depleted, an accumulation of sodium ions causes the cell to swell. Along with increasing acidosis, this swelling further impairs the cell's ability to function. It leads to deterioration of the cell membranes. Eventually, the membranes of the cells begin to leak. This contributes to cellular destruction, autolysis, and stimulation of the inflammatory response in surrounding tissues.

Vascular Response to Injury. Localized hyperemia (an increase in bloodflow in the area) develops after cellular injury. This produces edema. Leukocytes collect inside the vessels. There they release **chemotactic factors** (chemicals that attract more leukocytes to the area). These factors eventually migrate to the injured tissue.

CRITICAL THINKING
What physical examination finding is related to this infection fighting property?

Phagocytosis. Through phagocytosis, leukocytes engulf, digest, and destroy the invading pathogens. Circulating macrophages clear the area of dead cells and other debris. The ingestion of bacteria and dead cells (internal phagocytosis) releases chemicals that destroy leukocytes.

STAGES OF INFECTIOUS DISEASE

The progression from exposure to an infectious agent to the onset of clinical disease follows specific stages. The duration of each stage and the potential outcomes vary, depending on the infectious agent and individual host factors. These stages are the latent period, the incubation period, the communicability period, and the disease period (Table 28-2). The risk of infection may be *theoretical*. That is, transmission is acknowledged to be possible but has not actually occurred. The risk of infection is considered *measurable* when infection is confirmed or deduced from reported data.

Latent Period

The **latent period** begins when the pathogen invades the body. During this period, infection has occurred but the infectious agent cannot be passed (or "shed") to someone

else or cause clinically significant symptoms. In some diseases (e.g., HIV), the latent period is quite stable and can last several years. In others (e.g., influenza), the latent period may last only 24 to 72 hours. The latent period as a stage of infectious disease is distinct from a latent infection. A *latent infection* is an inactive infection that can still shed and produce symptoms; a *latent disease* is characterized by periods of inactivity either before signs and symptoms appear or between attacks. Herpes viruses are examples of pathogens that readily enter a latent stage. During this stage, symptoms disappear. They reappear at a later time upon reactivation of the latent infection.

Incubation Period

The **incubation period** is the interval between exposure to the pathogen and the first onset of symptoms. Like the latent period, the incubation period varies in length. It can range from hours to 15 years or longer, as is seen with some individuals with HIV infection. During the incubation period, the infectious organism reproduces in the host. The body is stimulated to produce antibodies specific for the disease or antigen. A person's blood may test positive (seroconversion) for exposure to the disease. A *window phase*, however, follows infection. In this phase, the antigen is present but there is no detectable antibody. A person whose blood is tested for disease-specific antibodies in the window phase may test negative, even when infection is present.

Communicability Period

The **communicability period** follows the latent period. It lasts as long as the agent is present and can spread to other hosts. (Clinically significant symptoms from the infection may manifest during this period.) This stage is variable. It often is the major determining factor in ease of transmission. The communicability period and the method of transmission can be altered in some diseases (e.g., tuberculosis, syphilis, gonorrhea). This depends on the stage of the disease and the primary site of infection.

TABLE 28-2	Stages of Infectious Disease	
Stage	**Begins**	**Ends**
Latent period	With invasion	When agent can be shed
Incubation period	With invasion	When disease process begins
Communicability period	When latent period ends	Continues as long as agent is present and can spread to others
Disease period	Follows incubation period	Variable duration

Disease Period

The **disease period** follows the incubation period. It varies in duration, depending on the specific disease. This stage may be free of symptoms or it may produce overt symptoms. These symptoms can arise directly from the invading organism or from the body's response to the disease. During the disease period, the body may be able to rid itself of the disease entirely. On the other hand, the organism may become incorporated and lie inactive inside certain cells (a latent disease). Several viruses (e.g., HIV and hepatitis) can lead to latent infection. The resolution of symptoms does not mean the infectious agent has been destroyed.

CRITICAL THINKING
Which of the four stages of infectious disease can overlap? What problems can the overlap (or overlaps) pose?

HUMAN IMMUNODEFICIENCY VIRUS

Human immunodeficiency virus (HIV) is present in the blood and serum-derived body fluids (semen, vaginal or cervical secretions) of people infected with the virus. The disease is directly transmitted person to person. It is passed through anal or vaginal intercourse, across the placenta, or by contact between infected blood or body fluids and mucous membranes or open wounds. It also can be transmitted indirectly. This occurs through transfusion with contaminated blood or blood products, transplantation of tissues and organs, and the use of contaminated needles or syringes. The incidence of HIV is highest in people with the following risk factors:

- High-risk sexual behavior
- Intravenous drug abuse
- Transfusion recipient between 1978 and 1985
- Hemophilia or other coagulation disorders requiring blood products
- Infant born to an HIV-positive mother

Other factors that may affect susceptibility to HIV include concurrent sexually transmitted diseases (STDs). This is especially true for those that cause skin ulcerations.

Pathophysiology

HIV infection results from one of two retroviruses that convert genetic ribonucleic acid (RNA) to deoxyribonucleic acid (DNA) after entering the host cell. The two types are known as *HIV-1* and *HIV-2*. Once the retrovirus is inside the cell, the cell's genetic material is altered into a hybrid of part virus and part cell. The virus basically takes over the cell to make more viral particles. When enough of the viral particles have been produced, the host cell ruptures. This destroys the cell and releases the virus into the blood to seek new target cells. The cell receptor sought by HIV is a T cell that has molecules called CD4 on its surface (CD4 T cell). When HIV attaches itself to the CD4 molecule, it allows the virus to enter and infect the cells, damaging them in the process. The CD4 T-cell count is used to determine how active the disease is; a very low count suggests severe disease. These CD4 molecules are also found on the surface of certain nerve cells, and monocytes and phagocytes, which probably carry the disease to other parts of the body. Even though the body develops antigen-specific antibodies to HIV, these antibodies do not protect against HIV. Secondary complications generally are caused by **opportunistic infections** that develop as the immune system deteriorates. These infections include the following:

- Pulmonary tuberculosis
- Recurrent pneumonia
- *Pneumocystis carinii* pneumonia
- Kaposi sarcoma
- Wasting syndrome
- HIV dementia
- Sensory neuropathy
- Toxoplasmosis of the central nervous system

NOTE
The two types of HIV (HIV-1 and HIV-2) are serologically and geographically distinct. However, they have similar epidemiological characteristics. HIV-1 is much more pathogenic than HIV-2. Most cases worldwide and in the United States are caused by HIV-1. HIV-2 seems to be more restricted to West Africa.[13] Some blood screening procedures test only for HIV-1.

Classification and Categories

The average interval from transmission of HIV to the development of serious complications is about 10 years if the condition is untreated. However, this time frame can vary greatly (Table 28-3).

The CDC has devised a classification system for HIV (revised in 1993) with three categories based on the CD4 T-cell count[14]:

Category 1: Cell count of 500/μL or higher
Category 2: Cell count of 200 to 499/μL
Category 3: Cell count below 200/μL

As the number of CD4 T cells decreases, the risk and severity of opportunistic illness increase. After viral transmission, the progression of HIV in adolescents and adults can be divided into three clinical categories: A, B, and C.

CATEGORY A

- *Acute retroviral infection:* This syndrome generally occurs 2 to 4 weeks after exposure. Clinical features include an infectious mononucleosis–like illness with fever, adenopathy, and sore throat. The febrile illness is self-limited. It usually lasts 1 to 2 weeks. During this stage, a transient decrease is observed in the CD4 T-cell count.

TABLE 28-3 Incubation and Communicability Periods of Various Infectious Diseases

Incubation Period	Communicability Period
Childhood Diseases	
Chickenpox	
2 to 3 weeks (average 13 to 17 days)	Occurs 1 or 2 days before onset of rash and until lesions have crusted over and not more than 6 days after appearance of vesicles
Mumps	
2 to 3 weeks (average 18 days)	Occurs 6 days before parotid symptoms to 9 days after; disease is most communicable 48 hours after parotid swelling develops
Pertussis	
7 to 14 days, commonly 7 to 10 days	Occurs 7 days after exposure and lasts 3 weeks after onset; highly communicable in early stage before cough; not communicable after 3 weeks, although cough may be present
Rubella	
14 to 23 days (average 16 to 18 days)	Occurs from 1 week before to 4 days after appearance of rash; infants with congenital rubella syndrome may shed virus for months after birth
Rubeola	
Commonly 10 days, 8 to 13 days until fever, 14 days until rash	Occurs a few days before fever to 5 to 7 days after appearance of rash
Hantavirus	
3 days to 6 weeks	No known human-to-human transmission
Hepatitis Virus	
Hepatitis A Virus (HAV)	
15 to 50 days (average 28 to 30 days)	Usually occurs in latter half of incubation period and continues for several days after onset of jaundice
Hepatitis B Virus (HBV)	
45 to 180 days (average 60 to 90 days)	Occurs during incubation period and lasts throughout clinical course (carrier state may persist for years)
Hepatitis C Virus (HCV)	
2 weeks to 6 months (average 6 to 9 weeks)	Occurs 1 or more weeks before onset of symptoms and indefinitely during chronic and carrier states
Human Immunodeficiency Virus (HIV)	
Varies: 6 to 12 weeks from exposure to seropositivity, up to 20 years for symptomatic immune suppression and to diagnosis of acquired immunodeficiency syndrome (AIDS)	Is lifelong from presence of HIV in serum until death; degree of communicability may vary during course of HIV infection
Influenza	
24 to 72 hours	Occurs 3 days after onset of symptoms; infection produces immunity to specific strain of virus, but duration of immunity varies
Meningitis	
2 to 10 days	Varies; lasts as long as infectious agents remain in nasal and oral secretions; microorganisms disappear from upper respiratory tract within 24 hours of antibiotic therapy
Mononucleosis	
4 to 6 weeks	Prolonged; pharyngeal excretion may last for years; 15% to 20% of adults are carriers

Continued

TABLE 28-3—cont'd

Incubation Period	Communicability Period
Pneumonia	
1 to 3 days	Occurs until organisms have been eliminated from respiratory discharges (24 to 48 hours after antibiotic treatment)
Rabies	
Usually 2 to 16 weeks	Human-to-human transmission by bite, scratch, or aerosolization has not been documented; theoretical transmission from contact with secretions of infected person
Severe Acute Respiratory Syndrome (SARS)	
10 days	Information to date suggests that people are most likely to be infectious when they have symptoms, such as fever or cough; however, it is not known how long before or after symptoms appear that disease can be transmitted
Sexually Transmitted Diseases	
Chlamydia	
5 to 10 days	Unknown
Gonorrhea	
2 to 7 days	Occurs for months if disease is untreated
Herpes Simplex Virus (HSV)	
HSV-1: 2 to 12 days	Occurs when lesions are present; virus is found in saliva as long as 7 weeks after recovery from lesions; transient shedding of virus is common
HSV-2: 2 to 12 days (average 6 days)	Occurs in 7 to 12 days with lesion; transient shedding of virus in absence of lesions probably occurs
Syphilis	
10 days to 10 weeks (average 3 weeks)	Varies; occurs during primary and secondary stages and in mucocutaneous recurrences (2 to 4 years if disease is untreated)
Tetanus	
3 to 21 days, commonly 10 days	Not directly transmitted; recovery from tetanus does not confer permanent immunity
Tuberculosis (TB)	
4 to 12 weeks after exposure or any time disease is in a latent stage	Occurs as long as bacilli are present in sputum, sometimes intermittently for years

- *Seroconversion:* The serological response with antigen-specific antibodies to HIV generally occurs 6 to 12 weeks after transmission. During this stage, the CD4 T-cell count returns to normal.

CRITICAL THINKING
What will probably happen if a sample is drawn for a blood test for HIV antibodies during the third week after exposure?

- *Asymptomatic infection:* The individual with HIV may have persistent generalized lymphadenopathy (enlarged lymph nodes involving two noncontiguous sites other than inguinal nodes) and a gradual decline in the CD4 T-cell count.

CATEGORY B

- *Early symptomatic HIV:* The usual CD4 T-cell count in this group is 100 to 300/μL. At this stage, common complications include localized candidal infections (thrush, *Candida* esophagitis, *Candida* vaginitis), oral lesions, shingles, pelvic inflammatory disease, peripheral neuropathy, and constitutional symptoms such as fever or diarrhea that last longer than 1 month.

CATEGORY C

- *Late symptomatic HIV:* This stage represents all acquired immunodeficiency syndrome (AIDS)-defining diagnoses found primarily with CD4 T-cell counts of 0 to 200/μL, including severe opportunistic infections; bacterial pneumonia (e.g., *P. carinii* pneumonia); pulmonary

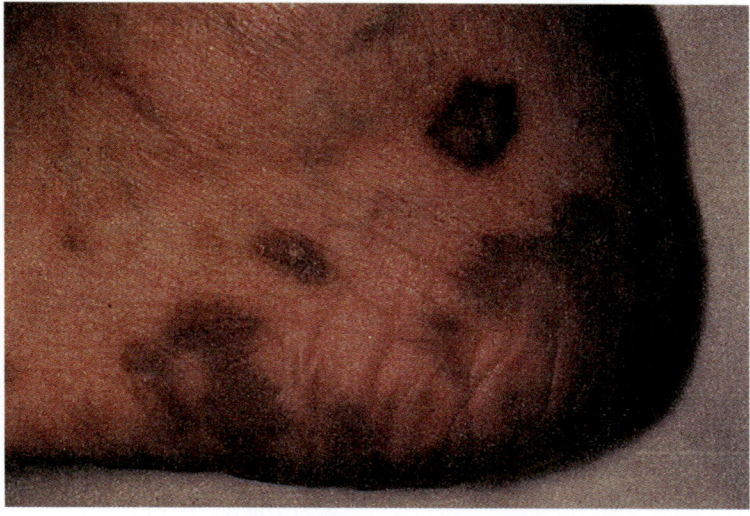

FIGURE 28-5 Kaposi sarcoma of the heel and lateral foot. (Courtesy Centers for Disease Control and Prevention, 1990. In Grimes D: *Infectious diseases,* St Louis, 1991, Mosby.)

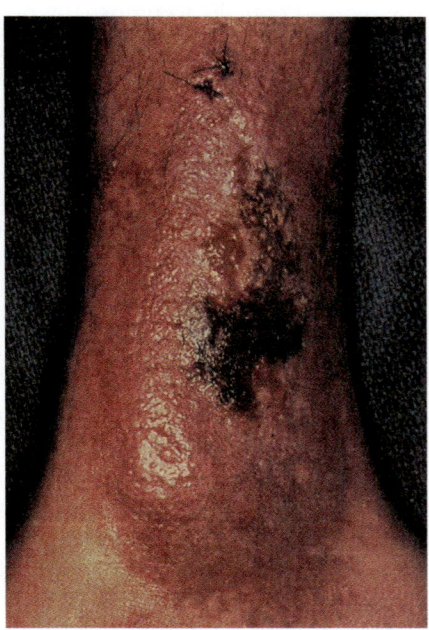

FIGURE 28-6 Kaposi sarcoma of the distal leg and ankle. (Courtesy Centers for Disease Control and Prevention, 1990. In Grimes D: *Infectious diseases,* St Louis, 1991, Mosby.)

tuberculosis; debilitating diarrhea; tumors in any body system, including Kaposi sarcoma (Figures 28-5 and 28-6); HIV-associated dementia; and neurological manifestations.

■ *Advanced HIV:* In this stage, the person has a CD4 T-cell count of 0 to 50/μL. These patients have a limited life expectancy, and most of them die of AIDS-related complications.

Personal Protection

Strict compliance with universal precautions is the only preventive measure health care workers can take against HIV. However, the chance of EMS personnel acquiring the infection through exposure to infected blood appears to be low (0.2% to 0.44%).[6] HBV exposure is a much greater occupational hazard. The risk to health care workers increases under the following circumstances:

1. The exposure involves a large amount of blood. This can occur when a piece of equipment is visibly contaminated with blood; when care of the patient involves placing a needle in a vein or an artery; and when the patient has deep injuries. The needle size and type (hollow bore or suture) and the depth of penetration influence the volume transferred to the skin. Health care workers suffer 600,000 to 800,000 injuries from conventional needles and sharps each year.[15]

 CRITICAL THINKING
Why would testing within 2 to 3 weeks of exposure be needed?

2. The exposure involves a patient with a terminal illness, possibly reflecting a higher dose of HIV in the late course of AIDS. The risk of exposure must be understood in terms of how the exposure occurred and what factors were involved. Although the potential may appear high, the probability actually may be quite low. Paramedics should follow agency protocol for notification and reporting of significant exposures to any infectious disease.

Postexposure Prophylaxis

If exposure is confirmed or suspected, the paramedic should immediately notify the DO (per protocol). This allows elective postexposure prophylaxis (PEP) to begin. Information on primary HIV indicates that systemic infection does not occur immediately; this leaves a narrow window of opportunity in which postexposure antiretroviral intervention may modify viral replication.[13] Several antiretroviral agents from at least four classes of drugs are available for the treatment of HIV. Examples include fusion inhibitors, nucleoside/nucleotide reverse transcriptase inhibitors (NRTIs), nonnucleoside reverse transcriptase inhibitors (NNRTIs), and protease inhibitors (PIs). After PEP, testing for HIV is performed 2 to 3 weeks after the exposure. It is performed again at 6 weeks, 3 months, 6 months, and 1 year.

> **NOTE**
> An important goal of PEP is to encourage and facilitate compliance with a 4-week PEP regimen of two drugs used for most HIV exposures. Combinations that can be considered for PEP include zidovudine (ZDV) and lamivudine (3TC) or emtricitabine (FTC); stavudine (d4T) and 3TC or FTC; and tenofovir (TDF) and 3TC or FTC. Moreover, an expanded regimen that includes the addition of a third drug is used for cases of HIV exposures that have an increased risk of transmission. When the patient's virus is known or suspected to be resistant to one or more of the drugs considered for the PEP regimen, the selection of drugs to which the virus is unlikely to be resistant is recommended.[16] All antiretroviral drugs have been associated with side effects (mainly gastrointestinal). In addition, some of these drugs (especially protease inhibitors) cause potentially serious drug interactions. Paramedics should receive counseling regarding evaluation and treatment after an exposure.

Psychological Reactions to HIV

HIV is almost always a progressive disease with morbid late consequences. Throughout the course of the infection, patients are likely to feel and express anger about many aspects of their illness. These include pain, dying prematurely and without dignity, and the social rejection and prejudice that the person may experience. Patient care should include helping these patients feel that they can obtain acceptance and compassion from health care workers.

Although no vaccine exists for HIV, many clinical trials are underway. Despite current limitations, the progression of the illness can be delayed with drug therapy and other strategies. This allows time for access to new therapeutic options.

HEPATITIS

As described in Chapter 30, **hepatitis** is a viral disease that produces pathological changes in the liver. The hepatitis viruses are divided into three main classes: **hepatitis A** (viral hepatitis), **hepatitis B** (serum hepatitis), and **hepatitis C** (non-A/non-B hepatitis) (Table 28-4).

> **NOTE**
> Hepatitis non-ABC is a fourth class of hepatitis caused by infection with the hepatitis D (delta) virus. HDV cannot sustain infection without the help of HBV. Two newer hepatitis viruses (E and G) can also cause infection of the liver. HVE and HVG (also known as GBV-C) are rare viruses. The routes of transmission for these viruses are thought to be similar to those for the hepatitis C virus (HCV).

Hepatitis A Virus

Hepatitis A (HAV) is the most common type of viral hepatitis in the United States, accounting for 42,000 infections in 2005.[14] The disease is acquired by ingesting HAV-contaminated food or drink. It also is acquired by the fecal/oral route. The virus localizes in the liver, reproduces, enters the bile, and is carried to the intestinal tract. From there it is shed in the feces. (Fecal shedding usually occurs before the onset of clinical symptoms.) Antibodies (anti-HAV) develop during acute disease. They also develop late in convalescence. Once infected, the person is immune to HAV for life. Hepatitis A is the only hepatitis virus that does not lead to chronic liver disease or a chronic carrier state. Many HAV infections are subclinical. They often manifest with influenza-like symptoms. About 1 in 100 patients with HAV suffers from a sudden and severe infection that may require a liver transplant.[17]

Immune globulin (IG) can provide temporary immunity to the virus (i.e., 2 to 3 months). It must be given before exposure to HAV or within 2 weeks after contact. Hepatitis A vaccines approved for people 2 years of age or older are recommended for the following groups:

- People who have close physical contact with those who live in areas with poor sanitary conditions or who are traveling or working in developing countries
- Employees in certain job classes, such as the foodservice industry (may be required in some communities)
- Men who have sex with other men
- Users of illicit drugs
- Children in populations that have repeated epidemics of hepatitis A (Native Alaskans, Native Americans, Pacific Islanders, and certain closed religious communities)
- People who have chronic liver disease or clotting factor disorders

The safety of the vaccine during pregnancy has not been determined.

Hepatitis B Virus

Infectious HBV particles are found in blood and in secretions containing serum (e.g., oozing, cutaneous lesions). They also are found in secretions derived from serum (e.g., saliva, semen, vaginal secretions). Like other viral types of

TABLE 28-4 The ABC's of Hepatitis

	Hepatitis A (HAV)	Hepatitis B (HBV)	Hepatitis C (HCV)	Hepatitis D (HDV)	Hepatitis E (HEV)
What Is It?	HAV is a virus that causes inflammation of the liver. It does not lead to chronic disease.	HBV is a virus that causes inflammation of the liver. It can cause liver cell damage, leading to cirrhosis and cancer.	HCV is a virus that causes inflammation of the liver. It can cause liver cell damage, leading to cirrhosis and cancer.	HDV is a virus that causes inflammation of the liver. It only infects those persons with HBV.	HEV is a virus that causes inflammation of the liver. It is rare in the U.S. Rarely it can cause chronic disease
Incubation Period	2 to 7 weeks. Average 4 weeks.	6 to 23 weeks. Average 17 weeks.	2 to 25 weeks. Average 7 to 9 wks.	2 to 8 weeks.	2 to 9 weeks. Average 40 days.
How Is It Spread?	Transmitted by fecal/oral (anal/oral sex) route, close person-to-person contact or ingestion of contaminated food and water. Hand to mouth after contact with feces, such as changing diapers.	Contact with infected blood, seminal fluid, vaginal secretions, contaminated needles, including tattoo and body-piercing tools. Infected mother to newborn. Human bite. Sexual contact.	Contact with infected blood, contaminated IV needles, razors, and tattoo and body-piercing tools. Infected mother to newborn. Not easily spread through sex.	Contact with infected blood, contaminated needles. Sexual contact with HDV infected person.	Transmitted through fecal/oral route. Outbreaks associated with contaminated water supply in other countries.
Symptoms	Children may have none. Adults usually have light stools, dark urine, fatigue, fever, nausea, vomiting, abdominal pain, and jaundice.	May have none. Some persons have mild flulike symptoms, dark urine, light stools, jaundice, fatigue, and fever.	Same as HBV	Same as HBV	Same as HAV
Treatment of Chronic Disease	Not applicable	Peginterferon, entecavir, and tenofovir are first-line treatment options.	Peginterferon with ribavirin and serine protease adjuncts.	Peginterferon with varying success.	Ribavirin for chronic hepatitis E but needs confirmation
Vaccine	Two doses of vaccine to anyone over 1 year of age.	Three doses may be given to persons of any age.	None for HCV. Should receive Hepatitis A and B vaccines	HBV vaccine prevents HDV infection.	None commercially available
Who Is at Risk?	Household or sexual contact with an infected person or living in an area with HAV outbreak. Travelers to developing countries, persons engaging in anal/oral sex, and injection drug users.	Infants born to infected mother, having sex with an infected person or multiple partners, injection drug users, emergency responders, health care workers, persons engaging in anal/oral sex, and hemodialysis patients.	Blood transfusion recipients before 1992, health care workers, injection drug users, hemodialysis patients, infants born to infected mother, multiple sex partners.	Injection drug users, persons engaging in anal/oral sex, and those having sex with an HDV-infected patient.	Travelers to developing countries, especially pregnant women.
Prevention	Vaccination or immune globulin within 2 weeks of exposure. Washing hands with soap and water after going to the toilet. Use household bleach (10 parts water to 1 part bleach) to clean surfaces contaminated with feces, such as changing tables. Safer sex.	Vaccination provides protection for 20 plus years. Clean up blood with household bleach and wear protective gloves. Do not share razors, toothbrushes, or needles. Safer sex. Hepatitis B immune globulin for vaccine non-responders after exposure.	Clean up spilled blood with household bleach. Wear gloves when touching blood. Do not share razors, toothbrushes, or needles with anyone. Safer sex.	Hepatitis B vaccine to prevent HBV/HDV infection, Safer sex.	Avoid drinking or using potentially contaminated water.

Hepatitis Foundation International, 504 Blick Drive, Silver Spring, Md 20904, 1-800-891-0707, www.HepatitisFoundation.org

hepatitis, HBV affects the liver and causes the signs and symptoms described previously. The virus may produce chronic infection. This can lead to cirrhosis and other complications. Although HBV usually lasts less than 6 months, the carrier state may persist for years.

> **NOTE**
> HBV is 100 times more infectious than HIV. One in 20 Americans will become infected with HBV at some time in their lives. There are an estimated 350 million people infected with the disease worldwide.[17]

The effects of HBV vary. Only a low-grade fever and malaise (influenza-like illness) may occur, with complete resolution of symptoms. On the other hand, extensive liver necrosis may develop that can lead to death. Other complications associated with HBV include coagulation defects, impaired protein production, impaired bilirubin elimination, pancreatitis, and hepatic cancer. Exposure generally occurs in one of five ways:

1. Direct percutaneous inoculation of infectious serum or plasma by needle or transfusion of infected blood or blood products
2. Indirect percutaneous introduction of infective serum or plasma (e.g., skin cuts or abrasions, tattoo/body piercing)
3. Absorption of infective serum or plasma through mucosal surfaces (e.g., the eyes or mouth), transplacentally, or through contamination from the mother's infected blood at birth
4. Absorption of infective secretions (e.g., saliva or semen) through mucosal surfaces, as might occur during vaginal, anal, or oral sexual contact (but never fecal transmission), and straws shared in snorting drugs
5. Transfer of infective serum or plasma via inanimate environmental surfaces

HBV is stable on environmental surfaces and can remain infective in visible blood for longer than 7 days.[17]

> **CRITICAL THINKING**
> Why is information about exposure risks important to paramedics?

PREEXPOSURE PROPHYLAXIS

With regulatory and legislative efforts and the publication of OSHA's *Bloodborne Pathogen Standard,* cases of HBV in health care workers have dropped dramatically. (The exposure risk for health care providers working with HBV-positive patients is estimated to be 2% to 40%.) Yet, even with this decline, HBV is a serious concern to all health care workers. The CDC recommends and OSHA requires that HBV vaccines be offered to all health care workers. The vaccine sometimes is given to newborns. Several states now require immunization of children who are middle school age.

Blood is the most important potential source of HBV in the workplace. The risk of infection is directly proportional to the probability that the blood contains HBV, the recipient's immunity status, and the efficacy of transmission. HBV vaccinations are available that provide protection for 18 years in those who respond to the inoculation.[16] The HBV vaccination schedule generally requires three doses over 6 months. These are intramuscular (deltoid) doses. For the best protection against HBV, the series should be completed before an exposure occurs. Vaccinations currently available include Recombivax HB and Engerix-B.

POSTEXPOSURE PROPHYLAXIS

Postexposure prophylaxis may be indicated if an unvaccinated person or a person who has not completed the vaccination schedule is exposed to HBV. Before treatment, a blood test is performed to determine immunity to HBV. People who are not immune generally receive the HBV vaccine and hepatitis B immune globulin. (This is an antibody used in postexposure treatment to provide passive immunity to HBV.)

Hepatitis C Virus

Hepatitis C virus (HCV) is a blood-borne virus. It causes a disease similar to HBV. The virus was associated with receipt of contaminated blood during transfusion before 1992. (It accounts for more than 90% of posttransfusion hepatitis cases in the United States.) Currently, about 4 million Americans are believed to be infected with the virus. Hepatitis C is the infection that most often results from needle-stick and sharps injury.[18,19] Of health care workers who become infected, 85% become chronic carriers. About one half to two thirds of those infected with HCV develop chronic hepatitis; one in five suffers severe liver disease, such as cirrhosis and liver cancer. No vaccine is available for HCV.

Although HCV is transmitted in the same manner as other forms of hepatitis, it is not easily spread through sexual contact. Signs and symptoms of the disease, when they occur, are similar to those of other types of hepatitis. Most people infected with HCV are asymptomatic.

Signs and Symptoms

Infection with any of the causative viruses may not produce any symptoms. On the other hand, it may cause a typical hepatitis with an abrupt onset of flulike illness that is followed by jaundice or dark urine, or both. A patient is most infectious during the first week of symptoms (see Table 28-3). Within 2 to 3 months of infection, the patient usually develops nonspecific symptoms. These may include anorexia, nausea and vomiting, fever, joint pain, and generalized rashes. About 1% of patients hospitalized with HBV develop full-blown liver crisis and die (Box 28-9).

BOX 28-9 Antiviral Therapy With Interferons

Interferons are proteins produced naturally by body cells in response to viral infection and other stimuli. Interferon alfa (Intron A and others) is effective at controlling the spread of common colds caused by rhinoviruses. It may be effective at treating chronic infections caused by the hepatitis B and C viruses (HBV and HCV, respectively) and the human immunodeficiency virus (HIV). The U.S. Food and Drug Administration (FDA) has approved combination therapy with Pegasys (peginterferon alfa-2a) and Copegus (ribavirin) for the treatment of adults with chronic hepatitis C who have compensated liver disease and have not previously been treated with interferon alpha.

Interferons work by attaching to the membranes of host cells and stimulating the host cells to attack the virus. If a virus invades a cell primed by interferon, enzymes are produced that impair viral copying. This nullifies the virus. Interferons also increase the activity of natural killer cells to stop or shorten the effects of the virus. Side effects of interferon include fever, malaise, headache, fatigue, hair loss, and bone marrow suppression.

Patient Management and Protective Measures

The management of patients out of the hospital is mainly supportive. The goal is to maintain circulatory status and prevent shock. All health care workers involved in the patient's care must follow careful personal protective measures. This includes effective hand washing. It also involves proper care in the use of diagnostic and therapeutic equipment (e.g., high-level disinfection of laryngoscope blades) and appropriate disposal of sharps.

TUBERCULOSIS

Each year, 9 million new cases of **tuberculosis** (TB) occur worldwide, and 2 million people die of the disease.[20] Reports of TB in the United States had declined continually since the turn of the twentieth century. However, in 1985 this trend reversed (attributed to the epidemic of HIV). The incidence of tuberculosis (TB) among patients with HIV is 40 times the incidence among people who are not infected with HIV. TB is the leading killer of people infected with HIV.[20] Other risk factors for TB include:

- Immigration of people from areas with a high prevalence of TB
- Transmission of TB in high-risk environments, such as correctional facilities, homeless shelters, hospitals, and nursing homes
- Deterioration of the TB public health care infrastructure

CRITICAL THINKING
Why is TB more prevalent in patients with HIV?

Pathophysiology

As described in Chapter 24, TB is a chronic pulmonary disease. It is acquired through inhalation of a dried-droplet nucleus containing tubercle bacilli (*Mycobacterium tuberculosis, Mycobacterium bovis,* or a variety of atypical mycobacteria). TB is passed mainly by infected persons coughing or sneezing the bacteria into the air. It can also be passed through contact with the sputum of an infected person. People who share the same air space as those who have infectious TB are at highest risk for infection. Transmission also may occur by ingestion or through the skin or mucous membranes. However, this is less common.

The pathology of TB is related to the production of inflammatory lesions throughout the body. It also is related to the ability of the TB bacillus to break through the body's natural defenses. This leads to the formation of caseating granulomas (necrotic inflammatory cells) and TB cavities. These may cause chronic and debilitating lung disease. Susceptibility to mycobacterial infection generally is highest in children younger than 3 years of age; in adults older than 65; and in chronically ill, malnourished, and immunosuppressed or immunocompromised individuals. The infection may remain dormant for an indefinite time (often not causing disease), or it may lead to active, contagious disease. As a result, two TB-related conditions exist. They are **latent TB infection** (LTBI) and **TB disease** (Table 28-5).

Signs and symptoms of TB include cough, fever, night sweats, weight loss, fatigue, and hemoptysis. The organ systems affected and the associated complications include the following:

1. Cardiovascular system
   - Pericardial effusions
   - Lymphadenopathy (cervical lymph nodes are usually involved)
2. Skeletal system
   - Intervertebral disk deterioration
   - Chronic arthritis of one joint
3. Central nervous system (CNS)
   - Subacute meningitis
   - Brain granulomas
4. Systemic miliary TB (extensive dissemination by the bloodstream of tubercle bacilli)

In the United States, an estimated 10 million to 15 million people are infected with *M. tuberculosis.* Without intervention, approximately 10% of these people will develop TB disease at some point in their lives.[21] Paramedics should maintain a high degree of suspicion for TB in individuals with undiagnosed lung disease, especially patients who are HIV positive.

TABLE 28-5 TB Disease: The Difference Between Latent TB Infection and TB Disease

A Person With Latent TB Infection	A Person With TB Disease
• Has no symptoms	• Has symptoms that may include: — a bad cough that lasts 3 weeks or longer — pain in the chest — coughing up blood or sputum — weakness or fatigue — weight loss — no appetite — chills — fever — sweating at night
• Does not feel sick	• Usually feels sick
• Cannot spread TB bacteria to others	• May spread TB bacteria to others
• Usually has a skin test or blood test result indicating TB infection	• Usually has a skin test or blood test result indicating TB infection
• Has a normal chest x-ray and a negative sputum smear	• May have an abnormal chest x-ray, or positive sputum smear or culture
• Needs treatment for latent TB infection to prevent active TB disease	• Needs treatment to treat active TB disease

From Centers for Disease Control and Prevention: *The difference between latent TB infection and TB disease,* Atlanta, www.cdc.gov/tb/topic/basics/default.htm, accessed 10-15-10.

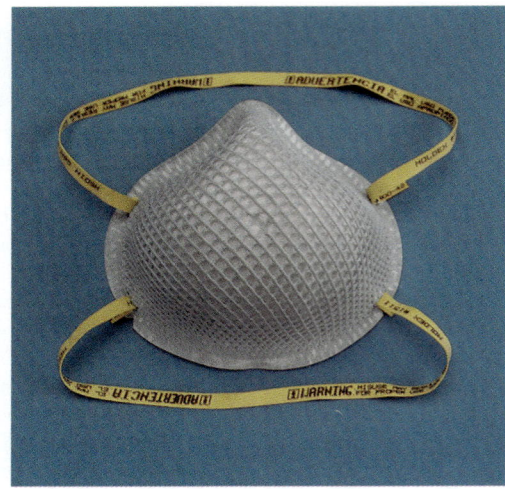

FIGURE 28-7 High-efficiency particulate air (HEPA) respirator.

Tuberculosis Testing

The signs and symptoms of initial infection may be minimal. However, early infection can be detected using the Mantoux tuberculin skin test (purified protein derivative [PPD]). A positive reaction to the PPD test indicates past infection and the presence of antibodies. Patients with positive test results usually have a chest x-ray and an acid-fast bacilli (AFB) sputum culture before treatment. Counseling and HIV antibody testing should be offered to all people infected with TB. This is because medical management may be altered if HIV is present. By law, every state is required to report cases of TB. A negative TB skin test result does not fully rule out TB infection. This is especially the case in people with TB-like symptoms, HIV, or AIDS. In these cases, a repeat skin test may be warranted 10 weeks after exposure.

Because identification and early treatment of TB are important, all health care workers should receive a routine evaluation consisting of PPD test and, in some cases, a chest x-ray and AFB culture. A negative immune response does not preclude reinfection with subsequent exposure.

Patient Care and Protective Measures

Paramedics should be aware of areas with a high incidence of active TB in their service region. (This information is reported by the local health authorities.) Prehospital care for patients with infectious TB is mainly supportive. As with any other infectious disease, universal precautions should be taken during patient care. This includes respiratory barriers for the patient and the paramedic. Surgical masks are insufficient for preventing inhalation of tuberculosis bacteria. However, they do reduce the number of droplet nuclei escaping from the patient. Therefore they should be placed on the patient during transport. NIOSH recommends that health care workers use particulate filter respirators that filter at least 95% of airborne particles when caring for patients with tuberculosis (Figure 28-7 and Box 28-10).[22] Ambulance ventilation systems that include high-efficiency particulate air (HEPA) filtration and a non-recirculating ventilation cycle are another measure for preventing exposure to TB during patient transport. After each call, disinfection of all patient care equipment should be performed.

Treatment

If effective treatment is begun without delay, TB is usually curable. Multidrug-resistant TB is on the rise (Box 28-11). For this reason, most patients with TB are started on a lengthy, four-drug regimen of isoniazid (INH), rifampin (RIF), pyrazinamide (PZA), and ethambutol (EMB) or streptomycin (SM) until the drug susceptibility results are known. (Patients who undergo preventive therapy should be monitored for drug side effects. They should be watched especially for signs and symptoms of hepatitis.) Sputum and cultures usually become negative 3 to 8 weeks after the start of therapy.

BOX 28-10 Tuberculosis-Protective Respirators

The federal Occupational Safety and Health Administration (OSHA), in conjunction with guidelines established by the Centers for Disease Control and Prevention (CDC), currently requires the use of respirators. OSHA is enforcing their use while developing specific standards for preventing the exposure of health care workers to tuberculosis (TB). The required respirator certified by the National Institute for Occupational Safety and Health (NIOSH) must have a disposable (or replaceable) high-efficiency particulate air (HEPA) filter capable of trapping airborne particles. Whenever respirators (including disposables) are required, a complete respiratory protection program must be implemented in accordance with federal regulations.*

Elements of the required respiratory protection program include the following:

1. Permissible practices for respirator use
2. Respirator program administration
3. Selection of respirators
4. Inspection of respirators
5. Cleaning and maintenance of respirators
6. Storage of respirators
7. Training in respiratory protection
8. Fit testing of respirators (to ensure accurate sizing)
9. Respirator program evaluation
10. Medical surveillance of respirator users

Modified from U.S. Department of Health and Human Services, National Institute of Occupational Safety and Health: *NIOSH guide to the selection and use of particulate respirators,* certified under 42 CFR 84, Washington, DC, Publication No. 96-101, 1996, Author.
*These specifications are found in 29 Code of Federal Register (CFR) 1910.134.

BOX 28-11 Multidrug-Resistant Tuberculosis

During the resurgence of tuberculosis (TB) in the United States that began in 1985, outbreaks of multidrug-resistant TB (MDR-TB) occurred in hospitals and prisons. This resulted in high death rates. It also resulted in transmission to health care workers.

MDR-TB is resistant to conventional drugs (isoniazid and rifampin). It is a very serious form of TB, because preventive therapy is limited. People at high risk for MDR-TB include the following:

• Those recently exposed to MDR-TB (especially if they are immunocompromised)
• TB patients who fail to take medications as prescribed
• TB patients who were prescribed an ineffective treatment regimen
• Patients previously treated for TB

A major cause of treatment failure and drug-resistant TB is failure to follow the treatment regimen. This threatens the health of TB patients and poses a serious public health risk. It also leads to prolonged infectivity and the spread of TB in the community.

PROPHYLACTIC ISONIAZID

For individuals younger than 35 years of age who have a positive result on a PPD skin test and who have not previously been treated, administration of INH is recommended. Isoniazid is not routinely recommended for those younger than 35 years old because it may damage the liver. However, the drug is used if one or more of the following factors is present.[23]

■ Recent infection, as evidenced by PPD skin test conversion
■ Close or household contact with a known case of infectious TB
■ Abnormal chest x-ray
■ Prolonged therapy with immunosuppressive drugs
■ HIV or other immunosuppressive disease

Patients who are receiving INH should avoid alcohol. This reduces the chance for chemical- or drug-induced hepatitis. (Patients who are receiving INH should also avoid pregnancy.) Side effects of INH include paresthesias, seizures (toxic reaction), orthostatic hypotension, nausea and vomiting, hepatitis, and hypersensitivity to the drug.

MENINGOCOCCAL MENINGITIS

Meningococcal meningitis is also known as *spinal meningitis*. It is inflammation of the membranes that surround the spinal cord and brain. Meningococcal meningitis can be caused by a variety of different bacteria, viruses, and other microorganisms. A major cause of bacterial meningitis is *Neisseria meningitidis*. Like *M. tuberculosis*, it is spread by airborne pathogens. The usual mode of transmission is prolonged, direct contact with upper respiratory tract secretions (discharge from the nose and throat) from an infected person or carrier. Once inhaled, the bacteria invade the respiratory passages. They travel by way of the blood to the brain and spinal cord. As the infecting agent spreads to more organs, it causes toxic effects in the involved organ system.

Meningitis strikes an estimated 15,000 Americans each year[24] and an estimated 2% to 10% of the population may carry meningococci at any one time. The throat's epithelial lining generally prevents the germ from invading the meninges and the cerebrospinal fluid. Although the conversion from carrier to clinical disease is rare in developed countries, outbreaks of disease in the United States have increased since the 1990s, partly because of increased rates of disease in people who may have a common organizational affiliation or who live in the same community.[25]

Other Infectious Agents Known to Cause Meningitis

Other common pathogens that cause meningitis include *Streptococcus pneumoniae* and *Haemophilus influenzae* type b (Hib), and some viruses. *S. pneumoniae* is the second most common cause of bacterial meningitis in adults, the most common cause of pneumonia in adults, and the most common cause of otitis media (middle ear infection) in children. This bacterium is spread by droplets, prolonged personal contact, or extended contact with linen soiled with respiratory discharges.

H. influenzae has the same mode of transmission as *N. meningitidis*. Vaccines for children were introduced in 1981. Before that time, *H. influenzae* was the leading cause of bacterial meningitis in children 6 months to 3 years of age. (This bacterium is also responsible for conditions such as pediatric epiglottitis, septic arthritis, and generalized sepsis.) This type of meningitis can be treated with antibiotics. However, 50% of infected children have lasting damage to the nervous system.[26]

Fortunately, none of the bacteria that cause meningitis are as contagious as the common cold or flu. In addition, they are not spread by casual contact or by simply breathing the air where a person with meningitis has been.

Viral meningitis (aseptic meningitis) is a syndrome generally associated with an existing systemic viral disease (e.g., enteroviral infection, herpes virus infection, mumps, and, less commonly, influenza). Symptoms are similar to those of bacterial meningitis (described later). However, they are usually less severe. In most cases viral meningitis is self-limited, and the patient recovers fully. The patient may experience muscle weakness and malaise during prolonged convalescence.

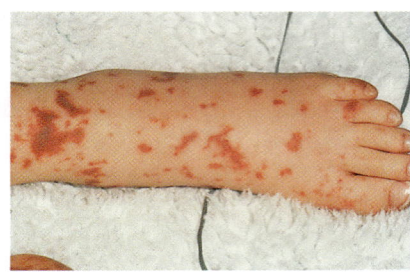

FIGURE 28-8 Petechial rash in meningococcal infection. (From Lissauer T, Clayden G: *Illustrated textbook of pediatrics,* ed 2, St Louis, 2001, Mosby.)

CRITICAL THINKING
What does a petechial rash look like?

> ### NOTE
> Viral meningitis that is caused by enteroviruses can be spread by direct contact with an infected person's stool. Examples of possible exposures include small children who are toilet training and adults who handle soiled diapers of infected infants. Enteroviruses and other viruses (such as mumps and varicella-zoster virus) can also be spread through direct or indirect contact with respiratory secretions (saliva, sputum, or nasal mucus). Although there are risks for infection through exposure, there is only a small chance of developing meningitis as a complication of the illness.[27]

Signs and Symptoms

The signs and symptoms of meningitis depend on the patient's age and general health. In infants, for example, signs of meningeal irritation may be absent. On the other hand, they may include only irritability, poor feeding or vomiting, a high-pitched cry, and fullness of the fontanelle. (Maternal antibodies generally protect neonates to 6 months of age.) In older infants and children, signs of meningitis may include malaise, low-grade fever, projectile vomiting, petechial rash (Figure 28-8), headache, and stiff neck from meningeal irritation (nuchal rigidity). Diagnostic signs of meningitis in older children include the *Brudzinski sign* (involuntary flexion of the arm, hip, and knee when the neck is passively flexed) and the *Kernig sign* (loss of the ability in a seated or supine patient to completely extend the leg when the thigh is flexed on the abdomen; the patient usually can extend the leg completely when the thigh is not flexed on the abdomen).

The risk of **bacterial meningitis** is most significant in neonates and in children 6 months to 2 years of age. However, infection should be suspected in any patient with fever, headache, stiff neck, altered mental status, the presence of petechiae and purpura, or underlying health problems (e.g., recent neurosurgery, trauma, or immunocompromise). If extensive meningeal involvement develops in a toxic or debilitated patient, the illness may be accompanied by acute adrenal insufficiency, convulsions, coma, and disseminated intravascular coagulation (*Waterhouse-Friderichsen syndrome*). In this case, death can occur in 6 to 8 hours. Other conditions and long-term complications associated with severe meningitis include blindness and deafness (from cranial nerve damage), arthritis, myocarditis, and pericarditis. Death can follow overwhelming infection.

Immunization and Control Measures

Vaccines are available for Hib, some strains of *N. meningitidis*, and many types of *S. pneumoniae*. The vaccines against Hib are very safe and highly effective. By 6 months of age, infants should have received at least three doses of Hib vaccine; a fourth dose ("booster") is recommended between 12 and 18 months of age. Vaccine against some strains of *N. meningitidis* is not routinely used in the United States and is not effective in children under 18 months of age.[27] However, the vaccine is sometimes used to control outbreaks of some types of meningococcal meningitis. Vaccines to prevent meningitis caused by *S. pneumoniae* also can prevent other forms of infection arising from the bacterium. This vaccine is ineffective for children under 2 years of age. However, it is recommended for all people over age 65. It also is recommended for younger people with certain chronic medical problems. Vaccines against meningitis have been instrumental in preventing outbreaks of the disease among military recruits in the United States. Before 1971, such outbreaks were a common occurrence.

Patient Management and Protective Measures

Patient management focuses on ensuring an adequate airway and ventilatory and circulatory support. The paramedic must take protective measures when caring for patients who have signs and symptoms of meningitis. Universal precautions (with surgical masks on the patient) should be used during care and transport. The EMS agency should have an exposure control plan for meningitis.

Early diagnosis and treatment of bacterial meningitis are essential. The diagnosis usually is confirmed by finding the bacteria in a sample of the patient's spinal fluid. This is obtained through a spinal tap (lumbar puncture). The disease is then treated using several antibiotics. Drugs to prevent the disease are available for those who may have intimate contact with the patient (e.g., family members).

> **NOTE**
> Meningitis is a true medical emergency. A chief goal of emergency care is administration of a bacteria-specific antibiotic. The drug should be given 30 to 60 minutes after arriving at the emergency department.

Bacterial endocarditis (also known as *infective endocarditis*) is inflammation of the endocardium and one or more heart valves. The condition can be caused by a variety of diseases that permit bacteria to enter the bloodstream. (There are nonbacterial causes of endocarditis as well.) These bacteria settle in the heart and grow on the valves of the heart in structures called *vegetation*.

These structures damage the heart valves and may cause them to leak. In severe cases, heart failure develops. If the bacteria dislodge from the valves and enter the bloodstream, they can cause stroke, vision impairment, and severe damage to other organ systems. Bacterial endocarditis is most common in patients older than 60 years of age as a result of degenerative valve disease; about 20% of people die of the disease within 5 years of diagnosis.[28] Other factors associated with the development of endocarditis include intravenous drug use, recent dental surgery, permanent central venous access lines, and prior heart valve surgery.

Signs and symptoms of endocarditis may develop slowly or be acute. The disease can be difficult to diagnose, as early symptoms may resemble the flu or other illnesses. These signs and symptoms include:

- Fatigue
- Weakness
- Fever
- Chills
- Night sweats
- Weight loss
- Muscle aches and pains
- Excessive sweating
- Joint pain

Other signs and symptoms of endocarditis include red, painless skin spots located on the palms and soles (*Janeway lesions*); red, painful nodes in the pads of the fingers and toes (*Osler's nodes*); jaundice, and splinter hemorrhages under the nails. If the patient's heart valves are seriously affected, a heart murmur, shortness of breath, chest discomfort, and dysrhythmias may be present. Other findings during the physical examination may include retinal hemorrhages, petechiae in the conjunctiva, and an enlarged spleen. Diagnosis of endocarditis is made through blood cultures to identify the bacteria and transesophageal echocardiograms. Hospitalization is usually required along with long-term antibiotic therapy (4 to 6 weeks) and sometimes heart valve replacement. Following recovery, prophylactic antibiotic therapy is often prescribed for these patients before dental procedures and surgeries. Those who have had endocarditis are at a higher risk of contracting the disease again. Some patients will carry an endocarditis wallet card issued by the American Heart Association or other organizations to provide information to the health care personnel.

PNEUMONIA

As described in Chapter 24, **pneumonia** is an acute inflammation of the bronchioles and alveoli. It can be spread by droplets and by direct and indirect contact with respiratory secretions. Etiologic agents responsible for this disease may be bacterial (*S. pneumoniae, M. pneumoniae, Staphylococcus aureus, H. influenzae, Klebsiella pneumoniae, Moraxella catarrhalis, Legionella* sp.), viral, or fungal. These organisms may affect several body systems. They include the respiratory system (pneumonia); the CNS (meningitis); and the ears, nose, and throat (otitis, pharyngitis media). The signs and symptoms of pneumonia include the following:

- Sudden onset of chills, high-grade fever, chest pain with respirations, and dyspnea
- Tachypnea and chest retractions (an ominous sign in children)
- Congestion caused by the development of purulent alveolar exudates in one or more lobes
- A productive cough with yellow-green phlegm

Susceptibility and Resistance

Susceptibility to pneumonia is increased by processes such as smoking, pulmonary edema, influenza, exposure to inhaled toxins, chronic lung disease, and aspiration of any form (postalcohol ingestion, near drowning, regurgitation caused by gastric distention from bag-valve-mask ventilation). Extremes of age also appear to increase susceptibility to the disease (e.g., elderly individuals and infants with a low birth weight and/or malnourishment). Other high-risk groups for pneumonia include the following conditions:

- Sickle cell disease
- Cardiovascular disease
- Chronic respiratory disease (e.g., chronic obstructive pulmonary disease [COPD], asthma, cystic fibrosis)

- **Asplenia** (congenital absence or surgical removal of the spleen)
- Diabetes
- Chronic renal failure (or other kidney disease)
- HIV
- Organ transplantation
- Multiple myeloma, lymphoma, Hodgkin's disease, lung cancer

Patient Management and Protective Measures

Prehospital care for patients with pneumonia includes providing airway support, oxygen, ventilatory assistance (as needed), intravenous (IV) fluids, cardiac monitoring, and transport for evaluation by a physician. Bacterial pneumonia is usually managed with analgesics, decongestants, expectorants, and antibiotic therapy. Patients generally do not need to be isolated from others. In hospitals, pneumonia patients may be isolated from other patients who may be more susceptible to infection.

CRITICAL THINKING

Which locations in your area are at high risk for influenza outbreaks?

Measures for protecting health care workers include BSI precautions and effective hand washing. Airway barriers (described earlier) should be used if TB is suspected. Immunizations exist for some causes of pneumonia. However, they generally are not recommended for people who come in contact with patients who have the disease.

TETANUS

Tetanus is a serious, sometimes fatal, disease of the central nervous system. It is caused by infection of a wound with spores of *Clostridium tetani*. Tetanus spores live mainly in soil and manure. However, they are also found in the human intestine. If the spores enter tissue (e.g., through a puncture wound or burn), they multiply and produce a toxin that acts on the nerves controlling muscular activity. (Dead or necrotic tissue is a favorable environment for *C. tetani*.) About 500,000 cases of tetanus occur worldwide each year, with a mortality rate of 45%. These deaths often occur from wounds that appear too trivial for medical evaluation. Only about 100 cases of tetanus are reported annually in the United States. They occur most often in patients 50 years of age or older. The relatively low number of tetanus cases in the United States is a result of immunization of the general population with tetanus vaccines.[28]

Signs and Symptoms

The most common symptom of tetanus is *trismus* (stiffness of the jaw); it is also known as *lockjaw* because of the accompanying difficulty in opening the mouth (Figure 28-9). Other symptoms include the following:

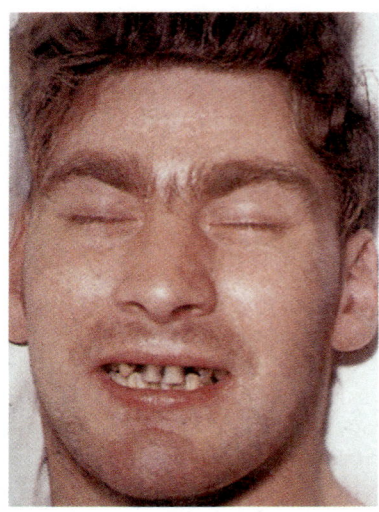

FIGURE 28-9 Trismus as a result of mild tetanus that developed 10 days after the individual received a benign-looking leg wound. (From London PS: *A colour atlas of diagnosis after recent injury,* Ipswich, England, 1990, Wolfe Medical Publications, Ltd.)

- Muscular tetany (muscle spasms and twitching)
- Painful muscular contractions in the neck, moving to the trunk
- Abdominal rigidity (often the first sign in pediatric patients)
- Painful spasms (contortions) of the face (*risus sardonicus*), which produce a grotesque smile
- Respiratory failure

Patient Management and Protective Measures

The prehospital care goals are to support vital functions. This may include aggressive airway management (intubation and surgical or needle cricothyrotomy). Muscle spasms should be treated with **diazepam** or **lorazepam** (i.e., benzodiazepines) or paralytic agents (per medical direction). Other drugs that may be indicated include IV fluids, **magnesium sulfate,** narcotics, and antidysrhythmics. After evaluation by a physician and stabilization of the patient's condition, care for individuals with tetanus includes administration of antitoxin (tetanus immune globulin [TIG]) to provide postexposure passive immunity, treatment to eliminate the toxin, active immunization with tetanus toxoid, and wound care. Most patients recover fully if they receive prompt treatment.

CRITICAL THINKING

When a patient with an open skin wound refuses care, should you explain the risks of tetanus infection?

Immunization

Immunization against tetanus usually is started in children. It is achieved using diphtheria-pertussis-tetanus (DPT) vaccination. This is a combined immunization against diphtheria (laryngitis, pharyngitis with discharge), pertussis (whooping cough), and tetanus. After the initial immunization, children receive a booster shot before starting elementary school. After that, a booster shot is recommended every 10 years.

Patients who have a recent wound should be counseled about postinjury tetanus prophylaxis and effective wound care. If it is suspected that a wound could carry tetanus, the tetanus vaccination will not adequately prevent infection; the patient will need tetanus immunoglobulin. The "tetanus shot" (tetanus immunization) only prevents tetanus exposure in future wounds. All patients should be questioned about their tetanus immunization status. (Boosters should be given every 10 years; 5 years for a "dirty" wound.) Recovery from infection does not confer immunity.

RABIES

Rabies (*hydrophobia*) is an acute viral infection of the central nervous system. The disease mainly affects animals. However, it can be transmitted from an infected animal to a human through virus-laden saliva (e.g., by a bite or scratch). (Transmission from person to person is theoretical but has never been documented.[29]) In the United States, wildlife rabies is common in skunks, raccoons, bats, foxes, dogs, wolves, jackals, mongooses, and coyotes. Healthy wild animals (e.g., skunks) are seldom seen by casual observance. A high degree of suspicion for rabies is indicated for all animals found outside their natural habitat. Hawaii is the only rabies-free state in the United States.

Humans are highly susceptible to the rabies virus after exposure to saliva in a bite or scratch from an infected animal. Several factors govern the severity of infection, including the following:

- Severity of the wound
- Richness of nerve supply close to the wound
- Distance from the wound to the CNS
- Amount and strain of the virus
- Degree of protection provided by clothing

Signs and Symptoms

The incubation period between a bite and the appearance of symptoms ranges from 9 days to 7 years. Initial symptoms include low-grade fever, headache, loss of appetite, hyperactivity, disorientation, and, in some cases, seizures. Often the patient has an intense thirst, but attempts to drink result in violent, painful spasms in the throat (hence the name *hydrophobia*). Eye and facial muscles may become paralyzed as the disease progresses. Without medical intervention, the disease lasts 2 to 6 days, often resulting in death secondary to respiratory failure.

Patient Management and Protective Measures

Physicians treat the signs and symptoms of the disease and provide respiratory and cardiovascular support (as needed). Patients also are treated with sedatives and analgesics. Thorough debridement of the wound without sutures (if possible) is indicated. This allows free bleeding and drainage. Human rabies immune globulin may be given to provide passive immunization. Also, a rabies vaccine (Human Diploid Rabies Vaccine, Rabies Vaccine) is given by injections spread over several weeks. (Injections are no longer given in the stomach.) Tetanus prophylaxis and antibiotics may be indicated for treatment of the bite wound.

CRITICAL THINKING

Has a case of rabies ever occurred in your community? What animal was implicated?

Most cases of rabies in humans are the result of a bite from a rabid dog. However, the possibility of rabies must be considered with *all* mammal bites. Scene safety and use of BSI precautions during wound management are paramount. Law enforcement personnel and animal control authorities should be contacted to assist in scene control.

If given within 2 days of the bite, immunizations almost always prevent rabies. Immunizations should be given for contact with open wounds or for exposure of mucous membranes to saliva. Immunizations also should be given to people with a high probability of contact with animal reservoirs (e.g., animal care workers, animal shelter personnel, and outdoor workers). If an animal is suspected of being rabid, it should be killed by the proper authorities and its brain should be examined for rabies inclusion bodies. If no inclusion bodies are found, the patient's rabies treatment is stopped.

HANTAVIRUS

Hantavirus was previously known to be associated with hemorrhagic fever with renal syndrome that occurs in Asia. Hantaviruses also are associated with a syndrome of severe respiratory distress and shock. This syndrome has occurred in several areas of the United States.[30] The virus is carried by rodents. It is transmitted by inhalation of aerosol material contaminated with rodent urine and feces (see Table 28-3). Many forms of this disease occur in specific geographical areas.

Hantavirus can cause significant disease in humans. Patients are usually healthy adults who experience an onset of fever and malaise. This is followed several days later by respiratory distress. (The severity of the illness is determined by the strain of the virus.) Other signs and symptoms may include fever, chills, headache, GI upset, and capillary hemorrhage. With severe infection, oliguria, kidney failure, and hypotension occur. Death typically results from decreased cardiac output and eventual cardio-vascular collapse. Treatment is supportive and guided by medical direction. Body substance isolation precautions are indicated because of the infectious nature of these viruses.

VIRAL DISEASES OF CHILDHOOD

The childhood infectious diseases presented in this chapter include rubella (German measles), rubeola (red measles or hard measles), mumps (parotitis), chickenpox (varicella), and pertussis (whooping cough). These infectious diseases are preventable with immunization for chickenpox and with the triple immunization measles, mumps, and rubella (MMR) vaccine. The incidence of these childhood diseases has declined because of widespread immunization of children. Immunization provides long-lasting immunity. It is known to be 98% to 99% effective.

All health care workers should use personal protective measures when caring for children with viral infections. Protective immunization, effective hand washing, BSI (including the use of surgical masks for both the paramedic and the patient), and careful handling of linens, supplies, and equipment that may be contaminated are important in preventing the spread of these diseases.

Rubella

Rubella is a mild, febrile, and highly communicable viral disease caused by the rubella virus. It is characterized by a diffuse, punctate, macular rash (Figure 28-10). The disease usually is transmitted by direct contact with nasopharyngeal secretions or droplet spray from an infected person. It also may be passed transplacentally (producing active infection in the fetus) and by contact with articles contaminated with blood, urine, or feces. After inoculation, the virus invades the lymph system. From there it enters the blood and produces an immune response. The subsequent rash

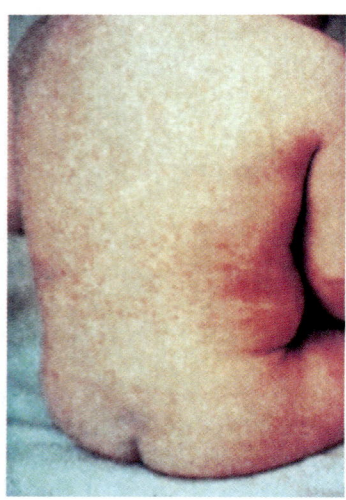

FIGURE 28-10 Acquired rubella (German measles) in an 11-month-old infant. (Courtesy Centers for Disease Control and Prevention, 1990. In Grimes D: *Infectious diseases,* St Louis, 1991, Mosby.)

spreads from the forehead to the face to the torso to the extremities (lasting 3 days). (A rash that lasts longer than 3 days indicates the presence of rubeola.) Maximal communicability appears to be the first few days before and 5 to 7 days after the onset of the rash. Complications from the disease are rare. However, young females sometimes develop a self-limiting arthritis.

CRITICAL THINKING
Is there any way a paramedic can avoid rubella other than being immunized for it?

Congenital rubella syndrome (CRS) affects approximately 90% of infants born to women who were infected with rubella during the first trimester of pregnancy.[31] The disease is associated with multiple congenital anomalies, mental retardation, deafness, and an increased risk of death from congenital heart disease and sepsis during the first 6 months of life. Infants with CRS shed large numbers of the virus in their secretions. The CDC recommends that all health care personnel receive immunization if they are not immune from previous rubella infection. This helps to reduce the risk of exposure to themselves and those they treat. Immunization is not recommended for pregnant women. This is due to the theoretical risk that the vaccine could cause developmental defects. As a precaution, pregnant EMS workers should not be exposed to patients with rubella.

Rubeola

Rubeola is an acute, highly communicable viral disease. It is caused by the measles virus. It is characterized by fever, conjunctivitis, cough, bronchitis, and a blotchy red rash (Figure 28-11). The virus is found in the blood, urine, and pharyngeal secretions. It usually is passed directly or indirectly through contact with infected respiratory secretions. With exposure, the virus invades the respiratory epithelium. It spreads via the lymph system. Rubeola may predispose a person to secondary bacterial complications such as otitis media, pneumonia, and myocarditis. The most serious life-threatening complication is *subacute sclerosing panencephalitis.* (This is a slowly progressing neurological disease. It is marked by loss of mental capacity and muscle coordination.)

Early (prodromal) symptoms that mark the onset of disease include high fever, nasal discharge, conjunctivitis, photophobia, and cough. About 1 or 2 days before the rash emerges, white spots are usually noted on the inside of the cheek (*Koplik spots*). The dermal rash begins a few days after respiratory tract involvement. The rash is red and maculopapular. It spreads from the forehead to the face, neck, and torso and eventually to the feet, usually by the third day. (The onset of the rash coincides with the production of serum antibodies.) Uncomplicated cases of rubeola usually last 6 days. Recovery from the illness confers lifelong immunity.

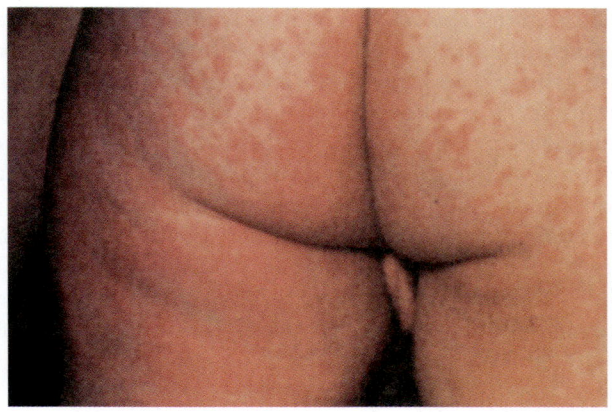

FIGURE 28-11 Rubeola (measles) rash on the third day. (Courtesy Centers for Disease Control and Prevention, 1990. In Grimes D: *Infectious diseases,* St Louis, 1991, Mosby.)

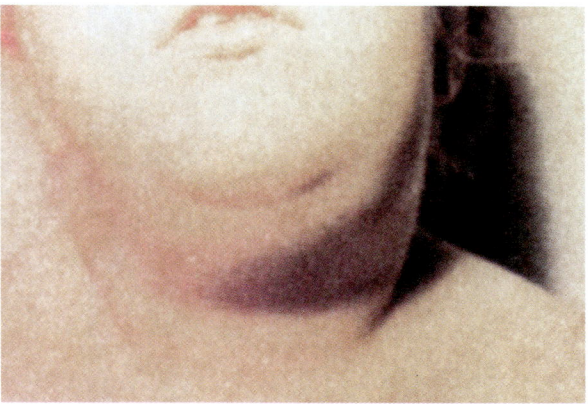

FIGURE 28-12 Submaxillary mumps in an infant. (Courtesy Centers for Disease Control and Prevention, 1990. In Grimes D: *Infectious diseases,* St Louis, 1991, Mosby.)

Mumps

Mumps is an acute, communicable systemic viral disease caused by the mumps virus. It is characterized by localized edema of one or more of the salivary glands (usually the parotid). The swelling may affect both or only one side of the neck (Figure 28-12). In some cases involvement of other glands also occurs. The virus is passed through direct contact with the saliva droplets of an infected person.

The virus invades and multiplies in the parotid gland or the upper respiratory tract passages. From there it enters the bloodstream and localizes in glandular or nervous tissue. The parotid, testes, and pancreas are the most frequently involved glands. When mumps occurs after the onset of puberty, it may cause a painful inflammation of the testicle (orchitis) and testicular atrophy; however, sterility is rare. The intensity of symptoms in mumps varies; 30% of infections are asymptomatic. Immunity after recovery is lifelong. Placental transfer of antibodies sometimes occurs.

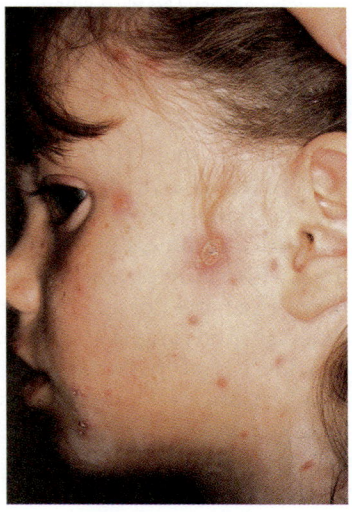

FIGURE 28-13 Chickenpox skin lesions. (Courtesy Gary Quick, MD.)

> ### CRITICAL THINKING
> Why are some viral diseases of childhood still seen despite widespread immunization?

Chickenpox

Chickenpox is a common childhood disease caused by the *varicella-zoster virus.* (Varicella-zoster is a member of the herpes virus family.) The virus is passed by direct and indirect contact with droplets (mainly airborne) from the respiratory passages of an infected person. Exposure to linen tainted with vesicular or mucous membrane discharges of infected people has been implicated.

Chickenpox is highly communicable. It is characterized by a sudden onset of low-grade fever, mild malaise, and a skin eruption that is maculopapular for a few hours and vesicular for 3 to 4 days, leaving a granular scab (Figure 28-13). At first, the skin lesions appear on the trunk. They usually progress to the extremities. The crops of skin eruptions (each associated with itching) usually are more abundant on covered areas of the body. The scalp, conjunctivae, and upper respiratory tract may also be affected. The appearance of crops of vesicles (fresh vesicles appearing while other lesions are scabbed) differentiates chickenpox from smallpox. (Smallpox has vesicles of the same age.) Treatment is symptomatic. Moreover, the disease is self-limited. Complications may include secondary bacterial infections, aseptic meningitis, mononucleosis, and Reye syndrome. Children with chickenpox should be isolated from schools, medical offices, emergency departments, and public places until all lesions are crusted and dry.

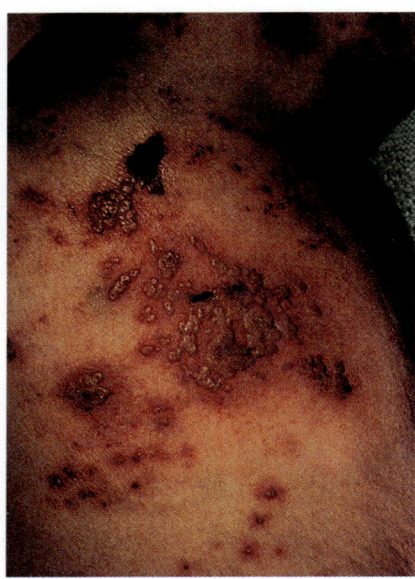

FIGURE 28-14 Vesicles associated with shingles. (From Epsetein O, et al: *Clinical examination,* ed 4, St Louis, 2008, Mosby.)

After recovery, the virus is thought to remain in the body in an asymptomatic latent stage. (It is possibly localized in the dorsal root ganglia.) The virus may reactivate during periods of stress or immunosuppression. During these periods, it may produce an illness known as **shingles.** The vesicles associated with shingles appear on the skin area supplied by the sensory nerves of a single group or associated groups of dorsal root ganglia (Figure 28-14). Unlike chickenpox, shingles is not passed through respiratory droplets. However, it can cause chickenpox in susceptible individuals who come in contact with open skin lesions (lesions that are not yet scabbed).

Antiviral drugs may shorten the duration of symptoms and pain in older patients. EMS personnel who have not had chickenpox should consider receiving the vaccine. Data indicate that adult antibody production occurs in 78% of patients after one dose. It occurs in 99% of patients after two doses.[32] (The vaccine should not be given to people who received high doses of systemic steroids in the previous month.) About 5% of those who receive the vaccine develop a rash. Some develop frank chickenpox, which is very debilitating in adults. To protect the fetus, varicella-zoster immune globulin (VZIG) is recommended for pregnant women with significant exposure to chickenpox who do not have a history of previous exposure.

Pertussis

Pertussis is an infectious disease that mainly affects infants and young children. It is caused by *Bordetella pertussis* and is spread by direct contact with discharges from mucous membranes contained in airborne droplets. The disease causes inflammation of the entire respiratory tract. It also causes a subtle onset of cough that becomes paroxysmal in 1 to 2 weeks. This cough can last 1 to 2 months.

The coughing episodes are violent (sometimes without an intervening inhalation, causing the high-pitched inspiratory "whoop") and end with expulsion of clear mucus and vomiting. (The whoop often is not present in children younger than 6 months of age.) Before the introduction of a vaccine against pertussis in the 1950s, the disease killed more children in the United States than all other infectious diseases combined. The incidence of the disease has increased since 1990, with a disproportionate increase in adolescents and adults.[33] Pertussis vaccine usually is given in combination with diphtheria and tetanus (DPT) vaccines to children at 2, 4, and 6 months of age; a booster dose is given at age 5.

The ability to spread pertussis is thought to be greatest before the onset of paroxysmal coughing. (This explains the need for BSI and surgical mask protection for the paramedic and the patient.) Erythromycin is known to shorten the communicability period, but it can reduce symptoms only if given during the incubation period. (This is before the onset of paroxysmal cough.) Infection with pertussis usually provides immunity. However, attacks after immunization in older children and adults indicate that immunity may diminish over time.

OTHER VIRAL DISEASES

Other viral diseases easily transmitted during the course of patient care include influenza, mononucleosis, and herpes simplex type 1 (HSV-1) infection (described later in this chapter). As with all other contacts with patients who may have infectious disease, BSI precautions are indicated during patient care.

Influenza

As described in Chapter 24, **influenza** is a respiratory infection that is spread by influenza viruses A, B, and C. The disease is popularly known as "the flu." It is spread by virus-infected droplets that are coughed or sneezed into the air. Influenza usually occurs in small outbreaks or, every few years, in epidemics. Resistance is normally conferred after recovery. However, this resistance is only to the specific strain or variant (Box 28-12).

> **NOTE**
> The 2009 H1N1 virus sickened about 50 million Americans and was responsible for more than 10,000 deaths. The virus is known to spread rapidly and is expected to reach all countries worldwide. This virus was originally referred to as "swine flu." This was because laboratory tests showed that many of the genes in this new virus were very similar to influenza viruses that normally occur in pigs (swine) in North America. Further studies showed that the virus is very different from what normally circulates in North American pigs. The H1N1 virus has two genes from flu viruses that normally circulate in pigs in Europe and Asia, and bird (avian) genes and human genes. Scientists call this a "quadruple reassortant" virus.[34] The seasonal influenza vaccination does not protect against new strains of flu such as H1N1.

DID YOU KNOW?

CDC Recommendations for EMS and Medical First Responder Personnel Including Firefighter and Law Enforcement First Responders During an Outbreak of Influenza (H1N1)

Patient Assessment: Interim Recommendations:

If there HAS NOT been swine-origin influenza reported in the geographical area, EMS personnel should assess all patients as follows:

1. EMS personnel should stay more than 6 feet away from patients and bystanders with symptoms and should exercise appropriate routine respiratory droplet precautions while assessing all patients for suspected cases of swine-origin influenza.

2. Assess all patients for symptoms of acute febrile respiratory illness (fever plus one or more of the following: nasal congestion/rhinorrhea, sore throat, or cough).
   - If no acute febrile respiratory illness, proceed with normal EMS care.
   - If symptoms of acute febrile respiratory illness, then assess all patients for travel to a geographical area with confirmed cases of swine-origin influenza within the last 7 days or close contact with someone with travel to these areas.
   - If travel exposure, don appropriate PPE for suspected case of swine-origin influenza.
   - If no travel exposure, place a standard surgical mask on the patient (if tolerated) and use appropriate PPE for cases of acute febrile respiratory illness without suspicion of swine-origin influenza (as described in PPE section).

If the CDC confirmed swine-origin influenza in the geographical area:

1. Address scene safety:
   - If Public Safety Answer Point (PSAP) advises potential for acute febrile respiratory illness symptoms on-scene, EMS personnel should don PPE for suspected cases of swine-origin influenza before entering scene.
   - If PSAP has not identified individuals with symptoms of acute febrile respiratory illness on-scene, EMS personnel should stay more than 6 feet away from patient and bystanders with symptoms and should exercise appropriate routine respiratory droplet precautions while assessing all patients for suspected cases of swine-origin influenza.

2. Assess all patients for symptoms of acute febrile respiratory illness (fever plus one or more of the following: nasal congestion/rhinorrhea, sore throat, or cough).
   - If no symptoms of acute febrile respiratory illness, provide routine EMS care.
   - If symptoms of acute febrile respiratory illness, don appropriate PPE for suspected case of swine-origin influenza.

Personal Protective Equipment (PPE): Interim Recommendations[35]:

- When treating a patient with a suspected case of swine-origin influenza as defined above, the following PPE should be worn:
  - Fit-tested disposable N95 respirator and eye protection (e.g., goggles, eye shield), disposable nonsterile gloves, and gown, when coming into close contact with the patient.
- When treating a patient that is not a suspected case of swine-origin influenza but who has symptoms of acute febrile respiratory illness, the following precautions should be taken:
  - Place a standard surgical mask on the patient, if tolerated. If not tolerated, EMS personnel may wear a standard surgical mask.
  - Use good respiratory hygiene—use nonsterile gloves for contact with patient, patient secretions, or surfaces that may have been contaminated. Follow hand hygiene including hand washing or cleansing with alcohol-based hand disinfectant after contact.
- Encourage good patient compartment vehicle airflow/ventilation to reduce the concentration of aerosol accumulation when possible.

BOX 28-12 Influenza Virus Types A, B, and C

People infected with certain strains of influenza type A or type B acquire immunity to that strain. However, the type A and type B viruses occasionally alter to produce new strains. This leads to a new infection. Type B virus is relatively stable. However, it occasionally changes to overcome resistance and may lead to small outbreaks of infection. Type A virus is highly unstable. It has caused worldwide flu epidemics. These variants are named for the geographical site and year of isolation (e.g., the Spanish flu in 1918, Asian flu in 1957, and Hong Kong flu in 1968) and the culture number (e.g., A/Japan/305/57).

Type C virus stimulates antibodies that provide immunity for life.

Signs and symptoms typically include chills, fever, headache, muscular aches, loss of appetite, and fatigue. These symptoms are followed by upper respiratory tract infection and a cough (often severe and drawn out) that lasts for 2 to 7 days. Patient management is mainly supportive. Mild cases of viral infection usually are not treated.

Severe cases (especially in the elderly and those with lung or heart disease) may result in secondary bacterial infection (e.g., *S. pneumoniae*). These cases can be fatal. Other viral respiratory diseases that can lead to bacterial complications include acute afebrile viral respiratory disease (excluding influenza) and acute febrile respiratory disease. Both diseases may cause illnesses in the upper and lower respiratory tracts. These illnesses include pharyngitis, laryngitis, croup, bronchitis, and bronchiolitis (Box 28-13).

Flu vaccines contain killed strains of type A and type B virus that are known to be currently in circulation. These vaccines may help prevent infection. A nasal spray flu

BOX 28-13 Bird Flu: The Next Pandemic?

A **pandemic** is an infectious disease outbreak that infects large numbers of people in a large geographical region and may occur worldwide. One occurs three to four times each century when new virus subtypes emerge and are easily transmitted from person to person. Any infectious disease may become a pandemic, but influenza is of great concern because it spreads easily and can kill many people. There were three influenza pandemics in the 20th century. They were the 1918 Spanish flu, which killed about 20 million people; the 1957 Asian flu, which killed as many as 4 million people; and the 1968 Hong Kong flu, which killed up to 2 million people. The World Health Organization (WHO) has predicted that the next pandemic influenza could kill between 2 million and 8 million people worldwide. The 2009 H1N1 virus was a pandemic.

Avian influenza (bird flu) is an infectious disease of birds, and less commonly pigs. It is caused by the A strain of the influenza virus, and is considered by many health officials as most likely to become the next pandemic. There are several strains and subtypes of avian influenza. One highly pathogenic strain of the virus (H5N1) began circulating in migratory birds in Southeast Asia in 2003 and more recently in parts of Europe. The virus is similar in makeup to the 1918 variety (believed by many to be a mutation of an avian virus) and can mutate rapidly. It also causes severe disease in humans who have come in contact with infected birds. The virus is easily spread among birds but has not yet acquired the ability to spread easily among humans. The fear is that as the virus continues to spread among migratory birds, it may mutate or merge with human strains of another virus, enabling the disease to be spread in humans. If this happens, the disease could sweep the world in as little as 3 months and could persist for years.

Because the virus has not mutated to easily spread infection among humans, a vaccine specific to the disease cannot be developed. Current vaccines under study may not be completely effective against the strain if it mutates. Two antiviral drugs, oseltamivir (Tamiflu) and zanamivir (Relenza), are clinically effective in interrupting the ability of the influenza A virus to replicate within the human body. The WHO recommends that nations stockpile enough of these antiviral drugs to cover 10% of their population. The prophylactic use of these antiviral drugs to prevent avian flu is not recommended. Doing so may result in a resistant strain of the virus. Annual flu vaccinations are not effective against bird flu. They are, however, effective against other flu viruses that may complicate the avian flu should an outbreak occur.

vaccine, FluMist (virus vaccine live, intranasal), has also been approved for protection against influenza A and B viruses in healthy people between 5 and 49 years of age. However, immunity does not last long. Therefore the vaccine must be repeated each year just before the start of the flu season (November to March in the United States). Health care workers should be immunized in the fall of each year with the current vaccine.

Amantadine, rimantadine, or zanamivir may be given to hospitalized patients to protect against influenza A. Despite advances in prevention and treatment, more than 36,000 people die each year in the United States from influenza and its complications.

CRITICAL THINKING

Will you get the influenza vaccine? What influenced your decision?

Mononucleosis

Mononucleosis is often referred to as "mono." It is caused either by the *Epstein-Barr virus* (EBV) or by *cytomegalovirus* (CMV) (Box 28-14). Both of these are members of the herpes virus family. Mononucleosis is spread from person to person via the oropharyngeal route and saliva (hence the name *kissing disease*). Blood transfusions also can be a mode of transmission. However, resultant clinical disease is rare. Most people with a healthy immune system are able to fend off the infection even after significant exposure.

Transmission from caregivers to young children is common. About 90% of people over age 35 have antibodies to CMV or EBV. This is probably the result of mild, childhood infection, often attributed to a common cold or the flu. Previous infection with EBV generally confers a high degree of resistance to future exposures.

Signs and symptoms of mononucleosis appear gradually. They are characterized by fever (which may last for weeks), sore throat, oropharyngeal discharges, lymphadenopathy (especially posterior cervical), and splenomegaly with abdominal tenderness. About 10% of people also develop a generalized rash or darkened areas in the mouth that resemble bruises. Recovery usually occurs in a few weeks. However, some people take months to regain their former level of energy. The patient may remain a carrier for several months after symptoms disappear. No immunization is available for mononucleosis.

SEXUALLY TRANSMITTED DISEASES

A **sexually transmitted disease** (STD) is a disease that can be passed from person to person through sexual activity. It may be transmitted to another person even when the infected person has no symptoms. More than 20 pathogens have been identified as belonging to this group of diseases (including HBV and HIV). Other common STDs are syphilis, gonorrhea, chlamydia, and herpes virus infections.

Several pathogenic agents are responsible for the host of STDs. These include bacteria, viruses, protozoa, fungi, and ectoparasites. These pathogens can produce multiple disease syndromes. Also, patients with STD syndromes often have multiple STDs. These infections usually cause a

BOX 28-14 Facts about CMV

General Information[36]:

Between 50% and 80% of adults in the United States are infected with CMV by 40 years of age.

CMV is the most common virus transmitted to a pregnant woman's unborn child.

Approximately 1 in 150 children is born with congenital CMV infection.

Approximately 1 in 750 children is born with or develops permanent disabilities attributable to CMV.

Approximately 8000 children each year suffer permanent disabilities caused by CMV.

Congenital CMV (meaning present at birth) is as common a cause of serious disability as Down syndrome, fetal alcohol syndrome, and neural tube defects.

About the Virus

CMV is found throughout the world in all geographical and socioeconomic groups, but, in general, it is more widespread in developing countries and in areas of lower socioeconomic conditions.

CMV is a member of the herpes virus family, which includes the herpes simplex viruses and the viruses that cause chickenpox (varicella-zoster virus) and infectious mononucleosis (Epstein-Barr virus).

CMV is found in body fluids, including urine, saliva (spit), breast milk, blood, tears, semen, and vaginal fluids.

Once CMV is in a person's body, it stays there for life.

Most CMV infections are "silent," meaning they cause no signs or symptoms in an infected person.

CMV can cause disease in unborn babies and in people with a weakened immune system.

Transmission and Prevention (How People Become Infected With CMV)

Transmission of CMV occurs from person to person, through close contact with body fluids (urine, saliva [spit], breast milk, blood, tears, semen, and vaginal fluids), but the chance of getting CMV infection from casual contact is very small.

In the United States, about 1% to 4% of uninfected mothers have primary (or first) CMV infection during a pregnancy.

About 33% of women who become infected with CMV for the first time during pregnancy pass the virus to their unborn babies.

No actions can totally eliminate all the risks of getting CMV, but there are simple measures that can reduce spread of the disease. The CDC recommends that pregnant women:

- Wash hands often with soap and water, especially after changing diapers. Wash well for 15 to 20 seconds.
- Do not kiss young children under the age of 5 or 6 on the mouth or cheek. Instead, kiss them on the head or give them a big hug.
- Do not share food, drinks, or utensils (spoons or forks) with young children. If you are pregnant and work in a day care center, reduce your risk of getting CMV by working with children who are older than $2\frac{1}{2}$ years of age, especially if you have never been infected with CMV or are unsure if you have been exposed.[37]

---

short-lived cellular immune response. They also can produce longer-lasting humoral antibody response. Neither of these protects against future exposures.

Syphilis

Syphilis is a systemic disease. It is characterized by a primary lesion, a secondary eruption involving the skin and mucous membranes, long latency periods, and late, seriously disabling lesions of the skin, bones, viscera, CNS, and cardiovascular system. The disease results from penetration of the skin, whether intact or broken, by the bacterium *Treponema pallidum*. Common modes of transmission include direct contact with fluid or pus from lesions on the skin and mucous membranes, blood transfusions or needlesticks (rare), and congenital transmission. After penetration, the organisms travel (within hours) to the lymph nodes. From there they are carried throughout the body. After the initial infection, syphilis follows well-defined stages of disease. It can be treated with antibiotic therapy. No immunization is available. It is estimated that 30% of exposures result in infection.

PRIMARY STAGE

Within 10 to 90 days of exposure, a primary lesion, or chancre, develops at the site of initial invasion (Figure 28-15). The surface of the chancre is usually crusted or ulcerated. It varies in size from 1 to 2 cm in diameter. The lesion usually is single and painless. In addition, it generally heals spontaneously within 1 to 5 weeks. Syphilis is highly communicable during this stage.

SECONDARY STAGE

The secondary stage begins about 2 to 10 weeks after the appearance of the primary lesion. This stage lasts for 2 to 6 weeks. It is heralded by systemic symptoms. These include headache, malaise, anorexia, fever, sore throat, lymphadenopathy, and bald spots in the area of infection. In addition, the patient may develop a rash, which usually is bilaterally symmetrical and often involves the palms and soles. Painless, wartlike regions (*condylomata lata*), which are extremely infectious, may also be found in moist, warm sites (e.g., the inguinal area). The CNS, eyes, bones, joints, or kidneys may be affected during this stage.

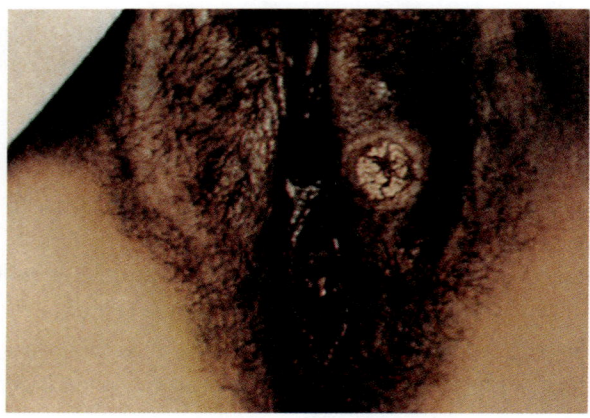

FIGURE 28-15 Primary syphilis chancre on the labia.

CRITICAL THINKING

Why do you think a patient in the secondary stage of syphilis would call EMS?

LATENCY

A latency period follows the secondary stage in untreated individuals. (This may range from 1 to 40 years or more.) During this period, recurrent episodes of secondary stage symptoms with subclinical infection may occur. This happens in about 25% of cases. About 33% of these patients progress to tertiary syphilis; the remainder remain free of symptoms. Tertiary syphilis is infectious involvement of the skin, CNS, and cardiovascular systems and may include the following manifestations:

1. Skin
   - Granulomatous lesions (gummas) on skin (painless) and bone (painful)
2. Central nervous system
   - Paresis
   - **Tabes dorsalis** (spinal column degeneration characterized by a wide gait and ataxia ["syphilitic shuffle"])
   - Loss of reflexes, pain, and temperature sensation
   - Meningitis
   - Psychosis
3. Cardiovascular
   - Cerebrovascular occlusion
   - Dissecting aneurysm of the ascending aorta
   - Myocardial insufficiency; aortic necrosis (which can lead to aortic rupture and death)

Gonorrhea

Gonorrhea is caused by the bacterium *Neisseria gonorrhoeae*. It is transmitted between individuals by fluids and pus from infected mucous membranes. It can also be spread from an infected mother to her baby during pregnancy and delivery. The disease occurs in both men and women. However, it differs in course, severity, and ease of recognition.

Gonorrhea often is treatable with antibiotics. However, some strains brought into the United States from other countries are resistant to the usual antibiotic therapy. Immunization is not available. Antibodies develop after exposure, but the antibodies are specific to the strain of gonorrhea that caused the infection. Consequently, future reinfection with other strains can occur.

Affected areas of the male anatomy are the urethra, Littre's gland, Cowper's gland, prostate gland, seminal vesicles, and epididymis. A sudden onset of dysuria and urinary urgency and frequency is seen several days after exposure. The associated urethral discharge rapidly becomes purulent and profuse. Direct spread of the infection may result in prostatitis, epididymitis, and seminal vesiculitis. Primary gonorrheal infections may also affect the pharynx, conjunctivae, and anus.

LOOK AGAIN

See Chapter 10: Review of Human Systems, pp. 201-205.

Affected areas of the female anatomy are the Bartholin glands, Skene glands, urethra, cervix, and fallopian tubes. More than 50% of infected women remain free of symptoms; others have a mucopurulent discharge that varies from scant to profuse. Contiguous spread of the disease may lead to endometritis, salpingitis, and parametritis (pelvic inflammatory disease) and the formation of tuboovarian abscesses. Complete or partial occlusion of the fallopian tubes may result in sterility and increased risk for ectopic pregnancy.

Between 1% and 3% of gonococcal infections become disseminated in the blood. This extension of the disease may produce septicemia, arthritis, endocarditis, meningitis, and skin lesions. In the bacteremic stage, the patient may complain of fever, chills, and malaise. Erythematous lesions are common, especially on the extremities. They may occur in clusters or singly.

Chlamydia

Chlamydia (*Chlamydia trachomatis*) is a major cause of sexually transmitted nonspecific urethritis (NSU) or nongonococcal genital infection. The disease is the most common sexually transmitted disease in the United States. (An estimated 25% of men are carriers.) It is a leading cause of preventable blindness.[38] The signs and symptoms are similar to those of gonorrhea. This makes differentiation difficult. No immunization is available.

In men, NSU may cause a penile discharge. It also may cause complications such as swelling of the testes, which, if untreated, may lead to infertility. In women, NSU usually is symptomless. However, it may cause a vaginal discharge or pain with urination, salpingitis, and cervicitis. Transmission occurs secondary to direct contact with exudates,

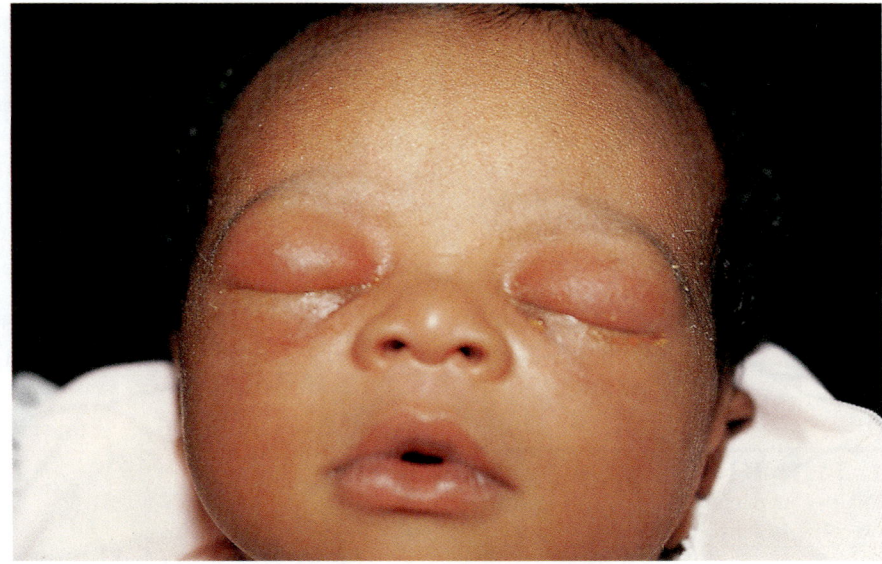

FIGURE 28-16 Conjunctivitis from a chlamydial infection in an 8-day-old infant. (From Lissauer T, Clayden G: *Illustrated textbook of pediatrics,* ed 2, St Louis, 2001, Mosby.)

either sexually or during birth (Figure 28-16). Chlamydial infections are treated with antibiotics.

Herpes Virus Infections

Four herpes viruses have been described. One is the herpes simplex virus. The others are CMV, which is associated with mononucleosis, hepatitis, and severe systemic disease in the immunosuppressed host; EBV, which causes mononucleosis; and varicella-zoster virus, which causes chickenpox and shingles. This section of the text addresses only the herpes viruses associated with STDs.

HERPES SIMPLEX VIRUS

The two antigenically distinct herpes simplex viruses responsible for STDs are **herpes simplex virus type 1** (HSV-1) and **herpes simplex virus type 2** (HSV-2). Both pathogens can cause herpes infection. Also, both can cause infection anywhere in the body. As a rule, HSV-1 most often is associated with herpes above the waist. In contrast, HSV-2 generally is associated with genital herpes. However, either type can cause disease in the genital area. Immunization is not available for either virus.

HSV is common in the United States. It causes 300,000 to 500,000 new infections each year; about 42 million Americans are thought to carry the virus.[39] It is estimated that 70% to 90% of adults have antibodies against HSV-1. The mode of transmission for HSV is strictly skin-to-skin contact with an infected area of the body. The virus enters through a break in the skin or through mucous membranes. Sexual contact is not required for transmission. For example, touching the herpes virus may result in finger infection (*herpetic whitlow*). Many young children who develop oral herpes (HSV-1) probably contract the virus

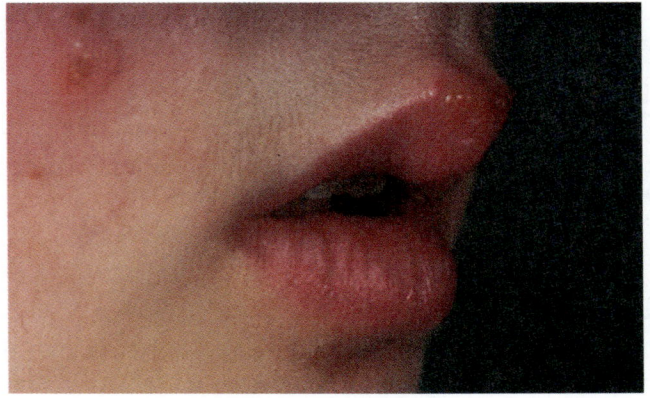

FIGURE 28-17 "Fever blister" caused by the herpes simplex virus. (From Epsetein O, et al: *Clinical examination,* ed 4, St Louis, 2008, Mosby.)

through a casual kiss from a parent or relative. The virus also may be spread to other external body sites by autoinoculation (e.g., it may be spread from lip to finger to genitalia). Initial HSV-1 transmission usually occurs by 4 years of age. It is manifested by gingivostomatitis ("cold sores" or "fever blisters") (Figure 28-17). Initial HSV-2 infection generally results from sexual activity. It is manifested by painful vesicular lesions of the cervix, vulva, penis, rectum, anus, and mouth (depending on sexual practices).

Once present in tissue, HSV produces an acute infection, with tissue destruction limited to one site. This primary infection produces a vesicular lesion (blister). The lesion heals spontaneously from the outside in without lasting scarring. However, the virus remains alive in the body despite circulating antibodies.

After the primary infection, the HSV enters the central nervous system nearest to the site of initial infection. It travels along sensory nerve pathways to a sensory nerve ganglion. There it remains in a latent stage until reactivated. When triggered by another infectious disease, menstruation, emotional stress, trauma, or immunosuppression, the virus reaches the epidermis by way of peripheral nerves. It reproduces a recurrent infectious disease state. This state usually lasts 4 to 10 days. The lesions usually appear in the area of initial inoculation. The number of lesions a person might experience during any given episode varies considerably.

CRITICAL THINKING
Why do you think the incidence of herpetic whitlow in health care workers has declined over the last 10 years?

HSV can remain inactive for a long time. It is unknown why many infected people never develop the disease, whereas others experience a lifetime of periodic outbreaks. Antiviral agents such as acyclovir may shorten the duration of an outbreak. They also may be used as prophylactic agents in instances of frequent recurrence.

LICE AND SCABIES

Lice and scabies are potential health hazards for all health care providers. Both can transmit communicable skin diseases and systemic illness, as well as dermatitis and discomfort. (Other vector-borne illnesses [e.g., Lyme disease] were described in Chapter 34.)

Lice

Lice are small, wingless insects that are ectoparasites of birds and mammals. Most are host specific. Two of the species are human parasites. One is *Phthirus pubis,* the pubic, or crab, louse. The other is *Pediculus humanus,* which has two forms: *Pediculus capitis* (the head louse) and *Pediculus corporis* (the body louse, which was involved in outbreaks of epidemic typhus and trench fever in World War I) (Figure 28-18). Lice have a three-stage life cycle. The eggs hatch in 7 to 10 days; the nymph stage lasts 7 to 13 days; and the egg-to-egg cycle lasts about 3 weeks.

Lice subsist on blood from the host and have mouths modified for piercing and sucking. During biting and feeding, secretions from the louse cause a small, red macule and pruritus. Long infestation periods may result in a decrease in pruritus and often a thick, dry, scaly appearance to the skin. In severe cases, oozing and crusting may be present. If sensitization to lice saliva and feces occurs, inflammation may develop. Secondary infection may result from scratching of lesions. Lice spread through close personal contact, and sharing of clothing and bedding may result in outbreaks (e.g., at schools, in day care facilities, and in families).

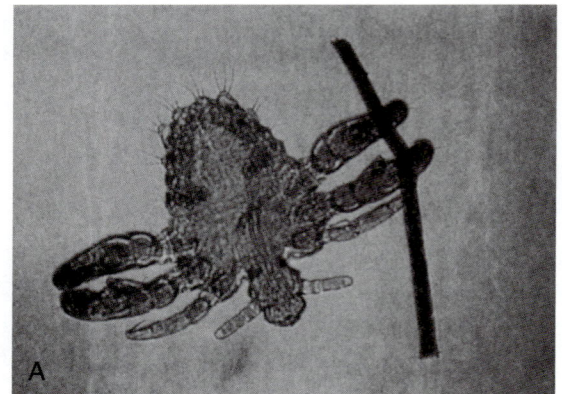

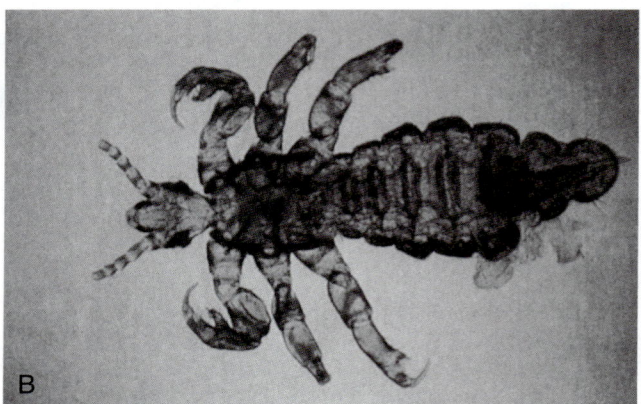

FIGURE 28-18 **A,** The pubic, or crab, louse. **B,** Male of the human head louse.

Pubic lice have a distinctive appearance, suggestive of miniature crabs. Gray-blue spots may be observed on the abdomen and thighs of infested patients. The eggs (*nits* or *ova*) often are evident on the shaft of pubic hairs. They are sometimes seen in the eyelashes, eyebrows, and axillary hairs. Pubic lice usually are acquired during sexual activity or from unchanged bedding in which egg-infested pubic hairs have been shed. Although primary bite lesions seldom are evident, the patient normally complains of intense pruritus and pubic scratching.

Head lice have an elongated body with a head that is slightly narrower than the thorax. Each louse has three pairs of legs, which possess delicate hooks at the distal extremities. The white ova of head lice (usually one nit to a shaft) are easily mistaken for dandruff, but the nits cannot be brushed out. These parasites most frequently affect children.

Body lice are slightly larger than head lice and concentrate around the waist, shoulders, axillae, and neck. Body lice and their nits usually are found in seams and on the fibers of clothing. The lesions from their bites begin as small, noninflammatory red spots, which quickly become papular wheals that resemble linear scratch marks (parallel scratch marks on the shoulders are a common finding). Head lice and body lice interbreed.

The treatment for all types of lice is designed to eradicate the parasites and nits and to prevent reinfestation. Patients usually are advised to wash all clothing, bedding, and personal articles thoroughly in hot water. They also are advised to wash the infected body area with gamma benzene hexachloride shampoo (Kwell), crotamiton (Eurax), Rid, or Nix. (Overtreatment should be avoided to prevent toxicity.)

> ### ? DID YOU KNOW
> **Bed Bugs**
>
> Bed bug infestations were common in the United States before World War II but were mostly eradicated in the 1940s and 1950s from the widespread use of DDT. In recent years, the common bed bug, *Cimex lectularius*, has made a comeback. It is increasingly being encountered in homes, apartments, hotels, motels, health care facilities, dormitories, shelters, schools, and modes of transport. Their resurgence may be the result of international travel since bed bugs are prevalent in other regions of the world. The most common place to find bed bugs is in bedding where they often hide within seams, tufts, and crevices of the mattress, box spring, bed frame, and headboard. The adult bed bug is reddish-brown, has a flattened body, and is easy to see. They can move quickly, but do not fly, and are commonly mistaken for ticks. Bed bugs usually bite at night while people are sleeping. The bites (which often occur in clusters) may cause an itchy welt or localized swelling, similar to a mosquito bite. These localized skin reactions may be immediate or delayed for several days after the bite. Scratching the bites can lead to skin infections. Although bed bugs can harbor pathogens in and on their bodies, transmission to humans is considered unlikely. Bed bugs require a blood meal to molt and can live 12-18 months. Visible signs of bed bugs include blood stains or fecal spots on bedding, furniture, and walls. If infestation is severe, there may be a sweet and musty odor in the room. Bed bug infestations require professional extermination.
>
> EMS personnel should take the following precautions when faced with possible bed bug infestation:
> - Tuck pant legs inside socks or boots.
> - Wear disposable shoe covers while at the scene and dispose of them in a sealed, plastic bag. Inspect work shoes before entering the ambulance or EMS base. Infested gear should not be taken into living quarters.
> - Place any clothing item with visible bed bugs in a plastic, sealed bag. Do not use the clothing again until it has been placed in a hot clothes dryer for at least 15 minutes to destroy the bed bugs.

From Potter M: Bed Bugs, University of Kentucky College of Agriculture, http://www.ca.uky.edu/entomology/entfacts/ef636.asp, accessed June 7, 2011.

Scabies

The human **scabies** mite (*Sarcoptes scabiei* var. *hominis*) is a parasite. It completes its entire life cycle in and on the epidermis of its host. Scabies infestation resembles a lice infestation. However, scabies bites generally are concentrated around the hands and feet, especially in the webs of the fingers and toes (Figure 28-19). Other common infestation

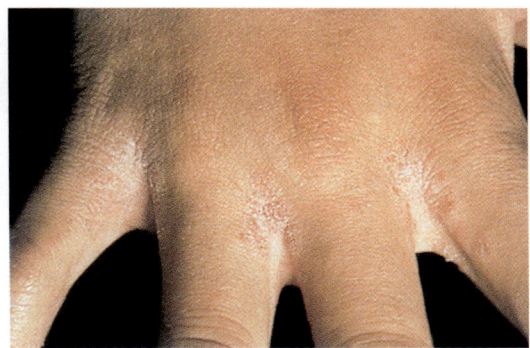

FIGURE 28-19 Common site of burrows in scabies.

areas include the face and scalp of children, the nipples in females, and the penis in males. The scabies mite usually is passed by intimate contact or acquired from infested bedding, furniture, and clothing. The mite can burrow into the skin within minutes.

Scabies infestation often is manifested by severe nocturnal pruritus. However, it takes 4 to 6 weeks for sensitization to develop and itching to begin. The adult female mite is responsible for symptoms. After impregnation, she burrows into the epidermis to lay her eggs. She remains in the burrow for a life span of about 1 month. Although vesicles and papules form at the surface, they often are disguised by the results of scratching. In severe cases (e.g., Norwegian scabies), oozing, crusting, and secondary infection may result. Susceptibility is general. However, people with a previous exposure usually develop fewer mites on later exposures and experience symptoms earlier (within 1 to 4 days).

The treatment is similar to that prescribed for lice infestation. Symptoms may persist for longer than 1 month until the mite and mite products are shed with the epidermis. (Mites are communicable until all mites and eggs have been destroyed.) Reinfestation is common; therefore the patient should be reexamined if the itching has not abated after several weeks. Antibiotic therapy may be needed to treat secondary bacterial infection. Immunization is not available. Protective measures against lice and scabies infestation are presented in Box 28-15.

REPORTING AN EXPOSURE TO AN INFECTIOUS OR A COMMUNICABLE DISEASE

An **exposure incident** (significant exposure) is any specific contact of the eyes, the mouth, other mucous membranes, or nonintact skin, or parenteral contact, with blood, blood products, bloody body fluids, or other potentially infectious materials. Exposures and all suspected exposures to an infectious or communicable disease must be reported to the DO. Reporting a possible exposure is important for the following reasons:

BOX 28-15 Protective Measures Against Lice and Scabies

1. Observe body substance isolation (BSI) and bag linen separately.
2. Spray the patient compartment of the ambulance with an effective insecticide. (Most commercial sprays contain effective pyrethrins, malathion, or carbamates.)
3. Spray the floor, gurney, and immediate areas where the patient's head was positioned (lice do not jump great distances).
4. Remove all insecticide residues with an appropriate solution.
5. Wear gloves during all steps and wash hands thoroughly when finished.
6. To treat a lice or scabies infestation:
   - Use an appropriate body or hair pediculicide; repeat in 7 to 10 days.
   - Launder personal clothing in hot water in a washer and dry on high heat in the dryer (of questionable benefit).

- Counseling regarding the risks, signs and symptoms, probability of developing clinical disease, and how to prevent future spread of the potential infection
- Appropriate treatment in line with current U.S. Public Health Service recommendations
- A discussion of medications offered and their side effects and contraindications
- Evaluation of any reported illness to determine whether the symptoms are related to HIV or hepatitis

STEPS INVOLVED

Blood tests of exposed employees are always contingent on employee agreement. Employees have the option to provide blood samples. However, they can refuse permission for HIV testing at the time the sample is drawn. The employer must maintain the blood samples for 90 days in case employees change their mind regarding testing if HIV-like or hepatitis-like symptoms develop.

1. It permits immediate medical follow-up. This allows identification of infection and immediate intervention.
2. It enables the DO to evaluate the circumstances of the incident. It also allows the DO to determine what changes to make to prevent future exposures.
3. It aids follow-up testing of the source person if permission for testing can be obtained.

Reporting also ensures that if the health care worker is infected, it has been documented that the disease occurred from a work-related exposure.

CRITICAL THINKING
How do you think you would feel if you were stuck by a contaminated needle and the patient refused HIV testing?

As an agent of the health care worker, the employer must take the following steps: (1) provide counseling to the employee based on test results; (2) provide informed consent regarding prophylaxis and therapeutic regimens; and (3) implement those regimens after receiving approval from the employee. Vaccines also should be made available to all employees who are exposed to blood and other potentially infectious materials during their work.

Written Report and Confidentiality

The agent of the employer will send a written report to the DO of the employer. This states whether vaccination was offered to the exposed employee. It also states whether the employee received it. The written report also must note that the employee was informed of the results of the evaluation and told of any medical conditions resulting from the exposure that may require further evaluation or treatment. A copy of this report must be provided to the employee and to the DO for the agency's files.

All other elements of the employee's medical record are confidential. They cannot be supplied to the employer. The employee must give written consent for anyone to view the records. The records must be maintained for the duration of employment plus 30 years. This complies with OSHA standards regarding access to employee exposure and medical records. (States who are not governed by OSHA must also follow these guidelines.)

NOTE
As described earlier in this chapter, under provisions of the Ryan White Act, an exposed employee has the right to request the infection status of the source patient from the patient's health care provider. Neither the agency nor the employee, however, can force testing of the source patient. As part of a good exposure control plan, employees must know what to do if an exposure incident occurs.

Submitting the Report

The Ryan White Act requires employers to appoint someone in the organization to whom an exposed employee can report. That person or officer follows the exposure control plan. The plan must comply with standards and guidelines relative to the exposure and must meet any local reporting requirements.

Medical Evaluation and Follow-Up

By law, employers must provide free medical evaluation and treatment to exposed employees. This would include the following:

PARAMEDIC'S ROLE IN PREVENTING DISEASE TRANSMISSION

Paramedics will have to deal with patients who have infectious diseases. It is important for them to be vigilant about the consequences to themselves and to their patients and co-workers. Part of this professional duty in preventing the spread of disease is knowing when *not* to go to work. A health care worker should not go to work if the following conditions are present:

- Fever
- Diarrhea
- Draining wound or any type of wet lesion
- Jaundice
- Mononucleosis
- Treatment with a medication and/or shampoo for lice or scabies
- Strep throat (unless antibiotics have been taken for longer than 24 hours)
- Cold with productive cough (unless the paramedic wears a surgical mask)

Health care workers also should ensure that their personal immunization status is current for MMR, hepatitis B, DPT, polio, chickenpox, and influenza.

CRITICAL THINKING
Have you come to school or work with any of these conditions?

Other Considerations in Disease Prevention

When called to provide emergency care, paramedics should always approach the scene with caution. They must keep in mind that an uncontrolled scene increases the likelihood of transmission of body fluids. Universal precautions should be observed at all times. These include wearing gloves, protective eyewear, a face shield, and a gown (if splash or spray is possible) and wearing an appropriate particulate mask when airborne disease is suspected. As mentioned previously, universal precautions are based on the premise that all body fluids, in any situation, may be infectious.

As a rule, if a patient has a productive cough, headache, general weakness, recent weight loss, nuchal rigidity, or high fever, the paramedic should immediately suspect an infectious process. Regardless of the patient's infectious status, however, the paramedic should do the following:

- Provide the same level of care to all patients.
- Disinfect equipment and the patient compartment with the proper disinfectant solution.
- Practice effective hand washing.
- Report any infectious exposure to the agency's DO.

CRITICAL THINKING
Imagine that you are on a call and get a small splash of blood in your eyes. What do you think would prevent you from reporting it immediately so that your postexposure care could begin?

SUMMARY

- National concerns about communicable disease and infection control have resulted in public laws, standards, guidelines, and recommendations to protect health care providers and emergency responders against infectious diseases. Paramedics must be familiar with these guidelines. They also must take personal protective measures against exposure to these pathogens.
- The chain of elements needed to transmit an infectious disease includes the pathogenic agent, a reservoir, a portal of exit from the reservoir, an environment conducive to transmission of the pathogenic agent, a portal of entry into the new host, and susceptibility of the new host to the infectious disease.
- The human body is protected from infectious disease by external and internal barriers. These serve as lines of defense against infection. External barriers include the skin, GI system, upper respiratory tract, and genitourinary tract. Internal barriers include the inflammatory response and the immune response.
- The progression of infectious disease from exposure to the onset of symptoms follows four stages. These are the latent period, the incubation period, the communicability period, and the disease period.

- The human immunodeficiency virus is directly transmitted person to person. This occurs through anal or vaginal intercourse, across the placenta, by contact with infected blood or body fluids on mucous membranes or open wounds, through blood transfusion or tissue transplant, or by the use of contaminated needles or syringes. The virus affects the CD4 T cells. Secondary complications are usually related to opportunistic infections that arise as the immune system deteriorates. Progression of the disease can be divided into category A (acute retroviral infection, seroconversion, and asymptomatic infection); category B (early symptomatic HIV); and category C (late symptomatic HIV and advanced HIV). Paramedics should observe strict compliance with universal precautions for protection against HIV. Patient care should include helping these patients feel that they can obtain acceptance and compassion from health care workers.
- Hepatitis is a viral disease. It produces pathological changes in the liver. The three main classes of hepatitis virus are hepatitis A, hepatitis B, and hepatitis C. Infection with hepatitis may cause mild symptoms, liver failure, or death.

Continued

- Tuberculosis is a chronic pulmonary disease. It is acquired through inhalation of tubercle bacilli. The infection is passed mainly when infected people cough or sneeze the bacteria into the air or by contact with sputum that contains virulent TB bacilli. The infection is characterized by stages of early infection (frequently asymptomatic), latency, and a potential for recurrent postprimary disease.

- Meningococcal meningitis is an inflammation of the membranes that surround the spinal cord and brain. It can be caused by bacteria, viruses, and other microorganisms.

- Bacterial endocarditis is inflammation of the endocardium and any one or more heart valves. The disease can be rapidly fatal if left untreated.

- Pneumonia is an acute inflammatory process of the respiratory bronchioles and alveoli. Bacteria, viruses, and fungi can cause this disease.

- Tetanus is a serious, sometimes fatal, disease of the CNS. It is caused by infection of a wound with spores of the bacterium *C. tetani*. The most common symptom is trismus (difficulty opening the mouth, lockjaw).

- Rabies is an acute viral infection of the CNS. Humans are highly susceptible to the rabies virus after exposure to saliva from the bite or scratch of an infected animal.

- Hantaviruses are carried by rodents. They are transmitted through inhalation of material contaminated with rodent urine and feces. Many forms of this disease occur in specific geographical areas.

- Rubella is a mild, febrile, highly communicable viral disease. It is characterized by a diffuse, punctate, macular rash. The CDC recommends that all health care providers receive immunization if they are not immune as a result of previous rubella infection.

- Rubeola is an acute, highly communicable viral disease caused by the measles virus. It is characterized by fever, conjunctivitis, cough, bronchitis, and a blotchy red rash.

- Mumps is an acute, communicable systemic viral disease. It is characterized by localized unilateral or bilateral edema of one or more of the salivary glands. Occasionally other glands are also involved.

- Chickenpox is highly communicable. It is characterized by a sudden onset of low-grade fever, mild malaise, and a maculopapular skin eruption that lasts for a few hours. This is followed by a vesicular eruption that lasts for 3 to 4 days, leaving a granular scab. The virus may reactivate during periods of stress or immunosuppression. At that time, it may cause an illness known as shingles.

- Pertussis is an infectious disease that leads to inflammation of the entire respiratory tract. It causes an insidious cough. The cough becomes paroxysmal in 1 to 2 weeks and lasts 1 to 2 months.

- Influenza is mainly a respiratory tract infection. It is spread by influenza viruses A, B, and C.

- Mononucleosis is caused either by the Epstein-Barr virus or by cytomegalovirus. Both of these are members of the herpes virus family.

- Syphilis is a systemic disease. It is characterized by a primary lesion; a secondary eruption involving skin and mucous membranes; long latency periods; and eventually by seriously disabling lesions of the skin, bone, viscera, CNS, and cardiovascular system.

- Gonorrhea is caused by the sexually transmitted bacterium *N. gonorrhoeae*. Gonorrhea can be treated with antibiotics. However, some strains brought into the United States from other countries do not respond to the usual antibiotic therapy.

- Chlamydia is a major cause of sexually transmitted nonspecific urethritis or genital infection. Signs and symptoms are similar to those of gonorrhea.

- Herpes simplex virus is transmitted by skin-to-skin contact with an infected area of the body. The primary infection produces a vesicular lesion (blister). This lesion heals spontaneously. After the primary infection, the virus travels to a sensory nerve ganglion. It remains there in a latent stage until reactivated.

- Lice are small, wingless insects that are ectoparasites of birds and mammals. During biting and feeding, lice secrete a substance that causes small, red macules and pruritus.

- The human scabies mite is a parasite. It completes its life cycle in and on the epidermis of the host. Scabies bites are usually concentrated around the hands and feet, especially in the webs of the fingers and toes.

- Reporting a possible communicable disease exposure permits immediate medical follow-up. It also enables the DO to make changes that might prevent exposures in the future. Moreover, it helps employees to obtain the proper evaluation and testing.

- Part of the paramedic's professional duty with regard to infectious disease transmission is to know when not to go to work. Paramedics also have a duty to use the proper BSI precautions at all times.

REFERENCES

1. Centers for Disease Control and Prevention: HIV in the United States: An overview, www.cdc.gov/hiv/topics/surveillance/resources/factsheets/incidence-overview.htm, accessed 9-2-11.
2. Joint United Nations Programme on HIV/AIDS: *AIDS epidemic update 2009*, www.unaids.org/en/KnowledgeCentre/HIV Data/EpiUpdate/EpiUpdArchive/2009/default.asp, accessed 9-2-10.
3. The Ryan White HIV/AIDS Treatment Modernization Act of 2006 (Public Law 109-415; 120 Stat. 2767), www.govtrack.us/congress/bill.xpd?bill=h109-6143, accessed 10-15-10.
4. Occupational Safety and Health Administration: *Final rule on protecting health care workers from occupational exposure to*

bloodborne pathogens (29 CFR 1910.1030), Washington, DC, March 1993 (revised 2008).

5. Text of S. 1793: *Ryan White HIV/AIDS Treatment Extension Act of 2009*, October 22, 2009, www.govtrack.us/congress/billtext. xpd?bill=s111-1793, accessed 10-15-10.

6. Centers for Disease Control and Prevention: Perspectives in disease prevention and health promotion update: universal precautions for prevention of transmission of immunodeficiency virus, hepatitis B virus, and other bloodborne pathogens in health care settings, *MMWR Morb Mortal Wkly Rep* 37(24):377, 1988.

7. U.S. Department of Health and Human Services, Centers for Disease Control and Prevention: *A curriculum guide for public-safety and emergency response workers*, Atlanta, 1989, Author.

8. National Institute of Allergy and Infectious Diseases: *Emerging and re-emerging infectious diseases*, www3.niaid.nih.gov/topics/emerging/, accessed 9-2-10.

9. McCance K, Huether S: *Pathophysiology: the biologic basis for disease in adults and children*, ed 6, St Louis, 2006, Mosby.

10. Grimes D: *Infectious diseases*, St Louis, 1991, Mosby.

11. World Health Organization: *Index of graphs*, www.who.int/infectious-disease-report/pages/grfindx.html, accessed 9-2-10.

12. *Community associated MRSA information for the public*, http://www.osha.gov/SLTC/bloodbornepathogens/index.html, Accessed May 5, 2011.

13. Eohlié S, Anglaret X: Decline of HIV-2 prevalence in West Africa: good news or bad news? *Int J Epidemiol* 5(5):1329-1330, 2006.

14. National Center for Infectious Diseases of HIV/AIDS: 1993 revised classification system for HIV infection and expanded surveillance case definition for AIDS among adolescents and adults, *MMWR* 41(RR-17), 1992, www.cdc.gov/mmwr/preview/mmwrhtml/00018871.htm, accessed 9-2-10.

15. United States Department of Labor, Occupational Safety and Health Administration: *Bloodborne Pathogens and Needlestick Prevention, Needlestick Safety and Prevention Act*, http://frwebgate.access.gpo.gov/cgi-bin/getdoc.cgi?dbname=106_cong_public_laws&docid=f:publ430.106.

16. U.S. Department of Health and Human Services Public Health Service Task Force: Updated U.S. Public Health Service guidelines for the management of occupational exposures to HBV, HCV, and HIV and recommendations for postexposure prophylaxis, *MMWR* 54(RR-09):1, 2005.

17. Hepatitis Foundation: *Hepatitis International on-line*, http://hepfi.org, accessed 9-3-10.

18. Bloodborne Pathogens and Needlstick Prevention, Occupational Safety and Health Administration, United States Department of Labor, CFR 1910.1030, rev 2001.

19. Recommendations for preventing transmission of human immunodeficiency virus and hepatitis B virus to patients during exposure-prone invasive procedures, *MMWR* 40(RR08):1, 1991.

20. Centers for Disease Control and Prevention: *Tuberculosis, data and statistics*, www.cdc.gov/tb/statistics/default.htm, accessed 12-11-09.

21. Centers for Disease Control and Prevention: *The difference between latent TB infection and TB disease*, Atlanta, www.cdc.gov/tb/topic/basics/default.htm, accessed 10-15-10.

22. Centers for Disease Control and Prevention: *NIOSH-approved particulate filtering facepiece respirators*, www.cdc.gov/niosh/npptl/topics/respirators/disp_part/, accessed 9-2-10.

23. Baldeep S: *Tuberculosis: review of PPD testing and prophylaxis*, www.med.ucla.edu/modules/wfsection/article.php?articleid=144, accessed 9-3-10,

24. National Meningitis Association: *Overview, meningitis*, www.nmaus.org/meningitis/, accessed 9-2-10.

25. Meningitis Research Foundation: *Meningococcal disease*, www.meningitis.org/disease-info/types-causes/meningococcal-disease, accessed 9-2-10.

26. National Institute of Neurological Disorders and Stroke: *Meningitis and encephalitis fact sheet*, www.ninds.nih.gov/disorders/encephalitis_meningitis/detail_encephalitis_meningitis.htm, accessed 9-2-10.

27. Centers for Disease Control and Prevention: *Meningitis: questions and answers*, www.cdc.gov/meningitis/about/faq.html, accessed 9-1-10.

28. Marx J, Hockberger R, Walls R: *Rosen's emergency medicine: concepts and clinical practice*, St Louis, 2006, Mosby.

29. World Health Organization: *Current WHO guide for rabies pre and post-exposure treatment in humans*, Geneva, 2002, Author.

30. Centers for Disease Control and Prevention: *All about hantaviruses*, www.cdc.gov/ncidod/diseases/hanta/hps/, accessed 9-5-10.

31. Centers for Disease Control and Prevention: Control and prevention of rubella: evaluation and management of suspected outbreaks, rubella in pregnant women, and surveillance of congenital rubella syndrome, *MMWR* 50(RR12):1-23, 2001.

32. Centers for Disease Control and Prevention: Prevention of varicella: recommendations of the Advisory Committee on Immunization Practices (ACIP), *MMWR* 56(RR-4):1-40, 2007.

33. Centers for Disease Control and Prevention: *Pertussis*, www.cdc.gov/ncidod/dbmd/diseaseinfo/pertussis_t.htm, accessed 3-1-10.

34. Centers for Disease Control and Prevention: *H1N1 flu (swine flu)*, www.cdc.gov/h1n1flu/general_info.htm, accessed 12-14-09.

35. Centers for Disease Control and Prevention: *Interim guidance for emergency medical services (EMS) systems and 9-1-1 Public Safety Answering Points (PSAPs) for management of patients with confirmed or suspected swine-origin influenza A (H1N1) infection*, www.cdc.gov/h1n1flu/guidance_ems.htm, accessed 10-16-2010.

36. Centers for Disease Control and Prevention: *Cytomegalovirus (CMV) and congenital CMV infection*, www.cdc.gov/cmv/facts.htm, accessed 10-16-2010.

37. Centers for Disease Control and Prevention: *About cytomegalovirus*, www.cdc.gov.cmv/facts.htm, accessed 10-16-10.

38. Carabeo RA, Grieshaber SS, Hasenkrug KJ, et al: Requirement for the Rac GTPase in chlamydia trachomatis invasion of non-phagocytic cells, *Traffic* 5:418-425, 2004.

39. Centers for Disease Control and Prevention: *Genital herpes, CDC Fact Sheet*, www.cdc.gov/STD/Herpes/STDFact-Herpes.htm#common, accessed 12-14-09.

CHAPTER
29 Abdominal and Gastrointestinal Disorders

OBJECTIVES

Upon completion of this chapter, the paramedic student will be able to:

1. Label a diagram of the abdominal organs.
2. Describe the function of the abdominal organs.
3. Outline the prehospital assessment of a patient complaining of abdominal pain.
4. Distinguish between pain characteristics in abdominal pain.
5. Describe general prehospital management techniques for a patient complaining of abdominal pain.

6. Describe signs and symptoms, complications, and prehospital management for the following abdominal and gastrointestinal disorders: gastrointestinal bleeding, acute and chronic gastroenteritis, ulcerative colitis, diverticulosis, appendicitis, peptic ulcer disease, bowel obstruction, Crohn's disease, pancreatitis, esophagogastric varices, hemorrhoids, cholecystitis, acute hepatitis, and hereditary hemochromatosis.

KEY TERMS

acute gastroenteritis Inflammation of the stomach and intestines with an associated sudden onset of vomiting, diarrhea, or both.

acute hepatitis An inflammatory condition of the liver associated with the sudden onset of malaise, weakness, anorexia, intermittent nausea and vomiting, and dull right upper quadrant pain, usually followed within 1 week by the onset of jaundice, dark urine, or both.

acute mesenteric ischemia An abrupt interruption of intestinal blood flow; it may result from an embolism, thrombosis, or a low-flow state (decreased perfusion).

anal fistula An abnormal opening of the cutaneous surface near the anus.

appendectomy Surgical removal of the appendix.

appendicitis Acute inflammation of the appendix.

ascites An abnormal accumulation of fluid in the space between the tissues lining the abdomen and abdominal organs.

bowel obstruction An occlusion of the intestinal lumen that results in blockage of normal flow of intestinal contents.

cholecystectomy Surgical removal of the gallbladder.

cholecystitis Inflammation of the gallbladder, most often associated with the presence of gallstones.

chronic gastroenteritis Inflammation of the stomach and intestines that accompanies numerous gastrointestinal disorders.

cirrhosis A chronic degenerative disease of the liver.

Crohn's disease A chronic, inflammatory bowel disease of unknown origin that usually affects the ileum, the colon, or both.

diverticulitis Inflammation of one or more diverticula.

diverticulosis The presence of pouchlike herniations through the muscular layer of the colon.

diverticulum A pouchlike herniation through the muscular wall of a tubular organ; it may be present in the stomach, small intestine or, most commonly, the colon.

emesis The forceful expulsion of stomach contents.

esophagitis Inflammation of the esophagus.

esophagogastric varices A complex of longitudinal, tortuous veins at the lower end of the esophagus that become enlarged and swollen as a result of portal hypertension.

fecalith A hard, impacted mass of feces in the colon.

gangrenous Necrosis or death of tissue.

gastroesophageal reflux disease (GERD) A condition in which the stomach contents leak backward from the stomach into the esophagus.

hematemesis Vomiting of bright red blood, indicating upper gastrointestinal bleeding.

hematochezia The passage of red blood through the rectum.

hemorrhoids Swollen, distended veins (internal, external, or both) in the rectoanal area.

hepatic encephalopathy A type of brain damage caused by liver disease and consequent ammonia intoxication.

hepatitis An inflammatory condition of the liver characterized by jaundice, hepatomegaly, anorexia, abdominal and gastric discomfort, abnormal liver function, clay-colored stools, and dark urine. The viruses responsible for hepatitis are hepatitis A virus (HAV), HBV, HCV, HDV, and HEV.

hereditary hemochromatosis An inherited condition in which the body absorbs and stores too much iron. The extra iron accumulates in several organs, especially the liver, heart, and pancreas.

hernia Protrusion of any organ through an abdominal opening in the muscle wall of the cavity that surrounds it.

hiatal hernia An anatomical abnormality in which part of the stomach protrudes through the diaphragm and up into the chest.

ileus An obstruction of the intestines.

involuntary guarding An unconscious rigid contraction of the abdominal muscles; a sign of peritoneal inflammation.

lactose intolerance A sensitivity disorder that results in the inability to digest lactose because of a deficiency of or defect in the enzyme lactase.

Mallory-Weiss syndrome A condition characterized by massive bleeding after a tear in the mucous membrane at the junction of the esophagus and the stomach.

melena Abnormal black, tarry stools containing digested blood.

pancreatitis Inflammation of the pancreas, which causes severe epigastric pain.

paralytic ileus A decrease in or the absence of intestinal peristalsis; it may occur after abdominal surgery, illness, or injury, and it is the most common cause of intestinal obstruction.

peptic ulcer disease An illness that results from a complex pathological interaction among the acidic gastric secretions and proteolytic enzymes and the mucosal barrier.

permissive hypotension A fluid resuscitation strategy in which fluid and red cell products are withheld until bleeding has been surgically controlled.

rebound tenderness Pain caused by the sudden release of fingertip pressure on the abdomen; it is a sign of peritoneal inflammation.

rectal abscess An infected, pus-filled cavity near the anus.

referred pain Pain felt at a site distant from its origin.

somatic pain Pain that arises from skeletal muscles, ligaments, vessels, or joints.

ulcerative colitis An inflammatory condition of the large intestine characterized by severe diarrhea and ulceration of the mucosa of the intestine.

visceral pain Deep pain that arises from smooth vasculature or organ systems.

---

*A*cute abdominal pain is a common chief complaint in emergency care that may reflect serious illness. The condition accounts for up to 10% of all visits to the emergency department each year.[1] This chapter reviews the gastrointestinal anatomy and disorders that produce gastrointestinal bleeding and abdominal pain. Appropriate evaluation and management in the prehospital setting may prevent the development of life-threatening complications.

(Courtesy Ray Kemp, St. Charles, Mo.)

REVIEW OF GASTROINTESTINAL ANATOMY

As described in Chapter 10, the gastrointestinal (GI) system provides the body with water, electrolytes, and other nutrients used by the cells. The major organs of the GI system are the esophagus, stomach, small and large intestines, liver, gallbladder, and pancreas (Figure 29-1 and Box 29-1). The genitourinary system (see Chapters 30 and 31) also can produce abdominal pain and bleeding.

ASSESSMENT OF THE PATIENT WITH ACUTE ABDOMINAL PAIN

When caring for a patient with abdominal pain, the paramedic should begin the primary survey by ensuring that the scene is safe. This should include an initial scene size-up. The paramedic should determine whether the abdominal pain is a result of trauma or a medical condition. This may be evident from the initial scene survey. The nature of the pain also may become evident through information obtained from the patient, family, or bystanders. The paramedic should inspect the nearby area for medication bottles and signs of alcohol or other drug use. These signs may offer clues to the cause of the patient's condition. If alcohol or other drug use is suspected, any containers of **emesis**

 LOOK AGAIN
See Chapter 10: Review of Human Systems, pp. 196-199.

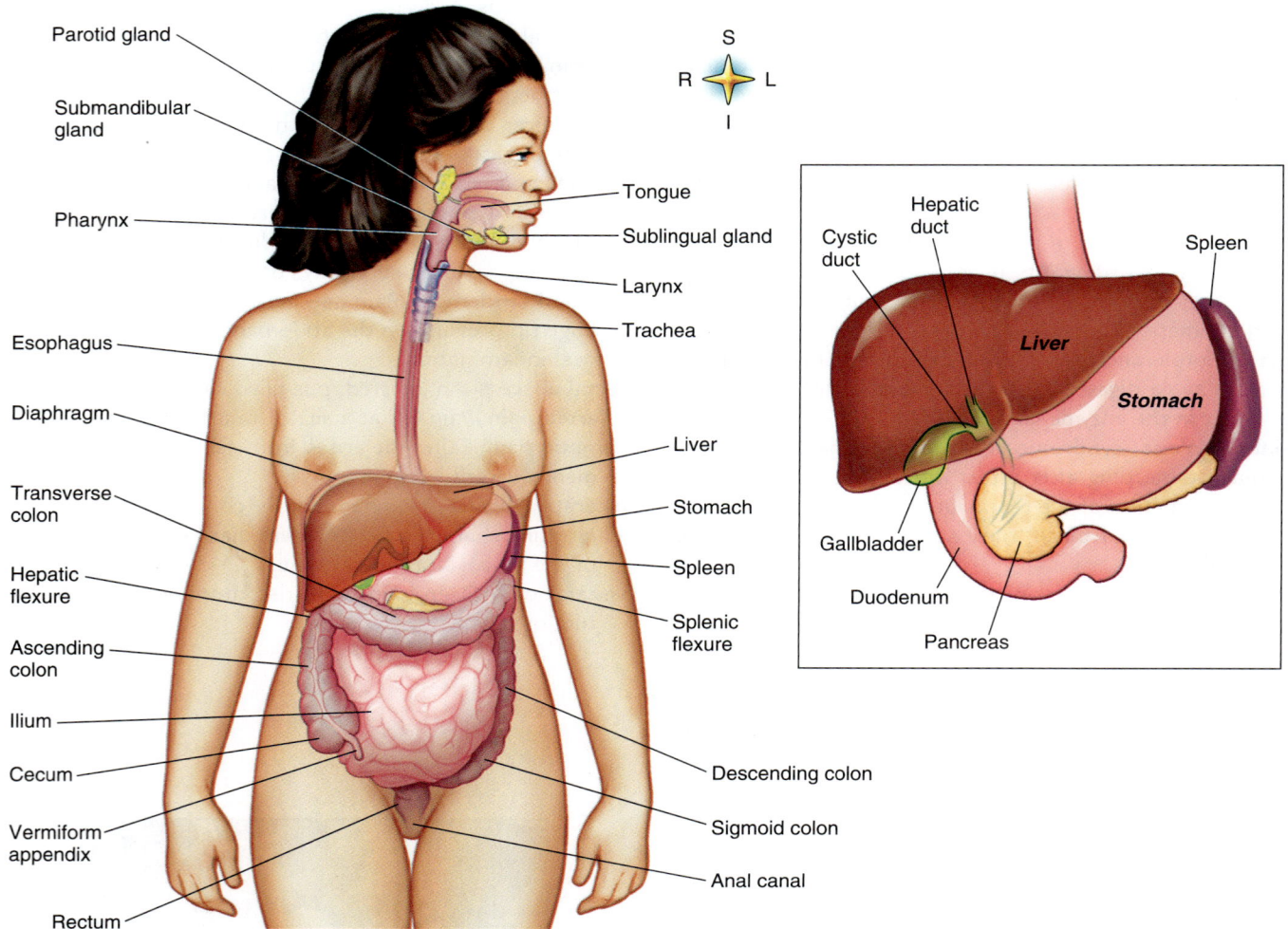

Parotid gland
Submandibular gland
Pharynx
Esophagus
Diaphragm
Transverse colon
Hepatic flexure
Ascending colon
Ilium
Cecum
Vermiform appendix
Rectum

Tongue
Sublingual gland
Larynx
Trachea
Liver
Stomach
Spleen
Splenic flexure
Descending colon
Sigmoid colon
Anal canal

S
R L
I

Hepatic duct
Cystic duct
Spleen
Liver
Stomach
Gallbladder
Duodenum
Pancreas

FIGURE 29-1 Location of the gastrointestinal system organs. (Patton KT, Thibodeau GA: *Anatomy and physiology,* ed 7, St Louis, 2010, Mosby.)

BOX 29-1 Organs of the Gastrointestinal System

Esophagus: The muscular canal extending from the pharynx to the stomach.

Stomach: The major organ of digestion, located in the right upper quadrant of the abdomen.

Small intestine: The largest portion of the digestive tract; it is divided into the duodenum, jejunum, and ileum.

Large intestine: The portion of the digestive tract comprising the cecum; appendix; ascending, transverse, and descending colons; and rectum.

Liver: The largest and most complex gland of the body. It is located in the upper right quadrant of the abdomen. It produces and secretes bile; stores glucose as glycogen, synthesizes proteins and fats, stores vitamins; processes hemoglobin; filters harmful substances from the blood; metabolizes drugs; and converts poisonous ammonia to urea.

Gallbladder: A pear-shaped excretory sac on the visceral surface of the right lobe of the liver. It serves as a reservoir for bile.

Pancreas: A fish-shaped, nodular gland located across the posterior abdominal wall in the epigastric region of the body. It secretes various substances, including digestive enzymes and the hormones insulin and glucagon.

should be transported with the patient for laboratory analysis.

SHOW ME THE EVIDENCE

Kennedy and colleagues studied the protocols of medical priority dispatch systems to evaluate the protocols' ability to predict patients who needed advanced life support (ALS) skills. They included patients with a chief complaint of abdominal pain who were transported to selected study hospitals. Of the 343 patients with a complaint of abdominal pain, 67% met the inclusion criteria. Eighty-four percent of the patients did not meet ALS criteria. The researchers concluded that significant overtriage of patients with abdominal pain occurs.

Kennedy JD et al: Effectiveness of a medical priority dispatch protocol for abdominal pain, *Prehosp Emerg Care* **7**:89-93, 2003.

After the primary survey to ensure adequacy of airway, breathing, and circulation, assessment of the patient with acute abdominal pain begins with a thorough history focused on the chief complaint. The paramedic should assess and document baseline vital signs and perform a systematic physical examination. This exam helps the paramedic identify abdominal emergencies. These may indicate the development of shock or the need for immediate transport for surgical intervention.

NOTE

Abdominal surgery may be necessary for the treatment of many conditions. These include inflammatory bowel disease (e.g. Crohn's disease or ulcerative colitis), diverticulitis, small bowel obstruction, or malignant diseases, including colon cancer and rectal cancer. Other common types of abdominal surgery include weight-loss surgery; hernia repair; liver, pancreatic, or stomach cancer surgery; **appendectomy, cholecystectomy,** and adhesiolysis (removal of scar tissue). Persistent abdominal pain that lasts several hours or longer warrants transport of the patient for evaluation by a physician.

History

When obtaining a history of abdominal pain, the paramedic should attempt to identify the location and type of pain and any associated signs and symptoms. As described in Chapter 18, the mnemonic OPQRST or a similar method can help the paramedic organize this information. Sample questions that might be included in the OPQRST evaluation include the following:

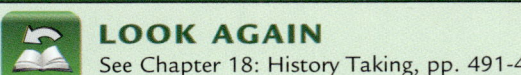

LOOK AGAIN

See Chapter 18: History Taking, pp. 491-495.

O (Onset): Was the onset of pain sudden? What were you doing when it started?

P (Provocative/palliative): What makes the pain better? What makes the pain worse? Does a sitting or lying position affect your discomfort? Does a deep breath increase the pain? Does the pain change after you eat or drink?

Q (Quality): What does the pain feel like? Is it sharp, dull, burning, tearing?

R (Region): Where is the pain located? Does it travel (radiate) to another area of the body or does it stay in the same place?

S (Severity): Is the pain mild, moderate, or severe? What is the degree of discomfort on a scale of 0 to 10 (with 10 being the worst)?

T (Time): When did the pain begin? Is it constant or intermittent? If intermittent, how long does the pain episode last?

Other key elements of a patient history can be obtained through a SAMPLE history (*s*igns and symptoms, *a*llergies, *m*edications, *p*ast medical history, *l*ast meal or oral intake, and *e*vents before the emergency). This helps identify symptoms, allergies, the medical history, the last oral intake, and important events that preceded the chief complaint. Other important elements of a patient history include any recent illness and past significant medical history. Of particular importance are hypertension or cardiac or respiratory disease that may manifest in abdominal pain; medication use; alcohol or other drug use; the last bowel movement and any significant changes in the patient's bowel habits; and previous abdominal surgeries. Women of childbearing age also should be questioned about menstrual periods (including regularity and the date of the last menstrual period) and the possibility of pregnancy.

CRITICAL THINKING

What factors can influence a patient's perception and description of pain?

Location and Type of Abdominal Pain

To assess a specific disorder, the paramedic can use a method that relates the anatomical location of GI organs and structures to the origin of the pain. Table 29-1 lists locations of abdominal pain and possible causes of illness. The types of abdominal pain that may result from chronic or acute episodes may be classified as *visceral, somatic,* or *referred.*

VISCERAL PAIN

Visceral pain (or organ pain) is caused by the stimulation of autonomic nerve fibers that surround an organ. Visceral pain also can be caused by compression and inflammation of solid organs and by distention or stretching of hollow organs or the ligaments. The patient usually describes the

TABLE 29-1 Common Conditions That Cause Acute Abdominal Pain

Condition	Usual Pain Characteristics	Possible Associated Findings
Appendicitis	Initially periumbilical or epigastric; colicky; later becomes localized to RLQ, often at McBurney's point	Guarding tenderness; positive iliopsoas and obturator signs; RLQ skin hyperesthesia; anorexia, nausea, or vomiting after onset of pain; low-grade fever; positive Aaron, Rovsing, Markle, and McBurney signs
Peritonitis	Sudden or gradual onset; generalized or localized, dull or severe and unrelenting; guarding; pain on deep inspiration	Shallow respirations; positive Blumberg, Markle, and Balance signs; reduced or absent bowel sounds; nausea and vomiting; positive obturator and iliopsoas tests
Cholecystitis	Severe, unrelenting RUQ or epigastric pain; may be referred to right subscapular area	RUQ tenderness and rigidity; positive Murphy sign; palpable gallbladder; anorexia; vomiting; fever; possible jaundice
Pancreatitis	Dramatic, sudden, excruciating LUQ, epigastric, or umbilical pain; may be present in one or both flanks; may be referred to left shoulder	Epigastric tenderness; vomiting; fever; shock; positive Grey Turner and Cullen signs (both signs occur 2 to 3 days after onset)
Salpingitis	Lower quadrant; worse on left	Nausea, vomiting, fever, suprapubic tenderness, rigid abdomen, pain on pelvic examination
Pelvic inflammatory disease	Lower quadrant; increases with activity	Tender adnexa and cervix, cervical discharge, dyspareunia
Diverticulitis	Epigastric, radiating down left side of abdomen especially after eating; may be referred to back	Flatulence, borborygmus, diarrhea, dysuria, tenderness on palpation
Perforated gastric or duodenal ulcer	Abrupt onset in RUQ; may be referred to shoulders	Abdominal free air and distention with increased resonance over liver; tenderness in epigastrium or RUQ; rigid abdominal wall; rebound tenderness
Intestinal obstruction	Abrupt, severe, spasmodic; referred to epigastrium, umbilicus	Distention, minimal rebound tenderness, vomiting, localized tenderness, visible peristalsis; bowel sounds absent (with paralytic obstruction) or hyperactive high pitched (with mechanical obstruction)
Volvulus	Referred to hypogastrium and umbilicus	Distention, nausea, vomiting, guarding; sigmoid loop volvulus may be palpable
Leaking abdominal aneurysm	Steady throbbing midline over aneurysm; may radiate to back, flank	Nausea, vomiting, abdominal mass, bruit
Biliary stones, colic	Episodic, severe, RUQ, or epigastrium lasting 15 min to several hours; may be referred to subscapular area, especially right	RUQ tenderness, soft abdominal wall, anorexia, vomiting, jaundice, subnormal temperature
Renal calculi	Intense; flank, extending to groin and genitals; may be episodic	Fever, hematuria; positive Kehr's sign
Ectopic pregnancy	Lower quadrant; referred to shoulder; agonizing with rupture	Hypogastric tenderness, symptoms of pregnancy, spotting, irregular menses, soft abdominal wall, mass on bimanual pelvic examination; ruptured: shock, rigid abdominal wall, distention; positive Kehr and Cullen signs
Ruptured ovarian cyst	Lower quadrant, steady, increases with cough or motion	Vomiting, low-grade fever, anorexia, tenderness on pelvic examination
Splenic rupture	Intense; LUQ, radiating to left shoulder; may worsen with elevation of foot of bed	Shock, pallor, lowered temperature

From Seidel H, et al: *Mosby's guide to physical examination,* ed 6, St Louis, 2006, Mosby.
LUQ, Left upper quadrant; *RLQ,* right lower quadrant; *RUQ,* right upper quadrant.

pain as cramping or gas-type pain. Patients often describe the pain as varying in intensity, increasing to severe and then subsiding. Visceral pain generally is diffuse; therefore, the pain is difficult to localize. Often the pain is centered at the umbilicus or lower in the midline. Visceral pain often is associated with other symptoms of autonomic nerve involvement, such as tachycardia, diaphoresis, nausea, or vomiting. Common causes of visceral abdominal pain include early appendicitis, pancreatitis, cholecystitis, and intestinal obstruction (described later in this chapter).

SOMATIC PAIN

Somatic pain is produced by bacterial or chemical irritation of nerve fibers in the peritoneum (peritonitis). Unlike visceral pain, somatic pain usually is constant. Moreover, the pain is localized to a specific area. The patient often describes the pain as sharp or stabbing. Patients with somatic abdominal pain generally are hesitant to move about. They may lie on the back or side with the legs flexed to prevent additional pain from stimulation of the peritoneal area. These patients often show **involuntary guarding** of the abdomen during the physical examination and **rebound tenderness** (signs of peritoneal inflammation). Common causes of somatic pain are appendicitis and an inflamed or a perforated viscus (ulcer, gallbladder, or small or large intestine).

> **NOTE**
> Ask the patient to take a deep breath as you palpate the upper right quadrant (URQ) of the abdomen. An inflamed gallbladder descends during inspiration and causes discomfort. This is known as *Murphy's sign.* Other physical signs in patients with acute abdominal pain are presented in Table 29-2.[2]

REFERRED PAIN

Referred pain is pain in a part of the body considerably removed from the tissues that cause the pain. This mechanism results from branches of visceral fibers that synapse in the spinal cord with the same second-order neurons that receive pain fibers from the skin. When these pain fibers are stimulated intensely, pain sensations spread. The patient experiences the pain in areas distant from the source.

A knowledge of referred pain is important, because many visceral ailments cause no symptoms except referred pain (Figure 29-2). For example, cardiac pain may be referred to the neck and jaw, shoulders, and pectoral muscles and down the arms; biliary pain to the right subscapular area; renal colic to the genitalia and flank area; uterine and rectal pain to the lower back; and a leaking aortic aneurysm to the lower back or buttocks.

> **NOTE**
> Providing analgesics to manage abdominal pain in the prehospital setting is controversial. Some medical experts believe the drugs may mask serious signs and symptoms. Others believe that these medications do not alter the diagnosis and that they may produce a more reliable physical examination.[3] The paramedic should follow established protocol as provided by medical direction.

Signs and Symptoms

Although numerous signs and symptoms may be associated with acute abdominal pain, the following, along with possible causes, are common:

1. Nausea, vomiting, anorexia
   - Appendicitis
   - Biliary tract disease
   - Gastritis
   - High intestinal obstruction
   - Pancreatitis
2. Diarrhea
   - Inflammatory process (gastroenteritis, ulcerative colitis)
3. Constipation
   - Dehydration
   - Obstruction
   - Medication-induced decreased intestinal motility (codeine, morphine)

TABLE 29-2 Physical Signs in Patients With Acute Abdominal Pain

Sign	Characteristics
Murphy's sign	Cessation of inspiration during examination of the right upper quadrant (may indicate acute cholecystitis)
McBurney's sign	Tenderness midway between the anterior-superior iliac spine and the umbilicus (may indicate acute appendicitis)
Cullen's sign	Periumbilical bluish discoloration (may indicate retroperitoneal hemorrhage, pancreatic hemorrhage, or rupture of an abdominal aortic aneurysm [AAA])
Grey Turner's sign	Bluish discoloration of the flanks (may indicate retroperitoneal hemorrhage, pancreatic hemorrhage, or AAA rupture)
Kehr's sign	Severe left shoulder pain (may indicate splenic rupture or rupture of an ectopic pregnancy)
Obturator sign	Pain with flexed right hip rotation (may indicate appendicitis)
Psoas sign	Pain when raising a straight leg against resistance (may indicate appendicitis, right-side AAA)

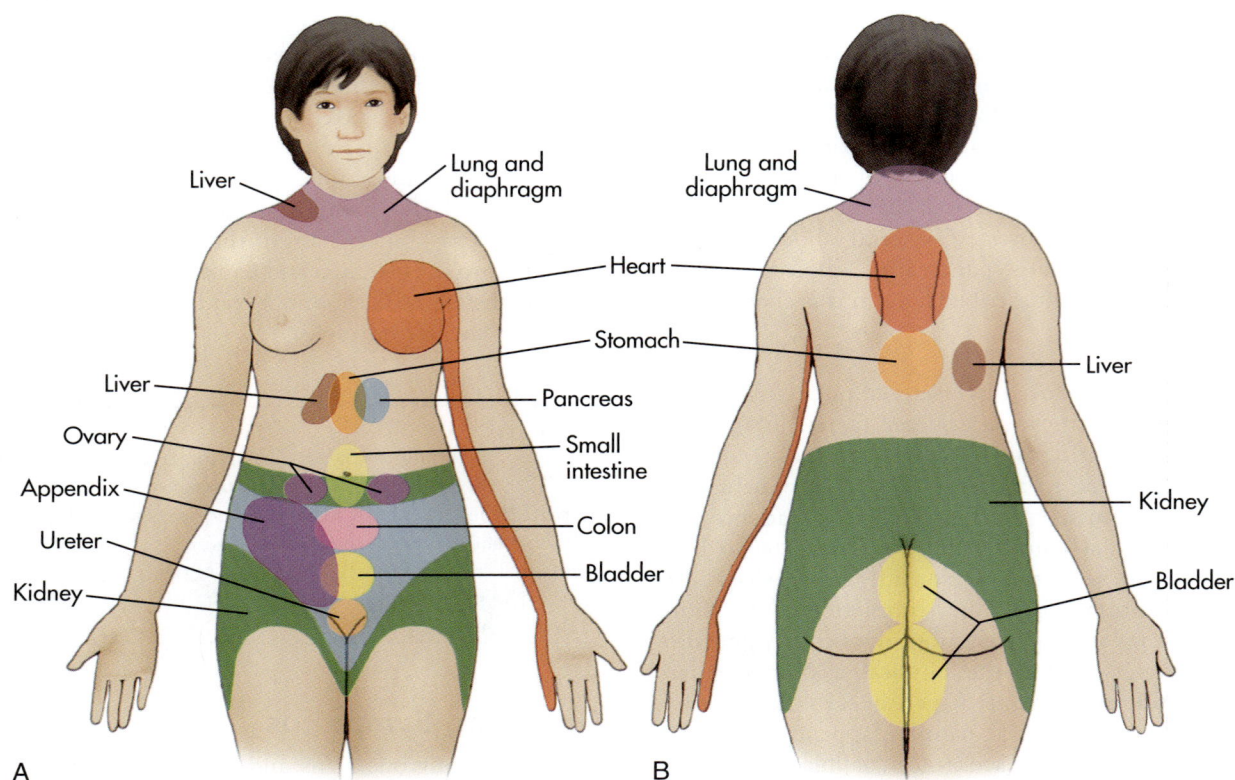

Liver

Lung and diaphragm

Lung and diaphragm

Heart

Stomach

Liver

Liver

Pancreas

Ovary

Small intestine

Appendix

Colon

Ureter

Bladder

Kidney

Kidney

Bladder

A

B

FIGURE 29-2 Referred pain. **A,** Anterior view. **B,** Posterior view.

4. Change in stool color
   - Biliary tract obstruction (clay-colored stools)
   - Lower intestinal bleeding (black, tarry stools)
5. Chills and fever
   - Appendicitis
   - Bacterial infection
   - Cholecystitis
   - Pyelonephritis

Vital Signs

Vital sign assessment should include evaluation and documentation of the patient's blood pressure, pulse rate (including electrocardiographic assessment), and respiratory rate and the color, moisture, temperature, and turgor of the skin. The presence or absence of orthostatic pulse and blood pressure changes should be noted if possible. As described in Chapter 22, rising from a recumbent position to a sitting or standing position, with an associated fall in systolic pressure (after 1 minute) of 10 to 15 mm Hg and/or a concurrent rise in the pulse rate (after 1 minute) of 10 to 15 beats/minute, indicates significant volume depletion and a decrease in perfusion status. The paramedic also should assess the blood pressure, pulses, and capillary refill in each extremity as a consideration for aortic dissection.

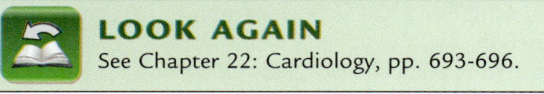

LOOK AGAIN
See Chapter 22: Cardiology, pp. 693-696.

Physical Examination

The physical examination of a patient with acute abdominal pain involves the skills of inspection, auscultation, percussion, and palpation. If a life-threatening illness is suspected, rapid stabilization and transportation of the patient are the first priorities. Further examination can be completed en route to the receiving hospital. The physical examination of a patient's abdomen is described in Chapter 20. The following discussion serves as a review. (Female physical examinations to evaluate genitourinary complaints are discussed in Chapter 31.)

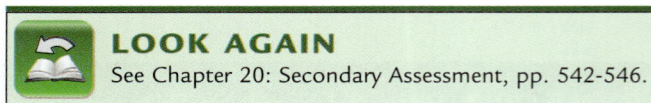

LOOK AGAIN
See Chapter 20: Secondary Assessment, pp. 542-546.

INSPECTION

In the initial patient encounter, the paramedic should note the position in which the patient is lying. As stated previously, many patients with abdominal peritoneal irritation lie on the side. The knees often are flexed and pulled in toward the chest. Other visual clues that may indicate abdominal pain are skin color, facial expressions (e.g., grimacing), and the presence or absence of voluntary movement. The paramedic should remove the patient's clothing (while ensuring privacy) and inspect the abdominal wall for bruises, scars, ascites (Figure 29-3), abdominal distention, or abdominal masses.

> **NOTE**
>
> **Ascites** is an abnormal accumulation of fluid in the space between the tissues lining the abdomen and abdominal organs (the peritoneal cavity). The fluid contains large amounts of protein and electrolytes. Ascites is caused by high pressure in the blood vessels of the liver (portal hypertension) and low albumin levels. A person with ascites usually has severe liver disease. Other disorders associated with ascites include congestive heart failure and pancreatitis.

AUSCULTATION

Determining the presence or absence of bowel sounds by auscultation usually is reserved for assessment in the emergency department. However, if auscultation is to be done, the paramedic should perform it for about 2 minutes in each quadrant before deciding that bowel sounds are absent. (Auscultation should always precede palpation and percussion, because these procedures may alter the intensity of bowel sounds.) An increase in the number, duration, or intensity of bowel sounds indicates the possibility of gastroenteritis or intestinal obstruction. A considerable decrease in the number and intensity of bowel sounds (or their absence) may indicate peritonitis or ileus (obstruction of the intestine).

PALPATION

The paramedic should begin palpation of the abdomen gently and avoid the painful area until the remainder of the abdomen has been examined. Signs of rigidity or spasm, tenderness or masses, and the patient's facial expressions should be noted. These may provide clues to the severity of the pain. In addition, the paramedic should identify the abdomen as soft or rigid.

PERCUSSION

If time permits, a general assessment of tympany and dullness by percussion may be performed. This is to detect the presence of fluid, air, or solid masses in the abdomen. The paramedic should use a systematic approach and move from side to side or clockwise. Tenderness and the temperature and color of the abdominal skin should be noted. To review, tympany is the major sound that should be noted during percussion because of the normal presence of air in the stomach and intestines. Dullness should be heard over organs and solid masses.

MANAGEMENT OF THE PATIENT WITH AN ABDOMINAL EMERGENCY

Patients with acute abdominal pain or GI bleeding cannot be managed effectively in the prehospital setting. Most require extensive evaluation in the emergency department, including laboratory analysis, radiological imaging, fluid and medication therapy, and perhaps surgical intervention. The role of the paramedic is to support the patient's airway and ventilatory status; to perform and document an initial patient assessment, including a thorough history; to monitor vital signs and cardiac rhythm; to initiate intravenous (IV) therapy for fluid replacement or fluid resuscitation; to administer analgesics and antiemetics per protocol; and to transport the patient rapidly for evaluation by a physician (Figure 29-4).

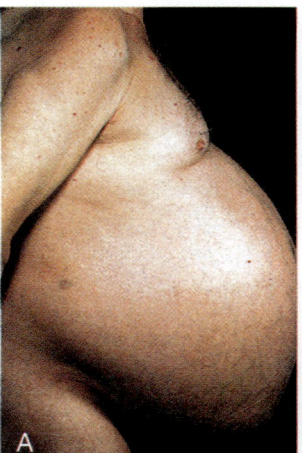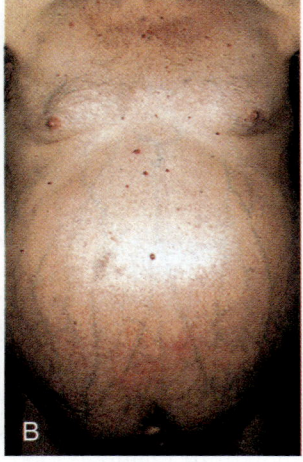

FIGURE 29-3 Gross ascites in a male patient. (Epstein O, et al: *Clinical examination,* ed 4, St Louis, 2008, Mosby.)

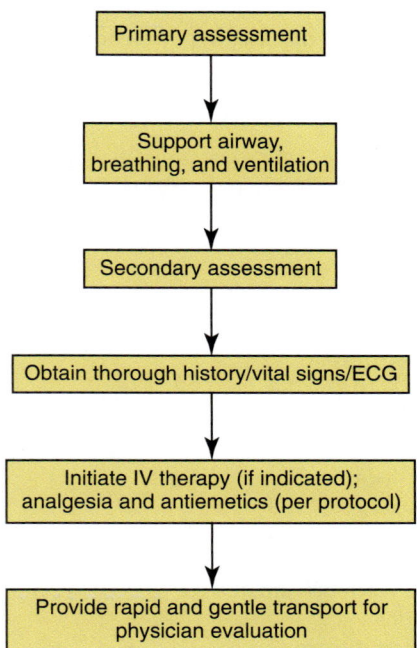

FIGURE 29-4 Abdominal pain algorithm.

SPECIFIC ABDOMINAL EMERGENCIES

Abdominal emergencies can result from inflammation, infection, and obstruction. Some disorders may be associated with upper gastrointestinal bleeding. (Examples of such disorders include lesions, peptic ulceration, and esophagogastric varices.) Some disorders may be associated with lower gastrointestinal bleeding. (Examples of these disorders include colonic lesions, diverticulosis, and hemorrhoids.) Other disorders, such as pancreatitis and cholecystitis, more often are associated with acute abdominal pain in the absence of bleeding. Box 29-2 lists the specific gastrointestinal disorders discussed in this chapter.[4]

Gastrointestinal Bleeding

Gastrointestinal bleeding is a common clinical problem seen by paramedics. It often requires hospitalization. It can vary from chronic blood loss to a massive, life-threatening hemorrhage. Massive hemorrhage may be difficult to control. Many bleeding episodes resolve spontaneously. However, evaluation by a physician to identify the bleeding site is crucial to help prevent a recurrence. Bleeding from the GI tract can be classified by site of origin as *upper* or *lower* gastrointestinal bleeding.

The most common causes of upper gastrointestinal bleeding are peptic ulcer disease and variceal rupture (e.g., esophageal varices that result from underlying chronic liver disease, such as cirrhosis). Another cause of upper gastrointestinal bleeding is **Mallory-Weiss syndrome** (an esophageal laceration that usually results from repeated vomiting or retching.) Other causes are tumors or cancers of the esophagus or stomach. Factors that may aggravate upper gastrointestinal bleeding include use of nonsteroidal antiinflammatory drugs (NSAIDs) such as *aspirin* and other antiarthritic drugs, chronic liver disease, blood-thinning medications (e.g., warfarin), and underlying medical conditions, such as renal disease, hypertension, and cardiorespiratory diseases. Upper gastrointestinal bleeding accounts for more than 300,000 hospitalizations each year and has a mortality rate of about 10%.[1] Risk factors include advancing age, alcohol and tobacco use, and coexisting illnesses, such as hypertension, diabetes, and cardiorespiratory disease.

The most common cause of lower gastrointestinal (colon) bleeding is diverticulosis. Other causes include colon cancers, colon polyps, and inflammatory bowel disorders, such as ulcerative colitis and Crohn's disease. Like upper gastrointestinal bleeding, lower gastrointestinal bleeding may be mild or it may be brisk and difficult to control. Common complaints include cramping abdominal pain, diarrhea (which may be bloody), nausea, vomiting, and changes in the patient's stool and bowel habits.

The seriousness of gastrointestinal bleeding depends on the acuteness and the source of the blood loss. Mild chronic gastrointestinal blood loss may present without any noticeable bleeding. It can result in an iron deficiency anemia. These patients often are unaware that they are bleeding and may or may not notice small amounts of blood with their bowel movements. Patients with severe cases of chronic or acute bleeding can have signs of anemia, such as weakness, pallor, dizziness, shortness of breath, or angina. (The hematocrit of these patients may be within normal range in the early phase of the hemorrhage [see Chapter 32].)

More serious gastrointestinal bleeding may occur with **hematemesis** (bloody vomitus). Vomit may be red or may have a dark, coffee ground–like appearance. Blood in the stool could present as bright red, dark and clotted, or black and tarry. The presentation depends on the location of the bleeding source. A black, tarry stool **(melena)** often indicates an upper gastrointestinal source of bleeding where blood has been partially digested. However, bleeding also could originate from the small intestine or right colon. Bright red blood from the rectum **(hematochezia)** after a bowel movement usually signifies a bleeding source close to the rectal opening. Such bleeding often results from hemorrhoids. However, conditions such as rectal cancers, polyps, ulcerations, or infections also can cause this type of bleeding.

Any source of gastrointestinal bleeding that is active or severe usually requires hospitalization. With hospitalization the hypovolemia can be managed with IV fluids or blood transfusions if needed. Attempts to identify and stop the source of hemorrhage may include the use of medications, diagnostic tests (e.g., barium GI studies, nuclear scans, angiography, endoscopy, and colonoscopy), and other therapeutic measures, such as gastric lavage, placement of a *Sengstaken-Blakemore tube* (to tamponade bleeding in the esophagus) and, in some cases, surgery.

Prehospital care for patients with active and severe gastrointestinal bleeding includes provision of emotional support, administration of high-concentration oxygen, and airway and ventilatory management. IV fluid resuscitation should begin with a 2 L fluid bolus in adults (20 mL/kg in children) to maintain blood pressure.[1] A pneumatic anti-shock garment should be considered (per protocol). All patients require rapid transport for physician evaluation.

BOX 29-2 Gastrointestinal Disorders

- Acute gastroenteritis
- Acute hepatitis
- Acute mesenteric ischemia
- Appendicitis
- Bowel obstruction
- Hemorrhoids
- Cholecystitis
- Chronic gastroenteritis
- Crohn's disease
- Diverticulosis
- Esophagogastric varices
- Gastrointestinal bleeding
- Hereditary hemochromatosis
- Pancreatitis
- Peptic ulcer disease
- Ulcerative colitis

> **NOTE**
> GI bleeding often is uncontrollable in the prehospital setting. In some cases hypotension can be protective, because a reduced blood pressure can allow the bleeding site to stabilize.[5] Medical direction may recommend that the patient's systolic blood pressure be maintained between 80 and 90 mm Hg (**permissive hypotension**) until the patient has been delivered to the emergency department for definitive care (see Chapter 36).[6]

cannot be changed, the symptoms of lactose intolerance can be managed with dietary changes. Most people with lactose intolerance can tolerate some amount of lactose in their diet. The Dietary Guidelines for Americans 2005 recommended that people with lactose intolerance choose milk products with lower levels of lactose than regular milk, such as yogurt and hard cheese. Other options include over-the-counter lactase enzyme drops or tablets that may make foods more tolerable.[8]

Acute Gastroenteritis

Acute gastroenteritis is inflammation of the stomach and intestines accompanied by the sudden onset of vomiting or diarrhea or both. The condition is a common problem worldwide and is responsible for more than 4 million deaths per year in developing countries.[7] It may be caused by bacterial or viral infection, parasites (e.g., organisms that cause "traveler's diarrhea," *Giardia lamblia* and *Cyclosporidium cayetanensis,* which is reported to be transmitted through ingestion of contaminated water), chemical toxins, and other conditions, such as allergies, lactose intolerance, and immune disorders. The inflammation causes hemorrhage and erosion of the mucosal layers of the gastrointestinal tract. Inflammation also can affect the way water and nutrients are absorbed.

> **? DID YOU KNOW?**
> **Lactose Intolerance**
> **Lactose intolerance** is the inability or insufficient ability to digest lactose, a sugar found in milk and milk products. (Lactose intolerance should not be confused with cow's milk allergy.) Lactose intolerance is caused by a deficiency of the enzyme *lactase,* which is produced by the cells lining the small intestine. Lactase breaks down lactose into two simpler forms of sugar called *glucose* and *galactose,* which then are absorbed into the bloodstream.
>
> The cause of lactose intolerance is best explained by describing how a person develops lactase deficiency. *Primary lactase deficiency* develops over time and begins after about age 2 when the body begins to produce less lactase. Most children who have lactase deficiency do not experience symptoms of lactose intolerance until late adolescence or adulthood. A genetic link may be involved in primary lactase deficiency. *Secondary lactase deficiency* results from injury to the small intestine that occurs with severe diarrheal illness, celiac disease, Crohn's disease, or chemotherapy. This type of lactase deficiency can occur at any age but is more common in infancy. Infants born prematurely are more likely to have lactase deficiency, because an infant's lactase levels do not increase until the third trimester of pregnancy.
>
> People with lactose intolerance may feel uncomfortable 30 minutes to 2 hours after consuming milk and milk products. Symptoms range from mild to severe, based on the amount of lactose consumed and the person's level of tolerance. Common symptoms include abdominal pain and bloating, gas, diarrhea, and nausea. Although the body's ability to produce lactase

Infectious forms of acute gastroenteritis usually are caused by exposure to rotavirus, adenovirus, astrovirus, Norwalk virus, or a group of noroviruses (see Chapter 28). The condition often is called the "stomach flu," although it is not caused by the influenza viruses. Typically, children under 5 years of age are most vulnerable to rotaviruses. (These are the most common cause of watery diarrhea in children.) Adenoviruses and astroviruses cause diarrhea mostly in young children, although older children and adults also can be affected. The Norwalk virus and noroviruses are more likely to cause diarrhea in older children and adults. Infectious acute gastroenteritis usually is transmitted through the fecal-oral route and by ingestion of infected food or contaminated water. The condition is common in institutional settings (e.g., schools, day care centers, and nursing homes) and other group settings (e.g., banquet halls, cruise ships, dormitories, and campgrounds), where it can spread quickly.

Infectious acute gastroenteritis also can arise among travelers in endemic areas (native populations generally are resistant) and in populations in disaster areas where water supplies are contaminated. Bacteria that may be responsible for acute gastroenteritis include *Salmonella* spp., *Escherichia coli, Campylobacter* spp., and *Staphylococcus* spp. Contamination generally results from poor sanitation, a lack of safe drinking water, or contaminated food.

As the name implies, acute gastroenteritis often is abrupt and violent in onset. It involves rapid loss of fluids and electrolytes from constant vomiting and diarrhea. Fluid loss and dehydration may be severe in pediatric patients, the elderly, and immunosuppressed individuals. Hypokalemia, hyponatremia, acidosis (from prolonged diarrhea), or alkalosis (from prolonged vomiting) may develop. Treatment mainly is supportive, requiring IV fluid replacement, sedation, bed rest, and medications to control vomiting and diarrhea. Bacterial causes of gastroenteritis can be treated with antibiotic therapy.

Emergency medical services (EMS) personnel working in disaster areas should observe the following guidelines:

- Avoid patient contact if you are ill.
- Know the source of water supplies, or drink hot beverages that have been boiled or disinfected.
- Avoid habits that aid fecal-oral/mucous membrane transmission.
- Observe body substance isolation precautions. Also observe good hand-washing procedures.

Chronic Gastroenteritis

Chronic gastroenteritis results from inflammation of the stomach and intestines. This can produce long-term changes or damage to the gastric mucosa. The condition usually is due to microbial infection, hyperacidity, or chronic use of alcohol, **aspirin,** and other nonsteroidal anti-inflammatory medications. Chronic gastroenteritis commonly results from *Helicobacter pylori* infection but also may be caused by other bacteria, such as *E. coli, Klebsiella pneumoniae, Enterobacter* spp., *Campylobacter jejuni, Vibrio cholerae, Shigella* spp., and *Salmonella* spp. Many of the bacteria responsible for chronic gastroenteritis are part of the normal intestinal flora, which precludes effective vaccination against these strains. Other causes of chronic gastroenteritis include Norwalk virus and rotavirus infection and parasitic infection from protozoa such as *G. lamblia* and *Cryptosporidium parvum.* The pathogenic agents responsible for the disease may be contracted through fecal-oral transmission and from contaminated food and water. EMS personnel should follow the same guidelines for personal safety as described previously.

NOTE
The bacterium *Helicobacter pylori* resides between the epithelial surface and the overlying mucosa in the human stomach. It is more prevalent in developing countries with contaminated water. It may be spread in adults and children through the fecal-oral route. The presence of *H. pylori* is believed to cause mucosal inflammation. This inflammation disrupts the normal defense mechanism of the stomach and can lead to ulceration.

Signs and symptoms of chronic gastroenteritis include epigastric pain, nausea and vomiting (which may be severe), fever, anorexia, mucosal bleeding *(erosive gastritis),* and epigastric tenderness on palpation. In severe cases the patient may have hypovolemia and shock. The condition is treated with dietary regulation, medications (antibiotics, antacids), and fluid replacement or fluid resuscitation if hypovolemia or dehydration occurs.

Ulcerative Colitis

Ulcerative colitis also is known as *colitis* or *proctitis.* Ulcerative colitis is an inflammatory condition of the large intestine. It is classified as an inflammatory bowel disease. Ulcerative colitis is characterized by ulceration of the mucosa of the intestine. This usually occurs in the rectum and lower part of the colon but may affect the entire colon. The inflammation makes the colon empty often (causing diarrhea). In addition, the ulceration causes bleeding and produces pus. Ulcerative colitis can occur at any age, although it most often starts between ages 15 and 30 or, less often, between ages 50 and 70. The condition affects men and women equally. A family history of the disease is present in 10% to 15% of cases. The cause of ulcerative colitis is unknown. The disorder may be related to the way the immune system reacts to a virus or bacterium that causes chronic inflammation in the intestinal wall. Other possible causes include allergies to certain foods (e.g., lactose intolerance) and environmental and psychological factors.

The most common signs and symptoms of ulcerative colitis are fatigue, weight loss, anorexia, rectal bleeding, and loss of body fluids and nutrients. Some patients have only mild symptoms. Other patients experience frequent fever, bloody diarrhea, nausea, and severe abdominal cramping. Some patients with the disease have remissions that last for months or years; in most patients, the symptoms eventually return. After evaluation by a physician and stabilization of the condition, ulcerative colitis usually is managed with steroids, electrolytes, antibiotics, and dietary regulation. Few patients require surgery, although surgical removal of the diseased colon may be indicated in severe cases. Prehospital care is dictated by the severity of the patient's condition. The care may vary from providing only emotional support and transportation for evaluation by a physician to providing airway, ventilatory, and circulatory support to manage hypovolemia and shock.

NOTE
In patients with acquired immunodeficiency syndrome (AIDS), the chronic diarrhea and diffuse colonic involvement of Kaposi's sarcoma (see Chapter 28) may mimic chronic ulcerative colitis. Undiagnosed signs of human immunodeficiency virus (HIV) infection also may be the cause. In some cases surgical bowel resection may be required in these patients.

Diverticulosis

A **diverticulum** is a sac or pouch that develops in the wall of the colon (Figure 29-5). Diverticula are a common development with advancing years and is associated with diets low in fiber. Diverticular outpouchings (a condition known as **diverticulosis**) tend to develop because of the high pressure in the contracting sigmoid colon that regulates movement of stool into the rectum. The outpouchings are most common at the weakest point in the colon wall. This is on the left side, just above the rectum. As a diverticulum expands, it develops a thin wall compared to the rest of the colon. The thin wall may allow bacteria to seep through and cause infection. Often a small artery or arteriole is present in the neck of the diverticulum from which subsequent bleeding may occur.

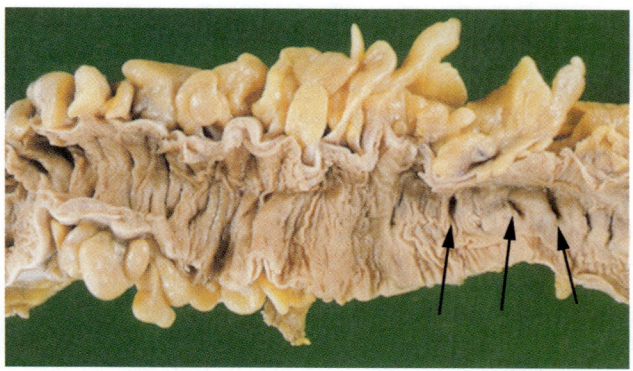

FIGURE 29-5 Diverticular disease. The outpouches of mucosa *(arrows)* in the sigmoid colon appear as slitlike openings from the mucosal surface of the opened bowel. (Modified from Stevens A, Lowe J: *Pathology,* London, 1995, Mosby.)

BOX 29-3 Abdominal Signs of Appendicitis

Rebound tenderness: Exert pressure in the right lower quadrant at McBurney's point and then release. Sharp abdominal pain when the pressure is released suggests appendicitis.
Iliopsoas muscle test: With the patient supine, ask the patient to raise the right leg and flex at the hip as you press down on the lower thigh. Lower quadrant pain may indicate appendicitis.
Obturator muscle test: With the patient supine, flex the right leg at the hip and knee. Then rotate the leg laterally and medially. Pain in the hypogastric region may indicate a ruptured appendix.

Most patients with diverticula are completely symptom free. However, up to 30% of these patients experience **diverticulitis** when one or more diverticula become obstructed with fecal matter. Mild complications of diverticulitis include irregular bowel habits (alternating constipation and diarrhea), fever, and lower left quadrant pain. Diverticulitis tends to recur within the first 5 years after the onset of symptoms. Definitive care for these patients includes dietary regulation, a high-fiber diet to stimulate daily bowel movements, antibiotic therapy and, in some cases, surgical repair.

Serious complications of diverticular disease are associated with perforation of the bowel. These complications include massive bright red rectal bleeding (or dark stools if bleeding is from a diverticulum in the right colon). Hemorrhage from a diverticulum can occur rapidly, is often painless, and is the most common cause of massive rectal bleeding in older adults. If bacteria escape into the abdomen, peritonitis or an abscess may develop. The hemorrhage often stops spontaneously. However, if the bleeding does not stop, emergency surgery may be necessary.

Appendicitis

Appendicitis is a common abdominal emergency. It occurs in 7% to 10% of the U.S. population.[9] The condition may present at any age, but most patients are 8 to 25 years old. Appendicitis is rare in children younger than 2 years.

Appendicitis occurs when the passageway between the appendix and the cecum is obstructed by fecal matter **(fecalith).** Appendicitis also may be due to inflammation of the area caused by a viral or bacterial infection. Obstruction of the passageway leads to distention of the appendix. Poor lymphatic and venous drainage allows bacterial infection to develop. If the condition continues, the inflamed organ eventually becomes **gangrenous.** The appendix then ruptures into the peritoneal cavity. This results in peritonitis (which may progress to shock) or the development of abscesses.

Because of variations in the position of the appendix, the patient's age, and the degree of inflammation, the clinical presentation of appendicitis often is inconsistent (Box 29-3). Also, many other disorders have similar signs and symptoms. Young children and older adults may have atypical illness because of a reduced inflammatory response associated with extremes of age. This makes appendicitis more difficult to diagnose in these age groups. The classic presentation of appendicitis is abdominal pain or cramping, nausea, vomiting, chills, low-grade fever, and anorexia. At first the pain is periumbilical and diffuse. Later it becomes intense and localized to the right lower quadrant just medial to the iliac crest *(McBurney's point).* If the appendix ruptures, the patient's pain diminishes before the development of peritoneal signs. The goal of definitive care for appendicitis is surgical removal of the appendix (appendectomy) before the organ ruptures.

CRITICAL THINKING
What other illness presents with similar signs or symptoms?

Peptic Ulcer Disease

Peptic ulcer disease results from a complex pathological interaction among the acidic gastric secretions and proteolytic enzymes and the mucosal barrier. As described in Chapter 10, digestion occurs as food passes through the GI tract. The stomach produces hydrochloric acid and an enzyme called pepsin to digest the food. From the stomach, food passes into the duodenum, where digestion and nutrient absorption continue. The stomach normally protects itself from the digestive fluids by producing mucus to shield stomach tissues. The stomach also produces

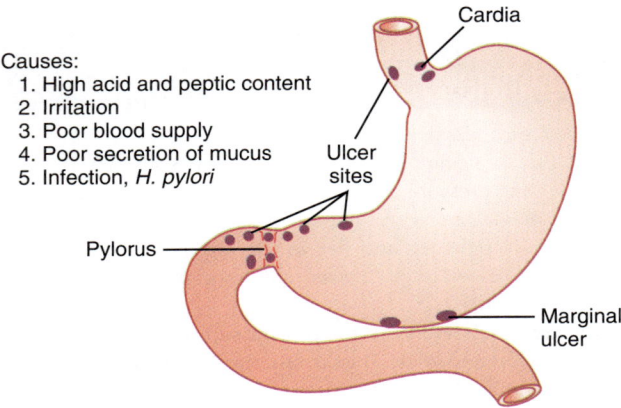

Causes:
1. High acid and peptic content
2. Irritation
3. Poor blood supply
4. Poor secretion of mucus
5. Infection, *H. pylori*

Cardia

Ulcer sites

Pylorus

Marginal ulcer

FIGURE 29-6 Peptic ulcer. *Helicobacter pylori (H. pylori).* (Hall J: *Guyton and Hall textbook of medical physiology,* ed 12, Philadelphia, 2011, Saunders.)

bicarbonate to neutralize and break down digestive fluids into substances less harmful to stomach tissue. Blood circulation to the stomach lining, cell renewal, and cell repair also help protect the stomach (Figure 29-6).

Ulcers can form in the lining of the stomach or duodenum, where acid and pepsin are present. These sores cause the disintegration and death of tissue as they erode the mucosal layers in the affected areas. If the sores are left untreated, massive hemorrhage or perforation may result. The two main causes of peptic ulcer disease are *H. pylori* infection and the use of NSAIDs. Another and less common cause is increased circulatory gastrin from gastrin-secreting tumors *(Zollinger-Ellison syndrome).*[1] All of these circumstances can cause the defense mechanisms of the stomach to fail. Ulcers can develop at any age but are rare among teenagers and even more uncommon in children. Duodenal ulcers occur for the first time usually between the ages of 30 and 50. They occur more often in men than in women.

A patient with a peptic ulcer usually is aware of the condition. The patient often uses over-the-counter antacids. The ulcer pain often is described as a burning or gnawing discomfort in the epigastric region or left upper quadrant (in the case of gastric ulcer). The discomfort develops before meals (classically, early morning) or during stressful periods, when the production of gastric acids increases. The pain usually is sudden in onset. Pain often is relieved by eating, taking antacids, or vomiting. In addition to pain and vomiting of blood, the patient may experience melena as a result of blood passing through the GI tract.

Prehospital care for patients with peptic ulcer disease includes obtaining a pertinent history, evaluating for hypotension, and providing circulatory support as needed. After evaluation by a physician, definitive care may involve antibiotics, antacids, H_2-receptor antagonists or other medications and, occasionally, dietary regulation (the benefit of which is controversial). Some patients with acute peptic ulcer disease require hospitalization for fluid or blood replacement or for surgery if medications are not effective or blood loss continues.

Bowel Obstruction

Bowel obstruction is an occlusion of the intestinal lumen. It results in blockage of normal flow of intestinal contents. Bowel obstruction may be caused by an **ileus,** a condition in which the bowel does not work properly. However, bowel obstruction more commonly results from mechanical obstruction, such as adhesions, **hernia** (Box 29-4), fecal impaction, polyps, and tumors. Other causes of bowel obstruction are *intussusception* (telescoping of one portion of the intestine into another, which results in decreased blood supply of the involved segment), *volvulus* (twisting of the intestines), ingested foreign bodies, and foreign bodies introduced from the anus (sexual or intentional insertion). Most bowel obstructions occur in the small bowel (accounting for 20% of all hospital admissions for abdominal complaints) and usually are caused by adhesions or hernias.[11] Large bowel obstructions most often result from tumors or fecal impactions.

Signs and symptoms of intestinal obstruction include nausea and vomiting, abdominal pain, diarrhea, constipation (a late finding), and abdominal distention. The speed of onset and degree of symptoms depend on the anatomical

BOX 29-4 Hernia

A hernia is the protrusion of an organ from its normal position through a congenital or acquired opening. Herniation most often occurs through the musculature of the groin or abdominal wall. Increases in intraabdominal pressure can cause the peritoneum to push outward through such an opening. (Examples of such increases in pressure include straining, coughing, or lifting.) When this occurs a sac is formed, into which various organs in the peritoneal cavity may enter.

Most hernias are uncomplicated and can be placed back into the peritoneal cavity by a physician. If the hernia cannot be returned to its proper position, the trapped contents of the peritoneal sac (usually a portion of bowel) can become strangulated. Patients with this condition often have acute abdominal pain and systemic signs, such as fever and tachycardia. Incarcerated or strangulated hernias can lead to serious complications, including intestinal obstruction, perforation, and peritonitis. Definitive care for complicated hernias is in-hospital observation, intravenous rehydration, pain medication, and surgical repair.

BOX 29-5 Acute Mesenteric Ischemia

Acute mesenteric ischemia is the abrupt interruption of intestinal blood flow. It may result from an embolism, thrombosis, or a low-flow state (decreased perfusion). The ischemia disrupts the mucosal barrier, allowing the release of bacteria, toxins, and vasoactive mediators. This in turn leads to myocardial depression and a systemic inflammatory response. If the condition goes unrecognized and untreated, the ischemia can result in multisystem organ failure and death. Acute mesenteric ischemia should be suspected whenever a patient presents with abdominal pain that is out of proportion to the physical findings (especially in patients over age 50). Definitive care may include surgery (embolectomy, revascularization, resection), infusion of vasodilators, and long-term therapy with anticoagulation and antiplatelet drugs.

CRITICAL THINKING

Have you ever responded to a call for "constipation"? Did the paramedics consider this diagnosis a possibility? What was their attitude toward the patient?

NOTE

Paralytic ileus can closely mimic bowel obstructions. (**Paralytic ileus** is a decrease in or the absence of intestinal peristalsis.) This pseudo-obstruction may result from a number of localized or systemic conditions, such as medications (especially narcotics), intraperitoneal infection, complications of abdominal surgery, and metabolic disturbances (e.g., decreased potassium levels).

site of obstruction (small versus large bowel). The most significant danger is perforation of the bowel with generalized peritonitis and sepsis.

A patient with bowel obstruction often has abdominal pain; dehydration may result from vomiting, decreased intestinal absorption, and fluid loss into the lumen and interstitium (bowel wall edema). As the affected portion of the bowel distends, its blood supply is decreased and the segment becomes ischemic (Box 29-5). The wall is weakened and perforates, producing peritonitis. If the intestine becomes strangulated, blood or plasma also may be lost from the affected intestinal segment. Definitive care involves fluid replacement, antibiotics, placement of a nasogastric tube for decompression (see Chapter 15) and, frequently, surgery to correct the obstructing lesion.

LOOK AGAIN

See Chapter 15: Airway Management, Respiration, and Artificial Ventilation, pp. 433-435.

Crohn's Disease

Crohn's disease is a chronic inflammatory bowel disease that usually affects the ileum, the colon, or both. Crohn's disease may occur in individuals of all ages but is primarily a disease of young adults. (Most cases are diagnosed before age 30.) The disease is thought to be autoimmune in origin and tends to run in families and in certain ethnic groups. More than 20,000 cases are reported annually in the United States.[12]

The inflammation associated with Crohn's disease may cause blockage of the intestine. Blockage occurs because the disease tends to thicken the intestinal wall with swelling and scar tissue, narrowing the passage. The disease also may cause ulcers that tunnel through the affected area into surrounding tissues, such as the bladder, vagina, or skin. The areas around the anus and rectum often are involved. The tunnels, called *fistulae,* are a common complication and often become infected. Other complications associated with Crohn's disease include arthritis, skin problems, inflammation of the eyes or mouth, kidney stones, gallstones, or other diseases of the liver and biliary system.

Crohn's disease can be difficult to diagnose, because its symptoms are similar to those of irritable bowel syndrome and ulcerative colitis. Crohn's disease is characterized by frequent attacks of diarrhea, severe abdominal pain, nausea, fever, chills, weakness, anorexia, and weight loss. (Patients with Crohn's disease and like disorders often suffer from depression because of the relentless and painful characteristics of these conditions.) The paramedic should suspect the disease in any patient with chronic inflammatory colitis and a history of rectal fistulae or abscesses. These patients frequently are hospitalized. Once the patient's condition has been stabilized, it may be managed with antibiotics, steroids, and antimotility agents in an attempt to induce remission, as well as with dietary regulation.

> **NOTE**
> The term *irritable bowel syndrome*, or *spastic colon*, is used to describe abnormally increased motility of the small and large intestines. Unlike inflammatory bowel disease, the abdominal pain of irritable bowel syndrome generally is associated with emotional and physical stress. The pain generally is also relieved by bowel movement.

Pancreatitis

As described in Chapter 10, the pancreas lies behind the stomach. This gland secretes digestive enzymes into the duodenum to help break down food into small molecules. These small molecules can be absorbed by the body. The pancreas also secretes insulin and glucagon into the bloodstream. These hormones help maintain an adequate glucose concentration. When the pancreas becomes inflamed (**pancreatitis**), it releases pancreatic enzymes into the blood, the pancreatic duct, and the pancreas itself. This causes further inflammation and autodigestion of the gland. Pancreatitis occurs in two stages, acute and chronic.

Acute pancreatitis is sudden in onset. It occurs soon after the pancreas becomes damaged or irritated by its own enzymes. Acute pancreatitis usually results from obstruction by gallstones in the bile duct or by alcohol abuse. Other, less common causes of acute pancreatitis include elevated serum lipids, thromboembolism, drug toxicity, infection, and some surgeries. Acute pancreatitis affects about 80,000 Americans each year.[13]

Chronic pancreatitis begins as acute pancreatitis. It becomes chronic when the pancreas becomes scarred. This condition usually results from long-term and excessive alcohol consumption. However, chronic pancreatitis also may develop from other causes of pancreatitis. Chronic pancreatitis can lead to exocrine and endocrine failure. In rare cases, pancreatitis leads to pancreatic cancer.

Pancreatitis may cause severe epigastric pain. It often is associated with nausea, vomiting, and abdominal tenderness and distention. The abdominal pain usually is described as severe, radiating from midumbilicus to the patient's back and shoulders. In severe cases the patient has fever, tachycardia, and signs of generalized sepsis and shock. These patients often are hospitalized. They are treated with IV fluids, pain medication, and placement of a nasogastric tube if the patient is vomiting.

Esophagogastric Varices

Esophagogastric varices are a complex of longitudinal, tortuous veins at the lower end of the esophagus that become enlarged and swollen as a result of portal hypertension. They are common in patients with liver disease and often result from portal hypertension caused by cirrhosis of the liver. Obstruction to blood flow in the liver, produced by the fibrosis in the liver, increases pressure. Obstruction also dilates vessels that drain into the liver. This subsequent dilation of thin-walled veins around the lower esophagus and upper end of the stomach produces esophagogastric varices (Figure 29-7). Varices can rupture. This results in life-threatening hemorrhage. Other causes of esophageal bleeding include **esophagitis** (associated with chronic use of alcohol and antiinflammatory nonsteroidal medications), malignancy, and episodes of prolonged, violent vomiting that produce a tear or laceration in the mucosa of the upper esophagus (Mallory-Weiss syndrome).

Clinically, a patient with esophageal bleeding has bright red hematemesis. This condition may be severe. If bleeding is profuse, melena may be evident. The patient also may manifest the classic signs of shock. Variceal bleeding usually is massive and generally difficult to control. Therapeutic intervention includes ensuring a patent airway and fluid resuscitation. (The placement of a nasogastric tube for gastric lavage is controversial.) Definitive care may include placement of a Sengstaken-Blakemore tube to tamponade bleeding vessels, surgical ligation of the bleeding varices, or transendoscopic injection of a sclerosing agent into the bleeding vessels. The mortality rate for patients with variceal bleeding is about 30%.[14]

Hemorrhoids

Hemorrhoids are swollen, distended veins inside the anus (internal) or under the skin around the anus (external). Hemorrhoids are common during pregnancy; they result from fetal pressure in the abdomen and hormonal changes that cause hemorrhoidal vessels to enlarge. Hemorrhoids are present in 50% of all individuals by age 50. Irritation of the distended veins is worsened by straining during bowel movements and by rubbing or cleaning around the anus, which may produce itching, bleeding, or both. As a rule, hemorrhoidal symptoms subside within a few days.

Pain from hemorrhoids is infrequent unless thrombosis, ulceration, or infection is present. If the patient has rectal pain, the paramedic should consider other possible causes (Box 29-6). Slight bleeding is the most common symptom. (Rarely do hemorrhoids cause significant hemorrhage.) The bleeding usually occurs during or after defecation. Blood dripping into the toilet after defecation or blood-streaked toilet tissue after wiping are common indications. Blood loss from hemorrhoids usually is slight. However, recurrent episodes of bleeding may be significant enough to produce anemia. Definitive care includes dietary modification, stool softeners, tissue fixation techniques, and operative hemorrhoidectomy for severe cases.

Cholecystitis

Cholecystitis is inflammation of the gallbladder. The disease is common in the United States. Cholecystitis occurs in 15% to 20% of the population and is more common

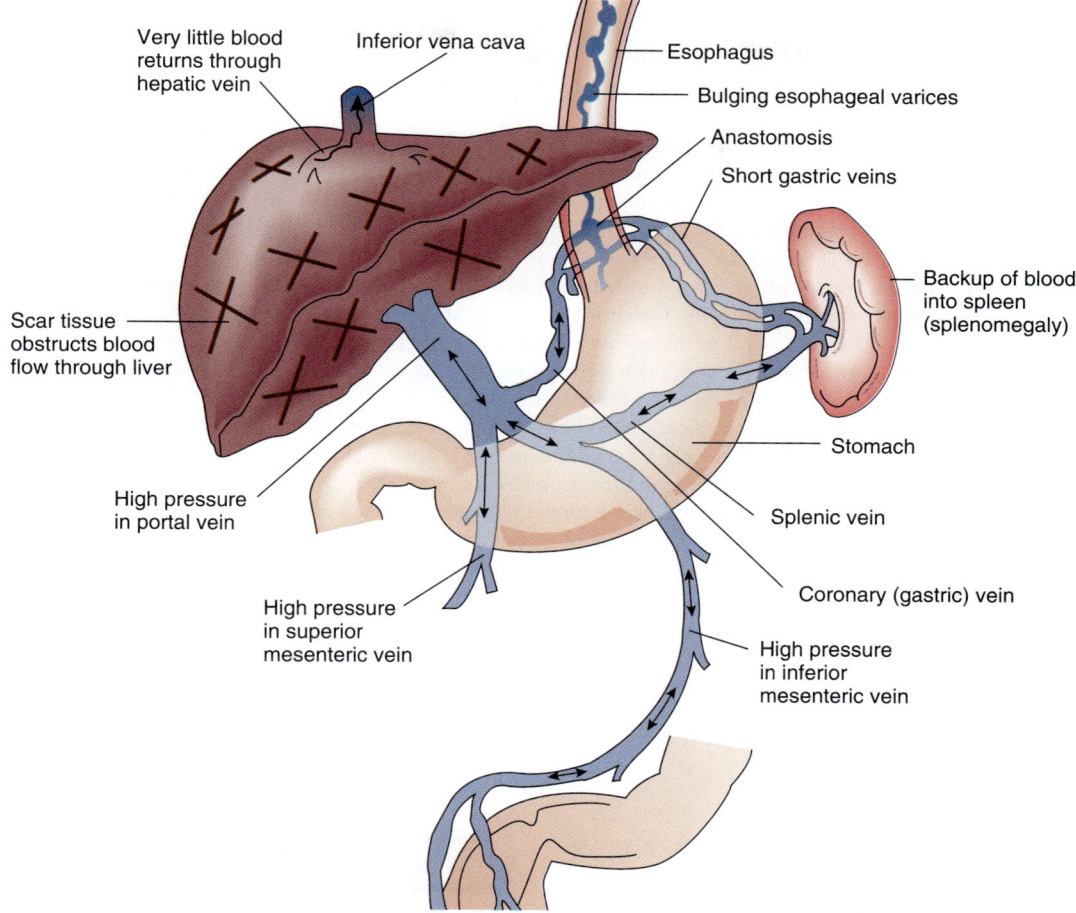

Very little blood returns through hepatic vein

Inferior vena cava

Esophagus

Bulging esophageal varices

Anastomosis

Short gastric veins

Backup of blood into spleen (splenomegaly)

Scar tissue obstructs blood flow through liver

Stomach

High pressure in portal vein

Splenic vein

Coronary (gastric) vein

High pressure in superior mesenteric vein

High pressure in inferior mesenteric vein

FIGURE 29-7 Development of esophageal varices. (Gould BE: *Pathophysiology for the health professional,* ed 3, St Louis, 2006, Saunders.)

BOX 29-6 Rectal Pain

Pain in the rectal area also may result from a rectal abscess, anal fistula, or foreign body. A **rectal abscess** is an infected cavity near the anus that is filled with pus. The condition results from blockage of the anal glands just inside the anus. Treatment consists of surgical drainage of the pus from the infected cavity. An incision also may be made near the anus to relieve pressure.

An **anal fistula** is an abnormal passage between the anal canal or rectum and the skin surface. Most fistulas begin as an abscess that opens spontaneously. This condition also is associated with some diseases, such as tuberculosis, cancer, and irritable bowel disorders. Pain occurs when the fistula becomes blocked, leading to recurrence of an abscess. Symptoms include discharge of pus and fecal material. The fistula requires surgical removal.

Foreign bodies placed in the rectum may result from self-exploration, sexual practices, or abuse. If a foreign body has been inserted in the rectum, no attempt should be made to remove it in the prehospital setting. Treatment by a physician is required.

in women 30 to 50 years of age than in men. The disease becomes more common with age in both men and women. Risk factors for cholecystitis include female gender, oral contraceptive use, increasing age, obesity, diabetes mellitus, chronic alcohol ingestion, and African American or Asian ethnicity. The condition may be chronic, with recurrent subacute symptoms, or acute as a result of gallstone obstruction.

In 90% of cases, acute cholecystitis is caused by gallstones (composed mainly of cholesterol) in the gallbladder. On occasion the gallstones completely obstruct the neck or cystic duct of the gallbladder, which leads to the common bile duct that empties into the small intestine. The trapped bile becomes concentrated. The bile causes irritation and pressure buildup in the gallbladder, which can lead to bacterial infection and perforation. The increased pressure causes a sudden onset of pain *(biliary colic),* which radiates to the right upper quadrant or right scapula. Patients with gallbladder disease commonly have episodes of pain at night. Generally, the episodes are associated with recent ingestion of fried or fatty foods. Severe illness, alcohol abuse and, in rare cases, tumors of the gallbladder also can cause cholecystitis.

Other associated hallmarks of cholecystitis include previous episodes, a family history of gallbladder disease, low-grade fever, nausea, vomiting that may be bile stained and described as bitter (variable), and pain and tenderness on palpation in the right upper quadrant. Passage of stones into the common bile duct with subsequent obstruction may cause shaking chills, high fever, jaundice, and acute pancreatitis. Treatment may include hospitalization, IV fluid therapy, antibiotics, and placement of a nasogastric tube. Definitive treatment is surgical removal of the gallbladder.

Acute Hepatitis

Hepatitis is inflammation of the liver. Hepatitis is the single most important cause of liver disease in the United States and worldwide (Box 29-7).

Acute hepatitis is associated with the sudden onset of malaise, weakness, anorexia, intermittent nausea and vomiting, and dull right upper quadrant pain. These signs usually are followed within 1 week by the onset of jaundice, dark urine, or both. Many viruses can infect the liver. However, the three classes of viruses that are of main concern as causes of acute infectious hepatitis are hepatitis A virus (HAV), hepatitis B virus (HBV), and hepatitis C virus (HCV, formerly known as *non-A/non-B hepatitis virus*). All types produce similar pathological changes in the liver. These viruses also stimulate an antibody response that is specific to the type of virus causing the disease (Box 29-8).

BOX 29-8 Risk Factors for Hepatitis

Hepatitis A (spread by fecal-oral route)
- Health care practice without body substance isolation precautions
- Household or sexual contact with an infected person
- Living in an area with a hepatitis A virus outbreak
- Travel to developing countries
- Engaging in sex with infected partners or multiple partners
- Drug use by injection

Hepatitis B (spread by infectious blood)
- Health care practice without body substance isolation precautions
- Infant born to mother infected with hepatitis B virus
- Engaging in sex with infected partners or multiple partners
- Drug use by injection
- Receiving hemodialysis

Hepatitis C (spread by infectious blood)
- Health care practice without body substance isolation precautions
- Receiving a blood transfusion before July, 1992
- Infant born to mother infected with the hepatitis C virus
- Engaging in sex with infected partners or multiple partners
- Drug use by injection; blood-contaminated straws used to snort drugs
- Receiving hemodialysis

Many hepatitis infections are subclinical; they often present with influenza-like symptoms. Serious conditions associated with hepatitis are cirrhosis (scarring of the liver; Figure 29-8), hepatic encephalopathy (brain and nervous system damage that occurs as a complication of liver disease), and liver cancer. These conditions are discussed in Chapters 28 and 34.

The inflammation of hepatitis has many possible causes, including alcohol or other drug use, autoimmune disorders, and toxic bacterial, fungal, parasitic, and viral infections. Patients with hepatitis require a physician's evaluation and care. Proper immunization of paramedics against HAV and HBV is important. Strict adherence to body substance isolation procedures also is crucial when paramedics are caring for these patients.

Hereditary Hemochromatosis

Hereditary hemochromatosis is one of the most common genetic disorders in the United States.[15] It is an inherited condition in which the body absorbs and stores too much iron. The extra iron accumulates in several organs, especially the liver, heart, and pancreas. Many people with the disease have no symptoms, even in advanced stages. Joint pain is the most common complaint of people with hemochromatosis. Other common symptoms include fatigue, abdominal pain, decreased libido, and heart problems. Symptoms tend to occur in men between the ages of 30 and 50 and in women over age 50. If the disease is not detected early and treated by ridding the body of excess iron with regular phlebotomy, serious illness (including death) may result. Systemic illness that develops from hemochromatosis includes[16]:

- Arthritis
- Liver disease, including an enlarged liver, cirrhosis, cancer, and liver failure
- Damage to the pancreas, possibly causing diabetes mellitus
- Heart abnormalities, such as irregular heart rhythms or congestive heart failure
- Impotence
- Early menopause
- Abnormal pigmentation of the skin, making it look gray or bronze
- Pituitary damage
- Damage to the adrenal gland

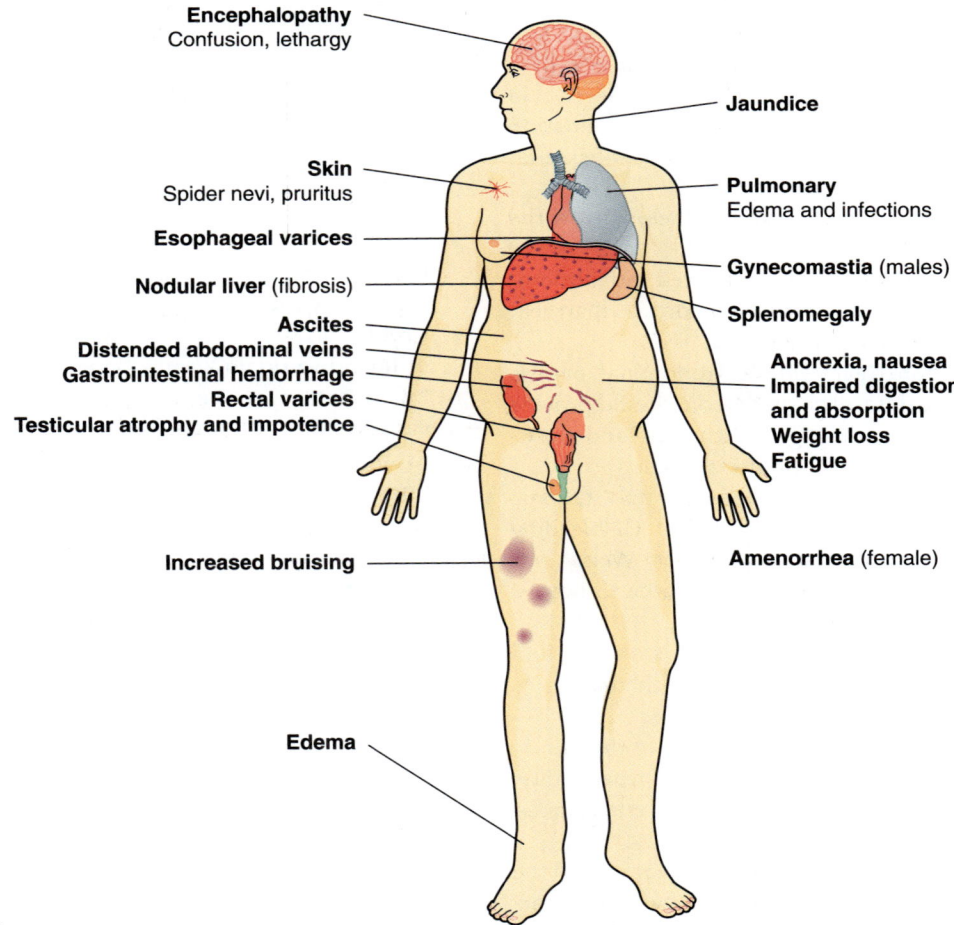

FIGURE 29-8 Effects of advanced cirrhosis. (Gould BE: *Pathophysiology for the health professional,* ed 3, St Louis, 2006, Saunders.)

To develop hemochromatosis, a person must inherit the defective gene from both parents. Those who inherit the defective gene from only one parent are carriers of the disease but usually do not develop it. Siblings of people who have hemochromatosis should have their blood tested to determine if they have the disease or are carriers. Parents, children, and other close relatives of people who have the disease should consider being tested.[15]

AGE-RELATED VARIATIONS IN ABDOMINAL PAIN

As discussed in Chapter 20, many physiological and anatomical differences exist among infant, child, and adult patients. The way in which these groups experience abdominal pain may also be quite different. For example, causes of abdominal pain in the elderly are more likely to be diseases that require surgical treatment; a vascular catastrophe; ischemic heart disease; or sepsis. Infants and young children are unable to communicate their history or degree of pain. As a result, they can become dehydrated and septic more quickly than adults. Vital signs in these groups often do not accurately reflect their degree of illness (see Chapters 48 and 49).[17]

> **CRITICAL THINKING**
> Why do you think a person would refuse the chance to be vaccinated against this deadly disease?

SUMMARY

- The major organs associated with the GI system include the esophagus, stomach, small and large intestines, liver, gallbladder, and pancreas.
- After the scene survey and primary assessment of a patient with abdominal pain, the paramedic should obtain a thorough history. The physical examination may help determine whether the pain is visceral, somatic, or referred.
- The type and location of the pain may help narrow the differential diagnosis.
- Important signs and symptoms associated with abdominal pain include nausea, vomiting, anorexia, diarrhea, constipation, stool color, and fever.
- The most common treatment for abdominal pain is provided at the hospital. The paramedic should provide supportive treatment, manage life threats, and transport the patient to an appropriate facility.
- Gastrointestinal bleeding can be slow and chronic or rapid and life threatening. Causes of GI bleeding include esophagogastric varices, Mallory-Weiss syndrome, cancer, medication use, and other systemic diseases.
- Gastroenteritis is inflammation of the stomach and intestines caused by infectious agents, chemicals, or other conditions.
- Gastritis is acute or chronic inflammation of the gastric mucosa. Gastritis commonly results from hyperacidity, alcohol or other drug ingestion, bile reflux, and *H. pylori* infection.
- Ulcerative colitis is an inflammatory condition of the large intestine. Colitis is characterized by severe diarrhea and ulceration of the mucosa of the intestine (ulcerative colitis).

- Diverticulosis may result in bright red rectal bleeding if perforation occurs.
- Diverticulitis results when a diverticulum becomes obstructed with fecal matter.
- Appendicitis occurs when the passageway between the appendix and cecum is obstructed by fecal material or by inflammation caused by infection.
- Peptic ulcer disease occurs when open wounds or sores develop in the stomach or duodenum.
- Bowel obstruction is an occlusion of the intestinal lumen. It results in blockage of the normal flow of intestinal contents.
- Crohn's disease is a chronic inflammatory bowel disease of unknown origin.
- Inflammation of the pancreas is called *pancreatitis*. It causes severe abdominal pain.
- Esophagogastric varices arise from obstruction of blood flow to the liver as a result of liver disease. Rupture of the varices can cause hemorrhage and death.
- Hemorrhoids are distended veins in the rectoanal area.
- Cholecystitis is inflammation of the gallbladder. It most often is associated with the presence of gallstones.
- Hepatitis is characterized by the sudden onset of malaise, weakness, anorexia, intermittent nausea and vomiting, and dull right upper quadrant pain. These signs usually are followed within 1 week by the onset of jaundice or dark urine or both.
- Hereditary hemochromatosis is a condition in which the body absorbs and stores too much iron. This can causes severe damage when the iron collects in the liver, heart, and pancreas.

REFERENCES

1. Rosen P, Barkin R: *Emergency medicine: concepts and clinical practice*, ed 6, St Louis, 2006, Mosby.

2. Goldman L: *Cecil medicine*, ed 23, Philadelphia, 2008, Saunders.

3. Alonso-Serra HM, Wesley K: *Prehospital pain management:* position paper. www.naemsp.org/pdf/Prehospital_Pain_Management.pdf. Accessed November 10, 2010.

4. National Highway Traffic Safety Administration: *The National EMS Education Standards.* Washington, DC, 2009, U.S. Department of Transportation/National Highway Traffic Safety Administration, DOT.

5. Graham CA, Parke TR: Critical care in the emergency department: shock and circulatory support, *Emerg Med J* 22:17-21. 2005.

6. NAEMT: *PHTLS prehospital trauma life support*, ed 6, St Louis, 2006, Mosby.

7. Bonheur JL, et al: Bacterial gastroenteritis, http://emedicine. medscape.com/article/176400-overview, Accessed May 5, 2011.

8. National Digestive Diseases Information Clearinghouse: *Lactose intolerance.* http://digestive.niddk.nih.gov/ddiseases/pubs/lactoseintolerance/. Accessed September 13, 2010.

9. Marx J, Hockberger R, Walls R: *Rosen's emergency medicine*, ed 7, St Louis, 2009, Mosby.

10. Fass R: Epidemiology and pathophysiology of symptomatic gastroesophageal reflux disease, *Am J Gastroenterol* 98:S2-S7, 2003.

11. Nobie BA: Obstruction, small bowel. www.emedicine.com/emerg/topic66.htm. Accessed February 21, 2005.

12. Crohn's & Colitis Foundation of America: About Crohn's Disease, http://www.ccfa.org/info/about/crohns, Accessed May 5, 2011

13. American Gastroenterological Association: Pancreatitis. Understanding pancreatitis, http://www.gastro.org/patient-center/digestive-conditions/pancreatitis, Accessed May 5, 2011.

14. Garcia-Tsao G, et al: Prevention and management of gastroesophageal varices and variceal hemorrhage in cirrhosis, *Am J Gastroenterol* 102:2086-2102, 2007.

15. National Digestive Diseases Information Clearinghouse: Hemachromatosis. http://digestive.niddk.nih.gov/diseases/pubs/hemochromatosis/index.htm. Accessed September 13, 2010.

16. American Liver Foundation: *Hemachromatosis.* www.liverfoundation.org/education/info/hemochromatosis/. Accessed September 13, 2010.

17. Hamilton GC, et al: *Emergency medicine: an approach to clinical problem-solving*, ed 2, Philadelphia, 2002, Saunders.

RECOMMENDED READING

Mistovich J, Krost W, Limmer D: Beyond the basics: acute abdominal pain, *EMS Magazine* 37:68-71, 2008.

30 Genitourinary and Renal Disorders

OBJECTIVES

Upon completion of this chapter, the paramedic student will be able to:

1. Label a diagram of the urinary system.
2. Distinguish between acute and chronic renal failure.
3. Outline the pathophysiology of renal failure.
4. Identify the signs and symptoms of renal failure.
5. Describe the process of hemodialysis and peritoneal dialysis.
6. Describe the signs and symptoms and care of emergency conditions associated with dialysis.
7. Describe the pathophysiology, signs and symptoms, assessment, and prehospital management of a patient with urinary retention, urinary tract infection, pyelonephritis, urinary calculus, epididymitis, Fournier's gangrene, phimosis, paraphimosis, priapism, benign prostatic hypertrophy, testicular masses, and testicular torsion.
8. Outline the physical examination of patients with genitourinary disorders.
9. Discuss the general prehospital management of a patient with a genitourinary disorder.

KEY TERMS

acute prostatitis Inflammation of the prostate gland that develops suddenly.

acute renal failure (ARF) A clinical syndrome that results from a sudden, significant decrease in filtration through the glomeruli, leading to the accumulation of salt, water, and nitrogenous wastes in the body.

acute tubular necrosis The death of tubular cells, which form the tubule that transports urine to the ureters.

anuria Inability to urinate; the cessation of urine production; a diminished urinary output (less than 100 to 250 mL a day).

arteriovenous fistula An internal anastomosis between an artery and a vein.

arteriovenous graft A synthetic material grafted between the patient's artery and vein.

autonomic hyperreflexia Overactivity of the autonomic nervous system that causes an abrupt onset of extremely high blood pressure.

azotemia A condition marked by retention of excessive amounts of nitrogenous compounds in the blood.

benign prostatic hypertrophy (BPH) Enlargement of the prostate gland.

chronic renal failure (CRF) A progressive, irreversible systemic disease, caused by kidney dysfunction, that leads to abnormalities in blood counts and blood chemistry levels.

circumcision Surgical removal of the penile foreskin.

creatinine A chemical waste molecule generated by muscle metabolism.

cystitis Inflammation of the urinary bladder and ureters.

dialysate A solution used in dialysis.

dialysis A technique used to normalize blood chemistry in patients with acute or chronic renal failure and to remove blood toxins in some patients who have taken a drug overdose.

disequilibrium syndrome A group of neurological findings that sometimes occur during or immediately after dialysis; they are thought to result from a disproportionate decrease in the osmolality of the extracellular fluid compared with that of the intracellular compartment in the brain or cerebrospinal fluid.

dysuria Difficult urination.

end-stage renal disease Complete or near complete failure of the kidneys to function.

epididymitis Inflammation of the epididymis, a tubular section of the male reproductive system that carries sperm from the testicle to the seminal vesicles.

Fournier's gangrene A bacterial infection of the skin that affects the genitals and perineum in both men and women.

genitourinary system The system comprising the genital and reproductive organs.

hematuria The abnormal presence of blood in the urine.

hemodialysis A procedure in which impurities or wastes are removed from the blood; it is used to treat renal insufficiency and various toxic conditions.

hydrocele A fluid-filled sac along the spermatic cord in the scrotum.

intrarenal disease Disease or damage within the kidney.

nephron The functional unit of the kidney.

nocturia Excessive urination at night.

oliguria A condition marked by diminished capacity to form or pass urine.

orchitis Painful inflammation of the testicle.

overflow incontinence Overflow of urine from the bladder.

paraphimosis A condition in uncircumcised men marked by the inability to pull the retracted foreskin back over the head of the penis.

peritoneal dialysis A dialysis procedure that uses the peritoneum as a diffusible membrane; it is performed to correct an imbalance of fluid or electrolytes in the blood or to remove toxins, drugs, or other wastes normally excreted by the kidney.

phimosis Tightness of the prepuce (foreskin) of the penis.

postrenal disease Disease that blocks the system that collects urine; it usually is caused by urinary tract obstruction.

prepuce In males, the free fold of skin that covers the glans penis; the foreskin. In females, the external fold of the labia minora that covers the clitoris.

prerenal disease Disease that compromises renal perfusion.

priapism Painful, persistent erection of the penis.

pseudoaneurysm A condition resembling an aneurysm that is caused by enlargement and tortuosity of a vessel.

pyelonephritis Inflammation of the kidney parenchyma caused by microbial infection.

spermatocele A benign cystic accumulation of sperm that arises from the head of the epididymis.

testicular mass An enlargement or growth on one or both testicles.

testicular torsion The twisting of a testicle on its spermatic cord, disrupting its blood supply.

urea A nitrogen-containing waste product.

uremia A condition marked by an excess of urea and other nitrogenous wastes in the blood.

urethritis Inflammation of the urethra.

urinary calculi Solid particles in the urinary system, commonly known as "kidney stones."

urinary retention Inability to urinate.

urinary tract infection (UTI) Infection of one or more structures of the urinary tract.

varicocele An abnormal enlargement of the veins that drain the testicle.

*L*ike gastrointestinal disorders, many genitourinary and renal disorders can produce acute abdominal pain and systemic illness. Treatment for these patients frequently begins in the prehospital setting. Successful outcomes often are determined in large part by the assessment skills of the paramedic.

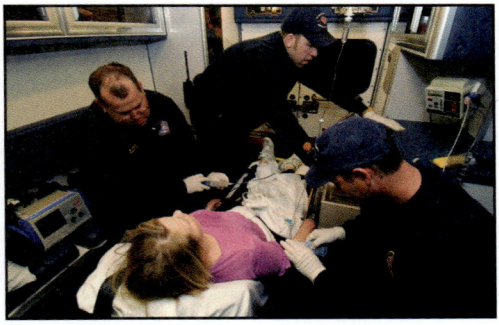

(Courtesy Ray Kemp, St. Charles, Mo.)

ANATOMY AND PHYSIOLOGY REVIEW

As described in Chapter 10, the genitourinary and renal systems work with other body systems to maintain homeostasis. The **genitourinary system** actually refers to two different body systems. *Genito* refers to genital organs and the reproductive system. This system is responsible for perpetuation of our species. The genital system is composed of the male and female reproductive organs (Figures 30-1 and 30-2 and Box 30-1). *Urinary* refers to the system responsible for the removal of metabolic waste products from the blood, the removal of concentrated urine, and the conservation of water. This system plays a primary role in the following processes[1]:

- Regulation of water and electrolytes
- Regulation of the acid-base balance
- Excretion of waste products and foreign chemicals
- Regulation of the arterial blood pressure
- Production of red blood cells
- Stimulation of glucose production

BOX 30-1 Reproductive Organs

Male Reproductive Organs

Testes
Epididymis
Ductus deferens
Seminal vesicles
Prostate gland
Bulbourethral glands
Scrotum
Penis

Female Reproductive Organs

Ovaries
Uterine (fallopian) tubes
Uterus
Vagina
External genital organs
Internal reproductive organs
Mammary glands

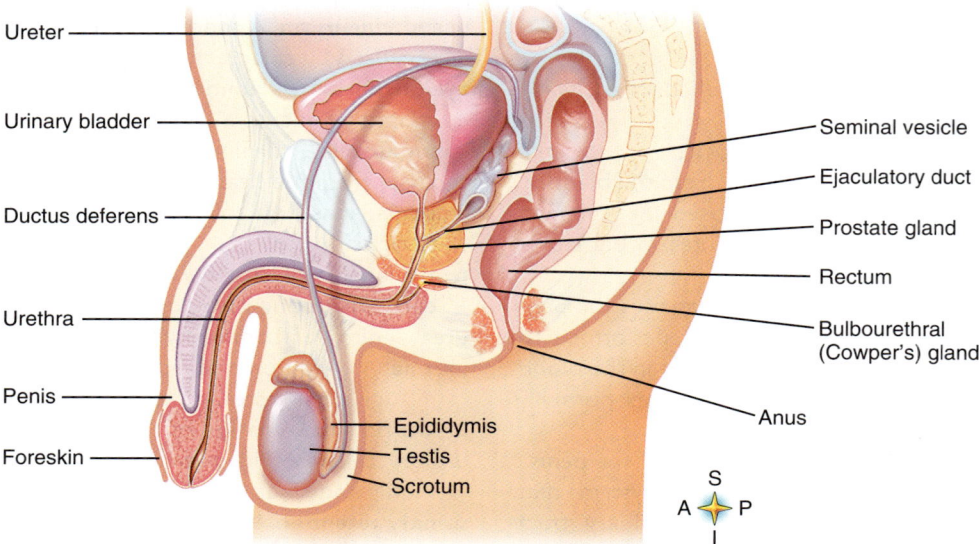

FIGURE 30-1 Male reproductive organs. (Thibodeau GA, Patton KT: *Structure and function of the body,* ed 13, St Louis, 2008, Mosby.)

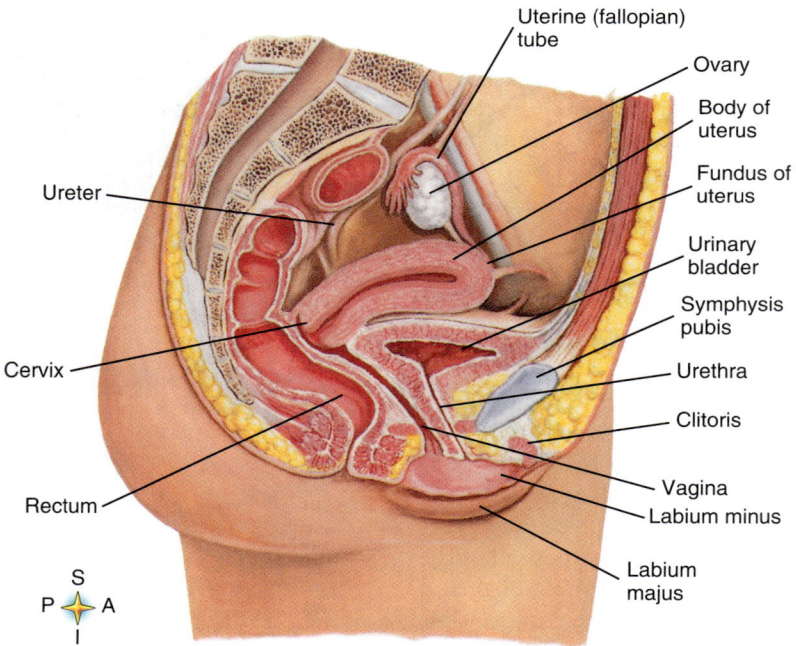

FIGURE 30-2 Female reproductive organs. (Thibodeau GA, Patton KT: *Structure and function of the body,* ed 13, St Louis, 2008, Mosby.)

The urinary system is made up of two kidneys, two ureters, the urinary bladder, and the urethra (Figure 30-3). The renal structures are the kidneys and their related structures (Figure 30-4). This chapter addresses renal diseases, urinary system conditions, and male genital tract conditions. Conditions that affect the female reproductive system are presented in Chapter 31.

LOOK AGAIN
See Chapter 10: Review of Human Systems, pp. 199-201.

is protected by the rib cage. As described in Chapter 10, the basic functional unit of the kidney is the **nephron.** There are millions of nephrons inside each kidney. The roles of the nephron are to filter blood, remove waste products, and produce urine. Damage to the nephrons results in renal (kidney) disease.

NOTE
Renal and urinary diseases affect an estimated 20 million Americans. They directly cause more than 95,000 deaths a year.[2] Diabetes is a major risk factor for renal disease.[3]

RENAL DISEASES

The kidneys are two bean-shaped organs about the size of a person's fist. They lie on the posterior abdominal wall behind the peritoneum. The superior border of the kidney reaches the level of the twelfth thoracic vertebra. The inferior border lies just above the horizontal plane of the umbilicus, typically level with the third lumbar vertebra. The inferior border is one finger's breadth superior to the iliac crest. The center of the kidney, where the ureter is attached, is level with the intervertebral disc between the first and second lumbar vertebrae. The superior pole of each kidney

The causes of renal failure can be classified as *prerenal, intrarenal,* and *postrenal* (Table 30-1). **Prerenal disease** occurs before the kidney is reached. It is characterized by inadequate blood flow (perfusion) to the kidneys. **Intrarenal disease** *(intrinsic disease)* refers to disease or damage within the kidney. **Postrenal disease** refers to disease that blocks the system that collects urine. All of these conditions can result in acute or chronic renal failure, leading to end-stage renal disease. The classification of disease depends on the duration of renal failure and the potential for reversibility. Assessment findings and symptoms of renal failure are listed in Table 30-2.

CRITICAL THINKING
Think about why a patient would develop the complications just described.

Acute Renal Failure

Acute renal failure (ARF) (also known as *acute kidney injury* [AKI]) is a clinical syndrome that results from a sudden, significant decrease in filtration through the glomeruli. This leads to the buildup of high levels of uremic toxins in the blood. Acute renal failure occurs when the kidneys are unable to excrete the daily load of toxins in the urine. Patients with ARF can be divided into two groups, based on the amount of urine excreted in 24 hours. One group is *oliguric;* these patients excrete less than 500 mL a day. The other is *nonoliguric;* these patients excrete more than 500 mL a day. Acute renal failure is a life-threatening condition. The mortality rate for patients hospitalized for the disease is 40% to 50%.[4] However, if ARF is recognized early and treated appropriately, it may be readily reversible. A variety of conditions can cause ARF, such as trauma, shock, infection, urinary obstruction, and multisystem diseases.

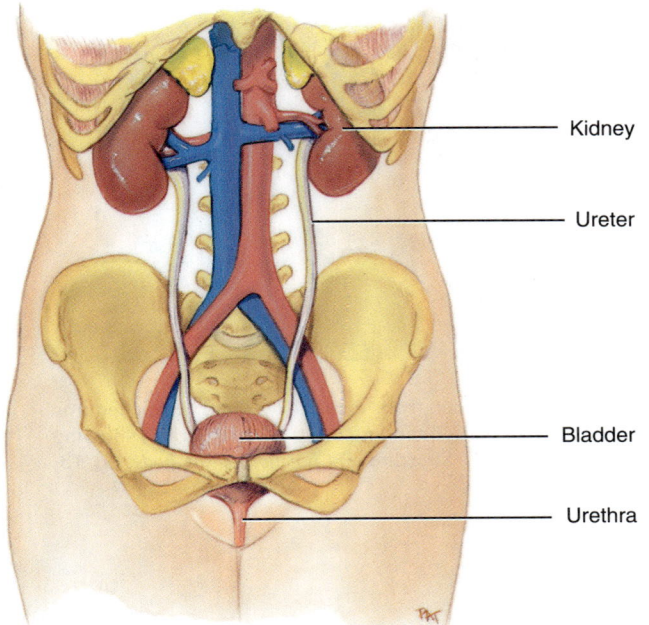

FIGURE 30-3 Components of the urinary system. (Applegate E: *The anatomy and physiology learning system,* ed 3, St Louis, 2006, Saunders.)

Kidney

Ureter

Bladder

Urethra

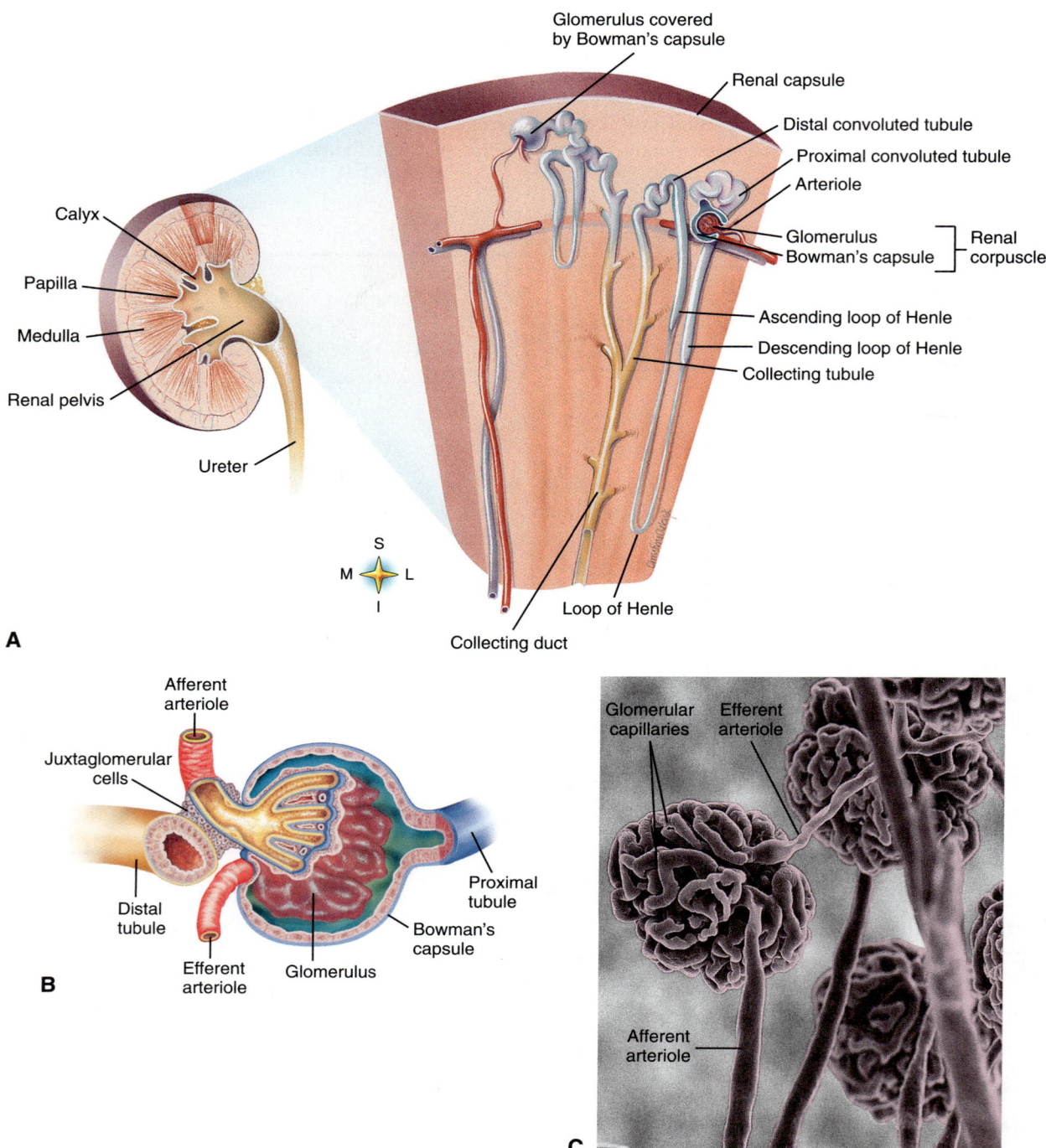

FIGURE 30-4 Location and components of the nephron. **A,** Magnified wedge cut from a renal pyramid. **B,** Schematic showing relationship of glomerulus to Bowman's capsule and adjacent structures. **C,** Scanning electron micrograph showing several glomeruli and their associated blood vessels. (Thibodeau GA, Patton KT: *Structure and function of the body,* ed 13, St Louis, 2008, Mosby.)

TABLE 30-1 Classification of Acute Renal Failure

Area of Dysfunction	Possible Causes

Prerenal	• Hypovolemia
	  • Hemorrhagic blood loss (trauma, GI bleeding, complications of childbirth)
	  • Loss of plasma volume (burns, peritonitis)
	  • Water and electrolyte losses (severe vomiting or diarrhea, intestinal obstruction, uncontrolled diabetes mellitus, inappropriate use of diuretics)
	• Hypotension or hypoperfusion
	• Septic shock
	• Cardiac failure or shock
	• Massive pulmonary embolism
	• Stenosis or clamping of renal artery

Intrarenal	• Acute tubular necrosis (postischemic or nephrotoxic) • Glomerulopathies • Malignant hypertension • Coagulation defects
Postrenal	• Obstructive uropathies (usually bilateral) • Ureteral obstruction (edema, tumors, stones, clots) • Bladder neck obstruction (enlarged prostate)

From McCance KL, Huether SE: *Pathophysiology: the biologic basis for disease in adults and children,* ed 4, St Louis, 2002, Mosby.

TABLE 30-2 Assessment Findings and Symptoms of Renal Failure[1]

Acute Renal Failure
- Reduced or no urinary output
- Excessive urinary output at night
- Lower extremity swelling
- Neuropathy of the hands and feet
- Anorexia
- Altered mental status
- Metallic taste in mouth
- Tremors or seizures
- Easy bruising or prolonged bleeding
- Flank pain
- Tinnitus
- Hypertension
- Abdominal pain or discomfort

Chronic Renal Failure
- Headache
- Weakness
- Anorexia
- Vomiting
- Increased urination
- Rusty-colored or brown urine
- Increased thirst
- Hypertension
- Pruritus

End-Stage Renal Disease
- Confusion
- Altered level of consciousness
- Shortness of breath
- Chest pain
- Bone pain
- Pruritus
- Nausea, vomiting, diarrhea
- Bruising
- Muscle twitching, tremors, seizures
- Hallucinations

The onset of ARF can occur within hours. As normal kidney function rapidly deteriorates, urine output frequently decreases **(oliguria)** or stops completely **(anuria).** This results in **uremia.** Uremia is an excess of **urea** and other nitrogenous wastes in the blood. The condition generally results from kidney malfunction. Uremia may be associated with the following (Table 30-3):

- Generalized edema from water and salt retention
- Acidosis from failure of the kidneys to rid the body of normal acidic products
- High concentrations of nonprotein nitrogens (especially urea) from failure of the body to secrete metabolic end products
- High concentrations of other products of renal excretion (e.g., uric acid and potassium).

Uremia must be recognized early and treated appropriately. If it is not, renal dysfunction leads to the development of heart failure, volume overload, hyperkalemia, and metabolic acidosis.

PRERENAL ACUTE RENAL FAILURE

Prerenal ARF results from inadequate perfusion of the kidneys. The damaged kidneys are unable to rid the blood of waste products such as urea and **creatinine.** This condition may be caused by hypovolemia or impaired cardiac output. Obstruction of renal arteries results in decreased blood flow to the kidneys. It also causes an increase in renal vascular resistance that effectively shunts blood away from the kidneys. Many patients with prerenal ARF are critically ill. They may have a number of preexisting medical conditions, such as atherosclerosis, chronic liver disease, and heart failure. (Dehydration caused by the use of diuretics in patients with heart failure is a major cause of prerenal ARF.) In addition, perfusion often is poor in many organs, and this may lead to multiple organ failure.

Signs and symptoms of prerenal ARF include dizziness, dry mouth, thirst, hypotension, tachycardia, and weight loss. The goal of treatment is to improve kidney perfusion and function by treating the underlying condition (e.g.,

TABLE 30-3   Systemic Effects of Uremia

System	Manifestations	Mechanisms	Treatment
Skeletal	Osteitis fibrosa (bone inflammation with fibrous degeneration); bone demineralization (principally subperiosteal loss of cortical bone in the fibers, lateral ends of the clavicles, and lamina dura of the teeth); spontaneous fractures, bone pain; osteomalacia (rickets) with end-stage renal failure	Bone resorption associated with hyperparathyroidism, vitamin D deficiency, and demineralization; lowered calcium and elevated phosphate levels	Control of hyperphosphatemia to reduce hyperparathyroidism; administration of calcium and aluminum hydroxide antacids, which bind phosphate in the gut, together with a phosphate-restricted diet; vitamin D replacement; avoidance of magnesium antacids because of impaired magnesium excretion
Cardiopulmonary	Hypertension, pericarditis with fever, chest pain, and pericardial friction rub, pulmonary edema, Kussmaul respirations	Extracellular volume expansion as cause of hypertension; hypersecretion of rennin also associated with hypertension; fluid overload associated with pulmonary edema and acidosis leading to Kussmaul respirations	Volume reduction with diuretics that are not potassium sparing (to avoid hyperkalemia); angiotensin-converting enzyme (ACE) inhibitors; combination of propranolol, hydralazine, and minoxidil for those with high levels of rennin; bilateral nephrectomy with dialysis or transplantation
Neurological	Encephalopathy (fatigue, loss of attention, difficulty problem solving); peripheral neuropathy (pain and burning in the legs and feet, loss of vibration sense and deep tendon reflexes); loss of motor coordination, twitching, fasciculations, stupor, and coma with advanced uremia	Uremic toxins associated with end-stage renal disease	Dialysis
Endocrine	Retarded growth in children	Decreased growth hormone	Exogenous recombinant human growth hormone
	Osteomalacia	Elevated parathyroid hormone levels	Same as for skeletal system manifestations
	Higher incidence of goiter	Decreased thyroid hormone	Hormone replacement when indicated
Hematological	Anemia, usually normochromic normocytic; platelet disorders with prolonged bleeding times	Reduced erythropoietin secretion associated with loss of renal mass, leading to reduced red cell production in the bone marrow; uremic toxins associated with shortened red cell survival	Dialysis; recombinant human erythropoietin and iron supplementation; conjugated estrogens; 1-desamino-8-D-arginine vasopressin (DDAVP); transfusion
Gastrointestinal	Anorexia, nausea, vomiting; mouth ulcers, stomatitis, ruinous breath (uremic fetor); hiccups, peptic ulcers, gastrointestinal bleeding, and pancreatitis associated with end-stage renal failure	Retention of urea, metabolic acids, and other metabolic waste products, including methylguanidine	Protein-restricted diet for relief of nausea and vomiting
Integumentary	Abnormal pigmentation and pruritus	Retention of urochromes, contributing to sallow, yellow color; high plasma calcium levels associated with pruritus	Dialysis with control of serum calcium levels
Immunological	Increased risk of infection that can cause death	Suppression of cell-mediated immunity; reduction in number and function of lymphocytes, diminished phagocytosis	Routine dialysis
Reproductive	Sexual dysfunction: menorrhagia, amenorrhea, infertility, and decreased libido in women; decreased testosterone levels, infertility, and decreased libido in men	Elevated hormones: luteinizing hormone (LH), follicle-stimulating hormone (FSH), prolactin, and LH-releasing hormone; decreased testosterone, estrogen, and progesterone	No specific treatment

From McCance KL, Huether SE: Pathophysiology: the biologic basis for disease in adults and children, ed 4, St Louis, 2002, Mosby.

infection, congestive heart failure, or liver failure). Fluids are administered intravenously to most patients to treat dehydration. After this, urine output generally increases and renal function improves.

INTRARENAL ACUTE RENAL FAILURE

Intrarenal ARF is also known as *intrinsic ARF*. It results from conditions that damage or injure both kidneys. Examples include glomerular and other microvascular diseases, tubular diseases, and interstitial diseases that directly damage the kidney parenchyma. Nearly 90% of cases are caused by ischemia or toxins. Both of these causes can lead to **acute tubular necrosis** (death of tubular cells).[5] Ischemic causes of intrarenal ARF are associated with renal hypoperfusion. These occur most often as a result of hemorrhage, trauma, and sepsis, and in patients undergoing cardiovascular surgery. Nephrotoxic causes of intrarenal ARF occur most often in the elderly and in patients with chronic renal failure. Drugs and other compounds that can trigger intrarenal ARF include antibiotics, nonsteroidal antiinflammatory drugs (NSAIDs), anticancer drugs, radiocontrast dyes, alcohol, and other drugs (e.g., cocaine). The condition also is associated with hypertension, autoimmune diseases (e.g., systemic lupus erythematosus), and pyelonephritis (described later in this chapter).

Signs and symptoms of intrarenal ARF include fever, flank pain, joint pain, headache, hypertension, confusion, seizure, and oliguria. The goal of treatment is to restore adequate renal blood flow. This is done by resolving the underlying cause and its complications. In severe cases, renal dialysis (described later) or kidney transplantation may be needed to manage the disease.

POSTRENAL ACUTE RENAL FAILURE

Postrenal ARF is caused by obstruction to urine flow from both kidneys. This form of renal failure may be caused by ureteral and urethral obstructions (e.g., bilateral calculi, prostatic enlargement, urethral strictures). It also can result from obstruction of a urinary catheter. The blockage of urine causes pressure to build in the renal nephrons and ultimately can cause the nephrons to shut down. The degree of renal failure corresponds directly to the degree of obstruction. Signs and symptoms of postrenal ARF include urine retention; a distended bladder; gross **hematuria;** pain in the lower back, abdomen, groin, or genitalia; and peripheral edema. The condition can be reversed by removing the obstruction to urine flow.

Chronic Renal Failure

Chronic renal failure (CRF) is a progressive, irreversible systemic disease. It develops over months to years as internal structures of the kidney are slowly damaged. As renal function steadily declines, CRF leads to **end-stage renal disease,** which eventually requires dialysis or kidney transplantation. CRF may be caused by congenital disorders or prolonged pyelonephritis. In the industrialized world, however, CRF more often results from systemic diseases (e.g., diabetes and hypertension) and autoimmune disorders. The kidneys try to make up for renal damage by hyperfiltration in the remaining working nephrons. Over time, hyperfiltration causes further nephron damage and loss of kidney function. Chronic loss of function causes generalized wasting and progressive scarring in all parts of the kidney. This damage results in a reduction in nephron mass and renal mass.

> **NOTE**
> Chronic renal failure and end-stage renal disease affect more than 2 in 1000 people in the United States. More than 50,000 Americans die each year from the disease.[6]

As does ARF, CRF results in the buildup of fluid and waste products in the body. This causes **azotemia** (the retention of excessive amounts of nitrogenous compounds in the blood). It also causes uremia. Most body systems are affected by CRF. Complications of the disease may include hypertension, congestive heart failure, anemia, electrolyte abnormalities, and others. Once CRF has been diagnosed and the cause has been identified, treatments are started to delay or possibly stop the progressive loss of kidney function. In its final stages, CRF often requires treatment with dialysis (hemodialysis or peritoneal dialysis) or kidney transplantation for the patient to survive. In addition to oliguria, a patient with CRF may show the following six systemic manifestations.

1. Gastrointestinal manifestations
   a. Anorexia
   b. Nausea
   c. Vomiting
   d. Metallic taste in the mouth
2. Cardiopulmonary manifestations
   a. Hypertension
   b. Pericarditis
   c. Pulmonary edema
   d. Peripheral, sacral, and periorbital edema
   e. Myocardial ischemia
3. Nervous system manifestations
   a. Anxiety
   b. Delirium
   c. Progressive obtundation
   d. Hallucinations
   e. Muscle twitching
   f. Neuropathies of the hands and feet
   g. Tremors or seizures
4. Metabolic or endocrine manifestations
   a. Glucose intolerance
   b. Electrolyte disturbances
   c. Anemia
5. Personality changes
   a. Fatigue
   b. Mental dullness
   c. Confusion

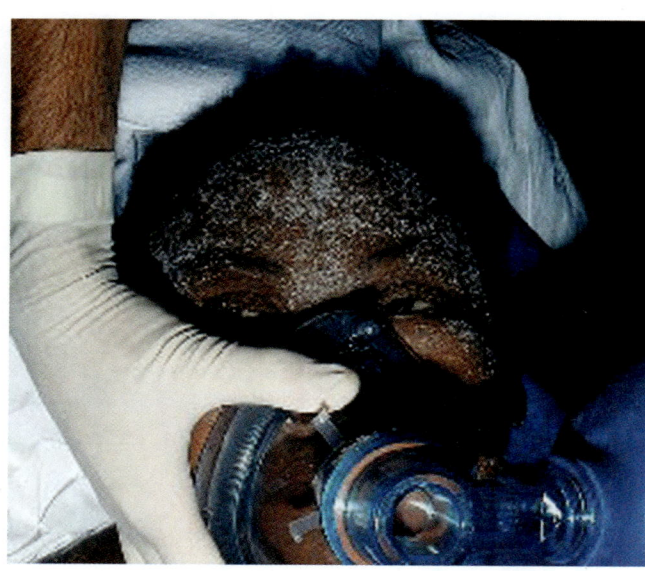

FIGURE 30-5 Uremic frost. Note the fine white powder on the skin of this patient with kidney failure. (Marx J, et al: *Rosen's emergency medicine: concepts and clinical practice,* ed 6, Philadelphia, 2006, Mosby.)

6. Signs of uremia
   a. Pasty, yellow skin and thin extremities from protein wasting
   b. Uremic frost (Figure 30-5), caused by the formation of urea crystals on the skin (late finding)

Renal Dialysis

Dialysis is a technique used to normalize blood chemistry and remove excess fluid in patients with acute or chronic renal failure. Dialysis also removes blood toxins in some patients who have taken a drug overdose. The two types of dialysis are *hemodialysis* and *peritoneal dialysis*. Both of these techniques bring the patent's blood into contact with a semipermeable membrane, across which water-soluble substances diffuse into a dialyzing fluid **(dialysate).** Eventually electrolytes are balanced between the patient's blood and the dialysis fluid, and waste products are eliminated.

The amount of substance that transfers during dialysis depends on the difference in the concentrations of solutions on the two sides of the semipermeable membrane, the molecular size of the substance, and the length of time the blood and the dialysate remain in contact with the membrane. In patients with end-stage renal disease, hemodialysis usually is performed three times a week. Each session may last 4 to 5 hours.

HEMODIALYSIS

In **hemodialysis** the patient's heparinized blood is pumped through a surgically constructed **arteriovenous fistula** (an internal anastomosis between an artery and a vein) or an **arteriovenous graft** (a synthetic material grafted between the patient's artery and vein [Figure 30-6]). These internal shunts usually are located in the inner aspect of the patient's

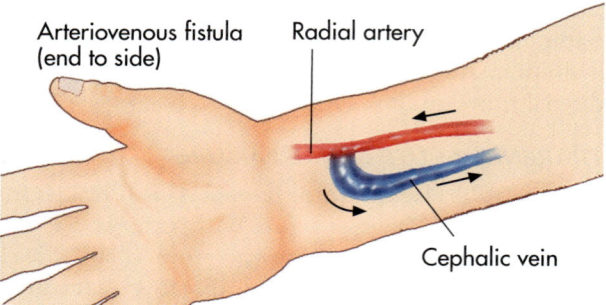

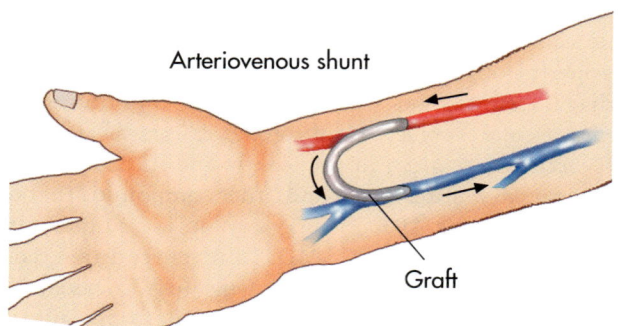

FIGURE 30-6 Arteriovenous shunts. (Ferguson DG, Fodden DI: *Accident and emergency medicine,* New York, 1998, Churchill Livingstone.)

forearm. Less often, they may be located in the upper arm or medial aspect of the lower extremity (see Chapter 52).

PERITONEAL DIALYSIS

In **peritoneal dialysis** the dialysis membrane is the patient's own peritoneum (Figure 30-7). The dialysate is infused into the peritoneal cavity by a temporary or permanently implanted catheter. Fluid and solutes diffuse from the blood in the peritoneal capillaries into the dialysate. Equilibration occurs after 1 to 2 hours. At this point, the dialysate is drained and fresh fluid is infused. Peritoneal dialysis works much more slowly than hemodialysis. Over time, however, it is just as effective. In addition, peritoneal dialysis does not require chronic blood access. A major complication of peritoneal dialysis is peritonitis. This usually results when the proper aseptic technique is not used. Peritoneal dialysis may be performed regularly in the home by the patient or by the family caregiver.

DIALYSIS EMERGENCIES

Emergencies the paramedic may encounter when caring for a patient with acute or chronic renal failure may result from the disease process itself or from complications of the dialysis. For example, these patients may experience problems associated with vascular access, hemorrhage, hypotension, chest pain, severe hyperkalemia, disequilibrium syndrome (described later), and the development of an air embolism. In addition, the paramedic should be aware of problems that may result from concurrent medical illness and its

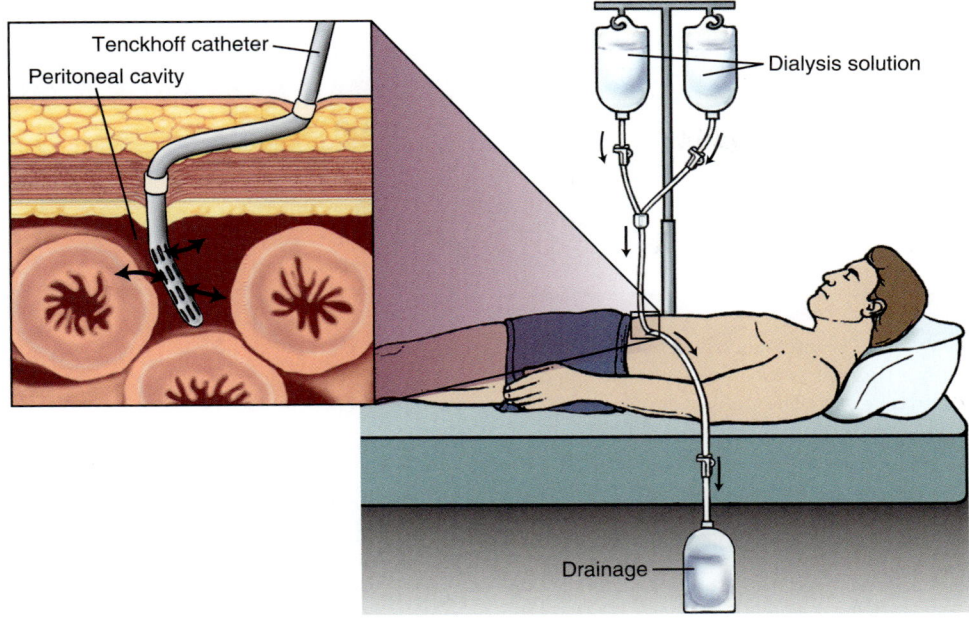

FIGURE 30-7 Peritoneal dialysis. (Linton AD: *Introduction to medical surgical nursing,* ed 4, St Louis, 2007, Saunders.)

treatment. Examples include decreased ability to tolerate the stress of significant illness or trauma, inadvertent over-administration of IV fluid, and altered metabolism and unpredictable action of drugs.

 NOTE
Renal failure is a common cause of pericardial disease, including pericarditis and pericardial effusions.[2] These conditions may result from uremia *(uremic pericarditis)* and may also occur in patients on maintenance dialysis. Most patients with pericardial disease complain of fever and pleuritic chest pain. The chest pain often is worsened by movement or breathing and may intensify when the patient is lying down. A pericardial friction rub may be audible. Signs of cardiac tamponade may be seen, particularly in patients with rapid accumulation of pericardial fluid.[7]

SHOW ME THE EVIDENCE
More than 50% of dialysis patients experience cardiac arrest in the first 5 years of hemodialysis. Davis and colleagues sought to describe the outcome of cardiac arrests at hemodialysis centers to which EMS responded. They examined the records of 110 patients who had a cardiac arrest that met their criteria between 1990 and 2004. Of that group, 104 patients suffered an arrest before EMS providers arrived. Four had return of spontaneous circulation (ROSC) before EMS providers arrived after dialysis center personnel defibrillated the patient with an automatic external defibrillator (AED). Ventricular fibrillation (VF) and pulseless ventricular tachycardia (VT) were reported in 67% of cases. When an AED was available, it was used in only 53% of arrests.

Davis TR, et al: Outcome of cardiac arrests attended by emergency medical services staff at community outpatient dialysis centers, *Kidney Int* 73:933-939, 2008.

CRITICAL THINKING
Which of these complications could pose an immediate threat to life?

Vascular Access Problems. Problems associated with vascular access include bleeding at the site of puncture for dialysis, thrombosis, and infection. Bleeding from the fistula or graft usually is minimal. The bleeding usually can be controlled by direct pressure at the site. (However, excessive pressure can cause thrombosis in the graft or fistula.) A rare but potential complication of an internal shunt is the development of a **pseudoaneurysm** (a dilation resembling an aneurysm that occurs at the site of the graft). The pseudoaneurysm can rupture and may cause a large hematoma and possible hypovolemia. If this occurs, the paramedic should apply direct pressure to the hematoma and assess and treat the patient for significant blood loss. This situation requires rapid transport for care by a physician.

Fistulae and grafts that become occluded as a result of thrombus formation usually require surgical intervention or the administration of a thrombolytic agent to restore flow. Patients with a surgical anastomosis are instructed to check periodically for a bruit or "thrill," which verifies unobstructed circulation. Attempts to clear the graft by irrigation or aspiration generally are not advised. If thrombosis occurs while the patient is undergoing dialysis, the dialysis should be stopped. Fluids then should be given intravenously in an alternative site. Decreased blood flow is a common trigger for thrombosis and is the main reason the blood pressure should not be taken in the arm with a vascular access.

An infection at the site of vascular access usually is the result of the puncture made during dialysis. Therefore, careful sterile technique is the rule when caring for these patients. Routine vascular access using the dialysis route should be discouraged. Vascular access infection should be considered when a dialysis patient has unexplained fever, malaise, or other signs of systemic infection.

> **NOTE**
> When drawing blood or intravenously infusing fluids in a patient with a surgical anastomosis, the paramedic should choose an alternative site. The paramedic also should avoid taking blood pressure measurements and using tourniquets in an extremity with an arteriovenous fistula or graft. In rare cases medical direction may advise using the internal shunt to obtain vascular access. If so, the paramedic must be careful not to puncture the back wall of the vessel. Careful, aseptic technique must be used during the procedure. IV infusions must be monitored closely to prevent a "runaway IV." Also, the IV catheter should be taped securely in place.

Hemorrhage. Patients undergoing dialysis are at increased risk of hemorrhage. This risk arises from their regular exposure to anticoagulants during hemodialysis and from the decrease in their platelet function. Therefore, a patient who experiences hemorrhage from trauma or a medical condition (e.g., gastrointestinal bleeding) should be monitored closely for signs of hypovolemia. Most patients on dialysis have anemia related to a decrease in the production of erythropoietin. This lowers their ability to compensate for blood loss when they have acute hemorrhage. Any significant blood loss (whether external or internal) may produce dyspnea or angina. If hemorrhage from trauma occurs in an extremity with a fistula or graft, the paramedic should control the bleeding and immobilize the extremity. Special care must be taken not to obstruct circulation in the anastomosis.

Hypotension. Hypotension can occur with hemodialysis. This may result from the rapid reduction in intravascular volume, abrupt changes in electrolyte concentrations, or vascular instability that may occur during the procedure. In addition, the patient's mechanisms for coping with these physiological changes may be impaired. This may result in an inability to maintain normal blood pressure. Patients with hypotension caused by dialysis must be managed cautiously with the administration of volume-expanding fluids. The paramedic should be careful not to produce a fluid overload. This may manifest as hypertension and the classic signs of congestive heart failure (Box 30-2). Most patients respond to a small fluid challenge (200 to 300 mL). If they do not, other potentially serious causes should be considered.

Chest Pain. The episodes of hypotension and mild hypoxemia that often occur during dialysis may result in

---

> ### BOX 30-2 Classic Signs of Congestive Heart Failure
>
> - Crackles
> - Engorged neck veins
> - Liver congestion and engorgement
> - Pitting edema
> - Pulmonary edema
> - Shortness of breath

myocardial ischemia and chest pain. The patient also may complain of other symptoms associated with decreased oxygen delivery, such as headache and dizziness. These complaints may indicate an evolving myocardial infarction. They often are relieved by the administration of oxygen, fluid replacement, and antianginal medications. Regardless, all patients with chest pain should be treated as though a myocardial infarction has occurred.

Dysrhythmias that result from myocardial ischemia also may be associated with dialysis. The most common ischemic rhythm disturbances are premature ventricular contractions. If dialysis is in progress, the procedure should be stopped and the paramedic should confer with medical direction.

Severe Hyperkalemia. Severe hyperkalemia is an emergency that poses a serious threat to life. It can occur rapidly in patients with acute renal failure. Severe hyperkalemia often results from poor dietary regulation and missed dialysis treatments. Patients with severe hyperkalemia may have weakness but often are asymptomatic. As described in Chapter 22, typical electrocardiographic (ECG) changes seen with hyperkalemia initially demonstrate a tall or tented T wave. As the potassium levels rise, conduction slows. This results in a prolonged P-R interval, depressed ST segments, and sometimes the loss of P waves. This may be followed by a widened QRS complex and delayed conduction in the interventricular conducting system. The ECG patterns resemble bundle branch blocks (Figure 30-8). Hyperkalemic disturbances may not become apparent until dangerous levels of potassium are present. Therefore, any patient with renal failure who is in cardiac arrest should be suspected of having severe hyperkalemia. Based on the patient history, medical direction may recommend separate administration of **calcium** and **sodium bicarbonate** during resuscitation. High-dose nebulized **albuterol** to reduce the plasma potassium concentration also has been reported to be effective.[8]

> 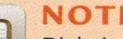 **NOTE**
> Dialysis patients with chronic renal failure tolerate increased potassium levels better than do patients with normal kidney function.

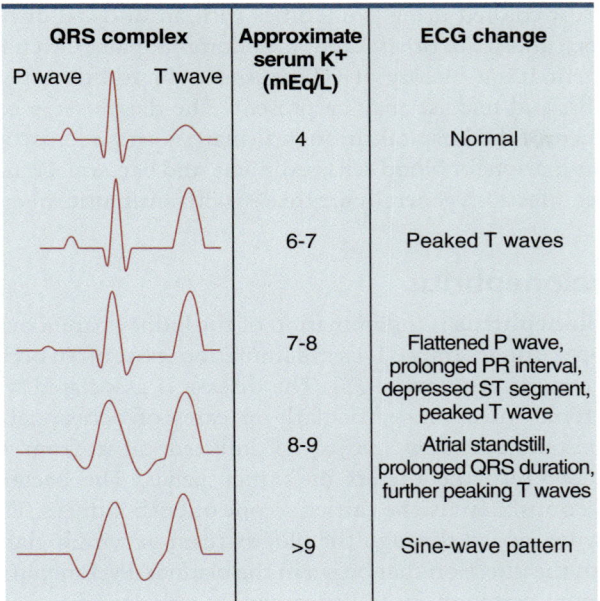

QRS complex	Approximate serum K⁺ (mEq/L)	ECG change
P wave T wave	4	Normal
	6-7	Peaked T waves
	7-8	Flattened P wave, prolonged PR interval, depressed ST segment, peaked T wave
	8-9	Atrial standstill, prolonged QRS duration, further peaking T waves
	>9	Sine-wave pattern

FIGURE 30-8 Electrocardiographic (ECG) changes seen in hyperkalemia. (Sole ML: *Introduction to critical care nursing*, ed 5, St Louis, 2009, Saunders.)

Disequilibrium Syndrome. Disequilibrium syndrome refers to a group of neurological findings that sometimes occur during or immediately after dialysis. These symptoms usually are mild (e.g., headache, restlessness, nausea, and fatigue), but they may be severe (confusion, seizures, and coma). The syndrome is thought to result from a disproportionate decrease in the osmolality of the extracellular fluid compared with that of the intracellular compartment in the brain or cerebrospinal fluid.[9] This results in an osmotic gradient between the blood and the brain. This in turn causes the movement of water into the brain and then cerebral edema and increased intracranial pressure. If seizures occur, an anticonvulsant may be indicated.

Air Embolism. Negative pressure on the venous side of the dialysis tubing or a malfunction in the machine can allow an air embolus to enter the patient's bloodstream. This is a rare occurrence. If air embolism occurs, the embolus may be carried to the right ventricle of the heart, where it may block the passage of blood to the left myocardium. The patient may experience severe dyspnea, cyanosis, hypotension, and respiratory distress. A patient with an air embolus requires high-concentration oxygen and rapid transport to a medical facility. In an effort to trap the embolism where it will be least likely to obstruct blood flow, the paramedic should position the patient on the left side. The patient should be transported in the modified Trendelenburg position.[10]

Management. To review, the prehospital management of patients with chronic or acute renal failure includes the following:

- Airway and ventilatory support with supplemental high-concentration oxygen
- Vascular access for fluid replacement, medication therapy (diuretics, antidysrhythmics, vasopressors), or fluid resuscitation if needed
- Meticulous aseptic technique during intravenous access
- ECG and other vital sign monitoring
- Rapid transport to an appropriate medical facility

URINARY SYSTEM CONDITIONS

There are many types of urinary tract diseases, which can range from mild to severe. Urinary system disorders that may cause acute pain include urinary retention, urinary tract infection (cystitis, urethritis), pyelonephritis, and renal calculi. As do disorders of the abdomen, urinary system disorders may produce visceral, somatic, and referred pain.

Urinary Retention

Urinary retention is the inability to urinate. Possible causes include urethral stricture, an enlarged prostate (benign or malignant *prostatic hypertrophy*), central nervous system (CNS) dysfunction, foreign body obstruction, and use of certain drugs, such as parasympatholytic or anticholinergic agents. Men develop urinary retention more often than women do, most commonly because of an enlarged prostate. However, other common causes can be found in both genders.

The signs and symptoms of urinary retention include severe abdominal pain associated with an urgent need to urinate and a distended bladder. The distended bladder often is palpable. Patients with a progressive obstruction, such as prostatic hypertrophy, often have a history of urinary hesitancy, a poor urine stream, a sense of incomplete emptying of the bladder, **nocturia** (excessive urination at night), and **overflow incontinence** (an overflow of urine from the bladder). The condition may also cause delirium, especially in elderly patients. In the emergency department, passage of a urethral catheter to empty the bladder often is required. Urinary retention is painful for the patient. Prehospital care for these patients mainly is supportive. If abdominal pain is present, an IV line to keep the vein open may be indicated. The cause of the retention should be sought; if it is not easily correctable after examination by a physician, the patient may require hospitalization. Some EMS systems may permit urinary catheterization in the prehospital setting to empty the patient's bladder (see Chapter 52).

> **CRITICAL THINKING**
> Have you ever been in a situation in which you needed to urinate urgently but could not because of the circumstances? How did you feel?

Urinary Tract Infection

Urinary tract infections (UTIs) account for 7 million to 8 million visits to physicians' offices each year and for 100,000 hospitalizations.[2] UTIs are the second most common problem seen by physicians, after respiratory tract infections. These infections usually develop first in the lower urinary tract (the urethra or bladder.) If left untreated, they can progress to the upper urinary tract (ureters or kidneys.) Upper tract infections often are associated with kidney infection (pyelonephritis, described later in this chapter) or abscesses that form in the kidney tissue. These conditions can lead to reduced kidney function, and untreated, severe cases can be fatal.

The more common lower UTI of the urethra **(urethritis)** and bladder **(cystitis)** occurs when enteric flora (particularly *Escherichia coli*, normally found in the bowel) enter the opening of the urethra and colonize the urinary tract. These infections are more common in women, because the urethra is short and close to the vagina and rectum. The infection also occurs in men (as a result of urethritis, prostatitis, and cystitis) and children. However, urethritis and prostatitis in young men most often results from venereal disease rather than a true UTI. Other factors that may contribute to a lower UTI include the use of contraceptive devices (women who use a diaphragm develop infections more often; condoms with spermicidal foam may cause the growth of *E. coli* in the vagina, which may enter the urethra), unsafe sexual practices, the presence of renal stones, bladder catheterization, and a suppressed immune system. In addition, men and women infected with *Chlamydia trachomatis* or *Mycoplasma hominis* can transmit the bacteria to their partner during sexual intercourse. These bacteria then could cause a UTI.

Signs and symptoms of UTI include painful or difficult urination **(dysuria),** urinary frequency, hematuria, cloudy or rust-colored urine (sometimes with an unusual or foul odor), and flank or suprapubic abdominal pain. Often the patient has a history of UTI episodes. In addition, fever, chills, and malaise may be present. The diagnosis is confirmed in the hospital through urinalysis and microscopic examination for blood cells, sediment, and bacteria. Urinary tract infections generally are treated with antibiotic therapy.

Pyelonephritis

Pyelonephritis is inflammation of the kidney parenchyma (upper urinary tract). This inflammation most often occurs as a result of a lower UTI. The disease is associated with bacterial infection, particularly in cases of occasional or persistent backflow (reflux) of infected urine from the bladder into the ureters or kidney pelvis. The bacterial infections may also be carried to one or both kidneys. They may be carried through the bloodstream or lymph glands from the infection that began in the bladder. Pyelonephritis is more common in adult women, but the condition can affect individuals of any age and either gender. Acute episodes can be severe in the elderly and in immunosuppressed people (e.g., those with cancer or acquired immunodeficiency syndrome [AIDS]).

The onset of signs and symptoms of pyelonephritis usually is abrupt. Patients often mistake the pain of pyelonephritis for lower back strain. The condition may be complicated by systemic infection, with signs and symptoms that include fever, chills, flank pain, cloudy or bloody urine, nausea, and vomiting. Left untreated, pyelonephritis can progress to a chronic condition that can last for months or years. It may lead to scarring and possible loss of kidney function. Therapeutic intervention consists primarily of antibiotics, fluid replacement, and sometimes hospitalization.

CRITICAL THINKING

How would you examine the patient for flank pain?

Urinary Calculus

Urinary calculi (kidney stones) are pathological concretions that originate in the renal pelvis. They are one of the most painful and most common disorders of the urinary tract, accounting for about 250,000 hospitalizations each year. It is estimated that 7% of men and 3% of women in the United States will have a kidney stone at some point in their lives.[2] Kidney stones result from supersaturation of the urine with insoluble salts. When the level of insoluble salts or uric acid in the urine is high, the urine lacks *citrate* (a chemical that normally inhibits the formation of stones). Kidney stones also can form if insufficient water is present in the kidneys to dissolve waste product,. Kidney stones are more common in men than in women; they most often occur in men between the ages of 20 and 50, and the disease is recurrent. Associated risk factors for this condition include dehydration, CNS disorders (absent sensory/motor impulses from injury or disease), drug use (anesthetics, opiates, psychotropic agents, some herbal medicines), and surgery (postoperative complication).

SHOW ME THE EVIDENCE

Safdar and coworkers conducted a randomized, controlled study to evaluate pain management in 130 patients presumed to have kidney stones. One group was treated with IV morphine, another with IV ketorolac, and the third group received both drugs. The group that receive the combination of morphine and ketorolac had better pain relief. This group also experienced less nausea and vomiting than the morphine group.

Safdar B et al: Intravenous morphine plus ketorolac is superior to either drug alone for treatment of acute renal colic, *Ann Emerg Med* 48:173-181, 2006.

The chemical composition of the kidney stones depends on the chemical imbalance in the urine. The four most common types of stones are composed of calcium, uric acid, struvite, and cystine. Calcium stones are calcium compounds that are chemically bound to oxalate (most common) or phosphate; they account for about 85% of all kidney stones. Calcium stones typically occur in patients with metabolic (e.g., gout) or hormonal disorders (e.g., hyperparathyroidism). Stones composed of uric acid account for about 10% of kidney stones; their formation is more common in men. These stones may have a heritable component. Struvite stones (also known as infection stones) are more common in women. These stones often are linked to chronic bacterial UTI or frequent bladder catheterization. Cystine stones are the least common and result from a rare congenital condition that results in large amounts of cystine (an amino acid) in the urine. Cystine stones are difficult to treat and may require lifelong therapy.

Signs and symptoms of urinary calculus vary according to the location of the stones. Most stones obstruct the ureters at points where they narrow in their passage from the kidneys to the bladder. This produces acute, excruciating pain. The pain originates in the flank area and radiates to the right or left lower abdominal quadrant, groin, and testes (in males). Renal or ureteral colic produces severe cyclical pain. The pain occurs as the ureter tries to use forceful contractions to push the stone into the bladder. This pain often has been described as having the same intensity as labor pain. The pain may be accompanied by restlessness, nausea and vomiting, urinary urgency or frequency, diaphoresis, low-grade fever, hematuria, dysuria, and elevated blood pressure (because of the pain). Prehospital care may include IV fluids, transport in a position of comfort,

BOX 30-3 Strategies for Preventing the Recurrence of Renal Calculi

The composition of a kidney stone determines the strategy used to prevent the formation of more stones. Patients may be advised to do the following:

- Increase water consumption
- Avoid foods containing calcium oxalate (e.g., chocolate, celery, grapes, strawberries, beans, and asparagus)
- Take daily supplements of vitamin B_6 and magnesium (to reduce the formation of oxalates)
- Avoid foods that raise uric acid levels (e.g., anchovies and sardines)
- Reduce uric acid by eating a low-protein diet
- Limit salt intake to reduce the level of calcium oxalate in the urine

antiemetics, and pain management as needed (***nitrous oxide, ketorolac,*** narcotic analgesics). Care by a physician may include analgesics (anesthetics, opiates, psychotropics), fluid replacement, antiemetics, and possibly hospitalization. If the calculus does not pass spontaneously, surgical intervention may be required (Box 30-3).

NOTE

It is not uncommon for "drug seekers" to feign symptoms of kidney stones to obtain narcotics. Most hospitals check the patient's urine for blood before providing narcotics. Blood in the urine in a symptomatic patient indicates that a kidney stone is passing through the ureters.

CRITICAL THINKING

Have you cared for or known someone who had a urinary calculus? How did that person describe the pain? What was the level of discomfort?

MALE GENITAL TRACT CONDITIONS

Paramedics encounter numerous genital tract conditions in the prehospital setting. Some may be related to disease; others may be the result of trauma (traumatic conditions are presented in Chapter 43: Abdominal and Genitourinary Trauma). Disorders of the male genital tract discussed in this chapter include epididymitis, Fournier's gangrene, and various structural conditions (phimosis, priapism, benign prostatic hypertrophy, testicular masses, and testicular torsion). The anatomy of the male genital tract is presented in Chapter 10.

LOOK AGAIN

See Chapter 10: Review of Human Systems, pp. 201-202.

Epididymitis

Epididymitis is inflammation of the epididymis, a tubular section of the male reproductive system that carries sperm from the testicle to the seminal vesicles. Epididymitis often is caused by a bacterial infection associated with other structures of the genitourinary tract. Infection tends to occur in sexually active young men. The most common type of epididymitis in young men results from venereal disease. In men older than age 35, urinary tract pathogens are the most common cause.[2]

The signs and symptoms of epididymitis include a gradual onset of unilateral scrotal pain that radiates to the spermatic cord. At times, tender swelling of the scrotum and testicle occurs. This swelling produces inflammation of one or both testes (**orchitis**). The patient may have a recent history of UTI, fever, and malaise, and a urethral discharge may be present. After evaluation by a physician, therapeutic intervention includes antibiotics, bed rest, analgesics, and elevation of the scrotum.

Fournier's Gangrene

Fournier's gangrene is a bacterial infection of the skin that affects the genitals and perineum in both men and women. It is a urological emergency that results after a wound or an abrasion becomes infected. A combination of microorganisms (e.g., staphylococci) and fungi (e.g., yeast) causes the infection to spread. It can lead to necrosis of the skin, subcutaneous tissue, and muscle. Fournier's gangrene can be fatal if the infection enters the bloodstream, causing sepsis, shock, and organ failure. Men are 10 times more likely to develop the disease. Men 60 to 80 years of age who have predisposing conditions are the most susceptible. Predisposing factors and conditions include alcoholism, IV drug use, genital piercing, obesity, diabetes, leukemia, and immune system disorders. The condition also can develop as a complication of surgery. Hallmarks of the disease are intense pain and tenderness in the genitalia (Figure 30-9).

Depending on the stage of disease, assessment findings in the genital area may include crepitus of the skin, gray-black coloration from decay (gangrene), drainage of pus, and fever.[1] Fournier's gangrene usually progresses through five stages[11]:

1. Prodromal symptoms of fever and lethargy, which may be present for 2 to 7 days
2. Intense genital pain and tenderness, usually associated with edema of the overlying skin
3. Increasing genital pain and tenderness with progressive erythema of the overlying skin
4. Dusky appearance of the overlying skin; subcutaneous crepitation
5. Obvious gangrene of a portion of the genitalia; purulent drainage from wounds

Prehospital care may range from providing only emotional support and rapid transport to full resuscitation measures to manage shock. After the patient's condition has been stabilized, care by a physician includes various methods to restore normal organ perfusion and function. These methods may include antibiotic therapy, hyperbaric oxygen therapy, and surgery (including reconstruction).

Phimosis

Phimosis is tightness of the **prepuce** (foreskin) of the penis. The condition prevents retraction of the foreskin over the glans (Figure 30-10). It can be caused by failure of the foreskin to loosen during growth, infection, genital disease, and trauma. Phimosis usually is a painless condition. However, infection can occur with ineffective cleaning of the penis, resulting in swelling, redness, and discharge. In rare cases a patient may complain of problems with urination or intercourse.

> **? DID YOU KNOW?**
>
> Circumcision is the surgical removal of the foreskin. The procedure often is performed on healthy boys for cultural or religious reasons. In the United States, if a newborn is to be circumcised, the procedure usually is done before the infant leaves the hospital. Jewish boys, however, are circumcised when they are 8 days old. In other parts of the world, including Europe, Asia, and South and Central America, circumcision is rare in the general population. The merits of circumcision have been debated. Opinions about the need for circumcision in healthy boys vary among health care professionals. Some believe there is great value to having an intact foreskin, such as allowing for a more natural sexual response during adulthood. Rather than routinely recommending circumcision for healthy boys, the American Academy of Pediatrics and the American Medical Association recommend that parents make an informed decision based on accurate, nonbiased information.[12]

Paraphimosis is inability to pull the retracted foreskin back over the head of the penis. This condition can restrict blood flow and requires emergency care. A hallmark sign of paraphimosis is a "doughnut" of swollen skin around the

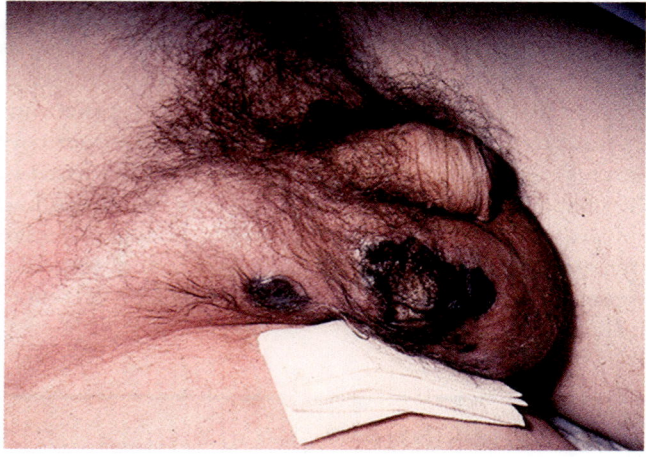

FIGURE 30-9 Fournier's gangrene. (Courtesy Mark Dropkin, M.D., Newton Wellesley Hospital, Newton, Mass.)

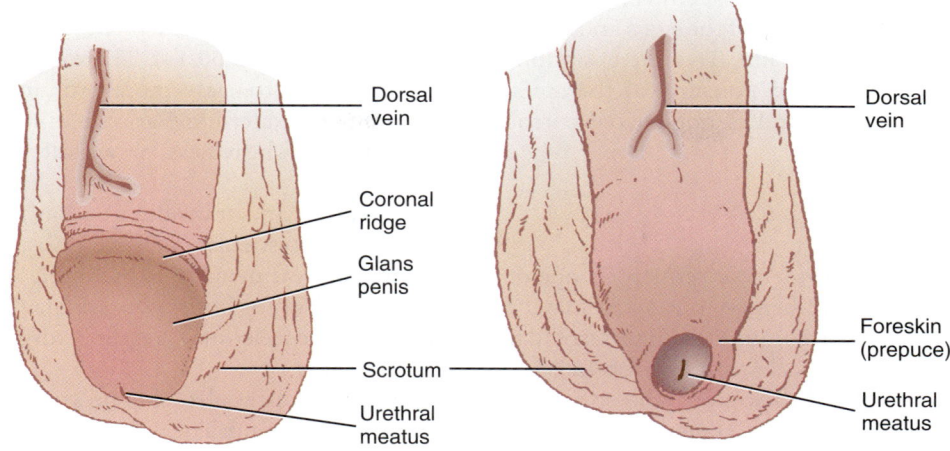

FIGURE 30-10 Appearance of the penis. **A,** Circumcised. **B,** Uncircumcised. (Linton AD: *Introduction to medical surgical nursing,* ed 4, St Louis, 2007, Saunders.)

shaft, near the head of the penis. Paraphimosis occurs most often in children and the elderly. If left untreated, it can disrupt blood flow to the tip of the penis.[13] In severe cases this can lead to damage of the tip of the penis, gangrene, and loss of the penis tip. Emergency care may include gentle compression of the head of the penis while pushing the foreskin forward or wrapping the penis in plastic and applying ice to reduce swelling, allowing the foreskin to return to its extended position. If this fails, the patient may require hospitalization and surgical circumcision.

Priapism

Priapism is a persistent, usually painful, erection that lasts 4 hours or longer and occurs without sexual stimulation. The condition develops when blood in the penis becomes trapped and unable to drain. If the condition is not treated immediately, it can lead to scarring and permanent erectile dysfunction. Priapism can occur in all age groups, including newborns. However, it usually affects male children between 5 and 10 years of age and men between 20 and 50 years of age. Priapism is subcategorized into two types, low flow and high flow.

- *Low-flow priapism* results when blood is trapped in the erection chambers of the penis. It often occurs for unknown reasons in men who are otherwise healthy. This type also affects men with sickle cell disease, leukemia and other cancers, or malaria.
- *High-flow priapism* is less common than the low-flow type and usually less painful. The condition results from a ruptured artery, which occurs because of an injury to the penis or the perineum. The rupture prevents blood in the penis from circulating normally.

> **NOTE**
> Sickle cell disease (see Chapter 32) is a common cause of priapism in men. About 42% of men with the disease eventually develop priapism.[2]

Some medications can cause priapism. Examples include antidepressants (e.g., Desyrel), antipsychotics (e.g., Thorazine), injection drugs used to treat erectile dysfunction (ED), and oral ED drugs (e.g., Viagra). Other causes of priapism include trauma to the spinal cord or genital area, black widow spider bites, carbon monoxide poisoning, and illicit drug use (e.g., marijuana and cocaine). Prehospital care for a patient with priapism is primarily supportive. All patients should be transported and evaluated by a physician.

Benign Prostatic Hypertrophy

Benign prostatic hypertrophy (BPH) is enlargement of the prostate gland. As described in Chapter 10, the prostate gland is the male organ that produces prostatic fluid, a component of semen. It sits beneath the bladder and surrounds the urethra. Most men have a period of prostate growth in their middle to late 40s, when cells in the central portion of the gland reproduce rapidly. As tissues in the area enlarge, they often compress the urethra and may partly block the flow of urine.

> **NOTE**
> The prostate gland is assessed during a rectal examination. The physician palpates the gland for size, consistency, nodularity, and tenderness. In benign prostatic hypertrophy (BPH), the gland is smooth, symmetrical, and feels slightly rubbery. In contrast, a cancerous prostate may feel asymmetrical and have a stony-hard consistency. Discrete nodules may be palpable. Marked prostatic tenderness suggests **acute prostatitis**. If a patient has signs and symptoms of prostate irregularities, his blood may be tested for prostate-specific antigen (PSA); if this value is elevated, the prostate may be biopsied to rule out cancer.

Not all men with BPH are symptomatic. However, some complain of urinary frequency, a weak urine stream, difficulty starting and stopping urination, overflow incontinence, hematuria, and urinary tract infection. Treatment of BPH depends on the severity of the signs and symptoms and how they affect daily life. Treatment options include medications, surgery, and nonsurgical therapies. Enlargement of the prostate gland is not related to the development of prostate cancer.

Testicular Masses

A **testicular mass** is an enlargement or growth on one or both testicles. Most masses are benign, but some may be malignant. Three of the most common benign testicular masses are hydroceles, spermatoceles, and varicoceles.

A **hydrocele** is a fluid-filled sack along the spermatic cord in the scrotum (Figure 30-11). A **spermatocele** is a benign cystic accumulation of sperm that arises from the head of the epididymis (Figures 30-12 and 30-13). Both conditions result in collections of fluid in the scrotal sac. These masses are generally soft and painless. Their size can change rapidly as fluid enters or leaves the scrotum. A **varicocele** is an enlargement of the veins that drain the testicles (Figure 30-14). These masses are soft, scrotal swellings that often are more prominent when the man is standing or exercising. Varicoceles sometimes may cause a sensation of heaviness or a dull ache in the genital area.

Ultrasound and transillumination techniques are used to diagnose testicular masses. Most testicular masses require no treatment. If a hydrocele or spermatocele is large or painful (or both), surgery may be needed to drain fluid. A varicocele may require surgery to tie off the affected veins.

Testicular cancer also may present as a testicular mass, with or without pain. The mass usually feels firm and arises from the testicle. The diagnosis is made using blood tests and scrotal ultrasound. Treatment involves surgery to remove the affected testicle, chemotherapy, and/or radiation. Testicular cancer is the most common cause of cancer

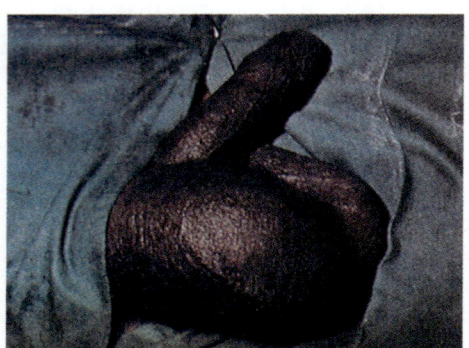

FIGURE 30-11 Hydrocele.

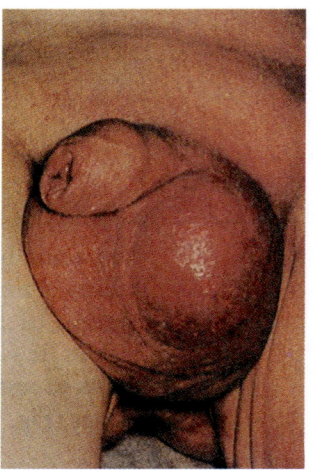

FIGURE 30-13 Epididymis.

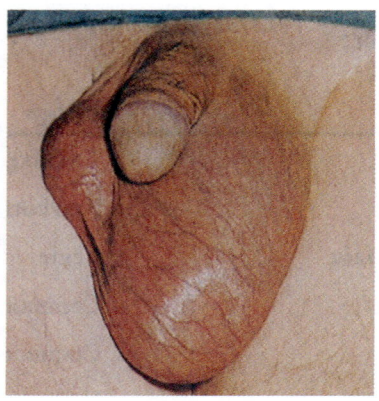

FIGURE 30-12 Spermatocele.

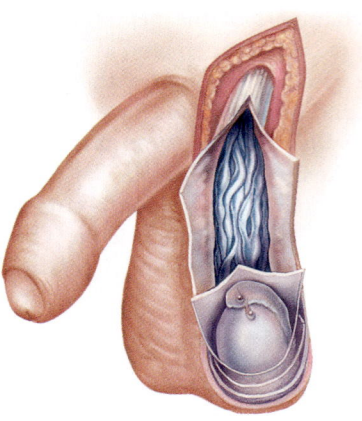

FIGURE 30-14 Varicocele.

TABLE 30-4 Abnormalities in the Scrotum

Disorder	Clinical Findings	Comments
Testicular torsion 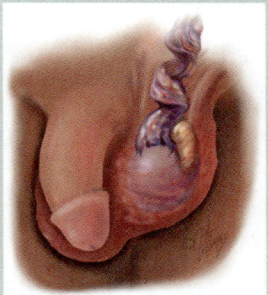 From Jarvis C: *Physical examination and health assessment,* ed 5, St Louis, 2007, Saunders.	S: Sudden onset of excruciating pain in testicle, often during sleep or after trauma; patient may also have lower abdominal pain, nausea and vomiting, no fever O: Inspection—Red, swollen scrotum, one testis (usually left) higher because of rotation and shortening Palpation—Cord feels thick, swollen, tender; epididymis may be anterior; cremasteric reflex absent on side of torsion A: Testicular torsion	Sudden twisting of the spermatic cord usually occurs in late childhood, early adolescence; it is rare after age 20. Torsion usually occurs on the left side. Faulty anchoring of the testis on the scrotal wall allows the testis to rotate. The anterior part of the testis rotates medially toward the other testis. Blood supply is cut off, resulting in ischemia and engorgement. This is an emergency that requires surgery; the testis can become gangrenous in a few hours.
Epididymitis 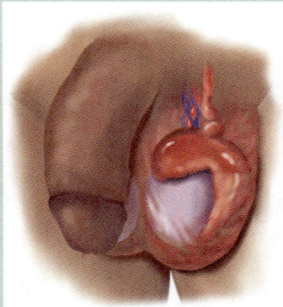 From Jarvis C: *Physical examination and health assessment,* ed 5, St Louis, 2007, Saunders.	S: Sudden onset of severe pain in scrotum, which is somewhat relieved by elevation (positive Phren's sign); also, rapid swelling, fever O: Inspection—Enlarged, reddened scrotum Palpation—Exquisitely tender; epididymis enlarged, indurated, and may be difficult to distinguish from testis; overlying scrotal skin may be thick and edematous Laboratory—White blood cells and bacteria in urine A: Tender swelling of epididymis	Acute infection of the epididymis commonly occurs as a result of prostatitis; after prostatectomy because of the trauma of urethral instrumentation; or because of a chlamydial, gonorrheal, or other bacterial infection. Differentiating between epididymitis and testicular torsion often is difficult.
Spermatic cord varicocele 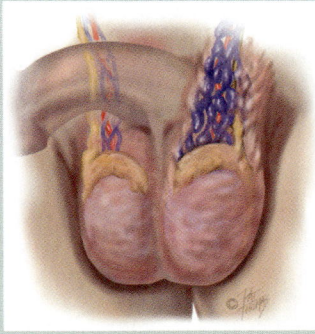 From Jarvis C: *Physical examination and health assessment,* ed 5, St Louis, 2007, Saunders.	S: Dull pain; constant pulling or dragging feeling; or may be asymptomatic O: Inspection—Usually no sign; may show bluish color through light scrotal skin Palpation—When patient is standing, a soft, irregular mass is felt posterior to and above the testis; this mass collapses when the patient is supine and refills when he is upright; mass feels distinctive, like a "bag of worms"; testis on the side of the varicocele may be smaller because of impaired circulation A: Soft mass on spermatic cord	A varicocele is dilated, tortuous varicose veins in the spermatic cord resulting from incompetent valves in the vein; this permits the reflux of blood. Varicoceles are found most often on the left side, perhaps because the left spermatic vein is longer and inserts at a right angle into the left renal vein. The condition is common in young men. Screening should be done in early adolescence; early treatment is important to prevent the possibility of infertility in adulthood.

Continued

TABLE 30-4—cont'd

Disorder	Clinical Findings	Comments
Spermatocele 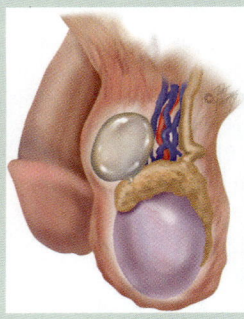 From Jarvis C: *Physical examination and health assessment,* ed 5, St Louis, 2007, Saunders.	*S:* Painless, usually found on examination *O:* Inspection—Transilluminates higher in the scrotum than a hydrocele; sperm may fluoresce Palpation—Round, freely movable mass lying above and behind testis; if large, feels like a third testis *A:* Free cystic mass on epididymis	Retention cyst in the epididymis. The cause is unclear but may be obstruction of tubules. Cyst is filled with thin, milky fluid that contains sperm. Most spermatoceles are small (about 1 cm); occasionally they may be larger, and they then are mistaken for a hydrocele.
Diffuse tumor 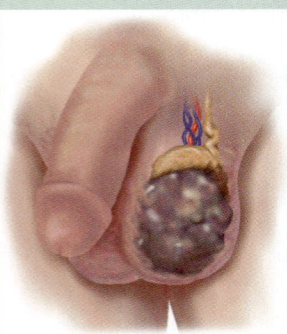 From Jarvis C: *Physical examination and health assessment,* ed 5, St Louis, 2007, Saunders.	*S:* Enlarging testis (most common symptom); when enlarged, it has the feel of increased weight *O:* Inspection—Enlarged testis, does not transilluminate Palpation—Enlarged, smooth, ovoid, firm Important—Firm palpation does *not* cause usual sickening discomfort seen with normal testis *A:* Nontender swelling of testis	Diffuse tumor maintains the shape of the testis.
Hydrocele 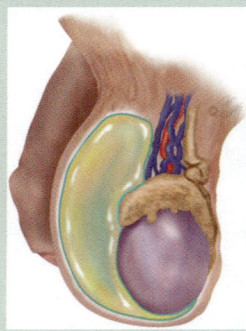 From Jarvis C: *Physical examination and health assessment,* ed 5, St Louis, 2007, Saunders.	*S:* Painless swelling, although the patient may complain of weight and bulk in the scrotum *O:* Inspection—Enlarged; mass transilluminates with a pink or red glow (in contrast to a hernia) Palpation—Nontender mass; able to get fingers above mass (in contrast to scrotal hernia) *A:* Nontender swelling of testis	Cystic, circumscribed collection of serous fluid in the tunica vaginalis, surrounding the testis. It may occur after epididymitis, trauma, hernia, or tumor of the testis, or spontaneously in the newborn.

TABLE 30-4—cont'd

Disorder	Clinical Findings	Comments
Scrotal hernia 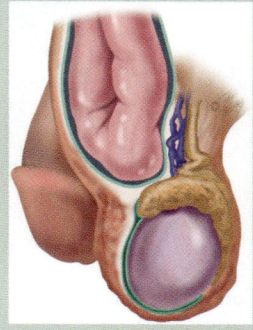 From Jarvis C: *Physical examination and health assessment*, ed 5, St Louis, 2007, Saunders.	S: Swelling; may have pain with straining O: Inspection—Enlarged; may reduce when patient is supine; does not transilluminate Palpation—Soft, mushy mass; palpating fingers cannot get above mass; mass is distinct from normal testicle A: Nontender swelling of scrotum	Scrotal hernia usually is due to indirect inguinal hernia (see Table 24-6).
Orchitis 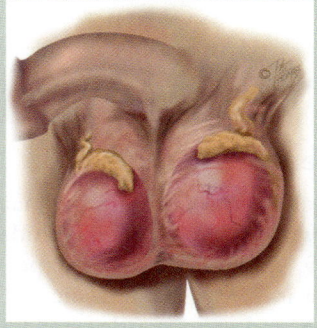 From Jarvis C: *Physical examination and health assessment*, ed 5, St Louis, 2007, Saunders.	S: Sudden onset of acute or moderate pain; swollen testis; feeling of weight; fever O: Inspection—Enlarged, edematous, reddened; does not transilluminate Palpation—Swollen, congested, tense, and tender; difficult to distinguish testis from epididymis A: Tender swelling of testis	Acute inflammation of testis. Most common cause is mumps, although it can occur with any infectious disease. Patient may have an associated hydrocele that transilluminates.

From Jarvis C: *Physical examination and health assessment*, ed 5, St Louis, 2007, Saunders.
S, Subjective data; O, objective data; A, assessment.

in men 15 to 34 years of age; it occurs most often between the ages of 20 and 39. Monthly self-examination of the testicles is recommended for men in this age group. Each year more than 8000 new cases of testicular cancer are diagnosed in the United States, and about 380 men die of the disease.[14]

Testicular Torsion

Testicular torsion is a true urological emergency. In this condition, a testicle (usually the left) twists on its spermatic cord, disrupting the blood supply of the testicle. The condition may result from blunt trauma to the scrotal area, but more often it is spontaneous. The two peak periods in which torsion is likely to occur are the first year of life and puberty[2] (the age range is 5 months to 41 years, and the average age of occurrence is 14 years).

Like epididymitis, testicular torsion results in a tender epididymis and painful swelling of the scrotal sac (Figure 30-15). Unlike in epididymitis, however, the patient usually is afebrile. The pain is sudden in onset and usually severe. It often is preceded by vigorous physical activity or an athletic event. The pain sometimes radiates to the ipsilateral left quadrant; is unrelieved by rest or scrotal elevation; and often is associated with nausea and vomiting. Testicular torsion must be diagnosed and treated within 6 hours to prevent loss of the testis from ischemic infarction.[15] Therapeutic intervention includes the application of ice packs to the scrotum and manual manipulation by a physician to reduce the torsion. The patient must undergo surgical repair within 4 to 6 hours of onset of the torsion. Therefore, rapid transport to the emergency department and early recognition are critical for treatment.

PHYSICAL EXAMINATION OF PATIENTS WITH GENITOURINARY OR RENAL DISORDERS

As described in Chapter 20, assessment of the abdomen and genitalia of either gender can be awkward and uncomfortable for the patient and the paramedic. The paramedic should protect the patient's privacy with proper drapes to ensure privacy. When possible, paramedics of the same gender as the patient should perform these examinations. If this is not possible, a chaperone should be present. The paramedic should proceed with a calm, caring, and competent attitude. The patient and significant others should be informed of all actions. As in the care of a patient with an abdominal complaint (see Chapter 29), the examination should include the following:

- Primary assessment
- Focused history
  - OPQRST (*o*nset/origin, *p*rovokes, *q*uality, *r*egion, *s*everity, *t*ime)
  - Previous history of similar event
  - Nausea or vomiting
  - Change in bowel habits or stool (constipation, diarrhea)
  - Change in urinary voiding pattern
  - Weight loss
  - Last oral intake
  - Last bowel movement
- Physical examination
  - Appearance
  - Posture
  - Level of consciousness
  - Apparent state of health
  - Skin color
  - Vital signs
  - Abdominal examination (inspection, auscultation, percussion, palpation)
  - Examination of the genitalia (if indicated)

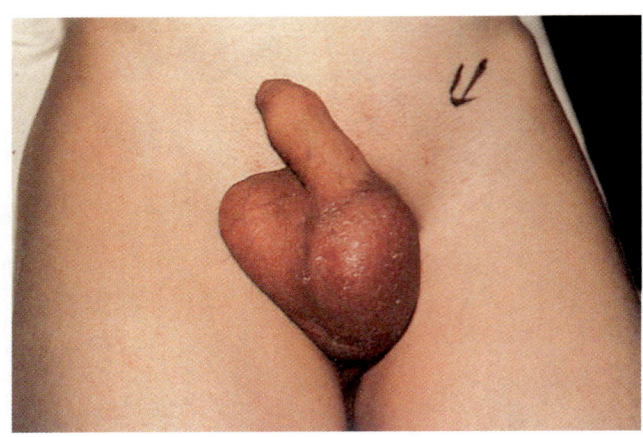

FIGURE 30-15 Four-day old torsion of the left testis.

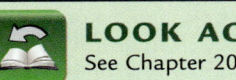
LOOK AGAIN
See Chapter 20: Secondary Assessment, pp. 542-546.

Management and Treatment Plan

The paramedic should manage patients with genitourinary disorders as any other patient with acute pain. This includes providing airway, ventilatory, and circulatory support; administering high-concentration oxygen (if indicated); ECG and vital sign monitoring; and rapid, gentle transportation for evaluation by a physician in the patient's position of comfort. Patients should not be permitted to eat or drink, because surgery may be indicated. All patients who have had persistent genitourinary pain or discomfort for several hours should be transported for evaluation by a physician.

SUMMARY

- The urinary system removes waste products from the blood. It also helps maintain a constant body fluid volume and composition.
- The nephron is the functional unit of the kidney. It filters blood, removes waste products, and produces urine.
- Renal failure may result in uremia, hyperkalemia, acidosis, hypertension, and volume overload with congestive heart failure.
- Acute renal failure occurs when the kidneys are unable to excrete the daily load of toxins in the urine. Its onset may be within hours.

- Prerenal ARF results from poor perfusion of the kidneys. Intrarenal ARF is caused by conditions that damage the tissues of the kidney. Postrenal ARF is caused by obstruction of urine flow from both kidneys.
- Dialysis is a technique used to normalize blood chemistry in patients with acute or chronic renal failure. It also is used to remove blood toxins. The two dialysis techniques are hemodialysis and peritoneal dialysis. Dialysis emergencies may include problems with vascular access, hemorrhage, hypotension, chest pain, severe hyperkalemia, disequilibrium syndrome, air embolism, or cardiac arrest.

- Urinary retention is the inability to urinate.
- Urinary tract infections can involve the upper or lower urinary tract.
- Pyelonephritis is inflammation of the kidney parenchyma. It can lead to chronic renal problems.
- Urinary calculi are stones that originate in the kidney.
- Epididymitis is inflammation of the epididymis. The epididymis is the tube that carries sperm from the testicle to the seminal vesicles.
- Fournier's gangrene is a bacterial infection of the genitals that can lead to death of skin tissue and systemic sepsis.
- Phimosis is tightness of the foreskin of the penis. Paraphimosis occurs when a male is unable to retract the foreskin over the head of the penis.

- Priapism is a painful, sustained erection.
- Benign prostatic hypertrophy is enlargement of the prostate gland. It may be associated with urinary difficulty and urinary tract infections.
- Testicular masses may be benign or cancerous.
- In testicular torsion a testicle twists on its spermatic cord, disrupting the blood supply to the testicle. This is a true emergency
- The physical examination for a patient with a urinary tract problem is similar to that for abdominal pain. Patients with genitourinary pain should be managed in the same way as any other patient with acute pain.

REFERENCES

1. National Highway Traffic Safety Administration: *The National EMS Education Standards*, Washington, DC, 2009, U.S. Department of Transportation/National Highway Traffic Safety Administration, DOT.
2. Marx J, Hockberger R, Walls R: *Rosen's emergency medicine: concepts and clinical practice*, St Louis, 2006, Mosby.
3. National Diabetes Information Clearinghouse: *Diabetes, heart disease and stroke*. http://diabetes.niddk.nih.gov/dm/pubs/stroke/. Accessed September 6, 2010.
4. Goldberg R, Dennen P: Long-term outcomes of acute kidney injury, *Adv Chronic Kidney Dis* 15:297-307, 2008.
5. Humes D, editor: *Kelly's essentials of internal medicine*, ed 2, Philadelphia, 2001, Lippincott Williams & Wilkins.
6. Kurokawa K, Nangaku M, Saito A, et al: Current issues and future perspectives of chronic renal failure, *J Am Soc Nephrol* 13:S3-S6, 2002.
7. Alpert MA, Ravenscraft MD: Pericardial involvement in end-stage renal disease, *Am J Med Sci* 325:228-236, 2003.
8. American Heart Association. 2010 American Heart Association Guidelines for Cardiopulmonary Resuscitation and Emergency Cardiovascular Care. *Circulation* 122(18 Supplement 3):S639-S946, 2010.
9. Im L, Atabay C, Eller AW: Papilledema associated with dialysis disequilibrium syndrome, *Semin Ophthalmol* 22:133-135, 2007.
10. Ahmad S: *Manual of clinical dialysis*, ed 2, New York, 2009, Springer Verlag.
11. Santora T: *Fournier gangrene*. http://emedicine.medscape.com/article/438994-overview. Accessed September 13, 2010.
12. American Academy of Pediatrics, Task Force on Circumcision: *Circumcision policy statement*. http://aappolicy.aappublications.org/cgi/content/full/pediatrics;103/3/686. Accessed September 13, 2010.
13. Jordan GH, Schlossberg SML: Surgery of the penis and urethra. In Wein AJ, editor: *Campbell-Walsh urology*, ed 9, Philadelphia, 2007, Saunders.
14. National Cancer Institute: Testicular cancer. www.cancer.gov/cancertopics/types/testicular. Accessed November 13, 2009.
15. Ringdahl E, Teague L: Testicular torsion, *Am Fam Physician* 74:1739-1743, 2006.

SUGGESTED READING

Davis TR, et al: Outcome of cardiac arrests attended by emergency medical services staff at community outpatient dialysis centers, *Kidney Int* 73:933-939, 2008.

31 Gynecology

OBJECTIVES

Upon completion of this chapter, the paramedic student will be able to:

1. Describe the physiological processes of menstruation and ovulation.
2. Describe the pathophysiology of the following nontraumatic causes of abdominal pain in females: pelvic inflammatory disease, Bartholin's abscess, vaginitis, ruptured ovarian cyst, ovarian torsion, cystitis, dysmenorrhea, mittelschmerz, endometriosis, ectopic pregnancy, vaginal bleeding, uterine prolapse, and vaginal foreign body.
3. Outline the prehospital assessment and management of a female with abdominal pain or bleeding.
5. Outline the specific assessment and management of a patient who has been sexually assaulted.
6. Describe specific prehospital measures to preserve evidence in sexual assault cases.

KEY TERMS

Bartholin's abscess An accumulation of pus that forms a lump in one of the Bartholin's glands; it results when blockage of the gland's duct allows infection to develop.

cesarean delivery A surgical procedure in which the abdomen and uterus are incised and the baby is delivered transabdominally.

cystitis Inflammation of the urinary bladder and ureters.

date rape Nonconsensual sex between people who are already acquainted (e.g., friends, acquaintances, or people who are dating).

dilation and curettage (D & C) A gynecological procedure in which the uterine cervix is widened and the endometrium of the uterus is scraped away.

dysfunctional uterine bleeding (DUB) Abnormal bleeding that occurs because of changes in hormone levels.

dysmenorrhea Pain associated with menstruation.

dyspareunia Pain with intercourse.

ectopic pregnancy An abnormal pregnancy in which the conceptus implants outside the uterine cavity.

endometriosis An abnormal gynecological condition characterized by ectopic growth and function of endometrial tissue. It is thought to result when fragments of endometrium from the lining of the uterus are regurgitated during menstruation backward through the fallopian tubes into the peritoneal cavity; there, they attach and grow as small cystic structures.

endometritis An inflammatory condition of the endometrium, usually caused by bacterial infection.

endometrium The mucous membrane lining of the uterus, which changes in thickness and structure with the menstrual cycle.

external genital organs The outer parts of the female genitalia; they consist of the labia majora, the labia minora, Bartholin's glands, and the clitoris. Also known as the *vulva.*

fallopian tubes A pair of ducts that open at one end into the uterus and at the other end into the peritoneal cavity, over the ovaries; also known as *uterine tubes.*

hysterectomy The surgical removal of the uterus.

mammary glands External accessory sex organs in females; breasts.

menarche The first menstruation and commencement of the cyclic menstrual function.

menopause The cessation of menses.

menstruation The periodic discharge through the vagina of a blood secretion containing tissue debris from the shedding of the endometrium from the nonpregnant uterus.

mittelschmerz Abdominal pain in the region of the ovary during ovulation; it usually occurs midway through the menstrual cycle.

oocytes Incompletely developed ova.

ovarian torsion Twisting of an ovary around its vascular pedicle.

ovaries A pair of female gonads, one on each side of the lower abdomen beside the uterus.

ovulation The release of an ovum or secondary oocyte from the vesicular follicle.

pelvic inflammatory disease (PID) Any inflammatory condition of the female pelvic organs, especially one caused by bacterial infection.

rape Nonconsensual sex or an attempt to force another person to have sex against his or her will; it includes intercourse in the vagina, anus, or mouth.

ruptured ovarian cyst A ruptured globular sac filled with fluid or semisolid material that develops in or on the ovary.

sexual assault The forcible perpetration of an act of sexual contact on the body of another person, male or female, without his or her consent.

uterine prolapse The falling or sliding of the uterus from its normal position in the pelvic cavity into the vaginal canal.

uterus The hollow, pear-shaped internal female organ of reproduction.

vagina The part of the female genitalia that forms a canal from the orifice through the vestibule to the uterine cervix.

vaginal bleeding The loss of blood from the uterus, cervix, or vagina.

vaginitis Inflammation of the vaginal tissues.

zygote The developing ovum from the time it is fertilized until it is implanted in the uterus as a blastocyst.

A number of disorders can occur in the female reproductive system. Some of these can lead to gynecological emergencies. This chapter discusses the causes of and emergency care for problems associated with the female reproductive system and the treatment of victims of sexual assault.

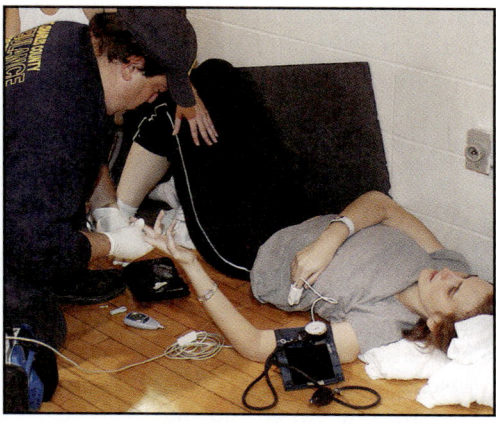

(Courtesy Ray Kemp, St. Charles, Mo.)

ORGANS OF THE FEMALE REPRODUCTIVE SYSTEM

The female reproductive organs include the ovaries, fallopian (uterine) tubes, uterus, vagina, external genital organs, and mammary glands (Figure 31-1; also see Chapter 10). The following is a brief review of these structures.

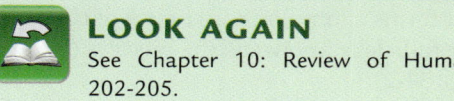

LOOK AGAIN
See Chapter 10: Review of Human Systems, pp. 202-205.

The **ovaries** are small, oval-shaped glands on either side of the uterus. Each ovary consists of a dense outer portion *(cortex)* and a less dense inner portion *(medulla)*. The ovaries produce eggs (ova) and hormones, especially estrogen and progesterone. The **fallopian tubes** are the uterine ducts for the ovaries. An ovum that is fertilized in the fallopian tube normally implants in the lining of the uterus *(endometrium)*. This signals the beginning of pregnancy.

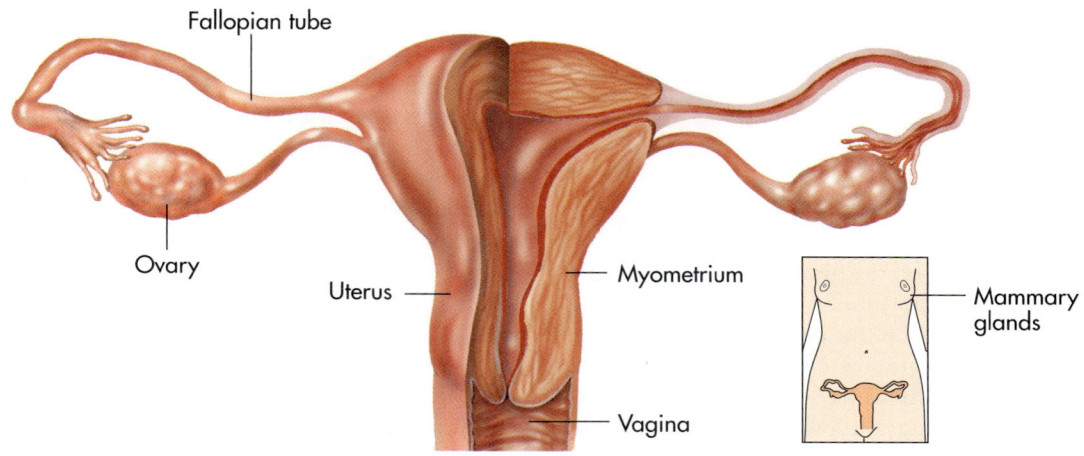

FIGURE 31-1 Female organs.

The **uterus** (womb) is a muscular organ the size and shape of a medium-sized pear. The main function of the uterus is to accept and nourish a fertilized ovum. A fertilized ovum that is not implanted in the uterus is shed from the body through menstruation.

The **vagina** (birth canal) is the female organ of copulation. It is a canal that joins the *cervix* (the lower portion of the uterus) to the outside of the body. It receives the penis during intercourse.

The **external genital organs** (*vulva*) are the outer parts of the female genitalia. They also protect the internal organs from infectious disease. The external genital organs consist of the *labia majora,* the *labia minora, Bartholin's glands.* and the *clitoris.*

The **mammary glands** are the organs of milk production. They are located in the breasts (*mammae*). Under the influence of hormones, the glands secrete milk during nursing.

MENSTRUATION AND OVULATION

Menstruation

In women of reproductive age, the body prepares for a possible pregnancy about once a month. If pregnancy does not occur (i.e., a fertilized ovum does not implant in the uterine wall), menstruation follows. **Menstruation** is the normal, periodic discharge of blood, mucus, and cellular debris from the uterine mucosa. The normal menstrual cycle lasts about 28 days. It occurs at more or less regular intervals from puberty to menopause (except during pregnancy and lactation). The average menstrual flow is 25 to 60 mL. The flow usually lasts 4 to 6 days and is fairly constant from cycle to cycle. The onset of menses **(menarche)** generally begins between ages 12 and 13. Menstruation ends permanently **(menopause)** at an average age of 47 years. However, the normal age for menopause can range from 35 to 60 (Box 31-1). Menstruation occurs in three phases: the follicular phase, the ovulatory phase, and the luteal phase.

> **NOTE**
> All phases of the menstrual cycle are affected by the release of hormones. These hormones include follicle-stimulating hormone (FSH), luteinizing hormone (LH), estrogen, and progesterone.

FOLLICULAR PHASE

The follicular phase begins on the first day of the menstrual cycle. Follicle-stimulating hormone (FSH) and luteinizing hormone (LH) are released from the brain and make contact with the ovaries. This stimulates each ovary to produce about 15 to 20 oocytes (immature ova). Each oocyte is surrounded by a layer of cells (granulosa cells). The structure is known as a *primary follicle.* FSH and LH also cause an increase in the production of estrogen. The rise in estrogen

BOX 31-1 Hysterectomy

A **hysterectomy** is the surgical removal of the uterus. Hysterectomy is one of the most frequently performed surgeries in the United States. It most often is performed to treat fibroid tumors that have caused symptoms and cancer of the uterus or cervix. Other indications for the surgery include heavy menstrual bleeding, endometriosis, pelvic inflammatory disease, and the removal of a prolapsed uterus. Depending on the type of hysterectomy, the surgery may be performed through the abdomen or vagina or laparoscopically.

In a *subtotal hysterectomy,* only the upper part of the uterus is removed; the cervix is not. (The fallopian tubes and ovaries may or may not be removed.) In a *total hysterectomy* (also called a *complete hysterectomy*), the body of the uterus, the cervix, the fallopian tubes, and the ovaries are removed. If cancer is present or in an advanced stage, a *radical hysterectomy* may be required in which the pelvic lymph nodes and lymph channels also are removed. After a hysterectomy, a woman is unable to bear children, does not menstruate, and needs no contraception.

Serious complications can occur from the surgery. These include blood clots, infection, adhesions, postoperative hemorrhage, bowel obstruction, or injury to the urinary tract. In addition to the direct surgical risks, long-term physical and psychological effects are possible. Examples of these include depression and loss of sexual pleasure. If the ovaries are removed along with the uterus before menopause, the risk of osteoporosis and heart disease may be increased.

levels stops the production of FSH, limiting the number of primary follicles that mature into *secondary follicles.* A mature secondary follicle continues to enlarge and produce estrogen. Eventually it forms a lump on the surface of the ovary. The fully mature follicle is known as the *vesicular* (or *graafian) follicle* (Figure 31-2).

OVULATORY PHASE

Cellular secretions of the graafian follicle cause it to swell more rapidly than can be accommodated by follicular growth. The rise in estrogen during this phase triggers the release of LH. This causes the follicle to expand and rupture and forces a small amount of blood and follicular fluid out of the vesicle. Shortly after this initial burst of fluid, an oocyte escapes from the follicle. The release of this secondary oocyte is called **ovulation.** Ovulation starts about 14 days after the follicular phase. It is the midpoint in the menstrual cycle. The egg is captured in the fallopian tube, where it may or may not be fertilized.

LUTEAL PHASE

After ovulation the empty follicle is transformed into a yellow glandular structure called the *corpus luteum.* The cells of this structure secrete large amounts of progesterone and some estrogen. If pregnancy occurs, the fertilized

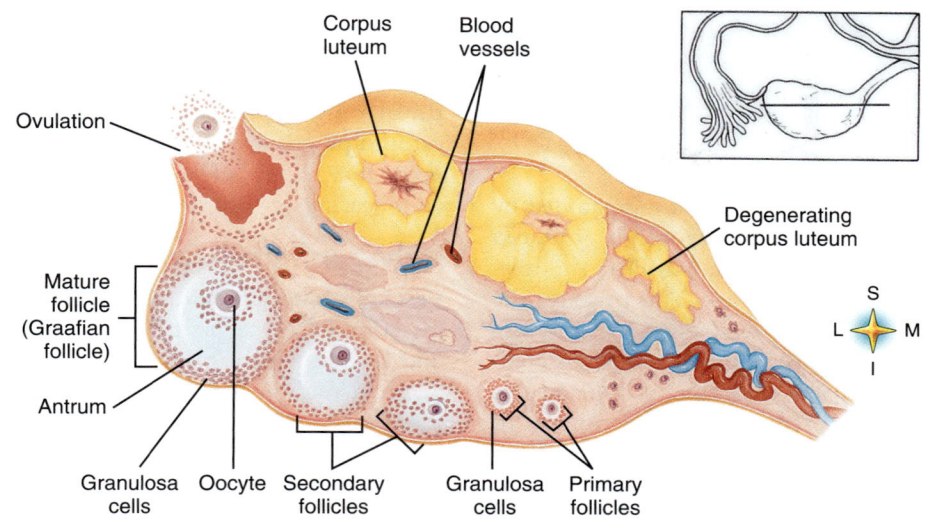

FIGURE 31-2 Diagram of the ovary and oogenesis. A cross section of the mammalian ovary shows successive stages of the ovarian (graafian) follicle and ovum development. The process begins with the first stage, the primary follicle, and (following clockwise) proceeds to the final stage, degeneration of the corpus luteum. (Thibodeau GA, Patton KT: *Structure and function of the body,* ed 13, St Louis, 2008, Mosby.)

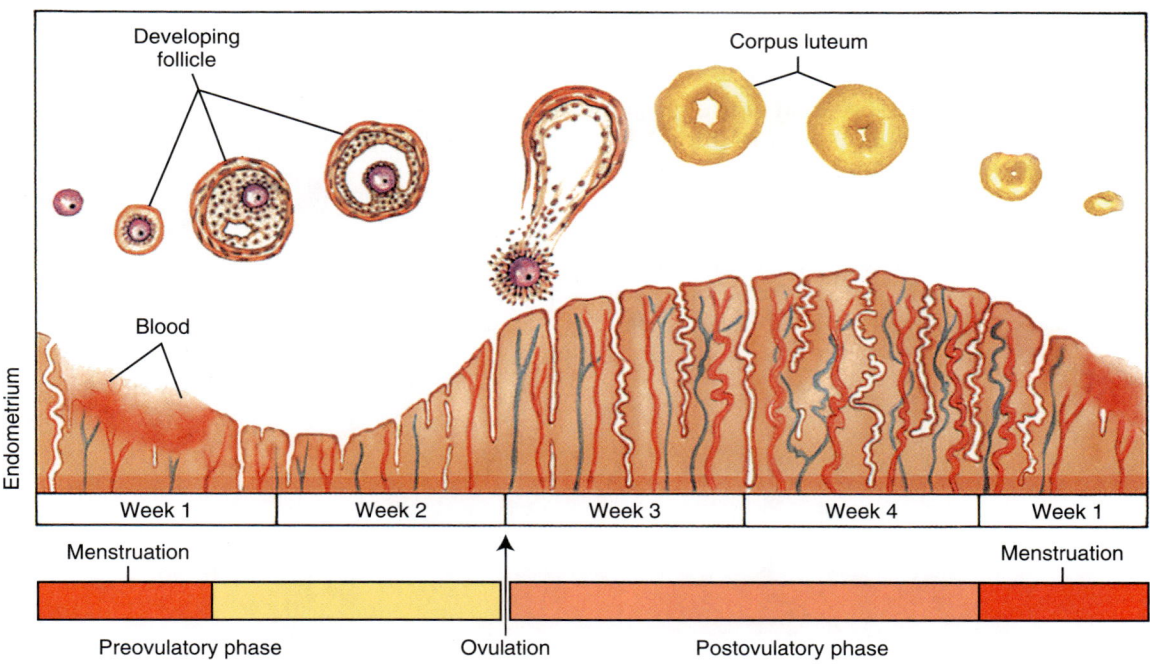

FIGURE 31-3 The female reproductive cycle. (Solomon EP: *Introduction to human anatomy and physiology,* ed 3, St Louis, 2009, Saunders.)

oocyte **(zygote)** travels through the fallopian tube to implant in the uterus. Chorionic gonadotropin is released to prevent the corpus luteum from degenerating. As a result, blood levels of estrogen and progesterone do not decrease and the menstrual period does not occur. If pregnancy does not occur, the corpus luteum degenerates and no longer produces progesterone; the estrogen level decreases, and the top layers of the lining are shed with the menstrual flow.

Hormonal Control of Ovulation and Menses

As described previously, hormones released from the hypothalamus and anterior pituitary control ovulation and menses. Under the influence of the ovarian hormones, the lining of the uterus **(endometrium)** goes through two phases of development: the proliferative phase and the secretory phase (Figure 31-3).

CRITICAL THINKING
What might happen to a woman's menstrual cycle if her hormonal balance were off?

The proliferative phase starts with and is sustained by increasing amounts of estrogen. This estrogen is produced by the maturing follicle. Estrogen stimulates the endometrium to grow and increase in thickness. This prepares the uterus for implantation of a fertilized ovum. The secretory phase begins after ovulation. This phase is under the combined influence of estrogen and progesterone. During this phase, the endometrium is prepared for implantation of the fertilized ovum. Within 7 days after ovulation (about day 21 of the menstrual cycle), the endometrium is ready to receive the developing embryo if fertilization has occurred.

If fertilization does not occur, the ovum can survive only 6 to 24 hours. After this time, the hormone levels drop and the endometrium is shed as menstrual flow. This process usually takes place on day 28 of the cycle. (This is about 14 days after ovulation.) The oocyte can be fertilized for up to 24 hours after ovulation (see Chapter 46).

GYNECOLOGICAL EMERGENCIES

Gynecological emergencies to be discussed in this chapter are medical conditions (Box 31-2) and sexual assault. (Other traumatic injuries are addressed in Chapter 43; genitourinary causes of abdominal pain are described in Chapter 30; and obstetrical emergencies are presented in Chapter 46.)

Acute or chronic infection involving a patient's uterus, ovaries, fallopian tubes, and adjacent structures may be a source of severe abdominal pain. Abdominal pain associated with the female reproductive system can cover a wide range. The pain may mark simply minor episodes of difficult menstruation, or it may indicate potentially life-threatening hemorrhage from a ruptured ovarian cyst or ectopic pregnancy. Regardless of the type of emergency, pregnancy should always be considered in any woman of childbearing age until a physician determines otherwise.

Pelvic Inflammatory Disease

Pelvic inflammatory disease (PID) is a general term for infection of the cervix, uterus, fallopian tubes, and ovaries and their supporting structures (Figure 31-4). PID affects about 1 million women annually and is responsible for more than 250,000 hospitalizations each year.[1] Pelvic

BOX 31-2 Gynecological Emergencies

- Gynecological disorders
  - Cystitis
  - Ectopic pregnancy
  - Endometriosis
  - Endometritis
  - Mittelschmerz
  - Pelvic inflammatory disease
  - Ruptured ovarian cyst
  - Vaginal bleeding
  - Bartholin's abscess
  - Vaginitis
  - Ovarian torsion
  - Dysfunctional uterine bleeding
  - Uterine prolapse
  - Vaginal foreign body
- Sexual assault

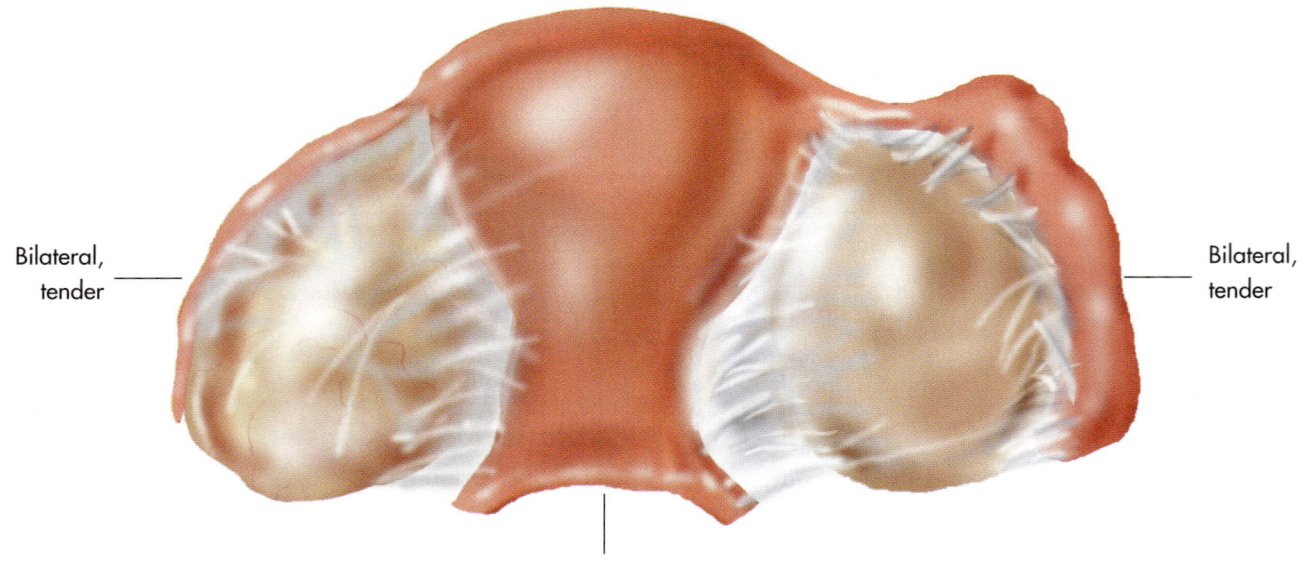

Bilateral, tender

Bilateral, tender

Movement of cervix painful

FIGURE 31-4 Symptoms of pelvic inflammatory disease.

inflammatory disease usually is caused by sexually transmitted bacteria, most commonly *Neisseria gonorrhoeae* (gonorrhea) and *Chlamydia trachomatis* (chlamydia). Staphylococci, streptococci, and other pathogens also may cause infection. However, these organisms usually are transmitted by instruments used during medical procedures.

Pathogens ascending from the vaginal area may infect the cervix initially (cervicitis). This may be followed by infection of the uterus proper (endometritis) and the fallopian tubes (salpingitis). Finally, the supporting structures around the uterus and fallopian tubes (parametritis) may become infected. Because the infection is polymicrobial, it can produce diffuse lower abdominal pain associated with low-grade fever (variable), vaginal discharge, and dyspareunia (pain with sexual intercourse). The inflammation often follows the onset of menstrual bleeding by 7 to 10 days. At that time, the reproductive organs are vulnerable to bacterial infection because the lining of the uterus has been shed during menstruation.

PID often is accompanied by pain on ambulation; the patient bends forward and takes short, slow steps, often guarding the abdomen ("PID shuffle"). Consequences of PID include secondary infertility, ectopic pregnancies, and tubo-ovarian abscesses. In severe cases the reproductive organs may need to be removed surgically. Definitive treatment usually consists of antibiotic therapy, which helps control the infection and prevent damage to the fallopian tubes.

Prehospital care is primarily supportive for all infections that affect the female reproductive system. In most cases, evaluation and care by a physician are required.

Bartholin's Abscess

Bartholin's abscess is an accumulation of pus that forms a lump (swelling) in one of the Bartholin glands. It occurs when blockage of the duct of the gland allows an infection to develop. The abscess can take years to form, or it may

arise quickly, over several days. Signs and symptoms include swelling and inflammation of the gland and a visible lump on one side of the vaginal opening. Fever also may be present. Any activity that puts pressure on the vulva (including walking, sitting, and sexual intercourse) can cause severe pain and discomfort.

After examination by a physician, treatment may include a biopsy to rule out malignancy; surgical incision to drain the infected gland; and oral antibiotic therapy. About 10% of infections recur. Surgery sometimes is required for recurrent infections.

Vaginitis

Vaginitis *(vulvovaginitis)* is inflammation and infection of the vulva and vagina. It can occur in young girls and women of all ages but is most common in postmenopausal and postpartum women. It is a very common disease that affects millions of women each year. Most cases of vaginitis result from *Candida* (yeast) infections, bacterial infections *(bacterial vaginosis)*, and the sexually transmitted disease *trichomoniasis* (see Chapter 28). Vaginitis also can be caused by parasites, viruses, and poor personal hygiene. Regardless of the cause of the infection, patients with vaginitis often complain of irritation and itching of the genital area, in addition to the following:

- Inflammation (redness and swelling) of the labia majora, labia minora, or perineal area
- Vaginal discharge
- Foul vaginal odor
- Discomfort or burning with urination

> **NOTE**
>
> *Noninfectious vaginitis* usually is caused by an allergic reaction (e.g., to detergents, soaps) or irritation from vaginal sprays, douches, and spermicidal products. This form of vaginitis can cause the same signs and symptoms as the infectious form.

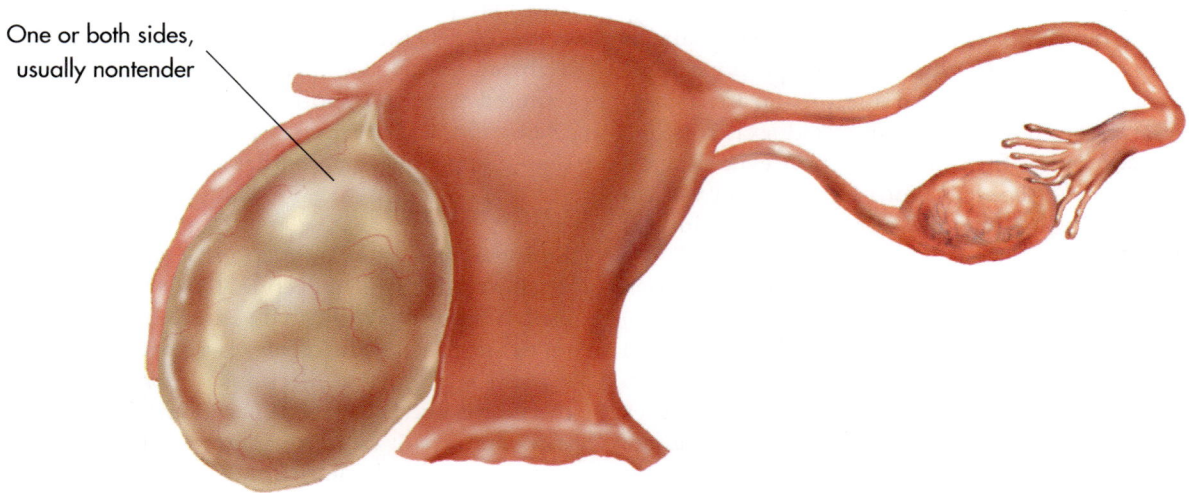

One or both sides, usually nontender

FIGURE 31-5 Ovarian cyst.

Depending on the cause of the infection, treatment for vaginitis may include antiyeast or antifungal creams, vaginal suppositories, and antibiotics. Most patients are advised not to engage in sexual activity until the infection has resolved. Vaginitis can be spread to sexual partners, who also may require treatment.

Ruptured Ovarian Cyst

A **ruptured ovarian cyst** can be a gynecological emergency that may result in significant internal hemorrhage. An ovarian cyst is a thin-walled, fluid-filled sac on the surface of the ovary (Figure 31-5). The abdominal pain caused by an ovarian cyst may result from rapid expansion, torsion that produces ischemia (described later), or acute rupture. The type of cyst most prone to rupture is the *corpus luteum cyst*. This cyst forms as a result of hemorrhage in a mature corpus luteum. The corpus luteum develops after ovulation (day 14 of the 28-day cycle). Therefore, most ruptures occur about 1 week before menstrual bleeding is to begin. However, some patients with a ruptured ovarian cyst have vaginal bleeding or report a late or missed period at the time of rupture.

 CRITICAL THINKING
Consider a patient you suspect has a ruptured ovarian cyst. How would you assess for the possibility of bleeding?

A ruptured ovarian cyst can result in localized, one-sided lower abdominal pain. A ruptured cyst also can result in generalized signs of peritonitis if massive hemorrhage has occurred. The onset of pain often is associated with minimal abdominal trauma, sexual intercourse, or exercise.

Ovarian Torsion

Ovarian torsion is the twisting of the ovary. Numerous conditions can cause such torsion, including congenital abnormalities, ovarian cysts or tumors, disease that affects the fallopian tube or ovary, adhesions from previous pelvic surgeries, trauma, and others. As a rule, torsion affects only one ovary and commonly the oviduct (adnexal torsion). Ovarian torsion is the fifth most common gynecological surgical emergency. About 70% of cases occur in women under 30 years of age. About 20% of reported cases involve pregnant women.[2]

Signs and symptoms of ovarian torsion include a sudden onset of lower abdominal pain (usually on the right side) that may radiate to the back, pelvis, or thigh. The pain often begins with exercise. The patient usually describes the pain as sharp or stabbing. Often the patient complains of nausea and vomiting. Fever may be present but is usually a late sign. Care by a physician may include pain management and fluid replacement. Surgery may be indicated to manage vascular compromise, peritonitis, or necrosis.

Cystitis

Cystitis is inflammation of the inner lining of the bladder. It usually is caused by a bacterial infection. Both males and females can develop infection. However, cystitis is more common in women, because the urethra is shorter. The main symptom of cystitis is a frequent urge to pass urine, with only a small amount of urine passed each time. Other signs and symptoms may include painful (burning) urination, fever, chills, and lower abdominal pain. The urine occasionally may be foul smelling or contain blood. Cystitis also can occur as a result of a structural abnormality of the ureters (this is common in children) or compression of the urethra as a result of inflammation. Indwelling urinary catheters are another cause. Prompt treatment of cystitis with a complete course of antibiotics usually settles the infection within 24 hours.

Dysmenorrhea and Mittelschmerz

Dysmenorrhea is pain during menstruation. The condition may include headache, faintness, dizziness, nausea, diarrhea, backache, and leg pain. In severe cases, chills, headache, diarrhea, nausea, vomiting, and syncope can occur. Dysmenorrhea occurs more often in women who are not sexually active and women who have not borne children. The lower abdominal pains associated with dysmenorrhea are thought to be related to muscular contraction of the myometrium (the muscular layer of the uterus). These muscle contractions are mediated by local prostaglandins. Other factors associated with dysmenorrhea include infection, inflammation, and the presence of an intrauterine contraceptive device.

Mittelschmerz is German for "middle pain." This pain may occur from the rupture of the graafian follicle and bleeding from the ovary during the menstrual cycle. Mittelschmerz is characterized by pain in the right or left lower quadrant of the abdomen. The pain occurs in the normal midcycle of a menstrual period (after ovulation) and lasts about 24 to 36 hours. The hormones produced by the ovary also may produce slight endometrial bleeding and low-grade fever. Dysmenorrhea and mittelschmerz do not pose a threat to life. However, evaluation by a physician is required to rule out more serious causes of menstrual pain. Evaluation also is required to differentiate the pain from that of appendicitis and other surgical emergencies.

Endometritis

Endometritis is inflammation of the uterine lining. It usually results from infection. Often it occurs after childbirth or abortion and usually is caused by retained placental tissue. (The condition also is a feature of PID and other sexually transmitted infections.) Endometritis may affect the uterus and fallopian tubes. If left untreated, endometritis may result in sterility, sepsis, and death. Signs and symptoms of endometritis include fever, purulent vaginal discharge, and lower abdominal pain. Treatment includes removal of any foreign tissue and antibiotic therapy.

Endometriosis

Endometriosis is an abnormal gynecological condition characterized by the growth of endometrial tissue outside the uterus. This may occur because fragments of endometrium have been regurgitated backward (during menstruation) through the fallopian tubes into the peritoneal cavity, where the fragments attach and grow as small cystic structures. The endometrial tissue of endometriosis functions cyclically and undergoes periodic menstrual breakdown. This can result in bleeding within cysts, stretching of the cyst wall, and pain.

Endometriosis is more common in women who defer pregnancy. The average age of women found to have endometriosis is 37 years. Characteristic symptoms of endometriosis are pain (particularly dysmenorrhea), painful defecation, and suprapubic soreness. Other common symptoms include vaginal spotting of blood before the start of a period and infertility. After evaluation by a physician, treatment may consist of drug therapy with analgesics or hormones and, in some cases, surgery.

CRITICAL THINKING
Why do you think these patients with endometriosis tend to be infertile?

Ectopic Pregnancy

An **ectopic pregnancy** is a pregnancy that develops outside the uterus (Figure 31-6). It is the third leading cause of maternal death and accounts for 6% of maternal mortality.[3] The pregnancy most commonly develops in the fallopian tube or ovary. In rare cases, it develops in the abdominal cavity or cervix. An ectopic pregnancy can be a life-threatening emergency. Most ectopic pregnancies are discovered in the first 2 months, often before the woman realizes she is pregnant. Signs and symptoms include severe abdominal pain that may radiate to the neck or shoulder (and which worsens on inspiration) and vaginal spotting. If rupture occurs, internal hemorrhage, sepsis, and shock may develop.[4] Once an ectopic pregnancy has been confirmed, surgery is performed to remove the developing fetus, placenta, and any damaged tissue at the site of the pregnancy. Ectopic pregnancy is common; it occurs in 2% of all pregnancies.[3] Ectopic pregnancy should be considered in any female of reproductive age who has abdominal pain. (Ectopic pregnancy is described further in Chapter 46.)

Vaginal Bleeding

Vaginal bleeding is the loss of blood from the uterus, cervix, or vagina. The most common source of nontraumatic vaginal bleeding is menstruation. (This bleeding

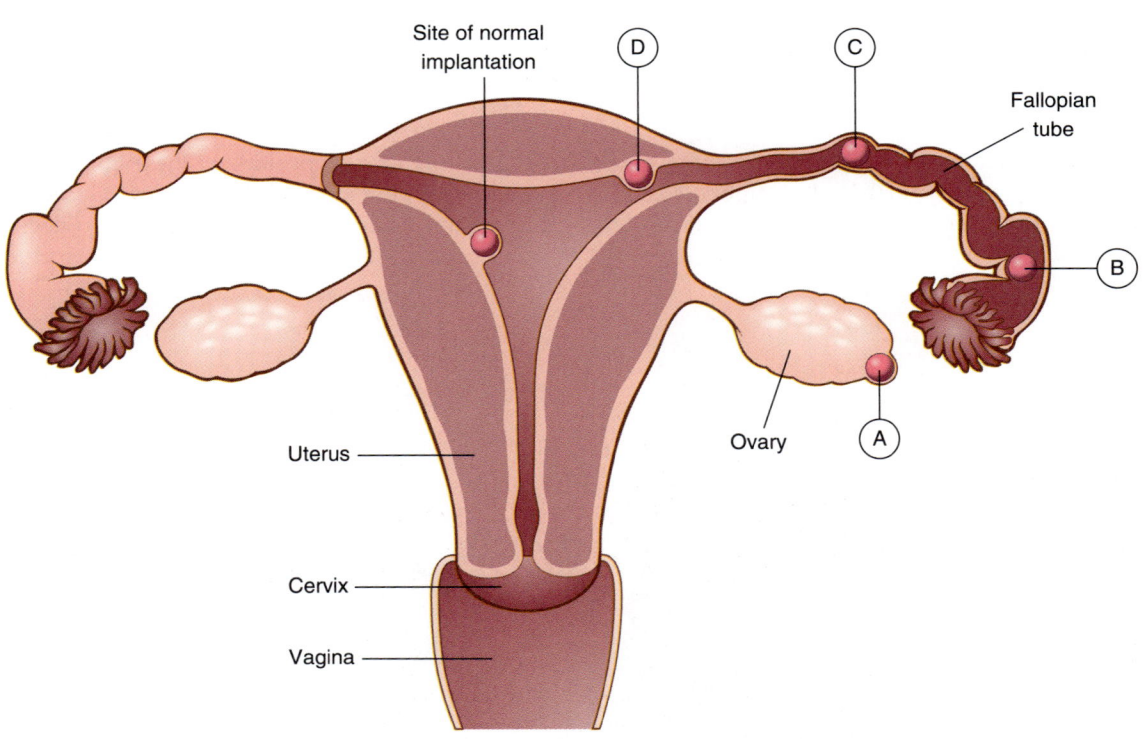

FIGURE 31-6 Ectopic pregnancy. *A, B, C,* and *D* are ectopic sites. The fallopian tube is the most common site for ectopic pregnancies (95%), but they also can occur on the ovary or on the surface of the peritoneum. Normal implantation takes place on the inner lining (endometrium) of the uterus. (Chabner DE: *Medical terminology: a short course,* ed 5, St Louis, 2009, Saunders.)

rarely results in a request for emergency care.) Possible causes of serious nonmenstrual bleeding include the following:

- Spontaneous abortion
- Disorders of the placenta
- Hormonal imbalances (especially menopause)
- Lesions
- PID
- Onset of labor

The paramedic should never assume that vaginal hemorrhage is due to *normal* menstruation. Some causes of vaginal bleeding may be life threatening and can lead to hypovolemic shock and death. (Vaginal passage of clots usually indicates bleeding at a rate greater than menstrual flow.)

Dysfunctional Uterine Bleeding

Dysfunctional uterine bleeding (DUB) is abnormal bleeding that occurs because of changes in hormone levels. The most common cause of the bleeding is failure of an ovary to release an oocyte *(anovulation);* consequently, ovulation does not take place. This results in continuous, unopposed production of estradiol, which stimulates overgrowth of the endometrium. Without progesterone, the endometrium proliferates and eventually outgrows its blood supply, leading to necrosis. The end result is overproduction of uterine blood flow. With symptoms of DUB, a patient may notice changes in her menstrual cycle, such as the following[5]:

- Vaginal bleeding or spotting that occurs between periods
- Menstrual periods less than 28 days or longer than 35 days apart
- Timing of menstrual periods that changes with each cycle
- Heavier than normal bleeding (passing large clots; changing protection during the night; soaking through a sanitary pad or tampon every hour for 2 to 3 hours in a row)

- Bleeding that lasts for more days than normal or for more than 7 days
- Tenderness and dryness of the vagina

DUB is most common at the extreme ages of a woman's reproductive years, either at the beginning or near the end, but it may occur at any time during reproductive life. Care by a physician may include a pregnancy test, IV hormone therapy, methods to tamponade the bleeding, and sometimes surgery.

Uterine Prolapse

Uterine prolapse is the falling or sliding of the uterus from its normal position in the pelvic cavity into the vaginal canal. As described in Chapter 10, the main portion of the uterus (the body) is positioned between the fundus and the cervix. The uterus is held in place by connective tissue, muscles, and the broad ligament, round ligaments, and uterosacral ligaments. If these muscles and ligaments stretch and weaken, the uterus has inadequate support and descends into the vaginal cavity (Figure 31-7). Factors that may cause uterine prolapse include the following:

- Trauma during vaginal childbirth
- Large babies and difficult vaginal delivery
- Loss of muscle tone associated with aging
- Menopause and reduced amounts of circulating estrogen
- Pelvic cavity tumors

Obesity, chronic constipation, and chronic obstructive pulmonary disease (COPD) can put a strain on the muscles and connective tissue in the pelvis. These conditions may also play a role in the development of uterine prolapse.

If the uterine prolapse is mild and the patient is asymptomatic, treatment may not be necessary. In these cases, patients often are advised to make lifestyle changes to slow progression of the prolapse. These may include losing weight, stopping smoking, and preventing coughing. Heavy lifting and straining also should be avoided. Signs and symptoms of a more severe prolapse include patient

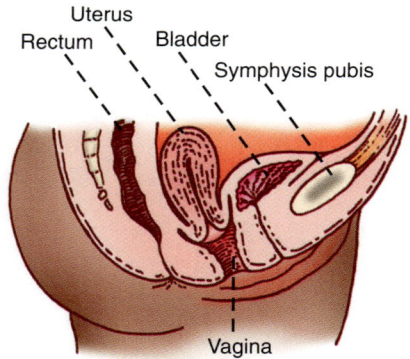
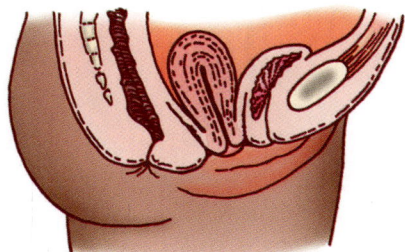
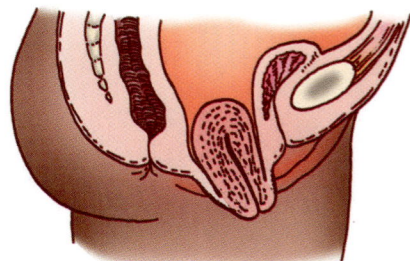

FIRST-DEGREE PROLAPSE   SECOND-DEGREE PROLAPSE   THIRD-DEGREE PROLAPSE

FIGURE 31-7 Degrees of uterine prolapse. (From Black JM, Hawks JH: *Medical-surgical nursing: clinical management for positive outcomes,* ed 8 Philadelphia, 2009, Saunders, p. 930.)

TABLE 31-1 Characteristics of Abdominal Pain in Gynecological Emergencies

Onset	Location	Quality	Radiation	Vaginal Discharge	Menstrual History
Ruptured Ectopic Pregnancy					
Rapid (can become generalized)	Unilateral (can become generalized)	Cramplike, then steady	Shoulder (may indicate intraperitoneal bleeding)	Vaginal bleeding (75% of cases)	Amenorrhea, 6 weeks or more since last period
Ruptured Ovarian Cyst					
Sudden	Unilateral (can become generalized)	Steady	Shoulder (may indicate intraperitoneal bleeding)	Possible vaginal bleeding	Usually 1 week before period
Pelvic Inflammatory Disease					
Gradual (can become generalized)	Diffuse, bilateral	Steady ache	Right upper quadrant	Watery, foul-smelling discharge	Usually within 1 week after period

complaints of feeling like she is "sitting on a small ball," heaviness in the vaginal area, low back pain, difficult or painful intercourse, and vaginal bleeding. In these cases, placement of a *vaginal pessary* (a device similar to a diaphragm) or surgery may be needed to hold the uterus in place.

Vaginal Foreign Body

It is not uncommon to find a foreign body inserted in the vagina. This is especially true of children, who may insert a foreign body during self-exploration and not tell their parents or caregivers. The foreign body can cause a foul-smelling, purulent discharge with or without vaginal bleeding. Vaginal foreign bodies also may be a result of a psychiatric disorder, unusual sexual practices, or an episode of abuse. Occasionally a tampon, broken portions of condoms, or a pessary is forgotten or lost and causes discomfort and a vaginal discharge. Less common symptoms may include pain or urinary discomfort. No attempt should be made in the prehospital setting to remove a foreign body in the vagina. The patient should be transported for evaluation by a physician.

ASSESSMENT AND MANAGEMENT OF GYNECOLOGICAL EMERGENCIES

Finding the cause of lower abdominal pain is difficult in both men and women. It can be especially challenging in women, because many gynecological conditions produce common characteristics. For example, a ruptured ectopic pregnancy, ruptured ovarian cyst, and PID can have identical presentations (Table 31-1). The goal of prehospital care is to quickly identify the conditions that require aggressive therapy and to rapidly transport the patient for definitive care. Prehospital care includes obtaining a history of the present illness (including a thorough gynecological history); providing airway, ventilatory, and circulatory support as needed; and transporting the patient for evaluation by a physician.

History of Present Illness and Obstetrical History

The paramedic should obtain a history of the present illness to better understand the patient's chief complaint (see Chapter 18). Important associated symptoms include fever, diaphoresis, syncope, diarrhea, constipation, and abdominal cramping. The interview should include a thorough obstetrical history. The obstetrical history includes the following 10 components.[6]

1. *Pregnancy.* The paramedic should determine the total number of pregnancies the patient has had and the number of pregnancies that were carried to term (see Chapter 46).
2. *Previous cesarean deliveries.* A **cesarean delivery** is a surgical procedure in which the abdomen and uterus are incised and the baby then is delivered through the abdomen. Cesarean delivery usually is done when maternal or fetal conditions might make vaginal delivery risky. A history of a previous cesarean delivery may indicate a high-risk pregnancy.
3. *Last menstrual period.* The paramedic should obtain information about the patient's last menstrual period. Questions to ask include the following:
   - When did it start (the date)? When did it end (the duration)? Have your menstrual periods occurred regularly?

- Was your last menstrual period normal for you? Was the menstrual flow heavier or lighter than other periods?
- Did any bleeding occur between periods?

4. *Possibility of pregnancy.* Some patients may hesitate to disclose a possible pregnancy. They may not answer a direct question honestly (e.g., "Could you be pregnant?"). If pregnancy is suspected (but not confirmed by the patient), the paramedic should ask specific questions about missed or late periods, breast tenderness, urinary frequency, morning sickness (nausea and/or vomiting), and unprotected sexual activity to determine the likelihood of a pregnancy.

CRITICAL THINKING

Does a patient always give you accurate information about whether she is pregnant? Why?

5. *History of previous gynecological problems.* The paramedic should identify any previous gynecological problems. Knowledge of these problems can be helpful to others who may be involved in the patient's care. Examples of important previous gynecological problems include infections, bleeding, painful intercourse **(dyspareunia),** miscarriage, abortion, **dilation and curettage (D & C),** and ectopic pregnancy.

NOTE

Dilation and curettage (D & C) is a gynecological procedure. It involves widening of the uterine cervix and scraping away of the endometrium of the uterus. The procedure is used for a variety of conditions. These include diagnosing disease of the uterus, correcting heavy or prolonged vaginal bleeding, and emptying the uterus of the products of conception after delivery or abortion.

6. *Present blood loss.* If the patient is actively bleeding, the paramedic should ask questions about the color (bright versus dark red blood), the amount of blood loss (estimated by the number of pads or tampons soaked per hour), and the duration of the bleeding episode.
7. *Vaginal discharge.* If the patient has a discharge, the paramedic should question her about the color, amount, and odor of the discharge. These findings may indicate the presence of infection, venereal disease, or other illness.

8. *Use and type of contraceptive.* The use and type of contraception is a key part of the obstetrical history. For example, the use of birth control pills has been associated with hypertension and pulmonary embolus. Also, intrauterine devices can cause intrauterine bleeding and infection. Other methods of contraception include the withdrawal or rhythm method (which may increase the likelihood of pregnancy), the use of spermicides and condoms, contraceptive systems (e.g., Norplant and Depo-Provera), and *surgical tubal ligation* (a permanent form of female sterilization in which the fallopian tubes are severed and sealed).
9. *History of trauma to the reproductive system.* The paramedic should question all patients about any injury to the reproductive tract. Such an injury may be responsible for vaginal bleeding or discharge. The paramedic should ask a sexually active patient whether pain or bleeding has occurred during or after intercourse.
10. *Degree of emotional distress.* The paramedic should evaluate the patient's emotional distress. Factors that may be responsible for a patient's emotional distress include personal health issues, depression, an unwanted pregnancy, and financial worries.

PHYSICAL EXAMINATION

The physical examination should be conducted in a comforting, professional manner with consideration shown for the patient's modesty, privacy, and discomfort. When evaluating the potential for serious blood loss, the paramedic should assess the patient's skin and mucous membranes for color, cyanosis, or pallor. Assessment of vital signs should include orthostatic measurements. If indicated, the vaginal area should be inspected for bleeding or discharge, and the color, amount, and presence of clots or tissue (or both) should be noted. The patient's abdomen should be palpated to assess for masses, areas of tenderness, guarding, distention, and rebound tenderness.

PATIENT MANAGEMENT

Management includes support of the patient's vital functions and administration of high-concentration oxygen during transport. Intravenous access usually is not needed unless the patient is showing signs of impending shock or has excessive vaginal bleeding. Many patients prefer to be transported in a left lateral recumbent, knee-chest position. Others may prefer a hips raised, knees bent position for comfort. Vaginal bleeding should be controlled with the application of sanitary pads or trauma dressings. The vagina should never be packed with dressings or tampons. The paramedic should count the number of soaked pads and should record the number on the patient care report.

During transport, the paramedic should monitor the patient for the onset of serious bleeding. If this occurs, or if the patient's condition begins to deteriorate, the paramedic should establish one or two large-bore intravenous lines with normal saline or lactated Ringer solution. At this point, electrocardiographic (ECG) and pulse oximetry monitoring are indicated. Analgesics should be considered.

SEXUAL ASSAULT

Sexual assault is a crime of violence with serious physical and psychological implications. Anyone of either gender at any age can be sexually assaulted (see Chapter 50). However, women and girls are most often the victims. Estimates indicate that one in six women will experience a completed or attempted rape during their lifetimes and that many of these crimes will go unreported.[7]

Often the paramedic is first to encounter these patients. Tact, kindness, and sensitivity during the patient care episode are essential.

CRITICAL THINKING

How do you feel about rape? How would you manage a patient who has been raped?

DID YOU KNOW?

Rape and Date Rape

Rape occurs when sex is nonconsensual (not agreed upon) or when a person forces or attempts to force another person to have sex against his or her will. Rape includes intercourse in the vagina, anus, or mouth. It is a felony offense that can happen to men, women, and children. Rape can cause physical or emotional harm, or both, to the victim.

Date rape is nonconsensual sex between people who are already acquainted (e.g., friends, acquaintances, people who are dating). The difference between rape and date rape is that in cases of date rape, the victim agreed to spend time with the attacker. Date rape often occurs in the context of domestic violence. It sometimes involves the use of illegal "date rape drugs" that produce amnesia and anesthesia in the victim. These drugs include ketamine, gamma hydroxybutyrate (GHB), and flunitrazepam (Rohypnol). Date rape is still rape. It is a felony offense. A nationally representative survey found that[8]:

- In the first rape experience of female victims, perpetrators were reported to be intimate partners (30.4%), family members (23.7%), and acquaintances (20%).
- In the first rape experience of male victims, perpetrators were reported to be acquaintances (32.3%), family members (17.7%), friends (17.6%), and intimate partners (15.9%).

Initially, paramedics should care for a victim of sexual assault as they would any other injured patient. The first priority is to manage any injury that poses a threat to life.

After that, however, the approach should be modified with regard to history taking and the physical examination. Before taking a history or performing an examination, the paramedic should move the patient to a private area. If possible, the patient should be interviewed and examined by a paramedic of the same gender.

SHOW ME THE EVIDENCE

Feldhaus and colleagues interviewed women who reported to the emergency department of an urban level I trauma center for any cause during random periods in 1997. These women were not critically ill. The patients were asked if they had ever been sexually assaulted at any time in their lives. During that time, 360 patients who were eligible for the researchers' study consented to be enrolled in it. Of that group 39% said they had been sexually assaulted at some point in their life, and an additional 12% reported an attempted sexual assault. When the sexual assault occurred during adulthood, 70% of the time the victim knew the perpetrator. Another 8% of the assaults involved multiple attackers. A weapon was used or threatened to be used during the assault 40% of the time. Of this adult assault group, only 45% reported the assault to the police. A report was more likely to be filed if the woman did not know her attacker. Those who were assaulted sought medical aid less than half the time. This study revealed a high lifetime incidence of sexual assault in this group of women.

Feldhaus KM, Houry D, Kaminsky R: Lifetime sexual assault prevalence rates and reporting practices in an emergency department population, *Ann Emerg Med* 36:23-27, 2000.

History Taking

As a rule, victims of sexual assault should not be questioned in detail about the incident in the prehospital setting. The history should be limited to the elements needed to provide emergency care. For example, questions about penetration, sexual history, or sexual practices are irrelevant to prehospital care. They only add to the patient's emotional stress. The patient should be allowed to speak openly, and all information should be recorded accurately and thoroughly. Common reactions to sexual assault include anxiety, withdrawal and silence, denial, anger, and fear.

Assessment

The physical examination should identify any physical trauma, including trauma outside the pelvic area, that needs immediate attention. Facial fractures, human bites of the hands and breasts, long-bone fractures, broken ribs, and trauma to the abdomen are not unusual. The paramedic should examine the genitalia only if a severe injury is present or suspected. When possible, the paramedic should explain all procedures before initiating them. All examination findings should be documented, including the patient's emotional state, the condition of the patient's clothing, obvious injuries, and any patient care provided. A professional attitude is important. Feelings and prejudices about the victim or the assault should not affect the delivery of care.

Management

After the management of life-threatening injuries, emotional support is the most important patient care procedure paramedics can offer a victim of sexual assault. The paramedic should provide a safe environment for the patient and should respond appropriately to the victim's physical and emotional needs. Paramedics also should be aware of the need to preserve evidence from the crime scene (further described in Chapter 56). Special considerations include the following:

- Handle clothing as little as possible.
- Do not clean wounds unless absolutely necessary.
- Do not allow the patient to drink or brush the teeth.
- Do not use plastic bags for blood-stained articles.
- Bag each clothing item separately.
- Ask the victim not to change clothes or bathe.
- Disturb the crime scene as little as possible.

SUMMARY

- Menstruation is the normal, periodic discharge of blood, mucus, and cellular debris from the uterine mucosa. Ovulation is the release of a secondary oocyte from the ovary.
- Pelvic inflammatory disease results from infection of the cervix, uterus, fallopian tubes, and ovaries and their supporting structures.
- Bartholin's abscess is a buildup of puss in one of Bartholin's glands.
- Vaginitis is inflammation and infection of the vulva and vagina.
- A ruptured ovarian cyst occurs when a thin-walled, fluid-filled sac on the ovary ruptures. This can cause internal hemorrhage.
- Ovarian torsion is twisting of the ovary caused by another condition or disease.
- Cystitis is inflammation of the inner lining of the bladder. It usually is caused by a bacterial infection.
- Dysmenorrhea is characterized by painful menses. It may be associated with headache, faintness, dizziness, nausea, diarrhea, backache, and leg pain.
- Mittelschmerz is German for "middle pain." This pain may occur from the rupture of the graafian follicle and bleeding from the ovary during the menstrual cycle.
- Endometritis is inflammation of the uterine lining. Endometriosis is characterized by endometrial tissue growing outside the uterus.

- An ectopic pregnancy is a pregnancy that develops outside the uterus. Rupture of an ectopic pregnancy can cause life-threatening hemorrhage.
- Vaginal bleeding is the loss of blood from the uterus, cervix, or vagina.
- Uterine prolapse occurs when the uterus descends into the vagina.
- Vaginal foreign bodies can cause vaginal discharge, pain, and urinary discomfort.
- The history obtained from a patient with a gynecological emergency should include the pregnancy history; history of cesarean births; last menstrual period; possibility of pregnancy; history of previous gynecological problems; blood loss; vaginal discharge; contraceptives used; history of trauma to the reproductive system; and degree of emotional distress.
- The goal of prehospital care of lower abdominal pain in the female is to obtain a history (including a gynecological history); provide airway, ventilatory, and circulatory support as needed; and provide transport for evaluation by a physician.
- Sexual assault is a crime of violence. It can have serious physical and psychological effects.
- Paramedics should be aware of the need to preserve evidence from a sexual assault crime scene.

REFERENCES

1. Centers for Disease Control and Prevention: Pelvic inflammatory disease. CDC Fact Sheet. www.cdc.gov/std/PID/STDFact-PID.htm#common. Accessed September 7, 2010.
2. Hasson J, Tsafrir Z, Azem F, et al: Comparison of adnexal torsion between pregnant and nonpregnant women, *Am J Obstet Gynecol* 202:536, 2010.
3. Rosen P, Barkin R: *Emergency medicine: concepts and clinical practice*, ed 6, St Louis, 2006, Mosby.
4. American College of Emergency Physicians: Clinical policy for the initial approach to patients presenting with a chief complaint of vaginal bleeding, *Ann Emerg Med* 293:435-458, 1997.
5. National Library of Medicine: Dysfunctional uterine bleeding (DUB). www.nlm.nih.gov/medlineplus/ency/article/000903.htm. Accessed September 7, 2010.
6. National Highway Traffic Safety Administration. *The National EMS Education Standards*, Washington, DC, 2009, U.S. Department of Transportation/National Highway Traffic Safety Administration, DOT.

7. Centers for Disease Control: Understanding sexual violence. Fact Sheet 2007. www.cdc.gov/ncipc/pub-res/images/SV%20 Factsheet.pdf. Accessed September 7, 2010.

8. Basile KC, Chen J, Black MC, et al: Prevalence and characteristics of sexual violence victimization among US adults, 2001-2003, *Violence Vict* 22:437-448, 2007.

SUGGESTED READING

Centers for Disease Control and Prevention: Sexual violence prevention, *Injury Center* 2010. www.cdc.gov/ncipc/factsheets/ svfacts.htm.

OBJECTIVES

Upon completion of this chapter, the paramedic student will be able to:
1. Describe the physiology of blood and its components.
2. Discuss pathophysiology and signs and symptoms of specific hematological disorders.
3. Outline general assessment and management of patients with hematological disorders.

KEY TERMS

acute chest syndrome A new abnormal consolidation on a chest radiograph in a patient with sickle cell disease.

albumin A water-soluble protein containing carbon, hydrogen, oxygen, nitrogen, and sulfur.

anemia A decrease in blood hemoglobin level.

basophil A white blood cell that promotes inflammation.

bilirubin The orange-yellow pigment of bile, formed principally from the breakdown of hemoglobin in red blood cells after termination of their normal life span.

blood clot The end result of the clotting process in blood; a blood clot normally consists of red cells, white cells, and platelets enmeshed in an insoluble fibrin network.

clotting cascade The blood clotting system or coagulation pathway.

clotting factors Substances in the blood that act in sequence to stop bleeding by forming a clot.

differential count A laboratory test that identifies the different types of leukocytes present in blood; also called the *diff.*

disseminated intravascular coagulopathy A grave coagulopathy that results from the overstimulation of the clotting and anticlotting processes in response to disease or injury.

eosinophil A white blood cell that inhibits inflammation; thought to deactivate leukotrienes.

fibrinogen A soluble blood protein converted into insoluble fibrin during clotting.

globulin One of a broad category of simple proteins classified by solubility, mobility, and size.

hematology The scientific study of blood and blood-forming organs.

hemoglobin A complex protein-iron compound in the blood that carries oxygen to the cells from the lungs and carbon dioxide away from the cells to the lungs.

hemolysis The breakdown of red blood cells and the release of hemoglobin.

hemolytic anemia A condition in which delivery of oxygen to tissues is reduced because of an increase in hemolysis of erythrocytes.

hemophilia A group of hereditary bleeding disorders in which one of the factors necessary for blood coagulation is deficient.

hemophilia A A condition caused by a deficiency of coagulation factor VIII; it is considered the classic type of hemophilia.

hemophilia B A condition caused by a deficiency of coagulation factor IX.

hemostasis The cessation of bleeding by mechanical or chemical means or by substances that arrest the blood flow.

Hodgkin's disease A malignant disorder characterized by pain and progressive enlargement of lymphoid tissue.

iron deficiency anemia Anemia caused by inadequate supplies of iron needed to synthesize hemoglobin.

leukemia A malignant neoplasm of blood-forming organs.

leukopenia A decrease in the number of white blood cells (most commonly neutrophils).

lymphocyte A type of white blood cell formed in lymphoid tissue.

lymphoma A group of diseases that range from slowly growing chronic disorders to rapidly evolving acute conditions.

macrophage A phagocytic cell in the immune system.

malignant Very dangerous or virulent; likely to cause death; a cancerous tumor that tends to metastasize.

monocyte A type of white blood cell found in lymph nodes, spleen, bone marrow, and loose connective tissue.

multiple myeloma A malignant neoplasm of the bone marrow.

neutrophil A small, phagocytic white blood cell with a lobed nucleus and small granules in the cytoplasm.

Non-Hodgkin's lymphoma Cancer of the lymphoid tissue, which includes the lymph nodes, spleen, and other organs of the immune system.

pernicious anemia Anemia that results from a vitamin B_{12} deficiency.

plasma The fluid portion of blood.

platelet A fragment of a cell; it contains granules in the central part and clear protoplasm peripherally but has no definite nucleus.

platelet plug A plug consisting of a mass of linked platelets that seals an injured vessel; part of the clotting cascade.

polycythemia A condition characterized by an unusually large number of red cells in the blood as a result of their increased production by the bone marrow.

primary polycythemia A rare disorder of the bone marrow where an increased production of red blood cells (RBCs) causes the blood to thicken; also known as *polycythemia vera*.

prothrombin A chemical that is part of the clotting cascade; the precursor of thrombin.

prothrombin activator A substance that combines with an enzyme to increase its catalytic activity; converts prothrombin to thrombin.

red bone marrow Specialized soft tissue found in many bones of infants and children, in the spongy bone of the proximal epiphyses of the humerus and femur, and in the sternum, ribs, and vertebral bodies of adults. It is essential in the manufacture of red blood cells; also known as *red marrow*.

secondary polycythemia A condition of increased production of RBCs caused by reduced air pressure and low oxygen concentration; may be a natural response to chronic hypoxia.

sickle cell anemia An inherited blood disorder that affects red blood cells; the most common type of sickle cell disease.

sickle cell crisis An acute episodic condition that occurs in individuals with sickle cell anemia.

sickle cell disease A debilitating and unpredictable recessive genetic illness that produces an abnormal type of hemoglobin with an inferior oxygen-carrying capacity.

thrombin An enzyme formed in plasma as part of the clotting process; it causes fibrinogen to change to fibrin, which is essential in the formation of a clot.

thrombocytopenia An abnormal hematological condition in which the number of platelets is reduced; the most common cause is a bleeding disorder.

yellow marrow Specialized soft tissue (mainly adipose) found in the compact bone of most adult epiphyses.

***H**ematology is the study of blood and blood-forming organs. Dysfunction in the hematological system can affect other body systems. This can result in a variety of clinical manifestations that characterize hematological disorders. Prehospital care for most patients with hematological disorders is mainly supportive. However, the paramedic's knowledge of these diseases enhances assessment skills. It also provides an understanding of the treatment these patients need.*

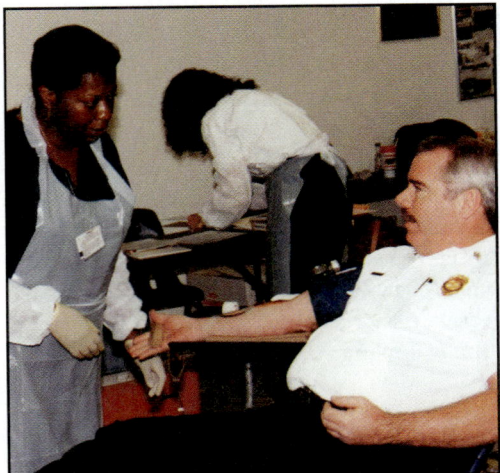

(Courtesy Florissant Valley Fire Protection District, St. Louis, Mo.)

BLOOD AND BLOOD COMPONENTS

As described in Chapter 10, blood is composed of cells and formed elements surrounded by plasma. About 95% of the volume of formed elements consists of red blood cells (RBCs; erythrocytes). The remaining 5% consists of white blood cells (WBCs; leukocytes) and cell fragments (platelets) (Figures 32-1 and Table 32-1). The continuous movement of blood keeps the formed elements dispersed throughout the plasma, where they are available to carry out their chief functions[1]: (1) delivery of substances needed for cellular metabolism in the tissues; (2) defense against invading microorganisms and injury; and (3) acid-base balance.

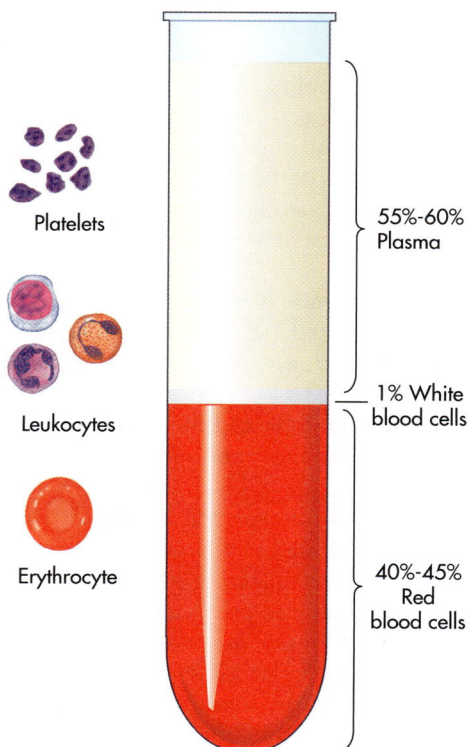

Platelets

Leukocytes

Erythrocyte

55%-60%
Plasma

1% White
blood cells

40%-45%
Red
blood cells

FIGURE 32-1 Blood will settle into three distinct, proportional layers when treated with salt. The transparent yellow layer at the top is plasma—the liquid portion of blood through which solid elements travel. White blood cells (WBCs) settle in the narrow white band in the center, and red blood cells (RBCs), which give blood its crimson color, fall to the bottom of the flask. Red blood cells outnumber white blood cells 600 to 1.

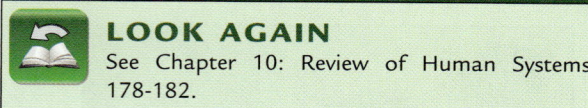

LOOK AGAIN
See Chapter 10: Review of Human Systems, pp. 178-182.

All types of blood cells are formed within the red bone marrow, which is present in all tissues at birth. In the adult the **red bone marrow** primarily is found in membranous bone such as the vertebrae, pelvis, sternum, and ribs. **Yellow marrow** produces some white cells but is composed mainly of connective tissue and fat. Other blood-forming organs include the following:

- Lymph nodes, which produce lymphocytes and antibodies
- The spleen, which stores large quantities of blood and produces lymphocytes, plasma cells, and antibodies
- The liver, a blood-forming organ only during intrauterine life, which plays an important role in the coagulation process

Plasma

Plasma, the clear portion of blood, is about 92% water. It contains three important proteins: albumin, globulins, and fibrinogen. **Albumin** is the most plentiful protein. Albumin

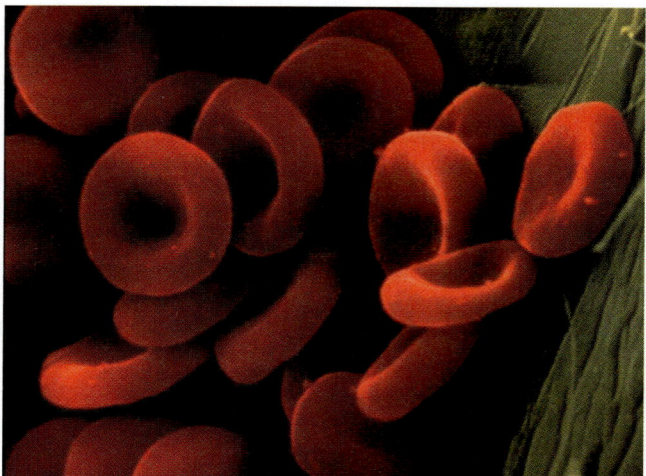

FIGURE 32-2 Mature erythrocytes. (Copyright Dennis Kunkel Microscopy, Inc. From McCance KL, Huether SE: *Pathophysiology: the biologic basis for disease in adults and children,* ed 6, St Louis, 2010, Mosby.)

is similar to egg white and gives blood its gummy texture. These large proteins keep the water concentration of blood low so that water diffuses readily from tissues into the blood. The **globulins** (alpha, beta, and gamma) transport other proteins and provide immunity to disease. **Fibrinogen** is responsible for blood clotting. Plasma proteins perform various functions that include maintaining blood pH (acting as either an acid or a base); transporting fat-soluble vitamins, hormones, and carbohydrates; and allowing the body to digest them temporarily for food. Plasma also contains salts, metals, and inorganic compounds.

Red Blood Cells

Red blood cells are the most abundant cells in the body. They are primarily responsible for tissue oxygenation. They appear as small rounded disks with nearly hollowed-out centers (Figure 32-2). They are composed mainly of water and the red protein **hemoglobin.** Red blood cell production continues throughout life to replace blood cells that grow old and die, are killed by disease, or are lost through bleeding. After RBC production occurs in the bone marrow, the new cell divides until there are 16 RBCs. The cells produce hemoglobin protein until the concentration of the protein becomes 95% of the dry weight of the cell. At this time, the cell expels its nucleus, giving the cell its characteristic pinched look. The new shape of the RBC increases the surface area of the cell and thus its oxygen-carrying potential. Red blood cells have a life span of about 120 days. As the cells age, their internal chemical machinery weakens; they lose elasticity; and they become trapped in small blood vessels in the bone marrow, liver, and spleen. They then are destroyed by specialized WBCs (**macrophages**). Most components of destroyed hemoglobin molecules are used again. However, some are broken down to the waste product **bilirubin.**

TABLE 32-1 Cellular Components of the Blood

Cell	Structural Characteristics	Normal Amounts of Circulating Blood	Function	Life Span
Erythrocyte (red blood cell)	Nonnucleated cytoplasmic disk containing hemoglobin	4.2-6.2 million/mm³	Gas transport to and from tissue cells and lungs	80-120 days
Leukocyte (white blood cell)	Nucleated cell	5000-10,000/mm³	Body defense mechanisms	Described below
Lymphocyte	Mononuclear immunocyte	25-33% of leukocyte count (leukocyte differential)	Humoral and cell-mediated immunity	Days or years depending on type
Monocyte and macrophage	Large mononuclear phagocyte	3-7% of leukocyte differential	Phagocytosis; mononuclear phagocyte system	Months or years
Eosinophil	Segmented polymorphonuclear granulocyte	1-4% of leukocyte differential	Phagocytosis, antibody-mediated defense against parasites, allergic reactions, associated with Hodgkin's disease, recovery phase of infection	Unknown
Neutrophil	Segmented polymorphonuclear granulocyte	57-67% of leukocyte differential	Phagocytosis, particularly during early phase of inflammation	4 days
Basophil	Segmented polymorphonuclear granulocyte	0-0.75% of leukocyte differential	Unknown, but associated with allergic reactions and mechanical irritation	Unknown
Platelet	Irregularly shaped cytoplasmic fragment (not a cell)	140,000-340,000/mm³	Hemostasis after vascular injury; normal coagulation and clot formation/retraction	8-11 days

Adapted from McCance KL, Huether SE: *Pathophysiology: the biologic basis for disease in adults and children*, ed 7, St Louis, 2006, Mosby.

Each RBC contains about 270 million hemoglobin molecules. Each hemoglobin molecule carries 4 oxygen molecules. The normal amount of hemoglobin in blood is about 15 g/100 mL. This normally is a little higher in males than in females. The number of RBCs is about 4.2 to 6.2 million cells/mm² (Box 32-1).

White Blood Cells

As described in Chapter 10, white blood cells arise from the bone marrow and are released into the bloodstream. White blood cells destroy foreign substances (e.g., bacteria and viruses) and clear the bloodstream of debris. Leukocyte production increases in response to infection. This causes an elevated WBC count in the blood. Chapters 27 and 28 provide a discussion of blood groups, the inflammatory process, and the immune response, respectively.

LOOK AGAIN

See Chapter 10: Review of Human Systems, pp. 178-182.

The bone marrow and lymph glands continually produce and maintain a reserve of WBCs. However, there are not many WBCs in the healthy bloodstream. The normal WBC count is about 5000 to 10,000 cells/mm². **Monocytes** make up about 5% of the total WBC count and increase with

BOX 32-1 Laboratory Tests

Hematocrit is the fraction of the total volume of blood that consists of red blood cells (RBCs), normally about 45%. For example, a value of 46% implies that there are 46 mL of RBCs in 100 mL of blood. The normal hematocrit for males is 40% to 54%. In females a normal hematocrit is 38% to 47%. A low hematocrit value indicates anemia that may result from trauma, surgery, internal bleeding, nutritional deficiency (e.g., iron or vitamin B_{12}), bone marrow disease, or sickle cell disease. A high hematocrit value may be caused by dehydration, lung disease, certain tumors, and disorders of the bone marrow.

Hemoglobin is reported in grams per 100 mL of blood. The normal hemoglobin level for males is 13.5 to 18 g/100 mL. In women a normal hemoglobin measurement is 12 to 16 g/100 mL.

Reticulocyte count offers details about the rate of RBC production. A reticulocyte count of less than 0.5% of the RBC count usually indicates a deceleration in the process of RBC formation. A reticulocyte count greater than 1.5% usually indicates an acceleration of RBC formation.

chronic infections. **Lymphocytes** account for about 27.5%, **neutrophils** about 65%, and **eosinophils** and **basophils** together about 2.5% of the total WBC count. A rise in the number of WBCs aids in the diagnosis of some diseases. An increased WBC count is specific for various illnesses such as bacterial infection, inflammation, leukemia, trauma, and stress.

The **differential count** (also called the *diff*) identifies the different types of leukocytes (WBCs) present in blood. The test is performed by spreading a drop of blood on a microscope slide, staining the slide, and examining it under a microscope. Cells are identified by the shape and appearance of the nucleus, the color of cytoplasm (the background of the cell), and the presence and color of granules. The percentage of each cell type is reported. At the same time, red cells and platelets are examined for abnormalities in appearance.

Platelets

Platelets (thrombocytes) are small, sticky cell fragments. They play an important role in blood clotting. When a blood vessel is cut, platelets travel to the site and swell into odd, irregular shapes and adhere to the damaged vessel wall. Platelets plug the leak and allow other cells to stick to them and to form a clot. However, if the damage to the vessel is too great, the platelets chemically signal the complex clotting process or **clotting cascade** (described later). Platelets repair millions of ruptured capillaries each day. They often make the rest of the clotting cascade unnecessary (Box 32-2).

CRITICAL THINKING
What body functions are impaired if the white blood cell number or function is diminished?

HEMOSTASIS

Hemostasis is the initial physiological response to wounding that causes bleeding to cease. Hemostasis is initiated when there is a break in the integrity of the vascular endothelium. The vascular reaction or physiology of hemostasis involves vasoconstriction, formation of a platelet plug, coagulation, and the growth of fibrous tissue into the blood clot that permanently closes and seals the injured vessel.

Vasoconstriction resulting from injury is rapid but temporary. In response to injury, severed blood vessels constrict and retract with the aid of the surrounding subcutaneous tissues. This vessel spasm slows blood loss immediately. Vasoconstriction may close the ends of the injured vessels completely. This response usually is sustained for as long as 10 minutes. During this time, blood coagulation mechanisms are activated to produce a blood clot.

Platelets adhere to injured blood vessels and to collagen in the connective tissue that surrounds the injured vessel. As platelets contact collagen, they swell, become sticky, and secrete chemicals that activate other surrounding platelets. This process causes the platelets to adhere to one another. The process creates a **platelet plug** in the injured vessel. If the opening in the vessel wall is small, the plug may be sufficient to stop blood loss completely. If the opening in the vessel is large, however, a **blood clot** is necessary to arrest the flow of blood.

BOX 32-2 Clotting Measurements

Clotting time is normally 7 to 10 minutes. The patient bleeds if the clotting time is prolonged. The patient develops intravascular clots if the clotting time is less than normal. Prothrombin (PT) time measures the clotting time of plasma (the extrinsic clotting cascade). The PT test is used to monitor patients taking certain medications and to diagnose clotting disorders. The PT test specifically evaluates the presence of factors VIIa, V, and X and of prothrombin and fibrinogen. A drop in the concentration of any of these factors will cause the blood to take longer to clot. A prolonged PT time is considered abnormal. The PT test is used in combination with the partial thromboplastin time (PTT) to screen for hemophilia and other hereditary clotting disorders.

The PTT uses blood to which a chemical has been added to prevent clotting before the test begins. The PTT measures the integrity of the extrinsic clotting cascade, which is affected by blood-thinning medications (e.g., heparin and warfarin). The PTT time can help determine a possible cause of abnormal bleeding or bruising. Increased PTT time in a person with a bleeding disorder may indicate that a clotting factor is missing or defective.

Blood coagulation occurs as a result of a chemical process that begins within seconds of a severe vessel injury. Coagulation progresses rapidly; within 3 to 6 minutes after the rupture of a vessel, the entire end of the vessel is filled with a clot. Within 30 minutes the clot retracts and the vessel is sealed further. The blood-clotting mechanism is a complex process and includes the following three mechanisms (Figure 32-3):

1. **Prothrombin activator** is formed in response to rupture or damage of the blood vessel.
2. Prothrombin activator stimulates the conversion of **prothrombin** to **thrombin.**
3. Thrombin in the presence of calcium ions acts as an enzyme to convert fibrinogen into *fibrin threads*. These threads entrap platelets, blood cells, and plasma to form the clot.

The process of hemostasis usually is protective and is required for survival. In some instances, though, hemostasis can result in responses that threaten life and function. Examples include myocardial infarction or stroke.

NOTE
Certain diseases or genetic factors that interrupt the clotting cascade can impair hemostasis. Thus they retard the process of clot formation. Examples include hemophilia, thrombocytopenia (low platelet count), and liver disease, which affects the production of **clotting factors** (substances in the blood that act in sequence to stop bleeding by forming a clot). Various drugs also can impair coagulation. *Aspirin* decreases platelet activity. Warfarin suppresses the ability of the liver to make certain clotting factors. In any patient with impaired hemostasis, even minor trauma can result in uncontrollable and life-threatening hemorrhage.

SPECIFIC HEMATOLOGICAL DISORDERS

Hematological disorders presented in this chapter are anemia, leukemia, leukopenia, lymphomas, polycythemia, disseminated intravascular coagulopathy, hemophilia, sickle cell disease, and multiple myeloma (Box 32-3).

Anemia

Anemia is a condition in which the concentration of hemoglobin or erythrocytes in the blood is below normal. Precipitating causes of anemia include chronic or acute blood loss, decreased production of erythrocytes, and increased destruction of erythrocytes. One should note that anemia is not a disease. Rather, anemia is a symptom of a disease. Those at greatest risk are persons with chronic kidney disease, diabetes, heart disease, and cancer; chronic inflammatory conditions such as rheumatoid arthritis or inflammatory bowel disease; and persistent infections such as

---

BOX 32-3 Hematological Disorders by Cell Type

Disorders of Red Blood Cells
Anemia
Polycythemia
Sickle cell disease

Disorders of White Blood Cells
Hodgkin's disease
Non-Hodgkin's lymphomas
Leukemia
Leukopenia
Multiple myelomas

Disorders of Hemostasis
Disseminated intravascular coagulation
Hemophilia
Thrombocytopenia

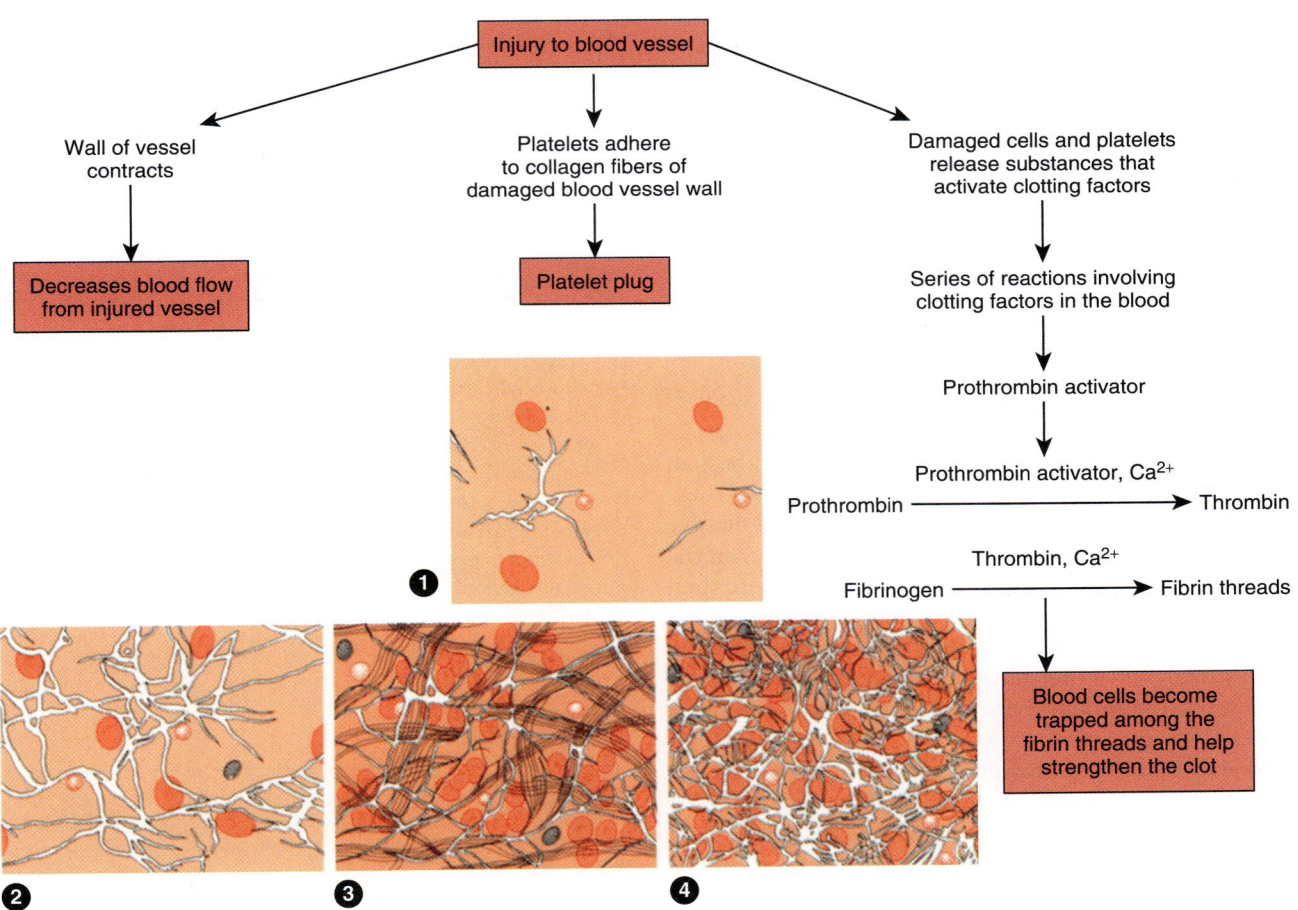

FIGURE 32-3 Overview of blood clotting. Fibrin threads form the webbing of the clot. Blood cells, platelets, and plasma become trapped among the fibrin threads and help strengthen the clot. (From Solomon EP: *Introduction to human anatomy and physiology,* ed 3, St Louis, 2009, Saunders.)

human immunodeficiency virus (HIV). These conditions can cause anemia by interfering with the production of oxygen-carrying RBCs. In the case of cancer and chemotherapy, anemia sometimes can be caused by the treatment itself. Two common forms of anemia are **iron deficiency anemia** and **hemolytic anemia.**

IRON DEFICIENCY ANEMIA

Iron is the critical part of a hemoglobin molecule, giving it the ability to bind oxygen (Figure 32-4). The lack of iron in iron deficiency anemia prevents the bone marrow from making enough hemoglobin for the RBCs. The RBCs produced are small and have a pale center. They also have a reduced oxygen-carrying capacity. The most common cause of iron deficiency anemia in adults is blood loss from menstrual bleeding or intestinal bleeding.[2] A diet that is low in iron usually is the cause of iron deficiency anemia in children. Vitamin deficiencies also can produce anemia. Lack of folic acid (one of the B vitamins) is the most common form of vitamin-deficiency anemia (Box 32-4).

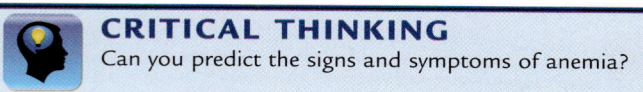

CRITICAL THINKING
Can you predict the signs and symptoms of anemia?

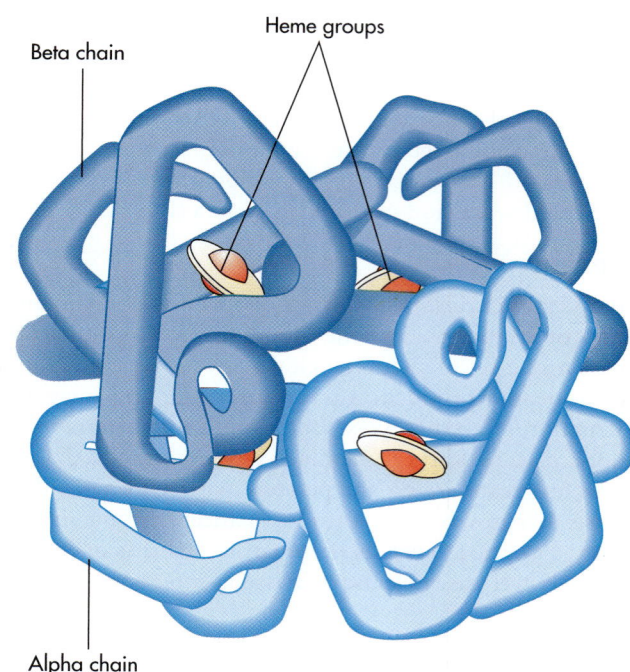

FIGURE 32-4 The 4-chained hemoglobin molecule is made from more than 10,000 atoms. Yet when fully laden, the molecule will carry only 4 pairs of oxygen atoms. Hemoglobin is built around 4 atoms of iron that act like oxygen magnets. Each red blood cell holds 300 million of these vital protein molecules.

Labels: Beta chain, Heme groups, Alpha chain

HEMOLYTIC ANEMIA

Premature destruction of RBCs in the blood (**hemolysis**) causes hemolytic anemia. This destruction can result from an inherited disorder inside the RBC. It also can result from a disorder outside the cell. The condition usually is acquired later in life.

Inherited Disorders. Hemolysis can occur as a result of abnormal rigidity of the cell membrane. This rigidity causes the cell to become trapped at an early stage of its life span in the smaller blood vessels (usually of the spleen). In these smaller blood vessels the RBC is destroyed by macrophages. This type of anemia can occur from a genetic defect in the hemoglobin within the cell (e.g., sickle cell anemia and thalassemia). It also can occur from a defect in one of the enzymes in the cell that helps protect the cell from chemical damage during infectious illness. A deficiency of one of the enzymes, glucose-6-phosphate dehydrogenase, is common in African Americans.

Acquired Disorders. Acquired hemolytic anemia results from one of three conditions:

1. Disorders in which normal RBCs are disrupted as a result of mechanical forces (e.g., abnormal blood vessel linings or blood clots)
2. Autoimmune disorders, which can destroy RBCs with antibodies that are produced by the immune system (e.g., drug-induced hemolytic anemia, an incompatible blood transfusion, described in Chapter 11).

BOX 32-4 Pernicious Anemia

Pernicious anemia results from a vitamin B_{12} deficiency. Pernicious anemia has a number of causes including surgery, infection, medication use, and poor diet. The condition can also result from a lack of *intrinsic factor* (a protein in the stomach), which is needed for the absorption of vitamin B_{12} from food. The deficiency of vitamin B_{12} prevents the body from making an adequate number of healthy RBCs. Severe vitamin B_{12} deficiency can cause neurological problems, such as confusion, dementia, depression, and memory loss.[3] The condition is usually treated with vitamin B_{12} supplements or injections.

NOTE
Drug-induced hemolytic anemia is a blood disorder that occurs from an autoimmune response. This autoimmune response can be triggered by a number of drugs, including cephalosporins, penicillin and its derivatives, NSAIDs, and others. The immune system attacks RBCs and causes their early breakdown and destruction. The condition usually resolves with good outcome when the drug responsible for the disorder is discontinued.

3. Conditions that can cause hemolytic anemia when RBCs are destroyed by microorganisms in the blood (e.g., malaria)

SIGNS AND SYMPTOMS OF ANEMIA

All forms of anemia share signs and symptoms. These signs and symptoms include fatigue and headaches, sometimes a sore mouth or tongue, brittle nails, and, in severe cases, breathlessness and chest pain (Table 32-2). Other patient complaints are related to an abnormal decrease in the number of WBCs (leukopenia) or a reduction in platelets (thrombocytopenia) and may include the following:

- Bleeding from mucous membranes
- Cutaneous bleeding
- Fatigue
- Fever
- Lethargy

DIAGNOSIS AND TREATMENT

The patient's signs and symptoms, patient history, and examination of the patient's blood through blood tests and bone marrow biopsy indicate a diagnosis of most forms of anemia. For example, iron deficiency anemia usually reveals RBCs that are smaller than normal. Hemolytic anemia shows RBCs that are immature and abnormally shaped. Treatment should be indicated to correct, modify, or diminish the mechanism or process that is leading to defective RBC production or reduced RBC survival.

NOTE

A bone marrow biopsy specimen taken from the sternum or pelvis offers details about the various parts of blood. The specimen also provides information about the presence of cells foreign to the marrow. Bone marrow biopsy is useful in diagnosing many hematological disorders such as anemia, leukemia, and certain infections. A bone marrow transplant sometimes is used to treat these and other diseases.

Leukemia

Leukemia refers to any of several types of cancer in which an abnormal proliferation of WBCs usually occurs in the bone marrow (Figure 32-5). The excess production of leukemic cells crowds and impairs the normal production of RBCs, WBCs, and platelets. Leukemia is more common in males than in females. Leukemia is also more common in Caucasians than in African Americans. In 2008, about 46,000 Americans (2500 of them children) were diagnosed with the disease.[4]

The exact cause of leukemia is not known; however, genetics may play a role. Abnormal chromosomes associated with congenital disorders (e.g., Down syndrome) and human immunodeficiency type (HIV-type) viruses are associated with a rare form of this disease. Other factors that may play a role in the development of leukemia include exposure to radiation, viral infections, immune defects, and exposure to various chemicals in home and work environments.

TABLE 32-2 Causes, Signs and Symptoms, and Treatment for Specific Forms of Anemia

Form of Anemia	Causes	Signs and Symptoms	Treatment
Iron deficiency anemia	Insufficient intake of iron Gastrointestinal disorders (e.g., ulcer disease) External and/or internal bleeding Prolonged aspirin or NSAID therapy Gastrectomy (surgical removal of part or all of stomach)	Those related to underlying cause (e.g., bleeding) Those common to all forms of anemia	Correction of underlying cause Supplemental iron tablets or injections
Hemolytic anemia	Genetic red blood cell disorder Autoimmune disorders Malaria and other infections	Jaundice Those common to all forms of anemia	Splenectomy Immunosuppressant drugs Avoidance of drugs or foods that precipitate hemolysis Antimalarial drugs Blood transfusions

NSAID, Nonsteroidal antiinflammatory drug.

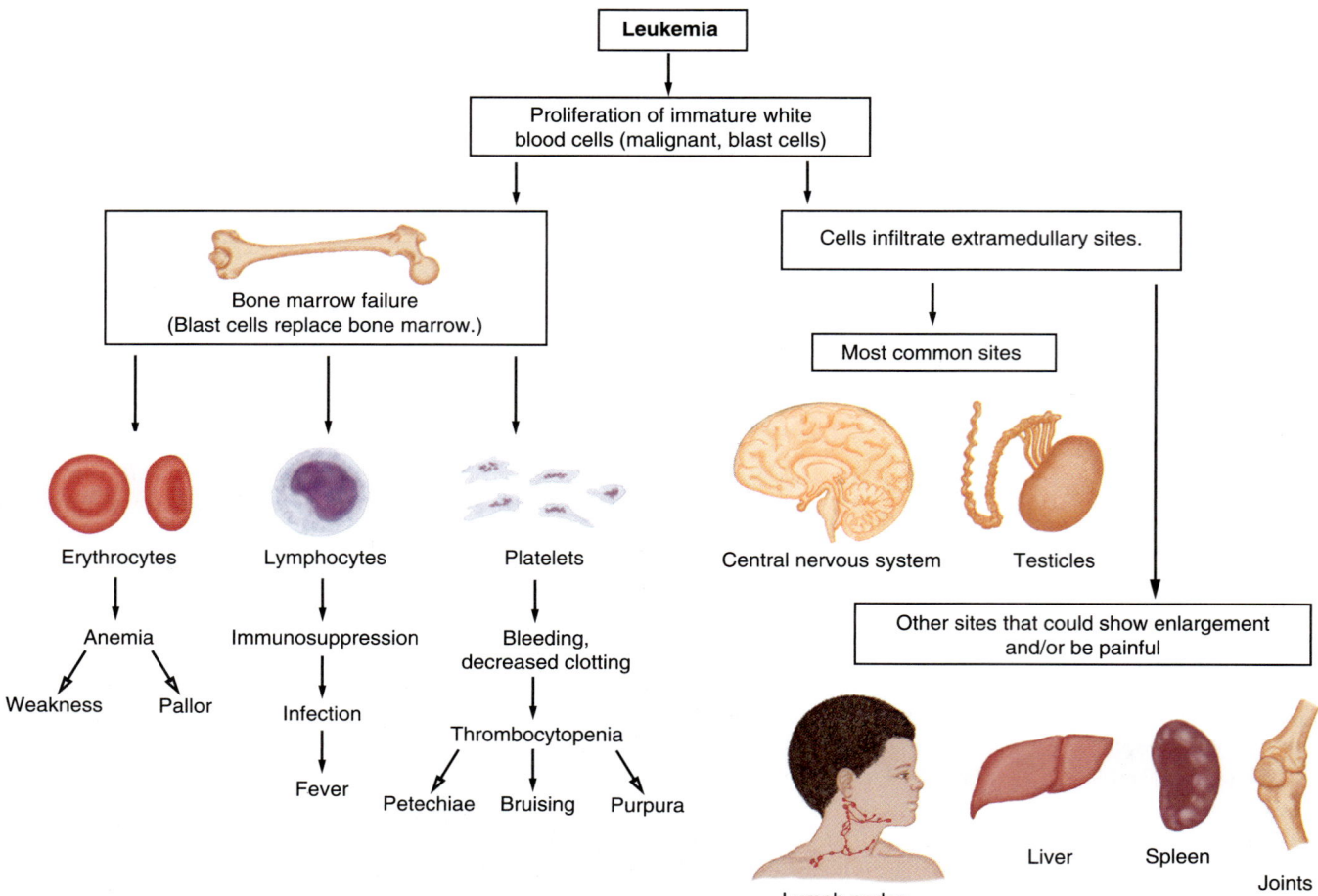

FIGURE 32-5 Pathophysiology of leukemia. (From McKinney ES et al: *Maternal-child nursing,* ed 2, St Louis, 2005, Saunders.)

NOTE

Leukopenia is a decrease in the number of white blood cells (most commonly neutrophils). When white cells are depleted, it weakens the immune system and places the person at risk for developing infection. Leukopenia has many causes including chemotherapy, radiation therapy, posttransplant medications, leukemia, various anemias, and other diseases. The condition is diagnosed with blood testing (complete blood count).

BOX 32-5 Types of Leukemia

The terms *lymphocytic* or *lymphoblastic* indicate that the cancerous change takes place in a type of marrow cell that forms lymphocytes. The terms *myelogenous* or *myeloid* indicate that the cell change takes place in a type of marrow cell that normally matures to form red cells, some types of white cells, and platelets.

Acute lymphocytic leukemia and acute myelogenous leukemia are each composed of *blast cells,* respectively known as lymphoblasts or myeloblasts. Acute leukemias progress rapidly without treatment.

Chronic leukemias have few or no blast cells. Chronic lymphocytic leukemia and chronic myelogenous leukemia usually progress slowly compared to acute leukemias.

CLASSIFICATIONS

Leukemia is classified as *acute* or *chronic.* Cancer cells in acute leukemia begin proliferating at an early stage of their development (arrested as immature cells). Chronic leukemia implies an abnormal proliferation of more mature but not fully differentiated cells. Leukemias are classified further according to the type of WBC involved (Box 32-5). Two common forms of leukemia are *acute lymphocytic leukemia* and *acute myelogenous leukemia.* The first affects mostly children younger than age 15. (It sometimes is called *childhood leukemia.*) The latter affects mostly middle-aged adults. In both types, abnormal WBCs are produced in such large amounts that they eventually accumulate in the vital organs (liver, spleen, lymph, and brain). This impedes the function of these organs and leads to death. Chronic forms of leukemia can develop slowly, often over many years. Cases of disease often are discovered by chance during routine blood analysis.

SIGNS AND SYMPTOMS

The proliferation of leukemic cells or the resulting inadequate production of other normal blood cells makes the patient highly susceptible to serious infections, anemia, and bleeding episodes. Signs and symptoms of leukemia include the following:

- Abdominal fullness
- Bleeding
- Bone pain
- Elevated body temperature and diaphoresis (i.e., sweating)
- Enlargement of lymph nodes
- Enlargement of the liver, spleen, and testes
- Fatigue
- Frequent bruising
- Headache
- Heat intolerance
- Night sweats
- Weight loss

 CRITICAL THINKING
If a child has a lot of odd bruises, what would you suspect if a diagnosis of leukemia is not known?

DIAGNOSIS AND TREATMENT

The diagnosis of leukemia is confirmed by bone marrow biopsy. The severity of the disease is assessed by the degree of liver and spleen enlargement, extent of anemia, and lack of platelets in the blood. Treatment for acute leukemia can include the transfusion of blood and platelets, antibiotic therapy to manage anemia and infection, and the use of anticancer drugs and sometimes radiation to destroy the leukemic cells. In some cases the leukemia is treated with a bone marrow transplant (Box 32-6). Patients with chronic leukemia can be managed effectively with medication. Many patients require no treatment in its early stages.

? DID YOU KNOW?
Blood Transfusion Complications
Each year, almost 5 million Americans receive a blood transfusion. The transfusion may be of whole blood (containing RBCs, WBCs, platelets, and plasma). More commonly, an individual component of whole blood is transfused (RBCs [most common], plasma, or platelets and clotting factors). Blood is usually obtained through blood banks. These facilities collect, test, and store the blood to ensure its safety and availability. The blood is typed as A, B, AB, or O, and Rh status is determined (described in Chapter 11). The blood is also tested for viral or bacterial infection (HIV, hepatitis B and C, variant Creutzfeldt-Jakob disease). Complications of blood transfusions (if any) are usually mild. Some, however, can be serious and life threatening. Possible complications include[5]:

- Allergic reaction: An allergic reaction to a transfusion may be mild or severe. Signs and symptoms include anxiety, nausea, pain in the chest or back, dyspnea, fever and chills, tachycardia, and hypotension.
- Viral or infectious disease from tainted blood (rare).

- Fever: May occur within 24 hours of the transfusion. This is usually a response to the white blood cells in donated blood. (These cells are sometimes removed by the blood bank to avoid this complication.)
- Circulatory overload: Occurs from a rapid transfusion of a large volume of blood. Risk increases in patients older than 60 years of age and in those who have cardiac or pulmonary failure or anemia. Primary signs and symptoms are dyspnea, orthopnea, peripheral edema, and a rapid rise in blood pressure.
- Iron overload: Often a result of frequent blood transfusions. The iron may accumulate and damage the heart, lung, and other organs.
- Lung injury: Usually a complication only in very ill patients. Although rare, injury usually occurs within 6 hours of the transfusion. Cause is unknown, but may be related to proteins found in the donated plasma of women who have been pregnant. The donated plasma of men is sometimes preferred.
- Acute immune hemolytic reaction: A rare and serious complication that results from type-and-cross-mismatch of patient and donor blood. Signs and symptoms of the reaction are usually sudden in onset and include fever, chills, chest pain, nausea, and dark urine. Hemolytic reactions attack new red blood cells and can lead to kidney damage.
- Delayed hemolytic reaction: A slower version of the acute immune hemolytic reaction that may not be noticed until the patient's RBC count is quite low.
- Graft versus host disease (GVHD): An often fatal illness caused by WBCs in donated blood. The disease causes destruction of host tissue. Symptoms usually begin within 1 month of the transfusion and include fever, rash, and diarrhea. GVHD is most common in patients with immune suppression.

Signs and symptoms of the reactions and complications listed above require that the transfusion be immediately stopped. In-hospital care for these patients will be dictated by the severity and cause of the adverse reaction.

Lymphomas

Lymphoma is a general term applied to any neoplastic disorder of the lymphoid tissue. Hodgkin's disease is one type; all others, despite their diversity, are called *non-Hodgkin's lymphomas*. All lymphomas are **malignant** (cancerous tumors that tend to metastasize).

 NOTE
Blood cancers such as leukemia, Hodgkin's lymphoma, non-Hodgkin's lymphoma, myeloma, and myelodysplastic syndromes are cancers that originate in the bone marrow or lymphatic tissues. They are considered to be related cancers because they involve the uncontrolled growth of cells with similar functions and origins. The diseases result from an acquired genetic injury to the DNA of a single cell, which becomes abnormal (malignant) and multiplies continuously. The accumulation of malignant cells interferes with the body's production of healthy blood cells. Every 4 minutes one person is diagnosed with a blood cancer. An estimated 139,860 people in the United States will be diagnosed with leukemia, lymphoma, or myeloma in 2009. New cases of leukemia, Hodgkin's and non-Hodgkin's lymphoma, and myeloma account for 9.5% of the more than 1.4 million new cancer cases diagnosed in the United States each year.[7]

BOX 32-6 Blood and Marrow Stem Cell Transplantation

A stem cell is a cell whose daughter cells may develop into other cell types. Some cells can develop into several different types of mature cells, including lymphocytes, granulocytes, thrombocytes, and erythrocytes. Stem cells reside in marrow and also circulate in the blood. They also circulate in large numbers in fetal blood. They can be recovered from umbilical cord and placental blood after childbirth. Stem cells can be harvested, frozen, and stored for future transplantation.

Stem cell transplantation is standard therapy for selected patients with leukemia, lymphoma, and myeloma. The two major types of stem cell transplants are *autologous* and *allogenic.* An autologous transplant uses the patient's own marrow. The marrow is collected while the patient is in remission. Before it is given back to the patient, the marrow may be treated with chemotherapeutic agents or antibodies to cleanse it of cancer cells that may be present in the marrow. An allogenic transplant uses marrow from a donor. The donor is usually a brother or sister with the same tissue type. If a sibling is not available, a search of bone marrow registries for tissue-typed volunteers can be made for an unrelated donor. In addition to treating some cancers and other blood disorders, stem cells may play a key role in the future in treating diseases such as Alzheimer's, Parkinson's, and heart disease.

Adapted from Leukemia and Lymphoma Society: *Blood and marrow stem cell transplantation,* White Plains, NY, Feb 2008, Author.

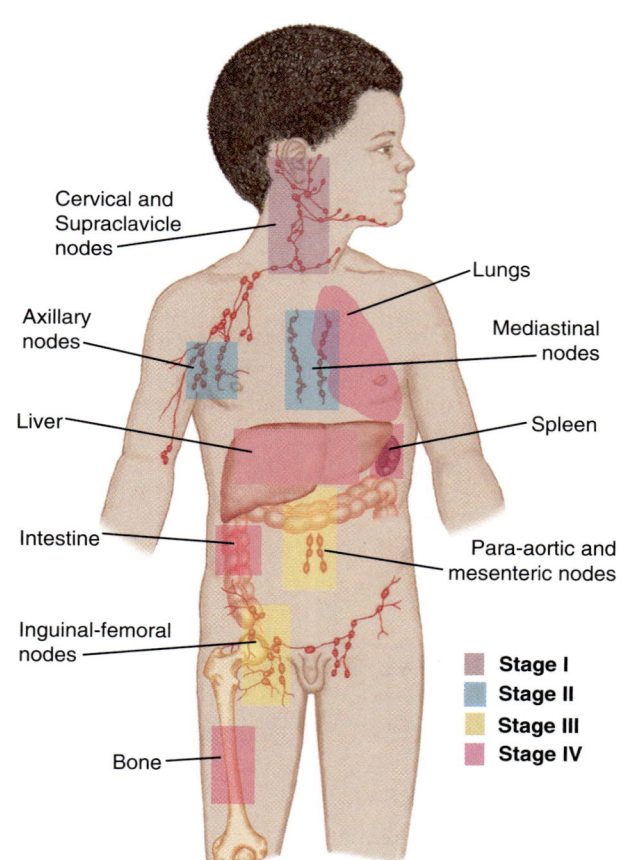

FIGURE 32-6 Pathophysiology of Hodgkin's disease. (From McKinney ES, et al: *Maternal-child nursing,* ed 2, St Louis, 2005, Saunders.)

HODGKIN'S DISEASE

Hodgkin's disease is characterized by painless, progressive enlargement of lymphoid tissue found mainly in the lymph nodes and spleen (Figure 32-6). Left unchecked, these cancer cells multiply and eventually displace healthy lymphocytes, suppressing the immune system. Signs and symptoms include swollen lymph nodes in the neck, axillae, or groin; fatigue; chills; and night sweats. Some patients also experience severe itching, persistent cough, weight loss, shortness of breath, and chest discomfort.

Hodgkin's disease is a rare cancer of unknown cause that may have a heritable component. The disease is more common in males than in females, with a peak incidence at age 20 to 29 as well as in persons between 55 and 70 years of age.[1] The disease is confirmed by the identification of *Reed-Sternberg cells* in lymph nodes or organs affected by the cancer. Treatment depends on the level of lymph node and organ system involvement (the *stage* of the disease) and can consist of radiation and chemotherapy with anticancer drugs. Hodgkin's disease is one of the most curable cancers.

NON-HODGKIN'S LYMPHOMAS

Non-Hodgkin's lymphomas vary in their malignancy according to the nature and activity of the abnormal cells. At least 10 types of non-Hodgkin's lymphoma have been identified. Each type is ranked as low, intermediate, or high grade. This ranking is based on how aggressively the disease behaves. Low-grade diseases usually progress slowly. They

also tend not to spread beyond the lymphatic system. High-grade diseases can spread to distant organs within a few months. Signs and symptoms include painless swelling of one or more groups of lymph nodes, enlargement of the liver and spleen, fever, and, in rare cases, abdominal pain and gastrointestinal bleeding.

The cause of these cancers is largely unknown. One form, *Burkitt's lymphoma,* is a childhood cancer. In Africa, it is strongly associated with infection by Epstein-Barr virus. Other types worldwide have been linked to infection by HIV-type viruses and other conditions that affect the immune system (e.g., organ transplantation, radiation and chemotherapy, lupus, and rheumatoid arthritis). Treatment consists of radiation therapy, administration of anticancer drugs, and sometimes bone marrow transplantation.

Polycythemia

Polycythemia is an increase in the total RBC mass of the blood. The condition may be a natural response to chronic hypoxia (*secondary polycythemia*). Polycythemia also may occur for unknown reasons (*primary polycythemia*). Polycythemia also can result from dehydration (*apparent polycythemia*). In this instance, the RBC production does not exceed the upper limits of normal.

SECONDARY POLYCYTHEMIA

Secondary polycythemia can be naturally present in persons who live in or visit areas of high altitude. Polycythemia is due to reduced air pressure and low oxygen concentration. When the oxygen supply to the blood is reduced, the kidneys produce the hormone *erythropoietin*. This hormone stimulates RBC production in the bone marrow to compensate for the reduced oxygen supply. The result is an increase in the oxygen-carrying efficiency of the blood. The RBC numbers return to normal when the person returns to sea level. Secondary polycythemia also can be present in heavy smokers. The disease can be caused by chronic bronchitis and conditions that increase erythropoietin production (e.g., liver cancer and some kidney disorders).

PRIMARY POLYCYTHEMIA

Primary polycythemia is also known as *polycythemia vera*. Primary polycythemia is a rare disorder of the bone marrow. In this disorder the increased production of RBCs causes the blood to thicken. This condition primarily develops in persons older than 50 years of age and can lead to several physiological problems that include the following:

- Blurred vision
- Dizziness
- Generalized itching
- Headache
- Hypertension
- Red hands and feet; red-purple complexion
- Splenomegaly

Other complications associated with primary polycythemia include platelet disorders, which cause bleeding or clot formation; stroke; and the development of other bone marrow diseases (e.g., leukemias). Treatment consists of phlebotomy. (This is the slow removal of blood through a vein.) Treatment also consists of anticancer drug therapy. The therapy controls the overproduction of RBCs in the marrow.

Disseminated Intravascular Coagulopathy

Disseminated intravascular coagulopathy (DIC) is a complication of severe injury, trauma, or disease. Disseminated intravascular coagulopathy is a common abnormal clotting disorder. The disease most often is seen in the critical care setting. It disrupts the balance among procoagulants, inhibitors, thrombus formation, and lysis. Signs and symptoms of DIC include dyspnea and bleeding and symptoms associated with hypotension and hypoperfusion.

Disseminated intravascular coagulopathy occurs in two phases.[8] The first phase is characterized by free thrombin in the blood, fibrin deposits, and aggregation of platelets. The second phase is characterized by hemorrhage caused by the depletion of clotting factors. The clinical consequences of these processes predispose the patient to multiple-system organ failure from bleeding and coagulation disorders caused by the following (Figure 32-7):

- Loss of platelets and clotting factors
- Fibrinolysis
- Fibrin degradation interference
- Small vessel obstruction, tissue ischemia, RBC injury, and anemia from fibrin deposits

DIC is confirmed through laboratory tests. Then the treatment is aimed at reversing the underlying illness or injury that triggered the event. In an effort to control the depletion of clotting factors, in-hospital care includes the replacement of platelets, coagulation factors, and blood. At the same time, attempts are made to manage the primary process.

Hemophilia

Hemophilia refers to a medical condition that causes uncontrolled bleeding and involves the loss of bleeding control mechanisms. The disease is a group of inherited bleeding disorders (Box 32-7). Hemophilia A is due to a deficiency in factor VIII. This factor is essential to the process of blood clotting (Table 32-3). Another less common form of hemophilia, caused by a deficiency of factor IX, is known as hemophilia B. This hemophilia also is known as *Christmas disease* (named for a man first diagnosed with the disease in 1952). All types of hemophilia present

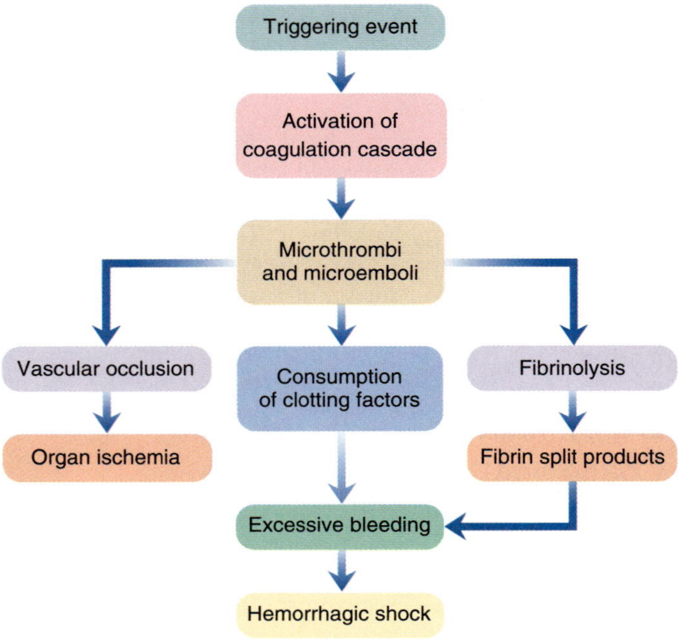

FIGURE 32-7 Pathophysiology of disseminated intravascular coagulation. Clotting and bleeding occur simultaneously, resulting in organ ischemia and hemorrhagic shock. (From Copstead-Kirkhorn LE, Banasik JL: *Pathophysiology*, ed 4, St Louis, 2010, Saunders.)

TABLE 32-3 Clotting Factors and Synonyms

Factor	Synonyms
I	Fibrinogen
II	Prothrombin
III	Thromboplastin
IV	Calcium
V	Proaccelerin
VI	None in use
VII	Serum prothrombin conversion accelerator
VIII	Antihemophilic globulin, antihemophilic factor
IX	Plasma thromboplastin component, Christmas factor
X	Stuart factor
XI	Plasma thromboplastin antecedent
XII	Hageman factor
XIII	Fibrin-stabilizing factor

BOX 32-7 Hereditary Characteristics of Hemophilia

Chromosomes from the mother link with an equal number from the father, and each pair determines the type of information that genes carry. Females have two X chromosomes. Males have an X and a Y chromosome. The mother passes on the X chromosome to her child, and the father passes on an X or a Y. Two X chromosomes produce a female child; an X and a Y produce a male child.

Hemophilia stems from an abnormal gene on the X chromosome. A female with an abnormal X chromosome usually is spared the disease because, although she received one abnormal X chromosome from one parent, the normal X chromosome passed on from her other parent counteracted the abnormal gene. However, she is a carrier of the disease and can pass it on to her children. A woman can have hemophilia only if her mother is a carrier and her father has hemophilia, which is rare. Affected males do not pass the defective gene to sons, but they pass it on to all of their daughters. A male, however, receives only one X chromosome. If his mother is a carrier, the male child will have a 50% chance of having hemophilia.

with similar problems. Yet the specific factor involved determines the severity of bleeding. About 18,000 people in the United States have hemophilia; about 400 are born with the disorder each year.[9]

Bleeding from hemophilia can occur spontaneously, even after minor injury. It also can occur during some medical procedures (e.g., tooth extraction). Hemorrhage can occur anywhere in the body. However, bleeding into joints, deep muscles, the urinary tract, and intracranial sites is the most common. Head trauma is potentially life threatening in these patients. Central nervous system bleeding is the major cause of death for patients with hemophilia in all age groups.[10]

Hemophilia is controlled by infusions of concentrates of factor VIII. These infusions can be administered by the patient. However, serious or unusual bleeding often requires hospitalization. Persons with hemophilia are advised to avoid activities that may increase their risk of injury. These include, for example, contact sports. Most patients with hemophilia are knowledgeable about their disease. Most seek emergency care only when complicated problems and trauma-related issues arise.

CRITICAL THINKING

Imagine that you are caring for a patient with hemophilia who has fallen 15 feet from a ladder. This patient refuses care and transportation. What should you do?

NOTE

Factor VIII is made from large pools of donor blood. During the first few years of the acquired immunodeficiency syndrome epidemic, many persons with hemophilia and their sexual partners became infected with human immunodeficiency virus through factor VIII infusions. There are careful screening protocols for blood now. However, infusions still carry a minute risk of transmitting hepatitis B virus, hepatitis C virus, and human immunodeficiency virus to factor VIII recipients. Another factor VIII product, recombinant factor VIII (Recombinate), is produced by inserting cloned factor VIII into animal tissues. Recombinate is not made from human plasma, is the purest form of factor VIII, does not transmit viral contamination, and is as effective as plasma-derived factor VIII.[11]

Thrombocytopenia

Thrombocytopenia is a low platelet count. In healthy people, the blood normally contains 150,000 to 450,000 platelets/microliter of blood. At levels of 20,000 to 30,000 platelets/microliter of blood, bleeding can occur with relatively minor trauma. At levels below 20,000 platelets/microliter of blood, spontaneous bleeding can occur, increasing the risk for shock and death. This is especially true if bleeding occurs in the brain. Bleeding on the skin is usually the first sign of a low platelet count. This may appear as:

- Small red or purple spots on the skin (petechiae), often on the lower legs
- Purple, brown, and red bruises (purpura) that happen easily and often
- Prolonged bleeding, even from minor cuts
- Bleeding or oozing from the mouth or nose, especially nosebleeds or bleeding from brushing teeth
- Unusually heavy menstrual flow

Thrombocytopenia can occur if the body does not produce enough or destroys too many platelets, or if the spleen retains too many platelets. The disease is often associated with leukemia or lymphoma, aplastic anemia, vitamin B_{12} or folic acid deficiency anemias, an enlarged spleen, infectious diseases such as HIV/acquired immunodeficiency syndrome (AIDS), and massive blood transfusions. Two diseases that occur because of increased destruction of platelets are[12]:

- Idiopathic thrombocytopenic purpura (ITP)—ITP occurs when antibodies attack and destroy the body's platelets for unknown reasons. In children, ITP can be an acute condition that occurs after infection. Acute ITP is rare in adults. More common is chronic ITP, a condition that may persist for years and most frequently affects women ages 20 to 40 years.
- Thrombotic thrombocytopenic purpura (TTP)—TTP is a life-threatening disease that occurs when small blood clots form suddenly throughout the body. It can result in cardiac hemorrhage and death. It occurs more often in women and is associated with pregnancy, metastatic cancer, chemotherapy, HIV/AIDS, and some prescription drugs. Patients with TTP experience kidney failure or decreased kidney function, fever, and neurological complications.

Treatment for thrombocytopenia depends on cause and severity. Some patients will only require careful monitoring of their platelet counts. Other more serious cases may be treated with administration of corticosteroids (prednisone), transfusion of platelets, and, rarely, surgical removal of the spleen.

Sickle Cell Disease

Sickle cell disease is an inherited blood disorder that affects red blood cells. There are several types of sickle cell disease. The most common type is **sickle cell anemia.** Sickle cell disease is a debilitating and unpredictable genetic illness. It affects persons of African descent and, less

BOX 32-8 Characteristics of Sickle Cell Trait

A person must inherit two sickle cell genes—one from each parent—to develop sickle cell disease. When only one gene is present, the condition is known as a *sickle cell trait*. Persons with sickle cell trait usually do not experience symptoms except occasionally under low-oxygen conditions (e.g., scuba diving or traveling at high altitudes). However, these persons can pass the gene, and possibly the disease, on to their children. If both parents have sickle cell trait, the child has a 25% chance of developing the disease, a 50% chance of having sickle cell trait, and a 25% chance of having neither. Genetic counseling should be considered for carriers of the disease who plan to become parents. Many states require sickle cell screening of newborns. Some colleges and universities also screen young athletes for the sickle cell trait as part of the athlete's health assessment.

commonly, persons of Mediterranean origin. One in 12 African Americans and more than 70,000 Americans of different ethnic origins are estimated to suffer from sickle cell disease. In the United States, about 1000 persons are born with the disease each year. It is estimated that 12.5 million Americans have *sickle cell trait*.[13] (Box 32-8). Signs and symptoms of sickle cell disease include the following:

- Delayed growth, development, and sexual maturation in children
- Jaundice
- Priapism in adolescent and adult males
- Splenomegaly
- Stroke

SHOW ME THE EVIDENCE

Researchers asked patients older than 16 years with sickle cell disease to maintain a diary for 6 months that outlined pain incidence and severity, opioid use, and frequency of emergency department (ED) visits. At entry they completed a survey of other pertinent information and blood and urine samples were analyzed. The goal of this study was to describe characteristics of patients who frequently seek emergency care for sickle cell disease versus those who do not. Because it is common for frequent ED users to be labeled as drug seekers these researchers sought to describe their characteristics. Of the patients included in the study 35% were identified as high ED users. These frequent users had more severe disease as evidenced by higher pain levels, lower hematocrit levels, and increased need for transfusions.

From Aisiku IP, Smith WR, McClish DK, et al: Comparisons of high versus low emergency department utilizers in sickle cell disease, *Ann Emerg Med* 53(5):587-593, 2009.

PATHOPHYSIOLOGY

Sickle cell disease produces an abnormal type of hemoglobin called *hemoglobin S*. This abnormal type has an inferior oxygen-carrying capacity. When hemoglobin S is exposed to low oxygen states, it crystallizes. This distorts the RBCs into a sickle shape (Figure 32-8). The sickle-shaped cells are fragile and easily destroyed. They also are unable to pass

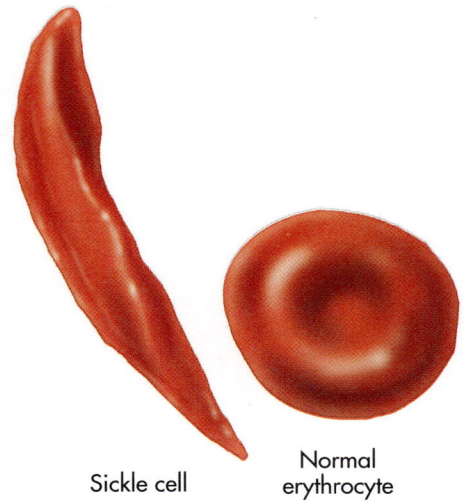

Sickle cell   Normal erythrocyte

FIGURE 32-8 Sickle cell versus normal erythrocyte. (From McKinney ES, et al: *Maternal-child nursing,* ed 2, St Louis, 2005, Saunders.)

easily through tiny blood vessels and consequently block flow to various organs and tissues. This causes a vasoocclusive **sickle cell crisis** that can be life threatening. As fewer RBCs pass through congested vessels, tissues and joints become starved for oxygen and other nutrients. This causes excruciating pain. Other signs and symptoms of sickle cell disease are increased weakness, aching, chest pain with shortness of breath, sudden and severe abdominal pain, bony deformities, icteric (jaundice) sclera (Figure 32-9), fever, and arthralgia (joint pain) (Figure 32-10).

NOTE
Acute chest syndrome (ACS) is defined as a new abnormal consolidation on a chest radiograph in a patient with sickle cell disease. The condition is usually caused by pulmonary infarction from a sickle crisis in adults, and infection in children. The syndrome may be associated with acute pleuritic chest pain, fever, and leukocytosis. ACS is a common medical emergency for patients with sickle cell disease. It often requires hospitalization.

CRITICAL THINKING
How do you think a patient with such chronic pain must feel at the beginning of a sickle cell crisis?

Sickle cell crisis can occur in any part of the body and can vary in intensity from one person to the next and from one crisis to the next. Over time the crises can destroy the spleen, kidneys, gallbladder, and other organs. Sickle cell crisis may occur for no apparent reason. It also may be triggered by conditions such as the following:
- Dehydration
- Exposure to extremes in temperature
- Infection

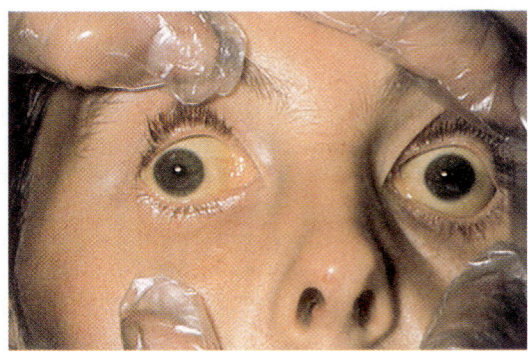

FIGURE 32-9 Jaundice of the sclera.

BOX 32-9 Care Objectives for Sickle Cell Crisis

The main care objectives of patients in sickle cell crisis are to provide (1) supplemental oxygen by facemask or nasal cannula to help counter tissue hypoxia and reduce cell clumping; (2) rest to minimize energy expenditure and oxygen use; (3) hydration through oral and IV therapy; (4) electrolyte replacement, because hypoxia results in metabolic acidosis, which also promotes sickling; (5) analgesics for the severe pain from vasoocclusion; and (6) blood replacement to treat anemia and to reduce the viscosity of the sickled blood.[14]

- Lack of oxygen
- Strenuous physical activity
- Stress
- Trauma

Three less common types of sickle cell crisis are aplastic, hemolytic, and splenic sequestration. In *aplastic crisis* the bone marrow temporarily stops producing RBCs. In *hemolytic crisis* the RBCs break down too rapidly to be replaced adequately. *Splenic sequestration* usually is a childhood difficulty that occurs when blood becomes trapped in the spleen. This causes the organ to enlarge and possibly may lead to death.

MANAGEMENT

At this time, no cure exists for sickle cell disease. Because of the eventual damage that occurs to the spleen, patients with sickle cell disease are at increased risk for septicemia if infected by certain types of bacteria. Children with the disease should be current with all immunizations. When in crisis, these patients require prompt treatment with oxygen if hypoxic, intravenous therapy to manage dehydration, antibiotics to manage infection, and analgesics (e.g., ***morphine***) to manage pain (Box 32-9). In severe cases a blood transfusion may be indicated to effect a temporary replacement of hemoglobin S. Blood transfusions also can be advised during pregnancy to reduce the risk of a crisis, which can be fatal to the mother and fetus. Transfusions also may be advised before surgery because anesthesia can be hazardous to those with the disease.

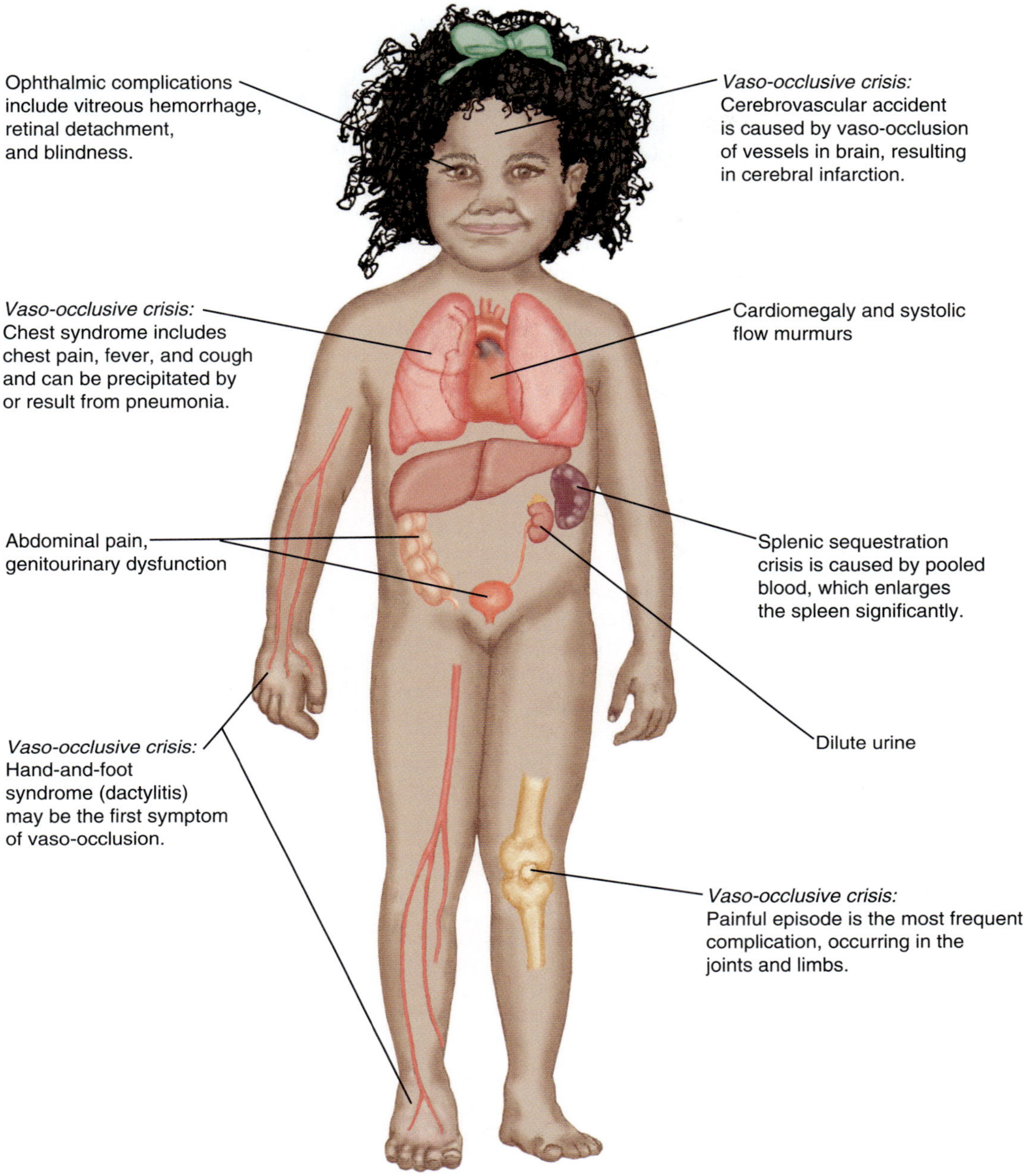

Ophthalmic complications
include vitreous hemorrhage,
retinal detachment,
and blindness.

Vaso-occlusive crisis:
Cerebrovascular accident
is caused by vaso-occlusion
of vessels in brain, resulting
in cerebral infarction.

Vaso-occlusive crisis:
Chest syndrome includes
chest pain, fever, and cough
and can be precipitated by
or result from pneumonia.

Cardiomegaly and systolic
flow murmurs

Abdominal pain,
genitourinary dysfunction

Splenic sequestration
crisis is caused by pooled
blood, which enlarges
the spleen significantly.

Vaso-occlusive crisis:
Hand-and-foot
syndrome (dactylitis)
may be the first symptom
of vaso-occlusion.

Dilute urine

Vaso-occlusive crisis:
Painful episode is the most frequent
complication, occurring in the
joints and limbs.

FIGURE 32-10 Pathophysiology of sickle cell disease. (From Ferguson DG, Fodden DI: *Accident and emergency medicine,* London, 1998, Churchill Livingstone.)

Multiple Myeloma

Multiple myeloma is a malignant neoplasm of the bone marrow. The tumor, composed of plasma cells, destroys bone tissue (especially in flat bones). This causes pain, fractures, hypercalcemia, and skeletal deformities. In myeloma the neoplastic cells produce large amounts of protein (*M protein*) that affect the viscosity of the blood. Masses of coagulated protein can accumulate within the tissues and impair function. Some patients with this disease die of kidney failure. The kidneys fail because of the buildup of proteins that infiltrate the kidneys and block the renal tubules. In many ways, multiple myeloma resembles leukemia. However, the plasma cell proliferation generally is confined to the bone marrow.

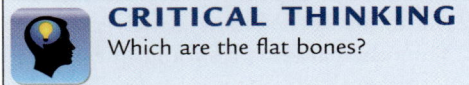

CRITICAL THINKING
Which are the flat bones?

Other disorders associated with multiple myeloma include proteinuria, anemia, weight loss, pulmonary complications from rib fracture, and recurrent infections from suppression of the immune system. Patient complaints associated with multiple myeloma may include weakness, skeletal pain, hemorrhage, hematuria, lethargy, weight loss, and frequent fractures.

Multiple myeloma occurs rarely before 40 years of age and then occurs increasingly with age. The disease is more common in males than in females and may have a heritable component.[1] Multiple myeloma is diagnosed through x-ray films, blood studies, and tumor biopsy. Treatment consists of chemotherapy with anticancer drugs, radiation therapy, plasma exchange, and bone marrow transplantation.

GENERAL ASSESSMENT AND MANAGEMENT OF PATIENTS WITH HEMATOLOGICAL DISORDERS

As stated previously, most patients with hematological disorders are knowledgeable about their disease. Often they call emergency medical services to help manage a "change" in their condition. They also may call to arrange for transportation to an emergency department for physician evaluation. The situations that invoke a call for emergency care vary by patient and disease. Common chief complaints can be classified by body system (Table 32-4).

Prehospital Care

In many cases the prehospital care for a patient with a hematological disorder will be mainly supportive. As with any other patient care encounter, however, the paramedic should perform a general assessment, a focused history, and focused physical examination. These measures will guide patient care. They also will help to determine the appropriateness of emergency transport. Some patients with hematological disorders will have complex medical histories. When possible, these patients should be transported to the primary hospital where they usually receive their medical care.

As referenced in Table 32-4, a patient with a hematological disorder may have a variety of complaints and physical findings. Some patient complaints may be vague as well. (Examples include fever, fatigue, and headache.) This can further complicate the paramedic's assessment. After ensuring adequate airway, ventilatory, and circulatory status, the paramedic should assess vital signs and perform a physical examination. The patient's skin should be assessed for color and turgor, noting any cyanosis or jaundice, warmth or coolness, bruising, edema, or ulcerations. The paramedic also should ascertain any new onset of fever, weakness, cough, rash, spontaneous bleeding (e.g., bleeding gums, epistaxis), vomiting, or diarrhea. Some hematological disorders can involve the ability of the blood to deliver enough oxygen to tissues. Thus the paramedic should question all patients with hematological disorders specifically about

recent dizziness, syncope, difficulty breathing, and heartbeat irregularities.

Other key elements of the patient assessment and history include identifying existing hematological disease (including any family history of hematological disease), any significant medical history or recent injury, the patient's medication use (prescriptions and over-the-counter medications, herbal supplements), allergies, and alcohol or illicit drug use.

Based on the patient's condition, prehospital care measures may include oxygen administration, intravenous fluid replacement, the use of antidysrhythmics, and the administration of analgesics for pain management. Some of these patients will be gravely ill; calming and comfort measures for the patient and family should be provided.

TABLE 32-4 Chief Complaints of Patients with Hematological Disorders Classified by Body System

Body System	Complaints	Possible Causes
Central nervous system	Altered level of consciousness	Anemia, sickle cell disease
	Increased weakness, numbness	Autoimmune disease
	Visual disturbances/ loss of vision	Unilateral sensory deficits
Cardiorespiratory	Dyspnea/crackles	Heart failure
	Anemia	Bleeding disorders
	Pulmonary edema	Hemoptysis
	Chest pain	Tachycardia
Integumentary	Prolonged bleeding	Hemolytic anemia; polycythemia
	Bruising	Sickle cell disease; liver disease
	Itching/petechiae	Jaundice
	Pallor	
Musculoskeletal	Bone or joint pain	Autoimmune disease
	Fracture	Hemophilia
Gastrointestinal	Abdominal pain	Hemolytic anemia, viral disease
	Bleeding of gums/ gingivitis	Blood-clotting abnormalities
	Epistaxis	Autoimmune disease
		Generalized sepsis
	Ulceration	Melena/ hematemesis
Genitourinary	Hematuria	Sickle cell disease, bleeding disorders
	Menorrhagia/ amenorrhagia	
	Priapism	Infection
		Sexually transmitted disease

SUMMARY

- Blood is composed of cells and formed elements surrounded by plasma. About 95% of the volume of formed elements consists of RBCs (erythrocytes). The remaining 5% consists of WBCs (leukocytes) and cell fragments (platelets).

- Anemia is a condition in which the amount of hemoglobin or erythrocytes in the blood is below normal. Two common forms of anemia are iron deficiency anemia and hemolytic anemia. All forms of anemia share signs and symptoms. These signs and symptoms include fatigue and headaches, sometimes a sore mouth or tongue, brittle nails, and, in severe cases, breathlessness and chest pain. Diagnosis is made by history and from blood tests and bone marrow biopsy results.

- Leukemia refers to any of several types of cancer in which an abnormal proliferation of WBCs usually occurs in the bone marrow. The proliferation of leukemic cells crowds and impairs the normal production of RBCs, WBCs, and platelets. Leukemia is classified as acute or chronic. The proliferation of leukemic cells makes the patient highly susceptible to serious infections, anemia, and bleeding episodes. The diagnosis is confirmed by bone marrow biopsy.

- Lymphoma refers to a group of diseases that range from slowly growing chronic disorders to rapidly evolving acute conditions. Hodgkin's disease is one type; all others are called non-Hodgkin's lymphomas.

- Polycythemia is characterized by an unusually large number of RBCs in the blood as a result of their increased production by the bone marrow. Polycythemia may be a natural response to hypoxia. (This is known as secondary polycythemia.) Polycythemia also may occur for unknown reasons. (This is known as primary polycythemia.)

- Disseminated intravascular coagulopathy is a complication of severe injury, trauma, or disease. It disrupts the balance among procoagulants, thrombin formation, inhibitors, and lysis. Signs and symptoms of disseminated intravascular coagulation include dyspnea, bleeding, and symptoms associated with hypotension and hypoperfusion. The treatment is aimed at reversing the underlying illness or injury that triggered the event.

- Hemophilia A is caused by a deficiency of a blood protein called factor VIII. Hemophilia B is caused by a deficiency of factor IX. Bleeding from hemophilia can occur spontaneously, after even minor injury, or during some medical procedures.

- Thrombocytopenia is a low platelet count. It can occur when the body does not produce enough or destroys too many platelets, or if the spleen retains too many platelets. Bleeding is the chief complication of thrombocytopenia.

- Sickle cell disease is a debilitating and unpredictable recessive genetic illness. It affects persons of African descent. Less often, it affects persons of Mediterranean origin. Sickle cell anemia produces an abnormal type of hemoglobin. This is called hemoglobin S. This abnormal type has an inferior oxygen-carrying capacity. Complications of sickle cell disease include episodes of severe pain, fatigue, pallor, jaundice, stroke, delayed growth, hematuria, priapism, and splenomegaly.

- Multiple myeloma is a malignant neoplasm of the bone marrow. The tumor destroys bone tissue (especially flat bones). This causes pain, fractures, hypercalcemia, and skeletal deformities.

- In many cases of hematological disorders, the prehospital treatment is supportive. Treatment includes ensuring adequate airway, ventilatory, and circulatory support.

REFERENCES

1. McCance KL, Huether SE: *Pathophysiology: the biologic basis for disease in adults and children*, ed 7, St Louis, 2006, Mosby.

2. Rosen P, Barkin R: *Emergency medicine: concepts and clinical practice*, ed 6, St Louis, 2006, Mosby.

3. National Heart, Lung, and Blood Institute, National Institutes of Health: *Pernicious anemia*, www.nhlbi.nih.gov/health/dci/Diseases/prnanmia/prnanmia_what.html, accessed 9-7-10.

4. Leukemia and Lymphoma Society: *Leukemia*, www.leukemia-lymphoma.org/all_page?item_id=7026, accessed 9-7-10.

5. National Heart, Lung, and Blood Institute, National Institutes of Health: *Blood transfusion*, www.nhlbi.nih.gov/health/dci/Diseases/bt/bt_risk.html, accessed 9-7-10.

6. Krishnan K: *Tumor lysis syndrome*, http://emedicine.medscape.com/article/282171-overview, accessed 5-1-10.

7. Leukemia and Lymphoma Society: *Facts and statistics. Leukemia, lymphoma, myeloma facts 2009-2010*, June 2009, White Plains, New York.

8. Saba HI, Morelli GA: The pathogenesis and management of disseminated intravascular coagulation, *Clin Adv Hematol Oncol* 4(12):919-926, 2006.

9. National Heart, Lung, and Blood Institute, National Institutes of Health: *Hemophilia*, www.nhlbi.nih.gov/health/dci/Diseases/hemophilia/hemophilia_what.html, accessed 9-7-10.

10. Bitting RL, Bent S, Li Y, et al: The prognosis and treatment of acquired hemophilia: a systematic review and meta-analysis, *Blood Coagul Fibrinolysis* 20(7):517-523, 2009.

11. www.clinicalpharmacology.com (Gold Standard), accessed 9-7-10.
12. National Heart, Lung, and Blood Institute, National Institutes of Health: *Thrombocytopenia*, www.nhlbi.nih.gov/health/dci/Diseases/thcp/thcp_signs.html, accessed 9-7-10.
13. Sickle Cell Disease Association of America: *Sickle cell FAQs*, www.sicklecelldisease.org/about_scd/faqs.phtml, accessed 9-7-10.
14. Hockenberry MJ: *Wong's essentials of pediatric nursing*, ed 8, St Louis, 2008, Mosby.

SUGGESTED READINGS

Abbott J: Even "frequent flyers" die, *Ann Emerg Med* 54(6):840, 2009.
Tanabe P, Myers R, Zosel A, et al: Emergency department management of acute pain episodes in sickle cell disease, *Acad Emerg Med* 14(5):419-425, 2007.

33 Nontraumatic Musculoskeletal Disorders

OBJECTIVES

Upon completion of this chapter, the paramedic student will be able to:

1. Outline musculoskeletal structure and function.
2. Describe how to perform a detailed assessment of the extremities and spine.
3. Specify questions in the patient history that help identify musculoskeletal problems.
4. Describe assessment and management of specific nontraumatic musculoskeletal disorders based on an understanding of the pathophysiology.

KEY TERMS

appendicular skeleton The bones of the upper and lower extremities.

arthritis An inflammatory condition of the joints, characterized by pain and swelling.

atrophy Decrease in size (shrinkage) of a cell, which adversely affects cell function.

axial skeleton The bones of the head, neck, and torso.

benign A noncancerous tumor or harmless condition.

bone spurs Bony growths formed on normal bone.

bone tumor An abnormal growth of cells within a bone; may be malignant or benign.

bursa A small sac containing synovial fluid that helps ease friction between a tendon and skin or between a tendon and bone.

bursitis An inflammation of the bursa, the connective tissue structure surrounding a joint.

carpal tunnel syndrome An entrapment neuropathy that occurs when the median nerve becomes pressed or squeezed at the wrist in the carpal tunnel.

cartilaginous joints Joints that are slightly movable.

cauda equina syndrome A rare disorder of the lumbar spine that affects the bundle of nerve roots at the lower end of the spinal cord; a surgical emergency.

chronic fatigue syndrome A debilitating and complex disorder, characterized by profound fatigue that is not improved by bed rest and that may be worsened by physical or mental activity.

dermatomyositis An inflammatory myopathy characterized by a skin rash that precedes or accompanies progressive muscle weakness.

diskectomy The surgical removal of a disk.

epiphyseal plate The site of bone elongation; also known as the *growth plate*.

fascia The loose areolar connective tissue found beneath the skin or dense connective tissue that encloses and separates muscle.

fasciitis Inflammation of the fascia.

fibromyalgia A disorder that causes extreme fatigue; associated with "tender points" on the neck, shoulders, back, hips, arms, and legs.

fibrous joints Joints that are immovable.

flexor tenosynovitis A pathological state that causes a disruption of tendon function in the hand; usually the result of infection.

gait A manner of walking or moving on foot.

gangrene Dead or dying body tissues attributable to blood supply that is lost or inadequate.

gout A disease associated with an inborn error of uric acid metabolism that increases production of or inter-feres with excretion of uric acid; also known as *hyperuricemia*.

herniated disk Occurs when all or part of a spinal disk is forced through a weakened part of the disk.

inflammatory myopathies A group of diseases that involve chronic muscle inflammation accompanied by muscle weakness.

joint Any one of the connections between bones that are classified according to structure and mobility as fibrous, cartilaginous, or synovial. *Fibrous joints* are immovable, *cartilaginous joints* are slightly movable, and *synovial joints* are freely movable.

joint disorder Any disease or injury that affects human joints.

kyphosis An abnormal condition of the vertebral column characterized by increased convexity in the curvature of the thoracic spine as viewed from the side.

ligament A band of white, fibrous tissue that connects bones.

lordosis An inward curvature in the lumbar spine that is normally present to some degree.

malignant Very dangerous or virulent; likely to cause death; a cancerous tumor that tends to metastasize—the ability of cancer cells to move or spread from one organ or tissue to distant locations in the body.

muscle strain A slight tear in a muscle or tendon.

muscle tone The constant tension produced by muscles of the body for long periods of time.

muscular system The body system responsible for execution of movement and postural maintenance.

musculoskeletal system The body system comprises bones, muscles, tendons and ligaments, and articulating surfaces (e.g., joints, bursae, disks).

myalgia Diffuse muscle pain, usually accompanied by malaise; it occurs in many infectious diseases.

myositis A muscular disorder characterized by progressive muscle weakness and wasting; also known as *inclusive body myositis*.

necrotizing fasciitis A rare infection of the deep layers of the skin and subcutaneous tissues.

osteoarthritis A form of arthritis in which one or many joints undergo degenerative changes.

osteomyelitis Local or generalized infection of bone and bone marrow, usually caused by bacteria introduced by trauma or surgery.

paronychia A common skin infection that occurs around the nails and that allows for an invasion of bacteria, yeast, or fungus.

pathological fracture A fracture that results from weakness in the bone caused by trauma, metabolic disease (such as osteoporosis), or tumor.

piriformis syndrome A neuromuscular disorder associated with irritation or compression of the sciatic nerve.

point-to-point movements Refers to methods used to evaluate a patient's coordination.

polymyositis Slow, but progressive muscle weakness that affects skeletal muscle on both sides of the body.

postural maintenance The result of muscle tone responsible for keeping the back and legs straight, the head in an upright position, and the abdomen from bulging; also balances the distribution of body weight.

primary tumor A malignant tumor in the original site where it first arose.

pseudogout Inflammation caused by *calcium pyrophosphate* (CPP) crystals; often clinically indistinguishable from gout.

rheumatoid arthritis A chronic, sometimes deforming destructive collagen disease that has an autoimmune component.

sciatica Inflammation of the sciatic nerve.

scoliosis A lateral curvature of the spine.

secondary tumor A malignant tumor that originates in one area of the body and spreads to another area of the body.

septic arthritis A condition that results from direct invasion of the joint space by various microorganisms; also known as *infectious arthritis*.

skeletal muscle Muscle tissue that appears microscopically to consist of striped myofibrils; also known as *striated muscle* and *voluntary muscle*.

skeletal system The body system comprises bones, muscles, tendons and ligaments, and articulating surfaces (e.g., joints, bursae, disks).

slipped capital femoral epiphysis A separation of the ball of the hip joint from the femur at the upper, growing end (growth plate) of the bone.

spinal stenosis Narrowing of the spinal canal.

sprain A partial tearing of a ligament caused by a sudden twisting or stretching of a joint beyond its normal range of motion.

stance The position of the body while standing.

strain An injury to the muscle or its tendon from overexertion or overextension.

synovial joints Joints that are freely movable.

tendon A band or cord of dense connective tissue that connects muscle to bone or other structures; it is characterized by strength and nonstretchability.

tendonitis An inflammatory condition of a tendon, usually caused by a sprain.

ulnar nerve entrapment An injury that occurs when the ulnar nerve in the arm becomes compressed.

Nontraumatic musculoskeletal disorders are common afflictions. These diseases cause pain in the bones, joints, muscles, and surrounding structures. Although the disorders are often associated with aging, they can affect all age groups and frequently cause impairments, disabilities, and handicaps. Nontraumatic musculoskeletal disorders are rarely life threatening. Paramedics, however, should be familiar with these common ailments and the supportive care required for these patients. Box 33-1 lists the musculoskeletal disorders discussed in this chapter.[1]

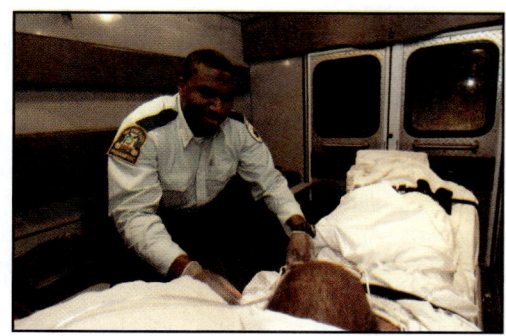

(Courtesy Ray Kemp, St. Charles, Mo.)

BOX 33-1 Musculoskeletal Disorders

Bony abnormalities
Disorders of the spine
Joint abnormalities
Muscle abnormalities
Overuse syndromes
Soft tissue infections

NOTE

Approximately 33% of adults in the United States are affected by musculoskeletal disorders that limit range of motion or cause pain in a joint or an extremity.[2]

ANATOMY AND PHYSIOLOGY REVIEW

As described in Chapter 10, the musculoskeletal system comprises bones, muscles, tendons and ligaments, and articulating surfaces (e.g., joints, bursae, disks). This discussion will provide a brief review of the skeletal system and the muscular system.

LOOK AGAIN

See Chapter 10: Review of Human Systems, pp. 158-171.

The Skeletal System

The **skeletal system** contains the bony structures that provide support and protection for the body. It also provides a system of levers on which muscles act to produce body movement. The skeletal system contains 206 individual bones. These bones are divided into two categories: the **axial skeleton** and the **appendicular skeleton**. The axial skeleton contains the skull, hyoid bone, vertebral column, and thoracic cage. The appendicular skeleton contains the bones of the upper and lower extremities and their girdles, by which they are attached to the body (Figure 33-1).

Body movement is made possible by bones that are connected to other bones. With the exception of the hyoid bone, every bone in the body connects to at least one other bone by way of **joints.** The three major classes of joints are fibrous, cartilaginous, and synovial. **Fibrous joints** consist of two bones that have little or no movement and are united by fibrous tissue. An example of a fibrous joint is the suture in skull bones. **Cartilaginous joints** unite two bones by means of hyaline cartilage and fibrocartilage. These types of joints are slightly movable. Examples of cartilaginous joints are the **epiphyseal plate** of a growing bone and junctions of the intervertebral disks. **Synovial joints** contain synovial fluid that allows for considerable movement. Most joints that unite the bones of the appendicular skeleton are synovial. Examples of synovial joints are the hinge joint of

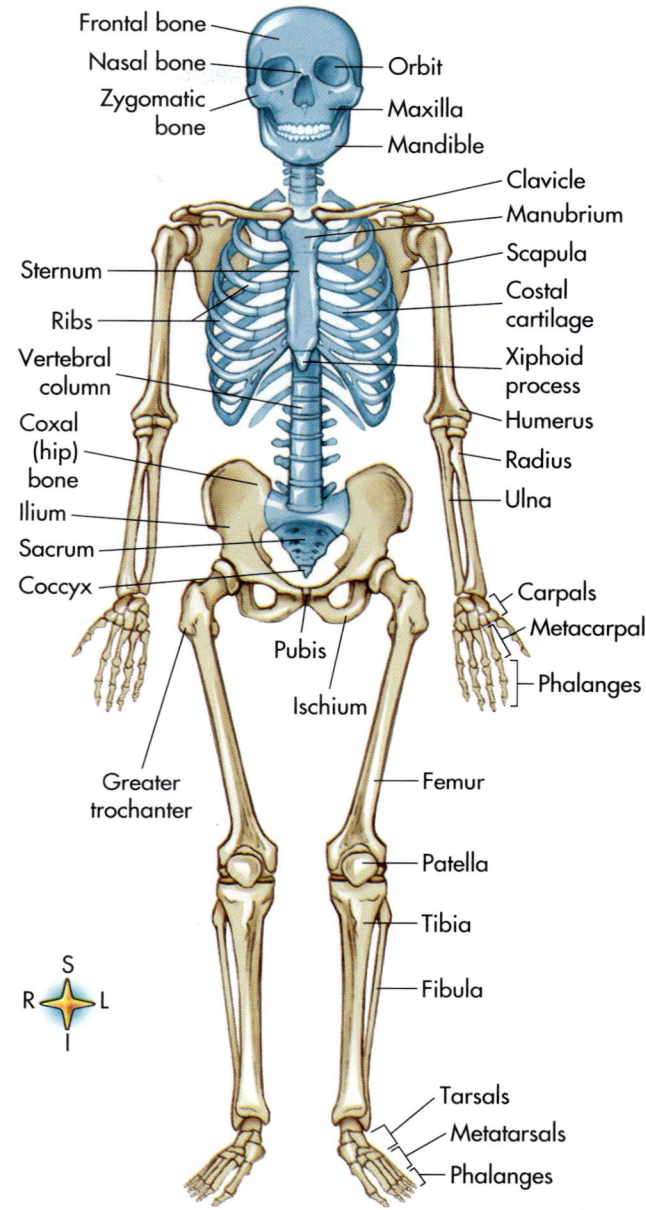

FIGURE 33-1 Skeleton. (From McCance KL, Huether SE: *Pathophysiology: the biologic basis for disease in adults and children,* ed 5, St Louis, 2006, Mosby.)

the elbow and knee and the ball-and-socket joints of the shoulder and hip. Figure 33-2 illustrates the movement found in different kinds of joints.

The Muscular System

The **muscular system** is responsible for execution of movement and postural maintenance. The major types of muscles are skeletal, cardiac, and smooth muscle. Of the three types, skeletal muscle is most common and is the focus of this chapter. It is also the muscle type most involved in musculoskeletal disorders. Skeletal muscles are attached to bones

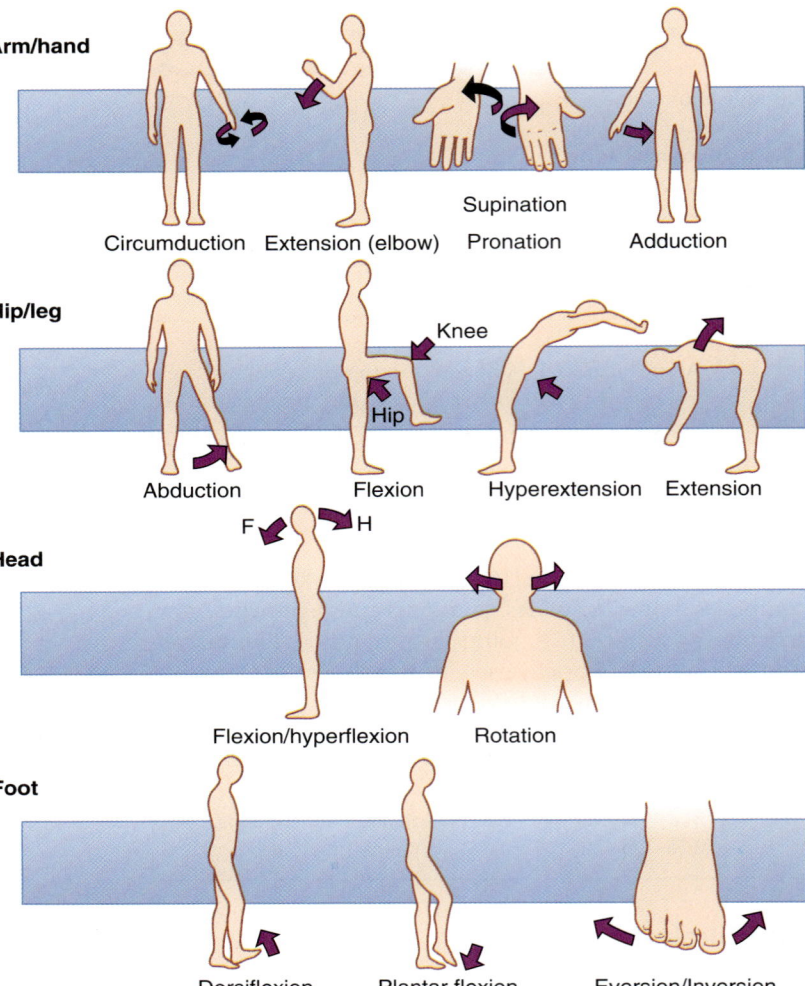

FIGURE 33-2 Joints.

by **tendons**. **Ligaments** connect bone or cartilage and help strengthen and support joints.

Skeletal muscle has specialized contractile cells known as *muscle fibers*. When a nerve impulse passes through the muscle fiber, specialized chemicals cause the muscle to contract. Most skeletal muscles extend from one bone to another and cross at least one joint. The contraction of some muscles and the simultaneous relaxation of other muscles produce body movement. These movements are made possible by pulling one of the bones toward the other across a movable joint.

Postural maintenance is the result of muscle tone. **Muscle tone** is the constant tension produced by muscles of the body for long periods of time. This tone is responsible for keeping the back and legs straight, the head in an upright position, and the abdomen from bulging. Postural maintenance also balances the distribution of body weight. This balance puts less strain on muscles, tendons, ligaments, and bones.

GENERAL ASSESSMENT STRATEGIES

As described in Chapter 20, the general assessment of a patient's musculoskeletal system includes an examination of the extremities, spine, vascular system, and motor system. The purpose of the assessment is to identify abnormal findings, which may include[1]:

- Pain or tenderness
- Swelling
- Abnormal or loss of movement
- Decreased sensation
- Circulatory changes
- Deformity

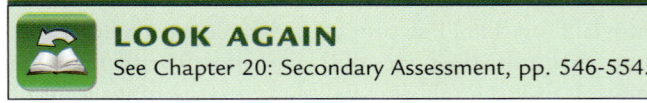

LOOK AGAIN
See Chapter 20: Secondary Assessment, pp. 546-554.

Extremity Exam

The patient's extremities should be examined for function and structure. General appearance, body proportions, and ease of movement should be noted. Other important observations are limitation in the range of motion, or an unusual increase in the mobility of a joint. Abnormal findings may include signs of inflammation (swelling, tenderness, increased heat, redness, decreased function), asymmetry, crepitus, deformities, decreased muscular strength, and **atrophy** (muscle wasting).

An assessment of the upper and lower extremities should include an evaluation of the skin and tissue overlying the muscles, cartilage, and bones. It should also include an assessment of the joints for soft tissue injury, discoloration, and swelling (Chapter 38). The upper and lower extremities should be reasonably symmetrical in structure and muscularity. Skin color, temperature, sensation, and the presence of distal pulses will help determine the circulatory status of each extremity. The patient's joints should be assessed for full range of motion. All movement should be made without pain, deformity, limitation, or instability.

Hands and wrists: The patient's hands and wrists should be inspected for contour and positional alignment. The hands, wrists, and joints of each finger should be assessed for tenderness, swelling, and deformity.

Elbows: The patient's elbows should be assessed and palpated in both flexed and extended positions. All movement should be made without pain or discomfort.

Shoulders: Both shoulders should be symmetrical and should be palpated for integrity of the clavicles, scapulae, and humeri. In addition, the patient should be able to shrug the shoulders and raise and extend both arms without pain or discomfort.

Pelvis and hips: Structural integrity of the patient's iliac crest and symphysis pubis should be assessed to determine stability. There should be no deformity or point tenderness during palpation.

Knees: The knees should be inspected and palpated for swelling and tenderness. The patella should be nontender and in midline position. The patient should be able to bend and straighten each knee without pain.

Ankles and feet: The ankles and feet should be inspected for contour, position, and size. Tenderness, swelling, and deformity are abnormal findings. The patient's toes should be straight and aligned with each other. The surface of the ankles and feet should be free of deformities, nodules, swelling, and calluses.

Spine Exam

A visual assessment should be made of the patient's cervical, thoracic, and lumbar curves. Abnormal findings may include curvature of the spine from abnormal **lordosis**, **kyphosis**, and **scoliosis**. In addition, there should be no major differences in the height of the shoulders or iliac crest that might result from abnormal spinal curvature.

The patient's neck should be in a midline position. The posterior neck should be free of point tenderness and swelling. In addition, the patient should be able to bend the head forward, backward, and from side to side without pain or discomfort.

The patient's thoracic lumbar spine should be inspected for signs of injury, swelling, or discoloration. In a normal exam, the spine is nontender to palpation.

Vascular Exam

As described in Chapter 10, the peripheral vascular system includes arteries, veins, the lymphatic system, and the fluids exchanged in the capillary beds. An assessment of the vascular system should be part of the general assessment strategy. The patient's upper and lower extremities should be assessed for color and texture and for arterial insufficiency. Lymph nodes should be nonswollen and nontender. Abnormal findings in a vascular exam include:

- Pale or cyanotic skin
- Weak or diminished pulses
- Skin that is cold to the touch
- Absence of hair growth
- Pitting edema

Motor Exam

The patient should be observed while moving and while at rest. Any abnormal or involuntary movements should be noted, as well as the patient's posture, level of activity, and fatigue. Muscle strength should be equal on both sides of the body. Patients should be assessed for agility and tested for flexion, extension, and abduction of the upper and lower extremities.

Coordination can be evaluated for point-to-point movements, gait, and stance. Examples of **point-to-point movements** include touching the finger to the nose and touching each heel to the opposite shin. Methods to evaluate **gait** include asking the patient to walk toe to toe, walk on the toes, and walk on the heels. As described in Chapter 20, **stance** and balance can be evaluated though the *Romberg test* and the *pronator drift test*.

Finally, a healthy patient should be responsive to sensations of pain, temperature, position, vibration, and touch. These are conducted by the sensory pathways of the nervous system. Sensory exams can be performed on conscious patients by using light touch on each hand and each foot. The exam should proceed from head to toe and be symmetrical on both sides of the body.

GENERAL MANAGEMENT STRATEGIES

General management strategies for a patient with a musculoskeletal disorder are the same as those for most other patient care encounters. Prehospital care will be guided by the patient's chief complaint and the severity of the patient's condition. General management strategies include:

- Scene size-up to ensure personal safety
- A primary survey to ensure airway, ventilation, and circulation
- Secondary assessment and reassessment
- Pharmacological and nonpharmacological measures to ensure comfort
- Transport considerations
- Effective therapeutic communications

The Patient History

The patient history should be thorough and focused on the patient's chief complaint. In addition to the general medical history described in Chapter 18, specific questions to ask a patient with a musculoskeletal disorder are listed in Box 33-2.

Management Guidelines

Prehospital care for most musculoskeletal disorders will be primarily supportive. Management most often is limited to immobilization of the affected area or body part; application of ice and/or elevation of an extremity to reduce pain and swelling; administration of analgesics to relieve pain; and gentle transport for physician evaluation.

BOX 33-2 Questions to Ask for Musculoskeletal Disorders

Complaint: Joint Pain
Where is the specific site of pain?
Does the pain change during the course of the day?
Have you had a recent injury?
How long has there been pain in the joint?
Does the pain get better or worse with movement?

Complaint: Muscle Weakness
Is the weakness widespread or isolated to one area?
Is the weakness related to a painful extremity?
Does the weakness fluctuate or is it constant?
Is the weakness increasing in severity?
Is the weakness associated with sensory changes?
Is there a family history of muscle disease?
Is the weakness the same on both sides of the body?

Complaint: Back Pain
Is the pain confined to the back or does it radiate to the upper or lower limbs?
Is the pain made worse by coughing or sneezing?
Was the pain sudden or gradual in onset?

Complaint: Gait or Balance Issues
Do you trip when walking?
Do you stagger to one particular side?
Do you ever injure yourself when walking?

OSTEOMYELITIS

Osteomyelitis is an acute or chronic bone infection; it affects 2 out of every 10,000 people.[3] The infection can be caused by a number of microbial agents, most commonly *Staphylococcus aureus*. Osteomyelitis also can develop from an open fracture or minor wound infection. It can also result from systemic infection (e.g., urinary tract infection, pneumonia) that allows bacteria to spread in the bloodstream and enter the bone. If left untreated, the infection can become chronic, resulting in a decreased blood supply to the bone and eventual death of the bone tissue. Osteomyelitis affects both children and adults and can affect any bone. In adults the vertebrae and pelvis are most often affected by the disease; in children the long bones are most often involved. Those at increased risk for developing osteomyelitis include:

- People who have undergone recent orthopedic surgery
- The elderly
- Intravenous (IV) drug abusers
- People with sickle cell disease
- People receiving hemodialysis
- People with compromised immune systems

Signs, Symptoms, and Patient Care

Signs and symptoms of osteomyelitis are listed in Box 33-3. The disease is diagnosed using blood tests to confirm infection, and blood cultures to identify the bacteria. Other diagnostic tools include needle aspiration, biopsy, and bone scans. Once the diagnosis has been made, patients are treated with oral or IV antibiotics to manage the infection and to prevent reinfection. Other care may include surgical drainage of a wound or abscess, immobilization of the affected bone or surrounding joints, and sometimes surgery to scrape the infection from the affected bone. In rare cases, amputation of an affected limb may be required.

BONE TUMORS

A **bone tumor** is an abnormal growth of cells within a bone. The tumor can be **malignant** (cancerous) or **benign** (noncancerous). Most bone tumors are benign and not life threatening. Common bone tumors that are benign include *nonossifying fibroma unicameral bone cyst, osteochondroma, giant cell tumor, enchondroma*, and *fibrous dysplasia*.

Malignant tumors can spread cancer cells throughout the body (**metastasize**) via blood or the lymphatic system. A malignant tumor that is in the original site where it first arose is a **primary tumor** (Figure 33-3). A malignant tumor that originates in another area of the body and spreads to the bone is a **secondary tumor.** The four most common types of primary bone tumors are[4]:

Multiple myeloma: Multiple myeloma is the most common primary bone cancer. It is a malignant tumor of bone marrow. Multiple myeloma affects approximately 20 people per million each year. Most cases are seen in patients between the ages of 50 and 70 years old. Any bone can be involved.

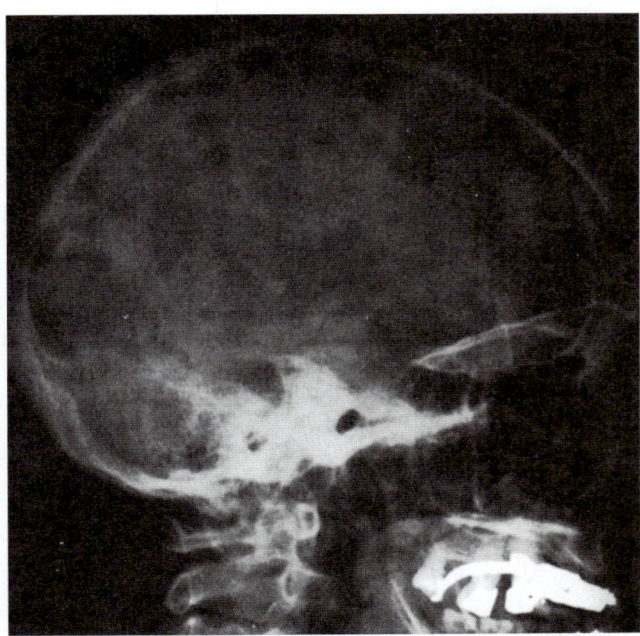

FIGURE 33-3 Multiple myeloma of the skull. Radiograph shows punched-out bone lesions filled with soft tumor. (From Gould BE, Dyer R: *Pathophysiology for the health professional,* ed 4, St Louis, 2011, Saunders.)

BOX 33-3 Signs and Symptoms of Osteomyelitis

- Pain and/or tenderness in the infected area
- Swelling and warmth in the infected area
- Fever, chills
- General malaise
- Drainage of pus through the skin
- Excessive sweating
- Back or neck pain (if the spine is involved)
- Swelling of the ankles, feet, and legs
- Walking that is painful or with a limp

Osteosarcoma: Osteosarcoma is the second most common bone cancer. It occurs in two or three new people per million people each year. Most cases occur in teenagers. Most tumors occur around the knee. Other common locations include the hip and shoulder.

Ewing's sarcoma: Ewing's sarcoma most commonly occurs between 5 and 20 years of age. The most common locations are the upper and lower leg, pelvis, upper arm, and ribs.

Chondrosarcoma: Chondrosarcoma occurs most commonly in patients between 40 and 70 years of age. Most cases occur around the hip and pelvis or the shoulder.

Signs, Symptoms, and Patient Care

Most patients with a bone tumor experience a dull or aching pain in the area of the tumor. The pain is sometimes made worse with physical activity and often awakes the patient at night. Other patients will not complain of pain, but will have discovered a painless mass on self-examination. Pathological fractures are common in these patients. These fractures result from trauma or a metabolic disease, such as osteoporosis, in which the bone weakened by the tumor breaks.

> **NOTE**
> A *pathological fracture* is a break at the site of a preexisting abnormality, usually by force that would not fracture a normal bone. Any disease process that weakens a bone (especially the cortex) predisposes the bone to pathological fracture. Pathological fractures are commonly associated with tumors, osteoporosis, infections, and metabolic bone disorders.[5] In some of these patients very minor trauma or even no apparent trauma (e.g., turning over in bed) can cause a pathological fracture.

Benign tumors may or may not require treatment (depending on the specific tumor). Some benign tumors can be aggressive and quickly destroy bone. Malignant tumors may require medication therapy or surgical removal. Still other tumors resolve on their own (especially some bone tumors in children). Most malignant tumors are surgically removed and treated with radiation. If the cancer has metastasized, other treatment may include additional radiation, chemotherapy, and *cryosurgery* (the freezing and killing of cancer cells with liquid nitrogen). In some patients, a bone implant or amputation of an affected limb will be needed. Patient follow-up with regular blood tests and x-ray is required because bone cancer can recur. People who have had bone cancer, particularly children and adolescents, have an increased likelihood of developing another type of cancer, such as leukemia, later in life.[6]

LOW BACK PAIN

Most everyone at some point has back pain that interferes with work, routine daily activities, or recreation. Americans spend at least $50 billion each year on low back pain, the most common cause of job-related disability and a leading contributor to missed work. Back pain is the second most common neurological ailment in the United States. Only headache is more common.[7]

As described in Chapter 10, the vertebral column consists of 26 bones that are divided into 5 regions: 7 cervical vertebrae, 12 thoracic vertebrae, 5 lumbar vertebrae, 1 sacral bone, and 1 coccygeal bone. Together, the vertebrae protect the spinal cord, the rootlets, and the 31 pairs of spinal nerves that convey sensation. The weight-bearing portion of the vertebra is a bony vertebral body. Intervertebral disks are located between the bodies of adjacent vertebrae and serve as shock absorbers (Figure 33-4). The disks allow for flexibility of the back. They also prevent the vertebral bodies from rubbing against each other.

Low back pain may be classified as *acute* or *chronic*. Acute back pain is usually of short duration, lasting only a few days to a few weeks. Most acute back pain is caused by trauma to the lower back (e.g., a sports injury or heavy lifting). It can also be caused by arthritis or other degenerative joint disease of the spine, viral infections, and congenital abnormalities. Chronic back pain is back pain that persists for 3 or more months. Although the cause of chronic back pain can be difficult to determine, it can be progressive and debilitating. The conditions discussed in this chapter are disorders of the intervertebral disks, cauda equina syndrome, and sprains and strains of the muscles and supporting structures of the back.

> **NOTE**
> Prehospital care for patients with low back pain is primarily supportive. Most care is focused on obtaining a thorough history and providing comfort measures and gentle transport for physician evaluation. Physicians investigate most cases of low back pain through x-rays, MRI (magnetic resonance imaging) scans, and CT (computed tomography) scans.

Disorders of the Intervertebral Disks

As stated previously, the intervertebral disks are found between the bodies of the vertebrae. They act as shock absorbers, prevent the bones of the spine from grinding against each other, and allow for flexibility of the back. Each disk has a central area composed of a jelly-like substance, called the *nucleus pulposus*. This structure is surrounded by concentric rings of fibrous tissue (*annulus*

fibrosus). Undue stress (along with degenerative disease) on a disk can force the gel against the inner ring and crack it. From there, the gel pushes outward, cracking successive rings in its path. If stress on the back is severe enough, the vertebral disks and fibrous tissues can be damaged, causing the disk to bulge or protrude. If the gel eventually breaks through the outer ring, it can pinch the nerve root leading from the vertebra. This can result in a "slipped" or **herniated disk** (Figure 33-5).

Disk injury most often affects the lumbar spine in patients 25 to 45 years of age. The most common risk factor for developing lumbar disk disease is lack of exercise that allows the muscles of the back to weaken. Symptoms of a herniated disk vary greatly depending on the position of the herniated disk and the size of the herniation. Common signs and symptoms may include:

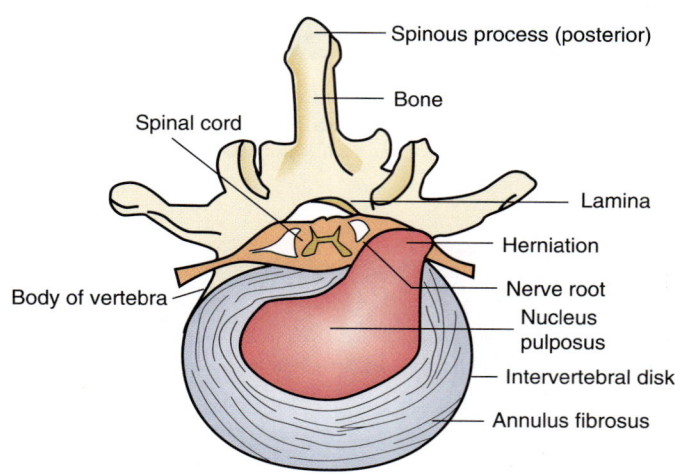

FIGURE 33-5 Herniated intervertebral disk. (From Gould BE, Dyer R: *Pathophysiology for the health professional*, ed 4, St Louis, 2011, Saunders.)

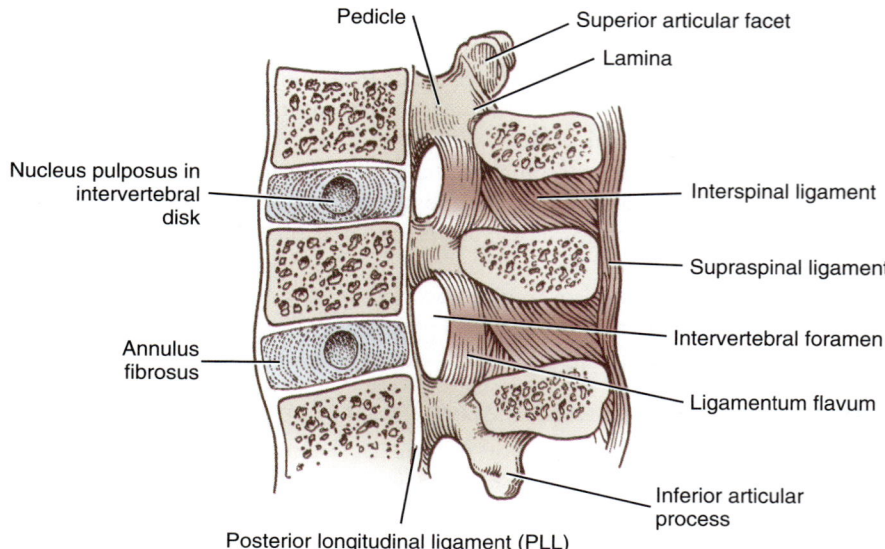

FIGURE 33-4 Median section through three lumbar vertebrae, showing intervertebral disks (nuclei pulposi). (From Rothrock JL: *Alexander's care of the patient in surgery*, ed 13, St Louis, 2007, Mosby.)

- Low back ache
- Numbness or weakness in the lower extremities
- Deep muscle pain and muscle spasms
- Acute or gradual leg pain (usually in only one leg)
- "Shooting" pain in the leg when sneezing, coughing, or straining; may be aggravated by sitting, prolonged standing, bending, or twisting
- Nerve-related symptoms, including muscle weakness in one or both legs, pain in the front of the thigh, and sciatica (Box 33-4)

The goals of treatment for a herniated disk are to relieve pain, weakness, or numbness in the leg caused by pressure on the spinal nerve root or spinal cord. Most patients are first treated with bed rest, analgesics, antiinflammatories, muscle relaxants, and corticosteroids. Physical therapy and exercise programs can help strengthen the back and prevent recurrent injury. Most herniated disks heal without surgery to remove the herniated disk (**diskectomy**).

Cauda Equina Syndrome

Cauda equina syndrome is a rare disorder of the lumbar spine that affects the bundle of nerve roots at the lower end of the spinal cord. It is a surgical emergency that occurs when the nerve roots are compressed and paralyzed, cutting off sensation and movement. If not treated, the syndrome can result in permanent paralysis, impaired bladder and bowel function, and loss of sexual sensation. Even with surgery to relieve the pressure on nerve roots, nerve damage may be irreversible.

Cauda equina syndrome can be caused by a herniated disk, spinal tumor, infection, and **spinal stenosis** (narrowing of the spinal canal). It can also result from spinal trauma, including direct trauma, falls, gunshot wounds, and stabbings. (Children born with spinal abnormalities also can develop the syndrome.) Signs and symptoms of cauda equina syndrome vary in intensity and may evolve slowly over time. These include:

- Bladder and/or bowel dysfunction (loss of control; inability to urinate or defecate)
- Severe or progressive weakness in the lower extremities
- Loss of sensation or an altered sensation between the legs, over the buttocks, the inner thighs and back of the legs (saddle area), and feet and heels
- Pain, numbness, or weakness that spreads to one or both legs and may cause a stumbling gait or difficulty rising from a sitting position

Sprains and Strains of the Lower Back

The lower back carries much of the body's weight during walking, running, lifting, and other activities. Because muscles, ligaments, and bones of the spine provide control and strength for many movements, sprains and strains of the lower back (especially the lumbar spine) are common injuries. They are often caused by twisting or pulling and from improper lifting that puts the back at risk for injury. It is estimated that 50% of all EMS personnel develop back pain every year and that one in four will have a career-ending back injury within the first 4 years of service.[9,10]

BOX 33-4 Sciatica

Sciatica *(sciatic neuralgia)* is a symptom of inflammation of the sciatic nerve. The sciatic nerve is the largest nerve in the body. It runs from the spinal cord to the buttock and hip area and down the back of each leg. This nerve innervates muscles in the back of the knee and lower leg. It also provides sensation to the back of the thigh, lower leg, and sole of the foot. Inflammation of the sciatic nerve causes pain, weakness, numbness, and tingling along its path. Sciatica usually affects only one leg.

Sciatica is a common condition that occurs in about 40% of adults.[8] It is often caused by a herniated disk or spinal stenosis. It can also be caused by injury (e.g., pelvic fracture) or piriformis syndrome (a neuromuscular disorder associated with irritation or compression of the sciatic nerve). Although the discomfort of sciatica can be severe and debilitating, it usually resolves without treatment or surgery in 4 to 8 weeks.

A **strain** is an injury to a muscle or tendon. A **sprain** is the stretching or tearing of a ligament beyond its normal range of movement. Differentiating a sprain from a strain is difficult and unnecessary in the prehospital setting. The signs, symptoms, treatment, and prognosis for both conditions are the same. Signs and symptoms include pain, warmth, muscle spasms, and swelling of the affected area. Most muscle sprains and strains of the lower back are successfully treated with bed rest for 24 to 48 hours to allow the back to heal. Analgesics, muscle relaxants, and antiinflammatories may be prescribed. Physical therapy and exercise programs can help to strengthen the back muscles and prevent future injury. Back pain that does not resolve with these measures will require further evaluation.

JOINT DISORDERS

A **joint disorder** is any disease or injury that affects human joints. These disorders may be short-lived or chronic. The joint disorders discussed in this chapter are those that produce inflammation as a result of disease. These include various forms of arthritis. Joint disorders that result from trauma are discussed in Chapter 44.

Arthritis

Arthritis is an inflammatory condition of the joint, characterized by pain and swelling. The disease limits the activity of nearly 19 million adults and is the most common cause of disability in the United States.[11] Although there are many kinds of arthritis, the disease can be grouped into three general categories: osteoarthritis, rheumatoid arthritis, and gout.

NOTE

Like most other nontraumatic musculoskeletal disorders, prehospital care is primarily supportive. Care is often limited to providing comfort measures and gentle transport for physician evaluation. Physician care for most joint disorders includes a combination of patient education, physical therapy, weight control, and medications to reduce pain and inflammation. In some cases, surgery or joint replacement may be indicated.

OSTEOARTHRITIS

Osteoarthritis is a chronic, degenerative joint disease, most often seen in people more than 40 years old. The onset of the disease is gradual and affects women more often than men. Osteoarthritis is mechanical in nature, resulting from normal wear-and-tear on joints over the course of a person's life. It is marked by the breakdown of cartilage that covers the surfaces of joints, and the formation of **bone spurs** (bony growths formed on normal bone). The wearing away of cartilage and the overgrowth of bone lead to pain and stiffness. As the disease progresses, bone rubs against bone, causing severe pain and reduced mobility. The joints most commonly affected are those in the knees, hips, hands, and the cervical and lumbar spine (Box 33-5).

> **NOTE**
> *Osteoarthritis* and *osteoporosis* have similar names, but are very different conditions. Osteoporosis is a preventable disease characterized by the loss of bone tissue, causing the bones to weaken and easily fracture. Osteoporosis is not a form of arthritis, although the two can occur together. The two diseases develop differently, have different symptoms, and are diagnosed and treated differently. Osteoporosis affects mainly postmenopausal women. It will be described in Chapter 49.

RHEUMATOID ARTHRITIS

Rheumatoid arthritis (RA) is an inflammatory disease of the joints that causes pain, swelling, stiffness, and loss of function. It is estimated that about 1.3 million people in the United States have the disease.[13] It occurs in all races and ethnic groups. Symptoms of the disease usually become apparent in middle and later life, but can also develop in young adults and children (Box 33-6). RA develops when lymphocytes travel to the synovium in the joints, causing inflammation (**synovitis**). During this process, the normally thin synovium becomes thick and makes the joint

---

BOX 33-5 Slipped Capital Femoral Epiphysis

Slipped capital femoral epiphysis is a separation of the ball of the hip joint from the femur at the upper, growing end (growth plate) of the bone. It occurs in about 2 of every 100,000 children. It is most common in boys 11 to 15 years of age, in children who are obese, in those who have hormone imbalances, and in those having growth spurts.[12] The condition may affect one or both hips and can occur after even minor trauma (e.g., jumping from a small height). Signs and symptoms include pain and tenderness in the thigh and hip. The affected limb may be slightly rotated in an outward position. A slipped capital femoral epiphysis most often requires surgery to stabilize the hip joint. The condition is associated with early arthritis of the hip joint and a greater risk for osteoarthritis later in life.

---

swollen and puffy to the touch. As the disease progresses, the inflamed synovium invades and damages the cartilage and bone of the joint. Surrounding muscles, ligaments, and tendons become weakened. Rheumatoid arthritis also can cause more generalized bone loss that may lead to osteoporosis. Unlike other forms of arthritis where only a specific joint is affected, RA generally occurs in a symmetrical pattern (e.g., both hands, both knees). A hallmark of the disease is visible swelling and inflammation of the finger joints closest to the affected hand (Figure 33-6). RA may also affect other areas of the body (neck, shoulder, elbows, feet), and is often associated with fatigue, occasional fever, and general malaise.

> **NOTE**
> *Juvenile rheumatoid arthritis* (JRA) and *juvenile idiopathic arthritis* (JIA) are classification systems for chronic arthritis in children. Most forms of juvenile arthritis are autoimmune disorders. Children with the disease are thought to have a genetic predisposition to it. Development of the disease is then triggered by an environmental factor, such as a virus. The most common symptoms of all types of juvenile arthritis are persistent joint swelling, pain, and stiffness that is typically worse in the morning or after a nap. The pain may limit movement of the affected joint, although many children, especially younger ones, will not complain of pain. Other symptoms include high fever and rash. Children with RA require multidisciplinary treatment and specialty care.

> **SHOW ME THE EVIDENCE**
> This retrospective review examined patient records from 1996 to 2005. The researchers reviewed mechanism of injury; prehospital, emergency, and hospital care; and neurological outcome of spinal cord injured (SCI) patients with a history of ankylosing spondylitis. Of the 18 patients identified, SCI in 15 was associated with trauma and the other 3 cases were related to surgery. Four patients died before discharge whereas four were able to walk assisted and seven were in a wheelchair. The researchers concluded that neurological deficits were initially subtle in this group of SCI patients. They also found that extension of the spine during care caused neurological deficits. They recommend cervical alignment in the patient's normal kyphotic flexed position during care.

Thumbikat P, Hariharan R, McClelland M: Spinal cord injury in patients with ankylosing spondylitis: a 10-year review, *Spine* 32(26):2989-2995, 2007.

Patients with RA have varying degrees of the disease. Some patients have only limited bouts, followed by remission and little damage. In other patients the disease is regularly active, lasting many years to a lifetime. This form of RA often leads to severe joint damage and disability. Physician care may include antiinflammatories to reduce pain

BOX 33-6 Ankylosing Spondylitis

Ankylosing spondylitis (AS) is a form of arthritis that primarily affects the spine, although other joints can become involved. It causes inflammation of the vertebrae that can lead to severe, chronic pain and discomfort. In the most advanced cases, this inflammation can lead to new bone formation on the spine, causing the spine to fuse in a fixed, immobile position. This sometimes creates a forward-stooped posture (*kyphosis*). AS can cause inflammation, pain, and stiffness in other areas of the body (e.g., the shoulders, hips, ribs, heels, and small joints of the hands and feet). The eyes can also be involved. Rarely, the lungs and heart can be affected. Unlike other forms of arthritis and rheumatic diseases, general onset of AS commonly occurs in younger people, between the ages of 17 and 35. It also can affect children and the elderly. The disease is more common in men than in women. The severity of the disease varies from person to person and may lead to permanent disability.[14]

Paramedics and other emergency personnel must remember that patients with AS have inflexible spines that cannot be moved. EMS procedures must be modified to accommodate these patients to prevent further injury. These include modifying splinting procedures, airway procedures, and transport considerations. For example, patients with AS will require additional padding with splinting techniques. Airway procedures must be performed without flexing the neck. If possible, advanced airway devices that do not require visualization of the airway (e.g., King L&D, laryngeal mask airway [LMA]) should be used instead of endotracheal intubation. Padding with pillows to support the patient's head, neck, and upper back will need to be applied during transport. Special training is available to EMS personnel for managing patients with this condition.[14]

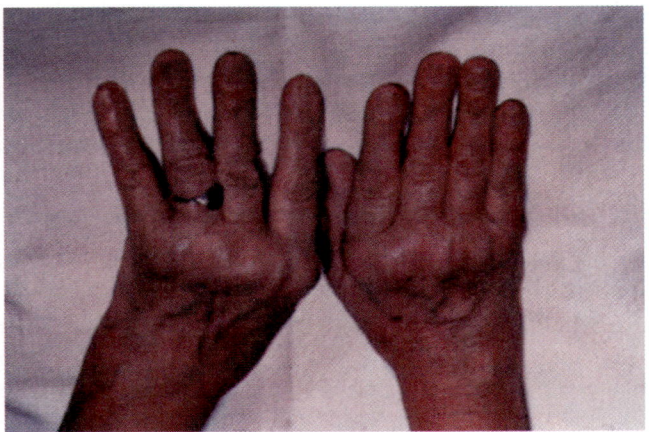

FIGURE 33-6 Rheumatoid arthritis of hands. (From Christensen BL et al: *Adult health nursing,* ed 6, St Louis, 2010, Mosby.)

common), viruses, mycobacteria, and fungi. Septic arthritis affects about 20,000 people in the United States each year.[16] It can occur in both children and adults.

> **NOTE**
> In the past, septic arthritis was more frequently caused by the bacterium *Neisseria gonorrhoeae,* which causes the sexually transmitted disease gonorrhea. Safer sex practices have led to a decline in gonorrhea and its complications, including septic arthritis. Still, in younger sexually active people, gonorrhea is a potential cause of septic arthritis.

The disease process begins when the infectious agent (most commonly *Staphylococcus aureus*) enters the joint. This usually occurs from active infection elsewhere in the body, such as a respiratory tract infection or urinary tract infection. Infection also can occur from direct invasion (e.g., an open wound near the joint; joint surgery). When the bacterium reaches the synovium in the joint, the immune system is activated, and cartilage begins to be destroyed. This results in inflammation and reduced blood flow to the joint and surrounding structures. Previously damaged joints, especially from rheumatoid arthritis, are the most susceptible to infection. The most commonly involved joint is the knee, followed by the hip, shoulder, ankle, and wrist. Signs and symptoms of septic arthritis include fever; shaking chills; and severe pain, warmth, and swelling in the affected joint. Septic arthritis is treated with antibiotics to resolve the infection. In severe cases, the joint may need surgical reconstruction or replacement.

and inflammation, disease-modifying antirheumatic drugs (DMARDs) to slow the course of the disease, analgesics, and physical therapy. Commonly performed surgical procedures include joint replacement, tendon reconstruction, and synovectomy.

> **NOTE**
> *Biologic response modifiers* are a new class of drugs used for the treatment of rheumatoid arthritis.[15] They help reduce inflammation and damage to the joints by blocking the action of cytokines (proteins of the body's immune system that trigger inflammation during normal immune responses). Examples of these drugs include etanercept (Enbrel), infliximab (Remicade), adalimumab (Humira), and anakinra (Kineret).

> **CRITICAL THINKING**
> When caring for a patient with severe rheumatoid arthritis or ankylosing spondylitis, how might you have to modify your care if you suspect spine injury?

SEPTIC ARTHRITIS

Septic arthritis is also known as *infectious arthritis*. The condition results from direct invasion of the joint space by various microorganisms. These include bacteria (most

> **SHOW ME THE EVIDENCE**
> Researchers cultured synovial fluid from 109 patients. Of those that were diagnosed with septic arthritis, 50% grew methicillin-resistant *Staphylococcus aureus* (MRSA). In this patient sample MRSA was the most common causative organism in septic arthritis.

Frazee BW, Fee C, Lambert L: How common is MRSA in adult septic arthritis? *Ann Emerg Med* 54(5):695-700, 2009.

GOUT

Gout is a form of arthritis marked by the deposit of uric acid crystals (monosodium urate) in and around a joint. Gout affects mostly men and is thought to be hereditary. It affects about 2.7 of every 1000 adults. For unknown reasons, gout surfaces most often in the metatarsophalangeal joint of the big toe. Gout may also present anywhere in the lower or upper extremities. In the elderly, many joints may be affected. People with gout may also develop tophi (masses of urate crystals deposited in soft tissue). This usually affects cooler areas of the body such as the elbows, ears, and distal finger joints. The disease is also associated with an increased risk for developing kidney stones.[17]

> **NOTE**
>
> **Pseudogout** is inflammation caused by *calcium pyrophosphate* (CPP) crystals. It is often clinically indistinguishable from gout. Both conditions are treated the same. Like gout, pseudogout is associated with a variety of metabolic disorders. However, unlike gout, there is no specific therapeutic regimen to treat the underlying cause of the disease. The most common sites for pseudogout are the knees, wrists, and shoulders. The symptoms often occur gradually over several days.

In acute gout, the affected joint and surrounding tissues appear hot, red, and swollen. The pain is usually intense and made worse by stimulation or light touch (e.g., covering the toe with a blanket). Gout may remit for long periods, followed by flares that last days to weeks. Chronic gout can lead to a degenerative form of arthritis called *gouty arthritis*. Risk factors for gout include joint injury, obesity, hypertension, alcohol use, diuretics that lead to hyperuricemia, and diets that are rich in meat and seafood. Of the forms of arthritis discussed here, gout is the most treatable form of the disease. It is managed with pain medicine, antiinflammatories, and intramuscular (IM) and oral corticosteroids. An acute episode usually subsides within 24 hours after treatment begins.

MUSCLE DISORDERS

As described in Chapter 10, the muscles of the body fulfill many purposes, such as movement, postural maintenance, and heat production. Inflammation of skeletal muscle can result from injury, infection, or autoimmune disease. Skeletal muscle disorders discussed in this chapter include myalgia and chronic fatigue syndrome. Trauma-related causes of muscle weakness, such as *rhabdomyolysis* and *compartment syndrome,* are described in Chapter 38.

Myalgia

Myalgia means muscle pain or pain in multiple muscles. There are many causes and various types of myalgia. The condition can be acute and temporary, or it can be chronic. Myalgia most often results from overuse, muscle injury, or stress (described later in this chapter). It can also result from a virus, an infection, and an autoimmune disorder. Myalgia can be an indication of serious illness. Serious illness associated with myalgia includes inflammatory myopathies and chronic fatigue syndrome.

INFLAMMATORY MYOPATHIES

Inflammatory myopathies refer to a group of diseases that involve chronic muscle inflammation accompanied by muscle weakness. Causes of these disorders may include injury, infection, autoimmune disease, alcohol and illicit drug use (e.g., cocaine), and some prescribed medications (e.g., some statins). The three main types of inflammatory myopathies are polymyositis, dermatomyositis, and myositis. These are rare disorders that can affect both children and adults. General symptoms that are common to these disorders include[18]:

- Slow and progressive muscle weakness that begins in the muscles closest to the trunk of the body
- Fatigue after walking or standing
- Frequent trips and falls
- Difficulty swallowing or breathing

Dermatomyositis is characterized by a skin rash that precedes or accompanies progressive muscle weakness. The rash looks patchy, with bluish-purple or red discolorations. It characteristically develops on the eyelids and on muscles used to extend or straighten joints, including knuckles, elbows, heels, and toes. Red rashes and swelling may also occur on the face, neck, shoulders, upper chest, back, and other locations. The rash sometimes occurs without obvious muscle involvement. Dermatomyositis may be associated with collagen-vascular or autoimmune diseases, such as lupus.

Polymyositis affects skeletal muscle on both sides of the body. It is rarely seen in persons younger than age 18; most cases are in adults between the ages of 31 and 60. Slow but progressive muscle weakness leads to difficulties climbing stairs, rising from a sitting position, lifting objects, or reaching overhead. People with polymyositis may also experience arthritis, shortness of breath, difficulty swallowing and speaking, and cardiac dysrhythmias. In some cases of polymyositis, muscles farther away from the trunk of the body, such as those in the forearms and around the ankles and wrists, may be affected as the disease progresses. Polymyositis may be associated with collagen-vascular or autoimmune diseases (e.g., lupus) and with infectious disorders, such as human immunodeficiency virus/acquired immunodeficiency syndrome (HIV/AIDS).

Myositis is also known as *inclusive body myositis* (IBM). The disorder is characterized by progressive muscle weakness and wasting. Myositis often begins with weakness in the wrists and fingers that causes difficulty with pinching, buttoning, and gripping objects. There may be weakness of the wrist and finger muscles and atrophy of the muscles in the forearms and legs. Difficulty swallowing occurs in about half of the patients.[19] Symptoms of the disease usually begin after the age of 50, although the disease can occur much earlier.

MANAGEMENT

There is no cure for inflammatory myopathies. Options for dermatomyositis and polymyositis include medications to reduce inflammation, physical therapy, exercise, heat therapy, orthotics, assistive devices, and rest. The standard treatment for these conditions includes oral or IV corticosteroid drugs and immunosuppressant drugs. Periodic treatment using intravenous immunoglobulin may also improve recovery.

There is no standard course of treatment for myositis. The disease is generally unresponsive to corticosteroids and immunosuppressive drugs. Physical therapy may be helpful in maintaining mobility. Other therapy is symptomatic and supportive.

Chronic Fatigue Syndrome

Chronic fatigue syndrome (CFS) is a debilitating and complex disorder. It is characterized by profound fatigue that is not improved by bed rest and that may be worsened by physical or mental activity. CFS affects between 1 and 4 million Americans, 25% of whom are unemployed or on disability because of the illness. According to the Centers for Disease Control and Prevention (CDC), about 40% of people in the general population who report symptoms of CFS have a serious, treatable, previously unrecognized medical or psychiatric condition (such as diabetes, thyroid disease, substance abuse)[20] (Box 33-7).

> **NOTE**
>
> **Fibromyalgia** (FM) is another disorder that causes extreme fatigue. In addition to fatigue, FM is associated with "tender points" on the neck, shoulders, back, hips, arms, and legs. The distinction between FM and CFS is not clear. Some experts believe they are one and the same disorder, with slightly different manifestations. The cause of both FM and CFS is unknown, although there may be a viral or heritable component.[21] Both FM and CFS have pain and fatigue as symptoms, and both disorders are treated in the same manner.

SIGNS AND SYMPTOMS OF CFS

The primary signs and symptoms of CFS are difficulties with memory and concentration, problems with sleep, and persistent muscle pain that lasts 6 months or more. In addition, the person may experience joint pain (without redness and swelling), headache, tender lymph nodes, sore throat, and malaise following exertion. Other symptoms may include[22]:

- Irritable bowel
- Depression, irritability, mood swings, anxiety, panic attacks
- Chills and night sweats
- Visual disturbances (blurring, sensitivity to light, eye pain)
- Allergies or sensitivities to foods, odors, chemicals, medications, or noise
- Brain fog (feeling like one is in a mental fog)

> ### BOX 33-7 Risk Groups for CFS[20]
>
> - CFS occurs up to four times more frequently in women than in men, although people of either gender can develop the disease.
> - The illness occurs most often in people between the ages of 40 and 59, but people of all ages can have CFS.
> - CFS is less common in children than in adults. Studies suggest that CFS is more prevalent in adolescents than in children.
> - CFS occurs in all ethnic and racial groups worldwide. Research indicates that CFS is at least as common among African Americans and Hispanics as it is among Caucasians.
> - People of all income levels can develop CFS, although there is evidence that it is more common in lower-income than affluent individuals.
> - CFS is sometimes seen in members of the same family, but there is no evidence that it is contagious. Instead, there may be a familial or genetic propensity. Further research is needed to explore this.
> - CFS can be as disabling as multiple sclerosis, lupus, rheumatoid arthritis, heart disease, end-stage renal disease, chronic obstructive pulmonary disease, and similar chronic conditions.

- Difficulty maintaining upright position, dizziness, balance problems, or fainting

CFS often follows a cyclical course, alternating between periods of illness and relative well-being. Some patients experience partial or complete remission of symptoms during the course of the illness, but symptoms often reoccur.

MANAGEMENT

Prehospital care is primarily supportive. Diagnosis of CFS and fibromyalgia (FM) is based on history and clinical signs and symptoms. (There is no laboratory marker to confirm the disorders.) Most patients are managed with a combination of therapies tailored to the severity of the illness. These may include counseling and behavioral therapy, drug therapy to relieve symptoms, relaxation therapy to reduce anxiety, and support groups with others who have the illness. There is no cure for the illness.

OVERUSE SYNDROMES

The overuse of muscles, tendons, ligaments, and supporting structures can result in numerous injuries and ailments (**overuse syndromes**). The specific disorders discussed in this chapter are bursitis, muscle strain, and tendonitis.

Bursitis

Bursitis is an inflammation of one or more bursae often caused by excessive use of a joint. A **bursa** is a small sac containing synovial fluid that helps ease friction between a tendon and skin or between a tendon and bone (Figure 33-7). Inflammation from injury, compression, overuse, or

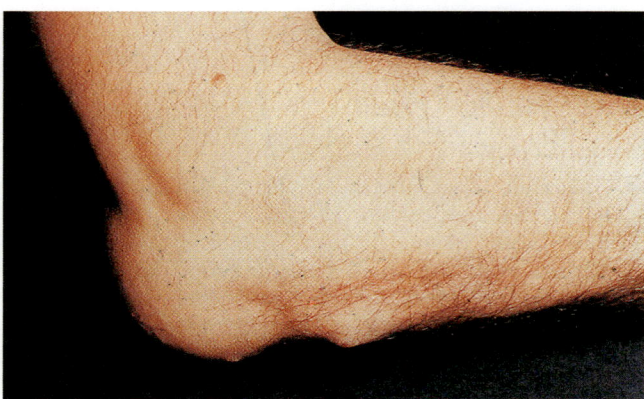

FIGURE 33-7 Bursitis. (From Epstein O, et al: *Clinical examination,* ed 4, St Louis, 2008, Mosby Ltd.)

infection is the most common cause of bursitis. Crystal deposits (uric acids) associated with some diseases such as gout, rheumatoid arthritis, and scleroderma can also lead to bursitis. Areas most commonly affected include the elbow, shoulder, hip, knee, and Achilles tendon. Risk factors for developing bursitis include[23]:

- *Overuse or repetitive use:* Overuse or repetitive actions, such as running, stair climbing, bicycling, or standing for prolonged periods, can cause bursitis.
- *Disease:* Various diseases, such as arthritis, thyroid disease, and diabetes, can lead to bursitis.
- *Leg-length inequality:* When one leg is shorter than the other by 1 inch or more it affects walking and could lead to irritation of hip bursa.
- *Previous surgery:* Surgery around the hip or prosthetic implants in the hip can irritate the bursae.
- *Bone spurs or calcium deposits:* Bone spurs or calcium deposits can develop within the tendons that attach to the trochanter, causing irritation and inflammation to the bursa.
- *Crystal deposits:* Uric acid, a normal byproduct of daily metabolism, may be deposited as crystals in joints, causing bursitis.

Bursitis most commonly affects people more than 40 years of age. The primary symptom of bursitis is pain, which may be sudden and severe. Loss of motion in a joint caused by crystal deposits can also indicate bursitis. Initial self-care for bursitis is listed in Box 33-8. Other treatment options may include corticosteroids, antibiotics, physical therapy, needle aspiration of bursal fluid, and surgical removal or drainage of an infected bursal sac.

Muscle Strains

Muscle strains, or "pulled muscles," are slight tears in muscles or tendons. They usually result from excessive stretching or use. The tiny tears in the damaged muscle cause muscle fibers to spasm. This results in pain that can last for days to weeks. When strained muscles heal, scar tissue replaces the injured muscle fibers. The scar tissue may cause some weakening of the muscle and may allow muscle injury to recur. Two commonly injured muscles in athletes are the *hamstring* and *quadriceps,* both of which cross the hip and knee joints. Another common site for muscle strains is the lower back.

> **NOTE**
> A person who experiences a muscle strain in the thigh will frequently describe a "popping" or "snapping" sensation as the muscle tears. Pain is sudden and may be severe. The area around the injury may be tender to the touch, with visible bruising.

Muscle strains are graded according to their severity. A grade 1 strain is mild and usually heals readily, whereas a grade 3 strain is a severe tear of the muscle that may take months to heal.[19] Most muscle strains can be successfully treated using the PRICEM formula, described in Box 33-8. Some injuries may require *therapeutic ultrasound,* a procedure in which torn muscles are broken down to allow them to heal properly. More severe injury may require surgical repair of torn ligaments, muscles, and tendons.

Tendonitis

Tendonitis is inflammation of a tendon. As described in Chapter 10: Review of Human Systems, a tendon is a tough and flexible band of fibrous tissue that connects muscles to bones. Tendons most often become inflamed from overuse. This may result in the tendon and surrounding tissues becoming swollen and tender. Movement may be painful or limited. Almost any tendon can become inflamed. The most common areas affected by tendonitis are the wrist, ankle and heel, knee, and the rotator cuff of the shoulder (Figure 33-8). Risk factors associated with tendonitis include

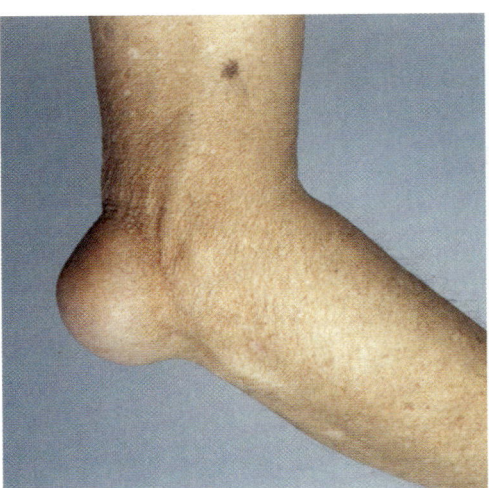

FIGURE 33-8 Abnormalities of the elbow: tendonitis. (From Jarvis C: *Physical examination and health assessment,* ed 5, St Louis, 2008, Saunders.)

advancing age; occupations that involve repetitive motions, forceful exertion, or awkward positions; and certain sports, such as bowling, swimming, tennis, baseball, and basketball.

Tendonitis is usually diagnosed by a history and physical examination. As a rule, x-rays or other imaging tests are not needed unless there is suspicion of fracture or underlying illness. Treatment usually consists of PRICEM (see Box 33-8). Some patients (for example, those with arthritis and gout) may be prescribed exercise and physical therapy to prevent recurrent injury.

PERIPHERAL NERVE SYNDROMES

As described in Chapter 10, the peripheral nervous system consists of all the nerves that exit the brain and spinal cord. Two common peripheral nerve syndromes are carpal tunnel syndrome and ulnar nerve entrapment. Both of these conditions can cause pain, tingling, and numbness in the arms, wrists, and fingers.

Carpal Tunnel Syndrome

Carpal tunnel syndrome is an *entrapment neuropathy* that occurs when the median nerve becomes pressed or squeezed at the wrist in the carpal tunnel. The *carpal tunnel* is a narrow, rigid passageway of ligament and bones at the base of the hand. This tunnel houses the median nerve and tendons (Figure 33-9). The median nerve controls sensations to the palm side of the thumb and fingers (although not the little finger). This nerve also provides impulses to small muscles in the hand that allow the fingers and thumb to move. Compression of the median nerve can cause pain, weakness, or numbness in the hand and wrist, radiating up the arm. Compression can be caused by any condition that decreases the space in the carpal tunnel (e.g., irritated tendons or other swelling).

Carpal Tunnel Syndrome

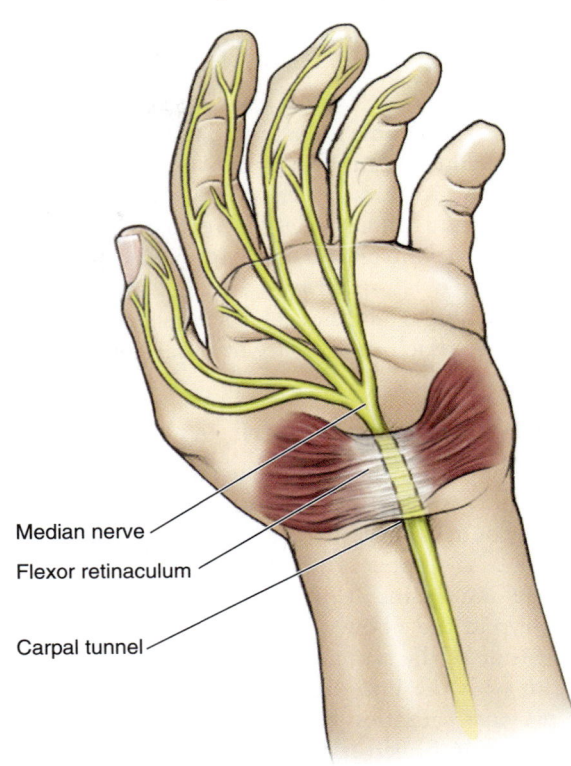

Median nerve
Flexor retinaculum
Carpal tunnel

FIGURE 33-9 Carpal tunnel syndrome. (From Herlihy B: *The human body in health and illness,* ed 3, St Louis, 2007, Saunders.)

There are few clinical data to prove whether repetitive and forceful movements of the hand and wrist during work or leisure activities can cause carpal tunnel syndrome.[25] The condition is most likely due to a congenital predisposition; that is, the carpal tunnel is simply smaller in some people than in others. Women are three times more likely than men to develop carpal tunnel syndrome. This is perhaps because the carpal tunnel itself may be smaller in women than in men. Other contributing factors include:

- Trauma or injury to the wrist that causes swelling (e.g., sprain or fracture)
- Overactivity of the pituitary gland
- Hypothyroidism
- Rheumatoid arthritis
- Mechanical problems in the wrist joint
- Repeated use of vibrating hand tools
- Fluid retention during pregnancy or menopause
- Cyst or tumor in the canal

SIGNS AND SYMPTOMS

The symptoms of carpal tunnel syndrome usually begin gradually, often during sleep. Complaints include frequent burning, tingling, or itching numbness in the palm of the hand and the fingers. Sleep is often interrupted with the need to "shake out" the wrist or hand. As symptoms worsen, tingling may occur during the day. The patient may have decreased grip strength, making it difficult to form a fist, grasp small objects, or perform other manual tasks. Early diagnosis and treatment are important in preventing permanent damage to the median nerve.

MANAGEMENT

Carpal tunnel syndrome is diagnosed through various tests that may include percussion of the median nerve (*Tinel's sign*), wrist-flexion tests (*Phalen's test*), compression tests, and nerve conduction studies.[26] Treatment may include drug therapy to control pain, decrease swelling, and reduce inflammation; wrist splinting to maintain correct wrist position; exercise and physical therapy to restore wrist strength; and sometimes surgery to release pressure in the carpal tunnel.

Ulnar Nerve Entrapment

Ulnar nerve entrapment occurs when the ulnar nerve in the arm becomes compressed. The ulnar nerve (often called the "funny bone") travels from under the clavicle and along the inside of the upper arm. It passes through the cubital tunnel, behind the inside of the elbow, where it can be palpated. Beyond the elbow, the nerve travels under muscles on the inside of the arm and into the hand on the side of the palm with the little finger (Figure 33-10). The ulnar nerve provides sensation to the little finger and the palm half of the ring finger. It also controls most of the small muscles in the hand that help with fine movements, and some larger muscles in the forearm that help a person make strong grips. Entrapment of the ulnar nerve most commonly occurs behind the elbow. The syndrome may be associated with previous injury to the elbow, bone spurs, and swelling. Cysts may also be a cause of the entrapment.

Signs and symptoms of ulnar nerve entrapment are similar to those caused by compression of the medial nerve. They include numbness, pain, and tingling in the elbow, forearm, wrist, and fingers. Often the patient complains that the hand has "fallen asleep." Symptoms frequently occur during sleep when the elbows are commonly flexed, and during daytime activities that involve bending of the elbow. Ulnar nerve entrapment is diagnosed and treated with tests and therapies similar to those for carpal tunnel syndrome. Surgery is sometimes used to reposition the ulnar nerve to avoid compression and entrapment.

SOFT TISSUE INFECTIONS

There are soft tissue infections that can destroy muscles, skin, and underlying tissue. Most are rare and are caused by a bacterial infection. Soft tissue infections specific to nontraumatic musculoskeletal disorders discussed in this chapter include fasciitis, gangrene, paronychia, and flexor tenosynovitis of the hand.

> **NOTE**
> The occurrence of serious and rare skin infections is on the rise. This is because of an increase in immunocompromised patients with diabetes, cancer, alcoholism, vascular insufficiencies, organ transplants, and HIV.[19]

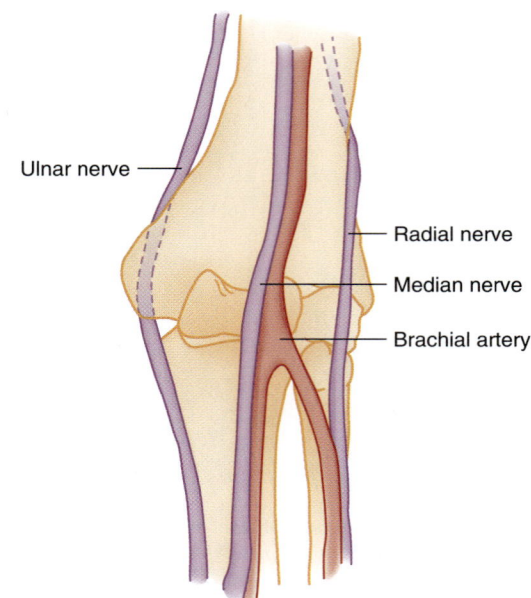

FIGURE 33-10 Ulnar nerve. (From Marx J et al: *Rosen's emergency medicine: concepts and clinical practice,* ed 6, St Louis, 2006, Mosby.)

Fasciitis

Fasciitis refers to inflammation of the fascia. **Fascia** is a strong connective tissue that forms under the skin. The tissue performs a number of functions. It envelops and isolates muscles, and sometimes groups of muscles, in the body. It also provides support and protection for body organs and structures.

Necrotizing fasciitis (also called "flesh-eating bacteria") is a rare infection of the deep layers of the skin and subcutaneous tissues. It rapidly spreads in the deep fascial plane with secondary necrosis (tissue death) in the subcutaneous tissue. Necrotizing fasciitis is most likely to occur in people with compromised immune systems. Many bacteria can cause the disease, some of which are resistant to antibiotics (Box 33-9).

The infection begins slowly, usually at a site of broken skin (minor or major trauma or surgery). Often the patient will complain of intense pain that is out of proportion to

---

BOX 33-9 Bacteria That Cause Necrotizing Fasciitis*

Streptococcus pyogenes
Staphylococcus aureus
Vibrio vulnificus
Clostridium perfringens
Bacteroides fragilis

***NOTE:** The term *flesh-eating bacteria* is a misnomer. The bacteria do not actually eat the tissue. Skin and muscle are destroyed by the release of toxins, which causes the overproduction of cytokines.

the appearance of the injury. As the disease progresses, the affected area quickly becomes red, hot, and swollen. The skin color may become violet-purple, and blisters may form as necrosis develops in the subcutaneous tissues. Fever, diarrhea, and vomiting are common. If left untreated, the infection may become systemic, leading to death.

> **NOTE**
> Since 1883, more than 500 cases of necrotizing fasciitis have been reported in the literature. Overall morbidity and mortality is as high as 75%. The mean age of survivors is 35 years. The mean age of nonsurvivors is 49 years. The disease rarely occurs in children.[27]

Patients with necrotizing fasciitis are managed with surgical debridement of the affected area, IV antibiotics, and support of vital functions. Aggressive surgical removal of the infected tissue is usually necessary. The need for skin grafts is not uncommon. Most patients require intensive care monitoring. Hyperbaric oxygen therapy may be an option in caring for these patients. Hyperbaric oxygen can increase the oxygen within the body's tissues, force oxygen into hypoxic tissue, decrease edema, destroy anaerobic bacteria, and promote the growth of new blood vessels within soft tissue.

> **DID YOU KNOW?**
> **Hyperbaric Oxygen Therapy**
> Altering the surrounding air pressure for medical treatment is a practice that dates back to the seventeenth century. At that time, "fevers and inflammations" were treated in crude chambers that were pressurized using hand bellows. Today, hyperbaric oxygen therapy (HBOT) is carried out in single-person chambers. These are monoplace chambers. The treatment also can be done in larger multiplace chambers, which can house several patients and the attending hyperbaric health care workers. HBOT has proved to be effective in the treatment of a wide variety of medical disorders. These include air embolism and decompression sickness; carbon monoxide poisoning and smoke inhalation; carbon monoxide poisoning complicated by cyanide poisoning (controversial); clostridial myonecrosis (gas gangrene); crush injury, compartment syndrome, and other acute traumatic ischemias; intracranial abscesses; and thermal burns. It also has been shown to enhance the healing of certain problem wounds, including tissue necrosis.[28] HBOT works to[29]:
> - Greatly increase oxygen concentration in all body tissues, even with reduced or blocked blood flow.
> - Stimulate the growth of new blood vessels to locations with reduced circulation, thereby improving blood flow to areas with arterial blockage.
> - Cause a rebound arterial dilation after HBOT, resulting in a blood vessel diameter that is greater than that before therapy, improving blood flow to compromised organs.
> - Aid in the treatment of infection by enhancing white blood cell action and potentiating germ-killing antibiotics.

Gangrene

Gangrene is a complication of tissue necrosis. It is characterized by the decay and death of body tissue, which becomes black (and/or green) and malodorous (foul smelling) (Figure 33-11). Gangrene results from decreased blood supply to a body part or organ, most commonly the toes, fingers, feet, and hands. It can also result from infection, disease, frostbite, and other soft tissue injury. Two major types of gangrene exist:

1. *Dry gangrene:* Caused by a reduction of blood flow through the arteries (not infection). It appears gradually and progresses slowly. Dry gangrene is associated with arteriosclerosis, diabetes, cigarette smoking, genetics, and other factors. In this type of gangrene, tissues appear dry and discolored and will eventually slough away.
2. *Wet gangrene (moist gangrene):* Develops as a complication of an untreated, infected wound. Swelling results from the bacterial infection that causes a sudden decrease in blood flow. (*Gas gangrene* is a type of wet gangrene caused by the bacteria *Clostridia,* which produce poisonous toxins and gas.) In this type of gangrene, tissues appear moist and produce oozing fluid or pus.

MANAGEMENT

Treatment of gangrene depends upon the type of gangrene (dry versus wet) and upon how much tissue is compromised. Immediate treatment is needed in all cases of wet gangrene and in some cases of dry gangrene. Treatment for both types of gangrene usually involves surgery, antibiotic therapy, anticoagulant therapy, pain management, supportive care, and rehabilitation (especially with surgical or autoamputation). If available, hyperbaric oxygen therapy (HBOT) may be indicated as additional therapy for gas gangrene.

Paronychia

Paronychia is a common skin infection that occurs around the nails. It is usually caused by an injury (e.g., nail biting, pulling a hangnail, trimming a cuticle) that allows for an

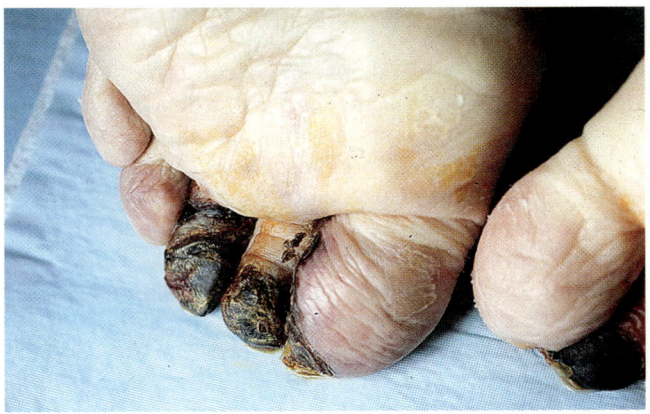

FIGURE 33-11 Gangrene of toes. Dry gangrene. (From Damjanov I: *Pathology for the health-related professions,* ed 2, Philadelphia, 2000, Saunders.)

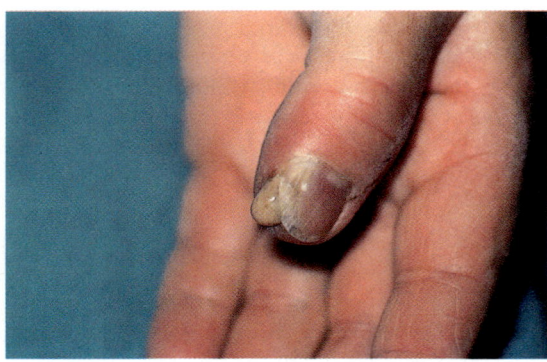

FIGURE 33-12 Paronychia. (From Callen J, Greer K, Hood A, et al: *Color atlas of dermatology,* ed 2, Philadelphia, 2000, Saunders.)

invasion of bacteria, yeast, or fungus (Figure 33-12). The condition is also common in persons with diabetes and in those who have their hands submerged in water for long periods of time. Symptoms include:

- Pain and redness around the nail
- Puss-filled blisters (especially with bacterial infection)
- Nails that are abnormally shaped or have an unusual color

MANAGEMENT

Physician care for patients with paronychia may include incision and drainage of the infection, nail removal, and antibiotic therapy. Warm hand soaks may also relieve discomfort. The condition usually responds well to treatment. Rarely, some infections can be prolonged, requiring additional therapy. Signs of systemic infection from paronychia include chills, red streaks proximal to the infection, fever, malaise, joint pain, and muscle spasm.[30]

Flexor Tenosynovitis

Flexor tenosynovitis is a pathological state that causes a disruption of tendon function in the hand. Most cases are the result of infection. The condition can also be secondary to acute or chronic inflammation as a result of overuse or disease (e.g., diabetes, arthritis). When infectious agents enter the closed space of a tendon sheath, the immune response causes swelling. This interferes with the gliding mechanism of the wrist, hand, and fingers, and can result in disruption of the tendon sheath. It may also lead to tendon necrosis. Flexor tenosynovitis is considered an orthopedic emergency. If left untreated, the infection may become systemic, spreading to fascia, synovial joint spaces, and skin. Subsequent osteomyelitis may result.[19]

The primary cause of infectious flexor tenosynovitis is penetrating trauma that allows native skin flora (both *Staphylococcus* and *Streptococcus*) to invade the tendon sheath. The patient may present with fever and chills. Other signs and symptoms include *Kanavel's sign*:

- Severe pain on passive range of motion
- Swollen digits ("sausage links")
- Fingers that are held slightly flexed
- Swelling and tenderness along the flexor sheath

MANAGEMENT

In most cases of infectious flexor tenosynovitis, surgical drainage is required. Other treatment may include prescribing antibiotics, splinting, and elevating the hand. All patients require physician care and follow-up. Prehospital care is primarily supportive.

SUMMARY

- Although more common in advanced age, nontraumatic musculoskeletal disorders affect patients of all ages.
- The musculoskeletal system is composed of bones, muscles, tendons, ligaments, and articulating surfaces. Three types of joints are fibrous, cartilaginous, and synovial. Muscles are responsible for movement, posture, and heat production.
- The extremities and spine should be examined to determine structure and function. Specific assessments include range of motion, vascular evaluation, and a motor and sensory exam.
- Prehospital management of nontraumatic musculoskeletal disorders includes routine care and pain management.
- Important historical data to gather on a patient with this type of disorder should relate to onset of signs and symptoms, nature and location of pain, presence of weakness or other alteration in motor function, and presence of sensory abnormalities.
- Osteomyelitis is a bone infection. It may result from an open fracture, wound infection, or systemic infection. Signs and symptoms include pain, signs of inflammation, fever, pus, and other functional alterations.
- Bone tumors are benign or malignant abnormal cell growth within a bone. Multiple myeloma is the most common type of primary bone cancer. This disorder is characterized by pain and fractures.
- Acute or chronic low back pain is common. It may be caused by trauma, arthritis, infections, or congenital abnormalities.
- Intervertebral disks can herniate and compress adjacent nerves, causing severe pain and weakness.

- Cauda equina syndrome is caused by compression of the nerve roots at the distal end of the spine. If the compression is not relieved promptly, permanent paralysis and incontinence can occur.
- A strain is an injury to a muscle or tendon. A sprain is stretching or tearing of a ligament. Both conditions cause pain.
- Arthritis is an inflammatory condition of a joint characterized by pain and swelling. Osteoarthritis is a chronic degenerative joint disease that has a gradual onset. Rheumatoid arthritis is an autoimmune disease that affects synovial joints. It causes severe pain, disability, and deformity. Ankylosing spondylitis is a form of arthritis that primarily affects the spine. It requires modifications in prehospital care. Septic arthritis is infection of a joint. Gout is a type of arthritis caused by deposits of uric acid in the joint space.
- Myalgia is pain in one or more muscles. It can be caused by an autoimmune disorder, overuse, or infection.
- Inflammatory myopathies are a group of diseases characterized by muscle inflammation and weakness. They can be caused by autoimmune disease, injury, infection, or drugs.

- Chronic fatigue syndrome is characterized by severe fatigue not improved by rest.
- Fibromyalgia causes fatigue and "tender points" on the neck, shoulders, back, hips, arms, and legs.
- Bursitis is inflammation of one or more bursae. It is often caused by overuse.
- Muscle strains are slight tears in the muscle caused by overuse or by injury.
- Tendonitis is inflammation of a tendon.
- Carpal tunnel syndrome is a type of neuropathy caused by entrapment of the median nerve after repetitive movement. It causes pain, numbness, and weakness.
- Ulnar nerve entrapment occurs when the ulnar nerve (funny bone) is compressed.
- Fasciitis is inflammation of the connective tissue that lies under the skin. Necrotizing fasciitis ("flesh-eating bacteria") is a rare infection that begins in the fascia and can become systemic.
- Gangrene is a complication of tissue necrosis. It occurs when tissue decays.
- Paronychia is a skin infection around the nails.
- Flexor tenosynovitis is often caused by infection. It can lead to dysfunction, necrosis, and systemic infection.

REFERENCES

1. National Highway Traffic Safety Administration: *The National EMS Education Standards*, Washington, DC, 2009, U.S. Department of Transportation/National Highway Traffic Safety Administration, DOT.
2. Felson D: *Encyclopedia of public health*, New York, 2002, Macmillan.
3. Cleveland Clinic: *Osteomyelitis*, http://my.clevelandclinic.org/disorders/osteomyelitis/hic_osteomyelitis.aspx, accessed 9-8-10.
4. American Academy of Orthopaedic Surgeons: *Bone tumor*, http://orthoinfo.aaos.org/topic.cfm?topic=A00074, accessed 9-8-10.
5. McCance KL, Brashers VL, *Pathophysiology: the biologic basis for disease in adults and children*, ed 6, St Louis, 2010, Mosby.
6. National Cancer Institute: *Bone cancer*, www.cancer.gov/cancertopics.factsheet/sites-types/bonem, accessed 9-8-10.
7. National Institute of Neurological Disorders and Strokes, National Institutes of Health: *Low back pain fact sheet*, www.ninds.nih.gov/disorders/backpain/detail_backpain.htm, accessed 9-8-10.
8. Panagiotopoulos EC, Syggelos SA, Ployas A, et al: Sciatica due to extrapelvic heterotopic ossification: a case report, *J Med Case Reports* 10(2):298, 2008.
9. Vallfors B: Acute, subacute and chronic low back pain: clinical symptoms, absenteeism and working environment, *Scand J Rehab Med Suppl* 11:1-98, 1985.
10. *Facts about EMS back and musculoskeletal disorders*, www.mytactical.com/downloads/SAM_S_EMS_BACK_INJURY_FACTS.doc, accessed 10-16-10.
11. Centers for Disease Control and Prevention: *Arthritis*, www.cdc.gov/arthritis, accessed 9-8-10.
12. MedlinePlus: *Slipped capital femoral epiphysis*, www.nlm.nih.gov/medlineplus/ency/article/000972.htm, accessed 9-8-10.
13. National Institute of Arthritis and Musculoskeletal and Skin Diseases, National Institutes of Health: *Rheumatoid arthritis*, www.niams.nih.gov/Health_Info/Rheumatic_Disease/default.asp, accessed 9-8-10.
14. Spondylitis Association of America: *About ankylosing spondylitis*, www.spondylitis.org/about/as.aspx, accessed 9-8-10.
15. Goronzy J, editor: *Rheumatoid arthritis: current directions in autoimmunity*, Basel, Switzerland, 2001, Karger.
16. Brusch J: *Septic arthritis*, http://emedicine.medscape.com/article/236299-overview, accessed 9-8-10.
17. Kramer HJ, Choi HK, Atkinson K, et al: The association between gout and nephrolithiasis in men: The Health Professionals' Follow-Up Study, *Kidney Int* 64(3):1022-1026, 2003.
18. National Institute of Neurological Disorders and Stroke, National Institutes of Health: *NINGS inclusion body myositis information*, www.ninds.nih.gov/disorders/inclusion_body_myositis/inclusion_body_myositis.htm, accessed 9-8-10.
19. Marx J, Hockberger R, Walls R: *Rosen's emergency medicine: concepts and clinical practice*, St Louis, 2006, Mosby.
20. Centers for Disease Control and Prevention: *CFS basic facts*, www.cdc.gov/cfs/cfsbasicfacts.htm, accessed 9-8-10.
21. Abeles AM, Pillinger MH, Solitar BM, et al: Narrative review: the pathophysiology of fibromyalgia, *Ann Intern Med* 146(10):726-734, 2007.
22. National Chronic Fatigue Syndrome and Fibromyalgia Association: www.ncfsfa.org, accessed 9-8-10.

23. American Academy of Orthopaedic Surgeons: *Hip bursitis*, http://orthoinfo.aaos.org/topic.cfm?topic=a00409, accessed 9-8-10.

24. Omnimedicalsearch.com: *Conditions and diseases: bones, muscles, and joints*, www.omnimedicalsearch.com/conditions-diseases/bursitis-introduction.html, accessed 9-8-10.

25. National Institute of Neurological Disorders and Stroke, National Institutes of Health: *Carpal tunnel syndrome fact sheet*, www.ninds.nih.gov/disorders/carpal_tunnel/detail_carpal_tunnel.htm, accessed 9-8-10.

26. Spinner RJ: Outcomes for peripheral nerve entrapment syndromes, *Clin Neurosurg* 53:285-294, 2006.

27. Cheng NC, Su YM, Kuo YS, et al: Factors affecting the mortality of necrotizing fasciitis involving the upper extremities, *Surg Today* 38(12):1108-1113, 2008.

28. Riseman JA, Zamboni WA, Curtis A, et al: Hyperbaric oxygen therapy for necrotizing fasciitis reduces mortality and the need for debridements, *Surgery* 108(5):847-850, 1990.

29. Neubauer R, Walker M: *Hyperbaric oxygen therapy*, New York, 1998, Avery Publishing Group.

30. Habif TP: *Clinical dermatology*, ed 4, St Louis, 2004, Mosby.

SUGGESTED READING

Spondylitis Association of America: *Ankylosing spondylitis: managing patients in an emergency setting, a primer for first responders*, 2009, www.spondylitis.org/physician_resources/ems_video.aspx, accessed 9-18-10.

34 Toxicology

OBJECTIVES

Upon completion of this chapter, the paramedic student will be able to:

1. Define poisoning.
2. Describe general principles for assessment and management of the patient who has ingested poison.
3. Describe the causative agents and pathophysiology of selected ingested poisons and the management of patients who have taken them.
4. Describe how physical and chemical properties influence the effects of inhaled toxins.
5. Distinguish among the three categories of inhaled toxins: simple asphyxiants, chemical asphyxiants and systemic poisons, and irritants or corrosives.
6. Describe general principles of managing the patient who has inhaled poison.
7. Describe the signs, symptoms, and management of patients who have inhaled cyanide, ammonia, or hydrocarbon.
8. Describe the signs, symptoms, and management of patients injected with poison by insects, reptiles, and hazardous aquatic creatures.
9. Describe the signs, symptoms, and management of patients with organophosphate or carbamate poisoning.
10. Outline the general principles of managing patients with drug overdose.
11. Describe the effects, signs and symptoms, and specific management for selected therapeutic and illegal drug overdoses.
12. Describe the short- and long-term physiological effects of ethanol ingestion.
13. Describe signs, symptoms, and management of alcohol-related emergencies.
14. Identify general management principles for the most common toxic syndromes based on a knowledge of the characteristic physical findings associated with each syndrome.

KEY TERMS

adsorb To accumulate on a surface in a condensed layer.

alcohol dependence A disorder characterized by chronic, excessive consumption of alcohol that results in injury to health or in inadequate social function and the development of withdrawal symptoms when the person stops drinking suddenly.

antidote A drug or other substance that opposes the action of a poison.

botulism An often fatal form of food poisoning caused by the bacillus *Clostridium botulinum*.

cathartic A substance that accelerates defecation.

cirrhosis A chronic degenerative disease of the liver.

delirium tremens An acute and sometimes fatal psychotic reaction caused by cessation of excessive intake of alcohol over a long period of time; also known as DTs.

disulfiram-ethanol reaction A potentially life-threatening physiological response caused by disulfiram and ethanol that produces ill effects on the gastrointestinal (GI), cardiovascular, and autonomic nervous systems; disulfiram is prescribed to some alcoholic patients to help them maintain abstinence.

drug abuse Self-medication or self-administration of a drug in chronically excessive amounts, resulting in psychological or physical dependence (or both), functional impairment, and deviation from approved social norms.

envenomation The injection of snake, arachnid, or insect venom into the body.

food poisoning Poisoning that results from food contaminated by toxic substances or by bacteria containing toxins.

gastric lavage Irrigation of the stomach with sterile water or normal saline.

gastrointestinal decontamination The use of medical methods to empty the stomach of ingested toxins to prevent absorption.

Korsakoff's psychosis A form of amnesia often seen in alcoholics, characterized by a loss of short-term memory and an inability to learn new skills.

liquefaction Conversion of solid tissues to a fluid or semi-fluid state.

Lyme disease An acute, recurrent inflammatory infection transmitted by a tick.

mediastinitis Inflammation of the mediastinum.

methemoglobin Hemoglobin with ferrous iron in the oxidized (Fe^{3+}) state.

methemoglobinemia The presence of methemoglobin in the blood, causing cyanosis as a result of the inability of the red blood cells to release oxygen.

nematocyst A capsule containing threadlike, venomous stinging cells found in some coelenterates.

nystagmus Involuntary rhythmic movements of the eyes.

pneumoperitoneum The presence of air or gas within the peritoneal cavity of the abdomen.

poison Any substance that produces harmful physiological or psychological effects.

Rocky Mountain spotted fever A serious tick-borne infectious disease, characterized by chills, fever, severe headache, mental confusion, and rash.

serotonin syndrome A potentially life-threatening drug reaction; most often occurs when two or more drugs that affect serotonin levels are taken together.

surface tension The tendency of the surface of a liquid to minimize the area of its surface by contracting.

tick paralysis A rare, progressive, reversible disorder caused by several species of ticks that release a neurotoxin that causes weakness, incoordination, and paralysis.

toxidromes Clinical syndromes grouped together for the successful recognition of poisoning patterns.

volatility The ability of a liquid to vaporize.

Wernicke-Korsakoff syndrome A disease that results from chronic thiamine deficiency combined with an inability to use thiamine because of a heritable disorder or because of a reduction in intestinal absorption and metabolism of thiamine by alcohol.

Wernicke's encephalopathy A stage of Wernicke-Korsakoff syndrome that usually develops suddenly with the clinical manifestations of ataxia, nystagmus, disturbances of speech and gait, signs of neuropathy, stupor, or coma.

West Nile virus A potentially serious mosquito-borne illness that affects the central nervous system.

whole-bowel irrigation An in-hospital method of GI decontamination; involves the rapid administration of large amounts of a specially balanced fluid to flush the GI tract.

Our environment contains a large number of potentially harmful substances that are both natural and synthetic. These substances can be accidentally or deliberately introduced into the body. These include animal and plant toxins, industrial and household chemicals, prescription medications, and drugs of abuse. Early identification of these agents and rapid transport for definitive care are crucial in managing patients with toxicological emergencies.

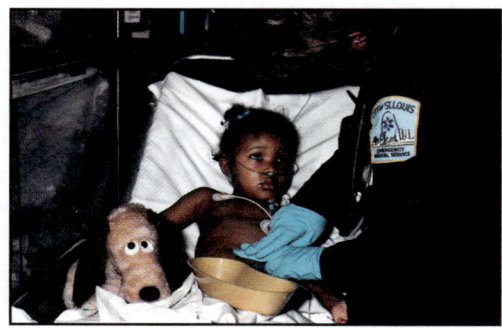

(Courtesy Monroe Yancey, St. Louis, Mo.)

SECTION ONE
Poisonings

A poison can be defined as any substance that produces harmful physiological or psychological effects. Emergencies that involve poisons are a major cause of morbidity and mortality in the United States. In 2006, there were more than 2 million unintentional poisonings reported by poison control centers, resulting in more than 700,000 emergency department visits. An additional 200,000 emergency department visits were caused by intentional poisoning; 75% of these patients had to be hospitalized or transferred to another medical facility.[1] According to the National Safety Council, poisoning by solids and liquids was the second leading cause of unintentional death in the United States in 2005, and the second leading cause of unintentional death for all persons ages 17 to 39.[2]

NOTE
Unintentional poisoning is poisoning that occurs when a person takes or gives a substance without the intent to harm. *Intentional poisoning* results when there is intent to cause harm.

CRITICAL THINKING
How many substances that fit the definition of a poison are there in or around your home?

POISON CONTROL CENTERS

More than 60 poison control centers exist across the United States to help treat poisoning emergencies. Most centers are based in major medical centers or teaching hospitals. Each one belongs to regional centers designated by the American Association of Poison Control Centers. Medical professionals staff regional centers. They offer 24-hour telephone access (1-800-222-1222) to population bases of at least 1 million. In 2007, an estimated 4.2 million poisonings were reported to poison control centers throughout the United States. More than 90% of these poisonings happen in the home; 51.2% of poisoning victims are children younger than 6 years of age.[3] By helping persons manage emergencies at home, these centers prevent about 1.6 million hospitalizations and visits to physicians' offices each year.

By request, information and treatment advice is given immediately by the poison control center. They provide this information through a large database of references on more than 350,000 toxic substances. These substances include drugs (legal, illicit, foreign, and veterinary), chemicals, plants, animals, insects, fish, snakes, cosmetics, and hazardous materials. Each request for information is followed up to determine the effectiveness and outcome of the treatment. In addition, the centers are responsible for the following elements of an organized poison system[4]:

1. Treatment information and toxicological consultation with health care providers (e.g., hospitals, physicians, EMS agencies) and the public, using a toll-free number with linkage into various 911 systems
2. Professional education to train those involved in care of poisoned patients
3. Data collection on all poisonings in the region for epidemiological and evaluation purposes
4. Public education and prevention
5. Research
6. Regional EMS poison system development (e.g., patient classification criteria, triage and management protocols, and regional transfer agreements)

Use by Emergency Medical Services Agencies

Regional poison control centers are a ready source of information for any toxicological emergency. Depending on local communications' protocol, poison control centers may be contacted directly by EMS and other public service agencies through telephone, cellular phone, a dispatching center, or medical direction. The immediate determination of potential toxicity is based on the specific agent or agents. It also is based on the amount ingested, the time of exposure, the patient's weight and medical condition, and any treatment given before EMS arrival. The poison center also can coordinate treatment protocol by notifying the receiving hospital while the patient is en route to the emergency department.

GENERAL GUIDELINES FOR MANAGING A POISONED PATIENT

Poisons may enter the body through ingestion, inhalation, injection, and absorption. Box 34-1 lists three types of toxicological emergencies that may result in poisoning. With the exception of administering lifesaving antidotes for specific poisons described later in this chapter, most poisoned patients require only supportive therapy to recover. The poisoned patient often can be managed properly in the prehospital setting using the following guidelines:

1. Ensure adequate airway, ventilation, and circulation. Take action to prevent or reduce the risk of aspiration by carefully monitoring the patient's airway.
2. Obtain a thorough history, and perform a focused physical examination.

3. Consider hypoglycemia in a patient who has an altered level of consciousness or is convulsing. Confirm through serum glucose testing.
4. Administer **naloxone** or **nalmefene** to a patient with respiratory depression.
5. If overdose is suspected, obtain an overdose history from the patient, family, or friends.
6. Consult with medical direction or a poison control center for specific management to prevent further absorption of the toxin or antidote therapy.
7. Frequently reassess the patient; monitor vital signs and electrocardiogram (ECG).
8. Safely obtain any substance or substance container of a suspected poison. Transport it along with the patient. The paramedic should collect a sample of the patient's vomitus (if present) for laboratory analysis.
9. Employ universal precautions for personal protection, especially if the substance can be absorbed through the skin.
10. Transport the patient for physician examination.

When caring for a patient who has been poisoned, personal safety remains the top priority. A toxicological emergency response may involve hazardous materials. It also may involve patient behavior that is unpredictable or violent. If the scene is not safe, the paramedic crew should retreat to a safe staging area and wait there until the scene has been secured by the proper personnel.

POISONING BY INGESTION

About 80% of all accidental ingestion of poisons occurs in children 1 to 3 years of age.[2] The most common poison exposures in this group result from household products. Such products include petroleum-based agents, cleaning agents, and cosmetics; medications; toxic plants; and contaminated foods. Poisoning in adults, however, usually is intentional. Deliberate poisonings may occur from:

- Attempts at suicide
- Recreational or experimental drug use
- Chemical warfare or acts of terrorism
- Assault and homicide

BOX 34-1 Types of Toxicological Emergencies

Unintentional Poisoning
Childhood poisoning
Dosage errors
Environmental exposure
Idiosyncratic reactions
Occupational exposure

Drug and Alcohol Abuse
Intentional Poisoning/Overdose
Assault/homicide
Chemical warfare
Suicide attempts

The toxic effects of ingested poisons may be immediate or delayed, depending on the substance that was ingested. For example, corrosive substances such as strong acids and alkalis may produce immediate tissue damage. This is evidenced by burns to the lips, tongue, throat, and upper gastrointestinal tract. Other substances, such as medications and toxic plants, usually require absorption and distribution through the bloodstream. They also may require alterations by different organs to produce toxic effects. Because only minimal absorption occurs in the stomach, poisons may take several hours to enter the bloodstream through the small intestine. Therefore early management of the ingested poisoning is focused on treating the patient's symptoms and providing supportive care.

Assessment and Management

The primary survey and initial management of a poisoned patient begins with ensuring scene safety. Then the paramedic should manage immediate threats to the patient's life. During scene size-up, the paramedic crew should be alert for specific clues or details that suggest a toxicological emergency. Examples include open medication bottles, scattered pills, vomitus, and open containers of household products. Patient findings that may suggest poisoning include a decreased level of consciousness, airway compromise/injury (e.g., vomitus or pills in the mouth, burns in the oral cavity), abnormal respiratory patterns, and dysrhythmias such as tachycardia and bradycardia.

> **NOTE**
> The paramedic must consider the possibility of poisoning whenever the patient's signs and symptoms cannot be attributed to other explainable conditions (e.g., hypoglycemia/hyperglycemia or cardiac dysfunction).

The primary goal of physical assessment of poisoned patients is to identify effects on the three vital organ systems most likely to produce morbidity or death. These organ systems are the respiratory system, the cardiovascular system, and the central nervous system. Obtaining a detailed history of the event and any significant medical or psychiatric history also is important. This information may help to direct treatment in the field or in the emergency department. For example, preexisting cardiac, liver, or renal disease and some psychiatric illnesses may be worsened by a toxic ingestion. These conditions may require care in addition to managing the toxic ingestion.

RESPIRATORY COMPLICATIONS

The first priority in managing a poisoned patient after ensuring scene safety is to secure a patent airway. The paramedic should provide adequate ventilatory support as needed. This includes providing high-concentration oxygen, monitoring pulse oximetry, and possibly implementing advanced airway management to protect the airway and prevent aspiration. Other respiratory complications that may be associated with poisoning include the early development of noncardiogenic pulmonary edema or the later development of adult respiratory distress syndrome (see Chapter 24). Bronchospasm may result from direct or indirect toxic effects.

LOOK AGAIN
See Chapter 24: Respiratory, pp. 757-758.

CARDIOVASCULAR COMPLICATIONS

The most common cardiovascular complication of poisoning by ingestion is the development of cardiac dysrhythmias. Thus the paramedic should assess the patient's circulatory status and continually monitor it by electrocardiogram and frequent blood pressure measurements. The presence of tachydysrhythmias or bradydysrhythmias may indicate serious metabolic disorders such as hypoxia and acidosis. Another cardiovascular complication is the development of hypotension associated with decreased vascular tone.

NEUROLOGICAL COMPLICATIONS

The paramedic should perform and document a baseline neurological examination. Deviations from a normal level of consciousness may range from mild drowsiness and agitation to hallucinations, seizures, coma, and death. Neurological complications may result from the toxin itself, such as lead poisoning in children who have ingested paint chips. Alternatively, the complications may result from a metabolic or perfusion disorder, such as poor cardiac output from dysrhythmias.

HISTORY

A thorough history of the exposure and any significant medical history should be obtained from the patient, family members, or bystanders. Although this information may be unreliable (as in cases involving pediatric patients, drug abuse, or suicide attempts), the following should be ascertained if possible:

- What was ingested? Obtain the poison container and remaining contents unless doing so poses a threat to rescuer safety.
- When was (were) the substance(s) ingested? This may affect the decision to use **activated charcoal** or gastric lavage, or to administer an antidote.
- How much of the substance was ingested?
- Was an attempt made to induce vomiting? Did the patient vomit?
- Has an antidote or **activated charcoal** been administered?
- Does the patient have a psychiatric history pertinent to suicide attempts? Has the patient had episodes of recent depression?

Gastrointestinal Decontamination

Gastrointestinal (GI) decontamination is the use of medical methods to empty the stomach of ingested toxins to prevent absorption. These methods include the administration of *activated charcoal,* gastric lavage, and whole-bowel irrigation. Before attempting to remove poison from the gastrointestinal tract, the paramedic should consult with medical direction or a poison control center. Although once a mainstay in the management of ingested toxins, GI decontamination plays a less important role in poison treatment today. With rare exceptions, gastric lavage and whole bowel irrigation are no longer recommended.[5,6]

> **NOTE**
> It should be noted that gastric decontamination rarely affects the clinical outcome of poisoned patients.[5] GI decontamination is only useful for patients who have ingested a poison within 1 hour of being seen. After 1 hour, the toxin most likely will have passed from the stomach into the small intestine where it will be absorbed. Therefore, care for most poisoned patients is primarily supportive. Decisions regarding the use of gastric decontamination are made by medical direction or a poison control center on a case-by-case and drug-by-drug basis.

ACTIVATED CHARCOAL

Activated charcoal is an inert, nontoxic product of wood material that has been heated to an extremely high temperature. Single-dose *activated charcoal* is generally recommended for patients who have ingested a life-threatening poison when no antidotes are available and when the charcoal can be administered within one hour of poisoning. The surface characteristics of *activated charcoal* enable it to **adsorb** (collect in a condensed form) molecules of chemical toxins while in the intestinal tract. *Activated charcoal* is indicated for some toxic ingestions, or for drugs that have delayed emptying. It should be given only when directed by medical direction or a poison control center.[5] It should not be given in cases where strong acid, strong alkali, or ethanol is the toxicant. It also should not be given when specific oral antidotes (e.g., *N*-acetylcysteine [Mucomyst] for acetaminophen overdose) are available. Box 34-2 lists the agents for which activated charcoal generally should and should not be given.[7]

    Activated charcoal comes mixed in an aqueous solution with or without a **cathartic** (most commonly sorbitol). A cathartic is an agent that causes bowel evacuation. It decreases the transit time and expels the charcoal within a short period (Box 34-3). Complications of *activated charcoal* are poor patient acceptance in consuming the charcoal and vomiting. EMS personnel should protect themselves, the patient, and the immediate area from the staining properties of the charcoal. Personal protective measures also should be taken when administering this agent.

BOX 34-2 Activated Charcoal: Indications and Contraindications

Agents for Which Activated Charcoal Generally Should Be Given*

Carbamazepine
Dapsone
Drugs with anticholinergic effects
Opioids
Phenobarbital
Quinine
Sustained-release drugs
Theophylline
Drug packets in "body stuffers"

Agents for Which Activated Charcoal Generally Should Not Be Given†

Cyanide
Ethanol intoxication
Ferrous sulfate or other iron salts
Lithium
Mineral acid ingestion
Methanol
Strong acids or alkalis

*When drugs have a delayed emptying.
†When specific antidotes are available.

BOX 34-3 Dosage of Activated Charcoal

1 to 2 g/kg body mass
30 to 100 g in adults
15 to 30 g in children
Prepared in a slurry and administered orally or by gastric tube

---

> **CRITICAL THINKING**
> Why might a patient be reluctant to take activated charcoal?

GASTRIC LAVAGE

Gastric lavage is a method of gastrointestinal decontamination that can immediately recover a portion of gastric contents. It sometimes is used in the emergency department when a highly toxic substance, such as a calcium channel blocker or tricyclic antidepressant (TCA), has been ingested within the past hour. To perform gastric lavage, a large-bore orogastric tube is inserted through the patient's mouth into the stomach. This is followed by instillation of normal saline through the tube, lavaging the stomach of gastric contents until the fluid returned is clear. Gastric lavage is contraindicated in patients who cannot protect their airway and who have an altered level of consciousness. The procedure also is contraindicated in those who have ingested low-viscosity hydrocarbons (e.g., gasoline, kerosene, furniture polish, mineral spirits) where the risk of aspiration is increased.

WHOLE-BOWEL IRRIGATION

Whole-bowel irrigation is another in-hospital method of GI decontamination. It involves the rapid administration of large amounts of a specially balanced fluid to flush the GI tract. It is administered either orally or via a nasogastric tube. Although rarely indicated, the procedure may be useful in cases of severe, recent ingestion of lithium or metals, such as iron or lead, and in patients who have ingested large amounts of sustained-release formulations of highly toxic drugs. Whole-bowel irrigation also may be useful in the evacuation of drug packets from "body packers."

> **NOTE**
> Syrup of ipecac is an over-the-counter liquid medication used to induce vomiting. It was once the treatment of choice in preventing the absorption of poisons. However, studies showed that ipecac-induced emesis reduced drug absorption by only about 30%. The drug also may interfere with the effectiveness of other methods of decontamination and can increase the risk of aspiration. In 2004 the Federal Drug Administration withdrew approval of syrup of ipecac because of its abuse by patients with bulimia (see Chapter 35). Although the drug may be found in a patient's home, it should not be administered to manage an ingested poison. Patients should be advised to remove syrup of ipecac from their home and to call 9-1-1 or a poison control center if needed.[7]

Antidotes

An antidote is an agent used to neutralize or counteract the effects of a specific poison. Some antidotes work by aiding the elimination of the toxin. Others reactivate enzymes that have been altered by the poison. With a few exceptions described in this chapter, most antidotes are given under physician supervision in the hospital setting (Table 34-1).

Management of Specific Ingested Poisons

Specific ingested poisons discussed in this section include strong acids and alkalis, hydrocarbons, methanol, ethylene glycol, isopropanol, metals (iron, lead, and mercury), and poisons from food and plants. Few effective antidotes are available for ingested poisons. Thus managing the patient's symptoms is the main goal in caring for the poisoned patient.

STRONG ACIDS AND ALKALIS

Strong acids and alkalis include those found in toilet-bowl cleaners, rust remover, ammonia, and most liquid drain cleaners (Box 34-4). These acids and alkalis may cause burns to the mouth, pharynx, esophagus, and sometimes the

TABLE 34-1 Antidotes to Common Toxins*

Toxin	Antidote
Acetaminophen	N-Acetylcysteine
Anticholinergic agents	Physostigmine
Benzodiazepines	Flumazenil
Beta blockers	Glucagon
Calcium channel blockers	Calcium
Cyanide	Amyl nitrate, sodium nitrate, hydroxocobalamin; sodium thiosulfate
Tricyclic antidepressants	Bicarbonate
Digoxin	Digoxin immune Fab
Iron	Deferoxamine
Methanol	Ethanol
Opioids	Naloxone
Organophosphates	Atropine, pralidoxime

*See the *Emergency Drug Index.*

BOX 34-4 Common Acid and Alkali Substances

Acids	Alkalis
Acetic acid	Ammonia
Battery acid	Bleach
Bleach disinfectants	Disk (button) batteries
Hydrochloric acid	Drain pipe and toilet-bowl cleaners
Metal cleaners	Hair dyes and tints
Phenol	Jewelry cleaners
Sulfuric acid	Metal cleaners or polishes
Swimming pool cleaners	Paint removers
Toilet bowl cleaners	Sodium or potassium hydroxide (lye)
	Washing powders

upper respiratory and gastrointestinal tracts. Perforation of the esophagus or stomach may result in vascular collapse, **mediastinitis** (inflammation of the mediastinum), or **pneumoperitoneum** (air or gas in the peritoneal cavity of the abdomen). The frequency of caustic ingestions (most commonly lye) is highest in small children, accounting for 5000 to 8000 accidental exposures each year.[2]

The ingestion of caustic and corrosive substances generally produces immediate damage to the mucous membrane and the intestinal tract. Acids generally complete their damage within 1 to 2 minutes. Alkalis, however, may continue to cause **liquefaction** of tissue and damage for minutes to hours. (Liquefaction is the conversion of solid tissue to a fluid or semifluid state.) Thus the prehospital care usually is limited to airway and ventilatory support, intravenous (IV) fluid replacement, and rapid transport to an appropriate medical facility.

In some cases, medical direction or poison control may recommend diluting the acid or alkali if the patient is conscious. This is done with the oral administration of milk or water: 200 to 300 mL for an adult, 15 mL/kg maximum for a child.[8] Efforts to neutralize the ingested agent with other fluids such as fruit juice, lemon juice, or vinegar are contraindicated. These fluids have the potential to induce intense heat-releasing reactions that can cause severe thermal burns.

> **CRITICAL THINKING**
> What is a risk of administering milk or water to a patient with this type of ingestion?

HYDROCARBONS

Hydrocarbons are a group of compounds that are derived mainly from crude oil, coal, or plant sources. Mixtures vary in their viscosity, surface tension, and volatility. **Viscosity** is the resistance of a liquid to flow; **surface tension** is the ability of a liquid to be attracted to another surface; **volatility** is the ability of a liquid to vaporize. These attributes determine the toxic effects of these agents. Other contributing factors include the presence of other chemicals in the product, total amount of product, and route of exposure.

Hydrocarbons are found in many household products. Examples include cleaning and polishing agents, spot removers, paints, cosmetics, pesticides, and hobby and craft materials. Baby oil is a hydrocarbon that is particularly dangerous if ingested. Hydrocarbons also are found in petroleum distillates, such as turpentine, kerosene, gasoline, lighter fluids, and pine oil products. In addition, a large group of halogenated hydrocarbons and aromatic hydrocarbons exists. Examples of halogenated hydrocarbons include carbon tetrachloride, trichloromethane, trichloroethylene, and methyl chloride. Examples of aromatic hydrocarbons are toluene, xylene, and benzene. Hydrocarbon poisonings are common, accounting for 7% of all ingestions in children younger than 5 years of age.[2] Most ingestions occur between May and September. It is during these months when home use of petroleum products allows children the greatest opportunity for exposure (e.g., cleaning and yard machinery).

The most important physical characteristic in the potential toxicity of ingested hydrocarbons is its viscosity. The lower the viscosity, the higher is the risk of aspiration and associated complications. For example, an ingested hydrocarbon product with a low viscosity, such as gasoline or turpentine, rapidly spreads over the surface of the mouth and throat. The more volatile components become gases on contact with the warm mucous membranes. This exposure causes irritation, coughing, and possible aspiration. If aspiration occurs, it may allow a toxic amount of hydrocarbons to enter the lungs. Hydrocarbons with high viscosity (e.g., asphalt, grease, tar) are not aspirated or absorbed in the gastrointestinal tract. Thus they do not have significant toxicity.

> **NOTE**
> A mnemonic for remembering hydrocarbons is CHAMP: *camphor*, *halogenated* hydrocarbons, *aromatic* hydrocarbons, (heavy) *metal*-containing hydrocarbons, and *pesticide*-containing hydrocarbons.

The clinical features of hydrocarbon ingestion vary widely, depending on the type of agent involved (Box 34-5). If the patient is not displaying symptoms on EMS arrival, the chances of serious complications usually are low. These patients generally are observed in the emergency department for several hours. They often require no treatment. However, any patient suspected of hydrocarbon ingestion who coughs, chokes, cries, or has spontaneous emesis on swallowing should be assumed to have aspirated the hydrocarbon until proven otherwise. Hydrocarbon ingestion may involve the patient's respiratory, gastrointestinal, and neurological systems. The clinical features may be immediate or delayed. Emergency care for symptomatic patients who have ingested hydrocarbon products includes the following:

1. Ensure a patent airway. Provide adequate ventilatory and circulatory support as needed.
2. Identify the substance. Contact medical direction or a poison control center.
3. Decontamination of the stomach generally is avoided in these patients because of the risk of aspiration. The use of **activated charcoal** or diluents has not been shown to be effective in managing hydrocarbon ingestion.[7]
4. Initiate intravenous fluid therapy.

BOX 34-5 Clinical Features of Hydrocarbon Ingestion

Immediate: Up to 6 Hours

Gastrointestinal System
Abdominal pain
Belching
Irritation
Mucous membrane hyperemia
Nausea and vomiting

Respiratory System
Cough and choking
Cyanosis
Dyspnea
Inspiratory stridor
Tachypnea

Neurological System
Coma
Fever
Lethargy
Malaise
Seizures
Systemic factors

Delayed: Days to Weeks

Gastrointestinal System
Diarrhea
Hepatic toxicity

Respiratory System
Atelectasis
Bacterial pneumonia
Dyspnea
Hemolytic and aplastic anemias
Pulmonary edema
Spontaneous hemorrhage
Sputum production
Systemic factors

5. Monitor cardiac rhythm.
6. Transport the patient for physician evaluation.

CRITICAL THINKING
Will the potential lethal effects of this ingestion always be visible on the scene?

METHANOL

Methanol (wood alcohol) is a poisonous alcohol found in a variety of products. Some of these include gas line antifreeze, windshield washer fluid, paints, paint removers, varnishes, canned fuels such as Sterno, and many shellacs. Methanol is a colorless liquid. It has an odor that is distinct from that of ethanol, the form of alcohol in alcoholic beverages. Poisonings may result from intentional or unintentional ingestions, absorption through the skin, or inhalation. Examples include deliberate use of the agent by chronic alcoholics to maintain an inebriated state, unintentional ingestion resulting from misuse or distribution of methanol for ethanol (as in contraband liquor), and accidental ingestions in children.

The metabolites of methanol are extremely toxic. As methanol is absorbed, it rapidly is converted in the liver to formaldehyde and then to formic acid. The accumulation of formic acid in the blood affects the central nervous system (lethargy, confusion, seizure) and the gastrointestinal tract (abdominal pain, nausea and vomiting) and leads to the development of metabolic acidosis (shock, multisystem failure, death). The patient's vision also may be affected (blurred vision, photophobia). The ingestion of as little as 4 mL can cause blindness.[9] The symptoms of methanol poisoning correlate with the degree of acidosis. The onset of symptoms after ingestion ranges from 40 minutes to 72 hours.

CRITICAL THINKING
Do you think this could have been the origin of the expression "blind drunk"?

Emergency care for methanol poisoning is as follows:
1. *Supportive care:* Secure a patent airway and monitor pulse oximetry. Provide adequate ventilatory and circulatory support as needed. Adequate ventilation is essential to ensure adequate oxygenation, to help correct the profound metabolic acidosis, and to maximize respiratory excretion. Establish an intravenous line. The patient should be placed on a cardiac monitor to detect rhythm disturbances.
2. *Gastrointestinal decontamination:* If the patient is seen within 1 hour after ingestion, gastric lavage may be indicated. **Activated charcoal** is ineffective and should not be given. Consult with medical direction or a poison control center.

3. *Correction of metabolic acidosis:* Medical direction may recommend an attempt to correct the metabolic acidosis with **sodium bicarbonate.** Large or repeated doses may be necessary. Serum formic acid may be neutralized with bicarbonate administration. However, hemodialysis will likely be necessary to remove toxic levels of methanol and formate.
4. *Prevention of the conversion of methanol to formic acid:* The conversion of methanol to formic acid may be prevented by the administration of ethanol. (Ethanol has 9 times greater affinity for the enzyme that converts methanol to formic acid.[10] If authorized by online medical direction or protocol, give the conscious patient 30 to 60 mL of 80-proof ethanol by mouth or gastric lavage tube. Unconscious patients should have their airway protected with an endotracheal tube before gastric tube administration of ethanol.
5. *Transport:* Rapidly transport the patient to a proper medical facility for definitive treatment.

ETHYLENE GLYCOL

Ethylene glycol is a colorless, odorless, water-soluble liquid. It is commonly used in windshield deicers, detergents, paints, radiator antifreeze, and coolants. The accidental ingestion of ethylene glycol is common in young children because of the brilliant colors added to these preparations. Ingestion also is due to the widespread availability of products containing ethylene glycol and the warm, sweet taste. The agent also is sometimes consumed by alcoholics as a substitute for ethanol. Without treatment, ingestion of as little as 0.2 mL/kg has been reported to be lethal to an adult.[7]

Early signs and symptoms of central nervous system (CNS) depression usually are caused by the ethanol-like effects of ethylene glycol. However, toxicity from ethylene glycol, as from methanol, is caused by the accumulation of glycolic and oxalic acids after metabolism. This occurs primarily in the liver and kidneys. The metabolic molecules may affect the CNS and cardiopulmonary and renal systems. The initial signs and symptoms of ethylene glycol poisoning may include slurred speech, nausea and vomiting, hallucinations, seizure, stupor, and coma. This can be followed by pulmonary edema and cardiac failure.

Emergency care for ethylene glycol poisoning is similar to that used for methanol poisoning. In addition, the paramedic should anticipate orders from medical direction or a poison control center for the following medications:
- **Thiamine** to degrade glycolic acid to nontoxic metabolites
- **Calcium gluconate** or **calcium chloride** to manage hypocalcemia
- **Diazepam** or **lorazepam** to control seizure activity

CRITICAL THINKING
The effects in stage one of ethylene glycol poisoning could be mistaken for what condition?

ISOPROPANOL

Isopropanol (isopropyl alcohol) is a volatile, flammable, colorless liquid. It has a characteristic odor and bittersweet taste. Rubbing alcohol is the most common household source of this agent. It also is used in disinfectants, degreasers, cosmetics, industrial solvents, and cleaning agents. Common routes of toxic exposure to isopropanol include intentional ingestion as a substitute for ethanol, accidental ingestion, and inhalation of high concentrations of local vapor. Isopropanol is more toxic than ethanol, but less toxic than methanol or ethylene glycol. A lethal dose in adults is rare.[8] In children, any amount of ingestion should be considered potentially toxic.

Isopropanol poisoning affects several body systems, including the central nervous, gastrointestinal, and renal systems. The signs and symptoms often occur within 30 minutes after ingestion. They include CNS and respiratory depression, abdominal pain, gastritis, hematemesis, and hypovolemia. Isopropanol poisoning causes acids to accumulate in the blood (*acetonemia*) and ketones to accumulate in the urine (*ketonuria*). However, associated metabolic acidosis usually does not occur unless the patient develops hypotension.

Emergency care for isopropanol poisoning mainly is supportive. Care includes airway and ventilatory support to ensure adequate respiratory elimination of acetone, fluid resuscitation as needed, and rapid transport to an appropriate medical facility, where dialysis may be necessary. Gastric lavage and ***activated charcoal*** are not effective.[8] Administration of ethanol has not proven to inhibit the toxic metabolite to the same degree as in methanol or ethylene glycol poisoning.

METALS

Infants and children are high-risk groups for unintentional iron, lead, and mercury poisoning. Their immature immune systems and increased absorption as a function of age contribute to this risk.

Iron Poisoning. About 10% of ingested iron (mainly ferrous sulfate) is absorbed each day from the small intestine. After absorption, the iron is converted and is stored in iron storage protein. Then the iron is transported to the liver, spleen, and bone marrow for incorporation into hemoglobin. When ingested iron exceeds the ability of the body to store it, the free iron circulates in the blood. The iron then is deposited into other tissues. Most iron poisonings result from the ingestion of pediatric multivitamins by children younger than 6 years of age.[3]

Unintentional or intentional ingestion of iron may be fatal. Ingested iron is corrosive to the lining of the gastrointestinal tract. Iron may produce gastrointestinal hemorrhage, bloody vomitus, painless bloody diarrhea, and dark stools. Severe cases involve the ingestion of more than 20 mg/kg. Ingestion of more than 60 mg/kg can produce cardiovascular collapse and death.[7] Prehospital care includes supportive measures and rapid transport for physician evaluation and possible gastric decontamination to

> ### BOX 34-6 Places Where Lead Can Be Found
>
> Homes in the city, country, or suburbs
> Apartments, single-family homes, and private and public housing painted before 1978
> Soil around a home (soil contaminated from exterior paint, or other sources such as past use of leaded gasoline in cars)
> Painted windows and window sills
> Doors and door frames
> Stairs, railings, and banisters
> Porches and fences
> Paint surfaces that have been scraped, dry-sanded, or heated (lead dust)
> Old painted toys and furniture
> The air after vacuuming or sweeping contaminated surfaces
> Food and liquid stored in lead crystal or lead-glazed pottery or porcelain
> Lead smelters or other industries
> Hobbies that use lead (e.g., making pottery or stained glass)
> Folk remedies (greta or azarcon used to treat an upset stomach)

prevent further absorption. The use of ***activated charcoal*** generally is not recommended because it adsorbs iron poorly. Most patients with iron poisoning survive the episode. The long-term prognosis is favorable.

Lead Poisoning. Metallic lead has been used by human beings for thousands of years. In 1978 lead-based paint was recognized as a major health hazard and was banned from household paints in the United States (Box 34-6). Children are the most common victims of lead poisoning; an estimated 250,000 children in the United States have levels of lead in their bloodstream of 10 mg/dL or greater.[11] Most pediatric poisonings result from ingestion of lead-based paint chips and contaminated house dust. Lead toxicity in adults most commonly results from exposure by inhalation. If not detected early, children with high levels of lead in their bodies can suffer from damage to the brain and nervous system. This can result in behavioral and learning problems, hyperactivity, slowed growth, hearing problems, and headaches. Even children who appear healthy can have dangerous levels of lead in their bodies. Adults with high levels of lead in their systems can experience difficult pregnancies, reproductive problems, hypertension, nerve disorders, muscle and joint pain, and problems with memory and concentration.

Most lead poisoning is slow in onset and results from chronic ingestion or inhalation. This eventually results in toxicity. The metal is excreted by the body slowly and tends to accumulate in body tissues (mainly bone). Lead exposure that results in acute intoxication may lead to paralysis, seizures, coma, and death. Patients who survive are likely to sustain brain damage. Prehospital care is focused on recognizing the potential for lead poisoning and transporting the patient for physician evaluation. If lead poisoning is confirmed through x-ray and laboratory testing, care may include gastric decontamination or whole-bowel irrigation. Following treatment, all patients must be discharged to a lead-free environment. Outpatient *chelation therapy* may be indicated to detoxify the lead and excrete the metal from the body.

CRITICAL THINKING

Paramedics play a key role in the emergency management of lead poisoning. What other role can they play in the management of this problem?

Mercury Poisoning. Mercury is the only metal that is liquid at room temperature. It has been used in thermometers, sphygmomanometers, and dental fillings. Various compounds of mercury also are used in some paints, pesticides, cosmetics, drugs, and in certain industrial processes. All forms of mercury (except those in dental fillings) are poisonous.

Inhalation of mercury vapor is the most common route of mercury poisoning. It may cause shortness of breath and lung damage. Mercury also may be absorbed through the skin, causing severe inflammation, and through the intestines after ingestion. After mercury enters the body, it passes into the bloodstream. It later accumulates in various organs, mainly the brain and kidneys. This causes a wide range of symptoms that may include the following:

- Malaise
- Incoordination
- Excitability
- Tremors
- Numbness in the limbs
- Vision impairment
- Nausea and emesis (symptoms of renal failure)
- Mental status changes

Prehospital care mainly is supportive. Following physician evaluation, patients are managed with gastrointestinal decontamination if the ingestion was recent, and with chelating agents. In severe cases, hemodialysis may be indicated.

FOOD POISONING

Food poisoning is a term used for any illness of sudden onset suspected of being caused by food eaten within the previous 48 hours. It is usually associated with stomach pain, vomiting, and diarrhea. Food poisoning can be classified as infectious (bacterial and viral) or noninfectious.

Infectious (Bacterial) Types. One of the common types of bacteria responsible for food poisoning is *Salmonella*. This organism is found in many animals (especially poultry) and in human beings. *Salmonella* bacteria also may be transferred to food from the excrement of infected animals or humans, and by an infected person handling food. Other bacteria (e.g., strains of staphylococcal bacteria) cause formation of toxins. These toxins may be difficult to destroy

even with thorough cooking of the food. Other bacteria that commonly cause diarrhea are certain strains of *Escherichia coli* (traveler's diarrhea) and *Campylobacter* and *Shigella* organisms.

Botulism is a rare but life-threatening form of food poisoning. It may result from eating improperly canned or preserved food that is contaminated with the bacterium *Clostridium botulinum*. This organism is found in soil and untreated water in most parts of the world. It also is harmlessly present in the intestinal tracts of many animals, including fish. Its spore-forming properties resist boiling, salting, smoking, and some forms of pickling. This allows the bacterium to thrive in improperly preserved or canned foods. Although foodborne botulism is rare, the disease is more common in the United States because of the popularity of preserving food in the home. Botulism is associated with severe CNS symptoms. These symptoms appear in a characteristic head-to-toe progression: headache, blurred or double vision, dysphagia, respiratory paralysis, and quadriplegia. Respiratory failure occurs in 50% of patients.[8] Death, however, is rare with treatment.

NOTE

Infant botulism is the most common form of illness in the United States, accounting for 72% of all cases.[8] It occurs in children younger than 1 year of age, with a peak incidence between 2 and 6 months of age. The illness often is caused by consuming infected spores from honey and, to a lesser degree, corn syrup.

Infectious (Viral) Types. The viruses that most often cause food poisoning are the Norwalk virus (a common contaminant of shellfish) and rotavirus. Both agents may be responsible for illness when raw or partly cooked foodstuffs have been in contact with water contaminated by human excrement.

Noninfectious Types. Noninfectious types of food poisoning may result from consuming mushrooms and toadstools. Food poisoning also can result from eating fresh foods and vegetables that are accidentally contaminated with large amounts of insecticide. Chemical food poisoning may result from eating food stored in a contaminated container (e.g., a container that previously was used to store poison). It also can result from improperly preparing and cooking various exotic foods.

Management Guidelines. The onset of signs and symptoms from food poisoning varies by cause and by how heavily the food was contaminated. As a rule, symptoms usually develop within 30 minutes in the case of chemical poisoning; in 1 to 12 hours in the case of bacterial toxins; and in 12 to 48 hours with viral and bacterial infections.[8] General principles of the management for patients with suspected food poisoning include the following:

- Use precautions to avoid contamination of self and equipment. Wear gloves, a gown, or both if appropriate.
- Ensure adequate airway, ventilatory, and circulatory support.
- Gather a complete history. This should include time and onset of symptoms, recent travel, the relation of symptoms to ingestion of a particular food, and effects on others who ate the same food. In addition, the paramedic should obtain information on the consistency, frequency, and odor of stool (including the presence of mucus or blood). Fever should be noted as well. Any patient history also should include significant medical history, allergies, and use of medications.
- Initiate intravenous therapy with a crystalloid solution. This will help to manage dehydration and electrolyte disturbances resulting from vomiting and diarrhea.
- Transport the patient for physician evaluation.

PLANT POISONING

Toxic plant ingestion is a frequently reported category of poisonings, second only to ingestion of cleaning substances.[2] The majority of these exposures occur in children less than 6 years of age.

CRITICAL THINKING
What features of a plant would make it attractive for children to eat?

Signs and Symptoms. The signs of toxicity following the ingestion of major poisonous plants are predictable. They are categorized by the chemical and physical properties of the plant. Most signs and symptoms tend to be consistent with the type of major toxic chemical component in the plant. They usually appear within several hours after ingestion, but may be delayed 1 to 3 days. Box 34-7 lists common poisonous plants. Paramedics should be familiar with common poisonous plant life in their response area.

Management. Several hundred species of green plants and more than 100 varieties of mushrooms in the United States contain toxic compounds. These plants and mushrooms have widely varying potencies and combinations of toxins. In addition, such factors as the age of the plant and soil conditions may influence the severity of toxic symptoms. Thus management guidelines should be customized to the patient's symptoms rather than to one type of ingestion. Identification of the plant is important if possible. However, the inability to do so should not delay patient care. The paramedic should consult with medical direction or a poison control center regarding appropriate management. Emergency care for toxic plant ingestion generally includes gastrointestinal decontamination and/or the administration of *activated charcoal* in conscious patients, IV fluids, and ensuring adequate airway, ventilatory, and

---

BOX 34-7 Common Poisonous Plants, Trees, and Shrubs

House Plants
Dieffenbachia
Hyacinth
Mistletoe
Narcissus
Oleander
Poinsettia

Flower-Garden Plants
Daffodil
Foxglove
Iris
Larkspur
Lily of the valley

Ornamental Plants
Azaleas
Daphne

Jasmine
Rhododendron
Wisteria

Other Plants
Buttercups
Jack-in-the-pulpit
Mayapple
Nightshade
Water and poison hemlock

Trees and Shrubs
Elderberry
Oaks
Wild and cultivated cherries

---

circulatory support. Most patients are hospitalized for observation and treatment as indicated for the toxin involved. Dialysis has not been shown to be effective in removing most plant toxins.[12]

POISONING BY INHALATION

The unintentional or intentional inhalation of poisons can lead to a life-threatening emergency. The type and location of injury caused by toxic inhalation depend on the specific actions and behaviors of the chemical involved.[13] Respiratory difficulty may not appear for several hours after exposure to toxic fumes and smoke. All patients should be encouraged to seek physician evaluation. This includes even those who are asymptomatic.

CRITICAL THINKING
Do you think that situations involving toxic gas inhalation are likely to involve one patient or multiple patients? Why?

Classifications

Toxic gases can be classified in three categories: simple asphyxiants, chemical asphyxiants, and irritants/corrosives. **Simple asphyxiants** (e.g., methane, propane, inert gases) cause toxicity by displacing or lowering the amount of oxygen in the air. **Chemical asphyxiants** (e.g., carbon monoxide, cyanide) can cause a number of local and pulmonary reactions when inhaled. Their toxic systemic effects prevent the uptake of oxygen by the blood and can interfere with tissue oxygenation. **Irritants/corrosives** (e.g., chlorine, ammonia) cause cellular destruction and inflammation as they come into contact with moisture. Table 34-2 provides an overview of toxic gases and their clinical features.

TABLE 34-2 Clinical Features of Toxic Gases and Fumes

Class of Toxin	Toxin	Source	Clinical Features	Management
Simple asphyxiants	Propane Methane Carbon dioxide Inert gases (nitrogen, argon)	Cooking gas Cooking gas All fires Industry (especially welding)	Displacement of normal air and lower fractional inspired oxygen concentration, symptoms of hypoxemia without airway irritation	Remove patient from source; give oxygen.
Chemical asphyxiants	Carbon monoxide	Fires	Formation of carboxyhemoglobin; inhibition of oxygen transport (headache is earliest symptom)	Give 100% oxygen.
	Hydrocyanic acid	Industry, burning plastics, furniture, fabrics	Highly toxic cellular asphyxiant	Use cyanide antidote.
	Hydrogen sulfide	Liquid manure pits, decaying organic materials	Highly toxic cellular asphyxiant similar to cyanide; sudden collapse; ability to smell characteristic odor of rotten eggs; rapid fatigue	Use sodium nitrite for cyanide (makes sulfmethemoglobin). Do not use thiosulfate.
Irritants: high solubility in water	Chlorine gas Hydrochloric acid	Industry, swimming pool chemicals, bleach mixed with acid at home	Early onset of lacrimation, sore throat, stridor, tracheobronchitis; with heavy exposure, pulmonary edema in 2-6 hr	Use humidified oxygen, bronchodilators, and airway management.
Irritants: low solubility in water	Ammonia Nitrogen dioxide Ozone Phosgene	Industry, burning fabrics Burning cellulose, fabrics Grain silos (acrid red gas) Inert gas arc welding, industry Burning of chlorinated organic material	Sweet "electric" smell; delayed onset (12-24 hr) of tracheobronchitis, pneumonitis, and pulmonary edema; late chronic bronchitis	Give oxygen: observe for 24-48 hr; give steroids (controversial).
Allergenic	Toluene diisocyanate	Manufacture of polyurethanes	Reactive bronchoconstriction; possible long-term effects (chronic obstructive pulmonary disease) in susceptible persons	Use bronchodilators.
Metal fumes	Zinc Copper Tin Teflon	Welding (especially galvanized metal welding)	"Metal fumes fever"; chills, fever, myalgias, headache, nonproductive cough, leukocytosis 4-8 hr after exposure	Is self-limited (12-24 hr).
	Arsine	Burning arsenic-containing ores, electronics industry	Highly toxic effect; hemolysis, pulmonary edema, renal failure; chronic arsenic toxicity	Perform exchange transfusion; use dimercaprol (BAL) for chronic arsenic toxicity only.
	Mercury Lead	Industry, welding	See specific metals	

From Ho MT: *Current emergency diagnosis and treatment*, ed 3, Norwalk, Conn, 1990, Appleton & Lange.

General Management

The general principles of managing patients who have inhaled poisons are the same as those for any other hazardous materials incident (see Chapters 57 and 58). These principles include the following:

1. Scene safety
2. Personal protective measures (protective clothing and appropriate respiratory protective apparatus)
3. Rapid removal of the patient from the poison environment

4. Surface decontamination
5. Adequate airway, ventilatory, and circulatory support
6. Initial assessment and physical examination
7. Irrigation of the eyes (as needed)
8. Intravenous line with a saline solution
9. Regular monitoring of vital signs, ECG, and pulse oximetry
10. Rapid transport to an appropriate medical facility

Management of Specific Inhaled Poisons

The specific inhaled poisons discussed in this section include cyanide, ammonia, and hydrocarbons. Carbon monoxide poisoning is described in Chapter 39. Other gases associated with atmospheres with low oxygen levels and chemical and biological warfare are discussed in Chapters 57 and 58.

CYANIDE

Cyanide refers to any of a number of highly toxic substances that contain the cyanogen chemical group. Because of its toxicity, cyanide has few applications. The agent sometimes is used in industry in electroplating ore extraction, fumigation of buildings, and as a fertilizer. Cyanide has been used in gas chambers as a means of execution. It is one of the byproducts of combustion from burning many substances, including nylon and polyurethane. Thus cyanide is a hazard in fire environments.

Cyanide poisoning may result from the inhalation of cyanide gas; the ingestion of cyanide salts, nitriles, or cyanogenic glycosides (e.g., amygdalin, a substance found in the seeds of cherries, apples, pears, and apricots, and the principal constituent of Laetrile); or the infusion of nitroprusside. Cyanide also can be absorbed across the skin. Regardless of the route of entry, cyanide is a rapidly acting poison. It combines and reacts with ferric ions (Fe^{3+}) of the respiratory enzyme cytochrome oxidase to inhibit cellular oxygenation. The cytotoxic hypoxia produces a rapid progression of symptoms from dyspnea to paralysis, unconsciousness, and death (Box 34-8). Large doses usually are fatal within minutes from respiratory arrest.

After ensuring personal safety, emergency care for a patient with cyanide poisoning begins with securing an open airway and providing adequate ventilatory support with high-concentration oxygen. Oxygen displaces cyanide from cytochrome oxidase and increases the effectiveness of drug administration. After these measures, one type of treatment of cyanide poisoning converts (oxidizes) ferrous ions in hemoglobin (Fe^{2+}) to ferric ions (Fe^{3+}). This forms **methemoglobin:** hemoglobin with ferrous ion in the oxidized (Fe^{3+}) state. Cyanide, which has a greater attraction to iron in the ferric state, is released from the cytochrome oxidase and combines with methemoglobin. This allows cytochrome oxidase to resume its function in normal cellular respiration. Cyanide antidotes (Box 34-9), such as those found in the Pasadena cyanide antidote kit (also known as the *Lilly Cyanide Poison Kit* and *Taylor Kit*), are thought to be effective because they induce methemoglobin production.

? DID YOU KNOW?

Methemoglobin (MetHb) is a dysfunctional form of hemoglobin that cannot transport oxygen. An increased level of methemoglobin in the blood is known as **methemoglobinemia**. This condition reduces blood oxygenation and produces a "functional anemia." Methemoglobinemia causes a leftward shift of the oxyhemoglobin dissociation curve. This impedes the unloading of oxygen from normal hemoglobin, reduces the amount of oxygen available to tissues, and leads to tissue hypoxia.

Methemoglobinemia may be congenital. It also may be acquired from exposure to industrial toxins (e.g., nitrites in grain silos) and the ingestion and overuse of some medications such as nitrates, nitrites, and sulfonamides. Signs and symptoms of methemoglobinemia include shortness of breath, cyanosis, mental status changes, headache, fatigue, dizziness, and loss of consciousness. The Rad 57 is an oximetry device that can be used in the prehospital setting to measure SaO_2, carboxyhemoglobinemia, and, in some cases, methemoglobin levels. In the emergency setting, methemoglobinemia is treated with oxygen and in-hospital administration of methylene blue. Methylene blue restores the iron in hemoglobin to its normal (reduced) oxygen-carrying state.

Because methemoglobin cannot transport oxygen, it must be reconverted to hemoglobin. This is accomplished in a three-part process. The goal of the first two steps is the formation of methemoglobin through the administration of **amyl nitrate** by inhalation, and IV sodium nitrite. These drugs convert ferrous hemoglobin into methemoglobin. The goal of the third part of the process is to detoxify the cyanide so that it can be eliminated. This is accomplished by giving IV **hydroxocobalamin**, with or without sodium thiosulfate (See the Emergency Drug Index). These drugs help detoxify cyanide so that it can be eliminated by the kidneys.[8] Prehospital care for patients with cyanide poisoning includes the following:

BOX 34-8 Early and Advanced Signs and Symptoms of Cyanide Poisoning

Early Effects	Advanced Effects
Agitation	Acidosis
Anxiety	Dysrhythmias
Confusion	Hypotension
Dyspnea	Intractable hypotension
Hypertension with reflex bradycardia	Lactic acidosis
	Pulmonary edema
	Seizures
	Coma

BOX 34-9 Three-Step Cyanide Antidote

Two Amyl Nitrite Inhalants in Gauze

Administer by inhalation for 15 to 30 seconds; may be repeated as necessary.

3% Sodium Nitrite (Stop Amyl Nitrite)

Adults: 10-mL slow intravenous administration over 2 to 4 minutes

Children: 0.2 mL/kg (up to 10 mL) slow intravenous administration over 5 minutes

Note: If hypotension develops, stop nitrite, treat for shock, and consider administration of *dopamine* (per medical direction).

Hydroxocobalamin

- Adults: 5 g IV
- Children: 70 mg/kg IV (do not exceed adult dose)
- Dilute in 100 mL normal saline; infuse over 15 minutes; may follow with sodium thiosulfate (separate IV)

25% Sodium Thiosulfate

Adults: 12.5 g (50 mL of 25% solution) IV over 10 minutes

Children: 400 mg/kg (1.65 mL/kg of 25% solution) IV over 10 minutes (do not exceed adult dose)

NOTE

The cyanide antidote described in Box 34-9 should not be given to patients with cyanide poisoning that resulted from smoke inhalation. Carbon monoxide limits the amount of oxygen that hemoglobin can carry. This, coupled with formation of methemoglobin from the antidote, leaves little hemoglobin that can carry oxygen to sustain life. The patient may die from anoxia.

Hydroxocobalamin (Cyanokit) is a vitamin B_{12} precursor that can be used to treat cyanide poisoning. It has a central cobalt atom that binds to cyanide in the blood and forms cyanocobalamin (vitamin B_{12}). Detoxification with hydroxocobalamin does not create methemoglobin, so it does not lower the oxygen-carrying capacity of the blood. Rare cases of allergic reaction have been reported. It does not cause hypotension.[14] This makes it possible to use hydroxocobalamin to treat all types of cyanide poisoning, including smoke inhalation (see the *Emergency Drug Index*).

---

1. Don personal protective equipment as needed. This will help to prevent rescuer contamination.
2. Remove the patient from the cyanide source. Rapid decontamination and removal of the patient's contaminated clothing is essential.
3. Ensure a patent airway and provide adequate ventilatory support.
4. Administer high-concentration oxygen and monitor pulse oximetry.
5. Administer the cyanide antidote. Consult with medical direction or a poison control center and follow the instructions provided by the manufacturer.
6. Initiate intravenous fluid therapy with a volume-expanding solution.
7. Monitor cardiac rhythm by electrocardiogram.
8. Rapidly transport the patient for physician evaluation.

Hypotension should be anticipated as a side effect of antidote therapy. The patient should remain lying down, if possible, and blood pressure must be monitored closely. If hypotension develops, medical direction may recommend the administration of vasopressors.

AMMONIA INHALATION

Ammonia is a toxic irritant that causes local pulmonary complications after inhalation. These complications include inflammation and irritation and, in severe cases, destruction of the mucosal tissue of all respiratory structures. Injury occurs as the ammonia vapor combines with water, producing a highly caustic alkaline compound. Patients usually develop coughing, choking, congestion, burning, and tightness in the chest and a feeling of suffocation. These respiratory symptoms often are associated with burning eyes and tearing. In severe cases, bronchospasm and pulmonary edema may develop. In addition to the general management principles, emergency care may include positive-pressure ventilation and the administration of diuretics and bronchodilators.

HYDROCARBON INHALATION

The hydrocarbons that pose the greatest risk for injury have low viscosity, high volatility, and high surface tension or adhesion of molecules along a surface. These characteristics allow hydrocarbons to enter the pulmonary tree. This causes aspiration pneumonitis and creates the potential for systemic effects as well. Examples of such effects include CNS depression and liver, kidney, or bone marrow toxicity.

Most hydrocarbon inhalations result from "recreational use" of halogenated hydrocarbons (e.g., carbon tetrachloride and methylene chloride) or aromatic hydrocarbons (e.g., benzene and toluene). These agents may produce a state of inebriation or euphoria through "sniffing" or "huffing." (This involves placing the solvent on a rag and inhaling the vapors through a plastic bag.) The onset of these effects usually is rapid, typically occurring within seconds. It may be followed by CNS depression, respiratory failure, or cardiac dysrhythmias. Other signs and symptoms of hydrocarbon inhalation include the following:

- Burning sensation on swallowing
- Nausea and vomiting
- Abdominal cramps
- Weakness
- Anesthesia
- Hallucinations
- Changes in color perception
- Blindness
- Seizures
- Coma

Emergency care for hydrocarbon inhalation generally is supportive and includes airway, ventilatory, and circulatory support; intravenous fluid therapy; vital sign and electrocardiogram monitoring; and transport for physician evaluation.

POISONING BY INJECTION

In addition to poisoning from the injection of drug misuse or abuse (described earlier), poisoning by injection also may result from bites and stings from arthropods, reptiles, and hazardous aquatic life. In contrast to most chemical compounds described previously, poisons from envenomation are mixtures of many different substances. These mixtures may produce several different toxic reactions in human beings. Thus the paramedic must be prepared to manage reactions in many organ systems at the same time. General management guidelines for most poisonings from bites and stings include the following:

1. Ensure personal safety.
2. Provide adequate airway, ventilatory, and circulatory support as needed. Watch for signs of a serious allergic reaction.
3. Clean the affected area with saline. Cover it with a sterile dressing. Intermittently apply ice to it. Obstruction tourniquets or suction devices do not help to delay absorption and should not be used. Commercially prepared antivenin (if available) sometimes is given in the emergency department after appropriate sensitivity testing.
4. Moderate to severe symptoms may require aggressive management. According to medical direction, muscle spasm, severe headache, vomiting, and paresthesia may be managed with benzodiazepines, antiemetics, and pain medication.
5. Transport the patient for physician evaluation. Most patients recover fully. Those at greatest risk for morbidity are the very young, older adults, and those with underlying hypertension or other medical problems.

Arthropod Bites and Stings

Arthropods are invertebrates with segmented bodies and jointed limbs. Some arthropods bite, some sting, and a few bite and sting. Arthropod venoms are complex and diverse in their chemistry and pharmacology. They may produce major toxic reactions in sensitized persons. Such reactions include anaphylaxis and upper airway obstruction. The various reactions to venoms are classified as local, toxic, systemic, and delayed[15-17] (Boxes 34-10 and 34-11).

HYMENOPTERA (WASPS, BEES, ANTS)

Hymenoptera is the name of a large, highly specialized order of insects that includes wasps, bees, and ants. Their venom contains mixtures of toxins, enzymes, and other compounds such as histamines, serotonin, acetylcholine, and dopamine. A single wasp, bee, or ant sting in an unsensitized person usually causes instant pain. This is followed by a wheal-and-flare reaction with variable edema. Anaphylaxis is the most serious complication of Hymenoptera stings. An estimated 0.4% of the U.S. population has some degree of chemical allergy to insect venoms; 40 to 100 deaths caused by anaphylaxis from Hymenoptera stings are reported annually.[7] Persons with a history of allergic reactions to stings often wear medical alert identification. These persons also often carry an emergency kit that contains a preloaded syringe of *epinephrine* (EpiPen). The ant species of greatest concern in the United States is the imported fire ant. Stings or bites from fire ants may produce systemic reactions, including anaphylaxis.

Honey bees (and other Hymenoptera) often leave their stingers in the wound. If a stinger is present, it should be scraped or brushed off the skin. Stingers should not be removed with forceps. This is because squeezing the attached venom sac may worsen the injury. Severe allergic reactions should be managed as described in Chapter 27. Hypovolemia (if present) should be treated in the conventional manner with a volume-expanding crystalloid infusion.

LOOK AGAIN
See Chapter 27: Immune System Disorders, pp. 835-836.

ARACHNIDA (SPIDERS, SCORPIONS, TICKS)

Arachnida is a large class of arthropods. These organisms usually have four pairs of legs and a body divided into a cephalothorax (a combined head and thorax) and abdomen. This discussion will be limited to spiders, scorpions, and ticks.

Spider Bites. Most spiders have venom glands. Two major types of reactions occur from spider venom. These are neurotoxic reactions resulting from the black widow bite and local tissue necrosis resulting from the bites of most other spiders.

Black Widow Spider. The female black widow spider is shiny and black with a red hourglass marking on the undersurface of the abdomen (Figure 34-1). The male is about half the size of the female, brown, and nonvenomous to human beings. The spider generally is found in undisturbed areas (under stones, logs, and clumps of vegetation). They rarely inhabit occupied dwellings. Most black widow bites occur in rural and suburban areas of southern and western states between April and October.

The bite of a black widow generally is described by patients as a slight pinprick that is initially painless. As a rule, the only physical findings are two small fang marks. These are about 1 mm apart and surrounded by a small papule. Multiple bites usually rule out any type of spider envenomation because spiders rarely bite more than once. Within 1 hour of envenomation, the neurotoxin produces characteristic muscle spasms and cramps. These may result in abdominal rigidity and intense pain. Associated symptoms include paresthesia (frequently described as a burning

BOX 34-10 Types of Reactions to Venoms

Local Reaction
- Marked and prolonged edema at the sting site
- Possible involvement of one or more neighboring joints
- Possible occurrence in the mouth or throat, producing airway obstruction
- Severe local reactions that may increase the likelihood of future systemic reactions
- Symptoms that usually subside within 24 hours

Toxic Reaction*
- Gastrointestinal disturbances
  - Diarrhea
  - Light-headedness
  - Vomiting
- Other symptoms
  - Convulsions (rare)
  - Edema without urticaria (hives)
  - Fever
  - Headache
  - Involuntary muscle spasms
  - Symptoms that usually subside within 48 hours
  - Syncope (common finding)

Systemic (Anaphylactic) Reaction†
- Reactions that can progress to death within minutes
- Immediate symptoms

- Facial flushing
- Generalized urticaria
- Itching eyes or generalized itching
- Subsequent symptoms
  - Bloody and frothy sputum production
  - Chest or throat constriction, or both
  - Chills and fever
  - Cyanosis
  - Dyspnea
  - Hypotension
  - Laryngeal stridor
  - Loss of bowel or bladder control
  - Loss of consciousness
  - Nausea and vomiting
  - Respiratory failure, cardiovascular collapse, or both
  - Shock
  - Wheezing

Delayed Reaction‡
- Serum sickness symptoms
  - Fever
  - Headache
  - Malaise
  - Polyarthritis
  - Urticaria

*Should be considered with a history of 10 or more stings.
†May occur in response to single or multiple stings.
‡Usually occurs 10 to 14 days after a sting.

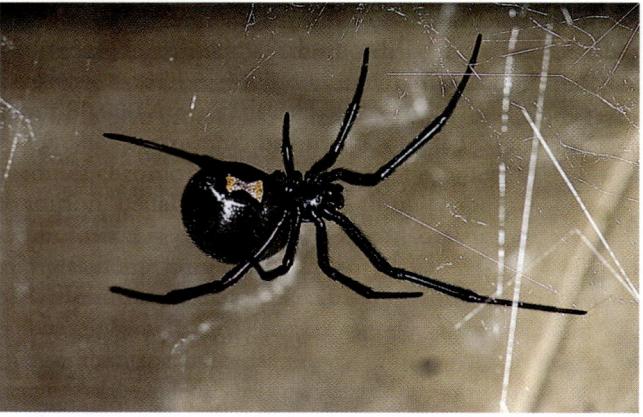

FIGURE 34-1 Black widow spider. (Courtesy Michael Cardwell and Associates, 1993. From Auerbach PS: *Wilderness medicine,* ed 5, Philadelphia, 2007, Mosby.)

NOTE
Abdominal rigidity in the absence of palpable tenderness is a crucial finding. This helps to distinguish envenomation from an acute abdominal condition.

sensation in the soles of the feet or entire body); pain in the muscles of the shoulders, back, and chest; headache; dizziness; nausea and vomiting; edema of the eyelids; and increased perspiration and salivation. Most patients recover fully within 36 to 72 hours.

Brown Recluse Spider. The brown recluse spider is also known as the fiddle-back spider. The spider is most prevalent in the Mississippi-Ohio-Missouri river basin and the southwestern United States. The species prefers hot, dry, and abandoned environments such as vacant buildings. The spider often is found in clothing closets. The spider is fawn to dark brown and is between 1 and 2 cm long (Figure 34-2). Identifying characteristics of the brown recluse are six white eyes arranged in a semicircle on the head (versus the usual eight eyes of most other spiders) and the presence of a dark, violin-shaped marking on the top of the cephalothorax. The brown recluse is considered shy. It generally does not attack unless threatened. Like black widows, these spiders are most active from April to October.

The venom of the brown recluse initially causes little pain and often is overlooked by the victim. Approximately 1 to 2 hours later, localized pain and erythema develop (Figure 34-3). This often is followed within 2 days by a blister or vesicle. The lesion may be surrounded by an ischemic ring that is outlined further by an irregular red halo, producing the classic bull's-eye appearance seen with this bite. Over the next 72 hours, the area often becomes larger and the center of the lesion may become purple or develop

BOX 34-11 West Nile Virus*

Mosquitoes are insects of the order Diptera (two-winged flies). Although they have long been associated with the spread of some diseases (e.g., malaria), some species recently have gained notoriety for spreading the West Nile virus. Mosquitoes become carriers of West Nile virus when they feed on infected birds. The mosquitoes then spread the virus to human beings and other animals when they bite.

West Nile virus was first isolated in Uganda in 1937. The virus was first reported in the United States (in Queens, New York) in 1999. In 2008 there were more than 1400 cases reported in the United States, none of which resulted in death.[16]

West Nile virus is a potentially serious illness. It affects the central nervous system. The virus was a major cause of illness in the United States. The symptoms (if present) usually develop within 3 to 14 days after being bitten by an infected mosquito. Most patients (about 80%) are asymptomatic after being bitten. About 20% of infected patients develop mild symptoms that include fever, headache, body aches, nausea and vomiting, and skin rash that lasts from a few days to several weeks. About 1 in 150 infected persons develops serious illness that can lead to seizures, coma, vision loss, numbness, paralysis, and other clinical manifestations such as West Nile fever, West Nile encephalitis, and West Nile meningitis. The neurological effects of the disease may be permanent.[17]

*No specific treatment exists for West Nile virus. Care is mainly supportive. Prevention of the disease is best achieved by avoiding mosquito bites, applying insect repellent containing *N,N*-diethyl-*meta*-toluamide (DEET) to exposed skin when outdoors during peak mosquito hours (evening and early morning), and participating in community mosquito control programs.

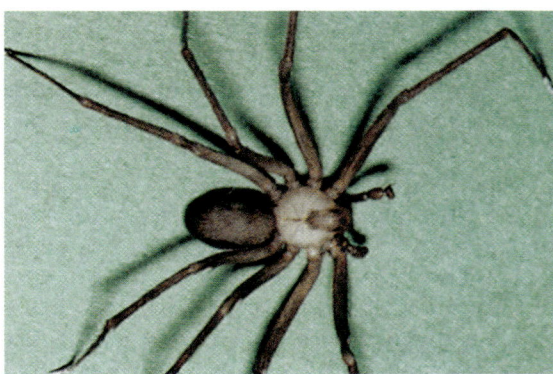

FIGURE 34-2 Brown recluse spider. (From Auerbach PS: *Wilderness medicine,* ed 5, Philadelphia, 2007, Mosby.)

a black eschar (dead tissue). The eschar eventually sloughs, leaving an ulcer of variable size and depth. The wound typically is slow to heal and may be visible for months to years after the bite. Occasionally, excision and skin grafting are necessary. Systemic involvement may occur with signs and symptoms that include fever, chills, malaise, nausea and vomiting, generalized rash, and the development of hemolytic anemia, hemoglobinuria, and hypotension. Death occasionally occurs, usually from disturbance of the coagulation system or hepatic injury.

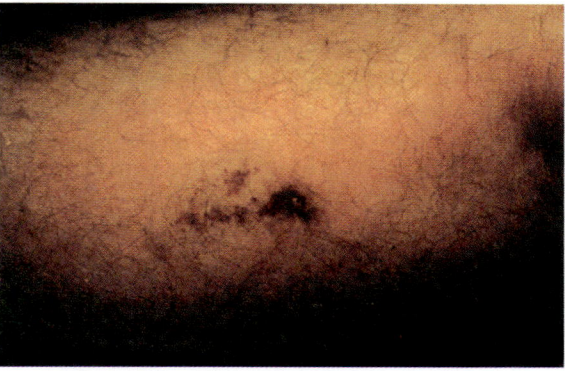

FIGURE 34-3 Brown recluse spider bite at about 6 hours with central hemorrhagic vesicle and gravitational pattern of venom spread. (From Auerbach PS: *Wilderness medicine,* ed 5, Philadelphia, 2007, Mosby.)

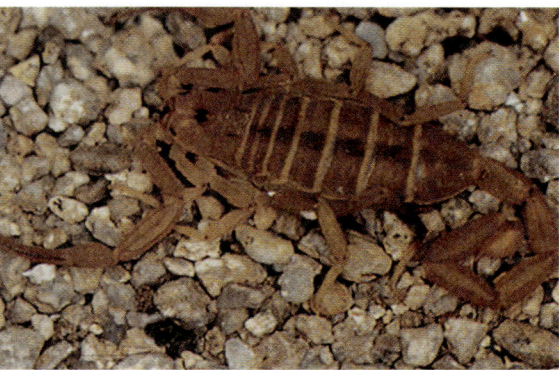

FIGURE 34-4 The sculptured scorpion commonly found in the deserts of Arizona, New Mexico, and California. (From Auerbach PS: *Wilderness medicine,* ed 5, Philadelphia, 2007, Mosby.)

CRITICAL THINKING
For which type of spider bite is a patient most likely to call an ambulance? Why?

Scorpion Stings. Only a few of the more than 650 species of scorpions produce human envenomation. In North America the sculptured or bark scorpion is the only species that is dangerous to human beings. This scorpion is found in the southwestern United States and Mexico. The scorpion is nocturnal and favors wooded areas along the edges of desert washes. Occasionally the scorpion invades homes, especially adobe houses. The sculptured scorpion is small and yellow to brown, and some have tail stripes (Figure 34-4). The species is most active from April to August, hibernating during the winter.

The venom of the scorpion is delivered by a stinger on the telson. The venom is a mixture of proteins that causes the release of acetylcholine. It also stimulates sympathetic nerves and directly stimulates the CNS, causing hyper-activity. This particular scorpion venom does not contain enzymes that cause tissue destruction. Thus local inflammation is not a feature. If swelling, ecchymosis, or redness is present, the scorpion was not of the neurotoxic type. Box 34-12 lists the signs and symptoms of sculptured scorpion stings. Despite the potential for life-threatening systemic effects, mild analgesics, cool compresses, and in-hospital observation are all that are required for these patients.

Tick Bites. Tick bites seldom require emergency care. However, they are capable of causing human disease. They can transmit microorganisms or secrete toxins or venoms. In North America, hard ticks are the most familiar type, although soft ticks also are common to Western states. Local reactions to tick bites vary from the formation of a small pruritic nodule to the development of extensive areas of ulceration. Some of the more important diseases for which ticks are vectors include Rocky Mountain spotted fever, Lyme disease, and tick paralysis.

Rocky Mountain Spotted Fever. **Rocky Mountain spotted fever** is an infectious disease transmitted from rabbits and other small mammals to human beings by the bites of the wood tick and dog tick. The disease occurs more commonly on the Atlantic seaboard and accounts for about 40 deaths in the United States each year.[8] Signs and symptoms usually develop within 1 week of the tick bite and include headache, high fever, and loss of appetite. This may be followed with small pink spots that appear on the wrists and ankles. Eventually the rash spreads over the entire body, and the spots darken and enlarge and become petechial. In mild cases, recovery occurs within 20 days. The mortality rate, if untreated, is between 8% and 25%.[15]

Lyme Disease. **Lyme disease** is the most commonly reported tick-borne disease in the United States. The disease is caused by the bite of an *Ixodes* tick known to infect deer and dogs. The course of the disease follows several stages. Initially a red dot appears at the site of the tick bite that gradually expands into a reddened rash. During this stage, fever, lethargy, muscle pain, and general malaise may develop. This may be followed by a second stage that is manifested by cardiac abnormalities (including various atrioventricular [AV] blocks) and neurological effects such as cranial nerve palsies. Still later, a third stage may develop, with arthritis as the primary symptom. Unless the disease is diagnosed and treated, symptoms may continue for several years, gradually declining in severity.

Tick Paralysis. **Tick paralysis** results from a prolonged bite by a female wood tick. The disease occurs sporadically during the spring and summer months. The paralysis is caused by a neurotoxin secreted from the salivary glands of the tick after the tick attaches to the host. At first the patient is restless and complains of paresthesia in the hands and feet. Over the next 48 hours, a flaccid paralysis may develop with loss of deep tendon reflexes. The paralysis begins at the feet and travels upward, affecting both sides of the body. In severe cases, death may result from respiratory paralysis. Removal of the tick usually results in rapid improvement and complete resolution within several days.

BOX 34-12 Signs and Symptoms of Scorpion Envenomation

- Hyperesthesia at the site of bite
- Pain, tingling, and a burning sensation radiating along the nerves at the location of the bite
- SLUDGE: *s*alvation, *l*acrimation, *u*rination, *d*efecation, *g*astrointestinal upset, and *e*mesis
- Initial bradycardia followed by tachycardia
- Cardiac dysrhythmias
- Muscle twitching
- Convulsions
- Roving eye movements (cranial nerve dysfunction)

If undiagnosed, the disease may be fatal, especially in young and older patients.

 CRITICAL THINKING
How can you distinguish tick paralysis from other conditions that cause progressive paralysis?

Management. The principal treatment of tick bites is proper removal of the tick. The paramedic should grasp the tick as close to the skin surface as possible with forceps, tweezers, or protected fingers and pull it out with steady pressure. Care should be taken not to crush or squeeze the body of the tick, which can transmit disease from infective tick fluid. Other methods of tick removal, such as applying fingernail polish, isopropanol, or a hot match head, should be avoided. These traditional methods are ineffective and may induce the tick to salivate or regurgitate into the wound. After removal, the bite should be disinfected with soap and water and should be covered with a sterile dressing.

Reptile Bites

The American Association of Poison Control Centers National Data Collection System listed a total 6343 bites from poisonous and nonpoisonous snakes in 2007.[3] Of these exposures, 3267 were known to be poisonous, and the rest were from unidentified snakes. According to these records, two deaths were reported. This reflects the high morbidity and low mortality associated with snake venom poisoning. Of the 115 species of snakes in the United States, only 19 are venomous. The two main families of venomous snakes indigenous to the United States are pit vipers and coral snakes.

PIT VIPERS

The pit viper family that inhabits the United States consists of rattlesnakes, the cottonmouth or water moccasin, the copperhead, the pigmy rattlesnake, and the Massasauga rattlesnake. The vast majority of snakebites in the United States are caused by the rattlesnake family. The identifying features of pit vipers are vertical elliptical pupils and a triangular head that is distinct from the rest of the body. The rattlesnake is characterized further by interlocking horny segments (rattles) formed on the tail that sometimes vibrate in direct relation to environmental temperatures (Figure 34-5).

The venom apparatus of pit vipers is connected to one or more elongated hollow fangs on each side of the head. The venom is designed to immobilize, kill, and digest prey. Depending on the species and the amount of venom injected, the venom may be capable of producing various toxic effects on blood and other tissues, including hemolysis, intravascular coagulation, convulsions, and acute renal failure (Box 34-13). Bleeding caused by coagulation defects and massive swelling can lead to hypovolemic shock. On

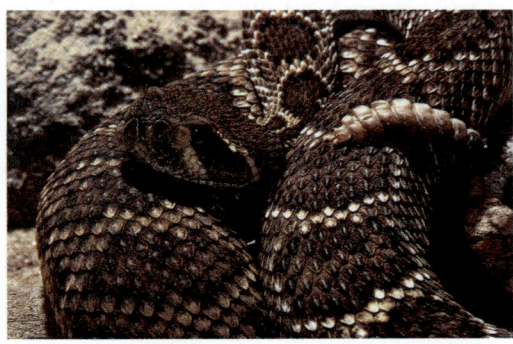

FIGURE 34-5 Pit viper. (Courtesy Saint Louis Zoo, St Louis, Mo.)

BOX 34-13 Signs and Symptoms of Pit Viper Envenomation

Mild Envenomation
Presence of one or more fang marks
Local swelling and pain
Lack of systemic symptoms

Moderate Envenomation
Presence of one or more fang marks
Pain and edema beyond the site
Systemic signs and symptoms
Weakness
Diaphoresis
Nausea and vomiting
Paresthesias

Severe Envenomation
Presence of one or more fang marks
Massive edema
Subcutaneous ecchymosis
Severe systemic symptoms
Shock

any given strike, the snake may release a quantity of venom varying from little or none to almost the entire contents of the glands.

CORAL SNAKES

Two members of the coral snake family are found in the United States: the Arizona coral snake and the Eastern coral snake. In contrast to the pit viper, the coral snake has round pupils and small, fixed fangs located near the anterior end of the maxilla. Most coral snakes have a three-color pattern with red, black, and yellow or white bands that completely encircle the body, along with a black snout (Figure 34-6). Many nonpoisonous snakes in the United States mimic the appearance of the coral snake. The coral snake is identified by the sequence of colors: red bands bordered by yellow indicate a venomous species. Thus there is a mnemonic: "red on yellow, kill a fellow; red on black, venom lack."

Most coral snakes are shy and docile and seldom bite unless threatened. The small mouth and fangs of the snake make it difficult to bite anything larger than a finger, toe, or fold of skin. The coral snake tends to hang on and chew rather than to strike and release like the pit viper. The venom of the coral snake mainly is neurotoxic. The bite generally produces little or no pain and no necrosis or edema. Early signs and symptoms of a coral snake bite are slurred speech, dilated pupils, and dysphagia (usually delayed several hours after the bite). If untreated, the venom produces flaccid paralysis and death within 24 hours. Death is caused by respiratory failure, following nervous system dysfunction.

MANAGEMENT OF SNAKE ENVENOMATION

Venom, like any drug or toxin, has absorption, distribution, and elimination phases. Tissue damage increases as venom spreads into the lymphatics and blood. Thus emergency care is directed at retarding the systemic spread of the venom. Prehospital management of snake bites includes the following:
1. Stay clear of the striking range of the snake (about the length of the snake), and move the patient to a safe area. If the snake has been killed before EMS arrival, it should

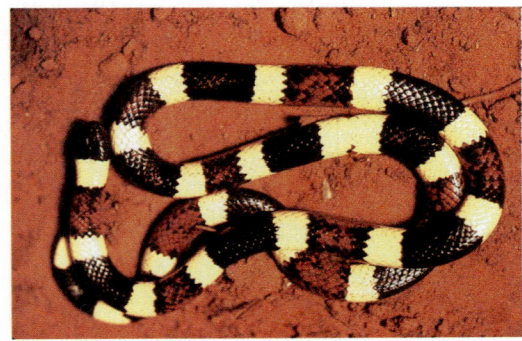

FIGURE 34-6 Coral snake. (Courtesy Saint Louis Zoo, St Louis, Mo.)

be transported in a closed container to the emergency department with the patient. EMS personnel should make no attempt to capture or kill the snake; doing so may result in a paramedic being bitten. Identification of the snake is not necessary to manage the patient appropriately.

2. Provide adequate airway, ventilatory, and circulatory support to the patient as needed. Continually monitor vital signs and the electrocardiogram. Also establish an intravenous line in an unaffected extremity with a volume-expanding fluid.

3. Medical direction may recommend that a bitten extremity be immobilized in a neutral position. Immobilization by splinting may delay systemic absorption and may diminish local tissue necrosis. Every effort should be made to keep the patient at rest. Applying a pressure immobilizaton bandage (as tightly as one would wrap an acute strain) along the entire length of the bitten extremity is an effective and safe way to slow dissemination of venom by slowing lymph flow Application of ice or chemical cold packs should be avoided. Their use may further damage tissue.[18]

4. Prepare the patient for immediate transport to a proper medical facility.

5. Methods to remove the venom (e.g., making an incision and performing suction) are potentially harmful and should not be used. In severe cases, administration of antivenin to neutralize the venom may be required. This is provided in the hospital after the patient has been tested for allergies to the antivenin.

CRITICAL THINKING

What strategies can you use to calm the emotional state of a patient who has sustained a snake bite?

Hazardous Aquatic Life

The marine animals most likely to be involved in human poisonings in U.S. coastal waters are the coelenterates, echinoderms, and stingrays. The specialized venom apparatuses of these animals are used for defense and for capturing prey. In addition to venom produced by the animal, aquatic life may contain other poisonous substances as a result of toxic ingestions. Exposures to hazardous aquatic life result from recreational, industrial, scientific, and military oceanic activities.

After stabilizing the patient with adequate airway, ventilatory, and circulatory support, the two primary goals of managing all envenomations from hazardous aquatic life are preventing further venom discharge and relieving pain by neutralizing the effects of the venom.[15,18]

COELENTERATES (JELLYFISH, SEA ANEMONES, FIRE CORAL)

Coelenterates are a group of species that may be encountered in the ocean (Figure 34-7). Some of these species carry venomous stinging cells (nematocysts). The nematocyst is

venom-filled and contains a long, coiled, hollow, threadlike tube that serves as a tiny hypodermic needle. The severity of envenomation is related to the type and toxicity of the venom, the number of nematocysts discharged, and the physical condition of the victim.

Jellyfish occur throughout the Atlantic and Pacific oceans. The Portuguese man-of-war is the largest jellyfish. The nematocyst-bearing tentacles of this jellyfish may be up to 100 feet long, and a single envenomation may involve several hundred thousand nematocysts. A swimmer who comes in contact with these tentacles may suffer enough envenomation to produce systemic signs and symptoms. Nematocysts often remain embedded in the tissues of the

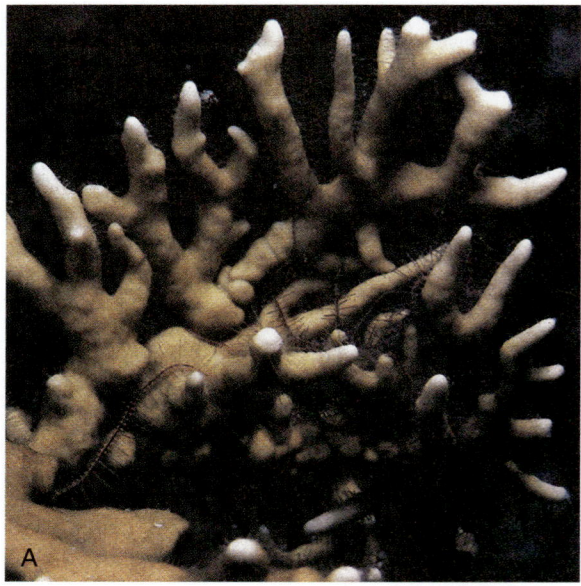

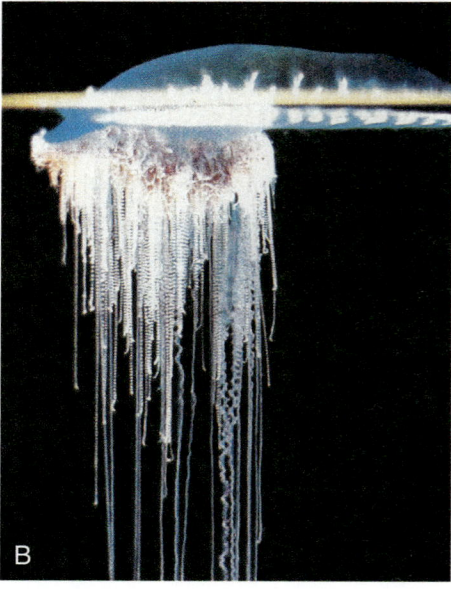

FIGURE 34-7 Coelenterates. **A,** Fire coral. **B,** Man-of-war. (From Uerbach JS: *A medical guide to hazardous marine life,* ed 2, St Louis, 1991, Mosby.)

victim. Detached tentacle fragments can retain their potency for months.

Sea anemones are colorful bottom dwellers; they are sometimes found in tidal pools. They have a flowerlike appearance and possess slender projections that are used to sting and paralyze passing fish. These nematocyst-type projections are capable of producing mild to moderate pain in human beings.

Fire corals are not true, stony corals, but rather ocean-bottom dwellers. They often are mistaken for seaweed because they commonly are attached to rocks, shells, and corals. These stinging corals may grow up to 2 meters high and have a razor-sharp exoskeleton with thousands of protruding nematocyst-bearing tentacles.

Management. Coelenterate envenomation ranges in severity from irritant dermatitis to excruciating pain, respiratory depression, anaphylaxis, and life-threatening cardiovascular collapse. Envenomation most often is mild and usually is characterized by a stinging sensation, paresthesias, pruritus, and reddish-brown linear wheals or "tentacle prints." If a potent venom or a large body surface area is involved, systemic symptoms may include nausea, vomiting, abdominal pain, headache, bronchospasm, pulmonary edema, hypotension, and respiratory arrest. Emergency care includes the following:

- Remove visible tentacle fragments with forceps. Avoid touching the tentacles.
  - Immediately wash the stings with liberal amounts of vinegar (4% to 6% acetic acid solution) or a baking soda slurry for at least 30 seconds. (Wet sand or freshwater usually causes the nematocysts to discharge their venom. Thus these are contraindicated.)
  - Instruct the patient to take a hot shower or immerse the affected body part in hot water when possible. The water should be as hot as can be tolerated without scalding, but no warmer than 45°C (113°F). The immersion should last for as long as pain persists. If hot water is not available, dry hot or cold packs may be helpful in decreasing pain.
  - Administer analgesics as needed.
- Transport the patient for physician evaluation.

ECHINODERMS (SEA URCHINS, STARFISH, SEA CUCUMBERS)

Echinoderms are marine animals with a water-vascular system. They usually have a hard, spiny skeleton and radial body (Figure 34-8).

Sea urchins have a globular, dome-shaped body and are found on rocky bottoms or burrowed in sand or crevices. These animals have tiny spines, some of which are venomous. Some also have small pincer-like organs that are thought to discharge a poisonous substance. The spines are dangerous to handle and may break off easily in the flesh, lodging deeply and making removal difficult.

Some starfish are covered with thorny spines that secrete toxins. As the spine enters the skin, it carries venom into the wound with immediate pain, copious bleeding, and mild edema. Multiple puncture wounds may result in acute systemic reactions.

Sea cucumbers are sausage-shaped animals found in shallow and deep water. They produce a liquid toxin in a tentacle-shaped organ. This organ can be projected and extended anally. Generally the liquid is secreted into the surrounding ocean. It usually produces only a minor dermatitis or conjunctivitis in swimmers and divers.

Management. Emergency management for echinoderm envenomation usually involves caring for puncture wounds caused by spines and inactivating the venom. The paramedic should remove embedded spines with forceps. Protective gloves should be worn to avoid self-contamination. Larger spines may require surgical removal by a physician.

Echinoderm toxins may cause immediate intense pain, swelling, redness, aching in the affected extremity, and nausea. Delayed toxic effects may include respiratory distress, paresthesia of the lips and face, and, in severe cases, respiratory paralysis and complete atonia. The paramedic must be prepared to deal with a variety of physical reactions.

Most marine venoms lose their toxicity when exposed to changes in temperature or humidity. The recommended management for stable patients is to immerse the affected area (usually the foot or hand) in hot water before and during transport.. As a safety precaution, it generally is recommended that both hands or feet not be immersed at the same time. This protects against thermal injury that may be unnoticed by the patient because of numbness or pain in the affected part.

STINGRAYS

Stingrays are responsible for about 1800 injuries each year in the United States.[15] These marine animals vary in size from 2 inches to 14 feet. They often are found half-buried in mud or sand in shallow water (Figure 34-9). The venom organ of stingrays consists of two to four venomous barbs on the dorsum of a whiplike tail. Envenomation generally occurs from stepping on the sand-buried ray. This causes the tail to thrust up and forward, driving the barb into the victim's leg or foot. The defensive barb produces a large, severe laceration that may be more than 15 to 20 cm long. In addition to injecting venom into the wound, the entire barb tip of the venom apparatus sometimes is detached and embedded in the tissue.

Stingray venom has local and systemic complications. Locally, the venom produces a traumatic injury that causes immediate, intense pain; edema; variable bleeding; and necrosis. Systemic manifestations include weakness, nausea, vomiting, diarrhea, vertigo, seizures, cardiac conduction abnormalities, paralysis, hypotension, and death. Prehospital care is directed to life support, alleviation of pain, inactivation of venom, and prevention of infection. The wound should be irrigated with normal saline or tap water.[15] If the venom apparatus is visible, it should be carefully removed. The affected part should be immersed in hot (but not scalding) water and remain there until pains subside or until the

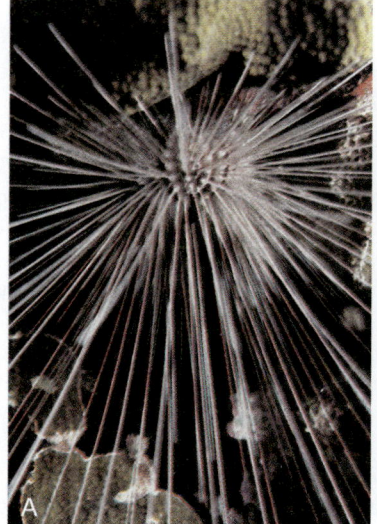
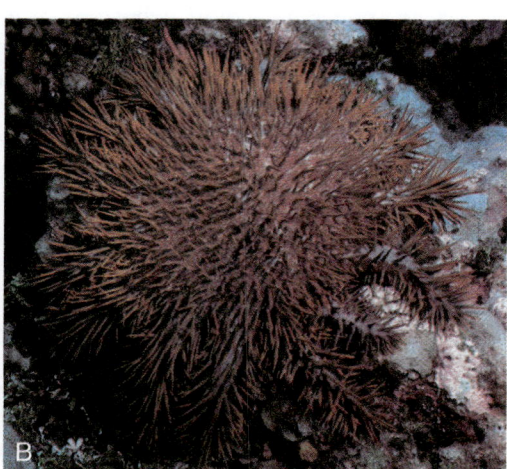
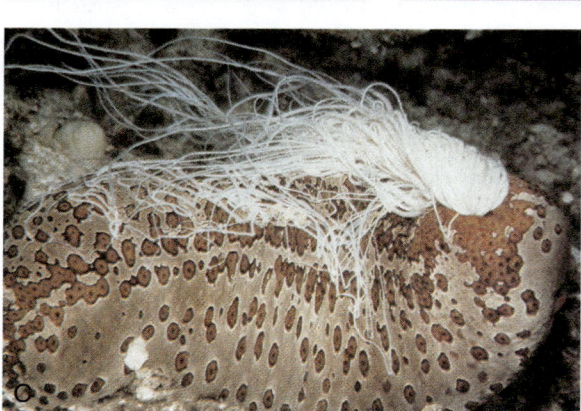

FIGURE 34-8 Echinoderms. **A,** Black sea urchin. **B,** Crown-of-thorns starfish. **C,** Sea cucumber with extended tentacles. (From Uerbach JS: *A medical guide to hazardous marine life*, ed 2, St Louis, 1991, Mosby.)

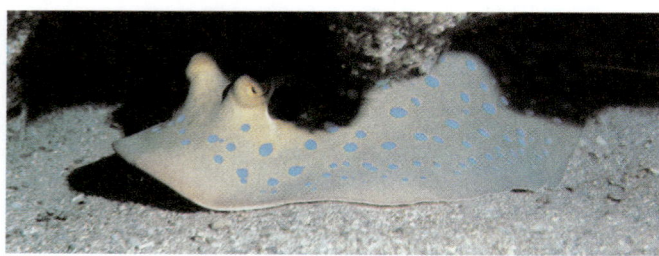

FIGURE 34-9 Stingray. (From Uerbach JS: *A medical guide to hazardous marine life*, ed 2, St Louis, 1991, Mosby.)

patient reaches the emergency department. Analgesics may be needed to manage pain.

POISONING BY ABSORPTION

Many poisons can be absorbed through the skin. Two compounds, organophosphates and carbamates, are responsible for a large number of skin-absorbed poisonings each year. Organophosphates and carbamates are commonly available for commercial and public use in the form of pet, home, and commercial insecticides. Organophosphates also are used in the development of military nerve agents

such as sarin and soman (see Chapter 58). Because of the widespread availability of insecticides that contain organophosphate/carbamate compounds, paramedics must be aware of the nature of these chemicals, the necessary precautions for personal safety, and the immediate management that may be required before symptoms or signs of illness occur.

Organophosphates and carbamates are highly toxic. In addition, they are well absorbed by ingestion, inhalation, and dermal routes. Both classes have similar pharmacological actions, inhibiting the effects of acetylcholinesterase, an enzyme that degrades acetylcholine at nerve terminals. To review, acetylcholine is a cholinergic neurotransmitter for preganglionic autonomic fibers, somatic nerves to skeletal muscle, and many synapses in the CNS. When acetylcholinesterase is inhibited, acetylcholine accumulates at the synapses. This results in a cholinergic "overdrive." The signs and symptoms resulting from cholinergic overdrive are seen in organophosphate and carbamate poisoning.

Signs and Symptoms

Early signs and symptoms of organophosphate or carbamate poisoning may be nonspecific, including headache, dizziness, weakness, and nausea. As overstimulation and disruption of transmission in the central and peripheral nervous systems occur, signs and symptoms begin to develop. These signs and symptoms result from a wide range of physiological and metabolic derangements (Box 34-14).

The rapidity and sequence in which these signs and symptoms develop depend on the particular compound and on the amount and route of exposure. The onset of symptoms is probably quickest after inhalation. Onset is slowest after a primary skin exposure and may be delayed for several hours. There are helpful mnemonics to recognize the signs of poisoning. One is *SLUDGE—s*alivation, *l*acrimation, *u*rination, *d*efecation, *g*astrointestinal upset, and *e*mesis. Another is *DUMBBELLS—d*iarrhea or *d*iaphoresis, *u*rination, *m*iosis or *m*uscle fasciculations, *b*ronchospasm, *b*radycardia, *e*mesis, *l*acrimation, *l*ethargy, and *s*alivation. Rapidly changing pupils with miosis are common with vapor exposure of organophosphates. Muscle twitching (fasciculations) can follow rapidly. Individual muscle twitching can result from liquid contact and local skin absorption at the site.

 CRITICAL THINKING
Consider a person who does not suspect poisoning. What condition might that person think he or she is suffering from with this clinical presentation?

Management

Emergency care begins with scene safety, personal protection, and decontamination procedures. The scene should be secured by qualified personnel. Personal protective actions include wearing protective clothing and using respiratory protection. The patient should be removed safely from the contaminated area as soon as possible so that decontamination can begin (see Chapter 58). After these measures are completed, patient care can be initiated. The general principles of management for poisoning by absorption include respiratory support, drug administration, and electrocardiogram monitoring. Organophosphates and carbamates produce similar physiological effects. However, carbamates have a shorter duration of action. Thus they have a more rapid decrease in their effect.

RESPIRATORY SUPPORT

Respiratory tract symptoms usually are first to appear after exposure to organophosphates or carbamates. In addition, respiratory paralysis may occur suddenly without warning. The need for advanced airway management and ventilatory support should be anticipated. Copious bronchial secretions may require suctioning. Bronchoconstriction also may necessitate positive-pressure ventilation and positive end-expiratory pressure.

DRUG ADMINISTRATION

Drug therapy in organophosphate or carbamate poisoning is directed at blocking the effects of acetylcholine, separating cholinesterase from the chemical compound, and

BOX 34-14 Signs and Symptoms of Organophosphate or Carbamate Poisoning

Cardiovascular System
Bradycardia
Variable blood pressure (usually hypotensive)

Respiratory System
Bronchoconstriction
Dyspnea
Rhinorrhea
Wheezing

Gastrointestinal System
Blurred vision
Cramps
Defecation
Emesis
Increased bowel sounds

Central Nervous System
Anxiety
Coma
Convulsions
Dizziness
Respiratory depression

Musculoskeletal System
Fasciculations
Flaccid paralysis

Skin
Diaphoresis

Other Signs and Symptoms
Lacrimation
Miosis
Rapidly changing pupil size
Salivation
Urination

suppressing seizure activity if present. The drugs currently used as antidotes include *atropine, pralidoxime chloride,* and *diazepam* or *lorazepam.*

 NOTE
Drug therapy should be initiated only if the patient has two or more signs or symptoms of poisoning and/or respiratory distress is present. Drug therapy should be initiated only after consulting with medical direction or a poison control center.

Atropine reverses the muscarinic effects (bradycardia, bronchoconstriction, increased respiratory secretions, and miosis) of moderate to severe organophosphate or carbamate poisoning. The drug competitively antagonizes the actions of acetylcholine. This results in a decrease in the hyperactivity of smooth muscles and glands. The drug is indicated to dry the patient's secretions. It also helps to decrease pulmonary resistance to ventilation. Potentially hypoxic patients may require the administration of large doses of *atropine* (see the *Emergency Drug Index*). The electrocardiogram should be monitored for dysrhythmias (other than tachycardia). Supplemental oxygen should be given to minimize the risk of ventricular fibrillation. *Atropine* is the drug of choice for carbamate poisonings.

> **NOTE**
> As a rule, cholinergic poisoning causes the patient to be "wet." This is manifested by profuse sweating, lacrimation, salivation, vomiting, diarrhea, and incontinence. Anticholinergic poisoning generally causes the patient to be "dry." This is manifested by dry, flushed skin; elevated temperature; and urinary retention. Being cognizant of this "wet vs. dry" symptomatology can be lifesaving for the poisoned patient. The wet-appearing patient will require atropine.

Pralidoxime is the treatment of choice for organophosphate poisoning after the administration of *atropine*. *Pralidoxime* should be used for nearly all patients with significant exposures, particularly those with muscular twitching and weakness. *Pralidoxime* has the primary effect of reactivating acetylcholinesterase. The adult and pediatric doses for *pralidoxime* can be found in the *Emergency Drug Index*.

Diazepam or *lorazepam* may be indicated if seizures are present. The need for seizure control may arise before decontamination is complete. In this case, the drugs can be administered intramuscularly to control seizure activity (see the *Emergency Drug Index*). As a safety precaution, IV therapy usually is not initiated in a patient in a contaminated area. The paramedic should be alert to the risk for respiratory and CNS depression.

> **CRITICAL THINKING**
> Consider that you give diazepam or lorazepam for seizures in this case. Will that eliminate the need for atropine?

ELECTROCARDIOGRAM MONITORING

Electrocardiogram monitoring may reveal a variety of abnormalities, including idioventricular rhythms, multifocal premature ventricular contractions, ventricular tachycardia, torsades de pointes, ventricular fibrillation, complete heart block, and asystole These dysrhythmias usually occur in two phases. The first phase begins with a transient episode of intense sympathetic tone. This results in sinus tachycardia. This phase is followed by a period of extreme parasympathetic tone. It may manifest as sinus bradycardia, atrioventricular block, and ST segment and T wave abnormalities. As described in Chapter 22, slow ventricular

dysrhythmias that do not respond to the usual therapy may need to be treated with overdrive pacing.

SECTION TWO
Drug Abuse

The term **drug abuse** refers to the use of prescription drugs for nonprescribed purposes. It also refers to the use of drugs that have no prescribed medical use (Box 34-15). Emergencies that result from drug abuse include adverse effects caused by the drug or impurities or contaminants mixed with the drug, life-threatening infections from intravenous or intradermal injection of drugs with unsterile equipment, injuries during intoxication, and drug dependence or withdrawal syndrome resulting from the habit-forming potential of many drugs (see Chapter 13).

Because of the widespread use and misuse of drugs (Box 34-16), the paramedic should maintain a high degree of suspicion and consider the possibility for a drug-related problem in *any patient* of *any age* who has seizures, behavioral changes, or decreased level of consciousness. In addition, consideration of the visibility, accessibility, and careful handling of all medications carried on an EMS vehicle should be a part of any EMS policy and procedure.

> **CRITICAL THINKING**
> Why might a patient (or their friends) delay calling for help in a situation involving drug overdose?

BOX 34-15 Drug Abuse Terminology

Drug abuse: Self-medication or self-administration of a drug in chronically excessive amounts, resulting in psychological and/or physical dependence, functional impairment, and deviation from approved social norms

Drug dependence: Condition marked by an overwhelming desire to continue taking a drug for its desired effect, usually an altered mental activity, attitude, or outlook

Physical dependence: An adaptive physiological state occurring after prolonged use of many drugs (Discontinuation causes withdrawal syndromes that are relieved by readministering the same drug or a pharmacologically related drug.)

Psychological dependence: Emotional reliance on a drug (manifestations range from a mild desire for a drug to craving and drug-seeking behavior to repeated compulsive use of a drug for its subjectively satisfying or pleasurable effects.)

Tolerance: A tendency to increase drug dosage to experience the same effect formerly produced by a smaller dose

Withdrawal syndrome: A predictable set of signs and symptoms that occurs after a decrease in the amount of the usual dose of a drug or its sudden cessation

BOX 34-16 Initiation of Substance Use (Incidence, or First-Time Use) Within the Past 12 Months: 2008 Data

- In 2008 an estimated 2.9 million persons ages 12 or older used an illicit drug for the first time within the past 12 months. This averages to almost 8000 initiates per day. A majority of these past year illicit drug initiates reported that their first drug was marijuana (56.6%). Nearly one third initiated with psychotherapeutics (29.6%), including 22.5% with pain relievers, 3.2% with tranquilizers, 3.0% with stimulants, and 0.8% with sedatives. A sizable proportion reported inhalants (9.7%) as their first illicit drug, and a small proportion used hallucinogens as their first drug (3.2%).
- In 2008 the illicit drug categories with the largest number of past year initiates among persons ages 12 or older were marijuana use (2.2 million) and nonmedical use of pain relievers (2.2 million).
- In 2008 there were 729,000 persons ages 12 or older who had used inhalants for the first time within the past 12 months; 70.4% were younger than age 18 when they first used.
- The number of past year initiates of methamphetamine among persons ages 12 or older was 95,000 in 2008.
- Between 2003 and 2008, the number of Ecstasy initiates increased from 642,000 to 894,000 and the number of LSD initiates increased from 200,000 to 394,000.
- Most (84.6%) of the 4.5 million past year alcohol initiates were younger than age 21 at the time of initiation.

From U.S. Department of Health and Human Services, Substance Abuse and Mental Health Services Administration, Office of Applied Studies: *2008 National Survey on Drug Use and Health: National Findings,* http://oas.samhsa.gov/nsduh/2k8nsduh/2k8Results.cfm#Ch5.

BOX 34-17 Common Agents Involved in Poisoning

Acetaminophen
Cardiac medications
Drugs abused for sexual purposes/sexual gratification
Hallucinogens
Lithium
Metals (iron, lead, and mercury)
Monoamine oxidase inhibitors
Nonprescription pain medicines
Opioids
Phencyclidine
Salicylates
Sedatives-hypnotics
Stimulants
Tricyclic antidepressants

TOXIC EFFECTS OF DRUGS

EMS personnel often encounter persons who are suffering from the toxic effects of drugs. Toxicity may be the result of an overdose, a potential suicide attempt, polydrug administration, or an accident (accidental ingestion,

miscalculation, changes in drug strength). Box 34-17 lists the drugs discussed in this chapter.

Common drugs of abuse, along with their names and uses, vary widely in different geographical areas. Also, the drugs of abuse often change over time. Table 34-3 is a partial list of common drugs of abuse, their street names, and miscellaneous terminology relating to drug use.

DID YOU KNOW?

Dextromethorphan (DXM) is an ingredient found in more than 100 over-the-counter cough medicines and cold remedies, such as Robitussin. When consumed in excessive doses, the drug can cause euphoria and dysphoria. It also may cause cardiac irregularities, seizure, loss of consciousness, and brain damage.[19] In 2008 there were nearly 8000 emergency department visits in the United States from the abuse of cough medicines. This reflects a 73% rise from cases reported in 2004. Paramedics should consider the possibility of DXM abuse in any patient who appears to be "high."

General Management Principles

The following are general principles for managing drug abuse and the overdose that may result:

1. Ensure that the scene is safe. Be prepared for unpredictable behavior from the patient. Consider the need for help from law enforcement.
2. Ensure adequate airway, ventilatory, and circulatory support as needed.
3. Obtain a history of the event. This should include the self-administration of other drugs that may have been taken by another route. Obtain any significant medical or psychiatric history.
4. Identify the substance. Consult with medical direction or a poison control center.
5. Perform a full, focused physical examination. Continually monitor the patient's vital functions and electrocardiogram.
6. Start intravenous therapy. Draw a blood sample for laboratory analysis and administer the proper drug antidote, such as ***naloxone*** if an opioid overdose is suspected. Pay special attention to personal protection because many of these patients are at high risk of harboring infectious disease. The nasal administration of ***naloxone*** should be considered in these patient groups.
7. Administer ***activated charcoal*** (per protocol) for orally administered drugs taken within the previous hour.
8. Rapidly transport the patient for physician evaluation.

When examining any patient suspected of abusing drugs, the paramedic should always look for track marks. These may be in the antecubital space, under the tongue, or on top of the feet. The possibility of "body packing" (concealing packets of drugs in body cavities of the stomach, rectum, and vagina) and "body stuffing" (swallowing drugs to avoid arrest) should be considered when a person who abuses drugs appears ill for no apparent reason.

TABLE 34-3 Commonly Abused Drugs and Their Street Names*

Substances: Category and Name	Examples of Commercial and Street Names	DEA Schedule†/ How Administered‡	Intoxication Effects/Potential Health Consequences
Tobacco			
Nicotine	Found in cigarettes, cigars, bidis, and smokeless tobacco (snuff, spit tobacco, chew), drug patches	Not scheduled/ smoked, snorted, chewed	Increased blood pressure and heart rate/ chronic lung disease; cardiovascular disease; stroke; cancers of mouth, pharynx, larynx, esophagus, stomach, pancreas, cervix, kidney, bladder, and acute myeloid leukemia; adverse pregnancy outcomes; addiction
Alcohol			
Alcohol (ethyl alcohol)	Found in liquor, beer, and wine	Not scheduled/ swallowed	In low doses, euphoria, mild stimulation, relaxation, lowered inhibitions; in higher doses, drowsiness, slurred speech, nausea, emotional volatility, loss of coordination, visual distortions, impaired memory, sexual dysfunction, loss of consciousness/increased risk of injuries, violence, fetal damage (in pregnant women); depression; neurologic deficits; hypertension; liver and heart disease; addiction; fatal overdose
Cannabinoids			
Hashish	Boom, gangster, hash, hash oil, hemp	I/swallowed, smoked	Euphoria; relaxation; slowed reaction time; distorted sensory perception; impaired balance and coordination; increased heart rate and appetite; impaired learning, memory; anxiety; panic attacks; psychosis/ cough, frequent respiratory tract infections; possible mental health decline; addiction
Marijuana	Blunt, dope, ganja, grass, herb, joint, bud, Mary Jane, pot, reefer, green, trees, smoke, sinsemilla, skunk, weed	I/swallowed, smoked	
Opioids			
Heroin	Diacetylmorphine: smack, horse, brown sugar, dope, H, junk, skag, skunk, white horse, China white; cheese (with OTC cold medicine and antihistamine)	I/injected, smoked, snorted	Euphoria; drowsiness; impaired coordination; dizziness; confusion; nausea; sedation; feeling of heaviness in body; slowed or arrested breathing/constipation; endocarditis; hepatitis; HIV; addiction; fatal overdose
Opium	Laudanum, paregoric: big O, black stuff, block, gum, hop	II, III, V/swallowed, smoked	
Stimulants			
Cocaine	Cocaine hydrochloride: blow, bump, C, candy, Charlie, coke, crack, flake, rock, snow, toot	II/snorted, smoked, injected	Increased heart rate, blood pressure, body temperature, metabolism; feelings of exhilaration; increased energy, mental alertness; tremors; reduced appetite; irritability; anxiety; panic; paranoia; violent behavior; psychosis/weight loss, insomnia; cardiac or cardiovascular complications; stroke; seizures; addiction
Amphetamine	Biphetamine, Dexedrine: bennies, black beauties, crosses, hearts, LA turnaround, speed, truck drivers, uppers	II/swallowed, snorted, smoked, injected	
Methamphetamine	Desoxyn: meth, ice, crank, chalk, crystal, fire, glass, go fast, speed	II/ swallowed, snorted, smoked, injected	Also, for cocaine—nasal damage from snorting. Also, for methamphetamine—severe dental problems
Club Drugs			
MDMA (methylenedioxy- methamphetamine)	Ecstasy, Adam, clarity, Eve, lover's speed, peace, uppers	I/swallowed, snorted, injected	**MDMA**—mild hallucinogenic effects; increased tactile sensitivity; empathic feelings; lowered inhibition; anxiety; chills; sweating; teeth clenching; muscle cramping/sleep disturbances; depression; impaired memory; hyperthermia; addiction
Flunitrazepam§	Rohypnol: forget-me pill, Mexican Valium, R2, roach, Roche, roofies, roofinol, rope, rophies	IV/swallowed, snorted	**Flunitrazepam**—sedation; muscle relaxation; confusion; memory loss; dizziness; impaired coordination/addiction
GHB§	Gamma-hydroxybutyrate: G, Georgia home boy, grievous bodily harm, liquid Ecstasy, soap, scoop, goop, liquid X	I/swallowed	**GHB**—drowsiness; nausea; headache; disorientation; loss of coordination; memory loss/unconsciousness; seizures; coma

Continued

TABLE 34-3—cont'd

Substances: Category and Name	Examples of Commercial and Street Names	DEA Schedule[†]/ How Administered[‡]	Intoxication Effects/Potential Health Consequences
Dissociative Drugs			
Ketamine	Ketalar SV: cat Valium, K, Special K, vitamin K	III/injected, snorted, smoked	Feelings of being separate from one's body and environment; impaired motor function/ anxiety; tremors; numbness; memory loss; nausea
PCP and analogs	Phencyclidine: angel dust, boat, hog, love boat, peace pill	I, II/swallowed, smoked, injected	
Salvia divinorum	Salvia, Shepherdess's Herb, Maria Pastora, magic mint, Sally-D	Not scheduled/ chewed, swallowed, smoked	Also, for ketamine—analgesia; impaired memory; delirium; respiratory depression and arrest; death
Dextromethorphan (DXM)	Found in some cough and cold medications: Robotripping, Robo, Triple C	Not scheduled/ swallowed	Also, for PCP and analogs—analgesia; psychosis; aggression; violence; slurred speech; loss of coordination; hallucinations
			Also, for DXM—euphoria; slurred speech; confusion; dizziness; distorted visual perceptions
Hallucinogens			
LSD	Lysergic acid diethylamide: acid, blotter, cubes, microdot, yellow sunshine, blue heaven	I/swallowed, absorbed through mouth tissues	Altered states of perception and feeling; hallucinations; nausea
			Also, LSD and mescaline—increased body temperature, heart rate, blood pressure; loss of appetite; sweating; sleeplessness; numbness, dizziness, weakness, tremors; impulsive behavior; rapid shifts in emotion
Mescaline	Buttons, cactus, mesc, peyote	I/swallowed, smoked	
Psilocybin	Magic mushrooms, purple passion, shrooms, little smoke	I/swallowed	**Also, for LSD**—flashbacks, hallucinogen persisting perception disorder
			Also for psilocybin—nervousness; paranoia; panic
Other Compounds			
Anabolic steroids	Anadrol, Oxandrin, Durabolin, Depo-Testosterone, Equipoise: roids, juice, gym candy, pumpers	III/injected, swallowed, applied to skin	Steroids—no intoxication effects/hypertension; blood clotting and cholesterol changes; liver cysts; hostility and aggression; acne; in adolescents—premature cessation of growth; in males—prostate cancer, reduced sperm production, shrunken testicles, breast enlargement; in females—menstrual irregularities, development of beard and other masculine characteristics
Inhalants	Solvents (paint thinners, gasoline, glues); gases (butane, propane, aerosol propellants, nitrous oxide); nitrites (isoamyl, isobutyl, cyclohexyl): laughing gas, poppers, snappers, whippets	Not scheduled/ inhaled through nose or mouth	Inhalants (varies by chemical)—stimulation; loss of inhibition; headache; nausea or vomiting; slurred speech; loss of motor coordination; wheezing/cramps; muscle weakness; depression; memory impairment; damage to cardiovascular and nervous systems; unconsciousness; sudden death

*For more information on prescription medications, please visit www.nida.nih.gov/DrugPages/PrescripDrugsChart.html
[†]Schedule I and II drugs have a high potential for abuse. They require greater storage security and have a quota on manufacturing, among other restrictions. Schedule I drugs are available for research only and have no approved medical use; Schedule II drugs are available only by prescription (unrefillable) and require a form for ordering. Schedule III and IV drugs are available by prescription, may have five refills in 6 months, and may be ordered orally. Some Schedule V drugs are available over the counter.
[‡]Some of the health risks are directly related to the route of drug administration. For example, injection drug use can increase the risk of infection through needle contamination with staphylococci, HIV, hepatitis, and other organisms.
[§]Associated with sexual assaults.

CRITICAL THINKING

For what illnesses is the patient who uses intravenous narcotics at risk?

Opioid Overdose

Heroin accounts for about 90% of the opioid abuse in the United States. Pure heroin is a bitter-tasting white powder. Heroin usually is adulterated or "cut" for street distribution. A typical "bag" is the single-dose unit of heroin and may weigh 100 mg. On average, heroin is only 20% to 30% pure and often is mixed with other drugs such as *fentanyl*. Other opioid drugs include *morphine*, hydromorphone, methadone, *meperidine*, codeine, oxycodone, propoxyphene, hydrocodone, and "designer opioids" that have been chemically modified such as alpha-methylfentanyl ("China white").

> **NOTE**
> Vicodin (hydrocodone) is one of the most commonly prescribed and most commonly abused pain medications today. Vicodin and its related medications, Lorcet, Lortab, Percodan, and OxyContin, are opioid-based drugs. Vicodin is a derivative of opium, which is also used to manufacture heroin. Vicodin successfully diminishes pain, but it is highly addictive. The drug can be taken orally in pill form, chewed, or crushed and sniffed like cocaine. Physical effects from misusing these drugs include dizziness, blurred vision, constipation, fluctuations in heart rate, hallucinations, nausea, vomiting, sedation, and respiratory depression. Signs and symptoms of withdrawal from these drugs are similar to those of other opioids. Overdose is not uncommon, and higher doses of *naloxone* may be required to manage these patients.

Depending on the preparation, these drugs may be taken orally, injected intradermally ("skin popping") or intravenously ("mainlining"), taken intranasally ("snorted"), or smoked. All opioids are CNS depressants. They can cause life-threatening respiratory depression. In severe intoxication, hypotension, profound shock, and pulmonary edema may be present. Signs and symptoms of narcotic/opioid overdose include the following:

> **SHOW ME THE EVIDENCE**
> Researchers reviewed records retrospectively to see the clinical response to intranasal (IN) versus intramuscular (IM) naloxone administration. Patients whose respiratory rate increased or whose Glasgow Coma Scale score reached 6 were responders. Although the mean time from administration to response was longer in the IN group, the time from patient contact to response was not significantly different. Three patients who received IN naloxone were later given IM or IV naloxone. The authors concluded that IN naloxone may be a safer alternative for prehospital naloxone administration.
>
> Robertson T, Hendey G, Stroh G, et al: Intranasal naloxone is a viable alternative to intravenous naloxone for prehospital narcotic overdose, *PEC* 13(4):512-515, 2009.

- Euphoria
- Arousable somnolence ("nodding")
- Nausea
- Pinpoint pupils (except with *meperidine*, under hypoxic conditions, or in combination with other types of drugs)
- Slow and shallow respirations
- Coma
- Seizures

ANTIDOTE THERAPY

As described in Chapter 13, *naloxone* is a pure opioid antagonist effective for virtually all opioid and opioid-like substances. The drug reverses the three major symptoms of opioid overdose: respiratory depression, coma, and miosis. Its use should be considered when opioid intoxication is suspected.[18] *Naloxone* also is indicated for use when a coma of unknown origin is present. The EMS crew should be prepared to restrain the patient. The patient's behavior may be unpredictable when the effects of the drug are reversed and the patient experiences withdrawal symptoms. Medical direction may recommend that the *naloxone* be given in small amounts. The amount should be enough to restore airway reflexes and adequate breathing, without fully awakening the patient. The patient should be ventilated with a bag mask before *naloxone* administration. If the patient does not respond to treatment with *naloxone*, intubation should be considered. (*Note:* In the absence of respiratory depression, the use of *naloxone* is controversial; seizure activity is a possible side effect of the drug.)

>
> **NOTE**
> Two other pure opioid antagonists are available. *Naltrexone* is an oral medication used in long-term programs for opioid addiction. *Nalmefene* appears to be as effective as *naloxone* in acute opioid intoxications. Moreover, *nalmefene* has a longer duration of action (4 to 8 hours) than *naloxone*.

Some opioids (e.g., heroin) and some narcotics (e.g., methadone) have a longer duration than *naloxone*. Thus the patient must be monitored closely during antidote therapy. Repeated doses of *naloxone* may be needed as well. In communities where abuse of naloxone-resistant opioids or the use of China white is common, larger initial doses of *naloxone* may be needed. The desired signs of reversal of opioid intoxication are adequate airway reflexes and ventilations, not complete arousal.

Naloxone can cause a withdrawal syndrome in opioid-dependent patients. Slowly administer a smaller dose of the drug for these patients. Withdrawal usually can be managed by symptomatic and supportive care. Box 34-18 lists signs and symptoms of opioid withdrawal.

Sedative-Hypnotic Overdose

Sedative-hypnotic agents include benzodiazepines and barbiturates. These drugs usually are taken orally. Yet they may be diluted and injected intravenously. Taking these drugs

BOX 34-18 Signs and Symptoms of Opioid Withdrawal

Abdominal cramps
Anorexia
Cold sweats or chills
Diaphoresis
Diarrhea
Fever
General malaise
Gooseflesh
Insomnia
Irritability
Nausea and vomiting
Pulmonary edema
Severe agitation
Ventricular dysrhythmias
Tachycardia
Tremors

BOX 34-19 Methamphetamine

Methamphetamine is a synthetically manufactured central nervous system stimulant. Methamphetamine is legally manufactured for medicinal purposes (Methedrine and Desoxyn). Yet illicit production of methamphetamine as a street drug in the United States is on the rise. Common names for methamphetamine include meth, speed, crank, crystal, water, or ice.

Illegal methamphetamine can be produced inexpensively in clandestine meth labs with common chemical methods (hydriodic acid, phenyl-2-propane, sodium ammonia, thionyl chloride). The drug then can be smoked, injected, snorted, or taken orally. Once methamphetamine enters the body, it can produce skeletal muscle tremors, sleeplessness, and euphoria that can last up to 10 days. During these drug-induced sleepless "binges," users may become hostile and paranoid. This is followed by a "crash" (an emotionally depressed state) that can last for several days.

In addition to ensuring personal safety when dealing with these patients, the paramedic crew should be keenly aware of potential hazards associated with clandestine labs. These hazards include the production of highly explosive toxic gases (e.g., phosphine) that can be absorbed readily through the skin in quantities that can be fatal; the presence of an oxygen-depleted environment; the use of toxic solvents that can lead to lab explosions; and exposure to other dangerous chemicals. Any time a meth lab is suspected, the emergency medical services crew should withdraw. Patients and bystanders should be evacuated. Law enforcement and specialized hazardous materials personnel should be summoned to the scene. Drug-making paraphernalia that should alert the paramedic to the presence of a meth lab include the following*:

- Amber stains on walls, furniture, and counters
- Equipment that has a red or amber color
- Two large, round-bottom flasks (with stoppers) connected by a hose
- Pyrex-type meatloaf container
- Various measuring and funnel devices
- A heat source

*From Goss J: Meth labs, *J Emerg Med Serv* 23:1, 1998.

with alcohol greatly increases their effects. Sedative-hypnotic drugs commonly are known as *downers*.

Benzodiazepines are among the best-known and most widely prescribed drugs used to control symptoms of anxiety, stress, and insomnia. These drugs sometimes are used to manage alcohol withdrawal and to control seizure disorders as well. They promote sleep and relieve anxiety by depressing brain function. Often they are abused for their sedative effects. Individually, these drugs are somewhat nontoxic. They may accentuate the effects of other sedative-hypnotic agents. Common benzodiazepines are *diazepam* (Valium), alprazolam (Xanax), and *lorazepam* (Ativan).

Barbiturates are general CNS depressants that inhibit impulse conduction in the brainstem. These drugs once were widely used to treat anxiety and insomnia. Their addictive properties and potential for abuse have led to their replacement by benzodiazepines and other nonbarbiturate drugs. Barbiturates that commonly are abused include phenobarbital, amobarbital, and secobarbital.

Signs and symptoms of sedative-hypnotic overdose chiefly are related to the central nervous and cardiovascular systems. Adverse effects include excessive drowsiness, staggering gait, and, in some cases, paradoxical excitability. In cases of severe toxicity the patient may become comatose, with respiratory depression, hypotension, and shock. The pupils may be constricted. More often, though, they become fixed and dilated even in the absence of significant brain damage. Airway control and ventilatory management are the most important actions in managing significant sedative-hypnotic overdose. *Flumazenil* is a benzodiazepine antagonist that can be used to reverse the effects of benzodiazepines.[18] The drug, however, can produce seizure activity, dysrhythmias, and hypotension.[18] *Flumazenil* is contraindicated in patients who are prone to seizures and in those with tricyclic antidepressant overdose. It is generally only used to reverse benzodiazepine effects after procedural sedation.

Stimulant Overdose

Commonly abused stimulant drugs are those of the sympathomimetic family (e.g., amphetamine sulfate, dextroamphetamine, cocaine, methamphetamine) (Box 34-19).

Sympathomimetic drugs often are used to produce general mood elevation, improve task performance, suppress appetite, and prevent sleepiness. Structurally, the amphetamines are similar to the catecholamines epinephrine and norepinephrine. Yet they differ in their more pronounced effects on the CNS. Adverse effects include tachycardia, hypertension, tachypnea, agitation, dilated pupils, tremors, and disorganized behavior. In severe intoxication the patient may exhibit psychosis and paranoia and may experience hallucinations. Sudden withdrawal or cessation of amphetamine use may result in a "crash" stage. In this stage the patient becomes depressed, suicidal, incoherent, or nearly comatose. As a rule, these drugs are taken orally. They also may be smoked or injected for a more rapid onset of action. Amphetamines commonly are known as *speed* or *uppers.*

COCAINE

Cocaine is one of the most popular illegal drugs in the United States. Cocaine is a fine, white crystalline powder. Like heroin, street forms of cocaine usually are adulterated. They vary in purity from 25% to 90%; doses vary from near 0 to 200 mg. This form of cocaine generally is taken intranasally by snorting a "line" containing 10 to 35 mg of the drug (depending on purity). After absorption through the mucous membranes, the effects of the drug begin within minutes. Peak effects occur 15 to 60 minutes after use, with a half-life of 1 to 2½ hours. Cocaine also is used by the subcutaneous, intramuscular, and intravenous routes; the intravenous route provides immediate absorption and intense stimulation. Taken IV, the peak occurs within 5 minutes and with a half-life of about 50 minutes. *Speedballing* refers to an injection of a cocaine-heroin combination.

Freebase or "crack" cocaine is a more potent formulation of the drug. Crack is prepared by mixing powdered street cocaine with an alkaline solution and then adding a solvent such as ether. The combination separates into two layers. The top layer contains the dissolved cocaine. Evaporation of the solvent results in pure cocaine crystals, which are smoked and absorbed via the pulmonary route. Cocaine in this form is called rock or crack because of the popping sound produced when the crystals are heated. Freebase cocaine generally is combined with marijuana or tobacco and is smoked in a pipe or a cigarette. The reactions are similar to those experienced in intravenous use, with equal intensity and effects.

> ### NOTE
> In recent years, a synthetic substitute for marijuana began to be distributed and sold throughout the United States. The product usually is packaged and marketed as an herbal product intended to be burned as incense. It is available under various names, including K2 and Spice. The active ingredient in the synthetic substitute is a cannabinoid, a class of drug that includes tetrahydrocannabinol (THC; the active ingredient in marijuana). As a result, the effects of the product are similar to those of marijuana when smoked or inhaled. Many local jurisdictions throughout the United States have banned the sale of these products. Synthetic THC also may be legally prescribed for medicinal use (Marinol). The "marijuana pill" has been found to relieve the nausea and vomiting associated with chemotherapy for cancer patients and to assist with loss of appetite with acquired immunodeficiency syndrome (AIDS) patients.
>
> Bath salts are also being sold in the United States, that when snorted, inhaled, or injected, produce effects similar to methamphetamine. These powders are sold under names such as Ivory Wave, White Lightning, and Hurricane Charlie. They contain mephedrone and methylenedioxypyrovalerone (also known as MDPV), and can cause hallucinations, paranoia, tachycardia, and suicidal thoughts. Many U.S. states are banning the sale of these products.

Cocaine is a major CNS stimulant. It causes profound sympathetic discharge. The increased levels of circulating catecholamines result in excitement, euphoria, talkativeness, and agitation. The effects of the drug can cause significant cardiovascular and neurological complications such as cardiac dysrhythmias, myocardial infarction, seizures, intracranial hemorrhage, hyperthermia, and psychiatric disturbances. Cocaine overdose can occur with any form of the drug and any route of administration. The adult fatal dose is thought to be about 1200 mg (1.2 g), but fatalities from cocaine-induced cardiac dysrhythmias have been reported with single doses of as little as 25 to 30 mg.[8]

Prehospital management of the cocaine-intoxicated patient may be difficult. Cocaine toxicity may range from minor symptoms to life-threatening overdose. Emergency care may require a full spectrum of basic and advanced life-support measures, including aggressive airway management, ventilatory and circulatory support, drug therapy, and rapid transport to an appropriate medical facility. Benzodiazepines are the mainstay of treatment initially in cocaine toxicity. For cocaine-induced hypertension or chest discomfort, **nitroglycerine** and/or **morphine** can be beneficial.[18]

PHENCYCLIDINE OVERDOSE

Phencyclidine (PCP) is a dissociative analgesic originally used as a veterinary tranquilizer. The drug has sympathomimetic and CNS stimulant and depressant properties. Phencyclidine is a potent psychoactive drug illegally sold in liquid, tablet, or powder form to be taken orally, intranasally, intravenously/intramuscularly, or with other drugs to be smoked (a "Sherman"). Most tablets contain about 5 mg of PCP. As a rule, PCP in its powder form is purer (50% to 100% PCP). Chronic use can result in permanent memory impairment and loss of higher brain functions. The pharmacological effects are dose-related. They can be divided into low-dose and high-dose toxicity. Ketamine is a derivative of PCP and has identical actions.

Low-Dose Toxicity. In low doses that are less than 10 mg, PCP intoxication produces an unpredictable state that can resemble drunkenness. The user may have a sense of euphoria or confusion, disorientation, agitation, or sudden rage. An intoxicated patient often has a blank stare and a stumbling gait. The patient often is in a dissociative state. The patient's pupils generally are reactive. The patient may experience flushing, diaphoresis, facial grimacing, hypersalivation, and vomiting. **Nystagmus** with a burstlike quality is characteristic of low-dose PCP use. In this range of toxicity, death usually is related to behavioral disturbances resulting from spatial disorientation, drug-induced immobility, and insensitivity to pain. This insensitivity to pain leads to bold acts of strength. This is because the

CRITICAL THINKING
Why does this type of drug intoxication put the patient at a high risk for injury?

normal muscle activity limitation resulting from pain is inhibited.

In low-dose toxicity sensory stimulation should be avoided. Verbal and physical stimuli will likely make the clinical symptoms worse. Violent and combative patients require protection from self-injury. Safeguards also must be provided for the emergency crew and bystanders. The paramedic should monitor the patient's vital signs and level of consciousness closely. The patient should be observed for increasing motor activity and muscle rigidity as well. These may precede seizures.

High-Dose Toxicity. Patients with high-dose PCP intoxication from more than 10 mg may be in a coma that can last from hours to several days. These patients often are unresponsive to painful stimuli. Respiratory depression, hypertension, and tachycardia also may be present, depending on the dosage. In severe cases a hypertensive crisis causing cardiac failure, hypertensive encephalopathy, seizures, and intracerebral hemorrhage may result. Prehospital care is directed at managing respiratory and cardiac arrest, controlling status seizures, and rapidly transporting the patient for physician evaluation.

PHENCYCLIDINE PSYCHOSIS

Phencyclidine psychosis is a true psychiatric emergency that may mimic schizophrenia. The psychosis usually is of acute onset. It may not become apparent until several days after drug ingestion. Psychosis can occur after a single low-dose exposure to PCP. Psychosis also may last from several days to weeks. Signs and symptoms may range from a catatonic and unresponsive state to bizarre and violent behavior. The patient often appears agitated and suspicious, and may experience auditory hallucinations and paranoia. Appropriate management usually requires involuntary hospitalization, control of violent behavior, and administration of antipsychotic agents. When dealing with these patients in the prehospital setting, personal safety is of prime importance; law enforcement personnel should be called upon for assistance.

Hallucinogen Overdose

Hallucinogens are substances that cause perceptual distortions. The most common hallucinogen in use today is lysergic acid diethylamide (LSD). Other hallucinogens include mescaline, found in the buttons of peyote cactus, which can be used legally in some religious settings; psilocybin mushrooms, found in the United States and Mexico; marijuana, the active agent of the plant *Cannabis sativa;* morning glory plant; nutmeg; mace; and some amphetamines, such as methylenedioxymethamphetamine (Ecstasy) and 3,4-methylenedioxyamphetamine (MDEA Eve).

Depending on the agent, the effects of hallucinogens may range from minor visual to more serious complications associated with lysergic acid diethylamide use. The more serious effects include respiratory and CNS depression (rare). Prehospital management usually is limited to supportive care, minimal sensory stimulation, calming measures, and transportation to a medical facility. After arrival at the emergency department, these patients generally are placed in a quiet environment for observation.

Tricyclic Antidepressant Overdose

Tricyclic antidepressants often are prescribed to help manage depression and certain pain syndromes. These drugs work by blocking the uptake of norepinephrine and serotonin into the presynaptic neurons. They also alter the sensitivity of brain tissue to the actions of these chemicals. Serious tricyclic antidepressant toxicity results in sodium channel blockade in the myocardium. Other toxicities include potassium efflux blockade and blockade of blood vessels, anticholinergic effects, and seizures. Commonly prescribed antidepressant drugs include the tricyclic antidepressants amitriptyline, desipramine, imipramine, and nortriptyline. The newer *selective serotonin reuptake inhibitors* such as fluoxetine, sertraline, and paroxetine are chemically unrelated to tricyclic antidepressants. These are considered safe and effective compared with tricyclic antidepressants (Box 34-20).

Early symptoms of tricyclic antidepressant overdose are dry mouth, blurred vision, confusion, inability to concentrate, and occasionally visual hallucinations. More severe symptoms include delirium, depressed respirations,

---

BOX 34-20 Serotonin Syndrome

Serotonin syndrome is a potentially life-threatening drug reaction. The reaction most often occurs when two or more drugs that affect serotonin levels are taken together. The drugs then cause too much serotonin to be released or to remain within brain tissue. Drug combinations that are associated with serotonin syndrome include migraine medicines (triptans) together with selective serotonin reuptake inhibitors (SSRIs) and selective serotonin/norepinephrine reuptake inhibitors (SNRIs). Popular SSRIs include Celexa, Zoloft, Prozac, Paxil, and Lexapro. SNRIs include Cymbalta and Effexor. Brand names of triptans include Imitrex, Zomig, Frova, Maxalt, Axert, Amerge, and Relpax. Drugs of abuse, such as Ecstasy and LSD, have also been associated with serotonin syndrome. Symptoms occur within minutes to hours and may include[20]:

- Agitation or restlessness
- Diarrhea
- Tachycardia
- Hallucinations
- Increased body temperature
- Loss of coordination
- Nausea
- Overactive reflexes
- Rapid changes in blood pressure
- Vomiting

Patients with serotonin syndrome usually require hospitalization for close observation and supportive care. Treatment may include benzodiazepines to decrease agitation, seizure-like movements, and muscle stiffness; cyproheptadine (Periactin) to block serotonin production; IV fluids; and the withdrawal of medicines that caused the syndrome.

hypertension, hypotension, hyperthermia, hypothermia, seizures, and coma (Box 34-21). Cardiac effects may range from tachycardia to bradycardia and various dysrhythmias caused by atrioventricular block. A prolonged QRS complex, right bundle branch block, and a Glasgow Coma Scale score less than 8, are characteristic findings that should alert the paramedic to a major toxicity with potentially serious complications. Sudden death from a cardiac arrest may occur several days after an overdose.

Prehospital management for major toxicity of a tricyclic antidepressant overdose is basic supportive care for the patient and rapid transport. About 25% of patients who ultimately die as a result of the overdose are alert and awake, and 75% have normal sinus rhythm when EMS personnel arrive.[3] Tachycardia, especially with a wide QRS complex greater than 100 ms, is an early sign of toxicity. **Sodium bicarbonate,** per medical direction, may begin to reverse cardiac toxicity.[18] Any patient with a history of tricyclic antidepressant ingestion should receive airway, ventilatory, and circulatory support; intravenous access; electrocardiogram monitoring; and rapid transport for physician evaluation. Treatment for specific problems such as seizures and ventricular dysrhythmias is complex. These conditions may require a combination of alkalinization and anticonvulsant medications. Rapid transport to the emergency department is the most prudent course of action.

CRITICAL THINKING

How can you ensure rapid transport of these patients?

Lithium

Lithium is a mood-stabilizing drug that is sometimes prescribed for the management of bipolar disorders (see Chapter 35). The drug has a low toxic-to-therapeutic dose ratio. Thus lithium overdose is common. Patients who are prescribed lithium have frequent blood tests to monitor the level of lithium in the body.

Lithium helps to prevent mood swings. It does this by interfering with hormonal responses to cyclic adenosine monophosphate and by increasing the reuptake of norepinephrine. This produces an antiadrenergic effect. As a result of these actions, lithium has many effects on the body. These include muscle tremor, thirst, nausea, increased urination, abdominal cramping, and diarrhea. With toxic ingestion, signs and symptoms may include the following:

- Muscle weakness
- Slurred speech
- Severe trembling
- Blurred vision
- Confusion
- Seizure
- Apnea
- Coma

BOX 34-21 Five Signs of Major Tricyclic Antidepressant Toxicity

Cardiac dysrhythmias
Coma
Gastrointestinal disturbances
Hypotension or hypertension
Respiratory depression

Prehospital care for patients with suspected lithium overdose should focus on airway management, ventilatory and circulatory support, and the control of seizure activity if present. **Activated charcoal** does not effectively bind lithium and should not be administered. In-hospital care may include restoring intravascular volume, maintaining urine output, correcting hyponatremia, and sometimes undergoing dialysis.

Cardiac Medications

Cardiac drugs are a common cause of poisoning deaths in children and adults. The drugs responsible for the majority of these fatalities are **digoxin,** beta blockers, and calcium channel blockers (Box 34-22). As in all other cases of

---

BOX 34-22 Toxic Effects of Common Cardiac Drugs

Digoxin
Atrial fibrillation
Atrial tachycardia
Bigeminal and multifocal premature ventricular contractions
First- and second-degree atrioventricular block
Sinus bradycardia
Ventricular tachycardia/ventricular fibrillation

Beta Blockers
Bradycardia
Hypotension
Respiratory arrest
Seizure
Unconsciousness
Ventricular tachycardia/ventricular fibrillation (rare)

Calcium Channel Blockers
Acute respiratory distress syndrome
Asystole
Atrioventricular dissociation
Coma
Confusion
Hypotension
Lactic acidosis
Mild hyperglycemia/hyperkalemia
Pulmonary edema
Respiratory depression
Sinus arrest
Sinus bradycardia
Slurred speech

poisoning, patients with toxic ingestion of cardiac drugs require high-concentration oxygen administration, intravenous access, and careful monitoring of vital signs and electrocardiogram.

Digoxin exerts direct and indirect effects on sinoatrial and atrioventricular nodal fibers. At toxic levels the drug can halt impulses in the sinoatrial node, depress conduction through the atrioventricular node, and increase sensitivity of the sinoatrial and atrioventricular nodes to catecholamines.[8] *Digoxin* affects the Purkinje fibers as well. It decreases the resting potential and action potential duration of the heart and increases automaticity. This can cause an increase in premature ventricular contraction formation. Unlike most cardiovascular drugs, *digoxin* can produce almost any dysrhythmia or conduction block. In addition to dysrhythmias, common signs and symptoms of *digoxin* toxicity include nausea, anorexia, fatigue, visual disturbances, and a variety of disorders of the gastrointestinal, ophthalmological, and neurological systems. Oral overdoses sometimes are managed with *activated charcoal* and drugs to treat life-threatening dysrhythmias. Severe overdoses are managed with intravenous digoxin-specific Fab. This is a drug that decreases the morbidity and mortality associated with *digoxin* overdose.

CRITICAL THINKING

Why is it possible that this type of overdose would not be noticed immediately?

Beta blockers are absorbed rapidly after ingestion. Toxicity impairs sinoatrial and atrioventricular node function. This leads to bradycardias and atrioventricular blocks. The associated depression in ventricular conduction and sodium channel blockade may cause the QRS complex to widen. Occasionally, patients become susceptible to ventricular dysrhythmias. However, rarely will these patients exhibit ventricular tachycardia or ventricular fibrillation. Other signs and symptoms include CNS and respiratory depression, hypotension, and seizures. Treatment for patients with beta-blocker overdose may include administration of *activated charcoal* and drugs to manage hypotension and dysrhythmias. The in-hospital care may include infusions of *glucagon,* high-dose *insulin,* or IV calcium salts.[18] Hemodialysis may be necessary, depending on the particular agent involved.

Toxic ingestion of calcium channel blockers can lead to myocardial depression and peripheral vasodilation with negative inotropic, chronotropic, dromotropic, and vasotropic effects. Hypotension and bradycardia are early signs of toxicity. Overdose may result in serious dysrhythmias that include atrioventricular block of all degrees, sinus arrest, atrioventricular dissociation, junctional rhythm, and asystole. (Calcium channel blockers have little effect on ventricular conduction; ventricular dysrhythmias are uncommon.) Other signs and symptoms of calcium channel toxicity include nausea and vomiting, hypotension, and CNS and respiratory depression. In addition to airway, ventilatory, and circulatory support, emergency care may include the use of antidysrhythmics, vasopressors, high-dose *insulin*, and *calcium chloride* (in shock refractory to other measures).[18]

Monoamine Oxidase Inhibitors

As described in Chapter 13, monoamine oxidase (MAO) inhibitors block the breakdown of monoamines (norepinephrine, dopamine, serotonin). These CNS transmitters are distributed throughout the body. The highest concentration is in the brain, liver, and kidneys. Monoamine oxidase inhibitors are prescribed as antidepressants, antineoplastics, antibiotics, and antihypertensives. Some monoamine oxidase inhibitors (e.g., the antidepressants phenelzine and tranylcypromine) have active metabolites. Signs of monoamine oxidase inhibitor toxicity usually are delayed, presenting 6 to 24 hours after ingestion. The duration of effects also may last for several days (Box 34-23). These effects include CNS depression and various neuromuscular and cardiovascular system manifestations.

LOOK AGAIN

See Chapter 13: Principles of Pharmacology and Emergency Medications, pp. 309-311.

The prehospital care is mainly supportive. Care includes airway, ventilatory, and circulatory support; cardiac medications as needed; and rapid transport for physician evaluation. *Activated charcoal* may be indicated.

Nonsteroidal Antiinflammatory Drugs

Nonsteroidal antiinflammatory drugs (NSAIDs) are a group of drugs that have an analgesic and antipyretic action. They also reduce inflammation of joints and soft tissues such as muscles and ligaments. They work by

BOX 34-23 Effects of Monoamine Oxidase Inhibitor Toxicity

Agitation
Bradysystolic rhythms
Cardiovascular system manifestations
Central nervous system depression
Hallucinations
Hyperreflexia
Hypertension
Hypotension with vascular collapse
Neuromuscular system manifestations
Nystagmus
Rigidity
Seizure
Sinus tachycardia

blocking the production of prostaglandins, which are chemicals that cause inflammation and trigger transmission of pain signals to the brain. Nonsteroidal antiinflammatory drugs are used widely to relieve symptoms caused by types of arthritis (rheumatoid arthritis, osteoarthritis, gout) and to treat back pain, menstrual pain, headaches, minor postoperative pain, and soft tissue injuries. Common nonsteroidal antiinflammatory drugs include diflunisal, fenoprofen, ibuprofen, and naproxen. Ibuprofen and naproxen are available over the counter.

IBUPROFEN OVERDOSE

Ibuprofen is one of the most commonly ingested nonsteroidal antiinflammatory drugs in overdose. The effects usually are reversible and are seldom life threatening. However, significant toxicity may result in coma, seizure, hypotension, and acute renal failure. Chronic and acute ingestion is usually more than 300 mg/kg. In such an ingestion, common symptoms include mild gastrointestinal and CNS disturbances. These usually resolve within 24 hours after ingestion. Other less common effects include mild metabolic acidosis, muscle fasciculations, chills, hyperventilation, hypotension, and asymptomatic bradycardia. Emergency care for patients who have ingested toxic amounts of ibuprofen may consist of gastric decontamination. These patients require careful monitoring for secondary complications such as hypotension and dysrhythmias.

SALICYLATE OVERDOSE

Salicylates are widely available in prescription and over-the-counter products such as acetylsalicylic acid (*aspirin*), many cold preparations, and oil of wintergreen (methyl salicylate) and in combination with some analgesics such as propoxyphene and oxycodone. Table 34-4 contains general guidelines for salicylate toxicity.

> ### NOTE
> At one time, the ingestion of colorful and tasty children's aspirin was the most common cause of pediatric poisoning. In response to this problem, the number of tablets now is limited to 36 per container. Because of the association of aspirin with Reye's syndrome, aspirin is not recommended for children younger than 16 years of age who have viral symptoms.

The process of toxicity with salicylate poisoning is complex. Toxicity includes direct CNS stimulation, interference with cellular glucose uptake, and inhibition of Krebs cycle enzymes that affect energy production and amino acid metabolism. The volume of distribution is dose-dependent and usually small. With toxic ingestion, however, redistribution of the drug into the CNS occurs. This prolongs elimination of the drug from the body. Complications that may result from chronic or acute ingestion of salicylates include CNS stimulation, gastrointestinal irritation, inhibition of glucose metabolism, fluid and

TABLE 34-4 Toxicity Guidelines to Salicylate	
Toxicity	**Amount Ingested**
Mild	<150 mg/kg
Moderate to severe	150-300 mg/kg
Severe	>300 mg/kg
Fatal	>500 mg/kg

From Clark J: *Pharmacological basis of nursing*, ed 10, St Louis, 2001, Mosby.

electrolyte imbalance, neurological symptoms, and coagulation defects. Confusion, lethargy, convulsions, respiratory arrest, coma, and brain death can occur in severe salicylate poisoning.

In addition to general supportive measures, prehospital care for salicylate poisoning may include the administration of **activated charcoal** for decontamination of the gastrointestinal tract. Treatment also may include intravenously administered glucose to manage hypoglycemia. Salicylates are weak acids that can be excreted by the kidney. Thus medical direction may recommend the administration of **sodium bicarbonate** in an effort to produce alkaline urine. Definitive care includes in-hospital intensive care observation, continued support of vital functions, and perhaps hemodialysis.

> **CRITICAL THINKING**
> Would you predict tachypnea or bradypnea in these patients? Why?

ACETAMINOPHEN OVERDOSE

Acetaminophen is a commonly prescribed analgesic and antipyretic agent. Acetaminophen is available in many prescription and nonprescription preparations (e.g., Tylenol and Panadol). The widespread availability of acetaminophen accounts for its high incidence in unintentional and intentional poisoning. Acetaminophen is 1 of the 10 most commonly used drugs for intentional self-poisoning and is associated with significant morbidity and mortality.[8] Acetaminophen overdose can cause life-threatening liver damage from toxic metabolites if it is not managed within 16 to 24 hours of ingestion. As few as 30 standard-size (325-mg) acetaminophen tablets are toxic in an average adult. Acetaminophen also is present in many drug combinations including Darvocet-N, Excedrin, and Sinutab.

Acute acetaminophen ingestion includes doses of 140 mg/kg or greater. The toxic effects of such an ingestion can be classified in four stages (Box 34-24). The course of toxicity begins with mild symptoms that may be overlooked or masked by more dramatic effects of other agents followed by temporary clinical improvement and finally peak liver

BOX 34-24 Stages of Acetaminophen Poisoning

Stage I: Gastrointestinal Irritability (0 to 24 hours)

Anorexia
Diaphoresis
General malaise
Nausea
Pallor
Vomiting

Stage II: Abnormal Laboratory Findings (24 to 48 hours)

Possible abdominal pain and tenderness in the right abdominal quadrant
Resolution of stage I symptoms

Stage III: Hepatic Damage (72 to 96 hours)

Dysrhythmias
Hepatotoxicity with significant increase in hepatic enzymes
Hypoglycemia
Jaundice
Lethargy
Vomiting

Stage IV: Recovery (4 to 14 days) or Progressive Hepatic Failure*

Resolution of hepatic dysfunction
Lack of permanent effects in patients who recover

*NOTE: The percentage of patients who recover in stage IV depends on the amount of acetaminophen ingested and whether effective therapy (activated charcoal, acetylcysteine, or both) was given. Patients with serum levels in the hepatotoxic range have mortality rates up to 25% if untreated.

BOX 34-25 Uppers, Downers, and All-Arounders

Uppers

Anabolic steroids
Coke/crack
Ecstasy
Speed/meth/crystal

Downers

Alcohol
Benzodiazepines (diazepam, temazepam, Rohypnol)
Gamma-hydroxybutyrate (GHB)
Heroin

All-Arounders

Cannabis/skunk
Ketamine
Lysergic acid diethylamide (LSD)
Poppers (alkyl nitrates)

damage. (If acetaminophen was the only drug taken and a dangerously high dose was ingested, the first two stages may be asymptomatic.) If antidote management is started within 8 hours of ingestion, full recovery should occur.

CRITICAL THINKING

Do you think most laypersons realize that acetaminophen overdose can be fatal?

Emergency care includes respiratory, cardiac, and hemodynamic support in critically ill patients. If ingestion is within 1 hour and the patient is alert, medical direction may recommend the administration of *activated charcoal.* Patients with progressive acetaminophen toxicity require in-hospital administration of its antidote, *N*-acetylcysteine.

Drugs Abused for Sexual Purposes/ Sexual Gratification

Some drugs are abused for sexual purposes or for sexual gratification. These drugs commonly are classified by users as "uppers," "downers," and "all-arounders" (those that have more than one primary effect). Box 34-25 gives a

sampling of these drugs. These drugs generally are taken alone or in combination to produce one or more of the following effects:

- A sense of euphoria
- Excitation ("rush")
- Relaxation ("blissed out")
- A loss of inhibition

Each of these drugs has different chemical structures, mechanisms of action, and side effects. So the problems associated with their use can vary greatly. Signs and symptoms of use of these drugs can range from mild nausea and vomiting to life-threatening respiratory depression, hypotension, **methemoglobinemia** (elevated serum hemoglobin level), coma, and death. The emergency care for these patients mainly is supportive. Care includes airway, ventilatory, and circulatory support, and rapid transport for physician evaluation. As with all other cases of patients who use mood-altering agents, personal safety is of primary importance.

SECTION THREE
Alcoholism

Alcohol and related illness continue to be a major problem in the United States. In 2008, 51.6% of Americans age 12 years and older reported current use of alcohol; 23.3% of the population admitted to binge drinking (5 or more drinks within 2 hours); and 23.3% of the population reported drinking 5 or more drinks per occasion on 5 or more days per month.[21] In addition, the most recent statistics report that alcohol is a key factor in 41% of vehicle fatalities, 68% of manslaughters, 62% of assaults, 54% of murder attempts, and 48% of robberies. The economic cost of alcohol and other drug-related crime is $61.8 billion annually.[2]

ALCOHOL DEPENDENCE

Alcohol dependence is a disorder characterized by chronic, excessive consumption of alcohol that results in injury to health or in inadequate social function and the development of withdrawal symptoms when the patient stops drinking suddenly. An estimated 5 million alcohol-dependent persons (1 in 50) live in the United States. Another 10 million have a difficult time controlling their consumption of the drug.[22] Alcohol dependence should be considered a chronic, progressive, potentially fatal disease characterized by remissions, relapses, and cures.

The development of alcohol dependence can be divided into four main stages.[23] These stages merge imperceptibly. The time frame of these stages may range from 5 to 25 years, but the average is about 10 years. In the first stage, tolerance of the drug develops in the heavy social drinker. This allows a person to consume larger quantities of alcohol before experiencing its ill effects. On entering the second stage, the drinker experiences memory lapses relating to events occurring during the drinking episodes. The third stage is characterized by loss or lack of control over alcohol; the drinker can no longer be certain of discontinuing alcohol consumption at will. The final stage begins with prolonged binges of intoxication. This is associated with mental and physical complications. Some drinkers halt their consumption for a brief time or permanently during one of the first three stages. The active ingredient in all alcoholic beverages is ethanol, a colorless, flammable liquid produced from the fermentation of carbohydrates by yeast.

Metabolism

About 80% to 90% of ingested alcohol is absorbed within 30 minutes. (Twenty percent is absorbed in the stomach, the rest in the small intestine.) Once absorbed, the drug is distributed rapidly throughout the vascular space. Alcohol reaches virtually every organ system. About 3% to 5% of alcohol is excreted unchanged via the lungs and kidneys; the rest is metabolized in the liver to carbon dioxide and water. The actual rate at which alcohol is metabolized depends on individual variation (e.g., physical and mental state, body weight, and size). Metabolism also depends on whether the drinker is alcohol-dependent.

Blood Alcohol Content

The alcohol content of blood is measured in terms of mass (milligrams) of alcohol per given volume of blood (deciliter). Blood alcohol content is used widely to evaluate the CNS status of an intoxicated person. In most states the legal limit of intoxication is 80 mg/dL. (This is equivalent to 0.08%.) Some states have laws that allow paramedics to assist in conducting breathalyzer or blood tests to detect alcohol or drug intoxication. EMS personnel should be well versed in the laws of their state before assisting with these tests and follow established protocols carefully.

MEDICAL CONSEQUENCES OF CHRONIC ALCOHOL INGESTION

Alcohol affects nearly every organ system of the body. Thus persons who consume large amounts of alcohol are at risk for a number of physical and mental disorders. These include neurological disorders, nutritional deficiencies, fluid and electrolyte imbalances, gastrointestinal disorders, cardiac and skeletal muscle myopathy, and immune suppression. In addition, alcohol may affect a patient's ability to tolerate traumatic injury.

Neurological Disorders

Alcohol is a potent CNS depressant. When consumed in moderate amounts, the drug reduces anxiety and tension. Alcohol gives most drinkers a feeling of relaxation and confidence. Initial feelings of well-being develop into impaired judgment and discrimination, prolonged reflexes, and incoordination and drowsiness. This ultimately may progress to stupor and coma. The long-term neurological effects of chronic alcohol abuse are similar to those of the aging process. They include short-term memory deficit, problems with coordination, and difficulty with concentration and abstraction.

Nutritional Deficiencies

Alcohol can satisfy the caloric requirements of the body for a brief time. Yet alcohol does not have essential vitamins, proteins, or fats. Thus alcohol-dependent persons may have a decreased dietary intake and malabsorption. This leads to multiple vitamin and mineral deficiencies that can cause altered immunity, poor wound healing, anorexia, cardiac dysrhythmias, and seizures.

WERNICKE-KORSAKOFF SYNDROME

Alcohol-dependent persons are at particular risk of developing **Wernicke-Korsakoff syndrome.** This results from a reduction in intestinal absorption and metabolism of thiamine caused by alcohol. The disease affects the brain and nervous system. The syndrome disrupts central and peripheral nerve function. The disease may consist of two stages: Wernicke's encephalopathy and Korsakoff's psychosis, or a combination of the two.

Wernicke's encephalopathy usually develops suddenly with the clinical manifestations of ataxia, nystagmus, disturbances of speech and gait, signs of neuropathy (paresthesias, impaired reflexes), stupor, and (rarely) coma.[24] Because the body needs thiamine to metabolize glucose, the syndrome may be caused by the intravenous administration of glucose or glucose-containing fluids in the malnourished patient. Coma may be the sole manifestation of Wernicke's encephalopathy. Therefore medical direction may recommend the intravenous administration of *thiamine* before giving IV glucose in patients with altered mental status or coma of unknown origin.

CRITICAL THINKING
Why do you think recognizing this syndrome is delayed in alcoholic patients?

Many chronic alcoholic patients also display signs of **Korsakoff's psychosis**. This is a mental disorder often found with Wernicke's encephalopathy. Signs include apathy, poor retentive memory, retrograde amnesia, confabulation (invention of stories to make up for gaps in memory), and dementia. Korsakoff's psychosis usually is considered irreversible. It leaves the patient permanently handicapped by memory loss, requiring continual supervision.

Fluid and Electrolyte Imbalances

Urinary output increases after ingesting alcohol, over and above that expected from the amount of fluid ingested. This diuresis results because alcohol blocks the secretion of antidiuretic hormone. This can lead to dehydration and electrolyte imbalances.

Gastrointestinal Disorders

The effects of alcohol on the gastrointestinal system can produce several types of alcohol-related illnesses and diseases. The alcohol-related gastrointestinal disorders most likely to initiate an EMS response include gastrointestinal hemorrhage, cirrhosis, and acute or chronic pancreatitis.

GASTROINTESTINAL HEMORRHAGE

Four primary causes of gastrointestinal hemorrhage in patients who drink alcohol are gastritis, ulcer formation, esophageal tear (Mallory-Weiss syndrome), and variceal hemorrhage (see Chapter 39).

Gastritis results from the toxic effects of ethanol on the gastric mucosa. This leads to diffuse or localized areas of erosion. In the chronic form of gastritis, blood may ooze continually from the mucosal lining, and ulcers may develop.

Esophageal tears of the gastroesophageal junction, stomach, or esophagus usually follow severe or protracted vomiting or retching. The injury results when gastric contents are forced against an unrelaxed gastroesophageal junction. This produces a sudden increase in pressure and a mucosal tear with subsequent bleeding. The bleeding can be worsened by clotting abnormalities. Such abnormalities are common in patients with alcoholic liver disease.

Varices are a result of portal hypertension caused by cirrhosis. Any of these thin-walled, blood-engorged veins are subject to rupture and hemorrhage. But the most common site is the varices of the esophagus. Bleeding esophagogastric varices remain one of the most difficult conditions to manage. Severe blood loss through vomiting requires aggressive supportive care with large-bore intravenous lines and fluid resuscitation. Like other forms of GI bleeding described in Chapter 29, permissive hypotension to maintain a systolic blood pressure of 80 to 90 mm Hg may be prudent.[25] The paramedic should consult with medical direction or follow established protocol.

LOOK AGAIN
See Chapter 29: Abdominal and Gastrointestinal Disorders, pp. 894-895.

CIRRHOSIS

Cirrhosis of the liver is caused by chronic damage to liver cells and eventual necrosis. In the disease process, bands of fibrous scar tissue develop and disturb the normal structure of the liver. The distortion and fibrosis of the liver lead to portal hypertension. This results in complications such as ascites, splenomegaly, and bleeding esophageal and gastric varices. In addition, cirrhosis may lead to **hepatic encephalopathy.** This is caused by the accumulation of toxic metabolic waste products that normally would be detoxified by a healthy liver. Cirrhosis is the twelfth leading cause of death by disease, accounting for 27,000 deaths each year.[26]

ACUTE OR CHRONIC PANCREATITIS

Alcohol is the most common cause of acute and chronic pancreatitis. Chronic pancreatitis usually produces the same symptoms as the acute form (described in Chapter 29). The pain, however, may last from several hours to several days. The attacks also become more frequent as the condition progresses. The effects of chronic pancreatitis include malabsorption and electrolyte imbalances. Diabetes mellitus also may develop from insufficient insulin production. Complications of pancreatitis are hemorrhagic pancreatitis, sepsis, and pancreatic abscess. These complications are associated with high mortality.

Cardiac and Skeletal Muscle Myopathy

Cardiac and skeletal muscle damage related to alcohol abuse is thought to result from a direct toxic effect of alcohol or its metabolites. In heart muscle, these toxic effects can result in a decreased force of contraction, dysrhythmias, and a tendency to develop congestive heart failure. In skeletal muscle the major symptoms are weakness and muscle wasting.

Immune Suppression

Long-term alcohol abuse renders the immune system less effective. Alcohol abuse suppresses bone marrow production of white blood cells. In addition, production of red blood cells and platelets is often decreased. Alcohol has direct, specific effects on lung tissue. These effects may impair macrophage mobilization and protective ciliary function. As a result, the ability of the body to fight pulmonary infection is lowered. This makes the alcoholic more susceptible to viral and bacterial pneumonia.

CRITICAL THINKING

For what other pulmonary disease is the immune-suppressed alcoholic patient at risk?

Trauma

Alcohol suppresses clotting factors that are produced in the liver. This blood-clotting deficiency makes alcoholics prone to bruising and internal hemorrhage. The deficiency also adds to the frequency of subdural bleeding, even after relatively minor head trauma[27] (see Chapter 40).

ALCOHOL EMERGENCIES

Several other conditions caused by consumption or abstinence from alcohol may require emergency care. These include acute alcohol intoxication, alcohol withdrawal syndromes, and disulfiram-ethanol reaction. Alcohol-induced ketoacidosis and hypoglycemia were discussed in Chapter 26.

LOOK AGAIN

See Chapter 26: Endocrine, pp. 813-814.

Acute Alcohol Intoxication

The ingestion of alcohol may cause acute poisoning if consumed in large amounts over a short period. At toxic levels, hypoventilation (including respiratory arrest), hypotension, and hypothermia may develop. The patient who has signs and symptoms of acute alcohol intoxication should be evaluated for hidden trauma and coexisting medical conditions. These conditions include hypoglycemia, cardiac myopathy and dysrhythmias, gastrointestinal bleeding, polydrug abuse, and ethylene glycol or methanol ingestion. Because the patient is prone to injury and usually has other medical problems, the paramedic should never assume that an intoxicated patient is merely inebriated.

MANAGEMENT

A patient who is mildly intoxicated may need to be transported for physician evaluation. In most cases, management requires patient observation in the emergency department only until the patient is sober. The paramedic should monitor the patient's vital signs and level of consciousness carefully en route. A thorough physical examination is warranted to rule out illness or injury masked by alcohol ingestion.

Care of the acutely intoxicated patient is aimed at protecting the patient from further injury and maintaining vital functions. If the patient is conscious and agitated, restraints may be necessary. If physical restraint becomes necessary, the police should be summoned. After scene safety has been established, the primary survey and resuscitation should include the following:

1. Rapidly evaluate airway patency with spinal precautions. Assess the patient's ventilatory and hemodynamic status while obtaining a history. The patient's account of the event may be unreliable because of the alcohol ingestion.
2. Initiate intravenous therapy. Draw blood samples for laboratory analysis. If hypoglycemia is confirmed, administer **thiamine, dextrose 50%** (per protocol). Give **naloxone** if opioid overdose is suspected.
3. Continually monitor the patient's airway and provide adequate ventilatory and circulatory support as needed. Be prepared to provide suction and aggressive airway management.
4. Monitor the electrocardiogram for dysrhythmias.
5. Rapidly transport the patient for physician evaluation.

Alcohol Withdrawal Syndromes

A period of relative or full abstinence from alcohol may cause withdrawal in an alcoholic. Alcohol withdrawal syndromes are mediated by several mechanisms that result in CNS hyperexcitability. Biochemical changes such as respiratory alkalosis and hypomagnesemia may also play a role. Alcohol withdrawal syndromes can be divided into four general categories: minor reactions, hallucinations, alcohol withdrawal seizures, and delirium tremens.[28]

SHOW ME THE EVIDENCE

These researchers sought to identify factors that predicted mortality in patients with delirium tremens (DT). They investigated 36 deaths related to DT that occurred between 2000 and 2006. Hyperthermia and the use of restraints were associated with an increased risk of death.

Khan A, Levy P, DeHorn S, et al: Predictors of mortality in patients with delirium tremens, *Acad Emerg Med* 15(8):788-790, 2008.

MINOR REACTIONS

Minor reactions begin about 6 to 12 hours after cessation or reduction of alcohol intake. These symptoms peak within 24 to 36 hours. They may persist for 10 to 14 days. When alcohol withdrawal is confined to minor reactions, the prognosis for full recovery is excellent with the proper management. Minor reactions include facial flushing, diaphoresis, nausea and vomiting, slight disorientation, and generalized tremor made worse by agitation. Mild tachycardia, hypertension, and hyperreflexia also may be present.

CRITICAL THINKING
What kinds of feelings do you think the patient and the patient's family may be having during withdrawal reactions?

HALLUCINATIONS

Hallucinations usually occur 12 to 24 hours after the patient stops drinking alcohol. Disorders of perception are common. They may vary from auditory and visual illusions to frank hallucinations. The latter can produce agitation, fear, and panic. During this period, the patient may show signs of suicidal and homicidal tendencies, and minor reactions may be more pronounced. The prognosis for hallucinations is the same as that for minor reactions with appropriate care.

ALCOHOL WITHDRAWAL SEIZURES

Alcohol withdrawal seizures (or "rum fits") usually occur 24 to 48 hours after ethanol cessation. They most often are grand mal of short duration; status seizures are rare.[8] This category of withdrawal may be self-limiting or may progress to delirium tremens with or without a lucid interval. Because of the high drug tolerance level of the alcoholic patient, seizure activity may require intravenous administration of large doses of *diazepam* or *lorazepam.* These drugs may synergistically interact with any ethanol still in the patient's system. Thus vital signs, respirations, and mental status should be monitored closely.

DELIRIUM TREMENS

Delirium tremens is the most dramatic and serious form of alcohol withdrawal. It affects about 5% of all alcoholics hospitalized for withdrawal.[29] Delirium tremens usually occurs 48 to 72 hours after cessation of alcohol. Yet it may be delayed up to 14 days. The syndrome is characterized by psychomotor, speech, and autonomic hyperactivity; profound confusion; disorientation; delusion; vivid hallucinations; tremor; agitation; and insomnia. A single episode may last 1 to 3 days and, with multiple recurrences, may last up to 1 month. Delirium tremens is a true medical

emergency. It has a mortality rate that approaches 15%.[30] Associated alcohol-related illnesses such as pneumonia, pancreatitis, and hepatitis are frequent contributing causes of death.

MANAGEMENT

The care for patients with alcohol withdrawal syndromes mainly is supportive. After scene safety is ensured, the paramedic should carefully monitor the patient's airway, ventilatory, and circulatory status. Intravenous therapy should be initiated with a saline solution for rehydration. Pharmacological therapy may be indicated for an altered level of consciousness, dysrhythmias, or seizure activity. In addition, these patients need calm reassurance and frequent reorientation. All patients with signs and symptoms of alcohol withdrawal syndrome require physician evaluation. Benzodiazepines (e.g., oxazepam, *lorazepam,* and *diazepam*) are often prescribed at regular intervals to help control the withdrawal symptoms.

Disulfiram-Ethanol Reaction

Disulfiram (tetraethylthiuram disulfide [Antabuse]) is a medication prescribed to some alcoholic patients to help them abstain. The drug works by inhibiting ethanol metabolism and by allowing the accumulation of the metabolite acetaldehyde. Acetaldehyde produces ill effects on the gastrointestinal, cardiovascular, and autonomic nervous systems. Acetaldehyde is the metabolic product that is thought to be responsible for the common "hangover." Patients who take disulfiram and then drink alcohol experience an unpleasant and potentially life-threatening physiological response.

The **disulfiram-ethanol reaction** begins 15 to 30 minutes after the ingestion of two to five alcoholic drinks. The reaction continues for 1 to 2 hours. It causes the patient to experience vertigo, headache, vomiting, and flushing, which may give the skin a "lobster-red" appearance. Other effects include dyspnea, diaphoresis, abdominal pain, and sometimes chest pain. More serious reactions include hypotension, shock, and dysrhythmias. Sudden death, myocardial and cerebral infarction, and cerebral hemorrhage also have been reported after as little as one drink of ethanol in patients taking high doses of disulfiram.[31] Acute overdose of disulfiram is now uncommon with current dosing regimens.[8]

MANAGEMENT

Prehospital care for a disulfiram-ethanol reaction involves airway, ventilatory, and circulatory support; administration of intravenous fluids to manage hypotension; pharmacological therapy as needed to manage dysrhythmias; and rapid transport for physician evaluation. Most patients recover from these episodes. Supportive care and in-hospital observation are usually all that are required.

SECTION FOUR
Management of Toxic Syndromes

GENERAL MANAGEMENT PRINCIPLES FOR TOXIC SYNDROMES

As stated before, most poisoned patients require only supportive therapy to recover, regardless of the toxic agent (Box 34-26). However, grouping toxic agents and physical findings into toxic syndromes, or **toxidromes,** can give the paramedic important clues to what type of poison or toxin is involved. This will aid the paramedic in remembering assessment and management strategies as well (Table 34-5). The five toxic syndromes presented in this chapter are the following[3]:

1. Cholinergic
2. Anticholinergic
3. Hallucinogenic
4. Opioid
5. Sympathomimetic

NOTE

Toxic syndrome classification does not consider how or why the toxin was introduced into the body. Thus the paramedic should consider route of entry in addition to specific treatments.

Cholinergics

Exposure to cholinergics is uncommon. However, it is important to recognize cholinergic poisoning so that lifesaving care can be initiated. Causative agents include pesticides (organophosphates, carbamates) and nerve agents (e.g., sarin and soman). Assessment findings include headache, dizziness, weakness, bradycardia, nausea, and a "wet" presentation manifested by profound *s*alivation, *l*acrimation, *u*rination, *d*efecation, *g*astrointestinal upset, and *e*mesis (SLUDGE). In severe cases, coma and convulsions may be present. In addition to airway, ventilatory, and circulatory support and decontamination, drug therapy may include administration of **atropine, pralidoxime, diazepam** or **lorazepam,** and **activated charcoal.**

Anticholinergics

Exposure to anticholinergics is fairly common because so many medications and plants have anticholinergic properties. Examples include drugs such as antihistamines, antipsychotics, antispasmodics, and tricyclic antidepressants; and plants such as jimson weed, night blooming jessamine, panther mushroom, and angel's trumpet. The signs and symptoms include tachycardia; dry, flushed skin; dilated pupils; and facial flushing. This "dry" patient presentation usually is managed with airway, ventilatory, and circulatory support. Physostigmine may be given as an antidote in rare cases, in the absence of tricyclic antidepressant overdose.[7]

TABLE 34-5 Toxicological Syndromes

Common Signs	Causative Agents	Specific Treatment
Cholinergic ("Wet" Patient Presentation)		
Confusion, CNS depression, weakness, SLUDGE (salivation, lacrimation, urination, defecation, gastrointestinal upset, emesis), bradycardia, wheezing, bronchoconstriction, miosis, coma, convulsions, diaphoresis, seizures	Organophosphate and carbamate insecticides, nerve agents, some mushrooms	**Atropine, pralidoxime** (2-PAM chloride), **diazepam** or lorazepam, **activated charcoal**
Anticholinergic ("Dry" Patient Presentation)		
Delirium, tachycardia, dry and flushed skin, dilated pupils, seizures, and dysrhythmias (in severe cases)	Antihistamines, antiparkinson medications, atropine, antipsychotic agents, antidepressants, skeletal muscle relaxants, many plants (e.g., Jimson weed and *Amanita muscaria*)	**Diazepam** or lorazepam, activated charcoal, rarely physostigmine (Antilirium)
Hallucinogens		
Visual illusions, delusions, bizarre behavior, flashbacks, respiratory and CNS depression	LSD, PCP, mescaline, some mushrooms, marijuana, Jimson weed, nutmeg, mace, some amphetamines	Minimal sensory stimulation, calming measures, **diazepam** or lorazepam if necessary
Opioids		
Euphoria, hypotension, respiratory depression/arrest, nausea, pinpoint pupils, seizures, coma	Heroin, **morphine,** codeine, **meperidine** (Demerol), propoxyphene, fentanyl	**Naloxone** (Narcan), **nalmefene** (Revex)
Sympathomimetics		
Delusions, paranoia, tachycardia or bradycardia, hypertension, diaphoresis; seizures, hypotension, and dysrhythmias in severe cases	Cocaine, amphetamine, methamphetamine, over-the-counter decongestants	Minimal sensory stimulation, calming measures, **diazepam** or lorazepam if necessary; manage dysrhythmias

LSD, Lysergic acid diethylamide; *PCP,* phencyclidine.

BOX 34-26 General Management Guidelines for the Poisoned Patient

1. Ensure scene and personal safety.
2. Provide adequate airway, ventilation, and circulation.
3. Obtain a thorough history, and perform a focused physical examination.
4. Consider hypoglycemia in a patient who is unconscious, convulsing, drowsy, or combative..
5. Administer naloxone or nalmefene to a patient with respiratory depression and suspected opioid ingestion.
6. If overdose is suspected, obtain an overdose history from the patient, family, or friends.
7. Consult with medical direction or a poison control center for specific treatment to prevent further absorption of the toxin (or antidote therapy).
8. Frequently monitor vital signs and electrocardiogram.
9. Safely obtain any substance or substance container of a suspected poison. Transport it with the patient.
10. Transport the patient for physician evaluation.

Hallucinogens

Common hallucinogens include lysergic acid diethylamide (LSD), PCP, peyote, mushrooms, and mescaline. Depending on the agent and dose, signs and symptoms may include CNS stimulation and/or depression, behavioral disturbances, delusions, hypertension, chest pain, tachycardia, seizures, and respiratory and cardiac arrest. Prehospital care for these patients is focused on ensuring personal safety and providing airway, ventilatory, and circulatory support.

Opioids

The opioid syndrome carries a hallmark triad of depressed level of consciousness, respiratory depression, and pinpoint pupils. Common causative agents include heroin, *morphine,* codeine, *meperidine,* oxycodone, hydrocodone, and *fentanyl.* Drugs in this class often are mixed with alcohol or other drugs (e.g., benzodiazepines). This leads to increased respiratory depression, hypotension, and bradycardia. Other signs and symptoms may include euphoria, nausea, pinpoint pupils, and seizures. In addition to ensuring airway, ventilatory, and circulatory support, drug therapy may include the administration of *naloxone* or another opioid-specific antidote agent.

Sympathomimetics

The sympathomimetic syndrome usually results from acute overdose of amphetamines or cocaine. Signs and symptoms include elevated blood pressure, tachycardia, dilated pupils, and altered mental status, including paranoid delusions. In severe cases, cardiovascular collapse can occur. Management consists of ensuring personal safety and providing airway, ventilatory, and circulatory support.

 CRITICAL THINKING
Why is it important to be able to identify these toxic syndromes?

SUMMARY

- A poison is any substance that produces harmful physiological or psychological effects.
- The toxic effects of ingested poisons may be immediate or delayed. This depends on the substance that is ingested. The main goal is to identify effects on the three vital organ systems most likely to produce immediate morbidity and mortality. These are the respiratory system, the cardiovascular system, and the central nervous system. In some cases, serious poisonings by ingestion are managed by preventing the toxic substance from reaching the small intestine. This limits its absorption.
- Strong acids and alkalis may cause burns to the mouth, pharynx, esophagus, and sometimes the upper respiratory and GI tracts. Prehospital care is usually limited to airway and ventilatory support, IV fluid replacement, and rapid transport to the appropriate medical facility.
- The most important physical characteristic in the potential toxicity of ingested hydrocarbons is its viscosity. The lower the viscosity, the higher the risk of aspiration and associated complications. Hydrocarbon ingestion may involve the patient's respiratory, gastro-

intestinal, and neurological systems. The clinical features may be immediate or delayed in onset.
- Methanol is a poisonous alcohol. It is found in a number of products. Methanol itself is no more toxic than ethanol. Yet its metabolites (formaldehyde and formic acid) are very toxic. Ingestion can affect the central nervous system, the gastrointestinal tract, and the eyes. It also can cause the development of metabolic acidosis.
- Ethylene glycol toxicity is caused by the buildup of toxic metabolites, especially glycolic and oxalic acids after metabolism. This occurs mainly in the liver and kidneys. This toxicity may affect the central nervous system and cardiopulmonary and renal systems. It may result in hypocalcemia as well.
- The majority of isopropanol (isopropyl alcohol) is metabolized to acetone after ingestion. Isopropanol poisoning affects several body systems, including the central nervous, gastrointestinal, and renal systems.
- Infants and children are high-risk groups for accidental iron, lead, and mercury poisoning. This is due to their immature immune systems or increased absorption as a function of age. Ingested iron is corrosive to

Continued

gastrointestinal tract mucosa. It may produce lethal GI hemorrhage, bloody vomitus, painless bloody diarrhea, and dark stools.

- Food poisoning is a term used for any illness of sudden onset (usually associated with stomach pain, vomiting, and diarrhea) suspected of being caused by food eaten within the previous 48 hours. Food poisoning can be classified as infectious. This results from a bacterium or virus. It also can be classified as noninfectious. This results from toxins and pollutants.

- The toxic effects of major poisonous plant ingestions are predictable. They are categorized by the chemical and physical properties of the plant. Most responses are consistent with the type of major toxic chemical component in the plant.

- The concentration of a chemical in the air helps to predict the severity of an inhalation injury. The duration of exposure helps to determine this as well. Solubility also influences the extent of an inhalation injury. Highly reactive chemicals cause more severe and rapid injury than less reactive chemicals. Properties that determine chemical reactivity are chemical pH; direct-acting potential of chemicals; indirect-acting potential of chemicals; and allergic potential of chemicals.

- Cyanide refers to any of a number of highly toxic substances that contain the cyanogen chemical group. Regardless of the route of entry, cyanide is a rapidly acting poison. It combines and reacts with ferric ions of the respiratory enzyme cytochrome oxidase. This inhibits cellular oxygenation. This can produce a rapid progression from dyspnea to paralysis, unconsciousness, and death.

- Ammonia is a toxic irritant. It causes local pulmonary complications after inhalation. In severe cases, bronchospasm and pulmonary edema may develop.

- Hydrocarbon inhalation may cause aspiration pneumonitis. It also has the potential for systemic effects such as CNS depression and liver, kidney, or bone marrow toxicity.

- Simple asphyxiants cause toxicity by lowering ambient oxygen concentration. Chemical asphyxiants possess intrinsic systemic toxicity. This toxicity occurs after absorption into the circulation. Irritants or corrosives cause cellular destruction and inflammation as they come into contact with moisture in the respiratory tract.

- The general principles of managing inhaled poisons are the same as those for any other hazardous materials incident.

- Hymenoptera and Arachnida cause the highest incidence of need for emergency care. Arthropod venoms are complex and diverse in their chemistry and pharmacology. They may produce major toxic reactions in sensitized persons. Such reactions include anaphylaxis and upper airway obstruction.

- The two main families of venomous snakes indigenous to the United States are pit vipers and coral snakes. Pit viper venom can produce various toxic effects on blood and other tissues. These effects include hemolysis, intravascular coagulation, convulsions, and acute renal failure. The venom of the coral snake is mainly neurotoxic. Signs and symptoms range from slurred speech, dilated pupils, and dysphagia to flaccid paralysis and death.

- The marine animals most likely to be involved in human poisonings in U.S. coastal waters are coelenterates, echinoderms, and stingrays. Coelenterate envenomation ranges in severity from irritant dermatitis to excruciating pain, respiratory depression, and life-threatening cardiovascular collapse. Echinoderm toxins may cause immediate intense pain, swelling, redness, aching in the affected extremity, and nausea. Delayed effects may include respiratory distress, paresthesia of the lips and face, and, in severe cases, respiratory paralysis and complete atonia. Locally, stingray venom produces a painful traumatic injury. It may cause bleeding and necrosis. Systemic manifestations range from weakness and nausea to seizures, paralysis, hypotension, and death.

- Organophosphates and carbamates inhibit the effects of acetylcholinesterase. A mnemonic that may help the paramedic to recognize this type of poisoning is SLUDGE. (This stands for *s*alivation, *l*acrimation, *u*rination, *d*efecation, *g*astrointestinal upset, and *e*mesis.) The most specific findings, however, are miosis, rapidly changing pupils, and muscle fasciculation.

- General principles for managing drug abuse and overdose include providing scene safety; ensuring adequate airway, breathing, and circulation; obtaining a history; identifying the substance; performing a focused physical exam; initiating an IV; administering an antidote if needed; preventing further absorption; and providing rapid patient transport.

- Narcotics are CNS depressants. They can cause life-threatening respiratory depression. In severe intoxication, hypotension, profound shock, and pulmonary edema may be present. Naloxone is a pure narcotic antagonist effective for virtually all narcotic and narcotic-like substances.

- Sedative-hypnotic agents include benzodiazepines and barbiturates. Signs and symptoms of sedative-hypnotic overdose are chiefly related to the central nervous and cardiovascular systems. Flumazenil (Romazicon) is a benzodiazepine antagonist. It is useful in reversing the effects of these agents if they were given in a clinical setting.

- Commonly used stimulant drugs are those of the amphetamine family. Adverse effects include tachycardia, hypertension, tachypnea, agitation, dilated pupils, tremors, and disorganized behavior. With sudden withdrawal, the patient becomes depressed, suicidal, incoherent, or nearly comatose.

- Phencyclidine (PCP) is a dissociative analgesic with sympathomimetic and CNS stimulant and depressant effects. In low doses, PCP intoxication produces an unpredictable state that can resemble drunkenness (and rage). High-dose intoxication may cause coma. This may last from several hours to days. Respiratory depression, hypertension, and tachycardia may be present. PCP psychosis is a psychiatric emergency. It may mimic schizophrenia.

- Hallucinogens are substances that cause distortions of perceptions. Depending on the agent, overdose may range from visual hallucinations and anticholinergic syndromes to more serious complications, including psychosis, flashbacks, and respiratory and CNS depression.

- Tricyclic antidepressant (TCA) toxicity is thought to result from central and peripheral, atropine-like anticholinergic effects and direct depressant effects on myocardial function. A prolonged QRS complex, a GCS score less than 8, or both, should alert the paramedic to a major TCA toxicity.

- Lithium is a mood-stabilizing drug. Toxic ingestion can include CNS effects that can range from blurred vision and confusion to seizure and coma.

- Cardiac drugs are a common cause of poisoning deaths in children and adults. The drugs responsible for the majority of these fatalities are digitalis, beta blockers, and calcium channel blockers.

- MAO inhibitors block or diminish the activity of the monoamines (norepinephrine, dopamine, serotonin). Toxic effects include CNS depression and various neuromuscular and cardiovascular system manifestations.

- Nonsteroidal antiinflammatory drugs (NSAIDs) work by blocking the production of prostaglandins. The effects of overdose of ibuprofen are usually reversible, are seldom life threatening, and include mild GI and CNS effects. Salicylate poisoning may cause CNS stimulation, GI irritation, inhibition of glucose metabolism, fluid and electrolyte imbalance, and coagulation defects.

- Acetaminophen overdose may cause life-threatening liver damage. This results from formation of a hepatotoxic intermediate metabolite if it is not managed within 16 to 24 hours of ingestion.

- Some drugs are abused for sexual purposes or for sexual gratification. These are commonly classified by users as "uppers," "downers," and those that have more than one primary effect ("all-arounders"). Problems associated with their use vary widely.

- Alcohol dependence is a disorder characterized by chronic, excessive consumption of alcohol that results in injury to health or in inadequate social function and the development of withdrawal symptoms when the patient stops drinking suddenly. Alcohol causes multiple systemic effects. These include neurological disorders, nutritional deficiencies, fluid and electrolyte imbalances, gastrointestinal disorders, cardiac and skeletal muscle myopathy, and immune suppression. Several conditions caused by consumption or abstinence from alcohol that may require emergency care are acute alcohol intoxication, alcohol withdrawal syndromes, and disulfiram-ethanol reaction.

- The most common toxic syndromes are cholinergic, anticholinergic, hallucinogenic, opioid, and sympathomimetic. Using these classifications allows the paramedic to group similar toxic agents together. It allows the paramedic to more easily remember how to assess and treat the poisoned patient.

REFERENCES

1. Centers for Disease Control and Prevention: *Poisonings in the United States: fact sheet*, www.cdc.gov/ncipc/factsheets/poisoning.htm, accessed 9-8-10.
2. National Safety Council: *Injury facts*, Chicago, 2010, The Council.
3. Bronstein AC, Spyker DA, Cantilena LR Jr, et al: 2007 Annual Report of the American Association of Poison Control Centers' National Poison Data System (NPDS): 25th Annual Report, *Clin Toxicol (Phila)* 46(10):927-1057, 2007.
4. National Academy of Sciences: *Forging a poison prevention and control system*, Washington, DC, 2004, National Academic Press.
5. American Heart Association: 2010 American Heart Association Guidelines for Cardiopulmonary Resuscitation and Emergency Cardiovascular Care, *Circulation* 122(18 Supplement 3):S840, 2010.
6. Chyka, PA, Seger D, Krenzelok EP, Vale JA: Position paper: Single-dose activated charcoal, *Clin Toxicol* 43:61-87, 2005.
7. www.goldstandard.com.
8. Marx JA, Hockberger RS, Walls RM, et al: *Rosen's emergency medicine: concepts and clinical practice*, ed 6, St Louis, 2006, Mosby.
9. OSHA: *Occupational Exposure Standards: Methanol*, CASRN: 67-56.
10. Albrecgt G: MRI of the brain in methanol intoxication, *Clin Neuroradiol* 18(2):122-126, 2006.
11. Centers for Disease Control and Prevention: *Lead*, www.cdc.gov/nceh/lead, accessed 9-8-10.
12. Brent J, Wallace K, Burkhart K: *Critical care toxicology: diagnosis and management of the critically poisoned patient*, St Louis, 2004, Mosby.
13. Borak J, Callan M, Abbott W, et al: *Hazardous materials exposure*, Englewood Cliffs, NJ, 1991, Prentice Hall.
14. Cyanokit package insert, Columbia, Md, 2009, Meridian Medical Technologies, Inc.
15. Auerbach PS, editor: *Wilderness medicine*, ed 5, St Louis, 2007, Mosby.

16. West Nile Virus Update—United States January-July 22, 2008, *MMRW* 57(29):801, 2008.

17. Centers for Disease Control and Prevention: *West Nile virus: what you need to know,* www.cdc.gov/ncidod/dvbid/westnile/wnv_factsheet.htm, accessed 9-11-10.

18. American Heart Association: 2010 American Heart Association Guidelines for Cardiopulmonary Resuscitation and Emergency Cardiovascular Care, *Circulation* 122(18 Supplement 3):S639-S946, 2010.

19. U.S. Food and Drug Administration: *Report to the FDA Drug Safety and Risk Management Advisory Committee on evaluating and scheduling recommendations for dextromethorphan,* www.fda.gov/downloads/advisorycommittees/drugs/ucm224446.pdf, accessed 10-16-10.

20. National Institutes of Health: *Serotonin syndrome,* www.nlm.nih.gov/medlineplus/ency/article/007272.htm, accessed 2-15-10.

21. National Institute on Drug Abuse, The Science of Drug Abuse and Addiction: *Alcohol,* www.drugabuse.gov/DrugPages/Alcohol.html, accessed 12-1-09.

22. National Institute on Alcohol Abuse and Alcoholism: Alcohol use disorders surpass drug use disorders, *Spectrum* 1(1), Sept 2009, www.spectrum.niaaa.nih.gov/media/pdf/NIAAA_Spectrum_Dec_12_tagged_wbleed.pdf, accessed 10-16-10.

23. Jellinek EM: *The disease concept of alcoholism,* New Haven, 1960, Hillhouse.

24. Caine D, Halliday GM, Krill JJ, et al: Operational criteria for the classification of chronic alcoholics: identification of Wernicke's encephalopathy, *J Neurosurg Psychiatr* 62(1):51-60, 1997.

25. McSwain NE: *PHTLS: Prehospital Trauma Life Support,* ed 6, St Louis, 2007, Mosby.

26. National Institute of Diabetes and Digestive and Kidney Disease, National Institutes of Health: *Cirrhosis,* http://digestive.niddk.nih.gov/ddiseases/pubs/cirrhosis/, accessed 9-11-10.

27. Saito T, Kushi H, Makino K, et al: The risk factors for the occurrence of acute brain swelling in acute subdural hematoma, *Acta Neurochir Suppl* 86:351-354, 2003.

28. American Psychiatric Association: *Diagnostic and statistical manual of mental disorders,* ed 4, Washington, DC, 2000.

29. Fiellin DA, O'Connor PG, Holmboe ES, et al: Risk for delirium tremens in patients with alcohol withdrawal syndrome, *Subst Abus* 23(2):83-94, 2002.

30. McCowan C, Marik P: Refractory delirium tremens treated with propofol: a case series, *Crit Care Med* 28(6):1781-1784, 2000.

31. Soghoiam S, Wiener WS: *Toxicity, disulfiram,* http://emedicine.medscape.com/article/814525-overview, accessed 9-11-10.

SUGGESTED READINGS

Baud FJ, Barriot P, Toffis V, et al: Elevated blood cyanide concentrations in victims of smoke inhalation, *N Engl J Med* 325(25):1761-1766, 1991.

Centers for Disease Control and Prevention: Emergency department visits involving nonmedical use of selected prescription drugs—United States, 2004-2008, *MMWR* 59(23):705-709, 2010.

Clark J: Isopropyl alcohol intoxication, *J Emerg Nurs* 36(1):81-82, 2010.

Koschel MJ: Where there's smoke, there may be cyanide, *Am J Nurs* 102(8):39-42, 2002.

Lopez DP: Emergency: acetaminophen poisoning, *Am J Nurs* 109(9):48-51, 2009.

Perrone J, DeRoos F: Clinical alert: the new high, *JEMS online* 32(1), 2007.

United States National Library of Medicine: *TOXNET,* retrieved 3-19-10 from http://toxnet.nlm.nih.gov/.

35 Behavioral and Psychiatric Disorders

Upon completion of this chapter, the paramedic student will be able to:

1. Define what constitutes a behavioral emergency.
2. Identify potential causes for behavioral and psychiatric illnesses.
3. List three critical principles that should be considered in the prehospital care of any patient with a behavioral emergency.
4. Outline key elements in the prehospital patient examination during a behavioral emergency.
5. Describe effective techniques for interviewing a patient during a behavioral emergency.
6. Distinguish between key symptoms and management techniques for selected behavioral and psychiatric disorders.
7. Identify factors that must be considered when assessing suicide risk.
8. Formulate appropriate interview questions to determine suicidal intent.
9. Explain prehospital management techniques for the patient who has attempted suicide.
10. Describe assessment of the potentially violent patient.
11. Outline measures that may be used in an attempt to safely diffuse a potentially violent patient situation.
12. List situations when patient restraints can be used.
13. Discuss key principles in patient restraint.
14. Describe safety measures taken when patient violence is anticipated.
15. Explain variations in approach to behavioral emergencies in children.

KEY TERMS

acute psychosis A condition that refers to a patient who presents with one or more of the following criteria: a sudden onset of delusions that rapidly change; hallucinations; bizarre behavior and posture; or disorganized speech.

affect An outward manifestation of a person's feelings or emotions.

agitated delirium Describes a person with delirium who has (1) acute onset and fluctuating course, (2) reduced clarity of awareness of the environment, (3) perceptual disturbance, disorientation, or memory disturbance, and (4) underlying general medical condition.

anhedonia The inability to enjoy what is usually pleasurable.

anorexia nervosa A disorder characterized by a prolonged refusal to eat, resulting in emaciation, amenorrhea, emotional disturbance concerning body image, and an abnormal fear of becoming obese.

anxiety A state or feeling of apprehension, uneasiness, agitation, uncertainty, and fear resulting from the anticipation of some threat or danger.

autism spectrum disorder A range of neurodevelopmental disorders characterized by three sets of behavioral features: (1) impairment in social interaction, (2) communication deficits (both verbal and nonverbal), and (3) restricted, repetitive behaviors, including decreased imaginative play, stereotyped behaviors, and inflexible adherence to routines.

behavioral emergency A change in mood or behavior that cannot be tolerated by the involved person or others and that requires immediate attention.

biological disturbances Mental disorders that result from a physical rather than a purely psychological cause.

bipolar disorder A disorder marked by alternating periods of mania and depression; also known as manic-depressive disorder.

bulimia nervosa A disorder characterized by an insatiable craving for food, often resulting in episodes of binge eating followed by purging (through self-induced vomiting or use of laxatives), depression, and self-deprivation.

chemical restraint The use of drugs to control behavior.

clinical depression A disabling condition that adversely affects a person's family, work or school life, sleeping and eating habits, and general health; also known as *major depression.*

cognitive disorder A disorder that results in a disturbance of cognitive functioning.

conversion disorder A mental illness in which painful emotions are repressed and unconsciously converted into physical symptoms.

delirium An abrupt disorientation for time and place, usually with delusions and hallucinations.

delusions Persistent beliefs or perceptions held by a person despite evidence that refutes them (i.e., false beliefs).

dementia A slow, progressive loss of awareness of time and place. It usually involves an inability to learn new things or recall recent events.

depression A mood disturbance characterized by feelings of sadness, despair, and discouragement.

dissociative disorders A group of psychological illnesses. In these illnesses, a particular mental function is separated (dissociated) from the mind as a whole.

dyskinesia An impairment of the ability to execute voluntary movements; often an adverse effect of prolonged use of antipsychotic medications.

dysthymia A form of depression that is chronic in nature, lasting as long as 2 years or more.

factitious disorders A group of disorders in which symptoms mimic a true illness. However, the symptoms have actually been invented.

hallucinations The apparent perception of sights, sounds, and other sensory phenomena that are not actually present.

impulse control disorders A group of psychiatric conditions characterized by the inability to resist an impulse or a temptation to perform some act that is unlawful, socially unacceptable, or self-harmful.

mania A mood disorder characterized by extreme excitement, hyperactivity, agitation, and sometimes violent and self-destructive behavior.

mental status examination An evaluation tool that includes an assessment of appearance and behavior,

speech and language, emotional stability, and cognitive abilities.

mood disorder Refers to changes in emotions that a person experiences in life (e.g., happiness, depression, fear, and anxiety).

Munchausen syndrome A factitious disorder in which the patient makes routine pleas for treatment and hospitalization for a symptomatic, but imaginary, acute illness.

Munchausen syndrome by proxy A factitious disorder in which a person injures or induces illness in others (usually children) in order to gain sympathy.

obsessive-compulsive disorder A psychiatric disorder in which a person feels stress or anxiety about thoughts or rituals over which the individual has little control.

panic disorder An anxiety disorder characterized by unexpected and repeated episodes of intense fear accompanied by physical symptoms that may include chest pain, heart palpitations, shortness of breath, dizziness, or abdominal distress.

paranoia A condition characterized by an elaborate, overly suspicious system of thinking.

personality disorder A large group of conditions distinguished by a failure to learn from experience or to adapt appropriately to changes; results in personal distress and impairment of social functioning.

phobia An anxiety disorder characterized by an obsessive, irrational, and intense fear of a specific object or activity.

posttraumatic stress disorder An anxiety reaction to a severe psychosocial event; also known as *posttraumatic syndrome.*

psychosis Maladaptive behavior involving major distortions of reality.

schizophrenia A group of disorders characterized by recurrent episodes of psychotic behavior.

somatization disorder A condition in which an individual has complaints (lasting several years) of various physical problems for which no physical cause can be found.

somatoform disorder Any of a group of neurotic disorders characterized by symptoms suggesting physical illness or disease, for which there are no organic or physiological causes.

suicide The act of a human being intentionally causing his or her own death.

*C*aring for a patient with a behavioral or psychiatric emergency can be challenging, even for the most experienced practitioner. These emergencies call for strong diagnostic skills and a good understanding of pharmacology and toxicology. They also require thorough assessment skills to identify organic illness that can masquerade as a psychiatric condition. Behavioral and psychiatric emergencies demand excellent communication skills, a compassionate and caring approach, and supportive measures to prevent a crisis from escalating.

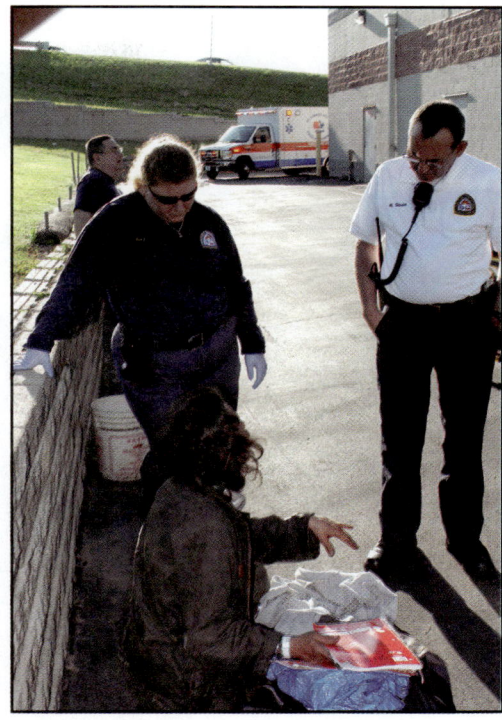

(Courtesy Ray Kemp, St. Charles, Mo.)

UNDERSTANDING BEHAVIORAL EMERGENCIES

An estimated 26.2% of Americans age 18 and older (1 in 4 adults) suffer from a diagnosable mental disorder in a given year. This number translates to about 57.7 million people.[1]

The National Institute of Mental Health has estimated that one in seven individuals will need treatment at some point in life for an emotional disturbance. Mental health problems are the leading cause of disability in the United States and Canada for people 15 to 44 years of age.

There is no clear agreement or ideal model for "normal" behavior. It generally is considered to be adaptive behavior that is accepted by society. (This can vary by culture and ethnic group.) The concept of "abnormal" (maladaptive) behavior also is defined by society when behavior:

- Deviates from society's norms and expectations
- Interferes with well-being and ability to function
- Harms the individual or group

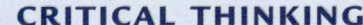

CRITICAL THINKING
Can you think of a time in your life when you, a family member, or a close friend had a behavior that fit the definition of abnormal behavior? How did it make you feel?

A **behavioral emergency** can be defined as a change in mood or behavior that cannot be tolerated by the involved person or others and that requires immediate attention. Behavioral emergencies may range from a brief inability to cope with stress or anxiety to more intense situations in which patients may be dangerous to themselves and others. However, most people with mental illness function well on a daily basis. Common conditions such as depression, anxiety disorders, and mild personality disorders often are effectively managed with medication and counseling in outpatient mental health centers. Most behavioral emergencies have a biological/organic, psychosocial, or sociocultural cause. Mental illness also may be the result of more

than one of these factors (Figure 35-1). Ten common myths about mental illness are listed in Box 35-1.

Biological Causes

Physical or biochemical disturbances in the brain can result in significant changes in behavior. In mental health care, **biological disturbances** are mental disorders that result from a physical rather than a purely psychological cause. Examples of biological causes include genetic factors, prenatal and postnatal factors (including infection, and endocrine, metabolic, and vascular disorders), an imbalance in brain chemistry (which may have a heritable component), and alterations in neurotransmission. An example of a biological mental illness is schizophrenia, described later in this chapter. In this illness, specific genes have been identified that may influence the balance of chemicals in the brain. As described in Chapter 13: Principles of Pharmacology and Emergency Medications, neurotransmitters are responsible for communication among the brain cells. To review, the predominant neurotransmitters in the brain include glutamate, γ-aminobutyric acid (GABA), **serotonin,** dopamine, and norepinephrine. Most scientists believe that mental illnesses result from problems with communication between these neurotransmitters and the neurons in the brain.

LOOK AGAIN
See Chapter 13: Principles of Pharmacology and Emergency Medications, pp. 308-310.

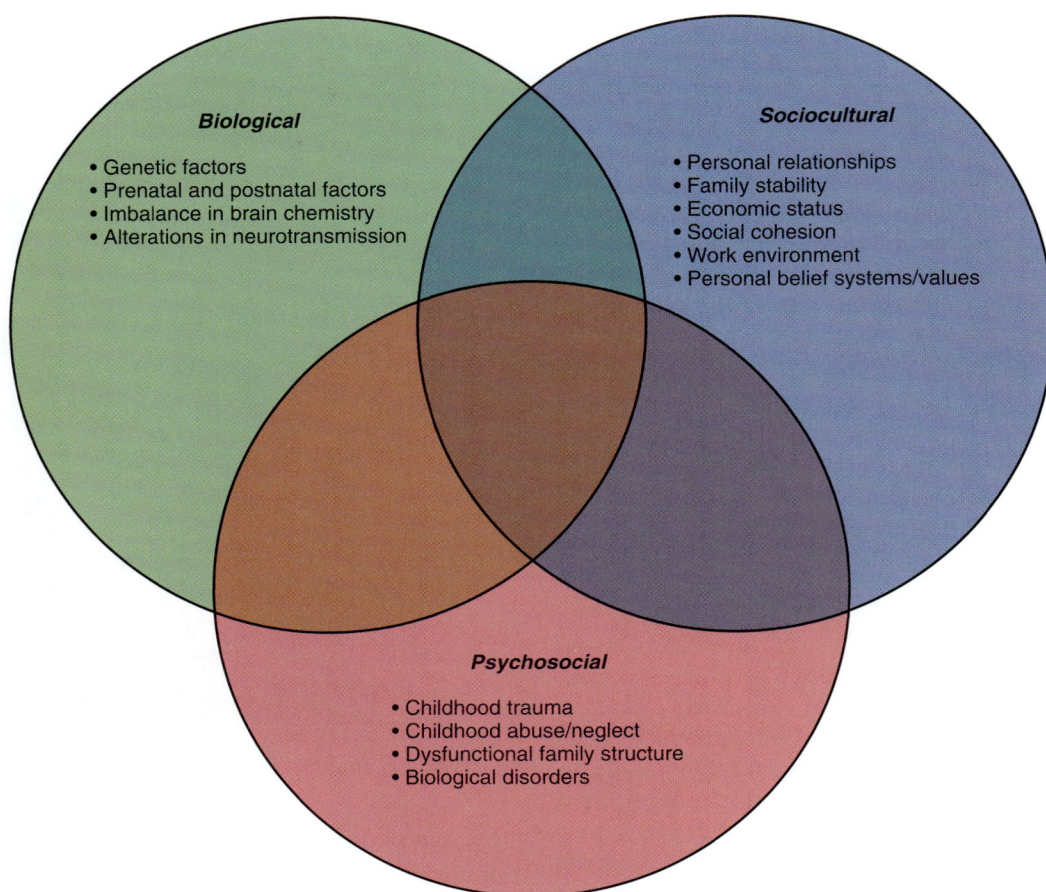

FIGURE 35-1 Common causes of behavioral emergencies.

Organic causes of behavioral emergencies that are discussed throughout this text include substance abuse, trauma, illness (e.g., diabetes, electrolyte imbalance), infections, tumors, and dementia (Box 35-2). It is important that the paramedic consider the possibility of these medical conditions as part of a differential diagnosis in all behavioral emergencies.

Psychosocial Causes

Psychosocial mental illness often is related to an individual's personality type. It also may be related to the person's ability to resolve situational conflict in life. For example, psychosocial mental illness may result from childhood trauma, child abuse or neglect, or a dysfunctional family structure that affects relationships with parents and siblings. Biological disorders may contribute to psychosocial causes of mental illness.

Sociocultural Causes

Sociocultural causes of mental illness are related to the way a person balances emotions, thoughts, and interactions in society. When this balance shifts rapidly, a person may experience emotional turmoil that results in crisis. Factors that may be related to sociocultural causes of behavioral emergencies include personal relationships, family stability, economic status, social cohesion, work environment,

and personal belief systems and values. Changes in behavior caused by personal or situational stress often are linked to a specific event (e.g., the death of a loved one) or a series of events. Examples include environmental violence related to society (e.g., war, terrorism, riots), personal violence (e.g., rape, assault), ongoing discrimination or prejudice, and economic and employment problems.

ASSESSMENT AND MANAGEMENT OF BEHAVIORAL EMERGENCIES

The initial assessment and management of a patient with a behavioral emergency are similar to those used in any other EMS response. These steps include ensuring scene safety, containing the crisis, providing proper emergency medical care, and transporting the patient to an appropriate health care facility. In addition, most EMS services have protocols that call for law enforcement personnnel to evaluate the scene for possible danger and to control any acts of aggression by the patient.

Assessment

Paramedics should begin the assessment by creating a rapport with the patient. They can do this while gathering information needed for immediate management of life-threatening conditions. On arrival, paramedics should survey the scene for any relevant details. These may include

BOX 35-1 Top 10 Myths About Mental Illness

Myth: 1: Psychiatric disorders are not true medical illnesses like heart disease and diabetes. People who have a mental illness are just "crazy."

Fact: Brain disorders, like heart disease and diabetes, are true medical illnesses. Research shows that psychiatric disorders have genetic and biological causes. Also, these diseases can be treated effectively.

Myth: 2: People with a severe mental illness, such as schizophrenia, are usually dangerous and violent.

Fact: Statistics show that the incidence of violence among people who have a brain disorder is not much higher than it is in the general population. Individuals suffering from a psychosis such as schizophrenia are more often frightened, confused, and despairing than violent.

Myth: 3: Mental illness is the result of bad parenting.

Fact: Most experts agree that genetic factors, along with other risk factors, lead to psychiatric disorders. In other words, mental illnesses have a physical cause.

Myth: 4: Depression results from a personality weakness or character flaw. People who are depressed could just snap out of it if they tried hard enough.

Fact: Depression has nothing to do with being lazy or weak. It results from changes in brain chemistry or brain function. Medication and/or psychotherapy often help people to recover.

Myth: 5: Schizophrenia means that the person has a split personality, and there is no way to control it.

Fact: Schizophrenia is often confused with multiple personality disorder. Actually, schizophrenia is a brain disorder that robs people of their ability to think clearly and logically. An estimated 2.5 million Americans have schizophrenia. Their symptoms range from social withdrawal to hallucinations and delusions. Medication has helped many of these people to lead fulfilling, productive lives.

Myth: 6: Depression is a normal part of the aging process.

Fact: It is not normal for older adults to be depressed. Signs of depression in older people include a loss of interest in activities, sleep disturbance, and lethargy. Depression in the elderly is often undiagnosed. Older adults and their family members need to recognize the problem and seek professional help.

Myth: 7: Depression and other illnesses, such as anxiety disorders, do not affect children or adolescents. Any problems they have are just a part of growing up.

Fact: Children and adolescents can develop severe mental illnesses. In the United States, 1 in 10 children and adolescents has a mental disorder severe enough to cause impairment. Yet only about 20% of these children receive treatment. Left untreated, these problems can worsen. *Anyone who talks about suicide should be taken very seriously.*

Myth: 8: If you have a mental illness, you can will it away. Being treated for a psychiatric disorder means an individual has in some way "failed" or is weak.

Fact: A serious mental illness cannot be willed away. Ignoring the problem does not make it go away, either. It takes courage to seek professional help.

Myth: 9: Addiction is a lifestyle choice and shows a lack of willpower. People with a substance abuse problem are morally weak or "bad."

Fact: Addiction is a disease that generally results from changes in brain chemistry. It has nothing to do with being a "bad" person.

Myth: 10: Electroconvulsive therapy (ECT), formerly known as "shock treatment," is painful and barbaric.

Fact: ECT has given a new lease on life to many people who suffer from severe and debilitating depression. It is used when other treatments such as psychotherapy or medication fail or cannot be used. Patients who receive ECT are asleep and under anesthesia; therefore they do not feel anything.

National Alliance for Research on Schizophrenia and Depression: *Top 10 myths about mental illness based on a nationwide survey,* Great Neck, NY, 2003.

evidence of substance abuse, a suicide attempt, or other clues that may shed light on the patient's state. The patient should be observed for emotional response, such as fear, anger, confusion, or hostility. While providing patient care, the paramedic should focus the evaluation on the patient's level of cognitive functioning. This includes alertness, orientation, speech patterns, **affect,** and the way in which the patient interacts with friends, loved ones, and family members. When possible, the number of people around the patient should be limited. This helps to control the scene. Anyone who interferes with the scene or the patient assessment or who adversely affects the patient's condition should be removed from the area.

Other information can be volunteered by the patient, obtained from the patient interview, or provided by family members, bystanders, and first responders. The patient's family or caregiver should be interviewed about the patient's usual level of functioning, about recent stress in the patient's life, and about approaches that may help the paramedic to gain the patient's trust and cooperation. Information that should be obtained for a full background and history of the event include significant medical history, medications the patient has taken (Table 35-1), past psychiatric problems, and any precipitating factors that may have contributed to the behavioral emergency.

Interview Techniques

After managing any life-threatening illness or injury, the patient should be interviewed if possible. The paramedic should not ask for more details than are needed. A limited

BOX 35-2 Common Medical Conditions That Manifest as Behavioral Disorders

Metabolic Disorders
Glucose, sodium, calcium, or magnesium imbalance
Acid-base imbalance
Acute hypoxia
Renal failure
Hepatic failure

Endocrine Disorders
Thyroid disease
Parathyroid disease
Adrenal hormone imbalance

Infectious Diseases
Encephalitis
Meningitis
Brain abscess
Severe systemic infection

Trauma
Concussion
Intracranial hematoma (especially subdural hematoma)

Cardiovascular Disorders
Cardiac dysrhythmia
Hypotension
Transient ischemic attack
Cerebrovascular accident (or stroke)
Hypertensive encephalopathy

Neoplastic Diseases
Central nervous system tumors or metastases

Degenerative Diseases
Dementia of the Alzheimer's type
Other dementias

Drug Abuse
Alcohol
Barbiturates
Narcotics
Sedative-hypnotics
Amphetamines and other stimulants
Hallucinogens

Drug Reactions
Beta-adrenergic blockers
Antihypertensives
Cardiac drugs
Bronchodilators
Beta-adrenergic agonists
Anticonvulsants

DID YOU KNOW?
Unemployment: Link to Mental Illness[2]
The U.S. recession that began in 2007 resulted in a national unemployment rate of nearly 10%. Following are key findings of a survey done by the National Alliance on Mental Illness:
- 13% of unemployed individuals report that they have thought of harming themselves, which is four times more than reported by persons with full-time work.
- People who are unemployed are approximately six times as likely to have difficulty paying household expenses—22% report great difficulty paying their utilities and almost 50% have significant difficulty in obtaining health care, further compounding their situation.
- People who are unemployed are also twice as likely to report concern with their mental health or use of alcohol or drugs within the last 6 months than individuals working full time.
- Of those who have not spoken to a health professional about these concerns, 42% cited cost or lack of insurance coverage as the main reason.
- Nearly 20% of the sample reported that they had experienced a forced change (e.g., pay cuts, reduced hours) in their employment during the last year.
- Although most of these individuals are employed, individuals with a forced change in employment are twice as likely to report symptoms consistent with severe mental illness than would be expected. They are also five times more likely to report feeling hopeless most or all of the time than individuals who had not experienced a forced change.

support and empathy, preventing interruptions, and respecting the patient's personal space by limiting physical touch (Box 35-3).

MENTAL STATUS EXAMINATION

A **mental status examination** (MSE) is an evaluation tool that can help the paramedic during the patient assessment. Although many variations of an MSE are available (Box 35-4), most include an assessment of appearance and behavior, speech and language, cognitive abilities, and emotional stability.[3] The following factors should be assessed in each of these areas.

Appearance and Behavior
- How does the patient look? Is the person neatly dressed and well groomed?
- Is the patient pleasant and cooperative or agitated?
- Is the patient's behavior appropriate for the particular situation?
- What is the patient's body language?
- Do body movements or posture suggest tension, anxiety, hostility, or aggression?
- Does the patient maintain eye contact during the patient interview?

Speech and Language
- Is the patient's speech intelligible and normal in tone, volume, and rate?

and supportive interview strengthens the paramedic's rapport with the patient. It also can help to establish and maintain a relationship during the provision of patient care. As described in Chapter 17 and Chapter 18, effective interview techniques include active listening, showing

TABLE 35-1 Examples of Drugs Used to Treat Psychiatric Disorders

Trade Name(s)	Generic Name	Drug Class
Abilify	Aripiprazole	Antipsychotic
Adderall	(amphetamine/ dextroamphetamine)	ADHD
Akineton	Biperiden	Antiparkinson agent
Anafranil	Clomipramine	Antidepressant
Asendin	Amoxapine	Antidepressant
Ativan	Lorazepam	Antianxiety
Aventyl	Nortriptyline	Antidepressant
Thorazine, Largactil, Chlorpromanyl, Novo-Chlorpromazine	Chlorpromazine	Antipsychotic
Celexa	Citalopram	SSRI
Clozaril	Clozapine	Antipsychotic
Cogentin, Apo-Benztropine, PMS Benztropine	Benztropine mesylate	Antiparkinson agent
Cymbalta	Duloxetine	Antidepressant
Desyrel	Trazodone	Antidepressant
Effexor	Venlafaxine	Antidepressant
Elavil, Levate, Apo-Amitriptyline, Novo-Triptyn, PMS Amitriptyline	Amitriptyline	Antidepressant
Eldepryl, SD Deprenyl	Selegiline	Antiparkinson agent
Fluanxol	Flupenthixol dihydrochloride	Antipsychotic
Geodon	Ziprasidone	Antipsychotic
Lexapro	Escitalopram	SSRI antidepressant
Modecate, Apo-Fluphenazine, Permitil, Moditen	Fluphenazine	Antipsychotic
Haldol, Apo-Haloperidol, Novo-Peridol, Peridol, PMS Haloperidol	Haloperidol	Antipsychotic
Kemadrin, PMS Procyclidine, Procyclid	Procyclidine	Antiparkinson agent
Lithium, Lithane, Carbolith, Duralith, Lithizine	Lithium carbonate	Antipsychotic
Luvox	Fluvoxamine maleate	Antidepressant
Marplan	Isocarboxazid	Antidepressant
Mellaril, Apo-Thioridazine, Novo-Ridazine, PMS Thioridazine	Thioridazine	Antipsychotic
Nardil	Phenelzine	Antidepressant
Neuleptil	Pericyazine	Antipsychotic
Norpramin, Pertofrane	Desipramine	Antidepressant
Nozinan	Methotrimeprazine	Antipsychotic
Orap	Pimozide	Antipsychotic
Parnate	Tranylcypromine	Antidepressant
Parsitan, Profenamine	Ethopropazine	Antiparkinson agent
Paxil	Paroxetine	SSRI
Piportil L4	Pipotiazine	Antipsychotic
Promazine	Promazine	Antipsychotic
Prozac	Fluoxetine	Antidepressant
Remeron	Mirtazapine	Antidepressant
Ritalin	Methylphenidate	Cerebral stimulant
Risperdal	Risperidone	Antipsychotic
Seroquel	Quetiapine	Antipsychotic
Serentil	Mesoridazine	Antipsychotic
Serzone	Nefazodone	Antidepressant
Sinequan, Novo-Doxepin, Triadapin	Doxepin	Antidepressant
Stelazine, Apo-Trifluoperazine, PMS Trifluoperazine, Terfluzine, Novo-Flurazine, Solazine	Trifluoperazine	Antipsychotic
Stemetil, Prorazin, PMS Prochlorperazine	Prochlorperazine	Antipsychotic
Surmontil, Apo-Trimip, Novo-Trimpramine, Rhotrimine	Trimipramine	Antidepressant
Tegretol, Apo-Carbamazepine, Mazepine, Novo-Carbamaz PMS	Carbamazepine	Antipsychotic
Tofranil, Apo-Imipramine, Impril, Novopramine, PMS Imipramine	Imipramine	Antidepressant
Trilafon, Apo-Perphenazine, PMS Perphenazine	Perphenazine	Antipsychotic
Triptil	Protriptyline	Antidepressant
Valium, Apo-Diazepam, Diazemuls, Novodipam, PMS Diazepam, Vivol	Diazepam	Antianxiety
Wellbutrin	Bupropion	Antidepressant
Xanax, Apo-Alpraz, Novo-Alprazol, Nu-Alpraz	Alprazolam	Antianxiety
Zoloft	Sertraline	SSRI Antidepressant
Zyprexa	Olanzapine	Antipsychotic

ADHD, Attention-deficit/hyperactivity disorder; *SSRI,* selective serotonin reuptake inhibitor.

- Does the tone of the patient's voice change?
- Is speech spontaneous, with ease of expression?
- Do the patient's words and sentences proceed in an orderly fashion?

Cognitive Abilities
- Is the patient oriented to person, time, and place?
- Does the patient know who and where he or she is?
- Does the patient know who you are?
- Can the patient remain focused on your questions and conversation?
- What is the patient's attention span?

- Can the patient follow a series of short commands?
- Does the patient respond to directions appropriately?
- Are the patient's comments logical and presented in an organized fashion?

Emotional Stability
- Is the patient aware of his or her environment?
- Can the patient describe or rate his or her mood using a scale of 1 to 10?
- Does the patient appear happy, sad, depressed, or angry?
- Is the patient's mood appropriate for the specific situation?
- Does the patient show mood swings or behaviors that indicate anxiety, depression, anger, or hostility?
- Does the patient stay focused during the interview or stray quickly to related topics?
- Is the patient experiencing perceptual distortions or hallucinations?

CRITICAL THINKING
Think about interviewing techniques that you have seen EMS crews use when caring for patients with behavioral emergencies. Were the techniques effective? Could the paramedics have improved their patient care by using any of the techniques listed in Box 35-3?

DIFFICULT PATIENT INTERVIEWS

Some patients with behavioral or psychiatric disorders are difficult to interview. For example, a patient may refuse to talk to the paramedic. (This may be the case especially if the family requested EMS assistance without the patient's consent.) A patient may be extremely talkative and have disorganized speech. In addition, a patient may be confrontational. If a patient refuses to be interviewed, paramedics should speak to the patient in a quiet voice. They should avoid questions that the patient may see as an "interrogation." Also, paramedics should allow the patient extra time to respond. Patients who are too talkative need to have their attention focused on the interview. To do this, the paramedic can raise a hand or call the person's name. With a confrontational patient, additional help may be required to ensure scene safety.

Other Patient Care Measures

After the initial assessment and history taking, the remainder of the examination is determined by the patient's overall condition and the nature of the psychiatric problem. The benefits of a thorough physical examination must be weighed against the risks of a patient who might construe the exam as a physical violation. If there is reason to suspect an organic cause for the patient's condition, a physical examination should be performed. Otherwise, patient care for a person with a behavioral emergency may be limited to maintaining an effective rapport with the patient during transfer to the hospital.

SPECIFIC BEHAVIORAL AND PSYCHIATRIC DISORDERS

More than 250 psychiatric conditions have been identified by mental health professionals. In addition, some patients may have symptoms that are associated with more than one condition. The following are common classifications of mental disorders discussed in this chapter[4]:

- Cognitive disorders
- Schizophrenia
- Anxiety disorders
- Mood disorders
- Substance-related disorders
- Somatoform disorders
- Factitious disorders
- Dissociative disorders
- Eating disorders
- Impulse-control disorders
- Personality disorders

NOTE

The American Psychiatric Association (APA) also has identified major classes of psychiatric disorders. These are known as *DSM-IV-TR* groups.[5] (*DSM-IV-TR* refers to the APA's *Diagnostic and Statistical Manual of Mental Disorders,* edition 4, text revision, which was published in 2000.) Many mental health professionals use these classifications for diagnostic purposes. In addition to the disorders listed in the text, other *DSM-IV* classes of psychiatric disorders include the following:

Disorders First Diagnosed in Infancy, Childhood, and Adolescence
- Delirium, dementia, amnesia, and other cognitive disorders
- Psychotic disorders other than schizophrenia
- Mental disorders caused by a general medical condition
- Sexual and gender identity disorders
- Sleep disorders
- Adjustment disorders
- Other conditions that may be the focus of clinical attention

---

Patient care for most behavioral emergencies is mainly supportive. It usually involves providing emotional support, assessing and managing coexisting emergency medical problems, and transporting the patient for evaluation by a physician. In some cases paramedics may need to take measures to protect the patient and others from harm. This includes the possible use of physical and chemical restraint (described later in this chapter).

Cognitive Disorders

Cognitive disorders may have an organic cause (e.g., a disease process). They also may be a result of physical or chemical injury, such as trauma or drug abuse. All cognitive disorders result in a disturbance of cognitive functioning. This may manifest as delirium or dementia (previously described in Chapter 25) or autism spectrum disorder.

DELIRIUM

Delirium is an abrupt disorientation of time and place. It usually involves delusions and hallucinations. **Delusions** are false beliefs. **Hallucinations** are the perception of sights, sounds, and other sensory phenomena that are not actually present. The symptoms vary according to an individual's personality, the environment, and the severity of the illness. Common signs and symptoms of delirium include inattention, memory impairment, disorientation, clouding of consciousness, and vivid visual hallucinations. Treatment of delirium is aimed at correcting the underlying physical disorder to reduce anxiety (Box 35-5). Sedatives may be required to manage the patient. The exact occurrence rate of delirium is unknown. However, some groups of people are more susceptible to delirium than others. These groups include the following:

- Older adults
- Children

BOX 35-5 Agitated Delirium

Agitated delirium or excited delirium describes a person with delirium who has (1) acute onset and fluctuating course, (2) reduced clarity of awareness of the environment, (3) perceptual disturbance, disorientation, or memory disturbance, and (4) an underlying general medical condition. Agitated delirium is not currently recognized as a medical or psychiatric condition by the America Psychiatric Association or the World Health Organization. It is a label assigned to the state of acute behavioral disinhibition manifested in a cluster of behaviors that may include bizarreness, aggressiveness, agitation, ranting, hyperactivity, paranoia, panic, violence, public disturbance, surprising physical strength, profuse sweating attributable to hyperthermia, respiratory arrest, and death.[6] Excited delirium has been reported to result from substance intoxication, psychiatric illness, alcohol withdrawal, head trauma, or a combination of these factors. The condition has gained public notice because it often is blamed for the deaths of persons being restrained by law enforcement personnel or who have died while in custody.[7]

- Burn patients
- Patients who have had major heart surgery
- Patients who have had a previous brain injury (e.g., stroke)
- Patients with acquired immunodeficiency syndrome (AIDS)

DEMENTIA

Dementia is a clinical state characterized by loss of function in multiple cognitive domains. It is a slow, progressive loss of awareness of time and place. It usually involves an inability to learn new things or to remember recent events. About 75 types of dementia have been identified (Box 35-6). However, most cases result from cerebrovascular disease (including stroke) and Alzheimer's disease (described in Chapter 25). Dementia is a major health problem in the United States because of Americans' long life spans. The disorder affects about 10% of those over age 65 and nearly 50% of those over age 85.[8] The personal habits of patients with dementia often deteriorate. Speech may become incoherent. Also, many of these patients revert to a "second childhood." These patients need total care for feeding, toileting, and physical activities. Treatment of certain illnesses may help to slow the mental decline associated with this disease.

Delirium and dementia may be difficult to differentiate. This is because both may cause disorientation and impaired memory, thinking, and judgment. Dementia usually occurs in people without diminished alertness, appears slowly, and worsens over time. Sleeping and waking problems occur less often in people with dementia than in those with delirium. People with dementia may have difficulty with short- and long-term memory, as well as impairment of judgment and abstract thinking. Delirium sometimes may occur at the same time as dementia. This is especially the case in older adults or people with chronic illnesses.

CRITICAL THINKING
Besides auditory hallucinations, think of other sensory hallucinations that can occur in these patients.

AUTISM SPECTRUM DISORDER

Autism spectrum disorder (ASD) is a range of neurodevelopmental disorders that include *autistic disorder* (classic autism), *Asperger's syndrome*, and *Pervasive Developmental Disorder-Not Otherwise Specified* (PDD-NOS, or atypical autism) (Box 35-7). Each of these disorders is characterized by three sets of behavioral features: (1) impairment in social interaction, (2) communication deficits (both verbal and nonverbal), and (3) restricted, repetitive behaviors, including decreased imaginative play, stereotyped behaviors, and inflexible adherence to routines. The degree to which these behaviors are manifested may vary between

---

BOX 35-6 Some Causes of Dementia

Degenerative Diseases
Huntington's disease
Parkinson's disease (not in all cases)
Cerebellar degenerations
Amyotrophic lateral sclerosis (not in all cases)
Rare genetic and metabolic diseases

Vascular Dementia
Multiinfarct dementia
Microinfarct dementia
Large infarct dementia
Cerebral embolic disease

Anoxic Dementia
Cardiac arrest
Cardiac failure (severe)
Carbon monoxide poisoning

Traumatic Dementia
Dementia pugilistica (boxer's dementia)
Head injury (open or closed)

Infectious Dementia
Acquired immunodeficiency syndrome (AIDS) dementia
Opportunistic infection
Postencephalitic dementia
Herpes dementia
Fungal meningitis or encephalitis
Bacterial meningitis or encephalitis
Parasitic encephalitis
Brain abscess
Neurosyphilis (general paresis)

Space-Occupying Lesions
Chronic or acute subdural hematoma
Primary brain tumor
Metastatic tumor

Autoimmune Disorders
Disseminated lupus erythematosus
Vasculitis

Toxic Dementia
Alcohol
Metals (e.g., lead, mercury, arsenic)
Organic poisons (e.g., solvents, some insecticides)

---

the disorders as well as between each individual. The symptoms of ASD can usually be observed in infants by 18 months of age, but often are unnoticed and therefore undiagnosed (Box 35-8). Autism spectrum disorders are more common in boys; in siblings of those with autism; and in people with certain developmental disorders (e.g., inherited mental retardation).

Children and adults with autism may engage in self-injurious behaviors such as hitting themselves, head

BOX 35-7 Forms of Autism

Autistic disorder: Generally classified by impairment in social interactions and communication and includes some restrictive or repetitive behaviors.

Asperger's syndrome: A syndrome characterized by impairments in social interactions and the presence of restricted interests and activities, with no clinically significant general delay in language, and testing in the range of average to above average intelligence.

Pervasive Developmental Disorder-Not Otherwise Specified: A general category of disorders characterized by severe and pervasive impairment in several areas of development, including having communication and social deficits.

BOX 35-8 Possible Red Flags for Autism[11]

- The child does not respond to his/her name.
- The child cannot explain what he/she wants.
- The child's language skills are slow to develop or speech is delayed.
- The child does not follow directions.
- At times, the child seems to be deaf.
- The child seems to hear sometimes, but not other times.
- The child does not point or wave "bye-bye."
- The child used to say a few words or babble, but now he/she does not.
- The child throws intense or violent tantrums.
- The child has odd movement patterns.
- The child is overly active, uncooperative, or resistant.
- The child does not know how to play with toys.
- The child does not smile back when you smile at him/her.
- The child has poor eye contact.
- The child gets "stuck" doing the same things over and over and cannot move on to other things.
- The child seems to prefer to play alone.
- The child gets things for himself/herself only.
- The child is very independent for his/her age.
- The child does things "early" compared to other children.
- The child seems to be in his/her "own world."
- The child seems to tune people out.
- The child is not interested in other children.
- The child walks on his/her toes.
- The child shows unusual attachments to toys, objects, or schedules (e.g., always holding a string or having to put socks on before pants).
- The child spends a lot of time lining things up or putting things in a certain order.

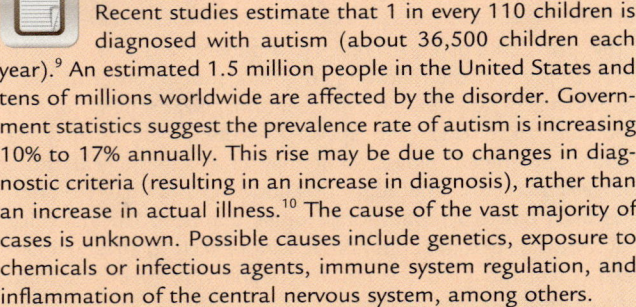

NOTE

Recent studies estimate that 1 in every 110 children is diagnosed with autism (about 36,500 children each year).[9] An estimated 1.5 million people in the United States and tens of millions worldwide are affected by the disorder. Government statistics suggest the prevalence rate of autism is increasing 10% to 17% annually. This rise may be due to changes in diagnostic criteria (resulting in an increase in diagnosis), rather than an increase in actual illness.[10] The cause of the vast majority of cases is unknown. Possible causes include genetics, exposure to chemicals or infectious agents, immune system regulation, and inflammation of the central nervous system, among others.

There is no cure for ASD. Therapies and early behavioral interventions to manage specific symptoms can result in substantial improvement in some patients. There are many different types of treatments available for ASD. These treatments may include auditory training, discrete trial training, and vitamin therapy. Other treatments may include facilitated communication, music therapy, occupational therapy, physical therapy, sensory integration, and applied behavioral analysis. The different types of treatments can generally be broken down into the following categories[9]:

- Behavior and communication approaches
- Dietary approaches
- Medication
- Complementary and alternative medicine

banging, biting or scratching themselves, and picking at skin or sores. In addition, a person with autism may not respond in a normal fashion to pain. This, combined with an impaired ability to communicate, can present the paramedic with challenges in assessment and patient care. Paramedics should employ the therapeutic communications techniques described in Chapter 27. They should also be prepared to provide gentle restraint to ensure personal safety, and the safety of the patient and others.

Schizophrenia

Schizophrenia is a group of disorders characterized by recurrent episodes of **psychotic behavior.** Psychotic behavior can be defined as an inability or unwillingness to recognize and acknowledge reality and to relate with others (Box 35-9). Although the exact cause of the disease has not yet been identified, it may result from a combination of genetics (a family history of schizophrenia often exists), chemical and hormonal changes, autoimmune illness, viral infection, and other stress factors.[12] Schizophrenia usually becomes apparent during adolescence or early adulthood (Box 35-10).[13] Signs and symptoms of the illness appear slowly over time. They become more pronounced and bizarre as the disease progresses. These patients often develop abnormalities of thought processing, thought content, perception, and judgment. Hallmarks of the disease are **paranoia** (intense and irrational feelings of mistrust or suspicions), delusions, and auditory hallucinations (e.g., hearing voices that insult or make demands) (Box 35-11).

Many patients with schizophrenia function quite well with drug therapy. Others function poorly between frank psychotic episodes. These episodes often are the result of failure to comply with drug therapy. Most patients require lifelong therapy with antipsychotic drugs and medications that block the action of dopamine. Compliance with drug therapy often controls symptoms of the disease. (Noncompliance with medications is common in these patients.)

BOX 35-9 Acute Psychosis

The term acute psychosis refers to a patient who presents with one or more of the following criteria: a sudden onset of delusions that rapidly change; hallucinations; bizarre behavior and posture; or disorganized speech.[5] Acute psychosis may be related to mental illness, or it may have a biological cause (*organic psychosis*). The acute psychotic episode may be brief, lasting 1 day to 1 month, or of longer duration. The incidence of the disorder is not common. It is more likely to affect women than men, and is most common in people who are in their third and fourth decades of life.[14]

BOX 35-10 Facts About Schizophrenia

- More than 2.4 million adult Americans are affected by schizophrenia.
- In men, schizophrenia usually appears in the late teens or early twenties.
- In women, schizophrenia usually appears in the twenties to early thirties.
- Schizophrenia affects men and women with equal frequency.
- Most people with schizophrenia suffer chronically throughout their lives.
- One in 10 people with schizophrenia eventually commits suicide.
- Schizophrenia costs the United States more than $48 billion annually.

However, the drugs may produce side effects, especially **dyskinesia** (abnormal muscular movements) and tremor.

Anxiety Disorders

A certain amount of anxiety is useful and necessary for adapting constructively to stress (see Chapter 2: Well-Being of the Paramedic). However, a patient who suffers from an anxiety disorder has a persistent, fearful feeling that cannot be consciously related to reality (Box 35-12).[13] This type of illness can be disabling. The patient may withdraw from daily activities. This is usually an unsuccessful attempt to avoid the episodes of intense activity. Severe anxiety disorders may manifest in a **panic disorder** ("panic attack"). As compared to anxiety disorders that may result from acute grief or various phobias, for example, panic disorders often have no precipitating cause of the attack. Signs and symptoms of panic disorders include (Box 35-13)[13]:

- Hyperventilation
- Feeling of breathlessness or smothering
- Blurred vision
- Perioral and hand and foot paresthesias
- Fear of losing control
- Fear of dying

BOX 35-11 Responding to Paranoia, Delusions, and Hallucinations

1. First, assess whether the problem is troublesome or frightening to the person experiencing it. If not, ignoring it may be the best approach.
2. If a person seems to be hallucinating, leave the individual alone or approach slowly so as not to frighten the person. Respond with caution.
3. Do not try to argue or rationalize. Realize that hallucinations and delusions seem very real to the person who is experiencing them. Arguing does not build trust.
4. Offer reassurance and validation. You might say, "I know this is troubling for you. Let me see if I can help."
5. Check out the reality of the situation; maybe what the person sees or thinks is true.
6. Sometimes things in the environment may be misinterpreted (i.e., a glare or shadow in the window, a noisy furnace). These may be frightening. Explain the potential or actual misinterpretation (e.g., that the noise is the furnace turning on).
7. Modify the environment if necessary. (A mirror may become distracting or confusing; adding more lights may be helpful at night.)
8. Assess whether the person is having problems with hearing or vision. Resolving such problems can reduce the degree of disability.
9. Recall that whispering or laughing around the person may be misinterpreted.
10. Do not take any accusations personally.
11. Use distraction to try to pull the person's focus from the delusion or hallucination.
12. If the person asks you directly whether you see or hear something, be honest. However, do not struggle to convince or reason with the individual about what is real.
13. Try to respond to what the person may be feeling: insecurity, fear, and confusion.
14. Rule out any illnesses or the use of any medicines that could be contributing to the problem.
15. Use tact and firmness in persuading a patient to be transported to the hospital.

Modified from the Alzheimer's Association handout: *Hallucinations and delusions and understanding difficult behaviors*, Anne Robinson, Beth Spencer, Laurie White, Geriatric Education of Michigan University, Ypsilanti, Mich, 1991.

BOX 35-12 Facts About Anxiety Disorders

- About 40 million adults 18 years and older in the United States suffer from anxiety disorders.
- Most people have their first episode by 21.5 years of age.
- Anxiety disorders often are complicated by depression, eating disorders, or substance abuse.
- Anxiety disorders cost the nation more than $46 billion each year.

BOX 35-13 Facts About Panic Disorders

- Panic disorders affect about 6 million people in the United States each year.
- Panic disorders usually strike in young adulthood; about half of those affected develop the condition before age 24.
- Women are twice as likely as men to develop a panic disorder.
- People with a panic disorder also may suffer from depression and substance abuse. About 30% of people with panic disorder abuse alcohol; 17% abuse other drugs (e.g., cocaine, marijuana).
- About one third of those with a panic disorder develop agoraphobia.

BOX 35-14 Facts About Obsessive-Compulsive Disorder

- About 2.2 million American adults have obsessive-compulsive disorder (OCD) in a given year.
- First symptoms often begin in childhood and adolescence; median age of onset is 19.
- OCD affects men and women with equal frequency.
- The nation's social and economic losses caused by OCD total more than $8 billion each year.

- Somatic complaints
- Chest discomfort
- Palpitations or tachycardia
- Dyspnea
- Choking
- Faintness
- Syncope
- Vertigo
- Trembling and sweating
- Urinary frequency and diarrhea

Patient management is mainly supportive. The paramedic should assure these patients that although they may feel as if they are dying, they are not. Also, the paramedic should assure them that effective treatment is available. Panic attacks may mimic a number of medical emergencies, including myocardial infarction. Therefore any patient who shows the signs and symptoms described in the preceding list should be fully assessed at the scene and transported for evaluation by a physician. Sedation may be required. Patients with anxiety disorders should not be left alone.

PHOBIA

A **phobia** is a type of anxiety disorder. A person with a phobia has transferred anxiety onto a situation or an object in the form of an irrational, intense fear, such as a fear of heights, closed spaces, water, or other people. As the object or situation comes closer, the person's anxiety increases. If the crisis is allowed to continue, the patient's anxiety may escalate into a panic attack. These patients usually recognize that their fear is unreasonable. However, they cannot overcome the phobia. In some cases the phobia does not initiate the EMS response but becomes a secondary complication in emergency care. An example is a person who is phobic of water being trapped in a submerged vehicle.

When caring for patients with a phobia, the paramedic should take care to explain each step of an emergency or rescue procedure. The key is a careful rehearsal with the patient, in which the paramedic explains exactly what care will be given and how it will be performed. In addition, the EMS crew should show patience and understanding of the phobia. They should assure the patient that no forceful steps will be taken to place the person in an unwilling position.

OBSESSIVE-COMPULSIVE DISORDER

Obsessive-compulsive disorder (OCD) is a psychiatric disorder in which a person feels stress or anxiety about thoughts or rituals over which the individual has little control (Box 35-14).[13] The disorder can take many forms. These include excessive hand washing or showering, or upsetting thoughts (e.g., violence, vulgarities, harm to oneself or others). Obsessions also may involve special numbers, colors, single words or phrases, and sometimes melodies.

Although most adults realize to some degree that these obsessions and compulsions are without merit, they have great difficulty stopping them. Children with OCD may not realize that their behavior is unusual. OCD affects men and women equally, can start at any age, and may have a heritable component. People with OCD often cleverly hide their condition from family, friends, and co-workers. Medications and behavior therapy are often effective in controlling the symptoms of this disorder.

POSTTRAUMATIC SYNDROME

Posttraumatic stress disorder (PTSD) (*posttraumatic syndrome*) is an anxiety reaction to severe psychosocial events (Box 35-15).[13] These events often are life threatening. Examples include events associated with military service, natural and man-made disasters, and rape. The events often result in repetitive, intrusive memories. Manifestations of this illness may include depression, sleep disturbances, nightmares, and survivor guilt. The syndrome often is complicated by substance abuse.[14]

EMS personnel and other emergency responders may be subject to this syndrome as a result of their work. Examples include responding to major incidents with a large number of injured people, the death of a co-worker, a sudden infant

CRITICAL THINKING

Do you know someone with an intense fear of a situation or object? How does this person behave when subjected to the object of the phobia?

BOX 35-15 Facts About Posttraumatic Syndrome

- About 7.7 million people in the United States have posttraumatic syndrome during the course of a given year.
- Posttraumatic syndrome can develop at any age, including childhood; median age of onset is 23 years.
- Posttraumatic syndrome is more common in women than men.
- About 30% of men and women who have spent time in a war zone experience this disorder.
- Posttraumatic syndrome often occurs after violent personal assaults, such as rape, mugging, or domestic violence; terrorism; natural or human-caused disasters; and accidents.
- Depression, alcohol or other substance abuse, or another anxiety disorder often accompanies posttraumatic syndrome.

BOX 35-16 Facts About Depression

- More than 14.8 million adult Americans suffer from depression each year. Many are unnecessarily unable to function normally for weeks or months because their illness remains untreated.
- Almost twice as many women (12%) as men (7%) are affected by depressive illness each year.
- Depression is a frequent and serious complication of heart attack, stroke, diabetes, and cancer.
- Depression increases the risk of heart attack.
- Depression costs the nation more than $30 billion a year in direct and indirect costs.
- Major depression is the leading cause of disability in the United States.

? DID YOU KNOW?
PTSD

In the annual meeting of the American Public Health Association (APHA) in 2007, it was estimated that PTSD in veterans returning from Iraq and Afghanistan ranged from 12% to 20%. Other studies have reported as many as 10% of Gulf War veterans and as many as 30% of Vietnam veterans also suffer from PTSD.[15] The APHA meeting also estimated a minimum of 300,000 psychiatric casualties, and a lifetime cost of treatment in excess of $660 billion for veterans returning from Iraq and Afghanistan. The official 17 symptoms of PTSD associated with these veterans can be placed into 3 broad groups[16]:
- Reexperiencing: intrusive memories, nightmares, flashbacks, triggered distress
- Avoidance: isolation, withdrawal, emotional numbing, detachment, memory gaps
- Hyperarousal: insomnia, irritability, anger outbursts, poor concentration, hypervigilance, exaggerated startle response

either a gradual or a rapid onset, and at times a clustering of episodes. The depressed patient may show feelings of hopelessness, extreme isolation, tenseness, and irritability. In severe cases the depression may be followed by **anhedonia,** which is the inability to feel pleasure or happiness from experiences that ordinarily are pleasurable. Other effects of severe depression include insomnia or hypersomnia, weight loss from diminished appetite, weight gain from overeating, decreased libido, and deep feelings of worthlessness and guilt. The mnemonic *IN SAD CAGES* identifies the major features of depression.[17]

Interest
Sleep
Appetite
Depressed mood
Concentration
Activity
Guilt
Energy
Suicide

death syndrome (SIDS) death, and the stress associated with responding to emergency calls (see Chapter 2: Well-Being of the Paramedic).

Mood Disorders

The term **mood disorder** is used to describe changes in emotions that a person experiences in life. (For example, these may include happiness, depression, fear, and anxiety.) Two conditions commonly associated with mood disorders are depression and bipolar disorder, both of which are associated with an increased risk of suicide.[4]

DEPRESSION

Depression is a mood disturbance characterized by feelings of sadness, despair, and discouragement. It is one of the most prevalent major psychiatric conditions, affecting 10% to 15% of the general population (Box 35-16).[13] Depression is usually episodic (episodes usually last longer than 1 month) with periods of remission. It is known to have

📋 NOTE
Depression can be classified as dysthymia or clinical (major) depression. **Dysthymia** is a less severe form of depression that is chronic in nature, lasting as long as 2 years or more. In contrast to major depression (**clinical depression**), the symptoms of dysthymia may not always result in clinically significant distress. They are not always associated with impairment in social, occupational, academic, or other major areas of functioning (as is more common with clinical depression). Both forms of depression share similar symptoms, including depressed mood, disturbed sleep, low energy, and poor concentration. Parallel symptoms include poor appetite, low self-esteem, and hopelessness in dysthymia. The more severe symptoms of weight change, excessive guilt, and thoughts of death or suicide are associated with major depression. Dysthymia can often be treated effectively with counseling. Clinical depression usually requires medication therapy.

Depression is common in the elderly. It also is associated with an increased risk of suicide for all age groups (described

The balance of emotions

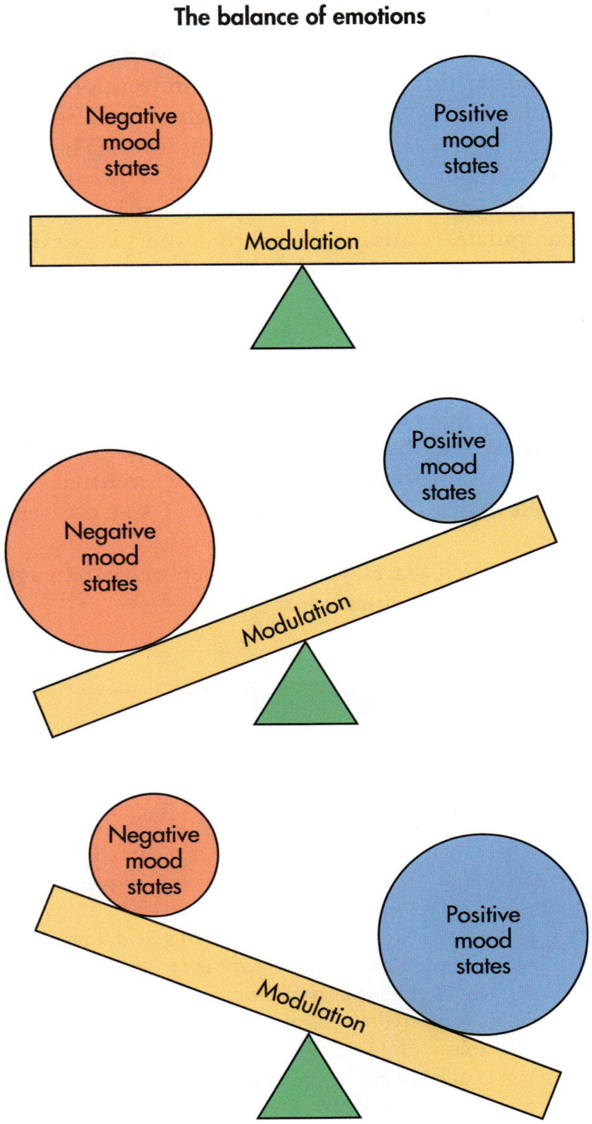

FIGURE 35-2 Bipolar disorder.

later in this chapter). Care for depressed patients is directed at quietly talking to the patient about things that appear to be of interest and trying to gain responsiveness. Depression may be treated with antidepressant drug therapy, counseling, psychotherapy, and, in a small number of cases, **electroconvulsive therapy** (ECT).

BIPOLAR DISORDER

Bipolar disorder is a biphasic emotional disorder in which depressive and manic episodes alternate (Figure 35-2). **Mania** is characterized by excessive elation, talkativeness, flight of ideas, motor activity, irritability, accelerated speech, and, often, delusions that center around personal grandeur. Bipolar disorders sometimes develop slowly over time. However, they may occur abruptly and may be instigated by a single event. The manic phase can be very brief or can last weeks to months. Compared with depression, mania is rare.[14] The most frequent age for initial episodes is 20 to 35 years, with initial bouts of depression occurring about 10 years later (Box 35-17).[13] Many patients with bipolar disorder are treated with lithium. As described in Chapter 13:

Principles of Pharmacology and Emergency Medications, lithium has a narrow therapeutic index; a common illness, such as influenza with diarrhea and/or vomiting, can result in lithium toxicity.

Emergency care should consist of calm, firm emotional support. It also should include transport for evaluation by a physician. If this is the patient's first manic episode, the paramedic should consider the possibility of drug abuse as a differential diagnosis. Stimulation should be kept to a minimum. If the patient's condition allows, EMS transport should proceed without using emergency lights and audible warning devices.

BOX 35-17 Facts About Bipolar Disorder

- More than 5.7 million Americans age 18 or older suffer from bipolar disorder in a given year. (This is about 2.6% of the U.S. population.)
- As many as 20% of people with bipolar disorder die by suicide.
- Men and women are equally likely to develop bipolar disorder.

CRITICAL THINKING

Do you think patients would be at higher risk for suicide during the depressive or the manic phase of bipolar disorder? Why?

SUICIDE AND SUICIDE THREATS

A threat of **suicide** is an indication that a patient has a serious crisis that calls for immediate intervention. In many cases suicide attempts are a cry for help. They also may be a form of direct or indirect communication. (The patient may be saying, "I don't want to live" or "I am angry with you.") Other suicide attempts are an effort by the patient to manipulate relationships so that the patient is surrounded by people who are ready and willing to provide advice and support (Box 35-18). In assessing the risk of suicide, the paramedic should consider these seven facts[19]:

1. In 2006 suicide was the eleventh leading cause of death for people of all ages; the seventh leading cause of death in males; and the sixteenth leading cause of death in females. More than 30,000 suicides occurred in the United States (91 suicides per day; 1 suicide every 16 minutes).

2. In the United States, Caucasian men older than age 75 have the highest suicide rate.

3. Women *attempt* suicide two to three times the rate at which men do.

4. Men *commit* suicide four times the rate at which women do (79% of all U.S. suicides).

5. Firearms are the most commonly used method for suicide in men. Poisoning is the most common method for suicide in women.

6. Among young adults 15 to 24 years of age, there are about 100 to 200 attempts for every completed suicide. Among adults older than 65 years of age, there are about 4 suicide attempts for every completed suicide.

7. The more specific and detailed the suicide plan, the greater the suicide potential.

Other factors associated with suicide threats include the recent death of a loved one or loss of a significant relationship, a financial setback or job loss, chronic or debilitating illness, social isolation, alcohol or other drug abuse, depression, and schizophrenia. If a suicide attempt is suspected, the paramedic should discuss these intentions with the patient. Questions such as the following are appropriate:

BOX 35-18   Myths About Suicide

Myth: People who talk about killing themselves rarely commit suicide.
Fact: Most people who commit suicide have given some clue or warning of their intent. *Suicidal threats and attempts should always be treated seriously.*
Myth: The tendency to commit suicide is inherited. It is passed from generation to generation.
Fact: Suicide does tend to run in families. However, the tendency does not appear to be transmitted genetically.
Myth: All suicidal people are deeply depressed.
Fact: Depression is often associated with suicidal feelings. However, not all people who kill themselves are obviously depressed. In fact, some suicidal people appear to be happier than they have been in quite a while because they have decided to "resolve" all their problems at the same time.
Myth: There is a very low correlation between alcoholism and suicide.
Fact: Alcoholism and suicide often go hand in hand. Alcoholics are prone to suicide. Even people who do not normally drink often ingest alcohol shortly before killing themselves.
Myth: Suicidal people are mentally ill.
Fact: Many suicidal people are depressed and distraught. However, most of them would not be diagnosed as mentally ill.
Myth: If a person attempts suicide, that individual will always entertain thoughts of suicide.
Fact: Most people who are suicidal are that way for only a brief period in their lives. An attempter who receives the proper assistance and support probably will never be suicidal again. Only about 10% of attempters later complete the act.
Myth: Asking a person about his or her suicidal intentions encourages the individual to act.
Fact: Actually, the opposite is true. Asking a person directly about suicidal intent often lowers the individual's anxiety level. In fact, it often acts as a deterrent to suicidal emotions.
Myth: Suicide is more common among the lower classes.
Fact: Suicide occurs in all socioeconomic groups. No one class is more susceptible to it than another.
Myth: Suicidal people rarely seek medical attention.
Fact: Research has consistently shown that about 75% of suicidal people visit a physician within 3 months of killing themselves.
Myth: Suicide is basically a problem limited to young people.
Fact: The suicide rate rises with age and reaches a peak among older Caucasian men.
Myth: Professional people do not kill themselves.
Fact: Physicians, lawyers, dentists, and pharmacists have high suicide rates.
Myth: When a person's depression lifts, the danger of suicide disappears.
Fact: The greatest danger of suicide exists during the first 3 months after a person recovers from a deep depression.
Myth: Suicide is a spontaneous activity that occurs without warning.
Fact: Most people plan their self-destruction. Then they give clues that they have become suicidal.
Myth: Because it includes the Christmas season, December has a high suicide rate.
Fact: No rash of suicides occurs at Christmas. In fact, December has the lowest rate of any month.

From Suicide Prevention Allied Regional Effort (SPARE): *The mythology of suicide,* Denver, www.mhaem.org/myths.htm, accessed 9-12-10.

"Do you have thoughts about killing yourself or others?" "Have you ever tried to kill yourself?" Many depressed patients are willing to discuss their suicidal (or homicidal) thoughts. During the patient interview, the paramedic should try to determine three important factors: (1) whether the patient has a plan (how and when the suicide will be done); (2) whether the plan is intended to be successful; and (3) whether the patient has the means or method to follow through with the plan.

CRITICAL THINKING

How would you feel about asking a patient, "Have you ever thought about killing yourself?"

When responding to a suicide attempt, paramedics should request police protection before approaching the scene. (Armed patients must be considered homicidal as well as suicidal.) After scene safety has been ensured and paramedics have gained access to the patient, the scene should be surveyed for the presence of dangerous objects (see Chapter 56).

The first priority in patient management is medical care. Unconscious patients should be managed with airway, ventilatory, and circulatory support and rapid transport. If the patient is conscious, creating rapport as soon as possible is essential. The paramedic should conduct a brief interview to assess the situation and determine the need for and direction of further action. To help reduce the potential for suicide, paramedics can take the following six steps:

1. Provide support and honest assurance about the patient's well-being.
2. Provide for physical safety as well as emotional security. Establish protective limits and measures. This helps to prevent injury to the patient or others. It also conveys to these patients that the paramedic will help them control their behavior until they can gain self-control.
3. Listen to the person, even if the speech seems bizarre, inappropriate, or unrealistic. Do not feel that every statement must be answered or that advice or opinions must be given. During the interview, acknowledge the patient's feelings; do not argue with the patient's wish to die. Explain alternatives to suicide that the patient may not have considered (e.g., counseling, support groups, pastoral care).
4. Determine the patient's support system or significant others when possible. Others may be better able to communicate with and calm the patient.
5. Encourage and reassure the patient during the crisis.
6. Transport the patient to the proper facility for emergency intervention.

Substance-Related Disorders

Some patients with a behavioral emergency may also be using alcohol or illegal drugs. This may cause difficulties during the physical examination. (Substance-related

disorders are described in Chapter 34.) Often these patients are trying to "self-medicate" to improve their mood or lessen the anxiety associated with mental illness. Other patients self-medicate before receiving a diagnosis for their illness or before seeking professional help. Signs that may indicate alcohol or illicit drug use include a breath odor of alcohol, the presence of drug paraphernalia, and needle tracks on the extremities.

PATIENTS WITH A DUAL DIAGNOSIS

Some people struggle both with serious mental illness and with substance abuse. This *dual diagnosis* may be difficult to identify, because one disorder may mimic the symptoms of the other (Box 35-19).[20] It therefore is easy to attribute the patient's symptoms to only one of the two afflictions. It is estimated that as many as 50% of mentally ill individuals have a substance abuse problem. The drug most often used is alcohol. The next most commonly used drugs are marijuana and cocaine. Prescription drugs such as tranquilizers and sleeping medicines may also be abused. Factors associated with a dual diagnosis include the following:

- Recreational use of alcohol or other drugs
- Misguided attempts to self-medicate to relieve anxiety or depression
- Susceptibility to mental illness *and* substance abuse
- Environmental and social influences

Patients who have a dual diagnosis may alternate between requesting EMS assistance for mental illness and for substance abuse. Most psychiatric and drug counseling organizations agree that the two disorders must be treated at the same time.[20]

Somatoform Disorders

Somatoform disorders are conditions that suggest a medical disorder when no physical cause can be found for the patient's symptoms. Two of the most common disorders in this group are somatization disorder and conversion disorder. Both are associated with anxiety, depression, and threats of suicide. Treatment for both disorders often requires psychotherapy, which can address the emotional conflicts that manifest in these illnesses. No definitive causes for most of the somatoform disorders have been established. Contributing factors may include[21]:

- Genetic and environmental influences appear to contribute to somatization.
- Children raised in homes with a high degree of parental somatization may model somatization.
- Sexual abuse may be associated with an increased risk of somatization later in life.
- Poor ability to express emotions may result in somatization.

SOMATIZATION DISORDER

Somatization disorder is a condition in which an individual has complaints (lasting several years) of various physical problems for which no physical cause can be found (Box 35-20).[13] The condition is more common in women than men. It sometimes results in unnecessary surgery and other treatments. These patients most often complain of neurological symptoms (double vision, seizure, weakness), gynecological symptoms (painful menstruation, painful intercourse), and gastrointestinal symptoms (abdominal pain, nausea).

CONVERSION DISORDER

Conversion disorder is a mental illness in which painful emotions are repressed and unconsciously converted into physical symptoms (Box 35-21).[13] A loss of sensory or motor capabilities or of special senses may occur. For example, the person suddenly may not be able to speak, hear, see, or feel, or an arm or a leg may be paralyzed. In many cases the areas of the body affected do not correspond to the actual arrangement of neural pathways. The symptoms also may be intermittent or may appear at different times and in different areas of the body.

MANAGEMENT

Paramedics should manage symptoms of somatoform disorders as if they are real, because differentiating these disorders from an organic ailment may be difficult. The paramedic should recognize that these patients are not "faking"; they believe their illness or loss of function to be factual. These patients require evaluation by a physician.

Factitious Disorders

Factitious disorders are a group of disorders in which symptoms mimic a true illness. However, the symptoms have actually been invented. The symptoms are under the control of the patient, who is attempting to gain attention. The most common disorder in this group is **Munchausen syndrome.** With this disorder, the patient makes routine pleas for treatment and hospitalization for a symptomatic, but imaginary, acute illness. Other complaints that may be associated with factitious disorders include bereavement, Cushing syndrome, dental problems, infection with the human immunodeficiency virus (HIV), hypoglycemia, and stroke. **Munchausen syndrome by proxy** is a form of this disorder in which a person injures or induces illness in others (usually children) in order to gain sympathy. Munchausen syndrome by proxy is often considered to be a form of child abuse.

The symptoms of a factitious disorder are often dramatic but plausible. They usually resolve with treatment. After the treatment, the person seeks treatment for another invented disease. Once the factitious disorder is diagnosed, treatment is aimed at protecting these people from unnecessary surgeries and other treatments they do not need.

Dissociative Disorders

Dissociative disorders are a group of psychological illnesses. In these illnesses, a particular mental function is separated (dissociated) from the mind as a whole. These disorders include the following:

- *Dissociative amnesia:* A disorder characterized by the blocking out of critical personal information, usually of a traumatic or stressful nature. Dissociative amnesia, unlike other types of amnesia, does not result from other medical trauma.
- *Dissociative fugue:* A rare disorder in which an individual suddenly and unexpectedly takes physical leave of the surroundings.

BOX 35-20 Facts About Somatization Disorders

- The lifetime prevalence rate for somatization disorder is 0.2% to 2% of the U.S. population.
- Somatization disorders are rare in men.
- Somatization disorders tend to run in families. They occur in 10% to 20% of the primary female relatives of somatization disorder patients.
- Most somatization disorders begin in adolescence or early adulthood. Most are chronic in nature.
- The symptoms sometimes increase and decrease in severity over time. Usually, though, the individual has a few symptom-free episodes.
- Anxiety and depression often accompany the disorder.
- Suicide threats are common in these patients, but suicide is rarely carried out.

BOX 35-21 Facts About Conversion Disorder

- True conversion disorder is rare in the United States.
- The disorder is seen more often in lower socioeconomic groups. It may be more common in military personnel exposed to combat.
- Conversion disorder may appear at any age. However, it is rare before age 10 or after age 35.
- In pediatric patients, the incidence of conversion disorder is higher after physical or sexual abuse. The incidence also rises among children whose parents are very ill or have chronic pain.
- About 64% of adult patients with conversion disorder have evidence of organic brain disorder.

- *Dissociative identity disorder:* A disorder that has been called "multiple personality disorder."
- *Depersonalization disorder:* A condition marked by a feeling of detachment or distance from one's own experience, body, or self.

Dissociative disorders usually are associated with emotional conflicts. These conflicts are so repressed that a split in the personality occurs. This results in an altered state of consciousness or confusion in identity. The condition also may be caused by an inability to cope with severe stress or conflict. Dissociation can occur soon after a catastrophic event, such as the traumatic death of a child or spouse. People with dissociative disorders often are unable to remember their names or personal histories. However, they can still speak, read, and learn new material. Treatment may include antianxiety medications, hypnosis, and psychotherapy.

Eating Disorders

The two most common eating disorders considered to be forms of psychiatric illness are anorexia nervosa and bulimia nervosa (Box 35-22).[22] Both of these eating disorders can lead to serious dehydration, starvation, and electrolyte imbalances. They also may cause critical illness or death. The disorders are best managed with supervision and regulation of eating habits, psychotherapy, and, sometimes, antidepressants. Most patients require hospitalization.

ANOREXIA NERVOSA

Anorexia nervosa is an eating disorder characterized by an intense fear of being obese, severe weight loss, malnutrition, and, eventually, amenorrhea (absence of menstrual bleeding). A patient feels intensely hungry, even though hunger pains are denied. Signs and symptoms include weight loss, obsession with exercise, fatigue, binge eating, induced vomiting, and use of laxatives to promote weight loss. The condition mainly is seen in adolescents, mostly girls. It usually is associated with emotional stress or conflict. It often is difficult to identify an exact underlying cause for this disease.

BOX 35-22 Facts About Eating Disorders

- More than 5 million Americans suffer from eating disorders.
- Anorexia, bulimia, and binge-eating disorders are diseases that affect the mind and body at the same time.
- Three percent of adolescent and adult women have an eating disorder. One percent of men have an eating disorder.
- A young woman with anorexia is 12 times more likely to die than another woman her age without anorexia.
- Fifteen percent of young women have substantially poor eating attitudes and behaviors.

BULIMIA NERVOSA

Bulimia nervosa is sometimes considered a form of anorexia. It is an insatiable craving for food. This craving often results in episodes of binge eating followed by purging (through self-induced vomiting or use of laxatives), depression, and self-deprivation. Like anorexia, bulimia is most common in adolescent girls and young women. Anorexic and bulimic patients often worry about their compulsive behavior. As a result, they may become depressed and suicidal.

> **NOTE**
> *Binge-eating disorder* is similar to anorexia and bulimia, but with slightly different characteristics. It involves recurrent binge-eating episodes during which a person feels loss of control over eating. Unlike bulimia, binge-eating episodes are not followed by purging, excessive exercise, or fasting. As a result, people with binge-eating disorder often are overweight or obese. They also experience guilt, shame, and/or distress about the binge eating, which can lead to more binge eating. Obese people with binge-eating disorder often have coexisting psychological illnesses including anxiety, depression, and personality disorders. In addition, links between obesity and cardiovascular disease and hypertension are well documented.[23]

Impulse Control Disorders

Impulse-control disorders are a group of psychiatric conditions. They are characterized by the inability to resist an impulse or a temptation to perform some act that is unlawful, socially unacceptable, or self-harmful. Disorders in this category include the following:

- *Intermittent explosive disorder:* A condition marked by frequent and often unpredictable episodes of extreme anger or physical outbursts. Between episodes there is usually no evidence of violence or physical threat.
- *Kleptomania:* The failure to resist impulses to steal things that are not needed either for personal use or for their monetary value.
- *Pathological gambling:* A persistent and maladaptive pattern of gambling that causes difficulties with interpersonal, financial, and vocational functioning.
- *Pyromania:* Deliberate and purposeful fire-setting for nonmonetary gain. This condition typically is associated with tension or heightened arousal before the act and with gratification or relief afterward.
- *Trichotillomania:* The recurrent pulling out of one's own hair, which results in significant hair loss.

Impulse-control disorders often are difficult to treat. Most are managed with behavior modification and drug therapy. Failure to control these disorders may result in violent behavior or unlawful activities (e.g., road rage). Incarceration is common.

PERSONALITY DISORDERS

Personality disorders are a large group of conditions distinguished by a failure to learn from experience or to adapt appropriately to changes. This failure results in personal distress and impairment of social functioning. These disorders may have an environmental component. They also may be genetic. Personality disorders become especially obvious during times of stress.

The symptoms of a personality disorder usually are first recognized in early adolescence. They continue throughout the person's life. The symptoms may vary in frequency and intensity. Generally, however, they are relatively constant. They usually affect most aspects of a patient's life. This includes thoughts, emotions, relationships and interpersonal skills, and impulse control. Personality disorders have been classified in a number of ways. However, the following are three common disorders:

- *Antisocial personality disorder:* A long-standing pattern (after the age of 15) of disregard for the rights of others. It often is associated with irresponsible behavior and a lack of remorse for wrongdoing.
- *Borderline personality disorder:* A pattern of unstable relationships, poor or negative self-image, mood swings, and poor impulse control. It may be associated with destructive and self-harming behaviors (e.g., suicide attempts, self-mutilation), an intense fear of abandonment, and displays of sudden anger.
- *Narcissistic personality disorder:* A pattern of grandiosity, need for admiration, and sense of entitlement. It often is associated with exaggerated achievements and fantasies about unlimited success, power, love, or beauty.

Many factors are associated with the development of a personality disorder. These may include unstable relationships during childhood, family violence, and childhood abuse or neglect (see Chapter 50). Treatment involves behavior modification techniques, counseling, drug therapy, and individual psychotherapy.

SPECIAL CONSIDERATIONS FOR PATIENTS WITH BEHAVIORAL PROBLEMS

In addition to caring for the immediate needs of patients with behavioral problems, paramedics may have to deal with complications arising from the situation or other factors affecting the patient. Among these factors are the patient's age and the possibility of violent behavior. This section presents special considerations for pediatric patients, elderly patients, and the potentially violent patient.

Behavioral Problems in Children

Young children who are victims of emotional crisis need to be managed with techniques that are different from those used to care for older children and adults. The following suggestions may be helpful to the paramedic in dealing with some children:

1. Gain the child's trust and try to convince the child that you are a friend who can help.
2. Make it clear that you are strong enough to be in control but will not hurt the child.
3. Keep the interview questions brief; the child's attention span may be extremely short.
4. Never lie; be honest.
5. Use all available resources to communicate (e.g., drawing pictures, telling stories).
6. Involve parents or caregivers in the interview or examination if appropriate.
7. Take any threat of violence seriously.

If the child's behavior or physical condition makes restraint necessary, the paramedic should use only humane and reasonable force (the minimum force necessary to ensure the patient's safety and the safety of the EMS crew). Sufficient manpower should be available. Calming measures may fail to work. If so, wrapping the child in a full body blanket secured to the stretcher with straps often is sufficient during transport for evaluation by a physician. As with any method of restraint, the paramedic should monitor the child's airway and circulation and ensure that they are not compromised. Documentation should be thorough and complete.

Behavioral Problems in Elderly Patients

An estimated 15% to 25% of elderly people in the United States suffer from significant symptoms of mental illness. More than 6.5 million elderly individuals are clinically depressed.[24] Most of these disorders can be diagnosed and treated successfully. However, many of these people do not seek care. Problem behavior in an elderly patient can be a sign of a long-standing psychiatric disorder, a newly emerging psychiatric problem, a medical illness, substance abuse, drug noncompliance or drug interactions, and other factors (see Chapter 49). The following suggestions may be helpful to the paramedic in communicating with some elderly patients:

1. Identify yourself and speak at eye level to make sure the patient can see you.
2. Address the patient by surname (e.g., "Mr. Jones" or "Miss [or Mrs.] Smith") unless directed otherwise.
3. Speak slowly, distinctly, and respectfully.
4. Ask one question at a time and allow time for complete answers.
5. Listen closely.
6. Explain what you are doing and why.
7. Provide reassuring physical touch.
8. Be patient.

CRITICAL THINKING

When responding to a behavioral emergency that involves a child or an adolescent, do you use the same safety guidelines that you use with an adult?

9. Permit family members and caregivers to remain with the patient if appropriate.
10. Preserve the patient's dignity.

Assessing the Potentially Violent Patient

Only a small number of people with mental health problems are potentially violent. Nonetheless, assessment and management of the potentially violent patient should be part of an EMS protocol. The following four factors may help the paramedic determine the potential for a violent episode[25]:

1. *Past history:* Has the patient previously shown hostile, aggressive, or violent behavior?
2. *Posture:* Is the patient sitting or standing? Does the patient appear to be tense or rigid?
3. *Vocal activity:* Loud, obscene, and erratic speech indicates emotional distress.
4. *Physical activity:* Is the patient pacing or agitated or protecting his or her physical boundaries?

If any of these signs of potentially violent behavior are present, efforts should be taken to reduce the effect of the stress while avoiding confrontation. Paramedics should prepare a way to cope with the crisis that reduces the potential for a life-threatening incident. It also should reduce the chance for psychologically damaging consequences.

> **NOTE**
> Paramedics should retreat from the scene if they anticipate violence that would threaten their personal safety or the safety of the crew. They should wait for law enforcement personnel to ensure that the scene is safe.

CONTROLLING VIOLENT SITUATIONS

Severely disturbed patients who pose a threat to themselves or others may need to be restrained, transported, and hospitalized against their will. Each state has a law establishing the criteria for involuntary commitment. The paramedic should be familiar with all relevant laws. The premise on which most state laws are based suggests that one person may restrain another to protect life or prevent injury.

When a psychiatric patient refuses care, EMS personnel should consult with medical direction. The decision to restrain, treat, or release the patient is a medical direction decision. If violent behavior must be contained, "reasonable force" should be used to restrain the patient. It should be used as humanely as possible and with respect for the patient's dignity. In most cases the restraint duty (if needed) should be given to law enforcement personnel. As in all other aspects of health care, details of the incident should be carefully documented for future reference. When dealing with a patient who may require restraint, the paramedic should do the following:

1. Provide a safe environment.
2. Gather a significant medical and psychiatric history.
3. Attempt to gain the patient's cooperation.
4. Be confident but not confrontational.

>
> **CRITICAL THINKING**
> Have you ever seen an EMS crew member or a police officer lose control of his or her own behavior when dealing with a violent patient? How did it affect the patient's physical or psychological state?

> **? DID YOU KNOW?**
> **Tasers**
> Tasers (stun guns) are electronic-control devices designed for self-defense and to subdue unruly or violent individuals. Tasers are used by many law enforcement, military, and security personnel. In most states, the devices are legal for civilian use (though some states or municipalities restrict or ban them). Tasers deliver a high-voltage, low-amperage electrical charge (about 3 milliampere [mA] or 0.3 joule [J]). The charge is delivered through two small dartlike electrodes tethered to the device by conductive wires. The electrodes in most devices can be quickly launched about 15 feet. The darts are pointed to penetrate clothing and barbed to prevent removal once in place. (Other styles of taser devices are available and use different methods.) The delivered current disrupts the voluntary control of muscles and produces neuromuscular incapacitation. Once the electricity stops flowing (preset time sequences up to 30 seconds in each cycle), the subject regains immediate control of all muscular activity. The use of tasers is considered highly controversial by some in the medical community and other groups.

RESTRAINT GUIDELINES

The following guidelines can help paramedics to use restraint appropriately:

- If the patient is homicidal, do not attempt restraint without assistance from law enforcement personnel. If the patient is armed, move everyone out of range and retreat from the scene. Wait for law enforcement personnel.
- Remember that the patient may not be responsible for his or her actions.
- When planning the restraining action, include a backup plan in case the initial attempt fails.
- Make sure that adequate help is available. This means that at least four capable people should be available to help restrain an adult patient.
- Keep in mind that the potential for personal injury and legal liability is always present.

RESTRAINT METHODS

A number of restraint methods can be used to manage a violent patient. A gentle, nonthreatening, low-profile technique should be attempted first. The approach should move to more direct intervention as needed. The options of physical restraint should always be explained to the patient before force is applied. If still unwilling to cooperate, the patient should be informed that restraint is required to protect against injury and to ensure the safety of others.

Before approaching a violent patient, the paramedic should be aware of the patient's surroundings. Seemingly harmless items should be noted, such as ashtrays, lighted cigarettes, hot coffee, letter openers, soda bottles, cans, and furniture. No attempt should be made to enter the patient's physical space until the other members involved in the restraint action are ready to proceed. (The patient's physical space usually is considered to be one arm's length.)

The patient's muscle groups and potential range of motion should be considered before restraint is initiated. The paramedic should plan to position the patient in a way that limits strength and range of motion. Each member of the restraint team should be assigned a specific body part or responsibility before the actual restraint procedure begins.

Paramedics must be familiar with the restraint devices available and should be able to improvise if the need arises. The preferred method is to use commercially manufactured wrist/waist/ankle padded leather or Velcro straps, or full jacket restraints (Figure 35-3). Effective restraints also may be improvised using common materials such as the following:

- Small towels that can be wrapped around the patient's wrists and ankles and secured with tape to the stretcher
- Cravats
- Webbed straps ordinarily used to secure patients to spine boards
- Roller bandage
- Blanket roll

Regardless of the types used, restraints should be strong enough to achieve the desired effect. However, they should not compromise circulatory or respiratory status.

SEQUENCE OF RESTRAINT ACTIONS

Trained personnel can use many restraint techniques. The following sequence is an example of a restraint action that may be used to contain violent behavior.

1. The paramedic offers the patient one final chance to cooperate.
2. If the patient does not respond, at least four rescuers move swiftly toward the person. They position themselves close to and slightly behind the patient. Two rescuers should then position an inside leg in front of the patient's leg to force the patient to the ground if necessary (Figure 35-4). Swift movement by several rescuers minimizes the patient's ability to focus on restraint actions. It also reduces the accuracy of kicks or blows. During the restraint procedure, the patient should be continually reassured by a rescuer not involved in the physical maneuver.

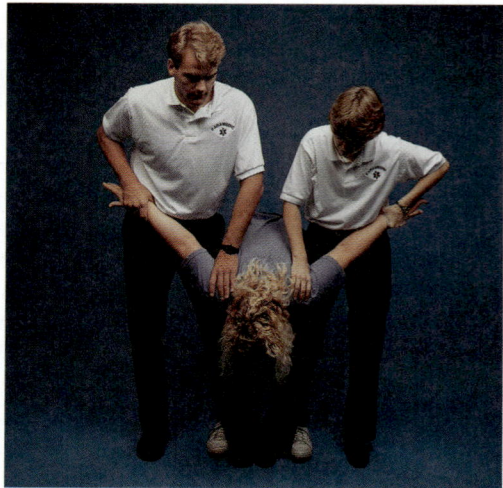

FIGURE 35-4 Control position. Rescuers face the same direction. The rescuers' inside legs are placed in front of the patient. The rescuers' outside hands hold the patient's wrists. The rescuers' inside hands form a C on the patient's shoulders.

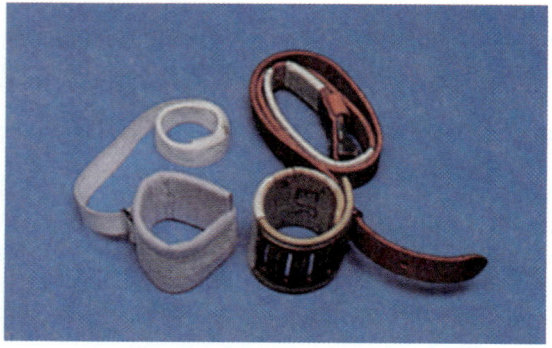

FIGURE 35-3 Restraint devices.

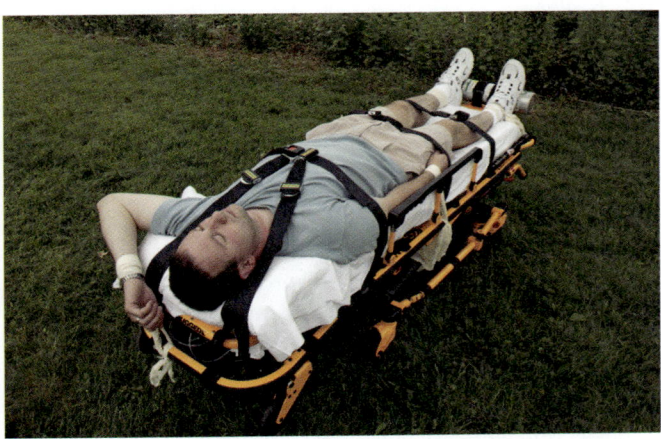

FIGURE 35-5 Patient restrained in supine position.

3. If the patient calms and agrees to be transported without restraints, the paramedic positions the patient lateral or supine on a stretcher (if not contraindicated by the mechanism of injury or medical condition). The paramedic secures the patient with straps to limit range of motion (Figure 35-5). If the patient becomes dangerous en route to the hospital, restraints should be used.

4. Once applied, restraints should not be removed until the patient is delivered to the emergency department or there are adequate resources to control the situation. The patient's respiratory and circulatory status should be assessed frequently and documented. This ensures that the restraint action has not compromised vital functions. If a change in the restraints is required, additional manpower must be available for assistance. Also, only one limb should be repositioned at a time.

Restraint procedures should be fully documented on the patient care report. Any attempts at negotiation and a description of the patient's behavior before restraint should be clearly described. Paramedics should document that circulatory evaluation and continued monitoring of the patient were performed after restraint. Again, physical restraint is advised only when all verbal and nonverbal techniques have been exhausted and only when a person presents a danger to self or others.

PERSONAL SAFETY

Paramedics' personal safety should be considered in any emergency response. However, behavioral emergencies are more likely to require that paramedics protect themselves and the crew from hostile injury. The following measures for preventing personal injury should be considered:

- When possible, remain a safe distance from the patient.
- Do not allow the patient to block the exit.
- Keep large furniture between you and the patient. Do not allow a single paramedic to remain alone with the patient.
- Do not make statements that the patient might perceive as threatening.
- Use folded blankets or cushions to absorb the impact of thrown objects.

Various training programs have been developed to provide safety and security to the rescuer and the violent patient. Paramedics should learn nonviolent personal protection maneuvers. They also should practice these maneuvers under the supervision of a qualified instructor.

CHEMICAL RESTRAINT

The term **chemical restraint** refers to the use of drugs to control behavior. Drug treatment varies. However, it generally is intended to provide sedation. Two groups of drugs that are effective for chemical restraint are benzodiazepines and antipsychotics (see Chapter 13).

Benzodiazepines bind to specific receptors in the cerebral cortex and limbic system (a major integrating system that governs emotional behavior). These drugs are popular because of their very high therapeutic index. They have four main actions: anxiety reducing, sedative-hypnotic, muscle relaxing, and anticonvulsant. Benzodiazepines commonly used for chemical restraint include **diazepam, midazolam,** and **lorazepam.**

Antipsychotics block dopamine receptors in specific areas of the central nervous system. These drugs are primarily used to treat schizophrenia. They also are used to treat other conditions that produce disturbed behavior (e.g., Tourette's syndrome and senile dementia associated with Alzheimer's disease). A well-known antipsychotic used for chemical restraint is **haloperidol.** The benzodiazepine **lorazepam** is also administered for this purpose. Short-term use of antipsychotics rarely produces extrapyramidal reactions. However, if such reactions occur, administration of **diphenhydramine** may reverse these side effects.

Benzodiazepines and antipsychotics can be very effective at controlling hostile or combative patients. As with all other restraint methods, paramedics should consult with medical direction, follow protocol, and carefully document the event.

> **NOTE**
>
> As described in Chapter 13, extrapyramidal reactions are neuromuscular effects that can be caused by some antipsychotic medications. These effects include Parkinson-like symptoms (e.g., tremor, muscle rigidity, pill-rolling motion, shuffling gait), akathisia (abnormal restlessness, agitation), dystonias (abnormal muscle tone or posturing), and tardive dyskinesia (involuntary, repetitive movement). The occurrence and severity of extrapyramidal reactions frequently are dose-related. They often subside when the dose is reduced or the drug is discontinued. However, in some patients tardive dyskinesia persists even after drug therapy is stopped. (This is especially the case for patients prescribed long-term drug therapy.) These rhythmical, involuntary movements are most evident in the tongue, face, mouth, or jaw. They are characterized by protrusion of the tongue, puffing of the cheeks, puckering of the mouth, chewing movements, and sometimes involuntary movements of the extremities.

SUMMARY

- A behavioral emergency is a change in mood or behavior. This change cannot be tolerated by the involved person or others. It calls for immediate attention.
- Physical or biochemical disturbances can result in significant changes in behavior. Psychosocial mental illness is often the result of childhood trauma, parental deprivation, or a dysfunctional family structure.
- Changes in behavior caused by interpersonal or situational stress are often linked to specific incidents, such as environmental violence, death of a loved one, economic or employment problems, or prejudice and discrimination.
- When dealing with behavioral emergencies, the paramedic should contain the crisis. It begins by establishing a rapport with the patient. He or she should provide the proper emergency care as well. Also, the paramedic should transport the patient to an appropriate health care facility.
- During the patient assessment, an attempt should be made to determine the patient's mental state, name and age, significant medical history, medications (and compliance), and past psychiatric problems, as well as the precipitating situation or problem.
- Effective interviewing techniques include active listening, being supportive and empathetic, limiting interruptions, and respecting the patient's personal space.
- A mental status exam includes assessment of appearance and behavior; speech and language; cognitive abilities; and emotional stability.
- All cognitive disorders result in a disturbance in thinking that may manifest as delirium or dementia.
- Schizophrenia is characterized by recurrent episodes of psychotic behavior. This behavior may include abnormalities of thought process, thought content, perception, and judgment.
- Anxiety disorders may cause a panic attack. Anxiety disorders include phobias, obsessive-compulsive disorders, and posttraumatic syndrome.
- Depression is a mood disorder. A person with depression may have feelings of hopelessness, loss of appetite, decreased libido, and feelings of worthlessness and guilt.
- Bipolar disorder is a manic-depressive illness. In this illness, depressive and manic episodes alternate.
- Suicide threats or attempts indicate the patient has a serious crisis. Certain factors increase the risk of suicide. Patients who express the wish to harm or kill themselves should be transported.
- Somatoform disorders are conditions in which there are physical symptoms for which no physical cause can be found. The cause is thought to be psychological. These include somatization disorder and conversion disorder.

- Factitious disorders are disorders in which symptoms mimic a true illness. However, the symptoms have been invented. They are under the control of the patient.
- Dissociative disorders are a group of psychological illnesses. In these disorders, a particular mental function is separated from the mind as a whole.
- The most common eating disorders considered to be forms of psychiatric illness are anorexia nervosa and bulimia nervosa.
- Impulse control disorders are characterized by the inability to resist an impulse or temptation to perform an act that is unlawful, socially unacceptable, or self-harmful.
- Personality disorders are conditions characterized by failing to learn from experience or adapt appropriately to changes. This results in personal distress and impairment of social functioning.
- A threat of suicide is an indication that a patient has a serious crisis. This crisis requires immediate intervention.
- Questions that determine the patient's ideation, plan, intent, and means to commit suicide should be asked.
- After ensuring scene safety, the first priority in patient management after a suicide attempt is medical care. If the patient is conscious, developing rapport as soon as possible is crucial.
- Assessment of a potentially violent patient should include history of violence, posture, vocal activity, and physical activity.
- When trying to defuse a situation involving a potentially violent patient, the paramedic should ensure a safe environment, gather the patient's history, try to gain the patient's cooperation, avoid threats, and explain the paramedic's role in providing care.
- Severely disturbed patients who pose a threat to themselves or others may need to be restrained.
- Reasonable force to restrain a patient should be used as humanely as possible. An adequate number of personnel is needed. This will ensure patient and rescuer safety during restraint. The risk of personal injury and legal liability is always present.
- Personal safety measures while responding to a behavioral emergency should include not allowing the patient to block the exit, keeping large furniture between you and the patient, working as a team, avoiding threatening statements, and using soft objects to absorb the impact of thrown objects.
- When caring for children with behavioral emergencies, the paramedic should attempt to gain the child's trust, tell the child he or she will not be hurt, keep questions brief, be honest, involve parents (if appropriate), and take threats of violence seriously.

REFERENCES

1. National Institute of Mental Health, National Institutes of Health: *Statistics*, www.nimh.nih.gov/health/topics/statistics/index.shtml, accessed 9-12-10.
2. National Alliance on Mental Health Illness: *Economic downturn taking a toll on Americans' mental health*, www.nami.org/Template.cfm?Section=press_room&template=/ContentManagement/ContentDisplay.cfm&ContentID=87096, accessed 11-10-10.
3. Seidel HM, Ball JW, Dains JE, et al: *Mosby's guide to physical examination*, ed 6, St Louis, 2006, Mosby.
4. National Highway Traffic Safety Administration: *The National EMS Education Standards*, Washington, DC, 2009, U.S. Department of Transportation/National Highway Traffic Safety Administration, DOT.
5. American Psychiatric Association: *Diagnostic and statistical manual of mental disorders–IV, text revision*, Washington, DC, 2000, The Association.
6. Samuel E, Williams RB, Ferrell RB: Excited delirium: consideration of selected medical and psychiatric issues, *Neuropsychiatr Dis Treat* 5:61-66, 2009.
7. Pollanen MS, Chiasson DA, Cairns JT, et al: Unexpected death related to restraint for excited delirium: a retrospective study of deaths in police custody and in the community, *CMAJ* 158(12):1603-1607, 1998.
8. National Institute of Mental Health, National Institutes of Health: *Mental disorders in America: the numbers count*, www.nimh.nih.gov/health/publications/the-numbers-count-mental-disorders-in-america/index.shtml#Alzheimer, accessed 9-12-10.
9. Centers for Disease Control and Prevention: *Autism spectrum disorder: data and statistics*, www.cdc.gov/ncbddd/autism/data.html, accessed 9-12-10.
10. Bishop DV, Whitehouse AJ, Watt HJ, et al: Autism and diagnostic substitution: evidence from a study of adults with a history of developmental language disorder, *Dev Med Child Neurol* 50(5):341-345, 2008.
11. National Institute of Child Health and Human Development, National Institutes of Health: *Autism and what we know*, www.nichd.nih.gov/publications/pubs/upload/autism_overview_2005.pdf#page=3, accessed 9-12-10.
12. American Psychiatric Association: *Schizophrenia and other psychotic disorders*, www.psych.org/MainMenu/Research/DSMIV/DSMIVTR/DSMIVvsDSMIVTR/SummaryofTextChangesInDSMIVTR/SchizophreniaandOtherPsychoticDisorders.asp, accessed 9-12-10.
13. National Institute of Mental Health: *The numbers count: mental disorders in America*, www.nimh.nih.gov/health/publications/the-numbers-count-mental-disorders-in-america/index.shtml, accessed 9-12-10.
14. Marx J, Hockberger R, Walls R: *Rosen's emergency medicine*, ed 7, St Louis, 2009, Mosby.
15. Tanielian T, Jaycoxx LH: *Invisible wounds of war: psychological and cognitive injuries, their consequences and services to assist recovery*, Santa Monica, Calif, 2008, Rand.
16. American Public Health Association 135th Annual Meeting: Abstract 165759, presented 11-05-07.
17. Hoyer D, David E: Screening for depression in emergency department patients, *J Emerg Med* Nov 18, 2008.doi:10.1016/j.jemermed.2008.05.004
18. Jaffe D, *Alliance for the Mentally Ill, Advocates for the Mentally Ill*, NY: *All about ECT*, www.medhelp.org/lib/ect.htm, accessed 9-12-10.
19. Centers for Disease Control and Prevention: *Suicide*, www.cdc.gov/violenceprevention/pdf/Suicide-DataSheet-a.pdf, accessed 9-12-10.
20. National Alliance on Mental Illness: *Dual diagnosis and integrated treatment of mental illness and substance abuse disorder*, www.nami.org/Template.cfm?Section=By_Illness&Template=/TaggedPage/TaggedPageDisplay.cfm&TPLID=54&ContentID=23049, accessed 9-12-10.
21. Smith RC, Gardiner JC, Lyles JS, et al: Exploration of DSM-IV criteria in primary care patients with medically unexplained symptoms, *Psychosom Med* 67(1):123-129, 2005.
22. South Carolina Department of Mental Health: *Eating disorder statistics*, www.state.sc.us/dmh/anorexia/statistics.htm, accessed 9-12-10.
23. National Institute of Mental Health, National Institutes of Health: *Eating disorders*, www.nimh.nih.gov/health/publications/eating-disorders/complete-index.shtml, accessed 9-12-10.
24. National Alliance on Mental Illness: *Depression in older persons fact sheet*, www.nami.org/Template.cfm?Section=By_Illness&template=/ContentManagement/ContentDisplay.cfm&ContentID=7515, accessed 9-12-10.
25. Judd R, Peszke M: Psychological and behavioral emergencies, *Top Emerg Med* 4(4):7, 1983.

SUGGESTED READINGS

AAP Committee on Pediatric Emergency Medicine: *Pediatric mental health emergencies in the emergency medical services system [Policy Statement]*, Ann Emerg Med 48(4):484-486, 2006, doi: 10.1016/j.annemergmed.2006.08.015.

Cuddeback G, Patterson PD, Moore C, et al: Utilization of emergency medical transports and hospital admissions among persons with behavioral health conditions, *Psychiatr Serv* 61(4):412-415, 2010.

Dunn T: *Handle with care: the challenges of transporting suicidal patients*, JEMS.com Oct 2008.

Larimer ME, Malone D, Garner M, et al: Health care and public service use and costs before and after provision of housing for chronically homeless persons with severe alcohol problems, *JAMA* 301(13):1349-1357, 2009.

Shock and Resuscitation

Chapter 36: Shock

CHAPTER

36 Shock

OBJECTIVES

Upon completion of this chapter, the paramedic student will be able to:

1. Define shock.
2. Outline the factors necessary to achieve adequate tissue oxygenation.
3. Describe how the diameter of resistance vessels influences preload.
4. Calculate mean arterial pressure when given a blood pressure.
5. Outline the changes in the microcirculation during the progression of shock.
6. List the causes of hypovolemic, cardiogenic, neurogenic, anaphylactic, and septic shock.
7. Describe pathophysiology as a basis for signs and symptoms associated with the progression through the stages of shock.
8. Describe key assessment findings that distinguish the etiology of the shock state.
9. Outline the prehospital management of the patient in shock based on knowledge of the pathophysiology associated with each type of shock.
10. Discuss how to integrate the assessment and management of the patient in shock.
11. Describe principles of fluid administration in shock.

KEY TERMS

anaphylactic shock Shock that occurs when the body is exposed to a substance that produces a severe allergic reaction.

cardiac output The volume of blood pumped each minute by the ventricle.

cardiogenic shock Shock that results when cardiac action is unable to deliver sufficient circulating blood volume for tissue perfusion.

colloid solutions Solutions that contain molecules (usually protein) that are too large to pass through the capillary membrane.

compensated shock A stage of shock associated with some decreased blood flow and perfusion to the tissues.

crystalloid solutions Solutions created by dissolving crystals such as salts and sugars in water.

disseminated intravascular coagulation A grave coagulopathy that results from the overstimulation of the clotting and anticlotting processes in response to disease or injury.

distributive shock Shock that occurs when peripheral vasodilation causes a decrease in systemic vascular resistance.

hemodilution Diluting the blood of elements.

hemostasis The cessation of bleeding by mechanical or chemical means or by substances that arrest the blood flow.

hypertonic solutions Solutions that have higher osmotic pressure than that of body cells.

hypoperfusion Severely inadequate circulation that results in insufficient delivery of oxygen and nutrients necessary

for normal tissue and cellular function. Also known as *shock.*

hypovolemic shock A form of shock most frequently caused by hemorrhage but also caused by dehydration.

irreversible shock A stage of shock that results in cellular ischemia and necrosis and subsequent organ death, even with oxygenation and perfusion restored.

leaky capillary syndrome A syndrome that occurs when the capillary lining permits protein-containing fluid to leak into the interstitial spaces.

mean arterial pressure The arithmetic mean of the blood pressure in the arterial portion of the circulation.

microcirculation Refers to circulation of blood from the heart to the arteries, capillaries, and veins.

microinfarcts A small infarct caused by obstruction of circulation in capillaries, arterioles, or small arteries.

neurogenic shock Shock resulting from vasomotor paralysis below the level of injury; also known as *spinal cord shock.*

obstructive shock Shock that results from obstruction to blood flow.

perfusion The circulation of blood to the tissues.

peripheral vascular resistance The total resistance against which blood must be pumped; also known as *afterload.*

pneumatic antishock garment A garment used to manage some forms of hypovolemia and to stabilize some fractures.

pulse pressure The difference between the systolic and diastolic blood pressures.

refractory shock A stage of shock that is resistant to treatment, but still reversible.

relative hypovolemia Inadequate preload as a result of vasodilation.

rouleaux formation An aggregation of red cells in what looks like a stack of coins or checkers.

septic shock A form of shock that most often results from a serious systemic bacterial infection.

shock An abnormal condition of inadequate blood flow to the body's peripheral tissues that is associated with life-threatening cellular dysfunction; also known as *hypoperfusion*.

uncompensated shock A stage of shock that occurs when the body is no longer able to maintain systemic blood pressure.

viscosity The physical property of a liquid. It is characterized by the degree of friction between its component molecules.

Severe illnesses and injury can threaten the normal internal environment of the body. During such events, the protective systems of the body try to compensate. They work to maintain cellular oxygenation. The paramedic must be able to integrate pathophysiological principles and assessment findings to form a field impression and to implement a treatment plan for the patient in shock.

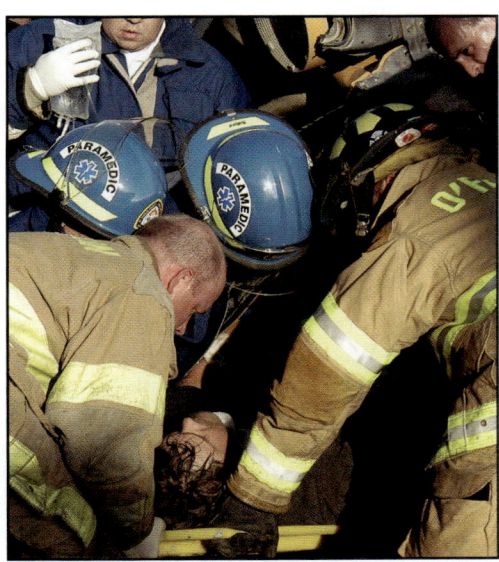

(Courtesy Ray Kemp, St. Charles, Mo.)

SHOCK

Shock was defined by Gross in 1850 as a "rude unhinging of the machinery of life"[1] and since has been redefined by many others. Robert M. Hardaway, professor of surgery at Texas Tech University School of Medicine in El Paso, Texas, defines shock this way[2]:

> I believe that the best definition of shock is inadequate capillary perfusion. As a corollary of this broad definition, almost anyone who dies, except one who is instantly destroyed, must go through a stage of shock—a momentary pause in the act of death.

Shock is not a single event. It does not have one specific cause and treatment. Rather, it is a complex group of physiological abnormalities. It can result from a variety of disease states and injuries[3] (Box 36-1). There are many complexities involved in shock. Thus, it is not adequately defined by pulse rate, blood pressure, or cardiac function. Moreover, it cannot be reduced to loss of circulating blood or loss of pressure in the vascular system. Shock may affect the entire body, or it may occur at a tissue or cellular level, even with normal hemodynamics. An understanding of cellular physiology is needed to recognize the subtle aspects of shock. This also will aid in properly assessing the severity of various stages of shock.

TISSUE OXYGENATION

The adequate oxygenation of tissue cells is known as **perfusion.** To achieve adequate oxygenation, three distinct components of the cardiovascular system must work properly. These components are the heart, vasculature, and lungs. When any one of these malfunctions, a decrease in cellular oxygenation can occur. This is known as **hypoperfusion.**

BOX 36-1 Possible Causes of Shock

Healthy Patient (Adult)
Coronary syndromes
Respiratory arrest
Anaphylaxis
Drowning
Traumatic hemorrhage
Spinal cord injury
Electrocution
Hypothermia
Toxic exposures
Pulmonary embolus

Unhealthy Patient (Adult)
Congestive heart failure
Renal failure

Uncontrolled hypertension
Uncontrolled diabetes
Obesity
Electrolyte imbalance
Drug toxicity
Stroke

Pediatric Patient
Trauma
Chest wall injury
Fluid loss
Spinal cord injury
Anaphylaxis
Heart disease

Heart

The pumping action of the heart produces pressure changes that circulate blood through the body. This repetitive pumping action is known as the *cardiac cycle*. **Cardiac output** (described in Chapter 22) is a crucial determinant of organ perfusion. Cardiac output depends on several factors, including strength of contraction, rate of contraction, and amount of venous return available to the ventricle (preload). The formula to determine cardiac output is as follows:

$$\text{Cardiac output (CO)} = \text{Heart rate (HR)} \times \text{Stroke volume (SV)}$$

LOOK AGAIN
See Chapter 22: Cardiology, pp. 578-580.

PRELOAD, AFTERLOAD, AND MAP

Important terms in understanding cardiac physiology and shock are *preload, afterload,* and *mean arterial pressure (MAP)*. To review, **preload** is the amount of venous return to the ventricle (the ventricular volume at the end of diastole). It is the "load" that must be given to the left ventricle before contraction. **Afterload** is the total resistance against which blood must be pumped. It is the "load" that must be given to the heart to overcome the resistance to ventricular ejection. Total peripheral vascular resistance is determined by the volume of blood in the vascular system and by the diameter of the vessel walls (described below).

Mean arterial pressure (MAP) is a function of total cardiac output and total peripheral resistance. MAP represents the average pressure in the vascular system that perfuses the tissues. Because more time is spent in diastole than in systole, MAP is not the average of diastolic and systolic pressure. Rather, MAP reflects the relative time spent in each portion of the cardiac cycle.[4] MAP can be calculated in several ways. A common formula used in prehospital care uses the diastolic pressure and the pulse pressure (the difference between the systolic and diastolic pressures)[5]:

$$\text{MAP} = \text{diastolic pressure} + \frac{1}{3} \text{pulse pressure}$$

Example

Patient with blood pressure of 120/80 mm Hg

$$\text{MAP} = 80 + ([120 - 80]/3)$$
$$= 80 + (40/3)$$
$$= 80 + 13.3$$
$$= 93.3, \text{rounded down to 93}$$

A systolic pressure of 80 to 90 mm Hg (MAP of 60 to 65 mm Hg) is needed to maintain adequate tissue

perfusion. MAP is further discussed later in this chapter and in Chapter 40.

Vasculature

The entire vascular system is lined with smooth, low-friction endothelial cells. All vessels larger than capillaries have layers of tissue surrounding the endothelium. These layers of tissue are known as *tunicae*. They provide supporting connective tissue to counter the pressure of blood contained in the vascular system. The layers have elastic properties to dampen pressure pulsations and minimize flow variations throughout the cardiac cycle. The layers also have muscle fibers to control the vessel diameter. The vascular system maintains blood flow by changes in pressure and peripheral vascular resistance.

PERIPHERAL VASCULAR RESISTANCE

As stated previously, peripheral vascular resistance (afterload) is the total resistance against which blood must be pumped. It is determined primarily by a change in the diameter of the arterioles: arteriolar constriction raises mean arterial pressure by preventing the free flow of blood into the capillaries. Dilation has the opposite effect. Reflex control of vasoconstriction and vasodilation is mediated by the sympathetic nervous system.[6]

Peripheral vascular resistance is a measure of friction between the vessel walls and fluid, and between the molecules of the fluid themselves, both of which oppose flow. When the resistance to flow increases, blood pressure must increase for the flow to remain constant. Resistance to blood flow increases with increased fluid viscosity or vessel length and decreased vessel diameter.

Viscosity is the physical property of a liquid. It is characterized by the degree of friction between its component molecules (e.g., between the blood cells and between the plasma proteins). Viscosity normally plays a minor role in blood flow regulation because it remains fairly constant in healthy persons. Vessel length in the human body also remains fairly constant. Vessel diameter is the main factor affecting the resistance to blood flow.

CRITICAL THINKING
How do firefighters use these principles of viscosity and vessel diameter when fighting a fire?

Major arteries are large. They offer little resistance to flow unless they have an abnormal narrowing (stenosis). Arterioles have a much smaller diameter than arteries. They offer the major resistance to blood flow. The smooth muscle in the arteriole walls can relax or contract, changing the diameter of the inside of the arteriole as much as fivefold. Thus the vasoconstriction or vasodilation of these vessels primarily regulates arterial blood pressure.

Fluid flows through a tube in response to pressure gradients between the two ends of the tube. The difference in pressure between the two ends determines flow, not the absolute pressure in the tube. In many animals and human beings the two ends are the aorta and the venae cavae.

Systemic pressure (left-sided pressure) and pulmonic pressure (right-sided pressure) are the measurements of pressure in the vascular system. Systemic pressure, like pulmonic pressure, has two phases: systolic and diastolic. As described earlier, the difference between these two pressures is the **pulse pressure.** Pulse pressure reflects the tone of the arterial system. This pressure is greatest at its origin (the heart) and is least at its terminating point (the venae cavae). Pulse pressure is more sensitive to changes in perfusion than the systolic or diastolic pressures alone.

> **SHOW ME THE EVIDENCE**
> This retrospective look at trauma registry data evaluated prehospital systolic blood pressure (PSBP) and patient injury severity and mortality to determine if a threshold for trauma triage greater than the current 90 mm Hg should be considered. The authors reviewed 32,266 trauma patients seen at a level I trauma center from 1995 to 2003. Their findings suggest that mortality risk increased when the PSBP dropped below 110 mm Hg. The risk of death increased substantially when the PSBP was less than 100 mm Hg. They recommend further study to determine if the systolic blood pressure threshold for trauma triage should be altered based on these data.

From Bruns B, Gentilello L, Elliott A, et al: Prehospital hypotension redefined, *J Trauma* 65(6):1217-1221, 2008.

MICROCIRCULATION

Microcirculation refers to circulation of blood from the heart to the arteries, capillaries, and veins. The microcirculation of the body is divided into *pulmonary microcirculation* and *peripheral microcirculation*. Separate pumps, the right side and left side of the heart, respectively, produce pressure in each of these divisions.

At any given moment, about 5% of the total circulating blood is flowing through the capillaries.[7] This 5% is exchanging nutrients and picking up the waste from cellular metabolism. The muscular arterioles are the major resistance vessels. They regulate regional blood flow to the capillary beds. The venules and veins serve as collecting channels and storage vessels. These are known as *capacitance vessels*. Capacitance vessels normally contain about 70% of the blood volume. The mechanisms that control blood flow to the tissues were described in Chapter 11 and include the following:

- Local control of blood flow by the tissues
- Nervous control of blood flow
- Baroreceptor reflexes
- Chemoreceptor reflexes
- Central nervous system ischemia response
- Hormonal mechanisms
- Adrenal-medullary mechanism
- Renin-angiotensin-aldosterone mechanism
- Vasopressin mechanism
- Reabsorption of tissue fluid

> **LOOK AGAIN**
> See Chapter 11: General Principles of Pathophysiology, pp. 238-240.

Lungs

Tissue cells require adequate oxygen to function. Adequate oxygen must be available to the red blood cells as they pass through the capillary membranes in the lungs. The high partial pressure of oxygen in inspired air, adequate depth and rate of ventilation, and matching of pulmonary ventilation and perfusion make adequate oxygenation possible.

> **CRITICAL THINKING**
> What might impair each of these components of adequate oxygenation?

THE BODY AS A CONTAINER

The healthy body can be viewed as a smooth-flowing fluid delivery system inside a container. The container must be filled to achieve adequate preload and tissue oxygenation. The external size of the container of any human body is relatively constant, yet the volume of the vascular component in the container is related directly to the diameter of the resistance vessels. This diameter can change rapidly. Any change in the diameter of the vessels changes the volume of fluid that the container holds. Thus this affects preload.

An example of this principle is a 5-L container. This is the normal container size for a 70-kg adult male (Figure 36-1). If the fluid volume is 5 L, preload is adequate. With a strong heart, cardiac output and perfusion also are adequate. If 2 L of this fluid has been lost, externally or internally, the 3 L that remain are inadequate to supply an effective preload. Because cardiac output depends on preload, a decrease in preload notably decreases cardiac output.

If the patient is hypovolemic and the 5-L container has remained the same size despite the 3-L volume, the patient becomes hypotensive or loses pressure in the container because of decreased cardiac output. However, if the container is reduced to 3 L by compensatory mechanisms (e.g., vasoconstriction), the 3-L container can provide adequate preload to the heart with the 3 L of available fluid. This is at the expense of certain tissues that are not perfused in this constricted state.

If fluid is adequate for a 5-L container but the container size has been enlarged to 7 L by illness or injury that results in vasodilation, the 5 L of fluid does not provide adequate preload for the container (**relative hypovolemia**). Factors that occasionally are responsible for vasodilation include cardiac and blood pressure medications,

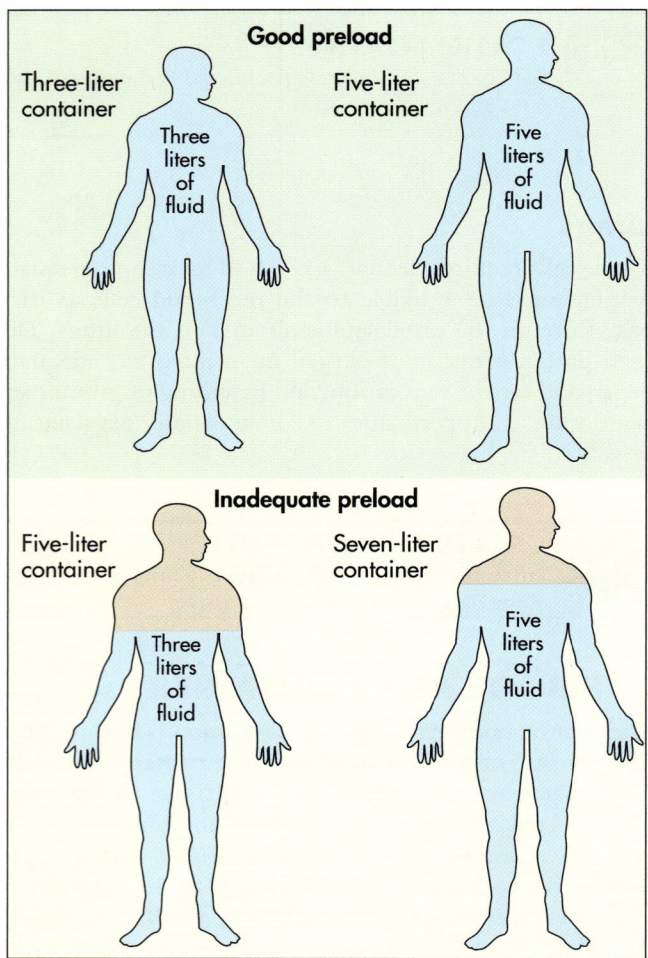

Good preload

Three-liter container — Three liters of fluid

Five-liter container — Five liters of fluid

Inadequate preload

Five-liter container — Three liters of fluid

Seven-liter container — Five liters of fluid

FIGURE 36-1 Fluid volume versus container volume.

allergic reaction, heat- and cold-related injuries, and alcohol or other drug use.

CAPILLARY-CELLULAR RELATIONSHIP IN SHOCK

The progression of shock in the microcirculation follows a sequence of stages related to changes in capillary perfusion and cellular necrosis (Figure 36-2).[1]

Stage 1: Vasoconstriction

In response to intravascular volume depletion (hypovolemia), the precapillary arterioles and postcapillary venules constrict. This constriction helps to maintain systemic blood pressure. Because of the narrowing of the entrance to the microcirculation, the velocity of blood passing through it increases. This leads to an increase in hydrostatic pressure in the capillaries and allows fluid to be reabsorbed into the circulation. Fluid is reabsorbed as it shifts from the extravascular space (*transcapillary refill*). As shock progresses, oxygen and nutrient delivery to the cells supplied by these capillaries decreases; anaerobic metabolism replaces aerobic

metabolism; and production of hydrogen ions and lactate increases. Shortly thereafter, the lining of the capillaries can begin to lose the ability to hold large molecules within the capillary. Thus the capillary lining permits protein-containing fluid to leak into the interstitial spaces. This is known as the **leaky capillary syndrome.**

CRITICAL THINKING
If this leak persists, what effect will it have on preload and cardiac output?

Arteriovenous (AV) shunts open, particularly in the skin, kidneys, and gastrointestinal tract. The shunts cause less flow to the arterioles and thus less flow through the capillaries. Sympathetic stimulation produces pale, sweaty skin; a rapid, thready pulse (caused by hypovolemia and vasoconstriction); and an elevation in blood glucose level. The release of epinephrine dilates coronary, cerebral, and skeletal muscle arterioles and constricts other arterioles. As a result, blood is shunted to the heart, brain, and skeletal muscle. Moreover, capillary flow to the kidneys and abdominal organs decreases. The vasoconstriction stage of shock must be treated by prompt restoration of circulatory fluid volume. Otherwise, shock progresses to the next stage.

NOTE
Stage 1 of hypovolemic shock occurs when intravascular blood volume is decreased by about 15%. Blood pressure and heart rate usually are normal at this stage of compensation. This stage is reversible if the hemorrhage is controlled.

Stage 2: Capillary and Venule Opening

As shock progresses, the precapillary sphincter relaxes. This results in some expansion of the vascular space. Postcapillary sphincters resist the relaxation effects. Thus they remain closed. This causes blood to pool or stagnate in the capillary system. The capillaries become engorged with fluid. Arterial hypotension, secondary arteriolar vasoconstriction, and opening of arteriovenous shunts result in less blood flow through arterioles. These conditions also contribute to the stagnation of blood flow in the capillaries.

The vascular space expands greatly as increasing hypoxemia and acidosis lead to the opening of more venules and capillaries. When this occurs, even normal blood volume may be inadequate to fill the container. The capillary and venule capacity can increase to the point that the volume of available blood returning to the great veins and venae cavae is reduced. This in turn results in decreased venous return and a drop in cardiac output. In addition, the viscera (lungs, liver, kidneys, and gastrointestinal mucosa) can become congested with fluid. The low arterial blood pressure, extremely constricted arterioles, presence of

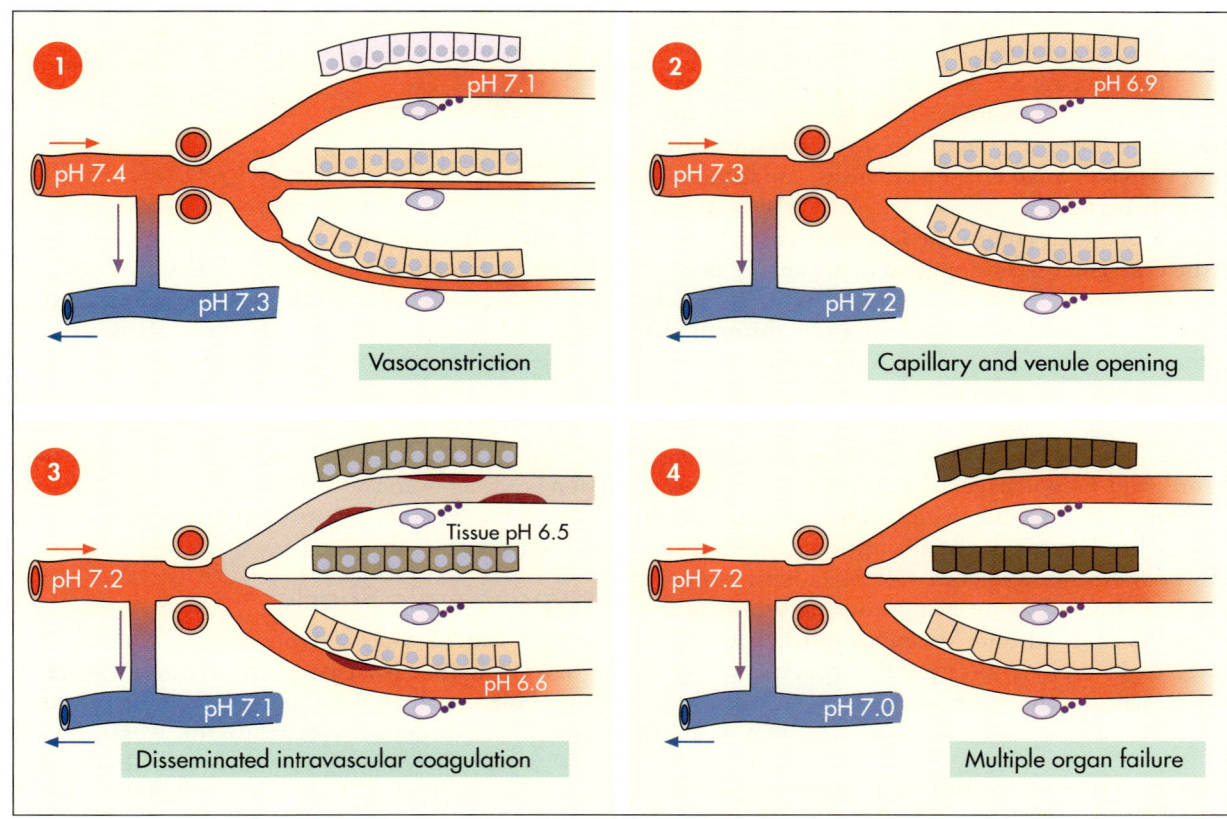

FIGURE 36-2 Diagram of the microcirculation in shock, progressing from (*1*) vasoconstriction, (*2*) capillary and venule opening, (*3*) disseminated intravascular coagulation, and (*4*) multiple organ failure. (Adapted from Hardaway R, editor: *Shock: the reversible stage of dying*, Littleton, Mass, 1988, PSG Publishing.)

arteriovenous shunts, and many open capillaries result in stagnant capillary flow.

CRITICAL THINKING
What happens to the function of the heart as acidosis increases?

Sluggish blood flow and a decrease in the amount of oxygen delivered to the cell result in cell metabolism occurring without oxygen (anaerobic metabolism). As described in Chapter 11, when tissue hypoxia is present, pyruvate oxidation decreases, lactate production increases, and adenosine triphosphate (ATP) formation continues via glycolysis. This results in metabolic acidosis. The respiratory system attempts to compensate for the acidosis by increasing ventilation to release carbon dioxide. This produces a partially compensated metabolic acidosis. As the acidosis increases and the pH decreases, the red blood cells may cluster. (This is known as *rouleaux formation*.) **Rouleaux formation** halts perfusion in the vital organ capillaries. In turn, this affects nutritional flow and prevents the removal of waste products of metabolism. Clotting mechanisms also are affected; this leads to hypercoagulability. This stage

of shock often advances to the third stage if fluid resuscitation is inadequate or delayed. This stage also may progress if the shock state is complicated by trauma or infection (sepsis).

LOOK AGAIN
See Chapter 11: General Principles of Pathophysiology, pp. 227-230.

NOTE
Stage 2 of hypovolemic shock occurs with a 15% to 25% decrease in intravascular blood volume. Heart rate, respiratory rate, and capillary refill time are increased, and pulse pressure is decreased at this stage. Blood pressure readings may still be normal.

Stage 3: Disseminated Intravascular Coagulation

Stage 3 of shock is resistant to treatment. (This is **refractory shock**.) However, stage 3 shock is still reversible early on with fluid replacement and support of vital functions. Blood begins to coagulate in the microcirculation, clogging capillaries. This is referred to as **disseminated intravascular coagulation.** Clumps of red blood cells may occlude the capillaries. This occlusion decreases capillary perfusion, prevents delivery of oxygenated substrates such as glucose, and prevents removal of metabolites. As a result, distal tissue cells switch to anaerobic metabolism, and lactic acid production increases.

As stage 3 of shock continues, lactic acid accumulates around the cell. The cell no longer has the energy needed to maintain homeostasis, or the balance to function normally. Water and sodium leak into the cell through the cellular membrane. Potassium leaks out. Lastly, the cells swell and die (also known as the *washout phase*). **Microinfarcts** (small areas of dead cells) develop in the organs. Microthrombi produce capillary congestion, fluid leakage, cell rupture, and hemorrhage. The pulmonary capillaries become permeable to fluid, which leads to pulmonary edema. The edema decreases the absorption of oxygen and results in possible alterations in carbon dioxide elimination. This can lead to acute respiratory failure or acute respiratory distress syndrome (described in Chapter 24). If shock and disseminated intravascular coagulation continue, the patient progresses to multiple organ failure.

> **NOTE**
> Stage 3 of hypovolemic shock occurs with a 25% to 35% decrease in intravascular blood volume. At this stage, hypotension occurs. This stage of shock usually requires blood replacement.

Stage 4: Multiple Organ Failure

The amount of cellular necrosis (death) required to produce organ failure varies with each organ. Cellular necrosis also depends on the underlying condition of the organ. Usually hepatic failure occurs first, followed by renal failure and heart failure. But if any given area of capillary occlusion persists for more than 1 to 2 hours, the cells nourished by that capillary undergo changes that rapidly become irreversible. In this stage of shock, blood pressure falls dramatically (to levels of 60 mm Hg or less). Even if blood pressure is returned to normal after a couple of hours, the ability of the cell to obtain energy through aerobic metabolism fails. Thus the cell dies from inadequate capillary perfusion. Inadequate tissue perfusion and cell death are the results of irreversible shock.

If cellular necrosis damages a critical amount of a vital organ, the organ soon fails. Failure of the liver and kidneys is common and often presents early in this stage. Capillary blockage can cause heart failure. Gastrointestinal bleeding and sepsis can result from gastrointestinal mucosal necrosis. In addition, pancreatic necrosis can lead to further clotting disorders and severe pancreatitis. Pulmonary thrombosis can produce hemorrhage and fluid loss into the alveoli. This can lead to death from respiratory failure.

>
> **NOTE**
> Stage 4 of hypovolemic shock occurs when intravascular blood volume is decreased by 35% to 40%.

CLASSIFICATIONS OF SHOCK

Many types of shock have been discussed in the medical literature. In emergency care, shock commonly is classified based on the initiating cause. (For example, the cause may be hypovolemia.) Although these classifications are separate and distinct, two or more types often are combined. For example, hypovolemia may occur in septic shock. Elements of cardiogenic shock may occur in hypovolemic shock. Regardless of the classification, the underlying defect is inadequate tissue perfusion. The following discussion is a brief overview of common classifications of shock. *Note:* A more detailed discussion can be found throughout this chapter by subject matter.

Hypovolemic Shock

In the United States, **hypovolemic shock** (shock that occurs from fluid loss) most often is caused by hemorrhage. Hypovolemic shock also can result from dehydration (commonly seen with severe diarrhea and vomiting). In either case, a loss of circulating volume occurs. Illnesses and injuries that can lead to hypovolemic shock include hemorrhage, burns, severe or prolonged diarrhea, vomiting, endocrine disorders, and internal third-space loss, as in peritonitis. In addition to loss of circulating volume, tissue injury resulting from trauma can worsen shock. Tissue injury causes microemboli and further activates the inflammatory and coagulation responses (Figure 36-3).

> **NOTE**
> Most patients with shock have hypovolemia. Thus shock is assumed to be hypovolemic in origin until it is proved otherwise. The paramedic should first manage the patient in shock by administering normal saline or lactated Ringer's solution (per protocol)[8] to stabilize blood pressure. This is the case unless the lungs are wet (identified by crackles). Crackles on physical examination indicate cardiogenic shock.

Cardiogenic Shock

Cardiogenic shock (described in Chapter 22) results when the cardiac pump cannot deliver adequate circulating blood volume for tissue perfusion. Cardiogenic shock can result from inadequate filling of the heart, poor contractility of the heart, and obstruction of blood flow from the heart to central circulation (Figure 36-4). The patient in cardiogenic shock usually suffers from an acute myocardial infarction, a serious cardiac rhythm disturbance, cardiac tamponade, tension pneumothorax, cardiac contusion, severe valvular heart disease, cardiomyopathy, pulmonary embolism, or dissecting aortic aneurysm. Cardiogenic shock occurs in 5% to 10% of patients hospitalized for myocardial infarction. The associated mortality rate in these patients approaches 80%.[9]

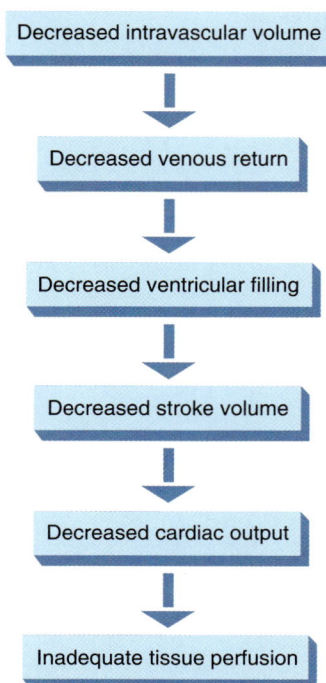

FIGURE 36-3 Pathophysiology of hypovolemic shock.

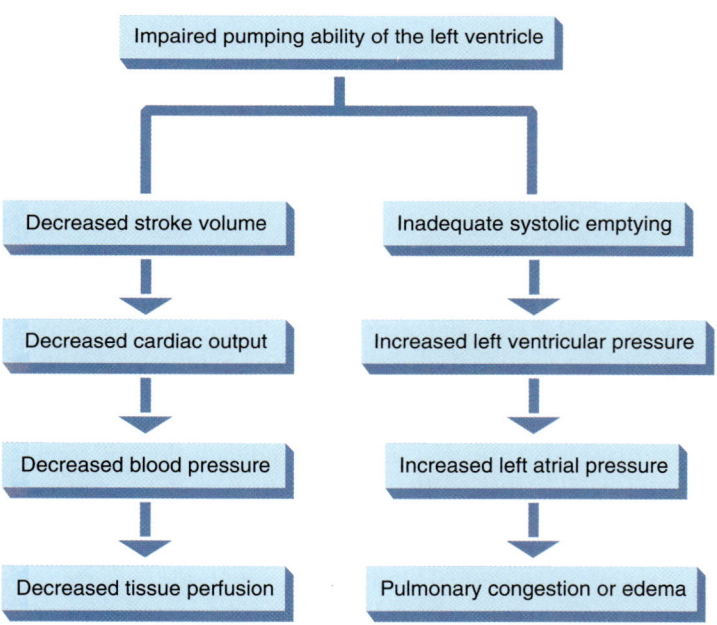

FIGURE 36-4 Cardiogenic shock.

> **NOTE**
> Cardiogenic shock that develops from extrinsic causes, such as cardiac tamponade, tension pneumothorax, or pulmonary embolism, is known as **obstructive shock**. This term is used because the common pathophysiology in these conditions is obstruction to blood flow. **Distributive shock** occurs when peripheral vasodilation causes a fall in systemic vascular resistance. The most common causes of distributive shock are septic shock, anaphylactic shock, and neurogenic shock.

> **CRITICAL THINKING**
> Why does cardiogenic shock develop in a patient who has had a severe myocardial infarction?

Neurogenic Shock

Neurogenic shock is also known as *spinal cord, distributive,* or *vasogenic shock*. Neurogenic shock results from vasomotor paralysis below the level of injury. Normal vasomotor tone through sympathetic nervous system control is lost. This results in a decrease in peripheral vascular resistance. The loss of sympathetic impulses causes vasodilation and increases the size of the container (so to speak) (Figure 36-5). Therefore, even normal intravascular volume is inadequate to fill the enlarged vascular compartment and perfuse the tissues. Because of the mechanism of injuries responsible for this syndrome, respiratory insufficiency, head injury, or both also may be present.

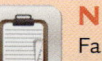

> **NOTE**
> Fainting may be due to mild, readily reversible vasogenic shock. This shock can occur in the absence of injury. This shock results from a temporary bradycardia and vasodilation that produce a drop in cardiac output.

Anaphylactic Shock

Anaphylactic shock (described in Chapter 27) occurs when the body is exposed to an antigen that produces a severe allergic reaction. To review, common causes include antibiotic agents (especially penicillins), venoms, and insect stings. The body responds to the release of histamine and other mediators. Histamine and other mediators act on receptors in the systemic and pulmonary microcirculation. They also produce an effect on bronchial smooth muscle. Histamine causes arterioles and capillaries to dilate and increases capillary membrane permeability. Intravascular fluid leaks into the interstitial space and results in a decrease in intravascular volume (Figure 36-6). In addition, many of the mediators released cause constriction of the upper and lower airways. This creates the potential for complete airway obstruction.

Septic Shock

Septic shock most often results from a serious systemic bacterial infection. Septic shock is thought to be caused by toxins that are a part of the microorganism (endotoxin: gram-negative sepsis) or are released by the organism (exotoxin: gram-positive shock). These toxins stimulate the release of complex vasoactive agents. The agents affect arterioles, capillaries, and venules. They alter pressure in the microcirculation and increase capillary permeability (Figure 36-7). Septic shock can result from staphylococcal and streptococcal infections, pneumonia, postoperative

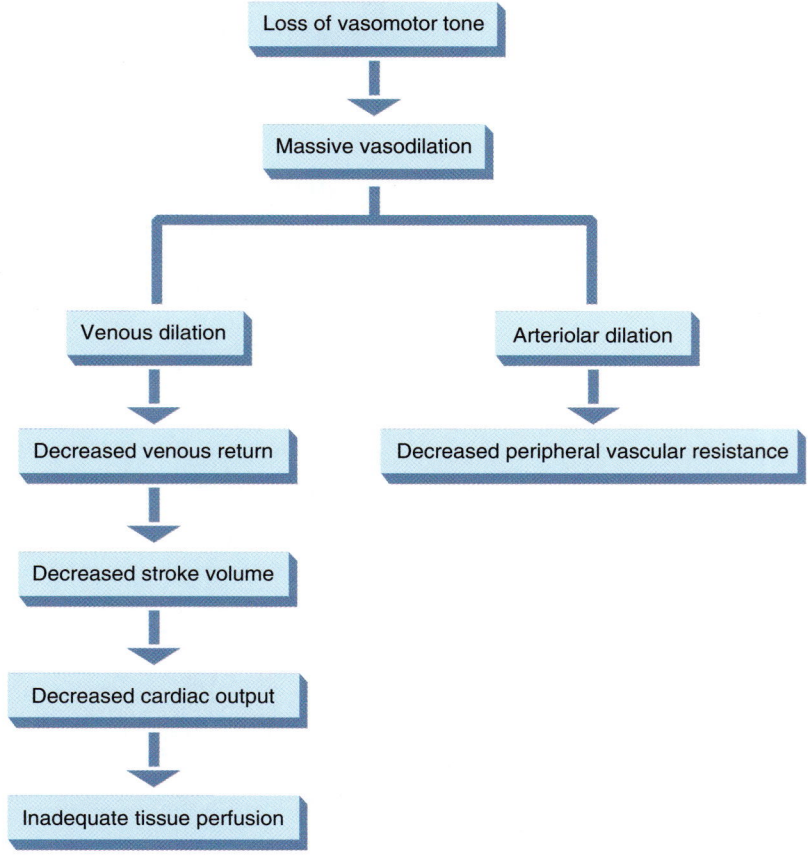

FIGURE 36-5 Pathophysiology of neurogenic shock.

infections, and infections from indwelling urinary catheters. Between 40,000 and 100,000 persons develop septic shock each year; septic shock is the leading cause of death in intensive care units.[10] Septic shock most often occurs in older adults (particularly nursing home residents), alcoholics, neonates, and patients who are immunosuppressed (e.g., patients with cancer, human immunodeficiency virus [HIV] infection, or sickle cell disease).

STAGES OF SHOCK

The degree of hypoperfusion and anaerobic metabolism can be categorized by stages of the response of the body to the shock syndrome. The three stages are (1) compensated shock, (2) uncompensated (or decompensated) shock, and (3) irreversible shock.[3] Table 36-1 lists the stages of shock and the signs and symptoms of each.

Compensated Shock

Compensated shock (Figure 36-8) is associated with some decreased blood flow and perfusion to the tissues. However, the compensatory responses of the body can overcome a decrease in available fluid. An increase in catecholamine production maintains cardiac output and a normal systolic blood pressure.

The decrease in perfusion and subsequent increase in acidosis lead to a chemoreceptor response. This response increases the rate and depth of ventilation. (This helps correct the acidosis by decreasing PCO_2.) Sympathetic stimulation increases heart rate and contractility. In addition, it causes bronchodilation, leads to increases in peripheral vascular resistance, and decreases capillary flow in some capillary beds, such as the gastrointestinal tract. The patient may exhibit delayed capillary refill and cool skin as the blood is shunted from the skin to the vital organs. In spite of maintaining normal blood pressure and urinary output, some patients may show signs of decreased central nervous system (CNS) perfusion (lethargy, confusion, combativeness), even at this stage. If the underlying cause of shock is untreated, the compensatory mechanisms collapse.

Uncompensated Shock

Uncompensated shock (Figure 36-9) occurs when the body is no longer able to maintain systemic blood pressure. The systolic pressure usually drops before the diastolic pressure because the systolic pressure depends more on blood volume. Diastolic pressure may rise at first because of vasoconstriction. The decrease in systolic pressure, along with maintained or increased diastolic pressure, can lead to a

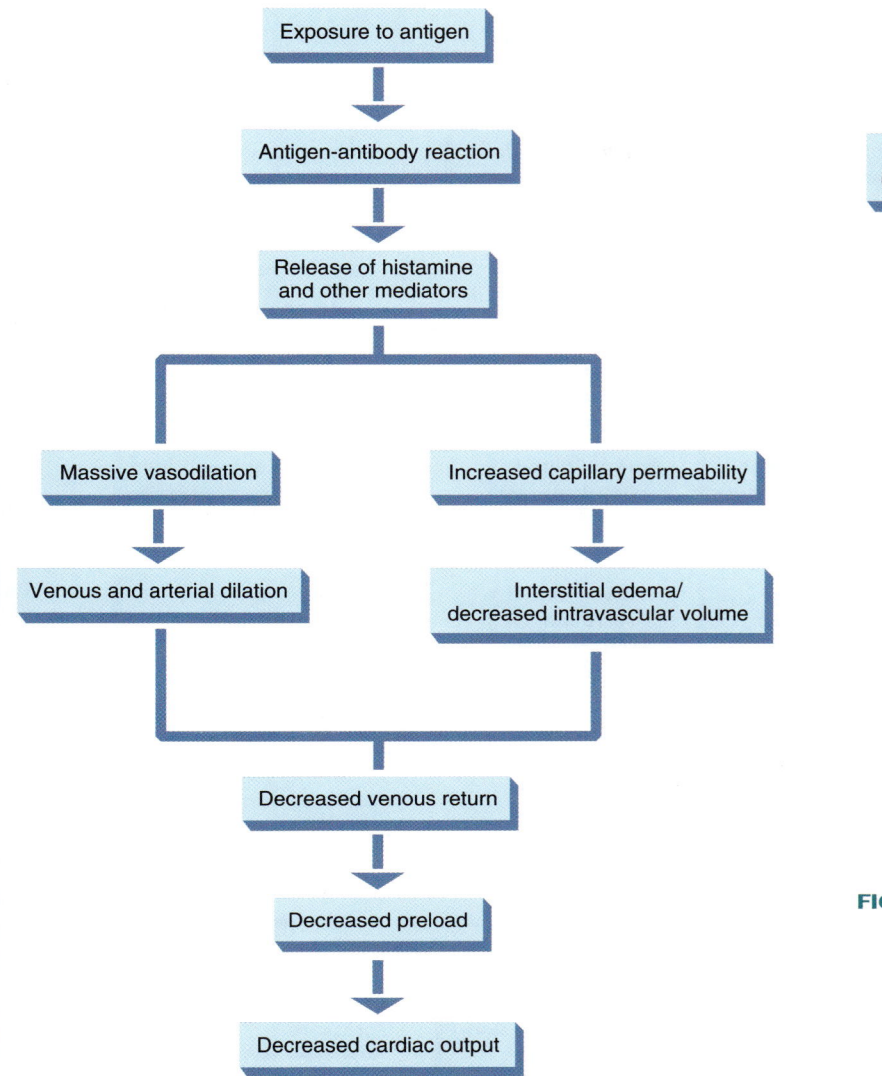

FIGURE 36-6 Pathophysiology of anaphylactic shock.

FIGURE 36-7 Pathophysiology of septic shock.

TABLE 36-1 Stages of Shock

| Vital Signs | SIGNS AND SYMPTOMS | | |
	Compensated Shock	Uncompensated Shock	Irreversible Shock
Heart rate	Mild tachycardia	Moderate tachycardia	Bradycardia, severe dysrhythmias
Level of consciousness	Lethargy, confusion, combativeness	Confusion, unconsciousness	Coma
Skin	Delayed capillary refill, cool skin	Delayed capillary refill, cold extremities, cyanosis	Pale, cold, clammy skin
Blood pressure	Normal or slightly elevated measurement	Decreased systolic and diastolic pressure	Frank hypotension

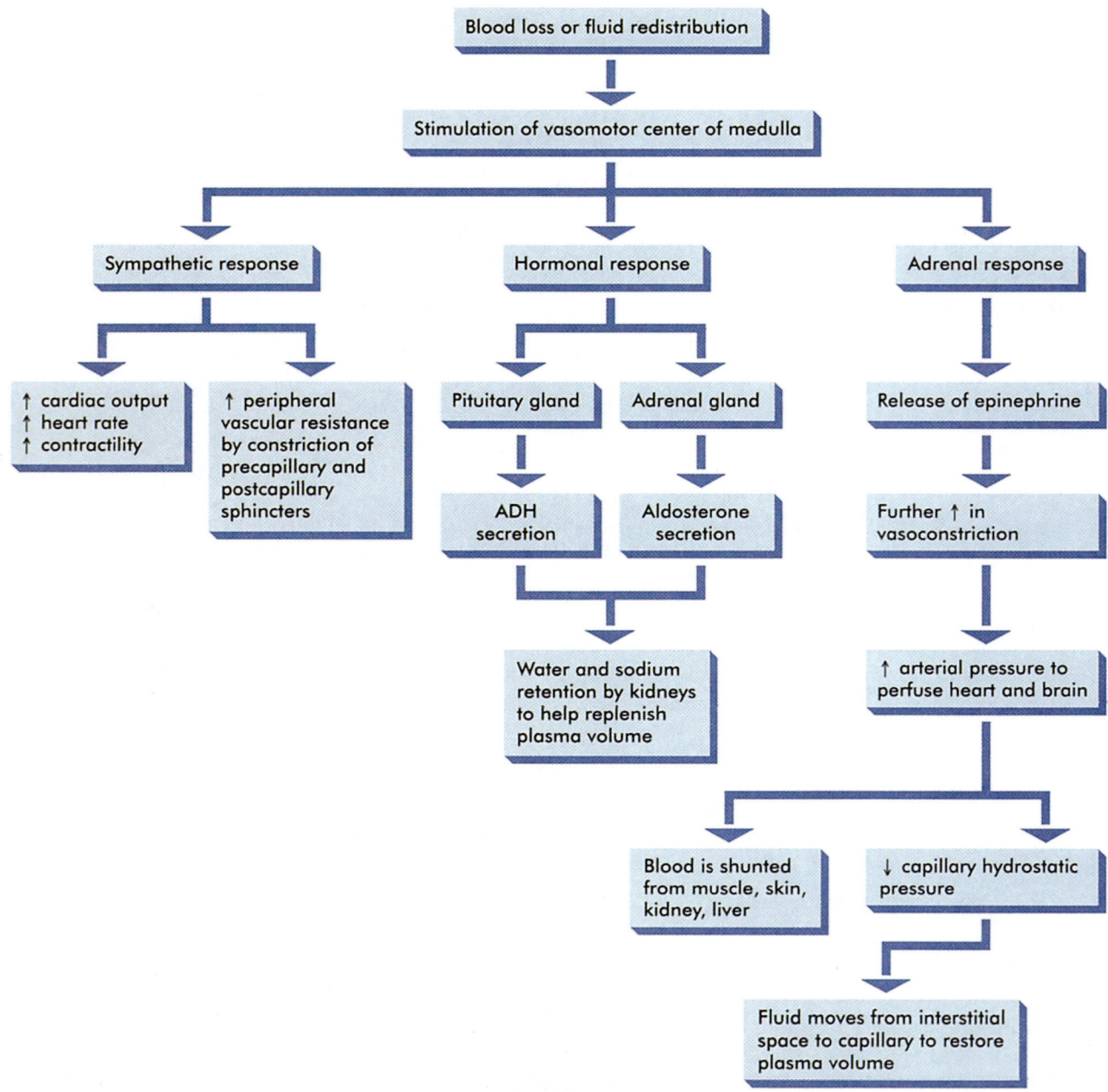

FIGURE 36-8 Compensated shock. This stage of shock is reversible.

narrow pulse pressure. The pulse pressure can be narrowed to such an extent that it is not detectable with a blood pressure cuff.

As the compensatory mechanisms of the body begin to fail, systolic and diastolic pressures drop and cerebral blood flow decreases. PO_2 may drop; however, PCO_2 usually remains normal or low unless the patient has a head or chest injury that leads to hypoventilation. The clinical signs of uncompensated shock include hypotension, tachycardia, tachypnea, delayed capillary refill, and decreased urinary output. Shunting of blood and tissue hypoxia may cause the patient

to have cold extremities and cyanosis. Effects on the cardiovascular system include a decreased preload and an increased rate of contraction caused by catecholamine stimulation. Myocardial contractions initially can be stronger as a result of catecholamine release. However, in the latter phases of uncompensated shock, myocardial strength may decrease as a result of the following factors:

1. Ischemia can result from a reduction of circulating red blood cells, a lower oxygen saturation pressure (PO_2), and decreased coronary perfusion because of hypotension (especially diastolic hypotension).

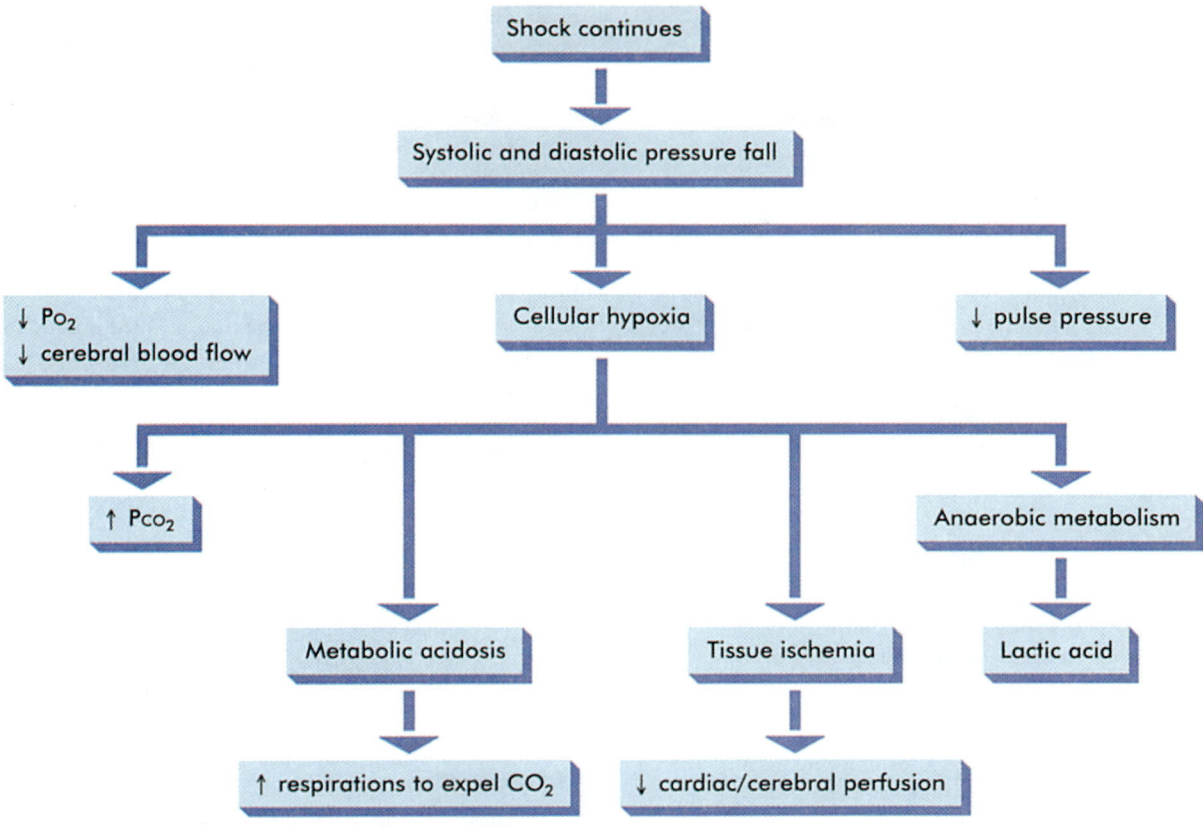

FIGURE 36-9 Uncompensated shock. This stage of shock is reversible.

2. Cardiodepressant substances (e.g., myocardial toxin released from the ischemic pancreas) can depress heart function in late shock.
3. Necrosis of myocardium (essentially simulating myocardial infarction) can result from associated ischemia.
4. Decreased preload can lead to decreased contractility.
5. Acidosis can lead to decreased contractility.
6. Cardiac rhythm disturbances can result from hypoxia.

Irreversible Shock

The progression of cellular ischemia and necrosis and subsequent organ death, even with oxygenation and perfusion restored, indicate **irreversible shock** (the third stage of shock) (Figure 36-10). Despite a return to normal perfusion, patients with irreversible shock as a result of massive cellular damage do not survive. Cells and the vital organs begin to die from the lack of energy. The membrane pumps fail. The various organelles in the cells sequentially break down. Thus necrosis is inevitable even if cell perfusion is restored.

Decompensation may occur suddenly or may be delayed from 1 day to 3 weeks after the onset of shock. The clinical signs of irreversible shock include bradycardia; serious dysrhythmias; frank hypotension; evidence of multiple organ failure; and pale, cold, and clammy skin. Cardiopulmonary collapse usually is imminent in these patients.

NOTE

During the prehospital management of shock, it is impossible to distinguish between uncompensated and irreversible shock. Therefore management of the shock victim should always focus on resuscitation. This is especially true because irreversible shock usually occurs over a longer period of time. Rapid resuscitation and transportation to an appropriate medical facility can prevent the development of irreversible shock. Fluid resuscitation in these patients should be guided by medical direction and established protocol.

Variations in Physiological Response to Shock

Many variations in physiological response occur among patients who are in shock. Determining factors include the following:

- Age
  - Older adults are less able to compensate
  - Children compensate longer but deteriorate faster
- General health
  - Preexisting disease
  - Other injuries
- Ability to activate compensatory mechanisms
- Medications, some of which can interfere with compensatory mechanisms
- Specific organ system(s) affected

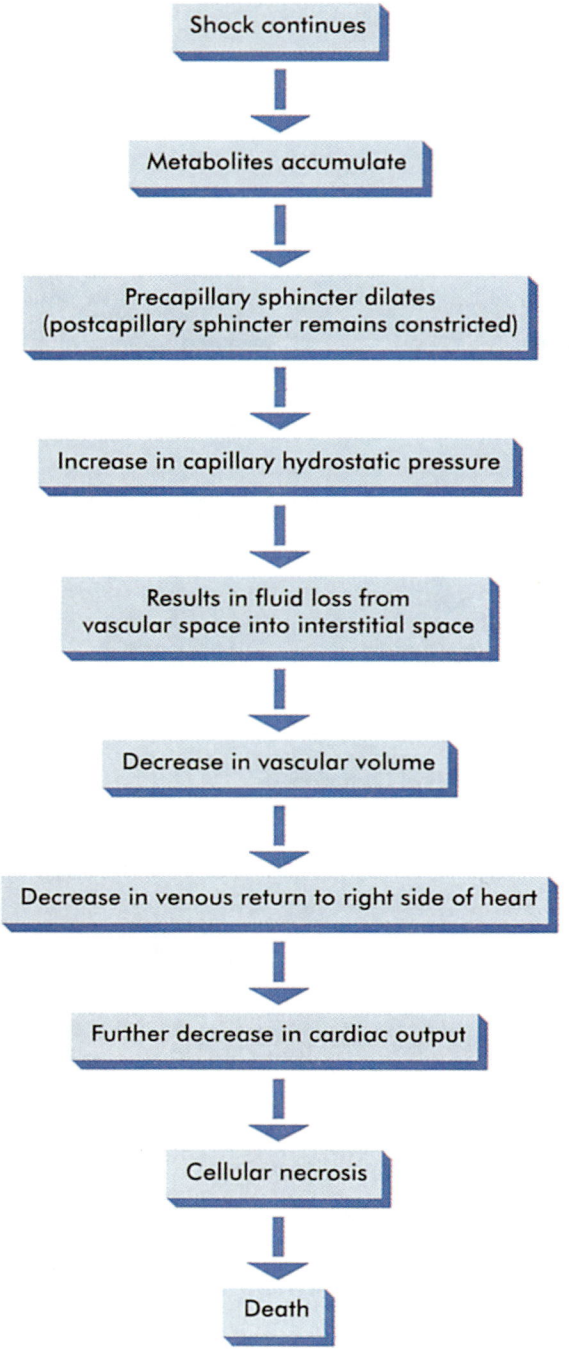

FIGURE 36-10 Irreversible shock.

 CRITICAL THINKING
What diseases can influence a patient's response to shock?

MANAGEMENT AND TREATMENT PLAN FOR THE PATIENT IN SHOCK

The management and treatment plan for the patient in shock focuses on assessment of oxygenation and perfusion of the body organs. The goals of the treatment plan are to ensure a patent airway, to provide adequate oxygenation and ventilation, and to restore perfusion.

Primary Survey

The primary survey can help to identify whether cell perfusion is adequate. The following five-step description of the primary survey focuses on evaluating the shock victim, but the paramedic should be aware of common objectives in evaluating any patient with other types of serious illness or injury:

1. *Airway.* The airway must be opened and patency must be maintained to ensure adequate air movement.
2. *Breathing.* The respiratory pattern often reflects the adequacy of ventilation. Respiration can offer clues to the presence of shock. For example, if the patient is acidotic, the rate and depth of ventilation increase in an attempt to reduce carbon dioxide content of the blood and compensate for the metabolic acidosis. Pulse oximetry should be closely monitored.
3. *Circulation.* The paramedic should assess the patient's circulatory status. The first step is to check the patient for any uncontrolled arterial bleeding. In cases of external hemorrhage, applying direct pressure almost always helps to control bleeding. If direct pressure does not immediately control vigorous bleeding in an extremity, a tourniquet should be applied. (See Chapter 38 for methods to control external bleeding.) This usually will control external hemorrhage until the patient can be taken to the emergency department for definitive care. Pressure dressings can be applied to maintain control of hemorrhage. (Examples of such are bandages or a pneumatic antishock garment [PASG], per protocol.) If the paramedic suspects internal bleeding, after securing the airway and ensuring adequate ventilation, rapid transport to a proper facility is the highest priority. Internal bleeding should be suspected in any trauma patient with signs of shock, especially trauma patients without evidence of external blood loss. Treatment for internal hemorrhage must be directed at definitive care to stop the bleeding. Thus rapid transport to a proper facility is critical. Intravenous fluid therapy, if initiated in the field, should be performed en route to avoid a delay of definitive care.

 CRITICAL THINKING
Consider a patient with early signs and symptoms of shock. However, the patient's SaO2 reading is normal. Should you administer oxygen?

The paramedic should evaluate the rate, character, and location of the patient's pulse as part of the circulatory assessment. Pulse rates increase fairly early in shock. The increase helps to maintain an adequate cardiac output. The strength of contraction also may increase. However, both of these attempts to maintain cardiac output may be negated by the decrease in preload. Tachycardia usually will not occur until the patient has suffered a 10% to 15% volume depletion (relative to container size) as a result of blood loss or an increase in container size. The character of the pulse can be strong or weak. The strength of the pulse provides an estimate of the filling volume of the artery being palpated and an indirect measurement of systolic pressure.

Tissue perfusion sometimes can be estimated by evaluating the color, moisture, and temperature of the skin. These guidelines, however, can be unreliable in older patients and in those who have been exposed to extremes of temperature. They also can be unreliable in those suffering from septicemia and shock caused by neurological injury. An evaluation of the fingers and toes (the most distal points of circulation) is crucial. These areas can be the first to show signs of inadequate tissue perfusion (cyanosis, cool skin). If ambient temperatures are moderate and tissue perfusion is adequate, these areas will be pink, warm, and dry.

The capillary refill test (described in Chapter 19) can offer useful details on the pediatric patient's tissue perfusion. These measurements should be used only as a guide. The accuracy of this test can be affected by the environment and by the patient's general health, age, and gender.

LOOK AGAIN
See Chapter 19: Primary Assessment, pp. 508-509.

4. *Disability.* The evaluation of the patient's level of consciousness is crucial in assessing cerebral oxygenation. The patient can become restless, agitated, and confused as cerebral ischemia develops. In addition to shock, cerebral edema and intracranial hemorrhage from head injury can compromise cerebral perfusion. Any significant change in the patient's sensorium should be considered an indicator of a critical perfusion deficit. This is true whether the decrease in cerebral circulation is from shock or from an increase in intracranial pressure. The paramedic can measure the patient's level of consciousness with the AVPU scale or other evaluation methods (see Chapter 40).

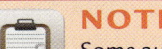
NOTE
Some authorities believe that the level of consciousness and other indicators of adequate brain functions are the best way to determine appropriate blood pressure for the trauma patient. They contend that the brain is the organ most sensitive to changes in physiological state. The goals of this patient-focused method of shock management are to ensure that systolic pressure is at least 90 mm Hg and that the patient has positive peripheral pulses and is awake or responsive to stimuli.[8]

5. *Exposure of the body surfaces.* The paramedic should expose the body surfaces in the primary survey as indicated by scenario or mechanism of injury. A visual inspection can reveal conditions that may be life threatening. These conditions can be hidden by clothing.

Differential Shock Assessment Findings

Shock is assumed to be hypovolemic until it is proved otherwise. However, assessment findings that can help the paramedic to differentiate between hypovolemic shock and other causes of shock include the following (Figure 36-11):
1. *Cardiogenic shock.* The patient often has a chief complaint of chest pain, dyspnea, or extreme heart rates (tachycardia, bradycardia, and other dysrhythmias). Some patients also show signs of congestive heart failure such as jugular vein distention (described in Chapter 22 and 42).
2. *Distributive shock* (neurogenic shock, anaphylactic shock, septic shock). The patient's history or scene assessment may reveal a mechanism that suggests vasodilation as the cause of the shock state. Signs and symptoms of distributive shock that are unusual in the presence of hypovolemic shock include warm, flushed skin (especially in dependent areas). Those of neurogenic shock include a normal pulse rate (*relative bradycardia*).
3. *Obstructive shock* (caused by obstruction to blood flow). These patients often are the victims of a major chest injury (usually a penetrating type of injury). Or they have a history that is consistent with pulmonary embolism. (For example, they have had a recent surgery or long bone fracture.) Patients with cardiac tamponade or tension pneumothorax often have jugular vein distention. Also, patients with tension pneumothorax almost always have decreased breath sounds on the affected side (see Chapter 42).

Detailed Physical Examination

As discussed, the first action is the primary survey and management of any life-threatening conditions. Then the paramedic should evaluate the patient further. A systematic approach offers a way to evaluate potentially life-threatening conditions and allows the paramedic to further assess the patient's perfusion status. This assessment should begin with baseline measurements of the patient's vital signs and evaluation of the patient's electrocardiogram.

CRITICAL THINKING
Can blood donation cause a fluid deficit large enough to cause shock? If so, how is that fluid deficit managed?

The paramedic should expect the pulse rate to increase above normal limits after fluid volume drops 10% to 15%. Some patients continue to have normal pulse rates even though a volume deficit of this extent exists. Thus the patient's pulse rate should be only one factor in evaluating the patient's level of perfusion.

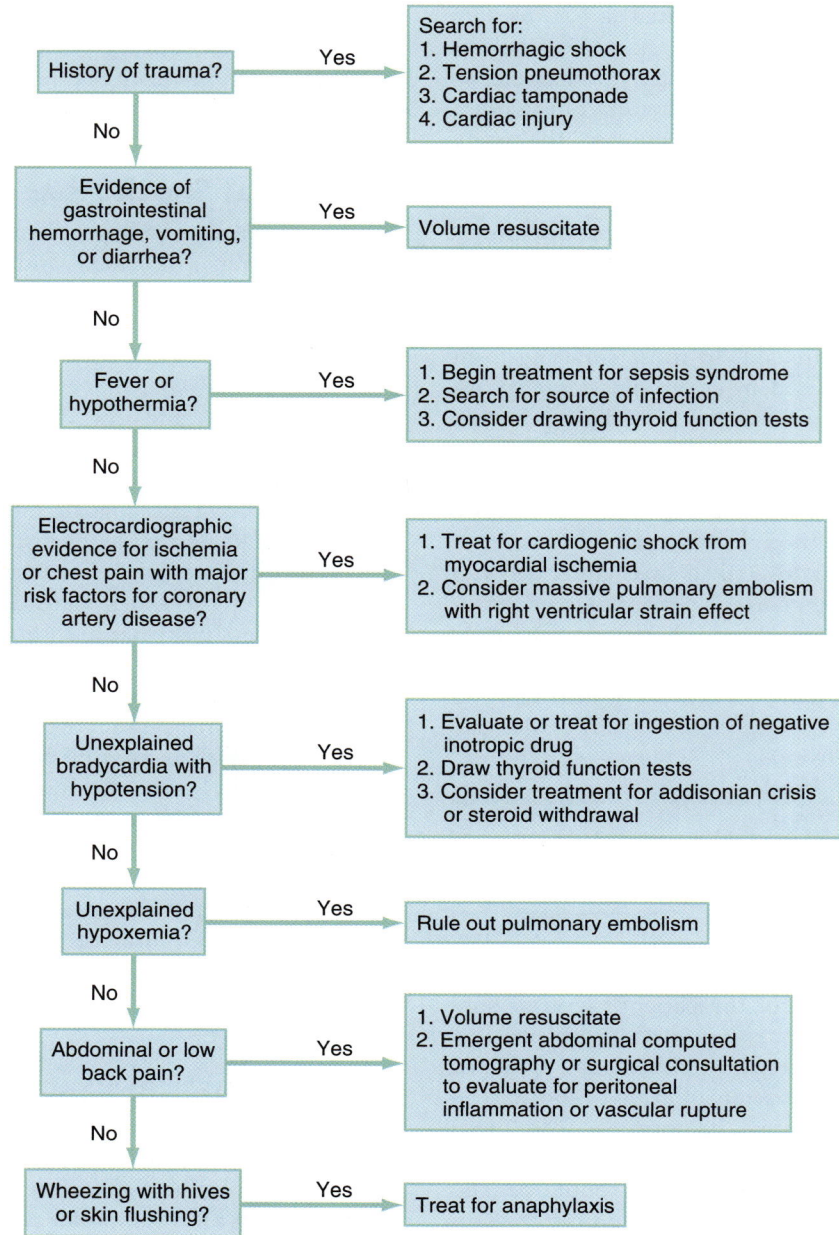

FIGURE 36-11 Flow diagram to classify undifferentiated shock. (From Marx J, et al: *Rosen's emergency medicine: concepts and clinical practice*, ed 6, St Louis, 2006, Mosby.)

Bradycardia, which can result from hypoxemia, existing neurological injury, increased vagal tone, preexisting illness, or prior medication use, also can indicate severe myocardial ischemia (a primary cause of cardiogenic shock). Bradycardic rhythms often occur just before cardiac arrest. If the rhythm is bradycardic, the paramedic should optimize oxygenation by increasing the fraction of inspired oxygen (FiO_2) and by assisting ventilations if needed.

The diastolic pressure at first rises as peripheral vascular resistance increases with increased vascular tone. These changes decrease the container size. Blood also is shunted away selectively from certain portions of the body. When

the heart can no longer pump blood to keep the container full on the arterial side, the diastolic pressure begins to drop. The paramedic should expect this when blood loss is greater than 20% to 25% of normal circulating blood volume.

The systolic pressure falls when the heart can no longer pump enough blood to fill the container at the end of cardiac contraction. Systolic pressure usually is more sensitive to volume depletion than is diastolic pressure. Therefore systolic pressure drops first. However, as the fluid deficit approaches 25%, systolic and diastolic pressures both begin to drop.

The paramedic should consider evaluation of orthostatic vital signs in conscious patients suspected of having lost circulating blood volume. This evaluation should only be performed in the absence of suspected spinal injury or another condition that precludes this assessment. As discussed in Chapter 20, a change from a recumbent position to a sitting or standing position that is associated with a decrease in systolic pressure (after 1 minute) of 10 to 15 mm Hg or a concurrent rise in pulse rate (after 1 minute) of 10 to 15 beats per minute indicates a significant (at least 10%) volume depletion (postural hypotension) and a decrease in perfusion status.

A fluid deficit still can exist even after the systolic pressure returns to normal following fluid replacement. However, continuing IV fluids after indicators of adequate tissue perfusion are present (e.g., improved skin color, capillary refill time of less than 2 seconds in pediatric patients, and normal pulse oximetry readings) is controversial. Aggressive fluid resuscitation can result in **hemodilution** (diluting the blood of elements), the disruption of clots, and renewed hemorrhage.[8] As a rule, patients who have suspected internal hemorrhage in their chest, abdomen, or pelvis should have fluids titrated to maintain a systolic blood pressure of 90 mm Hg (MAP of 60 to 65 mm Hg). This *permissive hypotension* can be protective and may prevent further blood loss. The paramedic should follow local protocol established by medical direction.

RESUSCITATION

Resuscitation of the shock victim is aimed at restoring adequate peripheral tissue oxygenation as quickly as possible. As previously stated, this is accomplished by ensuring adequate oxygenation, maintaining an effective ratio of volume to container size, and rapidly transporting the victim to an appropriate medical facility.

> **NOTE**
> The over-resuscitation of trauma patients can occur. In patients with closed head injury or pulmonary or cardiac contusion, one must avoid fluid overload. As stated before, medical direction and protocol should guide fluid resuscitation for the shock patient.

Red Blood Cell Oxygenation

Adequate oxygenation of red blood cells is required for adequate tissue oxygenation. For red blood cell oxygenation to be adequate, the patient must have a patent airway. Ventilation also must be supported with a high fraction of inspired oxygen. If needed, the paramedic can assist ventilation with positive pressure. Any abnormality that interferes with adequate ventilation should be corrected if possible. Examples include obstructed airway, pneumothorax,

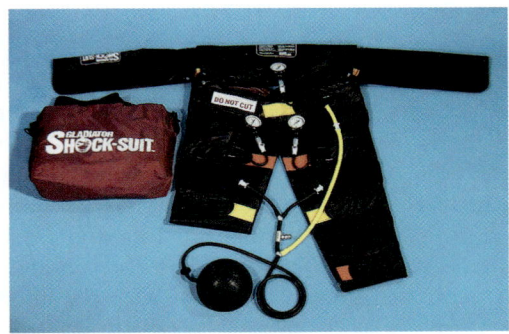

FIGURE 36-12 Jobst Gladiator shock suit. (Courtesy Jobst Institute, Inc., Toledo, Ohio.)

hemothorax, open chest wound, and an unstable chest wall (see Chapter 42).

Ratio of Volume to Container Size

The second component necessary to maintain adequate oxygen-carrying capacity requires that the container be full of fluid. The paramedic can achieve this by decreasing the size of the container. This is especially the case in shock states not associated with hemorrhage. In addition, in some cases of distributive shock, vasoconstricting drugs can be used to manage the shock when reduction of container size is the main concern. Volume replacement also may be necessary in these patients. One should note that vasoconstricting drugs are not recommended to treat patients in hypovolemic shock until fluid volume replacement is complete. Complete volume replacement rarely occurs in the prehospital setting.

Pneumatic Antishock Garment

The **pneumatic antishock garment** (PASG) (Figure 36-12) is thought by some to be effective in managing shock. The theory is that when the PASG is applied to the legs and abdomen, pressure is transmitted directly through the skin, fat, muscle, and other soft tissues to the blood vessels themselves. Hemorrhage is then controlled in a similar fashion as any other compression device or bandage.[8] The PASG device may be useful in managing hemorrhagic shock with hypotension (a systolic blood pressure <90 mm Hg) in cases of:

- Suspected pelvic fracture
- Suspected intraperitoneal hemorrhage
- Suspected retroperitoneal hemorrhage

Decisions to use the PASG are left to local protocol and medical direction. However, penetrating thoracic trauma, evisceration of abdominal organs, impaled objects in the abdomen, pregnancy, traumatic arrest, and coexisting medical conditions (congestive heart failure, pulmonary edema) generally are considered contraindications for the PASG.[8] The PASG is also not recommended as a splinting device for isolated lower extremity fractures in the absence of shock.[8]

GENERAL PNEUMATIC ANTISHOCK GARMENT GUIDELINES

The paramedic should apply the PASG when indicated after the lower extremities and abdomen have been inspected for major wounds. The garment must always be positioned below the level of the patient's lowest rib. The patient's blood pressure and lung sounds should be monitored before, during, and after inflation. Inflation is stopped when an adequate blood pressure has been obtained. The compartments are inflated before or with the abdominal compartment. *The paramedic should never inflate the abdominal section before inflating the leg sections.* Doing so can cause the abdominal compartment to act as a constrictive band that reduces venous return from the legs.

CRITICAL THINKING

Consider that the abdominal compartment of the pneumatic antishock garment is inflated mistakenly before the leg segments. What effect can this have on cardiac output?

After PASG inflation the garment should seldom if ever be deflated in the prehospital setting and only with a physician's direction. The abdominal section is deflated before the leg sections. The patient should be monitored closely during the deflation process. Removal of the garment before fluid replacement commonly results in a rapid fall of blood pressure and cardiac output, which can lead to cardiac arrest.

Changes in temperature and atmospheric pressure can cause a notable change in the pressure within the PASG. The paramedic should monitor the patient constantly when the patient is moved from a cold environment to a warm one or when transported by air. The relationship among temperature, atmospheric pressure, and pressure within the PASG is as follows:

- A rise in temperature raises the pressure within the PASG; a fall in temperature decreases the pressure.
- A fall in atmospheric pressure causes an increase in PASG pressure; a rise in atmospheric pressure produces a decrease in garment pressure.

The PASG is not without complications even with appropriate use. Sustained inflation of the garment for more than 1 to 2 hours can lead to decreased tissue perfusion, ischemia of the underlying tissues, and loss of the limb, even without underlying fracture.

Fluid Resuscitation in Shock

Almost every shock victim, except for patients in cardiogenic shock, requires volume expanders as part of resuscitation. The selection of intravenous (IV) fluids for initial volume replacement varies according to medical direction. In prehospital care, the most common emergency requiring fluid replacement is loss of volume caused by hemorrhage or dehydration. The type of fluid replacement needed depends on the nature and extent of the volume loss. The two main categories of fluids used in resuscitation are crystalloids and colloids. The paramedic should follow the recommendations for fluid resuscitation provided by medical direction.

CRYSTALLOIDS

Crystalloid solutions are created by dissolving crystals such as salts and sugars in water. These solutions do not have as much osmotic pressure as colloid solutions. They can be expected to equilibrate more quickly between the vascular and extravascular spaces. Two thirds of the infused crystalloid fluid leaves the vascular space within 1 hour. So 3 mL of a crystalloid solution is needed to replace 1 mL of blood. Examples of crystalloid solutions are lactated Ringer's solution, normal saline, and glucose solutions in water.

Hypertonic solutions have higher osmotic pressure than that of body cells. They include 5% dextrose in 0.9% sodium chloride, 7.5% saline, and 5% dextrose in 0.45% sodium chloride. Hypotonic solutions have a lower osmotic pressure than that of body cells (e.g., distilled water and 0.45% sodium chloride).

Lactated Ringer's solution is the fluid of choice for resuscitating patients in shock.[8] The solution is well balanced and contains many of the chemicals found in human blood. Lactated Ringer's solution contains sodium chloride, small amounts of potassium and calcium, and 28 mEq of lactate, which can act as a buffer to neutralize acidity when metabolized by the liver. One third of the infused solution remains in the vascular space after 1 hour.

Normal saline contains 154 mEq/L of sodium. Normal saline has no buffering capabilities. Although preferred by some physicians, the higher chloride content of normal saline is less desirable than the more balanced lactated Ringer's solution. As in lactated Ringer's solution, nearly one third of the infused normal saline remains in the vascular space after 1 hour. This makes it an equally effective volume expander. Paramedic should follow local protocol when choosing IV fluids.

Glucose-containing solutions (e.g., 5% dextrose in water) have immediate volume expansion effects. However, the glucose leaves the intravascular compartment rapidly with a resultant free water increase. The volume-replacement benefits of glucose solutions only last 5 to 10 minutes while the glucose is metabolized. Thus 5% dextrose in water should not be used to replace a volume deficit. Glucose solutions most often are used to maintain vascular access for administration of IV medications.

NOTE

Five percent dextrose in water is an isotonic solution. When administered, however, the dextrose molecules leave the circulation so rapidly that its effect is that of a hypotonic solution.

COLLOIDS

Colloid solutions contain molecules (usually protein) that are too large to pass through the capillary membrane. These solutions exhibit osmotic pressure. They remain within the vascular compartment for a considerable time. Examples of colloid solutions are whole blood, packed red blood cells, blood plasma, and plasma substitutes. Colloids generally are reserved for in-hospital use and are not recommended for prehospital management of shock.[8]

Whole blood replacement is rarely given in the United States for management of shock and is usually unavailable in the emergency department. Rather, packed red cells are transfused, and other blood components are transfused as necessary. (Packed red blood cells have a volume of hemoglobin per unit that is almost twice that of whole blood.) In addition, because there is no plasma in packed red cells, circulatory overload is less likely and transfusion reactions are less frequent.

A type and crossmatch should be obtained when possible before a patient is given blood products to determine the patient's ABO group and Rh type (described in Chapter 11). Typing and crossmatching also will determine whether other antibodies are present that may cause a transfusion reaction. Type-specific blood should be used for resuscitation when the patient's condition and time permit. However, uncrossmatched blood is usually given immediately for patients with hypotension and uncontrolled hemorrhage.[11] Group O universal donor blood does not have A or B antigens on their surface; they are not agglutinated by anti-A or anti-B antibodies. O-negative blood is used for women of childbearing age who are at risk for Rh complications with future pregnancies. O-positive blood is used in all other patients.

LOOK AGAIN
See Chapter 11: General Principles of Pathophysiology, pp. 245-246.

NOTE
Several types of blood transfusion reactions may occur during or up to 96 hours after infusion. Symptoms may range from mild fever to life-threatening shock. If a reaction is suspected (e.g., during an interhospital transfer), the paramedic should stop the transfusion and contact medical direction. The blood bag or tubing should not be discarded.

Blood plasma may be given without concern for ABO compatibility. Blood plasma contains fibrinogen, albumin, gamma globulins, *hemagglutinins* (an agglutinin that clumps red blood corpuscles), prothrombin (a chemical that is part of the clotting cascade, further described in Chapter 38), other clotting factors, sugar, and salts. Blood plasma sometimes is used to restore effective blood volume in circulatory failure associated with burns, traumatic shock, and hemorrhage. Blood plasma more commonly is used to correct clotting deficiencies. It is often supplied as *fresh frozen plasma*.

Plasma substitutes do not increase oxygen-carrying capacity by replacing red blood cells. They also do not improve clotting by the addition of plasma protein. Yet at times they are used to restore circulating blood volume as an emergency treatment for hypovolemia caused by blood loss. Plasma substitutes such as dextran and hetastarch have osmotic properties similar to those of plasma. Thus they stay in the intravascular space longer than crystalloid solution. Plasma substitutes do not carry the human immunodeficiency virus or hepatitis viruses. They also do not require typing and crossmatching before administration. They are readily available as well. Plasma substitutes do have some adverse effects, including increased bleeding tendencies and immune suppression. Emergency vehicles can carry plasma substitutes, but expense and storage issues make them impractical for general use in the prehospital setting.

NOTE
Oxygen-carrying blood substitutes (e.g., PolyHeme) are being studied. They may have future application in prehospital care for severely injured patients. These solutions contain hemoglobin from red blood cells (treated to destroy viruses). In addition, they are compatible with all blood types. They do not require refrigeration and can be stored up to several months.

Theory of Fluid Flow

The flow of fluid through a catheter is related directly to its diameter (to the fourth power) and inversely related to its length. Therefore, a catheter with a large diameter has a much greater flow rate than a catheter with a small diameter. This also means that short catheters provide faster flow rates than longer catheters of equal diameter. Other factors that affect the flow of fluid include the diameter and length of the tubing, the size of the vein, the height of the fluid bag, and the viscosity and temperature of the IV fluid. (Temperature affects viscosity; warm fluids generally flow better than cold ones.) Pressure bags are available that pressurize the IV system to 300 mm Hg to maximize the rate of fluid administration. Table 36-2 lists the maximum rate of fluid flow for various gauges of 2-inch Medicut catheters without pressure on the bag at a height of 1 m above the patient.[12] When aggressive fluid resuscitation is indicated, the paramedic should do the following:

- Use short, large-diameter catheters.
- Use warm fluids of low viscosity (if possible).
- Keep the tubing short, and pressurize the IV system.

CRITICAL THINKING
Aside from improved flow, what other benefits do warmed fluids offer for the patient in shock who needs a large-volume fluid bolus?

TABLE 36-2 Needle Gauges and Maximum Fluid Flow

Needle Gauge*	Maximum Fluid Flow
18 gauge	4.81 L/hr or 80 mL/min
16 gauge	7.45 L/hr or 124 mL/min
14 gauge	9.67 L/hr or 161 mL/min

*Inside diameter.

Key Principles in Managing Shock

The paramedic should follow these key principles as part of the plan for managing shock (Figure 36-13):
1. Establish and maintain an open airway.
2. Administer high-concentration oxygen. Assist ventilation as needed.
3. Control external bleeding (if present).
4. By order of medical direction or per protocol, initiate IV fluid replacement if appropriate. Two large-bore IV lines of a volume-expanding fluid commonly are established in cases of hypovolemia. *The IV administration of fluids in the prehospital setting should not delay patient transportation because crystalloid solutions cannot restore the oxygen-carrying capacity of blood.* Generally, the patient is best served by rapid assessment, airway stabilization, immobilization, and rapid transportation to an appropriate medical facility. Many emergency medical services authorities recommend that IV therapy for shock resuscitation be initiated en route to the hospital.
5. Consider the use of a PASG (per protocol).
6. Maintain the patient's normal body temperature. Patients in shock often are unable to conserve body heat. They can become hypothermic easily.
7. Transport the patient in the supine position, immobilized on a long spine board.
8. Monitor cardiac rhythm and oxygen saturation.
9. Frequently reassess vital signs en route to the emergency department.

MANAGEMENT OF SPECIFIC FORMS OF SHOCK

In addition to the general management appropriate for all shock victims, certain management guidelines are specific to each shock classification (Box 36-2).

Hypovolemic Shock

The management of hypovolemic shock is not considered complete until the volume is replaced and the cause or causes of shock are corrected. This includes crystalloid fluid replacement in cases of simple dehydration or volume replacement because of hemorrhage, definitive surgery,

critical care support, and postoperative rehabilitation. The amount of fluid replaced in trauma is controversial and should be guided by medical direction.

Trauma patients who are stable should not receive aggressive fluid resuscitation.[8] The volume of fluid that should be given to trauma patients will depend on the type of trauma and the patient's condition. Large volumes of fluid to maintain a systolic blood pressure ≥90 mm Hg (MAP 60 to 65 mm Hg) should only be given to patients with isolated head or extremity injuries. As stated earlier, aggressive fluid resuscitation may increase blood loss and can delay arrival to surgical care at a trauma center.

Cardiogenic Shock

The management of cardiogenic shock focuses on improving the pumping action of the heart and on managing cardiac rhythm irregularities. The paramedic should initiate fluid resuscitation in the adult with 100 to 200 mL of a volume-expanding fluid. Fluid resuscitation should be initiated as long as the patient has no crackles in the lung fields that would indicate pulmonary edema. If the patient improves, fluid therapy should be continued cautiously. Fluid therapy should continue until the blood pressure stabilizes and the pulse rate decreases. The paramedic should assess lung sounds often. If the patient shows signs of increased lung congestion, the paramedic should adjust the rate of infusion to keep the vein open.

Drug therapy for cardiogenic shock varies according to cause. Drug therapy can include vasopressors, vasodilators, inotropic drugs, and antidysrhythmics (usually after fluid infusion) (see Chapter 22). Patients with cardiogenic shock caused by myocardial ischemia or infarction require reperfusion strategies (clot-busting drugs or surgery) and possible circulatory support. The paramedic must manage obstructive causes of cardiogenic shock immediately, including tension pneumothorax and cardiac tamponade (see Chapter 42).

Neurogenic Shock

The management of neurogenic shock is similar to the management for hypovolemia. However, the paramedic must take care during fluid therapy to avoid circulatory overload. Throughout the resuscitation phase, the paramedic should monitor the patient's lung sounds closely for signs of pulmonary congestion. In addition, patients in neurogenic shock may respond to the administration of vasopressors (e.g., *dopamine*).

Anaphylactic Shock

As described in Chapter 27, intramuscular administration of *epinephrine* is the treatment of choice in acute anaphylactic reactions. Depending on the severity of reaction, other treatment modalities can include IV or intramuscular administration of antihistamines such as *diphenhydramine.* The paramedic can administer bronchodilators to treat

SHOCK MANAGEMENT ALGORITHM

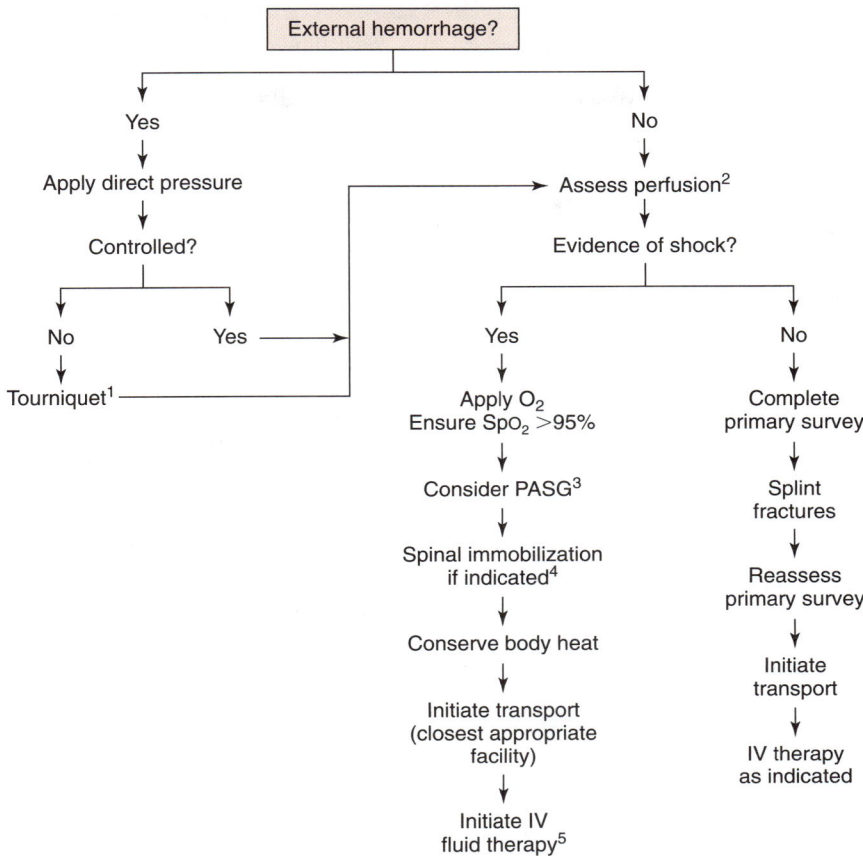

Notes:

[1] A manufactured tourniquet, blood pressure cuff, or cravat should be placed just proximal to the bleeding site and tightened until bleeding stops. The application time is marked on the tourniquet.

[2] Assessment of perfusion includes, presence, quality, and location of pulses; skin color, temperature, and moisture; and capillary refilling time.

[3] PASG should be considered for decompensated shock (SBP <90 mm Hg), and suspected pelvic, intraperitoneal, or retroperitoneal hemorrhage, and in patients with profound hypotension (SBP <60 mm Hg). PASG is contraindicated in penetrating thoracic trauma, abdominal evisceration, pregnancy, impaled object in the abdomen, and traumatic cardiopulmonary arrest, or for splinting the lower extremity fractures.

[4] See Indications for Spinal Immobilization algorithm (p. 235)

[5] Initiate two large-bore (14- or 16-guage) IV catheters en route. See Managing Volume Resuscitation algorithm (p. 188).

FIGURE 36-13 Shock management algorithm. (Courtesy Jobst Institute, Inc., Toledo, Ohio.)

bronchospasm that persists after administration of *epinephrine.* Steroids can be used to reduce the inflammatory response.

Crystalloid volume replacement also is indicated. Crystalloids may compensate for the increased container size caused by vasodilation resulting from histamine release during an anaphylactic reaction. Administration of 1 to 3 L of normal saline may be indicated in patients who have signs of shock after administration of

epinephrine. Paramedics should anticipate the need for aggressive airway management in any allergic reaction (see Chapter 27).

Septic Shock

The management of septic shock in the prehospital setting can include the management of hypovolemia (if present) and the correction of metabolic acid-base imbalance. Depending on the patient's response to the infection,

BOX 36-2 Categories of Shock According to Primary Treatment

Causes That Require Primarily the Infusion of Volume

Hemorrhagic shock
Traumatic
Gastrointestinal
Body cavity
Hypovolemia
Gastrointestinal losses
Dehydration from insensible losses
Third-space sequestration from inflammation

Causes That Require Improvement in Pump Function by Either Infusion of Inotropic Support or Reversal of the Cause of Pump Dysfunction

Myocardial ischemia
Coronary artery thrombosis
Arterial hypotension with hypoxemia
Cardiomyopathy
Acute myocarditis
Chronic diseases of heart muscle (ischemic, diabetic, infiltrative, endocrinological, congenital)
Cardiac rhythm disturbances
Atrial fibrillation with rapid ventricular response
Ventricular tachycardia
Supraventricular tachycardia
Hypodynamic septic shock (late sepsis)
Overdose of negative inotropic drug
Beta blocker
Calcium channel antagonist overdose (e.g., verapamil)

Structural cardiac damage
Traumatic (e.g., flail mitral valve)
Ventriculoseptal rupture
Papillary muscle rupture

Causes That Require Volume Support and Vasopressor Support

Hyperdynamic sepsis syndrome (early sepsis)
Anaphylactic shock
Central neurogenic shock
Drug overdose (dihydropyridines, α_1-antagonists)

Problems That Require Immediate Relief From Obstruction to Cardiac Output

Pulmonary embolism
Cardiac tamponade
Pneumothorax
Valvular dysfunction
Acute thrombosis of prosthetic valve
Critical aortic stenosis
Congenital heart defects in newborn (e.g., closure of patent ductus arteriosus with critical aortic coarctation)
Critical idiopathic subaortic stenosis

Cellular Poisons That Require Specific Antidotes

Carbon monoxide
Methemoglobinemia
Hydrogen sulfide
Cyanide

From Marx J, et al: *Rosen's emergency medicine: concepts and clinical practice*, ed 6, St Louis, 2006, Mosby.

prehospital care may involve fluid resuscitation, respiratory support, and the administration of vasopressors to improve cardiac output. If possible, the paramedic should obtain a thorough patient history to help identify the cause of sepsis. Any immunocompromised group of patients has an increased risk of septic shock. Examples of such groups include those with human immunodeficiency virus infection, some cancer patients receiving chemotherapy, and patients with indwelling urinary or vascular catheters.

INTEGRATION OF PATIENT ASSESSMENT AND THE TREATMENT PLAN

Complications of shock are many[3] (Box 36-3). The goals of prehospital care for the patient with severe hemorrhage or shock include rapid recognition of the event, initiation of treatment, prevention of additional injury, rapid transport to an appropriate medical facility by ground or air ambulance, and advanced notification of the receiving facility.

BOX 36-3 Complications of Shock

Acute renal failure
Acute adult respiratory distress syndrome
Hematologic failure
Multiple organ dysfunction syndrome (MODS)
Sepsis
Acute respiratory distress syndrome
Death of organs
Death of organism
Disseminated intravascular coagulation (DIC)

The paramedic should follow guidelines established by local protocol and medical direction in determining the appropriate prehospital level of care for patients and in identifying the appropriate medical facility for patient transport.

SUMMARY

- Shock is inadequate tissue perfusion. It is not a single event but rather the culmination of a complex group of physiological abnormalities.
- Perfusion is the adequate oxygenation of tissue cells. The heart, lungs, and blood vessels (and blood volume) must all be working effectively to achieve normal perfusion.
- The blood vessels form the body's container. This container must be able to shrink and grow and must be filled with an adequate volume to achieve normal tissue perfusion.
- Uncorrected shock progresses through a series of stages. These are vasoconstriction, capillary and venous opening, disseminated intravascular coagulation, and multiple organ failure.
- Shock can be categorized using many methods. Hypovolemic shock occurs when excess blood or body fluid is lost.
- Cardiogenic shock results from pump failure related to a heart muscle, valve, or rhythm problem.
- Neurogenic shock occurs when there is vasomotor paralysis high on the spinal cord.
- Anaphylactic shock is a type of severe allergic reaction that causes impaired vasomotor tone, fluid volume loss, airway obstruction, and bronchospasm.

- Septic shock occurs as a result of a systemic infection. Chemical toxins released from the infectious agent cause a cascade of events that impair cardiac output.
- The three stages of shock are compensated, uncompensated, and irreversible shock.
- Treatment of the patient in shock aims to ensure a patent airway, provide adequate oxygenation, and restore perfusion. The means to achieve each of those objectives varies according to the type of shock and the condition of the patient.
- Fluid resuscitation in shock varies according to the cause. If the patient has uncorrected internal hemorrhage isotonic crystalloid solution should be infused to maintain a systolic blood pressure of 90 mm Hg.
- Treatment of cardiogenic shock is aimed at normalizing heart rate and improving pumping action of the heart.
- During neurogenic shock fluids should be administered cautiously with frequent monitoring of lung sounds.
- Anaphylactic shock is treated with epinephrine, diphenhydramine, and fluid bolus.
- Treatment for patients with septic shock will include fluid resuscitation and possibly administration of vasopressors.

REFERENCES

1. Mann FC: Systems of surgery, *Bull Johns Hopkins Hosp* 25:205, 1914.
2. Hardaway R, editor: *Shock: the reversible stage of dying*, Littleton, Mass, 1988, PSG Publishing.
3. National Highway Traffic Safety Administration. The National EMS Education Standards. Washington, DC, 2009, U.S. Department of Transportation/National Highway Traffic Safety Administration, DOT.
4. Copstead-Kirkhorn C, Banasik JL: *Pathophysiology*, ed 4, Philadelphia, 2009, Saunders.
5. McSwain NE: *PHTLS: Prehospital Trauma Life Support*, ed 7, St Louis, 2011, Mosby.
6. McCance KL, Huether S: *Pathophysiology: the biologic basis for disease in adults and children*, ed 5, St Louis, 2005, Mosby.
7. Patton KT, Thibodeau GA: *Anatomy and physiology*, ed 7, St Louis, 2010, Mosby.
8. National Association of Emergency Medical Technicians: *PHTLS: basic and advanced prehospital trauma life support*, ed 7, St Louis, 2011, Mosby.
9. Sharma S: *Cardiogenic shock*, http://emedicine.medscape.com/article/152191-overview, accessed 9-14-10.
10. Annane D, Bellissant E, Cavaillon JN: Septic shock, *Lancet* 365(9453):63-78, 2005.
11. Marx JA, Hockberger RS, Walls RM, et al: *Emergency medicine: concepts and clinical practice*, ed 6, St Louis, 2006, Mosby.
12. Haynes BE, Carr FJ, Niemann JT: Catheter introducers for rapid fluid resuscitation, *Ann Emerg Med* 12(10):606, 1983.

SUGGESTED READINGS

Lieberman P, Nicklas R, Oppenheimer J, et al: The diagnosis and management of anaphylaxis practice parameter: 2010 update, *J Allergy Clin Immunol* 126(3):477-480.e442, 2010, doi: 10.1016/j.jaci.2010.06.022.

Revell M, Greaves I, Porter K: Endpoints for fluid resuscitation in hemorrhagic shock, *J Trauma* 54(5):S63-S67, 2003.

Sampson HA, Muñoz-Furlong A, Campbell RL, et al: Second symposium on the definition and management of anaphylaxis: summary report—second National Institute of Allergy and Infectious Disease/Food Allergy and Anaphylaxis Network Symposium, *Ann Emerg Med* 47(4):373-380, 2006.

Seymour CW, Kahn JM, Cooke CR, et al: Prediction of critical illness during out-of-hospital emergency care [Research], *JAMA* 304(7):747-754, 2010.

Wang HE, Yealy D: (2010). Assessing critical illness during emergency medical services care [Editorial], *JAMA* 304(7):797-798, 2010.

PART NINE

Trauma

Trauma Overview and Mechanism of Injury

OBJECTIVES

Upon completion of this chapter, the paramedic student will be able to:

1. Describe the incidence and scope of traumatic injuries and deaths.
2. Identify the role of each component of the trauma system.
3. Predict injury patterns based on knowledge of the laws of physics related to forces involved in trauma.
4. Describe injury patterns that should be suspected when injury occurs related to a specific type of blunt trauma.
5. Describe the role of restraints in injury prevention and injury patterns.
6. Discuss how organ motion can contribute to injury in each body region depending on the forces applied.
7. Identify selected injury patterns associated with motorcycle and all-terrain vehicle collisions.
8. Describe injury patterns associated with pedestrian collisions.
9. Identify injury patterns associated with sports injuries, blast injuries, and vertical falls.
10. Describe factors that influence tissue damage related to penetrating injury.

KEY TERMS

acceleration An increase in the velocity of a moving object.

blunt trauma An injury produced by the wounding forces of compression and change of speed, both of which can disrupt tissue.

cavitation A temporary or permanent opening produced by a force that pushes body tissues laterally away from the track of a projectile.

deceleration A decrease in the velocity of a moving object.

incident phase The phase of trauma that refers to the trauma event.

kinematics The process of predicting injury patterns that can result from the forces and motions of energy.

penetrating trauma An injury produced by crushing and stretching forces of a penetrating object that results in some form of tissue disruption.

postincident phase The phase of trauma where emergency care is delivered to injured patients.

preincident phase The phase of trauma that refers to the prevention of intentional and unintentional trauma deaths.

trauma center A specialized hospital distinguished by the immediate availability of specialized personnel, equipment, and services to treat most severe and critical injuries.

T rauma is a major cause of morbidity (nonfatal injury), mortality (death), and years of life lost from normal life expectancy. The paramedic must have an appreciation of trauma systems and how they impact patient care. The paramedic also must be able to recognize how mechanisms of injury predict injury patterns and severity. With these two abilities, the paramedic will be able to enhance patient assessment and emergency care. The purpose of this chapter is to provide an overview of trauma. Care considerations are addressed in later chapters by subject matter.

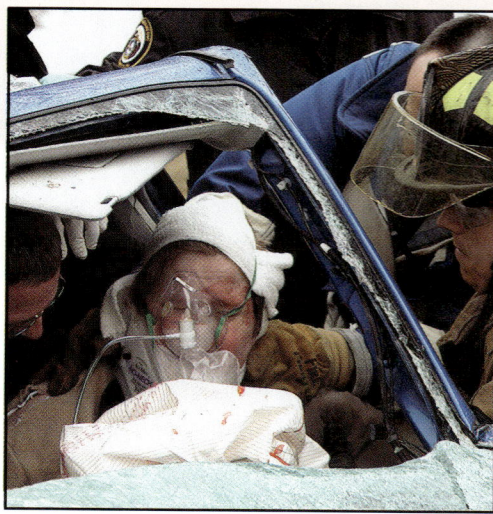

(Courtesy Ray Kemp, St. Charles, Mo.)

EPIDEMIOLOGY OF TRAUMA

Unintentional injury is a devastating medical and social problem. Unintentional injury is the leading cause of death among persons 1 to 44 years of age and the fifth leading cause of death among all Americans.[1] Trauma deaths in 2006 were exceeded only by deaths attributable to heart disease, cancer, stroke, and chronic lower respiratory tract diseases. In 2006, about 120,000 unintentional injury deaths occurred in the United States. The National Safety Council estimates that the total number of unintentional injuries in the United States approaches 61 million annually. Of these injuries, 9 million are disabling, 350,000 result in permanent impairment, and 8.4 million result in permanent disabilities. The economic effect of unintentional injuries in the United States exceeds $700 billion each year.

NOTE
In any given 10-minute period in the United States, 2 persons are killed. In that same time period, about 490 persons suffer a disabling injury. Costs in these 10-minute periods amount to more than $13.3 million.[1]

Trends in Trauma Deaths

Deaths from unintentional injury are increasing yearly. However, most deaths from trauma can be prevented. The increase in deaths points to the need for increased safety and health efforts to reverse the trend. After motor vehicle crashes, poisoning by solids and liquids, falls, fire and flames, drowning, and choking have been the top five causes of trauma deaths since 1970[1] (Fig. 37-1) (Box 37-1).[2]

NOTE
More than 3000 deaths resulted from the terrorist attacks of September 11, 2001. These deaths are not included in these statistics.

BOX 37-1 Classifications of Deaths Attributable to Trauma in the United States[2]

All external causes of mortality
Motor vehicle crashes
Pedestrian injury
Motorcycle crashes
Falls
Mechanical forces (struck by object or machinery)
Drowning
Electrical current
Intentional self-harm
Assaults (firearms)

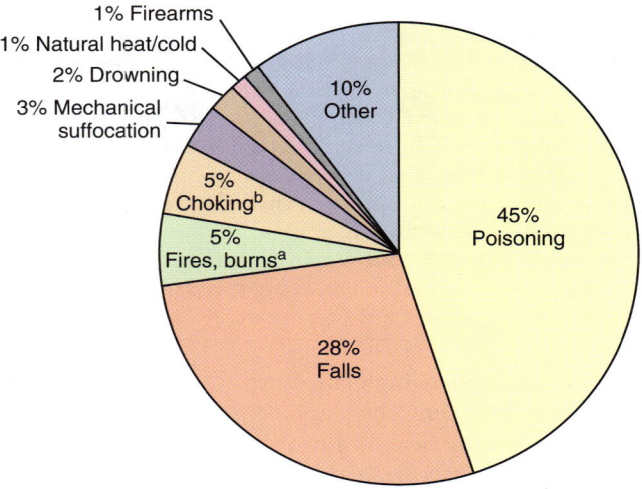

FIGURE 37-1 Deaths from unintentional injury by event. [a]Includes deaths resulting from conflagration, regardless of nature of injury. [b]Inhalation and indigestion of food or other object that obstructs breathing. (From National Safety Council: *Injury facts 2010 Edition.*)

Phases of Trauma Care

Trauma care is divided into three phases. The three phases are preincident, incident, and postincident.[3] The **preincident phase** refers to the prevention of intentional and unintentional trauma deaths. Paramedics and other health care professionals play a key role in this phase. A part of this phase includes participating in public education. (For example, paramedics may educate the public on the use of personal restraint systems, motorcycle helmets, and the proper use of 9-1-1.) Paramedics also promote legislation that supports injury prevention programs (see Chapter 3).

LOOK AGAIN
See Chapter 3: Injury Prevention and Public Health, pp. 56-58.

The **incident phase** is the trauma event. The paramedic can prevent many of these events through education and by practicing personal safety. Thus the paramedic's role in this phase is to "practice what you preach" and to teach by example. The paramedic can achieve this by driving safely and by using personal restraint systems while on and off duty. During the incident phase, the application of active (e.g., seat belts) and passive (e.g., air bags) systems can alter the outcome of a trauma event significantly.

The **postincident phase** is when the paramedic uses his or her expertise and skills. (This is the delivery of emergency care to injured patients.) Important responsibilities for the paramedic in this phase include the following:

BOX 37-2 The Golden Hour

The first hour after severe injury is known as the golden hour and is a critical period. In this period, surgical intervention for the trauma patient can enhance survival and reduce complications. The paramedic must recognize patients who are in this group. The paramedic also must ensure that prehospital care does not delay patient transportation. The paramedic can best serve these patients through rapid assessment, stabilization of life-threatening injuries, and rapid transportation to an appropriate medical facility for definitive care.

- Performing lifesaving maneuvers
- Properly preparing the patient for transportation to an appropriate medical facility
- Promptly transporting the patient to the appropriate medical facility (Box 37-2)

The factor most critical to any severely injured patient's survival is the length of time that elapses between the incident and definitive care[3,4] (Box 37-3).

Trauma Systems

A comprehensive trauma system consists of many different components. These components are integrated and coordinated to provide cost-effective services for injury prevention and patient care. At the center of this system is the continuum of care, which includes injury prevention, prehospital care, acute care facilities, and posthospital care.[5] The following is a sampling of these components:

1. Injury prevention
2. Prehospital care, including management, transportation, and trauma triage guidelines
3. Emergency department care
4. Interfacility transportation if needed
5. Definitive care
6. Trauma critical care
7. Rehabilitation
8. Data collection and trauma registry

 CRITICAL THINKING
How can you learn more about the components of the trauma system during your career as a paramedic?

The paramedic plays a crucial role in the trauma system. One aspect of this role is being involved in injury prevention programs. Another aspect includes entering appropriate patients into the trauma care system while providing appropriate patient care. Lastly, the paramedic fulfills this role by taking part in data collection and research. As described in Chapter 3: Injury Prevention and Public Health, this research can influence health care improvements in caring for injured patients (Box 37-4).

Trauma Centers

As described in Chapter 1, the U.S. Department of Health and Human Services released the *Position Paper on Trauma Center Designation* in 1980. Since then, states have developed

BOX 37-3 Prevention of Trauma Deaths

Deaths from trauma occur in three periods: immediate, early, and late. Each period presents its own unique problems.[4]

Immediate

Immediate death occurs within seconds or minutes of the injury. Lacerations of the brain, brainstem, upper spinal cord, heart, aorta, or other large vessels usually cause these deaths. Few if any patients in this category can be saved. Effective injury prevention programs are the only way to reduce the number of these deaths.

Early

The second peak of death occurs within the first 2 to 3 hours after injury. The causes of these deaths usually are major head injury, hemopneumothorax, ruptured spleen, lacerated liver, pelvic fracture, or multiple injuries associated with significant blood loss. Most of these injuries can be treated with available techniques. However, the time lapse between injury and definitive care is critical.

Late

The third peak of death occurs days or weeks after the injury. These deaths most often result from sepsis, infection, or multiple organ failure. Prehospital emergency care focused on early recognition and management of life-threatening injuries is critical to the prevention of late deaths from trauma.

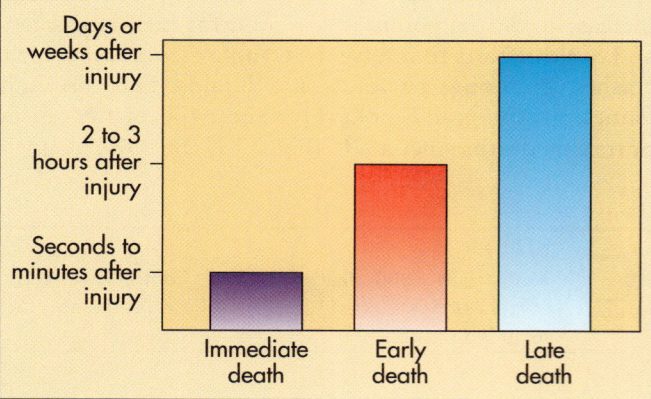

comprehensive trauma systems. As of 2010, 225 hospitals have a designated specialty in trauma.[6]

The American Medical Association recommended categorization of hospital emergency services in the early 1970s.[7] In 1990 (revised in 1999) the Task Force of the American College of Surgeons (ACS) Committee on Trauma published *Resources for Optimal Care of the Injured Patient*. The paper described three levels of trauma centers. These levels are based on resources (essential and desired), admissions, staff, research, and education involvement.

A level I trauma center has a full range of specialists and equipment available 24 hours a day and admits a minimum required annual volume of severely injured patients.

BOX 37-4 Trauma Registries

Trauma registries allow for the collection of injury data by individual hospitals or groups of hospitals on a local, regional, or state level. The American College of Surgeons funded these registries and the data collection software programs. (An example of a registry is the National Trauma Data Bank. An example of a software program is NATIONAL TRACS.) The registries and programs are meant to provide online data management. They also are intended to provide national exchange of injury data for a variety of commercial registry programs. Trauma registries generate periodic standard reports. These reports offer statistical data. The data allow facilities to compare the trends and to compare other key details regarding trauma care.

BOX 37-5 Trauma Centers

A trauma center is a specialized hospital distinguished by the *immediate* availability of *specialized* personnel, equipment, and services to *treat* most severe and critical injuries. This includes ready-to-go teams that perform immediate surgery and other necessary procedures for people with serious or life-threatening injuries, for example, due to a car crash, a long fall, or gunshot wounds. The mission of a trauma center is to ensure continuity and quality of care for injured patients from the scene of injury through treatment at the trauma center and ultimately physical rehabilitation. Currently, less than 10% of hospitals have a trauma center.

Trauma centers are classified by levels dependent upon the amount of equipment, staff, and care provided[8]:

- *Level I.* Has a full range of specialists and equipment available 24 hours a day. Admits a minimum required annual volume of severely injured patients. Has a research program. Is a leader in trauma education and injury prevention, and is a referral resource for communities in neighboring regions. Has a required program for substance abuse screening and provides brief intervention to patients.
- *Level II.* Usually works in collaboration with a level I center but may be the only resource in a rural state. Provides comprehensive trauma care and supplements the clinical expertise of a level I institution. Provides 24-hour availability of all essential specialties, personnel, and equipment. Has no minimum volume requirements. Provides an injury prevention program and also conducts substance screening, but is not required to have an ongoing program of research or a surgical residency program.
- *Level III.* Has resources for the emergency resuscitation, stabilization, emergent surgery, and intensive care of most trauma patients. Has transfer agreements with level I and/or level II trauma centers to ensure back-up resources for the care of patients with severe injuries. Has an injury prevention program. Does not have the full availability of specialists, except surgery and orthopedics, in most states.
- *Level IV.* Provides initial evaluation, emergency resuscitation, and stabilization of trauma patients, but most patients will require transfer to higher level trauma centers. Has 24-hour emergency coverage by a physician.

Additionally, a level I center has a program of research, is a leader in trauma education and injury prevention, and is a referral resource for communities in neighboring regions through community outreach. The level I trauma center must have a program for substance abuse screening and provide brief intervention to patients as appropriate.[6] A level I trauma center can provide total care for every aspect of injury. The level I center is followed by level II and III facilities. (A level IV trauma center exists in some states where the resources do not exist for a level III trauma centers [Box 37-5].) The assignment of category to a trauma center also enables emergency medical services personnel to transport patients rapidly to the most appropriate facility. Other specialized care facilities—such as pediatric trauma centers, burn centers, hyperbaric centers, and poison treatment centers—provide care for critically ill or injured patients with special needs. The ACS Committee on Trauma also established guidelines for field triage, interhospital triage to specialized care facilities, and mass casualty triage. These criteria are based on the patient's condition, mechanism of injury, injury severity indexes, and available patient care resources (Figure 37-2).

CRITICAL THINKING

Where can you find the trauma triage criteria for your area?

Transportation Considerations

Determining the proper level of care and hospital destination is based on the patient's needs and condition, and sometimes the advice of medical direction. (The Centers for Disease Control and Prevention along with key experts in trauma care have developed guidelines to assist EMS personnel in identifying patients who need trauma center care. Other methods of triage will be addressed in Chapter 54.) Once the paramedic determines the level of care needed and the destination facility, decisions can be made about the mode of transportation. (For example, the paramedic chooses between ground or air ambulance.)

SHOW ME THE EVIDENCE

Researchers reviewed previously collected data on selected trauma patients 16 years of age and older with a physiological abnormality. Patients were included if they had any of the following conditions: systolic blood pressure (SBP) ≤90 mm Hg; respiratory rate (RR) ≤10 or ≥29 breaths/min, Glasgow Coma Scale score (GCS) ≤12, or advanced airway intervention. The researchers examined the correlation between field times and patient deaths. Of their sample 22% died. The analyses found no significant association between time and mortality for any EMS interval (activation, response, on-scene, transport, or total EMS time).

From Newgard CD, Schmicker RH, Hedges JR, et al: Emergency medical services intervals and survival in trauma: assessment of the "Golden Hour" in a North American prospective cohort, *Ann Emerg Med* 55(3):235-246, 2010.

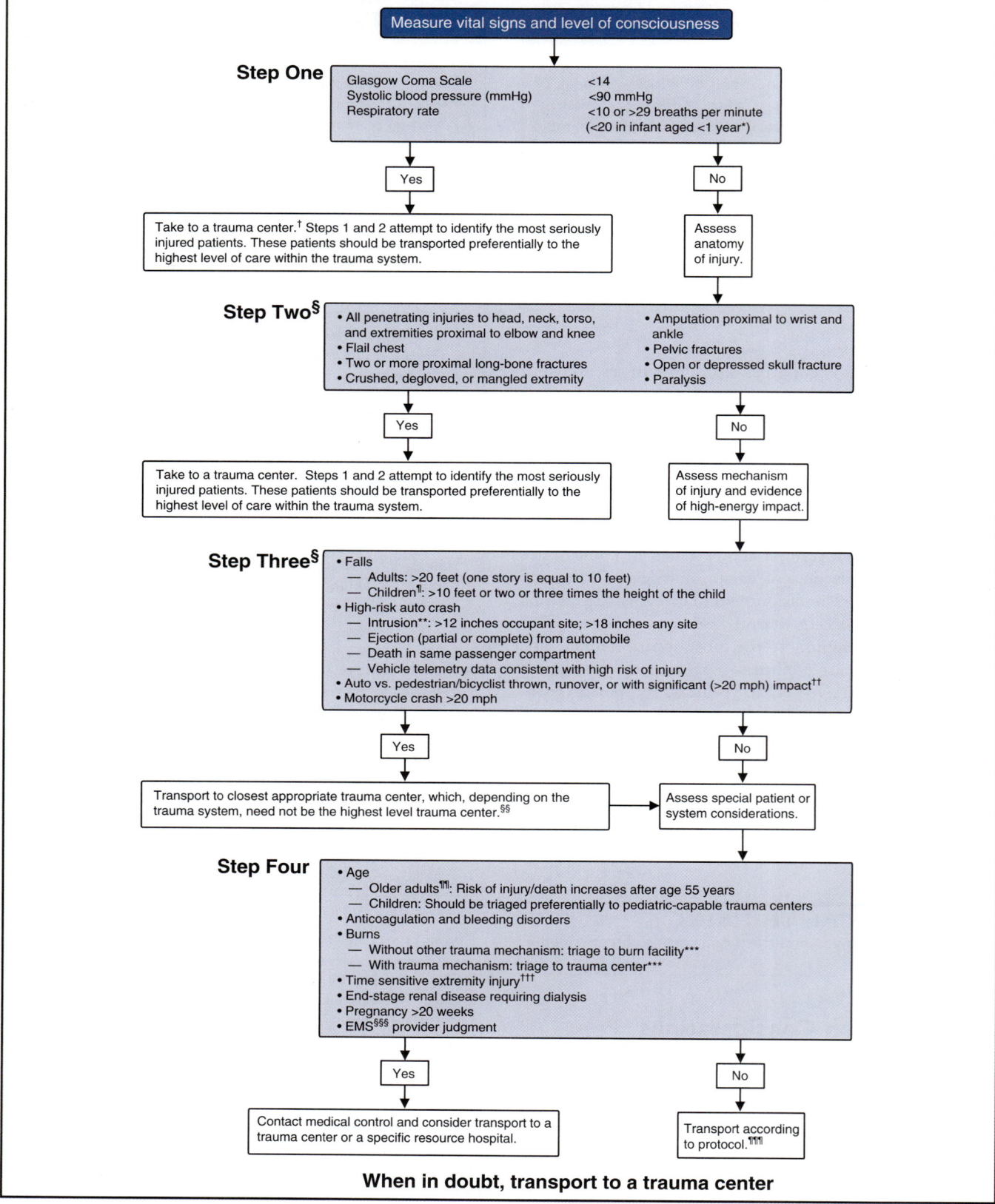

Measure vital signs and level of consciousness

Step One

Glasgow Coma Scale	<14
Systolic blood pressure (mmHg)	<90 mmHg
Respiratory rate	<10 or >29 breaths per minute (<20 in infant aged <1 year*)

Yes → Take to a trauma center.† Steps 1 and 2 attempt to identify the most seriously injured patients. These patients should be transported preferentially to the highest level of care within the trauma system.

No → Assess anatomy of injury.

Step Two§

- All penetrating injuries to head, neck, torso, and extremities proximal to elbow and knee
- Flail chest
- Two or more proximal long-bone fractures
- Crushed, degloved, or mangled extremity

- Amputation proximal to wrist and ankle
- Pelvic fractures
- Open or depressed skull fracture
- Paralysis

Yes → Take to a trauma center. Steps 1 and 2 attempt to identify the most seriously injured patients. These patients should be transported preferentially to the highest level of care within the trauma system.

No → Assess mechanism of injury and evidence of high-energy impact.

Step Three§

- Falls
  — Adults: >20 feet (one story is equal to 10 feet)
  — Children¶: >10 feet or two or three times the height of the child
- High-risk auto crash
  — Intrusion**: >12 inches occupant site; >18 inches any site
  — Ejection (partial or complete) from automobile
  — Death in same passenger compartment
  — Vehicle telemetry data consistent with high risk of injury
- Auto vs. pedestrian/bicyclist thrown, runover, or with significant (>20 mph) impact††
- Motorcycle crash >20 mph

Yes → Transport to closest appropriate trauma center, which, depending on the trauma system, need not be the highest level trauma center.§§

No → Assess special patient or system considerations.

Step Four

- Age
  — Older adults¶¶: Risk of injury/death increases after age 55 years
  — Children: Should be triaged preferentially to pediatric-capable trauma centers
- Anticoagulation and bleeding disorders
- Burns
  — Without other trauma mechanism: triage to burn facility***
  — With trauma mechanism: triage to trauma center***
- Time sensitive extremity injury†††
- End-stage renal disease requiring dialysis
- Pregnancy >20 weeks
- EMS§§§ provider judgment

Yes → Contact medical control and consider transport to a trauma center or a specific resource hospital.

No → Transport according to protocol.¶¶¶

When in doubt, transport to a trauma center

Figure 37-2 Field Triage Decision Scheme—United States, 2006. *The upper limit of respiratory rate in infants is >29 breaths per minute to maintain a higher level of overtriage for infants. †Trauma centers are designated level I to IV, with level I representing the highest level of trauma care available. §Any injury noted in steps 2 and 3 triggers a "yes" response. ¶Age <15 years. **Intrusion refers to interior compartment intrusion, as opposed to deformation, which refers to exterior damage. ††Includes pedestrians or bicyclists thrown or run over by a motor vehicle or those with estimated impact >20 mph with a motor vehicle. §§Local or regional protocols should be used to determine the most appropriate level of trauma center; appropriate center need not be level I. ¶¶Age >55 years. ***Patients with both burns and concomitant trauma for whom the burn injury poses the greatest risk for morbidity and mortality should be transferred to a burn center. If the nonburn trauma presents a greater immediate risk, the patient may be stabilized in a trauma center and then transferred to a burn center. †††Injuries such as an open fracture or fracture with neurovascular compromise. §§§Emergency medical services. ¶¶¶Patients who do not meet any of the triage criteria in steps 1 to 4 should be transported to the most appropriate medical facility as outlined in local EMS. (Adapted from American College of Surgeons: *Resources for the optimal care of the injured patient,* Chicago, Ill, 2006, Author. Footnotes have been added to enhance understanding of field triage by persons outside the acute injury care field.) (From CDC (2009): Guidelines for field triage of injured patients: Recommendations of the National Expert Panel on Field Triage, Jan. 29, 2009, V. 58 # RR-1.)

GROUND TRANSPORTATION

As a rule the paramedic should use ground transportation by ambulance if the appropriate facility can be reached within a "reasonable time." Reasonable time is defined by national standards (e.g., definitive care within 60 minutes after the injury for severe trauma) and local protocol. Factors that affect the decision to use ground or air transportation include geographical location, topographical area, population, weather, availability of resources, traffic conditions, and time of day.

AEROMEDICAL TRANSPORTATION

The availability and use of aeromedical services vary throughout the United States. Aeromedical services can provide rapid response time, high-quality medical care, and rapid transportation to appropriate care facilities. Helicopters also can provide aerial surveillance and transportation of additional personnel and equipment to the emergency scene. Paramedic crews should consult with medical direction and follow local protocol regarding the use of aeromedical services. (Use of aeromedical services is addressed further in Chapter 53.) The paramedic should consider air transportation in the following situations:

- The time needed to transport a patient by ground to an appropriate facility poses a threat to the patient's survival and recovery.
- Weather, road, or traffic conditions would seriously delay the patient's access to definitive care.
- Critical care personnel and equipment are needed to adequately care for the patient during transportation.

SECTION ONE
Kinematics

ENERGY

A transfer of energy from an external source to the human body causes injuries. The extent of injury is determined by (1) the type and amount of energy applied, (2) the speed with which energy is applied, and (3) the part of the body to which energy is applied.

Physical Laws

Knowledge of four basic laws of physics is required to understand the wounding forces of trauma:

1. *Newton's first law of motion.* An object, whether at rest or in motion, remains in that state unless acted upon by an outside force.
2. *Conservation of energy law.* Energy cannot be created or destroyed; it can only change form. (Energy can take mechanical, thermal, electrical, chemical, and nuclear forms.)
3. *Newton's second law of motion.* Force (F) equals mass (M) multiplied by acceleration (a) or deceleration (d):

$$F = M \times a \ or \ F = M \times d$$

4. *Kinetic energy.* Kinetic energy (KE) equals half the mass (M) multiplied by the velocity squared (V^2).

$$KE = \frac{1}{2}m \times V^2$$

As the kinetic energy formula shows, velocity is much more critical than mass in determining total kinetic energy. For example, a car and its unrestrained 150-lb driver are traveling 60 miles per hour. According to Newton's first law of motion, the car remains in motion until acted upon by an outside force. If the driver gradually applies the brakes, the friction of the brakes slowly converts the mechanical energy of the car to thermal energy (conservation of energy law); the energy transfer occurs gradually through the slow deceleration. If the car strikes a tree, though, and is stopped instantly, the tree absorbs the mechanical energy, the car, and the driver. When the front of the car has stopped, the rear of the car continues forward until all of the energy of its motion is absorbed. The driver is traveling in the same direction and at the same speed as the car before impact. So, like the rear of the car, the driver continues forward. The driver suffers injuries in areas of the body that strike the vehicle.

In this sequence the tree stops the motion of the front of the car. The steering column continues forward and stops against the dashboard. The driver's sternum stops against the steering column. The driver's chest cavity and its contents hit the sternum and are crushed from behind by the posterior thorax, deforming the entire chest. The kinetic energy in this example is calculated as follows:

KE = one half of the mass times the velocity squared,

$$\text{or KE} = \frac{1}{2}m \times V^2$$

$$\text{KE} = \frac{150}{2} \times 60^2$$

$$\text{KE} = 270,000 \text{ units of energy}$$

As shown in this calculation, the 150-lb driver traveling 60 miles per hour must change 270,000 units of kinetic energy (known as *foot-pounds,* calculated as pounds multiplied by miles per hour) into another form of energy when he or she stops. In addition, recall that force equals mass multiplied by acceleration (Newton's second law of motion). Thus the 150-lb driver is moving forward in the car with about 9000 ft-lb of force when stopped by the steering column. The energy of the motion of the body causes tissue destruction as this energy is absorbed into the body cells when the body stops. This example illustrates the principle. However, the actual total force also is determined by the true rate of deceleration, or "g" force, and several other factors. Lap and shoulder restraints and air bags increase the distance over which the body stops its movement. This can decrease the deceleration force a great deal. New car construction is also designed to absorb some of this energy and lessen the force applied to the vehicle occupants.

> **CRITICAL THINKING**
> Can you apply these same four laws of physics to another traumatic situation, such as a fall onto concrete? What force is applied? What factors influence the kinetic energy?

Kinematics

Kinematics is the process of predicting injury patterns. Specific types and patterns of injuries are associated with certain mechanisms. In addition to individual factors (such as age) and protective factors (such as restraint systems, helmets, and air bags), the paramedic should consider the following when evaluating the trauma patient:

- Mechanism of injury
- Force of energy applied
- Anatomy
- Energy (for example, mass; velocity; distance; and thermal, electrical, and chemical forms)

SECTION TWO
Blunt Trauma

BLUNT TRAUMA

Blunt trauma is an injury produced by the wounding forces of compression and change of speed (usually deceleration). These forces can disrupt tissue. Direct compression is the pressure on a structure and is the most common type of force applied in blunt trauma. The amount of injury depends on the length of time of compression, the force of compression, and the area compressed. For example, compression of the thorax can lead to rib fracture or pneumothorax. Other compression injuries include contusions and lacerations of solid organs and rupture of hollow (air-filled) organs.

Acceleration is an increase in the velocity of a moving object. **Deceleration** is a decrease in the velocity of a moving object. Both can produce major injury. For example, consider a car that comes to a stop abruptly. The occupant's body continues its constant velocity after the impact until it decelerates as a result of striking the steering wheel, restraint system, or dashboard. The external aspect of the body is stopped forcibly. However, the contents of the cranial, thoracic, and peritoneal cavities remain in motion because of inertia. As a result, tissues can be stretched, crushed, ruptured, lacerated, or sheared from their points of attachment. Examples of injuries caused by a change of speed include concussion, cardiac or pulmonary contusion, organ laceration, and aortic tear.

Motor Vehicle Collision

The various injuries produced by blunt trauma are illustrated best through examination of vehicle collisions. Forces that cause blunt trauma, however, can result from a variety of impacts. As described in the previous example, a vehicle collision involves three separate impacts as the energy is transferred. In the first impact, the vehicle strikes an object. In the second, the occupant collides with the inside of the car. In the third, the internal organs collide inside the body. The injuries that result depend on the type of collision and the position of the occupant inside the vehicle. The injuries also depend on the use or nonuse of active or passive restraint systems.

>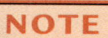
> **NOTE**
> Inattention to driving is a contributing factor in 78% of motor vehicle crashes and in 65% of near-crashes, according to data from observational studies by NHTSA.[9] Distracted driving includes being fatigued, glancing at a rear-view mirror, eating, smoking, and talking and listening on a wireless device. At any given time, about 5% of all drivers use a hand-held cell phone; 0.6% use headsets; and 0.4% manipulate a hand-held device.

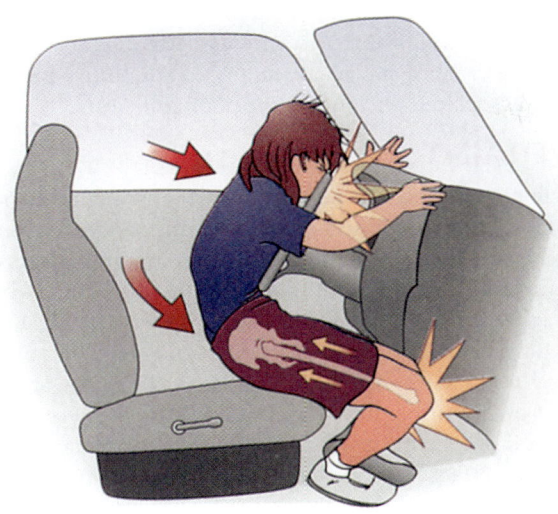

FIGURE 37-3 Down-and-under pathway. (From NAEMT: *Prehospital trauma life support,* ed 7, St Louis, 2011, Mosby.)

A vehicle collision is classified by the type of impact: head-on, lateral, rear-end, rotational, and rollover. The forces of compression and change of speed produce predictable injury patterns in each type of collision.

HEAD-ON (FRONTAL) IMPACT

Head-on collisions result when forward motion stops abruptly. (For example, one vehicle collides with another one traveling in the opposite direction.) The first collision occurs when the vehicle hits the second vehicle, resulting in damage to the front of the car. As the vehicle abruptly stops, the occupant continues to move at the speed of the vehicle before impact. The front seat occupant continues forward into the restraint system, steering column, or dashboard. This results in the second collision. The occupant who is not restrained usually travels in one of two pathways in relationship to the dashboard. The two pathways are down-and-under or up-and-over. The precise course of this pathway determines how the organs collide inside the body and the extent of tissue damaged.

In the down-and-under pathway the occupant travels downward into the vehicle seat and forward into the dashboard or steering column (Figure 37-3). The knees become the leading part of the body, striking the dashboard. The upper legs absorb most of the impact. Predictable injuries include knee dislocation, patellar fracture, femoral fracture, fracture or posterior dislocation of the hip, fracture of the acetabulum, vascular injury, and hemorrhage. After the initial impact of the knees into the dashboard, the body rotates forward. As the chest wall hits the steering column or dashboard, the head and torso absorb energy as indicated in the description of the up-and-over pathway.

CRITICAL THINKING

How does the use of lap and shoulder restraints influence the patterns of injury described here?

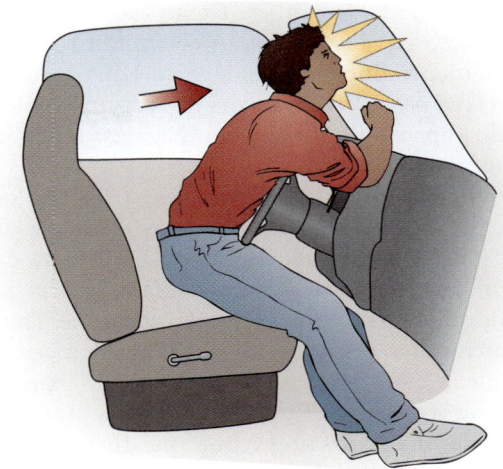

FIGURE 37-4 Up-and-over pathway. (From NAEMT: *Prehospital trauma life support,* ed 7, St Louis, 2011, Mosby.)

In the up-and-over pathway the body in forward motion strikes the steering wheel. As this occurs, the ribs and underlying structures absorb the momentum of the thorax (Figure 37-4). Predictable injuries from this transfer of energy include rib fracture, ruptured diaphragm, hemopneumothorax, pulmonary contusion, cardiac contusion, myocardial rupture, and vascular disruption (most notably aortic rupture).

If the abdomen is the point of impact, compression injuries can occur to the hollow abdominal organs, solid organs, and lumbar vertebrae. The kidneys, liver, and spleen are subject to vascular tears from supporting tissue. Such injuries may include the tearing of renal vessels from their points of attachment to the inferior vena cava and descending aorta. Predictable injuries include liver laceration, spleen rupture, internal hemorrhage, and abdominal organ incursion into the thorax (ruptured diaphragm).

If the head absorbs most of the impact, the cervical vertebrae absorb the continued momentum of the body. Cervical flexion, axial loading, and hyperextension (further described in Chapter 41) can result in fracture or dislocation of the cervical vertebrae. In addition, severe angulation of the cervical vertebrae can damage the soft tissues of the neck. This may cause spinal cord injury and spinal instability, even without fracture. Other predictable injuries include trauma to the brain (e.g., concussion, contusion, shearing injury, and edema) and disruption of vessels inside the head (intracranial vascular disruption), resulting in subdural or epidural hematoma (see Chapter 40).

LATERAL IMPACT

Lateral impact occurs when a vehicle is struck from the side. Injury patterns depend on whether the damaged vehicle remains in place or moves away from the point of impact. The external shell of a vehicle that remains in place after impact usually intrudes into the passenger compartment and usually directs force at the lateral aspect of the person's body. Predictable injuries result from compression to the torso, pelvis, and extremities. Examples of these injuries include fractured ribs, pulmonary contusion, ruptured liver or spleen (depending on the side involved), fractured clavicle, fractured pelvis, and head and neck injury. Vehicles that have side-impact air bags can guard against injury in some lateral impacts.

If the damaged vehicle moves away from the point of impact, the occupant accelerates away from the point of impact. The occupant moves laterally with the car. The effects of inertia on the head, neck, and thorax produce lateral flexion and rotation of the cervical spine. This movement can result in neurological injury. Such movement also can result in tears or strains of the lateral ligaments and supporting structures of the neck. Injuries also can occur on the side of the passenger opposite the impact as the occupant is propelled toward the other side of the car. If other occupants are in the vehicle, secondary collision with other passengers is likely.

REAR-END IMPACT

A vehicle that is struck from behind rapidly accelerates, causing it to move forward under the occupant. The greater the difference in the forward speed of the two vehicles, the greater the force and damaging energy of the initial impact. For example, consider a vehicle that is traveling 50 mph and hits a stationary vehicle. The damaging energy is greater than that of a vehicle traveling 50 mph that hits another vehicle going 30 mph. Thus in forward collisions, the sum of the speeds of both vehicles is the velocity that produces damage. In rear-end collisions the difference between the two speeds is the damaging velocity.

Predictable injuries in rear-end collisions include back and neck injuries and cervical strain or fracture caused by hyperextension. The cervical portion of the spine is susceptible to secondary hyperextension caused by the rapid forward acceleration of the vehicle and subsequent relative rearward movement of the occupant. If the vehicle collides with an object in front of it, the paramedic should suspect injuries associated with frontal impact.

ROTATIONAL IMPACT

Rotational impacts occur when an off-center portion of the vehicle (usually the front quarter) strikes an immovable object or one that is moving more slowly or in the opposite direction. The part of the vehicle striking the object stops during impact. The rest of the vehicle continues in forward motion until the energy is transformed completely. The occupant moves inside the vehicle with the forward motion. The occupant usually is struck by the side of the car as the vehicle rotates around the point of impact. A rotational impact results in injuries common to those found in head-on and lateral collisions.

ROLLOVER CRASHES

In rollover crashes or collisions the person tumbles inside the vehicle. The occupant is injured wherever his or her body strikes the vehicle. The various impacts occur at many different angles, which can cause multiple-system injuries. Predicting injury patterns from rollover collisions is difficult. These crashes can produce any of the injury patterns that are associated with other types of collisions.

RESTRAINTS

In recent years, public awareness programs and various state laws have increased the use of personal restraints. According to the National Safety Council, among passenger vehicle occupants more than 4 years of age, safety belts saved an estimated 15,383 lives in 2006.[1] Another 5541 lives could have been saved if *all* passengers older than 4 years of age had worn safety belts. At this time, all states and the District of Columbia have child safety seat laws. Forty-nine states and the District of Columbia have mandatory belt use laws in effect (the one exception is New Hampshire).

A serious hazard to unrestrained occupants is ejection from the vehicle after impact. Among crashes in which a fatality occurred in 2005, only 1% of restrained passenger car occupants were ejected, compared with 31% of those who were unrestrained.[1] In addition, 1 of every 13 ejection victims suffers a spinal fracture, and ejected victims are killed 6 times more often than those who are not ejected.[3] The mortality rate among ejected victims is high. This results in part from the occupant being subjected to a second impact as the body strikes the ground or another object outside the vehicle.

CRITICAL THINKING

How can you apply this knowledge about ejection statistics to your practice in each of the phases of trauma care (preincident, incident, and postincident)?

Four restraining systems are available in the United States. These are lap belts, diagonal shoulder straps, air bags, and child safety seats. All of these restraints significantly reduce injuries. If they are used inappropriately, however, these protective devices also can produce injuries.

Lap Belts

The lap belt, used alone or with a shoulder strap, is the most commonly used active restraint system. A person should direct the lap belt at a 45-degree angle to the floor between the anterior-superior iliac spine and the femur (Figure 37-5). A lap belt worn tightly enough to stay in this position absorbs energy forces. The belt protects the abdominal cavity by transferring energy to the strong, bony pelvis.

However, the lap belt often is worn incorrectly. If the lap belt is worn above the anterior iliac spine, the forward motion of the body during impact is absorbed by vertebrae T12, L1, and L2. As the thorax is propelled forward, the abdominal organs are compressed between the vertebral column and the lap belt. This compression can cause injury to the liver, spleen, duodenum, and pancreas. A sign of

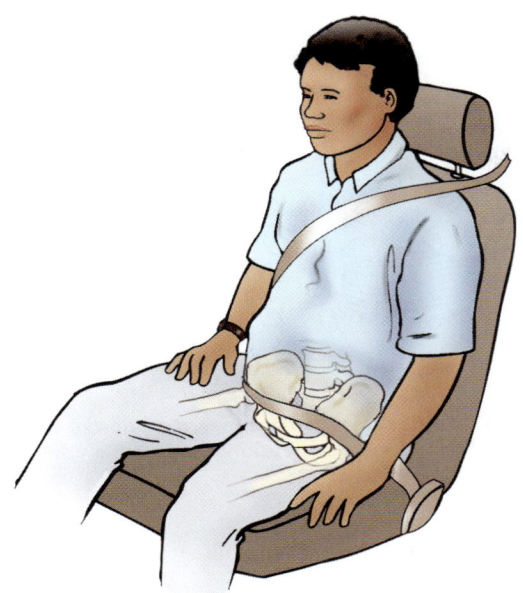

FIGURE 37-5 Properly positioned seat belt. (From NAEMT: *Prehospital trauma life support,* ed 7, St Louis, 2011, Mosby.)

these abdominal injuries is abrasions or a lap belt imprint over the abdomen.

Major injury can result even when a person uses a lap belt correctly. These injuries occur from angulation of the lumbar spine, pelvis, thorax, and head around the restraint system. Injuries also occur from failure of the restraint system to decrease the impact forces. Injuries that can occur during high-speed impacts include sternal fractures, chest wall injuries, lumbar vertebral fractures, head injuries, and maxillofacial trauma.

Diagonal Shoulder Straps

Use of a shoulder strap helps absorb the forward motion of the thorax after impact. When a person wears the shoulder strap with the lap belt, the shoulder strap prevents the thorax, face, and head from striking the dashboard, windshield, or steering column. Clavicular fracture can result from the position of the shoulder strap. Organ collision inside the body with resultant internal organ injury, cervical fracture, and spinal cord injury still can occur during high-speed impacts, even when personal restraint systems are used.

Air Bags

Some vehicles are equipped with side-impact air bags, curtain air bags, knee air bags, safety belt air bags, and rear-curtain air bags to protect against impacts. However, the more common air bag is a frontal air bag that inflates from the center of the steering wheel and from the dashboard during frontal impact. These devices cushion the forward motion of the occupant when used with a lap and shoulder belt. Frontal air bags deflate rapidly. They are effective only with initial frontal and near-frontal collisions. They are ineffective in multiple collisions, rear-impact collisions,

and lateral or rollover impacts. These systems do not prevent movement in the down-and-under pathway. Thus the occupant's knees still may be the point of impact. This may result in leg, pelvis, and abdominal injuries.

An air bag can produce significant injury if it is deployed in proximity (10 inches or closer) to the occupant. Deployment in these situations can produce spinal fractures, hand and eye injury, and facial and forearm abrasions. The following groups are at higher risk of injury from air bag deployment[10]:

- Infants and children less than 12 years of age
- Adults of short stature (less than 5 feet 2 inches)
- Older adults
- Persons with special medical conditions

Most air bag injuries are minor cuts, bruises, or abrasions. Most of these injuries are far less serious than the head, neck, and chest injuries that air bags prevent. According to the National Highway Traffic Safety Administration, frontal air bags saved more than 28,000 lives in 2009.[11] Although deaths do sometimes occur from air bag deployment, most are a result of the occupant being too close to the air bag when it deployed. This problem occurred more commonly from the child not being restrained adequately with lap/shoulder devices or child safety seats during precrash braking. To protect against injury from air bag deployment, the driver of the vehicle should be positioned at least 10 inches from the air bag cover; the front seat passenger should be positioned at least 18 inches away from the air bag cover; and children under 12 years of age should always ride in the back seat and be in the proper restraint device for their size.

Child Safety Seats

The leading cause of death in children younger than 4 years of age is injuries sustained in motor vehicle crashes. For each of these deaths, the U.S. Department of Health, Education, and Welfare estimates that thousands more suffer debilitating injury. The National Center for Statistics and Analysis reports that an estimated 4877 lives were saved by child restraints between 1975 and 1998, and 425 lives were saved by child restraints in 2006 alone.[12]

Child safety seats are available in several shapes and sizes. This variety accommodates the different stages of physical development. These seats include infant carriers, booster seats, and toddler seats. Child safety seats use a combination of lap belts, shoulder belts, full-body harnesses, and harness-and-shield apparatus to protect the child during vehicle collision. Predictable injuries likely to occur even with the appropriate use of child safety seats include blunt abdominal trauma, change-of-speed injuries from deceleration forces, and neck and spinal injury. A large amount of misuse of child safety seats occurs. (For example, common issues include location, installation, and strapping.) Public education on the correct use of child safety seats is a key prevention measure. For information on transporting children in an ambulance, see Box 37-6.

BOX 37-6 Transportation of Children in an Ambulance

Although no formal regulations have been established, it is recommended that child safety seats be available in emergency vehicles. In addition to practicing safe driving in all patient transports, the paramedic should observe the following guidelines.*

The method or device used to secure children during transport must provide effective restraint without compromising the safety of others on board.

Younger children and infants who do not require spinal immobilization should be transported in child safety seats appropriate for their size. If an appropriate safety seat is not available, the paramedic should ask to borrow one from family members (preferably one that has not been in a motor vehicle collision).

Any time a child is secured to a device such as a safety seat or spine board, the paramedic must ensure that the device is secured to the stretcher.

For any patient where medically appropriate, position the patient on the stretcher with the back of the stretcher placed upright at least at a 45-degree angle. This angle optimizes transportation safety in the event of an impact or deceleration.

If the child is secured in a safety seat, the seat should be secured to the stretcher using at least two belts placed at a 90-degree angle to each other; that is, one strap is oriented vertically and the other strap is oriented horizontally to secure the child seat to the upright stretcher. A child safety seat secured to the stretcher with the stretcher back in the upright position has performed well in the crash testing conducted to date.

Restraint systems applied to a flat stretcher are less secure in a crash. If a suboptimal restraint technique such as this must be used, the paramedic should notify the driver to exert additional caution during transport to minimize the risk.

Older children who do not require special positioning should be secured on a stretcher that has had the back elevated to an angle of at least 45 degrees.

The paramedic should use shoulder harnesses to restrain patients who must be immobilized in the supine position on a backboard and therefore cannot have the back of the stretcher elevated for protection. The paramedic should *never* secure the parent and child together on the stretcher. The paramedic also should *never* allow infants or young children to ride in the arms or lap of a parent or rescuer.

*The Center for Pediatric Emergency Medicine: *Teaching resource for instructors in prehospital pediatrics for paramedics: safe transport of children,* www.cpem.org/trippals/38TRANSP.PDF, accessed 3-15-10.

ORGAN COLLISION INJURIES

Organs can be injured as a result of movement caused by deceleration and compression forces. The paramedic must maintain a high degree of suspicion regarding injuries to organs based on the principles of kinematics. (In-depth discussions of these injuries are presented in later chapters by subject matter.)

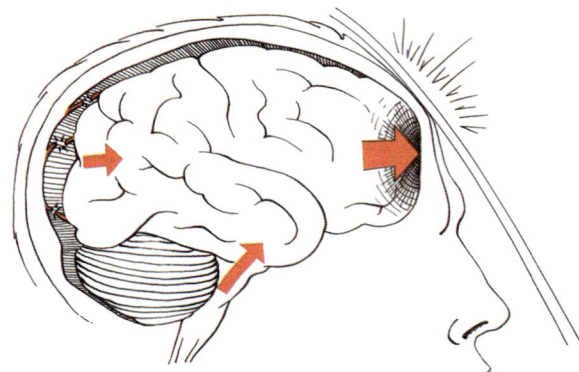

FIGURE 37-6 After cessation of forward motion of the skull the brain continues its motion, resulting in possible contusion and intracerebral hemorrhage.

Deceleration Injuries

When body organs are put into motion after an impact, they continue to move. They move in opposition to the structures that attach them to the body. Thus a risk exists of separation of body organs from their attachments. Injury to the vascular pedicle or mesenteric attachment can lead to brisk or exsanguinating hemorrhage.

HEAD INJURIES

When the head strikes a stationary object, the cranium comes to an abrupt stop. However, brain tissue inside the cranium continues to move. The brain moves until it is compressed against the skull (Figure 37-6). This movement can cause brain tissue to be bruised, crushed, or lacerated. Such movement also can cause blood vessels attached to the brain and skull to be torn, producing intracranial hemorrhage. Other injuries associated with deceleration of the head include central nervous system injury, caused by stretching of the spinal cord and its attachments, and cervical fracture.

THORACIC INJURIES

The aorta often is injured by severe deceleration forces. The aorta is affixed at several points. Proximally the aorta is affixed by the aortic valve in the descending portion of the aortic arch by the ligamentum arteriosum. The descending aorta also is attached to the thoracic spine. As the thorax hits a stationary object, the heart and aorta continue in motion. This motion is in opposition to their attachment at the lower end of the aortic arch. The aorta usually is sheared at the level of its ligamentum arteriosum attachment (Figure 37-7). Frank rupture of the aorta leads to rapid exsanguination. However, transection and dissection through to the internal lining (intima and media of the aorta) can result in cardiac tamponade. This can allow patients to arrive at an emergency department and survive the injury.

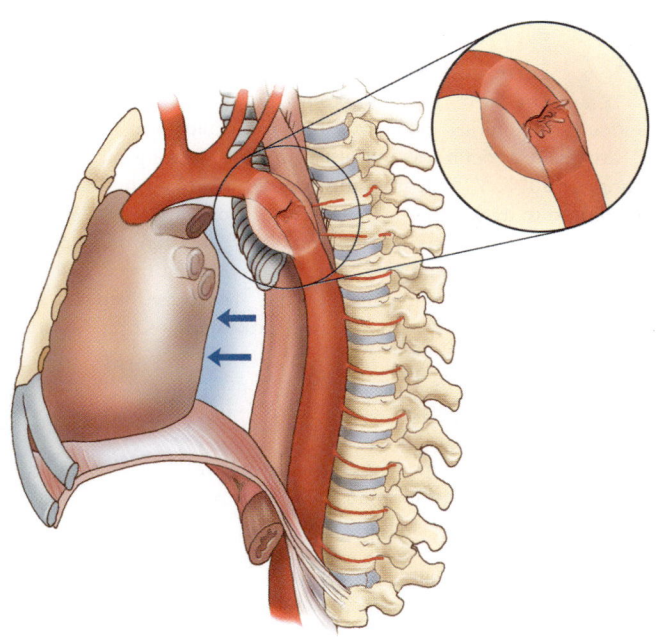

FIGURE 37-7 Shearing forces along the descending aorta move in opposition to the attachments at the lower end of the aortic arch. (From NAEMT: *Prehospital trauma life support,* ed 7, St Louis, 2011, Mosby.)

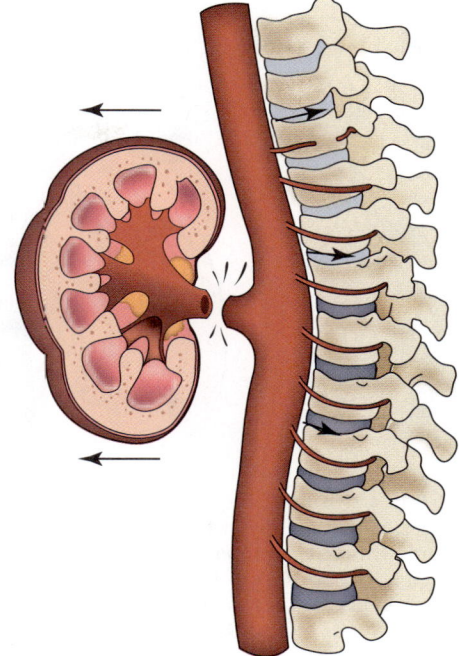

FIGURE 37-8 Forward motion of the kidney can cause separation at its midpoint from its vascular pedicle.

ABDOMINAL INJURIES

When deceleration forces are applied to the abdomen, intraabdominal organs and retroperitoneal structures (most commonly the kidneys) are affected. The forward motion of the kidneys can shear them away from their vascular pedicle attachments (Figure 37-8). The forward motion of the small and large intestines can result in mesenteric tears. The downward and forward motion of the liver can cause separation at its midpoint from its vascular and hepatic duct pedicle. The spleen is restrained by the diaphragm and abdominal wall attachments. The forward motion of the spleen can result in a tear of the splenic capsule.

Compression Injuries

Compressive forces can injure any portion of the body. This discussion is limited to injuries of the head, thorax, and abdomen.

HEAD INJURIES

Compression injuries to the head can result in open fractures, closed fractures, and bone fragment penetration (depressed skull fracture). Associated injuries include brain contusion and lacerations of brain tissue. Compression forces to the skull also can produce hemorrhage from fractured bone, meningeal vessels, or the brain itself. If facial structures are involved in the injury, soft tissue trauma and facial bone fractures can occur. The paramedic also should consider central nervous system injury. The paramedic should assume cervical fracture when evaluating injuries to

the head. Compression injury to the vertebral bodies can result in compression fracture, hyperextension, and hyperflexion injury.

THORACIC INJURIES

Compression injury to the thorax often involves the lungs and heart. Associated injuries to external structures include fractured ribs and sternum, which can lead to an unstable chest wall, open pneumothorax, or both.

A serious lung injury that can occur from compression forces is called the paper bag effect. This injury occurs when increased intrathoracic pressure causes rupture of the lungs. For example, a driver of a car is threatened by an approaching vehicle. The driver notes the potential collision. Thus the driver instinctively takes a deep breath and holds it. This protective inhalation fills the lungs (paper bag) with air against the closed glottis and creates a closed container (Figure 37-9). As the thorax strikes the steering column, the inward motion of the chest wall causes an increase in lung pressure. This increased pressure results in alveolar rupture (as when a hand strikes the paper bag). This phenomenon is thought to be the cause of most pneumothoraces after vehicle trauma.[8] Penetration of a fractured rib through the pleura and laceration of the lung also contribute to pneumothorax after blunt trauma to the chest.

During compression injury to the thorax, the heart can become trapped between the sternum and the thoracic spine. Depending on the amount of energy applied, the compression of the contents of the abdomen, and an

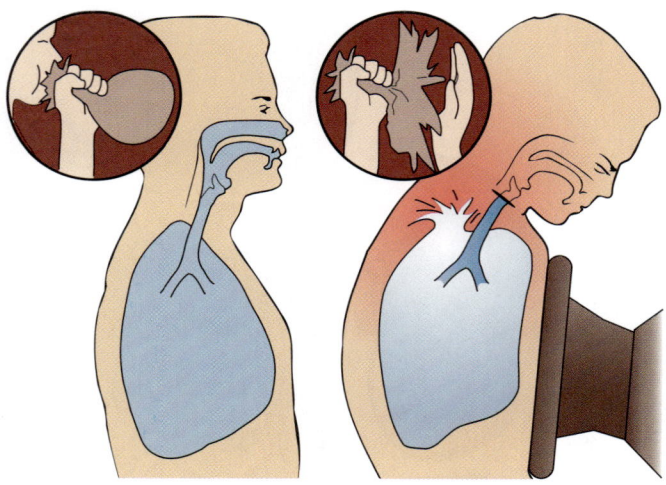

FIGURE 37-9 In a crash or collision, the lungs are similar to an air-filled paper bag held tightly at the neck and compressed with the other hand. Thoracic compression against the closed glottis causes the lungs to pop. (From NAEMT: *Prehospital trauma life support,* ed 7, St Louis, 2011, Mosby.)

increase in the pressure in the aorta, the aortic valve could rupture. Compression of the patient's heart between the sternum and the vertebral column can cause cardiac dysrhythmias, myocardial contusion, or atrial or ventricular rupture.

ABDOMINAL INJURIES

Compression injuries to the abdominal cavity can have serious effects. Some of these effects include solid organ rupture, vascular organ hemorrhage, and hollow organ perforation into the peritoneal cavity. Common injuries include rupture of the bladder, especially if it is full, and lacerations to the spleen, liver, and kidneys.

Just as the paper bag effect produces a pneumothorax in thoracic injury, compression of the abdominal cavity can cause increases in intraabdominal pressure. This increase in pressure can exceed the tensile strength (resistance to lengthwise stretch) of the walls of hollow organs or the diaphragm. Predictable injuries include rupture or herniation of the diaphragm and rupture of hollow organs such as the gallbladder, urinary bladder, duodenum, colon, stomach, and small bowel.

OTHER MOTORIZED VEHICULAR COLLISIONS

Injuries from other motorized vehicular collisions include those involving motorcycles, all-terrain vehicles (ATVs), motorized personal transportation devices, snowmobiles, motorboats, water bikes, jet skis, and farm machinery. This text discusses only motorcycles and ATVs because of their common recreational use and popularity. According to the National Highway Traffic Safety Administration, about 88,000 motorcycle riders and passengers are injured each year. More than 2000 die from their injuries.

> ### ? DID YOU KNOW?
> **Farm and Agricultural Injury**
>
> The farm as a workplace is dangerous. Farm and agricultural injuries also have high mortality and morbidity. Death from agricultural injuries ranks first among all occupations. In 2007, 715 deaths and 80,000 disabling injuries were attributed to agriculture.[13] In addition, approximately 100 unintentional injury deaths occur annually to children and adolescents on U.S. farms, and an additional 22,000 injuries to children younger than 20 years occur on farms.[14] Motorized vehicles and other machinery that are associated with many of these injuries include[15] the following:
> - *Tractors.* Overturns are a common cause of severe injury with traumatic brain injury, spinal cord injury, and major thoracoabdominal injuries.
> - *PTO (power take-off).* These devices deliver energy from the tractor to run other machines. The protective housing is often removed or becomes jammed, providing a site for entanglement.
> - *ROPS (rollover protection structures).* These devices are often lacking or removed to provide access in low-clearance situations.
> - *ATVs.* These vehicles are often used on farms and are a common cause of injury.
>
> In addition to trauma caused by motorized vehicles and machinery, there are multiple other causes of injury common in farm or agricultural settings. Some of these include:
> - *Animals.* Agricultural animals pose a threat because of size and unpredictability, resulting in a high incidence of injury. Animals also pose problems by causing cars to swerve and by their presence when using equipment at night.
> - *Falls.* Farmers often work at heights without the use of protective gear.
> - *Weather.* Impaired visibility, cold distraction, and equipment malfunction contribute to trauma in agricultural settings.
> - *Suffocation.* Silos and pits present common risks.
> - *Delayed discovery.* Farmers often work alone and at a distance from help or traffic.
>
> Injury forces and kinematics for farm and agricultural injuries are the same as those for other injuries and injury patterns described in this chapter. In addition to patient care measures, some of the injuries will require specialized forms of rescue (see Chapter 55).

Small motorized vehicles are thought to be more dangerous than other motor vehicles because they offer little protection to the rider. They offer minimum protection from the transfer of energy associated with collisions. The injuries from small motor vehicle crashes usually are more severe than those from car crashes. As with other types of motor vehicle collision, predictable injuries depend on the type of collision that occurs.

Motorcycle Collision

Common motorcycle collisions result from impact that is head-on or at an angle. They also result from laying the motorcycle down.

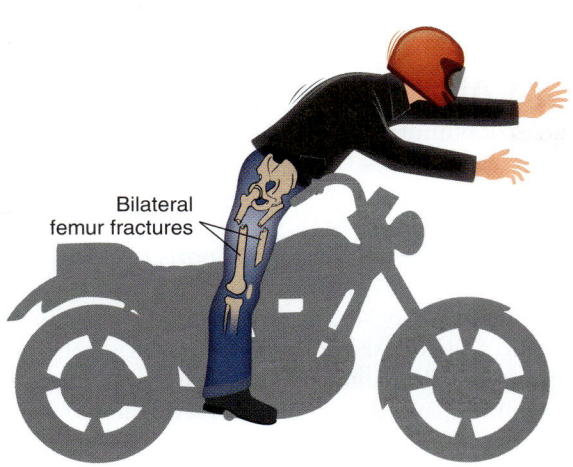

FIGURE 37-10 Head-on impact motorcycle collision. (Modified from NAEMT: *Prehospital trauma life support,* ed 7, St Louis, 2011, Mosby.)

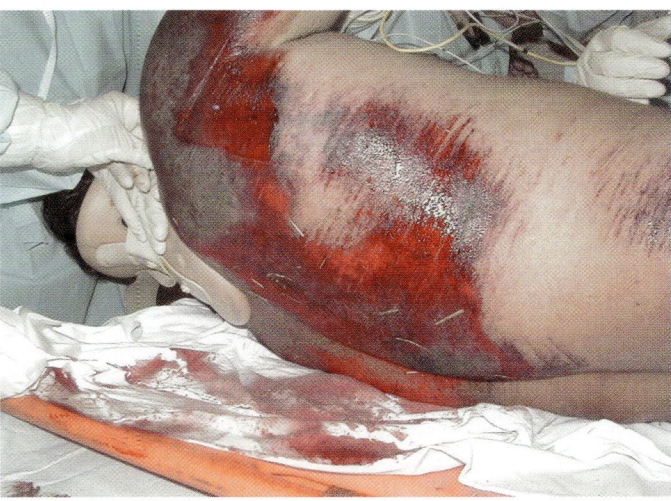

FIGURE 37-11 Road rash (abrasions). (From NAEMT: *Prehospital trauma life support,* ed 7, St Louis, 2011, Mosby.)

HEAD-ON IMPACT

The center of gravity of a motorcycle is above the front axle, forward of the rider's seat. When the motorcycle strikes an object that stops its forward motion, the rest of the bike and the rider continue forward until acted on by an outside force. Usually, the motorcycle tips forward. At that point, the rider is propelled over the handlebars. Secondary impacts with the handlebars or other objects stop the forward motion of the rider. Predictable injuries caused by these secondary impacts include head and neck trauma and compression injuries to the chest and abdomen. If the feet remain on the foot rests during impact, the midshaft of the femur absorbs the rider's forward motion (Figure 37-10). This can result in bilateral fractures to the femur and lower leg. Severe perineal injuries can result if the rider's groin strikes the tank or handlebars of the motorcycle.

ANGULAR IMPACT

A motorcycle may strike an object at an angle. When this occurs, the rider often is caught between the motorcycle and the second object. Predictable injuries include crush-type injuries to the patient's affected side. Examples of such are open fractures to the femur, tibia, and fibula and fracture and dislocation of the malleolus.

LAYING THE MOTORCYCLE DOWN

Professional racers and recreational riders often use the strategy of laying the motorcycle down before striking an object. This protective maneuver separates the rider from the motorcycle and the object. The maneuver allows the rider to slide away from the bike. Predictable injuries include massive abrasions (road rash) and fractures to the affected side as the rider slides on the ground or pavement (Figure 37-11). These injuries can be severe. However, they usually are less serious than those that occur from other types of impacts.

All-Terrain Vehicles

Injuries from crashes involving ATVs are different from those seen in motorcycle collisions. All-terrain vehicles have a higher center of gravity than motorcycles. They also have a large, flat front tire that makes them difficult to steer. A specific balance different than that required for riding motorcycles or bicycles is necessary to keep the ATV from overturning.

A natural tendency is for the rider to put a foot down to support the ATV when stopping. This can lead to the rear tire running over the rider's foot, catching the leg, and throwing the rider forward off the vehicle and onto his or her shoulder or crushing the rider. Predictable injuries from ATV collisions include extremity injury and fracture, clavicular fracture, and serious head and neck injuries.

Personal Protective Equipment

Protective equipment for riders of small motor vehicles includes boots, leather clothing, eye protection, and helmets. Helmets are structured to absorb the energy of an impact, thereby reducing injuries to the face, skull, and brain, and are estimated to be 37% effective in preventing fatal injuries.[1] Nonuse of helmets increases head injuries by more than 300%.[3]

PEDESTRIAN INJURIES

In 2006, 70,000 persons were injured in auto-pedestrian collisions in the United States. Of those injuries, 6100 were fatal.[1] All collisions of this nature can cause serious injuries. They require a high degree of suspicion for multiple-system trauma.

Three main mechanisms of injury (multiple impacts) exist in auto-pedestrian collisions. The first impact occurs when the bumper of the vehicle strikes the body. The second occurs as the pedestrian strikes the hood of the vehicle. The third occurs when the pedestrian strikes the ground or another object.

Predictable injuries depend on whether the pedestrian is an adult or a child. Variations in the height of the pedestrian in relation to the bumper and hood of the car affect the injury pattern. The velocity of the vehicle also is a major factor. However, even low speeds can result in serious trauma because of the mass of the vehicle and the transfer of energy. Another consideration in evaluating an auto-pedestrian collision is the possibility the patient may have been hit by another vehicle.

Adult Pedestrian

Most adult pedestrians who are threatened by an oncoming vehicle try to protect themselves by turning away from the vehicle. Therefore injuries often are a result of lateral or posterior impacts. During the initial impact, the adult usually is struck by the vehicle bumper in the lower legs. This often produces lower-extremity fractures.

The second impact occurs as the pedestrian falls toward the hood of the vehicle. This impact can result in fractures to the femur, pelvis, thorax, and spine. The impact also can produce intraabdominal or intrathoracic injury. In addition, the head and spine can be injured if the victim strikes the hood or windshield.

The third impact occurs as the victim strikes the ground or is thrown against another object. This can result in serious damage to the hip and shoulder of the affected side as the body makes contact with the landing surface. Sudden deceleration and compression forces are associated with this impact. These forces can cause fractures, internal hemorrhage, and head and spinal injury.

Child Pedestrian

As noted, adults try to protect themselves from auto-pedestrian injury. However, children tend to face the oncoming vehicle. Therefore their injuries often are the result of a frontal impact. Because children are smaller than most adults, the initial impact of the vehicle occurs higher on the body. Impact usually occurs above the knees or pelvis. Predictable injuries from the initial impact include fractures to the femur and pelvic girdle and internal hemorrhage.

The second impact occurs as the front of the hood of the vehicle continues forward, making contact with the victim's thorax. The victim instantly is thrown backward, forcing the head and neck to flex forward. Depending on the position of the patient in relation to the vehicle, the child's head and neck may contact the hood of the vehicle. Predictable injuries include abdominopelvic and thoracic trauma, facial trauma, and head and neck injury.

The third impact occurs as the child is thrown downward to the ground or another landing surface. Because of the child's smaller size and weight, the child can fall under the vehicle and be dragged for some distance. The child also can fall to the side of the vehicle and be run over by the front or rear wheels. Predictable injuries consist of

those previously described and may include traumatic amputation.

OTHER CAUSES OF BLUNT TRAUMA

Other causes of blunt trauma include sports injuries, vertical falls, and blast injuries.

Sports Injuries

Persons of all ages take part in sports. Sports that often are associated with injuries include contact sports, such as football, basketball, hockey, and wrestling; high-velocity sports, such as downhill skiing, water skiing, bicycling, rollerblading, and skateboarding; racquet sports; water sports, such as swimming and diving; and recreational and competitive equestrian sports. Sports offer a range of health benefits. However, they also can produce severe injury.

> **NOTE**
> Each year in the United States, an estimated 30 million people ride horses. In 2008 there were 77,328 horseback riding injuries and more than 14,000 upper extremity fractures (the single most common site and type of injury).[1]

Injuries related to sports are caused by forces of acceleration and deceleration, compression, twisting, hyperextension, and hyperflexion. The paramedic can use the general principles of kinematics to predict injuries by determining the following:

- What energy forces were transferred to the patient?
- To what part of the body was the energy transferred?
- What associated injuries should be considered as a result of the energy transfer?
- How sudden was the acceleration or deceleration?
- Was compression, twisting, hyperextension, or hyperflexion involved in the injury?

> **CRITICAL THINKING**
> Injuries related to sports often occur outside. What other considerations will you have for patient care based on the environment?

If the patient used protective equipment, the paramedic should evaluate it. This will help the paramedic determine the mechanism of injury. For example, the condition and structural stability of a helmet can provide clues concerning the amount of energy transferred to the patient during the injury. Other examples include broken skis, broken hockey sticks, and structural deformities of bicycles.

Blast Injuries

Blast injury is damage to a patient who is exposed to a pressure field that is produced by an explosion of volatile substances. Explosions of this nature mainly have been a

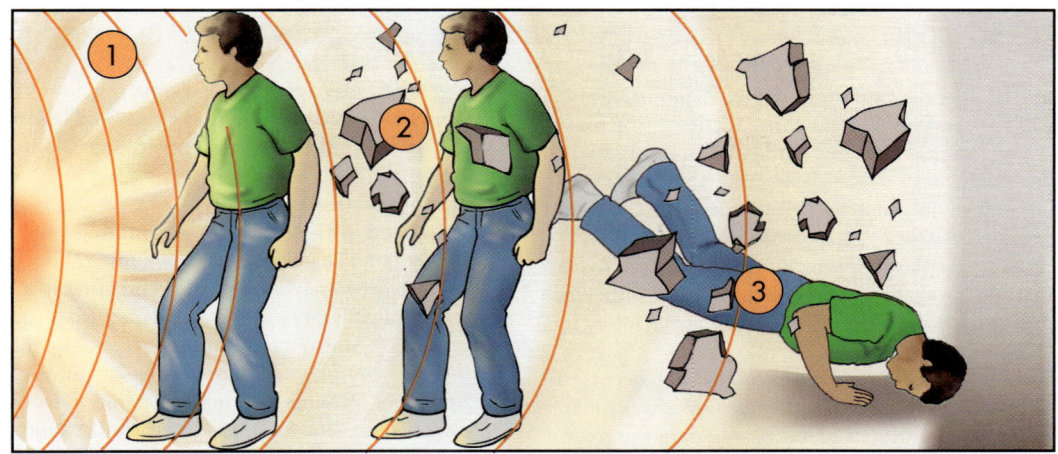

FIGURE 37-12 Three phases of injury occur during a blast. First, the pressure wave strikes the patient. Then flying debris can produce injury. In the third phase, the patient is thrown and is injured after impact with the ground or other objects.

wartime concern. However, in recent years the number of blast injuries has increased. These result from homemade bombs used in social protests and terrorist activities. Other causes include exploding car batteries, industrial use of volatile substances, chemical reactions in clandestine drug laboratories, explosions in mining, and transportation incidents or crashes involving hazardous materials.

 CRITICAL THINKING
In all incidents related to blast injury, what is your first consideration on the scene?

Blasts release large amounts of energy. This energy is in the form of pressure and heat. If this release of energy is confined in a casing (e.g., a bomb), the pressure ruptures the casing and ejects fragments of the housing at a high velocity. The remaining energy is transmitted to the surrounding environment. This energy can severely injure bystanders. Blast injuries are classified as *primary, secondary, tertiary,* and *quaternary* (Figure 37-12).

PRIMARY BLAST INJURIES

Primary blast injuries result from sudden changes in environmental pressure. These injuries usually occur in gas-containing organs. The most severe damage occurs when poorly supported tissue is displaced beyond its elastic limit. The organs and tissues most vulnerable to primary blast injury are the ears, lungs, blast lung injury (BLI) (Box 37-7), central nervous system, and gastrointestinal tract. Predictable damage to these areas includes hearing loss, pulmonary hemorrhage, cerebral air embolism, abdominal hemorrhage, and bowel perforation. Thermal burns also can result from the release of energy in the form of heat. These injuries are likely to occur on unprotected areas that are close to the source of explosion (see Chapter 39). (For

example, thermal burns might occur on the face and hands.) In closed spaces, because of blast reflection, victims farther from the explosion may be injured as severely as those close to the explosion.

SECONDARY BLAST INJURIES

Secondary blast injuries usually result when bystanders are struck by flying debris. (Examples of such debris include glass, metal, or falling mortar.) Obvious injuries are lacerations and fractures. Flying debris also can cause high-velocity missile-type injuries. This type of injury can result if nails, screws, or casing fragments are part of the debris.

TERTIARY BLAST INJURIES

Tertiary blast injuries occur when victims are propelled through space by an explosion and strike a stationary object. These injuries are similar to those from vertical falls. They also are similar to those from ejections from cars or small motor vehicles. In most cases, the sudden deceleration from the impact causes more damage than the acceleration through space because the deceleration is more sudden. Injuries from these forces include damage to the abdominal viscera, central nervous system, and musculoskeletal system.

QUATERNARY BLAST INJURIES

Quaternary blast injuries are all explosion-related injuries, illnesses, or diseases that are not caused by primary, secondary or tertiary mechanisms. This classification includes exacerbation or complications of existing conditions. Quaternary blast injuries can affect any body part. Types of injuries include burns (flash, partial- and full-thickness); radiation injuries, crush injuries; closed and open brain injuries; asthma, COPD, or other breathing problems from dust, smoke, or toxic gases (further described in Chapter 58); angina; hyperglycemia; and hypertension.

BOX 37-7 Blast Lung Injury: What Clinicians Need to Know

Blast lung injury (BLI) presents unique triage, diagnostic, and management challenges and is a direct consequence of the blast wave from high-explosive detonations upon the body. BLI is a major cause of morbidity and mortality for blast victims both at the scene and among initial survivors. The blast wave's impact upon the lung results in tearing, hemorrhage, contusion, and edema with resultant ventilation-perfusion mismatch. BLI is a clinical diagnosis and is characterized by respiratory difficulty and hypoxia, which may occur without obvious external injury to the chest.

Current patterns in worldwide terrorist activity have increased the potential for casualties related to explosions, yet few civilian health care personnel in the United States have experience treating patients with explosion-related injuries. Emergency care personnel are urged to learn more about the physics of explosions and other types of injuries that can result. Basic clinical information is provided here to inform practitioners of the presentation, evaluation, management, and outcomes of BLIs.

Clinical Presentation
- Symptoms may include dyspnea, hemoptysis, cough, and chest pain.
- Signs may include tachypnea, hypoxia, cyanosis, apnea, wheezing, decreased breath sounds, and hemodynamic instability.
- Associated pathology may include bronchopleural fistula, air emboli, and hemothoraces or pneumothoraces.
- Other injuries may be present.

Diagnostic Evaluation
- Chest radiography is necessary for anyone who is exposed to a blast.
- A characteristic "butterfly" pattern may be revealed upon x-ray.
- Arterial blood gases, computed tomography, and Doppler technology may be used.
- Most laboratory and diagnostic testing can be conducted per resuscitation protocols and further directed based upon the nature of the explosion (e.g., confined space, fire, prolonged entrapment or extrication, suspected chemical or biological event).

Management
- Initial triage, trauma resuscitation, treatment, and transfer should follow standard protocols; however, some diagnostic or therapeutic options may be limited in a disaster or mass casualty situation.

- In general, managing BLI is similar to caring for pulmonary contusion, which requires judicious fluid use and administration, ensuring tissue perfusion without volume overload.

Clinical Interventions
- All patients with suspected or confirmed BLI should receive supplemental high-flow oxygen sufficient to prevent hypoxemia (delivery may include nonrebreather masks, continuous positive airway pressure, or endotracheal intubation).
- Impending airway compromise, secondary edema, injury, or massive hemoptysis requires immediate intervention to secure the airway. Patients with massive hemoptysis or significant air leaks may benefit from selective bronchus intubation.
- Clinical evidence of or suspicion for a hemothorax or pneumothorax warrants prompt decompression.
- If ventilatory failure is imminent or occurs, patients should be intubated; however, caution should be used in the decision to intubate patients, because mechanical ventilation and positive end-expiratory pressure may increase the risk of alveolar rupture and air embolism.
- High-flow oxygen should be administered if air embolism is suspected, and the patient should be placed in prone, semi-left lateral, or left lateral position. Patients treated for air emboli should be transferred to a hyperbaric chamber.

Disposition and Outcome
- There are no definitive guidelines for observation, admission, or discharge following emergency department evaluation for patients with possible BLI following an explosion.
- Patients diagnosed with BLI may require complex management and should be admitted to an intensive care unit. Patients with any complaints or findings suspicious for BLI should be observed in the hospital.
- Discharge decisions will also depend upon associated injuries and other issues related to the event, including the patient's current social situation.
- In general, patients with normal chest radiographs and arterial blood gases (ABGs), who have no complaints that would suggest BLI, can be considered for discharge after 4 to 6 hours of observation.
- Data on the short- and long-term outcomes of patients with BLI are currently limited. However, in one study conducted on survivors 1 year after injury, no patients had pulmonary complaints, all had normal physical examinations and chest radiographs, and most had normal lung function tests.

From http://emergency.cdc.gov/masscasualties/blastlunginjury_prehospital.asp, accessed 3-6-10.

Vertical Falls

Falls accounted for 21,200 deaths in 2006 and were the third leading cause of accidental death in the United States.[1] (Nearly 8 million people were treated in an emergency department for fall-related injuries in 2005.) In predicting injuries associated with falls, the paramedic should evaluate three things: the distance fallen, the body position of

the patient on impact, and the type of landing surface struck. Injuries associated with vertical falls are a result of deceleration and compression. More than half of all falls occur in homes; nearly four out of five involve a person 65 years of age or older.

Falls from some levels rarely are associated with fatal injury. However, falls from distances greater than 3 times the height of an individual (15 to 20 feet) are more likely to be associated with severe injuries. As a point of reference for these distances, the roof of a one-story house is about 15 feet from the ground, and the roof of a two-story house is about 30 feet from the ground.

CRITICAL THINKING
What patients may be susceptible to serious injury from a fall that is from a low level?

Adults who have fallen more than 15 feet usually land on their feet. A predictable injury from this vertical fall is bilateral calcaneus fractures. As the energy dissipates from the initial impact, the head, torso, and pelvis push downward. The body is forced into flexion. When this occurs, hip dislocations and compression fractures of the spinal column in the thoracic and lumbar areas are seen. About 10% of patients with calcaneal fracture have associated spinal fractures. If the patient leans forward or tries to break the fall with outstretched hands, bilateral Colles' fractures to the wrists (clinically evident by the so-called silver fork deformity) are likely.

If the distance fallen is less than 15 feet, most adults land in the position in which they fell. For example, an adult who falls head first strikes the landing surface with the head, arms, or both. Predictable injuries depend on the body part that strikes the landing surface and the route of transfer of energy through the body. The paramedic should suspect internal injuries if the trunk of the body is the initial impact area. The ability of the landing surface to absorb energy influences the severity of injury. For example, less damage is expected from a fall on a soft, grassy surface than from a fall on asphalt or concrete.

Children tend to fall head first, regardless of distance fallen or body position during the fall. They fall head first because their heads are proportionally larger and heavier. For this reason, children who experience a vertical fall usually are victims of head injury. Older adult patients sustain a high number of low-distance falls, often resulting in hip fracture.

SECTION THREE
Penetrating Trauma

PENETRATING TRAUMA

Penetrating trauma is an injury that occurs when an object pierces the skin and enters a tissue of the body, creating an open wound. All penetrating objects, regardless of velocity, cause tissue disruption. This damage occurs as a result of two types of forces: crushing and stretching. The character of the penetrating object, its speed of penetration, and the type of body tissue it passes through or into determine which of the two mechanisms of injury predominates.

Cavitation

Cavitation is an opening produced by a force that pushes body tissues laterally away from the tract of a projectile. The amount of cavitation produced by a projectile is related directly to the density of tissue it strikes. Cavitation also is related directly to the ability of the body tissue to return to its original shape and position. For example, consider a person who receives a high-velocity blow to the abdomen. This person experiences abdominal cavitation at the moment of impact. However, because of the lower density of the abdominal musculature, the cavitation is temporary. (Cavitation lasts only a few microseconds.) Cavitation is temporary even in the presence of severe intraabdominal injury (Figure 37-13).

Permanent cavities are produced by penetrating injuries in which the force of the projectile exceeds the tensile strength of the tissue. Tissues with high water density (e.g., liver, spleen, and muscle) or solid density (e.g., bone) are more prone to permanent cavitation. Certain injuries (e.g., a stab wound to the abdomen) can produce cavitations as tissues are displaced in frontal and lateral directions.

Ballistics

The energy created and dissipated by the object into surrounding tissues determines the effect of a projectile on the body. The paramedic should consider the principles of

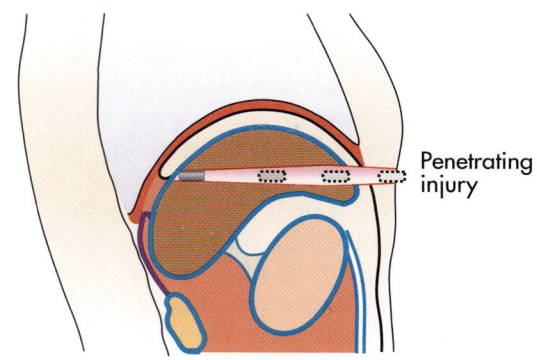

Permanent cavitation

Penetrating injury

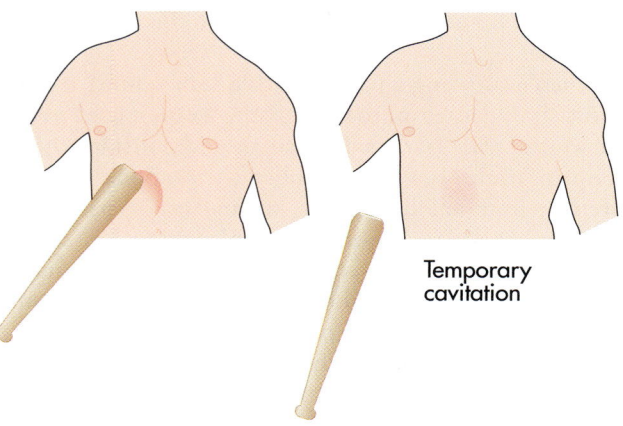

Temporary cavitation

FIGURE 37-13 Permanent and temporary cavitation.

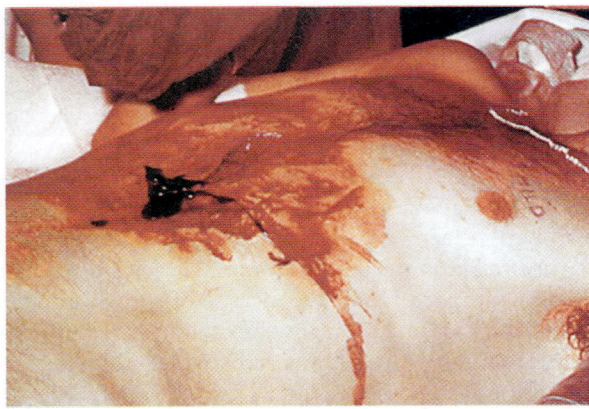

FIGURE 37-14 Stab wound in which a knife has pierced the liver and pancreas and entered the splenic vein.

CRITICAL THINKING

Your patient has a stab wound in the midaxillary line, lateral to the left nipple. What organs may be affected by this mechanism? What else would you like to know about this injury?

kinematics when dealing with injuries from penetrating trauma. To review, kinetic energy equals half the mass of an object multiplied by the square of its velocity. With reference to ballistic trauma, doubling the mass doubles the energy. However, doubling the velocity quadruples the energy. Therefore a small-caliber bullet traveling at a high speed can produce more serious injury than a large-caliber bullet traveling at a lower speed. This is the case as long as the large-caliber bullet does not strike a major vessel or organ.

DAMAGE AND ENERGY LEVELS OF PROJECTILES

Injuries caused by penetrating trauma result from three energy levels. The levels are low, medium, and high. This discussion considers hand-driven weapons as low-energy projectiles and bullets as medium- and high-energy projectiles.

Low-energy projectiles such as knives, needles, and ice picks cause tissue damage by their sharp, cutting edges (Figure 37-14). The amount of tissue crushed in these injuries usually is minimal because the amount of force applied in the wounding process is small. The more blunt the penetrating object, the more force that must be applied to cause penetration. The more force needed to cause penetration, the more tissue crushed. The damage of tissue from low-energy injuries usually is limited to the pathway of the projectile.

When evaluating a patient with a stab wound, the paramedic should attempt to identify the weapon used to cause the wound. The paramedic also should consider the possibility of multiple wounds, embedded weapons, hidden yet extensive internal damage to organs of the thorax and abdomen, and penetration of multiple body cavities. A high degree of suspicion of serious injury is also indicated for stab wounds to areas of the back and flank. These wounds may be associated with penetrating injuries to hollow organs and injuries to retroperitoneal organs, specifically the kidneys. Penetrating injuries of the thorax can involve the abdomen, just as abdominal injuries can involve the thorax.

Firearms can be labeled as medium- and high-energy weapons. Medium-energy weapons include handguns and some rifles. The injury tract produced by medium-energy weapons usually is 2 to 3 times the diameter of the projectile. Examples of high-energy weapons include military/assault rifles such as AR-15s, M-16s, and AK 47/74s and some hunting rifles. As with medium-energy injuries, the injury tract produced by high-energy weapons usually is 2 to 3 times the diameter of the projectile.

IMPLICATIONS OF SOFT BODY ARMOR

Some emergency medical services agencies have adopted soft body armor policies. The armor offers extra protection for paramedics against blunt and penetrating trauma. Most agencies follow U.S. Department of Justice guidelines to determine the type of body armor protection for the types of weapons most commonly found in their community. There are seven levels of body armor protection. Authorities generally recommend a type III or higher protection level for emergency medical services personnel. These soft vests protect against low-velocity and some medium-velocity and high-velocity weapons (see Chapter 56).

WOUNDING FORCES OF MEDIUM- AND HIGH-ENERGY PROJECTILES

A firearm cartridge is composed of a bullet made of metal, gunpowder to propel the bullet, a primer to explode and ignite the gunpowder, and a cartridge case that surrounds these components. When the trigger is pulled, the metal hammer strikes the firing pin, which ignites the primer. The gunpowder ignites and forces the bullet to exit the cartridge case.

The mechanism of injury from firearms is related to the energy created and dissipated by the bullet into the surrounding tissues. When a firearm is discharged, several events affect this dissipation of energy and ultimately the wounding forces of the missile:

1. As the missile travels through air, it experiences wind resistance, or *drag*. The greater the drag, the greater the slowing effect on the missile. Therefore a firearm discharged at close range usually produces a more severe injury than the same firearm discharged at a greater distance.

2. As the missile travels through air, a sonic pressure wave spreads out behind the missile. Because the speed of sound in tissue is about 4 times the speed of sound in air, the sonic pressure wave jumps ahead and precedes the missile through the tissue. This pressure wave displaces tissue and sometimes stretches it dramatically.

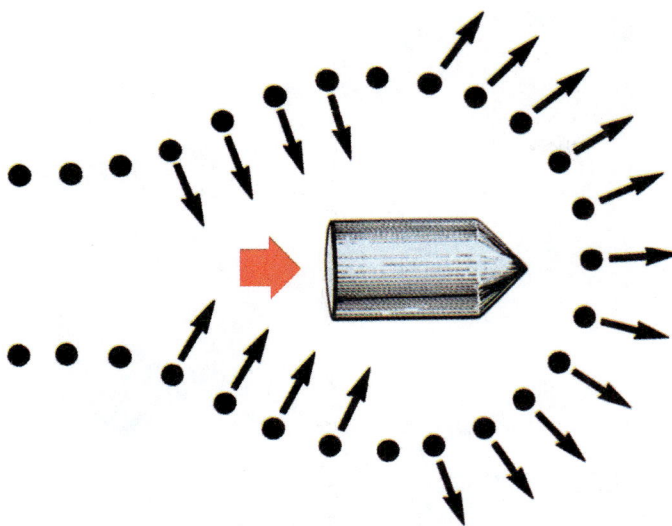

FIGURE 37-15 Bullet passing through tissue. Outward stretching of the permanent cavity as the tissue particles move away from the penetrating missile cause the temporary cavity. (From Moylan J: *Principles of trauma surgery*, ed 2, New York, 1992, Gower Medical Publishing.)

3. The localized crush of tissue in the path of the missile and the momentary stretch of the surrounding tissue cause tissue disruption.

When a projectile strikes a body, tissue stretches at the point of impact to allow entry of the penetrating object (*temporary cavitation*). The energy of the projectile exceeds the tensile strength of the tissue. Thus tissue crush occurs, forcing surrounding tissues outward from the path of the projectile (*permanent cavitation*). The differences in wounds caused by projectiles vary with the amount and location of crushed and stretched tissue (Figure 37-15). The wounding forces of a missile depend on the projectile mass, deformation, fragmentation, type of tissue struck, striking velocity, and range.[16]

Projectile Mass. Tissue crush is limited by the physical size or profile of the projectile. If the missile strikes point first, the crushed area is no larger than the diameter of the bullet. If the missile is tilted as it strikes the body, the amount of crushed tissue is no larger than the length and longitudinal cross section of the bullet.

Deformation. Some firearm missiles deform when striking tissue (e.g., expanding hollow-point or soft-point hunting bullets). The points of these projectiles typically flatten on impact. The diameter of the bullet expands, creating a larger area of crushed tissue. Military use of these bullets in war is forbidden.

Fragmentation. Each piece of missile crushes its own path through tissue, causing extensive tissue damage. These fragments produce a larger frontal area than a single, solid bullet and disperse energy into the surrounding tissues rapidly. Tissues weaken from the multiple fragment tracts and increase the subsequent stretch of the temporary cavity. The higher the velocity, the more likely the bullet is to fragment. If a bullet fragments, there may be no exit wound.

Type of Tissue Struck. Tissue disruption varies greatly with tissue type. For example, elastic tissues such as the bowel wall, lung, and muscle tolerate stretch much better than nonelastic organs such as the liver.

Striking Velocity. The velocity of a missile determines the extent of cavitation and tissue damage. Low-velocity missiles localize injury to a small radius from the center of the injury tract. These missiles have little disruptive effect, pushing the tissue aside. High-velocity missiles produce more serious injuries because they lose more energy to the tissues and produce more cavitation.

Bullet yaw, or tumble, in tissue also contributes to cavitation and tissue damage. The center of gravity of a wedge-shaped bullet is nearer to the base than to the nose. As the missile strikes body tissue, it slows rapidly. Momentum carries the base of the bullet forward; the center of gravity becomes the leading part of the missile. This forward rotation around the center of mass causes an end-over-end motion. This movement in turn produces more energy exchange and more tissue damage.

Range. The distance of the weapon from the target is a key factor in the severity of ballistic trauma. Air resistance (drag) slows the missile significantly; therefore increasing the distance of the projectile from the target decreases the velocity at the time of impact.

If the firearm is discharged at close range (within 3 feet), cavitation can occur from the combustion of powder and the forceful expansion of gases. The gas and powder can enter the body cavity and cause internal explosion of tissue. This is common with shotgun wounds. Internal explosion of tissue is less common with handguns because they produce a small amount of gas and create a small entrance wound. The expansion of only gas can cause extensive tissue destruction, especially in an enclosed area (e.g., the skull).

> **NOTE**
> Blanks are ammunition without projectiles. The explosion of gas explains how blanks can cause injury or death when fired at short range.

SHOTGUN WOUNDS

Shotguns are short-range, low-velocity weapons. They fire multiple lead pellets. These pellets are encased in a larger shell. Each pellet (there may be 9 to 400 or more, depending on pellet size and gauge of gun) is considered a missile capable of producing tissue damage. Each shell contains pellets, gunpowder, and a plastic or paper wad that separates the pellets from the gunpowder. This wad of unsterile material increases the potential for infection in shotgun wounds.

The energy transferred to body tissue and the tissue damage that results depend on several factors: gauge of the gun, size of the pellets, powder charge, and distance from the victim. For example, a 12-gauge, full-choke shotgun with number 6 shot (275 pellets) concentrates 95% of the

BOX 37-8 Forensic Considerations in Managing Gunshot Wounds

Lifesaving procedures always take precedence over forensic considerations. However, the paramedic should not touch or move weapons or other environmental clues unless it is absolutely necessary for patient care. Other forensic considerations follow:

- Document the exact condition of the patient and wound appearance on arrival at the scene. This should include environment of the patient and body position in relation to objects and doorways.
- Disturb the scene as little as possible.
- If possible, cut or tear clothing along a seam to avoid altering tears made by a penetrating object.
- Avoid cutting through a bullet hole in the clothing.
- Do not shake clothing.
- Keep all clothing in a paper bag rather than a plastic bag that may alter evidence. Do not give clothing to the victim's family members.
- Save any avulsed tissue for forensic pathological examination.
- If the bullet is retrieved, place it in a padded container to prevent marring and secure the evidence until it is delivered to the authorities (obtain a receipt).

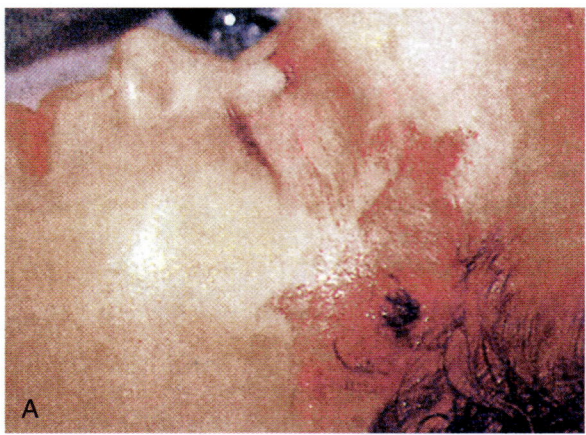

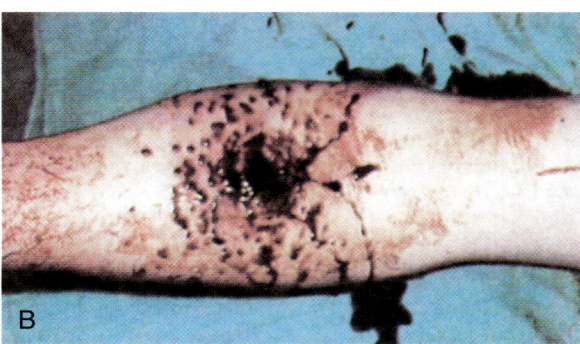

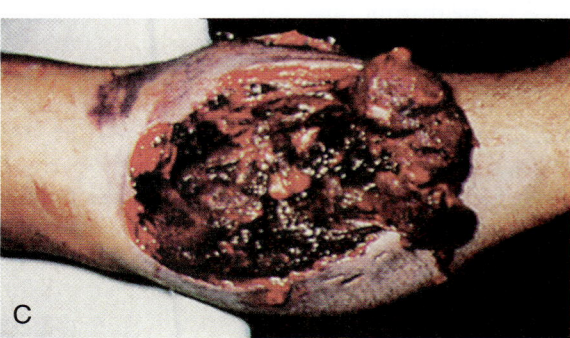

FIGURE 37-16 A, The powder marks show that this .22-caliber bullet wound was inflicted at close range. **B,** A short-range shotgun wound to the forearm. **C,** Exit wound caused by a powerful shotgun fired at close range. (From London PS: *A colour atlas of diagnosis after recent injury,* Ipswich, England, 1990, Wolfe Medical Publications, Ltd.)

pellets into a 7-inch circle at 10 yards. At close range a shotgun injury can create extensive tissue damage similar to that from a high-velocity missile weapon.

ENTRANCE AND EXIT WOUNDS

The presence of entrance and exit wounds is affected by several factors, including range, barrel length, caliber, powder, and weapon (Figure 37-16). In general, an entrance wound over soft tissue is round or oval and may be surrounded by an abrasion rim or collar. If the firearm is discharged at intermediate or close range, powder burns (tattooing) may be present (Box 37-8).

Exit wounds, if present, are generally larger than entrance wounds because of the cavitational wave that occurs as the bullet passes through the tissues. As the bullet exits the body, the skin can explode, resulting in ragged and torn tissue. This splitting and tearing often produces a starburst or stellate wound.

 CRITICAL THINKING

You locate an entrance wound but no exit wound on a patient who was shot. Does this mean that the injury is not serious?

If the muzzle is in direct contact with the skin at the time of firearm discharge, expanding gases can enter the tissue. These gases can produce crepitus. The burning gases also can produce thermal injury at the entrance site and along the injury tract.

NOTE

The paramedic should describe and document the appearance of all wounds. However, the paramedic should refrain from commenting or speculating on which is the entry or exit wound. Such speculation can result in the paramedic being served a subpoena. The paramedic may be subpoenaed to testify in court in an area that is beyond the scope of paramedic practice.

SPECIAL CONSIDERATIONS FOR SPECIFIC INJURIES

Locating ballistic injuries requires a thorough physical examination of the patient because the resulting trauma from high- and medium-velocity missiles is unpredictable. The impact of any projectile is critical in determining the type and severity of injury. Fractions of an inch can make a significant difference in the amount of trauma the patient suffers. These differences often are impossible to distinguish in the field.

Head Injuries. Gunshot wounds to the head typically are devastating because of the direct destruction of brain tissue and subsequent swelling. Patients with head wounds often sustain severe face and neck injuries as well. These can result in major blood loss, difficulty in maintaining airway control, and spinal instability.

As a medium-energy projectile penetrates the skull, the energy is absorbed within the closed space of the cranium. The force of the injury compresses brain tissue against the cranial cavity, often fracturing orbital plates and separating the dura from the bone. Depending on the qualities of the missile, the bullet may not have enough force to exit the skull after penetration. This is what occurs with .22- and .25-caliber handguns. In these injuries the bullet follows the curvature of the interior of the skull. As it follows this curvature, it produces significant damage.

High-velocity wounds to the skull produce massive destruction. Pieces of the skull and brain typically are destroyed. At close range, high-velocity wounds result in part from the large quantities of gas produced by combustion of the propellant. If the weapon is held in contact with the head, the gas follows the bullet into the cranial cavity, producing an explosive effect.

Thoracic Injuries. Gunshot wounds to the thorax can result in severe injury to the pulmonary and vascular systems. If the lungs are penetrated by a missile, the pleura and pulmonary parenchyma (the tissue of an organ, as distinguished from supporting and connective tissue) are likely to be disrupted, producing a pneumothorax. On occasion, the pulmonary defect allows air that cannot be expelled to continue to flow into the thoracic cavity. The subsequent increase in pressure eventually can cause collapse of the lung and a shift in the mediastinum to the unaffected side (tension pneumothorax).

Vascular trauma from penetrating injuries can result in massive internal and external hemorrhage. For example, if the pulmonary artery or vein, venae cavae, or aorta is injured, the patient can bleed to death within minutes. Other vascular injuries from penetrating trauma to the thorax can result in hemothorax and, if the heart is involved, myocardial rupture or pericardial tamponade.

Penetrating injury can cause thoracic trauma in the absence of visible chest wounds. For example, a bullet can enter the abdomen and travel upward through the diaphragm and into the thorax. The paramedic should evaluate all victims of abdominal gunshot wounds for thoracic injury. Likewise, the paramedic should evaluate all victims of thoracic gunshot wounds for abdominal injury.

Abdominal Injuries. Gunshot wounds to the abdomen usually require surgery to determine the extent of injury. Penetrating trauma can affect multiple organ systems, causing damage to air-filled and solid organs, vascular injury, trauma to the vertebral column, and spinal cord injury. The paramedic should assume a serious injury when managing victims of penetrating abdominal trauma. This should be the rule even if a patient appears to be stable.

Extremity Injuries. At times, gunshot wounds to the extremities are life threatening. Sometimes such wounds can result in lifelong disability. Special considerations with these injuries include vascular injury with bleeding into soft tissues and damage to nerves, muscles, and bones. The paramedic should evaluate any extremity that has sustained penetrating trauma for bone injury, motor and sensory integrity, and the presence of adequate blood flow (e.g., pulses and capillary refill).

Vessels can be injured by being struck by the bullet or by temporary cavitation. Either mechanism can damage the lining of the blood vessel, producing hemorrhage or thrombosis. Penetrating trauma can damage muscle tissue by stretching it as the muscle expands away from the path of the missile. Stretching that exceeds the tensile strength of the muscle produces hemorrhage.

Bone struck by a penetrating object can be deformed and fragmented. If this occurs, the transfer of energy causes pieces of bone to act as secondary missiles, crushing their way through surrounding tissue.

TRAUMA ASSESSMENT

Assessment and management of the trauma patient will be presented in depth throughout this textbook by subject matter. For most injury scenes, there are nine major components of assessment for trauma patients. The order of assessment is[2]:

1. Standard precautions
2. Scene size-up
3. General impression
4. Mechanism of injury
5. Primary survey
6. Baseline vital signs
7. Patient history and history of the event
8. Secondary assessment
9. Reassessment

Assessment Strategies Using Mechanism of Injury

Mechanism of injury (MOI) can be used to guide assessment for trauma patients.[2] MOI can be categorized as *significant* or *nonsignificant*. Examples of significant and non-significant MOI are provided in Box 37-9.

Using MOI as a guide for the potential for severe injury allows the paramedic to make decisions about on-scene assessment and care. For example, if the MOI is significant, the patient usually is in serious or critical condition. These

BOX 37-9 Mechanism of Injury

Significant MOI—Adult (Including, but Not Limited to):

- Injuries to multiple body systems
- Vehicle crashes with intrusion into the driver/passenger compartments
- Falls from heights >20 feet
- Pedestrian-vehicle collisions
- Motorcycle crashes >20 mph
- Death of an occupant in the same vehicle
- Ejection
- Vehicle telemetry system indicates high risk of injury
- Intrusion >12 inches near occupant; intrusion >18 inches anywhere

Significant MOI—Child (Including, but Not Limited to):

- Falls >10 feet without loss of consciousness
- Falls <10 feet with loss of consciousness
- Bicycle collision
- Medium to high-speed vehicle collision (<25 mph)

Nonsignificant MOI—All Ages (Including, but Not Limited to):

- Isolated trauma to a body part
- Falls without loss of consciousness

By comparison, on-scene assessment and care for patients with nonsignificant MOI can be modified as needed. After completing the primary survey, it may be appropriate to perform a thorough secondary assessment while at the scene. This assessment is focused on the patient's chief complaint or on findings in the initial assessment. Then the patient is transported for definitive care.

> **NOTE**
> MOI must be reevaluated during the patient care encounter. For example, the paramedic may initially find the patient to have a nonsignificant MOI. However, findings in the secondary assessment might indicate a more serious injury requiring rapid assessment and transport.

ROLE OF DOCUMENTATION IN TRAUMA

As described in Chapter 4, findings at the scene and the provision of patient care should be well documented on the patient care report. A thorough written record of the EMS response will help "paint a picture," or recreate the injury event for others who will be involved in the patient's care. A complete report is essential and will be referred to by hospital personnel. Documentation should include notations on an anatomical drawing for the location of wounds. It also should include a description of the scene and history of the event. Other important components of the patient care report are:

- Mechanism of injury
- Response time
- Time on-scene
- Initial findings
- Trauma scoring scales
- Changes in assessment findings
- Care provided
- Important negative findings
- Bystander care before EMS arrival

patients need to be rapidly assessed; stabilized if possible; and quickly transported to an appropriate facility for definitive care. Scene time should be limited to that required for airway, breathing, and circulatory support; spinal immobilization; and control of severe hemorrhage.

> **NOTE**
> In some cases even low-impact MOI can cause injury. For example, an infant improperly restrained in the front seat of a car that crashes or a low-speed collision with air bag deployment can result in serious injury. Every patient requires careful evaluation.

SUMMARY

- Trauma is the leading cause of death among persons 1 to 44 years of age and is the fifth leading cause of death among all Americans.
- Trauma care is divided into three phases: preincident, incident, and postincident.
- Components of the trauma system include injury prevention, prehospital care, emergency department care, interfacility transportation (if needed), definitive care, trauma critical care, rehabilitation, data collection, and trauma registry.

- Transport decisions for trauma patients should be made based on structured triage guidelines.
- Injuries are caused by a transfer of energy from some external source to the human body. The extent of injury is determined by the type of energy applied, by how quickly it is applied, and by the part of the body to which the energy is applied.
- Four laws of physics describe energy and forces that produce injury. They are Newton's first law of motion; conservation of energy law; Newton's

- second law of motion; and the formula for kinetic energy.
- Kinematics is the process of predicting injuries based on mechanism of injury, forces involved, anatomy, and energy.
- Blunt trauma is an injury produced by the wounding forces of compression and change of speed, which can disrupt tissues.
- Four restraining systems are available in the United States. These are lap belts, diagonal shoulder straps, child safety seats, and air bags. All of these significantly reduce injuries. However, if they are used inappropriately, these protective devices also can produce injuries.
- Organ injuries can result from sudden movement caused by deceleration and compression forces. The recognition of these injuries requires a high degree of suspicion. The paramedic must use the principles of kinematics.
- Small motorized vehicles such as motorcycles, all-terrain vehicles, snowmobiles, motorboats, water bikes, and farm machinery are considered to be more dangerous than other motor vehicles. They are more dangerous because they offer little protection to the rider. They offer minimal protection from the transfer of energy associated with collisions.

- All auto-pedestrian collisions can produce serious injuries. They require a high degree of suspicion for multiple-system trauma.
- Sports provide a variety of health benefits. However, they also can produce severe injury. Sports injuries are related to acceleration/deceleration, compression, twisting, hyperextension, and hyperflexion mechanisms of injury.
- Blast injury is damage to a patient exposed to a pressure field that is produced by an explosion of volatile substances. Blasts release large amounts of energy in the form of pressure and heat. Blast injuries are classified as primary, secondary, tertiary, and miscellaneous.
- Falls from greater than 3 times the height of a person (15 to 20 feet) are associated with an increased incidence of severe injuries. In predicting injuries associated with falls, the paramedic should evaluate three factors: the distance fallen, the body position of the patient on impact, and the type of landing surface struck.
- All penetrating objects, regardless of velocity, cause tissue disruption. The character of the penetrating object, its speed of penetration, and the type of body tissue it passes through or into determine whether crushing or stretching forces will cause injury.

REFERENCES

1. National Safety Council: *Injury facts*, Chicago, 2010, The Council.
2. National Highway Traffic Safety Administration: *The National EMS Education Standards*, Washington, DC, 2009, U.S. Department of Transportation/National Highway Traffic Safety Administration, DOT.
3. National Association of Emergency Medical Technicians: *PHTLS: basic and advanced prehospital life support*, ed 6, St Louis, 2007, Mosby.
4. Baker CC, Oppenheimer L, Stephens B, et al: Epidemiology of trauma deaths, *Am J Surg* 140:144, 1980.
5. National Highway Traffic Safety Administration: *Trauma system agenda for the future*, Washington, DC, 2002.
6. The Trauma Center Association of America, National Foundation for Trauma Care: *Trauma centers*, www.traumafoundation.org/trauma_centers/index.php, accessed 9-17-10.
7. Kuehl A, editor: *EMS medical director's handbook*, St Louis, 1989, Mosby.
8. The Trauma Center Association of America: Trauma Foundation: *Fact sheet*, www.traumafoundation.org/restricted/tinymce/jscripts/tiny_mce/plugins/filemanager/files/About%20Trauma%20Care_Trauma%20Fact%20Sheet.pdf, accessed 9-17-10.
9. National Highway Traffic Safety Administration: www.nhtsa.dot.gov, accessed 9-17-10.
10. Wallis LA, Greaves I: Injuries associated with airbag deployment, *Emerg Med J* 19:490-493, 2002.
11. Insurance Institute for Highway Safety: *Highway loss data institute*, www.iihs.org/research/qanda/airbags.html, accessed 9-17-10.
12. National Highway Traffic Safety Administration: *Safety facts 2006, occupant protection, DOT HS 810 807*, www-nrd.nhtsa.dot.gov/Pubs/810807.PDF, accessed 10-16-10.
13. U.S. Department of Labor, Bureau of Labor Statistics: *National census of fatal occupational injuries in 2008*, www.bls.gov/news.release/archives/cfoi_08202009.pdf, accessed 10-16-10.
14. American Academy of Pediatrics: *Prevention of agricultural injuries among children and adolescents*, http://aappolicy.aappublications.org/cgi/content/full/pediatrics;108/4/1016, accessed 9-17-10.
15. American College of Surgeons Committee on Trauma, Subcommittee on Injury Prevention and Control: *Farm injury prevention*, www.facs.org/trauma/farm.html, accessed 9-17-10.
16. McSwain N, Kerstein M: *Evaluation and management of trauma*, Norwalk, Conn, 1987, Appleton-Century-Crofts.

SUGGESTED READINGS

Champion HR, Holcomb JB, Young LA: Injuries from explosions: physics, biophysics, pathology, and required research focus, *J Trauma* 66:5, 2009; doi: 10.1097/TA.0b013e3181a27e7f.

Chapleau W: *Mechanism of injury and outcomes*, *JEMS.com*, 8-14-07, www.jems.com/news_and_articles/columns/Chapleau/Mechanism_of_Injury_Outcomes.html, accessed 4-3-10.
Minei JP, Schmicker RH, Kerby J, et al: Severe traumatic injury: regional variations in incidence and outcome, *Ann Surg* 252(1):149-153, 2010.

38 Bleeding and Soft Tissue Trauma

Upon completion of this chapter, the paramedic student will be able to:

1. Describe the normal structure and function of the skin.
2. Describe the pathophysiological responses to soft tissue injury.
3. Discuss pathophysiology as a basis for key signs and symptoms, and describe the mechanism of injury and signs and symptoms of specific soft tissue injuries.
4. Outline management principles for prehospital care of soft tissue injuries.
5. Describe, in the correct sequence, patient management techniques for control of hemorrhage.
6. Identify the characteristics of general categories of dressings and bandages.
7. Describe prehospital management of specific soft tissue injuries not requiring closure.
8. Discuss factors that increase the potential for wound infection.
9. Describe the prehospital management of selected soft tissue injuries.

KEY TERMS

abrasion A partial-thickness injury caused by scraping or rubbing away of a layer or layers of skin.

amputation A complete or partial loss of a limb caused by mechanical force.

avulsion A full-thickness skin loss in which the wound edges cannot be approximated.

compartment syndrome The result of a crush injury, usually caused by compressive forces or blunt trauma to muscle groups confined in tight fibrous sheaths with minimal ability to stretch.

contusion A closed, soft tissue injury characterized by swelling, discoloration, and pain.

crush injury Injury from exposure of tissue to a compressive force sufficient to interfere with the normal structure and metabolic function of the involved cells and tissues.

crush syndrome A life-threatening and sometimes preventable complication of prolonged immobilization; a pathological process that causes destruction, alteration, or both of muscle tissue.

deep fascia The dense layer of fibrous tissue beneath the dermis; provides for insulation, cushioning, caloric reserve, and body substance and shape.

degloving injury An injury usually involving the hand or finger in which the soft tissue is removed down to the bone.

dermis Dense, irregular connective tissue that forms the deep layer of the skin.

ecchymosis Skin discoloration (bruising) caused by the escape of blood into the tissues from ruptured blood vessels.

epidermis The outer portion of skin; it is formed of epithelial tissue that rests on or covers the dermis.

fasciotomy Incision of fascia to relieve elevated intracompartmental pressure.

hematoma A closed injury characterized by blood vessel disruption and swelling beneath the epidermis.

hemorrhage Flowing of blood.

hypertrophic scar An excess accumulation of scar tissue within the original wound borders.

keloid An excessive accumulation of scar tissue that extends beyond the original wound borders.

laceration A torn or jagged wound.

puncture wound An open injury that results from contact with a penetrating object.

rhabdomyolysis An acute, sometimes fatal, disease characterized by destruction of skeletal muscle.

tourniquet A constricting or compressing device used to control venous and arterial bleeding in an extremity.

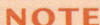The skin and its accessory organs are the primary defensive structures of the body. These structures perform many functions that are critical to survival. The paramedic must fully understand hemorrhage and soft tissue trauma. This knowledge allows the paramedic to quickly assess life-threatening injury and to intervene to promote normal healing and function.

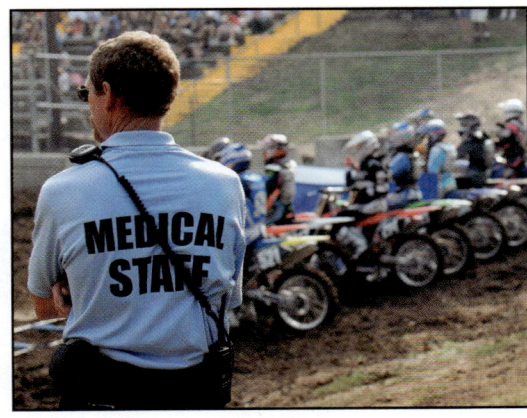

(Courtesy Ray Kemp, St. Charles, Mo.)

> **NOTE**
> Each year about 40 million persons in the United States seek care in emergency departments for soft tissue injuries that result from falls, motor vehicle crashes, blunt and penetrating trauma, and burns. Although most soft tissue injuries are not life threatening, more than 70,000 people die each year as a result of these injuries.[1]

HEMORRHAGE

Hemorrhage occurs when there is a disruption, or "leak," in the vascular system. Sources of hemorrhage can be external or internal.

External Hemorrhage

External hemorrhage results from soft tissue injury. External hemorrhage accounted for about 2.3 million emergency department visits in the United States in 2005.[1] Most soft tissue trauma is accompanied by mild hemorrhage and does not pose a threat to life. However, even mild soft tissue trauma can carry major risks of morbidity and disfigurement. The seriousness of the injury depends on three factors: the anatomical source of the hemorrhage (arterial, venous, capillary), the degree of vascular disruption, and the amount of blood loss that the patient can tolerate.

> **NOTE**
> Education and prevention before the event are the best ways to avoid significant trauma. One strategy to this effect is to educate the public. (For example, the use of personal restraint systems can be emphasized.) Another strategy is the enforcement of laws. (An example is the enactment of helmet laws.) A third strategy involves modifications to the environment and engineering strategies. (For example, walk signals at busy intersections can be installed.) These and other strategies can help reduce the occurrence of significant injury (see Chapter 3: Injury Prevention and Public Health).

Internal Hemorrhage

Internal hemorrhage can result from a blunt or penetrating trauma. Internal hemorrhage also can result from acute or chronic illnesses. Internal bleeding that leads to an insufficient amount of circulating blood can occur in one of four body cavities: the chest, abdomen, pelvis, or retroperitoneum. Intracranial hemorrhage also can cause grave hemodynamic instability from loss of blood. Internal hemorrhage is associated with higher morbidity and mortality rates than external hemorrhage. Signs and symptoms that can indicate significant internal hemorrhage include the following:

- Bright red blood from mouth, rectum, or other orifice
- Coffee-ground appearance of vomitus
- Melena (black, tarry stools)
- Hematochezia (passage of red blood through the rectum)
- Dizziness or syncope on sitting or standing
- Orthostatic hypotension (described later in this chapter)

> **CRITICAL THINKING**
> Internal hemorrhage is associated with an increase in morbidity and mortality rates. Why do you think this is the case?

ANATOMY AND PHYSIOLOGY OF THE SKIN

The anatomy and physiology of the skin was described in Chapter 10. The following discussion will serve as a review.

The skin is a tough, supple membrane that covers the entire body. The skin constitutes the largest and most dynamic organ of the body, covering more than 20 square feet and making up 16% of total body weight. The skin comprises two distinct layers of tissue: the outer layer (epidermis) and the inner layer (dermis) (Figure 38-1).

> **LOOK AGAIN**
> See Chapter 10: Review of Human Systems, pp. 155-158.

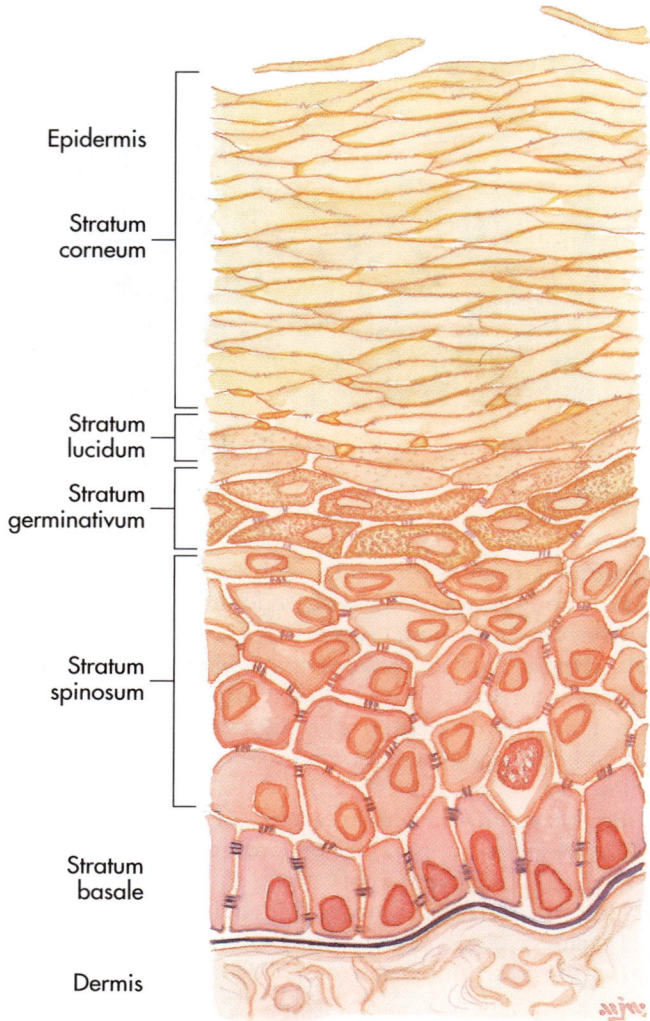

Epidermis

Stratum corneum

Stratum lucidum

Stratum germinativum

Stratum spinosum

Stratum basale

Dermis

FIGURE 38-1 · Tissue layers of the skin.

Epidermis

The **epidermis** is a thin, nonvascular epithelial tissue that derives its nourishment from the capillaries of the dermis. Although the epidermis is only as thick as a page of this text, the epidermis is composed of five layers: stratum basale, the innermost layer; stratum spinosum; stratum granulosum; stratum lucidum; and stratum corneum, the most superficial layer of the epidermis. The stratum corneum is composed of about 20 layers of dead skin cells that are filled with the waterproofing protein keratin.

Dermis

The **dermis** lies beneath the epidermis. The dermis contains connective tissue, elastic fibers, blood vessels, lymph vessels, and motor and sensory fibers. The dermis also houses other structures of the integumentary system. These other structures include hair, nails, and sebaceous and

sweat glands. This layer of skin offers protection against bacterial invasion and helps maintain fluid balance as well.

Connective tissue and elastic fibers in the dermis give skin its strength and elasticity. Blood vessels in the dermis nourish all skin cells. They also aid in body temperature regulation through vasoconstriction or vasodilation. Nerves in the dermis generate impulses to dermal muscles and glands. These nerves also are responsible for carrying impulses away from sensory receptors in the skin in response to pain, touch, heat, and cold.

> ### CRITICAL THINKING
> Predict the effects of destruction of a large segment of skin, which includes the dermis, based on your knowledge of its functions.

The dermis has a reservoir of defensive and regenerative elements. These elements combat infection and repair deep wounds. They do this by use of specialized white blood cells, lymphatics, and other cellular components.

The dense layer of fibrous tissue beneath the dermis is the **deep fascia.** This layer provides for insulation, cushioning, caloric reserve, and body substance and shape. The primary function of this tissue is to support and protect underlying structures.

PATHOPHYSIOLOGY

Surface trauma can disrupt the normal distribution of body fluids and electrolytes. Surface trauma also can interfere with the maintenance of body temperature. The two physiological responses to surface trauma are vascular and inflammatory reactions. These reactions can lead to healing, scar formation, or both. The extent and success of these responses are influenced by the amount of tissue that has been disrupted.

Hemostasis of Wound Healing

As described in Chapter 32: Hematology, *hemostasis* is the initial physiological response to wounding. This vascular reaction involves vasoconstriction, formation of a platelet plug, coagulation, and the growth of fibrous tissue into the blood clot that permanently closes and seals the injured vessel. To review, vasoconstriction resulting from injury is rapid but temporary. In response to injury, severed blood vessels constrict and retract with the aid of the surrounding subcutaneous tissues. This vessel spasm slows blood loss immediately and may completely close the ends of the injured vessels. The vasoconstriction usually is sustained for as long as 10 minutes. During this time, blood coagulation mechanisms are activated to produce a blood clot.

Platelets adhere to injured blood vessels and to collagen in the connective tissue that surrounds the injured vessel. As platelets contact collagen, they swell, become sticky, and secrete chemicals that activate other surrounding platelets.

This process creates a platelet plug in the injured vessel. If the opening in the vessel wall is small, the plug may be sufficient to completely stop blood loss. For larger wounds, however, a blood clot is necessary to stop the flow of blood (Figure 38-2).

Blood coagulation occurs as a result of a chemical process that begins within seconds of a severe vessel injury and within 1 to 2 minutes of a minor wound. Coagulation progresses rapidly; within 3 to 6 minutes after the rupture of a vessel, the entire end of the vessel is filled with a clot. Within 30 minutes the clot retracts and the vessel is sealed further. As described in Chapter 32: Hematology, the clotting cascade is a complex process and includes the following three mechanisms:

1. Prothrombin activator is formed in response to rupture or damage of the blood vessel.
2. Prothrombin activator stimulates the conversion of prothrombin to thrombin.
3. Thrombin acts as an enzyme to convert fibrinogen into fibrin threads. These threads entrap platelets, blood cells, and plasma to form the clot.

The process of hemostasis usually is protective and is required for survival. However, hemostasis also can result in responses that threaten life and function. Examples include blood clots that form in atherosclerotic vessels that lead to myocardial infarction or stroke (see Chapter 22).

CRITICAL THINKING
List some drugs that may impair the normal clotting functions.

Inflammatory Response

The release of chemicals from the injured vessel and various blood components (platelets, white blood cells) causes localized vasodilation of arterioles, precapillary sphincters, and venules. This response increases the permeability of the affected capillaries and vessels. Plasma, plasma proteins, electrolytes, and chemical substances from the leaking venules accumulate in the extracellular space for about 72 hours after the injury. Blood flow increases to the area of injury to supply the metabolic demands of the tissues during healing. This results in the redness, swelling, and pain associated with inflammation.

The transportation of granulocytes, lymphocytes, and macrophages to the injured area also increases local blood flow. These specialized cells prepare the wound for healing. They clear foreign bodies and dead tissue. They trigger new vessel formation as well. Within 12 hours of the injury, new epithelial cells are regenerated. (This is the *epithelialization phase*.) These cells begin the process of healing through the reestablishment of skin layers (Figure 38-3).

Collagen is the main structural protein of most body tissues. The normal repair of tissues depends on collagen synthesis and deposition. In the healthy body, fibroblasts synthesize and deposit collagen within 48 hours after injury. Collagen increases the tensile strength of the tissue. However, most injured tissue will not regain its full strength and function until at least 4 months later.[2]

Alterations of Wound Healing

Many factors can affect or alter wound healing. These include anatomical factors, concurrent drug use, medical condition and disease, and wounds that are high risk.

ANATOMICAL FACTORS

Some tissues of the body heal better and faster than others because of the body region and the amount of tension on the tissues (lines of tension). The elasticity of the skin and lines of tension vary in different areas of the body. Moreover, they are affected by muscular contraction and the body movements of flexion and extension. Thus these factors affect wound healing and scar formation. For example, a soft tissue injury to the forearm generally heals better and faster than one over a joint. Other anatomical factors that may adversely affect wound healing and scar formation include oily skin and pigmentation.

CONCURRENT DRUG USE, EXISTING MEDICAL CONDITIONS, AND DISEASE

Certain factors can delay or interfere with the normal wound-healing process through various mechanisms.[3] For instance, a patient's concurrent drug use can interfere with or delay this process. Existing medical conditions also may have this effect. In addition, disease can delay or interfere with the process. Common drugs that can alter wound healing include corticosteroids, nonsteroidal antiinflammatory drugs (*aspirin*), penicillin, colchicine, anticoagulants, and antineoplastic agents. Medical conditions and diseases that can result in delayed healing include the following:

- Advanced age
- Severe alcoholism
- Acute uremia
- Diabetes
- Hypoxia
- Peripheral vascular disease
- Malnutrition
- Advanced cancer
- Hepatic failure
- Cardiovascular disease

HIGH-RISK WOUNDS

High-risk wounds have an increased potential for infection because of the location of the wound or the nature of the wounding force. Examples of high-risk wounds include those located on or near the hands, feet, and perineal areas. Wound forces that are associated with a high risk for infection include those produced by human and animal bites, foreign bodies, and injection (e.g., high-pressure grease guns). Other high-risk wounds are those contaminated with organic material or that have a significant amount of

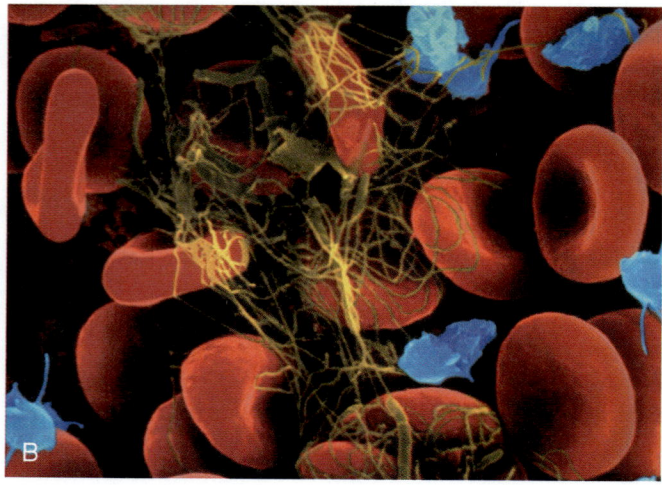

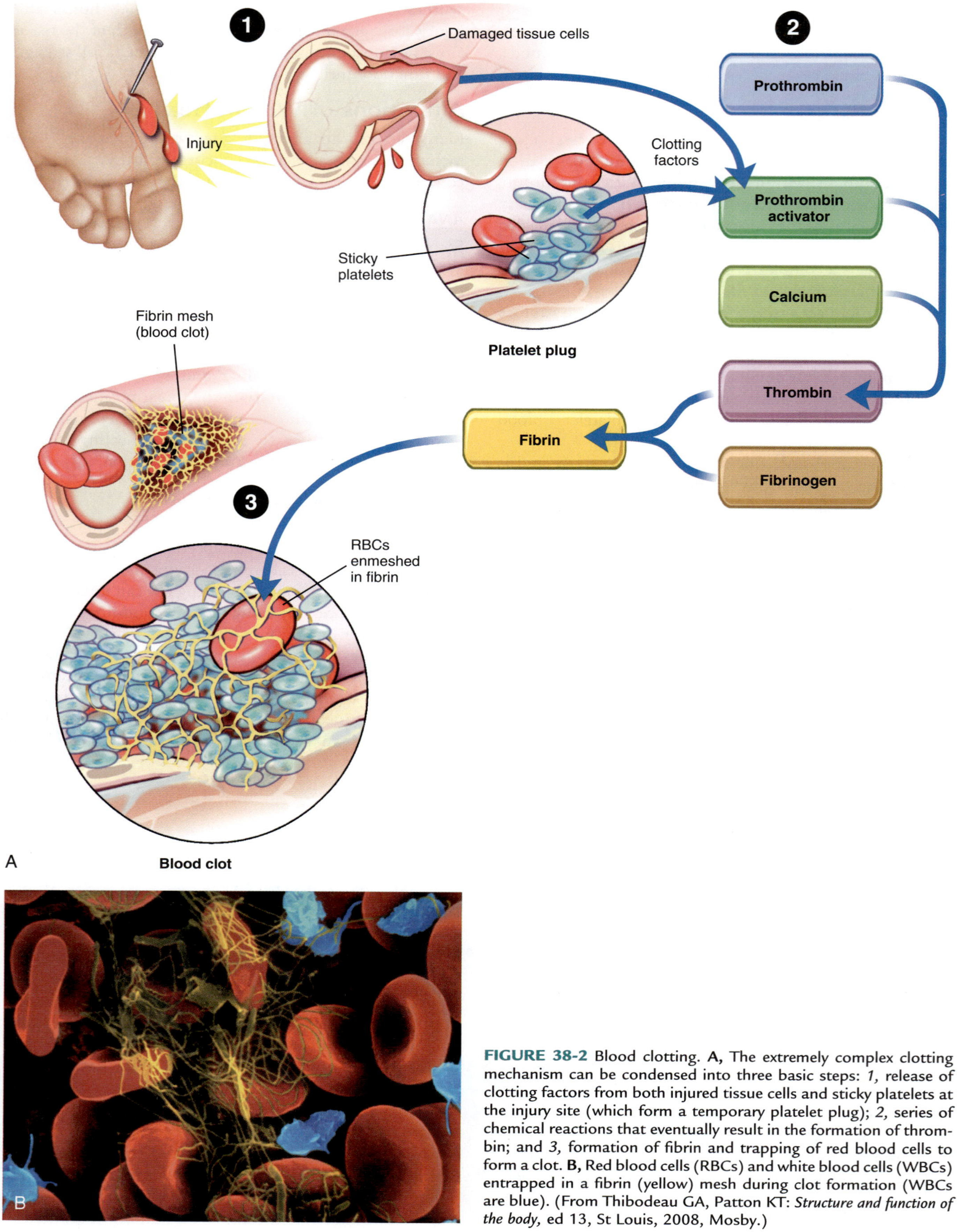

① Injury — Damaged tissue cells

Clotting factors

Sticky platelets

Platelet plug

② Prothrombin

Prothrombin activator

Calcium

Thrombin

Fibrinogen

Fibrin

Fibrin mesh (blood clot)

③ RBCs enmeshed in fibrin

Blood clot

A

B

FIGURE 38-2 Blood clotting. **A,** The extremely complex clotting mechanism can be condensed into three basic steps: *1,* release of clotting factors from both injured tissue cells and sticky platelets at the injury site (which form a temporary platelet plug); *2,* series of chemical reactions that eventually result in the formation of thrombin; and *3,* formation of fibrin and trapping of red blood cells to form a clot. **B,** Red blood cells (RBCs) and white blood cells (WBCs) entrapped in a fibrin (yellow) mesh during clot formation (WBCs are blue). (From Thibodeau GA, Patton KT: *Structure and function of the body,* ed 13, St Louis, 2008, Mosby.)

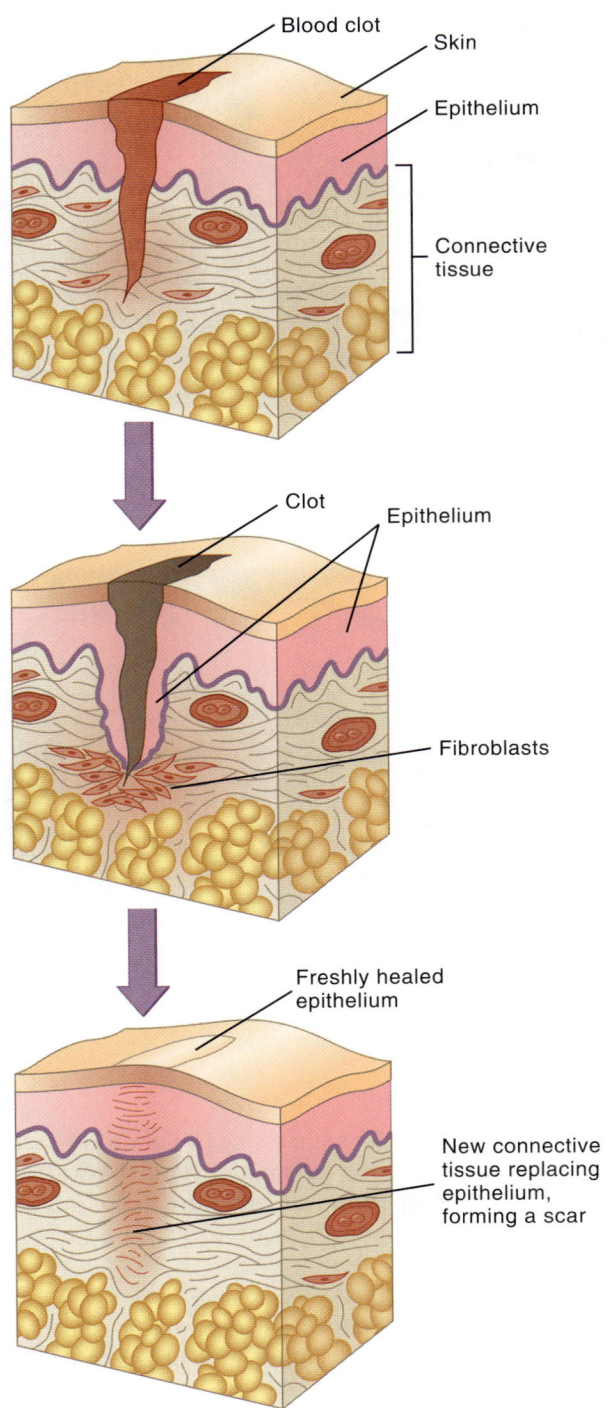

Blood clot

Skin

Epithelium

Connective tissue

Clot

Epithelium

Fibroblasts

Freshly healed epithelium

New connective tissue replacing epithelium, forming a scar

FIGURE 38-3 Healing of a minor wound. (From Thibodeau GA, Patton KT: *Structure and function of the body,* ed 13, St Louis, 2008, Mosby.)

dead (devitalized) tissue; crush wounds; and any wounds in patients who are immunocompromised or who have poor peripheral circulation.

ABNORMAL SCAR FORMATION

Abnormal scar formation can result in a keloid or hypertrophic scar. A **keloid** is the excessive accumulation of scar tissue that extends beyond the original wound borders. This abnormal scar is more common in darkly pigmented patients. The scar also is more common in those who have injuries to the ears, upper extremities, lower abdomen, or sternum. A **hypertrophic scar** has an excess accumulation of scar tissue within the original wound borders. This scar is more common in areas of high tissue stress such as the flexion creases across joints.

WOUNDS REQUIRING CLOSURE

Although all serious wounds should be evaluated by a physician, the paramedic should expect the following types of wounds to require closure:

- Wounds to cosmetic regions (e.g., face, lips, and eyebrows)
- Gaping wounds
- Wounds over tension areas (e.g., joints)
- Degloving injuries (described later in this chapter)
- Ring finger injuries
- Skin tearing

Many techniques are used to close a wound, including suture, tape, staples, and tissue adhesives.

PATHOPHYSIOLOGY AND ASSESSMENT OF SOFT TISSUE INJURIES

Soft tissue injuries are classified as closed or open. This classification depends on the absence or presence of a break in the continuity of the epidermis. Soft tissue wounds often are the most evident injury. However, they generally are considered low-priority injuries, unless life-threatening hemorrhage or associated airway compromise is present.

Closed Wounds

Closed soft tissue injuries usually are associated with little blood loss. However, some of these injuries can cause significant hemorrhage in the cavities of the thorax, abdomen, pelvis, or soft tissues of the legs. This text classifies closed wounds as contusion, hematoma, and crush injury.

CONTUSIONS AND HEMATOMATA

Blunt trauma causes contusions and hematomata. A **contusion** is characterized by blood vessel disruption beneath the epidermis. A contusion results in swelling, pain, and **ecchymosis** (bruising) that can occur 24 to 48 hours after the injury. A **hematoma** is a collection of blood beneath the skin. A hematoma may occur with a contusion. However, the hematoma represents a larger amount of tissue damage and the disruption of larger vessels (Figure 38-4). These

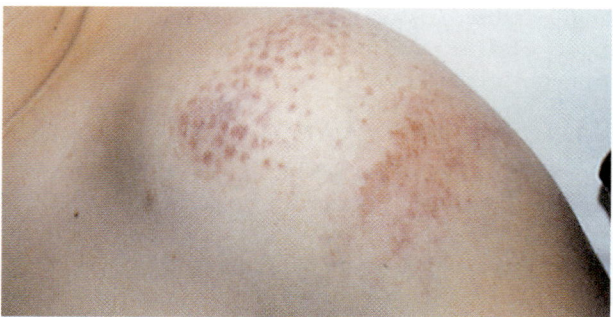

FIGURE 38-4 Spotty bruising in a well-padded part of the shoulder. (From London PS: *A colour atlas of diagnosis after recent injury,* Ipswich, England, 1990, Wolfe Medical Publications, Ltd.)

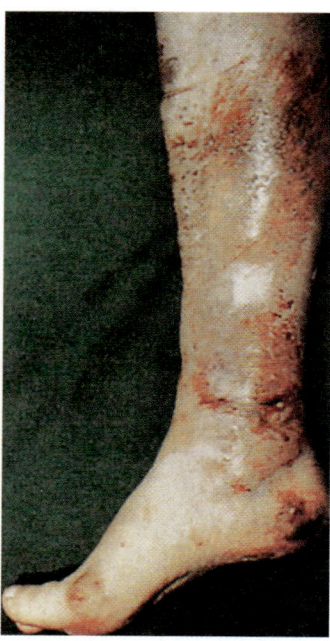

FIGURE 38-5 Appearance of a woman's leg after it had been run over by the wheel of a milk van. (From London PS: *A colour atlas of diagnosis after recent injury,* Ipswich, England, 1990, Wolfe Medical Publications, Ltd.)

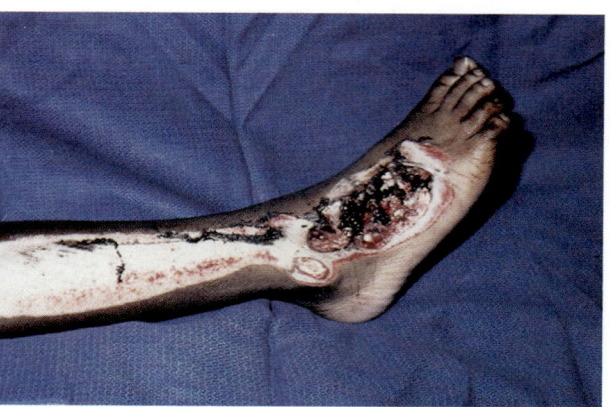

FIGURE 38-6 Deep abrasion caused by a fall from a bicycle. (From Henry MC, Stapleton ER: *EMT prehospital care,* ed 4, St Louis, 2009, Mosby.)

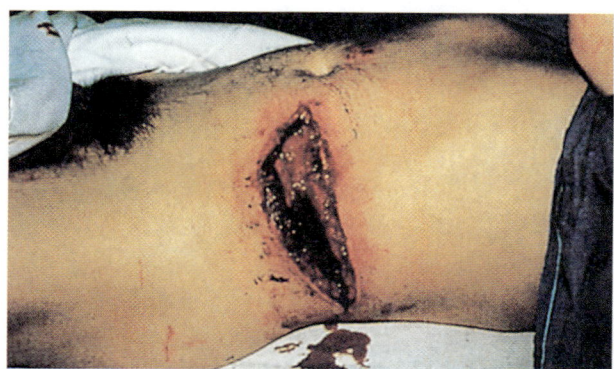

FIGURE 38-7 Large wound caused by a broken power saw. (From London PS: *A colour atlas of diagnosis after recent injury,* Ipswich, England, 1990, Wolfe Medical Publications, Ltd.)

wounds usually are superficial. Sometimes, though, they are associated with underlying fractures, vascular involvement, and significant hemorrhage.

CRUSH INJURY

Crush injury can occur when a crushing force is applied to a body area (Figure 38-5). These injuries can be severe. Sometimes they are associated with internal organ rupture, major fractures, and hemorrhagic shock. Overlying skin may remain intact with crush injury, even in the presence of severe injury and shock. Crush injuries are further described later in this chapter.

> **CRITICAL THINKING**
> What are some mechanisms of crush injury?

Open Wounds

Open soft tissue injuries are classified as abrasion, laceration, puncture, avulsion, amputation, and bites. (*NOTE:* Burns that include open and closed injury are addressed in Chapter 39.)

ABRASION

An **abrasion** is a partial-thickness skin injury. Abrasion is caused by the scraping or rubbing away of a layer or layers of skin (Figure 38-6). The wound usually results from friction with a hard object or surface. (For example, abrasions occur in sports injuries and motorcycle crashes.) Although these wounds often are superficial, they are painful and are at high risk for infection from contamination.

LACERATION

A **laceration** results from a tear, a split, or an incision of the skin (Figure 38-7). Lacerations most often are caused by a knife or other sharp object, resulting in a linear wound or incision. The sizes and depths of lacerations vary greatly depending on the injury sites and wounding mechanism. Lacerations can be sources of significant bleeding.

PUNCTURE

Contact with a sharp, pointed object commonly causes a **puncture wound** (Figure 38-8). (Examples of such objects include a wooden splinter, needle, staple, glass, or nail.) The entrance wound generally is small. Yet these injuries often may be associated with deep penetration and injury to underlying tissues. Punctures can be difficult to assess in the prehospital setting. Even an injury that appears to be minor can conceal a considerable amount of internal damage.

In some penetrating injuries, the object remains embedded or impaled in the wound (Figure 38-9). If the chest or abdomen is involved, severe bleeding and major underlying damage to internal organs can occur. Examples include the following:

- Chest injury
- Pneumothorax (simple, open, tension)
- Hemothorax
- Pericardial tamponade
- Penetrating heart wound
- Rupture of the esophagus, aorta, diaphragm, main stem bronchus
- Abdominal injury
- Hollow and solid organ damage
- Peritonitis (bacterial, chemical)
- Evisceration

CRITICAL THINKING

Why should a person always seek medical care to have a penetrating object removed?

The injection of a substance into the body under high pressure also can cause a puncture wound (Figure 38-10). (Examples include grease, paint, turpentine, dry-cleaning fluids, and molten plastics.) These injuries often have life- or limb-threatening potential. They often require rapid surgical decompression and debridement. These injuries usually are associated with minimal bleeding. In addition, they may not appear serious. Numbness and blanching of the involved area often occur because of increased tissue pressure of the injected substance. Most patients with injection injuries are surgical emergencies. Moreover, most of these patients are at high risk for developing compartment syndrome (described later in this chapter). Definitive care for injection injuries usually requires surgery and hospitalization to prevent infection. Amputation may be needed if treatment is delayed.

AVULSION

An **avulsion** is a full-thickness skin loss (Figure 38-11) in which the wound edges cannot be approximated. Frequently involved body areas are the earlobes, nose tip, and fingertips. A common cause of avulsion injury is industrial equipment, such as meat slicers or sawing devices. Another common cause is domestic violence, such as human bites.

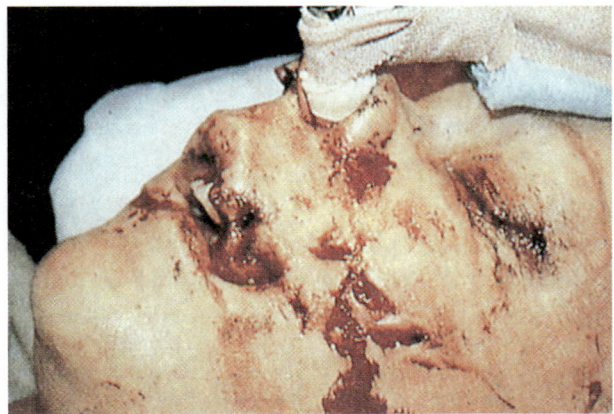

FIGURE 38-8 Puncture wounds caused by broken glass from a shattered windshield. (From London PS: *A colour atlas of diagnosis after recent injury,* Ipswich, England, 1990, Wolfe Medical Publications, Ltd.)

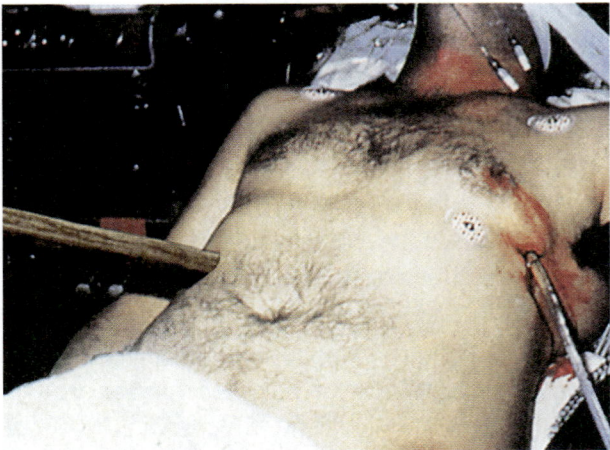

FIGURE 38-9 Piece of wood impaled in the right side of the chest, piercing the diaphragm and lacerating the spleen, stomach, and liver. (From London PS: *A colour atlas of diagnosis after recent injury,* Ipswich, England, 1990, Wolfe Medical Publications, Ltd.)

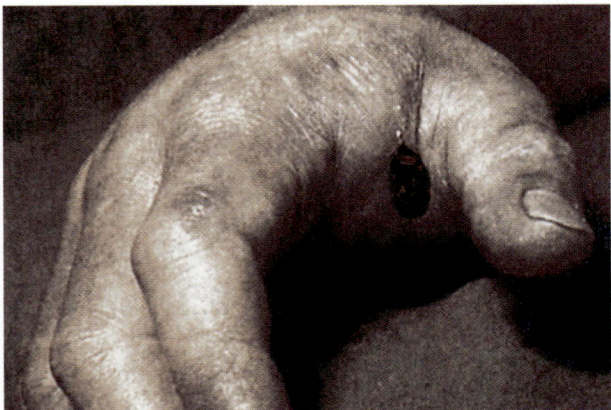

FIGURE 38-10 Injection of paraffin into the hand resulted in amputation of the index finger. (From London PS: *A colour atlas of diagnosis after recent injury,* Ipswich, England, 1990, Wolfe Medical Publications, Ltd.)

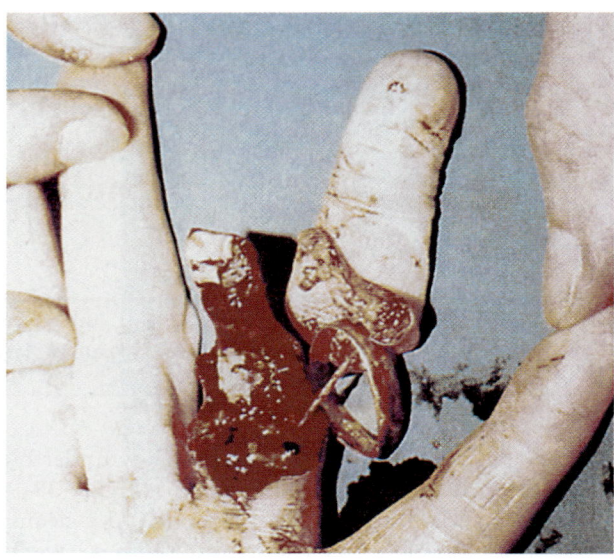

FIGURE 38-11 Ring avulsion injury. (From London PS: *A colour atlas of diagnosis after recent injury,* Ipswich, England, 1990, Wolfe Medical Publications, Ltd.)

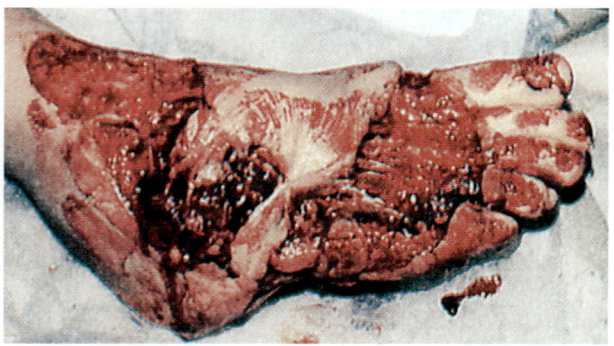

FIGURE 38-12 Degloving injury of the foot. (From London PS: *A colour atlas of diagnosis after recent injury,* Ipswich, England, 1990, Wolfe Medical Publications, Ltd.)

A **degloving injury** is a type of avulsion. In this injury, shearing forces separate the skin from the underlying tissues (Figure 38-12). A common cause of such an injury is industrial machinery. This machinery may entangle an extremity, producing circumferential tearing. Another common cause is finger jewelry that gets caught on a stationary object. This can produce a shearing of the soft tissue and possibly of the bone of the digit. Another common cause is machinery that entraps hair, resulting in scalp avulsion. Degloving injuries sometimes are associated with underlying skeletal damage. They also sometimes are associated with massive loss of tissue in the affected area. Bleeding can be significant.

AMPUTATION

Traumatic **amputation** involves a complete or partial loss of a limb by a mechanical force (Figure 38-13). The digits, lower leg, hand and forearm, and the distal part of the foot most often are injured in this way. Bleeding is a possible

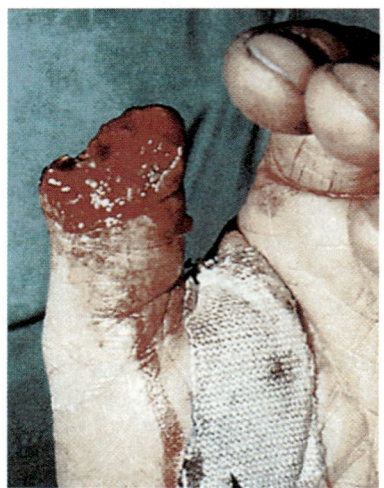

FIGURE 38-13 Amputation of the fingertip. (From London PS: *A colour atlas of diagnosis after recent injury,* Ipswich, England, 1990, Wolfe Medical Publications, Ltd.)

fatal complication of an amputation injury. In cases in which a complete amputation has occurred, injured arteries often retract. Hemorrhage may be less severe than in partial amputation injuries.

BITES

An animal or human bite wound frequently is a combination of puncture, laceration, avulsion, and crush injury (Figure 38-14). (Insect bites and stings also are a source of soft tissue injury. They are addressed in Chapter 34: Toxicology.) The pressure from a bite can be as great as 400 psi. The bite can involve deep structures such as tendons, muscles, and bones. Complications from bite wounds, particularly human bites, include abscesses, lymphangitis, cellulitis, osteomyelitis, tenosynovitis, tuberculosis, hepatitis B, and tetanus. Although it is theoretically possible for a human bite to transmit human immunodeficiency virus, the Centers for Disease Control and Prevention suggest that the potential for salivary transmission of the virus is remote.[4] Other less common complications of mammalian bites include the transmission of diseases such as actinomycosis, syphilis, and, rarely, rabies. All patients who have been bitten should seek physician evaluation.

> **NOTE**
>
> There is a common misperception that dog bites are "clean" bites, and that a dog's mouth has less germs than a human mouth. In reality, the mouths of dogs (and cats) are filled with bacteria, many of which can cause disease if they enter broken skin. Over 130 disease-causing microbes have been isolated from dog and cat bite wounds.[5] Animal saliva is also heavily contaminated with bacteria. Diseases that can be transmitted to humans through a bite from a dog or cat include pasteurellosis, streptococcal and staphylococcal infections, and *Capnocytophaga* infection (among others).

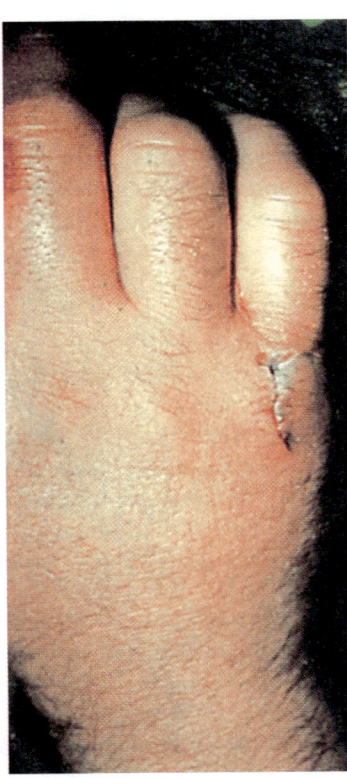

FIGURE 38-14 Human bite to the hand. (From London PS: *A colour atlas of diagnosis after recent injury,* Ipswich, England, 1990, Wolfe Medical Publications, Ltd.)

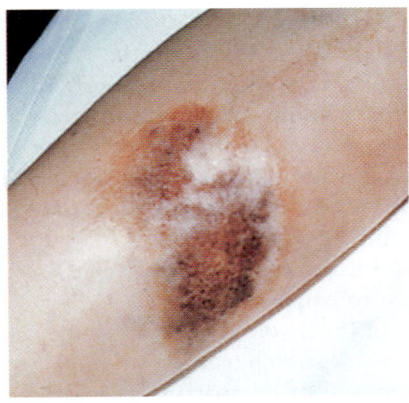

FIGURE 38-15 Appearance that can follow prolonged crushing, as when an unconscious person lies on a body part for several hours.

- Warfare injuries
- Industrial incidents
- Prolonged application of a pneumatic antishock garment and improperly applied casts

COMPARTMENT SYNDROME

Compartment syndrome is a result of crush injury and is a surgical emergency (Figure 38-15). Compartment syndrome usually results from compressive forces or blunt trauma to muscle groups confined in tight fibrous sheaths with minimal ability to stretch (below the knee, above the elbow). Other less common causes of compartment syndrome include the following[2]:

- Extreme exertional exercise
- Low-level repetitive injury
- Electrical injury
- Hemorrhage into a compartment (e.g., coagulopathy among hemophiliacs)
- Circumferential deep burns and electrical burns
- Vascular occlusion
- High-pressure injection injuries
- Immobility with the development of pressure necrosis (e.g., among alcoholics, drug addicts, and victims of stroke)

>
> **CRITICAL THINKING**
> Why would alcoholics, drug addicts, and stroke victims be at risk for compartment syndrome?

Compartment syndrome develops as associated hemorrhage and edema increase pressure in the closed fascial space (compartment). This results in ischemia to the muscle. This ischemia causes further muscle cell swelling. The intracompartmental pressure continues to rise. As this occurs, circulation is compromised. Irreversible tissue damage from lack of oxygen develops within several hours

> **CRITICAL THINKING**
> Consider that you are caring for a person who has sustained an animal bite. Aside from caring for the patient's wounds and documenting that care, what other concerns and responsibilities do you have?

Crush Injury

Crush injury is one of the three injuries that occurs when tissue is exposed to a compressive force. This force can be sufficient to interfere with the normal structure and metabolic function of the involved cells and tissues. The degree of injury produced by the crushing force depends on the amount of pressure applied to the body, the amount of time the pressure remains in contact with the body, and the specific body region in which the injury occurs. A massive crush injury to vital organs can cause immediate death.

Crush injury usually involves the upper or lower extremities, torso, or pelvis. Crush injury can result from entrapment under a heavy object, as in a foundation collapse, or from some other massive compressive force. Examples of situations that can cause crush injury include the following:

- Collapse of masonry or steel structures
- Collapse of earth (e.g., mud slides and earthquakes)
- Motor vehicle crashes

to several days after injury. In addition to muscular damage, any nerves that travel through the compartment can undergo necrosis if the condition remains untreated. Signs and symptoms of compartment syndrome in an extremity include those of vascular insufficiency (the five P's; Box 38-1). Other signs and symptoms that can indicate the presence of compartment syndrome include the following:

- Pain seemingly out of proportion to injury
- Swelling (tautness of the compartment)
- Tenderness to palpation
- Weakness of the involved muscle groups
- Pain on passive stretch (earliest finding)

The recognition of compartment syndrome calls for a high degree of suspicion based on patient history and mechanism of injury. Compartment syndrome most often is associated with tibial fracture of the lower leg. Yet compartment syndrome also can occur with crush injury or fracture of the femur, forearm, or upper arm. Delayed treatment can result in nerve death, muscle necrosis, and crush syndrome.

CRUSH SYNDROME

Crush syndrome is a life-threatening and sometimes preventable complication of prolonged immobilization or compression. The syndrome is a pathological process that causes destruction or alteration of muscle tissue. Crush syndrome is rare and is most likely to occur in catastrophic events in which patient rescue and extrication are delayed beyond 4 to 6 hours. (Examples of such events are earthquake or building collapse.) The prehospital management of crush syndrome often determines patient outcome.

The compressive forces of entrapment are believed to produce crush syndrome.[6] The pathological process disrupts vascular integrity and causes loss of structure of the cell and the cell membranes. Patients with crush syndrome may appear stable for hours or days, as long as the compressive forces remain in place. But when the patient is released from the entrapment, three harmful processes occur at the same time that can lead to death:

1. Oxygen-rich blood returns to the ischemic extremity. This produces a pooling of intravascular volume into crushed tissue. This reperfusion reduces total circulating volume, which in turn often leads to shock.
2. With the return of oxygen-rich blood, various toxic substances and waste products of anaerobic metabolism are released into the systemic circulation. This causes

metabolic acidosis. High levels of intracellular solutes and water are released from damaged cells. This results in hyperkalemia, hyperuricemia, hypocalcemia, and hyperphosphatemia.

3. Myoglobin is released from the damaged muscle cells of the injured extremity. Myoglobin is filtered through the kidneys (**rhabdomyolysis**) and results in acute renal failure.

Blast Injuries

As described in Chapter 36, severe injuries can result from an initial air blast, from flying debris, and from secondary contact with another object as the victim is thrown by the blast. Examples of situations that can result in blast injury include natural gas or gasoline explosions, fireworks explosions, explosions in grain elevators, and terrorist bombs. Scene and personal safety is of the highest priority. Paramedics should not enter the scene where a blast injury occurred until the scene has been made safe by the authorities. (The appropriate authorities include, for example, law enforcement, fire service, specialized rescue teams, hazardous materials teams, and other public service agencies.)

Injuries from blasts can be superficial or deep (Figure 38-16). The deep injuries can damage internal organs. Patients who suffer blast injury require rapid stabilization (airway and ventilatory support with spinal precautions; circulatory support) and rapid transportation for physician evaluation. Blast injuries and associated trauma can be difficult to identify in the prehospital setting. These patients

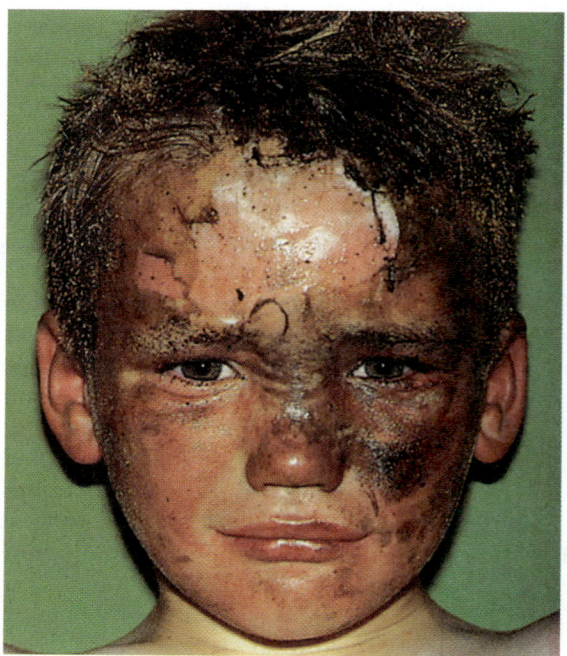

FIGURE 38-16 Blast injury to the face. His eardrums were normal. He was admitted because of the risk of swelling to his face and airway with potential airway obstruction. (From Beattie T, et al: *Pediatric emergencies,* London, 1997, Mosby-Wolfe.)

BOX 38-1 Five P's of Vascular Insufficiency

1. **P**ain
2. **P**aresis (late finding)
3. **P**aresthesia
4. **P**allor (variable)
5. **P**ulselessness (late finding)

will need extensive evaluation in a trauma center. Compression injuries that occur to air-filled organs include rupture of the eardrum, sinuses, lungs, stomach, and intestines.

> ### CRITICAL THINKING
> What injury do you suspect if a patient who has suffered a blast injury has a sudden onset of hearing loss?

MANAGEMENT PRINCIPLES FOR SOFT TISSUE INJURIES

Personal and scene safety is always the priority in any emergency response. If indicated, law enforcement and rescue personnel should advise the EMS crew that the scene is relatively safe to enter and that any perpetrators have been apprehended. Even so, the paramedic must always be alert for possible hazards at the scene (e.g., a second perpetrator or secondary explosive device). Help from other public service agencies also may be needed if other types of dangers exist. Examples of such dangers may include hazardous materials or bombs.

Treatment Priorities

The assessment of life-threatening injuries and resuscitation precedes evaluation and intervention of non–life-threatening soft tissue injuries. The paramedic should evaluate wounds that do not pose a threat to life later in the physical exam. General wound assessment should include a history of the wounding event and a careful examination of the injury. Figure 38-17 shows a treatment plan based on assessment findings for a patient with soft tissue injury.

Wound History

A wound history should include the following:

- Time of injury
- Environment where the injury occurred (risk of infection is greater in unclean environments)
- Mechanism of injury and likelihood of concurrent or associated injuries
- Volume of blood loss
- Severity of pain
- Medical history, including use of medications that may impair hemostasis
- Tetanus immunization

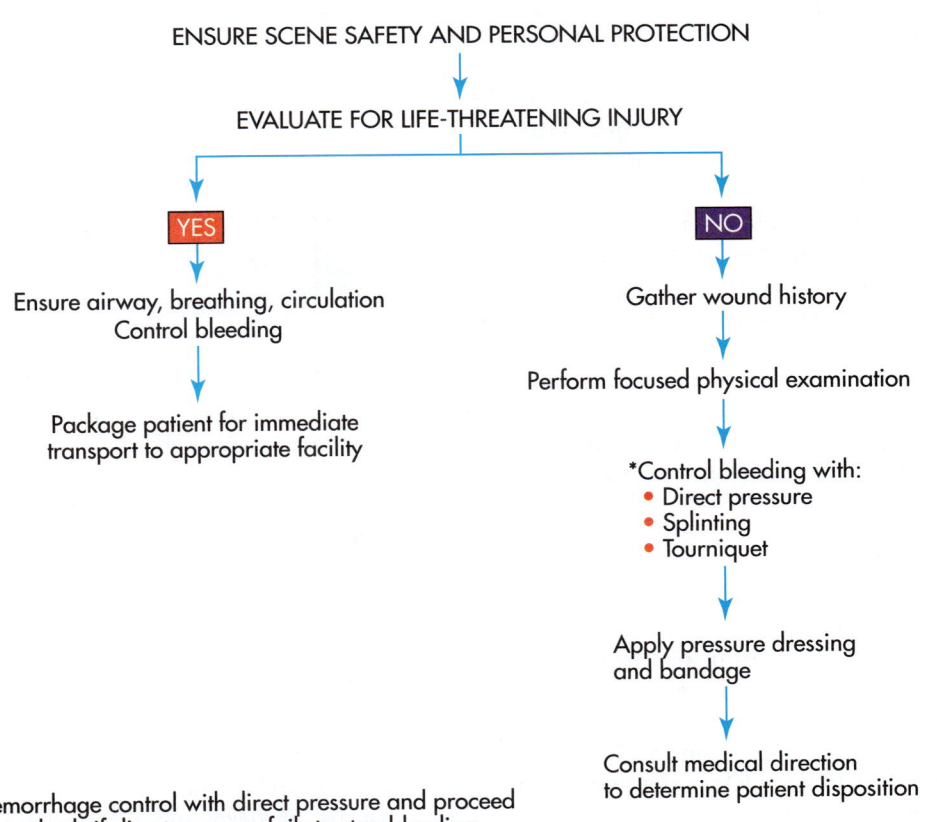

ENSURE SCENE SAFETY AND PERSONAL PROTECTION

EVALUATE FOR LIFE-THREATENING INJURY

YES

Ensure airway, breathing, circulation
Control bleeding

Package patient for immediate
transport to appropriate facility

NO

Gather wound history

Perform focused physical examination

*Control bleeding with:
- Direct pressure
- Splinting
- Tourniquet

Apply pressure dressing
and bandage

Consult medical direction
to determine patient disposition

*Begin hemorrhage control with direct pressure and proceed
to other methods if direct pressure fails to stop bleeding.

FIGURE 38-17 Treatment plan for a patient with soft tissue injury.

Physical Examination

Physical examination of a wound should include the following:

- Inspection of the wound for bleeding, size, depth, presence of foreign bodies, amount of tissue lost, edema, and deformity
- Inspection of the area surrounding the wound for damage to underlying structures, arteries, nerves, tendons, or muscle

CRITICAL THINKING
Will you perform this physical examination on every wound in the prehospital setting?

- Assessment of sensory or motor function of the extremity
- Evaluation of the perfusion status of the wound and tissue distal to the wound
- Palpation of the injury and associated structures to evaluate capillary refill, distal pulses, tenderness, temperature, edema, and crepitus (if underlying bony injury is suspected)

HEMORRHAGE AND CONTROL OF BLEEDING

Blood loss often is associated with soft tissue injury. The blood loss may result from damage to arteries, veins, capillaries, or a combination of these. Generally, arterial bleeding is characterized as bright red and spurting. Venous bleeding is dark reddish-blue and flowing. Capillary bleeding is bright red and oozing. But differentiation among the types of vessel hemorrhage often is difficult. In the prehospital setting the main concern in hemorrhage, regardless of origin, is to control bleeding.

Methods of hemorrhage control include direct pressure, immobilization by splinting, pneumatic pressure devices (air splints, pneumatic antishock garment), and the use of tourniquets. As in any patient encounter in which contact with body fluids is likely, the paramedic must take personal protective measures. (The use of pressure on an artery proximal to a wound and elevation of an extremity to control hemorrhage is no longer recommended as part of prehospital care.[3] There are insufficient data to support the effectiveness of these measures.[7])

Direct Pressure

The paramedic can control external hemorrhage by applying direct pressure over the injury site (Figure 38-18). Direct pressure controls most types of hemorrhage within 4 to 6 minutes. To maintain control, a pressure dressing can be applied over the site and held in place with an elastic bandage. The paramedic must continue direct pressure, even with a pressure dressing. Once the dressing has been applied, the paramedic should not remove it because removal can disrupt the fresh blood clot. If bleeding resumes and the dressing becomes soaked with blood, a

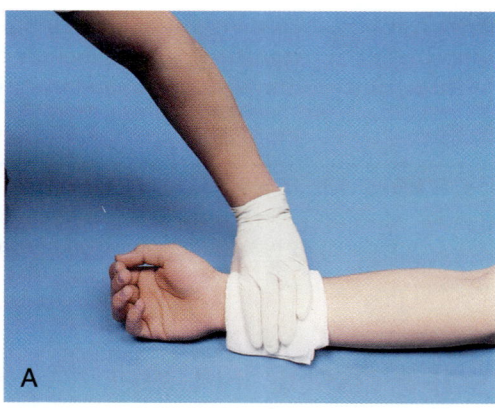

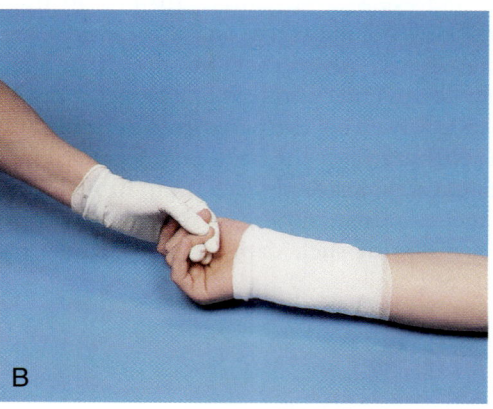

FIGURE 38-18 A, Application of direct pressure to control hemorrhage. **B,** Pressure dressing.

second dressing should be applied on top of the first one and held in place with direct pressure until the bleeding is controlled.

CRITICAL THINKING
Why should the pressure point chosen to control hemorrhage be proximal to the injury?

Immobilization by Splinting

Patient movement promotes the flow of blood. This movement can disrupt the clot or increase vascular injury. Thus patients should be immobilized whenever possible (Figure 38-19). The paramedic can immobilize extremity injuries with appropriate splinting devices. The patient can be immobilized fully with a long spine board. Immobilization is not effective alone as a method to control bleeding. Immobilization should be used as an adjunct.

Pneumatic Pressure Devices

Pneumatic pressure devices can provide uniform direct pressure to an immobilized injury site. (Examples of such devices are inflatable air splints applied to an extremity or the use of the pneumatic antishock garment.) These devices should be applied over a dressed wound only after other methods have controlled the bleeding (Figure 38-20).

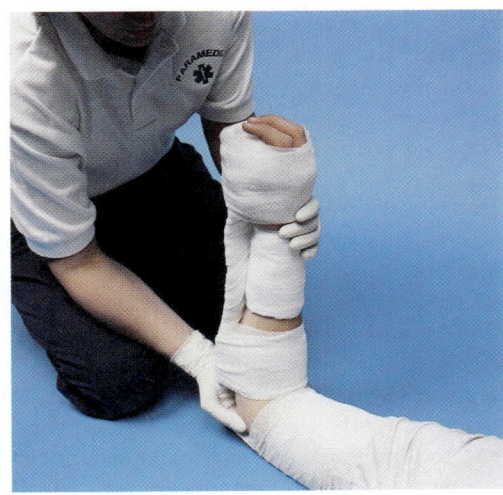

FIGURE 38-19 Immobilization by splinting to control hemorrhage.

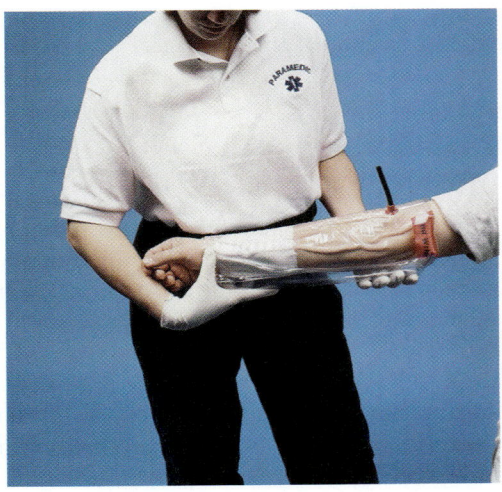

FIGURE 38-20 Application of pneumatic pressure device to control hemorrhage.

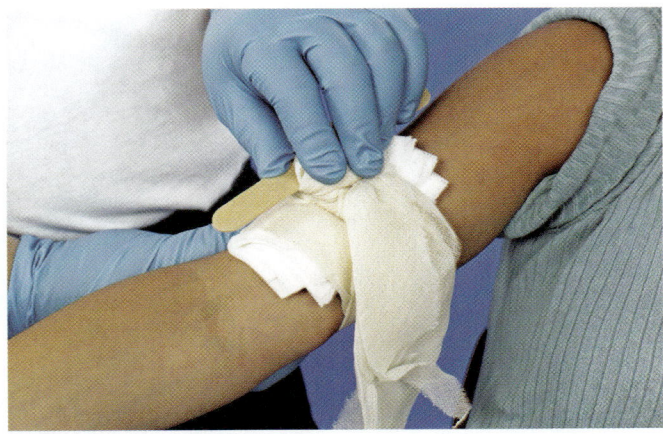

FIGURE 38-21 Application of a tourniquet to control hemorrhage.

Tourniquet

The use of a **tourniquet** to control bleeding was once considered a "last resort" in bleeding control. However, recent studies based on wartime injuries in Iraq and Afghanistan have proven tourniquets to be safe and effective when properly applied.[8] Guidelines for application of a tourniquet are as follows (Figure 38-21)[9]:

1. Consult with medical direction.
2. Select a site for the tourniquet. The site should be about 2 inches proximal to the wound and over the supplying brachial or femoral artery. A blood pressure cuff applied over the brachial artery also can act as a tourniquet. If a blood pressure cuff is used, note the time of application on the cuff itself.
3. Place the commercial tourniquet (e.g., Combat Application Tourniquet [C-A-T], Emergency Military Tourniquet [EMT], Special Operations Force Tactical Tourniquet [SOFTT]) or 4-inch wide, flat material just above the wound and over the artery to be compressed. Never use thin material such as rope or twine because it may damage underlying tissue. If a blood pressure cuff is used as a tourniquet, inflate the cuff until the cuff pressure exceeds the arterial pressure or to the point at which the hemorrhage stops.
4. Place the pad (a roll of gauze or thick folded dressings) over the artery to be compressed.
5. Encircle the tourniquet twice around the extremity and pad, and tie it in a half knot over the pad.
6. Place a windlass (stick, pen, or similar object) on the half knot, and secure it in place with a square knot.
7. Tighten the windlass by twisting *only* until hemorrhage stops. Secure the windlass in that position. Never loosen the tourniquet once it is tightened.
8. Note the time of tourniquet application and secure it to the patient, or clearly mark "TK" on the patient's forehead. Document the tourniquet procedure on the patient care report (Figure 38-22).

> **NOTE**
> The improper application of a tourniquet may cause damage to nerves and blood vessels and result in the eventual loss of an extremity. A poorly applied tourniquet can produce venous occlusion, only restricting the outflow but not the inflow of blood and producing an increase in blood loss. Use of a tourniquet should be considered only when other methods have failed to control bleeding and when its use is essential to save the patient's life. An example of such an extreme circumstance is a partial or complete traumatic amputation of a limb. Other indications for tourniquet use include mass casualty incidents with multiple bleeding injuries that overwhelm rescuer capabilities, tactical or combat situations in which the scene is not safe to render care, and when a greater priority exists, such as airway or respiratory management or initiating the treatment for shock.[10]

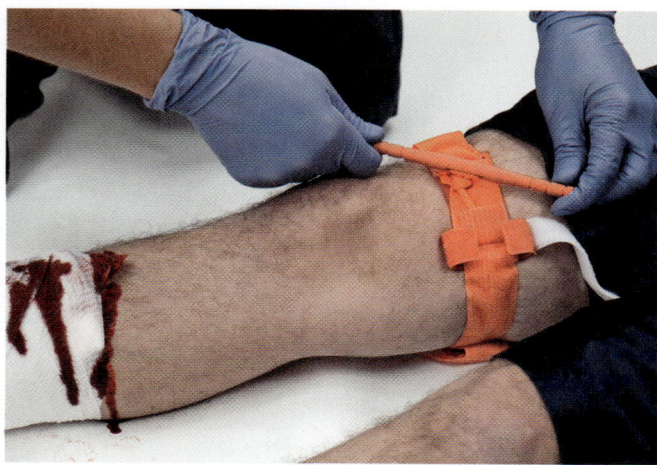

FIGURE 38-22 Commercial tourniquet application.

DRESSING MATERIALS USED WITH SOFT TISSUE TRAUMA

A variety of bandages and dressings are used in trauma care. The six general categories of dressings are as follows:

1. *Sterile dressings* are processed to eliminate bacteria. They should be used whenever infection of the wound is a concern.
2. *Nonsterile dressings* are not sterilized. They can be used when infection is not a prime concern.
3. *Occlusive dressings* do not allow the passage of air through the material. These dressings are useful in treating wounds of the thorax and major vessels where negative pressure can cause air to enter the body, resulting in a pneumothorax or air embolism, respectively (see Chapter 42).
4. *Nonocclusive dressings* allow air to pass through the material and are indicated for managing most soft tissue injuries.
5. *Adherent dressings* attach to the wound surface by incorporating wound exudate into the dressing mesh. Use of these dressings sometimes can assist in controlling acute bleeding.
6. *Nonadherent dressings* allow the passage of wound exudate and do not adhere to the wound surface. These dressings do not damage the wound when removed and often are used after wound closure.

Bandages hold dressings in place. Bandages are classified as absorbent, nonabsorbent, adherent, and nonadherent. Like dressings, bandages are sterile or nonsterile.

Complications of Improperly Applied Dressings and Bandages

Improperly applied dressings and bandages can harm the patient and can cause discomfort. For example, dressings that are applied too loosely often do not stop bleeding.

Bandages that are applied too tightly can cause tissue ischemia and structural damage to vessels, nerves, tendons, muscles, and skin.

Basic Concepts of Open Wound Dressing

The basic concepts of open wound dressing include the following steps:

1. Assess the wound for size, depth, location, and contamination.
2. Properly prepare the wound for dressing. Prehospital care usually is limited to cleaning the injured surface of gross contaminants by irrigation of the wound with sterile water or normal saline. Do not attempt extensive debridement in the prehospital setting. Apply antibacterial ointment if the patient is not allergic (per protocol).
3. Apply the appropriate dressing.
4. Secure the dressing in place with bandages or gauze wrappings.
5. Tape the loose ends of the bandage.

MANAGEMENT OF SPECIFIC SOFT TISSUE INJURIES NOT REQUIRING CLOSURE

The paramedic will encounter many minor open wounds that do not require closure or the evaluation by a physician. In these cases, basic first aid and instructions for self-care should be provided to the patient.

Dressings and Bandages

Depending on the nature and location of the patient's injury, dressings, bandages, and immobilization may be indicated to care for the wound properly. (Figure 38-23 illustrates basic dressing and bandaging procedures for various wounds.) Open wounds that usually require physician evaluation include those with the following:

- Neural, muscular, or vascular compromise
- Tendon or ligament compromise
- Heavy contamination
- Cosmetic complications (e.g., facial trauma)
- Foreign bodies
- Animal bites with deep punctures

Patients with soft tissue injuries that pose a threat to life or limb require rapid assessment, stabilization, and rapid transportation for physician evaluation.

> **NOTE**
> Some EMS agencies carry hemostatic dressings for wound care. These special dressings have multiple layers of resorbable materials and fibrin patches that contain coagulation proteins. Examples of these dressings include CELOX, QuikClot, and HemCon.

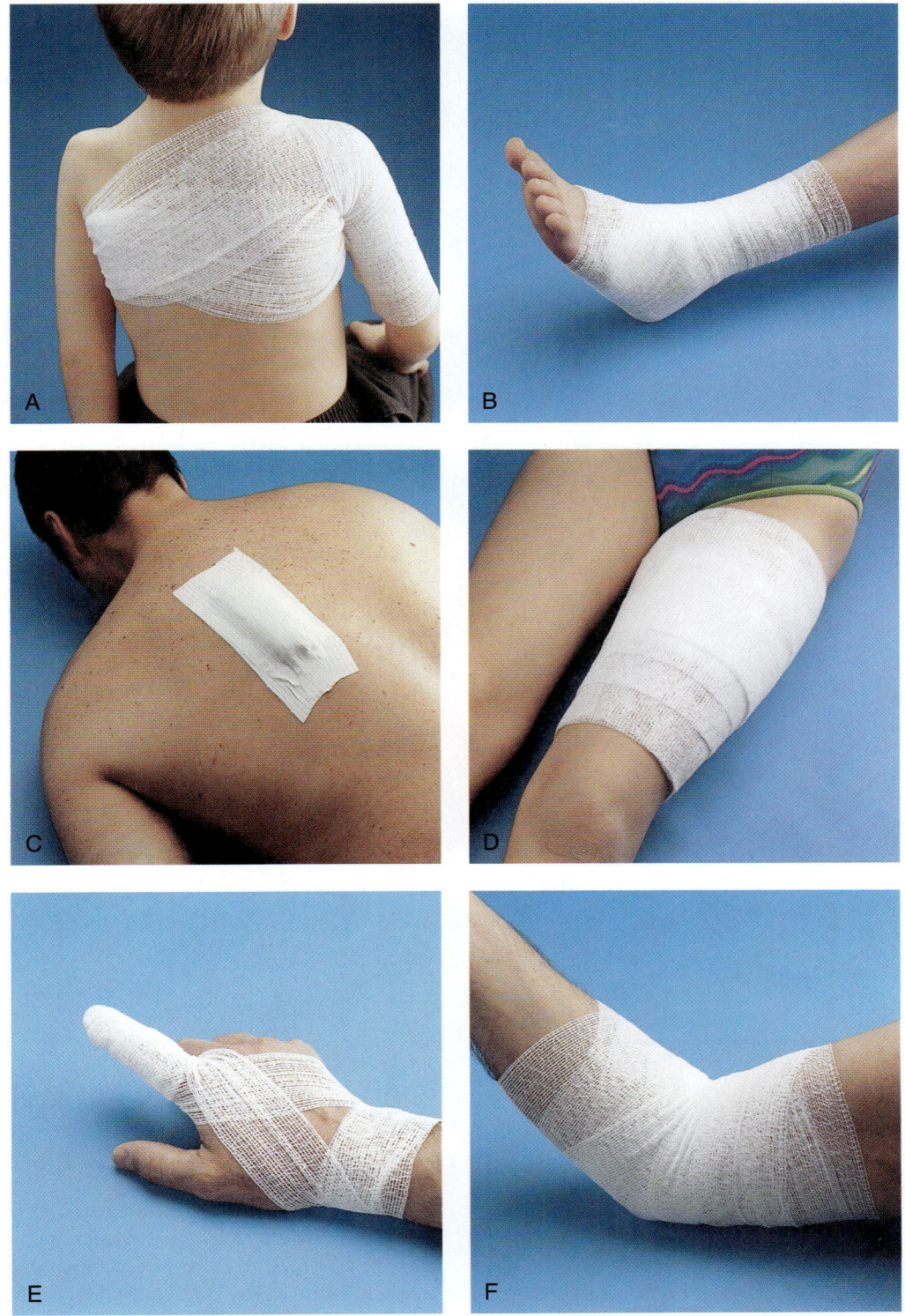

FIGURE 38-23 Types of dressings. **A,** Shoulder dressing. **B,** Ankle dressing. **C,** Torso dressing. **D,** Thigh dressing. **E,** Finger dressing. **F,** Elbow dressing.

Continued

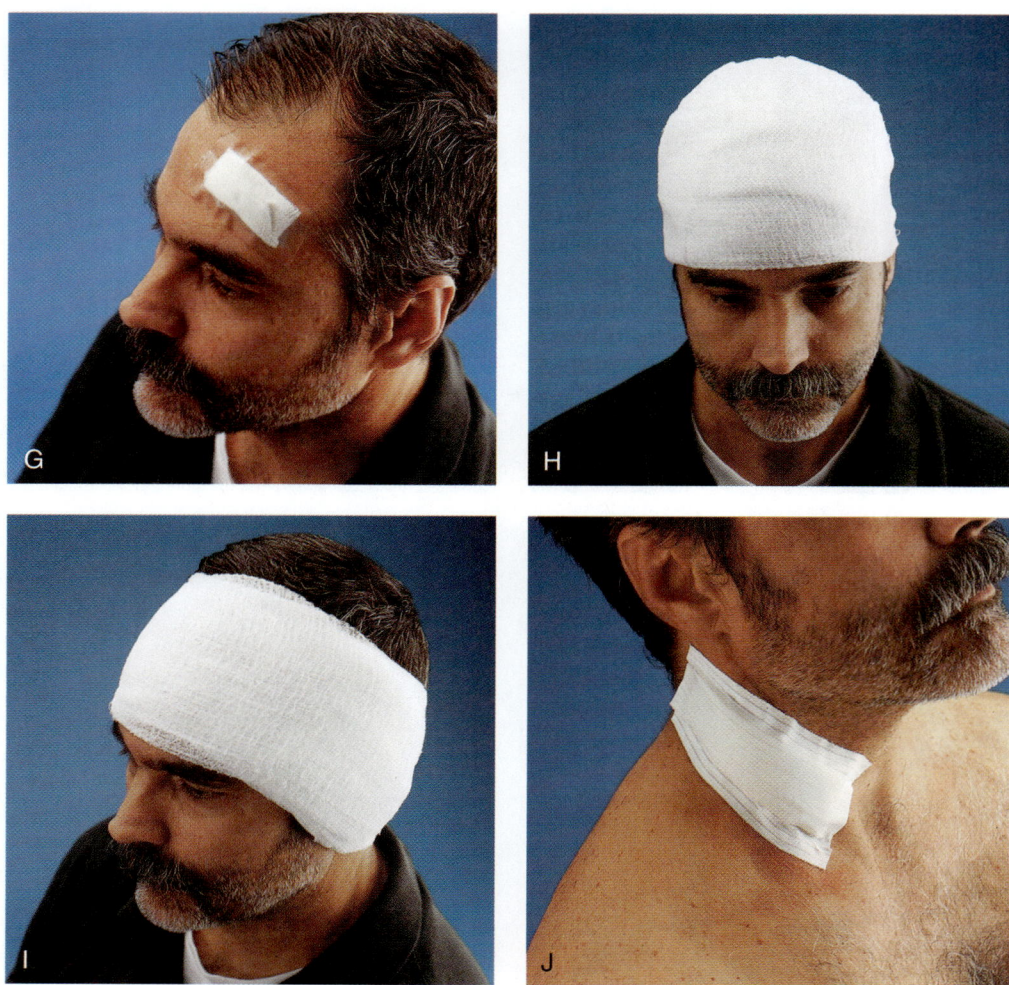

FIGURE 38-23, cont'd **G,** Forehead dressing. **H,** Scalp dressing. **I,** Ear/mastoid dressing. **J,** Neck dressing.

SHOW ME THE EVIDENCE

Amylopectin (Chitosan) dressings have been in use since the 1990s. These researchers sought to determine the effectiveness of amylopectin powder when directly poured into a wound. Using a pig model, the researchers induced femoral artery hemorrhage. In one group pressure was applied with gauze. In the other 100 g of powder was applied to the bleeding and then pressure was applied with gauze.

Additional powder was applied after 3 minutes in the intervention group if bleeding was not controlled.

The researchers concluded that the amylopectin group had less blood loss and higher mean arterial pressure at 180 minutes, and needed less fluid volume for resuscitation. In the amylopectin group the mean time to hemostasis was 9.0 minutes and hemostasis was never achieved in the control group. All animals in the amylopectin group survived whereas none survived in the control group.

From Kilbourne M, Keledjian K, Hess J, et al: Hemostatic efficacy of modified amylopectin powder in a lethal porcine model of extremity arterial injury, *Ann Emerg Med* 53(6):804-810, 2009.

Evaluation

Local protocol may permit the paramedic to manage and release the patient with minor soft tissue injury to the patient's own care. Local protocol also may allow the paramedic to manage and refer the patient to the patient's private physician for follow-up care. Some EMS systems allow paramedics to provide tetanus vaccine. Paramedics also may be permitted to give written and verbal instructions regarding care to patients who will not be transported by ambulance for physician evaluation.

TETANUS VACCINE

Tetanus is a serious and at times fatal disease. Tetanus is a disease of the central nervous system caused by the infection of a wound with spores of the bacterium *Clostridium tetani*. The patient can be protected against tetanus by periodic immunization with a tetanus vaccine. About half a million cases of tetanus occur across the world each year. In the United States only about 50 or fewer cases are reported each year. All cases occur in nonimmunized persons. Tetanus infection occurs mostly in those more than 50 years of age. Deaths are most likely to occur in people 60 years or older and in people with diabetes.[11]

Children and adults in the United States routinely receive a combined immunization against diphtheria, tetanus, and pertussis (whooping cough). (*Acellular pertussis* [TDaP] is given to those older than 7 years of age; *whole-cell pertussis* [DTaP] is given to infants and toddlers.) After initial immunization during childhood, children receive booster vaccines every 5 to 10 years. Patients who have not been previously immunized against tetanus receive tetanus immune globulin because it confers instant immunity. During wound care, the paramedic should ascertain the patient's last tetanus immunization. The paramedic also should determine any prior allergic reactions to tetanus preparations. Normal side effects from the vaccine include slight fever, sore injection site, or minor rash. The tetanus vaccine is contraindicated in infants less than 6 weeks of age, in pregnant patients, and in those who are hypersensitive to the vaccine.

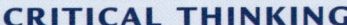

> ### CRITICAL THINKING
> Why is it crucial for you to be knowledgeable about tetanus and to ask the patient about tetanus vaccination if the vaccine is not carried on your ambulance?

PATIENT INSTRUCTIONS

Verbal and written instructions sometimes are referred to as a "patient instruction sheet." These instructions relate to wound care (Figure 38-24). Paramedics should give instructions to all patients who are not transported for physician evaluation. These instructions should include the following:

- Protection and care of wounded area
- Dressing change and follow-up
- Wound cleansing recommendations
- Signs of wound infection

Wound Infection

Infection is a common complication of soft tissue injury. It results from a break in the continuity of the skin and subsequent exposure to the nonsterile external environment. Most infections are minor. However, some can be serious. The goals of wound care are to prevent infection and protect from infection. Factors that influence the likelihood of infection include unclean wounds and wound mechanisms

(e.g., wounds contaminated by soil, dirt, or grease) and a patient's poor state of health. These factors can have both local and systemic complications and can affect the patient's general recovery.

Causes of Wound Infection

Many factors can cause wound infection. Nine of the most common factors are[4]:

1. *Time.* The risk of infection can be reduced greatly if the wound is cleaned and repaired within 8 to 12 hours after injury. Bacterial proliferation to a level that can result in infection can occur as early as 3 hours after injury.
2. *Mechanism.* Lacerations caused by fine cutting forces resist infection better than crush injuries. High-velocity missile injuries can produce internal damage that may not be apparent for several days.
3. *Location.* Injuries of the foot, lower extremity, hand, and perineum have a higher-than-normal risk for infection.
4. *Severity.* The more tissue damage produced by the injury, the higher the risk for infection.
5. *Contamination.* The presence of foreign matter in a wound decreases resistance to infection. Of particular concern are wounds contaminated by soil, saliva, and feces.
6. *Preparation.* Body, facial, and head hair removed by clipping versus shaving is less likely to result in wound infection. Shaving can cause additional injury by abrading the skin and potentially moving skin flora into the larger wound.
7. *Cleansing.* Wound cleansing should be performed with normal saline and a high-pressure syringe.
8. *Technique of repair.* Wounds at high risk for infection (e.g., animal bites) may need to be cleaned, debrided, left open for 4 to 5 days, and then closed through traditional techniques.
9. *General patient condition.* Elderly patients and patients with concurrent illness or preexisting disease (e.g., diabetes) often are less able to ward off infection.

Assessment of Wound Healing

A paramedic can assess a wound for proper healing by doing the following:

- Examine dressings for excess drainage. Change saturated dressings to prevent contamination of the wound.
- Examine wounds for early signs of infection or delayed healing. Inflammation, edema, and bloody drainage are normal during the first 3 days but should subside gradually as the wound heals.

Signs of wound infection include increasing inflammation or edema, purulent drainage, foul odor, persistent pain, delayed healing, enlarged lymph nodes proximal to the wound, and fever. If any of these is present, the paramedic should consult with medical direction. Medical

WOUND CARE INSTRUCTION SHEET

Patient name: _____

1. Call your physician. He/she may have further instructions to offer for your care.
2. Keep the wound and dressing as dry as reasonably possible, since water aids bacterial growth.
3. Remove the dressing applied after 2 days.
4. Check for signs of infection:
   a. Swelling
   b. Excessive redness
   c. Pain
   d. Heat—either locally or systemically as reflected by a fever
   e. Excessive drainage from wounds
5. Reapply a sterile gauze dressing, taping it down at the edges. Repeat this every 2 days until the wound heals.
6. Wounds in areas of high mobility, such as around joints, are subject to excessive tension. Appropriate precautions should be taken to decrease the motion of the affected joint to assist in healing.

Other instructions: _____

_____

_____

Treatment rendered: _____

Tetanus: Yes / No   Type: _____

I hereby acknowledge that I have read the instructions above, that they have been explained to me, that I understand them, and that I have received a copy of them.

I understand that I have had emergency treatment only and that I may be released before all of my medical problems are known and treated. I will arrange for the follow-up care as instructed.

_____   _____
Responsible Party's Signature   Relationship

_____   _____
Witness   Title

Original to Patient Care Report   _____
Copy to Patient   Date/Time

FIGURE 38-24 Sample instruction sheet for wound care.

direction may advise patient transport to the emergency department or may direct patient referral to a private physician for follow-up care.

SPECIAL CONSIDERATIONS FOR SOFT TISSUE INJURIES

As stated before, assessment of life-threatening injuries and resuscitation precede evaluation of and intervention for non–life-threatening soft tissue injuries. The paramedic can proceed with wound care after ensuring adequate airway, breathing, and circulatory status (with spinal precautions if indicated); controlling severe hemorrhage; and maintaining normal body temperature. Special considerations for specific wounds are described in the following sections.

Penetrating Chest or Abdominal Injury

Open wounds to the chest and upper abdomen must be covered properly with sterile and occlusive dressings. (Open wounds to the neck must also be covered with occlusive dressings to prevent air embolism, described in Chapter 40: Head, Face, and Neck Trauma.) Open chest wounds can involve severe pulmonary injuries. These injuries can include pneumothorax and tension pneumothorax (described in Chapter 42). Major complications of penetrating abdominal injury include hemorrhage from a major vessel or solid organ and perforation of a segment of bowel (see Chapter 43). The paramedic should observe the following guidelines in managing a penetrating wound to the chest or abdomen in which an impaled object is present:

1. Do not remove the impaled object; severe hemorrhage or damage to underlying structures can occur.
2. Do not manipulate the impaled object unless it is necessary to shorten the object for extrication or for patient transportation.
3. Control bleeding with direct pressure applied around the impaled object.
4. Stabilize the object in place with bulky dressings; immobilize the patient to prevent movement.

Avulsion

Prehospital management of avulsed tissue varies by protocol, but two guidelines generally apply:

1. If the tissue is still attached to the body, do the following:
   a. Clean the wound surface of gross contaminants with sterile saline.
   b. Gently fold the skin back to its normal position.
   c. Control bleeding, dress the wound with bulky pressure dressings, and maintain direct pressure.
2. If the tissue is completely separated from the body, do the following:

a. Control the bleeding with application of direct pressure.
b. Retrieve the avulsed tissue if possible, but do not delay transport to locate amputated body parts.
c. Wrap the tissue in gauze, either dry or moistened with lactated Ringer's or saline solution (per protocol).
d. Seal the tissue in a plastic bag.
e. Place the sealed bag on crushed ice; never place tissue directly on ice.

CRITICAL THINKING
Why should you use normal saline or lactated Ringer's solution instead of sterile water to wrap or clean avulsed tissue?

Amputations

As with other open wounds, hemorrhage control for amputation should be managed initially with direct pressure. (A severe amputation may require the use of a tourniquet. However, a tourniquet can cause tissue damage and may interfere with reimplantation attempts. Therefore direct pressure is the preferred method to control bleeding.) An amputated limb should be retrieved and managed in the same manner as avulsed tissue.

Crush Syndrome

Crush syndrome is complex and is difficult to diagnose and treat because of the many variables involved. These variables include the extent of tissue damage, duration and force of compression, patient's general health, and associated injuries. The management of crush syndrome is controversial. A medical direction physician who is familiar with this pathological process must supervise the prehospital care. Scenarios where crush injury may occur include earthquakes where victims are trapped in collapsed buildings, and people who have lain immobile in one position (e.g., from stroke or alcohol intoxication) for long periods of time.

Paramedics should consider possible crush syndrome when prolonged immobilization or compression occurs. The emergency care must be coordinated with rescue efforts so that the timing of the release from entrapment follows medical treatment. This will help to prevent hypovolemic shock and crush syndrome. After ensuring adequate airway and ventilatory support, initial prehospital care is focused on aggressive IV hydration to manage hypotension and to prevent renal failure. Other care at the scene should be guided by on-scene or online medical direction. Box 38-2 lists patient care measures for crush syndrome.[6]

BOX 38-2 Patient Care Measures for Crush Syndrome

Initial Management: Prehospital Setting

- Administer intravenous fluids before releasing the crushed body part. This step is especially important in cases of prolonged crush (more than 4 hours); however, crush syndrome can occur in crush scenarios of less than 1 hour.
- If this procedure is not possible, consider short-term use of a tourniquet on the affected limb until intravenous hydration can be initiated.

Initial Management: Hospital Setting

Hypotension

- Initiate (or continue) IV hydration—up to 1.5 L/hour.

Renal Failure

- Prevent renal failure with appropriate hydration, using IV fluids and mannitol to maintain diuresis of at least 300 mL/hr.
- Triage to hemodialysis as needed.

Metabolic Abnormalities

- Acidosis: Alkalinization of urine is critical; administer IV **sodium bicarbonate** until urine pH reaches 6.5 to prevent myoglobin and uric acid deposition in kidneys.
- Hyperkalemia/hypocalcemia: Consider administering the following (adult doses): **calcium gluconate** 10% 10 mL or **calcium chloride** 10% 5 mL IV over 2 minutes; **sodium bicarbonate** 1 mEq/kg IV slow push; regular insulin 5 to 10 units and D_{50} 1 to 2 ampules IV bolus; Kayexalate 25 to 50 g with sorbitol 20% 100 mL PO or rectally.
- Cardiac dysrhythmias: Monitor for cardiac dysrhythmias and cardiac arrest, and treat accordingly.

Secondary Complications

- Monitor casualties for compartment syndrome; monitor compartmental pressure if equipment is available; consider emergency **fasciotomy** (surgical relief of tension or pressure) for compartment syndrome.
- Treat open wounds with antibiotics, tetanus toxoid, and debridement of necrotic tissue.
- Apply ice to injured areas and monitor for the 5 P's: pain, pallor, paresthesias, pain with passive movement (i.e., paresis), and pulselessness.
- Observe all crush casualties, even those who look well.
- Delays in hydration of greater than 12 hours may increase the incidence of renal failure; delayed manifestations of renal failure can occur.

Disposition

- Patients with acute renal failure may require up to 60 days of dialysis treatment; unless sepsis is present, patients are likely to regain normal kidney function.

SUMMARY

- Hemorrhage can be internal or external.
- The skin and its accessory organs are the main cosmetic structures of the body. These structures perform many functions that are critical to survival. The skin is composed of two distinct layers of tissue: the outer layer (epidermis) and the inner layer (dermis).
- Surface trauma can disrupt the normal distribution of body fluids and electrolytes. Surface trauma also can interfere with the maintenance of body temperature. The two physiological responses to surface trauma are vascular and inflammatory reactions. These can lead to healing, scar formation, or both. Many factors can affect or alter wound healing.
- Soft tissue injuries are classified as closed or open. Classification is determined by the absence or presence

of a break in the continuity of the epidermis. Closed wounds include contusions, hematoma, and crush injury. Open wounds are classified as abrasions, lacerations, punctures, avulsions, amputations, and bites.

- Assessment of life-threatening injuries and resuscitation precedes evaluation and intervention of non–life-threatening soft tissue injuries. General wound assessment should include a history of the event that caused the wound and a careful examination of the injury.
- Methods of hemorrhage control include direct pressure, immobilization by splinting, pneumatic pressure devices, and the use of tourniquets.
- The general categories of dressings used in trauma care are sterile, nonsterile, occlusive, nonocclusive, adherent, and nonadherent. The general categories of

bandages are absorbent, nonabsorbent, adherent, and nonadherent.

- Depending on the nature and location of the patient's injury, cleansing, dressings, bandages, and immobilization may be indicated to care for a wound properly.
- The goals of wound care are to prevent infection and protect from infection. Factors that influence the

likelihood of infection include unclean wounds and wound mechanisms and a patient's poor state of health.

- Special considerations for specific wounds include penetrating chest or abdominal injury, avulsion, amputation, and crush syndrome.

REFERENCES

1. National Safety Council: *Injury facts*, Itasca, Ill, 2010, The Council.
2. Rosen P, Barkin R: *Emergency medicine: concepts and clinical practice*, ed 6, St Louis, 2006, Mosby.
3. National Highway Traffic Safety Administration: *The National EMS Education Standards*, Washington, DC, 2009, U.S. Department of Transportation/National Highway Traffic Safety Administration, DOT.
4. Centers for Disease Control and Prevention: HIV transmission, www.cdc.gov/hiv/resources/qa/transmission.htm, accessed 10-4-10.
5. Talan DA, Citron DM, Abrahamian FM, et al: Bacteriologic analysis of infected dog and cat bites, *N Engl J Med* 340:85-92, 1999.
6. Centers for Disease Control and Prevention: Blast injury: crush injury and crush syndrome, www.bt.cdc.gov/masscasualties/pdf/CrushInjury.pdf, accessed 10-16-10.
7. PHTLS and First Aid Science Advisory Board: *Circulation* 112(III):115, 2005.
8. Beekley AC, Sebesta JA, Blackborne LH, et al: Prehospital tourniquet use in Operation Iraqi Freedom: effect on hemorrhage control and outcomes, *J Trauma* 64(2 suppl):S28-S37, 2008.
9. McSwain NE: *PHTLS: Prehospital Trauma Life Support*, ed 7, St Louis, 2011, Mosby.
10. Cain J: Appropriate prehospital tourniquet use, www.jems.com/resources/supplements/the_war_on_trauma/appropriate_prehospital_tourniquet_use.html, accessed 3-06-10.
11. National Foundation for Infectious Diseases: Facts about tetanus for adults, www.nfid.org/pdf/factsheets/tetanusadult.pdf, accessed 10-16-10.

SUGGESTED READING

Kalish J, Burke P: The return of tourniquets: original research evaluates the effectiveness of prehospital tourniquets for civilian penetrating extremity injuries, July 29, 2008, www.jems.com, accessed 1-13-11.

Taillac P, Doyle G: Tourniquet first! Safe and rational protocols for prehospital tourniquet use, Oct 1, 2008, www.jems.com, accessed 1-13-11.

Zeller J, Fox A, Pryor J: Beyond the battlefield: the use of hemostatic dressings in civilian EMS, Mar 1, 2008, www.jems.com, accessed 1-13-11.

CHAPTER
39   Burns

OBJECTIVES

Upon completion of this chapter, the paramedic student will be able to:

1. Describe the incidence, patterns, and sources of burn injury.
2. Describe the pathophysiology of local and systemic responses to burn injury.
3. Classify burn injury according to depth, extent, and severity based on established standards.
4. Discuss the pathophysiology of burn shock as a basis for key signs and symptoms.
5. Outline the physical examination of the burned patient.
6. Describe the prehospital management of the patient who has sustained a burn injury.
7. Discuss pathophysiology as a basis for key signs, symptoms, and management of the patient with an inhalation injury.
8. Outline the general assessment and management of the patient who has a chemical injury.
9. Describe specific complications and management techniques for selected chemical injuries.
10. Describe the physiological effects of electrical injuries as they relate to each body system based on an understanding of key principles of electricity.
11. Outline assessment and management of the patient with electrical injury.
12. Describe the distinguishing features of radiation injury and considerations in the prehospital management of these patients.

KEY TERMS

burn shock Shock that results from local and systemic responses to thermal trauma.

carboxyhemoglobin A compound produced by the exposure of hemoglobin to carbon monoxide.

circumferential burns Burns that encircle a body part, producing a tourniquet-like effect that may quickly compromise circulation.

consensus formula A formula used to calculate the fluid needs of a burn-injured patient over the first 24 hours after injury.

contracture deformity An abnormal, usually permanent condition of a joint characterized by flexion and fixation and caused by atrophy and shortening of muscle fibers or by loss of elasticity of the skin.

eschar A scab or dry crust resulting from a thermal or chemical burn.

escharotomy Surgical incision into necrotic tissue caused by a severe burn; escharotomy sometimes is necessary to prevent edema from building up sufficient interstitial pressure to impair capillary filling and cause ischemia.

full-thickness burn A burn injury in which the entire thickness of the epidermis and dermis is destroyed; also known as a third-degree burn.

inhalation injury An upper and/or lower airway injury that results from thermal and/or chemical exposure.

Lund and Browder chart A method to estimate burn injury that assigns specific numbers to each body part and that

accounts for developmental changes in percentages of body surface area.

partial-thickness burn A burn injury that extends through the epidermis to the dermis; considered a deep partial-thickness injury if it extends to the basal layers of the skin; also known as a second-degree burn.

rule of nines A method to estimate burn injury that divides the total body surface area into segments that are multiples of 9%.

skin graft A portion of skin implanted to cover areas where skin has been lost through burns or injury or by surgical removal of diseased tissue.

smoke inhalation injury Inhalation injury caused by the accumulation of toxic by-products of combustion.

superficial burn A burn injury in which only a superficial layer of epidermal cells is destroyed; also known as a first-degree burn.

zone of coagulation In a burn wound, the central area that has sustained the most intense contact with the thermal source; in this area coagulation necrosis of the cells has occurred and the tissue is nonviable.

zone of hyperemia An area in which blood flow is increased as a result of the normal inflammatory response to injury; it lies at the periphery of the zone of stasis.

zone of stasis The area of burn tissue that surrounds the critically injured area; it consists of tissue that is potentially viable despite the serious thermal injury.

The management of burns often poses a challenge for the paramedic. Understanding the long-term results of a serious burn injury is important. Appropriate prehospital management can reduce morbidity and mortality for burn patients.

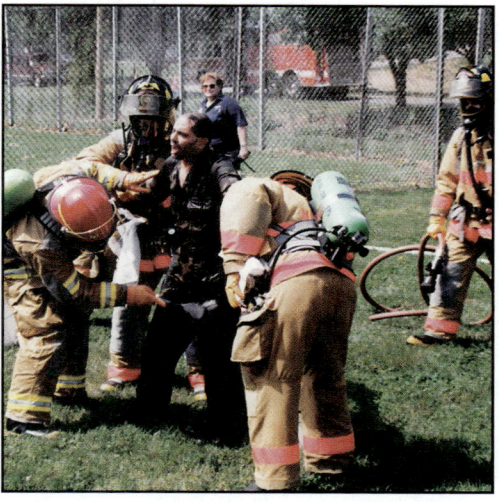

INCIDENCE AND PATTERNS OF BURN INJURY

Burns are a devastating form of trauma. They are associated with high mortality rates, lengthy rehabilitation, cosmetic disfigurement, and permanent physical disabilities. Each year, more than 2 million Americans seek medical attention for burns. Of these, 40,000 persons are hospitalized and about 3500 die as a result of thermal injury or burn-related infection.[1] Box 39-1 lists common complications that contribute to thermal injury deaths.

Morbidity and mortality rates from burn injury follow significant patterns regarding gender, age, and socioeconomic status. For example, two thirds of all fire fatalities are men; the death rate from thermal injury is highest among children and older adults; and three fourths of all fire deaths occur in the home, with the highest incidence in lower-income households.[2] A key part of the professional role of the paramedic is community education. This education should stress prevention as the most effective management of these injuries (see Chapter 3: Injury Prevention and Public Health) (Box 39-2).

Major Sources of Burns

A burn injury is caused by contact between energy and living cells. The source of this energy may be thermal, chemical, electrical, or radiation.

THERMAL BURNS

The majority of burns are thermal. These burns commonly result from flames, scalds, or contact with hot substances. (*Frostbite* is also a thermal injury. Frostbite is addressed in Chapter 45.) Studies have shown that surface temperatures of 44° C (111° F) do not produce burns unless exposure time exceeds 6 hours.[3] At temperatures between 44° and 51° C (111° and 124° F), the rate of epidermal necrosis approximately doubles with each degree of temperature increase. At 70° C (185° F) or greater, the exposure time required to cause transepidermal necrosis is less than 1 second.[4] The degree of tissue destruction depends on the temperature and on the duration of exposure. Factors that influence the ability of the body to resist burn injury

---

BOX 39-1 Physiological and Systemic Complications of Thermal Injuries

Depending on the severity of thermal injury, physiological and systemic complications may include the following:

- Acidosis
- Anoxia
- Dysrhythmias
- Electrolyte loss
- Fluid loss
- Heart failure
- Hypothermia
- Hypovolemia
- Hypoxia
- Infection
- Liver failure
- Renal failure

BOX 39-2 Burn Facts: Selected Statistics on Admissions to Burn Centers, 1999-2008

Survival rate: 96%

Total body surface area (TBSA) burned: more than one third of admissions (33%) exceeded 10% TBSA, 10% exceeded 30% TBSA, and only 4.8% exceeded 40% TBSA. Most included severe burns of such vital body areas as the face, hands, and feet

Gender: 71% male, 29% female

Ethnicity: 63% Caucasian, 17.4% African American, 13% Hispanic, 3.7% other, 2.2% Asian, 0.8% Native American

Burn cause: 41.8% fire/flame, 30.1% scald, 8.5% hot object contact, 3.8% electrical, 2.9% chemical, 9% other

Place of occurrence: 65.5% home, 7.2% street/highway, 11.1% industrial, 16.2% other

From American Burn Association National Burn Repository 2009 Report, Version 5.0, database includes information on more than 127,000 acute burn admissions from 79 hospitals from 33 states. http://www.ameriburn.org/2009NBRAnnualReport.pdf, accessed 6-17-11.

include the water content of the skin tissue; thickness and pigmentation of the skin; presence or absence of insulating substances such as skin oils or hair; and peripheral circulation of the skin, which affects dissipation of heat. Anatomy and physiology of the skin is presented in Chapter 38. The reader should refer to those chapters for review.

LOOK AGAIN
See Chapter 38: Bleeding and Soft Tissue Trauma, pp. 1101-1102.

CRITICAL THINKING
Based on these facts and your knowledge of life span development, would you predict a deeper burn from the same energy source in an 18-year-old or a 75-year-old patient? Why?

SHOW ME THE EVIDENCE
In this descriptive study, researchers in Arizona measured pavement temperatures over 24 hours. They also retrospectively reviewed cases of pavement burns. During the test period, pavement reached temperatures high enough to cause burns within 35 seconds between 10 AM and 5 PM. The patients who sustained pavement burns had neurological compromise (seizures, neuropathy) or were restrained, very young or old, or intoxicated. The mean burn size was 6% (range 1% to 13%). Air temperature ranged from 101° to 112° F (38.3° to 44.4° C) at the time of injury.

From Harrington WZ, Strohschein B, Reedy D, et al: Pavement temperature and burns: streets of fire, *Ann Emerg Med* 26(5):563-568, 1995.

CHEMICAL BURNS

Chemical burns are caused by a substance capable of producing chemical changes in the skin. These chemical changes disrupt the protein structure of the skin, with or without the production of heat. Heat may be generated during the burning process. Yet the chemical changes in the skin, not the heat, produce the greatest injury. Chemical burns differ from thermal burns. With chemical burns, the topical agent usually adheres to the skin for prolonged periods, producing continuous tissue destruction. The severity of the chemical injury is related to the tissue affected, the type of agent, the concentration and volume of the agent, and the duration of contact. Chemical agents that often cause burn injury include acids and alkalis. These agents are found in many household cleaning products and organic compounds. Chemical burns are associated with high morbidity. This is especially the case when they involve the eyes. Inhalation injury (described later in this chapter) may also result from thermal and/or chemical exposure.

NOTE
There are more than 25,000 chemicals used in industry, farming, and in homes that are known to cause burns. These chemicals constitute only about 3% of all burns. However, they have high morbidity (often needing surgery), often involve cosmetic areas of the body, and have a high mortality (about 30%).[5]

ELECTRICAL BURNS

Electrical injuries (including lightning injuries) result from direct contact with an electrical current. Electrical injuries can also result from the arcing of electricity between two contact points near the skin. In a direct contact injury the current itself is not considered to have any thermal properties. The potential energy of the current, however, is changed into thermal energy. This transformation occurs when electricity meets the electrical resistance of biological tissue interposed between the entrance and exit sites. Arc injuries are localized at the termination of current flow. They are caused by the intense heat or flash that occurs when the current "jumps," making contact with the skin. Flame burn also may occur as a result of arcing if the heat generated ignites clothing or another fuel source near the patient.

CRITICAL THINKING
Electrical energy is transformed to heat, causing tissue damage in a human being. Then why does an electrical cord not feel hot when you touch it?

RADIATION BURNS

Radiation injury is caused by ionizing and nonionizing radiation (described later in this chapter). Burns may result from a high level of radiation exposure to a specific body area. However, radiation injuries make up a small percentage of burn injuries.

Local Response to Burn Injury

Burn injury immediately destroys cells or so fully disrupts their metabolic functions that cellular death ensues. Cellular damage is distributed over a spectrum of injury. Some cells are destroyed instantly. Others are irreversibly injured. Some injured cells, though, may survive if rapid and appropriate intervention is provided in the prehospital setting and in-hospital care.

Major thermal burns have three distinct zones of injury (*Jackson's thermal wound theory*). These zones usually appear in a bull's-eye pattern (Figure 39-1). The central area of the burn wound, which has sustained the most intense contact with the thermal source, is the **zone of coagulation.** In this area, coagulation necrosis of the cells has occurred, and the tissue is nonviable. The **zone of stasis** surrounds the critically injured area. It consists of potentially viable tissue

Burn zones

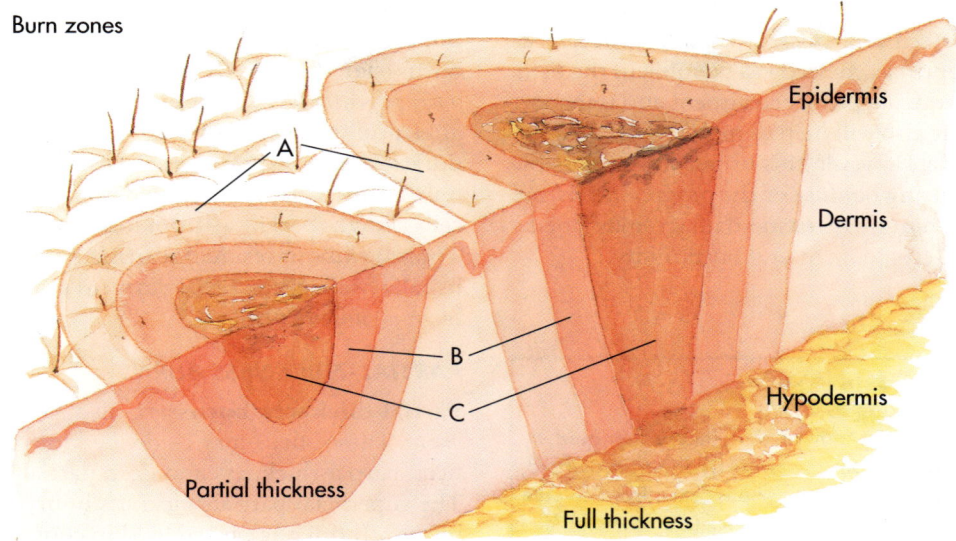

FIGURE 39-1 Three zones of intensity: **(A)** zone of hyperemia (peripheral); **(B)** zone of stasis (intermediate); and **(C)** zone of coagulation (central).

despite the serious thermal injury. In this zone, cells are ischemic because of clotting and vasoconstriction. The cells die within 24 to 48 hours after injury if no supportive measures are undertaken. At the periphery of the zone of stasis is the **zone of hyperemia.** This zone has increased blood flow as a result of the normal inflammatory response. The tissues in this area recover in 7 to 10 days if infection or profound shock does not develop.

Tissue damage from burns depends on the degree of heat and on the duration of exposure to the thermal source. As a rule, the burn wound swells rapidly because of the release of chemical mediators. These mediators cause an increase in capillary permeability and a fluid shift from the intravascular space into the injured tissues. The increased permeability is accentuated by injury to the sodium pump in the cell walls. As sodium moves into the injured cells, it causes an increase in osmotic pressure. This increase in osmotic pressure increases the influx of vascular fluid into the wound. Finally, the normal process of evaporative loss of water to the environment is accelerated (5 to 15 times that of normal skin) through the burned tissue. In a small wound, these physiological alterations produce a classic local inflammatory response (pain, redness, swelling) without major systemic effects. If the wound covers a large area, however, these local tissue responses can produce effects throughout the body and life-threatening hypovolemia.

Systemic Response to Burn Injury

As local events occur at the injury site, other organ systems become involved in a general response to the stress caused by the burn. One of the earliest manifestations of the systemic effects of a large thermal injury is hypovolemic shock. This hypovolemic shock is known as *burn shock* (described

BOX 39-3 Systemic Responses to Major Burn Injury

- Pulmonary response
  Hyperventilation to meet increased metabolic needs
- Gastrointestinal response
  Decrease in splanchnic perfusion that may lead to mucosal hemorrhage and transient adynamic ileus
  Vomiting and aspiration
  Stress ulcers
- Musculoskeletal response
  Decreased range of motion from immobility and edema
  Possible osteoporosis and demineralization (late)
- Neuroendocrine response
  Increased amounts of circulating epinephrine and norepinephrine and transient elevation of aldosterone levels
- Metabolic response
  Elevated metabolic rate, particularly with infection or surgical stress
- Immune response
  Altered immunity, resulting in increased susceptibility to infection
  Depressed inflammatory response
- Emotional response
  Physical pain
  Isolation from loved ones and familiar surroundings
  Fear of disfigurement, deformities, and disability
  Altered self-image
  Depression

later in this chapter). Burn shock is associated with a decrease in venous return, decreased cardiac output, and increased vascular resistance. Burn shock can lead to renal failure. Box 39-3 lists other systemic responses to major burn injury.

CLASSIFICATIONS OF BURN INJURY

Burns must be assessed and classified (body surface area involvement and depth) as correctly as possible in the field. This will help to ensure the proper treatment and transport to a proper facility. It also will help to monitor the progression of tissue damage. However, this usually is not possible in the prehospital setting because of the progressive nature of the injury. The amount of tissue damage may not be evident for hours or even days after a burn injury.

? DID YOU KNOW?

Skin Grafts

   A skin graft is a patch of skin that is removed by surgery from one area of the body (*autografting*) and transplanted, or attached, to another area. Healthy skin is taken from an area on the patient's body called the *donor site*. (Commercial skin substitutes [*heterografts*] or temporary skin substitutes [*cadaver allografts*] are used in some patients instead of autografting.) Most grafts are split-thickness skin grafts; that is, the epidermis and dermis are transplanted from the donor site. The donor site can be any area of the body (most often an area that is hidden by clothes, such as the buttock or inner thigh). The transplanted graft is held in place by special pressure dressings, staples, fibrin glue, synthetic adhesives and/or tapes, or small sutures. The donor site area is covered with a sterile dressing for 3 to 5 days.

   Patients with deeper tissue loss may need a full-thickness skin graft; that is, the entire thickness of the skin is transplanted from the donor site. The flap of skin from the donor site includes the epidermis, dermis, and the muscles and blood supply. New blood supply is established within 36 hours following transplantation. Common donor sites for full-thickness grafts include skin and muscle flaps from the back or the abdominal wall. Full-thickness grafts require a longer recovery period than split-thickness grafts. Most patients will be hospitalized for 1 to 2 weeks following the procedure. Possible complications of skin grafts include:

- Bleeding (which can be severe)
- Infection
- Loss of grafted skin (poor graft take)
- Scarring
- Reduced or lost skin sensation and/or increased sensitivity
- Chronic pain (rarely)
- Uneven skin surface, discoloration, and disfigurement

   Excision and grafting of large areas of burns is stressful. The surgery is tolerated poorly by patients with advanced age, other severe injuries (especially smoke inhalation injury and blunt trauma), and preexisting or coexisting medical conditions (especially diabetes or cardiovascular and peripheral vascular disease).[7]

Depth of Burn Injury

Burns are classified in terms of depth as superficial, partial-thickness, and full-thickness.[6] Superficial and **partial-thickness burns** usually heal without surgery, if the burns are uncomplicated by infection or shock. **Full-thickness burns** usually require **skin grafts.** Other depth classifications may be preferred by medical direction.

SUPERFICIAL BURNS

Superficial burns are also known as *first-degree burns*. These burns characteristically are painful, red, and dry and blanch with pressure (Figure 39-2). Superficial burns usually occur after prolonged exposure to low-intensity heat or a short-duration flash exposure to a heat source. In these burns, only a superficial layer of epidermal cells is destroyed. The cells slough (peel away from healthy tissue underneath the wound) without residual scarring. Superficial burn injuries usually heal within 2 to 3 days. An example of a superficial burn is *sunburn*.

PARTIAL-THICKNESS BURNS

Partial-thickness burns are also known as *second-degree burns*. These burns may be divided into two groups: superficial partial-thickness and deep partial-thickness wounds. The superficial partial-thickness injury is characterized by blisters. It often is caused by skin contact with hot but not boiling water or other hot liquids, explosions producing flash burns, hot grease, and flame.

   In superficial partial-thickness and deep partial-thickness burns (Figure 39-3), injury extends through the epidermis

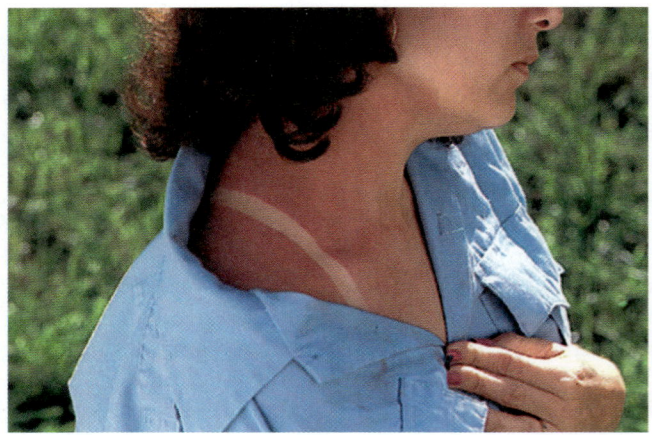

FIGURE 39-2 Superficial burn. (From Shade BR: *Mosby's EMT-intermediate for the 1999 national standards curriculum,* ed 3, St Louis, 2007, Mosby.)

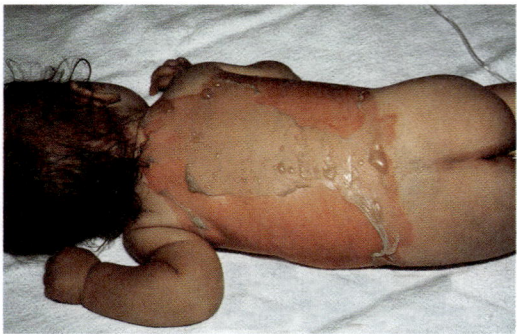

FIGURE 39-3 Superficial partial-thickness second-degree burn. (Courtesy St John's Mercy Medical Center, St Louis, Mo.)

to the dermis. However, the basal layers of the skin are not destroyed, and the skin regenerates within a few days to a week. Edematous fluid infiltrates the dermal-epidermal junction, creating the blisters characteristic of this depth of wound. Intact blisters provide a seal. This seal protects the wound from infection and excessive fluid loss. (For this reason, blisters should not be broken in the prehospital setting unless it is a chemical burn.) The injured area usually is red, wet, and painful and may blanch when the tissue around the injury is compressed. In the absence of infection, these wounds heal without scarring, usually within 14 days.

> **NOTE**
> The dermal layer of skin in children and the elderly is significantly thinner than in the average adult. Therefore, a burn that "looks like" a partial-thickness burn may actually be a more serious full-thickness burn in these patients.

If the depth of the partial-thickness burn involves the basal layer of the dermis, the burn is considered a deep partial-thickness burn (Figure 39-4). As in superficial partial-thickness burns, edema forms at the epidermal-dermal junction. Sensation in and around the wound may be diminished because of the destruction of basal layer nerve endings. The injury may appear red and wet or white and dry. The appearance depends on the degree of vascular injury. Wound infection and subsequent sepsis and fluid loss are major complications of these injuries. If uncomplicated, deep partial-thickness burns generally heal within 3 to 4 weeks. Skin grafting may be needed to promote timely healing and minimize thick scar tissue formation. The formation of thick scar tissue may severely restrict joint movements and may cause persistent pain and disfigurement.

FULL-THICKNESS BURNS

In **full-thickness burns** (also known as *third-degree burns*), the entire thickness of the epidermis and dermis is destroyed; thus skin grafts are necessary for timely and proper healing (Figure 39-5). The wound is characterized by coagulation necrosis of the cells. The wound appears pearly white, charred, or leathery. A definitive sign of a full-thickness burn is a translucent surface in the depths of which thrombosed veins are visible. **Eschar,** a tough, non-elastic coagulated collagen of the dermis, is present in these injuries.

> **NOTE**
> **Escharotomy** is the surgical incision through the eschar to release constricting tissues. This surgery is sometimes performed to allow body tissue and organs to maintain normal perfusion and function. Escharotomy releases the constriction caused by burns, but does not remove the eschar. Additional surgery may be required.

Sensation and capillary refill are absent in full-thickness burns because small blood vessels and nerve endings are destroyed. This often results in large plasma volume loss, infection, and sepsis. Natural wound healing may produce **contracture deformity** (a fixed tightening of the muscles, bones, ligaments, and skin that prevents normal movement). Severe scarring also may develop. Surgical intervention with skin grafting is necessary to close full-thickness wounds, minimize complications, and allow restoration of maximal function.

Some burn classifications also describe a full-thickness injury (sometimes called a *fourth-degree burn*) that penetrates the subcutaneous tissue, muscle, fascia, periosteum, or bone. These burns often result from incineration-type exposure and electrical burns in which the heat is great enough to destroy tissues below the skin.

Extent and Severity of Burn Injury

There are several methods to evaluate the extent of burn injury. Two common methods include the **rule of nines** and the **Lund and Browder chart.** The paramedic should use a method for determining the extent of burn injury

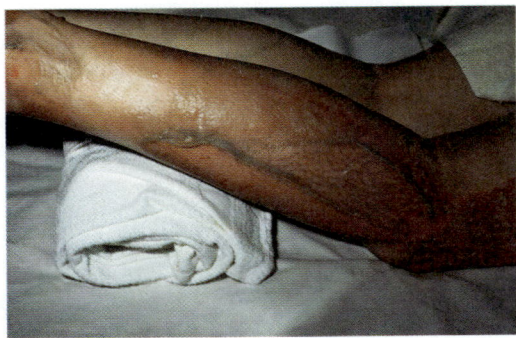

FIGURE 39-4 Deep partial-thickness burn. (Courtesy St John's Mercy Medical Center, St Louis, Mo.)

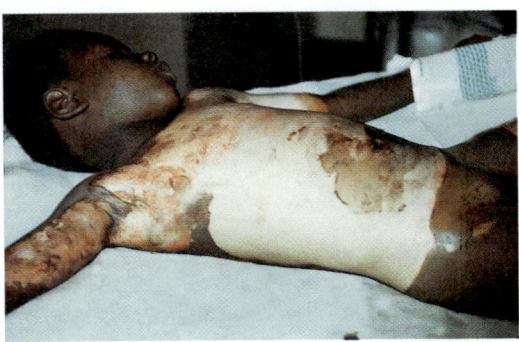

FIGURE 39-5 Full-thickness burn. (Courtesy St John's Mercy Medical Center, St Louis, Mo.)

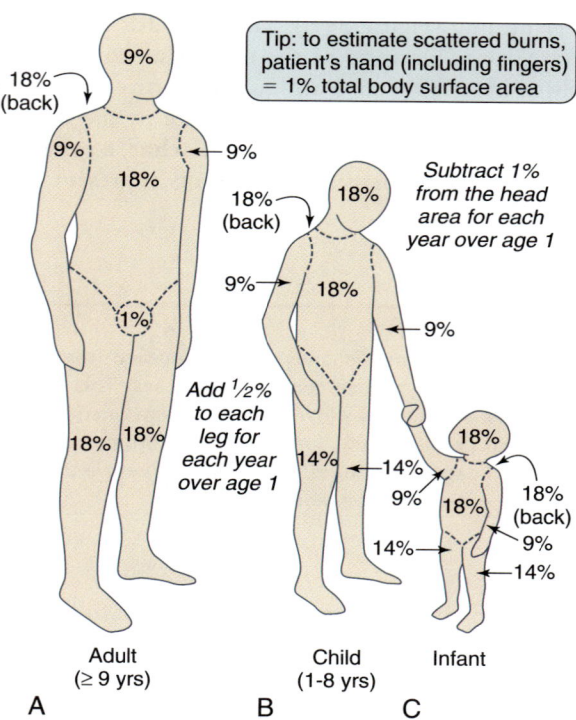

Tip: to estimate scattered burns, patient's hand (including fingers) = 1% total body surface area

FIGURE 39-6 The rule of nines. **A,** Adult; **B,** child; **C,** infant. (Modified from Sole ML: *Introduction to critical care nursing,* ed 5, Philadelphia, 2009, Saunders. Courtesy University of Michigan Trauma Burn Center, Ann Arbor, Mich.)

approved by medical direction. Use of any method to evaluate a burn injury should never delay patient care or transport.

RULE OF NINES

The rule of nines commonly is used in the prehospital setting. The measurement divides the total body surface area (TBSA) into segments that are multiples of 9%. This method provides a rough estimate of burn injury size and is most accurate for adults and children older than 10 years of age. Figure 39-6 explains the rule of nines.

> **CRITICAL THINKING**
> Why is the calculation of body surface area different for children less than 10 years of age?

If the burn is irregularly shaped or has a scattered distribution throughout the body, the rule of nines is difficult to apply. In these cases, burn size can be estimated by visualizing the patient's hand as an indicator of percentage. (This is the *rule of palms.*) The surface of the patient's hand, including fingers, equals about 1% of the TBSA.

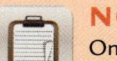

> **NOTE**
> Only partial- and full-thickness burns are included when calculating total body surface area. For large burns, total body surface area may be calculated more easily by subtracting the percentage of unburned area from 100.

LUND AND BROWDER CHART

The Lund and Browder chart (Figure 39-7) is a more accurate method of determining the area of burn injury because it assigns specific numbers to each body part. The chart allows for developmental changes in percentages of body surface area. For example, the adult head is 9% of TBSA, but the newborn head is 18% of TBSA.

AMERICAN BURN ASSOCIATION CATEGORIZATION

The American Burn Association has devised a method of categorizing burns to determine severity. The method is based on extent, depth, and location of burn injury; age of the patient; etiological agents involved; presence of inhalation injury; and coexisting injuries or preexisting illness. Using these criteria, burn injuries are categorized as *major, moderate,* and *minor* (Box 39-4).

> **BOX 39-4   Classification of Burn Severity**
>
> **Major Burns**
> 1. Partial-thickness burns greater than 25% of body surface area (BSA) in adults or greater than 20% of BSA in children or the elderly
> 2. Full-thickness burns greater than 10% of BSA
> 3. All burns involving the face, eyes, ears, hands, feet, or perineum that may result in functional or cosmetic impairment
> 4. Burns caused by caustic chemical agents
> 5. High-voltage electrical injury
> 6. Burns complicated by inhalation injury, major trauma, or in poor-risk patients
>
> **Moderate Burns**
> 1. Partial-thickness burns 15% to 25% of BSA in adults and 10% to 20% of BSA in children or the elderly
> 2. Full-thickness burns less than 10% of BSA
> 3. Not involving risk to areas of specialized function such as the face, eyes, ears, hands, feet, or perineum
>
> **Minor Burns**
> 1. Burns less than 15% of BSA in adults or 10% of BSA in children or the elderly
> 2. Full-thickness burns less than 2% of BSA
> 3. No functional or cosmetic risk to areas of specialized function

Adapted from the American Burn Association Injury Severity Grading System. American Burn Association, *J Burn Care Rehabil* 11:98-104, 1990, with additional information from Hartford CE: Care of outpatient burns. In Herndon DN, editor. *Total burn care,* pp. 71-80, Philadelphia, 1996, Saunders.

Age	0-1	1-4	5-9	10-14	15
A—$1/2$ of head	$9^1/_2$%	$8^1/_2$%	$6^1/_2$%	$5^1/_2$%	$4^1/_2$%
B—$1/2$ of one thigh	$2^3/_4$%	$3^1/_4$%	4%	$4^1/_4$%	$4^1/_2$%
C—$1/2$ of one leg	$2^1/_2$%	$2^1/_2$%	$2^3/_4$%	3%	$3^1/_4$%

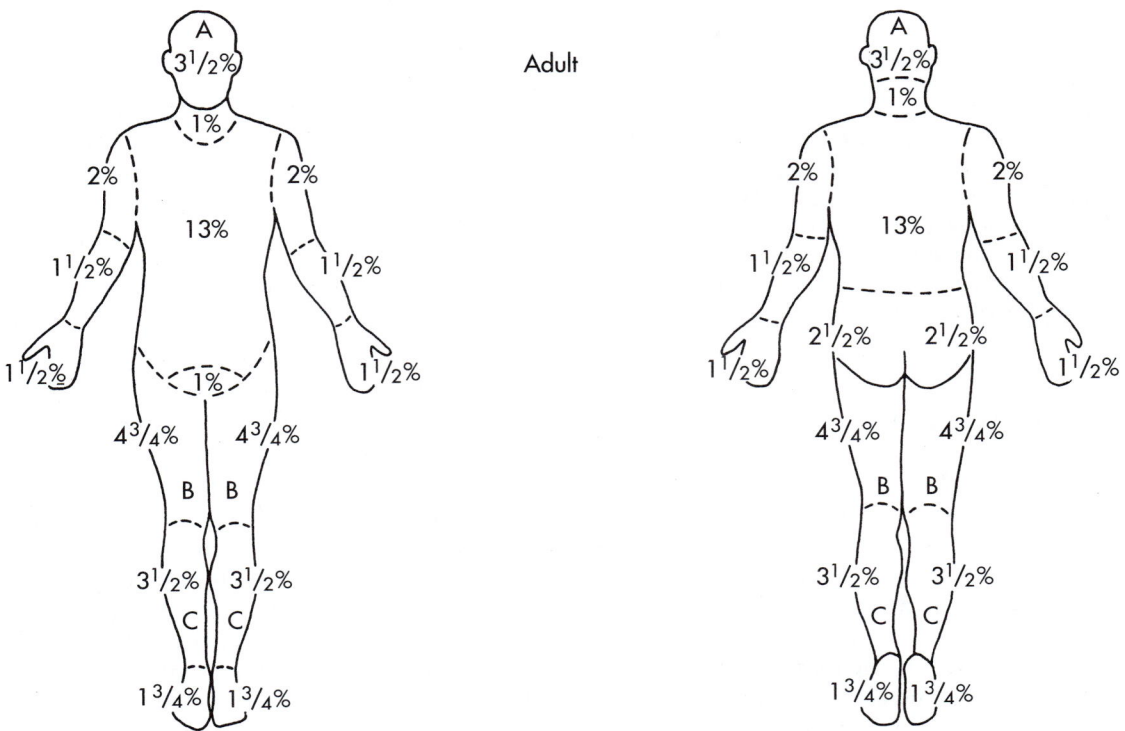

Adult

FIGURE 39-7 Lund and Browder chart. (From Lee G: *Flight nursing: principles and practice,* St Louis, 1991, Mosby.)

In determining severity, the paramedic also must consider factors such as the patient's age, the presence of concurrent medical or surgical problems, and the complications that accompany certain types of burns, such as those of the face and neck, hands and feet, and genitalia. For example, burns of the face and neck may cause respiratory compromise. They also may interfere with the ability to eat or drink. Burns of the hands and feet may interfere with ambulation and activities of daily living. Perineal burns present a high risk of infection because of the contaminants in this region. These burns may disrupt the normal patterns of elimination.

Burn Center Referral Criteria

Many emergency medical services use categories or other criteria determined by medical direction as the basis for determining which patients need transport to specialized burn centers. (See the CDC Triage Guidelines, described in Chapter 37.) According to the Committee on Trauma of the American College of Surgeons and the American Burn Association, burn injuries usually requiring referral to a burn center include the following[8]:

1. Partial-thickness burns greater than 10% total body surface area
2. Burns that involve the face, hands, feet, genitalia, perineum, or major joints
3. Third-degree burns in any age group
4. Electrical burns, including lightning injury
5. Chemical burns
6. Inhalation injury
7. Burn injury in patients with preexisting medical disorders that could complicate management, prolong recovery, or affect mortality
8. Any patients with burns and concomitant trauma (such as fractures) in which the burn injury poses the greatest risk of morbidity or mortality. In such cases, if the trauma poses the greater immediate risk, the patient may be initially stabilized in a trauma center before being transferred to a burn unit. Physician judgment will be necessary in such situations and should be in

concert with the regional medical control plan and triage protocols

9. Burned children in hospitals without qualified personnel or equipment for the care of children
10. Burn injury in patients who will require special social, emotional, or long-term rehabilitative intervention

> **NOTE**
> Verification of burn centers is a joint program of the American Burn Association (ABA) and the American College of Surgeons (ACS). It is a rigorous review program designed to verify a burn center's resources that are required for the provision of optimal care to burn patients from the time of injury through rehabilitation. About 55% of the 45,000 U.S. hospitalizations for burn injury each year are now admitted to the 125 hospitals with specialized burn centers.[9]

PATHOPHYSIOLOGY OF BURN SHOCK

As stated previously, shock can occur from large body surface area burns. **Burn shock** results from local and systemic responses to thermal trauma. The trauma leads to edema and accumulation of vascular fluid in the tissues in the area of injury. Locally, a brief initial decrease in blood flow to the area occurs (this is the *emergent phase*). This is followed by a considerable increase in arteriolar vasodilation. A concurrent release of vasoactive substances from the burned tissue causes increased capillary permeability. This in turn produces intravascular fluid loss and wound edema (the *fluid shift phase*). The fluid shifts cause cardiovascular changes such as a compromised cardiac output, increased systemic vascular resistance, and reduced peripheral blood flow.

> **NOTE**
> Hypovolemia caused by burn trauma usually is not seen in the prehospital setting. This is because burn edema develops over the first several hours after the burn. A hypovolemic patient with burns should be evaluated at the scene for other injuries that may be responsible for the volume loss.

Hypovolemia results from fluid loss in the injured tissues and fluid that evaporates from the body because of the loss of the skin. Despite the compensatory effort of the body to retain sodium and water, sodium is lost and potassium is released into the extracellular fluid. The blood becomes concentrated. In severe burns, red blood cells may burst (hemolyze). When combined with hemolysis, rhabdomyolysis, and subsequent hemoglobinuria and myoglobinuria seen with major burns and electrical injury, this

hypovolemic state can lead to renal failure (see Chapter 11: General Principles of Pathophysiology). Impaired peripheral blood flow can damage tissue further and can result in metabolic acidosis.

The greatest loss of intravascular fluid occurs in the first 8 to 12 hours. This loss is followed by a continued, moderate loss over the next 12 to 16 hours. At some point within 24 hours, the leaking of fluid from the cells greatly diminishes (this is the *resolution phase*). At this point, a balance between the intravascular space and the interstitial space is reached. Peripheral vascular resistance will increase in response to hypovolemia and the resulting decrease in cardiac output. With volume replacement, cardiac output can increase to levels above normal (this is the *hypermetabolic phase* of thermal injury) (Figure 39-8).

Fluid Replacement

Within minutes of a major burn injury, all capillaries in the circulatory system (not just those in the area of the burn) lose the ability to retain fluid. This increase in capillary permeability prevents the creation of an osmotic gradient between the intravascular and extravascular space. This change allows colloid solutions to equilibrate quickly across the capillaries and into the surrounding tissue. The process of burn shock continues for about 24 hours, at which time the normal capillary permeability is restored.[10] Therefore therapy for burn shock is aimed at supporting the patient's vital organ function through the period of hypovolemic shock. Crystalloid solution (e.g., lactated Ringer's solution or normal saline) usually is considered the fluid of choice in initial resuscitation.

> **NOTE**
> Fluid resuscitation in burn-injured persons is controversial. As a rule, fluid resuscitation should be initiated in the prehospital setting in patients with >20% TBSA burns if IV access can be quickly accomplished.[11] Transport should not be delayed to initiate intravenous therapy.

Several fluid resuscitation formulae consider body size and extent of burned body surface area. These formulae have proved clinically useful in replacing fluids. The two most common formulae for estimating fluid replacement are the *Parkland formula* and the *modified Brooke formula*. These formulae have been combined into the **consensus formula**. All three formulae stipulate that half of the total calculated amount of fluid should be infused over the first 8 hours from the time of the injury. The second half should be infused over the following 16 hours. Fluid resuscitation must be guided by regular monitoring of measures of hemodynamic function, including the patient's vital signs, respiratory rate, lung sounds, capillary refill, and, in some cases, urinary output. *When determining the percentage of burn for fluid resuscitation, the paramedic should calculate only partial- and full-thickness burns.*

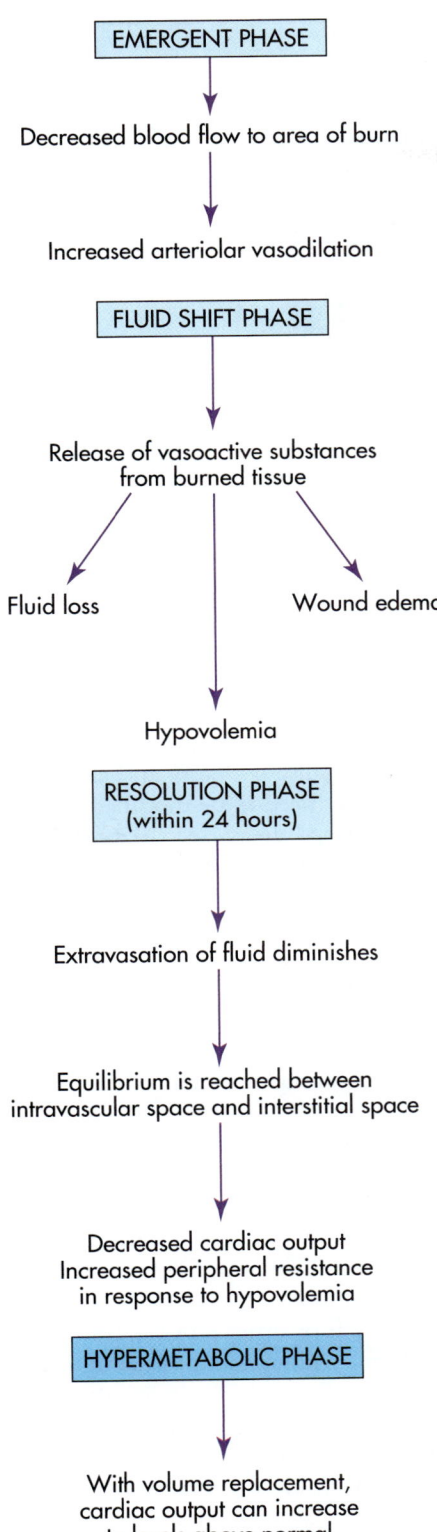

EMERGENT PHASE

↓

Decreased blood flow to area of burn

↓

Increased arteriolar vasodilation

FLUID SHIFT PHASE

↓

Release of vasoactive substances
from burned tissue

↓ ↘

Fluid loss   Wound edema

↓

Hypovolemia

RESOLUTION PHASE
(within 24 hours)

↓

Extravasation of fluid diminishes

↓

Equilibrium is reached between
intravascular space and interstitial space

↓

Decreased cardiac output
Increased peripheral resistance
in response to hypovolemia

HYPERMETABOLIC PHASE

↓

With volume replacement,
cardiac output can increase
to levels above normal

FIGURE 39-8 Phases of burn shock.

CONSENSUS FORMULA

The consensus formula is applied as follows:

1. The first 24 hours: 4 mL/kg lactated Ringer's solution or normal saline multiplied by percent of TBSA burned
   a. 50% of the calculated amount infused in the first 8 hours
   b. 25% of the calculated amount infused in the second 8 hours
   c. 25% of the calculated amount infused in the third 8 hours

   Example:

   A patient who weighs 100 kg has 30% body surface area (BSA) burns. Total fluid to be infused in the first 24 hours at 4 mL/kg is calculated as follows: 4 mL × 30% BSA × 100 kg = 12,000 mL. Of the 12,000 mL, 6000 mL should be infused in the first 8 hours at a rate of 750 mL/hr. Note that the volume of fluid actually infused may be adjusted according to patient needs as prescribed by medical direction.

The amount and type of fluids required after the first 24 hours are vastly different from those administered during the first 24 hours. Fluid replacement is dictated by the patient's response to the burn and the treatment regimen.

ASSESSMENT OF THE BURN PATIENT

As with any other trauma patient, emergency care for a burn patient begins with scene safety and the primary survey. In this assessment the paramedic should recognize and treat injuries that pose a threat to life. In burn patients, however, the dramatic appearance of burns, the patient's intense pain, and the characteristic odor of burnt flesh may distract the paramedic from life-threatening problems. A confident assessment by the paramedic and direction of efforts away from the burn wound and toward the patient as a whole are crucial.

Primary Survey

The evaluation of the patient's airway is a major concern, particularly for the patient with an inhalation injury (described later in this chapter). The paramedic should observe for stridor (an ominous sign of airway narrowing), facial burns, soot in the nose or mouth, singed facial or nasal hair, edema of lips and the oral cavity, coughing, inability to swallow secretions in the pharynx, hoarse voice, and **circumferential burns** around the neck or thorax. Airway management should be aggressive with these patients (Figure 39-9).

> **CRITICAL THINKING**
> Consider a patient who has a large burn. Your initial assessment reveals that the airway is patent. Why should you perform frequent reassessment of the airway?

The paramedic should evaluate breathing for rate, depth, and the presence of wheezes, crackles, or rhonchi. The patient's circulatory status is evaluated by assessing the presence, rate, character, and rhythm of pulses; capillary

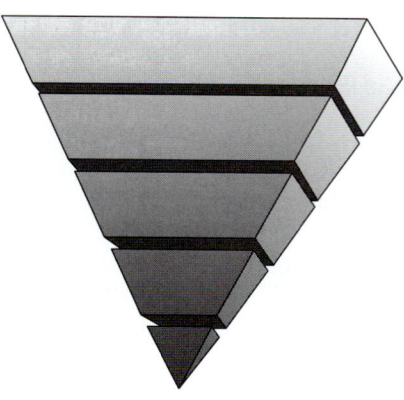

- Burns around nose or mouth

- Soot in mouth or nose: singed nasal hairs

- Intraoral burns: burned tongue

- Intraoral swelling (no stridor)

- Hoarseness of voice

- Visible pharyngeal edema

- Inspiratory stridor

FIGURE 39-9 Decreasing probability of upper airway obstruction.

refill; skin color and temperature; pulse oximetry, which may be inaccurate in the presence of carbon monoxide; and obvious arterial bleeding. The paramedic should determine the patient's neurological status by using the AVPU scale or similar method. The paramedic should evaluate carefully any deviations from normal for underlying cause. Abnormalities include hypoxia, decreased cerebral perfusion from hypovolemia, and cerebral injury resulting from head trauma. After the primary survey, a history of the event should be obtained while performing the secondary assessment.

An accurate history from the patient or bystanders can help the paramedic to determine the potential for inhalation injury, concomitant trauma, or preexisting conditions that may influence the physical examination or patient outcome. When obtaining the patient history, the paramedic should ascertain the following information:

1. What is the patient's chief complaint (e.g., pain or dyspnea)?
2. What were the circumstances of the injury?
   - Did the injury occur in an enclosed space?
   - Were explosive forces involved?
   - Were hazardous chemicals involved?
   - Is there related trauma?
3. What was the source of the burning agent (e.g., flame, metal, liquid, or chemical)?
4. Does the patient have any significant medical history?
5. What medications does the patient take (including recent ingestion of illegal drugs or alcohol)?
6. Did the patient lose consciousness at any time? (Suspect inhalation injury.)
7. What is the status of tetanus immunization?

Physical Examination

At the start of the physical exam, the paramedic should obtain a full set of vital signs. The paramedic should obtain a blood pressure measurement from an unburned extremity, if available. If all extremities are burned, the paramedic may place sterile gauze under the blood pressure cuff and attempt to auscultate a blood pressure. Patients with severe burns or preexisting cardiac or medical illness should be monitored with pulse oximetry and electrocardiogram. Lead placement may need to be modified to avoid placing electrodes over burned areas (see Chapter 22). Field care and hospital destination are determined by the depth, size, location, and extent of burned tissue and the presence of associated illness or injury.

GENERAL PRINCIPLES IN BURN MANAGEMENT

Goals for prehospital management of the severely burned patient include preventing further tissue injury, maintaining the airway, administering oxygen and ventilatory support, managing pain, providing fluid resuscitation (per protocol), providing rapid transport to an appropriate medical facility, using clean technique to minimize the patient's exposure to infectious agents, and providing psychological and emotional support. Patients with burns also should be evaluated for other types of trauma that pose a threat to life. Some will have additional injuries associated with the burn event. Examples include blunt or penetrating trauma sustained in automobile crashes, blast injury, and skeletal or spinal injury from attempts to escape the thermal source or contact with electrical current.

> **NOTE**
> Some burns will be very painful for the patient. Medications used to manage pain may include **morphine, fentanyl,** hydromorphone, and others. The presence or absence of IV access directly influences analgesic drug choice, particularly in children in whom IV access may be problematic.

Stopping the Burning Process

The first step in managing any burn is to stop the burning process. This step must be achieved with the safety of the emergency crew in mind because it often occurs in proximity to the source that caused the burn. With superficial burns the burning process can be terminated by cooling the local area with cool tap water.[11] Ice-cold water, ice, snow, or ointments should not be applied to the burn. These agents may increase the depth and severity of thermal injury. In addition, ointments may impair or delay assessment of the injury when the patient arrives in the emergency department.

In cases of severe burns the paramedic should move the patient rapidly and safely from the burning source to an area of safety if possible. A person whose clothing is in flames or smoldering should be placed on the floor or ground and rolled in a blanket to smother the flames or should be doused with large quantities of the cleanest available room-temperature water. (Cool water to decrease skin temperature rapidly is preferred.) Contaminated water sources, such as lakes or rivers, should be avoided. These patients should never be allowed to run or remain standing. Running may fan the flame, and an upright position may increase the likelihood of the patient's hair being ignited.

> **NOTE**
> The National Fire Protection Association developed a training program called *Stop, Drop, and Roll*. The program was designed to teach children and adults that in the event their clothing catches fire, they should *stop* (do not run); *drop* (cover your face with your hands and drop to the ground in a prone position); and *roll* (to smother the fire until the flames are extinguished).

The paramedic should remove the patient's clothing completely while cooling the burn so that heat is not trapped under the smoldering cloth. If pieces of smoldering cloth have adhered to the skin, the paramedic should cut, not pull, the clothing and gently remove it. Melted synthetic fabrics that cannot be removed should be soaked in water to stop the burning process. After the burn is cooled, the patient with a large body surface area injury should be covered with a clean, preferably sterile sheet to prevent hypothermia. Blankets may be placed over the sheet when ambient temperatures are low. The duration of cooling is controversial; cooling should continue at least until pain is relieved[12] and probably for a total duration of 15 to 30 minutes. Local cooling of less than 9% TBSA can be continued longer than 30 minutes to relieve pain.

Airway, Oxygen, and Ventilation

The paramedic should evaluate the adequacy of airway and breathing in all burn patients. Humidified high-concentration oxygen (if available) should be given to any patient with severe burns. Breathing should be assisted as needed. Use of continuous pulse oximetry is indicated in these patients. If inhalation injury is suspected, the paramedic should observe the patient closely for signs of impending airway obstruction. Life-threatening laryngeal edema may be progressive and may make tracheal intubation difficult if not impossible. The decision to intubate these patients should not be delayed. The paramedic should make every attempt to intubate the patient's trachea with a normal (not smaller) size endotracheal tube. The lungs of these patients often are difficult to ventilate, even with an appropriately sized tube. The decision to intubate in the field should be guided by transport time to the receiving hospital and indications of impending airway obstruction.

Circulation

The need for fluid resuscitation is based on the severity of the injury, the patient's vital signs, and the transport time to the receiving hospital. Some authorities contend that prompt intervention of intravenous therapy in the critically burned patient is essential to prevent long-term complications such as burn shock and renal failure. (The paramedic should consult with medical direction and follow local protocol regarding fluid replacement via the intravenous [IV] or intraosseous [IO] route.)

If intravenous therapy is to be performed, it should be initiated with a large-bore catheter in a peripheral vein in an unburned extremity. (The arm is the preferred site.) If an unburned site is not available, the paramedic may insert the catheter through burned tissue, although the risk of subsequent infection is greater. Care should be taken to secure the catheter with a dressing; tape may not adhere to the injured area as the tissue begins to leak fluid.

The administration of pain medication is an early intervention. Medical direction may recommend that patients with painful burns be given IV *morphine* or *fentanyl,* or other analgesic agents (e.g., *nitrous oxide*). Some of these medications can cause vasodilation and respiratory depression. Thus fluid resuscitation and ventilation support must be adequate. Other pharmacological therapy that may be given after arrival in the emergency department includes topical applications (e.g., silver sulfadiazine or special synthetic dressings), oral analgesics, and tetanus immunization.

> **CRITICAL THINKING**
> How should you administer pain medicine to a patient with a large burn? Why did you choose this route?

At times, transport of the burn patient is delayed. A lengthy interfacility transport may be anticipated as well. In either case, other patient care procedures may be required. One such procedure includes the placement of a nasogastric tube to prevent gastric distention or vomiting. Another procedure is the placement of an indwelling urinary catheter. This will measure urine output and maintain patency of the urethra in patients with burns to the genitalia (see Chapter 52).

> **NOTE**
> Urine output is a means to evaluate the effectiveness of fluid resuscitation. When the Parkland consensus formula is used, the patient is titrated to maintain urine output of 0.3 to 1.0 mL/kg/hr and a mean arterial pressure of 60 mm Hg or greater.[13]

Special Considerations

All burn injuries warrant good patient assessment and care. However, burns of specific body regions require special consideration. These include burns to the face and extremities and circumferential burns.

Burns of the face swell rapidly. These burns may be associated with airway problems. The head of the ambulance stretcher should be elevated at least 30 degrees, if not contraindicated by spinal trauma, to minimize the edema. If the patient's ears are burned, the paramedic should avoid use of a pillow to minimize additional injury to the area.

If burns involve the extremities or large areas of the body, the paramedic should remove all rings, watches, and other jewelry as soon as possible. This will help to prevent vascular compromise with increased wound edema. Peripheral pulses should be assessed frequently and burned limbs should be elevated above the patient's heart if possible.

> **CRITICAL THINKING**
> What life- or limb-threatening problems can develop from this swelling?

Burn injuries that encircle a body region can pose a threat to the patient's life or limbs. Circumferential burns that occur to an extremity may produce a tourniquet-like effect that may quickly compromise circulation. The effect can cause irreversible damage to the limb. Circumferential burns of the chest can severely restrict movement of the thorax. These burns may impair chest wall compliance significantly. If this occurs, the depth of respirations is reduced; tidal volume is decreased; and the patient's lungs may become difficult to ventilate, even by mechanical means. Definitive treatment for circumferential burns involves an in-hospital escharotomy to reduce compartment pressure and allow adequate blood volume to flow to and from the affected limb or thorax.

INHALATION BURN INJURIES

Smoke inhalation injury affects between 5% and 35% of all patients admitted to hospitals. The presence of inhalation injury increases the mortality from burns by 20%, and when combined with pneumonia by 60%.[11] Prehospital considerations in caring for patients with inhalation injury include recognition of the dangers inherent in the fire environment, awareness of the pathophysiological principles of inhalation injury, and early detection and treatment of impending airway or respiratory problems.

Smoke inhalation most often occurs in a closed environment such as a building, a vehicle, or an airplane. Such injury is caused by the accumulation of toxic by-products of combustion. Inhalation injury also can occur in an open space. Therefore all burn victims should be evaluated for this injury. Dangers that contribute to inhalation injury in a fire environment are:

- Heat
- Consumption of oxygen by the fire
- Production of carbon monoxide
- Production of other toxic gases such as cyanide and hydrogen sulfide

Inhalation injury also may occur in the absence of significant thermal injury from exposure to toxic gases (e.g., carbon monoxide).

> **NOTE**
> Responding to a scene with a possibility of smoke inhalation injury also poses a threat to EMS personnel. Carbon monoxide meters and other testing devices to measure dangerous gases should be used to ensure scene safety.

Pathophysiology

Smoke inhalation and inhalation injury can produce a large number of complications. For this text, these complications are classified as carbon monoxide poisoning, inhalation injury above the glottis (*supraglottic*), and inhalation injury below the glottis (*infraglottic*).

Carbon Monoxide Poisoning

Carbon monoxide is a colorless, odorless, tasteless gas produced by incomplete burning of carbon-containing fuels. Carbon monoxide does not harm lung tissue physically. However, it displaces oxygen from the hemoglobin molecule, forming **carboxyhemoglobin.** The result is low circulating volumes of oxygen despite normal partial pressures. In addition, the presence of carboxyhemoglobin requires that tissues be hypoxic before oxygen is released from the hemoglobin to fuel the cells. This condition is reversible.

Carbon monoxide has about 250 times the attraction to hemoglobin that oxygen has. Therefore small concentrations of carbon monoxide in inspired air can result in severe physiological impairments, including tissue hypoxia, inadequate cellular oxygenation, inadequate cellular and organ function, and eventually death. The physical effects of carbon monoxide poisoning are related to the level of carboxyhemoglobin in the blood (Box 39-5).

BOX 39-5 Physical Effects of Carbon Monoxide Blood Levels

Carbon monoxide levels less than 10% usually do not cause symptoms; they are common in smokers, traffic police, truck drivers, and others who are exposed to carbon monoxide chronically. At carbon monoxide levels of 20% a healthy patient may complain of headache, nausea, vomiting, and loss of manual dexterity. At 30% the patient may become confused and lethargic, and electrocardiogram abnormalities may be present. At levels between 40% and 60%, coma may develop. Levels above 60% often are fatal. Tachypnea and cyanosis usually are not present in these patients because arterial oxygen tension is normal. Patients with high carboxyhemoglobin levels may have a skin appearance that is bright red. More commonly, though, the patient has normal or pale skin and lip coloration.

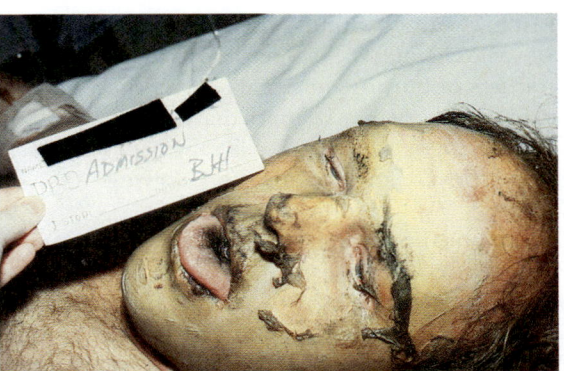

FIGURE 39-10 Signs of inhalation injury.

NOTE
As discussed in Chapter 15, the pulse oximeter is unreliable in determining effective oxygenation in a patient with carbon monoxide poisoning.

Prehospital care for the patient with carbon monoxide poisoning includes ensuring a patent airway, providing adequate ventilation, and administering high-concentration oxygen. The half-life of carbon monoxide at room air is about 4 hours. This half-life can be reduced to 30 to 90 minutes if 100% oxygen and adequate ventilations are provided.[14] The use of hyperbaric oxygen therapy may be recommended in treating carbon monoxide poisoning. This therapy promotes increased oxygen uptake by hemoglobin molecules that have not yet been bound to carbon monoxide. The paramedic should follow local protocol.

In addition to carbon monoxide, other gases (e.g., cyanide and hydrogen sulfide) may be released when some materials are burned. The inhalation of these toxic gases can result in inhalation poisoning (e.g., *thiocyanate intoxication*). This may require pharmacological therapy (e.g., *hydroxycobalamin,* cyanide antidote kit) as described in Chapter 34.

LOOK AGAIN
See Chapter 34: Toxicology, pp. 993-994.

CRITICAL THINKING
Can carbon monoxide poisoning be ruled out if the patient does not have these signs or symptoms?

Inhalation Injury Above the Glottis

The structure and function of the airway superior to the glottis make it susceptible to injury if exposed to high temperatures. The upper airway is vascular and has a large surface area. This allows the upper airway to normalize temperatures of inspired air. Because of this design, actual thermal injury to the lower airway is rare. The upper airway sustains the impact of injury when environmental air is superheated.

Thermal injury to the airway can result in immediate edema of the pharynx and larynx (above the level of the true vocal cords). This can progress rapidly to complete airway obstruction. Signs and symptoms of upper airway inhalation injury include the following (Fig. 39-10):

- Facial burns
- Singed nasal or facial hairs
- Carbonaceous sputum
- Edema of the face, oropharyngeal cavity, or both
- Signs of hypoxemia
- Hoarse voice
- Stridor
- Brassy cough
- Grunting respirations

Prompt assessment of the airway is critical in these patients. The paramedic must establish and protect the airway. If impending airway obstruction is suspected, early nasotracheal or orotracheal intubation may be warranted because progressive edema can make intubation hazardous if not impossible.

Inhalation Injury Below the Glottis

The two main mechanisms of direct injury to the lung tissue are heat and toxic material inhalation. Thermal injury to the lower airway is rare. One cause of such injury is the inhalation of superheated steam. This steam has 4000 times the heat-carrying capacity of dry air.[15] Another cause is the aspiration of scalding liquids. Explosions are another cause. These occur as the patient is breathing high concentrations of oxygen under pressure.

Most lower airway injuries in fires result from the inhalation of toxic chemicals. Such chemicals include the gaseous by-products of burning materials. Signs and symptoms of lower airway injury may be immediate, but more often they are delayed. Signs and symptoms may begin several hours after the exposure and include the following:

- Wheezes
- Crackles or rhonchi
- Productive cough
- Signs of hypoxemia
- Spasm of bronchi and bronchioles

Prehospital care should be directed at maintaining a patent airway providing high-concentration oxygen and ventilatory support. Specific airway and ventilatory management should be guided by online/direct medical direction. This may include nasal or oral tracheal intubation and drug therapy with bronchodilators.

 SHOW ME THE EVIDENCE
These researchers used data from a trauma registry to compare burn patients injured in methamphetamine-related incidents to another group of burn patients.

Body surface area burned was similar in both groups. Methamphetamine-injured patients needed endotracheal intubation more often and required a larger fluid volume for resuscitation than the controls. The methamphetamine group was more likely to have inhalation injury and to develop pneumonia than the control group.

From Blostein PA, Plaisier B, Sheldon BM, et al: Methamphetamine production is hazardous to your health, *J Trauma* 66(6):1712-1717, 2009.

CHEMICAL BURN INJURIES

Caustic chemicals often are present in the home and workplace. Unintentional exposure is common. Three types of caustic agents often are associated with burn injuries. These are alkalis, acids, and organic compounds. Alkalis are strong bases with a high pH. Alkalis include hydroxides and carbonates of sodium, potassium, ammonium, lithium, barium, and calcium. These compounds commonly are found in oven cleaners, household drain cleaners, fertilizers, heavy industrial cleaners, and the structural bonds of cement and concrete. Strong acids are in many household cleaners, such as rust removers, bathroom cleaners, and swimming pool acidifiers (Figure 39-11).

Organic compounds are chemicals that contain carbon. Most organic compounds, such as wood and coal, are harmless chemicals. However, several organic compounds produce caustic injury to human tissue. These compounds include phenols and creosote and petroleum products such as gasoline. In addition to their role in producing chemical burns, organic compounds may be absorbed by the skin. As described in Chapter 34, absorption in turn may cause serious systemic effects. The severity of chemical injury is related to the type of chemical agent, concentration and volume of the chemical, and duration of contact.

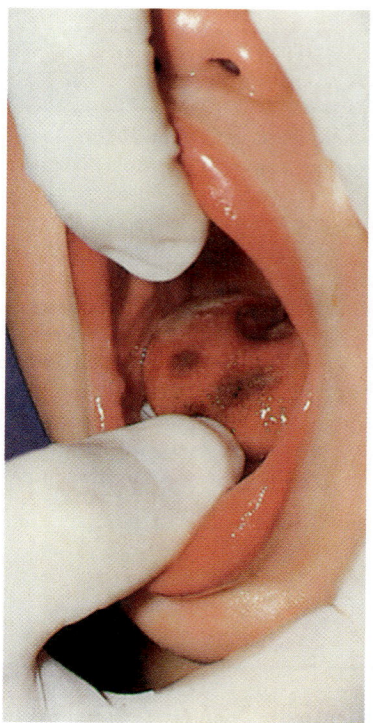

FIGURE 39-11 Intraoral chemical burns sustained by a boy who had ingested bleach. (From Beattie T, et al: *Pediatric emergencies*, London, 1997, Mosby-Wolfe.)

 **LOOK AGAIN**
See Chapter 34: Toxicology, pp. 1002-1004.

Assessment

While obtaining the patient history, the paramedic should collect facts regarding the exposure. When dealing with a chemical exposure, the paramedic should determine the following:

- Type of chemical substance. If the container is available and can be transported safely, it should be taken to the medical facility
- Concentration of chemical substance
- Volume of chemical substance
- Mechanism of injury (e.g., local immersion of a body part, injection, splash)
- Time of contamination
- First aid administered before EMS arrival
- Appearance (chemical burns vary in color)
- Pain

Management

As with all burn injuries, the safety of the rescuers must be the first priority in managing the victim of chemical injury. (Law enforcement, fire service, and special rescue personnel may be needed to secure the scene before entry.) The paramedic must consider the use of protective gear before entering the scene. Depending on the scene and the chemical agent(s), decontamination may be required. Personal protection may include gloves, eye shields, protective garments, and appropriate breathing apparatus. A response to a hazardous materials incident requires special safety considerations and trained rescue personnel (see Chapter 57). The treatment of chemical injuries varies little from that of thermal burns during the primary survey. Treatment is directed at stopping the burning process. This can best be achieved by the following actions:

1. Remove all clothing, including shoes. These can trap concentrated chemicals.
2. Brush off powdered chemicals.
   a. Break open and irrigate under blisters that may contain chemical.[16]
3. Irrigate the affected area with vast amounts of water.
   a. In otherwise stable patients, irrigation takes priority over transport. That is the case unless irrigation can be continued en route to the emergency department.
   b. If a large body surface area is involved, a shower should be used for irrigation, if available.

CHEMICAL BURN INJURY TO THE EYES

Chemical exposure to the eyes (e.g., from mace, pepper spray, or other irritants) may cause damage ranging from superficial inflammation (*chemical conjunctivitis*) to severe burns. Patients with these conditions have local pain, visual disturbance, lacrimation (tearing), edema, and redness of surrounding tissues. Management guidelines include flushing the eyes with water. This can be done by using a mild flow from a hose, intravenous tubing, or water from a container. (The affected eye should be irrigated from the medial to the lateral aspect. This will help to avoid flushing the chemical into the unaffected eye.) Irrigation should be continued during transport. If contact lenses are present, they should be removed. When retracting the lids to irrigate the eyes, the paramedic should take care to apply pressure only to the bony structures surrounding the eye. Pressure on the globe should be avoided.

Some EMS services use nasal cannulas to irrigate both eyes simultaneously. The cannula is placed over the bridge of the nose; the nasal prongs are pointing down toward the eyes. The cannula is attached to an intravenous administration set using normal saline or lactated Ringer's solution, and the fluid is run continually into both eyes (Figure 39-12). Irrigation lenses (e.g., *Morgan therapeutic lens*) may be useful for prolonged eye irrigation in adults, provided that edema is absent and there are no lacerations or penetrating wounds of the globe or eyelids (Figure 39-13). The use of these devices in the prehospital setting is controversial. Their use requires special training and authorization from medical direction. A chemical burn to the eye can be frightening for the patient. The patient may fear loss of sight from the injury. The paramedic should attempt to calm the

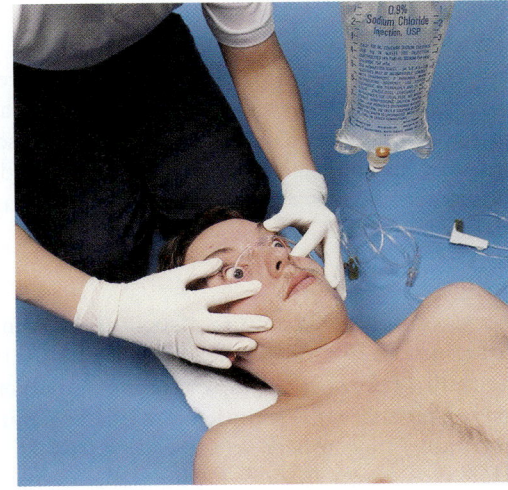

FIGURE 39-12 Use of nasal cannula for eye irrigation.

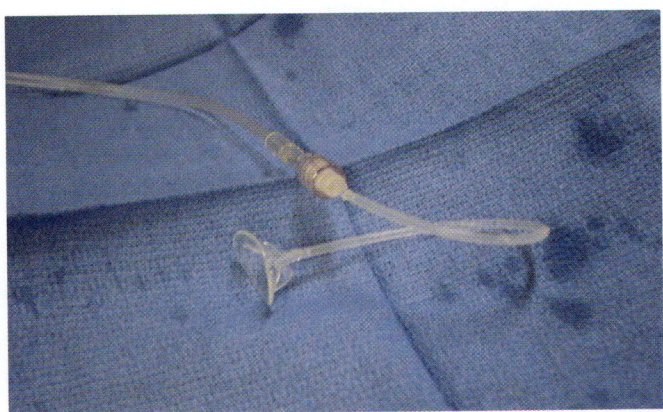

FIGURE 39-13 Commercial irrigation lens.

patient and explain the importance of thorough eye irrigation, which may be uncomfortable. This often improves the patient's cooperation.

USE OF ANTIDOTES OR NEUTRALIZING AGENTS

According to the American Burn Association, no agent has been found to be superior to water for treating most chemical burns.[16] Thus the use of antidotes or neutralizing agents should be avoided in initial prehospital management of most burn injuries. Many neutralizing agents produce heat. They may increase injury when applied to the wound.

In special circumstances, such as when an industrial complex within a response area is known to use a chemical agent with a specific antidote, medical direction may elect to have the EMS stock the neutralizer. In this case, paramedics should receive special training on the indications, contraindications, use, and side effects of these agents.

Specific Chemical Injuries

The main treatment for most chemical burns is copious irrigation with water. However, a number of chemical injuries necessitate further discussion and include those from petroleum, hydrofluoric acid, phenols, ammonia, and alkali metals. Personal safety is a priority when working around any of these chemicals.

PETROLEUM

In the absence of flame, products such as gasoline and diesel fuel can cause significant chemical burns if prolonged contact occurs. (This may occur, for example, with entrapment in a vehicle that is surrounded by spilled gasoline.) At first, the injury may appear to be only a superficial or partial-thickness burn. In fact, though, it may be a full-thickness injury. Systemic effects such as central nervous system depression, organ failure, and death may result from the absorption of various hydrocarbons. In addition, lead toxicity can occur if the exposure was from gasoline that contained tetraethyl lead.

HYDROFLUORIC ACID

Hydrofluoric acid is one of the most corrosive materials known. The acid is used in industry for cleaning fabrics and metals, for glass etching, and in the manufacture of silicone chips for electronic equipment. The hydrogen ion and fluoride ion are damaging to tissue. Fluoride hinders several chemical reactions that are required for cell survival. Fluoride also continues to penetrate and kill cells even when it is neutralized by binding to calcium or magnesium. Thus endogenous or exogenous hydrofluoric acid has the potential to produce deep, painful, and severe injuries. If large body surface areas are involved, the patient may experience severe hypocalcemia and even death. This is true with exposure to high concentrations of the acid also. Even the most minor-appearing wounds that involve hydrofluoric acid should be evaluated at a proper medical facility.

Irrigation of the exposed area with large amounts of water should be started immediately. On arrival in the emergency department, treatment may include subcutaneous injection of 10% calcium gluconate directly into the burn site.

PHENOL

Phenol (*carbolic acid*) is an aromatic hydrocarbon. Phenol is derived from coal tar and is used widely in industry as a disinfectant in cleaning agents. Phenol also is used in the manufacture of plastics, dyes, fertilizers, and explosives. Skin contact with phenol can result in local tissue coagulation and systemic toxicity if the agent is absorbed. A soft tissue injury from phenol exposure may be painless because of the anesthetic properties of the agent. Minor exposures may cause central nervous system depression and dysrhythmias. Patients with significant exposures (10% to 15% TBSA) may require systemic support. These patients should be observed carefully for signs of respiratory failure.

Wounds should be irrigated with large volumes of water. After irrigation, medical direction may advise that the wound be swabbed with a suitable solvent such as glycerol, vegetable oil, or soap and water to bind phenol and prevent its systemic absorption.

AMMONIA

Ammonia is a noxious, irritating gas. Ammonia also is a strong alkali that is very soluble in water. Ammonia is hazardous if introduced into the eye and may result in tissue necrosis and blindness. The patient with an ammonia burn to the eye probably will have swelling or spasm of the eyelids. These injuries must be irrigated with water or a balanced salt solution for up to 24 hours.

> **NOTE**
> Anhydrous ammonia burns may be encountered as a result of methamphetamine lab explosions (see Chapter 34).

Respiratory injury from ammonia vapors depends on two factors: the concentration and duration of exposure. For example, short-term, high-concentration exposure usually results in upper airway edema. However, long-term, low-concentration exposure may damage the lower respiratory tract. The initial care for patients with respiratory injury includes high-concentration oxygen administration, ventilatory support as needed, and rapid transport to an appropriate medical facility.

ALKALI METALS

Sodium and potassium are highly reactive metals. They can ignite spontaneously. Water generally is contraindicated when these metals are imbedded in the skin because they react with water and produce large amounts of heat. Physically removing the metal or covering it with oil minimizes the thermal injury.

ELECTRICAL BURN INJURIES

Electrical injuries account for 4% to 6.5% of admissions to burn centers and are responsible for about 500 deaths each year.[2] Good patient care and personal safety at the scene of an electrocution depend on understanding how electricity flows (current) through the body (Box 39-6).

Types of Electrical Injury

Three basic types of injury may occur as a result of contact with electrical current. These are *direct contact burns, arc injuries,* and *flash burns.* Direct contact burns occur when electrical current directly penetrates the resistance of the skin and underlying tissues. The hand and wrist are common entrance sites. The foot is a common exit site (Figure 39-14). Although the skin may initially resist current flow, continued contact with the source lessens resistance and permits

BOX 39-6 Principles of Tissue Damage Caused by Electricity

Tissue damage produced by electrical current is a function of six factors: amperage, voltage, resistance, type of current, current pathway, and duration of current flow.

1. *Amperage*. Amperage is a measure of the current flow (intensity) per unit of time. One ampere is a passage of 1 coulomb of charge per second past any point in the circuit. Thus a 10-amp flow means that 10 coulombs of electricity are passing a point per second.

2. *Voltage*. Voltage is a continuous force (tension) applied to any electrical circuit that produces a flow of electricity. Volts are the driving force for electrical current. One volt is the force needed to drive 1 amp of current in a circuit with 1 ohm of resistance. High-voltage electrical injuries result from contact with a source of 1000 volts or greater. High-tension accidents usually range from 7200 to 19,000 volts. Yet they may involve current with as high as 100,000 to 1 million volts.

3. *Ohm*. An ohm is a measure of the resistance of an electrical conductor. Electrical resistance is composed of four factors: (1) resistivity, the capacity of a material to resist current flow; (2) the size of the object pathway; (3) the length of the object pathway; and (4) temperature. Resistance to the flow of electricity varies greatly within the body because various tissues have different resistance to current flow. Tissue resistance to electrical flow in the body is highest in bone and decreases progressively through the fat, skin, muscle, blood, and nerve tissue.

4. *Type of current*. Two basic forms of electrical current are in common usage: direct current (DC) and alternating current (AC). The type of current can influence patterns and severity of injury. Direct current flows in one direction only. Direct current often is used in industry; it is the type of current produced by batteries. Direct current commonly is used in electrosurgical devices and defibrillators and is characterized by high amperage and low voltage.

   Alternating current reverses the direction of flow at regular intervals (60-cycle current has 60 reversals per second). These alterations in current direction can cause tetanic muscle contractions. These contractions may "freeze" the victim to the source until the current is terminated. Household current in the United States generally is alternating current and either 120 or 220 volts. Alternating current is a more common cause of electrical injury.

5. *Current pathway*. Electricity normally flows along a continuous pathway. This pathway is known as an electrical circuit. The current pathway can be unpredictable. However, as a rule, low-voltage current (less than 1000 volts) follows the path of least resistance. High-voltage current follows the shortest path. In either case, the greater the current flow, the greater the heat generated.

   The pathway of the current through the body is important because it gives a clue as to what anatomical structures are damaged. For example, if the current travels from one hand to the other, it may flow across the heart and provoke ventricular fibrillation or other dysrhythmias.

6. *Duration of flow*. Tissue injury results from the conversion of electrical energy into heat. The amount of heat produced is directly proportional to the square of the current strength multiplied by the resistance of the tissue multiplied by the duration of the current flow (Joule's law). Therefore injury is directly proportional to the duration of contact with the electrical source.

---

increased current flow. The greatest tissue damage occurs directly under and adjacent to the contact points and may include fat, fascia, muscle, and bone. Tissue destruction may be massive at the entrance and exit sites; however, injury to the area between these wounds is what poses the greatest threat to the patient's life.

Arc injuries occur when a person is close enough to a high-voltage source that the current between two contact points near the skin overcomes the resistance in the air, passing the current flow through the air to the bystander. Temperatures generated by these sources can be as high as 2000° to 4000° C (3632° to 7232° F). The arc may jump as far as 10 feet.

Flame and flash burn injuries can occur when the heat of electrical current ignites a nearby combustible source. Common injury sites include the face and eyes (*welder's flash*). Flash burns also may ignite a person's clothing or cause fire in the surrounding environment. No electrical current passes through the body in this type of burn.

Effects of Electrical Injury

Electrical injuries often are unpredictable. They vary according to the parameters that have been described. Yet certain physiological effects should be expected by the paramedic crew.

The skin is almost always the first point of contact with electrical current. Direct contact and passage of the current through tissue may cause wide areas of coagulation necrosis. The entrance site is often a bull's-eye wound. The site may appear dry, leathery, charred, or depressed. The exit wound may be ulcerated and may appear exploded. Areas of tissue may be missing.

Oral burns often are seen in children younger than 2 years of age. These wounds usually are caused by chewing or sucking on a low-tension electrical cord. Oral burns may be associated with injury to the tongue, palate, and face.

Hypertension and tachycardia associated with a large release of catecholamines is a common finding in electrical injury. Electrical current also may cause significant dysrhythmias (including ventricular fibrillation and asystole) and damage to the myocardium as it passes through the body. The patient may have suffered cardiac arrest. If early rescue and resuscitation can be initiated, success rates are high.

Nerve tissue is a good conductor of electrical current. Thus nerve tissue often may be affected in electrical injuries. Central nervous system damage may result in seizures or coma with or without focal neurological findings. Peripheral nerve injury may lead to motor or sensory deficits. These deficits may be permanent. If the current passes

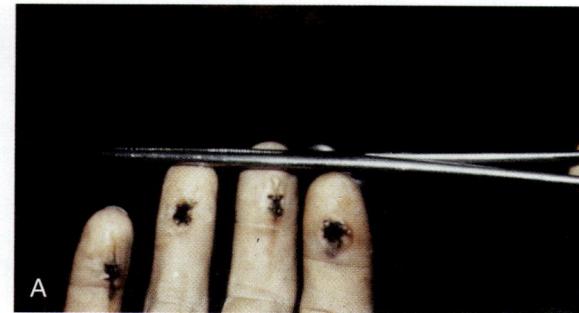

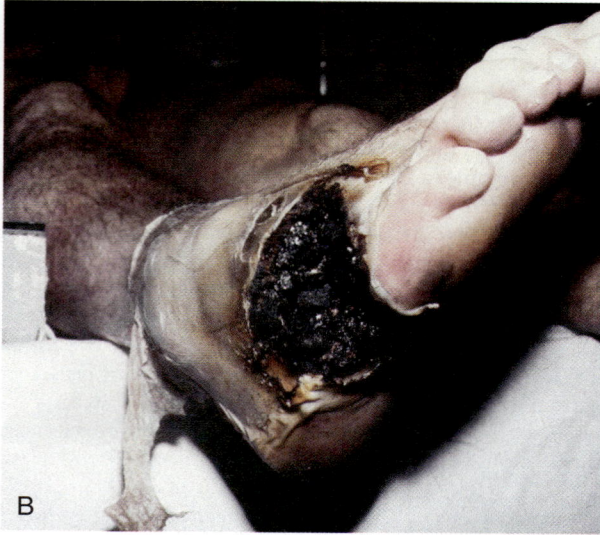

FIGURE 39-14 Direct contact burn. **A,** Entry wound (hand). **B,** Exit wound (foot).

through the brainstem, respiratory arrest or depression, cerebral edema, or hemorrhage may rapidly lead to death.

Electrical injury can cause extensive necrosis of blood vessels. This may not be evident upon the arrival of EMS. However, such injuries can cause immediate or delayed internal hemorrhage or arterial or venous thrombosis and embolism with subsequent complications.

Damage within the extremities after an electrical burn is similar to that sustained by crush injury (described in Chapter 38). Severe muscle necrosis releases myoglobin. Bursting of the red blood cells (hemolysis) releases hemoglobin. Both of these large molecules can precipitate in the renal tubules, producing acute renal failure. Some patients may require amputation of the affected extremity. This results from decreased circulation and compartment syndrome. In the electrocuted patient, severe muscle spasms can produce bony fractures. These spasms also may produce dislocations, even of major joints. A patient may fall after the electrical shock and sustain skeletal trauma (including damage to the cervical spine).

Acute renal failure can be a serious complication from significant direct contact electrical **injuries.**[17] Acute renal

failure may result from a combination of myoglobin or hemoglobin sludging in the renal tubules, disseminated intravascular coagulation caused by tissue damage, hypovolemic shock, and direct current damage. Acute renal failure is not of immediate consequence in the prehospital setting. Yet prompt fluid resuscitation and management of shock may have a positive impact on a number of these patients.

Ventilation may be impaired when electrical burns produce central nervous system injury or chest wall dysfunction. If the respiratory center is disrupted, hypoventilation can lead to immediate patient death. Contact with any alternating current sources also has been known to produce respiratory arrest and death from tetany of the muscles of respiration.

Conjunctival and corneal burns and ruptured tympanic membranes may be found in some electrical injuries. Cataracts and hearing loss also may appear as late as 1 year after the event.

A number of other internal structures may be damaged from electrical injury. These structures include the abdominal organs and urinary bladder. Submucosal hemorrhage may occur in the bowel; various forms of ulceration are possible. Each patient requires a thorough physical assessment and a high degree of suspicion for associated trauma.

Assessment and Management

Patient assessment should begin by ensuring that no hazards exist for the rescuers or bystanders. If the patient is still in contact with the electrical source, the paramedic should summon the electric company, fire department, or other specially trained personnel before approaching the patient. Once the scene is safe, the patient intervention may begin.

> ### CRITICAL THINKING
> What will you do if you respond to a scene and there is a child still in contact with electrical current and having tetanic movements? A large crowd has gathered and is screaming at you to help. The fire department is 3 minutes away. How will you feel?

PRIMARY SURVEY

The primary survey should proceed as it does for all other trauma patients. The paramedic should take care to immobilize the cervical spine. If the patient is not breathing, assisted ventilation should begin immediately. The paramedic should perform intubation as soon as possible because apnea may persist for lengthy periods. A patient who is breathing should have a patent airway maintained. Respirations should be supported with supplemental high-concentration oxygen as well. If the patient is in cardiac arrest, the paramedic should initiate resuscitation efforts according to protocol. If possible, a history of the event should be obtained that includes the following:

- Patient's chief complaint (e.g., injury or disorientation)
- Source, voltage, and amperage of the electrical injury
- Duration of contact
- Level of consciousness before and after the injury
- Significant medical history

NOTE
The source, voltage, and type of current (alternating current versus direct current) are essential information for the attending physician to estimate internal damage from electrical current.

PHYSICAL EXAMINATION

The physical exam should be thorough. The paramedic should search for entrance and exit wounds or any associated trauma caused by tetany or a fall. The paramedic should recall that there may have been multiple pathways of current. This would mean multiple wounds. The paramedic should remove all of the patient's clothing and jewelry and examine the areas between the patient's fingers and toes for sites of entry or exit. Distal pulses, motor function, and sensation in all extremities should be assessed and documented to monitor for possible development of compartment syndrome. The paramedic should cover entrance and exit wounds with sterile dressings and should manage any associated trauma appropriately.

Internal damage from electrical current may be much more significant than external wounds. Frequent reassessment is necessary because of the progressive nature of electrical injury. In addition, electrocardiogram monitoring should be implemented at the scene and continued during patient transport. As previously discussed, electrical injury may cause a variety of dysrhythmias, some of which can be lethal.

MANAGEMENT

Early administration of fluids is critical for patients with severe electrical injury. Fluid administration helps to prevent hypovolemia and subsequent renal failure. If possible, the paramedic should establish two large-bore intravenous lines. These should be in an extremity without entry or exit wounds. The fluid of choice generally is lactated Ringer's solution or normal saline without glucose. The flow rate should be determined by the patient's clinical status.

In the emergency department or during interhospital transfer, the patient's intravenous fluid rates will be regulated to maintain a urine output of 1 to 1.5 mL/kg/hr.[11] This rate decreases the potential for renal damage caused by myoglobin accumulation. Emergency department management may include the administration of **sodium bicarbonate** to help maintain an alkaline urine. Alkalinity in turn increases the solubility of hemoglobin and myoglobin and decreases the risk of renal failure.

Lightning Injury

Lightning strikes the earth about 7.4 million times each year and accounts for about 70 deaths each year.[2] Lightning can deliver direct current of up to 200,000 amps at a potential of 100 million or more volts, with temperatures that vary between 16,000° and 60,000° F (8871° and 33,315° C). Lightning injuries can occur from a direct strike or by a side flash (splash) between a victim and a nearby object that has been struck by lightning. About 30% of those struck by lightning die.[18] Lightning strikes are most common in Florida, Texas, and North Carolina.

Lightning strikes produce tissue injuries that differ from other types of electrical injury because the pathway of tissue damage often is over rather than *through* the skin (Figure 39-15). The duration of the lightning is short ($\frac{1}{100}$ to $\frac{1}{1000}$ second). Thus skin burns are less severe than those seen with other high-voltage current (full-thickness burns are rare). Common lightning burns are linear, feathery, and punctate (pinpoint). In addition, depending on the severity of the strike, 30% of those struck by lightning suffer cardiac and respiratory arrest.[12]

Lightning injuries may be classified as minor, moderate, or severe. The patients with minor lightning injuries usually are conscious. These patients often are confused and amnesic. Burns or other signs of injury are rare. The vital signs of these patients usually are stable.

The patients with moderate injury may be combative or comatose. These patients may have associated injuries from the impact of the lightning strike. Superficial and partial-thickness burns are common, as is tympanic membrane rupture. These patients may have serious internal organ damage. They should be observed carefully for signs and symptoms of cardiorespiratory dysfunction.

Severe lightning injuries include those that cause immediate brain damage, seizures, respiratory paralysis, and cardiac arrest. The prehospital care is directed at basic and advanced life support measures and rapid transport to a proper facility.

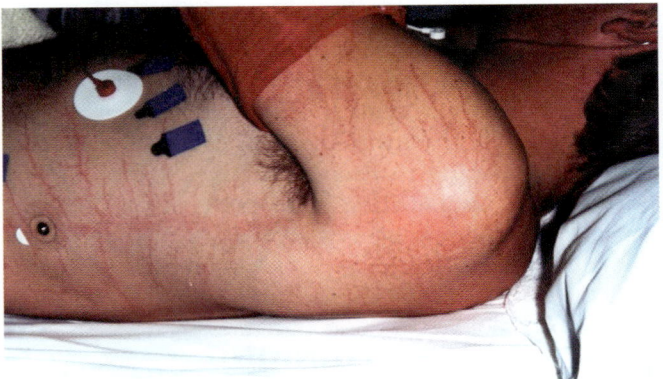

FIGURE 39-15 Lightning injury.

ASSESSMENT AND MANAGEMENT

Like all other emergency responses, scene safety is the first priority. If the electrical storm is still in progress, all patient care should take place in a sheltered area. To prevent injury from subsequent lightning strikes, the paramedic crew should stay away from objects that project from the ground. Such objects include trees, fences, and high buildings. The crew also should avoid areas of open water. If rescue attempts in an open area are necessary, the paramedic should stay low to the ground.

The prehospital management of lightning injuries is the same as that for other severe electrical injuries. Initial patient care is directed at airway and ventilatory support; basic and advanced life support; patient immobilization; fluid resuscitation to prevent hypovolemia and renal failure; pharmacological therapy (per protocol) to manage seizures (if present), promote excretion of myoglobin, and treat dysrhythmias; wound care; and rapid transport to a proper facility.

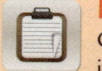

NOTE
Cardiopulmonary resuscitation should be initiated immediately for patients who are pulseless because resuscitation is possible after lightning injury.[19]

RADIATION EXPOSURE

The most common radiation incidents involve sealed radioactive sources used in industrial radiography and nondestructive testing. The victims of these types of incidents rarely require emergency care. However, EMS may be called to building fires and crashes that may involve radioactive materials. Thus an understanding of the hazards of radiation exposure is important. As with all incidents involving hazardous materials, the paramedic crew should never enter the scene until it has been made safe by the proper authorities.

Generally, safety issues regarding radiation have been minor because of excellent adherence to radiation regulations throughout the world. However, hazards associated with radiation became well known as a result of several incidents. First, the serious potential for disaster occurred at Three Mile Island in Pennsylvania in 1979. Second, a disastrous incident occurred at the Chernobyl Nuclear Power Station in the Soviet Union in 1986. Most recently, the earthquake and tsunami that struck Japan in 2011 caused a serious radiation event when the Fukushima Daiichi nuclear power plant was damaged.

CRITICAL THINKING
What industries in your area use radioactive materials? Is there a preplan for incidents at those sites?

Characteristics of Radioactive Particles

Radioactive particles generally are classified into three types: *alpha, beta,* and *gamma.* Alpha particles are large. They travel only a few millimeters. They have little penetrating ability. In fact, alpha particles may be stopped by paper, clothing, or skin. These particles are considered the least dangerous external radiation source. However, if alpha particles enter the body through inhalation, ingestion, or absorption, they can damage internal organs and interfere with the chemical functions of the body. Alpha radiation is considered the most dangerous form of internal radiation exposure.

Beta particles are 0.017 (one seven thousandth) the size of alpha particles. Yet beta particles have much more energy and penetrating power. Beta particles can penetrate subcutaneous tissue. They usually enter the body through damaged skin, ingestion, or inhalation. Protection from alpha and beta radiation requires full protective clothing, including a positive-pressure self-contained breathing apparatus.

Gamma rays and x-rays are the most dangerous forms of penetrating radiation. They require lead shields for protection. Gamma rays have 10,000 times the penetrating power of alpha particles. They have 100 times the penetrating power of beta particles.[20] Protective clothing does not stop gamma rays. Gamma rays pose internal and external hazards. They may produce localized skin burns and extensive internal damage.

Harmful Effects From Radiation Exposure

Nonionizing radiation includes radio waves and microwaves. Nonionizing radiation usually is considered safe. Ionizing radiation is produced by nuclear weapons, reactors, radioactive material, and x-ray machines. Although rare, the exposure to ionizing radiation poses a threat to victims and rescue workers.

The amount of emitted radiation is expressed in *roentgens* and indicates the ionization produced in the air by gamma or x-ray radiation. Other units used to measure radiation are the *rad* (radiation absorbed dose) and the *rem* (roentgen equivalent man). A rad is a measure of the amount of ionized radiation being emitted and the amount that has been absorbed and is active within the body tissues. A rem is used to assess the biological effects of the various types of radiation. For emergency purposes, rescue workers should assume that 1 roentgen equals 1 rad equals 1 rem.

Doses of less than 100 rem usually do not cause significant acute problems. Doses from 100 to 200 rem may cause symptoms. Yet the doses are not life threatening. When an exposure of 200 rem is neared, nausea, vomiting, and diarrhea begin within 2 to 4 hours. After an exposure of 450 rem, 50% mortality can be expected within 30 days if no medical care is given.[21] Victims of radiation rarely show immediate signs or symptoms of exposure. Thus all victims

BOX 39-7 Types of Radiation Injury

The harmful effects from radiation may be classified as external irradiation, contamination by radioactive materials, incorporation of radioactive materials, and combined radiation injury.

External irradiation occurs when all or part of the body is exposed to penetrating radiation from an external source. An example of external irradiation is a medical x-ray. The degree of radiation injury depends on the intensity of radiation, which in turn depends on the duration of exposure. Degree of injury also depends on the distance from the source. A patient who has been exposed to large amounts of radiation may have nausea, vomiting, and diarrhea. In severe cases, additional symptoms may include weight loss, hair loss, fever, bleeding, mouth and throat sores, skin burns, lowered body resistance, vesiculation, and ulceration. The effects from this type of radiation are not contagious; there are no risks to the rescuer in providing care.

Contamination occurs when radioactive materials in the form of gases, liquids, or solids are released into the environment. These materials contaminate persons internally, externally, or both. When radioactive material remains on the patient's clothing or skin or in open wounds, a potential hazard is present for the rescuer and the patient. Patients who have been contaminated should be considered medical emergencies. They may pose significant risk to emergency providers.

Incorporation refers to the uptake of radioactive materials by body cells, tissues, and target organs such as bone, liver, thyroid, or kidney. Incorporation is impossible unless contamination has occurred.

A combination radiation injury involves external irradiation, contamination, incorporation, or some combination of these. This type of exposure usually is the result of a major incident. Exposure may be complicated by a patient's physical injury.

After exposure to radiation, a person may be at risk for delayed complications. Such complications include cell and chromosomal changes, subsequent reproductive genetic aberrations, cell death, and sterility. Diseases such as anemia and forms of cancer may develop as well.

site. Emergency workers should not eat, drink, or smoke at the site or in any rescue vehicle. The proper local authorities should be contacted (state radiological health office, local specialists). Medical direction should be notified as well. Protective clothing suitable for other hazardous material releases should be worn by all emergency workers. In addition, dose meters should be available for all rescue personnel. Self-contained breathing apparatus should be used if fire, smoke, or gas is present.

Personal Protection From Radiation

The Federal Emergency Management Agency recommends that basic radiation protection for the rescuer and the patient include the following four factors[22]:
1. *Time:* The less time spent in a radiation field, the less radiation exposure. If adequate personnel are available, a rotating team approach can be used to keep individual radiation exposure to a minimum.
2. *Distance:* The farther a person is from the source of radiation, the lower the radiation dose. Even moving several feet away from a radioactive source greatly reduces the level of exposure.
3. *Shielding:* The general principle of shielding is that the denser the material, the greater its ability to stop the passage of radiation. Lead shields provide the best protection from exposure. However, vehicles, mounds of dirt, and pieces of heavy equipment placed between the radiation source and the rescuer and victim also can diminish exposure levels. Protective clothing and self-contained breathing apparatus may provide adequate protection from all alpha and some beta radiation, but protective clothing does not prevent penetration of gamma rays. If adequate shielding is not readily available, rescuers should use the time and distance factors to reduce radiation exposure.
4. *Quantity:* Limiting the amount of radioactive material in a specific area lessens the radiation exposure. Examples include removing contaminated clothing, bagging all contaminated items, and moving containers of radioactive material from the area.

of possible exposure should be presumed to have a radiation injury until proved otherwise (Box 39-7).

NOTE

An object or a person who has been exposed to radiation is not radioactive. Only the presence of the radioactive residue poses a threat to rescuers.

Emergency Response to Radiation Accidents

If the EMS crew has been advised that radioactive materials are present at an emergency scene, they should approach the site with caution. They should not enter the scene until it has been secured by proper authorities (see Chapter 57). Rescue personnel, emergency vehicles, and the command post should be positioned 200 to 300 feet upwind of the

Emergency Care for Victims of Radiation Exposure

A patient who has been irradiated is not radioactive. But when external contamination occurs and radioactive material remains on the patient's clothing and skin or in open wounds, the rescuer should consult with medical direction and follow agency protocol. The effects of radiation exposure may be instant (e.g., burns) or delayed.

With the exception of dealing with contaminants and containing their spread, there are no emergency care procedures specific to radiation injury. All external bleeding should be controlled, the spine immobilized, open wounds covered, and fractures stabilized in normal fashion. The EMS crew should move the patient away from the source of radiation as soon as possible. Lifesaving care should not be delayed for patient transfer or decontamination procedures. Intravenous fluid replacement should be initiated if indicated. (Strict aseptic technique should be used.) If an intravenous line is not needed for specific therapy, its use should be avoided to prevent introducing contaminants into the body.

Radiation Decontamination Procedures

Radiation emergencies involving patients may be defined in two ways: clean and dirty. *Clean* means that the patient was exposed but not contaminated. *Dirty* means that the patient was contaminated. Only properly trained personnel (e.g., hazardous materials teams and qualified county, state, or federal health department personnel) should attempt to decontaminate radiation victims at the scene. A patient who is to be transported to a hospital for decontamination should be isolated from the environment (described in Chapter 57). Also, all patient effects should be transported with the patient.

SUMMARY

- Each year more than 2 million Americans seek medical attention for burns. Morbidity and mortality rates from burn injury follow significant patterns regarding gender, age, and socioeconomic status. A burn injury is caused by an interaction between thermal, chemical, electrical, or radiation energy and biological matter.

- Tissue damage from burns depends on the degree of the heat and on the duration of exposure to the thermal source. As local events occur at the injury site, other organ systems become involved in a general response to the stress caused by the burn.

- Burns are classified in terms of depth as superficial, partial-thickness, and full-thickness. The rule of nines provides a rough estimate of burn injury size (extent) and is most accurate for adults and for children older than age 10. The Lund and Browder chart is a more accurate method of determining the area of burn injury. Severity of burn injury and burn center referral guidelines are based on standards that take into account the depth, extent, and severity of the burn wound; the source of injury; the age of the patient; the presence of concurrent medical or surgical problems; and the body region that is burned.

- Shock after thermal injury results from edema and accumulation of vascular fluid. These tissue changes occur in the area of injury and can produce systemic hypovolemia if the burn area is large.

- Emergency care for a burn patient begins with the initial assessment. The goal is to recognize and treat life-threatening injuries.

- Goals for prehospital management of the severely burned patient include preventing further tissue injury, maintaining the airway, administering oxygen and ventilatory support, providing fluid resuscitation, providing rapid transport to an appropriate medical facility, using aseptic (clean) technique to minimize the patient's exposure to infectious agents, managing pain, and providing psychological and emotional support.

- Prehospital considerations in caring for patients with inhalation injury include recognition of the dangers inherent in the fire environment, awareness of the pathophysiological principles of inhalation injury, and early detection and treatment of impending airway or respiratory problems.

- The severity of chemical injury is related to three factors: the chemical agent, the concentration and volume of the chemical, and the duration of contact. Treatment is directed at stopping the burning process by using copious irrigation.

- Three types of injury may occur as a result of contact with electrical current: direct contact burns, arc injuries, and flash burns. Once the scene is safe, patient intervention may begin. Internal damage from electrical current may be much more significant than external wounds.

- Persons who are injured by radiation rarely require emergency care. Radioactive particles are classified into three types: alpha, beta, and gamma. The Federal Emergency Management Agency recommends that basic radiation protection for the rescuer and the patient include four factors: minimize time in the radiation field; maintain a safe distance from the source; place shielding between the rescuers and the source; and limit the amount of radioactive material in a specific area.

REFERENCES

1. American Burn Association: Burn incidents and treatment in the US: 2011 fact sheet, www.ameriburn.org/resources_factsheet.php, accessed 6-17-11.
2. National Safety Council: *Injury facts*, Itasca, Ill, 2010, The Council.
3. Weaver AM, Himel HN, Edlich RF: Immersion scald burns: strategies for prevention, *J Emerg Med* 11(4):397-402, 1993.
4. Orgill D: Excision and skin grafting of thermal burns, *N Engl J Med* 360:893-901, 2009.
5. Palao R, Monge I, Ruiz M, et al: Chemical burns: pathophysiology and treatment, *Burns* 36(3):295-304, 2009.

6. National Highway Traffic Safety Administration: *The National EMS Education Standards*, Washington, DC, 2009, U.S. Department of Transportation/National Highway Traffic Safety Administration, DOT.

7. National Institutes of Health: Skin graft, www.nlm.nih.gov/medlineplus/ency/article/002982.htm, accessed 10-6-10.

8. Kagan RJ, Peck MD, Ahrenholz DH, et al: American Burn Association White Paper: surgical management of the burn wound and use of skin substitutes, American Burn Association, www.ameriburn.org/WhitePaperFinal.pdf, accessed 10-16-10.

9. American Burn Association: Burn center fact sheet 2010 Report, www.ameriburn.org/resources_factsheet.php, accessed 6-17-11.

10. Faldmo L, Kravitz M: Management of acute burns and shock resuscitation, *AACN Clin Issues Crit Care Nurs* 4(2):351, 1993.

11. Marx JA, Hockberger RS, Walls RM, et al: *Rosen's emergency medicine: concepts and clinical practice*, ed 6, St Louis, 2006, Mosby.

12. American Heart Association: 2010 American Heart Association guidelines for cardiopulmonary resuscitation and emergency cardiovascular care, *Circulation* 122(18 suppl):S639-S946, 2010.

13. Sole ML, Klein D, Moseley MJ: *Introduction to critical care nursing*, ed 5, Philadelphia, 2008, Saunders.

14. Shochat GN, Lucchesi M: Toxicity: carbon monoxide, http://emedicine.medscape.com/article/819987-overview, accessed 10-6-10.

15. Murray M, Coursin DB, Pearl RG, et al: *Critical care medicine: perioperative management*, ed 2, Philadelphia, 2002, Lippincott Williams & Wilkins.

16. American Burn Association: *Advanced burn life support provider manual*, Chicago, Ill, 2005.

17. Gabrielli A: *Civetta, Taylor and Kirby's critical care*, ed 4, Philadelphia, 2009, Lippincott Williams & Wilkins.

18. National Weather Service: Medical aspects of lightning, www.lightningsafety.noaa.gov/medical.htm, accessed 10-6-10.

19. American Heart Association: 2010 American Heart Association Guidelines for Cardiopulmonary Resuscitation and Emergency Cardiovascular Care, *Circulation* 122(18 Supplement 3):S639-S946, 2010.

20. U.S. Environmental Protection Agency: Radiation protection: gamma rays, www.epa.gov/rpdweb00/understand/gamma.html, accessed 10-6-10.

21. National Resources Defense Council: Grim blueprints: snapshots from the U.S. playbook for nuclear attack, www.nrdc.org/nuclear/planphoto/planphoto4.asp, accessed 10-6-10.

22. Federal Emergency Management Agency: Radiological emergency management, www.fema.gov, accessed 10-6-10.

SUGGESTED READINGS

Bloom GR, Suhail F, Hopkins-Price P, et al: Acute anhydrous ammonia injury from accidents during illicit methamphetamine production, *Burns* 34:713-718, 2007.

Khodabukus R, Tallouzi M: Chemical eye injuries 1: presentation, clinical features, treatment and prognosis, *Nursing Times* 105 (22):28-29, 2009.

Palao R, Monge I, Ruiz M, et al: Chemical burns: pathophysiology and treatment, *Burns* 36(3):295-304, 2010.

Usatch B: When lightning strikes: bolting down the facts and fiction, JEMS.com, April 2009, www.jems.com/news_and_articles/articles/jems/3404/when_lightning_strikes.html, accessed 4-8-10.

CHAPTER

40

Head, Face, and Neck Trauma

OBJECTIVES

Upon completion of this chapter, the paramedic student will be able to:

1. Describe the mechanisms of injury, assessment, and management of maxillofacial injuries.
2. Describe the mechanisms of injury, assessment, and management of ear, eye, and dental injuries.
3. Describe the mechanisms of injury, assessment, and management of anterior neck trauma.
4. Describe the mechanisms of injury, assessment, and management of injuries to the scalp, cranial vault, or cranial nerves.
5. Distinguish between types of traumatic brain injury based on an understanding of pathophysiology and assessment findings.
6. Outline the prehospital management of the patient with cerebral injury.
7. Calculate a Glasgow Coma Scale, trauma score, Revised Trauma Score, and pediatric trauma score when given appropriate patient information.

KEY TERMS

antegrade amnesia The loss of memory for events that occurred immediately after recovery of consciousness.

astigmatism An abnormal condition of the eye in which the light rays cannot be focused clearly on a point on the retina because the spherical curve of the cornea is not equal in all meridians.

barotitis An inflammation of the ear caused by changes in atmospheric pressure.

basilar skull fracture A fracture that may occur when the mandibular condyles perforate the base of the skull but that more commonly results from extension of a linear fracture into the floor of the anterior and middle fossae.

Battle's sign Ecchymosis over the mastoid process caused by a fracture of the temporal bone.

blowout fracture A fracture of the floor of the orbit caused by a blow that suddenly increases the intraocular pressure.

central vision The vision that results from images falling on the macula of the retina.

cerebral contusion Bruising of the brain in the area of the cortex or deeper within the frontal (most common), temporal, or occipital lobes.

cerebral perfusion pressure A measure of the amount of blood flow to the brain calculated by subtracting the intracranial pressure from the mean systemic arterial blood pressure.

concussion A head injury that results from violent jarring or shaking, such as that caused by a blow or explosion.

consensual movement The movement of one eye acting in concert with the other.

contrecoup An injury that occurs at a site opposite the side of impact.

corneal abrasion The rubbing off of the outer layers of the cornea.

coup Local damage that occurs at the site of impact.

Cushing's triad Increased systolic pressure, widened pulse pressure, and decrease in pulse and respiratory rates, which result from increased intracranial pressure.

decerebrate posturing A position in which a comatose patient's arms are extended and internally rotated and the legs are extended with the feet in forced plantar flexion; usually observed in patients who have compression of the brainstem.

decorticate posturing A position in which the comatose patient's upper extremities are rigidly flexed at the elbows and at the wrists; usually observed in patients who have a lesion in the mesencephalic region of the brain.

dental malocclusion A misalignment of the teeth.

depressed skull fracture Any fracture of the skull in which fragments are depressed below the normal surface of the skull.

epidural hematoma Accumulation of blood between the dura mater and the cranium.

focal injuries Specific, grossly observable brain lesions.

Glasgow Coma Scale A standardized system for assessing the degree of conscious impairment in the critically ill and for predicting the duration and ultimate outcome of coma.

hemotympanum Blood behind the tympanic membrane from fractures of the temporal bone.

intracerebral hematoma An accumulation of blood or fluid within the tissue of the brain.

Le Fort fracture A fracture pattern that can be produced in the midface region.

linear skull fracture A skull fracture that does not displace the bone tissue.

mean arterial pressure The arithmetic mean of the blood pressure in the arterial portion of the circulation.

moderate diffuse injury A head injury that results in minute petechial bruising of brain tissue.

open vault fracture A fracture that results in direct communication between a scalp laceration and cerebral substance.

pediatric trauma score An injury severity index that grades six components commonly seen in pediatric trauma patients: size (weight), airway, central nervous system, systolic blood pressure, open wound, and skeletal injury.

peripheral vision The ability to see objects that reflect light waves on areas of the retina other than the macula.

photophobia Abnormal sensitivity to light.

primary brain injury The direct trauma to the brain and the associated vascular injuries that occurred from the initial injury.

raccoon's eyes Ecchymosis of one or both orbits caused by fracture of the base of the sphenoid sinus.

retrograde amnesia The loss of memory for events that occurred before the event that precipitated the amnesia.

Revised Trauma Score An injury severity index that uses the Glasgow Coma Scale and measurements for systolic blood pressure and respiratory rate.

secondary brain injury Brain injury results from intracellular and extracellular derangements that probably were initiated at the time of the injury.

severe diffuse axonal injury Brain injury that involves severe mechanical shearing of many axons in both cerebral hemispheres extending to the brainstem.

stellate wound A star-shaped wound.

subarachnoid hematoma A collection of blood or fluid in the subarachnoid space.

subdural hematoma A collection of blood in the subdural space.

subgaleal hematomata A collection of blood beneath the strong sheet of fibrous connective tissue that joins the frontal and occipitofrontal muscles.

traumatic brain injury A traumatic insult to the brain capable of producing physical, intellectual, emotional, social, and vocational change.

traumatic hyphema A hemorrhage into the anterior chamber of the eye; it usually is a result of blunt trauma.

traumatic perforation A tear or puncture of the tympanic membrane.

visual acuity A measurement of the clarity or sharpness of vision.

vitreous humor The transparent, jellylike material that fills the space between the lens and the retina.

---

*E*ach year, an estimated 1.5 million people sustain head injury in the United States, and about 52,000 patients with severe head trauma die each year from traumatic brain injury.[1] The categories of head trauma discussed in this chapter include maxillofacial trauma; ear, eye, and dental trauma; anterior neck trauma; and trauma to the skull and brain.

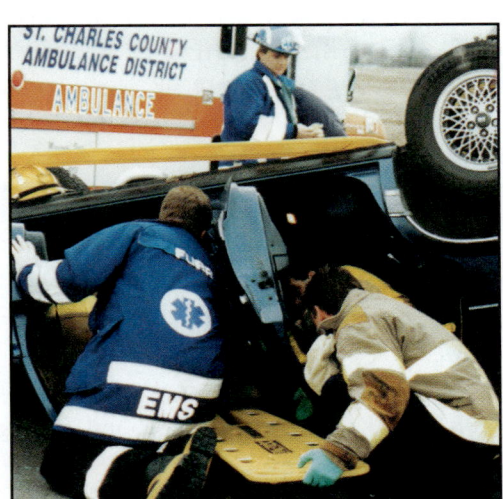

(Courtesy Ray Kemp, St. Charles, Mo.)

MAXILLOFACIAL INJURIES

In descending order of frequency, major causes of maxillofacial trauma are motor vehicle crashes, home injuries, athletic injuries, animal bites, intentional violent acts, and industrial injuries. Maxillofacial trauma may include soft tissue injuries and facial fractures.

Soft Tissue Injuries

The face receives its blood supply from the branches of the internal and external carotid arteries. These branches provide a rich vascular supply (Figure 40-1). As a result, soft tissue injuries to the face often appear to be serious (Figure 40-2). With the exception of a compromised upper airway

and the potential for heavy bleeding, however, damage to the tissues of the maxillofacial area is seldom life threatening. Depending on the mechanism of injury, facial trauma may range from minor cuts and abrasions to more serious injuries. The more serious injuries may involve extensive soft tissue lacerations and avulsions. If possible, the

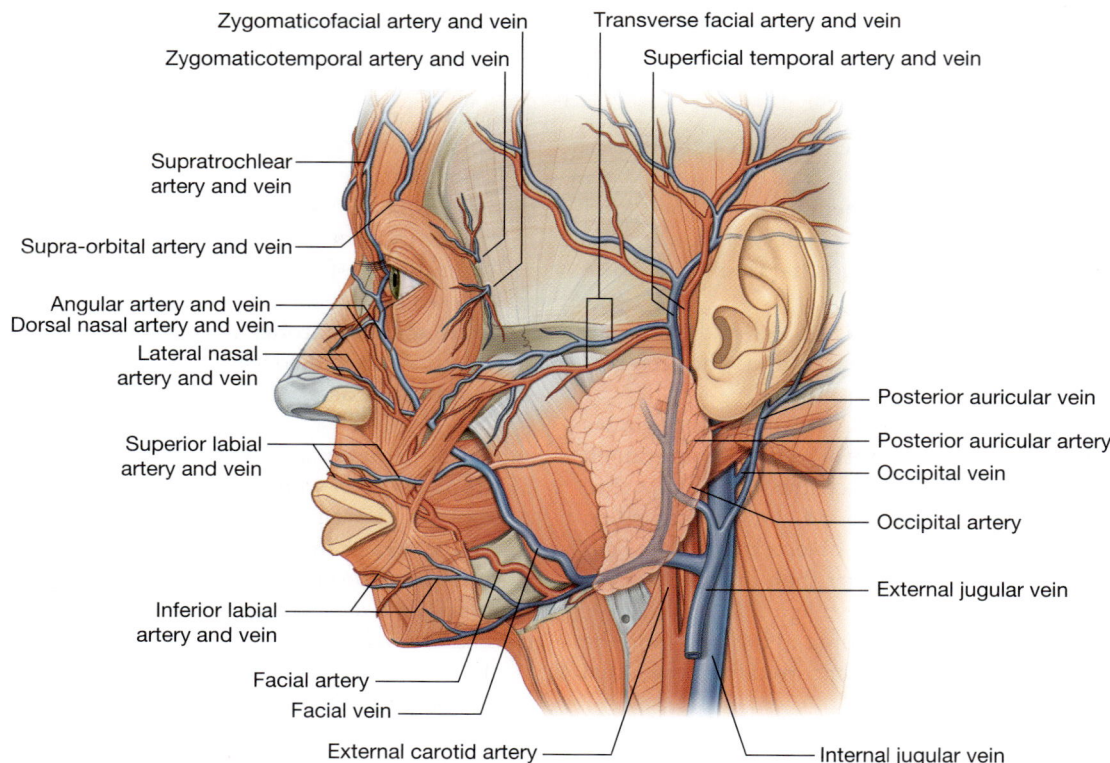

Zygomaticofacial artery and vein

Zygomaticotemporal artery and vein

Transverse facial artery and vein

Superficial temporal artery and vein

Supratrochlear artery and vein

Supra-orbital artery and vein

Angular artery and vein

Dorsal nasal artery and vein

Lateral nasal artery and vein

Superior labial artery and vein

Inferior labial artery and vein

Facial artery

Facial vein

External carotid artery

Posterior auricular vein

Posterior auricular artery

Occipital vein

Occipital artery

External jugular vein

Internal jugular vein

FIGURE 40-1 Arterial blood supply to the face. (From Drake R, et al: *Gray's anatomy for students,* ed 2, Philadelphia, 2010, Churchill Livingstone.)

paramedic should obtain a thorough history from the patient. The history should include mechanism of injury; events leading up to the injury; time of injury; associated medical problems; and allergies, medications, and last oral intake.

CRITICAL THINKING

Why might it be difficult to obtain a history from a patient with this type of injury?

MANAGEMENT

The management of soft tissue injuries was described in Chapter 38. The key principles of wound management include the control of bleeding with direct pressure and pressure bandages. The paramedic should use spinal precautions if indicated by mechanism of injury (described in Chapter 41). The paramedic also should pay close attention to airway management. Soft tissue injuries to the nose and mouth are common with facial injuries. The paramedic should assess the patient's airway for obstruction caused by blood, vomitus, bone fragments, broken teeth, dentures, and damage to the anterior neck. Suction may be needed to clear the patient's airway. Also, oral or nasal adjuncts, tracheal intubation, or cricothyrotomy may be required to ensure adequate ventilation and oxygenation.

Facial Fractures

Facial bones can withstand tremendous forces from the impact of energy. However, facial fractures are common after blunt trauma. The anatomical structure of the facial bones allows a stepwise fracture to absorb the impact of blunt trauma. Blunt trauma injuries may be classified anatomically as fractures to the mandible, midface, zygoma, orbit, and nose. Signs and symptoms of facial fractures include the following:

- Asymmetry of cheek bone prominences
- Crepitus
- Dental malocclusion
- Discontinuity of the orbital rim
- Displacement of the nasal septum
- Ecchymosis
- Lacerations and bleeding
- Limitation of forward movement of the mandible
- Limited ocular movements
- Numbness
- Pain
- Swelling
- Visual disturbances

FRACTURES OF THE MANDIBLE

The mandible is the single facial bone in the lower third of the face (see Chapter 10: Review of Human Systems). Because of its prominence, fractures to this bone rank

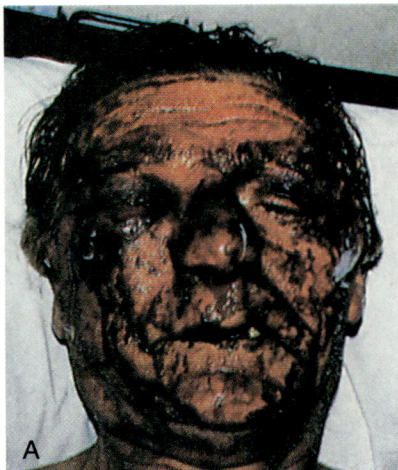

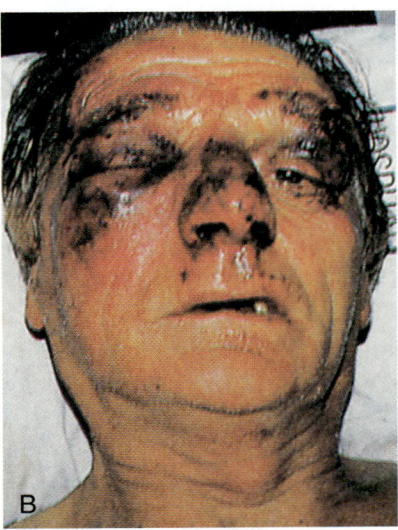

FIGURE 40-2 A, Appearance of a patient after being attacked. **B,** Appearance of same man after cleansing. (From London PS: *A colour atlas of diagnosis after recent injury,* Ipswich, England, 1990, Wolfe Medical Publications, Ltd.)

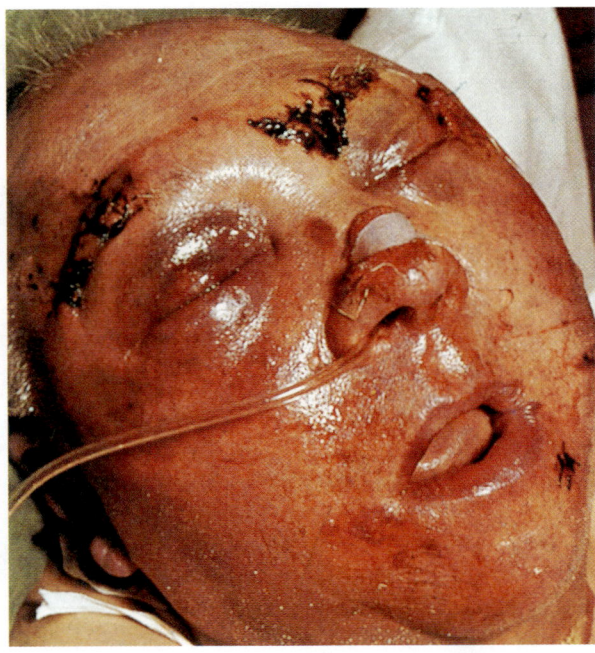

FIGURE 40-3 Fracture of the middle third of the face. (From London PS: *A colour atlas of diagnosis after recent injury,* Ipswich, England, 1990, Wolfe Medical Publications, Ltd.)

wide-open position. The patient usually feels severe pain from the spasm. The patient also experiences anxiety and discomfort that perpetuate the spasm. Mandibular dislocations are reduced manually in the emergency department with the aid of a muscle relaxant or sedative or in the operating room with a general anesthetic.

 CRITICAL THINKING
What will be your patient care priority with these patients?

second in frequency after nasal fractures. The mandible is a hemicircle of bone. It may break in multiple locations, often distant from the point of impact. Signs and symptoms specific to mandibular fractures include **dental malocclusion** (patients may complain that their teeth do not "feel right" when their mouths are closed), numbness in the chin, and inability to open the mouth. The patient also may have difficulty swallowing and may have excessive salivation. Most patients with mandibular fractures require hospitalization.

Anterior dislocation of the mandible in the absence of fracture also may occur as a result of blunt trauma to the face (rare), an abnormally wide yawn, and dental treatment requiring that the jaws remain open for long periods. In these cases, the condylar head advances forward beyond the articular surface of the temporal bone. The jaw-closing muscles spasm. As a result, the mouth becomes locked in a

FRACTURES OF THE MIDFACE

The middle third of the face includes the maxilla, zygoma, floor of the orbit, and nose. Fractures to this region result from direct or transmitted force. (For example, fractures may result from blunt trauma to the mandible with the energy transmitted to produce fractures to the maxilla.) These injuries often are associated with central nervous system injury and spinal trauma (Figure 40-3).

In 1901 a cadaver study done by Le Fort described three patterns of injuries (**Le Fort fractures).** These injuries occur in the midface region (Figure 40-4). The *Le Fort I fracture* involves the maxilla up to the level of the nasal fossa. The *Le Fort II* involves the nasal bones and medial orbits. The fracture line generally is shaped like a pyramid. The *Le Fort III* is a complex fracture in which the facial bones are separated from the cranial bones. Depending on

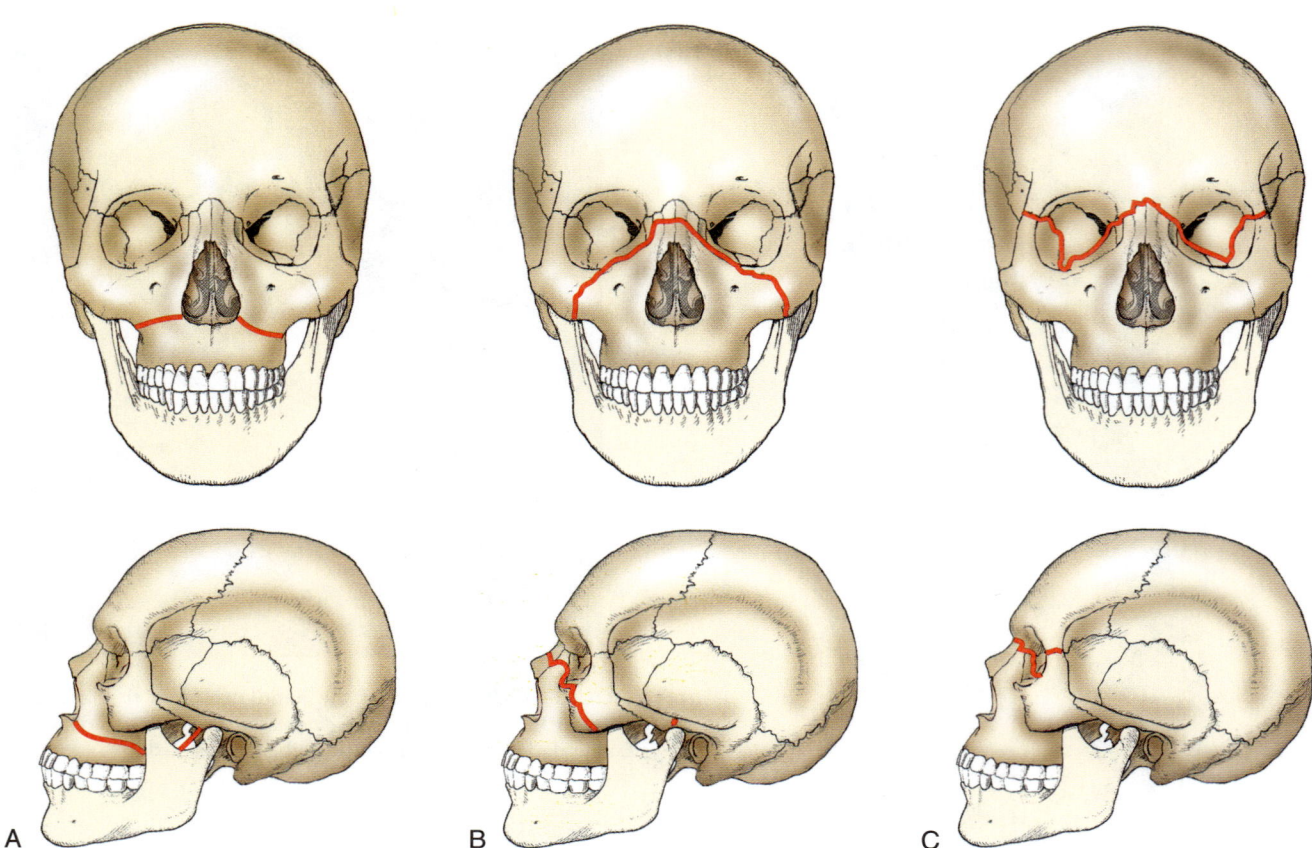

FIGURE 40-4 A, Le Fort I facial fractures (lateral and frontal views). **B,** Le Fort II fractures (lateral and frontal views). **C,** Le Fort III fractures (lateral and frontal views). (Modified from ENA: *Sheehy's emergency nursing,* ed 6, St Louis, 2010, Mosby.)

the severity of injury, different combinations of Le Fort fractures may be present.

Signs and symptoms specific to midface fractures include midfacial edema, unstable maxilla, lengthening of the face (donkey face), epistaxis, numb upper teeth, nasal flattening, and cerebrospinal fluid rhinorrhea (cerebrospinal fluid leakage from the nose caused by ethmoid cribriform plate fracture). Patients with midface fractures require hospitalization. These patients (particularly those with Le Fort II and III fractures) are at risk of having serious airway problems related to swelling and bleeding. Because of the extent of the fractures, placing nasogastric or even nasotracheal tubes into the brain tissue is a possibility.

> **NOTE**
> As described in Chapter 15, nasal airways, nasogastric tubes, and nasotracheal intubation are contraindicated in patients who have fractures of the basal skull or facial bones. Cerebrospinal fluid leakage from the ear or nose should be allowed to drain freely. The paramedic should make no attempts to control cerebrospinal fluid leakage with direct pressure.

FRACTURES OF THE ZYGOMA

The zygoma (malar eminence) articulates with the frontal, maxillary, and temporal bones. The zygoma commonly is called the *cheek bone*. It is rarely fractured because of its sturdy construction. When fractures occur, they usually are a result of physical assaults and vehicle crashes. Zygomatic fractures often are associated with orbital fractures and manifest similar clinical signs (Figure 40-5). The two are distinguished by x-ray exam. Signs and symptoms specific to zygomatic fractures include flatness of a usually rounded cheek area; numbness of the cheek, nose, and upper lip (particularly if an orbital fracture is involved); epistaxis; and altered vision.

FRACTURES OF THE ORBIT

The orbital contents are protected by a bony ring. The ring resembles a pyramid, with the apex pointed toward the back of the head. The bones of the walls, floor, and roof of the orbit are thin and are fractured easily by direct blows and transmitted forces. In addition, many orbital fractures are associated with other facial injuries, such as Le Fort II and III fractures.

A **blowout fracture** to the orbit can occur when an object of greater diameter than that of the bony orbital rim strikes the globe of the eye and surrounding soft tissue (Figure 40-6). This impact pushes the globe into the orbit and in turn compresses the orbital contents. The sudden increase in intraocular pressure is transmitted to the orbital floor. The orbital floor is the weakest part of the orbital structure. If the orbital floor fractures, the orbital contents may be forced into the maxillary sinus, where soft tissue and extraocular muscles may be trapped in the defect. Signs and symptoms of blowout fractures include periorbital edema, subconjunctival ecchymosis, diplopia (double vision), enophthalmos (recessed globe), epistaxis, anesthesia in the region of the infraorbital nerve (anterior cheek), and impaired extraocular movements.

 CRITICAL THINKING
How do you assess a patient's eye movement?

Orbital fractures often are associated with other fractures, including the Le Fort II and III injuries and those of the zygomatic complex. In addition, injury to the orbital contents is common. The paramedic should suspect such injury with any facial fracture.

FRACTURES OF THE NOSE

Of all the facial bones the nasal bones have the least structural strength. They are fractured most frequently. The external portion of the nose, formed mostly of hyaline cartilage, is supported mainly by the nasal bones and the frontal processes of the maxillary bones. Injuries to the nose may depress the dorsum of the nose, displace it to one side, or result only in epistaxis and swelling without apparent skeletal deformity. Fractures to the orbit also may be present. In children, minimal displacement of nasal bones can result in growth changes and ultimate deformity.

Management of Facial Fractures

When caring for a patient with facial fractures, the paramedic should assume that the spine has been injured and should use spinal precautions. Facial fractures are associated with a high percentage of related cervical spine

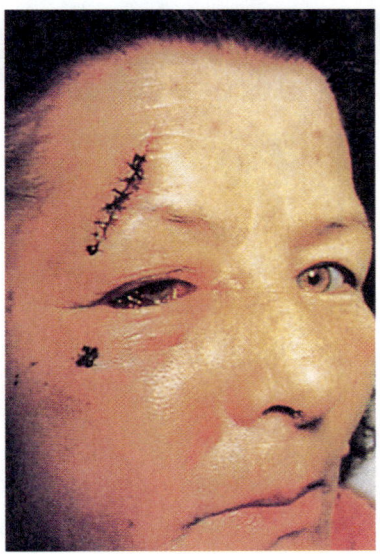

FIGURE 40-5 Fracture of the zygomatic bone. (From London PS: *A colour atlas of diagnosis after recent injury,* Ipswich, England, 1990, Wolfe Medical Publications, Ltd.)

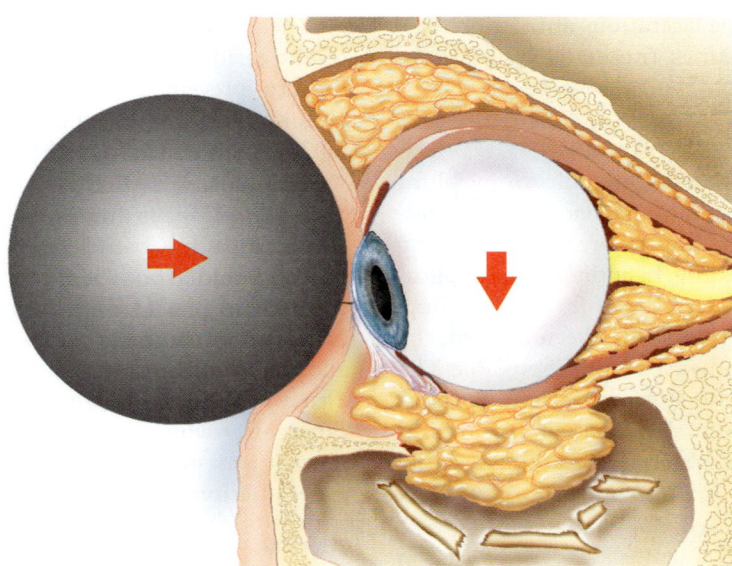

FIGURE 40-6 Artist's impression of a blowout fracture caused by the impact of a ball. (From Ragge N: *Immediate eye care,* London, 1990, Wolfe Medical Publications, Ltd.)

fractures.[1] The paramedic should assess the patient's airway for obstruction caused by blood, vomitus, bone fragments, broken teeth, dentures, and damage to the anterior neck. Suction may be needed to clear the airway of debris and fluid. The paramedic may need to maintain the airway with a nasal (in the absence of suspected midface or basal skull fracture) or oral adjunct, tracheal intubation, or cricothyrotomy if indicated.

Bleeding usually can be controlled by direct pressure and pressure bandages. Epistaxis may be severe and should be controlled by applying external pressure to the anterior nares. To prevent blood from draining down the throat, mild epistaxis is best controlled in the conscious patient by instructing the patient to sit upright or to lean forward (in the absence of spinal injury) while compressing the nares. An unconscious patient should be positioned on the side (if not contraindicated by injury). If bleeding is severe, the paramedic should evaluate the patient for hemorrhagic shock.

 CRITICAL THINKING
Why should the blood not drain posteriorly?

EAR, EYE, AND DENTAL TRAUMA

The ears, eyes, or teeth may be injured separately or along with other forms of head and facial trauma. Injury to these regions may be minor. Yet such injuries may result in permanent sensory function loss and disfigurement. Regardless of the severity, the paramedic should evaluate ear, eye, and dental trauma and treat it only after identifying and managing life-threatening problems.

Ear Trauma

Trauma to the ear may include lacerations and contusions, thermal injuries, chemical injuries, traumatic perforations, and barotitis.

LACERATIONS AND CONTUSIONS

Lacerations and contusions usually result from blunt trauma. They are particularly common in victims of domestic violence (Figure 40-7). These injuries are treated by using direct pressure to control bleeding. In addition, the application of ice or cold compresses decreases soft tissue swelling. If a portion of the outer ear (pinna) has been avulsed, the paramedic should retrieve the avulsed tissue if possible. The tissue should be wrapped in moist gauze, sealed in plastic, placed on ice, and transported with the patient for surgical repair. Cartilage tears often heal poorly and are easily infected.

THERMAL INJURIES

Thermal injuries may occur from prolonged exposure to extreme cold. They also may occur from exposure of lesser duration to extreme heat. Contact with hot liquids or

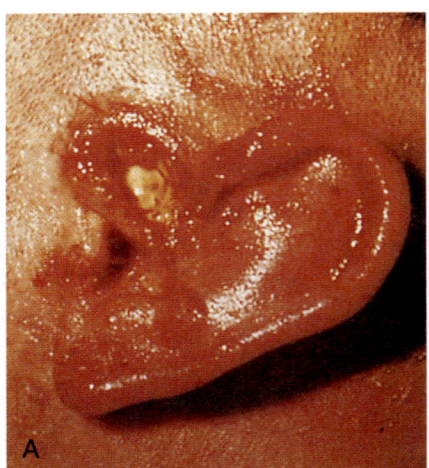

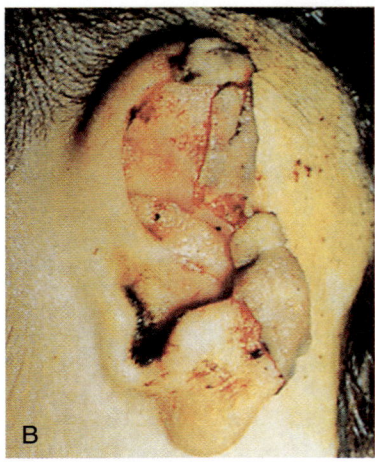

FIGURE 40-7 A, Partially detached pinna. **B,** Loss of rim. (From London PS: *A colour atlas of diagnosis after recent injury,* Ipswich, England, 1990, Wolfe Medical Publications, Ltd.)

electrical currents also can lead to thermal injury. Prehospital treatment usually is limited to application of dressings to prevent contamination and transportation for evaluation by a physician. (Thermal injuries are discussed in Chapter 39 and Chapter 45.)

CHEMICAL INJURIES

As described in Chapter 39: Burns, strong acids or alkalis produce burns on contact. Emergency care consists of copious irrigation. After irrigation, the paramedic should bathe the ear and ear canal with saline or sterile water, allowing the irrigation liquid to remain in the ear canal for 2 to 3 minutes. This procedure should be repeated 3 or 4 times, after which the ear should be dried and covered to prevent contamination. The patient should be transported for evaluation by a physician.

TRAUMATIC PERFORATIONS

The tympanic membrane can be perforated. **Traumatic perforation** can occur by objects such as a cotton-tipped applicator and by changes in pressure. Pressure injuries may result from explosions (blast injuries) or scuba diving (barotrauma). These injuries usually heal spontaneously without treatment. Still, evaluation by a physician is advised.

If the injury is caused by a penetrating object, the paramedic should stabilize the object in place and cover the ear to prevent further contamination. The inner or middle ear canal may have been contaminated (e.g., by swimming water or a foreign object). In that case, antibiotic therapy usually is prescribed. Serious complications that may result from perforations include facial nerve palsy (described in Chapter 23) frequently accompanied by temporal bone fractures, hearing loss, and vertigo.

BAROTITIS

Barotitis occurs when a person is exposed to changes in barometric pressure great enough to produce inflammation and injury to the middle ear. Barotitis can result, for example, from flying at high altitudes and from scuba diving.

Gas pressure in the air-filled spaces of the middle ear normally equals that of the environment. Boyle's law (further described in Chapter 45) states that at constant temperature, the volume of a gas is inversely proportional to the pressure. On ascent, gas expands. On descent, it contracts. Therefore when gases become trapped or partially trapped, they expand in direct proportion to the decrease in pressure. When trapped gas cannot reach equilibrium with environmental pressure, pain and the sensation of a blocked ear may develop. To equalize the pressure in the middle ear, the patient can be directed to bear down (Valsalva's maneuver), yawn, swallow, and move the lower jaw. These methods may cause the eustachian tube to open, which will equalize the pressure in the middle ear cavity.

Eye Trauma

More than 2000 eye and orbital injuries are estimated to occur each day in the United States.[2] Common causes of eye injury are blunt and penetrating trauma from motor vehicle crashes, sport and recreational activities, and violent altercations; chemical exposure from household and industrial accidents; foreign bodies; and animal bites and scratches.

EVALUATION

Acute eye injuries may be difficult to identify because a patient with normal vision may have a serious underlying injury. Symptoms requiring a high degree of suspicion include the following:

- Obvious trauma with eye injury
- Visual loss or blurred vision that does not improve with blinking, indicating possible damage to the globe, ocular contents, or optic nerve
- Loss of a portion of the visual field, indicating possible detachment of the retina, hemorrhage into the eye, or optic nerve injury

Evaluation of eye injury should include a thorough history and measurement of visual acuity, pupillary reaction, and extraocular movements (see Chapter 20: Secondary Assessment). Assessing the patient's vision will be a rough estimation at best. The patient's vision will be reevaluated in the emergency department under controlled circumstances.

CRITICAL THINKING

Aside from trauma, what are some other causes of visual disturbances?

History. A thorough history should include the following information:

- Exact mode of injury
- Previous ocular, medical, and drug history, including cataracts, glaucoma, and presence of hepatitis or human immunodeficiency virus
- Use of eye medications
- Use of corrective glasses or contact lenses
- Presence of ocular prostheses
- Duration of symptoms and treatment interventions that may have been attempted before emergency medical services arrival

Visual Acuity. The measurement of **visual acuity** is usually the first step in any examination of the patient's eyes. (The exception is a chemical burn to the eye. In this case, irrigation should be performed before measurement of visual acuity.) Visual acuity can be measured with a hand-held visual acuity chart (e.g., Snellen chart), or any printed material with small, medium, and large point sizes (e.g., an intravenous fluid bag). The paramedic should record the distance that the printed item was held from the patient's face.

The vision of each eye should be assessed separately while covering the other eye. (No pressure should be applied.) The paramedic should test the injured eye first for acuity comparison to the uninjured eye. If the patient wears corrective lenses, acuity should be measured with lenses first and then without lenses. Illiterate or non–English-speaking patients require an alternative method of evaluation. Such methods may include finger counting, hand motion, and presence or absence of light perception. Abnormal responses to any of these methods indicate significant loss of vision.

CRITICAL THINKING

The assessment of visual acuity may be difficult on some calls. What factors in the prehospital setting may make it difficult?

NOTE

The two types of vision are central and peripheral. **Central vision** results from images falling on the macula of the retina. **Peripheral vision** is the ability to see objects that reflect light waves on areas of the retina other than the macula.

PUPILLARY REACTION

Pupils should be black, round, and equal in size. The pupils also should react to light in the same way and at the same time. Both eyes should constrict in response to light and dilate in response to dark. (A *direct response to light* refers to constriction of the illuminated pupil. A *consensual response to light* refers to constriction of the opposite pupil.) Abnormal pupillary responses after blunt trauma to the eye are common and may be caused by tearing. More commonly, though, they are caused by direct trauma to the pupillary sphincter muscle. Abnormal responses also may suggest a more serious injury involving the optic nerve or globe. As described in Chapter 20, causes of pupil abnormalities in the absence of recent injury include drug use, cataracts, previous surgical procedures, ocular prosthesis, anisocoria (normal or congenital unequal pupil size), central nervous system disease, strokes, and previous injury. The paramedic should document all of the patient's pupil abnormalities.

> ### DID YOU KNOW?
> When the eyes are open, the central nervous system is exposed. This happens nowhere else in the human body. Because of this vulnerability, the brain is well wired to provide protection. A sudden movement near the face, a flash of bright light, or a loud noise will cause the eyelids to slam shut, forming a waterproof, airtight shield. Strong tarsal plates shield support and protect the eyelids. Eyelashes are rooted in nerve cells so sensitive that a particle of grit caught by one lash will close the both eyelids automatically.

EXTRAOCULAR MOVEMENTS

Extraocular muscles are responsible for movements of the globe, or eyeball. Voluntary muscles are innervated by cranial nerves III, IV, and VI. The muscles are attached to the outside of the eyeball and bones of the orbit and move the globe in any desired direction. Involuntary eye muscles are innervated by sympathetic nerves. These muscles are located within the eye. Examples of involuntary eye muscles are the iris and the ciliary muscle. These muscles dilate and constrict the pupil and change the shape of the lens, respectively.

To evaluate the extraocular movement of the eyes (described in Chapter 20), the paramedic should instruct the patient to visually track the movement of an object. (For example, the object may be a finger, pencil, or penlight.) The patient should be asked to track the object up, down, to the right, and to the left. Abnormalities in movement may indicate orbital content edema, cranial nerve injury, contusions or lacerations of extraocular muscles, or muscle entrapment in a fracture. Patients with limited or abnormal extraocular movements often complain of double vision in one or more directions of gaze. The paramedic should document all findings.

EVALUATION AND MANAGEMENT OF SPECIFIC EYE INJURIES

Few eye injuries are truly urgent. However, all victims of ocular trauma should be evaluated by a physician. Some patients need specialized care by an ophthalmologist. If the paramedic suspects a serious injury that may require specialized care, medical direction should be advised as soon as possible. That way, services will be ready when the patient arrives in the emergency department (Figure 40-8).

Foreign bodies in the cornea, conjunctiva, or eyelid usually cause the patient to complain of the sensation of something in the eye (especially when opening and closing the eyelids) and to have profuse tearing. If a foreign body is suspected, the inner surface of the upper and lower lids and conjunctivae should be inspected. The paramedic should remove the foreign body by gentle, copious irrigation with clear fluid. (For example, tap water, normal saline, or sterile water are appropriate.) Medical direction may recommend that an ophthalmic anesthetic such as **tetracaine** be applied for patient comfort. The paramedic should advise and remind the patient not to touch or rub the eye after the administration of **tetracaine.** Serious eye injury can result.

Corneal abrasion occurs when the outer layers of the cornea are avulsed. The injury often results from a foreign body scratching the cornea and is common in those who wear some types of contact lenses. Patients with a corneal abrasion usually complain of pain and foreign body sensation under the upper eyelid, **photophobia** (abnormal light sensitivity), excessive tearing, and sometimes a decrease in visual acuity. Often these signs and symptoms are delayed. The prehospital management of corneal abrasion is gentle irrigation with clear fluid. Management also involves the application of a double patch to eyes to prevent the injured eye from moving when the uninjured eye moves, causing aggravation (Figure 40-9). Corneal abrasions generally heal within 24 to 48 hours.

>
> ### CRITICAL THINKING
> Will the patient with a suspected corneal abrasion need to be evaluated by a physician?

Blunt trauma to the eye or its adjacent structures may result in a contusion injury, **traumatic hyphema** (bleeding into the anterior chamber), or globe or scleral rupture. Box 40-1 lists the signs and symptoms of these injuries.

Blunt injury to the eye may be associated with other serious injuries. Such injuries include orbital fracture, vitreous hemorrhage, and dislocation of the lens. The prehospital care should be limited to the control of any bleeding by application of gentle, direct pressure; protection of the eye with a metal shield or cardboard cup; and rapid transport for physician evaluation. If the paramedic suspects a traumatic hyphema or globe or scleral rupture, the paramedic should place the patient on a spine board and elevate the

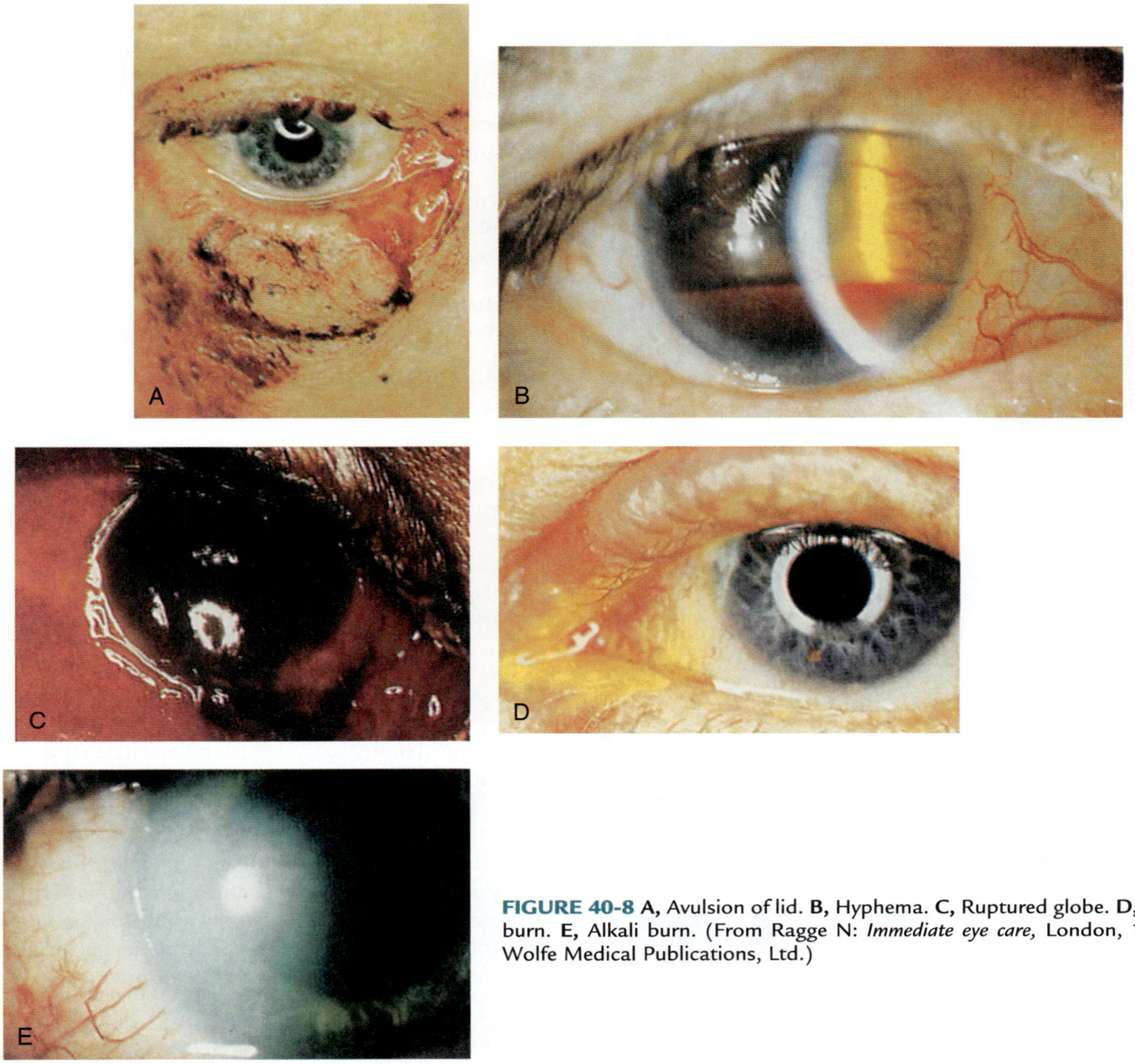

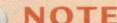

FIGURE 40-8 A, Avulsion of lid. **B,** Hyphema. **C,** Ruptured globe. **D,** Acid burn. **E,** Alkali burn. (From Ragge N: *Immediate eye care,* London, 1990, Wolfe Medical Publications, Ltd.)

head of the spine board 40 degrees to decrease intraocular pressure. The patient should also be instructed to avoid any activity that might increase intraocular pressure. Analgesics and antiemetics may be indicated for pain relief and nausea. These drugs can reduce movement, straining, coughing, and retching that may increase intraocular pressure.

Penetrating injury to the eye may be associated with embedded foreign bodies, lid avulsions, and lacerations to the lids, sclera, or cornea. Penetrating globe injuries can damage retinal structures and can cause a loss of **vitreous humor** (the jellylike fluid in the eye that fills the space between the lens and the retina) and subsequent blindness. The paramedic should control any bleeding by applying gentle, direct pressure. The globe should be protected from dehydration or contamination from foreign material. One way is to cover the orbital area with plastic or damp, sterile dressings and an eye shield.

> **NOTE**
> Eye drops should not be used when globe rupture is suspected. Aggressive pain management is crucial to prevent or decrease expulsion of intraocular contents. If the patient is nauseated, antiemetics should be given.[3]

The paramedic should stabilize foreign bodies protruding from the eye and should cover these with a cardboard cup and secure the cup with tape. The unaffected eye should also be covered to prevent **consensual movement** (one eye acting in concert with the other). The paramedic should not attempt to remove the object. If needed, the penetrating object may be shortened for transport (*after* consulting with medical direction). Oxygen and intravenous fluids also may be recommended in these cases.

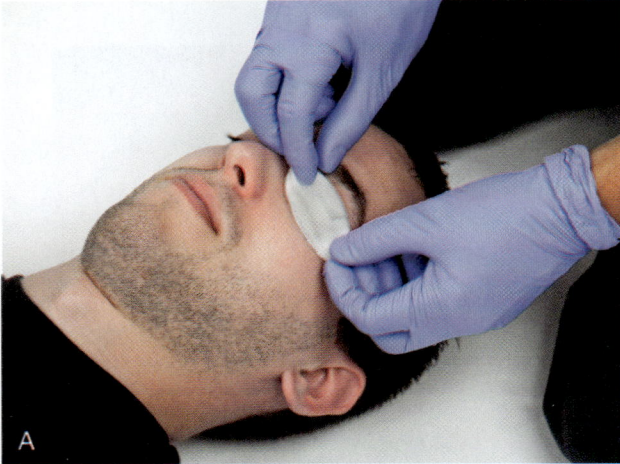

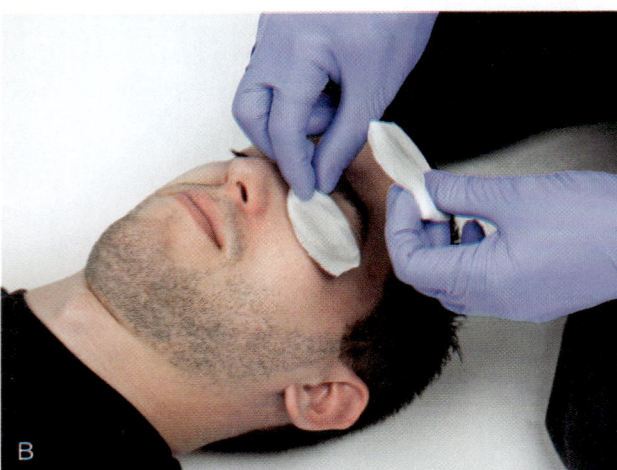

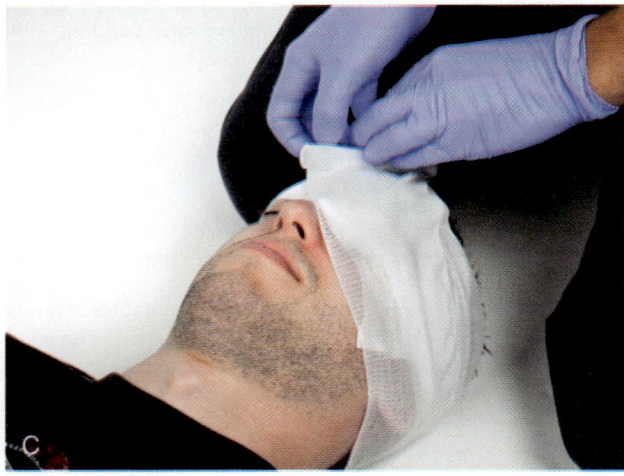

FIGURE 40-9 Application of a double patch. **A,** A folded pad is placed over the closed eye. **B,** A second unfolded pad is placed over the top of the first pad. **C,** The pads are secured firmly in place.

BOX 40-1 Signs and Symptoms of Eye Injuries

Contusion Injury
- Traumatic dilation or constriction of the pupil
- Pain
- Photophobia
- Blurred vision
- Tears of the iris (tear-shaped pupil)

Traumatic Hyphema
- Traumatic dilation or, less commonly, constriction of the pupil
- Decrease in visual acuity
- Blood in the anterior chamber (may be visible with penlight)

Globe or Scleral Rupture
- Decrease in visual acuity to hand movements or light perception
- Lowered intraocular pressure (soft eye)
- Pupil irregularity
- Hyphema

Chemical injury to the eye (described in Chapter 39) may be associated with loss of corneal epithelial tissue, globe perforation, and scarring and deformation of eyelids and conjunctivae. These injuries are true emergencies. They require immediate intervention. A chemical exposure generally mandates extensive, continuous irrigation of both eyes with a neutral fluid for 20 minutes before patient transport (if effective irrigation can be performed) and while en route to the emergency department.

 LOOK AGAIN
See Chapter 39: Burns, pp. 1136-1137.

 CRITICAL THINKING
Should you wait until contacting medical direction before you begin irrigation of the eye?

CONTACT LENSES

Contact lenses are of three general types: hard, soft hydrophilic, and rigid gas-permeable. Hard lenses are microlenses that sometimes are prescribed for **astigmatism** (these lenses rarely are used today). Soft (hydrophilic) lenses usually are large in diameter (extending onto the conjunctiva). Soft lenses may be designed for daily or extended wear. Rigid gas-permeable lenses are similar in size to microlenses. These lenses have a low water content and high oxygen permeability.

As a rule, paramedics should not attempt to remove contact lenses in patients with eye injuries. To do so may cause more damage and may aggravate the injury. If management of an eye injury is complicated by the presence of contact lenses (e.g., chemical burns to the eyes), medical direction may recommend that the lenses be removed. If the patient is unable to remove the lenses, the paramedic may be instructed to do so (Box 40-2).

Dental Trauma

The adult normally has 32 teeth. Each tooth consists of two sections: the *crown,* which projects above the *gingiva* (the portion of the oral mucosa surrounding the tooth), and the *root,* which fits into the bony socket (alveolus) of the maxilla or mandible. Three layers make up the hard tissues of the teeth: the *enamel,* the *dentin* (ivory), and the *cementum.* The soft tissues of the teeth include the *pulp* and the *periodontal membrane* (Figure 40-10).

The teeth and associated alveolar process may be injured alone or along with fractures of the jaw or facial bones. The two most common types of dental trauma involve fractures and avulsions of the anterior teeth. If a tooth is fractured, the paramedic should examine the oral cavity carefully for tooth fragments. Removal of fragments reduces the risk of aspiration and obstruction of the airway. Lacerations and avulsions to the tongue and surrounding mucous membranes often occur with dental trauma. These injuries often are painful and may bleed profusely. They may compromise the patient's airway as well.

BOX 40-2 Removal of Contact Lenses

Removal of Hard and Rigid Gas-Permeable Lenses

1. With gloved hands, separate the eyelids so that the margins of the lids are beyond the top and bottom edges of the lens.
2. Gently pass the eyelids down and forward to the edges of the lens.
3. Move the eyelids toward each other, forcing the lens to slide out between them.
4. Store the lens in a container with water or saline, and label the container with the patient's name. If a contact lens container is not available, store each lens in a separate container and label as left or right.
5. If lens removal is difficult, gently move the lens downward from the cornea to the conjunctiva overlying the sclera until arrival in the emergency department.

NOTE: Special suction cups are also available for the removal of hard and rigid contact lenses. This device should be moistened with saline or sterile water before contacting the lens.

Removal of Soft Lenses

1. With gloved hands, pull down the lower eyelid.
2. Gently slide the soft lens down onto the conjunctiva.
3. Using a pinching motion, compress the lens between the thumb and index finger.
4. Remove the lens from the eye.
5. Store the lens in a container (marked right or left) with water or saline, and label the container with the patient's name.

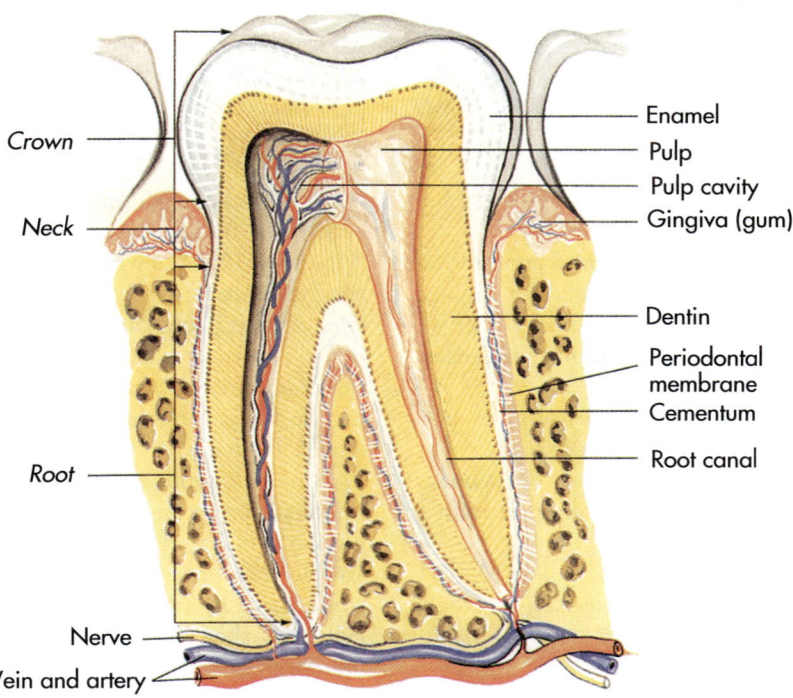

FIGURE 40-10 Longitudinal section of a tooth. (From Thibodeau GA, Patton KT: *Structure and function of the body,* ed 13, St Louis, 2008, Mosby.)

Tooth avulsions are common, and many teeth can be saved with proper emergency treatment.[4] Permanent teeth that have been avulsed have a good survival rate if reimplanted and stabilized within 1 hour. (Deciduous teeth [milk or baby teeth] generally are not reimplanted. They may become fused to the bone, delaying formation and eruption of the permanent tooth.) If the avulsed tooth has been out of the patient's mouth for less than 15 minutes, medical direction may recommend reimplanting the tooth into the original socket. The paramedic should take care not to reimplant the tooth backward and also should be alert for possible aspiration. If reimplantation is impossible, the paramedic should follow the guidelines established by the American Dental Association and the American Association of Endodontists:

1. Never place an avulsed tooth in anything that can dry or crush the outside of the tooth.
2. Do not handle the tooth roughly. Do not rinse it off or rub, scrape, or disinfect the outside of the tooth in any way. (Any adherent membrane or fibrous tissue should be left in place to avoid stripping off the periodontal membrane and ligament, which are critical to the survival of a reimplanted tooth.)
3. Place the tooth in a nurturing, break-resistant storage device (e.g., Emergency Tooth Preserving System). This device should have a tightly fitted top and soft inner walls.
4. Store the tooth in a pH-balanced, isotonic, glucose-, calcium-, and magnesium-enriched cell-preserving fluid (e.g., Hank's solution). Use refrigerated fresh whole milk as the best alternative storage medium. (Powdered milk is not suitable.) For short periods (1 hour or less), use sterile saline. Do not use tap water because it damages the periodontal ligament.
5. Advise medical direction of avulsed teeth so that appropriate services will be available when the patient arrives in the emergency department.

ANTERIOR NECK TRAUMA

Anterior neck injuries are caused by blunt and penetrating trauma (Figure 40-11). These injuries may result in damage to the skeletal structures, vascular structures, nerves, muscles, and glands of the neck. Common mechanisms of injury to the anterior neck are as follows:

- Strangulation injuries from clothing, jewelry, or personal equipment getting caught in machinery
- All-terrain vehicles and other small motor vehicles (clothesline injuries to the neck from running into wires, ropes, or fences)
- Blows to the neck
- Contact sports (boxing, karate, basketball, football, hockey)
- Hangings
- Horseback riding
- Hyperextension and hyperflexion injuries
- Industrial injuries

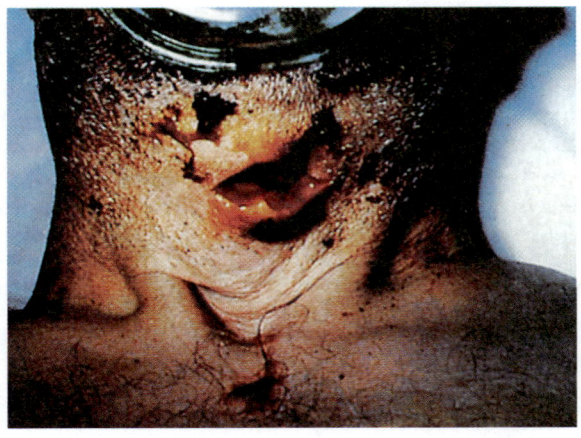

FIGURE 40-11 A self-inflicted stab wound that had entered the pharynx. (From London PS: *A colour atlas of diagnosis after recent injury,* Ipswich, England, 1990, Wolfe Medical Publications, Ltd.)

- Missile injury from firearms
- Motor vehicle crashes
- Neck striking dashboard or steering column
- Snow skiing
- Sport and recreational activities
- Stab wounds (knives, screwdrivers, ice picks)
- Violent altercations
- Water sports (jet skiing, water skiing)

With blunt and penetrating neck injuries, the paramedic should assume the patient has a cervical spine injury also. The paramedic must assume such injury until ruled out by clinical examination and x-ray films (radiography) of the cervical region of the neck. Radiographic examination alone does not rule out cervical spine injury (see Chapter 41).

Evaluation

For purposes of evaluating the trauma patient, the neck can be divided into three zones defined by horizontal planes (Figure 40-12).[5] Zone I represents the base of the neck. This zone extends from the sternal notch to the top of the clavicles or the cricoid cartilage. Injuries to this zone have the highest mortality rate because of the risk of injury to major vascular and thoracic structures (subclavian vessels and jugular veins, lungs, esophagus, trachea, cervical spine, cervical nerve roots).

Zone II extends from the clavicles or cricoid cartilage cephalad to the angle of the mandible. The carotid artery, jugular vein, trachea, larynx, esophagus, and cervical spine are the vital structures in this zone. Because of the relative size of zone II, injuries to this zone are the most common. However, they have a lower mortality rate than zone I injuries.

Zone III is the part of the neck above the angle of the mandible. The risk of injury to the distal carotid artery, salivary glands, and pharynx is greatest in this zone.

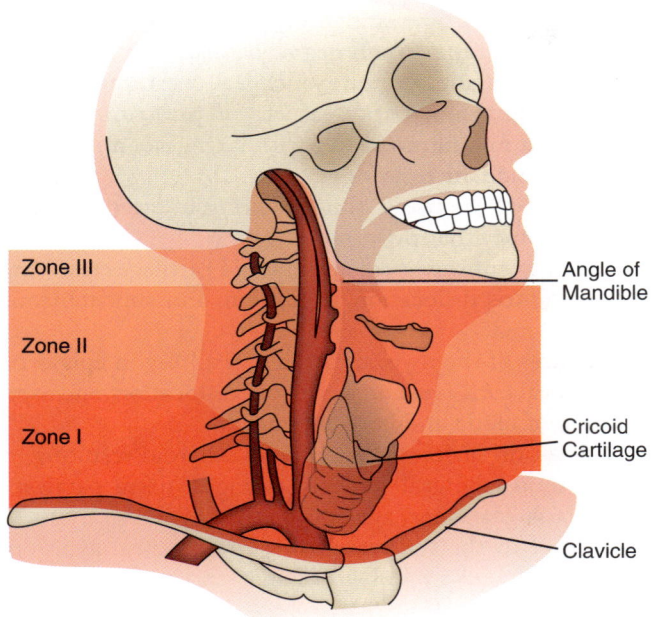

FIGURE 40-12 Zones of the neck. The junction of zone I and zone II is described variously as the cricoid cartilage or top of the clavicles.

Soft Tissue Injuries

Soft tissue injuries to the neck from blunt trauma often produce hematomata and associated edema or direct laryngeal or tracheal injury. Both of these injuries can result in airway compromise. Penetrating trauma may produce lacerations and puncture wounds with resultant vascular, laryngotracheal, or esophageal injury. Blunt trauma may cause vascular injuries as well. However, this is uncommon. As with all trauma victims, initial evaluation and resuscitation must begin with rapid assessment, control of the airway, and consideration for spinal injury.

CRITICAL THINKING
Is prehospital airway control always possible in patients with anterior neck injuries?

HEMATOMATA AND EDEMA

Edema of the pharynx, larynx, trachea, epiglottis, and vocal cords may produce enough pressure in the neck tissues to obstruct the airway completely. If the airway is compromised (evidenced by dyspnea, inspiratory stridor, cyanosis, or changes in voice quality), the paramedic should consider oral or nasal intubation with spinal precautions. Intubation stabilizes damaged areas of the neck, protects the airway, and provides a means for ventilatory support.

(A slightly smaller endotracheal tube may be needed to ensure passage through the airway.)

NOTE
Crushed or severed airways can be blocked totally or partially by attempts at oral or nasal intubation. In these cases (if the patient is moving air), rapid transport with high-concentration oxygen is perhaps the most prudent course.

When direct intubation is impossible because of blood, vomitus (that cannot be removed by suction), or progressive edema, a cricothyrotomy or translaryngeal cannula ventilation (described in Chapter 15) may be indicated. Another measure that may help in treating edematous airways includes the administration of cool, humidified oxygen. Yet another measure is the slight elevation of the patient's head. (This can be done if it is not contraindicated by the injury.)

LACERATIONS AND PUNCTURE WOUNDS

Lacerations and puncture wounds may be superficial or deep. Superficial wounds usually can be managed by covering the wound. The covering helps to prevent further contamination. Deep wounds are associated with more serious injuries to underlying structures. These injuries may require aggressive airway therapy and ventilatory support, suction, hemorrhage control by direct pressure, and fluid replacement. Signs and symptoms of significant penetrating neck trauma include the following:

- Active bleeding
- Dysphagia
- Dyspnea
- Hematemesis
- Hemoptysis
- Hoarseness
- Large or expanding hematoma
- Mobility and crepitus
- Neurological deficit (stroke, brachial plexus injury, spinal cord injury)
- Pulse deficit
- Shock
- Stridor
- Subcutaneous emphysema
- Tenderness to palpation

CRITICAL THINKING
Why is rapid transport crucial when caring for a patient who has anterior neck injuries?

VASCULAR INJURY

Blood vessels are the most commonly injured structures in the neck; they may be injured by blunt or penetrating trauma. Vessels at risk of injury include the carotid, vertebral, subclavian, innominate, and internal mammary arteries and the jugular and subclavian veins. Laceration of these major vessels can result in rapid exsanguination (death from extensive blood loss) if bleeding is not controlled.

Securing the airway (with spinal precautions) and providing adequate ventilatory support is the first priority. The next priority is to control hemorrhage. This can be achieved with constant, direct pressure. The paramedic should apply pressure only to the affected vessels. Thus blood flow to the brain will not be obstructed completely. If bleeding cannot be controlled in this manner, medical direction may advise applying direct pressure with a gloved finger to the vessel.

> **NOTE**
> Under no circumstances should cervical vessels be clamped with hemostats in the prehospital setting. Doing so may traumatize critical vascular structures and may produce permanent nerve injury.

If the paramedic suspects a venous injury, the patient should be kept supine or in a slight Trendelenburg position. This will help to prevent air embolism (a rare but lethal complication). If the paramedic suspects an air embolism (described in Chapter 14), the paramedic should turn the immobilized patient on the left side. The patient's head should be lower than the feet in an attempt to trap the air embolus in the right ventricle. Venous neck wounds should be dressed with an occlusive dressing.

Fluid replacement for hypovolemia should be guided by medical direction. Fluid replacement may include using large-bore catheters and isotonic crystalloid (lactated Ringer's solution or normal saline). If penetrating injury to the base of the neck (zone I) has occurred, upper extremity venous drainage may be compromised by the laceration. In this event, placement of at least one intravenous line in a lower extremity should be considered. Medical direction may advise that a second intravenous line be placed in the upper extremity on the side opposite the injury.

> **CRITICAL THINKING**
> Why might application of a pneumatic antishock garment be harmful with this type of injury?

LARYNGEAL OR TRACHEAL INJURY

Injury from blunt or penetrating trauma to the anterior neck may cause fracture or dislocation of the laryngeal and tracheal cartilages, hemorrhage, or swelling of the air passages. All of these injuries can compromise the airway and cause respiratory distress. Airway injury can lead to death in head and neck trauma patients. Thus rapid and judicious control of the airway and prevention of aspiration are crucial. In addition, a high degree of suspicion for associated vascular disruption and esophageal, chest, and intraabdominal injury is a critical aspect of preventing death. Injuries that may be associated with laryngeal and tracheal trauma include the following:

- Fracture of the hyoid bone resulting in laceration and distortion of the epiglottis
- Separation of the hyoid and thyroid cartilages resulting in epiglottis dislocation, aspiration, and subcutaneous emphysema
- Fractures of the thyroid cartilage resulting in epiglottis and vocal cord avulsion, arytenoid dislocation, and aspiration of blood and bone fragments
- Dislocation or fracture of the cricothyroid resulting in long-term laryngeal stenosis, laryngeal nerve paralysis, and laryngotracheal avulsion
- Fracture to the trachea resulting in tracheal avulsion, complete airway obstruction, and subcutaneous emphysema

The management of laryngeal and tracheal trauma is controversial. Some medical direction agencies recommend oral or nasal intubation. Other agencies believe that intubation attempts may contribute to the potential for injury resulting from lack of oxygen during the procedure. These attempts also may damage the airway structures further. Alternative methods of airway management include use of bag-mask ventilation, cricothyrotomy, and translaryngeal cannula ventilation.

> **NOTE**
> Airway procedures that involve entry through the neck generally are avoided in the field because of the associated risks. As a rule, these patients should be well ventilated with a bag-mask device. They should be transported rapidly to the receiving facility for surgical tracheotomy as well. As described in Chapter 15, translaryngeal cannula ventilation is hazardous in the presence of complete airway obstruction. Incorrectly used, this technique does not provide adequate exhalation of gases and air. The technique may result in carbon dioxide retention and significant injury from high pressure developing in the chest and airways (barotrauma).

If penetrating trauma causes complete disruption of the laryngotracheal structure, medical direction may recommend dissection through the wound. That way, the exposed distal trachea can be cannulated directly with a cuffed endotracheal tube. Regardless of the method chosen, emergency care is directed at securing the airway with spinal precautions, providing adequate ventilatory support, controlling hemorrhage, treating for shock, and providing rapid transport to an appropriate medical facility for definitive surgical care.

ESOPHAGEAL INJURY

Esophageal injuries should be suspected in patients with trauma to the neck or chest. Specific injuries that require a high degree of suspicion for associated esophageal injury include tracheal fractures, penetrating trauma from stab or gunshot wounds, and ingestion of caustic substances.

Esophageal injury is difficult to diagnose. It may be overlooked as the paramedic focuses on more obvious injuries that pose a threat to life. Signs and symptoms may include subcutaneous emphysema, neck hematoma, and bleeding from the mouth and nose.

Esophageal perforation is associated with a high mortality rate. Death results from mediastinitis caused by the release of gastric contents into the thoracic cavity. If not contraindicated by mechanism of injury, the paramedic should place the patient with a suspected esophageal tear in a semi-Fowler position. (This is an inclined position. The upper half of the body is raised by elevating the head or stretcher about 30 degrees.) This position will help to prevent reflux of gastric contents.

CRITICAL THINKING
Are these signs and symptoms so unique that you will be able to distinguish esophageal injury as the cause, versus other kinds of traumatic conditions?

HEAD TRAUMA

As described in Chapter 10: Review of Human Systems, the anatomical components of the skull are the scalp followed by the cranial vault, under which are the dural membrane, the arachnoid membrane, the pia mater, and brain substance. Injuries to the skull may be classified as soft tissue injuries to the scalp and as skull fractures.

LOOK AGAIN
See Chapter 10: Review of Human Systems, pp. 171-176.

NOTE
All patients with head or neck trauma must be assumed to have a spinal injury. This must be the case until injury is ruled out by clinical examination and x-ray films in the emergency department. (Spinal precautions [including helmet removal] are presented in Chapter 41.) This text assumes that spinal precautions will be used for all patients with a significant mechanism of injury.

Soft Tissue Injuries to the Scalp

The most common scalp injury is an irregular linear laceration. Like the face, the scalp is very vascular. Thus scalp lacerations may bleed heavily (Figure 40-13). They also may

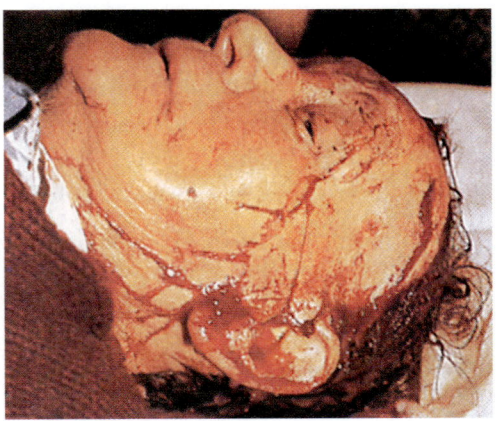

FIGURE 40-13 Even small wounds from the scalp can bleed profusely. (From London PS: *A colour atlas of diagnosis after recent injury,* Ipswich, England, 1990, Wolfe Medical Publications, Ltd.)

result in hypovolemia, particularly in infants and children. Other, less frequent scalp injuries include **stellate wounds** (ballistic wounds that are star-shaped), avulsions, and **subgaleal hematomata** (bleeding in the potential space between the skull and scalp).

Management of soft tissue injuries to the scalp includes efforts to prevent contamination of open wounds, use of direct pressure or pressure dressings to decrease blood loss, and replacement of fluids if needed. The potential for underlying skull fracture and brain and spinal trauma also exists with these injuries. Scalp lacerations that are the only injury rarely produce life-threatening complications. However, such lacerations can result in excessive blood loss. If not contraindicated by injury, the paramedic should position all patients with head or facial trauma on a stretcher or spine board with the head elevated 30 degrees (semi-Fowler position).

Skull Fractures

Skull fractures may be classified as *linear fractures, basilar fractures, depressed fractures,* and *open vault fractures* (Figure 40-14). Complications associated with these injuries are cranial nerve injury, vascular involvement (e.g., meningeal artery and dural sinuses), infection, underlying brain injury, and dural defects caused by depressed bone fragments. As with all injuries to the head, the paramedic should consider the possibility of a spinal injury. Proper spinal precautions should be maintained.

LINEAR FRACTURES

Linear fractures (seen as straight lines on x-ray film) account for 80% of all fractures to the skull.[6] Such fractures usually are not depressed. Often linear fractures occur without an overlying scalp laceration. As an isolated injury, these fractures usually have a low rate of complication. But if the fracture is associated with scalp laceration, infection is possible. Linear fractures that cross the meningeal groove

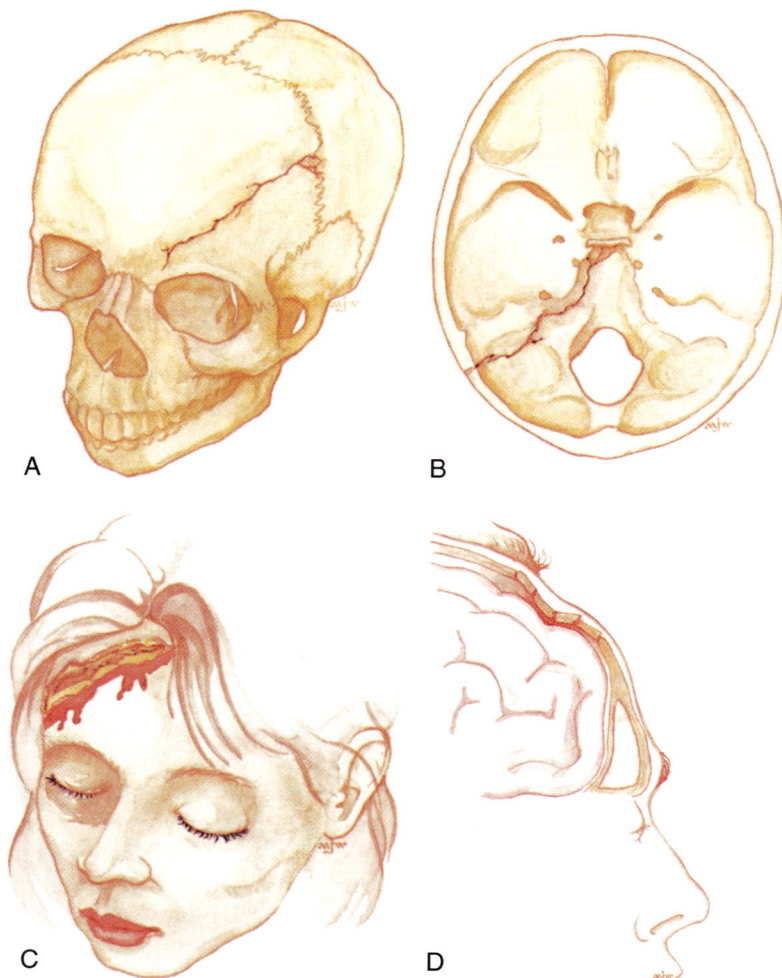

FIGURE 40-14 Skull fractures. **A,** Linear skull fracture. **B,** Basilar skull fracture. **C,** Open vault fracture. **D,** Depressed skull fracture.

in the temporal-parietal area, midline, or occipital area may lead to epidural bleeding from the middle cerebral artery.

CRITICAL THINKING

Will you be able to detect linear skull fractures during a physical examination in the prehospital setting?

BASILAR SKULL FRACTURES

Basilar skull fractures usually are associated with major impact trauma. These injuries may occur when the mandibular condyles perforate into the base of the skull. More commonly, though, they result from an extension of a linear fracture into the floor of the anterior and middle fossae. Basilar skull fractures can be difficult to see on x-ray films. They usually are diagnosed clinically by the following signs and symptoms:

- Ecchymosis over the mastoid process resulting from fracture to the temporal bone **(Battle's sign)** (Figure 40-15, *A*)

- Ecchymosis of one or both orbits caused by fracture of the base of the sphenoid sinus **(raccoon's eyes)** (Figure 40-15, *B*)
- Blood behind the tympanic membrane caused by fractures of the temporal bone **(hemotympanum)**
- Cerebrospinal fluid leakage, which can result in bacterial meningitis

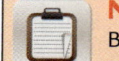

NOTE

Battle's sign and raccoon's eyes usually do not occur until some time after the injury. If they are present on the arrival of emergency medical services, the bruising is most likely the result of a prior injury.

Other complications associated with basilar skull fractures include cranial nerve injuries and massive hemorrhage from vascular involvement of the carotid artery. Treatment for basilar skull fractures includes bed rest, in-hospital observation, and evaluation for hearing loss caused by acoustic nerve injury.

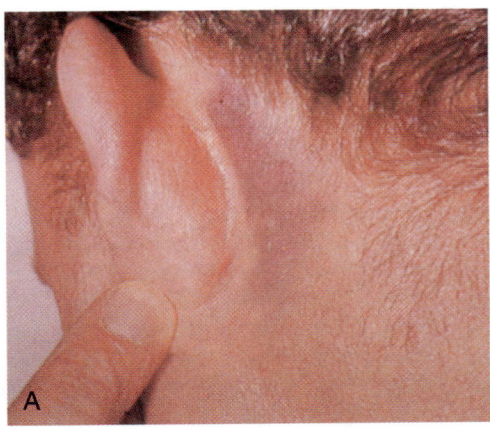

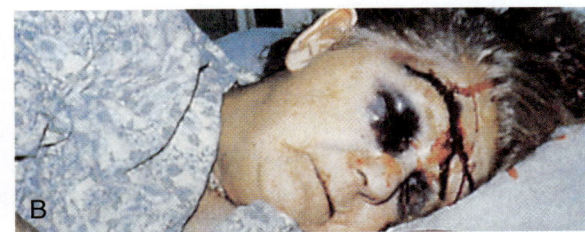

FIGURE 40-15 **A,** Battle's sign. **B,** Raccoon's eyes. (From London PS: *A colour atlas of diagnosis after recent injury,* Ipswich, England, 1990, Wolfe Medical Publications, Ltd.)

DEPRESSED SKULL FRACTURES

Depressed skull fractures usually result from a relatively small object striking the head at high speed. Thus they commonly are associated with scalp lacerations (Figure 40-16). The frontal and parietal bones most often are affected by these fractures. Thirty percent of patients with depressed skull fractures are estimated to have associated hematomata and cerebral contusions.[7] If the depression is greater than the thickness of the skull, dural laceration also is likely. Patients with depressed skull fractures often require surgical removal of the bone fragments (craniectomy).

OPEN VAULT FRACTURES

Open vault fractures result when an opening exists between a scalp laceration and brain tissue (Figure 40-17). Because of the nature of these injuries and the force required to produce them, they often are associated with multiple trauma to other systems. They have a high mortality rate. Exposure of brain tissue to the external environment may lead to infection (meningitis). Open vault fractures require surgical repair. Prehospital management usually is limited to spinal immobilization, ventilatory support, efforts to prevent contamination, and rapid transportation to an appropriate medical facility.

Cranial Nerve Injuries

As described in Chapter 10, 12 pairs of cranial nerves leave the brain and pass through openings in the skull called *foramina.* Injury to cranial nerves usually is associated with skull fractures. Signs and symptoms of common cranial nerve injuries are as follows:

Cranial nerve I (olfactory nerve)
- Loss of smell
- Impaired taste (dependent on food aroma)
- Hallmark of basilar skull fracture

Cranial nerve II (optic nerve)
- Blindness in one or both eyes
- Visual field defects

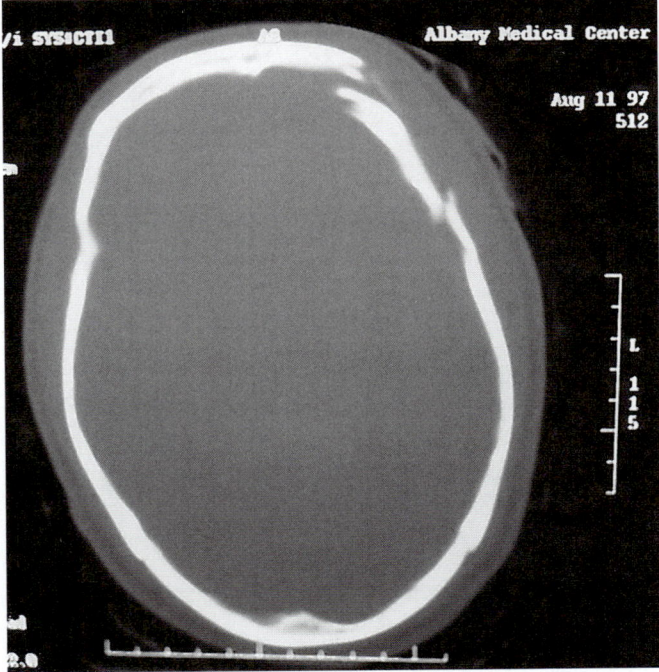

FIGURE 40-16 Head computed tomography scan showing a depressed skull fracture. (From Ferrera PC, Colucciello SA, Marx J, et al: *Trauma management: an emergency medicine approach,* St Louis, 2001, Mosby.)

Cranial nerve III (oculomotor nerve)
- Ipsilateral (same side), dilated, fixed pupil
- Especially compression by the temporal lobe
- Mimics direct ocular trauma

Cranial nerve VII (facial nerve)
- Immediate or delayed facial paralysis
- Basilar skull fracture

Cranial nerve VIII (auditory nerve)
- Deafness
- Basilar skull fracture

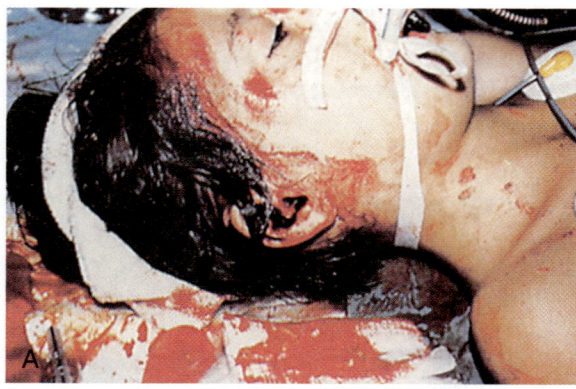

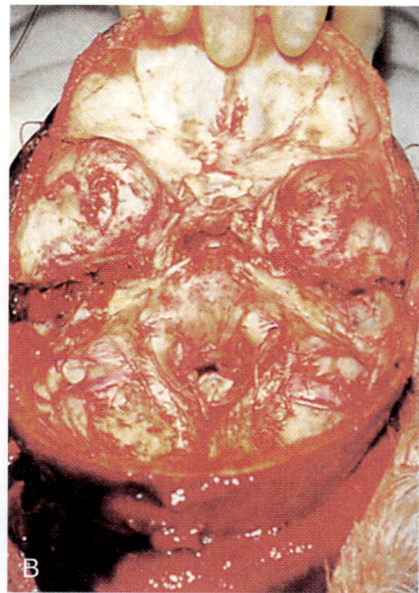

FIGURE 40-17 Severe fracture of the base of the skull. (From London PS: *A colour atlas of diagnosis after recent injury,* Ipswich, England, 1990, Wolfe Medical Publications, Ltd.)

 **LOOK AGAIN**
See Chapter 10: Review of Human Systems, pp. 177-180.

TRAUMATIC BRAIN INJURY

A **traumatic brain injury** (TBI) is defined by the Brain Injury Association as "a traumatic insult to the brain capable of producing physical, intellectual, emotional, social, and vocational change"[8] (Box 40-3). Traumatic brain injury can be divided into two categories: **primary brain injury** and **secondary brain injury.** Primary brain injury refers to direct trauma to the brain and to the associated vascular injuries that occurred from the initial injury. Secondary brain injury results from intracellular and extracellular derangements that probably were initiated at the time of the injury. These derangements may include hypoxia, hypocapnia, and hypercapnia from airway compromise,

aspiration of gastric contents, and thoracic injury; anemia and hypotension from external and internal hemorrhage; and hyperglycemia or hypoglycemia that can further injure ischemic brain tissue. The adverse effects of secondary brain injury can be minimized. They perhaps can be reversed, if they are recognized and properly managed in the prehospital setting. Brain injuries can be classified as *diffuse* (moderate or severe) or *focal.* (The two forms are commonly found together.[9])

Diffuse injuries (usually caused by acceleration-deceleration forces)
 Diffuse axonal injury (DAI)
 Hypoxic-ischemic damage
 Meningitis
 Vascular injury
Focal injuries (generally caused by contact)
 Scalp injury
 Skull fracture
 Surface contusions
 Brain hemorrhage

Diffuse Injuries

Diffuse injuries include concussion and diffuse axonal injury. The major cause of damage in diffuse injury is the disruption of axons—the neural processes that allow one nerve to communicate with another.

CONCUSSION

Concussion is sometimes called a *mild diffuse axonal injury.* Concussion is caused by a mild to moderate impact to the skull, movement of the brain within the cranial vault, or both. Concussion occurs when the function of the brainstem (particularly the reticular activating system) or both cerebral cortices is temporarily disturbed. This results in a brief altered level of consciousness, but not always a loss of consciousness. (If a loss of consciousness occurs, it is usually less than 5 minutes in duration.) A concussion may be a serious injury (*no concussion is minor*). Concussions can be assigned into one of three grades as defined by the American Academy of Neurology (AAN)[12]:

- Grade 1:
  - Transient confusion
  - **No** loss of consciousness
  - Concussion symptoms **clear in less than 15 minutes**
- Grade 2:
  - Transient confusion
  - **No** loss of consciousness
  - Concussion symptoms or mental status abnormalities **last longer than 15 minutes**
- Grade 3:
  - Any loss of consciousness, either brief (seconds) or prolonged (minutes)

> **NOTE**
> According to the American Academy of Neurology (AAN), permanent brain injury can occur with either grade 2 or grade 3 concussion. A concussion may have permanent consequences if the acute symptoms of the concussion continue for more than 15 minutes.[12]

The altered level of consciousness or loss of consciousness usually is followed by periods of drowsiness, restlessness, and confusion, with a fairly rapid return to normal behavior. The patient may have no recall of the events before the injury **(retrograde amnesia).** In addition, amnesia may exist after recovery of consciousness **(antegrade amnesia).** This short-term memory loss may produce anxiety. The patient may ask repetitive questions (e.g., "Where am I? What happened?"). Other signs and symptoms of concussion are vomiting; combativeness; transient visual disturbances (e.g., light flashes and wavy lines); defects in equilibrium and coordination; and changes in blood pressure, pulse rate, and respiration (rare). After physician evaluation, treatment usually consists of in-hospital or home observation by a reliable observer for 24 to 48 hours.

> **CRITICAL THINKING**
> Consider the patient with a new onset of retrograde or antegrade amnesia. Why should the patient not be considered a reliable historian?

A concussion injury affects the patient most severely at the time of impact but is followed by improvement.

Concussion is the most common type of brain injury. *Any patient whose condition worsens over time or whose level of consciousness deteriorates rather than improves must be suspected of having a more serious injury.* Therefore documentation of baseline measurements of level of consciousness, memory status, and neurological function (e.g., Glasgow Coma Scale or AVPU scale) in any victim of head injury is important. If a patient with a concussion has a loss of consciousness more than 5 minutes, the paramedic should suspect a more serious injury caused by contusion or hemorrhage.

MODERATE DIFFUSE AXONAL INJURY

A moderate diffuse injury is a head injury that results in minute petechial bruising of brain tissue. The involvement of the brainstem and reticular activating system leads to unconsciousness. These injuries account for 20% of all severe head injuries and 45% of all cases of diffuse injury.[13] Often these patients will have basilar skull fracture. Most patients will survive the injury, yet permanent neurological impairment is common.

A patient with moderate diffuse injury initially will be unconscious, followed by persistent confusion, disorientation, and amnesia of the event. During recovery, these patients often experience an inability to concentrate, frequent periods of anxiety, uncharacteristic mood swings, and sensorimotor deficits (e.g., an altered sense of smell). Patients with moderate diffuse injury are managed similar to those patients with concussion: frequent reassessments of the level of consciousness and assurance of an adequate airway and tidal volume are necessary. If possible, patients with head injury should be moved to a quiet, calm area. Exposure to bright lights should be avoided. (Patients often are photophobic.) Also, constant reorientation of the patient may be necessary.

SEVERE DIFFUSE AXONAL INJURY

As the name implies, a **severe diffuse axonal injury** is the severest form of brain injury. Severe DAI was once known as a *brainstem injury.* Severe DAI involves severe mechanical shearing of many axons in both cerebral hemispheres extending to the brainstem. Severe DAI occurs in approximately 16% of patients with severe head trauma.[6] These patients often are unconscious for prolonged periods. They may exhibit abnormal posturing and other signs of increased intracranial pressure (ICP), described later in this chapter. The prehospital care for these patients is focused on ensuring an adequate airway and tidal volume. Hypoxia must be prevented in all patients with head injury. (This helps to avoid secondary injury to brain tissue.)

> **CRITICAL THINKING**
> Can a patient with a diffuse axonal injury die as a result of that injury?

Focal Injury

Focal injuries are specific, grossly observable brain lesions. Included in this category are lesions that result from skull fracture (previously described), contusion, edema with associated increased ICP, ischemia, and hemorrhage. As described in Chapter 10, the brain occupies 80% of the intracranial space. The brain is divided into four areas: the brainstem (consisting of the medulla, pons, and midbrain), the diencephalon (including the thalamus and hypothalamus), the cerebrum, and the cerebellum. The intracranial contents consist of brain water (58%), brain solids (25%), cerebrospinal fluid (7%), and intracranial blood (10%).

CEREBRAL CONTUSION

A **cerebral contusion** is bruising of the brain in the area of the cortex or deeper within the frontal (most common), temporal, or occipital lobes (Figure 40-18). This bruising produces a structural change in the brain tissue. Bruising results in greater neurological deficits and abnormalities than are seen with concussions. These abnormalities may include seizures, hemiparesis, aphasia, and personality changes. If the brainstem also is contused, the patient may lose consciousness. In some cases, the comatose state may be prolonged. It may last hours to days or longer. Of the patients who die from head injury, the majority have cerebral contusions at autopsy.

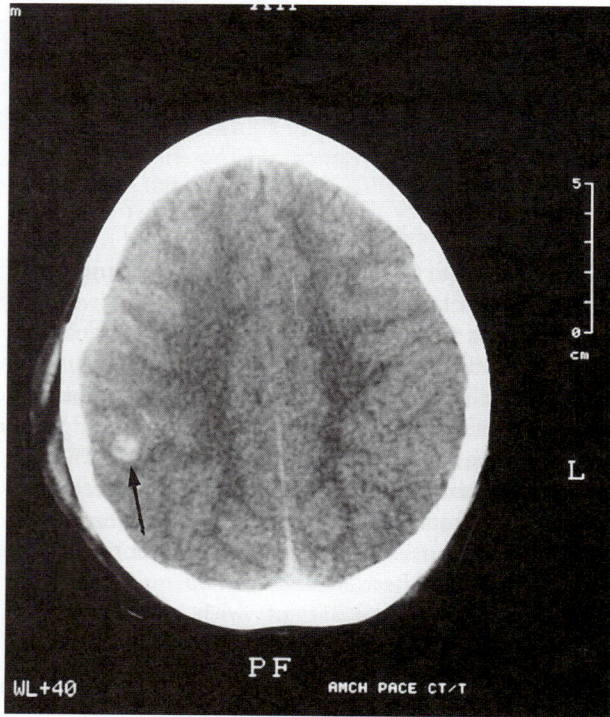

FIGURE 40-18 Head CT scan demonstrating a cerebral contusion (*arrow*). (From Ferrera PC, Colucciello SA, Marx J, et al: *Trauma management: an emergency medicine approach,* St Louis, 2001, Mosby.)

If applied force is enough to cause the brain to be displaced against the irregular surfaces of the skull, tiny blood vessels in the pia mater may rupture. The brain substance may be damaged locally at the site of impact **(coup)**. Or the brain may be damaged on the opposite, or contralateral, side **(contrecoup)**. Contrecoup injuries often are caused by deceleration of the head. This may occur, for example, in a fall or motor vehicle crash.

As a rule, cerebral contusions usually heal without intervention. As with patients with concussion, these patients usually improve. However, the time to heal and level of improvement differ in these two conditions. The most important complication associated with cerebral contusion is increased ICP manifested by headache, nausea, vomiting, seizures, and a declining level of consciousness. These signs usually are delayed responses to the injury. Therefore they usually are not seen in the prehospital emergency setting.

EDEMA

Major injuries to the brain often result in swelling of the brain tissue with or without associated hemorrhage. The swelling results from humoral and metabolic responses to injury. Swelling leads to considerable increases in ICP. This in turn can lead to decreased cerebral perfusion (described later) or herniation.

ISCHEMIA

Ischemia can result from vascular injuries, secondary vascular spasm, or increased ICP. In any case, focal or more global infarcts can result.

HEMORRHAGE

The same forces that result in concussion and contusion also may cause serious vascular damage. This damage may result in hemorrhage into or around brain tissue. These injuries may cause epidural or subdural hematomata. The hematomata compress the underlying brain tissue, or produce intraparenchymal hemorrhage (bleeding directly into the brain tissue). This bleeding often results from cerebral contusions and skull fractures.

Cerebral Blood Flow. Although the brain accounts for only 2% of adult weight, 20% of total body oxygen use and 25% of total body glucose use are devoted to brain metabolism. Oxygen and glucose delivery are controlled by cerebral blood flow.

As described in Chapter 25, cerebral blood flow is a function of cerebral perfusion pressure (CPP) and resistance of the cerebral vascular bed. Cerebral blood flow is determined by the mean arterial pressure (MAP) (the diastolic pressure plus one third pulse pressure) minus the intracranial pressure (CPP = MAP − ICP). Normal mean arterial pressure ranges from 85 to 95 mm Hg. Intracranial pressure is normally 10 to 15 mm Hg or less. Thus normal CPP is between 70 and 80 mm Hg. (A cerebral perfusion pressure of 60 mm Hg is the critical minimum threshold to adequately perfuse the brain.) As ICP approaches mean arterial pressure, the gradient for flow decreases and cerebral blood flow decreases. That is, when ICP increases, CPP decreases. As CPP decreases, vessels in the brain dilate (cerebral vasodilation). This results in increased cerebral blood volume (increasing ICP) and further cerebral vasodilation. In most emergency medical services systems, CPP is not calculated because mean arterial pressure and ICP are not measured in the prehospital setting. However, maintaining a systolic blood pressure of at least 90 mm Hg also may help maintain adequate mean arterial pressure.[1,14]

> ### CRITICAL THINKING
> What happens to the flow of oxygen to the brain, and carbon dioxide from the brain to the capillaries, when intracranial pressure is increasing and cerebral perfusion pressure is decreasing?

Vascular tone in the normal brain is regulated by carbon dioxide pressure (PCO_2), oxygen pressure (PO_2), and autonomic and neurohumoral control; PCO_2 has the greatest effect on intracerebral vascular diameter and subsequent resistance. For example, if PCO_2 is increased from 40 to 80 mm Hg, cerebral blood flow is doubled. This results in increased brain blood volume and ICP.

Intracranial Pressure. The normal range of ICP is 10 to 15 mm Hg or less. When ICP rises above this level, the body has difficulty maintaining adequate CPP, usually because of an expanding mass or diffuse swelling. Cerebral blood flow is diminished when the CPP is not adequate. As the cranial vault continues to fill (because of brain edema or expanding hematoma), the body tries to compensate for the decline in CPP by an increase in mean arterial pressure (*Cushing reflex*). Yet this increase in cerebral blood flow further elevates the ICP. As pressure continues to increase, cerebrospinal fluid is displaced to make up for the expansion. If unresolved, the brain substance may herniate over the edge of the tentorium. (This is one of three extensions of the dura mater that separates the cerebellum from the occipital lobe of the cerebrum.) Alternatively, it may herniate through the foramen magnum (Figure 40-19).

Early signs and symptoms of increased ICP include headache, nausea and vomiting, and altered level of consciousness (Box 40-4). These signs and symptoms eventually are followed by increased systolic pressure, widened pulse pressure, and decreased pulse rate and irregular respiratory pattern **(Cushing's triad).** As the volume continues to expand in the cranial vault, herniation of the temporal lobe of the brain through the tentorium may occur. The herniation causes compression of cranial nerve III. This produces a dilated pupil and loss of the light reflex on the

BOX 40-4 Levels of Increasing Intracranial Cerebral Pressure

Cortex and Upper Brainstem
Blood pressure rises; pulse rate slows.
Pupils remain reactive.
Cheyne-Stokes respirations may be present.
Patient initially will try to localize and remove painful stimuli (eventually withdraws and flexion occurs).
All effects are reversible at this stage.

Middle Brainstem
Wide pulse pressure and bradycardia are present.
Pupils become nonreactive or sluggish.
Central neurogenic hyperventilation develops.
Abnormal posturing (extension) occurs.
Few patients function normally with injury at this level.

Lower Portion of Brainstem/Medulla
Pupil is "blown" (fixed and dilated) on same side of injury.
Respirations become ataxic.
Patient will be flaccid.
Pulse rate is irregular.
QRS, S-T, and T wave changes will be present.
Blood pressure will fluctuate.
These patients generally do not survive.

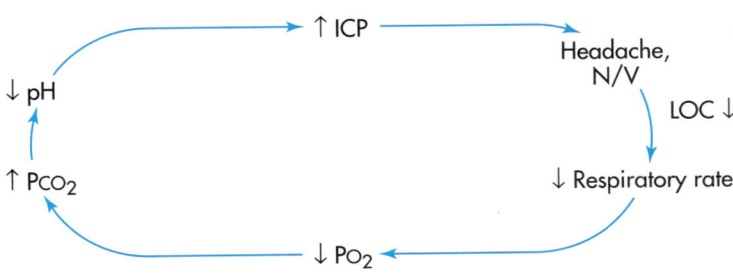

FIGURE 40-19 Effects of increased intracranial pressure.

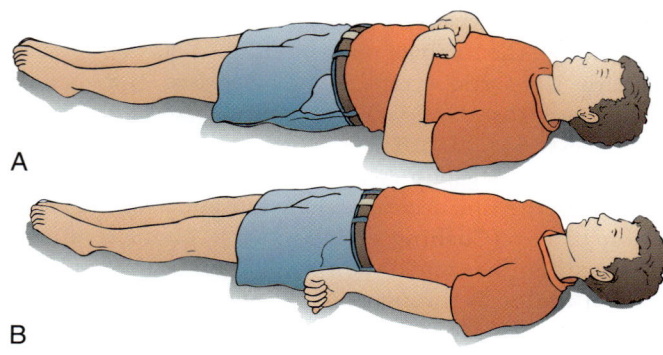

FIGURE 40-20 A, Abnormal flexion (decorticate posturing). **B,** Abnormal extension (decerebrate posturing). (Modified from ENA: *Sheehy's emergency nursing,* ed 6, St Louis, 2010, Mosby.)

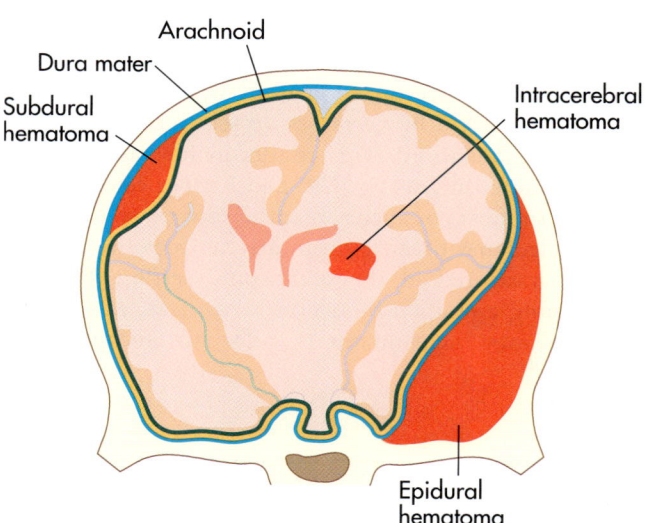

FIGURE 40-21 Varieties of intracranial hemorrhage.

side of compression. The patient rapidly becomes unresponsive to verbal and painful stimuli. The patient may exhibit the ominous sign of **decorticate posturing**. (This is characterized by extension of the legs and flexion of the arms at the elbows.) Or the patient may exhibit **decerebrate posturing**. (This is characterized by extension of all four extremities [Figure 40-20].)

CRITICAL THINKING
Why is cranial nerve III affected by this shift in brain tissue?

Respiratory Patterns. As ICP continues to rise, abnormal respiratory patterns (described in Chapter 15) may develop. Respiratory abnormalities associated with increased ICP and significant brainstem injury include hypoventilation, *Cheyne-Stokes breathing* (which may accompany decorticate posturing), *central neurogenic hyperventilation* (which may accompany decerebrate posturing), and *ataxic breathing*. The presence of decorticate (flexion) or decerebrate (extension) posturing and abnormal respiratory patterns is not of major clinical importance other than to identify the need for intervention and treatment (intubation and consideration of immediate neurosurgical intervention).

> **NOTE**
> Some motion of the limbs, albeit abnormal, is better than no motion of the limbs. (No motion indicates a worse level of neurological function.)

TYPES OF BRAIN HEMORRHAGE

Traditionally, brain hemorrhages are classified according to their location as epidural, subdural, subarachnoid, or cerebral (intraparenchymal) (Figure 40-21).

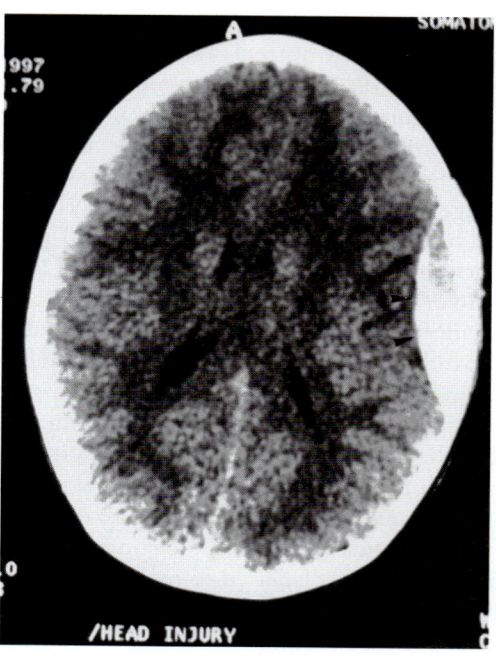

FIGURE 40-22 Head computed tomography scan showing an epidural hematoma. (From Ferrera PC, Colucciello SA, Marx J, et al: *Trauma management: an emergency medicine approach,* St Louis, 2001, Mosby.)

Epidural Hematoma. An **epidural hematoma** (accounting for 0.5% to 1% of all head injuries[1]) is a collection of blood between the cranium and the dura in the epidural space (Figure 40-22). The hematoma usually is a rapidly developing lesion. Usually the hematoma is associated with a laceration or tear of the middle meningeal artery. This hemorrhage often occurs as a result of a linear or depressed skull fracture in the temporal bone. Yet bleeding from other sites can produce epidural hemorrhage as well. If the source of hemorrhage is mostly venous, deterioration usually is not as rapid because low-pressure vessels bleed more slowly.

Fifty percent of patients with epidural hematoma have a transient loss of consciousness, followed by a lucid interval in which neurological status returns to normal. (The remaining 50% of patients with acute epidural hematoma never recover consciousness.) The lucid interval usually lasts between 6 and 18 hours. During this time the hematoma enlarges. As ICP rises, the patient develops a headache with lethargy, decreasing level of consciousness, and contralateral hemiparesis. In the early stages of an epidural hematoma, the patient may complain only of headache and drowsiness. Definitive treatment includes immediate recognition and rapid transport to a proper facility for surgery. Common causes of epidural hematoma include low-velocity blows to the head, violent altercations, and deceleration injuries. About 20% of these patients who are comatose die.[1]

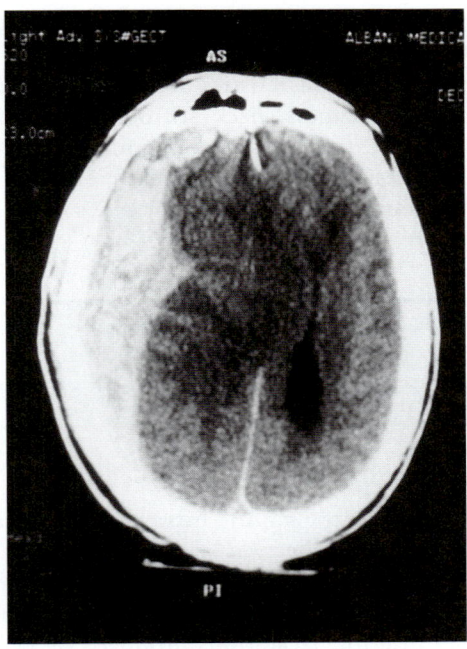

FIGURE 40-23 Head computed tomography scan showing an acute subdural hematoma. (From Ferrera PC, Colucciello SA, Marx J, et al: *Trauma management: an emergency medicine approach,* St Louis, 2001, Mosby.)

> ### CRITICAL THINKING
> What could account for delays in surgical treatment, causing subsequent death, in patients who have an epidural hematoma?

Subdural Hematoma. A **subdural hematoma** is a collection of blood between the dura and the surface of the brain in the subdural space (Figure 40-23). This injury usually results from bleeding of the veins that bridge the subdural space. Associated contusion or laceration of the brain often is present. The hematoma often results from blunt head trauma. Commonly the hematoma is associated with skull fracture. Subdural hematomata are classified as *acute, subacute,* and *chronic.* Classification depends on the time lapse between the injury and development of symptoms. As a general rule, if symptoms occur within 24 hours, the hematoma is considered acute; between 2 and 10 days, subacute; and after 2 weeks, chronic.[1] Subdural hematomata are more common than epidural hematomata.

Signs and symptoms of subdural hematoma are similar to those of epidural hematoma and include headache, nausea and vomiting, decreasing level of consciousness, coma, abnormal posturing, paralysis, and, in infants, bulging fontanelles. These findings may be subtle because of the slow development of the hematoma in the subacute and chronic phases. Definitive care consists of surgery to remove the blood from the hematoma. Individuals at increased risk of developing subdural hematoma include older adults, patients with clotting deficiencies (e.g., alcoholics, hemophiliacs, and persons who take anticoagulants), and patients with cortical atrophy (older adults, alcoholics).

Subarachnoid Hematoma. A **subarachnoid hematoma** refers to intracranial bleeding into the cerebrospinal

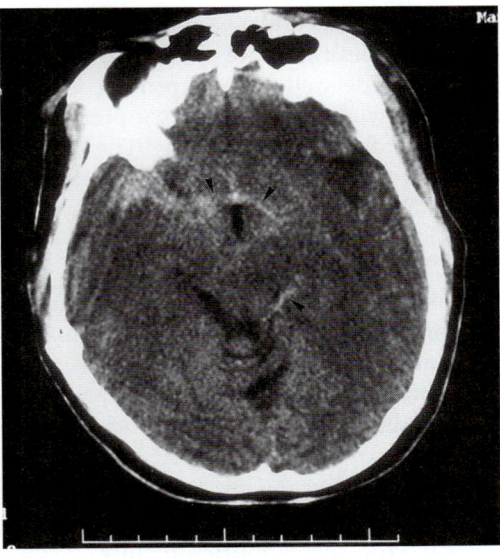

FIGURE 40-24 Head computed tomography scan showing a traumatic subarachnoid hemorrhage. (From Ferrera PC, Colucciello SA, Marx J, et al: *Trauma management: an emergency medicine approach,* St Louis, 2001, Mosby.)

fluid. This results in bloody cerebrospinal fluid and meningeal irritation (Figure 40-24). Bleeding that results from trauma, rupture of an aneurysm, or arteriovenous anomaly may extend into the brain if the force of the bleeding from the broken vessel is sudden and severe. Patients with this injury often complain of a sudden and severe headache. The headache initially may be localized. Then the headache spreads (from meningeal irritation) and becomes dull and throbbing. Other characteristics of a subarachnoid hemorrhage include dizziness, neck stiffness, unequal pupils, vomiting, seizures, and loss of consciousness. Severe hemorrhage may result in coma and death. Permanent brain damage is common in those who survive.

> ### CRITICAL THINKING
> What causes the vomiting, seizures, and loss of consciousness in a patient with subarachnoid hemorrhage?

Cerebral Hematoma. An **intracerebral hematoma** may be defined as a collection of more than 5 mL of blood somewhere within the substance of the brain, most commonly in the frontal or temporal lobe.[15] This injury can result from multiple lacerations produced by penetrating head trauma (gunshot wound). The injury also may result from a high-velocity deceleration injury (automobile crash) in which vessels are torn as the brain moves across rough surfaces of the skull. Increased ICP can produce an intracerebral hematoma as the result of the brain being compressed.

Cerebral hematoma often is associated with subdural hemorrhage and skull fracture. Signs and symptoms may be immediate or delayed. This depends on the size and location of the hemorrhage. Once symptoms appear, the patient usually deteriorates rapidly. The mortality rate after surgical evacuation of the hematoma (if possible) approaches 45%.[1]

PENETRATING INJURY

Penetrating injuries to the brain usually are caused by missiles fired from handguns and stab wounds caused by sharp objects. Such objects include knives, scissors, screwdrivers, and nails. Less often, penetrating trauma may result from falls and high-velocity vehicle crashes. Associated injuries include skull fracture; damage to cerebral arteries, veins, or venous sinuses; and intracranial hemorrhage. Complications include infection and posttraumatic epilepsy. Definitive care for these injuries requires neurosurgical intervention.

ASSESSMENT AND NEUROLOGICAL EVALUATION

Prehospital management of the patient with a head injury is determined by a number of factors, including the mechanism and severity of injury and the patient's level of consciousness. Associated injuries affect the priorities of emergency care.

Airway and Ventilation. The initial step in treating all patients with head trauma is to ensure an open airway with spinal precautions. The next step is to provide adequate ventilation with high-concentration oxygen. Airway management may include oral or nasal adjuncts, multilumen devices, or nasal or tracheal intubation to maintain and protect the airway. Tracheal intubation and ventilatory support usually are recommended in all patients with head injuries who have a Glasgow Coma Scale (GCS) score ≤8[11] (described later in the chapter).

> ### CRITICAL THINKING
> Imagine the appearance of a patient with a Glasgow Coma Scale score of 8 or less. Why should these patients be intubated? What if the Glasgow Coma Scale score improves rapidly?

Patients with head injuries are likely to vomit. If the patient has a decreased level of consciousness after the airway is secured, a nasogastric tube should be inserted to empty the stomach. In the presence of facial fractures, rhinorrhea (cerebrospinal fluid discharge from the nose), or otorrhea (cerebrospinal fluid discharge from the ear), an orogastric tube rather than a nasogastric tube should be inserted. Use of this tube helps to avoid possible intubation of the cranial cavity through the fracture site. In addition, the patient should be well stabilized on a long spine board for safe repositioning. Suction equipment with large-bore suction catheters should be available as well.

Ventilatory support should be focused on maintaining adequate oxygenation and optimizing cerebral perfusion. Capnography and pulse oximetry should be used to ensure that oxygen saturation is at a level of 95% or greater. Aggressive hyperventilation reduces carbon dioxide concentration; it can lead to secondary brain injury through cerebral vasoconstriction and a decrease in cerebral blood flow. (Routine prophylactic hyperventilation should be avoided.) Thus in the absence of capnography to guide ventilatory support, normal ventilations should be provided at 10 breaths/min for adults, 20 breaths/min for children, and 25 breaths/min for infants. With evidence of herniation (Box 40-5), the patient should be hyperventilated at the

> ### BOX 40-5 Indicators of Herniation for Hyperventilation
>
> Cushing's triad: increased systolic blood pressure, widened pulse pressure, and decrease in the pulse rate and irregular respiratory pattern
> *Or*
> An unresponsive patient with the following:
> Bilateral, dilated, unresponsive pupils or asymmetrical pupils (>1 mm)
> *And*
> Abnormal extension (decerebrate) posturing or no motor response to painful stimuli

following rates: 20 breaths/min for adults, 30 breaths/min for children, and 35 breaths/min for infants. These rates should yield a PCO_2 of about 35 mm Hg.[14,16]

Circulation. After the airway has been secured (maintaining spinal protection), support of the patient's cardiovascular function becomes the next priority. The paramedic should control major external bleeding and should assess the patient's vital signs. Assessment establishes a baseline for future evaluations. A cardiac monitor will detect changes in rhythm (particularly bradycardia and tachycardia) that can occur with increasing ICP and brainstem injury. The blood pressure of every patient should be maintained at normal levels with fluid replacement (per medical direction). A single episode of hypotension doubles mortality and increases morbidity in the patient with traumatic brain injury.[14] Therefore the paramedic should administer intravenous fluids to support oxygen delivery and to avoid hypertension or limit hypotension to the shortest duration possible. Systolic blood pressure thresholds that can be used to define hypotension in head-injured patients are listed in Box 40-6.

Persistent hypotension from an isolated head injury is a rare and terminal event. The exception is head injury in infants and small children. *Closed head injury in the adult does not produce hypovolemic shock.* Thus a patient with head injuries who also is hypotensive should be evaluated for other injuries that could cause hemorrhage. The paramedic also should evaluate the patient for the possibility of neurogenic shock from spinal cord trauma. Infusion of isotonic fluids (lactated Ringer's solution or normal saline) may be indicated for hemorrhagic shock. However, these fluids probably should be used cautiously in patients with hypotension caused by neurogenic shock. In the latter patient group, vasopressors also may be helpful in maintaining blood pressure. Neurogenic shock may be distinguished from hemorrhagic shock by the following:

- A relatively bradycardic response (e.g., a pulse rate of 80 beats/min with a blood pressure of 80 mm Hg)
- Skin that often is warm and dry (not cool and clammy)
- No evidence of significant blood loss or hypovolemia
- Paralysis and loss of spinal reflexes

Neurological Examination. Conscious patients should be interviewed to determine their memory status before and after the injury and establish significant medical history (e.g., heart disease, hypertension, diabetes, epilepsy, medication use, alcohol or other drug use, and allergies). The history also should include the mechanism of injury and the events that led up to the injury. (For example, the history may detail a loss of consciousness before or after the injury incident.)

The paramedic should evaluate the motor skills of conscious patients. Evaluation determines the patient's ability to follow commands and helps the paramedic to note any paralysis. (Hemiparesis or hemiplegia, especially with a sensory deficit on the same side, indicates brain damage rather than spinal trauma.) If the patient is unconscious on emergency medical services arrival, the paramedic should interview bystanders about the history of the event. The paramedic also should ask bystanders about the length of time the patient has been unconscious. The most important indicator of increasing ICP is deterioration in the patient's sensorium. Thus the paramedic should evaluate the level of consciousness using the GCS every 5 minutes. A decrease of 2 points with a GCS score of 9 or lower is significant; it indicates significant injury.[14]

NOTE

When assessing and managing an adult with a severe head injury, remember the Brain Trauma Foundation's "90-90-9 rule"[17]:

- A single drop in the patient's arterial oxygen saturation (SaO_2) to less than 90% doubles his or her chance of death.
- A single drop in the patient's systolic blood pressure to less than 90 mm Hg doubles his or her chance of death.
- A single drop in the patient's GCS score to less than 9 doubles his or her chance of death. A drop in the GCS score of 2 or more points, at any time, also doubles mortality.

CRITICAL THINKING

How reliable will the patient be regarding the duration of his or her loss of consciousness?

After the patient has been resuscitated and stabilized, the paramedic should assess the patient's pupils for symmetry, size, and reactivity to light. Abnormal pupillary responses may indicate an increase in ICP and cranial nerve involvement. *Asymmetrical pupils* differ more than 1 mm in size. *Dilated pupils* are greater than or equal to 4 mm in adults. A *fixed pupil* shows less than 1-mm change in response to bright light. (The paramedic should evaluate pupil size every 5 minutes.) Alcohol and some other drugs can cause abnormal pupillary reactions, but the reactions commonly are bilateral (except for certain eye drops, if placed in one eye). If the patient is conscious, the paramedic also should evaluate extraocular movement (see Chapter 20: Secondary Assessment).

BOX 40-6 Systolic Blood Pressure Thresholds Defining Hypotension in Head-Injured Patients

<65 mm Hg in patients from birth to 1 year of age
<75 mm Hg in patients 2 to 5 years of age
<80 mm Hg in patients 6 to 12 years
<90 mm Hg in patients 13 years or older

From Brain Trauma Foundation: *Guidelines for the management of severe head injury*, ed 3, New York, 2007.

Fluid Therapy. In the absence of hypotension, fluid therapy normally should be restricted in a patient with head injury to minimize cerebral edema. If the patient is hemodynamically stable, the paramedic should establish an intravenous line of crystalloid fluid to keep the vein open. If significant hypovolemia is present from another injury, the paramedic should give the patient an isotonic fluid bolus. (This should be guided by medical direction.) The patient also should be transported rapidly to a proper facility. In this case, the injury causing hypovolemia usually is more immediately life threatening than the head injury. As a rule, hypotension in the presence of head injury initially should be managed with fluid boluses to maintain a systolic blood pressure of at least 90 mm Hg.[1]

Drug Therapy. Prehospital use of drugs for the treatment of head injuries is controversial. Drugs that may be prescribed by medical direction to decrease cerebral edema or circulating blood volume may include **mannitol** and hypertonic saline. (Both are controversial.) Medical direction may require the insertion of an indwelling urinary catheter for careful monitoring of urine output before starting diuretic therapy. Hypotension leading to hypoperfusion may occur as a complication of diuretic use in patients with head injuries.

Anticonvulsant agents such as **lorazepam** and **diazepam** are used to control seizure activity in head-injured patients. As a rule, these drugs are not used in the initial management of head injuries because of their sedating effects. Prevention of seizures avoids the rise in ICP that often accompanies sudden seizure activity. Intravenously administered **lidocaine** has been shown to control increases in ICP that normally occur during endotracheal intubation.[1]

In addition, the use of sedatives and paralytics for some patients with head injuries may be indicated for airway management. These drugs also may be used to aid in the transport of combative patients (especially in aeromedical transport). The paramedic should follow local protocol and consult with medical direction regarding the use of these drugs.

INJURY RATING SYSTEMS

Several injury rating systems are used to triage, guide patient care, predict patient outcome, identify changes in patient status, and evaluate trauma care in epidemiological studies and quality assurance reviews. (These also are known as *indexes* or *scales*.) These indexes are important to prehospital personnel. They aid in determining patient care needs with reference to hospital resources. Rating systems commonly used in emergency care include the Glasgow Coma Scale, trauma score, Revised Trauma Score, and pediatric trauma score.

Glasgow Coma Scale

The **Glasgow Coma Scale** (GCS) evaluates eye opening, verbal and motor responses, and brainstem reflex function. The scale is considered one of the best indicators of eventual clinical outcome[11] and should be part of any neurological examination for patients with head injury (Table 40-1). A GCS score of 9 to 13 indicates moderate traumatic brain injury; a GCS score of 8 or less indicates a severe traumatic brain injury. (*NOTE:* The lowest possible score is 3; the highest possible score is 15.) Hypoxemia and hypotension have been shown to affect GCS scoring negatively. Thus GCS should be measured after the primary survey. The score should be measured after a clear airway is established. Also, the GCS should be measured after necessary ventilation and circulatory resuscitation have been performed. Unresponsive patients with a GCS score of 3 to 8 should be transported to a trauma center with traumatic brain injury capabilities.[14]

Trauma Score/Revised Trauma Score

The trauma score was developed in 1980 to predict outcome for patients with blunt or penetrating injuries. This score has limited use in the prehospital setting. The trauma score does not predict adequately the mortality for isolated, severe head injury.

The **Revised Trauma Score** was published in 1989. The Revised Trauma Score uses the GCS with measurements for systolic blood pressure and respiratory rate that are

TABLE 40-1 Glasgow Coma Scale*

Criteria	Points Assigned to Score
Eye Opening	
Spontaneous eye opening	4
Eye opening on command	3
Eye opening to painful stimulus	2
No eye opening	1
Best Verbal Response	
Answers appropriately (oriented)	5[†]
Gives confused answers	4
Gives inappropriate response	3
Makes unintelligible noises	2
Makes no verbal response	1
Best Motor Response	
Follows commands	6
Localizes painful stimuli	5
Withdraws from pain	4
Responds with abnormal flexion to painful stimuli (decorticate)	3
Responds with abnormal extension to painful stimuli (decerebrate)	2
Gives no motor response	1
TOTAL	—

From National Association of Emergency Medical Technicians: *PHTLS basic and advanced prehospital trauma life support,* St Louis, 2006, Mosby.
*Example: A head-injured patient with an eye opening response to pain would be assigned 2 (E2); with no verbal response would be assigned 1 (V1); and with decerebrate posturing would be assigned 2 (M2). The Glasgow Coma Scale score for this patient would be 5.
†It generally is agreed that a full verbal score of 5 should be assigned to a child less than 2 years of age who cries after stimulation.

TABLE 40-2 Revised Trauma Score*

Variable	Score (Points)	Start of Transport	End of Transport
A. Ventilatory Rate			
10-29 breaths/min	4		
>29 breaths/min	3		
6-9 breaths/min	2		
1-5 breaths/min	1		
0	0		
B. Systolic Blood Pressure			
>89 mm Hg	4		
76-89 mm Hg	3		
50-75 mm Hg	2		
1-49 mm Hg	1		
No pulse	0		
C. Glasgow Coma Scale Score			
13-15	4		
9-12	3		
6-8	2		
4-5	1		
<4	0		
Trauma score total = A + B + C	—		

Adapted from Champion HR, et al: A revision of the trauma score, *J Trauma* 29(5):624, 1989.
*Example: At the start of transport, a head-injured patient has spontaneous ventilations at 30 breaths/min (score of 3), a systolic pressure of 80 mm Hg (score of 3), and a Glasgow Coma Scale score of 12 (score of 3), providing a Revised Trauma Score of 9. At end of transport, the patient has spontaneous ventilations of 18 breaths/min (score of 4), a systolic pressure of 62 (score of 2), and a Glasgow Coma Scale score of 7 (score of 2), providing a Revised Trauma Score of 8.

TABLE 40-3 Pediatric Trauma Score

Component	+2	+1	−1
Size	Child/adolescent >20 kg	Toddler 11-20 kg	Infant <10 kg
Airway	Normal	Assisted: O_2 mask, cannula	Intubated: endotracheal tube, cricothyroidotomy
Consciousness	Awake	Obtunded, lost consciousness	Coma, unresponsive
Systolic blood pressure	90 mm Hg	51-90 mm Hg	<50 mm Hg
	Good peripheral pulses, perfusion	Carotid, femoral pulse palpable	Weak or no pulse
Fracture	None seen or suspected	Single closed fracture anywhere	Open or multiple fractures
Cutaneous	No visible injury	Confusion, abrasion, laceration <7 cm through fascia	Tissue loss, any gunshot wound or stab through fascia

From National Association of Emergency Medical Technicians: *PHTLS basic and advanced prehospital trauma life support,* ed. 7, St Louis, 2011, Mosby.

divided into five intervals. A range of values for these physiological measurements is assigned a number between 0 and 4. These numbers then are added to give a total between 0 and 12. (A score of 0 indicates the most critical. A score of 12 indicates the least critical [Table 40-2].) Calculating the Revised Trauma Score en route to the receiving hospital provides baseline measurements. This can be helpful to the physician in managing the patient's care. In some emergency medical services systems, this score is calculated after arrival at the emergency department using data from radio reports and the prehospital care report.

Pediatric Trauma Score

The **pediatric trauma score** grades six characteristics commonly seen in pediatric trauma patients. These are size (weight), airway, consciousness, systolic blood pressure, fracture, and cutaneous injury (Table 40-3). The pediatric trauma score has a significant inverse linear relationship with patient mortality. A child with a pediatric trauma score less than 8 should be cared for in an appropriate pediatric trauma center.[14]

Patient size (weight) is one of the first parameters to assess. The smaller the child, the greater the risk for severe injury because of an increased ratio of body surface to volume. The risk also is greater because of the potential for limited physiological reserve.

The child's airway is scored by potential difficulty in management. Scoring also is by the type of care required to ensure adequate ventilation and oxygenation. Respiratory failure is the main cause of death in most pediatric patients. Aggressive management to control the airway should be started without delay.

As with adult patients, the most critical factor in assessing the central nervous system of a child is a change in the level of consciousness. Any change in the level of consciousness will reduce this score—no matter how brief the time.

The assessment of systolic blood pressure in the pediatric patient is critical because the circulating volume is notably less than that of the adult. Because of a normal child's healthy heart and excellent reserve capacity, children often do not show classic signs of shock until they have lost about 25% of their circulating volume. Any child who has a systolic blood pressure less than 50 mm Hg is in obvious jeopardy.[18]

A child's skeleton is more pliable than that of the adult. It allows traumatic forces to be sent through the body and to the organs. Thus a fracture in the pediatric patient is a sign that serious injury likely has occurred.

Like fractures, cutaneous injury in the pediatric patient is a potential contributor to mortality and disability. These injuries include open and visible wounds and penetrating trauma.

For example, a head-injured child who is 8 years of age weighs 34 kg (+2); has spontaneous respirations (+1); is unresponsive (+1); has a systolic pressure of 86 mm Hg with palpable femoral pulses (+1); has no visible fractures (+2); and has an abrasion on the head with minimal bleeding (+1). The pediatric trauma score for this patient is 8.

SUMMARY

- Major causes of maxillofacial trauma are motor vehicle crashes, home accidents, athletic injuries, animal bites, intentional violent acts, and industrial injuries.
- With the exception of compromised airway and the potential for significant bleeding, damage to the tissues of the maxillofacial area is seldom life threatening. Some facial fractures are associated with basilar skull fracture. Blunt trauma injuries may be classified as fractures to the mandible, midface, zygoma, orbit, or nose.
- Injury to the ears, eyes, or teeth may be minor or may result in permanent sensory function loss and disfigurement. Trauma to the ear may include lacerations and contusions, thermal injuries, chemical injuries, traumatic perforation, and barotitis. Evaluation of the

eye should include a thorough history. Assessment also should include measurement of visual acuity, pupillary reaction, and extraocular movements.

- Anterior neck injuries may result in damage to the skeletal structures, vascular structures, nerves, muscles, and glands of the neck. The patient should be assessed for airway compromise, bleeding, and cervical spine injury.
- Injuries to the skull may be classified as soft tissue injuries to the scalp and skull fractures. Skull fractures may be classified as linear fractures, basilar fractures, depressed fractures, and open vault fractures.
- The categories of brain injury include DAI and focal injury. Diffuse axonal injury may be mild (concussion), moderate, or severe. Focal injuries are specific, grossly observable brain lesions. Included in this category are lesions that result from skull fracture, contusion, edema with associated increased ICP, ischemia, and hemorrhage.

- The prehospital management of a patient with head injuries is determined by a number of factors. One factor is the mechanism of injury. A second factor is the severity of injury. A third factor is the patient's level of consciousness. Associated injuries affect the priorities of care.
- Several injury rating systems are used to triage, guide patient care, predict patient outcome, identify changes in patient status, and evaluate trauma care. Rating systems commonly used in emergency care include the Glasgow Coma Scale, trauma score/Revised Trauma Score, and pediatric trauma score.

REFERENCES

1. Marx JA, Hockberger RS, Walls RM, et al: *Rosen's emergency medicine: concepts and clinical practice*, ed 6, St Louis, 2006, Mosby.
2. National Safety Council: *Injury facts*, Itasca, III, 2010, The Council.
3. Emergency Nurses Association: *Sheehy's emergency nursing: principles and practice*, ed 6, St Louis, 2005, Mosby.
4. American Association of Endodontists: *Treating the avulsed permanent tooth*, Chicago, 1998, The Association.
5. Wilson WC, Grande CM, Hoyt B, editors: *Trauma: emergency resuscitation, perioperative anesthesia, surgical management*, vol 1, New York, 2007, Informa Healthcare.
6. Brust J: *Current diagnosis and treatment: Neurology*, New York, 2007, McGraw-Hill.
7. Marini J, Wheeler AP, et al: *Critical care medicine: the essentials*, ed 4, Philadelphia, 2010, Lippincott Williams & Wilkins.
8. Adopted by the Brain Injury Association Board of Directors, Feb 22, 1986. This definition is not intended as an exclusive statement of the population served by the Brain Injury Association of America.
9. National Highway Traffic Safety Administration: *The National EMS Education Standards*, Washington, DC, 2009, U.S. Department of Transportation/National Highway Traffic Safety Administration, DOT.
10. Langlois JA, Rutland-Brown W, Thomas KE: *Traumatic brain injury in the United States: emergency department visits, hospitalizations, and deaths*, Atlanta, 2006, Centers for Disease Control and Prevention.
11. TBI facts and stats, www.neuroskills.com/tbi/facts.shtml, accessed 10-6-10.
12. Practice parameters: the management of concussion in sports, www.aan.com/professionals/practice/pdfs/pdf_1995_thru_1998/1997.48.581.pdf, accessed 10-6-10.
13. Chua KS, Ng YS, Yap SG, et al: A brief review of traumatic brain injury rehabilitation, *Ann Acad Med Singapore* 36(1): 31-42, 2007.
14. Brain Trauma Foundation: *Guidelines for the management of severe head injury*, ed 3, New York, 2007, Author.
15. Nelson JS, Mena H, Parisi JE, et al, editors: *Principles and practice of neuropathology*, ed 2, New York, 2003, Oxford University Press.
16. McSwain NE: *PHTLS: prehospital trauma life support*, ed 6, St Louis, 2007, Mosby.
17. American Academy of Orthopedic Surgeons: *Advanced assessment and treatment of trauma*, Boston, 2010, Jones and Bartlett.
18. National Association of Emergency Medical Technicians: *PHTLS: basic and advanced prehospital trauma life support*, ed 7, St Louis, 2011, Mosby.

SUGGESTED READINGS

Badjatia N, Carney N, Crocco T, et al: Guidelines for prehospital management of traumatic brain injury, *PEC* 12(1 suppl): S1-S52, 2007.

Brain Trauma Foundation: Brain Trauma Foundation, 2010, retrieved 4-10-10 from www.braintrauma.org.

Kraus J, Rice T, Peek-Asa C, et al: Facial trauma and the risk of intracranial injury in motorcycle riders, *Ann Emerg Med* 41(1):18-26, 2003.

Salomone JP, Ustin JS, McSwain N, et al: Opinions of trauma practitioners regarding prehospital interventions for critically injured patients, *J Trauma* 58(3):509-517, 2005.

Smith S: Ocular injuries. In McQuillan K, Truter K, Von Rueden R, et al, editors: *Trauma nursing: from resuscitation to rehabilitation*, ed 3, Philadelphia, 2002, Saunders.

Spine and Nervous System Trauma

Upon completion of this chapter, the paramedic student will be able to:

1. Describe the incidence, morbidity, and mortality related to spinal injury.
2. Predict mechanisms of injury that are likely to cause spinal injury.
3. Describe the anatomy and physiology of the spine and spinal cord.
4. Outline the general assessment of a patient with suspected spinal injury.
5. Distinguish between types of spinal injury.
6. Describe prehospital evaluation and assessment of spinal cord injury.
7. Identify prehospital management of the patient with spinal injuries.
8. Distinguish between spinal shock, neurogenic shock, and autonomic hyperreflexia syndrome.
9. Describe selected nontraumatic spinal conditions and the prehospital assessment and treatment of them.

KEY TERMS

anterior cord syndrome A spinal cord injury usually seen in flexion injuries; caused by pressure on the anterior aspect of the spinal cord by a ruptured intervertebral disk or fragments of the vertebral body extruded posteriorly into the spinal canal.

autonomic hyperreflexia syndrome Overactivity of the autonomic nervous system that causes an abrupt onset of extremely high blood pressure.

axial loading Vertical compression of the spine that results when direct forces are transmitted along the length of the spinal column.

Brown-Séquard syndrome A hemitransection of the spinal cord. In the classic presentation, pressure on half of the spinal cord results in weakness of the upper and lower extremities on the ipsilateral (same) side and loss of pain and temperature sensation on the contralateral (opposite) side.

central cord syndrome A spinal cord injury commonly seen with hyperextension or flexion cervical injuries; characterized by greater motor impairment of the upper than lower extremities.

degenerative disk disease A condition caused by the deterioration of the tissue of the intervertebral disk that occurs with aging.

dermatome The skin surface area supplied by a single spinal nerve.

distraction A spinal injury that occurs if the cervical spine is stopped suddenly while the weight and momentum of the body pull away from it.

herniated intervertebral disk Occurs when all or part of a spinal disk is forced through a weakened part of the disk.

mechanism of injury The means by which an injury event occurs.

neurogenic hypotension Hypotension following spinal shock; caused by a loss of sympathetic tone to the vessels.

quadriplegia A weakness or paralysis of all four extremities and the trunk.

spinal cord injury Damage to the spinal cord; may result from direct injury to the cord itself or indirectly from damage to surrounding bones, tissues, or blood vessels.

spinal shock A temporary loss of all types of spinal cord function distal to a cord injury.

spondylosis A condition of the spine characterized by fixation or stiffness of the vertebral joint.

subluxation A partial dislocation.

transection A complete or incomplete lesion to the spinal cord.

M ore than 250,000 victims of **spinal cord injury** (SCI) currently are living in the United States, and more than 12,000 new spinal cord injuries will occur this year.[1] Of these, more than 4800 persons will die before they are admitted to a hospital.[2] Education in injury prevention, prehospital assessment, and proper handling and transportation of these patients can decrease morbidity and mortality.

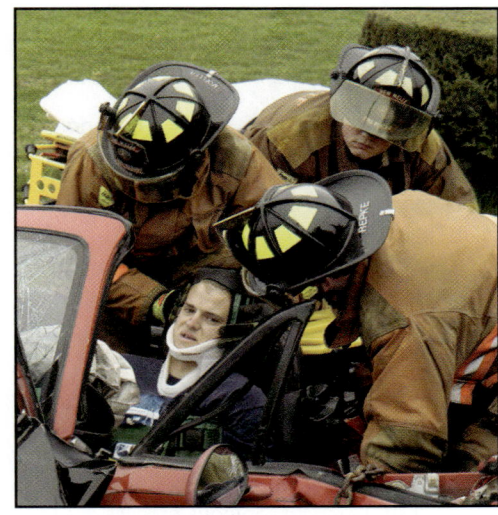

(Courtesy Ray Kemp, St. Charles, Mo.)

SPINAL TRAUMA: INCIDENCE, MORBIDITY, AND MORTALITY

Most spinal cord injuries (SCIs) result from motor vehicle crashes (42.1%). The next largest cause is falls (26.7%). Penetrating injuries from acts of violence (15.1%) and injuries from sports (7.6%) follow (Figure 41-1). The median age of spinal injury victims is 38 years; about 80% of victims are male.[3]

CRITICAL THINKING
Why do you think this group is at increased risk for spinal injuries?

Forty percent of trauma patients with neurological deficit will have a temporary or permanent SCI. In addition to the devastating emotional and psychological impact on victims and their families, the annual cost to society exceeds $5 billion. The average yearly costs that can be attributed

to SCI vary greatly by the severity of injury. The cost of lifelong care for a 25-year-old victim with a permanent and severe SCI is estimated at more than $3.1 million.[1] Injury prevention strategies can have a positive effect on incidence, morbidity, and mortality associated with spinal trauma (see Chapter 3).

REVIEW OF SPINAL ANATOMY

Anatomy of the spine was presented in Chapter 10. The following discussion will serve as a brief review.

The Spinal Column

The spinal column is composed of 33 bones (vertebrae). These bones are divided into five sections. The sections include 7 cervical, 12 thoracic, 5 lumbar, 5 sacral (fused), and 4 coccygeal (fused) vertebrae. The anterior elements of the spine include vertebral bodies, intervertebral disks, and anterior and posterior longitudinal ligaments that connect the vertebral bodies anteriorly and inside the canal (Figure 41-2).

Each vertebra consists of a solid body (bearing most of the weight of the vertebral column), a posterior and anterior arch, a posterior spinous process, and, in some vertebrae, a transverse process. Ligaments between the spinous processes provide support for the movements of flexion and extension. Those between the laminae provide support during lateral flexion. The spinal cord lies in the spinal canal.

The Spinal Cord and Spinal Nerves

The spinal cord runs from the base of the brain down through the cervical and thoracic spine. The cord ends at about L2. Below that area, a collection of nerve roots continues, looking somewhat like a horse's tail (*cauda equina*)

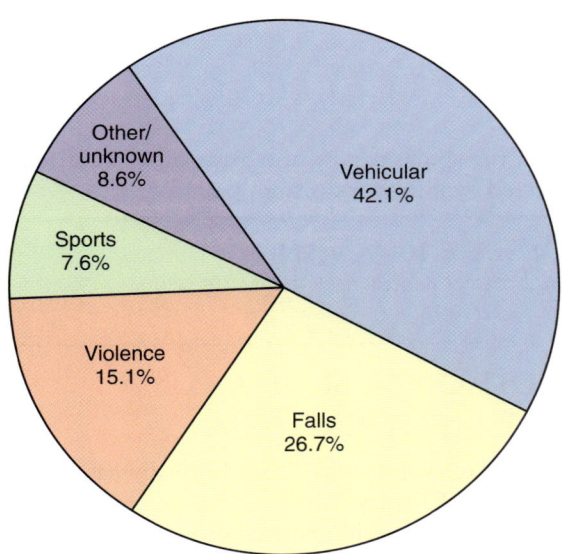

FIGURE 41-1 Mechanism of spine injury.[1]

(Pie chart labels:)
Other/unknown 8.6%
Vehicular 42.1%
Sports 7.6%
Violence 15.1%
Falls 26.7%

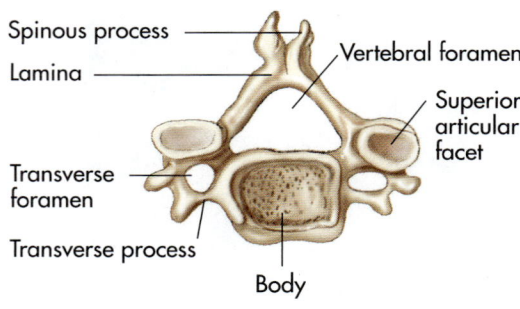

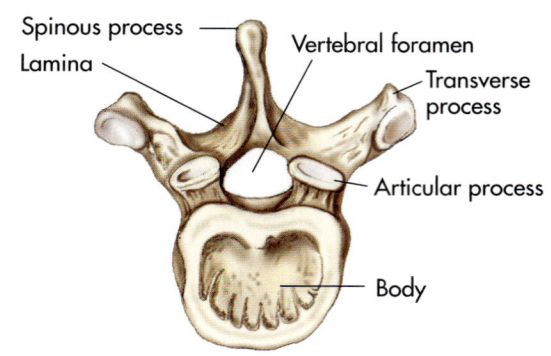

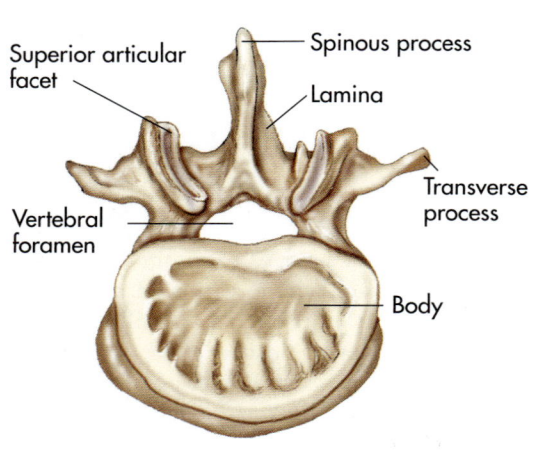

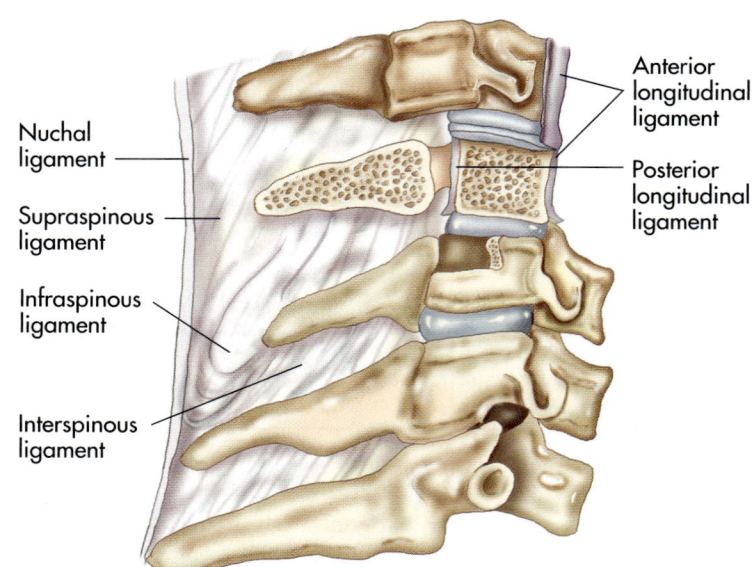

 FIGURE 41-2 Vertebral bodies and elements of the spine. (From Marx J, et al: *Rosen's emergency medicine: concepts and clinical practice,* ed 6, St Louis, 2006, Mosby.)

(Figure 41-3). The nerve roots pass out of the spinal canal through the intervertebral foramen, where they innervate the body either anteriorly (motor) or posteriorly (sensory). *Ascending nerve tracts* carry sensory impulses from various parts of the body through the cord up to the brain. *Descending nerve tracts* carry motor impulses from the brain through the spinal cord and down to the body. As described in Chapter 10, the levels of nerve functions in the spinal cord are represented by **dermatomes** (the sensory area on the body innervated by a nerve root). The anterior divisions of the nerves supply the front of the spine including the limbs. The posterior divisions of the nerves are distributed to the muscles behind the spine. The spinal cord provides a means of communication between the brain and peripheral nerves. Figure 41-4 shows the relationship between the spinal column, the spinal nerves, and areas of the body that can be affected by injury or disease.

LOOK AGAIN
See Chapter 10: Review of Human Systems pp. 176-178.

TRADITIONAL SPINAL ASSESSMENT CRITERIA

Assessment of suspected SCIs traditionally has focused on **mechanism of injury** (MOI). Spinal immobilization was required for two specific patient groups: (1) unconscious injury victims and (2) any patient with a motion injury. This MOI standard covers all patients with a potential for

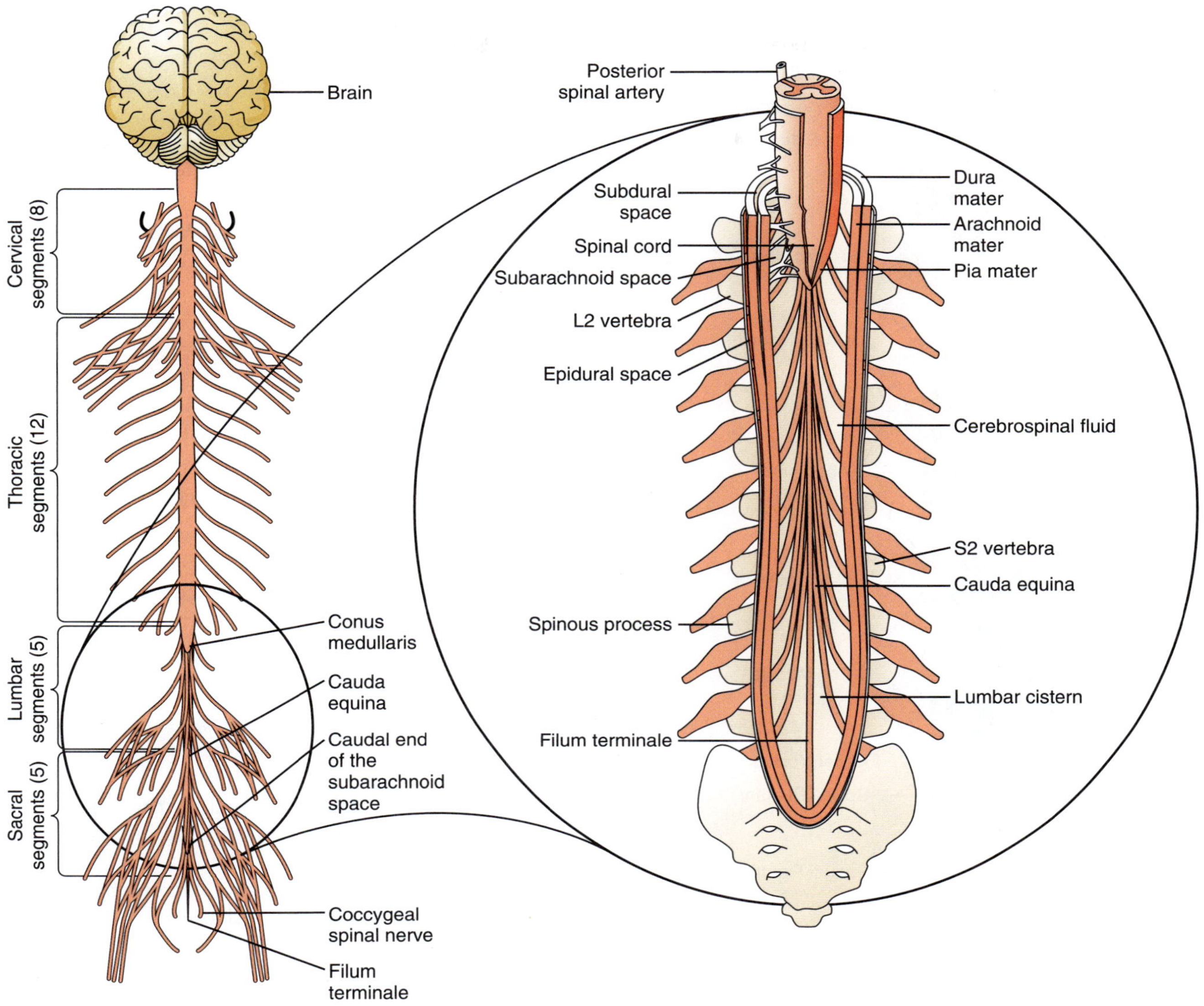

FIGURE 41-3 The spinal cord, spinal nerves, and meninges. Spinal meninges are similar to cranial membranes. Spinal meninges end at S2, creating a cerebrospinal fluid (CSF)–filled cistern below the spinal cord. The cauda equina (horse tail) is formed by the lumbar and sacral nerves, which protrude from the end of the spinal cord. (From Copstead-Kirkhorn LE, Banasik JL: *Pathophysiology,* ed 4, St Louis, 2010, Saunders.)

spinal injury, yet the standard is not always practical in the prehospital setting. The accuracy of prehospital assessment can be strengthened by applying clear, clinical guidelines (clinical criteria) for evaluating SCI, which includes the following signs and symptoms[4]:

- Altered level of consciousness (Glasgow Coma Scale score less than 15)
- Spinal pain or tenderness
- Neurological deficit or complaint
- Anatomical deformity of spine
- Evidence of alcohol or other drugs
- Distracting injury
- Inability to communicate

Mechanism of Injury

When determining MOI in a patient who may have spinal trauma, the paramedic can classify the MOI as *positive, negative,* or *uncertain.*[5] This method, combined with the clinical criteria for spinal injury listed previously, can help the paramedic identify situations in which spinal immobilization is appropriate. When in doubt, the paramedic should use full spinal precautions (Figure 41-5).

CRITICAL THINKING

What are the disadvantages of immobilizing a patient on a long spine board?

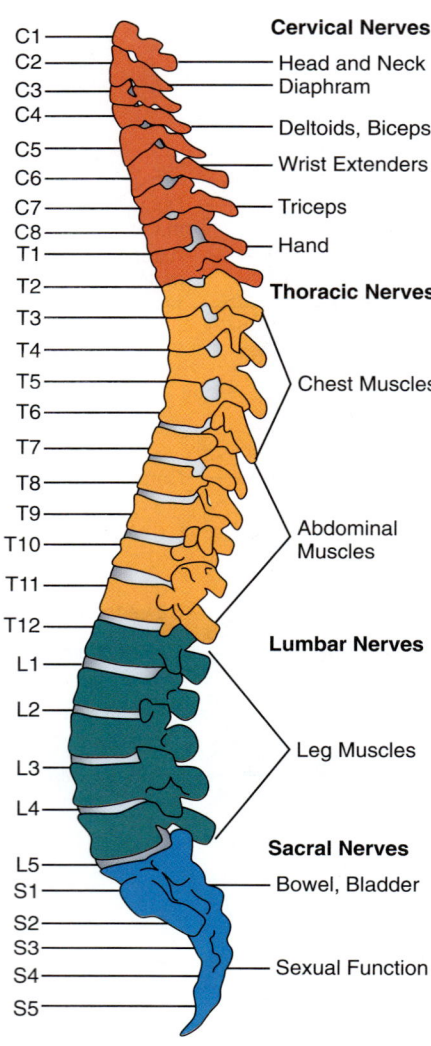

C1
C2
C3
C4
C5
C6
C7
C8
T1
T2
T3
T4
T5
T6
T7
T8
T9
T10
T11
T12
L1
L2
L3
L4
L5
S1
S2
S3
S4
S5

Cervical Nerves
Head and Neck
Diaphram
Deltoids, Biceps
Wrist Extenders
Triceps
Hand

Thoracic Nerves

Chest Muscles

Abdominal Muscles

Lumbar Nerves

Leg Muscles

Sacral Nerves
Bowel, Bladder

Sexual Function

FIGURE 41-4 Nerve tracts.

POSITIVE MECHANISM OF INJURY

In a positive MOI, the forces exerted on the patient are highly suggestive of SCI. A positive MOI with physiological findings for spinal injury requires full spinal immobilization. Examples of positive MOIs include the following:

- High-speed motor vehicle crashes
- Falls from greater than 3 times the patient's height
- Violent situations occurring near the patient's spine (e.g., blunt and penetrating injuries)
- Sports injuries
- Other high-impact situations

In the absence of signs and symptoms of SCI, some medical direction agencies may recommend that a patient with a positive MOI not be immobilized.[4] Medical direction bases this action on the paramedic's assessment, a reliable patient history, and the absence of distracting injuries (described later in this chapter).

NEGATIVE MECHANISM OF INJURY

A negative MOI includes events in which force or impact does not suggest a likely spinal injury. In the absence of SCI signs and symptoms, negative MOI injuries do not require spinal immobilization. Examples of negative MOIs include the following:

- Dropping an object on the foot
- Twisting an ankle while running
- Isolated soft tissue injury

UNCERTAIN MECHANISM OF INJURY

At times, the impact or force involved in the injury is unknown or uncertain. Thus clinical criteria must be the basis used to determine the need for spinal immobilization (Box 41-1).

Examples of uncertain MOIs include the following:

- Tripping or falling to the ground and hitting the head
- Falls from 2 to 4 feet
- Low-speed motor vehicle crashes ("fender benders")

Assessment of Uncertain Mechanism of Injury. When evaluating the need for spinal immobilization in which the MOI is uncertain, the paramedic must ensure that the patient is reliable. A reliable patient is one who is calm, cooperative, sober, alert, and oriented. Patients who would be considered unreliable include those who:

- Have acute stress reactions from sudden stress of any type
- Have brain injury
- Are intoxicated
- Have abnormal mental status
- Have distracting injuries
- Have problems communicating

CRITICAL THINKING
The reliability of a patient is not always easy to assess quickly in the prehospital setting. Why is this?

NOTE
Any patient who has altered mental status or altered pain perception should be considered unreliable. Examples include patients with Alzheimer's disease, a psychiatric illness, and those under the influence of alcohol or other drugs.

INDICATIONS FOR SPINAL IMMOBILIZATION

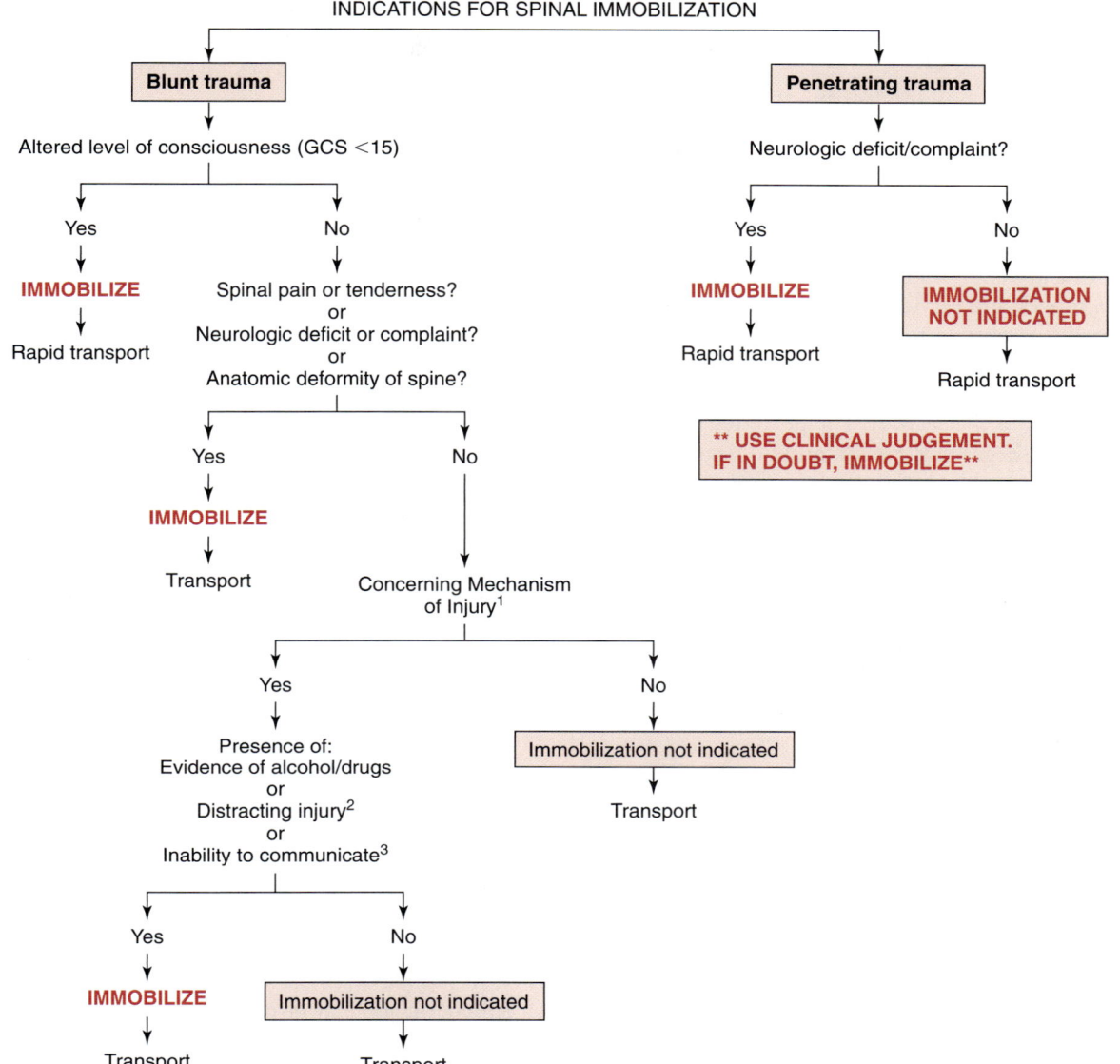

Notes:
[1]Concerning Mechanisms of Injury
• Any mechanism that produced a violent impact to the head, neck, torso, or pelvis (e.g., assault, entrapment in structural collapse, etc.)
• Incidents producing sudden acceleration, deceleration, or lateral bending forces to the neck or torso (e.g., moderate- to high-speed MVC, pedestrian struck, involvement in an explosion, etc.)
• Any fall, especially in the elderly
• Ejection or fall from any motorized or human-powered transportation device (e.g., scooters, skateboards, bicycles, motor vehicles, motorcycles or recreational vehicles)
• Victim of shallow-water diving incident

[2]Distracting Injury
   Any injury that may have the potential to impair the patient's ability to appreciate other injuries. Examples of distracting injuries include a) long bone fracture; b) a visceral injury requiring surgical consultation; c) a large laceration, degloving injury, or crush injury; d) large burns, or e) any other injury producing acute functional impairment.
   (Adapted from Hoffman JR, Wolfson AB, Todd K. Mower WR: Selective cervical spine radiography in blunt trauma: methodology of the National Emergency X-Radiography Utilization Study [NEXUS], *Ann Emerg Med* 461, 1998.)

[3]Inability to communicate. Any patient who, for reasons not specified above, cannot clearly communicate so as to actively participate in their assessment. Examples: speech or hearing impaired, those who only speak a foreign language, and small children.

FIGURE 41-5 Indications for spinal immobilization. (From National Association of Emergency Medical Technicians: *PHTLS: prehospital trauma life support,* ed 7, St Louis, 2011, Mosby.)

GENERAL ASSESSMENT OF SPINAL INJURY

Spinal injury most often results from the spine being forced beyond its normal range and limits of motion (Figure 41-6). The adult skull weighs 16 to 22 lb. The skull sits on top of the first cervical vertebra (C1), or the *atlas*. The second cervical vertebra (C2), or the *axis*, and its odontoid process allow the head to move with about a 180-degree range of motion. Because of the weight and position of the head in relation to the thin neck and cervical vertebrae, the cervical spine is particularly susceptible to injury (27% to 33% of all SCIs occur in the C1 to C2 region).[1] Other spinal components that affect physiological limits of motion are the posterior neck muscles and the sacrum. The posterior neck muscles allow up to 60 degrees of flexion and 70 degrees of extension without stretching of the spinal cord. The sacrum is joined to the pelvis by immovable joints.

The specific MOIs that often cause spinal trauma are axial loading; extremes of flexion, hyperextension, or hyperrotation; excessive lateral bending; and distraction. These mechanisms may result in stable and unstable injuries. This is based on the extent of damage to spinal structures and the relative strength of the structures remaining intact.

Axial Loading

Axial loading (vertical compression) of the spine results when direct forces are sent down the length of the spinal column. Examples include striking the head against the windshield of a car, shallow diving injuries, vertical falls, and being struck on the head or a helmet with a heavy object. These forces may produce compression fracture or a crushed vertebral body without SCI and most commonly occur from T12 to L2.[3]

Flexion, Hyperextension, and Hyperrotation

Extremes in flexion, hyperextension, or hyperrotation may result in fracture, ligament injury, or muscle injury. Spinal cord injury is caused when one or more of the cervical vertebrae dislocate **(subluxation)** and are forced into the spinal canal. This injures the spinal cord. Examples of these motion extremes include rapid acceleration or deceleration forces from motor vehicle crashes, hangings, and midfacial skeletal or soft tissue trauma. Serious injuries often are the result of a combination of loading and rotational forces. These forces produce displacement or fracture of one or more vertebrae.

Lateral Bending

Excessive lateral bending may result in dislocations and bony fractures to the cervical and thoracic spine. The injury occurs as a sudden lateral impact moves the torso sideways. Initially, the head tends to remain in place. Then the head is pulled along by the cervical attachments. Examples of lateral bending include side or angular collisions from motor vehicle crashes and injuries from contact sports. The mechanism of this lateral force requires less movement to produce an injury than flexion or extension forces in frontal or rear impacts.

Distraction

Distraction may occur if the cervical spine is stopped suddenly while the weight and momentum of the body pull away from it. This force or stretching may result in tearing and laceration of the spinal cord. Examples of distraction injuries include intentional or unintentional hangings (e.g., suicide or school yard or playground injuries).

Other Mechanisms

Other less common mechanisms of spinal injury include blunt and penetrating trauma and electrical injury. The spinal cord, like the brain, may suffer concussions, contusions, and lacerations. The spinal cord may develop hematomata and edema in response to blunt trauma. Examples include spinal injuries that result from direct blows such as from falling tree limbs or other heavy objects.

Penetrating trauma to the spine may be caused by missile-type injuries or stab wounds to the neck, chest, or abdomen. These forces may result in laceration of the spinal cord or nerve roots over a wide area. At times penetrating trauma may produce a complete **transection** (lesion). In addition, areas of edema or contusion adjacent to the laceration may disrupt cord tissue.

Spinal trauma may occur from direct electrical injury. Trauma also may occur from the violent muscle spasms that accompany electrical shock (described in Chapter 39: Burns).

CLASSIFICATIONS OF SPINAL INJURY

Spinal injuries may be classified as sprains and strains, fractures and dislocations, sacral and coccygeal fractures, and cord injuries. Regardless of the specific injury, all patients with suspected spinal trauma and signs and symptoms of SCI should be immobilized. Unnecessary movement should be avoided until injury to the spine or spinal cord can be excluded by clinical examination and radiography. An unstable spine can be ruled out only by radiography or lack of any potential mechanism for the injury. As a guideline, the paramedic should assume the presence of spine injury and an unstable spine with the following[4]:

- Any mechanism that produced a violent impact on the head, neck, torso, or pelvis (e.g., assault, entrapment in a structural collapse)
- Incidents that produce sudden acceleration, deceleration, or lateral bending forces to the neck or torso (e.g., moderate- to high-speed motor vehicle collisions; pedestrian struck by a vehicle; involvement in an explosion)
- Any fall, especially in elderly persons
- Ejection or a fall from any motorized or otherwise powered transportation device (e.g., scooters, skateboards, bicycles, motor vehicles, motorcycles, recreational vehicles)

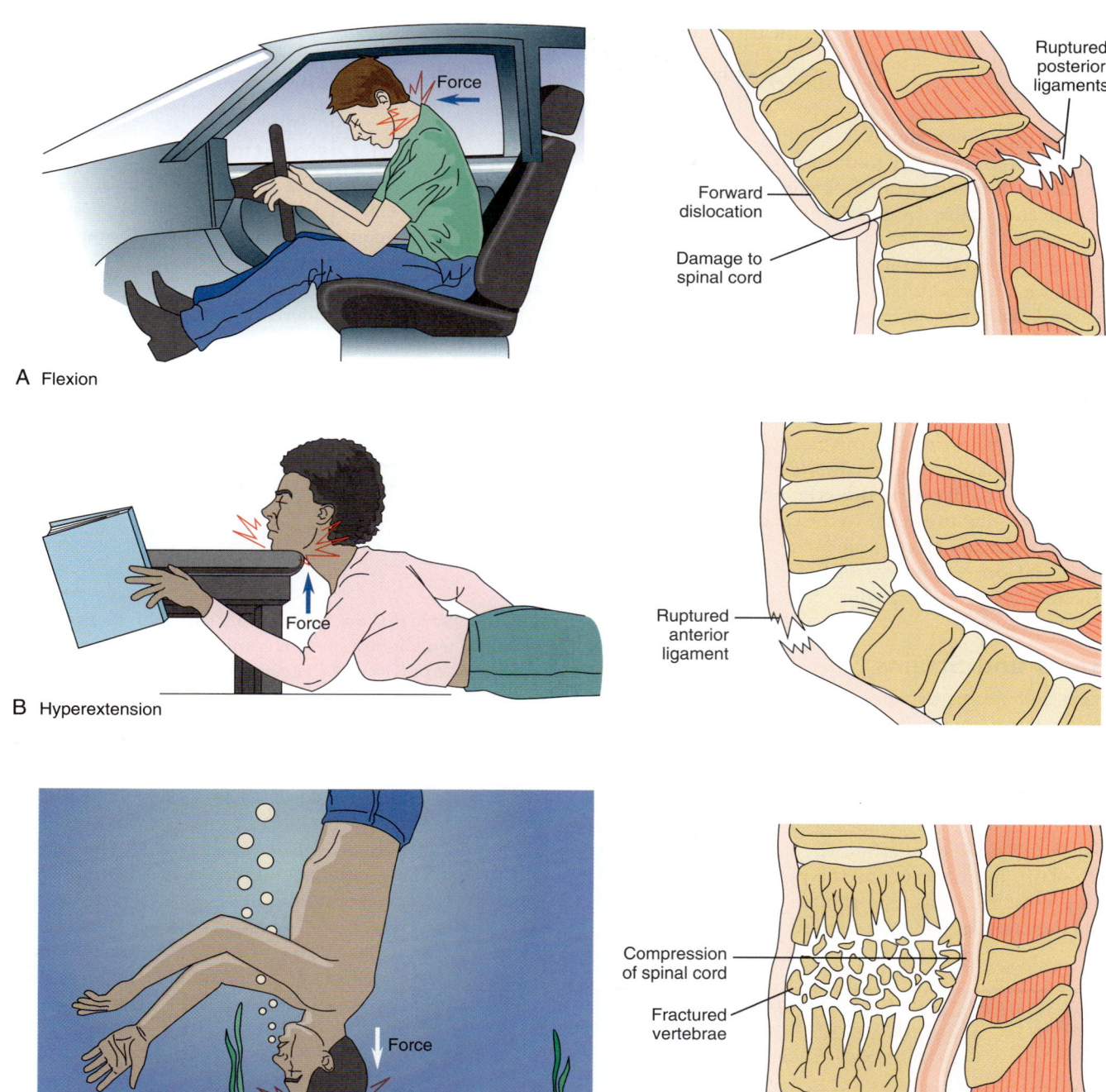

FIGURE 41-6 Mechanisms of spinal cord injury. Many situations may produce these consequences. This figure shows examples only. **A,** Flexion injury of the cervical spine ruptures the posterior ligaments. **B,** Hyperextension injury of the cervical spine ruptures the anterior ligaments. **C,** Compression fractures crush the vertebrae and force bony fragments into the spinal canal. (From Copstead-Kirkhorn LE, Banasik JL: *Pathophysiology,* ed 4, St Louis, 2010, Saunders.)

- Any victim of a shallow-water incident (e.g., diving, body surfing)
- Head injuries with any alteration in level of consciousness
- Significant helmet damage
- Significant blunt injury to the torso
- Impact or other deceleration fractures of the legs or hips
- Significant localized injuries to the area of the spinal column

Spinal injury (bony injury) can occur with or without SCI. Likewise, a patient may have SCI without bony injury. *Spinal cord injury without radiological abnormality* is a more common finding in children.[6]

The damage produced by the injury forces can be complicated further by the patient's age (calcification from the aging process), preexisting bone diseases (osteoporosis, spondylosis, rheumatoid arthritis, Paget's disease), and congenital spinal cord anomalies (e.g., fusion or narrow spinal canal). Spinal cord neurons do not regenerate to any great extent. Thus any injury to the central nervous system that causes destruction of tissue often results in irreparable damage and permanent loss of function. The role of the paramedic in protecting this critical area cannot be overemphasized.

Sprains and Strains

Sprains and strains usually result from hyperflexion and hyperextension forces. A *hyperflexion sprain* occurs when the posterior ligamentous complex tears at least partially. This sprain also can result in tears of the joint capsules. The sprain may allow partial dislocation (subluxation) of the intervertebral joints. *Hyperextension strains* are common in low-speed, rear-end car crashes. They are known commonly as whiplash. Injury occurs as the person is thrown backward against the posterior thorax during impact. This action damages anterior soft tissues of the neck.

CRITICAL THINKING

How can the paramedic distinguish between cervical sprain/strain and spinal fracture in the prehospital setting?

With sprains and strains, local pain may be produced by spasms of the neck muscles and injury to the vertebrae, intervertebral disks, and ligamentous structures. The pain usually is described as a nonradiating, aching soreness of the neck or back muscles. The discomfort often varies in intensity and with changes in posture.

On examination, a deformity of the spine may be palpable if dislocation (subluxation) has occurred. The patient may complain of associated point tenderness and swelling. Until the SCI is ruled out by x-ray exam, the paramedic should treat these patients as having unstable cervical spine injuries with a potential for damage to the spinal cord. After the diagnosis is confirmed, treatment of cervical

sprain or strain usually is symptomatic. Following physician evaluation, treatment occasionally may include a cervical collar to decrease neck movement, heat application, and analgesics.

Fractures and Dislocations

The most frequently injured spinal regions in descending order are C5 to C7, C1 to C2, and T12 to L2.[3] Of these injuries, the most common are wedge-shaped compression fractures and teardrop fractures or dislocations. Neurological deficits associated with these fractures and dislocations vary with the location. They also vary with the extent of injury. Although the spine and spinal cord are close to each other, the spine can be fractured without SCI and vice versa. In addition, spinal injuries at multiple levels are common.

CRITICAL THINKING

Look at an illustration of the spinal column. Why do you think these areas are susceptible to fractures?

Wedge-shaped fractures (Figure 41-7) are hyperflexion injuries. They usually result from compressive force applied to the anterior portion of the vertebral body. This results in stretching of the posterior ligaments. (These injuries often result from injuries and falls in industrial settings.) These fractures usually occur in the mid or lower cervical segments or at T12 and L1. They generally are considered stable because the posterior ligaments rarely are disrupted totally.

Teardrop fractures and dislocations (Figure 41-8) are unstable injuries. They result from a combination of severe hyperflexion and compression forces and often are seen in motor vehicle crashes. During impact, the vertebral body is fractured. The anterior-inferior corner of the vertebral body is pushed forward. Unlike simple wedge fractures, these

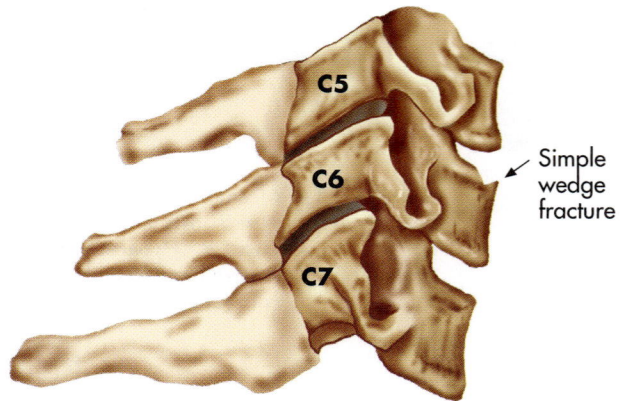

FIGURE 41-7 Lateral view of simple wedge fracture. (From Marx J, et al: *Rosen's emergency medicine: concepts and clinical practice,* ed 6, St Louis, 2006, Mosby.)

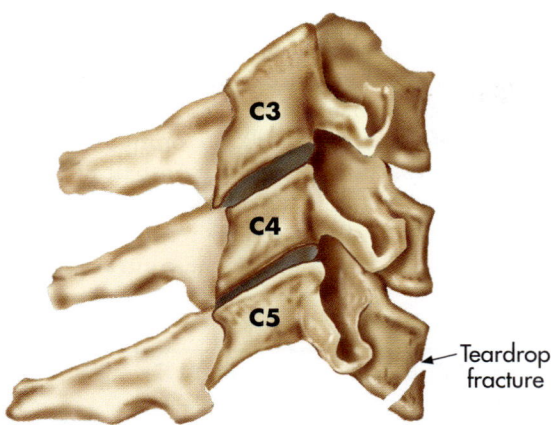

FIGURE 41-8 Lateral view of teardrop fracture. (From Marx J, et al: *Rosen's emergency medicine: concepts and clinical practice,* ed 6, St Louis, 2006, Mosby.)

fractures may be associated with neurological damage. These are among the most unstable injuries of the spine. A number of other spinal injuries are associated with the mechanisms of flexion, extension, rotation, and axial loading. Most of these are unstable and require careful immobilization.

Sacral and Coccygeal Fractures

The majority of serious spinal injuries occur in the cervical, thoracic, and lumbar regions. One reason for this is the location of the spinal cord and its termination in the adult spine at about L2. Another reason is the protection provided by the ring structure of the pelvis and the musculature of the buttocks and lower back. However, fractures through the foramina of S1 and S2 are fairly common. They may compromise several sacral nerve elements. Such fractures may result in loss of perianal sensory motor function. They also may result in damage to the bladder and bladder sphincters.

The sacrococcygeal joint also may be injured as a result of direct blows and falls. Patients often complain that they have "broken their tailbone." They often experience moderate pain from the mobile coccyx. Diagnosis usually is confirmed by a physician through a rectal examination.

Cord Injuries

Spinal cord injuries may be classified further as *primary* and *secondary* injuries.[1] Primary injuries occur at the time of impact. Secondary injuries occur after the initial injury. This type of injury can include swelling, ischemia, and movement of bony fragments. Like other tissues, the spinal cord can be concussed, contused, compressed, and lacerated. All of these mechanisms can cause temporary or permanent loss of cord-mediated functions distal to the injury from compression or ischemia. Bleeding from damaged blood vessels also can occur in the tissue of the spinal cord. Bleeding can cause an obstruction to spinal blood supply.

BOX 41-2 Complete Cord Lesions[7]

C1-C4 tetraplegia* (high tetraplegia): Individuals with complete C1-C4 (high) tetraplegia have little or no movement of upper and lower extremity muscles. They have movement of the head and neck, as well as, possibly, shoulder elevation (shrug). Persons with an injury at the C4 level have innervation of the diaphragm (the primary muscle for respiratory inspiration). They should not need long-term ventilatory assistance, although it is not uncommon to receive ventilation support initially after injury.

C5-C6 tetraplegia: Individuals with C5-C6 tetraplegia have functional use of elbow flexion and wrist extension. With the help of specialized assistive devices (such as wrist or hand orthotics to allow them to hold objects), these persons can achieve independence in feeding and grooming.

C7-C8 tetraplegia: Individuals with C7-C8 tetraplegia have the functional ability to extend their elbow and functional finger flexion, which greatly enhances their mobility and self-care skills. (C7 is usually the highest level at which patients can have an injury and still be able to live independently.) These patients can achieve independence in feeding, grooming, upper and lower extremity dressing, bathing, bed-mobility transfers, manual wheelchair propulsion, and bladder and bowel care, as well as in typing, writing, answering phones, and using computers. These persons can also drive independently using a van or a car adapted with hand controls.

Thoracic and lumbar paraplegia (below T1): Individuals with paraplegia have innervation and function of all upper extremity muscles, including those for hand function. They can achieve functional independence in self-care (including light housekeeping and meal preparation), in bladder and bowel skills, and, at the wheelchair level, in all mobility needs. Patients with this injury can drive independently by using a car adapted with hand controls.

*Tetraplegia is also known as **quadriplegia** (paralysis of four limbs).

The severity of these injuries depends on the amount and type of force that produced them and the duration of the injury.

CORD LESIONS

Lesions (transections) to the spinal cord are classified as *complete* or *incomplete*. Complete lesions usually are associated with spinal fracture or dislocation. Patients have total absence of pain, pressure, and joint sensation. They also have complete motor paralysis below the level of injury (Box 41-2). Autonomic nervous system dysfunction may be associated with complete cord lesions. This depends on the level of cord involvement. Manifestations of autonomic dysfunction include the following:

- Bradycardia caused by loss of sympathetic autonomic activity
- Hypotension caused by loss of vasomotor control and peripheral vascular resistance
- Priapism

- Loss of sweating and shivering
- Poikilothermy (body temperature varying with ambient temperature)
- Loss of bowel and bladder control

CRITICAL THINKING

Why should you immobilize a patient who already is showing signs and symptoms of a complete cord lesion?

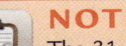

NOTE

The 31 pairs of spinal nerves are numbered according to the vertebra at which they exit the spinal column. From the first thoracic vertebra downward, all spinal nerves exit *below* their equivalent numbered vertebrae. For example, the spinal nerve T4 exits the spinal column through the foramen in the fourth thoracic vertebra; the spinal nerve L5 exits the spinal cord through the foramen in the fifth lumbar vertebra. In the cervical region of the spinal cord, the spinal nerves exit *above* the vertebrae. A change occurs at the C7 vertebra, however, where the C8 spinal nerve exits the vertebra below the C7 vertebra. Therefore, there is an eighth cervical spinal nerve, even though there is no eighth cervical vertebra. In descending order, the cervical nerves supply feeling and movement to the arms, neck, and upper trunk; thoracic nerves supply the trunk and abdomen; and lumbar and sacral nerves supply the legs, bladder, and sexual organs.

The paramedic should be familiar with signs and symptoms of several incomplete spinal cord syndromes. Knowledge of these rare syndromes helps the paramedic to understand the potential for further injury. The three syndromes indicating incomplete lesions of the spinal cord are as follows:

1. **Central cord syndrome:** Central cord syndrome commonly occurs with hyperextension or flexion cervical injuries. The syndrome is characterized by greater motor impairment of the upper than lower extremities. Signs and symptoms of central cord syndrome are as follows:
   - Paralysis of the arms
   - *Sacral sparing* (the preservation of sensory or voluntary motor function of the perineum, buttocks, scrotum, or anus)
2. **Anterior cord syndrome:** Anterior cord syndrome usually is seen in flexion injuries. The syndrome is caused by pressure on the anterior aspect of the spinal cord by a ruptured intervertebral disk or fragments of the vertebral body forced posteriorly into the spinal canal. Signs and symptoms include the following:
   - Decreased sensation of pain and temperature below the level of the lesion (including lesions of the sacral region)
   - Intact light touch and position sensation
   - Paralysis

3. **Brown-Séquard syndrome:** Brown-Séquard syndrome is a hemitransection of the spinal cord. This syndrome may result from a ruptured intervertebral disk or the pushing of a fragment of vertebral body on the spinal cord. This often occurs after knife or missile injuries. In the classic presentation, pressure on half of the spinal cord results in weakness of the extremities on the ipsilateral (same) side. Pressure also results in loss of pain and temperature sensation on the contralateral (opposite) side.

CRITICAL THINKING

How will the prehospital care differ for a patient who has signs or symptoms of one of these syndromes?

PHARMACOLOGICAL THERAPY FOR INCOMPLETE CORD INJURY

The benefits of pharmacological agents (glucocorticoids, *naloxone,* calcium channel blockers, GM-1 ganglioside, and others) in the management of incomplete cord injury are controversial. These drugs are thought to provide some type of damage control following some SCIs. Some of the drugs are thought to work by reducing the toxicity of excitatory amino acids that cause cells to die; others, by encouraging the growth of new neurons or by reducing inflammation of the injured spinal cord and the bursting open of damaged cells.[1] Of these, only *methylprednisolone* currently is used routinely for human victims of SCI.[3]

Methylprednisolone is a synthetic steroid that is sometimes given to reduce posttraumatic spinal cord edema and inflammation. Studies have found that patients treated with large doses of this drug (30 mg/kg IV bolus, followed by a maintenance drip) within 8 hours of injury had improved recovery.[8] *Methylprednisolone* and other steroids have known adverse effects and complications, including suppression of adrenal glands and immune functioning.[4] Therefore the use of these drugs in managing SCI is controversial. Paramedics should consult with medical direction and follow local protocol.

EVALUATION AND ASSESSMENT OF SPINAL CORD INJURY

Spinal cord trauma should be evaluated only after all injuries that pose a threat to life have been assessed and treated. As with any scenario of serious illness or injury, the paramedic's first priority must be scene survey, including ensuring personal safety. The primary survey and assessment and management of the patient's airway, breathing, and circulation must be performed in a way that minimizes further damage. The second priority is to preserve spinal cord function and avoid secondary injury to the spinal cord.

The primary injury to the spine occurs at impact. Thus the critical role of paramedics is to prevent secondary injury. A secondary injury could result from unnecessary movement of an unstable spinal column, hypoxemia, edema, or shock (which may reduce perfusion of the injured cord). These goals are best met by maintaining a high degree of suspicion for the presence of spinal trauma (based on scene survey, kinematics, and history of the event), providing early spinal immobilization, and rapidly correcting any volume deficit through fluid replacement, pneumatic antishock garment application (per protocol), and oxygen administration.

After any life-threatening problems found in the initial assessment are treated, the paramedic should perform a neurological examination. This examination may be done in the field. The exam also may be done en route to the receiving hospital if the patient's condition requires rapid transport. Any movement of the patient for performing a general or neurological examination must be accompanied by continuous, manual protection and in-line stabilization of the spine. Once the spine is stabilized, the paramedic should palpate the entire spine. Any report of pain on palpation indicates the need to immobilize the spine. Full documentation of the paramedic's findings provides an important baseline. This information will be useful for further assessment and evaluation of the patient in the emergency department. The components of the neurological examination include evaluation of motor and sensory findings and reflex responses.

Motor Findings

The paramedic should question conscious patients about pain in the neck or back with and without palpation. The paramedic also should ask patients about their ability to move their arms and legs. If possible, the paramedic should test the strength and motion of all four extremities. This can be done by asking the patient to flex the elbows (biceps, C6), extend the elbows (triceps, C7), and abduct/adduct the fingers (C8, T1). In unconscious patients, painful stimuli in the hands and lower extremities may initiate an involuntary muscle reflex unless the patient is in profound coma.

UPPER EXTREMITY NEUROLOGICAL FUNCTION ASSESSMENT

To test interosseous muscle function (controlled by T1 nerve roots), the paramedic should instruct the patient to spread the fingers of both hands. Then the patient should be instructed to keep the fingers apart while the paramedic squeezes the second and fourth fingers. Normal resistance should be springlike and equal on both sides.

To test the extensors of the hands and fingers (controlled by C7 nerve roots), the paramedic should instruct the patient to hold his or her wrists or fingers straight out and to keep them out while the paramedic presses down on the fingers. (The arm should be supported at the wrist to avoid testing arm function and other nerve roots.) Moderate resistance will normally be felt with moderate pressure. Both sides of the patient should be evaluated if not contraindicated by injury.

LOWER EXTREMITY NEUROLOGICAL FUNCTION ASSESSMENT

To test plantar flexors of the foot (controlled by S1 and S2 nerve roots), the paramedic should place his or her hands at the sole of each foot and instruct the patient to push against the hands. Both sides should feel equal and strong.

To test dorsal flexors of the foot and great toe (controlled by L5 nerve roots), the paramedic should hold the patient's foot (with fingers on toes) and instruct the patient to pull the feet back or toward the nose. Both sides should feel equal and strong.

Sensory Findings

In conscious patients, sensory examination should be performed with light touch on each hand and each foot (while the patient's eyes are closed) to evaluate the ability to feel this type of stimulus. (Light touch is carried by more than one nerve tract.) Sensation should be equal on both sides. The paramedic also should question the patient about weakness, numbness, paresthesia, or radicular pain (shooting pain that travels along a nerve).

If the patient cannot feel light touch or is unconscious, the paramedic may evaluate sensation by gently pricking the hands and soles of the feet. A sharp object that will not penetrate the skin is useful. (For example, the end of a pen or broken cotton-tipped applicator can be used.) One method of evaluation moves from head to toe, recording the level at which sensation stops or the unconscious patient ceases to respond to a painful stimulus by marking that location on the patient's skin with ink or a marker. Another method is to begin the sensory assessment by moving from an area of no sensation to an area where sensation begins. The paramedic would note the area where sensation begins with ink or marker. (These marks make it possible to compare sensory level accurately after repeated examinations.) Lack of response to stimulation in the upper extremities indicates cord damage in the cervical region; failure of only the lower extremities to respond indicates cord injury in the thoracic region, lumbar region, or both.

CRITICAL THINKING

How will you respond to the patient who fearfully asks you, "Why can't I move or feel my arms or legs?"

Dermatomes (described in Chapter 10) correspond to spinal nerves (Table 41-1), so the following four landmarks may be useful for a quick sensory evaluation in the prehospital setting:

1. C2 to C4 dermatomes provide a collar of sensation around the neck and over the anterior chest to below the clavicles.
2. T4 dermatome provides sensation to the nipple line.

TABLE 41-1 Common Nerve Root and Motor/Sensory Correlation

Nerve Root	Motor	Sensory
C3, C4	Trapezius (shoulder shrug)	Top of shoulder
C3 to C5	Diaphragm	Top of shoulder
C5, C6	Biceps (elbow flexion)	Thumb
C7	Triceps (elbow extension), wrist/finger extension	Middle finger
C8, T1	Finger abduction/adduction	Little finger
T4	Nipple	
T10	Umbilicus	
L1, L2	Hip flexion	Inguinal crease
L3, L4	Quadriceps	Medial thigh/calf
L5	Great toe/foot dorsiflexion	Lateral calf
S1	Knee flexion	Lateral foot
S1, S2	Foot plantar flexion	
S2 to S4	Anal sphincter tone	Perianal

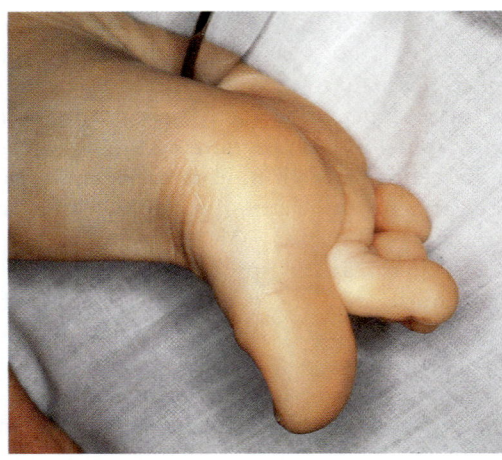

FIGURE 41-9 Babinski's sign: dorsiflexion of the great toe with or without fanning of the toes. (Courtesy Gary Quick, MD.)

3. T10 dermatome provides sensation to the umbilicus.
4. S1 dermatome provides sensation to the soles of the feet.

Reflex Responses

Reflex responses seldom are evaluated in the prehospital setting. However, some abnormal responses are observed easily. These responses may indicate autonomic nerve injury. These responses include loss of temperature control, hypotension, bradycardia, and priapism. Another pathological reflex includes the presence of Babinski's sign (the plantar reflex). This is a reflex movement in which the great toe bends upward when the outer edge of the sole of the foot is scratched (Figure 41-9). Babinski's sign (which may indicate a spinal cord lesion in the older child or adult) is a normal and expected response in children younger than 2 years of age.

Other Methods of Evaluation

A visual inspection of the spine may reveal the presence of injury and its level. For example, transection of the cord above C3 often results in respiratory arrest. Lesions that occur at C4 may result in paralysis of the diaphragm. However, transections that occur at C5 to C6 usually spare the diaphragm, allowing diaphragmatic breathing. This occurs because the intercostal muscles are innervated sequentially between C4 to C5 and T12. As a result, intercostal muscle groups may be paralyzed with cervical or thoracic spinal cord lesions below the level where diaphragmatic nerves are located. (The higher the lesion, the greater the loss of intercostal muscle function.)

The patient's body position also may offer clues about neurological injury. For example, a patient with a SCI at C6 may lie with the arms flexed at the elbows and wrists (the "holdup" position).

GENERAL MANAGEMENT OF SPINAL INJURIES

A significant spinal injury still may be present, even though the patient may not show signs of spinal injury.[9] Some patients with cervical spinal injuries have normal responses to motor, sensory, and reflex examinations. Thus if the paramedic suspects a spinal injury for any reason, the paramedic must protect the patient's spine. In addition, the patient's ability to walk does not rule out the need for spinal precautions. As previously stated, an unstable spine can be ruled out only by clinical examination, radiography, and the lack of any potential mechanism for spinal injury. General principles of spinal immobilization include the following:

1. The primary goal is to prevent further injury.
2. The spine should be treated as a long bone with a joint at either end (the head and pelvis).
3. The paramedic should always use complete spinal immobilization. (Splinting and isolation of a specific injury site is impossible. Having spine fractures in more than one location also is common.)
4. Spinal immobilization begins in the initial assessment and must be maintained until the spine is immobilized completely on a long spine board.
5. The patient's head and neck must be placed in a neutral, in-line position unless contraindicated by condition or MOI. (Neutral positioning allows for the most space for the spinal cord, thereby reducing cord hypoxia and excess pressure.)

Spinal Stabilization/Immobilization Techniques

As soon as a potential spine injury is recognized, the paramedic should manually protect the patient's head and neck. The basic principle to follow is that the head and neck must be maintained in line with the long axis of the body. If other injuries need treatment, the paramedic must maintain the patient's head and neck position without interruption.

A number of devices for immobilizing the spinal column are designed for prehospital use. When properly applied to patients who are sitting, standing, or lying, these devices can provide adequate spinal protection. However, no device should be considered for use until the head and neck have been stabilized with manual in-line immobilization.

> **NOTE**
> All spinal immobilization techniques discussed in this text follow the guidelines recommended by the Prehospital Trauma Life Support Committee of the National Association of Emergency Medical Technicians in cooperation with the Committee on Trauma of the American College of Surgeons.[4]

MANUAL IN-LINE IMMOBILIZATION

Manual in-line immobilization can be done from almost any patient position. It should be applied without traction on the head. Only enough tension should be applied to relieve the weight of the head from the cervical spine. After manual immobilization has been initiated, it must be continued without stopping until the head and spine are immobilized to a proper device (short spine board or vest, long spine board).

Contraindications for moving the patient's head to an in-line position follow. If any of these contraindications exist, all manual movement of the patient's head should stop. At that point, the head and neck should be stabilized in the position found. Contraindications include:

- Resistance to movement
- Neck muscle spasm
- Increased pain
- The presence or increase in neurological deficits during movement (e.g., numbness, tingling, and loss of motor function)
- Compromise of the airway or ventilation
- Severe misalignment of the head away from the midline of the shoulders and body axis (rare)

Manual Immobilization From the Sitting or Standing Patient's Side
1. Stand alongside the patient, holding the back of the head with one hand. Place the thumb and first finger of the other hand on each cheek, just below the zygomatic arch (Figure 41-10).
2. Tighten the position of both hands without moving the head or neck.
3. Move the head to an in-line position if needed. Maintain this position by bracing the elbows against your torso for support.

Manual In-Line Immobilization From the Front of the Sitting or Standing Patient
1. Stand in front of the patient and place the thumb of each hand on the patient's cheeks, just below the zygomatic arch.
2. Place the little fingers of each hand on the posterior aspect of the patient's skull.
3. Spread the remaining fingers of each hand on the lateral planes of the head and increase the strength of the grip (Figure 41-11).
4. Move the head to an in-line position if needed. Maintain this position by bracing the elbows against your torso for support.

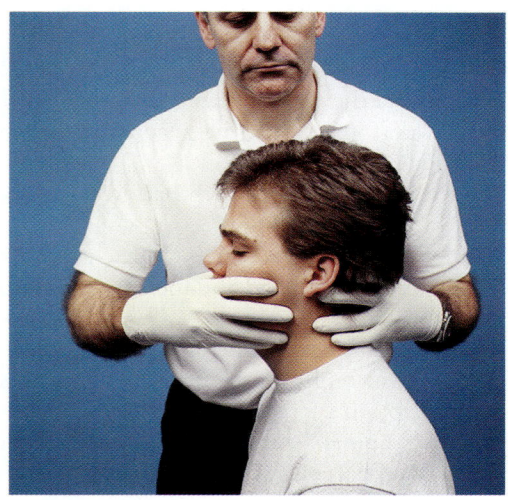

FIGURE 41-10 Manual in-line immobilization from the side.

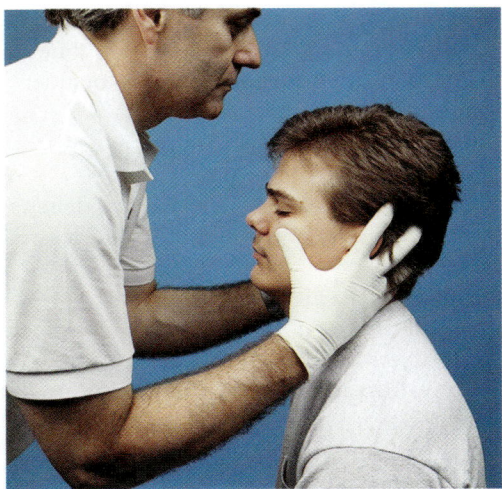

FIGURE 41-11 Manual in-line immobilization from the front.

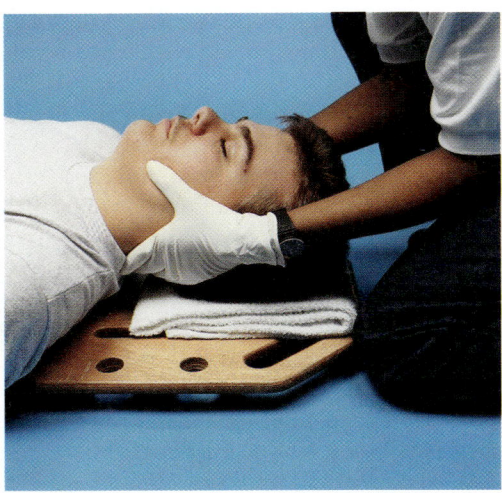

FIGURE 41-12 Manual in-line immobilization with a supine patient.

Manual In-Line Immobilization With a Supine Patient

1. Kneel or lie at the patient's head and place the thumbs of each hand just below the zygomatic arch of each cheek (Figure 41-12).
2. Place the little fingers of each hand on the posterior aspect of the patient's skull.
3. Spread the remaining fingers of each hand on the lateral planes of the head and increase the strength of the grip.
4. Move the head to an in-line position if needed. Maintain this position by bracing the elbows against your torso or ground surface for support.

Logroll With Spinal Precautions. Logrolling methods are used to move patients with a possible spinal injury. Examples include moving patients onto a mechanical immobilization device and turning patients from a prone

to a supine position. Logrolling maneuvers require at least four rescuers for adequate spinal protection. The position of the patient's arms during a logrolling maneuver may affect thoracic-lumbar motion and further compromise the stability of the spine. One method that may minimize lateral motion and help to maintain neutral alignment of the pelvis and legs is to position the patient with arms extended at the side. The patient's palms should be on the lateral thighs.

Logroll of the Supine Patient. The following steps should be used for logrolling of patients in the supine position (Figure 41-13).

1. Rescuer 1 should be positioned at the patient's head. Rescuer 1 should provide in-line manual stabilization. Another rescuer should apply a rigid cervical collar and place a long spine board at the patient's side. (If a spinal injury with paralysis is obvious or if shock is suspected, the pneumatic antishock garment should be prepared on the spine board per protocol.)
2. Rescuers 2 and 3 should be positioned at the patient's midthorax and knees. The patient's arms should be extended at the sides, palms on lateral thighs. The legs should be brought together for neutral alignment.
3. Rescuer 2 grasps the far side of the patient at the shoulder and wrist. Rescuer 3 grasps the hips (just distal of the wrists) and both lower extremities at the ankles.
4. In one organized move, the rescuers slowly logroll the patient onto his or her side. At the same time, they slide the spine board under the patient. In-line support of the patient's head must be maintained. This is done by rotating the head exactly with the torso to avoid flexion or hyperextension. In addition, the ankles must be elevated slightly to maintain lateral and anterior-posterior alignment.
5. Rescuer 4 positions the long spine board by placing the device flat on the ground or at a 30- to 40-degree angle against the patient's back.
6. In one organized move, the rescuers slowly logroll and center the patient on the long spine board.

Logroll of the Prone Patient. The basic principles used in logrolling supine patients can be applied to a patient who is in a prone or semiprone position. The procedure uses the same initial alignment of the patient's arms and legs. The rescuers have the same responsibilities for maintaining alignment. There are two major differences in this logroll maneuver. These are Rescuer 1's hand position during the logroll and the application of the rigid cervical collar, which can be applied only after the patient is in a supine position (Figure 41-14).

1. Rescuer 1 places his or her hands in a position that provides in-line stabilization and that accommodates rotation of the patient with the torso.
2. In one organized move, the rescuers rotate the patient away from the direction of the initial prone position.
3. A rescuer places the long spine board on a flat surface or positions it between the patient's back and the rescuers at the patient's side.

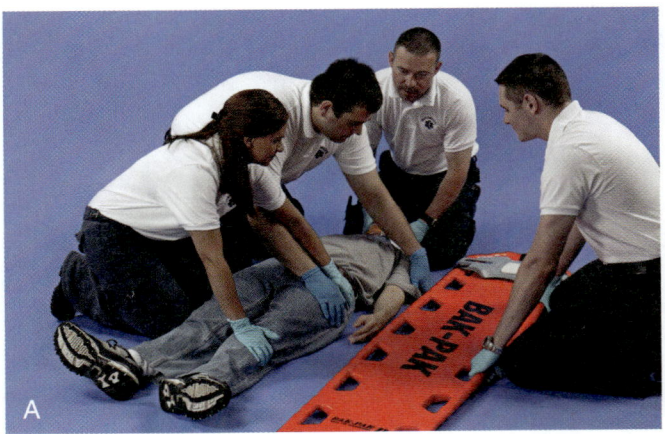

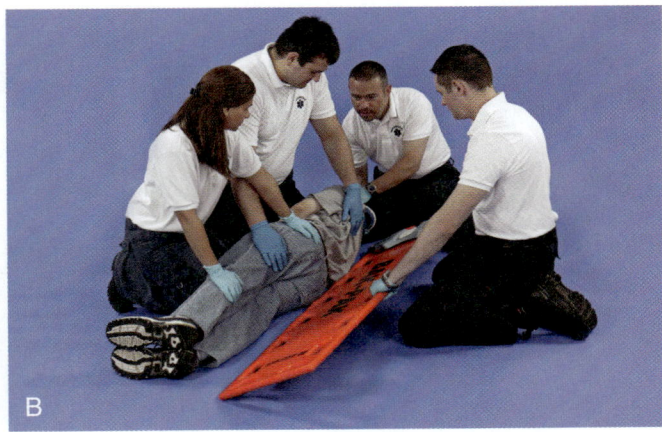

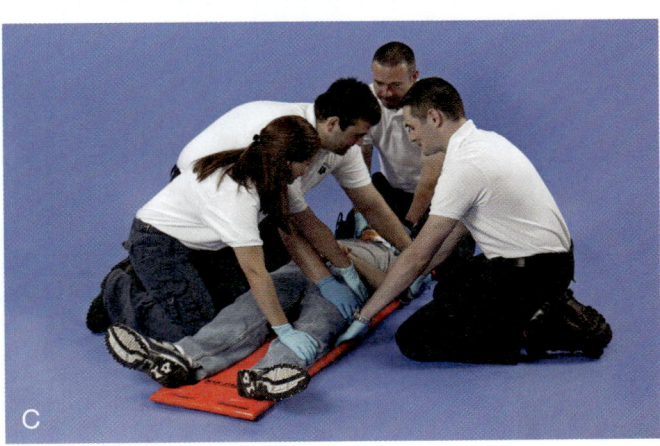

FIGURE 41-13 A, To logroll a supine patient, Rescuer 1 is positioned at the patient's head, providing in-line manual stabilization. Rescuers 2 and 3 are positioned at the patient's midthorax and knees. **B,** While maintaining immobilization, the rescuers slowly logroll the patient onto his or her side perpendicular to the ground in one organized move. Rescuer 4 positions the long spine board by placing the device flat on the ground or at a 30- to 40-degree angle against the patient's back. **C,** In one organized move the rescuers slowly logroll and center the patient onto the long spine board.

4. In one organized move, the rescuers slowly logroll and center the patient on the long spine board.
5. A rescuer applies a rigid cervical collar.

MECHANICAL DEVICES

Spinal immobilization equipment covered includes rigid cervical collars, short spine boards, and long spine boards. This text presents only general principles of spinal immobilization by mechanical devices. The specific methods of application vary by device. Paramedics should become familiar with the equipment used in their locale. They also should follow the application guidelines of the manufacturer.

Rigid Cervical Collars. Rigid cervical collars are designed to protect the cervical spine from compression. These devices may reduce movement and some range of motion of the head. However, they do not by themselves provide adequate immobilization of the spine. These devices must always be used along with manual in-line stabilization or immobilization by a suitable device (e.g., vest, short spine board, or long spine board). An effective rigid collar sits on the chest, posterior thoracic spine and clavicle, and trapezius muscles where tissue movement is at a minimum.[4] The

collar also must be correctly sized for the patient. To apply a rigid cervical collar, the paramedic should follow these general steps, which demonstrate the application of the Stifneck™ collar (Figure 41-15):

1. Rescuer 1 applies manual in-line immobilization from behind the patient and maintains this position throughout the procedure.
2. Rescuer 2 properly angles the collar for placement.
3. Rescuer 2 positions the collar bottom.
4. Rescuer 2 sets the collar in place around the patient's neck.
5. Rescuer 2 secures the collar with the Velcro straps.
6. Rescuer 1 spreads his or her fingers and maintains support until the patient is secured to a short or long spine board.

Rigid cervical collars are available in a number of sizes (or they are adjustable). They can accommodate the range of physical characteristics of patients. Choosing the proper size reduces flexion or hyperextension of the neck. These movements may occur during patient extrication and packaging. These movements also may result from acceleration and deceleration forces that normally occur during patient transport. The following guidelines apply to the use of rigid cervical collars[4]:

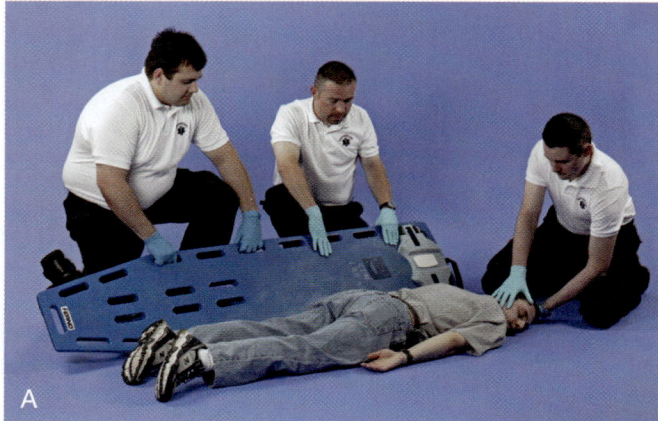
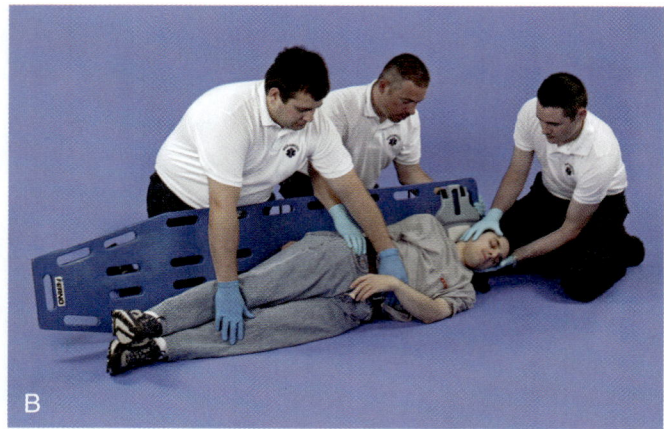
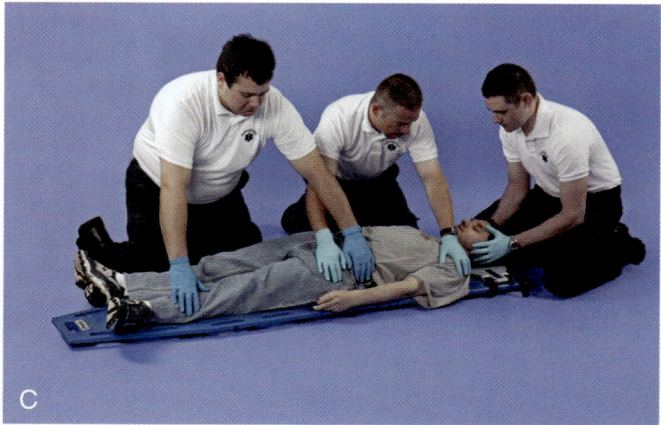
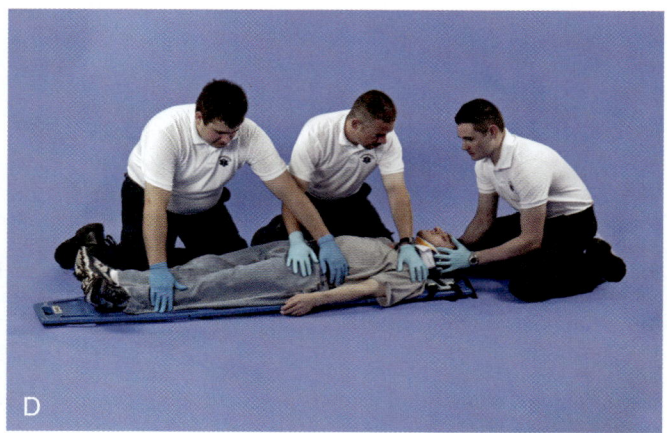

FIGURE 41-14 A, Rescuer 1 places his or her hands in a position that provides in-line stabilization and that accommodates the rotation of the patient with the torso. Rescuer 2 positions the long spine board. **B,** In one organized move the rescuers rotate the patient away from the direction of his or her initial prone position. **C,** In one organized move the rescuers slowly logroll and center the patient onto the long spine board. **D,** Another rescuer then applies a rigid cervical collar.

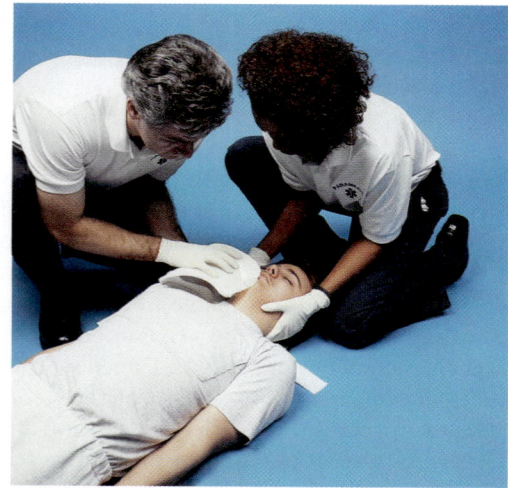

FIGURE 41-15 Rescuer 2 positions the collar and secures it with Velcro straps.

- They do not adequately immobilize by their use alone.
- They must be properly sized to the patient.
- They must not inhibit the patient's ability to open the mouth or the paramedic's ability to open the patient's mouth if vomiting occurs.
- They must not obstruct or hinder ventilation in any way.

Short Spine Boards. Short spine boards or other short spine extrication devices are used to splint the cervical and thoracic spine. These devices vary in design. They are available from a number of manufacturers. In general, short spine boards are used to provide spinal immobilization when the patient is sitting or is in a confined space. After short spine board immobilization, the patient is moved to a long spine board device for complete spinal immobilization. Examples of short spine boards include the plastic or synthetic half backboard, the Kendrick extrication device, the Oregon Spine Splint II, and the Hare extrication device. General principles of short spine board application,

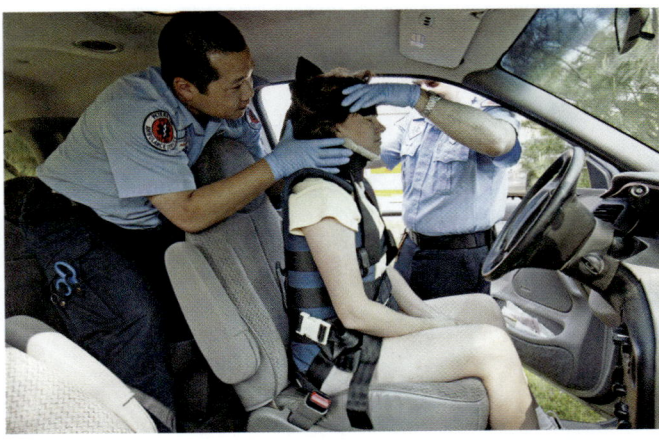

FIGURE 41-16 Application of the Kendrick extrication device.

demonstrated with the Kendrick extrication device, are as follows (Figure 41-16):

CRITICAL THINKING

When would the use of the short board *not* be indicated for spinal column immobilization?

1. After manual in-line immobilization and the application of a rigid cervical collar, place the short spine board device behind the patient. The board should be positioned snugly beneath the patient's axillae; this will prevent it from moving up the torso.
2. Immobilize the upper and middle torso by fastening the chest straps, starting with the middle chest straps and followed by the lower chest straps. The upper chest strap (if used) should not be so tight that it impedes patient ventilation.[4] The middle and lower straps should be snug so that fingers cannot be slipped beneath the straps. Readjust as needed.
3. Position and fasten each groin strap separately, forming a loop. These straps prevent the Kendrick extrication device from moving up and the lower end from moving laterally.
4. Pad the device as needed and secure the head to the short spine board.
5. Carefully move the patient as a unit to a long spine board by rotating the patient and Kendrick extrication device onto the board. Hold the legs proximal to the knees and lift them during the transition.
6. Center the patient on the long spine board, release the leg straps, and slowly lower the patient's legs to an in-line position.
7. Secure the patient and Kendrick extrication device to the long spine board, maintaining a neutral in-line position with the long axis of the body. Then slightly loosen the Kendrick extrication device leg straps.

NOTE

The use of a short spine board should be considered only if the patient's condition allows. If the patient is unstable because of life-threatening injury or the need for immediate resuscitation or if the time required to apply the device would jeopardize the patient's life (e.g., a patient with a carotid pulse, but absent radial pulse), the patient's head and neck should be stabilized with manual, in-line support, and the patient should be moved as a unit to a long spine board.

RAPID EXTRICATION

The steps required for rapid extrication may vary depending on the size and make of the vehicle. They also may vary based on the patient's location inside the vehicle. A general description of the steps required for rapid extrication are listed:

Three or More Rescuers (Figure 41-17)

1. Rescuer 1 supports the patient's head and neck. Rescuer 1 uses manual in-line stabilization from behind the patient or from the patient's side. Rescuer 1 maintains this stabilization throughout the extrication process.
2. After a rapid initial assessment, Rescuer 2 applies a rigid cervical collar and positions a long spine board near the vehicle.
3. Rescuer 3 manually stabilizes and controls movement of the patient's upper and lower torso and legs during extrication.
4. The rescuers then rotate the patient in a series of short, controlled movements so that the patient's back faces the open doorway. Rescuer 2 exits the vehicle. Rescuer 2 assumes control of manual stabilization from outside the vehicle. Rescuer 1 assumes control of the patient's lower torso and legs. Each movement during the rotation of the patient should be coordinated, stopping so that the rescuers and the patient can be repositioned as needed to limit unwanted patient movement.
5. A rescuer should insert the foot end of the long spine board on the car seat at the patient's buttocks and should position the head end on the ambulance stretcher. Rotation of the patient continues until the patient can be positioned onto the long spine board.
6. The rescuers center and secure the patient on the long spine board as described later.

Two Rescuers (Figure 41-18)

1. Rescuer 1 supports the patient's head and neck. Rescuer 1 uses manual in-line stabilization from behind the patient or from the patient's side. Rescuer 1 maintains this stabilization throughout the extrication process.
2. After a rapid initial assessment, Rescuer 2 applies a rigid cervical collar and places a prerolled blanket around the patient. Rescuer 2 places the center of the blanket roll at the patient's midline on the rigid

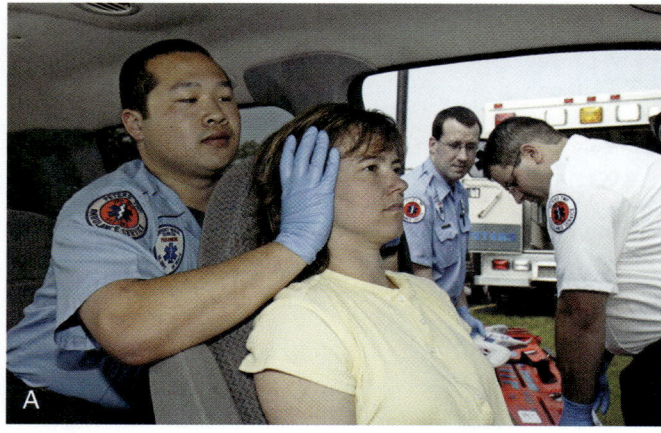
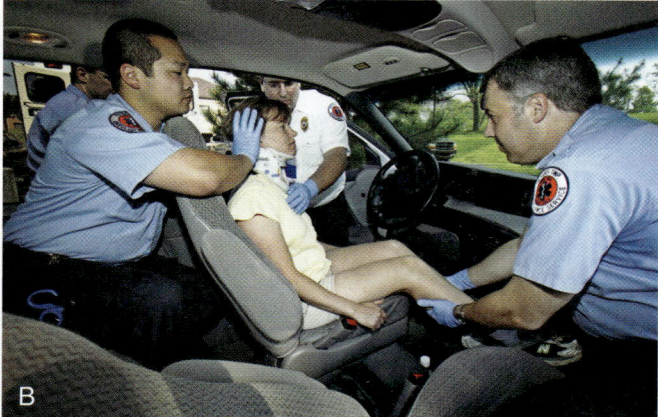
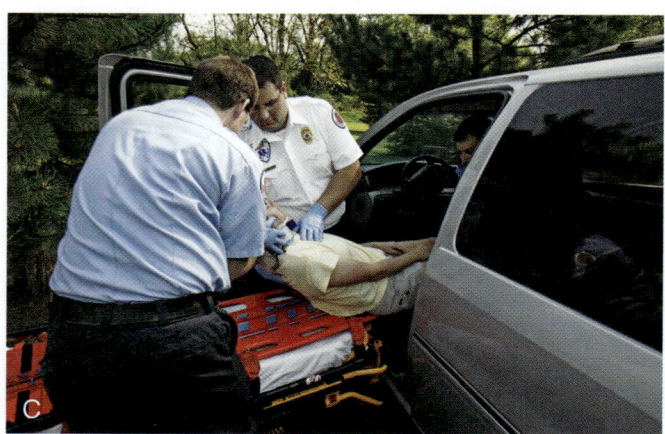
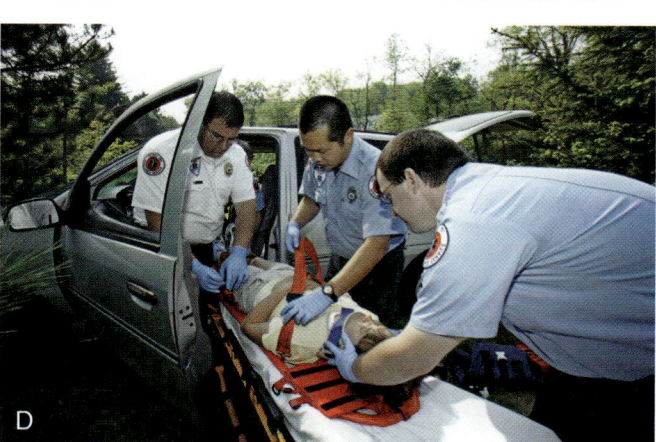

FIGURE 41-17 **A,** Rescuer 1 supports the patient's head and neck and uses manual in-line stabilization throughout the procedure. **B,** After a rapid primary assessment, Rescuer 2 helps support the patient's midthorax while Rescuer 3 frees the patient's lower extremities for extrication. **C,** The rescuers carefully lower the patient onto the long spine board. **D,** The rescuers center and secure the patient on the long spine board.

cervical collar. Rescuer 2 then wraps the ends of the blanket roll around the cervical collar and places them under the patient's arms. Rescuer 2 positions a long spine board near the vehicle.

3. Using the ends of the blanket roll, the rescuers rotate the patient in a series of short, controlled movements so that the patient's back faces the open doorway. Each movement during the rotation of the patient should be coordinated, stopping so that the rescuers and the patient can be repositioned as needed to limit unwanted patient movement.

4. Rescuer 1 takes control of the blanket ends, moving them under the patient's shoulders, and moves the patient by the blanket while Rescuer 2 controls the patient's lower torso, pelvis, and legs.

5. The rescuers center and secure the patient on the long spine board as described next.

Long Spine Board With Supine Patient. Like short spine boards, long spine boards are available in a variety of configurations. These include plastic and synthetic spine boards, metal alloy spine boards, vacuum mattress splints, and split litters (scoop stretchers) that must be used along with a long spine board. The following description of securing patients on a long spine board may be applied to any long spinal immobilization device.

Immobilization of the torso to a long spine board must be done before immobilization of the head. This will prevent angulation of the cervical spine. The torso must not be allowed to move up, down, or to either side. Straps should be placed at the shoulders or upper chest below the axillae to avoid compression and lateral movement of the thorax, around the midtorso, and across the iliac crest to prevent movement of the lower torso. The paramedic should take care not to tighten the straps to the point of reducing chest wall movement.

After immobilization of the torso, the head and neck should be immobilized in a neutral, in-line position. When most adults are placed on a long or short spinal device, a large space is produced between the back of the head and the spine board. Therefore noncompressible padding (e.g.,

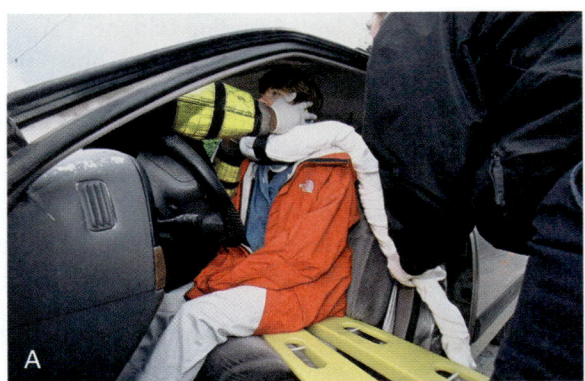
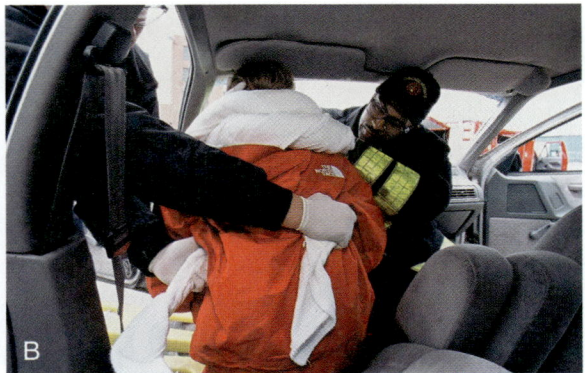
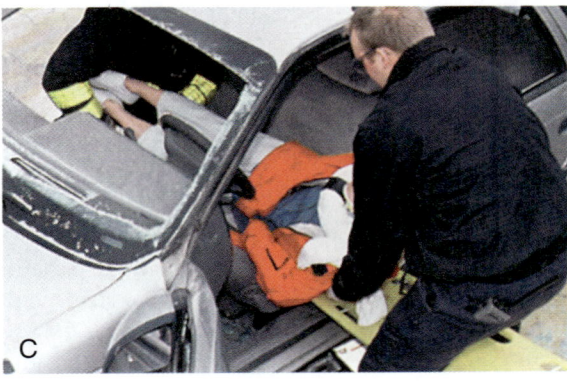

FIGURE 41-18 A, Rescuer 1 supports the patient's head and neck and uses manual in-line stabilization throughout the procedure. **B,** After assessment and application of a cervical collar, a rescuer positions the center of a blanket roll at the patient's midline on the cervical collar. The rescuer wraps the ends of the blanket roll around the cervical collar and places them under the patient's arms. **C,** The rescuers rotate the patient using the ends of the blanket roll until the patient's back faces the open doorway. (From National Association of Emergency Medical Technicians: *PHTLS: prehospital trauma life support,* ed 7, St Louis, 2011, Mosby.)

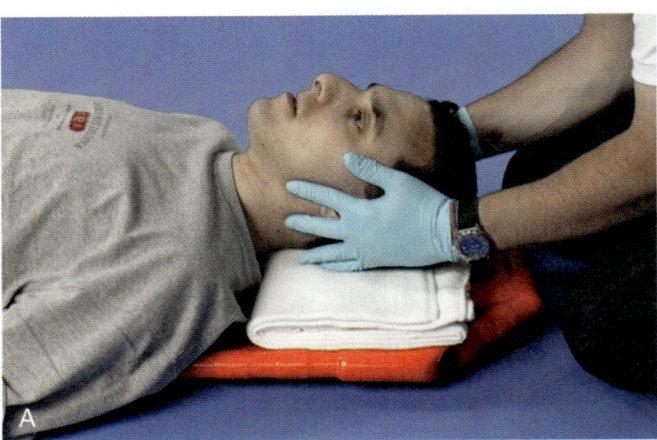
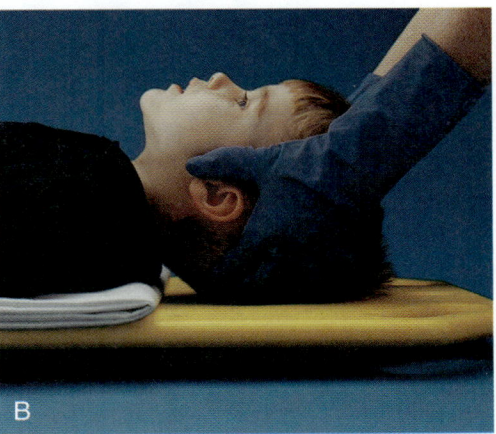

FIGURE 41-19 Padding requirements for adult (A) and pediatric (B) patients.

commercial padding or folded towels) should be added (body shims). This can be done before securing the head (Figure 41-19, *A*). The amount of padding required for in-line immobilization varies by patient and must be evaluated on an individual basis. Too little padding may cause hyperextension of the head, and too much padding may cause flexion; both may increase spinal cord damage. Children have proportionally larger heads than adults and may require padding under the torso to allow the head to lie in a neutral position on the board (Fig. 41-19, *B*). The padding (if needed) should be firm and should extend the full length and width of the torso from the buttocks to the top of the shoulders to prevent movement and misalignment of the spine. In addition to providing enhanced stabilization, padding also improves patient comfort during transport.

The head is secured to the spinal device by placing commercial pads or rolled blankets on both sides of the head and securing them with the included straps, 2- to 3-inch tape strips, or a self-adhering firm wrap (e.g., Coban, Medi-Rip, or Elastoplast). (Elastic or gauze bandages do not prevent movement.) The upper forehead should be secured across the supraorbital ridge. The lower portion of the head should be secured across the anterior portion of the rigid cervical collar. Chinstraps, sandbags, and intravenous bags are considered less optimal in immobilizing the head to a spinal device.

The patient's legs should be secured to the long spine board. Two or more straps can be applied above and below the knees. Towels, blankets, or suitable padding may be placed on both sides of the patient's lower legs. This will minimize movement and will help to maintain the patient's central position on the spinal device (Figure 41-20).

Before moving the patient, the patient's arms should be secured to the spinal device for safety. This is best achieved by placing the patient's arms at his or her side. (The patient's palms should be facing the body.) The arms should be secured with a separate strap placed across the forearms and torso.

Long Spine Board with Standing Patient. Patients who are standing also may be secured to a long spine board using the following technique (Figure 41-21):

1. Rescuer 1 applies manual in-line immobilization from behind the patient or in front of the patient. Rescuer 1 maintains this position throughout the procedure. Rescuer 2 applies a rigid cervical collar.
2. Rescuer 2 slides the long spine board behind the patient from the side and presses it against the patient.
3. Rescuers 2 and 3 stand on either side of the patient and insert the hand that is closest to the patient under the patient's axilla and grasp the nearest handhold of the backboard without moving the patient's shoulders. The rescuers grab the higher handhold on the board with their other hands and lower the patient and backboard to the ground while maintaining manual in-line immobilization.
4. Once on the ground, the rescuers secure the patient to the long backboard as described.

IMMOBILIZING PEDIATRIC PATIENTS

As with adult patients, prehospital care of a pediatric patient with suspected spine trauma should be managed with manual in-line immobilization, a rigid cervical collar, and a long spinal immobilization device. Many different pediatric immobilization devices are available from

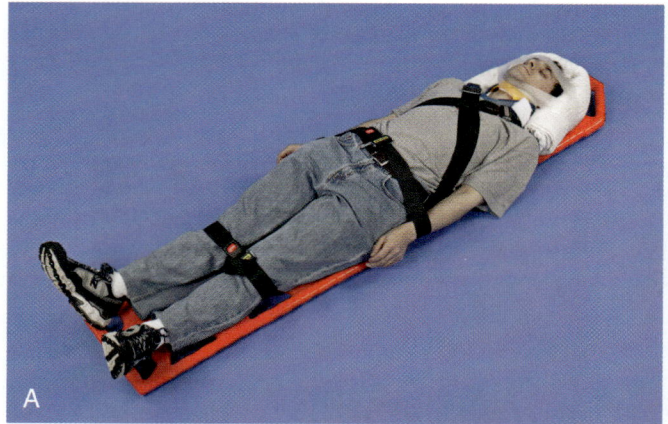

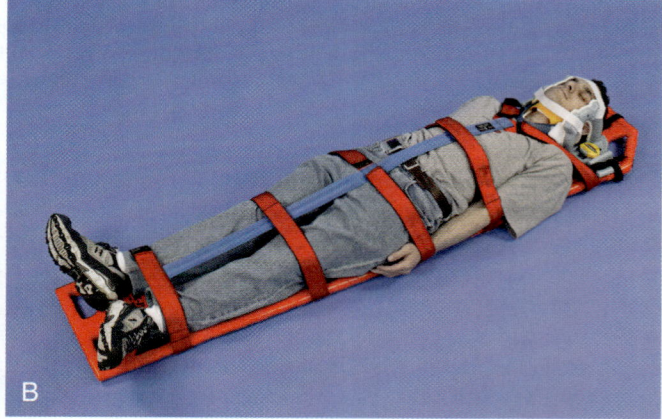

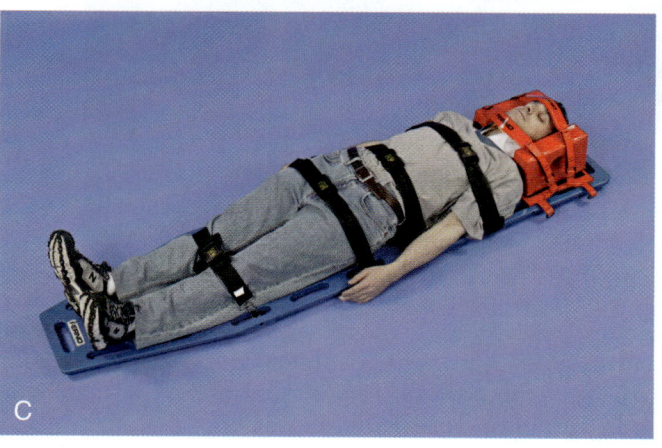

FIGURE 41-20 Long spine board immobilization (supine patient).

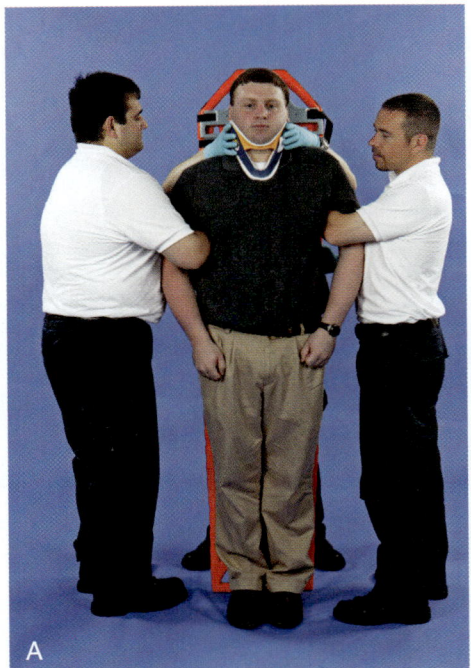 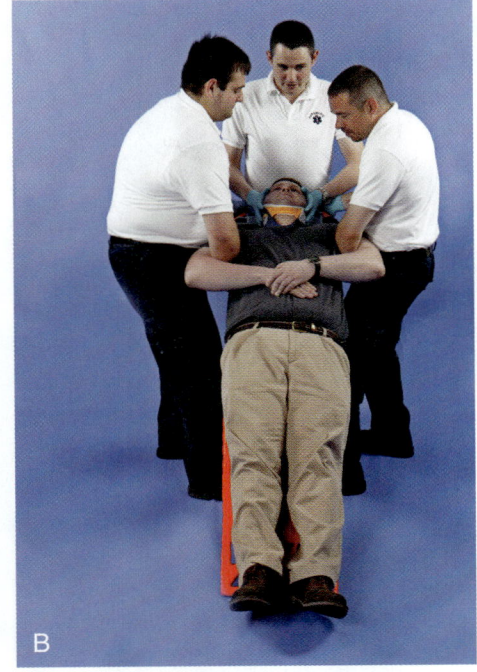

FIGURE 41-21 A, While Rescuer 1 maintains manual in-line stabilization, Rescuers 2 and 3 support the patient. **B,** In one organized move the rescuers lower the patient to the ground onto the long spine board for further immobilization.

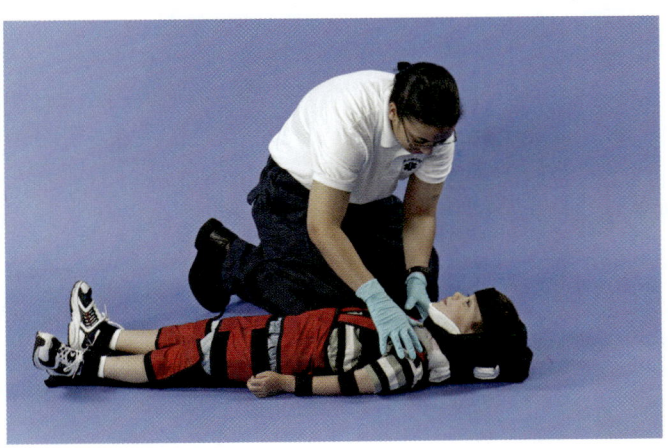

FIGURE 41-22 Infant and pediatric immobilization board.

manufacturers (Figure 41-22). If pediatric immobilization devices are not available, children may be secured on an adult long spine board. (A great deal of padding, however, is needed to fill voids. The padding also helps to prevent movement.)

Helmet Issues

The purpose of helmets is to protect the head and brain. Helmets are not intended to protect the neck. (This leaves the cervical spine open to injury.) The various types of helmets include full-face or open-face designs (used in motorcycling, bicycling, in-line skating, and other activities), and helmets designed for sports such as football and motocross. Factors that the paramedic should consider when determining the need to remove a helmet from an injured patient who requires airway management and spinal immobilization include the following:

- Athletic trainers may have special equipment (and training) to remove face pieces from sports helmets, allowing easier access to the patient's airway.
- Sports garb (e.g., shoulder pads) could compromise the cervical spine further if only the helmet were removed.
- The firm fit of a helmet may provide firm support for the patient's head.

Helmet Removal

Patients who are wearing full-face helmets must have the helmet removed early in the assessment process. Removing the helmet allows the rescuers to assess and manage a patient's airway and ventilatory status completely. In addition, rescuers can look for bleeding. The bleeding may be hidden by the helmet. They also can move the patient's head (from the flexed position caused by large helmets) into neutral alignment. The paramedic should consult with medical direction if the patient complains of increased pain during removal of the helmet or if the helmet is hard to remove in the field. The following steps in full-face helmet removal are recommended by the American College of Surgeons Committee on Trauma[4]:

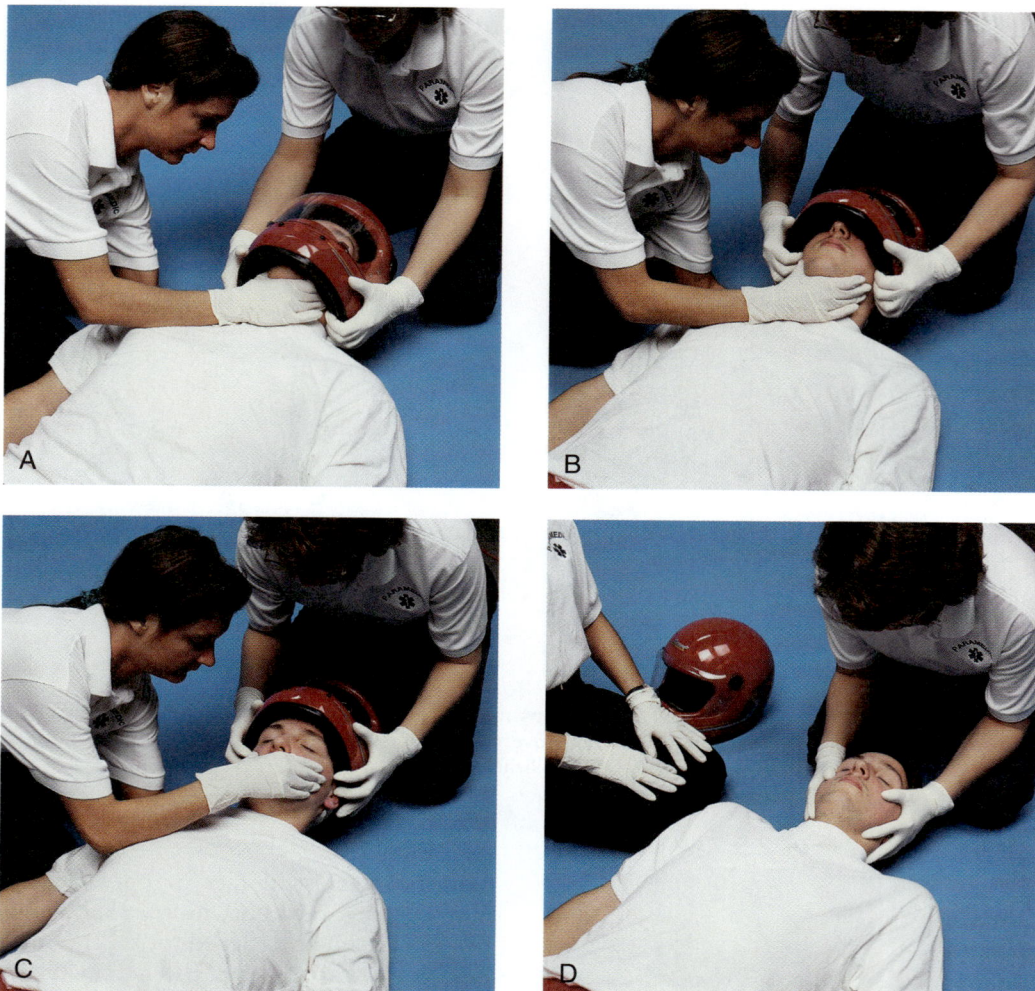

FIGURE 41-23 A, Rescuer 1 immobilizes the helmet and head in an in-line position. Rescuer 2 grasps the patient's mandible by placing the thumb at the angle of the mandible on one side and two fingers at the angle on the other side. Rescuer 2 places the other hand under the patient's neck at the base of the skull, producing in-line immobilization of the patient's head. **B,** Rescuer 1 carefully spreads the sides of the helmet away from the patient's head and ears. **C,** Rescuer 1 then rotates the helmet toward the rescuer to clear the nose and remove it from the patient's head in a straight line. **D,** After the removal of the helmet, Rescuer 1 applies in-line immobilization. Rescuer 2 applies a rigid cervical collar and places padding under the head.

1. Rescuer 1 immobilizes the helmet and head in an in-line position (Figure 41-23). Rescuer 1 presses his or her palms on each side of the helmet with the fingertips curled over the lower margin of the helmet.
2. Rescuer 2 removes the face shield and chinstrap. Rescuer 2 assesses the patient's airway and ventilatory status.
3. Rescuer 2 grasps the patient's mandible by placing the thumb at the angle of the mandible on one side and two fingers at the angle on the other side. Rescuer 2 places his or her other hand under the neck at the base of the skull, taking over in-line immobilization of the patient's head.
4. Rescuer 1 carefully spreads the sides of the helmet away from the patient's head and ears. Rescuer 1 then rotates

the helmet toward the rescuer to clear the patient's nose. Rescuer 1 then removes the helmet from the patient's head in a straight line. Just before removing the helmet from under the patient's head, Rescuer 1 assumes in-line immobilization by squeezing the sides of the helmet against the patient's head.
5. Rescuer 2 repositions his or her hands to support the head and to prevent it from dropping as the helmet is removed completely. This is accomplished by the rescuer placing a hand farther up on the occipital area of the head and by grasping the maxilla with the thumb and first fingers of the other hand on each side of the nose. After securing this position, Rescuer 2 takes over in-line immobilization.

6. Rescuer 1 rotates the helmet about 30 degrees, following the curvature of the patient's head. Rescuer 1 completely removes the helmet by carefully pulling it in a straight line.

7. After removal of the helmet, Rescuer 1 applies in-line immobilization, and Rescuer 2 applies a rigid cervical collar.

> ### NOTE
> A key point to remember during helmet removal is that in-line immobilization must be maintained throughout the procedure. Thus the rescuers should never remove their hands from the patient at the same time. In addition, the helmet must be rotated in one direction to clear the nose. The helmet must be rotated in the opposite direction to clear the back of the patient's head.

Spinal Immobilization in Diving Incidents

Most diving incidents involve injury to the patient's head, neck, and spine. If the patient is still in the water when EMS arrives, the patient should be managed as follows:

1. Ensure scene and personal safety. Only rescuers trained in water rescue should enter the water (Figure 41-24).

2. Float a supine patient to a shallow area without unnecessary movement of the spine.

3. Approach a prone patient from the top of the head. Position one arm under the patient to support the head, neck, and torso. Place the other arm across the patient's head and back, splinting the head and neck between the rescuer's arms. Carefully turn the patient to a supine position and quickly assess airway and breathing. (The

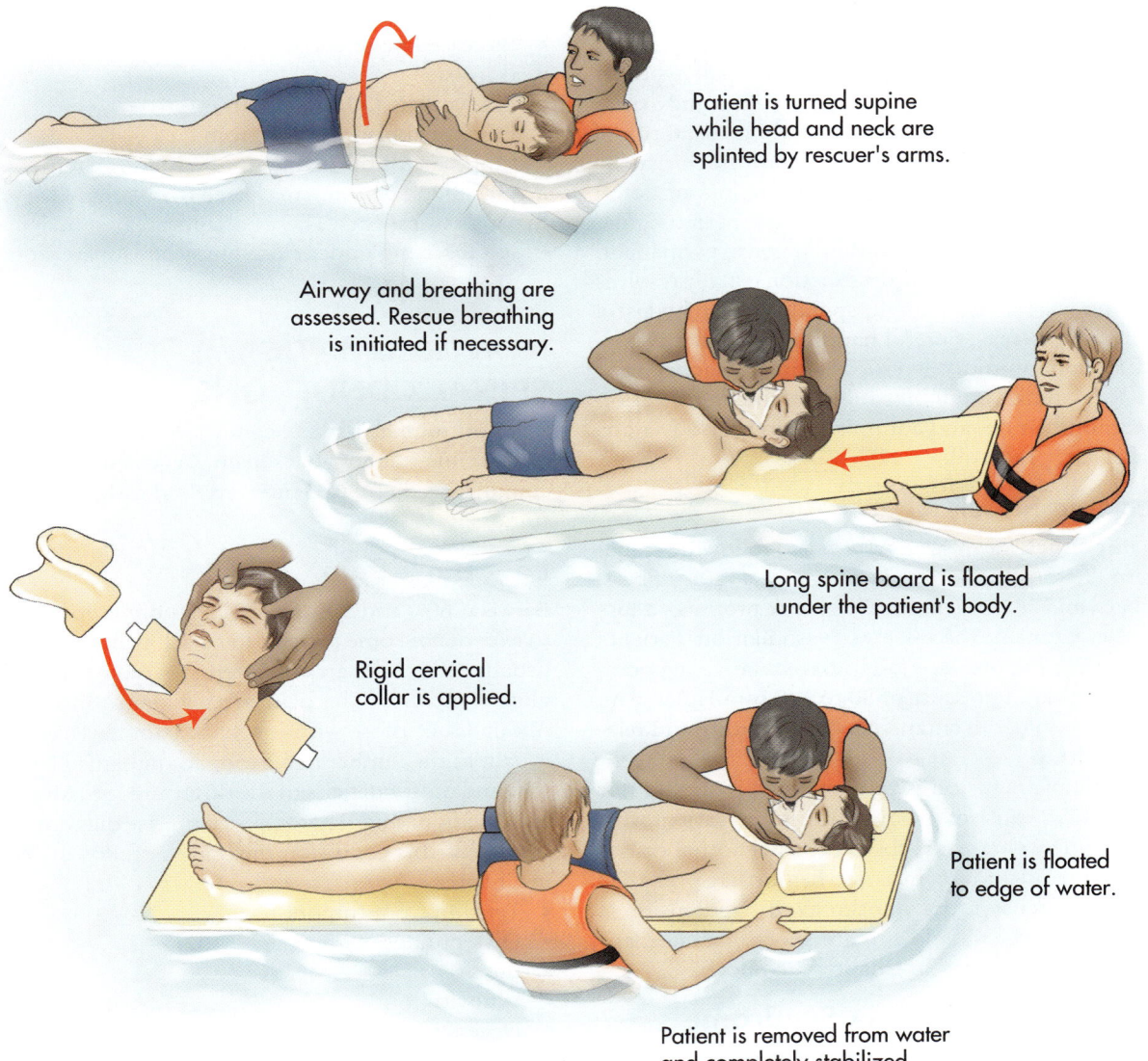

Patient is turned supine while head and neck are splinted by rescuer's arms.

Airway and breathing are assessed. Rescue breathing is initiated if necessary.

Long spine board is floated under the patient's body.

Rigid cervical collar is applied.

Patient is floated to edge of water.

Patient is removed from water and completely stabilized.

FIGURE 41-24 Extrication of a diving accident victim. Rescue breathing with barrier protection can begin in the water.

paramedic may initiate rescue breathing while in the water.[10])

4. A second rescuer slides a long spine board or other rigid device under the patient's body while the first rescuer continues to support the patient's head and neck without flexion or extension. Apply a rigid cervical collar. Maintain manual in-line immobilization throughout the rescue.
5. Float the spinal immobilization device to the edge of the water and lift it out.
6. The patient should be immobilized completely on the long spine board as previously described.

CORD INJURY PRESENTATIONS

Three cord injury presentations deserve special mention. These include spinal shock, neurogenic hypotension, and autonomic hyperreflexia syndrome.

Spinal Shock

Spinal shock refers to a temporary loss of all types of spinal cord function distal to the injury. Signs and symptoms of spinal shock include flaccid paralysis distal to the injury site and loss of autonomic function, which may be demonstrated by hypotension, vasodilation, loss of bowel and bladder control, priapism, and loss of thermoregulation. Spinal shock does not always involve permanent, primary injury. The autonomic dysfunction usually resolves within 24 hours. Rarely, though, spinal shock may last a few days to a few weeks. Careful handling of these patients to avoid secondary injury is crucial. Initial management includes full spinal immobilization, high-concentration oxygen administration, and administration of intravenous crystalloids (per protocol).

Neurogenic Shock

Neurogenic shock (*neurogenic hypotension*) following spinal shock results from the blockade of vasoregulatory fibers, motor fibers, and sensory fibers. This block produces a loss of sympathetic tone to the vessels or vasodilation. Patients with neurogenic hypotension often have relative hypotension (a systolic blood pressure of 80 to 100 mm Hg); warm, dry, and pink skin (from cutaneous vasodilation); and relative bradycardia.

Neurogenic hypotension is rare. Initially, it should not be considered as a cause of hypovolemia in the patient with a spine injury. The paramedic should consider other causes of hypotension, including internal hemorrhage, cardiac tamponade, and tension pneumothorax. If hypotension is severe, the paramedic should initiate shock management (per protocol), as described in Chapter 36: Shock.

Autonomic Hyperreflexia Syndrome

Autonomic hyperreflexia syndrome may occur after resolution of spinal shock and is associated with chronic SCI in patients who have injuries at T6 or above.[5] (The syndrome often is caused by a distended bladder or rectum.) The effects of this syndrome result from a massive, uncompensated cardiovascular response that stimulates the sympathetic nervous system. The stimulation of sensory receptors below the level of cord injury causes the intact autonomic nervous system to respond with spasms of the arterioles. These spasms in turn increase blood pressure. The baroreceptors sense the rise in blood pressure. They stimulate the parasympathetic nervous system. This decreases heart rate and sends the message to the peripheral and visceral vessels to dilate. Because of the cord injury, however, vasodilation is not possible. Thus blood pressure continues to rise and could pose a threat to life. The characteristics of this syndrome include the following:

- Paroxysmal hypertension (up to 300 mm Hg)
- Pounding headache
- Blurred vision
- Sweating (above the level of injury) with flushing of the skin
- Increased nasal congestion
- Nausea
- Bradycardia (30 to 40 beats/min)
- Distended bladder or rectum

Emptying of the bladder or bowel often relieves the syndrome. Blood pressure may need to be controlled with antihypertensive agents. These patients are best managed in the hospital setting under close physician supervision.

NONTRAUMATIC SPINAL CONDITIONS

The nontraumatic spinal conditions to be discussed in this chapter include low back pain, degenerative disk disease, spondylosis, herniated intervertebral disk, and spinal cord tumors.

Low Back Pain

Between 60% and 90% of the U.S. population is estimated to experience some form of low back pain.[11] Low back pain usually affects the area between the lower rib cage and the gluteal muscles. The pain often radiates into the thighs. About 1% of those with low back pain have sciatica. (This is pain in the lumbar nerve root accompanied by neurosensory and motor deficits in the thigh and leg.) Most low back pain is idiopathic. That makes a precise diagnosis difficult. Causes of this condition include the following (described in Chapter 33):

- Tension from tumors
- Disk prolapse
- Bursitis
- Synovitis
- Degenerative joint disease
- Abnormal bone pressure
- Inflammation caused by infection (e.g., osteomyelitis)
- Fractures
- Ligament strains

CRITICAL THINKING

What are some other medical conditions that may cause the patient to have a chief complaint of low back pain?

Risk factors associated with low back pain include occupations that require repetitive lifting or exposure to vibrations from vehicles or industrial machinery and also osteoporosis (elderly women report more symptoms than men).

Low back pain must come from innervated structures. However, deep pain and the way it is referred to other parts of the body vary by individual. Although the disk has no specific innervation, irritation of surrounding membranes that have pain receptors often develops. (This occurs especially in the presence of disk prolapse.) The source of most low back pain is at L3, L4, L5, and S1. Other areas of abundant pain receptors are found in anterior and posterior longitudinal ligaments that are vulnerable to strains and sprains.

Degenerative Disk Disease

Degenerative disk disease is a common finding in persons older than 50 years of age. The causes of this condition include deterioration of the tissue of the intervertebral disk that occurs with aging. The associated narrowing of the disk results in instability of the spine and can cause occasional low back pain.

Spondylosis

Spondylosis is a structural defect of the spine. It involves the lamina or vertebral arch. Spondylosis usually occurs in the lumbar spine between superior and inferior articulating surfaces. (Rotational stress fractures are common at the affected site.) Heredity appears to be a key factor for this condition.

Herniated Intervertebral Disk

Herniated intervertebral disk (*herniated nucleus pulposus*) refers to a tear in the posterior rim of the capsule that encloses the gelatinous center of the disk. Rupture of the disk usually is caused by trauma, degenerative disk disease, and improper lifting (most common). Men between the ages of 30 and 50 are more prone to develop this condition. Disks that most commonly are affected are L5-S1 and L4-L5. (Herniated intervertebral disk also at times occurs in the cervical area at C5-C6 and C6-C7.) These injuries may have an immediate onset. They also may develop over months to years.

Spinal Cord Tumors

Tumors in the spinal cord may develop from cord compression, from degenerative changes in bones and joints, or from an interruption in the blood supply to the cord. These tumors are classified by cell type, growth rate, and structure of origin. Clinical manifestations depend on tumor type and location. The manifestations may include bilateral or asymmetrical motor dysfunction, paresis, spasticity, pain, temperature dysfunction, sensory changes, and other abnormalities.

ASSESSMENT AND MANAGEMENT OF NONTRAUMATIC SPINAL CONDITIONS

As stated before, nontraumatic spinal conditions such as low back pain are difficult to diagnose. The assessment and management are based on the patient's chief complaint, the physical examination, and the evaluation of associated risk factors. Signs and symptoms that commonly are seen with nontraumatic spinal conditions include the following:

- Discomfort
- Difficulty in standing erect
- Pain with straining (e.g., coughing, sneezing)
- Limited range of motion
- Alterations in sensation, pain, and temperature
- Upper extremity pain or paresthesia that increases with motion
- Motor weakness

The management of patients with back pain in the prehospital setting mainly is supportive. Management focuses on decreasing the patient's pain and discomfort. Some patients are best managed with immobilization on a full spine board or vacuum-type stretcher. These devices prevent movement. Full spinal immobilization is not required unless the condition is a result of trauma. The in-hospital evaluation may include various testing such as computed tomography, electromyelography, and magnetic resonance imaging.

SUMMARY

- Most SCIs are the result of motor vehicle crashes. Other causes are falls, penetrating injuries from acts of human violence, and sport injuries.
- The spinal column is composed of 33 vertebrae. These are divided into five sections. The sections are 7 cervical,

12 thoracic, 5 lumbar, 5 sacral (fused), and 4 coccygeal (fused).
- The paramedic can classify the MOI as positive, negative, or uncertain. This classification is combined with the clinical guidelines for evaluating SCI, which include

Continued

the following signs and symptoms: pain, tenderness, painful movement, deformity, cuts/bruises over spinal area, paralysis, paresthesias, and weakness. This system can help to identify cases in which spinal immobilization is appropriate.

- The specific mechanisms of injury that frequently cause spinal trauma are axial loading; extremes of flexion, hyperextension, or hyperrotation; excessive lateral bending; and distraction.

- Spinal injuries may be classified as sprains and strains, fractures and dislocations, sacral and coccygeal fractures, and cord injuries. The spinal cord may sustain a primary or a secondary injury. Lesions (transections) of the spinal cord are classified as complete or incomplete.

- With spinal injuries, the first priority is to evaluate and manage any threats to life. The second priority is to preserve spinal cord function. This includes avoiding secondary injury to the spinal cord. These goals are best met by maintaining a high degree of suspicion for the presence of spinal trauma, by providing early spinal immobilization, by rapidly correcting any volume deficit, and by administering oxygen.

- General principles of spinal immobilization include prevention of further injury; treating the spine as a long bone with a joint at either end (the head and pelvis); always using complete spinal immobilization; beginning spinal immobilization in the initial assessment and maintaining it until the spine is immobilized completely on the long spine board; and placing the patient's head in a neutral, in-line position, unless contraindicated.

- Spinal shock refers to a temporary loss of all types of spinal cord function distal to the injury.

- Neurogenic shock produces a loss of sympathetic tone to the vessels. This causes relative hypotension; warm, dry, and pink skin; and relative bradycardia.

- Autonomic hyperreflexia syndrome results from a massive, uncompensated cardiovascular response that stimulates the sympathetic nervous system. This response in turn causes an increase in blood pressure and other symptoms.

REFERENCES

1. Spinal Cord Injury: *Facts & figures at a glance 2009, National Spinal Cord Injury Statistical Center,* www.nscisc.uab.edu/public_content/facts_figures_2009.aspx, accessed 10-7-10.
2. National Spinal Cord Injury Association Resource Center: *Spinal cord injury statistics,* www.makoa.org/nscia/fact02.html, accessed 10-17-10.
3. Rosen P, Barkin R: *Emergency medicine: concepts and clinical practice,* ed 6, St Louis, 2006, Mosby.
4. National Association of Emergency Medical Technicians: *PHTLS: prehospital trauma life support,* ed 6, St Louis, 2006, Mosby.
5. U.S. Department of Transportation, National Highway Traffic Safety Administration: *EMT paramedic national standard curriculum,* Washington, DC, 1998, The Department.
6. Wolfson AB, Hendey GW, Ling LJ, et al, editors: *Harwood-Nuss' clinical practice of emergency medicine,* ed 5, Philadelphia, 2010, Lippincott Williams & Wilkins.
7. McKinley W, Silver TM, Santos KG, et al: *Functional outcomes per level of spinal cord injury,* Feb 11, 2008, http://emedicine.medscape.com/article/322604-overview, accessed 10-7-10.
8. National Institute of Neurological Disorders and Stroke: *Spinal cord injury: emerging concepts,* www.ninds.nih.gov/news_and_events/proceedings/sci_report.htm, accessed 10-7-10.
9. Clark C, editor: *The cervical spine,* ed 4, Philadelphia, 2005, Lippincott Williams & Wilkins.
10. American Heart Association: *2010 American Heart Association guidelines for cardiopulmonary resuscitation and emergency cardiovascular care science,* vol 122, issue 18, suppl 3, Nov 2, 2010.
11. McCance K, Huether S: *Pathophysiology: the biological basis for disease in adults and children,* ed 5, St Louis, 2006, Mosby.

SUGGESTED READINGS

Bledsoe BE, Salomone JP For the National Association of EMS Physicians Standards and Clinical Practice Committee: High-dose steroids for acute spinal cord injury in emergency medical services, *PEC* 8(3):313-316, 2004.

Domeier RM, Frederiksen SM, Welch K: Prospective performance assessment of an out-of-hospital protocol for selective spine immobilization using clinical spine clearance criteria, *Ann Emerg Med* 46(2):123-131, 2005.

Domeier RM for The National Association of EMS Physicians Standards and Clinical Practice Committee: Indications for prehospital spinal immobilization, *PEC* 3(3):251-253, 1999.

Stroh G, Braude D: Can an out-of-hospital spinal clearance protocol identify all patients with injuries? An argument for selective immobilization, *Ann Emerg Med* 37(6):609-615, 2001.

CHAPTER

42 Chest Trauma

OBJECTIVES

Upon completion of this chapter, the paramedic student will be able to:

1. Discuss the mechanism of injury associated with chest trauma.
2. Describe the mechanism of injury, signs and symptoms, and management of skeletal injuries to the chest.
3. Describe the mechanism of injury, signs and symptoms, and prehospital management of pulmonary trauma.
4. Describe the mechanism of injury, signs and symptoms, and prehospital management of injuries to the heart and great vessels.
5. Outline the mechanism of injury, signs and symptoms, and prehospital care of the patient with esophageal and tracheobronchial injury and diaphragmatic rupture.

KEY TERMS

atelectasis An abnormal condition characterized by the collapse of lung tissue, which prevents the respiratory exchange of oxygen and carbon dioxide.

Beck's triad A combination of three symptoms that characterize cardiac tamponade: elevated central venous pressure, muffled heart sounds, and hypotension.

closed pneumothorax A collection of air or gas in the pleural space that causes the lung to collapse without exposing the pleural space to atmospheric pressure.

commotio cordis Sudden death that follows a blow to the chest.

costochondral separation Separation of the costochondral cartilages.

crepitus A grating sound associated with rubbing of bone fragments.

diaphragmatic rupture Traumatic rupture of the diaphragm that results from sudden compression of the abdomen.

electrical alternans Refers to a change in the amplitude of a patient's ECG waveforms that decrease with every other cardiac cycle; it is a rare finding in cardiac tamponade.

flail chest A chest wall injury in which three or more adjacent ribs are fractured in two or more places.

hemopneumothorax A collection of air and blood in the pleural space; also known as a *pneumohemothorax*.

hemothorax The accumulation of blood and other fluids in the pleural space caused by bleeding from the lung parenchyma or damaged vessels.

jugular notch The superior margin of the manubrium; it is palpated easily at the anterior base of the neck; also known as the *suprasternal notch*.

manubrium One of the three bones of the sternum; it has a broad, quadrangular shape that narrows caudally at its articulation with the superior end of the body of the sternum.

mediastinal shift A shift in a patient's mediastinum that moves tissue and organs within the chest cavity to one side.

myocardial rupture Traumatic rupture of the myocardium that occurs when blood-filled chambers of the ventricles are compressed with enough force to rupture the chamber wall, septum, or valve.

open pneumothorax A chest wall injury that exposes the pleural space to atmospheric pressure.

paradoxical motion Contrary movement of an injured segment of the chest wall with inspiration and expiration.

pericardial tamponade Compression of the heart produced by the accumulation of fluid or blood in the pericardial sac.

pulmonary contusion Bruising of the lung tissue that results in rupture of the alveoli and interstitial edema.

pulsus paradoxus An abnormal decrease in systolic blood pressure that drops more than 10 to 15 mm Hg during inspiration compared with expiration.

sternal angle The point at which the manubrium joins the body of the sternum; also known as the *angle of Louis*.

sternal fracture Fracture of the sternum.

sternoclavicular joint The double gliding joint between the sternum and the clavicle.

tension pneumothorax An accumulation of air or gas in the pleural cavity that can lead to collapse of the lung.

tracheal deviation Movement of the trachea from its midline position to the right or left.

traumatic aortic rupture Rupture of the aorta that is thought to be a result of shearing forces.

traumatic asphyxia A severe crushing injury to the chest and abdomen that causes an increase in the intrathoracic pressure. The increased pressure forces blood from the right side of the heart into the veins of the upper thorax, neck, and face.

---

*C*hest injuries are directly responsible for more than 20% of all traumatic deaths (regardless of mechanism) and account for about 16,000 deaths per year in the United States.[1] Chest injuries are caused by blunt trauma, penetrating trauma, or both.[2] They often are the result of motor vehicle crashes, falls from heights, blast injuries, blows to the chest, chest compression, gunshot wounds, and stab wounds. Thoracic trauma may be classified as skeletal injury, pulmonary injury, heart and great vessel injury, and diaphragmatic injury. (Anterior neck trauma is presented in Chapter 40.)

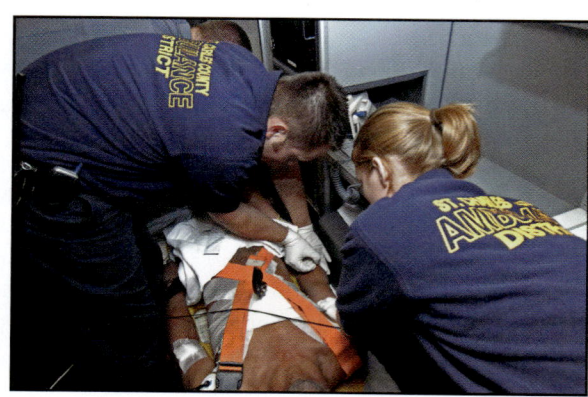

(Courtesy Ray Kemp, St. Charles, Mo.)

SKELETAL INJURIES

Skeletal injuries may be caused by blunt and/or penetrating trauma. The injuries discussed in this chapter include clavicular fractures, rib fractures, flail chest, and sternal fractures. Chest anatomy was presented in Chapter 10. To review, the thoracic cage protects vital organs within the chest. It also prevents the collapse of the thorax during respiration. The skeletal components of the thoracic cage include the 12 thoracic vertebrae, 12 ribs (with their associated costal cartilages), and the sternum. The superior 7 ribs (the *true ribs*) are attached by cartilage to the sternum. The inferior 5 ribs (the *false ribs*) articulate with the vertebrae, but do not attach directly to the sternum. Ribs 8, 9, and 10 are joined to a common cartilage, which is attached to the sternum. Ribs 11 and 12 are "floating ribs." These ribs have no attachment to the sternum.

The sternum has three parts: the **manubrium,** the *body,* and the **xiphoid process.** The **jugular notch** is located at the superior end of the manubrium. The manubrium joins the body of the sternum at the **sternal angle.** (The sternal angle is also known as the *angle of Louis*.) The **clavicles** are part of the appendicular skeleton. They attach the upper limbs to the axial skeleton. This attachment is made at the **sternoclavicular joint** between the clavicles and the sternum (Figure 42-1).

LOOK AGAIN

See Chapter 10: Review of Human Systems, pp. 158-162.

Clavicular Fractures

The clavicle accounts for 5% of all fractures and is the most frequently fractured bone in children.[1] An isolated clavicular fracture is seldom a significant injury (Figure 42-2). It is common in children who fall on their shoulders or outstretched arms. It also is common in athletes involved in contact sports. Treatment usually involves applying a clavicle strap or a sling and swathe that immobilizes the affected shoulder and arm (see Chapter 44). These injuries usually heal well within 4 to 6 weeks.

Signs and symptoms of clavicular fractures include pain, point tenderness, and evident deformity. A rare complication that may be associated with a clavicular fracture is injury to the subclavian vein or artery. Vascular injury can occur when bony fragments from the fracture puncture a vessel, resulting in a hematoma or venous thrombosis.

Rib Fractures

Rib fractures most often occur on the lateral aspect of the third through eighth ribs, where the ribs are least protected by musculature (Figure 42-3). Fractures are more likely to occur in adults than in children. This is because younger patients have more resilient cartilage that is not fully calcified. (When blunt forces are applied to the ribs of children, the energy is transmitted to the lung, where pulmonary contusion is a more frequent injury than rib fracture.) Morbidity or mortality from rib fractures depends on the patient's age and the number and location of the fractures.

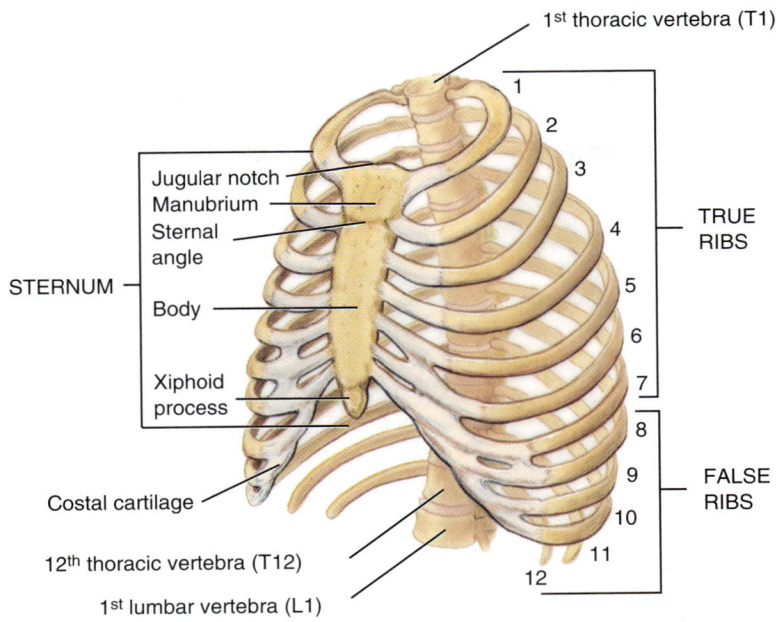

1st thoracic vertebra (T1)

Jugular notch
Manubrium
Sternal angle
STERNUM
Body
Xiphoid process

1
2
3
4
5
6
7

TRUE RIBS

8
9
10
11
12

FALSE RIBS

Costal cartilage

12th thoracic vertebra (T12)
1st lumbar vertebra (L1)

FIGURE 42-1 Thoracic cage. (From Applegate E: *The anatomy and physiology learning system,* ed 3, St Louis, 2006, Saunders.)

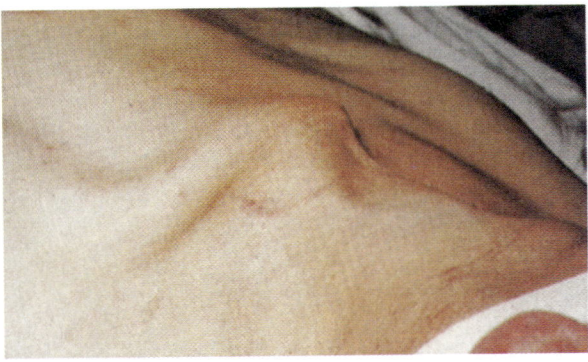

FIGURE 42-2 Fracture of the left clavicle seen from above the left shoulder. (From London PS: *A colour atlas of diagnosis after recent injury,* Ipswich, England, 1990, Wolfe Medical Publications, Ltd.)

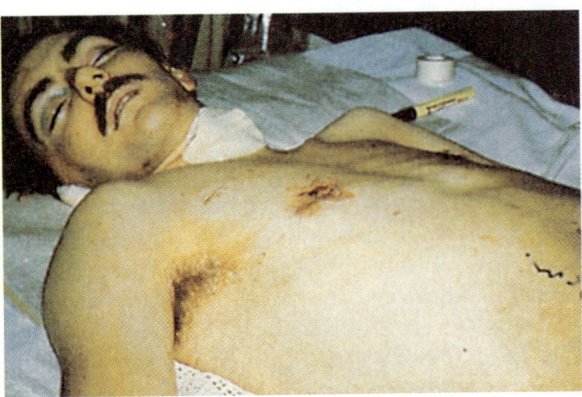

FIGURE 42-3 Chest wall asymmetry caused by rib fractures. (From London PS: *A colour atlas of diagnosis after recent injury,* Ipswich, England, 1990, Wolfe Medical Publications, Ltd.)

CRITICAL THINKING
Why would you expect greater underlying pulmonary injury in a child versus an adult with rib fractures?

NOTE
Separation of the costochondral cartilages also can occur from blunt anterior chest trauma. Signs and symptoms are similar to those for rib fracture. In addition, the patient may complain of a "snapping" sensation with deep respiration. These patients should be evaluated by a physician to rule out cardiac contusion. The pain associated with **costochondral separation** can persist for several weeks.

Simple rib fractures usually are very painful. However, they rarely are life threatening. Most patients can localize the fracture by pointing to the area. (This is confirmed by palpation.) Sometimes movement or grating of the bone ends (**crepitus**) can be felt. One complication of rib fracture is *respiratory or diaphragmatic splinting.* This occurs when the patient uses breath holding or minimizes chest wall movement to lessen pain. This splinting can lead to **atelectasis** (the collapse of lung tissue). Another complication is ventilation-perfusion mismatch (perfused alveoli that are not ventilated).

The goals of treatment for rib fractures are to relieve the pain and maintain pulmonary function to prevent atelectasis. (The paramedic should encourage the patient to cough and to breathe deeply.) Pain may be relieved by splinting the patient's arm against the chest wall with a sling and swathe. (Circumferential splinting should not be used because it may not allow complete expansion of the chest wall during respiration.) Administration of analgesics (per protocol) also may be helpful. Based on the mechanism of injury, the paramedic should consider the possibility of more serious trauma, such as closed pneumothorax and internal bleeding. Fractures to the lower ribs (8 through 12) may be associated with injuries to the spleen, kidneys, or liver.

Great force is required to fracture the first and second ribs. This is because of their shape and the protection provided by the scapulae, clavicles, and upper chest musculature. Fractures of the first and second ribs may be associated with myocardial contusion, bronchial tears, and vascular injury.

> ### NOTE
> The true danger of a fractured rib is not the injured rib. Rather, it is the potential for penetrating injury to the pleura, lung, liver, or spleen. Elderly patients or patients with preexisting respiratory disease are often unable to compensate for even minor trauma to the chest wall. These patients require careful monitoring for respiratory distress or fatigue.

Flail Chest

A **flail chest** may occur when three or more adjacent ribs are fractured in two or more places[1] (Figure 42-4). This injury may be difficult to detect in the prehospital setting because of the muscle spasm that often accompanies the injury. Within 2 hours after the injury, however, the muscle spasm subsides. At that point, the injured segment of the chest wall may begin to move in a contrary fashion (**paradoxical motion**) with inspiration and expiration. This interrupts the normal mechanics of breathing and decreases effective ventilation.

Causes of flail chest include vehicle crashes, falls, industrial accidents, assault, and birth trauma. The mortality rate is 8% to 35% because of underlying, associated injuries.[1] The mortality rate increases with advanced age, seven or more rib fractures, three or more associated injuries, shock, and head injury.

As described in Chapter 15, the diaphragm descends during inspiration. This lowers the intrapleural pressure. The unstable chest wall is pushed ("sucked") inward by the negative intrathoracic pressure as the rest of the chest wall expands. During expiration, the diaphragm rises, and the intrapleural pressure exceeds atmospheric pressure. This causes the unstable chest wall to move outward. Patients with flail chest often develop hypoxia. This is because of the lung contusions usually related to this injury. Bleeding from the alveoli and the lung tissue causes the contusion. It is associated with decreased vital capacity and vascular shunting of deoxygenated blood. Signs and symptoms of flail chest include bruising, tenderness, and bony crepitus on palpation and paradoxical motion (a late sign).

Prehospital management of patients with flail chest includes assisting ventilation with high-concentration supplemental oxygen and providing fluid replacement as

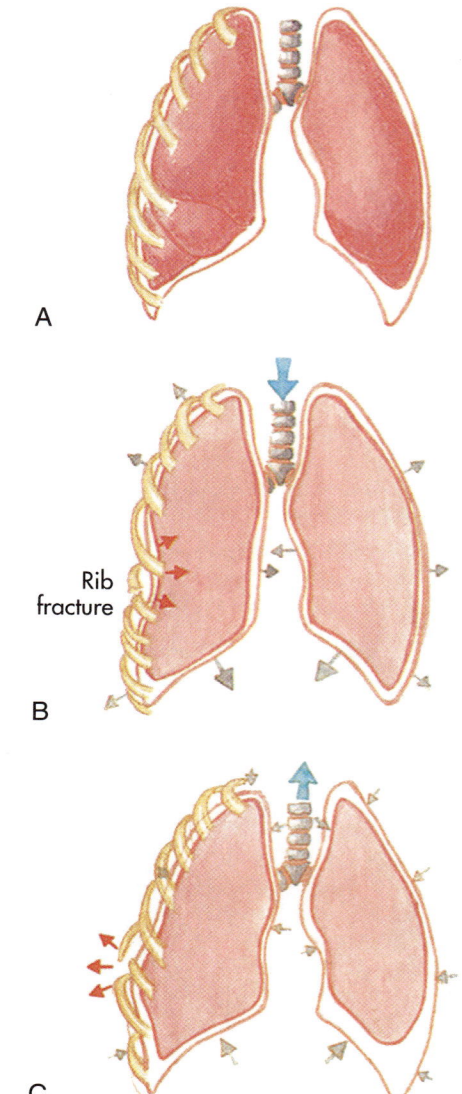

Rib fracture

FIGURE 42-4 Flail chest. **A,** Normal lungs. **B,** Flail chest during inspiration. **C,** Flail chest during expiration.

>
> ### LOOK AGAIN
> See Chapter 15: Airway Management, Respiration, and Artificial Ventilation, pp. 391-393.

needed. Field stabilization of the flail segment is not recommended.[3] Many authorities recommend intubation and positive-pressure ventilation (internal splinting) in patients with severe respiratory distress and a flail chest. Intubation also may be indicated if the chest injury is associated with shock, other severe injuries, head injury, or pulmonary disease, or if it occurs in a patient older than 65 years of age.

As a rule, the most conservative methods for obtaining adequate oxygenation and ventilation should be used to manage patients with flail chest.[1] A large percentage of patients with significant chest injury will progress to respiratory failure. This requires long-term ventilatory support and hospitalization.

CRITICAL THINKING
Why is positive-pressure ventilation the treatment of choice for this injury?

Sternal Fractures

A **sternal fracture** is an uncommon but serious injury. The fracture usually results from a direct blow to the chest (e.g., striking a steering column or dashboard) or from a massive crush injury (Figure 42-5). Sternal fractures usually are very painful. They may be associated with an unstable chest wall, myocardial injury, or cardiac tamponade. They occur in only 5% to 8% of patients with blunt chest trauma. However, the mortality rate is 25% to 45%.[4] Signs and symptoms include a history of significant anterior chest trauma, tenderness, and abnormal motion or crepitation over the sternum. Prehospital management includes maintaining a high degree of suspicion for associated injuries. These patients are best managed with airway maintenance, ventilatory support, pulse oximetry and electrocardiographic (ECG) monitoring, and rapid transport to an appropriate medical facility. Associated injuries that often contribute to serious disability or death include the following:

- Pulmonary and myocardial contusion
- Flail chest
- Vascular disruption of thoracic vessels (rare)
- Intraabdominal injuries
- Head injury

PULMONARY INJURIES

Pulmonary injuries may be classified as closed pneumothorax, tension pneumothorax, open pneumothorax, hemothorax, pulmonary contusion, and traumatic asphyxia. Any of these injuries can result in difficulty in breathing and respiratory insufficiency. Prehospital treatment must be directed at ensuring an open airway, providing ventilatory support, correcting immediately life-threatening ventilatory problems (e.g., tension pneumothorax), and arranging rapid transport for definitive care.

Closed Pneumothorax

A **closed pneumothorax** (*simple pneumothorax*) is caused by the presence of air in the pleural space. This air causes the lung to partially or totally collapse (Figure 42-6). A common cause of pneumothorax is a fractured rib that penetrates the underlying lung. Pneumothoraces also may occur without rib fractures. They may be caused by excessive pressure on the chest wall against a closed glottis (paper bag effect; see Chapter 37: Trauma Overview and Mechanism of Injury). They also may be caused by rupture or tearing of the lung tissue and visceral pleura from no apparent cause (e.g., spontaneous pneumothorax). Closed pneumothorax occurs in 15% to 50% of patients with severe blunt chest trauma, and in almost 100% of patients with penetrating chest trauma.[1]

CRITICAL THINKING
How does high-flow oxygen promote faster resolution of a closed pneumothorax?

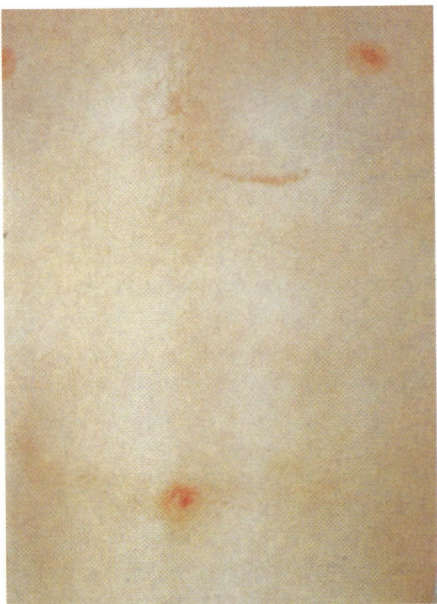

FIGURE 42-5 Well-marked band of spotty bruising caused by steering wheel impact. (From London PS: *A colour atlas of diagnosis after recent injury,* Ipswich, England, 1990, Wolfe Medical Publications, Ltd.)

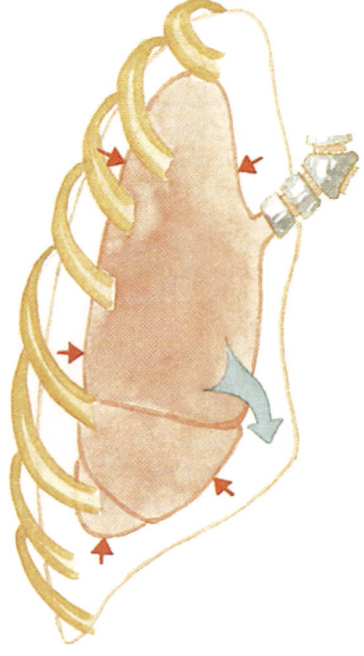

FIGURE 42-6 Closed (simple) pneumothorax.

The signs and symptoms of a closed pneumothorax are dependent on the severity of hypoxia, the degree of impairment of ventilation, and the percentage of the lung that has collapsed. These signs and symptoms may include chest pain, dyspnea, and tachypnea. Breath sounds may be diminished or absent on the affected side. Treatment includes ventilatory support with high-concentration oxygen. The patient should be carefully monitored for signs of a tension pneumothorax (described later). Patients should be transported in a semisitting position of comfort unless this position is contraindicated by the mechanism of injury. If the patient's respiratory rate is below 12 or above 28 breaths per minute, ventilatory assistance with a bag-valve-mask (BVM) may be indicated.[3]

Most healthy patients have large circulatory and ventilatory reserve capacities. Therefore closed pneumothoraces usually do not pose a threat to life. However, life-threatening consequences may develop if the pneumothorax is a tension pneumothorax, if it occupies more than 40% of the hemithorax, or if it occurs in a patient with shock or preexisting pulmonary or cardiovascular diseases.

Open Pneumothorax

An **open pneumothorax** (*communicating pneumothorax*) develops when a chest injury exposes the pleural space to atmospheric pressure (Figure 42-7). The severity of the injury is directly proportional to the size of the wound. When a chest wound is larger than the normal pathway for air through the nose and mouth, atmospheric pressure forces the air through the open wound and into the thoracic cavity during inspiration. As the air accumulates in the pleural space, the lung on the injured side collapses. The lung begins to shift toward the uninjured side. Very little air enters the tracheobronchial tree to be exchanged with intrapulmonary air on the affected side. This results in decreased alveolar ventilation and decreased perfusion. The normal side also is adversely affected. That is because expired air may enter the lung on the collapsed side. It then is rebreathed into the functioning lung with the next ventilation. This may result in severe ventilatory dysfunction, hypoxemia, and death unless the condition is quickly recognized and corrected.

> **NOTE**
> A small open chest wound may function like a ball-valve mechanism. That is, it may allow air in but not out. The accumulation of air may result in a shift in the patient's mediastinum, moving the tissue and organs within the chest cavity to one side. A **mediastinal shift** can lead to reduced preload and a reduction in cardiac output (Figure 42-8).

Signs and symptoms of open pneumothorax include shortness of breath, pain, and a sucking or gurgling sound as air moves in and out of the pleural space through the open chest wound (thus the term *sucking chest wound*).

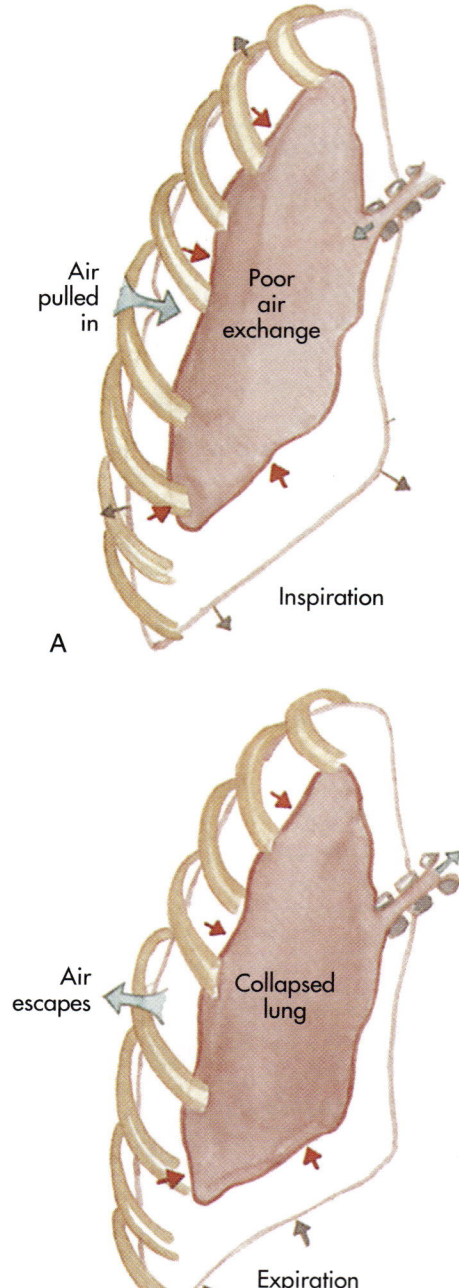

FIGURE 42-7 Open pneumothorax. **A,** Air enters the pleural cavity during inspiration. **B,** Air exits the pleural cavity during expiration.

Prehospital treatment of an open pneumothorax proceeds as follows (Figure 42-9):

1. Close the chest wound by first applying direct pressure with a gloved hand. The chest wound can then be sealed by applying an occlusive dressing of petroleum gauze[1] or a dressing of foil or plastic, and securing it with tape.[3] Medical direction may advise that only three sides of the dressing be taped. This provides a venting mechanism (or one-way valve). It also may allow spontaneous

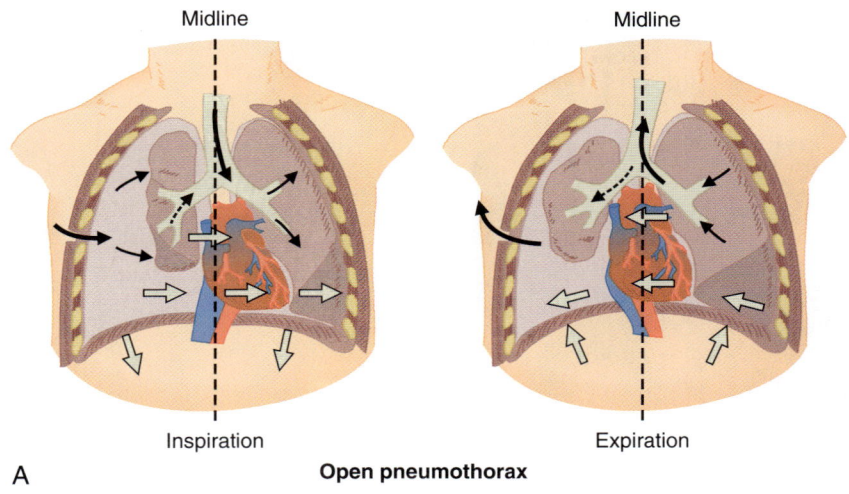

A, **Open pneumothorax**

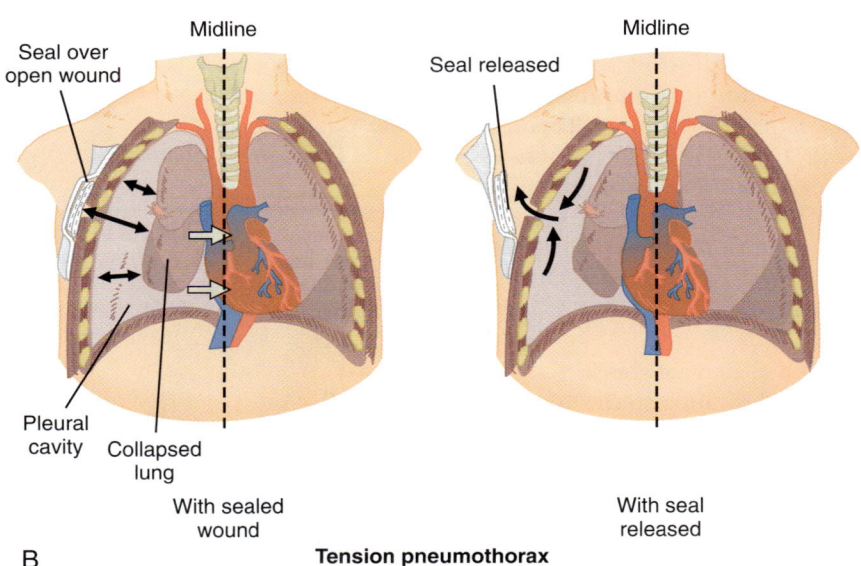

B, **Tension pneumothorax**

FIGURE 42-8 **A,** Open pneumothorax. Solid and dashed arrows represent air movement; open arrows represent structural movement. On inspiration, air is sucked into the pleural space through the open chest wound and the lung on the affected side collapses. The mediastinal contents shift toward the unaffected side. On expiration, air exits through the open wound and the mediastinal contents swing back toward the affected side (mediastinal flutter). **B,** An airtight dressing can cause a tension pneumothorax when air accumulates in the pleural space through a tear in the lung tissue. The air cannot exit if there is no open chest wound, and pressure builds, shifting the contents of the mediastinum toward the unaffected side and impairing circulatory and respiratory function (mediastinal shift). (From Linton AD: *Introduction to medical surgical nursing,* ed 4, St Louis, 2007, Saunders.)

decompression of a developing tension pneumothorax. The paramedic should closely monitor for the development of a tension pneumothorax if the patient's dressing does not provide a venting mechanism.

2. Provide ventilatory support with high-concentration oxygen and monitor oxygen saturation. Airway management includes assisting ventilations with a bag-mask device and intubation.
3. Treat the patient for shock by administering crystalloid (per protocol).

4. Rapidly transport the patient to an appropriate medical facility.

Tension Pneumothorax

When air in the thoracic cavity cannot exit the pleural space, a **tension pneumothorax** may develop (Figure 42-10). This is a true emergency. It results in profound hypoventilation and impaired perfusion. Tension pneumothorax may result in death if it is not immediately recognized and managed.

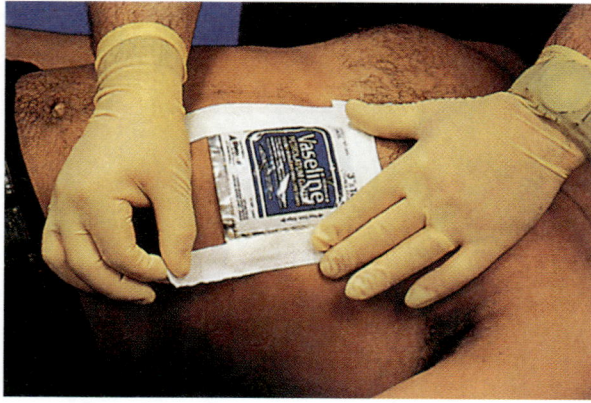

FIGURE 42-9 Sealing a chest wound.

When air is allowed to leak into the pleural space during inspiration and becomes trapped during expiration, the pleural pressure increases. This increase in pressure produces a shift in the mediastinum. It further compresses the lung on the uninjured side. In addition, compression of the vena cava reduces venous return to the heart. This results in a decrease in cardiac output. The signs and symptoms of a tension pneumothorax include the following:

- Anxiety
- Cyanosis
- Increasing dyspnea
- Tracheal deviation (a late sign)
- Tachycardia
- Hypotension or unexplained signs of shock
- Diminished or absent breath sounds on the injured side
- Distended neck veins (unless the patient is hypovolemic)
- Unequal expansion of the chest (tension does not fall with respiration)
- Subcutaneous emphysema

NOTE
Tracheal deviation may result from the displacement of mediastinal structures. However, tracheal deviation is an inconsistent finding with pneumothorax. If it occurs, it is often a late finding.[5] Tracheal deviation that results from chest injury is seldom seen in the prehospital setting.

CRITICAL THINKING
Why might the neck veins be distended in a patient with a tension pneumothorax?

A suspected tension pneumothorax should be managed aggressively. It is evidenced by increasing dyspnea, compromised ventilation, tachycardia, tachypnea, unilateral decreased or absent breath sounds, and hyperresonance on percussion. Emergency care is directed at reducing the pressure in the pleural space, that is, returning the intrapleural pressure to atmospheric or subatmospheric levels.

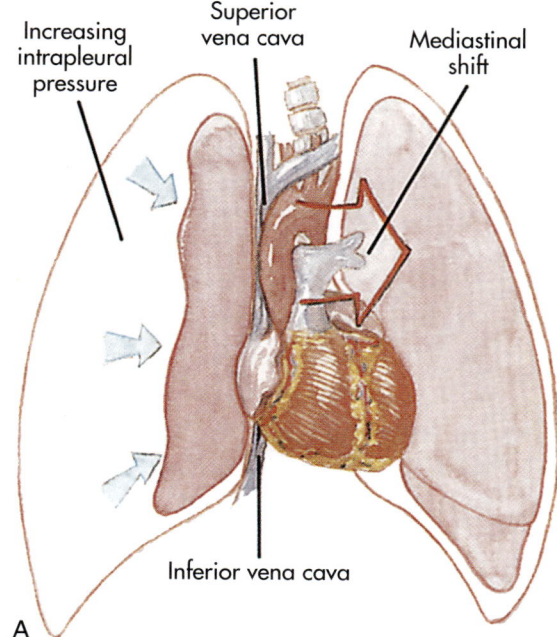

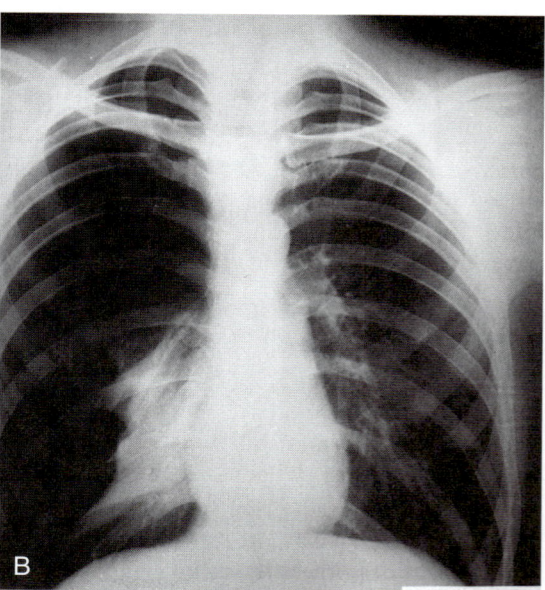

FIGURE 42-10 A, Tension pneumothorax. **B,** Tension pneumothorax of the right lung after a stab wound in this 25-year-old man. The collapsed lung has almost no air in it and is seen as a soft tissue density adjacent to the heart. (B from Kowalczyk N, Mace JD: *Radiographic pathology for technologists,* ed 5, St Louis, 2009, Mosby.)

NOTE
The value of chest percussion in the prehospital setting is questionable. In the field, it should not be the only method used to identify a tension pneumothorax or hemothorax.[3] As a rule, hyperresonance on percussion points to the presence of air (*pneumothorax*) or dullness on percussion pointing to the presence of blood and other fluids (*hemothorax*) should be used as identifiers.

needle should be inserted just above the rib. (This point is used to avoid the nerve, artery, and vein that lie just beneath each rib.) After insertion of the needle, an audible rush of air should be noted. This is pressure escaping from the pleural space (confirming the tension pneumothorax). At this point, the patient should show signs of improvement (i.e., the patient's lungs will be easier to ventilate or the patient's breathing will be less labored). The needle should be withdrawn and the catheter secured in place with tape. Needle decompression may need to be repeated if the catheter becomes occluded with a blood clot and tension pneumothorax recurs.[3]

CRITICAL THINKING

Put your finger on the point on your chest where a needle would be inserted for decompression of a tension pneumothorax. Is it easy to identify?

TENSION PNEUMOTHORAX ASSOCIATED WITH PENETRATING TRAUMA

As mentioned previously, sealing an open pneumothorax with an occlusive dressing may produce a tension pneumothorax. In such cases the increased pleural pressure can be relieved by momentarily removing the dressing. When the dressing is lifted from the wound, an audible release of air from the thoracic cavity should be noted. If this does not occur and the patient's condition remains unchanged, the wound should be gently spread open with gloved fingers. This may allow the trapped air to escape. After the pressure has been released, the wound should again be sealed. The dressing may need to be removed more than once to relieve pleural pressure during transport. If the tension is not relieved with this procedure, needle decompression of the thorax (*needle thoracentesis; needle thoracostomy*) should be performed. Needle decompression should be performed when three findings are present[3]:

1. Worsening respiratory distress or increasing difficulty ventilating with a BVM device
2. Unilateral decreased or absent breath sounds
3. Decompensated shock (systolic blood pressure <90 mm Hg)

TENSION PNEUMOTHORAX ASSOCIATED WITH CLOSED TRAUMA

A tension pneumothorax that develops in a patient with closed chest trauma must be relieved through thoracic decompression. This can be done with a large-bore needle or a commercially available thoracic decompression kit.

For needle decompression, a large-bore, 10- or 14-gauge hollow catheter-over-needle (8 cm or longer)[3] is inserted into the affected pleural space. The needle can be inserted anteriorly in the second intercostal space in the midclavicular line. It may also be placed in the fourth or fifth intercostal space laterally on the involved side[1] (Figure 42-11). The

HEMOTHORAX

A **hemothorax** is the accumulation of blood in the pleural space. It is caused by bleeding from the lung parenchyma or damaged vessels (Figure 42-12). If this condition is associated with a pneumothorax, it is called a **hemopneumothorax.** Blood loss may be massive in these patients; each side of the thorax can hold 30% to 40% (2000 to 3000 mL) of the patient's blood volume.[6] (A severed intercostal artery can easily bleed 50 mL per minute.) Thus patients with a hemothorax often have hypovolemia and hypoxemia. Hemothorax is commonly associated with pneumothorax (25%) and extrathoracic injuries (73%).[1]

As blood continues to fill the pleural space, the lung on the affected side may collapse. In rare cases the mediastinum may even shift away from the hemothorax. This would compress the unaffected lung. The resultant effects of respiratory and circulatory compromise are responsible for the following signs and symptoms:

- Tachypnea
- Dyspnea
- Cyanosis (often not evident in hemorrhagic shock)
- Diminished or decreased breath sounds (dullness on percussion)
- Hypovolemic shock
- Narrow pulse pressure
- Tracheal deviation to the unaffected side (rare)

Prehospital care for patients with a hemothorax is directed at correcting ventilatory and circulatory problems. This involves administration of high-concentration oxygen; implementation of ventilatory support with a bag-mask device or intubation, or both; administration of volume-expanding fluids to correct the hypovolemia; and rapid transport to an appropriate medical facility. Hemothorax associated with great vessel or cardiac injury has a high mortality rate: 50% of these patients die within 1 hour of their injury.[7]

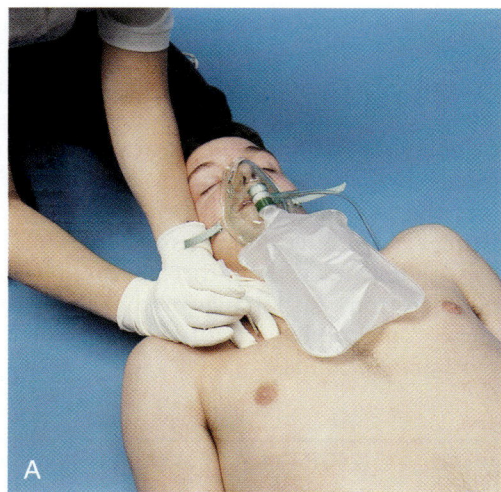
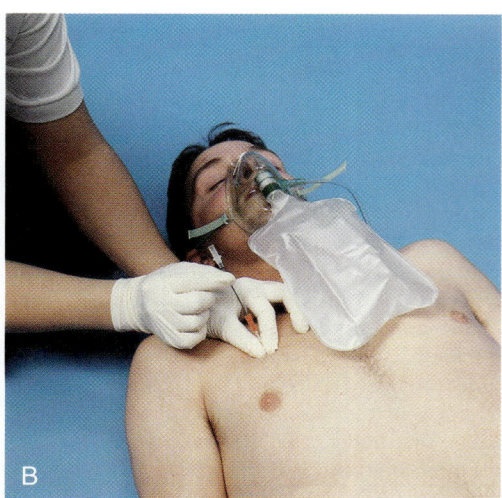
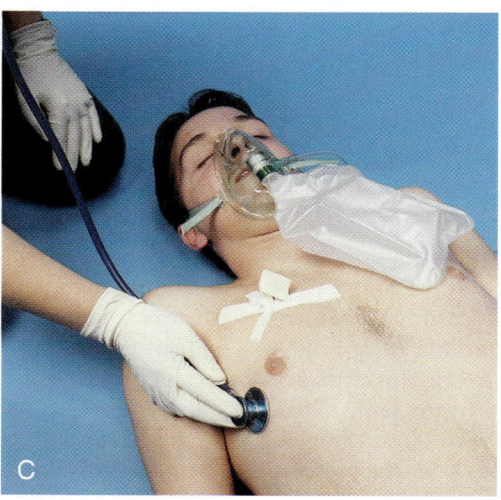

FIGURE 42-11 Needle decompression. **A,** A 2-inch, 10- or 14-gauge hollow needle or catheter is inserted into the affected pleural space, usually in the second intercostal space in the midclavicular line. **B,** After insertion of the needle, an audible rush of air should be noted as pressure escapes from the pleural space. **C,** The catheter is secured in place with tape. Care is taken to prevent reentry of air into the pleural space. The patient's respiratory status is monitored carefully.

CRITICAL THINKING

Hemothorax is associated with a higher mortality rate than a simple (closed) pneumothorax. Why is that the case?

Pulmonary Contusion

Pulmonary contusion most often is caused by rapid deceleration forces. (Such forces may be created by motor vehicle crashes and by injuries that result in a flail chest.) These forces push the lung against the chest wall. This results in rupture of the alveoli, with hemorrhage and swelling of the lung tissue. More than 50% of patients with blunt chest trauma have pulmonary contusion.[1]

During sudden inertial deceleration and direct impact, fixed and mobile parts of the lung move at varying speeds. The result is stretching and shearing of alveoli and intravascular structures. (This is the *inertial effect*.) This kinetic wave of energy is partly reflected at the alveolar membrane surface. The remainder causes a localized release of energy. (This is the *Spalding effect*.) Overexpansion of air in the lungs occurs after the primary energy wave has passed (*implosion effect*). Then low-pressure rebound shock waves cause overstretching and damage to lung tissue. The combination of these events results in alveolar and capillary damage with bleeding into the lung tissue and alveoli. The contused area of the lung is unable to function properly after injury. Therefore profound hypoxemia may develop. The degree of respiratory complication is directly related to the size of the contused area.

The signs and symptoms of pulmonary contusion are subtle at first. They should be suspected based on the kinematics of the event and the presence of associated injuries. Common signs and symptoms include the following:

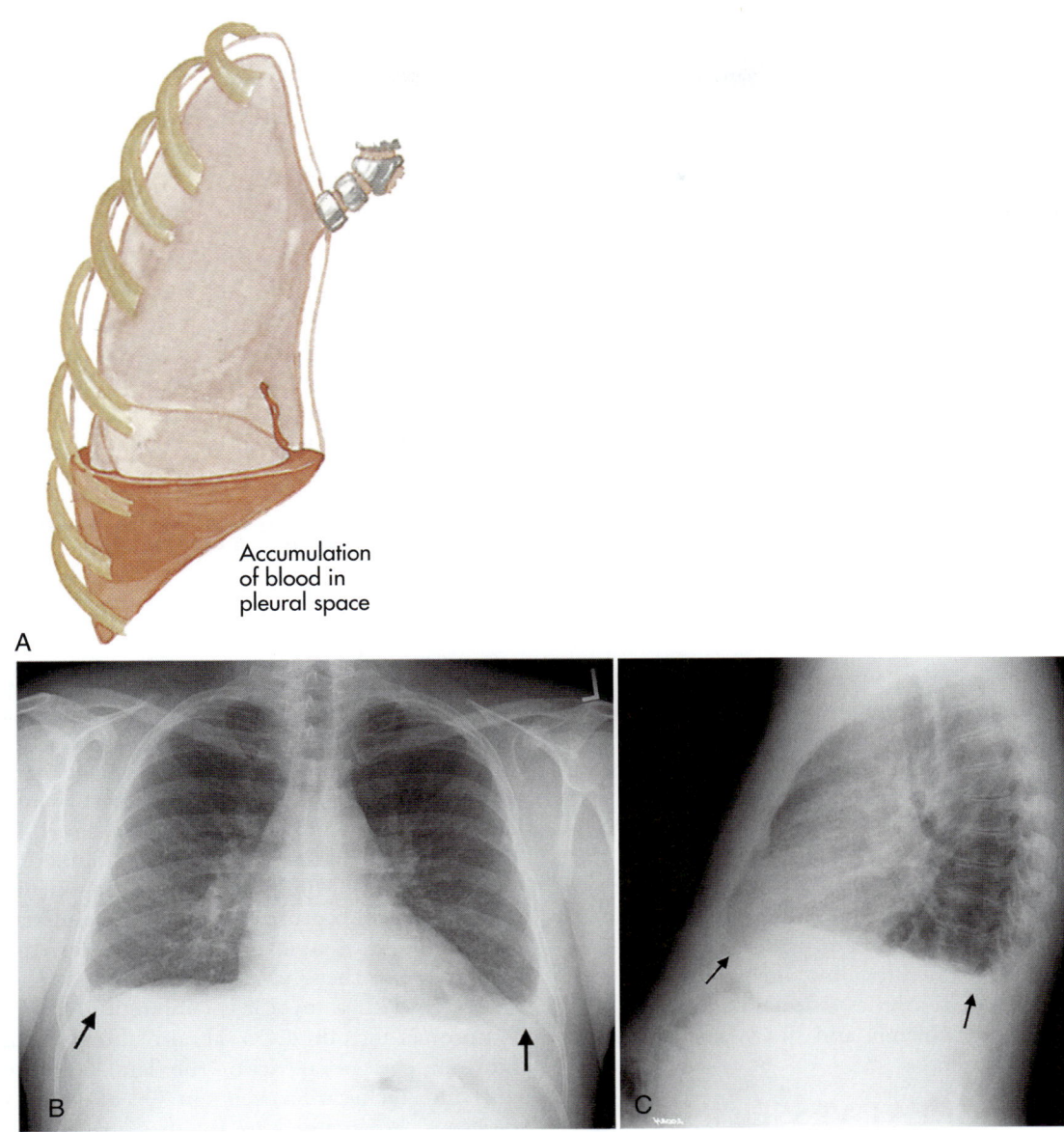

Accumulation
of blood in
pleural space

A

B

C

FIGURE 42-12 **A,** Hemothorax. **B,** Posteroanterior view. **C,** Left lateral chest radiograph demonstrating bilateral pleural effusions. (**B, C** from Kowalczyk N, Mace JD: *Radiographic pathology for technologists,* ed 5, St Louis, 2009, Mosby.)

- Tachypnea
- Tachycardia
- Cough
- Hemoptysis
- Apprehension
- Respiratory distress
- Dyspnea
- Evidence of blunt chest trauma
- Cyanosis

CRITICAL THINKING

Will you always be able to distinguish between simple pneumothorax and pulmonary contusion in the prehospital setting? Why or why not?

Emergency care for pulmonary contusion includes ventilatory support and administration of high-concentration oxygen. Patients with associated injuries or preexisting pulmonary or cardiovascular disease should be closely monitored in case ventilations need to be assisted with a bag-valve device, intubation, or both. Pulmonary contusions may be associated with a major chest injury. However, they generally heal spontaneously over several weeks.

Traumatic Asphyxia

The term **traumatic asphyxia** is used to describe a severe crushing injury to the chest and abdomen (Figure 42-13). It results from an increase in intrathoracic pressure. This pressure increase forces blood from the right side of the heart into the veins of the upper thorax, neck, and face. The

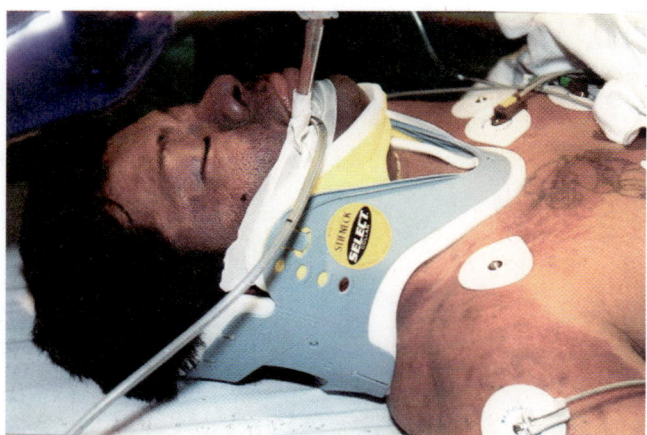

FIGURE 42-13 A victim of traumatic asphyxia displays ecchymosis and swelling above the level of the heart. A truck with a rear tire removed had slipped off the jack, trapping the patient underneath. At rescue the patient was in cardiac arrest. Prompt cardiopulmonary resuscitation by bystanders and early EMS response restored his circulation. He survived the injury. (From Henry MC, Stapleton ER: *EMT prehospital care*, ed 4, St Louis, 2009, Mosby.)

> **NOTE**
> The clinical findings in blunt cardiac trauma are often subtle and frequently overlooked for several reasons: (1) multiple injuries direct attention elsewhere; (2) often little evidence of thoracic injury is present; and (3) signs of cardiac injury may not be present on initial examination. The goals of prehospital care are to recognize the potential for cardiac trauma (based on mechanism of injury) and to monitor the patient for potentially fatal complications that may arise.

common.) Therefore a deformed dashboard or steering column should alert the paramedic to the possibility of a cardiac injury. Blunt myocardial injury occurs in as many as 55% of patients who suffer blunt trauma to the chest.[1]

> **CRITICAL THINKING**
> How would you manage a cardiac rhythm disturbance resulting from a myocardial contusion?

forces involved in this phenomenon may cause lethal injury, but traumatic asphyxia alone is not life threatening[1] (although brain hemorrhages, seizures, coma, and death have been documented to occasionally occur).

Signs and symptoms of traumatic asphyxia include reddish purple discoloration of the face and neck (the skin below the area remains pink), jugular vein distention, and swelling or hemorrhage of the conjunctiva (subconjunctival petechiae may appear). Emergency care is directed at ensuring an open airway, providing adequate ventilation, and caring for associated injuries. The paramedic should be ready to manage hypovolemia and shock when the compressive force is released.

HEART AND GREAT VESSEL INJURIES

Trauma to the heart and great vessels (i.e., the aorta, pulmonary arteries and veins, and superior and inferior venae cavae) may result from blunt or penetrating trauma and associated forces. The injuries discussed in this section include myocardial contusion, pericardial tamponade, myocardial rupture, and traumatic aortic rupture. Potentially fatal complications of these injuries include:

- Life-threatening dysrhythmias
- Conduction abnormalities
- Congestive heart failure
- Cardiogenic shock
- Cardiac tamponade
- Cardiac rupture
- Coronary artery occlusion

Myocardial Contusion

Myocardial contusions usually are caused by a vehicle collision. In these cases the chest wall strikes the dashboard or steering column. (Sternal and multiple rib fractures are

The extent of injury may vary. The injury may be only a localized bruise. It also may be a full-thickness injury to the wall of the heart with hemorrhage and edema. Blood may accumulate in the pericardium (*hemopericardium*) as a result of a tear in the epicardium or endocardium. This, in turn, may result in cardiac rupture or a traumatic myocardial infarction. The fibrinous reaction at the contusion site may lead to delayed rupture or ventricular aneurysm.

Patients with a myocardial contusion may have no symptoms, or they may complain of chest pain similar to that seen with a myocardial infarction. Other signs and symptoms include ECG abnormalities, a new cardiac murmur, pericardial friction rub (late), persistent tachycardia (sinus tachycardia occurs in 70% of patients[1]), and palpitations. Emergency care for these patients is similar to that for myocardial infarction: oxygen administration, ECG monitoring, and pharmacological therapy for dysrhythmias and hypotension (see Chapter 22). Any intervention that increases myocardial oxygen demand should be avoided (Box 42-1).

Pericardial Tamponade

Penetrating trauma (and, in rare cases, blunt trauma) may cause tears in the heart chamber walls. This allows blood to leak from the heart. If the pericardium has been torn sufficiently, blood can leak into the thoracic cavity and the patient rapidly dies from hemorrhage. Often, however, the pericardium remains intact. In such cases the blood enters the pericardial space. This causes an increase in pericardial pressure and volume (**pericardial tamponade**). The increased pressure prevents the heart from expanding and refilling with blood (60 to 100 mL of blood and clots in the pericardial sac can cause tamponade). This results in a decrease in stroke volume and cardiac output. Myocardial

BOX 42-1 Commotio Cordis

Commotio cordis is a Latin term that means *commotion or disturbance of the heart*. The condition describes sudden death that follows a blow to the chest.[8] Cardiac arrest is thought to be secondary to ventricular fibrillation (VF) when the chest trauma coincides with the cardiac T wave. It may also be associated with coronary vasospasm or changes in mycoardial contractility as a result of the chest trauma. Although commotio cordis can happen to anyone, victims are overwhelmingly young male athletes. Despite the fact that it is very rare, commotio cordis is the leading cause of death in youth baseball (accounting for 2 to 20 deaths per year).[3,9]

Commotio cordis has also been documented in hockey, lacrosse, karate, and soccer.

Commotio cordis is managed in a manner similar to that used for cardiac arrests resulting from myocardial infarction rather than those resulting from trauma. The cardiac rhythm should be determined quickly and rapid defibrillation should be administered if VF is identified.[3]

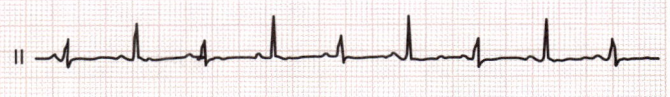

FIGURE 42-14 Lead II rhythm strip taken from a patient with acute pericarditis complicated by a large pericardial effusion and tamponade physiology. Note the resting sinus tachycardia with relatively low voltage and electrical alternans. (Courtesy Ary L. Goldberger, MD.)

- Narrow pulse pressure
- Cyanosis of the head, neck, and upper extremities

> **NOTE**
> It is important to stress that injuries other than pericardial tamponade can cause hypotension and elevated central venous pressure. These are most notably tension pneumothorax in trauma victims and cardiogenic shock. Patients with tamponade and hemorrhage may not initially have an elevated central venous pressure. In the field, a good indication of cardiac tamponade is the presence of jugular vein distention along with hypotension and tachycardia.

perfusion decreases because of pressure effects on the walls of the heart and decreased diastolic pressures. Associated ischemic dysfunction may result in myocardial infarction. Pericardial tamponade occurs in fewer than 2% of patients who suffer blunt chest trauma; 60% to 80% of patients with stab wounds involving the heart develop tamponade.[1]

> **NOTE**
> Penetrating injuries to the heart, such as those caused by some knife and gunshot wounds, may result in death from hemorrhage rather than tamponade. This happens when the wound in the heart is so large that the blood in the pericardial space cannot be contained.

At first, most patients with pericardial tamponade have peripheral vasoconstriction. (The diastolic blood pressure rises more than the systolic blood pressure. This causes a decrease in pulse pressure.) These patients are also tachycardic. The increase in heart rate compensates for the decrease in cardiac output. Up to this point, pericardial tamponade and hemorrhagic shock have similar signs. Yet a key clinical finding often allows differentiation of the two forms of shock. This clinical finding was first described by Beck in 1935. It and two other clinical clues compose **Beck's triad.** Beck's triad consists of elevated central venous pressure (evidenced by jugular vein distention), muffled heart sounds, and hypotension. The first element of Beck's triad, elevated central venous pressure, is the single best way to distinguish pericardial tamponade from hemorrhagic shock.[1] Other signs and symptoms of pericardial tamponade include the following:

- Tachycardia
- Respiratory distress

Two other findings in pericardial tamponade may include *pulsus paradoxus* and *electrical alternans*. **Pulsus paradoxus** is a systolic blood pressure that drops more than 10 to 15 mm Hg during inspiration compared with expiration. (Normally this drop is minimal.) The excessive decline in systolic pressure occurs in cardiac tamponade when pleural pressure is reduced during inspiration. The reduction of pleural pressure provides some relief from the tamponade and causes the inspiratory fall in arterial flow and systolic pressure. (Pulsus paradoxus is difficult to measure in the prehospital setting, especially if the patient is hypotensive.) **Electrical alternans** refers to a change in the amplitude of a patient's ECG waveforms that decrease with every other cardiac cycle (Figure 42-14). It is a rare finding in cardiac tamponade.

Pericardial tamponade is a true emergency. Pericardial blood must be removed in these patients. Also, the bleeding must be stopped if the patient is to survive the injury. Prehospital management includes careful monitoring, oxygen administration, aggressive fluid replacement to maintain adequate preload (if transport time is short), and rapid transport to an appropriate medical facility. Treatment at the medical facility involves *needle pericardiocentesis* to remove blood from the pericardial sac. Removal of as little as 20 mL may drastically improve cardiac output.[1]

Myocardial Rupture

Myocardial rupture occurs when blood-filled chambers of the ventricles are compressed with enough force to rupture the chamber wall, septum, or valve. The injury is nearly always immediately fatal. However, about 20% of patients will survive 30 minutes or longer, allowing time for surgical repair.[1] This may allow time for rapid transport and surgical repair. Motor vehicle crashes are responsible for most cases of myocardial rupture, accounting for 15% of fatal thoracic injuries. Other proposed mechanisms include the following:

- Deceleration or shearing forces that disrupt the inferior and superior venae cavae
- Upward displacement of blood (causing an increase in intracardiac pressure) after abdominal trauma
- Direct compression of the heart between the sternum and vertebrae
- Laceration from a rib or sternal fracture
- Complications of myocardial contusion

These patients often present with a significant mechanism of injury. Signs and symptoms of congestive heart failure and cardiac tamponade may be present. (The patient should be closely monitored for signs of pericardial tamponade.) Prehospital care for these patients is mainly supportive. It includes airway and ventilatory support and rapid transport for definitive care. It is crucial that paramedics also consider the possibility of a tension pneumothorax in these patients. The signs and symptoms of tension pneumothorax mimic those of myocardial rupture with tamponade.

Traumatic Aortic Rupture

Traumatic aortic rupture is thought to be a result of shearing forces. These forces develop between tissues that decelerate at different rates. Common mechanisms of injury include rapid deceleration in high-speed motor vehicle crashes, falls from great heights, and crushing injuries. It has been estimated that one in six people who die in motor vehicle crashes has a rupture of the aorta.[1] Of these patients, 80% to 90% die at the scene as a result of massive hemorrhage. About 10% to 20% survive the first hour. This is because the bleeding is tamponaded by the surrounding adventitia of the aorta and intact visceral pleura. Of these individuals, 30% have ruptures within 6 hours. For these reasons, rapid and pertinent evaluation and transport to an appropriate medical facility are critical. Aortic rupture is responsible for 15% of all deaths from blunt trauma.

The usual site of damage to the aorta is in the distal arch. This is just beyond the branching of the left subclavian artery and proximal to the ligamentum arteriosum (Figure 42-15). The ligamentum arteriosum and descending thoracic arch are somewhat fixed. On the other hand, the transverse portion of the arch is somewhat mobile. If shearing forces exceed the tensile strength of the arch, the junction of the mobile and fixed points of attachment may be partly torn. If the outer layer of tissue around the aorta remains intact, the patient may survive long enough for surgical repair.

Aortic rupture is a severe injury. About 85% of patients die before reaching a hospital.[10] Any trauma patient who has unexplained shock and an appropriate mechanism of injury (rapid deceleration) should be suspected of having a ruptured aorta. Blood pressure may be normal or elevated, with a significant difference between the two arms. In

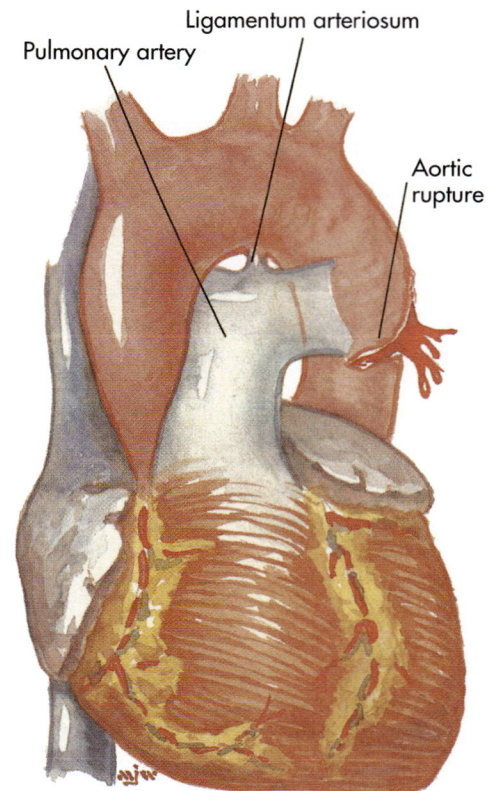

FIGURE 42-15 Aortic rupture.

addition, upper extremity hypertension with absent or weak femoral pulses can occur in these patients. (This is thought to result from compression of the aorta by the expanding hematoma.) Other patients have hypertension because of increased activity of the sympathetic nervous system. About 25% of these patients have a harsh systolic murmur that can be heard over the pericardium or between the scapulae. In rare cases these patients may have paraplegia without a cervical or thoracic spine injury. This occurs as a consequence of decreased blood flow through the anterior spinal artery. The anterior spinal artery is in the thoracic region. It is composed of branches from the posterior intercostal arteries. These in turn are branches of the thoracic aorta.

> **NOTE**
> A difference in pulse quality between the arms and lower torso or between the left and right arms is sometimes detected with aortic rupture. Therefore checking both radial and femoral pulses is important.[3]

Prehospital management of these patients includes advising medical direction of the suspected rupture, administering high-concentration oxygen, providing ventilatory support with spinal precautions, replacing fluids judiciously (avoiding overhydration), and ensuring rapid transport for surgical repair.

NOTE
Fluid replacement should be limited in patients who have a stable blood pressure. This helps to prevent an increase in pressure in the remaining aortic wall tissue.

Penetrating Wounds of the Great Vessels

Penetrating wounds of the great vessels usually involve injury to the chest, abdomen, or neck. These wounds often are accompanied by massive hemothorax, hypovolemic shock, cardiac tamponade, and enlarging hematomas that may cause compression of the vena cava, trachea, esophagus, great vessels, and heart. Prehospital care for patients with penetrating injury to the great vessels is directed at providing airway and ventilatory support, managing hypovolemia with judicious fluid therapy (guided by medical direction), and ensuring rapid transport for definitive care.

OTHER THORACIC INJURIES

Other injuries that may be associated with blunt or penetrating trauma to the thorax include esophageal and tracheobronchial injuries and diaphragmatic rupture.

Esophageal and Tracheobronchial Injuries

As discussed in Chapter 40, esophageal injuries most often are caused by penetrating trauma. (For example, these may be caused by projectile or knife wounds.) They also can result from spontaneous perforation caused by cancer and from anatomical distortions caused by diverticula or gastric reflux, both of which can lead to violent vomiting. Assessment findings may include pain, fever, hoarseness, dysphagia, respiratory distress, and shock. If esophageal perforation occurs in the cervical region, local tenderness, subcutaneous emphysema, and resistance to neck movement may be noted. Esophageal perforation that occurs lower in the thoracic region may result in mediastinal and subcutaneous emphysema, inflammation of the mediastinum, and splinting of the chest wall.

 LOOK AGAIN
See Chapter 40: Head, Face, and Neck Trauma, pp. 1158-1161.

Tracheobronchial injuries (*tracheobronchial disruptions*) are rare. They occur in fewer than 3% of victims of blunt or penetrating chest trauma. The mortality rate for these injuries is about 10%, depending on associated injuries, early diagnosis, and surgical repair.[1] Most injuries occur within 3 cm (about 1½ inches) of the carina. However, they can occur anywhere along the tracheobronchial tree. Signs

and symptoms of tracheobronchial injury include the following:

- Severe hypoxia
- Tachypnea
- Tachycardia
- Massive subcutaneous emphysema
- Dyspnea
- Respiratory distress
- Hemoptysis

Emergency care for patients with an esophageal or a tracheobronchial injury is directed at providing airway, ventilatory, and circulatory support and ensuring rapid transport for definitive care at an appropriate medical facility.

NOTE
A tension pneumothorax that does not improve after needle decompression or the absence of a continuous flow of air from the needle after decompression should alert the paramedic to the possibility of a tracheobronchial injury.

Diaphragmatic Rupture

As described in Chapter 10, the diaphragm is a sheet of dome-shaped muscle. This sheet of muscle separates the abdominal cavity from the thoracic cavity. Sudden compression of the abdomen (such as with blunt trauma to the trunk) results in a sharp increase in intraabdominal pressure. When this occurs, the pressure differences may cause abdominal contents to rupture through the thin diaphragmatic wall and enter the chest cavity (Figure 42-16). **Diaphragmatic rupture** is detected more often on the left side

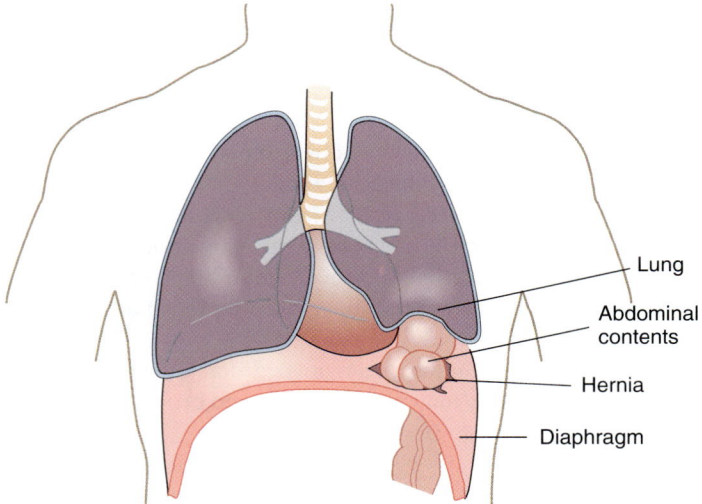

FIGURE 42-16 Diaphragmatic rupture. Sudden compression of the abdomen may increase intraabdominal pressure, causing the abdominal contents to rupture through the thin diaphragmatic wall and enter the chest cavity. (From National Association of Emergency Medical Technicians: *PHTLS: prehospital trauma life support,* ed 6, St Louis, 2007, Mosby.)

than on the right side. However, rupture on either side may allow intraabdominal organs to enter the thoracic cavity, where they may compress the lung, resulting in reduced ventilation, decreased venous return, decreased cardiac output, and shock. Because of the mechanical forces involved, patients with diaphragmatic rupture often have multiple injuries.

Signs and symptoms of a ruptured diaphragm include abdominal pain, shortness of breath, and decreased breath sounds. If most of the abdominal contents are forced into the chest, the abdomen may have a hollow or empty appearance. Also, bowel sounds may be heard in the chest. Prehospital management includes oxygen administration, ventilatory support as needed (positive-pressure ventilation may worsen the injury), use of volume-expanding fluids, and rapid transport with the patient in a supine position to an appropriate medical facility for surgical repair. Some medical direction agencies also may recommend that a nasogastric tube be placed to empty the stomach and reduce abdominal pressure.

SUMMARY

- Chest injuries are caused by blunt or penetrating trauma. Such trauma often results from motor vehicle crashes, falls from heights, blast injuries, blows to the chest, chest compression, gunshot wounds, and stab wounds.
- Fractures of the clavicle, ribs, or sternum as well as flail chest may be caused by blunt or penetrating trauma. Complications of skeletal trauma of the chest may include cardiac, vascular, or pulmonary injuries.
- Closed pneumothorax may be life threatening if (1) it is a tension pneumothorax, (2) it occupies more than 40% of the hemithorax, or (3) it occurs in a patient in shock or with a preexisting pulmonary or cardiovascular disease.
- Open pneumothorax may result in severe ventilatory dysfunction, hypoxemia, and death unless it is quickly recognized and corrected.
- Tension pneumothorax is a true emergency. It results in profound hypoventilation. It may result in death if it is not quickly recognized and managed.
- Hemothorax may result in massive blood loss. These patients often have hypovolemia and hypoxemia.
- Pulmonary contusion results when trauma to the lung causes alveolar and capillary damage. Severe hypoxemia may develop. The degree of hypoxemia is directly related to the size of the contused area.
- Traumatic asphyxia results from forces that cause an increase in intrathoracic pressure. When it occurs alone, it is often not lethal. However, brain hemorrhages, seizures, coma, and death have been reported after these injuries.
- The extent of injury from myocardial contusion may vary. The injury may be only a localized bruise. However,

it also may be a full-thickness injury to the wall of the heart. The full-thickness injury may result in cardiac rupture, ventricular aneurysm, or a traumatic myocardial infarction.
- Pericardial tamponade occurs if 150 to 200 mL of blood enters the pericardial space suddenly. This results in a decrease in stroke volume and cardiac output. *Myocardial rupture* refers to an acute traumatic perforation of the ventricles or atria. It is nearly always immediately fatal. However, death may be delayed for several weeks after blunt trauma.
- Aortic rupture is a severe injury. There is an 80% to 90% mortality rate in the first hour. The paramedic should consider the possibility of aortic rupture in any trauma patient who has unexplained shock after a rapid deceleration injury.
- Esophageal injuries most frequently are caused by penetrating trauma (e.g., missile projectile and knife wounds). Tracheobronchial injuries are rare. (They occur in fewer than 3% of victims of blunt or penetrating chest trauma, but the mortality rate is more than 30%.) A tension pneumothorax that does not improve following needle decompression or the absence of a continuous flow of air from the needle following decompression should alert the paramedic to the possibility of a tracheobronchial injury.
- Diaphragmatic ruptures may allow abdominal organs to enter the thoracic cavity. There they may cause compression of the lung, resulting in a reduction in ventilation, a decrease in venous return, a decrease in cardiac output, and shock.

REFERENCES

1. Rosen P, Barkin R: *Emergency medicine: concepts and clinical practice*, ed 6, St Louis, 2006, Mosby.
2. U.S. Department of Transportation, National Highway Traffic Safety Administration: *EMT paramedic national standards curriculum*, Washington, DC, 1998, The Department.
3. National Association of Emergency Medical Technicians: *PHTLS: prehospital trauma life support*, ed 7, St Louis, 2011, Mosby.
4. Recinos G, Inaba K, Dubose J, et al: Epidemiology of sternal fractures, *Am Surg* 75(5):401-404, 2009.

5. Bowman J: *Pneumothorax, tension and traumatic*, http://emedicine.medscape.com/article/827551-overview, accessed 10-8-10.
6. Wilson WC, Grande CM, Hoyt DB, editors: *Trauma, critical care*, vol 2, New York, 2006, Informa Health Care USA.
7. Lloyd D: *Thoracic trauma*, www.doh.wa.gov/hsqa/emstrauma/OTEP/thoracictrauma.ppt, accessed 3-21-10.
8. Maron BJ, Estes NA III: Commotio cordis, *N Engl J Med* 362(10):917-927, 2010.
9. Kirchhoffer JB, Ginsburg SH, Paris YM, et al: *Cardiac manifestations of a rare survivor*, http://chestjournal.chestpubs.org/content/114/1/326.full.pdf, accessed 3-21-10.
10. Sammet E: *Aorta: Trauma*, http://emedicine.medscape.com/article/416939-overview, accessed 10-8-10.

SUGGESTED READINGS

De Brito D, Challoner KR, Sehgal A, et al: The injury pattern of a new law enforcement weapon: the police bean bag, *Ann Emerg Med* 38(4):383-390, 2001.

Holmes JF, Sokolove PE, Brant WE, et al: A clinical decision rule for identifying children with thoracic injuries after blunt torso trauma, *Ann Emerg Med* 39(5):492-499, 2008.

43 Abdominal Trauma

OBJECTIVES

Upon completion of this chapter, the paramedic student will be able to:

1. Identify mechanisms of injury associated with abdominal trauma.
2. Describe mechanisms of injury, signs and symptoms, and complications associated with abdominal solid organ, hollow organ, retroperitoneal organ, and pelvic organ injuries.
3. Outline the significance of injury to intraabdominal vascular structures.
4. Describe the prehospital assessment priorities for the patient suspected of having an abdominal injury.
5. Outline the prehospital care of the patient with abdominal trauma.

KEY TERMS

Cullen's sign The appearance of irregularly formed hemorrhagic patches on the skin around the umbilicus.

Grey Turner's sign Bruising of the skin of the flanks or loin in acute hemorrhagic pancreatitis; also known as *Turner's sign.*

hematuria The abnormal presence of blood in the urine.

hemodilution The dilution of the blood of elements.

hemoperitoneum The presence of extravasated blood in the peritoneal cavity.

Kehr's sign Pain in the left shoulder thought to be caused by referred pain secondary to irritation of the adjacent diaphragm.

peritonitis Inflammation of the serous membrane that covers the abdominal wall.

ultrasound A diagnostic test that uses sound waves to make images of internal organs and structures; often used in the emergency department to view the peritoneal cavity for the presence of fluid or blood. Also known as a *sonogram.*

A bdominal trauma may be difficult to evaluate in the prehospital setting because of the wide spectrum of potential injuries to multiple organs. In addition, physical findings may be absent, minimal, or exaggerated. Patients may also have altered levels of pain perception as a result of preexisting conditions, shock, alcohol or other drug use, head injury, or other factors. Therefore the paramedic must have a high degree of suspicion based on the mechanism of injury and kinematics. Death from abdominal trauma usually is a result of ongoing hemorrhage and the delay of surgical repair.

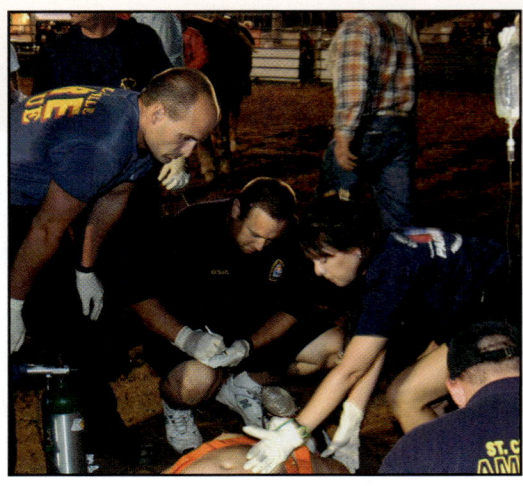

(Courtesy Ray Kemp., St. Charles, Mo.)

REVIEW OF ABDOMINAL ANATOMY

The structures of the abdomen were presented in Chapter 10. To review, organs in the abdomen include the intestines, kidneys, liver, gallbladder, pancreas, spleen, and stomach (Figures 43-1 and 43-2). In addition to these organs, the abdomen has many vascular structures. Some of these structures include[1]:

- Abdominal aorta
- Superior and inferior mesenteric arteries
- Renal artery
- Splenic artery
- Hepatic artery
- Iliac arteries
- Hepatic portal system
- Inferior vena cava

All abdominal organs and vascular structures are susceptible to injury. Quick recognition of injury, emergency care, and rapid transport for definitive care can tremendously alter morbidity and mortality.

LOOK AGAIN
See Chapter 10: Review of Human Systems, pp. 196-199.

MECHANISMS OF ABDOMINAL INJURY

Abdominal injury may result from blunt or penetrating trauma. Regardless of the organ injured, management usually is limited to securing the airway with spinal

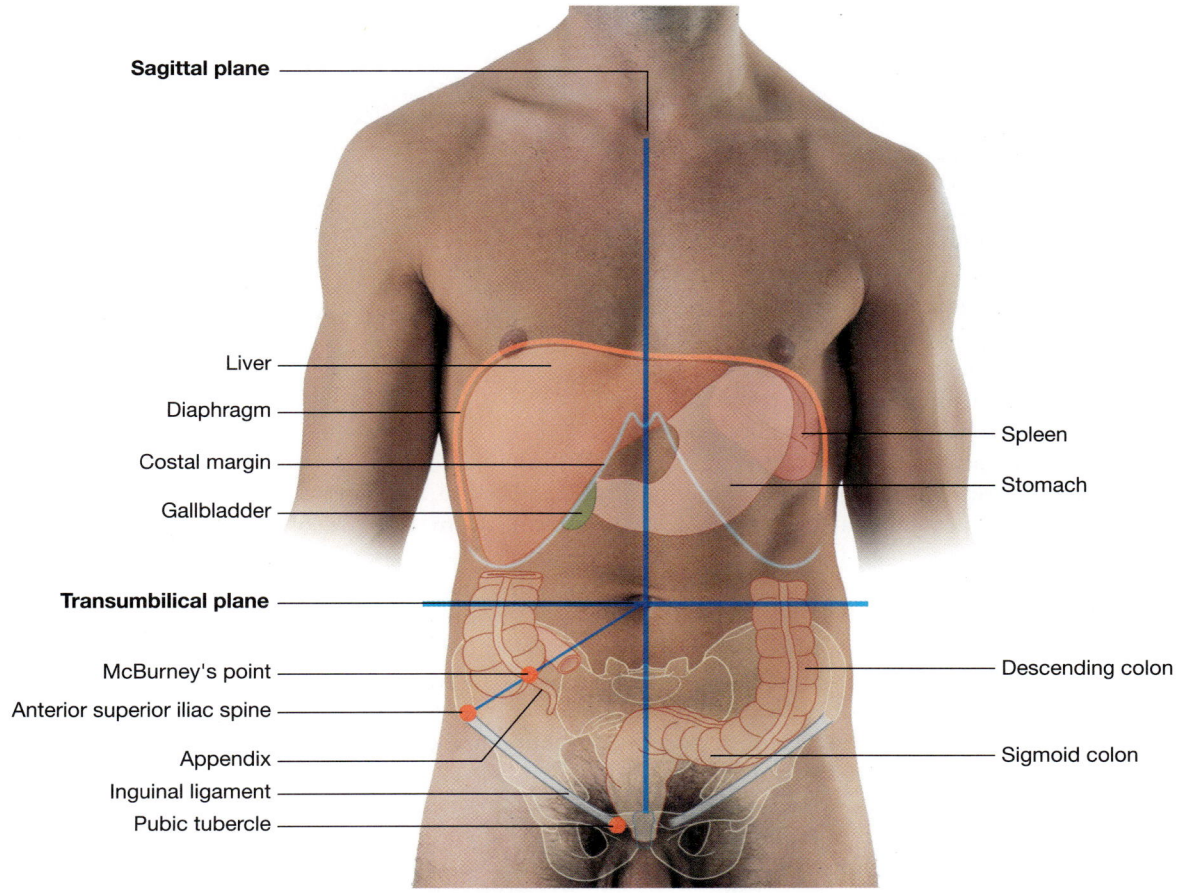

FIGURE 43-1 Abdominal quadrants and the positions of major viscera. Anterior view of a man. (From Drake R, et al: *Gray's anatomy for students,* ed 2, Philadelphia, 2010, Churchill Livingstone.)

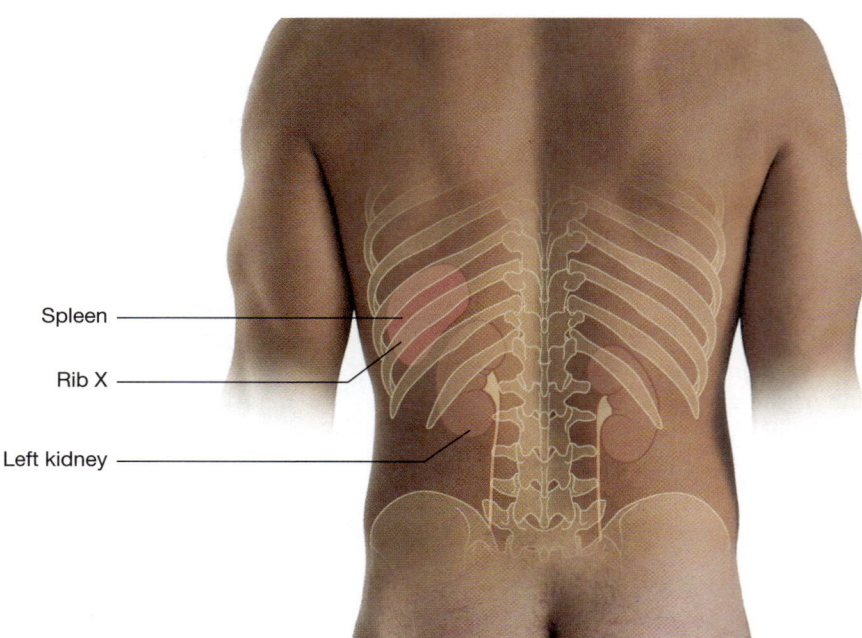

Spleen

Rib X

Left kidney

FIGURE 43-2 Surface projection of the spleen. Posterior view of a man. (From Drake R, et al: *Gray's anatomy for students,* ed 2, Philadelphia, 2010, Churchill Livingstone.)

precautions, providing ventilatory support, providing wound management, managing shock with fluid replacement and application of a pneumatic antishock garment (PASG) (per protocol), and rapidly transporting the patient for definitive care (Box 43-1).

The paramedic should be keenly aware of the kinematics and the mechanism of injury (described in Chapter 37) when evaluating a patient with abdominal trauma. For example, in the cases of a motor vehicle collision, the paramedic should note the extent of damage to the car; the patient's location within the car; whether the patient struck the steering wheel or dash; and if personal restraints were used properly. In the case of penetrating injury, the type, size, and direction of the penetrating object; the posture or position of the victim during the injury; and the amount of blood loss at the scene can provide valuable information to the receiving hospital.

Blunt Trauma

Blunt trauma to abdominal organs usually is caused by compression or shearing forces. Compression forces may cause the abdominal organs to be crushed between solid objects (e.g., between the steering column and the spinal vertebrae). Shearing forces may cause a tear or rupture of the solid organs or blood vessels. This occurs when the tissues are stretched at their points of attachment (stabilizing ligaments or blood vessels). The severity of injury usually is related to the degree and duration of force applied. It also is related to the type of abdominal structure injured (fluid filled, gas filled, solid, or hollow).

BOX 43-1 Prehospital Care for Abdominal Injury

1. Secure the airway with spinal precautions.
2. Provide ventilatory support.
3. Provide wound management.
4. Manage shock with fluid replacement and pneumatic anti-shock garment (per protocol).
5. Rapidly transport the patient for definitive care.

Blunt abdominal trauma may be caused by motor vehicle and motorcycle collisions (including injuries that result from the use of personal restraints), pedestrian injuries, falls, assaults, and blast injuries. The automobile is the major cause of blunt abdominal trauma (Figure 43-3). Automobile-automobile and automobile-pedestrian crashes have been cited as causes in 50% to 75% of cases, blows to the abdomen in about 15% of cases, and falls in 6% to 9% of cases.[2] Box 43-2 lists some signs of abdominal trauma.

CRITICAL THINKING
Young children are more susceptible to abdominal injuries than adults. Why?

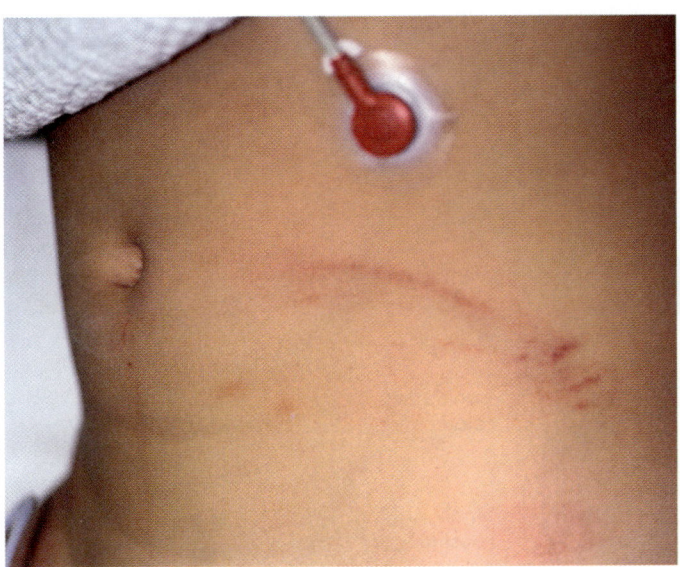

FIGURE 43-3 Marks of impact on the front-seat passenger in a car crash. (From National Association of Emergency Medical Technicians: *PHTLS: Prehospital trauma life support,* ed 7, St Louis, 2011, Mosby.)

BOX 43-2 Signs of Abdominal Trauma

Findings that raise the suspicion for abdominal trauma include[3]:
- Mechanism of injury consistent with rapid deceleration or significant compression forces
- Bent steering wheel
- Soft tissue injuries to the abdomen, flank, or back
- Shock without an obvious cause
- Level of shock greater than explained by other injuries
- "Seat belt signs"
- Peritoneal signs

Penetrating Trauma

Penetrating injury may result from stab wounds, gunshot wounds, or impalement. A major complication of this type of trauma is hemorrhage from a major vessel or solid organ. The amount of internal bleeding is related to the type and number of blood vessels injured and the vascularity of the solid organ. Penetrating injury also may cause perforation of a segment of bowel. As a rule, injuries caused by penetrating trauma do not have as high a mortality rate as those caused by blunt trauma. This is because injuries from blunt trauma are more difficult to diagnose. They are also often accompanied by injury to multiple organ systems.

SPECIFIC ABDOMINAL INJURIES

An abdominal injury may be classified as a solid organ, hollow organ, retroperitoneal organ, pelvic organ, or vascular injury (Figure 43-4).

Solid Organ Injury

Injury to solid organs usually results in rapid and significant blood loss. The two solid organs most often injured are the liver and spleen. Both of these organs are primary sources of life-threatening hemorrhage.

 CRITICAL THINKING

When does shock associated with injury to the liver or spleen develop?

LIVER

The liver is the largest organ in the abdominal cavity. Because of its location, it often is injured by trauma to the eighth through twelfth ribs on the right side of the body. It also is often injured by trauma to the upper central part of the abdomen. Injury to the liver should be suspected in any patient with a steering wheel injury, lap belt injury, or history of epigastric trauma. After an injury to the liver, blood and bile escape into the peritoneal cavity. This results in the signs and symptoms of shock and peritoneal irritation (abdominal pain, tenderness, rigidity). The liver is the second most commonly injured intraabdominal organ (the spleen is first). The liver is damaged in about 15% to 20% of blunt abdominal trauma cases, and in about 37% of cases of penetrating trauma.[4] The mortality rate for liver injury is 10%.[5]

SPLEEN

The spleen lies in the upper left quadrant of the abdomen. It is slightly protected by the organs that surround it medially and anteriorly. It also is protected by the lower portion of the rib cage. Injury to the spleen often is associated with other intraabdominal injuries. Splenic injury should be suspected in motor vehicle crashes and in falls or sports injuries involving an impact to the lower left chest or flank or to the upper left abdomen. About 40% of patients with splenic injuries have no symptoms. However, the patient may complain of pain in the left shoulder **(Kehr's sign)**. Pain in the left shoulder or left upper abdomen or generalized abdominal pain is thought to be caused by referred pain that occurs as a result of irritation of the adjacent diaphragm by a splenic hematoma or **hemoperitoneum.** The spleen is damaged in about 25% of cases of blunt abdominal trauma and in about 7% of cases of penetrating trauma.[6]

Hollow Organ Injury

Injuries to the hollow organs of the abdomen may result in sepsis, wound infection, and abscess formation, particularly if trauma to the intestine remains undiagnosed for an extended period. With injuries to solid organs, hemorrhage is the major cause of symptoms. In contrast, injury to the hollow organs results in symptoms from spillage of their contents (this spillage results in **peritonitis**) (Box 43-3).

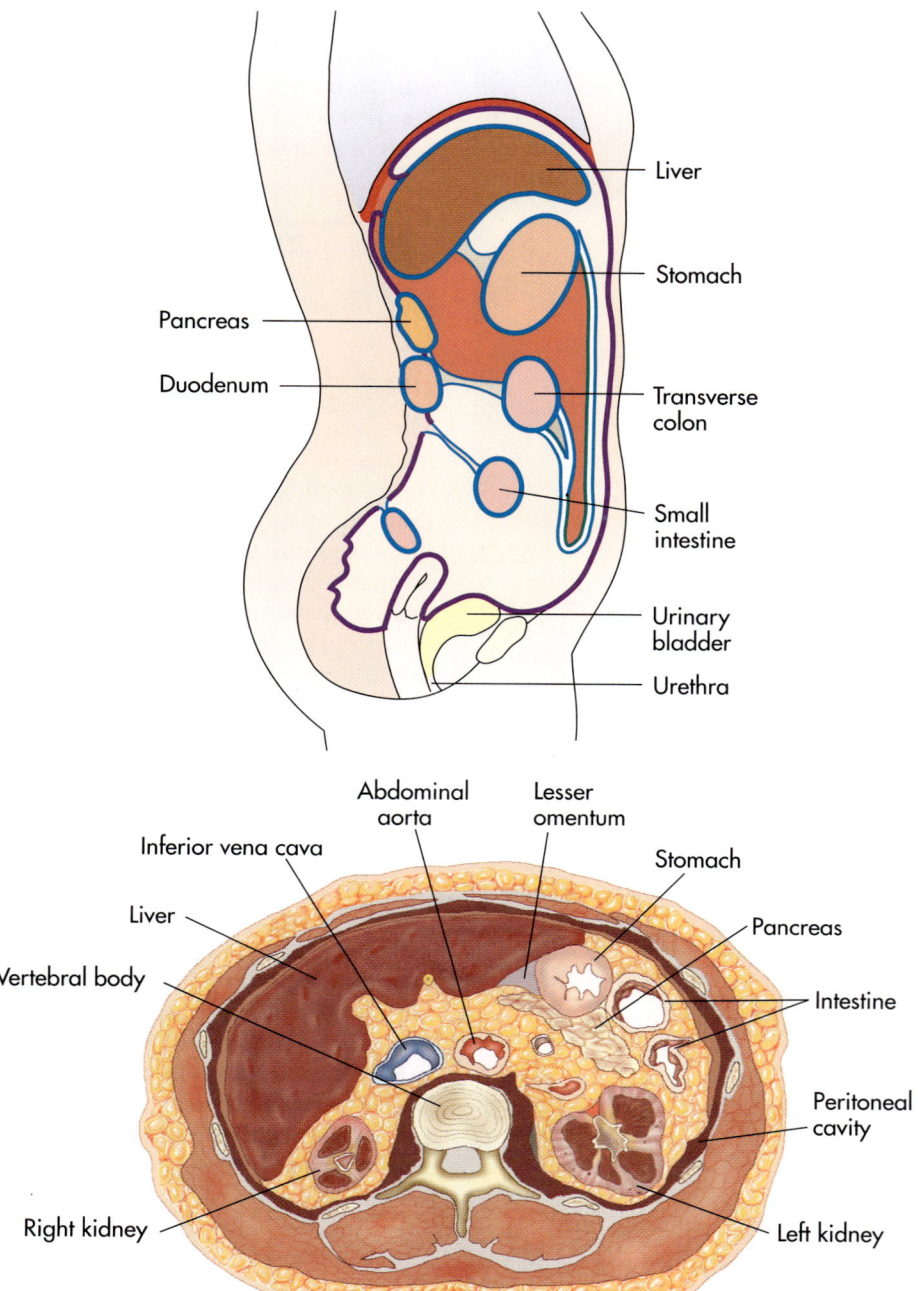

FIGURE 43-4 Hollow, solid, retroperitoneal, and pelvic organs.

STOMACH

Because of its protected location in the abdomen, the stomach is not often injured by blunt trauma. However, penetrating trauma may cause gastric transection or laceration. Patients with either of these injuries may show signs of peritonitis rather quickly as a result of leakage of acidic gastric contents. The diagnosis of injury to the stomach usually is confirmed during surgery or when nasogastric drainage returns blood. The stomach is damaged in about 1% of cases of blunt abdominal trauma and in 10% to 15% of cases of penetrating trauma.[5]

COLON AND SMALL INTESTINE

The colon and small intestine, like the stomach and duodenum, are more likely to be injured as a result of penetrating trauma than blunt trauma. (For example, the injury may be caused by a gunshot wound to the abdomen or buttocks.) However, the large bowel and small bowel also may be injured by compression forces in high-speed motor vehicle crashes. They also may sustain deceleration injuries associated with the wearing of personal restraints. Considerable force is required to cause an injury to the colon or small intestine. Therefore other injuries usually are present.

BOX 43-3 Peritoneal Irritation

Peritonitis usually is acute and quite painful. It may be delayed for hours or days after injury to a hollow viscus organ. It results from the spillage of enzymes, acids, and bacteria into the abdominal cavity. The spillage causes chemical irritation of the peritoneum. The peritoneum is the membrane that lines the wall of the abdomen and covers the abdominal organs. (Blood is not a chemical irritant to the abdomen.) The pain of peritonitis usually is localized (via somatic nerve fibers). However, it also may be diffuse. Signs and symptoms of peritonitis include the following:

- Pain
- Tenderness on percussion or palpation
- Guarding, rigidity
- Fever (if untreated)
- Distention (a late finding)

NOTE: The adult abdomen can accommodate 1.5 L of fluid without the belly looking bloated (abdominal distention).

Peritoneal contamination with bacteria is a common problem. With blunt abdominal trauma, the colon is damaged in about 2% to 5% of cases and the small intestine in about 5% to 15% of cases. The colon is damaged in about 25% of gunshot wounds and in about 5% of stab wounds. The small intestine is damaged in about 26% of these cases.[5]

Retroperitoneal Organ Injury

Injury to the retroperitoneal organs (kidneys, ureters, pancreas, duodenum) may occur as a result of blunt or penetrating trauma to the anterior abdomen, posterior abdomen (particularly the flank area), or thoracic spine. Hemorrhage within the retroperitoneal area may be massive (Figure 43-5). Most retroperitoneal hemorrhages result from pelvic or lumbar fractures. Retroperitoneal structures are damaged in about 9% of cases of blunt abdominal injuries and in about 11% of cases of penetrating trauma.[5]

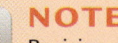 **NOTE**
Bruising of the flanks (**Grey Turner's sign**) or around the umbilicus (**Cullen's sign**) indicates retroperitoneal hemorrhage (Figure 43-5). However, these signs usually are delayed 12 hours to several days.

KIDNEYS

The kidneys are solid organs that lie in the retroperitoneal space. They may be injured by abdominal trauma. The trauma may cause minor lacerations and contusions (Figure 43-6) as well as major lacerations and fractures to the organ (Figure 43-7). These injuries can result in hemorrhage, extravasation of urine, or both. Contusions usually are self-limiting and usually heal with bed rest and forced fluids. Organ fractures and lacerations are more severe. They may require surgical repair, depending on which part of the kidney is damaged.

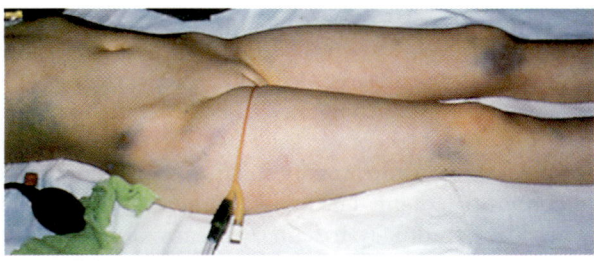

FIGURE 43-5 Bruising caused by rupture of the liver and right kidney. (From London PS: *A colour atlas of diagnosis after recent injury,* Ipswich, England, 1990, Wolfe Medical Publications, Ltd.)

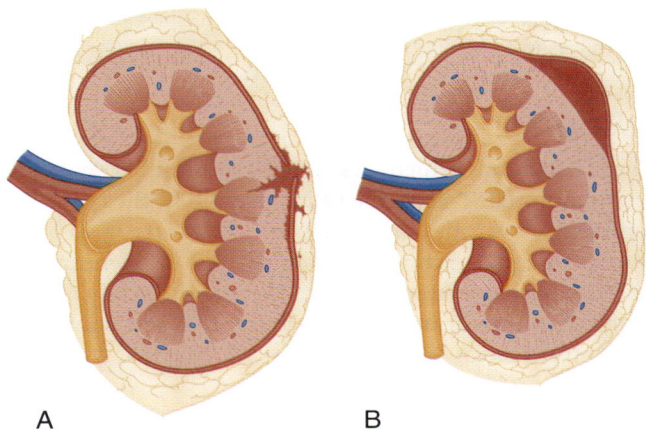

A   B

FIGURE 43-6 Minor renal injuries. **A,** Minor renal laceration. **B,** Renal contusion. (From Nicolaisen GS, McAninch JW, Marshall GA, et al: Renal trauma: re-evaluation of the indication for radiographic assessment, *J Urol* 133[2]:183, 1985.)

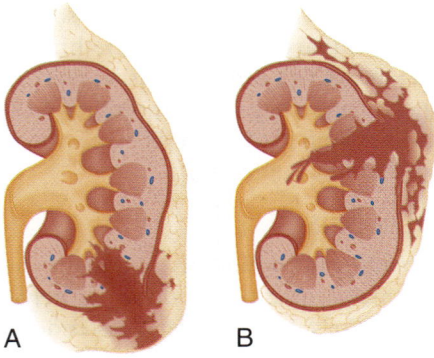

A   B

FIGURE 43-7 Major renal lacerations. **A,** Deep medullary laceration. **B,** Laceration into collecting system. (From Nicolaisen GS, McAninch JW, Marshall GA, et al: Renal trauma: re-evaluation of the indication for radiographic assessment, *J Urol* 133[2]:183, 1985.)

URETERS

The ureters are hollow organs that are rarely injured by blunt trauma. This is because of their flexible structure. When injury occurs, it usually is the result of penetrating abdominal or flank wounds (e.g., stab wounds, firearm injuries).

PANCREAS

The pancreas is a solid organ that lies within the retroperitoneal space. Injury to the pancreas is rare. When it occurs, it usually is caused by compressive or penetrating forces on the upper left quadrant, as in steering wheel and bicycle handlebar impalement. The pancreas more often is injured by penetrating trauma (particularly firearms) than by blunt trauma.

> **CRITICAL THINKING**
> What functions of the pancreas may be disrupted after injury? What might be the effects of spillage of pancreatic juices into the abdominal cavity?

DUODENUM

The duodenum, which lies across the lumbar spine, is seldom injured. This is due to its location in the retroperitoneal area, near the pancreas. When great force from blunt trauma or a penetrating injury occurs, the duodenum may be crushed or lacerated. Injury to this organ usually is associated with concurrent pancreatic trauma; it is confirmed through surgery.

Pelvic Organ Injury

Injury to pelvic organs (bladder, urethra) usually results from motor vehicle crashes that cause pelvic fractures. Other, less frequent causes of pelvic organ injury are penetrating trauma, straddle-type injuries from falls, pedestrian injuries, and some sexual acts. The pelvis supports and protects multiple organ systems. Therefore the risk of associated injury is high. The most common associated injuries are those to the urinary bladder and urethra. Fractures of the pelvis (Figure 43-8) often are associated with severe retroperitoneal hemorrhage. The mortality rate for pelvic fractures ranges from 6.4% to 19%[5] (pelvic fractures are further described in Chapter 44).

URINARY BLADDER

The urinary bladder is a hollow organ that may be ruptured by blunt trauma, penetrating trauma, or pelvic fracture. Rupture is more likely if the bladder is distended at the time of injury. With rupture, the integrity of the peritoneum may be disrupted. Urine may enter the peritoneal cavity. Bladder injury should be suspected in inebriated patients who suffer trauma to the lower abdomen. Gross hematuria (blood in the urine) may be present. The patient also may complain of being unable to void. The urinary bladder and surrounding structures are damaged in about 6% of cases of abdominal trauma.[5]

URETHRA

A tear in the urethra occurs more often in men than in women. It usually occurs as a result of blunt trauma associated with pelvic fracture. The patient may complain of

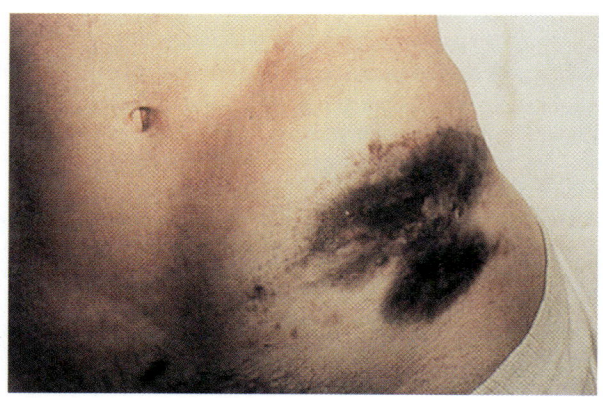

FIGURE 43-8 Massive swelling and bruising from a pelvic fracture. (From London PS: *A colour atlas of diagnosis after recent injury,* Ipswich, England, 1990, Wolfe Medical Publications, Ltd.)

abdominal pain and of being unable to urinate. Blood at the meatus indicates urethral injury. Passage of an indwelling urinary catheter is contraindicated in these patients.

VASCULAR STRUCTURE INJURIES

Injuries to arterial and venous vessels in the abdomen can be life threatening because of their potential for massive hemorrhage. These injuries usually are caused by penetrating trauma. However, they may also be the result of compression or deceleration forces on the abdomen. As in solid organ injury, vascular injury usually is marked by hypovolemia. In some cases vascular injuries are associated with a palpable abdominal mass. The major vessels most often injured are the aorta, the inferior vena cava, and the renal, mesenteric, and iliac arteries and veins. Injury to major vessels in the abdomen has a high mortality rate. Immediate surgical repair is often required.

> **CRITICAL THINKING**
> How can you attempt to manage shock when major vessels have been injured as a result of a severe pelvic fracture?

ASSESSMENT OF ABDOMINAL TRAUMA

The most significant sign of severe abdominal trauma is unexplained shock. The mechanism of injury and the classic presentation of hypovolemia are important indicators. Other signs and symptoms that should alert the paramedic to the possibility of severe abdominal trauma are abdominal wall injuries (e.g., bruising and discoloration of the abdomen, abrasions) and the following:

- Obvious bleeding
- Pain and abdominal tenderness or guarding
- Abdominal rigidity and distention
- **Evisceration** (Box 43-4)

BOX 43-4 Evisceration

Evisceration is the protrusion of an internal organ or the peritoneal contents through a wound or surgical incision, especially in the abdominal wall (Figure 43-9). The presence of an evisceration from abdominal trauma generally is associated with major abdominal injury. In the prehospital setting the wound is managed by covering the eviscerated contents with moist, sterile gauze or a dressing with an outer cover that is occlusive to prevent further contamination and drying. No attempt should be made to replace eviscerated organs into the peritoneal cavity; this would increase the risk of infection. It also would complicate surgical evaluation of the injury.

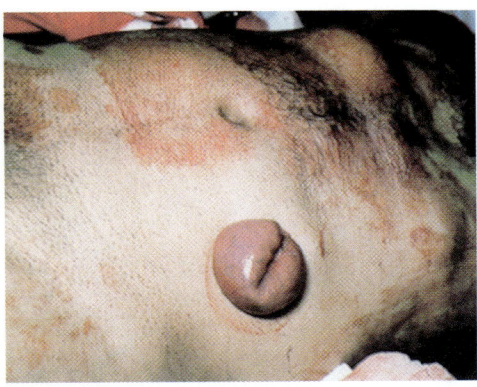

FIGURE 43-9 A loop of gut that emerged through a stab wound to the abdomen. (From London PS: *A colour atlas of diagnosis after recent injury,* Ipswich, England, 1990, Wolfe Medical Publications, Ltd.)

- Rib fractures
- Pelvic fractures

However, the absence of these signs and symptoms does not rule out an abdominal injury. The paramedic must maintain a high degree of suspicion based on the mechanism of injury.

NOTE

Assessment and management of abdominal trauma in children and older adults basically follow the same principles outlined in this chapter. Specific care considerations for pediatric and geriatric patients will be presented in Chapter 48 and Chapter 49. Trauma care considerations for pregnant patients will be presented in Chapter 46. Trauma that results from sexual assault will be presented in Chapter 50.

Focused History

When possible, a focused history should be obtained from the patient or a reliable source. Historical facts that may be important include events before the injury (e.g., use of seat belts; location in the vehicle), alcohol or other drug use, and underlying medical problems such as diabetes, cardiovascular disease, respiratory disease, or seizure disorder. Medication use (e.g., anticoagulants) and drug allergies can also be important in the course of the patient's care.

MANAGEMENT OF ABDOMINAL TRAUMA

Emergency care of patients with abdominal trauma usually is limited to two courses of action: (1) stabilizing the patient's condition and (2) rapidly transporting the patient to a hospital for physician evaluation and surgical repair of the injury.

The following are the most important components of on-scene care:

- A thorough scene survey to identify forces involved in abdominal trauma
- Rapid evaluation of the patient and the mechanism of injury

DID YOU KNOW?

An **ultrasound** uses sound waves to make images of internal organs and structures. Also known as a *sonogram,* the technology is often used in the emergency department to view the peritoneal cavity for the presence of fluid or blood. Advantages of a sonogram are that it can be rapidly performed at the patient's bedside, it does not interfere with resuscitation, and it is noninvasive and less costly than a CT scan. It also does not use ionizing radiation.

Although the test cannot differentiate the types of fluids that are present in the peritoneal cavity, any fluid in the trauma patient is presumed to be blood. The presence of fluid in one or more areas is considered a positive scan. These areas appear black on the monitor screen (Figure 43-10).

Note: Studies are underway to evaluate the efficacy of sonogram technology in the prehospital setting.

SHOW ME THE EVIDENCE

This multicenter study conducted in Frankfurt, Germany, sought to evaluate whether prehospital focused abdominal sonography for trauma (PFAST) was feasible and accurate. In 2002 to 2003 physicians and paramedics on ground and air ambulance performed PFAST on all patients with suspected abdominal trauma. The goal was to detect blood in the peritoneum. A total of 230 patients with a wide variety of mechanisms of injury were included in the study. In 219 (95%) cases, rescuers stated the exam could be performed without exceeding target on-scene times. In the other cases, the crews indicated the procedure extended scene times by 4 minutes. PFAST exams in 214 (93%) of the cases provided good or acceptable diagnostic images. Free blood was detected in the abdomen in 28 (14%) cases. There were 26 (11%) true positives, 1 false positive, and 2 false negatives. PFAST findings changed prehospital care in 42 (21%) cases. In 44 (22%) of the patients with positive findings the transport destination decision changed. Following this study, one air ambulance service in Germany implemented PFAST.

From Walcher F, Weinlich M, Conrad G et al: Prehospital ultrasound imaging improves management of abdominal trauma, *Br J Surg* 93:238-242, 2006.

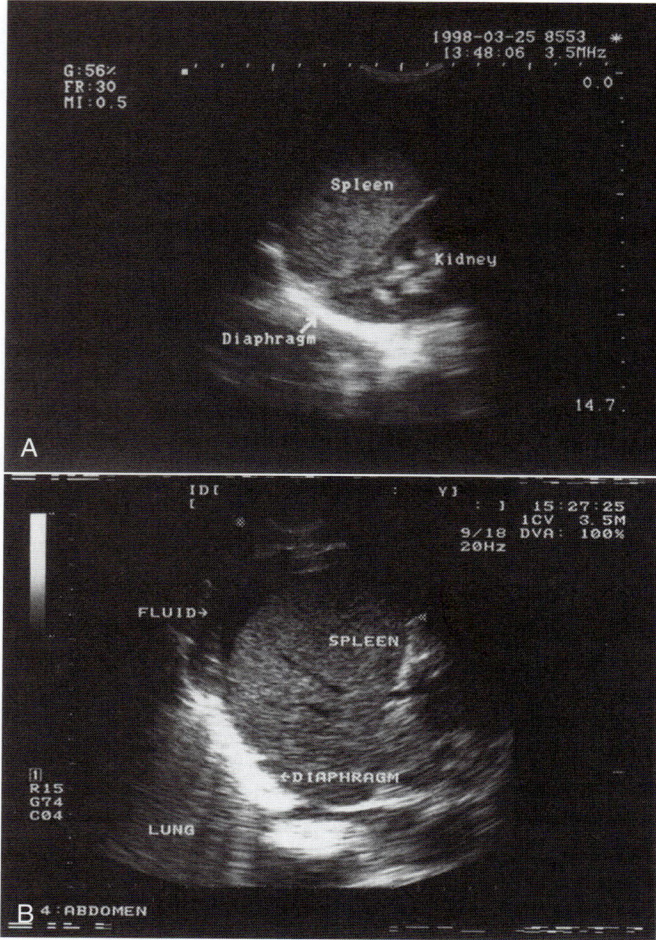

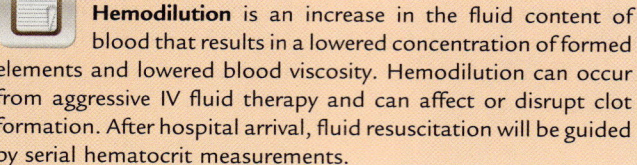

FIGURE 43-10 Abdominal ultrasound indicating trauma. **A,** Normal splenorenal view. **B,** The presence of fluid blood (black stripe next to spleen). (From National Association of Emergency Medical Technicians: *PHTLS: Prehospital trauma life support,* ed 7, St Louis, 2011, Mosby.)

- Airway maintenance with spinal precautions
- Administration of high-concentration oxygen ≥85%
- Ventilatory support as needed
- Reduction of hemorrhage by application of pressure

- Fluid replacement with volume expanders
- Use of a PASG (per protocol)
- Cardiac monitoring

Oxygen saturation should be maintained at or above 90%. The goal of fluid resuscitation for a patient with abdominal injury and hypotension is to maintain a systolic blood pressure between 80 and 90 mm Hg (mean arterial pressure of 60 to 65 mm Hg).[3] Aggressive fluid replacement in these patients can reinitiate bleeding in the abdomen from sites that had stopped bleeding from blood clots and hypotension. Therefore paramedics should strive to balance perfusion to vital organs without restoring blood pressure to normal limits.

> **NOTE**
>
> **Hemodilution** is an increase in the fluid content of blood that results in a lowered concentration of formed elements and lowered blood viscosity. Hemodilution can occur from aggressive IV fluid therapy and can affect or disrupt clot formation. After hospital arrival, fluid resuscitation will be guided by serial hematocrit measurements.

En route to the hospital, a full physical examination and ongoing assessment can be performed. These procedures should include vital sign assessment (and reassessment), and inspection, percussion, and palpation of the abdomen (see Chapter 20). Auscultation of the abdomen for the presence of bowel sounds can establish a baseline measurement for hospital personnel. This assessment is difficult and time-consuming in the prehospital setting and should never delay patient transport.

> **LOOK AGAIN**
>
> See Chapter 20: Secondary Assessment, pp. 542-546.

SUMMARY

- Blunt trauma to abdominal organs usually results from compression or shearing forces.
- Penetrating injury may result from stab wounds, gunshot wounds, or impaled objects.
- The two solid organs most commonly injured are the liver and the spleen. Both of these organs are primary sources of death from hemorrhage. Injuries to the hollow abdominal organs may result in sepsis, wound infection, and abscess formation.
- Injury to the retroperitoneal organs (kidneys, ureters, pancreas, duodenum) may cause massive hemorrhage.

- Injury to the pelvic organs (bladder, urethra) usually results from motor vehicle crashes that produce pelvic fractures.
- Injuries to abdominal vascular structures may be life threatening. This is due to their potential for massive hemorrhage.
- The most significant sign of severe abdominal trauma is the presence of unexplained shock.
- Emergency care of patients with abdominal trauma usually is limited to two courses of action. One is to stabilize the patient. The other is to rapidly transport the patient to a hospital for surgery to repair the injury.

REFERENCES

1. National Highway Traffic Safety Administration: *The National EMS Education Standards*, Washington, D.C., U.S. Department of Transportation/National Highway Traffic Safety Administration, 2009, DOT.

2. Rosen P, Barkin R: *Emergency medicine: concepts and clinical practice*, ed 6, St Louis, 2006, Mosby.

3. National Association of Emergency Medical Technicians: *PHTLS: prehospital trauma life support*, ed 7, St Louis, 2011, Mosby.

4. Khan AN, Vadeyar H, MacDonald S, et al: *Liver: trauma*, http://emedicine.medscape.com/article/370508-overview, accessed 10-8-10.

5. Peitzman A, Rhodes M, Schwab CW et al, editors: *The trauma manual: trauma and acute care surgery*, ed 3, Philadelphia, 2005, Lippincott.

6. Bjerke HS, Bjerke JS: *Splenic rupture*, http://emedicine.medscape.com/article/432823-overview, accessed 10-8-10.

SUGGESTED READINGS

Cotton BA, Jerome R, Collier BR, et al: Guidelines for prehospital fluid resuscitation in the injured patient, *J Trauma* 67(2):389-402, 2009.

Ruesseler M, Kirschning T, Breitkreutz R, et al: Prehospital and emergency department ultrasound in blunt abdominal trauma, *Eur J Trauma Emerg Surg* 35:341-346, 2009.

Zygowicz WM: *Anything but routine: responders answer unprecedented evisceration call*, JEMS.com, www.jems.com/news_and_articles/articles/jems/3301/anything_but_routine.html, accessed 4-17-10.

OBJECTIVES

Upon completion of this chapter, the paramedic student will be able to:

1. Describe the features of each class of musculoskeletal injury.
2. Describe the features of bursitis, tendonitis, and arthritis.
3. Given a specific patient scenario, outline the prehospital assessment of the musculoskeletal system.
4. Outline general principles of splinting.
5. Describe the significance and prehospital management principles for selected upper extremity injuries.
6. Describe the significance and prehospital management principles for selected lower extremity injuries.
7. Identify prehospital management priorities for open fractures.
8. Describe the principles of realignment of angular fractures and dislocations.

KEY TERMS

Achilles tendon The largest tendon in the body; connects the calf muscle to the heel bone; also known as the *tendon calcaneus.*

Achilles tendon rupture A complete tear through the Achilles tendon.

appendicular skeleton The bones of the upper and lower extremities.

axial skeleton The bones of the head, neck, and torso.

boxer's fracture Fracture of the fifth metacarpal bone from direct trauma to a closed fist.

Colles' fracture A fracture of the radius at the epiphysis within 1 inch of the joint of the wrist; it is easily recognized by the resultant dorsal and lateral position of the hand.

epiphyseal fracture A fracture involving the epiphyseal plate of a long bone.

epiphyseal plate The site of bone elongation; also known as the *growth plate.*

false movement An unnatural movement of an extremity, usually associated with fracture.

first-degree sprain An injury in which there is partial tearing of a ligament without joint disability.

fracture A break in the continuity of bone or cartilage.

joint dislocation An injury that occurs when the normal articulating ends of two or more bones are displaced.

luxation A complete dislocation.

nursemaid's elbow Subluxation of the radial head.

open fracture A break in a bone that has penetrated the soft tissue or skin; also known as *compound fracture.*

rigid splint A splint in which the shape cannot be changed.

second-degree sprain An injury that results from some stretching and tearing of ligaments.

soft splint A splint that can be molded into a variety of shapes and configurations to accommodate the injured body part.

sprain A partial tearing of a ligament caused by a sudden twisting or stretching of a joint beyond its normal range of motion.

strain An injury to the muscle or its tendon from overexertion or overextension.

subluxation A partial dislocation.

third-degree sprain An injury that results from severe stretching and tearing of ligaments.

torus The buckling of the cortex of bone.

traction splint A splint specifically designed for midshaft femoral fractures.

Volkmann's contracture A serious, persistent flexion contraction of the forearm and hand caused by ischemia.

*O*rthopedic trauma and related complications are very common complaints. These injuries account for a large number of the more than 100 million patients in the United States who seek emergency department care each year.[1] Trauma to an extremity is seldom life threatening. However, early recognition and management may prevent long-term disability.

>
> ### NOTE
> Extremity trauma usually results from motor vehicle crashes, falls, acts of violence, and contact sports. Prevention strategies include proper sports training (working with athletic trainers on the use of protective equipment), use of personal restraints, gun safety education, and fall prevention (e.g., high-rise window guards) (see Chapter 3).

REVIEW OF THE MUSCULOSKELETAL SYSTEM

As described in Chapter 10, the musculoskeletal system and associated neurovascular structures are made up of bones, nerves, vessels, muscles, tendons, ligaments, and joints. To review, the skeletal system contains 206 individual bones. These bones are divided into two categories: the axial skeleton and the appendicular skeleton (Figure 44-1, *A, B*). The axial skeleton consists of the skull, hyoid bone, vertebral column, and thoracic cage. The appendicular skeleton consists of the bones of the upper and lower extremities. It also includes the *girdles*, by which the extremities are attached to the body.

The muscular system provides for movement, postural maintenance (muscle tone), and heat production. The major types of muscles are skeletal, cardiac, and smooth muscle. Skeletal muscle is the most common type of muscle in the body and will be the focus of this chapter (Figure 44-2).

> ### LOOK AGAIN
> Chapter 10: Review of Human Systems, pp. 167-171.

CLASSIFICATIONS OF MUSCULOSKELETAL INJURIES

Injuries that result from traumatic forces to the musculoskeletal system include fractures, sprains, strains, and joint dislocations. Patients suspected of having trauma to an extremity should be managed as though a fracture exists. Problems associated with musculoskeletal injuries include the following:

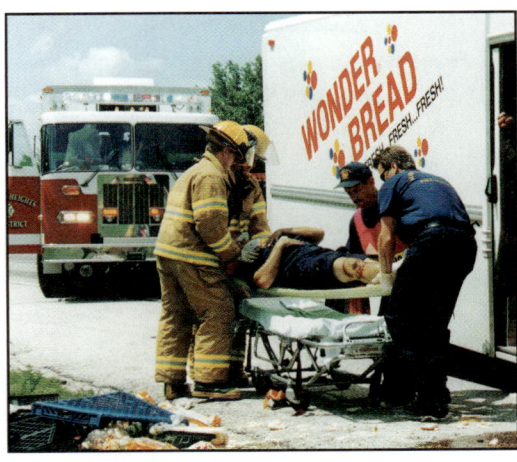

- Hemorrhage
- Instability
- Loss of tissue
- Simple laceration and contamination
- Interruption of blood supply
- Nerve damage
- Long-term disability

>
> ### CRITICAL THINKING
> How could long-term disability result from a musculoskeletal injury?

Musculoskeletal injuries can result from direct trauma (e.g., blunt force applied to an extremity), indirect trauma (e.g., a vertical fall that produces a spinal fracture distant from the site of impact), or pathological conditions such as some forms of arthritis and malignancy (described in Chapter 33). Paramedics should consider kinematics when caring for a patient with a musculoskeletal injury and carefully evaluate the scene (see Chapter 37).

Fractures

A **fracture** is any break in the continuity of bone or cartilage (Figure 44-3). It may be *complete* or *incomplete*, depending on the line of fracture through the bone. Fractures also are classified as *open* or *closed*, depending on the integrity of the skin near the fracture site (Box 44-1). Fractures of long bones may result in moderate to severe hemorrhage within the first 2 hours. As much as 550 mL of blood may be released in the lower leg from a tibial or fibular fracture, 1000 mL of blood in the thigh from a femoral fracture, and 2000 mL of blood from a pelvic fracture.[1]

As described in Chapter 10, the head of long bones in children is separated from the shaft of the bone by the **epiphyseal plate** until the bone stops growing. Fractures

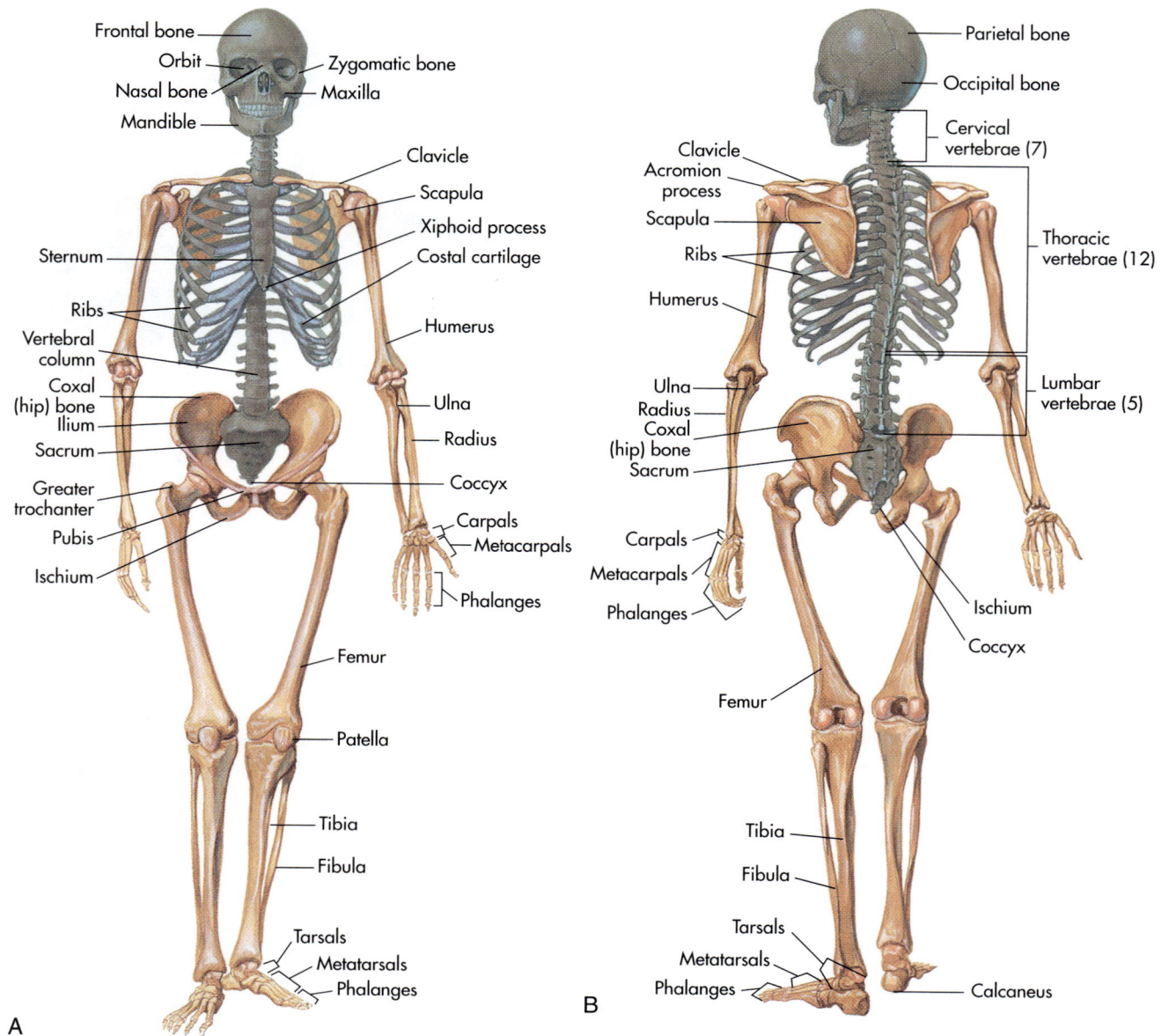

FIGURE 44-1 A, Skeleton, anterior view. Axial skeleton is shown in blue. Appendicular skeleton is bone colored. **B,** Skeleton, posterior view. Axial skeleton is shown in blue. Appendicular skeleton is bone colored. (From Christensen BL, et al: *Adult health nursing*, ed 6, St Louis, 2010, Mosby.)

that involve the epiphyseal plate are called **epiphyseal fractures.** These are serious injuries that may result in separation or fragmentation of the growth plate. They also may result in permanent bending or deformity of an extremity. This is known as **torus** (buckling of the cortex of bone) (Figure 44-4).

Sprains

A **sprain** is a partial tearing of a ligament (Figure 44-5). It is caused by sudden twisting or stretching of a joint beyond its normal range of motion (Figure 44-6). Two common

areas for sprains are the knee and the ankle. Sprains are graded by severity (Box 44-2). A **first-degree sprain** has no joint instability. This is because only a few fibers of the ligament are torn. Swelling and hemorrhage are minimal. (Repeated first-degree sprains can result in stretching of the ligaments.) A **second-degree sprain** causes more disruption than a first-degree injury. The joint usually is still intact, but swelling and bruising are increased. In a **third-degree sprain** the ligaments are completely torn. If third-degree sprains are accompanied by dislocation, nerve or blood vessel compromise to the extremity is possible. Some

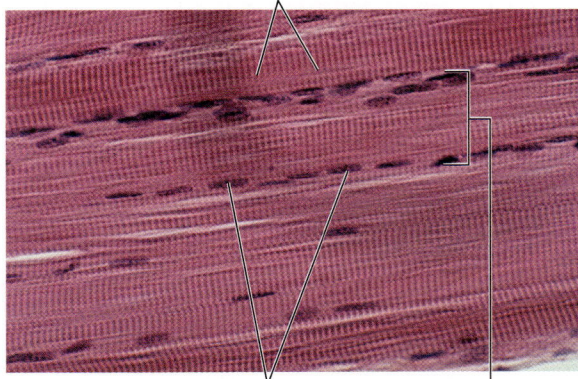

Cross striations of muscle cell

Nuclei of muscle cell   Muscle fiber

FIGURE 44-2 Skeletal muscle. (From Patton KT, Thibodeau GA: *Anatomy and physiology,* ed 7, St Louis, 2010, Mosby.)

second-degree sprains and most third-degree sprains have the same presentation as a fracture.

The application of ice to an injury during the first 24 hours generally reduces pain and swelling. After that time, heat (e.g., warm soaks) often is prescribed to increase circulation.

> **NOTE**
> Orthopedic injuries, including sprains, strains, fractures, and dislocations, can be quite painful for the patient. Per protocol, prehospital care may include the use of analgesics (*morphine, fentanyl, nitrous oxide*) before splinting or moving an injury.

Strains

A **strain** is an injury to the muscle or its tendon from over-exertion or overextension. Strains commonly occur in the back and arms and may be accompanied by a significant loss of function. Severe strains may cause an avulsion of bone from the tendon attachment site.

Joint Dislocations

A **joint dislocation** occurs when the normal articulating ends of two or more bones are displaced (Figure 44-7). Joints that often are dislocated are those of the shoulders, elbows, fingers, hips, knees, and ankles. Dislocation should be suspected when a joint is deformed or does not move with normal range of motion. A complete dislocation is called a **luxation;** an incomplete dislocation is called a **subluxation.** All dislocations can result in great damage and instability.

>
> **CRITICAL THINKING**
> Why do dislocations have a high rate of vascular or nerve damage?

BOX 44-1 Classification of Fractures

Open: A break in which a protruding bone or penetrating object causes a soft tissue injury
Closed: A break in the bone that has not yet penetrated the soft tissue or skin
Comminuted: A fracture that involves several breaks in the bone, resulting in multiple bone fragments
Greenstick: A break in which the bone is bent but only broken on the outside of the bend (common in children)
Spiral: A break caused by a twisting motion
Oblique: A break at a slanting angle across a bone
Transverse: A break that occurs at right angles to the long axis of the bone
Stress: A break (especially in one or more of the foot bones) caused by repeated, long-term, or abnormal stress
Pathological: A break resulting from weakness in bone tissue caused by neoplasm or malignant growth
Epiphyseal: A break that involves the epiphyseal growth plate of a child's long bone; may result in permanent angulation or deformity and may cause premature arthritis

---

BOX 44-2 Grading of Sprains by Severity

First-Degree Sprain
No joint instability
Minimal swelling/hemorrhage

Second-Degree Sprain
Joint usually intact
Increased swelling/ecchymosis

Third-Degree Sprain
Total disruption of ligaments
Possible nerve or vascular compromise

SIGNS AND SYMPTOMS OF EXTREMITY TRAUMA

The signs and symptoms of trauma to an extremity vary. They may be subtle complaints of discomfort. However, they also may include obvious deformity or open fracture. Field evaluation should be rapid, assuming significant injury. Common signs and symptoms of extremity trauma include the following:

- Pain on palpation or movement
- Swelling, deformity
- Crepitus
- Decreased range of motion
- **False movement** (unnatural movement of an extremity)
- Decreased or absent sensory perception or circulation distal to the injury (evidenced by alterations in skin color and temperature, distal pulses, and capillary refill)

>
> **CRITICAL THINKING**
> How can a paramedic differentiate a serious sprain from a fracture in the prehospital setting?

Pediatric fractures are seldom complete breaks. Rather, children's bones tend to bend or buckle because of increased flexibility. This flexibility is due to a thicker periosteum and increased amounts of immature bone.

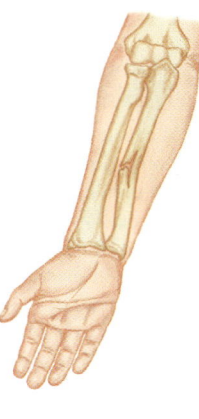

Greenstick

Break occurs through the periosteum on one side of the bone while only bowing or buckling on the other side. Seen most frequently in forearm.

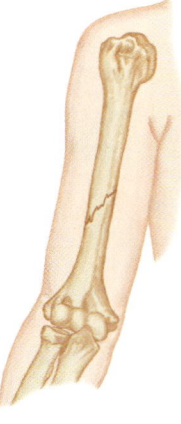

Spiral

Twisted or circular break that affects the length rather than the width. Seen frequently in child abuse.

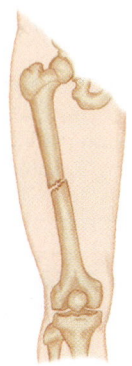

Oblique

Diagonal or slanting break that occurs between the horizontal and perpendicular planes of the bone.

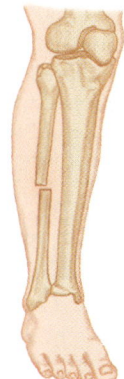

Transverse

Break or fracture line occurs at right angles to the long axis of the bone.

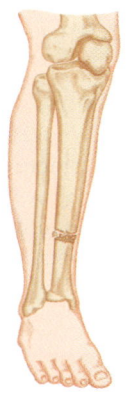

Comminuted

Bone is splintered into pieces. This is a rare occurrence in children.

Physeal growth plate injuries: Salter-Harris classification. Epiphyseal fractures are common in children.

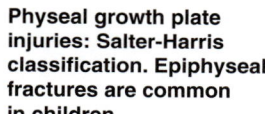

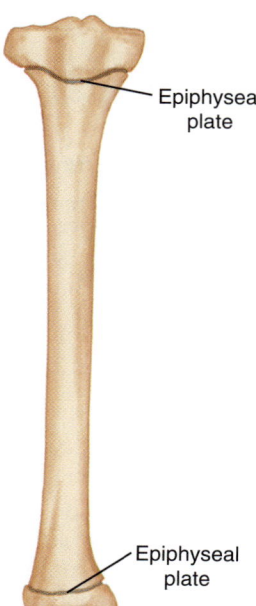

Epiphyseal plate

Epiphyseal plate

Type I

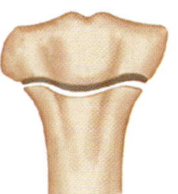

Epiphysis is completely separated from the metaphysis without fracture.

Type II

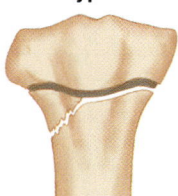

Transverse fracture extends through the separated epiphyseal plate, producing triangular break.

Type III

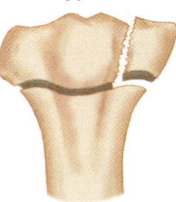

Fracture extends through part of the epiphyseal plate into the joint.

Type IV

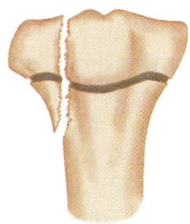

Fracture extends through the epiphyseal plate and through the metaphysis.

Type V

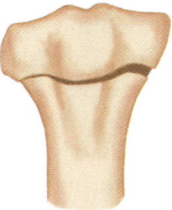

Epiphyseal plate is crushed, causing cell death in growth plate.

FIGURE 44-3 Bone fractures. **A,** Complete and incomplete. **B,** Comminuted and transverse. **C,** Impacted. **D,** Oblique and spiral. (Courtesy David J. Mascaro and Associates; from McKinney ES, et al: *Maternal-child nursing,* ed 3, St Louis, 2009, Saunders.)

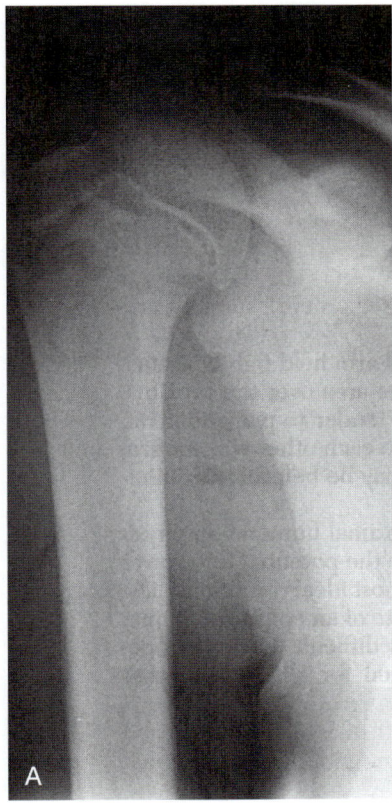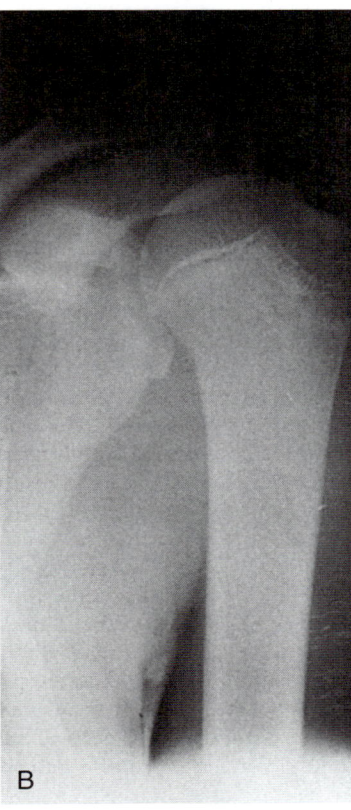

FIGURE 44-4 **A,** Fracture of the proximal humeral epiphysis. Normal left side (**B**) is included for comparison. (From Ferrera PC, Colucciello SA, Marx JA, et al: *Trauma management—an emergency medicine approach,* St Louis, 2001, Mosby.)

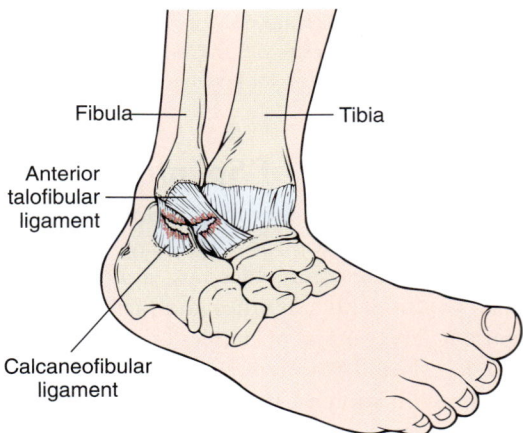

FIGURE 44-5 Ankle sprain. (From Frazier MS, Drzymkowski J: *Essentials of human diseases and conditions,* ed 4, Philadelphia, 2008, Saunders.)

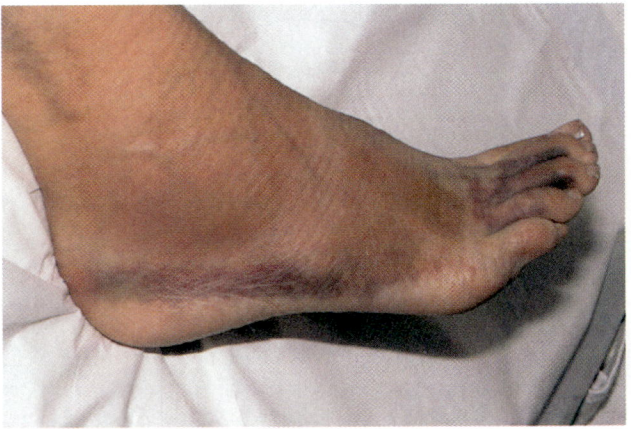

FIGURE 44-6 Swelling and bruising from a sprain of a lateral ligament. (From Ferguson DG, Fodden DI: *Accident and emergency medicine,* London, 1998, Churchill Livingstone.)

ASSESSMENT OF MUSCULOSKELETAL INJURIES

For the purposes of musculoskeletal assessment, patients can be divided into four classes:

- Those with life- or limb-threatening injuries or conditions, including life- or limb-threatening musculoskeletal trauma
- Those with other life- or limb-threatening vascular injuries and only simple musculoskeletal trauma
- Those with no other life- or limb-threatening injuries but with life- or limb-threatening musculoskeletal trauma
- Those with only isolated injuries that are not life or limb threatening

The paramedic should perform a primary survey to determine whether the patient has any conditions that pose a threat to life. Such conditions must be dealt with first. Paramedics must never overlook musculoskeletal trauma. In addition, a grotesque, but noncritical,

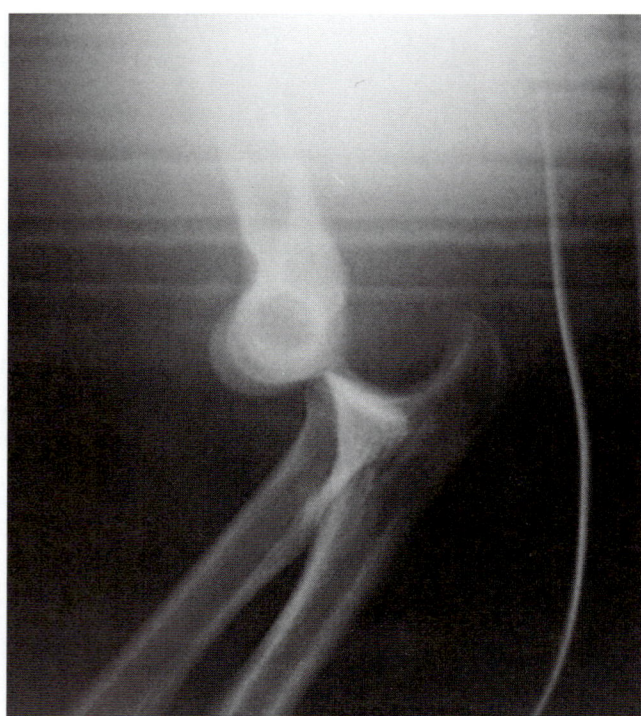

FIGURE 44-7 Posterior elbow dislocation. (From Ferrera PC, Colucciello SA, Marx JA, et al: *Trauma management—an emergency medicine approach*, St Louis, 2001, Mosby.)

musculoskeletal injury should never distract from the priorities of care.

> **NOTE**
> Orthopedic trauma can be a very painful injury. The paramedic should follow protocol established by medical direction for the use of analgesics to manage pain.

> **SHOW ME THE EVIDENCE**
> Researchers aimed to evaluate the effect of ethnicity, age, income, and gender on the administration of prehospital analgesia for isolated extremity injuries. This was a retrospective cohort study conducted in California in 2005. Of the 953 cases that met inclusion criteria and had complete data, 279 (29%) of the patients received morphine. The researchers found that patients were more likely to receive medication as their income increased. Women were less likely than men to receive prehospital analgesia. They also found a correlation between pain score and transport time—the higher the score and the longer the transport time, the more likely it was for patients to be medicated for pain.

From Michael G, Sporer KA, Youngblood GM: Women are less likely than men to receive prehospital analgesia for isolated extremity injuries, *Am J Emerg Med* 25(8):901-906, 2007.

Evaluation of an injured extremity should always include checking the *"six Ps": pain, pallor, paresthesia, pulses, paralysis,* and *pressure* (Box 44-3). The paramedic also should evaluate

> **BOX 44-3 Six P's of Musculoskeletal Assessment**
>
> **P**ain or tenderness
> **P**allor (pale skin or poor capillary refill)
> **P**aresthesia (pins-and-needles sensation)
> **P**ulses (diminished or absent)
> **P**aralysis (inability to move)
> **P**ressure

an extremity's neurovascular status by assessing the distal pulse, motor function, and sensation (before and after movement or splinting). In addition, the injury should be inspected and palpated for surface trauma, tenderness, and swelling. If possible, the assessment should include comparison with the opposite, uninjured extremity. If trauma to an extremity is suspected, the extremity should be splinted (Figure 44-8).

> **NOTE**
> This text presents methods to immobilize fractures and dislocations for isolated extremity injuries. Again, seldom does trauma to an extremity pose a threat to life. Therefore patients with multiple-system traumatic injury should first be managed for conditions that compromise the airway, breathing, and circulation (including internal and external hemorrhage in the extremities) and spinal stability. Rapid transport may be indicated by the patient's condition or mechanism of injury. If this is the case, injured extremities can be stabilized by fully immobilizing the patient on a long spine board.

General Principles of Splinting

The goal of splinting is immobilization of the injured body part. Immobilization by splinting helps alleviate pain; decreases tissue injury, bleeding, and contamination of an open wound; and simplifies and facilitates transport of the patient. The general principles of splinting are listed in Box 44-4. It should be noted that the principles of splinting and immobilization are the same for both children and adults. Special considerations for managing pediatric and geriatric patients will be addressed in Chapter 48 and Chapter 49.

TYPES OF SPLINTS

A wide variety of splints and splinting materials are available. Splints can be broadly categorized as rigid splints, soft or formable splints, and traction splints.

The shape of a **rigid splint** cannot be changed. The body part must be positioned to fit the splint's design. Examples of rigid splints include board splints, contoured metal and plastic splints, and some cardboard splints (Figure 44-9). Rigid splints should be padded before use to accommodate for shape and patient comfort.

A **soft splint** or *formable splint* can be molded into a variety of shapes and configurations to accommodate the

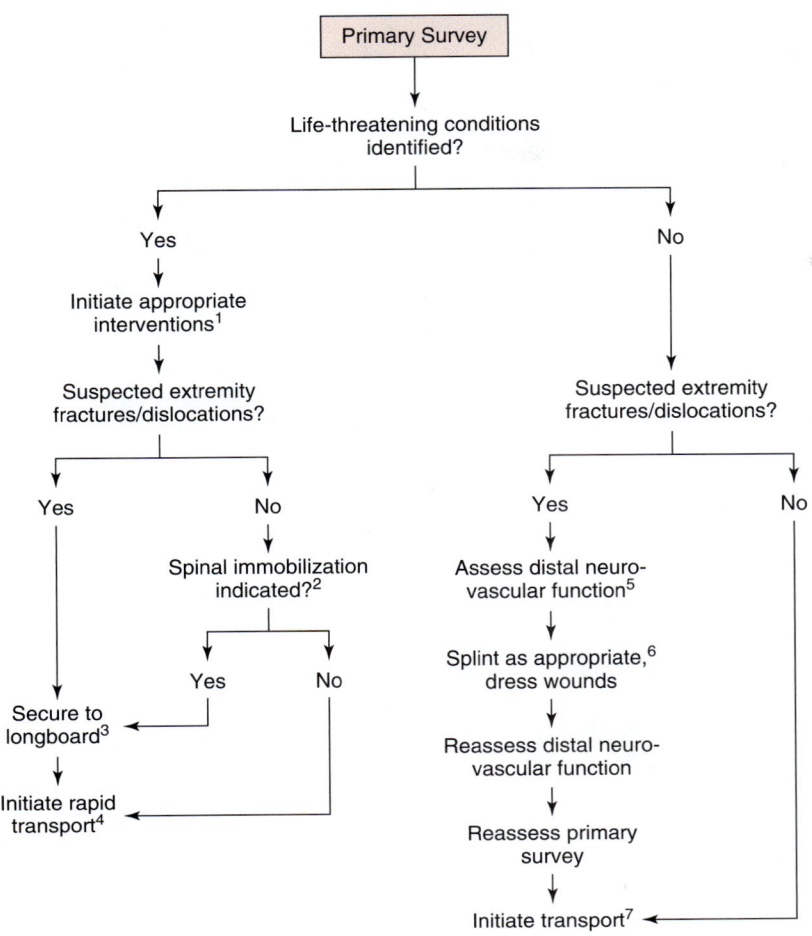

FIGURE 44-8 Evaluating extremity trauma. (From National Association of Emergency Medical Technicians: *PHTLS: prehospital trauma life support,* ed 5, St Louis, 2003, Mosby.)

[1]Airway management, ventilatory support, shock therapy.

[2]See Indications for Spinal Immobilization algorithm.

[3]Injured extremities are immobilized in anatomic position by securing to longboard.

[4]Transport to closest appropriate facility (trauma center, if available); assess distal neurovascular function and apply traction splint (if suspected femur fracture) as time permits.

[5]Assess perfusion (pulses and capillary refilling) and neurologic function (motor and sensory) distal to the suspected fracture or dislocation.

[6]Use appropriate splinting technique to immobilize suspected fracture or dislocation; if suspected midshaft femur fracture, apply traction splint.

[7]Transport to closest appropriate facility.

injured body part. Examples of soft or formable splints include pillows, blankets, slings and swathes, vacuum splints, some cardboard splints, wire ladder splints, and padded, flexible aluminum splints (Figure 44-10). Inflatable air splints also are considered soft or formable splints. However, they are not designed to be used for injuries to the knee or elbow.

A **traction splint** is specifically designed for midshaft femoral fractures. These splints do not apply or maintain enough traction to reduce a femoral fracture. However, they provide enough traction to stabilize and align it. They also are useful to tamponade bleeding and reduce pain. Examples include Thomas half-ring, Hare traction, and Sager traction splints (Figure 44-11).

UPPER EXTREMITY INJURIES

Upper extremity injuries can be classified as fractures or dislocations to the shoulder, humerus, elbow, radius and ulna, wrist, hand, and finger (Figure 44-12). Clavicular injury was discussed in Chapter 42. Most upper extremity vinjuries can be adequately immobilized with a sling and swathe.

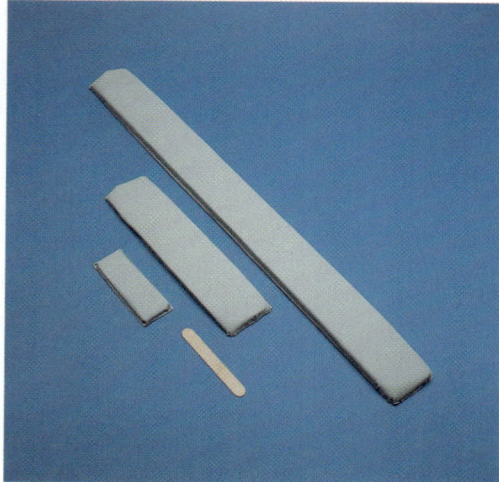

FIGURE 44-9 Rigid splints.

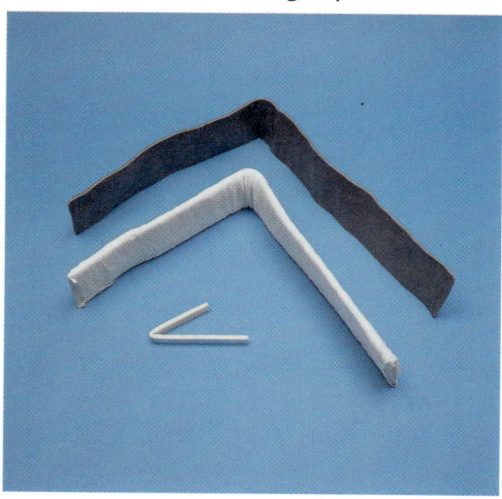

FIGURE 44-10 Formable splints.

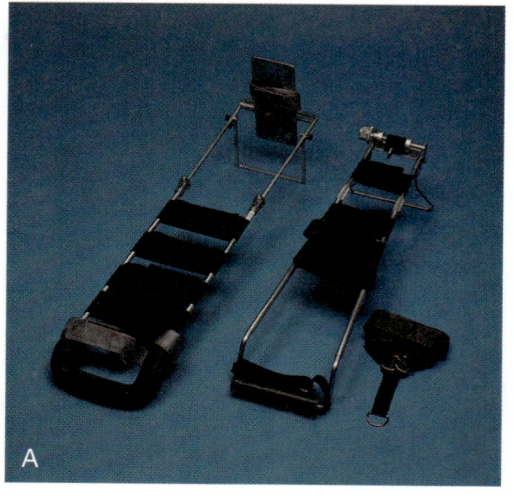

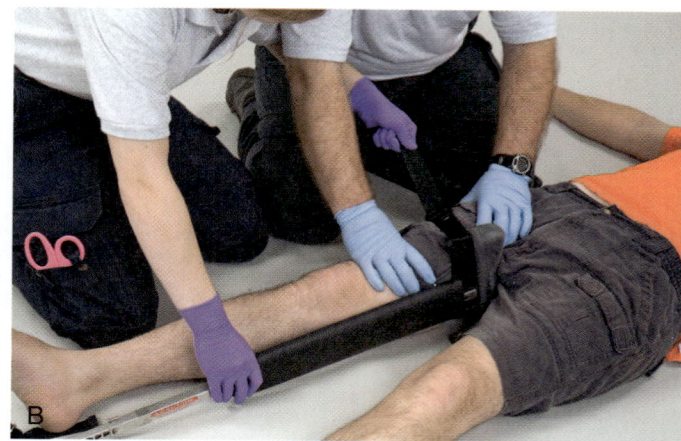

FIGURE 44-11 A, Traction splints. **B,** Unipolar traction splint. (B from Aehlert B: *Paramedic practice today: above and beyond,* St Louis, 2010, Mosby.)

BOX 44-4 General Principles of Splinting

1. Splint joints and bone ends above and below the injury.
2. Immobilize open and closed fractures in the same manner.
3. Cover open fractures to minimize contamination.
4. Check and document pulses, sensation, and motor function before and after splinting. Recheck frequently.
5. Stabilize the extremity with gentle in-line traction to a position of normal alignment.
6. Immobilize a long bone extremity in a straight position that can be splinted easily.
7. Immobilize dislocations in a position of comfort; ensure good vascular supply.
8. Immobilize joints as found; joint injuries are aligned only if no distal pulse is felt.
9. Apply cold to reduce swelling and pain. Give analgesics per protocol.
10. Apply compression to reduce swelling.
11. Elevate the extremity if possible.

NOTE: Immobilization requires a minimum of two rescuers. All splints should be well padded for patient comfort.

Shoulder Injury

Shoulder injuries are common in older adults. This is due to a weaker bone structure. Shoulder injuries often result from a fall on an outstretched arm. Patients with an anterior fracture or dislocation (accounting for 90% of cases) often have the affected arm and shoulder close to the chest (with the lateral aspect of the shoulder appearing flat instead of rounded). In addition, a deep depression between the head of the humerus and the acromion laterally ("hollow shoulder") may be visible. Patients with posterior fracture or dislocation may be found with the arm above the head. Other injuries that may affect the shoulder include *sternoclavicular strain* (that results from a direct blow or twisting of an extended arm) and *rotator cuff tendon injuries*. Rotator cuff injuries can be acute or chronic and usually involve the deltoid muscle. Injury to the rotator cuff can occur from a violent pull on the arm or abnormal rotation of the shoulder. They can also result from falls on an outstretched arm that tears and ruptures shoulder tendons. Management of shoulder injuries includes the following:

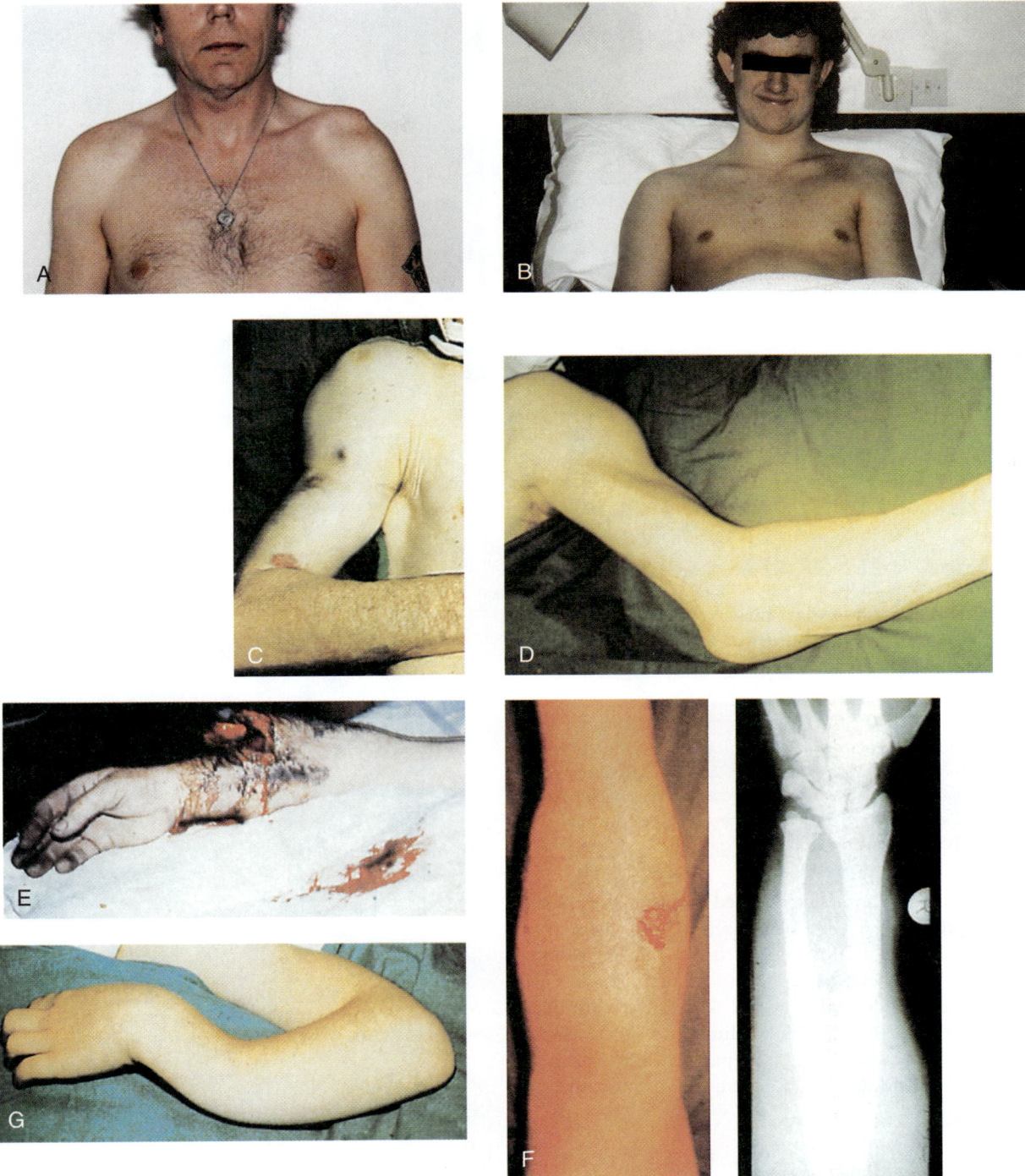

FIGURE 44-12 **A,** Complete separation of the left acromioclavicular joint. **B,** Anterior dislocation of the left shoulder. **C,** Fracture of the proximal humerus. **D,** Posterior dislocation of the elbow joint with marked deformity. **E,** Severe open fracture of the forearm. **F,** Penetration of the forearm caused by a nail gun. **G,** Greenstick fracture with marked deformity.

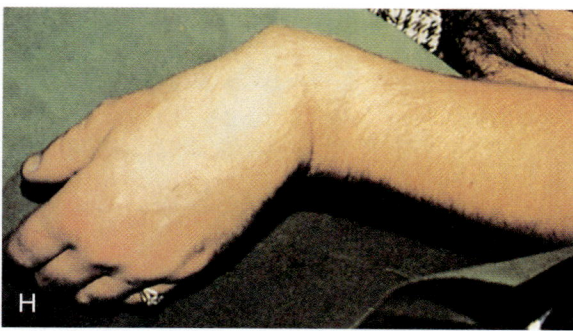

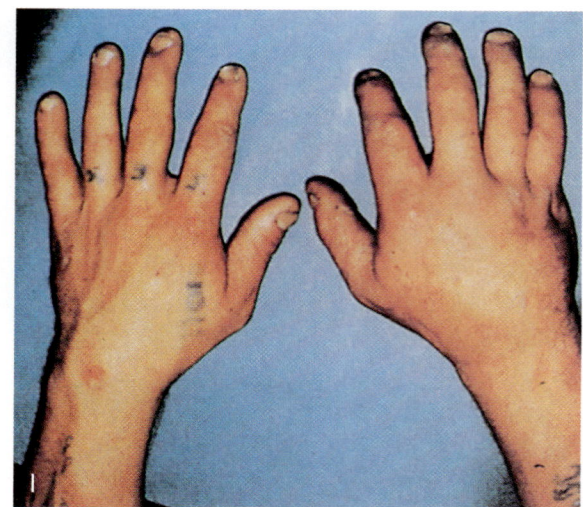

FIGURE 44-12, cont'd   **H,** Fracture of the distal radius. **I,** Hand injury from a motorcycle crash. (From Ferguson DG, Fodden DI: *Accident and emergency medicine,* London, 1998, Churchill Livingstone; C-H from London PS: *A colour atlas of diagnosis after recent injury,* Ipswich, England, 1990, Wolfe Medical Publications, Ltd.)

1. Assessment of neurovascular status
2. Application of a sling and swathe (Figure 44-13)
3. Application of ice

> **NOTE**
> Ice should be placed in a plastic bag and applied for 20-minute periods to the injury site, removed for 20 minutes, and then reapplied. If ice is not available, refreezable packs of gelled solution can be used in the short term, and may provide some comfort and reduce swelling.

Based on the position of the affected arm and shoulder, a makeshift splint may need to be devised to hold the injury in place. For example, with some fractures or dislocations, the paramedic may need to use a rolled blanket with a cravat at the center. The blanket roll is positioned under the elevated arm and secured like a sling. The arm is then swathed to prevent movement. If the patient's arm is positioned above the head, it should be splinted in position.

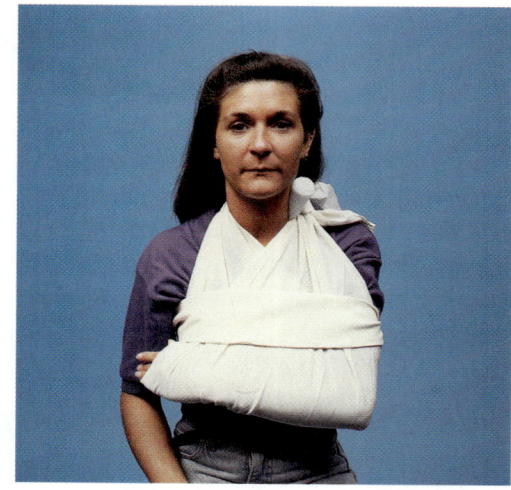

FIGURE 44-13 Immobilization of the shoulder.

Humeral Injury

Upper arm fractures are common in older adults and children. They often are difficult to stabilize. Radial nerve damage may be present if a fracture occurs in the middle or distal portion of the humeral shaft. A fracture of the humeral neck may cause axillary nerve damage. Internal hemorrhage into the joint also may be a complication. Management includes the following measures:

1. Assessment of neurovascular status
2. Realignment if vascular compromise is present
3. Application of a rigid splint and sling and swathe (Figure 44-14) or splinting of the extremity with the arm extended
4. Application of ice

Elbow Injury

Elbow injuries are common in children and athletes. They are especially dangerous in children. They may lead to ischemic contracture (**Volkmann's contracture**) with serious deformity of the forearm and a claw-like hand. The mechanism of injury usually involves falling on an outstretched arm or flexed elbow. Also, laceration of the brachial artery and radial nerve damage can occur. Management includes the following measures:

1. Assessment of neurovascular status
2. Splinting in the position found with a pillow, blanket, rigid splint, or sling and swathe (Figure 44-15)
3. Application of ice

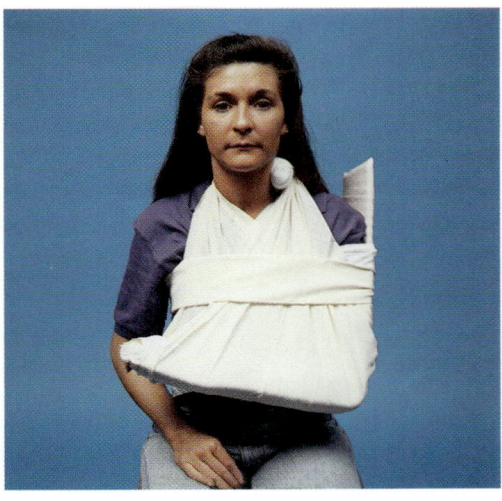

FIGURE 44-14 Immobilization of the humerus.

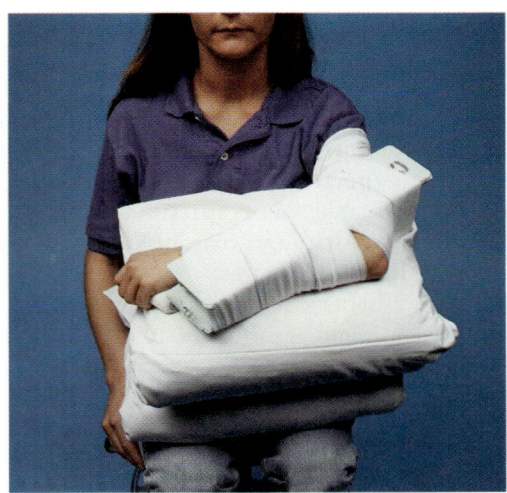

FIGURE 44-15 Immobilization of the elbow.

Radial, Ulnar, or Wrist Injury

As with most other upper extremity injuries, injuries to the radius, ulna, and wrist usually are the result of a fall on an

> **NOTE**
> Subluxation of the radial head (**nursemaid's elbow**) accounts for about 20% of upper extremity injuries in children and is seen in children ages 6 months to 5 years, most often in children in the 1- to 3-year-old age group. History of a pull on the arm or a fall is often reported. The child usually refuses to use the arm but does not seem in pain or distress.[2]

outstretched arm. Wrist injuries may involve the distal radius, the ulna, or any of the eight carpal bones. The most common wrist injury is a fracture with a "silver fork" deformity of the distal radius with dorsal angulation (**Colles' fracture**) (Figure 44-16). Forearm injury is common in both children and adults. Management includes the following measures:

1. Assessment of neurovascular status
2. Splinting in the position found with rigid or formable splints or a sling and swathe (Figure 44-17)
3. Application of ice and elevation

> **CRITICAL THINKING**
> What effect does a cold pack have on musculoskeletal injuries?

Hand (Metacarpal) Injury

Injury to the hand often results from contact sports, violence (fighting), and work-related crushing injuries. A common metacarpal injury is **boxer's fracture.** This results from direct trauma to a closed fist, resulting in fracture of

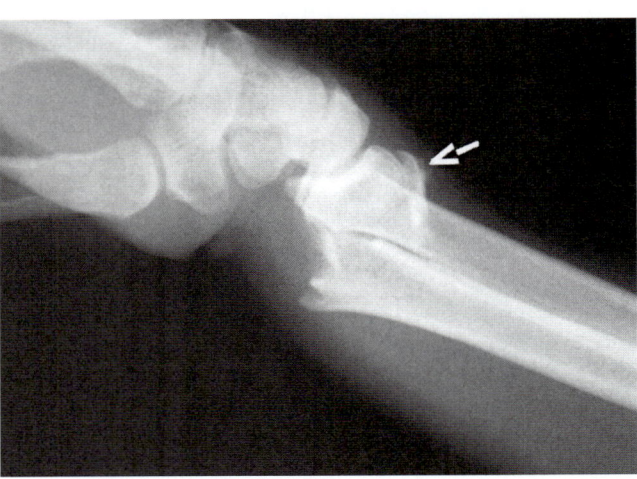

FIGURE 44-16 Colles' fracture (arrow shows dorsal angulation of distal radius fragment).

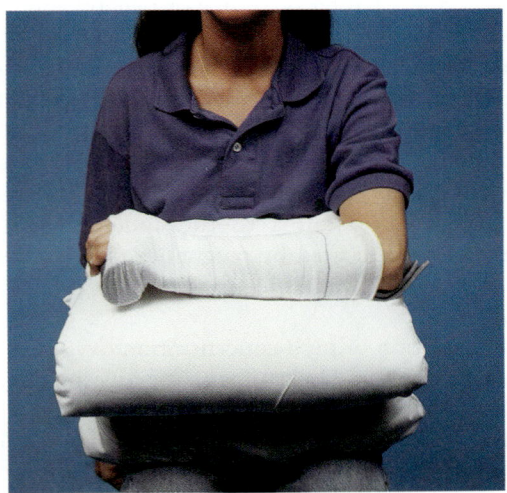

FIGURE 44-17 Immobilization of the forearm.

the fifth metacarpal bone (Figure 44-18). These injuries also may be associated with hematomas and open wounds. Boxer's fracture is the most common metacarpal fracture, but any of the metacarpals can be fractured, depending on the mechanism of injury. Hand injuries should be splinted in the position of function (as with a hand grasping a football). Rigid or formable splints (previously described for a radial, ulnar, or wrist injury) may be used. Management includes the following measures:

1. Assessment of neurovascular status
2. Splinting with a rigid or formable splint (pillow, blanket) in the position of function
3. Application of ice and elevation

Finger (Phalangeal) Injury

Injured fingers may be immobilized with foam-filled aluminum splints or tongue depressors. They also may be immobilized simply by taping the injured finger to an adjacent one ("buddy splinting") (Figure 44-19). Finger injuries are common. However, they should not be considered trivial. Serious injuries include fractures of the thumb. Also, any open or markedly comminuted fractures of the hand or fingers are serious. Management includes the following measures:

1. Assessment of neurovascular status
2. Splinting as previously described
3. Application of ice and elevation

LOWER EXTREMITY INJURIES

Lower extremity injuries include fractures of the pelvis and fractures or dislocations of the hip, femur, knee and patella, tibia and fibula, ankle and foot, and phalanx (Figure 44-20). Compared with upper extremity injuries, lower extremity injuries are associated with greater forces. They also are associated with more significant blood loss. They are more difficult to manage in patients with multiple injuries, and they may be life threatening (e.g., femoral and pelvic fractures).

Pelvic Fracture

As described in Chapter 43, blunt or penetrating injury to the pelvis may result in fracture, severe hemorrhage, and associated injury to the urinary bladder and urethra. The pelvis is surrounded by heavy muscles and other soft tissues. Therefore deformity may be difficult to see (Figure 44-21). Injury to the pelvis should be suspected based on the mechanism of injury or tenderness on palpation of the iliac crests (see Chapter 20). Trauma to the abdomen and pelvic area may be complicated by pregnancy (further described in Chapter 46). Management includes the following measures:

1. Administration of high-concentration oxygen
2. Management for shock (pneumatic antishock garment [PASG] per protocol)
3. Full-body immobilization on a long spine board or scoop stretcher (adequately padded for comfort)
4. Regular monitoring of vital signs
5. Rapid transport (essential)

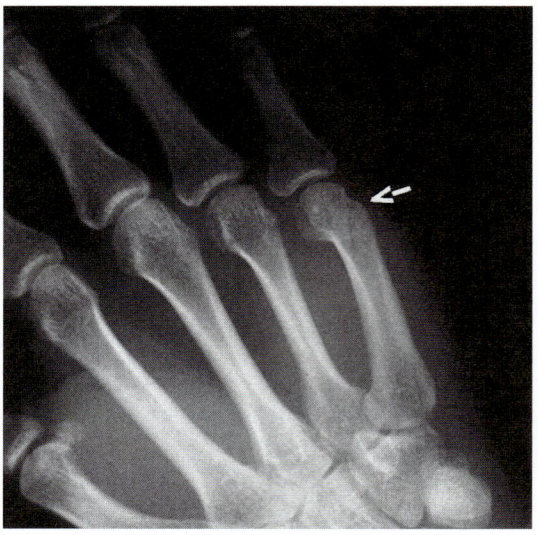

FIGURE 44-18 Boxer's fracture (*arrow*).

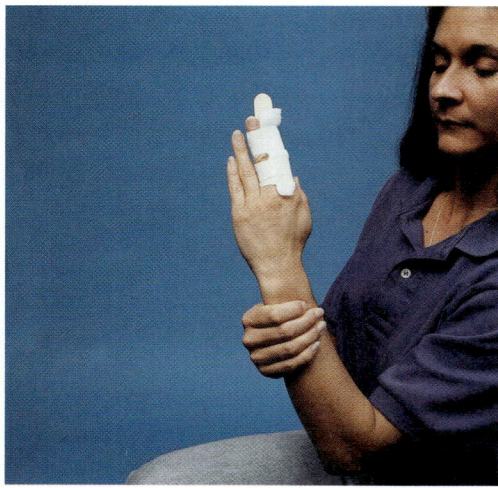

FIGURE 44-19 Immobilization of the finger.

> **NOTE**
>
> As described in Chapter 36, the pneumatic antishock garment (PASG) may help to arrest hemorrhage by tamponading bleeding vessels in the pelvis or lower extremities. It also may be used to stabilize pelvic and lower extremity fractures in the presence of hypotension (SBP < 90 mm Hg).[3] Decisions on the use of the PASG are made per local protocol and according to medical direction. Commercial pelvic stabilization devices ("pelvic binders") are also available to immobilize unstable pelvic fractures. Examples include the Trauma Pelvic Orthotic Device (T-POD) and the SAM Pelvic Sling (Figure 44-22). Pelvic binders are most appropriate to stabilize pelvic fractures that have been confirmed by x-ray.[6]

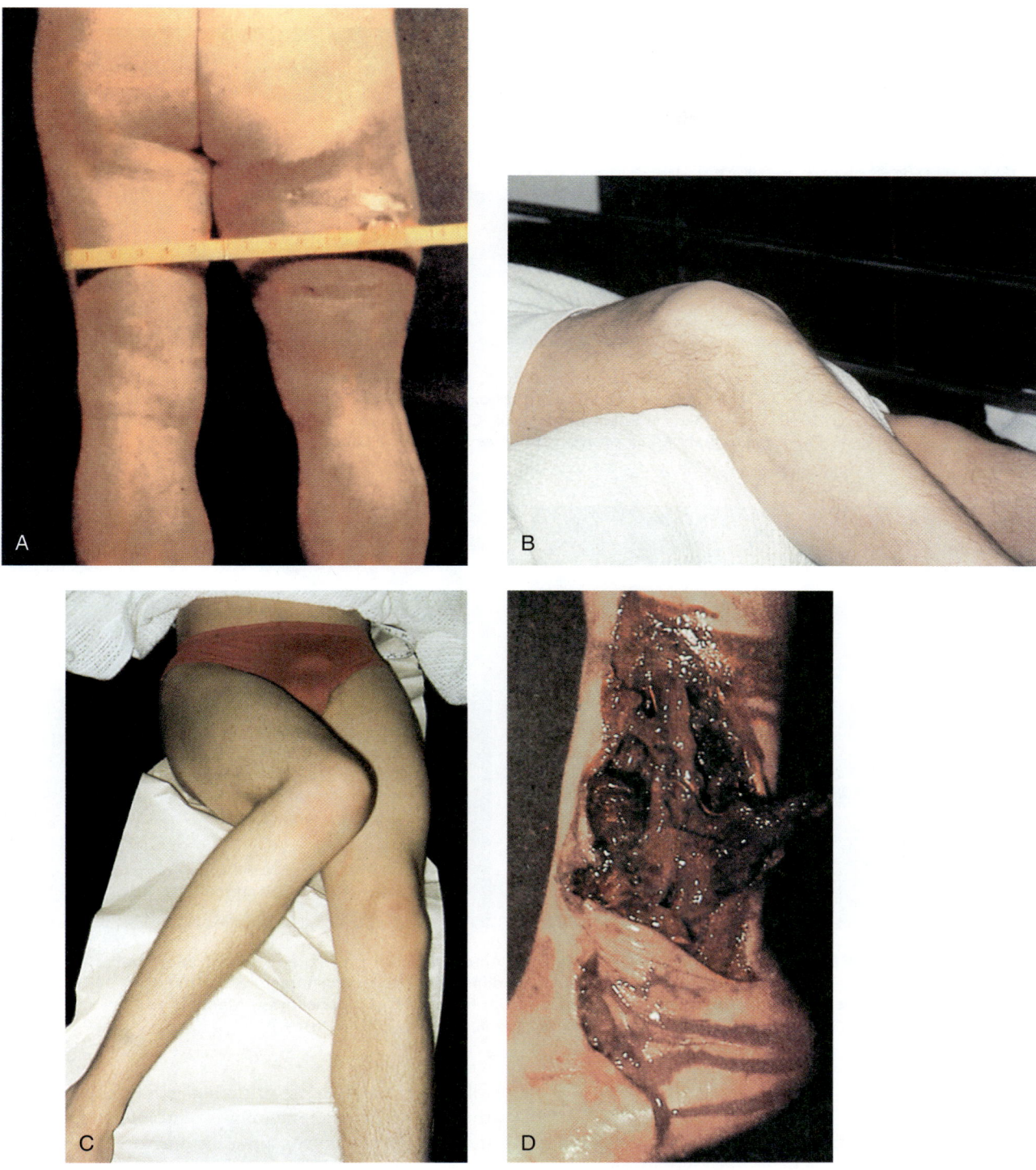

FIGURE 44-20 A, The diameter of the right thigh represents an increase in volume of 2 to 3 L of blood. **B,** Lateral dislocation of the right patella. **C,** Posterior dislocation of the right hip. **D,** Open fracture of the lower leg.

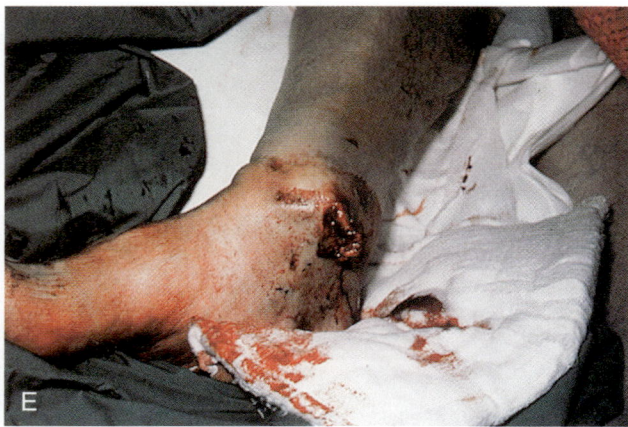

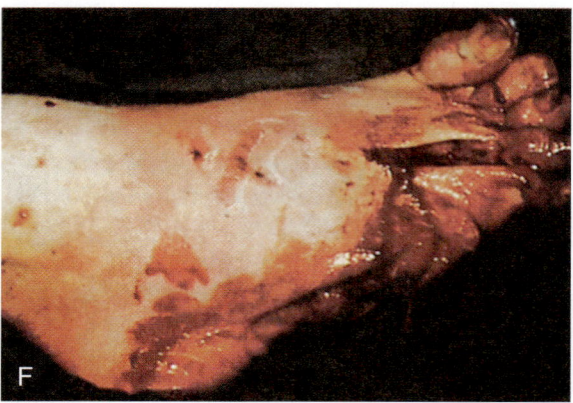

FIGURE 44-20, cont'd E, Subtalar dislocation. F, Foot that was run over by the wheel of a railway coach. (A, B, D, F from London PS: *A colour atlas of diagnosis after recent injury,* Ipswich, England, 1990, Wolfe Medical Publications, Ltd.; C, E from Ferrera PC, Colucciello SA, Marx JA, et al: *Trauma management—an emergency medicine approach,* St Louis, 2001, Mosby.)

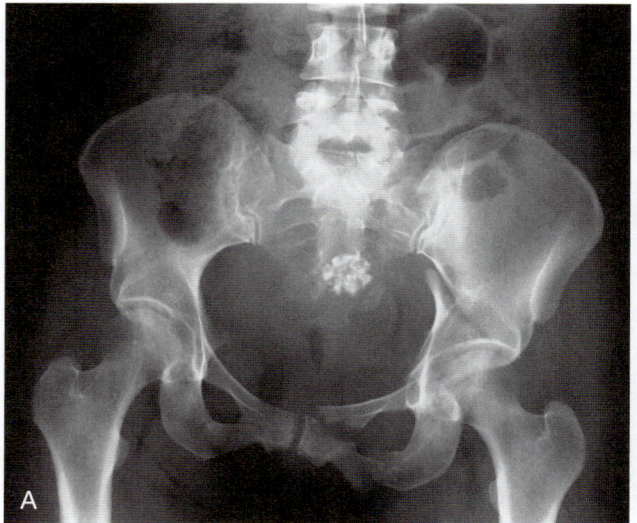

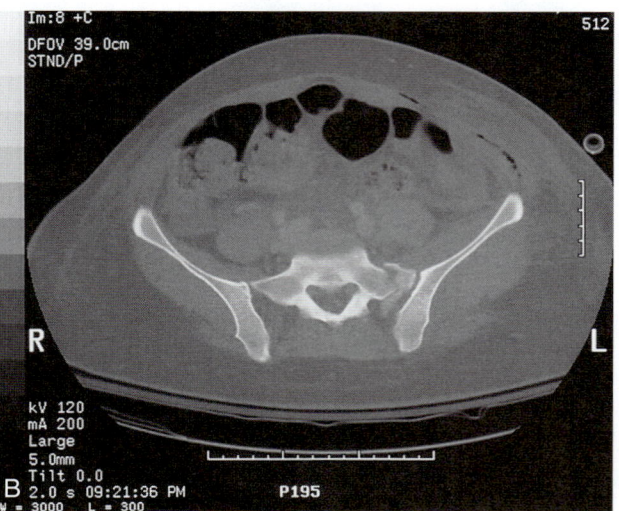

FIGURE 44-21 Lateral compression injury. A, Anteroposterior projection demonstrating the characteristic horizontal anterior ring fracture and ipsilateral sacral crush fracture. B, The sacral fracture is well visualized on the pelvic CT. (From Ferrera PC, Colucciello SA, Marx JA, et al: *Trauma management—an emergency medicine approach,* St Louis, 2001, Mosby.)

Hip Injury

Hip injuries commonly occur in older adults as a result of a fall. They also are common in younger patients as a result of major trauma. If the hip is fractured at the femoral head and neck, the affected leg usually is shortened and externally rotated. By comparison, with hip dislocation the affected leg is usually shortened and internally rotated (Figure 44-23). (Fractures closer to the head of the femur may manifest similar to an anterior hip dislocation, with a shortened and internally rotated leg.)

Hip fractures are serious injuries, especially in older patients. Complications from the injury can be life threatening. About 25% of older patients die within the first year following injury.[1] Most of these deaths result from venous thromboembolism, pneumonia, and infection. The majority of patients who sustain a hip fracture will require prolonged specialized care, such as a long-term nursing or rehabilitation facility. Less than 30% of patients who sustain a fractured hip will return to their preinjury level of activity.[4] Prehospital management of hip fracture includes the following measures:

1. Assessment of neurovascular status
2. Splinting with a long spine board or scoop stretcher (Figure 44-24) and generously padding the patient for comfort during transport (slight flexion of the knee or padding beneath the knee may improve comfort)
3. Frequent monitoring of vital signs

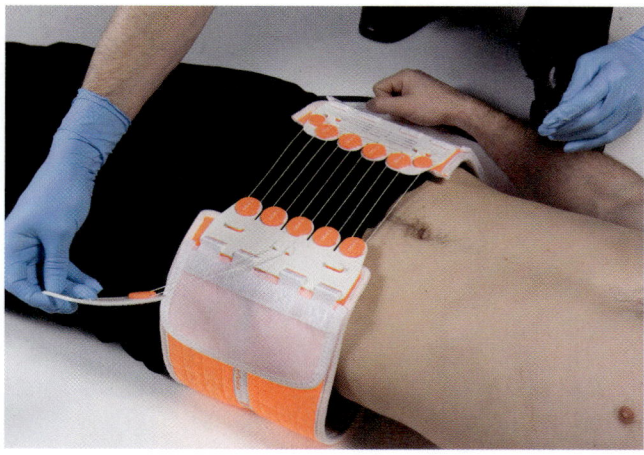

FIGURE 44-22 Pelvic stabilization device. (Courtesy Ray Kemp, St Charles, Mo.)

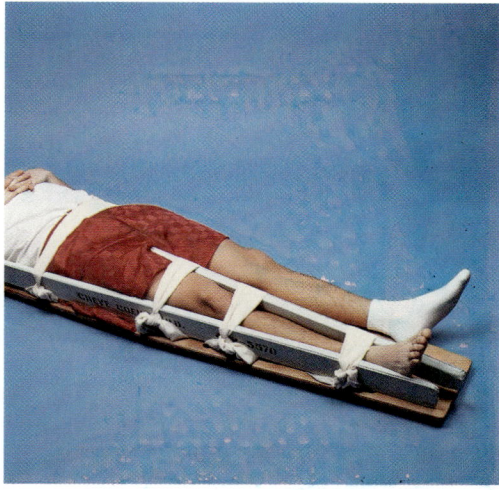

FIGURE 44-24 Immobilization of the hip.

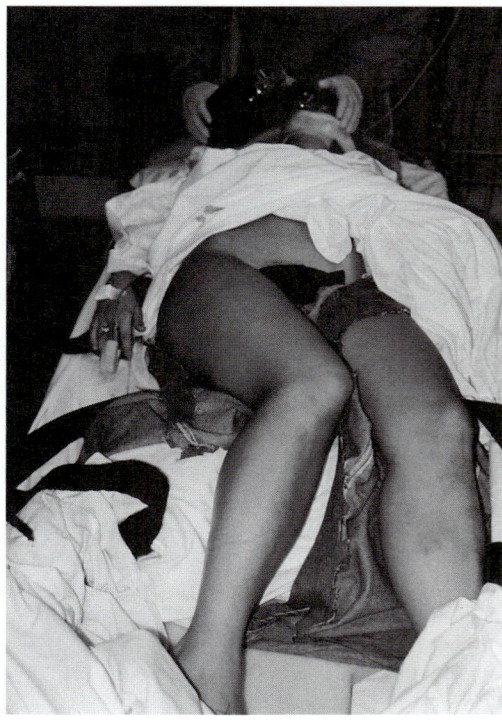

FIGURE 44-23 Young woman with internal rotation, adduction, and shortening of right femur, consistent with her right posterior hip dislocation. (From Ferrera PC, Colucciello SA, Marx JA, et al: *Trauma management—an emergency medicine approach,* St Louis, 2001, Mosby.)

Femoral Injury

Injury to the femur usually results from major trauma, such as may occur with motor vehicle crashes and pedestrian injuries. It also is a fairly common result of child abuse, accounting for 30% of femur fractures in children younger than 4 years of age.[5]

Fractures of the femur result in powerful thigh muscle contractions. These contractions cause the bone fragments to move back and forth over each other. The patient generally has a shortened leg that is externally rotated and midthigh swelling from hemorrhage, which can be life threatening (Figure 44-25). These fractures should be immobilized in the field with a traction splint. Management includes the following measures:

1. Administration of high-concentration oxygen
2. Management for shock
3. Assessment of neurovascular status
4. Application of a traction splint (Figure 44-26)
5. Regular monitoring of vital signs

> **NOTE**
> Traction splints should be used only to immobilize midshaft femoral fractures. They should not be used with fractures of the lower third of the leg, pelvic fractures, hip injury, knee injury, or avulsion or amputation of the ankle and foot. These splints should not be applied if the patient has life-threatening injuries. Rather, the patient should be secured on a long spine board and rapidly transported for definitive care.[6]

When more than one injury contributes to the development of shock, the PASG and traction splint may be used together (per local protocol for the use of the PASG). The traction splint should be applied over the PASG only after it has been inflated. Traction devices placed under the PASG may promote continued hemorrhage, tissue damage, and compromised circulation to the injured extremity.

Knee and Patellar Injury

Fractures of the knee (supracondylar fracture of the femur, intraarticular fracture of the femur or tibia) and fractures and dislocations of the patella commonly result from

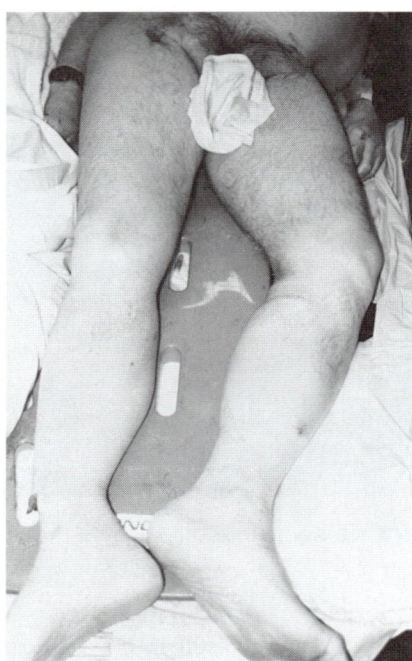

FIGURE 44-25 Young man with external rotation, abduction, and shortening of the left femur, consistent with his midshaft fracture. Also note right tibia fracture. (From Ferrera PC, Colucciello SA, Marx JA, et al: *Trauma management—an emergency medicine approach,* St Louis, 2001, Mosby.)

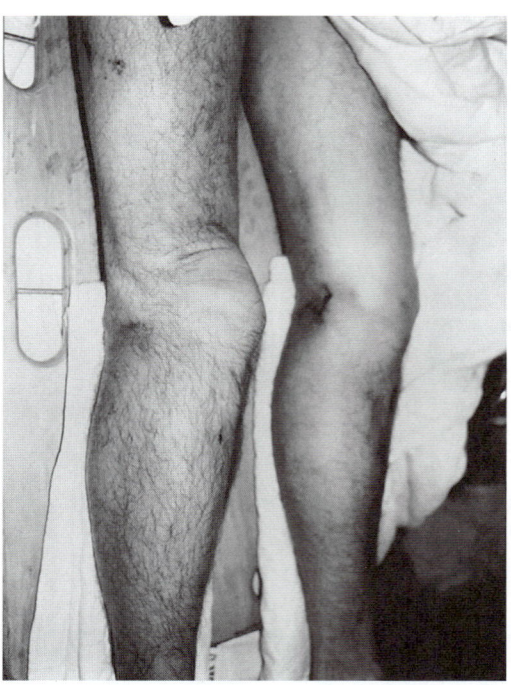

FIGURE 44-27 Right anterior knee dislocation with overriding of tibia on femur. (From Ferrera PC, Colucciello SA, Marx JA, et al: *Trauma management—an emergency medicine approach,* St Louis, 2001, Mosby.)

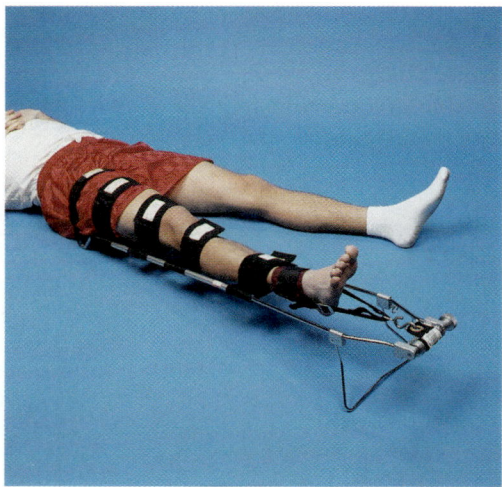

FIGURE 44-26 Application of a traction splint.

BOX 44-5 Ligament Injuries of the Knee

Injuries to the ligaments around the knee can result from direct blows, from hyperextension, and (more commonly) from twisting or torsion of the knee (e.g., in sports activities). The ligaments outside the knee are the medial collateral ligament and the lateral collateral ligament. They provide the stability for the knee and limit the amount the knee can move from side to side. The medial collateral ligament is on the inner side of the knee and is taut when the leg is straight. It is a strong ligament but can be sprained or completely ruptured (torn) if the straightened knee is twisted at the same time the knee is forced sideways (e.g., during a football tackle). The lateral collateral ligament runs on the outer side of the knee. It connects the distal end of the femur to the top of the fibula. Injury to this ligament seldom occurs as an isolated event. If injured, it is usually associated with another damaged ligament.

The ligaments inside the knee are the anterior cruciate ligament and the posterior cruciate ligament. These ligaments cross over each other. The crisscross formation provides additional stability to the knee, particularly in forward and backward movements of the knee joint (Figure 44-29).

Ligament injuries are managed with rest, ice, compression, and elevation (R-I-C-E); anti-inflammatories and analgesics; and physical therapy. In some cases, surgical repair is required.

motor vehicle crashes, pedestrian injuries, contact sports, and falls on a flexed knee (Figure 44-27). (The popliteal artery is close to the knee joint and may therefore be an associated injury. This is particularly true with posterior dislocations.) Other common knee and patella injuries involve nearby ligaments and tendons (Box 44-5). Management includes the following measures:

1. Assessment of neurovascular status

2. Splinting in the position found with a rigid or formable splint (Figure 44-28) that effectively immobilizes the hip and ankle (traction splints should not be used to immobilize a knee or patellar injury)

3. Application of ice and elevation, if possible

Tibial and Fibular Injury

Injuries to the tibia and fibula may result from direct or indirect trauma. They also may result from twisting injury (Figures 44-29 and 44-30). If the injury is associated with the knee, popliteal vascular injury should be suspected. Management includes the following measures:

1. Assessment of neurovascular status
2. Splinting with a rigid or formable splint (Figure 44-31)
3. Application of ice and elevation

Foot and Ankle Injury

Fractures and dislocations of the foot and ankle may result from a crush injury, a fall from a height, or a violent rotating or twisting force (Figure 44-32). Injuries to nearby tendons also can occur (Box 44-6). The patient with foot or ankle injury usually complains of point tenderness. The person also often is hesitant to bear weight on the extremity. Management includes the following measures:

1. Assessment of neurovascular status
2. Application of a formable splint, such as a pillow, blanket, or air splint (Figure 44-33)
3. Application of ice and elevation

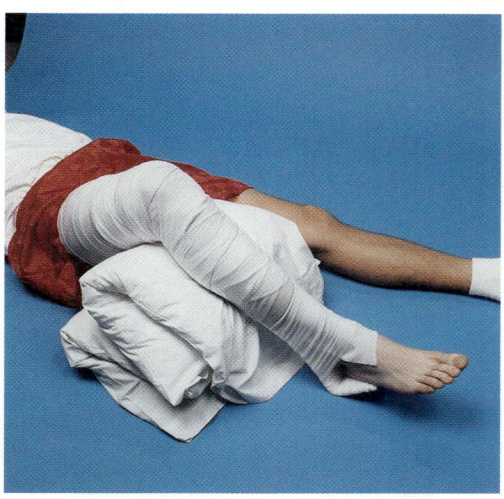

FIGURE 44-28 Immobilization of the knee.

> **? DID YOU KNOW?**
> **Ottawa Ankle Rules**
>
> In medicine, the *Ottawa ankle rules* are a set of guidelines used by physicians and other health care professionals to evaluate injuries to the ankle and midfoot. The rules also are used to determine the need for x-rays to identify fractures. (The rules were initially developed for foot and ankle injuries, but similar guidelines have been developed to evaluate the knees [*Ottawa knee rules*].) The Ottawa rules consider bone tenderness and the ability to bear weight when walking four steps. The risk of fracture is highest when there is any pain in the malleolar zone and any one of the following[8]:
>
> - Bone tenderness along the distal 6 cm of the posterior edge of the tibia or tip of the medial malleolus
> or
> - Bone tenderness along the distal 6 cm of the posterior edge of the fibula or tip of the lateral malleolus
> or
> - An inability to bear weight both immediately and in the emergency department for four steps

Note: Clinical judgment should prevail over the rules if the patient is under the influence of alcohol or other drugs; has other distracting or painful injuries; has diminished sensation in the legs; or has gross swelling that prevents palpation of malleolar bones. The rules have a 98.5% sensitivity for ankle and midfoot fracture in patients 6 years of age and older.[9]

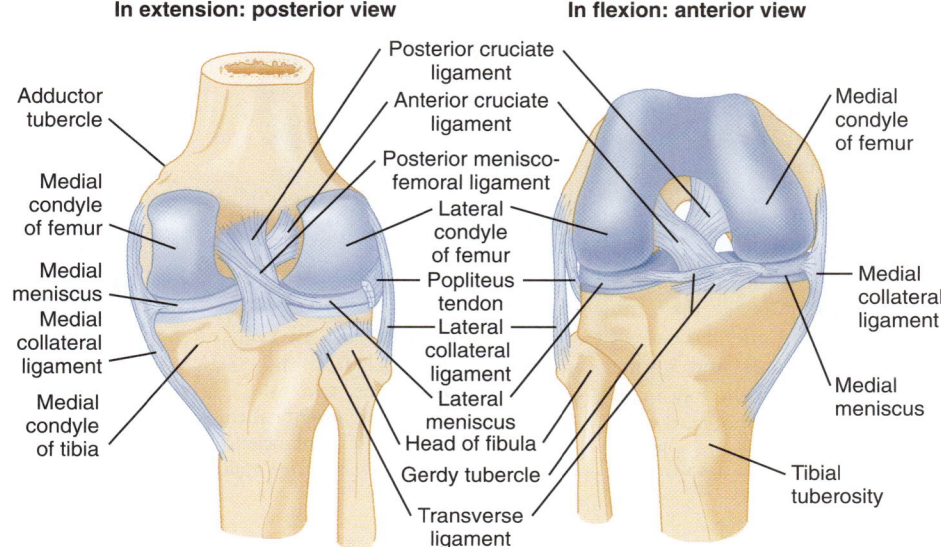

FIGURE 44-29 Anterior and posterior view of the right knee. (From Marx J et al: *Rosen's emergency medicine: concepts and clinical practice,* ed 6, St Louis, 2006, Mosby.)

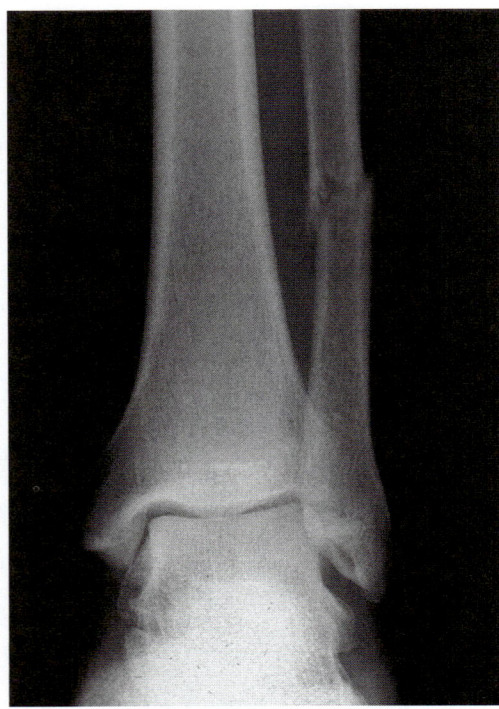

FIGURE 44-30 Isolated fibular shaft fracture. This patient sustained a direct blow to the lateral leg to produce this transverse fracture. A fracture in this location should arouse suspicion of associated injury to knee ligaments or ankle injury. (From Ferrera PC, Colucciello SA, Marx JA, et al: *Trauma management—an emergency medicine approach,* St Louis, 2001, Mosby.)

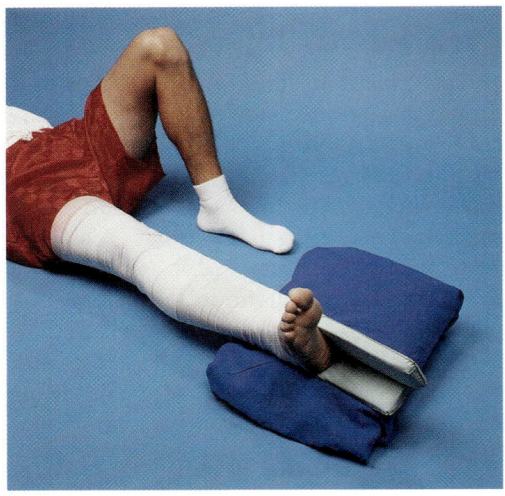

FIGURE 44-31 Immobilization of the lower leg.

BOX 44-6 Achilles Tendon Rupture

A common injury to the ankle is a tear or rupture of the Achilles tendon. The Achilles tendon, or *tendon calcaneus,* is the largest tendon in the human body. It is a large ropelike band of fibrous tissue that connects the powerful calf muscles to the calcaneus (heel bone). When the calf muscles contract, the Achilles tendon is tightened, pulling the heel. This allows a person to point the foot and stand on tiptoe. The Achilles tendon is vital to activities, such as walking, running, and jumping. Therefore, it is often a sports-related injury.

A complete tear through the tendon, which usually occurs about 2 inches above the heel, is called an Achilles tendon rupture. This injury usually results from excessive dorsiflexion of the foot. It is common in middle-age male athletes (the "weekend warrior"), in older people, and in those with arthritis and diabetes. Use of corticosteroids and antibiotics also increases the risk for this injury. Treatment may include surgical and nonsurgical therapies as well as foot and ankle casts or braces to prevent movement while the tendon heals.[7]

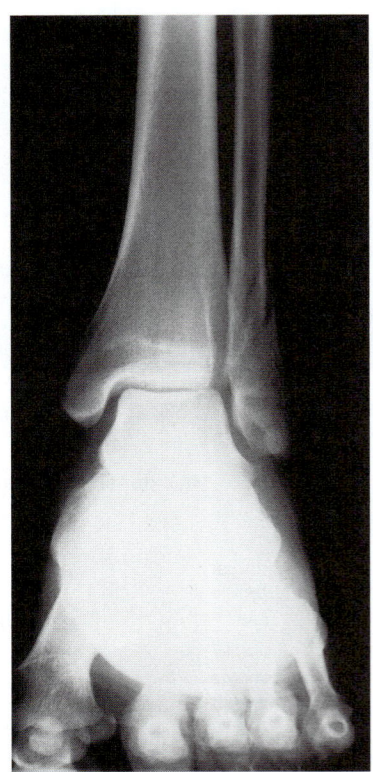

FIGURE 44-32 Weber B ankle fracture. The fracture lines extend obliquely from the mortise. The medial joint line (between medial malleolus and talus) is somewhat widened. This patient had deltoid ligament rupture and was later treated with surgery. (From Ferrera PC, Colucciello SA, Marx JA, et al: *Trauma management—an emergency medicine approach,* St Louis, 2001, Mosby.)

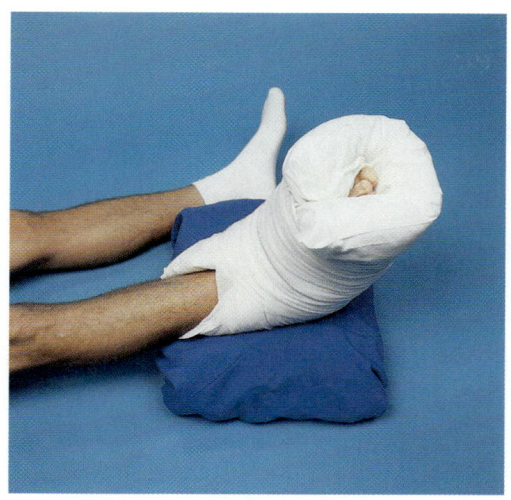

FIGURE 44-33 Immobilization of the foot and ankle.

Phalangeal Injury

Toe injuries often are caused by "stubbing" the toe on an immovable object. These injuries usually are managed by buddy taping the toe to an adjacent toe. This helps to support and immobilize the injury. Management includes the following measures:

1. Assessment of neurovascular status
2. Buddy splinting
3. Application of ice and elevation

OPEN FRACTURES

Patients with an **open fracture** require special care and evaluation by the paramedic. Fractures may be opened in two ways. They may be opened *from within,* as when a bone fragment pierces the skin, or they may be opened *from without* (e.g., after a gunshot wound). An open fracture also may have made contact with the skin some distance from the fracture site.

Although most open fractures are obvious because of associated hemorrhage, a small puncture wound may not be immediately apparent, and bleeding may be minimal. Therefore the paramedic must consider any soft tissue wound in the area of a suspected fracture to be evidence of an open fracture.

Open fractures are considered a true surgical emergency because of the potential for infection. Most authorities agree that open wounds associated with fractures should be covered with sterile, dry dressings. They should not be irrigated in the field or soaked with any type of antiseptic solution. Hemorrhage should be controlled with direct pressure and pressure dressings.

If a bone end or bone fragment is visible, it should be covered with a dry, sterile dressing and splinted. Bone ends that slip back into the wound during immobilization should be noted and reported to the receiving hospital so that the bone can be cleaned in surgery.

Stages of Fracture Healing

The healing of a fracture proceeds in several different stages. The time required for fracture healing depends on its severity and size. In the earliest stage following the fracture, a hematoma forms at the fracture site. This is followed by the formation of fibrovascular tissue (scar tissue) that replaces the hematoma and stabilizes the fracture area. Genes and proteins in the bone marrow then signal the production of osteoblasts (immature bone cells) and chondrocytes (cartilage cells). Next, the membrane around the bone and the immature bone cells form a callus at the fracture site. Newly formed cartilage cells begin to replace the scar tissue. In the final stage of healing, the immature bone cells held in place by the membrane grow and mature. This newly formed bone replaces the cartilage (*remodeling*) and the healing is completed (Figure 44-34).

The time required for fracture healing depends on how severe and how large it is, where it occurs, how the broken bone is used, and how strong the bone was before the fracture. Some small fractures in the hands heal in a few weeks. Large fractures in the legs or pelvis may take many months to heal (partly because these bones must bear the person's weight). Most fractured bones are immobilized with casts, braces, or surgical fixation devices while they heal. Even after healing, possible complications of fractures include the formation of a fat embolism, nonunion, and osteomyelitis.

STRAIGHTENING ANGULAR FRACTURES AND REDUCING DISLOCATIONS

Angular fractures and dislocations may pose significant problems in splinting and, in some situations, patient extrication and transport. When manipulation of a fracture is required to aid in transport or to improve circulation to the injured extremity, the paramedic should consult with medical direction.

 NOTE
Limb-threatening injuries include knee dislocation, fracture or dislocation of the ankle, and subcondylar fractures of the elbow. These serious injuries require rapid transport for evaluation by a physician.

 CRITICAL THINKING
Aside from narcotic analgesics, what other drugs may be indicated to relieve muscle spasm, provide anesthesia, and relax the patient while a dislocation or fracture is reduced?

As a rule, fractures and dislocated joints should be immobilized in the position of injury, and the patient should be transported as quickly as possible to the emergency department for x-ray films and realignment (reduction). (Radiographs are often taken of the affected limb to

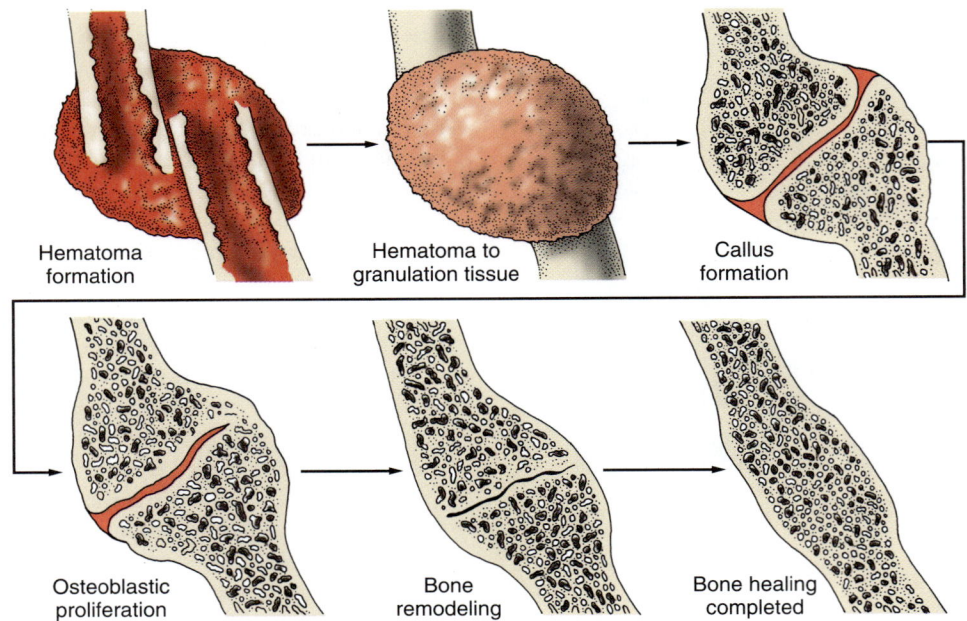

Hematoma formation

Hematoma to granulation tissue

Callus formation

Osteoblastic proliferation

Bone remodeling

Bone healing completed

FIGURE 44-34 Stages of fracture healing. (From Linton AD: *Introduction to medical surgical nursing*, ed 4, St Louis, 2007, Saunders.)

rule out bone fragments or other fractures that may complicate reduction.) However, if transport is delayed or prolonged, and if circulation is impaired, an attempt should be made to reposition a grossly deformed fracture or dislocated joint. The exception is the elbow. The elbow should never be manipulated in the prehospital setting. A grossly deformed fracture or dislocation elsewhere often can be realigned if required. This usually can be done without causing more damage or extreme discomfort to the patient. The injury should be handled carefully. Gentle, firm traction should be applied in the direction of the long axis of the extremity. If obvious resistance to alignment is felt, the extremity should be splinted without repositioning.

> ### NOTE
> The National Association of EMS Physicians (NAEMSP) recommends reduction of dislocations when transport time is prolonged.[10] The rationale of the Association is that joints are more difficult to reduce if they are left in a dislocated position for a prolonged period; therefore the prehospital care provider can attempt reduction in the field. Before attempting reduction of dislocation in the prehospital setting, the paramedic should be properly trained in appropriate techniques. Attempted reduction should only be undertaken when permitted by written protocols or online medical direction. The procedures should be properly documented.[6]

Specific Techniques for Specific Joints

A brief description of specific techniques for realigning extremity injuries is provided in the following discussion. (Additional training and authorization from medical direction is required.) Only *one* attempt at realignment should be made in the prehospital setting, and *only* if severe neurovascular compromise is present (e.g., extremely weak or absent distal pulses). Moreover, the attempt should be made *only* after consultation with medical direction. Manipulation (if indicated) should be performed as soon as possible after the injury. It should not be performed if the patient has other severe injuries, including the potential for an associated fracture. If not contraindicated by other injuries, IV analgesics (e.g., *fentanyl, morphine*) and benzodiazepines (e.g., *midazolam*) should be used before realignment. The paramedic should always assess and document pulse, sensation, and motor function before and after manipulating any injured extremity or joint.

FINGER REALIGNMENT

1. Apply in-line traction along the shaft of the finger.
2. Continue with slow, steady traction until the finger is realigned and the patient feels relief from pain.
3. Immobilize the finger with a splint device or by buddy splinting.

SHOULDER REALIGNMENT

1. Attempt realignment only in the absence of severe back injury.
2. Check circulatory and sensory status.
3. Apply slow, gentle longitudinal traction, with counter-traction exerted on the axilla.
4. Slowly bring the extremity to the midline. (Do not apply force.) Realign in the anatomical position while maintaining traction (Figure 44-35).
5. Immobilize with a sling and swathe.

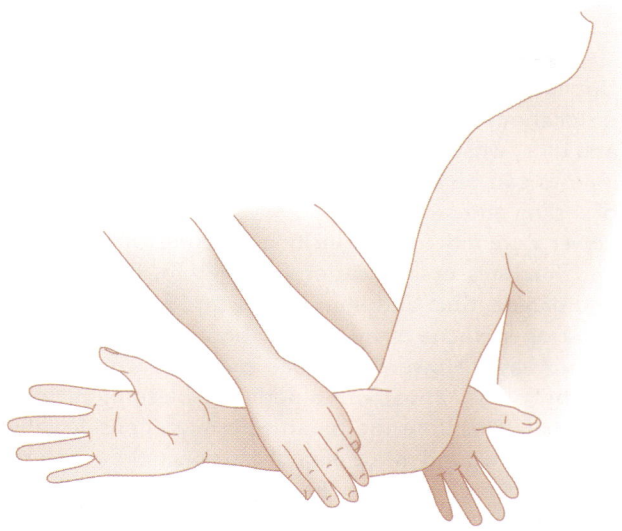

FIGURE 44-35 Traction-countertraction method for reducing anterior shoulder dislocation (From Marx J et al: *Rosen's emergency medicine: concepts and clinical practice*, ed 6, St Louis, 2006, Mosby.)

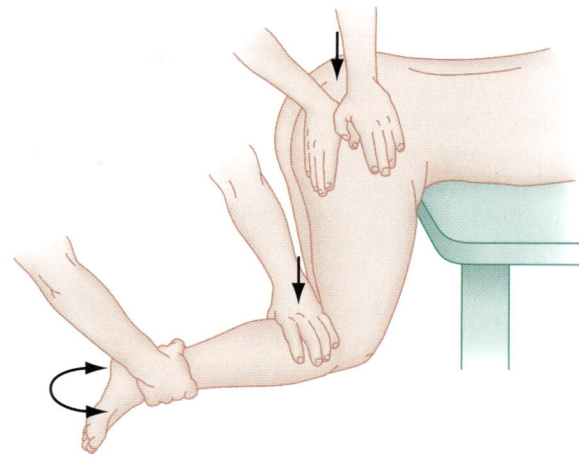

FIGURE 44-36 The Allis technique for hip reduction. (From Marx J et al: *Rosen's emergency medicine: concepts and clinical practice*, ed 6, St Louis, 2006, Mosby.)

HIP REALIGNMENT

1. Place the patient supine and stabilize the pelvis.
2. With the knee flexed, apply steady traction in-line with the deformity.
3. Slowly bring the hip to 90 degrees of flexion with slow, steady traction and gentle rotation to relax the muscle spasm (Figure 44-36). Successful realignment is indicated by a "pop" into the joint, a sudden relief of pain, and easy manipulation of the leg to full extension.
4. Immobilize the leg in full extension with the patient positioned on a long spine board. Reevaluate pulses and neurovascular status.
5. If full extension is not achieved, immobilize the leg at a flexion not to exceed 90 degrees with pillows or blankets. Place the patient supine.

KNEE REALIGNMENT

1. Apply gentle, steady traction while moving the injured joint into normal position.
2. Successful realignment is indicated by a "pop" into the joint, resolution of deformity, relief of pain, and increased mobility.
3. Immobilize the leg in full extension (or slight flexion for comfort). Position the patient supine on a long spine board.

NOTE

There is a high incidence of popliteal artery injury with knee dislocation. Therefore, a dislocated knee requires immediate reduction. Placing the hip in flexion and applying longitudinal traction to the leg will facilitate the realignment of the tibia and femur. Angiography *after reduction* is indicated to rule out arterial injury.[11]

ANKLE REALIGNMENT

1. Apply in-line traction on the talus while stabilizing the tibia.
2. Successful realignment is noted by a sudden rotation to a normal position.
3. Immobilize the ankle in the same manner as for a fracture.

REFERRAL OF PATIENTS WITH MINOR MUSCULOSKELETAL INJURY

Some patients with a minor musculoskeletal injury (e.g., a minor sprain) do not require transport by emergency medical services. To make this determination, the paramedic should follow these guidelines:

- Evaluate the need for immobilization.
- Evaluate the need for radiography. This is based on the patient's condition and the mechanism of injury.

 CRITICAL THINKING

What should be documented for calls involving minor musculoskeletal injuries?

- Evaluate the need for emergency department assessment versus the patient going to his or her private physician. This is based on the patient's condition and the mechanism of injury.
- Consult with medical direction.

Patients who are not transported to the hospital should be given advice on how to care for the injury. (An instruction sheet should explain techniques for immobilization, elevation, cold or heat application, rest, use of analgesics, and indications for physician follow-up.) If any doubt exists about the seriousness of the patient's injury, the person should be transported to the emergency department for evaluation by a physician.

SUMMARY

- Injuries that can result from traumatic force on the musculoskeletal system include fractures, sprains, strains, and joint dislocations. Problems associated with musculoskeletal injuries include hemorrhage, instability, loss of tissue, simple laceration and contamination, interruption of blood supply, and long-term disability.

- Common signs and symptoms of extremity trauma include pain on palpation or movement, swelling or deformity, crepitus, decreased range of motion, false movement, and decreased or absent sensory perception or circulation distal to the injury.

- Once the paramedic has assessed for life-threatening conditions, the extremity injury should be examined for pain, pallor, paresthesia, pulses, paralysis, and pressure.

- Immobilization by splinting helps alleviate pain; reduces tissue injury, bleeding, and contamination of an open wound; and simplifies and facilitates transport of the patient. Splints can be categorized as rigid, soft or formable, and traction splints.

- Upper extremity injuries can be classified as fractures or dislocations of the shoulder, humerus, elbow, radius and ulna, wrist, hand, and finger. Most upper extremity injuries can be adequately immobilized by application of a sling and swathe.

- Lower extremity injuries include fractures of the pelvis and fractures or dislocations of the hip, femur, knee and patella, tibia and fibula, ankle and foot, and toes.

- Most open fractures are obvious because of associated hemorrhage. However, a small puncture wound may not be initially apparent. In addition, bleeding may be minimal. Therefore the paramedic must consider any soft tissue wound in the area of a suspected fracture to be evidence of an open fracture. Open fractures are considered a true surgical emergency. This is due to the potential for infection.

- Only *one* attempt at realignment should be made. This should be done *only* if severe neurovascular compromise is present (e.g., extremely weak or absent distal pulses). Moreover, it should be done *only* after consultation with medical direction.

REFERENCES

1. Marx J, Hockberger R, Walls R: *Rosen's emergency medicine*, ed 7, St Louis, 2009, Mosby.

2. Emergency Nurses Association: *Sheehy's emergency nursing: principles and practice*, ed 6, St Louis, 2010, Mosby.

3. Wilson WC, Grande CM, Hoyt DB, editors: *Trauma, critical care*, vol 2, New York, 2006, Informa Health Care USA.

4. Rosencher N, Vielpeau C, Emmerich J, et al: Venous thromboembolism and mortality after hip fracture surgery: the ESCORTE Study, *J Thromb Haemost* 3(9):2006-2014, 2005.

5. Halkala BE: *Pediatric femoral shaft fractures*, www.medscape.com/viewarticle/408516, accessed 10-9-10.

6. National Association of Emergency Medical Technicians: *PHTLS: prehospital trauma life support*, ed 7, St Louis, 2011, Mosby.

7. Nannini C: *Achilles tendon rupture*, emedicine health, www.emedicinehealth.com/achilles_tendon_rupture/article_em.htm, accessed 10-8-10.

8. Stiell I, McKnight RD, Greenberg GH, et al: Implementation of the Ottawa Ankle Rules, *JAMA* 271:827-832, 1994.

9. Dowling S, Spooner CH, Liang Y, et al: Accuracy of Ottawa ankle rules to exclude fractures of the ankle and midfoot in children: a meta-analysis, *Acad Emerg Med* 16(4):277-287, 2009.

10. Goth P, Garnett G: Clinical guidelines for delayed or prolonged transport. II, Dislocations, Rural Affairs Committee, National Association of Emergency Medical Services Physicians, *Prehosp Disaster Med* 8(1):77, 1993.

11. Hamilton GC, Sanders AB, Strange G, et al: *Emergency medicine: an approach to clinical problem-solving*, ed 2, Philadelphia, 2003, Saunders.

SUGGESTED READINGS

Caine D, Cain C, Maffulli N: Incidence and distribution of pediatric sport-related injuries, *Clin J Sport Med* 16(6):500-513, 2006.

Cuske J: *The lost art of splinting: how to properly immobilize extremities and relieve pain*, www.jems.com/news_and_articles/articles/jems/3307/the_lost_art_of_splinting.html, accessed 4-17-10.

45 Environmental Conditions

OBJECTIVES

Upon completion of this chapter, the paramedic student will be able to:

1. Describe the physiology of thermoregulation.
2. Discuss the risk factors, pathophysiology, assessment findings, and management of specific hyperthermic conditions.
3. Discuss the risk factors, pathophysiology, assessment findings, and management of specific hypothermic conditions and frostbite.
4. Discuss the risk factors, pathophysiology, assessment findings, and management of submersion and drowning.
5. Identify the mechanical effects of atmospheric pressure changes on the body based on knowledge of the basic properties of gases.
6. Discuss the risk factors, pathophysiology, assessment findings, and management of diving emergencies and high-altitude illness.

KEY TERMS

acute mountain sickness A common high-altitude illness that results when an unacclimatized person rapidly ascends to high altitudes.

afterdrop phenomenon A sudden return of cold blood and waste products to the core of the body as a result of rewarming methods used to treat hypothermia.

air embolism The presence of air bubbles in the bloodstream.

barotrauma A physical injury sustained as a result of exposure to increased environmental pressure; also known as *dysbarism.*

barotrauma of ascent A diving illness that occurs through the reverse process of descent; also known as "reverse squeeze."

barotrauma of descent A diving illness that results from the compression of gas in enclosed spaces as the ambient pressure increases with descent under water; also known as "squeeze."

Boyle's law A law pertaining to the properties of gas; it states that if temperature remains constant, the volume of a given mass of gas is inversely proportional to the absolute pressure; that is, when the pressure is doubled, the volume of gas is halved (compressed into a smaller space), and vice versa.

central thermoreceptors Nerve endings located in or near the anterior hypothalamus that are sensitive to heat.

conduction The direct movement of heat from a warmer object to a cooler one (simple transfer).

convection The transfer of heat by mass motion of a fluid such as air or water.

core body temperature The temperature of deep structures of the body as compared with the temperatures of peripheral tissues.

Dalton's law A law pertaining to the pressure of gas; it states that the pressure exerted by each gas in a mixture of gases is the same pressure that the gas would exert if it alone occupied the same volume.

decompression sickness A multisystem disorder that results when nitrogen in compressed air converts back from solution to gas, forming bubbles in the tissues and blood.

demarcation The visible boundary between living tissue and necrotic tissue.

drowning A mortal event in which a submersion victim is pronounced dead at the scene of the attempted resuscitation or within 24 hours after arrival in the emergency department or hospital.

dysbarism Describes illnesses that result directly or indirectly from changes in ambient atmospheric pressure and the pressure of gases within the body.

frostbite A localized injury that results from environmentally induced freezing of body tissues.

frostnip A cold injury manifested by transient numbness and tingling that resolves after rewarming.

heat cramps Brief, intermittent, and often severe muscular cramps that frequently occur in muscles fatigued by heavy work or exercise.

heat exhaustion A form of heat illness characterized by minor aberrations in mental status, dizziness, nausea, headache, and a mild to moderate increase in the core body temperature.

heat stroke A syndrome that occurs when the thermoregulatory mechanisms normally in place to meet the demands of heat stress break down entirely. As a result, the body temperature increases to extreme levels. Multisystem tissue damage and physiological collapse also occur.

Henry's law A law of gas pressure that states that, at a constant temperature, the solubility of a gas in a liquid solution is proportionate to the partial pressure of the gas.

high-altitude cerebral edema The most severe form of acute high-altitude illness. It is characterized by a progression of global cerebral signs in the presence of acute mountain sickness.

high-altitude illness Refers to illness that principally occurs at altitudes 8200 feet or more above sea level.

high-altitude pulmonary edema A high-altitude illness thought to be caused at least partly by an increase in pulmonary artery pressure that develops in response to hypoxia.

hyperthermia Abnormal elevation of body temperature.

hypothermia An abnormal body temperature below 95° F (35° C).

mammalian diving reflex A reflex stimulated by cold water that shunts blood to the brain and heart from the skin, gastrointestinal tract, and extremities.

nitrogen narcosis An illness associated with scuba diving in which nitrogen becomes dissolved in solution as a result of greater than normal atmospheric pressure; also known as rapture of the deep.

Osborn wave A positive deflection at the J point on an ECG, characteristically seen in hypothermia; also known as a J wave.

peripheral thermoreceptors Nerve endings sensitive to heat, located in the skin and some mucous membranes; they usually are categorized as cold or warm receptors.

pulmonary overpressurization syndrome A condition that results from expansion of trapped air in the lungs; it may lead to alveolar rupture and extravasation of air into extraalveolar locations.

radiation The direct release of body heat to cooler surroundings.

recompression The use of elevated pressure (including hyperbaric oxygen therapy) to treat conditions within the body caused by a rapid decrease in pressure.

submersion An incident in which a person experiences some swimming-related distress that is sufficient to require support in the prehospital setting and transportation to a medical facility for further observation and treatment.

thermogenesis The production of heat, especially by the cells of the body.

thermolysis The dissipation of heat by means of radiation, evaporation, conduction, or convection.

thermoregulation The maintenance of body temperature, even under a variety of external conditions.

trench foot An injury that occurs from prolonged exposure to cold, but not freezing, water.

Exposure to elements in the environment can produce many types of emergencies. Paramedics must be prepared to recognize and manage these conditions. This requires being knowledgeable about the causative factors and the pathophysiology of specific disorders.

THERMOREGULATION

Thermoregulation is the maintenance of body temperature, even under a variety of external conditions. Body temperature is regulated in the brain by a thermoregulatory center.

This center is located in the posterior hypothalamus. It receives information from **central thermoreceptors** in or near the anterior hypothalamus and from **peripheral thermoreceptors** in the skin and some mucous membranes. Peripheral thermoreceptors are nerve endings usually categorized as cold receptors and warm receptors. Cold receptors are stimulated by lower skin-surface temperatures. Warm receptors are stimulated by higher skin-surface temperatures. Information from these receptors is transmitted

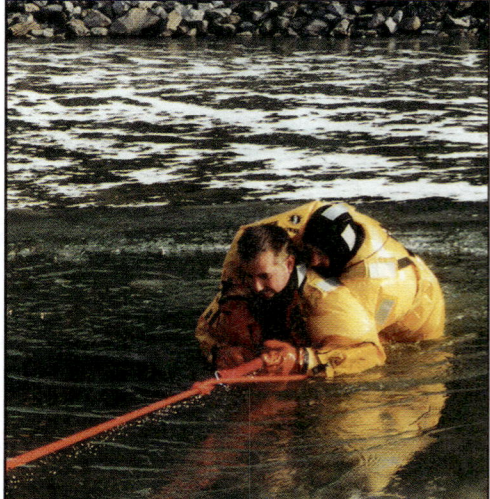

(Courtesy Creve Coeur Fire Protection District.)

by the spinal cord to the posterior hypothalamus. The posterior hypothalamus responds with appropriate signals to help the body reduce heat loss and increase heat production (cold receptor stimulation) or increase heat loss and reduce heat production (warm receptor stimulation).

CRITICAL THINKING
The body has many more cold receptors than heat receptors. Why do you think this is true?

Central thermoreceptors are neurons that are sensitive to changes in temperature. These neurons react directly to changes in the temperature of the blood. They send messages to the skeletal muscle through the central nervous system (CNS). They affect vasomotor tone, sweating, and the metabolic rate through sympathetic nerve output to skin arterioles, sweat glands, and the adrenal medulla.

As discussed in Chapter 20, the thermoregulatory center has an inherent set point. This maintains a relatively constant **core body temperature** (CBT) of 98.6° F (37° C). To maintain an optimum environment for normal cell metabolism (homeostasis), the body must keep the CBT fairly constant, even when external and internal conditions tend to raise or lower it. Body temperature can be increased or decreased in two ways. One way is through the regulation of heat production **(thermogenesis).** The other way is through the regulation of heat loss **(thermolysis).**

Regulating Heat Production

The body can generate heat in response to cold. It does this through mechanical, chemical, metabolic, and endocrine activities. Several physiological and biochemical factors affect the direction and magnitude of these compensatory responses. Such factors include the person's age, general health, and nutritional status.

Heat is controlled chemically by cellular metabolism (oxidation of energy sources). Every tissue contributes to this type of heat production. However, skeletal muscles produce the largest amount of heat, particularly when shivering occurs. Along with shivering, which is often associated with chattering of the teeth, vasoconstriction occurs to conserve as much heat as possible. Shivering is the body's best defense against cold. It can increase heat production by as much as 400%.[1]

CRITICAL THINKING
What fuels does the body need to increase heat production through the mechanism of shivering?

Endocrine glands also regulate heat production. They do this through the release of hormones from the thyroid gland and adrenal medulla. Sympathetic discharge of epinephrine and norepinephrine (along with the activity of sympathetic nerves that lead to adipose tissue) increases metabolism. This results in an increase in heat production. Box 45-1 presents examples of ways the body regulates heat production.

Regulating Heat Loss

Heat is lost from the body to the external environment through the skin, lungs, and excretions. The skin is the most important of these in regulating heat loss. Radiation,

BOX 45-1 Compensatory Mechanisms for Regulating Heat Production

Mechanisms That Decrease Heat Loss
Peripheral vasoconstriction
Reduction of surface area by body position (or clothing)
Piloerection (not effective in humans)

Mechanisms That Increase Heat Production
Shivering
Increased voluntary activity
Increased hormone secretion
Increased appetite

conduction, **convection**, and evaporation are the major mechanisms of heat loss (Figure 45-1).

Radiation is the direct release of body heat to cooler surroundings. The surface of the human body constantly emits heat in the form of infrared rays. If the surface of the body is warmer than the environment, heat is lost through radiation.

Conduction is the direct movement of heat from a warmer object to a cooler one (simple transfer). Heat moves from a higher temperature to a lower temperature. Thus the body surface loses or gains heat by direct contact with cooler or warmer surfaces, including air. If the ambient air temperature is lower than the skin temperature, body heat is lost to the surrounding air by conduction. The greater the temperature difference between two objects, the more quickly heat is transferred between them.

Convection is similar to conduction; however, in convection the two objects in contact are also moving relative to one another. It is heat transfer by mass motion of a fluid such as air or water. For example, if air or water next to the body is heated, moves away, and is replaced by cool air or water, heat loss occurs by convection. Convection can be greatly aided by external forces such as wind or fans. It promotes conductive heat exchange by continuously maintaining a supply of cool air. Factors that contribute to the cooling effects of convection are the speed of air currents and the temperature of the air.

CRITICAL THINKING
How does wearing the fully enclosed hazardous materials suit affect your body's ability to regulate temperature?

Evaporation is a process by which fluid changes from a liquid to a gas, and lowers the temperature on the surface where the evaporation occurred. When fluid evaporates, it absorbs heat from surrounding objects and air. The temperature of the surrounding air and the relative humidity greatly affect the amount of heat lost as a result of evaporation of moisture from the skin or the respiratory tract (breathing). The relative humidity is 100% when the air is fully saturated with moisture. Sweating can markedly increase evaporative heat loss as long as the humidity is low enough to allow the sweat to evaporate. At humidity levels above 75%, evaporation decreases. At levels approaching 90%, evaporation essentially ceases.[2] Box 45-2 presents other examples of ways the body regulates heat loss.

External Environmental Factors

Some factors in the environment can contribute to a medical emergency. They also may affect rescue and transport. These elements include the climate, season, weather, atmospheric pressure, and terrain. When the potential for an environmental emergency exists, the paramedic must consider the following factors:

- Localized prevailing weather norms and any deviations
- Characteristics of seasonal variation in climate
- Weather extremes (wind, rain, snow, humidity)
- Barometric pressure (e.g., at altitude or under water)
- Terrain that can complicate injury or rescue

The patient's health also is a factor related to environmental stressors. It can also worsen other medical or traumatic conditions. Examples include the patient's age, predisposing medical conditions, use of prescription and over-the-counter medications, use of alcohol or recreational drugs, and previous rate of exertion.

BOX 45-2 Compensatory Mechanisms for Regulating Heat Loss

Mechanisms That Increase Heat Loss
Vasodilation of skin vessels
Sweating

Mechanisms That Decrease Heat Production
Decreased muscle tone and voluntary activity
Decreased hormone secretion
Decreased appetite

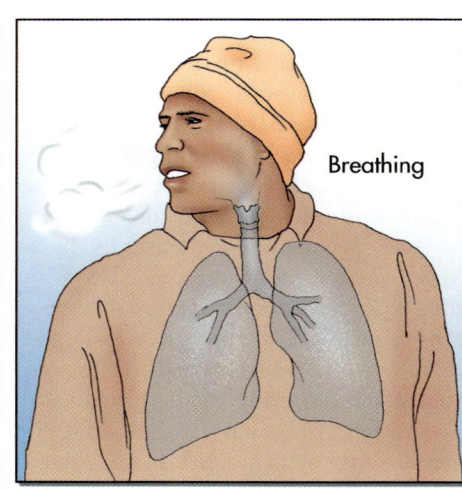

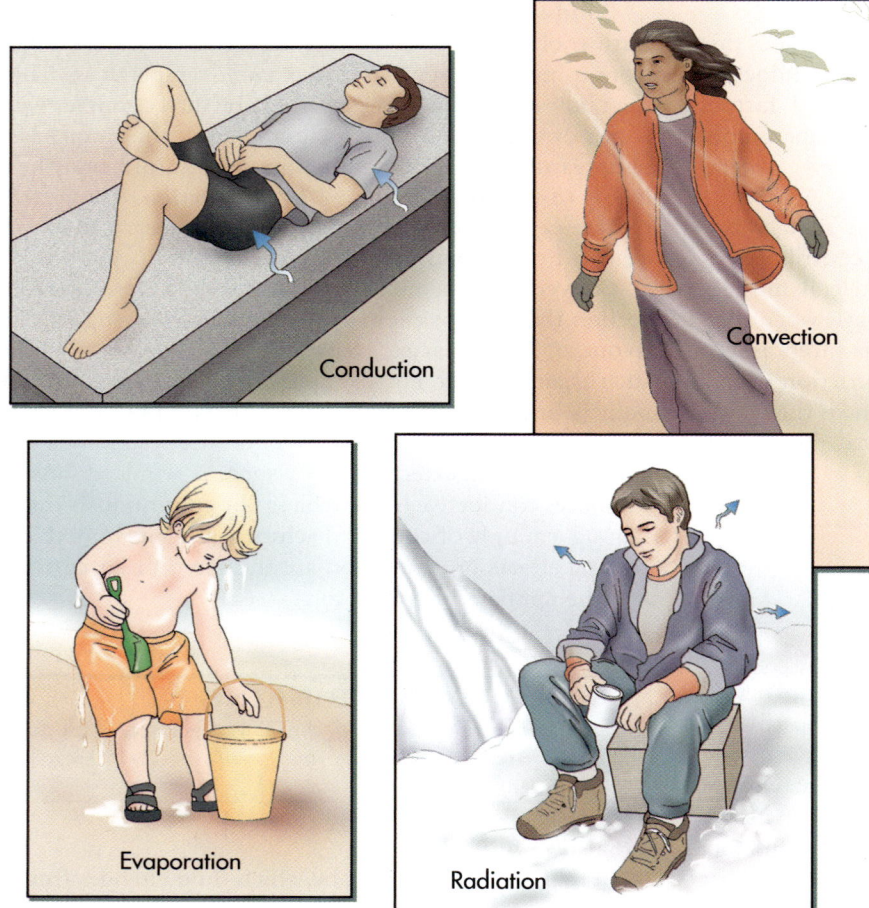

FIGURE 45-1 Mechanisms of heat loss. (From McSwain N, Paturas J: *The basic EMT: comprehensive prehospital patient care,* ed 2, St Louis, 2001, Mosby.)

HYPERTHERMIA

Hyperthermia, or heat illness, results from one of two basic causes: One cause is temperature-regulating mechanisms that are overwhelmed by high temperatures in the environment or, more commonly, by excessive exercise in moderate to extremely high temperatures. The second cause is temperature-regulating centers that fail, usually in older adults or in ill or incapacitated patients. Either cause can result in heat illness such as heat cramps, heat exhaustion, and heat stroke.

Heat Cramps

Heat cramps are brief, intermittent, and often severe muscular cramps that occur in hot environments. They often affect muscles fatigued by heavy work or exercise. The primary cause of heat cramps is sodium and water loss.

People who suffer from heat cramps sweat profusely and drink water without adequate salt. During times of high environmental temperatures, 1 to 3 L of water per hour can be lost through sweating. Each liter contains 30 to 50 mEq of sodium chloride. The water and sodium deficiency together cause muscle cramping. This normally occurs in the most heavily exercised muscles, including the calves and arms, although any muscle can be involved. The patient is usually alert and has hot, sweaty skin, tachycardia, and a normal blood pressure. The CBT is normal.

Heat cramps are easily managed by removing the patient from the hot environment. Also, sodium and water should be replaced. In more serious cases, medical direction may recommend intravenous (IV) infusion of a balanced sodium chloride solution. Oral salt additives (e.g., salt tablets) can cause gastrointestinal irritation, ulceration, and vomiting. This worsens the electrolyte imbalance. Paramedics should follow local protocol with regard to providing a carbohydrate- and salt-containing beverage (e.g., Gatorade and Powerade) to help rehydrate patients.

Heat Exhaustion

Heat exhaustion is a more severe form of heat illness. It is characterized by dizziness, nausea, headache, and mild to moderate elevation of the CBT (up to 103° F [39° C]). In severe cases, dizziness caused by significant intravascular volume loss, as well as fainting, may occur. This orthostatic dizziness occurs when the patient changes from a lying position to a sitting or standing position.

Like heat cramps, heat exhaustion more often is associated with a hot environment and results in profuse sweating. Loss of water and salt, electrolyte imbalance, and difficulty maintaining blood pressure contribute to inadequate peripheral and cerebral perfusion. The person usually recovers rapidly when removed from the hot environment, given replacement fluids, and cooled with a cool water spray. Patients with significant fluid loss or orthostatic hypotension may require IV administration of a balanced sodium chloride solution. Heat exhaustion can progress to heat stroke if left untreated.[2]

Heat Stroke

Heat stroke occurs when the body's temperature-regulating mechanisms break down entirely. As a result of this failure, the body temperature rises to 105.8° F (41° C) or higher. This damages tissue in all the body systems and results in total body collapse. Heat stroke is a true medical emergency. The syndrome commonly is classified into two types: classic heat stroke and exertional heat stroke.

> **NOTE**
> Increased body temperature caused by failure of the temperature-regulating mechanisms should not be confused with fever associated with a response to inflammation or infection. With fever, the effect on the hypothalamus is caused by endogenous pyrogens released by phagocytic leukocytes. Antipyretic drugs can reverse these effects, returning the set point of the hypothalamus to normal.

Classic heat stroke occurs during periods of sustained high ambient temperatures and humidity. The illness commonly affects the very young, older adults, and those who live in poorly ventilated homes without air conditioning. An example is a young child left in an enclosed car on a hot afternoon. Another example is an older person confined to a hot room during a heat wave. Victims of classic heat stroke also often suffer from chronic diseases. Some of these include diabetes, heart disease, alcoholism, or psychiatric disorders. These diseases predispose the individual to the syndrome. Many patients who are susceptible to classic heat stroke take prescribed medications for other conditions. These may include diuretics, antihypertensives, psychotropics (antipsychotics, phenothiazines), antihistamines, and anticholinergics. These drugs further impair a person's ability to tolerate heat stress. In these patients the illness develops from poor dissipation of environmental heat.

> **NOTE**
> The autoimmune neuropathy associated with diabetes can interfere with vasodilation, perspiration, and thermoregulatory input. Some cardiac drugs (e.g., anticholinergics, beta blockers, diuretics) can predispose a patient to dehydration, can interfere with vasodilation, and can reduce the body's ability to increase the heart rate in response to a volume loss.

In contrast to patients with classic heat stroke, patients with *exertional heat stroke* are usually young and healthy. Athletes, military recruits, and firefighters who work or exercise in the heat and humidity often are affected. In these situations, heat builds up more rapidly in the body than it can be dispersed into the environment. Preventive measures to reduce the risk of exertional heat illness for all age groups include the following:

- Avoiding or limiting exercise in hot environments, especially on consecutive days
- Maintaining an adequate fluid intake

- Achieving acclimatization, which results in more perspiration with a lower salt concentration, thereby increasing fluid volume in the body

CLINICAL MANIFESTATIONS

As described previously, the temperature-regulating centers in the brain receive their information largely from the temperature of circulating blood in the deep and superficial veins and from the skin. In response to hypothalamic stimulation, a number of physiological events occur: (1) the respiratory rate quickens to increase heat loss through exhaled air; (2) cardiac output increases to provide more blood flow through skin and muscle to enhance heat radiation; and (3) sweat gland activity increases to enhance evaporative heat loss. These compensatory mechanisms require a normally functioning CNS to properly respond to the temperature extreme. They also require a working cardiovascular system to move excess heat from the core to the surface of the body. Problems in either or both of these systems lead to a rapidly increasing CBT.

Central Nervous System Manifestations. The CNS manifestations of heat stroke vary. Some patients may be in frank coma. Others may show confusion and irrational behavior before collapse. Convulsions are common. They can occur early or late in the course of the illness. Because the brain stores little energy, it depends on a constant supply of oxygen and glucose. Decreased cerebral perfusion pressure results in cerebral ischemia and acidosis. Increased temperatures markedly increase the metabolic demands of the brain as well. The extent of brain damage depends on the severity and duration of the hyperthermic episode. Fever from illness (e.g., infection) and an increased CBT from heat stroke produce similar symptoms, especially in the central nervous system. The paramedic should obtain a thorough history (if available) so as to distinguish between the two syndromes. If unsure of the cause, the paramedic should treat the patient for heat stroke.

CRITICAL THINKING
What other conditions can demonstrate the types of mental status changes seen with heat stroke?

Cardiovascular Manifestations. A rise in skin temperature reduces the thermal gradient between the core and the skin. This causes an increase in skin blood flow (peripheral vasodilation), which gives the skin a flushed appearance. About 50% of victims of exertional heat stroke have persistent sweating,[2] which results from increased release of catecholamines. In classic heat stroke, sweating usually is absent. This is due to dehydration, drug use that impairs sweating, direct thermal injury to sweat glands, or sweat gland fatigue. Therefore the presence of sweating does not rule out the diagnosis. Also, the cessation of sweating is not the cause of heat stroke. Peripheral vasodilation results in decreased vascular resistance and shunting as the illness

progresses. High-output cardiac failure is common. It is manifested by extreme tachycardia and hypotension. Cardiac output initially can be four to five times normal. However, as temperatures continue to rise, myocardial contractility begins to decrease. Also, the central venous pressure rises. In any age group, the presence of hypotension and decreased cardiac output points to a poor prognosis. Other systemic manifestations associated with heat stroke include:

- Pulmonary edema (accompanied by systemic acidosis, tachypnea, hypoxemia, and hypercapnia)
- Myocardial dysfunction
- Gastrointestinal bleeding
- A reduction in renal function (secondary to hypovolemia and hypoperfusion)
- Hepatic injury
- Clotting disorders
- Electrolyte abnormalities

MANAGEMENT

Heat stroke almost invariably leads to death if left untreated. The factors most important to a successful outcome are initiation of basic life support (BLS) and advanced life support (ALS) measures, rapid recognition of the heat illness, and rapid cooling of the patient. After ensuring an adequate airway and ventilatory and circulatory support, the paramedic should manage the patient with heat stroke as follows[3]:

1. Move the patient to a shady environment and remove restrictive clothing. If available, use hyperthermic thermometers (e.g., rectal probes) to monitor the CBT. Take and record the temperature at least every 5 minutes during the cooling process. This ensures adequate rates of cooling. It also helps to prevent inadvertent (rebound) hypothermia. Rebound hypothermia can best be avoided by stopping the cooling measures when the patient's CBT reaches about 102° F (39° C).

2. Begin cooling by fanning the patient while keeping the skin wet. Continue lowering the body temperature by this method en route to the hospital. If transport is delayed, complete immersion (victim is placed in cold water up to the chin) or spraying tepid water (60° F [16° C]) over the body surface is recommended. Shivering should be controlled with IV *diazepam*.

> **NOTE**
> **Submersion** in ice water or cold water is an effective means to rapidly lower core body temperature.[3] The use of these methods is controversial. Some authorities believe they may lead to patient discomfort, shivering, frank shaking, peripheral vasoconstriction, and convulsions, which act to increase the CBT as the body temperature is lowered. Other authorities recommend ice water submersion after other methods prove unsuccessful within 30 minutes of treatment.[4] Paramedics should follow the recommendations established by medical direction.

3. If hypovolemia is present, administer IV fluids per medical direction. (Ideally, 1 to 2 L of fluid should be administered during the first hour after collapse and additional fluids administered according to the level of hydration.) In most patients the blood pressure rises to a normal range during the cooling process. This occurs as large volumes of blood from the skin move back to the central circulation. Rapid cooling directly improves cardiac output. Be very cautious with fluid replacement. Also, closely monitor the patient for signs of fluid overload. The administration of too much fluid can cause pulmonary edema, especially in older adults.

4. Administer medications as prescribed by medical direction. Depending on the patient's status and response to cooling methods, these drugs may include *diazepam* or *lorazepam* for sedation and seizure control, *mannitol* to promote renal blood flow and diuresis, and glucose to manage hypoglycemia.

HYPOTHERMIA

Hypothermia (CBT less than 95° F [35° C]) can result from a decrease in heat production, an increase in heat loss, or a combination of these two processes.

Hypothermia can have metabolic, neurological, traumatic, toxic, and infectious causes. However, it most often is seen in cold climates and in exposure to extremely cold conditions in the environment. Failure to recognize and properly treat hypothermia can increase the rate of morbidity and mortality.

Pathophysiology

Exposure to cold produces a chain of events in the body aimed at conserving core heat. Initially, immediate vasoconstriction in the peripheral vessels occurs. At the same time, the rate of metabolism by the CNS increases. The blood pressure and the heart and respiratory rates also increase dramatically. As cold exposure continues, muscle tone increases. The body generates heat in the form of shivering. Shivering continues until the CBT reaches about 86° F (30° C), glucose or glycogen is depleted, or insulin is no longer available for glucose transfer. When shivering stops, cooling is rapid. A general decline then begins in the function of all body systems.

With continued cooling, respirations decline slowly; the pulse rate and blood pressure decrease; the blood pH drops; and significant electrolyte imbalances emerge. Hypovolemia can develop from a shift of fluid out of the vascular space, with increased loss of fluid through urination (*cold diuresis*). After early tachycardia, progressive bradycardia develops. This often does not respond to **atropine.** Significant electrocardiographic (ECG) changes occur. These include prolonged PR, QRS, and QT intervals; and obscure or absent P waves.[2] In addition, the J point (**Osborn wave**) may be present at the junction of the QRS complex and ST segment (Figure 45-2). These events generally are followed by cardiac and respiratory arrest as the CBT approaches 68° F (20° C).

The progression of clinical signs and symptoms of hypothermia is divided into three classes based on the CBT[5]: mild, moderate, and severe. *Mild hypothermia* is classified as a CBT between 93.2° and 96.8° F (34° and 36° C); *moderate hypothermia* as a CBT between 86° and 93° F (30° and 34° C); and *severe hypothermia* as a CBT below 86° F (30° C). The signs and symptoms of the three classes of hypothermia are listed in Table 45-1.

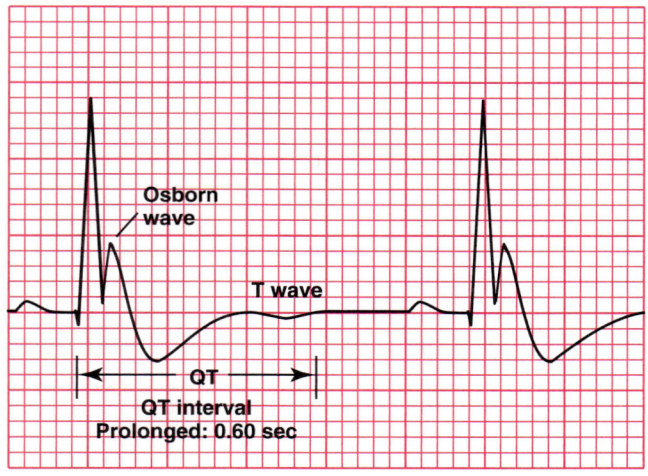

FIGURE 45-2 Osborn wave of hypothermia. (From Wesley K: *Huszar's basic dysrhythmias and acute coronary syndromes: interpretation and management,* ed 4, St Louis, 2012, Mosby.)

TABLE 45-1 Progression of Clinical Signs and Symptoms of Hypothermia*

Classification	Core Body Temperature	Signs and Symptoms
Mild	96.8° F (36° C)	Increased metabolic rate, maximum shivering, thermogenesis
	93.2° F (34° C)	Impaired judgment, slurred speech
Moderate	86° F (30° C)	Respiratory depression, myocardial irritability, bradycardia, atrial fibrillation, Osborn waves
Severe	<86° F (<30° C)	Basal metabolic rate 50% of normal, loss of deep tendon reflexes, fixed and dilated pupils, spontaneous ventricular fibrillation

*Often no reliable correlation is seen between clinical signs and symptoms and a specific core body temperature.

Those at increased risk for developing unintentional hypothermia are outdoor enthusiasts (e.g., campers, hikers, hunters, and fishermen), older adults, the very young, and individuals with concurrent medical or psychiatric illness. Thermoregulatory mechanisms also can be impaired by brain damage caused by trauma, hemorrhage, hypoxia, and CNS depression from drug overdose or intoxicants. Drugs known to impair thermoregulation include alcohol, antidepressants, antipyretics, phenothiazines, sedatives, and various pain medicines (including *aspirin,* acetaminophen, and nonsteroidal antiinflammatory drugs [NSAIDs]). Acid-base imbalances, such as those that occur during ketoacidosis, also can affect the body's ability to stabilize body temperature. This occurs when the imbalances cause a decrease in heat production or an increase in heat loss.

> **CRITICAL THINKING**
> What group of people is especially vulnerable to hypothermia as a result of their environmental, medical, and social situation?

Management

The first step in managing hypothermia is to maintain a high degree of suspicion for its presence. When the exposure is obvious (e.g., a victim involved in an avalanche or cold water immersion), diagnosis is simple. However, in some situations, signs and symptoms may be subtle (e.g., hunger, nausea, chills, and dizziness). When hypothermia is suspected, the paramedic's immediate action is to extricate and evacuate the patient to a site of warm shelter; remove cold, wet clothing; prevent a further drop in the victim's CBT; survey for traumatic injuries; cover the patient with warm blankets and increase the temperature in the ambulance; and rapidly and gently transport the patient for definitive care.

Rewarming techniques for managing patients with hypothermia are classified as *passive, active external,* and *active internal.* Passive rewarming includes measures such as moving the patient to a warm environment, removing wet clothing, and applying warm blankets. Active rewarming techniques refer to heating methods or devices such as radiant heat, forced hot air, and warm water packs. Active internal rewarming is invasive. Some of these procedures can be performed in the field, such as administering warmed IV fluids and providing warm, humidified oxygen. Other procedures are reserved for in-hospital care. Examples include peritoneal and/or pleural lavage with warm fluids; use of esophageal rewarming tubes; cardiopulmonary bypass (active core rewarming); and extracorporeal circulation (blood warming with partial bypass).

> **NOTE**
> Rewarming methods such as hot water immersion can cause hypotension from peripheral vasodilation (rewarming shock) and a sudden return of cold, acidotic blood and waste products to the body's core **(afterdrop phenomenon).** Therefore active rewarming techniques in the prehospital setting generally are avoided unless patient transportation is to be delayed.

Mild Hypothermia

In mild cases of hypothermia, removal of the victim from the cold environment and passive rewarming may be all that is necessary to manage the cold exposure. The paramedic can accomplish this by removing wet clothing (wet clothes allow five times as much heat loss as dry clothes) and wrapping the victim in a dry blanket to prevent further chilling and help retain the patient's body heat. If the victim is conscious, warm drinks and sugar sources can support a gradual rise in CBT and help correct any dehydration present. Patients should not be permitted to smoke, which causes vasoconstriction; to drink alcoholic beverages, which produce peripheral vasodilation and increase heat loss from the skin; or to drink caffeine-containing beverages, which cause vasoconstriction and diuresis. These patients may be lethargic and somewhat dulled mentally but generally are oriented with no marked mental derangements.

Moderate Hypothermia

At CBTs below 93° F (34° C), mental derangements are invariably present and include disorientation, confusion, and lethargy proceeding to stupor and coma. Patients with moderate hypothermia usually have lost their ability to shiver, and their uncoordinated physical activity renders them unable to perform meaningful tasks. Management of patients with moderate hypothermia begins with ensuring adequate airway, ventilatory, and circulatory support and maintaining body temperature. The paramedic should first employ passive rewarming techniques and should not permit these patients to move about independently or physically exert themselves. Even minor physical activity can trigger dysrhythmias, including ventricular fibrillation. External rewarming (e.g., heated blankets, forced air, and warmed IV infusion) and rapid and gentle transportation for definitive care are indicated for these patients. Careful monitoring of the patient's mental status, ECG, and vital functions is crucial.

> **NOTE**
> Paramedics should not delay urgent procedures in patients who are hypothermic. Airway management should begin with basic manual procedures (head-tilt, chin-lift) and ventilatory assistance. The use of oral or nasal adjuncts, including oral and nasal intubation, may be necessary to control the airway and provide ventilatory support.

Severe Hypothermia

If the patient's CBT is below 86.4° F (30° C), he or she usually is unconscious. The patient should be gently moved to a warm environment if vital signs are present. The paramedic should institute passive and external rewarming, administer oxygen, and transport the patient to an appropriate medical facility.

If the patient with moderate-to-severe hypothermia is in cardiac arrest (ventricular fibrillation [VF] or pulseless ventricular tachycardia [VT]), the paramedic should begin CPR and attempt defibrillation once. If the patient does not respond to one shock, further defibrillation attempts should be deferred. Care should be focused on providing effective CPR, rewarming the patient, and ensuring rapid transport to the emergency department. In-hospital active internal rewarming will be required for these patients. If a patient with severe hypothermia is pulseless, cyanosis, fixed and dilated pupils, and stiff and rigid muscles (simulating rigor mortis) may be present. Prolonged resuscitation can be beneficial in these patients, and CPR is indicated even if signs of death are present.[6] (Resuscitation may be withheld, however, if the victim has obvious lethal injuries or if the body is frozen so that the nose and mouth are blocked by ice and chest compression is impossible.) Some physicians will not presume a hypothermic patient to be dead until a near-normal CBT has been achieved and resuscitation efforts are still unsuccessful.

SPECIAL CARE CONSIDERATIONS FOR PATIENTS WITH HYPOTHERMIA

Prehospital care for patients with hypothermia should focus on airway, breathing, and circulation with some modification in approach. These modifications are listed below[6]:

1. Pulse and respirations may be difficult to detect. These vital signs (including ECG readings) should be assessed for 30 to 45 seconds to confirm the need for CPR. If there is any doubt about the presence of a pulse, begin CPR immediately.
2. For unresponsive patients and those in arrest, advanced airway management is indicated. This will serve two purposes: (1) it will enable provision of effective ventilation with warm, humidified oxygen (if available); and (2) it will isolate the airway to reduce the likelihood of aspiration.
3. The hypothermic heart may be unresponsive to cardiovascular drugs. In addition, drug metabolism may be reduced, allowing for toxic accumulation of the drug in the peripheral tissues. For these reasons, IV drugs were often withheld when the CBT was less than 30°C. Without sufficient data to support these theories, the American Heart Association has stated it may be reasonable to consider administration of a vasopressor during cardiac arrest according to the standard ACLS algorithm, concurrent with rewarming strategies (Class IIb).
4. Sinus bradycardia may be protective in severe hypothermia. This rhythm may maintain sufficient oxygen delivery when hypothermia is present. Cardiac pacing usually is not indicated or successful.

FROSTBITE

Frostbite is a localized injury. It results from environmentally induced freezing of body tissues. It often occurs in the lower extremities, particularly the toes and feet. Less often it occurs in the upper extremities (the fingers and hands). Frostbite also occurs on the ears, nose, and other body areas not protected from environmental extremes.

Pathophysiology

Frostbite occurs as ice crystals form in tissue. This produces macrovascular and microvascular damage and direct cellular injury. The freezing depth depends on the intensity and duration of cold exposure. Severe freezing can also occur in tissue exposed to volatile hydrocarbons (e.g., from industrial injuries) at low temperatures.

Under most conditions of frostbite, ice crystals form in the extracellular tissue. This draws water out of the cells and into the extravascular spaces. As a result, the electrolyte concentration in the cell can reach toxic levels. The ice crystals can also expand and cause direct mechanical destruction of tissue. This leads to damage to blood vessels (particularly the endothelial cells), partial shrinkage and collapse of the cell membrane, loss of vascular integrity, local edema, and disruption of nutritive blood flow. Ischemia often produces the most damaging effects of frostbite.

When frozen tissue thaws, blood flow through the capillaries is initially restored. However, blood flow declines within minutes after thawing. This occurs as the arterioles and venules constrict and release emboli, which travel through the small vessels. Progressive tissue loss results from thrombosis and hypoxia. The endothelium is damaged and results in deterioration of the microvasculature and dermal necrosis. The process of thawing and refreezing is more harmful to tissue than allowing the frostbitten part to remain frozen until it can be warmed with minimal risk of refreezing. In addition to extreme temperature, wind, and humidity, predisposing factors for frostbite include the following:

- Lack of protective clothing
- Poor nutrition
- Preexisting injury or medical or psychiatric illness
- Fatigue
- Decrease in local tissue perfusion
- Tobacco use
- Atherosclerosis
- Tight, constrictive clothing (especially socks and boots)
- Increased vasodilation
- Alcohol or other drug consumption in hypothermic patients
- Use of medications
- History of previous cold injury

Classifications and Symptoms

Cold injury can be subdivided into a number of classifications. For example, cold injury commonly is divided into two categories: frostnip and frostbite. Initial evaluation of the severity of the frostbite is difficult. This is because the injury does not always reflect the underlying vascular changes.[2] Regardless of the depth of injury, the area may appear to be frozen. Palpation may help the paramedic to distinguish between superficial and deep injury. With superficial injury, the underlying tissue springs back on compression. With deep injury, the underlying tissue is hard and cannot be compressed.

FROSTNIP

Frostnip is manifested by transient numbness and tingling that resolves after rewarming. This cold injury does not represent true frostbite, because no tissue destruction occurs. The initial symptoms are coldness and numbness in the affected area.

FROSTBITE

Frostbite can be graded as first-, second-, and third-degree injuries, based on the severity of exposure. Affected areas may include the dermal and shallow subcutaneous layers as well as the subdermal layers and deep tissues. All grades involve at least some tissue loss. The disrupted nutritional capillary flow is never restored to the damaged tissue. With severe injuries, the affected area remains cold, mottled, and blue or gray after rewarming. After rewarming, edema usually appears within 3 hours. This is followed by the formation of vesicles within 3 to 24 hours (Figure 45-3). The blisters begin to resolve within 1 week, after which the skin blackens into a hard eschar. Eventually the blackened tissue peels away **(demarcation)** (Figure 45-4). This reveals shiny, red skin beneath. This tissue is sensitive to heat and cold and often remains susceptible to repeated frostbite injury.

Management

Prehospital care for frostbite is limited to support of the patient's vital functions, elevation and protection of the affected extremity (jewelry should be removed), pain management, and rapid transport to a medical facility. Vigorous rubbing or massage is ineffective and harmful. Partial, slow

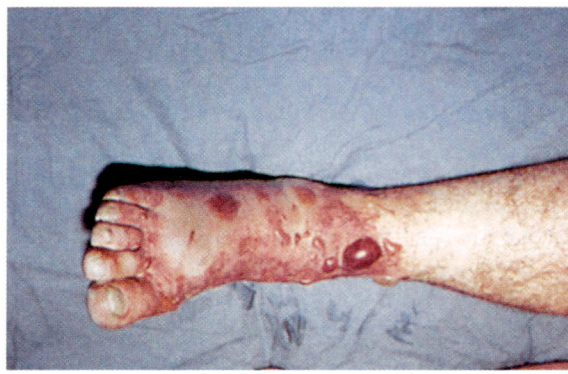

FIGURE 45-3 Edema and blister formation 24 hours after frostbite injury in an area covered by a tightly fitting boot. (From Auerbach PS: *Management of wilderness and environmental emergencies*, ed 5, St Louis, 2007, Mosby.)

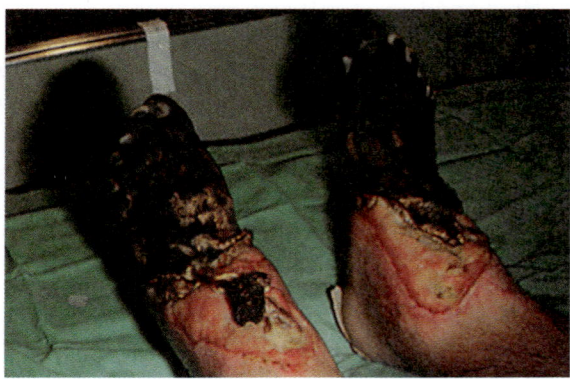

FIGURE 45-4 Gangrenous necrosis 6 weeks after a frostbite injury. (From Auerbach PS: *Management of wilderness and environmental emergencies*, ed 5, St Louis, 2007, Mosby.)

> **NOTE**
> **Trench foot** (immersion foot) is similar to frostbite. However, it occurs from prolonged exposure to cold, but not freezing, water. The signs and symptoms of this condition are similar to those of frostbite. They include pain and the formation of blisters with rewarming. The paramedic should cover the affected area with sterile dressings and keep it dry and warm.

rewarming with blankets or other warm objects can worsen the injury. If the frostbite involves the patient's lower extremities, the person should not be allowed to walk. During transport, all restrictive and wet clothing should be removed from the patient. These should be replaced with warm, dry clothing and blankets to guard against hypothermia. The patient should not be permitted to consume alcohol or smoke tobacco. Rapid rewarming of the frozen part by immersion in hot water (maximum of 104° F [40° C]) is the most effective therapeutic measure for preserving viable tissue. Because of the risk of refreezing, this method of rewarming should not be used in the prehospital setting if transport to a medical facility will be delayed (e.g., backwoods rescue, natural disasters).

SUBMERSION

Drowning was the fifth leading cause of unintentional death in the United States in 2006. It was the second leading cause of unintentional injury or death among children and youths. About 80,000 submersion incidents are reported each year. Of these, 85% of the victims are male, and two thirds of the victims are nonswimmers.[7]

Classifications

As recommended by the American Heart Association, the World Health Organization, and the Utstein definition and style of data reporting, the term drowning is defined as "a process resulting in primary respiratory impairment from submersion/immersion in liquid."[5,8] (The term *submersion* usually refers to the head being below water, whereas *immersion* refers to the head being above water. The two terms often are used interchangeably.[9]) The definition further requires that a liquid/air interface be present at the entrance of the victim's airway, preventing the victim from breathing air. According to this definition, the victim may live or die after this process, but whatever the outcome, he or she has been involved in a drowning event. Victims of submersion incidents usually fall into one of two categories:

- Conscious patients, such as nonswimmers, exhausted swimmers, river canoeists who become trapped by roots or strong currents, individuals who fall overboard or off a dock, and motor vehicle crash victims who are trapped in submerged vehicles; also included in this category are conscious patients who fall into extremely cold water and who do not resurface (*sudden submersion syndrome*)
- Unconscious patients, such as those who suffer a stroke or cardiac arrest while swimming and those who fall into water and die as a result of hypothermia

Pathophysiology

Drowning begins with intentional or unintentional submersion. After submersion, the victim realizes he or she is in distress. An example of this is a nonswimmer who panics or a swimmer who becomes fatigued. Drowning begins with the conscious victim taking in several deep breaths. This is an attempt to store oxygen before breath-holding (Figure 45-5). The victim holds the breath until breathing reflexes override the breath-holding effort. As water is aspirated, laryngospasm occurs. Laryngospasm and aspiration produce severe hypoxia. This results in serious hypoxemia and acidosis, which lead to cardiac dysrhythmias and CNS anoxia. The physiological events that follow are partly determined by the type and amount of water aspirated. Regardless of the type of water aspirated, the pathophysiology of drowning is characterized by hypoxia, hypercapnia, and acidosis, which result in cardiac arrest.

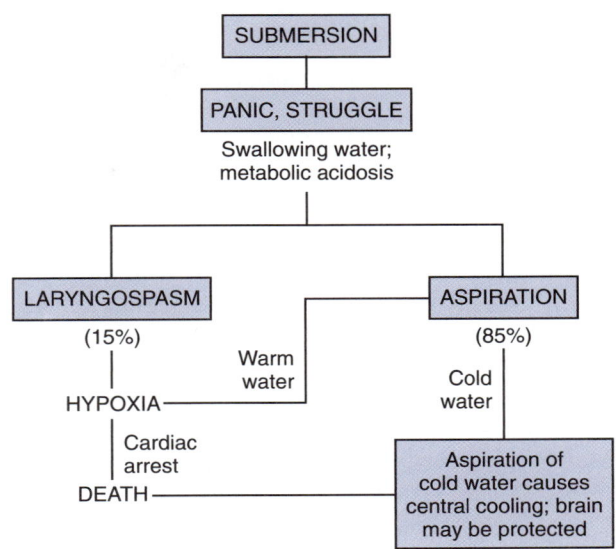

FIGURE 45-5 Progression of the drowning incident. (Modified from Auerbach PS: *Management of wilderness and environmental emergencies,* ed 5, St Louis, 2007, Mosby.)

Drowning can occur in almost any type of water. Victims of submersion aspirate salt water or fresh water, tap water, or contaminated water (such as water containing sewage, chemicals, algae, bacteria, or sand). In theory, different fluids have different effects. However, these differences are not clinically significant in prehospital care. They should not be considered in the initial management of submersion patients. The single most important factors that determine outcome are the duration of submersion and the duration and severity of hypoxia.[1]

Pulmonary Pathophysiology Secondary to Drowning

Respiratory failure, hypoxia, and acidosis are the life-threatening complications of submersion. Hypoxia can result from the following factors:

- Fluid in the alveoli and interstitial spaces
- Loss of surfactant
- Contaminant particles in the alveoli and tracheobronchial tree
- Damage to the alveolar-capillary membrane and vascular endothelium

Poor perfusion and hypoxemia lead to metabolic acidosis in most patients. In those who survive the incident, acute respiratory failure may occur. This includes the development of acute respiratory distress syndrome (ARDS). ARDS (described in Chapter 24) reduces lung compliance and increases ventilation-perfusion mismatches and intrapulmonary shunting. The onset of symptoms can be delayed for as long as 24 hours after the submersion (*secondary drowning*).

CRITICAL THINKING
Do other swimmers or onlookers often "hear" a person who is drowning?

LOOK AGAIN
See Chapter 24: Respiratory, pp. 757-758.

In addition to pulmonary effects, submersion can affect other body systems. For example, cardiovascular derangements can occur as a result of hypoxia and acidosis, leading to dysrhythmias and decreased cardiac output. CNS dysfunction and nerve damage result from cerebral edema and anoxia. The paramedic also must be suspicious of spinal injury in drowning victims. Renal dysfunction is not a common complication. However, when it does occur, it can progress to acute renal failure. This is usually the result of hypoxic injury or hemoglobinuria, leading to acute tubular necrosis.

Factors That Affect the Clinical Outcome

The following four factors can affect the clinical outcome of a submersion incident:

1. *Duration of submersion.* The longer the time submersed, the less likely the patient is to survive. When rescue takes longer than 30 minutes, victims rescued from warm water in summer months or in warm southern waters usually do not survive. Submersion in cold water for up to 66 minutes in children has been associated with survival, including intact brain function. (Most children rescued from cold water should receive resuscitation even with prolonged submersion.) Resuscitation is indicated for all patients unless physical evidence of death is present (e.g., putrefaction, dependent lividity, and rigor mortis). Submersion victims who have spontaneous circulation and breathing when they reach the hospital usually recover, with good outcomes.[5]
2. *Cleanliness of the water.* Contaminants in water have an irritant effect on the pulmonary system. This may lead to bronchospasm and poor gas exchange. These can cause a secondary pulmonary infection with delayed severe respiratory compromise.
3. *Temperature of the water.* Submersion in cold water can have beneficial and negative effects. The rapid onset of hypothermia can serve a protective function. This is especially the case with brain viability in patients who have undergone prolonged submersion. An incident in which a child was submerged for 66 minutes in a creek with a water temperature of 37° F (5° C) is the longest documented submersion with a good neurological outcome.[10] This phenomenon is not fully understood. A contributing factor may be the **mammalian diving reflex** in infant and child submersions. This is a reflex stimulated by cold water. It shunts blood to the brain and heart from the skin, gastrointestinal tract, and extremities. This reflex occurs in seals and lower mammals. It also occurs in humans to some extent. As described in Chapter 22, hypothermia may slow brain

cell death and organ demise that can lead to permanent neurological damage. Likewise, hypothermia can also contribute to neurological recovery after prolonged submersion by reducing the metabolic needs of the brain. (Hypothermia also may develop secondary to submersion and later heat loss through evaporation during attempts at resuscitation. In these cases, the hypothermia is not protective.) The relative contributions of the diving reflex and hypothermia are not clear. The adverse effects of submersion in cold water include severe ventricular dysrhythmias.

4. *Age of the victim.* The younger the patient or victim, the better the chance for survival.

Management

At the site of a submersion incident, the safety of the EMS crew is paramount. Only personnel trained in water rescue should try to intervene (see Chapter 55). Depending on the type and duration of submersion, the patient's symptoms may vary from an asymptomatic presentation to cardiac arrest. After gaining access to the victim, the paramedic should take spinal precautions while the victim is still in the water only if spinal injury is suspected (e.g., diving injury, obvious injury, alcohol consumption) (see Chapter 41). Rescue breathing (if needed) should be initiated as soon as possible. The use of subdiaphragmatic thrusts to remove water from the airways is ineffective and dangerous and may cause vomiting and aspiration. Subdiaphragmatic thrusts are indicated, however, if foreign body airway obstruction is suspected.[2]

After removing the patient from the water, the paramedic should evaluate the patient to ensure an adequate airway. Ventilatory and circulatory support should be provided as needed. Other forms of initial patient care include administration of high-concentration oxygen, pulse oximetry, ECG monitoring, and establishment of an IV line. Patients who are in cardiac arrest should be managed with standard BLS and ALS protocols.

Victims of submersion incidents often are at risk for hypothermia; heat loss in water can be up to 32 times greater than that in air. Hypothermia can make resuscitation more difficult. It requires special consideration with regard to gentle handling, the administration of drugs, and defibrillation. As with all other victims of hypothermia, the paramedic should remove the patient's wet clothing. The patient then should be dried and wrapped in blankets to conserve body heat. External warming and the administration of heated, humidified oxygen at the scene and during transport should be considered. All patients suspected of having hypothermia should be managed as described earlier.

According to the AHA, "all victims of drowning who require any form of resuscitation (including rescue breathing alone) should be transported to the hospital."[5] Asymptomatic patients also require transport for physician evaluation. They should be given oxygen and carefully monitored to guard against aspiration pneumonia and undetected hypoxia that can result from submersion. Oxygen is the most important treatment needed by submersion victims.

CRITICAL THINKING
What are the risks to rescuers on a call involving submersion victims?

DIVING EMERGENCIES

The United States has more than 4 million recreational scuba divers,[11] and more than 400,000 new sport divers are certified each year. Emergencies unique to pressure-related diving include those caused by the mechanical effects of pressure (barotrauma), air embolism, and the breathing of compressed air (decompression sickness and nitrogen narcosis).

NOTE
The term *scuba* is actually an acronym. It stands for self-contained underwater breathing apparatus. This equipment allows divers to breathe underwater. Scuba gear typically consists of one or two compressed air tanks. These are strapped to the diver's back and connected by a hose to a regulator.

Basic Properties of Gases

The weight of the atmosphere exerts a pressure of 14.7 pounds per square inch (psi) of force at sea level. (14.7 psi is equal to 760 mm Hg.) This means that a 1-inch column of air as tall as the atmosphere would weigh 14.7 pounds. This weight is commonly referred to as *1 atmosphere of pressure* (1 atm). Water weighs considerably more than air and can exert much more pressure. For example, a 1-inch column of seawater needs to be only 33 feet tall to weigh 14.7 pounds. This means that at a depth of 33 feet, the total pressure is 29.4 psi, or 2 atm of pressure (1 atm from the air and 1 atm from the 33 feet of water [2 × 14.7 = 29.4]). This is referred to as *ambient pressure* or *absolute pressure*. Every additional 33 feet of seawater adds another 14.7 pounds of pressure, or another 1 atm.

LAWS PERTAINING TO GASES

Three laws of the properties of gases underpin all pressure diving-related emergencies (and some high-altitude illnesses). These are Boyle's law, Dalton's law, and Henry's law. The following properties of gases can aid comprehension of these laws: *increased pressure dissolves gases into the blood; oxygen metabolizes, and nitrogen dissolves.*

NOTE
The term **dysbarism** describes illnesses that result directly or indirectly from changes in ambient atmospheric pressure and the pressure of gases within the body.

Boyle's Law. Boyle's law states that, if temperature remains constant, the volume of a given mass of gas is inversely proportional to the absolute pressure; that is, when the pressure is doubled, the volume of gas is halved (compressed into a smaller space), and vice versa. This can be expressed by the equation $PV = K$, in which P is pressure, V is volume, and K is a constant. Boyle's law explains the "popping" or "squeezing" sensation in the ears that a person may feel when traveling by air. It is the basic mechanism for all types of barotrauma: *trapped gases expand as pressure decreases.* For example, when a diver uses a scuba tank of pressurized air, the lung volumes remain constant at various depths. If the diver ascends but does not exhale, water pressure decreases and the gas in the lungs expands. This greatly increases the pressure in the lungs.

NOTE
Gas expands as pressure decreases. This fact applies to increases in altitude that occur during air transportation. For example, in a patient transported by air, gas can expand in the respiratory system, gastrointestinal system, or sinuses as altitude increases and pressure decreases. Medical equipment also can be affected by an increase in air volume. Examples include endotracheal tube cuffs and air splints.

Dalton's Law. Dalton's law states that the pressure exerted by each gas in a mixture of gases is the same pressure that the gas would exert if it alone occupied the same volume. On the other hand, the total pressure of a mixture of gases equals the sum of the partial pressures that make up the mixture. This law is expressed by the equation $P_t = PO_2 + PN_2 + P_x$, where P_t is the total pressure, PO_2 is the partial pressure of oxygen, PN_2 is the partial pressure of nitrogen, and P_x is the partial pressure of the remaining gases in the mixture.

To simplify, the air we breathe is about 80% nitrogen and 20% oxygen; that is, about 80% of the pressure of the air (i.e., the gas mixture) is exerted by the nitrogen in the mixture. About 20% of the pressure is exerted by the oxygen in the mixture. This means that at sea level, the pressure exerted on us by the nitrogen in the air is 80% of 14.7, or 11.76 psi; the pressure from the oxygen is 20% of 14.7, or 2.94 psi. Together, these account for the 14.7 psi of pressure at the surface. Even though the gas mixtures remain with normal percentages of nitrogen and oxygen, the partial pressures of these gases change at different altitudes above sea level or at depths below sea level. The principles of this law explain problems that can arise from the breathing of compressed air: *gas expansion causes the partial pressure of oxygen to drop as gas molecules move farther apart, reducing the available oxygen.*

Henry's Law. Henry's law states that, at a constant temperature, the solubility of a gas in a liquid solution is proportionate to the partial pressure of the gas. This means that more gas can be dissolved into a liquid at a higher pressure, and less gas can be dissolved into the liquid when that pressure is released. For example, when a container of a carbonated beverage (pressurized with dissolved carbon dioxide gas) is opened, a "pop" is heard and bubbles form on the liquid. This occurs because the pressure in the container is no longer great enough to hold the dissolved gas inside. Henry's law is expressed by the equation: $\% X = P_x / P_t \times 100$, where $\% X$ is the amount of gas dissolved in a liquid, P_x is the partial pressure of the gas, and P_t is the total atmospheric pressure. This law explains why more nitrogen, which makes up almost 80% of air, dissolves in a diver's body as ambient pressure increases with descent. This dissolved nitrogen is released from the tissues on ascent as pressure decreases.

Barotrauma

Barotrauma is tissue injury caused by a change in pressure, which compresses or expands gas contained in various body structures. The type of barotrauma depends on whether the diver is in descent or ascent. Barotrauma is the most common injury of scuba divers.

BAROTRAUMA OF DESCENT

Barotrauma of descent (also known as *squeeze*) results from the compression of gas in enclosed spaces as the ambient pressure increases with descent under water. Air trapped in noncollapsible chambers is compressed. This leads to a vacuum-type effect that results in severe, sharp pain caused by the distortion; vascular engorgement; edema; and hemorrhage of the exposed tissue (Box 45-3). As a rule, squeeze usually results from a blocked eustachian tube or from failure of the diver to clear (open) the eustachian tube with exhalation during descent. The ears and paranasal sinuses are most likely to be affected. Squeeze occurs in the ears, sinuses, lungs and airways, gastrointestinal tract, thorax, teeth (pulp decay, recent extraction of sockets or fillings), or added air spaces (face mask or diving suit).

The management of barotrauma of descent involves slowly returning the diver to shallower depths. Prehospital care is mainly supportive. After the patient has been evaluated by a physician, definitive care may include bed rest with the head elevated, avoidance of strain and strenuous activity, use of decongestants and possibly antihistamines and antibiotics, and perhaps surgical repair.

 CRITICAL THINKING

What preexisting illness can make a diver more susceptible to squeeze?

BAROTRAUMA OF ASCENT

Barotrauma of ascent occurs through the reverse process of descent ("reverse squeeze"). Assuming that the air-filled cavities of the body have equalized pressure during the diver's descent, the volume of air trapped in this pressurized space expands as ambient pressure decreases with ascent (Boyle's law). If air is not allowed to escape because

---

BOX 45-3   Signs and Symptoms of Diving-Related Conditions

Squeeze
Pain
Sensation of fullness
Headache
Disorientation
Vertigo
Nausea
Bleeding from the nose or ears

Pulmonary Overpressurization Syndrome (POPS)
Gradually increasing chest pain
Hoarseness
Neck fullness
Dyspnea
Dysphagia
Subcutaneous emphysema

Air Embolism
Focal paralysis or sensory changes (strokelike symptoms)
Aphasia
Confusion
Blindness or other visual disturbances
Convulsions
Loss of consciousness
Dizziness
Vertigo
Abdominal pain
Cardiac arrest

Decompression Sickness
Shortness of breath
Itching
Rash
Joint pain
Crepitus
Fatigue
Vertigo
Paresthesias
Paralysis
Seizures
Unconsciousness

Nitrogen Narcosis
Impaired judgment
Sensation of alcohol intoxication
Slowed motor response
Loss of proprioception
Euphoria

---

of obstruction (e.g., breath-holding, bronchospasm, or mucous plug), the expanding gases distend the tissues surrounding them. The most common cause of this type of barotrauma is breath-holding during ascent.

Problems from reverse squeeze are rare. However, one type of reverse squeeze (**pulmonary overpressurization** syndrome [POPS]) can occur as a result of the expansion of trapped air in the lungs and can lead to alveolar rupture. It also can lead to leakage of air into areas outside the alveoli. The clinical syndromes associated with barotrauma of ascent include pneumomediastinum, subcutaneous emphysema, pneumopericardium, pneumothorax, pneumoperitoneum, and systemic arterial air embolism. Except for tension pneumothorax (a rare complication that may require needle or tube decompression) and air embolism, which may require hyperbaric recompression therapy (Box 45-4), POPS usually requires only administration of oxygen, observation, and transport for evaluation by a physician.

AIR EMBOLISM

Air embolism is the most serious complication of pulmonary barotrauma. It is a major cause of death and disability among sport divers. Divers risk this condition when they ascend too rapidly or hold their breath during ascent. The classic description of a dive causing an air embolism is rapidly ascending to the surface because of panic.

Air embolism results as the expanding air disrupts tissues and air is forced into the circulatory system. The air bubbles pass through the left side of the heart and become lodged in small arterioles. This occludes distal circulation. The syndrome usually manifests as the diver surfaces and exhales. Exhaling releases the high intrapulmonic pressure that resulted from lung overexpansion. With the decrease in intrathoracic pressure, bubbles advance into the left side of the heart and enter the systemic arterial supply. This results in a dramatic presentation. The clinical manifestations depend on the site of systemic arterial occlusion. The most common presentation of air embolism is similar to that of stroke and includes vertigo, confusion, loss of consciousness, visual disturbances, and focal neurologic deficits.

Air embolism should be suspected if a diver suddenly loses consciousness immediately after surfacing.

Paramedics should begin BLS and ALS measures, and the patient should be rapidly transported for recompression treatment. Also, the patient should be thoroughly evaluated for signs of POPS, such as a pneumothorax.

A patient suspected of having an air embolism should be transported in a horizontal, neutral position.[2,12] This position helps to avoid aggravating cerebral edema that may develop. If air transport is to be used, the patient should be transported by an aircraft that is pressurized to sea level. The patient also can be transported by a rotary wing aircraft that flies at low altitude. This prevents existing intraarterial air bubbles from expanding further. The flight altitude must be as low as possible if the internal cabin pressure cannot be maintained at sea level. Ideally, it should never be over 1000 feet above sea level.

Recompression. **Recompression** is the use of elevated pressure (including hyperbaric oxygen therapy) to treat conditions within the body caused by a rapid decrease in pressure (e.g., air embolism). Recompression takes place in a hyperbaric oxygen chamber (Figure 45-6). As described in Chapter 33, hyperbaric chambers allow for the delivery of oxygen at a higher than normal atmospheric pressure. The process is used to overcome the natural limit of oxygen solubility in blood. It thus reduces the intravascular bubble volume and restores tissue perfusion. Slow decompression helps to prevent bubbles from re-forming. Paramedics should know the location of the nearest hyperbaric treatment facility and should follow the protocol established by medical direction. Ground transportation to a hyperbaric facility is preferred over air transportation. This is because the increase in altitude lowers the ambient pressure and allows microbubbles to expand. Recompression is not required for diving injuries such as ear or facial barotrauma, nitrogen narcosis, pneumothorax, pneumomediastinum, or subcutaneous emphysema.[2]

CRITICAL THINKING
Where is the nearest hyperbaric chamber in your area?

BOX 45-4 Hyperbaric Oxygen Therapy

Altering the surrounding air pressure for medical treatment is a practice that dates back to the seventeenth century. At that time, "fevers and inflammations" were treated in crude chambers that were pressurized using hand bellows. Today, hyperbaric oxygen therapy (HBOT) is carried out in single-person chambers (mono chamber). These are monoplace chambers. The treatment also can be done in larger multiplace chambers (dual chamber), which can house several patients and the attending hyperbaric health care workers. HBOT has proved to be effective in the treatment of a wide variety of medical disorders. These include air embolism and decompression sickness; carbon monoxide poisoning and smoke inhalation; carbon monoxide poisoning complicated by cyanide poisoning; clostridial myonecrosis (gas gangrene); crush injury, compartment syndrome, and other acute traumatic ischemias; intracranial abscesses; and thermal burns. It also has been shown to enhance the healing of certain problem wounds.

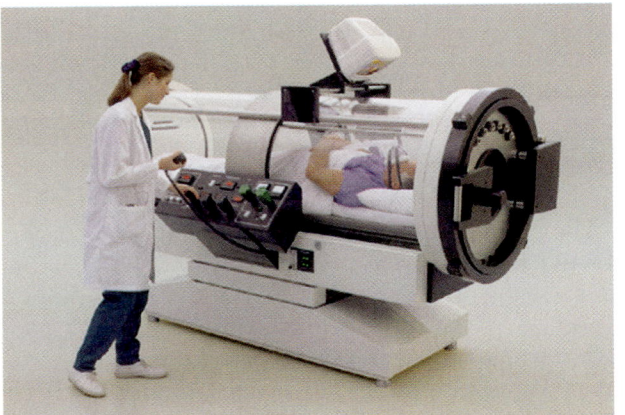

FIGURE 45-6 Hyperbaric oxygen chamber. (From Auerbach PS: *Management of wilderness and environmental emergencies,* ed 5, St Louis, 2007, Mosby.)

> **NOTE**
> The Diver's Alert Network, a nonprofit organization operated by Duke University Medical Center, specializes in diving-related illnesses. It offers consultation and referral services. The telephone number is 1-800-446-2671.

DECOMPRESSION SICKNESS

Decompression sickness is also known as *the bends, dysbarism, caisson disease,* and *diver's paralysis.* It is a multisystem disorder. It results when nitrogen in compressed air (dissolved into tissues and blood from the increase in the partial pressure of the gas at depth) converts back from solution to gas. This results in the formation of bubbles in the tissues and blood. The syndrome occurs when the ambient pressure decreases (Henry's law). The cause is an ascent that is too rapid. In such an ascent, the balance between the dissolved nitrogen in tissue and blood and the partial pressure of nitrogen in the inspired gas cannot be reached. Because the nitrogen bubbles can form in any tissue, *lymphedema* (the accumulation of lymph in soft tissues), cellular distention, and cellular rupture also can occur. The net effect of all these processes is poor tissue perfusion and ischemia. The joints and the spinal cord are most often affected. Signs and symptoms of decompression sickness may initially include rashes, itching, and a complaint of "bubbles under the skin." Pulmonary complaints may include chest pain, cough, and shortness of breath.

Failure to make recommended decompression "stops" during ascent usually causes decompression sickness. (Stops are based on diving tables and charts that consider depth, the duration of the dive, and previous dives completed.) Making stops during the ascent allows more time for safe *off-gassing.* Many hyperbaric professionals advise a 3- to 5-minute safety stop at 15 to 20 feet for any dive.[13] For dives below 60 feet, another safety stop at 30 feet may be of value. If possible, the paramedic should ask the diver about safety stops made during ascent.

> **NOTE**
> Compressed gas at 33 feet (2 atmospheres) doubles in volume when the diver moves to the surface (1 atmosphere). This is because the pressure is half of 33 feet. The last 6 feet of ascent have the greatest potential for volume expansion. This is considered the most dangerous depth.

The paramedic should suspect decompression sickness in any patient who has symptoms within 12 to 36 hours after a scuba dive. These will be symptoms that cannot be explained by other conditions. (An example is a patient with unexplained joint pain who had been diving within the previous 24 hours.) Prehospital care includes support of vital functions, administration of high-concentration oxygen, fluid resuscitation, and rapid transportation for recompression. The patient transport and air evacuation guidelines described for air embolism should also be used with these patients.

NITROGEN NARCOSIS

Nitrogen narcosis ("rapture of the deep") is a condition in which nitrogen becomes dissolved in the blood. This is caused by a higher than normal partial pressure of nitrogen. Dissolved nitrogen crosses the blood-brain barrier. It produces depressant effects similar to those of alcohol. This can seriously impair the diver's thinking and lead to lethal errors in judgment. Symptoms of nitrogen narcosis usually become evident at depths of 75 to 100 feet. At depths below 300 feet, with standard air (an oxygen-nitrogen mixture), the diver loses consciousness. Nitrogen narcosis affects all divers, but is better tolerated by experienced divers. It is more likely to occur if the diver is cold, fatigued, or frightened. Helium-oxygen mixtures are used to improve the nitrogen complication (improving mental clarity) for deep dives. (Examples of these mixtures are TriMix and Heliox.) The narcotic effects of nitrogen are reversed with ascent.

> **NOTE**
> The depressant effect of pressurized nitrogen has been compared to drinking one dry martini on an empty stomach every 10 minutes (the "martini rule"). The theory is that being 15 meters under water is equivalent to drinking one martini; at 30 meters, two martinis; at 45 meters, three martinis, and so on.

Nitrogen narcosis is a common factor in diving accidents, and it may be responsible for memory loss. Prehospital care is mainly supportive. The paramedic should assess the patient for injuries that may have occurred during the dive, and the patient should be transported for evaluation by a physician.

> **NOTE**
> Less common diving-related illnesses may result from oxygen toxicity (usually seen with prolonged exposure to oxygen or exposure to excessive concentrations of oxygen), breathing of contaminated gases (e.g., carbon monoxide in the compressed air), hypercapnia, and hyperventilation.

HIGH-ALTITUDE ILLNESS

High-altitude illness principally occurs at altitudes 8200 feet or more above sea level.[2] It is attributed directly to exposure to reduced atmospheric pressure (described previously), which results in hypobaric hypoxia. Activities associated with these syndromes include mountain climbing, aircraft or glider flight, riding in hot air balloons, and the use of low-pressure or vacuum chambers.

> **NOTE**
> Worldwide, it is estimated that about 40 million people live above 8000 feet, and 25 million live above 12,000 feet.[14] Most cases of high-altitude illness are not associated with these groups who are acclimated to high altitudes. Those most affected by illness from high altitudes are people who occasionally ascend into mountainous regions, such as mountain sport enthusiasts and tourists.[2]

> **? DID YOU KNOW?**
> **Normal PaO$_2$ at High Altitude**
> Altitude also affects the normal, expected PaO$_2$. High altitude decreases barometric pressure and therefore the inspired PO$_2$. Up to an altitude of 10,000 feet above sea level, barometric pressure decreases about 24 mm Hg per 1000 feet of elevation. For example, in Denver, where the elevation is 5280 feet, barometric pressure is about 633 mm Hg. At 10,000-feet elevation barometric pressure is only 523 mm Hg. The general formula for changing observed sea-level PaO$_2$ values to PaO$_2$ values at a different barometric pressure is as follows:
>
> Expected PO$_2$ at high altitude =
>
> (High-altitude barometric pressure/760 mm Hg)×sea level PO$_2$
>
> According to this calculation, if a normal person's sea-level PaO$_2$ is 95 mm Hg, the PaO$_2$ in Denver is about 79 mm Hg; at 10,000-feet elevation, it is only 65 mm Hg.[15]

The high-altitude syndromes discussed in this chapter are acute mountain sickness (AMS), high-altitude pulmonary edema, and high-altitude cerebral edema. Emergency care for all forms of high-altitude illness includes airway, ventilatory, and circulatory support and descent to a lower altitude. In addition, a physician should evaluate all patients with high-altitude illness. Strategies for preventing high-altitude illness include the following[16]:

1. Gradual ascent (days)
2. Limited exertion
3. Decreased sleeping at altitude
4. Adequate fluid intake to prevent dehydration
5. High-carbohydrate diet
6. Medications (all are controversial)
   - Acetazolamide (to speed acclimatization and reduce the incidence of AMS)
   - Nifedipine (used solely by those with a history of high-altitude pulmonary edema [HAPE] to prevent recurrence upon ascent)
   - Steroids

Exposure to high altitude can worsen chronic medical conditions. This is the case even without apparent altitude sickness. (Examples of such conditions include angina pectoris, congestive heart failure [CHF], chronic obstructive pulmonary disease [COPD], sickle cell disease, and hypertension.) These conditions can worsen as a result of a low partial pressure of oxygen. A low partial pressure of oxygen means that less oxygen is inhaled with each normal respiratory volume.

Acute Mountain Sickness

Acute mountain sickness (AMS) is a common high-altitude illness. It results when an unacclimatized person ascends rapidly to high altitudes. The illness usually develops within 4 to 6 hours of reaching a high altitude and reaches maximum severity within 24 to 48 hours (Box 45-5). It abates on the third or fourth day after exposure with gradual acclimatization.

BOX 45-5 Signs and Symptoms of High-Altitude Illness

Acute Mountain Sickness (AMS)
Headache (most common symptom) attributed to subacute cerebral edema or to spasm or dilation of cerebral blood vessels secondary to hypocapnia or hypoxia
Malaise
Anorexia
Vomiting
Dizziness
Irritability
Impaired memory
Dyspnea on exertion

High-Altitude Pulmonary Edema (HAPE)
Shortness of breath
Dyspnea
Cough (with or without frothy sputum)
Generalized weakness
Lethargy
Disorientation

High-Altitude Cerebral Edema (HACE)
Headache
Ataxia
Altered consciousness
Confusion
Hallucinations
Drowsiness
Stupor
Coma

The physical findings with AMS vary. They include tachycardia, bradycardia, postural hypotension, and ataxia (impaired ability to coordinate movement). Ataxia is a key sign of the progression of the illness. As AMS becomes severe, the victim may experience alterations in consciousness, disorientation, and impaired judgment. Emergency care includes administration of oxygen. It also includes descent to as low an altitude as needed to achieve relief. Definitive treatment after evaluation by a physician may involve the use of diuretics to treat fluid retention associated with AMS, steroids to reduce associated cerebral edema, and hyperbaric therapy.

High-Altitude Pulmonary Edema

High-altitude pulmonary edema (HAPE) is caused at least partly by increased pulmonary artery pressure that develops in response to hypoxia. The increased pressure results in the release of leukotrienes. These increase the permeability of pulmonary arterioles. The increased pressure also results in the leakage of fluid into extravascular space. The initial symptoms of HAPE usually begin 24 to 72 hours after the exposure to high altitudes. The symptoms often are preceded by vigorous exercise.

Physical findings in patients with HAPE include hyperpnea, crackles, rhonchi, tachycardia, and cyanosis. Emergency care includes administration of oxygen to increase arterial oxygenation and reduce pulmonary artery pressure. It also includes descent to a lower altitude. After evaluation by a physician, the patient may be hospitalized for observation.

Portable hyperbaric chambers (e.g., the Gamow bag and Gamow tent) are commercially available. These may temporarily reverse the effects of high-altitude pulmonary and cerebral edema. They are used by some EMS agencies in high-risk areas when immediate descent is not possible.

High-Altitude Cerebral Edema

High-altitude cerebral edema (HACE) is the most severe form of acute high-altitude illness. It is characterized by a progression of global cerebral signs in the presence of AMS. These signs probably are related to an increase in intracranial pressure caused by cerebral edema and swelling.

Therefore the distinctions between AMS and HACE are inherently blurred. The progression from mild AMS to unconsciousness associated with HACE can occur quickly (i.e., within 12 hours). However, it usually requires 1 to 3 days of exposure to high altitudes.

> **NOTE**
> The symptoms of mild AMS are similar to a "hangover," and usually include headache and slurred speech. Patients with HACE will have symptoms of mild AMS plus ataxia (an impaired ability to coordinate movements) and mental status changes.[17]

HACE must be managed promptly, because without treatment the syndrome rapidly progresses to stupor, coma, and death. As with other forms of high-altitude illness, emergency care focuses on airway, ventilatory, and circulatory support and descent to a lower altitude.

SUMMARY

- Body temperature is regulated by a thermoregulatory center in the posterior hypothalamus. The body temperature can be increased or decreased in two ways. One of these ways is through the regulation of heat production. (This is known as thermogenesis.) The other way is through the regulation of heat loss. (This is known as thermolysis.)
- Heat illness results from one of two basic causes. First, the normal temperature-regulating functions can be overwhelmed by conditions in the environment. These conditions can include heat stress. More often, though, they involve excessive exercise in moderate to extreme environmental conditions. The other cause is failure of the body's thermoregulatory mechanism. This may occur in older adults or ill or debilitated individuals. Heat cramps are brief, intermittent, and often severe. They are muscular cramps that occur in muscles fatigued by heavy work or exercise. Heat exhaustion is characterized by minor aberrations in mental status, dizziness, nausea, headache, and a mild to moderate rise in the core body temperature (CBT) (up to less than 103° F [39° C]). Heat stroke occurs when the temperature-regulating functions break down entirely. This failure results in body temperature increasing to 105.8° F (41° C) or higher. Temperatures this high damage all tissues and lead to collapse.
- Hypothermia (a CBT lower than 95° F [35° C]) can result from a decrease in heat production, an increase in heat loss, or a combination of these two factors. The progression of clinical signs and symptoms of hypothermia is divided into three classes based on the CBT: mild (CBT between 93.2° and 96.8° F [34° and 36° C]), moderate (CBT between 86° and 93° F [30° and 34° C]), and severe (CBT below 86° F [30° C]). Severely hypothermic patients have no vital signs, including respiratory effort, pulse, and blood pressure.
- Frostbite is a localized injury. It results from environmentally induced freezing of body tissues. This freezing leads to the damage to blood vessels. Ischemia often produces the most damaging effects of frostbite. In deep frostbite this can include mummification and sloughing of nonviable skin and deep structures.
- Drowning is a process that results in primary respiratory impairment from submersion/immersion in a liquid medium that prevents the person from breathing air. Regardless of the type of water aspirated, the pathophysiology of drowning is characterized by hypoxia, hypercapnia, and acidosis, which result in cardiac arrest.
- The three laws pertaining to the basic properties of gases that are involved in all pressure-related diving emergencies are Boyle's law, Dalton's law, and Henry's law. Increased pressure dissolves gases into blood; oxygen metabolizes, and nitrogen dissolves.
- Barotrauma is tissue damage. It results from compression or expansion of gas spaces when the gas pressure in the body differs from the ambient pressure. The type of barotrauma depends on whether the diver is in descent or ascent. Air embolism is the most serious complication of pulmonary barotrauma. It is a major cause of death and disability among sport divers.
- High-altitude illness results from exposure to reduced atmospheric pressure, which results in hypoxia. Forms of high-altitude illness include acute mountain sickness, high-altitude pulmonary edema, and high-altitude cerebral edema.

REFERENCES

1. Venable CL, UTMB Anesthesiology: *Shivering*, www.anesth.utmb.edu/Venable/Students/Postop/03shivering.html, accessed 10-9-10.

2. Marx J, Hockberger R, Walls R: *Rosen's emergency medicine*, ed 7, St Louis, 2009, Mosby.

3. Auerbach PS: *Wilderness medicine*, ed 4, St Louis, 2005, Mosby.

4. Casa DJ, McDermott BP, Lee EC, et al: Cold water immersion: the gold standard for exertional heatstroke treatment, *Exerc Sport Sci Rev* 35(3):141-149, 2007.

5. American Heart Association: Cardiac arrest in special situations 2010 American Heart Association guidelines for cardiopulmonary resuscitation and emergency cardiovascular care science, 122:S829-S861, Nov 2, 2010.

6. American Heart Association: 2010 American Heart Association Guidelines for Cardiopulmonary Resuscitation and Emergency Cardiovascular Care, *Circulation* 122(18 Supplement 3): S639-S946, 2010.

7. National Safety Council: *Injury facts*, Itasca, Ill, 2010, The Council.

8. van Beeck EF, Branche CM, Szpilman D, et al: A new definition of drowning: towards documentation and prevention of a global public health problem, *Bull World Health Organ* 83(11):853-856, 2005.

9. Ambulance Service: *Association, UK Ambulance Service Clinical Practice Guidelines. Trauma emergencies: the immersion incident*, Oct 2006, available at www2.warwick.ac.uk/fac/med/research/hsri/emergencycare/guidelines/the_immersion_incident_2006.pdf, accessed 5-25-11.

10. Bolte RG, Black PO, Bowers RS, et al: The use of extracorporeal rewarming in a child submerged for 66 minutes, *JAMA* 260:377, 1988.

11. Lynch J, Bove AA: Diving medicine: a review of current evidence, *J Am Board Fam Med* 22(4):399-407, 2009.

12. Berrill S: *Arterial gas embolism. Royal Perth hospital*, 2006, available at www.rph.wa.gov.au/anaesth/downloads/arterial_gas_embolism.pdf, accessed 5-25-11.

13. Richardson R: *PADI open water diver manual*, Rancho Santa Margarita, Calif, 2009, Professional Association of Diving Instructors.

14. Moore LG: Altitude aggravated illness: examples from pregnancy and prenatal life, *Ann Emerg Med* 16:965, 1986.

15. Beachey W: *Respiratory care anatomy and physiology: foundations for clinical practice*, ed 2, St Louis, 2007, Mosby.

16. Frazier MS, Drzymkowski J: *Essentials of human diseases and conditions*, ed 4, Philadelphia, 2008, Saunders.

17. The Lake Louise Consensus on the Definition and Quantification of Altitude Illness. In Sutton JR, Coates G, Houston CS, editors: *Hypoxia and mountain medicine*, Burlington, Vt, 1992, Queen City Printers.

PART TEN

Special Patient Populations

46 Obstetrics

OBJECTIVES

Upon completion of this chapter, the paramedic student will be able to:

1. Describe the basic anatomy and physiology of the reproductive system during pregnancy.
2. Outline fetal development from ovulation through birth.
3. Explain normal maternal physiological changes that occur during pregnancy and describe how they influence prehospital patient care and transportation.
4. Describe appropriate information to be elicited during the obstetrical patient's history.
5. Describe specific techniques for assessment of the pregnant patient.
6. Describe the general prehospital care of the pregnant patient.
7. Discuss the special implications of trauma in pregnancy.
8. Outline principles of care for a pregnant patient in cardiac arrest.
9. Recognize and begin treatment for complications of pregnancy such as hyperemesis gravidarum, Rh sensitization, diabetes mellitus, and infection.
10. Describe the assessment and management of patients with preeclampsia and eclampsia.
11. Explain the pathophysiology, signs and symptoms, and management of vaginal bleeding in pregnancy.
12. Outline the physiological changes that occur during the stages of labor.
13. Describe the role of the paramedic during normal labor and delivery.
14. Compute an Apgar score.
15. Describe assessment and management of postpartum hemorrhage.
16. Discuss the identification, implications, and prehospital management of complicated deliveries.

KEY TERMS

abruptio placentae A partial or full detachment of a normally implanted placenta at more than 20 weeks' gestation.

amniotic fluid Fluid in the amniotic sac; primarily produced by the fetal urine and placenta.

amniotic fluid embolism An embolism that occurs when particulate matter in amniotic fluid forms an embolus and gains access to maternal circulation during labor or delivery or immediately after delivery.

amniotic sac A thin-walled bag that contains the fetus and amniotic fluid during pregnancy.

Apgar score The evaluation of a newborn's physical condition, usually performed at 1 minute and 5 minutes after birth, including heart rate, respiratory effort, muscle tone, reflex irritability, and color.

Braxton-Hicks contractions Irregular tightening of the pregnant uterus that begins in the first trimester and increases in frequency, duration, and intensity as pregnancy progresses.

breech presentation The intrauterine position of the fetus in which the buttocks or feet present, rather than the head.

cephalopelvic disproportion An obstetrical condition in which a newborn's head is too large or a mother's birth canal too small to permit a normal vaginal delivery.

cesarean delivery A surgical procedure in which the abdomen and uterus are incised and the baby is delivered transabdominally.

Chadwick's sign The bluish coloration of the vulva and vagina that develops after the sixth week of pregnancy as a normal result of local venous congestion; an early sign of pregnancy.

chorioamnionitis An inflammatory reaction in the amniotic membranes caused by infection in the amniotic fluid.

cord presentation A presentation that occurs when the cord slips down into the vagina or appears externally after the amniotic membranes have ruptured.

crowning The phase at the end of labor in which the fetal head is seen at the opening of the vagina.

ductus arteriosus A vascular channel in the fetus that joins the pulmonary artery directly to the descending aorta.

eclampsia A grave form of pregnancy-induced hypertension, characterized by convulsions, coma, proteinuria, and edema.

ectopic pregnancy A pregnancy that occurs when a fertilized ovum implants anywhere other than the uterus.

embryo In human beings the stage of prenatal development between the time of implantation of the fertilized ovum until the end of the seventh or eighth week.

erythroblastosis fetalis A life-threatening blood disorder caused by maternal antibodies directed against the fetus' erythrocytes, secondary to ABO or Rh incompatibility between the mother and the fetus.

estimated date of confinement Delivery date for the fetus.

fetus Unborn young, from the third month of the intrauterine period until birth.

first stage of labor The stage of labor that begins with contractions and ends when the cervix is fully dilated at 10 cm; divided into *early labor*, *active labor*, and *transition*.

foramen ovale An opening in the septum between the right and left atria in the fetal heart; it provides a bypass for blood that would otherwise flow to the fetal lungs.

fundal massage The application of external pressure to the uterus to stop postpartum bleeding.

gestation The period from fertilization of the ovum until birth.

gestational diabetes mellitus A disorder characterized by impaired ability to metabolize carbohydrates, usually caused by a deficiency of insulin; it occurs in pregnancy and disappears after delivery but in some cases returns years later.

gestational hypertension Hypertension that occurs during the latter stages of pregnancy (>20 weeks) without any other features of preeclampsia, and resolves during the postpartum period; recognized by a new blood pressure reading of 140/90 mm Hg or higher.

gravida The number of all current and past pregnancies.

HELLP syndrome A severe form of preeclampsia with *H*, hemolysis; *EL*, elevated liver enzymes; and *LP*, low platelet count.

hydrops fetalis A fetal condition characterized by the accumulation of fluid throughout body tissues, including the lungs, heart, and abdominal organs.

hyperemesis gravidarum A condition of pregnancy characterized by severe nausea, vomiting, weight loss, and electrolyte disturbance; sometimes referred to as "a severe case of morning sickness."

iatrogenic Caused by treatment or diagnostic procedures.

lochia A normal postpartum vaginal discharge that contains blood, mucus, and placental tissue from the lining of the uterus.

mucous plug A collection of cervical mucus that fills and seals the cervical canal during pregnancy. It is discharged from the vagina during childbirth.

multiple gestation A pregnancy with more than one fetus.

ovum An egg in the ovary of a female.

para The number of past pregnancies that have remained viable to delivery.

parturition The process by which an infant is born.

placenta A highly vascular fetal-maternal organ through which the fetus absorbs oxygen, nutrients, and other substances and excretes carbon dioxide and other wastes.

placenta previa Placental implantation in the lower uterine segment partially or completely covering the cervical opening.

postpartum hemorrhage Blood loss of more than 500 mL after delivery of the newborn.

precipitous delivery A rapid, spontaneous delivery of less than 3 hours from onset of labor to birth; it results from overactive uterine contractions and little maternal soft tissue or bony resistance. Childbirth that occurs with such speed that usual preparations cannot be made.

preeclampsia An abnormal disease of pregnancy characterized by the onset of acute hypertension associated with proteinuria after the twentieth week of gestation.

premature infant An infant who is born before 37 weeks' gestation.

premature rupture of the membranes Rupture of the amniotic sac before the onset of labor, regardless of gestational age.

prolapsed umbilical cord An umbilical cord that protrudes beside or ahead of the presenting part of the fetus.

Rh disease An immune disorder that develops in a fetus, when IgG antibodies directed against Rh-positive red blood cells are produced by the mother and pass through the placenta.

Rh sensitization A condition that can occur during pregnancy if an Rh-negative woman is pregnant with a baby who has Rh-positive blood. If this occurs, the immune system reacts to the Rh factor by producing antibodies to destroy it.

second stage of labor The stage of labor that is measured from full dilation of the cervix to delivery of the infant.

shoulder dystocia An obstacle to delivery that occurs when the fetal shoulders press against the maternal symphysis pubis, blocking shoulder delivery.

shoulder presentation The presentation that results when the long axis of the fetus lies perpendicular to that of the mother; also known as *transverse presentation*.

spontaneous abortion The nontherapeutic termination of pregnancy that usually occurs before 20 weeks' gestation; the lay term is *miscarriage*.

third stage of labor The stage of labor that begins with delivery of the infant and ends when the placenta is expelled and the uterus has contracted.

third-trimester bleeding Vaginal bleeding that occurs in the third trimester of pregnancy.

TORCH infections An acronym for a special group of infections that may be acquired by a woman during pregnancy: **T**oxoplasmosis, **O**ther infections (namely, hepatitis B, syphilis, and herpes zoster), **R**ubella, **C**ytomegalovirus, **H**erpes simplex virus.

trimester One of three periods of approximately 3 months into which pregnancy is divided.

umbilical cord A flexible structure connecting the umbilicus of the fetus with the placenta and giving passage to the umbilical arteries and vein.

uterine atony The lack of uterine tone.
uterine inversion A rare event in which the uterus turns inside out after birth.

uterine rupture A spontaneous or traumatic rupture of the uterine wall.
zygote The developing ovum from the time it is fertilized until it is implanted in the uterus as a blastocyst.

Childbirth is common in the prehospital setting. Most often, paramedics only assist in this natural process. However, obstetrical emergencies can develop suddenly and have life-threatening consequences. The paramedic must be prepared to recognize and manage these events and sometimes assist in abnormal deliveries. This chapter presents the causes and treatment of obstetrical emergencies. It also discusses the normal and abnormal events associated with childbirth.

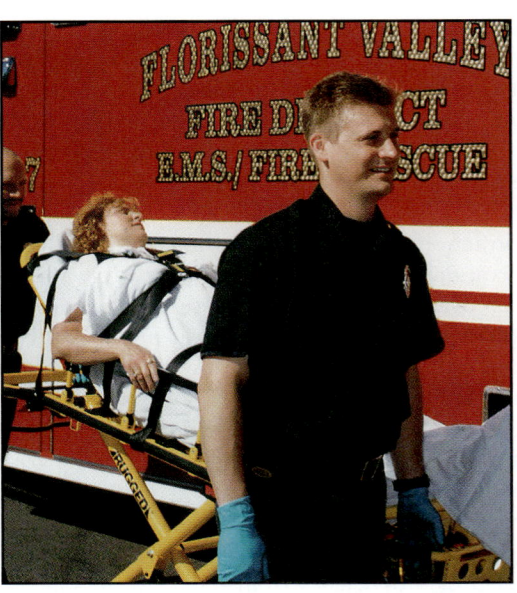

(Courtesy Florissant Valley Protection District.)

REVIEW OF FEMALE REPRODUCTIVE ANATOMY

As described in Chapter 10 and in Chapter 31, the female reproductive system is composed of external and internal anatomical structures that allow for pregnancy. To review, the external genitalia are the labium minora and majora, the vagina, and the clitoris. The internal organs that lie within the pelvis include the uterus, ovaries, uterine (or fallopian) tubes, and cervix (Figure 46-1).

The female reproductive cycle (described in Chapter 31) is under the control of the endocrine system and its hormones. For women of child-bearing age, the cycle usually is a monthly event that begins with menstruation (shedding of the endometrium or uterine lining). The cycle ends with pregnancy or, in the absence of fertilization, with another menstrual cycle.

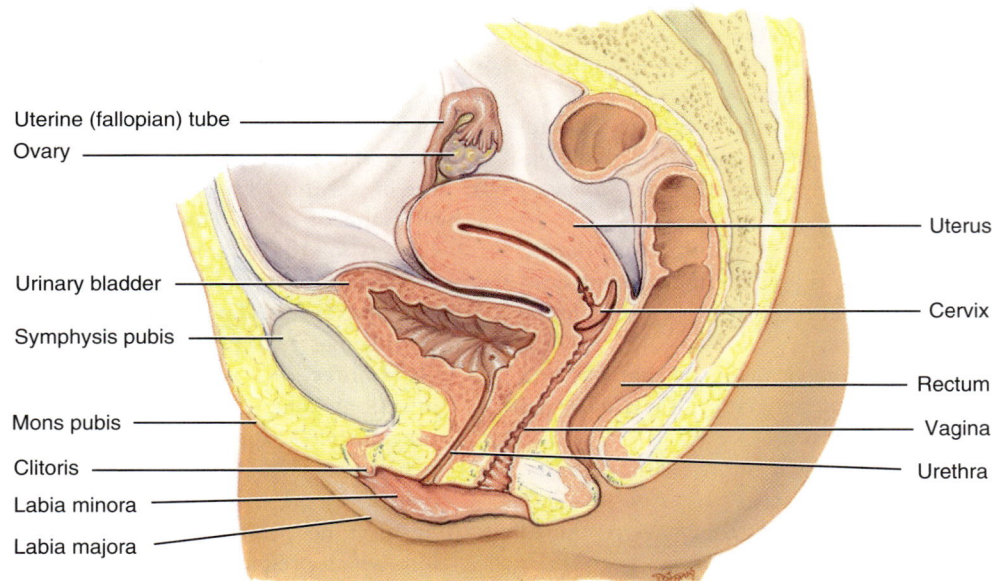

FIGURE 46-1 Organs of the female reproductive system. (From Applegate E: *The anatomy and physiology learning system,* ed 3, St Louis, 2006, Saunders.)

LOOK AGAIN

See Chapter 10: Review of Human Systems, pp. 202-205, and Chapter 31: Gynecology, pp. 930-931.

NOTE

In 2006, there were 435,436 births to mothers ages 15 to 19 years in the United States (a birth rate of 41.9 per 1000 women in this age group). Nearly two thirds of these births were to mothers under 18 years of age; more than half were among mothers ages 18 to 19 years; most births were unintended. Teen pregnancy, birth, and abortion rates in the United States are considerably higher than most other developed countries.[1] The possibility of pregnancy should always be considered when caring for patients of child-bearing age.

DID YOU KNOW?

Cultural Values That May Affect Pregnancy

Pregnancy is a universal event that is embedded in a cultural context, both from expectant parents and from surrounding family members. Common to all cultures is the fear that there may be a negative outcome from the pregnancy or that the baby or the mother may die during childbirth. A universal ideal of pregnancy is that the baby will be born healthy and eager to thrive. Although cultural values rarely affect medical care, the beliefs of all pregnant mothers should be respected. Below is a sampling of cultural values about pregnancy[2]:

- The predominant U.S. culture treats pregnancy like an illness, with frequent visits to a physician, many laboratory tests, and hospitalization for delivery with various medical interventions. Other cultures, however, may see pregnancy as a natural condition that does not require medical care.
- Some Hispanic women believe that wearing proper clothing will ensure a safe birth.
- Some Puerto Rican women are indulged by their families during pregnancy. Exercise is considered inappropriate.
- Some American Indian women avoid tying knots or braids during pregnancy to prevent complications involving the umbilical cord.
- Some Sephardic Jewish women delay having baby showers until after birth to prevent a stillbirth.
- Some Cuban women avoid loud noises or looking at people with deformities during pregnancy.
- Some Japanese women may believe that if they are happy during pregnancy it will cause good fortune for the fetus (who is learning from the mother).
- Some Cambodian women may avoid standing in doorways to prevent the baby from becoming stuck in the birth canal.
- In many cultures, women must avoid contact with illness and death and may not attend funerals during pregnancy.
- Many Navajo families do not choose a name for the baby until after birth because they fear it will harm the infant.
- Some Jewish families select items needed for the new baby, but do not bring them into the home until after the birth.

NORMAL EVENTS OF PREGNANCY

Fertilization normally occurs in the fallopian tube when the head of a sperm penetrates a mature **ovum.** After penetration the nuclei of the sperm and ovum fuse. At this time the newly fertilized ovum becomes a **zygote.** The zygote undergoes repeated cell divisions as it passes down the fallopian tube. After a few days of rapid cell division, a ball of cells called a *morula* is formed with cell differentiation between the inner layer of cells (blastocyst cells) and the outer layer of cells (trophoblast cells). Trophoblast cells attach to the endometrium lining of the uterus. Implantation begins within 7 days after fertilization. Implantation is completed when the trophoblast cells make contact with maternal circulation. (This is about day 12.) Trophoblast cells go on to make various life support systems for the embryo (placenta, amniotic sac, umbilical cord); blastocyst cells develop into the embryo itself (Figure 46-2).

SPECIALIZED STRUCTURES OF PREGNANCY

The placenta, the umbilical cord, and the amniotic sac and its fluid provide nutrients for the developing embryo. They also are part of fetal circulation.

Placenta

The trophoblast cells continue to develop and form the placenta for about 14 days after ovulation. The **placenta** is a disklike organ composed of interlocking fetal and maternal tissues. The placenta is the organ of exchange between the mother and fetus and is responsible for the following five functions:

1. *Transfer of gases.* The diffusion of oxygen and carbon dioxide through the placental membrane is similar to the diffusion that occurs in the lungs. Dissolved oxygen in maternal blood passes through the placenta into fetal blood. This takes place as a result of the increase in the partial pressure of oxygen in the mother's blood compared to that of the fetus. Conversely, as fetal carbon dioxide pressure (PCO_2) increases, a low-pressure gradient of carbon dioxide develops across the placental membrane. The carbon dioxide then diffuses from fetal blood to maternal blood.

CRITICAL THINKING

What happens to diffusion of gases if the mother becomes hypoxic?

2. *Transport of nutrients.* Other metabolic substrates that the fetus needs diffuse into fetal blood in the same manner as oxygen. For example, glucose levels in fetal blood are about 20% to 30% lower than those in maternal blood. This results in a rapid diffusion of glucose to the fetus. Diffusion also transports other substrates, such as fatty acids, potassium, sodium, and chloride. The placenta also actively absorbs some nutrients from maternal blood.

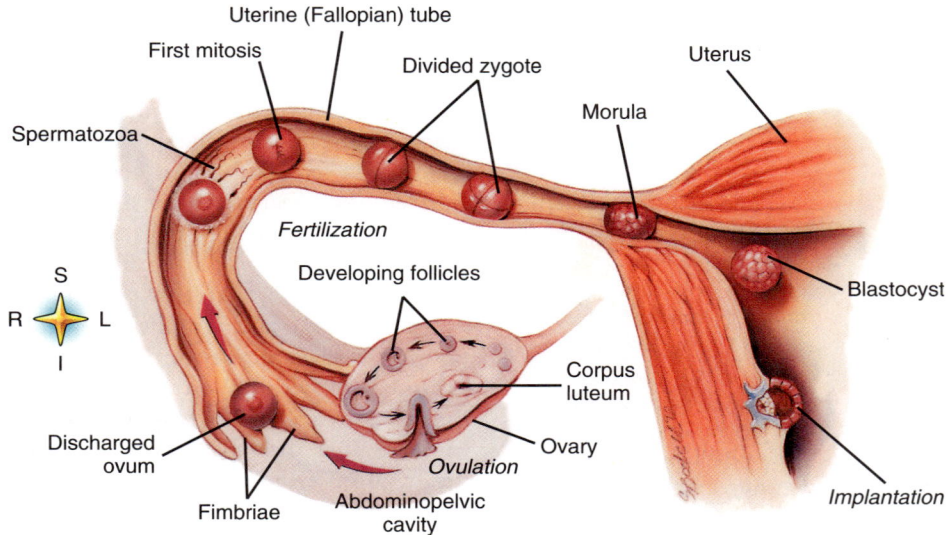

FIGURE 46-2 Fertilization and implantation. At ovulation the ovary releases an ovum, which begins its journey through the uterine tube. While the ovum is in the tube, a sperm fertilizes the ovum to form the single-celled zygote. After a few days of rapid cell division, a ball of cells called a *morula* forms. After the morula develops into a hollow ball (blastocyte), implantation occurs. (From Thibodeau G, Patton K: *Anatomy and physiology,* ed 5, St Louis, 2003, Mosby.)

3. *Excretion of wastes.* Waste products diffuse from fetal blood into maternal blood. Examples of such products are urea, uric acid, and creatinine. They are excreted with the waste products of the mother. Wastes transfer from fetal circulation to maternal circulation by moving osmotically from a higher concentration to a lower concentration, in the same manner as carbon dioxide.

4. *Hormone production.* The placenta becomes a temporary endocrine gland. It secretes estrogen and progesterone. By the third month of fetal development the corpus luteum (described in Chapter 31) on the ovary no longer is needed to sustain the pregnancy. Estrogen, progesterone, and other hormones maintain the uterine lining, prevent the occurrence of menses, and stimulate changes in the pregnant woman's breasts, vagina, cervix, and pelvis that prepare her body for delivery and lactation.

5. *Formation of a barrier.* The placenta forms a barrier against some harmful substances in the mother's circulation (e.g., bacteria and certain drugs). The placental barrier is only partially selective and does not fully protect the fetus. Certain medications easily cross the placenta. Among these are steroids, narcotics, anesthetics, and some antibiotics.

Umbilical Cord

The umbilical cord connects the umbilicus with the placenta. (The average umbilical cord is about 55 cm long with a diameter of 1 to 2 cm.) Blood flows from the fetus to the placenta through two umbilical arteries in the cord. These arteries carry deoxygenated blood. Oxygenated blood returns to the fetus through the umbilical vein. Fetal circulation is independent of and separated from the maternal circulation. Anatomical structures unique to fetal circulation are the ductus venosus, the foramen ovale, and the ductus

arteriosus. The ductus venosus is a continuation of the umbilical cord. It serves as a shunt to allow most blood returning from the placenta to bypass the immature liver of the embryo. The ductus venosus allows blood to empty directly into the inferior vena cava. The foramen ovale and the ductus arteriosus allow blood to bypass the embryo's lungs. The lungs remain collapsed until birth.

The **foramen ovale** is a shunt from the right atrium into the left atrium. The **ductus arteriosus** connects the pulmonary artery to the aorta. Thus the well-oxygenated blood from the placenta enters the left side of the heart directly from the right side, bypassing the lungs. The left ventricle pumps the oxygenated blood mainly into vessels of the head and forelimbs. The blood entering the right atrium from the superior vena cava progresses downward through the tricuspid valve into the right ventricle. Most of this blood is deoxygenated blood from the head of the fetus. The blood is pumped by the right ventricle into the pulmonary artery. The deoxygenated blood passes from the pulmonary artery, through the ductus arteriosus, into the descending aorta, through the two umbilical arteries, and into the placenta for oxygenation. At birth the various arteriovenous shunts close in most infants (Figure 46-3).

Amniotic Sac and Amniotic Fluid

The **amniotic sac** completely surrounds the embryo. It contains **amniotic fluid,** which is primarily produced by the fetal urine and by the placenta. The fluid is continually produced. It amounts to about 175 to 225 mL by the fifteenth week of pregnancy and about 1 L at birth. The amniotic sac may rupture before or at the time of delivery. There may be a large loss of fluid (gross rupture) or a small trickle (leaking of membranes).

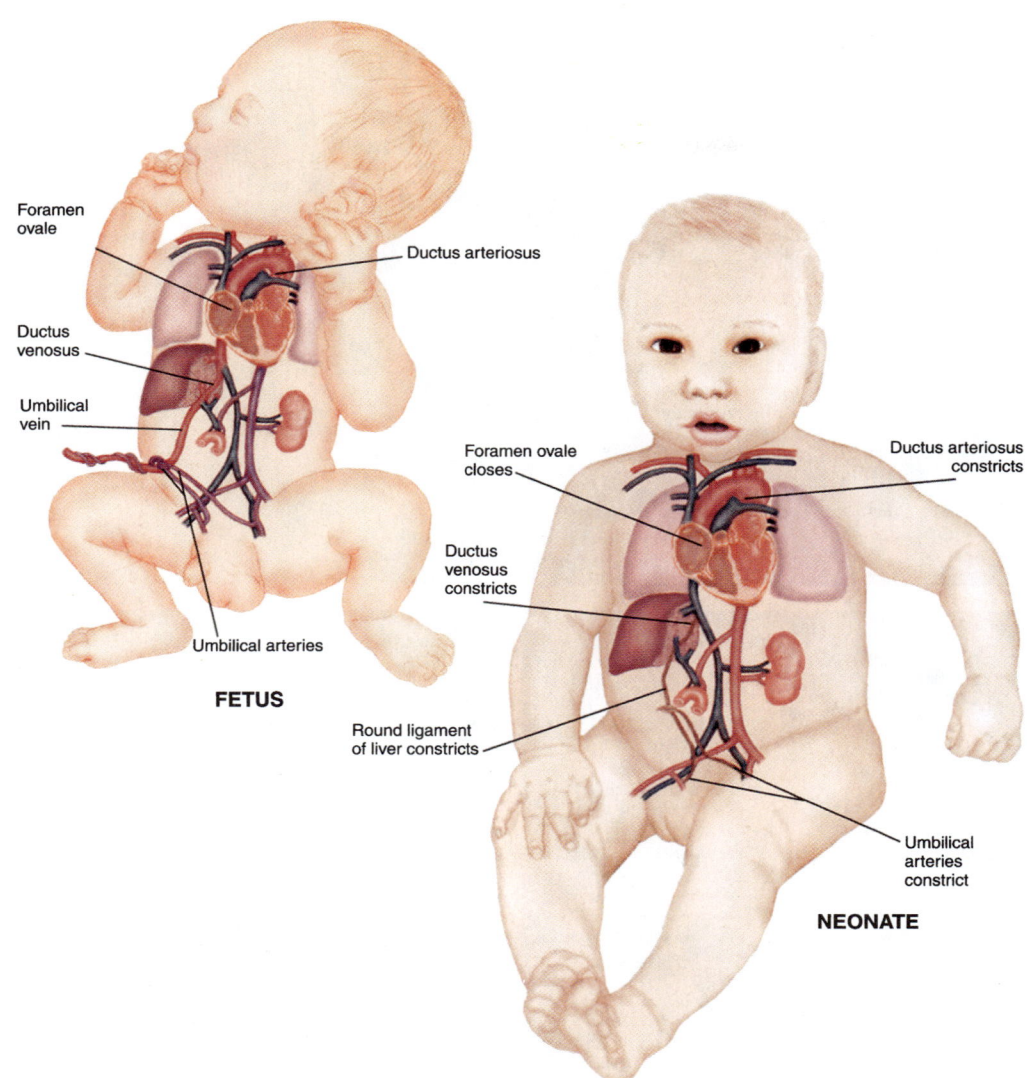

FIGURE 46-3 Fetal circulation and changes in circulation after birth. (From McKinney ES, Ashwill JW, et al: *Maternal-child nursing*, Philadelphia, 2000, Saunders.)

FETAL GROWTH AND DEVELOPMENT

The developing ovum is called an **embryo** during the first 8 weeks of pregnancy. Thereafter and until birth, it is called a **fetus.** The period during which the fetus grows and develops within the uterus is known as **gestation.** Gestation averages 40 weeks from the time of fertilization to delivery of the newborn. Gestation is divided into **trimesters.** The calculated *delivery date* is referred to as the **estimated date of confinement** (EDC). Rapid fetal growth and development characterize the period of gestation (Figure 46-4 and Box 46-1).

Infant Adaptations After Birth

At birth, the infant loses the placental connection with the mother. The fetal circulation changes almost immediately to permit adequate blood flow through the lungs (see later).

A newborn usually begins to breathe spontaneously at birth. This occurs when the chest exits the birth canal or with some external stimulation. At birth, the surface tension of the viscid fluid that fills the alveoli holds the walls of the alveoli together. The newborn's first breaths need to be powerful enough to open the alveoli and to allow subsequent respirations to occur with less effort.

The ductus venosus, ductus arteriosus, and foramen ovale allow blood flow to bypass the immature liver and lungs of the developing fetus. When blood flow through the placenta ceases at birth, there is a resultant increase in systemic vascular resistance and an increase in pressure in the aorta, left ventricle, and left atrium. In addition, pulmonary vascular resistance decreases greatly because of lung expansion. This reduces the pulmonary arterial, right ventricular, and right atrial pressures. As a result of these changes in pressure, the arteriovenous shunts close normally within a few hours after birth. They eventually

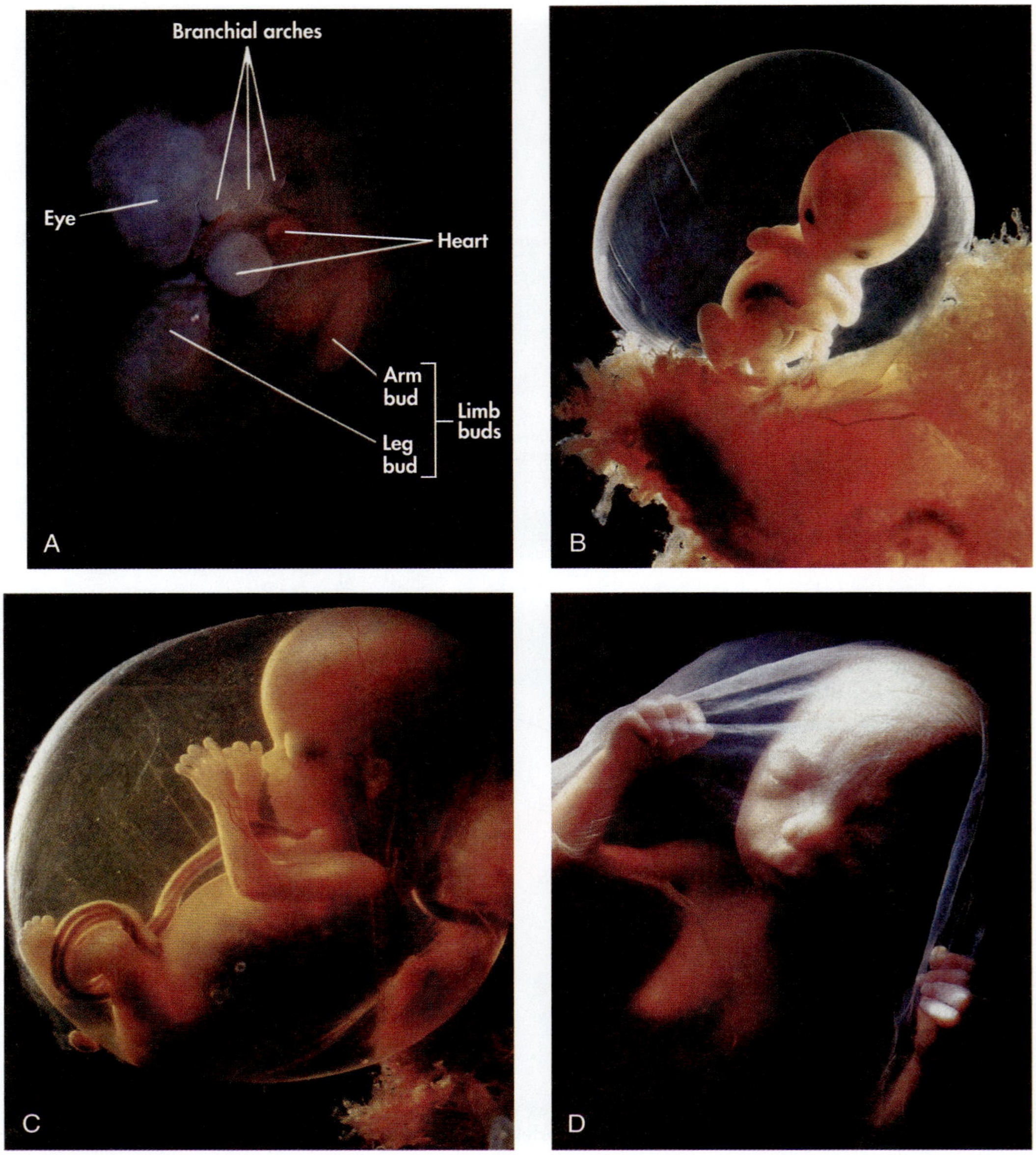

FIGURE 46-4 Human embryos and fetuses. **A,** At 35 days. **B,** At 49 days. **C,** At the end of the first trimester. **D,** At 4 months. (From Thibodeau G, Patton K: *Structure and function of the body,* ed 9, St Louis, 1992, Mosby.)

close completely and are covered with a growth of fibrous tissue.

> **CRITICAL THINKING**
> Do newborn heart tones sound normal if you auscultate them immediately after birth?

PREGNANCY TERMINOLOGY (GTPAL)

GTPAL is an acronym that stands for *Gravida, Term, Preterm, Abortions,* and *Living.* Gravida is the number of times a woman has been pregnant. Term is the number of term deliveries. Preterm is the number of preterm deliveries. Abortions is the number of spontaneous or induced abortions. Living is the number of living children.

Pregnant patients are described by their gravid and parous states. As just stated, gravida refers to the number of times the woman has been pregnant, including the present pregnancy. Para refers to the number of infants born after 20 weeks' gestation. For example, a woman who is pregnant for the first time is gravida 1, para 0 (Box 46-2). A woman who has had two or more deliveries is multipara. A woman who has never delivered a child is nullipara.

PATIENT ASSESSMENT

The paramedic must be familiar with the normal physiological changes that occur in the pregnant woman. This will help the paramedic to assess a pregnant patient.

BOX 46-1 Embryo and fetal Development in Utero for Each Lunar Month (28 Days)

First Lunar Month
- Foundations form for the nervous system, genitourinary system, skin, bones, and lungs.
- Buds of arms and legs begin to form.
- Rudiments of eyes, ears, and nose appear.

Second Lunar Month
- The head is disproportionately large because of brain development.
- Gender differentiation begins.
- The centers of bones begin to ossify.

Third Lunar Month
- Fingers and toes are distinct.
- The placenta is complete.
- Fetal circulation is complete.

Fourth Lunar Month
- Gender is differentiated.
- Rudimentary kidneys secrete urine.
- Heartbeat is present.
- Nasal septum and palate close.

Fifth Lunar Month
- Fetal movements are felt by the mother.
- Heart sounds are perceptible with a fetoscope.

Sixth Lunar Month
- The skin appears wrinkled.
- Eyebrows and fingernails develop.

Seventh Lunar Month
- The skin is red.
- The pupillary membrane disappears from the eyes.
- If born, the infant cries and breathes but frequently dies.

Eighth Lunar Month
- The fetus is viable if born.
- The eyelids open.
- Fingerprints are set.
- Vigorous fetal movement occurs.

Ninth Lunar Month
- The face and body have a loose, wrinkled appearance because of subcutaneous fat deposits.
- Amniotic fluid decreases slightly.

Tenth Lunar Month
- Skin is smooth.
- Eyes are uniformly slate colored.
- The bones of the skull are ossified and nearly together at sutures.

BOX 46-2 Obstetrical Terminology

Antepartum: The maternal period before delivery
Grand multipara: A woman who has had seven deliveries or more
Multigravida: A woman who has had two or more pregnancies
Multipara: A woman who has had two or more deliveries
Nullipara: A woman who has never delivered
Perinatal: Occurring at or near the time of birth
Postpartum: The maternal period after delivery
Prenatal: Existing or occurring before birth
Primigravida: A woman who is pregnant for the first time
Primipara: A woman who has given birth only once
Term: A pregnancy that has reached 40 weeks' gestation

Maternal Changes During Pregnancy

In addition to cessation of menstruation and obvious enlargement of the uterus, the pregnant woman undergoes many other physical changes. These changes affect the genital tract, breasts, gastrointestinal system, cardiovascular system, respiratory system, and metabolism.[3]

GENITAL TRACT

Uterus
- Uterine size increases from 70 g (nongravid) to 1000 g by term.
- The uterus triples in size and weight by 8 weeks of pregnancy.
- The uterus occupies the entire pelvic cavity. It may be palpated suprapubically by 12 weeks of pregnancy.
- The uterus becomes an abdominal organ and the top of the uterus (fundus) reaches the level of the umbilicus by 20 weeks' gestation.
- The uterine fundus descends a little when the fetus descends into the pelvis. This occurs close to term between 38 and 40 weeks' gestation.

Cervix
- Increased uterine blood volume and lymphatic fluid cause pelvic congestion and edema. This results in softening and bluish discoloration of the cervix (**Chadwick's sign**).

Vagina
- The vagina develops a violet color from increased vascularity.
- The vaginal mucosa increases in thickness and vaginal secretions increase.
- The pH of vaginal secretions decreases to about 3.5 because of the increased production of lactic acid from glycogen in the vaginal epithelium. Acidic pH reduces the growth of some pathogens.

Bladder
- Early in the first trimester, frequency of urination occurs mainly from pressure of the expanding uterus on the bladder. Physiological increases in blood volume and cardiac output of the mother may also play a role. Urinary frequency disappears when the

uterus rises out of the pelvis. It returns once again when the fetal head engages in the pelvis near term.

BREASTS

- The breasts become tender in the early weeks of pregnancy.
- The breasts increase in size as a result of hypertrophy of the mammary alveoli by the second month of pregnancy.
- The nipples become larger, more deeply pigmented, and usually more erectile early in pregnancy.
- As breast glands proliferate, the nipples may secrete a clear fluid by the tenth week of pregnancy if stimulated.

GASTROINTESTINAL SYSTEM

- Morning sickness and nausea may occur at any time. They usually begin by the sixth and abate by the fourteenth week of pregnancy. The cause of morning sickness is unknown but may be related to the high serum levels of chorionic gonadotropin in early pregnancy.
- The enlarging uterus displaces the mother's stomach and intestines upward and laterally. This may cause indigestion and gastroesophageal reflux disease (GERD) and may increase the risk for aspiration in unconscious patients.
- The liver is displaced backward, upward, and to the right.
- The tone and motility of the gastrointestinal tract decrease, leading to prolonged gastric emptying and relaxation of the pyloric sphincter. Heartburn and constipation are common.

CRITICAL THINKING

Consider an unconscious pregnant woman who has sustained trauma. What are problems associated with the gastrointestinal changes of pregnancy?

CARDIOVASCULAR SYSTEM

Heart

- Elevation of the diaphragm displaces the heart to the left and upward. Flat or negative T waves may be present in lead III on the electrocardiogram.
- Cardiac output increases by 30% by the thirty-fourth week of pregnancy.
- The pulse rate may increase 15 to 20 beats/min above baseline late in the third trimester.
- Pulmonic systolic and apical systolic murmurs are common. This is because lowered blood viscosity and increased flow lead to turbulence in the great vessels.

Circulation

- Total blood volume increases by 30%. Plasma volume increases by 50%. As a result, hemodilutional anemia is possible beginning at 28 weeks.
- Blood pressure decreases 10 to 15 mm Hg during the second trimester. This is because of the reduction in peripheral resistance. Blood pressure gradually increases to prepregnancy levels toward term.

- The enlarged uterus interferes with venous return from the legs, resulting in peripheral edema in the ankles. Hemorrhoids and varicose veins may be present.
- The supine position may cause the uterus to compress the inferior vena cava. This can produce decreased cardiac filling and decreased cardiac output (*supine hypotension syndrome*). The patient may become faint and hypotensive while lying on her back after the first or second trimester.

Blood

- The leukocyte count increases.
- Fibrinogen levels increase by 50% because of the influence of estrogen and progesterone.

RESPIRATORY SYSTEM

- Tidal volume and minute ventilation increase by 30% to 40% in late pregnancy.
- Functional residual capacity decreases by about 25%.
- The respiratory rate may be normal or may increase because of elevation of the diaphragm by the enlarged uterus.
- PCO_2 normally decreases because of an increased respiratory rate. PCO_2 changes from 40 to 30 torr to provide a gradient for fetal carbon dioxide. This may cause dizziness and a sensation of shortness of breath for the pregnant woman.

METABOLISM

- The mother normally will experience a weight gain of 15 to 30 pounds.
- Increased water retention produces an increase in hydrostatic pressure within the capillaries. This favors filtration from the vascular bed and can result in edema.
- The metabolic rate and caloric demand (especially for protein) increase.
- Glucose escapes into the urine because of increased glomerular filtration.
- Maternal gestational diabetes mellitus (GDM) may result from an impaired ability to metabolize carbohydrates. Gestational diabetes mellitus is further described later in this chapter.
- Fetal demands for calcium and iron may deplete maternal stores if the patient does not supplement them through diet.

History

When obtaining a history from an obstetrical patient, the paramedic first should gather details about the chief complaint. This complaint may not be related to the pregnancy. If possible, paramedics should solicit information about the onset of signs and symptoms and examine the patient in privacy. After ruling out life-threatening illness or injury, the paramedic should interview the patient to obtain relevant information. The history for a pregnant patient must incorporate the following eight points:

1. Obstetrical history
   a. Length of gestation
   b. Parity and gravidity
   c. Previous cesarean delivery
   d. Maternal lifestyle (alcohol or other drug use, smoking history)
   e. Infectious disease status
   f. History of previous gynecological or obstetrical complications (e.g., eclampsia, GDM, premature labor, or ectopic pregnancy)
2. Presence of pain
   a. Onset (gradual or sudden)
   b. Character
   c. Duration and evolution over time
   d. Location and radiation
3. Presence, quantity, and character of vaginal bleeding
4. Presence of abnormal vaginal discharge
5. Presence of "show" (expulsion of the mucous plug in early labor) or rupture of membranes
6. Current general health and prenatal care (none, physician, nurse, midwife)
7. Allergies and medications taken (especially the use of narcotics in the last 4 hours)
8. Maternal urge to bear down or sensation of imminent bowel movement, indicating imminent delivery

> **NOTE**
> Pregnancy may aggravate some preexisting medical conditions. Examples are diabetes, heart disease, hypertension, and seizure disorders. And some medications (e.g., antihypertensive agents and oral hypoglycemic drugs) used to manage these disorders cannot be taken by the mother during her pregnancy. This is due to the potential harm to the fetus. Thus a thorough patient history is vital. The history will help the paramedic anticipate care that may be required at the scene and during patient transport.

Physical Examination

The patient's chief complaint determines the extent of the examination. The goal in examining an obstetrical patient is to identify acute life-threatening conditions rapidly. A part of this goal is to identify imminent delivery. If delivery is near, the paramedic must take the proper management steps.

The paramedic should assess the patient's general appearance and skin color. If she is very pale, hemorrhage should be suspected. Sunken cheeks, cracked lips, or hollow eyes with a history of vomiting indicate dehydration. Vital signs should be monitored often during the care. Orthostatic vital signs may indicate the early presence of significant bleeding or fluid loss. The paramedic should recall that normal physiological changes in the pregnant patient can produce variations in vital signs. Examples are mild tachycardia, a slight fall in systolic and diastolic blood pressures, and an increase in respiratory rate.

The patient's abdomen should be examined for scars and gross deformities. Gentle palpation may reveal the presence of masses, enlarged organs, intestinal distention, or a distended bladder. In late pregnancy, though, these may be difficult to recognize. During the examination, it may be possible to discern peritoneal irritation. Peritoneal irritation is diagnosed by the presence of tenderness, guarding, or rebound tenderness. If the patient is obviously pregnant, the paramedic may need to assess uterine size and monitor the fetus.

EVALUATION OF UTERINE SIZE

The uterine contour usually is irregular between 8 and 10 weeks' gestation. Thus early uterine enlargement may not be symmetrical and may be deviated to one side. The uterus is above the symphysis pubis at 12 to 16 weeks' gestation. The uterus is at the level of the umbilicus at 20 weeks and near the xiphoid process at term. Figure 46-5 shows changes in fundal height at the various weeks of gestation.

FETAL MONITORING

Fetal heart sounds can be auscultated beginning at 12 weeks' gestation. (They may be difficult to hear in a noisy environment.) They can be auscultated by use of a

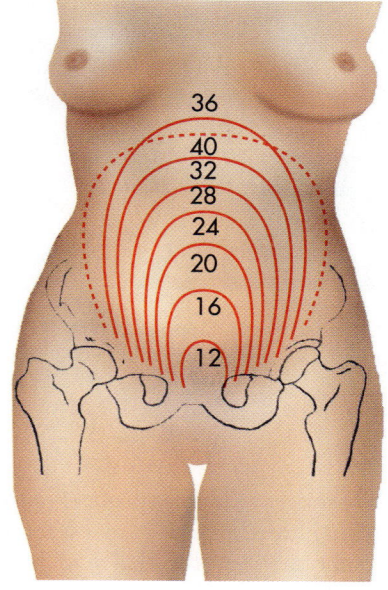

FIGURE 46-5 Changes in fundal height during pregnancy. *Weeks 10 to 12:* The uterus is within the pelvis, and fetal heartbeat can be detected with a Doppler probe. *Week 12:* The uterus is palpable just above the symphysis pubis. *Week 16:* The uterus is palpable just between the symphysis pubis and umbilicus. *Week 20:* The uterine fundus is at the lower border of the umbilicus. A fetal heartbeat can be auscultated with a fetoscope. *Weeks 24 to 26:* The uterus becomes ovoid, and the fetus is palpable. *Week 28:* The uterus is about halfway between the umbilicus and xiphoid process, and the fetus is easily palpable. *Week 32:* The uterine fundus is just below the xiphoid. *Week 40:* Fundal height drops as the fetus begins to engage in the pelvis. (From Seidel HM, et al: *Mosby's guide to physical examination,* ed 2, St Louis, 1991, Mosby.)

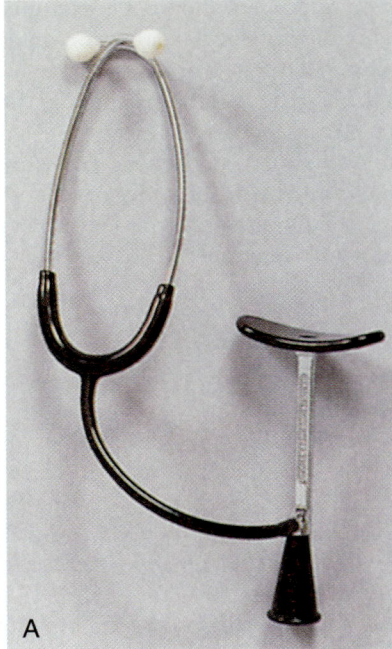

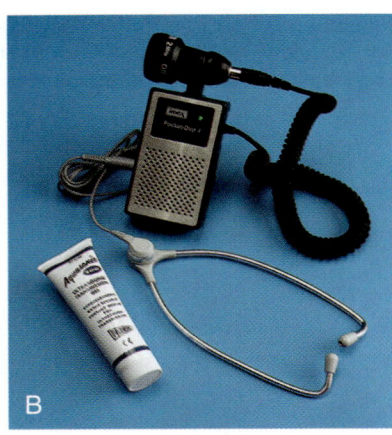

FIGURE 46-6 A, Fetoscope. **B,** Doppler probe. (From Seidel HM, et al: *Mosby's guide to physical examination,* ed 2, St Louis, 1991, Mosby.)

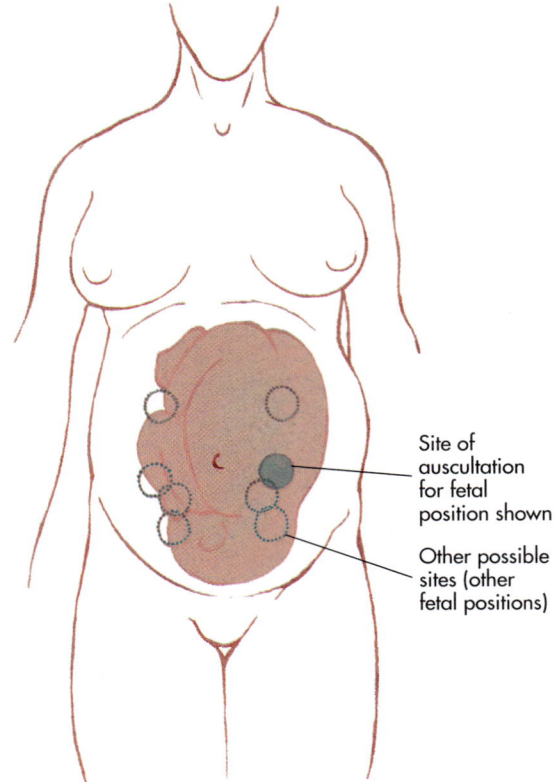

Site of auscultation for fetal position shown

Other possible sites (other fetal positions)

FIGURE 46-7 Sites for auscultation of fetal heart tones.

stethoscope, fetoscope, or Doppler probe (Figure 46-6). The purpose of checking heart tones is to assess fetal well-being. The paramedic should monitor the fetal heart rate and maternal vital signs every 5 to 10 minutes.

When auscultating the fetal heart rate (FHR), the paramedic should position the high-intensity diaphragm of the stethoscope (the bell of the fetoscope or the microphone of the Doppler probe) firmly on the mother's abdominal wall. If more than 20 weeks' gestation, the paramedic should palpate for the fetal back (defined by a structure that is firm and hard versus small body parts). The diaphragm is then moved in a circular pattern of 6 to 8 inches in diameter around the woman's umbilicus until fetal heart tones can be heard (Figure 46-7). If using a Doppler, it should be placed below the umbilicus on the

side of the fetal back. Once the paramedic locates the tones, the fetal heart rate is measured in beats per minute. Because fetal heart tones can often be difficult to hear, one should not spend too much time trying to find them, particularly in a patient who is seriously sick, in active labor, or otherwise unstable.

> **NOTE**
> At 12 to 15 weeks' gestation, the fetal heart rate can be heard directly above the mother's symphysis pubis, or slightly to the right or left. At 15 to 26 weeks' gestation, fetal heart rate should be monitored halfway between the mother's symphysis pubis and umbilicus.

The normal fetal heart rate is 120 to 160 beats/min. A fetal heart rate that remains above 160 beats/min (*fetal tachycardia*) or below 110 beats/min (*fetal bradycardia*) for more than 60 seconds may be an early sign of fetal distress. It also may be a sign of fetal or maternal hypoxia. Intermittent, short-term increases or decreases in the fetal heart rate usually are normal. Variation can occur at any time and is a sign of fetal suckling. Short-term periodic changes in fetal heart rate are common during fetal sleep, fetal movement, and contractions associated with labor and delivery.

General Management of the Obstetrical Patient

If birth is not imminent, care for the healthy patient should be limited to basic treatment modalities (airway, ventilatory, and circulatory support) and transportation for physician evaluation. In the absence of distress or injury, the patient should be transported in a comfortable position. (This is usually left lateral recumbent.) The paramedic may need to monitor the electrocardiogram, administer oxygen (5 to 7 L/min), and monitor the fetus based on patient assessment and vital sign determinations. Medical direction may advise intravenous (IV) access in some patients. Most drugs usually are inappropriate because they can mask symptoms of a worsening condition.

> **NOTE**
> Complications associated with pregnancy can result from trauma (including abuse), medical conditions, prior disease processes that the pregnancy can aggravate or mask, the pregnancy itself (vaginal or intraperitoneal hemorrhage), spontaneous abortion, or problems associated with labor and delivery. Often the patient with gynecological or obstetrical complaints is embarrassed, apprehensive, and, if pregnant, concerned about the unborn child. Tact, understanding, and a caring, supportive attitude from the paramedic are important when managing these patients.

TRAUMA DURING PREGNANCY

About 1 in every 12 pregnancies is complicated by physical trauma.[4] When a pregnant woman is severely injured, the fetus is at high risk for death. The anatomical and physiological changes of pregnancy can alter the pregnant woman's response to injury. This may necessitate modified assessment, treatment, and transportation strategies.

Maternal Injury

The causes of maternal injury in decreasing order of frequency are vehicular crashes, falls, and penetrating objects. These injuries can result in trauma to the gravid uterus and to the maternal bladder, liver, and spleen. In addition, an injury that results in a pelvic fracture can produce massive hemorrhage and damage to the fetal skull. As described in Chapter 37, the severity of any injury depends on many factors and may involve multiple organ systems.

During pregnancy, the fetus is well protected within the uterus; amniotic fluid surrounds the fetus. This fluid serves as an excellent shock absorber. Because of this protection the fetus rarely experiences physical trauma except as a result of direct penetrating wounds or extensive blunt trauma to the maternal abdomen. The greatest risk of fetal death is from interruption of blood flow to the placenta from trauma to or death of the mother. This can cause fetal distress and intrauterine demise. Thus when dealing with a pregnant trauma patient, the paramedic promptly should assess and intervene on behalf of the mother. Severe abdominal injury can result in premature separation of the placenta, premature labor or abortion, rupture of the uterus, and fetal death. Causes of fetal death from maternal trauma include death of the mother, separation of the placenta, maternal shock, uterine rupture, and fetal head injury. Although direct life-threatening fetal injury is uncommon in blunt trauma, in penetrating trauma direct injury to the fetus can cause fetal death, even if the mother's injuries are not life threatening.

Assessment and Management

The priorities in assessing and managing a pregnant trauma patient are the same as those for a nonpregnant patient: adequate airway, ventilatory, and circulatory support with spinal precautions; hemorrhage control; and rapid assessment, stabilization, and rapid transportation to a medical facility. Resuscitating the mother is key to the survival of the mother and fetus. Thus during the first stages of assessment and management, the mother's status should be the focus. Despite the severity, all pregnant trauma patients should be given high-concentration oxygen and transported for physician evaluation.

The examination should be thorough. The paramedic must detect, identify, and manage injuries that contribute to hypovolemia or hypoxia. With the normal increase in maternal blood volume, the mother can tolerate more blood loss before showing signs and symptoms of shock. A 30% to 35% reduction in blood volume can produce minimal changes in blood pressure but reduce uterine blood flow by 10% to 20%.[5] Thus the mother may maintain adequate blood pressure at the expense of the fetus. The true amount of blood loss may be difficult to detect. Fetal monitoring is the best available indicator of fetal well-being after trauma. However, patient transport should never be delayed to assess fetal heart rate.

> **NOTE**
> Any traumatic injury to the uterus causing blood loss can result in massive hemorrhage much more quickly than in nonpregnant patients. Any vaginal bleeding after injury should be addressed immediately.

Accelerations of fetal heart rate above baseline are associated with fetal movement and contractions. However, this also may be an early sign of fetal distress. Decreased fetal movement and increased fetal heart rate can indicate maternal shock.

Decelerations in fetal heart rates (below the baseline) result from a decrease in cardiac output and hypoxia. A hypoxic fetus in metabolic acidosis cannot accelerate his or her heart rate. Thus the fetus becomes bradycardic (a heart rate of less than 100 beats/min). Sustained fetal bradycardia (lasting 10 minutes or more) may be a response to increased parasympathetic tone. The fetus can tolerate this only for a short time before becoming acidotic. Fetal bradycardia may be a late sign of maternal hypotension, hypoxia, or decreased maternal circulating volume. It also is a sign of fetal distress attributable to umbilical cord compression or prolonged decelerations in heart rate.

CRITICAL THINKING
What might be some common feelings of traumatized pregnant females?

Special Management Considerations

Special considerations in managing the pregnant trauma patient include oxygenation, volume replacement, and hemorrhage control. Labor is a complication of trauma in pregnancy. The paramedic crew should be ready to manage delivery or spontaneous abortion (described later in this chapter).

Oxygenation

- Adequate maternal airway maintenance and oxygenation are essential to prevention of fetal hypoxemia.
- Oxygen requirements are 10% to 20% greater than in the normal, nonpregnant patient. Fetal hypoxia may occur with even small changes in maternal oxygenation. The paramedic should administer oxygen at 5 to 7 L/min.
- Pulse oximetry should be used to monitor oxygen saturation.

Volume Replacement

- Signs and symptoms of hypovolemia may not be present until the blood loss is large.
- Blood is shunted preferentially from the uterus to preserve maternal blood pressure.
- Bleeding also may occur inside the uterus. The pregnant uterus can sequester up to 2000 mL of blood after separation of the placenta with little or no evidence of vaginal bleeding.[5]
- Crystalloid fluid replacement is indicated, even when blood pressure remains normal.
- Vasopressors generally are not recommended. They decrease uterine blood flow and fetal oxygen delivery. Vasodilators sometimes are given to patients with severe preeclampsia who are hypertensive.

Hemorrhage Control

- External hemorrhage should be controlled by using the same techniques as for a nonpregnant patient.
- The use of the pneumatic antishock garment is controversial in trauma, and is rarely used today. Most studies suggest that the role of the pneumatic antishock garment for internal hemorrhage is very limited.[8] If the pneumatic antishock garment is to be applied, only the leg compartments should be inflated. This is because use of the abdominal compartment may increase blood loss from pelvic injury. The abdominal

compartment can be inflated (by order of medical direction) when maternal and fetal deaths are imminent. However, this is rarely done.

- Vaginal bleeding may point to placental separation, placenta previa, or uterine rupture.
- Avoid a vaginal examination. It may increase bleeding and trigger delivery. This may be the case especially if unsuspected placenta previa is present (described later in this chapter).
- Document the amount and color of vaginal bleeding.
- Collect and transport any expelled tissue with the patient to the facility.

Transportation Strategies

Pregnant patients more than 3 to 4 months' gestation should not be transported in a supine position because of the potential for supine hypotension. In the absence of suspected spinal injury, the patient should be transported in a left lateral recumbent position. If spinal injury is suspected, the patient should be prepared for transportation in the following manner:

1. Fully immobilize the patient on a long spine board.
2. After immobilization, carefully tilt the board on its left side by logrolling the secured patient 10 to 15 degrees.
3. Place a blanket, pillow, or towel under the right side of the board to move the uterus to the left side.

CRITICAL THINKING
Which facilities in your community are prepared to manage high-risk deliveries?

CARDIAC ARREST IN THE PREGNANT PATIENT

Cardiac arrest can occur in pregnant women from a number of causes (Box 46-3). However, many cardiovascular problems associated with pregnancy are related to changes in anatomy that produce a decrease in the return of venous blood.[6] Key interventions to prevent cardiac arrest in a distressed or compromised pregnant patient include placing the patient in the left lateral position or *manually* and *gently* displacing the uterus to the left, administering 100% oxygen, and giving a fluid bolus. The key to resuscitation of the fetus is often resuscitation of the mother. The mother cannot be resuscitated until blood flow to her right ventricle is restored.

An aggressive resuscitation effort is justified in patients who are near term. This can allow for a **cesarean delivery** at the hospital. Fetal survival improves if the time between maternal death and delivery is less than 5 minutes. Survival is poor if the time is longer than 20 to 25 minutes.[6] Alerting the emergency department staff of the possibility of the need for an emergency cesarean section is critical to infant survival.

BOX 46-3 Causes of Cardiac Arrest Associated With Pregnancy

Events That Occur at the Time of Delivery
Amniotic fluid embolism
Drug toxicity (e.g., because of magnesium sulfate or epidural anesthetic)
Eclampsia

Events That Occur from Complex Physiological Changes Associated with Pregnancy
Possible Contributing Factors (BEAU-CHOPS)
 Bleeding/DIC
 Embolism: coronary/pulmonary/amniotic fluid embolism
 Anesthetic complications
 Uterine atony
 Cardiac disease (MI/ischemia/aortic dissection/cardiomyopathy
 Hypertension/preeclampsia/eclampsia
 Other: differential diagnosis of standard ACLS guidelines
 Placenta abruptio/previa
 Sepsis

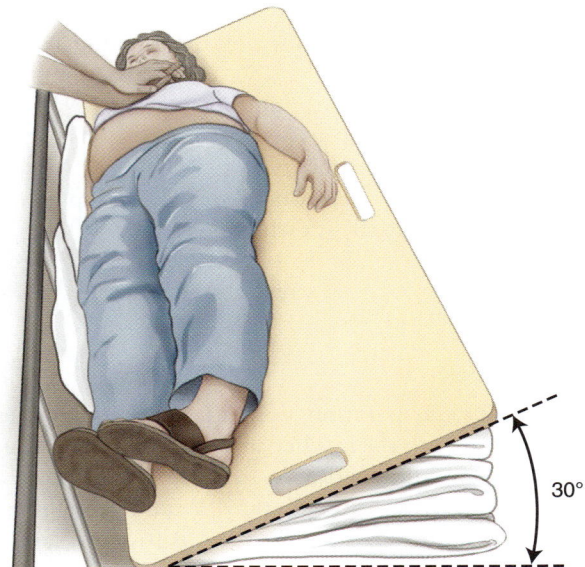

FIGURE 46-8 Patient positioning to displace the uterus.

> **NOTE**
> A cesarean delivery or *C-section* is the delivery of a newborn through a surgical incision in the abdominal wall and uterus. A cesarean delivery is performed for a variety of fetal and maternal indications that can complicate childbirth. It may also be the preferred method of delivery by the mother. Cesarean delivery occurs in about 27% of deliveries in the United States.[7]

> **NOTE**
> Magnesium sulfate toxicity in pregnant patients may result in prolonged PR, QRS and QT intervals, nodal block, bradycardia, hypotension, and cardiac arrest. Should this occur, the magnesium sulfate drip should be discontinued and calcium chloride should be given.[6]

If cardiac arrest occurs, the paramedic should institute cardiopulmonary resuscitation (CPR) with a few modifications[6]:

- Relieve pressure on the aorta and the inferior vena cava. This can be done by placing the hands on the abdomen to move the uterus to the patient's right or left side. Displacement can also be accomplished by placing the patient in a left lateral tilt of 20 to 30 degrees, using blankets, pillows, or a wedge to support the pelvis and thorax (Figure 46-8).
- Generally perform chest compressions higher on the sternum (that ensures a palpable pulse wave) to adjust for the shifting of the pelvic and abdominal contents toward the head.

Other patient management considerations that are unique to the pregnant patient in cardiac arrest include establishing intravenous access above the diaphragm to enhance the systemic circulation of fluids and drugs, and managing maternal hypotension (systolic blood pressure <100 mm Hg or <80% of baseline) to avoid reduced placental perfusion. In addition, the paramedic should anticipate a difficult airway because of changes in airway mucosa that occur during pregnancy. Standard drug doses and defibrillation therapies are recommended.[6]

MEDICAL CONDITIONS AND DISEASE PROCESSES THAT CAN COMPLICATE PREGNANCY

Pregnancy can mask or worsen certain medical conditions and diseases. These include hypertension, diabetes, infection, neuromuscular disorders, and cardiovascular disease. These conditions and diseases should be considered as part of the paramedic's differential diagnosis. Pregnancy can also cause certain conditions to present atypically, such as acute appendicitis and acute cholecystitis. Specific medical conditions and disease processes discussed in this section include hyperemesis gravidarum, Rh sensitization, hypertensive disorders specific to pregnancy, and infection.

Hyperemesis Gravidarum

Hyperemesis gravidarum (HG) is a condition of pregnancy characterized by severe nausea, vomiting, weight loss, and electrolyte disturbance. It is sometimes referred to as "a severe case of morning sickness." In women who have HG, symptoms begin within 2 to 5 weeks after conception. The nausea and vomiting generally eases after the first trimester and typically stops before 20 weeks' gestation. About 10% to 20% of mothers will have nausea and vomiting until delivery, though it is usually less severe. HG in previous pregnancies often follows a similar pattern of duration and severity in future pregnancies. The exact cause of HG is unknown. However, it is likely due to several factors that may include[9]:

- Sensitivity of the brain to motion
- Slow gastric emptying
- Insufficient fluids or nutrition
- Rapidly changing hormone levels during pregnancy, because of the rapidly growing placenta
- Gastrointestinal reflux
- Physical and emotional stress of pregnancy
- Vitamin deficiencies

MANAGEMENT

HG can lead to dehydration, weight loss, and malnutrition that can harm both the mother and the fetus. HG is usually managed with antiemetics to control the nausea and vomiting and rehydration therapy. Vitamin and mineral supplements also may be prescribed. Antidepressants are sometimes needed to manage depression that may accompany the illness. Severe cases may require hospitalization and fluid therapy to manage dehydration. Prehospital care is primarily supportive.

Rh Sensitization

As described in Chapter 11, people with Rh-negative blood do not carry the Rh marker on their red blood cells; people with Rh-positive blood do carry the marker. Rh sensitization can occur during pregnancy if an Rh-negative woman is pregnant with a baby who has Rh-positive blood. If this occurs, the immune system reacts to the Rh factor by producing antibodies to destroy it (Rh sensitization). During the first pregnancy, Rh sensitization usually does not pose a problem for the mother or baby. This is because the first exposure of fetal blood to maternal blood normally does not occur until delivery, which then becomes the sensitizing event. Maternal antibodies take some time to develop. However, if the mother was sensitized before the pregnancy (e.g., as a result of a previous abortion, ectopic pregnancy, or amniocentesis that caused bleeding into the uterus) or if there is a subsequent pregnancy with an Rh-positive fetus, maternal antibodies can destroy fetal red blood cells.

LOOK AGAIN
See Chapter 11: General Principles of Pathophysiology, pp. 245-246.

NOTE
If the mother is Rh-negative and the father is Rh-positive, the baby has a 50% chance of being Rh-positive, and blood Rh sensitization can occur.
If both parents have Rh-negative blood, the baby will have Rh-negative blood. Sensitization will not occur.

Women are tested early in pregnancy for their Rh factor and to determine if they have been sensitized. Women who have Rh-negative blood and who are not sensitized will require antibody tests until delivery; the newborn will have blood tested at birth. Injections of Rh immune globulin (e.g., RhoGAM) are usually given to prevent Rh sensitization. (This will need to be repeated with each pregnancy.) Women who are sensitized will need careful monitoring and serial blood testing to measure antibody levels during their pregnancy. Doppler studies and amniocentesis may be performed to monitor the fetus. If fetal anemia is severe, the baby may need blood transfusions before birth (intrauterine transfusion) and immediately after birth. Early cesarean delivery is common in these cases.

Rh DISEASE

An infant born with Rh disease may have no symptoms of the illness. Other newborns can have a serious and life-threatening blood disorder known as erythroblastosis fetalis. (The most common form of erythroblastosis fetalis is ABO incompatibility. The less common form is Rh incompatibility.) Symptoms of the disease include anemia, jaundice, edema, an enlarged liver or spleen, and hydrops fetalis (the accumulation of fluid throughout body tissues, including the lungs, heart, and abdominal organs). Rh disease is treated with blood transfusion.

Pregnancy-Induced Hypertensive Disorders

Pregnancy-induced hypertensive (PIH) disorders occur in about 6% to 8% of pregnancies in the United States; they increase the risk to the mother and the fetus. PIH disorders are generally divided into three categories: gestational hypertension, preeclampsia, and eclampsia.[5]

GESTATIONAL HYPERTENSION

Gestational hypertension (GH) occurs during pregnancy and resolves during the postpartum period. It is recognized by a new blood pressure reading of 140/90 mm Hg or higher. This condition is thought to result from rejection of the pregnancy by the immune system and can be an early sign of preeclampsia.

PREECLAMPSIA AND ECLAMPSIA

Preeclampsia is gestational hypertension with proteinuria. The hypertension can be *mild* or *severe* (a diastolic blood pressure that exceeds 110 mm Hg). The progression of preeclampsia to eclampsia is unpredictable and can occur rapidly.[10] The pathophysiology of preeclampsia, which does not reverse until after delivery, is characterized by vasospasm, endothelial cell injury, increased capillary permeability, and activation of the clotting cascade. The signs and symptoms of preeclampsia result from hypoperfusion to the tissue or organs involved (Box 46-4). Generalized edema is a possible sign of preeclampsia although it may occur both in a normal pregnancy and in a pregnancy

BOX 46-4 Signs and Symptoms of Preeclampsia

Cerebrum
Headache
Hyperreflexia

Retina
Blurred vision
Diplopia

Gastrointestinal System
Right upper quadrant or epigastric pain and tenderness

Renal System
Proteinuria
Azotemia
Oliguria
Anuria

Vasculature or Endothelium
Hypertension
Edema
Activation of the clotting cascade

Placenta
Abruptio placentae
Fetal distress

postpartum renal biopsy. When preeclampsia is suspected, most patients are hospitalized.

> ### ? DID YOU KNOW?
> **HELLP Syndrome**
> The most severe form of preeclampsia is **HELLP syndrome** (*H*, hemolysis; *EL,* elevated liver enzymes; *LP,* low platelet count). HELLP syndrome is a true obstetrical emergency that affects about 10% of pregnant women who have preeclampsia or eclampsia.[11] Signs and symptoms of HELLP syndrome include headache, worsening nausea and vomiting, upper abdominal pain, and vision disturbances. When the disease is not treated early, up to 25% of women develop serious complications. Without treatment, a small number of women die. The death rate among babies born to mothers with HELLP syndrome varies and depends on birth weight and the development of the baby's organs, especially the lungs. Definitive treatment is to deliver the newborn as soon as possible. The disease affects blood clotting abilities and liver function with consequences that can be harmful to both mother and child.
>
> HELLP syndrome often is asymptomatic with vague complaints made by the patient of "feeling unwell," related to severe preeclampsia. (It often presents without elevated blood pressure or proteinuria.) The prominent symptom of HELLP syndrome is pain in the right upper quadrant, the lower chest, or epigastric area. There also may be tenderness because of liver distention. It is important to avoid traumatizing the liver by abdominal palpation and to use care in transporting the patient. A sudden increase in intraabdominal pressure, including a seizure, could lead to rupture of a subcapsular hematoma, resulting in internal bleeding and hypovolemic shock.[12]

complicated by another disorder (Figure 46-9, *A* and *B*). In addition to a first-time pregnancy, factors associated with preeclampsia include advanced maternal age, chronic hypertension, chronic renal disease, vascular diseases such as diabetes and systemic lupus, and multiple gestation. Preeclampsia is a clinical diagnosis that can be confirmed by

Eclampsia is the occurrence of seizures in a patient with other signs of preeclampsia. It is most common in patients with severe preeclampsia. It is a disease of unknown origin that primarily affects previously healthy, normotensive

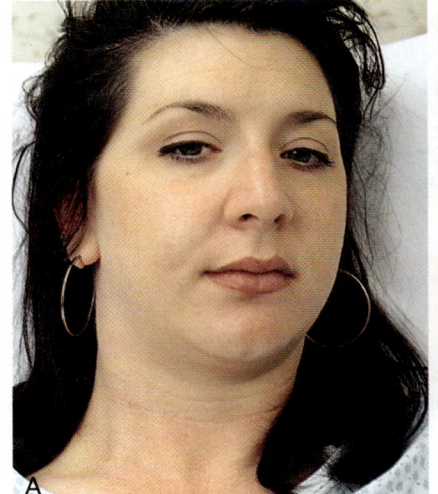
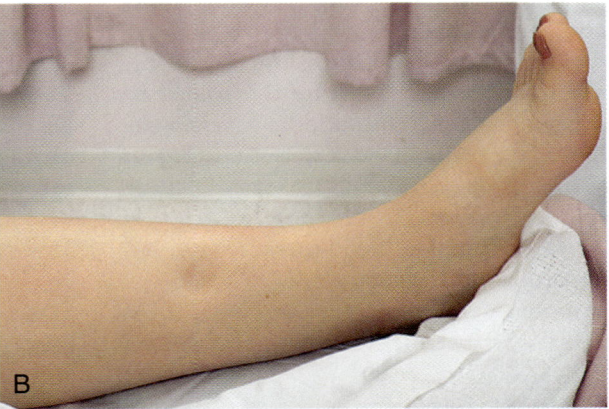

FIGURE 46-9 Generalized edema is a possible sign identified with preeclampsia although it may occur both in a normal pregnancy and in a pregnancy complicated by another disorder. **A,** Facial edema may be subtle. **B,** Pitting edema of the lower leg. (From McKinney ES, et al: *Maternal-child nursing,* ed 3, St Louis, 2009, Saunders.)

women in their first pregnancy. The disease occurs after 20 weeks' gestation, often near term, but may occasionally be seen postpartum. Preeclampsia is dangerous for the expectant mother and fetus for two reasons[2]: (1) it can develop and progress rapidly; and (2) the early symptoms are often unnoticed by the woman or may be attributed to other causes.

MANAGEMENT

Not all hypertensive patients have preeclampsia. Also, not all preeclamptic patients have hypertension. The illness has many serious complications. Thus the paramedic should always suspect preeclampsia or eclampsia when hypertension or headache, visual changes, or epigastric pain present in late pregnancy or within 2 weeks' postpartum. If preeclampsia or eclampsia is suspected, prehospital care is directed at preventing or controlling seizures and treating hypertension (under the guidance of medical direction).

Seizure activity in eclampsia most often is characterized by tonic-clonic activity (described in Chapter 25). The seizure often begins around the mouth in the form of twitching. Eclampsia may be associated with apnea during the seizure. Labor can begin suddenly and progress rapidly. The regimen for managing severe preeclampsia is as follows:

1. Place the patient in a left lateral recumbent position to help maintain or improve uteroplacental blood flow. It also will help to lessen the risk of insult to the fetus.
2. Handle the patient gently and minimize sensory stimulation. (For example, darken the ambulance.) This will help to avoid seizures.
3. Administer high-concentration oxygen and monitor O_2 saturation. Assist respirations as needed.
4. Initiate IV therapy per protocol.
5. Anticipate seizures at any moment. Be prepared to provide airway, ventilatory, and circulatory support.
6. Be ready to administer the following medications per medical direction and local protocol:
   a. *Magnesium sulfate* 10%. The loading dose is normally 4 grams over 20 minutes. It is rare for this to make a patient hypermagnesemic. The antidote (*calcium gluconate*) should be close at hand if necessary to treat respiratory depression.
   b. *Diazepam* or *lorazepam*
      (1) May precipitate a fall in blood pressure.
      (2) May jeopardize fetal circulation.
      (3) Closely monitor vital signs.
7. Gently transport the patient to a proper medical facility.

Gestational Diabetes Mellitus

Gestational diabetes mellitus (GDM) is diabetes caused by pregnancy. The condition occurs in about 4% of all pregnancies, affecting 135,000 women in the United States each year.[13] GDM is thought to be related to an inability of the mother to metabolize carbohydrates. This may be caused by a deficiency of the mother's insulin or from placental

hormones that block the action of the mother's insulin (*insulin resistance*). As a result, the mother's body is not able to produce or use all of the insulin it needs during the pregnancy. Excessive amounts of her glucose are transmitted to the fetus where it is stored as fat. Treatment for GDM includes regular glucose monitoring, dietary modification, and exercise. In some cases, pregnant women will need insulin injections to manage the condition. Gestational diabetes mellitus usually subsides after pregnancy. However, it may return in later years or with future pregnancies.

Most women with GDM are aware of their condition through prenatal care and have healthy pregnancies and healthy babies. Without treatment, however, mothers with GDM often have very large babies. This results in a more difficult labor and delivery (with increased risk for fetal and maternal injury) and a longer recovery. In addition, children whose mothers had GDM are at higher risk for certain health problems. Examples of such are respiratory distress syndrome, obesity, and related health issues as children or adults. These children also have an increased risk for developing type 2 diabetes during their lifetime.[13]

MANAGEMENT

Prehospital care for patients with insulin-dependent GDM may include airway, ventilatory, and circulatory support; glucose testing; management of hypoglycemia with IV fluids and **dextrose;** or management of hyperglycemia with the administration of IV fluids and **insulin** (per medical direction) (see Chapter 26).

Infection

Numerous infections can pose problems for the pregnant mother and some can be spread to the developing fetus and newborn. One example is the HIV infection (described in Chapter 28). Another is TORCH infection, described below. Infectious diseases that may affect a woman's pregnancy, fetus, or newborn are listed in Box 46-5.

TORCH INFECTION

TORCH is an acronym for a special group of infections (**TORCH infections**) that may be acquired by a woman during pregnancy. "TORCH" stands for the following infections:

BOX 46-5 Pregnancy and Infection

Urinary tract infection
Vaginal infection
Sexually transmitted infections
Bacterial vaginosis
   Candidiasis
   Chlamydial infection
   Gonorrhea
   Human papillomavirus
   Syphilis
   Trichomoniasis

T: Toxoplasmosis

O: Other infections: namely, hepatitis B, syphilis, and herpes zoster (the virus that causes chickenpox)

R: Rubella (formerly known as German measles)

C: Cytomegalovirus (CMV)

H: Herpes simplex virus (the cause of genital herpes)

TORCH infections can be passed to the fetus in the womb, resulting in fetal death or serious complications for the newborn. These complications include[14]:

- Miscarriage
- Congenital heart disease or heart defects (rare)
- Hearing impairment, including deafness
- Mental retardation or other learning, behavioral, or emotional problems
- Anemia
- Liver or spleen enlargement
- Pneumonia
- Microcephaly (small head and brain size)
- Jaundice
- Low birth weight or poor growth inside the womb
- Blindness or other vision problems, such as cataracts (a clouding of the lens of the eye)
- Skin rash or scarring

Most TORCH infections can be prevented through immunization, good personal hygiene, and safe sex practices. In the case of toxoplasmosis, prevention includes avoidance of raw meat and exposure to cats, which can sometimes carry the disease.

BLEEDING COMPLICATIONS RELATED TO PREGNANCY

Although most pregnancies are successful events, complications can and do occur. Vaginal bleeding during pregnancy can result from spontaneous abortion (miscarriage), ectopic pregnancy, abruptio placentae, placenta previa, uterine rupture, or postpartum hemorrhage. Patients with vaginal bleeding have varying degrees of blood loss. Some require aggressive resuscitation.

CRITICAL THINKING

When a mother loses blood from vaginal hemorrhage, what effect does that have on her fetus?

Spontaneous Abortion

Spontaneous abortion is the nontherapeutic termination of pregnancy from any cause before 20 weeks' gestation. (Between 21 and 36 weeks' gestation, it is known as a *preterm birth.*) Abortion is the most frequent cause of vaginal bleeding in pregnant women. It occurs in about 1 in 10 pregnancies. Box 46-6 lists common classifications of abortion.[3]

Most spontaneous abortions occur in the first trimester, usually before the tenth week. The patient often is anxious and apprehensive and complains of vaginal bleeding with

---

BOX 46-6 Classifications of Abortion

Complete abortion: An abortion in which the patient has passed all of the products of conception

Criminal abortion: An intentional ending of any pregnancy under any condition not allowed by law

Elective abortion: The elective termination of a pregnancy for nonmedical reasons

Habitual abortion: Three or more consecutive pregnancies that end in abortion

Incomplete abortion: An abortion in which the patient has passed some but not all of the products of conception

Induced abortion: An abortion in which the pregnancy is terminated intentionally

Missed abortion: The retention of the fetus in utero for 4 or more weeks after fetal death

Septic abortion: An abortion complicated by fever, endometritis, parametritis, pelvic disease, often leading to sepsis

Spontaneous abortion: An abortion that usually occurs before the twelfth week of gestation (the lay term is *miscarriage*). (Predisposing factors include acute or chronic illness in the mother, abnormalities in the fetus, and abnormal attachment of the placenta. Often the cause is unknown)

Therapeutic abortion: A pregnancy legally terminated for reasons of maternal well-being

Threatened abortion: An abortion in which a patient has some uterine bleeding with an intrauterine pregnancy in which the internal cervical os is closed. A threatened abortion may stabilize and end in normal delivery or progress to an incomplete or complete abortion

---

pain. Bleeding may be slight (dime- or quarter-sized spotting) or profuse. The pain may be referred to the lower back and is often described as cramp-like and similar to the pain of labor or menstruation. In addition, the patient may have suprapubic pain. When obtaining a history, the paramedic should ascertain the time of onset of pain and bleeding, the amount of blood loss (a soaked sanitary pad suggests 20 to 30 mL of blood loss), and whether the patient passed any tissue with the blood. If the patient passed tissue during bleeding episodes, the tissue should be collected and transported with the patient for analysis.

MANAGEMENT

The assessment of all first-trimester bleeding should include close observation for signs of significant blood loss and hypovolemia. The paramedic should measure vital signs often during transport. Depending on the patient's hemodynamic status, IV fluid therapy may be indicated. All patients with suspected abortion should receive oxygen, emotional support, and transportation for physician evaluation.

Ectopic Pregnancy

An **ectopic pregnancy** occurs when a fertilized ovum implants anywhere other than the uterus. Ectopic gestation occurs in about 2% of all pregnancies; it is the leading cause of first-trimester death and accounts for more than 6% of all maternal deaths in the United States.[5] Death from ectopic pregnancy usually results from hemorrhage.

Ectopic pregnancy has many causes. Most involve factors that delay or prevent the passage of the fertilized ovum to its normal site of implantation. Predisposing factors include pelvic inflammatory disease, adhesions from previous surgery, tubal ligation, previous ectopic pregnancy, and possibly the presence of intrauterine contraceptive devices. Thus obtaining a full gynecological history is important in risk assessment. Although the time from fertilization to rupture varies, most ruptures occur by 2 to 12 weeks' gestation.

The signs and symptoms of ectopic pregnancy often are difficult to distinguish from those of a ruptured ovarian cyst, pelvic inflammatory disease, appendicitis, or abortion (thus the name the *great imitator*). The classic triad of symptoms includes abdominal pain, vaginal bleeding, and amenorrhea (absence of menstruation); however, vaginal bleeding may be absent, spotty, or minimal, and amenorrhea may be replaced by oligomenorrhea (scanty flow). The variable presentation of this type of pregnancy is one reason for its high-risk profile. Other symptoms of ectopic pregnancy include signs of early pregnancy. These include referred pain to the shoulder, nausea, vomiting, syncope, and the classic signs of shock.

MANAGEMENT

A ruptured ectopic pregnancy is a true emergency. It calls for initial resuscitation measures and rapid transport for surgical intervention. The patient may become unstable quickly. If the paramedic suspects an ectopic pregnancy, the patient should be managed like any victim of hemorrhagic shock—with airway, ventilatory, and circulatory support and IV fluid resuscitation.

Third-Trimester Bleeding

Third-trimester bleeding occurs in 4% of all pregnancies and is never normal.[5] About half of bleeding episodes are a result of abruptio placentae, placenta previa, or uterine rupture. Table 46-1 differentiates among abruptio placentae, placenta previa, and uterine rupture.

ABRUPTIO PLACENTAE

Abruptio placentae is partial or full detachment of a normally implanted placenta at more than 20 weeks' gestation. It occurs in about 1% of all pregnancies and is severe enough to result in fetal death in about 15% of cases of abruption.[15] Predisposing factors to abruptio placentae include maternal hypertension, preeclampsia, multiple pregnancies, trauma, and previous abruption.

NOTE

Maternal use of cocaine, which causes vasoconstriction in the endometrial arteries, is a leading cause of abruptio placentae.[2]

CRITICAL THINKING

Why is abruptio placentae associated with such a high fetal death rate?

TABLE 46-1 Differentiation of Abruptio Placentae, Placenta Previa, and Uterine Rupture

History	Bleeding	Abnormal Pain	Abdominal Examination
Abruptio Placentae Association with severe hypertension, toxemia of pregnancy, and methamphetamine or cocaine use	Often absent or scant episode of dark vaginal bleeding	Present	Localized uterine tenderness Fetal heart rate slows after contractions Absent fetal heart tones
Placenta Previa Previous cesarean section Grand multiparity	Bleeding after intercourse Classic bleeding pattern: 1 bleed in early second trimester 1 bleed in late second or early third trimester 1 severe bleed after onset of labor	Usually absent	Lack of uterine tenderness Labor Fetal heart tones
Uterine Rupture Previous cesarean section Tetanic contraction	Possible vaginal bleeding	Severe pain usually present and associated with sudden onset of nausea and vomiting	Diffuse abdominal tenderness Sudden cessation of labor Bradycardia

The common presentation of abruptio placentae is sudden third-trimester vaginal bleeding and pain. The vaginal bleeding may be minimal. The degree of shock is often out of proportion to the visible blood loss because much of the hemorrhage is concealed behind the placenta. The more extensive the separation, the greater the uterine irritability, resulting in a tender abdomen and rigid uterus. Contractions may be present. The absence of fetal heart tones or a bradycardic fetal heart rate suggests severe abruptio placentae, and fetal death is likely.

PLACENTA PREVIA

Placenta previa is placental implantation in the lower uterine segment partially or completely covering the cervical opening. It occurs in about 5 in 1000 deliveries.[16] The incidence is higher in preterm births. The condition is characterized by painless, bright red bleeding with or without uterine contraction. The bleeding may occur in episodes and may be slight to moderate. In addition, bleeding may become more profuse if active labor begins. Fetal heart rate slows because of hypoxia.

Placenta previa is associated with increasing maternal age, multiple pregnancies, previous cesarean section, and previous placenta previa episodes. Recent sexual intercourse can lead to bleeding.

UTERINE RUPTURE

Uterine rupture is a spontaneous or traumatic rupture of the uterine wall. It most frequently results from reopening of a previous uterine scar (e.g., a previous cesarean section). It also may result from a prolonged or obstructed labor, or direct trauma. Uterine rupture occurs in about 1 in 1500 pregnancies. It carries a 0% to 1% maternal mortality rate and a 2% fetal mortality rate in developed countries. The fetal mortality rate, which had been about 65% in the 1960's and 1970's, has steadily declined in the last 2 decades to less than 5%.[17]

Uterine rupture is characterized by sudden abdominal pain described as steady and "tearing," active labor, early signs of shock (complaints of weakness, dizziness, anxiety), and bleeding, which may not be visible. On examination, the abdomen usually is rigid. The patient complains of diffuse abdominal pain. Fetal parts may be felt easily through the abdominal wall.

MANAGEMENT

The prehospital management of a patient with third-trimester bleeding is aimed at preventing shock. The paramedic should not try to examine the patient vaginally; doing so may increase hemorrhage and precipitate labor. Emergency care measures should include the following:

1. Provide adequate airway, ventilatory, and circulatory support as needed (with spinal precautions if indicated).
2. Place the patient in a left lateral recumbent position.
3. Begin transport immediately.
4. Initiate IV therapy with volume-expanding fluid.

5. Apply a fresh perineal pad. Note the time of application to assess bleeding during transport.
6. Check fundal height. Document it for baseline measurement.
7. Closely monitor the patient's vital signs en route to the medical facility.
8. Closely monitor fetal heart rate.

LABOR AND DELIVERY

Parturition is the process by which the infant is born. Near the end of pregnancy the uterus becomes increasingly irritable and exhibits occasional contractions. These contractions become stronger and more frequent until parturition begins. During and as a result of these contractions, the cervix begins to dilate. As uterine contractions increase, complete cervical dilation occurs to about 10 cm; the amniotic sac usually ruptures; and the fetus, and shortly thereafter the placenta, is expelled from the uterus through the vaginal canal (Figure 46-10).

Stages of Labor

Labor follows several distinct stages.[3] The lengths of these stages vary depending on whether the mother is nullipara or multipara (Box 46-7). Thus the paramedic should use the stages of labor only as a guideline in assessing labor progression in the average pregnancy.

FIRST STAGE OF LABOR

The **first stage of labor** begins with contractions and ends when the cervix is fully dilated at 10 cm. This stage of labor is divided into early labor, active labor, and transition.

> **NOTE**
> About 2 to 3 weeks before the onset of *active labor*, the cervix undergoes the process of softening, effacement (thinning), and dilation. During this timeframe, the fetus may move into the mother's pelvis. This is commonly called *lightening*. Lightening is characterized by relief of pressure in the mother's upper abdomen and a simultaneous increase in pressure in her pelvis. **Braxton-Hicks contractions** refer to irregular tightening of the pregnant uterus. These begin in the first trimester (before 30 weeks' gestation). They are usually benign and painless. They often subside with walking or other exercise. Many patients are not aware of Braxton-Hicks contractions. They may perceive them as a slight uterine hardening. As the pregnancy continues, the Braxton-Hicks contractions increase in frequency and duration.

Early labor is defined by cervical dilation of 0 to 3 cm and contractions occurring every 5 to 20 minutes and lasting 30 to 45 seconds. In this stage of labor, the mother typically notices backache and mild discomfort. The contractions progress over time, becoming longer, stronger, and closer together. Between contractions, the mother feels relatively normal and pain free.

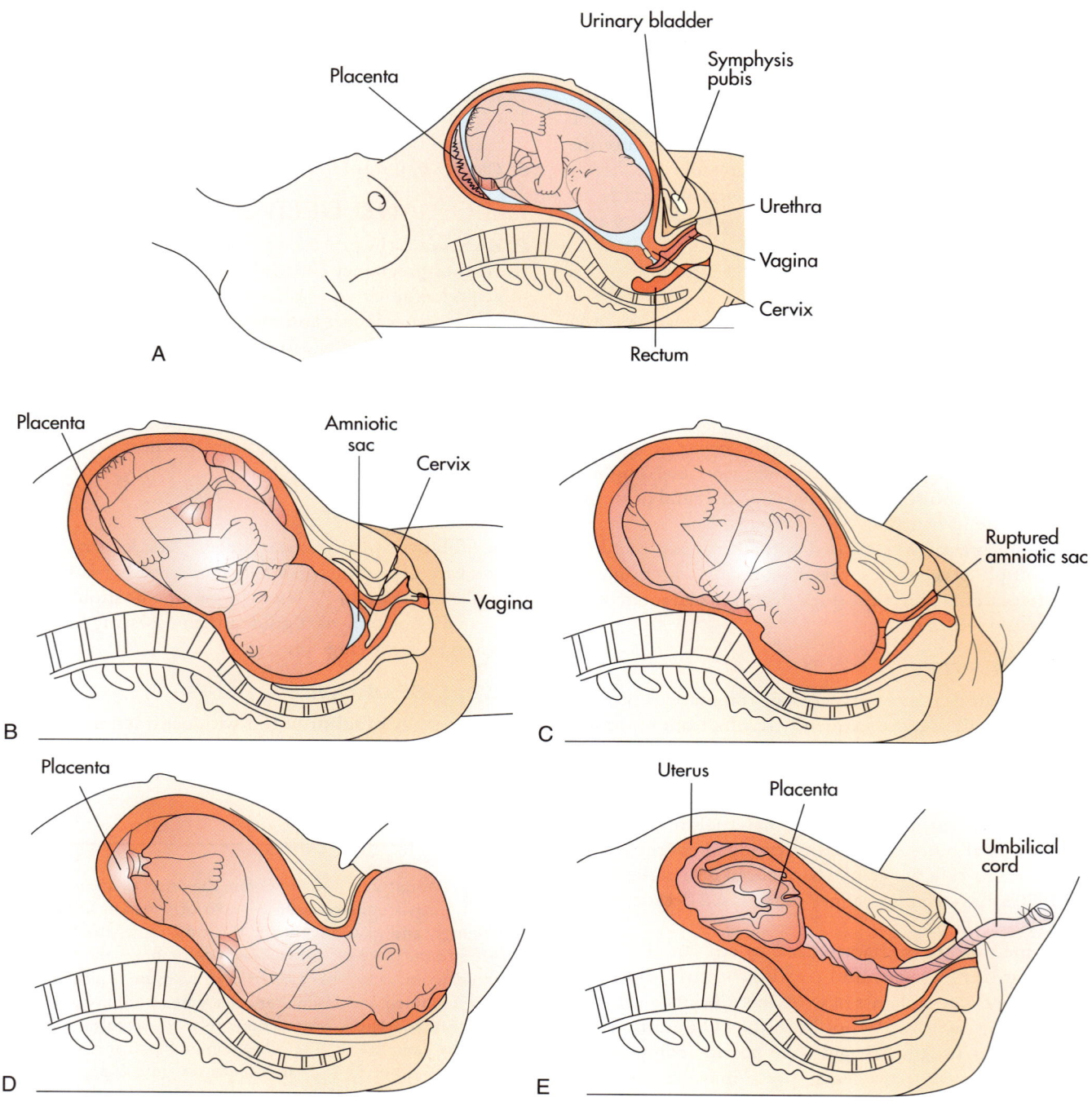

FIGURE 46-10 Parturition. **A,** The relation of the fetus to the mother. **B,** The fetus moves into the birth canal. **C,** Dilation of the cervix is complete. **D,** The fetus is expelled from the uterus. **E,** The placenta is expelled.

For first-time mothers, this stage of labor may last 8 to 20 hours. With subsequent births, the stage lasts 6 to 8 hours or less.

Active labor is defined by cervical dilation of 4 to 8 cm, and contractions 4 to 5 minutes apart, lasting about 60 seconds. This stage marks the beginning of intense contractions. Between contractions, the mother may experience trembling, nausea, and vomiting. Coached relaxation and slowed breathing between contractions

often is comforting to the mother. This stage of labor usually lasts 1 to 2 hours.

Transition is defined by cervical dilation of 8 to 10 cm. During transition, contractions are about 2 to 3 minutes apart and last for about 60 to 90 seconds. The contractions are intense and may occur with little rest for the mother. They may be accompanied by rectal pressure if the baby's head is positioned low. In many pregnancies, the amniotic sac ruptures (*rupture of membranes*) toward the end of the

BOX 46-7 Stages of Labor

Stage I
- Onset of regular contractions to complete cervical dilation
- Average time: Early labor 8-20 hours in primipara, 6-8 hours or less in multipara
- Active labor 1-2 hours
- Transition 15-30 minutes on average

Stage II
- Full dilation of cervix to delivery of the newborn
- Average time: 1-2 hours in primipara, 30 minutes or less in multipara

Stage III
- Immediately after delivery of the infant until expulsion of the placenta
- Average time: 5 to 60 minutes regardless of parity

BOX 46-8 Premonitory Signs of Labor

Lightening
Braxton-Hicks contractions
Cervical changes
Bloody show
Rupture of membranes

BOX 46-9 Cardinal Movements: Positional Changes During Birth

Infants must make several positional changes (*cardinal movements*) during the birth process. These movements are deliberate and precise changes made by the infant so that passage through the bony pelvis can occur. These positional changes are descent, flexion, internal rotation, extension, external rotation, and expulsion.

Descent is the movement of the baby's head into the pelvic cavity. Babies enter the birth canal with their head in the transverse position, with the occiput either to the right or to the left. *Flexion* occurs during descent as the head encounters resistance. This causes the baby's head to flex so that the chin meets the chest. As the head reaches the pelvic floor, it rotates to an anterior-posterior position (*internal rotation*) to accommodate for the smallest diameter of the birth canal between the ischial spines. *Extension* occurs as the fetus stops flexion of the head when the baby's head, face, and chin are born. Following extension, the baby must rotate (*external rotation*) from an anterior-posterior position to a transverse position (facing one of the mother's thighs). This movement (also known as *restitution*) allows for the shoulders to pass under the mother's pubic arch. After external rotation, the shoulders are born. This is followed by full delivery of the newborn (*expulsion*).

first stage of labor. The period of transition lasts only 15 to 30 minutes on average (Box 46-8).

CRITICAL THINKING
What comfort measures can you use during transportation for the patient who is in the first stage of labor?

SECOND STAGE OF LABOR

The **second stage of labor** is measured from full dilation of the cervix to delivery of the infant. During this stage, the fetal head enters the birth canal. The mother's contractions become more intense and frequent (usually 2 to 3 minutes apart). Often the mother becomes diaphoretic and tachycardic during this stage. She experiences an urge to bear down with each contraction. In addition, she may express the need to have a bowel movement. This is a normal sensation caused by pressure of the fetal head against the mother's rectum. During this stage a **mucous plug** (sometimes mixed with blood, thus the name *bloody show*) is expelled from the dilating cervix and discharged from the vagina. (The mother may not notice passage of the plug.) The presenting part of the fetus (usually the head) emerges from the vaginal opening. This process, known as **crowning,** indicates that delivery is imminent. The second stage of labor usually lasts 1 to 2 hours in the nullipara mother. It usually lasts 30 minutes or less in the multipara mother (Box 46-9).

THIRD STAGE OF LABOR

The **third stage of labor** begins with delivery of the infant and ends when the placenta is expelled and the uterus has contracted (described later in this chapter). The length of this stage varies from 5 to 60 minutes, regardless of parity.

Signs and Symptoms of Imminent Delivery

The following signs and symptoms indicate that delivery is imminent. With these, the paramedic should prepare for childbirth at the scene:

- Regular contractions lasting 45 to 60 seconds at 1- to 2-minute intervals. Intervals are measured from the beginning of one contraction to the beginning of the next. If contractions are more than 5 minutes apart, there generally is time to transport the mother to a receiving hospital.
- The mother has an urge to bear down or has a sensation of a bowel movement.
- There is a large amount of bloody show.
- Crowning occurs.
- The mother believes that delivery is imminent.

If any of these signs and symptoms are present, the EMS crew should prepare for delivery. With the exception of cord presentation (described later in this chapter), the paramedic should not try to delay delivery. If complications are anticipated or an abnormal delivery occurs, medical direction may recommend expedited transport of the patient to a medical facility.

Preparation for Delivery

When preparing for delivery, the paramedic should try to provide an area of privacy. The mother should be positioned on a bed, stretcher, or table. The surface should be long enough to project beyond the mother's vagina. The delivery area should be as clean as possible. It should be covered with absorbent material to guard against staining and contamination by blood and fecal material.

The mother should be placed on her back. Her knees should be flexed and widely separated (or in another position preferred by the mother). The vaginal area should be draped appropriately. If delivery occurs in a car, the mother should be instructed to lie on her back across the seat with one leg flexed on the seat and the other leg resting on the floorboard. A pillow or blanket, if available, should be placed beneath the mother's buttocks. This will aid in the delivery of the infant's head. The paramedic should evaluate the mother's vital signs for baseline measurements. The fetal heart rate may be monitored for signs of fetal distress. Per protocol and medical direction, the paramedic should consider maternal oxygen administration and IV access for fluid administration or postdelivery administration of *oxytocin* if needed.

The mother should be coached to bear down and push during contractions and to rest between contractions to conserve strength. If the mother finds it difficult to refrain from pushing, she should be encouraged to breathe deeply or "pant" through her mouth between contractions. Deep breathing and panting help decrease the force of bearing down and promote rest.

DELIVERY EQUIPMENT

Prehospital delivery equipment ("OB kit") generally includes the following components (Figure 46-11):
- Surgical scissors
- Cord clamps or umbilical tape
- Towels

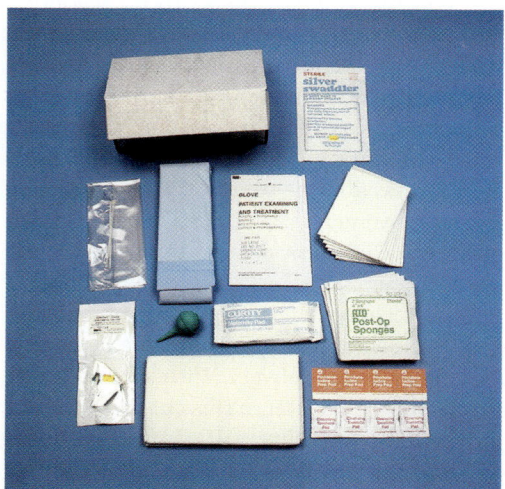

FIGURE 46-11 Prehospital delivery equipment.

- Surgical masks
- 4 × 4 inch gauze sponges
- Sanitary napkins
- Bulb syringe and DeLee suction kit
- Baby blanket and baby stocking cap
- Plastic bag for placental transportation
- Neonatal resuscitation equipment
- IV fluid supplies

Personal protective measures should be used when assisting in a delivery. Sterile technique should be used when handling equipment.

Assistance With Delivery

In most cases the paramedic only assists in the natural events of childbirth. The chief duties of the EMS crew are to prevent an uncontrolled delivery and protect the infant from cold and stress after the birth. The following are steps to be taken in assisting the mother with a normal delivery (Figure 46-12):

1. Observe standard precautions.
2. When crowning occurs, apply gentle palm counterpressure to the infant's head to prevent an explosive delivery and tearing of the mother's perineum. If membranes are still intact, tear the sac with finger pressure to allow escape of amniotic fluid.
3. After delivery of the head, examine the infant's neck for a looped (*nuchal*) umbilical cord. If the cord is looped around the neck, gently slip it over the infant's head.
4. Suction the infant's mouth and nose with a bulb syringe to clear the airway. Perform suction after the head appears but before the next contraction. The next contractions deliver the shoulders and chest. The risk of aspiration is minimal.
5. Support the infant's head as it rotates for shoulder presentation. Most infants present face down. The infant usually rotates to the left or right so that the shoulders present in an anterior-posterior position.
6. If the shoulders do not spontaneously deliver with the next contraction, using gentle pressure, guide the infant's head downward to deliver the anterior shoulder and then upward to release the posterior shoulder. The rest of the infant is delivered quickly by smooth uterine contraction.
7. Be careful to grasp and support the infant as he or she emerges, using a dry towel or clean piece of clothing. Hold the infant with his or her head dependent to aid drainage of secretions. Place the infant on the mother's abdomen if she is able to hold her infant.
8. Clear the infant's airway of any secretions with sterile gauze. Suction the infant's nose and mouth if there is coarse gurgling.
9. Dry the infant with sterile towels, and cover the infant (especially the head) to reduce heat loss.
10. Record the infant's gender and time of birth.

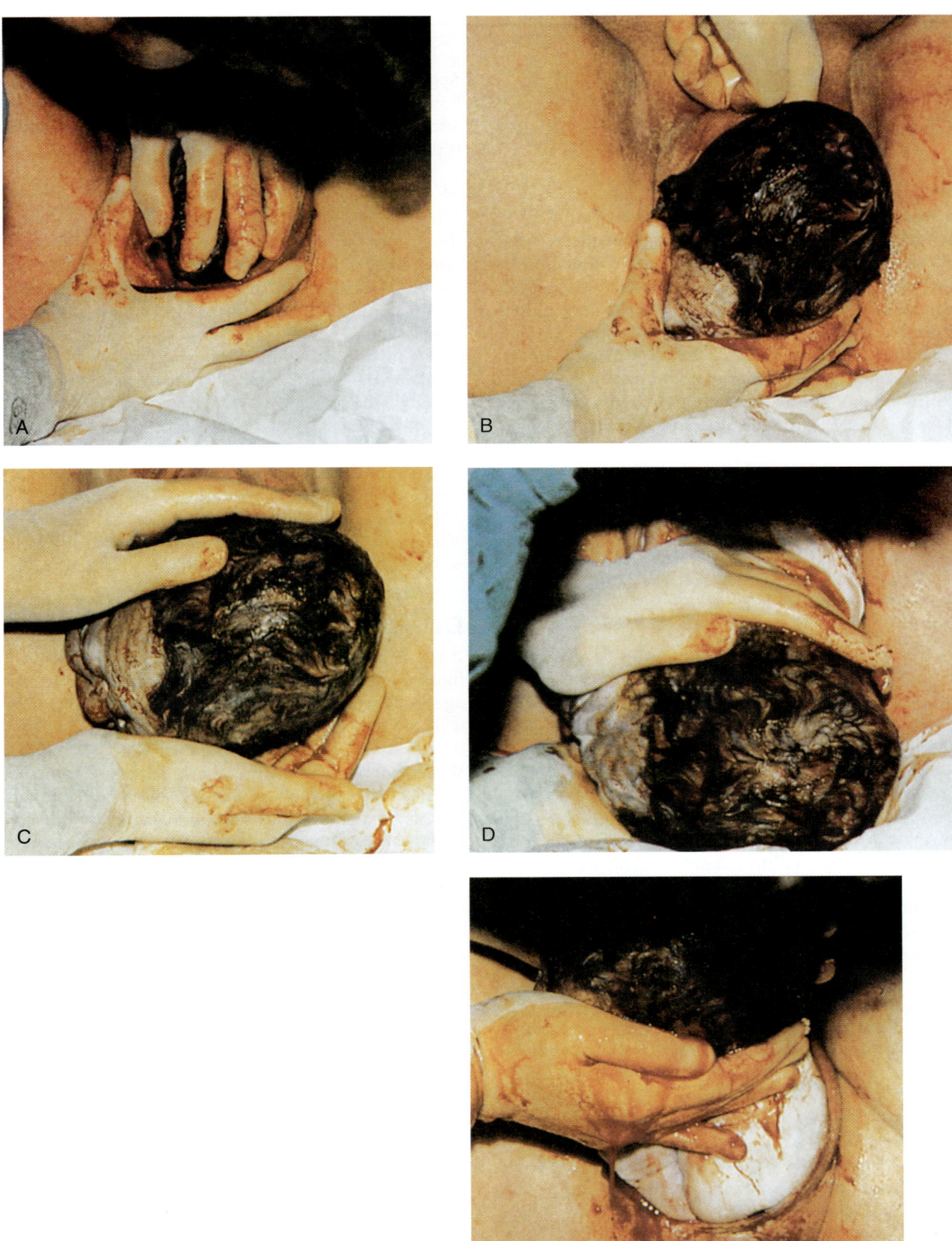

FIGURE 46-12 Normal delivery. **A,** When crowning occurs, apply gentle palm pressure to the infant's head. **B,** Examine the neck for the presence of a looped umbilical cord. **C,** Support the infant's head as it rotates for shoulder presentation. **D,** Guide the infant's head downward to deliver the anterior shoulder. **E,** Guide the infant's head upward to release the posterior shoulder. (From Al-Azzawi F: *Color atlas of childbirth and obstetric techniques,* London, 1990, Wolfe.)

CRITICAL THINKING
How do you think you will feel after attending a birth of a healthy infant?

Evaluation of the Infant

After delivery, the infant should be positioned on the side or with padding under the back if needed. The paramedic should clear the airway and provide tactile stimulation to initiate respirations. If there is no need for resuscitation, the paramedic should assign an **Apgar score** at 1 minute and 5 minutes to evaluate the infant (Table 46-2). Criteria for computing the Apgar score include *appearance* (color), *pulse* (heart rate), *grimace* (reflex irritability to stimulation), *activity* (muscle tone), and *respiratory effort*. Each criterion is rated from 0 to 2. The numbers are added for a total Apgar score.

NOTE
Newly born infants who do not require resuscitation can generally be defined by a rapid assessment of the following four characteristics:
- Was the baby born after a full-term gestation?
- Is the amniotic fluid clear of meconium and evidence of infection?
- Is the baby breathing or crying?
- Does the baby have good muscle tone?

If the answer to all four of these questions is "yes," the baby does not need resuscitation and should not be separated from the mother. If the answer to any of these questions is "no," the infant should be resuscitated (see Chapter 47).

An Apgar score of 10 indicates that the infant is in the best possible condition, 7 to 9 indicates that the infant is slightly depressed (near normal), 4 to 6 indicates that the infant is moderately depressed, and 0 to 3 indicates that the infant is severely depressed. Most newborns have an Apgar score of 8 to 10 at 1 minute after birth. Newborns with an Apgar score of less than 6 generally require resuscitation; however, *the paramedic should not solely use the Apgar score to determine the need for resuscitation.*[18] (Neonatal resuscitation is presented in Chapter 47.)

CUTTING THE UMBILICAL CORD

After the paramedic delivers and evaluates the infant and the cord has stopped pulsing, the umbilical cord should be clamped (or tied with umbilical tape) and cut (Figure 46-13). Clamping or cutting the cord may be delayed for at least 1 minute in term and preterm infants not requiring resuscitatioin.[18] The paramedic should take the following steps to manage the umbilical cord:

1. Clamp the cord about 4 to 6 inches away from the infant in two places.
2. Cut between the two clamps with sterile scissors or a scalpel.
3. Examine the cut ends of the cord to ensure that there is no bleeding. If the cut end attached to the infant is bleeding, clamp the cord proximal to the previous clamp and reassess for bleeding. Do not remove the first clamp.
4. Handle the cord carefully at all times because it can tear easily.

Delivery of the Placenta

If the baby and mother are in good condition and if the mother is agreeable, place the baby at her breasts to encourage suckling. This will stimulate the release of oxytocin that will lead to decreased blood loss. The placenta normally is delivered within 20 minutes of the infant. Thus transport should not be delayed for placental delivery. Placental delivery is characterized by episodes of contractions, a palpable rise of the uterus within the abdomen, lengthening of the umbilical cord protruding from the vagina, and a sudden gush of vaginal blood.

TABLE 46-2 The Apgar Scoring System			
SIGN	**0**	**1**	**2**
Appearance (skin color)	Blue, pale	Body pink, blue extremities	Completely pink
Pulse rate (heart rate)	Absent	<100 beats/min	>100 beats/min
Grimace (irritability)	No response	Grimace	Cough, sneeze, cry
Activity (muscle tone)	Limp	Some flexion	Active motion
Respirations (respiratory effort)	Absent	Slow, irregular	Good, crying

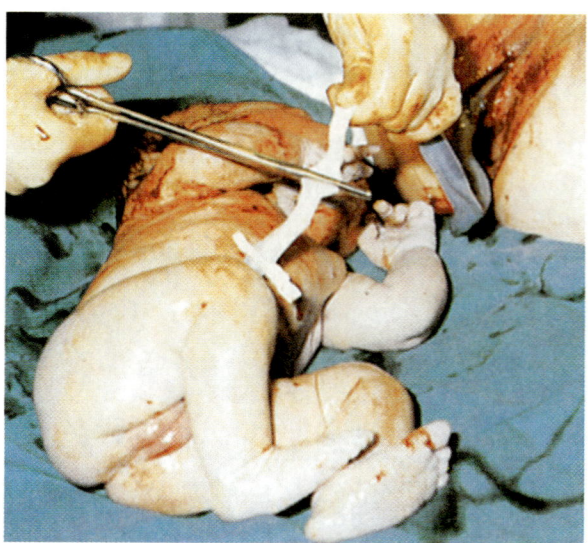

FIGURE 46-13 After delivery and evaluation of the infant, the paramedic clamps and cuts the cord. (From Al-Azzawi F: *Color atlas of childbirth and obstetric techniques,* London, 1990, Wolfe.)

After birth of the infant and clamping of the cord, the mother should be told to bear down with contractions. The paramedic should place one hand lightly on the mother's abdomen and the other hand should apply steady traction to the cord. This is not a pulling motion. Traction is used to keep the cord taut until there is a gush of vaginal blood or lengthening of the cord.

> **NOTE**
> The hand that is placed on the mother's abdomen *may* feel the rise of the uterus with cord lengthening or the gush of vaginal blood. This can indicate that the placenta is ready to deliver or only partly separated from the uterine wall. At this time, the paramedic should gently increase traction on the cord and ask the mother to bear down with the next contraction. As she pushes, gently pull down and out on the cord. If there is no immediate progress (further lengthening of the cord), stop pulling and reinstate steady cord traction and wait for spontaneous cord lengthening to occur. Again, placental delivery should not delay patient transport.

When the placenta is expelled, it should be placed in a plastic bag or other container and transported with the mother and infant to the receiving hospital. At the hospital the placenta will be examined for abnormality and completeness. Pieces of placenta retained in the uterus can cause persistent hemorrhage and infection. After the delivery of the placenta, the paramedic should assess the mother's perineum for tears. If tears are present, the bleeding should be managed by applying sanitary napkins to the area and maintaining direct pressure. The paramedic should initiate fundal massage (described later) to promote uterine contraction, and monitor the mother during transport for signs of hemorrhage or shock. Medical direction also may prescribe oxytocin to manage postpartum bleeding, if needed.

> **SHOW ME THE EVIDENCE**
> These authors attempted to distinguish characteristics of planned versus unplanned home births. They reviewed data from 11,787 home births from 19 states that occurred in 2006. Of these home births, 9810 (83.2%) were planned. Of the unplanned birth group, 26% reported no prenatal care. Women who had an unplanned delivery at home were more likely to be non-white, to smoke, to have no prenatal care, and to be younger than those who planned home delivery. Prematurity was present in 3% of planned versus 26% of unplanned home births. A significant limitation of the study was that the authors could not identify cases that were planned for home delivery but were instead taken to the hospital. They conclude that although there are only about 4000 unplanned home births in the United States each year, this group is high-risk and effort should be made to identify their characteristics during prenatal care.

From Declercq E, MacDorman MF, Menacker F, et al: Characteristics of planned and unplanned home births in 19 states, *Obstet Gynecol* 116(1):93-99, 2010.

Postpartum Hemorrhage

Postpartum hemorrhage is characterized by more than 500 mL of blood loss after the delivery of the newborn. (The actual volume of blood loss is difficult to estimate with accuracy.) Hemorrhage often occurs within the first few hours after delivery. Yet it can be delayed up to 24 hours. Postpartum hemorrhage occurs in about 5% of all deliveries and accounts for up to 25% of obstetrical deaths.[5] Hemorrhage often results from ineffective or incomplete contraction of the interlacing uterine muscle fibers. Other causes of postpartum hemorrhage include retained pieces of placenta or membranes in the uterus. Hemorrhage can also be caused by vaginal or cervical tears during delivery. Risk factors associated with postpartum hemorrhage include **uterine atony** (lack of uterine tone) from prolonged or tumultuous labor, grand multiparity, twin pregnancy, placenta previa, and a full bladder.

> **NOTE**
> **Lochia** is postpartum vaginal discharge that contains blood, mucus, and placental tissue from the lining of the uterus. This discharge is normal, and typically continues for about 2 to 4 weeks after childbirth. Lochia is similar to menstrual bleeding, but initially heavier, and then diminishes. The discharge usually begins as bright red, and will later become pink or yellow-white in color.

MANAGEMENT

Postpartum hemorrhage can occur in the prehospital setting after a field delivery, home delivery, or delivery at an independent birthing center. The assessment and management are similar to those described for third-trimester bleeding. In addition, the paramedic should take the following measures to encourage uterine contraction:

1. *Massage the uterus.* Palpate the uterus for firmness or loss of tone. If the uterus does not feel firm, apply fundal pressure by supporting the lower uterine segment with the edge of one hand just above the symphysis and massaging the fundus with the other hand. Continue massaging until the uterus feels firm. Reevaluate the patient every 10 minutes; note the location of the fundus in relation to the level of the umbilicus, the degree of firmness, and vaginal flow.
2. *Encourage the infant to breastfeed.* If the mother and infant are stable and the mother is agreeable, place the newborn to her breast to encourage breastfeeding. Stimulation of the breasts may promote uterine contraction.
3. *Administer oxytocin.* Per medical direction and after ensuring that a second fetus is not present in the uterus, add 10 units of *oxytocin* to 1000 mL of lactated Ringer's solution. Infuse at 20 to 30 drops/min via microdrip tubing (titrated to the severity of hemorrhage and uterine response or as ordered by medical direction). Continue

with fluid resuscitation as indicated by the patient's vital signs.

> **NOTE**
>
> The paramedic should manage external bleeding from a perineal tear with direct pressure. There should be no attempts at vaginal examination or vaginal packing to control hemorrhage. These patients should be rapidly transported for physician evaluation.

DELIVERY COMPLICATIONS

As stated previously, most women have uncomplicated pregnancies. Prehospital deliveries seldom present any significant problems for the mother, newborn, or paramedic crew. The delivery complications discussed in this chapter include cephalopelvic disproportion, abnormal presentation, premature birth, multiple gestation, precipitous delivery, uterine inversion, pulmonary embolism, and fetal membrane disorders. Box 46-10 lists factors that should alert the paramedic to anticipate an abnormal delivery.

BOX 46-10 Factors Associated With High-Risk Delivery

Maternal Factors
- Maternal age: very young or very old
- Absence of prenatal care
- Maternal lifestyle: alcohol, tobacco, or drug usage
- Preexisting maternal illness, including diabetes, chronic hypertension, or Rh sensitization
- Previous obstetrical history of the following:
  Premature delivery
  Previous malformed neonate
  Previous multiple births
  Previous cesarean delivery
- Intrapartum disorders
  Preeclampsia
  Prolonged rupture of membranes
  Prolonged labor
  Abnormal presentation
  Abruptio placentae
  Placenta previa

Fetal Factors
- Lack of fetal well-being
  History of decreased fetal movement
  Hydramnios (excess amniotic fluid)
  History of heart rate abnormalities
  Evidence of fetal distress
- Fetal immaturity: prematurity as established by dates, ultrasound, uterine size, amniocentesis
- Fetal growth: history of poor intrauterine growth or post-date delivery; fetal macrosomia (birth weight more than 4000 g [8 lb])
- Specific fetal malformation detected by ultrasound: diaphragmatic hernia or omphalocele

---

Cephalopelvic Disproportion

Cephalopelvic disproportion is a condition in which the newborn's head is too large or the mother's birth canal is too small to allow normal labor or birth. The mother often is primigravida and having strong, frequent contractions for a prolonged period. Prehospital care is limited to maternal oxygen administration, IV access for fluid resuscitation if needed, and rapid transport to the receiving hospital.

Abnormal Presentation

Most infants are born head first (cephalic or vertex presentation). But sometimes a presentation is abnormal. These include a breech presentation, shoulder dystocia, shoulder presentation, and a cord presentation **(prolapsed umbilical cord)**.

BREECH PRESENTATION

In a **breech presentation** the largest part of the fetus (the head) is delivered last. Breech presentation occurs in 3% to 4% of deliveries at term.[5] Breech presentation is more frequent with multiple births and when labor occurs before 32 weeks' gestation. Categories of breech presentation include the following (Figure 46-14)[5]:

- *Frank breech.* The fetal hips are flexed and the legs extend in front of the fetus. The buttocks are the presenting part. Frank breech accounts for about 60% to 65% of breech presentations.
- *Complete breech.* The fetus has both knees and hips flexed. The buttocks are the presenting part. Complete breech accounts for about 5% of breech presentations.
- *Incomplete breech.* The fetus has one or both hips incompletely flexed. This results in presentation of one or both lower extremities (often a foot). Incomplete breech accounts for about 25% to 30% of breech presentations.

CRITICAL THINKING

What resources can you use to assist in a delivery with an abnormal presentation?

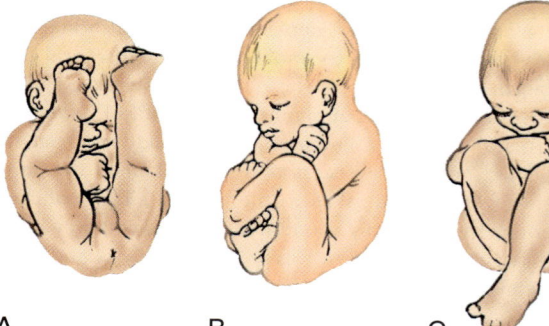

FIGURE 46-14 Types of breech presentation. **A,** Front or back. **B,** Complete. **C,** Incomplete.

Management. An infant in a breech presentation is best delivered in a hospital where emergency cesarean section is an alternative to vaginal delivery. Sometimes, however, the paramedic must assist in a breech delivery. If delivery is imminent, the EMS crew should proceed as follows:

1. Prepare the mother for delivery as described earlier in this chapter.
2. Provide supplemental oxygen and IV access; continuously monitor the fetal heart rate.
3. Allow the fetus to deliver spontaneously up to the level of the umbilicus. If the fetus is in a frank breech presentation, gently extract the legs downward after the buttocks are delivered.
4. After the infant's legs are clear, support his or her body with the palm of the hand and volar surface of the arm.
5. After the umbilicus is visible, gently extract a 4- to 6-inch loop of umbilical cord to allow delivery without excessive traction on the cord. Gently rotate the fetus to align the shoulders in an anterior-posterior position. Continue with gentle traction until the axilla is visible.
6. Gently guide the infant upward to deliver the posterior shoulder.
7. Gently guide the infant downward to deliver the anterior shoulder.
8. Be aware that the head often is delivered without difficulty after shoulder delivery. Be careful to avoid excessive head and spine manipulation or traction.

If the head does not deliver immediately, action must be taken to prevent suffocation of the infant. The paramedic should maintain the fetal head in a flexed position by placing the index and middle fingers on either side of the infant's nose (the *Mauriceau maneuver*).[19] The fetal body should be supported in a neutral position, using care not to overextend the baby's neck. During this maneuver a second rescuer should apply suprapubic pressure. If the head does not deliver quickly, poor fetal outcome is likely.[5] The mother should be transported rapidly to the hospital.

SHOULDER DYSTOCIA

Shoulder dystocia occurs when the fetal shoulders are wedged against the maternal symphysis pubis. This blocks shoulder delivery. In this presentation the head delivers normally but then pulls back tightly against the maternal perineum (the *turtle sign*). Shoulder dystocia is a common condition in pregnancy, occurring in 1 in 300 deliveries.[5] Complications include brachial plexus damage, fractured clavicle, and fetal anoxia from cord compression. Fifty percent of shoulder dystocia cases occur in women without risk factors.

Management. Shoulder dystocia delivery requires dislodging one shoulder and then rotating the fetal shoulder girdle at an angle into the wider part of the pelvic opening. Because the shoulder is pressing against the pelvis, there is a potential for cord compression. Thus the paramedic should deliver the anterior shoulder immediately after the head. Several maneuvers can help the paramedic successfully deliver an infant when shoulder dystocia arises. The following steps represent one approach to shoulder dystocia:

1. Position the mother on her left side in a dorsal-knee-chest position. This increases the diameter of the pelvis.
2. Try to guide the infant's head downward to allow the anterior shoulder to slip under the symphysis pubis. Avoid excessive force or manipulation.
3. Gently rotate the fetal shoulder girdle at an angle to the wider pelvic opening. The posterior shoulder usually delivers without resistance. Medical direction may recommend that the paramedic try to deliver the posterior shoulder first by rotating the posterior shoulder downward and into the left posterior quadrant. The anterior shoulder usually follows.
4. After delivery, continue with resuscitative measures as needed.

SHOULDER PRESENTATION

Shoulder presentation (*transverse presentation*) results when the long axis of the fetus lies perpendicular to that of the mother. This position usually results in the fetal shoulder lying over the pelvic opening. The fetal arm or hand may be the presenting part. This abnormal presentation occurs in only 0.3% of deliveries but occurs in 10% of second twins.[5]

Management. Normal delivery of a shoulder presentation is not possible. The paramedic should provide the mother with adequate oxygen, ventilatory, and circulatory support and then provide rapid transport to the hospital. A cesarean delivery is required regardless of the condition of the fetus.

CORD PRESENTATION

Cord presentation (prolapsed cord) occurs when the cord slips down into or out of the vagina after the amniotic membranes have ruptured. The umbilical cord is compressed against the presenting part of the fetus. This diminishes fetal oxygenation from the placenta. A prolapsed cord occurs in about 0.3% to 0.6% of all deliveries.[5] When fetal distress is present, the paramedic should suspect a prolapsed cord. Predisposing factors include breech presentation, premature rupture of membranes (described later), multiple gestation, a long cord, and preterm labor.

Management. Fetal asphyxia can ensue rapidly if circulation through the cord is not reestablished and maintained until delivery. If the paramedic can see or feel the umbilical cord in the vagina, the following steps should be taken:

1. With a gloved hand, gently push the infant back into the vagina. Elevate the presenting part to relieve pressure on the cord. The cord may retract spontaneously. However, the paramedic should not try to reposition the cord.
2. Maintain this hand position during rapid transport to the hospital. The definitive treatment is a cesarean delivery.
3. Position the mother with hips elevated as much as possible. The Trendelenburg or knee-chest position may relieve pressure on the cord.
4. Administer oxygen to the mother.

5. If help is available, apply moist sterile dressings to the exposed cord. This will minimize temperature changes that may cause umbilical artery spasm.

6. Instruct the mother to pant with each contraction to prevent bearing down.

OTHER ABNORMAL PRESENTATIONS

Other abnormal presentations include *face* or *brow (military) presentation* and *occiput posterior presentation*. In these presentations the infant's head is delivered face up instead of face down. Face-up presentations result in increased risks to the fetus because of difficult labor and delivery. Sometimes the fetus has other associated abnormalities. These presentations may require cesarean delivery. Thus early recognition of potential complications, maternal support and reassurance, and rapid transport for definitive care are the goals of prehospital management.

Premature Birth

A **premature infant** is an infant born before 37 weeks' gestation (Figure 46-15). Low birth weight (less than 2.5 kg [5.5 lb]) also determines prematurity, although the conditions are not synonymous. Premature deliveries occur in 8% to 10% of all pregnancies.[20] After a preterm labor the newborn is at increased risk for hypothermia because of a large body surface/body mass ratio and at increased risk for cardiorespiratory distress because of the prematurely developed cardiovascular system. Therefore these infants require special care and observation. After delivery, prehospital management for a premature infant includes the following:

- Keep the infant warm. Dry the infant, wrap the infant in a warm blanket, place the infant on the mother's abdomen, and cover the mother and infant. If transport time is delayed, very small (<1500 g) infants should be wrapped in food-grade heat-resistant plastic wrap and placed under radiant heat in addition to other warming methods.[21]
- Frequently suction secretions from the infant's mouth and nares.
- Carefully monitor the cut end of the umbilical cord for oozing. If bleeding is present, manage as described before.
- Administer humidified free-flow oxygen through a makeshift oxygen tent. Aim oxygen flow toward the top of the tent; do not allow it to flow directly into the infant's face.
- Protect the infant from contamination. Don a mask and gown and minimize family member and bystander contact with the infant.
- Gently transport the mother and infant to the receiving hospital.

One should note that *tocolytic agents* (drugs used to inhibit labor) are used widely today by some mothers who are at risk for a premature birth. These drugs may be administered in the home setting. They include magnesium sulfate, nicardipine, nifedipine, ritodrine, terbutaline, indomethacin, and others.[2] The paramedic should ask the patient about any recent medication use, including the use of tocolytic agents.

Multiple Gestation

A **multiple gestation** is a pregnancy with more than one fetus. Historically, twin births usually occurred in only 1% of all deliveries. Because of the increasing use of fertility treatments, about 30% of every 1000 live births are now multiple births[5] (Box 46-11). Multiple gestation places more stress on the maternal system and also is accompanied by an increased complication rate. Associated complications include premature labor and delivery (30% to 50% of twin deliveries are premature), premature rupture of membranes, abruptio placentae, postpartum hemorrhage, and abnormal presentation. A mother who has not received prenatal care may be unaware of her multiple pregnancy.

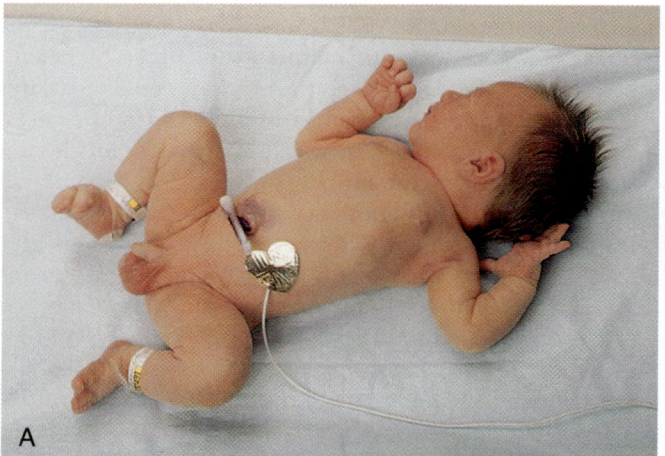 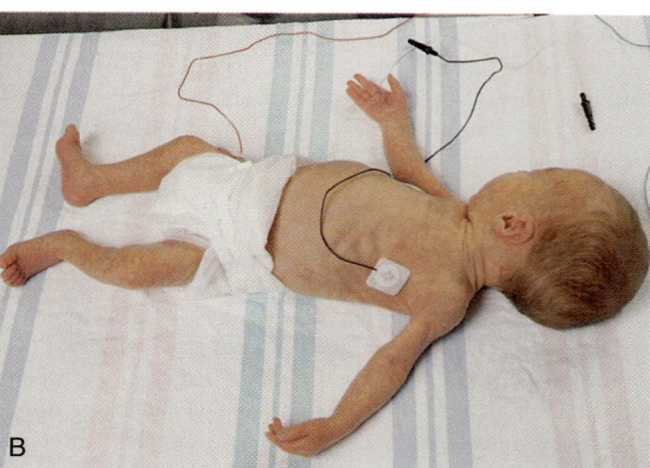

FIGURE 46-15 Posture in newborns. **A,** The healthy full-term infant remains in a strongly flexed position. **B,** The preterm infant's extremities are extended. (From Murray SS, McKinney ES: *Foundations of maternal newborn nursing,* ed 5, Philadelphia, 2010, Saunders.)

BOX 46-11 Twin Terminology

Fraternal twins result from the fertilization of two ova by two spermatozoa. Each fraternal twin has a separate placenta. Each also is separated by individual amniotic membranes. Fraternal twins are not identical in appearance. They are often of different gender.

Identical twins result from the fertilization of a single ovum. They may share a common placenta and amniotic sac or have separate placental structures. Identical twins are less common than fraternal twins. (They occur in one out of three twin conceptions.) Unlike fraternal twins, identical twins look alike, are of the same gender, and are genetically identical.

CRITICAL THINKING

Do you have enough supplies on your ambulance to manage more than one delivery?

DELIVERY PROCEDURE

First-twin delivery is identical to single delivery with the same presentation. However, up to 50% of second-twin deliveries are not in a normal presentation position. Fetuses are smaller in multiple births.

After the delivery of the first twin, the paramedic should cut and clamp (or tie) the umbilical cord as described earlier. Within 5 to 10 minutes after delivery of the first twin, labor begins again. The delivery of the second twin usually occurs within 30 to 45 minutes. Medical direction may recommend transport before the delivery of the second twin. Usually both twins are born before the delivery of the placenta.

Infants in multiple births often are smaller than infants in single term births. The paramedic should give special attention to keeping these infants warm, well oxygenated, and free from unnecessary contamination as described for premature infants. Postpartum hemorrhage may be more severe after multiple births. Hemorrhage may require fluid resuscitation, uterine massage, and **oxytocin** infusion to control bleeding.

Precipitous Delivery

A **precipitous delivery** is a rapid spontaneous delivery with less than 3 hours from onset of labor to birth. Precipitous delivery results from overactive uterine contractions and insignificant maternal soft tissue or bony resistance. A precipitous delivery most often occurs in a mother who is grand multipara. It can be associated with soft tissue injury and uterine rupture (rare). Precipitous delivery has an increased perinatal mortality rate because of trauma and hypoxia. The main danger to the fetus during this kind of delivery is from cerebral trauma or tearing of the umbilical cord.

If the paramedic expects a precipitous delivery, attempts should be made to prevent an explosive one. This can be done by providing gentle counterpressure to the infant's head; however, the paramedic should not attempt to detain fetal head descent. After delivery, the infant should be kept dry and warm to prevent heat loss. The mother should be examined for perineal tears that often accompany a rapid birth.

Uterine Inversion

Uterine inversion is an infrequent complication of childbirth where the uterus turns "inside out." The condition is thought to occur in about 1 in 2000 deliveries.[5] Uterine inversion is a serious condition. The resultant postpartum hemorrhage is associated with a maternal mortality rate of around 15%.

Uterine inversion may occur suddenly after a contraction or with increased abdominal pressure caused by coughing or sneezing. However, uterine inversion more often is caused by medical personnel or a medical procedure (**iatrogenic**) secondary to excessive pulling on the umbilical cord and fundal massage. The risk is elevated when the placenta has implanted high in the uterus. Uterine inversion is *incomplete* if the uterine fundus does not extend beyond the cervix; it is *complete* if the fundus does protrude through the cervix; and it is *prolapsed* if the entire uterus protrudes through the vaginal ring. Signs and symptoms of uterine inversion include postpartum hemorrhage and sudden and severe lower abdominal pain. The hemorrhage may be profuse. Hypovolemic shock may develop quickly.

MANAGEMENT

Prehospital care for a patient with uterine inversion includes airway, ventilatory, and circulatory support and rapid transportation for physician evaluation. Medical direction may recommend that the paramedic attempt manual replacement of the uterus only if the cervix has not yet constricted. The technique for manual replacement is as follows:

1. Place the patient in a supine position.
2. Do not attempt to remove the placenta, if it has not already been delivered. Doing so is likely to increase hemorrhage.
3. Apply pressure with the fingertips and palm of a gloved hand and push the fundus upward and through the cervical canal. If this is ineffective, cover all protruding tissues with moist sterile dressings and rapidly transport the patient.

Manual replacement of the uterus may be painful to the patient. Medical direction may indicate the use of analgesics. The paramedic should explain the need for the procedure to the patient.

Pulmonary Embolism

The development of pulmonary embolism during pregnancy, labor, or the postpartum period is a significant cause of maternal death.[22] The embolus often results from a blood clot in the pelvic circulation (venous thromboembolism). There is a slight increased risk of pulmonary embolus with cesarean versus vaginal delivery. The patient often has classic signs and symptoms. These include sudden dyspnea;

sharp, focal chest pains; tachycardia; tachypnea; and sometimes hypotension. If the embolism occurs in the prehospital setting, emergency care should be focused on airway, ventilatory, and circulatory support; electrocardiogram monitoring; and rapid transportation for physician evaluation (see Chapter 24).

> **NOTE**
>
> Thromboembolism is 2 times as likely to occur in pregnancy and 5.5 times as likely to occur during the postpartum period. Pregnancy causes changes in the coagulation and fibrinolytic systems that persist into the postpartum period. During pregnancy, the levels of many coagulation factors are elevated. In addition, the fibrinolytic system is suppressed. Together, this hinders clot disintegration (lysis). The result is that factors that promote clot formation are increased to prevent maternal hemorrhage and factors that prevent clot formation are decreased. This results in a higher risk for thrombus formation during pregnancy and the postpartum period.[2]

Fetal Membrane Disorders

The fetal membrane disorders discussed in this chapter include premature rupture of membranes and amniotic fluid embolism. Another fetal membrane disorder, meconium staining, is described in Chapter 47).

PREMATURE RUPTURE OF MEMBRANES

Premature rupture of the membranes is a rupture of the amniotic sac before the onset of labor. The condition is termed *premature* regardless of fetal age. Premature rupture occurs in about 3% of pregnancies. In 10% to 15% of all cases, the fetus is at or near term.[5] Signs and symptoms include a history of a trickle or sudden gush of fluid from the vagina. The paramedic should transport patients for physician evaluation. The medical facility will prepare for delivery if the patient begins labor. Delivery is required if an infection of fetal membranes is diagnosed **(chorioamnionitis).**

Chorioamnionitis is linked to premature rupture of membranes occurring 24 hours before labor begins. It also can occur with a prolonged labor, in part as a result of multiple vaginal exams. The infection generally is accompanied by maternal fever, chills, and uterine pain. Infection is treated with antibiotics. The definitive treatment for this infection is the delivery of the fetus.

AMNIOTIC FLUID EMBOLISM

When amniotic fluid enters the maternal circulation during labor or delivery or immediately after delivery, an **amniotic fluid embolism** can occur. Probable routes of entry include lacerations of the endocervical veins during cervical dilation, the lower uterine segment or placental site, and uterine veins at sites of uterine trauma. Particulate matter in the amniotic fluid (e.g., meconium, lanugo hairs, and fetal squamous cells) forms an embolus and obstructs the pulmonary vasculature. Amniotic fluid embolism is rare, occurring in 6 to 14.8 per 100,000 primigravid and multiparous deliveries, respectively.[5] The condition most often is seen in multiparous women late in the first stage of labor. Other conditions that can increase the incidence of this severe complication are placenta previa, abruptio placentae, and intrauterine fetal death. The maternal mortality rate is high.

The signs and symptoms of amniotic fluid embolism are the same as those described for pulmonary embolism. They may include cardiopulmonary arrest. These patients are managed with airway, ventilatory, and circulatory support; fluid resuscitation; and rapid transportation.

SUMMARY

- Cultural differences may influence a woman's response to pregnancy and childbirth. The paramedic should be sensitive to these cultural beliefs.
- Fertilization of an ovum by a sperm forms a zygote that divides as it passes through the fallopian tube to become a morula. The trophoblast cells of the morula implant within 7 days after fertilization and transform into the life support systems of the embryo. The blastocyst cells develop into the embryo.
- The placenta is a disklike organ. It is composed of interlocking fetal and maternal tissues. It is the organ of exchange between the mother and fetus. Blood flows from the fetus to the placenta through two umbilical arteries. These arteries carry deoxygenated blood. Oxygenated blood returns to the fetus through the umbilical vein. The amniotic sac is a fluid-filled bag. It completely surrounds and protects the embryo.

- The developing ovum is known as an embryo during the first 8 weeks of pregnancy. After that time and until birth it is called a fetus. Gestation (fetal development) usually averages 40 weeks from the time of fertilization to the delivery of the newborn.
- At birth, in the normal newborn the arteriovenous shunts present in the fetus close.
- Gravida is the total number of current and past pregnancies. Para refers to past pregnancies that resulted in a live birth.
- The pregnant woman undergoes many physiological changes that affect the genital tract, breasts, gastrointestinal system, cardiovascular system, respiratory system, and metabolism.
- The patient history should include obstetrical history; presence of pain; presence, quantity, and character of vaginal bleeding; presence of abnormal vaginal

discharge; presence of "bloody show"; current general health and prenatal care; allergies and medicines taken; and maternal urge to bear down.

- The goal in examining an obstetrical patient is to rapidly identify acute life-threatening conditions. A part of this involves recognizing imminent delivery. Then the paramedic must take the proper management steps. In addition to the routine physical examination, the paramedic should assess the abdomen, uterine size, and fetal heart sounds.

- If birth is not imminent, the paramedic should limit prehospital care for the healthy patient. It should be limited to basic treatment modalities. It should include transport for physician evaluation as well.

- Causes of fetal death from maternal trauma include death of the mother, separation of the placenta, maternal shock, uterine rupture, and fetal head injury.

- To treat a critically ill pregnant patient, administer high-concentration oxygen. Tilt the patient left lateral. Administer IV fluid if there are signs of shock. Aggressively resuscitate the mother in an attempt to save the baby. Cardiac arrest can occur from a number of causes. Rapid transport is indicated.

- Hyperemesis gravidarum presents with severe nausea, vomiting, weight loss, and electrolyte disturbance. Fluid therapy is indicated if there are signs of dehydration.

- Rh sensitization occurs if the mother has Rh-negative blood and the baby Rh-positive blood. It can cause anemia, jaundice, edema, enlarged liver or spleen, and hydrops fetalis.

- Gestational hypertension is onset of blood pressure greater than 140/90 mm Hg during pregnancy. It can indicate preeclampsia.

- Preeclampsia occurs after 20 weeks' gestation. The criteria for diagnosis include hypertension, protein in the urine, and excessive weight gain with edema. Eclampsia is characterized by the same signs and symptoms with the addition of seizures or coma.

- Gestational diabetes mellitus is diabetes caused by pregnancy.

- Infection during pregnancy can place the mother and fetus at risk. TORCH is an acronym for infections the mother can pass to the fetus that cause fetal death or complications.

- Vaginal bleeding during pregnancy can result from abortion (miscarriage), ectopic pregnancy, abruptio placentae, placenta previa, uterine rupture, or postpartum hemorrhage. Abortion is the termination of pregnancy from any cause before 20 weeks' gestation. Ectopic pregnancy occurs when a fertilized ovum implants anywhere other than the uterus. Abruptio placentae is partial or complete detachment of the placenta at more than 20 weeks' gestation. Placenta previa is placental implantation in the lower uterine segment partially or completely covering the cervical opening.

Uterine rupture is a spontaneous or traumatic rupture of the uterine wall.

- The first stage of labor begins with the onset of regular contractions. It ends with complete dilation of the cervix. The second stage of labor is measured from full dilation of the cervix to delivery of the infant. The third stage of labor begins with delivery of the infant and ends when the placenta is expelled and the uterus has contracted.

- One of the primary responsibilities of the EMS crew is to prevent an uncontrolled delivery. The other is to protect the infant from cold and stress after birth.

- Criteria for computing the Apgar score include appearance (color), pulse (heart rate), grimace (reflex irritability), activity (muscle tone), and respiratory effort.

- More than 500 mL of blood loss after the delivery of the newborn is called a postpartum hemorrhage. It often results from ineffective or incomplete contraction of the uterus.

- Paramedics should be alert to factors that point to a possible abnormal delivery.

- Cephalopelvic disproportion produces a difficult labor because of the presence of a small pelvis, an oversized uterus, or fetal abnormalities. Most infants are born head first (cephalic or vertex presentation). However, sometimes a presentation is abnormal. In breech presentation, the largest part of the fetus (the head) is delivered last. Shoulder dystocia occurs when the fetal shoulders impact against the maternal symphysis pubis. This blocks shoulder delivery. Shoulder presentation (transverse presentation) results when the long axis of the fetus lies perpendicular to that of the mother. The fetal arm or hand may be the presenting part. Cord presentation occurs when the cord slips down into the vagina or presents externally.

- A premature infant is born before 37 weeks' gestation.

- A multiple gestation is a pregnancy with more than one fetus. It is accompanied by an increased complication rate.

- A precipitous delivery is a rapid spontaneous delivery with less than 3 hours from onset of labor to birth. The main danger to the fetus is from cerebral trauma or tearing of the umbilical cord.

- Uterine inversion is a rare complication of childbirth. It is a serious complication. With this condition, the uterus turns "inside out."

- The development of pulmonary embolism during pregnancy, labor, or the postpartum period is a significant cause of maternal death.

- Premature rupture of the membranes is a rupture of the amniotic sac before the onset of labor, regardless of gestational age.

- An amniotic fluid embolism may occur when amniotic fluid enters the maternal circulation during labor or delivery or immediately after delivery.

REFERENCES

1. Centers for Disease Control and Prevention: *Adolescent reproductive health: about teen pregnancy: an update in 2009*, www.cdc.gov/reproductivehealth/AdolescentReproHealth/AboutTP.htm, accessed 4-8-10.
2. McKinney ES, James SR, Murray SS, et al: *Maternal-child nursing*, ed 3, Philadelphia, 2008, Saunders.
3. U.S. Department of Transportation, National Highway Traffic Safety Administration: *EMT-Paramedic national standards curriculum*, Washington, DC, 1998, The Department.
4. American Academy of Pediatrics: *Guidelines for perinatal care*, ed 6, 2007, The Academy.
5. Rosen P, Barkin R: *Emergency medicine: concepts and clinical practice*, ed 7, St Louis, 2010, Mosby.
6. American Heart Association, (2010): *2010 American Heart Association guidelines for cardiopulmonary resuscitation and emergency cardiovascular care, Circulation* 122(18 suppl):S639-S946, 2010.
7. Centers for Disease Control and Prevention: *CDC NCHS data brief*, www.cdc.gov/nchs/data/databriefs/db35.htm, accessed 5-7-10.
8. National Association of Emergency Medical Technicians: *PHTLS: prehospital trauma life support*, ed 7, St Louis, 2011, Mosby.
9. HER Foundation: *Hyperemesis education and research*, www.helpher.org, accessed 10-13-10.
10. Erogul M: *Preeclampsia, pregnancy*, http://emedicine.medscape.com/article/796690-overview, accessed 10-12-10.
11. National Institutes of Health: *HELPP syndrome*, www.nlm.nih.gov/medlineplus/ency/article/000890.htm, accessed 10-12-10.
12. Sibai BM: Hypertension. In Gabbe SG, Niebyl JR, Simpson JL, editors: *Obstetrics: normal and problem pregnancies*, ed 5, Philadelphia, 2007, Churchill Livingstone.
13. American Diabetes Association: *Gestational diabetes*, www.diabetes.org/diabetes-basics/gestational/what-is-gestational-diabetes.html, accessed 10-12-10.
14. Boyer SG, Boyer KM, et al: *Update on TORCH infections in the newborn infant*, www.medscape.com/viewarticle/472409, accessed 10-12-10.
15. Slava V: *Abruptio placentae*, http://emedicine.medscape.com/article/795514-overview, accessed 10-13-10.
16. Oppenheimer L: Diagnosis and management of placenta previa, *J Obstet Gynaecol Can* 29(3):261-273, 2007.
17. Nahum G, Pham KQ: *Uterine rupture in pregnancy*, http://emedicine.medscape.com/article/275854-overview, accessed 10-13-10.
18. American Heart Association: *Pediatric advanced life support*, Dallas, 2005, The Association.
19. Fisher F: *Breach presentation*, http://emedicine.medscape.com/article/262159-overview, accessed 10-25-10.
20. National Library of Medicine, National Institutes of Health: *Premature babies*, www.nlm.nih.gov/medlineplus/prematurebabies.html, accessed 10-13-10.
21. American Heart Association: *Textbook of neonatal resuscitation*, Dallas, 2005, The Association.
22. Stone S, Morris TA: Pulmonary embolism during and after pregnancy, *Crit Care Med* 33(10 suppl):S294-S300, 2005.

SUGGESTED READINGS

Aboutanos MB, Aboutanos SZ, Dompkowski D, et al: Significance of motor vehicle crashes and pelvic injury on fetal mortality: a five-year institutional review, *J Trauma* 65(3):616-620, 2008.

Brunette D, Sterner S: Prehospital and emergency department delivery: a review of eight years experience, *Ann Emerg Med* 18(10):1116-1118, 1989.

Criddle LM: Trauma in pregnancy, *Am J Nurs* 109(11):41-47, 2009.

Edgerly D: It's a boy, *Jems.com*, www.jems.com/article/patient-care/its-boy, accessed 5-28-10.

47 Neonatal Care

OBJECTIVES

Upon completion of this chapter, the paramedic student will be able to:

1. Identify risk factors associated with the need for neonatal resuscitation.
2. Describe physiological adaptations at birth.
3. Describe the pathophysiology and implications of selected genetic anomalies present in some neonates.
4. Outline the prehospital assessment and management of the neonate.
5. Describe resuscitation of the distressed neonate.
6. Discuss postresuscitative management and transport.
7. Describe signs and symptoms and prehospital management of specific neonatal resuscitation situations.
8. Identify injuries associated with birth.
9. Describe appropriate interventions to manage the emotional needs of the neonate's family.

KEY TERMS

antepartum The period before labor and delivery.

apnea An absence of spontaneous respirations.

atrial septal defect A congenital anomaly in which an opening exists between the heart's two upper chambers.

central cyanosis Cyanosis of the tongue and mucous membranes; usually reflects decreased saturation of the hemoglobin in arterial blood.

choanal atresia A bony or membranous occlusion that blocks the passageway between the nose and pharynx; it can result in serious ventilation problems in the neonate.

cleft lip An incomplete closure of the infant's lip that occurs when one or more fissures fail to fuse in the embryo.

cleft palate An incomplete closure in the hard palate of the roof of the mouth that runs along its midline; occurs when one or more fissures fail to fuse in the embryo.

coarctation of the aorta A congenital defect in which there is narrowing or constriction of the aorta.

cold stress A condition that occurs when the body is unable to warm itself.

congenital anomalies Defects that occur during fetal development.

diaphragmatic hernia A herniation in the diaphragm caused by the improper fusion of structures during fetal development.

Dubowitz score A scoring method of clinical assessment in the newborn from birth until 5 days old. The score includes 10 neurological signs for the infant's maturity and 12 physical signs (external signs of development) to determine apparent gestational age.

esophageal atresia The incomplete formation of the esophagus.

hypoplastic left heart syndrome A condition in which the heart's left side, including the aorta, aortic valve, left ventricle, and mitral valve, is underdeveloped.

intestinal malrotation A congenital defect caused by abnormal rotation of the intestine around the superior mesenteric artery during embryological development.

intrapartum The period during labor and delivery.

meconium staining The inhalation of meconium by the fetus or newborn; this can block air passages and result in failure of the lungs to expand or cause other pulmonary dysfunction.

neonate An infant in the first 28 days of life.

newborn An infant in the first few hours of life.

omphalocele A type of hernia in which the infant's intestines or other abdominal organs protrude through the umbilicus; results during fetal development when the muscles in the abdominal wall do not close properly.

peripheral cyanosis Cyanosis that is confined to the extremities (common in the first few minutes of life); also known as *acrocyanosis*.

Pierre Robin syndrome A complex of congenital anomalies including a small mandible, a tongue that falls back into the airway, and a cleft palate.

preterm infant An infant born before 37 weeks' gestation.

pulmonary atresia A congenital anomaly in which no pulmonary valve exists; blood cannot flow from the right ventricle into the pulmonary artery and on to the lungs.

pulmonary hypoplasia A congenital malformation characterized by incomplete development of lung tissue.

pyloric stenosis A congenital defect in which there is narrowing of the pylorus (the opening from the stomach into the small intestine). It is the most common cause of intestinal obstruction in infancy.

single-ventricle defects Complex defects that occur in the embryonic stage and result when one of the ventricles is underdeveloped.

tetralogy of Fallot A congenital cardiac anomaly that consists of four defects: pulmonic stenosis, ventricular septal defect, malposition of the aorta so that it rises from the septal defect or the right ventricle, and right ventricular hypertrophy.

total anomalous pulmonary venous return A congenital heart defect in which the four pulmonary veins that transport oxygen-rich blood back to the heart from the lungs are not properly attached to the left atrium.

tracheoesophageal fistula An abnormal connection between the esophagus and trachea that results from a failed fusion of the tracheoesophageal ridges during fetal development.

transposition of the great arteries A congenital defect in which the positions of the great arteries are reversed; the aorta arises from the right ventricle and the pulmonary artery from the left ventricle.

tricuspid atresia A congenital defect in which there is absence or abnormal development of a tricuspid valve.

truncus arteriosus A rare type of congenital heart disease characterized by a large ventricular septal defect over which a large, single great vessel (truncus) arises.

ventricular septal defect A congenital anomaly in which an opening exists between the heart's two lower chambers.

About 10% of newborns require some assistance to begin breathing at birth, and about 1% require extensive resuscitation.[1] This chapter addresses risk factors that may lead to the need for resuscitation in newborns. It also describes initial care that may be required for the newborn and neonate.

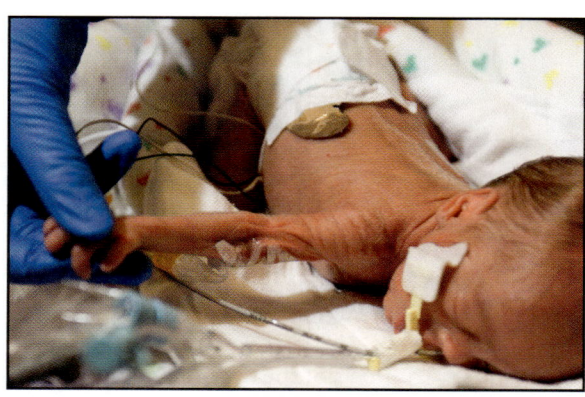

RISK FACTORS ASSOCIATED WITH THE NEED FOR RESUSCITATION

The vast majority of term newborns require no resuscitation beyond maintenance of temperature, and mild stimulation.[2] The incidence of complications, however, increases as birth weight decreases. In fact, resuscitation is required for about 80% of the 30,000 babies who weigh less than 1500 g (3½ lb) at birth.[3]

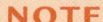

> **NOTE**
> The term **newborn** refers to a recently born infant in the first few hours of life. The term **neonate** refers to a newly born infant in the first 28 days of life.

The average term newborn weighs about 3600 g (7.5 lb). The baby's birth weight depends on a number of factors, including the size and racial origin of the parents. For example, small parents tend to have small babies. Also, Asian babies tend to be smaller than Caucasian babies. Newborn boys usually weigh about 8 oz more than do baby girls. Causes of low birth weight include premature birth, undernourishment in the uterus, and certain maternal factors. These factors include, for example, preeclampsia and cigarette smoking during pregnancy.

In addition to low birth weight, various **antepartum** (before labor and delivery) and **intrapartum** (during labor and delivery) risk factors may affect the need for resuscitation. (See Chapter 46 for review of the obstetrical history.) These include the following[4]:

- Antepartum
  Multiple gestation
  Inadequate prenatal care
  Mother's age (less than age 16 or older than age 35)
  History of perinatal morbidity or mortality
  Postterm gestation
  Drugs/medications
  Toxemia, hypertension, diabetes
  Perinatal infections
  Known fetal malformations
- Intrapartum
  Premature labor
  Meconium-stained amniotic fluid
  Rupture of membranes greater than 18 hours before delivery
  Use of narcotics within 4 hours of delivery
  Abnormal presentation
  Prolonged labor or precipitous delivery
  Prolapsed cord
  Bleeding (abruptio placentae)

BOX 47-1 Neonatal Resuscitation Equipment and Drugs

In addition to a standard obstetrics kit, neonatal resuscitation equipment should include the following:

- Endotracheal tube stylets for full-term infants
- Endotracheal tubes (2.5, 3.0, 3.5, 4.0)
- Meconium aspirator attachment
- Laryngoscope blades (straight, 0, and 1)
- Laryngoscope handles
- Face masks (premature, newborn, and infant sizes)
- Orogastric/nasogastric tubes
- Multiple blankets
- Medications and fluids
  Dextrose 10%
  Epinephrine 1:10,000
  Naloxone
  Sodium bicarbonate (0.5 mEq/mL; 4.2% solution)
  Volume expanders (normal saline, lactated Ringer's solution)
- Self-inflating bag (450 to 750 mL)
- Umbilical vessel catheterization equipment
- Suction catheters (5, 8, and 10 French)
- Syringes (1, 3, 10, and 20 mL)
- Three-way stopcocks

When any of the foregoing risk factors are present during delivery, the paramedic should prepare equipment and drugs that may be needed for neonatal resuscitation (Box 47-1). Medical direction also should be advised of the situation so the appropriate destination hospital can be determined.

CRITICAL THINKING

Does your ambulance have the right size equipment for resuscitation of the newborn?

CONGENITAL ANOMALIES

Congenital anomalies are defects that occur during fetal development. (They develop usually within the first trimester.) They are present in about 2% of all births. These defects are responsible for 20% of all infant deaths.[5] Thus the presence of congenital anomalies may be a factor in the need for neonatal resuscitation. Congenital anomalies may be heritable, caused by maternal infection, alcohol or other drug use during pregnancy (*teratogens*), and other factors.[4] Congenital defects presented in this chapter include anomalies of the airway, heart, and the abdomen and lower back. Spina bifida was described in Chapter 25.

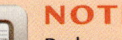

NOTE
Prehospital care for infants born with congenital anomalies requires early assessment to control and protect the airway, positioning to improve respirations, suction to clear the airway, oxygen administration, and careful monitoring with pulse oximetry to ensure adequate ventilation. Advanced airway equipment should be kept close at hand.

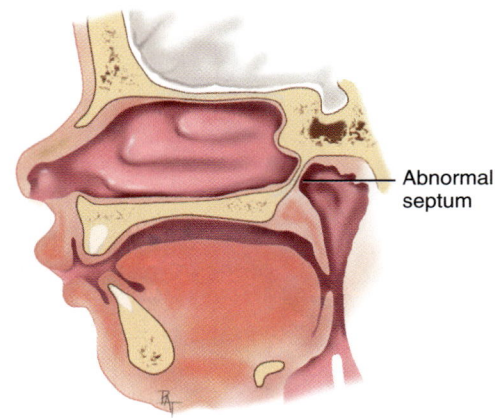

FIGURE 47-1 Choanal atresia. (From Jarvis C: *Physical examination and health assessment,* ed 6, Philadelphia, 2012, Saunders.)

Anomalies of the Airway

CHOANAL ATRESIA

Choanal atresia is a bony or membranous occlusion that blocks the passageway between the nose and pharynx (Figure 47-1). The defect is thought to occur during fetal development when the thin tissue that separates the nose and mouth remains after birth. Choanal atresia is the most common nose abnormality in newborn infants, affecting about 1 in 7000 live births.[5] It commonly is associated with other congenital anomalies.

NOTE
Newborns generally breathe through their nose unless they are crying. Therefore, babies born with choanal atresia have difficulty breathing unless they are crying. Resuscitation, including tracheal intubation, may be required.

Choanal atresia may affect one or both sides of the nasal cavity and may require surgical repair. Bilateral obstruction can result in serious ventilation problems. Depending on the degree of obstruction, symptoms may include:

- Chest wall retraction (unless the infant is breathing through the mouth or crying)
- Dyspnea, which may result in cyanosis (unless infant is crying)
- Inability to nurse and breathe at same time
- Persistent one-sided nasal blockage or discharge

TRACHEOESOPHAGEAL FISTULA

Tracheoesophageal fistula is a congenital disorder that occurs in about 1 in every 4000 live births.[5] It is an abnormal connection between the esophagus and trachea that results from a failed fusion of the tracheoesophageal ridges during fetal development. It commonly occurs along with **esophageal atresia** (the incomplete formation of the esophagus) (Figure 47-2). If not surgically corrected, both conditions can allow for food and fluid in the esophagus

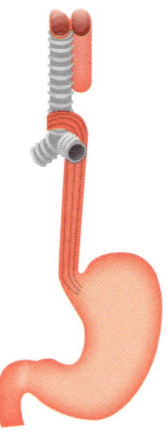

Esophageal Atresia with Distal TEF

Incidence: 85%–88%
Clinical Manifestations: Feeding causes regurgitation and coughing. Constant flow of saliva. Gastric distention.
Diagnostic Findings: Contrast reveals blind pouch. Air on abdominal x ray.
Surgical Treatment: One-stage surgical repair to ligate fistula and anastomose esophagus.

FIGURE 47-2 Esophageal atresia. (Modified from McKinney ES et al: *Maternal-child nursing,* ed 3, St Louis, 2009, Saunders.)

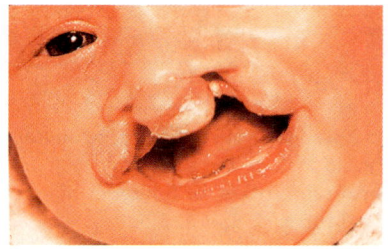

FIGURE 47-3 Cleft lip. (From Lissauer T, Clayden G: *Illustrated textbook of paediatrics,* ed 2, St Louis, 2001, Mosby.)

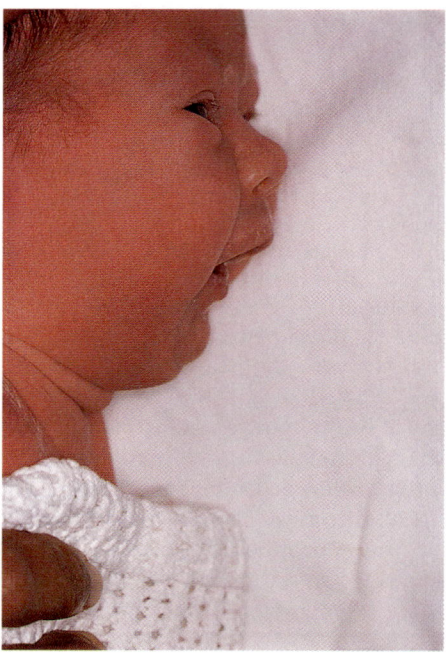

FIGURE 47-4 Pierre Robin syndrome. (From Lissauer T, Clayden G: *Illustrated textbook of paediatrics,* ed 2, St Louis, 2001, Mosby.)

to enter the trachea and lungs. The defect can also allow for air in the trachea to enter the esophagus. Signs and symptoms of both disorders in the newborn include:

- Copious salivation
- Choking
- Coughing
- Regurgitation during feeding
- Cyanosis

Many infants born with tracheoesophageal fistula or esophageal atresia have other congenital anomalies, including heart, kidney, and limb deformities (often occurring together). These infants are unable to feed properly. Once diagnosed, early surgery is required.

CLEFT LIP AND CLEFT PALATE

A **cleft lip** is incomplete closure of the infant's lip. It occurs when one or more fissures fail to fuse in the embryo. It is visible at birth as a vertical, usually off-center split in the upper lip that may extend to the nose (Figure 47-3). A **cleft palate** is a fissure in the hard palate of the roof of the mouth that runs along its midline. Both conditions can occur with other congenital anomalies. A cleft palate may involve one or both sides of the roof of the mouth and can extend through the hard and soft palates into the nasal cavity. A cleft lip or cleft palate can cause nasal deformity and difficulty in feeding and speech, and is associated with frequent ear infections. The condition affects 1 in every 2500 live births.[5] A cleft lip or cleft palate can lead to failure to thrive, misaligned teeth, and difficulties with speech. The

defect is corrected with one or more surgeries, usually beginning in the first year of life.

PIERRE ROBIN SYNDROME

Pierre Robin syndrome is a complex of congenital anomalies including a small mandible, a tongue that falls back into the airway, and a cleft palate. Additional craniofacial abnormalities and defects of the eyes and ears may be present with this syndrome (Figure 47-4). Symptoms of the disorder include a high-arched palate, a receding chin, a tongue that appears large for the jaw, and teeth that are present at birth (*natal teeth*). Pierre Robin syndrome occurs in 1 in every 2000 live births.[5]

Complications associated with Pierre Robin syndrome include breathing difficulties, poor feeding early in life, cerebral hypoperfusion, pulmonary hypertension, and congestive heart failure. Death can result from respiratory failure, secondary to airway obstruction. The condition is managed with surgical repair of the cleft palate and other methods to prevent breathing difficulties and episodes of choking. Most children have some relief from the effects of the syndrome as the jaw grows and allows more space for the tongue.

> ### NOTE
> As a rule, oral airways are rarely indicated for airway control in neonates. However, in infants born with birth defects that affect the airway, an oral airway should be inserted. Examples include newborns with bilateral choanal atresia, Pierre Robin syndrome, and unusual enlargement of the tongue (*macroglossia*). Infants born with these and other craniofacial defects are prone to airway obstruction and choking. They should not be placed supine.

Anomalies of the Heart

Congenital heart abnormalities refer to defects in the heart's structure. These defects occur during embryonic development and are present at birth (Box 47-2). Congenital heart defects are the most common type of birth defect. They affect 8 of every 1000 newborns, 50% of which produce hemodynamic effects from altered cardiac function. Each year, more than 35,000 babies in the United States are born with congenital heart defects. About 1 million American adults live with a congenital heart abnormality.[6]

Causes of congenital heart defects are often unknown. Heredity may play a role in some heart defects. For example, a parent who has a congenital heart defect may be more likely than other people to have a child with the condition. In rare cases, more than one child in a family is born with a heart defect. Children who have genetic disorders, such as Down syndrome, often have congenital heart defects. (Half of all babies who have Down syndrome have congenital heart defects.) Smoking during pregnancy also has been linked to several congenital heart defects, including septal defects.[6] Other possible causes of congenital heart defects include[4]:

> ## BOX 47-2 Congenital Heart Diseases
>
> Congenital heart disease can be an underlying cause of congestive heart failure. These include:
>
> ### Cyanotic Disease
> Hypoplastic left heart syndrome (HLHS)
> Tricuspid atresia
> Transposition of the great arteries (TGA)
> Tetralogy of Fallot (ToF)
> Total anomalous pulmonary venous return (TAPVR)
> Truncus arteriosus
>
> ### Noncyanotic Disease
> Coarctation of the aorta (CoA)
> Atrial septal defect (ASD)
> Ventricular septal defect (VSD)
> Patent ductus arteriosus (PDA)

- Maternal rubella
- Maternal ingestion of alcohol
- Maternal ingestion of drugs or certain medications

Congenital heart defects can involve the interior walls of the heart, the heart valves, or the arteries and veins that carry blood to the heart and other body tissues. These defects can range from "simple defects" with no signs or symptoms to "complex defects" that are life threatening. There are many types of congenital heart defects. Specific diseases discussed in this section include left-to-right shunt abnormalities, valvular defects, single-ventricle defects, transposition, and congenital dysrhythmias. Prehospital care for these patients may be limited to providing only comfort measures and transport to an appropriate medical facility. In some cases, complete support of vital functions will be needed. Infants who are born with congenital heart defects often require surgery within the first week of life. Additional surgeries may also be needed through adulthood. Medication therapy and long-term physician care are required.

> ### NOTE
> Signs and symptoms of congenital heart defects depend on the number, type, and severity of the defects. In infants, signs and symptoms may include tachypnea, cyanosis, poor circulation, and fatigue (e.g., tiring easily when feeding). Older children who have congenital heart defects may tire easily or be short of breath during physical activity. In severe cases (and in adults) signs and symptoms of heart failure may develop. Congenital heart defects do not cause chest pain. A heart murmur may or may not be present and is not diagnostic. (Many healthy children have heart murmurs.)

LEFT-TO-RIGHT SHUNT

The most common physiology seen in patients with congenital heart disease involves a **left-to-right shunt.** The physiological effect of a left-to-right shunt is that oxygenated blood is shunted from the left (systemic) side to the right (pulmonary) side to be oxygenated again, creating a redundant circulation. This leads to an increased venous return from the lungs, via the pulmonary veins, to the left atrium and the left ventricle. The associated volume overload on the left ventricle and the pulmonary circulation decreases cardiac output. Left-to-right shunts are classified according to their hemodynamic effects.

Coarctation of the Aorta. Coarctation of the aorta (CoA) is a narrowing or constriction of the aorta. The defect usually occurs in a short segment of the aorta known as the *juxtaductal part*. The location of this segment is just beyond where the arteries branch to the head and arms, close to where the ductus arteriosus attaches. (The ductus arteriosus is a blood vessel that is normally present in a fetus and that normally closes or contracts in the first hours of life [Figure 47-5].) Coarctation may be caused by the presence of extra ductal tissue that extends into the adjacent aorta, which results in aortic narrowing as the ductal tissue

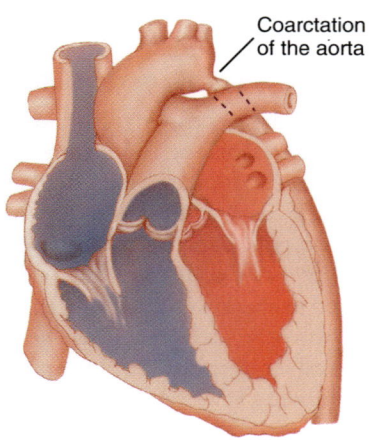

FIGURE 47-5 Coarctation of the aorta. (From McKinney ES, et al: *Maternal-child nursing*, ed 3, St Louis, 2009, Saunders.)

contracts. Coarctation may also occur along with other cardiac defects, typically involving the left side of the heart (e.g., left septal defect). In the presence of a coarctation, the left ventricle has to work harder, because it must generate a higher pressure than normal to force blood through the narrow segment of the aorta to the lower part of the body.

CoA is common in children with some chromosomal abnormalities, such as Turner's syndrome. Coarctation usually presents in the first month of life. It is suspected when the physician is unable to feel (or feels weak) pulses in the groin or the legs of an infant or when the lower body is cyanotic. (A murmur may also be present.) Patients with CoA are at increased risk for hypertension, ruptured aorta, aortic aneurysm, and stroke. Care is aimed at improving ventricular function and improving circulation to the lower extremities with various drugs. Surgical repair is sometimes needed.

Septal Defects. Septal defects (a "hole in the heart") may involve the atrium or ventricle. With **atrial septal defect** (ASD) an opening exists between the heart's two upper chambers. This lets some blood from the left atrium return via the hole to the right atrium instead of flowing through the left ventricle, out the aorta and to the body. Many children with ASD have few, if any, symptoms. Closing the atrial defect by open-heart surgery in childhood can prevent serious problems later in life.

With **ventricular septal defect** (VSD), an opening exists between the heart's two lower chambers. Some blood that has returned from the lungs and been pumped into the left ventricle flows to the right ventricle through the hole instead of being pumped into the aorta. Because the heart has to pump extra blood and is overworked, the heart may become enlarged. Pulmonary hypertension also can develop. If a septal defect is large, surgery may be needed to close the hole. The hallmark of a septal defect is a loud heart murmur.

Patent Ductus Arteriosus. Patent ductus arteriosus (PDA) allows blood to mix between the pulmonary artery and the aorta. As described previously, before birth an open

passageway (the ductus arteriosus) exists between these two blood vessels. Normally this closes within a few hours of birth. When closure does not occur, some blood that should flow through the aorta and on to nourish the body returns to the lungs. (This is quite common in premature infants but rather rare in full-term **babies.**[7]) If the ductus arteriosus is large, a child may become fatigued quickly, grow slowly, and be prone to pulmonary infection, especially pneumonia. If the ductus arteriosus is small, the child often seems healthy. Surgery is sometimes needed to close the ductus arteriosus and restore normal circulation.

Truncus Arteriosus. Truncus arteriosus is a rare type of congenital heart disease. It is characterized by a large ventricular septal defect over which a large, single great vessel (truncus) arises. It occurs when a single blood vessel (the truncus) arises from the right and left ventricles, instead of the normal two vessels (the pulmonary artery and the aorta). This single great vessel carries blood both to the body and to the lungs. The truncus sits over a large opening or hole in the wall between the two pumping chambers (ventricular septal defect). A decrease in peripheral vascular resistance at birth causes a left-to-right shunt with evidence of congestive heart failure early in life. These children have a very high incidence of pulmonary hypertension and vascular disease. Children with this defect may experience shortness of breath, decreased exercise endurance, and sometimes headaches and dizziness. Surgical repair is needed to close the ventricular septal defect and separate blood flow to the body from blood flow to the lungs. Long-term follow-up care is required.

VALVULAR DEFECTS

Some children are born with defective heart valves that occurred during embryonic development. These defects may present at birth or during childhood, or not become apparent until adulthood. Common valvular defects include stenosis of the tricuspid and mitral valves (on the left side of the heart) and stenosis of the aortic and pulmonic valves (on the right side of the heart). The narrowing (caused by valvular lesions) of one or more of these valves leads to a pressure gradient across the valve during the time blood is flowing through the valve opening.[8]

Mitral valve stenosis results from a narrowing of the mitral valve orifice when the valve is open. The high resistance across the stenotic mitral valve causes blood to back up into the left atrium, thereby increasing left atrial pressure. This results in the left atrial pressure being much greater than the left ventricular pressure during diastolic filling. Mitral valve stenosis is associated with a diastolic murmur because of turbulence that occurs as blood flows across the stenotic valve.

Tricuspid valve stenosis is similar to mitral valve stenosis except that the pressure and volume changes occur on the right side of the heart.

Aortic valve stenosis is characterized by the left ventricular pressure being much greater than the aortic pressure during left ventricular ejection. Left ventricular pressure is greatly elevated and the aortic pressure is slightly reduced. The pressure gradient across the stenotic lesion results from both increased resistance (related to narrowing of the valve opening) and turbulence distal to the valve (associated with a systolic murmur).

Pulmonic valve stenosis is similar to aortic valve stenosis except that the changes in pressure are on the right side of the heart. This leads to an increased resistance to outflow. In turn, this elevates right ventricular pressure and limits pulmonary blood flow. Pulmonary valve stenosis accounts for about 8% to 12% of all congenital defects in children.[9] A stenotic pulmonary valve may occur without associated congenital abnormalities, although it is most often associated with other structural abnormalities of the heart.

SINGLE-VENTRICLE DEFECTS

Single-ventricle defects are complex and rare. They occur in the embryonic stage and result when one of the ventricles is underdeveloped. The most common types of single-ventricle defects are tricuspid atresia, pulmonary atresia, and hypoplastic left heart syndrome.[10] In the prehospital setting, standard resuscitation procedures should be followed in infants and children with single-ventricle anatomy. It should be noted, however, that end-tidal CO_2 measurements in these children may not be a reliable indicator of cardiopulmonary resuscitation (CPR) quality. This is because in children with single-ventricle anatomy, pulmonary blood flow changes rapidly and will not always reflect cardiac output during CPR.[1a] Modifications in the care of these patients will be provided in the in-hospital setting.

Tricuspid Atresia. Tricuspid atresia is the absence or abnormal development of a tricuspid valve. This prevents the normal flow of blood from the right atrium to the right ventricle and results in a right ventricle that is small and not fully developed. Ultimately, the blood cannot enter the lungs for oxygenation. The survival of these patients depends on the presence of an atrial septal defect and usually a ventricular septal defect. Because there is no atrioventricular pathway, an atrial septal defect must be present to maintain blood flow. Likewise, because there is an underdeveloped right ventricle, there must be a way to pump blood into the pulmonary arteries through a ventricular septal defect. (A patent ductus arteriosus is also usually formed to increase pulmonary flow.) Cyanosis and shortness of breath are usually present in these infants until surgical repair is made. Surgery is required to repair the connection between the arteries to the body and the arteries to the lungs.

Pulmonary Atresia. In **pulmonary atresia,** no pulmonary valve exists. Blood cannot flow from the right ventricle into the pulmonary artery and on to the lungs. (The right ventricle and tricuspid valve also are often poorly developed.) In these patients, an opening in the atrial septum lets blood exit the right atrium, so low-oxygen blood mixes with the oxygen-rich blood in the left atrium. The left ventricle pumps this mixture of oxygen-poor blood into the aorta and out to the body. As a result, the infant appears cyanotic. Often, the only source of blood flow to the lung is the patent ductus arteriosus. Surgical repair is required.

Hypoplastic Left Heart Syndrome. Hypoplastic left heart syndrome (HLHS) is a condition in which the heart's left side, including the aorta, aortic valve, left ventricle, and mitral valve, is underdeveloped. Blood returning from the lungs must flow through an opening in the wall between the atria (atrial septal defect). The right ventricle pumps the blood into the pulmonary artery, and blood reaches the aorta through a patent ductus arteriosus. Surgical repair is required.

TETRALOGY OF FALLOT

Tetralogy of Fallot (ToF) is a rare congenital heart defect that affects about 5 out of every 10,000 babies.[11] Tetralogy of Fallot involves four heart defects:

1. A large ventricular septal defect (VSD)
2. Pulmonary stenosis
3. Right ventricular hypertrophy
4. An overriding aorta

The VSD allows oxygen-rich blood from the left ventricle to mix with oxygen-poor blood from the right ventricle. Pulmonary stenosis causes the heart to work harder than normal to pump blood through the narrowed pulmonary valve, causing right ventricular hypertrophy. In tetralogy of Fallot, the aorta is between the left and right ventricles (*an overriding aorta*), directly over the VSD. (In healthy hearts, the aorta is directly attached to the left ventricle.) As a result, oxygen-poor blood from the right ventricle flows directly into the aorta instead of into the pulmonary artery to the lungs. Together, these four defects prevent blood from reaching the lungs for oxygenation. As a result, oxygen-poor blood flows out to the body, resulting in cyanosis. (Other signs and symptoms of ToF include a heart murmur, delayed growth and development, and clubbing of the fingers.) Although the cause of the defect is often unknown, contributing factors that may occur during pregnancy include:

- German measles (rubella) and some other viral illnesses
- Poor nutrition
- Overuse of alcohol
- Age (mother older than 40 years)
- Diabetes

Heredity may also play a role in causing tetralogy of Fallot. An adult who has tetralogy of Fallot is at an increased risk of having a baby with the condition. Children who have certain genetic disorders, such as Down syndrome and DiGeorge syndrome, often have congenital heart defects, including tetralogy of Fallot. Surgical repair of the four defects is required early in life. Babies who have unrepaired tetralogy of Fallot sometimes have "tet spells" when blood oxygen level suddenly drops. This is often in response to an activity such as crying or having a bowel movement (Figure 47-6). The drop in oxygen level causes severe cyanosis. The baby also may:

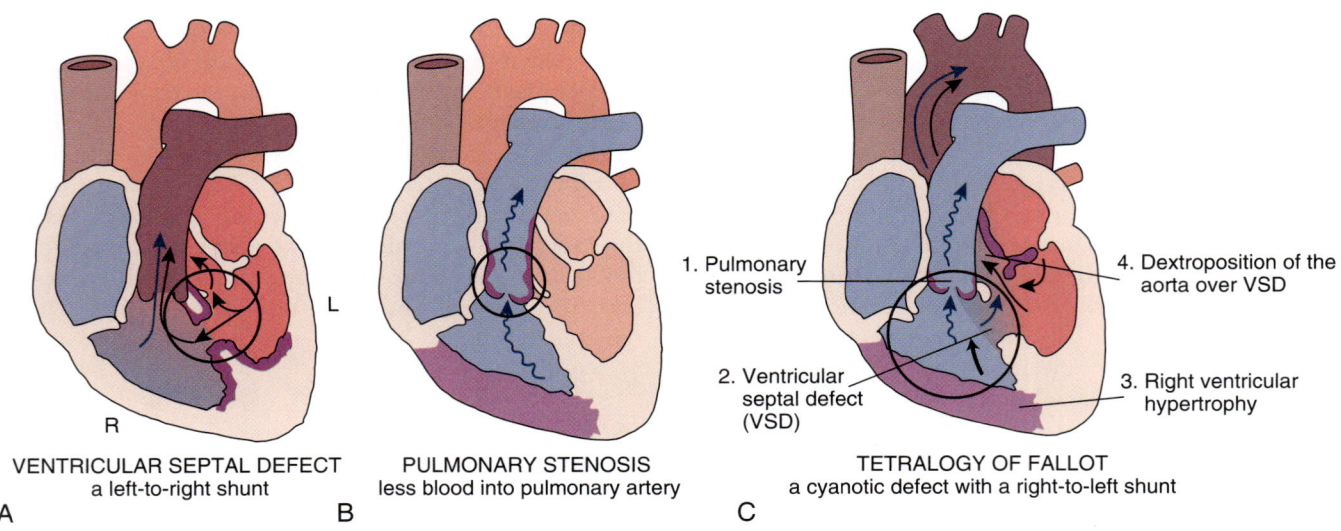

VENTRICULAR SEPTAL DEFECT
a left-to-right shunt

A

L

R

PULMONARY STENOSIS
less blood into pulmonary artery

B

1. Pulmonary stenosis

2. Ventricular septal defect (VSD)

4. Dextroposition of the aorta over VSD

3. Right ventricular hypertrophy

TETRALOGY OF FALLOT
a cyanotic defect with a right-to-left shunt

C

FIGURE 47-6 Congenital heart defects. (From Gould BE, Dyer R: *Pathophysiology for the health professional*, ed 4, St Louis, 2011, Saunders.)

- Have difficulty breathing
- Become very tired and limp
- Not respond to a parent's voice or touch
- Become irritable and fussy
- Lose consciousness

TRANSPOSITION OF THE GREAT ARTERIES

In a healthy heart, the aorta and pulmonary artery are properly positioned and aligned with the appropriate ventricle. If this is reversed (transposed), the aorta arises from the right ventricle and the pulmonary artery from the left ventricle. This congenital heart defect is known as **transposition of the great arteries** (TGA). TGA results in the systemic and pulmonary circulations being in parallel rather than in series. As a result, oxygen-poor blood returning from the body to the right atrium and right ventricle is pumped out to the aorta and to the body. Oxygen-rich blood returning from the lungs to the left atrium and ventricle is sent back to the lungs via the pulmonary artery. Like other heart defects, survival of these patients before surgical repair depends on the presence of an ASD, a VSD, or PDA. Untreated, more than 50% of infants with transposition will die in the first month of life, 90% in the first year.[12]

TOTAL ANOMALOUS PULMONARY VENOUS RETURN

Total anomalous pulmonary venous return (TAPVR) is a congenital heart defect in which the four pulmonary veins that carry oxygen-rich blood back to the heart from the lungs are not properly attached to the left atrium. Instead, they are improperly attached to another area (usually the superior vena cava). With this defect, oxygen-rich blood that should return to the left atrium—and then the left ventricle, the aorta, and the body—instead mixes with the oxygen-poor blood flowing into the right side of the heart.

In other words, blood simply circles to and from the lungs, and never to the body.

To survive before corrective surgery, a large ASD or patent foramen ovale (a passage between the left and right atria) must exist to allow oxygenated blood to flow to the left side of the heart and the rest of the body. Infants with TAPVR may appear critically ill with the following symptoms[13]:

- Lethargy
- Poor feeding
- Rapid breathing
- Poor growth
- Frequent respiratory tract infections
- Cyanosis

CONGENITAL DYSRHYTHMIAS

Many children born with congenital heart disease (CHD) now live well into adulthood. It has been estimated that there are more than 800,000 adults with CHD living in the United States.[14] Of these, approximately 45% are considered to have mild forms of CHD (e.g., atrial septal defect, valvular pulmonary stenosis), 40% are classified as having moderate disease (e.g., tetralogy of Fallot), and 15% are considered to have complex disease (e.g., single ventricle, transposition of the great arteries). Although dysrhythmias can develop within any of these groups, the incidence is highest for patients in the moderate and severe categories.

Malfunctions in embryonic development that are responsible for congenital heart defects can directly impact the development of the heart's conduction system (especially displacement of the atrioventricular [AV] node and bundle of His). This makes these patients more vulnerable to many dysrhythmias, including atrial fibrillation, atrial flutter, reentry tachycardias, and heart blocks. Standards of care for patients with dysrhythmias that result from CHD

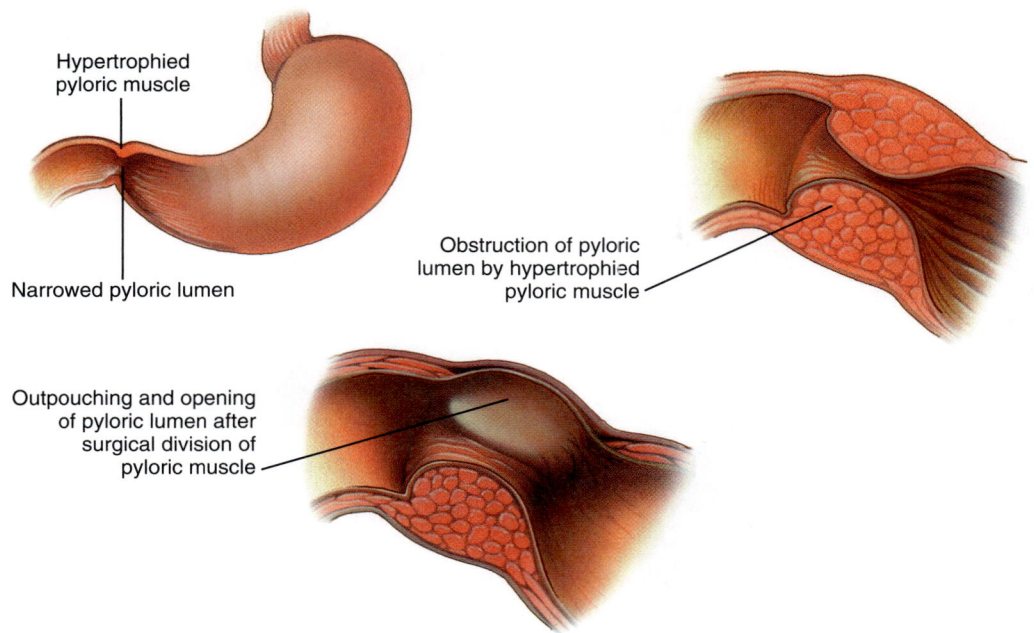

Hypertrophied pyloric muscle

Narrowed pyloric lumen

Obstruction of pyloric lumen by hypertrophied pyloric muscle

Outpouching and opening of pyloric lumen after surgical division of pyloric muscle

FIGURE 47-7 In pyloric stenosis, the pyloric muscle hypertrophies and obstructs the passage of stomach contents into the intestines. (From Price DL, Gwin JF: *Pediatric nursing: an introductory text,* ed 10, St Louis, 2008, Saunders.)

follow the same treatments guidelines as for other patients (see Chapter 48).

Anomalies of the Abdomen and Lower Back

INTESTINAL MALROTATION

Intestinal malrotation is caused by abnormal rotation of the intestine around the superior mesenteric artery during embryological development. It is a congenital defect that can cause a serious bowel obstruction. The condition occurs in about 1 in every 500 live births.[15] Malrotation is commonly seen with other birth defects such as omphalocele, diaphragmatic hernia, and Hirschsprung's disease. The condition usually becomes evident within the first week of life; 75% of cases are diagnosed within the first 12 months. The illness may be acute or chronic. The primary presenting sign in acute malrotation is emesis that contains bile. Features of chronic malrotation include recurrent bouts of abdominal pain and diarrhea (alternating with constipation), intolerance of solid food, jaundice, lower gastrointestinal (GI) tract bleeding, and gastroesophageal reflux. If symptoms persist, the child may develop shock, including poor perfusion, decreased urine output, and hypotension. Malrotation requires surgical repair.

PYLORIC STENOSIS

Pyloric stenosis is narrowing of the pylorus (the opening from the stomach into the small intestine). It is the most common cause of intestinal obstruction in infancy.[16] The narrowing occurs from muscles around the pylorus that have grown too large (Figure 47-7). The diagnosis is usually made when an infant presents with a history of progressive, forceful vomiting. This usually begins within the second or third week of life. Parents may complain that the baby is "spitting up." They often have tried a different formula in formula-fed babies without any change being noted. Signs and symptoms are related to dehydration and may include dry mucous membranes, slow capillary refill, sunken fontanelles, and decreased urine output (dry diapers for several hours). After diagnosis, surgery will be required to dilate the muscles around the pyloric valve of the stomach.

DIAPHRAGMATIC HERNIA

Diaphragmatic hernia is caused by the malformation of the diaphragm during fetal development. The condition affects 1 in every 2500 to 5000 live births.[5] Diaphragmatic hernia may occur on the right, left, or both sides, but the left side is most common. It results from a defect (hole) in the diaphragm muscle. The opening allows abdominal organs, such as the stomach, bowel, liver, and spleen, to enter the chest cavity (Figure 47-8). As a result, the lung on the affected side does not develop normally **(pulmonary hypoplasia),** and this reduces lung capacity. Other organs can be damaged as well, including the heart. A significant prenatal shift in the mediastinum may indicate some degree of pulmonary hypoplasia on the contralateral side.[4] The infant's head and thorax should be elevated to assist with downward displacement of the abdominal organs and to help improve ventilation.

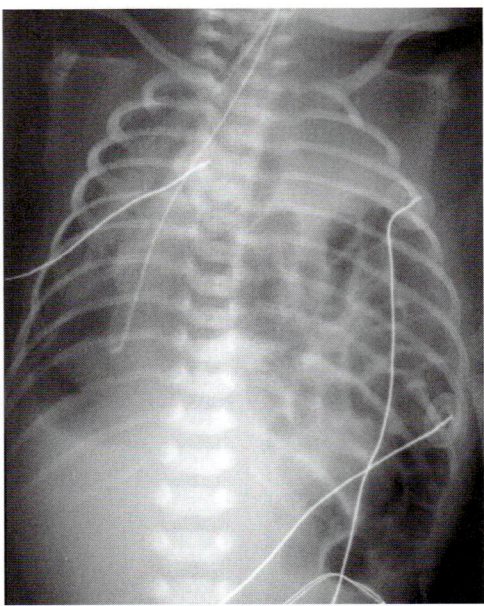

FIGURE 47-8 Left-sided congenital diaphragmatic hernia. Note the loops of bowel present in the thoracic cavity. (From Kacmarek RM, Dimas S: *The essentials of respiratory care,* ed 4, St Louis, 2005, Mosby.)

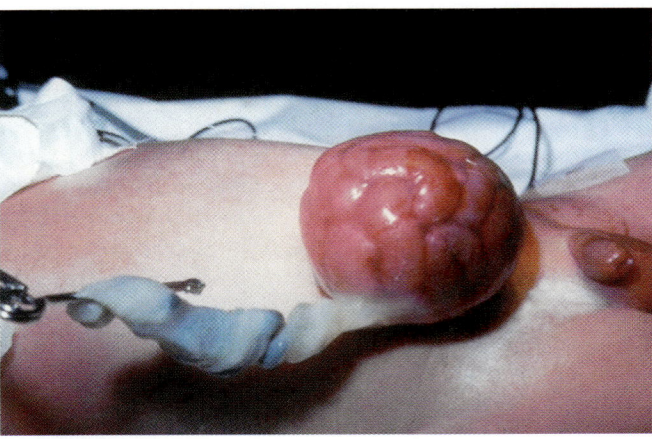

FIGURE 47-9 Omphalocele in membranous sac. (From Hockenberry MJ: *Wong's nursing care of infants and children,* ed 9, St Louis, 2011, Mosby.)

> **NOTE**
> Diaphragmatic hernia is a true emergency that requires surgical repair. Newborns who do not survive usually die within the first days or weeks of life. Survival for the infant who requires mechanical ventilation in the first 18 to 24 hours of life is about 50%. If there is no respiratory distress within the first 24 hours of life, survival approaches 100%.[4]

Respiratory distress usually develops shortly after birth. Other symptoms include cyanosis that is unresponsive to ventilations, tachypnea, and tachycardia. On examination, the infant born with this disorder may have irregular chest wall movement, displaced heart sounds, absent breath sounds on the affected side, and bowel sounds in the chest cavity. In addition, the abdomen may be scaphoid (flat) and feel "full" on palpation. Medical direction may recommend placement of an orogastric tube, with low periodic suction to improve ventilations. In some cases, tracheal intubation may be needed. The use of a bag device or aggressive positive-pressure ventilation may cause gastric distention and worsen the condition. (The use of a bag device is contraindicated.) Surgery is required to repair the hernia and to place the abdominal organs in their normal location. If the condition is diagnosed during pregnancy, fetal surgery may be indicated.

OMPHALOCELE

An **omphalocele** is a type of hernia in which the infant's intestines or other abdominal organs protrude through the umbilicus. It results during fetal development when the muscles in the abdominal wall (umbilical ring) do not close properly. As a result, the intestines remain outside the umbilical cord (Figure 47-9). The defect affects 1 in every 5000 to 6000 live births. Up to 25% to 40% of infants with an omphalocele will have another (often more serious) congenital anomaly.[5] The omphalocele usually is first seen on ultrasound during prenatal care.

Most omphaloceles will be quite visible at birth. The omphalocele may be small (containing only a small section of intestines) or large (containing the liver and spleen). The protruding organs will usually be covered by a thin sac of peritoneum (*intact omphalocele*). The umbilical vessels are usually present within the sac. Exposed tissue should be protected and covered with moist, sterile gauze pads to prevent injury and infection. Rupture of an omphalocele (*nonintact omphalocele*) may occur immediately before or during delivery.

> **NOTE**
> An umbilical cord that appears unusually large in diameter should be examined for the presence of a small omphalocele before it is clamped and cut as part of the delivery process. If suspected, the cord should not be clamped or cut. The paramedic should consult with medical direction.

An omphalocele usually is successfully repaired with surgery. As part of the surgery, the exposed tissues of a small omphalocele will be covered and held in place with a special plastic pouch (*silo*) that over time squeezes the exposed tissue back into the infant's abdomen. Surgical repair of the infant's abdominal muscles may be needed as well. Surgery for a larger omphalocele with an intact sac is often delayed. The tissue will eventually be covered by the growth of surrounding skin, after which surgery can be performed to improve cosmetic outcome.

PHYSIOLOGICAL ADAPTATIONS AT BIRTH

Newborns make three major physiological adaptations at birth that are necessary for survival: (1) emptying fluids from their lungs and beginning ventilation, (2) changing their circulatory pattern, and (3) maintaining body temperature.[17]

During vaginal delivery, the newborn's chest usually is compressed. This forces fluid from the lungs into the mouth and nose. As the chest wall recoils, air is drawn into the lungs. The newborn takes the first breath in response to chemical changes and changes in temperature.

When the cord is cut and placental circulation ceases, the circulatory system must function on its own. This involves the immediate and permanent closure of the pathways that allowed the fetus to receive oxygen without the use of lungs (described in Chapter 46). As the lungs expand with initial breaths, the resistance to blood flow in the lungs decreases, and the newborn's blood begins to be oxygenated.

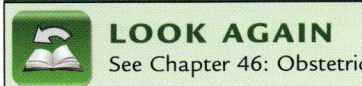
LOOK AGAIN
See Chapter 46: Obstetrics, pp. 1279-1280.

Newborns are sensitive to hypoxia. Permanent brain damage will occur from prolonged hypoxemia. Causes of hypoxia include compression of the cord, difficult labor and delivery, maternal hemorrhage, airway obstruction, hypothermia, newborn blood loss, and immature lungs in the premature newborn. Cardiovascular anomalies also may result in hypoxia.

Newborns are at risk for rapidly developing hypothermia. Thus they should be delivered in a warm, draft-free area when possible. This risk factor is due to their larger body surface area (BSA), decreased tissue insulation, and immature temperature regulatory mechanisms. The cool, wet environment of birth also increases heat loss for the newborn. Newborns try to conserve body heat through vasoconstriction and an increase in their metabolism. This places them at risk for hypoxemia, acidosis, bradycardia, and hypoglycemia.

ASSESSMENT AND MANAGEMENT OF THE NEONATE

The initial steps of assessment and management of any newborn should be accomplished within about 60 seconds (the "Golden Minute").[1] Following these steps enables the paramedic to immediately recognize an infant in need of resuscitation. It also leads to efficient and effective emergency care delivery. The initial steps in assessment and management of the neonate are (Figure 47-10)[1]:

1. Provide warmth by drying the baby to prevent heat loss and avoid hypothermia.

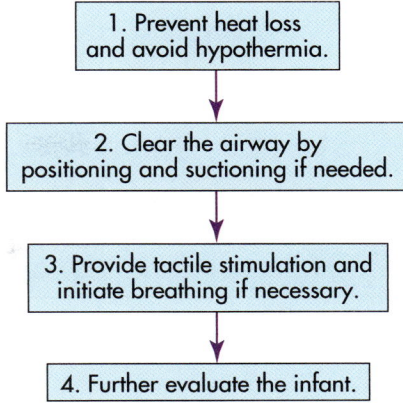

FIGURE 47-10 Steps in neonatal assessment and management.

2. Position the head in a sniffing position to open the airway.
3. Clear the airway if necessary with a bulb syringe or suction catheter.
4. Provide tactile stimulation to initiate breathing if necessary.
5. Further evaluate the infant.

NOTE
Body substance isolation (BSI) precautions are recommended during delivery of a newborn. Gloves and other appropriate protective barriers (including gowns and goggles) should be worn when handling the newborn or contaminated equipment.

SHOW ME THE EVIDENCE
In a case-control retrospective study conducted from 1995 to 1999, Scottish researchers investigated unplanned out-of-hospital deliveries in an attempt to identify risk factors associated with them. During that period 117 women delivered 121 babies accidentally in the prehospital setting. Each study birth was compared to the next woman who delivered in the hospital after spontaneous labor. Compared to hospital deliveries, the study group women were likely to be of greater parity and to have less prenatal care. Babies in the study group were more likely to be younger gestational age and lower birth weight, to deliver after a shorter labor, and to be admitted to the neonatal intensive care unit than the control group. The infant mortality rate in the accidental delivery group was six times higher than the controls.

From Rodie VA, Thomson A, Norman J: Accidental out-of-hospital deliveries: an obstetric and neonatal case control study, *Acta Obstet Gynecol Scand* 81(1):50-54, 2002.

Prevent Heat Loss and Avoid Hypothermia

Even healthy term newborns are limited in their ability to conserve heat when exposed to a cold environment and are at risk for developing hypothermia. Therefore, immediately after delivery, the infant's body and head should be dried

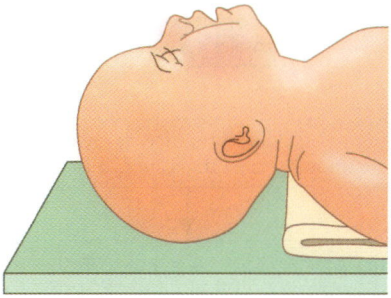

FIGURE 47-11 Positioning the neonate to open the airway.

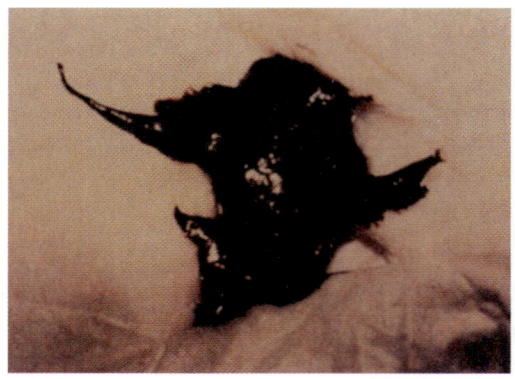

FIGURE 47-12 Meconium-stained birth.

to prevent evaporative heat loss and metabolic derangements that may be instigated by **cold stress** (when the body is unable to warm itself). The act of drying also provides gentle stimulation, which may initiate respirations. Care should be taken to remove any wet coverings from the infant and cover the infant with dry wrappings. The majority of heat loss can be prevented by covering the newborn's head (which accounts for 20% of the newborn's BSA). Covering the baby in plastic wrapping such as food wrap can prevent hypothermia.[1]

CRITICAL THINKING
What other measures can you take to warm the infant?

Clear the Airway by Positioning and Suctioning (If Needed)

After the newborn has been dried and covered, the next step is to establish an open airway. This is achieved by placing the infant supine, with the head in a sniffing position. Care should be taken to prevent hyperextension or underextension, which may compromise the airway. Placing a blanket or towel under the infant's shoulders (thereby elevating the torso ¾ to 1 inch) can help maintain the correct position (Figure 47-11).

CRITICAL THINKING
Do infants breathe through their noses or mouths?

Once the infant has been properly positioned, most newborns will breathe without difficulty. If the airway is obstructed by secretions, a bulb syringe or catheter can be used to suction the nose and mouth. It is preferable to suction the mouth first to prevent aspiration in case the infant gasps when the nose is cleared. Each application of suction should last no more than 5 seconds to prevent hypoxia. The newborn's heart rate should be monitored during suctioning, and time should be provided during suction attempts for spontaneous ventilation.

NOTE
Suctioning the airway at birth can stimulate the posterior pharynx and can produce a vagal response with resulting bradycardia, apnea, or both. Therefore, suctioning should be reserved for babies who have obvious obstruction to spontaneous breathing or who require positive-pressure ventilation. Supplemental oxygen delivery (described elsewhere) should be guided by pulse oximetry results.[1]

MECONIUM STAINING

Meconium staining is the presence of fetal stool in the amniotic fluid. It occurs in utero or intrapartum and in about 12% of all deliveries.[4] Meconium staining becomes more common in postterm and small-for-gestational-age newborns. It is also common in those infants who develop fetal distress during labor and delivery. Meconium staining is associated with increased perinatal mortality, hypoxemia, aspiration pneumonia, pneumothorax, and pulmonary hypertension.

The appearance of meconium depends on the amount of meconium particles and amniotic fluid. Meconium staining may appear as only a slight yellow or light green staining that is thin and watery. Or it may have a thick, pea-soup appearance that is dark green or black (Figure 47-12). When thick meconium is present in amniotic fluid, a chance exists that the particles will be aspirated into the infant's mouth, and potentially into the trachea and lungs. This can lead to partial or complete obstruction of the airways. Death can result from hypoxia, hypercapnia, and acidosis.

NOTE
Meconium can be used to test for maternal drug use. It has a greater sensitivity than urine and positive findings that persist longer. If time permits, a specimen should be collected and delivered to the emergency department.

If meconium (or evidence of infection) is observed and the newborn is vigorous (strong respiratory efforts, good muscle tone, and a heart rate greater than 100 beats per minute), no special care of the airway is required. If the newborn is not vigorous (absent or depressed respirations, decreased muscle tone, heart rate less than 100 beats per minute), endotracheal (ET) intubation and endotracheal suctioning are recommended immediately after birth.[1] Because the presence of meconium can be determined only after the membranes have ruptured, it is critical that the paramedic crew have airway equipment available. Emergency care for these newborns includes the following steps (Figure 47-13):

1. Prepare the necessary equipment (e.g., intubation equipment, bulb syringe, and DeLee suction, 12 F [French] or 14 F suction catheter, portable suction and irrigation solution, gauze pads, infant bag device). Intubation equipment should include padding for patient positioning, stethoscope, number 0 and number 1 laryngoscope blades, ET tubes (2.5, 3.0, 3.5, 4.0), stylet, meconium aspirator, and oxygen tubing. The procedure for endotracheal intubation of an infant is described in Chapter 15.

> **LOOK AGAIN**
> See Chapter 15: Airway Management, Respiration, and Artificial Ventilation, pp. 439-445.

2. After delivery, clear the infant's airway and thoroughly suction the nose, mouth, and pharynx. Remove residual meconium in the hypopharynx by suction under direct visualization.
3. Quickly intubate the trachea. Apply suction to the proximal end of the ET tube using the DeLee device while withdrawing the tube. During intubation and suctioning, aim 100% oxygen toward the infant's face and monitor the fetal heart rate for bradycardia. If bradycardia develops, ventilate the infant's lungs using a bag device after suctioning to prevent persistent bradycardia and hypoxia.
4. Repeat the intubation-suction-extubation cycle until no further meconium is obtained. Do not ventilate between intubations.
5. After tracheal suction is complete, continue resuscitative measures as needed. If respirations are adequate, manage the infant's airway in the normal fashion. Medical direction may recommend that an 8 F orogastric tube that is aspirated with a syringe and left open to air be placed to prevent aspiration of gastric contents after resuscitation is complete.

If tracheal suctioning cannot be achieved promptly and the infant is bradycardic, consider bag-mask ventilation.[1]

Provide Tactile Stimulation to Initiate Breathing

If drying does not induce respirations in the infant, additional tactile stimulation should be provided. The two safe and appropriate methods of tactile stimulation are slapping or flicking the soles of the infant's feet and rubbing the infant's back.

Further Evaluate the Infant

Drying and positioning are necessary in every infant at birth. These maneuvers are used to open the airway and initiate breathing. To further evaluate the infant the paramedic should follow these steps:

1. Observe and evaluate the infant's respirations. If they are normal (e.g., crying), continue the evaluation. If available, place a neonatal pulse oximetry probe on the right upper extremity (usually the infant's wrist or medial surface of the palm) to monitor oxygen saturation. Target SpO_2 readings after birth are provided in Box 47-3.
2. Evaluate the infant's heart rate by stethoscope or palpation of the pulse in the base of the umbilical cord. If it is greater than 100 beats/min, continue the evaluation.
3. Evaluate the infant's color. Peripheral cyanosis (*acrocyanosis*) is common in the first few minutes of life and does not indicate hypoxemia. If the infant's color is normal ("pinking up") and the SpO_2 readings are increasing, continue the evaluation by obtaining the Apgar score.

> **NOTE**
> Cyanosis can be divided into two types: central and peripheral. **Central cyanosis** (identified by cyanosis of the tongue and mucous membranes) usually reflects *decreased saturation* of the hemoglobin in arterial blood. The cause is most often from heart or lung disease. Less commonly, it results from an increased amount of abnormal hemoglobin. **Peripheral cyanosis** is confined to the extremities. This type of cyanosis reflects a *difference in the saturation* of hemoglobin between arterial and venous blood at a time when arterial hemoglobin saturation is normal. Peripheral cyanosis occurs when blood vessels in the hands and feet constrict and slow the flow of blood. As a result, more oxygen than usual is permitted to be extracted from hemoglobin by the surrounding tissues, thus desaturating it. Peripheral cyanosis is expected and considered normal in newborn infants.

APGAR SCORE

The Apgar score (described in Chapter 46) enables rapid evaluation of a newborn's condition at specific intervals after birth. It routinely is assessed at 1 and 5 minutes of age.

BOX 47-3 Target SpO_2 Readings After Birth[1]	
1 minute	60% to 65%
2 minutes	65% to 70%
3 minutes	70% to 75%
4 minutes	75% to 80%
5 minutes	80% to 85%
10 minutes	85% to 95%

Newborn Resuscitation

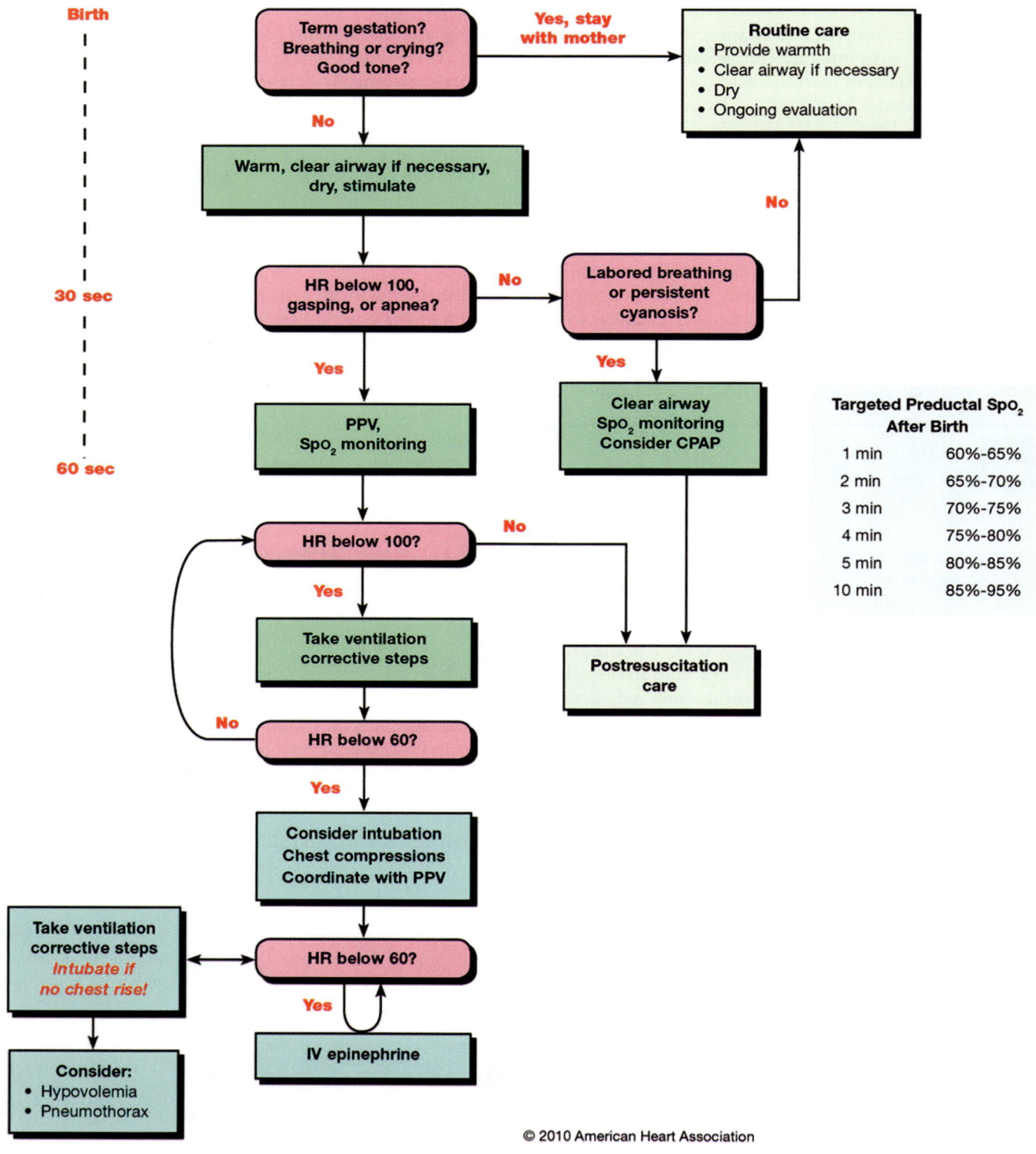

© 2010 American Heart Association

FIGURE 47-13 Neonatal flow algorithm. (Reprint with permission: American Heart Association Guidelines For CPR and ECC, *Circulation* 122 [suppl 3]: S685-S919, American Heart Association, Inc, 2010.)

Although the Apgar score is a useful tool to evaluate the newborn, it should not be used alone in determining the need for resuscitation. To review, an Apgar evaluates **a**ppearance, **p**ulse rate, **g**rimace, **a**ctivity, and **r**espirations. A score of 7 to 10 is considered normal; a score of 4 to 6 identifies a moderately distressed infant who requires oxygen and stimulation; and a score less than 4 identifies a severely distressed infant who requires resuscitation (Table 47-1).

RESUSCITATION OF THE DISTRESSED NEONATE

Newborns who are full term, who have an airway that is clear of meconium or have no evidence of infection, who are breathing and crying, and who have good muscle tone do not usually require resuscitation. As described earlier, this assessment should be completed within 60 seconds. If resuscitation is required because of inadequate respirations or heart rate, the infant will need one or more of the following interventions in sequence[1] (Figure 47-14):

> 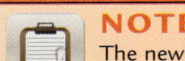 **NOTE**
> The newborn should have regular respirations that are sufficient to improve color, achieve target SpO_2 ranges, and maintain a heart rate of greater than 100 beats per minute.

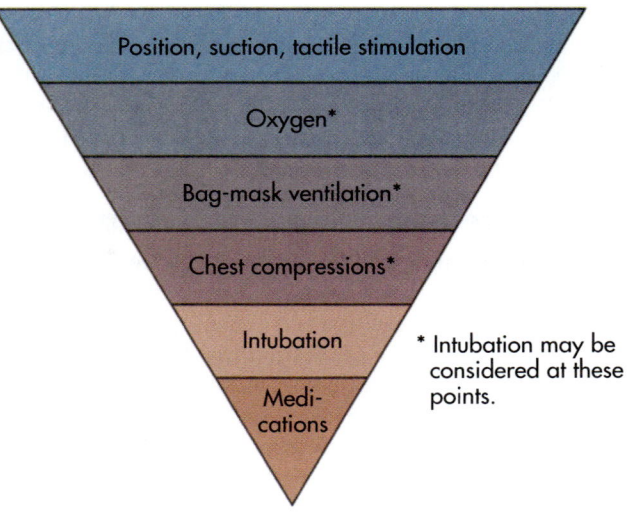

FIGURE 47-14 Inverted pyramid reflecting the approximate relative frequency of neonatal resuscitative efforts. Note that a majority of infants respond to simple measures.

1. Reevaluate initial steps in stabilization (provide warmth, position, clear airway if necessary, dry, and stimulate).
2. Provide ventilations.
3. Provide chest compressions at 120/min.
4. Administer *epinephrine* and/or volume expanders.

TABLE 47-1 APGAR Score*

	POINTS		
Assessment	**0**	**1**	**2**
Heart rate	Absent	Below 100 beats/min	100 beats/min or higher
Respiratory effort	No spontaneous respirations	Slow respirations or weak cry	Spontaneous respirations with strong, lusty cry
Muscle tone	Limp	Minimal flexion of extremities; sluggish movement	Flexed body posture; spontaneous and vigorous movement
Reflex	No response to suction	Minimal response (grimace) to suction or gentle slap on soles	Responds promptly to suction or gentle slap to sole with cry or active movement
Color	Pallor or cyanosis	Bluish hands and feet only	Pink (light skinned) or absence of cyanosis (dark skinned); pink mucous membranes
0 1 2 3 4		**5 6 7**	**8 9 10**
Infant needs resuscitation.		Gently stimulate by rubbing infant's back while administering oxygen. Determine whether mother received narcotics, which may have depressed infant's respirations. Have naloxone (Narcan) available for administration.	Provide no action other than support of infant's spontaneous efforts and continued observation.

From Murray SS, McKinney ES: *Foundations of maternal newborn nursing*, ed 5, St Louis, 2010, Saunders
*The Apgar score is a method for rapid evaluation of the infant's cardiorespiratory adaptation after birth. The nurse scores the infant at 1 minute and 5 minutes in each of five areas. The assessments are arranged from most important (heart rate) to least important (color). The infant is assigned a score of 0 to 2 in each of the five areas, and the scores are totaled. Resuscitation should not be delayed until the 1-minute score is obtained. However, general guidelines for the infant's care are based on three ranges of 1-minute scores. Note: Neonatal resuscitation measures, if needed, do not await 1-minute Apgar scoring but are instituted at once.

The need to progress in sequence from one intervention to the next is based on the simultaneous assessment of the infant's respirations, heart rate, and oximetry readings. About 30 seconds should be allotted to complete each step, to reevaluate, and to decide whether to progress to the next sequenced step in resuscitation.[1]

Reevaluate Initial Steps in Stabilization

The initial steps in stabilization should be reevaluated. The paramedic should ensure that the infant is dry and warm. (Cold stress can increase oxygen consumption and impede effective breathing.) Hypothermia can be associated with perinatal respiratory depression. Additional methods that can be used to warm a newborn include covering the baby in plastic wrap (food-grade, heat-resistant plastic) and placing the baby skin-to-skin with the mother and covering both with a blanket. Hyperthermia should be avoided. The goal is to achieve and maintain a normal body temperature for the newborn.

The head and neck of the newborn should be properly positioned (or repositioned) to ensure an open airway. In addition, the paramedic can make other attempts at stimulation to initiate breathing. If the infant is breathing, but color and SpO_2 do not improve within 90 seconds after birth or if there is central cyanosis, supplemental oxygen should be given. Free-flow oxygen mixed with air can be applied through a face mask and flow-inflating bag, an oxygen mask, or a hand cupped around the oxygen tubing (held 2 inches from the infant's nose). Oxygen therapy should be guided by pulse oximetry measurements and continued until the target SpO_2 range is achieved. Oxygen delivery should begin with bag-mask ventilation with room air and then be titrated to maintain SpO_2 in the target range. If the baby is bradycardic (heart rate less than 60 beats per minute) after 90 seconds of resuscitation, oxygen concentration should be increased to 100% until recovery of a normal heart rate.[1]

> **NOTE**
> Babies born at term should begin resuscitation with blended oxygen (oxygen mixed with air) guided by pulse oximetry, rather than giving 100% oxygen. Healthy babies born at term have an initial oxygen saturation of less than 60% and can require more than 10 minutes to reach saturations above 90%. Hyperoxia can be toxic to newborns, especially preterm infants.[1]

Provide Ventilations

As stated previously, the newborn should have regular respirations that are sufficient to maintain target SpO_2 and a heart rate greater than 100 beats per minute. Gasping and apnea indicate the need for assisted ventilations. Increasing or decreasing heart rate can also provide clues of improvement or deterioration in the newborn.

> **NOTE**
> Hypoxia is nearly always present in a newly born infant who requires resuscitation.

If respirations are inadequate (evidenced by low SpO_2 readings) or if the heart rate remains less than 100 beats per minute 30 seconds after completing the initial steps discussed earlier, positive-pressure ventilation should be initiated. Assisted ventilations should be provided at a rate of 40 to 60 breaths per minute to achieve or maintain a heart rate greater than 100 beats per minute.[1] Assisted ventilations can be delivered with a flow-inflating bag, with a self-inflating bag, or with a T-piece (a valved, mechanical device designed to control flow and limit pressure). Medical direction may recommend providing continuous positive airway pressure (CPAP) to infants who are breathing spontaneously, but with difficulty, following birth. Positive end-expiratory pressure (PEEP) may also be effective in supporting ventilations. The use of CPAP or PEEP should be guided by medical direction.

> **NOTE**
> The lungs of a preterm infant can be easily injured by large-volume inflations immediately after birth. Therefore, high pressures during assisted ventilations should be avoided with babies who are premature. High inflation pressures may be evident by excessive chest wall movement.

ENDOTRACHEAL INTUBATION

Endotracheal intubation may be indicated at several points during neonatal resuscitation. These include[1]:

- When tracheal suctioning of meconium is required
- If bag-mask ventilation is ineffective or prolonged
- When chest compressions are performed
- For special resuscitation circumstances, such as congenital diaphragmatic hernia or extremely low birth weight (less than 1000 g)

Before the paramedic considers intubation or pharmacological therapy, two components of the resuscitation process should be reevaluated:

1. Is chest movement adequate? Check for the adequacy of chest expansion and auscultate for bilateral breath sounds.
   a. Is the bag mask seal tight? A relatively large mask should be turned upside down for a better fit.
   b. Is the airway blocked from improper head position or secretions in the nose, mouth, or pharynx? Reassess head position and reexamine the airway for the presence of secretions.
   c. Is adequate ventilatory pressure being used? A bag mask pop-off valve may need to be disabled to allow for higher inspiratory pressures, especially for premature or meconium-aspiration delivery.[2]

d. Is air in the stomach interfering with chest expansion? Consider nasogastric or orogastric decompression per protocol.

2. Are target SpO_2 measurements within normal range?
   a. Is the oxygen tubing attached to the bag and flowmeter?
   b. If using a self-inflating bag, is the oxygen reservoir attached?

A prompt increase in heart rate and increased chest wall movement after endotracheal intubation and administration of intermittent positive-pressure ventilation are the best indicators of correct tube placement. However, the paramedic should verify tube placement visually during intubation and by using primary and secondary confirmation methods (described in Chapter 15). Exhaled carbon dioxide detection is effective and is the recommended method for confirmation of endotracheal tube placement in infants with adequate cardiac ouput.[1] (False-negative readings can occur, if the infant has poor or absent pulmonary flow.) The laryngeal mask airway (LMA) may be used to establish an airway in a newborn if bag-mask ventilation is ineffective or tracheal intubation has failed.

Provide Chest Compressions

Chest compressions are indicated if the newborn's heart rate is less than 60 beats per minute after 30 seconds of adequate ventilation with supplemental oxygen. (The paramedic should ensure that assisted ventilations are effective before initiating chest compressions.) As described in Chapter 22, chest compressions should be coordinated with ventilations to avoid simultaneous delivery. Compressions and ventilations should be delivered at a ratio of 3:1 at a rate of 120 per minute. This will achieve about 90 compressions and 30 breaths per minute.

To review, the two thumb–encircling hands' chest compression is the preferred technique for chest compressions for newly born infants and older infants who are full term. (Preterm infants and infants who are small for gestational age should have chest compressions performed using only two fingers.) Compressions should be performed on the lower third of the sternum. Depth of compression should be approximately one third of the anterior-posterior diameter of the chest and should be sufficiently deep to generate a palpable pulse.[1] Respirations, heart rate, and oxygenation

CRITICAL THINKING
Why would compressions be initiated when the infant still has a pulse?

should be reassessed frequently. Coordinated chest compressions and ventilations should continue until spontaneous heart rate is equal to or greater than 60 beats per minute.

Administer Epinephrine and/or Volume Expanders

Drugs are rarely indicated in the resuscitation of the newly born infant. As a rule, drugs should be administered only if the heart rate remains below 60 beats per minute, despite adequate ventilation with 100% oxygen and effective chest compressions.[1] Drug therapy that may be indicated includes the administration of *epinephrine* and volume expanders. Buffers, a narcotic antagonist, or vasopressors are rarely useful (Table 47-2).

Important points for the paramedic to remember when administering drugs or volume expanders include:

1. The IV route is preferred for drug administration. All drugs should be given intravenously as soon as venous access is obtained. *Epinephrine* may be administered through the ET tube (at higher doses) while obtaining IV access, but safety and efficacy have not been established (Class IIb, LOE C). The concentration of *epinephrine* for either route is 1:10,000 (0.1 mg/mL).

NOTE
Bradycardia in the newborn infant is usually the result of inadequate lung inflation or hypoxemia. Therefore, establishing adequate ventilation is the most important step to correct it.

2. Volume expanders should be considered when blood loss is suspected. They should also be considered if the infant appears to be in shock (pale skin, poor perfusion, weak pulse) and has not responded to other resuscitative measures. (End-organ perfusion should be evaluated by comparing the strength of central versus peripheral pulses and through capillary refill tests.) Volume expanders should be given slowly and with caution when resuscitating premature infants. The recommended dose is 10 mL/kg, which may need to be repeated. Rapid infusions of large volumes of volume expanders have been associated with intraventricular hemorrhage.[1]

ROUTES OF DRUG ADMINISTRATION

Although the IV route is the preferred route for drug therapy in the newborn, other methods that may be considered include the endotracheal route and the intraosseous (IO) route (described in Chapter 14). During CPR or treatment of severe shock, IO access should be established when venous access cannot be rapidly achieved.[18]

NOTE
Venous access through the umbilical cord is usually not an option in the prehospital setting or beyond the first several days of birth.[19] The procedure also requires special training and authorization from medical direction. Accessing the umbilical vein is described in the Appendix, Advanced Practice Procedures in Critical Care.

TABLE 47-2 Medications for Neonatal Resuscitation

Medication	Dose/Route	Concentration	Weight (kg)	Total (mL)	Precautions
Epinephrine*†	0.01-0.03 mg/kg IV/IO	1:10,000	1	0.1-0.3	Give rapidly
			2	0.2-0.6	Repeat every 3-5 min
			3	0.3-0.9	
			4	0.4-1.2	
Volume expanders Normal saline or blood	10 mL/kg IV over 5-10 min		1	10	Reassess after each bolus
			2	20	
			3	30	
			4	40	
Naloxone	0.1 mg/kg IV, ET, or IM/ subQ if perfusion is adequate	0.4 mg/mL	1	0.25	Repeat doses may be needed to prevent apnea
			2	0.50	
			3	0.75	
			4	1.00	
		1.0 mg/mL	1	0.1	Do not give if mother is suspected of abusing narcotics
			2	0.2	
			3	0.3	
			4	0.4	

*Epinephrine also may be given endotracheally 0.05-0.1 mg/kg.
†*Note:* The endotracheal tube dose may not result in effective plasma concentration of the drug, so vascular access should be established as soon as possible. Drugs administered by endotracheal tube should be diluted to a volume of 3 to 5 mL before instillation. Drugs given ET require higher dosing than when given IV/IO.

BOX 47-4 Dope Pneumonic

D: Dislodgement (ET tube is misplaced; right mainstem bronchus, esophagus)

O: Obstruction (secretions obstructing the tube)

P: Pneumothorax (decreased or absent breath sounds on the affected side)

E: Equipment failure (such as ventilator malfunction or disconnect)

LOOK AGAIN
See Chapter 14: Venous Access and Medication Administration, pp. 368-370.

POSTRESUSCITATION CARE

The three most common complications of the postresuscitation period are endotracheal tube migration (including dislodgment), tube occlusion by mucus or meconium, and pneumothorax (Box 47-4).[2] These complications should be suspected in the presence of the following:

- Decreased chest wall movement
- Diminished breath sounds
- Return of bradycardia
- Unilateral decrease in chest expansion
- Altered intensity to pitch of breath sounds
- Increased resistance to hand ventilation

Corrective management in the field for these postresuscitative complications may include adjustment of the endotracheal tube (exhaled carbon dioxide devices are recommended for monitoring tracheal tube placement), reintubation, and suction. Needle decompression to manage a suspected pneumothorax must be guided carefully by medical direction.

CRITICAL THINKING
How much movement would it take to dislodge an endotracheal tube from a neonate?

Induced Therapeutic Hypothermia

As described in Chapter 22, induced therapeutic hypothermia (33.5° to 34.5° C) can lower mortality and reduce neurological complications in some patients who have a return of spontaneous circulation (ROSC) following cardiac arrest. Protocols for this treatment in neonates ≥36 weeks' gestation generally include cooling within 6 hours following birth. The cooling is continued for 72 hours, after which the infant is slowly rewarmed over at least 4 hours.[1] Induced therapeutic hypothermia is not a prehospital consideration in neonatal resuscitation. The procedure is instituted in the hospital setting.

NEONATAL TRANSPORT

During transport of the neonate, it is important to maintain the infant's body temperature and prevent hypothermia. In addition, it is critical to maintain oxygen levels and

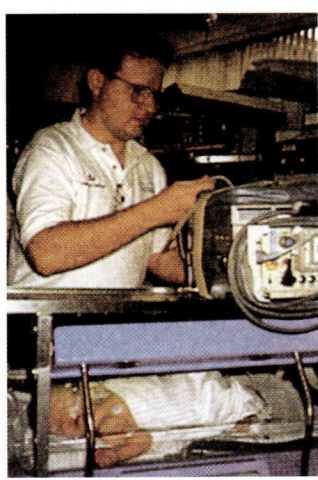

FIGURE 47-15 Neonatal transport. (Courtesy Nellcor Puritan Bennett, Minneapolis, Minn.)

to support the infant's ventilations. In the initial prehospital phase of care, transport strategies usually are limited to providing a warm ambulance, administering free-flow oxygen (warmed if available), covering the baby's head, and applying warm blankets to prevent hypothermic complications. Specialized transport equipment such as isolettes and radiant heating units often is used for interhospital transfers. These devices require special training. Highly trained neonatal transport teams consisting of paramedics, nurses, respiratory therapists, and physicians are part of well-organized regional referral systems throughout the United States (Figure 47-15).

SPECIFIC SITUATIONS

Specific situations may call for advanced life support for the neonate. These situations include apnea, bradycardia, prematurity, respiratory distress and cyanosis, hypovolemia, seizures, fever, hypothermia, hypoglycemia, vomiting and diarrhea, and common birth injuries. While providing advanced life support in these and other situations, the paramedic must consider the emotional needs of the mother and family. When possible, the paramedic should explain what is being done for the infant and why a procedure is necessary.

Apnea

Apnea is an absence of spontaneous respirations. *Primary apnea* is a self-limited condition controlled by P_{CO_2} levels. It is a common event immediately after birth. *Secondary apnea* is described as apnea that exceeds 20 seconds without spontaneous breathing occurring. This can lead to hypoxemia and bradycardia. Secondary apnea is common in the preterm infant. It often results from hypoxia or hypothermia. Secondary apnea also may be caused by conditions that include maternal use of narcotics or central nervous system depressants, prolonged or difficult labor and delivery, airway and respiratory muscle weakness,

septicemia, metabolic disorders, and central nervous system disorders.

Emergency care for an infant with prolonged apnea begins with stimulating the infant to breathe. This is done by flicking the soles of the feet or rubbing the back. If needed, a bag device (with a disabled pop-off valve) should be used, while applying the least amount of pressure that produces adequate chest rise. The paramedic should suction secretions from the infant's airway as needed and maintain the infant's body temperature to prevent hypothermia. Endotracheal intubation and circulatory support may be required if central cyanosis persists despite adequate ventilations. Drug therapy that may be appropriate in managing some infants with prolonged apnea includes *dextrose* (10% dextrose in water), if hypoglycemia is confirmed. Another is *naloxone* for reversal of respiratory depression in a newborn whose mother received narcotics within 4 hours of delivery.[1] (As discussed earlier, narcotic antagonists should not be given to the infant if the mother is a drug abuser. Doing so may induce drug withdrawal in the neonate.) Apnea that is treated early and aggressively normally results in a good outcome.

Bradycardia

Bradycardia is described as a heart rate less than 100 beats/min. In the neonate, bradycardia most commonly is caused by hypoxia. It also may result from increased intracranial pressure, hypothyroidism, acidosis, and congenital AV nodal block in infants of mothers who have systemic lupus erythematosus. Other risk factors include prolonged suctioning and the use of airway or any invasive procedures during resuscitation that may cause vagal stimulation (e.g., inadequately secured ET tube movement). Bradycardia is a minimal risk to life in neonates if it is corrected quickly.

The initial management for a neonate with bradycardia is to assess for upper airway obstruction. Such obstruction may be caused by airway secretions, foreign body, or the position of the tongue or soft tissues of the neck. Prehospital care to improve ventilation may include airway positioning, suction, positive-pressure ventilation with supplemental oxygen, and tracheal intubation. The paramedic should monitor ventilatory and circulatory status of the infant closely. This will determine the need for more advanced life support measures. Such measures may include chest compressions and drug therapy (described later in this chapter and in Chapter 48: Pediatrics).

Prematurity

A **premature infant** (*preemie*) refers to a baby who is born before 37 weeks' gestation. (The weight of these newborns often is between 0.6 and 2.2 kg [from 1½ to 5 lb].) Healthy premature infants who weigh more than 1700 g have a survivability and outcome about equal to those of full-term infants. The mortality rate decreases weekly with gestation beyond the onset of fetal viability (currently around 23 to 24 weeks' gestation).[4] Premature infants have an increased risk for respiratory depression, hypothermia, and brain injury from hypoxemia. They are also especially vulnerable to changes in blood pressure, intraventricular hemorrhage, and fluctuations in serum chemistry, such as changes in blood glucose and electrolyte levels. The degree of immaturity determines how the infant appears physically (based on maternal dates, expected date of confinement, size for gestational age). However, most premature infants will have a large trunk, short extremities, less subcutaneous fat than full-term infants, and skin that appears translucent. Premature infants have some telltale physical findings. These include lanugo (Fig. 47-16) and characteristic changes in the ears (Fig. 47-17) and in muscle tone (Fig. 47-18). Risk factors for prematurity are listed in Box 47-5.

The prehospital care for premature infants is the same as for any other newborn. It may include airway, ventilatory,

> **DID YOU KNOW?**
> **Dubowitz Score**
> The **Dubowitz score** or scale is a method of clinical assessment in the newborn from birth to 5 days old. The score includes 10 neurological signs for the infant's maturity and 12 physical signs (external signs of development) to determine apparent gestational age.[20] The two scores are added. The minimum score is 0. The maximum score is 72. Typically, the more neurologically mature, the higher the score.

and circulatory support. *The paramedic should attempt resuscitation if the infant has any signs of life.* Special care must be taken to maintain the infant's body temperature and to prevent hypothermia. Examples include wrapping the baby in food-grade resistant plastic and the application of radiant heat.[1] Transport to a facility with special services for low-birth-weight newborns may be indicated.

> **NOTE**
> Concern for eye damage (retinopathy of prematurity) from long-term oxygen use in premature infants is not a consideration in the emergency setting. Hypoxemia causes irreversible brain damage in these newborns. High-concentration oxygen is indicated.

Respiratory Distress and Cyanosis

Prematurity is the most common cause of respiratory distress and cyanosis in the neonate. These conditions occur most often in infants less than 1200 g (2½ lb) and less than 30 weeks' gestation.[4] These problems may be related to the infant's immature central respiratory control center. The center is affected more easily by environmental and metabolic changes than that of the full-term infant. Other

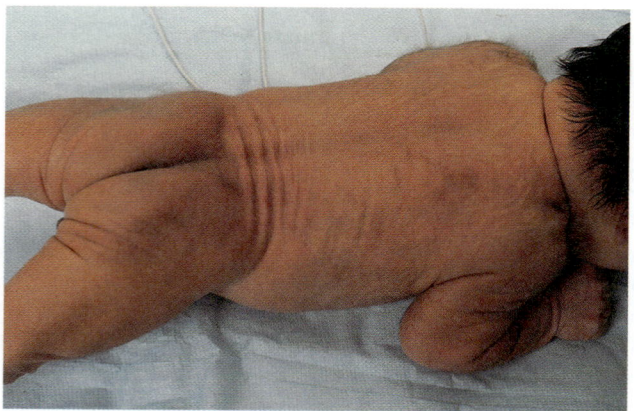

FIGURE 47-16 Infants at gestational age 20 to 28 weeks are covered with fine hair all over the body called lanugo. (From Gorrie T, McKinney E, Murray S: *Foundations of maternal newborn nursing,* Philadelphia, 1994, WB Saunders.)

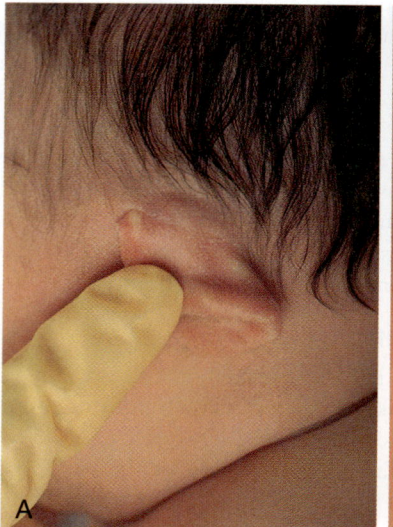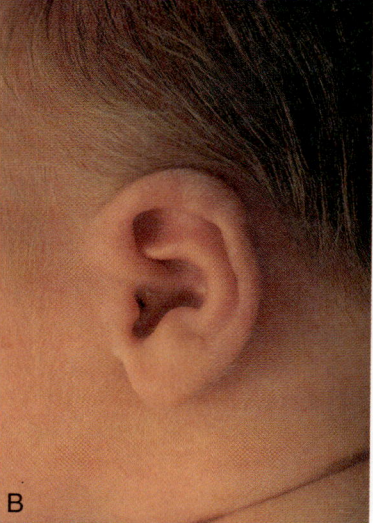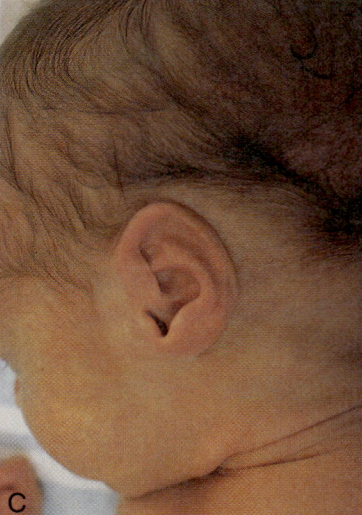

FIGURE 47-17 Ear maturation. **A** and **B,** Full-term infant. **C,** Preterm infant. (From Gorrie T, McKinney E, Murray S: *Foundations of maternal newborn nursing,* Philadelphia, 1994, WB Saunders.)

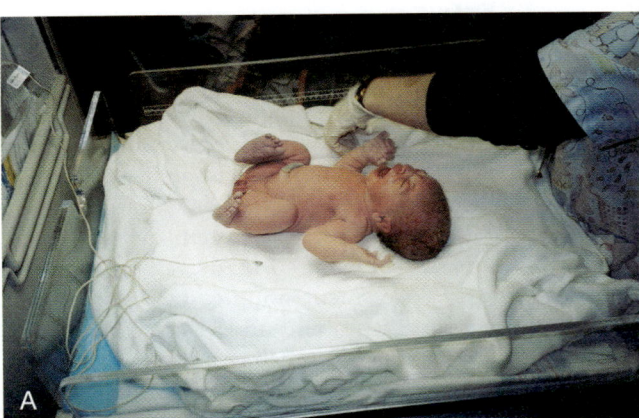
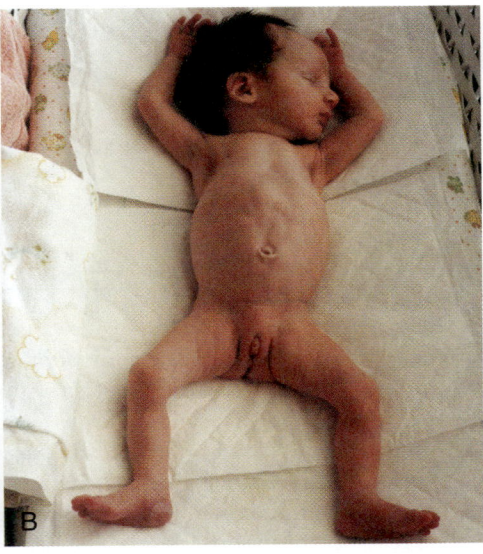

FIGURE 47-18 A, The term newborn shows flexion of the arms and legs. Note the acrocyanosis of the hands and feet. **B,** The preterm newborn holds extremities in extension, exposing more of the body surface area to the environment. This factor contributes to the development of cold stress and difficulty with thermoregulation. (From Leifer G: *Maternity nursing: an introductory text,* ed 10, St Louis, 2010, Saunders.)

BOX 47-5   Risk Factors for Prematurity

Factors Related to Comorbidity

Trauma
Neonatal sepsis
Maternal infection
Urinary tract infection
Chorioamnionitis (inflammation of fetal membranes)
Illness resulting in dehydration

Congenital Anomalies

Genetic disorders
Congenital malformations
Congenital heart defect
Spina bifida
Placental insufficiency
Oligohydramnios (deficiency of amniotic fluid)
Polyhydramnios (excess amniotic fluid)

Previous Premature Deliveries

Incompetent cervix
Relative large fetal size

Multiple Gestation

Eclampsia
Preeclampsia
Gestational hypertension

risk factors for respiratory distress and cyanosis in the neonate include multiple gestations, prenatal maternal complications, and infants born with the following conditions:

- Birth defects
- Central nervous system disorders

- Diaphragmatic hernia
- Esophageal atresia
- Lung immaturity
- Lung or heart disease
- Meconium or amniotic fluid aspiration
- Metabolic acidosis
- Mucous obstruction of nasal passages
- Pneumonia
- Primary pulmonary hypertension
- Shock and sepsis
- Tracheoesophageal fistula

Respiratory distress and cyanosis can lead to cardiac arrest in the neonate. The situation necessitates immediate actions to improve breathing and support respirations. Assessment findings may include tachypnea, paradoxical breathing, intercostal retractions, nasal flaring, expiratory grunting, and central cyanosis. As described earlier, respiratory insufficiency in the neonate generally is managed with stimulation, positioning of the airway, prevention of heat loss and hypothermia, oxygenation and ventilation, and suction and intubation with ventilatory support (if needed).

Hypovolemia

Hypovolemia in infants may result from dehydration, hemorrhage, trauma, or sepsis. It also may be associated with myocardial dysfunction. Signs and symptoms of hypovolemia include mottled or pale color, cool skin, tachycardia, diminished peripheral pulses, and delayed capillary refill despite normal ambient temperature. Shock may be present despite a normal blood pressure. Prompt and effective treatment of early signs of compensated shock may prevent the development of hypotension (decompensated shock) and associated high morbidity and mortality.[2] Prehospital

---

BOX 47-6 Causes of Neonatal Seizures

- Developmental abnormalities
- Drug withdrawal
- Hypoglycemia
- Hypoxic-ischemic encephalopathy
- Intracranial hemorrhage
- Meningitis or encephalopathy
- Metabolic disturbances

care is always directed at ensuring adequate airway, ventilatory, and circulatory support (including control of external hemorrhage) and providing rapid transport to an appropriate facility.

When signs of hypovolemia are present, the paramedic should give a fluid bolus (10 mL/kg over 5 to 10 minutes of isotonic crystalloid) immediately after obtaining IV access, and then reassess the infant. If signs of shock persist, the paramedic should give a second 10 mL/kg bolus. Further boluses should be given as needed and under the guidance of medical direction.

Seizures

Seizures occur in a small percentage of newborns. When present, they usually are a sign of an underlying abnormality (Box 47-6). Prolonged seizures or frequent seizures may result in metabolic changes and cardiopulmonary difficulties.

TYPES OF SEIZURES

Seizures in neonates usually are fragmented and not well sustained. They have been classified as subtle seizures, tonic seizures, multifocal seizures, focal clonic seizures, and myoclonic seizures.[4]

Subtle seizures involve eye deviation, blinking, sucking, swimming movements of the arms, and peddling movements of the legs. Apnea may be present during subtle seizures. *Tonic seizures* usually involve extension of the limbs. Less often, they involve flexion of the upper extremities and extension of the lower extremities. This type of seizure is more common in infants who are premature, especially in infants with intraventricular hemorrhage. *Multifocal seizures* usually involve clonic activity in one extremity that may migrate randomly to another area of the body. This type of seizure mainly occurs in full-term infants. *Focal clonic seizures* involve clonic, localized jerking. They have been known to occur in full-term and premature newborns. *Myoclonic seizures* involve flexion and jerking of the upper or lower extremities. These seizures may occur singly. They also may occur in a series of repetitive jerking cycles.

Emergency care for managing neonatal seizures includes providing airway, ventilatory, and circulatory support and maintaining the infant's body temperature. As described in Chapter 25, drug therapy that may be prescribed by medical direction includes **dextrose** to treat hypoglycemia, anticonvulsant agents, and perhaps benzodiazepines (for status epilepticus). Seizure activity is always considered pathological; rapid transport for physician evaluation is needed.

LOOK AGAIN
See Chapter 25: Neurology, pp. 785-788.

Fever

Fever in neonates is described as a rectal temperature greater than 100.4° F (38.0° C). Fever in neonates usually is a cause for concern and often is a response to an acute viral or bacterial infection. Fever also may result from a change in the infant's limited ability to control body temperature or be an effect of dehydration. The rise in core temperature increases oxygen demands and increases glucose metabolism. These increases may lead to metabolic acidosis. Assessment findings may include mental status changes (e.g., irritability and lethargy), a history of decreased intake, rashes and petechiae, and warm or hot skin.

NOTE
Term newborns produce beads of sweat on their brow but not over the rest of their bodies. Premature infants generally have no visible sweat.

The prehospital care for febrile infants mainly is supportive. As a rule, cooling procedures and the use of antipyretics will be delayed until the child has arrived at the hospital. Febrile seizures usually affect children between 6 months and 5 years of age. Generally they are not a concern in caring for the neonate (see Chapter 48). All febrile neonates require immediate transport for physician evaluation. These patients should be presumed to have systemic sepsis until it is proved otherwise.

Hypothermia

As described in Chapter 45, hypothermia is a core body temperature below 95° F (35° C). Hypothermia may result from a decrease in heat production, an increase in heat loss (through evaporation, conduction, convection, or radiation), or a combination of both. Neonates are sensitive to the effects of hypothermia because of their increased surface-to-volume ratio. This is especially the case when they are wet (e.g., after delivery). The associated increase in metabolic demand to maintain body temperature can cause metabolic acidosis, pulmonary hypertension, and hypoxemia. Hypothermia also may be a sign of sepsis in the neonate. Assessment findings may include the following:

- Pale color
- Cool skin (especially in the extremities)
- Respiratory distress
- Apnea
- Bradycardia
- Central cyanosis
- Acrocyanosis (cyanosis of the extremities)
- Irritability (initially)
- Lethargy (in the late stage)
- Absence of shivering (variable)

The prehospital care for these patients may include provision of basic and advanced cardiac life support. (This depends on the severity of hypothermia.) The care also consists of rapid transport to an appropriate facility. Other therapeutic measures include ensuring that the infant is dry and warm, warming the hands before touching the newborn, and perhaps administering *dextrose* to treat hypoglycemia and IV therapy with warm fluids. The patient should be transported in a heated ambulance (76° to 80° F [24° to 26.5° C]).

Hypoglycemia

A blood glucose measurement less than 40 mg/dL in the infant indicates hypoglycemia (described in Chapter 26).[1] The condition should be determined by blood glucose screening on all sick infants. Hypoglycemia may be due to inadequate glucose intake or increased use of glucose. Risk factors associated with hypoglycemia include asphyxia, toxemia, being the smaller twin, central nervous system hemorrhage, and sepsis. Assessment findings may include the following:

- Twitching or seizure
- Limpness
- Lethargy
- Irritability
- Eye rolling
- High-pitched crying
- Apnea
- Irregular respirations
- Cyanosis (possibly)

NOTE

Small infants and chronically ill children have limited glycogen stores. These may be depleted rapidly during stress events. If allowed to persist, hypoglycemia can depress myocardial function. Hypoglycemia may have catastrophic effects on the brain as well.

The prehospital care is directed at ensuring adequate airway, ventilatory, and circulatory support; maintaining body temperature; providing rapid transport; and perhaps IV administration of *dextrose 10%* (per medical direction) (Box 47-7). The paramedic should check the glucose level again if the infant fails to respond to initial resuscitative measures. All infants who do not respond normally and those who are hypoglycemic and fail to respond to the *dextrose* should be transported immediately to a medical facility.

Vomiting and Diarrhea

Occasional vomiting or diarrhea is not unusual in the neonate. For example, vomiting mucus (that may be streaked with blood) is common in the first few hours of life. Also, five to six stools per day is considered normal, especially if the infant is breastfeeding. Persistent vomiting and/or diarrhea, however, should be considered warning signs of serious illness.

VOMITING

Persistent vomiting in the first 24 hours of life suggests an obstruction in the upper digestive tract or perhaps increased intracranial pressure. Vomit that contains non–bile-stained

---

BOX 47-7 Glucose Administration

Dose: 0.5 to 1.0 g/kg intravenously over 20 minutes
Preparation: Dilute dextrose 50% 1:1 with sterile water, resulting in 25% dextrose in water solution; administer 2 to 4 mL/kg.
or
Dilute dextrose 50% 1:4 with sterile water, resulting in 10% dextrose in water solution; administer 5 to 10 mL/kg.
Precautions: Hypertonic glucose is hyperosmolar and may sclerose peripheral veins.

Note: Some sterile water has preservatives containing alcohol. This solution should not be used. It can cause profound hypoglycemia and death when administered to infants.

---

fluid is a sign of anatomical or functional obstruction. This obstruction is at or above the first portion of the duodenum. Vomiting also may indicate gastroesophageal reflux. Bile-stained vomit may result from obstruction below the opening of the bile duct. Vomit that contains dark blood usually is a sign of life-threatening illness. Assessment findings may include a distended stomach and signs of infection, dehydration, and increased intracranial pressure. The paramedic also should consider that the vomiting may be a result of drug withdrawal (from the mother's drug use).

The prehospital care usually requires maintaining an airway that is clear of vomit and ensuring adequate oxygenation. In severe cases, medical direction may advise that IV fluid therapy be started before transport. Fluid therapy treats dehydration and any bradycardia that may develop from vagal stimulation. If possible, infants should be transported on their sides. This will help prevent aspiration.

DIARRHEA

Persistent diarrhea can lead to serious dehydration and electrolyte imbalance in the neonate. The diarrhea often is associated with a bacterial or viral infection. Other possible causes include the following:

- Bacterial enteritis (*Clostridium difficile, Salmonella, Shigella*)
- Cystic fibrosis
- Lactose intolerance
- Neonatal abstinence syndrome (drug withdrawal)
- Phototherapy (a treatment for hyperbilirubinemia and jaundice in the newborn)
- Thyrotoxicosis
- Viral gastroenteritis (rotavirus)

Assessment findings often include the presence of loose stools, decreased urinary output, and signs of dehydration. Treatment consists of supporting the infant's vital functions, IV fluid therapy (per medical direction), and rapid transport to the receiving hospital.

Common Birth Injuries

Significant birth injury accounts for less than 2% of neonatal deaths and stillbirths in the United States. Of every 1000 live births, there is an average of 6 to 8 injuries. In general, larger infants are more susceptible to birth trauma. Higher rates are reported for infants who weigh more than 4500 g.[21]

An uncontrolled, explosive delivery (described in Chapter 46) is the greatest risk factor for birth injuries. Cranial injuries may include molding of the head and overriding of the parietal bones, soft tissue injuries from forceps delivery, subconjunctival and retinal hemorrhage, subperiosteal hemorrhage, and skull fracture. Intracranial hemorrhage can occur from trauma or asphyxia. Spine and spinal cord injury can result from strong traction or a lateral pull during delivery. Other birth injuries include peripheral nerve injury, liver or spleen injury, adrenal hemorrhage, clavicle or extremity fracture, and brain or soft tissue injury from hypoxia-ischemia. The assessment findings vary by the nature of the injury. They may include the following:

- Diffuse, sometimes ecchymotic, edematous swelling of the soft tissues of the scalp
- Paralysis below the level of spinal cord injury
- Paralysis of the upper arm with or without paralysis of the forearm
- Paralysis of the diaphragm
- Movement on only one side of the face when the newborn cries
- Inability to move the arm freely on the same side of a fractured clavicle
- Lack of spontaneous movement of an injured extremity
- Hypoxia
- Shock

The goal of prehospital care for an infant with a birth injury is to support the newborn's vital functions. This can be done by ensuring adequate oxygenation, ventilation, and circulatory support and administering fluid or drug therapy (if indicated). These infants are high-risk newborns. They require rapid transport to a proper medical facility.

Neonatal Resuscitation, Postresuscitation, and Stabilization

A neonate's heart generally is healthy and strong. However, disorders in the conduction system of the heart can and do occur. Most often the disorders occur as a result of hypoxemia and respiratory arrest. The outcome for these infants is poor if interventions are not initiated quickly. In addition, the likelihood for brain and organ damage is increased in infants who require resuscitation. The paramedic should continually assess and monitor neonates with respiratory distress for treatable causes of the distress.

Asystole and pulseless cardiac arrest are uncommon in the neonate. Like bradycardia, they usually are the result of hypoxia. Cardiac arrest also can be caused by primary and secondary apnea, unresolved bradycardia, and persistent fetal circulation (persistent pulmonary hypertension). Assessment findings may include peripheral cyanosis, inadequate respiratory effort, and ineffective or absent heart rate. Risk factors associated with cardiac arrest in the newborn include the following:

- Congenital malformations
- Congenital neuromuscular disease

- Drugs administered to or taken by the mother
- Intrapartum hypoxemia
- Intrauterine asphyxia

Emergency care for neonates with asystole or pulseless arrest was described earlier in this chapter and includes airway, ventilatory, and circulatory support; pharmacological therapy; and rapid transport to an appropriate medical facility.

NOTE
The decision to withhold resuscitation or to discontinue resuscitative efforts in the prehospital setting must be guided by medical direction. Infants without signs of life (no pulse or respiratory effort) after 10 minutes of resuscitation show either a high mortality or severe neurodevelopmental disability. Therefore, after 10 minutes of continuous and adequate resuscitative efforts, the discontinuation of resuscitation may be justified if there are no signs of life. Decisions to continue resuscitation beyond 10 minutes should be guided by medical direction. Factors that should be considered include presumed cause of the arrest, gestation of the baby, the presence or absence of complications, the potential role of therapeutic hypothermia, and the parents' wishes.[1]

CRITICAL THINKING
How will you feel if you deliver a critically ill or dead infant?

PSYCHOLOGICAL AND EMOTIONAL SUPPORT

The paramedic must be aware of the normal feelings and reactions of parents, siblings, other family members, and caregivers while providing emergency care to an ill or injured child. (These events also are often highly charged and emotional for the emergency crew.) The paramedic should keep those at the scene abreast of all procedures being performed and should inform family members of the necessity of the procedures.

NOTE
After delivery, the mother continues to be a patient herself. She still has certain physical and emotional needs.

As a rule, emergency responders should never discuss the infant's chances of survival with a parent or family member. They also should not give false hope about the infant's condition. The paramedic should assure the family that everything that can be done for the child is being done. The paramedic also should assure the family that their baby will receive the best possible care during transport and at the hospital. The hospital will have support personnel who can assist family members and loved ones.

SUMMARY

- Low birth weight and a variety of antepartum and intrapartum risk factors affect the need for resuscitation.
- Some of the more common congenital anomalies include choanal atresia, tracheobronchial fistula and atresia, Pierre Robin syndrome, cleft lip and cleft palate, congenital heart anomalies, pyloric stenosis, diaphragmatic hernia, omphalocele, and spina bifida.
- At birth, newborns make three major physiological adaptations necessary for survival: (1) emptying fluids from their lungs and beginning ventilation, (2) changing their circulatory pattern, and (3) maintaining body temperature.
- The initial steps of neonatal resuscitation (except for those born through meconium) are to prevent heat loss, clear the airway by positioning and suctioning, provide tactile stimulation and initiate breathing if necessary, and further evaluate the infant.
- If neonatal resuscitation is needed the paramedic should reevaluate the initial steps of stabilization (warm, position, clear airway, dry, stimulate, reposition). If there is no change, resuscitation proceeds in 30-second increments with ventilation, chest compressions, and, if needed, epinephrine administration.
- The three most common complications during the postresuscitation period are endotracheal tube position change (including dislodgment), tube occlusion by mucus or meconium, and pneumothorax. During transport of the neonate, it is important to maintain body temperature, oxygen administration, and ventilatory support.
- Specific situations that may require advanced life support for the neonate include meconium staining, apnea, diaphragmatic hernia, bradycardia, premature infants, respiratory distress and cyanosis, hypovolemia,

seizures, fever, hypothermia, hypoglycemia, vomiting and diarrhea, and birth injuries.

- Primary apnea is common immediately after birth and is self-limiting. Secondary apnea is a pause in breathing that exceeds 20 seconds.
- Bradycardia is a heart rate less than 100 beats/min. It is most often caused by hypoxia.
- Premature infants have an increased risk of respiratory suppression, hypothermia, and head and brain injury. In addition to low birth weight, various antepartum and intrapartum risk factors may affect the need for resuscitation.
- Prematurity is the most common cause of respiratory distress in the neonate.
- Hypovolemia in infants may result from dehydration, hemorrhage, trauma, or sepsis.
- Seizures in the newborn signal an underlying abnormality.
- A temperature greater than 100.4° F (38.0° C) is a fever and often signals viral or bacterial infection.
- Hypothermia is a core body temperature below 95° F (35° C). It increases metabolic demand and can cause metabolic acidosis, pulmonary hypertension, and hypoxemia.
- Blood glucose level less than 40 mg/dL indicates hypothermia in the neonate.
- Injuries at birth may include cranial trauma, intracranial hemorrhage or brain injury, spine and spinal cord injury, peripheral nerve injury, spleen or liver injuries, fractures or soft tissue injury.
- The paramedic should be aware of the normal feelings and reactions of parents, siblings, other family members, and caregivers while providing emergency care to an ill or injured child.

REFERENCES

1. American Heart Association: 2010 American Heart Association guidelines for cardiopulmonary resuscitation, *Circulation* 122(suppl 3):S909-S919, 2010.

1a. American Heart Association: *2010 American Heart Association guidelines for cardiopulmonary resuscitation, Circulation* 122(part 14):S876-S908, 2010.

2. American Heart Association: *Pediatric advanced life support*, Dallas, 2007, The Association.

3. American Heart Association: *Textbook of neonatal resuscitation*, ed 5, Dallas, 2006, American Academy of Pediatrics.

4. U.S. Department of Transportation, National Highway Traffic Safety Administration: *EMT paramedic national standards curriculum*, Washington, DC, 1998, The Department.

5. CDC: *Birth defects*, www.cdc.gov/ncbddd/bd/default.htm, accessed 10-14-10.

6. National Heart Lung and Blood Institute, U.S. Department of Health and Human Services, National Institutes of Health:

Congenital heart defects, www.nhlbi.nih.gov/health/dci/Diseases/chd/chd_what.html, accessed 10-15-10.

7. American Heart Association: *Congenital cardiovascular defects*, www.americanheart.org/presenter.jhtml?identifier=4565#pda, accessed 10-15-10.

8. Klabunde R: *Cardiovascular physiology concepts*, ed 1, New York, 2004, Lippincott.

9. Nadas A: Pulmonary stenosis. In Fyler DC, editor: *Nadas' pediatric cardiology*, pp 459-470, Philadelphia, 1992, Hanley & Belfus.

10. American Heart Association: *Single ventricle defects*, www.americanheart.org/presenter.jhtml?identifier=11072, accessed 10-15-10.

11. National Heart Lung and Blood Institute, National Institutes of Health: *Tetralogy of Fallot*, www.nhlbi.nih.gov/health/dci/Diseases/tof/tof_what.html, accessed 10-15-10.

12. Cincinnati Children's Hospital Medical Center: *Transposition of the great arteries*, www.cincinnatichildrens.org/health/heart-encyclopedia/anomalies/transposition.htm, accessed 10-15-10.

13. Zipes DP, Libby P, Bonow RO, et al, editors: *Braunwald's heart disease: a textbook of cardiovascular medicine*, ed 8, St Louis, 2007, WB Saunders.

14. Warnes CA, Liberthson R, Danielson GK, et al: Task force 1: the changing profile of congenital heart disease in adult life, *J Am Coll Cardiol* 37:1170-1175, 2001.

15. Parish A: *Intestinal malrotation, emedicine,* http://emedicine.medscape.com/article/930313-overview, accessed 10-15-10.

16. Marx J, Hockberger R, Walls R, editors: *Rosen's emergency medicine: concepts and clinical practice*, ed 6, St Louis, 2006, Mosby.

17. Barkin R, editor: *Pediatric emergency medicine: concepts and clinical practice*, ed 2, St Louis, 1997, Mosby.

18. American Academy of Pediatrics, American Heart Association, PALS Provider Manual, Dallas, 2005, American Heart Association.

19. American Academy of Pediatrics: *Worksheet for proposed evidence-based guideline recommendations,* www.aap.org/nrp/pdf/2005ilcor/interosseous/n.inteross.WAE.03Nov04.Final.pdf, accessed 4-26-10.

20. Dubowitz LMS, Dubowitz V, Goldberg C: Clinical assessment of gestational age in the newborn infant, *J Pediatr* 77:1-10, 1970.

21. Nirupama L: *Birth trauma, emedicine pediatrics: cardiac disease and critical care medicine,* March 16, 2010, http://emedicine.medscape.com/article/980112-overview, accessed 10-22-10.

SUGGESTED READINGS

Berglund S, Grunewald C, Petterson H, et al: Neonatal resuscitation after severe asphyxia—a critical evaluation of 177 Swedish cases, *Acta Paediatr* 97(6):714-719, 2008.

Heightman AJ: *JEMS editor-in-chief A.J. Heightman comments on this case and the jury award, JEMS,* 4-7-10, www.jems.com/news_and_articles/news/2010/04/jems_editor_in_chief_aj_heightman_comments_on_this_case_and_the_jury_award.html.

CHAPTER
48 Pediatrics

OBJECTIVES

Upon completion of this chapter, the paramedic student will be able to:

1. Identify the role of the Emergency Medical Services for Children program.
2. Identify age-related illnesses and injuries in pediatric patients.
3. Outline the general principles of assessment and management of the pediatric patient.
4. Identify modifications in patient assessment techniques that assist in the examination of patients at different developmental levels.
5. Describe the pathophysiology, signs and symptoms, and management of selected pediatric respiratory emergencies.
6. Describe the pathophysiology, signs and symptoms, and management of shock in the pediatric patient.
7. Describe the pathophysiology, signs and symptoms, and management of selected pediatric dysrhythmias.
8. Describe the pathophysiology, signs and symptoms, and management of pediatric seizures.
9. Describe the pathophysiology, signs and symptoms, and management of hypoglycemia and hyperglycemia in the pediatric patient.
10. Describe the pathophysiology, signs and symptoms, and management of infectious pediatric emergencies.
11. Identify common causes of poisoning and toxic exposure in the pediatric patient.
12. Describe special considerations for assessment and management of specific injuries in children.
13. Outline the pathophysiology and management of sudden infant death syndrome.
14. Describe the risk factors, key signs and symptoms, and management of injuries or illness resulting from child abuse and neglect.
15. Identify prehospital considerations for the care of infants and children with special needs.

KEY TERMS

apparent life-threatening events Clinical events in which young infants (usually less than 6 months of age) may experience abrupt changes in breathing, color, or muscle tone.

asthma A respiratory disorder characterized by recurring episodes of paroxysmal dyspnea, wheezing on expiration caused by constriction of the bronchi, coughing, and viscous mucoid bronchial secretions.

bacterial tracheitis A bacterial infection of the upper airway and subglottic trachea; it is characterized by expiratory wheezes, respiratory distress, inflammation, and obstruction at the level of the bronchioles.

bronchopulmonary dysplasia A chronic respiratory disorder characterized by scarring of lung tissue, thickened pulmonary arterial walls, and ventilation-perfusion mismatch; often occurs in infants who have dependence on long-term artificial ventilation.

child abuse The physical, sexual, or emotional maltreatment of a child.

croup An acute viral infection of the upper and lower respiratory tract that occurs primarily in infants and young children 3 months to 3 years of age; it is characterized by hoarseness, fever, a harsh and brassy cough, inspiratory stridor, and varying degrees of respiratory distress; also known as *laryngotracheobronchitis*.

emetic center An area located in the reticular formation of the brainstem; thought to be the control center for vomiting.

epiglottitis Inflammation of the epiglottis; a severe form of the condition that affects primarily children is characterized by fever, sore throat, stridor, croupy cough, and an erythematous epiglottis.

febrile seizure A seizure that results from fever.

hydrocephalus A pathological condition characterized by an abnormal accumulation of cerebrospinal fluid, usually under increased pressure, within the cranial vault, resulting in dilation of the ventricles.

jaundice A yellow discoloration of the skin, mucous membranes, and sclerae of the eyes caused by a greater than normal amount of bilirubin in the blood.

pathological jaundice A prolonged jaundice that results from illness in the newborn and a rapid rise in serum bilirubin concentration; usually appears within 24 hours after birth.

pertussis An acute, highly contagious respiratory disease characterized by paroxysmal coughing that ends in a loud, whooping inspiration; also known as *whooping cough*.

physiological jaundice A common jaundice that occurs during the first week of life; caused by the breakdown of fetal red blood cells, which release bilirubin into the blood, and by the immaturity of the newborn's liver,

which cannot effectively metabolize the bilirubin and prepare it for excretion into the urine.

pneumonia An acute inflammation of the lungs, usually caused by inhaled pneumococci of the species *Streptococcus pneumoniae*.

shunt A tube or device surgically implanted in the body to redirect body fluid from one cavity or vessel to another.

sudden infant death syndrome The unexpected and sudden death of an apparently normal and healthy infant that occurs during sleep.

Emergencies involving pediatric patients account for fewer than 10% of emergency medical services responses.[1] However, caring for these patients has unique challenges. The challenges are related to size, physical and intellectual maturation, and diseases specific to neonates, infants, and children. This chapter addresses the anatomical and physiological changes associated with normal growth and development, medical emergencies common to children, and initial assessment and management strategies that often are critical in the patient's survival.

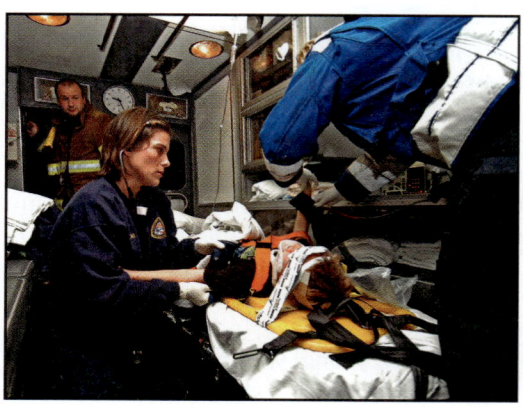

(Courtesy Ray Kemp, St. Charles, Mo.)

THE PARAMEDIC'S ROLE IN CARING FOR PEDIATRIC PATIENTS

Paramedics play an important role in the care of infants and children. This role involves the prehospital care and interfacility transfer. Emergency medical services personnel can help to reduce mortality and morbidity for children as well. They can become active participants in school, community, and parent education programs and provide thorough documentation appropriate for prehospital trauma registries, epidemiological research, and surveillance (see Chapter 3). For paramedics, improvement of their knowledge and clinical skills is important. They can do this through continuing education programs that are specific to the pediatric age group. A sampling of continuing education programs includes the following:

- Neonatal Resuscitation Program
- Neonatal Advanced Life Support
- Pediatric International Trauma Life Support
- Pediatric Advanced Life Support
- Pediatric Education for Prehospital Professionals
- Prehospital Pediatric Care
- Teaching Resource for Instructors of Prehospital Pediatrics

Other ways to enhance continuing education and clinical skills include reading textbooks and journals, participating in Internet study programs, attending regional conferences and seminars, and working or volunteering at pediatric emergency departments, pediatric hospitals, or a pediatrician's office.

EMERGENCY MEDICAL SERVICES FOR CHILDREN

In 1985 the Emergency Medical Services for Children (EMSC) Demonstration Program was established through grants provided by the Maternal and Child Health Bureau of the U.S. Department of Health and Human Services and by the National Highway Traffic Safety Administration, a division of the U.S. Department of Transportation. This program, which was designed to enhance and expand emergency medical services for acutely ill and injured children, defined 12 basic components of an effective Emergency Medical Services for Children system[2]:

1. System approach
2. Education
3. Data collection
4. Quality improvement
5. Injury prevention
6. Access
7. Prehospital care
8. Emergency care
9. Definitive care
10. Rehabilitation
11. Finance
12. Continual health care from birth to young adulthood

CRITICAL THINKING
Are you familiar with any Emergency Medical Services for Children injury prevention programs that are in your area?

EMSC grants and the organizational efforts aimed at improving emergency care for children have resulted in specific programs targeted to prehospital care providers. These include continuing education programs, educational resources for instructors, equipment guidelines, protocols for prehospital management, quality improvement procedures for evaluating prehospital care for children, and designation of facilities with special capabilities for pediatric care.

As stated in *Emergency medical services for children: a report to the nation,* published in 1991 by the National Center for Education in Maternal and Child Health: "The lives of many infants, children, and young adults ... can be saved through implementation of emergency medical services for children. Outcomes for critically ill and injured children can be influenced by the provision of timely care by health care professionals who are well trained and equipped for pediatric emergency and critical care."[3] In 2005 the EMSC program celebrated its twentieth anniversary. As stated in the Institute of Medicine's 2006 report *Future of emergency care, emergency care of children: growing pains*: "The program's accomplishments are numerous ... The program has broadly advanced the state of pediatric emergency care nationwide. It has improved the availability of child-size equipment in ambulances and EDs; initiated hundreds of programs to prevent injuries; and provided thousands of hours of training to EMTs, paramedics, and other emergency medical care providers ... to help achieve the program's goals. ..."[4]

GROWTH AND DEVELOPMENT REVIEW

As described in Chapter 12, children have unique anatomical, physiological, and psychological characteristics that change during their development. The following is a review of growth and development by age group. Special considerations and approach strategies that must be considered when caring for pediatric patients are provided in Box 48-1 (see Chapter 20).

LOOK AGAIN
See Chapter 20: Secondary Assessment, pp. 555-557.

CRITICAL THINKING
How comfortable are you with the "normal" well child?

Newborn (First Few Hours of Life)

Assessment and care for the newborn are described in Chapter 47. The method most commonly used to evaluate the newborn is the Apgar score. Resuscitation of the newborn (if needed) should follow the recommendations established by the American Heart Association, including those found in the curriculum for the Neonatal Resuscitation Program. To review, the newborn's heart rate during the first 30 minutes of life is between 120 and 160 beats/min. Respirations at birth are usually between 40 and 60 breaths/min. They average 30 to 40 breaths/min within a few minutes after delivery (Table 48-1). The full-term newborn normally weighs 3 to 3.5 kg (about 6 to 8 lb) (Figure 48-1).

Neonate (First 28 Days of Life)

Total body weight in the neonate may decrease 5% to 10% during the first few days of life because of the excretion of extracellular fluid. This lost weight is regained by the second week of life and generally exceeds the newborn weight. Most infants gain an average of 5 to 6 oz per week.

Neonates respond to their environment with a range of stereotypical reflexes. These reflexes are protective and include those associated with breathing, eating, and stress

TABLE 48-1 Average Vital Signs by Age Group*

Age	Pulse (beats/min)	Respirations (breaths/min)	Blood Pressure (mm Hg)
Newborn	120-160	40-60	80/40
1 year	80-140	30-40	82/44
3 years	80-120	25-30	86/50
5 years	70-115	20-25	90/52
7 years	70-115	20-25	94/54
10 years	70-115	15-20	100/60
15 years	70-90	15-20	110/64

*Note: Normal vital signs vary with age. Carry a reminder chart to ensure accuracy. Do not depend on your memory in an emergency. Blood pressure in a child older than 1 year may be estimated with the following formula: (age in years × 2) + 70 = minimum systolic blood pressure. Example for a 3-year-old child: (3 × 2 = 6) + 70 = 76 mm Hg.

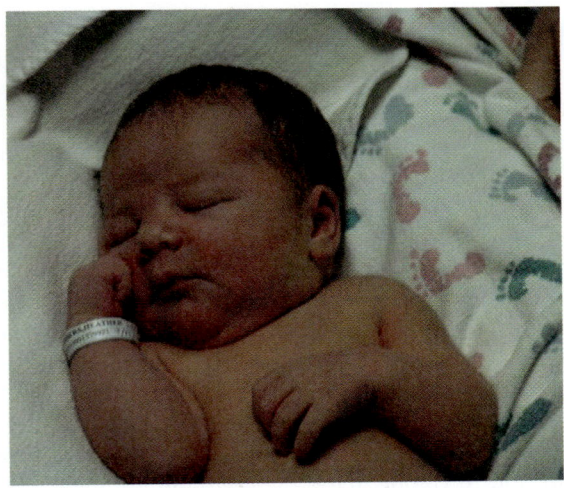

FIGURE 48-1 Newborn. (Courtesy the Sanders family, O'Fallon, Mo.)

BOX 48-1 Developmental Stages and Approach Strategies for Pediatric Patients

Infants

Major Fears
Separation and strangers

Approach Strategies
Provide consistent caretakers.
Reduce parents' anxiety, because it is transmitted to the infant.
Minimize separation from parents.

Toddlers

Major Fears
Separation and loss of control

Characteristics of Thinking
Primitive
Unable to recognize views of others
Little concept of body integrity

Approach Strategies
Keep explanations simple.
Choose words carefully.
Let toddler play with equipment (stethoscope).
Minimize separation from parents.

Preschoolers

Major Fears
Bodily injury and mutilation
Loss of control
The unknown and the dark
Being left alone

Characteristics of Thinking
Highly literal interpretation of words
Unable to abstract
Primitive ideas about the body (e.g., fear that all blood will "leak out" if a bandage is removed)

Approach Strategies
Keep explanations simple and concise.
Choose words carefully.
Emphasize that a procedure will help the child be healthier.
Be honest.

School-Age Children

Major Fears
Loss of control
Bodily injury and mutilation

Failure to live up to expectations of others
Death

Characteristics of Thinking
Vague or false ideas about physical illness and body structure and function
Able to listen attentively without always comprehending
Reluctant to ask questions about something they think they are expected to know
Increased awareness of significant illness, possible hazards of treatments, lifelong consequences of injury, and the meaning of death

Approach Strategies
Ask children to explain what they understand.
Provide as many choices as possible to increase the child's sense of control.
Reassure the child that he or she has done nothing wrong and that necessary procedures are not punishment.
Anticipate and answer questions about long-term consequences (e.g., what the scar will look like and how long activities may be curtailed).

Adolescents

Major Fears
Loss of control
Altered body image
Separation from peer group

Characteristics of Thinking
Able to think abstractly
Tendency toward hyperresponsiveness to pain (reactions not always in proportion to event)
Little understanding of the structure and workings of the body

Approach Strategies
When appropriate, allow adolescents to be a part of decision making about their care.
Give information sensitively.
Express how important their compliance and cooperation are to their treatment.
Be honest about consequences.
Use or teach coping mechanisms such as relaxation, deep breathing, and self-comforting talk.

---

or discomfort. Neonates sleep an average of 16 to 18 hours per day, with sleep and wakefulness evenly distributed over 24 hours. Infants are *obligate nose breathers* (breathing occurs mainly through the nose) during the first month of life. The horizontal position of the ribs produces the characteristic diaphragmatic breathing in this age group. Although crying is common in the neonate, the crying gradually decreases throughout infancy. Persistent crying may indicate physiological distress. Illnesses that may be encountered in this

age group are those that cause respiratory problems, jaundice, vomiting, fever, sepsis, meningitis, and problems of prematurity (Figure 48-2).

Infant (2 to 12 Months)

During infancy, major advances in physical and mental skills occur as the brain and nervous system gradually mature. Their response to their environment evolves from reflexes of purposeful movements. During this period of

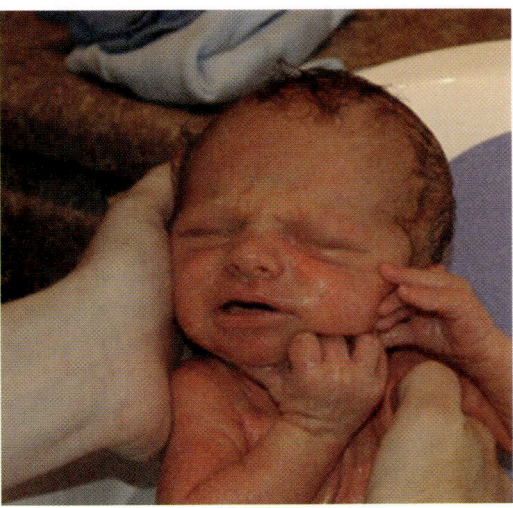

FIGURE 48-2 Neonate. (Courtesy the Sanders family, O'Fallon, Mo.)

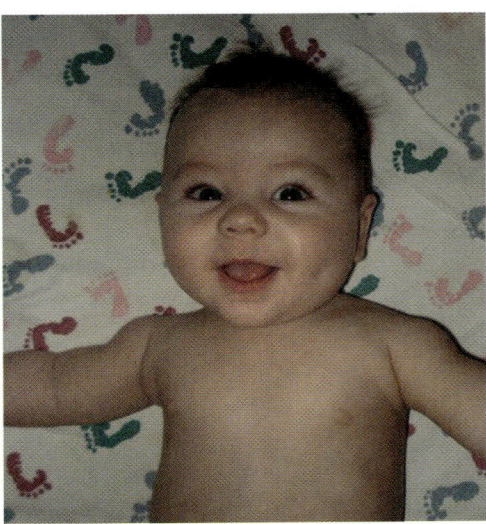

FIGURE 48-3 Infant. (Courtesy the Sanders family, O'Fallon, Mo.)

time, the musculature of the neck and back enables them to hold the head upright, sit, and babble (Figure 48-3). Between 4 and 6 months of age, most infants have doubled their birth weight, tripling it within 9 to 12 months. In the first year of life the heart also doubles in size, the heart rate gradually slows, and blood pressure begins to increase.

By 12 months of age the development of mature nerves is nearly complete and, along with muscle strength, enables many infants to stand and walk with little or no assistance. (Muscle weight in infants is about 25% of the entire musculoskeletal system.)

Common illnesses typically affect the respiratory, gastrointestinal, and central nervous systems. They manifest themselves as respiratory distress; nausea, vomiting, and diarrhea with dehydration; and seizures, respectively. Other illnesses that may be encountered in this age group include sepsis, meningitis, and sudden infant death syndrome (SIDS). (SIDS is also known as *sudden unexpected death in*

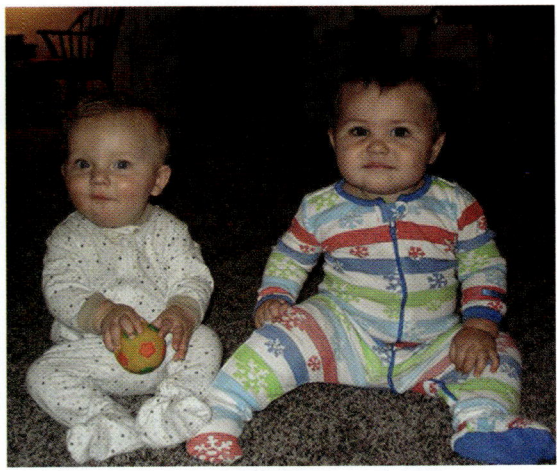

FIGURE 48-4 Toddlers.

infancy.) In addition, the older infant (6 to 12 months of age) may experience bronchiolitis, croup, foreign body airway obstruction, and physical injury from sexual abuse, neglect, falls, and motor vehicle crashes.

Toddler (1 to 3 Years)

Muscle mass and bone density increase during the toddler years (Figure 48-4). Most children gain an average of 2 kg (about 4 lb) each year. By age 2 years, much of the nervous system is fully developed. By this time, basic motor skills (e.g., balance and walking) and fine motor skills (e.g., stacking building blocks) also become visible. In addition, most children are capable of controlling bladder and bowel function by 2 to 3 years of age. By 2 years of age, toddlers have developed unique personality traits, moods, and specific likes and dislikes. Basic language skills are mastered by age 3. However, these skills continue to be refined through childhood. By 3 years of age toddlers and preschoolers also begin to recognize the difference between the sexes and start to model themselves after persons of their own gender. Illnesses in this age group may cause respiratory distress (e.g., from asthma, bronchiolitis, foreign body aspiration, or croup), vomiting and diarrhea with dehydration, febrile seizures, sepsis, and meningitis. Toddlers who are learning to walk are prone to falls. They also may find themselves in dangerous environments without proper supervision or barriers (e.g., baby gates). Physical injuries also occur from poisonings from accidental ingestions, physical/sexual abuse, drowning, and motor vehicle crashes (Table 48-2).

Preschooler (3 to 5 Years)

During the preschool years, children experience advances in gross and fine motor skills (Figure 48-5). Peer relationships also begin to form with other children near the same age and level of maturity. These relationships often begin with play that involves acting out fantasies or using imagination for new situations, all of which can lead to problem-solving skills and cognitive development. Illnesses and injuries that may be encountered in this age group include

TABLE 48-2 Unintentional Injury Deaths by Event, Ages Birth to 19 Years, United States, 2006*

Age	Population	Total	Rates†	Motor Vehicle	Falls	Poisoning	Drowning	Fires/Flames	Choking‡	Mechanical Suffocation	Firearms	All Others
<1 year	4,160	1,147	27.6	140	23	16	51	27	62	781	0	47
1-19 years	77,739	10,527	13.5	6,866	157	823	1,026	461	136	185	154	719
1 year	4,105	521	12.7	180	12	9	159	41	36	44	0	40
2 years	4,103	460	11.2	155	14	9	151	53	22	6	4	46
3 years	4,052	343	8.5	123	10	4	85	64	7	8	6	36
4 years	4,017	286	7.1	130	2	5	63	41	7	7	3	28
5 years	4,072	273	6.7	131	5	9	51	32	7	7	6	25
6 years	3,918	212	5.4	113	4	4	27	33	3	4	1	23
7 years	3,873	194	5.0	125	2	1	22	15	1	5	4	19
8 years	3,883	189	4.9	99	2	3	31	21	6	4	3	20
9 years	3,909	176	4.5	109	4	1	11	17	4	9	4	17
10 years	3,992	187	4.7	125	1	4	13	13	2	3	2	24
11 years	4,057	198	4.9	114	6	1	22	15	3	10	2	25
12 years	4,091	205	5.0	124	5	5	17	12	2	7	4	29
13 years	4,176	267	6.4	152	2	11	29	12	4	15	9	33
14 years	4,247	357	8.4	247	7	19	33	11	1	11	6	22
15 years	4,315	566	13.1	402	5	29	42	12	8	9	10	49
16 years	4,393	1,057	24.1	790	13	86	64	15	9	9	19	52
17 years	4,232	1,328	31.4	1,029	13	110	63	17	3	10	19	64
18 years	4,171	1,825	43.8	1,390	18	222	65	19	5	10	23	73
19 years	4,134	1,883	45.5	1,328	32	291	78	18	6	7	29	94
0-4 years	20,437	2,757	13.5	728	61	43	509	226	134	846	13	197
5-9 years	19,655	1,044	5.3	577	17	18	142	118	21	29	18	104
10-14 years	20,563	1,214	5.9	762	21	40	114	63	12	46	23	133
15-19 years	21,245	6,659	31.3	4,939	81	738	312	81	31	45	100	332

From National Safety Council tabulations of National Center for Health Statistics mortality data, Injury facts, National Safety Council, Itasca, Ill., 2010.
*Note: Data do not include "age unknown" cases, which totaled 57 in 2006.
†Deaths per 100,000 in each age group.
‡Suffocation by inhalation or ingestion of food or other object.

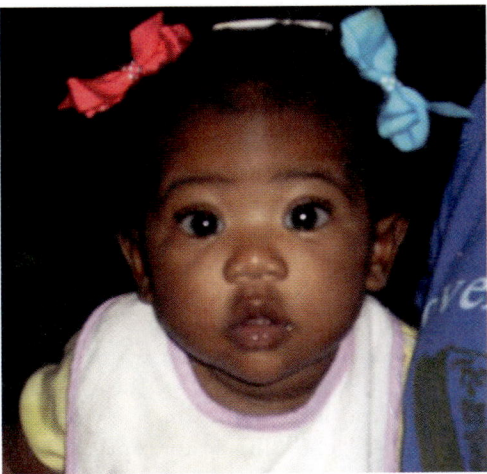

FIGURE 48-5 Preschooler. (Courtesy Norma Boozer, Florissant, Mo.)

those mentioned before for toddlers. As a result, preschoolers are more likely to experience injuries from thermal burns and pedestrian accidents, and be victims of submersion incidents or drowning. Preschoolers are curious and often have an urge to explore. Many have a minimal concept of danger.

School Age (6 to 12 Years)

The growth of school-age children is slower and steadier than during the infancy, toddler, and preschooler years (Figure 48-6). Most children gain about 3 kg (6.6 lb) per year. They average a yearly gain in height of about 2½ inches (6 cm). Most bodily functions reach adult levels in this age group. Two key areas of development during the school-age years include an increased ability to concentrate and learn quickly and the onset of puberty. Psychosocial development of school-age children varies by individual. As a rule, however, self-concept and moral traits and behavior begin to emerge during the school-age years. During these years, children spend more time with others outside their immediate family. Most illnesses in school-age children are caused by viral infection. Injuries become more common in this age group because of increased physical activity. These injuries include injuries from bicycle crashes, fractures from falls, and sport-related injuries.

> **NOTE**
> About 40,000 to 50,000 children are estimated to be injured permanently each year, and at least 1 million seek medical care because of unintentional injuries (the leading cause of death in children).[5]

Adolescent (13 to 18 Years)

During adolescence, the final phase of change in growth and development occurs (Figure 48-7). Organs rapidly increase in size, blood chemistry values become nearly equal to adult

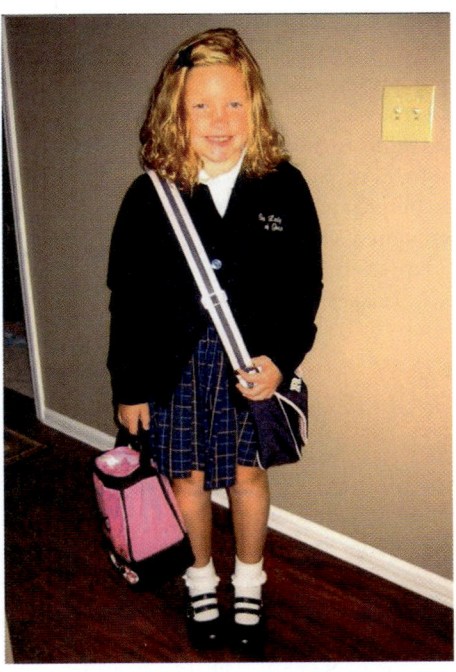

FIGURE 48-6 School-age child. (Courtesy Stephanie Gates, Indianapolis, Indiana.)

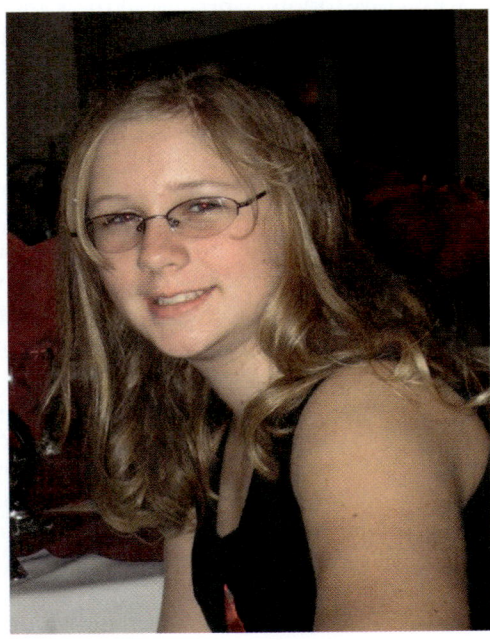

FIGURE 48-7 Adolescent. (Courtesy the Sanders family, O'Fallon, Mo.)

levels, and growth of bone and muscle mass becomes nearly complete. Also in adolescence a person reaches reproductive maturity. With the development of secondary sex characteristics in both genders comes a final period of rapid growth. Most boys gain an average of 8 inches in height before age 21, when growth usually stops. Growth in girls is less dramatic and is usually complete by age 18.

Along with the physical changes associated with adolescence, most teenagers begin to experiment with different identities. They begin to develop their personality into that of an adult. Many make dramatic moves away from parents and family members toward their peer groups. In their peer groups, they may experiment with alcohol and other drugs, sex, and extreme forms of behavior. In addition to those physical injuries mentioned for younger age groups, in this age group the paramedic may encounter behavioral emergencies associated with alcohol or other drug use, eating disorders, depression, suicide and suicide gestures, sexually transmitted diseases, pregnancy, and sexual assault.

ANATOMY AND PHYSIOLOGY REVIEW

As stressed throughout this text, physical differences in infants and children set them apart from the adult patient. The following is a review of anatomy and physiology by body region. Also included are special emergency care implications for the pediatric patient.

Head

Up until the age of 8 years, a child's head is proportionally large. It accounts for about 25% of the total body weight in newborns. Children also have a larger occipital region and a smaller face relative to adults. Because of these anatomical features, a high percentage of blunt trauma in children involves the head and face. The prominent occiput of the child predisposes the neck to slight flexion when the child is placed on a flat surface. To prevent this, a spine board with an occipital well or blankets placed under the child's torso should be used to maintain a neutral position of the neck.[1]

To accommodate for brain growth in the infant, the anterior fontanelle remains open for 9 to 18 months after birth. The anterior fontanelle is usually level or slightly below the surface of the skull. A tight or bulging fontanelle suggests increased intracranial pressure (ICP; as seen with meningitis or brain injury); a sunken fontanelle indicates possible dehydration. The paramedic should assess the anterior fontanelle in infants and young children who are ill or injured. The fontanelle is best assessed when the child is upright and not crying.

Airway

The airway structures of children are narrower and less stable at all levels than those of adults. This makes the airways of pediatric patients more easily blocked by secretions, obstructions, and injury or inflammation. In addition, the larynx is higher (at the level of cervical vertebrae C3 to C4) and more anterior, extending into the pharynx. The trachea is bifurcated at a higher level. The tracheal cartilage also is softer and smaller in length and diameter. The cricoid ring is the narrowest part of the airway in young children. The jaw is proportionally small, and the tongue is proportionally large. This increases the likelihood of airway obstruction by the tongue in the unconscious child. The epiglottis in infants is omega-shaped and extends into the

airway at a 45-degree angle. The epiglottic folds also have softer cartilage and can become "floppy," causing airway obstruction. As described in Chapter 15 and later in this chapter, management considerations for these patients include the following:

- Placing padding under the shoulders of small children to maintain a neutral position of the airway
- Avoiding hyperflexion or hyperextension of the neck, which can obstruct the airway
- Using suction to clear the airway if secretions and particulate matter are present
- Modifying tracheal intubation techniques by ensuring a gentle touch to the soft tissue of the airway, which is easily injured and inflamed; using a straight blade that lifts the epiglottis; choosing an appropriately sized endotracheal tube; and constantly monitoring the airway for proper endotracheal tube placement with continuous capnography[6,7]

> **NOTE**
> Both cuffed and uncuffed endotracheal tubes are acceptable for intubating infants and children. Cuffed endotracheal tubes may decrease the risk of aspiration. If cuffed endotracheal tubes are used, cuff inflating pressure should be monitored and limited according to manufacturer's instructions (usually less than 20 to 25 cm H_2O).[6]

The paramedic also should remember that infants breathe mainly through the nose during the first month of life. Obstruction of the small nares by secretions can result easily in respiratory insufficiency. Thus assessment and suction of the nares as needed are important, and especially important in infants less than 6 months of age.

Chest and Lungs

In infants and young children the chief support for the chest wall comes from muscles rather than bones. These chest muscles are immature. They can fatigue easily. The use of these muscles for breathing also requires higher metabolic and oxygen consumption rates than in older children and adults. This increases the pediatric patient's susceptibility to the accumulation of lactic acid in the blood. The ribs of a child are more pliable and are positioned horizontally, and the mediastinum is more mobile. Therefore the chest wall offers less protection to internal organs. It allows for significant internal injury to occur without external signs of trauma. Rib fractures are less common in children. Yet they can occur with child abuse and other forms of trauma.

The lung tissue of a pediatric patient is fragile. Because of this and the limited protection provided by the chest wall, pulmonary contusions from trauma and pneumothorax from barotrauma are common in this age group. When evaluating a pediatric patient who has suffered major trauma, the paramedic should remember that infants and children are diaphragmatic breathers and are prone to gastric distention; the mobile mediastinum may have a greater shift with a tension pneumothorax; and the thin chest wall easily transmits breath sounds, which may complicate the assessment of a pneumothorax or endotracheal tube placement. As a result, auscultation of breath sounds from the axillary regions in addition to the anterior and posterior thorax often is helpful.

Abdomen

Like the chest wall, the immature muscles of the abdomen in a child offer less protection to internal organs. In addition, the abdominal organs are closer together. The liver and spleen are proportionally larger and more vascular, as well. These features allow for multiple organ injuries to be more common following abdominal trauma. The liver and spleen also are injured more often than in the adult patient.

Extremities

As described in Chapter 10, bones in children are softer and more porous until adolescence. As long bones mature, hormones act on the cartilage in growing bones, replacing the soft cartilage with hard bones. Epiphyseal plates (growth plates) are located at the distal ends of the long bones. This is the area where new cartilage is laid down and ossified, thus lengthening the bones. It is a point of relative weakness. With age, long bones also thicken as additional layers of bone are laid down.

LOOK AGAIN
See Chapter 10: Review of Human Systems, pp. 153-155.

Because of the soft composition of bones in pediatric patients, at first all strains and sprains should be considered a fracture. They should be managed with full immobilization of the extremity. In addition, paramedics should be wary of injuries to the growth plate that may disrupt bone growth. Careful technique during intraosseous infusion procedures is critical. This is because improper insertion into the growth plate can affect future bone growth (see Chapter 14).

Skin and Body Surface Area

The skin in children is thinner and more elastic than the skin of adults. In addition, most children younger than 2 years of age have less subcutaneous fat.[8] The child also has a larger body surface area/body mass ratio. These factors can affect injury and illness in children in several ways. For example, the thinner skin of a child allows for deeper injury to occur from heat or cold exposure. The lack of subcutaneous fat and the larger body surface area/body mass ratio also increase a child's likelihood of hypothermia, hyperthermia, and dehydration from fluid loss.

Respiratory System

The tidal volume of infants and young children is proportionally smaller than that of adolescents and adults. The metabolic oxygen requirements for normal breathing are about double those of adolescents and adults. Pediatric patients also have smaller functional residual capacity. Thus they have proportionally smaller oxygen reserves. Because of these factors, hypoxia can develop rapidly in infants and young children. The paramedic also should remember that muscles are the main support for the chest wall. These muscles can tire easily during respiratory distress. This in turn can lead to respiratory failure and ultimately arrest. The paramedic should anticipate respiratory failure if any of the following signs are present[6]:

- An increased respiratory rate, particularly with signs of distress (e.g., increased respiratory effort including nasal flaring, retractions, seesaw breathing, or grunting)
- An inadequate respiratory rate, effort, or chest excursion (e.g., diminished breath sounds or gasping), especially if mental status is depressed
- Cyanosis with abnormal breathing despite supplementary oxygen

Cardiovascular System

Cardiac output is rate-dependent in infants and small children: The faster the heart rate, the greater the cardiac output. Children are not as able as adults to increase the contractility and stroke volume of the heart. The circulating blood volume in children is proportionally larger than that in adults. Yet the child's absolute blood volume is smaller. The ability of children to use vasoconstriction to decrease size of the vessels allows them to maintain blood pressure longer than adults. However, early intervention is required to prevent irreversible or decompensated shock. Special considerations in managing these patients include the following:

- Cardiovascular reserve is vigorous, but limited.
- Loss of small volumes of fluid and blood can cause shock.
- A child may be in shock despite a normal blood pressure.
- Bradycardia is often a response to hypoxia.

As described in Chapter 36, hypotension is a late sign of shock in the pediatric patient. Thus the assessment of shock must be based on clinical signs of tissue perfusion (e.g., level of consciousness, skin color, oxygen saturation, and capillary refill). The paramedic should suspect shock in any ill or injured child who has tachycardia and evidence of decreased perfusion. Hypotension in infants and children can be defined as a *systolic* blood pressure[6]:

- <60 mm Hg in term neonates (birth to 28 days)
- <70 mm Hg in infants (1 month to 12 months)
- <70 mm Hg + (2 × age in years) in children 1 to 10 years
- <90 mm Hg in children ≥10 years of age

Nervous System

As described in Chapter 12, the nervous system develops throughout childhood. Developing neural tissue is fragile. However, compared to adults, there is a greater cerebrospinal fluid (CSF) space around the neural tissues in children, which buffers blunt forces. Their spinal column also is more pliable. As a result, children suffer spinal cord injury less frequently than adults[9] (56% of spinal cord injuries in the United States occur between the ages of 16 and 30).[10] Children also may be free of injury, even after falls from a great distance.

The anterior and posterior fontanelles in young children remain open for 9 to 18 months after birth. Therefore direct trauma to the head can lead to brain injuries that are devastating in young children.

Metabolic Differences

The way in which children and adults expend energy differs in many ways. For example, infants and children have limited glycogen and glucose stores. Their blood glucose levels can drop quite low in response to illness or injury. Pediatric patients can experience significant volume loss from vomiting and diarrhea. Children are also prone to hypothermia because of their increased body surface area. Newborns and neonates also do not have the ability to shiver or sweat to maintain body temperature. For these reasons, it is important to assess a severely ill or injured child for hypoglycemia or hypoperfusion, to minimize heat loss, and to keep all children warm during treatment and transport.

CRITICAL THINKING
Why is it important to know what injuries and illnesses are commonly seen in specific age groups?

GENERAL PRINCIPLES OF PEDIATRIC ASSESSMENT

The general principles of assessment for the pediatric patient are very similar to those for adult patients. Approach strategies and medical equipment will differ in some ways because of the patient's age, maturity, and physical development. The following is a brief overview of the general principles of pediatric assessment, including evaluation of the scene (scene size-up), primary survey, vital functions, transition phase, focused history, secondary assessment, and reassessment. Specific differences in providing care to a child are presented later in this chapter by subject matter.

Evaluation of the Scene (Scene Size-Up)

As with all other patient care events, the paramedic should begin the physical assessment of a child with a quick scene survey, noting any potential hazards. The paramedic also

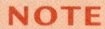

NOTE
Initial patient evaluation for children should include observing the patient and involving the parent or guardian in the assessment. The parent or guardian often can help make the child more comfortable during the assessment and can usually offer key details about the child's medical history. The parent also may know whether aspects of the child's behavior or response to the illness or injury are normal or abnormal.

should note any visible mechanism of injury or illness. For example, the presence of pills, medicine bottles, or household chemicals may indicate the possibility of toxic ingestion. Injury and a history that does not coincide with the stated mechanism of injury may indicate child abuse. In addition, the paramedic should observe the relationship between the parent, guardian, or caregiver and the child to determine the appropriateness of their interaction. For example, does the interaction demonstrate concern, anger, or indifference? Other important assessments the paramedic can make during the scene size-up include the orderliness, cleanliness, and safety of the home and the general appearance of other children in the family.

CRITICAL THINKING
Would you want to make a comment to the parents about an unsafe situation on the scene before transport? Why or why not?

Primary Survey

The primary survey begins with the paramedic forming a general impression of the patient. This assessment should focus on the details most valuable for determining whether life-threatening conditions exist. The pediatric assessment triangle (Figure 48-8) is a tool that can be used to quickly assess a child. The assessment triangle has three components: appearance (mental status and muscle tone); work of breathing (respiratory rate and effort); and circulation (skin signs and skin color). If the child's condition is urgent, care should proceed with rapid assessment of airway, breathing, and circulation; management; and rapid transport. If the child's condition is not urgent, care can proceed with a focused history and detailed physical examination.

CRITICAL THINKING
Think about one abnormal finding in each area of the assessment triangle. Would any single finding influence your triage decision?

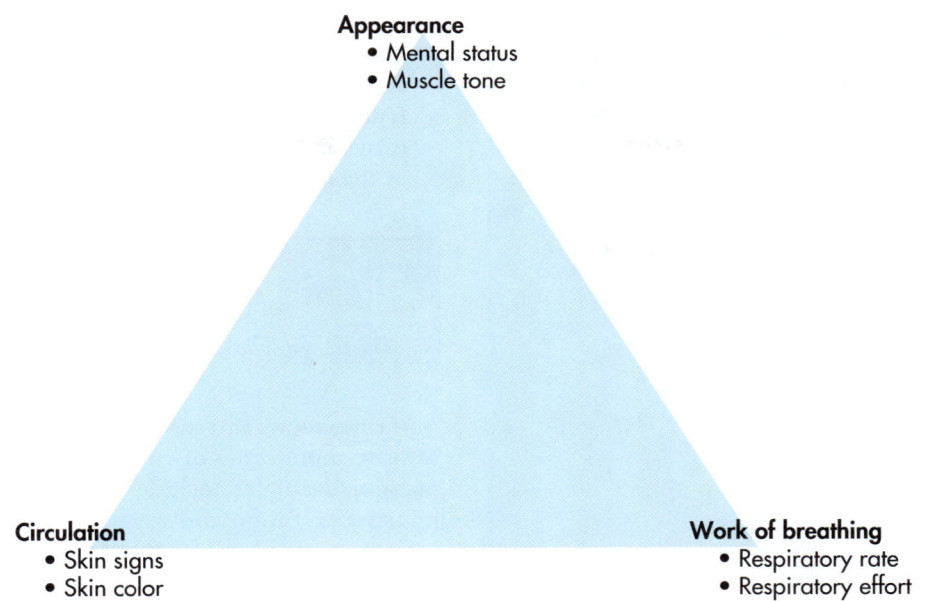

Appearance
- Mental status
- Muscle tone

Circulation
- Skin signs
- Skin color

Work of breathing
- Respiratory rate
- Respiratory effort

FIGURE 48-8 Pediatric assessment triangle.

Vital Functions

The AVPU scale (*alert*; responds to *verbal* stimuli; responds to *painful* stimuli; *unresponsive*) or the Modified Glasgow Coma Scale (Table 48-3) can be used to determine the child's level of consciousness and to assess for signs of inadequate oxygenation.

AIRWAY AND BREATHING

The child's airway should be patent, and breathing should proceed with adequate chest rise and fall. Signs of respiratory distress include the following:

- Abnormal breath sounds
- Absent breath sounds
- Apnea or bradypnea
- Grunting
- Head bobbing
- Irregular breathing pattern
- Nasal flaring
- Tachypnea
- Use of accessory muscles

CIRCULATION

The paramedic assesses circulation by comparing the strength and quality of central and peripheral pulses. Blood pressure should be measured in children over 3 years of age with an appropriately sized cuff, and in *all* children who are seriously ill or injured. The skin should be evaluated for color, temperature, moisture, turgor, and capillary refill. Any signs of visible hemorrhage should be noted and managed appropriately. See Table 48-1 for normal vital signs for each age group.

Transition Phase

The *transition phase* is integrated throughout assessment. This phase is used to allow the child to become more familiar with the paramedic crew and medical equipment (e.g., "get to know you" conversations and playing with stethoscope) (see Chapter 19). Use of this phase depends on the seriousness of the patient's condition and is only appropriate for a conscious child who is not acutely ill. If the patient is unconscious or acutely ill, management should proceed quickly to emergency care and transport.

Focused History

When obtaining the focused history for an infant, a toddler, or a preschooler, the paramedic often must elicit information from the parent, guardian, or caregiver. School-age and adolescent patients can provide most information by themselves. The paramedic should question patients in private (away from parents or family members) about sexual activity, pregnancy, alcohol or other drug use, or suspicion of child abuse (if appropriate for the complaint). The focused history can be obtained using the SAMPLE and OPQRST methods. (These methods are described in Chapter 18.) The paramedic should use these methods as appropriate for the patient's age. Important elements of the focused history are as follows:

1. Chief complaint
   - Nature of illness or injury
   - The length (duration) of illness or injury
   - Last meal
   - Presence of fever
   - Effects on behavior

TABLE 48-3 Pediatric Modification of Glasgow Coma Scale by Age of Patient*		
Glasgow Coma Scale Score		**Pediatric Modification**

Eye Opening

≥1 Year	Birth to 1 Year
4 Spontaneously	4 Spontaneously
3 To verbal command	3 To shout
2 To pain	2 To pain
1 No response	1 No response

Best Motor Response

≥1 Year	Birth to 1 Year
6 Obeys	5 Localizes pain
5 Localizes pain	4 Flexion withdrawal
4 Flexion withdrawal	3 Flexion abnormal (decorticate)
3 Flexion abnormal (decorticate)	2 Extension (decerebrate)
2 Extension (decerebrate)	1 No response
1 No response	

Best Verbal Response

>5 Years	Birth to 2 Years	2-5 Years
5 Oriented and converses	5 Cries appropriately, smiles, coos	5 Appropriate words and phrases
4 Disoriented and converses	4 Cries	4 Inappropriate words
3 Inappropriate words	3 Inappropriate crying/screaming	3 Cries/screams
2 Incomprehensible sounds	2 Grunts	2 Grunts
1 No response	1 No response	1 No response

*The Glasgow Coma Scale score is the sum of the individual scores from eye opening, best verbal response, and best motor response, using age-specific criteria. A Glasgow Coma Scale score of 13 to 15 indicates mild head injury; a score of 9 to 12 indicates moderate head injury; and a score of 8 or lower indicates severe head injury.

- Vomiting or diarrhea
- Frequency of urination
2. Medications and allergies
3. Medical history
   - Physician care
   - Chronic illnesses

Secondary Assessment

The paramedic should perform a detailed secondary assessment as described in Chapter 20. The exam should proceed from head to toe in older children. It should proceed from toe to head in younger children.[11] Depending on the patient's condition, some or all of the following assessments may be appropriate:

- *Pupils:* Are they equal and reactive to light?
- *Capillary refill* (most accurate in patients under 6 years of age): Is it less than 2 seconds (normal) or delayed?
- *Hydration:* Does the skin show normal resiliency (skin turgor)? Are there tears and saliva? Are the fontanelles in the infant sunken or flat?

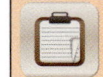

NOTE

When assessing a pediatric patient who is ill, it is important to note the presence or absence of fever, nausea, vomiting, diarrhea, and frequency of urination.

If time allows and the patient's condition warrants, non-invasive monitoring of vital signs can provide more information. Examples include the use of pulse oximetry to measure perfusion and oxygen saturation, blood pressure assessment, and measurement of body temperature. In addition, all seriously ill or injured children should receive continuous electrocardiogram monitoring. Measurement tools (e.g., blood pressure cuffs and electrodes) should be appropriate for the size of the child (Figure 48-9).

Reassessment

Reassessment should be ongoing and is appropriate for all patients. The purpose of reassessment is to monitor the patient for changes in respiratory effort, skin color and temperature, mental status, and vital signs (including pulse oximetry measurements). A key point to remember is that a child's condition can change rapidly. Thus vital signs should be assessed every 15 minutes in a child who is not critical. They should be assessed every 5 minutes in a child who is seriously ill or injured.

CRITICAL THINKING

Why is ongoing assessment critical when caring for the young child?

GENERAL PRINCIPLES OF PATIENT MANAGEMENT

The principles of patient management depend on the patient's condition. These principles may include basic airway management, advanced airway management, circulatory support, pharmacological therapy, nonpharmacological therapy, transport considerations, and psychological support, comfort measures, and communication strategies. Like the general principles of assessment discussed earlier in this chapter, the general principles of patient management for children are similar to those of adult patients. The following discussion will serve as a brief review.

Basic Airway Management

Basic and advanced airway management procedures for the pediatric patient are presented in detail in Chapter 15. These procedures may include manual positioning of the

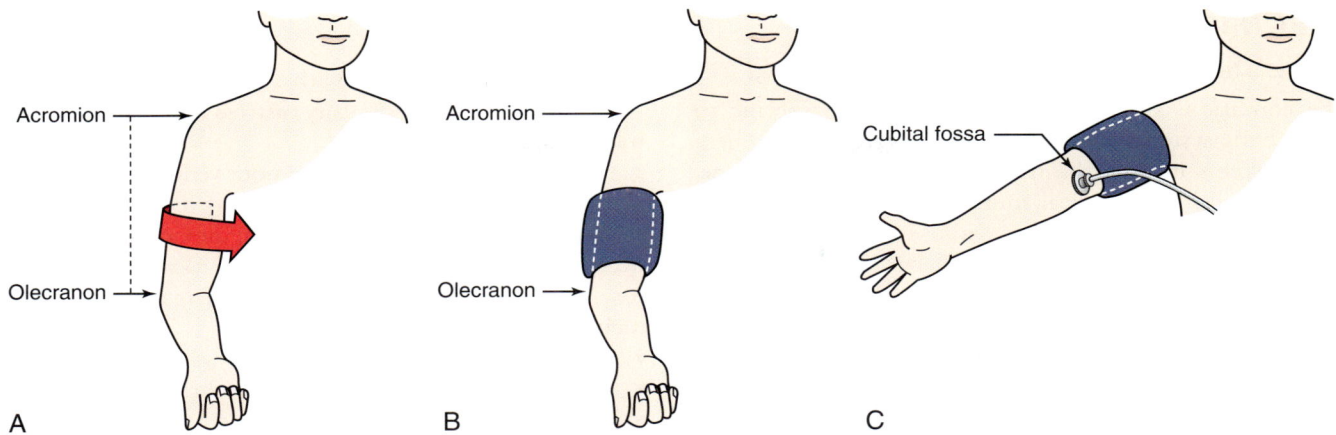

FIGURE 48-9 Determination of proper blood pressure cuff size. **A,** The cuff bladder width should be approximately 40% of the circumference of the arm measured at a point midway between the olecranon and acromion. **B,** Cuff bladder length should cover 80% to 100% of the circumference of the arm. **C,** Blood pressure should be measured with the cubital fossa at heart level. The arm should be supported. The stethoscope bell is placed over the brachial artery pulse, proximal and medial to the cubital fossa, and below the bottom edge of the cuff.

airway, removal of foreign body airway obstruction with chest compressions or abdominal thrusts, suctioning of secretions from the airway, providing supplemental oxygen, using oral or nasal airway adjuncts, and assisting ventilation with a bag-valve device.

Advanced Airway Management

Advanced airway management procedures may be needed when caring for a child who is acutely ill or seriously injured. These techniques include removing foreign body airway obstruction under direct visualization with Magill forceps, endotracheal intubation (including drug-assisted intubation), and cricothyroidotomy (per medical direction) when other methods to maintain a patent airway have failed.

Circulatory Support

Circulatory support may be required in an ill or injured child. In addition to providing basic life support with cardiopulmonary resuscitation, vascular access may be required for drug therapy and fluid resuscitation. Methods to obtain vascular access in pediatric patients are described in Chapter 14 and later in this chapter. These methods may include peripheral venous cannulation and intraosseous infusion.[6]

Pharmacological Therapy

At times, drug therapy will be required when caring for the pediatric patient. Examples include therapy for pain management; drug-assisted intubation; and patients with respiratory, cardiac, endocrinological, or neurological conditions. Drugs that are used in pediatric emergencies are described later in this chapter and in the Emergency Drug Index.

Additional Therapy

Additional therapies may be indicated depending on the type of illness or injury. These include spinal immobilization for trauma patients, hemorrhage control and bandaging and splinting, and electrical therapy (described later in this chapter). In addition, lowering body temperature with cooling methods or maintaining body temperature with blankets and warm clothing may be needed.

Transport Considerations

As described in Chapter 37, some pediatric patients will need transport to a specialty care medical facility. Examples of specialty care facilities are pediatric trauma centers, high-risk newborn care facilities, and pediatric burn centers. In addition to choosing a proper facility, the paramedic crew must consider the proper mode of caring for these patients. This includes decisions to provide rapid transport versus providing on-scene care, and the use of ground or air ambulance.

Psychological Support

It is important for the paramedic to provide psychological support to the pediatric patient and to the patient's family or caregivers. Pediatric emergencies often are emotionally charged events. Helpful strategies for approaching and communicating with pediatric patients and their caregivers are described in Chapter 17.

LOOK AGAIN
See Chapter 17: Therapeutic Communications, pp. 486-487.

SPECIFIC PATHOPHYSIOLOGY, ASSESSMENT, AND MANAGEMENT

The conditions discussed in this section are specific to major body systems and associated illness or injury. These body systems include the respiratory, cardiac, endocrine, hematological, neurological, immune, and gastrointestinal. In addition, shock, toxicology, abuse and neglect, and sudden infant death syndrome will be discussed. Other considerations for specialized care (e.g., children with cystic fibrosis, muscular dystrophy, cerebral palsy, Down syndrome) will be presented in Chapter 51.

Respiratory Compromise

Respiratory distress can be caused by many conditions that affect the upper and lower airways. These include upper and lower foreign body airway obstruction, upper airway disease (croup, epiglottitis, and bacterial tracheitis), and lower airway disease (asthma, bronchiolitis). Other causes of respiratory compromise include pneumonia, pertussis, cystic fibrosis, and bronchopulmonary dysplasia. It should be noted that most cases of cardiac arrest in children occur because of respiratory insufficiency (*asphyxial arrest*).[6] For this reason, respiratory emergencies require rapid assessment and management. The severity of respiratory compromise may be classified as respiratory distress, respiratory failure, and respiratory arrest.

> **NOTE**
>
> The paramedic should attempt to calm and reassure a child with respiratory compromise. It is important not to agitate the conscious patient or lay the child down (supine). Doing so may aggravate the airway condition and lead to life-threatening airway obstruction. When possible, allow the parent or other caregiver to stay with the child. The receiving hospital should be advised of the patient's status as soon as possible so that arrangements can be made for appropriate medical personnel.

Respiratory distress is the mildest form of respiratory compromise. Respiratory distress is evident by an increase in the rate and depth of breathing and by the use of accessory muscles to assist ventilation (Figure 48-10). These changes cause a slight decrease in arterial carbon dioxide levels in the blood as respiratory rate increases. As respiratory distress increases, the patient becomes exhausted. The partial pressure of carbon dioxide (PCO_2) gradually increases as the patient's condition worsens. Signs and symptoms of respiratory distress include the following:

- A change in mental status from normal to irritable or anxious
- Tachypnea
- Retractions (accessory muscle use)
- Nasal flaring
- Poor muscle tone
- Tachycardia

- Head bobbing
- Grunting
- Cyanosis that improves with supplemental oxygen

If left untreated, respiratory distress may lead to respiratory failure.

Respiratory failure results from poor ventilation or lack of oxygenation. It occurs when the heart and lungs do not exchange enough oxygen and carbon dioxide. This causes a decrease in PO_2 and an increase in PCO_2 (leading to respiratory acidosis). Signs and symptoms of respiratory failure include the following:

- Irritability deteriorating to lethargy
- Marked tachypnea deteriorating to bradypnea
- Marked retractions deteriorating to agonal respirations
- Marked tachycardia deteriorating to bradycardia
- Central cyanosis

Respiratory failure in any patient is an ominous sign. Without immediate help, respiratory arrest can occur.

Respiratory arrest is the cessation of breathing. Good outcomes can be expected with early treatment that protects the airway and provides adequate ventilation and oxygenation. However, failure to treat respiratory arrest can lead to cardiopulmonary arrest. Signs and symptoms of respiratory arrest include the following:

- Unresponsiveness
- Apnea
- Absent chest wall movement
- Limp muscle tone
- Bradycardia deteriorating to asystole
- Profound cyanosis

Providing aggressive ventilatory and circulatory support for patients in respiratory distress is critical. Airway interventions may include bag-valve-mask ventilation, endotracheal intubation, gastric decompression (if abdominal distention is impeding ventilation), needle decompression for pneumothorax, and cricothyrotomy for complete upper airway obstruction that cannot be relieved by other means. The success of emergency care is indicated by an improvement in the patient's color and oxygen saturation, an improvement in the pulse rate, and an improved level of consciousness. Box 48-2 provides assessment information that is important when caring for a child with respiratory compromise.

UPPER AND LOWER FOREIGN BODY AIRWAY OBSTRUCTION

Obstruction of the upper or lower airway by a foreign body may cause a partial or full obstruction. This usually occurs in toddlers and preschoolers (1 to 4 years of age). Children develop molars around age 3, but do not chew well. As a result, obstruction often is caused by foods such as hot dogs (most common food to cause obstruction), peanut butter, hard candy, popcorn, grapes, nuts, and seeds. Other causes of upper airway obstruction include small objects such as coins and balloons. The paramedic should suspect foreign body aspiration in an otherwise healthy child with sudden onset of respiratory compromise.

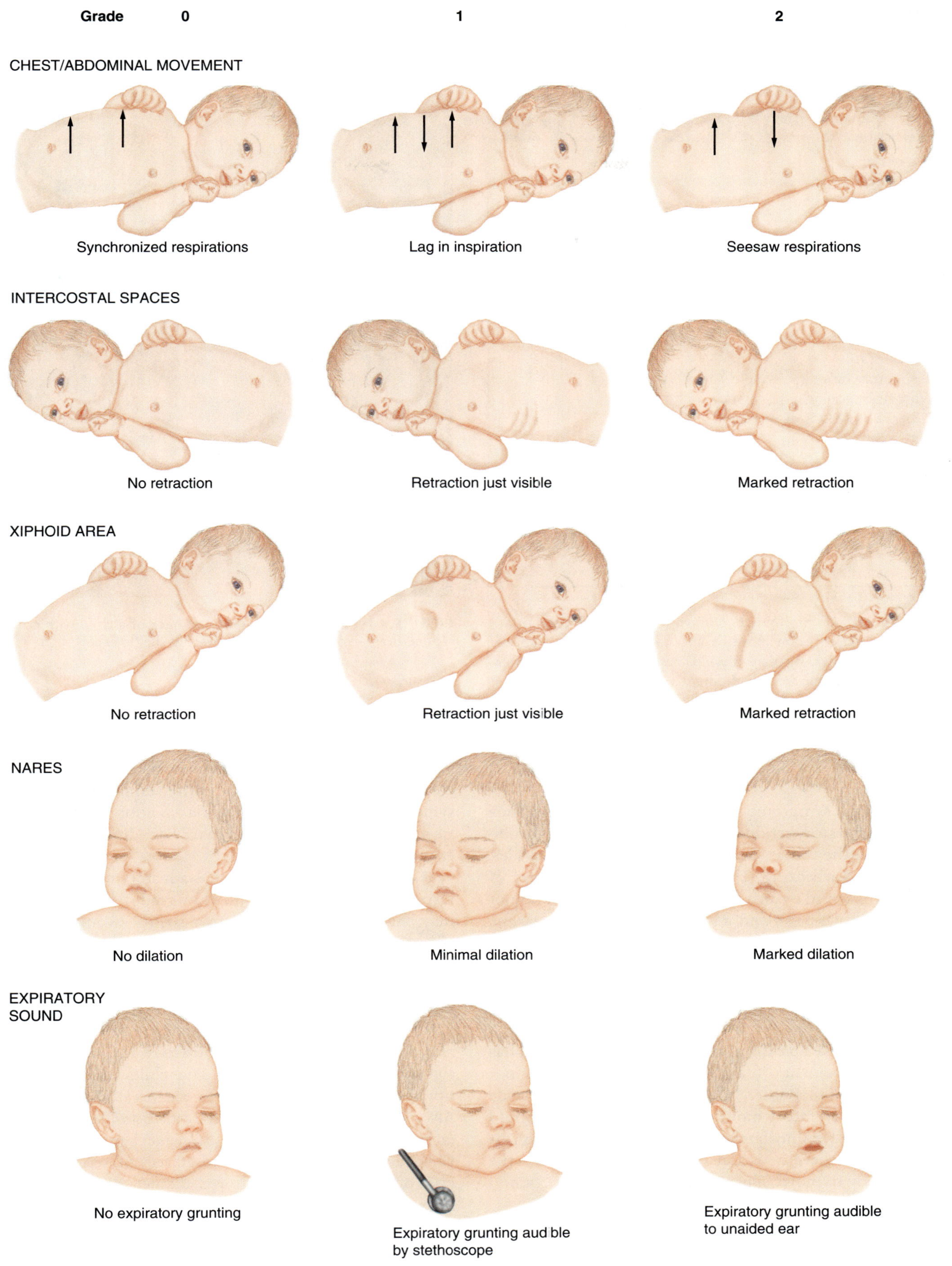

Grade	0	1	2

CHEST/ABDOMINAL MOVEMENT

Synchronized respirations | Lag in inspiration | Seesaw respirations

INTERCOSTAL SPACES

No retraction | Retraction just visible | Marked retraction

XIPHOID AREA

No retraction | Retraction just visible | Marked retraction

NARES

No dilation | Minimal dilation | Marked dilation

EXPIRATORY SOUND

No expiratory grunting | Expiratory grunting audible by stethoscope | Expiratory grunting audible to unaided ear

FIGURE 48-10 Assessment of respiratory distress. The Silverman-Anderson index is used to score the infant's degree of respiratory difficulty. The score for individual criteria matches the grade, with a total possible score of 10 indicating severe distress.

BOX 48-2 Assessment Information for Respiratory Compromise

History
Age
Preceding symptoms
Choking episode
Underlying disease
Recent exposure to illness
Exposure to toxins
Prematurity

Physical Findings
Mental status
Respiratory rate
Work of breathing
Presence of stridor or wheezes
Skin color
Heart rate
Tidal volume
Pulse oximetry
Capnography

NOTE
The common practice of using inflated balloons or an inflated exam glove to entertain or distract a young child while providing care should be avoided. This practice creates a choke hazard for children under 3 years of age.[12] In addition, parents and other caregivers should be advised to keep deflated balloons and broken balloon pieces away from children.

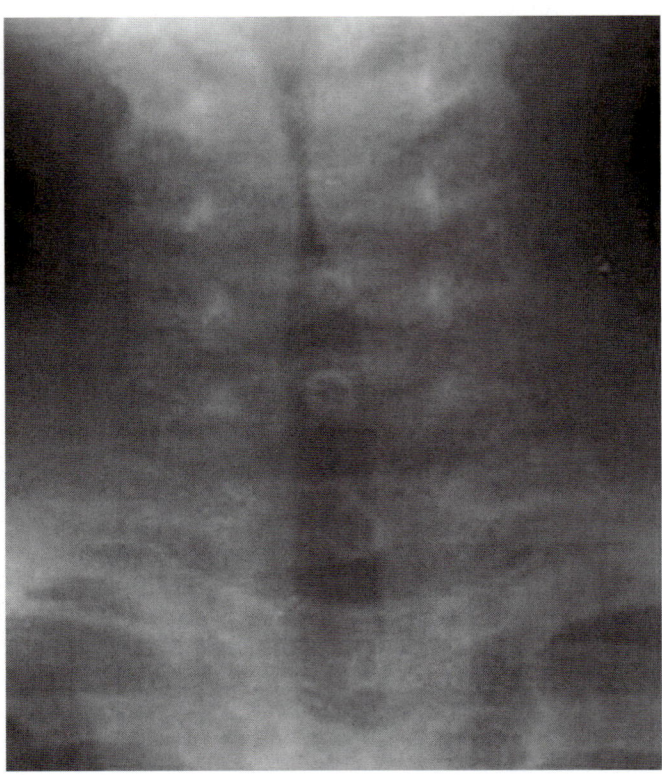

FIGURE 48-11 Frontal radiograph of neck of a child with croup. Notice the narrowing of airway showing the "steeple" sign.

Signs and symptoms of airway obstruction include anxiety, inspiratory stridor, muffled or hoarse voice, drooling, pain in the throat, decreased breath sounds, crackles, rhonchi, and wheezing. The child may have a history of choking (observed by an adult). If a full obstruction cannot be relieved with basic and advanced methods of clearing, direct laryngoscopy to identify the obstruction and removal with McGill forceps may be indicated. Full obstruction calls for immediate intervention to relieve the obstruction. Basic and advanced methods of clearing the airway are presented in Chapter 15.

If a child with a partial obstruction is conscious and has adequate movement of air, the paramedic should not agitate the child. Rather, the paramedic should provide continuous respiratory monitoring. Also, the child should be transported immediately to the hospital. Agitation or attempts to relieve a partial obstruction may cause the foreign body to move. This may lead to full obstruction.

CROUP

Croup (laryngotracheobronchitis) is a common viral infection of the upper airway. It usually occurs in children between the ages of 6 months and 4 years. It often occurs

during the late fall and early winter months. Croup usually is caused by the parainfluenza virus. However, respiratory syncytial virus, rubeola, and adenovirus also can cause croup. Croup may involve the entire respiratory tract with symptoms that are caused by inflammation in the subglottic region (at the level of the larynx extending to the cricoid cartilage) (Figure 48-11).

A child with croup usually has a history of recent upper respiratory tract infection and a low-grade fever. The patient may have hoarseness, inspiratory stridor (from subglottic edema), and a barking cough. Stridor mainly occurs on inspiration, but symptoms may be present on expiration if the lower airways are involved. However, symptoms occur mainly on inspiration. Most often, the emergency episode occurs at night after the child has gone to bed. On EMS arrival, a patient with severe croup may have all the classic signs of respiratory distress. The child may be sitting upright and leaning forward to aid breathing (variable). Also, nasal flaring, intercostal retractions, and cyanosis (a late sign of respiratory insufficiency) may be present. Children with severe croup are at risk of serious airway obstruction from the narrowed diameter of the trachea (Box 48-3).

Prehospital management of croup includes maintenance of airway, administration of cool mist or humidified or nebulized oxygen (per protocol), and transportation in a position of comfort. Symptoms may improve dramatically

BOX 48-3 Stages of Croup

Stage 1—Fever, hoarse, croupy cough, inspiratory stridor

Stage 2—Continuous stridor, intercostal retractions, labored breathing

Stage 3—Signs of hypoxia and hypercarbia with pallor, sweating, tachypnea

Stage 4—Cyanosis, apnea

Treatment

Nebulized racemic epinephrine—peak effect 20 minutes.[13] Signs and symptoms can reappear after 2 hours, when duration of effect is complete.

Cool mist therapy is controversial—not harmful as long as it does not make the child anxious.

Intubation is rarely needed.

Corticosteroids (dexamethasone) have proven to be helpful.[14]

TABLE 48-4 Comparison of the Symptoms of Croup and Epiglottitis

Characteristics	Croup	Epiglottitis
Occurrence	6 months to 4 years	Any age
Onset	Slow; frequently at night	Rapid
Comfortable position	Patient may lie down or sit upright	Patient prefers to sit upright
Cough	Barking cough; may have inspiratory stridor	No barking cough; may have inspiratory stridor
Drooling	No drooling	Drooling, pain on swallowing
Temperature	<104° F	>104° F
Cause	Viral	Bacterial (now uncommon because of Hib vaccination)

in patients with croup after the child is exposed to cool, humidified air. (For example, this may occur after moving the patient from the residence to the emergency vehicle.) Nebulized *racemic epinephrine* may be used to stimulate beta2 receptors in the lungs, resulting in relaxation of the bronchial smooth muscles, thereby relieving the bronchospasm. (See the EDI.) The paramedic should make all efforts to keep the child comfortable and at ease.

EPIGLOTTITIS

Epiglottitis is inflammation of the epiglottis caused by a bacterial infection of the upper airway. Although uncommon, epiglottitis can progress rapidly and become life threatening. It can occur at any age. The disease usually is associated with *Haemophilus influenzae* type B, but *Streptococcus, Pneumococcus,* and *Staphylococcus* organisms also have been implicated. The bacterial infection causes edema and occlusion from swelling of the epiglottis and supraglottic structures (pharynx, aryepiglottic folds, and arytenoid cartilage). Epiglottitis is a true emergency. It requires prompt, expert airway management.

NOTE

The *Haemophilus influenzae* type B (Hib) vaccine has dramatically reduced the number of cases of epiglottitis in children. Before the Hib vaccine was made available in 1985, the incidence of epiglottitis was 41 cases per 100,000 persons. In recent years, this figure has declined to 0.3 cases per 100,000 persons.[15] See Appendix Figures 48-1 and 48-2 for recommended childhood and adolescent immunizations.

Epiglottitis usually begins suddenly. Typically, the child goes to bed without any symptoms and wakes up complaining of a sore throat and pain on swallowing. The child may have fever, a muffled voice (from edema of the mucosal covering of the vocal cords), and drooling from the pooled

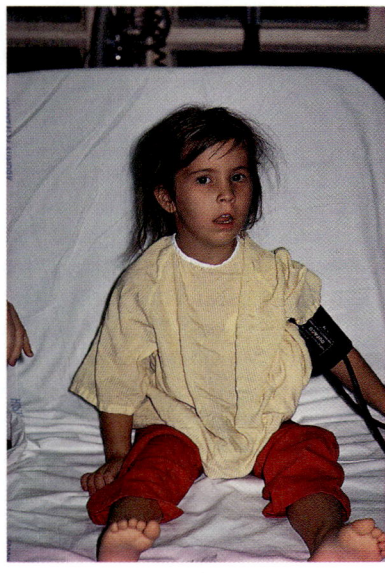

FIGURE 48-12 Acute epiglottitis at presentation.

saliva that occurs because of difficult and painful swallowing (an ominous sign of impending airway obstruction). Differentiating epiglottitis from croup in the prehospital setting may be difficult. Table 48-4 lists the different characteristics of these illnesses.

On arrival, the paramedic usually finds a child with epiglottitis sitting upright (Figure 48-12). Often the child is leaning forward with the head hyperextended. This position aids breathing (tripod position). The tongue may be protruding, or the child may have inspiratory stridor. These children usually do not cry or struggle because all of their attention and energy is being used to maximize air exchange. Inspiratory stridor with a characteristic rattle often is present. The child also may be gasping or gulping for air.

Classic signs of respiratory distress usually are present. The preferred and definitive care for epiglottitis is in-hospital intubation and parenteral antibiotic therapy.

CRITICAL THINKING
What other childhood respiratory problems (traumatic and nontraumatic) can manifest with stridor?

Children with acute epiglottitis are in danger of full airway obstruction and respiratory arrest. Occlusion of the airway can occur suddenly. Occlusion may be caused by minor irritation of the throat, stress, and anxiety. For these reasons, gentle handling of a child suspected of having epiglottitis is essential. The following guidelines in prehospital management should be observed:

- Do not attempt to lay the child down or to change the position of comfort.
- Do not attempt to visualize the airway if the child is still ventilating adequately.
- Advise medical direction of the suspicion of epiglottitis so that appropriate personnel and resources can be made available.
- Administer 100% humidified oxygen by mask unless it provokes agitation.
- Do not attempt vascular access.
- Have the correct-sized emergency airway equipment selected and ready.
- Transport the child to the hospital in the position of comfort.

If respiratory arrest occurs before arrival at the emergency department, the paramedic must attempt intubation. The child's lungs should be hyperventilated and preoxygenated with a bag-valve device before intubation. After the airway has been established, the paramedic should obtain intravenous (IV) access if time allows.

Intubation may be difficult because the vocal cords are likely to be hidden by swollen tissues. (An uncuffed endotracheal tube one to two sizes smaller than normal may be recommended by some medical direction physicians.) The paramedic should locate the opening to the larynx by looking for mucous bubbles in the cleft between the edematous aryepiglottic folds and the swollen epiglottis. (Chest compressions during glottic visualization may produce a bubble at the tracheal opening.) In the rare instance that intubation cannot be achieved and the child cannot be ventilated adequately by a bag-valve device, medical direction may advise needle cricothyrotomy. Often a child's lungs can be ventilated through the occlusive crisis of epiglottitis by bag-valve-mask ventilation using a tight facial seal. This may call for two persons—one to maintain the seal and the other to ventilate.

BACTERIAL TRACHEITIS

Bacterial tracheitis is an uncommon infection (often caused by staphylococcus) of the upper airway and subglottic trachea that may occur after a viral illness. It generally

---

BOX 48-4 Asthma Statistics in Children

- Approximately 40% of children who have asthmatic parents will develop asthma.
- An average of 1 out of every 10 school-aged children has asthma.
- Nine million U.S. children under 18 have been diagnosed with asthma at some point in their lifetime.
- Nearly 4 million children have had an asthma attack in the previous year.
- Asthma is the third leading cause of hospitalization among children under age 15.
- In 2006, 131 children under age 15 died from asthma.[18]

---

occurs in infants and toddlers (1 to 5 years of age), but also can occur in older children. Bacterial tracheitis can lead to airway obstruction that is severe enough to cause respiratory arrest.[16] The signs and symptoms of bacterial tracheitis are those of respiratory distress or failure (depending on the severity) and may include the following:

- Agitation
- Cough that produces pus or mucus
- High-grade fever
- Hoarseness
- Inspiratory and expiratory stridor
- Throat pain

Emergency care is directed at providing airway, ventilatory, and circulatory support and rapid transport for evaluation by a physician. If airway obstruction, respiratory failure, or respiratory arrest develops, tracheal intubation is required with tracheal suction to remove mucus or pus. (Bag-valve-mask ventilation may require high pressures.) In-hospital care includes intravenously administered antibiotics that are specific for the causative organism. These will be given after the child's airway has been stabilized.

ASTHMA

As described in Chapter 24, **asthma** is a chronic inflammatory disorder of the airways that may cause recurrent episodes of wheezing, breathlessness, chest tightness, and cough. Asthma is characterized by inflammation, bronchoconstriction, and mucus production that obstructs the lower airways. Asthma results from autonomic dysfunction or exposure to sensitizing agents. The hallmarks of an acute exacerbation are anxiety, dyspnea, tachypnea, and audible expiratory (and when severe, inspiratory) wheezes with a prolonged expiratory phase. (A silent chest indicates impending respiratory failure.) Asthma is common among children over 2 years of age, but can be difficult to diagnose. (Other respiratory conditions in children can cause similar signs and symptoms.) It affects about 10% of those under 10 years of age (Box 48-4). In 2008 there were an estimated 7 million children with asthma in the United States.[17] An acute exacerbation may be triggered by infection, changes in temperature, physical exercise, emotional response, and exposure to allergens.

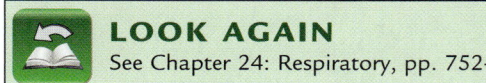

LOOK AGAIN
See Chapter 24: Respiratory, pp. 752-755.

CRITICAL THINKING
What other signs or symptoms would lead you to believe that a child with asthma is decompensating?

The goals of prehospital management include ventilatory assistance (as needed), administration of humidified oxygen, reversal of the bronchospasm, and rapid transport for evaluation and treatment. Severe asthma may be life threatening and can progress rapidly to respiratory failure. The paramedic should be ready to initiate aggressive airway management along with ventilatory and circulatory support. Depending on local protocol, prior medication use, and the recommendations of medical direction, drug therapy may include aerosolized bronchodilators (*albuterol, ipratropium,* or *levalbuterol*), subcutaneously administered *epinephrine* or *terbutaline* with severe respiratory distress or failure, and sometimes corticosteroids (e.g., *methylprednisolone*) during prolonged transports.[19] (See the Emergency Drug Index.) If the patient requires tracheal intubation, medical direction may advise the administration of *magnesium sulfate* and low tidal volumes (5 to 8 mL/kg) to reduce the potential for barotrauma.

BRONCHIOLITIS

Bronchiolitis (like asthma) manifests with tachypnea and wheezing. The illness is caused by viral infections that can cause inflammation of the lower airway. An example of such a virus is the respiratory syncytial virus (RSV). Bronchiolitis usually affects children under 2 years of age. It often occurs in the winter months and generally is associated with upper respiratory tract infection. Bronchiolitis sometimes is unresponsive to therapy aimed at relieving bronchospasm. Table 48-5 lists key features that may aid in the differential diagnosis.

NOTE
RSV is highly contagious, is most common in children under 1 year of age, and usually occurs epidemically in the winter months.[20]

Bronchiolitis generally is not serious and recovery is uneventful. However, sometimes it may become life threatening. Infants are at greater risk of developing respiratory failure from this condition because of the small diameter of the bronchioles. The prehospital care is aimed at providing ventilatory support with humidified oxygen. The patient should be transported rapidly for evaluation by a physician. A therapeutic trial of *albuterol* via nebulizer may

TABLE 48-5 Differentiation of Bronchiolitis and Asthma

Clinical Features	Bronchiolitis	Asthma
Occurrence	Usually <18 months	Any age
Season	Winter, spring	Any time
Family history of asthma	Usually absent	Usually present
Cause	Virus	Allergy, infection, exercise, virus
Response to drugs	Some reversal of bronchospasm with beta agonists	Reversal of bronchospasm

be used as a temporary measure to reduce respiratory distress.[21]

Pneumonia

Pneumonia (described in Chapter 24) is an acute infection of the lower airway and lungs that involves the alveolar walls or the alveoli. Pneumonia commonly is caused by a bacterial or viral infection. Children with pneumonia may have a history of recent airway infection, such as influenza or pertussis. They also may have respiratory distress or failure (depending on the severity) and any of the following:

- Decreased breath sounds in affected area
- Fever
- Pain in the chest
- Rales localized to the affected area
- Rhonchi (localized or diffuse)
- Tachypnea

Most children with pneumonia have only mild signs and symptoms and require no immediate treatment or airway support. However, when respiratory distress is present, stabilization of the airway and provision of oxygenation are the highest priority. In severe cases, bronchodilators may be indicated. Assisted ventilations via a bag-valve device or intubation of the trachea also may be required.

Pertussis

As described in Chapter 28, pertussis primarily affects infants and young children. It is an infectious disease caused by the bacterium *Bordetella pertussis*. It is spread by direct contact with discharges from mucous membranes contained in airborne droplets. Pertussis causes inflammation of the entire respiratory tract. The major complications of pertussis in infants are pneumonia (less than 6 months of age) and apnea (less than 2 months of age). Other possible complications include weight loss, sleep disturbance, and seizures. The incidence of complications is highest in children less than 1 year of age.

Pertussis is commonly associated with episodes of violent and productive coughing with an inspiratory "whoop" or gasp. (High coughing pressure may cause pneumothorax, epistaxis, subconjunctival hemorrhage, and rib fracture.) These coughing episodes can last 1 to 2 months. Most children are vaccinated for this through a series of pertussis vaccines given in combination with diphtheria and tetanus (DPT). (See Appendix, Advanced Practice Procedures in Critical Care.) Respiratory protection for both the patient and the EMS crew is required.

Bronchopulmonary Dysplasia

Bronchopulmonary dysplasia (BPD; formerly known as *chronic lung disease of infancy*) is a rare, chronic lung disease affecting about 12,000 babies in the United States each year.[22] BPD usually occurs in premature infants who receive lung damage from oxygen toxicity and barotrauma attributable to mechanical ventilation early in life. This use of supplemental oxygen can lead to overproduction of *oxygen radicals* (agents of oxygen toxicity). These include superoxide, hydrogen peroxide, and perhydroxyl radicals. Preterm infants are particularly susceptible to oxygen radicals because the antioxidant systems are developed in the last trimester of pregnancy. Prolonged hyperoxia begins a sequence of lung injury that leads to inflammation, diffuse alveolar damage, pulmonary dysfunction, and death.[23] The classic diagnosis of BPD may be assigned at 28 days of life if the following criteria are met[24]:

- Positive-pressure ventilation during the first 2 weeks of life for a minimum of 3 days
- Clinical signs of abnormal respiratory function
- Requirements for supplemental oxygen for longer than 28 days of age to maintain PaO_2 above 50 mm Hg
- Chest radiograph with diffuse abnormal findings characteristic of BPD

Children with BPD often suffer from recurrent respiratory tract infections and exercise-induced bronchospasm. The primary goal for infants with BPD is to promote growth and development. Cornerstones of treatment are utilizing pulmonary support to maintain optimal oxygen saturation and preventing complications. In addition, nutritional support is needed to promote growth. As infants grow, lung function improves and the risk of severe cardiopulmonary complications and morbidity and mortality attributable to respiratory tract infection decline.

Treatment therapies for children with BPD may include dietary and vitamin supplementation, fluid restriction, and use of diuretics, inhaled bronchodilators, and corticosteroids. Oxygen therapy through continuous positive airway pressure (CPAP) and bilevel positive airway pressure (BiPAP) to maintain oxygen saturation at or above 92% during eating, sleeping, and periods of crying is recommended. (Continuous pulse oximetry is often prescribed to monitor oxygen saturation levels.) While providing emergency care, airway management may include positioning of the airway, using oral or nasal

---

BOX 48-5 Signs and Symptoms of Compensated and Decompensated Shock

Compensated (Reversible)
Cool, pale extremities
Decreased urinary output
Delayed capillary refill
Irritability or anxiety
Normal systolic blood pressure
Tachycardia
Tachypnea
Weak peripheral pulses/full central pulses

Decompensated (Often Irreversible)
Absent peripheral pulses/weak central pulses
Cool, pale, dusky, mottled extremities
Hypotension
Lethargy or coma
Marked tachycardia or bradycardia
Marked tachypnea or bradypnea
Significantly decreased urinary output
Significantly delayed capillary refill

---

adjuncts, and providing suction and assisted ventilations. In severe cases, endotracheal intubation may be required. Following stabilization, treatment of infants with BPD involves steps to minimize additional lung damage and prevent pulmonary hypertension and cor pulmonale. Infants with severe disease may be dependent on supplemental oxygen or mechanical ventilation for months. Some will have symptoms of airway obstruction for years. Therapy usually is supportive throughout the course of the disease.

Shock

As described in Chapter 36, shock is an abnormal condition characterized by inadequate delivery of oxygen to meet the metabolic demands of tissues. The condition may occur with increased, normal, or decreased blood pressure. Shock is categorized as *compensated* (shock without hypotension) or *decompensated* (shock with hypotension) (Box 48-5), and is further categorized as cardiogenic and noncardiogenic. *Cardiogenic shock* is characterized by adequate intravascular volume, but myocardial dysfunction limits stroke volume and cardiac output. *Noncardiac shock* can be hypovolemic shock from loss of volume. It may also be distributive shock (septic, neurogenic, or anaphylactic).

The paramedic must take into account a number of special considerations when caring for a child in shock. These include circulating blood volume, body surface area and hypothermia, cardiac reserve, respiratory fatigue, vital signs, and assessment.

TABLE 48-6 Systolic Blood Pressure Characterizing Hypotension in the Pediatric Patient

Age	Systolic Blood Pressure
Term neonates (birth to 28 days of age)	<60 mm Hg
Infants (1 to 12 months)	<70 mm Hg
Children (1 to 10 years)	<70 mm Hg (2 × age in years)
Beyond 10 years	<90 mm Hg

CIRCULATING BLOOD VOLUME

In adults, blood volume accounts for 5% to 6% of total body weight, or 50 to 60 mL/kg of body weight; in children, blood volume accounts for 7% to 8% of total body weight, or 70 to 80 mL/kg of body weight.[25] Although the percentage of circulating blood volume in a child is greater than that in an adult, a child's actual blood volume is considerably lower than an adult's. Therefore a relatively small loss of blood may be devastating. For example, a blood loss of 100 mL in an adult is a 2% loss; a 100 mL loss in an infant is a 15% to 20% loss, resulting in shock.[1]

A child with a blood or fluid deficit will maintain stable hemodynamics until all compensatory mechanisms fail (i.e., the blood pressure may be normal or only slightly decreased) (Table 48-6). At that point, shock progresses rapidly, with serious deterioration. These efficient compensatory mechanisms can mask a potentially life-threatening condition. Thus the paramedic must maintain a high degree of suspicion, based on the patient's complaint or clinical presentation. Early recognition, stabilization (airway control, fluid replacement), and rapid transport to a proper facility are critical when caring for children in shock. Treatment must be focused on ventilation, fluid administration, and improvement of the pumping action of the heart.

CRITICAL THINKING

How comfortable are you with starting an intravenous infusion on an infant or young child?

BODY SURFACE AREA AND HYPOTHERMIA

Young children have a large body surface area in proportion to body weight. Their compensatory mechanisms (e.g., shivering and sweating) also are not well developed. Children in shock quickly can develop hypothermia from exposure and concurrent metabolic acidosis, increased vascular resistance, respiratory depression, and myocardial dysfunction. Hypothermia makes resuscitation and drug therapy less effective. Thus the paramedic should maintain the

patient's body temperature by using blankets, covering the child's head with towels, and using warming devices for IV fluids.

CARDIAC RESERVE

Infants and children already have high metabolic needs. As a result, they have less cardiac reserve than adults for stressful situations such as shock. An important step is to reduce the energy and oxygen requirements of a child in shock as much as possible. This can be accomplished by providing ventilatory support, reducing anxiety, and maintaining moderate ambient temperatures.

RESPIRATORY FATIGUE

Respiratory muscle fatigue may lead to hypoventilation, hypoxemia, and respiratory failure or arrest. Like other compensatory mechanisms of the child, respiratory compensation generally is at a maximum until it is depleted. At that time, deterioration can be sudden. For this reason, airway control and supplemental oxygen administration are essential in all children who are seriously ill or injured.

VITAL SIGNS AND ASSESSMENT

The paramedic must consider many factors when evaluating a child's vital signs. For example, blood pressure and pulse rate vary greatly with age, body temperature, and degree of agitation. The paramedic should measure vital signs as baseline assessments, even though they may be of limited value in assessing the circulation of a child in shock. The most effective assessment is constant monitoring of the child's mental and physical status and the response to therapy. The following nine evaluation components should be noted when assessing a child in shock:

1. Level of consciousness
   Ability to make eye contact
   Ability to recognize family members
   Agitation
   Anxiety
2. Skin
   Capillary refill (in children under 6 years of age)
   Color
   Moisture
   Temperature
   Turgor
3. Mucous membranes
   Color
   Moisture
4. Nail beds
   Capillary refill (in children younger than 6 years of age)
   Color
5. Peripheral circulation
   Collapse
   Distention
6. Cardiac
   Electrocardiogram findings
   Location of pulses

Quality of pulses
Rate
Rhythm
7. Respiration
Depth
Rate
8. Blood pressure (in children over 3 years of age) with appropriate sized cuff
9. Body temperature

> ### NOTE
> Sustained tachycardia in the absence of obvious causes such as fever, pain, and agitation may be an early sign of cardiovascular compromise. Bradycardia, however, may be a preterminal cardiac rhythm indicating advanced shock and often is associated with hypotension.[6]

HYPOVOLEMIA

One common cause of hypovolemia in children is dehydration resulting from vomiting and diarrhea. Another is blood loss resulting from trauma or internal bleeding. Children are also at risk of intravascular volume depletion as a result of burns (see Chapter 39).

Dehydration. Profound fluid and electrolyte imbalances can occur in children as a result of vomiting, diarrhea, poor fluid intake, fever, or burns. Dehydration compromises cardiac output and systemic perfusion. This occurs if the child loses the fluid equivalent of 5% or more of total body weight. For the adolescent, losses of 5% to 7% of total body weight can compromise perfusion (Figure 48-13). If allowed to progress, dehydration can result in renal failure, shock, and death. The severity of the dehydration and fluid loss can be estimated from a history of the child's weight loss and the physical examination (Figure 48-14). Table 48-7 provides signs and symptoms related to degrees of dehydration.

Airway and ventilatory support (if needed) are the initial steps in treatment for the dehydrated child. Next, treatment is directed at replacing and maintaining blood volume and perfusion. Intravenous therapy should be initiated with isotonic crystalloids such as lactated Ringer's solution or normal saline.[6] A fluid bolus of 20 mL/kg (administered in less than 20 minutes)[1] should be given even if blood pressure is normal.[6] Fluid boluses may be repeated if the patient's systemic perfusion fails to improve. After physician evaluation and initial shock resuscitation, the fluid administration rate and type of fluid replacement are determined by the volume and type of fluid deficit (isotonic,

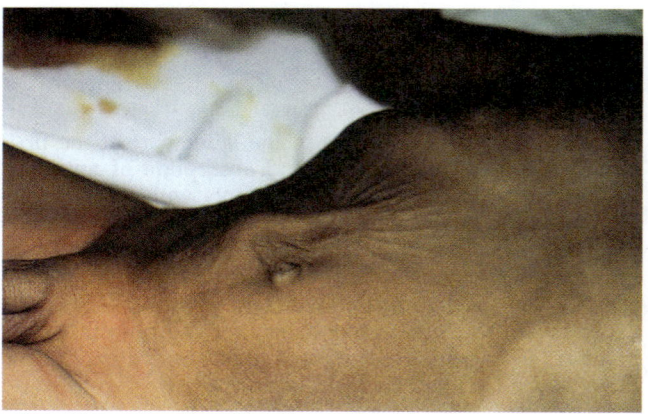

FIGURE 48-13 Severe dehydration.

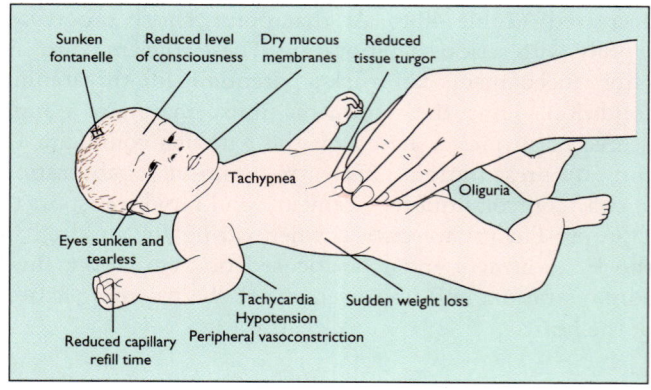

FIGURE 48-14 Clinical features of dehydration in an infant.

TABLE 48-7   Assessment of Degree of Dehydration

Clinical Parameters	Mild	Moderate	Severe
Body weight loss	Infant: 5% (50 mL/kg)	10% (100 mL/kg)	15% (150 mL/kg)
Skin turgor	Slightly decreased	Moderately decreased	Greatly decreased
Fontanelle (infant)	Possibly flat or depressed	Depressed	Significantly depressed
Mucous membranes	Dry	Very dry	Parched
Skin perfusion	Warm with normal color	Cool (extremities), pale	Cold (extremities), mottled or gray
Heart rate	Mildly tachycardic	Moderately tachycardic	Extremely tachycardic
Peripheral pulses	Normal	Diminished	Absent
Blood pressure	Normal	Normal	Reduced
Sensorium	Normal or irritable	Irritable or lethargic	Unresponsive

TABLE 48-8 Classification of Hemorrhagic Shock in Pediatric Trauma Patients Based on Systemic Signs

System	Very Mild Hemorrhage*	Mild Hemorrhage†	Moderate Hemorrhage‡	Severe Hemorrhage§
Cardiovascular	Normal or mildly increased heart rate	Tachycardia	Significant tachycardia	Severe tachycardia
	Normal pulse rate	Peripheral pulses may be diminished	Thready peripheral pulses	Thready central pulses
	Normal blood pressure	Normal blood pressure	Hypotension	Significant hypotension
	Normal pH	Normal pH	Metabolic acidosis	Significant acidosis
Respiratory	Normal rate	Tachypnea	Moderate tachypnea	Severe tachypnea
Central nervous system	Slight anxiousness	Irritability, confusion	Irritability or lethargy	Lethargy
		Combative affect	Diminished pain response	Coma
Skin	Warm, pink color	Cool extremities, mottling	Cool extremities, mottling or pallor	Cold extremities, pallor or cyanosis
	Brisk capillary refill	Delayed capillary refill	Prolonged capillary refill	Prolonged capillary refill
Kidneys	Normal urine output	Oliguria, increased specific gravity	Oliguria, increased blood urea nitrogen level	Anuria

*Indicates <15% blood volume loss.
†Indicates 15% to 25% blood volume loss.
‡Indicates 25% blood volume loss.
§Indicates 40% blood volume loss.

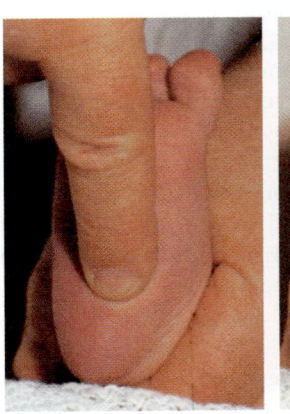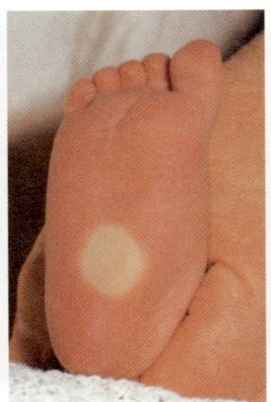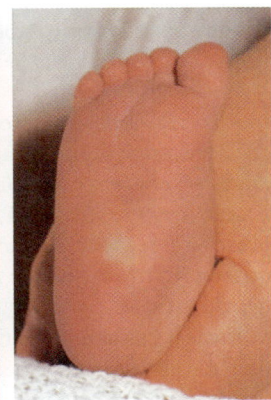

FIGURE 48-15 Capillary refill in a child in shock.

hypotonic, hypertonic) and the patient's response to therapy.

 CRITICAL THINKING
What are some ways to determine the child's weight for fluid and drug dosing?

Blood Loss. As stated before, even a small amount of blood loss can be serious for the pediatric patient (Table 48-8). After the paramedic achieves control of external hemorrhage (if present), secures the patient's airway, and provides high-concentration oxygen, the child's circulatory status may require support with IV therapy.

As with other causes of hypovolemia, volume replacement is needed. Isotonic crystalloid solutions such as normal saline or lactated Ringer's solution should be used.

The first bolus should be 20 mL/kg.[1] If the volume loss is in the 20% range, vital signs should improve after this infusion. If improvement occurs, IV therapy should be continued at a maintenance rate during patient transport. The child may show little response to the first bolus. For example, a slight improvement in color and capillary refill and a decreased heart rate may be evident (Figure 48-15). If this is the case or if the patient does not respond to the initial infusion, the paramedic should give a second bolus of 20 mL/kg.[6]

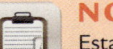 **NOTE**
Establishing an intravenous line in a child through a peripheral vein (described in Chapter 14) can be difficult even in the most controlled settings. As a result, medical direction may advise that the paramedic establish an intraosseous infusion for the child in shock.

DISTRIBUTIVE SHOCK

As described previously, distributive shock is used to refer to septic shock, neurogenic shock, and anaphylactic shock. This type of shock results in peripheral pooling because of loss of vasomotor tone. The vasodilation that occurs causes the blood pressure to fall. Vasodilation also allows plasma to leak from the vascular space. This type of shock is fairly uncommon in children.

Septic shock usually is caused by a systemic bacterial infection. Septic shock sometimes is associated with illnesses such as meningitis and pneumonia. Toxins released by the pathogen affect arterioles, capillaries, and venules, altering microcirculatory pressure and capillary permeability. These children usually appear very ill. They may have signs and symptoms that include those of decompensated shock. Characteristic findings in septic shock include skin that is warm in the early stages, and skin that is cool in the late stages of the illness.

Neurogenic shock results from sudden peripheral vasodilation caused by a traumatic injury. Most often this injury is to the spinal cord. The loss of sympathetic impulses and resultant vasodilation increase the size of the vascular compartment. The normal intravascular volume is not enough to fill the vascular compartment and to perfuse tissues. Characteristic findings in neurogenic shock include warm skin, bradycardia, and impaired neurological function.

Anaphylactic shock occurs when a person is exposed to a substance that produces a severe allergic reaction (see Chapter 27). Common causes of allergic reactions include antibiotic agents, foods, and insect stings. The bodily response to the antigen causes a release of histamine. This release results in peripheral vasodilation and the leakage of intravascular fluid into the interstitial space, resulting in a decrease in intravascular volume. Characteristic findings in anaphylactic shock include a rapid onset of skin signs (hives, allergic rash, and erythema), upper airway obstruction or dyspnea, signs of shock, and gastrointestinal distress.

Emergency care for patients with distributive shock is directed at ensuring the patient's vital functions through airway, ventilatory, and circulatory support, and rapid transport to an appropriate medical facility. Medical direction may advise IV fluid therapy and drugs to manage specific forms of distributive shock. (For example, *dopamine* may be given for neurogenic shock; *epinephrine* should be given for anaphylactic shock.) Aids that often are used to calculate drug and fluid doses for pediatric patients were described in Chapter 14. These aids include the Pedi-Wheel and the Broselow tape (Figure 48-16).

LOOK AGAIN

See Chapter 14: Venous Access and Medication Administration, pp. 345-347.

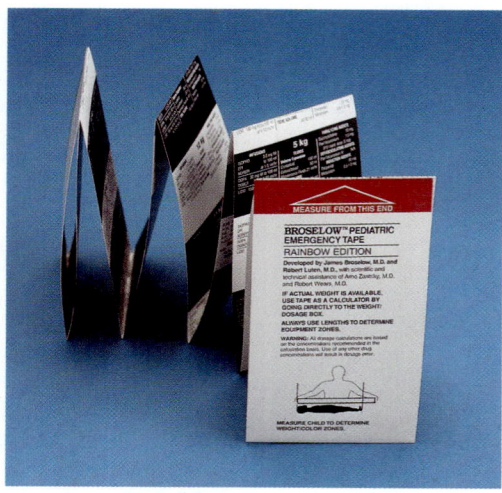

FIGURE 48-16 Pediatric Broselow tape.

Congestive Heart Failure. Congestive heart failure in children may result from cardiomyopathy, myocarditis, and congenital heart diseases. To review, *myocarditis* is inflammation of the heart. *Cardiomyopathy* refers to degeneration of the heart muscle that causes a reduction in the force of heart contractions. Both conditions decrease the force of contractions and the amount of blood circulated to the lungs and to the rest of the body. In children, congestive heart failure usually results from viral infection or congenital abnormalities that affect both ventricles of the heart (described in the following sections). Symptoms include fatigue, chest pain, and dysrhythmias. In severe cases, they include signs of heart failure and cardiogenic shock, such as the following:

- Crackles
- Hypotension
- Jugular vein distention (difficult to determine in young children)
- Peripheral edema
- Tachycardia
- Tachypnea

Patients in stable condition are managed with supportive care, oxygen administration, and transport for evaluation by a physician. Children who are hypotensive and show other signs and symptoms of decompensation may require vascular access for the administration of drugs (e.g., antidysrhythmics, diuretics, and vasopressors). Intravenous fluid therapy should be given to children in shock with signs of CHF in small boluses of 5 to 10 mL/kg.[1] This will help to avoid volume overload

Rhythm Disturbances

Most children are born with healthy hearts. (Congenital heart defects are presented in Chapter 47.) When rhythm disturbances occur, they usually are the result of hypoxia, acidosis, hypotension, or structural heart disease.[6] The most common dysrhythmias in pediatric patients are sinus tachycardia, supraventricular tachycardia, bradycardia, and asystole. Pulseless ventricular tachycardia or ventricular fibrillation is the initial rhythm in 5%-15% of pediatric cardiac arrests and is reported in up to 27% of pediatric in-hospital arrests at some point during the resuscitation.[6] The recommended management for these dysrhythmias is outlined in Figures 48-17 to 48-19. Drug treatments and specific guidelines for use of airway equipment during pediatric life support are listed in Tables 48-9 and 48-10.

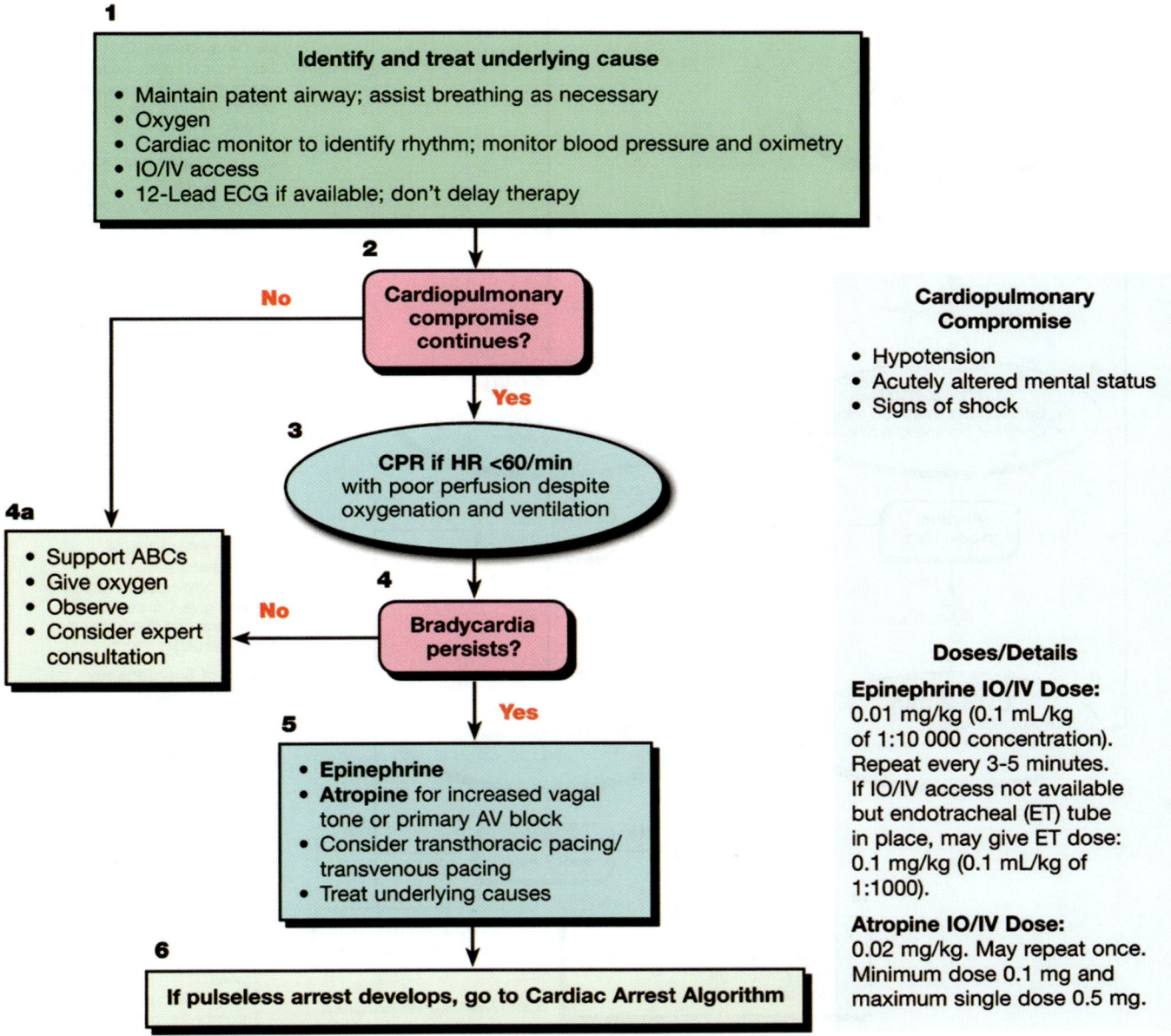

Pediatric Bradycardia
With a Pulse and Poor Perfusion

1
Identify and treat underlying cause
- Maintain patent airway; assist breathing as necessary
- Oxygen
- Cardiac monitor to identify rhythm; monitor blood pressure and oximetry
- IO/IV access
- 12-Lead ECG if available; don't delay therapy

2
Cardiopulmonary compromise continues?
— No
— Yes

3
CPR if HR <60/min with poor perfusion despite oxygenation and ventilation

4a
- Support ABCs
- Give oxygen
- Observe
- Consider expert consultation

4
Bradycardia persists?
— No
— Yes

5
- **Epinephrine**
- **Atropine** for increased vagal tone or primary AV block
- Consider transthoracic pacing/ transvenous pacing
- Treat underlying causes

6
If pulseless arrest develops, go to Cardiac Arrest Algorithm

Cardiopulmonary Compromise
- Hypotension
- Acutely altered mental status
- Signs of shock

Doses/Details

Epinephrine IO/IV Dose:
0.01 mg/kg (0.1 mL/kg of 1:10 000 concentration). Repeat every 3-5 minutes. If IO/IV access not available but endotracheal (ET) tube in place, may give ET dose: 0.1 mg/kg (0.1 mL/kg of 1:1000).

Atropine IO/IV Dose:
0.02 mg/kg. May repeat once. Minimum dose 0.1 mg and maximum single dose 0.5 mg.

© 2010 American Heart Association

FIGURE 48-17 Algorithm for bradycardia in a pediatric patient. (Reprinted with permission, American Heart Association Guidelines For CPR and ECC, *Circulation 122* [suppl 3]:S685-S919, American Heart Association, Inc, 2010.)

Pediatric Cardiac Arrest

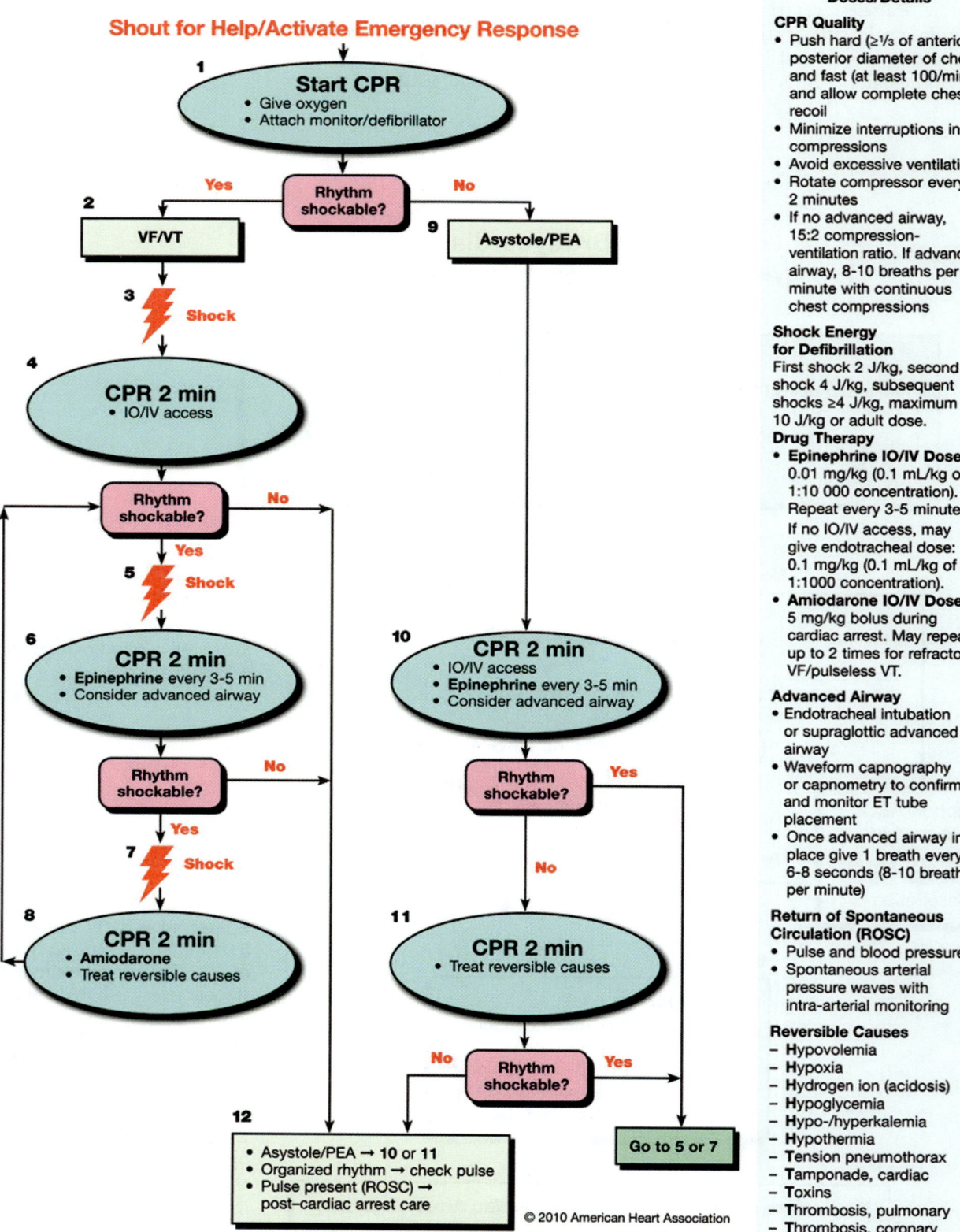

Shout for Help/Activate Emergency Response

1 **Start CPR**
- Give oxygen
- Attach monitor/defibrillator

Rhythm shockable? — Yes / No

2 VF/VT

3 Shock

4 CPR 2 min
- IO/IV access

Rhythm shockable? — No

5 Shock — Yes

6 CPR 2 min
- **Epinephrine** every 3-5 min
- Consider advanced airway

Rhythm shockable? — No

7 Shock — Yes

8 CPR 2 min
- **Amiodarone**
- Treat reversible causes

9 Asystole/PEA

10 CPR 2 min
- IO/IV access
- **Epinephrine** every 3-5 min
- Consider advanced airway

Rhythm shockable? — Yes

No

11 CPR 2 min
- Treat reversible causes

Rhythm shockable? — No / Yes

12
- Asystole/PEA → **10** or **11**
- Organized rhythm → check pulse
- Pulse present (ROSC) → post–cardiac arrest care

Go to 5 or 7

© 2010 American Heart Association

Doses/Details

CPR Quality
- Push hard (≥⅓ of anterior-posterior diameter of chest) and fast (at least 100/min) and allow complete chest recoil
- Minimize interruptions in compressions
- Avoid excessive ventilation
- Rotate compressor every 2 minutes
- If no advanced airway, 15:2 compression-ventilation ratio. If advanced airway, 8-10 breaths per minute with continuous chest compressions

Shock Energy for Defibrillation
First shock 2 J/kg, second shock 4 J/kg, subsequent shocks ≥4 J/kg, maximum 10 J/kg or adult dose.

Drug Therapy
- **Epinephrine IO/IV Dose:** 0.01 mg/kg (0.1 mL/kg of 1:10 000 concentration). Repeat every 3-5 minutes. If no IO/IV access, may give endotracheal dose: 0.1 mg/kg (0.1 mL/kg of 1:1000 concentration).
- **Amiodarone IO/IV Dose:** 5 mg/kg bolus during cardiac arrest. May repeat up to 2 times for refractory VF/pulseless VT.

Advanced Airway
- Endotracheal intubation or supraglottic advanced airway
- Waveform capnography or capnometry to confirm and monitor ET tube placement
- Once advanced airway in place give 1 breath every 6-8 seconds (8-10 breaths per minute)

Return of Spontaneous Circulation (ROSC)
- Pulse and blood pressure
- Spontaneous arterial pressure waves with intra-arterial monitoring

Reversible Causes
- **Hypovolemia**
- **Hypoxia**
- **Hydrogen ion (acidosis)**
- **Hypoglycemia**
- **Hypo-/hyperkalemia**
- **Hypothermia**
- **Tension pneumothorax**
- **Tamponade, cardiac**
- **Toxins**
- **Thrombosis, pulmonary**
- **Thrombosis, coronary**

FIGURE 48-18 Pediatric advanced life support pulseless arrest algorithm. (Reprinted with permission, American Heart Association Guidelines For CPR and ECC, *Circulation 122* [suppl 3]:S685-S919, American Heart Association, Inc, 2010.)

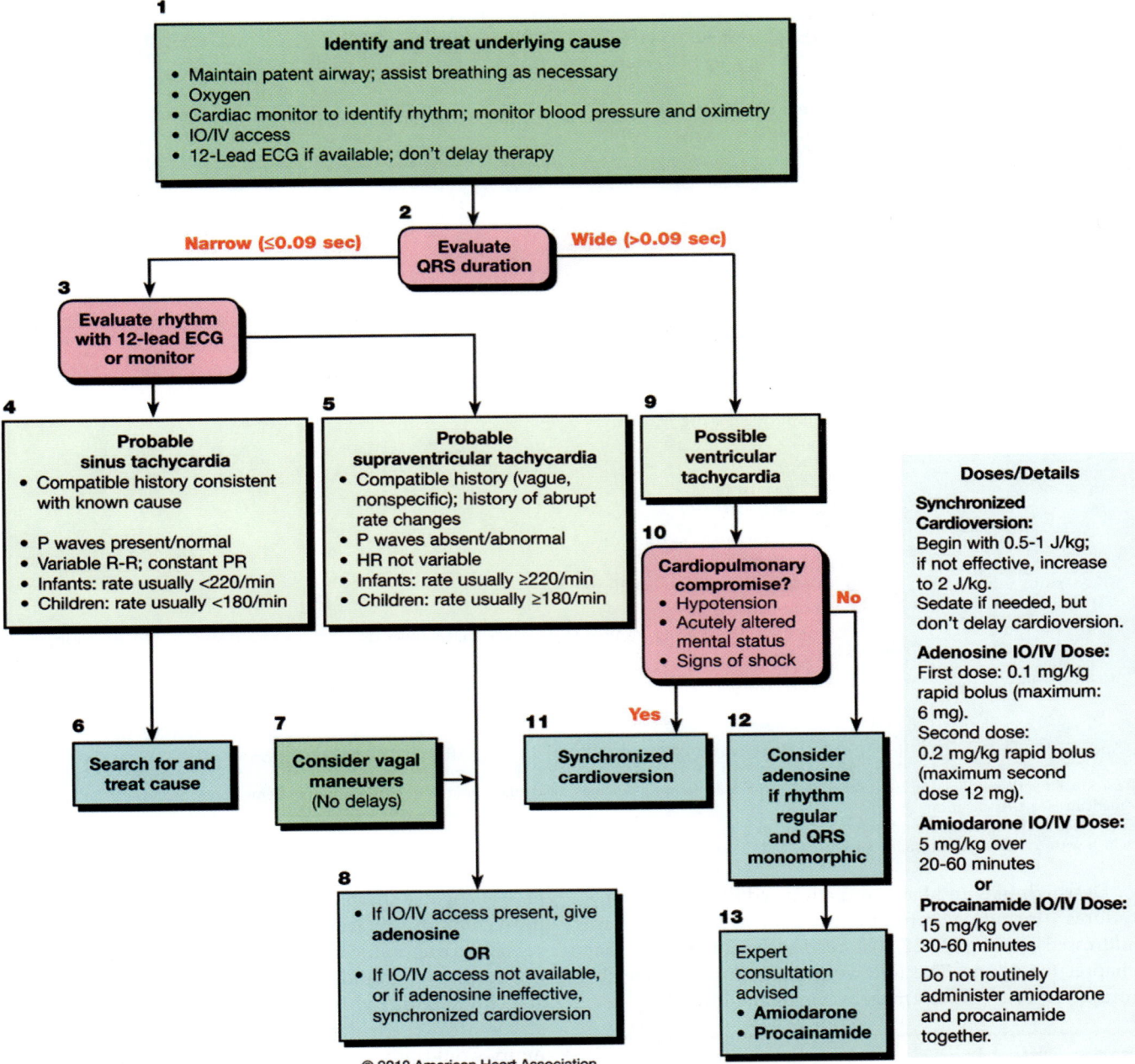

Pediatric Tachycardia
With a Pulse and Poor Perfusion

1

Identify and treat underlying cause
- Maintain patent airway; assist breathing as necessary
- Oxygen
- Cardiac monitor to identify rhythm; monitor blood pressure and oximetry
- IO/IV access
- 12-Lead ECG if available; don't delay therapy

2 Evaluate QRS duration

Narrow (≤0.09 sec)   **Wide (>0.09 sec)**

3 Evaluate rhythm with 12-lead ECG or monitor

4 Probable sinus tachycardia
- Compatible history consistent with known cause
- P waves present/normal
- Variable R-R; constant PR
- Infants: rate usually <220/min
- Children: rate usually <180/min

5 Probable supraventricular tachycardia
- Compatible history (vague, nonspecific); history of abrupt rate changes
- P waves absent/abnormal
- HR not variable
- Infants: rate usually ≥220/min
- Children: rate usually ≥180/min

9 Possible ventricular tachycardia

10 Cardiopulmonary compromise?
- Hypotension
- Acutely altered mental status
- Signs of shock

No

6 Search for and treat cause

7 Consider vagal maneuvers (No delays)

11 Synchronized cardioversion   **Yes**

12 Consider adenosine if rhythm regular and QRS monomorphic

8
- If IO/IV access present, give **adenosine**
  OR
- If IO/IV access not available, or if adenosine ineffective, synchronized cardioversion

13 Expert consultation advised
- **Amiodarone**
- **Procainamide**

Doses/Details

Synchronized Cardioversion:
Begin with 0.5-1 J/kg; if not effective, increase to 2 J/kg. Sedate if needed, but don't delay cardioversion.

Adenosine IO/IV Dose:
First dose: 0.1 mg/kg rapid bolus (maximum: 6 mg).
Second dose: 0.2 mg/kg rapid bolus (maximum second dose 12 mg).

Amiodarone IO/IV Dose:
5 mg/kg over 20-60 minutes
or
Procainamide IO/IV Dose:
15 mg/kg over 30-60 minutes

Do not routinely administer amiodarone and procainamide together.

© 2010 American Heart Association

FIGURE 48-19 Pediatric advanced life support tachycardia algorithm for infants and children with rapid rhythm and adequate perfusion. (Reprinted with permission, American Heart Association Guidelines For CPR and ECC, *Circulation 122* [suppl 3]:S685-S919, American Heart Association, Inc, 2010.)

TABLE 48-9 Medications for Pediatric Resuscitation and Dysrhythmias

Medication	Dose	Remarks
Adenosine	0.1 mg/kg (maximum 6 mg) Repeat: 0.2 mg/kg (maximum 12 mg)	Monitor ECG Rapid IV/IO bolus
Amiodarone	5 mg/kg IV/IO; repeat this dose up to total dose of 15 mg/kg Maximum (single dose): 300 mg	Monitor ECG and blood pressure Adjust administration rate to urgency (give more slowly when perfusing rhythm present) Use caution when administering with other drugs that prolong QT (consider expert consultation)
Atropine	0.02 mg/kg IV/IO 0.04-0.06 mg/kg ET* Repeat once if needed Minimum dose: 0.1 mg Maximum single dose: Child 0.5 mg	Higher doses may be used with organophosphate poisoning
Calcium chloride (10%)	20 mg/kg IV/IO (0.2 mL/kg)	Slowly
Epinephrine	0.01 mg/kg (0.1 mL/kg 1:10,000) IV/IO 0.1 mg/kg (0.1 mL/kg 1:1000) ET† Maximum dose: 1 mg IV/IO	May repeat every 3-5 min in arrest
Glucose	0.5-1 g/kg IV/IO	$D_{10}W$: 5-10 mL/kg $D_{25}W$: 2-4 mL/kg
Lidocaine	Bolus: 1 mg/kg IV/IO Maximum dose: 100 mg Infusion: 20-50 mcg/kg/min ET†: 2-3 mg/kg	
Magnesium sulfate	25-50 mg/kg IV/IO over 10-20 min; Maximum dose: 2 g	
Naloxone	<5 yr or ≤≤20 kg: 0.1 mg/kg IV/IO ≥≥5 yr or >20 kg: 2 mg IV/IO	Use lower doses to reverse respiratory depression associated with therapeutic opioid use (1-5 mcg/kg)
Procainamide	15 mg/kg IV/IO over 30-60 min	Monitor ECG and blood pressure Use caution when administering with other drugs that prolong QT (consider expert consultation)
Sodium bicarbonate	1 mEq/kg per dose IV/IO slowly	After adequate ventilation

Reproduced with permission. 2010 American Heart Association guidelines for cardiopulmonary resuscitation and emergency cardiovascular care, 2010, American Heart Association.

ECG, Electrocardiogram; *ET,* endotracheal tube; *mcg,* micrograms; *IO,* intraosseous; *IV,* intravenous.

*Flush with 5 mL of normal saline and follow with 5 ventilations.

Dysrhythmias and basic and advanced life support procedures (including cardiopulmonary resuscitation) are addressed in Chapter 22. The reader should refer to that chapter for review. The following discussions outline the unique aspects of abnormal rhythms in children.[6]

> **NOTE**
> Even though short-term initial resuscitation rates for infants and children in cardiac arrest have improved, survival to hospital discharge remains very low, at about 6%.[6]

BRADYDYSRHYTHMIAS

Clinically significant bradycardia is defined as a heart rate less than 60 beats/min (or a rapidly dropping heart rate) associated with poor systemic perfusion. This bradycardia occurs despite adequate oxygenation and ventilation. Bradydysrhythmias may be caused by hypoxemia, acidosis, hypotension, hypoglycemia, central nervous system injury, or excessive vagal stimulation (e.g., from endotracheal intubation or pharyngeal suctioning). In infants and children, sinus bradycardia, sinus node arrest with slow junctional or idioventricular rhythm, and atrioventricular block are the most common preterminal rhythms. The paramedic should consider drug-induced causes (e.g., digitalis toxicity) and myocarditis with bradycardia caused by heart block. Infants and children with a history of heart surgery may have injury at the atrioventricular node or conduction system. This injury would produce sick sinus syndrome or heart block. All symptomatic bradycardias require treatment. Important electrocardiogram findings include the following:

- Heart rate is less than 60 beats/min.
- P waves may or may not be visible.
- QRS complex duration may be normal or prolonged.
- The P wave and QRS complex often are unrelated.

Treatment. The initial management of bradycardia should ensure that breathing is adequate and the patient is receiving supplemental oxygen (Figure 48-17). (Mechanical problems with oxygen delivery should be assessed before drug administration.) If pulses, perfusion, and respirations are adequate, no emergency treatment is necessary.[6] Monitor and proceed with evaluation. If drug therapy is required, *epinephrine* is the drug of choice. Bradycardia

TABLE 48-10 Equipment Selection for Pediatric Tracheal Intubation

Age	Weight (kg)	Blade Size	Blade Type	Tracheal Tube Size (mm)	Tracheal Tube	Tracheal Tube Length (cm at lip)	Stylet (F)
Newborn/small infant (0-3 months)	3-5	0-1	Straight	2.5-3.5†	Uncuffed	10-10.5	6
Infant (3-6 months)	6-7	1	Straight	3.5 3.0	Uncuffed Cuffed	10-10.5	6
Infant (7-10 months)	8-9	1	Straight	3.5 3.0	Uncuffed Cuffed	10.5-12	6
Toddler (11-18 months)	10-11	1	Straight	4 3.5	Uncuffed Cuffed	11-12	6
Small child (19-35 months)	12-14	2	Straight	4.5 4.0	Uncuffed Cuffed	12.5-13.5	6
Child (3-4 years)	15-18	2	Straight or curved	5 4.5	Uncuffed Cuffed	14-15	6
Child (5-6 years)	19-22	2	Straight or curved	5.5 5.0	Uncuffed Cuffed	15.5-16.5	14
Large child (7-9 years)	24-30	2-3	Straight or curved	6	Cuffed	17-18	14
Adult (10-12 years)	32-40	3	Straight or curved	6.5	Cuffed	18.5-19.5	14

Based on Broselow Resuscitation Tape.
*Use 2.5 for premature infant. Use 3.0-3.5 for term infant.

caused by heart block or increased vagal tone (both of which are rare in pediatric patients) should be managed with *atropine.* In cases where bradycardia is caused by dysfunction in the sinus node, external cardiac pacing may be lifesaving. Pacing is not useful for asystole or bradycardia attributable to postarrest hypoxic/ischemic myocardial insult or respiratory failure.[6] External cardiac pacing is uncomfortable. Its use in children is reserved for profound symptomatic bradycardia that does not respond to advanced life support and basic life support treatments.

PULSELESS ELECTRICAL ACTIVITY

Pulseless electrical activity often precedes asystole. It usually is caused by prolonged periods of hypoxia, ischemia, or hypercarbia. Reversible causes of pulseless electrical activity include the *H's* and *T's* (described in Chapter 22). To review, the *H's* are hypovolemia, hypoxemia, hypothermia, hyper/hypokalemia, hydrogen ion excess (acidosis), and hypoglycemia. The *T's* are tension pneumothorax, pericardial tamponade, toxins, and thromboembolus (Box 48-6). Important electrocardiogram findings include the following:
- A slow, wide-complex rhythm
- The presence of some electrical activity (other than ventricular tachycardia/ventricular fibrillation) and the absence of a detectable pulse

Treatment. Pulseless electrical activity (PEA) is managed in the same way as asystole (Figure 48-18) with drug therapy (*epinephrine*) and cardiopulmonary resuscitation. Defibrillation is not effective in the treatment of PEA and asystolic

arrest.[6] Reversible causes of the condition should be considered and corrected if possible. Identification and treatment of the underlying cause is the only true means of reversal of pulseless electrical activity. Early recognition and treatment of pulseless electrical activity that results in a return of a pulse before arrival in the emergency department is associated with improved chances for survival.

> **NOTE**
> The survival of children under 18 years of age who suffer cardiac arrest in the out-of-hospital setting is rare. Of those who are discharged, only a small percentage remain neurologically intact.[26] Paramedics should be prepared to deal with intense emotion related to unsuccessful resuscitation and seek appropriate support services (see Chapter 2).

SUPRAVENTRICULAR TACHYCARDIA

Supraventricular tachycardia is the most common nonarrest dysrhythmia during childhood and is the most common dysrhythmia that produces cardiovascular instability during infancy.[6] Two factors can help distinguish supraventricular tachycardia from sinus tachycardia caused by shock. They include patient history (e.g., dehydration or hemorrhage associated with shock) and heart rate. (Sinus tachycardia is usually less than 220 beats/min in infants, usually less than 180 beats/min in children, and usually greater than those rates with supraventricular tachycardia.)

Important electrocardiogram findings in supraventricular tachycardia include the following:

- Heart rate is greater than 220 beats/min in infants and greater than 180 beats/min in children.
- The rhythm usually is regular because associated atrioventricular block is rare.
- P waves may not be identifiable, especially when the ventricular rate is high. If present, P waves usually are negative in leads II, III, and aV$_F$.
- QRS complex duration is normal in most children (<0.09 second).[6] Supraventricular tachycardia with aberrant

conduction (wide-complex supraventricular tachycardia) may be difficult to distinguish from ventricular tachycardia (but this form of ventricular tachycardia is rare in infants and children).

Treatment. Signs and symptoms during supraventricular tachycardia are affected by the child's age, duration of supraventricular tachycardia, prior ventricular function, and ventricular rate (see Figure 48-19). If the child is hemodynamically stable and cooperative, vagal maneuvers such as applying ice/water to the child's face for infants and young children, and blowing through a straw, vagal maneuvers or massaging the carotid sinus in older children may be successful in terminating the rhythm.[6] Unstable supraventricular tachycardia is best managed with synchronized cardioversion or drug therapy. (**Adenosine** is the drug of choice.)

Wide-complex tachycardias with signs of compromised tissue perfusion and impaired level of consciousness require immediate care. The paramedic should treat these tachycardias as if they are ventricular tachycardia. Urgent treatment includes synchronized cardioversion if pulses are present, and defibrillation if pulses are absent.

VENTRICULAR TACHYCARDIA AND VENTRICULAR FIBRILLATION

As stated before, ventricular tachycardia and ventricular fibrillation are uncommon in children. If present, the paramedic should consider causes of these dysrhythmias that include congenital heart disease, cardiomyopathies, myocarditis, reversible causes (e.g., drug toxicity), metabolic causes (e.g., hypoglycemia), or hypothermia. Important electrocardiogram findings include the following:

1. Ventricular tachycardia
   Ventricular rate at least 120 beats/min and regular
   Wide QRS complex
   P waves that often are unidentifiable
2. Ventricular fibrillation
   No identifiable P wave, QRS complex, or T wave
   Ventricular fibrillation waves that may be coarse or fine

NOTE

Automated external defibrillators (AEDs) with pediatric cable-pad systems with a dose attenuator have been approved by the Food and Drug Administration. They may be used in infants and children up to 25 kg (approximately 8 years of age). These children must have no signs of circulation (Class IIb) and shockable rhythms (ventricular fibrillation and pulseless ventricular tachycardia). The device also should be able specifically to identify pediatric dysrhythmias that require a shock. In infants less than 1 year of age, a manual defibrillator is preferred. If a manual defibrillator is not available, an AED with a dose attenuator may be used. An AED without a dose attenuator may be used if neither a manual defibrillator nor a defibrillator with a dose attenuator is available (Class IIb, LOE C).[6] For a lone rescuer responding to a child with no signs of circulation, 1 minute of cardiopulmonary resuscitation is still advised before any other action, such as activating EMS or using an automated external defibrillator.

BOX 48-7 Terminating Resuscitative Efforts

Most children who have a cardiac arrest will not survive, even with a transient return of spontaneous circulation. Clinical variables associated with survival include length of CPR, number of epinephrine doses, age, witnessed versus unwitnessed cardiac arrest, and the first and subsequent rhythm. Prolonged resuscitation is indicated, however, in infants and children with recurring or refractory ventricular fibrillation or ventricular tachycardia. Prolonged resuscitation is also recommended if the arrest resulted from toxic drug exposure or a primary hypothermic insult.[6] In the absence of these conditions, medical direction may advise that resuscitative efforts be discontinued. Family members should be given the option to be present during the resuscitation efforts, If possible, one person should be assigned to the family to answer questions and provide comfort measures. (As with adults, resuscitation should not be initiated in children who have obvious signs of death, such as rigor mortis.)

Treatment

Ventricular Tachycardia With a Pulse. Hemodynamically stable ventricular tachycardia should be managed under the advice of medical direction and with caution (see Figures 44-18 and 44-19). The initial efforts are aimed at determining the origin of the tachycardia and obtaining a thorough history. Drug therapy usually is delayed in the stable patient until arrival in the emergency department. In-hospital, administration of **amiodarone** or **procainamide,** may be considered. (These drugs should not routinely be administered together.) Ventricular tachycardia that produces a palpable pulse and signs of shock (low cardiac output, poor perfusion) requires immediate synchronized cardioversion.

Pulseless Ventricular Tachycardia and Ventricular Fibrillation. Pulseless ventricular tachycardia and ventricular fibrillation are managed with immediate defibrillation, cardiopulmonary resuscitation, intubation with ventilatory support, and drug therapy (e.g., **epinephrine** and **vasopressin, amiodarone,** and **lidocaine**). Infant patches (4.5 cm) generally should be used during defibrillation for infants up to about 1 year of age or weighing 10 kg. Adult patches (8 to 10 cm) generally should be used for patients older than 1 year of age or weighing more than 10 kg (Box 48-7).[6]

Postresuscitation Stabilization

The postresuscitation phase begins after initial stabilization of the patient with shock or respiratory failure or after return of spontaneous circulation in a patient who was in cardiac arrest. The goals of postresuscitation stabilization are as follows[6]:

- Preserve brain function.
- Maintain oxygen saturation to at least 94%.
- Avoid secondary organ injury.

TABLE 48-11 Summary of Postresuscitation Care

Vital Function	Intervention
Airway	Tracheal intubation with confirmation of tube position and repeat confirmation on movement/transport
	Secure tube before transport
	Gastric decompression
Breathing	Titrate inspired oxygen for $Spo_2 \geq 94\%$
	Provide mechanical ventilation targeting normal ventilation goals (Pco_2 35-40 mm Hg)
	Monitor continuous pulse oximetry and capnography, if available
Circulation	Ensure adequate intravascular volume (volume titration)
	Optimize myocardial function and systemic perfusion (inotropes, vasopressors, vasodilators)
	Monitor capillary refill, blood pressure, continuous electrocardiogram, urine output; measure arterial blood gas and lactate to assess degree of acidosis, if available
	Ideally maintain two routes of functional vascular access
Disability	Perform secondary assessment including brief neurological assessment
	Avoid hyperglycemia; treat hypoglycemia (monitor glucose)
	If seizures are observed, medicate with anticonvulsant agents
	Obtain laboratory studies (if available): arterial blood gases, glucose, electrolytes, hematocrit, chest radiograph
Exposure	Avoid and correct hyperthermia (monitor temperature)
	Consider therapeutic hypothermia (<32° C to 34°C)

From American Heart Association. 2010 American Heart Association Guidelines for Cardiopulmonary Resuscitation and Emergency Cardiovascular Care. *Circulation,* 122 (18 Supplement 3), S639-S946, 2010.

- Seek and correct causes of illness.
- Manage pain with analgesics (e.g., **morphine**) or sedatives (**lorazepam, midazolam**) as ordered by medical direction.[6]
- Enable the patient to arrive at an appropriate care facility in the best possible physiological state.

Postresuscitation stabilization focuses on preserving neurological function and avoiding multisystem organ failure (Table 48-11). Postresuscitation stabilization requires knowledge and experience in the evaluation of all organ systems. It includes stabilizing the airway and supporting oxygenation, ventilation, and perfusion;

BOX 48-8 Causes of Altered Mental Status in Children

Electrolyte or glycemic imbalance
Infection
Intracranial bleeding
Intracranial mass
Intussusception (telescoping intestines)
Seizure
Toxins
Trauma
Uremia
Important history to obtain: Age, fever, vomiting, photophobia, headache, prior seizures, extremity shaking, staring episodes, trauma, ataxia, ingestions, oral intake, bloody stool, urine output, baseline development level
Important physical findings: Vital signs, photophobia, nuchal rigidity, Glasgow Coma Scale score, palpation of ventricular shunt, full neurological examination

performing a thorough secondary assessment; and obtaining a medical history. Family members should be kept abreast of what has been done and how the patient is responding to care. Frequent reports also should be provided to the receiving hospital (Box 48-7).

Meningitis

As described in Chapter 28, *meningitis* is inflammation of the fluid-containing membranes (meninges) that surround the brain and spinal cord. Meningitis normally occurs as a complication of bacterial or viral infection. Meningitis can be life threatening (10% to 15% of cases of bacterial meningitis are fatal).[16] Meningitis can rapidly progress to permanent brain damage, impaired vision or hearing, neurological dysfunction, and death. The highest incidence of meningitis is 6 months to 2 years of age. The greatest time for risk is immediately after birth and again at 3 to 8 months of age.[27] Most commonly, meningitis develops over 1 to 4 days. However, in severe cases, a child who looks healthy can rapidly become seriously ill within a day.

The signs and symptoms of meningitis depend on the child's age and are not always obvious. Classic symptoms in infants younger than 3 months include decreased liquid intake, vomiting, irritability, lethargy, fever, bulging fontanelle, and seizures. Signs and symptoms for older children and adults include nausea and vomiting, headache, photophobia, fever, altered mental status, lethargy, seizures, and neck stiffness (nuchal rigidity) or pain. Other classic presentations which may aid in diagnosis are:

- *Brudzinski's sign:* Knees automatically brought up toward the body when the neck is bent forward or pain in the legs when bent
- *Kernig's sign:* Inability to straighten the lower legs when the thigh is flexed on the abdomen
- *Rash:* Petechial or purpuric rash may appear if meningococcus is the causative agent

Prehospital care is primarily supportive. Universal precautions should be employed. A surgical mask should be applied to the patient while providing care and during transport. In some cases, seizure control or IV fluid replacement will be necessary. In-hospital care will be based on the causative agent.

Seizure

A seizure (described in Chapter 25 Chapter 47) is an episode of sudden abnormal electrical activity in the brain. It results in abnormalities in motor, sensory, or autonomic function usually associated with abnormal behavior, changes in level of consciousness, or both (Box 48-8). Common causes of seizure in adults and children include noncompliance with a drug regimen for the treatment of epilepsy, head trauma, intracranial infection, brain tumor, metabolic disturbance, or poisoning. The most common cause of new onset of seizure in children is fever.

LOOK AGAIN
See Chapter 25: Neurology, pp. 785-788.

CRITICAL THINKING
Are you comfortable using the pediatric paddles on the defibrillators you will be using in clinicals and on the ambulance?

FEBRILE SEIZURES

A **febrile seizure** is a seizure associated with fever but without evidence of intracranial infection or other definable cause; such seizures usually occur between the ages of

6 months and 5 years.[33] About 2% to 5% of children under 7 years of age experience a febrile seizure. About 30% of those who have a seizure experience a recurrence. More than half of febrile seizures occur in children ages 9 to 20 months. In 60% of cases, a family history of febrile seizures is a factor.[33]

Febrile seizures usually are associated with an underlying viral infection (most often of the upper respiratory tract), gastroenteritis, roseola, otitis media, or another febrile illness. The seizures usually occur in vulnerable patients during a rapid rise in body temperature. However, the intensity of the seizure is not related to the severity of the fever.

Febrile seizures may manifest with generalized tonic-clonic activity. Or they may have a more subtle presentation. As a rule, classic febrile seizures are of short duration. (They usually last less than 5 minutes.) They also have an uncomplicated and short postictal period. Seizures that last longer than 20 minutes call for extensive investigation. These should never be considered benign. Regardless of the suspected cause, all children who have suffered a seizure should be transported for evaluation by a physician per protocol.

Assessment and Management. In most cases the seizure has stopped before emergency medical services arrives. In many instances, the child is in a postictal state. As in any emergency, the first priorities are airway management and ventilatory and circulatory support. This includes airway positioning, suctioning of the airway, and administration of oxygen. Repeated assessment of the adequacy of ventilation is necessary. Special emphasis should be placed on respiratory rate and depth. If the airway cannot be maintained with manual maneuvers, airway adjuncts should be used.

After initial stabilization of the patient's condition, the paramedic should assess vital signs and obtain a history. Important elements of the history include the following:

- Previous seizures
- Number of seizures in this episode
- Duration of seizure activity
  - Tonic-clonic—from onset of symptoms until clonic activity stops
  - Absence—time from loss of consciousness to return of consciousness
  - Complex partial—from loss of consciousness or start of motor activity, automatism until child is responsive
- Description of seizure activity
  - Areas of body involved
  - Area of the body the seizure activity originated (e.g., foot, mouth, generalized)
  - Positional change
  - Length of tonic and clonic phases
  - Absence of movement or muscle tone in selected body areas
- Presence of vomiting during the seizure (aspiration risk)
- Color change during seizure

- Appearance of face during the seizure
- Appearance of eyes during the seizure
  - Pupils
  - Gaze
- Condition of the child when first found
- Recent illness
- Potential for toxic ingestion
- Potential head injury (as primary cause or secondary complication)
- Significant medical problems
- Recent headache or stiff neck (which may suggest meningitis)
- Medication use and compliance with anticonvulsant medication

During transport to the emergency department, the paramedic should continuously monitor the child and be alert for recurrent seizures. The characteristics of the postictal period (level of consciousness, movement, speech, sensory or motor impairment) should be noted. Medical direction may advise that a febrile patient be given an antipyretic if the patient is alert. The antipyretic will reduce the fever en route to the receiving hospital. The paramedic should not apply ice or submerge the patient in a cool bath in an effort to reduce fever.

STATUS EPILEPTICUS

Status epilepticus is continuous seizure activity that lasts 30 minutes or longer or a recurrent seizure without an intervening period of consciousness. Such a seizure is a true emergency. It can lead to hypotension and cardiovascular, respiratory, and renal failure, in addition to permanent brain damage. Children in status epilepticus should be managed with the following initial interventions:

1. Provide adequate airway, ventilatory, and circulatory support. Intubation for airway protection or mechanical ventilation seldom is needed. Intubation should be withheld unless the child fails to respond to the initial management.

2. Per protocol, obtain vascular access through an IV or intraosseous route. Measure the blood glucose level to screen for hypoglycemia. If the value is less than 60 mg/dL (40 mg/dL in an infant[4]), administer **dextrose** 10%, or dextrose 25% (per medical direction). (Hypoglycemia also can be treated with an intramuscular injection of **glucagon** if IV or intraosseous access cannot be established.) If seizures do not stop, consult medical direction regarding IV, intraosseous, or rectal administration of the anticonvulsants **diazepam** or **lorazepam**. (*Lorazepam* may also be given intramuscularly [IM].)

3. Attach a cardiac monitor. Observe for rhythm or conduction abnormalities that may suggest hypoxia.

Diazepam. *Diazepam* breaks active seizures in 70% of cases.[33] The drug has a short duration of action (15 minutes). It may require repeat administration to a maximum of three doses. In addition, the paramedic should be ready for sudden respiratory depression or hypotension when using this drug. If IV or intraosseous access cannot be obtained,

BOX 48-9 Procedure for Rectal Administration of Diazepam

1. Carefully restrain the child. If possible, place the child in a knee-chest or decubitus position with the legs flexed at the hip and knee.
2. Draw the calculated diazepam dose into a syringe. A higher dose of 0.5 mg/kg is required because absorption is incomplete.
3. Introduce a lubricated 1-mL syringe just beyond the external sphincter (aimed just above the junction of the skin and mucous membranes and directed toward the rectal wall).
4. Inject the solution into the rectum and clear the syringe with 1 mL of normal saline.
5. Facilitate drug retention by squeezing the buttocks together with manual pressure.
6. Transport the patient for evaluation by a physician. Remove excessive clothing. En route, continually monitor the patient for recurrent seizures and the need for airway, ventilatory, and circulatory support.

diazepam may be administered rectally (Box 48-9) and *lorazepam* or *midazolam* may be given intramuscularly.[13] Transport of the patient should not be delayed so as to attempt vascular access.

Lorazepam. An alternative to the IV or intraosseous administration of *diazepam* is *lorazepam*. The drug has a long duration of action (6 to 8 hours), and is preferred by some physicians. *Lorazepam* may be injected intramuscularly. It also may be given intravenously, intraosseously, or rectally. The side effects are similar to those of *diazepam* in terms of cardiorespiratory and central nervous system depression. The paramedic should be alert for these complications.

NOTE

Midazolam is being used by some emergency medical services systems to treat status epilepticus and refractory seizures in pediatric patients. *Midazolam* also is used when seizures do not respond to *diazepam* or *lorazepam*. The drug may be administered intramuscularly, intravenously, buccally, or intranasally. The use of *midazolam* to control pediatric seizures is controversial; it has a short half-life; it may cause respiratory depression.[13]

Hypoglycemia

As described in Chapter 26, hypoglycemia is an abnormally low concentration of glucose in the blood. In children, hypoglycemia is usually the result of excessive response to glucose absorption, illness, physical exertion, or decreased dietary intake. In diabetic children, hypoglycemia usually is caused by too large an insulin dose, a delayed or missed meal, or vigorous physical activity. The condition most commonly occurs in the prehospital setting in infants and children with type 1 diabetes, a disease that affects about 0.2% of all school-age children; about 15,000 children in the United States under age 20 are diagnosed with type 1 diabetes each year.[28]

The signs and symptoms of hypoglycemia can be classified as *mild, moderate,* and *severe.* Mild symptoms include hunger, weakness, tachypnea, and tachycardia. Moderate symptoms include sweating, tremors, irritability, vomiting, mood disorders, blurred vision, stomachache, headache, and dizziness. Severe symptoms include decreased level of consciousness and seizure activity. This is an emergency that requires prompt treatment with **dextrose** to prevent brain damage.

The prehospital care is directed first at ensuring adequate airway, ventilatory, and circulatory support. A blood glucose measurement should be obtained in any child with an altered level of consciousness that has no explainable cause. Conscious children who are mildly hypoglycemic should receive an oral glucose solution or paste. Unconscious children or those with moderate or severe hypoglycemia require IV/intraosseous **dextrose** or intramuscular **glucagon** administration. This should be followed by a repeat blood glucose measurement in 10 to 15 minutes. All children with signs and symptoms of hypoglycemia should be transported for physician evaluation.

Hyperglycemia

Hyperglycemia is an abnormally high concentration of glucose in the blood. It results from an absence or resistance to insulin. The low insulin level prevents glucose from entering the cells. This causes glucose to build up in the blood. If not treated, hyperglycemia can lead to dehydration, diabetic ketoacidosis, and coma. In children with type 1 diabetes, the condition often is the result of too small an insulin dose in relation to food intake, failure to take **insulin,** illness, or a malfunctioning insulin-delivery system (e.g., insulin pump).

The signs and symptoms of hyperglycemia are classified as *early* or *late*. Early signs and symptoms include increased thirst (polydipsia), increased hunger (polyphagia), and increased urination (polyuria). (Weight loss also is considered an early sign of the illness.) Late signs and symptoms associated with dehydration and early ketoacidosis include weakness, abdominal pain, generalized aches, loss of appetite, nausea, vomiting, signs of dehydration (with the exception of urinary output), altered mental status (lethargy), fruity breath odor, tachypnea, hyperventilation, and tachycardia. If untreated, Kussmaul's respirations and coma may occur.

Children suspected of being hyperglycemic should receive adequate airway, ventilatory, and circulatory support. This should be followed by glucose testing. These patients often require IV fluid therapy if signs of dehydration are present (Figure 48-20). The administration of **insulin** usually is reserved as an in-hospital procedure.

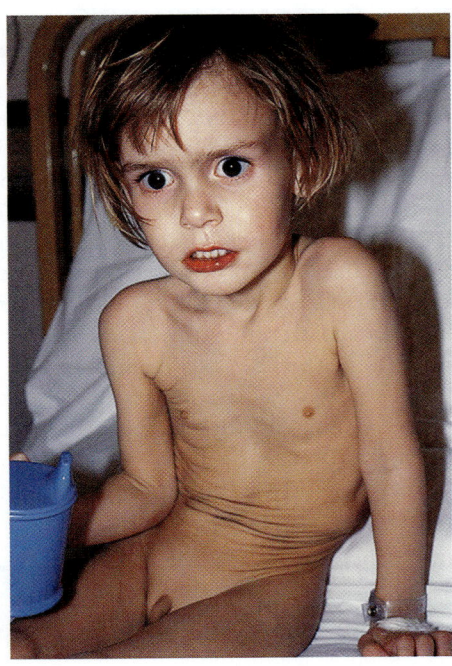

FIGURE 48-20 Severe dehydration and weight loss from diabetic ketoacidosis.

disorders (e.g, thrombocytopenia, hemophilia, von Willebrand's disease), leukemia, leukopenia, lymphoma, and others. After obtaining a thorough patient history (often provided by the parent or caregiver), important assessment findings include[20]:

- History of chest pain
- Weakness
- Abdominal pain
- Extremity pain
- Trauma
- Bleeding
- Swollen joints
- Swollen glands
- Fever
- Bruising

Depending on the condition of the patient and nature of the illness, prehospital care may include IV hydration, fluid resuscitation, bleeding control, pain control, and transport for physician evaluation. In children who have a high risk of infection (e.g., children with leukopenia and other white blood cell diseases), obtaining routine IV access should be avoided in the prehospital setting.

CRITICAL THINKING

Why do you think type 1 diabetes may stay undetected until a child is seriously ill?

NOTE

It is estimated that about 2 million children ages 12 to 19 (and 57 million adults) in the United States have a pre-diabetic condition linked to obesity and inactivity.[29] This condition, known as *pre-diabetes,* refers to blood glucose levels that are higher than normal but not yet high enough to be diagnosed as diabetes. Pre-diabetes increases risk for full-blown diabetes and cardiovascular disease. In addition, persons with pre-diabetes tend to have higher levels of bad (LDL) cholesterol and triglycerides. It has been suggested that intensive lifestyle interventions in this age group may prevent or delay pre-diabetes from progressing to type 2 diabetes. These interventions include physical activity and improvements in diet.

DID YOU KNOW?

Childhood Leukemia

Leukemia in children often is described as being acute or chronic. Almost all childhood leukemia is acute. The two main types of acute leukemia in children are *acute lymphocytic leukemia* (ALL) and *acute myelogenous leukemia* (AML), both of which can be further divided into subtypes. Of the estimated 3500 children (ages birth to 14 years) who will develop leukemia in the United States each year, about 3 out of 4 will be diagnosed with acute lymphocytic leukemia. Most of the remaining cases will be acute myelogenous leukemia. Chronic leukemias are rare in children.

Acute lymphocytic leukemia starts from the lymphoid cells in the bone marrow. Acute myelogenous leukemia (also called acute myeloid leukemia, acute myelocytic leukemia, or acute nonlymphocytic leukemia) accounts for most of the remaining cases. This leukemia originates from the cells that form white blood cells (other than lymphocytes), red blood cells, or platelets. ALL is most common in early childhood, peaking between 2 and 4 years of age. AML is most common during the first 2 years of life, and again during teenage years. The 5-year survival rate for children with ALL is now greater than 80%. The 5-year survival rate for children with AML is now 50% to 70%.[30]

Blood Disorders

As described in Chapter 32, there are a number of conditions and diseases that can cause blood disorders in children and adults. These disorders may affect the oxygen-carrying capacity of hemoglobin, blood clotting mechanisms, immune function, and infection risk. Common blood disorders presenting in children include sickle cell disease (presenting as acute chest syndrome, splenic sequestration, vasoocclusive crisis, and priapism), bleeding

Gastrointestinal Disorders

Abnormalities in the gastrointestinal (GI) tract can lead to illnesses in the pediatric patient that can cause vomiting and bleeding. These abnormalities may be the result of *gastrointestinal embryology* (the formation of the GI tract during fetal development). They may also result from illness and infection. Important components of the patient's history for children with GI disorders include[20]:

- Blood or bile in emesis
- Epistaxis
- Diarrhea
- Constipation
- Fever
- Medications
- Prematurity
- ABO incompatibility
- Liver disease

? DID YOU KNOW?
GI Embryology

The primitive gut forms during the fourth week of gestation into the *midgut, foregut,* and *hindgut.* The midgut gives rise to the distal duodenum, jejunum, ileum, appendix, ascending colon, and proximal transverse colon. Errors in midgut development include omphaloceles (protrusion of the intestines through the umbilicus), umbilical hernias, and gastroschisis (extrusion of the viscera without involving the umbilicus).

The foregut develops into the pharynx, lower respiratory system, esophagus, stomach, proximal duodenum, liver and biliary tree, and pancreas. Errors in foregut development include esophageal atresia and tracheoesophageal fistula.

The hindgut matures into the distal transverse colon, descending colon, sigmoid colon, rectum, and proximal anal canal. Although rare, the most common error in hindgut development is neonatal bowel obstruction (*Hirschsprung's disease*) attributable to improper muscle movement in the bowel.

Depending on the cause of the child's illness, physical findings may include an elevation or decrease in heart rate and blood pressure, signs of dehydration (dry mucous membranes, absence of tears, decreased urinary output, delayed capillary refill), icterus (jaundice), abdominal distention or abdominal mass, hepatomegaly (enlarged liver), and pallor.

NOTE

Jaundice (yellowing of the skin, mucous membranes, and sclera) is the most common condition that requires medical attention in newborns.[31] It develops from elevation in the level of bilirubin (the pigment of bile). Physiological jaundice can occur during the first week of life. It is due to two causes: (1) the breakdown of fetal red blood cells, which release bilirubin into the blood; (2) the immaturity of the newborn's liver, which cannot effectively metabolize the bilirubin and prepare it for excretion into the urine. Physiological jaundice is common and normally resolves with time. All other forms of jaundice in the neonate are considered pathological. Pathological jaundice is a prolonged jaundice that results from illness in the newborn and a rapid rise in serum bilirubin concentration. It usually appears within 24 hours after birth. Illnesses that can cause pathological jaundice include sepsis, rubella, toxoplasmosis, and erythroblastosis.

GI DISORDERS THAT CAUSE VOMITING

Vomiting is a protective mechanism that removes toxic materials from the GI tract before they are absorbed. Vomiting is controlled by the emetic center, located in the reticular formation of the brainstem. The emetic center can be stimulated by chemoreceptors, cranial nerves, vagal and enteric input, and the central nervous system. Three disorders that can cause vomiting in the pediatric patient are gastroenteritis, intestinal malrotation, and pyloric stenosis.

As described in Chapter 29, *gastroenteritis* is inflammation of the stomach and intestines that can accompany many conditions of the GI tract. In infants and children, gastroenteritis is most often due to viral infections that can cause diarrhea, with or without vomiting. In the very young and very old, gastroenteritis can cause life-threatening dehydration that may require volume replacement therapy.

LOOK AGAIN

See Chapter 29: Abdominal and Gastrointestinal Disorders, pp. 895-896.

GI DISORDERS THAT CAUSE BLEEDING

Bleeding can occur from the upper and lower GI tract in children of all ages (Box 48-10). For example, upper GI bleeding can occur in newborns who swallow maternal

---

BOX 48-10 Causes of GI Bleeding[16,20]

Neonate
Swallowed maternal or nasopharyngeal blood
Anal fissure
Necrotizing enterocolitis
Malrotation
Hirschsprung's disease
Coagulopathy

Infants and Toddlers
Allergic colitis
Infectious enteritis
Intussusception
Congenital diverticulum (*Meckel's diverticulum*)
GI duplication (congenital growth of a twin segment of intestine)

School-Age Children
Infectious enteritis
Juvenile polyps
Hemolytic uremic syndrome
Henoch-Schönlein purpura (systemic inflammation of blood vessels)

Adolescents
Infectious diarrhea
Juvenile polyps
Inflammatory bowel disease

BOX 48-11 Signs and Symptoms of Infection in Pediatric Patients

Bulging fontanelle (infants)
Chills
Cool or clammy skin
Cough
Dehydration
Fever
Hypoperfusion
Hypothermia (neonates)
Irritability
Lethargy
Malaise
Nasal congestion
Poor feeding
Respiratory distress
Seizure
Severe headache
Sore throat
Stiff neck
Tachycardia
Tachypnea
Vomiting or diarrhea (or both)

blood. Lower GI bleeding can occur in adolescents from inflammatory bowel disease. The child's condition, signs, and symptoms will be related to the site and cause of the bleeding. Prehospital care may range from supportive care and transportation for physician evaluation to providing advanced life support for the management of shock and hypovolemia. Following stabilization, patients with disorders that cause vomiting or bleeding are managed with bowel rest, antibiotics (if needed), and volume replacement.

Infection

Children with infection may have a variety of signs and symptoms. The symptoms depend on the source and extent of infection and the length of time since the patient was exposed (Box 48-11). Often the parent or caregiver provides a history of recent illness. (This may include, for example, fever, upper respiratory tract infection, or otitis media.) When caring for any patient who may have an infectious disease, the paramedic must strictly adhere to body substance isolation because of the unknown cause of the infection.

Most children with infection need only supportive care while being transported for evaluation by a physician. However, in very sick children, support of the airway, ventilation, and circulation may be needed. If signs of decompensated shock are present, IV therapy may be needed. Active seizure activity may require the use of anticonvulsant agents. When possible, a child in stable condition should be transported in the child's position of comfort. The child also should be transported in the company of the parent or caregiver.

Poisoning and Toxic Exposure

As discussed in Chapter 34, most poisoning in the United States involves children and is a major cause of preventable death in children under 5 years of age.[5] Common sources of poisoning (unintentional and intentional) include the following:

- Acetaminophen
- Alcohol
- Anticholinergics
- Aspirin
- Barbiturates
- Cold medicines
- Corrosives
- Digitalis, beta-blocker agents
- Hydrocarbons
- Narcotics
- Organic solvents (inhaled)
- Organophosphates
- Sedatives
- Vitamins (especially iron)

The signs and symptoms of poisoning vary, depending on the toxic substance and the length of time since the child was exposed. These signs and symptoms may include cardiac and respiratory depression, central nervous system stimulation or depression, gastrointestinal irritation, and behavioral changes. Emergency care should be directed first at ensuring adequate airway, ventilatory, and circulatory support (Box 48-12). The paramedic should contact medical direction and the poison control center for specific treatments. All pills, substances, and containers associated with the poisoning should be transported with the child to the receiving hospital. As described in Chapter 34, no efforts should be made in the prehospital setting to induce vomiting. Gastric lavage also is contraindicated unless ingestion of poison has been less than 1 hour before EMS arrival.

CRITICAL THINKING

For what critical signs or symptoms of poisoning should you be alert?

Pediatric Trauma

Blunt trauma and penetrating trauma are major causes of injury and death in children.[5] These and other significant injuries in children often result from falls, motor vehicle crashes, pedestrian-vehicle collisions, drowning/submersion incidents, penetrating injuries, burns, and abuse. The following common injuries highlight the value of injury prevention programs (see Chapter 3):

Falls: Falls are the single most common cause of injuries in children. Fortunately, serious injury or death from truly unintentional falls is uncommon, that is, unless the fall is from a significant height.

BOX 48-12 Toxicological Emergencies in Pediatric Patients

The most important agents associated with cardiac arrest or requiring advanced life support in children are cocaine, narcotics, tricyclic antidepressants, calcium channel blockers, beta-adrenergic blockers, and opioids. Regardless of the drug, the initial approach in toxicological emergencies is to ensure adequate oxygenation, ventilation, and circulation. Subsequent priorities include reversing the adverse effects of the toxin (if possible) and preventing further absorption of the agent (see Chapter 34). This is an overview of these drugs, their effects, and specific treatment that may be required in the prehospital setting. (*Note:* All drug therapy referenced in this box is based on patient presentation and should be guided by medical direction.)

Cocaine

Effects are complex and are related to route of administration and form of cocaine used.

Signs and Symptoms

May include tachycardia (including ventricular tachycardia/ventricular fibrillation [VT/VF]), tremor, diaphoresis, mydriasis, mood elevation, movement disorders, hypertension, and acute coronary syndrome (chest pain and dysrhythmias)

Specific Treatment

Cool to prevent hyperthermia
Oxygen administration and ventilatory support
Continuous electrocardiogram monitoring
Benzodiazepines (diazepam or lorazepam) for anticonvulsant and central nervous system depressant effect
Nitroglycerin to reduce coronary vasoconstriction
Sodium bicarbonate and lidocaine for ventricular dysrhythmias and cocaine-induced myocardial infarction
Epinephrine to increase coronary perfusion pressure during cardiac arrest
Do not give beta blockers

Cyclic Antidepressants (and Other Sodium Channel Blocking Agents)

Effects result from inhibition of fast sodium channels in the brain and myocardium.

Signs and Symptoms

May include cardiac rhythm disturbances, including preterminal sinus bradycardia and heart block with junctional or ventricular wide-complex escape beats

Specific Treatment

Oxygen administration and ventilatory support
Continuous electrocardiogram monitoring
Do not give amiodarone, sotalol, procainamide, quinidine, flecainide, propafenone
Sodium bicarbonate and lidocaine to increase myocardial contractility and to manage ventricular dysrhythmias
Normal saline boluses (10 mL/kg) to manage hypotension
Vasopressors (norepinephrine or epinephrine) to maintain vascular tone and blood pressure

Calcium Channel Blockers

Effects result from inhibiting the influx of calcium into cells, leading to bradydysrhythmias and hypotension.

Signs and Symptoms

May include bradycardia, hypotension, and altered mental status (including syncope, seizure, coma) from cerebral hypoperfusion

Specific Treatment

Oxygen administration and ventilatory support
Continuous electrocardiogram monitoring
Normal saline boluses (5 to 10 mL/kg) to manage hypotension (avoid pulmonary edema)
Calcium chloride 10% (Class IIb) and atropine to overcome channel blockade
High-dose vasopressor therapy with norepinephrine or epinephrine to treat bradycardia and hypotension
Insulin-glucose therapy to maintain serum glucose concentration (avoid hypoglycemia)

Beta-Adrenergic Blockers

Effects result from competition at beta-adrenergic receptors, resulting in bradycardia and decreased cardiac contractility.

Signs and Symptoms

May include hypotension with bradycardia, varying degrees of heart block, and altered mental status (including seizures and coma)

Specific Treatment

Oxygen administration and ventilatory support
Continuous electrocardiogram monitoring
Treat for shock
Epinephrine infusions and glucagon may be effective in managing beta-adrenergic blockade and overdose
Insulin-glucose therapy to maintain serum glucose concentration (avoid hypoglycemia)
Calcium chloride to improve heart rate if glucagon and catecholamine are not effective (Class IIb)

Opioids

Effects produce central nervous system depression.

Signs and Symptoms

May include altered level of consciousness, hypoventilation, apnea, and respiratory failure

Specific Treatment

Oxygen administration and ventilatory support
Continuous electrocardiogram monitoring
Naloxone to reverse narcotic toxicity (normalize partial pressure of PCO_2 with ventilations before administration)

Adapted from American Heart Association: Guidelines 2005 for Cardiopulmonary Resuscitation and Emergency Cardiovascolar Care, *Circulation* 112: IV-1 to IV-211, 2005.

CRITICAL THINKING
Why are children at risk for injuries related to falls?

Motor vehicle crashes: Motor vehicle crashes are the leading cause of permanent brain injury, serious injury, and death in children. Among infants less than 1 year old, death from motor vehicle crashes is second only to mechanical suffocation.[5]

Pedestrian-vehicle collisions: Pedestrian-vehicle collisions can result in serious injury or death in children. The initial injury is caused by impact with the vehicle. (The impact usually occurs to the extremity or trunk.) The child often is thrown from the force of the first impact. This causes additional injury (e.g., head and spine) upon a second impact with other objects. These objects may include the ground, another vehicle, or nearby objects (see Chapter 37).

Drowning/submersion: Drowning/submersion incidents are the third leading cause of death in children from birth to 4 years of age. Each year, about 1000 children die from drowning[12]; 5% to 20% of children who are hospitalized for submersion suffer severe, permanent brain damage.

Penetrating injuries: Although blunt trauma is more common, penetrating injuries are a major cause of trauma in children. They occur especially during adolescence. Penetrating injuries that are intentional (e.g., from violent crime) are more common in inner cities; however, unintentional penetrating injuries in rural areas also occur often. Stab wounds and firearm injuries make up about 10% to 15% of all pediatric trauma admissions. The risk of death from these injuries increases with the age of the patient. As with penetrating injuries to adults, the appearance of the external wounds cannot be used to determine the extent of internal injury in children.

Burns: Children less than 4 years of age and children with disabilities are at the greatest risk of burn-related death and disability.[32] Survival from burn trauma is determined by the size and depth of the burn, the presence of inhalation injury, and the nature of other injuries that may have occurred during the event (see Chapter 39).

CRITICAL THINKING
What types of situations cause burn injuries to children in the home?

Child abuse: Injuries to children may result from physical abuse, sexual abuse, emotional abuse, and child neglect. Physical abuse often is associated with domestic disturbances, younger-aged parents, substance abuse, and community violence. Abuse of children also occurs in all levels of society. When caring for a child who may have been abused, thorough documentation of pertinent findings, treatment, and interventions is critical for legal purposes. (Child abuse is described later in this chapter.)

SPECIAL CONSIDERATIONS FOR SPECIFIC INJURIES

Special considerations for managing pediatric injury are addressed in the chapters of Part 9: Trauma. The following is a review of some of the more important elements in assessment and management for children with head and neck injury, traumatic brain injury, chest injury, abdominal injury, extremity injury, and burns.

Head and Neck Injury
1. The larger relative mass of the head and lack of neck muscle strength provide increased momentum in acceleration-deceleration injuries.
2. The fulcrum of cervical mobility in the younger child is at the C2 to C3 level (70% of fractures in children younger than 8 years of age occur in C1 or C2).[33]
3. Head injury is the most common cause of death in pediatric trauma victims.[33]
4. Diffuse head injuries are common in children; focal injuries are rare.
5. Soft tissues, skull, and brain are more compliant in children than in adults.
6. Because of open fontanelles and sutures, infants up to 12 to 18 months of age may be more tolerant to increased intracranial pressure (ICP) and can have delayed signs.
7. Subdural bleeding in an infant can produce hypotension (rare).
8. Significant blood loss can occur through scalp lacerations, and such bleeding should be controlled immediately.
9. The modified Glasgow Coma Scale (GCS) should be used for assessing infants and young children.

Traumatic Brain Injury
1. Early recognition and aggressive management can reduce mortality and morbidity.
2. The modified Glasgow Coma Scale (GCS) should be used for assessing infants and young children.
3. Signs of increased ICP include elevated blood pressure, bradycardia, irregular respirations progressing to Cheyne-Stokes respirations, and bulging fontanelle in infants.
4. Signs of herniation include asymmetrical pupils and abnormal posturing.
5. Management includes the following:
   a. Administer high-concentration oxygen for mild to moderate head injury (GCS score of 9 to 15). Monitor pulse oximetry.
   b. Intubate and ventilate at normal breathing rate with 100% oxygen for severe head injury (GCS score less than 8).[6]
   c. Hyperventilate only with signs of increased ICP.
   d. Some authorities recommend the use of *lidocaine* before intubation to blunt the rise in ICP. This, however, is controversial. Use of *lidocaine* should be guided by medical direction.

CRITICAL THINKING
What are some early signs of increasing intracranial pressure in a child?

Chest Injury
1. Chest injuries in children less than 14 years of age usually are the result of blunt trauma.[33]
2. Because of flexibility of the chest wall, severe intrathoracic injury (such as severe pulmonary contusion) can be present without signs of external injury such as rib fractures.
3. Tension pneumothorax is poorly tolerated and is an immediate threat to life.
4. Flail segment is an uncommon injury in children; when noted without a significant mechanism of injury, child abuse should be suspected.
5. Many children with cardiac tamponade have no physical signs other than hypotension.

Abdominal Injury
1. Musculature is minimal and poorly protects the viscera.
2. Organs most commonly injured are the liver, kidneys, and spleen.
3. Onset of symptoms may be rapid or gradual.
4. Because of the small size of the abdomen, palpation should be performed in one quadrant at a time.
5. Any child who is hemodynamically unstable without an obvious source of blood loss should be considered to have an abdominal injury until it is proved otherwise.
6. The majority of children with abdominal injury have abdominal bruising or ecchymosis.

Extremity Injury
1. Extremity injury is relatively more common in children than adults.
2. Growth plate injuries are common.
3. Compartment syndrome is an emergency in children.
4. Management includes the following:
   a. Control any sites of active bleeding.
   b. Perform splinting to prevent further injury and blood loss.
   c. Use of a pneumatic antishock garment or pelvic binding with a sheet may be helpful for an unstable pelvic fracture with hypotension (per protocol).
5. Most femur fractures result from falls or other unintentional injuries; however, child abuse should be considered.

Burns
1. Burns may be thermal, chemical, or electrical.
2. Management priorities include the following:
   a. Prompt management of the airway is required because swelling can develop rapidly.
   b. If intubation is indicated, an endotracheal tube one half size smaller than expected may be required.
   c. Suspect musculoskeletal injuries in electrical burn patients, and perform spine immobilization. (Spinal cord injury can be present in children without vertebral abnormality.)

TRAUMA MANAGEMENT CONSIDERATIONS FOR PEDIATRIC PATIENTS

In addition to the general patient care guidelines appropriate for all injured persons, injured children require special consideration for airway control, immobilization techniques, fluid management, and pain relief. The following discussion reviews the highlights of management guidelines presented in the chapters of Part 9: Trauma.

Airway Control. The airway of an injured child should be maintained in an in-line or neutral position. (The sniffing position is appropriate for older children and adults.) (Padding may need to be placed under the shoulders in some children. This will help to maintain a neutral airway position.) High-concentration oxygen should be given to all patients. Jaw-thrust positioning and suctioning can be used to keep the airway open. Endotracheal intubation (followed by insertion of a gastric tube) should be performed when airway and ventilation remain inadequate. Cricothyroidotomy rarely is indicated for traumatic upper airway obstruction.

All paramedics who provide care for infants and children must be able to provide effective oxygenation and ventilation using the bag-mask technique. Endotracheal intubation sometimes may be needed when caring for injured children. When tracheal intubation is required, endotracheal tube placement should be confirmed by monitoring exhaled carbon dioxide, especially in children with a perfusing rhythm.

Immobilization. Spinal immobilization devices must be the right size for infants and children. Equipment that may be used includes the following:
- Child safety seat
- Long spine board
- Padding
- Pediatric immobilization device
- Rigid cervical collar
- Straps, cravats
- Tape
- Towel/blanket roll/sandbags
- Vest-type/short spine board

NOTE
Spine boards are extrication devices meant to assist emergency personnel in moving patients. As a stand-alone device, they do not provide adequate immobilization of the spine.

The patient should be placed supine (unless positioned in an infant carrier) and immobilized in a neutral in-line position. This is achieved most effectively by using a backboard with a recess for the head or by using padding under the back from the shoulders to the buttocks.[1]

Fluid Management. Management of the child's airway and breathing takes priority over management of circulation. Circulatory compromise is less common in children than adults. When vascular access is indicated, the paramedic should consider the following[1]:

- Large-bore IV catheters should be inserted into large peripheral veins.
- Transport should not be delayed to obtain vascular access.
- Intraosseous access in children can be used if IV access fails.
- An initial fluid bolus of 20 mL/kg of lactated Ringer's solution or normal saline should be given. This will help to manage volume depletion.
- Vital signs should be reassessed and the bolus (20 mL/kg) repeated if needed; vital signs that do not improve after a second bolus indicate the need for rapid surgical intervention.

Pain Relief. Injuries are often painful. Relief from pain should be a priority when providing care to an injured child (see Box 48-13 and Figure 48-21). Drugs that may be used to manage some forms of pain and to alter the emotional response in pediatric patients include *fentanyl, ketamine, ketorolac, morphine,* or *nitrous oxide* (in the absence of hemorrhage).[34] Other indications for pain relief or sedation in pediatric patients include some airway management procedures (e.g., drug-assisted intubation), entrapment requiring extended extrication time, and cardioversion or other uncomfortable procedures.

Sudden Infant Death Syndrome

Sudden infant death syndrome (SIDS) is the leading cause of death in American infants under 1 year of age.[35] The syndrome is defined as the sudden death of a seemingly healthy infant that remains unexplained by history and an autopsy. Sudden infant death syndrome affects about 0.57 per 1000 live births each year in the United States.[36] The syndrome cannot be predicted or prevented. However, positioning during sleep appears to be a factor (Box 48-14).

NOTE

Infants may experience episodes termed **apparent life-threatening events** (ALTEs). These are clinical events in which young infants (usually less than 6 months of age) may experience abrupt changes in breathing, color, or muscle tone. Common causes of ALTEs include viral respiratory tract infection (e.g., RSV), gastroesophageal reflux disease, or seizure. There is no scientific evidence that links ALTEs as events that may lead to SIDS.[37]

ALTE requires medical evaluation. Abusive head injury, intentional suffocation, and Munchausen syndrome by proxy have been associated with ALTEs. Medical disorders associated with an ALTE may be respiratory, metabolic, neurological, and endocrinological in origin. In about 50% of cases no cause is identified.[16]

BOX 48-13 Pain Management

Pain management is important when caring for children. It should be considered when indicated to relieve pain associated with traumatic injury such as fractures and burns. Children do not always express their pain as clearly as adults. As a result, they are less likely to receive appropriate pain therapy in an emergency situation. Thus the paramedic should perform a systematic pain assessment. A memory aid for one type of pain assessment is QUESTT*:

Q: Question the child about his or her pain, using age-appropriate language (e.g., "owie" or "boo-boo" for young children).

U: Use pain rating scales (e.g., the Faces Pain Rating Scale for young children; a numerical pain scale from 0 to 10 for older children).

E: Evaluate the child's behavior (e.g., facial grimace, rigidity, crying, and anxious behavior).

S: Secure the parent or caregiver's involvement in assessing the child's pain. (The parent will have seen the child in pain or discomfort before and will be aware of subtle changes.)

T: Take cause of the pain into account (e.g., type of injury and expected intensity of pain).

T: Take action to provide comfort and to relieve pain (e.g., narcotic and nonnarcotic drugs, comfort measures such as application of cold, elevation, and distraction techniques).

*From Wong D, Hess C: *Clinical manual of pediatric nursing,* ed 5, St Louis, 2000, Mosby.

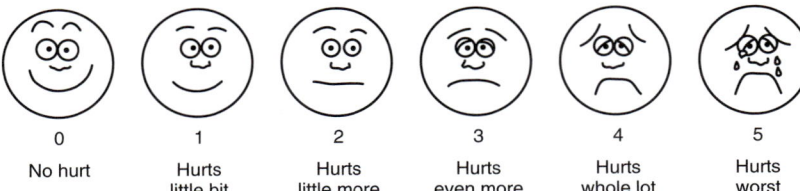

FIGURE 48-21 Wong-Baker Pain Scale. Explain to the child that each face is for a person who feels happy because there is no pain (hurt) or sad because there is some or a lot of pain. Face 0 is very happy because there is no hurt. Face 1 hurts just a little bit. Face 2 hurts a little more. Face 3 hurts even more. Face 4 hurts a whole lot, but Face 5 hurts as much as you can imagine, although you do not have to be crying to feel this bad. Ask child to choose the face that best describes the child's own pain. Record the number under chosen face on patient care report.

Sudden infant death syndrome occurs during periods of sleep. It usually occurs between midnight and 6 AM. The typical age for SIDS is the first year of life, but most SIDS deaths occur within the first 6 months.[35]

The seasonal distribution for SIDS is October through March (in the northern hemisphere). The infant often has a history of minor illness, such as a cold, within 2 weeks before death. Signs that may be present include lividity; frothy, blood-tinged drainage from the nose and mouth; and rigor mortis. With most SIDS cases, no external signs of injury are found. Often evidence indicates that the baby was active just before the death (e.g., rumpled bed clothes, unusual position or location in the bed).

PATHOPHYSIOLOGY

The cause of SIDS is unknown. Studies have failed to confirm a number of physiological, environmental, genetic, and social factors as causes. The studies have confirmed, however, that SIDS is not caused by external suffocation, regurgitation or aspiration of vomitus, hereditary factors, or allergies. (A small percentage of SIDS deaths are thought to be abuse related.[38]) Various physiological aspects that have been suggested to explain SIDS include immaturity of the central nervous system following a prenatal event, idiopathic apnea, brainstem abnormalities, upper airway obstruction, hyperactive upper airway reflexes, cardiac conduction disorders, abnormal responses to hypoxia and hypercarbia, abnormal responses to hyperthermia, and alterations in fat metabolism. Although no specific cause has been identified, a number of risk factors have been associated with the syndrome. These factors include the following[39]:

- Maternal smoking
- Young maternal age (under age 20)
- Infants of mothers who received poor or no prenatal care
- Infants born with low levels of serotonin
- Social deprivation
- Premature births and low-birth-weight infants
- Infants of mothers who used cocaine, methadone, or heroin during pregnancy

Sudden infant death syndrome is confirmed by excluding other causes of death. Autopsy findings that occur in most SIDS deaths include smooth muscle thickening in small pulmonary arteries and right ventricular hypertrophy. Both of these are thought to occur following hypoxia and constriction of the pulmonary vasculature. Other findings include brainstem tumors and low serotonin levels, which may be associated with respiratory center dysfunction. The presence of neuroepithelial bodies in the tracheobronchial tree along with distal atelectasis has also been found in SIDS victims. About 80% of SIDS victims also have intrathoracic petechiae, especially on the thymus, pleura, and pericardium.[38]

> **NOTE**
>
> It has recently been discovered that the brains of infants who die of sudden infant death syndrome produce low levels of serotonin. Researchers theorize that this newly discovered serotonin abnormality may reduce an infant's capacity to respond to breathing challenges, such as low oxygen levels or high levels of carbon dioxide. These high levels may result from rebreathing exhaled carbon dioxide that accumulates in bedding while sleeping face down.[40]

MANAGEMENT

EMS providers can do little to help the SIDS infant. The main role of the paramedic is to offer emotional support for parents or other caregivers and loved ones. If the infant possibly could be viable, resuscitation should proceed as for any other infant in cardiac arrest. Even though resuscitation most likely will be unsuccessful, it is important for the parents or other caregivers to see that everything possible is being done for their child. The paramedic should follow pediatric resuscitation protocols and should consult with medical direction on decisions to initiate or continue efforts.

A variety of grief reactions should be expected from those who witness the event (parents, family members, neighbors, babysitters). These reactions may vary from shock and disbelief to anger, rage, and self-blame. Arrangements should be made for a relative or neighbor to stay with the family or accompany them to the hospital so that they are not left alone. Many areas have SIDS resource services. These services provide immediate counseling and support for the family of an infant who dies of SIDS.

Sudden infant death syndrome victims may appear to have been abused or neglected. The mysterious nature of SIDS deaths and classic signs such as postmortem lividity and frothy fluid in the infant's nose and mouth give such an appearance. Regardless of the circumstances, the paramedic should avoid comments or questions that may imply a suspicion of improper child care. Determining the cause of death is not the duty of the emergency medical services crew. (However, careful scene observation is crucial.) The paramedic should document all findings objectively, accurately, and completely. Medical direction and other authorities (per protocol) should be advised if inappropriate child care is suspected.

The death of an infant has a powerful effect on all who are involved. Rescuers commonly have a range of emotional reactions after a SIDS death. Some emergency medical services, working with medical direction and SIDS resource agencies, provide counseling and formal debriefing programs. If these services are not available, the emergency medical services crew should discuss the event openly with others involved in the response (e.g., co-workers and law enforcement officers). This may help relieve normal feelings of anxiety and stress.

CRITICAL THINKING
What factors do you think influence the reactions of each crew member to a child who dies from sudden infant death syndrome?

Child Abuse and Neglect

More than 3 million cases of suspected child abuse and neglect are reported each year in the United States. (These reports can include multiple children.) In 2007, about 5.8 million children were involved in an estimated 3.8 million reports and allegations.[41] In the United States, child abuse and neglect results in about five deaths per day; the majority of deaths are children under 4 years of age. Paramedics should follow local protocol in reporting suspected abuse. They should discuss any suspicions of child abuse or neglect with medical direction as well. Agencies that may be involved in cases of child abuse or neglect include state, regional, and local child protection services. Also included are hospital-based social service departments and child protection programs.

Child abuse and neglect is a crime that must be reported by law in all 50 states. In some states persons have a legal duty to report child abuse or neglect (*mandated reporter*). Failure to report these cases may result in criminal prosecution and may be punishable by fine or imprisonment or both. As a rule, reporting in good faith provides immunity from legal liability as a consequence of reporting, which may be raised as a defense if one is sued for negligent reporting.

ELEMENTS OF CHILD ABUSE

Child abuse and neglect is the maltreatment of children by their parents, guardians, or other caregivers. Forms of maltreatment include infliction of physical injury (battered child syndrome, shaken baby syndrome), sexual exploitation, and infliction of emotional pain and neglect (medical neglect, safety neglect, nutritional and social deprivation). A number of factors come into play in the potential for child abuse. These include a caregiver with the potential to abuse, a child with particular characteristics that place him or her at risk for abuse, and an element of crisis.

Characteristics of Abusers. Child abuse usually reflects a pattern of unstable behavior. Child abuse is typically not a single act of violence. In many cases the abuser is the child's parent. However, other caregivers may be responsible. (For example, others may include family members, a boyfriend or girlfriend of the child's mother or father, an unrelated babysitter, or a sibling of the abused child.) In the case of physical abuse, most abusers tend to be unhappy, angry adults. They often are under extreme stress. They usually are isolated. Often they are incapable of using support agencies or an extended family in times of crisis. Often the abusers were the victim of physical or emotional abuse as children. Abusers come from all ethnic, geographical, religious, educational, occupational, and socioeconomic groups. Other factors that are characteristic of abusers include poverty and alcohol or other drug dependence. Other facts about child abuse are provided in Box 48-15.

CRITICAL THINKING
Can you make a determination that someone is not an abuser if they do not fit this profile based on your prehospital assessment?

Characteristics of an Abused Child. Abused children often have certain characteristics that increase their risk for abuse.[42] Common traits include demanding and difficult behavior, decreased level of functioning (e.g., a handicapped child or preterm infant requiring extra parenting), hyperactivity, and precociousness with intellectual ability equal to or superior to the parent. Often the parent sees the abused child as "special" or "different" from other siblings. Other factors that tend to increase the potential for child abuse are age (the child is usually under 5 years old), gender (boys are involved more often than girls), and illegitimacy.

BOX 48-15 Facts About Child Abuse and Neglect[41]

- It is estimated that between 60% and 85% of child fatalities attributable to maltreatment are not recorded as such on death certificates.
- 90% of child sexual abuse victims know the perpetrator in some way; 68% are abused by family members.
- 31% of women in prison in the United States were abused as children.
- Over 60% of people in drug rehabilitation centers report being abused or neglected as a child.
- About 30% of abused and neglected children will later abuse their own children, continuing the horrible cycle of abuse.
- The estimated annual cost of child abuse and neglect in the United States for 2009 is $104 billion.
- Abused children are 25% more likely to experience teen pregnancy.
- 14% of all men in U.S. prisons were abused as children.
- 36% of all women in prison were abused as children.
- Children who experience child abuse and neglect are 59% more likely to be arrested as a juvenile, 28% more likely to be arrested as an adult, and 30% more likely to commit violent crime.
- Abused teens are 3 times less likely to practice safe sex, placing them at greater risk for sexually transmitted infections (STIs).
- Children who have been sexually abused are 2.5 times more likely to abuse alcohol.
- Children who have been sexually abused are 3.8 times more likely to develop drug addictions.
- Nearly two thirds of the people in treatment for drug abuse reported being abused as children.

Crises That May Precipitate Abuse. Physical abuse or neglect can occur constantly during a child's life. More often, though, abuse and neglect are intermittent and unpredictable. The abuse often is triggered by stressors in the adult caregiver's life, especially when the caregiver expects the child to fill emotional needs created by the stress. Failure of the child to respond in an ideal way to the caregiver's needs may lead to abuse. Common crises associated with an episode of child abuse include the following:

- Financial stress
- Loss of employment
- Eviction from housing
- Marital or relationship stress
- Physical illness in a child that leads to intractable crying
- Death of a family member
- Diagnosis of an unwanted pregnancy
- Birth of a sibling

HISTORY OF INJURIES SUSPICIOUS FOR ABUSE

Physical abuse or neglect often is hard to determine. The ultimate diagnosis usually begins with suspicions based on unexplained injuries, discrepant history, delays in seeking medical care, and repeated episodes of suspicious injuries. If at any time an injured child indicates that an adult caused him or her physical harm, the paramedic should take this report seriously and advise medical direction. The paramedic should contact the proper authorities as well. In many cases these accusations are true. The following are 15 indicators of possible abuse[43]:

1. Any obvious or suspected fractures in a child under 2 years of age
2. Injuries in various stages of healing, especially burns and bruises
3. More injuries than are usually seen in other children of the same age
4. Injuries scattered on many areas of the body
5. Bruises or burns in patterns that suggest intentional infliction
6. Suspected increased intracranial pressure in an infant
7. Suspected intraabdominal trauma in a young child
8. Any injury that does not fit the description of the cause
9. An accusation that the child injured himself or herself intentionally
10. Long-standing skin infections
11. Extreme malnutrition
12. Extreme lack of cleanliness
13. Inappropriate clothing for the situation
14. Child who withdraws from parent
15. Child who responds inappropriately to the situation (e.g., quiet, distant, and withdrawn)

PHYSICAL FINDINGS SUGGESTIVE OF ABUSE

Some physical findings, such as multiple, widely dispersed bruises; welts; and burns, are suggestive of abuse. Such physical findings, along with a vague history or delays in seeking medical care for the child, should alert the paramedic to the possibility of abuse or neglect (Figure 48-22).

Bruises

- Bruises that predominate on the buttocks or lower back are almost always related to punishment.
- Genital area or inner thigh bruises may be inflicted for toileting mishaps.
- Facial bruises or a number of petechiae on the earlobe may be caused by slapping.
- Bruises of the upper lip and labial frenulum may be caused by forced feedings or from forcing a pacifier into the mouth of a screaming infant.
- Human hand marks resulting from squeezing are pressure bruises in shapes resembling fingertips, fingers, or the entire hand of the abuser.
- Human bite marks result in paired, crescent-shaped bruises. These bruises often contain individual teeth marks. The size of the arc distinguishes adult bites from child bites.

CRITICAL THINKING

Consider an infant under 3 months of age. Based on the physical capabilities of this age group, where would you expect to see "normal bruises"?

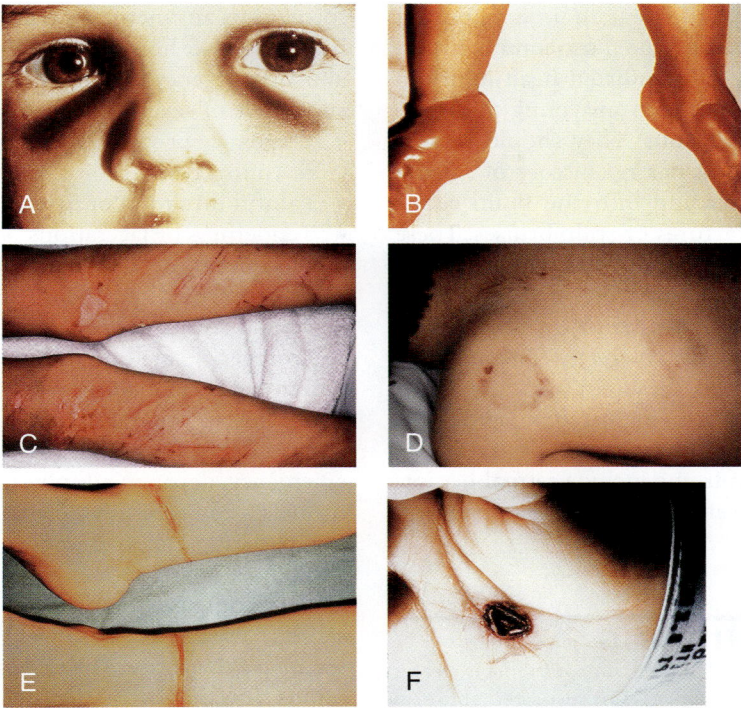

FIGURE 48-22 Cutaneous manifestations of child abuse. **A,** "Raccoon eyes," or periorbital bruising, is a possible indication of basilar skull fracture. **B,** Dunking/submersion burns of the feet. **C,** Welts and abrasions to legs as a result of an electrical cord. **D,** Human bites. **E,** Fresh abrasions of restraint injury. **F,** Fresh cigarette burn to palm.

> **NOTE**
>
> Identifying the age of bruises within 24 hours of the actual injury has been proven highly inaccurate, even among highly trained professionals.[44] Therefore, paramedics should not attempt to identify the age of a bruise or report the age of a bruise based on examination of the injured area. Doing so can lead to liability should litigation occur. The paramedic should, however, document what was observed, including color, size, location of any bruises, without reference to age.

Welts

- Strap marks 1 to 2 inches wide are almost always caused by a belt.
- Bizarre-shaped welts or bruises usually are inflicted by a blunt object that resembles its shape (e.g., a toy or shoe).
- Choke marks may be seen on the neck with or without associated petechiae of the face.
- Circumferential bruising or abrasions on the ankles or wrists may be caused by rope, cord, or a dog leash.

Burns

- Cigarette burns often are found on the palms, soles, or abdomen.
- A lighted cigarette, a hot match, or burning incense sometimes is applied to the hand to stop the child from sucking the thumb or to the genital area to discourage masturbation.
- Burns may be inflicted with lighters or other sources of open flame (e.g., a gas stove) to teach a child not to play with fire.
- Dry contact burns may result from forcibly holding a child against a heating device (e.g., a radiator, hot iron, or electric hot plate).
- The most common abusive hot-water burns or scalds occur from forcible immersion of the hands, feet, or buttocks in scalding water. These injuries often involve both arms or both legs, or they may be circular burns restricted to the buttocks; such burns are incompatible with falling or stepping into a tub of hot water.

Bites

- Human bites have different characteristics than animal bites and are usually more superficial injuries. For example, a human bite appears as 2 joined "c" shapes; a dog's bite has more of an oval or "u" shape.
- Human bites also may be seen with sexual assault.

Other less visible injuries may indicate child abuse. These include brain injury, abdominal visceral injury, and bone fractures.

Subdural Hematoma. Brain injury is the leading cause of death in battered children. The various pathological lesions include cerebral contusions, intraparenchymal hemorrhage, and subdural or even epidural hematomata. Subdural hematomata are among the most common injuries associated with intentionally inflicted head injury in children. They should be suspected in any young child who is in a coma or having convulsions. They should be suspected particularly if the child has no history of seizure disorder. In many cases, bleeding into the brain tissue occurs as a result of skull fractures or scalp bruises. These commonly result from a direct blow from a hand or by being thrown against a wall or door.

Subdural hematomata also can result from vigorous shaking of the child (*shaken baby syndrome*). The acceleration and deceleration forces on the brain associated with shaking cause tearing of the bridging cerebral veins. This leads to bleeding into the subdural space. Signs and symptoms of the shaken baby syndrome include retinal hemorrhages, irritability, altered level of consciousness, vomiting, and a full fontanelle.

CRITICAL THINKING

Why is it critical that your documentation be clear, objective, and complete in cases of suspected abuse?

Abdominal Visceral Injury. Intraabdominal injuries are the second most common cause of death in battered children. These injuries usually are produced by a blunt force such as a punch or blow to the abdomen. Children with an abdominal injury often have recurrent vomiting, abdominal distention, absent bowel sounds, and localized tenderness with or without abdominal bruising. Caregivers routinely deny a history of trauma to the child's abdomen in these cases.

Bone Injury. More than 20% of physically abused children have a positive result on radiological bone survey from previous abusive episodes.[33] Injuries that may be obvious only through radiography include fractures of the ribs, lateral portion of the clavicle, scapula, sternum, and extremities. Multiple fractures in various stages of healing are highly suspicious for physical abuse.

INJURIES FROM SEXUAL ABUSE

Sexual abuse of a child is a symptom of a seriously disturbed family relationship. Sexual abuse usually is associated with physical or emotional neglect or abuse. Often the sexually abusive adult received similar abuse as a child. The adult may justify this behavior in his or her mind. Family relationships are complex, and silent complicity by at least one parent often is involved.

Injuries from sexual abuse may be physical and psychological. Sexual abuse may include vaginal intercourse, sodomy (anal intercourse), oral-genital contact, or molestation (fondling, masturbation, or exposure). In many cases the victimized child is a girl. More than half of the victims are under 12 years of age at the time of the first offense.[45] Many of these incidents are chronic and occur without

force. Thus an emergency medical services response seldom is initiated. If, however, a physical injury results from the abuse, emergency care may be summoned. Physical findings suggestive of sexual abuse include the following:

- Pregnancy or venereal disease in a child 12 years of age or younger
- Painful urination or defecation
- Tenderness or lacerations of the perineal area
- Bleeding from the rectum or vagina
- Presence of dried blood, semen, or pubic hair in the genital area of a child

Emergency care for child victims of sexual abuse should be limited to managing injuries that pose a threat to life and giving emotional support during transport. These children undergo extensive interviews and examination by the emergency department physician and others. The paramedic should carefully document any statements made by the patient, family member, or caregiver. Any findings should be reported to medical direction. These children require compassionate support. A sexually abused child should never be made to feel that he or she is responsible for any of the abuse. The child also should not be given the impression that discussion of the event is inappropriate. If possible, a paramedic of the same gender should interview and care for the child.

All patients, regardless of age, who report sexual assault should be transported for physician evaluation to a medical facility staffed with nurses or physicians who are trained in forensic collection of evidence. Most regions coordinate an intensive interview by a social worker and a physical examination by a physician. This assessment is provided at hospital-based programs that have specialized training in the assessment and care of sexually abused children. Ideally, the paramedic should contact medical direction to identify a child protection center where these services can be provided. It is preferable that victimized children be interviewed and undergo physical examination only when needed.

INFANTS AND CHILDREN WITH SPECIAL NEEDS

Some infants and children are born with or develop conditions that pose special needs. These children may require special medical equipment to sustain life. Examples of these conditions include infants born prematurely, those who have altered functions from birth, and those who have chronic or acute disease of the lung, heart, or central nervous system. Often these children are cared for at home by family and home health services. Many are dependent on special medical equipment such as tracheostomy tubes, home artificial ventilators, central venous lines, gastrostomy tubes, and shunts (see Chapter 52). The parents and other family members of a child with special medical needs often are "experts" in caring for the child and maintaining the required medical equipment. Their knowledge, skills, and experience are valuable. The paramedic should use the

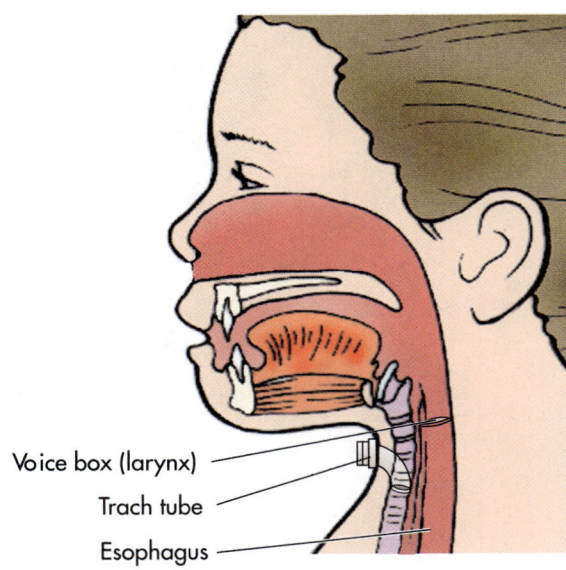

FIGURE 48-23 Pediatric tracheostomy tube.

Voice box (larynx)
Trach tube
Esophagus

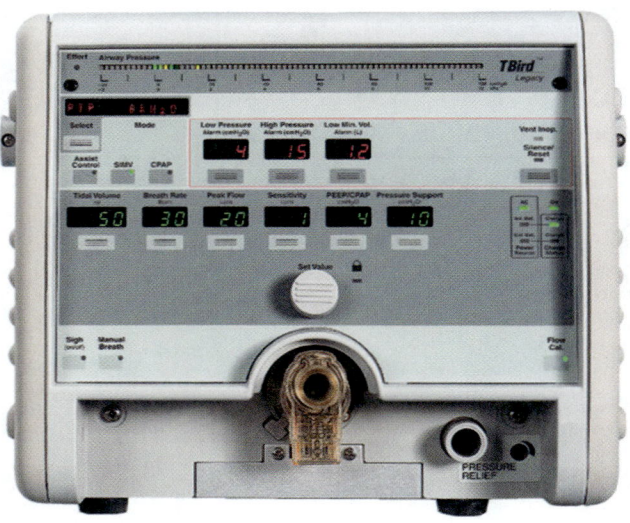

FIGURE 48-24 Home ventilator.

skills and expertise of these parents when managing these emergencies.

Tracheostomy Tubes

In a patient with a complete tracheostomy, the airway surgically bypasses the larynx at the level of the trachea. The larynx is no longer connected to the trachea. Modern tracheostomy tubes are flexible and relatively comfortable for the patient. They have few associated risks (Figure 48-23). Complications that can occur with the tracheostomy tube include obstruction, air leak, bleeding, dislodgment, and infection. All of these may lead to inadequate ventilation. (Bleeding around a tracheostomy usually occurs within 24 hours of the surgery and is not commonly seen in the prehospital setting.[33]) Aseptic technique and respiratory support are always high priorities in caring for these patients.

MANAGEMENT

The tracheostomy tube may become blocked or dislodged. In these cases, the paramedic must clear the tube with sterile water or saline or remove and reinsert it as described in Chapter 15. (Medical direction may advise that a tracheostomy tube be replaced with an endotracheal tube as a temporary measure.) Tracheal suctioning (using sterile technique) may be required to remove secretions and mucus. If tracheal intubation becomes necessary in these patients, it must be performed via the stoma.

NOTE

Tracheal suctioning is a difficult procedure and often is traumatic for the patient. It can easily lead to hypoxia. Tracheal suctioning should be performed only when absolutely necessary. It should be performed briefly, for only a period of 10 to 15 seconds. After that, high-concentration supplemental oxygen should be administered by mask to the stoma or via a bag-valve mask.

Home Artificial Ventilators

When a child needs help breathing, he or she may be put on a mechanical ventilator (Figure 48-24). This can simulate the normal movement of the diaphragm and thoracic cage. The type of home ventilator used depends on the patient's specific needs. Ventilators are classified by function. This is based on the amount of air and pressure they are set to deliver during certain phases of the respiratory cycle. Complications can occur from malfunction of the machine and alarms, airway obstruction, and respiratory distress (Table 48-12).

MANAGEMENT

Because of the variety of artificial ventilators, the paramedic should never try to troubleshoot a ventilator problem. The paramedic also should not try to adjust the settings of the ventilator. Rather, the emergency medical services crew should always treat the patient and not try to correct the malfunction of the machine. Steps in managing a patient with a home artificial ventilator problem are presented in Chapter 52.

TABLE 48-12 Complications Seen With Home Artificial Ventilators	
Complication	**Possible Cause**
Airway obstruction	Bronchospasm, mucus or secretions, tracheostomy or endotracheal tube malfunction, patient cough, fear, anxiety
Barotrauma Pneumothorax	High-pressure volumes
Atelectasis	Improper deep breathing, pneumothorax
Cardiovascular impairment	Reduction in venous return to heart caused by positive intrathoracic pressure, which compresses pulmonary circulation
Gastrointestinal complications	Swallowing air, gastrointestinal bleeding, gastric distention
Tracheal trauma	Cuff pressure on trachea
Respiratory tract infection	Bypass of natural defenses of upper airway, poor aseptic technique
Oxygen toxicity	High concentration of oxygen over prolonged periods

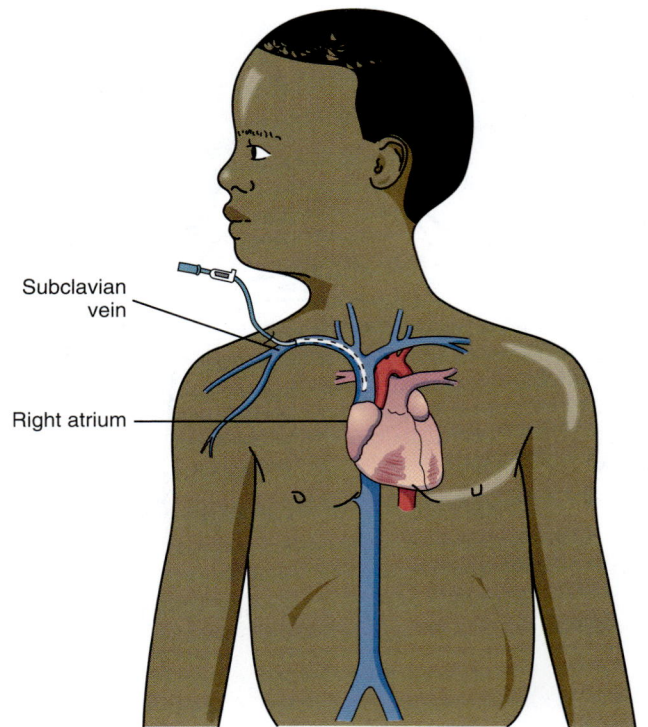

FIGURE 48-25 Central venous line.

Central Venous Lines

Some patients with chronic illnesses need prolonged and frequent access to venous circulation for drug or fluid therapy. This is made possible through vascular access devices. These devices are seen often in the prehospital setting in child and adult patients who are cared for in the home (Figure 48-25). These devices include surgically implanted medication delivery devices (e.g., Port-A-Cath), peripheral vascular access devices (e.g., peripherally inserted central catheters, Intracath), and central venous access devices (e.g., Broviac, Groshong, Hickman) (see Chapter 14 and Chapter 52). Complications that may occur with vascular access devices include a cracked line, air embolism, bleeding, obstruction, and local infection. Patients with vascular access devices often have a serious illness such as cancer or acquired immunodeficiency syndrome. The effects of these illnesses may complicate the assessment and management of emergencies associated with central venous lines.

MANAGEMENT

A torn or leaking catheter (cracked line) may allow fluids or drugs to infiltrate into the surrounding tissues. This can lead to an air embolism. A torn catheter is evidenced by leaking fluid, a complaint of a burning sensation, or swollen and tender skin near the insertion site. If a torn catheter is suspected, the paramedic should stop the infusion immediately and clamp the catheter between the tear and the patient. The patient who develops an altered level of consciousness (indicating a possible air embolism) should be positioned on the left side.[33] The patient's head should be slightly lowered to help prevent the embolism from traveling to the brain. High-concentration oxygen, IV access, and rapid transport for evaluation by a physician are indicated. Any bleeding at the site should be controlled with direct pressure.

Occasionally, the lumen port becomes obstructed by a blood clot that disrupts the flow of fluids or drugs. (Signs and symptoms of obstruction include a sluggish flow and swelling and tenderness at the site.) When this occurs, the patient should be transported to the hospital so that the catheter can be cleared with thrombolytics or replaced. Attempts to clear a vascular access device require special training and authorization from medical direction. The technique is described in Chapter 52.

Gastric Tubes and Gastrostomy Tubes

A gastric tube (Figure 48-26) is used as a temporary measure to provide liquid feeding to a patient who cannot swallow or absorb nutrients (often used for feeding premature infants). The tubes are inserted through the nose or mouth into the stomach and can cause irritation to the nasal and mucous membranes. They are designed for short-term use.

A gastrostomy tube (Figure 48-27) provides a permanent route for gastric feeding in patients who usually cannot be fed by mouth (e.g., a patient with facial burns or paralysis). The tube is surgically placed into the stomach. The tube can be visualized in the upper left quadrant of the abdomen. The opening (stoma) has a flexible, silicone "button." (This is covered with a protective cap.) The stoma allows for regular feedings.

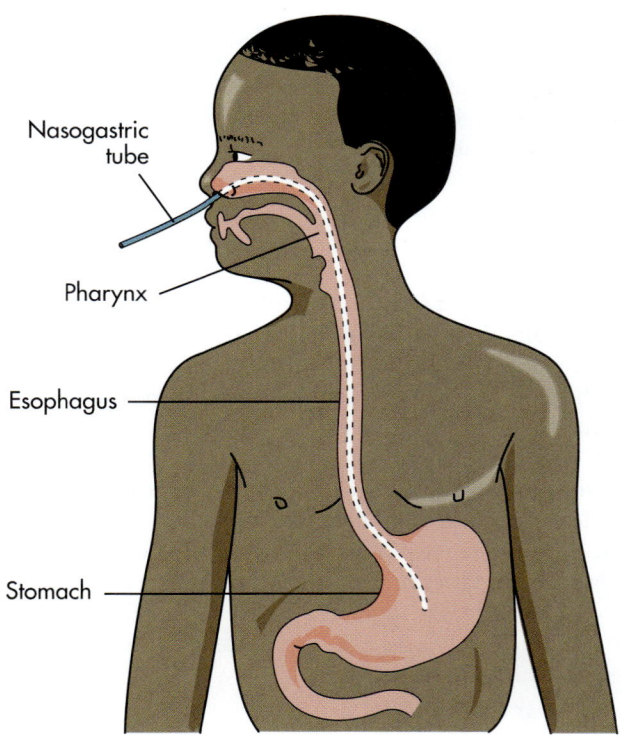

FIGURE 48-26 Nasogastric tube.

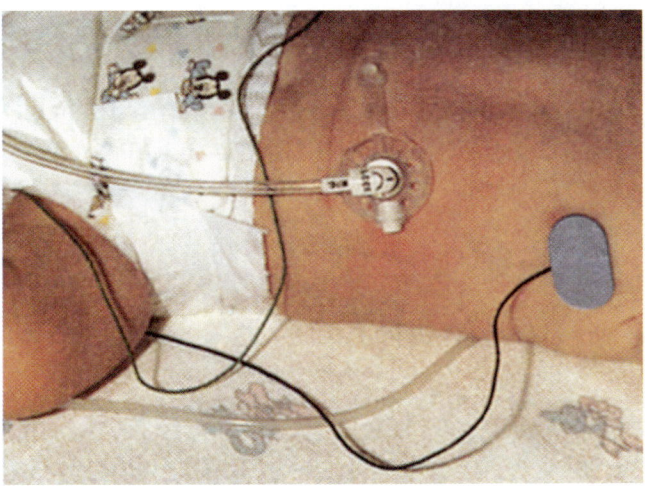

FIGURE 48-27 Gastrostomy tube.

MANAGEMENT

Serious complications with gastric or gastrostomy tubes are rare. They seldom require emergency care. Potential complications include obstruction, pulmonary aspiration, gastrointestinal disturbances (vomiting and diarrhea), irritation to the mucous membrane, and electrolyte imbalances. All of these can result in inadequate nutrition and fluid needs. Emergency care mainly is supportive. Care may include transport for evaluation by a physician. If not contraindicated, the patient will be most comfortable lying on the right side with the head elevated.

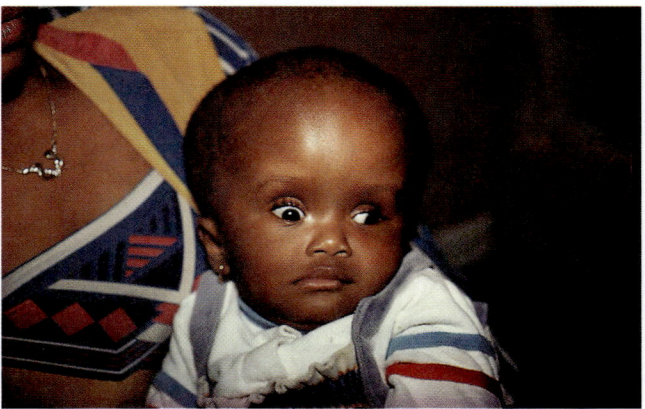

FIGURE 48-28 Untreated hydrocephalus.

Shunts

A **shunt** is a tube or device that is implanted surgically in the body. The shunt redirects body fluid from one cavity or vessel to another. An example of a shunt is one used to relieve abnormal fluid pressures from excess cerebrospinal fluid around the brain in children with **hydrocephalus** (Figure 48-28).

> **NOTE**
> The term hydrocephalus is derived from the Greek words "hydro" meaning water and "cephalus" meaning head. As the name implies, it is a condition in which the primary characteristic is excessive accumulation of fluid around the brain. (Although hydrocephalus was once known as "water on the brain," the "water" is actually cerebrospinal fluid.) The excessive accumulation of CSF results in an abnormal widening of the ventricles in the brain. This widening creates potentially harmful pressure on brain tissues. Hydrocephalus may be congenital or acquired. Congenital hydrocephalus (present at birth) may be caused either by events during fetal development or by genetic abnormalities. Acquired hydrocephalus develops at the time of birth or at some point afterward. This type of hydrocephalus can affect individuals of all ages and may be caused by injury or disease.

The shunt for hydrocephalus consists of two catheters, a reservoir, and a valve to prevent backflow (Figure 48-29). The first catheter is inserted through the skull. It drains fluid from the ventricles of the brain. The second catheter is passed into another body cavity (usually the abdomen or right atrium of the heart through the jugular vein), where the excess fluid is absorbed. The two catheters are connected by a reservoir and valve which is placed under the scalp. The reservoir usually can be palpated over the mastoid area, just behind the ear.

MANAGEMENT

Complications from this procedure include the need for catheter replacement as the child grows (requiring several surgeries in the first 10 years of life), obstruction from

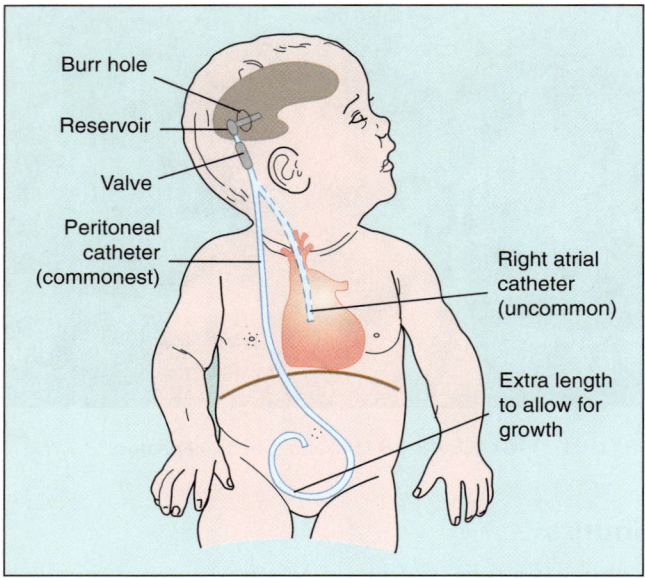

FIGURE 48-29 Ventricular shunt for drainage of symptomatic hydrocephalus.

clotted blood or fluid, and catheter displacement. Infection may occur, but is most common during the first 6 months after surgical placement. The signs and symptoms of obstruction or displacement are those of increased ICP. They include the following:

- Headache
- Nausea and vomiting
- Visual disturbances, in particular limitation in extraocular movements
- Cushing's triad (elevated systolic pressure, irregular respirations, bradycardia), which are signs of impending brainstem herniation

Children who have complications from a ventricular shunt need emergency surgery to prevent brainstem herniation. The paramedic first should ensure adequate airway, ventilatory, and circulatory support for these patients. Medical direction may recommend endotracheal intubation and hyperventilation to lower ICP, followed by IV access. These patients are prone to respiratory arrest. They need immediate transport to a proper facility for evaluation by a physician. If possible, the patient's head should be elevated during transport.

SUMMARY

- Paramedics must continually maintain their knowledge of pediatric emergency care.
- The Emergency Medical Services for Children (EMSC) program was designed to enhance and expand emergency medical services for acutely ill and injured children. The program has defined 12 basic components of an effective Emergency Medical Services for Children system.
- Children have unique anatomical, physiological, and psychological characteristics, which change during their development.
- Airway structures are narrower and less stable than those of adults. This increases the risk of upper and lower airway obstruction related to injury or illness.
- Principles of assessment are similar to those used for adults, but pediatric-sized equipment and specific adaptations to the examination should be made.
- Some childhood diseases and disabilities can be predicted by age group.
- Many elements of the initial evaluation can be done by observing the child. The child's parent or guardian also should be involved in the initial evaluation. The three components of the pediatric assessment triangle are appearance, work of breathing, and circulation.
- Paramedics must recognize and distinguish between respiratory distress, respiratory failure, and respiratory arrest.
- Obstruction of the upper or lower airway by a foreign body usually occurs in toddlers or preschoolers. Obstruction may be partial or complete.

- Croup is a common inflammatory respiratory illness. It usually is seen in children between the ages of 6 months and 4 years. Symptoms are caused by inflammation in the subglottic region.
- Epiglottitis is a rapidly progressive, life-threatening bacterial infection. It causes edema and swelling of the epiglottis and supraglottic structures. It often affects children between 3 and 7 years of age.
- Bacterial tracheitis is an infection of the upper airway and subglottic trachea usually seen in infants and toddlers; it often occurs with or after croup.
- Asthma is common in children over 2 years of age. Asthma is characterized by bronchoconstriction that results from autonomic dysfunction or sensitizing agents.
- Bronchiolitis is a viral disease frequently caused by respiratory syncytial virus infection of the lower airway; it usually affects children 6 to 18 months of age.
- Pneumonia is an acute infection of the lower airways and lungs involving the alveolar walls and the alveoli.
- Pertussis is a bacterial respiratory tract infection associated with a long course of illness, a violent cough with a characteristic "whoop," and a risk of pneumonia and death, especially in infants.
- Bronchopulmonary dysplasia is a chronic lung disease resulting from intervention with oxygen and ventilation in a neonate. It causes alveolar damage and chronic pulmonary dysfunction that can lead to death.
- Several special differences must be remembered when caring for a child in shock. These include circulating blood volume, body surface area and hypothermia,

cardiac reserve, and vital signs and assessment. A child in shock may appear normal and stable until all compensatory mechanisms fail. At that point, pediatric shock progresses rapidly, with serious deterioration.

- When dysrhythmias occur in children, they usually result from hypoxia or structural heart disease.
- Goals of postresuscitation stabilization in children include preserving brain function, avoiding secondary injury, identifying causes of illness, managing pain, and transporting to an appropriate facility.
- Meningitis is inflammation of the meninges. It can lead to neurological damage, hearing or vision impairment, and death.
- The most common causes of seizure in adult and pediatric patients are noncompliance with a drug regimen for the treatment of epilepsy, in addition to head trauma, intracranial infection, metabolic disturbance, or poisoning. The most common cause of new onset of seizure in children is fever.
- Hypoglycemia and hyperglycemia should be suspected whenever a child has an altered level of consciousness with no explainable cause. Consider diabetes as a possible cause in children even in the absence of a history of diabetes.
- Blood disorders that may affect children include sickle cell disease, leukemia, clotting disorders, and others.
- GI disorders in children can lead to serious illness including life-threatening dehydration and death.
- Children with infection may have a variety of signs and symptoms. These depend on the source and extent of infection and the length of time since the patient was exposed.
- Most poisoning events in the United States involve children. Signs and symptoms of accidental poisoning vary, depending on the toxic substance and the length of time since the child was exposed.
- Blunt and penetrating trauma is a chief cause of injury and death in children. Head injury is the most common cause of death in pediatric trauma patients. Early recognition and aggressive management can reduce morbidity and mortality caused by traumatic brain injury in children.
- Because of the pliability of the chest wall, severe intrathoracic injury can be present without signs of external injury. The liver, kidneys, and spleen are the most frequently injured abdominal organs. Extremity injuries are more common in children than adults.
- Sudden infant death syndrome is the leading cause of death in American infants under 1 year of age. The syndrome is defined as the sudden death of a seemingly healthy infant. The death cannot be explained by history and an autopsy.
- Child abuse and neglect is the maltreatment of children by their parents, guardians, or other caregivers. Forms of maltreatment include infliction of physical injury, sexual exploitation, and infliction of emotional pain and neglect.
- Some infants and children are born with or develop conditions that pose special needs. These children may require special medical equipment to sustain life. Often these children are cared for at home. Many are dependent on specialized medical equipment such as tracheostomy tubes, home artificial ventilators, central venous lines, gastrostomy tubes, and shunts. They may have emergencies associated with airway obstruction, impaired ventilation, infection, or increased intracranial pressure.

REFERENCES

1. American Heart Association: *Pediatric advanced life support,* Dallas, 2006, The Association.
2. Durch J, Lohr K, editors: *The Institute of Medicine Report, EMSC Report Summary,* Washington, DC: National Academy Press, 1993, p. 5.
3. National Center for Education in Maternal and Child Health: *Emergency medical services for children: a report to the nation,* Washington, DC, 1991, The Center.
4. Institute of Medicine: *Emergency care for children: growing pains,* http://iom.edu/Reports/2006/Emergency-Care-for-Children-Growing-Pains.aspx, accessed 10-26-10.
5. National Safety Council: *Injury facts,* Itasca, Ill, 2010, The Council.
6. American Heart Association: *2010 American Heart Association guidelines for cardiopulmonary resuscitation, Circulation* 122:S876-S908, 2010.
7. Weiss M, Dullenkopf A, Fischer JE, et al: Prospective randomized controlled multi-centre trial of cuffed or uncuffed endotracheal tubes in small children, *Br J Anaesth* 103(6):867-873, 2009.
8. Huang T, Johnson MS, Figueroa-Colon R, et al: Growth of visceral fat, subcutaneous abdominal fat, and total body fat in children, *Obesity Res* 9(5):283-289, 2001.
9. The National SCI Statistical Center: *Spinal Cord Injury Information Network, facts and figures at a glance: 2008,* www.spinalcord.uab.edu/show.asp?durki=116979, accessed 11-11-10.
10. National Spinal Cord Injury Statistical Center, Birmingham, Alabama. Spinal Cord Injury: *Facts and figures at a glance.* www.spinalcord.uab.edu, accessed July 22, 2011.
11. American Academy of Pediatrics, American College of Emergency Physicians: *APLS: the pediatric emergency medicine resource,* ed 4, Sudbury, Mass, 2007, Jones & Bartlett.
12. American Academy of Pediatrics: Policy Statement—prevention of choking among children, *Pediatrics* 125(3):601-607, 2010.
13. Gold Standard, Elsevier. http://www.clinicalpharmacology.com/?epm=2_1, accessed July 22, 2011.
14. Shah S, Sharieff G: Pediatric respiratory infections, *Emerg Med Clin N Am* 25(4):961-979, 2007.
15. Felter R, Waldrop R: *Pediatrics, epiglottitis,* http://emedicine.medscape.com/article/801369-overview, accessed 10-15-10.

16. Hockenberry MJ, Wilson D: *Wong's essentials of pediatric nursing,* ed 8, St Louis, 2009, Mosby.

17. Centers for Disease Control and Prevention: *Asthma,* www.cdc.gov/nchs/fastats/asthma.htm, accessed 10-15-10.

18. American Academy of Allergy, Asthma, and Immunology: *Asthma statistics,* www.aaaai.org/media/statistics/asthma-statistics.aspp, accessed 10-15-10.

19. National Heart, Lung and Blood Institute, National Institutes of Health: *Expert Panel Report 3 (EPR3): guidelines for the diagnosis and management of asthma,* www.nhlbi.nih.gov/guidelines/asthma/asthgdln.htm, accessed 10-15-10.

20. National Highway Traffic Safety Administration. *The National EMS Education Standards.* Washington, DC: U.S. Department of Transportation/National Highway Traffic Safety Administration, 2009, DOT.

21. American Academy of Pediatrics: Diagnosis and management of bronchiolitis, *Pediatrics* 18(4):1774-1793, 2006.

22. *Respiratory distress syndrome and bronchopulmonary dysplasia,* http://lungusa.org/assets/documents.ALA_LDD08_RDS_FINAL.PDF, accessed 10-15-10.

23. Wilkins RL, Stoller MD, Kacmarek RM: *Egan's fundamentals of respiratory care,* ed 9, St Louis, 2008, Mosby.

24. Rhoads GG, McNellis DC, Kessel SS: Bureau of Maternal and Child Health Resources Development: guidelines for the care of children with chronic lung disease, pediatric pulmonology, *Am J Obstet Gynecol* 3:3-13, 1989.

25. Thibodeau GA, Patton KT: *Anatomy & physiology,* ed 6, St Louis, 2006, Mosby.

26. Donoghue D, Nadkarni V, Berg RA, et al: Out of hospital pediatric cardiac arrest: epidemiologic review and assessment of current knowledge, *Ann Emerg Med* 46:523-524, 2006.

27. emedicine: *Meningitis in children,* www.emedicinehealth.com/meningitis_in_children/page3_em.htm, accessed 10-15-10.

28. National Diabetes Education Program: *Overview of diabetes in children and adolescents: a fact sheet from the National Diabetes Education Program,* http://ndep.nih.gov/media/Youth_FactSheet.pdf, accessed 10-14-10.

29. American Diabetic Association: *Diabetes statistics 2007,* www.diabetes.org/diabetes-basics/diabetes-statistics/, accessed 10-15-10.

30. American Cancer Society: *What are the key statistics about childhood leukemia?* www.cancer.org/docroot/CRI/content/CRI_2_4_1X_What_are_the_key_statistics_about_childhood_leukemia_24.asp?rnav=cri, accessed 10-15-10.

31. Hansen T: *Jaundice, neonatal,* http://emedicine.medscape.com/article/974786-overview, accessed 5-3-10.

32. National Safe Kids Campaign: *Burn injury fact sheet,* Washington, DC, 2004, The Campaign.

33. Rosen P, Barkin R: *Emergency medicine: concepts and clinical practice,* ed 7, St Louis, 2006, Mosby.

34. Hoekelman R et al, editors: *Primary pediatric care,* St Louis, 2001, Mosby.

35. Centers for Disease Control and Prevention: *Sudden infant death syndrome (SIDS) and sudden unexpected infant death (SUID),* www.cdc.gov/sids/, accessed 10-17-10.

36. Adams SM, Good MW, Defranco GM: Sudden infant death syndrome, *Am Fam Physician* 79(10):870-874, 2009.

37. Carolan P: *Sudden infant death syndrome,* http://emedicine.medscape.com/article/1004238-overview, accessed 10-16-10.

38. Stoker J, Dehner L: *Pediatric pathology,* ed 2, vol 1, Philadelphia, 2001, Lippincott.

39. McMillan J, editor: *Oski's pediatrics: principles and practice,* ed 4, Philadelphia, 2006, Lippincott.

40. U.S. Department of Health and Human Services, National Institutes of Health: *SIDS linked to low levels of serotonin,* Washington, D.C., 2010, NIH News.

41. National Child Abuse Statistics: *Child help, prevention and treatment of child abuse,* www.childhelp.org/pages/statistics, accessed 10-16-10.

42. Craighead E, Nemeroff C, editors: *Corsini encyclopedia of psychology and behavioral science,* ed 3, New York, 2001, John Wiley & Sons.

43. *Indicators of child abuse and maltreatment,* www.childabuse.com/help.htm, accessed 10-17-10.

44. Bariciak E, Benntt S, Gaboury I, et al: Dating of bruises in children: an assessment of physician accuracy, *Pediatrics* 112(4):804-807, 2003.

45. Pyrek K: *Forensic nursing,* Boca Raton, Fla, 2006, CRC Press.

SUGGESTED READINGS

Banasiak N: Pediatric asthma, *RN,* July:26-31, 2008.

Dieckmann RA, Brownstein D, Gausche-Hill M: The pediatric assessment triangle: a novel approach for the rapid evaluation of children [review article], *Pediatr Emerg Care* 26(4):312-315, 2009.

Shah S, Sharieff G: Pediatric respiratory infections, *Emerg Med Clin N Am* 25:961-979, 2007.

U.S. Department of Health and Human Services, Health Resources and Services Administration, EMSC National Resource Center: *Publications and resources,* 2010. Retrieved 5-17-10 from www.childrensnational.org/emsc/pubres/downloaddocs.aspx.

Recommended Childhood and Adolescent Immunization Schedules

Recommended Immunization Schedule for Persons Aged 0 Through 6 Years—United States • 2011
For those who fall behind or start late, see the catch-up schedule

Vaccine ▼ Age ▶	Birth	1 month	2 months	4 months	6 months	12 months	15 months	18 months	19–23 months	2–3 years	4–6 years
Hepatitis B[1]	HepB	HepB				HepB					
Rotavirus[2]			RV	RV	RV[2]						
Diphtheria, Tetanus, Pertussis[3]			DTaP	DTaP	DTaP	see footnote[3]	DTaP				DTaP
Haemophilus influenzae type b[4]			Hib	Hib	Hib[4]	Hib					
Pneumococcal[5]			PCV	PCV	PCV	PCV				PPSV	
Inactivated Poliovirus[6]			IPV	IPV		IPV					IPV
Influenza[7]						Influenza (Yearly)					
Measles, Mumps, Rubella[8]						MMR		see footnote[8]			MMR
Varicella[9]						Varicella		see footnote[9]			Varicella
Hepatitis A[10]						HepA (2 doses)				HepA Series	
Meningococcal[11]										MCV4	

Range of recommended ages for all children

Range of recommended ages for certain high-risk groups

This schedule includes recommendations in effect as of December 21, 2010. Any dose not administered at the recommended age should be administered at a subsequent visit, when indicated and feasible. The use of a combination vaccine generally is preferred over separate injections of its equivalent component vaccines. Considerations should include provider assessment, patient preference, and the potential for adverse events. Providers should consult the relevant Advisory Committee on Immunization Practices statement for detailed recommendations: **http://www.cdc.gov/vaccines/pubs/acip-list.htm**. Clinically significant adverse events that follow immunization should be reported to the Vaccine Adverse Event Reporting System (VAERS) at **http://www.vaers.hhs.gov** or by telephone, **800-822-7967**.

1. **Hepatitis B vaccine (HepB).** (Minimum age: birth)
   At birth:
   • Administer monovalent HepB to all newborns before hospital discharge.
   • If mother is hepatitis B surface antigen (HBsAg)-positive, administer HepB and 0.5 mL of hepatitis B immune globulin (HBIG) within 12 hours of birth.
   • If mother's HBsAg status is unknown, administer HepB within 12 hours of birth. Determine mother's HBsAg status as soon as possible and, if HBsAg-positive, administer HBIG (no later than age 1 week).
   Doses following the birth dose:
   • The second dose should be administered at age 1 or 2 months. Monovalent HepB should be used for doses administered before age 6 weeks.
   • Infants born to HBsAg-positive mothers should be tested for HBsAg and antibody to HBsAg 1 to 2 months after completion of at least 3 doses of the HepB series, at age 9 through 18 months (generally at the next well-child visit).
   • Administration of 4 doses of HepB to infants is permissible when a combination vaccine containing HepB is administered after the birth dose.
   • Infants who did not receive a birth dose should receive 3 doses of HepB on a schedule of 0, 1, and 6 months.
   • The final (3rd or 4th) dose in the HepB series should be administered no earlier than age 24 weeks.
2. **Rotavirus vaccine (RV).** (Minimum age: 6 weeks)
   • Administer the first dose at age 6 through 14 weeks (maximum age: 14 weeks 6 days). Vaccination should not be initiated for infants aged 15 weeks 0 days or older.
   • The maximum age for the final dose in the series is 8 months 0 days
   • If Rotarix is administered at ages 2 and 4 months, a dose at 6 months is not indicated.
3. **Diphtheria and tetanus toxoids and acellular pertussis vaccine (DTaP).** (Minimum age: 6 weeks)
   • The fourth dose may be administered as early as age 12 months, provided at least 6 months have elapsed since the third dose.
4. **Haemophilus influenzae type b conjugate vaccine (Hib).** (Minimum age: 6 weeks)
   • If PRP-OMP (PedvaxHIB or Comvax [HepB-Hib]) is administered at ages 2 and 4 months, a dose at age 6 months is not indicated.
   • Hiberix should not be used for doses at ages 2, 4, or 6 months for the primary series but can be used as the final dose in children aged 12 months through 4 years.
5. **Pneumococcal vaccine.** (Minimum age: 6 weeks for pneumococcal conjugate vaccine [PCV]; 2 years for pneumococcal polysaccharide vaccine [PPSV])
   • PCV is recommended for all children aged younger than 5 years. Administer 1 dose of PCV to all healthy children aged 24 through 59 months who are not completely vaccinated for their age.
   • A PCV series begun with 7-valent PCV (PCV7) should be completed with 13-valent PCV (PCV13).
   • A single supplemental dose of PCV13 is recommended for all children aged 14 through 59 months who have received an age-appropriate series of PCV7.
   • A single supplemental dose of PCV13 is recommended for all children aged 60 through 71 months with underlying medical conditions who have received an age-appropriate series of PCV7.

   • The supplemental dose of PCV13 should be administered at least 8 weeks after the previous dose of PCV7. See *MMWR* 2010:59(No. RR-11).
   • Administer PPSV at least 8 weeks after last dose of PCV to children aged 2 years or older with certain underlying medical conditions, including a cochlear implant.
6. **Inactivated poliovirus vaccine (IPV).** (Minimum age: 6 weeks)
   • If 4 or more doses are administered prior to age 4 years an additional dose should be administered at age 4 through 6 years.
   • The final dose in the series should be administered on or after the fourth birthday and at least 6 months following the previous dose.
7. **Influenza vaccine (seasonal).** (Minimum age: 6 months for trivalent inactivated influenza vaccine [TIV]; 2 years for live, attenuated influenza vaccine [LAIV])
   • For healthy children aged 2 years and older (i.e., those who do not have underlying medical conditions that predispose them to influenza complications), either LAIV or TIV may be used, except LAIV should not be given to children aged 2 through 4 years who have had wheezing in the past 12 months.
   • Administer 2 doses (separated by at least 4 weeks) to children aged 6 months through 8 years who are receiving seasonal influenza vaccine for the first time or who were vaccinated for the first time during the previous influenza season but only received 1 dose.
   • Children aged 6 months through 8 years who received no doses of monovalent 2009 H1N1 vaccine should receive 2 doses of 2010–2011 seasonal influenza vaccine. See *MMWR* 2010;59(No. RR-8):33–34.
8. **Measles, mumps, and rubella vaccine (MMR).** (Minimum age: 12 months)
   • The second dose may be administered before age 4 years, provided at least 4 weeks have elapsed since the first dose.
9. **Varicella vaccine.** (Minimum age: 12 months)
   • The second dose may be administered before age 4 years, provided at least 3 months have elapsed since the first dose.
   • For children aged 12 months through 12 years the recommended minimum interval between doses is 3 months. However, if the second dose was administered at least 4 weeks after the first dose, it can be accepted as valid.
10. **Hepatitis A vaccine (HepA).** (Minimum age: 12 months)
    • Administer 2 doses at least 6 months apart.
    • HepA is recommended for children aged older than 23 months who live in areas where vaccination programs target older children, who are at increased risk for infection, or for whom immunity against hepatitis A is desired.
11. **Meningococcal conjugate vaccine, quadrivalent (MCV4).** (Minimum age: 2 years)
    • Administer 2 doses of MCV4 at least 8 weeks apart to children aged 2 through 10 years with persistent complement component deficiency and anatomic or functional asplenia, and 1 dose every 5 years thereafter.
    • Persons with human immunodeficiency virus (HIV) infection who are vaccinated with MCV4 should receive 2 doses at least 8 weeks apart.
    • Administer 1 dose of MCV4 to children aged 2 through 10 years who travel to countries with highly endemic or epidemic disease and during outbreaks caused by a vaccine serogroup.
    • Administer MCV4 to children at continued risk for meningococcal disease who were previously vaccinated with MCV4 or meningococcal polysaccharide vaccine after 3 years if the first dose was administered at age 2 through 6 years.

The Recommended Immunization Schedules for Persons Aged 0 Through 18 Years are approved by the Advisory Committee on Immunization Practices (**http://www.cdc.gov/vaccines/recs/acip**), the American Academy of Pediatrics (**http://www.aap.org**), and the American Academy of Family Physicians (**http://www.aafp.org**).
Department of Health and Human Services • Centers for Disease Control and Prevention

APPENDIX FIGURE 48-1 Centers for Disease Control and Prevention—United States, 2011.

Recommended Immunization Schedule for Persons Aged 7 Through 18 Years—United States • 2011

For those who fall behind or start late, see the schedule below and the catch-up schedule

Vaccine ▼ Age ►	7–10 years	11–12 years	13–18 years	
Tetanus, Diphtheria, Pertussis[1]		Tdap	Tdap	Range of recommended ages for all children
Human Papillomavirus[2]	see footnote [2]	HPV (3 doses)(females)	HPV series	
Meningococcal[3]	MCV4	MCV4	MCV4	
Influenza[4]	Influenza (Yearly)			
Pneumococcal[5]	Pneumococcal			Range of recommended ages for catch-up immunization
Hepatitis A[6]	HepA Series			
Hepatitis B[7]	Hep B Series			
Inactivated Poliovirus[8]	IPV Series			
Measles, Mumps, Rubella[9]	MMR Series			Range of recommended ages for certain high-risk groups
Varicella[10]	Varicella Series			

This schedule includes recommendations in effect as of December 21, 2010. Any dose not administered at the recommended age should be administered at a subsequent visit, when indicated and feasible. The use of a combination vaccine generally is preferred over separate injections of its equivalent component vaccines. Considerations should include provider assessment, patient preference, and the potential for adverse events. Providers should consult the relevant Advisory Committee on Immunization Practices statement for detailed recommendations: **http://www.cdc.gov/vaccines/pubs/acip-list.htm.** Clinically significant adverse events that follow immunization should be reported to the Vaccine Adverse Event Reporting System (VAERS) at **http://www.vaers.hhs.gov** or by telephone, **800-822-7967.**

1. **Tetanus and diphtheria toxoids and acellular pertussis vaccine (Tdap).** (Minimum age: 10 years for Boostrix and 11 years for Adacel))
   - Persons aged 11 through 18 years who have not received Tdap should receive a dose followed by Td booster doses every 10 years thereafter.
   - Persons aged 7 through 10 years who are not fully immunized against pertussis (including those never vaccinated or with unknown pertussis vaccination status) should receive a single dose of Tdap. Refer to the catch-up schedule if additional doses of tetanus and diphtheria toxoid–containing vaccine are needed.
   - Tdap can be administered regardless of the interval since the last tetanus and diphtheria toxoid–containing vaccine.
2. **Human papillomavirus vaccine (HPV).** (Minimum age: 9 years)
   - Quadrivalent HPV vaccine (HPV4) or bivalent HPV vaccine (HPV2) is recommended for the prevention of cervical precancers and cancers in females.
   - HPV4 is recommended for prevention of cervical precancers, cancers, and genital warts in females.
   - HPV4 may be administered in a 3-dose series to males aged 9 through 18 years to reduce their likelihood of genital warts.
   - Administer the second dose 1 to 2 months after the first dose and the third dose 6 months after the first dose (at least 24 weeks after the first dose).
3. **Meningococcal conjugate vaccine, quadrivalent (MCV4).** (Minimum age: 2 years)
   - Administer MCV4 at age 11 through 12 years with a booster dose at age 16 years.
   - Administer 1 dose at age 13 through 18 years if not previously vaccinated.
   - Persons who received their first dose at age 13 through 15 years should receive a booster dose at age 16 through 18 years.
   - Administer 1 dose to previously unvaccinated college freshmen living in a dormitory.
   - Administer 2 doses at least 8 weeks apart to children aged 2 through 10 years with persistent complement component deficiency and anatomic or functional asplenia, and 1 dose every 5 years thereafter.
   - Persons with HIV infection who are vaccinated with MCV4 should receive 2 doses at least 8 weeks apart.
   - Administer 1 dose of MCV4 to children aged 2 through 10 years who travel to countries with highly endemic or epidemic disease and during outbreaks caused by a vaccine serogroup.
   - Administer MCV4 to children at continued risk for meningococcal disease who were previously vaccinated with MCV4 or meningococcal polysaccharide vaccine after 3 years (if first dose administered at age 2 through 6 years) or after 5 years (if first dose administered at age 7 years or older).
4. **Influenza vaccine (seasonal).**
   - For healthy nonpregnant persons aged 7 through 18 years (i.e., those who do not have underlying medical conditions that predispose them to influenza complications), either LAIV or TIV may be used.
   - Administer 2 doses (separated by at least 4 weeks) to children aged 6 months through 8 years who are receiving seasonal influenza vaccine for the first

time or who were vaccinated for the first time during the previous influenza season but only received 1 dose.
   - Children 6 months through 8 years of age who received no doses of monovalent 2009 H1N1 vaccine should receive 2 doses of 2010-2011 seasonal influenza vaccine. See *MMWR* 2010;59(No. RR-8):33–34.
5. **Pneumococcal vaccines.**
   - A single dose of 13-valent pneumococcal conjugate vaccine (PCV13) may be administered to children aged 6 through 18 years who have functional or anatomic asplenia, HIV infection or other immunocompromising condition, cochlear implant or CSF leak. See *MMWR* 2010;59(No. RR-11).
   - The dose of PCV13 should be administered at least 8 weeks after the previous dose of PCV7.
   - Administer pneumococcal polysaccharide vaccine at least 8 weeks after the last dose of PCV to children aged 2 years or older with certain underlying medical conditions, including a cochlear implant. A single revaccination should be administered after 5 years to children with functional or anatomic asplenia or an immunocompromising condition.
6. **Hepatitis A vaccine (HepA).**
   - Administer 2 doses at least 6 months apart.
   - HepA is recommended for children aged older than 23 months who live in areas where vaccination programs target older children, or who are at increased risk for infection, or for whom immunity against hepatitis A is desired.
7. **Hepatitis B vaccine (HepB).**
   - Administer the 3-dose series to those not previously vaccinated. For those with incomplete vaccination, follow the catch-up schedule.
   - A 2-dose series (separated by at least 4 months) of adult formulation Recombivax HB is licensed for children aged 11 through 15 years.
8. **Inactivated poliovirus vaccine (IPV).**
   - The final dose in the series should be administered on or after the fourth birthday and at least 6 months following the previous dose.
   - If both OPV and IPV were administered as part of a series, a total of 4 doses should be administered, regardless of the child's current age.
9. **Measles, mumps, and rubella vaccine (MMR).**
   - The minimum interval between the 2 doses of MMR is 4 weeks.
10. **Varicella vaccine.**
   - For persons aged 7 through 18 years without evidence of immunity (see *MMWR* 2007;56[No. RR-4]), administer 2 doses if not previously vaccinated or the second dose if only 1 dose has been administered.
   - For persons aged 7 through 12 years, the recommended minimum interval between doses is 3 months. However, if the second dose was administered at least 4 weeks after the first dose, it can be accepted as valid.
   - For persons aged 13 years and older, the minimum interval between doses is 4 weeks.

The Recommended Immunization Schedules for Persons Aged 0 Through 18 Years are approved by the Advisory Committee on Immunization Practices (**http://www.cdc.gov/vaccines/recs/acip**), the American Academy of Pediatrics (**http://www.aap.org**), and the American Academy of Family Physicians (**http://www.aafp.org**).
Department of Health and Human Services • Centers for Disease Control and Prevention

APPENDIX FIGURE 48-2 Centers for Disease Control and Prevention—United States, 2011.

49 Geriatrics

Upon completion of this chapter, the paramedic student will be able to:

1. Explain the physiology of the aging process as it relates to major body systems and homeostasis.
2. Describe general principles of assessment specific to older adults.
3. Describe the pathophysiology, assessment, and management of specific illnesses that affect selected body systems in the geriatric patient.
4. Identify specific problems with sensations experienced by some geriatric patients.
5. Discuss effects of drug toxicity and alcoholism in the older adult.
6. Identify factors that contribute to environmental emergencies in the geriatric patient.
7. Discuss prehospital assessment and management of depression and suicide in the older adult.
8. Describe epidemiology, assessment, and management of trauma in the geriatric patient.
9. Identify characteristics of elder abuse.

KEY TERMS

adverse drug event An injury resulting from the use of a drug.

Alzheimer's disease A disease characterized by confusion, memory failure, disorientation, speech disturbances, and inability to carry out purposeful movements.

biliary disease Disorders of the liver and gallbladder caused by abnormalities in bile composition, biliary anatomy, or function.

cataract A loss of transparency of the lens of the eye that results from changes in the delicate protein fibers within the lens.

cerebral atrophy Refers to brain issue that becomes smaller in size with age.

confabulation The invention of stories to make up for gaps in memory.

continence The ability to control bladder or bowel function.

decubitus ulcers Skin lesions caused by many factors, including unrelieved pressure, friction, humidity, shearing forces, temperature, age, incontinence, and medication.

delirium An abrupt disorientation for time and place, usually with illusions and hallucinations.

dementia A slow, progressive loss of awareness of time and place. It usually involves an inability to learn new things or recall recent events.

elder abuse The infliction of physical pain, injury, debilitating mental anguish, unreasonable confinement, or willful deprivation by a caregiver of services that are necessary to maintain mental and physical health of a geriatric person.

fecal impaction An accumulation of hardened feces in the rectum or sigmoid colon that the person is unable to move.

frailty A biological syndrome of decreased reserve and resistance to stressors, resulting from cumulative declines across multiple physiological systems, and causing vulnerability to adverse outcomes.

gerontology The study of the problems of all aspects of aging.

glaucoma A condition in which intraocular pressure increases and causes damage to the optic nerve.

hyperthyroidism A condition characterized by increased activity of the thyroid gland.

hypothyroidism A condition characterized by decreased activity of the thyroid gland.

incontinence The inability to control bladder or bowel function.

kyphosis An abnormal condition of the vertebral column characterized by increased convexity in the curvature of the thoracic spine as viewed from the side.

organic brain dysfunction Physical disorders that affect cognition.

osteoarthritis A form of arthritis in which one or many joints undergo degenerative changes.

osteoporosis A disorder characterized by a reduction in bone density; it occurs most often in postmenopausal women.

Parkinson's disease A disease caused by degeneration or damage (of unknown origin) to nerve cells within the basal ganglia in the brain.

pressure ulcers Sores or ulcers in the skin over a bony prominence that occur most frequently on the sacrum, elbows, heels, outer ankles, inner knees, hips, and shoulder blades of high-risk patients, especially those who are obese, elderly, or suffering from chronic diseases, infections, injuries, or a poor nutritional state.

retinopathy A group of inflammatory eye disorders often caused by diabetes, hypertension, and atherosclerotic vascular disease.

tinnitus A ringing sound in the ears.

The "graying" of American society includes the prospect that the health care needs of older adults will continue to increase in all areas. This includes prehospital care. About 25% of Americans will be 65 years of age or older by the year 2030 and will represent 70% of all ambulance transports.[1] This chapter addresses anatomical and physiological changes that accompany the aging process, special considerations in assessing and managing geriatric patients, and common emergencies that may result from normal aging and chronic illness.

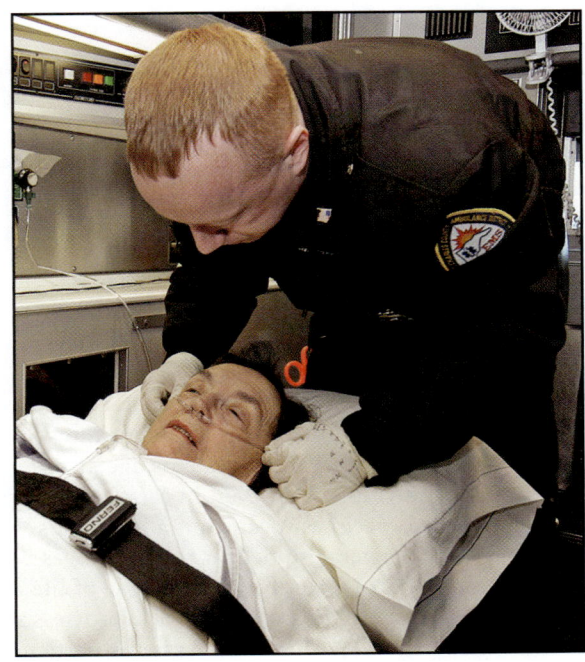

(Courtesy Ray Kemp, St. Charles, Mo.)

DEMOGRAPHICS, EPIDEMIOLOGY, AND SOCIETAL ISSUES

More than 34 million Americans (12% of the U.S. population) are 65 years of age or older. The size of this group has soared during the last 100 years. At the same time, fertility rates in the United States have dropped. Thus there will be fewer persons under 65 years of age to support the cost of health care and living expenses of those over 65 years of age.

By the year 2050, nearly 25% of Americans will be eligible for Medicare. Also, the population over 85 years of age will have grown from 4 million to 19 million. This creates many challenges. Society will need to provide quality, cost-effective health care and support the increasing health and living expenses for the elderly. To meet the needs of this aging population properly, society must achieve the following[2]:

- The public must become better educated about the needs of the elderly because caregiving often becomes the responsibility of families and friends.
- Current and new health care professionals must be educated on the special needs of the aging population.
- The aging of the U.S. population demands continued and expanded research efforts into chronic diseases that affect the elderly and their families.
- Health care professionals need to reform heath care financing, delivery, and administrative structures to accommodate the predominance of chronic illness among the aging population.
- Health care professionals must develop solutions for the long-term care needs of the growing aging population. These solutions must address the emotional and financial needs of older adults and their families. They also must address the financial influence of long-term care in the United States.

Other key issues to consider in caring for the aging population include legal ones such as advance directives, durable power of attorney, and do not resuscitate orders. These were discussed in Chapter 6.

LIVING ENVIRONMENTS AND REFERRAL SOURCES

Many older Americans enjoy independent living. They enjoy this lifestyle with the help of spousal or family support and home health care programs. Others live dependently in nursing care facilities, assisted-living environments, and nursing homes. The elderly often receive assistance in independent and dependent living environments. They receive this help through local, state, and national programs and other resource agencies (Box 49-1). The paramedic should be familiar with the programs in the community that offer assistance to the elderly.

BOX 49-1 Sampling of Support and Assistance Programs for the Geriatric Patient

Community-based services
Home health care services
Hospice programs
In-home services
Institutional services
Multipurpose senior centers
Nutrition services
Religious and pastoral services
State advisory councils
State and national aging organizations
Volunteer organizations

PHYSIOLOGICAL CHANGES OF AGING

Gerontology is the study of the problems of all aspects of aging. The aging process proceeds at different rates in different persons. In addition, organ systems age at differing rates within the individual. However, in certain areas, predictable functional declines occur in all persons with increasing age. As a general guideline, these changes begin to occur at a rate of 5% to 10% for each decade of life after 30 years of age. The aging process affects all body systems. However, the effects on specific organ systems particularly relevant to the older adult occur in the respiratory, cardiovascular, renal, nervous, and musculoskeletal systems (Table 49-1).

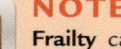

CRITICAL THINKING
Consider your family members and friends who are in their 40s, 60s, or 80s. What age-related changes have you noticed?

NOTE
Frailty can be defined as a biological syndrome of decreased reserve and resistance to stressors, resulting from cumulative declines across multiple physiological systems, and causing vulnerability to adverse outcomes.[3] This concept distinguishes frailty from physical disability that is associated with advancing age.

Characteristics of frailty are low physical activity, muscle weakness, slowed performance, fatigue or poor endurance, and unintentional weight loss. Most frail older adults are women (partly because women outlive men), are more than 80 years old, and often receive care from an adult child. Because of the rapid rate of growth in the population 65 years and older, the number of frail elderly persons is increasing every year.[4]

Respiratory System Changes

Respiratory function in the older adult generally declines as the lung tissue ages. Reduced pulmonary capacity results from changes in lung and chest wall compliance. With aging, the chest wall becomes stiffer as the bony thorax becomes more rigid. Lung elastic recoil also decreases. Despite the loss of elasticity, which would tend to increase total lung capacity, total lung capacity remains the same. This is due to the opposing loss of chest wall compliance and weakened respiratory muscles. The diameter of the alveoli increases. The distal airways tend to collapse on expiration. These changes lead to an increase in residual volume and a decrease in vital capacity. Consequently, by 75 years of age, vital capacity may decrease by as much as 50%, maximum breathing capacity by as much as 60%, and maximum work rate and maximum oxygen uptake by as much as 70%.[5]

The arterial partial pressure of oxygen (PaO_2) also slowly decreases with age. But arterial carbon dioxide pressure stays the same. (This is most likely related to the much greater reserve in carbon dioxide elimination than in oxygen absorption.) At 30 years of age the PaO_2 of a healthy person breathing ambient air at sea level is about 90 mm Hg (90 torr). At 70 years of age the expected PaO_2 is 70 mm Hg (70 torr). These findings, along with the normal decline in chemoreceptor function, produce a diminished ventilatory response to hypoxia and hypercapnia.

Other factors that affect the respiratory system are the loss of cilia in the airways and a diminished cough reflex and impaired gag reflex. These can impair the bodily defense against inhaled bacteria and particulate matter. The decline in these defense mechanisms makes infectious pulmonary diseases of the older adult more common. It also makes these infections harder to resolve.

Cardiovascular System Changes

Cardiac function declines with age as a result of nonischemic physiological changes and the high incidence of atherosclerotic coronary artery disease.[6] Differentiation of the changes that are solely due to aging from those associated with ischemia is difficult because coronary artery disease is so prevalent in the older adult. However, even with aging alone, structural and physiological changes occur that limit cardiac function in the cardiovascular system. These changes include a diminished ability to raise the heart rate even in response to exercise or stress, a decrease in compliance of the ventricle, a prolonged duration of contraction, and a decreased responsiveness to catecholamine stimulation. Between 30 and 80 years of age, resting cardiac output decreases about 30%. Combined with the progressive increase in peripheral vascular resistance that occurs after 40 years of age, this decrease in cardiac output yields a significant drop in organ perfusion.[3] Myocardial hypertrophy, coronary artery disease, and hemodynamic changes predispose the geriatric patient to dysrhythmias, heart failure, and sudden cardiac

TABLE 49-1 Physiological Changes of Aging

Change	Result
Overall Appearance	
Skin	
Loss of elasticity	Wrinkling, thinning of skin
Loss of collagen	Increased susceptibility to injury
Shrinking of sweat glands	Dryness
Pigment deposition	Age spots
Sun damage	Senile keratosis
Eyes	
Clouding of lens	Cataracts (decreased visual acuity)
	Poor peripheral vision
Pigment deposition	Arcus senilis (bluish circle that forms around outer edge of iris)
Cardiovascular System	
Increased internal thickening of arteries	Hypertension
	Increased risk of stroke or heart attack
	Varicosities and clots
	Dysrhythmias
Increased cholesterol deposits (atherosclerotic heart disease)	Coronary artery disease and peripheral vascular disease
Decreased rate of cardiac hypertrophy	Decreased cardiac output
Decreased cardiac output	Loss of exercise tolerance
	Diminished activity
	Increased work to heart
	Increased risk of myocardial infarction
Pulmonary System	
Decreased elasticity	Diminished breathing capacity
Decreased compliance and surface area	Decreased maximal oxygen uptake
Decreased ciliary activity	Increased risk of infection/toxicity
Gastrointestinal Tract	
Decreased hydrochloric acid production	Difficulty with digestion
	Food absorption problems and constipation
Delay in intestinal motility	Feeling full early, causing weight loss
Decreased saliva flow	Dry mouth, difficulty chewing
Fewer taste buds	Loss of food enjoyment, decreased appetite
Gum atrophy (shrinkage)	Tooth loss
Decreased liver function	Risk of toxicity from drugs
	Alcohol damage
	Loss of blood clotting
Central Nervous System	
Decreased cortical cell count	Memory impairment (dementia)
Increased synapse time	Decreased complex learning
Decreased nerve conduction velocity	Slower psychomotor skills
	Increased reflex time leading to risk of falling
Brain atrophy (shrinkage)	Prone to subdural hematomata
Vision	
Growth of lens	Decreased focusing ability
Cataract deposition	Hyperopia (farsightedness)
	Opacification of vision
Decreased pupil size	Decreased acuity and color perception
Loss of accommodation (focusing ability)	Decreased depth perception
	All cause increased risks of accidents and falls

TABLE 49-1 Physiological Changes of Aging—cont'd

Change	Result
Hearing	
Ossicle degeneration	Loss of high-frequency range of hearing
Atrophy (shrinkage) of auditory meatus	Loss of high-frequency range of hearing
Atrophy (shrinkage) of cochlear hair cells and auditory neurons	Decreased keenness and pitch discrimination
	Decreased sense of balance
	All cause increased risks of accidents and falls
Renal Function	
Decreased glomerular function	Decreased renal clearance
Decreased renal blood flow	Increased risk of toxicity from all drugs and toxins processed in kidneys
Genitourinary System	
Loss of bladder control	Urinary infections
Prostate enlargement	Tumors and urinary retention
Endocrine Function	
Decrease in thyroid, ovarian, and testicular function	Decreased energy, decreased metabolic rate
	Decreased heat/cold tolerance
	Decreased reproductive function
Increased insulin	Predisposition for hypoglycemia
Musculoskeletal System	
Decreased muscle mass	Loss of strength
Increased joint/tendon breakdown	Arthritis, stiffness, loss of flexibility
	Increased risk of falls
	Loss of bone strength and size
Bone demineralization	Increased risk of fracture
Psychological/Social	
Loss of physical function	Decreased activity
Loss of friends/family	Depression
Loss of social support	Increased isolation and anxiety
	Increased risk of suicide attempts
Immune System	
Loss of T-cell function	Increased infection

From MedicAlert: *Geriatric emergencies: an EMT teaching manual,* Turlock, Calif, 1994, MedicAlert Foundation.

arrest when the cardiovascular system is placed under unexpected stress.

Changes also occur in the electrical conduction pathways of the heart. These changes occur as cells in the sinoatrial and atrioventricular nodes and the rest of the conduction system lose the ability to function. These physiological changes often lead to dysrhythmias. These include chronic atrial fibrillation, sick sinus syndrome, and various types of bradycardias and heart blocks. All of these can contribute to the decline in cardiac output.

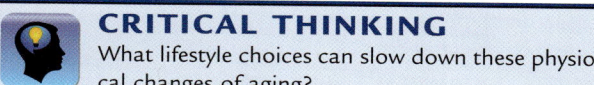

CRITICAL THINKING
What lifestyle choices can slow down these physiological changes of aging?

Renal System Changes

Structural and functional changes in the kidneys occur during the aging process. For example, renal blood flow decreases an average of 50% between 30 and 80 years of age.[5] This reduction in renal blood flow is associated with a proportional decrease in the glomerular filtration rate of about 8 mL/min per decade. Renal mass decreases by about 20% between 40 and 80 years of age. The steady decline in kidney function places the geriatric patient at greater risk for renal failure from trauma, obstruction, infection, and vascular occlusion.

As the patient ages, significant impairment develops in renal concentrating ability, sodium conservation, free water clearance (diuresis), glomerular filtration, and renal plasma flow. Hepatic blood flow decreases as well. This limits the effectiveness of liver metabolism. Decreases in kidney and liver function and loss of muscle and body water make the geriatric patient more susceptible to electrolyte disturbances. They also make the geriatric patient more likely to experience problems with medications or drugs.

> ### ? DID YOU KNOW?
> **Beers List**
> In 1993 a gerontologist named Mark H. Beers developed a national guideline and reference guide for pharmacists and physicians to improve medication use in the elderly. (The list is updated frequently.) This guide is known as the *Beers List*. In the guide, there are two tables developed by Dr. Beers. Table 1 lists 48 individual medications or classes of medications to avoid or use within specified dose and duration ranges in elderly patients. Examples of Table 1 drugs include flurazepam (Dalmane), amitriptyline (Elavil), and meperidine (Demerol). Table 2 lists medications to avoid in elderly patients with 20 different diseases or conditions, including specific concomitant diseases. For example, if the patient is diagnosed with blood clotting disorders or receiving anticoagulant therapy, aspirin has a high risk. If the patient is diagnosed with Parkinson's disease, metoclopramide (Reglan) has a high risk. The application of the Beers criteria for identifying potentially inappropriate medication use helps physicians and pharmacists to plan interventions for decreasing both drug-related costs and overall costs and thus minimize drug-related problems.[7]

ADVERSE DRUGS EVENTS IN OLDER ADULTS

Adverse drug events (ADEs), including reactions and interactions, in older people are a common cause of hospital admission, and are an important cause of morbidity and death. Even after excluding errors in drug administration, noncompliance, overdose, drug abuse, therapeutic failures, and possible ADEs, the overall incidence of serious ADEs in the general hospitalized population in the United States is believed to be between 6% and 7%.[8] Studies suggest that more than 80% of ADEs causing admission or occurring in the hospital are dose-related. Therefore, many ADEs are predictable and some are potentially **avoidable.**[9] Cardiovascular medications followed by diuretics, nonopioid analgesics, hypoglycemics, and anticoagulants are some of the most common medication categories associated with preventable ADEs. Electrolyte/renal, gastrointestinal tract, hemorrhagic, metabolic/endocrine, and neuropsychiatric events were the most common types of preventable adverse drug events.[10]

Nervous System Changes

Although it was long thought that mental dysfunction in the geriatric patient was caused solely by senility, it is now well known that intellectual functioning deteriorates selectively and may result from many organic causes.[11] For example, beginning at about 30 years of age, the total number of neurons in certain cortical areas decreases gradually, so by 70 years of age, a 10% reduction in brain weight

has occurred.[5] These factors, decreased cerebral blood flow, and changes in the location and amounts of specific neurotransmitters probably contribute to changes in the central nervous system (CNS). The velocity of nerve conduction in the peripheral nervous system decreases with aging as well. This may lead to changes in motor or position sense and delays in reaction time and motor responses. Other gradual changes in the patient's nervous system can result in decreased visual acuity and auditory keenness. They also can result in changes in sleep patterns.

Toxic or metabolic factors that can affect mental functioning include the use of medications (e.g., anticholinergics, antihypertensives, antidysrhythmics, and analgesics); electrolyte imbalances; hypoglycemia; acidosis; alkalosis; hypoxia; liver, kidney, and lung failure; pneumonia; congestive heart failure (CHF); cardiac dysrhythmias; infection; and the development of benign or malignant tumors.

Musculoskeletal System Changes

As the body ages, muscles shrink, muscles and ligaments calcify, and intervertebral disks become thin. Osteoporosis is common in geriatric patients (especially in women). An estimated 68% of geriatric patients show some degree of **kyphosis** ("humpback posture") (Figure 49-1). These musculoskeletal changes result in a decrease in total muscle mass, a decrease in height of 2 to 3 inches, widening and weakening of certain bones, and a posture that impairs mobility and alters the balance of the body. As a result, falls are common. Moreover, the falls often are associated with significant morbidity and mortality.

Prevention strategies (described in Chapter 3) that can decrease injuries associated with falls include the following:

- Using assistive devices (e.g., walker or cane)
- Removing scatter rugs and securing loose carpeting

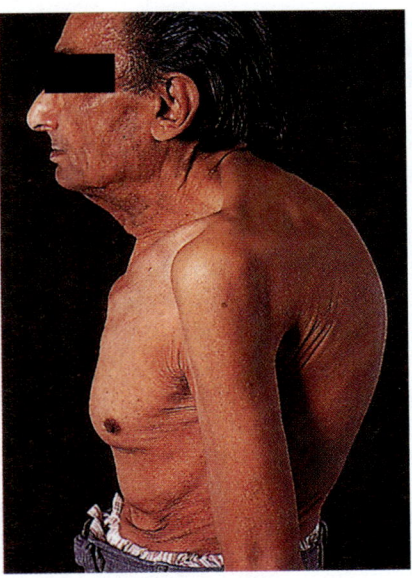

FIGURE 49-1 Kyphosis.

- Removing items that may cause tripping
- Providing and using handrails
- Ensuring adequate lighting
- Removing clutter from the environment
- Arranging furniture for walking ease
- Using nonslip decals in the bathtub or shower
- Providing handrails on bathtubs, showers, and commodes
- Suggesting patients consult with their physician regarding medicines if they are taking medication that increases the risk of falls

> **CRITICAL THINKING**
> Consider a patient who has significant kyphosis. What aspects of care will you need to alter to immobilize the spine of this patient?

Other Physiological Changes

Other physiological changes that occur with aging include a decrease in lean body mass, an increase in body fat, a decrease in total body water, a decreased ability to maintain internal homeostasis, a decrease in the function of immunological mechanisms, nutritional disorders, and decreases in hearing and visual acuity.

As an individual approaches 65 years of age, lean body mass may decrease as much as 25%, and fat tissue may increase as much as 35%.[5] These changes in body composition can affect the dosage and frequency of administration of fat-soluble drugs. This is because there is more drug per weight of metabolically active tissue and a larger reservoir for accumulation of the drug. Likewise, the decrease in total body water is likely to increase the concentration of water-soluble drugs.

The ability of the body to maintain normal temperature through thermoregulatory mechanisms declines over time. The decline begins at about 30 years of age. Because of this, the geriatric patient is at greater risk for cold- and heat-related conditions. These include hypothermia, heat exhaustion, and hyperthermia. Several factors contribute to the increased risk of thermoregulatory disorders, including impaired sympathetic nervous system function, causing decreased capacity for peripheral vasoconstriction, lowered metabolic rate, poor peripheral circulation, and chronic illness. Because of the decline in many body functions, including blood pressure, cardiac output, and temperature regulation, a specific illness or injury often puts the geriatric patient "over the edge" without adequate compensatory mechanisms to manage the event.

Aging causes a decrease in primary antibody response and cellular immunity and elevations in the amount of abnormal immunoglobulins and immune complexes.[5] These physiological changes increase the risk of infection, autoimmune disorders, and perhaps cancer. In addition, infections may not produce the usual signs and symptoms.

> **NOTE**
> Changes in the immunological systems of the elderly make them more prone to infections, and exacerbations of chronic disease processes. As the thymus ages, T-cell production is reduced and leukocytes are not activated. As a result, infections may not produce fever that would normally be seen in younger patients with viral, bacterial, or occult infection.

About one in eight deaths in geriatric patients results from cancer.[12] In younger patients, cancer often is the main or only disease from which they suffer. However, geriatric patients often have more than one disease and disability. Thus signs and symptoms such as a change in bowel habits, rectal bleeding, malaise, fatigue, weight loss, and anorexia may result from other maladies. Treatment with chemotherapy often results in immunosuppression. This increases the risk of infection and often masks the typical signs and symptoms associated with infection.

Many geriatric patients consume less than the minimum daily requirement of most vitamins,[13] which may be a result of loneliness and depression, decreased sensitivity to taste, decreased appetite, financial difficulties, physical infirmity, decreased vision, or a combination of these elements. All of these elements may act to reduce the motivation to shop for and prepare fresh food. Other factors associated with poor nutrition are poor dentition and reduced mastication, decreased esophageal motility, frequent hypochlorhydria (low stomach acid secretion), and decreased intestinal secretions that reduce absorption. Geriatric patients easily can become victims of malnutrition. Malnutrition in turn can cause dehydration, hypoglycemia, and numerous other complications.

> **CRITICAL THINKING**
> What effects can poor nutrition have on body function?

GENERAL PRINCIPLES IN ASSESSMENT OF THE GERIATRIC PATIENT

Normal physiological changes and underlying acute or chronic illness may make evaluation of an ill or injured geriatric patient a challenge. In addition to the components of a normal physical assessment (described in Chapter 20), the paramedic should consider special characteristics of geriatric patients that can complicate the clinical evaluation:

- Geriatric patients are likely to suffer from more than one illness at a time.
- Chronic problems can make assessment for acute problems difficult.
- Signs or symptoms of chronic illness can be confused with signs or symptoms of an acute problem.

- Aging can affect an individual's response to illness or injury.
- Pain may be diminished or absent.
- The patient or paramedic can underestimate the severity of a condition.
- Social and emotional factors may have a greater influence on health in geriatric patients than in any other age group.
- The patient fears losing autonomy.
- The patient fears the hospital environment.
- The patient has financial concerns about health care.

Patient History

Gathering a history from a geriatric patient usually requires more time than with younger patients (see Chapter 18). In addition to a longer medical history because of the patient's age, chronic illness, and medication use, the geriatric patient may have physical impediments such as hearing loss and visual impairment. Questioning a patient who is fatigued or easily distracted also may lengthen the interview process. The paramedic should use the following techniques when communicating with geriatric patients:

- Always identify yourself.
- Speak at eye level to ensure that the patient can see you as you communicate.
- Locate a hearing aid, eyeglasses, and dentures (if needed).
- Turn on lights.
- Speak slowly, distinctly, and respectfully.
- Use the patient's surname, unless the patient requests otherwise.
- Listen closely.
- Be patient.
- Preserve dignity.
- Use gentleness.

CRITICAL THINKING

Why should you ask geriatric patients to bring all of their medications to the hospital?

Physical Examination

When conducting the physical examination of a geriatric patient, the paramedic should consider the following six points:

1. The patient may tire easily.
2. Geriatric patients often wear many layers of clothing for warmth. This may hamper the examination.
3. Respect the patient's modesty and need for privacy unless it interferes with the care.
4. Explain actions clearly before examining all geriatric patients. This is important with patients with diminished sight.
5. Be aware that the patient may minimize or deny his or her symptoms. Denial may be due to a fear of being bedridden or institutionalized or losing self-sufficiency.

6. Try to distinguish symptoms of chronic disease from acute problems.

If time allows, the paramedic should assess the geriatric patient's immediate surroundings for evidence of alcohol or medication use (e.g., insulin syringes, "vial of life," or MedicAlert information), presence of food, general condition of housing, and signs of adequate personal hygiene. These and other observations help provide information to the physician about the patient's general health and ability for self-care after release from the hospital.

The paramedic should question friends or family members who are present about the patient's appearance and responsiveness *now* versus the patient's normal appearance, responsiveness, and other characteristics. The paramedic also should discreetly ask about advance directives and initiation of care for the patient (described in Chapter 6). If these documents are available, the paramedic should obtain them and convey the information to medical direction. Finally, the paramedic should ensure gentle handling and padding for patient comfort if transport is needed.

SYSTEM PATHOPHYSIOLOGY, ASSESSMENT, AND MANAGEMENT

The pathophysiology, assessment, and management of specific illnesses described in this section include those of the pulmonary system, cardiovascular system, CNS, endocrine system, gastrointestinal system, integumentary system, musculoskeletal system, and problems associated with special senses. Toxicology, environmental considerations, behavioral and psychiatric disorders, trauma, and elder abuse also are discussed in this section. Box 49-2 provides general assessment tools for patient evaluation.

Pulmonary System

Specific illnesses of the pulmonary system that are common in elderly patients include bacterial pneumonia, chronic obstructive pulmonary disease, and pulmonary embolism. These conditions were described in Chapter 24. They are presented here as a review.

BOX 49-2 General Assessment Tools for Patient Evaluation

Thorough neurological examination
Blood pressure
Evaluation of limb lead ECG
Interpretation of 12-lead ECG for signs of ischemia, injury, or anomalies
Auscultation of the heart to detect irregular, muffled, or extra heart sounds
Auscultation of the lungs to detect adventitious breath sounds
Capnography
Oxygen saturation
Evaluation of blood glucose level

BACTERIAL PNEUMONIA

Pneumonia is a leading cause of death in the geriatric age group and often is fatal in frail adults.[14] In addition, geriatric patients are more likely to develop bacteremia. They also are more susceptible to several respiratory pathogens (e.g., gram-negative bacilli). This susceptibility, associated with the presence of chronic disease, impairs respiratory tract clearance. It also allows germs to grow in the throat that then may travel to or be aspirated into the lungs. Because of the decreased lung function, pneumonia often may be associated with respiratory failure. Risk factors for bacterial pneumonia include institutional environments, feeding tubes, chronic diseases, and compromise of the immune system.

Unlike in younger patients with bacterial pneumonia, the usual clinical picture of fever, productive cough, pleurisy, and signs of pulmonary congestion often is absent in the geriatric patient. This atypical presentation is responsible for the common delay in diagnosis. The following are possible signs and symptoms:

- Alterations in mental status
- Cough
- Fever (variable)
- Shortness of breath
- Tachycardia
- Tachypnea

Geriatric patients with pneumonia may be too weak to cough or produce sputum. They also may not be able to breathe deeply. Therefore breath sounds may be misleading because of preexisting emphysema or chronic CHF. Tachycardia and tachypnea often are the most reliable indicators of bacterial pneumonia in the prehospital setting.

Emergency care for geriatric patients with bacterial pneumonia focuses on managing life threats, maintaining oxygenation, and providing transport for physician evaluation. Bacterial pneumonia is linked to a high rate of hospital admission. Pneumonia generally is managed with antibiotics.

CRITICAL THINKING

Why is flu season linked to an increase in pneumonia in the elderly?

CHRONIC OBSTRUCTIVE PULMONARY DISEASE

Chronic obstructive pulmonary disease (COPD) in the geriatric patient is a major health problem in the United States. Chronic obstructive pulmonary disease is a common finding in the geriatric patient with a history of smoking. It usually is associated with various diseases that result in reduced expiratory airflow. (Examples of such diseases are asthma, emphysema, and chronic bronchitis.) An exacerbation of COPD often follows an acute respiratory tract infection that causes airway edema, bronchial smooth muscle irritability, and increased mucus secretion. These airway abnormalities may lead to factors associated with acute decompensation, including the following:

- Limited airflow
- Increased work of breathing
- Dyspnea
- Ventilation-perfusion mismatching
- Hypoxemia
- Respiratory acidosis
- Hemodynamic compromise

Signs and symptoms of COPD in the geriatric patient include extreme anxiety, cyanosis, wheezing, and abnormal or diminished breath sounds associated with marked dyspnea and the use of accessory muscles. Other signs and symptoms include dysrhythmias, paradoxical breathing, jugular vein distention, and decreased oxygen saturation levels (per pulse oximetry). The paramedic should obtain a full history of the event, including any history of intubation or steroid therapy. The paramedic also should be prepared for aggressive airway management. The care for a patient with COPD is aimed at correcting life-threatening hypoxemia and improving airflow. To achieve these goals, the use of airway and ventilatory support with supplemental oxygenation and the administration of bronchodilators by inhalation or injection may be indicated. Failure to begin aggressive treatments to correct the acidosis and hypoxia from COPD can lead to a progressive decline in the patient's condition.

PULMONARY EMBOLISM

Pulmonary embolism is a life-threatening cause of dyspnea. The condition is associated with venous stasis, heart failure, COPD, malignancy, and immobilization. All of these are common in older adults. Most pulmonary emboli in geriatric patients form in the veins of the legs. From there they travel through the femoral veins to the inferior vena cava and the heart. The clinical presentation of pulmonary embolism often is misleading in geriatric patients and frequently is misdiagnosed.[5]

Signs and symptoms of pulmonary embolism can vary greatly. They may range from a presentation of left ventricular failure with sudden tachypnea, unexplained tachycardia (a hallmark sign), and atrial fibrillation to signs and symptoms solely of the underlying venous thrombosis. (These include calf discomfort without tenderness, mild calf or ankle edema, increased warmth, and dilation of superficial veins in one foot or leg.) Pulmonary embolism can precipitate CHF. Pulmonary embolism also may be mistaken for bacterial pneumonia in geriatric patients.

CRITICAL THINKING

What other conditions have similar cardiovascular signs and symptoms?

Emergency care focuses on ensuring adequate airway, ventilatory, and circulatory support; immobilizing and elevating an affected extremity; and rapidly transporting the patient for physician evaluation. In-hospital care may include analgesics, bed rest, hemodynamic stabilization with intravenously administered fluids and vasopressors to support blood pressure, and efforts to prevent further embolization. Thrombolytics are sometimes given to lyse the thrombus. The physician also may treat these patients with anticoagulants to prevent further emboli.

Cardiovascular System

Cardiovascular disorders were described in Chapter 22. Specific disorders reviewed in this section include myocardial infarction, heart failure, dysrhythmias, abdominal and thoracic aneurysm, and hypertension.

MYOCARDIAL INFARCTION

Chest pain as a symptom of myocardial infarction (MI) becomes less frequent by 70 years of age. Only 45% of patients over 85 years of age with MI have this complaint. Lack of typical chest pain can cause MI to be unrecognized in the geriatric patient.[6] The following are six major risk factors that the paramedic should evaluate when assessing a patient for MI:

1. Previous MI
2. Angina
3. Diabetes
4. Hypertension
5. High cholesterol level
6. Smoking

Some geriatric patients have chest pain or discomfort. However, many complain only of vague symptoms. Examples of such include dyspnea (the most common sign in patients over 85 years of age), abdominal or epigastric distress, and fatigue.

In patients older than 85 years, atypical presentation for MI should be anticiapted.[11] For many geriatric patients the event is totally "silent." This may be a result of decreased visceral sensory function or a higher incidence of mental deterioration in this age group. Silent MIs are almost always marked by an atypical complaint. This may include fatigue, breathlessness, nausea, or abdominal pain. Thus the paramedic must maintain a high index of suspicion for MI in elderly patients with unusual warning signs or symptoms. Consider performing a 12-lead electrocardiogram (ECG) if the patient has these complaints.

CRITICAL THINKING
What hormonal change in older women increases their risk for heart disease?

Emergency care includes airway, ventilatory, and circulatory support; oxygen administration and pain management therapy; management of serious dysrhythmias according to advanced life support protocol; and rapid and gentle transportation for physician evaluation.

HEART FAILURE

Heart failure is more frequent in geriatric patients, occurring in about 10% of people over the age of 80. It is also the most common reason for admission to an acute care hospital in patients age 65 and older.[15] Heart failure in this age group also has a larger incidence of noncardiac causes. Heart failure occurs when the ventricular output cannot meet the metabolic demands of the body. Heart failure often is caused by ischemic heart disease, valvular heart disease, cardiomyopathy, dysrhythmias, hyperthyroidism, and anemia. The following are common signs and symptoms of heart failure:

- Dyspnea
- Fatigue (often the first symptom of left-sided heart failure)
- Orthopnea
- Dry, hacking cough progressing to productive cough with frothy sputum
- Dependent edema caused by right-sided heart failure
- Nocturia
- Anorexia, hepatomegaly, ascites

NOTE
Differentiating among the causes of dyspnea is difficult in the prehospital setting. However, such differentiation is important. If the patient has a history of acute episodes of heart failure, the current emergency event also is likely to be heart failure.[16] A thorough patient history is important.

The emergency care is aimed at reversing the conditions associated with heart failure as soon as possible. This will help to prevent cardiac damage. In addition to oxygen administration and electrocardiograph monitoring, management may include intubation, intravenous (IV) therapy, and drug therapy (**nitroglycerin, morphine,** and perhaps **furosemide**).

CRITICAL THINKING
How do furosemide, nitroglycerin, and morphine work to relieve the signs and symptoms of heart failure?

DYSRHYTHMIAS

A common cause of dysrhythmias in the geriatric patient is hypertensive heart disease.[17] But any condition that decreases blood flow to the heart can cause rhythm irregularities. When assessing dysrhythmias in the geriatric patient, the paramedic should consider the following:

- Premature ventricular contractions are common in most adults over 80 years of age.

- Atrial fibrillation is the most common dysrhythmia.
- Dysrhythmias may result from electrolyte imbalances.

In addition to the serious implications of some dysrhythmias, associated complications may include traumatic injury from falls that result from cerebral hypoperfusion, transient ischemic attack, and heart failure. The paramedic should focus emergency care on ensuring adequate airway, ventilatory, and circulatory support; administering oxygen; and transporting the patient for physician evaluation. Serious dysrhythmias should be managed as described in Chapter 22.

ABDOMINAL AND THORACIC ANEURYSM

Atherosclerotic disease is a common cause of abdominal and thoracic aneurysm. Abdominal aortic aneurysm affects about 2% to 4% of the U.S. population in men over 50 years of age.[11] Acute dissecting aortic aneurysm is more common than abdominal aneurysm and is associated with a high mortality rate. Signs and symptoms vary according to the site of rupture or extent of dissection (Box 49-3).

The goals of prehospital care are relief of pain and immediate transport to a hospital. Airway, ventilatory, and circulatory support may be required if the patient's condition deteriorates. Other prehospital care measures include the following:

- Gentle handling of the patient
- Allaying anxiety
- High-concentration oxygen administration
- Small-bore IV access to restrict fluids unless severe hypotension is present
- Pain medication per medical direction

HYPERTENSION

Geriatric patients who have atherosclerosis also frequently have hypertension. Associated risk factors for hypertension include advanced age, diabetes, and obesity. Hypertension often is defined as a resting blood pressure consistently greater than 140/90 mm Hg. Chronic hypertension is associated with many medical conditions, including the following:

- Aneurysm formation
- Blindness
- Cardiac hypertrophy and left ventricular failure
- Kidney failure
- Myocardial ischemia and infarction
- Peripheral vascular disease
- Stroke

NOTE

Systolic blood pressure gradually increases with age. However, diastolic pressure often stays normal or slightly decreases. Thus in persons over age 50, systolic pressure is a better indicator of risk for heart disease and stroke.[18] Current guidelines recommend that physicians treat older patients who have systolic hypertension with antihypertensive drugs. The goal of treatment is to achieve a blood pressure less than 140/90 mm Hg or less than 130/80 mm Hg in patients with diabetes or kidney disease. For patients with stage I hypertension (systolic pressure of 140 to 159 mm Hg) and additional cardiovascular risk factors, a sustained reduction in systolic pressure for more than 10 years will decrease mortality rates.[19]

Hypertension in the geriatric patient may manifest only in nonspecific complaints such as headache, forgetfulness, and general malaise. Other signs and symptoms that may indicate chronic hypertension include epistaxis, tremors, and nausea and vomiting. Care is mainly supportive. In severe cases, medical direction may advise the use of antihypertensives (e.g., *metoprolol*). After physician evaluation, the patient with chronic hypertension often is managed with oral medications, dietary sodium reduction, weight loss, and exercise.

Nervous System

Neurological disorders were described in Chapter 25. Specific disorders described in this section for review include cerebral vascular disease, delirium, dementia, Alzheimer's disease, and Parkinson's disease. Possible assessment findings in patients with neurological disorders are provided in Box 49-4.

BOX 49-3 Signs and Symptoms of Abdominal and Thoracic Aneurysm

Absent or reduced pulses
Acute myocardial infarction
Chest pain
Diminished distal pulses
Heart failure
Hypotension
Low back pain or flank pain
Pericardial tamponade
Pulsatile, tender mass
Stroke
Sudden onset of abdominal or back pain
Syncope
Unexplained hypotension

BOX 49-4 Possible Assessment Findings in Patients with Neurological Disorders

Changes in peripheral, core, and neurovascular perfusion
Changes in response of pupils
Changes in response to motor tests
Dysrhythmias
Adventitious breath sounds

CEREBRAL VASCULAR DISEASE

Stroke is the third leading cause of death in most countries and the leading cause of brain injury in adults.[4] As described in Chapter 22, the neurological impairment is caused by an ischemic or hemorrhagic interruption in the blood supply to the brain. Associated risk factors for cerebral vascular disease in the older adult include smoking, hypertension, diabetes, atherosclerosis, hyperlipidemia, polycythemia, and heart disease. Box 49-5 provides a review of the signs and symptoms of stroke and transient ischemic attack.

Once the paramedic suspects stroke, the paramedic must *minimize time in the field* because there is limited time to initiate therapy. (In many cases, less than 3 hours from onset is recommended for fibrinolytic therapy.) The paramedic should focus on managing the patient's airway, breathing, and circulation and on monitoring vital signs. Aside from supporting vital functions, the most important element of prehospital care for a stroke victim is identification of the patient with stroke and rapid transportation of the patient to a stroke center that can provide treatment within 1 hour after arrival at the emergency department door.[20]

> ### CRITICAL THINKING
> What factors can cause a delay between the onset of signs and symptoms of stroke in the geriatric patient and when an emergency telephone call is made?

DELIRIUM

As described in Chapter 35, delirium is an abrupt disorientation to time and place. It usually includes illusions and hallucinations. The patient's mind may "wander;" speech may be incoherent; and the patient may be in a state of mental confusion or excitement. Delirium commonly is a result of physical illness. Signs and symptoms vary according to personality, environment, and severity of the illness. Causes of delirium are associated with organic brain dysfunction: physical versus psychological disorders that affect cognition. Examples of these disorders and risk factors include the following[21]:

BOX 49-5 Signs and Symptoms of Stroke and Transient Ischemic Attack

Ataxia
Diplopia
Facial droop
Language disturbance
Monocular blindness
Numbness
Slurred speech
Unilateral paralysis
Vertigo
Visual disturbance

- Alcohol intoxication or withdrawal
- Anticholinergic medications
- Cardiovascular disease
- Dehydration
- Depression
- Drug reactions
- Environmental emergencies
- Fever
- Hyper/hypoglycemia
- Malnutrition
- Metabolic disorders
- Psychiatric disorders
- Tumor
- Urinary tract infection/bowel obstruction
- Vitamin deficiencies
- Withdrawal from sedatives

Delirium can be life threatening. It requires emergency care. The condition may be reversible if it is diagnosed early. Yet delirium can progress to chronic mental dysfunction. Prehospital care includes the following measures:

1. Ensure adequate airway, breathing, and circulatory support.
   a. Manage hypoxia with oxygen.
   b. Manage hypotension with IV fluids if appropriate.
2. Reduce agitation and anxiety.
3. Avoid patient injury, and ensure personal safety.
   a. Restrain the patient if needed, per protocol.
   b. Sedate the patient as a last resort.
4. Consider hypoglycemia or a narcotic state.
   a. Measure blood glucose level.
   b. Administer **dextrose 50%** or **naloxone** per protocol.
5. Assess for CNS injury (e.g., trauma or stroke). Perform a careful neurological examination.
6. Look for signs of CNS infection (e.g., encephalitis).
7. Transport the patient for physician evaluation.

DEMENTIA

Dementia is a slow, progressive loss of awareness of time and place. It usually involves an inability to learn new things or recall recent events. Dementia often is a result of brain disease caused by strokes, genetic or viral factors, and Alzheimer's disease. Dementia generally is considered irreversible. It eventually results in full dependence on others as a result of the progressive loss of cognitive functioning. During the course of the disease, patients often try to "cover up" their memory loss by **confabulation** (making up stories to fill gaps in memory). Sudden outbursts or embarrassing conduct may be the first clear signs of dementia. Some patients eventually regress to a "second childhood." At that point, they need full care for feedings, toileting, and physical activity. Dementia is present in about 30% to 50% of persons over 85 years of age.[5] Possible causes of dementia include[21]:

- Alzheimer's disease
- Brain trauma
- Brain tumor
- Drug toxicity

- Huntington's chorea
- Infections
- Major depression
- Parkinson's disease
- Metabolic and endocrine disorders
- Multi-infarct dementia
- Psychiatric disorders

Dementia can be difficult to differentiate from delirium in the prehospital setting. The key difference between the two is that delirium is new with rapid onset, and dementia is progressive (Table 49-2). Thus a history of the event from a reliable witness (e.g., friend or family member) is the best source of information. A history provided by the patient may be unreliable. If a good witness is not available, the paramedic should manage the patient for delirium that may be a life-threatening emergency.

ALZHEIMER'S DISEASE

Alzheimer's disease is a condition in which nerve cells in the cerebral cortex die and the brain substance shrinks. The disease is the single most common cause of dementia and is responsible for the majority of cases in persons over 65 years of age.[22] Alzheimer's disease does not cause death directly; patients ultimately stop eating and become malnourished and immobilized. Then they are prone to intercurrent infections.

The exact cause of Alzheimer's disease is not known. Possible causes include abnormalities in glutamate metabolism, chronic infection, toxic poisoning by metals, reduction in brain chemicals (e.g., acetylcholine), and genetics. Atherosclerosis is *not* a cause of Alzheimer's disease. The primary disorder is in the nerve cells, not the blood vessels.

Early symptoms of Alzheimer's disease mainly are related to memory loss, especially the ability to make and recall new memories (Box 49-6). As the disease progresses, agitation, violence, and impairment of abstract thinking occur. Judgment and cognitive abilities begin to interfere with work and social relations. In the advanced stages of Alzheimer's disease, patients often become bedridden and totally unaware of their surroundings. Once the patient is bedridden, pressure ulcers (bed sores), feeding problems, and pneumonia shorten the patient's life.

No specific treatment exists for Alzheimer's disease. (Some medications such as cholinesterase inhibitors, antipsychotics, and antidepressants may help delay the disease and lessen associated symptoms.) Treatment primarily consists of nursing and social care for the patient and relatives. The paramedic manages Alzheimer's patients the same as dementia patients.

PARKINSON'S DISEASE

As described in Chapter 25, **Parkinson's disease** is a brain disorder caused by degeneration of or damage to nerve cells in the basal ganglia. The disease causes muscle tremor, stiffness, and weakness. Characteristic signs of Parkinson's disease are resting tremors and shaking (usually beginning in one hand, arm, or leg), a rigid posture and muscle stiffness, slow movements, and a shuffling, unbalanced walk. This increases the patient's risk for falls. Other signs and symptoms include:

- Difficulty swallowing and chewing
- Impaired speech
- Impaired cognitive function
- Urinary problems
- Excessive sweating
- Depression
- Sleep difficulties
- Mask-like facial expression

> **NOTE**
> Some patients with Parkinson's disease "freeze" when trying to walk or stand up from a sitting position. When assisting a patient to ambulate, the paramedic can have the patient rock from side to side to begin motion or have them count to begin their motor movement.

BOX 49-6 The Seven Warning Signs of Alzheimer's Disease

1. Asking the same question over and over again.
2. Repeating the same story, word for word, again and again.
3. Forgetting how to cook, or how to make repairs, or how to play cards—activities that were previously done with ease and regularity.
4. Losing one's ability to pay bills or balance one's checkbook.
5. Getting lost in familiar surroundings, or misplacing household objects.
6. Neglecting to bathe or wearing the same clothes over and over again even as patients insist that they have taken a bath or that their clothes are still clean.
7. Relying on someone else, such as a spouse, to make decisions or answer questions they previously would have handled themselves.

From Alzheimer's Disease Education & Referral Center: *The seven warning signs of Alzheimer's disease,* www.alzheimers.org/pubs/sevensigns.htm, accessed 9-23-03. Reprinted with the permission of the Suncoast Gerontology Center, University of South Florida. Revised 9-1-99.

TABLE 49-2 Differential Diagnosis for Delirium and Dementia

	Delirium	Dementia
Onset	Abrupt	Gradual
Characteristics	Reduced attention span	Impaired recent memory
	Disorganized thinking	Regression
	Hallucinations	Poor judgment

If left untreated, the disease progresses over 10 to 15 years to severe weakness and incapacity. One in 100 Americans over the age of 60 is afflicted with Parkinson's disease,[23] with 50,000 new cases diagnosed in the United States each year.

The emergency care for these patients mainly is supportive. It includes airway, ventilatory, and circulatory support and transport for physician evaluation. Parkinson's disease has no cure. However, counseling, exercise, special aids in the home, and drug therapy can improve the patient's morale, mobility, and quality of life.

Endocrine System

Two common endocrine disorders often are seen in geriatric patients. These disorders are type 2 diabetes and thyroid disease (described in Chapter 26). The following is a review of these conditions.

TYPE 2 DIABETES

About 20% of older adults have diabetes, and almost 40% have some impaired glucose tolerance.[24] Type 2 (non–insulin-dependent) diabetes is most common in geriatric patients, especially when the person is overweight. The following are associated risk factors in older adults for complications related to diabetes:

- Decreased ability to care for self
- Living alone
- Concurrent illness
- Decline in renal function
- Polydrug use

A combination of dietary measures, weight reduction, and oral hypoglycemic agents can usually keep type 2 diabetes under control. In most cases, insulin injections are not required for type 2 diabetes. However, if not controlled, diabetes can lead to complications. These include **retinopathy** (inflammatory eye disorders), peripheral neuropathy (ulcers on the feet are common), autonomic neuropathy (causes gastrointestinal [GI], genitourinary [GU], cardiovascular [CV] symptoms, and sexual dysfunction), and kidney damage.[25] Diabetic patients also have a higher-than-average risk for atherosclerosis, hypertension, and other cardiovascular disorders and for cataracts. Emergency care for diabetic patients is outlined in Chapter 26 and includes airway, ventilatory, and circulatory support; blood glucose level screening; IV *dextrose* (if indicated and in the absence of cerebral damage); and transport for physician evaluation. Possible assessment findings in diabetic patients are provided in Box 49-7.

Hyperglycemic hyperosmolar nonketotic syndrome (HHNS), described in Chapter 26, is a serious complication of elderly type 2 diabetic patients. It carries a mortality rate of 20% to 50%.[5] The paramedic often finds the type 2 diabetic patient comatose. If awake, the patient may complain of profound thirst and frequent urination. Frequent urination results from osmotic diuresis and leads to dehydration and electrolyte loss. Predisposing factors that make the geriatric patients susceptible to hyperglycemic

hyperosmolar nonketotic syndrome include infection, noncompliance with medications, polydrug use, pancreatitis, stroke, hypothermia, heat stroke, and MI. If HHNS is suspected, the paramedic should ensure adequate airway, ventilatory, and circulatory support; search vigorously for an underlying cause; initiate IV therapy to manage dehydration; and rapidly transport the patient for physician evaluation.

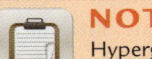
NOTE
Hyperglycemia is defined as a blood glucose level greater than 200 mg/dL or a fasting level greater than 126 mg/dL.[21]

NOTE
HHNS coma is a complication of type 2 diabetes in elderly patients. Unlike in diabetic ketoacidosis (DKA), the elevated blood glucose level in HHNS coma does not result in ketosis. Instead, it leads to osmotic diuresis and a fluid shift to the intravascular space that result in dehydration.

CRITICAL THINKING
What finding is present in the patient with diabetic ketoacidosis yet is absent in the patient with hyperglycemic hyperosmolar nonketotic coma?

THYROID DISEASE

Thyroid disease is common in geriatric patients. It may be related to the aging process. The classic signs and symptoms of thyroid disorders (e.g., fullness in the neck, goiter, muscle or joint pain) often are not present in the geriatric patient. Thus the paramedic should suspect thyroid dysfunction in any geriatric patient who is ill. Possible

---

BOX 49-8 Possible Assessment Findings in Patients With Thyroid Disease

Changes in peripheral, core, and neurovascular perfusion
Bradycardia
Respiratory failure or arrest
Hypercarbia
Changes in serum glucose levels
Nonpitting or pitting edema

BOX 49-9 Possible Assessment Findings in Patients With Gastrointestinal Disorders

Changes in peripheral, core, and neurovascular perfusion
Diffuse abdominal tenderness, distention, guarding or masses
Orthostatic blood pressure changes
Hypovolemia
Pale, thin skin
Jaundice
Frail musculoskeletal system
Peripheral, sacral, or periorbital edema
Hypertension
Fever
Tachycardia
Dyspnea

---

assessment findings in patients with thyroid disease are provided in Box 49-8.

As described in Chapter 26, **hypothyroidism** results from the destruction of thyroid tissue over time. The disease leads to an insufficient amount of thyroid hormone in the blood. The older patient often attributes the signs and symptoms of hypothyroidism to "growing old." Common complaints include nonspecific musculoskeletal complaints and confusion. More serious conditions associated with this disorder include CHF, anemia, hyponatremia, depression, dementia, seizures, and coma. Other signs and symptoms associated with hypothyroidism include:

- Cold intolerance
- Fatigue
- Weight gain
- Poor cognitive function
- Scaly dry skin and hair loss
- Peripheral and facial edema
- Paranoia

Hyperthyroidism is less common than hypothyroidism in elderly patients. Hyperthyroidism may result from medication errors (e.g., too many doses of a thyroid hormone replacement). Signs and symptoms of hyperthyroidism include weight loss, constipation, mental status changes, CHF, tachydysrhythmias, and lethargy.

LOOK AGAIN
See Chapter 26: Endocrinology, pp. 817-820.

The emergency care mainly is supportive to ensure vital functions. The physician evaluates the patient with thyroid disease and treats the patient with various thyroid drugs, radioactive iodine treatments, and sometimes surgery. Severe complications from thyroid disease include *thyroid storm* and *myxedema coma* (described in Chapter 26). These complications can be made worse in a patient who has coronary artery disease.

Gastrointestinal System

Gastrointestinal emergencies (described in Chapter 29) are common in the elderly. The paramedic should always consider abdominal pain a serious complaint in a geriatric patient. Life-threatening causes of abdominal pain in this age group include abdominal aortic aneurysm, gastrointestinal hemorrhage, ruptured viscus, dead or ischemic bowel, and acute bowel obstruction. Specific disorders discussed in this section are gastrointestinal hemorrhage, bowel obstruction, problems with continence, and problems with elimination. Possible assessment findings in patients with gastrointestinal disorders are provided in Box 49-9.

GASTROINTESTINAL HEMORRHAGE

Gastrointestinal bleeding most commonly affects patients between 60 and 90 years of age.[5] Possible causes of GI bleeding include peptic ulcer disease, esophageal varices, stomach and esophageal cancer, diverticulitis, bowel obstruction, and cirrhosis of the liver. GI bleeding in older patients has a mortality rate of about 10%. The older the patient, the higher the risk of death. This higher risk is because of the following[26]:

- Geriatric patients are less able to compensate for acute blood loss.
- They are less likely to feel symptoms and therefore seek treatment at later stages of disease.
- They are more likely to be taking *aspirin* or nonsteroidal antiinflammatory drugs (NSAIDs), which places them at higher risk for ulcer disease and bleeding.
- They are at higher risk for colon cancer, intestinal vascular abnormalities, and diverticulitis.
- They are more likely to be taking anticoagulants such as warfarin (Coumadin).

Signs and symptoms of gastrointestinal bleeding include vomiting of blood or coffee-ground emesis; blood-tinged or black, tarry stools; agitation; weakness; syncope; pain; jaundice; and constipation or diarrhea. If the paramedic suspects or confirms bleeding in a patient with signs and symptoms of shock, the paramedic should begin measures to ensure adequate airway, ventilatory, and circulatory support. The paramedic also should transport the patient rapidly for definitive care.

BOWEL OBSTRUCTION

Bowel obstruction generally occurs in patients with prior abdominal surgeries or hernias. Obstruction occurs in those with colonic cancer as well. Most complain of constipation, abdominal cramping, and an inability to pass gas. Other signs and symptoms include protracted vomiting of food or bile and vomiting of fecal material. The patient's heart rate and blood pressure measurements often are in normal ranges. The abdomen also may be mildly distended and tender in all four quadrants. (Abdominal pain is variable.)

The prehospital care mainly is supportive to ensure vital functions. After physician evaluation, patient care may include bowel rest, nasogastric suction, and volume replacement. Some patients may need surgery to lyse the offending adhesions. Surgery may result in a cycle of new scarring and obstruction. Patients also may need surgery for hernia repair (most often in men).

>
> **NOTE**
> **Biliary disease** refers to disorders of the liver and gallbladder. It describes a wide spectrum of disorders caused by abnormalities in bile composition, biliary anatomy, or function. The disease can result from primary liver disease, congestive heart failure, gallstones, cholecystitis, and medications that adversely affect the liver. Like other GI disorders, biliary disease may be accompanied by jaundice, fever, and vomiting. There often is right upper quadrant abdominal pain that radiates to the upper back and shoulder.

PROBLEMS WITH CONTINENCE

Continence is the ability to control bladder or bowel function. It requires anatomically correct gastrointestinal and genitourinary tracts, competent sphincter mechanisms, cognitive and physical function, and motivation. Some factors associated with continence are affected by age. These factors include a decrease in bladder capacity, involuntary bladder contractions, decreased ability to postpone voiding, and medications that can affect bladder and bowel control. **Incontinence** of urine or bowel is abnormal at any age.

Urinary incontinence can vary in severity. It can be only mild incontinence (the escape of small amounts of urine). Or it can be total incontinence, with complete loss of bladder control. Causes of urinary incontinence include injury or disease of the urinary tract, prolapse of the uterus, a decline in sphincter muscle control surrounding the urethra (common in the elderly), CNS injury or disease, pelvic fracture, prostate cancer, and dementia.

Bowel incontinence in the geriatric patient usually is the result of **fecal impaction.** This occurs when feces lodged in the rectum irritate and inflame the lining. This allows fecal fluid and small feces to pass involuntarily. Other causes of bowel incontinence include severe diarrhea, injury

---

to anal muscles (from childbirth or surgery), CNS injury or disease, and dementia.

All forms of incontinence usually are embarrassing for the patient. If incontinence is chronic, it can lead to skin irritation, tissue breakdown, and urinary tract infection (Box 49-10). Some cases are managed with surgery to restore sphincter function. Patients with mild cases often wear absorptive undergarments to relieve discomfort and embarrassment.

> **CRITICAL THINKING**
> Consider the incontinent patient. How can you minimize the patient's embarrassment and discomfort?

PROBLEMS WITH ELIMINATION

Causes of difficulty in urination usually result from enlargement of the prostate (in men), urinary tract infection, urethral strictures, and acute or chronic renal failure. Difficulty in bowel elimination often is associated with diverticular disease, constipation, and colorectal cancer. Problems with elimination can cause great pain and anxiety for geriatric patients. The paramedic should take their complaints seriously. These conditions call for physician evaluation to identify the cause and to select appropriate therapy.

>
> **NOTE**
> *Chronic renal failure* (the inability of the kidneys to excrete waste, concentrate urine, or control electrolyte balance in the body) was described in Chapter 30. Chronic renal failure may be the result of diabetes, congenital disorders, pyelonephritis, hypertension, autoimmune disorders, glomerulonephritis, or medications that have an adverse effect on the kidneys (e.g., antibiotics, NSAIDs, anticancer drugs). The paramedic should refer to Chapter 30 for review.

Integumentary System

As persons age, the skin gradually becomes dry, transparent, and wrinkled. These integumentary changes are associated with a loss of elasticity, uneven pigmentation, and various benign and malignant lesions. In addition, aging results in a gradual decrease in epidermal cellular turnover and a reduced rate of nail and hair growth. The associated loss of deep, dermal vessels and capillary circulation leads to common complaints such as dry, itchy skin; changes in thermal regulation; and skin-related complications. Some of these complications include the following:

- Slow healing
- Increased risk of secondary infection
- Increased risk of fungal or viral infections
- Increased susceptibility to abrasions and tears

The paramedic should always be gentle with the skin of a geriatric patient. Examples include use of aseptic technique during wound management, gentle placement and removal of electrocardiogram electrodes, and using careful taping procedures when securing IV catheters or tubing.

CRITICAL THINKING

Consider a geriatric patient who has a burn injury. How do these changes influence the patient's recovery?

PRESSURE ULCERS

Pressure ulcers are common in geriatric patients (Figure 49-2). They often develop on the skin of patients who are bedridden or immobile (e.g., **decubitus ulcers**). Most pressure ulcers occur in the lower legs, back, and buttocks, and over bony areas such as the greater trochanter or the sacrum. They often affect victims of brain or spinal cord injury, stroke, or other illnesses that result in a loss or change in the sensation of pain. Skin exposure to moisture (e.g., from incontinence), poor nutrition, and friction or shear also may be factors for developing pressure ulcers. Other causes of pressure ulcers in geriatric patients include vascular and metabolic disorders (e.g., venous stasis and diabetes), trauma, and cancer.

Pressure ulcers result from tissue hypoxia. They generally start as red, painful areas that become purple before the skin breaks down. Then they develop into open sores. Once the integrity of the skin has been breached, the sores often become infected. Then they are slow to heal. Pressure ulcers should be covered with sterile dressing using aseptic technique. The paramedic then should transport the patient for physician evaluation and wound care to facilitate healing.

Musculoskeletal System

As described in Chapter 12 and earlier in this chapter, musculoskeletal changes occur as part of the aging process. Two musculoskeletal conditions that are common in elderly patients are osteoarthritis and osteoporosis. (These and other forms of arthritis were described in Chapter 33.)

LOOK AGAIN

See Chapter 33: Nontraumatic Muscle Disorders, pp. 969-972.

OSTEOARTHRITIS

Osteoarthritis is a common form of inflammatory arthritis in geriatric patients. Osteoarthritis is a degenerative condition that results from cartilage loss and wear and tear on the joints (Figure 49-3). The condition leads to pain, stiffness, and sometimes loss of function of the affected joint. Often the affected joint becomes large and distorted from outgrowths of new bone (*osteophytes*) that tend to develop at the margins of the joint surface. Osteoarthritis evolves in the middle years. It occurs to some extent in almost all persons over 60 years of age. However, some persons have no symptoms. After physician evaluation, treatment may

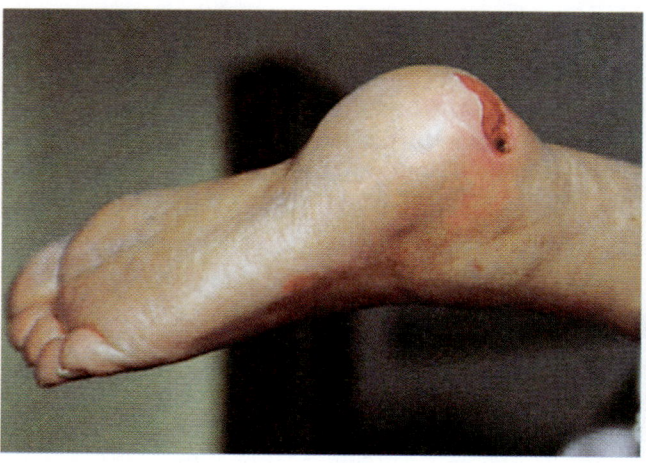

FIGURE 49-2 Pressure ulcers.

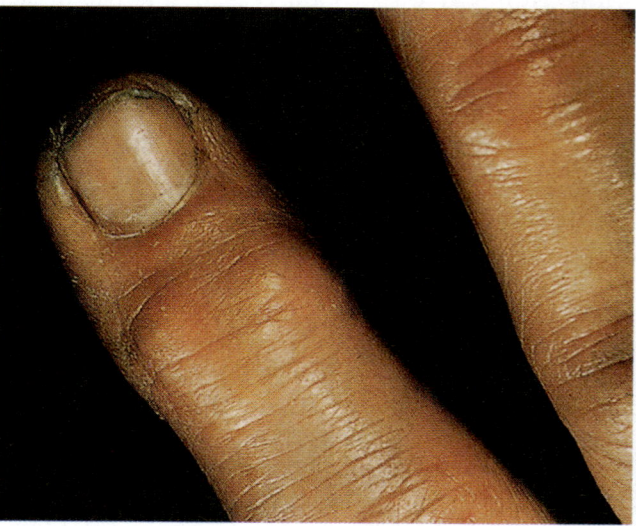

FIGURE 49-3 Osteoarthritis.

include medications (analgesics, nonsteroidal antiinflammatory drugs, corticosteroids), physical therapy, and sometimes joint replacement surgery. Newer drugs (cyclooxygenase-2 inhibitors) relieve the inflammation and pain associated with arthritis. These newer drugs have less risk of causing stomach irritation than traditional medications such as *aspirin,* nonsteroidal antiinflammatory drugs, and ibuprofen. An example of these newer drugs is celecoxib (Celebrex).

OSTEOPOROSIS

Osteoporosis is a disease that decreases bone density. It is a natural part of aging and is especially common in older women after menopause. This is because of a decrease in the hormone estrogen, which helps maintain bone mass. Osteoporosis is present in most persons by 70 years of age, by which time the density of the skeleton has diminished by one third. Most persons with osteoporosis have some degree of kyphosis. Risk factors that may affect the progression of the disease include genetics, smoking, exercise habits, and diets poor in calcium and vitamin D.

The loss of bone density causes bones to become brittle. Brittle bones can fracture easily, which often is the first sign of osteoporosis. Typical sites for fractures are just above the wrist, at the head of the femur, and at one of several vertebrae (often a spontaneous fracture). Osteoporosis is treated with preventive measures. These include a diet high in calcium, calcium supplements, exercise, and hormone replacement therapy after menopause (controversial).

Special Problems with Sensations

As persons age, they may experience problems with vision, hearing, and speech.

PROBLEMS WITH VISION

Vision changes begin to occur at around 40 years of age. They gradually increase over time. Vision impairments can severely limit daily activities. They can lead to a loss of independence in geriatric patients. The following are some effects of aging on vision:

- Reading difficulties
- Poor depth perception
- Poor adjustment of the eyes to variations in distance
- Altered color perception
- Sensitivity to light
- Decreased visual acuity

Two common eye conditions that develop with age are cataracts and glaucoma. A **cataract** is a loss of transparency of the lens of the eye. It results from changes in the delicate protein fibers within the lens (Figure 49-4). A cataract never causes full blindness. Yet clarity and detail of an image progressively are lost. Cataracts usually occur in both eyes. In most cases, though, one eye is affected more severely than the other. Almost everyone over 65 years of age has some degree of cataract. Also, most persons over 75 years of age have minor visual deterioration from the disorder.

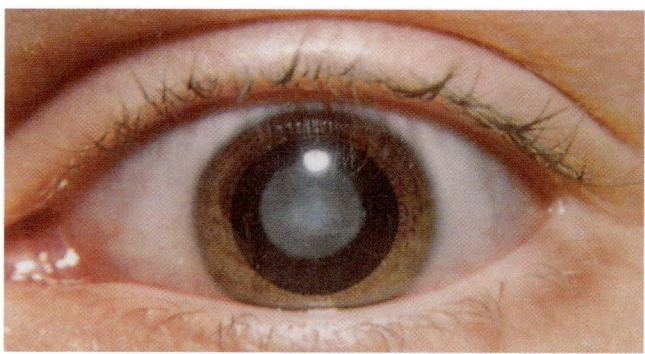

FIGURE 49-4 Appearance of an eye with a cataract.

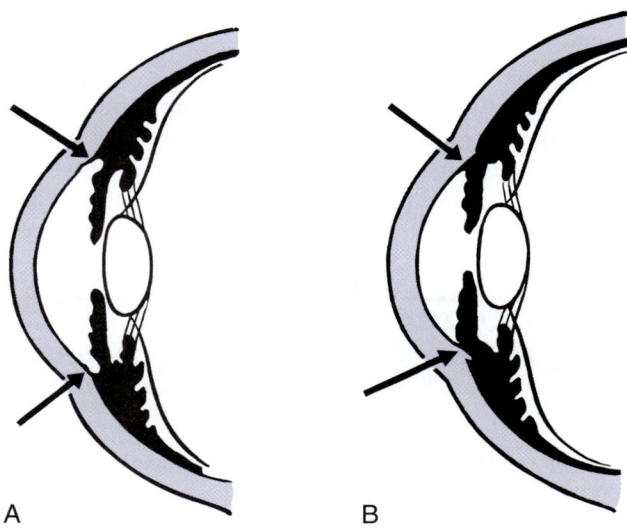

A   B

FIGURE 49-5 Glaucoma. **A,** Open-angle glaucoma. The obstruction to aqueous flow lies in the trabecular meshwork. **B,** Closed-angle glaucoma. The trabecular meshwork is covered by the root of the iris. (From Stein HA, Slatt BJ, Stein RM: *The ophthalmic assistant: fundamentals in clinical practice,* St Louis, 1988, Mosby.)

Surgery to remove the cataract is a common procedure in the United States.

Glaucoma is a condition in which intraocular pressure increases. This pressure causes damage to the optic nerve. The result is nerve fiber destruction and partial or full loss of peripheral and central vision (Figure 49-5). Glaucoma may result from aging (rarely seen before 40 years of age), a congenital abnormality, or trauma to the eye. Glaucoma is the most common major eye disorder in persons over 60 years of age and is the leading cause of preventable blindness in the United States.[27] Symptoms of acute glaucoma include dull, severe, aching pain in and above the eye; fogginess of vision; and the perception of "rainbow rings" (halos) around lights at night. Testing for glaucoma is part of most eye examinations in adults. If detected early, the condition can be treated with oral medications and eye drops to relieve pressure.

CRITICAL THINKING

Consider the patient who has glaucoma. What prehospital cardiac medication should not be given to this patient?

PROBLEMS WITH HEARING

Not all geriatric patients have hearing loss. However, overall hearing tends to decrease with age. This results from degeneration of the hearing mechanism (sensorineural deafness). Meniere's disease (increased fluid pressure in the labyrinth), certain drugs, tumors, and some viral infections also can cause hearing problems. Hearing loss can interfere with the ability to perceive speech. Thus it can limit the ability to communicate. Hearing aid devices and surgical implants sometimes can restore or improve hearing.

Tinnitus is the perception of noise in the ear (e.g., ringing, buzzing, or whistling). It can occur as a symptom of many ear disorders. The noise in the ear sometimes may change in nature and intensity. However, in most cases it is present at all times with intermittent awareness by the person. Tinnitus is almost always associated with hearing loss, especially hearing loss that develops from aging.

CRITICAL THINKING

What common analgesic, when taken in excess, can cause tinnitus?

PROBLEMS WITH SPEECH

Speech is the most often used method of communication. Common problems with speech in geriatric patients often are associated with difficulty in word retrieval, decreased fluency of speech, slowed rate of speech, and changes in voice quality. These disorders may occur from damage to the language centers of the brain (usually as a result of stroke, head injury, or brain tumor), degenerative changes in the nervous system, hearing loss, disorders of the larynx, and poor-fitting dentures.

Toxicology

As described in Chapter 13, geriatric patients are at increased risk for adverse drug reactions. This is the result of age-related changes in body composition as well as drug absorption, distribution, metabolism, and excretion.

LOOK AGAIN

See Chapter 13: Principles of Pharmacology and Emergency Medications, pp. 296-297.

Age-related changes that affect absorption include increased gastric pH and decreased gastrointestinal motility. Both of these may increase or decrease the absorption of various drugs (depending on the chemical properties of the drug). Drug distribution may be affected by decreased cardiac output (e.g., as seen in CHF), decreased total body water, changes in the ratio of lean mass to fat, and increased body fat. Metabolic changes may result from decreased liver blood flow; diseases such as thyroid disease, CHF, and cancer; smoking; and drug interactions. (Drug-induced metabolic changes are especially significant in the elderly. This is because they often take several different drugs for multiple diseases and conditions. This further increases their risk for adverse drug reactions.) Renal function decreases with age in the majority of adults. This can lead to an accumulation of drugs that normally are cleared through the renal system. In addition, the action of drugs affecting the CNS (e.g., benzodiazepines, anesthetics, and narcotics) and the cardiovascular system (e.g., beta blockers, calcium channel blockers, and diuretics) often is altered in older adults. Because of these changes, drugs may not produce the desired effect or may cause major drug toxicity in older adults. Drugs that commonly cause toxicity in the geriatric patient include the following:

- Analgesics
- Angiotensin-converting enzyme inhibitors
- Antidepressants
- Antihypertensives
- Beta blockers
- Digitalis
- Diuretics
- Psychotropics

The adverse reactions associated with these and other drugs often result from "accidents" or "mishaps" in the prescribed drug regimen. Other common reasons for drug-induced illness in the geriatric patient include dispensing errors, noncompliance, confusion, forgetfulness, vision impairment, and the self-selection of drugs. In addition, older adults commonly have several prescriptions from more than one physician; improperly resume an old medication in addition to a newly prescribed one; or take prescribed medications along with over-the-counter drugs that may have synergistic or cumulative effects. Finally, changes in habits regarding alcohol intake, diet, and exercise also can affect drug metabolism. These changes can increase the risk for adverse drug reactions. The emergency care for geriatric patients with adverse drug reactions varies. Care may range from transport only to full advanced cardiac life support measures. Box 49-11 lists symptoms of drug toxicity and adverse reactions that can occur in the geriatric patient.

Substance Abuse

As described in Chapter 34, substance abuse involving alcohol and other drugs is common in the elderly population. Up to 17% of U.S. citizens age 60 and older are estimated to be addicted to substances, and this number is expected to rise as the baby boomer population enters older age.[28]

BOX 49-11 Symptoms of Drug Toxicity and Adverse Drug Reactions in the Geriatric Patient

Acute delirium
Akathisia
Altered vision
Bradycardia
Cardiac dysrhythmias
Chorea
Coma
Confusion
Constipation
Fatigue
Glaucoma
Hypokalemia
Orthostatic hypotension
Paresthesias
Psychological disturbances
Pulmonary edema
Severe bleeding
Tardive dyskinesia
Urinary hesitancy

BOX 49-12 Signs of Substance Abuse

Alcohol Abuse

Anorexia
Confusion
Denial
Frequent falling
Hostility
Insomnia
Mood swings
Note: Ingestion of even small amounts of alcohol by the geriatric patient can cause intoxication.

Other Drug Abuse

Altered level of consciousness
Falling
Hallucinations
Memory changes
Orthostatic hypotension
Poor coordination
Restlessness
Weight loss

Note: Individuals often have a history of alcohol and other drug abuse.

Substance abuse in the geriatric patient often is attributed to severe stress as the primary risk factor. This stress may result from life changes such as age-related changes in health or appearance, loss of employment, loss of spouse or life partner, illness, malnutrition, loneliness, loss of independent living arrangements, and others. Box 49-12 lists signs of substance abuse.

If the paramedic suspects substance abuse, friends and family members at the scene should be discreetly interviewed about the patient's alcohol or other drug use. The cornerstones of therapy for these patients are identifying the problem and arranging referral to a physician for treatment. Treatment for the acutely intoxicated patient is described in Chapter 34 and may include resuscitative measures to manage the patient's airway, ventilation, and circulation. In addition, the paramedic should carefully assess the geriatric patient who has signs and symptoms of alcohol or other drug intoxication for occult trauma and any underlying medical conditions. These conditions may include hypoglycemia, cardiomyopathy and dysrhythmias (such as atrial fibrillation), gastrointestinal bleeding, polydrug use (especially barbiturates and tranquilizers), and ethylene glycol or methanol ingestion.

Environmental Considerations

Elderly patients are at risk for developing illness from extremes in the environment. This is a result of the aging process and other factors (see Chapter 45). Two emergencies that relate to the environment are most common in geriatric patients. These are hypothermia and hyperthermia.

HYPOTHERMIA

Patients who are younger often develop hypothermia from extremes in the environment. In contrast, an older patient may develop hypothermia while indoors. This may occur as a result of cold surroundings and/or an illness that alters heat production or conservation. This is due in part to the following characteristics of older adults:
- They are less able to compensate for environmental heat loss.
- They have a decreased ability to sense changes in temperature.
- They have less total body water to store heat.
- They are less likely to develop tachycardia to increase cardiac output in response to cold stress.
- They have a decreased ability to shiver to increase body heat.

In addition to these physical changes, geriatric patients are more prone to develop hypothermia as a result of socioeconomic factors. For instance, a fixed income may inhibit an older person from paying for the cost of properly heating and insulating his or her home. Poor nutrition that results in a decrease in fat stores may contribute to hypothermia in geriatric patients who live alone. The following are other medical causes of hypothermia in geriatric patients:
- Arthritis
- Drug overdose
- Hepatic failure
- Hypoglycemia
- Infection
- Parkinson's disease
- Stroke

- Thyroid disease
- Uremia

The signs and symptoms of hypothermia may be subtle. They may include an altered mental status, slurred speech, ataxia, and dysrhythmias. In severe cases, coma without signs of life may be present. Hypothermia in the geriatric patient carries a high mortality rate. The paramedic should manage these patients as described in Chapter 45. Rapid and gentle transport for in-hospital rewarming and life support measures is crucial for the patient's survival.

HYPERTHERMIA

Hyperthermia in the geriatric patient is less common than hypothermia. Yet hyperthermia carries a significant mortality rate. The condition most likely results from exposure to high temperatures. These temperatures most likely continue for several days (e.g., during a heat wave). As in hypothermia, geriatric patients are unable to control body temperature even in moderate heat. Hyperthermia also may result from medical conditions such as hypothalamic dysfunction and spinal cord injury. Certain medications (e.g., antidysrhythmics, beta blockers, and cyclic antidepressants) can lead to hyperthermia. They do this by inhibiting heat dissipation, increasing motor activity, and impairing cardiovascular function.

As described in Chapter 45, hyperthermic illness may present as heat cramps, heat exhaustion, or heat stroke. Emergency care includes removing the patient from the warm environment, cooling the patient, and ensuring the patient's vital functions through airway, ventilatory, and circulatory support. Rapid transport for physician evaluation is indicated to manage the problems resulting from serious heat-related illness.

Behavioral and Psychiatric Disorders

Fifteen million elderly persons are expected to suffer from some kind of psychiatric illness by the year 2030.[29] In addition to the neurological disorders such as dementia and Alzheimer's disease, depression and suicide are common in geriatric patients.

DEPRESSION

Depression is a serious illness that requires physician evaluation. In the geriatric patient, depression can result from physiological and psychological causes. Examples include cognitive disorders with physical causes (e.g., dementia) and various personality disorders such as schizophrenia (see Chapter 35). Box 49-13 lists other physiological and psychological causes of depression in the geriatric patient. The signs and symptoms of depression vary by individual. They may include the following:

- Decreased libido
- Deep feelings of worthlessness and guilt
- Extreme isolation
- Feelings of hopelessness
- Irritability
- Loss of appetite

BOX 49-13 Common Causes of Depression in the Geriatric Patient

Physiological
Dehydration
Electrolyte imbalance
Fever
Hyponatremia
Hypoxia
Medications
Metabolic disturbances
Organic brain disease
Reduced cardiac output
Thyroid disease

Psychological
Fear of dying
Financial insecurity
Loss of a spouse
Loss of independence
Significant illness

- Loss of energy (fatigue)
- Recurrent thoughts of death
- Significant weight loss
- Sleeplessness
- Suicide attempts

 CRITICAL THINKING
What endocrine disorder can produce signs or symptoms that are similar to those of depression?

A major goal of care is to identify the patient who may be depressed. These patients need to be evaluated by a physician. The physician will rule out medical illness—especially thyroid disease, stroke, malignancy, and dementia—or medication use (e.g., beta blockers) that may be responsible for the patient's depression. After determining that there are no physical threats to life, the paramedic should try to establish a rapport with the patient who is depressed. The patient should be encouraged to talk openly about his or her feelings, especially any thoughts of suicide. If possible, the paramedic should interview the family about the patient's mental state and question family members about any history of depression in the patient.

SUICIDE

The rate of completed suicides for geriatric patients is higher than that of the general population, and most of these persons visited their primary care physician in the month before the suicide.[30] Most were suffering from their first episode of major depression, which was only moderately severe, yet the depressive symptoms were unrecognized and untreated. Thus the paramedic should be aware of the increased risk for suicide when evaluating geriatric patients who are depressed. Clues and indicators for suicide in the geriatric patient that may be obtained through a patient history or observed by friends and family include[31]:

- Talking about or seemingly preoccupied with death and "getting affairs in order"
- Giving away prized possessions (e.g., family heirlooms, photographs, and keepsakes)
- Taking unnecessary risks (e.g., walking alone in unsafe areas or driving without personal restraints)
- Increased use of alcohol or other drugs
- Nonadherence to medical regimen (e.g., failure to take prescribed medications)
- Acquiring a weapon, especially firearms

As described in Chapter 35, there is no evidence that questions about suicidal thoughts and feelings increase the risk of suicide. Many depressed persons are willing to discuss their suicidal thoughts; therefore the paramedic should question the patient about suicidal thoughts if he or she suspects that the patient is at high risk. The following questions are appropriate for the paramedic to ask the patient:

1. Do you have thoughts about killing yourself?
2. Have you ever tried to kill yourself?
3. Have you thought about how you might kill yourself?

Most suicides committed by older adults involve firearms. Therefore, the safety of those at the scene and the emergency medical services crew is a priority when caring for a patient with suicidal tendencies. When indicated, law enforcement personnel should be available at the scene. After assessing the risk for suicidal tendencies, the patient should be transported for physician evaluation. While en route to the hospital, the paramedic should encourage the patient to discuss his or her feelings and reassure the patient that he or she can be helped through the crisis.

Trauma

Trauma (described in detail in Part 9: Trauma) is the fifth leading cause of death for persons over 65 years of age. One third of traumatic deaths in persons 65 to 74 years of age are caused by vehicular trauma, and 25% result from falls. In those older than 72 years of age, falls are the leading cause of unintentional injury or death.[32] Burns also are a major cause of disability and death in geriatric patients. Contributing factors that increase the severity of traumatic injury in geriatric patients include the following:

- Osteoporosis and muscle weakness that increase the likelihood of falls and fractures
- Reduced cardiac reserve that decreases the ability to compensate for blood loss
- Decreased respiratory function that increases the likelihood of adult respiratory distress syndrome
- Impaired renal function that decreases the ability to adapt to fluid shifts

SHOW ME THE EVIDENCE

Researchers in New England performed a retrospective record review of blunt trauma patients ages 17 to 35 years (young) and ages 65 and older (geriatric) seen at one level I trauma center between 2003 and 2008. They sought to correlate blood pressure and heart rate on arrival to the ED with mortality. During this period, 2194 geriatric and 2081 young patients were admitted. Mortality in the geriatric group was 11.4% (251) versus 2.4% (49) in the young group. Bradycardia on arrival was associated with increased mortality in both groups. There was a significant increase in mortality in geriatric patients whose heart rate was greater than 90 beats/min as opposed to 130 beats/min in the young group. Mortality correlated to a systolic blood pressure (SBP) less than 110 mm Hg in geriatric patients but was not significant until SBP declined below 95 mm Hg in the young patients. The authors suggest that new triage set points be considered for geriatric patients with blunt trauma.

From Heffernan DS, Thakkar RK, Monaghan SF, et al: Normal vital signs are unreliable in geriatric blunt trauma victims, *J Trauma* 69(4):813-820, 2010.

VEHICULAR TRAUMA

More than 15 million licensed drivers are over 65 years of age. In 2008 more than 2700 deaths in this age group were attributed to motor vehicle crashes.[32] Most of these vehicle collisions are not related to high speed or use of alcohol. Rather, they are related to errors in perception or judgment or to delayed reaction time. A large number of older adults are injured as drivers or passengers in moving vehicles. In addition, more than 2000 pedestrian fatalities among older adults occur each year in the United States. This accounts for 20% of all pedestrian deaths from trauma.

The risk of death from multiple trauma is estimated to be 3 times greater at 70 years of age than at 20 years of age. This is mainly because the geriatric patient is more susceptible to serious injury from equivalent degrees of trauma. This patient also is less capable of an appropriate, protective physiological response. Prompt identification of injuries and sources of hemorrhage is critical in any trauma patient but is especially important in the geriatric patient. The geriatric patient has much less cardiac reserve. The patient will succumb more quickly to shock.

HEAD TRAUMA

A head injury with loss of consciousness in geriatric patients often has a poor outcome. The brain becomes smaller in size with age (**cerebral atrophy**). This atrophy produces an increase in distance between the surface of the brain and the skull. As veins are stretched across this space, they are more easily torn. This results in subdural hematomata. The extra space within the skull often allows a large amount of bleeding to occur before signs and symptoms of increased intracranial pressure are seen.

Geriatric patients also are at high risk for injuries of the cervical spine because of the arthritic and degenerative changes associated with aging. These structural changes

CRITICAL THINKING
Consider geriatric patients with head trauma. What home medications also can lead to an increased risk of intracerebral bleeding in these patients?

lead to increased stiffening and decreased flexibility of the spine with narrowing of the spinal canal. This makes the spinal cord much more at risk for damage from fairly minor trauma.

CHEST INJURIES

Any mechanism of injury that produces thoracic trauma in a geriatric patient can be potentially lethal. The aged thorax is less elastic. Thus the thorax is more susceptible to injury. The pulmonary system also has marginal reserve because of a reduced alveolar surface area, decreased patency of small airways, and diminished chemoreceptor response.

Injuries to the heart, aorta, and major vessels are a greater risk to geriatric patients than they are to younger patients. Again, this is due to decreased functional reserve in older patients. It also is due to anatomical changes that make injury in these areas of greater significance. Myocardial contusion may be a complication of blunt injury to the chest. If severe, myocardial contusion may result in pump failure or life-threatening dysrhythmias. Rarely, cardiac tamponade occurs after blunt thoracic trauma. Cardiac rupture, valvular injury (e.g., flail valves), and aortic dissection also may occur with significant blunt chest injury. The first two entities are rare but rapidly fatal. When the mechanism of injury produces rapid deceleration, the paramedic should always consider the possibility of dissecting aortic aneurysm. Aortic dissections often are not immediately fatal. Proper evaluation and treatment can be lifesaving (see Chapter 22).

CRITICAL THINKING
Consider the patient who has a dissecting aortic aneurysm. What specific signs and symptoms may the paramedic see in this patient?

In the geriatric patient the heart cannot respond as effectively to increased demand for oxygen as in the younger person. This coupled with a slowed conduction system may cause ischemia and dysrhythmias when the geriatric patient has a significant trauma. These problems may occur even if the heart has not been damaged directly by the trauma. The patient's oxygenation and circulatory status must be closely monitored.

ABDOMINAL INJURIES

Abdominal injuries in geriatric patients have more serious consequences than injuries to any other body area. Abdominal injuries often are less obvious. Thus they require a high degree of suspicion. The geriatric patient is less likely to tolerate abdominal surgery well. This patient is more likely to develop pulmonary complications and infection following surgery.

MUSCULOSKELETAL INJURIES

The osteoporotic bones of geriatric patients are more at risk for fractures, even with mild trauma. Pelvic fractures are highly lethal in this age group. They can cause severe hemorrhage and soft tissue injury. When assessing for skeletal trauma, the paramedic should recall that the geriatric patient may have decreased pain perception. Often these patients have amazingly little tenderness with major fractures. Even with proper care, the mortality rate for geriatric patients with musculoskeletal injury is increased by delayed complications such as adult respiratory distress syndrome, sepsis, renal failure, and pulmonary embolism.

FALLS

Falls are a major cause of morbidity and mortality in older adults, with an overall fatality rate of 7.0%.[32] About one third of older adults living at home fall each year. One in 40 of these persons is hospitalized. A major cause of falls in older adults results from the use of prescribed sedative-hypnotics. These drugs affect balance and postural control. Some examples are alprazolam, *diazepam*, chlordiazepoxide, and flurazepam.

CRITICAL THINKING
Consider geriatric patients who have fallen. What common problems may contribute to an increased death rate in these patients?

Fractures are the most common fall-related injuries—the hip being the fracture that most often results in hospitalization. In those who survive hip fracture, most will have significant problems with walking and moving about. They may become more dependent on others for help. Falls that do not result in physical injury may lead to self-imposed immobility from the fear of falling again. When immobility is strict and prolonged, joint contractures, pressure sores, urinary tract infection, muscle atrophy, depression, and functional dependency may result.

The paramedic should assume that any fall indicates an underlying problem until it is proved otherwise. Attempts should be made to uncover any medical, psychological, and environmental factors that may have been responsible for the fall. Thus the patient history should include a full review of all medical problems and medications. It also should include precise details of the fall. (This includes history of falling, time and location of fall, symptoms experienced, activity in which the victim was engaged, use of devices, and presence of witnesses.) The paramedic also should evaluate the patient's cardiovascular, neurological, and musculoskeletal systems.

BURNS

More than 1000 older adults die from fires and burns in the United States each year.[32] The increased risk of morbidity and mortality from burn trauma in older adults is due to preexisting disease, skin changes that result in increased burn depth, impaired nutrition, and decreased ability to fight infection. The initial care and resuscitation of geriatric patients with thermal injury is described in Chapter 39. Geriatric burn patients need special approaches to fluid therapy to prevent damage to the kidneys. The patient's fluid status will need to be assessed in the initial hours after a burn injury by monitoring pulse and blood pressure, and striving to maintain a urine output of at least 50 to 60 mL per hour.

Trauma Management Considerations

The priorities of trauma care for geriatric patients are similar to those for all trauma patients described in Part Nine: Trauma. However, the paramedic should give special consideration to transport strategies and the geriatric patient's cardiovascular, respiratory, and renal systems.

CARDIOVASCULAR SYSTEM

Special considerations for cardiovascular problems include the following:

- Recent or past MI contributes to the risk of dysrhythmias and CHF.
- Adjustment of heart rate and stroke volume may be decreased in response to hypovolemia.
- Geriatric patients may need higher arterial pressures than younger patients for perfusion of vital organs. This is because of atherosclerotic peripheral vascular disease.
- Rapid IV fluid administration to geriatric patients may cause volume overload. The paramedic must take care not to overhydrate these patients. Older adults as a group are more susceptible to CHF. However, hypovolemia and hypotension are also poorly tolerated. The paramedic should consider hypovolemia in any geriatric patient whose systolic blood pressure is less than 120 mm Hg. Tachycardia may not occur if the patient takes beta blockers. The paramedic should monitor lung sounds and vital signs carefully and frequently during fluid administration.

RESPIRATORY SYSTEM

Special considerations for respiratory problems include the following:

- Physical changes decrease chest wall compliance and movement. Thus they diminish vital capacity as well.
- PaO_2 decreases with age.
- Lower PO_2 at the same fractional inspired oxygen concentration occurs with each passing decade.
- All organ systems have less tolerance to hypoxia.
- Chronic obstructive pulmonary disease (common in geriatric patients) requires that the paramedic carefully adjust airway management and ventilation support for appropriate oxygenation and carbon dioxide removal. High-concentration oxygen may suppress hypoxic drive in some patients. However, oxygen should never be withheld from a patient with clinical signs of cyanosis. The paramedic may need to remove the patient's dentures for adequate airway and ventilation management.

RENAL SYSTEM

Special considerations for renal problems include the following:

- The kidneys have decreased ability to maintain normal acid-base balance. They have decreased ability to compensate for fluid changes as well.
- Kidney disease may further decrease the ability of the kidneys to compensate.
- Decreased kidney function (along with decreased cardiac reserve) places the injured geriatric patient at risk for fluid overload and pulmonary edema following IV fluid therapy.

TRANSPORTATION STRATEGIES

Special considerations for transportation of geriatric patients include the following:

- Positioning, immobilization, and transport of a geriatric trauma patient may require modifications to accommodate physical deformities (e.g., arthritis or spinal abnormalities).
- Packaging should include bulk and extra padding to support and give comfort to the patient.
- The paramedic can prevent hypothermia by keeping the patient warm.

Elder Abuse

Elder abuse refers to the infliction of physical pain, injury, debilitating mental anguish, unreasonable confinement, or willful deprivation by a caregiver of services that are necessary to maintain mental and physical health of a geriatric person. Elder abuse has become more and more recognized as a growing problem in the United States. Elder abuse is estimated to affect between 1 and 2 million older adults each year.[33]

Elder abuse takes many forms. These include physical abuse, sexual abuse, emotional or psychological abuse, neglect, abandonment, financial or material exploitation, and self-neglect. Box 49-14 lists the signs and symptoms of each type of elder abuse as defined by the National Center on Elder Abuse.

All 50 states have elder abuse statutes. Also, reporting of suspected elder abuse is mandatory under law in most states. If the paramedic suspects abuse or neglect of an older adult, the medical direction should be advised. Moreover, the paramedic should follow the procedures that are established by local protocol. Emergency care is aimed at managing injuries that pose a threat to life and transporting the patient for physician evaluation. Abuse and neglect are discussed further in Chapter 50.

BOX 49-14 Signs and Symptoms of Elder Abuse and Neglect

Physical Abuse

Abandonment

Bruises, black eyes, welts, lacerations, and rope marks

Bone fractures, skull fractures

Open wounds, untreated injuries in various stages of healing

Sprains, dislocations, and internal injuries/bleeding

Broken eyeglasses/frames, physical signs of being subjected to punishment, and signs of being restrained

An elder's report of being hit, slapped, kicked, or mistreated

An elder's sudden change in behavior

The caregiver's refusal to allow examination of an elder without the caregiver being present

The desertion of an elder at a hospital, a nursing facility, or other similar institution

The desertion of an elder at a shopping center or other public location

An elder's own report of being abandoned

Financial or Material Exploitation

Sudden changes in bank account or banking practice, including an unexplained withdrawal of large sums of money by a person accompanying the elder

The inclusion of additional names on an elder's bank signature card

Unauthorized withdrawal of the elder's funds using the elder's automatic teller machine card

Sexual Abuse

Abrupt changes in a will or other financial documents

Bruises around the breasts or genital area

Unexplained venereal disease or genital infections

Unexplained vaginal or anal bleeding

Torn, stained, or bloody underclothing

An elder's report of being sexually assaulted or raped

Unexplained disappearance of funds or valuable possessions

Substandard care being provided or bills unpaid despite the availability of adequate financial resources

Discovery of an elder's signature being forged for financial transactions or for the titles of his or her possessions

Emotional or Psychological Abuse

Sudden appearance of previously uninvolved relatives

Being emotionally upset or agitated

Being extremely withdrawn and noncommunicative or nonresponsive

Unusual behavior usually attributed to dementia (e.g., sucking, biting, or rocking)

An elder's report of being verbally or emotionally mistreated claiming their rights to an elder's affairs and possessions

Unexplained sudden transfer of assets to a family member or someone outside the family

The provision of services that are not necessary

An elder's report of financial exploitation

Neglect

Self-Neglect

Dehydration, malnutrition, untreated bed sores, and poor personal hygiene

Unattended or untreated health problems

Hazardous or unsafe living conditions/arrangements (e.g., improper wiring and lack of heat or running water)

Unsanitary and unclean living conditions (e.g., dirt, fleas, body lice, soiled bedding, fecal/urine smell, and inadequate clothing)

An elder's report of being mistreated

Dehydration, malnutrition, untreated or improperly attended medical conditions, and poor personal hygiene

Hazardous or unsafe living conditions/arrangements (e.g., improper wiring, no indoor plumbing, and lack of heat or running water)

Unsanitary or unclean living quarters (e.g., animal/insect infestation, no functioning toilet, and fecal/urine smell)

Inappropriate and/or inadequate clothing, lack of the necessary medical aids (e.g., eyeglasses, hearing aids, and dentures)

Grossly inadequate housing or homelessness

Adapted from National Center on Elder Abuse: *The basics: major types of elder abuse,* www.elderabusecenter.org/default.cfm?p=basics.cfm, accessed 10-1-03.

SUMMARY

- The aging process proceeds at different rates in different persons. Respiratory function in the older adult generally is compromised. This is a result of changes in pulmonary physiology that accompany the aging process. Cardiac function also declines with age. This is a result of normal physiological changes and the high incidence of coronary artery disease. Renal blood flow falls an average of 50% between 30 and 80 years of age. A gradual decrease in the number of neurons, decreased cerebral blood flow, and changes in the location and amounts of specific neurotransmitters probably contribute to changes in the CNS. As the body ages, muscles shrink, muscles and ligaments calcify, and the intervertebral disks become thin. Other physiological changes that occur with aging include changes in body mass and total body water, a decreased ability to maintain internal homeostasis, a decrease in the function of immunological mechanisms, an increase in possible nutritional disorders, and decreases in hearing and visual acuity.

Continued

- Normal changes with aging and existing illnesses may make evaluation of an ill or injured geriatric patient a challenge.
- Pneumonia is a leading cause of death in the geriatric age group. It often is fatal in frail adults. Chronic obstructive pulmonary disease (COPD) is a common finding in the geriatric patient who has a history of smoking. The disease usually is associated with various other diseases that result in reduced expiratory airflow. Pulmonary embolism is a life-threatening cause of dyspnea. Pulmonary embolism is associated with venous stasis, heart failure, COPD, malignancy, and immobilization. All of these are common in older adults.
- A lack of typical chest pain can cause an MI to be unrecognized in the geriatric patient. Heart failure is more frequent in geriatric patients and has a larger incidence of noncardiac causes. The most common cause of dysrhythmias in the geriatric patient is hypertensive heart disease. Abdominal aortic aneurysm affects 2% to 4% of the U.S. population over 50 years of age. This aneurysm is most prevalent between 60 and 70 years of age. The incidence of hypertension in the geriatric patient increases when atherosclerosis is present.
- Risk factors for cerebral vascular disease in the older adult include smoking, hypertension, diabetes, atherosclerosis, hyperlipidemia, polycythemia, and heart disease.
- Delirium is an abrupt disorientation to time and place. Delirium is commonly a result of physical illness.
- Dementia is a slow, progressive loss of awareness of time and place. It usually involves an inability to learn new things or remember recent events. This condition often is a result of brain disease. Alzheimer's disease is the most common cause of dementia. Alzheimer's disease is a condition in which nerve cells in the cerebral cortex die and the brain substance shrinks.
- Parkinson's disease is a brain disorder. It causes muscle tremor, stiffness, and weakness.
- About 20% of older adults have diabetes. Almost 40% have some impaired glucose tolerance. Hyperglycemic hyperosmolar nonketotic coma is a serious complication of elderly type 2 diabetic patients. It has a mortality rate of 20% to 50%. Thyroid disease is more common

in geriatric patients. It may not present in the classic manner.
- Gastrointestinal bleeding most often affects patients between 60 and 90 years of age. It has a mortality rate of about 10%. Bowel obstruction generally occurs in patients with prior abdominal surgeries or hernias. It also occurs in those with colonic cancer. Some geriatric patients may have problems with continence or with elimination as well.
- Aging results in a gradual decrease in epidermal cellular turnover. It also results in loss of deep and dermal vessels. Alterations in capillary circulation lead to changes in thermal regulation and skin-related complications.
- Osteoarthritis is a common form of arthritis in geriatric patients. It results from cartilage loss and wear and tear on the joints. The loss in bone density from osteoporosis causes bones to become brittle. These bones may fracture easily.
- As persons age, they may experience problems with vision, hearing, and speech.
- Geriatric patients are at an increased risk for adverse drug reactions. This is due to age-related changes in body composition and drug distribution. It also is the result of metabolism and excretion. Moreover, the risk for adverse drug reactions often stems from multiple prescribed drugs. Alcohol abuse is a common problem in geriatric patients.
- The geriatric patient may develop hypothermia while indoors. This may be the result of cold surroundings and/or an illness that alters heat production or conservation. Hyperthermia most likely results from exposure to high temperatures that continue for several days.
- Depression is common in geriatric patients. It can result from physiological and psychological causes. The rate of completed suicides for geriatric patients is higher than that of the general population.
- One third of traumatic deaths in persons 65 to 74 years of age result from vehicular trauma. Twenty-five percent result from falls. In those older than 80 years of age, falls account for 50% of injury-related deaths. The risk of fatality from multiple trauma is estimated to be 3 times greater at 70 years of age than at 20 years of age.
- Elder abuse is classified as physical abuse, psychological abuse, financial or material abuse, and neglect.

REFERENCES

1. U.S. Department of Health and Human Services, U.S. Senate Special Committee on Aging: *Aging America: trends and projections*, Washington, DC, 1988, The Department.
2. American Geriatrics Society Foundation for Health in Aging: *2000-2010 decade of health in aging: the challenge—the aging of the U.S. population*, www.healthinaging.org/the challenge.html, accessed 11-3-04.
3. Freid L, Tangen CM, Walston J, et al: Frailty in older adults: evidence of a phenotype, *J Gerentol Biol Sci Med Sci* 56(3):M146-M156, 2001.
4. Torpy JM: JAMA patient page, frailty in older adults, *JAMA* 296(18):2280, 2006.
5. Bosker G, Schwartz GR, Jones JS, et al: *Geriatric emergency medicine*, St Louis, 1990, Mosby.

6. American Heart Association: *Advanced cardiac life support*, Dallas, 1997, The Association.

7. Fick DM, Cooper JW, Wade WE, et al: Updating the Beers criteria for potentially inappropriate medication use in older adults: results of a US consensus panel of experts, *Arch Intern Med* 163:2716-2724, 2003.

8. Routeledge P, O'Mahony MS, Woodhouse KW: Adverse drug reaction in elderly patients, *Br J Clin Pharmacol* 57(2):121-126, 2004.

9. Moore N, Lecointre D, Noblet C, et al: Frequency and cost of serious adverse drug reactions in a department of general medicine, *Br J Clin Pharmacol* 57(2):121-126, 2004.

10. Gurwitz JH, Field TS, Harrold LR, et al: Incidence and preventability of adverse drug events among older persons in the ambulatory setting, *JAMA* 289:110-116, 2003.

11. Rosen P, Barkin R: *Emergency medicine: concepts and clinical practice*, ed 6, St Louis, 2006, Mosby.

12. National Centers for Health Statistics, Centers for Disease Control and Prevention: *Health, United States, 1999 with health and aging chartbook*, www.cdc.gov/nchs/data/hus99.pdf, accessed 10-20-10.

13. McClatchey K, editor: *Clinical laboratory medicine*, ed 2, Philadelphia, 2002, Lippincott Williams & Wilkins.

14. Furman C, Rayner AV, Tobin EP: Pneumonia in older residents of long-term care facilities, *Am Fam Physician* 70:1495-1500, 2004.

15. American Geriatric Society, National Council of State EMS Training Coordinators, Snyder D, editor: *Geriatric education for emergency medical services*, Boston, 2003, Jones & Bartlett.

16. Ahmed A, Allman RM, Aronow WS, et al: Diagnosis of heart failure in older adults: predictive value of dyspnea at rest, *Arch Gerontol Geriatr* 38(3):297-307, 2004.

17. Ham R, Sloane PD, Warshaw GA, et al: *Primary care geriatrics: a case based approach*, Philadelphia, 2007, Mosby.

18. American Heart Association: *New high blood pressure guidelines say start early, treat aggressively*, www.americanheart. org/presenter.jhtml?identifier=3011728, accessed 10-26-04.

19. U.S. Department of Health and Human Services, National Institutes of Health, National Heart, Lung and Blood Institute: *Seventh report of the Joint National Committee on prevention, detection, evaluation, and treatment of high blood pressure (JNC 7)*, NIH Publ No. 04-5230, Washington, DC, Aug 2004, The Institute.

20. American Heart Association: Guidelines 2010 for cardiopulmonary resuscitation and emergency cardiovascular care, International Consensus on Science, *Circulation* 122(18):suppl 3, 2010.

21. National Highway Traffic Safety Administration: *The National EMS Education Standards*, Washington, DC: U.S. Department of Transportation/National Highway Traffic Safety Administration, 2009, DOT.

22. Raji MA, Brady SR: Mirtazapine for treatment of depression and comorbidities in Alzheimer disease, *Ann Pharmacother* 35(9):1024-1027, 2001.

23. Hermanns M: Parkinson's focus: Parkinson's is debilitating but new treatments are on the horizon, *RN* 71(10):24-28, 2008.

24. Odegard PS, Setter SM, Neumiller JJ: Considerations for pharmacological treatment in older adults, *Diabetes Spectrum* 20(4):239-247, 2007.

25. Wold GH: *Basic geriatric nursing*, ed 4, St Louis, 2004, Mosby.

26. Cassel C, Leipzig RM, Cohen HJ, et al: *Geriatric medicine: an evidence-based approach*, ed 4, New York, 2003, Springer-Verlag.

27. The Glaucoma Foundation: *What is glaucoma?* www.glaucomafoundation.org, accessed 10-15-10.

28. U.S. Department of Health and Human Services, Substance Abuse and Mental Health Services Administration: *Results from the 2009 National Survey on Drug Use and Health*, www.oas.samhsa.gov/NSDUH/2k9NSDUH/2k9Results.htm#2.4, accessed 10-14-10.

29. American Association of Geriatric Psychiatry: *Geriatric mental illness—the facts*, www.aagpgpa.org/prof/facts_mh.asp, accessed 10-15-10.

30. National Institute of Mental Health: *Older adults depression and suicide facts*, www.nimh.nih.gov/health/publications/older-adults-depression-and-suicide-facts-fact-sheet/index.shtml, accessed 10-15-10.

31. Snyder D, Christmas C, editors: *Geriatric education for emergency medical services*, American Geriatric Society, National Council of EMS Training Coordinators, Sudbury, Mass, 2003, Jones & Bartlett.

32. National Safety Council: *Injury facts*, Chicago, 2010, The Council.

33. National Center on Elder Abuse: *Fact sheet*, www.ncea.aoa.gov/ncearoot/Main_Site/pdf/publication/FinalStatistics050331.pdf, accessed 10-20-10.

SUGGESTED READINGS

Fick DM, Cooper JW, Wade WE, et al: Updating the Beers criteria for potentially inappropriate medication use in older adults: results of a US consensus panel of experts, *Arch Intern Med* 163(12):2716-2724, 2003.

Goldstein P: Assessment and treatment of hypoglycemia in elders: cautions and recommendations, *Medsurg Nurs* 18(4):215-223, 241, 2009.

Torpy JM: Frailty in older adults, *JAMA* 296(18):2280, 2006.

Weber JM, Jabolonski R, Penrod J: Missed opportunities: underdetection of trauma in elderly adults involved in motor vehicle crashes, *JEN* 36(1):6-9, 2010, doi: 10.1016/j.jen.2009.06.008.

CHAPTER
50 Abuse and Neglect

OBJECTIVES

Upon completion of this chapter, the paramedic student will be able to:
1. Define battering.
2. Describe the characteristics of abusive relationships.
3. Outline findings that indicate a battered patient.
4. Describe prehospital considerations when responding to and caring for battered patients.
5. Identify types of elder abuse.
6. Discuss legal considerations related to all forms of abuse.
7. Describe characteristics of abused children and their abusers.
8. Outline the physical examination of the abused child.
9. Describe the characteristics of sexual assault.
10. Outline prehospital patient care considerations for the patient who has been sexually assaulted.

KEY TERMS

battering Repeated physical violence and assault; may include establishing control and fear in a relationship through violence and other forms of abuse.

domestic violence A type of violence that occurs between opposite- and same-sex partners.

economic abuse Making or attempting to make an individual financially dependent by maintaining total control over financial resources, withholding one's access to money, or forbidding one's attendance at school or employment.

elder abuse The infliction of physical pain, injury, debilitating mental anguish, unreasonable confinement, or willful deprivation by a caregiver of services that are necessary to maintain mental and physical health of a geriatric person.

emotional abuse The infliction of anguish, pain, or distress through verbal or nonverbal acts.

financial/material exploitation The illegal or improper use of funds, properties, or assets.

neglect The refusal or failure of the caregiver to fulfill obligations or duties to a person.

patterned injuries Injuries that result from an identifiable object.

physical abuse The use of physical force that may result in bodily injury, physical pain, or impairment.

physical assault An intentional act by one person that creates apprehension in another of an imminent harmful or offensive contact.

self-neglect A type of elder abuse; behaviors of an older adult that intentionally threaten personal health or safety.

sexual abuse Nonconsensual sexual contact of any kind.

shaken baby syndrome A serious form of child abuse that describes injuries to infants that occur after being shaken violently.

stalking A pattern of repeated and unwanted attention, harassment, contact, or any other course of conduct directed at a specific person that would cause a reasonable person to feel fear.

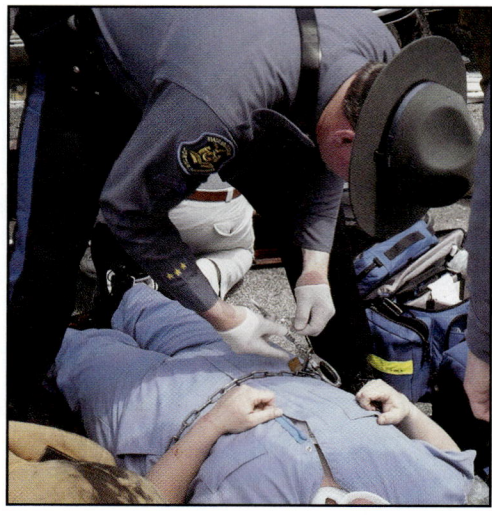

*P*artner, elder, and child abuse are growing problems in the United States. Paramedics will encounter victims of abuse in their careers. Abuse and neglect can result in mental and physical illness or injury, and even death. Education programs for paramedics must include information about these violent crimes. This information includes identification of victims, special aspects of care, scene safety, and documentation requirements. This chapter addresses the types of abuse and neglect, the personality traits of those who abuse, and legal considerations in providing emergency care.

BATTERING

Battering refers to repeated physical violence and assault. Battering often includes the establishment of control and fear in a relationship through violence and other forms of abuse. The batterer may use acts of violence and series of behaviors to coerce and control the other person. These behaviors include intimidation, threats, psychological abuse, and isolation (Figure 50-1). Battering can include many types of abuse and neglect. Examples include[1]:

- **Physical abuse:** Hitting, slapping, shoving, grabbing, pinching, biting, and hair-pulling, for example. Physical abuse also includes denying a partner medical care or forcing alcohol and/or drug use.
- **Sexual abuse:** Coercing or attempting to coerce any sexual contact or behavior without consent. Sexual abuse includes, but is not limited to, marital rape, attacks on sexual parts of the body, forcing sex after physical violence has occurred, or treating one in a sexually demeaning manner.
- **Emotional abuse:** Undermining an individual's sense of self-worth and/or self-esteem. This may include, but is not limited to, constant criticism, diminishing one's abilities, name-calling, or damaging one's relationship with his or her children.
- **Economic abuse:** Making or attempting to make an individual financially dependent by maintaining total control over financial resources, withholding access to money, or forbidding attendance at school or employment.

The violence associated with battering may not happen often. Yet battering is a hidden and constant terrorizing factor in some relationships. Over time the beatings usually become more severe and more frequent. They often occur without provocation. If children are present in a marriage or relationship, often the violence eventually turns toward them. Persons involved in abusive relationships often fail to see other options and feel powerless to change.

Domestic violence is also known as *intimate partner violence* (IPV). This type of violence occurs between opposite- and same-sex partners. Domestic violence follows a cycle of three phases[2] (Figure 50-2). Phase one involves arguing and verbal abuse; phase two progresses to physical and sexual abuse; and phase three consists of denial and apologies (the "honeymoon phase"). The paramedic best achieves intervention in phase two or three. The cycle repeats itself without intervention and usually increases in frequency and severity. Understanding this cycle of violence will help the paramedic assess the situation and care for the victim.

> ### NOTE
> Although not usually considered a form of abuse, **stalking** can be defined as a pattern of repeated and unwanted attention, harassment, contact, or any other course of conduct directed at a specific person that would cause a reasonable person to feel fear. Like domestic violence, stalking is a crime of power and control. In 2006, 3.4 million people in the United States were victims of stalking.[2] During their lifetimes, 1 in 12 women and 1 in 45 men will be stalked, for an average duration of almost 2 years.[3] During the course of their careers and when assisting law enforcement personnel at emergency scenes, paramedics will likely encounter victims who have been stalked.

> ### SHOW ME THE EVIDENCE
> Investigators evaluated the accuracy of EMTs as compared to a trained ride-along observer to complete a domestic violence screen on patients transported from their home. They also compared agreement between the Domestic Violence Scene Assessment Screen (DVSAS) and the Abuse Assessment Screen (AAS). Their sample was 43 patients. They found moderate to good agreement between the independent observer and EMT (kappa was 0.56 [0.29-0.83]). When compared to the AAS the DVSAS agreed in 60% of cases (sensitivity 75%; specificity 55%). The authors conclude that EMTs can reliably complete the DVSAS at the end of transport.
>
> From Weiss S, Garza A, Casaletto J, et al: The out-of-hospital use of a domestic violence screen for assessing patient risk, *PEC* 4(1): 24-27, 2000.

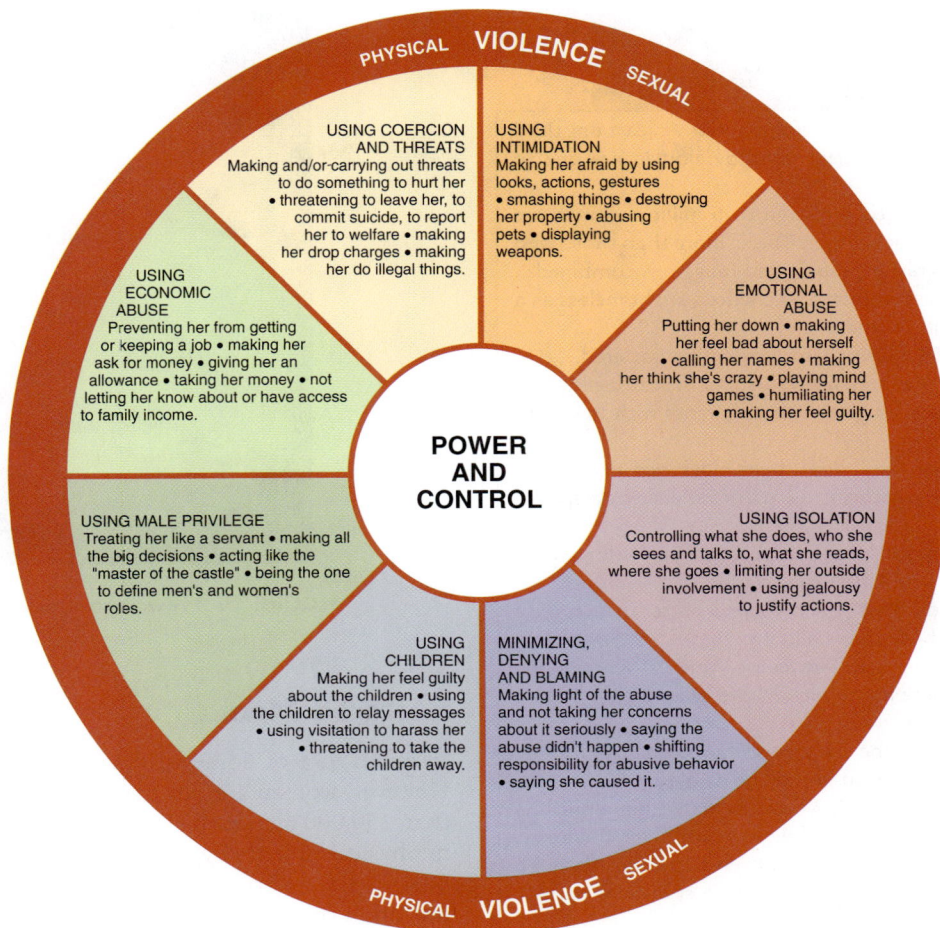

FIGURE 50-1 Relationship of violence to use of power and control. (From Domestic Abuse Intervention Project: *Wheel gallery,* retrieved 1-30-11 from www.duluth-model.org; Maurer FA, Smith CM: *Community/public health nursing practice,* ed 4, St Louis, 2009, Saunders.)

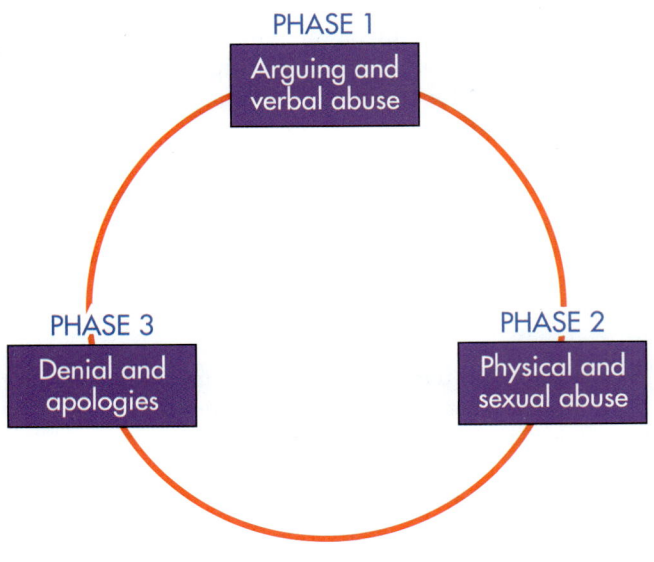

FIGURE 50-2 Cycle of violence.

Battered Women

An estimated 1.3 million women are battered by their husband, boyfriend, or intimate partner each year[4,5] (Box 50-1). Even so, less than 10% of women report battering incidents for reasons that include the following:

1. Personal fear or fear for her children
2. Belief that the offender's behavior will change (abusers often appear charming and loving after the battering incident)
3. Lack of financial and/or emotional support
4. Belief that she is the cause of the violent behavior
5. Belief that battering is "part of the marriage" and must be endured to keep the family together

Women of all cultures, races, occupations, income levels, and ages are battered by their past and present husbands, boyfriends, and intimate partners. Domestic violence is the leading cause of injury to women who are between 15 and 44 years of age in the United States.[6] Women who leave

BOX 50-1 Domestic Violence: Facts and Statistics

- Battered women often are severely injured. At least one third of all emergency department visits by women are due to battering.
- Every year an estimated 4 million to 6 million women are beaten by a spouse or partner. This is more than those who are hurt in auto crashes, rapes, and muggings combined.
- Half of all homeless women and children are homeless as a result of domestic violence.
- About 15% to 25% of pregnant women are battered.
- Battered women are more likely to suffer miscarriages. They also are more likely to give birth to infants with low birth weights.
- Living in suburban and rural areas does not decrease a woman's risk of experiencing an act of violence by a spouse or partner.
- Up to 75% of domestic assaults reported to law enforcement agencies were inflicted after the couples had separated.
- Between 50% and 70% of the men who batter their spouse or partner also abuse their children.
- About 63% of young men between 11 and 20 years of age who are serving time for homicide have killed their mother's abuser.
- Domestic violence is the sixth most dangerous call for law enforcement officers killed in the line of duty.
- The United States has nearly 3 times as many animal shelters as it does shelters for battered women and their children.
- Compared with males, females experience more than 10 times as many incidents of violence by a spouse or partner each year.
- Children are present in 40% to 55% of homes when police intervene in domestic violence calls.
- In 85% to 90% of domestic homicides, the police had been called to the home at least once during the 2 years before the incident. In more than half of these cases the police had been called 5 times or more.
- Almost 6 times as many women victimized by spouses or partners, compared with those victimized by strangers, did not report their violent victimization to police because they feared reprisal from the offender.

From Federal Bureau of Investigation, National Coalition Against Domestic Violence, National Woman Abuse Prevention Project, U.S. Senate, Committee on the Judiciary, U.S. Department of Justice, Bureau of Justice Statistics, May 2005.

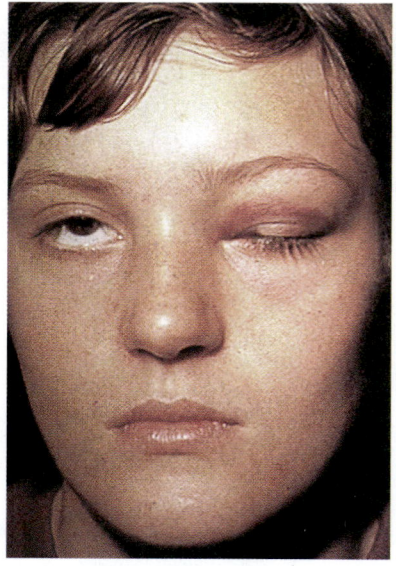

FIGURE 50-3 A woman struck in the face.

their batterers are at 75% greater risk of being killed by the batterer than those who stay in the abusive relationship. These women are also 25 times more likely to be seriously injured by their batterer when they leave than when they stay[7] (Figure 50-3).

> **NOTE**
> Intimate partner violence (IPV) in the United States resulted in nearly 2 million injuries and 1510 deaths in 2005. Of these deaths, 78% were women and 22% were men.[8]

Battered Men

In about 95% of domestic assaults the batterer is a man.[9] However, women are not the only battering victims. More than 150,000 men in the United States each year are victims of physical violence by a spouse or intimate partner (Figure 50-4).[4] Men report physical violence by a spouse or partner less often than women. This may be the result of humiliation, guilt, and/or fear to admit loss of control. In addition, society may seem to be less empathetic toward battered men than battered women. Communities generally have fewer resources for support.

Characteristics of Persons in Abusive Relationships

Certain personality traits may draw persons into abusive relationships. The following are characteristics of one or both persons in an abusive relationship[10]:

1. Intense need for love and affection
2. Low self-esteem
3. Alcohol or other drug dependence
4. Difficulty in finances, job security, and possible legal issues
5. Background of physical, emotional, or sexual abuse; abusers are often survivors of abuse
6. Belief that abuse is demonstrating discipline
7. Fear of being "out of control"
8. Uncontrolled temper, extreme jealousy, and insecurity
9. Inability to set and enforce personal boundaries
10. Unrealistic expectations of a relationship
11. Difficulty in expressing anger
12. Loyalty to the abuser that takes precedence over emotional or physical safety
13. Repeated attempts to leave the relationship

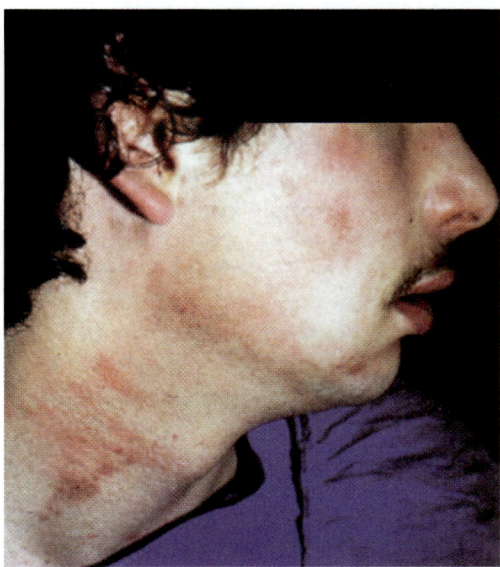

FIGURE 50-4 Soft tissue injury to the face from blows and to the neck from a firm grip.

14. Clinical depression
15. Suicidal ideation or attempts

Identification of the Battered Patient

The paramedic may have difficulty identifying the battered patient. Often the description of the injuries may be incorrect, inaccurate, and protective of the attacker. Injuries that are unintentional often involve the extremities and the periphery of the body. However, injuries from domestic violence often involve contusions and lacerations of the face, head, neck, breast, and abdomen. Bruises and lacerations may appear to be "old." This is because many victims of abuse do not seek medical help for their injuries. Other clues of domestic violence are the following:

- Excessive delays between injury and seeking treatment
- Repeated requests for emergency medical services assistance
- Injuries during pregnancy
- Substance abuse
- Frequent suicide gestures

Scene Safety

The paramedic must ensure scene and personal safety in domestic violence events. If dispatch reveals that the scene involves domestic violence, the paramedic should summon law enforcement personnel. The EMS crew also should not enter the scene until it has been secured. If domestic violence was not suspected until after arriving at the scene, the victim should be removed from the area as soon as possible. Violence often is directed at EMS personnel. This is especially the case if the abuser feels that the paramedic is giving too much empathy to the victim. Thus the paramedic should not question the victim about possible violence in the presence of the abuser. No display of sympathy should

be shown until the victim is in the ambulance or has been separated from the suspected batterer.

Care of the Victim

All injuries should be managed according to standard protocols. The paramedic should direct special attention to the emotional needs of the victim. The abuser often is unwilling to allow the victim to give a history or allow the victim to be alone with EMS personnel. Therefore, the paramedic should question the patient privately about the incident when possible.

 CRITICAL THINKING
If you suspect abuse, what can you say to encourage the victim to talk about it?

History of the events that led to physical injury should be obtained by using direct questions. Often the patient will avoid eye contact and be hesitant or evasive about details of an injury. Some may offer clues by saying, "Things haven't been going well lately," or "There have been problems at home" (Box 50-2). The paramedic should convey to the patient his or her suspicions of battering. The patient may be relieved to know that someone else is aware of the abuse.

During the patient interview, it is important to be nonjudgmental and to avoid comments such as "How awful" or "Why don't you leave?" The paramedic should listen carefully to the victim and offer emotional support. The patient should be encouraged to gain control of his or her life and to consider the best interests and needs of any children who may be involved in the abusive relationship. Access to community resources should be provided to the victim. These resources include battered spouse programs, victim-witness assistance programs, and other support agencies for abused victims and their families. Finally, the paramedic should discuss safety measures with the victim who elects not to be transported for evaluation. This may include helping the patient identify a quick way out of a dangerous situation (e.g., where to go and whom to call). It also may include giving the victim an approved written list

---

BOX 50-2 Lies Abusers Tell

- "I just need to be understood."
- "I had a bad childhood."
- "I can't control it."
- "I get angry."
- "She fights too."
- "She pushes my buttons."
- "If I don't control her, she will control me."
- "My smashing things isn't abusive, it's venting."
- "I have a lot of stress in my life."
- "I just have an anger management problem."
- "I just have a problem when I drink or use drugs."

BOX 50-3 National Domestic Violence Hotline

In 1996 the U.S. government established a nationwide 24-hour toll-free domestic violence hotline through the Violence Against Women Act of 1994. The voice number for the hotline is 1-800-799-SAFE. The TDD number for the hearing impaired is 1-800-787-3224. The hotline is available 365 days a year. It operates throughout the United States, Puerto Rico, and the Virgin Islands. The hotline is staffed by trained advocates. These advocates offer crisis intervention, support, and referrals to local services in the caller's community.

Other components of the act include allocating funds for training prosecutors and police, maintaining shelters, and providing educational programs in schools and communities. These programs work with the hotline to treat domestic violence as a serious crime. They also help to prevent domestic violence before it starts.

or a small card (that can be hidden easily from the abuser) of community resources, shelters, and hotline numbers (Box 50-3).

CRITICAL THINKING

How would you feel if you respond to a call in which a woman has been injured by a batterer but chooses not to leave?

Some patients who have suffered abuse eventually leave the abusive relationship. This often is made possible by health care providers and support agency personnel who do the following:

- Treat the victim in a sensitive and sympathetic manner.
- Confirm that the victim is not at fault and does not deserve to be abused.
- Ensure the victim's safety.
- Become "agents of change" in helping provide the support needed for the victim to leave the abusive environment.

Legal Considerations

Physical assault is an intentional act by one person that creates apprehension in another of an imminent harmful or offensive contact. Physical assault is a crime that may be a misdemeanor or a felony, depending on state law, the amount of injury inflicted, and devices that the attacker uses during the assault. Often the attacker is arrested but is released from custody within hours on his or her own recognizance. If early release from custody is likely, the patient must be made aware of this and encouraged to take personal safety precautions.

Most states do not have mandatory reporting requirements for acts of domestic violence.[11] Paramedics should be aware of the requirements in their state. Emergency medical services personnel are bound professionally to advise medical direction of their suspicions and observations about acts of violence.

Any act of physical abuse against a spouse, partner, elder, or child is a crime. Therefore, the scene must be treated as a crime scene. Paramedics should be careful not to disturb the scene or destroy possible evidence. Documentation is key. It should include a precise account of injuries, a description of the reported mechanisms of injuries, and a depiction of the behavior of the victim and alleged abuser. Using body diagrams in the patient care report may be helpful. The paramedic should record the victim's own words in the narrative when possible and record the names of police officers and witnesses at the scene. These details are important in cases of litigation (see Chapter 4).

LOOK AGAIN

See Chapter 4: Documentation, pp. 67-68.

ELDER ABUSE

Elder abuse (abuse, neglect, exploitation of the elderly) was described in Chapter 49. Elder abuse is a prevalent medical and social problem in the United States. Although it is difficult to estimate how many older Americans are abused, neglected, or exploited, studies suggest that there may be as many as 5 million victims every year.[12] Factors that contribute to elder abuse include the following:

- Increased life expectancy
- Physical and mental impairment
- Decreased productivity
- Increased dependence
- Limited resources for care of the elderly
- Economic factors
- Stress of the middle-age caregiver responsible for two generations

CRITICAL THINKING

Do you think that the problem of elder abuse will increase or decrease during your career in emergency medical services? Why?

Types of Elder Abuse

According to the National Center on Elder Abuse[13] elder abuse may be classified as *physical abuse* (Figure 50-5), *sexual abuse, emotional/psychological abuse, neglect, abandonment, financial or material exploitation,* and *self-neglect* (Box 50-4). (**Self-neglect** refers to behaviors of an older adult that intentionally threaten personal health or safety. Examples include poor nutrition and noncompliance with prescribed drugs.) Elder abuse also is classified by where it occurs. It occurs in domestic settings or in institutions.

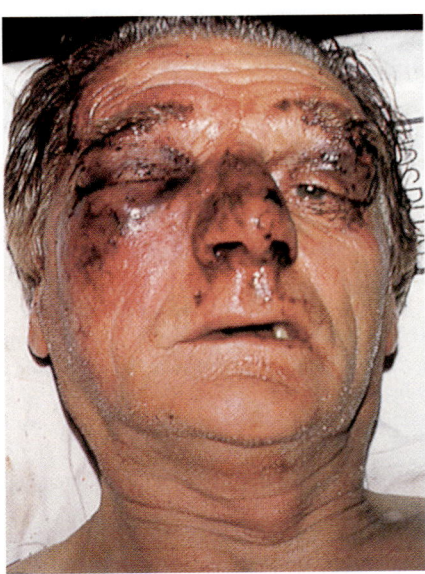

FIGURE 50-5 Injuries from facial blows to an older adult.

DOMESTIC SETTINGS

The average victim of elder abuse in domestic settings is about 78 years of age. The National Aging Resource Center on Elder Abuse provides data regarding types of elder abuse in domestic settings.[14] The abused elder usually has multiple, chronic health conditions that make him or her dependent on others for care. Widows over 75 years of age carry the greatest risk of elder abuse. Neglect is the most common form of elder abuse in domestic settings; unexplained trauma is the most common finding. Evidence suggests that elder abuse is associated more with the personality of the abuser than with the burden of caring for a sick, dependent person (Box 50-5).

Four major theories of causes of domestic elder abuse are as follows:
1. Elder abuse occurs in settings where the caregiver is under a great amount of stress. This stress is a result of personal problems and/or a lack of knowledge about how to provide care to an older adult.
2. Mental and/or physical impairments common in many older adults make them more likely to be abused than older adults who are in good health.
3. A "cycle of violence" often occurs in elder abuse. The cycle begins with ongoing tension. This tension escalates in a crisis in which abuse occurs. The abuse generally is followed by a period of calm, reconciliation, and denial, after which the cycle repeats.
4. Abusers of older adults often have more personal problems than nonabusers. (For example, they may have job insecurity and/or financial troubles.)

Older adults often are repeatedly abused by family members. The abusers most often are the children of the abused. Because of this familial relationship, many older adults do not report the abuse. Many also do not seek medical care for their injuries.

INSTITUTIONAL SETTINGS

About 5% of the U.S. population 65 years of age and older live in nursing homes, elder care facilities, assisted-living facilities, and board-and-care homes. Almost 50% of American who are 95 years of age and older reside in nursing homes. Based on Census Bureau projections, by 2030 it is estimated that 70% of patients 85 years of age and older will require some form of residential care.[15] These individuals are at risk for intentional harm, physical violence, verbal aggression, or neglect from other residents and paid caregivers, staff, and professionals. Clues that may indicate institutional abuse include the following:

- Burns caused by cigarettes, caustics, or acids
- Caregiver who cannot explain the victim's condition adequately
- Dehydration, malnutrition, or pressure sores
- Emotional abuse
- Loss of weight
- Neglect
- Open wounds, cuts, bruises, welts, or discoloration
- Physical abuse
- Unsanitary and unclean conditions (dirt, soiled bed, or fecal or urine odor)
- Unusual behavior by the victim (sucking, biting, or rocking)
- Victim who is begging for food
- Victim who is emotionally upset or agitated
- Victim who is extremely withdrawn and noncommunicative
- Victim with poor personal hygiene
- Victim's sudden change in behavior

Legal Considerations

All 50 states have elder abuse statutes. Reporting of suspected elder abuse is mandatory under law in most states. If the paramedic suspects any form of elder abuse, all findings should be carefully documented. Medical direction should be advised and procedures established by local protocol should be followed.

CHILD ABUSE

In 2007 child protective service agencies investigated more than 3 million reports alleging maltreatment of children. These agencies determined that an estimated 794,000 of these children were victims of substantiated or indicated abuse or neglect.[16] That same year, an estimated 1760 children died from child abuse.[17] As described in Chapter 48, various forms of child abuse—including physical injury, sexual exploitation, infliction of emotional pain, and neglect—can result in physical or emotional impairment.

Neglect is the most common form of child abuse. However, many children suffer more than one type of abuse. Neglect is the failure to provide physical care (e.g., medical care, nutrition, shelter, and clothing) or the failure to provide emotional care (i.e., indifference and disregard). Most substantiated reports of child abuse or neglect come from professional sources (educators, social services, law

BOX 50-4 Signs and Symptoms of Elder Abuse

Physical Abuse

- Bruises, black eyes, welts, lacerations, and rope marks
- Bone fractures, broken bones, and skull fractures
- Open wounds, cuts, punctures, untreated injuries in various stages of healing
- Sprains, dislocations, and internal injuries/bleeding
- Broken eyeglasses/frames, physical signs of being subjected to punishment, and signs of being restrained
- Laboratory findings of medication overdose or underutilization of prescribed drugs
- An elder's report of being hit, slapped, kicked, or mistreated
- An elder's sudden change in behavior
- The caregiver's refusal to allow visitors to see an elder alone

Sexual Abuse

- Bruises around the breasts or genital area
- Unexplained venereal disease or genital infections
- Unexplained vaginal or anal bleeding
- Torn, stained, or bloody underclothing
- An elder's report of being sexually assaulted or raped

Emotional/Psychological Abuse

- Being emotionally upset or agitated
- Being extremely withdrawn and noncommunicative or nonresponsive
- Unusual behavior usually attributed to dementia (e.g., sucking, biting, rocking)
- An elder's report of being verbally or emotionally mistreated

Neglect

- Dehydration, malnutrition, untreated bed sores, and poor personal hygiene
- Unattended or untreated health problems
- Hazardous or unsafe living conditions/arrangements (e.g., improper wiring, no heat, or no running water)
- Unsanitary and unclean living conditions (e.g., dirt, fleas, lice on person, soiled bedding, fecal/urine smell, inadequate clothing)
- An elder's report of being mistreated

Abandonment

- The desertion of an elder at a hospital, a nursing facility, or other similar institution
- The desertion of an elder at a shopping center or other public location
- An elder's own report of being abandoned

Financial or Material Exploitation

- Sudden changes in bank account or banking practice, including an unexplained withdrawal of large sums of money by a person accompanying the elder
- The inclusion of additional names on an elder's bank signature card
- Unauthorized withdrawal of the elder's funds using the elder's ATM card
- Abrupt changes in a will or other financial documents
- Unexplained disappearance of funds or valuable possessions
- Substandard care being provided or bills unpaid despite the availability of adequate financial resources
- Discovery of an elder's signature being forged for financial transactions or for the titles of his/her possessions
- Sudden appearance of previously uninvolved relatives claiming their rights to an elder's affairs and possessions
- Unexplained sudden transfer of assets to a family member or someone outside the family
- The provision of services that are not necessary
- An elder's report of financial exploitation

Self-Neglect

- Dehydration, malnutrition, untreated or improperly attended medical conditions, and poor personal hygiene
- Hazardous or unsafe living conditions/arrangements (e.g., improper wiring, no indoor plumbing, no heat, no running water)
- Unsanitary or unclean living quarters (e.g., animal/insect infestation, no functioning toilet, fecal/urine smell)
- Inappropriate and/or inadequate clothing, lack of the necessary medical aids (e.g., eyeglasses, hearing aids, dentures)
- Grossly inadequate housing or homelessness

From National Center on Elder Abuse: Major Types of Elder Abuse, U.S. Administration on Aging. http://www.ncea.aoa.gov/ncearoot/main_site/FAQ/Basics/Types_Of_Abuse.aspx, accessed July 21, 2011

BOX 50-5 Percentage of Those Who Abuse Elders

Adult children: 32.5%
Grandchildren: 4.2%
Intimate partners: 14.4%
Sibling: 2.5%
Other relative: 12.5%
Friend or neighbor: 7.5%
All others: 18.2%
Unknown: 2.0%

From The AGS Foundation for Health and Aging: *Preventing elder abuse and neglect in older adults,* New York, 2009, American Geriatric Society.

enforcement, and medical personnel). Persons in the family of the victim report only 18% of child abuse cases.[17]

Characteristics of Abusers

The characteristics of abusers are not related to social class, income, or level of education. Most child abusers are the child's parents (77%). Eleven percent are other relatives of the victim. Most abusers are under 40 years of age. Two thirds are female (usually the child's mother). Persons who are in other caregiving relationships to the victim (e.g., childcare providers, foster parents, and facility staff) account for only 2% of perpetrators. About 10% of all abusers are noncaregivers or unknown. Neglect often is

BOX 50-6 Characteristics of Child Abusers

- Demonstrate immature behavior
- Show personal preoccupation (self-centeredness)
- Have little perception of how a child feels (physically or emotionally)
- Are critical of the child
- Seldom touch or look at the child
- Are unconcerned about the child's injury, treatment, or prognosis
- Show no feeling of guilt or remorse
- Blame the child for the injury or illness

BOX 50-7 Who Are the Child Victims of Abuse?

- Nearly 50% are 7 years of age or younger.
- Thirty-three percent are younger than 4 years of age.
- Nearly 20% are 8 to 11 years of age.
- Twenty-one percent are 12 to 18 years of age.
- Fifty-one percent are female.
- Forty-eight percent of sexual abuse victims are boys.
- Children younger than 4 years of age account for 76% of fatalities from abuse.

From Child Maltreatment 2008, Administration for Children & Families, U.S. Department of Health and Human Services, Washington, DC.

attributed to female perpetrators, whereas sexual abuse most often is attributed to males.[17] Box 50-6 provides other characteristics of child abusers.

CRITICAL THINKING

How does it make you feel when you hear a story about child abuse on the news? Think about how you will manage those feelings when you are at a scene with such a child.

A family history of rigorous discipline accounts for the cyclical nature of child abuse. Because many abusers were severely punished and beaten as children by their parents, they often prefer to use other forms of discipline for their children. But the stresses of child rearing eventually culminate in some parents regressing to the earliest patterns of discipline that they experienced as a child. The abusive adult sometimes is aware of this cyclical nature. The adult may even try to seek help to prevent abusive behavior toward his or her children. During this pre-abuse state, the following pattern often occurs:

1. The adult makes several calls for help within a 24-hour period to 9-1-1 or support agencies.
2. The adult frequently calls EMS for inconsequential symptoms.
3. The adult begins to exhibit behavior of being unable to handle an impending crisis.

The pre-abuse state is important in identifying the potential for abuse. The pattern is often repetitive and results in frequent calls for EMS to visit the patient's home. The paramedic should remember that this behavior indicates the adult's awareness that child abuse is likely to occur. It also means that the adult is actively seeking help to prevent the abuse.

Characteristics of the Abused Child

Abused children often display behavior that provides important clues about abuse and neglect (Box 50-7). Although this behavior may be age-related, the paramedic should observe carefully the child under 6 years of age who is excessively passive, the child over 6 years of age who is excessively aggressive, and the child of any age with the following characteristics:

- Does not mind if his or her parents leave the room
- Cries hopelessly during treatment or cries very little
- Does not look at parents for reassurance
- Is wary of physical contact
- Is extremely apprehensive
- Appears constantly on the alert for danger
- Constantly seeks favors, food, or comfort items (e.g., blankets and toys)

Physical Examination

Injuries during childhood are common. Most injuries are unintentional and not the result of abuse. Distinguishing between an intentional and unintentional injury can be challenging for the paramedic. The most important clues can be obtained by observing the child and his or her relationship with the parent or caregiver and by matching the history of the event to the injury. If the child volunteers the history of the event without hesitation and matches the history that the parent provides (and the history is suitable for the injury), child abuse is unlikely.

LEGAL CONSIDERATIONS

When possible, the paramedic should partner with another colleague when performing the examination of a child who is a suspected victim of abuse. This will help verify that the note-taking is objective. The exam also will help ensure that assumptions and personal perceptions do not taint findings. The report must be succinct and legible. The paramedic should document all relevant findings and observations. Child abuse is a crime that is reportable under law in all 50 states. Paramedics should follow local protocol in reporting suspected child abuse. In addition, they should discuss any suspicions of child abuse or neglect with medical direction.

COMMON TYPES OF INJURIES

Common types of injuries associated with child abuse include the following:

Soft tissue injuries: Soft tissue injuries are the most common injury seen in cases of child abuse. They are often found in early abuse. They may present in various forms such as multiple bruises and ecchymosis, especially if bruises are extensive and are a mixture of old and new bruises. Defense wounds may be found on multiple body planes. They often are **patterned injuries** that result from an identifiable object. (For example, they might be bites, loop marks from a cord or belt [Figure 50-6], cigarette burns, or bristle marks from a hairbrush.) In addition, scalds are a common form of abuse in the young and old (Figure 50-7).

Fractures: Fractures are the second most common injury in cases of child abuse. They often are caused by twisting and jerking forces and may be different ages (new and healed), indicating repeated injury. Rib fractures and multiple fractures are common findings.

Head injuries: Head injury is the most common cause of death in cases of child abuse, and children who survive head injury often have permanent disability (Figure 50-8). Often there is a visible progression of injury that begins at the child's trunk and extremities and moves toward the head. Associated injuries include scalp wounds, skull fractures, subdural or subgaleal hematomata, and repeated concussions.

Abdominal injuries: Abdominal injuries in cases of child abuse are less common than those injuries just described. However, they often are serious. Blunt trauma to the abdomen may lead to rupture of the liver as well as injuries to the intestines and mesentery.

Children Who Die From Abuse and Neglect

As stated earlier in this chapter, more than 1700 children die from child abuse and neglect in the United States each year. Fatal injuries from maltreatment result from many different acts, including the following:

- Severe head trauma
- Shaken baby syndrome
- Trauma to the abdomen and thorax

> **NOTE**
> **Shaken baby syndrome** (SBS) is a serious form of child abuse. It describes injuries to infants that occur after being violently shaken for as little as 5 seconds.[18] These rapid shakes can cause cerebral hemorrhage, brain damage, blindness, paralysis, and death. Shaken baby syndrome most often occurs before 2 years of age but may be seen up to age 5. The shaking episode usually results from inconsolable crying. It is estimated that as many as 1000 to 1400 babies are severely injured or killed by shaking each year in the United States.[19]

- Scalding
- Drowning
- Suffocation
- Poisoning

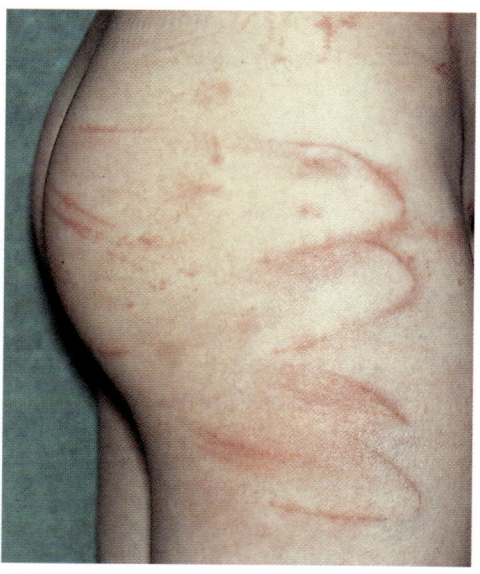

FIGURE 50-6 Patterned injury from being struck with a belt.

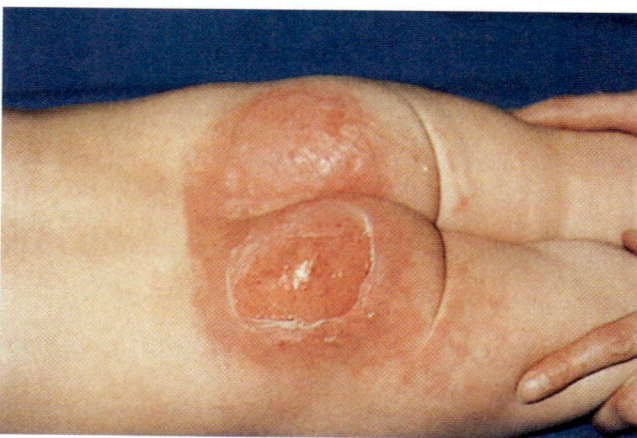

FIGURE 50-7 "Bath dipping" typically produces scalds on the buttocks and feet.

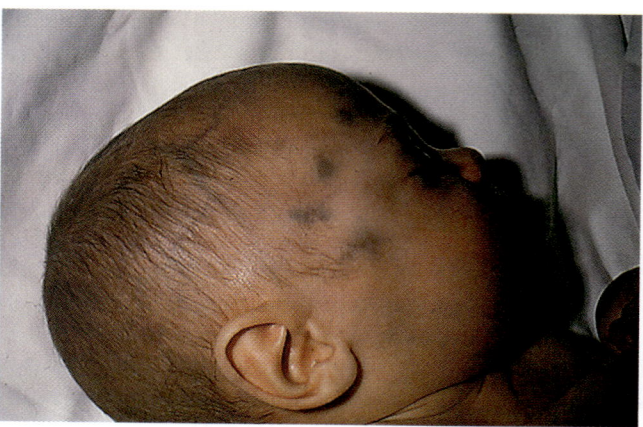

FIGURE 50-8 Multiple bruises on an infant's head from finger pressure.

Types of neglect that can result in death include the following:

1. *Supervision neglect* includes death that involves a critical moment in which the parent or caregiver is absent and the child is killed by a suddenly arising danger (e.g., leaving a child unattended in a bathtub).
2. *Chronic neglect* includes death that is caused by slowly building problems (e.g., malnutrition).
3. Deaths that result from *child physical abuse* involve fatal parental assaults on infants and children. These assaults are triggered by events such as inconsolable crying, feeding difficulties (Figure 50-9), failed toilet training, and the parent's exaggerated perceptions of acts of "disobedience." Parents may have unrealistic expectations for the child's behavior for the child's age group.

Another factor that increases a child's risk of death is living in a home where spouse or partner abuse occurs. Acts of domestic violence often are transferred to children living in the household. Studies have shown that frequently the following characteristics identify an abusive parent who kills a child[17]:

- Is a young male in his mid-twenties
- Lives near or below poverty level
- Has not finished high school
- Is depressed and unable to cope with stress
- Has experienced violence firsthand

CRITICAL THINKING

How can you calm yourself after caring for a child killed by abuse before writing a patient care report that likely will be called to account?

SEXUAL ASSAULT

Sexual assault is a serious crime. The number of sexual assaults has fallen by more than 60% in recent years. Even so, 248,300 victims age 12 years or older reported a sexual assault in 2007. (It is estimated that every 2 minutes someone in the United States is sexually assaulted.) Approximately 60% of all assaults are not reported to law enforcement personnel.[20] Sexual assault can result in mental or physical injury and death.[21]

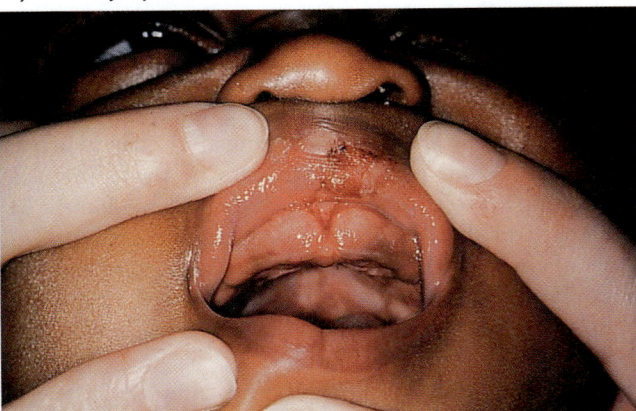

FIGURE 50-9 A torn frenulum that may have been caused by forced bottle-feeding.

DID YOU KNOW?
Who Are The Victims of Sexual Assault?

Women

1 out of every 6 American women has been the victim of an attempted or completed rape in her lifetime (14.8% completed rape; 2.8% attempted rape).

17.7 million American women have been victims of attempted or completed rape.

9 of every 10 rape victims were female in 2003.

Although about 80% of all victims are Caucasian, minorities are somewhat more likely to be attacked.

Lifetime rate of rape/attempted rape for women by race:
- All women: 17.6%
- Caucasian women: 17.7%
- African-American women: 18.8%
- Asian Pacific Islander women: 6.8%
- American Indian/Alaskan women: 34.1%
- Mixed race women: 24.4%

Men

About 3% of American men—or 1 in 33—have experienced an attempted or completed rape in their lifetime.
- In 2003, 1 in every 10 rape victims was male.
- 2.78 million men in the United States have been victims of sexual assault or rape.

Children

15% of sexual assault and rape victims are under age 12.
- 29% are ages 12-17.
- 44% are under age 18.
- Ages 12-34 are the highest risk years.
- Girls ages 16-19 are 4 times more likely than the general population to be victims of rape, attempted rape, or sexual assault.
- 7% of girls in grades 5-8 and 12% of girls in grades 9-12 said they had been sexually abused.
- 3% of boys in grades 5-8 and 5% of boys in grades 9-12 said they had been sexually abused.

In 1995 local child protection service agencies identified 126,000 children who were victims of either substantiated or indicated sexual abuse.
- Of these, 75% were girls.
- Nearly 30% of child victims were between the ages of 4 and 7.

93% of juvenile sexual assault victims know their attacker.
- 34.2% of attackers were family members.
- 58.7% were acquaintances.
- Only 7% of the perpetrators were strangers to the victim.

Effects of Rape
Victims of sexual assault are:
- 3 times more likely to suffer from depression.
- 6 times more likely to suffer from posttraumatic stress disorder.
- 13 times more likely to abuse alcohol.
- 26 times more likely to abuse drugs.
- 4 times more likely to contemplate suicide.

Adapted from Who Are the Victims of Rape, Abuse, and Incest National Network (RAINN), http://www.rainn.org.

Legal Aspects of Sexual Assault

Each state has different interpretations of sexual assault. The term generally refers to any genital, anal, oral, or manual penetration of the victim's body by way of force and without the victim's consent. Lack of consent includes the inability to give consent. This inability may be a result of impaired mental function caused by alcohol and other drugs (Rohypnol, gamma-hydroxybutyrate [GHB], ketamine), sleep, or unconsciousness. If a victim reports a sexual assault, the paramedic should accept the victim's story as accurate. The victim should be encouraged to seek medical care. Ideally the patient should be transported to a hospital with specialized personnel (sexual assault nurse examiner [SANE]) so that evidence of the assault can be collected. In addition, the patient should be accompanied by a local support advocacy group representative, if available.

In many cases, sexual assault is a felony crime that must be proved by evidence. Legal considerations for providing care to a patient who has been sexually assaulted include the following:

1. Take steps to preserve evidence.
2. Discourage the patient from urinating or defecating, douching, or bathing.
3. Do not remove evidence from any part of the body that was subjected to sexual contact unless necessary to provide urgent medical care.
4. Notify law enforcement personnel as soon as possible, if the victim consents.
5. Be aware that there will be a "chain of evidence" with specific requirements of proof.
6. Follow local and state requirements in reporting these cases. Consult with medical direction and follow established protocols.

> **NOTE**
> In most states, it is the prerogative of the patient whether to report a sexual assault (unless a firearm is involved). If the victim does not want police involved and the paramedic summons law enforcement, the patient's HIPAA rights may be violated (see Chapter 6).

Characteristics of Sexual Assault

Anyone can be a victim of sexual assault at any age. The victim often knows the assailant. Sometimes the victim feels shame and personal responsibility for the attack. The methods that the assailant uses to gain control over male and female victims include entrapment, intimidation, and physical force. The assailant commonly uses threats of harm and a weapon to gain submission. Male victims are more likely to suffer significant physical trauma from sexual assault by other men than are female victims (Box 50-8). The following are common injuries that result from sexual assault:

> ### BOX 50-8 Five Myths and Misconceptions About Sexual Assault
>
> *Myth:* All victims of sexual assault are women, and all perpetrators are men.
> *Fact:* Most sexual assaults are perpetrated by men. However, men can be assaulted by other men. Sometimes women perpetrate sexual assaults against men and other women.
> *Myth:* Rape is an impulsive act.
> *Fact:* About 58% to 71% of rapes clearly are planned.
> *Myth:* Rape is motivated by sexual desire.
> *Fact:* Rape is a crime of violence, motivated by anger and the desire for power and control.
> *Myth:* Most women are raped by strangers.
> *Fact:* Most women are victims of "acquaintance rape" by a known, trusted assailant.
> *Myth:* According to the law, a husband cannot be charged with rape against his wife.
> *Fact:* The law stipulates circumstances in which the husband can be charged with rape against his wife.

- Abrasions and bruises on the upper limbs, head, and neck
- Forcible signs of restraint (e.g., rope burns and mouth injuries)
- Petechiae of the face and conjunctiva caused by choking
- Human bites
- Broken teeth, swollen jaw or cheekbone, and eye injuries from being punched or slapped in the face
- Anogenital trauma (bruises, abrasions, lacerations)
- Muscle soreness or stiffness in the shoulder, neck, knee, hip, or back from restraint in postures that allow sexual penetration

> **CRITICAL THINKING**
> How do you feel when you hear others say, "That rape victim brought it on herself"?

Psychosocial Aspects of Care

The trauma of sexual assault creates physical and psychological distress. Victims may behave in various ways. Some may be surprisingly calm and seem in control of their emotions. In contrast, others may be agitated, apprehensive, distraught, or tearful. After managing all threats to life, the paramedic should proceed with care by providing emotional support to the victim. As described in Chapter 31, the paramedic should not question victims of sexual assault in detail about the incident in the prehospital setting. The paramedic should limit the patient history to only what is required to provide care. The initial contact with the victim should include the following:

- Nonjudgmental and supportive attitude
- Empathetic and sensitive comments
- Quiet speech
- Slow movements

- Considerate gestures (ensure privacy and respect modesty)
- Avoid "why" questions, such as "Why were you alone in that part of town?"

The paramedic should move the patient to a safe and quiet environment. This will help to avoid further exposure and embarrassment. When possible, a paramedic of the same gender should provide care. If this is not possible, a chaperone should be present. The patient should not be left unattended. The paramedic should ask for permission to call a friend, family member, or sexual assault crisis advocate. Concerns of the victim about pregnancy and contracting human immunodeficiency virus and other sexually transmitted diseases should be relayed to medical direction. After the patient recovers from physical injury, the goal of treatment is for the patient to regain control of his or her life. Often this takes long-term counseling and support.

Child Victims

Children are particularly vulnerable to sexual assault and usually have frequent contact with the assailant. Often the assault occurs in a trusted person's home. Most sexual assaults involve a male assailant and female victim. About 30% of acquaintance sexual assaults occur when the victim is between 11 and 17 years of age. Many young victims do not think of their experience as a sexual assault because they often are fondled or physically explored without intercourse. As a result, they rarely report the attack and often assume that they are to blame. (Many times, children will conceal sexual assault out of fear of punishment.) Victims involved in a same-sex assault also are unlikely to report the incident because of confusion or embarrassment. For these reasons, most victimized children do not receive proper treatment, including prophylaxis and counseling.

ASSESSMENT AND PATIENT CARE CONSIDERATIONS

Assessment for children of sexual assault should proceed as described before for other victims. The assessment should include age-related considerations that are appropriate for all children. The paramedic should be aware of the following symptoms when caring for any child. These symptoms may indicate behavior or physical manifestations as a result of sexual assault:

- Abrupt behavior changes
- Sleep difficulties, sleep disorders, and nightmares
- Withdrawal from and avoidance of friends and family
- Low self-esteem or desire to be invisible
- Phobias related to the offender
- Hostility
- Self-destructive behaviors
- Mood swings, depression, and anxiety
- Regression (e.g., bed-wetting)
- Truancy
- Eating disorders
- Alcohol or other drug use

The attitude and behavior of adults, including health care providers, greatly influence a child's impression of the assault. The paramedic should try to lessen the emotional influence of the assault by reassuring the child that he or she is not responsible for the attack. The child should also be assured that he or she did nothing wrong. The paramedic should encourage the child to talk openly about the assault and any concerns that he or she may have.

LEGAL CONSIDERATIONS

If sexual assault is suspected or confirmed, the paramedic must follow laws that apply to the crime. Local and state laws affect the confidentiality of children. Paramedics should be aware of the regulations in their community and consult with medical direction.

SUMMARY

- Battering is the establishment of control and fear in a relationship through violence and other forms of abuse.
- Domestic violence follows a cycle of three phases. Phase one involves arguing and verbal abuse. Phase two progresses to physical and sexual abuse. Phase three consists of denial and apologies. Certain personality traits may predispose a person to abusive relationships.
- The paramedic may have a hard time identifying the battered patient. Injuries from domestic violence often involve contusions and lacerations of the face, neck, head, breast, and abdomen.
- The paramedic must ensure scene and personal safety in domestic violence events. The paramedic should manage physical injuries according to standard protocols. The paramedic should direct special attention toward the emotional needs of the victim as well. Assault is a crime. The perpetrator is often released soon after arrest. This is a dangerous time for the victim.
- Elder abuse is classified into four categories: physical abuse, psychological abuse, financial or material abuse, and neglect.
- All 50 states have elder abuse statutes. Reporting of suspected elder abuse also is mandatory under law in most states.
- Most child abusers are the child's parents (77%). Eleven percent are other relatives of the victim. Abused children often exhibit behavior that provides key clues about abuse and neglect. The paramedic should observe carefully the child under 6 years of age who is passive or the child over 6 years of age who is aggressive.

Continued

- If the child volunteers the history of the event without hesitation and matches the history that the parent provides (and the history is suitable for the injury), child abuse is unlikely.
- Injuries may include soft tissue injuries, fractures, head injuries, and abdominal injuries.

- Sexual assault generally refers to any genital, anal, oral, or manual penetration of the victim's body by way of force and without the victim's consent.
- After managing all threats to life, the paramedic should provide emotional support to the victim. The paramedic should deliver care in a way that preserves evidence.

REFERENCES

1. U.S. Department of Justice: *About domestic violence*, www.ovw.usdoj.gov/domviolence.htm, accessed 10-20-10.
2. Bureau of Justice Statistics: *Stalking victimization in the United States, Bureau of Justice Statistics Special Report*, Washington, DC, 2009, U.S. Department of Justice.
3. National Institute of Justice: *Stalking in America*, Washington, DC, 1998, U.S. Department of Justice.
4. Bureau of Justice Statistics: *Crime data brief, intimate partner violence, 1993-2001*, Washington, DC, 2003, U.S. Department of Justice.
5. Bureau of Justice Statistics: *Crime data brief, intimate partner violence in the U.S. 1993-2004*, Washington, DC, 2003, U.S. Department of Justice.
6. Centers for Disease Control and Prevention: *Violence*, www.cdc.gov/women/pubs/violence.htm, accessed 10-20-10.
7. The Julian Center: www.juliancenter.org/more_facts.html, accessed 10-20-10.
8. Centers for Disease Control and Prevention: *Understanding intimate partner violence, fact sheet 2009*, www.cdc.gov/violenceprevention/pdf/IPV_factsheet-a.pdf, accessed 10-20-10.
9. American College of Emergency Physicians: *Guidelines for the role of EMS personnel in domestic violence (policy resource and education paper, October 2006)*, www.acep.org/1,443,0.html, accessed 5-8-10.
10. Alabama Coalition Against Domestic Violence: *Why do abusers batter?* www.acadv.org/abusers.html, accessed 10-20-10.
11. National Center for the Prosecution of Violence Against Women: *Reporting requirements for competent adult victims of domestic violence*, Alexandria, Va, 2006, American Prosecutors Research Institute.
12. Centers for Disease Control and Prevention: *Elder maltreatment: injury prevention and control: violence prevention*, www.cdc.gov/ViolencePrevention/eldermaltreatment/index.html, accessed 10-2-10.
13. National Center on Elder Abuse: *Major types of elder abuse*, www.ncea.aoa.gov/NCEAroot/Main_Site/FAQ/Basics/Types_Of_Abuse.aspx, accessed 10-20-10.
14. National Center on Elder Abuse: *Types of elder abuse in domestic settings*, www.ncea.aoa.gov/ncearoot/Main_Site/pdf/basics/fact1.pdf, accessed 10-10-10.
15. Administration on Aging: *Aging in the 21st century*, www.aoa.gov/AoARoot/Aging_Statistics/future_growth/aging21/health.aspx#Nursing, accessed 10-20-10.
16. Centers for Disease Control and Prevention: *Child maltreatment: facts at a glance*, Spring 2009, www.cdc.gov/violenceprevention/pdf/CM-DataSheet-a.pdf, accessed 10-20-10.
17. Child Welfare Information Gateway: *Child abuse and neglect fatalities: statistics and interventions*, 2008, www.childwelfare.gov/pubs/factsheets/fatality.cfm, accessed 10-20-10.
18. MedlinePlus: *Shaken baby syndrome*, www.nlm.nih.gov/medlineplus/ency/article/000004.htm, accessed 10-10-10.
19. National Center on Shaken Baby Syndrome: *Facts about SBS*, www.dontshake.org/sbs.php?topNavID=3&subNavID=21, accessed 10-10-10.
20. U.S. Department of Justice, Office on Violence Against Women: *Sexual assault*, www.ovw.usdoj.gov/sexassault.htm, accessed 10-10-10.
21. Rape, Abuse & Incest National Network (RAINN): Adapted from: *Who are the victims?* www.rainn.org/get-information/statistics/sexual-assault-victims, accessed 10-10-10.

SUGGESTED READINGS

Centers for Disease Control and Prevention: *Injury prevention & control: violence prevention*, www.cdc.gov/ViolencePrevention/index.html, accessed 5-31-10.

Davis JW: Domestic violence: the "rule of thumb": 2008 Western Trauma Association presidential address, *J Trauma* 65(5):969-973, 2008.

The Missouri Coalition Against Domestic and Sexual Violence: A framework for understanding the nature and dynamics of sexual violence, Jefferson City: Family Violence Prevention and Services Act Grant, 2007.

51 Patients with Special Challenges

OBJECTIVES

Upon completion of this chapter, the paramedic student will be able to:

1. Identify considerations in prehospital management related to physical challenges such as hearing, visual, and speech impairments; obesity; and patients with paraplegia or quadriplegia.
2. Identify considerations in prehospital management of patients who have mental illness, are developmentally disabled, or are emotionally or mentally impaired.
3. Describe special considerations for prehospital management of patients with selected pathological challenges.
4. Outline considerations in management of culturally diverse patients.
5. Describe special considerations in the prehospital management of terminally ill patients.
6. Identify special considerations in management of patients with communicable diseases.
7. Describe special considerations in the prehospital management of patients with financial challenges.

KEY TERMS

amblyopia The loss of one eye's ability to see details; the most common cause of eye vision problems in children; also known as "lazy eye."

astigmatism A vision condition that causes blurred vision attributable either to the irregular shape of the cornea (the clear front cover of the eye) or sometimes to the curvature of the lens inside the eye.

ataxia Failure of muscle coordination; a type of cerebral palsy.

athetosis A neuromuscular condition characterized by slow, continuous, and involuntary movement of the extremities; a type of cerebral palsy.

bariatrics The field of medicine that focuses on the treatment and control of obesity and diseases associated with obesity.

cataract A cloudy or opaque area in the normally clear lens of the eye; most common in people over age 55.

cerebral palsy A general term for nonprogressive disorders of movement and posture.

conductive deafness Refers to the faulty transportation of sound from the outer to the inner ear. This type of deafness often is curable.

cortical vision impairment A temporary or permanent visual impairment caused by the disturbance of the posterior visual pathways and/or the occipital lobes of the brain; the most common cause of permanent visual impairment in children.

cystic fibrosis An inherited metabolic disease of the lungs and digestive system that manifests in childhood; also known as *mucoviscidosis*.

deafness A complete or partial inability to hear.

diversity Differences of any kind: race, class, religion, gender, sexual preference, personal habitat, and physical ability.

Down syndrome A congenital condition characterized by varying degrees of mental retardation and multiple defects; also known as *trisomy 21*.

emotional/mental impairment Impaired intellectual functioning that results in an inability to cope with normal responsibilities of life.

glaucoma An eye disease in which the internal pressure in the eyes increases enough to damage the nerve fibers in the optic nerve, causing vision loss.

hyperopia A vision condition in which distant objects are seen clearly but close ones do not come into proper focus; also known as "farsightedness."

mental illness Any form of psychiatric disorder.

mental retardation A disorder characterized by below-average intellectual function with deficits or impairments in the ability to learn and adapt socially.

multiple sclerosis A progressive disease of the central nervous system in which scattered patches of myelin in the brain and spinal cord are destroyed.

muscular dystrophy An inherited muscle disorder of unknown cause marked by a slow but progressive degeneration of muscle fibers.

myasthenia gravis An autoimmune disorder in which muscles become weak and tire easily.

myopia A vision condition in which near objects are seen clearly, but distant objects do not come into proper focus; also known as "nearsightedness."

obesity A condition in which a person is 30% above ideal body weight.

optic nerve atrophy A permanent visual impairment caused by damage to the optic nerve.

optic nerve hypoplasia A congenital condition in which the optic nerve has not developed properly; it is too small.

paraplegia A weakness or paralysis of both legs and sometimes part of the trunk.

quadriplegia A weakness or paralysis of all four extremities and the trunk.

retinopathy A general term that refers to some form of non-inflammatory damage to the retina of the eye; one of many retinal diseases.

sensorineural deafness A type of deafness in which sounds that reach the inner ear fail to be transmitted to the brain because of damage to the structures within the ear or to the acoustic nerve; often incurable.

spastic paralysis A type of cerebral palsy that produces abnormal stiffness and contraction of groups of muscles.

spina bifida A congenital defect in which part of one or more vertebrae fail to develop completely, leaving a portion of the spinal cord exposed.

strabismus A condition that occurs when one or both eyes turn in, out, up, or down; usually caused by poor eye muscle control; also known as "crossed eye."

terminally ill patients Patients with advanced stage of disease with an unfavorable prognosis and no known cure.

trisomy 21 A genetic failure where there is a triplet of chromosomes 21 rather than the usual pair; the cause of Down syndrome.

---

*P*aramedics often provide care to patients with special challenges. The patient groups to be discussed in this chapter include those who have physical, emotional, or pathological challenges; patients who are culturally diverse, have terminal illness, and communicable diseases; and those with financial challenges that may hinder access to health care.

PHYSICAL CHALLENGES

Patients who are physically challenged may require special considerations in patient assessment and management. The physical challenges presented in this chapter include hearing, visual, and speech impairments; obesity; and patients with paraplegia or quadriplegia.

Hearing Impairments

Deafness is a complete or partial inability to hear. Total deafness is rare and usually congenital. Partial deafness may range from mild to severe. It most commonly results from an ear disease, injury, or degeneration of the hearing mechanism that occurs with age. All deafness is conductive or sensorineural and may be a combination of both (*mixed hearing loss*).

Conductive deafness refers to the faulty transportation of sound from the outer to the inner ear. This type of deafness often is curable. In adults, conductive deafness commonly results from the buildup of earwax that blocks the outer ear canal. Conductive deafness also may result from infection (e.g., otitis media) and from injury to the eardrum or middle ear (e.g., from barotrauma).

Sensorineural deafness often is incurable. In this type of deafness, sounds that reach the inner ear fail to be transmitted to the brain. This is because of damage to the structures within the inner ear or to the acoustic nerve, which connects the inner ear to the brain. Sensorineural deafness that is present in early life may be congenital. It also can

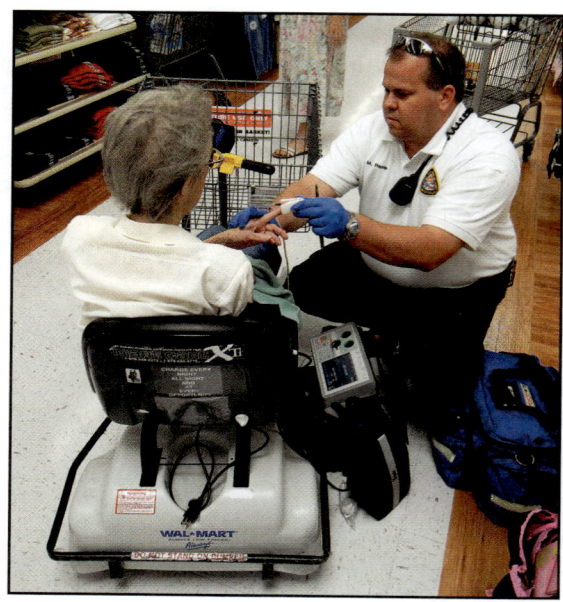

(Courtesy Ray Kemp. St. Charles, Mo.)

result from a birth injury or from damage to the developing fetus (e.g., from premature birth or a mother who has syphilis during pregnancy). Sensorineural deafness that occurs in later life may be caused by prolonged exposure to loud noise, disease (e.g., Meniere's disease), tumors, medications, viral infections, or natural degeneration of the cochlea or labyrinth in old age.

> **NOTE**
>
> *Auditory neuropathy/auditory dyssynchrony* (AN/AD) describes a diagnosis that affects a small group of patients with hearing loss and speech difficulties that are out of proportion with their hearing loss. The exact cause(s) of the disease is (are) unknown. Theories include axonal damage to the auditory nerve, abnormalities within the auditory brainstem, viral disease, seizure disorders, high fever, and others.[1] AN/AD is most common in children, but is also diagnosed in adults. In children, AN/AD may lead to developmental speech and language delays (*auditory processing deficit*) that can affect all levels of learning.

Special Considerations

The paramedic can use several helpful techniques for recognizing a patient who has a hearing impairment. One of these is noting the presence of hearing aids. Another is observing the patient for poor diction or the inability to respond to verbal communication in the absence of direct eye contact. Some accommodations may be needed. One includes retrieving the patient's hearing aid or other amplified listening device. Another is providing paper and pen to aid in communication.

When providing care to these patients, the paramedic should not shout or exaggerate lip movement. Rather, the paramedic should speak softly and directly into the patient's ear canal, using a low-pitched voice. (About 80% of hearing loss is related to the inability to hear high-pitched sounds.) Another method to aid in communication includes asking family members to assist. The paramedic also can use pictures to illustrate basic needs and routine medical procedures. Other communication assistance devices include American Sign Language, pictographs (laminated cards that show drawings of common activities), speech amplifiers, and wireless text communications.

Finally, the paramedic must notify the hospital as soon as possible if the patient has severe deafness. Some patients with severe hearing impairments will speak with unusual syntax. Some may use American Sign Language. Personnel with special training (e.g., an interpreter) may need to be summoned to assist with patient care.

Visual Impairments

Estimates indicate that more than 1 million Americans are blind and that 3 million are visually impaired, even with the best correction.[2] Normal vision depends on the uninterrupted passage of light from the front of the eye to the light-sensitive retina at the back. Any condition that obstructs the passage of light from the retina can cause vision loss. Vision impairment may be present at birth from a congenital disorder. It also may result from a number of other causes. These causes include the following:

- Cataracts
- Degeneration of the eyeball, optic nerve, or nerve pathways
- Diseases such as diabetes and hypertension
- Eye or brain injury (e.g., trauma, chemical burns, and stroke)
- Infections such as those that are caused by cytomegalovirus, herpes simplex virus, and bacterial ulcers
- Vitamin A deficiency in children living in developing countries

Patients with visual impairments may be totally blind or have a partial loss of vision that affects central vision, peripheral vision, or both (Box 51-1). A patient who has central loss of vision is usually aware of the condition. Those who have a loss of peripheral vision may be more

---

BOX 51-1 Types of Visual Impairments[3]

Amblyopia ("lazy eye"): The loss of one eye's ability to see details; the most common cause of eye vision problems in children.

Astigmatism: A vision condition that causes blurred vision attributable either to the irregular shape of the cornea (the clear front cover of the eye) or sometimes to the curvature of the lens inside the eye.

Cataract: A cloudy or opaque area in the normally clear lens of the eye; most common in people over age 55.

Cortical vision impairment: A temporary or permanent visual impairment caused by the disturbance of the posterior visual pathways and/or the occipital lobes of the brain; the most common cause of permanent visual impairment in children.

Glaucoma: An eye disease in which the internal pressure in the eyes increases enough to damage the nerve fibers in the optic nerve, causing vision loss.

Hyperopia (farsightedness): A vision condition in which distant objects are seen clearly but close ones do not come into proper focus.

Myopia (nearsightedness): A vision condition in which near objects are seen clearly but distant objects do not come into proper focus.

Optic nerve atrophy: A permanent visual impairment caused by damage to the optic nerve.

Optic nerve hypoplasia: A congenital condition in which the optic nerve has not developed properly; it is too small.

Retinopathy: A general term that refers to some form of non-inflammatory damage to the retina of the eye; one of many retinal diseases.

Strabismus (crossed eye): A condition that occurs when one or both eyes turn in, out, up, or down; usually caused by poor eye muscle control.

---

difficult to identify. This is because the loss often remains unnoticed by the person until it is well advanced.

SPECIAL CONSIDERATIONS

Techniques in assessing and managing patients with vision loss are described in Chapter 17. To review, accommodations that may be necessary for these patients include retrieving visual aids, describing all procedures before performing them, and providing sensory information (e.g., location of obstacles) as needed. The paramedic should guide ambulatory patients by "leading," not by "pushing." If possible and appropriate, a patient's guide dog should be permitted to accompany the patient to the hospital. The paramedic should advise medical direction of the patient's special needs. That way, the appropriate personnel can be made available.

LOOK AGAIN
See Chapter 17: Therapeutic Communications, pp. 486-488.

Speech Impairments

Speech impairments include disorders of language, articulation, voice production, or fluency (blockage of speech). All of these can lead to an inability to communicate well (Box 51-2).

Language disorders result from damage to the language centers of the brain. (They usually result from stroke, head injury, or brain tumor.) These patients often exhibit **aphasia** (loss of power of speech) with a slowness to understand speech and problems with vocabulary and sentence structure. Aphasia can affect children and adults. It may affect their ability to speak and to comprehend written or spoken words. Delayed development of language in a child may result from hearing loss, lack of stimulation, or emotional disturbance. It also may result from *pragmatic language impairment,* a developmental disorder related to autism and Asperger's syndrome (described in Chapter 35).

An articulation disorder is an inability to produce speech sounds. The disorder sometimes is referred to as *dysarthria* or *motor speech disorder.* These disorders result from damage to nerve pathways passing from the brain to the muscles of the larynx, mouth, or lips. Often the patient's speech will be slurred, indistinct, slow, or nasal. Disorders of articulation may result from brain injury. They also may result from diseases such as multiple sclerosis and Parkinson's disease. In children, articulation disorders commonly result from delayed development from hearing problems. *Phonological process disorder* is a type of articulation disorder in which there are difficulties with "rules of language," such as combinations of words and syllables. Examples include "top" for "stop," "daw" for "dog," and "tee" for "three."

CRITICAL THINKING

What may cause a paramedic to become impatient when caring for a patient with this type of disorder?

Voice production disorders are characterized by hoarseness, harshness, inappropriate pitch, and abnormal nasal resonance. They often result from disorders that affect closure of the vocal cords. Some disorders are caused by hormonal or psychiatric disturbances and by severe hearing loss.

Fluency disorders are not well understood. They are marked by repetitions of single sounds or whole words and by the blocking of speech. An example of a fluency disorder is stuttering.

SPECIAL CONSIDERATIONS

Once speech impairment has been identified, history taking and assessment need to be modified. Methods include allowing extra time for the patient to respond to questions, clarifying what the patient says or asking the patient to repeat an answer if it was not clearly understood, and offering appropriate aids (e.g., pen and paper) to assist in communications. If the patient lip-reads, the paramedic should face the patient at eye level and speak slowly and clearly. (Gum chewing should be avoided.) The hospital also should be advised if a patient has a severe speech impairment, so that appropriate personnel (e.g., audiologist or speech specialist) can be made available.

Obesity

Obesity is defined as being 30% above ideal body weight. The disease affects nearly one third of the adult American population and is responsible for at least 300,000 deaths in the United States each year.[4] In addition, obesity in U.S. children and teens ranges from about 10% in infants and toddlers, to about 18% in adolescents and teenagers.[5] As discussed in Chapter 2, the body mass index (BMI) is used to define ideal body weight, overweight, and obesity ranges. An adult who has a BMI between 25 and 29.9 is considered overweight; a BMI of 30 or higher is considered obese.[6]

Obesity is an abnormal increase in the proportion of fat and cells. The increase is mainly in the viscera and the subcutaneous tissues of the body. Although reasons for obesity in some persons are unclear, known causes for the condition include the following:

- Caloric intake that exceeds calories expended
- Low basal metabolic rate
- Genetic disposition for obesity

The complications of obesity are many (Box 51-3). Obesity increases a person's chance of becoming seriously ill. For example, obesity is associated with an increased risk for hypertension, stroke, heart disease, diabetes, and some cancers. Osteoarthritis also is aggravated by increased body weight. The condition is treated with weight loss programs, exercise, counseling, medications, and sometimes surgery.

BOX 51-2 Types of Speech Impairments

Language Disorders
Brain tumor
Delayed development
Emotional disturbance
Head injury
Hearing loss
Lack of stimulation
Stroke

Articulation Disorders
Damage to nerve pathways passing from the brain to muscles in the larynx, mouth, or lips
Delayed development from hearing problems
Slow maturation of nervous system

Voice Production Disorders
Disorders affecting closure of vocal cords
Hormonal or psychiatric disturbance
Severe hearing loss

Fluency Disorders
Stuttering (for example)
Patient is not fully understood

BOX 51-3 Medical Complications of Obesity[7]

- Blood lipid (fat) abnormalities
- Cancer, including cancer of the uterus, cervix, ovaries, breast, colon, rectum, and prostate
- Depression
- Gallbladder disease
- Gynecological problems, such as infertility and irregular periods
- Heart disease
- High blood pressure
- Metabolic syndrome
- Nonalcoholic fatty liver disease
- Osteoarthritis
- Skin problems, such as intertrigo and impaired wound healing
- Sleep apnea
- Stroke
- Type 2 diabetes

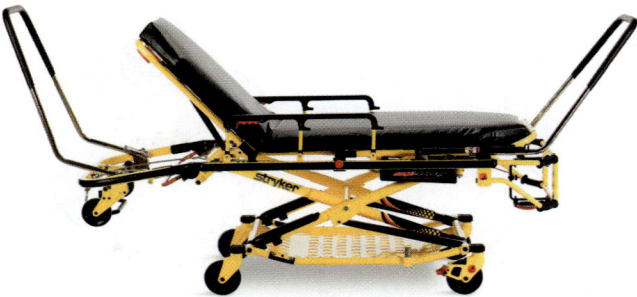

FIGURE 51-1 Device to move bariatric patient.

> **NOTE**
> One should note that weight limits vary widely for helicopters. When requesting an emergency rotary aircraft flight, the paramedic should inform the dispatcher if the patient is obese. This will help to determine whether the patient can be transported safely by air.

The goal of treatment is lasting weight loss. The field of medicine that focuses on the treatment and control of obesity and diseases associated with it is known as **bariatrics.**

> **CRITICAL THINKING**
> Consider this situation. A crew member makes an insensitive remark about a patient's obesity within hearing range of the patient or the patient's family. How will you respond?

SPECIAL CONSIDERATIONS

The paramedic needs to give special considerations to caring for an obese patient. These include the need to obtain a thorough history. The history often will be extensive because of associated health problems. The paramedic should be aware that symptoms the patient may credit to obesity (e.g., fatigue, shortness of breath at rest or on exertion) may be a sign of an acute illness. (For example, the illness may be congestive heart failure or myocardial infarction.)

The examination of an obese person also may require some modifications. These may include using large blood pressure cuffs, positioning the patient to better allow for hearing lung sounds, and placing electrocardiogram leads on areas of the body with less fat (e.g., the arms and thighs versus the chest wall). In addition, more personnel and special equipment may be needed to assist with moving the patient for transport (Figure 51-1). (For example, stretchers that can accommodate excessive weight and wide girth, ambulances equipped with a winch system, and ramps to load and offload the patient safely.) Obese patients often are self-conscious about their weight. They may worry about the hardships they place on the EMS crew and other

rescuers. Paramedics must maintain professionalism during these patient care encounters.

Patients With Paraplegia/Quadriplegia

Paraplegia is weakness or paralysis of both legs and sometimes part of the trunk; **quadriplegia** is weakness or paralysis of all four extremities and the trunk. The conditions result from nerve damage in the brain and spinal cord. These conditions usually are caused by a crash, sports injury, fall, or gunshot wound. (Medical illnesses such as lupus, multiple sclerosis, and stroke also can result in weakness and paralysis.) Paraplegia and quadriplegia are accompanied by a loss of sensation and loss of urinary control. Priapism may be present in some male patients.

> **NOTE**
> When performing the physical assessment, the application of pressure that would be appreciated by patients with normal sensation may not be recognized in patients who have weakness or paralysis.

SPECIAL CONSIDERATIONS

Patients with extremity and trunk paralysis may require accommodations in patient care. For example, the patient may have a halo traction device to stabilize the spine (Figure 51-2). Or the patient may rely on a home ventilator to assist with breathing. Both of these situations can complicate airway management. They also can make patient transport more difficult. Some patients who are paralyzed will have special equipment (e.g., walkers or wheelchairs); ostomies for the trachea, bladder, or colon; and medical devices that rely on electricity or a battery supply.

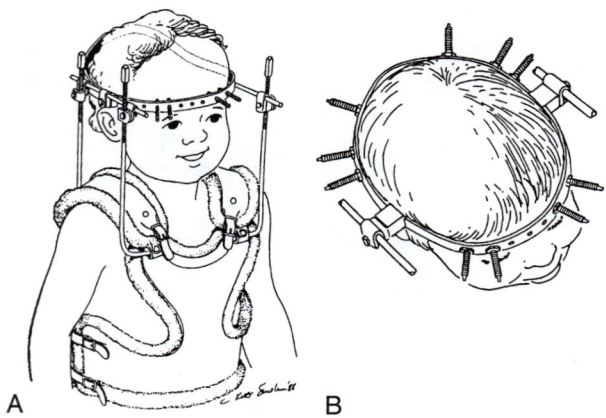

FIGURE 51-2 A, Custom halo vest and light superstructure. **B,** Ten pin placement sites for infant halo ring attachment using multiple-pin, low-torque technique. Usually, four pins are placed anteriorly, avoiding the temporal area, and the remaining six pins are placed in the occipital area.

(Technology-assisted devices will be presented in Chapter 52.) Additional personnel may be required to assist with moving special equipment and to prepare the patient for ambulance transport.

MENTAL CHALLENGES

Persons who have developmental, emotional, behavioral, or psychological and psychiatric problems are considered mentally challenged. The specific patient groups presented in this section include those with mental illness, developmental disabilities, emotional impairments, and emotional/mental impairments.

Mental Illness

Mental illness refers to any form of psychiatric disorder. As described in Chapter 35, most forms of mental illness result from biological, psychosocial, or sociocultural causes. A person's mental illness may result from more than one of these factors. To review, examples of biological causes of mental illness are schizophrenia and depression that result from biochemical imbalance; and organic causes such as trauma, illness, and dementia. Psychosocial causes of mental illness can result from childhood trauma, child abuse or neglect, a dysfunctional family structure, or other issues that cause an inability to resolve situational conflicts in a person's life. Sociocultural causes of mental illness may be related to personal relationships, family stability, economic status, and other factors that result in situational stress.

SPECIAL CONSIDERATIONS

Recognizing a patient with mental illness may be difficult, especially if the patient has only mild symptoms of the disease. Other patients with more serious disorders may have signs and symptoms that are consistent with mental illness. (An example is paranoid behavior in patients with schizophrenia.) When obtaining the patient history, the paramedic should not hesitate to ask about the following:

- History of mental illness
- Prescribed medications
- Compliance with prescribed medications
- Use of over-the-counter herbal products (e.g., St. John's wort)
- Concomitant use of alcohol or other drugs

If the patient is anxious, the paramedic should ask the patient's permission before performing any assessment or any procedure. This will help to establish rapport and trust during the care. Unless the call is related specifically to the mental illness, care should proceed in the same manner as for any other patient. Patients with mental illness experience medical illness and injury like all other patient groups. If the patient acts aggressively or combatively, the paramedic should retreat from the scene and request law enforcement personnel to secure the scene.

Developmentally Disabled

A person who is developmentally disabled has impaired or insufficient development of the brain. This causes an inability to learn at the usual rate (*developmental delay*). Developmental delay has many causes, including the following:

- Lack of stimulation (as seen with child abuse or neglect)
- Severe vision or hearing impairment
- Mental retardation
- Brain damage before, during, or after birth
- Severe diseases of body organs and systems

Persons who are developmentally disabled often function well with daily activities, hold jobs, and live independently (or with their family or in residential group homes). However, some development delays may be severe and may affect any or all of the major areas of human achievement: walking upright; fine eye-hand coordination; listening, language, and speech; and social interaction.

The accommodations that may be needed when caring for these patients will vary depending on the severity of disability. The paramedic should allow extra time for obtaining a history and performing an examination. Additional time should also be allotted for preparing the patient for transport. When possible, a member of the patient's family or a caregiver should remain with the patient during the care.

 CRITICAL THINKING
Do you think a patient with developmental delays should have any input into their care? Why?

Down Syndrome

Down syndrome results from an abnormal chromosome. This abnormality causes mild to severe mental retardation and a characteristic physical appearance (Figure 51-3). The child with Down syndrome has features that typically include the following:

- Eyes that slope upward at the outer corners
- Folds of skin on either side of the nose that cover the inner corners of the eyes
- A small face and small facial features
- A large and protruding tongue

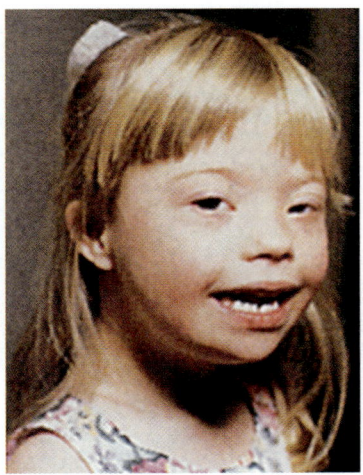

FIGURE 51-3 Child with Down syndrome.

- Flattening on the back of the head
- Hands that are short and broad

In most cases, Down syndrome occurs from the failure of the two chromosomes numbered 21 in a parent cell to go into separate daughter cells during the first stage of sperm or egg cell formation. This results in a triplet of chromosomes 21 (trisomy 21) rather than the usual pair. The extra number 21 chromosome is passed on to the child and leads to Down syndrome. The incidence of affected fetuses increases with increased maternal age (mothers over age 35). It also increases in those with a family history of Down syndrome.

> **NOTE**
> In the general population, trisomy 21 occurs in only 1 of about 600 live births. After age 35, a mother's chances of having a Down syndrome child increase dramatically to as high as 1 in 100 by age 40.[8] Because of this increased risk, pregnant mothers over age 35 usually are tested to assess for the abnormality.

Patients with Down syndrome usually do not survive past middle age. Many are cared for at home, and others live in long-term nursing care facilities. About 25% of children born with Down syndrome have a heart defect at birth. Many have congenital intestinal disorders, hearing defects, and other illnesses. The degree of mental disability varies with an intelligence quotient (IQ) that ranges from 30 to 80. (An IQ of 80 to 120 is considered average.) Persons with Down syndrome are capable of limited learning and often are affectionate and friendly. Extra time must be allowed for obtaining a history and for performing assessment and patient care procedures.

Emotionally Impaired

Persons with emotional problems often suffer from anxiety disorders. These disorders were described in Chapter 35. They can result in a wide range of physical or mental symptoms attributed to mental stress.

LOOK AGAIN
See Chapter 35: Behavioral and Psychiatric Disorders, pp. 1036-1038.

SPECIAL CONSIDERATIONS

Distinguishing between symptoms produced by stress and those that indicate serious medical illness may be difficult. Thus management should always focus on the presenting complaint. The paramedic also should assume the most serious cause. As described in Chapter 35, signs and symptoms that may result from emotional impairment include somatic complaints such as chest discomfort, tachycardia, dyspnea, choking, and syncope. Hence the paramedic must gather a full history from the patient. A thorough examination also is essential to rule out serious illness. The prehospital care for these patients (in the absence of serious illness) mainly is supportive. It includes calming measures and transport for physician evaluation.

Emotionally/Mentally Impaired

Emotional/mental impairment (EMI) refers to persons who have impaired intellectual functioning (**mental retardation**). This impairment results in an inability to cope with the normal responsibilities of life. Mental retardation can be classified further with IQ assessment as mild (IQ 55 to 70), moderate (IQ 40 to 54), severe (IQ 25 to 39), and profound (IQ less than 25).[9] The more severe grades of emotional/mental impairment usually have a specific physical cause (e.g., brain damage or Down syndrome). In contrast, mild emotional/mental impairment often has no specific cause. However, poverty, malnutrition, and heredity may play a role (Box 51-4). Mild mental retardation is the most common form of emotional/mental impairment. It accounts for about 85% of the retarded population.

SPECIAL CONSIDERATIONS

Changes to normal patient care vary based on the patient's level of retardation. Many with mild retardation show no symptoms other than slowness in carrying out mental tasks. Others with moderate to severe retardation may have limited to absent speech. Neurological problems are common. These patients may require extra time and care in patient assessment, management, and transportation.

PATHOLOGICAL CHALLENGES

Certain pathological conditions may require special assessment and management skills. Specific pathological conditions presented in this section include arthritis, cancer, cerebral palsy, cystic fibrosis, multiple sclerosis, muscular dystrophy, poliomyelitis, previous head injury, spina bifida, and myasthenia gravis. These conditions have been presented elsewhere in this text by subject matter. The following discussion will provide a brief review.

BOX 51-4 Causes of Mental Retardation

Genetic Conditions

Phenylketonuria (a single-gene disorder causing an enzyme deficiency)

Chromosomal disorder (e.g., Down syndrome)

Fragile X syndrome (a single-gene disorder on the Y chromosome; the leading inherited cause of mental retardation)

Problems During Pregnancy

Use of alcohol or other drugs by the mother

Use of tobacco

Illness and infection (toxoplasmosis, cytomegalovirus, rubella, syphilis, human immunodeficiency virus)

Problems at Birth

Brain injury

Prematurity

Low birth weight

Problems After Birth

Childhood diseases (whooping cough, chickenpox, measles, Hib disease)

Injury (e.g., head injury or near drowning)

Exposure to lead, mercury, and other environmental toxins

Poverty and Cultural

Deprivation

Malnutrition

Disease-producing conditions

Inadequate medical care

Environmental health hazards

Lack of stimulation

From Arc National Headquarters: *Introduction to mental retardation,* Arlington, Tex, 2004, The Association.

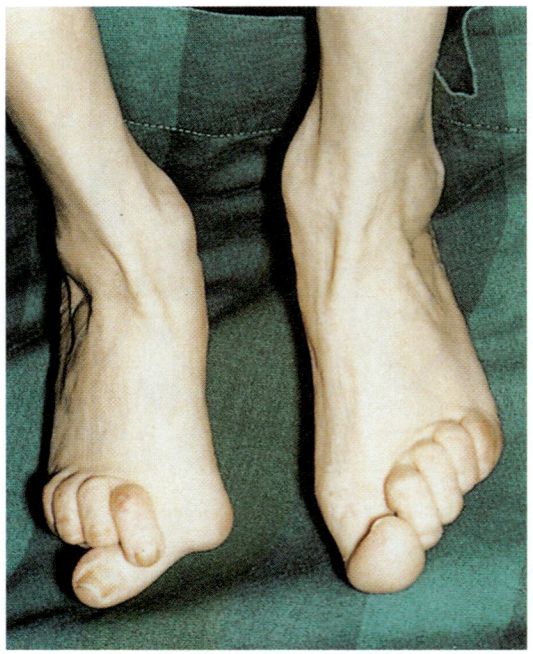

FIGURE 51-4 Rheumatoid arthritis of the feet.

Arthritis

As described in Chapter 26 and Chapter 49, arthritis is the inflammation of a joint, characterized by pain, stiffness, swelling, and redness. The disease has many forms and varies widely in its effects. Two forms of arthritis are common. One is osteoarthritis that results from cartilage loss and wear and tear of the joints (common in elderly patients). The other is rheumatoid arthritis (an autoimmune disorder that damages joints and surrounding tissues) (Figure 51-4).

SPECIAL CONSIDERATIONS

Patients with arthritis often have decreased range of motion and mobility. This may limit the physical exam. (It is important to ensure patient comfort whenever possible.) The paramedic also should determine current medication use (e.g., analgesics) before administering drugs to these patients. Transport strategies must take into account the patient's limited mobility. The paramedic also must adjust the equipment (e.g., backboards and splints) to fit the patient (not vice versa). This can be achieved by supplying adequate padding to fill all voids.

Cancer

Cancer is a group of diseases that allow for an unrestrained growth of cells in one or more of the body organs or tissues (see Chapter 32). The malignant tumors most often develop in major organs. These include the lungs, breasts, intestine, skin, stomach, and pancreas. However, they also may occur in cell-forming tissues of the bone marrow and in the lymphatic system, muscle, or bone.

SPECIAL CONSIDERATIONS

Patients with cancer often are very ill. The signs and symptoms of their disease depend on the site of origin of the cancer (Box 51-5). Often no signs of the disease are visible. However, medical treatment (e.g., chemotherapy or radiation) for many of the cancers can produce obvious signs and symptoms and various illnesses that may initiate an EMS response. (Patients with cancer are also at increased risk for pulmonary embolism.) Signs and symptoms associated with chemotherapy and radiation include the following:

- Anorexia
- Depression
- Fatigue
- Gastrointestinal upset
- General malaise
- Loss of appetite
- Loss of hair (alopecia)
- Pain

BOX 51-5 Common Examples of Site of Origin Classifications for Cancer

Adenocarcinoma: Originates in glandular tissue

Blastoma: Originates in embryonic tissue of organs

Carcinoma: Originates in epithelial tissue (i.e., tissue that lines organs and tubes)

Leukemia: Originates in tissues that form blood cells

Lymphoma: Originates in lymphatic tissue

Myeloma: Originates in bone marrow

Sarcoma: Originates in connective or supportive tissue (e.g., bone, cartilage, muscle)

BOX 51-6 Causes of Cerebral Palsy

Disorders During Pregnancy That May Cause Cerebral Palsy[11]

1. Multiple births (e.g., twins, triplets)
2. A damaged placenta that may interfere with fetal growth
3. Sexually transmitted infectious diseases (e.g., AIDS, herpes, syphilis, gonorrhea)
4. Poor nutrition
5. Exposure to toxic substances, including nicotine, alcohol, and drugs
6. Rh or ABO blood type incompatibility between mother and infant
7. Chromosome abnormalities
8. Biochemical genetic disorders
9. Chance malformations of the baby's brain
10. A labor that is too long or too abrupt; poor oxygen supply may destroy brain tissue
11. German measles during pregnancy
12. Small pelvic structure
13. Premature delivery
14. Cesarean or breech delivery
15. Effects of anesthetics, analgesics

Disorders During Early Childhood That May Cause Cerebral Palsy as a Result of Brain Injury

1. Infections such as meningitis
2. Brain hemorrhages
3. Head injury following falls, car accidents, or abuse
4. Drowning accidents
5. Poisoning

Requests for emergency services for patients with advanced cancer often are related to the patient's pain medication. An example is patients whose pain is no longer relieved by the medicine. Another example is patients who have taken an accidental overdose of pain medicine. This may result in an altered level of consciousness or respiratory depression. If the patient's pain is not being managed, the paramedic should consult with medical direction. (Larger than normal doses may need to be given to provide pain relief.) If an overdose is suspected, the paramedic should initiate the standard care for narcotic overdose.

A full patient history should be obtained, including a list of all medications. Many cancer patients take anticancer drugs and pain medications through transdermal skin patches that contain analgesic agents and through surgically implanted devices (e.g., MediPorts). If intravenous therapy is necessary, additional time should be allotted to access the patient's peripheral veins or medication port. (Strict aseptic technique is especially important in these patients. They often are immunocompromised as a result of the treatment for their disease.) As described in Chapter 14, paramedics should consult with medical direction and follow protocols before using a surgically implanted port for fluid or drug therapy. Special techniques are required to access these devices.

The course of the disease and the medical regimen of care for cancer patients can be devastating for the patient, family, and loved ones. The paramedic must provide emotional support for all involved. Also essential is to ensure the patient's comfort. Finally, patients should be transported to the hospital where they are being treated for their cancer, when possible.

Cerebral Palsy

Cerebral palsy (CP) is a general term for nonprogressive disorders of movement and posture. The disease results from damage to the fetal brain during later months of pregnancy, during birth, during the newborn period, or in early childhood (Box 51-6). The most common cause of cerebral palsy is cerebral dysgenesis (abnormal cerebral development) or cerebral malformations.[10] Other less common causes include fetal hypoxia, birth trauma, maternal infection, kernicterus (excessive fetal bilirubin, associated with hemolytic disease), and postpartum encephalitis, meningitis, or head injury. Cerebral palsy often is diagnosed during the child's first year of life when parents notice unusual muscle tone during holding. Sometimes they notice feeding difficulties. No cure exists for the disease. But those persons with moderate disability may live with relative independence and have a near-normal life expectancy.

TYPES OF CEREBRAL PALSY

Three distinct types of cerebral palsy exist. They are spastic paralysis, athetosis, and ataxia. **Spastic paralysis** produces abnormal stiffness and contraction of groups of muscles. With this type of cerebral palsy, the child may be categorized as *diplegic, hemiplegic,* or *quadriplegic.* With diplegic, all four limbs are affected. The legs are affected more severely than the arms. With hemiplegic, the limbs on only one side of the body are affected. The arm is usually more severe than the leg. With quadriplegic, all four limbs are severely affected, not necessarily symmetrically.

Athetosis produces involuntary writhing movements and a loss of coordination and balance. Hearing defects, epilepsy, and other central nervous system disorders are often present with the disease. Although some with athetosis and diplegia are highly intelligent, 30% to 50% of all persons with cerebral palsy have mental retardation.[12] Most persons with quadriplegia are severely retarded.

Ataxia is the least common form of cerebral palsy. People with ataxic CP have a disturbed sense of balance and depth perception. They usually have poor muscle tone (hypotonic), a staggering walk, and unsteady hands. Ataxia results from damage to the cerebellum, the brain's major center for balance and coordination.

> ### CRITICAL THINKING
> How can you determine the patient's normal level of functioning?

SPECIAL CONSIDERATIONS

Weakness, paralysis, and developmental delay vary by the type and severity of disease. For example, some children with mild cerebral palsy attend regular schools. Others with more severe forms of the disease never learn to walk or communicate well. They may require lifelong skilled nursing care. Accommodations that may be needed while providing care include allowing extra scene time for the physical examination and extra resources and personnel to aid transport.

Cystic Fibrosis

Cystic fibrosis (CF) (*mucoviscidosis*) is an inherited metabolic disease of the lungs and digestive system that manifests in childhood. The disease is caused by a defective, recessive gene that is inherited from each parent. The defective gene causes the glands in the lining of the bronchi to produce excessive amounts of thick mucus. This predisposes the person to chronic lung infections. In addition, the pancreas of a patient with cystic fibrosis fails to produce the enzymes required for the breakdown of fats and their absorption from the intestine. These alterations in metabolism cause classic symptoms of cystic fibrosis that include pale, greasy-looking, foul-smelling stools (often noticeable soon after birth); persistent cough and breathlessness; and lung infections that often develop into pneumonia, bronchiectasis, and bronchitis. Other features of the disease include stunted growth and sweat glands that produce abnormally salty sweat. In some cases the child with cystic fibrosis may fail to thrive; many patients survive into adulthood, although poor health is common.

> ### NOTE
> If only one defective gene is inherited, that person will be a carrier of the disease. However, the person will have no symptoms. Often, these persons are unaware that they carry the defective gene. Genetic counseling and testing are appropriate for persons who have a family history of cystic fibrosis.

SPECIAL CONSIDERATIONS

Older patients (and parents of children) with cystic fibrosis generally are aware of their disease. Some may be oxygen dependent. They may need respiratory support and suctioning to clear the airway of mucus and secretions. Many will use inhalants. The paramedic should expect a lengthy history and physical exam because of the nature of the disease and associated medical problems. Some patients will have received heart and lung transplants. They may require transfer to specialized medical facilities for treatment. If parents are unaware of the possibility of cystic fibrosis in the presence of signs and symptoms described previously, the paramedic should advise the physician at the hospital of his or her suspicions.

Multiple Sclerosis

Multiple sclerosis is a progressive and incurable autoimmune disease of the central nervous system that destroys patches of myelin in the brain and spinal cord. Scarring and destruction of the tissues cause symptoms that range from numbness and tingling to paralysis and incontinence. The cause of multiple sclerosis is unknown; however, it may have a heritable or viral component. (Many persons with multiple sclerosis lead active, normal lives between exacerbations of their illness.) The disease usually begins early in adult life, becomes active for a brief time, and then resumes years later. As described in Chapter 25, the symptoms of multiple sclerosis vary with the affected areas of the central nervous system. The symptoms may include the following:

Brain Involvement
- Ataxia
- Blurred or double vision
- Clumsiness
- Fatigue
- Muscle weakness
- Numbness, weakness, or pain in the face
- Slurred speech
- Vertigo

Spinal Cord Involvement
- Extremities that feel heavy and become weak
- Spasticity
- Tingling, numbness, or feeling of constriction in any part of the body

The symptoms of multiple sclerosis may occur singly or in combination. They may last from several weeks to several months. Attacks vary in intensity and may be precipitated by injury, infection, or physical or emotional stress. Some patients become disabled, bedridden, and incontinent early in middle life. Disabled patients also often suffer from painful muscle spasms, constipation, urinary tract infections, skin ulcerations, and mood swings. The disease is managed with medications, physical therapy, and counseling.

SPECIAL CONSIDERATIONS

Some patients with multiple sclerosis may be difficult to examine. They may be unable to provide a complete medical history because of the nature of their illness. The paramedic should allow extra time for patient assessment and to prepare the patient for transport. (The patient should not be expected to ambulate.) In severe cases, respiratory support may be indicated.

Muscular Dystrophy

Muscular dystrophy (described in Chapter 25) is an inherited muscle disorder that results in a slow but progressive degeneration of muscle fibers. The disease is classified according to the age that symptoms first appear, the rate at which the disease progresses, and the way in which the disease is inherited. Muscular dystrophy is incurable. Genetic counseling and testing is appropriate for persons with a family history of muscular dystrophy.

The most common form of the disease is *Duchenne's muscular dystrophy,* caused by a sex-linked recessive gene that affects only males. Duchenne's muscular dystrophy rarely is diagnosed before age 3. Signs and symptoms of the disease include a child who is slow in learning to sit up and walk; an unusual gait; curvature of the spine; and muscles that become bulky as they are replaced by fat. Eventually, most children will be unable to walk. Many do not live past their teenage years as a result of chronic lung infections and congestive heart failure. With other less common forms of muscular dystrophy, patients may live well into their middle years with varying degrees of muscle weakness.

SPECIAL CONSIDERATIONS

Accommodations that may be required during emergency care depend on the person's age, weight, and severity of disease. For example, young children may be fairly easy to examine and prepare for transport. When caring for older patients, extra personnel may be needed to move the patient to the ambulance. In severe cases the patient may need respiratory support.

Poliomyelitis

Poliomyelitis (polio) is an infectious disease caused by *Poliovirus hominis.* The virus is spread through direct and indirect contact with infected feces and by airborne transmission. Poliovirus attacks with variable severity. The severity can range from asymptomatic infection to a febrile illness without neurological complications to aseptic meningitis and finally to paralytic disease (including respiratory paralysis) and possible death.

As described in Chapter 25, the incidence of polio cases has declined since the Salk and Sabin vaccines were made available in the 1950s. The disease, however, may affect nonimmune adults and indigent children. Signs and symptoms of polio in the nonparalytic and paralytic forms include fever, malaise, headache, and intestinal upset. In the majority of cases, persons with the nonparalytic form of polio recover fully. In the paralytic form, extensive paralysis of muscles of the legs and lower trunk can occur.

SPECIAL CONSIDERATIONS

Caring for a patient with paralytic polio who has respiratory paralysis may necessitate advanced airway support to ensure adequate ventilation. (Patients on home ventilators typically have a tracheostomy.) If the lower body is paralyzed, catheterization of the bladder may be needed (see Appendix, Advanced Practice Procedures in Critical Care). Extra resources and personnel may be needed to prepare the patient for transport.

Previously Head-Injured Patients

Traumatic brain injury can result from many types of trauma (see Chapter 40). These injuries can affect many cognitive, physical, and psychological skills. Physical deficit can include ambulation, balance and coordination, fine motor skills, strength, and endurance. Cognitive deficits of language and communication, information processing, memory, and perceptual skills are common. Psychological status also often is altered (Table 51-1).

TABLE 51-1 Brain Injury Deficits	
Injury	**Injury Deficits**
Cerebral Cortex	
Frontal lobe	Paralysis of various body parts
	Inability to plan a sequence of complex movements
	Inability to focus on tasks
	Mood changes
	Personality changes
	Inability to express language
Parietal lobe	Inability to name an object
	Problems with reading and writing
	Difficulty in distinguishing right from left
	Difficulty with math skills
	Difficulty with eye and hand coordination
Occipital lobe	Defects in vision
	Production of hallucinations
	Visual illusions
	Inability to recognize words
	Difficulties in reading and writing
Temporal lobe	Difficulty in recognizing faces
	Difficulty in understanding spoken words
	Short-term memory loss
	Interference with long-term memory
	Persistent talking
	Aggressive behavior
Brainstem	Decreased vital capacity in breathing
	Difficulty in swallowing food and water
	Difficulty with organization
	Problems with balance and movement
	Dizziness and nausea
	Sleeping difficulties
Cerebellum	Loss of ability to coordinate fine movements
	Loss of ability to walk
	Tremors
	Dizziness
	Slurred speech

SPECIAL CONSIDERATIONS

Depending on the patient's area of brain injury, obtaining a history and performing assessment and care may be difficult. Some patients may need restraint. Family and other caregivers should be involved in managing the patient (when appropriate). The paramedic also should interview them to determine whether the patient's actions and responses are "normal" or "baseline" for the patient. Additional time should be allotted at the scene to provide care to these patients.

 CRITICAL THINKING
Why is this group of patients at high risk for injury?

Spina Bifida

Spina bifida (see Chapter 25) is a congenital defect. With this condition, part of one or more vertebrae fails to develop. This leaves a portion of the spinal cord exposed. The condition ranges in severity from that of minimal evidence of a defect to a child who is severely disabled. In severe cases the legs of some children may be deformed with partial or full paralysis and loss of sensation in all areas below the level of the defect. Associated abnormalities may include hydrocephalus with or without brain damage (Figure 51-5), cerebral palsy, epilepsy, and mental retardation.

SPECIAL CONSIDERATIONS

Because of the varying degrees of spina bifida, care must be tailored to the patient's specific needs. Some patients require no special accommodations. Others need extra on-scene time for assessment and management. Additional resources and personnel to prepare the patient for transport may be needed as well.

 NOTE
Between 18% and 73% of children and adolescents with spina bifida are estimated to be sensitive to latex.[13] Thus all patients with spina bifida should be considered at high risk for having an allergic reaction to rubber. These persons should avoid contact with rubber products, especially during medical procedures. The paramedic should use only nonlatex gloves. Alternative products can be substituted safely. These other products usually are made of silicone, plastic, or vinyl. Other common medical equipment that may contain latex includes:
- Oral and nasal airways
- Endotracheal tubes
- IV tubing
- Surgical masks
- Rubber aprons
- Catheters
- Injection ports
- Needle sheaths on medicines
- Wound drains
- Blood pressure cuffs
- Syringes
- Stethoscopes
- Tourniquets
- Electrode pads

Myasthenia Gravis

Myasthenia gravis is an autoimmune disorder in which muscles become weak and tire easily. The damage occurs to muscle receptors that are responsible for transmitting nerve impulses. The disease commonly affects muscles of the eyes, face, throat, and extremities (Figure 51-6). Myasthenia gravis is a rare disease that can begin suddenly or gradually. It can occur at any age but usually appears in

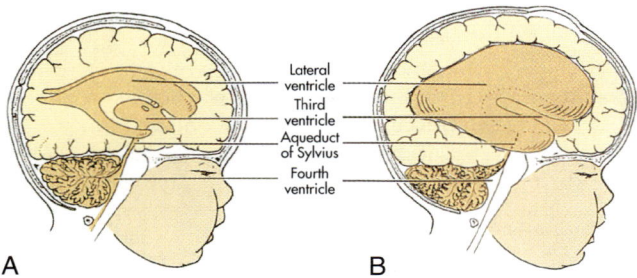

FIGURE 51-5 Hydrocephalus: a block in flow of cerebrospinal fluid. **A,** Patent cerebrospinal fluid circulation. **B,** Enlarged lateral and third ventricles caused by obstruction of circulation—stenosis of aqueduct of Sylvius.

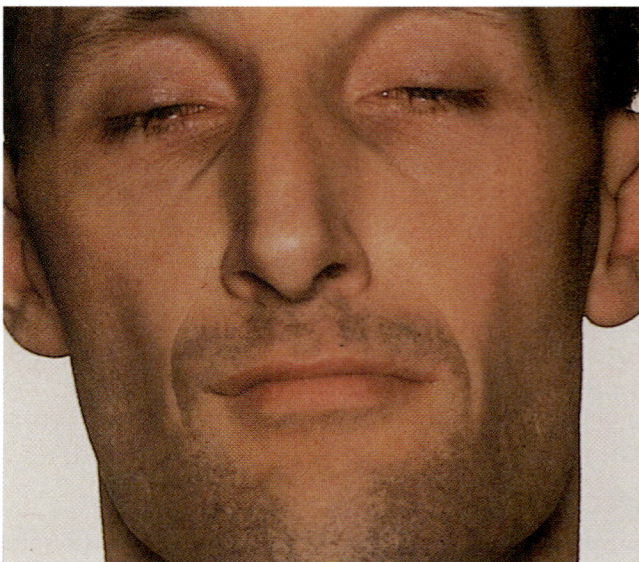

FIGURE 51-6 A patient with myasthenia gravis.

women between ages 20 and 30 and in men after 50 years of age.[14] Classic signs and symptoms include the following:

- Drooping eyelids, double vision
- Difficulty speaking
- Difficulty in chewing and swallowing
- Difficult extremity movement
- Weakened respiratory muscles

The affected muscles become fatigued with use. However, they may recover completely with rest. The condition may be worsened by infection, stress, medications, and menstruation. Myasthenia gravis often can be controlled with drug therapy to enhance the transmission of nerve impulses in the muscles. (Removal of the thymus gland may improve the condition.) In a small number of patients the disease will progress to paralysis of the throat and respiratory muscles and may lead to death.

SPECIAL CONSIDERATIONS

Accommodations required for care will vary based on the patient's presentation. In most cases, supportive care and transport will be all that is required. In the presence of respiratory distress, the paramedic should take measures to ensure adequate airway and ventilatory support.

CULTURALLY DIVERSE PATIENTS

As described in Chapter 17, individuals vary in many ways, and huge diversity exists in populations of all cultures. **Diversity** is a term that once was used mainly to describe "racial awareness." Now it refers to differences of any kind. These differences include age, race, class, religion, gender, sexual preference, personal habitat, and physical ability. Good health care depends on sensitivity toward these differences.

CRITICAL THINKING
What kinds of diversity are there in your classroom? How do you feel about that diversity?

Experiences of health and illness vary widely as a result of different beliefs, behaviors, and past experiences. These experiences may conflict with learned medical practice of the paramedic. By revealing awareness of cultural issues, the paramedic conveys interest, concern, and respect. When dealing with patients from different cultures, the paramedic should remember the following eight key points:

1. The individual is the "foreground" and the culture is the "background."
2. Different generations and individuals within the same family may have different sets of beliefs.
3. Not all persons identify with their ethnic cultural background.
4. All persons share common problems or situations.
5. Respect the integrity of cultural beliefs.
6. Realize that persons may not share your explanations of the causes of their ill health but may accept conventional treatments. (You do not have to "convert" a patient to your way of thinking to get the desired result.)
7. You do not have to agree with every aspect of another's culture, nor does the person have to accept everything about yours for effective and culturally sensitive health care to occur.
8. Recognize your personal cultural assumptions, prejudices, and belief systems. Do not let them interfere with patient care.

Special Considerations

Regardless of the patient's cultural background, education, occupation, or ability to speak English, most patients will be anxious during an emergency event. If the paramedic does not speak the patient's language, communication should begin using English first. The patient may understand or speak some English words or phrases. (Bystanders, co-workers, or family members may be available to assist.) In some areas, special translator devices (e.g., a telephone language line, a computer-generated Internet or cell phone application) for non–English-speaking patients are available. If the patient does not speak or understand English, the paramedic should try to communicate with signs or gestures. The hospital should be notified as soon as possible so that arrangements for an interpreter can be made.

If time allows, the paramedic should perform all assessment procedures slowly and with the patient's permission. The paramedic should be aware that "private space" is culturally defined (see Chapter 17). Therefore the best approach is to point to the area of the body to be examined before touching the patient. The paramedic must respect the patient's need for modesty and privacy at the scene and during transport. Women and men of some cultures have very strict religious beliefs regarding personal modesty and the appropriateness of being touched, especially by strangers. When possible, every effort should be made to honor their wishes, protect their privacy, and ensure their comfort.

TERMINALLY ILL PATIENTS

As health care professionals, paramedics will care for **terminally ill patients.** (These are patients with advanced stage of disease with an unfavorable prognosis and no known cure.) Often, these calls will be emotionally charged events. They will require a great deal of empathy and compassion for the patient and his or her loved ones. If emotions at the scene are out of control, the paramedic must take control and try to calm the persons involved.

If EMS has been called during the late stages of a patient's terminal illness or for a change in the patient's condition, a full history should be obtained. The patient or family should be asked about advance directives and the appropriateness of resuscitation procedures (see Chapter 6). The paramedic should review carefully any documentation made available concerning advance directives (e.g., a do not resuscitate order). Advance directives should be discussed with medical direction so that care decisions can be made.

NOTE

Not all patients receiving hospice care will have advance directives. Although advance directives are encouraged and sometimes required by hospice, there are variations between hospice programs and their requirements to participate.

LOOK AGAIN

See Chapter 6: Medical and Legal Issues, pp. 102-103.

Special Considerations

Care of a terminally ill patient often is mainly supportive and limited to calming and comfort measures. Care may include transport for physician evaluation. Many terminally ill patients and their families will be involved in hospice care (described in Chapter 2) to help them deal with death and dying. Pain assessment and the management of pain are important aspects of caring for these patients. The paramedic should try to gather a full pain medication history and examine the patient for the presence of transdermal drug patches or other pain-relief devices. Following an assessment of the patient's vital signs, level of consciousness, and medication history, medical direction may advise the use of analgesics or sedatives to ensure the patient's comfort.

PATIENTS WITH COMMUNICABLE DISEASES

As described in Chapter 28, exposure to some infectious diseases can be a significant health risk to paramedics. Thus it is crucial to ensure personal protection on *every* response. The required precautions depend on the mode of transmission and on the ability of the pathogen to cause disease. For example, in some cases gloves provide the required protection. In other cases, respiratory barriers also are needed. Although paramedics cannot be provided with a totally risk-free environment, simple measures of protection greatly reduce exposure to pathogens.

Special Considerations

Some infectious diseases (e.g., acquired immunodeficiency syndrome [AIDS]) are detrimental to the emotional well-being of affected patients, their families, and loved ones. The psychological aspects of providing care to these patients include an emphasis on recognizing each patient as an individual with unique health care needs, respecting each person's personal dignity, and providing considerate, respectful care focused upon the person's individual needs.

CRITICAL THINKING

How do you think you will feel when called to care for a patient who is positive for human immunodeficiency virus or has acquired immunodeficiency syndrome?

FINANCIAL CHALLENGES

More than 45.7 million Americans and one third of persons living in poverty are estimated to have no health insurance.[15] In addition, the insurance coverage held by many others would not carry them through a catastrophic illness. Financial challenges for health care can quickly result from loss of a job and depletion of savings. Financial challenges that are combined with medical conditions that require uninterrupted treatment (e.g., cancer, tuberculosis, HIV/AIDS, diabetes, hypertension, and mental disorders) or that occur in the presence of unexpected illness or injury can deprive the patient of basic health care. Most medical personnel and health care facilities recognize their ethical duty to provide services immediately, without regard to payment, in emergencies.

Poor health also is associated closely with homelessness. Many homeless persons have multiple health problems. In addition to chronic illness, frostbite, leg ulcers, and respiratory tract infections are common. These often are the direct result of homelessness. Homeless persons also are at greater risk for trauma from muggings, beatings, and rape. Homelessness precludes good nutrition, good personal hygiene, and basic first aid. In addition, some homeless persons with mental disorders may use alcohol or other drugs to self-medicate. Those with addictive disorders often are at risk of human immunodeficiency virus and other communicable diseases. Paramedics should be familiar with services in their community for the homeless. They should know where to refer the homeless for food and shelter.

NOTE

It is estimated that approximately 3.5 million people in the United States, 1.35 million of them children, are likely to experience homelessness in a given year.[16] In addition, in 2007, 12.5% of the U.S. population, or 37.3 million people, lived in poverty.[17]

CRITICAL THINKING

Consider patients with chronic illness and no insurance. How do you think that financial pressures influence medication compliance in these patients?

Special Considerations

Persons with financial challenges often are anxious about seeking medical care. Fortunately, the ability to pay for emergency care generally is not a concern for EMS personnel (see Chapter 7). According to *Emergency Medical Services: Agenda for the Future*, "the focus of public access is the ability to secure prompt and appropriate EMS care regardless of socioeconomic status, age, or special need. For all those who contact EMS with a perceived requirement for care, the subsequent response and level of care provided must be commensurate with the situation."[18] When caring for a patient with financial challenges who is concerned about the cost of receiving needed health care, the paramedic should explain the following:

1. The patient's ability to pay should never be a factor in obtaining emergency care.
2. Federal law requires that care be provided, regardless of the patient's ability to pay.
3. Payment programs for health care services are available in most hospitals.
4. Government services are available to help patients in paying for health care.
5. Free (or near-free) health care services are available through local, state, and federally funded organizations.

In cases in which no life-threatening condition exists, the paramedic should ask the patient which hospital is covered through the patient's health plan or insurance policy. When the patient does not have insurance coverage, the paramedic should tell the patient about alternative facilities for health care for the patient's present condition. The patent also should be counseled about future situations that do not require transport for emergency department evaluation. As an example, the paramedic should provide an approved list of alternative health care sites (e.g.,

a minor-emergency center or health clinic) that can provide medical care at costs that are much less than those charged by emergency departments.

SHOW ME THE EVIDENCE

From July 2006 to March 2007 researchers in San Francisco gathered data on adult patients who made a decision to come to the ED for care and met selected inclusion criteria. They asked homeless patients and a control group of patients who were not homeless a series of questions about their ED visit. Homeless patients were more likely to say they came to the ED because of hunger, fear for safety, or lack of shelter. Over half of the homeless patients reported being assaulted. Homeless patients interviewed spent an average of 3.5 nights per week sleeping on the street and only one third of the homeless patients felt they had adequate clothing. Although there were a number of limitations to this study, the authors conclude that nonmedical needs constitute a significant number of ED visits in homeless persons.

From Rodriguez RM, Fortman J, Chee C et al: Food, shelter and safety needs motivating homeless persons' visits to an urban emergency department, *Ann Emerg Med* 53(5):598-602, e591, 2008, doi: 10.1016/j.annemergmed.2008.07.046.

SUMMARY

- Certain accommodations may be needed for a hearing-impaired patient. These include helping with a patient's hearing aid, providing paper and pen to aid in communication, speaking softly into the patient's ear, and speaking in clear view of the patient.
- When caring for the visually impaired patient, the paramedic should help the patient use his or her glasses or other visual aids. The paramedic also should describe all procedures before performing them.
- Allow extra time for the history of a patient with speech impairment. If appropriate, provide aids such as a pen and paper to assist in communication.
- When caring for an obese patient, use the proper-sized diagnostic devices. Also, secure extra personnel if needed to move the patient for transport.
- When transporting patients with paraplegia or quadriplegia, extra personnel may be needed to move special equipment.
- Once rapport and trust have been established with a patient who has mental illness, the paramedic should proceed with care in the standard manner.
- When caring for a patient with developmental delays, the paramedic should allow enough time to obtain a history, perform an assessment, deliver care, and prepare for transport.

- The challenge in assessing patients with emotional impairments is distinguishing between symptoms produced by stress and those caused by serious medical illness.
- Pathological conditions may require special assessment and management skills. The paramedic should ask about current medications and the patient's normal level of functioning.
- Diversity refers to differences of any kind. These include race, class, religion, gender, sexual preference, personal habitat, and physical ability. Good health care depends on sensitivity toward these differences.
- Often, calls involving the care of a terminally ill patient will be emotionally charged. They require a great deal of empathy and compassion for the patient and his or her loved ones.
- Some infectious diseases will take a toll on the emotional well-being of affected patients, their families, and loved ones. Paramedics should be sensitive to the psychological needs of the patient and his or her family.
- Financial challenges can deprive a patient of basic health care services. These patients may be reluctant to seek care for illness or injury.

REFERENCES

1. Shaia T: *Auditory neuropathy,* http://emedicine.medscape.com/article/836769-overview, accessed 10-21-10.

2. American Academy of Ophthalmology: *Statistics on blindness,* www.aao.org/newsroom/press.../Eye-Health-Statistics-June-2009.pdf, accessed 10-21-10.

3. American Optometric Association: *Eye and vision problems,* www.aoa.org/x10295.xml, accessed 10-21-10.

4. Flegal K, Carroll MD, Ogden CL, et al: Prevalence and trends of obesity among US adults *1999-2008, JAMA* 303(3):235-241, 2010.

5. Ogden CL, Carroll MD, Curtin LR, et al: Prevalence of high body mass in US children and adolescents*, 2007-2008, JAMA* 303(3):242-249, 2010.

6. Centers for Disease Control and Prevention: *Defining overweight and obesity,* www.cdc.gov/obesity/defining.html, accessed 10-21-10.

7. Mayoclinic.com: *Obesity complications,* www.mayoclinic.com/health/obesity/DS00314/DSECTION=complications, accessed 10-21-10.

8. National Down Syndrome Society: *Incidences and maternal age,* www.ndss.org/index.php?option=com_content&view=article&id=61&Itemid=78, accessed 10-21-10.

9. Mash E, Wolfe D: *Abnormal child psychology,* ed 4, Belmont, Calif, 2010, Wadsworth Cengage.

10. Lissauer T, Clayden C: *Illustrated textbook of pediatrics,* revised ed 3, St Louis, 2007, Mosby.

11. Ontario Federation for Cerebral Palsy: *About cerebral palsy,* www.ofcp.on.ca/aboutcp.html, accessed 10-21-10.

12. Odding E, Roebroeck ME, Stam HJ: The epidemiology of cerebral palsy: incidence, impairments and risk factors, *Disabil Rehabil* 28(4):183-191, 2006.

13. Spina Bifida Association of America: *Latex (natural rubber) allergy in spina bifida,* www.spinabifidaassociation.org/site/c.liKWL7PLLrF/b.2700271/k.1779/Latex_Natural_Rubber_Allergy_in_Spina_Bifida.htm, accessed 10-21-10.

14. Howard JF Jr: *Myasthenia gravis: a summary,* St Paul, Minn, 2006, Myasthenia Gravis Foundation of America, www.myasthenia.org/hp_clinicaloverview.cfm, accessed 10-21-10.

15. National Coalition for the Homeless: *Healthcare and homelessness,* www.nationalhomeless.org/factsheets/health.html, accessed 11-7-10.

16. National Law Center on Homelessness and Poverty, 2007.

17. National Coalition for the Homeless: *Why are people homeless?* www.nationalhomeless.org/factsheets/why.html, accessed 10-21-10.

18. U.S. Department of Transportation, National Highway Traffic Safety Administration, U.S. Department of Health and Human Services: *Emergency medical services: agenda for the future,* Washington, DC, 1996, The Department.

SUGGESTED READINGS

Beebe R: *Treating and transporting bariatric patients, JEMS,* 2009, www.jems.com/article/patient-care/treating-and-transporting-bari, accessed 5-29-10.

Hines J: Communication problems of hearing impaired patients, *Nurs Standard* 14(19):33-37, 2000.

Stevens N: Special considerations in working with gastric bypass patients for the emergency nurse, *J Emerg Nurs* 35(5):434-436, 2009.

U.S. Department of Health and Human Services, Health Resources and Services Administration: *Common emergencies affecting children and youth with special health care needs,* EMSC National Resource Center, 2007, retrieved 5-16-10 from http://bolivia.hrsa.gov/emsc/Downloads/CommonEmergenciesCSHCN/CommonEmergenciesforCSHCN.htm.

Acute Interventions for Home Care

OBJECTIVES

Upon completion of this chapter, the paramedic student will be able to:

1. Discuss general issues related to the home health care patient.
2. Outline general principles of assessment and management of the home health care patient.
3. Describe medical equipment, assessment, and management of the home health care patient with inadequate respiratory support.
4. Identify assessment findings and acute interventions for problems related to vascular access devices in the home health care setting.
5. Describe medical equipment, assessment, and management of the patient with a gastrointestinal or genitourinary crisis in the home health care setting.
6. Identify key assessments and principles of wound care management in the home health care patient.
7. Outline maternal/child problems that may be encountered early in the postpartum period in the home health care setting.
8. Describe medical therapy associated with hospice and comfort care in the home health care setting.

KEY TERMS

bladder catheterization Drainage of the bladder using a urinary catheter.

bronchopulmonary dysplasia A chronic respiratory disorder characterized by scarring of lung tissue, thickened pulmonary arterial walls, and ventilation-perfusion mismatch; often occurs in infants who have long-term dependence on artificial ventilation.

colostomy A surgical opening into the large intestine.

failure to thrive The abnormal retardation of the growth and development of an infant resulting from conditions that interfere with normal metabolism, appetite, and activity.

gastric tube A device that is inserted into the stomach or intestines; used to remove fluids and gas by suction or gravity, to instill irrigation solutions or medications, and to administer enteral feedings.

hospice A type of care and philosophy of care that includes supportive social, emotional, and spiritual services for the terminally ill and their family.

ileostomy A surgical opening into the small intestine.

infantile apnea An unexplained episode of cessation of breathing for 20 seconds or longer, or a shorter respiratory pause associated with bradycardia, cyanosis, pallor, and/or marked hypotonia (diminished tone).

obstructive apnea A form of sleep apnea involving a physical obstruction of the upper airways that can lead to pulmonary failure, chronic fatigue, and cardiac abnormalities.

ostomy An artificial opening into the urinary tract, gastrointestinal tract, or trachea; any surgical procedure in which an opening is created between two hollow organs or between a hollow viscus and the abdominal wall.

palliative care A unique form of health care primarily directed at providing relief to terminally ill persons through symptom management and pain management; also known as comfort care.

sleep apnea A disorder characterized by abnormal pauses in breathing or episodes of abnormally slow breathing during sleep.

urosepsis Septic poisoning caused by retention and absorption of urinary products in the tissues.

vascular access device A device used to provide nutritional support and to administer medications in patients who need long-term vascular access.

T*he cost-driven allocation of health care resources and advances in technology have led to shortened hospital stays. This also has allowed many patients to be treated in the home setting. An estimated 7.6 million persons in the United States require home health care services because of acute illness, long-term health conditions, personal preference, permanent disability, or terminal illness.[1] Paramedics likely will play a key role in providing acute interventions to these patients.*

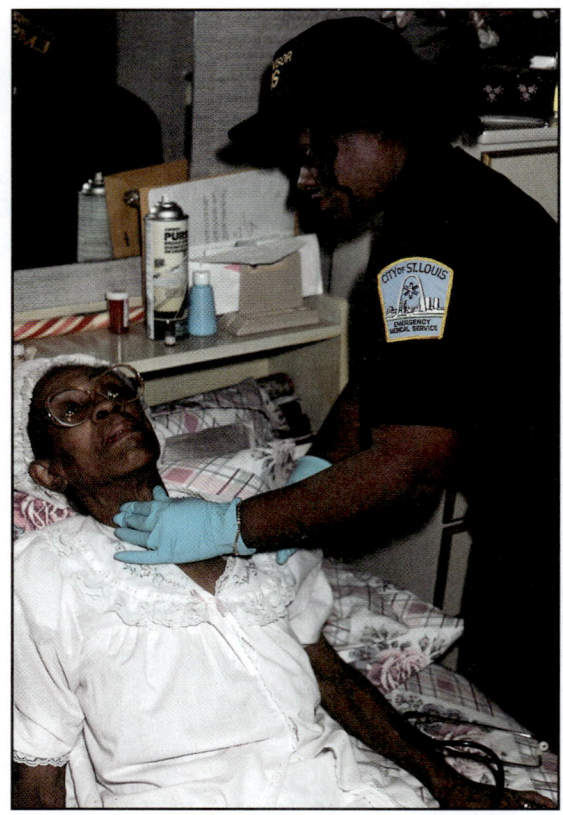

(Courtesy Monroe Yancie, St. Louis, Mo.)

OVERVIEW OF HOME HEALTH CARE

Home health care began in the United States in the late 1800s as a direct result of escalating city growth and an increase in the number of immigrants moving into large cities.[2] The emphasis of home health care at that time was personal hygiene and preventive care. The health services were provided by visiting nurses. These nurses worked in tenements to assist the poor. They also cared for wealthy and middle-class families after births or discharges from hospitals. At first, few physicians were associated with most of these home health care groups.

Until the mid-1960s, home health care continued to focus on the poor. The remainder of the population received care in hospitals and physicians' offices. With the passage of the Social Security Act Amendments (commonly known as Medicare) in 1965, home health care became a benefit to older adult patients receiving Medicare. This greatly accelerated growth of the industry. (In 1973 these services were extended to certain disabled younger Americans; hospice benefits were added in 1983.) By 1997 an estimated 38.5 million older adult and disabled Americans were enrolled in Medicare programs. In 2008, 7.6 million Medicare recipients received formal home care services.[3] Medicare is the single largest payer of home care services in the United States.[4] Other funding sources include Medicaid, the Older Americans Act, Title XX Social Services Block Grants, the Veterans Administration, TRICARE/CHAMPUS for military personnel, private insurance, and managed care organizations.

In recent years, federal health care reform has led to the development of managed care services that are provided to members by managed care organizations (see Chapter 1). These plans now cover about 95% of the U.S. population.[4] They have greatly influenced methods of health care delivery (including home health care services).

Today, home health care incorporates a wide variety of health and social services. These services are provided at home to recovering, disabled, or chronically ill and terminally ill persons in need of medical, nursing, social, or therapeutic treatment and help with the essential activities of daily living. The following is a sampling of services provided to home health care patients:

- Skilled nursing services
- Physical, speech, and occupational therapy
- Medical social services
- Home health aides
- Nutritional counseling

Advanced Life Support Response to Home Health Care Patients

About 21% of home health care patients have conditions related to diseases of the circulatory system as their primary diagnosis.[3] (Persons with heart disease, including congestive heart failure, constitute about half of this group.) Other common diagnoses of home health care patients include cancer, diabetes, chronic lung disease, renal failure/dialysis, and hypertension. Thus emergency responses for home health care patients likely will be more common for emergency medical services (EMS) agencies. Typical emergencies may include respiratory failure, cardiac decompensation, septic complications, equipment malfunction, and other conditions that worsen in the home health care setting (Box 52-1).

BOX 52-1 Examples of Home Health Care Problems

Home Care Services Requiring Intervention by a Home Health Care Practitioner or Physician
Acquired immunodeficiency syndrome
Cardiopulmonary care
Catheter management/intravenous therapy infusion
Chemotherapy
Dermatological and wound care
Gastroenterological and ostomy care
Hospice care
Organ transplantation
Orthopedic care
Pain management
Rehabilitative care
Specimen collection
Urological and renal care

Home Health Care Problems Requiring Acute Intervention
Acute cardiac events
Acute infections
Acute respiratory events
Gastrointestinal/genitourinary crisis
Hospice/comfort care
Inadequate respiratory support
Maternal/child conditions
Vascular access complications

CRITICAL THINKING
What factors decrease the risks of spreading infection within a home health care setting versus a hospital?

- Mask
- Gown
- Goggles, glasses, or face shield
- Resuscitation mask
- Specimen bags
- EPA-approved disinfectant effective against hepatitis B virus, human immunodeficiency virus, and tuberculosis
- Soap and water/hand sanitizers
- Disposable paper towels
- Impervious trash bags and labels

This text assumes that the proper personal protection will be used by paramedics. The nature of the emergency and the patient's condition will dictate what protection to use.

Types of Home Care Patients

The need to reduce the costs of health care and the technological advances in medicine have allowed many types of patients to receive home care. Many EMS agencies ask their communities to notify them when someone is part of a complex home health care program. Many of these agencies will visit the home before the onset of an emergency. This allows them to become familiar with the patient's condition and special equipment. There are many classifications of home health care patients. Examples include those with the following conditions:
- Pathological conditions of the airway causing inadequate pulmonary toilet or inadequate alveolar ventilation and/or oxygenation
- Circulatory pathological conditions causing alterations in central circulation (e.g., heart failure) or peripheral circulation (e.g., pressure ulcers, delayed healing, or infection)
- Neurological conditions such as stroke, traumatic brain injury, spinal cord injury
- Orthopedic trauma or surgery that requires rehabilitation (e.g., fractured hip, hip or knee replacement)
- Gastrointestinal/genitourinary conditions requiring special devices such as ostomies, feeding catheters, and special equipment needed for home dialysis
- Infection from cellulitis or systemic illness (e.g., sepsis)
- Wounds that require care (e.g., surgical wound closure, decubitus wounds, and surgical drains)

Other patient groups the paramedic may encounter in the home health care setting include patients receiving hospice care, expectant or new mothers, patients with dementia or other conditions that require psychological support for the patient or family, patients receiving

Injury Control and Prevention in the Home Health Care Setting

The scientific approach to illness and injury prevention as a means to minimize morbidity and mortality is discussed in Chapter 3. Readers should refer to that chapter to review primary prevention, acute care, and rehabilitation (tertiary prevention); their concepts; and their strategies.

INFECTION CONTROL

As with all other patient encounters, the paramedic should practice infection control in the home health care setting. Infection control includes using universal precautions and body substance isolation (or transmission-based precautions) when indicated. This practice, along with treating all patients as though they have an infectious disease, forms the basis for infection control guidelines recommended by the Centers for Disease Control and Prevention. The Occupational Safety and Health Administration, Centers for Disease Control and Prevention, and Environmental Protection Agency (EPA) recommend the same infection control standards for the treatment of home health care patients as for acute care patients. Equipment proposed by these agencies for infection control in the home setting includes the following:

chemotherapy or home care for chronic pain, and patients with organ transplants or those who are waiting for organ transplantation (*transplant candidate*).

GENERAL PRINCIPLES AND MANAGEMENT
Scene Size-Up

When paramedics arrive at the scene of a home health care patient, the scene size-up should include universal precautions, elements of scene safety, and an assessment of the patient's environment (environmental setting).

UNIVERSAL PRECAUTIONS

As described in Chapter 13 and Chapter 28, paramedics should use universal precautions to guard against communicable disease when caring for any patient. Equipment that may be found in the home health care setting includes containers of medical waste, ostomy collection bags, tracheostomy tubes, sharps, soiled dressings, and other equipment (e.g., emesis basins, walkers, and wheelchairs) that may be contaminated with the patient's body fluids. In addition to personal precautions, the EMS crew should ensure that any infectious waste found in the home is contained properly. The waste should be disposed according to protocol.

LOOK AGAIN
See Chapter 14: Venous Access and Medication Administration, pp. 380-381.

SCENE SAFETY

Whenever an EMS response is made to a person's home, the paramedic should evaluate the scene for the presence of dangerous pets, firearms and other home protection devices, and for any home hazards (e.g., inadequate lighting, icy sidewalks, or steep stairwells). For the safety of the EMS crew, the patient, and others at the scene, all potential hazards found in a home must be contained or remedied. For example, it may be necessary to request law enforcement personnel to help with unruly or hostile bystanders. In addition, extra personnel and equipment may be needed to help move a patient down a flight of steps for transport or to manage technology-assisted patient care devices.

ENVIRONMENTAL SETTING

The paramedic should assess the setting for the patient's ability to maintain a healthy environment. Examples include cleanliness of the home; evidence of basic nutritional support; and needs of heat, water, shelter, and electricity. The EMS crew also should note any signs of abuse or neglect. Other factors to note are the cleanliness and condition of any medical devices. (For example, this includes clean oxygen and ventilation equipment and wheelchairs and hospital beds that are in good repair.)

Patient Assessment

The primary survey should focus on life-threatening illness or injury, and appropriate measures should be taken as indicated (see Chapter 19). After the primary survey, a focused history should be obtained and secondary assessment performed. The paramedic should make use of any medical documents found in the home (e.g., patient records kept by home health care providers and do not resuscitate orders). In addition, information should be gathered from family and health care professionals (e.g., a home care nurse or physical or respiratory therapist) who may be present at the scene. Critical findings should alert the paramedic to forgo a detailed assessment and proceed with resuscitation measures and rapid transport for physician evaluation. If there are no critical findings, the paramedic should perform a physical examination that considers the possibility of medication interactions, compliance with the treatment regimen, and the possibility of dementia or a metabolic disturbance in a patient with an altered mental status.

A comprehensive assessment may include a physical examination using inspection, palpation, auscultation, and percussion (as indicated by the patient's condition and chief complaint). The reassessment (ongoing assessment) should evaluate any changes in the patient's status while at the scene or en route to the hospital. These assessment strategies can aid in differential diagnosis, treatment, and direction of patient management.

Management and Treatment Plan

Depending on the patient's condition, the home health care treatment may need to be replaced with advanced life support measures. These measures may include airway, ventilatory, and circulatory support and pharmacological and nonpharmacological therapy (e.g., electrical therapy).

Some patients with acute illness or injury need to be transported to the hospital for evaluation. When transport is needed, the paramedic must give special consideration for patient packaging and for moving the patient's equipment. Examples include properly securing intravenous (IV) catheters, urinary catheters, and feeding tubes; and ensuring available personnel to assist with moving patient care devices such as ventilation equipment. Family members at the scene often are well versed on the patient's medical devices. They usually will be eager to help when asked by the EMS crew. If there is no family at the scene, the paramedic should attempt to contact a family member or caregiver and advise this person of the patient's condition and hospital destination.

Other patients need only home care follow-up by home health care practitioners, or they may need a referral to other public service agencies. The paramedic should follow protocol and consult with medical direction about referrals and the need for notifying private physicians or home health care agencies. Regardless of the need for EMS transport, the paramedic should thoroughly document all findings and any care provided on the patient care report.

CRITICAL THINKING
What feelings may a patient's family member (or caregiver) in the home setting have if there is a problem and the patient's condition worsens?

SPECIFIC ACUTE HOME HEALTH CARE INTERVENTIONS

Acute home health care emergencies may occur from equipment failure or malfunction, drug reactions, complications related to home treatment, and worsening medical conditions. This section discusses acute interventions for respiratory support, cardiovascular support, vascular access devices, gastrointestinal/genitourinary crisis, acute infections, maternal/child conditions, and hospice/palliative care.

Respiratory Support

More than 630,000 patients are discharged to home health care with diseases of the respiratory system each year.[1] These patients are at increased risk for airway infections. The progression of some respiratory diseases also may lead to an increased respiratory demand, making current support inadequate. Examples of chronic pathological conditions that require home respiratory support include the following:

- Asthma
- Awaiting lung transplantation
- Bronchopulmonary dysplasia
- Chronic lung disease
- Cystic fibrosis
- Infection causing exacerbation of condition
- Sleep apnea

Acute interventions may be required for these patients. Any patient with respiratory distress should receive high-concentration oxygen, pulse oximetry monitoring, and ventilatory support as priorities in care. Problems that may lead to a request for EMS assistance include increased respiratory demand, increased bronchospasm, increased secretions, obstructed or malfunctioning respiratory devices, or improper application of medical devices to support respirations.

OXYGEN THERAPY IN THE HOME SETTING

Three common ways to provide oxygen therapy in the home are compressed gas, liquid oxygen, and oxygen concentrators. Compressed gas is oxygen stored under pressure in oxygen cylinders equipped with a regulator that controls flow rate. Liquid oxygen is cold and is stored in a container similar to a thermos. When released, the liquid converts to gas and is used like compressed gas. An oxygen concentrator is an electrically powered device that separates oxygen from air, concentrates it, and stores it (Figure 52-1). This system does not have to be resupplied and is not as costly as liquid oxygen. A cylinder

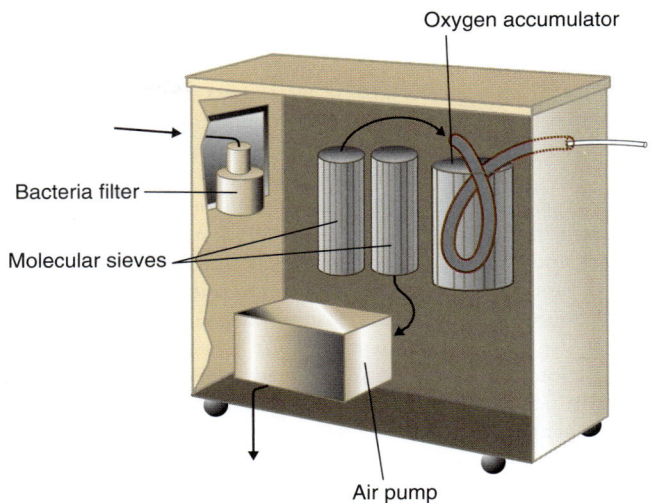

FIGURE 52-1 Oxygen concentrator.

of oxygen must be available as a backup, however, in case of power failure.

CRITICAL THINKING
What safety precautions for administering oxygen should be in place in the home setting?

Oxygen is delivered to patients via nasal cannulae, oxygen masks, tracheostomy collars (devices that deliver high humidity and oxygen to patients with surgical airways), and ventilators. Some patients may require continuous positive airway pressure (CPAP) delivered by ventilatory support systems through mask CPAP, nasal CPAP, or biphasic positive airway pressure (BiPAP). As described in Chapter 24, the BiPAP ventilatory support system (designed for mask-applied ventilation in the home) delivers two different levels of positive airway pressure. The system cycles spontaneously between a preset level of inspiratory positive airway pressure and expiratory positive airway pressure. The BiPAP ventilatory support system is intended only to augment the patient's breathing; it does not provide for total ventilatory requirements. The BiPAP system is used by some patients with sleep apnea or chronic obstructive pulmonary disease.

Supportive ventilator management may be indicated to achieve the following:
- Prevent nocturnal hypoxemia caused by sleep hypoventilation in patients with neuromuscular disorders (e.g., muscular dystrophy or myasthenia gravis).
- Prevent respiratory fatigue in patients with chronic obstructive pulmonary disease.
- Improve ventilation and oxygen saturation in patients with **obstructive apnea,** a form of **sleep apnea** involving a physical obstruction of the upper airways that can lead to pulmonary failure, chronic fatigue, and cardiac abnormalities.

Sleep apnea is a disorder characterized by abnormal pauses in breathing or episodes of abnormally slow breathing during sleep. The pauses often occur 5 to 30 times or more each hour. The condition is common, affecting about 12 million Americans.[5] Untreated, sleep apnea can increase the risk of hypertension, stroke, myocardial infarction, worsening heart failure, and dysrhythmias. It also is related to obesity and diabetes. Once diagnosed, the most common treatment in adults is application of continuous positive airway pressure (CPAP) during sleep. Other treatment therapies include lifestyle changes (weight loss, smoking cessation, limited alcohol use), alterations in sleep positioning, and the use of mouthpieces designed to maintain an open airway during sleep. Surgical alteration of the soft tissues of the airway may be indicated for some patients.

Home Ventilators. Home ventilators can be classified as *volume ventilators, pressure ventilators,* and *negative-pressure ventilators.* Most ventilators have a number of controls and ventilator settings. Box 52-2 describes some of these settings.

Volume ventilators (volume-preset) deliver a predetermined volume of gas with each cycle, after which inspiration is terminated. These types of ventilators deliver a constant tidal volume regardless of changes in airway resistance or compliance of the lungs and thorax. The volume remains the same unless very high peak airway pressures are reached. In that case, safety release valves stop the flow (Box 52-3 and Table 52-1).

Pressure ventilators (pressure-preset) are pressure-cycled devices that terminate inspiration when a preset pressure is achieved. When the preset pressure is reached, the gas flow stops, and the patient passively exhales. These ventilators most often are used for patients whose ventilatory resistance is not likely to change.

Negative-pressure ventilators have settings for the respiratory rate and pressure of the negative force exerted. These devices use negative pressure to raise the rib cage and lower the diaphragm. This creates negative pressure within the lungs so that air flows into the lungs. Negative-pressure ventilators often are used for patients with healthy lungs who have a muscular inability to inhale. (For example, this may include patients with spinal cord injury or neuromuscular disease.) Examples of this type of ventilator are the "iron lung" and plastic wrap, or poncho ventilators (Figure 52-2).

BOX 52-2 Standard Initial Ventilator Settings

FIO₂ (fraction of inspired oxygen)	100%
Tidal volume	10 to 15 mL/kg body mass
Respiratory rate	10 to 15 breaths/min
Inspiratory flow rate	40 to 60 L/sec
Sensitivity	12 cm H₂O
Sigh rate (optional)	1 to 2/min

BOX 52-3 Ventilator Alarms

Ventilators are equipped with alarms. These alarms signal that there are problems with ventilator function. There are alarms for loss of power, frequency alarms (indicating changes in respiratory rate), volume alarms (indicating low exhaled volume or low/high minute ventilation), and high-pressure alarms. If alarms are sounding, the paramedic should check for the following possible causes:
- Kinks in endotracheal tube
- Disconnected ventilator tubing or poor connections
- Water in ventilator tubing
- Excessive secretions
- Pneumothorax
- Patient anxiety

After consulting with medical direction, acute interventions may include providing temporary ventilation assistance with a bag-mask device, repositioning the endotracheal tube, correcting poor ventilator tube connections, emptying water from tube or water traps, suctioning the airway, decompressing the thorax, and possibly sedating the patient.

TABLE 52-1 Ventilator Alarms*

Alarm Type	Causes	Interventions
High pressure	Increased secretions	Suction secretions from patient.
High pressure	Kinked tubing	Unkink tubing.
High pressure	Water in tubing	Disconnect tubing and allow it to drain.
High pressure	Anxiety	Decrease anxiety by providing a calm environment.
Low pressure	Disconnected tubing	Reconnect tubing.
Low pressure	Cuff leak	Add 1 mL of air at a time to pilot balloon of tracheostomy tube.
Low pressure	Tracheostomy tube out	Reinsert new tracheostomy tube.
Oxygen	Insufficient oxygen supply	Manually ventilate patient's lungs and prepare for transport.
Ventilator not operating	Power failure	Manually ventilate patient's lungs and prepare for transport.

*Note: A memory aid useful for identifying possible causes of ventilator malfunction is DOPE. This stands for **d**isplacement of the tube, **o**bstruction of the tube, **p**neumothorax, and **e**quipment failure.

ASSESSMENT FINDINGS

When caring for a patient who requires oxygen therapy, the paramedic should evaluate the patient's work of breathing, tidal volume, peak flow, oxygen saturation, and quality of breath sounds. This assessment can be performed with visual inspection (chest rise and fall), peak flow meters, pulse oximetry, and auscultation (described in Chapter 15 and Chapter 24). The paramedic should be alert for signs and symptoms of hypoxia, including the following:

- Confusion and mental status changes
- Increased work of breathing
- Cyanosis
- Dyspnea
- Headache
- Hypertension
- Hyperventilation
- Restlessness
- Tachycardia

MANAGEMENT

Management goals for a patient receiving oxygen therapy who requires acute intervention are to improve airway patency, ventilation, and oxygenation.

Improving Airway Patency. To improve airway patency, the paramedic first should reposition airway devices (e.g., face masks and nasal cannulae) to ensure they are applied properly and are well fitted. Any secretions that obstruct airflow from the airway should be cleared with suction and sterile water should be used to clean airway devices. If needed, the home airway device should be replaced with a new device. A tracheostomy tube that has become blocked and cannot be cleared may need to be replaced with another tracheostomy tube to ensure adequate ventilation (Figure 52-3) or the tube can be replaced temporarily with an endotracheal tube (see Chapter 15).

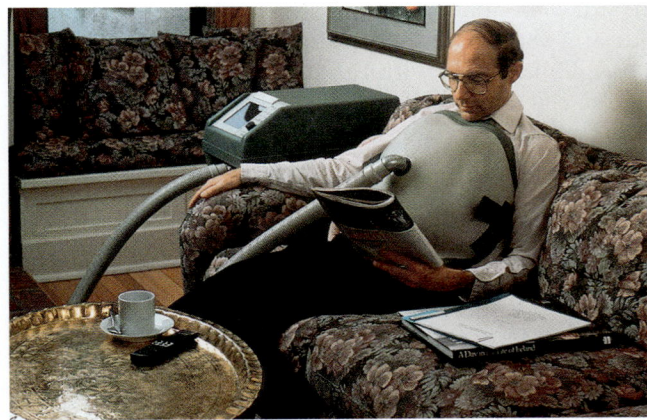

FIGURE 52-2 Home negative pressure ventilator.

> **NOTE**
> The paramedic should always ensure that powered airway equipment is working properly; that oxygen is flowing; and that the equipment is connected to the power source (battery or electrical current). Equipment that is connected properly and still not working may result from power outage in the home (e.g., failed fuse or circuit breaker).

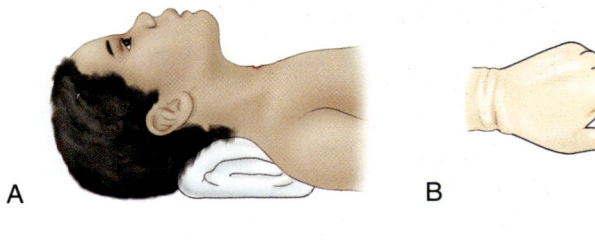
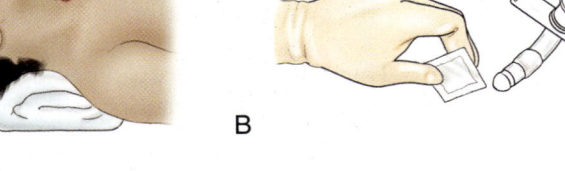

A

B

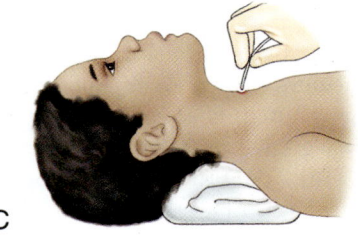
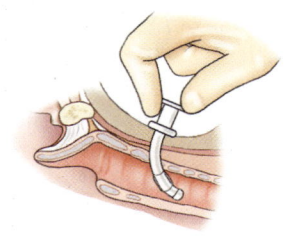

C

D

FIGURE 52-3 Replacement of a tracheostomy tube. **A,** Position the child with padding under the shoulders. **B,** Select a tube the same size or one size smaller than the one removed and moisten it with sterile, water-soluble lubricant. **C,** Suction the stoma and trachea before insertion of the new tube. **D,** Insert the tube gently into the trachea with the curve pointing downward. **E,** If the tube has an obturator, remove it; if it is a cuffed tube, inflate the cuff. **F,** Assess for correct tube placement and secure the tube.

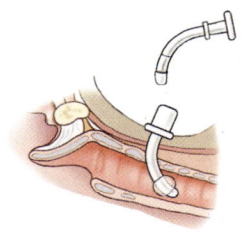
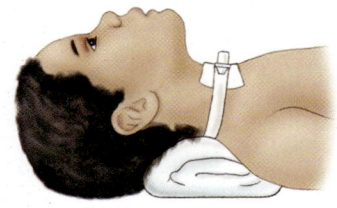

E

F

LOOK AGAIN
See Chapter 15: Airway Management, Respiration, and Artificial Ventilation, pp. 426-427.

Improving Ventilation and Oxygenation. If ventilation does not improve after providing a patent airway, the paramedic should remove the home ventilator care device. The patient's ventilations should then be assisted with positive-pressure ventilation via a bag-valve-mask device and supplemental oxygen. Oxygen saturation should be monitored with pulse oximetry. The paramedic also should administer supplemental oxygen as needed to maintain oxygen saturation at 90% or higher. Medical direction may advise adjusting the settings of a home care device or changing the flow rate of an oxygen delivery device to improve ventilation and oxygenation. Extra personnel may be needed to assist in moving the patient who has a ventilator device to the ambulance for transport.

On some ventilators the inspiratory flow rate is determined by tidal volume, respiratory rate, and the inspiratory/expiratory ratio. (This ratio is generally 1:2. This allows for complete exhalation and prevents air trapping.) On other ventilators the flow rate is set independently. This allows for adjustment of airflow to the flow wave pattern that is most comfortable for the patient. If the patient is having difficulty with spontaneous breathing, an increase in the flow rate may be indicated. However, a higher flow rate means a shorter inspiratory time and usually a higher respiratory pressure because of increased resistance. A lower flow rate requires a longer inspiratory time with a decreased inspiratory pressure. The paramedic should always consult with medical direction before changing the flow rate on any ventilator.

PSYCHOLOGICAL SUPPORT AND COMMUNICATION STRATEGIES

Difficulty breathing can be a horrifying experience for the patient, especially for a patient who depends on a ventilator. The paramedic crew should try to calm the patient and family. They should be assured that respirations will be supported adequately by other means while at the scene and during transport.

Some patients with tracheostomies have special valves attached to the tracheostomy tube ("talking trachs"). These valves redirect exhaled air around the tracheostomy tube, through the vocal cords, and out of the mouth and nose to allow for normal speech. Loss of verbal communication is a major source of anxiety in patients who have tracheostomies. The ability to communicate with these patients will be based on the patient's cognition, level of consciousness, language, and fine and gross motor skills. Methods of communication may include signing and writing on notepads. The paramedic should enlist the help of family and other caregivers in communicating with the patient.

Cardiovascular Support

As described in Chapter 22, it is likely that paramedics will encounter patients who have a left ventricular assist device (LVAD). The most common patient groups who use LVADs are heart transplant candidates, heart surgery patients during recovery, and patients with severe congestive heart failure. To review, an LVAD is a battery-operated, mechanical pump-type device that is surgically implanted. It helps maintain the pumping ability of a heart that cannot effectively function on its own. It essentially assumes or augments the pumping function of the left ventricle. LVADs can operate in fixed mode—the pump beats at a set rate, regardless of other conditions—and auto mode—the pump fills at a variable rate depending on the patient's activity and volume status. With either mode, there is no relationship to the rate or rhythm of the heart. Families and caregivers generally are advised to contact EMS if the patient:

- Is unconscious
- Is awake but nonresponsive
- Falls or suddenly collapses
- Has a severe sensory or motor deficit
- Experiences a severe dysrhythmia or cardiac arrest

TYPES OF LVADS

The two most common LVADs used today are pulsatile pumps and nonpulsatile pumps. A pulsatile LVAD pumps blood in a cycle similar to the normal heart (cycles of contraction-relaxation). Nonpulsatile pumps move blood continuously through the body. Both types of LVADs are controlled by battery packs and an electronic pump and system controller. (These are usually carried on a belt around the patient's waist or on a shoulder strap.) Both types of LVADs can malfunction, triggering an advisory or alarm. Therefore, home care patients and their families are trained to troubleshoot the device. Examples of malfunctions include a failure in the pumping device or system controller, and loss of power. Most malfunctions of an LVAD can be remedied by the patient or family member by checking cables, changing the power source, and changing the system controller. Some devices have emergency "hand pumps" in the event there is a system failure. Manufacturer recommendations for managing advisories and alarms should be closely followed. An LVAD that fails to provide the pumping action of the left ventricle can result in heart failure and cardiac arrest.

NOTE
There are a number of LVADs in use. Some models will produce a palpable pulse and blood pressure; other models do not (depending on the device). In addition, some patients with end-stage heart failure will also have a pacer or implanted defibrillation device in place.

MANAGEMENT

If the patient experiences pulseless ventricular tachycardia, ventricular fibrillation, or asystole, normal care protocols should be applied. Manufacturer guidelines regarding chest compressions and defibrillation must be followed. For example, performing chest compressions over some LVADs may damage the heart and cause severe bleeding. Some LVADs will need to have the power source disconnected before administering electrical therapy. The paramedic should consult with knowledgeable family members or caregivers and with medical direction (Figure 52-4).

Vascular Access Devices

Many patients in the home care setting have an indwelling **vascular access device** (VAD). Vascular access devices are used to provide nutritional support. They also are used to administer medications. In addition, VADs are used for patients who need long-term vascular access. (For example, this includes patients receiving dialysis or chemotherapy.) Those with indwelling vascular devices may experience problems, including the following:

- Anticoagulation associated with percutaneous or implanted devices
- Embolus formation associated with indwelling devices, stasis, and inactivity
- Air embolus associated with central venous access devices
- Obstructed or malfunctioning VADs
- Infection at the access site ("line sepsis")
- Infiltration and extravasation
- Obstructed dialysis shunts
- Bleeding if catheter is torn

> **NOTE**
> Congestive heart failure is a common reason for hospitalization. Attempts often are made to manage these patients at home when possible. Thus paramedics may find patients with congestive heart failure receiving medications (e.g., **dobutamine**) intravenously through a VAD in the home setting.

TYPES

As described in Chapter 14, there are a variety of vascular access devices. These include surgically implanted subcutaneous VADs, medication delivery devices (e.g., MediPorts), peripheral VADs (e.g., peripherally inserted central catheters [PICCs] and midline catheters), central venous tunneled catheters (e.g., Hickman, Groshong, or Broviac), and dialysis shunts (Figure 52-5).

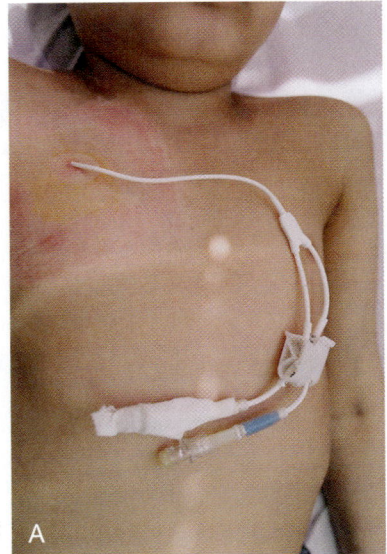

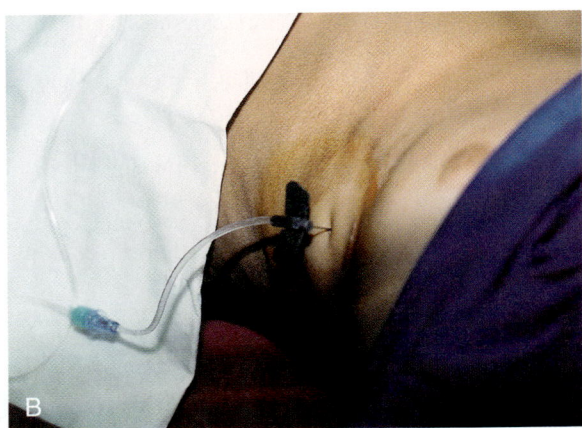

FIGURE 52-5 Vascular access devices. **A,** External venous catheter (note redness from dressing site). **B,** Implanted venous access device with Huber needle placement.

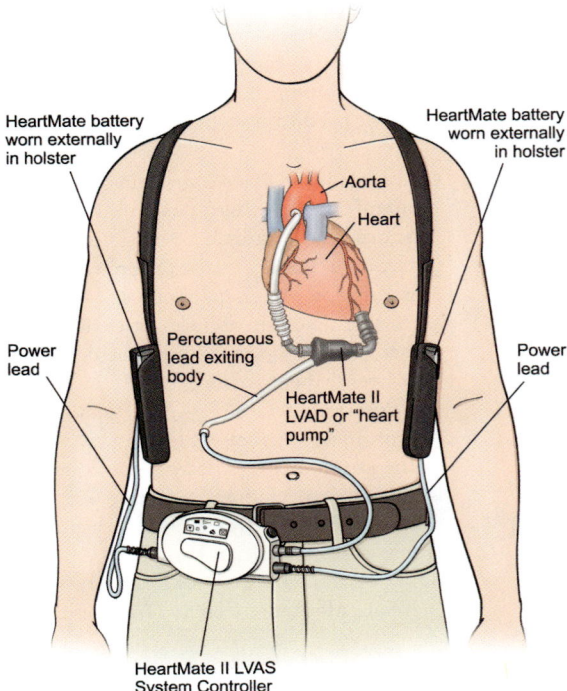

FIGURE 52-4 Ventricular assist device.

LOOK AGAIN

See Chapter 14: Venous Access and Medication Administration, pp. 367-368.

ASSESSMENT FINDINGS AND ACUTE INTERVENTIONS

Certain assessment findings may require acute interventions in patients with VADs. These findings include infection, hemorrhage, hemodynamic compromise from circulatory overload or embolus, obstruction of the vascular device, catheter breakage, and leakage of medication (e.g., chemotherapeutic agents) (Table 52-2).

Infection. Home health care patients who have VADs generally are instructed to regularly examine the area for infection. They also are instructed to change the dressings around their device often. As a rule, this is done by family members and home health care practitioners. All types of dressings must be changed immediately if they become wet, soiled, contaminated, or unocclusive. A common problem of VADs is infection near the exit site, tunnel, or port. Signs and symptoms of localized site infection include pain, redness, warmth, and purulence. Signs and symptoms of systemic infection (which may result from a site infection) include fever, tachycardia, general weakness, malaise, mental status changes, body aches, and possibly septicemia. If the patient has any evidence of systemic signs of infection, he or she should be transported to the hospital. General principles in managing the site of infection are as follows:

1. Wash your hands.
2. Put on nonsterile gloves and remove the old dressing.
3. Discard dressing and gloves.
4. Open the dressing change kit and don sterile gloves.
5. Inspect site for signs of swelling, redness, or other complications.
6. Clean the site vigorously.
   a. Chlorhexidine is gaining acceptance as the antiseptic of choice. Use a side-to-side cleaning motion.
   b. If using alcohol and povidone-iodine (in this order or iodine will be inactivated):
      i. Use the alcohol first to kill *Staphylococcus epidermidis* (organism most likely to cause catheter sepsis).
      ii. Then vigorously clean with povidone-iodine and let skin dry completely.

TABLE 52-2 Correcting Common Problems With Venous Access Devices

Complication	Signs and Symptoms	Prehospital Interventions
Mechanical Problems		
Clotted intravenous catheter	Interrupted flow rate, resistance to flushing and blood withdrawal	Attempt to aspirate clot. If unsuccessful, contact medical direction.
Cracked or broken tubing	Fluid leaking from tubing	Apply padded hemostat above break to prevent air from entering line and change tubing (with orders from medical direction).
Dislodged catheter	Catheter out of vein	Apply pressure to site with a sterile gauze pad.
Too-rapid infusion	Nausea, headache, lethargy, dyspnea	Adjust infusion rate, and if applicable, check infusion pump. Contact medical direction about need to transport.
Other Problems		
Air embolism	Apprehension, chest pain, tachycardia, hypotension, cyanosis, seizures, loss of consciousness, and cardiac arrest	Clamp catheter. Place patient in a steep, left lateral Trendelenburg position. Give oxygen as ordered. If cardiac arrest occurs, begin cardiopulmonary resuscitation.
Extravasation	Swelling and pain around insertion site	Stop infusion. Assess patient for cardiopulmonary abnormalities. Notify medical direction for further advice.
Phlebitis	Pain, tenderness, redness, and warmth	Apply gentle heat to area; elevate insertion site if possible.
Pneumothorax and hydrothorax	Dyspnea, chest pain, cyanosis, and decreased breath sounds	If signs and symptoms of tension pneumothorax are present, consider needle decompression after consulting with medical direction. Rapid transport is indicated.
Septicemia	Red and swollen catheter site, chills, fever	Transport for physician evaluation.
Thrombosis	Erythema and edema at insertion site; ipsilateral swelling of arm, neck, face, and upper chest; pain at insertion site and along vein; malaise; fever; tachycardia	Apply warm compresses to insertion site; elevate affected extremity. Transport patient.
Hemorrhage	Bleeding at site of venous access device or from broken device	Apply pressure to site. Clamp venous access device and treat for shock.

7. Do not apply ointment unless you are removing the catheter.
8. Cover with a gauze or transparent dressing (according to local medical direction protocol).

CRITICAL THINKING
Will it always be possible to identify the catheter as the source of sepsis while on the scene?

Hemorrhage. Bleeding at the site of a VAD should be controlled by applying gentle, direct pressure with aseptic technique. These patients need to be transported for physician evaluation. Blood loss from a broken or dislodged VAD can be significant. (Medical direction may recommend that the damaged catheter be clamped.) If blood loss is severe, the patient should be treated for hemorrhagic shock.

Hemodynamic Compromise. Hemodynamic compromise may result from circulatory overload or embolus. Circulatory overload can develop from too much IV fluid being delivered too fast. Signs and symptoms of circulatory overload include a rise in blood pressure, distended neck veins, pulmonary congestion (crackles and wheezes), and dyspnea. If circulatory overload is suspected, the paramedic should do the following:

1. Slow the infusion to a keep-open rate.
2. Provide high-concentration oxygen and monitor oxygen saturation.
3. Elevate the patient's head.
4. Maintain body warmth. This will promote peripheral circulation. It also will ease the stress on the central veins.
5. Monitor vital signs.
6. Consult with medical direction for patient management and disposition.

CRITICAL THINKING
What drug(s) may the physician order if this happens?

Displacement of a surgically implanted catheter or port is rare. However, an embolus that occurs from air, thrombus, or plastic or catheter tip entering the circulation can develop (Box 52-4). Signs and symptoms of an embolus include hypotension; cyanosis; weak, rapid pulse; and loss of consciousness. A patient suspected of having an embolism should be managed as follows (described in Chapter 14):

1. Stop the IV infusion.
2. Position the patient on the left side with the head down (in an attempt to keep the embolus in the right side of the heart).
3. Administer high-concentration oxygen and monitor oxygen saturation.
4. Notify medical direction.

BOX 52-4 Causes of Embolus Formation

Intravenous fluid containers that run dry
Air in intravenous tubing
Loose connections in catheter tubing
Catheter tears and breakage

Thrombus
Clot formation from inactivity or stasis

Plastic or Catheter Tip Migration
Plastic or catheter fragment from tugging or shearing forces
Wire from central line placement

If a plastic or catheter tip embolism is suspected, medical direction may advise that a constricting band be applied above the VAD site. This should stop the embolus from further movement.

Obstruction of the Vascular Device. An indwelling vascular device may become obstructed and disrupt the flow of fluids and medications. When this occurs, immediate intervention is needed. The device must be cleared by irrigation or the administration of fibrinolytic agents. The paramedic should always consult with medical direction before attempting to clear an obstruction from a VAD.

NOTE
Accessing a VAD requires special needles and adapters. Only paramedics with special training and authorization from medical direction should attempt to access these devices.

Flushing and Irrigation. Vascular access devices and medication ports need regular irrigation with normal saline and/or *heparin*. The solution used depends on the type of VAD (Table 52-3). The frequency of irrigation depends on the specific device and on the frequency of medication administration. If a VAD is obstructed, the paramedic should consult with medical direction and follow these steps[6]:

1. Explain the procedure to the patient.
2. Establish a sterile field and use strict aseptic technique.
3. Prepare prescribed irrigation solutions (normal saline or normal saline and *heparin*).
4. Clean the injection cap(s) with an antiseptic and alcohol wipe (per protocol) and allow to air-dry.
5. Release the clamp from the catheter (if present).
6. Irrigate the lumen with an appropriate volume of solution using a 10-mL syringe (no faster than 0.5 mL/sec). If resistance is persistent, stop the irrigation, or the catheter may rupture. *Note:* The paramedic must never try to force or dislodge a clot or other obstruction. Fibrinolytic agents may be required. The application of force could dislodge the obstruction and cause it to enter the circulatory system.

TABLE 52-3 Irrigation for Vascular Access Devices

Device	Syringe Size (mL)	Solution	Amount (mL)
Peripheral access devices	3	Heparin flush solution 10 units/mL	2.5-3.0
Central Venous Access Devices			
Groshong	10	0.9% sodium chloride (normal saline)	5; 10-20 following blood draws
MediPorts	10	Sodium chloride 0.9% (normal saline)	10
		Heparin 100 units/mL	5

From Terry J: *Intravenous therapy: clinical principles and practice*, Philadelphia, 1995, Saunders.

7. Aspirate blood back into the syringe; this removes clots or fibrin sheaths.
8. Flush with normal saline (10 to 20 mL) to clear the system.
9. Use a heparin lock if necessary (e.g., Broviac, Hickman, or peripherally inserted central catheter).
10. Clamp catheter if needed.
11. Loop the catheter with the cap pointing upward on the dressing. Secure with tape.
12. Properly dispose of all equipment.

Anticoagulant Therapy. At times, a medication port or other vascular device may require declotting with fibrinolytic agents (e.g., tissue plasminogen activator [t-PA]). Flushing with fibrinolytic agents should be performed by specialized personnel. An x-ray may be needed before administration of these agents.

Other Complications. If you are unable to aspirate blood from the central VAD, or the patient or family reports that the length of the catheter that was visible has changed, do not administer fluid or drugs through it. The patient will need transport for further evaluation.

A decrease in the length of catheter coupled with a sudden onset of tachycardia can mean that the catheter has moved into the right atrium. If the patient hears bubbling in the ear when the catheter is flushed, or has a sudden earache on the side of the body where the catheter is inserted, the catheter may have advanced into the jugular vein. In all of these situations, an x-ray will be needed to determine the location of the catheter.

Catheter Damage. A damaged (e.g., cracked or torn) catheter can allow fluids or medications to infiltrate into the surrounding tissues and lead to an air embolism. Signs and symptoms of a damaged catheter include leaking fluid, complaint of a burning sensation, or swollen and tender

skin near the insertion site. If catheter damage is suspected, the infusion should be stopped immediately. The catheter should be clamped between the crack or tear in the catheter and the patient. These patients are managed with high-concentration oxygen and pulse oximetry, IV access through a peripheral vein, and transport for physician evaluation. A patient who develops an altered level of consciousness (indicating a possible air embolism) should be positioned on the left side. The head should be slightly lowered. This positioning will help to prevent the embolism from traveling to the brain.[7]

Gastrointestinal/Genitourinary Crisis

More than 500,000 patients with diseases of the digestive or genitourinary system are discharged to home health care each year.[1] Some of these patients have medical devices such as urinary catheters or urostomies, indwelling nutritional support devices (e.g., percutaneous endoscopic gastrostomy tube or gastrostomy tube), colostomies, and nasogastric tubes (Box 52-5). Acute interventions that may be required for these patients can result from urinary tract infection (UTI), **urosepsis,** urinary retention, and problems with gastric emptying or feeding.

URINARY TRACT INFECTION, UROSEPSIS, AND URINARY RETENTION

Urinary tract infection is common. It occurs in all age groups and both genders (see Chapter 30). The organisms most often associated with UTI are gram-negative organisms normally found in the gastrointestinal tract. These include *Escherichia coli*, *Klebsiella*, *Proteus*, *Enterobacter*, and *Pseudomonas*. These frequently are introduced from the hands of health care personnel at the time of bladder catheterization.[7] (About 75% of UTIs are the result of urological instrumentation. Sterile technique during these procedures

BOX 52-5 Medical Therapy Found in the Home Setting for Patients With Gastrointestinal/Genitourinary Disease

Devices for Gastric/Intestinal Emptying or Feeding
Colostomy
Feeding tube
Nasogastric tube
Percutaneous endoscopic gastrostomy tubes, jejunostomy tubes, gastrostomy tubes

Devices for the Urinary Tract
External urinary catheters (e.g., condom catheter or Texas catheter)
Indwelling urinary catheter (e.g., Foley catheter or coudé catheter)
Surgical urinary catheters (e.g., suprapubic catheters)
Urostomy

is crucial.) Other factors that increase the risk of UTI include the following:

- Obstructions (e.g., urethral strictures, calculi, tumors, or blood clots)
- Trauma (e.g., abdominal injury, ruptured bladder, or local trauma related to sexual activity)
- Congenital anomalies (e.g., polycystic kidneys, horseshoe kidney, or spina bifida)
- Abdominal or gynecological surgery
- Acute or chronic renal failure
- Immunocompromised state (e.g., patients with human immunodeficiency virus or older adults)
- Postpartum state
- Aging changes, particularly in women

If UTI is allowed to progress, it may lead to septic complications (urosepsis). This disease is managed with antibiotics.

Urinary Retention. Urinary retention may result from urethral stricture, inflammation, enlarged prostate, central nervous system dysfunction, foreign body obstruction, and use of certain drugs, such as parasympatholytic or anticholinergic agents. These patients need to be evaluated by a physician to determine the cause of the retention. If the cause is not easily correctable, the patient may need to be hospitalized. Some patients may require **bladder catheterization** with an indwelling Foley catheter device. (See the Appendix, Advanced Practice Procedures in Critical Care.)

CRITICAL THINKING

What measure should you take to protect yourself legally when inserting a Foley catheter into a patient in a home?

PROBLEMS WITH GASTRIC EMPTYING OR FEEDING

Gastric tubes used in the home health care setting are devices that are inserted into the stomach or intestines (Figure 52-6). They are used to remove fluids and gas by suction or gravity, to instill irrigation solutions or medications, and to administer enteral feedings (through *feeding tubes*) (Table 52-4). Two common problems with gastric tubes are aspiration of gastric contents and malfunction of gastric devices.

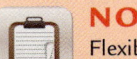

NOTE

Flexible feeding tubes (such as the Dobhoff feeding tube) are commonly used in patients who cannot take nourishment by mouth. The feeding tubes may be inserted orally or nasally so that the tip of the tube is placed in either the stomach or the duodenum. These tubes generally have a weighted tungsten tip and have a guidewire to prevent them from curling up in the back of the patient's throat.

Aspiration of Gastric Contents. Aspiration of gastric contents may occur in the home health care patient as a result of a nonpatent gastric tube, improper nutritional support via a feeding tube, or patient positioning with

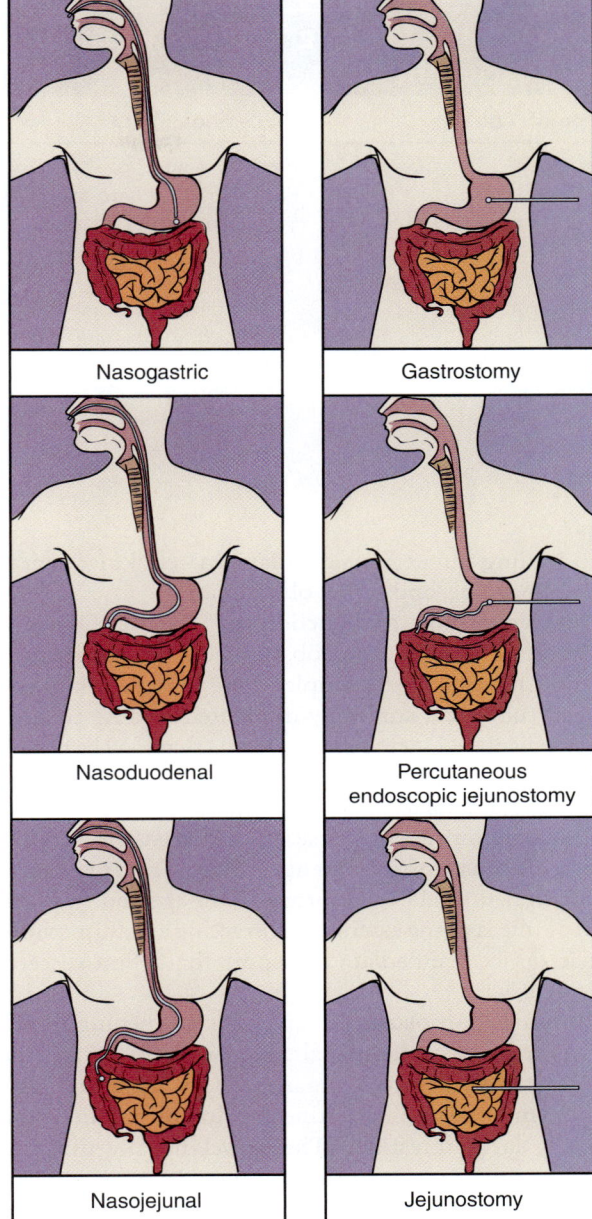

FIGURE 52-6 Tube feeding sites.

these medical devices. The patients at greatest risk for aspiration of tube feedings are those who:

- Are unconscious
- Are confused
- Are seriously debilitated
- Are older adults
- Have tracheostomies or large-bore feeding tubes
- Have impaired gag reflexes
- Cannot sit upright

The paramedic should monitor patients with feeding tubes closely for signs of increased respiratory effort. Lung sounds should be clear on auscultation. Respiratory difficulty or tachypnea may indicate developing aspiration pneumonitis. Other problems that can occur in patients

TABLE 52-4 Feeding Tubes: Types and Placement

Type of Tube	Placement
Nasogastric	Passed via nose into stomach
Nasointestinal	Passed via nose into intestine
Esophagostomy	Passed into esophagus through a surgically created opening in anterior neck
Gastrostomy	Passed directly into stomach through an opening created in abdominal wall
Jejunostomy, percutaneous endoscopic gastrostomy	Passed into jejunum through an opening created in abdominal wall

TABLE 52-5 Managing Tube-Feeding Problems*

Complication	Interventions
Aspiration of gastric secretions	Discontinue feeding immediately.
	Perform tracheal suction of aspirated contents if possible.
	Notify physician.
	Check tube placement before feeding to prevent complications.
Tube obstruction	Flush tube with warm water. If necessary, replace tube.
	Flush tube with 50 mL of water after each feeding to remove excess sticky formula, which could occlude tube.
Nasal or pharyngeal irritation or necrosis	Provide frequent oral hygiene using mouthwash or lemon-glycerin swabs. Use petroleum jelly on cracked lips.
	Change position of tube. If necessary, replace tube.
Vomiting, bloating, diarrhea, or cramps	Reduce flow rate.
	Warm formula.
	For 30 minutes after feeding, position patient on right side with head elevated to facilitate gastric emptying.
	Notify physician. Physician may want to reduce amount of formula being given during each feeding.
Constipation	Provide additional fluids if patient can tolerate them.
	Administer a bulk-forming laxative.
	Increase fruit, vegetable, or sugar content of feeding.

*This table lists some interventions that the nurse, paramedic, patient, or caregiver may use to solve home tube-feeding problems.

with feeding tubes include diarrhea, choking, irritable bowel syndrome, and bowel obstruction.

Obstruction or Malfunction of Gastric Devices. A gastric device may become obstructed or malfunction for different reasons. For example, there may be a kinked or clogged tube, or a surgically implanted feeding tube may become displaced. Acute interventions that may be required include unkinking a tube, irrigating a clogged tube, and reinserting a displaced tube (per medical direction; Table 52-5). When transporting a patient with a gastric device, the paramedic must ensure patient comfort. The device should be positioned to allow for proper drainage and to prevent reflux. Time is of the essence in correcting a malfunctioning gastric device. Immediate transport for definitive care is indicated.

Ostomies. An **ostomy** is an artificial opening into the urinary tract, gastrointestinal tract, or trachea. An ostomy may be temporary or permanent. (An **ileostomy** is an opening into the small intestine. A **colostomy** is an opening into the large intestine.) The bowel usually discharges liquid or solid feces into the bag (pouch) once or twice a day; the bag then is changed. Potential complications associated with ostomies include infection, hemorrhage, obstruction, and stoma problems (e.g., necrosis, retraction, stenosis, and prolapse).

Colostomy irrigation, ostomy care, and pouch changes usually are performed for home health care patients by the patients themselves, family members, and home health care practitioners. These procedures require special training. They usually are not considered an acute intervention for paramedic practice. Bowel perforation and significant fluid/electrolyte imbalances may accidentally occur from colostomy irrigation performed by the patient or caregiver.

ASSESSMENT AND MANAGEMENT OF PATIENTS WITH GASTROINTESTINAL/GENITOURINARY CRISIS

The paramedic should evaluate a patient with gastrointestinal/genitourinary complaints by obtaining a focused history and performing a physical examination to determine the need for immediate transport for physician evaluation. Depending on the patient's chief complaint, the physical examination may include assessment for the following:

- Abdominal distention
- Abdominal pain
- Aspiration
- Fever
- Intestinal obstruction
- Peritonitis
- Urinary tract infection
- Urinary retention

Acute Infections

More than 160,000 patients with infectious and parasitic diseases are discharged to home health care in the United States each year.[1] Home health care patients with acute infections have an increased death rate from sepsis and severe peripheral infections. They also may have a decreased ability to perceive pain or perform self-care. Patients with chronic diseases, poor nutrition, or an inability to perform self-care are at increased risk for infection and impaired healing. Conditions that may result in the need for acute interventions in the home health care population include the following[8]:

- Airway infections in the immunocompromised patient
- Delayed healing and increased peripheral infection from poor peripheral perfusion
- Skin breakdown and peripheral infections from immobility or sedentary lifestyle
- Infection and sepsis from implanted medical devices
- Wounds and incisions
- Abscesses
- Cellulitis

OPEN WOUNDS

Patients with open wounds who are discharged to home health care may have a variety of dressings, wound packings, and drains that permit drainage of fluid or air. They also may have a variety of wound closure devices (Box 52-6). (Dressings, packings, and wound closure devices can become contaminated; drains can become occluded or displaced.) Wound healing greatly depends on wound management. The patient must be made aware of the importance of taking all prescribed medications (especially antibiotics). The patient also should be informed of the importance of completing all wound care procedures. Wound repair generally is believed to be enhanced by the following:

- Moist environment
- Wound bed free of necrotic tissue, eschar, and environmental contamination or infection
- Adequate blood supply to meet metabolic demands for tissue generation
- Sufficient oxygen and nutrition for cellular metabolism and tissue generation

GENERAL PRINCIPLES IN WOUND CARE MANAGEMENT

Wound care requires assessment of the wound and the surrounding tissues. It also requires evaluation for infection or sepsis. General principles in wound care management include an assessment for the following[9]:

1. Location and size of wound.
2. Color of the wound bed. A red or pink granular wound bed indicates healing. A green, yellow, or black wound bed suggests infection or necrosis (tissue death).
3. Drainage. Clear or blood-tinged drainage is common in a healing wound. Green or yellow drainage suggests infection.
4. Wound odor. A sweet smell may indicate decay. A foul smell may indicate infection.
5. Surrounding skin. The paramedic should assess the skin for redness, inflammation, or signs of tissue breakdown. If the dressing is wet or contaminated, the paramedic should change it after wound evaluation. Medical direction may advise cleaning the wound with normal saline and/or antiseptic solution before redressing it. The debridement of necrotic tissue may be required. Mechanical debridement is achieved by gently rubbing the tissue with a gauze pad moistened with sterile, normal saline. Some patients may need transport for physician evaluation if severe infection or sepsis is suspected.

Maternal/Child Conditions

In the early 1990s, many insurance companies began paying only for 24-hour hospital stays for uncomplicated vaginal childbirth. (These sometimes were called "drive-by deliveries.") In the wake of complaints about inadequate care, states began passing laws in 1995 and 1996. These laws required insurance to pay for 52-hour stays. A similar federal law was passed in 1996. This law took effect in January 1998 and became a Final Rule in 2009. Under this law, health plans must cover hospital stays of at least 48 hours for women who give birth naturally and 96 hours following a cesarean delivery.[10] Problems that may be

---

BOX 52-6 Sampling of Wound Care Devices Found in Home Health Care Patients

Dressings and Wound Packing Material

Combination dressings
Cotton dressings (gauze)
Exudate absorptive dressings
Foam dressings
Hydrocolloid dressings
Hydrogel dressings
Hydrophilic powder dressings
Impregnated cotton dressings
Paste bandages
Transparent film (adhesive or nonadhesive)

Drains

Jackson-Pratt drains
Penrose drains

Wound Closure Techniques

Skin adhesive
Staples
Sutures
Tape
Wires

encountered when these patient groups return to the home health care setting include the following:

- Postpartum pathophysiologies (e.g., hemorrhage, infection, and pulmonary embolism)
- Postpartum depression
- Septicemia in the newborn
- Infantile apnea
- Failure to thrive
- Sudden infant death syndrome

POSTPARTUM PATHOPHYSIOLOGIES

Postpartum pathophysiologies include hemorrhage, infection, and pulmonary embolism. (Acute interventions for these patients are presented in Chapter 46) Postpartum hemorrhage occurs in about 5% of all deliveries. It frequently takes place within the first few hours after delivery, but it can be delayed up to 6 weeks.[7] Causes of postpartum hemorrhage include incomplete contraction of uterine muscle fibers, retained pieces of placenta or membranes in the uterus, and vaginal or cervical tears during delivery (which are rare).

Postpartum infection affects 2% to 8% of all pregnancies.[7] (The most common infection is endometritis.) The condition occurs when bacteria grow and invade the uterus or other tissues along the birth canal. The symptoms usually develop on the second or third day after delivery. Fever and abdominal pain are the most common signs of infection.

Pulmonary embolism during pregnancy, labor, or the postpartum period is one of the most common causes of maternal death. The embolus often results from a blood clot in the pelvic circulation; it more commonly is associated with cesarean section than with vaginal delivery.

CRITICAL THINKING
A mother is having a postpartum complication that requires urgent transport. What will you do with the baby if they are home alone?

POSTPARTUM DEPRESSION

Postpartum depression affects 10% to 15% of mothers. The depression most likely is caused by a combination of sudden hormonal changes and psychological and environmental factors. The disease can be a short-lived attack of mild depression ("baby blues). Or, in contrast, it can manifest as a depressive illness that requires in-hospital supervision. Risk factors for postpartum depression include the following:

- Adverse socioeconomic conditions
- Anxiety
- Complicated pregnancy or delivery
- Fetal complications
- Low self-esteem
- Poor marital adjustment

- Previous episodes of depression
- Recent life stressors

Recognizing and treating postpartum depression is important. The depression can interfere with the bonding between the mother and infant. It also can seriously affect the mother's ability to care for her newborn (Box 52-7). Many women with postpartum depression fear they will harm their babies. They often feel ashamed and guilty for these feelings. Sensitivity to the possibility of depression is crucial and necessary for successful diagnosis and treatment. (Interventions for depression are presented in Chapter 35)

SEPTICEMIA IN THE NEWBORN

As described in Chapter 47, healthy newborns are vulnerable to several conditions that can require hospital treatment. Examples include jaundice that results from physiological immaturity of bilirubin metabolism, dehydration that can lead to serious electrolyte abnormalities, and sepsis. In addition, neonates are highly susceptible to infection because of diminished nonspecific (inflammatory) and specific (humoral) immunity.

Septicemia in the newborn usually is caused by group B streptococci, *Listeria monocytogenes,* or gram-negative enteric organisms (especially *Escherichia coli*).[11] Signs and symptoms of sepsis may be minimal and nonspecific. ("In the newborn, anything can be a sign of anything.") Examples of signs and symptoms of sepsis in the newborn include the following:

BOX 52-7 Signs and Symptoms of Postpartum Depression

Anxiety
Change of appetite (loss of appetite or overindulgence)
Desire to leave or feelings of being trapped
Difficulty making decisions
Excessive concern or lack of concern for baby
Fantasies of disaster or bizarre fears
Fatigue or exhaustion
Fear of harming self or baby
Forgetfulness or memory loss
Hatred of spouse, self, or baby
Hopelessness
Hostility
Inability to care for baby
Increased alcohol consumption or other drug use
Irritability
Lack of interest in previously enjoyed activities
Lack of sexual interest
Loss of hope
Panic attacks
Rapid mood swings
Severe sleep disturbance
Unexplainable crying (in joy or sadness)

- Temperature instability
- Respiratory distress
- Apnea
- Cyanosis
- Gastrointestinal changes (e.g., vomiting, distention, diarrhea, and anorexia)
- Central nervous system features (e.g., irritability, lethargy, and weak suck)

Risk factors for sepsis include prematurity, prolonged rupture of membranes, and chorioamnionitis (an inflammatory reaction in the amniotic membranes caused by bacterial viruses in the amniotic fluid). The diagnosis generally is confirmed after physician evaluation by a positive blood, urine, or cerebrospinal fluid culture.

INFANTILE APNEA

Infantile apnea is defined by the American Academy of Pediatrics as "an unexplained episode of cessation of breathing for 20 seconds or longer, or a shorter respiratory pause associated with bradycardia, cyanosis, pallor, and/or marked hypotonia (diminished tone)."[12] Apnea often reflects the immature respiratory control centers in some infants. Other causes of infantile apnea include the following[13]:

- Metabolic derangements (e.g., hypoglycemia, hypocalcemia, or hypothermia)
- Infection (e.g., sepsis, pneumonia, or meningitis)
- Central nervous system damage (e.g., hemorrhage, hypoxic injury, or seizures)
- Pulmonary disorders (e.g., respiratory distress, hyaline membrane disease, pneumonia, obstruction, or upper respiratory tract abnormalities)
- Intentional poisoning (child abuse)

The paramedic must assess the presence of apnea carefully and document it. Most infants with the diagnosis of apnea will be hospitalized and observed closely. They are observed using electronic apnea monitoring devices. These devices detect changes in thoracic or abdominal movement and heart rate. Managing apnea in these patients may include the home health care use of apnea monitors, oscillating waterbeds, and CPAP with supplemental oxygen. Some patients also may be prescribed respiratory stimulants (e.g., doxapram or methylxanthines).

FAILURE TO THRIVE

Failure to thrive is an abnormally slow rate of growth and development of an infant. It results from conditions that interfere with normal metabolism, appetite, and activity. Causative factors include the following:

- Chromosomal abnormalities
- Major organ system defects that lead to deficiency or malfunction
- Systemic disease or acute illness
- Physical deprivation (primarily malnutrition related to insufficient breast milk, poverty, or poor knowledge of nutrition)
- Various psychosocial factors (e.g., maternal deprivation)

SHOW ME THE EVIDENCE

Researchers in Los Angeles County conducted this retrospective cohort outcome study to assess causes of 9-1-1 activation for apparent life-threatening events (ALTEs) in infants less than 12 months of age. In these cases the call was initiated for apnea or change in skin color or muscle tone. The mean age of the 60 infants enrolled was 3 months, and 83.3% of the infants did not appear to be in distress. However, the following conditions were identified in the overall group: pneumonia or bronchiolitis (12%), seizure (8%), sepsis (7%), intracranial hemorrhage (3%), bacterial meningitis (2%), dehydration (2%) and severe anemia (2%). Of the study group, two patients were not transported and one was subsequently admitted for failure to thrive. Of those transported to the ED, one was discharged and later readmitted with an intracranial hemorrhage related to child abuse. The authors conclude that when EMS is called for an ALTE the infant should be transported for a thorough medical evaluation.

From Stratton S, Taves A, Lewis R, et al: Apparent life-threatening events in infants: high risk in the out-of-hospital environment, *Ann Emerg Med* 43(6):711-717, 2004, doi: 10.1016/j.annemergmed.2003.10.038.

Failure to thrive can result in permanent and irreversible retardation of physical, mental, or social development. Any suspicions of failure to thrive should be documented carefully. The paramedic should report these suspicions to medical direction as well.

WELL-BABY CARE

Some infants and children have periodic health assessments through well-baby care programs. These programs specialize in medical supervision and services for healthy infants. Well-baby care promotes optimal physical, emotional, and intellectual growth and development. Such health care measures include the following:

- Routine immunizations to prevent disease
- Screening procedures for early detection and treatment of illness
- Parental guidance and instruction in proper nutrition, injury prevention, and specific care and rearing of the child at various stages of development

The recommended preventative health care schedule for children who are developing normally is monthly for the first 6 months of life, every 2 months until 1 year of age, every 3 months during the second year, and every 6 months during the third year, followed by annual visits. Well-baby care may be provided in a clinic ("well-baby clinics"), a physician's office, the office of a community health nursing center, or a school. Nurses or nurse practitioners often provide the care in these programs.

Hospice/Palliative Care

In 2006 **hospice** care served more than 1 million patients throughout the United States.[3] Hospice services include supportive social, emotional, and spiritual services for the

---

BOX 52-8 Essential Elements of a Palliative Care Program

Palliative care is an accepted specialty of medicine and nursing that concentrates on the total care of patients suffering from any form of terminal illness. Its development, as part of the health care services, is acknowledgment that dying is a normal consequence of living. The support of health professionals and use of modern medical technology can relieve much of the distress normally associated with dying. Essential elements of a palliative care program are the following:

1. The program involves the coordination of care for patients with a terminal illness, at home or in hospital, by a distinct service.
2. The unit of care is the patient and the patient's family, who have the right to make choices and decisions based on an understanding of the illness and to have those decisions respected.
3. The care is provided by an interdisciplinary team.
4. The care is coordinated and delivered by specifically selected and trained nurses.
5. The service is directed by a physician.
6. The emphasis is on control of symptoms, be they physical, social, or emotional.
7. The services are available on a 24 hours a day, 7 days a week, on-call basis.
8. The program must be sensitive to differences in faith and culture and must incorporate the patient's beliefs into decisions on his or her care.
9. Following the death of a patient, the program should ensure that grief support is available for the family. This may be provided by the program itself or by other community services.
10. There is a system of structured staff support and communication.
11. The program is integrated and coordinated with other services, and continuity of care for the patient is provided.
12. Evaluation of the program and its services must be regular. This evaluation may extend into the area of research.
13. The program will provide education for its own staff, other health care providers, and the public.

From Health Canada, Minister of Public Works and Government Services: *Essential elements of a palliative care program,* 2000, Ottawa, Canada.

---

terminally ill. They also provide support for the patient's family. Hospice care relies on the combined knowledge and skill of a team of professionals. This team includes physicians, nurses, medical social workers, therapists, counselors, chaplains, and volunteers. These persons work together to provide a personal plan of care for each patient and family. The need for hospices likely will continue to rise because of an aging population, the increasing number of persons with acquired immunodeficiency syndrome, and rising health care costs. Medical professionals and the general public are more frequently choosing hospice care over other forms of health care for terminally ill patients. The holistic, patient-family, in-home–centered philosophy is one reason for this.

PALLIATIVE CARE

Palliative care is a unique form of health care. It mainly is directed at providing relief to terminally ill persons through symptom management and pain management. (Palliative care also is called *comfort care*.) This specialty focuses on the needs of the patient and family when a life-threatening illness such as cancer or acquired immunodeficiency syndrome has reached the terminal stage. A chief goal of palliative care is to improve the quality of a person's life as death approaches and to help patients and their families move toward this reality with comfort, reassurance, and strength. Palliative care is not focused on death; it is about specialized care for the living. Well-rounded palliative care programs also address mental health and spiritual needs. Palliative care may be delivered in hospice, home care settings, and hospitals. Medical needs vary depending on the disease that is leading toward death. Thus specialized palliative care programs exist for common conditions such as cancer and acquired immunodeficiency syndrome (Box 52-8).

Emergency medical services and medical direction should work closely with the families and physicians of terminally ill patients in private homes and hospice programs so that they will make the best use of the EMS system. (For instance, they will know when to call 9-1-1.) Even though resuscitation may not be indicated, paramedics may be needed to manage pain, treat acute medical illness or traumatic injury, and provide transport to a hospital. If the patient is not to receive medical intervention to prolong life, the paramedic should provide measures of comfort to the patient and emotional support to family members and loved ones (see Chapter 2).

HOSPICE CARE IN THE HOME SETTING

A patient receiving hospice care may be receiving medication delivery for the relief of pain (e.g., narcotic infusion devices). The patient also will have medical and legal documents such as do not resuscitate orders and advance directives (see Chapter 6). The paramedic should discuss any concerns about effective pain management, overmedication, or interpreting medical or legal documents with medical direction (Box 52-9). It is important to note that not all patients who receive hospice care have "Do Not Resuscitate" orders.

BOX 52-9 Bill of Rights and Responsibilities for Terminally Ill Patients

A. Personal Dignity and Privacy

1. You have the right to considerate, respectful service and care, with full recognition of your personal dignity and individuality, without regard to gender, age, ethnicity, income level, lifestyle, educational background, or spiritual philosophy.
2. You have the right to be dressed as you wish and not to be disrobed or uncovered any longer than necessary for your care.
3. You have the right to privacy and the assurance of confidentiality when receiving care, to refuse visitors or persons not directly involved in your care, and to choose who will receive information about your condition.
4. You have the right to request the presence of a person of your choice during interactions with health care professionals.
5. You have the right to experience all emotions, including anger, sadness, confusion, guilt, depression, impatience, fear, and loss.
6. You have the right to have your end-of-life choices respected by health care professionals, including continuing or discontinuing treatment or requesting medications to self-administer for a hastened death.
7. You have the right to die with your loved ones present and to request the presence of a health care professional, if desired.
8. You have the responsibility to treat your caregiver with respect and to follow their directions when consistent with your wishes.
9. You have the responsibility to make certain that your right to privacy and confidentiality is clearly understood by all parties involved in your care and to communicate to your health care providers when you feel that your rights to privacy and confidentiality are in jeopardy.

B. Informed Participation

1. You have the right to honest, accurate, and understandable information about your current diagnosis and prognosis; the recommended treatment and what it is expected to do; the possibility of success; and the possible risks of complications and side effects, including the probability of their occurrence.
2. You have the right to be informed about alternative forms of treatment, including hospice and home care, and to participate in all decisions affecting your care.

3. You have the right to request and receive a second opinion. When curative care is no longer indicated or desired, you have the right to access palliative care, including pain medication in whatever dosage or schedule you deem necessary to alleviate pain and suffering, even at the risk of hastening death.
4. You have the right to make your own decisions regarding what constitutes your human dignity, as long as you are mentally competent and continue to have basic decision-making capacity. You will be considered mentally competent if you can understand the nature of your condition, the treatment alternatives available, and the likely outcomes of treatment versus nontreatment and can accept responsibility for your decisions.
5. You have the right to access information in your medical record and to know if your health care providers believe that your condition or course of disease will result in death. This information may be needed to make informed decisions about your future.
6. You have the right to forgo eating and drinking naturally in order to permit the process of dying to proceed unencumbered.
7. You have the right and responsibility to complete a directive to physicians (living will).
8. You have the right and responsibility to execute a durable power of attorney for health care so that someone you choose can make health care decisions for you, if needed.

C. Competent Care

1. You have the right to competent medical, nursing, and social services care.
2. You have the right to choose your personal physician and to change your physician at any time.
3. You have the right to know who is responsible for coordinating and supervising your care and to know how to contact that person.
4. You have the right to be informed about who owns and controls the agency or facility involved with your care and the right to referral to institutions, facilities, and practitioners who can provide the care you need.
5. You have the responsibility to choose a primary care physician who is able and willing to carry out your wishes.
6. You have the responsibility to communicate your end-of-life wishes to family, friends, and health care providers.

From Compassion in Dying Federation, Portland, Ore.

SUMMARY

- About 25% of home health care patients have heart and circulatory diseases as their primary diagnosis. Other common diagnoses of home health care patients include cancer, diabetes, and hypertension. Typical EMS calls to a home health care setting may include respiratory failure, cardiac decompensation, septic complications, equipment malfunction, and other medical problems.

- After arrival at the scene of a home health care patient, the scene size-up should include standard precautions, elements of scene safety, and environmental setting. The initial assessment should focus on illness or injury that poses a threat to life. The paramedic should take appropriate measures as indicated.

- Patients with diseases of the respiratory system being cared for at home are at increased risk for airway infections. In addition, the progression of their illnesses may lead to difficulty breathing, making current support equipment inadequate.

- Assessment findings that may require acute interventions in patients with VADs include infection, hemorrhage, hemodynamic compromise from circulatory overload or embolus, obstruction of the vascular device, and catheter damage with leakage of medication.

- Patients with diseases of the digestive or genitourinary system may have medical devices such as urinary catheters or urostomies, indwelling nutritional support devices (e.g., percutaneous endoscopic gastrostomy tube or gastrostomy tube), colostomies, and nasogastric tubes. Acute interventions required for these patients can result from UTI, urosepsis, urinary retention, and problems with gastric emptying or feeding.

- Home health care patients with acute infections have an increased death rate from sepsis and severe peripheral infections. Many also have a decreased ability to perceive pain or perform self-care.

- Maternal/child conditions that one may encounter in the home health care setting during the postpartum period include postpartum hemorrhage, infection, pulmonary embolism, postpartum depression, septicemia in the newborn, infantile apnea, and failure to thrive.

- Hospice services include supportive social, emotional, and spiritual services for the terminally ill. They also provide support for a patient's family. Palliative care is directed mainly at providing relief to a terminally ill person. They do this through symptom and pain management.

REFERENCES

1. National Association of Home Care: *Basic statistics about home care: updated 2008*, Washington, DC, 2009, The Association.
2. *Home health care: history and philosophy*, Kansas City, Kan, 1997, Spectrum Home Health Agency.
3. National Association for Home Care & Hospice: *Basic statistics about home care: updated 2008*, Washington, DC, 2009, The Association.
4. Department of Health and Human Services: *CMS overview, Centers for Medicare & Medicaid Services*, www.cms.gov/QualityInitiativesGenInfo/, accessed 10-24-10.
5. National Heart, Lung and Blood Institute, U.S. Department of Health and Human Services, National Institutes of Health: *Sleep apnea*, www.nhlbi.nih.gov/health/dci/Diseases/SleepApnea/SleepApnea_WhatIs.html, accessed 10-24-10.
6. Rice R: *Home health nursing procedures*, ed 2, St Louis, 1995, Mosby.
7. Rosen P, Barkin R: *Emergency medicine: concepts and clinical practice*, ed 7, St Louis, 2010, Mosby.
8. National Highway Traffic Safety Administration: *The National EMS Education Standards*, Washington, DC, 2009, U.S. Department of Transportation/National Highway Traffic Safety Administration, DOT.
9. Rice R: *Handbook of home health nursing procedures*, St Louis, 1995, Mosby.
10. Federal Register: EBSA final rules, rules and regulations, *Fed Regis* 73(203), 10-20-08.
11. McKinney ES, Ashwill J, James SR, et al: *Maternal-child nursing*, Philadelphia, 2000, Saunders.
12. Committee on Fetus and Newborn, American Academy of Pediatrics: *Apnea, sudden infant death syndrome, and home monitoring*, *Pediatrics* 111(4 pt 1):914-917, 2003.
13. Rocker JA, Israel J: *Pediatrics, apnea*, http://emedicine.medscape.com/article/800032-overview, accessed 10-24-10.

SUGGESTED READINGS

Hagan K: LVADs help mend a broken heart, *Nurse Pract* 35(6):29-36, 2010.

Patee A, Goss J: *Pediatric airway maintenance: choosing between the home ventilator & manual ventilation*, *Jems.com*, 2009, www.jems.com/article/patient-care/pediatric-airway-maintenance-c, accessed 5-31-10.

Stuban SL: Home mechanical ventilation, *Am J Nurs* 110(5):63-67, 2010.

PART ELEVEN

EMS Operations

53 Ground and Air Ambulance Operations

OBJECTIVES

Upon completion of this chapter, the paramedic student will be able to:

1. List standards that govern ambulance performance and specifications.
2. Discuss the tracking of equipment, supplies, and maintenance on an ambulance.
3. Outline the considerations for appropriate stationing of ambulances.
4. Describe measures that can influence safe operation of an ambulance.
5. Identify aeromedical crew members and training.
6. Describe the appropriate use of aeromedical services in the prehospital setting.

KEY TERMS

ambulance A generic term that describes the various land-based emergency vehicles used by emergency medical services (EMS) personnel, including basic and advanced life support units, paramedic units, mobile intensive care units, and others.

fend-off position Positioning the ambulance about 50 feet in front of the scene for safety; diverts and averts oncoming traffic.

KKK A-1822E standards The national standards that provide the foundation of uniformity for the design of ambulance vehicles.

landing zone An area prepared for the landing of an aircraft; generally 100 by 100 feet.

type I ambulance An ambulance design based on the chassis-cabs of light duty pickup trucks.

type II ambulance An ambulance design based on modern passenger/cargo vans.

type III ambulance An ambulance design based on chassis-cabs of light duty vans.

T*he modern ambulance is more than just a vehicle for transporting a patient to the hospital. Today's ambulance is a well-equipped and efficiently organized vehicle or aircraft. It has advanced communications and technology that bring needed medical supplies, personnel, and advanced life support care to the emergency scene.*

AMBULANCE STANDARDS

In 1968 the National Academy of Sciences–National Research Council (NAS-NRC) recommended ambulance design standards. These standards included the size, shape, color, electrical systems, and emergency equipment. They led to the development of the federal specifications that

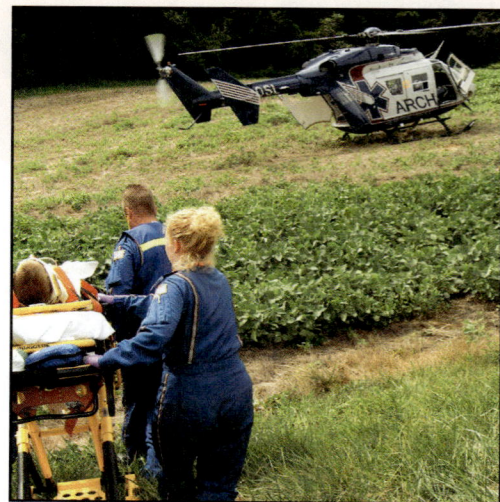

(Courtesy Ray Kemp. St. Charles, Mo.)

many states now use as ambulance standards. The national standards developed by NAS-NRC and the National Highway Traffic Safety Administration (NHTSA) are known as the **KKK A-1822E standards**. These standards and their revisions provide the basis for uniformity in the design of ambulance vehicles. They cover the three basic ambulance designs: type I, type II, and type III (Figure 53-1). Also, because of the extra weight of equipment used in rescue and emergency care and the space needed for this equipment, the standards include *additional duty* type I-AD and type III-AD (ambulances mounted on large chasses) (Box 53-1). Fire service vehicles (e.g., pumpers, rescue units, and fire trucks) also carry EMS equipment.

The federal standards of design and performance for ambulance vehicles are augmented by other federal standards, state statutes, administrative rules, and city, county, and district ordinances. These influence ambulance design,

equipment, and staffing. These additional requirements include the following:

- Air ambulance standards
- Operational staffing standards
- Operational driver standards
- Operational driving standards
- Operational equipment standards

CRITICAL THINKING
Consider your state or regional standards. What do they require for ambulance design, performance, and equipment?

CHECKING AMBULANCES

Completing an equipment and supply checklist at the beginning of every work shift is important. It is essential for safety, patient care, and risk management. It also helps to ensure proper handling and safekeeping of scheduled medications (Figure 53-2). Either paper checklists or special computer software can be used for this purpose. Some equipment (e.g., Glucometers and defibrillators) requires

> **Box 53-1 Ambulance Types**
>
> - **Type I ambulances** are based on the chassis-cabs of light duty pickup trucks.
> - **Type II ambulances** are based on modern passenger/cargo vans.
> - **Type III ambulances** are based on chassis-cabs of light duty vans.
>
>   There are also *AD* (additional duty) versions of both type I and type III designs. They include large-chassis vehicles that allow for increased storage and payload capacity.

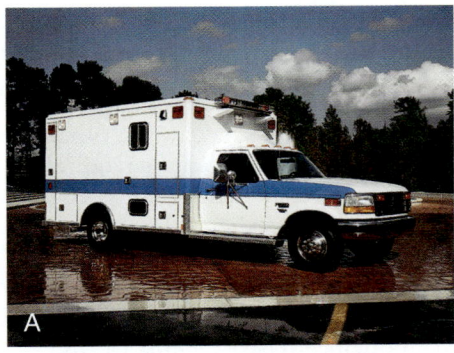

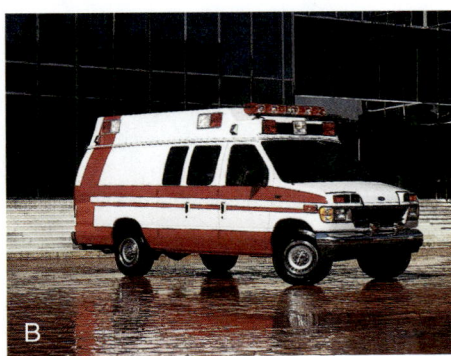

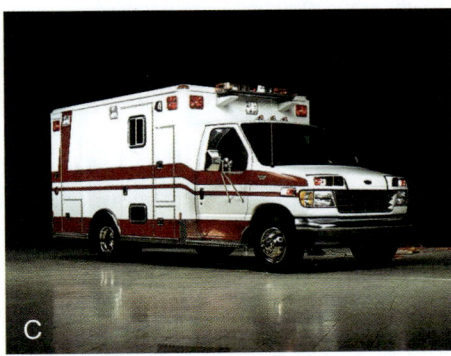

FIGURE 53-1 Basic ambulance designs. **A,** Type I. **B,** Type II. **C,** Type III.

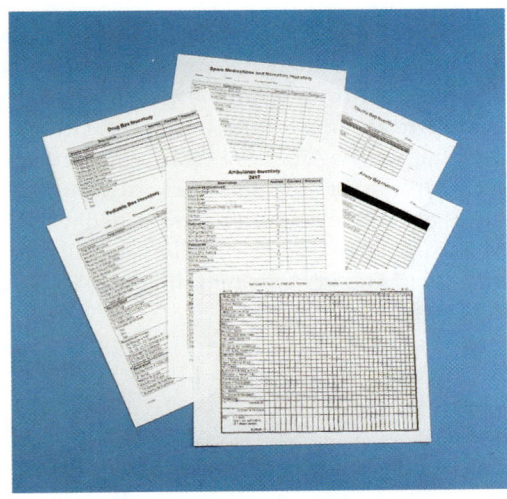

FIGURE 53-2 Ambulance checklists.

Box 53-2 Examples of Equipment Checks on an EMS Vehicle

General Operations
Airway equipment (basic and advanced)
Burn supplies
Drug inventory
Extrication/rescue supplies
Infection control supplies
Immobilization equipment
Obstetrical/childbirth supplies
Patient assessment equipment
Stretchers and related equipment
Vehicle safety and operations
Wound care supplies

Specific Medical Equipment
Automated transport ventilator (ATV)
Cardiac monitor/defibrillator
Glucometer
Pulse oximetry equipment
Telemetry equipment

routine maintenance, testing, and cleaning (Box 53-2). This ensures safe and effective operation. Some disposable items such as medications, electrocardiogram (ECG) patches, defibrillation pads, and glucose check strips expire and should be checked monthly to ensure they are still within their appropriate shelf life.

The procedures for vehicle maintenance vary by EMS agency. These procedures are in place to improve the vehicles' reliability and extended use of life. The paramedic should follow all agency guidelines and procedures for checking vehicles, equipment, and supplies.

AMBULANCE STATIONING

In the 1970s, the methods for estimating the need for ambulance service and where they should be stationed in a community were based on the availability of ambulances. They also were based on the average response time to the emergency scene. Methods for estimating needs have changed. They have shifted toward determining the percentage of compliance (*standard of reliability*) in providing EMS services within time frames that meet national guidelines. (For example, the American Heart Association reports that most neuro-intact survivors are resuscitated within 5 to 8 minutes of cardiac arrest. Therefore, defibrillation and advanced cardiac life support should be available within that time frame[1]) Factors that may affect an EMS system's standard of reliability include:

- Geographical area
- Population and patient demand
- Traffic conditions
- Time of day
- Appropriate placement of emergency vehicles

Strategies for ambulance stationing often are based on areas with the highest volume of calls (*peak load*). These strategies take into consideration the day of the week and the time of day. Computers, global positioning systems, and other technology may be used to formalize strategic unit deployment and reduce response times. Deployment strategies vary by EMS agency. They range from simple deployment of one vehicle stationed in the middle of a response area to comprehensive automated deployment plans for each hour of the day and each day of the week. The comprehensive plans include "mini-deployment" plans within each hour, depending on the number of ambulances left in the system (*system status management*). The optimal deployment system usually is a compromise between these two extremes.[2]

SAFE AMBULANCE OPERATION

Between 1991 and 2000, there were 300 fatal crashes involving occupied ambulances. These resulted in the deaths of 82 ambulance occupants and 275 occupants of other vehicles and pedestrians.[3] In addition, it has been reported that death for EMS employees attributable to transport-related fatalities is more than double that of other U.S. workers (Table 53-1).[4]

Safe operation of ambulances is crucial. It is essential for the safety of patients, the EMS crew, and others in the vicinity of a response. Most EMS agencies require their personnel to take an emergency driving course. Many also are required to undergo periodic evaluations of their emergency driving skills and knowledge (Box 53-3). In addition to the size and weight of the emergency vehicle and the driver's experience, a number of factors influence safe operation of an ambulance. These include the following:

- Appropriate use of personal restraints
- Appropriate use of escorts
- Environmental conditions
- Appropriate use of warning devices
- Proceeding safely through intersections
- Parking at the emergency scene
- Operating with due regard for the safety of others
- Safely moving a patient into and out of the ambulance

CRITICAL THINKING
How do you think you would feel if you struck another vehicle while driving an ambulance?

Appropriate Use of Personal Restraints

According to the National Safety Council there were more than 1800 ambulance crashes and more than 2700 injuries related to those crashes in 2008.[5] Many of these injuries might have been prevented with the appropriate use of personal restraints. Many EMS agencies incorporate into their standard procedures the following guidelines to protect patients, passengers, and EMS personnel:

- All operators and front-seat passengers of ambulance service vehicles must use seat belts when the vehicle is in motion.

TABLE 53-1 Crashes Involving Emergency Vehicles, United States, 2008

	AMBULANCE		FIRE TRUCK/CAR		POLICE CAR	
	Total	Emergency Use	Total	Emergency Use	Total	Emergency Use
Emergency vehicles in fatal crashes	27	14	24	13	103	52
Emergency vehicles in injury crashes	1,384	873	396	344	7,483	4,440
Emergency vehicles in all crashes	**5,998**	**3,136**	**2,719**	**2,008**	**28,994**	**11,467**
Emergency vehicle drivers killed	1	0	5	4	31	14
Emergency vehicle passengers killed	3	1	0	0	2	0
Other vehicle occupants killed	24	12	21	11	51	31
Nonmotorists killed	3	2	1	0	25	11
Total killed in crashes	**31**	**15**	**27**	**15**	**109**	**56**
Total injured in crashes	**2,770**	**1,852**	**702**	**443**	**11,684**	**7,226**

National Safety Council analysis of data from National Highway Traffic Safety Administration Fatality Analysis Reporting System (FARS) and General Estimates System (GES). Emergency lights and/or sirens in use.

Box 53-3 Guidelines for Safe Ambulance Driving

1. Be tolerant and observant of other motorists and pedestrians.
2. Always use occupant safety restraints (both driver and passenger).
3. Be familiar with the characteristics of the emergency vehicle.
4. Be alert to changes in weather and road conditions.
5. Exercise caution in the use of audible and visual warning devices.
6. Drive within the speed limit except in circumstances allowed by law.
7. Select the fastest and most appropriate route to and from the incident scene.
8. Maintain a safe following distance.
9. Drive with due regard for the safety of all others.
10. Always drive in a manner consistent with managing acceptable levels of risk.

- Any patient on a stretcher must be secured at all times when the vehicle is in motion or the stretcher is being moved.
- All equipment in the ambulance must be secured to prevent it from becoming a "missile" during a crash.
- All EMS personnel in the patient compartment must use seat belts when not attending to a patient and when the vehicle is in motion.
- All non-EMS personnel in the patient compartment must use seat belts when not attending to a patient and when the vehicle is in motion.

- Whenever possible, if a child is being transported and the child's own restraining device (child safety seat) is available, the child should be placed in the device and belted into the ambulance seat.
- If the child is the patient, he or she should be appropriately secured onto the stretcher with straps or a child seat.

Finally, the emergency vehicle should not be put in motion until the driver, EMS personnel, and all passengers are seated safely and wearing seat belts. (Every occupant of an emergency vehicle needs to be belted.) In addition, the emergency vehicle should be completely stopped before anyone unbuckles their seat belts and exits the ambulance.

Appropriate Use of Escorts

Police escorts during an emergency response can be dangerous and should be used sparingly. Collisions can occur as a result of confusion when motorists in the area may wrongly assume that only one emergency vehicle is on the road. As a rule, paramedics should use escorts only when the EMS crew is responding to a scene in an unfamiliar area. Even then the EMS driver should keep a safe distance between the ambulance and the escort. The use of audible and visual warning devices during escorts should be guided by local protocol. If the paramedic uses audible and visual warning devices, the ambulance and police escort should use different siren tones (per protocol). This alerts other motorists to the fact that a second emergency vehicle is in the area.

Some communities use a *tiered response system*. In such a system, several units and sometimes several agencies respond to emergency calls. The tiered response system allows for a safer emergency response. It also helps to ensure that the proper resources and personnel are available during an emergency. For example, a fire service unit staffed with basic-level EMTs responds to a car crash with full use of audible and visual warning devices. The EMTs determine that the patient's injury is minor. They request a basic life support (BLS) ambulance (either public or private) to respond to the scene in a nonemergency mode (at normal speed and without warning devices). The BLS ambulance assumes care and provides transport to the hospital.

Environmental Conditions

Poor weather conditions can create significant dangers when paramedics respond to a call. Factors that can affect safe ambulance operation include road and weather conditions, such as fog and heavy rain that reduce visibility, and slippery pavement caused by ice, snow, mud, oil, or water that can cause the ambulance to hydroplane.

When poor environmental conditions are present, the driver of the emergency vehicle should proceed at safe speeds. These speeds should be appropriate for the road and weather conditions. The driver should use low-beam headlights during all responses. This increases visibility for the EMS crew and makes it easier for other motorists to recognize the ambulance.

Dry roads and clear weather do not guarantee a safe response. About 69% of all emergency vehicle crashes occur on dry roads, and about 77% occur during clear weather.[5]

Appropriate Use of Warning Devices

As noted before, during an emergency response and patient transport, lights and sirens should be used according to protocol and state motor vehicle laws. Most EMS agencies authorize the use of these devices during all responses when the cause or severity of the emergency is unknown. In these cases, audible and visual warning devices should be used simultaneously. (If one is indicated, so is the other.) The use of warning devices during patient transport usually is reserved for patients with limb- or life-threatening illness or injury.

When using lights and sirens, paramedics should keep in mind that motorists who drive with the car windows rolled up or who are using an audio device, air conditioning, or the heating system may not be able to hear the sirens or air horns. Therefore the EMS crew should always proceed with caution. They should never assume that the vehicle's lights, sirens, and air horns provide an absolute right-of-way or privileged immunity to proceed. It should be noted that some state and motor vehicle laws grant privileged immunity only to drivers of emergency vehicles that respond using *all* available lights and sirens. Paramedics should be familiar with the motor vehicle laws in their state that cover an emergency response.

Proceeding Safely Through Intersections

Approximately 53% of ambulance crashes in the United States occur in intersections where an ambulance proceeds against a red light.[6] It is important that the driver of an emergency vehicle stop at all controlled intersections. The driver should try to make eye contact with all motorists before going through the intersection. Another safety measure for going through an intersection is making a secondary stop to assess the intersection before crossing. A final measure is using the siren's "yelp" mode or air horn to alert nearby traffic. Some emergency vehicles now have traffic signal preempting devices. These devices can change the traffic light at an intersection to green (in the ambulance's direction of travel).

SHOW ME THE EVIDENCE
These authors examined data from ambulance crashes in Denver from 1989 to 1997. Within that period there were 206 collisions, with 192 occurring when the ambulance was moving and the other 14 occurring while it was parked. Of that group, 39 (18%) resulted in injury or fatality to 81 individuals. There were two deaths, both civilian drivers in the study group. Factors that predicted injury were T-bone collision, intersection collision, and alcohol intoxication of the civilian driver. In 71% of crashes the emergency vehicle driver had a record of multiple crashes. Based on their findings the authors emphasize the need to visually ensure the intersection is clear before proceeding into it, to make eye contact with other drivers, and to use visual and audible warning signals.

From Custalow C, Gravitz C: Emergency medical vehicle collisions and potential for prevention, *PEC* 8(2):175-184, 2004.

Parking at the Emergency Scene

When parking the ambulance at a scene, the paramedic should make sure that the vehicle's location allows for traffic flow around the area. If law enforcement and fire service personnel have secured the scene, the paramedic should position the ambulance about 100 feet past the scene. (This should be on the same side of the road.) The ambulance should be positioned uphill (about 200 feet). It also should be positioned upwind if the presence of hazardous materials is suspected. If law enforcement and fire service personnel have not secured the scene, the paramedic should position the ambulance about 50 feet in front of the scene. This is the **fend-off position** (Figure 53-3). In this position, the emergency vehicle deflects and averts from the scene other vehicles that may strike the ambulance or providers.

Other safety precautions a paramedic can take when parking an ambulance at an emergency scene include the following[7]:

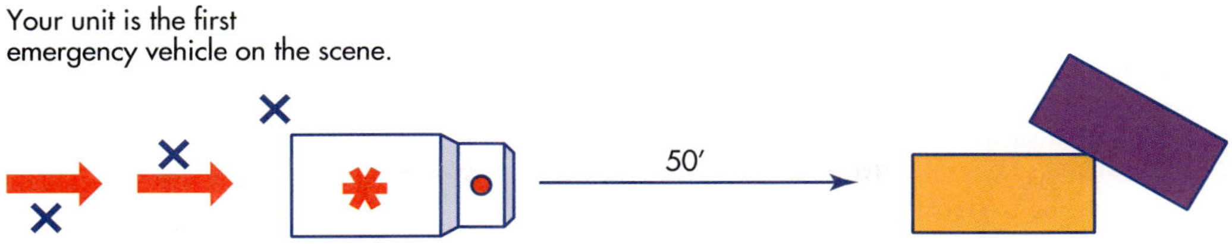

Your unit is the first
emergency vehicle on the scene.

50'

FIGURE 53-3 The "fend-off" position.

- Emergency lighting should be used when the vehicle blocks traffic.
- The parking brake should be set. (Setting the parking brake before putting the transmission in "Park" allows the entire weight of the vehicle to be shared between the emergency brake and the transmission.)
- Another person should be asked to help guide the vehicle when it is backing up. (This person should be visible in the vehicle mirrors at all times while the ambulance is slowly backing up.)
- Reflective gear should be worn when paramedics work near the roadway.

When choosing a parking area for the ambulance, the paramedic also should consider the possibility of collapsing structures, fires, explosive hazards, and downed electrical wires.

Operating With Due Regard for the Safety of All Others

Most states allow privileges for drivers of emergency vehicles. For instance, they are allowed to drive slightly above the speed limit. They also are allowed to proceed through a controlled intersection (after a stop) during an emergency response (Box 53-4). However, these privileges must take into consideration the safety of all people using the roads. This "due regard for the safety of all others" carries legal responsibility. The paramedic and the EMS agency can incur liability if damage, injury, or death results from failure to observe this principle (see Chapter 6). The paramedic should be aware of local and state laws and regulations that cover the operation of an emergency vehicle.

NOTE
An ambulance service is 10 times more likely to be sued for a motor vehicle crash than for a medical error.[8]

LOOK AGAIN
See Chapter 6: Medical and Legal Issues, pp. 101-102.

Safely Moving a Patient Into and Out of an Ambulance

After initial stabilization at the scene, the patient must be packaged and safely placed in the emergency vehicle for transport. The paramedic crew should use safe lifting

practices (see Chapter 2). These techniques help to prevent personal injury. They also ensure that the patient is positioned securely on the ambulance stretcher. The patient compartment of the ambulance is equipped with locking devices. These prevent the stretcher from moving while the ambulance is in motion. Unnecessary equipment should be stowed before transport. Also, objects such as monitors should be secured in a locking device to minimize the risk of injuries in a collision. All those traveling in the ambulance (except for the paramedic providing patient care) should have their personal restraints securely fastened. Before the vehicle leaves the scene, the driver of the ambulance should be signaled that it is safe to put the vehicle in motion.

NOTE
Whenever possible, children should be transported secured in a proper child safety seat. Except in the most critical cases, care can be delivered effectively when the child is restrained in this way.

During transport, the patient should be closely monitored for any changes in status. If emergency care is required while the ambulance is in motion (e.g., intubation, defibrillation), the driver of the vehicle should be advised to slow the vehicle. When possible, the driver should safely park the vehicle and stay parked until the procedure has been successfully performed.

Upon arrival at the hospital, the ambulance should come to a full stop. At that point, personal restraints can be removed and the vehicle can be exited. All patient care equipment must be secured before the stretcher is released from the locking device. (This includes, for example, immobilization devices, intravenous lines, and airway adjuncts.) Using safe lifting techniques, the patient's stretcher should be removed from the ambulance. The patient should be appropriately transferred to health care personnel at the facility.

AEROMEDICAL TRANSPORTATION

Like many other aspects of prehospital emergency care, air evacuation is rooted in military history. During the Prussian siege of Paris in 1870, soldiers and civilians were evacuated by a hot-air balloon. In 1928 a Marine pilot used an engine-powered aircraft to evacuate the wounded in

Box 53-4 The Two-Second Rule and Braking Distance Chart

Most rear-end collisions are caused by drivers who follow too closely behind the vehicle in front of them. Therefore it is important that the paramedic keep enough space (following distance) between the emergency vehicle and the vehicle in front to avoid a crash if the car in front brakes suddenly.

A quick method for gauging the recommended distance is the 2-second rule. It works like this:
1. You (the driver of the emergency vehicle) note an object by the side of the road (e.g., a tree or sign) that the vehicle in front of you will soon pass.
2. Count "one thousand and one, one thousand and two." If you reach the object before the phrase is complete, you are too close to the vehicle in front of you.
3. This rule applies with good road and weather conditions. If the road and weather conditions are not good, the following distance should be increased to a 4- or 5-second count.

Braking distance is based on average reaction time, average vehicle weight, average road conditions, and average brakes. Wet roadways, poor brakes, poor tires, heavy vehicle weight, and poor reaction times lengthen the braking distance. The following chart shows braking distance at various speeds.

NOTE: Larger emergency vehicles (e.g., those mounted on a freightliner-type chassis) have different handling characteristics and longer braking and stopping distances than conventional type I, II, or III emergency vehicles.

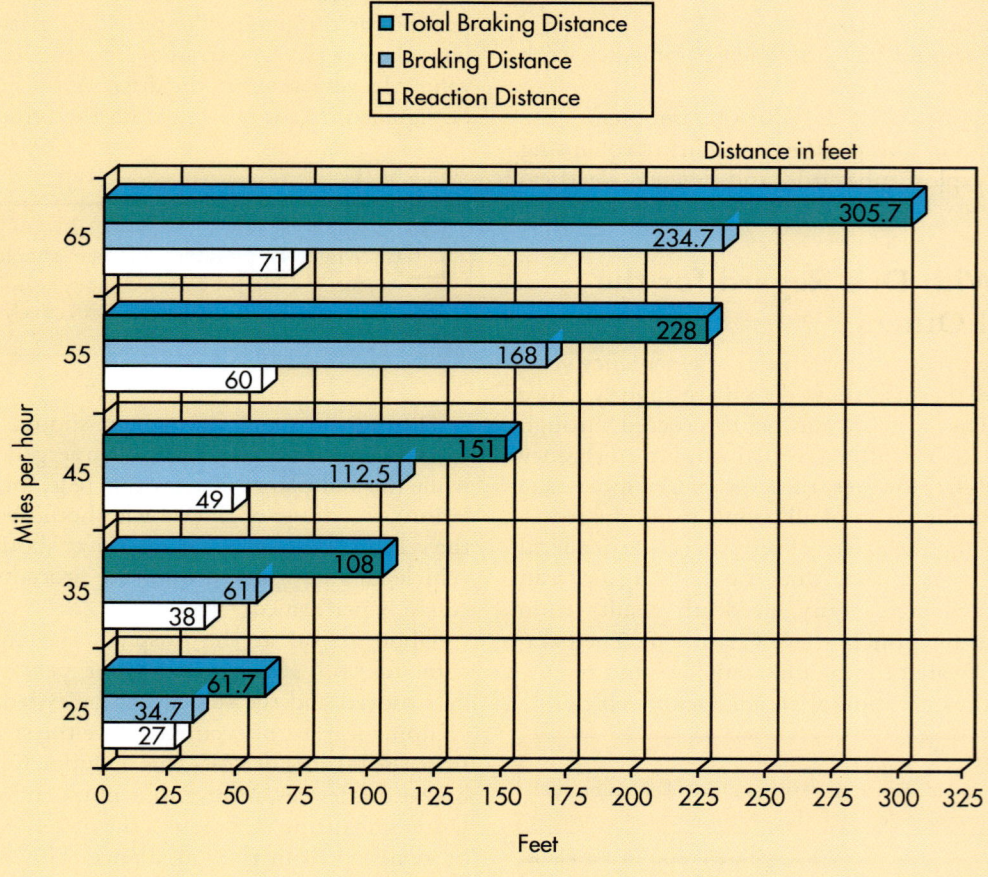

Miles per hour × 1.5 = feet per second
An average reaction time is about 3/4 or 0.75 of a second

From Los Angeles Unified School District Police Department: *Braking distance chart,* Los Angeles, Calif, 1999, Los Angeles Police Department.

Nicaragua.[9] However, the first full-scale use of aircraft for medical evacuation did not occur until 1950, during the Korean conflict. The experience gained in Korea formed the basis for helicopter rescue in Vietnam. In Vietnam, nearly 1 million casualties were transported by air. In the more recent military confrontations involving the United States in Panama, Grenada, and the Middle East, massive advanced aeromedical support capabilities and plans were on site before the conflicts began. Response times of 25 minutes were achieved for air evacuation of wounded soldiers in the Persian Gulf. Field surgical units were set up to handle the 1500 to 3000 casualties estimated to occur within the first 24 hours of the war; most of the injured soldiers arrived by air transportation.[10]

Currently, more than 390 air medical service programs using fixed wing aircraft (Figure 53-4) and/or rotary wing (helicopter) aircraft (Figure 53-5) have been established throughout the United States.[11] Fixed wing aircraft services are not usually as high profile as helicopters. Often they are used for interhospital transfer of patients and to deliver organs for transplantation when the distance is greater than 100 miles.

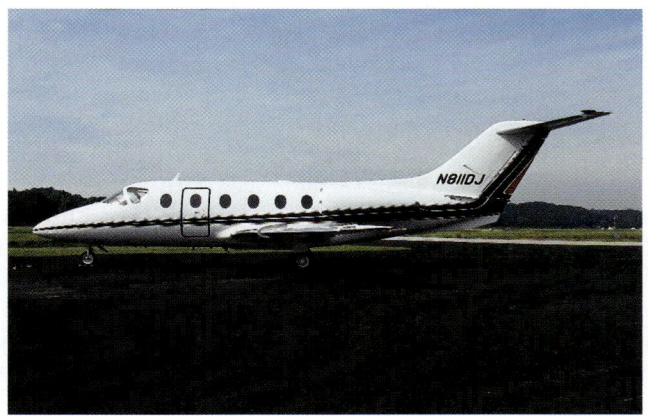

FIGURE 53-4 Fixed wing aircraft. (Courtesy Air Rescue Consortium of Hospitals, St. Louis, Mo.)

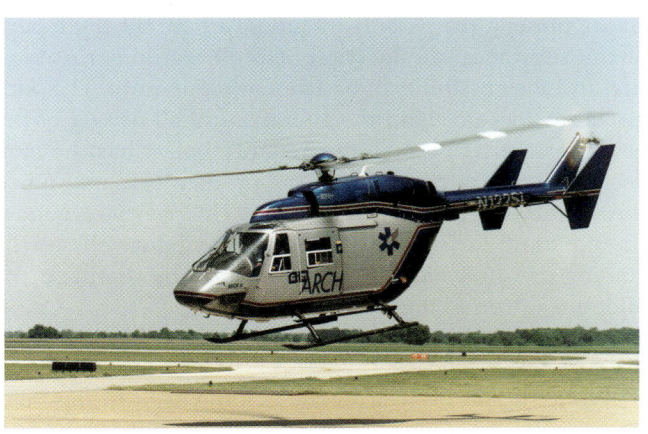

FIGURE 53-5 Rotary wing aircraft. (Courtesy Air Rescue Consortium of Hospitals, St. Louis, Mo.)

Aeromedical Crew Members and Training

The staffing of air ambulances includes a pilot and various health care professionals. (These may include EMTs, paramedics, respiratory therapists, nurses, physicians, and others.) Air ambulance crews undergo specialized training in flight physiology and advanced medical equipment and procedures. The American College of Surgeons (ACS) Committee on Trauma and the Association of Air Medical Services have established guidelines for personnel qualifications. The Department of Transportation (DOT) and the NHTSA funded the development of the *Air Medical Crew National Standard Curriculum* in 1988. Many flight programs have used this curriculum to teach flight physiology, aircraft components and construction, safety regulations, aviation and navigation terminology, and operational safety (Box 53-5).

> **NOTE**
> According to the National Transportation Safety Board, there were 55 EMS-related aviation accidents (fatal and nonfatal) in the United States between January 2002 and January 2005. It was reported that "many of these could have been prevented with simple corrective actions, including oversight, flight risk evaluations, improved dispatch procedures, and the incorporation of available technologies."[12] In 2008, 29 people died in air ambulances crashes.[13]

Use of Aeromedical Services

The local EMS system develops the criteria for requesting aeromedical services to the scene of an emergency. As described in Chapter 37, the paramedic generally should consider air transport when emergency personnel have determined that one or more of the following is a factor:

> **Box 53-5 Selected Organizations Associated With the Air Medical Industry**
>
> Air Medical Physicians Association (AMPA)
> Association of Air Medical Services (AAMS)
> Commission on Accreditation of Air Medical Services (CAAMS)
> Commission on the Accreditation of Medical Transport Services (CAMTS)
> International Association of Flight Paramedics (IAFP)
> International Society of Air Medical Services (Australasia) (ISAS)
> National Association of Air Medical Communications Specialists (NAACS)
> National EMS Pilots Association (NEMSPA)
> National Flight Nurses Association (NFNA)
> National Flight Paramedics Association (NFPA)
> Shock Trauma Air Rescue Society (STARS)

- The time needed to transport a patient by ground to an appropriate facility would pose a threat to the patient's survival and recovery.
- Weather, road, or traffic conditions would seriously delay the patient's access to advanced life support.
- Critical care personnel and specialized equipment are needed to care for the patient adequately during transport (Box 53-6).

LOOK AGAIN
See Chapter 37: Trauma Overview and Mechanism of Injury, pp. 1079-1081.

NOTIFICATION OF AEROMEDICAL SERVICES

Most aeromedical transportation providers accept requests for medical services from physicians, EMS and fire service personnel, or other on-scene public service agency personnel. Local and state guidelines cover aeromedical activation. The paramedic should consult with medical direction and follow all state laws, administrative rules, and city, county, and district ordinances and standards when using aeromedical services. When notified that an aeromedical response may be needed, the flight crews of some services move to the aircraft so that they are ready for the flight. (They are placed on *stand-by*.) If paramedics determine that the situation does not require an aeromedical response, the appropriate agency should be notified as soon as possible. This makes the crew available for other flights.

Box 53-6 Advantages and Disadvantages of Air Medical Services

Advantages
- Transports are rapid and usually smooth.
- Access to accident sites is quick.
- Traffic, trains, mountains, ship canals, and other barriers can be avoided.
- Travel is still possible when road conditions are poor.
- Sophisticated communication equipment is available.
- Quality of care is improved in rural areas where only basic life support is available.

Disadvantages
- In urban settings, ground ambulances are usually faster within a 30-mile range.
- If the helicopter is on another flight, no other aircraft may be available.
- Inclement weather may prevent the aircraft from traveling.
- Space and weight restrictions may limit access to the patient and restrict the crew, patients, and equipment that can be carried.
- Helicopter transports are more expensive than transports by ground ambulance.
- Helicopter crashes have fewer survivors.

If paramedics request air service for medical, trauma, or search and rescue events, they should advise the flight crew of the type of emergency response, the number of patients, the location of a **landing zone** (LZ), and any prominent landmarks and hazards (e.g., vertical structures or power lines). Direct ground to air communication must be available between a designated LZ officer and the aeromedical staff on the responding aircraft. If possible, the fire department should be dispatched to the LZ to provide fire-suppression support. Law enforcement personnel also should be available for securing the scene.

LANDING SITE PREPARATION

The space requirement for a helicopter LZ generally is 100 by 100 feet. The ideal LZ should have no vertical structures that can hamper takeoff or landing. It should be relatively flat and free of high grass, crops, or other factors that can conceal uneven terrain or hinder access. The LZ also should be free of debris that can injure people or damage structures or the helicopter. If patients are close to the LZ, the paramedic should provide protection by covering wounds and eyes. Rescue personnel close to the landing site should wear protective equipment such as reflective clothing, helmets with lowered face shields, and safety glasses.

If a nighttime LZ is used, emergency vehicles with lighted bar lights should be situated at the perimeters of the LZ. If white lights are used, they should be directed *down* to the center of the LZ as spotlights because white lights (spotlights or headlights) directed toward the aircraft can temporarily blind the pilot. Traffic cones with reflectors can help identify the LZ. Flares should not be used because the helicopter rotor wash can blow the flares from the site and create a fire hazard. A fire crew should wet down dusty LZs, especially if vehicle traffic is moving in the area. This prevents the pilot and vehicle drivers from being temporarily blinded by the dust.

Helpful radio communications with the pilot include notification of wind direction and any possible obstructions or hazards. Wind direction can be determined by throwing grass or dirt, by wetting a finger, or by observing smoke patterns from smoke canisters. If hazardous materials are present, the paramedic should advise the flight crew of the substance, the location of the hazardous materials site, and the possibility of patient contamination. The pilot generally does not land the aircraft until all danger of fire or explosion has been eliminated. (The pilot has the final decision to use or change an LZ to another location.) When the aircraft is coming in to land, one emergency responder should stand facing the LZ so that the pilot will see the landing area. LZ hand signals that may be useful to the pilot are shown in Figure 53-6.

SAFETY PRECAUTIONS

Everyone should be clear of the landing area during takeoffs and landings. A distance of 100 to 200 feet is best (Figure 53-7). In addition, paramedics should take the following precautions[14]:

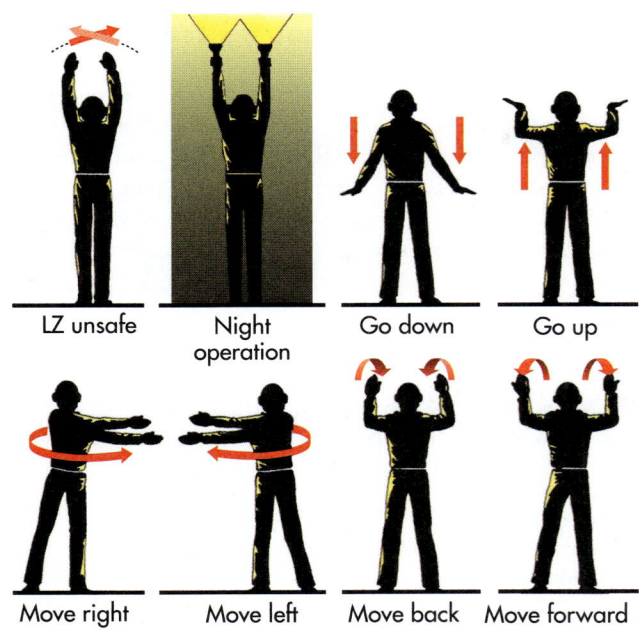

FIGURE 53-6 Landing zone hand signals.

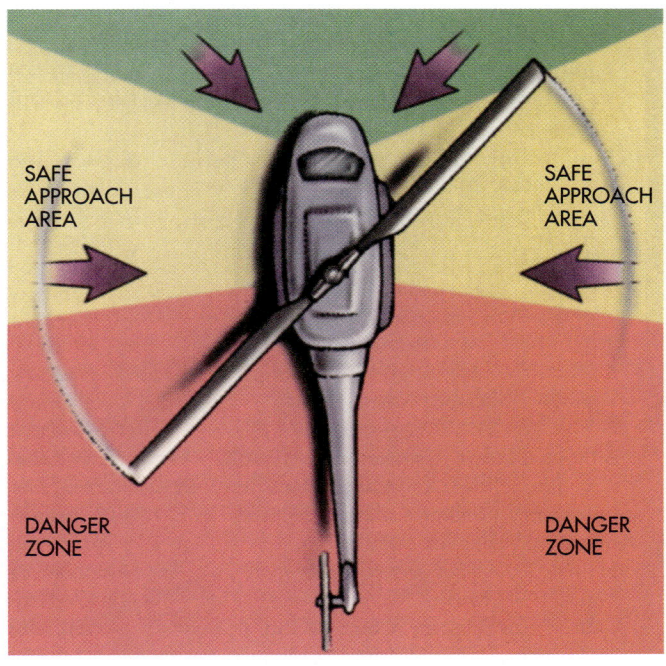

FIGURE 53-7 Safe-approach zones.

- Never allow ground personnel to approach the helicopter unless the pilot or flight crew asks them to do so.
- Allow only necessary personnel to help load or unload patients.
- Secure any loose objects or clothing that could be blown by rotor downwash (e.g., stretcher, sheets, or blankets).
- Do not allow smoking.
- After the aircraft is parked, make eye contact with the pilot, move to the front beyond the perimeter of the rotor blades, and *wait for a signal from the pilot* to approach.
- Approach the helicopter in a crouched position, staying in view of the pilot or other crew members.
- *Never approach the rear of the aircraft from any direction.* The tail rotors on most aircraft are near the ground and spin at 3400 revolutions per minute. This makes them virtually invisible. Tail rotor injuries are often fatal.
- Carry long objects horizontally and no higher than waist high.

- Depart the helicopter from the front and within view of the pilot.

PATIENT PREPARATION

Preparing a patient for air transport requires special measures. Some medical procedures must be done *before* the patient is loaded into the aircraft. For example, the patient's airway should be established and secured before loading. Also, application of a traction splint must be done before loading. Special equipment (e.g., automated chest compression devices) must be positioned according to the aircraft's configuration. Most aeromedical crews perform a brief patient assessment before liftoff. They do so to verify the patient's condition. Patients who are combative may require physical or chemical restraint during flight.

 CRITICAL THINKING
How do you think an alert patient would feel while waiting for helicopter transportation?

SUMMARY

- The federal KKK A-1822 standards provide the foundation of uniformity for the design of ambulance vehicles.
- Completing an equipment and supply checklist at the start of every work shift is important. It is essential for safety, patient care, and risk management. It also helps to ensure proper handling and safekeeping of scheduled medications.

- The methods for estimating ambulance service needs and placement in a community have changed. Compliance in providing EMS services within time frames that meet national standards is the method that now is commonly used.
- Factors that influence safe ambulance operation include proper use of escorts, awareness of environmental conditions, proper use of warning devices, proceeding

Continued

safely through intersections, correct parking at the emergency scene, and operating with due regard for the safety of all others. Moving patients safely in and out of the ambulance is also essential.

- The staffing of air ambulances includes a pilot and various health care professionals. These individuals undergo specialized training in flight physiology and the use of special medical equipment and procedures.

- When paramedics request aeromedical service, the flight crew should be advised of the type of emergency response, the number of patients, and the location of the landing zone as well as the presence of any prominent landmarks and hazards. Paramedics should always follow strict safety measures during helicopter landings. This helps to prevent injury to air medical crews, ground crews, the patient, and bystanders.

REFERENCES

1. American Heart Association: 2010 American Heart Association Guidelines for Cardiopulmonary Resuscitation and Emergency Cardiovascular Care, *Circulation* 122(18 Supplement 3):S639-S946, 2010.
2. Fitch J: *Prehospital care administration: issues, readings, cases*, St Louis, 1995, Mosby.
3. Centers for Disease Control and Prevention: Ambulance crash-related injuries among emergency medical services workers—United States, 1991-2002, *MMWR Mortal Wkly Rep* 52(08):154-156, 2003.
4. *EMS insider*, vol. 36, no.8, St Louis, Aug 2009, Elsevier.
5. National Safety Council: *Injury facts*, Itasca, Ill, 2010, The Council.
6. Kahn C: Characteristics of fatal ambulance crashes in the United States: an 11-year retrospective, *Prehosp Emerg Care* 5(3):261-269, 2001.
7. Federal Emergency Management Association: *Alive on arrival: tips for safe emergency vehicle operations*, www.usfa.dhs.gov/downloads/pdf/publications/fa-255.pdf, accessed 11-7-10.
8. *EMS insider*, vol. 33, no. 6, St Louis, June 2006, Elsevier.
9. Hurd WW, Thompson NJ, Jernigan JG, et al: *Aeromedical evacuation: management of acute and stabilized patients*, New York, 2003, Springer Verlag.
10. Burkle FM: Emergency medicine in the Persian Gulf. I. Preparations for triage and combat casualty care, *Ann Emerg Med* 23(4):742, 1994.
11. *Air medical transport registry*, www.flightweb.com/AMT-Registry, accessed 6-16-10.
12. National Transportation Safety Board: *Safety of Helicopter Emergency Medical Services (HEMS) operations public hearing*, Feb 3-6, 2009, ntsb.gov/events/hearing-HEMS/default.htm, accessed 6-17-10.
13. *EMS insider*, vol. 36, no. 3, St Louis, March 2009, Elsevier.
14. Federal Aviation Administration: *Rotorcraft flying handbook*, New York, 2007, Skyhorse Publishing.

SUGGESTED READINGS

Baker SP, Grabowski JG, Dodd R, et al: EMS helicopter crashes: what influences fatal outcome? *Ann Emerg Med* 47(4):251-356, 2006.

Isakov AP: Souls on board: helicopter emergency medical services and safety, *Ann Emerg Med* 47(4):357-360, 2006.

Maguire BJ, Hunting K, Smith G, et al: Occupational fatalities in emergency medical services, *Ann Emerg Med* 40(6), 2002.

Proudfoot SL, Romano M, Bobick TG, Division of Safety Research, National Institute for Occupational Safety and Health, et al: Ambulance crash-related injuries among emergency medical services workers—United States, 1991-2002, *MMWR* 52:154-156, 2003.

Medical Incident Command

Upon completion of this chapter, the paramedic student will be able to:

1. Outline the components that define a major incident.
2. Identify the components of an effective incident command system.
3. Outline the activities of the preplanning, scene management, and postdisaster follow-up phases of an incident.
4. Identify the five major functions of the incident command system.
5. List command responsibilities during a major incident response.
6. Describe the section responsibilities in the incident command system.
7. Identify situations that may be classified as major incidents.
8. Describe the steps necessary to establish and operate the incident command system.
9. Given a major incident, describe the groups and/or divisions that would need to be established and the responsibilities of each.
10. List common problems related to the incident command system and to mass casualty incidents.
11. Outline the principles and technology of triage.
12. Identify resources for the management of critical incident stress.

apparatus A vehicle used for fire suppression or rescue; this category does not include staff vehicles.

command The act of directing, ordering, or controlling by virtue of explicit, statutory, regulatory, or delegated authority.

command post The area from which command directs operations for an incident.

communications center A facility used to dispatch emergency equipment and coordinate communications between field units and personnel.

disaster A term that usually is associated with a man-made or natural event that involves damage across a large area or to a community's infrastructure.

disaster management The mobilization of resources and the methods used to meet the needs of a disaster response.

divisions Subdivisions of the incident command system that encompass specific geographical areas of responsibility as deemed necessary by the incident commander.

emergency operations center The main communications center where department heads, government officers and officials, and volunteer agencies gather to coordinate their response to an emergency event.

extrication/rescue group The group or division responsible for managing patients who are trapped at the scene. This involves search, rescue, initial triage, tagging, and treatment before transfer of the patients to the treatment group.

finance/administration section The section responsible for tracking costs and the way reimbursement is handled.

groups Subdivisions of the incident command system that encompass specific functional areas of responsibility as deemed necessary by the incident commander.

incident command system (ICS) A management program designed to control, direct, and coordinate emergency response operations and resources.

incident commander The person assuming command in the incident command system.

infrastructure The fundamental facilities and systems serving a country, city, or area, such as transportation and communication systems, power plants, and schools.

interoperability The ability of multiple organizations to communicate effectively.

lifesaving intervention Lifesaving care such as controlling major hemorrhage, opening the airway, and providing rescue breathing, chest decompression, and auto injector antidotes.

local/regional threshold Refers to when the number of casualties or the nature of the event overwhelms the available resources.

logistics section The section that is responsible for providing supplies and equipment, facilities, services, food, and communications support. The main function of this section is to provide gear and support to the responders.

major incident An event for which available resources are insufficient to manage the nature of the emergency.

mass casualty incident An event for which available resources are insufficient to manage the number of casualties.

medical direction A process of ensuring that actions taken on behalf of ill or injured people are medically appropriate, including prospective, concurrent, and retrospective aspects of emergency medical services quality improvement, hiring, and education.

METTAG system A method of triage that uses the international agreement on color coding and priorities to alert emergency care personnel and staff members of the receiving hospital to the patient's category.

mutual aid An agreement with neighboring emergency agencies to exchange equipment and personnel when necessary.

operations section A section that directs and coordinates all emergency scene operations. It also ensures the safety of all personnel. EMS operation areas generally fall under this section.

planning section The section responsible for providing past, present, and future information about the incident and the status of resources.

postdisaster follow-up An after-action review of an incident that includes the "lessons learned" from the incident; also includes methods of improvement.

preplan The element of preplanning for a major incident that addresses common goals and the specific duties of each group.

preplanning The first phase of preparing for a major incident or disaster.

primary triage Triage performed at the incident site to rapidly categorize patient conditions for treatment.

rehabilitation area A part of the major incident response plans of many fire and EMS agencies. This area usually is set up outside the operational area; allows rescue personnel to get physical and psychological rest.

SALT triage A method of triage that uses Sort-Assess-Lifesaving interventions-Treatment and/or Transport to categorize patients.

scene management The development of a strategy to manage the incident scene.

secondary triage The retriaging of patients in a treatment area.

section chiefs The managers or supervisors of ICS sections.

single command The type of command where one person is responsible for the entire operation.

SMART tag system A method of triage that uses five color triage coding cards that have military bar codes for tracking patients.

span of control The number of people one section chief can manage effectively.

staging area A designated area where incident-assigned vehicles are directed and held until needed.

standard operating procedures Established procedures and guidelines to be carried out in a certain operation or a given situation.

START field guide A method of triage that focuses on the patient's ability to walk, respiratory effort, pulses/perfusion, and mental status.

support branch The section that is in charge of gathering and distributing equipment and supplies at a major incident.

tracking log A system of recordkeeping that includes patient identification, transporting unit, patient priority, and hospital destination.

transportation group The group that communicates with the receiving hospitals, ambulances, and air medical services for patient transport during a major incident.

treatment group The group that provides advanced care and stabilization until the patients are transported to a medical facility. Most paramedics and hospital personnel are assigned to this group.

triage A method used to sort or categorize patients according to severity of injury.

triage tagging system A system of tags, tapes, ribbons, and labels is used to indicate a victim's triage category.

unified command A type of command where specialized organizations are identified (e.g., EMS, fire, police, health department, American Red Cross), and personnel unify to complement command.

A *major incident* is an event for which the available resources are insufficient to manage the number of casualties or the type of emergency. Major incidents include highway crashes, air crashes, major fires, train derailments, building collapses, acts of violence or terrorism, search and rescue operations, hazardous materials releases, and natural disasters. These incidents stress and may overwhelm local, regional, state, and even national and international resources.

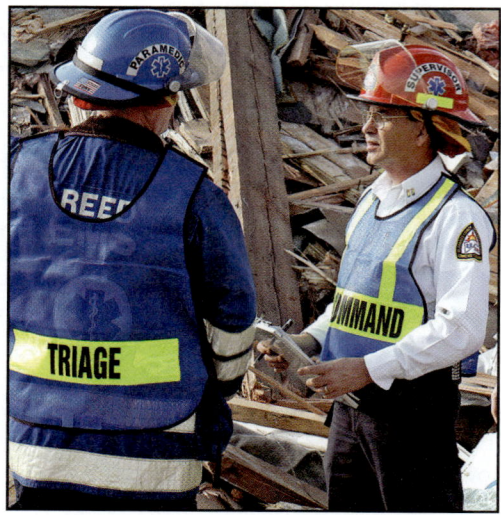

(Courtesy Ray Kemp, St. Charles, Mo.)

NOTE

The term **disaster** usually is associated with a man-made or natural event that involves damage across a large area or to a community's **infrastructure**. (For example, this may include roads, power, communications, or housing.) A subcategory of a disaster is a **mass casualty incident** (MCI), which involves many injuries and/or fatalities. The mobilization of resources and the methods used to meet the needs of a disaster response constitute **disaster management.**

CRITICAL THINKING

What effect do you think lack of organization could have on rescue operations, scene safety, patient care, and transportation in a major incident?

INCIDENT COMMAND SYSTEM

Historically, emergency management of a major incident often resulted in the response of many different agencies (EMS, fire service, rescue organizations, law enforcement, and others). Often times, each of these agencies operated independently with little or no interagency organization. This made it difficult to determine who was in charge of the scene. It also made it difficult to determine what emergency services were needed or were being provided.

The **incident command system** (ICS) was developed to address these concerns. This system organizes interagency functions and responsibilities. In 2004 the ICS was included as part of the National Incident Management System (NIMS) of the Department of Homeland Security (Box 54-1). All emergency response agencies at every level of government are required to use the incident command system at *all* incidents[1] regardless of the type, size, or complexity.

The ICS provides for a number of arrangements: (1) single jurisdiction and single agency involvement; (2) single jurisdiction and multiagency involvement; and (3) multi-jurisdiction and multiagency involvement. This allows the

ICS to be adapted to the needs of any agency or to the size, nature, or geographical location of a particular incident requiring emergency management. The ICS also must be capable of being expanded from dealing with a nonmajor incident to a major one in a logical way. Use of the ICS as standard operating procedure for small incidents allows a smooth transition when a major incident occurs. Other components of the ICS include common elements of organization, terminology (Box 54-2), and procedures. The system should be put into place with the least possible disruption to existing systems (EMS, fire, and law enforcement agencies). It should be simple enough to keep operating and upkeep costs to a minimum.

The ICS system can easily be used at a minor incident in which the units dispatched to the scene are sufficient to handle the event. It can be expanded if more units are needed for a minor incident that becomes a major one. Use of the ICS is critical whenever it becomes apparent that the need for extended operations will quickly overwhelm the responding units. (An example is an event that involves many patients or one that may last several hours to days.)

Federal law now requires use of the ICS in response to all types of incidents. The ICS is a flexible system. It is used in both public and private sectors in all incidents. Much of the success of the ICS is due to its application of a common

BOX 54-1 NIMS Concepts

NIMS provides an organized set of *scalable* and *standardized* operational structures, which is critical for allowing various organizations and agencies to work together in a predictable, coordinated manner. In summary, NIMS is[1]:

- A comprehensive, nationwide systematic approach to incident management.
- A core set of doctrine, concepts, principles, terminology, and organizational processes for all hazards. It is not a detailed operational or resource plan.
- Scalable, so it may be used for all incidents (from day-to-day to large-scale).
- Essential principles for a common operating picture and communications interoperability.
- Standardized resource management procedures for coordination among different jurisdictions and organizations.

BOX 54-2 Important Terminology for Medical Incident Command Systems

apparatus: A vehicle used for fire suppression or rescue; this category does not include staff vehicles.

command: The act of directing, ordering, or controlling by virtue of explicit, statutory, regulatory, or delegated authority.

command post: The area from which command directs operations for an incident.

communications center: A facility used to dispatch emergency equipment and coordinate communications between field units and personnel.

division: A subdivision of the incident command system (ICS) that encompasses a specific geographic area of responsibility as deemed necessary by the incident commander.

group: A subdivision of the ICS that encompasses a specific functional area of responsibility as deemed necessary by the incident commander.

medical direction: A process of ensuring that actions taken on behalf of ill or injured people are medically appropriate, including prospective, concurrent, and retrospective aspects of emergency medical services (EMS) quality improvement, hiring, and education.

mutual aid: An agreement with neighboring emergency agencies to exchange equipment and personnel when necessary.

staging area: A designated area where incident-assigned vehicles are directed and held until needed.

organizational structure and key principles in a standardized way. ICS organization is built around the following five major components (Figure 54-1)[2]:

1. Command
2. Finance/administration
3. Logistics
4. Operations
5. Planning

The five major components of ICS are also known as *C-FLOP* (*c*ommand, *f*inance/administration, *l*ogistics, *o*perations, *p*lanning). They are the foundation on which organization develops. They apply during a major event, in preparation for a major event, or in management of the response to a major event.

Command Function

At most incidents the responsibility of command should belong to *one* person who assumes the function of command. This should be an individual with the ability to coordinate a variety of emergency activities. This is the cornerstone of the ICS structure.

The initial command should be determined by a preplanned system of arriving emergency units and personnel (e.g., the first or second arriving EMS, fire, or law enforcement unit). The person assuming command is the **incident commander** (IC). This person must be familiar with the ICS structure. The IC also must be familiar with the operating procedures of other responding agencies. The IC need not be the person with the highest rank or the most medical training (although this is commonly the case). Rather, the IC should be the person best able to manage the emergency scene effectively.

Command must be established immediately. The commander must be clearly identified. Also, all others at the scene must be informed as to who is in command. As a more qualified person arrives, command may be transferred per **standard operating procedures** (SOPs). This transfer of command is usually done face to face. Once established, command should take the following steps:

- Assume an effective command mode and position.
- Transmit brief reports by radio to the communications center, identifying the location of the command post.
- Evaluate the situation quickly.
- Develop a management strategy.
- Request more resources and provide assignments as needed.
- Implement a personal accountability and safety system.
- Control and assign **divisions** and/or **groups** as required (these should be consistent with the needs of the incident, SOPs, or disaster plans); also, provide these units with operating objectives.
- Provide ongoing effective command and progress reports until relieved by a higher ranking person.
- Develop the command organization by delegating authority to subordinates (this helps to accomplish incident needs and objectives).
- Review and evaluate the effectiveness of site operations and revise these operations as needed.

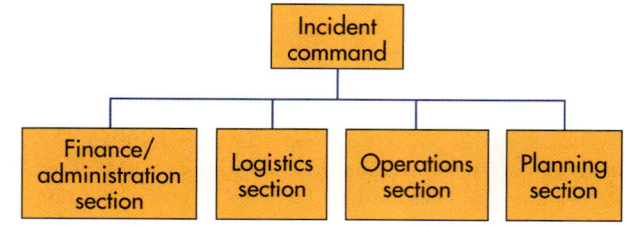

FIGURE 54-1 Incident command system organization (C-FLOP).

- Return units to service and end command when appropriate.

TYPES OF COMMAND

Command may take a single or unified form (Box 54-3). With **single command,** one person is responsible for the entire operation. This type of command often works well for incidents with limited jurisdictions or responsibilities. It also works best in small events of short duration.

Unified command may be needed in large events or as a small incident evolves. In unified command, specialized organizations are identified (e.g., EMS, fire, police, health department, American Red Cross), and personnel unify to complement command. This type of command stimulates cooperation (the "right" agency leads command at the "right" time) and provides for balanced decision making. It also facilitates **interoperability** (the ability of multiple organizations to communicate effectively) when many different communication frequencies and communications equipment are used by responding agencies. The concept of unified command allows agencies with different legal, geographical, and functional authorities and responsibilities to work together effectively. This is done without affecting individual agency authority, responsibility, or accountability[3] (Figure 54-2). Unified command may be indicated in incidents such as those with:

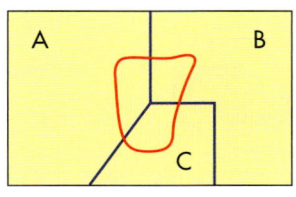

Incidents that affect more than one political jurisdiction

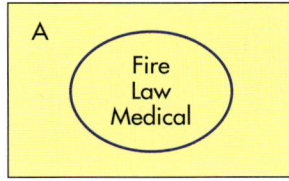

Incidents involving multiple agencies within a jurisdiction

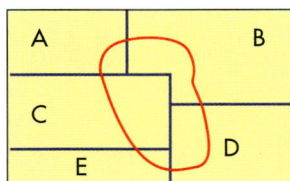

Incidents that have an impact on multiple geographic and functional agencies

FIGURE 54-2 Application of unified command.

- More than one political jurisdiction
- Multiple agencies within a jurisdiction
- Multiple geographical and functional agencies

 CRITICAL THINKING
Where do you think command should be located in a major incident that is confined to one area?

In either single or unified command, the IC may delegate authority for certain activities by activating additional **sections** (operations, planning, logistics, or finance/administration). These sections help to meet the needs of the situation. The incident commander bases the decision to expand (or contract) the ICS organization on three major incident priorities[4]:

1. *Life safety.* The IC's first priority is *always* the safety of the responders and the public.
2. *Incident stability.* The IC is responsible for deciding on strategies to minimize the effect of the incident on the area. These strategies also should maximize the response effort while using resources effectively.
3. *Property conservation.* The IC is responsible for minimizing damage to property while achieving the incident objectives.

When expansion of command is required, the IC establishes the other general staff positions (Figure 54-3).

Section Responsibilities

In the ICS, a manageable **span of control** (the number of people one section chief can manage effectively) falls within the range of three to seven, with five being the optimum.

In some cases the span of control indicates that the incident organization must be expanded to allow effective management of the situation. In such cases the IC assigns one or more of the general staff sections (planning,

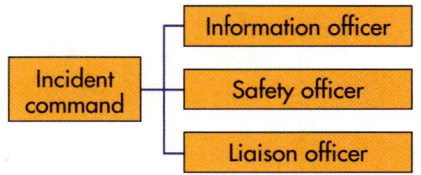

FIGURE 54-3 Command staff positions. The information officer handles all media inquiries and coordinates the release of information to the media with the public affairs officer at the emergency operations center (EOC). The safety officer monitors safety conditions and develops measures for ensuring the safety of all assigned personnel. The liaison officer is the on-scene contact for other agencies assigned to the incident.

operations, logistics, and/or finance/administration) to **section chiefs.** Section chiefs must be strong supervisors and managers. Their chief role in the ICS is to "make things happen." They enact the plans and strategies of the incident commander. They also ensure that all rescuers in their sections are working toward a common goal. Which of the four sections may be needed varies, depending on the scope of the incident. The IC makes this determination (Figure 54-4).

Section chiefs should not become involved in physical tasks. (Examples of such tasks are carrying litters or operating rescue equipment.) This allows them to maintain control and supervise the section. General responsibilities of section chiefs include the following:

- Accomplishing the objectives set by command
- Monitoring work progress
- Redirecting activities as necessary
- Coordinating related activities with other sections
- Requesting additional resources as needed for the section
- Monitoring the welfare of personnel from each section
- Providing command with frequent reports
- Reallocating resources within the section

The section chief should report to command when a job is assigned, when a job is accomplished, or if a job cannot be accomplished.

FINANCE/ADMINISTRATION SECTION

The **finance/administration section** (Figure 54-5) is important for tracking costs and the way reimbursement is handled. This section is seldom used in small-scale incidents. However, it is considered essential if the incident grows in magnitude and costs (e.g., a presidential declaration of a disaster). Functions of the finance/administration section during a major incident may include time accounting, procurement, payment of claims, and estimation of costs.

LOGISTICS SECTION

The **logistics section** (Figure 54-6) is responsible for providing supplies and equipment (including personnel to operate the equipment), facilities, services, food, and communications support. The main function of this section is to provide gear and support to the responders. The essential equipment for supporting a medical incident includes

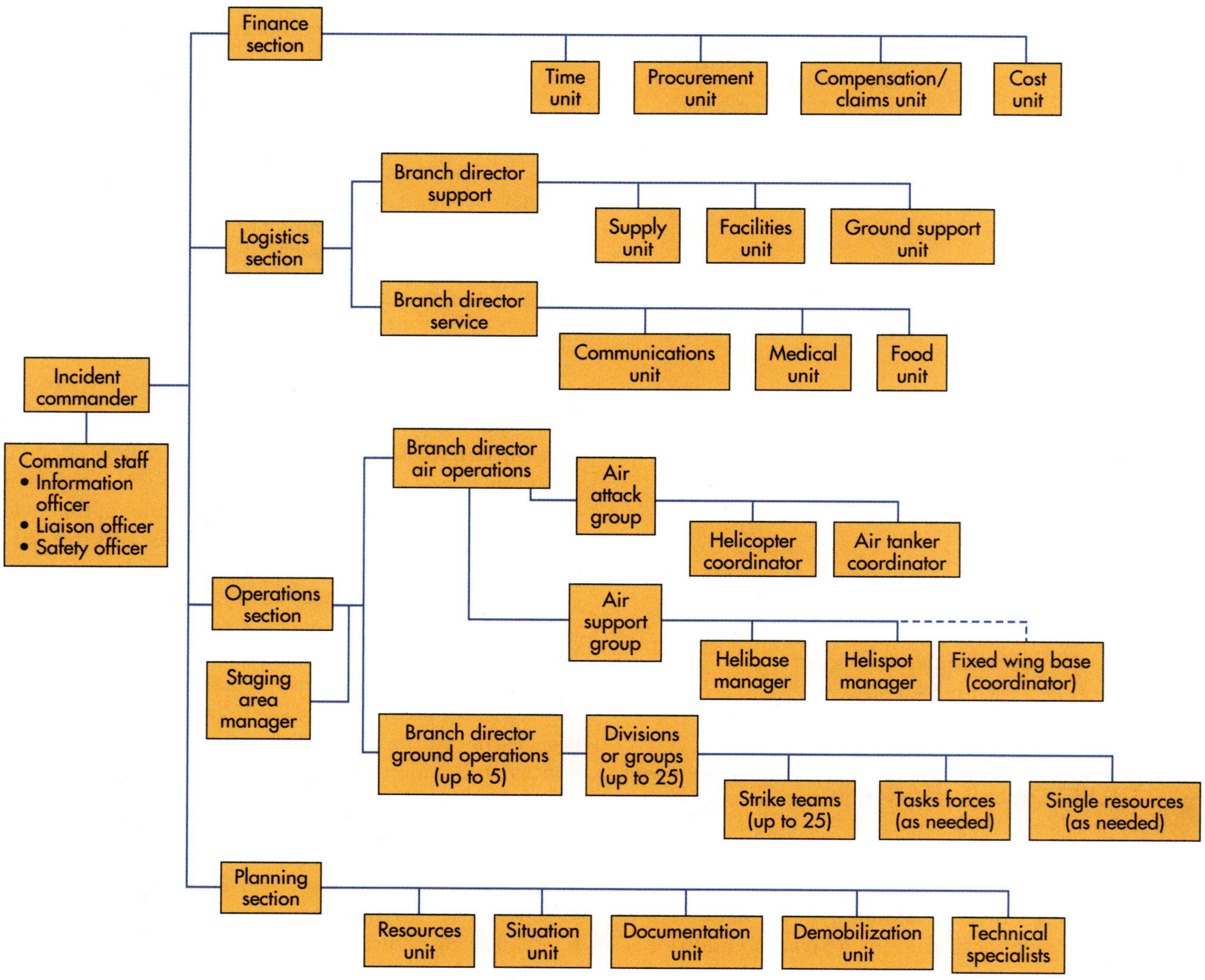

FIGURE 54-4 Command section organizational plan.

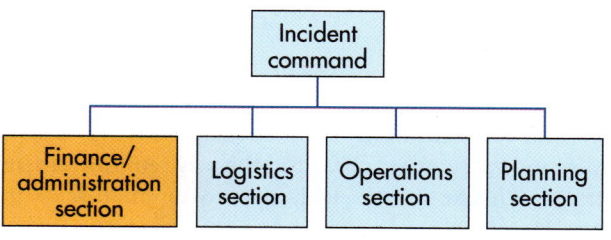

FIGURE 54-5 Finance/administration section.

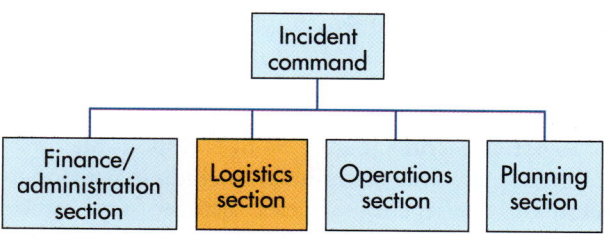

FIGURE 54-6 Logistics section.

supplies for airway, respiratory, and hemorrhage control, burn management, and patient packaging and immobilization. Resources for moving and transporting patients (people, ambulances, buses) also may be needed. *The medical unit* of the logistics section cares for the incident responders; it does not care for the civilian victims. Often part of the logistics section is used for routine daily incidents. For example, *responder rehabilitation* (described later in this chapter) and the *support branch* are parts of the logistics section.

OPERATIONS SECTION

The **operations section** (Figure 54-7) directs and coordinates all emergency scene operations. It also ensures the safety of all personnel. (EMS operation areas generally fall under this section.) The operations section chief is in charge of the tactical operations at an incident. This person is responsible for the following activities:

- Accomplishing tactical objectives
- Directing front-end activities

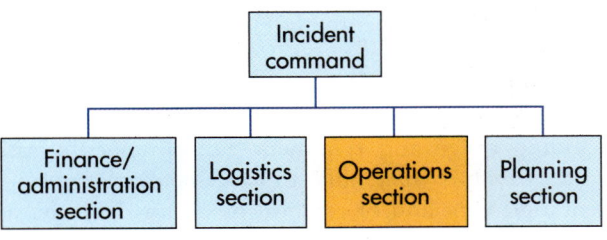

FIGURE 54-7 Operations section.

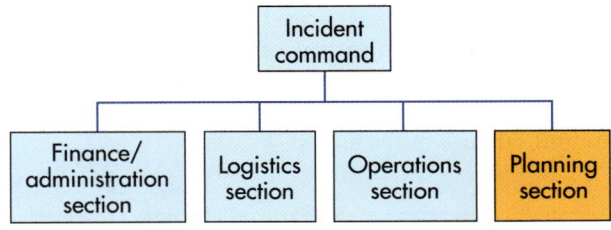

FIGURE 54-8 Planning section.

- Participating in planning
- Modifying action plans as needed
- Maintaining discipline
- Accounting for personnel
- Updating command on the progress or lack of progress of an operation

PLANNING SECTION

The staff function of the **planning section** (Figure 54-8) is to provide past, present, and future information about the incident and the status of resources. This section's duties also may include the creation of a written or verbal **incident action plan** (IAP). (The incident commander determines the need for an IAP.) The IAP defines the response activities and use of resources for a specified period. These operational periods can vary in length; however, they should be no longer than 24 hours (12-hour operational periods are common for large-scale incidents). IAPs may be indicated when (1) resources from several agencies are used; (2) several jurisdictions are involved; or (3) the incident is complex (e.g., changes in shifts or personnel are required).

Declaring a Major Incident

Declaring a major incident is a critical phase of the response. If an EMS unit is dispatched to a scene that has this potential, the crew should be advised or should declare (per established protocol) that they are responding to a possible major incident or mass casualty incident (MCI) and will confirm on arrival. This information allows other agencies to be contacted, and those agencies can be placed on standby. It also allows time for determination of the availability of other resources. Medical direction and area hospitals should also be alerted. The receiving hospitals need information on the number of patients and the severity of injuries as soon as possible. That way, they can begin to prepare for the patients' arrival. A possible major incident should be declared when:

- More than two ambulance units are required for adequate treatment, particularly in rural areas where communities may have only one ambulance
- Hazardous or radioactive materials or chemicals in significant quantity are involved
- An MCI results in a large number of patients and requires special EMS resources, such as helicopters, rescue teams, or several rescue or extrication units

PREPARING FOR A MAJOR INCIDENT

Preparation for a major incident involves three phases: preplanning, scene management, and postdisaster follow-up (or after-action review).[4]

Phase 1: Preplanning. Phase 1 of the preparation for a major incident is **preplanning.** Efforts by agencies to work together and to plan ahead are crucial to the management of a major incident. All agencies that will be called upon in an incident must agree to the **preplan.** The preplan also must address common goals and the specific duties of each group. Multiagency efforts succeed as a result of frequent meetings and practice sessions or exercises (drills or "tabletop" exercises). The preplan should include a system of sorting or prioritizing care, treatment, and transportation.

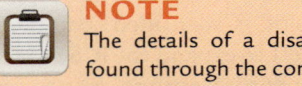

> **NOTE**
> The details of a disaster preparedness plan can be found through the community's local emergency disaster planning committee (LEPC).

Another component of the disaster is the identification of hazards in a community (a risk assessment). Such hazards may include the manufacture, storage, and transport of hazardous materials; fire threats; the population base at various times of the day; and violence and other potential social problems. An inventory of resources that may be needed during a major incident includes the following:

- Shelter and mass feeding
- Air evacuation
- Medical equipment and supplies
- Heavy equipment, power generators, and lighting
- Communications equipment
- Law enforcement personnel
- Specialized rescue services

Phase 2: Scene Management. Phase 2 of preparation involves the development of a strategy to manage the incident scene **(scene management).** Some major incidents can be managed with local resources and personnel (closed or contained incidents). However, other incidents may affect large geographical areas and many jurisdictions (open or uncontained incidents). In these incidents, many federal, state, and local agencies become involved. Regardless of the size of the incident or the number of agencies involved, scene management calls for a coordinated effort. This effort must ensure an effective response and the efficient and safe use of resources.

> **NOTE**
>
> The procedure for managing a major multiagency, multijurisdictional incident is outlined in the federal National Incident Management System (NIMS). This procedure should be adopted for local use.

Phase 3: Postdisaster Follow-Up. Phase 3 involves a **postdisaster follow-up** (or *after-action review*). This includes the "lessons learned" from the incident. It also includes methods of improvement. These may include improvement of emergency response, planning, and community protection. This phase also should assess stress-related anxiety and illness among emergency workers that may have resulted from the incident.

MASS CASUALTY INCIDENTS

The ICS at a mass casualty incident is expanded when the number of casualties or the nature of the event overwhelms the available resources (the **local/regional threshold**). In communities where the local threshold is low, frequent use of the ICS for practice is encouraged. (For example, it can be used when an incident involves more than one patient.) When a mass casualty incident is identified, command must quickly determine how best to expand the ICS to meet the needs of the event. In other words, sections, groups, and

divisions must be put into place according to the size and scope of the incident.

Typically, initial expansion of the ICS for a mass casualty incident requires the establishment of a *medical group* (including triage and treatment subcomponents, called *units*); a *transport group;* and an *extrication/rescue group* for disentanglement and/or removal of victims from hazardous areas. If more than five groups (or divisions, if assigned geographically) are activated, an operations section typically is established (Figure 54-9).

> **CRITICAL THINKING**
>
> How do you think you will feel when you arrive first on the scene of a mass casualty incident?

Scene Assessment

The first EMS unit to arrive at the scene should make a quick and rapid assessment (size-up) of the situation. If the arriving unit is a two-paramedic crew, one paramedic assumes the function of command; the second paramedic begins triage. A more precise and full assessment should be performed as soon as safety and time allow. This fuller assessment should include the following:

- The type of incident and the potential duration
- Whether entrapment or special rescue resources may be needed
- The number of patients in each triage category (described later in this chapter)
- Initial assignments for incoming units
- The need for any additional resources to manage the incident

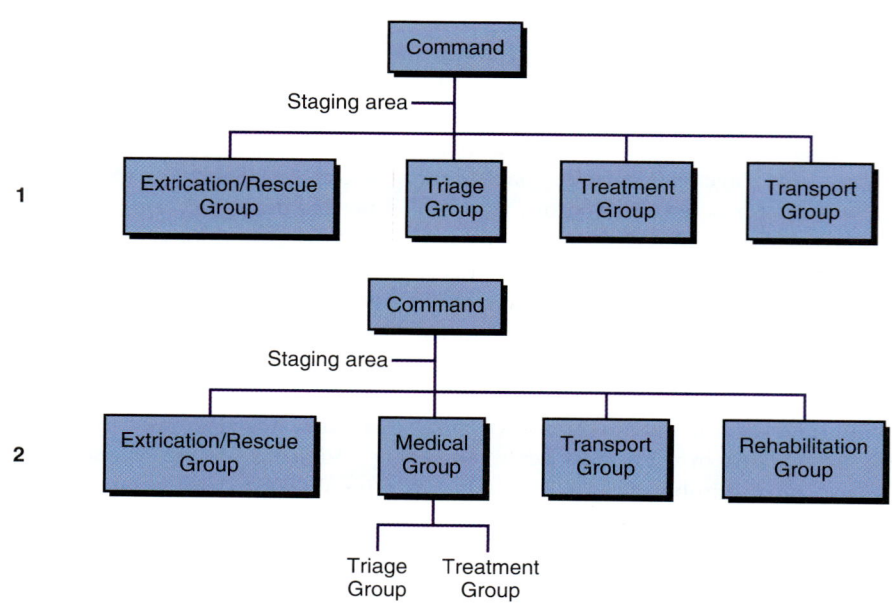

FIGURE 54-9 Two examples of ICS of mass casualty incidents.

NOTE
The scene assessment must be updated continually. This helps in the identification of specific or changing needs.

Communications

Command must immediately establish radio contact with the main communications center or the **emergency operations center** (EOC). Most jurisdictions maintain an EOC as part of their community's preparedness program. An EOC is where department heads, government officers and officials, and volunteer agencies gather to coordinate their response to an emergency event. Command and the EOC share similar goals. However, they function at different levels of responsibility. The incident commander is responsible for on-scene activities. The EOC is responsible for the entire community-wide response to the event. Radio traffic can be very distracting; therefore incident personnel must observe strict radio and/or phone procedures. Moreover, they should use clear, plain English. All transmissions should be short and to the point.

NOTE
Runners (messengers), cell phones, and satellite phones (SAT phones) are used when radio communications fail (e.g., in a large-scale disaster). Communications is often considered the #1 problem in major incidents.

Obtaining Resources

More units should be requested as soon as the need has been identified or anticipated. (The communications center should have a written SOP for requesting **mutual aid.**) Support may include obtaining food, shelter, and clothing for victims. The IC is responsible for providing instructions for the deployment of the resources. (Personnel should stay with their vehicle until instructions are received.) Staging techniques that may be used to deploy resources effectively include the following:

- Lining vehicles up at the scene to facilitate egress
- Staging away from a limited access highway
- Identifying a formal staging area with an assigned staging officer

The "tool box" theory of strategic deployment of resources can be used. It involves identifying the resources ("tools") specific to the incident, using only the needed resources, and issuing instructions for the deployment of resources.

Group or Division Functions

As stated previously, the number of groups or divisions needed at a major medical incident varies. Common groups and their responsibilities include extrication/rescue,

treatment, and transportation. The staging area, rehabilitation area, and support branch are also important parts of an incident organization.

EXTRICATION/RESCUE GROUP

The **extrication/rescue group** is responsible for managing patients who are trapped at the scene. This involves search, rescue, initial triage, tagging, and treatment before transfer of the patients to the treatment group. Patient care for this group includes only assessment and treatment of life-threatening injuries. Examples include the need to open the airway, control severe bleeding, and cover open chest wounds. In addition, the rescue/extrication group is responsible for site safety and personnel safety (e.g., supplying self-contained breathing apparatus; atmospheric monitoring if indicated for explosive or oxygen-deficient atmospheres; protective clothing) and for evaluating and directing the resources needed for extrication and rescue. Rescue/extrication group responsibilities include the following:

- Determining whether triage and the primary treatment will be conducted on site or in the treatment group area
- Attaching tagging assignments to injured patients
- Evaluating the resources needed for extrication of trapped patients and for their delivery to the treatment group
- Ensuring site safety
- Evaluating resources needed for triage and the primary treatment of patients
- Communicating resource requirements to command
- Allocating assigned resources
- Supervising assigned personnel and resources
- Collecting, assembling, and assessing the walking wounded
- Reporting progress to command
- Reporting "all clear" to command when all patients have been extricated and delivered to the treatment group
- Coordinating with other groups

CRITICAL THINKING
What dilemmas might you face in doing triage at a multiple casualty incident?

TREATMENT GROUP

The **treatment group** works closely with the rescue/extrication group in patient care. As patients are delivered, they are recategorized according to their medical needs. The treatment group provides advanced care and stabilization until the patients are transported to a medical facility. Most paramedics and hospital personnel are assigned to this group.

With a large number of patients, the area usually is further divided into *immediate* and *delayed treatment zones*. This helps in the determination of priorities for patient transport. Immediate treatment patients include those with life-threatening injuries; delayed treatment patients include the walking wounded and those whose care and transport can be delayed if necessary. It should be noted that triage monitoring is a function of all groups involving ill or injured patients. It is a continuing component of the ICS. Treatment group responsibilities include the following:

- Locating a suitable treatment area that satisfies hazardous material (hazmat) concerns, if applicable (e.g., uphill/upwind/upstream), and reporting that location to the rescue/extrication group and command
- Evaluating resources required for patient treatment and reporting these needs to command
- Providing secondary triage of patients arriving in the treatment area; tagging patients if not already done
- Providing suitable immediate and delayed treatment areas
- Allocating resources
- Assigning, supervising, and coordinating personnel in the group
- Reporting progress to command
- Coordinating with other divisions and groups

On-Scene Physicians. Physicians who are on-scene can provide valuable help during an MCI. The roles of the physicians may include providing on-scene medical direction, making difficult triage decisions and secondary triage decisions in a treatment area, and performing emergency surgery to facilitate extrication. Physicians also can perform specialized invasive procedures at the scene, as well as a more detailed patient assessment. In addition, they may provide direction for specific treatments that may be beyond the scope of normal paramedic practice.

Disposition of the Deceased. Depending on the scale of the incident, personnel may be assigned to disposition of the deceased. The duties of these individuals may include the following:

- Working with the medical examiner, coroner, law enforcement personnel, and other appropriate agencies to coordinate disposition
- Assisting in the establishment of an appropriate and secure area for a morgue, if needed

When possible, the deceased victims should be left in the location in which they were found until a plan has been made for removal and storage of the bodies.

TRANSPORTATION GROUP

The **transportation group** communicates with the receiving hospitals, ambulances, and air medical services for patient transport. This group must work closely with the treatment group. They help to determine appropriate destinations for injured patients. Also, the arrival and departure of transfer vehicles must be coordinated with the staging area. Transportation group responsibilities include the following:

- Determining patient transportation needs and obtaining appropriate transportation

- Evaluating resources required to manage patient transportation
- Establishing an ambulance staging area (if command has not already done so) and patient loading areas
- Establishing and operating a helicopter landing zone
- Communicating with hospitals to determine hospital surge capacity and capability to handle specialty patients
- Coordinating patient transportation allocations with the treatment group and hospitals
- Tracking patients leaving the site with a written log (including patient identification, the transporting unit, and the destination facility)
- Reporting resource requirements to command
- Coordinating with other divisions and groups
- Advising command when the last patient has been transported

Staging Area

Staging areas are needed for large incidents. They help to prevent vehicle congestion and delays in response. All emergency vehicles (fire, law enforcement, EMS) should report to this area for direction. Other agencies, such as disaster relief services and news media, also may be supervised by the staging area manager. The responsibilities of the staging area manager include the following:

- Coordinating with law enforcement personnel to block streets, intersections, and other areas to allow the establishment of a staging area
- Ensuring that all equipment and vehicles are parked in an appropriate manner
- Maintaining a log of all equipment in the staging area and an inventory of all specialized equipment and medical equipment that may be needed
- Reviewing with command the resources that must be maintained in staging, as well as coordinating this request with the dispatching center
- Assuming a visible position for incoming equipment and vehicles (e.g., leaving emergency lights operating on one vehicle and wearing an identification vest)
- Coordinating with other divisions and groups

Rehabilitation Area

A **rehabilitation area** (*rehab area*) is part of the major incident response plans of many fire and EMS agencies. This area usually is set up outside the operational area. It allows rescue personnel to get physical and psychological rest. With smaller incidents, the rehab unit leader usually reports directly to command. In large-scale incidents or whenever a logistics group is established, the rehab unit leader reports to the logistics chief. (In large-scale incidents, more than one rehab area may be needed.)

One duty of the rehab unit leader is to ensure that personnel receive medical care and treatment as needed. Another duty is to keep accurate logs of those who enter and leave the area. Records of medical care and treatments are kept for each person who enters the rehab area. (Medical care of rescue personnel is further addressed in Chapter 57.)

CRITICAL THINKING
Why do you think a rehabilitation area is important?

Support Branch

The **support branch** is in charge of gathering and distributing equipment and supplies. This branch may be responsible for obtaining medical supplies from area hospitals, rescue supplies, and other equipment needed at the incident. Support branch responsibilities include the following:

- Determining the medical supply needs of other divisions and groups
- Establishing a suitable location for supply operations
- Coordinating procurement of medical supplies from hospitals with the transportation group
- Coordinating procurement of medical supplies that are not available from hospitals
- Reporting additional resource requirements to command
- Allocating supplies and equipment as needed
- Reporting progress to command
- Coordinating with other divisions and groups

NOTE
Often only specific parts of the logistics group are needed at an incident. One of these is the rehabilitation unit; the other is the support branch. Depending on the span of control, these two units can be implemented without the establishment of a logistics group section chief; they report directly to command.

Identification and Communication

When an ICS is in place, all responders must know its organizational structure and the lines of radio communication. Although clothing and identification vary by system, the following guidelines usually apply:

- Color-coded vests identify personnel. For example, the commander may wear a white vest; EMS group managers, blue vests; fire group managers, red; law enforcement group managers, green; and so on.
- With the exceptions of command and division/group communications, most communications are face to face. Radio use is intended for command operations.
- Radio communications use operation titles instead of personal or unit names: "Treatment group to command" or "Rescue/extrication group to treatment group." This system ensures that all participants can reach the appropriate person by one radio designation.

RADIO COMMUNICATIONS

Communications is a key function during a major incident. Preplanning includes identifying the radio frequencies to be used in major incident responses. It also includes planning for the ways these frequencies are to be used. For example, all responding units should have multichannel radios that use a common frequency. Within this common frequency, separate frequencies should be used for EMS, fire, and other support operations. Division and group officers should have portable radios set on a channel that permits direct communication with command. These channels may be assigned in advance or by the dispatching agency at the time of the incident. In addition, state, regional, and local communications systems should undergo a periodic review. This review should include the controls for activating communications, system frequencies, and portable and mobile radio equipment. Other communications considerations include the following:

- Radio traffic must be clear, concise, and in plain English.
- Messages should be given thought and prepared before transmission.
- The speaker should clearly identify the unit number or division or group.
- All radio traffic should be minimized.
- Face to face communication is preferable and encouraged.

Common Problems at Mass Casualty Incidents

In addition to common failures of incident command systems (Box 54-4), there are common problems specific to mass casualty incidents. These include the following[4]:

- Failure to adequately provide widespread notification of the event
- Failure to provide rapid initial stabilization of all patients
- Failure to move, collect, and organize patients quickly in a treatment area
- Failure to provide proper triage
- Provision of overly time-consuming care
- Transport of patients prematurely
- Improper use of personnel in the field
- Failure to distribute patients to medical facilities properly
- Failure to communicate with local hospitals regarding patient flow and hospital capacity
- Lack of proper preplanning and of adequate training for all personnel

PRINCIPLES AND TECHNOLOGY OF TRIAGE

Triage is a method of categorizing patients according to priorities of treatment (Box 54-5). Assessment of the severity of injury is based on abnormal physiological signs, obvious anatomical injury (including the mechanism of injury), and concurrent disease factors that might affect the patient's prognosis. It should be stressed that triage is an ongoing process during a major incident. Constant monitoring of the patient's condition may reveal a need to change the initial grouping and priority of treatment. The

BOX 54-4 Common Failures Seen in the Incident Command System

Incident Command Failures
- To establish a single, unified command
- To establish staging
- To request additional resources early
- To delegate authority
- To wear identification vests

Dispatch Failure
- To coordinate the response of on-duty and off-duty emergency personnel to the scene

Communications Failures
- To designate a single radio channel for disaster operations
- To adopt standard operating procedures that limit radio traffic during incident operations

Staging Operation Failures
- To establish a central staging area (command)
- To select a large or easily accessible staging area (staging manager)
- To frequently inventory specialized equipment and personnel (staging manager)

General Division/Group Failures
- To provide adequate progress reports to command
- To become involved in physical tasks, such as carrying litters or operating rescue equipment (division/group supervisor)
- To control the perimeter (law enforcement)
- To advise command of available personnel

Extrication/Rescue Group Failures
- To triage and tag patients
- To treat patients where they are found (as opposed to stabilizing them and moving them to a treatment area) (rescuers)
- To provide adequate safety precautions

Treatment Group Failures
- To collect patients into an organized treatment area
- To establish a sufficiently large treatment area
- To organize the treatment area and monitor patients
- To effectively coordinate transportation arrangements with the transportation group

Transportation Group Failures
- To establish adequate access and egress routes for vehicles
- To have adequate personnel to assist in transportation
- To alert or update hospitals
- To advise hospitals when the last patient has been transported

Support Branch Failures
- To plan for the medical supply needs of mass casualty events
- To provide rapid transport of supplies to the scene

BOX 54-5 Primary Versus Secondary Triage

Triage may be classified as primary or secondary. **Primary triage** is used at the site to rapidly categorize patient conditions for treatment. During primary triage, the paramedic records the location of the patient and the transport needs. A triage label, tag, ribbon, or tape is then attached to the patient. No care is given during primary triage except for immediate lifesaving measures to ensure an airway or control hemorrhage. The goal is to sort patients quickly.

Secondary triage is used at the treatment area, where patients are triaged again. They are labeled (usually with paper tags) to assign priorities of care. Secondary triage often is not needed at small-scale incidents.

criteria for triage classifications are determined by the size of the incident, the number of injured patients, and the available personnel. National guidelines have been established for field triage (*SALT triage*).[5] Another widely recognized model is the **s**imple **t**riage **a**nd **r**apid **t**reatment (START) technique. The paramedic must be familiar with local methods of triage categorization.

SALT Triage

SALT triage (Sort-Assess-Lifesaving interventions-Treatment and/or Transport) was developed as a national all-hazards mass casualty initial triage standard for all patients (e.g., adults, children, special populations). SALT was designed to allow agencies to easily incorporate it into their current MCI triage protocol through simple modification.

Step 1: Sort

SALT begins with a global sorting of patients, prioritizing them for individual assessment. If possible, patients should be asked to walk to a designated area and should be assigned last priority for individual assessment. Those who remain should be asked to wave (i.e., follow a command) or be observed for purposeful movement. Those who do not move (i.e., are still) and those with obvious life threats should be assessed first since they are the most likely to need lifesaving interventions.

Step 1: Group sorting
- Priority 1: Still/obvious life threat
- Priority 2: Wave/purposeful movement
- Priority 3: Walk

Step 2: Assess

The individual assessment should begin with limited rapid lifesaving interventions:

- Controlling major hemorrhage through the use of tourniquets or direct pressure provided by other patients or other devices
- Opening the airway through positioning or basic airway adjuncts (no advanced airway devices should be used)
- If the patient is a child, consider giving two rescue breaths

- Chest decompression
- Auto injector antidotes

A **lifesaving intervention** (LSI) should only be performed within the responder's scope of practice and only if the equipment is immediately available. Patients should be prioritized for treatment and/or transport by assigning them to one of five categories: *immediate, expectant, delayed, minimal, dead*. Patients who have mild injuries that are self-limited if not treated and can tolerate a delay in care without increasing their risk of mortality should be triaged as *minimal* and should be designated with the color green. Patients who are not breathing even after lifesaving interventions are attempted should be triaged as *dead* and should be designated with the color black. Patients who do not obey commands, **or** do not have a peripheral pulse, **or** are in respiratory distress, **or** have uncontrolled major hemorrhage should be triaged as *immediate* and should be designated with the color red. Providers should consider if these patients have injuries that are likely to be incompatible with life given the currently available resources; if this is true, then the provider should triage these patients as *expectant* and should be designated with the color gray. The remaining patients should be triaged as *delayed* and should be designated with the color yellow.

This prioritization process is dynamic and may be altered by changing patient conditions, resources, and scene safety. Triage labeling systems should account for the dynamic nature of triage and be easily modifiable for a single patient. After *immediate* patients have received care, patients designated *expectant, delayed*, or *minimal* should be reassessed as soon as possible with the expectation that some patients will have improved and others will have decompensated. In general, treatment and/or transport should be provided for *immediate* patients first, then *delayed*, and then *minimal*. *Expectant* patients should be provided with treatment and/or transport when resources permit. Efficient use of transport assets may include mixing categories of patients and using alternate forms of transport. Some patients may only require treatment at the scene and not transport (Figure 54-10).

START Technique of Primary Triage

The *START Field Guide* was developed by Hoag Memorial Presbyterian Hospital in Newport Beach, California. It describes a 60-second assessment. This assessment focuses on the patient's ability to walk, respiratory effort, pulses/perfusion, and mental status (Figure 54-11). This assessment is used to classify a victim's status as *minor, delayed, immediate*, and *dead*. The *START Field Guide* allows rescuers to quickly identify victims at greatest risk of early death. Rescuers can then advise other rescuers of the patient's need for stabilization by tagging the patient with color-coded triage tags (described in the following section).

TRIAGE PROCEDURE

The paramedic should first assess the patient's ability to walk. Patients who can walk and understand basic

commands are categorized as *minor* ("walking wounded"). They will be further triaged and tagged as more rescuers arrive. Patients who are *minor* should be directed to remain in their location for further assistance or to walk to a treatment or transportation site. The initial START triage is directed toward patients who cannot walk.

> **NOTE**
> The mnemonic "30-2-can-do" is used as the START triage prompt. *30* refers to the patient's respiratory rate; *2* refers to capillary refill time; and *can-do* refers to the patient's ability to follow commands. A respiratory rate of fewer than 30 breaths/min, a capillary refill time of less than 2 seconds, and the ability to walk and follow commands is considered a minor patient.

Patients who meet the "30-2-can-do" criteria but who cannot walk are categorized as *delayed*. Patients who are unconscious, have rapid breathing, have delayed or absent capillary refill, or have an absent radial pulse are categorized as *immediate*. Patients who are not breathing should have their airway opened. If they resume spontaneous breathing, they are considered *delayed*. If breathing does not resume after opening the airway, the patient is categorized as *dead*.

> **CRITICAL THINKING**
> What conditions might a patient have if the respiratory rate is fewer than 10 or more than 30 breaths per minute?

As mentioned previously, repositioning the airway and controlling severe hemorrhage are the only treatments given in initial triage. However, in a mass casualty event, these measures should not delay the triage of other patients. Depending on the circumstances and the number of casualties, the walking wounded may be able to help provide airway support and control severe hemorrhage for more seriously wounded victims.

> **SHOW ME THE EVIDENCE**
> Researchers sought to determine the accuracy of START triage. They hypothesized that this triage tool would be 90% sensitive and specific for predicting injury. Of the 163 triaged on the scene at a 2003 train crash, they were able to find and retrospectively review 148 hospital records. On the scene patients were triaged 22 red, 68 yellow, and 58 green. Patient outcome records showed 2 red, 26 yellow, and 120 green. No level met their predicted criteria although the tool was 100% sensitive for determining red (immediate) patients and 89.3% specific for green patients. They felt that in this instance there was a sufficient amount of undertriage but it did produce a large amount of overtriage. They conclude that the tool was effective to prioritize patient transport to hospitals from the scene.

From Kahn CA, Schultz C, Miller K, et al: Does START triage work? An outcomes assessment after a disaster, *Ann Emerg Med* 54(3):424-430, 2009.

SALT Mass Casualty Triage

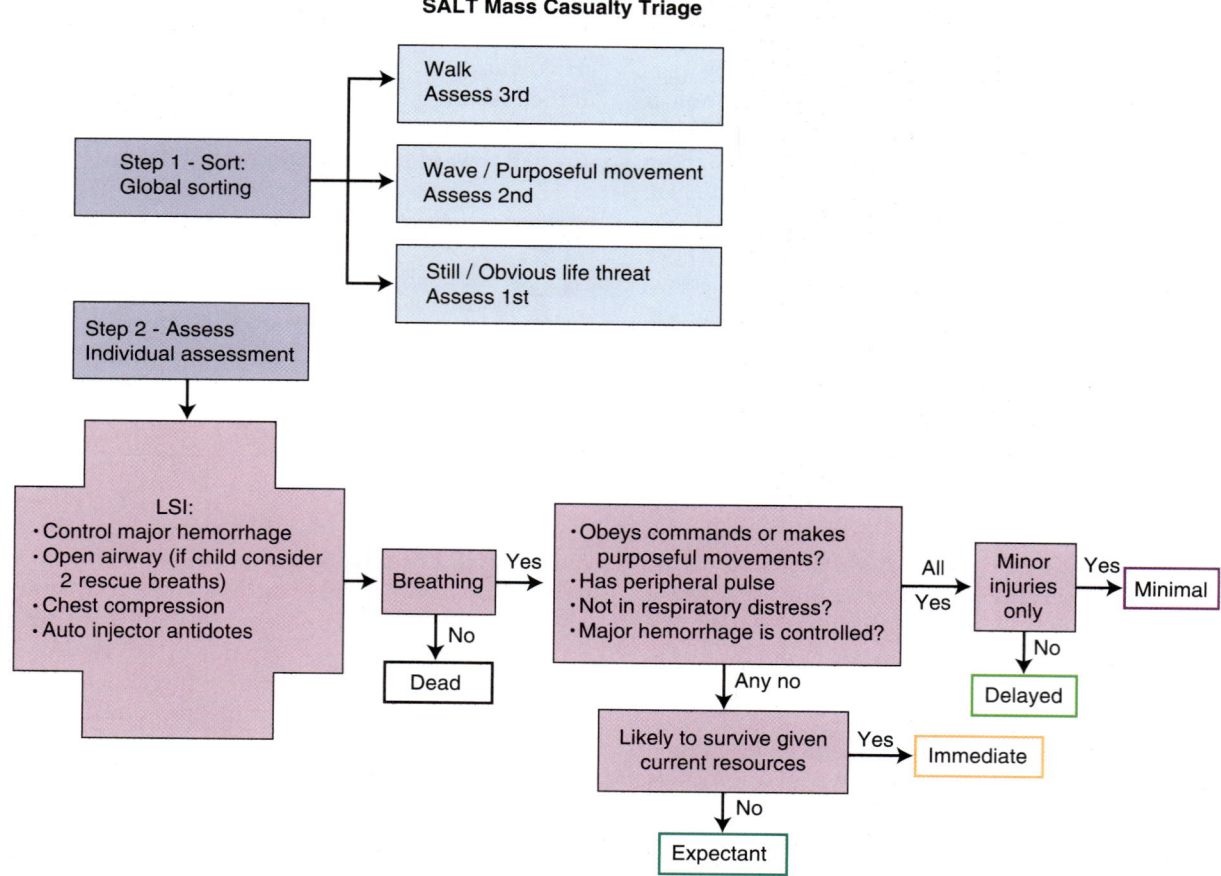

FIGURE 54-10 SALT Triage Scheme.*

---

*This field triage decision scheme, originally developed by the American College of Surgeons Committee on Trauma, was revised by an expert panel representing emergency medical services, emergency medicine, trauma surgery, and public health. The panel was convened by the Centers for Disease Control and Prevention (CDC), with support from the National Highway Traffic Safety Administration (NHTSA).

TABLE 54-1 International Color Coding and Priorities		
Patient Status	**Color Code**	**Priority**
Immediate	Red	Priority no. 1 (P-1)
Delayed	Yellow	Priority no. 2 (P-2)
Hold	Green	Priority no. 3 (P-3)
Deceased	Black	Priority no. 0 (P-0)

Triage Tagging/Labeling

Many types of tags, tapes, ribbons, and labels are used to indicate a victim's triage category (**triage tagging system**). Two commonly used labeling methods are the **METTAG system** and the **SMART tag system**. The METTAG system uses the international agreement on color coding and priorities to alert emergency care personnel and staff members of the receiving hospital to the patient's category (Table 54-1). *Red* identifies the victims who are most critically injured; *yellow,* those less critically injured; *green,* those with injuries that are not life or limb threatening; and *black,* patients who have died or whose injuries preclude survival (Figure 54-12). Triage tags and labels should be used routinely for practice so that EMS crews become familiar with their use. The SMART tag system uses four color triage coding cards that have military bar codes for tracking patients[6] (Figure 54-13):

1. Priority 1 (red) indicates immediate treatment.
2. Priority 2 (yellow) indicates urgent treatment.
3. Priority 3 (green) indicates delayed treatment.
4. Black cards indicate death.

Regardless of the labeling system used, categorization must identify the priority of the patient's condition, prevent retriage of the same patient, and serve as a tracking system during treatment and transport. Therefore all tags and labels should have the following characteristics:

- Be easy to use.
- Rapidly identify the patient's priority.
- Allow for easy tracking.

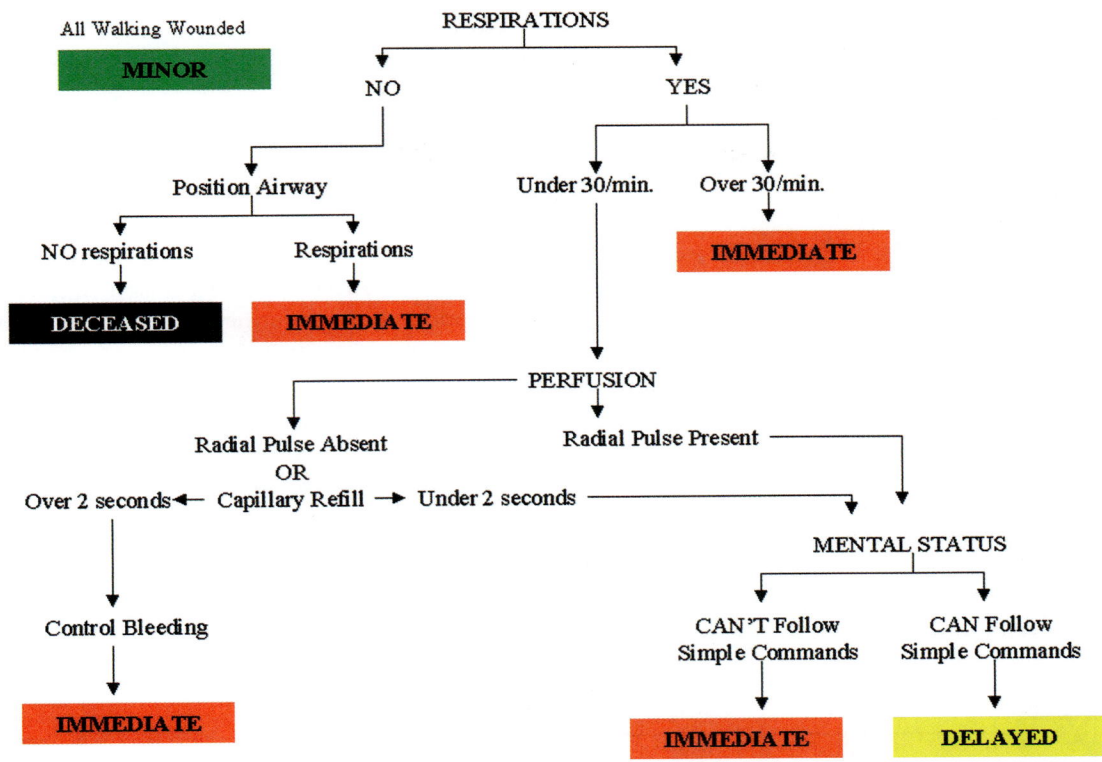

FIGURE 54-11 The simple triage and rapid treatment (START) system sorts patients into critical or delayed categories. Patients are quickly removed from the scene according to their triage group.

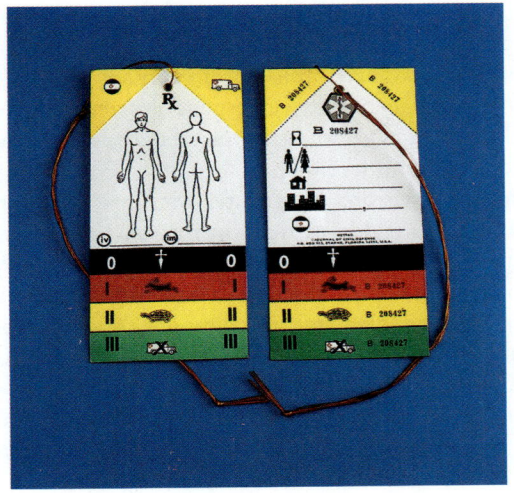

FIGURE 54-12 METTAG card.

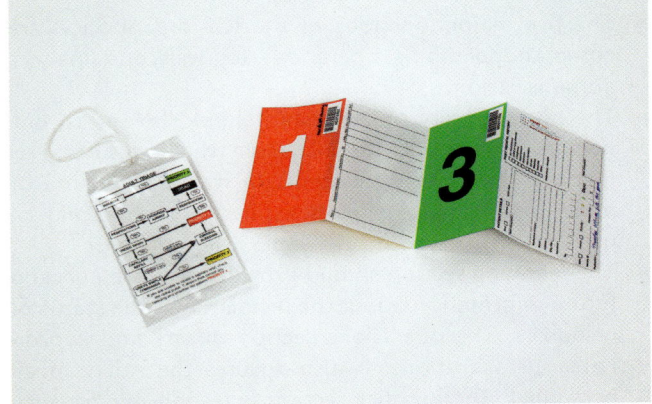

FIGURE 54-13   SMART triage tag with bar code.

- Allow room for some documentation.
- Prevent patients from retriaging themselves.

Tracking Systems for Patients

As described previously, the transportation group officer must keep a tracking or destination log that integrates the triage tagging system. In addition, the log should have the patient's name or triage label identification number. A **tracking log** is similar to a shipping manifest. It must have the following information:

- Patient identification
- Transporting unit
- Patient priority
- Hospital destination

Transportation of Patients

The way patients are transported depends on their triage priority and situation. Ambulances typically are used. However, buses may be used to transport a large number of stable patients. Air ambulances are usually reserved for the transport of patients in critical condition.

CRITICAL INCIDENT STRESS MANAGEMENT

As described in Chapter 2, *critical incident stress* is a potential hazard for rescue personnel. For this reason, critical incident stress debriefings often are conducted after a disaster. To review, the basic types of services that should be made available include the following[7]:

- Preincident stress training for all personnel
- On-scene support for obviously distressed personnel
- Individual consults when only one or two rescuers are affected by an incident

- Defusing services immediately after a large-scale incident
- Mobilization services after a large-scale incident
- Critical incident stress debriefing 24 to 72 hours after an event for any emergency personnel involved in a stressful incident
- Follow-up services to ensure that personnel are recovering
- Specialty debriefings to nonemergency groups when no other timely resources are available in the community
- Support during routine discussions of an incident by emergency personnel
- Advice to command staff during large-scale events

Other approaches that can aid stress management include employee assistance programs, counseling, spouse support programs, family life programs, pastoral services, and periodic stress evaluations.

SUMMARY

- Major incidents are events for which available resources are not adequate to manage the number of casualties or the type of emergency.
- The ICS organizational structure should be adaptable to any agency or to any incident requiring emergency management. The ICS also must be expandable. It must be able to expand from dealing with a nonmajor incident to a major one in a logical way.
- The five major functions of the ICS organization are command, planning, operations, logistics, and finance/administration.
- The responsibility of command should belong to one person. This should be a person who can effectively manage the emergency scene. In multiagency and/or multijurisdictional incidents, unified command may be used.
- The planning section should provide past, present, and future information about the incident and the status of resources. The operations section directs and coordinates all operations. It also ensures the safety of all personnel. The logistics section is responsible for providing supplies and equipment (including personnel to operate the equipment), facilities, services, food, and communications support. The finance/administration section tracks incident and reimbursement costs.
- All participating response agencies must agree to the preplan (phase 1 of the ICS). The preplan must address common goals and the specific duties of each group. Phase 2 requires the development of a strategy to manage the emergency scene. Phase 3 includes a post-disaster review of lessons learned from the incident and the determination of ways to improve the response effort.
- The need to expand the ICS at a medical incident is based on the number of casualties and the nature of the event.
- The first EMS unit to arrive at the scene should make a quick and rapid assessment of the situation. Command must immediately establish radio contact with the communications center or emergency operations center. Additional units should be requested as soon as the need has been identified.
- Common divisions or groups that may need to be established include extrication/rescue, treatment, and transportation. A staging area and support branch may also be needed. The rescue/extrication group is responsible for managing trapped patients at the scene. The treatment group provides advanced care and stabilization until the patients are transported to a medical facility. The transportation group communicates with the receiving hospital, ambulances, and aeromedical services for patient transport. The staging area is used in large incidents to prevent vehicle congestion and delays in response. The rehabilitation area allows rescue personnel to receive physical and psychological rest. The support branch coordinates the gathering and distribution of equipment and supplies for all divisions and groups.
- Problems of mass casualty incidents and incident command systems stem from numerous issues related to communication, resource allocation, and delegation.

- Triage is a method used to categorize patients for priorities of treatment. START triage uses a 60-second assessment. It focuses on the patient's ability to walk, respiratory effort, pulses/perfusion, and neurological status. The METTAG system is one of a number of tape, tag, and label systems used to categorize patients during triage.

- Critical incident stress debriefing is part of a critical incident stress management program. Such debriefing should be part of postdisaster standard operating procedures.

REFERENCES

1. *FEMA, National Incident Management System*, www.fema.gov/pdf/emergency/nims/NIMS_core.pdf, accessed 11-9-10.
2. Cittone G, editor: *Disaster medicine*, Philadelphia, 2006, Mosby.
3. National Fire Academy, U.S. Fire Administration: *ICS-400: Advanced ICS for command and general staff, complex incidents and MACS for operational first responders (H-467) student manual*, www.nctcog.dst.tx.us/ep/training/ICS_400_Student_Manual.pdf, accessed 11-9-10.
4. U.S. Department of Homeland Security: *National Incident Management System*, Washington, DC, 2008, Author.
5. MMWR: *Guidelines for field triage of injured patients: recommendations of the national expert panel on field triage*, www.cdc.gov/mmwr/pdf/rr/rr5801.pdf, accessed 11-9-10.
6. tagassociates.co.uk/English/civilian/products/smart_tag.htm, Accessed September 11, 2011.
7. Mitchell J, Bray G: *Emergency services stress*, Englewood Cliffs, NJ, 1990, Brady Publishing.

SUGGESTED READINGS

Annas GJ: Standard of care—in sickness and in health and in emergencies, *N Engl J Med* 362:2126-2131, 2010.

Lerner E, Swartz R, Coule P, et al: Use of SALT triage in a simulated mass casualty incident, *PEC* 14(1):21-25, 2010.

55 Rescue Awareness and Operations

supplied-air breathing apparatus A device that provides a nearly unlimited supply of air from a source located outside the confined space.

surface water rescue The rescue of a patient who is afloat on the surface of a body of water.

systems operations approach A form of rescue management where extrication is performed by fire service personnel, specialized units, or both—and where patient care is the duty of EMS personnel.

Rescue is defined as "the act of delivery from danger or imprisonment." Many of the day-to-day activities of EMS personnel and other public service agencies are embraced by this definition when they respond to an emergency where people have been traumatized or stranded. Rescue requires specialized medical and mechanical skills, with the right amount of each being applied at the appropriate time.

> **NOTE**
> Rescue skills have become highly specialized. Techniques have been devised and refined for farm rescue, high-angle rescue, rescue in confined spaces, search and recovery, and others. In addition, many rescue agencies require training and certification by an authority or jurisdiction. A number of rescue skills may be needed in a specific area. Also, many different techniques may be involved in a rescue. This chapter focuses on concepts that are basic to all rescue operations.

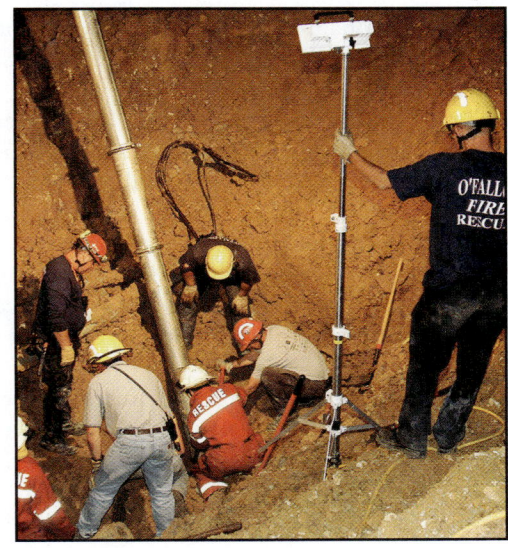

(Courtesy Ray Kemp. St. Charles, Mo.)

APPROPRIATE TRAINING FOR RESCUE OPERATIONS

Rescue work requires training and expertise so that medical and mechanical skills are carefully balanced. This helps to ensure that patients receive effective treatment and timely extrication. The rescue effort must be driven by the patient's needs, both medical and physical. The success of any rescue depends on a coordinated effort between medical care and specialized rescue efforts. A coordinated effort allows the following:

- Patient access and assessment for treatment needs
- Initiation of treatment at the site
- Release of the patient from entrapment or imprisonment
- Continuous medical care throughout the incident

Role of the Paramedic in Rescue Operations

Most rescues in the United States are accomplished through a **systems operations approach.** In this form of rescue management, extrication is performed by fire service personnel, specialized units, or both—patient care is the duty of EMS personnel. In another type of rescue system, rescue services are provided by fire, EMS, or law enforcement

agencies that have **cross-trained personnel.** In this system, the roles and responsibilities for rescue and patient care are shared.

The primary role of the paramedic in rescue operations is to have proper training and appropriate personal protective equipment (PPE) that allow for safe access to the patient and treatment at the site and throughout the incident. Paramedics often are the first responders to many scenes that require rescue. Therefore they should:

- Understand the hazards associated with various environments
- Know when it is safe to gain access or attempt rescue
- Have the skills to perform a rescue when it is safe and necessary
- Understand the rescue process and know when certain techniques are indicated or contraindicated
- Be skilled in patient packaging techniques to allow safe extrication and medical care

> **CRITICAL THINKING**
> What kind of emotions do you think you would see in a critical life-threatening rescue?

> **NOTE**
> Medical monitoring and rehabilitation (*rehab*) of other rescuers at the scene also is an important role for paramedics. Medical monitoring and rehab will be further addressed in Chapter 57.

Safety

Safety during any rescue operation is paramount because of the potential for associated risks. For example, rescues may involve hazardous materials, inclement weather, temperature extremes, fire, electrical hazards, toxic gases, unstable structures, heavy equipment, road hazards, and sharp edges and fragments. Initial scene assessment for hazards, use of personal protective measures, and constant monitoring throughout the operation are essential for every rescue response.

The priorities for safety in any rescue are (1) personal safety, (2) the safety of the crew, (3) the safety of bystanders, and (4) rescue of the trapped and injured. The reasons for this order of priority are as follows:

- When well-trained and properly equipped rescuers act safely, remaining vigilant for hazards, they minimize the risk of personal injury and of complicating the scene by becoming another patient who requires care and possibly extrication.
- The crew is the support team for the rescuer. Therefore crew safety is essential to ensure an effective rescue and to provide mutual support for each team member. Operating with disregard for the safety of fellow team members increases the risk of injuries. It also complicates the operation.
- Uninvolved people must be evacuated and kept clear of hazards. Bystanders or untrained "helpers" only increase the risk of additional injuries. They also complicate the rescue operation.
- Rescue of the trapped or injured is the last priority. These people are already trapped or injured. Carrying out the first three priorities safely maximizes the chance for a successful rescue.

Phases of a Rescue Operation

A rescue operation has seven phases: (1) arrival and scene size-up, (2) hazard control, (3) gaining access to the patient, (4) medical treatment, (5) disentanglement, (6) patient packaging, and (7) transportation. As is stressed throughout this text, paramedics should not enter a scene until it has been secured and made safe by trained personnel. Personal safety is always a priority.

Arrival and Scene Size-Up

The first phase of a rescue is the arrival and scene size-up. This phase requires the paramedic to determine what is needed at a specific emergency event. This involves quickly gathering facts about the situation, analyzing the problems, and determining the appropriate response. During this phase, the EMS crew must:

- Understand the environment and risks
- Establish command and conduct a scene assessment
- Determine the number of patients and triage as necessary
- Determine whether the situation is a search, rescue, or body recovery

- Perform a risk versus benefit analysis that considers personal safety before rescue is attempted
- Request additional information
- Make a realistic time estimate in accessing and evaluating patients or other people at the scene

Scene size-up is an ongoing evaluation of the emergency scene. It begins when the call is received and when information is obtained from the dispatch center. The paramedic must constantly be alert to situations that may change the needs of a particular incident. If power lines are downed during an extrication, for example, electrical utility services may be needed that were not initially required. Three elements of the assessment phase are response, other factors, and resources.

RESPONSE

During the initial response to a scene, information often is limited. En route, the EMS crew and the dispatcher should gather as much detail about the situation as possible. Essential information includes exact location, type of occupancy (manufacturing, mercantile, residence), number of victims, type of situation, and hazards involved. Weather conditions (e.g., extreme heat or cold, rising water, rain, high winds) also can affect rescue attempts, the patient's status, and the need to expedite the operation.

As described in Chapter 17, standardized dispatch protocols guide the initial emergency response. This predetermined system is based on the level of the reported emergency. For example, if the event is a single-car crash, a first-responder fire company and EMS unit may be dispatched. If the event involves a bus wreck with many patients, several fire companies and EMS units may respond. As the dispatch center receives information about the actual severity of the event, the dispatch protocol upgrades or downgrades the response as needed. The center advises the responding units of the updated reports.

CRITICAL THINKING
Is there any disadvantage to routinely sending too much emergency equipment to a scene?

OTHER FACTORS

Other factors to be considered in determining the type of response needed are the description of the scene and the time of day. An emergency in a highly populated area may call for special vehicles and equipment for extrication and fire suppression. Examples of such a scene would be a high-rise apartment, a school, or a shopping mall. An emergency in a rural or wilderness setting may require helicopter rescue or other resources. If hazardous materials are present, special response and decontamination equipment may be needed for bystanders, patients, and rescue personnel.

The time of day may affect on-scene needs. For example, rush-hour traffic and crowd control may be a concern; extra lighting may be needed for early morning, evening, or night rescue. These and other factors determine the personnel requirements and the scene management operations.

RESOURCES

The ability to assess an emergency quickly and correctly requires preplanning. It also requires the development of a systems approach to the response. The available resources are a critical part of any response. The responding crew may not have the personnel, training, or expertise to handle the event. Resources that may be required include the following:

- Additional emergency vehicles for a large number of patients
- Area hospital availability and personnel
- Aeromedical services
- Law enforcement personnel
- Fire service for automobile extrication, fire suppression, or lighting
- Water rescue, teams with self-contained underwater breathing apparatus (SCUBA), and other specialized rescue units
- Hazardous materials teams
- Urban search and rescue teams

Hazard Control

Hazard control is the phase of rescue in which on-scene dangers are quickly identified and managed by the first-arriving crew. This involves minimizing risks from uncontrollable hazards, making sure the scene is as safe as possible, and ensuring that all personnel are equipped with PPE appropriate for the incident. Examples of possible hazards at a scene include fire, unstable structures, confined spaces, swift water, poisonous substances, dangerous animals, and unruly crowds. Hazard control for specific types of incidents is discussed throughout this chapter.

Gaining Access to the Patient

Rapid access to an ill or injured patient who requires extrication or rescue can be critical to the patient's eventual outcome. For patients who have multisystem trauma, assessment, stabilization, and extrication should be rapid. However, these procedures must be accomplished with the safety of both the patient and the rescue team as a top priority. To safely gain access, the paramedic must determine the best method of reaching the patient, deploy appropriate personnel to the patient, and stabilize the patient's physical location.

Extrication tools and equipment (Figure 55-1) can cause injuries. To reduce the risk, paramedics should use the least amount of force needed. They should clear the area of unnecessary people. In addition, extraneous noise should be kept to a minimum. Also, a **safety officer** should remain alert to the stress of the operation on the rescuers. This

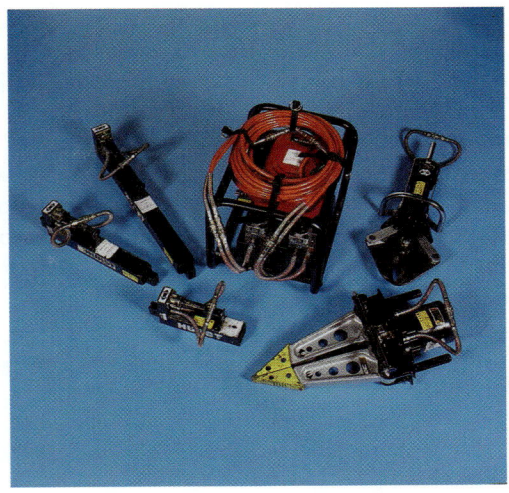

FIGURE 55-1 Extrication tools and equipment.

officer should rotate personnel to prevent heat exposure disorders and injuries resulting from fatigue. Rescuers should wear approved protective clothing. Also, protective covering for the patient should be supplied.

Paramedics may not directly take part in freeing the patient. However, they have chief responsibility for patient care. In addition, they serve a key role as observers for potentially hazardous procedures. The "team concept" is the most important element in any rescue system or operation. Teamwork maximizes safety, efficiency, and effectiveness. It is a basic element of prehospital care. In addition, it has powerful implications for the safety of responders.

Medical Treatment

After the team has gained access to the patient, medical treatment can begin. The paramedic should perform a rapid primary survey to identify and manage any life-threatening situations. Care may be limited by circumstances and the physical working area. However, the paramedic may be able to initiate some stabilization procedures, such as spinal immobilization, airway management, oxygen administration, and intravenous (IV) fluid therapy. If the paramedic recognizes rapidly fatal or potentially fatal conditions, a "load and go" approach must be taken. In these cases, rapid extrication and transport are indicated.

A physical examination should be performed after the primary survey has been completed and life-threatening conditions have been managed. Another crew member may perform the examination at the same time of the primary survey if it does not interrupt the initial assessment and emergency care.

Disentanglement

Disentanglement involves making a pathway through the wreckage of an incident and removing wreckage from patients. The main responsibilities of the paramedic during disentanglement are to release the patient from entrapment and to perform a **risk versus benefit analysis**. (*Does the risk outweigh the benefit or vice versa?*) This analysis should take personal safety into account. This phase of rescue is driven by the needs of the patient. It may call for specialized rescue personnel and equipment. Paramedics should be aware of the available resources in their area. They also should know how to mobilize these resources. Disentanglement often is time-consuming; the EMS crew should be prepared for extended scene time.

CRITICAL THINKING
What rescue teams are accessible to your community?

Patient Packaging

Stabilizing a patient physically and preparing the person for transport is known as **patient packaging.** This may require special rescue capabilities. For instance, the patient may need to be moved over hazardous terrain or lifted by hoist to a helicopter. As with all other aspects of rescue, the coordination of activities and the sharing of patient care responsibilities among the various agencies offer the greatest chance of a successful outcome.

It is the paramedic's responsibility to ensure the patient is ready to be removed from the scene. It also is the paramedic's duty to protect the patient from additional injury during disentanglement and **egress** (exit pathway). The patient should be covered with blankets or tarpaulins and provided with ear and eye protection. In addition, a face mask with supplemental oxygen or air should be applied. This protects the patient from toxic fumes, if present.

For minimum packaging for transport, the patient's airway and cervical spine must be stabilized, IV lines and oxygen tubing must be secured, and the patient must be immobilized on a long spine board. When time allows, extremity fractures should be immobilized and open wounds covered with sterile dressings and secured with bandages. A scene delay for patients who require rapid stabilization and transport may lessen the patient's chances of survival.

Use of other patient care equipment should be considered as the patient is removed from the area of entrapment. Communication and coordination with other rescuers must continue during this process. The exit pathway must be clear and secure. No additional danger for the patient or the rescuers should exist during the removal phase.

During disentanglement and patient packaging, the paramedic should consider the patient's emotional needs. Patients often are anxious and frightened by the rescue operations. When possible, paramedics should maintain a rapport with the patient. They should (1) provide reassurance that the patient is receiving good care; (2) prepare the patient for unexpected movements or procedures that may cause discomfort; and (3) explain all rescue maneuvers.

Transportation

If the patient is to be transported immediately to the ambulance, a wheeled stretcher, basket stretcher, scoop stretcher, or long spine board should be available. While the patient is transported to the emergency vehicle, the terrain, equipment, and personnel requirements for moving the patient should be considered (e.g., the need for air evacuation, specialized resources, and extra personnel). The ambulance should be appropriately warmed or cooled, based on the patient's needs and the rescue setting. The rescue is considered complete once the patient is en route to the hospital. As in any other patient transport, the EMS crew continues emergency care, and medical direction is advised of the patient's status.

RESCUER PERSONAL PROTECTIVE EQUIPMENT

Personal protective equipment for EMS personnel historically has been adapted from other fields (e.g., the fire service). The standards for protective clothing and PPE established by the National Fire Protection Association[1] and the federal Occupational Safety and Health Administration (OSHA)[2] have been adopted by many fire and EMS agencies, including a number of municipal and industrial fire services throughout the United States. It generally is agreed that, at minimum, EMS providers involved in rescue and other rescue personnel should have access to the following PPE:

- Impact-resistant protective helmet with ear protection and chinstrap
- Safety goggles with elastic strap and vents to prevent fogging
- Lightweight, puncture-resistant turnout coat
- Slip-resistant, waterproof gloves
- Boots with steel insoles and steel toe protection
- Self-contained breathing apparatus (SCBA)

The same PPE is not appropriate in all situations. Adequate protection depends on the level of rescuer involvement and the nature of the incident. Other PPEs may be appropriate in some rescue events (Box 55-1).

SHOW ME THE EVIDENCE
This research performed a retrospective review of the rate of injury or illness of Southern Arizona Rescue Association (SARA) volunteers during wilderness rescue over 30 years. This group averages 60 to 80 rescue operations per year. SARA volunteers had a similar number of lost work days for health services personnel as fire department personnel. Injuries were primarily musculoskeletal although there was one near drowning, one scorpion sting, and one chipped tooth reported. There were no deaths. The author cautions against generalizing this information to other rescue squads because of the uniqueness of the geographical terrain and because incident operations occurred mostly at night; in addition, SARA volunteers had an average of 8 years' experience.

From Iserson K: Injuries to search and rescue volunteers, *West J Med* 151:352-353, 1989.

Box 55-1 Supplemental Personal Protective Equipment

Head Protection That Meets Safety Standards for the Appropriate Use

- Compact firefighters' helmet that meets National Fire Protection Association (NFPA) standards for most vehicle/structural applications
- Climbing helmet for confined-space and technical rescue uses
- Padded rafting/kayaking helmet for water rescue

Eye Protection

- Adequate face shield (face shields on most fire helmets are inadequate)
- American National Standards Institute (ANSI)–approved safety glasses or goggles with solid shields (preferred)

Hearing Protection

- Required for high-noise areas
- Ear plugs or ear muffs should be available

Hand Protection

- Gloves that allow adequate dexterity and protect against cuts and punctures

Foot Protection

- Gear that provides ankle support to limit range of motion
- Tread that provides traction and prevents slips
- Insulation from environmental extremes
- Steel toe/shank that meets safety requirements

Flame/Flash Protection (When Fire Is Possible)

- Nomex/PBI/flame-retardant cotton to provide limited flash protection, turnout clothing, jumpsuits/flyers/coveralls (*Note:* This clothing does not provide complete protection from punctures or cuts. The thermal protection offered by turnout clothing may increase heat stress.)

Personal Flotation Device (When Operating on or Around Water)

- Meets Coast Guard standards for flotation
- Type II or type III (preferred for most water rescue work)
- Attached whistle and strobe light
- Attached knife for cutting

Visibility

- Reflective trim on all outerwear
- Orange clothing or safety vests for use during highway operations

Extended, Remote, or Wilderness Protection

- Additional or different personal protective equipment, if needed, for bad weather conditions not normally encountered (e.g., cold, rain, snow, wind)
- Personal drinking water and snacks
- Possible shelter needs

Personal Protection from Blood-Borne Pathogens

OSHA has established criteria for workplace protection from blood-borne and airborne diseases.[3,4] These measures for personal protection (described in Chapter 14) should be observed whenever the potential exists for exposure to a patient's body fluids or to communicable diseases.

 LOOK AGAIN
See Chapter 14: Venous Access and Medication Administration, pp. 380-381.

SURFACE WATER RESCUE

Surface water rescue is the rescue of a patient who is afloat on the surface of a body of water. People are drawn to moving water for recreation. Many, including rescuers, underestimate the power and hazards of water. The hydraulics of moving water are affected by several variables. These include the depth and velocity of water and any obstructions to flow. Water rescue is very dangerous and requires special training and skills. Water rescue should never be attempted by a single rescuer or by an untrained one.

Obstructions to Flow

Water that moves over a uniform obstruction can create recirculating currents ("drowning machines") (Figure 55-2). These can trap victims and make escape difficult. Recirculating currents commonly are found in rivers and on low-head dams and often appear harmless. (The height of the dam is no indication of the degree of hazard.) The force of the moving water is very deceptive and makes for a hazardous rescue. Trapped victims often succumb to fatigue, hypothermia, and drowning.

Strainers are obstructions (e.g., trees, grating wire, or mesh) that allow current to flow through but that can trap objects such as boats or people. The force of the water against the victim makes escape difficult. Rescue teams must approach strainers cautiously to avoid becoming entrapped themselves.

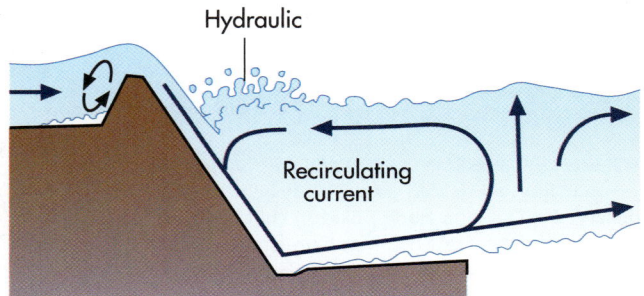

FIGURE 55-2 Low-head dams range in height from 6 inches to 10 feet. They can create dangerous hydraulics.

Foot or Extremity Pin

It generally is considered unsafe to walk in fast-moving water that is over knee-high depth. Doing so may lead to entrapment of an extremity in a strainer, and the victim can be dragged under the water's surface. With a foot or extremity pin, it is crucial to remember that *the body part must be extricated in the same way it became trapped.*

Flat Water

About 3600 deaths occur each year in flat (static) water (lakes, ponds, and marsh) as a result of drowning.[5] Factors that contribute to these deaths include alcohol or other drug use. Another factor is a cool water temperature, which leads to hypothermia. These factors can quickly incapacitate a victim and result in drowning. Most people who drown never planned on being in the water. **Personal flotation devices** (PFDs) that are worn routinely and fastened properly when a person is on or around the water can save lives by reducing the likelihood of drowning. PFDs are required during water rescue operations. Type I or type II PFDs are preferred for water rescue work. Specialty type III, IV, and V PFDs are suitable for some rescue situations.[6]

Water Temperature

As described in Chapter 45, immersion in water with a temperature below 98° F (37° C) can cause hypothermia. A person cannot maintain body heat when the water temperature is below 92° F (33° C). Water causes heat loss 25 times faster than exposure to air at the same temperature. (The colder the water, the faster the rate of heat loss.) At a water temperature of 35° F (1.7° C), a person immersed for 15 to 20 minutes likely will die of hypothermia and drowning.[7]

Sudden immersion in cold water may trigger laryngospasm. This can lead to aspiration, severe hypoxia, and unconsciousness. If hypothermia develops, the victim often is unable to follow directions (e.g., grab a safety device) or help himself or herself to safety. PFDs lessen heat loss and the energy required for flotation. In cases of sudden immersion, a single victim should assume a fetal position (the heat escape–lessening posture [HELP]).

Multiple victims should *huddle* together to reduce heat loss (Figure 55-3).

COLD PROTECTIVE RESPONSE

The cold protective response is the *mammalian diving reflex* (see Chapter 45). This response increases the chance of a victim's survival in cold water. To review, this protective response includes parasympathetic stimulation from immersion of the face in cold water. It leads to bradycardia, peripheral vasoconstriction that shunts blood to the core, and hypotension. The effectiveness of this protective response depends on the victim's age, posture in the water, and lung volume, as well as the water temperature.

The rapid development of hypothermia sometimes can improve brain viability in patients who suffer prolonged submersion. Therefore hypothermic patients should be presumed salvageable. ("A victim is never cold and dead—only warm and dead.") The patient must be rewarmed in a hospital before an accurate assessment can be made.

Rescue Versus Body Recovery

Rescue versus body recovery refers to the chance to save a human life (rescue) versus recovering a body without the goal of saving a human life. In addition to temperature, other factors affect the outcome of a patient who has been submerged in water. These include the length of time the victim has been submerged, known or possible trauma, environmental conditions, the victim's age and physical condition, and the time until rescue or removal is achieved. Because successful resuscitation with full neurological recovery has occurred in victims of prolonged submersion in extremely cold water, resuscitation should be initiated by rescuers at the scene unless physical evidence of death is obvious (e.g., putrefaction, dependent lividity, or rigor mortis).[8]

In-Water Spinal Immobilization

In-water spinal immobilization (see Chapter 41) requires special training. Only rescuers trained in water rescue should enter the water. To review, the steps required for in-water spinal immobilization are as follows[9]:

1. Turn the patient to a supine position by rotating the entire upper half of the body as a single unit.

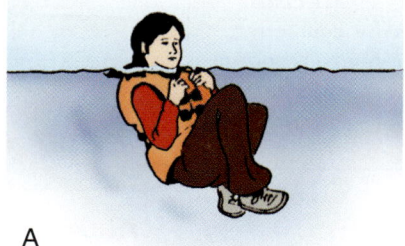
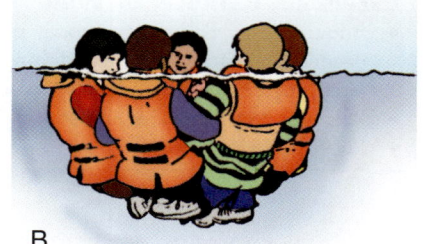

FIGURE 55-3 HELP and HUDDLE. When a person is floating in cold water, body heat can be conserved by using a body position that reduces the escape of heat. **A,** If the person is alone, the HELP position should be used. **B,** If several people are present, they should *huddle* together.

A   B

2. Using spinal precautions, begin artificial ventilation (if needed). Do not attempt to clear the airway of water.[10]
3. Float a long spine board under the patient's body.
4. Apply a rigid cervical collar.
5. Secure the patient to the spine board with straps, cravats, or other devices.
6. Float the patient to the edge of water and remove the patient from the water and completely stabilize. Cover the patient to prevent hypothermia. Begin cardiopulmonary resuscitation (CPR) if indicated.

Overview of Rescue Techniques

As previously stated, rescuers should never underestimate the power of moving water. Also, they should never attempt water rescue without highly specialized training. The recommended water rescue model is *reach-throw-row-go*.

- *Reach.* If the victim is close to shore, the paramedic should try to reach out to the person. An oar, a large branch, a pole, or some other rescue device should be used for this purpose. Before a rescue attempt, paramedics should don a PFD. They also should make sure their footing is secure so that they are not pulled into the water by the victim.
- *Throw.* While the paramedic remains on the shore, a flotation device (e.g., a water throw bag attached to polypropylene rope) should be thrown to the victim. That way, the victim can be pulled to shore.
- *Row.* If reach and throw methods are unsuccessful or if the victim is unconscious, trained rescuers should row out to the victim in a boat if one is available.
- *Go.* If a boat is unavailable and reach and throw methods are not viable options, trained rescuers should go to the patient by wading or swimming.

A shore-based rescue attempt by a first responder, either by coaching the victim in self-rescue or by reaching or throwing, is the method of choice. Boat-based or "go" techniques require specialized training.

SELF-RESCUE TECHNIQUES

If paramedics inadvertently enter dangerous water, they should use self-rescue techniques as follows:
1. Cover your mouth and nose during entry.
2. Protect your head and keep your face out of the water.
3. If in flat water, assume the HELP position.
4. If in moving water, do not attempt to stand up.
5. Float on your back with your feet downstream and your head pointed toward the nearest shore at a 45-degree angle.

HAZARDOUS ATMOSPHERES

Hazardous atmospheres are oxygen-deficient environments that may occur in **confined spaces.** (Confined spaces have limited access or egress and are not designed for human occupancy or habitation.) According to the National Institute of Occupational Safety and Health (NIOSH), nearly 60% of the deaths associated with confined spaces

are people attempting rescue of a **victim.**[11] Examples of confined spaces include the following:
- Grain bins and silos
- Wells and cisterns
- Storage tanks
- Manholes and pumping stations
- Drainage culverts
- Underground vaults
- Trenches and cave-ins

Hazards Associated With Confined Spaces

According to OSHA, there are six major hazards associated with confined spaces. These include oxygen-deficient atmospheres, chemical/toxic exposure or explosion, engulfment, machinery entrapment, electricity, and structural concerns.

OXYGEN-DEFICIENT ATMOSPHERES

Oxygen-deficient atmospheres are not a visible hazard. Therefore rescuers often presume that an atmosphere is safe. The available oxygen in confined spaces must be tested by trained personnel. They use an atmospheric monitoring meter at the top, middle, and bottom of a confined space before entry. Any confined space that has an oxygen concentration less than 19.5% must be considered an atmospheric hazard.[12] An oxygen level that is too high (above 22%) in a confined space may produce rapid combustion. This also is a serious safety hazard.

CHEMICAL/TOXIC EXPOSURE OR EXPLOSION

Oxygen can be removed from the atmosphere by certain chemical reactions. Examples include reactions that occur during the formation of rust on steel structures and while pouring concrete, and natural decaying processes that displace oxygen by producing dangerous gases (e.g., methane). In addition, the presence of some chemicals and gases can lead to toxic exposure (see Chapter 57) (Box 55-2). They also may pose a high risk of explosion. Some dusts and particulate materials found in grain bins, silos, and storage tanks can be highly explosive when mixed with air. Many gases are heavier than air. Therefore these gases are found in higher concentrations at the bottom of storage vessels. As

---

Box 55-2 Toxic Gases That May Be Found in Confined Spaces

Hydrogen sulfide (H_2S)
Carbon dioxide (CO_2)
Carbon monoxide (CO)
Chlorine (Cl)
Low or high oxygen (O_2) concentrations
Methane (CH_4)
Ammonia (NH_3)
Nitrogen dioxide (NO_2)

with oxygen content, trained personnel should monitor for toxic or explosive gases in confined spaces using an appropriate testing device.

CRITICAL THINKING
Why can workers easily become disabled in situations that may involve exposure to toxic gases?

NOTE
Some silos are designed to produce oxygen-limiting conditions. This aids the fermentation process. These silos usually can be identified by their blue exteriors.

ENGULFMENT

Mechanical entrapment can occur when earth, grain, coal, or any other dry material that can flow engulfs a person in a confined space. **Engulfment** can produce an oxygen-deficient atmosphere and subsequent suffocation. In addition, those trapped by engulfment may be victims of physical (crushing) injury. They also are at an increased risk from explosive hazards.

MACHINERY ENTRAPMENT

Some structures, such as grain bins and silos, often have augers, screws, conveyors, and other machinery to move material stored in them. These and other mechanical devices can entrap a person, requiring extrication. Before rescue is attempted, trained and experienced personnel should identify and secure all such devices.

DID YOU KNOW?
The Power Take-Off (PTO)
A power take-off (PTO) is a splined driveshaft, usually on a tractor or other farm machinery. The PTO is used to provide power to an attachment or separate machine. The power transfer shaft that connects to the PTO can be a safety hazard to farm workers and emergency responders at the scene. Rescue personnel should never approach a PTO shaft until the machinery has been shut off, disengaging the PTO. In addition, it is important never to step over a rotating PTO shaft, but to walk around the machinery instead. The PTO shaft is responsible for many farm injuries. Clothing, such as shirt sleeves and long pant legs, and long hair can easily get caught on the shaft, resulting in severe injury or death. The rotating PTO shaft has caused more farm workers to lose arms and legs than any other single farming accident.[13]

ELECTRICITY

Electrical hazards from the power supply of motors and materials-management equipment may be present in some situations. Like machinery, all electrical devices must be identified and secured by experienced personnel. (These devices include electrical boxes and switches.) This helps to ensure the safety of the rescuer. This **lock-out process**

must prevent any unauthorized person from entering the area or gaining access to the controls that have been disconnected. Motors and other electrical devices can "store" power that can lead to entrapment or injury. Chemical, steam, and water lines also must be secured or blocked by trained personnel during all rescues.

STRUCTURAL CONCERNS

The supporting structures of a confined space must be identified before entry to aid in safe rescue and extrication. For example, most cylindrical structures are supported by central I beams. These beams allow relatively easy maneuvering. However, noncylindrical structures may have L-, T-, and X-shaped spaces. These can affect entry and rescue procedures. They also can complicate the extrication pathway.

CRUSH COMPARTMENT SYNDROMES SECONDARY TO ENTRAPMENT

As described in Chapter 38, compartment syndrome can be caused by crushing mechanisms, which lead to ischemic muscle damage, tissue necrosis, and crush syndrome. These injuries can be severe. They are associated with rupture of internal organs, major fractures, and hemorrhagic shock. The degree of injury produced by the crushing force depends on three elements: (1) the amount of pressure applied to the body; (2) the length of time the pressure is exerted on the body; and (3) the specific body region where the injury occurs. A massive crush injury to vital organs may cause immediate death.

Patients with crush syndrome are victims of compressive forces that crush tissue. This causes prolonged hypoxia. The patient may appear stable for hours or days, as long as the compressive forces remain in place. When the patient is released from the entrapment, the reperfusion of the trapped body part may lead to detrimental processes. These include volume loss into the tissue and the release of myoglobin, lactic acid, and other toxins into the circulation. As described in Chapter 38, these events occur simultaneously and may ultimately lead to death. If the patient's condition or the mechanism of injury is suspicious for compartment syndrome or crush injury, the paramedic should consult with medical direction. Management of crush syndrome is controversial. Prehospital care must be supervised through a medical direction physician familiar with this pathological process.

LOOK AGAIN
See Chapter 38: Bleeding and Soft Tissue Trauma, pp. 1109-1110.

Emergencies in Confined Spaces

OSHA requires a permit before workers may enter a confined space.[12] This standard has forced industrial, municipal, and government response teams to be better prepared to manage confined-space incidents. Requirements for obtaining a permit include the following:

1. The area must be made safe or workers must wear PPE.
2. Fall-arresting and retrieval devices must be in place.
3. Environmental monitoring must be available at the site before entry.

Sites without permits at which no atmospheric monitoring is performed are likely locations for emergencies. At these sites, rescuers often may encounter oxygen-deficient atmospheres. Other types of emergencies that can occur in confined spaces (in both permitted and nonpermitted locations) include the following:

- Falls
- Medical emergencies
- Explosion
- Entrapment
- Exposure to toxic gases and chemicals

SAFE ENTRY FOR RESCUERS

As previously stated, safe entry for rescuers in a confined-space operation requires specialized training. No rescuer should enter the space until a rescue team has made the area safe. Safe entry cannot be made without the following[11]:

- Proper and thorough training in confined-space rescue
- Atmospheric monitoring to determine the oxygen concentration, hydrogen sulfide level, carbon monoxide level, explosive limits, flammable atmosphere, and toxic air contaminants
- Proper ventilation
- Secured electrical systems (lock-out/tag-out of all power)
- Dissipation of stored energy
- Disconnection of all pipes (blinding/blanking) to prevent flow into the site
- Appropriate respiratory protection

Supplied-Air Breathing Apparatus. Close quarters make access and extrication difficult in confined-space rescue. Because of this, use of the typical "bottle on back" SCBA is usually dangerous. The device provides a limited air supply, can cause entrapment, and may have to be removed in order to reach the victim. The **supplied-air breathing apparatus** (air-line SABA) is preferred in confined-space operations (Figure 55-4). These lightweight devices provide a nearly unlimited supply of air from a device located outside the confined space.

Potential complications of the SABA include equipment malfunction, damaged or entangled air lines, and limitations imposed by the length of the air hose. Trained rescuers carry a small, personal reserve air supply (escape bottle) that can be used for a short time if needed.

ARRIVING AT THE SCENE

An EMS crew that arrives at the scene of a confined-space emergency should proceed as follows:

1. Perform a scene size-up and determine the nature of the emergency by obtaining a copy of the OSHA permit (Figure 55-5) for the site from the permit/entry

supervisor. Determine the number of workers (victims) in the confined space.
2. Request specialized rescue teams.
3. Establish a safe perimeter away from the incident. Allow only rescue team members to enter the space.
4. Assist workers at the site with any remote retrieval devices they may be using.

NOTE: Scene safety is of prime importance for all involved in the rescue. Only specialized rescue personnel should directly perform rescue activities. EMS personnel who are not trained in specialized rescue should assist the rescue team only if they can do so safely without entering the space.

Rescue From Trenches and Cave-Ins

Most trench collapses occur in trenches less than 12 feet deep and 6 feet wide. Federal law requires either shoring or a trench box for evacuations that are 5 feet or deeper. Often these collapses occur when contractors forsake safety measures because of the increased cost of providing them. Factors that contribute to collapse include the following:

- Cave-in of lips on one or both sides of the trench
- Walls that shear away and cave in
- Piling of excavated dirt too close to the edge, causing collapse
- The presence of intersecting trenches
- Ground vibrations
- Water seepage

> **NOTE**
> One cubic foot of soil weighs 100 pounds; 2 feet of soil on a person's chest or back is equal to 700 to 1000 pounds of pressure, which can cause burial and can rapidly lead to suffocation.

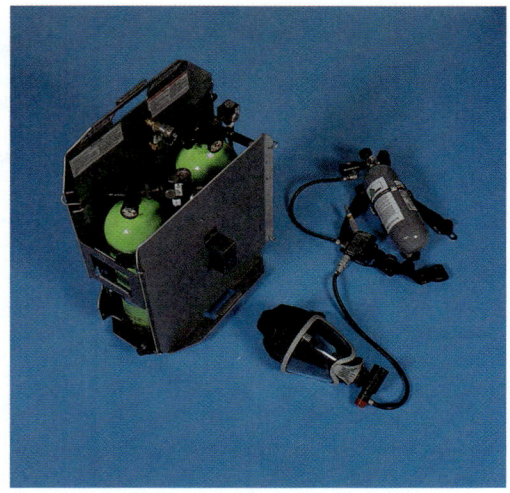

FIGURE 55-4 Supplied-air (air-line) breathing apparatus (SABA).

CONFINED SPACE ENTRY PERMIT

SCOPE

Effective date _____ 19 _____ Time _____ [AM / PM] Expiration date _____ Time _____ [AM / PM]

Permit Issued to _____

Description of Work _____

Lease or Area _____ Specific Location _____

PREP

- ☐ Equipment/piping depressurized & vented
- ☐ Powered(forced air) ventilation
- ☐ Other _____
  _____
- ☐ Equipment/piping blinded, blanked, or misaligned
- ☐ Electric, hydraulic,pneumatic & mechanical energy sources shut-off & locked out
- ☐ Vessel/space steamed,cleaned,or washed

ATMOSPHERE TESTING

Type	☐ Flammable		☐ Oxygen		☐ Hydrogen sulfide	☐ Other_____		☐ Continuous Monitoring	
Time								Instrument	
%, LEL or PPM								Most Recent Calibration date	
Tested by		CO. VERIFY		CO. VERIFY		CO. VERIFY		CO. VERIFY	Field Calibration O.K. ☐
Action Levels	10% L.E.L. <10% evaluate for toxicity		LESS THAN 19.5% MORE THAN 23%		10 PPM		Carbon Monoxide(35ppm),Aromatic Hydrocarbon(10ppm) Ammonia(25ppm),Mineral Spirits(100ppm),Methanol(200ppm)		

PROTECTIVE EQUIPMENT

OPERATIONAL AND PROTECTIVE EQUIPMENT

- ☐ Warning signs, barricades
- ☐ Barricade tape/cones
- ☐ Ventilation Fan or blower
- ☐ Fire extinguisher
- ☐ Ground fault circuit interupter
- ☐ Lighting(hazardous location rated)
- ☐ Static protection
- ☐ Ladder
- ☐ Other _____

PERSONAL PROTECTIVE EQUIPMENT

- ☐ Self Contained Breathing Apparatus
- ☐ Airline supplied respirator
- ☐ Chemical splash goggles
- ☐ Impervious gloves
- ☐ Impervious clothing
- ☐ Boots
- ☐ Hearing protection
- ☐ Safety glasses
- ☐ Fall protection/arresting equipment
- ☐ Other _____

EMERGENCY ACTION

RESCUE PROCEDURES AND EQUIPMENT

Emergency Phone Number [   ]   **Base Station** _____

Location of Phone/Radio _____

RESCUE EQUIPMENT NEEDED

- ☐ Full body harness/lifeline
- ☐ Rescue winch
- ☐ Wristlets
- ☐ Personal motion alarm
- ☐ Davit/Tripod
- ☐ Other _____

CSE COMMUNICATION

- ☐ Radio communication
- ☐ Rope signals
- ☐ Visual hand signals
- ☐ Other _____

POTENTIAL EMERGENCY SITUATION(S) _____
_____

ACTIONS TO BE TAKEN _____
_____

SIGNATURE

CONFINED SPACE ENTRANT(S)   We(I) have reviewed the potential emergency situations and actions to be taken. We(I) are familiar with all rescue equipment, and communication methods.

X _____   X _____   X _____

CONFINED SPACE OBSERVER/STANDBY   I have checked all rescue and communication equipment and reviewed all emergency actions to be taken with entrant personnel. X _____

CONTRACT SUPERVISOR   I have evaluated and completed all portions of this permit. All personnel have reviewed the conditions of the permit and are adequately trained to perform this job. I have reviewed the site to ensure compliance with the requirements of this permit. X _____

MOBIL REPRESENTATIVE   I have evaluated and completed all portions of this permit. All personnel have reviewed the conditions of the permit and are adequately trained to perform this job. I have reviewed the site to ensure compliance with the requirements of this permit. X _____

DEBRIEF

Were any Hazards or Potential Hazards Encountered During the CSE?   NO ☐   YES ☐   If yes, Explain
_____
_____

White - Local Safety Dept.   **Manila Tag - Post at Job Site**

BAKCSE 93

iv - xii

CMC Confined Space Rescue Manual

FIGURE 55-5 Example of a confined-space entry permit.

ARRIVAL AT THE SCENE

On arrival at the scene of a collapse that has resulted in burial, paramedics should keep in mind that a second collapse is likely and should not approach the lip. EMS personnel should not attempt a rescue unless the trench is less than waist deep. Instead, they should take the following steps in scene management:

1. Secure the scene, establish command, and secure a safe perimeter.
2. Shut down nonessential equipment that can cause vibrations.
3. Request specialized rescue teams.
4. Prevent entry into the trench or cave-in area.

Access to the patient should be attempted by trained personnel only after proper shoring is in place. The process of shoring and excavating can be labor and time intensive. However, scene safety is necessary for a successful recovery.

CRITICAL THINKING

Consider an EMS and rescue team that, for safety reasons, will be unable to go in after a person who is buried in a trench collapse. How do you think they will feel?

HIGHWAY OPERATIONS

Traffic flow is a major hazard in EMS highway operations. Factors associated with highway hazards include emergency responses to limited and unlimited access highways, emergency vehicle crashes, and the backup of traffic that impedes flow to and from the scene. Because of the potential problems in traffic flow, EMS personnel must work closely with law enforcement personnel to help ensure a safe response. Paramedics can take the following steps to reduce traffic hazards:

- Position an apparatus (pumper, rescue, or other emergency vehicle) across the traffic direction in the fend-off position. This protects the scene from traffic hazards.
- Stage unnecessary apparatus off the highway (this is essential on limited access highways); establish a staging area away from the scene.
- Position an apparatus to reduce traffic flow and provide for a safe ambulance loading area.
- Use only essential warning lights so that drivers are not distracted or confused. (Consider the use of amber scene lighting.) Turn off headlights that might blind nearby motorists.
- Use traffic cones and flares to redirect traffic away from workers and to create a safe zone. (Use flares safely in proximity to the scene. Do not extinguish them once they have been ignited.)
- Make sure that all rescuers wear high-visibility clothing (e.g., orange highway vests, reflective trim).

Other scene hazards associated with highway operations include fuel and fire hazards, electrical power, unstable vehicles, air bags and supplemental restraint systems (SRS), and hazardous cargoes.

Fuel and Fire Hazards

Gasoline spills from crashes are a common fire hazard encountered by EMS providers. The chances that flammable liquids will ignite can be reduced by turning off the vehicle ignition switch, forbidding smoking, and avoiding use of flares near the spill. EMS personnel should approach the scene with fire extinguishers and should keep the extinguishers ready throughout extrication (Box 55-3). Ideally, a fire apparatus with a charged hose line should be at the scene.

The vehicle should be put in park and the engine stopped immediately after gaining access. The battery of a crashed car generally should be left connected so that power electric door locks, windows, seat mechanisms, and trunks can be operated. However, if the battery is to be disabled, the ground cable should be disconnected first to reduce the chance of sparking. Sparking may ignite spilled fuel or leaking battery gases. Most newer American cars have positive ground cables that can be identified by battery markings or by locating the ground wires attached to the frame, engine, or body of the vehicle. The battery cable can be cut with wire cutters or disconnected with battery pliers. The disconnected cable should be folded back onto itself. Then it should be securely taped to insulate it from any bare metal contact that might reestablish the electrical ground to the system. Both cables should be disconnected and secured.

Box 55-3 Fire Extinguishers

Portable fire extinguishers are classified by their anticipated effectiveness in suppressing four classes of fires:

- Class A—Ordinary combustibles
- Class B—Flammable liquids
- Class C—Energized electrical equipment
- Class D—Combustible metals

ABC all-purpose extinguishers are suitable for more than one class of fire. They should be carried by EMS crews. These dry chemical extinguishers can be used to suppress fires of ordinary combustible materials, flammable liquids, and electrical equipment.

Class A and class B fire extinguishers are given a numerical rating in addition to the letter classification. This rating designates the size of fire the extinguisher can be expected to suppress. A 20-B extinguisher generally extinguishes 20 times as much fuel as a 1-B extinguisher.

Fire suppression agents work by reducing heat and eliminating the oxygen needed to maintain combustion. Eliminating oxygen may present a danger to the rescuer and patient; therefore paramedics must work carefully in confined spaces. In addition, crew members and patients should avoid undue exposure to the fumes of any fire suppression agent. All rescuers should use an appropriate breathing apparatus.

Vehicle fires associated with crashes usually are caused by ruptured fuel tanks and fuel lines ignited during the crash. (Catalytic converters are capable of igniting spilled fuel.) Paramedics should not try to fight fully involved vehicle fires unless they have been trained and are properly equipped to do so. If the fire service has not arrived and victims are in a burning vehicle, the EMS crew should quickly determine whether the victims can be safely removed. If the victims are trapped and the vehicle is not fully engulfed by flames, an attempt should be made to stop the fire from spreading. This should be done using fire extinguishers.

Burning vehicles present very serious potential hazards. They may explode with deadly force at any time. All actions must be directed toward rescuer safety and protection. When paramedics must approach a burning vehicle, they should crouch low and approach from the side, staying clear of bumpers that may fly off during explosions. PPE also should be worn to guard against dangerous and caustic smoke.

ALTERNATE FUEL SYSTEMS

Some automobiles operate with alternate fuel systems. Examples include cars that are powered by natural gas, high-voltage electrical storage cells, and hybrid vehicles that use a combination of fuel sources. These alternate fuel sources are capable of producing fire hazards and injury from explosion of high-pressure cylinders and storage cells. Electric vehicles also carry enough voltage to cause serious burns, electric shock, and death. Hybrid vehicles often can be identified by a hybrid label and the presence of orange sleeves that cover components under the hood, in the rear, and under the car. Each automobile manufacturer has specific guidelines for emergency personnel to follow when working at a crash scene. The following are general guidelines for rescue[14]:

- Remain a safe distance from the vehicle if it is on fire.
- Always power down windows, open locks and latches, and move electric seats before disabling any vehicle. Put the vehicle in park. Chock the wheels as soon as possible in case a car in the "sleep mode" has its gas pedal depressed inadvertently by a driver.
- Verify that the vehicle is absolutely not under any power. *Always assume the vehicle is powered up despite no engine noises.* Shutting the vehicle off shuts down the hybrid system, shuts down the fuel pump, stops the electrical flow to air bags, and isolates the high-voltage current from the battery pack. (Many conventional and hybrid vehicles use a keyless entry/start ignition/start system.) High-voltage capacitors can store a voltage current for up to 10 minutes, even after the vehicle is shut down. During this "drain time," the vehicle should be considered unsafe.
- Never touch, cut, or open any orange cable or components protected by orange sleeves. Always consider a high-voltage cable to be live or hot.

Electrical Power

Downed electrical wires are dangerous. Modern transformers are programmed to retest broken circuits at certain time intervals. The dead lines can suddenly surge with lethal current. Rescuers must be familiar with the power system in their area. They should check with the local power company for information and the availability of training sessions for the response team. Only utility workers and trained rescuers using proper equipment should secure downed electrical wires.

Rescuers should never approach the patient until the scene is safe. Rescuers who experience tingling sensations in the soles of the feet, legs, or thorax as they enter an area should not proceed. Rather, they should retreat from the area. Victims inside a vehicle that is in contact with downed wires should be advised to remain inside unless they are at additional risk of injury (e.g., explosion, fire). Leaving the vehicle is dangerous and poses a significant risk of electrical injury.

When it is absolutely necessary to touch a patient who is in contact with a source of electricity, trained personnel may use nonconductive equipment such as leather gauntlets, wooden poles, polypropylene rope, and other specially designed equipment. However, none of these measures provides absolute safety from electrical injury.

Unstable Vehicles

Unstable vehicles are a common hazard in rescue events. All unstable vehicles must be stabilized before access is gained. The mechanism of the crash, the position and number of vehicles, and the environment of the scene must all be considered when assessing the stability of vehicles.

Some vehicles are obviously unstable. (For example, a vehicle may be positioned on its side or on its roof.) However, even a car on its wheels that appears to be stable may be unstable from possible movement of the tires and swaying of the vehicle's suspension system. All wrecked vehicles should be approached cautiously. Standard methods of stabilizing vehicles include supporting the vehicle with wooden cribbing, wheel chocks, and air bags and securing the vehicle with ropes, cables, and chains to poles, trees, and other vehicles and structures (Figure 55-6). Figure 55-7 shows equipment used to stabilize vehicles. Specialized training is required for paramedics involved in this aspect of rescue management.

Air Bags and Supplemental Restraint Systems

Air bags as a **supplemental restraint system** (SRS) are required safety features in all cars manufactured in the United States. The three main types of air bags are frontal impact, side impact, and head protection bags. (These devices can be located in numerous places inside the vehicle.) Air bags generally are considered an effective safety device in crashes. However, children and small adults in the

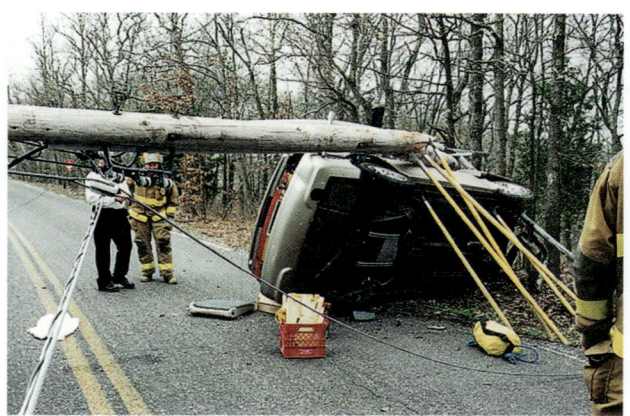
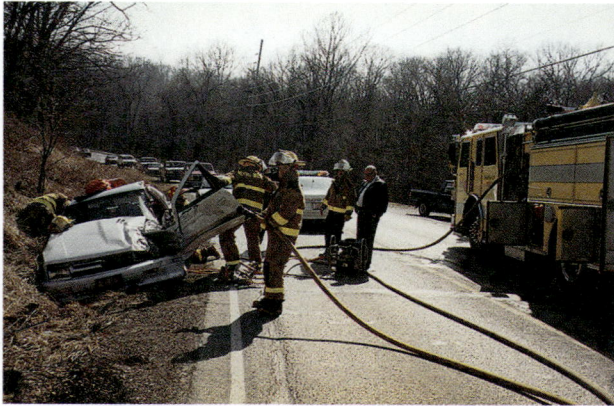
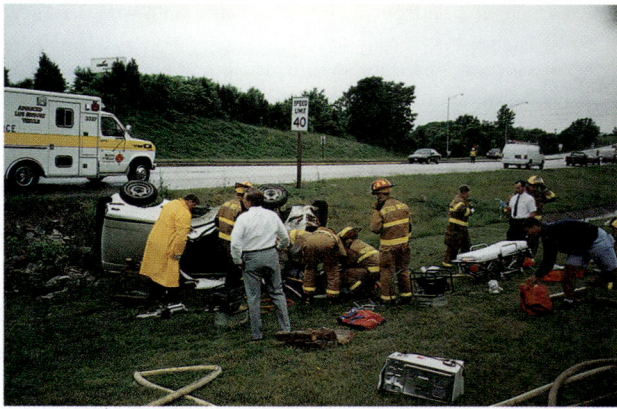
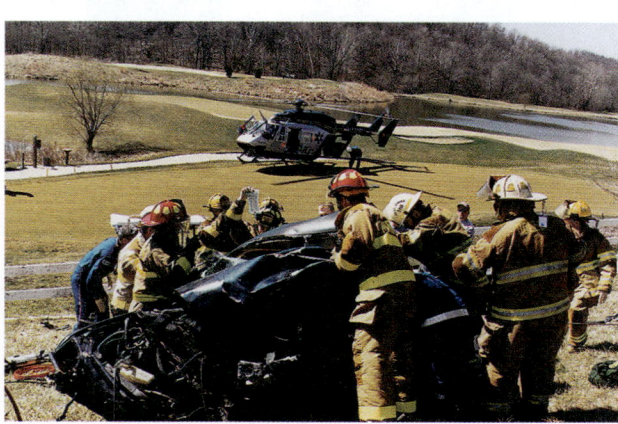
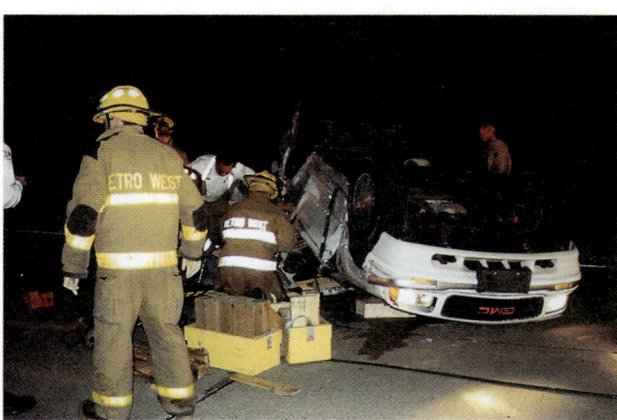
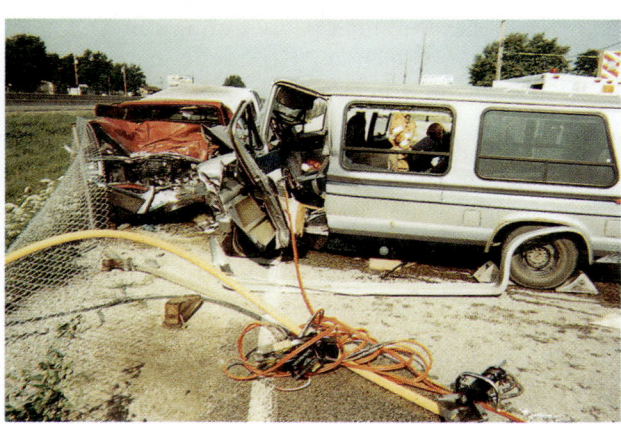

FIGURE 55-6 Vehicle stabilization.

passenger seat have been fatally injured after air bag deployment.[15]

> **NOTE**
>
> Most air bags are designed to automatically deploy in the event of a vehicle fire when temperatures reach 300° to 400° F. This safety feature helps to ensure that such temperatures do not cause an explosion of the inflator unit within the air bag module.

Once deployed, air bags are not dangerous. However, they do produce a residue that can cause minor skin or eye irritation. Irritation from this residue is temporary. It can be avoided by wearing gloves and eye protection; by keeping the residue away from the patient's eyes and wounds; and by thoroughly washing after exposure. Emergency personnel should be trained in detection and scene management of SRS equipment. Rescue guidelines for air bag–equipped cars have been provided by the National Highway Traffic Safety Administration and automobile and air bag

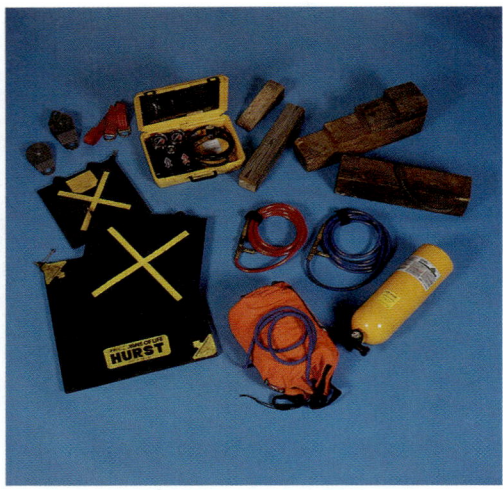

FIGURE 55-7 Equipment used to stabilize vehicles.

manufacturers and have been coordinated with the U.S. Fire Administration (Box 55-4).[16]

Hazardous Cargoes

Most hazardous substances transported in the United States travel by road. Therefore paramedics should be suspicious of crashes that involve commercial vehicles. Methods that can be used to identify carriers of hazardous cargoes (e.g., United Nations class identification number and North American number [UN/NA number] and placards) and the management of hazardous materials incidents are discussed in Chapter 57.

Automobile Anatomy

Vehicle rescue operations require a basic understanding of the anatomy of automobiles (Figure 55-8). The following are several important features:

- *Construction, roof,* and *support posts.* Most vehicles are of unibody rather than frame construction. The support posts (A, B, C, and D posts), floor fire wall, and trunk are integral to the integrity of unibody construction. Cutting the support posts can threaten the stability of these vehicles.
- *Fire wall* and *engine compartment.* A fire wall separates the engine and occupant compartments. The fire wall often collapses onto the occupant's legs during high-speed, head-on collisions. The car battery is usually located in the engine compartment.
- *Glass.* Safety glass is composed of glass-plastic and laminate glass and is usually found in the windshield. It is designed to stay intact when the glass is broken or shattered (it fractures into long strands). Tempered glass has high tensile strength and may not remain intact when it is shattered or broken (it fractures into small pieces).
- *Doors.* Most car doors contain a reinforcing bar. They are designed to provide structural integrity to the vehicle and protection to the occupants during front-impact and side-impact collisions. Doors also have a

---

Box 55-4 Rescue Guidelines for Air Bag–Equipped Cars

Incident With a Deployed Air Bag

Deployed air bags are not dangerous. However, not all air bags deploy during a crash. Also, side-impact air bags operate independently of the frontal air bags. Rescuers should practice the *5-10-20 rule* for safe distancing to reduce the severity and risk of injury should unintentional deployment occur. The rule is as follows:

- Side-impact curtain and air bags—Maintain a safe distance of 5 inches or more.
- Driver-side frontal air bags—Maintain a safe distance of 10 inches or more.
- Passenger-side frontal air bags—Maintain a safe distance of 20 inches or more.

In addition, rescuers should not place any hard board or device between an air bag and a patient or rescuer.

Once the air bag is deployed, it will not deploy again.

Incident With an Undeployed Air Bag

Undeployed air bags can suddenly deploy during a rescue. This releases a tremendous amount of energy. The energy can be dangerous to both the patient and the rescuer. If a patient is pinned behind an undeployed air bag, the car battery should be deactivated as soon as possible. Before they disconnect the battery, paramedics should determine whether they will need to move a power seat, unlock electric doors, or power down electric windows. The procedure for deactivating the battery is as follows:

1. Turn off all electrical units and the ignition switch. Carefully disconnect both battery cables (disconnect the negative cable first).
2. Cables that need to be cut should be cut twice to ensure that the cut ends will not touch and arc. Make sure the battery terminals cannot make contact with metal body parts that could reactivate an electrical circuit. Do not attempt to turn on the ignition switch to test a battery disconnect; verify it by attempting to turn on the lights.
3. For additional safety, maintain the 5-10-20 rule near air bags that have not deployed.

NOTE: If the incident involves fire, normal fire extinguishing procedures should be used. Heat may trigger an undeployed air bag. However, it will not cause the activating canister to explode.

---

case-hardened steel "Nader" pin or latch that is designed to prevent the car door from opening during impact. If the pin is engaged, it may be difficult to pry open the door; it must be disengaged first.

RESCUE STRATEGIES

Rescue strategies for vehicle crashes should begin during the initial scene size-up. They sometimes can be based on the details provided by the dispatching center before arrival. On arriving at the scene, the EMS crew should begin hazard control, establish command, and call for appropriate backup. Important elements of the scene size-up include the following:

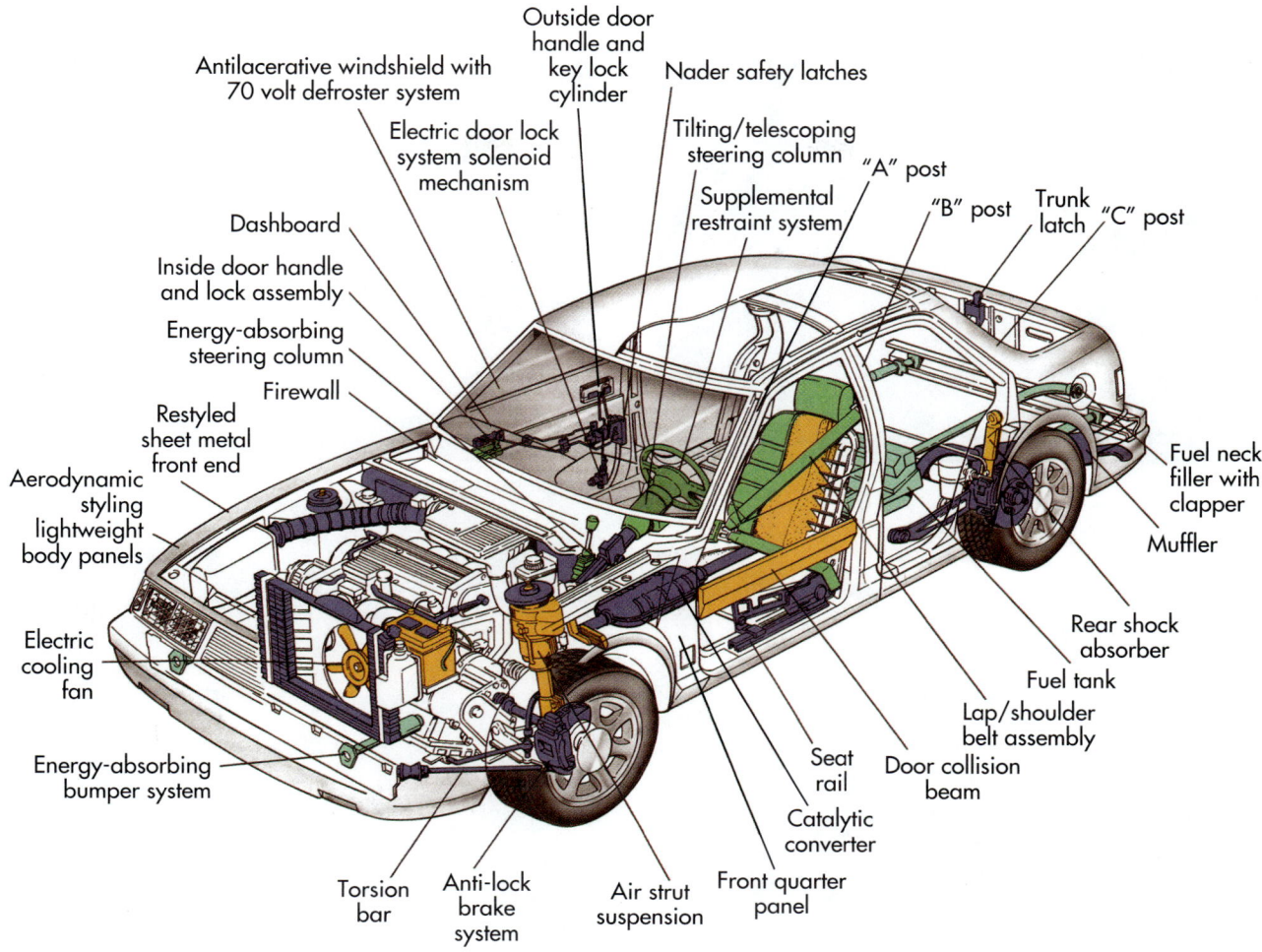

FIGURE 55-8 Anatomy of a car.

- Scene safety (including protecting the scene from traffic hazards)
- Location of the crash
- Vehicle stability
- Electrical hazards
- Fire hazards
- Hazardous materials
- Special rescue needs
- Number and location of patients

After performing the initial scene size-up and ensuring scene safety, the responding crew should assess the degree of entrapment and the fastest means of extrication. The paramedic should try to gain access to trapped victims by first trying to open all car doors. When a door cannot be readily opened by the patient or rescuer, another option is the side windows. (Glass windows can be shattered by striking the glass in a lower corner or by using a spring-loaded center punch.) Initial care can then be provided until the patient has been extricated. Trained rescue personnel with extrication tools can gain access to the patient by door removal, roof removal, front or rear windshield openings, or a dash roll-up maneuver (Figure 55-9). Paramedics

involved in the rescue or who are near the site should wear PPE that provides adequate hand, eye, and body protection. (Persons trapped in a vehicle should also be protected during extrication.) Clothing with reflective striping improves safety during day and night operations.

HAZARDOUS TERRAIN

Hazardous terrain can pose major difficulties during rescue operations. An example is a car crash that occurs on an embankment. Other examples are rescues for sport enthusiasts such as rock climbers, snow skiers, and mountain bikers. Three common classifications of hazardous terrain are low-angle, high-angle, and flat terrain with obstructions (Box 55-5). Highly specialized training and equipment are required for rescues in both low-angle (weight supported by ground) and high-angle (weight supported by rope) environments.

The term *low angle* (steep slope) refers to terrain that can be walked on without the use of the hands. However, secure footing may be difficult on steep slopes. This makes it hazardous to carry a litter even with several rescuers. In these situations, **low-angle rescue** is used to prevent falls and

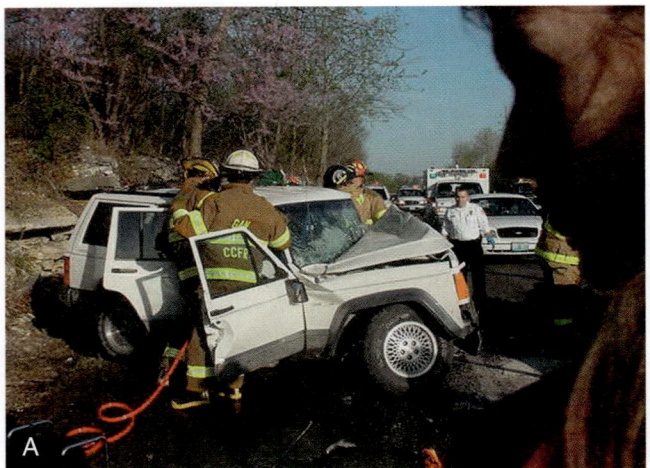
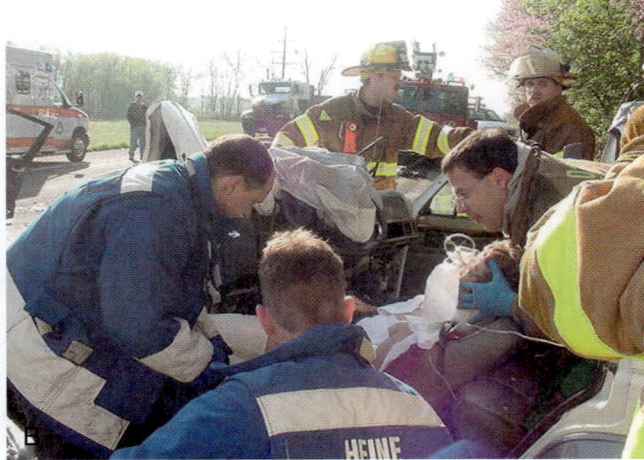
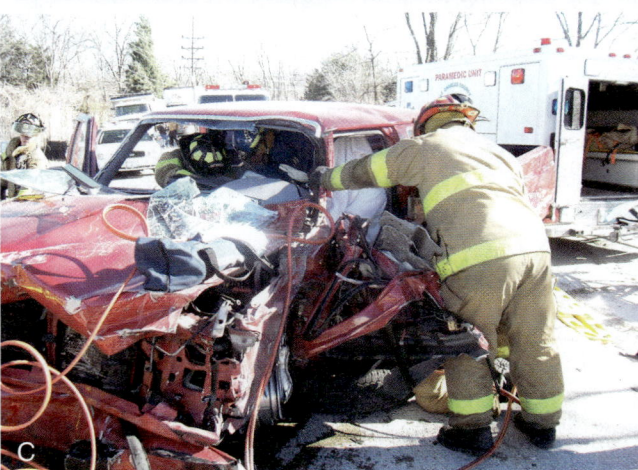
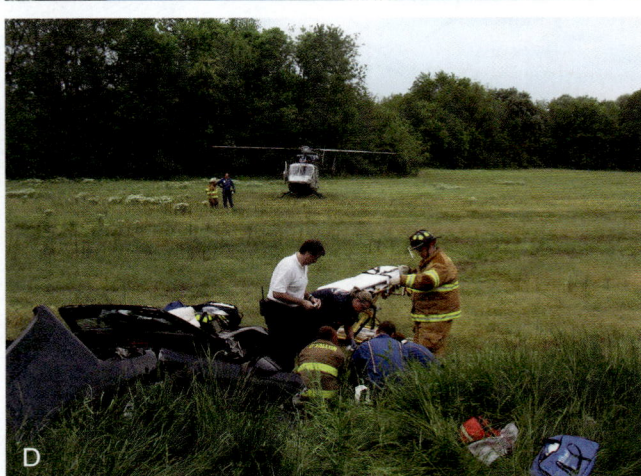

FIGURE 55-9 Extrication scenes. (Courtesy O'Fallon Fire Department, O'Fallon, Mo.)

Box 55-5 Terms and Definitions Related to Rescue Over Hazardous Terrain

anchoring: Attaching a high-angle rope to a secure point.

belay: A method of attaching a safety rope and controlling the rope so that if the person or load starts to fall, the belay rope prevents the fall.

high angle: An environment in which rescuers need to be secured with rope for safety. Most of the rescue load is supported by the rope system.

low angle: An environment in which the weight of the stretcher is supported primarily by the tender's legs, but rope systems are required to facilitate movement and for protection against falls.

rappelling: A method of descent that involves lowering oneself with a rope.

scrambling: Movement over rough terrain that is not steep enough to require the use of a rope.

tumbles through the use of ropes to counteract gravity during litter carrying (Figure 55-10).

The term *high angle* (vertical) refers to terrain (cliffs, sides of buildings) that is so steep the hands must be used to maintain balance (slopes of more than 40 degrees). In these situations, rescuers are completely dependent on rope or aerial apparatus for litter movement. **High-angle rescue** requires **rappelling** (controlled descent by a rope) by trained personnel to retrieve victims. Falls are likely to result in serious injury or death (Figure 55-11). Box 55-6 and Figure 55-12 discuss ropes and basic knots used in rescue.

CRITICAL THINKING
What factors in the environment can increase the danger of steep-slope rescue?

Flat terrain rescue may include various obstructions that can make rescue difficult. Examples include level land with large rocks, loose soil (scree), and waterbeds or creeks. In these situations, extra personnel and resources may be needed to extricate a victim safely and to ensure safe litter movement.

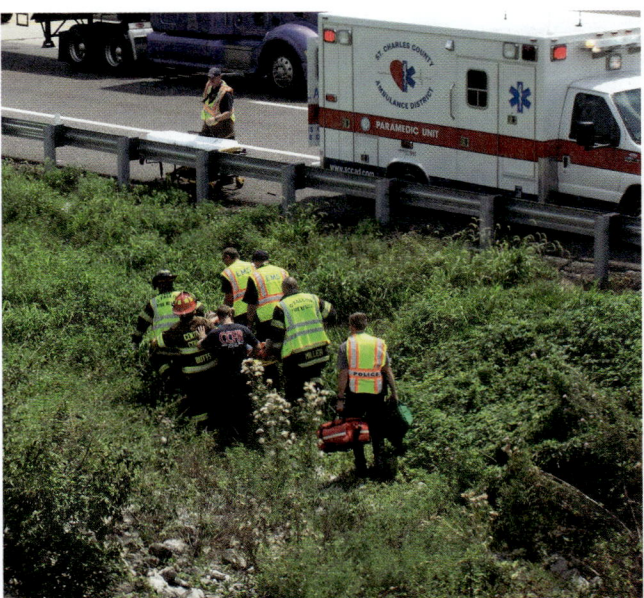

FIGURE 55-10 Low-angle rescue. (Courtesy O'Fallon Fire Department, O'Fallon, Mo.)

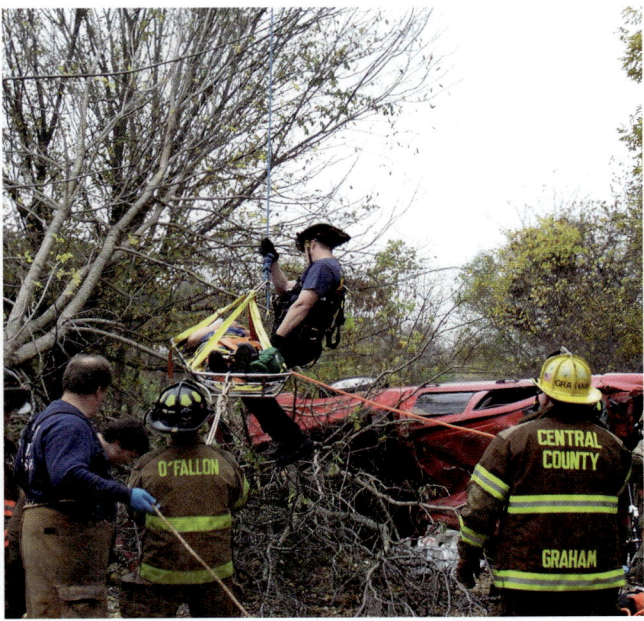

FIGURE 55-11 High-angle rescue. (Courtesy O'Fallon Fire Department, O'Fallon, Mo.)

Box 55-6 Ropes and Knots

There are generally two types of rope used for life safety rope: **static rope** and **dynamic rope.** The preferred rope used for life safety rescue operations is **static Kernmantle.** (Kern means core and mantle means sheath.) Dynamic rope is usually used when climbing toward or above an anchor point. Static rope provides for minimal stretch (a low elongation factor). Dynamic rope is designed to stretch (a higher elongation factor). All ropes used for rescue operations should meet the NFPA minimum standards for life safety rope. These ropes will have a minimum safety factor of 15:1 for a two-person **load**.[17]

Knots are used in rescue operations to fasten and secure a rope by tying or interweaving. Although there are many knots used in rescue operations, common knots often belong to the figure 8 family. These include (Figure 55-12):

Figure 8
Figure 8 on a bite
Figure 8 follow-through
Double-loop figure 8
Figure 8 bend
Inline figure 8
Note: A common phrase used by rescue personnel when teaching the tying of knots: *If you can't tie a knot—tie a lot!* Wrapping and re-wrapping ropes around a stable structure often can provide stability.

Patient Packaging With Litters

The **basket stretcher** is the standard for rough terrain evacuation. The rigid frame of this device offers protection for the victim. It also is relatively easy to carry with adequate personnel. Patients generally are immobilized on a long backboard and secured in the basket. Alternative spinal immobilization devices (e.g., vest-type devices) also can be used in conjunction with the basket stretcher. Using the basket stretcher itself as a spinal immobilization device should be considered a last resort. The older "military style" devices do not provide adequate spinal immobilization.

Basket stretchers have two basic designs: wire mesh (Stokes) and plastic. Wire mesh generally is the stronger of the baskets. It also is relatively inexpensive. The design allows for air and water to flow through the device. This makes it ideal in water rescue when used with supplemental flotation. Plastic basket stretchers generally are weaker than steel mesh. However, they provide better protection for the patient. (Plastic bottoms with steel frames are considered superior designs.) Most basket stretchers are equipped with adequate restraints. However, all require additional strapping or lacing (e.g., harness, leg stirrups) to prevent movement, as well as padding for rough-terrain evacuation or extraction. A plastic helmet or litter shield should be available to protect the patient.

PATIENT MOVEMENT

Methods of moving a patient over rough terrain may include evacuation and litter-carrying over flat terrain. However, special rescue equipment may be required for low-angle and high-angle evacuation. Such equipment may include load-lifting straps, anchors, and rope-lowering and rope-hauling systems. In addition, the use of aerial apparatus (e.g., tower-ladder or bucket trucks, aerial ladders) also may be required in some high-angle rescue operations. Moving a patient during low-angle and high-angle evacuations requires specialized knowledge and skills.

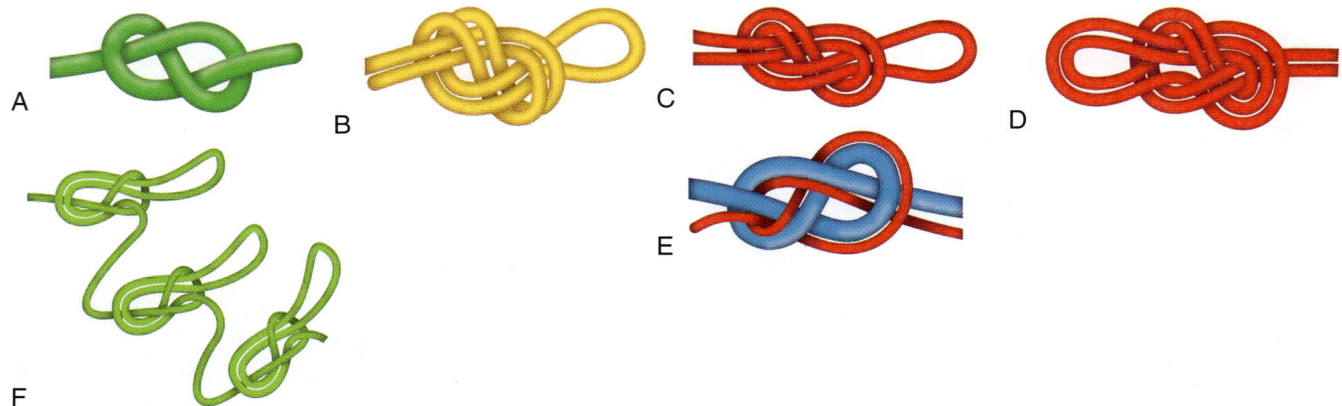

FIGURE 55-12 Knots. **A,** Figure 8. **B,** Figure 8 on a bite. **C,** Figure 8 follow-through. **D,** Double-loop figure 8. **E,** Figure 8 bend. **F,** Inline figure 8.

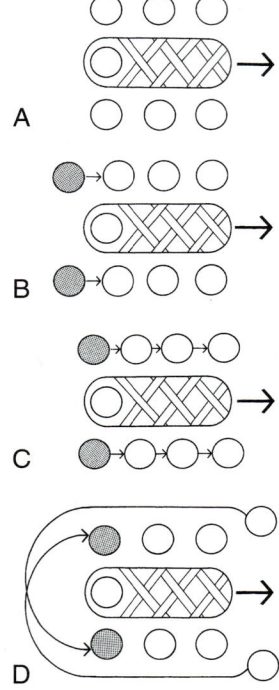

FIGURE 55-13 Litter-carrying sequence. **A,** Six rescuers are usually required to carry a litter; they may need relief over long distances (more than ¼ mile). **B,** Relief rescuers can rotate into position while the litter is in motion by approaching from the rear. As relief rescuers move forward, others progressively move forward **(C)** until the forward-most rescuers can release the litter (peel out) and move to the rear **(D).** Rescuers in the rear can rotate sides so that they can alternate carrying arms. Carrying straps (webbing) can also be used to distribute the load over the rescuers' shoulders. In most cases the litter is carried feet first with a medical attendant at the head monitoring airway, breathing, level of consciousness, and so on.

LITTER-CARRYING PROCEDURES

Carrying a litter across rough, flat terrain requires a minimum of six rescuers: four to carry the litter and two to observe or "scout" for potential hazards (e.g., loose rocks, holes, tree branches). Team members should be matched in height. This ensures that equal weight is shared and that the litter remains level. Load-lifting straps sometimes are used to spread the weight of the load over other parts of the rescuer's body (e.g., around the rescuer's shoulders and back). As described in Chapter 2, proper lifting techniques should be used to protect and support the rescuer's back. Figure 55-13 shows a basic litter-carrying sequence.

Helicopter Use in Hazardous Terrain Rescue

As described in Chapter 53, helicopters can be used for transport and for rescues. When they are used for rescue, the helicopter team (civilian and military) is geared toward performing the rescue rather than providing medical care and transport. The rescue helicopter team has specialized knowledge and skills. They are required to hover or land in tight places and to transport people and equipment. Special rescue techniques that these helicopters use may include cable hoisting to extract people from the ground, and short-haul (sling load) operations that allow personnel and equipment to be carried beneath the helicopter as an external load. Rescue helicopters have the same safety concerns and limitations as those used for medical transport described in Chapter 53. All personnel at the scene should be familiar with the elements of scene safety, hazards, and restrictions for helicopter use.

LOOK AGAIN
See Chapter 53: Ground and Air Ambulance Operations, pp. 1471-1475.

ASSESSMENT PROCEDURES DURING RESCUE

Patient assessment during rescue operations often is complicated by factors such as weather and temperature extremes, available access, equipment limitations, patient entrapment, and cumbersome PPE that affects rescuer mobility. Other factors that can affect the paramedic's ability to perform a thorough assessment and that can result in a compromised physical examination include the following:

- Difficulty completely exposing a patient
- Restrictive clothing and PPE required for personal safety
- Working in a cramped space
- Limited lighting
- Difficulty transporting medical equipment to the patient

Specific Assessment and Management Considerations

During rescues, paramedics may need to downsize medical equipment. They may not be able to carry the normal bags and "street packaging." Ideally, paramedics should be able to carry the equipment hands-free. In addition to ensuring adequate lighting to perform assessment and treatment, paramedics should have access to the equipment listed in Box 55-7.

EXPOSURE OF PATIENTS

Patients who need to be rescued may be at high risk for developing hypothermia. They should be covered to ensure thermal protection. Also, the patient should be protected with shields (e.g., backboards or blankets) to prevent injury from equipment and debris during the extrication.

ADVANCED LIFE SUPPORT MEASURES

Advanced life support (ALS) measures should be provided only if necessary. However, good basic life support (BLS) techniques are mandatory. As a rule, ALS equipment such as IV lines, endotracheal (ET) tubes, and electrocardiographic (ECG) leads will complicate the extrication process. (Advanced airway support and volume replacement, however, may be essential.) Airway control with administration of supplemental oxygen must always be a priority during the rescue.

PATIENT MONITORING

Monitoring of the patient's vital signs and level of consciousness is necessary throughout the rescue. In high-noise and tight spaces, blood pressure may need to be measured by palpation. It also may be necessary to use compact devices such as a pulse oximeter. Paramedics should create and continue a rapport with the patient when possible. They should explain the procedures performed and why they are necessary. Providing emotional support during the rescue is crucial.

Box 55-7 Paramedic Equipment

Airway
- Oral and nasal airways
- Manual suction device
- Intubation equipment

Breathing
- Thoracic decompression device
- Small oxygen tank and regulator
- Masks and cannulae
- Pocket mask and bag-valve-mask device

Circulation
- Bandages and dressings
- Triangular bandages
- Occlusive dressings
- Intravenous fluid administration set
- Blood pressure cuff and stethoscope

Disability
- Extrication collars

Exposure of Body Surface
- Scissors

Miscellaneous
- Headlamp and flashlight
- Space blanket
- Pneumatic splints

Personal Protective Equipment
- Leather gloves
- Latex gloves
- Eye shields
- Other equipment as indicated

IMPROVISATION

Because of space and equipment limitations, some patient care may have to be improvised during a rescue. For example, an upper extremity fracture can be temporarily stabilized by tying it to the patient's torso; a lower extremity fracture can be tied to the patient's uninjured leg (buddy splinting). Formable splints (e.g., structural aluminum malleable [SAM] splint) also can be very useful for securing extremity fractures or dislocations.

PAIN CONTROL

Pain control for patients who require rescue may include drug therapy (narcotics, analgesics) and other methods. Examples of nondrug therapy to manage pain includes splinting and positioning, distraction (talking to the patient and asking questions), and methods such as creating sensory stimuli (e.g., mildly scratching the patient) when a painful procedure or maneuver is performed. Pain medication can mask serious injury and alter a patient's level of consciousness. Therefore the paramedic should follow established protocol regarding the use of drug therapy in these situations.

SUMMARY

- Rescue is a patient-driven event. It requires specialized medical and mechanical skills. The right amount of each must be applied at the right time. The main role of the paramedic in rescues is to have the proper training and the appropriate PPE. These allow safe access to the patient and the provision of treatment at the site and throughout the incident.

- The seven phases of a rescue operation are arrival and scene size-up, hazard control, gaining access to the patient, medical treatment, disentanglement, patient packaging, and transportation.

- The standards for protective clothing and personal protection equipment established by the National Fire Protection Association and OSHA have been adopted by many fire and EMS agencies. The appropriate PPE depends on the level of rescuer involvement and the nature of the incident.

- Water rescue should never be attempted by a single rescuer or by one who is untrained.

- Water hazards include obstructions to flow and foot or extremity pins that can trap victims and drag them under water. Some factors that contribute to flat water drowning are alcohol or other drug use. Also, cool water temperatures contribute to such drownings.

- Hazardous atmospheres are environments with low oxygen. These environments can occur in confined spaces. The six major hazards associated with confined spaces are oxygen-deficient atmospheres, chemical/toxic exposure and explosion, engulfment, machinery entrapment, electricity, and structural concerns.

- Traffic flow is the biggest hazard in EMS highway operations. Other scene hazards associated with highway operations include fuel or fire hazards, electrical power, unstable vehicles, air bags and supplemental restraint systems, and hazardous cargoes.

- Hazardous terrain can create major difficulties during rescue events. Three common classifications of hazardous terrain are low-angle, high-angle, and flat terrain with obstructions.

REFERENCES

1. National Fire Protection Association: *Standard on protective clothing for medical operations (NFPA 1999)*, Quincy, Mass, 2008, The Association.

2. Occupational Safety and Health Administration: *Hazardous waste operations and emergency response (HAZWOPER)*, Standard 1910.120, Washington, DC, 2003 (rev. 2005), The Administration.

3. Occupational Safety and Health Administration: *Occupational exposure to bloodborne pathogens (29 CFR 1910.1030)*, Washington, DC, 2001 (rev. 2008), The Administration.

4. Occupational Safety and Health Administration: *Enforcement policy and procedures for occupational exposure to tuberculosis*, Washington, DC, 1995 (rev. 2004), The Administration.

5. National Safety Council: *Accident facts*, Itasca, Ill, 2010, The Council.

6. Cooper DC, editor: *Fundamentals of search and rescue*, Sudbury, Mass, 2005, Jones & Bartlett.

7. Marx J, Hockberger R, Walls R: *Rosen's emergency medicine*, ed 7, St Louis, 2009, Mosby.

8. American Heart Association: *Advanced cardiac life support*, Dallas, Tex, 2005, The Association.

9. Polack N, editor: *Care and transportation of the sick and injured, American Academy of Orthopedic Surgeons*, ed 9, Sudbury, Mass, 2005, Jones & Bartlett.

10. Markenson D, Ferguson JD, Chameides L, et al: Part 17: first aid: 2010 American Heart Association and American Red Cross Guidelines for First Aid, *Circulation* 122:S934-S946, 2010.

11. U.S. Department of Labor, OSHA: *Hazards II*, www.osha.gov/pls/oshaweb/owadisp.show_document?p_table=PREAMBLES&p_id=839, accessed 6-25-10.

12. Occupational Safety and Health Administration: *Permit required confined spaces for general industry (29 CFR 1910.146)*, Washington, DC, 1998, The Administration.

13. Lapraed J: *Hazards of the PTO on farm tractors*, www.aces.edu/pubs/docs/A/ANR-1262/, accessed 11-9-10.

14. General Motors Technical Service College: *First responder vehicle support information*, www.colonialparkfire.org/cmsAdmin/uploads/VehicleSupportInfoGuide_001.pdf, accessed 11-9-10.

15. National Highway Traffic Safety Administration: *Special crash investigation study*, Washington, DC, 2010, The Administration.

16. United States Government Printing Office: *Emergency response guidelines for air-bagged equipped vehicles*, Washington, DC, 2004, Author.

17. Frank JA, editor: *CMC rope rescue manual*, Columbia, Mo, 1998, CMC Rescue.

SUGGESTED READINGS

Burke G: Employee safety when working at heights, *AAOHN* 56(2):85-87, 2008.

Cook L: EMS operations at water aircraft crashes, *JEMS* 2009, www.jems.com/article/extrication-rescue/ems-operations-water-aircraft, accessed 7-7-10.

Ross P: Confined space entry, *AAOHN* 55(6):245-249, 2007.

OBJECTIVES

Upon completion of this chapter, the paramedic student will be able to:

1. Describe general techniques for determining whether a scene is violent and choosing the appropriate response to a violent scene.
2. Outline techniques for recognizing and responding to potentially dangerous residential calls.
3. Outline techniques for recognizing and responding to potentially dangerous calls on the highway.
4. Describe signs of danger and emergency medical services (EMS) response to violent street incidents.
5. Identify characteristics of and EMS response to situations involving gangs, clandestine drug labs, and domestic violence.
6. Outline general safety tactics that EMS personnel can use if they find themselves in a dangerous situation.
7. Describe special EMS considerations when providing tactical patient care.
8. Discuss EMS documentation and preservation of evidence at a crime scene.

KEY TERMS

audible and visual warning devices Safety devices used in emergency responses to make vehicle presence known; examples include lights, sirens, and horns.

avoidance The act of keeping away from someone, something, or a situation, or of preventing the occurrence of something; it requires the paramedic to continually be aware of the scene by remaining observant and being knowledgeable about warning signs that may indicate a dangerous situation.

backlighting Positioning oneself between the ambulance lights and residence; a safety hazard.

clandestine drug lab A place of illegal drug manufacturing.

concealment A means of keeping out of sight; it provides no ballistic protection.

contact provider The person who initiates and provides direct patient care.

cover A type of concealment that offers ballistic protection.

cover provider The person whose role is to ensure safe cover for the contact providers while they provide patient care.

crime scene A location where any part of a criminal act has occurred, or a location where evidence relating to a crime may be found.

distraction A self-defense measure in which a diversion is created to attract a person's attention.

evasive tactics A self-defense measure in which an aggressor's moves and actions are anticipated, and unconventional pathways are used during retreat for personal safety.

gang Any group of people who engage in socially disruptive or criminal behavior.

graffiti Gang markings that usually indicate territorial boundaries; also known as "tagging."

hot zone In tactical response, the area where patient care activities occur inside the scene perimeter.

soft body armor Clothing that provides protection from some blunt and penetrating trauma; also known as *"bullet-proof vests."*

special weapons and tactics operations Violent and dangerous incidents where specially trained emergency personnel teams respond; also known as "SWAT operations."

staging A tactical response to avoid danger by waiting at a safe distance from the scene until the area has been secured by the appropriate authorities.

tactical EMS Emergency medical support provided by EMS personnel who are specially trained and equipped to provide prehospital emergency care in tactical environments.

tactical patient care Patient care activities that occur inside the scene perimeter, or hot zone, of a dangerous scene.

tactical retreat Leaving the scene when danger is observed or when violence or indicators of violence are displayed; requires immediate and decisive action.

turf Refers to territorial boundaries established by gangs.

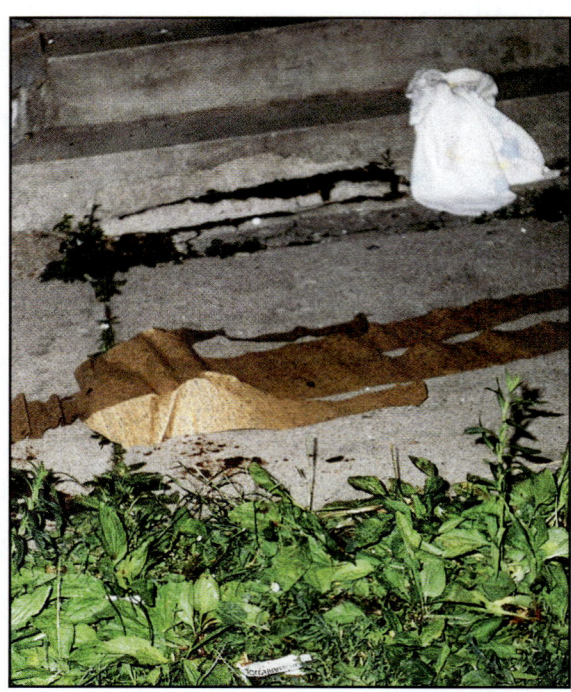

Many violent crimes require an EMS response, and often EMS crews arrive at the scene before law enforcement personnel. Consequently, awareness and avoidance of dangerous situations are issues of concern for emergency responders. Although national studies have reported a decline in violent crimes in recent years, violence against EMS personnel from street gangs, threat groups, domestic disputes, and drug users is on the rise.[1,2] Personal safety and crime scene awareness must be top priorities on every call of this nature.

(Courtesy Ronald Olschwanger, St. Louis, Mo.)

CRITICAL THINKING
Why is it not always possible to identify a dangerous scene before arriving at the scene?

APPROACHING THE SCENE

For paramedics and other responders, determining personal safety is a basic part of analyzing a scene. It begins before paramedics arrive at the scene with information provided by a dispatching center. *A key point in ensuring personal safety is to identify and respond to potential dangers before they threaten.* Information may be available from a dispatching center that should alert the EMS crew to possible dangers. Such information includes known locations of unsafe scenes (e.g., through computer-aided dispatch systems) and/or the presence of the following:

- Large crowds
- People under the influence of alcohol or other drugs
- On-scene violence
- Weapons

Other information can sometimes be gathered en route to the scene from crew members, dispatchers, and other emergency responders monitoring the call who have had previous experience with a particular area or address. The paramedic also should be aware of additional inherent hazards that may exist at the scene. Examples include downed power lines, busy roadways, toxic substances, the potential for fire, dangerous pets, and vehicle hazards and dangers. If the scene is not safe, the EMS crew should retreat. The crew should stage at a safe location to await the arrival of law enforcement and/or other rescuers.

When responding to a scene with a potential for danger, the EMS crew should begin observation several blocks from the scene. They also should use **audible and visual warning devices** (AVW devices) that are appropriate for the call. For example, responding with AVW devices to an urban scene may draw a crowd of bystanders; lights generally are required for safety at highway scenes. As described in Chapter 53, joint fire-EMS-law enforcement responses should be defined through preplanning (for example, a fire-EMS emergency response with full use of AVW devices, and law enforcement response without AVW devices and at normal speed).

Scene safety considerations for all types of danger must continue throughout the EMS response. A scene that has been made safe can become unsafe, even when the police are present. This can happen if violence resumes, crowds gather or turn violent, or other people enter the scene. Violence against EMS providers also may occur if they are mistaken for police officers (because of uniform colors or badges) or when they exit an emergency vehicle that has AVW devices. The paramedic crew must be familiar with local protocols when intervening in violent situations. They also must have a strategic escape plan ready.

Scenes Known to Be Violent

If the scene is known to be violent, the EMS crew should remain at a safe, out-of-sight distance from the area until it has been secured ("out of sight—out of scene"). Remaining at a safe staging area away from a violent scene is important for several reasons:

- If paramedics can be seen, people will come to them.
- Entering an unsafe scene adds one or more potential victims.
- Paramedics may be injured or killed.
- Paramedics may be taken hostage.
- Paramedics may become additional patients in a scene that is already a multiple casualty incident.

It must be stressed that if the scene is unsafe, the EMS crew should not enter. Rather, they should retreat to a staging area and wait for resource personnel who can provide scene safety.

🔍 SHOW ME THE EVIDENCE

In this abstract, the authors describe their investigation of the type and frequency of violence experienced by EMS personnel in a metropolitan system that served a population of nearly one-half million people. They performed a prospective direct observation study for 737 hours and 342 ambulance runs. Of the calls, 81% were rated nonviolent, 5% violent, and 14% postviolent. Of the violence observed, 88% involved verbal abuse solely, 38% demonstrated physical aggression solely toward objects or self, and 38% demonstrated both verbal and physical aggression against others.

From Fowlie EJ, Eustis SW, et al: Prospective field study of violence in EMS, *Ann Emerg Med* 23(3):620, 1994.

Weapons at the Scene

Most states (excluding Illinois and Wisconsin, and the District of Columbia) have enacted laws that permit some citizens to carry a handgun or other weapon.[3] Therefore, paramedics will likely respond to emergency calls where weapons are present.

All weapons should be secured by law enforcement personnel if officers are present at the scene. If law enforcement is not present, paramedics should request that the weapons be safely secured away from the scene. This request should be explained as an additional safety measure for the EMS crew, patient, and any bystanders.

DANGEROUS RESIDENCE

A response to a residence is an everyday occurrence for most EMS personnel. However, even calls that appear "routine" require a scene size-up that begins before the EMS crew leaves the emergency vehicle. Warning signs of danger in residential calls include the following:

- A history of problems or violence
- A known drug or gang area
- Loud noises (e.g., screams, items breaking, possible gunshots)
- Seeing or hearing acts of violence
- The presence of alcohol or other drug use
- The smell of chemicals or the presence of empty chemical containers
- Evidence of dangerous pets (e.g., exotic snakes and reptiles, breeds of dogs that are often trained to be vicious)
- Unusual silence or darkened residence

If any of these or other warning signs are present, the EMS crew should retreat from the scene and call for law enforcement assistance.

When approaching a suspicious residence, the EMS crew should choose tactics that match the threat or situation. For example, avoiding the use of AVW devices, taking unconventional pathways (rather than using the sidewalk, for example), and avoiding a position between the ambulance lights and residence **(backlighting)** are safety measures that should be considered. In addition, paramedics should listen for sounds indicating danger before announcing their presence or entering the home. They should stand on the side of the entry door opposite the hinges (doorknob side) (Figure 56-1). If danger becomes evident, paramedics should immediately retreat from the scene.

DANGEROUS HIGHWAY ENCOUNTERS

As with calls to residences, a response to a traffic incident should never be considered routine. Such calls involve inherent dangers associated with traffic flow, emergency vehicle positioning, and extrication. Also, the danger of violence may exist. For example, a vehicle's occupants may be armed, wanted, or fleeing felons; intoxicated or drugged; or violent and abusive because of an altered mental state (Box 56-1).

When approaching a vehicle, a one-person approach is recommended. This allows the partner who remains in the ambulance to notify dispatch of the situation, location, license plate number, and state registration of suspicious vehicles. (Because the ambulance is elevated, it provides greater visibility of the vehicle.) At night, ambulance lights

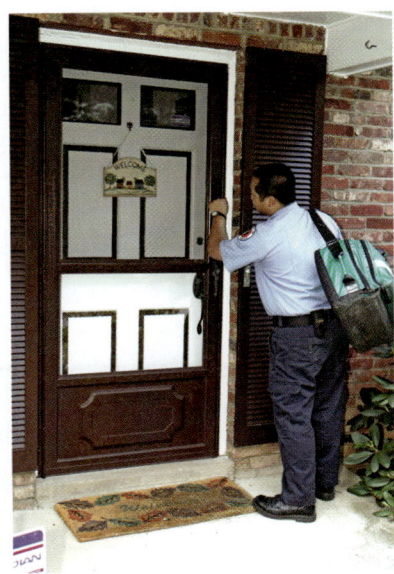

FIGURE 56-1 If danger from inside a residence is suspected, paramedics should stand on the side of an entry door opposite the hinges (i.e., the doorknob side).

BOX 56-1 Street-Smart Safety Tips

- When working in a traffic way, always wear reflective clothing and make sure you can leave the scene quickly and safely if required.
- At nighttime, use the ambulance lights to illuminate a vehicle's interior.
- Before approaching a vehicle, consider using the public address (PA) system to get a response from passengers in the car.
- If a passenger in the car is adjusting the side or rear view mirror as you approach, retreat to safety. (This is a sign of danger.)
- Open or unlatched trunks may indicate that people are hiding or have been restrained in the compartment. If the trunk is slightly open, slam it shut without opening it further.
- Retreat to the ambulance (or another place of safety) at the first sign of danger.

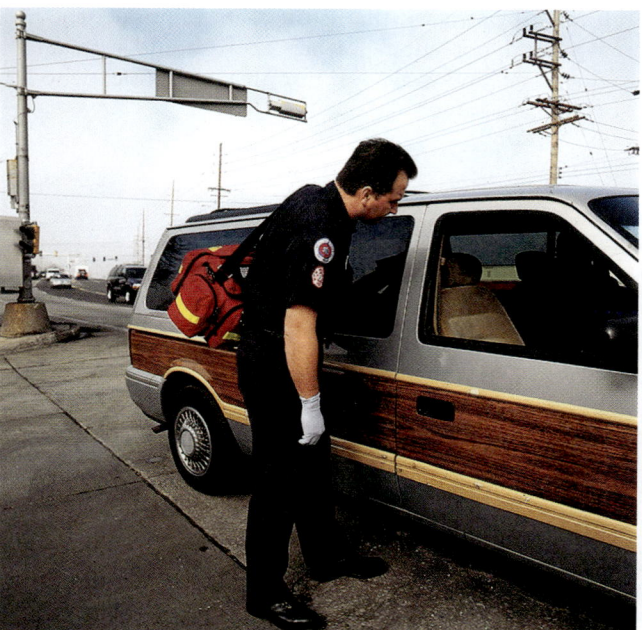

FIGURE 56-2 In approaching a car with potentially dangerous occupants, paramedics should observe the front seat from behind post B. They should move forward only after ensuring their safety.

should be used to illuminate the interior of the vehicle and the surrounding area.

The paramedic who approaches the car should do so from the passenger side of the vehicle. This provides protection from vehicular traffic. Furthermore, it usually is the opposite approach a driver would expect from law enforcement personnel. As another safety precaution, the paramedic should not walk between the ambulance and the other vehicle, to avoid being trapped and injured if the vehicle backs up. Also, the paramedic should walk around the rear of the ambulance and then to the passenger side of the vehicle.

Car posts A, B, and C (see Chapter 55) may provide the better ballistic protection as opposed to windows and doors. The paramedic should observe for unusual activity in the rear seat and not move forward of the post nearest the threat unless no threats exist in these areas. The paramedic should observe the front seat from behind post B and move forward only after ensuring it safe to do so (Figure 56-2). If signs of danger are present (e.g., weapons, suspicious behavior or movements in the vehicle, arguing or fighting among passengers), paramedics should immediately retreat to a safe staging area. From that area, they should request the help of law enforcement, if not already present at the scene.

LOOK AGAIN
See Chapter 55: Rescue Awareness and Operations, pp. 1508-1509.

CRITICAL THINKING
In your community, what type of EMS calls routinely merit a law enforcement response?

VIOLENT STREET INCIDENTS

Murder, assault, and robbery are common occurrences in the United States. Many of these crimes involve dangerous weapons. Violence may be directed toward EMS personnel from perpetrators at the scene (or who return to the scene). The violence may even come from injured and distraught patients. In addition, dangerous crowds and bystanders quickly can become large in number and volatile. They may direct violence toward everyone and everything in the surrounding area. Warning signs of potential danger in violent street incidents include the following:

- Voices that become louder, escalating in tone
- Pushing and shoving
- Hostility toward people at the scene (e.g., perpetrator, police, victim)
- A rapid increase in the size of the crowd
- The use of alcohol or other drugs by people at the scene
- Inability of law enforcement personnel to control the crowd

Paramedic crews should constantly monitor crowds and retreat from the scene if necessary. The location and careful parking of the emergency vehicle are important for personal safety. The EMS crew should position the ambulance so that it cannot be blocked by other vehicles (allowing for easy retreat from the scene). When possible and when it is safe to do so, the patient should be removed from the scene as the crew retreats. (This may eliminate the need to return to the scene.)

VIOLENT GROUPS AND SITUATIONS

According to a study completed by the Department of Justice's Office of Juvenile Justice and Delinquency Prevention (OJJDP), more than 770,000 gang members currently belong to more than 27,500 gangs throughout the United States[4] (Box 56-2). Most gangs and other threat groups operate through intimidation and extortion (Box 56-3).

Gang Characteristics

A **gang** can be defined as any group of people who engage in socially disruptive or criminal behavior. They usually are territorial, and often but not always of the same gender. Gangs also operate by creating an atmosphere of fear in a community. The gang may choose a name, logo, specific color, or method of dress to identify its own members and counterparts.

> ### CRITICAL THINKING
> In addition to consulting police sources and familiarizing yourself with gang markings, dress, and colors, how can you obtain information about gang activity in your community?

BOX 56-2 Short History of Gangs

Modern-era gangs first emerged in the United States in the late 1960s. Two of the best-known gangs, the Crips and the Bloods, started in Compton, California, when two rival high schools began to sport their school colors. The Bloods wore red to denote their gang affiliation; the Crips wore blue. Other gangs' ancestries originated in the prison system. The Black Gangster Disciples (now known as the Gangster Disciple Nation) was the most noteworthy of these. This gang started in the Chicago prison system and competed for the drug market in that city. In recent years, gangs have evolved to include all ethnic origins and backgrounds (e.g., Asian, Hispanic, Latin, and white threat groups). Most operate in secrecy with codes of honor and pledges that frequently involve acts of violence. Gang membership often is a lifetime commitment.

BOX 56-3 Some Gangs and Other Threat Groups in the United States

18th Street Gang	Latin Kings (Almighty Latin King & Queen Nation)
Bad Boy Club	
Banditos	Mara Salvatrucha 13 (MS-13)
Bloods	Mexican Posse (MP)
Crips	Norteños
Gangs for Disciples	Pagans
Hell's Angels	Skin Heads
	Sureños
	Outlaws

GRAFFITI AND CLOTHING

Graffiti ("tagging") is probably the most visible sign of gang criminal activity. It can be seen in neighborhood parks and on the backs and side walls of stores, fences, retaining walls, and any other prominent structure that is paintable (Figure 56-3). Gang graffiti usually marks territorial boundaries. (This is known as **turf**.) Gang-related clothing often is unique and specific to a group. It is worn to identify affiliation and rank. Common gang-related clothing and styles are listed in Box 56-4.

SAFETY ISSUES IN GANG AREAS

Common gang activities include fighting, vandalism, armed robbery, weapon offenses, automobile theft, battery, and drug dealing. (Not all gang members are engaged in illegal activities.) The criminal activity usually is committed for status or monetary benefit, either for the gang in general or for a single member. The likelihood for those violent acts and the fact that EMS personnel often "look like" law enforcement officials require that paramedics be very cautious about personal safety when working in gang areas.

Clandestine Drug Labs

As described in Chapter 34, the illegal manufacture of drugs can pose significant hazards for emergency personnel. Activities that take place in some **clandestine drug labs** include creating drugs (*synthesis*) from chemical precursors (e.g., lysergic acid diethylamide [LSD], methamphetamine). Also, a drug's form can be changed (*conversion*). For example, cocaine hydrochloride may be changed to a base form. The processes of drug synthesis and conversion can produce oxygen-depleted atmospheres. They also can create highly explosive and toxic gases (e.g., phosgene). These gases can readily be absorbed through the skin in amounts that can be fatal. Toxic solvents involved in drug-making processes also can lead to lab explosions and exposure to dangerous chemicals.

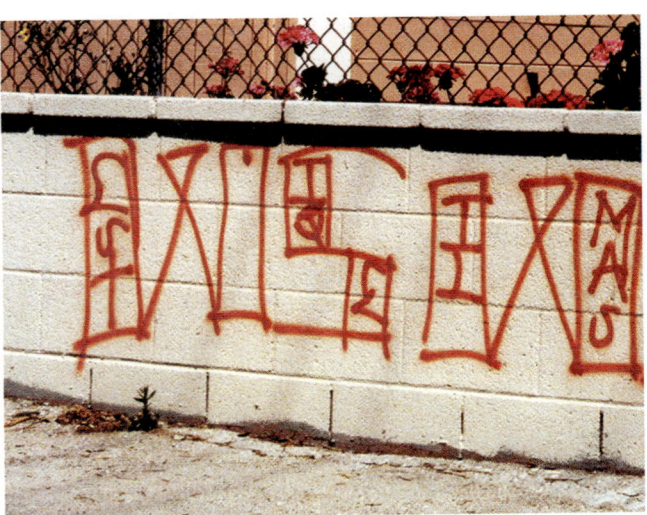

FIGURE 56-3 Blood graffiti on a wall in Los Angeles. (Courtesy Lisa Taylor-Austin, Milford, Conn.)

BOX 56-4 Gang Clothing and Styles

Male

- Shaved, bald head or extremely short hair; gang name or symbols shaved into hair
- Tattoos (variable) and jewelry
- Bandanas
- White, oversized T-shirt that is creased in the middle
- White, athletic-type undershirt
- Polo-type knit shirts (oversized), usually worn buttoned to the top and not tucked in; other types of oversized shirts
- Oversized Dickie, Ben Davis, or Solos pants
- Pants worn low, or "sagging," and cuffed inside at the bottom or dragging on the ground
- Baseball caps worn backward (usually black and sometimes having the gang's initials)
- Cutoff, below-the-knee short pants worn with knee-high socks
- A predominance of dark or dull clothing or clothing of one particular color
- Black stretch belt with chrome or silver gang initial belt buckle
- Clothing a mixture of gang colors, black and silver, or white

Female

- Exaggerated use of mousse, gel, or baby oil in the hair
- Tattoos (variable) and jewelry
- Black or dark clothing and shoes
- Black oversized jackets, sweatshirts, or athletic football jerseys
- Oversized shirts worn outside of pants
- Oversized T-shirts
- Dark jackets with lettering (cursive or Old English style)
- Baggy, long pants that drag on the ground
- Heavy makeup, dark and excessive eye shadow, shaved eyebrows, dark lipstick, dark fingernail polish
- Tank tops or revealing blouses
- Stretch belt with initial on belt buckle

From Texas Youth Commission: *Gang related clothing*, www.tyc.state.tx.us/prevention/clothing.html, accessed 10-31-10.

Other safety hazards that are associated with clandestine drug labs include *booby traps* that can maim or kill an intruder. Also, those who operate these labs are sometimes armed or otherwise violent. Clandestine labs usually are located in an area that ensures privacy. They generally are well ventilated. They also usually have access to water, electric, and gas utilities, which are required for the drug-making process. Suspicious individuals, activities, and deliveries often are at the site.

CRITICAL THINKING

What type of calls might EMS crews respond to at a drug lab?

DID YOU KNOW?

Shake n' Bake Meth

A new and popular way to manufacture small quantities of methamphetamine is called the *Shake n' Bake* or "one-pot method." The method uses one sealed container, such as a soft drink bottle. The container is usually flipped upside-down to cause the chemical reaction needed to turn the ingredients into meth. The chemical reaction causes an extremely high pressure inside the container after being shaken. This is one of the most dangerous ways to produce the drug because the pressure can cause a large explosion. The *Shake n' Bake* method is fast and portable. The method is often "cooked" while driving an automobile. Driving while making meth releases the fumes from the chemical process into the air. Once the drug is produced, the container is then thrown from the car. EMS personnel must be aware of the explosive danger of this method of meth production when approaching an automobile or the trunk of a car. Explosions also pose a hazard to children, who naturally want to explore things they find on the ground. EMS personnel should not investigate these containers and should alert law enforcement if found.

When responding to a scene that may be a site of illegal drug manufacture, EMS crews should be alert for suspicious signs. These may include chemical odors and the presence of chemical equipment (e.g., glassware, chemical containers, heating mantles, burners). If a drug lab is identified, the EMS crew should:

1. Leave the area at once.
2. Notify law enforcement and request appropriate agencies and personnel (e.g., hazardous materials [hazmat] teams, fire service personnel, U.S. Drug Enforcement Administration [DEA] personnel, chemistry specialists).
3. Initiate an incident management system and hazmat procedures per protocol.
4. Assist law enforcement personnel to evacuate the surrounding area in an orderly fashion to ensure public safety.

NOTE
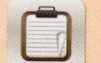
EMS crews should never touch anything found in or around a clandestine drug lab. Only specially trained personnel should try to alter drug-making equipment or stop chemical reactions in a drug lab.

Domestic Violence

As described in Chapter 50, *domestic violence* is violence that occurs between people in a relationship. The perpetrator may be male or female. The individuals may be in an opposite-sex or same-sex relationship. Domestic violence results in physical, emotional, sexual, verbal, or economic abuse. It may occur in several combinations. To review, many signs indicate domestic violence and abuse. Some of these include the following:

- Apparent fear of a household member
- Different or conflicting accounts by parties at the scene
- One party preventing another from speaking
- A patient who is reluctant to speak
- Injuries that do not match the reported mechanism of injury
- Unusual or unsanitary living conditions or personal hygiene

EMS personnel who respond to a scene of domestic violence should be aware that acts of violence may be directed toward them by the perpetrator. They should take all safety precautions. If the scene is considered safe for the EMS crew, paramedics should treat the patient's injuries. They also should notify medical direction and other authorities consistent per standard procedures and protocol. (Mandatory reporting may be required.) To help ensure scene safety for the crew and the abused person, paramedics should not be judgmental about the relationship. They should not direct accusations toward the abuser or the victim. When appropriate, paramedics should supply the victim with phone numbers for domestic violence hotlines, community support programs, and available shelters.

SAFETY TACTICS

Tactics that help ensure personal safety include avoidance, tactical retreat, cover and concealment, and distraction and evasive maneuvers. Many programs in the United States teach tactics for safety and patient care. Some EMS providers are specially trained and equipped to work in tactical law enforcement settings (Box 56-5).

Avoidance

Avoidance is the action of keeping away from a dangerous situation or preventing the development of a dangerous situation. Avoidance is always preferable to confrontation. To practice avoidance, paramedics must continually be aware of the scene. They can stay aware by being observant and by being knowledgeable about warning signs that may indicate a dangerous situation. In addition, they must be knowledgeable about tactical responses for avoiding danger or for dealing with danger that cannot be avoided. An example of avoidance is **staging.** With staging, the dispatching center learns of danger and advises the EMS crew not to approach the scene until it has been secured by the appropriate authorities.

Tactical Retreat

Tactical retreat describes leaving the scene when danger is observed or when violence or indicators of violence are displayed. Tactical retreat requires immediate and decisive action. Retreat on foot or by vehicle (in a calm, safe manner) involves choosing the mode and route of retreat that

---

BOX 56-5 Tactical EMS

The term *tactical EMS (TEMS)* refers to EMS personnel who are specially trained and equipped to provide prehospital emergency care in tactical law enforcement settings. Such settings may include hostage-barricaded situations, high-risk search warrants, and other adverse situations involving law enforcement and/or rescue operations in which standard EMS units may be inappropriate.

The concept of training emergency medical technicians (EMTs) and paramedics in TEMS started in the late 1980s. It has since expanded nationwide. Forward-thinking law enforcement departments have adopted TEMS programs as a way to increase the safety of their special weapons and tactics (SWAT) officers and the innocent hostage or bystander. They also are a means of addressing liability exposure. Tactical training for EMS personnel also is recognized as a valuable tool for personal safety when EMS personnel find themselves in an unsafe situation.

Many tactical medical teams use the Counter Narcotics and Terrorism Operational Medical Support (CONTOMS) program for initial training of their personnel. CONTOMS is a joint federal program supported by the U.S. Department of Health and Human Services, U.S. Department of Homeland Security, and U.S. Park Police, with assistance from the Department of Justice, as well as many state and local law enforcement agencies. The CONTOMS program leads to certification as an EMT-Tactical (EMT-T) or SWAT medic. The focus of the training is to integrate specific skills to complement an agency's standard operating procedures. These skills include the ability to:

- Assess and plan for preventive medicine needs in sustained operations
- Provide preventive medical care in sustained operations
- Recognize and treat unique wound patterns resulting from deliberate interpersonal aggression
- Use medical care skills appropriate to hostile and austere environments
- Explain medical and physiological parameters that lead to performance decrement and implement plans that minimize those effects
- Develop and apply injury control strategies
- Access and analyze medical information and make a medical threat assessment
- Apply special law enforcement principles to the delivery of medical care

See www.trueresearch.org/contoms/, accessed 10-27-10.

---

provides the least exposure to danger. During tactical retreat, the EMS crew should be aware that the risks they faced are now located behind them. They must stay alert for associated dangers. Of course, the required distance from danger for a safe tactical retreat must be guided by the nature of the incident. In general, a safe distance must:

- Protect the crew from any potential danger
- Keep the crew out of the immediate line of sight

- Protect the crew from gunfire (i.e., provide cover)
- Keep the crew far enough away to give them time to react if danger reappears

CRITICAL THINKING
Could the EMS crew be charged with abandonment if they make a tactical retreat and leave the patient?

Once tactical retreat has been achieved, the EMS crew must notify other responding units and agencies of the danger. They notify other units using interagency EMS and law enforcement standard operating procedures and agreements. (Interagency procedures that deal with violent situations should be established in the preplanning stages so that each agency is aware of its specific duties.)

Documentation also is essential to reducing liability if injuries or deaths occur. Thorough documentation should include observations of danger at the scene; names of persons notified of the danger; actions at the scene; and accurate times that retreat or return to the scene occurred. Most legal authorities do not consider tactical retreat for appropriate circumstances to be patient abandonment.

Cover and Concealment

Cover and **concealment** provide protection from injury. *Cover* provides ballistic protection and is often in the form of large, heavy structures. Examples of such structures include large trees, telephone poles, and a vehicle's engine block. *Concealment* hides the body. However, it offers little or no ballistic protection. Examples of concealment include bushes, wall-boards, and the doors of vehicles.

Cover and concealment should be integrated into tactical retreat or used when the EMS crew is "pinned down" (e.g., by gunfire) or in other dangerous settings. When the need for cover or concealment arises, paramedics should:

- Constantly be aware of their surroundings
- Be aware that "stepping off" cover may actually provide more protection than "hugging" your cover (Figure 56-4)
- Constantly look for ways to improve protection and location
- Be aware of reflective clothing (e.g., trim, badges) that may draw attention or serve as a target

CRITICAL THINKING
What parts of your ambulance provide cover?

Distraction and Evasive Tactics

Distraction and **evasive tactics** can be used as self-defense measures during retreat. They also can be used when retreat and cover and concealment are not available options (Box

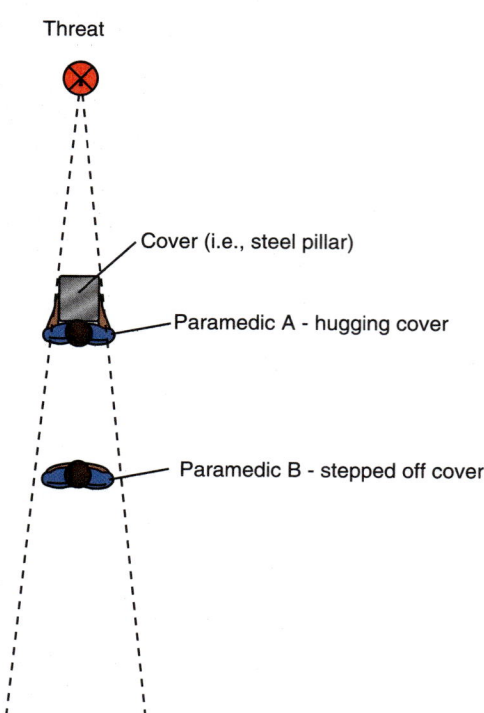

FIGURE 56-4 At times stepping-off cover provides more protection than hugging cover. Paramedic B is less exposed and must expose far less of him/herself to visualize the threat if needed as compared to paramedic A.

BOX 56-6 Self-Defense Measures

Training in self-defense is probably appropriate for all emergency responders. Avoidance is always superior to confrontation. However, some violent situations may call for self-defense. Examples include physical attacks that cannot be avoided, armed confrontation or robbery, hostage situations, and dangerous animals. A person can be controlled with physical or chemical restraints (see Chapter 35). Equipment (e.g., metal clipboards, jump kits, stretchers) or other items (e.g., furniture) can be used to block an aggressor. In addition to these techniques, self-defense measures may include training in the use of pepper sprays or other chemical deterrents and defensive physical maneuvers that can allow escape.

Sometimes escape is impossible, and paramedics may be caught in a dangerous situation. (For example, they may be held as a hostage.) In such cases paramedics should:

- Remain as calm as possible
- Avoid any confrontation
- Play an active role with the captor in resolving the incident
- Focus on a peaceful resolution and escape

56-6). For example, equipment may be used to provide distraction (e.g., a stretcher may be wedged in a doorway to block an aggressor) or equipment may be thrown to trip or slow a pursuer. These actions may allow the EMS crew to make a safe retreat or gain adequate cover and

BOX 56-7 Warning Signs of Possible Violent Aggression

People who are about to escalate to violence often give subtle warning signs of this development. Such a person may:

- Conspicuously ignore emergency responders
- Be verbally abusive
- Invade the responder's personal space
- Have a violent history or background
- Shift the body weight from side to side or foot to foot (boxer stance)
- Clench the fists
- Tighten the muscles (e.g., have stiff arms and/or shoulders)
- Maintain eye contact by staring

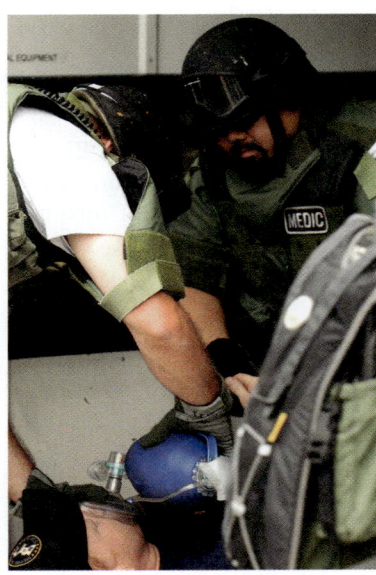

FIGURE 56-5 Tactical patient care. (Courtesy Ray Kemp. St. Charles, Mo.)

concealment. Evasive tactics involve anticipating the moves of the aggressor (Box 56-7) and using unconventional pathways during retreat.

Paramedic crews trained in **tactical EMS** often use pre-assigned roles for distraction and evasive maneuvers. One paramedic usually is the **contact provider,** who initiates and provides direct patient care. This includes patient assessment and most elements of interpersonal scene contact. Another crew member serves as the **cover provider.** In a tactical context, the cover provider's role is to ensure safe cover for the contact providers while they provide patient care. This role includes monitoring the scene for danger. The cover provider generally does not perform patient care duties that would prevent observation of the scene. The cover provider also may be responsible for ensuring the safekeeping of equipment, drugs, and supplies while at the scene.

Methods of communication between the contact and cover providers should be developed in advance. That way, they can alert team members of potential dangers without alerting the aggressor. This often can be done with subtle verbal and nonverbal signals, such as using coded terms, scratching the neck, or rubbing the nose. It is crucial in these situations to maintain radio contact with the dispatching center. The crew also should involve the dispatcher in the danger signal process. For example, if the dispatcher hears a coded term that means danger, a priority response of the proper personnel can be initiated.

TACTICAL PATIENT CARE

The term **tactical patient care** describes patient care activities that occur inside the scene perimeter. This is also known as the **hot zone.** The provision of EMS in the hot zone requires special training and authorization, body armor and a tactical uniform, compact and functional equipment, and, in some operations, personal defensive weapons. Tactical EMS in the hot zone often requires risks not taken in standard EMS situations. *Tactical medics*

provide immediate medical care to the injured during a **special weapons and tactics** (SWAT) **operation.** These medics treat the injured on-site or stabilize them and extract them from the scene. Tactical medics generally work alongside law enforcement officers. Some agencies use individuals who are cross-trained in law enforcement and tactical EMS (Fig. 56-5).

Body Armor

As described in Chapter 37, **soft body armor** (also known as *bulletproof vests*) offers protection from some blunt and penetrating trauma. It absorbs and distributes the impact of a ballistic missile or penetrating object. This equipment is effective against most handgun bullets. The equipment does not protect against knives or pointed, sharp objects.[5] However, they do not provide protection from high-velocity rifle bullets or thin or edged weapons (e.g., ice picks). Like all other protective clothing, body armor is effective only when it is properly worn. It also must be in good condition. Some body armor (e.g., Kevlar) degrades with age. This armor may carry a ballistic expiration date that should be observed. Wet or worn vests do not provide optimum protection. A type III or higher level of protection generally is recommended for tactical EMS providers.

When wearing body armor, paramedics should take care not to develop a false sense of security. *A general rule is: "Never try a maneuver that wouldn't normally be done without body armor."* Also, paramedics should keep in mind that body armor does not cover the entire body. Severe injury can still result from the forces of blunt trauma (in the absence of penetration) even when the vest is properly worn. This "back-face signature" (transmitted impact energy) is variable according to the type of vest and projectile.

EMS CARE IN THE HOT ZONE

As previously stated, the provision of EMS care in tactical situations calls for special training and authorization. Most tactical medics (EMT-Ts and SWAT medics) are trained in the following[6]:

- Team health and management
- Care under fire
- Officer rescue
- Medical operations planning and medical intelligence
- Responding to the active shooter
- Special medical gear for tactical operations
- Personal protective gear
- Special needs for extended operations
- Preventive medicine
- Management of weapons of mass destruction and toxic hazards

Most programs involve training exercises. Some of these include the following:

- Physical assessment under sensory deprivation/overload conditions
- Medical threat assessment
- Advanced medical-tactical techniques
- Field expedient decontamination
- New technologies for safe searches
- Management of dental injuries
- "Officer down" rescue and extraction
- Aeromedical evacuation
- Medical management of clandestine drug lab raids
- Safe search techniques
- Remote physical assessment

Patient care in dangerous settings involves a number of special concerns. These include the frequent need to remove a patient from the area safely; the frequent care of trauma patients; the need to modify patient care; and medical and transport actions that must be coordinated with the incident commander. Often tactical EMS providers work under protocols and standing orders that differ from those of "standard" EMS practice. These medical direction issues regarding patient care are dictated by the nature of the event. They also are determined by the uncontrolled and hazardous scene in which emergency medical services are provided. Awareness programs are available for those who supervise or manage personnel assigned to a tactical team. Programs are also available for physicians (and others) who provide medical direction for rescuers who work with tactical law enforcement teams. Quality assurance programs and direct physician involvement at the local level are recommended.

EMS AT CRIME SCENES

A **crime scene** is a location where any part of a criminal act has occurred. It also can be a location where evidence relating to a crime may be found. Important physical evidence that may be found at a crime scene includes fingerprints, footprints, and blood and other body fluids. Fingerprints and footprints are unique to an individual. No two people have identical prints. These ridge characteristics often are left behind on a surface, along with oil and moisture from the skin. Blood and other body fluids can be tested for deoxyribonucleic acid (DNA) and ABO blood typing; they also have characteristics that may be unique to the individual. In addition, particulate evidence (e.g., hair, carpet, and clothing fibers) can provide useful information and is considered valuable at a crime scene.

The paramedic's observations at a crime scene are important. They should be documented carefully on the patient care report or other appropriate form. For example, victims' positions and injuries and conditions at the scene may be helpful to law enforcement personnel in solving the crime. Documentation also should include any statements made by the patient or other people at the scene and any **dying declarations.** Paramedics should be careful to (1) record their observations objectively; (2) record patients' or bystanders' words in quotes; and (3) avoid personal opinions that are not relevant to patient care. Paramedics must keep in mind that patient care reports are legal documents; they may be used in court. Paramedics should avoid labeling ballistic injuries as "entrance" or "exit" wounds. Rather, the wound and characteristics of the wound should be described and documented in the patient care report.

> **NOTE**
>
> A *dying declaration* is a statement(s) made by a person who believes he or she is about to die. The statement concerns the cause or circumstance surrounding his or her impending death. An example is an assault victim who makes a dying declaration implicating a certain person as being her attacker.

Preserving Evidence

Patient care is the paramedic's ultimate priority, even at crime scenes. However, evidence can be protected while caring for the patient. This can be accomplished by being careful not to disturb the scene unnecessarily or destroy evidence. For example, paramedics should be observant of the scene and surroundings; they should touch only what is required for patient care; and they should wear latex gloves for infection control and to avoid leaving additional fingerprints at the scene. Other measures that aid crime scene preservation are listed in Box 56-8.

> **CRITICAL THINKING**
>
> If the main goal is caring for the patient, why should a paramedic be concerned about preserving evidence?

BOX 56-8 Considerations for Crime Scene Preservation

Paramedics should observe the following rules when called to a known or a possible crime scene:

1. Approach no crime scene until it has been secured for your safety.
2. Park your vehicle as far away as conveniently possible to preserve skid marks, tire prints, or other evidence.
3. Survey and assess the scene before proceeding to the victim.
4. Try to approach the victim from a route different from the assailant's probable route.
5. Follow the same path to and from the victim.
6. Avoid stepping on blood stains or spatter if possible.
7. Disturb the victim and the victim's clothing as little as possible while performing your assessment and during treatment.
8. When cutting clothing from a victim, try to do it in a way that preserves the points of wounding.
9. Report your actions and any disturbances you make to the crime scene investigator.
10. Keep all unnecessary people away from the victim.
11. Do not smoke or eat at the crime scene.
12. Do not touch any evidence if at all possible.
13. Make no comments to bystanders about the situation.
14. Save the victim's clothes and personal items in a paper bag. The bag should be labeled, sealed, and turned over to law enforcement personnel.
15. Be alert to any dying declarations the patient makes.
16. Keep accurate, detailed records.
17. Keep in mind that law enforcement personnel are in charge of the crime scene; you are in charge of the patient.

Modified from Vollrath R: Crime scene preservation: it's everybody's concern, *J Emerg Med Serv* 20(1):53, 1995.

SUMMARY

- A key point in ensuring scene safety is to identify and respond to dangers before they threaten. If the scene is known to be violent, the EMS crew should remain at a safe and out-of-sight distance from the area. They should remain at this distance until the scene has been secured.
- The paramedic should look for warning signs of violence during response to a residence. He or she should retreat from the scene if danger becomes evident.
- A response to a highway incident may present the dangers associated with traffic and extrication. However, it may present danger from violence as well. Occupants may be armed, wanted, or fleeing felons; intoxicated or drugged; or violent/abusive from an altered mental state.
- The paramedic should monitor for warning signs of danger in violent street incidents. He or she should retreat from the scene if necessary.
- A gang is any group of people who take part in socially disruptive or criminal behavior. Some gangs are involved in violent criminal activities. EMS personnel often look like law enforcement officers. Thus, they should be very cautious about personal safety when working in gang areas.

- Clandestine drug lab activities can produce explosive and toxic gases. Other risks include booby traps that can maim or kill an intruder, and armed or violent occupants.
- EMS personnel who respond to a scene of domestic violence should be aware that acts of violence may be directed toward them by the perpetrator; they should take all safety precautions.
- Tactics for safety include avoidance, tactical retreat, cover and concealment, and distraction and evasive maneuvers.
- Tactical patient care refers to care activities that occur inside the scene perimeter. This is known as the "hot zone." Providing care in this area calls for special training and authorization, body armor and a tactical uniform, compact and functional equipment, and, in some operations, personal defensive weapons.
- The paramedic's observations at a crime scene are important. They should be carefully documented. Evidence should be protected while caring for the patient. This can be done by not unnecessarily disturbing the scene or destroying evidence.

REFERENCES

1. Maguire BJ, Hunting KL, Smith GS, et al: Occupational fatalities in emergency medical services: a hidden crisis, *Ann Emerg Med* 40(6):625-632, 2002.
2. Archer K: *Health workers' safety in spotlight*, www.emsresponder.com/features/article.jsp?id=10230&siteSection=25, accessed 6-26-10.
3. National Rifle Association of America, Institute for Legislative Action: *Right-to-carry 2010*, www.nraila.org/Issues/FactSheets/Read.aspx?ID=18, accessed 10-27-10.
4. Egley A Jr: *Highlights of the 2008 National Youth Gang Survey*, Washington, DC, March 2010, U.S. Department of Justice, Office of Juvenile Justice and Delinquency Prevention, www.ojjdp.ncjrs.gov/publications/PubAbstract.asp?pubi=251276, accessed 6-26-10.

5. Office of Law Enforcement Standards, National Institute of Technology: *Ballistic resistance of body armor*, www.ojp.usdoj.gov/nij/pubs-sum/223054.htm, accessed 11-7-10.
6. U.S. Immigration and Customs Enforcement, Federal Protective Service Office of Protective Medicine, U.S. Department of

Homeland Security: *EMT-T tactical course*, www.trueresearch.org/CONTOMS, accessed 10-27-10.

SUGGESTED READINGS

Di Maio V: *Gunshot wounds: practical aspects of firearms, ballistics, and forensic techniques*, ed 2, Boca Raton, Fla, 1999, CRC Press.

Hammesfahr R, Collins D: *Tactical emergency medical support: the tactical medical handbook*, ed 2, 2009.

Sztajnkrycer M, et al: Excited delirium and sudden unexpected death, *Emerg Med Serv* 34(4):77-81, 2005.

57 Hazardous Materials Awareness

OBJECTIVES

Upon completion of this chapter, the paramedic student will be able to:

1. Define hazardous materials terminology.
2. Identify legislation about hazardous materials that influences emergency health care workers.
3. Describe resources to assist in identification and management of hazardous materials incidents.
4. Identify the protective clothing and equipment needed to respond to selected hazardous materials incidents.
5. Describe the pathophysiology and signs and symptoms of internal damage caused by exposure to selected hazardous materials.
6. Identify the pathophysiology, signs and symptoms, and prehospital management of selected hazardous materials that produce external damage.
7. Outline the prehospital response to a hazardous materials emergency.
8. Describe medical monitoring and rehabilitation of rescue workers who respond to a hazardous materials emergency.
9. Describe emergency decontamination and management of patients who have been contaminated by hazardous materials.
10. Outline the eight steps to decontaminate rescue personnel and equipment at a hazardous materials incident.

KEY TERMS

asphyxiants Gases that displace the oxygen in the air and also dilute the oxygen concentration of the air.

carcinogens Cancer-causing agents.

cardiotoxins Hazardous materials that can cause myocardial ischemia and dysrhythmias.

cold zone A safety zone in a hazmat response that encompasses the warm zone; usually considered safe, requiring only minimal protective clothing.

corrosives Hazardous materials that are either acids or bases (alkaline).

cryogenics Refrigerant liquid gases that can freeze human tissue on contact.

decontamination The process of making patients, rescuers, equipment, and supplies safe by eliminating harmful substances.

dose response The physical change or effect caused by exposure to a chemical; dependent on the concentration of the chemical to which the person was exposed.

formal product identification A method of identifying a hazardous material through written means.

hazard and risk assessment An analysis of the consequences and probability that exposure to a chemical may cause danger or peril.

hazardous material Any substance or material capable of posing an unreasonable risk to health, safety, and property.

hemotoxins Hazardous substances that may cause the destruction of red blood cells.

hepatotoxins Hazardous substances that damage the liver.

hot zone The area of a hazmat incident that includes the hazardous material.

informal product identification A method of identifying a hazardous material through unwritten means.

irritants Substances that affect the respiratory system, including the surfaces of the eyes, nose, mouth, and throat.

liquefaction Conversion of solid tissues to a fluid or semifluid state.

material safety data sheets Written product identification as required by OSHA for each chemical produced, stored, or used in the United States.

medical monitoring The ongoing evaluation of rescuers who are at risk for illness or injury from operations at the incident.

nephrotoxins Hazardous materials that are especially destructive to the kidneys.

nerve poisons Poisonous substances that act on the nervous system.

neurotoxins Poisons that affect the nervous system.

placards Four-sided, diamond-shaped signs displayed on hazardous materials containers that usually are yellow, orange, white, or green. They have a four-digit United

Nations identification number and a legend to indicate the contents of the container.

primary contamination Exposure to a hazardous substance that is harmful only to the person exposed and that poses little risk of exposure to others.

rehabilitation Activities that are provided at an incident to sustain the energy of rescuers, improve performance, and decrease the likelihood of on-scene injury or death; also known as rehab.

safe distance factor The minimum safe distance for personal safety from hazardous materials as outlined in the reference guides.

secondary contamination Exposure to a hazardous substance whereby liquid and particulate substances are transferred easily to others by touching.

self-contained breathing apparatus A respiratory protection device that provides an enclosed system of air.

shipping papers Descriptions of the hazardous materials that include the substance name, classification, and United Nations identification number.

supplied-air breathing apparatus A device that provides a nearly unlimited supply of air from a source located outside the confined space.

synergistic effects The effects of one chemical enhancing the effects of a second chemical.

UN/NA number The United Nations class (or division) identification number and North American number for a hazardous material.

warm zone In a hazmat incident, a buffer area that surrounds the hot zone with "cold" and "hot" end corridors; usually considered a safer environment for workers.

H*azardous materials incidents create added responsibilities for EMS personnel. Large incidents may involve a number of political jurisdictions. In addition, cooperation in mass evacuations and mass decontamination may be required. Specialized roles and responsibilities include, among others, recognition and identification of hazardous material, scene safety, responsibilities to stage at major scenes, containment and cleanup of the material, extrication and decontamination of exposed individuals, provision of emergency care, and continual medical monitoring of team members involved in the incident.*

SCOPE OF HAZARDOUS MATERIALS

A **hazardous material** is defined as "any substance or material capable of posing an unreasonable risk to health, safety, and property."[1] More than 50 billion tons of hazardous materials are made in the United States each year. About 2 billion tons are shipped within the United States. From 1998 to 2007, the U.S. Department of Transportation (DOT) reports there were 141 hazmat transportation-related fatalities, approximately 14 per year. Of these, 124 deaths were on the highways and 17 were rail-related.[2] Emergency responses to vehicular crashes are common; thus the potential for exposure to hazardous materials is great. Other possible causes of hazardous materials incidents include mishaps in the storage of materials and manufacturing operations, illicit drug manufacturing (e.g., "meth labs"), and acts of terrorism (see Chapter 58).

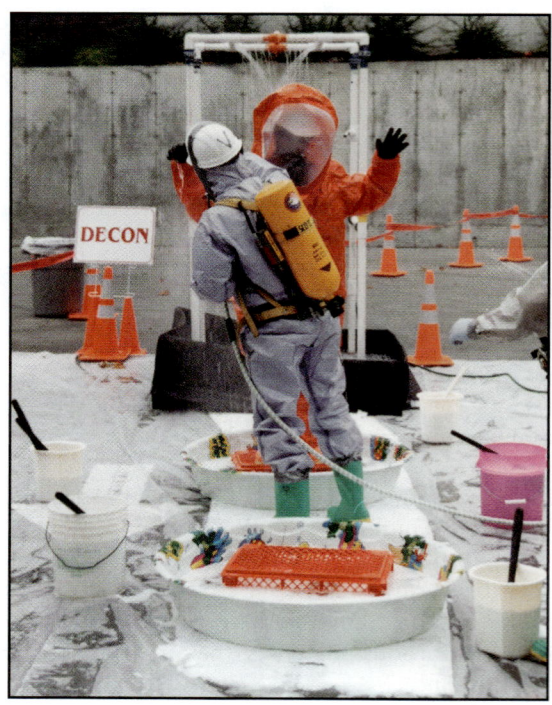

As described in Chapter 34, injury or illness can also result from exposure to household chemicals, pesticides, and industrial toxins. The following statistics emphasize the importance of emergency medical service (EMS) personnel knowing how to manage hazardous materials exposure[3]:

- About 9000 deaths occur each year from exposure to poisonous solids, liquids, and gases.
- An estimated 100,000 industrial workers are exposed to respiratory tract irritants each year.
- Pesticide poisoning accounts for more than 3000 hospitalizations each year.
- Most fire-related deaths result from inhalation of toxic products of combustion.

CRITICAL THINKING

Consider the industries in your area. Do any of these have the potential for a hazardous materials exposure?

LAWS AND REGULATIONS

In recent years much focus has been placed on the handling of hazardous materials. Major incidents have attracted the attention of employee and citizen groups. These incidents also have drawn the attention of local, state, and federal officials. Some of these incidents include the Union Carbide disaster in Bhopal, India (1984); the Chernobyl nuclear accident in the Soviet Union (1986); the Three Mile Island incident in the United States (1979); the Criticality accident in Tokaimura, Japan (1999); threats and acts of bioterrorism (e.g., the sarin gas attack on Tokyo subways in 1995); anthrax attacks in the United States (2001); and the need for proper disposal of hazardous wastes. This attention has resulted in more laws and regulations to ensure strict control of hazardous materials.

The Superfund Amendments and Reauthorization Act (the Superfund Act) of 1986 established requirements for federal, state, and local governments and industry regarding emergency planning and the reporting of hazardous materials–related incidents. This act was intended to help communities better manage a chemical emergency. The Superfund Act helped increase public knowledge about hazardous materials in communities and helped to improve public access to this information. The act required owners and operators of facilities using or storing any of the extremely hazardous substances identified by the Environmental Protection Agency (EPA) to notify the local fire department, the local emergency planning committee, and the state emergency response commission.

In 1989 the Occupational Safety and Health Administration (OSHA) and the EPA published rules to govern training requirements, emergency plans, medical checkups, and other safety precautions for workers at uncontrolled hazardous waste sites and for those responding to hazardous chemical releases or spills.[4] The Superfund Act mandates that states adopt these rules. The training requirements apply to five groups of persons who may respond to an emergency that involves hazardous materials (see chapter appendix).

In addition to these training levels outlined by OSHA, the National Fire Protection Association (NFPA) has published standards that address competencies for EMS personnel at hazardous materials (hazmat) scenes.[5] According to these standards, paramedics who transport patients who pose no risk of **secondary contamination** must be trained to NFPA standard 473 Level I. Paramedics who may have to decontaminate rapidly or assist in the **decontamination** area must be trained to NFPA standard 473 Level II.

IDENTIFICATION OF HAZARDOUS MATERIALS

At the center of dealing with hazardous materials is identifying the substance. Two methods used to identify such materials are **informal product identification** and **formal product identification.**

Informal Product Identification

Arriving emergency personnel may be able to determine the presence and type of hazardous materials at the scene. Informal methods of identification include the following:

- Visual inspection of the scene with binoculars before entering the site
- Verbal reports by bystanders or other responsible individuals
- Occupancy type (intended use of a particular structure such as fuel storage or pesticide plant)
- Incident location (probable location for presence of hazardous materials)
- Location within a building (what is stored in that area)
- Visual indicators (vapor clouds, smoke, leakage)
- Vehicle types (named carriers or company)
- Container characteristics (size, shape, color, deformed containers)
- Senses (peculiar smell reported by bystanders)
- Signs and symptoms of victims of exposure

These informal ways to identify a product should be used as a quick means to determine the presence of any hazardous materials. The paramedic should always identify a product formally before taking any action that may pose a threat to the safety of all responders.

> **NOTE**
> Personal safety is the number one priority when responding to a hazardous materials incident. If the scene is not safe, the EMS crew should retreat and not enter the scene until it has been made safe by trained personnel.

Formal Product Identification

Traditionally, hazardous materials have been labeled by one or more of the following six systems:

1. The American National Standards Institute uses a label to identify a specific hazard (e.g., explosives, flammable liquids, radioactive materials) rather than a specific chemical.
2. The U.S. Department of Transportation (DOT) uses labels and placards with pictographs and printed hazard categories. In addition, DOT requires specific information on shipping manifests.
3. The United Nations Labeling System uses pictographs, symbols, or both, similar to those used by DOT, to identify a specific hazard rather than a specific chemical.
4. The International Air Transport Association uses the United Nations pictographs and indicates written emergency precaution measures in case of an incident.
5. The National Fire Protection Association uses color and a numerical rating scale (NFPA 704 System) to identify the degree of hazard for health, fire, and reactivity. Many state and local fire codes require the diamond-shaped identification symbols on fixed facilities (Figure 57-1). The numbering system rates each category from 1 (least harmful) to 4 (most harmful).

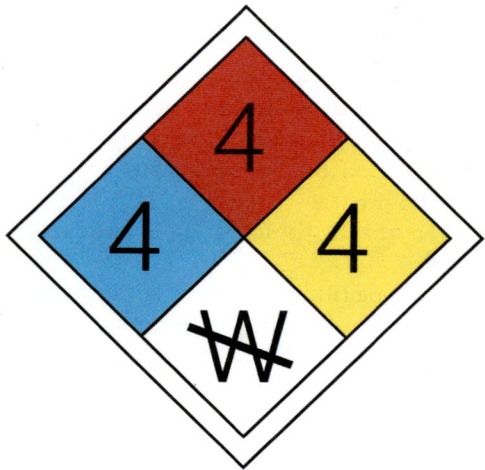

FIGURE 57-1 The National Fire Protection Association placard. It consists of four diamonds within a larger diamond. The red (flammability) diamond is at "12 o'clock"; the yellow (instability) diamond is at "3 o'clock"; the white (special hazards) diamond is at "6 o'clock"; and the blue (health hazard) diamond is at "9 o'clock." The degree of hazard severity is indicated by a numerical rating that ranges from 4, indicating the most severe hazard, to 0, indicating no hazard. Special hazards are indicated in the white section and refer to chemicals that react with water ($\mathcal{W}$) and those that are oxidizers (OX).

6. The U.S. Department of Labor requires material safety data sheets (also known as MSDSs) for hazardous chemicals that are stored, handled, or used in the workplace.

>
> **CRITICAL THINKING**
> The next time you are on the highway, see if you can easily spot the placards on large trucks.

PLACARDS AND SHIPPING PAPERS

A number of identification systems may be used. However, hazardous materials usually are identified by **placards** (Figure 57-2) and **shipping papers.**

The United Nations class (or division) identification number and the North American number **(UN/NA number)** may be displayed on the bottom of a placard. Or the number may be displayed on the shipping paper after the listed shipping name or names. In certain cases this class or division number may replace the written name of the hazard class in the shipping paper description. Box 57-1 shows the meanings of the class and division numbers.

The location and type of paperwork that identifies hazardous materials varies according to the mode of transport. Most shipping papers are kept near the operator (e.g., driver, pilot, or captain) of the vehicle, aircraft, train, or ship. Several chemical agents may have the same UN/NA number. Thus it is important to refer to specific guidelines for hazardous material by chemical name in addition to this number.

> **NOTE**
> Shippers are responsible for tracking hazardous loads in transit. If shipping papers are difficult to obtain or too dangerous to recover, law enforcement personnel or the dispatch agency can contact the shipper by phone with a description of the vehicle (e.g., truck or car number and license plate number). This will help identify the type of hazardous material.

BOX 57-1 International Classification System for Hazardous Materials

Class or division numbers may be displayed in the bottom of placards, or they may be displayed in the hazardous materials description on shipping papers. In certain cases a class or division number may replace the written name of the hazard class description on the shipping paper. The class and division numbers have the following meanings:

Class 1	**Explosives**
Division 1.1	Explosives with a mass explosion hazard
Division 1.2	Explosives with a projection hazard
Division 1.3	Explosives with predominantly a fire hazard
Division 1.4	Explosives with no significant blast hazard
Division 1.5	Very insensitive explosives
Division 1.6	Extremely insensitive explosive articles
Class 2	**Gases**
Division 2.1	Flammable gases
Division 2.2	Nonflammable gases
Division 2.3	Poison gases
Division 2.4	Corrosive gases (Canadian)
Class 3	**Flammable Liquids**
Division 3.1	Flashpoint below −18° C (0° F)
Division 3.2	Flashpoint −18° C and above but less than 23° C (73° F)
Division 3.3	Flashpoint of 23° C and up to 61° C (141° F)
Class 4	**Flammable Solids, Spontaneously Combustible Materials, Materials That Are Dangerous When Wet**
Division 4.1	Flammable solids
Division 4.2	Spontaneously combustible materials
Division 4.3	Materials that are dangerous when wet
Class 5	**Oxidizers and Organic Peroxides**
Division 5.1	Oxidizers
Division 5.2	Organic peroxides
Class 6	**Poisonous and Etiological (Infectious) Materials**
Division 6.1	Poisonous materials
Division 6.2	Etiological (infectious) materials
Class 7	**Radioactive Materials**
Class 8	**Corrosives**
Class 9	**Miscellaneous Hazardous Materials**

From U.S. Department of Transportation: *North American emergency response guidebook,* Washington, DC, 2008, The Department.

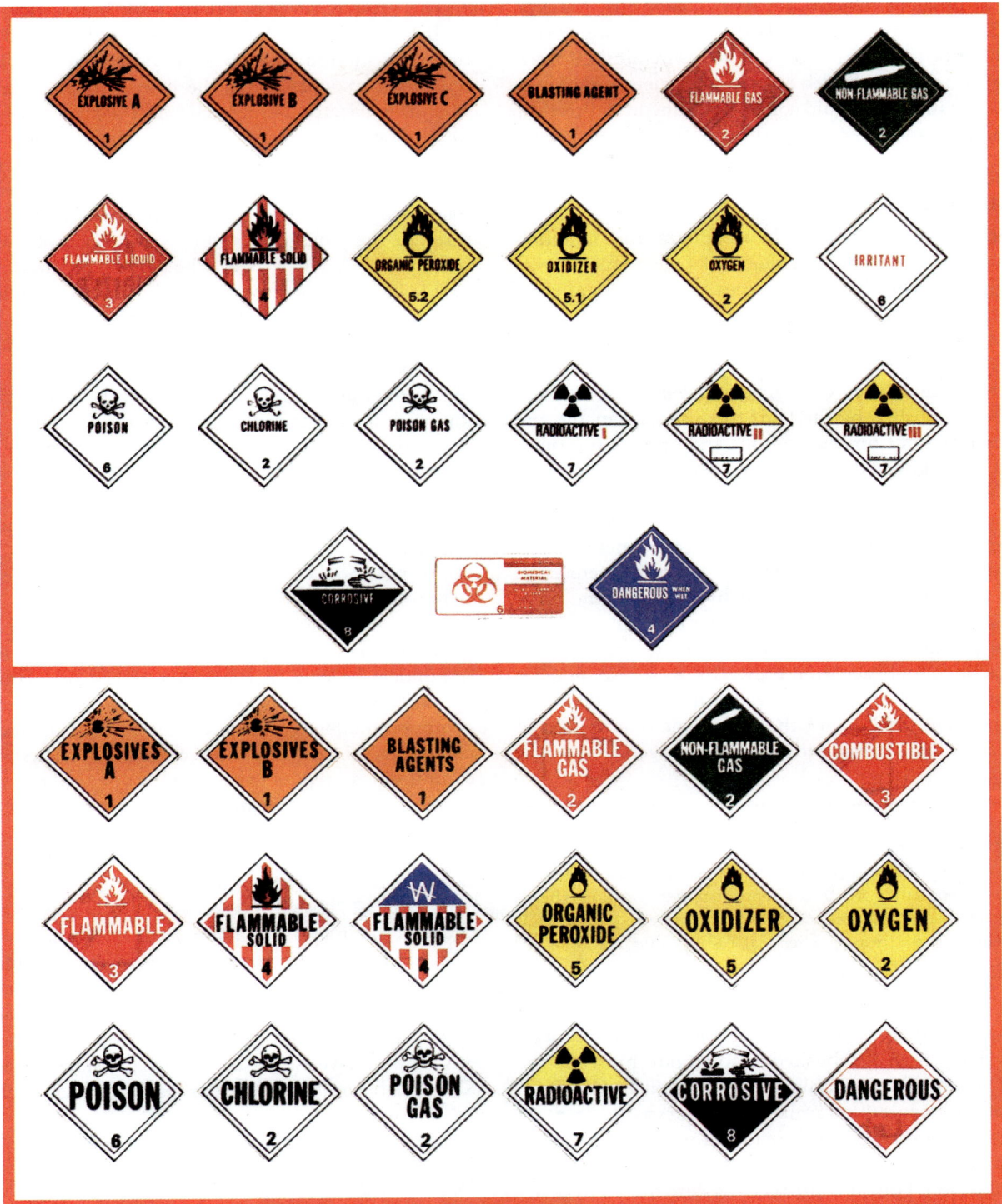

FIGURE 57-2 Hazardous materials warning placards and labels.

MATERIAL SAFETY DATA SHEETS

Material safety data sheets (MSDSs) are required by OSHA for each chemical produced, stored, or used in the United States. Material safety data sheets are supplied by the manufacturer. They contain information for the safe and proper handling and storage of the material. They also have information on emergency actions needed following exposure. Material safety data sheets also classify the potential of significant health hazards from exposure to a material.

The potential health hazard of a material may be defined in a number of different ways. This may depend on the degree of inherent toxicity and type of exposure. Material safety data sheets provide useful information. However, they should not be used as the sole source of chemical information, information on health risks, or treatment recommendations. Paramedics should consult with medical direction, a poison control center, or another appropriate authority.

OTHER SOURCES OF INFORMATION ON HAZARDOUS MATERIALS

A number of resources are available for hazardous materials reference. These references include books, telephone support through emergency hazmat agencies, computer databases, and Internet sources. Product information should be referenced through more than one source. (Preferably three sources should be used, if time and availability permit.) One such reference is the *North American Emergency Response Guidebook* published by the DOT, Transport Canada, and the Secretariat of Communications and Transportation of Mexico. This guidebook lists more than 1000 hazardous materials. It also lists the basic first aid procedures for managing an exposure. It includes names and identification numbers of substances. The book is cross-referenced in alphabetical and numerical order. This free reference is carried in emergency vehicles by many EMS, fire, and other public service agencies. One should note that the *Emergency Response Guidebook* is designed to assist first responders with initial actions for evacuation only. The book also includes the distance and area from the incident that should be evacuated. The book is not the only guide that should be referenced when dealing with hazmat emergencies.

> **NOTE**
>
> When a hazardous substance cannot be precisely identified, trained personnel may use sophisticated devices to ensure scene safety and to aid in product identification. These devices include air and gas monitoring equipment, and special equipment for pH testing, chemical testing, and colorimetric tube testing.

As described in Chapter 34, regional poison control centers have been established throughout most of the United States. They are a valuable asset in any EMS system. Many of these centers are available 24 hours a day. They are staffed with specialists who provide information, consultation, treatment recommendations, patient follow-up, and data collection. Poison control centers are linked to many agencies that deal with toxic substances. In addition, they are tied closely to all area hospitals. These centers maintain a listing of more than 350,000 drugs, toxic substances, and other products. The Universal Poison Control number is 1-800-222-1222.

> **LOOK AGAIN**
> See Chapter 34: Toxicology, pp. 982-983.

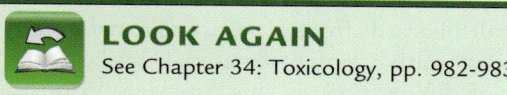

The Chemical Transportation Emergency Center (CHEMTREC) is a public service of the Chemical Manufacturers Association. The center provides immediate advice to on-scene personnel about the management of known or unknown hazardous materials. The agency also contacts the shipper of the material for more information or assistance when needed. The Chemical Transportation Emergency Center operates 24 hours a day, 7 days a week. The center can be reached in the United States and Canada through the emergency toll-free number 1-800-424-9300 (in Alaska 0-202-483-7616). The paramedic should contact CHEMTREC as soon as possible during a hazmat incident. EMS personnel should provide the center with the name of the substance, its identification number, and the nature of the problem. Involving CHEMTREC in the management of a hazmat incident is usually part of the standard operating procedure of any emergency response team.

ChemTel is an emergency response communications center. It serves the United States and Canada. The office can provide specific product information. It also can provide referral to the proper state and federal authorities for incidents that involve radioactive material. ChemTel can be reached 24 hours a day, 7 days a week, through the toll-free number 1-800-255-3924.

Computer-aided management of emergency operations (CAMEO) systems are designed to assist emergency responders quickly in the management of hazmat incidents. The program is available to municipalities. It uses computer modeling to predict the effects of chemical spills and toxins released in plumes of smoke. The system helps communities prepare emergency response plans. CAMEO currently provides information on more than 6000 chemicals. The systems also contain more than 80,000 chemical synonyms and identification numbers that can be quickly searched to identify unknown substances during an incident. Box 57-2 lists other government and private sector agencies that may assist in a hazmat incident.

There are many Internet sources for hazmat identification and management. These include federal, state, and local governmental agencies; colleges and universities; businesses and industry; trade associations; and nonprofit groups who have established easily accessible websites. Box 57-3 lists federal Internet websites for hazmat reference.

PERSONAL PROTECTIVE CLOTHING AND EQUIPMENT

The potential for injury from exposure to hazardous materials is related to the toxicity, flammability, and reactivity of a particular substance. Use of the right protection is crucial for anyone dealing with hazardous materials. This includes the use of the proper respiratory protection and personal protective equipment (PPE).

Protective Respiratory Devices

The potential for exposure of the respiratory system to hazardous materials is of paramount importance to the

BOX 57-2 Agencies That Assist in Hazardous Materials Incidents*

Federal Agencies
Centers for Disease Control and Prevention
Department of Transportation
Environmental Protection Agency
Federal Aviation Administration
National Response Center
- Armed Forces (Army, Navy, Air Force, Marines)
- Coast Guard
- Department of Energy

Regional and State Agencies
National Guard
State emergency management agencies
State environmental protection agency
State health departments
State police

Local Agencies
Emergency management
Fire service (hazardous materials units)
Law enforcement agencies
Poison control center
Public utilities
Sewage and treatment facilities

Commercial Agencies
American Petroleum Institute
Association of American Railroads and Hazardous Materials Systems
Chemical Manufacturers Association
Chevron (provides assistance with Chevron products)
HELP (the Union Carbide Emergency Response System for company shipments)
Local industry
Local contractors
- Local: carriers and transporters
- Railway industry

*This box lists only a sampling of the agencies; the list is not all-inclusive.

BOX 57-3 Federal Internet Websites for Hazmat Reference

Federal Agencies	Websites
U.S. EPA	www.epa.gov/epahome/text.htm
U.S. EPA Chemical Emergency Preparedness and Prevention Office (CEPPO)	www.epa.gov/ceppo
U.S. EPA Region 1	www.epa.gov/region01/
U.S. EPA Region 1 EPCRA Team	www.epa.gov/region01/steward/emerplan/
Chemical Safety and Hazard Investigation Board	www.csb.gov/
National Response Center: Home Page	www.nrc.uscg.mil/
National Response Team	www.nrt.org
DOT Hazmat Safety Homepage	http://hazmat.dot.gov/
Federal Emergency Management Agency	www.fema/gov
U.S. Fire Academy	www.usfa/fema/gov
U.S. Army Counterterrorism	www.cbdcom.apgea.army.mil
Emergency Response Notification System	www.epa.gov/ERNS/

emergency responder. The respiratory system can be protected by air purification devices and by equipment that supplies clean air (atmosphere supplying device).

Air purification relies on respirators or filtration devices. These devices remove particulate matter, gases, or vapors from the atmosphere. These devices do not use a separate source of air. They also require constant monitoring for contaminants and oxygen levels. As a rule, they are not recommended for use in a hazardous materials release and must be fitted to the wearer. Filtration devices are material-specific ("must match the gas"). They are not used in the presence of multiple types of chemicals. These devices cannot be used in an environment with a low oxygen concentration.

Atmosphere supplying devices rely on a separate source of positive pressure to supply air. They provide the highest level of respiratory protection. Two basic types are available. One is the **self-contained breathing apparatus** (SCBA). The other is the **supplied air breathing apparatus** (SABA), or air lines. The use of either requires training, recertification, and proper fit-testing as governed by regulations from OSHA.

The self-contained breathing apparatus provides respiratory protection in oxygen-deficient and toxic atmospheres. Only SCBAs that maintain positive pressure in the facepiece during inhalation and exhalation should be used when working with hazardous materials. The SCBA usually is considered excellent protection in hazardous environments. However, the rescuer should be aware of potential facepiece penetration and contamination by certain toxic substances, such as methyl bromide, Telone (1,3-dichloropropene and chloropicrin), and ethyleneimine.

The supplied air breathing apparatus supplies air to the rescuer via an air-line hose away from the scene. These devices often are used at hazardous material sites when extended working times are required. The SABA must have an escape capability for operations in atmospheres classified as immediately dangerous to life and health. Respiratory protection devices that combine SCBAs and air-line hose units are available. However, because of their dependence on air supply via a line, they limit the distance entry personnel can enter into a contaminated area (hot zone).

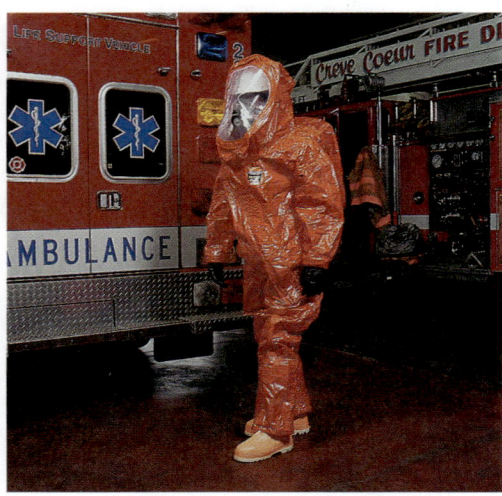

FIGURE 57-3 Level A protective clothing. (Courtesy Creve Coeur Fire District, Creve Coeur, Mo.)

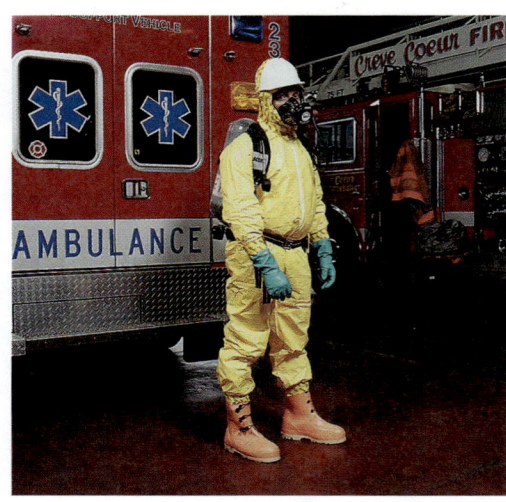

FIGURE 57-4 Level B protective clothing. It offers the highest level of respiratory protection and a higher level of skin protection than Level C protective clothing. (Courtesy Creve Coeur Fire District, Creve Coeur, Mo.)

BOX 57-4 Forms of Chemical Intrusion

Degradation: The physical destruction or decomposition of a clothing material caused by exposure to chemicals, use, or ambient conditions.
Penetration: The flow of a hazardous liquid chemical through zippers, stitched seams, pinholes, or other imperfections in a material.
Permeation: The process by which a hazardous liquid chemical moves through a material on a molecular level.

Classifications of Protective Clothing

Protective clothing is categorized in two ways: disposable or reusable. The clothing is made from a variety of materials that are designed specifically for certain chemical exposures. (Training in the use of this clothing should take place in a safe environment before it is used at emergency scenes.) Examples of this material include Tyvek/Saranex, nitrile rubber, Teflon, and Viton. No single material is compatible with all chemicals. Thus the manufacturer's guidelines and recommendations must be followed (Box 57-4). Protective clothing is classified in several ways. The classifications defined by OSHA and the EPA follow[6,6a]:

Level A: Level A provides the highest level of skin, respiratory, and eye protection (Figure 57-3). Level A equipment typically is used by hazmat teams for entry into the incident site. Level A equipment includes a positive-pressure (pressure demand), full-facepiece SCBA or positive-pressure supplied air respirator with escape SCBA, approved by the National Institute of Occupational Safety and Health (NIOSH). This level of protection also includes a totally encapsulating (gastight) chemical protective suit, coveralls and long underwear (optional), outer and inner gloves that are chemical resistant, an undersuit hard hat (optional), and a disposable protective suit (including gloves and steel-toed boots) that may be worn over a totally encapsulating suit. (Unless specified by the manufacturer, these disposable suits are not to be worn in flammable atmospheres.)

Level B: Level B provides the highest level of respiratory protection. However, it provides a lower level of skin protection (Figure 57-4). Level B protection typically is worn by the decontamination team. Level B equipment includes positive-pressure, full-facepiece SCBA or positive-pressure supplied air respirator with escape SCBA (NIOSH approved); hooded, chemical-resistant clothing (overalls, long-sleeved jacket, coveralls, one-or two-piece chemical splash suit, disposable chemical overalls); coveralls (optional); inner and outer chemical-resistant gloves; chemical-resistant boots with steel toe and shank; outer chemical-resistant boot covers (optional); an optional hard hat and face shield.

Level C: Level C protection is used during the transport of contaminated patients. Level C protection is used when the concentration and type of airborne substance (or substances) is known and the criteria for using air-purifying respirators are met. Level C equipment includes full face or half mask air-purifying respirators (NIOSH approved); hooded, chemical-resistant clothing (overalls, two-piece chemical splash suit, disposable chemical-resistant overalls); coveralls (optional); outer and inner chemical-resistant gloves; outer chemical-resistant boots with steel toe and shank (optional); disposable outer

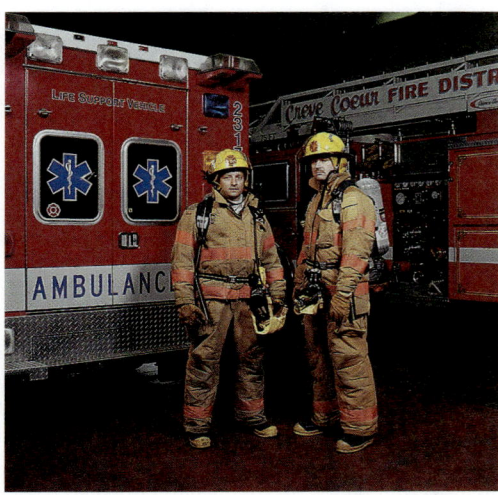

FIGURE 57-5 Level D protective clothing. (Courtesy Creve Coeur Fire District, Creve Coeur, Mo.)

chemical-resistant boot covers (optional); and optional escape mask and face shield.

Level D: Level D is a work uniform that affords minimal protection (used for nuisance contamination only; Figure 57-5). Level D protection commonly is known as firefighter "turnout" gear. (Turnout gear with SCBA may be considered level B protection for some chemicals that do not pose danger for skin contact or absorption.) Level D equipment includes coveralls; optional gloves, chemical-resistant boots or shoes with steel toe and shank; disposable outer chemical-resistant boots (optional); safety glasses or chemical splash goggles; and optional hard hat, escape mask, and face shield.

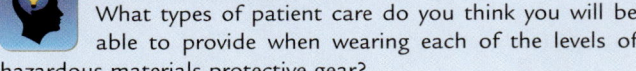

CRITICAL THINKING

What types of patient care do you think you will be able to provide when wearing each of the levels of hazardous materials protective gear?

Regardless of the type of PPE used during a hazmat incident, all avenues through which hazardous materials can enter the body must be protected. The following points should be of particular concern to any rescuer involved in hazmat response:

- Protective clothing should not be affected adversely by the hazardous materials involved.
- Protective clothing should seal all exposed skin.
- Contact with the hazardous materials should be of the absolute minimal duration required.
- Protective clothing and equipment should be decontaminated properly. Or it should be discarded properly.

- The safety standards and methods for cleaning and disposing of clothing and equipment should be followed strictly.
- Contaminated patient clothing should be left at the scene for proper and safe disposal. It should not be transported with the patient. This will limit the contamination of the ambulance.

HEALTH HAZARDS

As described in Chapter 34, hazardous materials may enter the human body by inhalation, ingestion, injection, and absorption. Entry by means of any of these routes may result in internal and external damage to the rescuer. Exposure to dangerous substances may affect the body in several different ways. It may produce numerous injuries or illnesses.

Exposure to poisons can produce acute toxicity, delayed toxicity, and local and systemic effects. The way that the body responds depends on the concentration of the chemical to which the body is exposed (also called the **dose response**). The paramedic also should be aware that drug treatment can result in **synergistic effects** (the effects of one chemical enhancing the effects of a second chemical). Thus all treatment methods must be guided by medical direction, a poison control center, or other appropriate authority.

Internal Damage

Internal damage to the human body from exposure to hazardous materials may involve the respiratory tract, the central nervous system (CNS), or other internal organs. Some substances injure all cells on contact. Others have a more direct effect on specific organs (target organs), such as the kidneys and liver.

Depending on the hazardous materials, the physical injury may vary. It may range from minor irritation to more serious complications, including cardiorespiratory compromise and death. Chronic illness (e.g., chronic obstructive pulmonary disease) and various forms of cancer also may result. Some substances can cause abnormal fetal development and changes in gene structure. For example, penetrating radiation (described in Chapter 39) can lead to cell and chromosomal changes and can cause genetic changes, cell death, and sterility.

IRRITANTS

Irritants that affect the respiratory system are a common complaint of rescuers and patients who have been exposed to hazardous materials. Chemical irritants emit vapors that affect the mucous membranes of the body. These include the surfaces of the eyes, nose, mouth, and throat. As these irritants combine with moisture, acidic or alkaline reactions may occur. Exposure to these irritants may result in damage to the upper, lower, and deep respiratory tract. Examples of chemical irritants are hydrochloric acid, halogens, and ozone.

Self-defense chemical sprays used by some civilians and law enforcement officers are common and can present a hazard to responders. These sprays are irritants and produce excessive tearing of the eyes. They include chloroacetophenone, *ortho*-chlorobenzalmalononitrile, and capsicum oleoresin (*pepper spray*).

ASPHYXIANTS

Asphyxiants are gases that displace the oxygen in the air and also dilute the oxygen concentration of the air. Examples of simple asphyxiants are carbon dioxide, methane, and propane. Other gases not only displace oxygen in the air but also interfere with tissue oxygenation; these are referred to as *blood poisons* or *chemical asphyxiants*. They tend to interrupt the transport or use of oxygen by tissue cells. Through various mechanisms, these toxic gases deprive body tissue of needed oxygen. Examples include hydrogen cyanide, carbon monoxide, and hydrogen sulfide (Box 57-5).

NERVE POISONS, ANESTHETICS, AND NARCOTICS

Nerve poisons, anesthetics, and narcotics act on the nervous system. These agents affect either the cardiorespiratory mechanisms of the brain or the ability to transmit impulses required for adequate heart and lung function.

Nerve poisons were developed by the military. They often are referred to as *war gases, nerve gases,* or *nerve agents* (see Chapter 58). Similar substances are used in solid pesticides. Exposure to these chemicals may result in fatal complications. Examples of these poisons include carbamates, organophosphates, parathion, and malathion. Anesthetics and narcotics are less hazardous than nerve poisons. However, continuous exposure or exposure to large concentrations may result in unconsciousness or death. Examples include ethylene oxide, nitrous oxide, and ethyl alcohol.

HEPATOTOXINS

Hepatotoxins are substances that damage the liver. The poisons accumulate in the body and destroy the ability of the liver to function. Examples include chlorinated and halogenated hydrocarbons.

CARDIOTOXINS

Cardiotoxins are hazardous materials that can cause myocardial ischemia and dysrhythmias. Examples include some nitrates and ethylene glycol. Acute myocardial infarction and sudden death have been reported in healthy young persons who were exposed to these substances. Short-term exposure to fluorocarbons and other halogenated hydrocarbons also has been known to cause cardiac abnormalities.

NEPHROTOXINS

Nephrotoxins are hazardous materials that are especially destructive to the kidneys. Examples include carbon disulfide, lead, high concentrations of organic solvents, and inorganic mercury. Exposure to carbon tetrachloride, used

---

BOX 57-5 Hydrogen Sulfide

Hydrogen sulfide (H_2S) is considered a poison that affects several systems of the body, mostly the nervous system. It is a colorless, flammable, and extremely hazardous gas with a rotten egg smell. Hydrogen sulfide is similar to cyanide, and it is five to six times more toxic than carbon monoxide.[7] Exposure to the gas can be lethal within a few minutes.

Hydrogen sulfide can be easily produced by combining common household chemicals. It is sometimes used as a method of suicide (*detergent suicide*). Most of these suicides in the United States have involved young adults who make the hydrogen sulfide in their cars.[8] All rescuers working in a confined space or who are responding to a possible suicide in a confined space (e.g., automobile, closet) should[9]:

- Be aware of the possibility of poisonous gas
- Remember that hydrogen sulfide has a pungent odor similar to rotten eggs
- Retreat to a safe area and use PPE and SCBA if hydrogen sulfide is suspected
- Be aware that confined spaces will temporarily continue to discharge noxious gas
- Know that a person and his or her clothing will release the gas for a brief period
- Expect the need for decontamination of the chemicals spilled
- Request hazmat support with a cyanide antidote kit

---

as a solvent for dry cleaning or as a fire-extinguishing agent, can damage the kidneys.

NEUROTOXINS

Neurotoxins are poisons that affect the nervous system. Neurological and behavioral toxicity may result from exposure to hazardous substances such as arsenic, lead, mercury, and organic solvents. In some cases, cerebral hypoxia may occur as a result of decreased oxygen in the blood.

HEMOTOXINS

Hemotoxins are hazardous substances that may cause the destruction of red blood cells. This destruction can result in hemolytic anemia (see Chapter 32). Substances that can produce hemolytic anemia include aniline, naphthol, quinones, lead, mercury, arsenic, and copper. Pulmonary edema and cardiac and liver injury also may be caused by hemotoxin exposure.

CARCINOGENS

Carcinogens are cancer-causing agents. Many hazardous materials are carcinogenic or are suspected carcinogens. The exact amount of hazardous materials exposure required for cancer to develop is unknown. However, short-term exposure to specific agents is known to produce long-term effects. Disease and complications have been reported 20 years after exposure to hazardous materials.[10]

Of particular interest to rescuers involved in firefighting is that all fossil and organic fuels produce dioxins when they are burned. **Dioxin** is a general term that describes a group of hundreds of chemicals that are highly persistent in the environment. These chemicals are an unintentional byproduct of many industrial processes (e.g., waste incineration, pesticide manufacturing).[11] Many of the dioxins are carcinogens. (For example, burning wood produces carcinogenic formaldehyde.) A positive-pressure SCBA is the most important piece of protective equipment to protect against these carcinogenic vapors and respiratory poisons. All rescuers should avoid exposure to smoke or clouds of fumes as a standard practice in scene safety.

>
> **NOTE**
>
> An important sign of a critical exposure is several persons having the same symptoms at the same time. Any time two or more members of the team report that they "feel" similar symptoms, a toxic gas or agent should be suspected. Emergency personnel should immediately report the onset of symptoms to their crew members and other emergency responders at the scene.

GENERAL SYMPTOMS OF EXPOSURE

Health effects from exposure to hazardous materials vary by individual. They also depend on the chemical involved, the concentration of the chemical, the duration of exposure, the number of exposures, and the route of entry (inhalation, ingestion, injection, absorption). In addition, a person's age, gender, general health, allergies, smoking habits, alcohol consumption, and medication use influence how that person is affected.

Various symptoms may result from exposure to hazardous materials. Some symptoms may be delayed or masked by common illnesses such as influenza or by smoke inhalation. If any of the following symptoms is present after exposure to hazardous materials, the rescuer or patient should seek immediate medical attention:

- Changes in skin color or blushing
- Chest tightness
- Confusion, light-headedness, anxiety, dizziness
- Coughing or painful respiration
- Diarrhea and involuntary urination or defecation (or both)
- Dim, blurred, or double vision; photophobia
- Loss of coordination
- Nausea, vomiting, abdominal cramping
- Salivation, drooling, rhinorrhea
- Seizure
- Shortness of breath, burning of the upper airway
- Tingling or numbness of extremities
- Unconsciousness

> **CRITICAL THINKING**
> Two rescuers complain of similar symptoms on the scene of a rescue that may involve hazardous materials. What actions should be taken immediately?

External Damage

Body surface tissue may be injured by hazardous materials. Many substances have corrosive properties or become corrosive when mixed with water. Exposure to these substances may produce chemical burns and severe tissue damage. Examples include hydrochloric acid, hydrofluoric acid, and caustic soda.

SOFT TISSUE DAMAGE

Corrosives are acids or bases (alkaline). Exposure to either may cause pain on contact. However, alkalis generally burn more extensively than acids. Exposing human tissue to a base corrosive such as lye may result in **liquefaction** (a breakdown of fatty tissue) that produces a greasy or slick feeling to the skin. These signs should alert the rescuer to decontaminate immediately and seek medical attention. Unless the substance is identified, decontamination should begin by brushing off the dry powder and flushing the skin with copious amounts of water. (Different areas of the skin absorb chemicals at different rates.) Paramedics should never try to neutralize an acid or base; doing so could produce great heat and cause further burns. The area should be flushed copiously with water, and the patient should be transported for care. Rescuers should be aware of possible "off-gassing" or fumes resulting from the decontamination of a wound site and take appropriate protective measures.

Cryogenics are refrigerant liquid gases that can freeze human tissue on contact. These liquids vaporize as soon as they are released from their containers. They may cause tissue damage. Extreme caution should be used when near any refrigerated liquids. They can produce freeze burns, frostbite, and other cold-related injuries. Examples include Freon, liquid oxygen, and liquid nitrogen.

CHEMICAL EXPOSURE TO THE EYES

Chemical exposure to the eyes (described in Chapter 39) may cause damage ranging from superficial inflammation to severe burns. Patients with these conditions have local pain, visual disturbance, tearing, edema, and redness of surrounding tissues. Basic management guidelines include immediately flushing the eyes with water. This should be done using a mild flow from a hose, intravenous tubing, water from a container, or irrigation lens (per protocol). A rapid assessment of visual acuity is important. However, assessment should not delay flushing or irrigation of the eyes.

>
> **LOOK AGAIN**
> See Chapter 39: Burns, pp. 1136-1137.

RESPONSE TO HAZARDOUS MATERIALS EMERGENCIES

When an EMS crew is dispatched to a scene involving the potential for hazardous materials, decisions must be made about rescuer safety, the type and degree of the potential hazard, the involvement of other agencies, and protection for the general public. As discussed in Chapter 54, preplanning and early coordination of activities in these major incidents is important. In addition, medical direction should be advised of the incident as soon as possible to prepare personnel and facilities. Not all hazmat incidents are large-scale events. Sometimes, a single event involving only one patient may require a full hazmat response.

The first rescue personnel to arrive at the scene of a hazmat incident may not be the most qualified or best equipped. However, most communities look to the first responders to provide immediate safety and direction. Thus the EMS crew must be capable of the initial management of hazmat incidents.

Hazard and Risk Assessment

While en route to the scene, EMS personnel should begin to research hazmat references. They also should begin a **hazard and risk assessment.** In hazmat incidents, *hazards* are the chemical properties of a material that may cause danger or peril (Box 57-6). *Risk* refers to the possibility of suffering harm or loss. Risk levels vary and are influenced by several factors, including the following[12] (Figure 57-6):

- Hazardous nature of the material involved
- Worst-case scenario situations
- Quantity of the material involved
- Weather conditions that might affect the scene adversely
- Containment system and type of stress applied to the container
- Proximity of exposures (e.g., schools, nursing homes, and shopping centers)
- Level of available resources
- Lead time for mutual aid

A hazard and risk assessment also includes consideration of the potential hazards to the public and environment, the potential risk of **primary contamination** to patients, and the potential risk for **secondary contamination** to rescuers (Box 57-7).

If the product can be identified through hazmat references, the EMS crew should familiarize themselves with potential health hazards, recommended PPE, initial first aid, and the **safe distance factor** (the minimum safe distance for personal safety) as outlined in the reference guides. Most emergency response guides offer only general management actions. After formal product identification, the appropriate hazmat agencies (e.g., CHEMTREC and poison control) can give more exact information.

BOX 57-6 Hazardous Materials Terminology and Definitions

Toxicological Terms Used to Determine Toxicity of a Compound

IDLH (immediately dangerous to life and health): Any atmosphere that poses an immediate hazard to life or that produces immediate, irreversible debilitating effects on health.

LD50 (lethal dose, 50% kill): The amount of a dose that, when administered to laboratory animals, kills 50% of them.

PEL (permissible exposure limit): The maximum time-weighted concentration at which 95% of exposed, healthy adults suffer no adverse effects over a 40-hour workweek.

ppm/ppb: Parts per million/parts per billion.

TLV-C (threshold limit value—ceiling level): The maximum concentration that should not be exceeded even instantaneously.

TLV-STEL (threshold limit value—short-term exposure limit): A 15-minute, time-weighted average exposure that should not be exceeded at any time or repeatedly more than 4 times a day, with 60-minute rest periods required between each STEL exposure.

Specific Terminology for Medical Hazardous Materials Operations

Alpha radiation: Large radioactive particles that have minimal penetrating ability.

Beta radiation: Small radioactive particles that can penetrate subcutaneous tissue and usually enter the body through damaged skin, ingestion, or inhalation.

Boiling point: The temperature at which a liquid changes to a vapor or a gas; the temperature at which the pressure of the liquid equals atmospheric pressure.

Flammable/exposure limits: The range of gas or vapor concentration that will burn or explode if an ignition source is present.

Flashpoint: The minimum temperature at which a liquid disperses enough vapors to ignite and flash-over but not to continue to burn without additional heat.

Gamma radiation: The most dangerous form of penetrating radiation, which can produce internal and external hazards.

Ignition temperature: The minimum temperature required to ignite gas or vapor without a spark or flame being present.

Specific gravity: The weight of a material as compared with the weight of an equal volume of water.

Vapor density: The weight of a pure vapor or gas compared with the weight of an equal volume of dry air at the same temperature and pressure.

Vapor pressure: The pressure exerted by the vapor within the container against the sides of a container.

Vapor solubility: The ability of a vapor to mix with water.

From Noll G, et al: *Hazardous materials: managing the incident,* Stillwater, Okla, 2004, Fire Protection Publications.

Approaching the Scene

The paramedic should approach the scene cautiously from uphill and upwind. The EMS crew should be alert to environmental clues. These include wind direction, unusual odors, leakage, and vapor clouds. Other environmental clues that are good indicators for the presence of hazardous

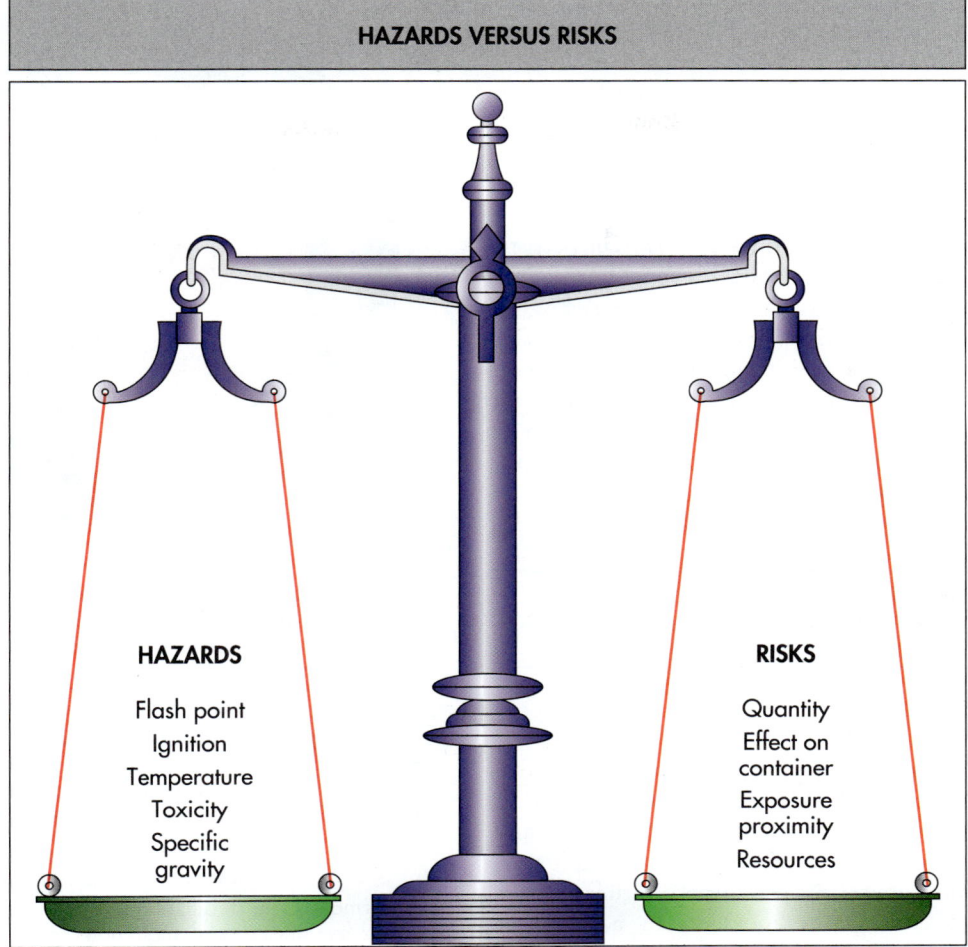

FIGURE 57-6 Hazards versus risk.

BOX 57-7 Types of Contamination

Primary Contamination
Exposure to substance
Substance only harmful to exposed person
Little chance of exposure to others

Secondary Contamination
Exposure to substance
Liquid and particulate substances easily transferred by touching

---

materials include affected or afflicted wildlife and plant life (e.g., dead birds and wilted or discolored plants). Paramedics can use binoculars initially to observe the scene from a safe distance. Emergency vehicles should never be driven through leakage or vapor clouds or smoke. In addition, personnel should not enter the incident area until it has been determined to be safe. In addition to these guidelines,

rescuers should do the following as recommended in the *Emergency Response Guidebook*[13]:

- *Approach cautiously.* Resist the urge to rush into the incident area; you cannot help others until you know what you are facing.
- *Identify the hazards.* Placards, container labels, shipping papers, and knowledgeable persons on the scene are valuable sources of information. Evaluate all of them and then consult the recommended guide page before you place yourself or others at risk. Do not be alarmed if new information from a CHEMTREC expert changes some of the emphasis or details of the guide page warnings. You must remember that the guide page provides only the most important information for your initial response with a family or class of hazardous materials. As more accurate, material-specific information becomes available, your response becomes more appropriate for the situation.
- *Secure the scene.* Without entering the immediate hazard zone, do what you can to isolate the area and ensure the safety of persons and the environment. Move and keep

persons away from the scene and the perimeter. Allow enough room to move and remove your own equipment.

■ *Obtain help.* Advise your headquarters to notify responsible agencies and call for assistance from trained experts through CHEMTREC and the National Response Center, which can be reached through CHEMTREC or dialed directly.

■ *Decide on site entry.* Any efforts you make to rescue persons or protect property or the environment must be weighed against the possibility that you could become part of the problem. Enter the area with the appropriate protective gear (if trained to do so). Above all, *do not walk into or touch spilled material.* Avoid inhaling fumes, smoke, and vapors, even if no hazardous materials are known to be involved. Do not assume that gases or vapors are harmless because of lack of smell.

 CRITICAL THINKING
Which of these guidelines would it be easy for the first arriving crew to miss?

Control of the Scene

The first agency to arrive at the scene has several responsibilities. Its members must detect and identify the materials involved, assess the risk of exposure to rescue personnel and others, consider the potential risk of fire or explosion, gather information from on-site personnel or other sources, and confine and control the incident. In addition, a command post should be established per the preplanned incident command structure. Members also must define the safety distances and zones.

Safety Zones

After the presence of hazardous materials has been confirmed, the scene should be separated into hot, warm, and cold zones (Figure 57-7). These zones should have access and egress corridors between them. (Corridors provide control points. They also allow responders working in the zones to know where they should exit and enter for decontamination, accountability, and debriefing.) Safety zones should be established and enforced early in the incident (Box 57-8). The dispatch center and responding units should be advised of the location of the hot zone and safe approach directions.

The **hot zone** is the area of the incident that includes the hazardous material. It also includes any surrounding area that may be exposed to gases, vapors, mist, dust, or runoff. All rescue personnel and vehicles should be stationed outside this zone. Anyone entering this zone must wear high-level PPE. Only specially trained EMS personnel should attempt patient care activities in this area. Some EMS agencies and incident command system structures refer to the hot zone as the *exclusion zone,* a *restricted area,* or the *red zone.*

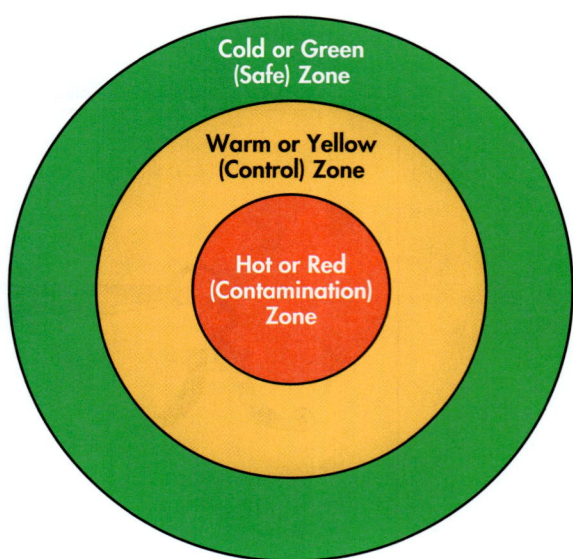

Hot or Red (Contamination) Zone
• Contamination is actually present.
• Personnel must wear appropriate protective gear.
• Number of rescuers limited to those absolutely necessary.
• Bystanders never allowed.

Warm or Yellow (Control) Zone
• Area surrounding the contamination zone.
• Vital to preventing spread of contamination.
• Personnel must wear appropriate protective gear.
• Life-saving emergency care and decontamination are performed.

Cold or Green (Safe) Zone
• Normal triage, stabilization, and treatment are performed.
• Rescuers must shed contaminated gear before entering the cold zone.

FIGURE 57-7 Zones at a hazmat incident.

BOX 57-8 Hazardous Materials Zones

Hot Zone
Contamination present
Site of incident
Entry with high-level personal protective equipment
Entry limited

Warm Zone
Buffer zone outside hot zone
Contains decontamination corridor with "hot" and "cold" end

Cold Zone
Safe area
Staging area for personnel and equipment
Site of medical monitoring
One end of corridor

The **warm zone** is a larger, buffer area that surrounds the hot zone with "cold" and "hot" end corridors. Although protective clothing is required, it usually is considered a safer environment for workers. However, if the hot zone becomes unstable, the warm zone may be exposed to the hazardous materials. This zone is where most EMS activities, such as decontamination and patient care, are performed. Some agencies refer to this zone as the *limited-access zone*, the *containment reduction corridor*, or the *yellow zone*.

The **cold zone** is the area that encompasses the warm zone. The cold zone also is restricted to emergency personnel. This area usually is considered safe, requiring only minimal protective clothing. The cold zone contains the command post and other support agencies necessary to control the incident. This area is referred to by some agencies as a *support zone* or the *green zone*.

REHABILITATION AND MEDICAL MONITORING

The safety of rescue personnel is of prime importance in any emergency. Thus a rehab and medical monitoring program should be part of any incident where rescue personnel may be at risk for physical and emotional stress. In addition, the United States Fire Administration (USFA) and the National Fire Protection Association (NFPA) recommend and require rehab and medical monitoring at all emergency scenes where personnel exceed a safe level of physical or mental endurance.[14,15]

Rehabilitation

The purpose of **rehabilitation** (*rehab*) is to sustain the energy of rescuers, improve performance, and decrease the likelihood of on-scene injury or death. As described in Chapter 54, rehab is part of the incident command structure and is a responsibility of command. The rehab area (or areas) usually is established near the incident, but away from operations. The location must ensure safety and must provide for rest and recuperation. Depending on weather and the nature of the incident, these areas may be outdoors, in a building, or in a specially designed rehab vehicle. Activities that may take place in a rehab sector include:

- Relief from environmental extremes (active or passive cooling or warming)
- Rest and recovery
- Rehydration
- Food and drink replacement

> **NOTE**
> In most management systems, emergency medical procedures are not performed in the rehab area. If emergency care is needed for a rescuer, that care is provided by EMS personnel in the treatment sector, located away from or in a separate part of the rehab area.

Medical Monitoring

Medical monitoring is the ongoing evaluation of rescuers who are at risk for illness or injury from operations at the incident. *Medical monitoring* should not be confused with *treatment*. The purpose of medical monitoring in the rehab area is to identify personnel who may need treatment (provided in the treatment sector) or transport. In hazmat operations, medical monitoring may also include accountability, record-keeping, and periodic evaluation of the surveillance program.

> **NOTE**
> OSHA requires medical examinations for members of hazmat response teams and employees who may have been exposed to hazardous substances during an emergency.

Medical monitoring should include assessment protocols that involve a "presuit" examination before entering a hazardous area. The purpose of the examination is to establish a health history and baseline vital signs for any rescuer who will be exposed to a hazardous substance. During the presuit exam, rescuers should be advised of the expected symptoms of illness or exposure before entering the hazardous area. In addition to injury from exposure, responders working in protective clothing and equipment can become dehydrated and develop heat illnesses. Rescue protective suits protect, but they also prevent cooling through evaporation, conduction, convection, or radiation. Heat-stress factors are affected by the prehydration of the rescuer, degree of physical fitness, ambient air temperature, and degree and duration of physical activity. The parameters of the presuit evaluation should include the following:

- Temperature, pulse, respiration, and blood pressure measurements
- Cardiac rhythm
- Body weight
- Cognitive and motor skills
- Hydration
- Significant recent medical history (e.g., medications or illnesses)

After entry into the hazardous area, medical monitoring should note the amount of time a rescuer has been in protective clothing. Rescuers should be observed for any signs of heat-related illness or exposure (described in Chapter 45). If illness or injury occurs to any team member, all entry team members should be removed from the hot zone for treatment. A backup team should be ready to assist the entry team members in the hot zone at all times.

After the incident, rescue personnel should be reevaluated in the "rehab sector," using the same parameters as in the presuit examination. This exam determines the rescuer's ability to be released to reenter the operation if needed. As a rule, rescuers are not allowed to reenter the site until vital signs and hydration level are normal. Body weight generally is used to estimate fluid loss and the need for oral or intravenous fluid replacement (per protocol) (Figure 57-8).

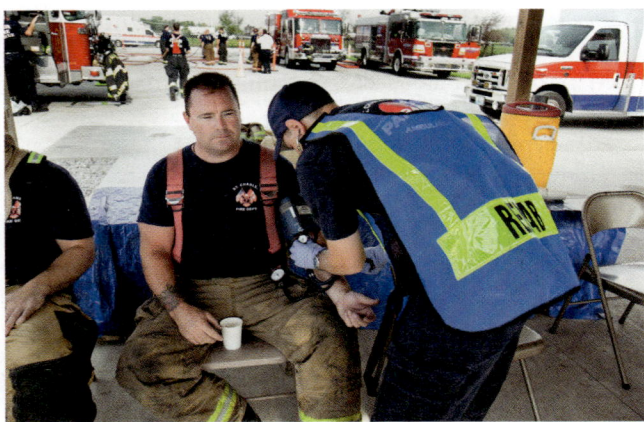

FIGURE 57-8 Rehabilitation branch.

CRITICAL THINKING

What might prevent personnel from seeking emergency medical services for medical monitoring unless there is a strict procedure to guarantee they are monitored?

SHOW ME THE EVIDENCE

Researchers in a mid-size southwestern metropolitan area retrospectively reviewed hazardous materials incidents fire departments responded to over 3 years. Their goal was to discover which chemicals were involved and identify patient needs. During the study period there were 6232 hazmat incidents, 11% of which met criteria for hazmat control team dispatch. Of these 428 incidents, there were 489 materials involved; 4.5% of incidents had more than 1 chemical involved. The most common chemical was methane gas (26%); automotive fluids accounted for 32% of incidents. Of the hazmat responses 7% involved patient exposure. Inhalation was the most common exposure route. Fourteen patients were firefighters, EMTs, or paramedics exposed after responding to the scene. A total of 45 patients were transported to the hospital. The researchers concluded that most incidents did not have contaminated patients. The patients exposed often had inhalation exposures and usually only needed oxygen administration.

From Walter FG, Bates G, Criss E, et al: Hazardous materials responses in a mid-size metropolitan area, *PEC* 7(2):214-218, 2003.

Documentation

Detailed records are a necessary part of hazmat medical monitoring and rehabilitation. At a minimum, records should include the following:

- The name of the hazardous substance
- The toxicity and danger of secondary contamination
- Use of appropriate PPE and any permeation ("breakthrough") that occurred
- The level of decontamination performed or required
- Use of antidotes and other medical treatment
- The method of transportation and destination

Baseline statistics from preentry and postentry screenings also should be included in the records. (Many agencies use preprinted forms for these.)

EMERGENCY MANAGEMENT OF CONTAMINATED PATIENTS

Patient care activities, triage, and evacuation should be part of a preplanned incident command system structure. Identifying a specific hazardous substance may take some time. Thus rescue efforts, decontamination, possible evacuation, and timely treatment of toxic exposures are important. The primary goals of decontamination are to reduce the patient's dosage of material, decrease the threat of secondary contamination, and reduce the risk of rescuer injury. The specific substance and route of contamination affect triage and decontamination methods. The following guidelines for rapid decontamination are general. They should not supersede any organizational approach in scene management of hazmat incidents or treatment recommendations for chemical exposures:

1. The paramedic should not enter a contaminated area or initiate care without adequate PPE. The paramedic also must possess training that is specific to the incident. Victims who can walk should be encouraged to extricate themselves from the scene. They should be advised to stay together for treatment or until they are escorted individually to decontamination.

2. Patients who cannot walk should be removed from the hot zone by trained personnel. Removal usually is performed by fire service personnel, specialized hazmat teams, or both. Patient care activities in the hot zone should be limited to gross airway management, spinal immobilization, and hemorrhage control. Decontamination and further patient care should be done in the warm zone by a properly equipped decontamination team.

3. All patients exposed to the hot zone should be considered contaminated. They should be treated as such until they have been properly assessed, triaged, and decontaminated.

4. Patient care provisions of airway, breathing, and circulatory support should begin as soon as the patient is contacted and conditions allow. The rescuer safety information received from hazmat agencies should be used when performing basic life support procedures.

5. Intravenous therapy should be administered only under a physician's direction. This and other invasive procedures may allow the hazardous materials to enter the patient.

6. Decontamination procedures should avoid any unnecessary exposure to the rescuer. EMS personnel assisting in decontamination should be well protected with two or three layers of gloves, head coverings, positive-pressure SCBA, and proper protective clothing. Decontamination teams or anyone working in the warm zone should be wearing the same PPE (or no less than one protection level down) as those working in the hot zone.

7. When the hazardous material is a dry agent, lightly brush the material from the patient. Ensure that the dry agent is not introduced into the patient's airway. Cutting or removing clothing often removes most of the contaminating material. After the dry agent has been removed, the decontamination should continue as follows:

a. Wash the patient with copious amounts of water and mild detergent soap. Make sure that all water and runoff is contained in the warm zone. Depending on the exposure, other patient decontamination procedures may be warranted. Pay special attention to irrigation of the eyes, hair, ears, underarms, and pubic areas and thorough cleaning of the body creases of the neck, groin, elbows, and knees. Be careful not to abrade the skin, which may promote absorption of the material involved.

b. Leave all patient clothing, rescuer clothing, and decontamination equipment in the decontamination area. Safely move the patient to the support zone for further triage, treatment, and transport.

> **NOTE**
> Water is considered the universal decontamination solution to dilute the concentration of a substance. Water generally does not alter the chemical structure of a compound. Degradation solutions may be recommended for some exposures. These include water and mild soap, isopropyl alcohol, and vegetable oil (among others). These solutions should be used only when advised by medical direction or other appropriate authority. They should not be applied directly to the skin, and should not be used for exposures to chemicals that react with water.

One should note that the field decontamination procedures described represent only a gross decontamination. The resources needed for full decontamination usually are not available at the scene. Thus the patient should be isolated from the environment. This will help to contain any contamination that has been missed during these procedures. This is accomplished by placing the patient in a body bag (or similar containment) to the neck and covering the patient's hair. In the absence of body bags, the victim may be packaged for transport by folding one side of a sheet or blanket over the patient and using the other side to overlap and package the patient. If necessary, the patient's arm may be exposed through an opening in the sheet for vital sign assessment and fluid and drug administration.

> **NOTE**
> Rapid decontamination is a two-step process. In the first step, remove the patient from danger. In the second step, provide gross decontamination.

Decontamination Decision Making

Hazardous materials incidents often are "fast breaking" and may require rapid decision making. For example, a group of walking, contaminated persons at the scene may be trying to reach rescuers; others self-rescue by walking out of the hot zone; and some may become impatient and leave the hot zone while waiting for rescue teams to arrive. In these situations the paramedic crew must be prepared for quick gross decontamination and treatment, rapid application of PPE, and quick transport and isolation procedures.

If the patient's condition is critical (and it is unknown if the exposure involved a life-threatening material), the paramedic should perform decontamination and treatment simultaneously. This is done by removing the patient's clothing, treating life-threatening problems, lavaging the patient with copious amounts of water, and providing for isolation and transportation. Patients who are not in critical condition can be managed in the same manner with a more contemplative approach, particularly if the hazardous substance is known.

A hazmat incident that is well controlled (not a fast-breaking event) can be managed over longer duration. In these cases, rescue should not be attempted for patients in the hot zone. Rather the paramedic crew should wait for a hazmat team and for a decontamination corridor to be established (Figure 57-9). (This may take an hour or more.) Longer-duration events allow for more thorough decontamination, better use of PPE, less chance of secondary contamination, and better environmental protection.

> **CRITICAL THINKING**
> What type of hazardous materials response resources does your community have?

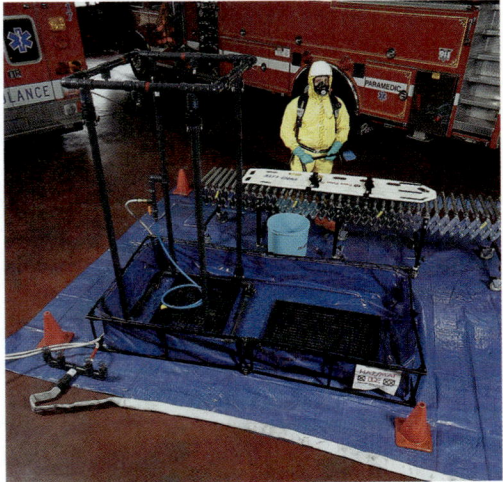

FIGURE 57-9 Patient decontamination area. (Courtesy Creve Coeur Fire District, Creve Coeur, Mo.)

Preparing the Ambulance for Patient Transfer

Contamination of ambulances and equipment can be minimized by preparing the vehicle before transporting a partly decontaminated patient. These measures include using as much disposable equipment as necessary. They also include removing all items from cabinets that will not be needed for patient use. Ideally, the patient should be isolated completely in a stretcher decontamination pool. This should be covered in plastic and secured to the stretcher. Immediate notification of the hospital staff that they will be receiving contaminated patients is crucial. The emergency department will need time to prepare and manage the patients adequately and efficiently.

On arrival at the hospital, the EMS crew should follow the decontamination protocols of the hospital. The crew should not return to regular service until rescue personnel, vehicle, and equipment have been monitored for contamination. Equipment decontamination should follow the recommendations of local, state, and federal authorities or standard operating procedures of medical direction. Specific solutions may be required for a particular hazmat exposure. However, most equipment can be cleaned adequately and made ready for use with soap and water.

DECONTAMINATION OF RESCUE PERSONNEL AND EQUIPMENT

Decontamination procedures of rescue personnel vary by agency and protocol. Decontamination typically involves eight steps and begins in the decontamination corridor (Figure 57-10). These steps include the following:

1. An entry point is established at the "hot" end of the corridor where "dirty" personnel and equipment are set up to start the decontamination process.
2. A tool drop is designated. Outer gloves and boots are removed and placed in a receptacle.
3. Gross surface contamination is removed. Generally this is done by washing with copious amounts of water.
4. Contaminated SCBA bottles are removed (doffed) for personnel who must reenter the dirty area; at this step they receive clean SCBA bottles.
5. Protective clothing is removed and handled (stored, decontaminated) as required.
6. Other clothing is removed. This step depends on the seriousness of the hazardous materials involved.
7. Personnel wash their bodies using overhead showers. Usually two washings are required. Personnel dry off and receive new or clean, uncontaminated clothing.
8. Personnel going through the decontamination system receive medical evaluation. The person is then transported to a medical facility for continued medical evaluation.

In addition, the following safety precautions should be followed by any rescuer exposed to hazardous materials:

- Do not touch your face, mouth, nose, or genital area before full body decontamination.
- Shower first with a cold rinse (no scrubbing) to wash off potential contaminants without opening pores of the skin and then thoroughly wash with warm water, surgical soap, sponge, and brush; pay particular attention to hair, body orifices (especially the ears), and any body parts that come in contact with each other (arms and chest, thighs, fingers, toes, and buttocks). Repeat shower and rinse.
- Shampoo hair several times and rinse thoroughly.

 CRITICAL THINKING
Why do you think that extensive preplanning and drills are needed to make this system work well?

Care and Maintenance of Clothing and Equipment

After the hazmat incident, the rescuer should take the following precautions:

- Properly dispose of any protective clothing that has been torn or worn through.
- Properly and thoroughly clean all clothing and equipment. This will reduce the risk of chemical reactions at future incidents. It also will lessen the potential for chronic exposure to absorbed chemicals. Some hazardous materials can destroy or penetrate protective clothing and equipment. For this reason, product compatibility tables should be evaluated during the decontamination procedure. Decontamination provides no assurance that protective clothing is clean or that the process of chemical penetration has stopped.
- Do not wash or dispose of clothing or equipment at home. This helps to avoid exposing family members and contaminating home articles.
- Follow all local codes and laws regarding disposal or decontamination of equipment and clothing.
- Carefully maintain personal SCBA.

When the incident is over, all personnel operating at the scene (in any capacity) should be debriefed. The debriefing session should include identification and explanation of the substances. It also should include information regarding possible acute and chronic health issues that may arise and any associated signs and symptoms. Information describing follow-up procedures for long-term effects also should be provided. The documentation for possible work-related exposures should follow standard department/company policies.

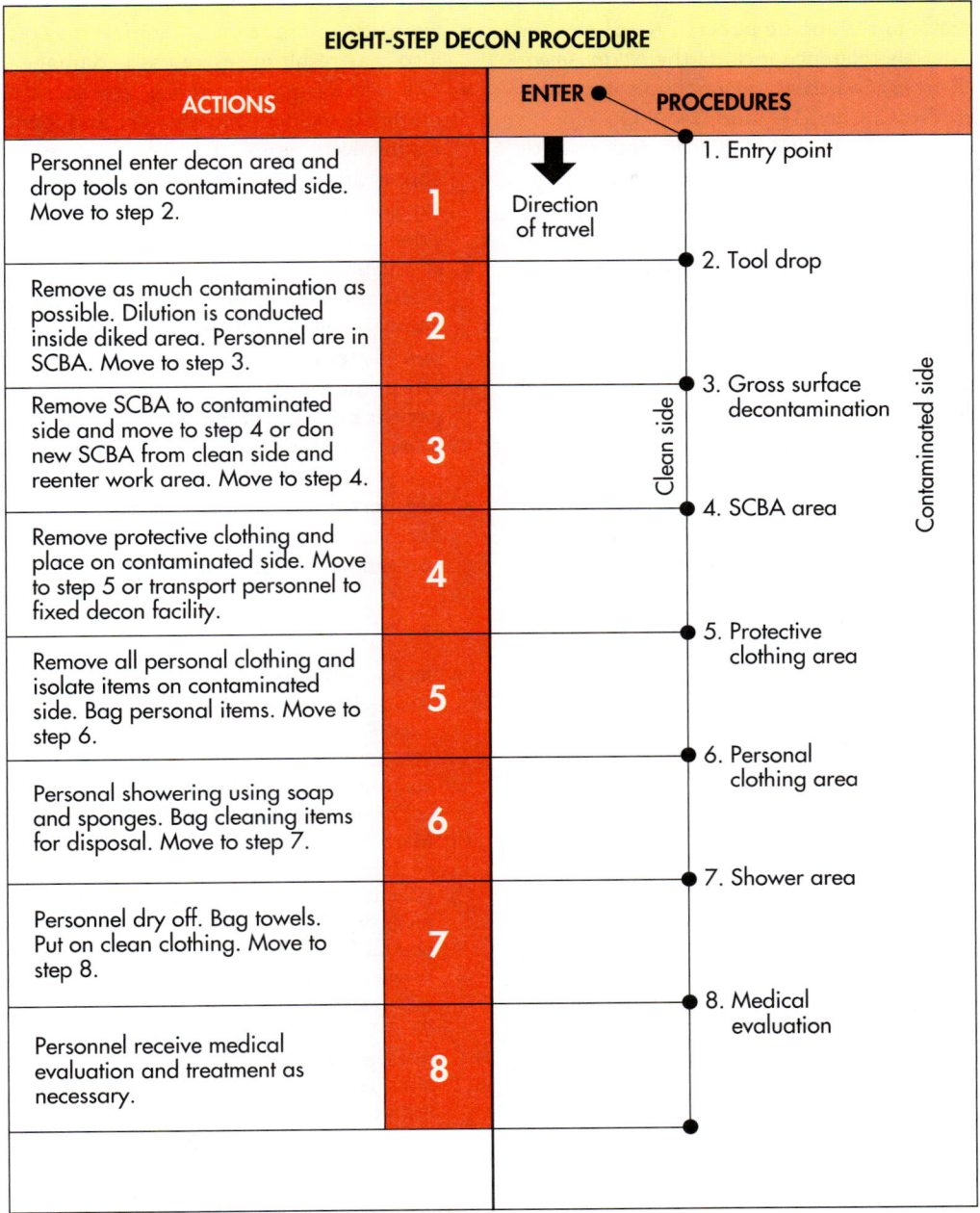

FIGURE 57-10 Eight-step decontamination process.

SUMMARY

- A hazardous material is any substance or material that is capable of posing an unreasonable risk to health, safety, and property.
- The Superfund Amendments and Reauthorization Act of 1986 established requirements for federal, state, and local governments and industry regarding emergency planning and the reporting of hazardous materials–related incidents. In 1989 OSHA and the EPA published rules to govern training requirements, emergency plans,

medical checkups, and other safety precautions for workers at uncontrolled hazardous waste sites and for those responding to hazardous chemical spills. In addition, the NFPA has published standards that address competencies for EMS workers at hazmat scenes.
- There are two methods used to identify hazardous materials. One is informal product identification. (This includes visual, olfactory, and verbal clues.) The other is formal product identification. (This includes, for

Continued

example, placards and shipping papers.) Resources for hazardous materials reference include the *North American Emergency Response Guidebook*, regional poison control centers, CHEMTREC, ChemTel, and CAMEO.

- It is crucial that anyone dealing with hazardous materials use proper protection. This includes using the proper respiratory devices. It also includes wearing protective clothing. This clothing is made of a variety of materials. The clothing is designed for certain chemical exposures. Thus, the manufacturer's guidelines must be followed.

- Hazardous materials may enter the body through inhalation, ingestion, injection, and absorption. Internal damage to the human body from hazardous materials exposure may involve the respiratory tract, CNS, or other internal organs. Chemicals producing internal damage include irritants, asphyxiants, nerve poisons, anesthetics, narcotics, hepatotoxins, cardiotoxins, nephrotoxins, neurotoxins, and carcinogens.

- Exposure to hazardous materials may result in burns. It also may result in severe tissue damage.

- The first agency to arrive at the scene of a hazardous materials incident must detect and identify the materials involved, assess the risk of exposure to rescue personnel and others, consider the potential risk of fire or explosion, gather information from on-site personnel or other sources, and confine and control the incident.

- A hazmat medical monitoring program may include medical examination for members of hazmat response teams, provision of medical care, record-keeping, and periodic evaluation of the surveillance program.

- The primary goals of decontamination are to reduce the patient's dosage of material, decrease the threat of secondary contamination, and reduce the risk of rescuer injury.

- Rescuers should follow strict protocols for proper decontamination of themselves, their clothing, and any contaminated equipment.

REFERENCES

1. General Services Administration, National Archives and Records Service, Office of the Federal Register: *Code of federal regulations*, 49 CFR, 173.500, parts 100-177, Washington, DC, 1981, The Administration.
2. American Chemistry Council: *Issue brief: hazmat transportation safety*, www.americanchemistry.com/s_acc/sec_article_acc.asp?CID=1695&DID=10020, accessed 10-28-10.
3. National Safety Council: *Injury facts*, Itasca, Ill, 2010, The Council.
4. General Services Administration: *Hazardous waste operations and emergency response standards*, 29 CFR, 1910.120, Washington, DC, 2003, The Administration.
5. National Fire Protection Association: *Standard for competencies for EMS personnel responding to hazardous materials incidents*, NFPA 473 (rev 2002), Quincy, Mass, 2002, The Association.
6. U.S. Department of Transportation, National Highway Traffic Safety Administration: *EMT-Paramedic national standard curriculum*, Washington, DC, 1998, The Department.
6a. U.S. Department of Health and Human Services, Occupational Safety and Health Administration: *General description and discussion of the levels of protection and protective gear*, 20 CFR, 1910.120, Appendix B, Washington, DC, 2004, The Administration.
7. Chemical Safety Associates Inc.: *Nonflammable gas mixtures MSDS 50018*, www.raesystems.com/-raedocs/Documentation/MSDS/MSDS-50018_4-gas_with_H2S.pdf, accessed 11-9-10.

8. Regional Organized Crime Information Center, Special Research Report: *Hydrogen sulfide suicide: latest technique hazardous to first responders and the public*, www.npstc.org/documents/H2S%20Report%20for%204112.pdf, accessed 11-9-10.
9. Hydrogen sulfide suicides threaten responders, *EMS insider*, vol 37, no. 4, St Louis, April 2010, Elsevier.
10. Marx J, Hockberger R, Walls R: *Rosen's emergency medicine*, ed 7, St Louis, 2009, Mosby.
11. Committee on EPA's Exposure and Human Health Reassessment of TCDD and Related Compounds, Board on Environmental Studies and Toxicology, Division on Earth and Life Studies, National Research Council of the National Academies: *Health risks from dioxin and related compounds: evaluation of the EPA reassessment*, Washington, DC, 2006, The National Academic Press.
12. Noll G, et al: *Hazardous materials: managing the incident*, Stillwater, Okla, 1988, Fire Protection Publications.
13. U.S. Department of Transportation: *North American emergency response guidebook*, Washington, DC, 2008, The Department.
14. U.S. Fire Administration: *Emergency incident rehabilitation*, www.usfa.dhs.gov/downloads/pdf/publications/fa_314.pdf, accessed 11-9-10.
15. NFPA 1584: *Recommended practices on the rehabilitation of members operating at incident scene operations and training exercises, 2008 standards*, www.pdftop.com/view/aHR0cDovL3d3dy5maXJlcmVzY3VlMS5jb20vZGF0YS9SZWhhYmlsaXRhdGlvbiUyME5GUEElMjAxNTg0LnBkA==, accessed 11-9-10.

SUGGESTED READINGS

Hostler D, McConachie S: Everyday hazmat risks: the top 10 hazardous chemicals every provider needs to understand, *JEMS* 31(4):50-59, 2006.

Oak Ridge Institute for Science and Education: *Radiation Emergency Assistance Center/Training Site (REAC/TS)*, 2010, retrieved 10-30-10 from https://orise.orau.gov/reacts/default.aspx

Zeitz P: Frequency and type of injuries in responders of hazardous substances emergency events, 1996 to 1998, *J Occup Environ Med* 42(11):115-1120, 2000.

Overview of Training Requirements for EMS Personnel Responding to a Hazardous Materials Incident as Established by OSHA/EPA and the NFPA*

OSHA/EPA TRAINING REQUIREMENTS

1. *First responder awareness*. This category pertains to individuals who are likely to witness or discover a hazardous substance release but who do not have emergency response duties pertaining to hazardous materials as part of their job functions. This applies to most law enforcement officers. Individuals in this category must have sufficient training to demonstrate the following:
   a. An understanding of what hazardous materials are and the risks associated with them in an accident
   b. An understanding of the possible outcomes of an emergency in which hazardous materials are present
   c. The ability to recognize the presence of hazardous materials in an emergency
   d. The ability to identify the hazardous materials (if possible)
   e. An understanding of the role of the first responder in the emergency response plan
   f. The ability to recognize the need for additional resources

2. *First responder operations*. Individuals are included in this category if they respond to hazardous materials incidents to protect nearby persons, property, or the environment without trying to stop the hazardous release. Firefighters and emergency medical services (EMS) personnel are in this category. In addition to the knowledge base of first responder awareness, these individuals must have training in the following:
   a. Basic hazard and risk assessment techniques
   b. Personal protective clothing and equipment
   c. Basic control, containment, and confinement operations
   d. Basic decontamination procedures

3. *Hazardous materials technicians*. Individuals in this category respond to hazardous materials emergencies for the purpose of stopping the release. Hazardous materials technicians usually are considered members of a hazardous materials response team. These individuals have additional training in the following:
   a. Emergency response plans
   b. The use of survey instruments and equipment to identify hazardous materials
   c. Incident command systems
   d. Specialized protective clothing and equipment
   e. Specialized containment and confinement operations

4. Hazardous materials specialists. The duties of these individuals require specific knowledge of the various hazardous substances. Hazardous materials specialists respond with and provide support to hazardous materials technicians and act as site liaisons with federal, state, and local government authorities. In addition to the knowledge base of the hazardous materials technician, hazardous materials specialists have training in the following:
   a. The use of advanced survey instruments and equipment
   b. In-depth hazard and risk assessment
   c. Implementation of decontamination procedures
   d. Site safety and control
   e. Chemical, radiological, and toxicological terminology relevant to hazardous substance behaviors

5. On-scene incident commander. The on-scene incident commander is trained to assume control of a hazardous materials event. In addition to the first responder awareness level of training, the on-scene incident commander's responsibilities include the following:
   a. Implementation of an incident command system
   b. Implementation of emergency response plans
   c. Knowledge of state and federal regional response teams
   d. Knowledge of medical hazards and risks for individuals working in protective clothing and equipment

NPFA 473: COMPETENCIES FOR EMS PERSONNEL RESPONDING TO HAZARDOUS MATERIALS INCIDENTS†

Level I Responders

The goal of the competencies at EMS/HM Level I shall be to provide the individual with knowledge and skills necessary to safely deliver emergency medical care in the cold zone (and meet the following requirements):

1. Analyze a hazardous materials emergency to determine what risks are present to the provider and the patient by completing the following tasks:
   a. Determine the hazards present to the Level I responder and the patient in a hazardous materials incident
   b. Assess the patient to determine the risk of secondary contamination
2. Plan a response to provide emergency medical care to persons involved in hazardous materials incidents by completing the following tasks:
   a. Describe the role of the Level I responder in a hazardous materials incident
   b. Plan a response to provide the appropriate level of emergency medical care in a hazardous materials incident
   c. Determine if the personal protective equipment provided is appropriate
   d. Determine if the equipment and supplies provided are adequate (that is, will meet the patient care needs)
3. Implement the planned response by completing the following tasks:
   a. Perform the necessary preparations for receiving the hazardous materials patient and preventing secondary contamination
   b. Treat the hazardous materials patient
   c. Transport the patient as appropriate
   d. Terminate the incident

Level II Responders

The goal of the competencies at EMS/HM Level II shall be to provide the Level II responder with the knowledge and skills necessary to perform and/or coordinate patient care activities and medical support of hazardous materials response personnel in the warm zone. The Level II responder should be able to perform the following:

1. Analyze a hazardous materials incident to determine the magnitude of the problem in terms of outcomes by completing the following tasks:
   a. Determine the hazards present to the Level II responder and the patient in a hazardous materials incident
   b. Assess the patient to determine the patient care needs and the risk of secondary contamination
2. Plan a response to provide the appropriate level of emergency medical care to persons involved in hazardous materials incidents and to provide medical support to hazardous materials response personnel by completing the following tasks:
   a. Describe the role of the Level II responder in a hazardous materials incident
   b. Plan a response to provide the appropriate level of emergency medical care in a hazardous materials incident
   c. Determine if the personal protective equipment provided to EMS personnel is appropriate
3. Implement the planned response by completing the following tasks:
   a. Perform the preparations for receiving the patient
   b. Provide treatment to the hazardous materials patient
   c. Coordinate and manage the EMS component of the hazardous materials incident
   d. Perform medical support of hazardous materials incident response personnel
4. Terminate the incident

---

*OSHA, Occupational Safety and Health Administration; *EPA*, Environmental Protection Agency; *NFPA*, National Fire Protection Association.
†From National Fire Protection Association: NFPA 473: Competencies for EMS personnel responding to hazardous materials incidents, Quincy, Mass, 1997, The Association.

58 Bioterrorism and Weapons of Mass Destruction

OBJECTIVES

Upon completion of this chapter, the paramedic student will be able to:

1. List five types of weapons of mass destruction.
2. Identify actions, signs and symptoms, methods of distribution, and management of biological weapons of mass destruction.
3. Identify actions, signs and symptoms, methods of distribution, and management of chemical weapons of mass destruction.
4. Identify actions, signs and symptoms, methods of distribution, and management of nuclear weapons of mass destruction.
5. Describe security threat alerts as defined by the Department of Homeland Security.
6. Identify measures to be taken by paramedics who respond to incidents with suspected weapons of mass destruction involvement.

KEY TERMS

anthrax An acute infectious disease caused by the spore-forming bacterium *Bacillus anthracis*.

bioterrorism The use of biological agents, such as pathogenic organisms or agricultural pests, for the express purpose of causing death or disease, to instill a sense of fear and panic in the victims, and to intimidate governments or societies for political, financial, or ideological gain.

B-NICE An acronym used for identifying categories of weapons of mass destruction: *Biological, Nuclear, Incendiary, Chemical,* and *Explosives.*

botulism An often fatal paralytic disease caused by the bacillus *Clostridium botulinum*.

CBREN An acronym used for identifying categories of weapons of mass destruction: *Chemical, Biological, Radiological, Explosive,* and *Nuclear* agents.

chlorine A poisonous, yellow-green gas with an odor that has been described as a mixture of pineapple and pepper.

cutaneous anthrax Anthrax that affects the skin, caused by the spore-forming bacterium *B. anthracis*.

Ebola An infectious viral hemorrhagic fever.

explosive Refers to bombs that can be made from a variety of dangerous materials.

foodborne botulism Illness that results from eating foods that contain the bacillus *Clostridium botulinum*.

improvised explosive device A "homemade" bomb constructed of explosives attached to a detonator; also known as a *roadside bomb*.

incendiary devices Firebombs.

infant botulism Illness caused by consumption of the spores of the botulinum bacteria, which then grow in the intestines and release toxin.

inhalational anthrax Anthrax caused by inhaling the spore-forming bacterium *B. anthracis*.

intestinal anthrax Anthrax caused from consuming meat contaminated with the bacterium *B. anthracis*.

Marburg An infectious viral hemorrhagic fever.

nerve agents Chemicals that disrupt the nerve transmissions in the central and peripheral nervous systems.

oropharyngeal anthrax A rare form of anthrax that occurs when the mouth and throat are infected with the spore-forming bacterium *B. anthracis*.

phosgene A poisonous gas that appears as a grayish white cloud and smells of newly mowed hay.

plague A disease caused by the bacteria *Yersinia pestis*, found in rodents (e.g., chipmunks, prairie dogs, ground squirrels, and mice) and their fleas in many areas around the world.

pneumonic plague An infectious pulmonary disease caused by exposure to the bacteria *Yersinia pestis*.

radiological dispersion device A nuclear explosive device; also called a "dirty nuke" or "dirty bomb."

ricin A potent protein cytotoxin derived from the beans of the castor plant (*Ricinus communis*).

riot control agents Chemicals that can produce sensory irritation or disabling physical effects that disappear within a short time after termination of exposure.

sarin A clear, colorless, and tasteless liquid that has no odor in its pure form; may be used as a nerve agent.

smallpox A highly contagious viral disease caused by the variola virus; characterized by fever, prostration, and a vesicular, pustular rash.

soman A clear, colorless, tasteless liquid with a slight camphor odor; may be used as a nerve agent.

tabun A clear, colorless, tasteless liquid with a faint fruity odor; may be used as a nerve agent.

tularemia A serious illness that is caused by the bacterium *Francisella tularensis* found in animals (especially rodents, rabbits, and hares).

vesicants Chemicals with severely irritating properties that produce fluid-filled pockets on the skin and damage to the eyes, lungs, and other mucous membranes.

viral hemorrhagic fevers A group of illnesses caused by several distinct families of viruses that include arenaviruses, filoviruses, bunyaviruses, and flaviviruses.

VX A thick, amber-colored, odorless liquid that resembles motor oil; may be used as a nerve agent.

weapons of mass destruction Large conventional biological, nuclear, incendiary, chemical, or explosive weapons.

wound botulism Botulism caused by toxins produced from a wound infected with *C. botulinum*.

*I*nternational conventions have long prohibited the use of chemicals and biological agents during war and bar any country from making or acquiring biological weapons.[1] A number of countries and terrorist groups, however, maintain them. This chapter serves as an overview of **bioterrorism** and **weapons of mass destruction** (WMD). Bioterrorism is the intentional release of biological products to cause illness or death. Weapons of mass destruction are weapons that can kill or bring harm to a large number of people. The chapter also provides general guidelines for emergency response.

> **NOTE**
> **B-NICE** is an acronym that can be used for identifying five categories of weapons of mass destruction. It stands for *Biological, Nuclear, Incendiary, Chemical,* and *Explosives.* Another acronym is **CBREN.** It stands for *Chemical, Biological, Radiological, Explosive,* and *Nuclear* agents.

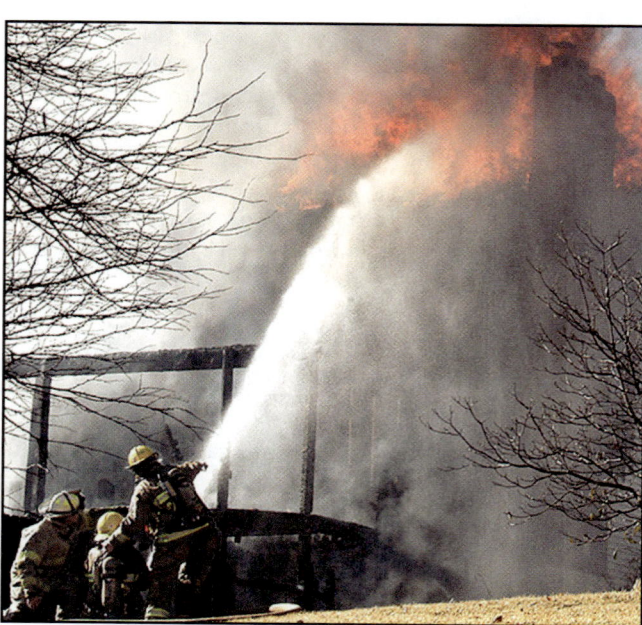

HISTORY OF BIOLOGICAL WEAPONS

The use of biological agents as weapons has occurred throughout history, dating back to 184 BC when Hannibal ordered that pots filled with venomous snakes be thrown onto the decks of enemy ships (Box 58-1).[2] However, many countries agreed to stop biological weapons research and development in 1972. Some of these countries included the United States, the former Soviet Union, Canada, and the United Kingdom. Some countries, however, continue to have biological warfare programs. In addition, the use of biological agents against civilians through acts of bioterrorism recently has appeared. The serious reality of bioterrorism became clear in the United States in 2001 when anthrax cases occurred following exposure to contaminated mail in New York, New Jersey, and Washington, DC.

CRITICAL BIOLOGICAL AGENTS AND RESPONDER DATABASES

The Centers for Disease Control and Prevention (CDC)[4] has published a list of critical biological agents. The list is divided into categories A, B, and C (Box 58-2).

> **NOTE**
> Acts of terrorism can pose significant risk to civilian populations. If airplanes sprayed chemical and biological agents on a city on a clear, breezy night, thousands and perhaps millions of persons would be killed. For example, 200 lb of anthrax sprayed over a city the size of Omaha would kill as many as 2.5 million persons; 200 lb of botulinum toxin would kill as many as 40,000 persons in an area the size of the Mall of America; and 200 lb of VX sprayed over an area the size of Disneyland would kill about 12,500 persons.[3]

Category A agents are the highest priority. They pose a risk to national security. They can be spread easily by person-to-person contact. They cause a high death rate and have the potential to cause a major public health problem. They might cause public panic and disruption. Category A agents require special action for public health preparedness. An example of a category A agent is *Bacillus anthracis* (anthrax).

Category B agents are the second highest priority. They are fairly easy to disseminate. They cause moderate illnesses and have a lower death rate than category A agents. These

In 2003 it was announced that the federal government was deploying an early warning network of sensors to detect biological attack (the "BioWatch Program"). The Department of Homeland Security (DHS) is responsible for the program, which has three main elements that are each coordinated by different agencies[5]:

1. The Environmental Protection Agency (EPA) maintains the sampling component—the sensors that collect airborne particles.
2. The Centers for Disease Control and Prevention (CDC) coordinates analysis—the laboratory testing of the samples.
3. The Federal Bureau of Investigation (FBI) is designated as the lead agency for the law enforcement response if a bioterrorism event is detected.

The installation of the sensor network is ongoing, with over 30 cities chosen as locations for these sensors. Selected cities include Philadelphia, New York City, Washington DC, San Diego, Boston, Chicago, San Francisco, St. Louis, Houston, and Los Angeles.

agents require specific enhancements of diagnostic capacity and disease surveillance. An example of a category B agent is *Coxiella burnetii* (Q fever).

Category C agents are the third highest priority. They include new pathogens that could be engineered for mass dissemination in the future. These agents are widely available. They also are easy to produce and dispense. They have the potential to cause a high rate of death and sickness. An example of a category C agent is Nipah virus.

Emergency Response Safety and Health Database

The CDC in conjunction with the National Institute of Occupational Safety and Health (NIOSH) has developed the Emergency Response Safety and Health Database (ERSH-DB). The ERSH-DB was developed for the emergency response community. The database contains accurate and concise information on high-priority chemical, biological, and radiological agents that could be encountered by

BOX 58-1 Time Line of Suspected or Reported Use of Biological Weapons

Early Examples
- The Tartar army catapulted bodies of plague victims into the city of Caffa in 1346.
- The British army provided the Delaware Indians in 1763 with blankets that had been used by smallpox patients.

Pre–World War II
- The Germans used various human and animal pathogens as agents of germ warfare in Europe during World War I. They are reported to have shipped horses, sheep, and cattle inoculated with *Bacillus anthracis* and *Pseudomonas pseudomallei* to the United States and other countries.
- Germany was accused of spreading cholera in Italy and plague in Russia in 1915.

World War II
- The Japanese used germ warfare against the Chinese and the Soviets by scattering *Yersinia pestis*-contaminated rice and fleas by airplane. This was followed by an outbreak of bubonic plague in those areas.
- The Japanese experimented with biological agents by exposing prisoners of war to anthrax, botulism, brucellosis, cholera, dysentery, gas gangrene, meningococcal infection, and plague. More than 1000 prisoners died from the experiments.
- The British performed trials with *Bacillus anthracis* off the coast of Scotland.
- The United States prepared about 5000 anthrax bombs at Camp Detrick, Maryland, in 1942 (although none were used during the war).

Post–World War II
- The United States dispersed stimulant aerosols over large areas around U.S. cities from 1949 to 1968.

- The United States exposed willing volunteer members of the Seventh Day Adventist Church (who were religious objectors to warfare) to aerosols of *Francisella tularensis* and *Coxiella burnetii* in 1953. (No deaths occurred and all recovered.)
- An unintentional release of anthrax spores from a biological warfare facility in the Soviet Union resulted in 66 deaths from inhalational anthrax in 1979.

The Gulf War
- The Iraqi government admitted that it had conducted research into the offensive use of *B. anthracis*, *Clostridium botulinum* toxin, and *C. perfringens* and had filled warheads with biological agents.

The Aum Shinrikyo
- The religious cult intentionally contaminated the Tokyo subway system with sarin in 1995, resulting in 5500 health care visits and 12 deaths.
- Several unsuccessful attempts were made to release anthrax or botulinum toxin to other areas around Tokyo.

Recent Terrorist Group Activities
- A religious commune deliberately contaminated several community salad bars in the United States with *Salmonella typhimurium*, resulting in more than 750 illnesses in 1984.
- Anthrax-laden envelopes were sent via U.S. mail in 2001, resulting to date in 11 cases of inhalational anthrax (including 5 deaths) and 12 cases of cutaneous anthrax.

From Darling R, et al: *Bioterrorism: the May 2002 issue of the Emergency Medicine Clinics of North America*, Philadelphia, 2002, Saunders.

BOX 58-2 Critical Biological Agents

Category A
Anthrax (*Bacillus anthracis*)
Botulism (*Clostridium botulinum* toxin)
Plague (*Yersinia pestis*)
Smallpox (variola major)
Tularemia (*Francisella tularensis*)
Viral hemorrhagic fevers (filoviruses [e.g., Ebola and Marburg] and arenaviruses [e.g., Lassa and Machupo])

Category B
Brucellosis (*Brucella* species)
Epsilon toxin of *Clostridium perfringens*
Food safety threats (e.g., *Salmonella* species, *Escherichia coli* O157:H7, and *Shigella*)
Glanders (*Burkholderia mallei*)
Melioidosis (*Burkholderia pseudomallei*)
Psittacosis (*Chlamydia psittaci*)
Q fever (*Coxiella burnetii*)
Ricin toxin from *Ricinus communis* (castor beans)
Staphylococcal enterotoxin B
Typhus fever (*Rickettsia prowazekii*)
Viral encephalitis (alphaviruses [e.g., Venezuelan equine encephalitis, eastern equine encephalitis, and western equine encephalitis])
Water safety threats (e.g., *Vibrio cholerae* and *Cryptosporidium parvum*)

Category C
Nipah virus
Hantaviruses
Tick-borne hemorrhagic fever viruses
Tick-borne encephalitis viruses
Yellow fever
Multidrug-resistant tuberculosis

From Centers for Disease Control and Prevention: *Bioterrorism agents/diseases*, www.bt.cdc.gov/agent/agentlist-category.asp#a, accessed 10-28-10.

BOX 58-3 Groups of Agents in the ERSH-DB

The database is composed of cards for the following groups of agents:
- Biotoxins
- Blister agents
- Incapacitating agents
- Lung damaging agents
- Nerve agents
- Riot control/tear agents
- Systemic agents
- Vomiting agents

DID YOU KNOW?

Riot Control/Tear Agents are solid chemicals with low vapor pressure that are dispersed in the air as fine particles. They produce sensory irritation or disabling physical effects that disappear within a short time after termination of exposure. Riot control agents often are referred to as "tear gas" and sometimes are used in military exercises, by law enforcement personnel for crowd control, and by individuals and the general public for personal protection (e.g., Mace and pepper spray). Paramedics and other emergency responders likely will encounter exposure to these agents during their careers. Personal protective equipment is needed to guard against the effects of these agents.

The most common riot control agent compounds are chloroacetophenone (CN) and chlorobenzylidenemalononitrile (CS). Other examples include chloropicrin (PS), bromobenzyl cyanide (CA), dibenzoxazepine (CR), and combinations of various agents. Riot control agents cause irritation to the area of contact (e.g., eyes, skin, and nose) within seconds of exposure. Signs and symptoms vary, depending on the location of exposure (open versus enclosed spaces) and the duration of contact with the agent, and may include some or all of the following:
- Eyes: excessive tearing, burning, blurred vision, redness
- Nose: runny nose, burning, swelling
- Mouth: burning, irritation, difficulty swallowing, drooling
- Lungs: chest tightness, coughing, choking sensation, wheezing, shortness of breath
- Skin: burns, rash
- Gastrointestinal system: nausea and vomiting

Although most effects from exposure to riot control agents are minor and last only 15 to 30 minutes, exposure to large doses or exposure in an enclosed area rarely may result in blindness, glaucoma, severe burns to airway structures, and life-threatening respiratory failure. Emergency care consists of moving persons away from the source to fresh air. In severe cases, oxygen administration, ventilatory support, burn care, and decontamination may be required.

From Centers for Disease Control and Prevention: *Facts about riot control agents*, www.bt.cdc.gov/agent/riotcontrol/factsheet.asp, accessed 10-28-10.

personnel responding to a terrorist event. The objectives of the ERSH-DB are[6]:
- To rapidly disseminate information to emergency response personnel on specific agents that may be used in terrorist events and that pose an occupational hazard of injury, illness, and death
- To provide information to be incorporated into management systems of emergency response operations for the purpose of reducing work-related injuries and illnesses
- To provide information that may be used in continuing education and training programs for the emergency response community

The information contained in the ERSH-DB represents a compilation of material from many sources. It is intended to address the safety and health information needs of a wide range of emergency response personnel. These groups include fire and rescue, emergency medicine, law enforcement, emergency management, public health, safety and health, and mortuary and funeral services. This central source of information allows different segments of the emergency response community to share information that is not readily accessible. It also helps to avoid duplication of effort (Box 58-3). Each response card includes information for:

- Agent Category
- Agent Characteristics
- Agent Name
- Agent Properties
- CAS #
- Common Names
- Emergency Response
- Decontamination (Environmental/Equipment)
- First Aid
- Decontamination (Human)
- Long-Term Implications
- Occupational Exposure Limits
- On-Site Fatalities
- Packaging and Labeling
- Personal Protective Equipment
- RTECS #
- Signs/Symptoms
- Trade Names and Other Synonyms

METHODS OF DISSEMINATION

Most biological agents used in bioterrorism are designed to enter the body through one of three ways. One of these is the inhalation of small particles into the lungs. Another is through the ingestion of contaminated food or water. The third way is by contamination of the skin that allows for absorption of the toxins. Because all category A agents can be disseminated through aerosolization, the inhalation route is of greatest concern.

Aerosols can be delivered in wet or dry form in closed or open spaces. Equipment that may be used to disseminate aerosols includes crop-dusting planes for open spaces, aerosol-generating devices for enclosed areas (e.g., subways and enclosed malls), ventilation systems in buildings, and contamination of items in the environment with fine powders that are aerosolized easily when disrupted. (The last example is the method of dispersal that occurred in the 2001 anthrax cases in the United States. Those were caused by opening contaminated mail.)

CRITICAL THINKING
Why would aerosolized agents of mass destruction pose a great risk to first responders?

SPECIFIC BIOLOGICAL THREATS

Hundreds of biological and chemical agents can be used in a bioterrorism attack. This section provides a brief overview of a few of these agents. The agents described in the following sections are considered most likely to be used as a threat to civilian populations. The most common biological threats are thought to be anthrax, botulism, plague, ricin, tularemia, smallpox, and viral hemorrhagic fevers.[7]

NOTE
Like all other hazardous materials incidents, it is assumed that all responders will wear the proper personal protective equipment. It also is assumed that they will use universal precautions at the scene and during patient care (see the chapter appendix). EMS personnel should not enter a scene with known or suspected biological or chemical threats until the scene has been made safe by the proper personnel.

Anthrax

Anthrax is an acute infectious disease caused by the spore-forming bacterium *Bacillus anthracis.* Anthrax most often occurs in warm-blooded animals. However, it also can infect human beings. Symptoms of disease vary. Usually, though, symptoms appear within 7 days after exposure. The most common form of anthrax is **cutaneous anthrax.** It results from direct contact with spores or bacilli. (Cutaneous anthrax also can occur from exposure to contaminated soil, and is not necessarily associated with a weapons of mass destruction [WMD] incident.) Cutaneous anthrax causes localized itching. This is followed by a papular lesion that turns vesicular and subsequent development of black eschar within 7 to 10 days of the initial lesion (Figure 58-1). Symptoms of **inhalational anthrax** often resemble a common cold in the initial stages. This is followed by severe respiratory distress and sepsis (Figure 58-2). (Inhalational

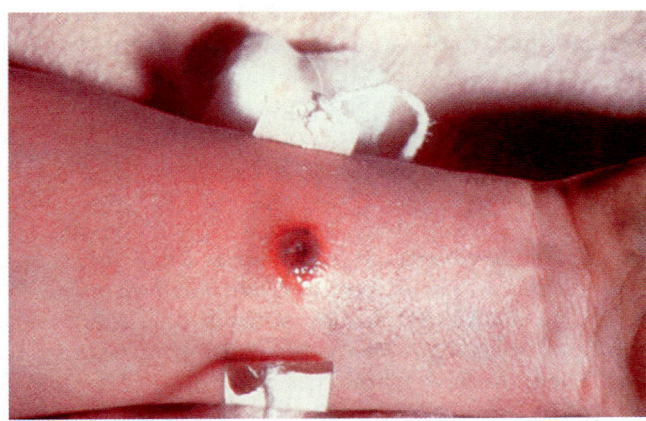

FIGURE 58-1 Cutaneous anthrax. (From Federal Emergency Management Agency: *Federal response plan, notice of change,* FEMA 229, Chapter 11, Feb 7, 1997, www.fas.org/irp/offdocs/pdd39_frp.htm, accessed 7-6-10.)

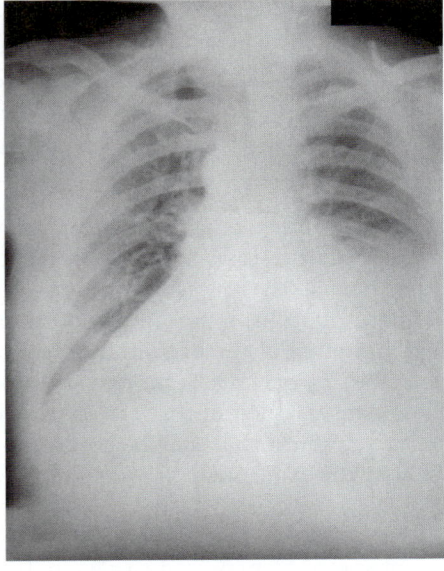

FIGURE 58-2 Respiratory distress and sepsis in anthrax.

anthrax usually results in death within 36 hours after onset of the acute symptoms.[8]) Other, less common forms of anthrax include **intestinal anthrax** from consuming contaminated meat and **oropharyngeal anthrax** when the mouth and throat are infected (rare).

TREATMENT

Direct person-to-person spread of anthrax most likely does not occur. Thus immunization or treatment of persons who have come in contact with a patient (e.g., household members, friends, and co-workers) is unnecessary. These persons do not need to be treated unless they also were exposed to the aerosol at the time of the attack. The disease is diagnosed by isolating *B. anthracis* from the blood, skin lesions, or respiratory tract secretions or by measuring specific antibodies in the blood of suspected cases. Treatment with antibiotics should be early; if left untreated, the disease can be fatal. Human anthrax vaccines (controversial) are available and are reported to be 93% effective against cutaneous anthrax.[9] Vaccination to protect against inhalational anthrax is recommended only for those at high risk.[10] This includes, for example, military personnel and workers in research laboratories that routinely handle anthrax bacteria.

Botulism

As described in Chapter 34, **botulism** is a rare but serious paralytic illness. The bacterium *Clostridium botulinum* produces a nerve toxin that causes paralysis. Botulinum toxin is one of the most potent and lethal substances known to man. There are three main types of botulism. One type is **foodborne botulism.** Eating foods that contain the botulism toxin causes it. The second type is **wound botulism** (Figure 58-3). This type is caused by toxin produced from a wound infected with *C. botulinum*. The third type is **infant botulism.** This type is caused by consumption of the spores of the botulinum bacteria, which then grow in the intestines and release toxin. All forms of botulism can be fatal and are considered medical emergencies.

 **LOOK AGAIN**
See Chapter 34: Toxicology, pp. 990-991.

In a bioterrorism attack, inhaling the toxin as an aerosol weapon or ingesting the toxin via contaminated food or water are the most likely routes of exposure for serious illness. Foodborne botulism can be especially dangerous because small amounts of the bacterium in contaminated food can poison many persons. Signs and symptoms of the illness include nausea, dry mouth, blurred vision, dysphagia, fatigue, and dyspnea that may begin several hours to several days after the exposure.

TREATMENT

Botulism is not spread from person to person. If diagnosed early, foodborne and wound botulism can be treated with

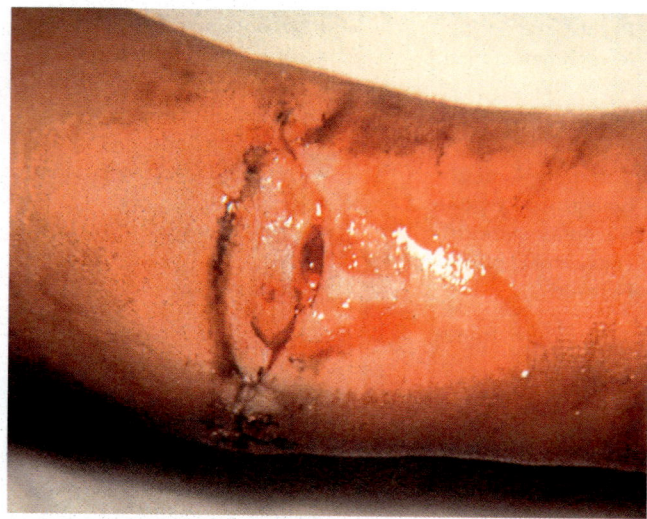

FIGURE 58-3 Wound botulism.

an antitoxin. The antitoxin blocks the action of toxin circulating in the blood. Recovery may take several weeks. As a result of the paralysis and respiratory failure that occur with botulism, the patient may be placed on a ventilator.

 CRITICAL THINKING
What kind of resources would your community need to support hundreds of patients who need care on a ventilator?

Plague

Plague is caused by the bacterium *Yersinia pestis*. The bacteria are found in rodents (e.g., chipmunks, prairie dogs, ground squirrels, and mice) and their fleas in many areas of the world. The bacteria also can be grown in large amounts and disseminated by aerosol in a bioterrorism attack. This would result in an epidemic of the pneumonic form of the disease **(pneumonic plague)** with the potential for secondary contamination. Signs and symptoms include fever, extreme weakness, shortness of breath, chest pain, cough, and bloody sputum. Gastrointestinal symptoms are often present, including nausea, vomiting, abdominal pain, and diarrhea. The illness can lead to septic shock within 2 to 4 days.[11] Without treatment, plague has a high mortality rate.

 NOTE
Pneumonic plague is one of three forms of the disease, all of which are caused by the bacteria *Yersinia pestis*. *Bubonic plague* is an infection of the buboes (lymph nodes). *Septicemic plague* is an infection of the bloodstream.

A bioterrorism attack with the bacteria would be characterized by pneumonic plague occurring at the same time in persons following a common exposure. A secondary outbreak of illness would occur in others who had close contact with an infected person's respiratory droplets.

TREATMENT

The disease is diagnosed through testing for the bacteria. Plague must be treated early (within 24 hours) with antibiotic or antimicrobial agents. Persons who have been in close contact with the patient should be identified. These persons must be evaluated for postexposure drug therapy. Pneumonic plague is spread through the respiratory droplets of an infected person. Thus patients with the disease should be isolated. Universal precautions and personal respiratory protection for all caregivers are critical.

> ### CRITICAL THINKING
> Your service notices a sudden increase in patients with severe respiratory distress. These patients also have pneumonia-like signs and symptoms. Would you initially consider bioterrorism as a cause of the outbreak?

Ricin

Ricin is a potent protein cytotoxin. Ricin is derived from the beans of the castor plant (*Ricinus communis*) (Figure 58-4). Castor beans are widely available throughout the world. The toxin also is relatively easy to extract. Ricin can be made into a mist, powder, or pellet. When ricin is inhaled as an aerosol, it results in pulmonary toxicity with severe respiratory symptoms within 8 hours. This is followed by acute hypoxic respiratory failure in 36 to 72 hours.[12] (Nonspecific findings of weakness, fever, vomiting, cough, hypoxemia, hypothermia, and hypotension in large numbers of patients might suggest exposure to several respiratory pathogens.) If ricin is ingested, severe gastrointestinal symptoms occur with rapid onset of nausea, vomiting, abdominal cramps, and severe diarrhea. This is followed by vascular collapse and death.

TREATMENT

No antidote exists for ricin poisoning. Treatment is aimed at avoiding exposure and eliminating the toxin from the body as quickly as possible. Patients who have inhaled ricin should be moved to an area with fresh air, clothing contaminated with the toxin should be removed, and the patient should be decontaminated (see Chapter 57). The prehospital care may include airway, ventilatory, and circulatory support. Seizures, hypotension, and respiratory failure should be anticipated.

Smallpox

Smallpox was declared extinct by the World Health Organization in 1980 because of near-universal vaccination. However, the virus could be used as a biological weapon. The variola virus that causes smallpox is fairly stable. The

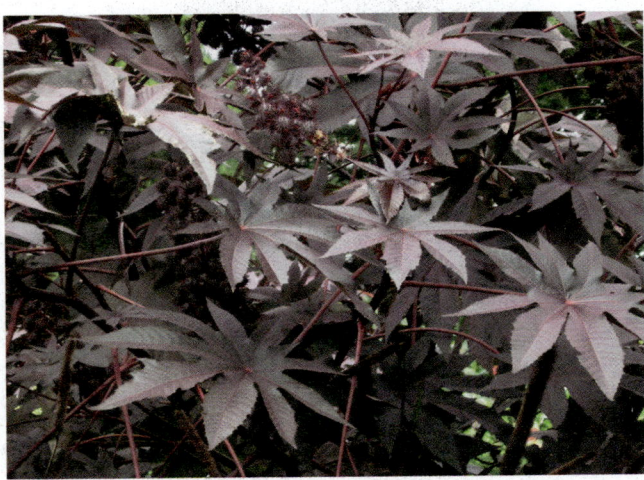

FIGURE 58-4 The seed pods of the castor bean plant are used to manufacture ricin.

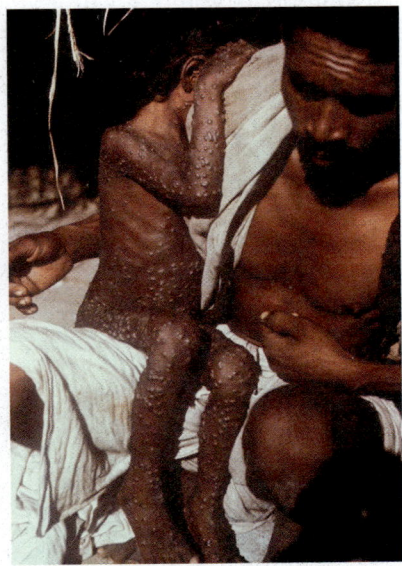

FIGURE 58-5 Smallpox lesions.

infectious dose also is small. Moreover, an aerosol release of the virus would be widely spread. The incubation period for smallpox is about 12 days following exposure. The virus usually is spread by an infected person releasing infected saliva from the mouth into the air. Persons in close or prolonged contact to the infected person inhale the virus. Smallpox also can be spread through direct contact with infected body fluids or contaminated objects such as bedding or clothing. Signs and symptoms of the disease include high fever, fatigue, headache, and backache. These are followed within 2 to 3 days with the smallpox rash and skin lesions. These lesions finally form crusts. Upon healing, the lesions leave depressed, depigmented scars (Figure 58-5). Permanent joint deformities and blindness may follow recovery. The death rate from smallpox is about 30% in unvaccinated persons.[13]

Vaccine immunity may prevent or modify the illness. At this time, however, the federal government does not recommend prophylactic vaccination for health care workers or the general public because of the possibility of toxic or allergic reactions.[14] If an attack is known or imminent, smallpox response teams whose members have received the vaccine will administer the vaccine to others. They also will care for victims who have been exposed. Currently, the United States has enough smallpox vaccine in storage to vaccinate everyone in the country who might need it in the event of an emergency.[15] Production of a new vaccine is also under way.

TREATMENT

There is no proven treatment for smallpox. However, several antiviral drugs are being studied. Patients with smallpox should receive supportive care provided by vaccinated personnel. The personnel must use universal precautions. (This includes appropriate respiratory protection.) Objects that come in contact with the patient require disinfection. (Examples of such objects are bed linens, clothing, ambulances, and equipment.) This disinfection must be by fire, steam, or sodium hypochlorite solution.

CRITICAL THINKING
Your employer asks you to get the smallpox vaccination. Where can you look to find information about the side effects and risks of immunization with this vaccine?

Tularemia

Tularemia is a serious illness caused by the bacterium *Francisella tularensis*. This bacterium is found in animals (especially rodents, rabbits, and hares). (The illness can be caused by skinning the fresh carcass of rabbits ["rabbit fever"], if the bacterium is introduced through broken skin. Rubber gloves should be worn when handling animals that might harbor the bacterium.) The disease is highly infectious. Some strains are resistant to antibiotics. The bacterium responsible for tularemia can be delivered in a bioterrorism attack by aerosol. Infection may result from inhalation of the aerosol. It also may result from the skin, mucous membranes, respiratory tract, or gastrointestinal tract (via contaminated soil, water, food, or animals) being exposed to the virus. Transmission of the disease from person to person does not occur. The development of signs and symptoms varies widely (from 1 day to 2 weeks). This is based on the strength of the strain and the route of exposure. Following a bioterrorism attack with the agent, patients may complain of an abrupt onset of an acute febrile illness (headache, chills, general malaise).

They also may complain of gastrointestinal illness that includes nausea, vomiting, and diarrhea. If left untreated, septic tularemia may lead to disseminated intravascular coagulation with bleeding, acute respiratory failure, and death.

TREATMENT

The disease is managed with antibiotics. The patient may require airway, ventilatory, and circulatory support. Although funding has been provided for the development of a vaccine for civilian use, one is not currently available in the United States. The U.S. Department of Defense has developed an experimental tularemia vaccine. To date, health officials have limited the use of this vaccine to laboratory and other high-risk workers.[16]

Viral Hemorrhagic Fevers

Viral hemorrhagic fevers (VHFs) refer to a group of illnesses caused by several distinct families of viruses that include arenaviruses, filoviruses, bunyaviruses, and flaviviruses. The VHFs have limited geographical ranges and are found mostly across eastern and southern Africa, South America, and the Pacific islands.[17] Most are highly infectious if spread as an aerosol. These viruses naturally reside in animals (e.g., cotton rat and deer mouse) or arthropods (e.g., ticks and mosquitoes). The viruses are fully dependent on these living hosts for reproduction and survival. Viruses that cause hemorrhagic fever usually are transmitted to human beings during contact with urine, fecal matter, saliva, or other body excretions from an infected rodent or by a bite from an infected mosquito or tick. Some VHFs (e.g., **Ebola** and **Marburg**) also can spread from person to person following an initial infection. This type of infection most often results from close contact with infected persons through their body tissues and fluids.

Viral hemorrhagic fevers cause a multisystem syndrome. The syndrome is characterized by hemorrhage and life-threatening disease. Signs and symptoms vary by the type of VHF. However, they often include fever, fatigue, dizziness, muscle aches, loss of strength, and exhaustion. Patients with severe cases of VHF may bleed from mucous membranes, from internal organs, or from the mouth, eyes, or ears. (Death rarely results from this blood loss.) Shock, renal failure, central nervous system dysfunction, coma, and seizures may develop with severe infection. These may lead to a fatal outcome.

TREATMENT

Therapy for patients with VHFs is supportive. With the exception of *yellow fever* and *Argentine hemorrhagic fever*, for which vaccines have been developed, no vaccines exist that can protect against these diseases. The goals of therapy are to maintain vital functions. This may allow for recovery in some patients.

NUCLEAR AND RADIOLOGICAL THREATS

Nuclear explosions can cause deadly effects from blinding light, intense heat (thermal radiation), initial nuclear radiation, blast, fires started by the heat pulse, and secondary fires caused by destruction. A **radiological dispersion device** (RDD) is also called a "dirty nuke" or "dirty bomb." The use of such a device as a terrorist weapon is considered far more likely than use of a true nuclear device. (A true nuclear device uses weapons-grade uranium or plutonium.)[18] These dirty bombs appeal to terrorists. They require little technical knowledge to build and deploy compared with that of a true nuclear device. These radioactive materials also are used widely in medicine, agriculture, industry, and research. They are readily available and easy to obtain.

> **NOTE**
> Radiological attacks are a credible threat. However, they would not result in the hundreds of thousands of deaths that could be caused by a crude nuclear weapon that requires a fission reaction. A radiological attack, however, could cause serious illness in persons in the immediate area, contaminate several city blocks, and require costly cleanup (if even possible).

The main type of RDD combines an explosive, such as dynamite, with a radioactive material. The extent of contamination would depend on a number of factors. These include the size of the explosive, the amount and type of radioactive material used, and weather conditions (e.g., wind). The detonation of an RDD releases radioactive fallout. This could cause radiation sickness, severe burns, and long-term cancer fatalities. In most cases the conventional explosive itself would result in more deaths than from exposure to the radioactive material.[19] A second type of RDD might involve a powerful radioactive source hidden in a public place. It may be hidden, for example, in a trash can in a busy train or subway station. In such a place, persons passing close to the source might receive a significant dose of radiation.

> **CRITICAL THINKING**
> What emergency medical services groups or divisions should you consider setting up if there is a report of a dirty bomb explosion?

Emergency Care

As described in Chapter 39, the principles of *time, distance,* and *shielding* should be used for personal protection and for the protection of others:

1. Limit the amount of *time* at a radiological scene. Fallout radiation loses its intensity fairly rapidly. Use or wear radiation detection monitors.
2. Increase the *distance* between you and the scene.
3. *Shield* yourself with appropriate personal protective equipment (PPE), geography, or structural materials whenever possible. Your protection increases in proportion to the number of heavy, dense materials located between you and the fallout particles.

After dealing with the initial blast, the top priorities are the treatment of radiation sickness, the containment and monitoring of radioactive fallout, evacuation, and decontamination.

>
> **LOOK AGAIN**
> See Chapter 39: Burns, pp. 1142-1144.

INCENDIARY THREATS

Incendiary devices are firebombs. These devices range from a simple Molotov cocktail (a bottle containing a rag soaked in gasoline that is ignited) to much larger and sophisticated devices. Their main use in terrorism is to generate panic (a *weapon of mass disruption*). However, they are also capable of causing loss of life and property damage from fire. Depending on the severity of the attack, primary concerns may include the following:

- The possibility for large numbers of injured victims and fatalities
- Significant damage to buildings and the infrastructure of a community
- Overwhelming of local resources (emergency response agencies, hospitals, mental health agencies)
- The involvement of law enforcement at local, state, and federal levels because of the criminal nature of the event
- The closing of workplaces and schools
- Possible restrictions on domestic and international travel
- The need for evacuation and extended cleanup
- Public fear that can continue for a prolonged period

Emergency Care

Emergency care depends on the nature of the attack. Care may include providing initial wound care for injured victims at a small-scale event. However, care also may include managing a scene with multiple patients at a large-scale event (see Chapter 54). As with any emergency response, EMS crews should not approach the scene until it has been made safe by the proper personnel. Following the initial explosion, detonation of a second device is possible. The second device may be designed to injure or kill emergency response personnel or bystanders. In addition,

BOX 58-4 Required Resource Guidelines and Recommendations for EMS Response to Terrorist Bombing Attacks[20]

- Personnel must:
  1. Be appropriately trained, equipped, and knowledgeable about chemical, biological, radiological, nuclear, and explosives (CBRNE) detection, personal protection, and decontamination.
  2. Be educated in the care of blast-related injuries for adult and pediatric patients.
  3. Be prepared to institute triage.
  4. Have the necessary resources and be capable of rapidly detecting CBRNE agents to assist with the decontamination plan.
  5. Be prepared to institute and participate in a unified incident command.
- An incident management process to address 72-hour operations.
- A communications system that is interoperable with the public safety disciplines (fire, law enforcement, EMS, and emergency management) and with receiving hospitals, other health care facilities, and local public health officials.
- Rapid access to a medical cache(s) sufficient to treat the volume of critically injured patients.
- Ambulance resources to transport critically injured patients.
- Alternative resources (e.g., buses) to transport noncritically injured persons.
- Decontamination equipment for ambulatory and nonambulatory patients. Equipment should be rapidly deployable to the explosion site, a secondary treatment site, or a hospital.
- Secondary triage and treatment sites that can be determined and implemented within the community.
- A demobilization plan that includes access to mental health professionals.

biological, chemical, or nuclear materials may have been used in the explosion. Thus it is critical to personal safety not to enter the scene until the area is determined to be safe. The CDC has issued required resource guidelines and recommendations for EMS response to terrorist bombing attacks (Box 58-4).

SPECIFIC CHEMICAL THREATS

Specific chemicals that may be used in war and acts of terrorism include nerve agents, poisonous gases, and blister agents. The deliberate release of these chemicals in the form of toxic gas, liquid, or solid can poison persons or the environment.

Nerve Agents

Nerve agents were used in military conflicts in the Persian Gulf in the 1980s. They also were used in terrorist attacks in Japan in 1995. They are the most toxic and rapidly acting

of the known chemical warfare agents.[21] Nerve agents are similar to organophosphates in terms of their mechanism of action and the kinds of harmful effects they cause. (However, they are more potent [see Chapter 34].) Nerve agents inhibit the effects of acetylcholinesterase, which causes a cholinergic "overdrive" (*cholinergic crisis*). This disrupts the nerve transmissions in the central and peripheral nervous systems. The extent of poisoning caused by nerve agents depends on the amount, route, and length of exposure. Mildly or moderately exposed persons usually recover fully. Severely exposed persons are not likely to survive. The nerve agents discussed in this chapter are sarin (BG), soman (GD), tabun (GA), and VX.

NOTE
Allied forces in World War II coined these nerve agents as "G" series. They were so named because they were first developed by German scientists during the war.[22]

CRITICAL THINKING
Would you expect a fast or slow heart rate if the patient has been exposed to a nerve agent?

Sarin (also known as "BG") is a clear, colorless, and tasteless liquid that has no odor in its pure form. However, sarin can evaporate into a vapor (gas) and spread into the environment. The agent also mixes easily with water. This allows for contamination by persons touching or drinking water. Symptoms may begin within minutes to hours after exposure. They may include headache, salivation, chest pain, abdominal cramps, wheezing, fasciculations (i.e., muscle twitching), seizure, and respiratory failure that possibly can lead to death.

Soman (also known as "GD") is a clear, colorless, tasteless liquid with a slight camphor odor. The odor is similar to the smell of Vicks VapoRub or a rotting fruit odor. The agent can vaporize if heated. Compared with other nerve agents, soman is more volatile than VX but less volatile than sarin. (The higher the volatility of a chemical, the more likely it will evaporate and disperse into the environment.) Persons can be exposed to the vapor even if they do not come in contact with the liquid form. Symptoms may begin within seconds to hours after exposure. They include headache, salivation, chest pain, abdominal cramps, wheezing, fasciculations, seizure, and respiratory failure that possibly can lead to death.

Tabun (also known as "GA") is a clear, colorless, tasteless liquid with a faint fruity odor. The chemical can vaporize if heated. Thus persons can be exposed to the nerve agent by skin or eye contact or by inhalation. The agent also mixes easily with water. This allows for possible cutaneous exposure and exposure to the gastrointestinal tract if contaminated food or water is ingested. Moreover, secondary contamination is possible. This would occur from clothing or personal articles that have been contaminated by tabun vapor. Symptoms generally appear within a few seconds after exposure to tabun vapor and within 18 hours after exposure to liquid tabun.[21] Signs and symptoms of mild to moderate exposure to tabun include watery eyes, blurred vision, headache, weakness, cough, drooling, polyuria, excessive sweating, fasciculations, hypotension or hypertension, and cardiac abnormalities. With severe exposure, patients may experience loss of consciousness, seizures, and cardiorespiratory arrest. Severely poisoned patients are not likely to survive.

VX

VX (O-ethyl S-[2-(diisopropylamino)ethyl]methylphosphonothioate) is a thick, amber-colored, odorless liquid. It resembles motor oil and is the most potent of all nerve agents. VX is considered to be much more toxic when absorbed through the skin and somewhat more toxic by inhalation than are other nerve agents. VX is primarily a liquid exposure hazard. However, if heated to very high temperatures, it can turn into small amounts of vapor. Following release of VX into the air, persons can be exposed through skin contact, eye contact, or inhalation. VX also can be released into the water. This allows for exposure by ingestion or absorption. Symptoms will appear within a few seconds after exposure to the vapor form of VX. They will appear within a few minutes to up to 18 hours after exposure to the liquid form. Signs and symptoms of exposure are the same as those for other nerve agents.

TREATMENT

Treatment for exposure to nerve agents consists of quickly removing the agent from the body and supporting the patient's vital functions. If vapor exposure has occurred, the patient should be moved quickly to an area of fresh air. If the exposure occurred in an open-air environment, the patient should be moved uphill and upwind from the contamination site. Many nerve agents are heavier than air and will settle in low-lying areas. The patient's clothing should be removed and the patient should be decontaminated by trained personnel. A person's clothing and other contaminated surfaces can release nerve agents for about 30 minutes after exposure.[23] Thus secondary contamination is possible.

Atropine and *pralidoxime chloride* are antidotes (available in autoinjector kits, e.g., MARK I and DuoDote kits) for nerve agent toxicity (Table 58-1). They work by blocking the effects of acetylcholine (see Chapter 34 and the Emergency Drug Index). Large doses of these drugs and repeated administration may be required. *Diazepam* or *lorazepam* may be indicated if seizures are present. (The paramedic should consult with medical direction before administering these drugs if muscle twitching is present.) Once seizures begin, they can be almost impossible to stop. Caring for patients who have ingested a nerve agent should be guided by medical direction, a poison control center, or other authority.

TABLE 58-1 Recommendations for Prehospital Nerve Agent Therapy

Patient's Age	Antidotes* Mild/Moderate Symptoms[†]	Severe Symptoms[‡]	Other Treatment
Infant (birth to 2 yr)	Atropine: 0.05 mg/kg IM; 2-PAM-Cl: 15 mg/kg IM	Atropine: 0.1 mg/kg IM; 2-PAM-Cl: 25 mg/kg IM	For severe exposures, assisted ventilation should be started after administration of antidotes.
Child (2-10 yr)	Atropine: 1 mg IM; 2-PAM-Cl: 15 mg/kg IM	Atropine: 2 mg IM; 2-PAM-Cl: 25 mg/kg IM	
Adolescent (>10 yr)	Atropine: 2 mg IM; 2-PAM-Cl: 15 mg/kg IM	Atropine: 4 mg IM; 2-PAM-Cl: 25 mg/kg IM	**Repeat atropine (2 mg IM)** at 5- to 10-min intervals until secretions have diminished and breathing is comfortable or airway resistance has returned to near normal.
Adult	Atropine: 2-4 mg IM; 2-PAM-Cl: 600 mg IM Or 1 MARK I kit IM	Atropine: 6 mg IM; 2-PAM-Cl: 1800 mg IM Or 3 MARK I kits IM	
Elderly, frail	Atropine: 1 mg IM; 2-PAM-Cl: 10 mg/kg IM	Atropine: 2-4 mg IM; 2-PAM-Cl: 25 mg/kg IM	

Modified from Agency for Toxic Substances and Disease Registry: *Medical management guidelines (MMGs) for nerve agents,* www.atsdr.cdc.gov.
*2-PAM-Cl (2-pralidoxime chloride) solution must be prepared from an ampule containing 1 g of desiccated 2-PAM-Cl: inject 3 mL of saline and 5% distilled or sterile water into the ampule and shake well. The resulting solution is 3.3 mL of 300 mg/mL 2-PAM-Cl.
[†]Mild to moderate symptoms include localized sweating, muscle fasciculations, nausea, vomiting, weakness, and dyspnea.
[‡]Severe symptoms include unconsciousness, convulsions, apnea, and flaccid paralysis.

Poisonous Gases

Poisonous gases were popular weapons in World War I. Although they have not been used as toxic pulmonary inhalants by the military since 1918,[21] they are produced in large quantities worldwide for use in the industrial sector. They are widely available. Thus use of these gases for acts of terrorism is a possibility. The gases described in this section are chlorine and phosgene.

Chlorine is a yellow-green gas with an odor that has been described as a mixture of pineapple and pepper. Chlorine gas can be pressurized and condensed to change it into a liquid. In liquid form, chlorine can be shipped and stored. When liquid chlorine is released, it quickly vaporizes into a gas that stays close to the ground and spreads rapidly. If chlorine is released into the air, persons may be exposed to chlorine gas through skin or eye contact or by inhalation. If chlorine liquid is released into water, exposure can occur by touching or drinking contaminated water or by ingesting food that was prepared with the contaminated water. Like other chemical agents, the extent of poisoning depends on the amount, route, and duration of exposure to the agent. Signs and symptoms may include cough; chest pain; burning sensation in the nose, eyes, or throat; watery eyes; blurred vision; gastrointestinal disturbances; dermal burns from skin contact; and shortness of breath and dyspnea. Pulmonary edema can develop within 2 to 4 hours following inhalation of the gas.[24]

Phosgene (also known as "CG") is a poisonous gas that appears as a grayish white cloud and smells of newly mowed hay. With cooling and pressure, the gas can be condensed into a liquid so that it can be shipped and stored. When liquid phosgene is released, it quickly vaporizes into a gas that stays close to the ground and spreads rapidly. Inhaled phosgene damages the lungs, producing a burning sensation, cough, and labored breathing. Pulmonary edema with frothy sputum production may develop. Cutaneous exposure to the gas can result in skin or eye injury. Exposure also can occur by touching or drinking water contaminated with the gas or by ingesting food that was prepared with the contaminated water. In addition to the signs and symptoms noted previously for chlorine exposure, phosgene poisoning may cause hypotension and heart failure. In lethal doses, death can occur within 48 hours.[25]

TREATMENT

No antidotes exist for chlorine or phosgene poisoning. Treatment for exposure to these gases consists of removing them from the body as soon as possible and providing supportive medical care. All patients should be moved to an area of fresh air and to the highest ground possible (if exposure occurred in an open air space). The patient's clothing should be removed. Then the patient should be decontaminated by trained personnel.

Blister Agents

Blister agents or **vesicants** are chemicals with highly irritating properties that produce fluid-filled pockets on the skin and damage to the eyes, lungs, and other mucous membranes. In addition to cutaneous effects from exposure to these agents, blister agents also can cause loss of vision, convulsions, and respiratory failure. The gastrointestinal system, central nervous system, and bone marrow also can be affected through systemic absorption. Symptoms of exposure may be delayed until hours after exposure. The major chemicals in this category are sulfur mustard (H, HD, HT), nitrogen mustard (HN-1, HN-2, HN-3), and lewisite (L, L-1, L-2, L-3). Phosgene oxime is more of an urticant, producing irritation without blisters. However, the gas still is classified as a vesicant.

Mustard (*sulfur mustard* and *nitrogen mustard*) is an oily liquid that comes in a variety of colors ranging from brown to yellow. It may smell like garlic, onion, horseradish, or mustard itself. *Lewisite* is an oily, odorless liquid. Lewisite is more volatile than mustard and smells like geraniums in its gaseous state. (Unlike mustard, in which symptoms may be delayed, lewisite causes immediate pain and irritation on contact.) *Phosgene oxime* is a colorless solid or yellowish brown liquid. It may have a peppery or pungent odor. Like lewisite, this agent causes immediate pain and irritation on contact with the skin or mucous membranes.

TREATMENT

After ensuring personal safety (including the use of appropriate personal protective equipment), the initial assessment and treatment of the patient should begin with airway, ventilatory, and circulatory support as needed. Immediate decontamination may reduce damage to tissue. All skin exposures should be treated with standard burn care. Advanced cardiac life support protocols should be followed for any patient with cardiac or respiratory problems. Advanced trauma life support protocols should be followed for any trauma patient. The signs and symptoms may not develop for several hours following exposure to some blister agents. Thus a patient with a significant exposure should be evaluated by a physician. Patients who have only mild symptoms should be advised to seek physician evaluation if signs and symptoms worsen.

EXPLOSIVE THREATS

An **explosive** is a bomb. Bombs can be made from a variety of dangerous materials and can be made in a variety of sizes weighing several ounces to several thousand pounds. Explosives used by terrorists are often classified by the following categories[26]:

- *Unconventional use:* A conventional object used in an unconventional way to create mass destruction. In the September 11, 2001, attacks on the World Trade Center and the Pentagon, hijackers flew passenger planes into their intended targets, relying on the impact of the planes and their full fuel tanks to create havoc.

- *Vehicle bomb:* Usually large powerful devices that consist of a large quantity of explosives fitted with a timer or a remotely triggered detonator packed onto a car or truck.
- *Pipe bomb:* A quantity of explosives sealed into a length of metal or plastic pipe. A timing fuse usually controls detonation, but other methods can be used, including electronic timers, remote triggers, and motion sensors. These are the most common explosive devices and are at the opposite end of the scale from vehicle bombs in terms of size and power.
- *Satchel charge:* An old military term for an explosive device in a canvas-carrying bag. In recent history, "daypacks" or knapsacks have been used for the carrying device, and the explosives have contained antipersonnel materials such as nails and glass to inflict more casualties.
- *Package or letter bomb:* Explosive material contained in a package or letter that usually is triggered by opening of the package (Figure 58-6).

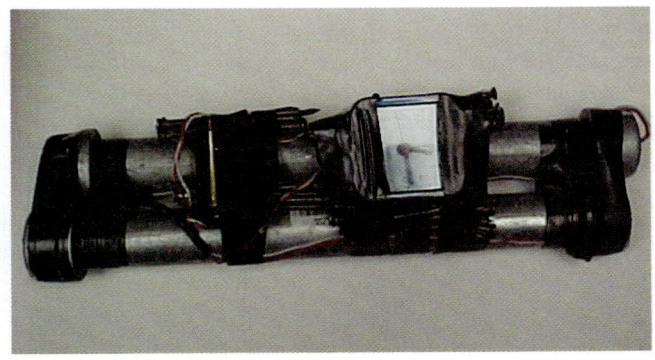

FIGURE 58-6 Pipe bomb.

> **NOTE**
>
> An **improvised explosive device** (IED) is also known as a *roadside bomb*. These devices are "homemade" bombs constructed of explosives attached to a detonator. IEDs are used in terrorist actions or in unconventional warfare. In 2007 they had become responsible for nearly two thirds of the American combat deaths in Iraq.[27]

> **SHOW ME THE EVIDENCE**
>
> The authors reviewed 35 research articles related to terrorist bombing incidents that involved 30 or more patients or that caused structural collapse of 1 or more floors. The 29 terrorist bombing incidents identified resulted in 8362 injured patients, and 903 died immediately. Deaths were highest (25%) in structural collapse bombings, followed by confined-space (8%) and open-air (4%) bombings. Most deaths occurred immediately with fewer deaths occurring in the ED or during hospital admission. Patients injured in structural collapse bombings had a higher incidence of fractures. Confined-space bombings produced a higher incidence of pressure-related injuries affecting the lungs and tympanic membranes, burns, and injuries to the spleen or liver. Soft tissue injury was more prevalent in open-air bombing patients. Although all injury types are found in all bombing locations, health care personnel should anticipate a higher incidence of specific injury based on the location of the bombing.

From Arnold JL, Hallpern P, Tsai M-C, et al: Mass casualty terrorist bombings: a comparison of outcomes by bombing type, *Ann Emerg Med* 43(2):263-273, 2004.

Emergency Care

Like the incendiary devices described earlier, the care for victims of an explosion may vary. Treatment may require only minor wound care to several persons. Or treatment could be a large-scale event. The larger events may have many patients and casualties. The incident may involve secondary explosions and chemical and biological threats. Thus it is critical to personal safety not to enter the scene

until the area is determined to be safe by the proper personnel. As described Chapter 37, there are many injuries that result from explosive forces, including *primary, secondary, tertiary, and quaternary blast injuries.*

> **LOOK AGAIN**
>
> See Chapter 37: Trauma Overview and Mechanism of Injury, pp. 1090-1092.

DEPARTMENT OF HOMELAND SECURITY

Following the terrorist attacks on the World Trade Center in New York City on September 11, 2001, the Department of Homeland Security was established through the Homeland Security Act of 2002 (H.R. 5005).[28] The three primary missions of the Department of Homeland Security are to (1) prevent terrorist attacks within the United States, (2) reduce America's vulnerability to terrorism, and (3) minimize the damage from potential attacks and natural disasters. To help meet these goals, a uniform national threat advisory system (NTAS) (Homeland Security Advisory System) was developed to inform federal agencies, state and local officials, and the private sector of terrorist threats and appropriate protective actions.

The Homeland Security Advisory System establishes two threat alerts that are issued when credible information is available. These alerts will include a clear statement that there is an **imminent threat** or **elevated threat**. Using available information, the alerts will provide a concise summary of the potential threat, information about actions being taken to ensure public safety, and recommended steps that individuals, communities, businesses and governments can take to help prevent, mitigate, or respond to the threat. The NTAS Alerts will be based on the nature of the threat: in some cases, alerts will be sent directly to law enforcement or affected areas of the private sector, while in others, alerts will be issued more broadly to the American people through both official and media channels.[29] NTAS

Alerts contain a **sunset provision** indicating a specific date when the alert expires—there will not be a constant NTAS Alert or blanket warning that there is an overarching threat. If threat information changes for an alert, the Secretary of Homeland Security may announce an updated NTAS Alert. All changes, including the announcement that cancels an NTAS Alert, will be distributed the same way as the original alert (Box 58-5).

GENERAL GUIDELINES FOR EMERGENCY RESPONSE

General guidelines for responding to a scene that may involve hazardous materials were described in Chapter 57. Many aspects of a WMD incident are comparable to other medical, trauma, and hazardous materials incidents. However, there are some significant differences. (1) Terrorists have been known to time secondary events (e.g., booby traps, additional bombs, and armed resistance) to injure

emergency responders. (2) A terrorist act is a criminal event. This means that the site becomes a crime scene. Thus everything is considered evidence of the crime. Fear and panic can be expected from the public, patients, and emergency responders. This makes scene safety, security, and crowd control major issues with which to contend. (3) Contingency plans for emergency responders at the scene and at destination facilities will need to be in place. These plans will help emergency responders to deal with the large numbers of upset, agitated, frightened, and injured patients. Large-scale events will likely involve local, state, and federal agency involvement.

CRITICAL THINKING

Why will correct, prompt information to the media be critical during a weapons of mass destruction event?

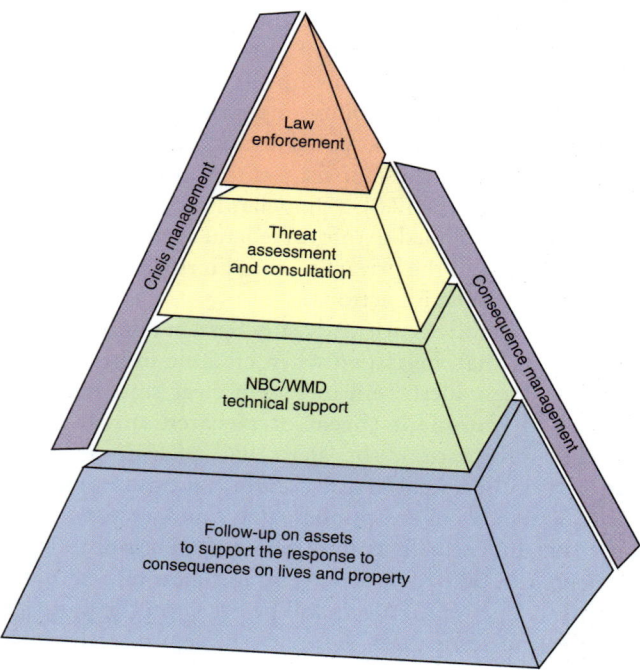

FIGURE 58-7 Relationship between crisis and consequence management.

Emergency Responder Guidelines

Emergency responder guidelines have been established by the Office of Justice Program, Office for Domestic Preparedness, to prepare for and respond to incidents of domestic terrorism. These incidents may involve chemical and biological agents and nuclear, radioactive, and explosive devices. Recommended guidelines for EMS providers are as follows[30]:

- Recognize hazardous materials incidents.
- Know the protocols used to detect the potential presence of WMD agents or materials.

■ Know and follow self-protection measures for WMD events and hazardous materials events.
■ Know procedures for protecting a potential crime scene.
■ Know and follow agency/organization scene security and control procedures for WMD and hazardous material events.
■ Possess and know how to use equipment properly to contact dispatchers or higher authorities to report information collected at the scene and to request

additional assistance or emergency response personnel. Know how to characterize a WMD event and be able to identify available response assets within the affected jurisdiction(s).

Finally, EMS agencies must be prepared to implement incident operations, provide personal and public safety measures, perform appropriate decontamination, and provide emergency medical care specific to the incident.

SUMMARY

■ There are five categories of weapons of mass destruction. These include biological, nuclear, incendiary, chemical, and explosive.
■ Biological agents include anthrax, botulism, plague, ricin, tularemia, and smallpox.
■ Person-to-person spread is possible in patients who are infected with plague or smallpox.
■ Nerve agents include sarin, soman, tabun, and VX. Exposure causes a cholinergic overdrive. The antidotes for nerve agent exposure are atropine and pralidoxime chloride.
■ Poisonous gases such as chlorine and phosgene cause severe respiratory problems. They also can cause skin

and eye injury. Move exposed patients to safety, remove their clothing, and treat their symptoms.
■ Dirty bombs could cause heat damage and radiation sickness, severe burns, and cancer.
■ The Department of Homeland Security has identified five terrorist threat levels. Each level has specific community-wide emergency preparedness activities to be taken.
■ Emergency responders at a WMD incident should recognize hazmat incidents, know protocols to detect WMD, use PPE, know crime-scene procedures, know how to activate more resources, and implement incident operations.

REFERENCES

1. Geissler E, editor: *Biological and toxin weapons today*, Oxford, England, 1986, Oxford University Press.
2. Osterholm MT, Schwartz J: *Living terrors: what America needs to know to survive the coming bioterrorist catastrophe*, New York, 2000, Delacorte Press.
3. Cowley G, Rogers A: The terrors of toxins, *Newsweek* Nov 1997.
4. Centers for Disease Control and Prevention: Biological and chemical terrorism: strategic plan for preparedness and response—recommendations of the CDC strategic planning workgroup, *MMWR* 49(RR04):1-14, 2000.
5. Congressional Research Service Report: *The BioWatch program: detection of bioterrorism*, no. RL 32152, www.fas.org/sgp/crs/terror/RL32152.html#1_2, accessed 10-28-10.
6. Centers for Disease Control and Prevention: *The Emergency Response Safety and Health Database (ERS-HD)*, www.cdc.gov/NIOSH/ershdb/about.html, accessed 10-28-10.
7. Kortepeter MG, Parker GW: *Potential biological weapons threats*, specialissue,www.cdc.gov/ncidod/eid/vol5no4/kortepeter.htm, accessed 10-28-10.
8. Dixon TC, Meselson M, Guillemin J, et al: Anthrax, *N Engl J Med* 341:815-826, 1999.
9. Centers for Disease Control and Prevention: *Fact sheet: anthrax information for health care providers*, www.bt.cdc.gov/agent/anthrax/anthrax-hcp-factsheet.asp#Cutaneous, accessed 12-30-03.
10. Centers for Disease Control and Prevention: Use of anthrax vaccine in response to terrorism: supplemental recommendations of the Advisory Committee on Immunization Practices, *MMWR* 51(45):1024-1026, 2002.
11. Dennis DT, Campbell GL: Plague and other Yersinia infections. In Fauci AS, Braunwald E, Kasper DL, et al, editors: *Harrison's principles of internal medicine*, ed 17, New York, 2008, McGraw-Hill Medical Publishing Division.
12. Centers for Disease Control and Prevention: *Facts about ricin*, www.bt.cdc.gov/agent/ricin/pdf/ricinfacts.pdf, accessed 7-6-10.
13. Wiser I, Balicer RD, Cohen D: An update on smallpox vaccine candidates and their role in bioterrorism related vaccination strategies, *Vaccine* 25(6):976-984, 2007.
14. Centers for Disease Control and Prevention: *Protecting Americans: smallpox vaccination program*, www.bt.cdc.gov/agent/smallpox/vaccination/vaccination-program-statement.asp, accessed 1-7-04.
15. Darling R, et al: *Bioterrorism: the May 2002 issue of the Emergency Medicine Clinics of North America*, Philadelphia, 2002, Saunders.
16. National Institute of Allergies and Infectious Diseases, Department of Health and Human Services, National Institutes of Health: *Tularemia treatment*, www.niaid.nih.gov/topics/tularemia/Pages/treatment.aspx, accessed 10-28-10.
17. Peterson AT, Lash RR, Carroll DS, et al: Geographic potential for outbreaks of Marburg hemorrhagic fever, *Am J Trop Med Hyg* 75(1):9-15, 2006.
18. Federal Emergency Management Agency: *Nuclear and radiological attack: are you ready? A guide to citizen preparedness*, www.fema.gov/areyouready/nuclear_blast.shtm, accessed 3-23-05.
19. U.S. Nuclear Regulatory Commission: *Fact sheet on dirty bombs*, www.nrc.gov/reading-rm/doc-collections/fact-sheets/dirty-bombs.html, accessed 1-13-04.

20. Centers for Disease Control and Prevention: *Updated in a moment's notice: surge capacity for terrorist bombings*, www.bt.cdc.gov/masscasualties/pdf/CDC_Surge-508.pdf, accessed 11-9-10.

21. Centers for Disease Control and Prevention: *Facts about tabun*, www.bt.cdc.gov/agent/tabun/basics/facts.asp, accessed 1-8-04.

22. Weinbroum A: Pathophysiological and clinical aspects of combat anticholinesterase poisoning, *Br Med Bull* 72:119-133, 2005.

23. Centers for Disease Control and Prevention: *Facts about tabun: emergency preparedness and response*, www.bt.cdc.gov/agent/tabun/basics/facts.asp, accessed 7-6-10.

24. Traub SJ: Respiratory agent attack (toxic inhalational injury). In Ciottone GR, editor: *Disaster medicine*, ed 3, Philadelphia, 2006, Mosby.

25. Leikin JB, Paloucek FP: *Poisoning and toxicology handbook*, New York, 2008, Informa Healthcare USA, Inc.

26. Virginia Department of Emergency Management: *Terrorist information: the facts—how to prepare, how to respond*, www.vaemergency.com/prepare/terrorismtoolkit/terrguide/weapons/incendiary.htm, accessed 11-9-04.

27. Atkinson R: The single most effective weapons against our deployed forces, *Washington Post* Nov 30, 2007.

28. Homeland Security Act of 2002 (HR 5005), Nov 25, 2002.

29. U.S. Department of Homeland Security: *NATS Public Guide*, http://www.dhs.gov/files/publications/ntas-public-guide.shtm, accessed 8-3-2011.

30. U.S. Department of Homeland Security, Office of Domestic Preparedness: *Emergency responder guidelines*, Washington, DC, August 2002, The Office.

SUGGESTED READINGS

CDC & EMS: Preparing for terrorist explosions, *JEMS* 31(4):26-29, 2006.

Crabtree J: Terrorist homicide bombings: a primer for preparation, *J Burn Care Res* 27(5):576-588, 2006.

Currance PL: *Medical response to weapons of mass destruction*, St Louis, 2005, Mosby.

Wightman JM, Gladish SL: Explosions and blast injuries, *PEC* 37(6):664-678, 2001.

Personal Protective Equipment for Chemical, Biological, Radiological, and Nuclear Agents

INTRODUCTION

Recent terrorist events in the United States underscore the importance of emergency response procedures for dealing with terrorist-related events involving chemical, biological, radiological, or nuclear (CBRN) agents. OSHA and NIOSH continue to work with other federal response agencies to provide accurate, current information to help prepare these on-scene responders.

PERSONAL PROTECTIVE EQUIPMENT (PPE) FOR CBRN RESPONSE

Emergency responses to hazardous substance releases including CBRNs are guided under OSHA's Hazardous Waste Operations and Emergency Response (HAZWOPER) Standard (29 CFR 1910.120[q]). Personal protective equipment is selected to meet the requirements of this standard and Subpart I. NIOSH has developed a respiratory protection approval specifically for CBRN exposures and the Department of Homeland Security also adopted guidelines for appropriate PPE. To use this guidance effectively, an employer must assess the risk of a hazardous substance release to the emergency responders and base the PPE selection on the level of knowledge relative to that risk. This kind of assessment is a typical safety and health evaluation with the unusual caveats that many of the agents are highly toxic by both skin contact and inhalation; typical indicators of exposure such as odor, smoke, or fumes may not be present; exposure monitoring is difficult for some of the compounds; and there may be a locally limited supply of CBRN-approved respirators for a large response during initial emergency operations. Based on the hazardous substances and conditions known to be present, the incident commander in charge of a response shall implement appropriate emergency operations, including selection of appropriate PPE for employees who respond. This includes, at a minimum, PPE meeting the criteria in 29 CFR 1910.156(e) for firefighting operations beyond the incipient stage, 29 CFR 1910.120(q)(3)(iii).

SITE CONTROL

Site control is an important part of managing any emergency response operation. Some guidance for zoning exists in 29 CFR 1910.120 Appendix C and in the NFPA 471 Standard (2002) (Hot, Warm, Cold) with hot denoting a contaminated area where adverse effects might be seen, warm being an initially clean area for close support and decontamination, and cold representing an area with no potential exposure. Other guidance from the DOT Emergency Response Guidebook (2004) provides for an "Initial Isolation Zone" where dangerous or life-threatening concentrations of a substance may exist or a "Protective Action Zone" where serious or irreversible health effects may be seen. The OSHA zones of Red, Yellow, and Green described below are available to be used by incident commanders as complementary guidance for personal protective equipment selection based on the level of knowledge about the WMD events. The use of the Red, Yellow, and Green zones is neither mandatory nor exclusionary of other site control concepts. It is intended to offer flexibility to an incident commander managing a large WMD event within the limitations of current first responder monitoring capabilities.

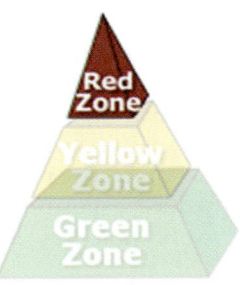

Red Zone. Areas where significant contamination with chemical, biological, radiological, or nuclear (CBRN) agents has been confirmed or is strongly suspected but area has not been characterized. The area is presumed to be life threatening from both skin contact and inhalation.

Level A protection is generally needed when the active release is still occurring, or the release has stopped but there is no information about the duration of the release or the airborne concentrations of CBRN agents. Respirators chosen initially for responders entering a known release area where CBRNs are suspected should be a positive-pressure self-contained breathing apparatus (SCBA) with a fully encapsulating protective suit until monitoring results allow for other decisions. Level A protection should be consistent with the description in HAZWOPER Appendix B and suits should be appropriate for CBRN agents—that is, they should meet the requirements of NFPA 1994-2001, have been tested by a third party such as the U.S. Army and Soldier and Biological Chemical

Command (SBCCOM), or have undergone other manufacturer testing. An NIOSH-certified CBRN SCBA respirator should be used, if available.

Other prudent work practices should include minimizing exposure time to that essential for lifesaving or initial monitoring, avoiding any unnecessary contact with surfaces or potentially contaminated material, and using natural ventilation flows to reduce exposure, mandatory decontamination, and postexit evaluation for signs and symptoms of exposure.

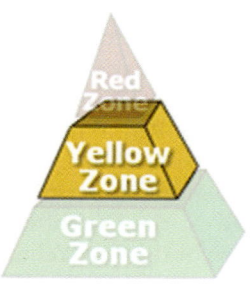

Yellow Zone. Areas where contamination with chemical, biological, radiological, or nuclear (CBRN) agents is possible but active release has ended and initial monitoring exists.

Areas in close proximity to the release area or that are known to be contaminated and certain job activities on the periphery of the event area should be considered for this zone. Risk factors that should be considered include determining the relative risk for job activities from inhalation based on available air monitoring results, skin contact and absorption potential, proximity to the event, and wind directions. Refer to the specific hazard information pages below to select personal protective equipment and limited work durations to reduce exposure to safe levels. Use the other prudent work practices listed for red zone exposures.

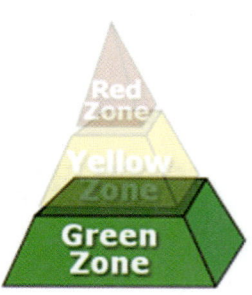

Green Zone. Areas where contamination with chemical, biological, radiological, or nuclear (CBRN) agents is unlikely. This zone covers the area beyond the expected significant dispersal range of the initial event and secondary contamination range caused by traffic and emergency responders.

Even in areas that are believed to be hazard-free, there may be a concern or potential for a minimal level of transient or unknown exposures in the aftermath of an event. The following suggestions for prudent work practices may reduce the amount of concern regarding this potential:

- Inform people of location of event and control zones.
- Provide information regarding signs and symptoms of exposure.
- Suggest a means for reporting suspected exposures.
- Suggest attention to general hygiene practices.
- Provide information on voluntary use of personal protective equipment.

Modified from U.S. Department of Labor, Occupational Safety and Health Administration: OSHA/NIOSH interim guidance—August 30, 2004: chemical-biological-radiological-nuclear (CBRN) personal protective equipment selection matrix for emergency responders, www.osha.gov/SLTC/emergencypreparedness/cbrnmatrix/index.html, accessed 2-4-11.

59 Putting It All Together: Assessment-Based Management

KEY TERMS

action plan A plan of action based on the patient's condition and the environment.

assessment-based management Comprehensive care that is based on patient assessment, the patient's history, and the physical examination.

contemplative approach An approach to patient care where a history is obtained and a physical examination is performed before providing patient care.

field impression An impression of the patient's condition that the paramedic makes from pattern recognition and gut instinct that results from experience.

labeling A form of assessment bias where a patient is assigned to a group or is stereotyped.

multitasking The ability to ask questions, take notes, and perform tasks while listening to the patient's answers.

pattern recognition The process of comparing gathered information with the paramedic's knowledge base of medical illness and disease.

presenting the patient The effective communication and transfer of patient information in the course of out-of-hospital and hospital care.

resuscitative approach An approach to patient care that recognizes the need for immediate intervention for patients with life-threatening illness or injury.

tunnel vision A narrow outlook; the focus of attention on a particular problem without proper regard for possible consequences or alternative approaches.

As has been stressed throughout this text, assessment is the foundation of patient care. To perform an effective assessment, the paramedic must be able to pull together many elements. These include pathophysiological principles and physical findings to formulate a field impression and implement a treatment plan for patients with common complaints. The paramedic gathers, evaluates, and synthesizes the information; makes appropriate decisions based on the information; and takes appropriate actions required for the patient's care. The purpose of this chapter is to review and emphasize how assessment-based management "puts it all together."

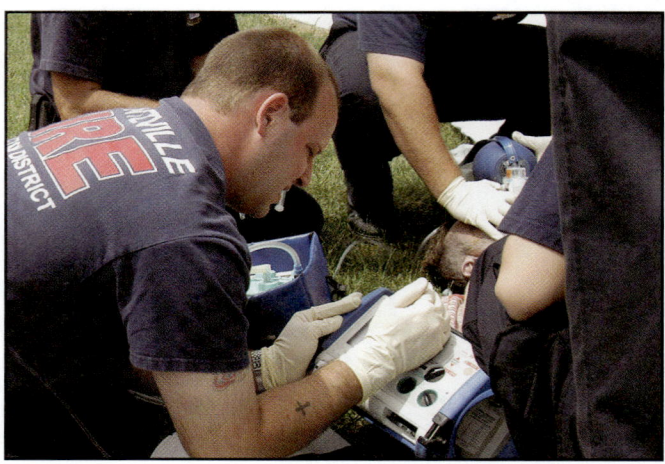

(Courtesy Ray Kemp, St. Charles, Mo.)

EFFECTIVE ASSESSMENT

Assessment-based management describes comprehensive care that is based on patient assessment. Effective assessment depends on the patient's history and the physical examination. The paramedic's knowledge of disease allows him or her to hold a high degree of suspicion for possible illness. This knowledge also helps the paramedic to focus the history toward the patient's complaint and associated problems. Likewise, the paramedic must focus the physical examination toward body systems associated with the complaint. Some field situations may impair the thoroughness of the examination. For example, unsafe scenes or entrapment may hinder this process. Still, the paramedic must not overlook the importance of the physical examination or perform it hastily.

Pattern Recognition

Once paramedics obtain the patient's history and perform the physical examination, they can compare the information gathered with their knowledge base of medical illness and disease. They must ask whether the history and physical examination match a recognized pattern of illness. This is known as **pattern recognition.** For example, consider a 55-year-old man with chest pain and shortness of breath. This person "matches" a recognized pattern for acute myocardial infarction. However, a 20-year-old woman with similar complaints and no family history of early myocardial events would not match this pattern. Other examples include a 4-year-old child who is in respiratory distress and drooling (matching a pattern for epiglottitis), and an elderly woman with distended neck veins and respiratory congestion who produces a pink, frothy sputum when she coughs. This person matches a pattern for congestive heart failure. Pattern recognition makes it possible for the paramedic to form a field impression and to begin a treatment plan (Box 59-1). Thus the greater the paramedic's knowledge base and quality of assessment, the greater the probability of appropriate decision making and quality patient care.

CRITICAL THINKING

How can pattern recognition lead you down the wrong path?

BOX 59-1 Pattern Recognition for Various Patient Presentations

Paramedics are trained in patient assessment and management priorities for patients with the following:

- Acute abdominal pain
- Allergic reactions
- Altered mental status
- Behavioral problems
- Chest pain
- Dyspnea
- Environmental or thermal problem
- Gastrointestinal bleeding
- Hazardous material or toxic exposure
- Medical and traumatic cardiac arrest
- Obstetrical or gynecological problems
- Seizures
- Syncope
- Trauma or multitrauma

Field Impression and Action Plan

The paramedic forms a **field impression** of the patient's condition from pattern recognition and from "gut instinct" that comes from experience (Figure 59-1). After making a field impression, it must be confirmed through the patient history and physical examination. Then, the paramedic can formulate an **action plan.** This plan is based on the patient's condition and the environment. Using the previous example of the two patients with chest pain, the field impression of the 55-year-old patient most likely leads to an action plan that includes electrocardiogram (ECG) monitoring, pulse oximetry, IV therapy, *aspirin* administration, pain relief measures, and perhaps drug therapy for dysrhythmias. The 20-year-old patient's action plan most likely includes ECG monitoring to evaluate and manage supraventricular tachycardia, pulse oximetry, and a more thorough assessment to detect a recent respiratory illness to rule out the possibility of pleurisy or pneumonia.

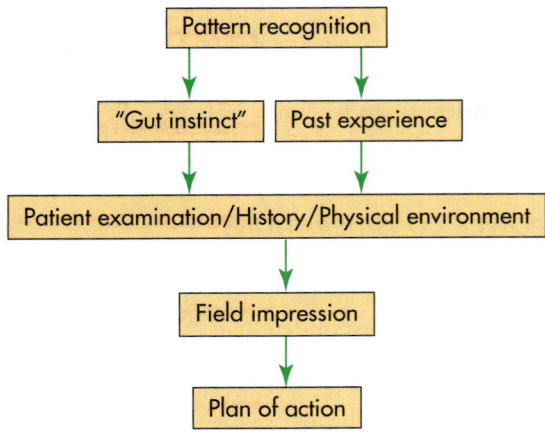

FIGURE 59-1 Matrix pattern.

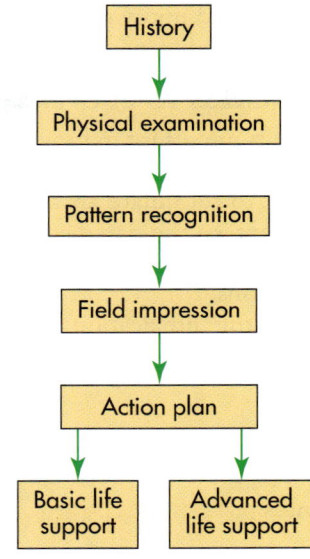

FIGURE 59-2 Effective assessment.

NOTE

The paramedic should not ignore a gut instinct. If something seems wrong, the paramedic should keep looking. Gut instincts often help the paramedic to identify subtle physical findings that are difficult to quantify (e.g., patient affect or dull and lackluster eyes).

Following the field impression and the action plan, the paramedic provides basic and advanced life support treatment (Figure 59-2). These treatments are based on knowledge of the protocols and on judgment—that is, knowing when and how to apply the protocols. Judgment also involves knowing when it is appropriate to deviate from the protocols. For example, consider the administration of *nitroglycerin* to a 58-year-old man complaining of ischemic chest pain. His blood pressure measurement is within normal range, but during the patient history he reveals he has taken Viagra within the past 18 hours. As described in Chapter 13, the administration of *nitroglycerin* can cause a lethal drop in blood pressure in these patients. Good judgment in this case would lead the paramedic to deviate from a common protocol used to manage normotensive patients with ischemic chest pain.

- Labeling and tunnel vision
- Environment
- Patient compliance
- Manpower considerations

CRITICAL THINKING

Have you ever seen any of these factors affect patient care?

SHOW ME THE EVIDENCE

These authors examined the elements of cognitive psychology involved in endotracheal intubation. They noted that this process is more complex than it may first appear because it is a psychomotor skill that not only involves skills-based processing but also sometimes requires algorithmic or rules-based processing; it can even encompass knowledge-based processing when unusual or difficult situations are present. They concluded that these findings have significant implications related to patient safety and EMS education.

From Wang HE, Katz S: Cognitive control and prehospital endotracheal intubation, *PEC* 11(2):234-239, 2007.

CRITICAL THINKING

How can you continue to improve your patient care judgment?

Factors That Affect Assessment and Decision Making

Many factors can affect the quality of assessment and decision making by the paramedic. The following factors are discussed in this section:
- Paramedic's attitude
- Patient's willingness to cooperate
- Distracting injuries

PARAMEDIC'S ATTITUDE

The paramedic must be professional and nonjudgmental in all actions. These traits are required to perform an effective assessment. A biased or judgmental attitude can "short circuit" the information-gathering process. This in turn can cause the paramedic to overlook important patient data. For example, a paramedic who assumes that an indigent patient is intoxicated may not consider complications from diabetes or drug use, head injury or hypoxia, or hypovolemia that may have resulted from an internal injury.

PATIENT'S WILLINGNESS TO COOPERATE

Patient cooperation is important in providing patient care. Patients who do not cooperate can complicate the patient assessment required to formulate an action plan. As discussed in earlier chapters, the paramedic should evaluate patients who are uncooperative, restless, or belligerent for the following conditions:

- Alcohol or other drug intoxication
- Head injury or concussion
- Hypoglycemia
- Hypothermia
- Hypovolemia
- Hypoxia
- Psychiatric illness
- Stroke

Distracting Injuries. Obvious but non–life-threatening injuries can distract the paramedic from performing a thorough assessment for more serious problems. Examples include open fractures and facial bleeding that is profuse. If necessary, these wounds should be covered with dressings during the assessment. This will help the paramedic to focus on the more serious problems.

LABELING AND TUNNEL VISION

Labeling and **tunnel vision** can lead to an inaccurate assessment and an incorrect field impression. For example, labeling a patient as "just another drunk" can lead to a biased assessment. Another example is labeling someone who has been transported by ambulance many times for minor complaints or imagined illness as a "frequent flyer." Tunnel vision is assuming an incorrect field impression based on a misplaced or an uneducated gut instinct, or focusing on only a portion of the presenting illness. Either of these assumptions can cause the paramedic to miss the "big picture." Like labeling, tunnel vision can result in a rushed judgment early in the patient assessment and an inappropriate action plan.

ENVIRONMENT

Factors in the environment can adversely affect assessment techniques and decision making at the scene. Examples include scene chaos, violent or dangerous situations, crowds of bystanders or other emergency workers, severe weather, and high noise levels. After ensuring personal safety, the paramedic should quickly establish control of the environment. This can include requesting the help of law enforcement personnel to control the scene so that appropriate assessment and care can be delivered without distraction.

PATIENT COMPLIANCE

The patient's willingness to cooperate and comply with the assessment may depend on his or her trust in the paramedic crew. For example, the patient who perceives the paramedic as competent and professional often provides a thorough history. The patient also often will agree to a complete physical examination. Other factors that can affect compliance are cultural and ethnic barriers. As described in Chapter 17 and Chapter 18, these may include language barriers and religious and social beliefs, among others.

MANPOWER CONSIDERATIONS

Depending on the EMS agency, crews may consist of a single paramedic and an EMT, two paramedics, or several types or groups of responders (e.g., EMS, fire and rescue, and police). In cases in which only EMS is involved and only one paramedic is at the scene, the paramedic will work with the EMT to develop a proper sequence for gathering information and providing care. If two paramedics are available, the information gathering and treatment often can occur simultaneously, with each paramedic assuming specific duties. If multiple responders and agencies are at the scene, roles and duties should be defined in advance. For example, one paramedic may be in charge of history taking and conferring with medical direction. Another paramedic may be in charge of treatment. The fire-rescue members may be in charge of extrication and gathering equipment. Finally, law enforcement personnel may be in charge of securing the scene.

CRITICAL THINKING

How can too many paramedics on the scene have a negative influence on patient assessment and care?

Assessment and Management Choreography

In cases where multiple responders are at the scene of an emergency, a coherent assessment can be difficult. A large emergency response may occur with multiple-tier response systems (e.g., EMS, fire, and police). The situation often is made more complex if the responders are trained at the same level (e.g., paramedic) without a clear direction for individual duties. Therefore members of the response team must have a preplan for deciding roles. The team can assign these predesignated roles by shift or crew, or they can rotate them among team members.

An example of a preplan for two paramedics is to assign one as the *team leader* and one as the *patient care person*. This type of plan must be flexible in rapidly changing field situations. However, the basic "game plan" allows others to participate and is important in preventing confusion at the scene. The following are sample responsibilities for each of the paramedics in this type of preplan:

1. Team leader responsibilities
   a. Accompanies the patient to definitive care
   b. Establishes contact and a dialogue with the patient
   c. Obtains the history
   d. Performs the physical examination

e. Presents the patient and gives verbal reports over the radio or after definitive care
f. Completes all documentation
g. Tries to maintain the overall patient perspective and provides leadership to the team by designating tasks and coordinating transportation
h. Designates and actively participates in critical interventions during the resuscitative phase of the primary survey
i. Acts as initial EMS command in multiple-casualty situations (see Chapter 54)
j. Interprets the electrocardiogram, communicates with medical direction and relays drug orders, controls access to bags, and documents drug administration and effects during advanced cardiac life support

2. Patient care person responsibilities
   a. Provides scene cover (watches the team leader's back)
   b. Gathers scene information and talks to family members and bystanders
   c. Obtains vital signs
   d. Performs skills and interventions as requested by the team leader (e.g., attaches monitor leads, provides oxygen, initiates intravenous access, administers drugs, and obtains transportation equipment)
   e. Acts as triage group leader in multiple-casualty situations
   f. Administers drugs; monitors endotracheal tube placement, pulse oximetry, and basic life support interventions during advanced cardiac life support

THE "RIGHT STUFF"

Having the "right stuff" means carrying the right equipment to the patient's side. Not having the "right stuff" can compromise care and also can cause panic and confusion. The paramedic crew should always be prepared for the worst event. They should carry essential equipment to manage every aspect of patient care, including cardiac monitoring and defibrillation (Box 59-2). The concept of having the "right stuff" can be compared with backpacking. A person who is backpacking must have essential items that are downsized to facilitate rapid movement with minimum weight and bulk.

OPTIONAL "TAKE-IN" EQUIPMENT

In addition to essential equipment for the EMS crew, other equipment can be carried to the patient's side. For example, most EMS systems require that the paramedic carry drug bags and kits for IV supplies. This includes those agencies that have nontransporting emergency vehicles staffed by paramedic personnel as well. Most EMS systems require that paramedics carry these supplies even though they are not appropriate for every patient contact. Other factors that can affect what equipment the paramedic carries to the patient's side depend on the following:

- Local protocol
- Standing order flexibility

BOX 59-2 Essential Items for All Aspects of Patient Care

Personal Protection
Eye shields
Gloves
Gowns
Masks

Airway Control
Endotracheal tubes, stylettes, and tape
Laryngoscope and blades
Nasal airways
Oral airways
Rigid Yankauer and flexible suction catheters
Suction (electrical or manual)

Breathing
Large-bore intravenous catheter for thoracic decompression
Manual ventilation bag-valve-mask device
Mouth-powered ventilation device (pocket mask)
Occlusive dressings
Oxygen masks, cannulae, and extension tubing
Pulse oximetry
Oxygen tank and regulator
Spare masks

Circulation
Bandages and tape
Blood pressure cuff and stethoscope
Dressings
Infection-control supplies (gloves and eye shields)
Intravenous fluids, catheters, and tubing
Note pad and pen or pencil or electronic device

Disability and Dysrhythmia
Cardiac monitor and defibrillator
Flashlight
Rigid collar

Exposure
Scissors
Space blanket or other device to cover and protect the patient

---

- Number of paramedic responders
- Difficulty in accessing patients

Other items that are essential on every call include patient care reports, worksheets, or computer notation devices. Personal items such as pens or pencils, wristwatches, flashlights, and portable radios or cellular phones will also be needed. Personal protective equipment should be readily available on every response.

> **CRITICAL THINKING**
> Have you been on ambulance calls when you did not have the right equipment? How did it affect patient care?

GENERAL APPROACH TO THE PATIENT

A calm and orderly manner is important for the paramedic when approaching a patient. As described in Chapter 1, the paramedic must look and act the part of a professional. This, in addition to a caring and confident bedside manner, will help gain the patient's trust and cooperation. Patients may not be able to rate medical performance; however, they generally are very good at rating "people skills" and service.

As previously described, a preplan should be in effect to prevent confusion at the scene and improve the accuracy of patient assessment. Ideally, one team member should be responsible for talking to the patient. This member should use an active and concerned dialogue that allows for careful listening. Taking notes when acquiring the history demonstrates a thorough assessment to the patient and prevents the paramedic from asking repetitive questions. All essential equipment should be at the patient's side, and the EMS crew should be ready to provide resuscitative care if needed. An initial survey of the scene can offer important clues to help the paramedic formulate an impression. Initial size-up information that is useful in all EMS responses includes hazards and potential hazards, mechanism of injury or illness, and the number of patients at the scene.

Setting the Tone for the Patient Encounter

Two approaches in the primary survey set the tone for the patient encounter. The first is the resuscitative approach. The second is the contemplative approach. The **resuscitative approach** recognizes the need for immediate intervention for patients who have life-threatening illness or injury such as the following:

- Cardiorespiratory arrest
- Coma or altered level of consciousness
- Major trauma
- Possible cervical spine injury
- Respiratory distress or failure
- Seizures
- Shock or hypotension
- Unstable cardiac rhythms

If a life-threatening problem is present, the paramedic crew must take resuscitative action. History taking and other details should be delayed until immediate resuscitation measures have been provided. If immediate intervention to manage life threats is not required, the paramedic can use the **contemplative approach.** With this approach, the patient history is obtained and physical examination is performed before providing patient care.

In any patient care encounter, the paramedic may need to move the patient immediately to the emergency vehicle if any of the following occur:

- The paramedic cannot provide lifesaving interventions at the patient's side.

- The scene is too unstable or unsafe.
- The scene is too chaotic to allow thorough assessment.
- Inclement weather hinders assessment and care.

"Looking to Find"

Paramedics must find something before they can treat or report it. To find something, it must be suspected. Therefore during the primary survey, the paramedic must actively look for any problems that pose a threat to life. The assessment must be systematic so that the patient's chief complaint can be rapidly determined. The paramedic must then assess the degree of distress, obtain baseline vital signs, and stay focused on the patient's history and physical findings. A mental "rule-out list" often is a good approach in "looking to find." This is a list that considers the most serious problems *first* that could cause the patient's signs and symptoms.

Experience assists the paramedic in developing the ability for multitasking. In relation to health care, **multitasking** is the ability to ask questions, take notes, and perform tasks while listening to the patient's answers. In time the paramedic will gain the level of experience required for multitasking. Until then it is best to ask direct questions and then carefully listen to the patient's response. Important clues can be lost by not listening. If a particular task is required while the paramedic is obtaining a patient history, a partner should provide the patient care measure if possible. The patient's ability to describe symptoms and the paramedic's ability to listen may greatly influence the assessment. The paramedic should remember that the severity and location of the patient's pain may not always correlate well with some potentially life-threatening conditions. For example, a patient with myocardial infarction may at first complain of pain only in the arm or shoulder or some other minor discomfort (e.g., indigestion). The paramedic's role is to rapidly assess and provide treatment for the worst-case scenario.

BOX 59-3 Discrete Areas of Information

1. Patient identification, age, gender, and degree of distress
2. Chief complaint
3. Present illness or injury
   a. Pertinent details about the present problem
   b. Pertinent negatives (expected findings that are absent)
4. Medical history, including allergies and medications
5. Physical findings
   a. Vital signs
   b. Pertinent positive findings
   c. Pertinent negative findings
6. Assessment, including paramedic impression
7. Plan
   a. What has been done
   b. Orders requested

PRESENTING THE PATIENT

Presenting the patient in the course of out-of-hospital and in-hospital care is twofold. It refers to the skills of effective communication and to the effective transfer of patient information. Patient presentation is often a weak link in the chain of patient care despite its importance in every patient encounter.

The paramedic routinely provides patient presentation face to face, over the phone or radio, and in writing. These communication skills are essential and help the paramedic to establish trust and credibility with co-workers and other members of the health care teams. Good presentations suggest effective patient assessment and care to the listener, and vice versa. Poor presentation can compromise patient care. This may occur when the paramedic does not convey patient needs and status effectively to medical direction. As described in Chapter 17, the following are characteristics of an effective patient presentation:

- The presentation is concise, usually lasting less than 1 minute.
- The presentation is usually free of extensive medical jargon.
- The presentation follows the same basic information pattern.
- The presentation generally follows a standard format.
- The presentation includes pertinent findings and pertinent negatives.

When communicating a patient presentation, the paramedic should *begin the report with the end in mind*. For instance, the paramedic should anticipate discrete areas of information that others will question and be ready to provide those details (Box 59-3). Communicating a patient presentation requires experience. Until then, it may be best to use a preprinted card or other memory device (e.g., the SOAP format or similar method). These aids will help the paramedic to organize information and assessment findings.

CRITICAL THINKING
Can you think of any areas of improvement for your skills in "presenting the patient"?

SUMMARY

- Assessment-based management "puts it all together." This means that the paramedic gathers, evaluates, and synthesizes information. The paramedic makes proper decisions based on the information. Then the paramedic takes the appropriate actions required for the patient's care.
- Factors that can affect the quality of assessment and decision making include the paramedic's attitude, the patient's willingness to cooperate, distracting injuries, labeling and tunnel vision, the environment, patient compliance, and considerations of personnel availability.
- Promoting a coherent assessment is the goal. Thus members of the response team should have a preplan for determining roles and responsibilities.

- The paramedic crew should always be prepared for the worst event. They should carry essential equipment to manage every aspect of patient care.
- A calm and orderly manner is essential for the paramedic. This is especially the case when approaching a patient. During the initial assessment the paramedic must look actively for problems that pose a threat to life.
- Presenting the patient in the course of prehospital and hospital care is twofold. Presentation refers to the skills of effective communication. Presentation also refers to the effective transfer of patient information.

SUGGESTED READINGS

Croskerry P: Achieving quality in clinical decision making: cognitive strategies and detection of bias, *Acad Emerg Med* 9(11):1184-1204, 2002.

Croskerry P: Cognitive forcing strategies in clinical decision making, *Ann Emerg Med* 41(1):110-120, 2003.

Croskerry P: Diagnostic failure: a cognitive and affective approach, *Adv Patient Safety* 2:241-254, 2008.

Jensen JL, Croskerry P, Ah T: Paramedic clinical decision making during high acuity emergency calls: design and methodology of a Delphi study, *BMC Emerg Med* 9:17, 2009.

Meisel ZF, Mathew R, Wydro G, et al: Multicenter validation of the Philadelphia EMS Admission Rule (PEAR) to predict hospital admission in adult patient using out-of-hospital data, *Acad Emerg Med* 16(6):519-525, 2009.

Emergency Drug Index

Abciximab
Activated charcoal
Adenosine
Albuterol
Alteplase
Amiodarone
Aspirin
Atenolol
Atropine sulfate
Calcium chloride
Dexamethasone
Dextrose 50%
Diazepam
Digoxin
Digoxin Immune Fab
Diltiazem
Diphenhydramine
Dobutamine
Dopamine
Epinephrine
Epinephrine racemic
Eptifibatide
Esmolol
Etomidate
Fentanyl
Flumazenil
Furosemide
Glucagon
Haloperidol lactate
Heparin sodium
Hydromorphone
Hydroxocobalamin
Ibutilide
Insulin
Ipratropium
Isoproterenol
Ketamine
Ketorolac tromethamine
Labetalol
Levalbuterol
Lidocaine
Lorazepam
Magnesium sulfate
Mannitol
Meperidine
Methylprednisolone
Metoclopramide
Metoprolol
Midazolam hydrochloride
Morphine sulfate

Naloxone
Nitroglycerin
Nitropaste
Nitroprusside
Nitrous oxide/oxygen
Norepinephrine
Ondansetron
Oxygen
Oxytocin
Pancuronium
Phenytoin
Pralidoxime
Procainamide
Promethazine
Propranolol
Reteplase
Sodium bicarbonate
Sotalol
Streptokinase
Succinylcholine
Tenecteplase
Tetracaine
Thiamine
Tirofiban
Vasopressin
Vecuronium
Verapamil

DRUG IDENTIFICATION GUIDE

The *Emergency Drug Index* is a list of commonly prescribed medications that are used in prehospital care; it is not intended to be a complete guide to all emergency medications. For additional drug information, consult other standard references. Drugs included in this index are listed alphabetically by generic name. Common trade names are shown in parentheses following the generic listing.

NOTE
The way in which drugs are packaged and supplied varies by manufacturer. It is important that paramedics verify how a particular drug is supplied by their EMS service. In addition, paramedics should verify the recommended dose or formula, know the indications and contraindications of any drug they administer, and take all safety precautions. Any concerns regarding the dose or administration of any drug should be guided by medical direction.

PREGNANCY CATEGORY RATINGS FOR DRUGS

Drugs have been categorized by the Food and Drug Administration according to the level of risk to the fetus. These categories are listed for each drug herein under "Pregnancy safety" and are interpreted as follows:

Category A: Controlled studies in women fail to demonstrate a risk to the fetus in the first trimester, and there is no evidence of risk in later trimesters; the possibility of fetal harm appears to be remote.

Category B: Either (1) animal reproductive studies have not demonstrated a fetal risk but there are no controlled studies in pregnant women or (2) animal reproductive studies have shown an adverse effect (other than decreased fertility) that was not confirmed in controlled studies on women in the first trimester and there is no evidence of risk in later trimesters.

Category C: Either (1) studies in animals have revealed adverse effects on the fetus and there are no controlled studies in women or (2) studies in women and animals are not available. Drugs in this category should be given only if the potential benefit justifies the risk to the fetus.

Category D: Positive evidence of human fetal risk exists, but the benefits for pregnant women may be acceptable despite the risk, as in life-threatening diseases for which safer drugs cannot be used or are ineffective. An appropriate statement must appear in the "Warnings" section of the labeling of drugs in this category.

Category X: Studies in animals or human beings have demonstrated fetal abnormalities, there is evidence of fetal risk based on human experience, or both; the risk of using the drug in pregnant women clearly outweighs any possible benefit. The drug is contraindicated in women who are or may become pregnant. An appropriate statement must appear in the "Contraindications" section of the labeling of drugs in this category.

ABCIXIMAB (REOPRO)

CLASS

Glycoprotein IIb/IIIa inhibitor

DESCRIPTION

Glycoprotein IIb/IIIa inhibitors inhibit the integrin GP IIb/IIIa receptor in the membrane of the platelets. As a result, they inhibit the common final pathway activation of platelet aggregation. Abciximab (in combination with aspirin and heparin) is indicated for use in patients undergoing PCI as well as for the treatment of unstable angina or NSTEMI infarction when PCI is planned within 24 hr.

ONSET AND DURATION

Onset: 2 hr
Duration: Platelet aggregation restored within 24-48 hr after infusion is stopped

INDICATIONS

Patients with NSTEMI, unstable angina, or PCI within 24 hr

CONTRAINDICATIONS

Active internal bleeding
Bleeding disorder
History of intracranial hemorrhage, neoplasm, AV malformation, aneurysm, or stroke within 2 years
Major surgical procedure or trauma within 6 weeks
Aortic dissection, pericarditis, and severe hypertension
Hypersensitivity to any GP IIb/IIIa inhibitor
Low platelet count (<100,000/mm^3)

ADVERSE REACTIONS

Anaphylactoid reaction/anaphylactic shock may occur
Bleeding (secondary to drug-induced platelet dysfunction)
GI bleeding
Hematemesis
Hematuria
Hypotension
Intracranial bleeding
Platelet dysfunction
Retroperitoneal bleeding
Stroke
Thrombocytopenia

DRUG INTERACTIONS

Concomitant use of other agents that may affect hemostasis, such as anticoagulants, other platelet inhibitors, NSAIDs, and thrombolytic agents, may be associated with an increased risk of bleeding.

HOW SUPPLIED

2 mg/mL (must be given with heparin)

DOSAGE AND ADMINISTRATION (ADULT)

PCI only: 0.25 mg/kg IV bolus (10-60 min before procedure); then 0.125 mcg/kg/min (max 10 mcg/min) IV infusion for 12 hr
ACS with planned PCI within 24 hr: 0.25 mg/kg IV bolus; then 10 mcg/min IV infusion for 18-24 hr, concluding 1 hr after PCI

SPECIAL CONSIDERATIONS

Pregnancy safety: Category C
Readministration may cause hypersensitivity reaction.

ACTIVATED CHARCOAL (ACTIDOSE-AQUA, ACTIDOSE, LIQUI-CHAR)

CLASS

Adsorbent, antidote

DESCRIPTION

Activated charcoal is a fine black powder that binds and adsorbs ingested toxins. Once the drug binds to the activated charcoal, the combined complex is excreted in the feces.

ONSET AND DURATION

Onset: Immediate
Duration: Continual while in gastrointestinal tract; reaches equilibrium once saturated

INDICATIONS

Many oral poisonings and medication overdoses

CONTRAINDICATIONS

Corrosives, caustics, petroleum distillates (relatively ineffective and may induce vomiting)

ADVERSE REACTIONS

May indirectly induce nausea and vomiting.
May cause constipation or mild, transient diarrhea.

DRUG INTERACTIONS

Syrup of ipecac (adsorbed by activated charcoal and will result in vomiting of the charcoal)

HOW SUPPLIED

25 g (black powder)/25g/125mL bottle (200 mg/mL)
50 g (black powder)/50g/240ml bottle (200 mg/mL)
Other sizes include 15 g and 30 g, bottles and squeeze tubes. Most products come premixed (not powder) with water (aqueous preparations) or with sorbitol, a cathartic.

DOSAGE AND ADMINISTRATION

From 1 to 2 g/kg body mass (larger amounts if food is also present), prepared in a slurry and administered PO or slowly via nasogastric or orogastric tube
Adult: 30-100 g
Pediatric (1-12 yr): 15-30 g or 1-2 g/kg
Infant (less than 1 yr): 1 g/kg

SPECIAL CONSIDERATIONS

Pregnancy safety: Category C
Charcoal frequently is administered to pregnant patients, and the potential benefit versus risk is very high. Because charcoal remains within the gastrointestinal tract, its risk to the fetus virtually is eliminated, unless the charcoal and other stomach contents are aspirated.
Activated charcoal also may be known as "AC."
Activated charcoal is relatively insoluble in water.
Activated charcoal may blacken feces.
Activated charcoal must be stored in a closed container.
Different charcoal preparations may have varying adsorptive capacity.
Activated charcoal does not adsorb all drugs and toxic substances (e.g., phenobarbital, aspirin, cyanide, lithium, iron, lead, and arsenic).

ADENOSINE (ADENOCARD)

CLASS

Endogenous nucleoside, miscellaneous antidysrhythmic

DESCRIPTION

Adenosine primarily is formed from the breakdown of adenosine triphosphate. Adenosine triphosphate and adenosine are found in every cell of the human body and have a wide range of metabolic roles. Adenosine slows supraventricular tachycardias by decreasing electrical conduction through the atrioventricular node without causing negative inotropic effects. It also acts directly on sinus pacemaker cells and vagal nerve terminals to decrease chronotropic (heart rate) activity. First drug of choice for most forms of stable, narrow-complex SVT. May be considered for unstable narrow-complex reentry tachycardia while preparing for cardioversion. Adenosine does not convert atrial fibrillation, atrial flutter, or VT.

ONSET AND DURATION

Onset: Immediate
Duration: 10 sec

INDICATIONS

First drug for most forms of narrow-complex paroxysmal supraventricular tachycardia and dysrhythmias associated with bypass tracts such as Wolff-Parkinson-White (WPW) syndrome in adults and pediatric patients.
In undifferentiated regular stable wide-complex tachycardia, IV adenosine may be considered relatively safe. It may convert the rhythm to sinus, and may help diagnose the underlying rhythm.

CONTRAINDICATIONS

Drug-induced tachycardia
Second- or third-degree atrioventricular block
Hypersensitivity to adenosine
Atrial flutter, atrial fibrillation, ventricular tachycardia, WPW with atrial fibrillation/flutter. (Adenosine is not effective in converting these rhythms to sinus rhythm.)

ADVERSE REACTIONS

Facial flushing
Light-headedness
Paresthesias
Headache
Diaphoresis
Palpitations
Chest pain
Flushing
Hypotension

Shortness of breath

Transient periods of sinus bradycardia, sinus pause, or bradyasystole

Ventricular ectopy (fibrillation, flutter, tachycardia, torsades de pointes)

Nausea

Metallic taste

DRUG INTERACTIONS

Methylxanthines (e.g., caffeine and theophylline) antagonize the action of adenosine.

Dipyridamole potentiates the effect of adenosine; reduction of adenosine dose may be required.

Carbamazepine may potentiate the atrioventricular-nodal blocking effect of adenosine.

HOW SUPPLIED

Parenteral for IV injection

3 mg/mL in 2-mL and 5-mL flip-top vials

DOSAGE AND ADMINISTRATION

Adult: Initial dose: 6-mg rapid IV bolus over 1-3 sec, followed by a 20-mL saline bolus; then elevate extremity. A second dose (12 mg) may be given in 1-2 min if needed.

Injection technique: Place patient in mild reverse Trendelenburg position before drug administration. Record ECG during drug administration. Draw up adenosine and flush in 2 separate syringes. Attach both syringes to the IV injection port closest to the patient. Clamp IV tubing above injection port. Push adenosine as quickly as possible (1-3 sec). Maintain pressure on adenosine plunger while pushing saline flush as rapidly as possible after adenosine. Unclamp IV tubing.

Pediatric: Initial dose 0.1 mg/kg IV/IO (max single dose: 6 mg); second dose 0.2 mg/kg IV/IO rapid push; followed with 5-10 mL NS flush[1]

SPECIAL CONSIDERATIONS

Pregnancy safety: Category C

A brief period of asystole (up to 15 sec) following conversion, followed by resumption of normal sinus rhythm, is common after rapid administration.

Reduce initial dose to 3 mg in patients receiving dipyridamole or carbamazepine, in heart transplant patients, or if given by central venous access.

Patients taking theophylline or caffeine may require larger doses of adenosine.

Deterioration (including hypotension) may result if given for irregular, polymorphic wide-complex tachycardia/VT.

Adenosine may produce bronchoconstriction in patients with asthma and in patients with bronchopulmonary disease.

ALBUTEROL (PROVENTIL AND OTHERS)

CLASS

Sympathomimetic, bronchodilator, beta$_2$ agonist

DESCRIPTION

Albuterol is a sympathomimetic that is selective for beta$_2$-adrenergic receptors. It relaxes smooth muscles of the bronchial tree and peripheral vasculature by stimulating adrenergic receptors of the sympathetic nervous system.

ONSET AND DURATION

Onset: 5-8 min after inhalation

Duration: 2-6 hr after inhalation

INDICATIONS

Relief of bronchospasm in patients with reversible obstructive airway disease

Prevention of exercise-induced bronchospasm

Anaphylaxis

Hyperkalemia

CONTRAINDICATIONS

Prior hypersensitivity reaction to albuterol or levalbuterol

Cardiac dysrhythmias associated with tachycardia (precaution)

ADVERSE REACTIONS

Usually dose-related

Restlessness, apprehension

Dizziness

Palpitations, tachycardia

Dysrhythmias

Tremors

DRUG INTERACTIONS

Other sympathomimetics may exacerbate adverse cardiovascular effects.

MAO inhibitors and tricyclic antidepressants may potentiate effects on the vasculature (vasodilation).

Beta blockers may antagonize albuterol.

Albuterol may potentiate diuretic-induced hypokalemia.

HOW SUPPLIED

Metered-dose inhaler: 90 mcg/metered spray (17-g canister with 200 inhalations)

Solution for aerosolization: 0.5% (5 mg/mL); 0.083% (2.5 mg) in 3-mL unit dose/nebulizer

DOSAGE AND ADMINISTRATION

Bronchial Asthma/Anaphylaxis/Hyperkalemia

Adult:

Metered-dose inhaler: 1-2 inhalations (90-180 mcg) q 4-6 hr (wait 5 min between inhalations); max 12 inhalations/day

Solution: 2.5 mg (0.5 mL of 0.5% solution) diluted to 3 mL with 0.9% NS (0.083% solution); administer over 5-15 min; 3-4 times/day by nebulizer

NOTE: In settings of severe asthma exacerbation, 4 inhalations or 5 mg in 2.5-3 mL is indicated.

Pediatric:

Metered-dose inhaler: 4-8 puffs (inhalation) as needed, with spacer if not intubated

Solution: 0.01-0.03 mL (0.05-0.15 mg)/kg/dose to max of 0.50 mL/dose diluted in 2 mL of 0.9% NS; may be repeated q 20 min

Nebulized albuterol: <20 kg: 2.5 mg/dose (inhalation); >20 kg: 5 mg/dose (inhalation)

SPECIAL CONSIDERATIONS

Pregnancy safety: Category C

Albuterol may precipitate angina pectoris and dysrhythmias.

Albuterol should be used with caution in patients with diabetes mellitus, hyperthyroidism, prostatic hypertrophy, seizure disorder, or cardiovascular disorder.

In prehospital emergency care, albuterol should be administered only via inhalation.

ALTEPLASE (t-PA)

CLASS

Fibrinolytic

DESCRIPTION

Tissue plasminogen activator is a naturally occurring enzyme that has been mass-produced using recombinant DNA technology. The enzyme binds to fibrin-bound plasminogen at the site of an arterial clot, thus converting plasminogen to plasmin. Plasmin digests the fibrin strands of the clot, causing clot lysis and restoration of perfusion to the occluded artery. In prehospital care, fibrinolytic agents are used in treating selected patients with acute evolving myocardial infarction. (Other indications include ischemic stroke, deep vein thrombosis, peripheral artery embolism, IV catheter occlusion.)

ONSET AND DURATION

Onset: Clot lysis often occurs within 30 min.
Duration: 30-45 min (80% cleared in 10 min)

INDICATIONS

Acute evolving myocardial infarction
Massive pulmonary emboli
Deep venous thrombosis
Arterial thrombosis and embolism
To clear arteriovenous cannulae
Acute stroke

CONTRAINDICATIONS

Active bleeding or known bleeding disorder
Recent surgery (within 2-3 weeks)
Recent cerebrovascular accident
History of intracranial hemorrhage
Prolonged cardiopulmonary resuscitation
Recent intracranial or intraspinal surgery
Recent significant trauma (particularly head trauma)
Seizure at onset of stroke symptoms
Uncontrolled hypertension
Recent gastrointestinal bleeding

ADVERSE REACTIONS

Bleeding (gastrointestinal, genitourinary, intracranial, other sites)
Allergic reactions
Hypotension
Chest pain
Reperfusion dysrhythmias
Abdominal pain

DRUG INTERACTIONS

Acetylsalicylic acid may increase risk of bleeding (and may be beneficial in improving overall effectiveness).
Heparin and other anticoagulants also may increase risk of bleeding and improve overall effectiveness.

HOW SUPPLIED

50, 100 mg/vial with 50, 100 mL, and 2 mg (Cathflo) of diluent, respectively. May dilute further with equal amounts of 0.9% sodium chloride or D_5W.

DOSAGE AND ADMINISTRATION (BASED ON PATIENT'S WEIGHT)

Adult STEMI: Give 15 mg IV bolus, then 0.75 mg/kg over next 30 min (not to exceed 50 mg), and then 0.5 mg/kg over 60 min (not to exceed 35 mg); maximum total dose 100 mg. (Other doses may be prescribed by medical direction; different dosing is indicated for stroke.)
Pediatric: Safety not established

SPECIAL CONSIDERATIONS

Pregnancy safety: Category C
Obtain blood sample for coagulation studies before administration.
Gently roll—do not shake—the vial to mix powder with liquid.
Closely monitor vital signs.
Observe for bleeding.
Do not administer IM injections to patients receiving fibrinolytic drugs.
No arterial blood gas specimens should be drawn on potential fibrinolytic therapy candidates due to bleeding tendency.
Use caution when moving patient to avoid bleeding or bruising.
Use one IV line exclusively for fibrinolytic administration.

AMIODARONE (CORDARONE)

CLASS

Class III antidysrhythmic

DESCRIPTION

Amiodarone is a unique antidysrhythmic agent with multiple mechanisms of action. The drug prolongs the duration of the action potential and the effective refractory period, and when given short-term IV, probably includes noncompetitive beta-adrenergic receptor and calcium channel blocker activity.

ONSET AND DURATION

Onset: Within minutes
Duration: Variable

INDICATIONS (IV USE)

Initial treatment and prophylaxis of frequently recurring ventricular fibrillation and hemodynamically unstable ventricular tachycardia in patients unresponsive to shock delivery, CPR, and vasopressors
Recurrent hemodynamically unstable VT
Treatment of some stable atrial and ventricular dysrhythmias

CONTRAINDICATIONS

Pulmonary congestion
Cardiogenic shock
Second- or third-degree AV block if no pacemaker present
Bradycardia
Sensitivity to amiodarone or iodine

ADVERSE REACTIONS

Hypotension
Headache
Dizziness
Bradycardia
Atrioventricular conduction abnormalities
Flushing
Abnormal salivation
Pain at IV site
Liver function abnormalities
Congestive heart failure
Abnormal thyroid function

DRUG INTERACTIONS

May potentiate bradycardia and hypotension with beta blockers and calcium channel blockers.
May increase risk of atrioventricular block and hypotension with calcium channel blockers.
May increase anticoagulant effects of warfarin.
May decrease metabolism and increase serum levels of phenytoin, procainamide, quinidine, and theophyllines.
Routine use in combination with drugs that prolong the Q-T interval is not recommended.
Y-site incompatibilities with furosemide, heparin, and sodium bicarbonate

HOW SUPPLIED

50 mg/mL vials

DOSAGE AND ADMINISTRATION

Adult:
   Pulseless arrest unresponsive to CPR, shock, and vasopressors: 300 mg IV/IO push. If needed, second dose of 150 mg IV/IO push
   Life-threatening dysrhythmias: Max cumulative dose: 2.2 g IV/24 hr. May be given as rapid infusion 150 mg IV over first 10 min (15 mg/min) repeated every 10 min as needed. Slow infusion: 360 mg IV over 6 hr (1 mg/min). Maintenance infusion: 540 mg IV over 18 hr (0.5 mg/min)
Pediatric:
   Refractory VF, pulseless VT: 5 mg/kg rapid IV/IO bolus; can be repeated to total dose of 15 mg/kg (2.2 g in adolescents) IV per 24 hr; max single dose: 300 mg
   Perfusing supraventricular and ventricular dysrhythmias: Loading dose 5 mg/kg IV/IO over 20-60 min (max single dose: 300 mg); can repeat to a max of 15 mg/kg (2.2 g in adolescents) per day IV

SPECIAL CONSIDERATIONS

Pregnancy safety: Category D
Rapid infusion may cause hypotension.
Continuous electrocardiogram monitoring is required.
Slow infusion or discontinue if bradycardia or atrioventricular block occurs.
Do not give with other drugs that prolong Q-T interval (e.g., procainamide).
Maintain at room temperature and protect from excessive heat.

ASPIRIN (ASA, BAYER, ECOTRIN, ST. JOSEPH, OTHERS)

CLASS

Analgesic, antiinflammatory, antipyretic, antiplatelet

DESCRIPTION

Aspirin decreases inflammation (analgesic effect not limited to effects in CNS), dilates peripheral vessels, and decreases platelet aggregation. The use of aspirin is strongly recommended for all patients with acute coronary syndrome.

ONSET AND DURATION

Onset: 15-30 min
Duration: 4-6 hr

INDICATIONS

Mild to moderate pain or fever
Prevention of platelet aggregation in ischemia and thromboembolism
All patients with ACS
Any patient with symptoms of ischemic chest pain

Unstable angina
Prevention of myocardial infarction or reinfarction

CONTRAINDICATIONS

Hypersensitivity to salicylates
Gastrointestinal bleeding
Active ulcer disease or acute asthma (relative contraindication)
Hemorrhagic stroke
Bleeding disorders
Children with flulike symptoms

ADVERSE REACTIONS

Stomach irritation
Heartburn or indigestion
Nausea or vomiting
Allergic reaction

DRUG INTERACTIONS

Decreased effects with antacids and steroids
Increased effects with anticoagulants, insulin, oral hypoglycemics, fibrinolytic agents

HOW SUPPLIED

Tablets (65, 81, 325, 500, 650, 975 mg)
Capsules (325, 500 mg)
Controlled-release tablets (800 mg)
Suppositories (varies from 60 mg to 1.2 g)

DOSAGE AND ADMINISTRATION

Adult: Mild pain and fever: 325-650 mg PO q 4 hr
ACS: 160-325 mg PO non–enteric-coated tablet (chewing is preferable to swallowing); may use rectal suppository for patients who cannot take orally
Pediatric: Not indicated in prehospital setting

SPECIAL CONSIDERATIONS

Pregnancy safety: Category D in third trimester, Category C in first and second trimesters
Should be given as soon as possible to the patient with ACS.

ATENOLOL (TENORMIN)

CLASS

Beta-blocking agent

DESCRIPTION

Atenolol competes with beta-adrenergic agonists for available beta-receptor sites on the membranes of cardiac muscle, bronchial smooth muscle, and the smooth muscle of blood vessels. The $beta_1$-blocking action on the heart decreases heart rate, conduction velocity, myocardial contractility, and cardiac output. Atenolol is used to control ventricular response in supraventricular tachydysrhythmias (paroxysmal supraventricular tachycardia, atrial fibrillation, atrial flutter). Atenolol is considered a second-line agent after adenosine, diltiazem, or digitalis derivative.

ONSET AND DURATION

Onset: Within 10 min (IV)
Duration: 2-4 hr

INDICATIONS

All patients with suspected MI and unstable angina in the absence of contraindications (can reduce the incidence of VF)
Useful as an adjunctive agent with fibrinolytic therapy (may reduce nonfatal reinfarction and recurrent ischemia)
To convert to normal sinus rhythm or to slow ventricular response (or both) in supraventricular tachydysrhythmias (reentry SVT, atrial fibrillation, or atrial flutter)
To reduce myocardial ischemia in AMI patients with elevated heart rate, blood pressure, or both

CONTRAINDICATIONS

Hemodynamically unstable patients
STEMI if signs of heart failure, low cardiac output, or increased risk for cardiogenic shock are present
Relative contraindications include P-R interval >0.24 sec, second- or third-degree heart block, active asthma, reactive airway disease, severe bradycardia, SBP <100 mm Hg.
Not available intravenously in the United States

ADVERSE REACTIONS

Bradycardia
Atrioventricular conduction delays
Hypotension
Bronchospasm

DRUG INTERACTIONS

Atenolol may potentiate antihypertensive effects when given to patients taking calcium channel blockers or MAO inhibitors; catecholamine-depleting drugs may potentiate hypotension; sympathomimetic effects may be antagonized; signs of hypoglycemia may be masked.

HOW SUPPLIED

5 mg in 10-mL ampules (injectable form is not available in the United States)

DOSAGE AND ADMINISTRATION

Adult: 5 mg slow IV (over 5 min); wait 10 min and then give second dose of 5 mg over 5 min
Pediatric: Not recommended

SPECIAL CONSIDERATIONS

Pregnancy safety: Category C
Atenolol must be given slowly IV over 5 min.
Concurrent IV administration with IV calcium channel blockers such as verapamil or diltiazem can cause severe hypotension.
Atenolol should be used with caution in persons with liver or renal dysfunction.

ATROPINE SULFATE (ATROPINE AND OTHERS)

CLASS

Anticholinergic agent

DESCRIPTION

Atropine sulfate (a potent parasympatholytic) inhibits actions of acetylcholine at postganglionic parasympathetic (primarily muscarinic) receptor sites. Small doses inhibit salivary and bronchial secretions; moderate doses dilate pupils and increase heart rate. Large doses decrease gastrointestinal motility, inhibit gastric acid secretion, and may block nicotinic receptor sites at the autonomic ganglia and at the neuromuscular junction. Blocked vagal effects result in increased heart rate and enhanced atrioventricular conduction with limited or no inotropic effect. In emergency care, atropine primarily is used to increase the heart rate in life-threatening or symptomatic bradycardia and to antagonize excess muscarinic receptor stimulation caused by organophosphate insecticides or chemical nerve agents (e.g., sarin and soman).

ONSET AND DURATION

Onset: Rapid
Duration: 2-6 hr

INDICATIONS

Hemodynamically significant bradycardia
Organophosphate or nerve gas poisoning

CONTRAINDICATIONS

Tachycardia
Hypersensitivity to atropine
Use with caution in patients with myocardial ischemia and hypoxia
Avoid in hypothermic bradycardia
Obstructive disease of gastrointestinal tract
Obstructive uropathy
Unstable cardiovascular status in acute hemorrhage with myocardial ischemia
Narrow-angle glaucoma
Thyrotoxicosis

ADVERSE REACTIONS

Tachycardia
Paradoxical bradycardia when pushed too slowly or when used at doses less than 0.5 mg
Palpitations
Dysrhythmias
Headache
Dizziness
Anticholinergic effects (dry mouth/nose/skin, photophobia, blurred vision, urinary retention, constipation)
Nausea and vomiting
Flushed, hot, dry skin
Allergic reactions

DRUG INTERACTIONS

Use with other anticholinergic agents may increase vagal blockade.
Potential adverse effects may occur when administered with digitalis, cholinergics, neostigmine.
The effects of atropine may be enhanced by antihistamines, procainamide, quinidine, antipsychotics and antidepressants, and thiazides.
Increased toxicity: amantadine

HOW SUPPLIED

Parenteral: There are various injection preparations.
In emergency care, atropine usually is supplied in prefilled syringes containing 1 mg in 10 mL of solution.

DOSAGE AND ADMINISTRATION

Bradydysrhythmia (With or Without ACS)
Adult: 0.5 mg every 3-5 min for desired response (max total dose: 3 mg); use shorter dosing intervals (3 min) and higher doses in severe clinical conditions
Pediatric: 0.02 mg/kg IV/IO; min dose: 0.1 mg; max single dose of 0.5 mg; may be repeated once; max total dose for a child: 1 mg; for adolescent: 3 mg; ET dose is 0.04-0.06 mg/kg
Anticholinesterase Poisoning
Adult: 1-2 mg IV push every 5-15 min until atropine effects are observed; then every 1-4 hr for at least 24 hr; extremely large doses (2-4 mg or more) may be needed
Pediatric: <12 years: 0.02-0.05 mg/kg/dose IV/IO; may be repeated every 20-30 min until muscarinic symptoms reverse; >12 years: 2 mg IV/IO; then 1-2 mg IV/IO every 20-30 min until muscarinic symptoms reverse
Rapid Sequence Intubation
0.01-0.02 mg/kg IV/IO; max single dose: 0.5 mg

SPECIAL CONSIDERATIONS

Pregnancy safety: Category C
Follow endotracheal tube administration with several positive pressure ventilations.
Atropine causes pupillary dilation, rendering the pupils nonreactive; pupil response may not be useful in monitoring central nervous system status.

CALCIUM CHLORIDE

CLASS

Electrolyte

DESCRIPTION

Calcium is an essential component for the functional integrity of the nervous and muscular systems, for normal cardiac contractility, and for the coagulation of blood. Calcium chloride contains 27.2% elemental calcium. Calcium chloride is a hypertonic solution and should be administered only IV (slowly, not exceeding 1 mL/min).

ONSET AND DURATION

Onset: 5-15 min
Duration: Dose-dependent (effects may persist for 4 hr after IV administration)

INDICATIONS

Hyperkalemia (except when associated with digitalis toxicity)
Hypocalcemia (e.g., after multiple blood transfusions)
Calcium channel blocker toxicity
Hypermagnesemia
To prevent hypotensive effects of calcium channel blocking agents (e.g., IV verapamil and diltiazem)

CONTRAINDICATIONS

Ventricular fibrillation during cardiac resuscitation
In patients with digitalis toxicity
Hypercalcemia

ADVERSE REACTIONS

Bradycardia (may cause asystole)
Hypotension
Metallic taste
Severe local necrosis and sloughing following intramuscular use or IV infiltration

DRUG INTERACTIONS

Calcium may worsen dysrhythmias caused by digitalis.
Calcium may antagonize the peripheral vasodilatory effects of calcium channel blockers.

HOW SUPPLIED

10% solution in 10-mL (100 mg/mL) ampules, vials, and prefilled syringes

DOSAGE AND ADMINISTRATION

Hyperkalemia and Calcium Channel Blocker Overdose
Adult: Typical dose is 500-1000 mg (5-10 mL of a 10% solution); may be repeated as needed
Pediatric: 20 mg/kg (0.2 mL/kg) IV of 10% solution slow IV/IO; may repeat if documented or clinical indication persists (e.g., toxicological problem); dose should not exceed adult dose

SPECIAL CONSIDERATIONS

Pregnancy safety: Category C
Calcium may produce vasospasm in coronary and cerebral arteries.
Do not use routinely in cardiac arrest.

Hypertension and bradycardia may occur with rapid administration.
Monitor heart rate during administration.

NOTE
It is important to flush the IV line between administration of calcium chloride and sodium bicarbonate to avoid precipitation.

DEXAMETHASONE (DECADRON, HEXADROL, AND OTHERS)

CLASS

Glucocorticoid

DESCRIPTION

Dexamethasone is a synthetic steroid that is related chemically to the natural hormones secreted by the adrenal cortex. The drug suppresses acute and chronic inflammation, potentiates the relaxation of vascular and bronchial smooth muscle by beta-adrenergic agonists, and possibly alters airway hyperreactivity. In emergency care, dexamethasone generally is used in the treatment of allergic reactions and asthma and to reduce swelling in the central nervous system.

ONSET AND DURATION

Onset: 4-8 hr after parenteral administration
Duration: 24-72 hr

INDICATIONS

Endocrine, rheumatic, hematological disorders
Allergic states
Septic shock
Chronic inflammation

CONTRAINDICATIONS

Hypersensitivity to the product
Active untreated infections (relative)

ADVERSE REACTIONS

Decreased wound healing
Hypertension
Gastrointestinal bleeding
Hyperglycemia

DRUG INTERACTIONS

Barbiturates and phenytoin can decrease dexamethasone effects.

HOW SUPPLIED

Common preparations used in emergency care are for IV administration and are as follows:
4 mg/mL in 1-, 5-, 10-, 25-, 30-mL vials
10 mg/mL in 10-mL vials, 1-mL syringe, 1-mL ampule

20 mg/mL in 5-mL vials (IV or IM), 5-mL syringe (IV)
24 mg/mL (IV only) in 5- and 10-mL vials

DOSAGE AND ADMINISTRATION

Adult: There is considerable variance in recommended dexamethasone doses. The usual range in emergency care is 4-24 mg IV. Some physicians may prefer significantly higher doses (up to 100 mg) for unusual indications.
Pediatric: 1 dose of 0.6 mg/kg PO/IM/IV (max dose: 16 mg)

SPECIAL CONSIDERATIONS

Pregnancy safety: Category C; dexamethasone crosses the placenta and may cause fetal damage.
Medication should be protected from heat.
Because of onset of action (4-8 hr), dexamethasone should not be considered a first-line medication for allergic reactions.

DEXTROSE 50%

CLASS

Carbohydrate, hypertonic solution

DESCRIPTION

The term *dextrose* is used to describe the six-carbon sugar *D-glucose*, the principal form of carbohydrate used by the body. 50% dextrose solution is used in emergency care to treat hypoglycemia and in the management of coma of unknown origin.

ONSET AND DURATION

Onset: 1 min
Duration: Depends on the degree of hypoglycemia

INDICATIONS

Hypoglycemia (documented or strongly suspected)
Altered level of consciousness
Coma of unknown origin
Seizure of unknown origin

CONTRAINDICATIONS

Intracranial hemorrhage
Increased intracranial pressure
Known or suspected stroke in the absence of hypoglycemia

ADVERSE REACTIONS

Warmth, pain, burning from medication infusion, hyperglycemia, thrombophlebitis

DRUG INTERACTIONS

None significant

HOW SUPPLIED

25 g/50 mL prefilled syringe (500 mg/mL)

DOSAGE AND ADMINISTRATION

Adult: 12.5-25 g slow IV; may be repeated once
Pediatric: 0.5-1 g/kg IV/IO (max recommended concentration: 25%)
2-4 mL/kg 25%
5-10 mL/kg 10%
10-20 mL/kg 5% if volume tolerated

SPECIAL CONSIDERATIONS

Pregnancy safety: Category C
Draw blood sample before administration if possible.
Perform blood glucose analysis before administration if possible.
Extravasation may cause tissue necrosis; use large vein and aspirate occasionally to ensure route patency.
50% dextrose solution sometimes may precipitate severe neurological symptoms (Wernicke's encephalopathy) in thiamine-deficient patients (for example, alcoholics). (This can be prevented by administering 100 mg of thiamine IV.)

DIAZEPAM (VALIUM AND OTHERS)

CLASS

Benzodiazepine

DESCRIPTION

Diazepam is a frequently prescribed medication to treat anxiety and stress. In emergency care, diazepam is used to treat alcohol withdrawal and grand mal seizure activity. Diazepam acts on the limbic, thalamic, and hypothalamic regions of the central nervous system to potentiate the effects of inhibitory neurotransmitters, raising the seizure threshold in the motor cortex. It also may be used in conscious patients during cardioversion and transcutaneous pacing to induce amnesia and sedation. Its use as an anticonvulsant may be short-lived because of rapid redistribution from the central nervous system. Rapid IV administration may be followed by respiratory depression and excessive sedation, particularly in elderly patients.

ONSET AND DURATION

Onset: (IV) 1-5 min; (IM) 15-30 min
Duration: (IV) 15 min-1 hr; (IM) 15 min-1 hr

INDICATIONS

Acute anxiety states
Acute alcohol withdrawal
Skeletal muscle relaxation
Seizure activity
Premedication before countershock or transcutaneous pacing

CONTRAINDICATIONS

Hypersensitivity to the drug
Substance abuse (use with caution)

Coma (unless the patient has seizures or severe muscle rigidity or myoclonus)

Shock

Central nervous system depression as a result of head injury

Respiratory depression

ADVERSE REACTIONS

Hypotension

Reflex tachycardia (rare)

Respiratory depression

Ataxia

Psychomotor impairment

Confusion

Nausea

Dizziness

Drowsiness

Blurred vision

DRUG INTERACTIONS

Diazepam may precipitate central nervous system depression and psychomotor impairment when the patient is taking other central nervous system depressant medications.

Diazepam should not be administered with other drugs because of possible precipitation (incompatible with most fluids; should be administered into an IV of NS solution).

HOW SUPPLIED

Parenteral: 5 mg/mL vials, ampules, Tubex

DOSAGE AND ADMINISTRATION

Seizure Activity

Adult: 5 mg over 2 min (up to 10 mg for most adults) IV q 10-15 min prn (max dose: 30 mg)

Pediatric: Dose for infants 30 days to 5 yr is 0.2-0.5 mg slow IV q 2-5 min to max 5 mg; children 5 yr or older is 1 mg q 2-5 min to max 10 mg slow IV

Premedication for Cardioversion or Transcutaneous Pacing

Adult: 5-15 mg IV, 5-10 min before procedure

Rapid Sequence Intubation in Children

0.2-0.3 mg/kg IV/IO; max single dose 10 mg

SPECIAL CONSIDERATIONS

Pregnancy safety: Category D

Diazepam may cause local venous irritation.

Diazepam has short duration of anticonvulsant effect.

Reduce dose by 50% in elderly patients.

Rectal administration may require higher dose because absorption is incomplete.

Resuscitation equipment should be readily available.

DIGOXIN (LANOXIN)

CLASS

Cardiac glycoside, miscellaneous antidysrhythmic

DESCRIPTION

Digoxin (digitalis) is a cardiac glycoside derived primarily from the foxglove plant. Its primary action involves alteration of ion transport across cardiac cell membranes. Increased intracellular calcium improves myocardial contractility. Digoxin increases vagal tone and therefore indirectly decreases sinus node rate, reduces sympathetic tone, and decreases atrioventricular node conduction velocity (with an increase in atrioventricular node refractory period). Sodium pumped out of cells may cause increased automaticity.

ONSET AND DURATION

Onset: (IV) 5-30 min

Duration: 3-4 days

INDICATIONS (MAY BE OF LIMITED USE)

Supraventricular tachycardias, especially atrial flutter and atrial fibrillation

Alternative drug for reentry SVT

CONTRAINDICATIONS

Ventricular fibrillation

Ventricular tachycardia

Atrioventricular block

Digitalis toxicity

Hypersensitivity to digoxin

Second- or third-degree heart block in the absence of artificial pacing

ADVERSE REACTIONS (MOSTLY RELATED TO DIGITALIS TOXICITY)

Headache

Weakness

Visual disturbances (blurred, yellow or green vision)

Confusion

Seizures

Dysrhythmias (virtually any disturbance, but junctional tachycardias are most common)

Nausea and vomiting

Skin rash

Hypotension

DRUG INTERACTIONS

Amiodarone, verapamil, and quinidine may increase serum digoxin concentrations by 50% to 70%.

Concurrent administration of IV digoxin and IV verapamil may lead to severe heart block.

Erythromycin and tetracycline may increase serum digoxin concentrations by reducing hepatic breakdown.

Diuretics may potentiate digoxin cardiotoxicity via loss of potassium.

Sympathomimetics may augment the inotropic and cardiotoxic effects of digoxin.

Concomitant administration of kaolin, pectin, and antacids may reduce digoxin absorption from the gastrointestinal tract.

HOW SUPPLIED

In emergency care, the common form of digoxin is supplied in 2-mL ampules, containing 0.5 mg of the drug (0.25 mg/mL)

DOSAGE AND ADMINISTRATION

Adult: Loading dose 0.004-0.006 mg/kg (4-6 mcg/kg) initially over 5 min; second and third boluses of 0.002-0.003 mg/kg (2-3 mcg/kg) to follow at 4-8 hr intervals (total loading dose 8-12 mcg/kg divided over 8-16 hr); maintenance dose affected by body mass and renal function

Pediatric: Not recommended in prehospital setting

SPECIAL CONSIDERATIONS

Pregnancy safety: Category C

Patient should be monitored constantly for signs of digitalis toxicity.

Patients with myocardial infarction and/or renal failure are prone to developing digitalis toxicity.

Digitalis toxicity is potentiated in patients with hypokalemia, hypomagnesemia, and hypercalcemia.

Avoid use in patients with Wolff-Parkinson-White syndrome because of possible ventricular dysrhythmias.

Avoid electrical cardioversion if patient is receiving digoxin unless condition is life threatening; use lower dose (10-20 J).

Reduce dose by 50% when used with amiodarone.

DIGOXIN IMMUNE FAB (DIGIBIND, DIGIFAB)

CLASS

Biologic response modifier; antidote

DESCRIPTION

Digoxin immune Fab (ovine) is a protein that consists of antibody fragments, which are used as an antidote for digitalis toxicity. Molecules of digoxin or digitoxin are removed from tissue binding sites and are sequestered in the extracellular fluid, shifting equilibrium away from binding of the drug to its tissue receptors.[2]

ONSET AND DURATION

Onset: Within minutes
Duration: Dose-dependent

INDICATIONS

Digoxin toxicity with:
    Life-threatening dysrhythmias
    Shock or congestive heart failure
    Hyperkalemia (potassium level >5 mEq/L)

CONTRAINDICATIONS

Ovine protein hypersensitivity

Use with caution in patients with renal failure or renal impairment.

ADVERSE REACTIONS

Anaphylaxis
Atrial fibrillation
Heart failure
Hypokalemia
Hypotension
Injection site reaction
Phlebitis

DRUG INTERACTIONS

None known

HOW SUPPLIED

38 mg (Digibind) and 40 mg (DigiFab) powder for IV injection

DOSAGE AND ADMINISTRATION

Adults and children: Dose varies according to amount of digoxin ingested. (Each vial binds about 0.5 mg of digoxin.) Average dose is 10 vials (400 mg); may require up to 20 vials (800 mg). For chronic intoxication 3-5 vials may be effective. Monitor children for volume overload.

SPECIAL CONSIDERATIONS

Pregnancy safety: Category C

Visually inspect parenteral products for particulate matter and discoloration before administration whenever solution and container permit.

Closely monitor the patient's temperature, blood pressure, and ECG.

DILTIAZEM (CARDIZEM) INJECTABLE

CLASS

Calcium channel blocker or calcium channel antagonist

DESCRIPTION

Diltiazem is a calcium channel blocking agent that slows conduction, increases refractoriness in the atrioventricular node, and causes coronary and peripheral vasodilation. The drug is used to control ventricular response rates in patients with atrial fibrillation or flutter, multifocal atrial tachycardias. Use after adenosine to treat refractory reentry SVT in patients with narrow QRS complex and adequate blood pressure.

ONSET AND DURATION

Onset: 2-5 min
Duration: 1-3 hr

INDICATIONS

To control ventricular rate in atrial fibrillation and atrial
flutter
Multifocal atrial tachycardias
Paroxysmal supraventricular tachycardia

CONTRAINDICATIONS

Wide QRS tachycardias of unknown origin or poison/drug-
induced tachycardia
Sick sinus syndrome
Second- or third-degree atrioventricular block (except with
a functioning pacemaker)
Hypotension (less than 90 mm Hg)
Cardiogenic shock
Hypersensitivity to diltiazem
Rapid atrial fibrillation or atrial flutter associated with
Wolff-Parkinson-White syndrome or a short P-R interval
syndrome
Ventricular tachycardia
Acute myocardial infarction

ADVERSE REACTIONS

Atrial flutter
First- and second-degree atrioventricular block
Bradycardia
Hypotension
Chest pain
Congestive heart failure
Peripheral edema
Syncope
Ventricular dysrhythmias
Sweating
Nausea and vomiting
Dizziness
Dry mouth
Dyspnea
Headache
Rash

DRUG INTERACTIONS

Caution is warranted in patients receiving medications that
affect cardiac contractility and/or sinoatrial or atrioventricular node conduction.
Diltiazem is incompatible with simultaneous furosemide
injection.

HOW SUPPLIED

25 mg (5-mL vial); 50 mg (10-mL vial)

DOSAGE AND ADMINISTRATION

Acute rate control: 0.25 mg/kg (15-20 mg for the average
patient) IV over 2 min; may be repeated in 15 min
(0.35 mg/kg; 20-25 mg for the average patient) IV over
2 min
Maintenance infusion: Dilute 125 mg (25 mL) in 100 mL
of solution (NS or D₅W); infuse 5-15 mg/hr, titrated to
heart rate
Pediatric: Safety not established

SPECIAL CONSIDERATIONS

Pregnancy safety: Category C
Use with caution in patients with impaired renal or hepatic
function.
Hypotension occasionally may result (more common with
verapamil); carefully monitor vital signs.
Concurrent IV administration with IV beta blockers can
cause severe hypotension and AV block. Use caution in
patients taking oral beta blockers.
Premature ventricular contractions may be present on conversion of paroxysmal supraventricular tachycardia to
sinus rhythm.
Shelf-life at room temperature is 1 month.

DIPHENHYDRAMINE (BENADRYL)

CLASS

Antihistamine

DESCRIPTION

Antihistamines prevent the physiological actions of histamine by blocking H₁ (e.g., diphenhydramine and cimetidine) and H₂ (e.g., cimetidine, ranitidine, and famotidine)
receptor sites. Antihistamines are indicated for conditions
in which histamine excess is present (e.g., acute urticaria)
and are used as adjunctive therapy (with epinephrine, for
example) in the treatment of anaphylactic shock. Antihistamines also are effective in the treatment of certain extrapyramidal (dystonic) reactions and for relief of upper
respiratory tract and sinus symptoms associated with allergic reactions.

ONSET AND DURATION

Onset: Max effects 1-3 hr
Duration: 6-12 hr

INDICATIONS

Moderate to severe allergic reactions (after epinephrine)
Anaphylaxis
Acute extrapyramidal (dystonic) reactions

CONTRAINDICATIONS

Patients taking non-selective MAO inhibitors
Hypersensitivity
Narrow-angle glaucoma (relative)
Newborns and nursing mothers

ADVERSE REACTIONS

Dose-related drowsiness
Disturbed coordination

Hypotension
Palpitations
Tachycardia, bradycardia
Thickening of bronchial secretions
Dry mouth and throat
Paradoxical excitement in children

DRUG INTERACTIONS

Central nervous system depressants may increase depressant effects.
MAO inhibitors may prolong and intensify anticholinergic effects of antihistamines.

HOW SUPPLIED

Parenteral: 10 and 50 mg/mL vials, prefilled syringe

DOSAGE AND ADMINISTRATION

Adult: The standard dose of diphenhydramine is 10-50 mg IM, slow IV q 6-8 hr (max: 400 mg/day)
Pediatric (greater than 10 kg): 1.25 mg/kg/dose q 6 hr (max: 300 mg/day)

SPECIAL CONSIDERATIONS

Pregnancy safety: Category C
Use cautiously in patients with central nervous system depression or lower respiratory tract diseases such as asthma.

DOBUTAMINE (DOBUTREX)

CLASS

Sympathomimetic

DESCRIPTION

Dobutamine is a synthetic catecholamine that primarily stimulates $beta_1$-adrenergic receptors, and has much less significant effects on $beta_2$- and alpha-adrenergic receptors. The clinical effects of this drug include positive inotropic effects with minimal changes in chronotropic activity or systemic vascular resistance. For these reasons, dobutamine is useful in the management of congestive heart failure when an increase in heart rate is not desired.

ONSET AND DURATION

Onset: 1-2 min; peak after 10 min
Duration: 10-15 min

INDICATIONS

Pump problems (CHF, pulmonary congestion) with SBP of 70-100 mm Hg and *no* signs of shock

CONTRAINDICATIONS

Tachydysrhythmias (atrial fibrillation, atrial flutter)
Severe hypotension with signs of shock
Idiopathic hypertrophic subaortic stenosis
Suspected or known drug-induced shock

ADVERSE REACTIONS

Anxiety
Headache
Nausea
Fluctuations in blood pressure
Dose-related tachydysrhythmias
Hypertension
Ventricular ectopy

DRUG INTERACTIONS

Beta-adrenergic antagonists may blunt inotropic responses.
Sympathomimetics and phosphodiesterase inhibitors may exacerbate dysrhythmia responses.
Dobutamine is incompatible with sodium bicarbonate and furosemide in same IV line; it may be given in separate IV lines.

HOW SUPPLIED

12.5 mg/mL injectable

DOSAGE AND ADMINISTRATION

Adult: Usual dose is 2-20 mcg/kg/min IV, based on inotropic effect; titrate so heart rate does not increase by >10% of baseline
Pediatric: 2-20 mcg/kg/min IV/IO, titrated to desired effect

SPECIAL CONSIDERATIONS

Pregnancy safety: Category C
Administer via an infusion pump to ensure precise flow rates.
Blood pressure should be monitored closely; hemodynamic monitoring is recommended for optimal use.
Dobutamine may be administered through a Y-site with concurrent dopamine, lidocaine, nitroprusside, and potassium chloride infusions; do not mix with sodium bicarbonate.
Increases in heart rate of more than 10% may induce or exacerbate myocardial ischemia.
Lidocaine should be readily available.
Correct hypovolemia before using dobutamine in hypotensive patients.
Elderly patients may have significantly decreased responses.

DOPAMINE (INTROPIN)

CLASS

Sympathomimetic

DESCRIPTION

Dopamine is related chemically to epinephrine and norepinephrine. It acts primarily on $alpha_1$- and $beta_1$-adrenergic receptors in a dose-dependent fashion. At moderate doses ("cardiac doses"), dopamine stimulates beta-adrenergic receptors, causing enhanced myocardial contractility, increased cardiac output, and a rise in blood pressure. At high doses ("vasopressor doses"), dopamine has an alpha-adrenergic effect, producing peripheral arterial and venous constriction. Dopamine is a second-line drug for symptomatic bradycardia (after atropine). It commonly is used in the treatment of hypotension (SBP <70-100 mm Hg) with signs and symptoms of shock.

ONSET AND DURATION

Onset: 2-4 min
Duration: 10-15 min

INDICATIONS

Hemodynamically significant hypotension in the absence of hypovolemia
Symptomatic bradycardia (second-line drug after atropine)

CONTRAINDICATIONS

Tachydysrhythmias
Ventricular fibrillation
Patients with pheochromocytoma

ADVERSE REACTIONS

Dose-related tachydysrhythmias
Hypertension
Increased myocardial oxygen demand (e.g., ischemia)
Headache
Anxiety
Nausea and vomiting

DRUG INTERACTIONS

Dopamine may be deactivated by alkaline solutions (sodium bicarbonate and furosemide).
MAO inhibitors may potentiate the effect of dopamine.
Sympathomimetics and phosphodiesterase inhibitors exacerbate dysrhythmia response.
Beta-adrenergic antagonists may blunt inotropic response.
When administered with phenytoin, hypotension, bradycardia, and seizures may develop.

HOW SUPPLIED

200, 400, 800 mg in 5-mL prefilled syringe and ampule for IV infusion (IV piggyback)

DOSAGE AND ADMINISTRATION

Adult: Usual infusion rate 2-20 mcg/kg/min; titrate to response; taper slowly
Pediatric: 2-20 mcg/kg/min IV/IO, titrated to patient response (not to exceed 20 mcg/kg/min); if infusion dose >20 mcg/kg/min is required, consider alternative adrenergic agent (e.g., epinephrine/norepinephrine)

SPECIAL CONSIDERATIONS

Pregnancy safety: Category C
Infuse through large, stable vein to avoid the possibility of extravasation injury.
Use infusion pump to ensure precise flow rates.

Monitor patient for signs of compromised circulation.
Correct hypovolemia before using dopamine in hypotensive patients.
Do not mix with sodium bicarbonate.

EPINEPHRINE (ADRENALIN)

CLASS

Sympathomimetic

DESCRIPTION

Epinephrine is an endogenous catecholamine that directly stimulates alpha-, beta$_1$-, and beta$_2$-adrenergic receptors in dose-related fashion. Epinephrine is the initial drug of choice for treating bronchoconstriction and hypotension resulting from anaphylaxis and all forms of cardiac arrest. Epinephrine is useful in the management of reactive airway disease, but beta-adrenergic agents usually are considered the drugs of choice because they are inhaled and have fewer side effects. Rapid injection produces a rapid increase in blood pressure, ventricular contractility, and heart rate. In addition, epinephrine causes vasoconstriction in the arterioles of the skin, mucosa, and splanchnic areas, and antagonizes the effects of histamine.

ONSET AND DURATION

Onset: (subQ) 5-10 min; (IV/endotracheal tube) 1-2 min
Duration: 5-10 min

INDICATIONS

Acute allergic reaction (anaphylaxis)
Cardiac arrest
Pulseless electrical activity
Ventricular fibrillation and pulseless ventricular tachycardia unresponsive to initial defibrillation
Symptomatic bradycardia
Severe hypotension accompanied by bradycardia when pacing and atropine fail
Bronchial asthma

CONTRAINDICATIONS

Hypersensitivity (not an issue especially in emergencies—the dose should be lowered or given slowly in non–cardiac arrest patients with heart disease)
Hypovolemic shock (as with other catecholamines, correct hypovolemia before use)
Coronary insufficiency (use with caution)

ADVERSE REACTIONS

Headache
Nausea and vomiting
Restlessness
Weakness
Dysrhythmias, including ventricular tachycardia and ventricular fibrillation
Hypertension
Precipitation of angina pectoris

Tachycardia
Tremors
Dyspnea

DRUG INTERACTIONS

MAO inhibitors may potentiate the effect of epinephrine.
Beta-adrenergic antagonists may blunt inotropic response.
Sympathomimetics and phosphodiesterase inhibitors may exacerbate dysrhythmia response.
May be deactivated by alkaline solutions (sodium bicarbonate, furosemide).

HOW SUPPLIED

Parenteral: 1 mg/mL (1:1000), 0.1 mg/mL (1:10,000) ampule and prefilled syringe
Autoinjector (EpiPen): 0.3 mg/mL (1:2000)

DOSAGE AND ADMINISTRATION

Profound Bradycardia or Hypotension
Adult: 2-10 mcg/min infusion; titrate to patient response
Pediatric: All IV/IO doses: 0.01 mg/kg (1:10,000, 0.1 mL/kg); continuous infusion: 0.1-1 mcg/kg/min; higher doses may be effective
All ET doses: 0.1 mg/kg (0.1 mL/kg of 1:1000)
Pulseless Arrest
Adult:[1]
   IV/IO dose: 1 mg (10 mL, 1:10,000) IV/IO push or endotracheal tube (2-2.5 mg diluted in 10 mL of NS), repeated every 3-5 min during resuscitation (follow each IV dose with a 20-mL saline flush); elevate arm for 20-30 sec after dose; higher doses (up to 0.2 mg/kg) may be used for specific indications (e.g., beta-blocker or calcium channel blocker overdose; poison/drug-induced shock)
Pediatric:
   IV/IO dose: 0.01 mg/kg (1:10,000, 0.1 mL/kg) every 3-5 min during arrest; max dose: 1 mg
   All ET doses: 0.1 mg/kg of 1:1000 (0.1 mL/kg) every 5 min of arrest until IV/IO access; then begin with first IV/IO dose
Continuous Infusions for Pulseless Arrest
Adult: Add 1 mg of epinephrine (1 mL of 1:1000 solution) to 500 mL of NS or D_5W; initial infusion rate of 0.1-0.5 mcg/kg/min; titrate to response
Anaphylactic Reaction or Bronchoconstriction
Adult:
   Mild: 0.3-0.5 mL (1:1000) IM/subQ; repeat in 15-20 min if needed
   Severe: 1 mL (1:10,000) slow IV over 5 min; IV infusion at rates of 1-4 mcg/min may prevent the need to repeat epinephrine injections frequently
Pediatric: Severe: 0.01 mg/kg (0.01 mL/kg of 1:1000) IM; max single dose: 0.3 mg; repeat as needed

SPECIAL CONSIDERATIONS

Pregnancy safety: Category C
Do not use prefilled syringes for epinephrine infusions.
Syncope has occurred following epinephrine administration to asthmatic children.
Epinephrine may increase myocardial oxygen demand.

> 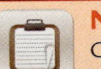 **NOTE**
> Complications of IV administration of epinephrine are significant and include the development of uncontrolled systolic hypertension, vomiting, seizures, dysrhythmias, and myocardial ischemia. This route should be used only in patients with a critical life-threatening condition. Intravenous administration of epinephrine rarely is performed in conscious patients. Intravenous administration is performed with extreme caution in rare circumstances and only with authorization from medical direction. *Epinephrine 1:1000 should never be given as an IV bolus.*

EPINEPHRINE RACEMIC (MICRONEFRIN)

CLASS

Sympathomimetic

DESCRIPTION

As with other forms of epinephrine, racemic epinephrine acts as a bronchodilator that stimulates $beta_2$ receptors in the lungs, resulting in relaxation of bronchial smooth muscle. This alleviates bronchospasm, increases vital capacity, and reduces airway resistance. Racemic epinephrine is also useful in treating laryngeal edema. Racemic epinephrine also inhibits the release of histamine.

ONSET AND DURATION

Onset: Within 5 min
Duration: 1-3 hr

INDICATIONS

Bronchial asthma
Treatment of bronchospasm
Croup (laryngotracheobronchitis)
Laryngeal edema

CONTRAINDICATIONS

Hypertension
Underlying cardiovascular disease
Epiglottitis

ADVERSE REACTIONS

Tachycardia
Dysrhythmias

DRUG INTERACTIONS

MAO inhibitors may potentiate the effect of epinephrine.
Beta-adrenergic antagonists may blunt the bronchodilating response.

Sympathomimetics and phosphodiesterase inhibitors may exacerbate dysrhythmia response.

HOW SUPPLIED

Metered-dose inhaler: 0.16-0.25 mg/spray
Solution: 7.5, 15, 30 mL in 1%, 2.25% solution

DOSAGE AND ADMINISTRATION

Metered-Dose Inhaler
Adult: 2-3 inhalations, repeat once in 5 min prn
Solution
Adult: Dilute 5 mL (1%) in 5 mL of saline, administer over 15 min
Pediatric: Dilute 0.25 mL (0.1%) in 2.5 mL of saline (if less than 20 kg); 0.5 mL in 2.5 mL of saline (if 20-40 kg); 0.75 mL in 2.5 mL of saline (if greater than 40 kg); administer by aerosolization

SPECIAL CONSIDERATIONS

Pregnancy safety: Category C
Racemic epinephrine may produce tachycardia and other dysrhythmias.
Monitor vital signs closely.
Excessive use may cause bronchospasm.
Rebound exacerbation of severe croup may occur following drug administration.

EPTIFIBATIDE (INTEGRILIN)

CLASS

Glycoprotein IIb/IIIa inhibitor

DESCRIPTION

Glycoprotein IIb/IIIa inhibitors inhibit the integrin GP IIb/IIIa receptor in the membrane of the platelets. As a result, they inhibit the common final pathway activation of platelet aggregation.

ONSET AND DURATION

Onset: Rapid
Duration: 30-45 min; platelet aggregation restored within 4 hr after infusion stopped

INDICATIONS

Eptifibatide (in combination with aspirin and heparin) is indicated for use in patients undergoing percutaneous coronary intervention (PCI) as well as for the treatment of unstable angina or non-STEMI myocardial infarction.

CONTRAINDICATIONS

Active internal bleeding
Bleeding disorder within the past 30 days
History of intracranial hemorrhage, neoplasm, AV malformation, aneurysm, or stroke within 30 days
Major surgical procedure or trauma within 1 month
Aortic dissection, pericarditis, and severe hypertension
Hypersensitivity to any GP IIb/IIIa inhibitor
Low platelet count

ADVERSE REACTIONS

Anaphylactoid reaction/anaphylactic shock
Bleeding
GI bleeding
Hematemesis
Hematuria
Hypotension
Intracranial bleeding
Platelet dysfunction
Retroperitoneal bleeding
Stroke
Thrombocytopenia

DRUG INTERACTIONS

Concomitant use of eptifibatide and other agents that may affect hemostasis, such as anticoagulants, other platelet inhibitors, NSAIDs, and thrombolytic agents, may be associated with an increased risk of bleeding.

HOW SUPPLIED

Solution: 0.75 mg/mL, 2.0 mg/mL

DOSAGE AND ADMINISTRATION (ADULTS)

Unstable angina and NSTEMI myocardial infarction (PCI): 180 mcg/kg IV (max: 22.6 mg) bolus over 1-2 min, followed by 2 mcg/kg/min (max: 15 mg/hr) continuous IV infusion; repeat bolus in 10 min. Decrease dose in patients with impaired renal function.

SPECIAL CONSIDERATIONS

Pregnancy safety: Category B
Bleeding risk may be increased in patients receiving eptifibatide concomitantly with heparin, other anticoagulant therapy, or thrombolytics.
Eptifibatide should not be used in patients with renal failure and is contraindicated in patients with dependency on renal dialysis.
Elderly patients may be at increased risk for bleeding while receiving eptifibatide.

ESMOLOL (BREVIBLOC)

CLASS

Beta$_1$ blocker

DESCRIPTION

Esmolol is an extremely short-acting cardioselective beta blocker. Unlike other beta$_1$-selective beta blockers (e.g., metoprolol, atenolol), esmolol is administered via continuous IV infusion. It has a short duration of action, making it useful for acute control of hypertension or certain supraventricular dysrhythmias, such as sinus tachycardia, atrial flutter and/or fibrillation in the emergency setting. Nonapproved indications include short-term control of perioperative hypertension, management of tachydysrhythmias complicating acute MI, and minimization of acute myocardial ischemia secondary to acute MI or unstable angina.

ONSET AND DURATION

Onset: Rapid
Duration: Less than 10 min

INDICATIONS

All patients with suspected MI and unstable angina in the absence of contraindications (can reduce the incidence of VF)
Useful as an adjunctive agent with fibrinolytic therapy (may reduce nonfatal reinfarction and recurrent ischemia)
To convert to normal sinus rhythm or to slow ventricular response (or both) in supraventricular tachydysrhythmias (reentry SVT, atrial fibrillation, or atrial flutter)
To reduce myocardial ischemia in AMI patients with elevated heart rate, blood pressure, or both

CONTRAINDICATIONS

Hemodynamically unstable patients
STEMI if signs of heart failure, low cardiac output, or increased risk for cardiogenic shock are present
Relative contraindications include P-R interval >0.24 sec, second- or third-degree heart block, active asthma, reactive airway disease, severe bradycardia, SBP <100 mm Hg

ADVERSE REACTIONS

Myocardial depression
AV block
Bradycardia
Cardiac arrest
Diaphoresis
Dizziness
Headache
Hyperglycemia
Hypoglycemia
Hypotension
Nausea
Vomiting

DRUG INTERACTIONS

A potentially clinically significant interaction between esmolol and digoxin may exist because of their additive effects on the AV node.
Esmolol can potentiate the suppressive effects of diltiazem and verapamil on AV nodal conduction.
Depression of AV nodal conduction and myocardial function are possible when used in combination with adenosine, disopyramide, or other antidysrhythmics or drugs, especially in patients with preexisting left ventricular dysfunction.

Careful titration of esmolol is prudent when given with morphine.

HOW SUPPLIED

Solution: 10 mg/mL; 20 mg/mL

DOSAGE AND ADMINISTRATION

0.5 mg/kg (500 mcg/kg) over 1 minute, followed by 0.05 mg/kg (50 mcg/kg) per minute infusion; maximum: 0.3 mg/kg (300 mcg/kg) per minute.
If inadequate response after 5 minutes, may repeat 0.5 mg/kg (500 mcg/kg) bolus and then titrate infusion up to 0.2 mg/kg (200 mcg/kg) per minute. Higher doses are unlikely to be beneficial.
Has a short half-life (2 to 9 minutes).

SPECIAL CONSIDERATIONS

Pregnancy safety: Category C
Administration of esmolol can exacerbate Raynaud's disease or peripheral vascular disease.
Use with caution in patients with poorly controlled diabetes mellitus or renal disease.
Avoid extravasation of esmolol during intravenous administration. Sloughing of the skin and necrosis have been reported following infiltration and extravasation of IV esmolol infusions.

ETOMIDATE (AMIDATE)

CLASS

Nonbarbiturate hypnotic, anesthetic

DESCRIPTION

Etomidate is a short-acting drug that acts at the level of the reticular activating system to produce anesthesia. Etomidate may be administered for conscious sedation to relieve apprehension or impair memory before tracheal intubation or cardioversion.

ONSET AND DURATION

Onset: Less than 1 min
Duration: 5-10 min

INDICATIONS

Premedication for tracheal intubation or cardioversion

CONTRAINDICATIONS

Hypersensitivity to etomidate
Labor/delivery

ADVERSE REACTIONS

Nausea and vomiting
Dysrhythmias
Breathing difficulties
Hypotension
Hypertension
Involuntary muscle movement

Pain at injection site
Cortisol suppression

DRUG INTERACTIONS

Effects may be enhanced when given with other central nervous system depressants.

HOW SUPPLIED

2 mg/mL vials

DOSAGE AND ADMINISTRATION FOR RSI

Adult: 0.2-0.4 mg/kg IV over 30-60 sec; limit to 1 dose
Pediatric (>10 years of age): 0.2-0.4 mg/kg for sedation infused over 30-60 sec; max dose: 20 mg

SPECIAL CONSIDERATIONS

Pregnancy safety: Category C
Carefully monitor vital signs.
Etomidate can suppress adrenal gland production of steroid hormones, which can cause temporary gland failure.
Avoid routine use in patients suspected to have septic shock.

FENTANYL (SUBLIMAZE)

CLASS

Opioid analgesic

DESCRIPTION

Fentanyl (like other opioids) combines with receptor sites in the brain to produce potent analgesic effects. The drug often is given in combination with benzodiazepines for conscious sedation.

ONSET AND DURATION

Onset: 1-2 min (IV)
Duration: ½ to 1 hr

INDICATIONS

Pain control
Sedation for invasive airway procedures (e.g., rapid sequence induction)

CONTRAINDICATIONS

Respiratory depression
Hypotension
Head injury
Cardiac dysrhythmias
Myasthenia gravis
Hypersensitivity to opiates

ADVERSE REACTIONS

Respiratory depression
Bradycardia

Hypotension or hypertension
Nausea and vomiting
Chest wall muscle rigidity

DRUG INTERACTIONS

Effects may be increased when given with other central nervous system depressants or skeletal muscle relaxants.

HOW SUPPLIED

0.05-0.1 mg/mL ampules

DOSAGE AND ADMINISTRATION

Adult: 0.05-0.1 mg IV slow IV over 1-2 min every 1-2 hr as needed to control pain
Child: 1-2 mcg/kg; rarely used in the prehospital setting
Rapid Sequence Intubation
2-5 mcg/kg IV/IO

SPECIAL CONSIDERATIONS

Pregnancy safety: Category C
Fentanyl is a schedule II drug with the potential for abuse.
Fentanyl should be used (if at all) with caution in elderly patients and in those with severe respiratory disorders, seizure disorders, cardiac disorders, or pregnancy.
Naloxone or nalmefene should be available to reverse respiratory depression.

FLUMAZENIL (ROMAZICON)

CLASS

Benzodiazepine receptor antagonist, antidote

DESCRIPTION

Flumazenil antagonizes the actions of benzodiazepines in the central nervous system. It has been shown to reverse sedation, impairment of recall, and psychomotor impairment produced by benzodiazepines. Flumazenil is not, however, as effective in reversing hypoventilation. Flumazenil does not antagonize central nervous system effects of ethanol, barbiturates, or opioids.

ONSET AND DURATION

Onset: 1-2 min
Duration: Related to plasma concentration of benzodiazepine

INDICATIONS

Reversal of respiratory depression and sedation from pure benzodiazepine overdose

CONTRAINDICATIONS

Hypersensitivity to flumazenil or to benzodiazepines
Tricyclic antidepressant overdose
Chronic benzodiazepine users or alcoholics
Cocaine or other stimulant intoxication
Known seizure disorder (relative)

ADVERSE REACTIONS

Nausea and vomiting
Dizziness
Headache
Agitation
Injection site pain
Cutaneous vasodilation
Abnormal vision
Seizures

DRUG INTERACTIONS

Toxic effects of mixed drug overdose (especially tricyclic antidepressants) may emerge with the reversal of the benzodiazepine effects.

HOW SUPPLIED

5- and 10-mL vials (0.1 mg/mL)

DOSAGE AND ADMINISTRATION

For Suspected Benzodiazepine Overdose
Adult:
    First dose: 0.2 mg IV over 15 sec
    Second dose: 0.3 mg IV over 30 sec
    Third dose: 0.5 mg over 30 sec at 1-min intervals until adequate response or max dose of 3 mg is given
Pediatric: Not recommended

SPECIAL CONSIDERATIONS

Pregnancy safety: Category C
To minimize the likelihood of injection site pain, administer through an IV infusion established in a large vein.
Be prepared to manage seizures in patients who are physically dependent on benzodiazepines to control seizures or who have ingested large doses of other drugs.
Flumazenil may precipitate withdrawal syndromes in patients who are dependent on benzodiazepines.
Patients should be monitored for possible resedation, respiratory depression, or other residual benzodiazepine effects.
Be prepared to establish and assist ventilation.

FUROSEMIDE (LASIX)

CLASS

Loop diuretic

DESCRIPTION

Furosemide is a potent diuretic that inhibits the reabsorption of sodium and chloride in the proximal tubule and loop of Henle. Intravenous doses also can reduce cardiac preload by increasing venous capacitance.

ONSET AND DURATION

Onset: (IV) Diuretic effects within 15-20 min; vascular effects within 5 min
Duration: 2 hr

INDICATIONS

Acute pulmonary edema in patients with a SBP >90-100 mm Hg (without signs and symptoms of shock)
Hypertensive emergencies
Hyperkalemia

CONTRAINDICATIONS

Anuria (though loop diuretics can be used in patients with reduced creatinine clearance)
Hypersensitivity
Hypovolemia/dehydration
Known hypersensitivity to sulfonamides (caution)
Severe electrolyte depletion (hypokalemia)

ADVERSE REACTIONS

Hypotension
Electrocardiogram changes associated with electrolyte disturbances
Dry mouth
Hypochloremia
Hypokalemia
Hyponatremia
Hypocalcemia
Hyperglycemia
Hearing loss can occur rarely after too rapid infusion of large doses especially in patients with renal impairment.

DRUG INTERACTIONS

Digitalis toxicity may be potentiated because of potassium depletion, which can result from furosemide administration.
Furosemide increases ototoxic potential of aminoglycoside antibiotics.
Lithium toxicity may be potentiated because of sodium depletion.
Furosemide may potentiate therapeutic effect of other antihypertensive drugs.

HOW SUPPLIED

Parenteral: 10 mg/mL in 2-, 4-, 8-mL ampule, 10 mg/mL in 10-mL vial

DOSAGE AND ADMINISTRATION

IV: 0.5-1 mg/kg over 1-2 min; if no response, double dose to 2 mg/kg given slowly over 1-2 min; for new-onset pulmonary edema with hypovolemia, give <0.5 mg/kg
Pediatric: 1 mg/kg/dose (max total dose: 6 mg/kg)
Hyperkalemia (adult): 40-80 mg IV

SPECIAL CONSIDERATIONS

Pregnancy safety: Category C
Furosemide has been known to cause fetal abnormalities.
Furosemide should be protected from light and stored at room temperature; do not use if solution is discolored or yellow.

GLUCAGON

CLASS

Pancreatic hormone, antihypoglycemic agent

DESCRIPTION

Glucagon is a protein secreted by the alpha cells of the pancreas. When released, glucagon results in blood glucose elevation by increasing the breakdown of glycogen to glucose (glycogenolysis) and stimulating glucose synthesis (gluconeogenesis). The drug is only effective in treating hypoglycemia if liver glycogen is available and therefore may be ineffective in chronic states of hypoglycemia, starvation, and adrenal insufficiency. In addition, glucagon exerts positive inotropic action on the heart and decreases renal vascular resistance. For this reason, glucagon also is used in managing patients with beta-blocker and calcium channel blocker cardiotoxicity who do not respond to saline infusions or other conventional therapy.

ONSET AND DURATION

Onset: Within 1 min
Duration: 60-90 min

INDICATIONS

Hypoglycemia
Calcium channel blocker or beta-blocker toxicity

CONTRAINDICATIONS

Hypersensitivity (allergy to proteins)

ADVERSE REACTIONS

Tachycardia
Hypotension
Nausea and vomiting
Urticaria

DRUG INTERACTIONS

Effect of anticoagulants may be increased if given with glucagon.
Do not mix with saline.

HOW SUPPLIED

Glucagon must be reconstituted (with provided diluent) before administration. Dilute 1 unit (1 mg) of white powder in 1 mL of diluting solution (1 mg/mL).

DOSAGE AND ADMINISTRATION

Hypoglycemia
Adult: 0.5-1 mg IM; may repeat in 7-10 min
Pediatric: For >20 kg, 0.5-1 mg IM
Calcium Channel Blocker or Beta-Blocker Toxicity
Adult: 3-10 mg slow IV over 3-5 min, followed by infusion at 3-5 mg/hr
Pediatric: Safety and efficacy have not been established.

SPECIAL CONSIDERATIONS

Pregnancy safety: Category B
Glucagon should not be considered a first-line choice for hypoglycemia.
May cause vomiting and hyperglycemia.
Intravenous glucose will need to be administered if the patient does not respond to a second dose of glucagon.
Do not use the provided diluent to mix continuous infusions.

HALOPERIDOL LACTATE (HALDOL)

CLASS

Antipsychotic/neuroleptic

DESCRIPTION

Haloperidol has pharmacological properties similar to those of the phenothiazines. The drug is thought to block dopamine (type 2) receptors in the brain, altering mood and behavior. In emergency care, haloperidol usually is administered IM.

ONSET AND DURATION

Onset: (IM) 30-60 min
Duration: 12-24 hr

INDICATIONS

Acute psychotic episodes
Emergency sedation of severely agitated or delirious patients

CONTRAINDICATIONS

Central nervous system depression
Coma
Hypersensitivity
Pregnancy
Severe liver or cardiac disease

ADVERSE REACTIONS

Dose-related extrapyramidal reactions:
Pseudoparkinsonism
Akathisia
Dystonias
Hypotension
Orthostatic hypotension
Nausea, vomiting
Allergic reactions
Blurred vision
Drowsiness

DRUG INTERACTIONS

Other central nervous system depressants may potentiate effects.
Haloperidol may inhibit vasoconstrictor effects of epinephrine.

HOW SUPPLIED

5 mg/mL

DOSAGE AND ADMINISTRATION

Adult: 2-5 mg IM every 4-8 hr as needed
Pediatric: Safety not established

SPECIAL CONSIDERATIONS

Pregnancy safety: Category C

HEPARIN

Low Molecular Weight Heparin (Enoxaparin)

CLASS

Anticoagulant

DESCRIPTION

Heparin is available as Low Molecular Weight Heparin (LMWH [Enoxaparin]) and Unfractionated Heparin (UFH). Both inhibit the clotting cascade by activating specific plasma proteins. Natural heparin (heparin sodium) consists of molecular chains of varying lengths or *molecular weights*. LMWHs consist of only short chains of molecular weight and produce a more predictable coagulation response than UFH.[2] The use of LMWH has been approved for both the prevention and treatment of acute deep vein thrombosis, acute pulmonary embolism, and for the treatment of acute coronary syndromes.

ONSET AND DURATION

Onset: (IV) Immediate
(SQ) 20-60 min
Duration: 4-8 hr

INDICATIONS

ACS,
Acute deep vein thrombosis
Acute pulmonary embolism

CONTRAINDICATIONS

Same as for fibrinolytic therapy
Renal insufficiency
Active bleeding or low platelet count
Hypersensitivity to heparin or pork products
Recent intracranial, intraspinal, or eye surgery
Severe hypertension
Heparin-induced thrombocytopenia

ADVERSE REACTIONS

Allergic reaction (chills, fever, back pain)
Thrombocytopenia
Hemorrhage
Bruising
Rash

DRUG INTERACTIONS

None noted
Salicylates, ibuprofen, dipyridamole, and hydroxychloroquine may increase risk of bleeding.

HOW SUPPLIED

Concentrations range from 30 mg to 150 mg in various mL of solution for SQ or IV administration

DOSAGE AND ADMINISTRATION

STEMI Protocol
    Age <75 years: initial bolus 30 mg IV with second bolus 15 min later of 1 mg/kg SQ (max 100 mg dose for first 2 doses).
    Age ≥75 years: Eliminate initial IV bolus; give 0.75 mg/kg SQ every 12 hours (max 75 mg dose for first 2 doses).
Should use UFH if early cardiac catheterization (within 12 hours) is planned.
UA/NSTEMI Protocol
Loading dose: 30 mg IV bolus; maintenance dose 1 mg/kg SQ every 12 hours.
Deep Vein Thrombosis (DVT) or Pulmonary Embolism Protocol
Adults: 1 mg/kg SQ every 12 hours or 1.5 mg/kg SC every 24 hours.

SPECIAL CONSIDERATIONS

Pregnancy safety: Category B
The platelet count should be monitored in patients receiving enoxaparin.
Always follow institutional protocol regarding heparin administration.
Multiple-dose vials of enoxaparin contain benzyl alcohol (1.5%) as a preservative and should be avoided in patients with benzyl alcohol hypersensitivity.
Do not administer IM.
Enoxaparin cannot be used interchangeably (unit for unit) with heparin sodium or other low molecular weight heparins.
Do not mix with other products or infusion fluids.

HEPARIN SODIUM

Unfractionated (UFH)

CLASS

Anticoagulant

DESCRIPTION

Heparin inhibits the clotting cascade by activating specific plasma proteins. The drug is used in the prevention and treatment of all types of thromboses and emboli, disseminated intravascular coagulation, arterial occlusion, and thrombophlebitis and is used prophylactically to prevent clotting before surgery. Heparin is considered part of the antithrombotic package (along with aspirin and fibrinolytic agents) administered to patients with STEMI, UA/NSTEMI, and acute coronary syndromes.

ONSET AND DURATION

Onset: (IV) Immediate
(SQ) 20-60 min
Duration: 4-8 hr

INDICATIONS

Acute myocardial infarction
UA/NSTEMI
STEMI
Prophylaxis and treatment of thromboembolic disorders (e.g., pulmonary emboli and deep venous thrombosis)

CONTRAINDICATIONS

Same as for fibrinolytic therapy
Hypersensitivity
Active bleeding
Recent intracranial, intraspinal, or eye surgery
Severe hypertension
Bleeding tendencies
Severe thrombocytopenia

ADVERSE REACTIONS

Allergic reaction (chills, fever, back pain)
Thrombocytopenia
Hemorrhage
Bruising
Rash

DRUG INTERACTIONS

Salicylates, ibuprofen, dipyridamole, and hydroxychloroquine may increase risk of bleeding.

HOW SUPPLIED

Concentrations range from 1000 to 40 000 units/mL

DOSAGE AND ADMINISTRATION

IV Infusion- STEMI and UA/NSTEMI
   Initial bolus of 60 units/kg (max bolus: 4000 units); continue 12 units/kg/hr, round to the nearest 50 units (max initial rate: 1000 units/hr).

SPECIAL CONSIDERATIONS

Pregnancy safety: Category C
Dosing should be guided by laboratory analysis of platelet count and partial thromboplastin time. Always follow institutional protocol regarding heparin administration.

HYDROMORPHONE (DILAUDID)

CLASS

Analgesic; opiate agonist

DESCRIPTION

Hydromorphone is a semisynthetic analog of morphine used to relieve moderate to severe pain in cancer, surgery, trauma, burn, and cardiac patients. The drug works at opioid receptors to produce analgesia and euphoria. It may also produce respiratory depression, miosis, decreased gastrointestinal motility, and physical dependence. Hydromorphone is a schedule II controlled substance.

ONSET AND DURATION

Onset (IV/IM): Within 15 min (dose related)
Duration: 4-5 hr in nondependent patients

INDICATIONS

Moderate to severe pain
Analgesia
Preoperative medication

CONTRAINDICATIONS

Asthma
GI obstruction
Hypersensitivity to narcotics
Ileus
Respiratory depression
Status asthmaticus

ADVERSE REACTIONS

Respiratory depression
Nausea and vomiting
Euphoria
Delirium
Agitation
Hallucination
Seizures
Headache
Hypotension
Visual disturbances
Coma
Facial flushing
Circulatory collapse
Dysrhythmias
Allergic reaction
Drowsiness
Rash

DRUG INTERACTIONS

Respiratory depression, hypotension, or sedation may be potentiated by central nervous system depressants.
Therapeutic doses of hydromorphone have caused additive CNS or respiratory depression and hypotension in patients taking MAO inhibitors.

HOW SUPPLIED

Solution for injection: 1 mg/mL, 2 mg/mL, 4 mg/mL

DOSAGE AND ADMINISTRATION

Adult: 1-2 mg subQ/IM or slow IV every 6 hr; titrate to pain relief

Pediatric (>50 kg): 1 mg IV/subQ every 4 hr; pediatric (<50 kg or >6 months of age): 0.015-0.02 mg/kg IV/subQ every 2-4 hr; titrate to pain relief

SPECIAL CONSIDERATIONS

Pregnancy safety: Category C

High potential for abuse

Use with extreme caution in patients with head trauma, increased intracranial pressure (ICP), or a preexisting seizure disorder.

Use with caution in patients with cardiac dysrhythmias, hypotension, circulatory shock, or hypovolemia.

Elderly patients may be more susceptible to adverse reactions.

Can induce vasovagal syncope or orthostatic hypotension.

Naloxone should be readily available.

HYDROXOCOBALAMIN (CYANOKIT)

CLASS

Vitamin; antidote

DESCRIPTION

Hydroxocobalamin is a parenteral preparation of vitamin B_{12}; specifically, it is the hydroxylated active form of vitamin B_{12}. Hydroxocobalamin is used to treat known or suspected cyanide toxicity.

ONSET AND DURATION

Onset: Rapid

Duration: Greater than 24 hr

INDICATIONS

Known or suspected cyanide poisoning

CONTRAINDICATIONS

Known hydroxocobalamin hypersensitivity

ADVERSE REACTIONS

Allergic reaction/anaphylaxis

Elevated blood pressure

Headache

Hypertension

Injection site reaction

Nausea

Photophobia

Red-colored urine

DRUG INTERACTIONS

None

HOW SUPPLIED

Powder for injection: 5 g

Solution: 1000 mcg/mL

DOSAGE AND ADMINISTRATION

Adults: Initially, 5 g (two 2.5-g vials) IV infused over 15 min (approximately 15 mL/min or 7.5 min per vial). A second 5-g dose infused over 15 min to 2 hr (depending on patient status), for a total of 10 g, may be administered based on clinical response and severity of cyanide poisoning

Children: Doses of 70 mg/kg IV have been used; not FDA approved

SPECIAL CONSIDERATIONS

Pregnancy safety: Category C

Before administration of the antidote, a blood sample should be taken to determine the cyanide concentration.

Treatment of cyanide poisoning includes supportive therapy, such as cardiovascular support, airway/ventilation management, control of seizure activity, and hydration in addition to the use of hydroxocobalamin.

Solution is bright red.

IBUTILIDE (CORVERT)

CLASS

Short-acting Class III antidysrhythmic

DESCRIPTION

Ibutilide prolongs the action potential duration and increases the refractory period of cardiac tissue. Ibutilide is recommended to convert acute supraventricular dysrhythmias, including atrial flutter and atrial fibrillation, when their duration is 48 hours or less. The drug may also be used as an adjunct to electrical cardioversion.

ONSET AND DURATION

Onset: $\frac{1}{2}$ to $1\frac{1}{2}$ hr

Duration: 10-12 hr

INDICATIONS

Supraventricular dysrhythmias

Conversion of atrial fibrillation and atrial flutter of brief duration

CONTRAINDICATIONS

History of heart failure or ventricular tachycardia

Patients with QTc >400 ms

Sensitivity to ibutilide

ADVERSE REACTIONS

Ventricular dysrhythmias, including polymorphic VT, torsades

Bradycardia

Hypotension and hypertension

Headache

DRUG INTERACTIONS

Avoid concurrent administration of ibutilide with other antidysrhythmics that prolong the refractory period (e.g., amiodarone) or drugs that induce Q-T interval prolongation (e.g., procainamide).

HOW SUPPLIED

1 mg in 10-mL ampules

DOSAGE AND ADMINISTRATION

Adult (60 kg or more): 1 mg (10 mL) diluted or undiluted IV over 10 min. A second dose may be administered at the same rate 10 min later. The initial dose for adults who weigh less than 60 kg is 0.01 mg/kg IV.
Pediatric: Not recommended

SPECIAL CONSIDERATIONS

Pregnancy safety: Category C
Ibutilide must be given slowly IV over 10 min. This may make it impractical for use in emergent situations.
Ventricular dysrhythmias develop in 2% to 5% of patients who are given ibutilide; continuous electrocardiogram monitoring is essential.
Use with caution in patients with impaired left ventricular function.

INSULIN (REGULAR, NPH, AND OTHERS)

CLASS

Antidiabetic agent

DESCRIPTION

Insulin is secreted by the beta cells (islets of Langerhans) of the pancreas and is required for proper glucose utilization by the body. If insulin secretion is diminished (as in diabetes mellitus), supplemental insulin must be obtained by injection. Insulin preparations are classified as *short-acting* (regular) and *intermediate-acting* (NPH). Insulin seldom is administered in the prehospital setting, even when ketoacidosis is present. (Large amounts of normal saline solution are considered the first-line treatment.) Insulin may be required for long transport times.

ONSET AND DURATION

Onset: ½ to 1 hr (short-acting); 1 to 1½ hr (intermediate-acting); 4-6 hr (long-acting)
Duration: 6-8 hr (short-acting); 18-24 hr (intermediate-acting)

INDICATIONS

Type 1 diabetes mellitus
Type 2 diabetes mellitus if oral hypoglycemic agents do not control blood glucose adequately
Diabetic ketoacidosis
Nonketotic hyperosmolar coma
Insulin and 50% dextrose solution are given together to lower potassium levels in hyperkalemia.

CONTRAINDICATIONS

Hypoglycemia

ADVERSE REACTIONS

Hypoglycemia
Fatigue
Weakness
Confusion
Headache
Tachycardia
Rapid, shallow breathing
Nausea
Diaphoresis
Allergic reaction

DRUG INTERACTIONS

Corticosteroids, dobutamine, epinephrine, and thiazide diuretics may antagonize (decrease) the hypoglycemic effects of insulin.
Alcohol, beta-adrenergic blockers, MAO inhibitors, and salicylates may potentiate (increase) the hypoglycemic effects of insulin.

HOW SUPPLIED

100 units/mL in 10-mL vials

DOSAGE AND ADMINISTRATION

Insulin may be administered subQ or IM. Regular insulin can be given IV, and dosage is governed by the clinical presentation of the patient. A standard dose of insulin administration is as follows:
Adult: 10-25 units of regular insulin IV, followed by an infusion of 0.1 unit/kg/hr
Pediatric: 0.1-0.2 unit/kg/hr IM
Infusion: 100 units of regular insulin mixed in 100 mL of NS (1 unit/mL), infused at a rate of 0.1-0.2 unit/kg/hr (use infusion pump)

SPECIAL CONSIDERATIONS

Pregnancy safety: Category B
Insulin is the drug of choice for control of diabetes in pregnancy.
Insulin injected into the abdominal wall is absorbed most rapidly, insulin in the arm is absorbed more slowly, and insulin is absorbed slowest when injected into the thigh.

IPRATROPIUM (ATROVENT)

CLASS

Anticholinergic, bronchodilator

DESCRIPTION

Ipratropium inhibits interaction of acetylcholine at receptor sites on bronchial smooth muscle, resulting in decreased levels of cyclic guanosine monophosphate and bronchodilation.

ONSET AND DURATION

Onset: 5-15 min
Duration: 4-6 hr

INDICATIONS

Persistent bronchospasm
Chronic obstructive pulmonary disease exacerbation

CONTRAINDICATIONS

Hypersensitivity to ipratropium, atropine, alkaloid, soybean
protein, peanuts

ADVERSE REACTIONS

Nausea and vomiting
Cramps
Coughing
Worsening of symptoms
Headache
Tachycardia
Dry mouth
Blurred vision
Anxiety

DRUG INTERACTIONS

None reported

HOW SUPPLIED

Aerosol 17-18—nebulizer
18 mcg—MDI

DOSAGE AND ADMINISTRATION

NOTE: When used in combination with beta agonists
(e.g., albuterol), the beta agonist is always administered
first with a 5-min wait before administering
ipratropium.
Adult: 1-2 inhalations
Pediatric: 250-500 mcg (by nebulizer or MDI) every 20 min
times 3 doses

SPECIAL CONSIDERATIONS

Pregnancy safety: Category B
Shake well before use.
Use with caution in patients with urinary retention.

ISOPROTERENOL (ISUPREL)

CLASS

Sympathomimetic

DESCRIPTION

Isoproterenol is a synthetic catecholamine that stimulates
both $beta_1$- and $beta_2$-adrenergic receptors (no alpha-
receptor stimulation). The drug affects the heart by increasing inotropic and chronotropic activity. In addition,
isoproterenol causes arterial and bronchial dilation
and sometimes is administered via aerosolization
as a bronchodilator to treat bronchial asthma and bronchospasm. (Because of the undesirable $beta_1$ cardiac effects, the
use of this drug as a bronchodilator is uncommon in the
prehospital setting.) Isoproterenol should be used cautiously as a temporizing measure if an external pacer is
not available for symptomatic bradycardia.

ONSET AND DURATION

Onset: 1-5 min
Duration: 15-30 min

INDICATIONS

Hemodynamically significant bradycardias secondary to
beta-blocker overdose
Management of refractory torsades de pointes, unresponsive to magnesium sulfate
Temporary control of bradycardia in heart transplant
patients, unresponsive to atropine

CONTRAINDICATIONS

Ventricular tachycardia
Ventricular fibrillation
Hypotension (relative)
Pulseless idioventricular rhythm
Ischemic heart disease/angina (relative)
Cardiac arrest
Acetylcholinesterase-induced bradycardias
Poison/drug-induced shock (other than beta-blocker
poisoning)

ADVERSE REACTIONS

Dysrhythmias
Hypotension
Precipitation of angina pectoris
Facial flushing
Restlessness
Dry throat
Discoloration of saliva (pinkish red)

DRUG INTERACTIONS

MAO inhibitors potentiate the effects of catecholamines.
Beta-adrenergic antagonists may blunt inotropic response.
Sympathomimetics and phosphodiesterase inhibitors may
exacerbate dysrhythmia response.
Do not give with epinephrine; can cause VF or VT.

HOW SUPPLIED

5-mL (0.2 mg/mL) vial; 0.02 mg/mL in 1- and 10-mL
vials

DOSAGE AND ADMINISTRATION

Adult: Dilute 1 mg in 250 mL of D_5W (4 mcg/mL);
infuse at 2-10 mcg/min or until the desired heart
rate is obtained; in torsades de pointes, titrate to
increase heart rate until ventricular tachycardia is
suppressed
Pediatric: Not recommended

SPECIAL CONSIDERATIONS

Pregnancy safety: Category C

Isoproterenol increases myocardial oxygen demand and can induce serious dysrhythmias (including ventricular tachycardia and ventricular fibrillation).

Administer via infusion pump to ensure precise flow rates.

Isoproterenol may exacerbate tachydysrhythmias caused by digitalis toxicity or hypokalemia.

Newer inotropic agents have replaced isoproterenol in most clinical settings.

If electronic pacing is available, it should be used instead of isoproterenol or as soon as possible after drug administration has been initiated.

KETAMINE (KETALAR)

CLASS

Nonbarbiturate anesthetic

DESCRIPTION

Ketamine acts on the limbic system and cortex to block afferent transmission of impulses associated with pain perception. It produces short-acting amnesia without muscular relaxation. Ketamine is a derivative of a drug of abuse, phencyclidine.

ONSET AND DURATION

Onset: Within 30 sec
Duration: 5-10 min

INDICATIONS

Pain control
As an adjunct to nitrous oxide

CONTRAINDICATIONS

Stroke
Increased intracranial pressure
Severe hypertension
Cardiac decompensation
Hypersensitivity to ketamine

ADVERSE REACTIONS

Hypertension
Increased heart rate
Hallucinations, delusions, explicit dreams
Less common side effects include hypotension, bradycardia, and respiratory depression

DRUG INTERACTIONS

No significant drug interactions have been reported.

HOW SUPPLIED

10, 50, and 100 mg/mL vials

DOSAGE AND ADMINISTRATION

Adult: 1-2 mg/kg IV over 1 min or 4-5 mg/kg IM
Child (>2 years of age): 1-2 mg/kg IV over 1 min or 3-5 mg/kg IM
Rapid Sequence Intubation
1-2 mg/kg IV/IO

SPECIAL CONSIDERATIONS

Pregnancy safety: Category C

Ketamine may increase blood pressure, muscle tone, and heart rate.

As with any anesthetic, the dosage needs to be assessed carefully and individualized.

Keep patient in a quiet environment (if possible).

KETOROLAC TROMETHAMINE (TORADOL)

CLASS

Nonsteroidal antiinflammatory

DESCRIPTION

Ketorolac tromethamine is an antiinflammatory drug that also exhibits peripherally acting nonnarcotic analgesic activity by inhibiting prostaglandin synthesis.

ONSET AND DURATION

Onset: Within 10 min
Duration: 6-8 hr

INDICATIONS

Short-term management (less than 5 days) of moderate to severe pain

CONTRAINDICATIONS

Hypersensitivity to the drug
Patients with allergies to aspirin or other nonsteroidal antiinflammatory drugs
Bleeding disorders
Renal failure
Active peptic ulcer disease

ADVERSE REACTIONS

Anaphylaxis from hypersensitivity
Edema
Sedation
Bleeding disorders
Rash
Nausea
Headache

DRUG INTERACTIONS

Ketorolac may increase bleeding time when administered to patients taking anticoagulants.
Effects of lithium and methotrexate may be increased.

HOW SUPPLIED

15 or 30 mg in 1 mL
60 mg in 2 mL

DOSAGE AND ADMINISTRATION

Adult:
  IM: 1 dose of 60 mg (for patients <65 years of age); 1 dose of 30 mg for patients >65 years of age, have renal impairment, and/or weigh less than 50 kg
  IV: 30 mg over 1 min (for patients <65 years of age or weigh less than 50 kg); one-half dose (15 mg) for patients >65 years of age, have renal impairment, and/or weigh less than 50 kg
Pediatric: Not recommended

SPECIAL CONSIDERATIONS

Pregnancy safety: Category C
Solution is clear and slightly yellow.
Use with caution and reduce dose when administering to elderly patients.

LABETALOL (TRANDATE)

CLASS

Alpha- and beta-adrenergic blocker

DESCRIPTION

Labetalol is a competitive alpha$_1$-receptor blocker and a nonselective beta-receptor blocker that is used for lowering blood pressure in hypertensive crisis. Labetalol is a more potent beta blocker than alpha blocker. Blood pressure is reduced without reflex tachycardia, and total peripheral resistance is decreased, helping maintain cardiac output. In emergency care, labetalol is administered IV.

ONSET AND DURATION

Onset: Within 5 min
Duration: 3-6 hr

INDICATIONS

Hypertensive emergencies
All patients with suspected MI and unstable angina in the absence of contraindications (can reduce the incidence of VF)
Useful as an adjunctive agent with fibrinolytic therapy (may reduce nonfatal reinfarction and recurrent ischemia)
To convert to normal sinus rhythm or to slow ventricular response (or both) in supraventricular tachydysrhythmias (reentry SVT, atrial fibrillation, or atrial flutter)
To reduce myocardial ischemia in AMI patients with elevated heart rate, blood pressure, or both

CONTRAINDICATIONS

Hemodynamically unstable patients
STEMI if signs of heart failure, low cardiac output, or increased risk for cardiogenic shock are present
Relative contraindications include P-R interval >0.24 sec, second- or third-degree heart block, active asthma, reactive airway disease, severe bradycardia, SBP <100 mm Hg

ADVERSE REACTIONS

Headache
Dizziness
Edema
Fatigue
Vertigo
Ventricular dysrhythmias
Dyspnea
Allergic reaction
Facial flushing
Diaphoresis
Dose-related orthostatic hypotension (most common)
Bradycardia
Nausea and vomiting
Tinnitus

DRUG INTERACTIONS

Bronchodilator effects of beta-adrenergic agonists may be blunted by labetalol.
Nitroglycerin may augment hypotensive effects.

HOW SUPPLIED

5 mg/mL in 4-, 8-, 20-, and 40-mL vials

DOSAGE AND ADMINISTRATION

Adult: 10 mg IV over 1-2 min. May repeat or double labetalol every 10 min to a max dose of 150 mg. Alternative dosing: Give initial dose as a bolus, and then begin infusion at 2-8 mg/min
Infusion: Mix 200 mg in 250 mL of D$_5$W (0.8 mg/mL); infuse at a rate of 2-8 mg/min, titrated to supine blood pressure
Pediatric: Safety has not been established; initiate cautiously with careful dosage adjustments and blood pressure monitoring

SPECIAL CONSIDERATIONS

Pregnancy safety: Category C
Blood pressure, pulse rate, and electrocardiogram should be monitored continuously.
Observe for signs of congestive heart failure, bradycardia, and bronchospasm.
Labetalol should be administered only with the patient in a supine position.

LEVALBUTEROL (XOPENEX)

CLASS

Sympathomimetic, bronchodilator, beta$_2$ agonist

DESCRIPTION

Levalbuterol is a relatively selective beta$_2$-adrenergic receptor agonist. It acts as a functional antagonist to relax the smooth muscles of all airways, from the trachea to the terminal bronchioles.

ONSET AND DURATION

Onset: 5-15 min after inhalation
Duration: 3-4 hr after inhalation

INDICATIONS

Treatment or prevention of bronchospasm in patients over 6 years of age with reversible, obstructive airway disease

CONTRAINDICATIONS

Prior hypersensitivity to levalbuterol or racemic albuterol
Cardiac dysrhythmias associated with tachycardia

ADVERSE REACTIONS

Usually dose related
Restlessness, apprehension, tremor
Chills, body pain, chest pain
Eye itch
Hypertension, hypotension, syncope
Palpitation, tachycardia
Dysrhythmias

DRUG INTERACTIONS

Other sympathomimetics may exacerbate adverse cardiovascular effects.
Antidepressants may potentiate effects on the vasculature (vasodilation).
Beta blockers may antagonize levalbuterol.
Levalbuterol may potentiate diuretic-induced hypokalemia.

HOW SUPPLIED

Solution for aerosolization: 3-mL unit dose (0.31, 0.63, 1.25 mg)
Solution packaged in color-coded foil pouches

DOSAGE AND ADMINISTRATION

Bronchospasm
Pediatric: 6-11 years old: 0.31 mg by nebulization q 6-8 hr. Dose not to exceed 0.63 mg every 6-8 hr
Adult: 12 or older: 0.63-1.25 mg by nebulization q 6-8 hr
NOTE: In settings of acute asthma, 1.25 mg of levalbuterol should be administered every 20 min for a total of 3 doses.

SPECIAL CONSIDERATIONS

Pregnancy safety: Category C
Levalbuterol should not be given to children younger than 6 years of age.
Levalbuterol may precipitate angina pectoris and dysrhythmias.

Levalbuterol is sometimes preferred over albuterol for patients with preexisting tachycardia.
Levalbuterol should be used with caution (if at all) in patients taking beta blockers, diuretics, digoxin, monamine oxidase inhibitors, or tricyclic antidepressants.

LIDOCAINE (XYLOCAINE)

CLASS

Antidysrhythmic (Class IB), local anesthetic

DESCRIPTION

Lidocaine decreases phase 4 diastolic depolarization (which decreases automaticity) and has been shown to be effective in suppressing premature ventricular complexes. In addition, lidocaine is used as an alternative to amiodarone to treat cardiac arrest from VT or VF. Lidocaine also raises the ventricular fibrillation threshold.

ONSET AND DURATION

Onset: 30-90 sec
Duration: 10-20 min

INDICATIONS

Cardiac arrest from ventricular tachycardia or ventricular fibrillation
Stable monomorphic VT with preserved ventricular function
Stable polymorphic VT with normal baseline Q-T interval and preserved LV function after correction of ischemia and electrolyte balance
Stable polymorphic VT with baseline-prolonged Q-T interval if torsades is suspected
Wide-complex tachycardia of uncertain origin
Significant ventricular ectopy in the setting of myocardial ischemia/infarction

CONTRAINDICATIONS

Prophylactic use in AMI
Hypersensitivity
Stokes-Adams syndrome
Second- or third-degree heart block in the absence of an artificial pacemaker

ADVERSE REACTIONS

Light-headedness
Confusion
Blurred vision
Hypotension
Bradycardia
Cardiovascular collapse
Bradycardia
Altered level of consciousness, irritability, muscle twitching, seizures with high doses
Headache
Seizures

DRUG INTERACTIONS

Metabolic clearance of lidocaine may be decreased in patients taking beta-adrenergic blockers or in patients with decreased cardiac output or liver dysfunction.

Apnea induced with succinylcholine may be prolonged with large doses of lidocaine.

Cardiac depression may occur if lidocaine is given concomitantly with IV phenytoin.

Additive neurological effects may occur with procainamide and tocainide.

HOW SUPPLIED

Prefilled syringes: 100 mg in 5 mL of solution; 1- and 2-g additive syringes

Ampules: 100 mg in 5 mL of solution; 1- and 2-g vials in 30 mL of solution; 5 mL containing 100 mg/mL

DOSAGE AND ADMINISTRATION

Cardiac Arrest From Ventricular Tachycardia/Ventricular Fibrillation

Adult: 1-1.5 mg/kg IV/IO bolus or endotracheal tube (at 2-2.5 times the IV dose); for refractory VF, may give additional 0.5-0.75 mg/kg IV push; repeat in 5-10 min; max 3 doses or total of 3 mg/kg

Pediatric: 1 mg/kg IV/IO loading dose; ET dose: 2-3 mg/kg

Perfusing Dysrhythmia (Stable VT; Wide-Complex Tachycardia of Uncertain Type; Significant Ectopy)

Adult: Doses may range from 0.5 to 0.75 mg/kg (up to 1-1.5 mg/kg may be used). Repeat 0.5-0.75 mg/kg every 5-10 min; max total dose 3 mg/kg

Pediatric: 1 mg/kg IV/IO. ET dose is 2-3 mg/kg

Maintenance Infusion After Resuscitation From Cardiac Arrest From Ventricular Tachycardia/Ventricular Fibrillation

Adult: 1-4 mg/min (30-50 mcg/kg/min); reduce maintenance dose (not loading dose) in presence of impaired liver function or LV dysfunction

Pediatric: 20-50 mcg/kg/min IV/IO; repeat bolus dose if infusion initiated >15 min after initial bolus therapy

Pediatric: Initial loading dose of 1 mg/kg IV/IO, followed by infusion of 20-50 mcg/kg/min

Rapid Sequence Intubation

1-2 mg/kg IV/IO (max 100 mg)

SPECIAL CONSIDERATIONS

Pregnancy safety: Category B

A 75-100 mg bolus will maintain adequate blood levels for only 20 min (in absence of shock).

If bradycardia occurs along with premature ventricular contractions, always treat the bradycardia first with atropine.

Discontinue infusion immediately if signs of toxicity develop.

Exceedingly high doses of lidocaine can result in coma or death.

Decrease dose in the elderly.

Avoid lidocaine for reperfusion dysrhythmias following fibrinolytic therapy.

Use extreme caution in patients with hepatic disease, heart failure, marked hypoxia, severe respiratory depression, hypovolemia or shock, incomplete heart block, or bradycardia and atrial fibrillation.

LORAZEPAM (ATIVAN)

CLASS

Benzodiazepine

DESCRIPTION

Lorazepam is a benzodiazepine with antianxiety and anticonvulsant effects. When given by injection, it appears to suppress the propagation of seizure activity produced by foci in the cortex, thalamus, and limbic areas.

ONSET AND DURATION

Onset: 5 min (IV)
Duration: 6-8 hr

INDICATIONS

Agitation requiring sedation

Initial control of status epilepticus or severe recurrent seizures (investigational)

CONTRAINDICATIONS

Hypersensitivity to the drug
Substance abuse (relative)
Coma (unless seizing)
Severe hypotension
Shock
Preexisting central nervous system depression

ADVERSE REACTIONS

Respiratory depression
Tachycardia/bradycardia
Hypotension
Sedation
Ataxia
Psychomotor impairment
Confusion
Blurred vision

DRUG INTERACTIONS

Lorazepam may precipitate central nervous system depression and psychomotor impairment when the patient is taking central nervous system depressant medications.

HOW SUPPLIED

2 and 4 mg/mL concentrations in 1-mL vials

DOSAGE AND ADMINISTRATION

Before IV administration, lorazepam must be diluted with an equal volume of sterile water or sterile saline. When given IM, lorazepam is not to be diluted.

Adult: 1-4 mg slow IM/IV over 2-10 min; may be repeated in 15-20 min to a max dose of 8 mg

Pediatric (not FDA-approved): 0.05-0.1 mg/kg slow IV/IO/IM over 2 min; may be repeated once in 5-10 min to a max dose of 4 mg; 0.1-0.2 mg/kg (rectal dose)

SPECIAL CONSIDERATIONS

Pregnancy safety: Category D

Monitor respiratory rate and blood pressure during administration.

Have suction and intubation equipment available.

Inadvertent intraarterial injection may produce arteriospasm, resulting in gangrene that may require amputation.

Lorazepam expires in 6 weeks when not refrigerated; do not use if discolored or if solution contains precipitate.

MAGNESIUM SULFATE

CLASS

Electrolyte, anticonvulsant

DESCRIPTION

Magnesium sulfate reduces striated muscle contractions and blocks peripheral neuromuscular transmission by reducing acetylcholine release at the myoneural junction. In emergency care, magnesium sulfate is used in the management of seizures associated with toxemia of pregnancy. Other uses of magnesium sulfate include uterine relaxation (to inhibit contractions of premature labor), as a bronchodilator after beta-agonist and anticholinergic agents have been used, and replacement therapy for magnesium deficiency. Magnesium sulfate is recommended for use in cardiac arrest only if torsades de pointes or suspected hypomagnesemia is present.

ONSET AND DURATION

Onset: (IV) Immediate; (IM) 3-4 hr
Duration: 30 min (IV); 3-4 hr (IM)

INDICATIONS

Seizures of eclampsia (toxemia of pregnancy)

Cardiac arrest only if torsades de pointes is suspected or hypomagnesemia is present

Life-threatening ventricular dysrhythmias attributable to digitalis toxicity

Suspected hypomagnesemia

Status asthmaticus not responsive to beta-adrenergic drugs

CONTRAINDICATIONS

Heart block or myocardial damage

ADVERSE REACTIONS

Diaphoresis
Facial flushing
Hypotension
Depressed reflexes
Hypothermia
Reduced heart rate

Circulatory collapse
Respiratory depression
Diarrhea
Nausea and vomiting

DRUG INTERACTIONS

Central nervous system depressant effects may be enhanced if the patient is taking other central nervous system depressants.

Serious changes in cardiac function may occur with cardiac glycosides (avoid excess magnesium administration).

HOW SUPPLIED

10%, 12.5%, 50% solution in 40, 80, 100, and 125 mg/mL

DOSAGE AND ADMINISTRATION

Seizure Activity Associated With Pregnancy

Adult: 1-4 g (8-32 mEq) IV; max dose of 30-40 g/day

Pulseless Arrest (for Hypomagnesemia or Torsades de Pointes), Status Asthmaticus

Adult: 1-2 g (2-4 mL of a 50% solution) diluted in 10 mL of D_5W IV/IO push

Pediatric: 25-50 mg/kg IV/IO (max 2 g) over 10-20 min; over 15-30 min for status asthmaticus

Torsades de Pointes With Pulse or AMI With Hypomagnesemia

Adult: Loading dose of 1-2 g in 50-100 mL of D_5W over 5-60 min IV; follow with 0.5-1 g/hr IV (titrate dose to control torsades)

Pediatric: Same as pulseless arrest

SPECIAL CONSIDERATIONS

Pregnancy safety: Category A

Magnesium sulfate is administered for the treatment of toxemia of pregnancy. It is recommended that the drug not be administered in the 2 hr before delivery, if possible. IV calcium gluconate or calcium chloride should be available as an antagonist to magnesium if needed

Convulsions may occur up to 48 hr after delivery, necessitating continued therapy.

The "cure" for toxemia is delivery of the baby.

Magnesium must be used with caution in patients with renal failure because it is cleared by the kidneys and can reach toxic levels easily in those patients.

MANNITOL (OSMITROL)

CLASS

Osmotic diuretic

DESCRIPTION

Because of the osmotic properties of mannitol, the drug promotes the movement of fluid from the intracellular into the extracellular space. In emergency care, mannitol most often is used to decrease cerebral edema and intracranial pressure caused by head injury or mass lesions.

ONSET AND DURATION

Onset: 1-3 hr for diuretic effect; within 15 min for reduction of intracranial pressure

Duration: 4-6 hr for diuretic effect; 3-8 hr for reduction of intracranial pressure

INDICATIONS

Cerebral edema

Other causes of increased intracranial pressure (space-occupying lesions)

Rhabdomyolysis (myoglobinuria)

Blood transfusion reactions

Promoting urinary excretion of toxic substances

CONTRAINDICATIONS

Severe hypotension

Active intracranial bleeding

Dehydration

Hyponatremia

Severe pulmonary edema or congestion

Profound hypovolemia

Severe renal disease (anuria)

ADVERSE REACTIONS

Transient volume overload

Pulmonary edema

Renal failure

Congestive heart failure

Hypotension (from excessive diuresis)

Sodium depletion

Nausea and vomiting

DRUG INTERACTIONS

When given concurrently with digitalis glycosides, an increase in digitalis toxicity may develop.

HOW SUPPLIED

250 and 500 mL of a 20% solution for IV infusion (200 mg/mL); 25% solution in 50 mL for slow IV push

DOSAGE AND ADMINISTRATION

Adult: 0.5-1 g/kg in a 20% solution over 5-10 min through an in-line filter; usual adult dose is 20-200 g/24 hr. Additional doses of 0.25-2 g/kg can be given every 4-6 hr as needed

Pediatric: 0.2-0.5 g/kg dose IV infusion over 30-60 min (max dose: 1 g/kg) every 4-6 hr

SPECIAL CONSIDERATIONS

Pregnancy safety: Category C

Mannitol may crystallize at low temperatures and may need to be warmed in boiling water until clear (cool to body temperature before use).

In-line filter should always be used.

Use with support of oxygenation and ventilation.

Effectiveness depends on large doses and an intact blood-brain barrier.

The use of mannitol and its dosages in emergency care are controversial.

MEPERIDINE (DEMEROL)

CLASS

Opioid analgesic

DESCRIPTION

Meperidine is a synthetic opioid agonist that works at opioid receptors to produce analgesia and euphoria. Excessive doses can cause respiratory and central nervous system depression and seizures. It has high potential for physical dependence and abuse and is classified as a schedule II drug.

ONSET AND DURATION

Onset: (IM) 10-15 min; (IV) within 5 min

Duration: 2-4 hr

INDICATIONS

Moderate to severe pain

Preoperative medication

Obstetrical analgesia

CONTRAINDICATIONS

Hypersensitivity to narcotics

Patients taking MAO inhibitors or selective serotonin reuptake inhibitors

During labor or delivery of a premature infant

Head injury

ADVERSE REACTIONS

Respiratory depression

Nausea and vomiting

Euphoria

Delirium

Agitation

Hallucination

Seizures

Headache

Hypotension

Visual disturbances

Coma

Facial flushing

Circulatory collapse

Dysrhythmias

Allergic reaction

Drowsiness

DRUG INTERACTIONS

Respiratory depression, hypotension, or sedation may be potentiated by central nervous system depressants.

Therapeutic doses of meperidine have caused fatal reactions in patients taking MAO inhibitors within the previous 14 days.

Phenytoin may decrease analgesic effects.

HOW SUPPLIED

Parenteral: 25, 50, 100 mg/mL in 1- and 5-mL prefilled syringe and tubex

DOSAGE AND ADMINISTRATION

Adult: 50-100 mg IM every 3-4 hr as needed; 15-35 mg IV per hour (dose should be individualized)
Elderly: 25 mg IM every 4 hr as needed
Pediatric: 1-2 mg/kg dose IM every 3-4 hr as needed; maximum single dose not to exceed 100 mg

SPECIAL CONSIDERATIONS

Pregnancy safety: Category B (if not used for prolonged periods or in high doses at term)
Use with caution in patients with asthma and chronic obstructive pulmonary disease.
Meperidine may aggravate seizures in those with convulsive disorders (especially in patients with renal insufficiency).
Use with caution in those susceptible to central nervous system depression.
Naloxone should be readily available.
Protect from light and freezing.
Use with caution in patients with SVT

METHYLPREDNISOLONE (SOLU-MEDROL)

CLASS

Glucocorticoid

DESCRIPTION

Methylprednisolone is a synthetic steroid that suppresses acute and chronic inflammation. In addition, it potentiates vascular smooth muscle relaxation by beta-adrenergic agonists and may alter airway hyperactivity. It currently is used for reduction of post-traumatic spinal cord edema, but this indication is controversial.[2]

ONSET AND DURATION

Onset: 1-2 hr
Duration: 8-24 hr

INDICATIONS

Anaphylaxis
Bronchodilator: unresponsive asthma
Shock (controversial)
Acute spinal cord injury (controversial)
Adrenal insufficiency (hydrocortisone [Solu-Cortef] also may be used)

CONTRAINDICATIONS

Use with caution in patients with gastrointestinal bleeding, diabetes mellitus, or severe infection.

ADVERSE REACTIONS

Headache
Hypertension
Sodium and water retention
Hypokalemia
Alkalosis

DRUG INTERACTIONS

Hypoglycemic responses to insulin and oral hypoglycemic agents may be blunted.
Potassium-depleting agents may potentiate hypokalemia induced by corticosteroids.

HOW SUPPLIED

20, 40, 80 mg/mL; 125 mg/2 mL

DOSAGE AND ADMINISTRATION

Adult: Variable; usually within the range of 40-125 mg IV. (Higher doses for spinal cord injury, per medical direction.)
Pediatric: Loading dose: 1-2 mg/kg IV

SPECIAL CONSIDERATIONS

Pregnancy safety: Category C

METOCLOPRAMIDE (METOZOLV ODT, OCTAMIDE, REGLAN)

CLASS

Antiemetic, GI stimulant

DESCRIPTION

Metoclopramide enhances GI motility. The drug is chemically related to procainamide, but has no anesthetic or antidysrhythmic properties. Metoclopramide was originally developed to treat nausea during pregnancy but is also useful in the treatment of chemotherapy-induced nausea and vomiting.

ONSET AND DURATION

Onset: 30-60 min (oral); 1-3 min (IV); 10-15 min (IM)
Duration: 1-2 hr

INDICATIONS

Nausea
Vomiting

CONTRAINDICATIONS

Hypersensitivity to the drug or procainamide
GI obstruction, bleeding, or perforation

ADVERSE REACTIONS

CNS effects may occur
Confusion
Depression
Drowsiness
Cardiac conduction disturbances

Fatigue
Headache
Hypotension
Hypertension
Nausea
Insomnia
Tardive dyskinesia

DRUG INTERACTIONS

Metoclopramide can increase the rate or extent of absorption of other drugs (acetaminophen, aspirin) because of accelerated gastric emptying.

Digoxin absorption and bioavailability may be diminished in some patients.

HOW SUPPLIED

Tablet: 5, 10 mg
Oral solution: 5 mg/mL
Solution for injection: 5 mg/mL

DOSAGE AND ADMINISTRATION

Pregnant women: 5 mg PO every 8 hr as needed
Chemotherapy-induced nausea and vomiting:
   IM: 10 mg; may be repeated in 4-6 hr as needed
   IV: 1-2 mg/kg; may be repeated twice at 2-hr intervals
Children: Not recommended

SPECIAL CONSIDERATIONS

Pregnancy safety: Category B

Use with caution in patients with renal disease, such as renal failure or renal impairment, attributable to possible accumulation and toxicity.

Not recommended for patients with Parkinson's disease.

Concurrent use of ethanol can increase the CNS depressant effects of metoclopramide. Combined use of metoclopramide and other CNS depressants, such as anxiolytics, sedatives, and hypnotics, can increase possible sedation.

METOPROLOL (LOPRESSOR)

CLASS

Beta-blocking agent

DESCRIPTION

Beta-adrenergic blocking agents compete with beta-adrenergic agonists for available beta-receptor sites on the membrane of cardiac muscle, bronchial smooth muscle, and the smooth muscle of blood vessels. The beta$_1$-blocking action on the heart decreases heart rate, conduction velocity, myocardial contractility, and cardiac output. Metoprolol is used to control ventricular response in supraventricular tachydysrhythmias (paroxysmal supraventricular tachycardia, atrial fibrillation, atrial flutter). Metoprolol is considered a second-line agent after adenosine, diltiazem, or a digitalis derivative.

ONSET AND DURATION

Onset: 1-2 min
Duration: 3-4 hr

INDICATIONS

All patients with suspected MI and unstable angina in the absence of contraindications (can reduce the incidence of VF)

Useful as an adjunctive agent with fibrinolytic therapy (may reduce nonfatal reinfarction and recurrent ischemia)

To convert to normal sinus rhythm or to slow ventricular response (or both) in supraventricular tachydysrhythmias (reentry SVT, atrial fibrillation, or atrial flutter)

To reduce myocardial ischemia in AMI patients with elevated heart rate, blood pressure, or both

CONTRAINDICATIONS

Hemodynamically unstable patients

STEMI if signs of heart failure, low cardiac output, or increased risk for cardiogenic shock are present

Relative contraindications include P-R interval >0.24 sec, second- or third-degree heart block, active asthma, reactive airway disease, severe bradycardia, SBP <100 mm Hg

ADVERSE REACTIONS

Bradycardia
Atrioventricular conduction delays
Hypotension
Palpitations
Nausea and vomiting

DRUG INTERACTIONS

Metoprolol may potentiate antihypertensive effects when given to patients taking calcium channel blockers or MAO inhibitors.

Catecholamine-depleting drugs may potentiate hypotension.

Sympathomimetic effects may be antagonized; signs of hypoglycemia may be masked.

HOW SUPPLIED

1 mg/mL, 5 mg/5 mL ampules

DOSAGE AND ADMINISTRATION

Adult: 5 mg slow IV at 5-min intervals to a total of 15 mg
Pediatric: Safety not established

SPECIAL CONSIDERATIONS

Pregnancy safety: Category C

Metoprolol must be given slowly IV over 5 min.

Concurrent IV administration with IV calcium channel blockers such as verapamil or diltiazem can cause severe hypotension.

Metoprolol should be used with caution in persons with liver or renal dysfunction.

MIDAZOLAM HYDROCHLORIDE (VERSED)

CLASS

Short-acting benzodiazepine

DESCRIPTION

Midazolam hydrochloride is a water-soluble benzodiazepine that may be administered for conscious sedation to relieve apprehension or impair memory before tracheal intubation or cardioversion. The drug may also be used in the management of seizures in children.

ONSET AND DURATION

Onset: 1-3 min (IV); dose dependent
Duration: 2-6 hr; dose dependent

INDICATIONS

Premedication for tracheal intubation, cardioversion, or other painful procedures
Seizures in children when other benzodiazepines are not effective

CONTRAINDICATIONS

Hypersensitivity to midazolam
Glaucoma (relative)
Shock
Coma
Alcohol intoxication (relative; may be used for alcohol withdrawal)
Depressed vital signs
Concomitant use of barbiturates, alcohol, narcotics, or other central nervous system depressants

ADVERSE REACTIONS

Respiratory depression
Hiccups
Cough
Oversedation
Pain at the injection site
Nausea and vomiting
Headache
Blurred vision
Fluctuations in vital signs
Hypotension
Respiratory arrest

DRUG INTERACTIONS

Sedative effect of midazolam may be accentuated by concomitant use of barbiturates, alcohol, or narcotics (and therefore should not be used in patients who have taken central nervous system depressants).

HOW SUPPLIED

2-, 5-, 10-mL vials (1 mg/mL)
1-, 2-, 5-, 10-mL vials (5 mg/mL)

DOSAGE AND ADMINISTRATION

Sedation
Adult: 1-2.5 mg slow IV (over 2-3 min); may be repeated if necessary in small increments (total max dose not to exceed 0.1 mg/kg)
Elderly: 0.5 mg slow IV (max: 1.5 mg in a 2-min period)
Pediatric: Loading dose: 0.05-0.2 mg/kg; then continue infusion 1-2 mcg/kg/min
Seizures in children: 0.1-0.15 mg/kg (max dose 5 mg) IV slow over 1-2 min or IM
Rapid Sequence Intubation
0.1-0.3 mg/kg IV/IO; max single dose: 10 mg

SPECIAL CONSIDERATIONS

Pregnancy safety: Category D
Never administer medication as IV bolus.
NOTE: Midazolam has been associated with respiratory depression and respiratory arrest when used for sedation. Its use requires continuous monitoring of respiratory and cardiac function. Emergency airway equipment should be readily available.

MORPHINE SULFATE (ASTRAMORPH/PF AND OTHERS)

CLASS

Opioid analgesic

DESCRIPTION

Morphine sulfate is a natural opium alkaloid that has a primary effect of analgesia. It also increases peripheral venous capacitance and decreases venous return (chemical phlebotomy). Morphine sulfate causes euphoria and respiratory and central nervous system depression. Secondary pharmacological effects of morphine include depressed responsiveness of alpha-adrenergic receptors (producing peripheral vasodilation) and baroreceptor inhibition. In addition, because morphine decreases preload and afterload, it may decrease myocardial oxygen demand. The properties of this medication make it extremely useful in emergency care. Morphine sulfate is a schedule II drug.

ONSET AND DURATION

Onset: 1-2 min after administration
Duration: 2-7 hr

INDICATIONS

Chest pain associated with ACS unresponsive to nitrates
Acute cardiogenic pulmonary edema (with adequate blood pressure), with or without associated pain
Moderate to severe acute and chronic pain

CONTRAINDICATIONS

Hypersensitivity to narcotics
Hypovolemia
Hypotension
Head injury or undiagnosed abdominal pain

Increased intracranial pressure
Severe respiratory depression
Patients who have taken MAO inhibitors within 14 days
Use with caution in RV infarction

ADVERSE REACTIONS

Hypotension in volume-depleted patients
Tachycardia
Bradycardia
Palpitations
Syncope
Facial flushing, diaphoresis, pruritus
Respiratory depression
Euphoria
Bronchospasm
Dry mouth
Allergic reaction

DRUG INTERACTIONS

Central nervous system depressants may potentiate effects of morphine (respiratory depression, hypotension, sedation).
Phenothiazines may potentiate analgesia.
MAO inhibitors may cause paradoxical excitation.

HOW SUPPLIED

Morphine is supplied in tablets, suppositories, and solution. In emergency care, morphine sulfate usually is administered IV.
Parenteral preparations are available in many strengths. A common preparation is 10 mg in 1 mL of solution, ampules and Tubex syringes.

DOSAGE AND ADMINISTRATION

Adult:
   STEMI: 2-4 mg IV; may give additional doses of 2-8 mg IV at 5- to 15-min intervals
   UA/NSTEMI: 1-5 mg IV only if symptoms not relieved by nitrates or if symptoms recur (use with caution)
   Pain: 2-4 mg slow IV over 1-5 min every 5-30 min; titrated to effect
Pediatric: 0.1-0.2 mg/kg dose IV (max total dose: 15 mg)

SPECIAL CONSIDERATIONS

Pregnancy safety: Category B (if not used for prolonged periods or in high doses at term); narcotics rapidly cross the placenta
Safety in neonates has not been established.
Use with caution in the elderly, in those with asthma, and in those susceptible to central nervous system depression.
Morphine should be used with caution in chronic pain syndromes.

Morphine may worsen bradycardia or heart block in inferior myocardial infarction (vagotonic effect).
Naloxone (0.4-2 mg IV) should be readily available.

NALOXONE (NARCAN)

CLASS

Opioid antagonist

DESCRIPTION

Naloxone is a competitive narcotic antagonist used in the management of known or suspected overdose caused by narcotics. Naloxone antagonizes all actions of morphine. Naloxone is the preferred first-line agent in suspected opioid overdose unresponsive to oxygen and support of ventilation.

ONSET AND DURATION

Onset: Within 2 min
Duration: 30-60 min

INDICATIONS

For the complete or partial reversal of central nervous system and respiratory depression induced by opioids including the following:
Narcotic Agonist
   Morphine sulfate
   Heroin
   Hydromorphone
   Methadone
   Meperidine
   Paregoric
   Fentanyl citrate
   Oxycodone
   Codeine
Narcotic Agonist/Antagonist
   Butorphanol tartrate
   Pentazocine
   Nalbuphine
Decreased Level of Consciousness
Coma of Unknown Origin

CONTRAINDICATIONS

Hypersensitivity
Use with caution in narcotic-dependent patients who may experience withdrawal syndrome (including neonates of narcotic-dependent mothers).
Avoid use in meperidine-induced seizures

ADVERSE REACTIONS

Tachycardia
Hypertension
Dysrhythmias
Nausea and vomiting
Diaphoresis
Blurred vision
Withdrawal (opiate)

DRUG INTERACTIONS

Incompatible with bisulfite and alkaline solutions

HOW SUPPLIED

0.4 mg/mL (1, 10 mL); 1 mg/mL (2-mL) vials

DOSAGE AND ADMINISTRATION

Adult:

Typical IV (or endotracheal tube diluted) dose: 0.4-mg; titrate until ventilation is adequate. Use higher doses (up to 2 mg) for complete narcotic reversal. Can administer up to 6-10 mg over short period (<10 min). For respiratory depression from sedation, smaller doses of 0.4 mg repeated every 2-3 min may be used. For chronic opioid-addicted patients use smaller doses and titrate slowly.

IM/subQ dose: 0.4-0.8 mg

Pediatric:

0.1 mg/kg IV/IO/ET (diluted) every 2 min as needed for total reversal of narcotic effects (max 2 mg); if total reversal is not required, smaller doses (0.001-0.005 mg/kg) may be used, titrated to effect.

Pediatric IV/IO infusion: 0.002-0.16 mg/kg (2-160 mcg/kg) per hour

SPECIAL CONSIDERATIONS

Pregnancy safety: Category C

Some research has demonstrated the efficacy of intranasal naloxone administration; however, the optimal dose for the intranasal route has not been established.

Seizures have been reported (no causal relationship has been established).

Naloxone may not reverse hypotension.

Exercise caution and use smaller doses when administering naloxone to narcotic addicts (may precipitate withdrawal with hypertension, tachycardia, and violent behavior).

Rare anaphylactic reactions have been reported.

NITROGLYCERIN (NITROSTAT AND OTHERS)

CLASS

Vasodilator

DESCRIPTION

Nitrates and nitrites dilate arterioles and veins in the periphery (and coronary arteries in high doses). The resultant reduction in preload, and to a lesser extent in afterload, decreases the workload of the heart and lowers myocardial oxygen demand. Nitroglycerin is lipid soluble and is thought to enter the body from the gastrointestinal tract through the lymphatics rather than the portal blood.

ONSET AND DURATION

Onset: 1-3 min
Duration: 30-60 min

INDICATIONS

Ischemic chest pain
Congestive heart failure
AMI (large anterior wall infarction, persistent or recurrent ischemia, hypertension)
Hypertensive emergencies with ACS

CONTRAINDICATIONS

Volume depletion
Hypersensitivity
Hypotension (SBP <90 mm Hg or ≥30 mm Hg below baseline)
Head injury
Extreme bradycardia (HR <50 beats/min)
Extreme tachycardia (HR >100 beats/min) in the absence of heart failure
Right ventricular infarction
Cerebral hemorrhage
Recent use of tadalafil (Cialis), vardenafil (Levitra), or sildenafil (Viagra)
Aortic stenosis

ADVERSE REACTIONS

Transient headache
Reflex tachycardia
Hypotension
Nausea and vomiting
Postural syncope
Diaphoresis
Flushing

DRUG INTERACTIONS

Other vasodilators may have additive hypotensive effects.
Do not mix with other drugs.

HOW SUPPLIED

Tablets: 0.15 mg (1/400 gr), 0.3 mg (1/200 gr), 0.4 mg (1/150 gr), 0.6 (1/100 gr), and extended-release capsules and transdermal preparations
Metered spray: 0.4 mg per spray (do not shake)
Parenteral: 5 mg/mL; 10, 20, 40 mg/100 mL

DOSAGE AND ADMINISTRATION

Adult:

Tablet: 0.3-0.4 mg sublingually; may repeat for a total of 3 doses at 5-min intervals

Metered spray: 1-2 sprays (0.4 mg/dose) for 0.5-1 sec at 5-min intervals; max 3 sprays within 15 min

Infusion: Begin at a rate of 10 mcg/min; increase by 10 mcg/min q 3-5 min until desired effect is achieved; ceiling dose of 200 mcg/min commonly used

Pediatric (continuous infusion): Initial dose 0.25-0.5 mcg/kg/min; titrate by 1 mcg/kg/min every 15-20 min; typical dose range: 1-5 mcg/kg/min

SPECIAL CONSIDERATIONS

Pregnancy safety: Category C

Nitroglycerin is associated with increased susceptibility to hypotension in the elderly.

Nitroglycerin decomposes when exposed to light or heat.

Nitroglycerin must be kept in airtight containers.

Active ingredient of nitroglycerin will "sting" when administered sublingually.

Use with extreme caution in patients with inferior acute myocardial infarction with possible right ventricular involvement.

Administer IV nitroglycerin by infusion pump to ensure precise flow rate.

PVC tubing may absorb up to 80% of available drug; non-PVC tubing should be used.

NITROPASTE (NITRO-BID OINTMENT)

CLASS

Vasodilator

DESCRIPTION

Nitropaste contains a 2% solution of nitroglycerin in an absorbent paste.

ONSET AND DURATION

Onset: 15-60 min
Duration: 2-12 hr

INDICATIONS

Angina pectoris

Chest pain associated with acute myocardial infarction (less easily titratable than IV nitroglycerin)

CONTRAINDICATIONS

Same as those for nitroglycerin
Hypersensitivity
Hypotension
Head injury
Cerebral hemorrhage

ADVERSE REACTIONS

Transient headache
Postural syncope
Reflex tachycardia
Hypotension
Nausea and vomiting
Allergic reaction

DRUG INTERACTIONS

Other vasodilators may have additive hypotensive effects.

HOW SUPPLIED

20-, 60-g tubes of 2% nitroglycerin paste (measuring applicators are supplied)

DOSAGE AND ADMINISTRATION

Adult: Apply 1-2 inches over 2- to 4-inch area of skin that is free of hair (usually the chest wall); cover with transparent wrap and secure with tape

Pediatric: Not recommended

SPECIAL CONSIDERATIONS

Pregnancy safety: Category C

Wear gloves when applying paste.

Do not massage or rub paste (rapid absorption will interfere with the sustained action of the drug).

Store paste in a cool place with the tube tightly capped.

Although the adverse effects for nitropaste are the same as those for sublingually administered nitroglycerin, their frequency and severity usually are considerably less with the sustained-release preparations because of the slower absorption and less erratic serum levels.

NITROPRUSSIDE

CLASS

Vasodilator

DESCRIPTION

Nitroprusside is an intravenous hypotensive agent effective in the acute management of hypertensive crisis and in the management of congestive heart failure. Nitroprusside-induced peripheral vasodilation results in a reduced left ventricular afterload. This, along with a reduced venous return to the heart, causes a slight increase in heart rate and decrease in cardiac output in hypertensive patients. In patients with congestive heart failure, nitroprusside improves left ventricular heart performance, increasing cardiac output and stroke volume. The peripheral vasodilatory effects of nitroprusside are due to a direct action of the drug on arterial and venous smooth muscle.

ONSET AND DURATION

Onset: Immediate
Duration: 1-10 min following infusion

INDICATIONS

Heart failure
Hypertensive emergency
Hypotension induction

CONTRAINDICATIONS

Aortic coarctation
AV shunt
High-output cardiac failure

Hypotension
Hypovolemia
Increased ICP
Pulmonary or renal disease
Cyanide toxicity
Recent ingestion of drugs for erectile dysfunction (e.g., sildenafil)

ADVERSE REACTIONS

Abdominal pain
Ataxia
Bradycardia
Coma
Confusion
Cyanide toxicity
Diaphoresis
Dizziness
Dyspnea
Flushing
Headache
Hyperreflexia
Hypotension
Increased ICP
Muscle cramps
Seizures
Syncope
Tachycardia
Vomiting

DRUG INTERACTIONS

Additive hypotensive effects may occur when nitroprusside is used concomitantly with other antihypertensive agents, general anesthetics, ganglionic blocking agents, and negative inotropic agents.
Sympathomimetics, such as cocaine, dobutamine, dopamine, norepinephrine, epinephrine, and others, may antagonize the antihypertensive effects of nitroprusside when administered concomitantly.
Additive hypotensive effects may be seen when MAOIs are combined with antihypertensives or medications with hypotensive properties.

HOW SUPPLIED

50 mg/2 mL for injection: Must be diluted with dextrose 5% in water (D_5W) before administration. Do not administer by direct injection. Administer diluted solution by IV infusion using a controlled infusion device.

DOSAGE AND ADMINISTRATION

Adults and children: Begin at 0.1 mcg/kg/min and titrate upward every 3-5 min to desired effect (usually up to 5 mcg/kg/min, but higher doses up to 10 mcg/kg/min

may be needed). Infusion is titrated to desired blood pressure and/or cardiac output.

SPECIAL CONSIDERATIONS

Pregnancy safety: Category C
Nitroprusside should be used only when appropriate monitoring equipment and personnel are available; blood pressure should be continuously monitored.
Use of infusion pump is strongly advised.
Cyanide toxicity or methemoglobinemia may occur with prolonged administration.
Use lower end dosage range for elderly patients.
Protect nitroprusside from light.

NITROUS OXIDE/OXYGEN (50:50) (NITRONOX)

CLASS

Gaseous analgesic/anesthetic

DESCRIPTION

Nitrous oxide/oxygen is a blended mixture of 50% nitrous oxide and 50% oxygen. When inhaled, nitrous oxide/oxygen depresses the central nervous system, causing anesthesia. In addition, the high concentration of oxygen delivered along with the nitrous oxide increases oxygen tension in the blood, thereby reducing hypoxia. Nitrous oxide/oxygen is self-administered.

ONSET AND DURATION

Onset: 2-5 min
Duration: 2-5 min

INDICATIONS

Moderate to severe pain
Anxiety
Apprehension

CONTRAINDICATIONS

Impaired level of consciousness
Head injury
Chest trauma (pneumothorax)
Inability to comply with instructions
Decompression sickness (nitrogen narcosis, air embolus, air transport)
Undiagnosed abdominal pain or marked distention
Bowel obstruction
Hypotension
Shock
Chronic obstructive pulmonary disease (with history or suspicion of CO_2 retention)

ADVERSE REACTIONS

Dizziness
Apnea
Cyanosis

Nausea and vomiting
Malignant hyperthermia (rare but dangerous)

DRUG INTERACTIONS

None significant

HOW SUPPLIED

D and E cylinders (blue and white in Canada, blue and green in United States) of 50% nitrous oxide and 50% oxygen compressed gas

DOSAGE AND ADMINISTRATION

Adult: Invert cylinder several times before use; instruct the patient to inhale deeply through a patient-held mask or mouthpiece
Pediatric: Same as adult

SPECIAL CONSIDERATIONS

Pregnancy safety: Nitrous oxide has been shown to increase the incidence of spontaneous abortion.
Nitrous oxide is 34 times more soluble than nitrogen and will diffuse into pockets of trapped gas in the patient (intestinal obstruction, pneumothorax, blocked middle ear).
As the nitrogen leaves and is replaced by larger amounts of nitrous oxide, increased pressures or volumes may cause serious damage, for example, intestinal rupture.
Nitrous oxide is a nonexplosive gas.
Patient must hold mask and self-administer.

> **NOTE**
> When delivering nitrous oxide and oxygen from a single tank, the paramedic must ensure that enough oxygen remains in the tank to provide adequate oxygenation. Inverting the cylinder several times to mix the gases is important for this reason. Monitoring of oximetry during administration of nitrous oxide also is reasonable.

NOREPINEPHRINE (LEVOPHED)

CLASS

Sympathomimetic

DESCRIPTION

Norepinephrine is an alpha- and beta$_1$-adrenergic agonist. Norepinephrine is a potent vasoconstrictor that also increases myocardial contractility. Because norepinephrine tends to constrict the renal and mesenteric blood vessels, it rarely is used in the prehospital setting. It is an agent of last resort for management of ischemic heart disease and shock.

ONSET AND DURATION

Onset: 1-3 min
Duration: 5-10 min

INDICATIONS

Severe cardiogenic shock
Neurogenic shock
Inotropic support
Hemodynamically significant hypotension (SBP <70 mm Hg) with low total peripheral resistance, refractory to other sympathomimetic amines

CONTRAINDICATIONS

Hypotensive patients with hypovolemia (relative contraindication)

ADVERSE REACTIONS

Headache
Dysrhythmias
Tachycardia
Reflex bradycardia
Angina pectoris
Hypertension

DRUG INTERACTIONS

Norepinephrine can be deactivated by alkaline solutions.
MAO inhibitors and bretylium may potentiate the effects of catecholamines.
Beta-adrenergic antagonists may blunt inotropic response.
Sympathomimetics and phosphodiesterase inhibitors may exacerbate dysrhythmia response.

HOW SUPPLIED

1 mg/mL, 4-mL ampule

DOSAGE AND ADMINISTRATION

Adult: Dilute 4 mg in 250 mL of D$_5$W or D$_5$NS (16 mcg/mL); begin infusion at 0.1-0.5 mcg/kg/min (up to 30 mcg/min) titrated to desired effect (average adult dose is 7-35 mcg/min); poison/drug-induced hypotension may require higher doses to achieve adequate perfusion
Pediatric: Begin at 0.1-2 mcg/kg/min IV/IO; adjust infusion rate to achieve desired change in blood pressure and systemic perfusion.

SPECIAL CONSIDERATIONS

Pregnancy safety: Category C
Norepinephrine may cause fetal anoxia when used in pregnancy.
Infuse norepinephrine through a large, stable vein to avoid extravasation and tissue necrosis.
Use infusion pump to ensure precise flow rate.
Do not administer in same IV line as alkaline solutions.
May induce dysrhythmias.

ONDANSETRON (ZOFRAN, ZUPLENZ)

CLASS

Antiemetic

DESCRIPTION

Ondansetron is an oral and parenteral antiemetic agent. It is the first selective serotonin blocking agent to be marketed. The primary use of the drug is to manage nausea and vomiting in postoperative patients and in those undergoing chemotherapy. Ondansetron preferentially blocks the serotonin 5-HT$_3$ receptors. These receptors are found centrally in the chemoreceptor trigger zone and peripherally at vagal nerve terminals in the intestines.

ONSET AND DURATION

Onset: Within 30 min
Duration: 3-6 hr

INDICATIONS

Nausea
Vomiting

CONTRAINDICATIONS

Hypersensitivity to the drug
Liver disease
GI obstruction

ADVERSE REACTIONS

Generally well tolerated
ECG irregularities (rare)
Hiccups
Pruritus
Flushing
Chills
Headache
Dizziness
Drowsiness
Extrapyramidal symptoms
Shivering
Hypoxia

DRUG INTERACTIONS

None significant in emergency care

HOW SUPPLIED

Tablet: 4, 8, 24 mg
Dissolving film and tablets: 4, 8 mg
Oral solution: 4 mg/5 mL
Solution for injection: 2 mg/mL

DOSAGE AND ADMINISTRATION (ADULT; PARENTERAL, ORAL)

IV: Up to 4 mg may be given undiluted; inject over 30 sec (2-5 min preferred)
Infusion (available in a premix or dilute dose in 50 mL of D$_5$W): Infuse over 15 min
IM: 4 mg, single injection in well-developed muscle
Oral film and tablets: Adults 4 mg PO
Safety in children not established.

SPECIAL CONSIDERATIONS

Pregnancy safety: Category B
The use of ondansetron may mask the symptoms of adynamic ileus, GI obstruction, or gastric distention after abdominal surgery.
Tablets should be gently removed from foil; not pushed through package. Allow to dissolve on tongue with saliva.

OXYGEN

CLASS

Naturally occurring atmospheric gas

DESCRIPTION

Oxygen is an odorless, tasteless, colorless gas that is present in room air at a concentration of approximately 21%. Oxygen is an important emergency drug used to reverse hypoxemia; in doing so, it helps oxidize glucose to produce adenosine triphosphate (aerobic metabolism). Oxygen may help reduce the size of infarcted tissue during an acute myocardial infarction (in patients who are hypoxemic on room air).

ONSET AND DURATION

Onset: Immediate
Duration: Less than 2 min

INDICATIONS

Any suspected cardiopulmonary emergency
Confirmed or suspected hypoxia
Ischemic chest pain
Respiratory insufficiency
Suspected stroke or ACS with hypoxemia (when oxygen saturation is unknown or <94%)
Prophylactically during air transport
Confirmed or suspected carbon monoxide poisoning and other causes of decreased tissue oxygenation (cardiac arrest)

CONTRAINDICATIONS

Oxygen should never be withheld in any critically ill patient.

ADVERSE REACTIONS

High-concentration oxygen may cause decreased level of consciousness and respiratory depression in patients with chronic carbon dioxide retention.

DRUG INTERACTIONS

None significant

HOW SUPPLIED

Oxygen cylinders (usually green and white) or wall-mounted delivery devices that supply 100% compressed oxygen gas

DOSAGE AND ADMINISTRATION

Adult and child:

Administer highest possible concentration during initial evaluation and stabilization; then administer to maintain oxygen saturation of 94-99%

High-concentration: 10-15 L/min via nonrebreather mask or high-flow oxygen delivery device

Low concentration: 1-4 L/min via nasal cannula

Venturi mask concentrations (e.g., 24%, 28%, 32%, 36%) for intermediate rates of oxygen administration in patients with chronic obstructive pulmonary disease

SPECIAL CONSIDERATIONS

Pregnancy safety: NA

Oxygen vigorously supports combustion.

OXYTOCIN (PITOCIN)

CLASS

Pituitary hormone

DESCRIPTION

Oxytocin means "rapid birth" and is a synthetic hormone named for the natural posterior pituitary hormone. It stimulates uterine smooth muscle contractions and helps expedite the normal contractions of a spontaneous labor. As with all significant uterine contractions, a transient reduction in uterine blood flow occurs. Oxytocin also stimulates the mammary glands to increase lactation, without increasing the production of milk. The drug is administered in the prehospital setting to control postpartum bleeding.

ONSET AND DURATION

Onset: (IV) Immediate; (IM) within 3-5 min

Duration: (IV) 20 min after the infusion is stopped; (IM) 30-60 min

INDICATIONS

Postpartum hemorrhage after infant and placental delivery

CONTRAINDICATIONS

Hypertonic or hyperactive uterus

Presence of a second fetus

Fetal distress

ADVERSE REACTIONS

Hypotension

Tachycardia

Hypertension

Dysrhythmias

Angina pectoris

Anxiety

Seizure

Nausea and vomiting

Allergic reaction

Uterine rupture (from excessive administration)

DRUG INTERACTIONS

Vasopressors may potentiate hypertension

HOW SUPPLIED

10 USP units/1-mL ampule (10 units/mL) and prefilled syringe 5 USP units/1-mL ampule (5 units/mL) and prefilled syringe

DOSAGE AND ADMINISTRATION

Control of Postpartum Hemorrhage

IM: 3-10 units IM following delivery of placenta

Bleeding Following Incomplete or Elective Abortion

IV: Mix 10-40 units (1-4 mL) in 1000 mL of NS or lactated Ringer's; infuse at 10-40 milliunits/min via microdrip tubing, titrated to severity of bleeding and uterine response

SPECIAL CONSIDERATIONS

Pregnancy safety: Category X

Vital signs and uterine tone should be monitored closely.

Oxytocin should be administered only in the prehospital setting after delivery of all fetuses.

PANCURONIUM

CLASS

Neuromuscular blocker (nondepolarizing)

DESCRIPTION

Pancuronium produces complete muscular relaxation by binding to the receptor for acetylcholine at the neuromuscular junction, without initiating depolarization of the muscle membrane. As the concentration of acetylcholine rises in the neuromuscular junction, pancuronium is displaced and muscle tone is regained. Neuromuscular blocking agents are used to provide muscle relaxation during surgery (particularly relaxation of the abdominal muscles) usually with general anesthesia and to prevent convulsive muscle spasms during electroconvulsive therapy. In emergency care, pancuronium is used to optimize conditions for endotracheal intubation and assisted ventilations.

ONSET AND DURATION

Onset: Paralysis in 3-5 min

Duration: 45-60 min

INDICATIONS

Induction or maintenance of paralysis after intubation to assist ventilations

CONTRAINDICATIONS

Known hypersensitivity to the drug

Inability to control airway and/or support ventilations with oxygen and positive pressure

Neuromuscular disease (e.g., myasthenia gravis)

ADVERSE REACTIONS

Transient hypotension
Tachycardia
Dysrhythmias
Hypertension
Excessive salivation
Pain, burning at IV injection site

DRUG INTERACTIONS

Positive chronotropic drugs may potentiate tachycardia.

HOW SUPPLIED

1, 2 mg/mL

DOSAGE AND ADMINISTRATION

Adult: 0.04-0.1 mg/kg slow IV; repeat q 30-60 min prn
Pediatric: 0.04-0.1 mg/kg slow IV
Newborn: 0.02 mg/kg dose

NOTE
If the patient is conscious, explain the effects of the medication before administration, and always sedate the patient before using a neuromuscular blocking agent.

SPECIAL CONSIDERATIONS

Pregnancy safety: Category C
Patients must be sedated completely and have an artificial airway during paralysis.
Carefully monitor the patient and be prepared to resuscitate.
The effects of pancuronium are antagonized by neostigmine (Prostigmin) 0.05 mg/kg and should be accompanied by atropine (0.6-1.2 mg IV).
Pancuronium has no effect on consciousness or pain.
Pancuronium will not stop neuronal seizure activity or decrease central nervous system damage caused by seizures.
Heart rate and cardiac output will be increased.
Pancuronium is excreted in the urine; doses should be decreased for patients with renal disease.

NOTE
Neuromuscular blocking agents produce respiratory paralysis. Therefore intubation and ventilatory support must be readily available.

Neuromuscular blocking agents produce respiratory paralysis. Therefore intubation and ventilatory support must be readily available.

PHENYTOIN (DILANTIN)

CLASS

Anticonvulsant

DESCRIPTION

Phenytoin (a hydantoin) is a drug used to control grand mal and focal motor seizure activity when other drugs are not successful. It was developed as an alternative anticonvulsant that would cause less sedation than barbiturates. Phenytoin appears to inhibit the spread of seizure activity by promoting sodium efflux from neurons, thereby stabilizing the threshold of the neuron against excitability caused by excess stimulation. Phenytoin also has been used to treat digitalis-induced atrial and ventricular dysrhythmias by stabilizing the sodium influx in Purkinje fibers of the heart, decreasing abnormal ventricular automaticity, and increasing atrioventricular node conduction.

ONSET AND DURATION

Onset: 20-30 min for seizure disorder
Duration: Several days

INDICATIONS

Major motor seizures (generalized grand mal, simple partial. and complex partial seizures)
Status epilepticus

CONTRAINDICATIONS

Hypersensitivity
Sinus bradycardia
Second- and third-degree heart block
Sinoatrial block

ADVERSE REACTIONS

Hypotension with rapid IV push (greater than 50 mg/min)
Cardiovascular collapse (with rapid IV use)
Dysrhythmias
Bradycardia
Respiratory depression
Central nervous system depression
Ataxia
Nystagmus
Thrombophlebitis
Nausea and vomiting
Pain from injection site

DRUG INTERACTIONS

Anticoagulants, cimetidine, sulfonamides, and salicylates may increase serum phenytoin levels.
Chronic alcohol consumption or use induces metabolism of the drug.
Lidocaine, propranolol, and other beta-blocking agents may increase cardiac depressant effects.
Xanthines may result in decreased phenytoin absorption.
Precipitation may occur when mixed with D_5W.
Phenytoin is incompatible with many solutions and medications.
Anticoagulation is enhanced with warfarin administration.

HOW SUPPLIED

50 mg/mL in 2- and 5-mL ampules, 2-mL prefilled syringe. May be diluted in NS (1-10 mg/mL, per protocol); use in-line filter

IV line should be flushed with 0.9% NS before and after the drug is administered

DOSAGE AND ADMINISTRATION

Seizures

Adult: 1000 mg or 15-20 mg/kg (usual loading dose) slow IV; not to exceed 1 g or rate of 50 mg/min; followed by 100-150 mg/dose at 30-min intervals (max of 1500 mg/24 hr)

Pediatric: 10-20 mg/kg slow IV (<0.5 mg/kg/min) loading dose

SPECIAL CONSIDERATIONS

Pregnancy safety: Category D

Phenytoin normally may have slight yellow color.

Carefully monitor vital signs.

Venous irritation can occur because of the alkalinity of the solution.

Use with caution in patients with pulmonary, cardiovascular, hepatic, or renal insufficiency.

Use large, stable vein for injection (extravasation may cause tissue necrosis).

PRALIDOXIME (2-PAM, PROTOPAM)

CLASS

Cholinesterase reactivator and antidote

DESCRIPTION

Pralidoxime reactivates the enzyme acetylcholinesterase, which allows acetylcholine to be degraded, thus relieving the parasympathetic overstimulation caused by excess acetylcholine. This drug is sometimes combined with atropine in an autoinjector such as the DuoDote autoinjector kit.

ONSET AND DURATION

Onset: Within minutes

Duration: Variable

INDICATIONS

Organophosphate poisoning (after atropine)

CONTRAINDICATIONS

Hypersensitivity to pralidoxime

ADVERSE REACTIONS

Tachycardia
Hypertension
Laryngospasm
Hyperventilation
Muscle weakness
Nausea

DRUG INTERACTIONS

Pralidoxime should not be mixed in the same syringe or solution with any other drug.

HOW SUPPLIED

Emergency single-dose kit containing a 20-mL vial of 1 g of the sterile drug, a 20-mL ampule of sterile diluent, and a 20-mL syringe with needle

DOSAGE AND ADMINISTRATION

Adult: 600 mg IM (usually by autoinjector) or 1-2 g IV over 15-30 min

Pediatric: 20-50 mg/kg IV over 15-30 min

SPECIAL CONSIDERATIONS

Pregnancy safety: Category C

Each 1 g of sterile powder is diluted with 20 mL of sterile water for injection.

Pralidoxime should be diluted further in 100 mL of NS and given as an IV infusion. Use promptly after reconstitution.

Medical direction may recommend the almost simultaneous administration of atropine.

Pralidoxime is not recommended in carbamate poisoning.

Reduce dosage in cases of known renal insufficiency.

PROCAINAMIDE

CLASS

Antidysrhythmic (Class IA)

DESCRIPTION

Procainamide suppresses phase 4 depolarization in normal ventricular muscle and Purkinje fibers, reducing the automaticity of ectopic pacemakers. It also suppresses reentry dysrhythmias by slowing intraventricular conduction. Procainamide may be effective in treating premature ventricular contractions and recurrent ventricular tachycardia that cannot be controlled with lidocaine.

ONSET AND DURATION

Onset: 10-30 min

Duration: 3-6 hr

INDICATIONS

Numerous dysrhythmias, including stable monomorphic VT with normal Q-T interval and preserved LV function

Reentry SVT uncontrolled by adenosine and vagal maneuvers if normotensive

Stable wide-complex tachycardia of unknown origin

Atrial fibrillation with rapid rate in WPW syndrome

CONTRAINDICATIONS

Second- and third-degree atrioventricular block (without functioning artificial pacemaker)

Digitalis toxicity
Torsades de pointes
Complete heart block
Tricyclic antidepressant toxicity

ADVERSE REACTIONS

Hypotension in patients with impaired LV function
Bradycardia
Reflex tachycardia
Atrioventricular block
Widened QRS complex
Prolonged P-R or Q-T interval
Premature ventricular contractions
Ventricular tachycardia, ventricular fibrillation, asystole
Central nervous system depression
Confusion
Seizure

DRUG INTERACTIONS

Increases effects of skeletal muscle relaxants.
Increases plasma/N-acetylprocainamide (active metabolites) concentrations with cimetidine, ranitidine, beta blockers, amiodarone, trimethoprim, and quinidine.
Use with caution with other drugs that prolong the Q-T interval (e.g., amiodarone).

HOW SUPPLIED

1 g in 10-mL vial (100 mg/mL)
1 g in 2-mL vials (500 mg/mL) for infusion

DOSAGE AND ADMINISTRATION

Adult: 20 mg/min slow IV infusion in recurrent ventricular fibrillation/pulseless ventricular tachycardia (max total: 17 mg/kg; max dose usually 1 g). In urgent situations, up to 50 mg/min may be given to a total dose of 17 mg/kg.
Other indications: 20 mg/min IV infusion until one of the following occurs: dysrhythmia resolves, hypotension, QRS widens by >50% of original width, total dose of 17 mg/kg
Maintenance: Infusion (after resuscitation from cardiac arrest): mix 1 g in 250 mL of solution in D_5W or NS (4 mg/mL), infuse at 1-4 mg/min
Pediatric: Loading dose 15 mg/kg IV/IO; infuse over 30-60 min

SPECIAL CONSIDERATIONS

Pregnancy safety: Category C
Procainamide has potent vasodilating and negative inotropic effects.
Rapid injection may cause procainamide-induced hypotension.
Carefully monitor vital signs and electrocardiogram (a small amount of QRS complex widening is expected).
Reduce dose in patients with cardiac or renal dysfunction to maximum total dose of 12 mg/kg and maintenance infusion to 1-2 mg/min.

Administer cautiously to patients with asthma, digitalis-induced dysrhythmias, acute myocardial infarction, or cardiac, hepatic, or renal insufficiency.

NOTE
Discontinue if the dysrhythmia is suppressed, hypotension develops, the QRS complex is widened by 50% of its original width, or a total of 1 g has been administered.

PROMETHAZINE (PHENERGAN)

CLASS

Phenothiazine, antihistamine

DESCRIPTION

Promethazine is an H_1-receptor antagonist that blocks the actions of histamine by competitive antagonism at the H_1 receptor. In addition to antihistaminic effects, promethazine also possesses sedative, antimotion, antiemetic, and considerable anticholinergic activity. Promethazine often is administered with analgesics, particularly narcotics, to potentiate their effects, although the occurrence of potentiation is controversial.

ONSET AND DURATION

Onset: IV (rapid)
Duration: 4-6 hr

INDICATIONS

Nausea and vomiting
Motion sickness
Preoperative and postoperative, obstetrical (during labor) sedation
To potentiate the effects of analgesics
Allergic reactions

CONTRAINDICATIONS

Hypersensitivity
Comatose states
Central nervous system depression from alcohol, barbiturates, or narcotics
Signs associated with Reye's syndrome

ADVERSE REACTIONS

Sedation
Dizziness
May impair mental and physical ability
Allergic reactions
Dysrhythmias
Nausea and vomiting
Hyperexcitability
Dystonias
Use in children may cause hallucinations, convulsions, and sudden death

DRUG INTERACTIONS

Concomitant use of central nervous system depressants may have an additive sedative effect.

Increased incidence of extrapyramidal effects occurs when given with some MAO inhibitors.

Concomitant use of epinephrine may decrease blood pressure further.

HOW SUPPLIED

25, 50 mg/mL in 1-mL ampules and Tubex syringes

DOSAGE AND ADMINISTRATION

Adult: 12.5-25 mg IV (dilute in 9 mL of NaCl and give 25 mg or less over 10-15 min) or deep IM (undiluted)

Pediatric: Not indicated in the prehospital setting

SPECIAL CONSIDERATIONS

Pregnancy safety: Category C (generally considered safe for use during labor)

Use caution in patients with asthma, peptic ulcer, and bone marrow depression.

Take care to avoid accidental intraarterial injection. IM injections are the preferred route of administration. (Avoid veins in the hands or wrists.) Give slow IV administration over 1 min.

PROPRANOLOL (INDERAL)

CLASS

Beta-adrenergic blocker, antidysrhythmic (Class II)

DESCRIPTION

Propranolol is a nonselective beta-adrenergic blocker that inhibits chronotropic, inotropic, and vasodilator response to beta-adrenergic stimulation. It slows the sinus rate, depresses atrioventricular conduction, decreases cardiac output, and reduces blood pressure. In addition, propranolol decreases myocardial oxygen demand and reduces the risk of sudden death in patients with acute myocardial infarction.

ONSET AND DURATION

Onset: Within 1-2 hr
Duration: 6-12 hr

INDICATIONS

Hypertension

Angina pectoris

Ventricular tachycardia, ventricular fibrillation, and rapid supraventricular dysrhythmias refractory to other therapies

All patients with suspected MI and unstable angina in the absence of contraindications (can reduce the incidence of VF)

Useful as an adjunctive agent with fibrinolytic therapy (may reduce nonfatal reinfarction and recurrent ischemia)

To convert to normal sinus rhythm or to slow ventricular response (or both) in supraventricular tachydysrhythmias (reentry SVT, atrial fibrillation, or atrial flutter)

To reduce myocardial ischemia in AMI patients with elevated heart rate, blood pressure, or both

CONTRAINDICATIONS

Hemodynamically unstable patients

STEMI if signs of heart failure, low cardiac output, or increased risk for cardiogenic shock are present

Relative contraindications include P-R interval >0.24 sec, second- or third-degree heart block, active asthma, reactive airway disease, severe bradycardia, SBP <100 mm Hg

DRUG INTERACTIONS

Adverse reactions:

Bradycardia

Second- or third-degree atrioventricular block

Asthma

Cardiogenic shock

Pulmonary edema

Uncompensated congestive heart failure

Chronic obstructive pulmonary disease (relative)

Cocaine intoxication

Catecholamine-depleting drugs may potentiate hypotension.

Sympathomimetic effects may be antagonized.

Verapamil may worsen atrioventricular conduction abnormalities.

Succinylcholine effects may be enhanced.

Isoproterenol, norepinephrine, dopamine, and dobutamine may reverse effects of propranolol.

Epinephrine may cause a rise in blood pressure, a decrease in heart rate, and severe vasoconstriction.

Signs of hypoglycemia may be masked.

HOW SUPPLIED

1 mg/mL vials

DOSAGE AND ADMINISTRATION

Adult: 1-3 mg IV over 2-5 min (not to exceed 1 mg/min); can be repeated after 2 min (total dose of 0.1 mg/kg)

Pediatric: Not recommended.

SPECIAL CONSIDERATIONS

Pregnancy safety: Category C

Propranolol may produce life-threatening side effects; closely monitor patient during administration.

Use with caution in elderly patients.

Use with caution in patients with impaired hepatic or renal function.

Atropine should be readily available.

NOTE
Beta₁-selective drugs now available are used more commonly for cardiac emergencies.

RETEPLASE (RETAVASE)

CLASS

Fibrinolytic

DESCRIPTION

Reteplase is a recombinant plasminogen activator. Fibrinolytic action occurs by generating plasmin from plasminogen. Plasmin degrades the fibrin matrix of a thrombus. The drug is used in the management of acute myocardial infarction in adults, for the improvement of ventricular function following acute myocardial infarction, and for a reduction in the incidence of congestive heart failure. Treatment with reteplase should be initiated as soon as possible after the onset of acute myocardial infarction symptoms.

ONSET AND DURATION

Onset: Causes reperfusion within 90 min for most patients
Duration: Variable

INDICATIONS

Management of acute myocardial infarction in adults (must be confirmed with 12-lead ECG)

CONTRAINDICATIONS

Active internal bleeding
History of stroke
Recent intracranial or intraspinal surgery or trauma
Intracranial neoplasm, atrioventricular malformation, or aneurysm
Bleeding disorders
Severe uncontrolled hypertension

ADVERSE REACTIONS

Bleeding (internal and at superficial sites)
Reperfusion dysrhythmias
Allergic reaction (rare)
Nausea and vomiting
Hypotension

DRUG INTERACTIONS

Risk of bleeding will be increased if used concurrently with drugs that alter platelet function.
Risk of bleeding with concomitant use of heparin, vitamin K antagonist (e.g., warfarin) is greatly increased.
Reteplase is incompatible with heparin; do not administer in the same IV line.

HOW SUPPLIED

Supplied in kit with components for reconstitution: single-use reteplase vials (10.8 units each), single-use diluent vials of sterile water (10 mL each), sterile 10-mL syringes with 20-gauge needles, sterile dispensing pins, sterile 20-gauge needles for administration, and alcohol swabs. Reconstitute by withdrawing 10 mL of diluent; open the package containing the dispensing pin; remove the needle from the syringe and discard the needle; remove the connective cap from the dispensing pin and connect the syringe to the pin; remove the flip cap from one vial of reteplase; remove the protective cap from the spike end of the dispensing pin and insert the spike into the vial of reteplase; transfer the diluent through the dispensing pin into the vial of reteplase; with the dispensing pin and syringe still attached, swirl (not shake) the vial gently to dissolve the reteplase; withdraw 10 mL of the reconstituted solution back into the syringe; detach the syringe from the dispensing pin, and attach a sterile 20-gauge needle; the 10-mL bolus dose is now ready to administer.

DOSAGE AND ADMINISTRATION

Adult: Administered 10 units as IV bolus over 2 min; administer a second 10-unit IV bolus in 30 min. (Give NS flush before and after each bolus.) Heparin and aspirin should be administered concomitantly.
Pediatric: Safety not established

SPECIAL CONSIDERATIONS

Pregnancy safety: Category C
Reteplase should be given in an IV line in which no other medication is being injected or infused simultaneously.
Protect contents of package from light.

SODIUM BICARBONATE

CLASS

Buffer, alkalinizing agent, electrolyte supplement

DESCRIPTION

Sodium bicarbonate reacts with hydrogen ions to form water and carbon dioxide and thereby can act to buffer metabolic acidosis. As the plasma hydrogen ion concentration decreases, blood pH rises.

ONSET AND DURATION

Onset: 2-10 min
Duration: 30-60 min

INDICATIONS

Tricyclic antidepressant overdose
Known preexisting hyperkalemia
Known preexisting bicarbonate responsive acidosis
Intubated patient with continued long arrest interval, pulseless electrical activity
Alkalinization for treatment of specific intoxications/ rhabdomyolysis
Management of metabolic acidosis
Diabetic ketoacidosis

CONTRAINDICATIONS

Not effective in hypercarbic acidosis (e.g., cardiac arrest and CPR without intubation)

In patients with chloride loss from vomiting and gastrointestinal suction

Metabolic and respiratory alkalosis

Severe pulmonary edema

Abdominal pain of unknown origin

Hypocalcemia

Hypokalemia

Hypernatremia

When administration of sodium could be detrimental

ADVERSE REACTIONS

Metabolic alkalosis

Hypoxia

Rise in intracellular PCO_2 and increased tissue acidosis

Electrolyte imbalance (hypernatremia)

Seizures

Tissue sloughing at injection site

DRUG INTERACTIONS

Sodium bicarbonate may precipitate in calcium solutions. Alkalinization of urine may shorten elimination half-lives of certain drugs.

Vasopressors may be deactivated.

HOW SUPPLIED

50 mEq in 50 mL; 0.5, 0.6 mEq/mL

DOSAGE AND ADMINISTRATION

Urgent Forms of Metabolic Acidosis/Severe Hyperkalemia

Adult: 1 mEq/kg IV

Pediatric: Same as adult; infuse slowly and only if ventilations are adequate

SPECIAL CONSIDERATIONS

Pregnancy safety: Category C

Not recommended for routine use in cardiac arrest patients.

When possible, blood gas analysis should guide bicarbonate administration.

Bicarbonate administration produces carbon dioxide, which crosses cell membranes more rapidly than bicarbonate (potentially worsening intracellular acidosis).

Sodium bicarbonate may increase edematous or sodium-retaining states.

Sodium bicarbonate may worsen congestive heart failure.

Maintain adequate ventilation (gas exchange).

SOTALOL (BETAPACE, SORINE)

CLASS

Beta blocker, Class III antidysrhythmic

DESCRIPTION

Sotalol is a nonselective beta-adrenergic blocking agent used to treat ventricular and supraventricular dysrhythmias in patients without structural heart disease. The drug has both type II (beta-blocking) and type III (cardiac action potential elongation) properties. Because of this, sotalol is used in the treatment of atrial dysrhythmias or life-threatening ventricular dysrhythmias, including sustained ventricular tachycardia. It should not be used for mild dysrhythmias because it is known to be proarrhythmic, with an increased risk for torsades de pointes. It should also be avoided in patients with poor perfusion because of its significant negative inotropic effects.

ONSET AND DURATION

Onset: Rapid

Duration: 8-16 hr

INDICATIONS

Ventricular and atrial dysrhythmias

SVTs in patients without structural heart disease

CONTRAINDICATIONS

Bronchial asthma

Sinus bradycardia

Second- and third-degree AV block (unless a functioning pacemaker is present)

Congenital or acquired long QT syndromes

Cardiogenic shock

Uncontrolled congestive heart failure

Hypersensitivity to sotalol

ADVERSE REACTIONS

Bradycardia

Heart blocks

Hypotension

QT prolongation

Syncope

Torsades de pointes

Ventricular dysrhythmias

DRUG INTERACTIONS

Most drug interactions with sotalol occur via enhanced pharmacological and electrophysiological effects (beta blockade, QT prolongation, AV blockade) with other drugs.

Proarrhythmic events are common. Use caution when administering sotalol together with calcium channel blockers such as verapamil and diltiazem because concomitant use may have additive effects on AV conduction, ventricular function, and blood pressure. Use caution when administering sotalol together with beta agonists such as albuterol, terbutaline, and isoproterenol.

HOW SUPPLIED

Tablet: 80, 120, 160, 240 mg
Solution for injection: 150 mg/10 mL

DOSAGE AND ADMINISTRATION (IV)

1-1.5 mg/kg; follow protocol for infusion rate

SPECIAL CONSIDERATIONS

Pregnancy safety: Category B
As with all beta blockers, sotalol may worsen congestive heart failure because of impaired ventricular contraction or decreased ejection fraction.
Doses should be reduced in patients with renal impairment.

STREPTOKINASE (STREPTASE)

CLASS

Fibrinolytic agent

DESCRIPTION

Streptokinase combines with plasminogen to produce an activator complex that converts free plasminogen to the proteolytic enzyme plasmin. The plasmin in turn functions as an enzyme that degrades fibrin threads and fibrinogen, causing lysis of the blood clot. Streptokinase is administered to selected patients with acute myocardial infarction.

ONSET AND DURATION

Onset: 10-20 min (fibrinolysis, 10-20 min; clot lysis, 60-90 min)
Duration: 3-4 hr (prolonged bleeding times up to 24 hr)

INDICATIONS

Acute myocardial infarction
Massive pulmonary emboli
Arterial thrombosis and embolism
To clear arteriovenous cannulae
Deep venous thrombosis (rare)

CONTRAINDICATIONS

Hypersensitivity
Active bleeding
Recent surgery (within 2-3 weeks)
Recent cerebrovascular accident
Prolonged cardiopulmonary resuscitation
Intracranial or intraspinal surgery
Recent significant trauma (particularly head trauma)
Uncontrolled hypertension (systolic pressure ≥180 mm Hg; diastolic pressure ≥110 mm Hg)

ADVERSE REACTIONS

Bleeding (gastrointestinal, genitourinary, intracranial, other sites)
Allergic reactions
Hypotension
Chest pain
Reperfusion dysrhythmias
Abdominal pain

DRUG INTERACTIONS

Acetylsalicylic acid may increase risk of bleeding (and may be beneficial in improving overall effectiveness).
Heparin and other anticoagulants may increase risk of bleeding and improve overall outcome.

HOW SUPPLIED

250,000, 750,000, and 1,500,000 unit vials
Reconstitute by slowly adding 5 mL of sodium chloride or D_5W, directing the stream toward the side of the vial, rather than into the powder. Gently roll—do not shake—the vial for reconstitution. Slowly dilute the entire contents of the vial to a total of 45 mL.

DOSAGE AND ADMINISTRATION

Acute Myocardial Infarction
Adult: 1.5 million units diluted to 45 mL (IV) over 1 hr (use infusion pump)
Pediatric: Safety not established

SPECIAL CONSIDERATIONS

Pregnancy safety: Category C
Do not administer IM injections to patients receiving fibrinolytic drugs.
Obtain blood sample for coagulation studies before administration.
Carefully monitor vital signs.
Observe the patient for bleeding.
Use caution when moving patient to avoid bruising or bleeding.
Do not draw arterial blood gas specimens in fibrinolytic therapy candidates.
Use one IV line exclusively for fibrinolytic administration.

SUCCINYLCHOLINE (ANECTINE)

CLASS

Neuromuscular blocker (depolarizing)

DESCRIPTION

Succinylcholine has the quickest onset and briefest duration of action of all neuromuscular blocking drugs, making it a drug of choice for procedures such as endotracheal intubation, electroconvulsive shock therapy, and terminating laryngospasm. Like nondepolarizing blockers, depolarizing drugs also bind to the receptors for acetylcholine. However, because they cause depolarization of the muscle membrane, they often lead to fasciculations and some muscular contractions.

ONSET AND DURATION

Onset: Less than 1 min
Duration: 5-10 min after single IV dose

INDICATIONS

To facilitate intubation
Terminating laryngospasm
Muscle relaxation

CONTRAINDICATIONS

Burns or injuries in the first 12 hr
Hypersensitivity
Skeletal muscle myopathies
Inability to control airway and/or support ventilations with oxygen and positive pressure
Personal or family history of malignant hyperthermia
Acute rhabdomyolysis
Intraocular (globe rupture) injuries

ADVERSE REACTIONS

Hypotension
Respiratory depression
Bradycardias
Dysrhythmias
Initial muscle fasciculation
Excessive salivation
Malignant hyperthermia
Allergic reaction
Succinylcholine may exacerbate hyperkalemia in trauma patients (hours after trauma).

DRUG INTERACTIONS

Oxytocin, beta blockers, chronic contraceptive use, and organophosphates may potentiate effects.
Diazepam may reduce duration of action.
Cardiac glycosides may induce dysrhythmias.

HOW SUPPLIED

20, 100 mg/mL; 1-g multidose vial

DOSAGE AND ADMINISTRATION

> **NOTE**
> If the patient is conscious, explain the effects of the medication before administration. Premedication with atropine should be strongly considered, particularly in the pediatric age group. Premedicating with lidocaine may blunt any increase in intracranial pressure associated with intubation. Finally, diazepam or another sedative should be used in any conscious patient before undergoing neuromuscular blockade.

Adult: 0.3-1.1 mg/kg (25-75 mg) over 10-30 sec IV; 0.04-0.07 mg/kg to maintain relaxation
Pediatric: 1-2 mg/kg dose rapid IV; max 150 mg
Rapid Sequence Intubation
1-1.5 mg/kg IV/IO for adults and children; 2 mg/kg IV/IO for infants

SPECIAL CONSIDERATIONS

Pregnancy safety: Category C

> **NOTE**
> Neuromuscular blocking agents will produce respiratory paralysis. Therefore intubation and ventilatory support must be readily available.

Carefully monitor the patient and be prepared to resuscitate. Administer with caution to patients with severe trauma, burns, and electrolyte imbalances (high potassium levels).
Brain or spinal cord injury may prolong effects.
Patients must have a patent or artificial airway and adequate sedation during paralysis. Children are not as sensitive to succinylcholine on a weight basis as adults and may require higher doses.
Succinylcholine has no effect on consciousness or pain.
Succinylcholine will not stop neuronal seizure activity.
Succinylcholine rarely may cause ventricular dysrhythmias/cardiac arrest in infants and children.

TENECTEPLASE (TNK-TPA)

CLASS

Fibrinolytic

DESCRIPTION

Tenecteplase is a modified form of human tissue plasminogen activator (tPA) that binds to fibrin and converts plasminogen to plasmin. The drug has been mass produced using recombinant DNA technology. The enzyme binds to fibrin-bound plasminogen at the site of an arterial clot, thus converting plasminogen to plasmin. Plasmin digests the fibrin strands of the clot, causing clot lysis and restoration of perfusion to the occluded artery. In prehospital care, fibrinolytic agents are used in treating selected patients with acute evolving myocardial infarction (STEMI).

INDICATIONS

AMI with ST-elevation (STEMI) attributable to coronary artery thrombosis

CONTRAINDICATIONS

Active bleeding or known bleeding disorder
Recent surgery (within 2-3 weeks)
Recent cerebrovascular accident
History of intracranial hemorrhage
Prolonged cardiopulmonary resuscitation
Recent intracranial or intraspinal surgery
Recent significant trauma (particularly head trauma)
Seizure at onset of stroke symptoms
Uncontrolled hypertension
Recent gastrointestinal bleeding

ADVERSE REACTIONS

Bleeding (gastrointestinal, genitourinary, intracranial, other sites)
Allergic reactions
Hypotension
Chest pain
Reperfusion dysrhythmias
Abdominal pain

DRUG INTERACTIONS

Use with caution in patients who have recently received glycoprotein IIb/IIIa inhibitors or anticoagulants (e.g., warfarin) because of the potential for enhanced effects on hemostasis.
Platelet aggregation may be impaired by serotonin norepinephrine reuptake inhibitors (SNRIs).

HOW SUPPLIED

50-mg powder for injection; reconstitute by using the diluent, syringe, needle, and dispensing system provided by the manufacturer. Reconstitute only with 10 mL of sterile water for injection without preservatives. Gently swirl the vial until contents are completely dissolved. Do not shake. The reconstituted vial will be a colorless to pale yellow transparent solution containing TNKase at 5 mg/mL.

DOSAGE AND ADMINISTRATION

Adult: IV bolus over 5 sec
Weight adjusted: <60 kg, give 30 mg; 60-69 kg, give 35 mg; 70-79 kg, give 40 mg; 80-89 kg, give 45 mg; ≥90 kg, give 50 mg
Pediatric: Not indicated

SPECIAL CONSIDERATIONS

Pregnancy safety: Category C
Incompatible with dextrose solutions.
Administer via a dedicated IV line in which no other medications are being simultaneously injected or infused.

TETRACAINE (PONTOCAINE)

CLASS

Topical ophthalmic anesthetic

DESCRIPTION

Tetracaine is used for rapid, brief superficial anesthesia. The agent inhibits conduction of nerve impulses from sensory nerves.

ONSET AND DURATION

Onset: Within 30 sec
Duration: 10-15 min

INDICATIONS

Short-term relief from eye pain or irritation
Patient comfort before eye irrigation

CONTRAINDICATIONS

Hypersensitivity to tetracaine
Open injury to the eye

ADVERSE REACTIONS

Burning or stinging sensation
Irritation

DRUG INTERACTIONS

Incompatible with mercury or silver salts often found in ophthalmic products

HOW SUPPLIED

0.5% solution

DOSAGE AND ADMINISTRATION

Adult: 1-2 drops
Pediatric: Same as adult

SPECIAL CONSIDERATIONS

Pregnancy safety: Category C
Tetracaine can cause epithelial damage and systemic toxicity.
Tetracaine is not recommended for prolonged use.

THIAMINE (BETAXIN)

CLASS

Vitamin (B_1)

DESCRIPTION

Thiamine combines with adenosine triphosphate to form thiamine pyrophosphate, a coenzyme necessary for carbohydrate metabolism. Most vitamins required by the body are obtained through diet; however, certain states such as alcoholism and malnourishment may affect the intake, absorption, and utilization of thiamine. The brain is extremely sensitive to thiamine deficiency.

ONSET AND DURATION

Onset: Rapid
Duration: Depends on the degree of deficiency

INDICATIONS

Coma of unknown origin (with administration of dextrose 50% or naloxone)
Delirium tremens

Beriberi (rare)
Wernicke's encephalopathy

CONTRAINDICATIONS

None significant

ADVERSE REACTIONS

Hypotension (from rapid injection or large dose)
Anxiety
Diaphoresis
Nausea and vomiting
Allergic reaction (usually from IV injection; rare); angioedema

DRUG INTERACTIONS

None significant

HOW SUPPLIED

1-, 2-mL vials (100 mg/mL)

DOSAGE AND ADMINISTRATION

Adult: 100 mg slow IV or IM
Pediatric: Not recommended in the prehospital setting

SPECIAL CONSIDERATIONS

Pregnancy safety: Category A (Category C if dose exceeds recommended daily allowance)
Large IV doses may cause respiratory difficulties.
Anaphylactic reactions have been reported.

TIROFIBAN (AGGRASTAT)

CLASS

Glycoprotein IIb/IIIa inhibitor

DESCRIPTION

Glycoprotein IIb/IIIa inhibitors inhibit the integrin GP IIb/IIIa receptor in the membrane of the platelets. As a result, they inhibit the common final pathway activation of platelet aggregation. Tirofiban (in combination with aspirin and heparin) is indicated for use in patients who have unstable angina or NSTEMI infarction.

ONSET AND DURATION

Onset: Within 30 min
Duration: Platelet aggregation restored within 4-8 hr after infusion is stopped

INDICATIONS

Patients with NSTEMI or unstable angina undergoing PCI

CONTRAINDICATIONS

Active internal bleeding
Bleeding disorder within the past 30 days
History of intracranial hemorrhage, neoplasm, AV malformation, aneurysm, or stroke within 30 days
Major surgical procedure or trauma within 1 month

Aortic dissection, pericarditis, and severe hypertension
Hypersensitivity to any GP IIb/IIIa inhibitor
Low platelet count

ADVERSE REACTIONS

Anaphylactoid reaction/anaphylactic shock
Bleeding (secondary to drug-induced platelet dysfunction)
GI bleeding
Hematemesis
Hematuria
Hypotension
Intracranial bleeding
Platelet dysfunction
Retroperitoneal bleeding
Stroke
Thrombocytopenia

DRUG INTERACTIONS

Concomitant use of other agents that may affect hemostasis, such as anticoagulants, other platelet inhibitors, NSAIDs, and thrombolytic agents, may be associated with an increased risk of bleeding.

HOW SUPPLIED

Premixed solution for injection: 50 mcg/mL

DOSAGE AND ADMINISTRATION (ADULT)

0.4 mcg/kg/min IV for 30 min; then 0.1 mcg/kg/min IV infusion over 18-24 hr after PCI

SPECIAL CONSIDERATIONS

Pregnancy safety: Category B
The 2004 ACCP guidelines recommend that tirofiban NOT be used in patients undergoing primary PCI.
Reduce dose in patients with impaired renal function.

VASOPRESSIN (PITRESSIN)

CLASS

Naturally occurring antidiuretic hormone

DESCRIPTION

Vasopressin acts by direct stimulation of smooth muscle V_1 receptors. When given in extremely high doses, it acts as a noradrenergic peripheral vasoconstrictor. Vasopressin may be used as an alternative pressor to epinephrine in adult shock-refractory VF; in asystole and PEA; and for hemodynamic support in septic shock.

ONSET AND DURATION

Onset: Immediate
Duration: Variable

INDICATIONS

As an alternative pressor to epinephrine in adult cardiac arrest
Vasodilatory shock

CONTRAINDICATIONS

Responsive patients with coronary artery disease

ADVERSE REACTIONS

Ischemic chest pain
Abdominal distress
Sweating
Nausea and vomiting
Tremors
Bronchial constriction
Uterine contraction

DRUG INTERACTIONS

No significant drug reactions have been reported.

HOW SUPPLIED

20 units/mL

DOSAGE AND ADMINISTRATION

Adult: Ventricular fibrillation/cardiac arrest: 40 units IV/IO push; may replace either first or second dose of epinephrine
Vasodilatory shock: Continuous infusion of 0.02-0.04 unit/min
Child and infant:
   Cardiac arrest: 0.4-1 unit/kg IV/IO bolus (max 40 units)
   Hypotension (continuous infusion): 0.0002-0.002 unit/kg/min (0.2-2 milliunits/kg/min)

SPECIAL CONSIDERATIONS

Pregnancy safety: Category C
Vasopressin may increase peripheral vascular resistance and provoke cardiac ischemia and angina.
Not recommended for responsive patients with coronary artery disease.

VECURONIUM

CLASS

Nondepolarizing neuromuscular blocker

DESCRIPTION

Vecuronium bromide is an intermediate-acting, nondepolarizing, neuromuscular blocking agent. Nondepolarizing agents produce skeletal muscle paralysis by blockade at the myoneural junction. Unlike depolarizing agents, vecuronium has little agonist activity, with no depolarizing effect at the motor endplate. Neuromuscular blockade progresses in a predictable order, beginning with muscles associated with fine movements (e.g., eyes, face, and neck); followed by muscles of the limbs, chest, and abdomen; and, finally, the diaphragm. Vecuronium is used to promote skeletal muscle relaxation during surgery, to aid controlled respiration by increasing pulmonary compliance, and to facilitate endotracheal intubation.

ONSET AND DURATION

Onset: Within 1 min
Duration: 25-40 min (dose related)

INDICATIONS

To facilitate intubation
Muscle relaxation

CONTRAINDICATIONS

Bromide hypersensitivity
Inability to control airway and/or support ventilations with oxygen and positive pressure
Bradycardias
Dysrhythmias
Hypotension
Respiratory depression
Muscular disease
Malignant hyperthermia

ADVERSE REACTIONS

Rare hypersensitivity reactions (e.g., bronchospasm, flushing, erythema, urticaria, hypotension, sinus tachycardia)
Excessive doses of vecuronium can cause prolonged apnea, dyspnea, respiratory depression, and/or profound muscular weakness (muscle paralysis).

DRUG INTERACTIONS

Can interact with opiate agonists by increasing the incidence and severity of bradycardia and hypotension.
Administration of IV phenytoin to patients currently receiving vecuronium has been noted to augment the neuromuscular activity of vecuronium.

HOW SUPPLIED

Powder for injection: 10, 20 mg

DOSAGE AND ADMINISTRATION

Neuromuscular Blockade
Adults, adolescents, and children >10 years: 80-100 mcg/kg IV; reconstitute by adding 10 or 20 mL of bacteriostatic water for injection to 10 or 20 mg, respectively, to give a parenteral solution containing 1 mg/mL
Rapid Sequence Intubation
0.1-02 mg/kg IV/IO for adults; 0.1-0.3 mg/kg IV/IO in children

SPECIAL CONSIDERATIONS

Pregnancy safety: Category C
Reconstituted vecuronium, which has an acid pH, should not be mixed with alkaline solutions (e.g., barbiturate solutions such as thiopental) in the same syringe or administered simultaneously during intravenous infusion through the same needle or through the same intravenous line.

VERAPAMIL (ISOPTIN)

CLASS

Calcium channel blocker (Class IV antidysrhythmic)

DESCRIPTION

Verapamil is used as an antidysrhythmic, antianginal, and antihypertensive agent. It works by inhibiting the movement of calcium ions across cell membranes. The slow calcium ion current blocked by verapamil is more important for the activity of the sinoatrial node and atrioventricular node than for many other tissues in the heart. By interfering with this current, calcium channel blockers achieve some selectivity of action. Verapamil decreases atrial automaticity, reduces atrioventricular conduction velocity, and prolongs the atrioventricular nodal refractory period. In addition, verapamil depresses myocardial contractility, reduces vascular smooth muscle tone, and dilates coronary arteries and arterioles in normal and ischemic tissues. Verapamil may be used as an alternative drug (after adenosine) to terminate reentry SVT with narrow QRS complex and adequate blood pressure and preserved LF function.

NOTE
Some physicians recommend slow IV administration of 500 mg of calcium chloride before the dose of verapamil to minimize the untoward results of hypotension and bradycardia.

ONSET AND DURATION

Onset: 1-5 min
Duration: 30-60 min (may persist longer)

INDICATIONS

Give only to narrow-complex reentry supraventricular tachycardias or known supraventricular dysrhythmias.
Atrial flutter with a rapid ventricular response
Atrial fibrillation with a rapid ventricular response
Multifocal atrial tachycardia
Vasospastic and unstable angina

CONTRAINDICATIONS

Hypersensitivity
Sick sinus syndrome (unless the patient has a functioning pacemaker)
Second- or third-degree heart block
Sinus bradycardia
Hypotension
Cardiogenic shock
Severe congestive heart failure
Wolff-Parkinson-White syndrome with atrial fibrillation or flutter
Patients receiving IV beta blockers
Give with extreme caution to patients receiving oral beta blockers.
Wide-complex tachycardias of uncertain origin (ventricular tachycardia can deteriorate into ventricular fibrillation when calcium channel blockers are given.)

ADVERSE REACTIONS

Dizziness
Headache
Nausea and vomiting
Hypotension
Bradycardia
Complete atrioventricular block
Peripheral edema

DRUG INTERACTIONS

Verapamil increases serum concentration of digoxin.
Beta-adrenergic blockers may have additive negative inotropic and chronotropic effects.
Antihypertensives may potentiate hypotensive effects.

HOW SUPPLIED

Parenteral: 5 mg/2 mL in 2-, 4-, 5-mL vials, or 2-, 4-mL ampules

DOSAGE AND ADMINISTRATION

Adult:
  Initial dose: 2.5-5 mg slow IV bolus over 2 min (over 3 min in older patients)
  Repeat dose: 5-10 mg bolus in 15-30 min after initial dose if needed; or 5 mg bolus every 15 min until a desired response is achieved (max dose 30 mg)
Pediatric: Not recommended in the prehospital setting

SPECIAL CONSIDERATIONS

Pregnancy safety: Category C
Closely monitor patient's vital signs.
Be prepared to resuscitate.
Atrioventricular block or asystole may occur because of slowed atrioventricular conduction.

REFERENCES

1. American Heart Association (2010). 2010 American Heart Association guidelines for cardiopulmonary resuscitation and emergency cardiovascular care, *Circulation* 122(18 suppl):S639-S946, 2010.
2. Gold Standard, Elsevier, www.clinicalpharmacology-ip.com/Default.aspx, accessed 11-18-10.
3. American College of Surgeons: *Steroids for spinal cord injury*, www.trauma.org/index.php/main/article/394/, accessed 11-2-10.

SUGGESTED READINGS

American Heart Association: *2005 Handbook of emergency cardiovascular care for healthcare providers*, Dallas, 2005, The Association.

American Heart Association: *Advanced cardiac life support*, Dallas, 2006, The Association.

American Heart Association: *Pediatric advanced life support*, Dallas, 2006, The Association.

AHA Circulation: 2010.

Eppert H, Goddard K: Administration of amiodarone during resuscitation of ventricular arrhythmias, *J Emerg Nurs* 36(1):26-28, 2010.

Gahart B, Nazareno AR: *2010 Intravenous medications: a handbook for nurses and health professionals*, ed 26, St Louis, 2010, Mosby.

Guy JS: *Pharmacology for the prehospital professional*, St Louis, 2009, Mosby/Jems.

Kee JL, et al: *Pharmacology*, ed 7, Philadelphia, 2012, Saunders.

Lehne RA: *Pharmacology for nursing care*, ed 7, St Louis, 2010, Saunders.

McKenry L, et al: *Mosby's pharmacology in nursing*, ed 22, St Louis, 2006, Mosby.

Physicians' desk reference, ed 64, Oradell, NJ, 2010, Medical Economics.

Salerno E: *Pharmacology for health professionals*, St Louis, 1999, Mosby.

Skidmore-Roth L: *Mosby's 2011 nursing drug reference*, St Louis, 2012, Mosby.

Glossary

abandonment Terminating medical care without legal excuse or turning care over to personnel who do not have training and expertise appropriate for the medical needs of the patient.

abdominal Pertaining to the abdomen.

abdominal aorta The portion of the descending aorta that passes from the aortic hiatus of the diaphragm into the abdomen, where it divides into the two common iliac arteries.

abdominal cavity The space within the abdominal walls between the diaphragm and the pelvic area; it contains the liver, stomach, intestines, spleen, kidneys, and associated tissues and vessels.

abdominopelvic cavity The space between the diaphragm and the groin.

abduction Movement away from the midline.

abnormal Deviating from the normal.

abnormal presentation A type of vaginal delivery in which the newborn's head does not deliver first.

abortion The spontaneous or induced termination of a pregnancy before the fetus has developed into a stage of viability.

abrasion A partial-thickness injury caused by scraping or rubbing away of a layer or layers of skin.

abruptio placentae Separation of the placenta implanted in a normal position in a pregnancy of 20 weeks or more; it occurs during labor or delivery of the fetus.

absence seizure A seizure that is characterized by brief lapses of consciousness without loss of posture; also known as *petit mal seizure*.

absolute refractory period The portion of the action potential during which the membrane is insensitive to all stimuli regardless of strength.

absorption The process by which drug molecules are moved from the site of entry into the body into the general circulation.

accelerated atrioventricular conduction See *anomalous conduction*.

accessory muscles Muscles that sometimes assist in breathing; includes the scalenes and the sternocleidomastoid (deep muscles of the neck and thorax), posterior neck and back muscles, and the abdominal muscles.

acclimatization Physical adjustment to a different climate or to changes in altitude or temperature.

acetabulum The large, cup-shaped articular cavity at the juncture of the ilium, the ischium, and the pubis that contains the ball-shaped head of the femur.

acetate A byproduct of fatty acids in the liver.

acetoacetic acid A colorless, oily ketone body produced by the metabolism of lipids and pyruvates; it is excreted in trace amounts in normal urine and in elevated amounts with diabetes mellitus, especially in ketoacidosis.

acetonemia The presence of acetone in the blood, characterized by the fruity breath odor of ketoacidosis.

acetylcholine A neurotransmitter, widely distributed in body tissues, with the primary function of mediating the synaptic activity of the nervous system.

acetylcholinesterase An enzyme found in the synaptic cleft that causes the breakdown of acetylcholine into acetic acid and choline, thereby limiting the stimulatory effect of acetylcholine.

acid A compound that yields hydrogen ions when dissociated in solution.

acid-base balance The body's balance between acidity and alkalinity.

acidosis A condition marked by a high concentration of hydrogen ions (i.e., a pH below 7.35).

acinus A small lobule of a compound gland; the exocrine portion of the pancreas that produces pancreatic juice.

acoustic neuroma A noncancerous tumor that involves the vestibular portion of the eighth (i.e., vestibulocochlear) cranial nerve.

acquired immunodeficiency syndrome A disease that results from infection with the human immunodeficiency virus; the syndrome impairs the immune system, giving rise to opportunistic infections and malignancies.

acquired immunity Immunity that develops after exposure to specific antigens; also known as *adaptive immunity*.

acromegaly A chronic metabolic condition characterized by a gradual, marked enlargement and elongation of the bones of the face, jaw, and extremities.

acromion process The lateral extension of the spine of the scapula; it provides attachment for the deltoideus and trapezius muscles.

actin A protein found in muscle fibers that acts with myosin to cause contraction and relaxation.

actinomycosis A chronic systemic disease characterized by deep, lumpy abscesses that extrude a granular pus through multiple sinuses.

action plan A plan of action based on the patient's condition and the environment.

action potential A change in membrane potential in an excitable tissue that acts as an electrical signal and is propagated in an all-or-none fashion.

active transport A carrier-mediated process that can move substances against a concentration gradient.

active tubular secretion Secretion that involves the transport of free drug from the blood across the proximal tubular cell and into the tubular urine by an active process against a concentration gradient.

acute chest syndrome A new abnormal consolidation on a chest radiograph in a patient with sickle cell disease.

acute dystonia A sudden impairment of muscle tone; it commonly involves the head, neck, or tongue and often occurs as an adverse effect of medication.

acute gastroenteritis Inflammation of the stomach and intestines with an associated sudden onset of vomiting, diarrhea, or both.

acute hepatitis An inflammatory condition of the liver associated with the sudden onset of malaise, weakness, anorexia, intermittent nausea and vomiting, and dull right upper quadrant pain, usually followed within 1 week by the onset of jaundice, dark urine, or both, characterized by jaundice.

acute mesenteric ischemia The abrupt interruption of intestinal blood flow; may result from an embolism, a thrombosis, or a low-flow state (decreased perfusion).

acute mountain sickness A common high-altitude illness that results when an unacclimatized person rapidly ascends to high altitudes.

acute pain Severe pain, such as that following trauma or accompanying myocardial infarction or other conditions and diseases.

acute prostatitis Inflammation of the prostate gland that develops suddenly.

acute psychosis A condition that refers to a patient who presents with one or more of the following criteria: a sudden onset of delusions that rapidly change; hallucinations; bizarre behavior and posture; or disorganized speech.

acute renal failure A clinical syndrome that results from a sudden and significant decrease in filtration through the glomeruli, leading to the accumulation of salt, water, and nitrogenous wastes within the body.

acute respiratory distress syndrome A fulminant form of respiratory failure characterized by acute lung inflammation and diffuse alveolar-capillary injury.

acute tubular necrosis A medical condition involving the death of tubular cells that form the tubule that transports urine to the ureters.

adaptation A cellular response to stress of any kind to escape and protect from injury; a central part of the response to changes in the physiological condition.

addiction A compulsive, uncontrollable dependence on a substance, habit, or practice to such a degree that cessation causes severe emotional, mental, or physiological reactions.

Addison's disease A rare and potentially life-threatening disorder caused by a deficiency of the corticosteroid hormones normally produced by the adrenal cortex.

adduction Movement toward the midline.

adenohypophysis The anterior lobe of the pituitary gland.

adenoma A tumor of glandular epithelium in which the cells of the tumor are arranged in a recognizable glandular structure.

adenosine A compound derived from nucleic acid and composed of adenine and a carbohydrate (i.e., sugar).

adenosine diphosphate A product of the hydrolysis of adenosine triphosphate.

adenosine monophosphate A compound that affects energy release in work done by muscles.

adenosine triphosphate Adenosine, an organic base, with three phosphate groups attached to it; it stores energy in muscles.

adhesion The quality of remaining in close contact with or stuck to another entity; also, a structure that joins several parts, sometimes abnormally.

adipose tissue A specialized connective tissue that stores lipids; also known as *fat tissue*.

adolescent A person 13 to 18 years of age.

adrenal gland Either of two secretory glands perched atop the kidneys; each gland consists of two parts, the cortex and medulla, which have independent functions.

adrenal medullary mechanism The mechanism by which epinephrine and norepinephrine are released from the adrenal medulla as a result of the same stimuli that increase sympathetic stimulation of the heart and blood vessels.

adrenaline An endogenous adrenal hormone that helps prepare the body for energetic action.

adrenergic Of or pertaining to the sympathetic nerve fibers of the autonomic nervous system, which use epinephrine or epinephrine-like substances as neurotransmitters.

adrenocorticotropic hormone A hormone of the anterior pituitary gland that stimulates growth of the adrenal gland cortex and secretion of corticosteroids.

adsorb To gather on a surface in a condensed layer.

adsorption The capacity of a substance to attract and hold other materials or particles on its surface.

adult respiratory distress syndrome A group of symptoms that accompany fulminant pulmonary edema, resulting in acute respiratory failure; also known as *non-cardiogenic pulmonary edema*.

advanced cardiac life support Clinical care or guidelines for care of life-threatening cardiovascular and respiratory disorders.

advanced life support The provision of care that paramedics or allied health professionals render, including advanced airway management, defibrillation, intravenous therapy, and medication administration.

aerobic Of or pertaining to the presence of air or oxygen.

aerobic oxidation A biochemical reaction that increases the positive charges on an atom or the loss of negative charges in the presence of oxygen.

aerosol Pressurized gas that contains a finely nebulized medication for inhalation therapy.

affect An outward manifestation of a person's feelings or emotions.

affective disorder Any of a group of psychotic disorders characterized by severe and inappropriate emotional responses, prolonged and persistent disturbances of mood and related thought distortions, and other symptoms associated with depressed or manic states.

afferent division The division of the peripheral nervous system that transmits impulses from the periphery to the central nervous system.

afferent neurons Nerve fibers that send impulses from the periphery to the central nervous system.

affinity The propensity of a drug to bind or attach itself to a given receptor site.

afterdrop phenomenon A sudden return of cold blood and waste products to the core of the body as a result of rewarming methods used to treat hypothermia.

afterload The total resistance against which blood must be pumped. Also known as *peripheral vascular resistance.*

agglutinated Reference to cells that have clumped together. See *agglutination.*

agglutination A clumping together of cells as a result of their interaction with specific antibodies called agglutinins.

agglutinin A kind of antibody; its interaction with antigens is manifested as agglutination.

agitated delirium Describes a person with delirium who has (1) acute onset and fluctuating course, (2) reduced clarity of awareness of the environment, (3) perceptual disturbance, disorientation, or memory disturbance, and (4) underlying general medical condition.

agonal rhythm A ventricular escape complex or rhythm that occurs when the electrical impulses from the sino-atrial node, atria, or atrioventricular junction fail to reach the ventricles because of sinus arrest or high-degree atrioventricular block; frequently seen as the last rhythm in an unsuccessful resuscitation.

agonists Drugs that combine with receptors and initiate the expected response.

air embolism The presence of air bubbles in the blood-stream.

air trapping The result of a prolonged but inefficient expiratory effort, usually caused by chronic obstruction of the pulmonary tree, as is seen commonly in chronic obstructive pulmonary disease or asthma.

akathisia An abnormal condition characterized by restlessness and agitation.

albumin A water-soluble protein containing carbon, hydrogen, oxygen, nitrogen, and sulfur.

alcohol dependence A disorder characterized by chronic, excessive consumption of alcohol that results in injury to health or in inadequate social function and the development of withdrawal symptoms when the person stops drinking suddenly.

aldosterone A steroid hormone produced by the adrenal cortex to regulate the sodium and potassium balance in the blood.

aliquot A sample that is representative of the whole.

alkaline Having the reactions of an alkali.

alkalosis A condition marked by a low concentration of hydrogen ions (i.e., a pH above 7.45).

allergens Substances that can produce hypersensitivity reactions in the body.

allergic reaction A hypersensitivity response to an allergen to which a person previously was exposed and to which the person has developed antibodies.

allergy A hypersensitivity reaction to intrinsically harmless antigens, most of which are environmental.

allografting The transplantation of cells, tissues, or organs between nonidentical (genetically unrelated) persons.

all-or-none principle The principle that when a stimulus is applied to a cell, an action potential is produced or is not produced.

alpha cell A constituent of the islets of Langerhans that produces glucagon.

alpha-adrenergic receptor Any one of the postulated adrenergic components of receptor tissues that responds to norepinephrine and to various blocking agents.

alveolar duct Part of the respiratory passages beyond a respiratory bronchiole; alveolar sacs and alveoli arise from it.

alveoli Small outpouchings of walls of alveolar space through which gas exchange takes place between alveolar air and pulmonary capillary blood.

alveolus A small cavity; the terminal ending of a secretory gland. Alveoli of the lungs are microscopic, saclike dilations of terminal bronchioles.

Alzheimer's disease A disease characterized by confusion, memory failure, disorientation, speech disturbances, and inability to carry out purposeful movements.

amaurosis fugax Unilateral vision loss as a result of internal carotid artery plaque emboli.

ambulance A generic term that describes the various land-based emergency vehicles used by emergency medical services personnel, including basic and advanced life support units, paramedic units, mobile intensive care units, and others.

amenorrhea The absence of menstruation.

amino acid An organic chemical compound composed of one or more basic amino groups and one or more acidic carboxyl groups.

ammonia A colorless, aromatic gas consisting of nitrogen and hydrogen.

ammonium ion The monovalent cation NH_4.

amnestic Causing amnesia.

amniocentesis An obstetrical procedure in which a small amount of amniotic fluid is removed for laboratory analysis; it aids in diagnosis of fetal abnormalities.

amniotic fluid embolism An embolism that occurs when particulate matter in amniotic fluid forms an embolus and gains access to maternal circulation during labor or delivery or immediately after delivery.

amniotic sac A thin-walled bag that contains the fetus and amniotic fluid during pregnancy.

amplitude modulation A transmitted radio frequency carrier fixed in frequency but increasing or decreasing in amplitude in accordance with the strength of the applied audio.

ampulla A round, saclike dilation of the uterine tube.

amputation A complete or partial loss of a limb caused by mechanical force.

amylase A starch-splitting enzyme.

amyotrophic lateral sclerosis One of a group of rare disorders in which the nerves that control muscular activity degenerate in the brain and spinal cord; also called Lou Gehrig's disease.

anabolic steroid Any of several compounds derived from testosterone or prepared synthetically to promote general body growth, to oppose the effects of endogenous estrogen, or to promote masculinizing effects.

anaerobic Of or pertaining to the absence of oxygen.

anaerobic metabolism Metabolism that occurs in the absence of oxygen.

anal canal The final portion of the alimentary tract between the rectal ampulla and the anus.

anal fissure A linear ulceration or laceration of the skin of the anus.

anal fistula An abnormal opening of the cutaneous surface near the anus.

anal triangle The posterior portion of the perianal region through which the anal canal opens.

anaphylactic shock Shock that occurs when the body is exposed to a substance that produces a severe allergic reaction.

anaphylactoid reaction An allergic reaction that is not mediated by an antigen-antibody reaction; presents exactly like anaphylaxis, but does not require previous exposure.

anaphylaxis An exaggerated, life-threatening hypersensitivity reaction to a previously encountered antigen.

anasarca Generalized, massive edema.

anastomosis The joining of two parts.

anatomical dead space The volume of the conducting airways from the external environment down to the terminal bronchioles.

anatomical position A position standing erect with the feet and palms facing the examiner.

anchoring Attaching a high-angle rope to a secure point.

androgen Any steroid hormone that increases male characteristics.

anemia A decrease in blood hemoglobin level.

anesthesia Without sensation.

aneurysm A localized dilation of the wall of a blood vessel.

angina pectoris Ischemic chest pain most often caused by myocardial anoxia as a result of atherosclerosis of the coronary arteries.

angioedema A localized edematous reaction of the deep dermal or subcutaneous or submucosal tissues that appears as giant wheals.

angiogram A study of vessels.

angioplasty Repair of damaged vessels.

angiotensin I The inactive form of angiotensin, formulated by the stimulation of renin, which is converted to angiotensin II.

angiotensin II A potent vasoconstrictor that also acts to stimulate the secretion of antidiuretic hormone.

angiotensin-converting enzyme A circulating enzyme that participates in the body's renin-angiotensin system, which mediates extracellular volume and arterial vasoconstriction.

angle-closure glaucoma A form of glaucoma associated with a physically obstructed anterior chamber angle; may be chronic or, rarely, acute.

angle of Louis See *sternal angle*.

anhedonia The inability to enjoy what is usually pleasurable.

anion An ion with a negative charge.

anisocoria Normal or congenital unequal pupil size.

anomalous conduction A preexcitation syndrome; a clinical condition associated with abnormal conduction pathways between the atria and ventricles that bypass the atrioventricular node and bundle of His and allow the electrical impulses to initiate depolarization of the ventricles earlier than usual. Also known as *accelerated atrioventricular conduction*.

anorexia Lack or loss of appetite, resulting in an inability to eat.

anorexia nervosa A disorder characterized by a prolonged refusal to eat, resulting in emaciation, amenorrhea, emotional disturbance concerning body image, and an abnormal fear of becoming obese.

anovulation Failure of the ovaries to produce, mature, or release eggs.

antagonism The opposition between two or more medications; it occurs when the combined (conjoint) effect of two drugs is less than the sum of the drugs acting separately.

antagonist muscle A muscle that works in opposition to another muscle.

antagonists Agents designed to inhibit or counteract the effects of other drugs or undesired effects caused by normal or hyperactive physiological mechanisms.

antecubital fossa See *antecubital space*.

antecubital space The depressed area in front of the elbow or at the bend of the elbow; also known as the *antecubital fossa*.

antegrade amnesia The loss of memory for events that occurred immediately after recovery of consciousness.

antenatal Occurring or formed before birth.

antepartum The period before labor and delivery.

anterior The front, or ventral, surface.

anterior chamber of the eye The chamber of the eye between the cornea and the iris.

anterior communicating artery The artery that connects with the anterior cerebral arteries and completes the circle of Willis.

anterior cord syndrome A spinal cord injury usually seen in flexion injuries; caused by pressure on the anterior aspect of the spinal cord by a ruptured intervertebral disk or fragments of the vertebral body extruded posteriorly into the spinal canal.

anterior superior iliac spine One of two bony segments that form the iliac crest.

anthrax An acute infectious disease caused by the spore-forming bacterium *Bacillus anthracis*.

antibodies Substances produced by the body that destroy or inactivate a specific substance (antigen) that has entered the body.

anticholinergic Of or pertaining to the blocking of acetylcholine receptors, resulting in inhibition of transmission of parasympathetic nerve impulses.

anticoagulant A substance that prevents or delays coagulation of the blood.

antidiuretic hormone A hormone produced in the posterior pituitary gland to regulate the balance of water in the body by accelerating the resorption of water.

antidote A drug or other substance that opposes the action of a poison.

antigen-antibody reaction The binding of an antibody with an antigen of the type that stimulated the formation of the antibody; results in greater susceptibility for ingestion and destruction by phagocytes, or neutralization of an exotoxin.

antigenic site A site capable of binding to and reacting with an antibody.

antigens Substances (usually proteins) that cause the formation of an antibody and react specifically with that antibody.

antiplatelet drug A drug that interferes with platelet aggregation.

antipyretic Something that works against fever.

antivenin A suspension of venom-neutralizing antibodies prepared from the serum of immunized horses.

anuria The inability to urinate; the cessation of urine production; a diminished urinary output of less than 100 to 250 mL per day.

anus The distal end or outlet of the rectum.

anxiety A state or feeling of apprehension, uneasiness, agitation, uncertainty, and fear resulting from the anticipation of some threat or danger.

aorta The main and largest artery in the body.

aortic aneurysm A localized dilation of the wall of the aorta.

aortic body Any of the specialized nerve cells located in the arch of the aorta, where they monitor levels of oxygen and hydrogen ions in the cardiovascular system.

aortic semilunar valve A valve that guards the orifice between the left ventricle and the aorta.

apex of the heart The top or tip of the heart opposite the base.

Apgar score The evaluation of a newborn's physical condition, usually performed at 1 minute and 5 minutes after birth, including heart rate, respiratory effort, muscle tone, reflex irritability, and color.

aphasia Loss of the power of speech.

apical impulse A pulsation of the left ventricle of the heart, palpable and sometimes visible at the fifth intercostal space to the left of the midline.

apnea An absence of spontaneous respirations.

apneustic center A group of neurons in the pons that has a stimulatory effect on the inspiratory center.

apocrine gland A gland that has cells that contribute cytoplasm to its secretion, such as a mammary gland.

apothecary A system of graduated liquid volumes arranged in order of heaviness; it is based on the grain.

apparatus A vehicle used for fire suppression or rescue that does not include staff vehicles.

appendectomy Surgical removal of the appendix.

appendicitis An acute inflammation of the appendix.

appendicular region The limbs or extremities.

appendicular skeleton The bones of the upper and lower extremities.

appendix A wormlike, blunt process extending from the cecum; also known as the *vermiform appendix*.

application of principle A component of critical thinking in which the examiner makes patient care decisions based on conceptual understanding of the situation and the interpretation of data gathered from the patient.

aqueous humor The clear, watery fluid circulating in the anterior and posterior chambers of the eye.

Arachnida A large class of arthropods that includes spiders, scorpions, mites, and ticks.

arachnoid layer A delicate, weblike middle membrane that covers the brain.

areflexia A neurological condition characterized by the absence of reflexes.

areola The circular, pigmented area surrounding the nipple.

areolar connective tissue A loose tissue that consists of delicate webs of fibers and a variety of cells embedded in a matrix of soft, sticky gel.

areolar gland A gland that forms small, rounded projections from the surface of the areola of the mamma.

arrector pili Smooth muscles of the skin attached to hair follicles; when contraction occurs, the hair rises, resulting in gooseflesh.

arterial capillary The ends of capillaries closest to arterioles.

arteriogram A study of arteries.

arteriole A small branch of an artery.

arteriovenous anastomosis A vessel that allows blood to flow from arteries to veins without passing through capillaries; also known as an *arteriovenous shunt*.

arteriovenous fistula An internal anastomosis between an artery and a vein.

arteriovenous graft A synthetic material grafted between the patient's artery and vein.

arteriovenous malformation An abnormal connection between veins and arteries; believed to arise during fetal development or soon after birth.

arteriovenous shunt See *arteriovenous anastomosis*.

artery A vessel that carries blood away from the heart.

arthritis An inflammatory condition of the joints, characterized by pain and swelling.

arthroscopy Surgical inspection of a joint.

artifact A deflection on the electrocardiogram display or tracing produced by factors other than the electrical activity of the heart.

arytenoid cartilages Small, pyramidal laryngeal cartilages that articulate with the cricoid cartilage.

asbestosis A chronic lung disease caused by the inhalation of asbestos fibers; it results in the development of alveolar, interstitial, and pleural fibrosis.

ascending colon The segment of the colon that extends from the cecum in the right lower quadrant of the abdomen to the transverse colon at the hepatic flexure on the right side; usually at the level of the umbilicus.

ascites An abnormal intraperitoneal accumulation of fluid containing large amounts of protein and electrolytes.

aseptic Sterile, without germs.

asphyxiation A state of suffocation, caused by severe hypoxia, that leads to hypoxemia and hypercapnia, loss of consciousness, and, if not corrected, death.

aspiration Inhalation of foreign substances into the pulmonary system.

aspiration pneumonia Inflammation of the lung tissue from foreign material that enters the tracheobronchial tree.

asplenia Congenital absence or surgical removal of the spleen.

assault Creating apprehension, or unauthorized handling and treatment of a patient.

asthma A respiratory disorder characterized by recurring episodes of paroxysmal dyspnea, wheezing on expiration caused by constriction of the bronchi, coughing, and viscous mucoid bronchial secretions.

asthma exacerbation An aggravation of asthma, usually associated with severe symptoms.

astigmatism An abnormal condition of the eye in which the light rays cannot be focused clearly on a point on the retina because the spherical curve of the cornea is not equal in all meridians.

astrocyte gliosis A tumor composed of glial cells within the nervous system; it may be associated with respiratory center dysfunction and neuroepithelial bodies in the tracheobronchial tree, along with distal atelectasis.

asystole A life-threatening cardiac condition characterized by the absence of electrical and mechanical activity of the heart.

ataxia Failure of muscle coordination.

ataxic breathing A type of cluster or irregular breathing pattern characterized by a series of inspirations and expirations.

atelectasis An abnormal condition characterized by the collapse of lung tissue, which prevents the respiratory exchange of oxygen and carbon dioxide.

atelectatic breathing A modified respiratory effort thought to be a protective reflex to hyperinflate the lungs and reexpand alveoli that might have been collapsed.

atheroma An abnormal accumulation of fat or lipids as a cyst or a deposit in an arterial wall; a hard, atherosclerotic plaque.

atherosclerosis A common arterial disorder characterized by yellowish plaques of cholesterol, lipids, and cellular debris in the inner layers of the walls of large and medium-sized arteries.

athetosis A neuromuscular condition characterized by slow, continuous, and involuntary movement of the extremities.

atlantooccipital joint One of a pair of condyloid joints formed by the articulation of the atlas of the vertebral column with the occipital bone of the skull.

atlas The first cervical vertebra, which articulates with the occipital bone and the axis.

atmospheric pressure The pressure exerted by the weight of the atmosphere; at sea level this pressure is 760 mm Hg.

atom The smallest division of an element that exhibits all the properties and characteristics of the element; atoms consist of neutrons, electrons, and protons.

atonic seizure A seizure that produces an abrupt loss of muscle tone, loss of posture, or sudden collapse ("drop attacks").

atony Weak muscle tone.

atria Chambers or cavities, such as the atria of the heart.

atrial natriuretic factor A peptide released from the atria when atrial blood pressure is increased; it lowers blood pressure by increasing urine production, thus reducing blood volume.

atrial natriuretic hormone A hormone secreted by specialized muscle fibers in the atrial wall of the heart that influences water reabsorption in the kidney; it acts as an antagonist of aldosterone.

atrial synchronous ventricular pacemaker An artificial pacemaker synchronized with the patient's atrial rhythm; it paces the ventricles only when an atrioventricular block occurs.

atrial-ventricular demand pacemaker An artificial pacemaker that paces the atria or ventricles when the intrinsic rate of the paced chamber drops dangerously low.

atrioventricular canal The path through which the atria open into the ventricles.

atrioventricular dissociation A conduction disturbance in which atrial and ventricular contractions occur rhythmically but are unrelated to each other.

atrioventricular node An area of specialized cardiac muscle that receives the cardiac impulse from the sinoatrial node and conducts it to the bundle of His.

atrioventricular sequential pacemaker An artificial pacemaker that paces the atria first and then the ventricles when spontaneous activity is absent or slowed in the atria and ventricles.

atrioventricular valve A valve in the heart through which blood flows from the atria to the ventricles.

atrophy Decrease in size (shrinkage) of a cell, which adversely affects cell function.

attachments Physical and emotional bonds that develop between infants and their family members or caregivers.

attention deficit disorder A syndrome that affects children, adolescents, and, in rare cases, adults and is characterized by learning and behavioral disabilities.

auditory Of or pertaining to hearing or the organs of hearing.

auditory meatus A tubelike channel of the external ear extending from the auricle to the tympanum of the middle ear.

auditory ossicles The incus, malleus, and stapes; small bones in the middle ear that articulate with each other and the tympanic membrane.

auditory tube The auditory canal; it extends from the middle ear to the nasopharynx; also known as the *eustachian tube*.

aura A sensation that may precede a migraine or seizure activity.

auricle The part of the external ear that protrudes from the head; also known as the *pinna*.

auscultation A technique that requires the use of a stethoscope and is used to assess body sounds produced by the movement of various fluids or gases in organs or tissues.

autism spectrum disorder A range of neurodevelopmental disorders characterized by three sets of behavioral features: (1) impairment in social interaction, (2) communication deficits (both verbal and nonverbal), and (3) restricted, repetitive behaviors, including decreased imaginative play, stereotyped behaviors, and inflexible adherence to routines.

autoimmune disease A condition that occurs when the immune system mistakenly attacks and destroys healthy body tissue.

autoimmune pericarditis Inflammation of the pericardium associated with the production of antibodies directed against one's own tissues.

autoimmunity An abnormal characteristic or condition in which the body reacts against constituents of its own tissues.

autolysis The spontaneous disintegration of tissues or cells by the action of their own autogenous enzymes.

autonomic hyperreflexia Overactivity of the autonomic nervous system that causes an abrupt onset of extremely high blood pressure.

autonomic nervous system The division of the peripheral nervous system that acts as a control system functioning largely below the level of consciousness, and controls visceral functions.

automatic external defibrillator A device used in cardiac arrest to perform a computer analysis of the patient's cardiac rhythm and deliver defibrillatory shocks when indicated.

automatic implantable cardioverter-defibrillator A surgically implanted device that monitors a person's heart rate; it is designed to deliver defibrillatory shocks as needed.

automatic vehicle location A radio communications subsystem that uses one or more electronic methods periodically to determine the position of a land, marine, or air vehicle and relay that information via radio to a communications center.

automaticity A property of specialized excitable tissue that allows self-activation through spontaneous development of an action potential.

automatism Abnormal repetitive motor behavior such as lip smacking, chewing, or swallowing during which the patient is amnestic.

autonomic hyperreflexia syndrome A neurological disorder characterized by a discharge of sympathetic nervous system impulses as a result of stimulation of the bladder, large intestine, or other visceral organs.

autonomic nervous system The part of the nervous system that regulates involuntary vital functions, including the activity of cardiac muscle, smooth muscle, and glands.

autophagia Nutrition of the body by consumption of its own tissues.

avascular The absence of blood vessels.

Avogadro's number The number of molecules in a gram mole of any chemical substance.

avoidance The act of keeping away from someone, something, or a situation, or of preventing the occurrence of something; it requires the paramedic to continually be aware of the scene by being observant and knowledgeable about warning signs that may indicate a dangerous situation.

avulsion A full-thickness skin loss in which the wound edges cannot be approximated.

axial loading Vertical compression of the spine that results when direct forces are transmitted along the length of the spinal column.

axial region The head, neck, thorax, abdomen, and pelvis.

axial skeleton The bones of the head, neck, and torso.

axillae Armpits.

axillary node One of the lymph glands of the axillae that help fight infections in the chest, armpit, neck, and arm and drain lymph nodes from those areas.

axis The second cervical vertebra about which the atlas rotates, allowing the head to be turned, extended, or flexed.

axon The main central process of a neuron that normally conducts action potentials away from the neuron cell body.

azotemia The retention of excessive amounts of nitrogenous compounds in the blood.

B lymphocytes The lymphocytes responsible for antibody-mediated immunity.

Babinski's sign A reflex movement in which the great toe bends upward when the outer edge of the sole is scratched; also known as *Babinski's reflex*.

bacteremia The presence of bacteria in the blood.

bacteria Single-celled microorganisms that cause an infection characteristic of that species.

bacterial endocarditis Inflammation of the endocardium and one or more heart valves; also known as *infective endocarditis*.

bacterial meningitis A life-threatening illness that results from bacterial infection of the meninges.

bacterial pneumonia A type of pneumonia associated with a bacterial infection.

bacterial tracheitis A bacterial infection of the upper airway and subglottic trachea.

bacteriocidal Destructive to bacteria.

bacteriophage Any virus that causes lysis of host bacteria.

bacteriostatic Tending to restrain the development or the reproduction of bacteria.

ball-and-socket joint A joint that consists of a ball (head) at the end of one bone and a socket in an adjacent bone into which a portion of the ball fits.

bariatrics The field of medicine that focuses on the treatment and control of obesity and diseases associated with obesity.

baroreceptor A sensory nerve ending in the walls of the atria of the heart, venae cavae, aortic arch, and carotid sinuses; it is sensitive to stretching of the walls caused by an increase in blood pressure.

barotitis An inflammation of the ear caused by changes in atmospheric pressure.

barotrauma A physical injury sustained as a result of exposure to increased environmental pressure.

Bartholin's abscess The accumulation of pus that forms a lump in one of the Bartholin's glands; results from the duct of the gland being blocked, thereby allowing infection to occur.

Bartholin's gland One of two small, mucus-secreting glands located on the posterior and lateral aspect of the vestibule of the vagina.

Barton's bandage A circumferential head dressing applied to restrict jaw movement and minimize pain.

base A chemical compound that combines with an acid to form a salt; also known as an *alkali*.

base of the heart The portion of the heart opposite the apex, directed to the right side of the body.

base station A grouping of radio equipment consisting of at least a transmitter, a receiver, a transmission line, and an antenna located at a specific, fixed location.

basic life support Care provided by persons trained in first aid, cardiopulmonary resuscitation, and other noninvasive care.

basilar artery The single arterial trunk formed by the junction of the two vertebral arteries at the base of the skull.

basilar fracture A fracture that may occur when the mandibular condyles perforate the base of the skull but that more commonly results from extension of a linear fracture into the floor of the anterior and middle fossae.

basophil A white blood cell that promotes inflammation.

battering A form of domestic violence that establishes control and fear in a relationship through violence and other forms of abuse.

battery Physical contact with a person without consent and without legal justification.

Battle's sign Ecchymosis over the mastoid process caused by a fracture of the temporal bone.

Beck's triad A combination of three symptoms that characterize cardiac tamponade: elevated central venous pressure, muffled heart sounds, and hypotension.

behavior indicator Nonspecific behavioral changes that may suggest that a child is being maltreated. Behavior indicators for sexual abuse are called nonspecific because children may display such behavior changes because of other traumatic conditions. Prompt evaluation is warranted when these nonspecific behavior indicators occur to rule out maltreatment; appropriate assistance for the child must be obtained.

behavioral emergency A change in mood or behavior that cannot be tolerated by the involved person or others and requires immediate attention.

belay Method of attaching a safety rope and controlling the rope so that if the person or load starts to fall, the belay rope will prevent the fall.

Bell's palsy A condition in which paralysis of the facial muscles is caused by inflammation of the seventh cranial nerve (i.e., facial nerve); usually is one-sided and temporary and often develops suddenly.

benign A noncancerous tumor or harmless condition.

beta cell A constituent of the islets of Langerhans that produces insulin.

beta-adrenergic receptor Any of the postulated adrenergic components of receptor tissues that respond to epinephrine and various blocking agents.

beta-hydroxybutyric acid One of the ketone bodies that occur in abnormal amounts in diabetic ketoacidosis as a result of fatty acid oxidation.

bicarbonate buffer system The principal mechanism for stabilizing acid-base balance.

biceps brachii The biceps muscle of the arm that flexes and supinates the forearm.

bicuspid valve One of the two atrioventricular valves located between the left atrium and ventricle; also known as the *mitral valve*.

bifurcate To divide into two branches.

bilateral Having or occurring on two sides.

bile A bitter, yellow-green secretion of the liver that is stored in the gallbladder.

bilirubin The orange-yellow pigment of bile, formed principally from the breakdown of hemoglobin in red blood cells after termination of their normal life span.

bioethics The systematic study of moral dimensions including moral vision, decisions, conduct, and policies of the life sciences and health care.

biological disturbances Mental disorders that result from a physical rather than a purely psychological cause.

biological half-life The time required to metabolize or eliminate half the total amount of a drug in the body.

biology The study of life.

biosynthesis A chemical reaction that continually occurs throughout the body in which molecules form more complex molecules.

Biot's respiration A respiratory pattern consisting of irregular respirations that vary in depth and that are interrupted by intervals of apnea.

bioterrorism The use of biological agents, such as pathogenic organisms or agricultural pests, for the express purpose of causing death or disease, to instill a sense of fear and panic in the victims, and to intimidate governments or societies for political, financial, or ideological gain.

biotransformation The process by which a drug is converted chemically to a metabolite.

biphasic complex A QRS complex that is partly positive and partly negative.

biphasic positive airway pressure Airway support that combines partial ventilatory support and continuous positive airway pressure; allows the pressure to vary during each breath cycle

biphasic reaction An anaphylactic reaction that resolves and then recurs hours later without further exposure to the trigger.

bipolar disorder A disorder marked by alternating periods of mania and depression; also known as *manic-depressive disorder.*

bipolar lead A lead composed of two electrodes of opposite polarity.

bivalent cation An ion with two positive charges.

blast injury A general term used to describe damage to a person exposed to a pressure field.

blastocyst The stage of mammalian embryos in which the embryo consists of the inner cell mass and a thin trophoblast layer.

bleb An accumulation of fluid under the skin.

blood The fluid and its suspended, formed elements that circulate through the heart, arteries, capillaries, and veins.

blood clot The end result of the clotting process in blood; a blood clot normally consists of red cells, white cells, and platelets enmeshed in an insoluble fibrin network.

blood colloid osmotic pressure Osmotic pressure caused by the presence of plasma proteins (mostly albumin) that are too large to pass through the wall of the capillary; also known as *oncotic pressure.*

blood-brain barrier An anatomical-physiological feature of the brain thought to consist of walls of capillaries in the central nervous system and surrounding glial membranes; its function is to prevent or slow the passage of chemical compounds from the blood into the central nervous system.

blowout fracture A fracture of the floor of the orbit caused by a blow that suddenly increases the intraocular pressure.

blunt trauma An injury produced by the wounding forces of compression and change of speed, both of which can disrupt tissue.

B-NICE An acronym used for identifying five categories of weapons of mass destruction: *B*iological, *N*uclear, *I*ncendiary, *C*hemical, and *E*xplosives.

body The largest or main part of any organ or structure.

body lice Tiny parasites that concentrate around the waist, shoulders, axillae, and neck.

Bohr effect A property of hemoglobin; it states that an increasing concentration of protons and/or carbon dioxide will reduce the oxygen affinity of hemoglobin.

bone A highly specialized form of hard, connective tissue; it consists of living cells and mineralized matrix.

bone marrow Specialized soft tissue that fills the spaces in the cancellous bone of the epiphyses.

bone spurs Bony growths formed on normal bone.

bone tumor An abnormal growth of cells within a bone; may be malignant or benign.

bony labyrinth Part of the inner ear; it contains the membranous labyrinth.

borderline personality disorder A pervasive pattern of instability of interpersonal relationships, self-image, and affect, in addition to considerable impulsivity that begins by early adulthood.

botulism An often fatal form of food poisoning caused by the bacillus *Clostridium botulinum.*

bowel obstruction An occlusion of the intestinal lumen that results in blockage of normal flow of intestinal contents.

Bowman's capsule The expanded beginning of a renal tubule.

boxer's fracture Fracture of the fifth metacarpal bone from direct trauma to a closed fist.

Boyle's law See *general gas law.*

brachial plexus A network of nerves in the neck that passes under the clavicle and into the axilla, originating in the fifth, sixth, seventh, and eighth cervical nerves and the first two thoracic spinal nerves; the brachial plexus innervates the muscles and the skin of the chest, shoulders, and arms.

bradycardia A heart rate of less than 60 beats per minute.

bradykinin A peptide of nonprotein origin that contains nine amino acid residues; a potent vasodilator.

bradypnea A persistent respiratory rate slower than 12 breaths per minute.

brain abscess An accumulation of purulent material (pus) surrounded by a capsule within the brain.

brain tumor A mass in the cranial cavity.

brainstem The midbrain, pons, and medulla.

brand name See *trade name.*

Braxton-Hicks contraction Irregular tightening of the pregnant uterus that begins in the first trimester and increases in frequency, duration, and intensity as pregnancy progresses.

breech presentation The intrauterine position of the fetus in which the buttocks or feet present.

broad ligament A folded sheet of peritoneum draped over the uterine tubes, uterus, and ovaries.

bronchial breath sounds Breath sounds heard only over the trachea and are the highest in pitch.

bronchial tree An anatomical complex of the bronchi and bronchial tubes.

bronchiectasis An abnormal dilation of the bronchi caused by a pus-producing infection of the bronchial wall.

bronchiole A small branch of a bronchus.

bronchiolitis An acute viral infection of the lower respiratory tract that occurs primarily in infants under 18 months of age; it is characterized by expiratory wheezes, respiratory distress, inflammation, and obstruction at the level of the bronchioles.

bronchopulmonary dysplasia A chronic respiratory disorder characterized by scarring of lung tissue, thickened pulmonary arterial walls, and ventilation-perfusion mismatch; often occurs in infants who have dependence on long-term artificial ventilation.

bronchovesicular breath sounds Normal breath sounds heard over the major bronchi and over the upper right posterior lung field.

brow presentation See *face presentation*.

Brown-Séquard syndrome A hemitransection of the spinal cord. In the classic presentation, pressure on half of the spinal cord results in weakness of the upper and lower extremities on the ipsilateral (same) side and loss of pain and temperature sensation on the contralateral (opposite) side.

bruit An abnormal sound or murmur heard while auscultating an artery, organ, or gland.

buccal Of or pertaining to the inside of the cheek.

buccal route A route for administering medication in which the agent is placed between the teeth and mucous membrane of the cheek.

bulbourethral glands Small glands located just below the prostate gland that lubricate the terminal portion of the urethra and contribute to seminal fluid; also known as *Cowper's glands*.

bulimia nervosa A disorder characterized by an insatiable craving for food, often resulting in episodes of binge eating followed by purging (through self-induced vomiting or use of laxatives), depression, and self-deprivation.

bullae Thin-walled blisters of the skin or mucous membranes that contain clear, serous fluid.

bullet tumble See *bullet yaw*.

bullet yaw The forward rotation of a bullet around its center of mass, which causes an end-over-end motion, producing a greater energy exchange and greater tissue damage; also known as *bullet tumble*.

bundle of His A band of fibers in the myocardium through which the cardiac impulse is transmitted from the atrioventricular node to the ventricles.

bundle of Kent Fibers that connect atrial muscle to ventricular muscle, bypassing the AV node; also known as *Kent fibers*.

burette An intravenous device used to deliver a wide range of accurate, specific volumes.

bursa A small sac containing synovial fluid that helps ease friction between a tendon and skin or between a tendon and bone.

bursitis An inflammation of the bursa, the connective tissue structure surrounding a joint.

C. *diff* colitis Inflammation of the colon caused by the bacterium *Clostridium difficile*.

calcaneus The heel bone, the largest of the tarsal bones.

calcium The fifth most abundant element in the human body; it occurs mainly in bone.

calipers An instrument with two hinged, adjustable legs used to measure components of the electrocardiogram.

canaliculus A very small tube or channel.

cancellous bone Latticelike tissue normally present in the interior of many bones where spaces usually are filled with marrow; also known as *spongy bone*.

cancer A neoplasm characterized by the uncontrolled growth of anaplastic cells that tend to invade surrounding tissue and to metastasize to distant body sites.

Candida A genus of yeastlike fungi.

candidiasis An infection caused by a species of *Candida* organisms that is characterized by pruritus, exudate, and easy bleeding.

cannulation The insertion of a cannula into a body duct or cavity.

capillaries Tiny vessels that connect arterioles to venules.

capillary network A complex, interconnected structure where a single blood cell traveling from an arteriole to a venule via a capillary bed passes through capillary segments.

capillary refill test A test used to evaluate the rate of blood flow through peripheral capillary beds.

capitation A method of payment to cover all health care expenses for each member of a managed care organization.

capitulum The lateral aspect of the humerus; it articulates with the head of the radius.

capnography The measurement of carbon dioxide concentrations in exhaled air.

capsid A protein coat that encloses a virus.

carbaminohemoglobin A chemical complex formed by carbon dioxide and hemoglobin after the release of oxygen by the hemoglobin to a tissue cell.

carbohydrate Any group of organic compounds composed of carbon, hydrogen, and oxygen; it is primarily obtained from plant foods.

carbonic acid An aqueous solution of carbon dioxide.

carbonic anhydrase The enzyme that converts carbon dioxide into carbonic acid.

carboxyhemoglobin A compound produced by the exposure of hemoglobin to carbon monoxide.

carcinogenic Cancer causing.

cardiac cycle The complete round of cardiac systole and diastole.

cardiac ejection fraction The percentage of ventricular blood volume released during a contraction.

cardiac muscle A special striated muscle of the myocardium that contains dark, intercalated disks at the junctions of the abutting fibers; cardiac muscle is characterized by special contractile abilities.

cardiac myopathy An abnormal condition of the heart characterized by weakness of the myocardium.

cardiac output The volume of blood pumped each minute by the left ventricle.

cardiac plexus One of several nerve complexes situated close to the arch of the aorta.

cardiac sphincter A ring of muscle fibers at the juncture of the esophagus and stomach.

cardiogenic shock Shock that results when cardiac action is unable to deliver sufficient circulating blood volume for tissue perfusion.

cardiography Recording the movements of the heart.

cardiomyopathy Any disease that affects the myocardium.

cardiopulmonary Of or pertaining to the heart and lungs.

cardiopulmonary resuscitation An emergency procedure for life support consisting of artificial respiration and manual external cardiac massage.

carina of the trachea A downward and backward projection of the lowest tracheal cartilage, forming a ridge between the openings of the right and left primary bronchi.

carotid body A small structure containing neural tissue at the bifurcation of the carotid arteries; it monitors the oxygen content of the blood and helps regulate respiration.

carotid sinus massage See *carotid sinus pressure*.

carotid sinus pressure A technique used to increase vagal tone to convert paroxysmal supraventricular tachycardia to sinus rhythm; also known as *carotid sinus massage*.

carpal Pertaining to the carpus, or wrist.

carpal tunnel syndrome An entrapment neuropathy that occurs when the median nerve becomes pressed or squeezed at the wrist in the carpal tunnel.

carpometacarpal joint The joint of the thumb.

carrier A radio signal of specific frequency generated by a transmitter without audio information imposed on it.

carrier molecule A protein that combines with solutes on one side of a membrane, transporting the solute to the other side; it is used in mediated transport mechanisms.

cartilage Firm, smooth, nonvascular connective tissue.

cartilaginous joint See *joint*.

catabolic Pertaining to the destruction of complex substances by living cells to form simple compounds.

cataract A loss of transparency of the lens of the eye that results from changes in the delicate protein fibers within the lens.

catecholamine Any of a group of sympathomimetic amines, including dopamine, epinephrine, and norepinephrine.

cathartic Causing evacuation of the bowel.

catheter fragment embolism The shearing or detachment of an IV catheter, allowing the embolus to travel in the bloodstream.

cation An ion with a positive charge.

cauda equina syndrome A rare disorder of the lumbar spine that affects the bundle of nerve roots at the lower end of the spinal cord; a surgical emergency.

cavitation A temporary or permanent opening produced by a force that pushes body tissues laterally away from the track of a projectile.

cecum A cul-de-sac constituting the first part of the large intestine.

cell The functional basic unit of life.

cell body The part of the cell that contains the nucleus and surrounding cytoplasm, exclusive of any projections or processes; it is concerned more with metabolism of the cell than with a specific function.

cell-mediated immunity Immunity characterized by the formation of a population of lymphocytes that attack and destroy foreign material.

cellular phone An 800- to 900-MHz radio communications system used to gain access to dial-up telephone circuits and vice versa. The system usually is divided into small coverage areas called cells, which are interconnected via microwave or dedicated telephone circuits.

cellulitis An inflammation of the skin characterized most commonly by local heat, redness, pain, swelling, and occasionally fever, malaise, chills, and headache.

cementum The bonelike connective tissue that covers the roots of the teeth and helps to support them.

centigram A metric unit of mass equal to $\frac{1}{100}$ of a gram.

centimeter A metric unit of length equal to $\frac{1}{100}$ of a meter, or 0.3937 inches.

central cord syndrome A spinal cord injury commonly seen with hyperextension or flexion cervical injuries; characterized by greater motor impairment of the upper than lower extremities.

central nervous system The brain and spinal cord.

central nervous system ischemic response An increase in blood pressure caused by vasoconstriction that occurs when oxygen levels are too low, carbon dioxide levels are too high, or pH is too low in the medulla.

central pain syndrome Infection or disease of the trigeminal nerve (cranial nerve V).

central retinal artery occlusion The blockage of blood supply to the arteries to the retina.

central thermoreceptors Nerve endings located in or near the anterior hypothalamus that are sensitive to heat.

centrifugation The process of separating components of different densities contained in a liquid by spinning them at high speeds.

centriole Usually paired organelles lying in the centrosome.

centrosome A specialized zone of cytoplasm close to the nucleus that contains two centrioles.

cephalic presentation A classification of fetal position in which the head of the fetus is at the uterine cervix; also known as *vertex presentation*.

cephalopelvic disproportion An obstetrical condition in which a newborn's head is too large or a mother's birth canal too small to permit normal labor or birth.

cephalothorax The united head and thorax of a spider.

cerebellar cortex The outer portion of the cerebellum.

cerebellum The second largest part of the brain, which plays an essential role in producing normal movements.

cerebral Pertaining to the brain.

cerebral aneurysm A weak or thin spot on a blood vessel in the brain that balloons and fills with blood; cerebral embolism.

cerebral aqueduct The narrow conduit between the third and fourth ventricles in the midbrain that conveys cerebrospinal fluid.

cerebral blood flow A function of cerebral perfusion pressure and resistance of the cerebral vascular bed.

cerebral cortex A thin layer of gray matter, made up of neuron dendrites and cell bodies, that composes the surface of the cerebrum.

cerebral edema An accumulation of fluid in the brain tissue.

cerebral palsy A general term for nonprogressive disorders of movement and posture.

cerebral perfusion pressure A measure of the amount of blood flow to the brain calculated by subtracting the intracranial pressure from the mean systemic arterial blood pressure.

cerebral thrombosis A blood clot (thrombus) forms in an artery that supplies blood to the brain.

cerebrospinal fluid Fluid that fills the subarachnoid space in the brain and spinal cord and in the cerebral ventricles.

cerebrospinal fluid rhinorrhea Leakage of cerebrospinal fluid caused by fracture of the ethmoid cribriform plate.

cerebrovascular accident An abnormal condition of the blood vessels of the brain characterized by occlusion by an embolus, thrombus, or cerebral hemorrhage; also known as *stroke and "brain attack."*

cerebrum The largest and uppermost part of the brain; it controls consciousness, memory, sensations, emotions, and voluntary movements.

certification (or registration) The process by which an agency or association grants recognition to an individual for meeting specific requirements to participate in an activity.

cerumen A yellowish or brownish waxy secretion produced in the external ear canal; also known as *earwax.*

ceruminous gland The gland that produces a waxy substance, cerumen (earwax).

cervical Pertaining to the neck.

cervical node One of the lymph glands in the neck.

cervical plexus The network of nerves formed by the ventral primary divisions of the first four cervical nerves.

cervical spondylosis A form of degenerative joint and disk disease that affects the cervical vertebrae and results in compression of the associated nerve roots.

cervical vertebrae The first seven segments of the vertebral column, designated C1 to C7.

cervicitis Acute or chronic inflammation of the uterine cervix.

cervix The lower part of the uterus.

cesarean delivery A surgical procedure in which the abdomen and uterus are incised and the baby is delivered transabdominally.

Chadwick's sign The bluish coloration of the vulva and vagina that develops after the sixth week of pregnancy as a normal result of local venous congestion; an early sign of pregnancy.

chalazion A small bump in the eyelid; caused by the blockage of a tiny oil gland in the upper or lower eyelid.

chancre A skin lesion, usually of primary syphilis, that begins at the site of infection as a papule and develops into a red, bloodless, painless ulcer with a craterlike appearance.

channel An assigned frequency or pair of frequencies used to carry voice or data communications or both. In emergency medical services, an advanced life support "MED" channel is a pair of radio frequencies, one used for transmitting, the other for receiving.

chemical name The exact designation of a chemical structure as determined by the rules of chemical nomenclature.

chemical restraint The use of drugs to control behavior.

chemoreceptor A sensory cell stimulated by a change in the concentration of chemicals to produce action potentials.

chemotactic factors Biochemical mediators that are important in activating the inflammatory response.

chemotaxis The response of leukocytes to products formed in immunological reactions; a part of the inflammatory response.

CHEMTREC (Chemical Transportation Emergency Center) A public service of the Chemical Manufacturers Association, the center provides immediate advice to on-scene personnel regarding management of hazardous materials.

Cheyne-Stokes respiration A regular, periodic pattern of breathing with equal intervals of apnea followed by a crescendo-decrescendo sequence of respirations.

chickenpox See *varicella.*

chief complaint A patient's primary complaint.

child abuse The physical, sexual, or emotional maltreatment of a child.

Chlamydia A genus of microorganisms that live as intracellular parasites; a common cause of sexually transmitted diseases and a frequent cause of sterility.

chlorine A poisonous, yellow-green gas with an odor that has been described as a mixture of pineapple and pepper.

choanal atresia A bony or membranous occlusion that blocks the passageway between the nose and pharynx; it can result in serious ventilation problems in the neonate.

cholecystectomy Surgical removal of the gallbladder.

cholecystitis Inflammation of the gallbladder, most often associated with the presence of gallstones.

cholecystokinin A hormone that stimulates the contraction of the gallbladder and the secretion of pancreatic juice.

cholesterol A fat-soluble compound found in animal fats and oils that is distributed widely in the body.

cholinergic Of or pertaining to the effects produced by the parasympathetic nervous system or drugs that stimulate or antagonize the parasympathetic nervous system.

chondrocytes Cartilage cells.

chorioamnionitis An inflammatory reaction in the amniotic membranes caused by organisms in the amniotic fluid.

chorionic gonadotropin A chemical component of the urine of pregnant women.

choroid The portion of the vascular tunic associated with the sclera of the eye.

choroid plexus A network of brain capillaries that are involved in producing cerebrospinal fluid.

chromatin granules The material within the cell nucleus from which chromosomes are formed.

chromosome An organized structure of DNA and protein that is found in cells.

chronic bronchitis Obstructive airway disease of the trachea and bronchi.

chronic fatigue syndrome A debilitating and complex disorder, characterized by profound fatigue that is not improved by bed rest and that may be worsened by physical or mental activity.

chronic gastroenteritis Inflammation of the stomach and intestines that accompanies numerous gastrointestinal disorders.

chronic obstructive pulmonary disease A progressive, irreversible condition characterized by diminished inspiratory and expiratory capacity of the lungs.

chronic pain Pain that continues or recurs over a prolonged period; it is caused by various diseases or by abnormal conditions.

chronic pulmonary hypertension A condition of abnormally high pressure within the pulmonary circulation.

chronic renal failure A progressive, irreversible systemic disease caused by kidney dysfunction that leads to abnormalities in blood counts and blood chemistry levels.

chronotropic Pertaining to agents that affect the heart rate; a drug that increases the heart rate is said to have a positive chronotropic effect.

chyme The semifluid mass of partly digested food passed from the stomach into the duodenum.

cilia Small, hairlike processes on the outer surfaces of some cells.

ciliary body A structure continuous with the choroid layer that contains smooth muscle cells and that functions in accommodation.

ciliated tissue Any tissue that projects cilia from its surface, such as portions of the epithelium in the respiratory tract.

circadian rhythm A pattern based on a 24-hour cycle, especially repetition of certain physiological phenomena, such as sleeping and eating.

circle of Willis The circle of interconnected blood vessels at the base of the brain.

circulatory shock Failure of the cardiovascular system to supply the cells with enough oxygenated blood to meet metabolic demands.

circumcision The surgical removal of the penile foreskin.

circumduction Movement in a circular motion.

circumflex artery The subdivision of the left coronary artery that feeds the lateral and posterior portions of the left ventricle and part of the right ventricle.

cirrhosis A chronic degenerative disease of the liver.

citrate Any salt or ester of citric acid.

classic heat stroke A severe, sometimes fatal condition resulting from the failure of the temperature-regulating capacity of the body; it is caused by prolonged exposure to the sun or to high temperatures.

claudication Cramplike pains in the calves caused by poor circulation of blood to the leg muscles.

clavicle A long, curved, horizontal bone just above the first rib that forms the ventral portion of the shoulder girdle.

clinical depression A disabling condition that adversely affects a person's family, work or school life, sleeping and eating habits, and general health; also known as *major depression*.

clinical perineum The portion of the perineum between the vaginal and anal openings.

clinical reasoning Use of the results of questions to think about associated problems and body system changes related to the patient's complaint.

clitoris Erectile tissue located in the vestibule of the vagina.

closed-ended questions Questions that are restrictive and can be answered with a "yes" or "no" response.

closed pneumothorax A collection of air or gas in the pleural space that causes the lung to collapse without exposing the pleural space to atmospheric pressure.

Clostridium difficile A bacterium that normally is present in small numbers in the intestines.

clotting cascade The blood-clotting system or coagulation pathway.

clotting factors Substances in the blood that act in sequence to stop bleeding by forming a clot.

cluster headache A type of headache that occurs in bursts (clusters); also known as *histamine headache*.

coagulation Formation of a clot.

coarse ventricular fibrillation Fibrillatory waves greater than 3 mm in amplitude.

coccygeal bone The four segments of the sacral vertebral column that fuse to form the adult coccyx.

coccygeal plexus A network of coccygeal nerves.

cochlea Part of the bony labyrinth of the inner ear.

cognitive development The construction of thought processes, including remembering, problem solving, and decision making, from childhood through adolescence to adulthood.

cognitive disorder A disorder that results in a disturbance of cognitive functioning.

coitus See *copulation.*

colitis An inflammatory condition of the large intestine characterized by severe diarrhea, bleeding, and ulceration of the mucosa of the intestine.

collagen The ropelike protein of the extracellular matrix.

collagen vascular disease Abnormal immune system activity with inflammation in the connective tissues; results in the accumulation of extra antibodies in the circulation.

collecting duct A straight tubule that extends from the cortex of the kidney to the tip of the renal pyramid.

Colles' fracture A fracture of the radius at the epiphysis within 1 inch of the joint of the wrist; it is easily recognized by the resultant dorsal and lateral position of the hand.

colloid A state of matter in which large molecules or aggregates of molecules that do not precipitate are dispersed in another medium.

colloid solutions Solutions that contain molecules (usually protein) that are too large to pass through the capillary membrane.

colon The portion of the large intestine that extends from the cecum to the rectum.

colorectal cancer A malignant disease of the large intestine characterized by a change in bowel habits and the passing of blood.

colostomy A surgical opening into the large intestine.

coma An abnormally deep state of unconsciousness where the patient cannot be aroused by external stimuli.

command The act of directing, ordering, or controlling by virtue of explicit, statutory, regulatory, or delegated authority.

command post The area from which command directs operations for an incident.

communicability period A stage of infection that begins when the latent period ends and continues as long as the agent is present and can spread to other hosts.

communicable disease An infectious disease that can be transmitted from one person to another.

communications The transmission and reception of information, resulting in common understanding.

communications center A facility used to dispatch emergency equipment and coordinate communications between field units and personnel.

community health assessment An assessment of a target community to identify needs and resources required to provide prevention and wellness promotion activities.

compact bone Hard, dense bone that usually is found at the surface of skeletal structures, as distinguished from cancellous bone.

compartment syndrome The result of a crush injury, usually caused by compressive forces or blunt trauma to muscle groups confined in tight fibrous sheaths with minimal ability to stretch.

compensated shock A stage of shock associated with some decreased blood flow and perfusion to the tissues.

competitive antagonist An agent with an affinity for the same receptor site as an agonist. The competition with the agonist for the site inhibits the action of the agonist; increasing the concentration of the agonist tends to overcome the inhibition.

complement One of 11 complex, enzymatic serum proteins; complement causes lysis in an antigen-antibody reaction.

complement system A group of proteins that coat bacteria; the proteins either help kill the bacteria directly or assist neutrophils (in the blood) and macrophages (in the tissues) to engulf and destroy the bacteria.

complete abortion An abortion in which the patient has passed all the products of conception.

complete breech A delivery presentation that occurs when the fetus has both knees and hips flexed; the buttocks are the presenting part.

complex partial seizure A seizure that originates in the temporal lobe; usually begins with an aura and is followed by repetitive motor behavior.

compliance The ease with which the lungs and thorax expand during pressure changes. The greater the compliance, the easier the expansion.

components of skeletal survey An x-ray study comprising a two-view chest with bone technique, two-view skull technique, views of the lateral lumbar spine and anteroposterior pelvis, and anteroposterior views of the upper and lower extremities, including anteroposterior views of the feet and posteroanterior views of the hands.

computer-aided dispatching An enhanced dispatch system in which computerized data are used to assist the dispatcher in selecting and routing emergency equipment and resources.

concealment A means of keeping out of site; it provides no ballistic protection.

concentration gradient The concentration difference between two points in a solution divided by the distance between the points.

concept formation A component of critical thinking that refers to all elements that are gathered to form a general impression of the patient.

concha The three bony ridges on the lateral wall of the nasal cavity.

concussion A head injury that results from violent jarring or shaking, such as that caused by a blow or explosion.

condyle A rounded projection on a bone, usually for articulation with another bone.

cone A photoreceptor in the retina of the eye; it is responsible for color vision.

confabulation The invention of stories to make up for gaps in memory.

congenital Present at birth.

congenital anomalies Defects that occur during fetal development.

congenital rubella syndrome A serious disease that affects about 25% of infants born to women infected with rubella during the first trimester of pregnancy; it is associated with multiple congenital anomalies, mental retardation, and an increased risk of death from congenital heart disease and sepsis during the first 6 months of life.

congestive heart failure An abnormal condition that reflects impaired cardiac pumping, usually a result of myocardial infarction, ischemic heart disease, or cardiomyopathy.

conjugate gaze Deviation of both eyes to either side at rest; the condition implies a structural lesion.

conjunctiva A mucous membrane that covers the anterior surface of the eyeball and the lining of the eyelids.

conjunctivitis Inflammation of the conjunctiva, caused by bacterial or viral infection, allergy, or environmental factors.

connective tissue Tissue that supports and binds other body tissues and parts.

conservation of energy law The principle that energy can be neither created nor destroyed; it can only change from one form (mechanical, thermal, electrical, or chemical) to another.

constipation Difficulty passing stools, or incomplete or infrequent passage of hard stools.

contact dermatitis Skin rash that results from exposure to an irritant or sensitizing antigen.

continence The ability to control bladder or bowel function.

continuous positive airway pressure Airway support that transmits positive pressure into the airways of a spontaneously breathing patient throughout the respiratory cycle.

continuous quality improvement A management approach to customer service and organizational performance that includes constant monitoring, evaluation, decisions, and actions.

contracture deformity An abnormal, usually permanent condition of a joint characterized by flexion and fixation and caused by atrophy and shortening of muscle fibers or by loss of elasticity of the skin.

contraindications Medical or physiological factors that make it harmful to administer a medication that would otherwise have a therapeutic effect.

contralateral Affecting or originating in the opposite side of the body.

contrastimulant A factor that works against stimulation.

contrecoup An injury that occurs at a site opposite the side of impact.

control console Typically, a desk-mounted, enclosed piece of equipment that contains the mechanical and electronic controls used to operate a radio base station.

controlled substance Any drug defined in the categories of the Comprehensive Drug Abuse Prevention and Control Act (also known as the Controlled Substances Act) of 1970.

contusion A closed, soft tissue injury characterized by swelling, discoloration, and pain.

conversion disorder A mental illness in which painful emotions are repressed and unconsciously converted into physical symptoms.

copulation The sexual union of two persons of the opposite sex in which the penis is introduced into the vagina; also known as *coitus*.

cor pulmonale An abnormal cardiac condition characterized by hypertrophy of the right ventricle of the heart as a result of hypertension of the pulmonary circulation.

cord presentation A presentation that occurs when the cord slips down into the vagina or appears externally after the amniotic membranes have ruptured.

core body temperature The temperature of deep structures of the body as compared with temperatures of peripheral tissues.

cornea The convex, transparent, anterior part of the eye.

corneal abrasion The rubbing off of the outer layers of the cornea.

corniculate cartilage A conical nodule of elastic cartilage that surrounds the apex of each arytenoid cartilage.

coronal plane See *frontal plane.*

coronary artery One of two arteries that arise from the base of the aorta and carry blood to the muscle of the heart.

coronary artery disease One of several abnormal conditions that affect the arteries of the heart and reduce the flow of oxygen and nutrients to the myocardium.

coronary sinus A short trunk that receives most of the veins of the heart and empties into the right atrium.

corpus callosum An arched mass of white matter in the depths of the longitudinal fissure; it is made up of the transverse fibers that connect the cerebral hemispheres.

corpus luteum A yellow endocrine body formed in the ovary at the site of a ruptured vesicular follicle immediately after ovulation.

corpus luteum cyst A type of cyst prone to rupture that forms as a result of hemorrhage in a mature corpus luteum.

cortisol A steroid hormone that occurs naturally in the body.

costal cartilages Cartilages that connect the sternum and the ends of the ribs; allow the chest to move in respiration.

costal margin The margin of the lower limit of the ribs.

costochondral Pertaining to the junction of the ribs and cartilage.

countershock A high-intensity, short-duration electrical shock applied to the area of the heart, resulting in total cardiac depolarization.

coup Local damage that occurs at the site of impact.

couplet Two premature ventricular contractions in a row.

cover A type of concealment that hides the body and offers ballistic protection.

coverage The area covered by radio communication. The generally accepted national emergency system standard is the "90/90" standard. This means that 90% of the coverage area will have communication 90% of the time. Coverage usually is expressed as dead (no coverage), marginal (spotty), good (few problems), or excellent (no problems).

Cowper's glands See *bulbourethral glands*.

coxae The hip joints; the head of the femur and the acetabulum of the innominate bone.

crackle A fine, bubbling sound heard on auscultation of the lung; it is produced by air entering distal airways and alveoli that contain serous secretions.

cranial nerve One of 12 pairs of nerves that originate from a nucleus within the brain.

cranial vault The eight skull bones that surround and protect the brain; the brain case.

craniectomy Surgical removal of bone fragments from the cranium.

creatinine A chemical waste molecule that is generated from muscle metabolism.

cremaster muscle A thin muscle layer spreading out over the spermatic cord in a series of loops; it functions to draw the testis up toward the superficial inguinal ring in response to cold or stimulation of the nerve.

crenate The shrinking of red blood cells caused by exposure to a hypertonic solution.

crepitus A grating sound associated with rubbing of bone fragments.

Creutzfeldt-Jakob disease A rare and fatal brain disorder characterized by rapidly progressive dementia.

cricoid cartilage The most inferior laryngeal cartilage.

cricothyroid membrane The membrane joining the thyroid and cricoid cartilages.

cricothyrotomy An emergency incision into the larynx.

crime scene A location where any part of a criminal act has occurred, or a location where evidence relating to a crime may be found.

Crohn's disease A chronic, inflammatory bowel disease of unknown origin, usually affecting the ileum, the colon, or both structures.

croup An acute viral infection of the upper and lower respiratory tract that occurs primarily in infants and young children 3 months to 3 years of age; it is characterized by hoarseness, fever, a harsh and brassy cough, inspiratory stridor, and varying degrees of respiratory distress; also known as *laryngotracheobronchitis*.

crown The portion of the human tooth covered by enamel.

crowning The phase at the end of labor in which the fetal head is seen at the opening of the vagina.

crush injury Injury from exposure of tissue to a compressive force sufficient to interfere with the normal structure and metabolic function of the involved cells and tissues.

crush syndrome A life-threatening and sometimes preventable complication of prolonged immobilization; a pathological process that causes destruction, alteration, or both of muscle tissue.

crystalloid A substance in a solution that can be diffused through a semipermeable membrane.

crystalloid solutions Solutions created by dissolving crystals such as salts and sugars in water.

crystalluria The presence of crystals in the urine.

cubic centimeter A metric unit of length equal to $\frac{1}{100}$ of a meter.

Cullen's sign The appearance of irregularly formed hemorrhagic patches on the skin around the umbilicus.

cultural imposition Forcing one's beliefs, values, and patterns of behavior on people from another culture.

cumulative action The effect that occurs when several doses of a drug are administered or when absorption occurs more quickly than removal by excretion or metabolism or both.

cuneiform cartilage A small rod of elastic cartilage above the corniculate cartilages in the larynx.

CUPS system A method of patient status coding that assigns patients to one of four categories: Cardiopulmonary resuscitation, Unstable, Potentially unstable, and Stable.

current health status A focus on the patient's current state of health, environmental conditions, and personal habits.

Cushing's disease A metabolic disorder resulting from the chronic and excessive production of cortisol by the adrenal cortex or by the administration of glucocorticoids in large doses for several weeks or longer; also known as *Cushing's syndrome*.

Cushing's reflex An attempt by the body to compensate for a decline in cerebral perfusion pressure by a rise in mean arterial pressure.

Cushing's syndrome A condition caused by an abnormally high circulating level of corticosteroid hormones, produced naturally by the adrenal glands.

cutaneous Of or pertaining to the skin.

cuticle The skinfold covering the root of the nail.

cyanotic Having bluish discoloration.

cystic medial necrosis Degenerative changes in the connective tissue of the aortic media.

cystitis Inflammation of the urinary bladder and ureters.

cytochrome oxidase A respiratory enzyme that functions in the transfer of electrons from cytochromes to oxygen, thus activating oxygen, which unites with hydrogen to form water.

cytochromes Proteins in the liver that play a role in drug detoxification.

cytology The study of cells.

cytomegalovirus A member of a group of large, species-specific, herpes-type viruses with a wide variety of disease effects.

cytoplasm All of the substance of a cell other than the nucleus.

cytoplasmic membrane The plasma membrane.

cytotoxic Pertaining to a pharmacological compound or other agent that destroys or damages tissue cells.

dartos muscle A layer of smooth muscle in the skin of the scrotum; it raises and lowers the testes in the scrotum in response to changes in ambient temperature.

data interpretation A component of critical thinking in which the examiner gathers the necessary data to form a field impression and working diagnosis.

date rape Nonconsensual sex between people who are already acquainted (e.g., friends, acquaintances, people who are dating).

DCAP-BTLS An acronym for wound assessment: *Deformity* Contusions, *Abrasions, Penetrations or punctures, Burns, Tenderness, Lacerations, and Swelling.*

deafness A complete or partial inability to hear.

debriefing An activity in which rescuers and others involved in an emergency event discuss their feelings to relieve emotions and anxiety; it usually takes place 24 to 72 hours after the event.

decerebrate posturing A position in which a comatose patient's arms are extended and internally rotated and the legs are extended with the feet in forced plantar flexion; usually observed in patients who have compression of the brainstem.

deciduous tooth Any of the 20 teeth that appear normally during infancy.

deciliter A metric unit of volume equal to $\frac{1}{10}$ of a liter.

decoding The act of interpreting symbols and format.

decompression sickness A multisystem disorder that results when nitrogen in compressed air converts back from solution to gas, forming bubbles in the tissues and blood.

decontamination The process of making patients, rescuers, equipment, and supplies safe by eliminating harmful substances.

decorticate posturing A position in which the comatose patient's upper extremities are rigidly flexed at the elbows and at the wrists; usually observed in patients who have a lesion in the mesencephalic region of the brain.

dedicated line A special telephone circuit designated for specific point-to-point communication purposes, such as alerting emergency medical services quarters.

deep frostbite A cold injury that results in significant tissue loss even with appropriate therapy; it is associated with subdermal layers and deep tissues.

deep tendon reflexes Reflexes elicited by sensory afferents from muscle rather than bone.

deep vein thrombosis A disorder involving a thrombus in one of the deep veins of the body, most commonly the iliac and femoral veins.

defecation The elimination of feces from the digestive tract through the rectum.

defense mechanism An unconscious, intrapsychic reaction to protect the self from a stressful situation.

defibrillation The delivery of direct electrical current in an attempt to terminate ventricular fibrillation or pulseless ventricular tachycardia.

defibrillator A device used to depolarize fibrillating myocardial cells, thus allowing them to repolarize uniformly.

deficient ambient oxygen An oxygen concentration that is less than 21%.

defusing An informal gathering of the persons involved in an emergency event to allow an initial release of feelings and an opportunity for persons to share their experiences.

degloving injury An injury usually involving the hand or finger in which the soft tissue is removed down to the bone.

degradation The physical destruction or decomposition of clothing material caused by use, ambient conditions, or exposure to chemicals.

degranulation A cellular process that releases antimicrobial substances from secretory vesicles (granules) found inside mast cells and basophils; plays a role in allergic reactions.

dehydration An excessive loss of water from the body tissues; it may follow prolonged fever, diarrhea, vomiting, acidosis, and other conditions.

delirium An abrupt disorientation for time and place, usually with illusions and hallucinations.

delirium tremens An acute and sometimes fatal psychotic reaction caused by cessation of excessive intake of alcohol over a long period of time; also known as *DTs.*

delta cell A constituent of the islets of Langerhans; it secretes somatostatin.

delta wave Widened, abnormal slurring or notching of the onset of the QRS complex; it indicates anomalous spread of the impulse and is a diagnostic finding for Wolff-Parkinson-White syndrome.

deltoid muscle A large, thick, triangular muscle that covers the shoulder joint.

delusions Persistent beliefs or perceptions held by a person despite evidence that refutes them (i.e., false beliefs).

dementia A slow, progressive loss of awareness of time and place. It usually involves an inability to learn new things or recall recent events.

dendrite The branching processes of a neuron that receive stimuli and conduct potentials toward the cell body.

dental abscess A bacterial infection in the center of the tooth.

dentalgia The medical term for toothache.

dentin The chief component of teeth, surrounding the pulp and situated inside the enamel and cementum.

deoxyribonucleic acid A type of nucleic acid that comprises the genetic material of cells.

dependent lividity A red or bluish purple tissue condition in dependent areas of the body caused by venous congestion.

depersonalization Forced emotional estrangement.

depolarization A change in electrical charge difference across the cell membrane that causes the difference to be smaller or closer to 0 mV; a phase of the action potential in which the membrane potential moves toward zero or becomes positive.

depressant A substance that decreases or lessens a body function or activity.

depressed skull fracture Any fracture of the skull in which fragments are depressed below the normal surface of the skull.

depression A mood disturbance characterized by feelings of sadness, despair, and discouragement.

dermatitis Inflammation of the skin.

dermatome The skin surface area supplied by a single spinal nerve.

dermatomyositis An inflammatory myopathy characterized by a skin rash that precedes or accompanies progressive muscle weakness.

dermis Dense, irregular connective tissue that forms the deep layer of the skin.

descending colon The segment of the colon that extends from the end of the transverse colon at the splenic flexure on the left side of the abdomen down to the beginning of the sigmoid colon in the pelvis.

desensitization Emotional insensitivity.

designated officer A person who serves as a liaison between the public safety agency and community health agencies involved in monitoring and responding to communicable diseases.

diabetes insipidus A metabolic disorder characterized by extreme polyuria and polydipsia, caused by deficient production or secretion of antidiuretic hormone or inability of the kidney tubules to respond to antidiuretic hormone.

diabetes mellitus A complex disorder of carbohydrate, fat, and protein metabolism that primarily results from partial or complete lack of insulin secretion by the beta cells of the pancreas or of defects of the insulin receptors.

diabetic ketoacidosis An acute, life-threatening complication of uncontrolled diabetes characterized by hyperglycemia, hypovolemia, electrolyte imbalance, and a breakdown of free fatty acids, causing acidosis; also known as *diabetic coma.*

diad The combination of sarcoplasmic reticulum and T tubules.

diagnosis Identification of a disease or condition by an evaluation of physical signs, symptoms, history, laboratory tests, and procedures.

dialysate A solution used in dialysis.

dialysis A technique used to normalize blood chemistry in patients with acute or chronic renal failure and to remove blood toxins in some patients who have taken a drug overdose.

dialysis fistula An artificial passage, as in an arteriovenous fistula, used to gain access to the patient's bloodstream for hemodialysis.

diaphoresis Profuse secretion of sweat.

diaphragm The dome-shaped, musculofibrous partition that separates the thoracic and abdominal cavities.

diaphragmatic hernia A herniation in the diaphragm caused by the improper fusion of structures during fetal development.

diaphysis The shaft of a long bone, consisting of a tube of compact bone that encloses the medullary cavity.

diarrhea The frequent passage of loose, watery stools; it is generally the result of increased motility in the colon.

diastolic blood pressure The minimum level of blood pressure measured between contractions of the heart.

diencephalon The parts of the brain between the cerebral hemispheres and the mesencephalon.

differential count A laboratory test that identifies the different types of leukocytes present in blood; also called the *diff.*

differential diagnosis The process of weighing the probability of one disease versus that of other diseases possibly accounting for a patient's illness.

differentiation A process in which cells become specialized in one type of function or act in concert with other cells to perform a more complex task.

diffusion The process in which solid, particulate matter in a fluid moves from an area of higher concentration to an area of lower concentration, resulting in an even distribution of the particles in the fluid.

dilation and curettage A gynecological procedure that refers to widening of the uterine cervix and scraping away of the endometrium of the uterus.

diphtheria An acute contagious disease characterized by the production of a systemic toxin and a false membrane lining of the mucous membranes of the throat.

diplopia Double vision.

direct laryngoscopy Visual examination of the larynx with a laryngoscope.

disease period A stage of infection that follows the incubation period; the duration of this period varies with the disease.

disentanglement The process of making a pathway through the wreckage of an accident and removing wreckage from patients.

disequilibrium Unstable equilibrium; motion sickness.

disequilibrium syndrome A group of neurological findings that sometimes occur during or immediately after dialysis; thought to result from a disproportionate decrease in osmolality of the extracellular fluid compared with that of the intracellular compartment in the brain or cerebrospinal fluid.

diskectomy The surgical removal of a vertebral disk.

disoriented Unaware of surroundings.

dispositional hearing The phase of the family court process in which appropriate placement for a child and appropriate treatment, if any, for the parent of a child are determined and ordered.

dissecting aortic aneurysm Localized dilation of the aorta characterized by a longitudinal dissection between the outer and middle layers of the vascular wall.

disseminated intravascular coagulation A grave coagulopathy that results from the overstimulation of the clotting and anticlotting processes in response to disease or injury.

dissociative disorders A group of psychological illnesses. In these illnesses, a particular mental function is separated (dissociated) from the mind as a whole.

dissolution The rate at which a solid drug goes into solution after ingestion; the faster the rate of dissolution, the more quickly the drug is absorbed.

distraction (1) A self-defense measure in which a diversion is created to draw a person's attention. (2) A spinal injury that occurs if the cervical spine is suddenly stopped while the weight and momentum of the body are pull away from it.

distress Negative, debilitating, or harmful stress.

distribution The transport of a drug through the bloodstream to various tissues of the body and ultimately to its site of action.

distributive shock Shock that occurs when peripheral vasodilation causes a fall in systemic vascular resistance.

disulfiram-ethanol reaction A potentially life-threatening physiological response caused by disulfiram and ethanol that produces ill effects on the gastrointestinal, cardiovascular, and autonomic nervous systems; disulfiram is prescribed to some alcoholic patients to help them maintain abstinence.

diuresis The increased formation and secretion of urine.

diversity Differences of any kind: race, class, religion, gender, sexual preference, personal habitat, and physical ability.

diverticulitis Inflammation of one or more diverticula.

diverticulosis The presence of pouchlike herniations through the muscular layer of the colon.

diverticulum A pouchlike herniation through the muscular wall of a tubular organ; it may be present in the stomach, small intestine, or, most commonly, the colon.

divisions Subdivisions of the incident command system that encompass specific geographical areas of responsibility as deemed necessary by the incident commander.

do not resuscitate A physician order instructing emergency care providers not to attempt resuscitation of a patient in the event of cardiac or respiratory failure; also known as a *"no code" order.*

dorsal root A sensory component that conveys afferent nerve processes to the spinal cord.

dorsal root ganglia See *spinal ganglia.*

dorsogluteal site An area made up of several gluteal muscles; it is used as an injection site.

Down syndrome A congenital condition characterized by varying degrees of mental retardation and multiple defects.

dram A unit of mass equal to an apothecary measure of 60 gr or ⅛ oz.

dromotropic Pertaining to agents that affect conduction velocity through the conducting tissues of the heart; a drug that speeds conduction is said to have a positive dromotropic effect.

drowning A mortal event in which a submersion victim is pronounced dead at the scene of the attempted resuscitation, or within 24 hours after arrival in the emergency department or hospital.

drug Any substance taken by mouth; injected into a muscle, blood vessel, or cavity of the body; or applied topically to treat or prevent a disease or condition.

drug absorption A process in which drug molecules move from the site of entry into the body to the general circulation.

drug abuse Self-medication or self-administration of a drug in chronically excessive amounts, resulting in psychological or physical dependence (or both), functional impairment, and deviation from approved social norms.

drug allergy A systemic reaction to a drug resulting from previous sensitizing exposure and the development of an immunological mechanism.

drug dependence A state in which intense physical or emotional disturbance is produced if a drug is withdrawn; previously called *habituation.*

drug interaction Modification of the effects of one drug by the previous or concurrent administration of another drug, thereby increasing or diminishing the pharmacological or physiological action of one or both drugs.

drug receptors Parts of a cell (usually an enzyme or large protein molecule) with which a drug molecule interacts to trigger its desired response or effect.

drug-protein complex A complex formed by the attachment of a drug to proteins, mainly albumin.

ductus arteriosus A vascular channel in the fetus that joins the pulmonary artery directly to the descending aorta.

ductus deferens A thick, smooth muscular tube that allows sperm to exit from the epididymis through the ejaculatory duct; also known as the *vas deferens.*

ductus venosus The continuation of the umbilical vein through the liver to the inferior vena cava.

duodenum The first subdivision of the small intestine.

duplex mode A communications mode with the ability to transmit and receive traffic simultaneously through two different frequencies, one to transmit and one to receive.

duplex/multiplex system A communications system with the ability to transmit and receive simultaneously with concurrent transmission of voice and telemetry.

dura mater The outermost layer of the meninges.

duration of action The period from the onset of drug action to the time when a drug effect is no longer seen.

dysarthria Difficult and poorly articulated speech resulting from poor control over the muscles of speech.

dysconjugate gaze Deviation of the eyes to opposite sides at rest; it implies a structural brainstem dysfunction in the pathways that traverse the brainstem from the upper midbrain to at least the level of the lower pons.

dysfunctional uterine bleeding Abnormal bleeding that occurs because of changes in hormone levels.

dyshemoglobinemia Hemoglobin saturated with compounds other than oxygen, such as carbon monoxide or methemoglobin.

dyskinesia An impairment of the ability to execute voluntary movements; often an adverse effect of prolonged use of antipsychotic medications.

dysmenorrhea Pain associated with menstruation.

dyspareunia Pain with intercourse.

dysphagia Inability or difficulty in swallowing because of medical or traumatic causes.

dysphonia An abnormality in the speaking voice, such as hoarseness.

dysplasia Abnormal cellular growth.

dyspnea Difficulty breathing.

dysrhythmia Variation from a normal rhythm.

dysthymia A form of depression that is chronic in nature, lasting as long as 2 years or more.

dystonia A condition characterized by local or diffuse changes in muscle tone, resulting in painful muscle spasms, unusually fixed postures, and strange movement patterns.

dysuria Difficult urination.

EACOM/HEAR The Emergency Administrative Communications (by General Electric) or Hospital Emergency Administrative Radio (by Motorola). These radio systems use 1500-Hz rotary-pulse dialing, which transmits specific groups of rotary tone pulses for the purpose of selectively addressing hospital-based receivers in particular regions throughout the United States. Most ambulance services have access to this system.

eardrum The cellular membrane that separates the external ear from the middle ear; also known as the *tympanic membrane.*

early adulthood Persons 20 to 40 years of age.

eating disorders A term referring to anorexia nervosa and bulimia nervosa, conditions in which dissatisfaction with weight and body shape cause an individual to develop disordered eating behaviors.

eclampsia A grave form of pregnancy-induced hypertension, characterized by convulsions, coma, proteinuria, and edema.

ectoparasite An organism that lives on the outside of the body of the host, such as a louse.

ectopic Out of place.

ectopic foci Cardiac dysrhythmias caused by irritation of an excitation impulse at a site other than the sinus node.

ectopic pregnancy An abnormal pregnancy in which the conceptus implants outside the uterine cavity.

eczema Superficial dermatitis of unknown cause.

edema The accumulation of fluid within the interstitial spaces.

effacement The shortening of the vaginal portion of the cervix and the thinning of its walls as it is stretched and dilated by the fetus during labor.

effective dose 50 The amount of drug that produces a therapeutic response in 50% of those who take it.

effector organ A muscle or gland that responds to nerve impulses from the central nervous system.

efferent division The division of the central nervous system that transmits action potentials to effector organs such as muscles and glands.

efferent neuron Nerve fibers that send impulses from the central nervous system to the periphery.

efficacy An intrinsic activity that refers to the ability of a drug to initiate biological activity as a result of such binding.

Einthoven's triangle An equilateral triangle formed by the patient's right arm, left arm, and left leg; it is used in electrode sensor placement for electrocardiogram monitoring.

ejaculatory duct A duct formed by the joining of the ductus deferens and the duct from the seminal vesicle that allows sperm to enter the urethra.

ejection The forceful expulsion of blood from the ventricle of the heart.

elastin The major connective tissue protein of elastic tissue; it has a structure like a coiled spring.

elder abuse The infliction of physical pain, injury, debilitating mental anguish, unreasonable confinement, or willful deprivation by a caregiver of services that are necessary to maintain mental and physical health of a geriatric person.

electroconvulsive therapy Induction of a brief convulsion by passing an electrical current through the brain to treat affective disorders.

electrolyte A cation or anion in solution that conducts an electrical current.

elevation Movement of a structure in a superior direction.

ellipsoid joint A modified ball-and-socket joint in which the articular surfaces are ellipsoid rather than spherical.

emaciated To be abnormally lean from disease or lack of nutrition.

embolectomy A surgical incision into an artery for the removal of an embolus or clot.

embolus A blockage or free-moving thrombus in a blood vessel.

embryo In human beings the stage of prenatal development between the time of implantation of the fertilized ovum until the end of the seventh or eighth week.

emergency medical services A national network of services coordinated to provide aid and medical assistance from primary response to definitive care; the network involves personnel trained in rescue, stabilization, transportation, and advanced management of traumatic and medical emergencies.

emissary veins The small vessels in the skull that connect the sinuses of the dura with the veins on the exterior of the skull through a series of anastomoses.

emotional abuse The infliction of anguish, pain, or distress through verbal or nonverbal acts.

emotional/mental impairment Impaired intellectual functioning that results in an inability to cope with normal responsibilities of life.

empathy The ability to see a situation from the viewpoint of the person experiencing it.

emphysema An abnormal condition of the pulmonary system characterized by overinflation and destructive changes in the alveolar walls, resulting in a loss of lung elasticity and a decrease in gases.

EMS communications The delivery of patient and scene information (either in person, in writing, or through communications technology) to other members of the emergency response team.

enamel A hard white substance that covers the dentin of the crown of the tooth.

encephalitis An inflammatory condition of the brain, usually caused by an infection transmitted by the bite of an infected mosquito; it also may result from lead or other poisoning or from hemorrhage.

encoding The act of placing a message in an understandable format (either written or verbal).

end-stage renal disease Complete, or near-complete, failure of the kidneys to function.

endocrine gland A gland that secretes chemicals and hormones directly into the blood, rather than through a duct.

endolymph Fluid found within the membranous labyrinth.

endometriosis An abnormal gynecological condition characterized by ectopic growth and function of endometrial tissue; it is thought to result when, during menstruation, fragments of endometrium from the lining of the uterus are regurgitated backward through the fallopian tubes into the peritoneal cavity, where they attach and grow as small cystic structures.

endometritis An inflammatory condition of the endometrium, usually caused by bacterial infection.

endometrium The mucous membrane lining of the uterus, which changes in thickness and structure with the menstrual cycle.

endoplasmic reticulum A network of connecting sacs or canals that wind through the cytoplasm of a cell and serve as a miniature circulatory system for the cell.

endorphin Any of several peptides secreted in the brain that have a pain-relieving effect like morphine.

endotoxin A toxin contained in the cell walls of some microorganisms, especially gram-negative bacteria.

endotracheal intubation An airway management procedure in which an endotracheal tube is inserted through the mouth or nose into the trachea. Intubation is used to maintain a patent airway, to prevent aspiration of material from the digestive tract, to permit suctioning of tracheobronchial secretions, to administer positive-pressure ventilation, and to administer certain medications when other means of vascular access are unavailable.

endotracheal route Refers to drugs administered through an endotracheal tube.

enhanced automaticity The cause of dysrhythmias in Purkinje fibers and other myocardial cells with a high resting membrane potential; it results from an acceleration of phase 4 depolarization commonly caused by abnormally high leakage of sodium ions into the cells, which causes the cells to reach threshold prematurely.

enophthalmos An abnormal condition characterized by recession of the eyeball within the orbit.

enteral route A route of drug administration along any portion of the gastrointestinal tract.

envenomation The injection of snake, arachnid, or insect venom into the body.

enzyme A protein produced by living cells that catalyzes chemical reactions in organic matter.

eosinophil A white blood cell that inhibits inflammation; thought to deactivate leukotrienes.

eosinophil chemotactic factor of anaphylaxis A group of active substances, including histamine and leukotrienes, that are released during an anaphylactic reaction.

epicardium See *visceral pericardium.*

epicondyle A projection on the surface of a bone above its condyle.

epidermis The outer portion of skin; it is formed of epithelial tissue that rests on or covers the dermis.

epididymis A tightly coiled tube that lies along the top of and behind the testes, where sperm mature.

epididymitis An inflammation of the epididymis, a tubular section of the male reproductive system that carries sperm from the testicles to the seminal vesicles.

epidural hematoma Accumulation of blood between the dura mater and the cranium.

epidural space The space above or on the dura.

epiglottis A lidlike cartilage that overhangs the entrance to the larynx.

epiglottitis Inflammation of the epiglottis; a severe form of the condition that affects primarily children is characterized by fever, sore throat, stridor, croupy cough, and an erythematous epiglottis.

epilepsy A condition characterized by a tendency of the individual to have recurrent seizures (excluding those that arise from correctable or avoidable circumstances).

epinephrine Adrenaline, a hormone secreted by the adrenal medulla.

epiphyseal line A dense plate in a bone that is no longer growing, indicating the former site of the epiphyseal plate.

epiphyseal plate See *growth plate.*

epiphysis The head of a long bone that is separated from the shaft of the bone by the epiphyseal plate until the bone stops growing, the plate is obliterated, and the shaft and the head are united.

epistaxis Bleeding from the nose.

epithelial tissue The cellular covering of internal and external surfaces of the body, including the lining of vessels and other small cavities.

Epstein-Barr virus The herpesvirus that causes infectious mononucleosis.

erection The condition of hardness, swelling, and elevation observed in the penis and to a lesser degree in the clitoris, usually caused by sexual arousal.

erythema Redness of the skin, caused by hyperemia of the capillaries in the lower layers of the skin.

erythrocyte A red blood cell.

escape beat An automatic beat of the heart that occurs after an interval longer than the duration of the dominant heartbeat cycle.

eschar A scab or dry crust resulting from a thermal or chemical burn.

escharotomy Surgical incision into necrotic tissue caused by a severe burn; escharotomy sometimes is necessary to prevent edema from causing sufficient interstitial pressure to impair capillary filling and lead to ischemia.

esophageal reflux A chronic disease manifested by various sequelae associated with reflux of the stomach and duodenal contents into the esophagus.

esophageal stricture An abnormal temporary or permanent narrowing of the esophagus caused by inflammation, external pressure, or scarring.

esophagitis Inflammation of the esophagus.

esophagogastric varices A complex of longitudinal, tortuous veins at the lower end of the esophagus that become large and swollen as a result of portal hypertension; also known as *esophageal varices*.

esophagus The muscular canal extending from the pharynx to the stomach.

estimated date of confinement Delivery date for the fetus.

estrogen One of a group of hormonal steroid compounds that promote the development of female secondary sex characteristics.

ethics The discipline relating to right and wrong, moral duty and obligation, moral principles and values, and moral character; a standard for honorable behavior designed by a group with expected conformity.

ethmoid bone The very light, spongy bone at the base of the cranium that forms most of the walls of the superior part of the nasal cavity.

ethmoid sinus One of the numerous small, thin-walled cavities in the ethmoid bone of the skull, rimmed by the frontal maxilla and the lacrimal, sphenoidal, and palatine bones.

ethnocentrism Seeing one's own life as the most acceptable or best; acting in a superior manner toward another culture's way of life.

ethylene glycol A chemical used in automobile antifreeze preparations.

eukaryote A cell with a true nucleus, found in all higher organisms and in some microorganisms.

eustachian tube See *auditory tube.*

eustress Positive, performance-enhancing stress.

evaluation A component of critical thinking in which the examiner assesses the patient's response to care.

evasive tactics A self-defense measure in which an aggressor's moves and actions are anticipated, and unconventional pathways are used during retreat for personal safety.

eversion Turning outward.

evisceration The protrusion of an internal organ through a wound or surgical incision, especially in the abdominal wall.

excitability The property of a cell that enables it to react to irritation or stimulation.

excretion The elimination of toxic or inactive metabolites, primarily by the kidneys; the intestines, lungs, and mammary, sweat, and salivary glands also may be involved.

excursion Movement from side to side.

exertional heat stroke An abnormal condition characterized by weakness, vertigo, nausea, muscle cramps, and loss of consciousness; caused by depletion of body fluid and electrolytes resulting from exposure to intense heat or inability to acclimatize to heat.

exocrine gland A gland that secretes chemicals and hormones into a duct.

exophthalmos An abnormal condition characterized by marked protrusion of the eyeballs.

exothermic Marked or accompanied by the evolution of heat.

exotoxin A toxin secreted or excreted by a living organism.

expiration Breathing out (exhalation), normally a passive process.

expiratory center The region of the medulla that is electrically active during nonquiet expiration.

expiratory reserve volume The maximum volume of air that can be exhaled after expiration of the normal tidal volume.

exposure incident Any specific contact of the eyes, the mouth, other mucous membranes, nonintact skin, or parenteral contact with blood, blood products, bloody body fluids, or other potentially infectious materials.

expressed consent Verbal or written consent to the treatment.

extended scope of practice The expansion of health care services provided by emergency medical technicians and paramedics in the prehospital setting.

extension Stretching out.

external anal sphincter A sphincter muscle located at the tip of the coccyx and surrounding fascia; it prevents the movement of feces out of the rectum until it is relaxed.

external auditory canal The passage for sound impulses passing through the ear.

external auditory meatus The canal of the external ear; also known as the *external auditory canal.*

external barriers The surface of the body that is exposed to the environment. This includes the skin and the mucous membranes of the digestive, respiratory, and genitourinary tracts; the body's first line of defense against infection.

external cardiac pacing The delivery of repetitive electrical currents to the heart, substituting for a natural pacemaker that has become blocked or dysfunctional; also known as *transcutaneous cardiac pacing.*

external ear The portion of the ear that includes the auricle and external auditory meatus; it terminates at the eardrum.

external genital organs The outer parts of the female genitalia; consist of the labia majora, the labia minora, Bartholin's glands, and the clitoris. Also known as *vulva.*

external jugular vein One of a pair of large vessels in the neck that receive most of the blood from the exterior of the cranium and deep tissues of the face.

external respiration The transfer (diffusion) of oxygen and carbon dioxide between the inspired air and pulmonary capillaries.

external urinary sphincter The smooth muscle that surrounds the urethra as the urethra extends through the pelvic floor; it controls the flow of urine through the urethra.

extracellular Occurring outside of a cell or cell tissues or in cavities or spaces between cell layers or groups of cells.

extracellular fluid The water found outside the cells, including that in the intravascular and interstitial compartments.

extracellular matrix Nonliving chemical substances located between connective tissue cells.

extrapyramidal reaction A response to a treatment or drug characterized by involuntary movement, changes in muscle tone, and abnormal posture.

extravasation The passage or escape of blood, serum, or lymph into the tissues.

extubation Removal of an endotracheal tube.

exudate Fluid, cells, or other substances that have been discharged slowly from cells or blood vessels through small pores or breaks in cell membranes.

face presentation An abnormal presentation in which the brow or forehead of the fetus is the first part of the body to enter the birth canal; also known as *brow presentation.*

facial bones The 14 bones that form the structure of the face in the anterior skull; they do not contribute to the cranial vault.

facial nerve palsy Partial or total loss of the functions of the facial muscles or loss of sensation in the face.

facies A facial expression or appearance.

facilitated diffusion A carrier-mediated process that moves substances into or out of cells from a high to a low concentration.

factitious disorders A group of disorders in which symptoms mimic a true illness. However, the symptoms have actually been invented.

failure to thrive The abnormal retardation of the growth and development of an infant resulting from conditions that interfere with normal metabolism, appetite, and activity.

fallopian tube See *uterine tube.*

false imprisonment Intentional and unjustifiable detention of a person.

false movement An unnatural movement of an extremity, usually associated with fracture.

false rib See *rib.*

false vocal cord See *vestibular fold.*

family court Sometimes referred to as juvenile court; the court is authorized to handle proceedings involving claims of abuse and neglect, dependency, delinquency, and requests for the termination of parental rights.

family function Refers to how a family deals with daily problems and conflicts, and whether this is done in a respectful, productive, and nonaggressive way.

family history Illness or disease in a patient's family or a family's background that may be relevant to the patient's complaint.

fascia The loose areolar connective tissue found beneath the skin or dense connective tissue that encloses and separates muscle.

fascicle A small bundle or cluster of nerve or muscle fibers that provides pathways for impulse conduction.

fasciculation A localized, uncoordinated, uncontrollable twitching of a single muscle group that can be palpated and seen under the skin.

fasciitis Inflammation of the fascia.

fasciotomy Incision of a fascia to relieve elevated intracompartmental pressure.

fat A substance composed of lipids or fatty acids.

Fc receptor A protein found on the surface of certain cells that contribute to the protective functions of the immune system. Fc receptors bind to antibodies that are attached to infected cells or invading pathogens.

febrile seizure A seizure that results from fever.

fecal impaction An accumulation of hardened feces in the rectum or sigmoid colon that the person is unable to move.

fecalith A hard, impacted mass of feces in the colon.

feces Waste material discharged from the intestines.

Federal Communications Commission A federal agency with jurisdiction over interstate and international telephone and telegraph services and satellite communications.

femoral vein A large vein in the thigh that originates in the popliteal vein and accompanies the femoral artery in the proximal two thirds of the thigh.

femur The thigh bone, which extends from the pelvis to the knee; the largest and strongest bone in the body.

fetal membrane disorder One of several disorders that pertain to the fetus or to the period during its development, including premature rupture of membranes, amniotic fluid embolism, and meconium staining.

fetus Unborn young, from the third month of the intrauterine period until birth.

fibrinogen A soluble blood protein converted into insoluble fibrin during clotting.

fibrocartilage Cartilage that consists of a dense matrix of white collagenous fibers.

fibromyalgia A disorder that causes extreme fatigue; associated with "tender points" on the neck, shoulders, back, hips, arms, and legs.

fibrosis An abnormal condition in which fibrous connective tissue spreads over or replaces normal smooth muscle or other normal organ tissue.

fibrous connective tissue A connective tissue that consists mainly of bundles of strong, white collagenous fibers arranged in parallel rows.

fibrous joint See *joint*.

fibrous pericardium Fibrous outer layer of the heart.

fibrous tunic The sclera and cornea.

fibula One of the two bones of the lower leg, lateral to and smaller than the tibia.

Fick principle The principle used to determine cardiac output. It assumes that the quantity of oxygen delivered to an organ is equal to the amount of oxygen consumed by that organ plus the amount of oxygen carried away from that organ.

field impression An impression of the patient's condition that the paramedic makes from pattern recognition and gut instinct that results from experience.

filtrate A filtered liquid.

filtration Movement caused by a pressure gradient of a liquid through a filter that prevents some or all of the substances in the liquid from passing through the filter.

fimbria A fringelike structure located at the border of the uterine tube.

financial/material exploitation The illegal or improper use of funds, properties, or assets.

fine ventricular fibrillation Fibrillatory waves less than 3 mm in amplitude.

first stage of labor The stage of labor that begins with the onset of regular contractions and ends with complete dilation of the cervix.

first-degree burn A burn injury in which only a superficial layer of epidermal cells is destroyed.

first-pass metabolism The initial biotransformation of a drug during passage through the liver from the portal vein that occurs before the drug reaches the general circulation.

fistula An abnormal passage from an internal organ to the body surface.

flail chest A chest wall injury in which three or more adjacent ribs are fractured in two or more places.

flat bones Bones that have a thin, flattened shape, such as certain skull bones, the ribs, the sternum, and scapulae.

flatulence Excessive air or gas in the stomach or intestinal tract, causing distention of the organs and in some cases mild to moderate pain.

flexion Bending.

flexor tenosynovitis A pathological state that causes a disruption of tendon function in the hand; usually the result of infection.

floating rib See *rib*.

flora Microorganisms that live on or in the body to compete with disease-producing microorganisms and provide a natural immunity against certain infections.

flutter waves Abnormal P waves in a sawtooth or picket fence pattern; they represent atrial depolarization in an abnormal direction followed by atrial repolarization.

focal seizure See *jacksonian seizure*.

focused history A component of patient assessment to ascertain the patient's chief complaint, history of present illness, medical history, and current health status.

fontanelle A space covered by a tough membrane between the bones of an infant's cranium.

food poisoning Poisoning that results from food contaminated by toxic substances or by bacteria containing toxins.

foramen ovale An opening in the septum between the right and left atria in the fetal heart; it provides a bypass for blood that would otherwise flow to the fetal lungs.

foreign body airway obstruction A disturbance in normal function or a pathological condition caused by an object lodged in the airway.

formed elements Cells and cell fragments of blood.

formic acid A colorless, pungent liquid found in nature in ants and other insects.

Fournier's gangrene A bacterial infection of the skin that affects the genitals and perineum in both men and women.

fourth ventricle The ventricle located in the superior region of the medulla; continuous with the central canal of the spinal cord.

fourth-degree burn A full-thickness burn injury that penetrates the subcutaneous tissue, muscle, fascia, periosteum, or bone.

fracture A break in the continuity of bone or cartilage.

frank breech See *front breech*.

fraternal twins Two offspring born of the same pregnancy from two ova released simultaneously from the ovary and fertilized at the same time.

French scale system A scale used to denote the size of catheters and other tubular instruments; each unit is roughly equivalent to 0.33 mm in diameter.

frequency The number of repetitive cycles per second completed by a radio wave.

frequency modulation A deviation of carrier frequency in accordance with the strength of applied audio. Frequency modulation is less susceptible to some types of interference than amplitude modulation and typically is used in emergency medical services communications.

front breech A presentation that occurs when the fetal hips are flexed and the legs extend in front of the fetus, making the buttocks the presenting part; also known as a *frank breech*.

frontal bone The single cranial bone that forms the front of the skull.

frontal lobe The largest of the five lobes that comprise each of the two cerebral hemispheres; it significantly influences personality and is associated with higher mental activities such as planning, judgment, and conceptualization.

frontal plane An imaginary plane that divides the body into front and back or anterior and posterior positions; also known as the *coronal plane*.

frontal sinus One of a pair of small cavities in the frontal bone of the skull that communicates with the nasal cavity.

frostbite A localized injury that results from environmentally induced freezing of body tissues.

frostnip The mildest form of cold injury; it may be treated without loss of tissue.

full-thickness burn A burn injury in which the entire thickness of the epidermis and dermis is destroyed; also known as a *third-degree burn.*

functional residual capacity The expiratory reserve volume plus the residual volume; it reflects the amount of gas remaining in the lungs at the end of a normal expiration.

fundus The bottom or rounded end of a hollow organ, such as the fundus of the uterus.

fusion beat A premature ventricular contraction that occurs at approximately the same time that an electrical impulse of the underlying rhythm is activating the ventricles, thereby causing ventricular depolarization to occur simultaneously in two directions; it results in a QRS complex that has the characteristics of the premature ventricular contraction and the QRS complex of the underlying rhythm.

gag reflex A normal neural response triggered by touching the soft palate or posterior pharynx.

gait A manner of walking or moving on foot.

gallbladder A pear-shaped excretory sac on the visceral surface of the right lobe of the liver; it serves as a reservoir for bile.

gallows humor Morbid or cynical humor.

ganglia A group of nerve cell bodies in the peripheral nervous system.

gangrene Dead or dying body tissues attributable to blood supply that is lost or inadequate.

gangrenous Necrosis or death of tissue.

gap junction A small channel between cells that allows the passage of ions and small molecules between cells.

gastric gland A gland located in the stomach mucosa.

gastric lavage Irrigation of the stomach with sterile water or normal saline.

gastrin A polypeptide hormone that stimulates the flow of gastric juice and contributes to the stimulus that causes bile and pancreatic enzyme secretion.

gastritis Inflammation of the lining of the stomach; it may be acute or chronic.

gastroenteritis The inflammation of the stomach and intestines that accompanies numerous gastrointestinal disorders.

gastroesophageal reflux disease A condition in which the stomach contents leak backward from the stomach into the esophagus.

gastrointestinal Of or pertaining to the organs of the gastrointestinal tract from the mouth to the anus.

gastrointestinal decontamination The use of medical methods to empty the stomach of ingested toxins to prevent absorption.

gastrostomy An artificial opening into the stomach.

gating protein A protein that controls the rate at which ions move through an ion channel.

general gas law The characteristic of gas that it flows from an area of higher pressure or concentration to an area of lower pressure or concentration; also known as *Boyle's law.*

general impression An immediate assessment of the environment and the patient's chief complaint used to determine if the patient is ill or injured and the nature of the illness or the mechanism of injury.

generalized seizure A seizure without an identifiable focus in the brain.

generic name The official, established name assigned to a drug.

genitalia Reproductive organs.

genitourinary Of or pertaining to the genital and urinary systems of the body, the organ structures, the organ functions, or both.

genitourinary system Refers to the genital organs and reproductive systems.

German measles See *rubella.*

gerontology The study of the problems of all aspects of aging.

gestation The period from fertilization of the ovum until birth.

gestational diabetes mellitus A disorder characterized by impaired ability to metabolize carbohydrates, usually caused by a deficiency of insulin; it occurs in pregnancy and disappears after delivery but in some cases returns years later.

gingiva The portion of the oral mucosa surrounding the tooth.

gingival hypertrophy Swelling of the gums; it often is associated with chronic phenytoin therapy.

gingivostomatitis Multiple, painful ulcers on the gums and mucous membranes of the mouth; the result of a herpesvirus infection.

Glasgow Coma Scale A standardized system for assessing the degree of conscious impairment in the critically ill and for predicting the duration and ultimate outcome of coma.

glaucoma A condition in which intraocular pressure increases and causes damage to the optic nerve.

glia limitans A supporting structure of nervous tissue consisting of large, star-shaped cells.

gliding joint See *plane joint.*

globule A small, spherical mass.

globulin One of a broad category of simple proteins classified by solubility, mobility, and size.

glomerular filtration rate The amount of plasma that filters into Bowman's capsule per minute.

glomerulus The mass of capillary loops at the beginning of each nephron.

glossopharyngeal nerve Either of a pair of cranial nerves essential to the sense of taste, to sensation in some viscera, and to secretion from certain glands; cranial nerve IX.

glossopharyngeal neuralgia Irritation of the ninth (IX) cranial nerve.

glottic opening The vocal cords and the space between them.

glottis The space between the vocal cords.

glucagon A hormone produced by the alpha cells in the islets of Langerhans that stimulates the conversion of glycogen to glucose in the liver.

glucocorticoid An adrenocortical steroid hormone that increases glyconeogenesis, exerts an antiinflammatory effect, and influences many body functions.

gluconeogenesis The formation of glycogen from fatty acids and proteins rather than carbohydrates.

glucosuria The abnormal presence of glucose in the urine resulting from large amounts of carbohydrates, from kidney disease, or from a metabolic disease such as diabetes mellitus.

gluteus medius muscle The muscle that originates between the anterior and posterior gluteal lines of the ilium and inserts into the greater trochanter of the femur.

glycogenolysis The breakdown of glycogen to glucose.

glycolysis An anaerobic process during which glucose is converted to pyruvic acid.

glycoprotein Any of a large group of conjugated proteins in which the nonprotein substance is a carbohydrate.

goblet cell One of the many specialized cells that secrete mucus and form glands of the epithelium of the stomach, intestine, and parts of the respiratory tract.

goiter A hypertrophic thyroid gland, usually evident as a pronounced swelling in the neck.

golden hour The critical period during which surgical intervention for a trauma patient can enhance survival and reduce complications.

Golgi apparatus Specialized endoplasmic reticulum that concentrates and packages materials for secretion from the cell.

gomphosis An articulation by the insertion of a conic process into a socket, such as the insertion of the root of a tooth into an alveolus of the mandible or maxilla.

gonad A gamete-producing gland, such as an ovary or testis.

gonorrhea A sexually transmitted disease that results from contact with the causative organism *Neisseria gonorrhoeae*.

gout A disease associated with an inborn error of uric acid metabolism that increases production of or interferes with excretion of uric acid; also known as *hyperuricemia*.

gouty arthritis A type of arthritis caused by excess concentration of uric acid, which is converted to sodium urate crystals that are deposited in the joints.

graafian follicle See *vesicular follicle*.

grain The smallest unit of mass in apothecary weights; equal to about 65 mg.

gram A metric unit of mass equal to $\frac{1}{1000}$ of a kilogram.

gram-negative sepsis Sepsis caused by gram-negative bacteria when the bacteria die and are broken down in the body.

grand mal seizure A seizure characterized by a generalized involuntary muscular contraction and cessation of respiration followed by tonic and clonic spasms of the muscles.

grand multipara A woman who has had seven or more deliveries.

granulosa cell A cell in the layer surrounding the primary follicle.

Graves disease A type of excessive thyroid activity characterized by generalized enlargement of the thyroid gland (goiter), which leads to a swollen neck and, often, protruding eyes (exophthalmos).

gravida The number of all current and past pregnancies.

gray matter The gray tissue that makes up the inner core of the spinal column.

great vessels The large arteries and veins entering and leaving the heart; they include the aorta, the pulmonary arteries and veins, and the superior and inferior venae cavae.

groups Subdivisions of the incident command system that encompass specific functional areas of responsibility as deemed necessary by the incident commander.

growth hormone A polypeptide hormone produced and secreted by the anterior pituitary gland; acts as an insulin antagonist.

growth plate The site of bone elongation; also known as the *epiphyseal plate*.

Guillain-Barré syndrome A rare disease that affects the peripheral nervous system, especially the spinal nerves, but also the cranial nerves; it is associated with a viral infection or immunization.

habituation See *drug dependence*.

hair follicle An invagination of the epidermis into the dermis that contains the root of the hair and receives the ducts of sebaceous and apocrine glands.

hair papilla A small, cup-shaped cluster of cells located at the base of the follicle where hair growth begins.

hair root The part of the hair that lies hidden in the follicle.

hair shaft The visible part of the hair.

half duplex The use of two different frequencies, one to transmit and one to receive, that cannot be used simultaneously.

half-life The amount of time required to reduce a drug level to one half its initial value.

hallucinations The apparent perception of sights, sounds, and other sensory phenomena that are not actually present.

Hantavirus A cause of several different forms of hemorrhagic fever with renal syndrome.

hard palate The floor of the nasal cavity that separates the nasal cavity from the oral cavity.

hazard control The phase of rescue that includes managing, reducing, and minimizing risks from uncontrollable hazards; ensuring scene safety; and providing personal protective equipment that is appropriate for the incident.

head lice Tiny parasites that concentrate around the scalp (sometimes including the eyebrows and eyelashes).

head of bone An eminence on a bone by which it articulates with another bone.

heart The muscular, cone-shaped organ that pumps blood throughout the body by coordinated nerve impulses and muscular contractions.

heart murmur An abnormal heart sound caused by altered blood flow into a chamber or through a valve.

heat cramps Brief, intermittent, and often severe muscular cramps that frequently occur in muscles fatigued by heavy work or exercise.

heat exhaustion A form of heat illness characterized by minor aberrations in mental status, dizziness, nausea, headache, and mild to moderate increase in core body temperature.

heat stroke A syndrome that occurs when the thermoregulatory mechanisms normally in place to meet the demands of heat stress break down entirely. As a result, the body temperature increases to extreme levels. Multisystem tissue damage and physiological collapse also occur.

hemasite A small, button-shaped indwelling vascular device usually placed in the upper arm or proximal, anterior thigh; it is similar to an arteriovenous graft but has an external rubber septum sutured to the skin through which a dialysis catheter is inserted for treatment.

hematemesis Vomiting of bright red blood, indicating upper gastrointestinal bleeding.

hematochezia The passage of red blood through the rectum.

hematology The scientific study of blood and blood-forming tissues.

hematoma A closed injury characterized by blood vessel disruption and swelling beneath the epidermis.

hematoma formation The collection of blood or fluids at the site of injection or cannulation.

hematuria The abnormal presence of blood in the urine.

hemiblock Failure in conduction of the cardiac impulse in either of two main divisions of the left branch of the bundle of His; interruption may occur in the anterior (superior) or posterior (inferior) division.

hemifacial spasm A neuromuscular disorder characterized by frequent involuntary contractions of the muscles on one side of the face.

hemiparesis One-sided weakness.

hemiplegia Paralysis of one side of the body.

hemitransection A cut across the long axis of tissue, such as the spinal cord.

hemoagglutinin An agglutinin that clumps red blood corpuscles.

hemochromatosis A disease of iron metabolism characterized by excess deposition of iron throughout the body.

hemodialysis A procedure in which impurities or wastes are removed from the blood; it is used in treating renal insufficiency and various toxic conditions.

hemodilution The dilution of the blood of elements.

hemoglobin A complex protein-iron compound in the blood that carries oxygen to the cells from the lungs and carbon dioxide away from the cells to the lungs.

hemolysis The breakdown of red blood cells and the release of hemoglobin.

hemolytic anemia A condition in which delivery of oxygen to tissues is reduced because of an increase in hemolysis of erythrocytes.

hemopericardium An accumulation of blood within the pericardial sac surrounding the heart.

hemoperitoneum The presence of extravasated blood in the peritoneal cavity.

hemophilia A group of hereditary bleeding disorders in which one of the factors necessary for blood coagulation is deficient.

hemophilia A A condition caused by a deficiency of coagulation factor VIII; it is considered the classic type of hemophilia.

hemophilia B A condition caused by a deficiency of coagulation factor IX.

hemopneumothorax See *pneumohemothorax*.

hemopoietic tissue Tissue related to the process of formation and development of various types of blood cells.

hemoptysis Coughing up of blood from the respiratory tract.

hemorrhage Flowing of blood.

hemorrhagic shock Hypoperfusion associated with the sudden and rapid loss of significant amounts of blood.

hemorrhagic stroke A stroke (cerebrovascular accident [CVA]) that is caused by bleeding.

hemorrhoids Swollen, distended veins (internal, external, or both) in the rectoanal area.

hemostasis The cessation of bleeding by mechanical or chemical means or by substances that arrest the blood flow.

hemostatic An agent that reduces bleeding by speeding clot formation.

hemothorax The accumulation of blood in the pleural space caused by bleeding from the lung parenchyma or damaged vessels.

hemotympanum Blood behind the tympanic membrane from fractures of the temporal bone.

heparin A substance that inhibits blood clotting; it is obtained from the liver.

heparin lock A peripheral vascular access device that has no attached intravenous tubing; it is used to ensure ready access to peripheral veins for brief administration of medications or when frequent intravenous therapy is indicated on an outpatient basis (e.g., chemotherapy).

hepatic artery The branch of the aorta that delivers blood to the liver.

hepatic encephalopathy A type of brain damage caused by liver disease and consequent ammonia intoxication.

hepatic portal system The system that transports blood from the digestive tract to the liver.

hepatitis An inflammatory condition of the liver characterized by jaundice, hepatomegaly, anorexia, abdominal and gastric discomfort, abnormal liver function, clay-colored stools, and dark urine. Viruses responsible for hepatitis are *hepatitis A virus, hepatitis B virus, hepatitis C virus, hepatitis D virus,* and *hepatitis E virus.*

hepatitis A Viral hepatitis. See *hepatitis.*

hepatitis B Serum hepatitis. See *hepatitis.*

hepatitis C Non-A/non-B hepatitis. See *hepatitis.*

hepatomegaly Enlargement of the liver.

hereditary hemochromatosis An inherited condition in which the body absorbs and stores too much iron. The extra iron accumulates in several organs, especially the liver, heart, and pancreas.

Hering-Breuer reflex A reflex in which afferent impulses from stretch receptors in the lungs arrest inspiration; expiration then occurs; inflation and deflation reflexes triggered to prevent overinflation of the lungs.

hernia Protrusion of any organ through an abdominal opening in the muscle wall of the cavity that surrounds it.

herniated disk Occurs when all or part of a spinal disk is forced through a weakened part of the disk.

herniation A protrusion of a body organ or portion of an organ through an abnormal opening in a membrane, muscle, or other tissue.

herpes Any of several acute inflammatory viral diseases characterized by the eruption of small blisters on the skin and mucous membranes.

herpes simplex virus type 1 An infection caused by the herpes simplex virus; it tends to occur in the facial area, particularly around the mouth and nose.

herpes simplex virus type 2 An infection caused by the herpes simplex virus; it usually is limited to the genital region.

hertz A unit of frequency equal to 1 cycle per second.

hexaxial reference system The system of intersecting lines of the standard limb leads and three other intersecting lines of reference: aV_R, aV_L, and aV_F leads.

hiatal hernia An anatomical abnormality in which part of the stomach protrudes through the diaphragm and up into the chest.

Hickman catheter A long indwelling catheter sometimes used by patients with cancer, gastrointestinal dysfunction, or debilitating disease and by those who need intermittent intravenous administration of antibiotics, nutritional supplements, or other intravenous medications.

high angle An environment in which rescuers need to be secured with rope for safety. The majority of the rescue load is supported by the rope system.

high-altitude cerebral edema The most severe form of acute high-altitude illness. It is characterized by a progression of global cerebral signs in the presence of acute mountain sickness.

high-altitude pulmonary edema A high-altitude illness thought to be caused at least partly by an increase in pulmonary artery pressure that develops in response to hypoxia.

high-grade atrioventricular block Occurs when at least two consecutive atrioventricular impulses (atrial P waves) fail to be conducted to the ventricles.

hilum A depression or pit at the part of an organ where the vessels and nerves enter.

hinge joint A joint that consists of a convex cylinder in one bone applied to a corresponding concavity in another bone; this type of joint allows movement in one plane only.

histamine An amine released by mast cells and basophils that promotes inflammation.

history taking Information gathered during the patient interview.

Hodgkin's disease A malignant disorder characterized by pain and progressive enlargement of lymphoid tissue.

homeopathic Pertaining to homeopathy, a system of therapeutics in which diseases are treated with small doses of drugs that, in larger doses, are capable of producing in healthy persons symptoms like those of the disease to be treated.

homeostasis A state of equilibrium in the body with respect to functions and composition of fluids and tissues.

hordeolum An acute infection of the oil gland; commonly known as a *sty.*

horizontal plane Any place of the erect body parallel to the horizon; dividing the body into upper and lower parts.

hormone A substance, usually a peptide or steroid, produced by one tissue and conveyed by the bloodstream to another tissue or organ to effect physiological activity, such as growth or metabolism.

hormone receptor A receptor on target organs and body tissues that is able to respond to a particular hormone.

host The human or animal exposed to an infectious agent.

host susceptibility Factors of the host that contribute to prevention or continuation of infection.

household system A common system of measure that includes the *glass, cup, tablespoon, teaspoon, drop, quart,* and *pint.*

human immunodeficiency virus The viral agent responsible for acquired immunodeficiency syndrome.

humerus The largest bone of the upper arm, consisting of a body, head, and condyle.

humoral immunity One of the two forms of immunity that respond to antigens such as bacteria and foreign tissue.

Huntington's disease A rare, hereditary disease characterized by quick, involuntary movements, speech disturbances, and mental deterioration; it is caused by degenerative changes in the cerebral cortex and basal ganglia; also known as *Huntington's chorea.*

hyaline cartilage Gelatinous, glossy cartilage tissue; it thinly covers the articulating ends of bones, connects the ribs to the sternum, and supports the nose, trachea, and part of the larynx.

hydrocele A fluid-filled sac along the spermatic cord within the scrotum.

hydrocephalus A pathological condition characterized by an abnormal accumulation of cerebrospinal fluid, usually under increased pressure, within the cranial vault, resulting in dilation of the ventricles.

hydrochloric acid The acid in gastric juice.

hydrogen ion The acidic element in a solution.

hymen A mucous membrane that may partly or entirely occlude the vaginal outlet.

Hymenoptera A large, highly specialized order of insects that includes wasps, bees, and ants.

hyoid bone The U-shaped bone between the mandible and the larynx.

hyperbilirubinemia Larger than normal amounts of the bile pigment bilirubin in the blood, often characterized by jaundice, anorexia, and malaise.

hypercalcemia A higher than normal concentration of calcium in the blood.

hypercholesterolemia Increased serum cholesterol level.

hypercoagulability A tendency of the blood to coagulate more rapidly than normal.

hyperglycemia A greater than normal amount of glucose in the blood.

hyperkalemia A higher than normal concentration of potassium in the blood.

hyperkaluria A high potassium concentration in the urine.

hyperlipidemia An excess of lipids in the plasma.

hypermagnesemia A higher than normal concentration of magnesium in the blood.

hypernatremia A greater than normal concentration of sodium in the blood.

hypernatremic dehydration The loss of more water than sodium.

hyperosmolar hyperglycemic nonketotic syndrome A diabetic state in which the level of ketone bodies is normal. It is caused by hyperosmolarity of extracellular fluid and results in dehydration of intracellular fluid.

hyperparathyroidism A condition of increased parathyroid function.

hyperphosphatemia High levels of alkaline phosphate in the blood.

hyperplasia An excessive increase in the number of cells.

hyperpolarization An increase in the charge difference across the cell membrane; it causes the charge difference to move away from 0 mV.

hypersensitivity reaction An altered immunological response to an antigen that results in a pathological immune response upon reexposure.

hypersomnia Excessive drowsiness; a sleep disorder of excessive depth or duration.

hypertension A disorder characterized by elevated blood pressure, which persistently exceeds 140/90 mm Hg.

hypertensive crisis A sudden, severe increase in blood pressure greater than 200/120 mm Hg.

hypertensive encephalopathy A set of symptoms—including headache, convulsions, and coma—that result solely from elevated blood pressure.

hyperthermia Abnormal elevation of body temperature.

hyperthyroidism A condition characterized by increased activity of the thyroid gland.

hypertonic A term used to describe a solution that causes cells to shrink.

hypertonic solutions Solutions that have higher osmotic pressure than that of body cells.

hypertrophy An increase in the size of a cell.

hyperuricemia See *gout*.

hyperventilation syndrome Abnormally deep or rapid breathing that results in excessive loss of carbon dioxide (producing respiratory alkalosis).

hyphema A hemorrhage into the anterior chamber of the eye; it usually is a result of blunt trauma.

hypocalcemia A lower than normal concentration of calcium in the blood.

hypocarbia A state of diminished carbon dioxide in the blood; also known as *hypocapnia*.

hypochlorhydria A deficiency of hydrochloric acid in the gastric juice of the stomach.

hypoglycemia A lower than normal amount of glucose in the blood.

hypokalemia A lower than normal concentration of potassium in the blood.

hypomagnesemia A lower than normal concentration of magnesium in the blood plasma.

hyponatremia A lower than normal concentration of sodium in the blood.

hyponatremic A term describing a lower than normal concentration of sodium in the blood.

hyponatremic dehydration The loss of more sodium than water.

hypoparathyroidism A condition of diminished parathyroid function.

hypoperfusion Severely inadequate circulation that results in insufficient delivery of oxygen and nutrients necessary for normal tissue and cellular function. Also known as *shock*.

hypophosphatemia Low levels of alkaline phosphate in the blood.

hypopituitarism An abnormal condition caused by diminished activity of the pituitary gland; it is marked by excessive deposits of fat or acquisition of adolescent characteristics.

hypopyon An accumulation of pus in the anterior chamber of the eye.

hypotension An abnormal condition in which the blood pressure is not adequate for normal perfusion and oxygenation of the tissues.

hypothalamus A portion of the diencephalon of the brain that activates, controls, and integrates the peripheral autonomic nervous system, endocrine processes, and many somatic functions such as body temperature, sleep, and appetite.

hypothermia An abnormal body temperature below 95° F (35° C).

hypothyroidism A condition characterized by decreased activity of the thyroid gland.

hypotonia A condition of diminished tone or tension that may involve any body structure.

hypotonic A term used to describe a solution that causes cells to swell.

hypotonicity of the muscles Decreased muscle tone or tension.

hypovolemia An abnormally low circulating blood volume.

hypovolemic shock A form of shock most frequently caused by hemorrhage but also caused by dehydration.

hypoxemia A state of decreased oxygen content of arterial blood.

hypoxia A state of decreased oxygen content at the tissue level.

hypoxic drive The low arterial oxygen pressure stimulus to respiration that is mediated through the carotid bodies.

hysterectomy The surgical removal of the uterus.

iatrogenic Caused by treatment or diagnostic procedures.

identical twins Two offspring born of the same pregnancy and developed from a single fertilized ovum that splits into equal halves during the early phase of embryonic development, giving rise to separate fetuses.

idiopathic Arising from an obscure or unknown cause.

idiopathic epilepsy See *primary epilepsy.*

idiosyncrasy An abnormal or peculiar response to a drug.

idioventricular rhythm A ventricular escape rhythm that results when impulses from higher pacemakers fail to reach the ventricles or when the rate of discharge of higher pacemakers becomes less than that of the ventricles.

IgA Immunoglobulin A is an antibody that plays a crucial role in mucosal immunity.

IgD Immunoglobulin D is an antibody that is present on the surface of most, but not all, B cells, early in their development; signals B cells to be activated.

IgE Immunoglobulin E is an antibody that plays an important role in allergies; especially associated with type I anaphylactic reactions.

IgG Immunoglobulin G is the most abundant antibody; equally distributed in blood and tissue liquids.

IgM Immunoglobulin M is a basic antibody that produces B cells; the first antibody to appear in response to initial exposure to an antigen.

ileocecal sphincter The valve between the ilium of the small intestine and the cecum of the large intestine.

ileostomy A surgical opening into the small intestine.

ileum The distal portion of the small intestine.

ileus An obstruction of the intestines.

iliac crest The upper free margin of the ilium of the hipbone.

iliac spine A portion of the iliac crest; the flaring portion of the hipbone.

ilium One of the three bones that make up the innominate bone.

immersion hypothermia Hypothermia from immersion in cold water.

immune response A defense function of the body that produces antibodies to destroy invading antigens and malignancies.

immune system A complex network of cells, tissues, and organs that work together to protect the body against "attacks" by foreign substances.

immunity Insusceptibility to a particular disease or condition.

immunization The process of rendering a person immune or of becoming immune.

immunogen Any agent or substance capable of an immune response or of producing immunity.

immunoglobulin Any of five structurally and antigenically distinct antibodies present in the serum and external secretions of the body; they are IgA, IgD, IgE, IgG, and IgM.

immunologic memory The ability to rapidly produce large quantities of specific immune cells after subsequent exposure to a previously encountered antigen.

immunology A broad branch of medical science that covers the study of the immune system.

immunosuppression The reduction in the activation or efficiency of the immune system often caused by drugs or radiation in order to prevent the rejection of grafts or transplanted tissues or to control autoimmune disease.

implied consent The presumption that an unconscious or incompetent person would consent to lifesaving care.

impulse control disorders A group of psychiatric conditions characterized by the inability to resist an impulse or a temptation to perform some act that is unlawful, socially unacceptable, or self-harmful.

inadvertent hyperventilation Excessive ventilation is thought to result in increased intrathoracic pressure and decreased coronary perfusion pressure; also known as *rescuer hyperventilation.*

incident command system A management program designed to control, direct, and coordinate emergency response operations and resources.

incomplete abortion An abortion in which the patient has passed some but not all of the products of conception.

incomplete breech The presentation that occurs when the fetus has one or both hips incompletely flexed, resulting in the presentation of one or both lower extremities, often a foot.

incontinence The inability to control bladder or bowel function.

incubation period The stage of infection during which an organism reproduces; it begins with invasion of an agent and ends when the disease process begins.

incus The middle of the three ossicles in the middle ear.

indigenous flora Agents found on various sites of the body that could produce disease if allowed access to the interior of the body.

induced abortion The intentional termination of a pregnancy.

infant A child 28 days to 1 year of age.

infarction Cell death.

infectious disease Any illness that is caused by a specific microorganism.

infectious pericarditis Inflammation of the pericardium associated with infection.

inferior Toward the feet; below a point of reference in the anatomical position.

inferior nasal concha One of three bony ridges on the lateral wall of the nasal cavity.

inferior vena cava The vein that returns blood from the lower limbs and the greater part of the pelvic and abdominal organs to the right atrium.

infertility The inability to produce offspring.

infiltration The process whereby a fluid passes into tissues.

inflammatory myopathies A group of diseases that involve chronic muscle inflammation accompanied by muscle weakness.

inflammatory response A tissue reaction to injury or an antigen; it may include pain, swelling, itching, redness, heat, and loss of function.

influenza A highly contagious infection of the respiratory tract transmitted by airborne droplet infection. Researchers have identified three main types of the virus (types A, B, and C).

informed consent Consent obtained from a patient after explaining all facts necessary for the patient to make a reasonable decision.

inguinal canal The passage through the lower abdominal wall that transmits the spermatic cord in the male and the round ligament in the female.

inguinal node One of approximately 18 nodes in the group of lymph glands in the upper femoral triangle of the thigh.

inhalation injury An upper and/or lower airway injury that results from thermal and/or chemical exposure.

initial assessment A component of the patient assessment to recognize and manage all immediate life-threatening conditions.

injury risk Real or potentially hazardous situations that put individuals at increased risk for sustaining an injury.

injury surveillance The ongoing systematic collection, analysis, and interpretation of injury data essential to the planning, implementation, and evaluation of public health practice.

inner ear The part of the ear that contains the sensory organs for hearing and balance.

inotropic Pertaining to the force or energy of muscle contraction, particularly contractions of the heart.

insertion The more movable attachment point of a muscle.

insomnia A chronic inability to sleep or to remain asleep throughout the night.

inspection A visual assessment of the patient and surroundings.

inspiration The act of drawing air into the lungs.

inspiratory capacity The sum of the tidal volume and the inspiratory reserve volume.

inspiratory center The region of the medulla that stimulates inspiration.

inspiratory reserve volume The maximum volume of air that can be inspired after a normal inspiration.

insulin A hormone secreted by the pancreatic islets.

integumentary system The largest organ system in the body, consisting of the skin and accessory structures.

interatrial septum Tissue that separates the right and left atria of the heart.

intercalated disk Cell-to-cell attachment with gap junctions between cardiac muscle cells.

intercellular Occurring between or among cells.

intercostal muscles Internal and external muscles between the ribs that contract to raise the ribs, thereby increasing the front-to-back (anterior-posterior) and side-to-side dimensions of the chest cavity.

interference Any undesired radio signal on a radio frequency. It may arise from other radio transmitters or other sources of electromagnetic radiation. "Nuisance interference" is interference that can be heard but does not override system signals. "Destructive interference" overrides system signals.

internal anal sphincter A sphincter muscle located at the caudal end of the rectum.

internal barriers Protection against germs provided by the inflammatory response and the immune response; the body's second line of defense against infection.

internal carotid artery Each of two arteries that enter the cranial vault through the carotid canals.

internal jugular vein One of a pair of veins in the neck; each collects blood from one side of the brain, the face, and the neck, and both unite with the subclavian vein to form the brachiocephalic vein.

internal mammary artery One of the pair of arteries that arise from the first portions of the subclavian arteries; it supplies the pectoral muscles, breasts, pericardium, and abdominal muscles; also known as the *internal thoracic artery*.

internal respiration The transfer (diffusion) of oxygen and carbon dioxide between the capillary red blood cells and the tissue cells.

internal thoracic artery See *internal mammary artery*.

internal urinary sphincter The smooth muscle of the bladder located at the junction of the urethra with the urinary bladder; it controls the flow of urine through the urethra.

interneuron See *motor neuron*.

internodal tract Pathways between the segments of a nerve fiber.

interpolated premature ventricular complex A premature ventricular contraction that falls between two sinus beats without interrupting the rhythm.

interstitial fluid Fluid that occupies the space outside the blood vessels and/or outside of cells of an organ or tissue.

interventricular foramen One of two passageways between the two lateral ventricles and the third ventricle.

interventricular septum The tissue that separates the right and left ventricles of the heart.

intervertebral disk One of the fibrous disks between all adjacent spinal vertebrae except the atlas and axis; it serves as a shock absorber for the vertebral column and provides additional support for the body; it also prevents the vertebral bodies from rubbing against each other.

intracellular Occurring within cell membranes.

intracellular fluid The fluid found in all body cells.

intracerebral hematoma An accumulation of blood or fluid within the tissue of the brain.

intracranial pressure The pressure inside the skull, brain tissue, and cerebrospinal fluid.

intradermal injection The introduction of a substance (e.g., serum or vaccine) with a hypodermic needle into the dermis.

intramuscular injection The introduction of medication with a hypodermic needle into muscle.

intraocular pressure Pressure within the eye that keeps the eye inflated.

intraosseous infusion Placement of a rigid needle into a bone and the infusion of fluid and medication directly into the bone marrow.

intraosseous injection The introduction of medication or fluid into the bone marrow.

intrapartum The period during labor and delivery.

intrapleural Within the pleura.

intrapleural pressure See *intrathoracic pressure*.

intrapulmonic pressure The pressure of the gas within the alveoli.

intrarenal disease Refers to disease or damage within the kidney.

intrathecal injection The introduction of medication with a hypodermic needle into the subarachnoid space.

intrathoracic pressure The pressure in the pleural space; also known as *intrapleural pressure*.

intravenous injection The introduction of medication with a hypodermic needle into a vein.

intrinsic factor The factor secreted by the parietal cells of the gastric glands; it is required for adequate absorption of vitamin B_{12}.

invagination Infolding or in-pocketing.

invasion of privacy Making public, without legal justification, details about a person's private life that might reasonably expose that person to ridicule, notoriety, or embarrassment.

inversion Turning inward.

involuntary Occurring without conscious control or direction.

involuntary consent Treatment that is granted by authority of law.

involuntary guarding An unconscious rigid contraction of the abdominal muscles; a sign of peritoneal inflammation.

involuntary muscle A muscle that is not normally consciously controlled; see *smooth muscle*.

ion An atom or group of atoms carrying a charge of electricity by virtue of having gained or lost one or more electrons.

ipsilateral Pertaining to the same side of the body.

iris The colored contractile membrane of the eye that can be seen through the cornea.

iritis Inflammation of the iris of the eye.

iron deficiency anemia Anemia caused by inadequate supplies of iron needed to synthesize hemoglobin.

irregular bones Bones that are not representative of the other three categories (long, short, or flat bones); examples include vertebrae and facial bones.

irreversible shock A stage of shock that results in cellular ischemia and necrosis and subsequent organ death, even with oxygenation and perfusion restored.

ischemia A state of insufficient perfusion of oxygenated blood to a body organ or part.

ischium One of the three parts of the hipbone, which joins the ilium and the pubis to form the acetabulum.

islets of Langerhans Clusters of cells within the pancreas that produce insulin, glucagon, and pancreatic polypeptide.

isoimmunity An immune response directed against beneficial foreign tissues.

isolette A self-contained incubator unit that provides controlled heat, humidity, and oxygen for the isolation and care of premature and low-birth-weight neonates.

isometric contraction A muscle contraction in which the length of the muscle does not change, but the tension produced increases.

isotonic A term used to describe a solution that causes cells neither to shrink nor to swell.

isotonic contraction A muscle contraction in which the tension produced by the muscle stays the same, but the muscle length becomes shorter.

isotonic dehydration Excessive loss of sodium and water in equal amounts.

J point The point at which the T wave takes off from the QRS complex.

jacksonian seizure A transitory disturbance in motor, sensory, or autonomic function resulting from abnormal neuronal discharges in a localized part of the brain; also known as a *focal seizure*.

jaundice A yellow discoloration of the skin, mucous membranes, and sclerae of the eyes caused by a greater than normal amount of bilirubin in the blood.

jejunum One of the three portions of the small intestine.

joint Any one of the connections between bones that are classified according to structure and movability as fibrous, cartilaginous, or synovial. *Fibrous joints* are immovable, *cartilaginous joints* are slightly movable, and *synovial joints* are freely movable.

joint capsule A well-defined structure that encloses a joint.

joint dislocation An injury that occurs when the normal articulating ends of two or more bones are displaced.

joint disorder Any disease or injury that affects human joints.

Joule's law The principle that the amount of heat produced is directly proportional to the square of the current strength times the resistance of the tissue times the duration of the current flow.

jugular notch The superior margin of the manubrium; it is palpated easily at the anterior base of the neck; also known as the *suprasternal notch.*

jugular vein distention Engorgement of jugular veins caused by an increase in central venous pressure; it is estimated by positioning the head of a supine patient at a 45-degree angle and observing the neck veins.

kallikrein/kinin system A proposed hormonal system that functions within the kidneys, mediating production of bradykinin, which acts as a vasodilator peptide.

Kaposi's sarcoma A malignant, multifocal neoplasm of reticuloendothelial cells that begins as soft, brownish or purple papules on the feet and slowly spreads in the skin, metastasizing to the lymph nodes and viscera; it is associated with diabetes, malignant lymphoma, acquired immunodeficiency syndrome, and other disorders.

Kehr's sign Pain in the left shoulder thought to be caused by referred pain secondary to irritation of the adjacent diaphragm.

Kent fibers See *bundle of Kent.*

keratitis Any inflammation of the cornea.

ketoacidosis Acidosis accompanied by the accumulation of ketones in the body, resulting from faulty carbohydrate metabolism.

ketoacids Compounds containing the carbonyl and carboxyl groups.

ketogenesis The formation or production of ketone bodies.

ketone bodies The normal metabolic products of lipids and pyruvate within the liver; excessive production leads to their excretion in urine.

ketonuria Presence in the urine of excessive amounts of ketone bodies.

kidney The organ that cleanses the body of the waste products continually produced by metabolism.

kilogram A metric unit of mass equal to 1000 grams or 2.2046 pounds.

kilohertz A unit of frequency equal to 1000 cycles per second.

kinematics The process of predicting injury patterns that can result from the forces and motions of energy.

kinin Serum protein that causes vasodilation and increases vascular permeability.

KKK standards The national standards that provide the foundation of uniformity among ambulance vehicles.

Koplik's spots Small red spots with bluish white centers on the lingual and buccal mucosa, characteristic of measles.

Korsakoff's psychosis A form of amnesia often seen in alcoholics, characterized by a loss of short-term memory and an inability to learn new skills.

Krebs cycle A sequence of enzymatic reactions involving the metabolism of carbon chains of sugar, fatty acids, and amino acids to yield carbon dioxide, water, and high-energy phosphate bonds.

Kussmaul's respiration An abnormally deep, rapid sighing respiratory pattern characteristic of diabetic ketoacidosis or other metabolic acidosis.

kyphosis An abnormal condition of the vertebral column characterized by increased convexity in the curvature of the thoracic spine as viewed from the side.

labia majora Two rounded folds of skin surrounding the labia minora and the vestibule.

labia minora Two longitudinal folds of mucous membrane enclosed by the labia majora and bounding the vestibule.

labial frenulum A medial fold of mucous membrane connecting the inside of each lip to the corresponding gum.

labyrinthitis An ear disorder that involves irritation and swelling of the inner ear structure called the *labyrinth.*

laceration A torn or jagged wound.

lacrimal bone One of the smallest and most fragile bones of the face; it is located in the anterior part of the medial wall of the orbit.

lacrimal canal The canal that carries excess tears away from the eye.

lacrimal gland The tear gland located in the superolateral corner of the orbit.

lacrimal sac An enlargement of the lacrimal canal that leads into the nasolacrimal duct.

lacrimation Excessive tear production.

lactate A salt of lactic acid.

lactation The secretion of milk from the breasts to nourish an infant or child.

lactic acid A three-carbon molecule derived from pyruvic acid as a product of anaerobic respiration.

lactic acidosis A disorder characterized by an accumulation of lactic acid in the blood, resulting in a lowered pH in muscle and serum.

lactiferous duct The duct that drains the grapelike cluster of milk-secreting glands in the breast.

lactose intolerance A sensitivity disorder resulting in the inability to digest lactose because of a deficiency of or defect in the enzyme lactase.

landing zone An area prepared for the landing of an aircraft; generally 100 by 100 feet.

lanugo hair Soft, downy hair covering a normal fetus.

laparoscopy Examination of the abdominal cavity with a laparoscope.

large intestine The portion of the digestive tract comprising the cecum, the appendix, the ascending, transverse, and descending colons, and the rectum.

laryngectomy Surgical removal of the larynx, performed to treat cancer of the larynx.

laryngitis Inflammation of the larynx.

laryngopharynx The lowest part of the pharynx.

laryngoscope An endoscope for visualization of the larynx.

laryngoscopy Examination of the larynx via a laryngoscope.

laryngotracheobronchitis See *croup*.

larynx The voice box, located just below the pharynx.

late adulthood Persons 61 years of age and older.

latent period A stage of infection that begins when a pathogenic agent invades the body and ends when the agent can be shed or communicated.

latent period of drug action See *onset of action*.

latent TB infection Tuberculosis that is not symptomatic or infectious; must be treated to prevent active TB disease.

lateral malleolus The rounded process on the lateral side of the ankle joint.

lateral recumbent position The position in which the patient is lying on his or her right or left side.

lateral ventricle A large, fluid-filled space in each cerebral hemisphere.

laxative A substance that causes evacuation of the bowel by increasing the bulk of the feces, by softening the stool, or by lubricating the intestinal wall.

lead An electrode sensor attached to the body to record electrical activity, especially of the heart and brain.

leaky capillary syndrome A syndrome that occurs when the capillary lining permits protein-containing fluid to leak into the interstitial spaces.

Le Fort fracture A fracture pattern that can be produced in the midface region.

left anterior descending artery The subdivision of the left coronary artery that supplies the left auricle and its appendix and supplies branches to both ventricles and numerous small branches to the pulmonary artery and commencement of the aorta.

left atrium One of the four chambers in the human heart; receives oxygenated blood from the lungs and pumps it into the left ventricle.

left coronary artery One of a pair of branches from the ascending aorta that supplies both ventricles and the left atrium.

left mainstem bronchus One of two main bronchi that branches from the trachea at the level of the carina.

legend A prescription drug.

legionellosis An acute bacterial pneumonia caused by infection with *Legionella pneumophila*; it is characterized by an influenza-like illness followed within a week by high fever, chills, muscle aches, and headache.

legionnaires' disease See *legionellosis*.

Lenègre's disease See *Lev's disease*.

lens The crystalline portion of the eye.

lethargy A state of indifference, apathy, or sluggishness.

leukemia A malignant neoplasm of blood-forming organs.

leukocyte White blood cell.

leukocytosis An abnormal increase in the number of circulating white blood cells.

leukopenia A decrease in the number of white blood cells (most commonly neutrophils).

leukotrienes A class of biologically active compounds that occur naturally in leukocytes and that produce allergic and inflammatory reactions.

Lev's disease Third-degree block in the elderly from chronic degenerative changes in the conduction system; it usually is not associated with increased parasympathetic tone or drug toxicity; also known as *Lenègre's disease*.

libel Publishing in writing false statements about someone, knowing them to be false, with malicious intent or with reckless disregard for their falsity.

libido The drive associated with sexual desire, pleasure, or creativity.

licensure The process by which a government agency grants permission to an individual to engage in an occupation or profession.

life threat An illness or injury that threatens survival.

ligament A band of white, fibrous tissue that connects bones.

ligamentum arteriosum A fibrous cord from the pulmonary artery to the branch of the aorta; the remains of the ductus arteriosus of the fetus.

limbic system The part of the brain involved with emotions and olfaction.

linear fracture A fracture that extends parallel to the long axis of a bone but does not displace the bone tissue.

lingual tonsil A collection of lymphoid tissue on the posterior portion of the dorsum of the tongue.

lipid Any of the free fatty acid fractions in the blood.

lipid bilayer The central layer of the cytoplasmic membrane; it is composed of a double layer of lipid molecules.

lipodystrophy Any abnormality in the metabolism or distribution of fats.

lipoprotein A conjugated protein in which lipids form an integral part of the molecule; it is synthesized primarily in the liver.

liquefaction Conversion of solid tissues to a fluid or semifluid state.

liter A metric unit of capacity equal to 1 cubic decimeter, 61.025 cubic inches, or 1.0567 liquid quarts.

Littre's gland The inner surface of the membrane lining the urethra.

liver An organ in the upper abdomen that aids in digestion and removes waste products and cellular debris from the blood; the largest solid organ in the human body.

loading dose A large quantity of drug that temporarily exceeds the capacity of the body to excrete the drug.

lobule A small lobe or subdivision of a lobe.

long bones Bones that are longer than they are wide, such as the humerus, ulna, radius, femur, tibia, fibula, and phalanges.

long saphenous vein See *saphenous vein*.

loop diuretic A group of powerful, short-acting agents that inhibit sodium and chloride reabsorption in the loop of Henle, resulting in an excessive loss of potassium and water and an increase in the excretion of sodium.

loop of Henle The U-shaped portion of the renal tubule.

lordosis An inward curvature in the lumbar spine that is normally present to some degree.

low angle An environment in which the weight of the stretcher is supported primarily by the tender's legs, but rope systems are required to facilitate movement and for fall protection.

lower airway Airway structures below the glottis.

lower esophageal sphincter The ring of muscle located at the inferior end of the esophagus that regulates the passage of materials out of the esophagus.

lucid interval A period of relative mental clarity between periods of decreased consciousness or irrationality.

Ludwig's angina A type of cellulitis that involves inflammation of the tissues of the floor of the mouth, under the tongue.

lumbar vertebrae The five largest segments of the movable part of the vertebral column; they are designated L1 to L5.

lumbosacral plexus The combination of all the ventral primary divisions of the lumbar, sacral, and coccygeal nerves.

lumen A cavity or channel within any organ or structure of the body.

Lund and Browder chart A method to estimate burn injury that assigns specific numbers to each body part and that accounts for developmental changes in percentages of body surface area.

lung One of a pair of light, spongy organs in the thorax; the main component of the respiratory system.

lung cancer A disease of uncontrolled cell growth in tissues of the lung.

lunula The crescent-shaped white area of the nail; it is most visible on the thumbnail.

luxation A complete dislocation.

Lyme disease An acute, recurrent inflammatory infection transmitted by a tick.

lymph node An encapsulated mass of lymph tissue found among lymph vessels.

lymph nodule Any of the small, densely packed spherical nodes or aggregations of lymph cells embedded in the reticular meshwork of the lymphatic system; found mainly in the tonsils, spleen, and thymus.

lymphangitis An inflammation of one or more lymphatic vessels.

lymphatic system The network of vessels, ducts, nodes, valves, and organs involved in protecting and maintaining the internal fluid environment of the body.

lymphocyte A type of white blood cell formed in lymphoid tissue.

lymphokine One of the chemical factors produced and released by T lymphocytes that attract macrophages to the site of infection or inflammation.

lymphoma A group of diseases that range from slowly growing chronic disorders to rapidly evolving acute conditions.

lyse To cause decomposition.

lysis The process by which a cell swells and ruptures.

lysosome A membranous-walled organelle that contains enzymes, which enable it to function as an intracellular digestive system.

macrodrip tubing An apparatus used to deliver measured amounts of intravenous solutions at specific flow rates based on the size of drops of the solution. The drops delivered by a macrodrip are larger than those delivered by a microdrip.

macromolecule A molecule of colloidal size, such as a protein, nucleic acid, or polysaccharide.

macrophage A phagocytic cell in the immune system.

macula A small pigmented area that appears separate or different than the surrounding tissue.

maintenance dose The amount of a drug required to keep a desired steady state of drug concentration in tissues.

major incident An event for which available resources are insufficient to manage the nature of the emergency.

malaise A vague feeling of weakness or discomfort.

malar eminence The zygomatic bone or cheekbone.

malaria A serious infectious illness caused by one or more of at least four species of the protozoan genus *Plasmodium;* it is characterized by chills, fever, anemia, and an enlarged spleen.

malignant Very dangerous or virulent; likely to cause death; a cancerous tumor that tends to metastasize.

malleolus A rounded, bony process, such as the protuberance on each side of the ankle.

malleus The largest of the three ossicles in the middle ear.

Mallory-Weiss syndrome A condition characterized by massive bleeding after a tear in the mucous membrane at the junction of the esophagus and the stomach.

mamma The breast; the organ of milk secretion.

mammalian diving reflex A reflex triggered by immersing the face in cold water; it diverts blood from the arms and legs to the central circulation and lowers the heart rate as a result of vagal stimulation.

mammary gland An external accessory sex organ in females; breasts.

managed care Patient care services that are provided to members by managed care organizations.

managed care organizations Networks that provide patient care services to their members, including health maintenance organizations and preferred provider organizations.

mandible A large bone that constitutes the lower jaw.

mania A mood disorder characterized by extreme excitement, hyperactivity, agitation, and sometimes violent and self-destructive behavior.

manic Pertaining to a specific psychosis.

manic-depressive disorder See *bipolar disorder.*

manubriosternal junction The point at which the manubrium joins the body of the sternum; the location of the second rib; also known as the *sternal angle.*

manubrium One of the three bones of the sternum; it has a broad, quadrangular shape that narrows caudally at its articulation with the superior end of the body of the sternum.

Marfan syndrome An abnormal condition characterized by elongation of the bones, often with associated abnormalities of the eyes and cardiovascular system.

mass casualty incident An event for which available resources are insufficient to manage the number of casualties.

mast cells Specialized cells of the inflammatory response.

mastectomy Surgical removal of one or both breasts, performed to remove a malignant tumor.

mastication Chewing, tearing, or grinding food with the teeth while it is mixed with saliva.

mastoid air cell One of several spaces within the mastoid process of the temporal bone; it is connected to the middle ear by ducts.

masturbation Sexual stimulation, especially of one's own genitals, often to the point of orgasm.

maxilla One of a pair of large bones that form the upper jaw.

maxillary sinus One of the pair of large air cells that form a pyramidal cavity in the body of the maxilla.

McBurney point A site of extreme sensitivity in acute appendicitis situated in the normal area of the appendix, approximately 2 inches from the right anterior-superior spine of the ilium, on a line between that part of the spine and the umbilicus.

mean arterial pressure The arithmetic mean of the blood pressure in the arterial portion of the circulation.

measles An acute, highly contagious viral disease involving the respiratory tract that is characterized by a spreading, maculopapular, cutaneous rash.

meconium aspiration syndrome Inhalation of meconium by the fetus or newborn; the meconium can block the air passages and result in failure of the lungs to expand or cause other pulmonary dysfunction.

meconium staining The presence of fetal stool in amniotic fluid.

medial malleolus The rounded process on the medial side of the ankle joint.

mediastinitis Inflammation of the mediastinum.

mediastinum A portion of the thoracic cavity in the middle of the thorax between the pleural sacs containing the two lungs; it extends from the sternum to the vertebral column and contains all the thoracic viscera except the lungs.

mediated transport mechanisms Mechanisms that use carrier molecules to move large, water-soluble molecules or electrically charged molecules across cell membranes.

medical asepsis The removal or destruction of disease-causing organisms or infected material.

medical direction A process of ensuring that actions taken on behalf of ill or injured persons are medically appropriate, including prospective, concurrent, and retrospective aspects of emergency medical services quality improvement, hiring, and education.

medulla The lowest part of the brainstem, which controls vital functions; an enlarged extension of the spinal cord; also known as the *medulla oblongata.*

medulla oblongata See *medulla.*

medullary cavity A large, marrow-filled cavity in the diaphysis of a long bone.

megahertz A unit of frequency equal to 1 million cycles per second; emergency medical services radios transmit and receive on frequencies measured in megahertz.

melanocyte A body cell capable of producing melanin.

melatonin The only hormone secreted in the bloodstream by the pineal gland; it lightens skin pigmentation and may inhibit numerous endocrine functions.

melena Abnormal black, tarry stools containing digested blood.

membrane channel A tunnel through which specific molecules may pass.

membrane permeability A quality of cell membranes that permits the passage of solvents and solutes into and out of cells.

membranous labyrinth A membranous structure within the inner ear; it forms the cochlea, vestibule, and semicircular canals.

memory cells Cells that remember the same pathogen for faster antibody production with future exposures; produced by the division of B cells.

menarche The first menstruation and the commencement of the cyclic menstrual function.

Meniere's disease An abnormality of the inner ear that causes vertigo and tinnitus; associated with fluctuations in hearing loss and a sensation of pressure or pain in the affected ear.

meninges Fluid-containing membranes surrounding the brain and spinal cord.

meningitis Inflammation of the meninges.

meningococcal meningitis Inflammation of the membranes that surround the spinal cord and brain; it can be caused by a variety of different bacteria, viruses, and other microorganisms; also known as *spinal meningitis.*

menopause The cessation of menses.

menstruation The periodic discharge through the vagina of a blood secretion containing tissue debris from the shedding of the endometrium from the nonpregnant uterus.

mental illness Any form of psychiatric disorder.

mental retardation A disorder characterized by below-average intellectual function with deficits or impairments in the ability to learn and adapt socially.

mental status examination An evaluation tool that includes an assessment of appearance and behavior, speech and language, emotional stability, and cognitive abilities.

merocrine gland A gland that secretes products with no loss of cellular material, such as a water-producing sweat gland.

mesencephalon See *midbrain*.

mesentery The double layer of peritoneum extending from the abdominal wall to the abdominal viscera; it conveys vessels and nerves.

mesovarium A short peritoneal fold connecting the ovary with the broad ligament of the uterus.

metabolic acidosis A disorder that results when excess acid is added to the body fluids or bicarbonate is lost from them.

metabolic alkalosis A disorder that results from a significant loss of acid in the body or increased levels of the base bicarbonate.

metabolism The culmination of all chemical processes that take place in living organisms.

metabolite A substance that is produced by metabolic action or that is necessary for the metabolic process.

metacarpal One of five bones extending from the carpus to the phalanges.

metaplasia A change from one cell type to another that is better able to tolerate adverse conditions; a conversion into a form that is not normal for that cell.

metarteriole One of the small peripheral blood vessels that contain scattered groups of smooth muscle fibers in their walls; they are located between the arterioles and the true capillaries.

metastasis The movement or spreading of cancer cells from one organ or tissue to distant locations in the body.

metastasize The ability of cancer cells to move or spread from one organ or tissue to distant locations in the body.

metatarsal Any one of the five bones comprising the metatarsus.

meter A metric unit of length equal to 1000 millimeters.

methanol A chemical widely used as a solvent and in the production of formaldehyde.

methemoglobin A form of hemoglobin in which the iron component has been oxidized from the ferrous to the ferric state.

methemoglobinemia The presence of methemoglobin in the blood, causing cyanosis as a result of the inability of the red blood cells to release oxygen.

metric system Units of measurement that include the meter, the liter, and the gram.

microcirculation Refers to circulation of blood from the heart to the arteries, capillaries, and veins.

microdrip tubing An apparatus for delivering relatively small amounts of intravenous solutions at specific flow rates; the drops delivered by a microdrip are smaller than those delivered by a macrodrip.

microgram A metric unit of mass equal to $\frac{1}{1,000,000}$ of a gram.

microinfarct A small infarct caused by obstruction of circulation in capillaries, arterioles, or small arteries.

microorganism Any tiny, usually microscopic entity capable of carrying on living processes, such as bacteria, fungi, protozoa, and viruses.

microthrombus A minute thrombus.

microtubule A hollow tube that helps to support the cytoplasm of the cell; a component of certain cell organelles such as centrioles, spindle fibers, cilia, and flagella.

microwave Radio waves with frequencies of 890 MHz and higher. The signals are generated by special equipment that depends on line of sight placement to operate properly. Microwave channels may have a wide band to carry a large number of simultaneous transmissions.

midbrain One of the three parts of the brainstem; also known as the *mesencephalon*.

middle adulthood Persons 41 to 60 years of age.

middle cerebral artery The artery that supplies a large portion of the lateral cerebral cortex.

middle ear An air-filled space within the temporal bone that contains the auditory ossicles.

migraine A severe, incapacitating headache that often is preceded by visual and/or gastrointestinal disturbances.

milliequivalent A unit of measure equal to $\frac{1}{1000}$ of a gram equivalent.

milligram A metric unit of mass equal to $\frac{1}{1000}$ of a gram.

milliliter A metric unit of capacity equal to $\frac{1}{1000}$ of a liter.

millimeter A metric unit of length equal to $\frac{1}{1000}$ of a meter.

mineral An inorganic substance usually referred to by the name of the compound of which it is a part; minerals are important in regulating many body functions.

mineralocorticoid A hormone secreted by the adrenal cortex that maintains normal blood volume, promotes sodium and water retention, and increases urine secretion of potassium and hydrogen ions.

minim A measure of volume in the apothecary system, originally 1 drop of water; 60 minims equal 1 fluid dram, and 1 minim equals 0.06 mL.

minimal effective concentration The lowest plasma concentration that produces the desired drug effect.

minute alveolar ventilation The amount of inspired gas available for gas exchange during 1 minute.

minute volume The amount of gas inhaled or exhaled in 1 minute. It is found by multiplying the tidal volume by the respiratory rate.

miscarriage See *spontaneous abortion*.

missed abortion The retention of the fetus in utero for 4 or more weeks after fetal death.

mitochondria Small, spherical, rod-shaped, or thin filamentous structures in the cytoplasm of cells; a site of adenosine triphosphate production.

mitosis Cell division resulting in two daughter cells with exactly the same number and type of chromosomes as the mother cell.

mitral valve See *bicuspid valve.*

mitral valve prolapse Protrusion of one or both cusps of the mitral valve back into the left atrium during ventricular systole, resulting in incomplete closure of the valve and mitral insufficiency.

mittelschmerz Abdominal pain in the region of the ovary during ovulation; it usually occurs midway through the menstrual cycle.

MMR vaccine The abbreviation for live measles, mumps, and rubella virus vaccine.

mobile data terminal A computer connected through a modem ("black box") with a radio that sends and receives pretyped messages to printers, computer screens, or both. Some mobile data terminals have graphics (floor plans) and database (hazardous materials) capabilities. Mobile data terminals rely on a host computer interfaced to a base station.

mobile relay station A fixed base station that automatically retransmits mobile or portable radio communications back to the receiving frequency of other portables, mobiles, and base stations operating in the same system; also known as a repeater.

mobile repeater A mobile radio unit capable of automatically retransmitting any radio traffic originated by a hand-held portable, by other mobiles, or by base stations. This repeater may be one-way or two-way and may be known as a PAC-RAT (Motorola) or an extender. Also known as a vehicle repeater.

mode of transmission The way in which diseases are transmitted; may be direct or indirect contact.

mole A standard unit used to measure the amount of a substance.

monocyte A type of white blood cell found in lymph nodes, spleen, bone marrow, and loose connective tissue.

monomorphic Existing only in one form.

mononucleosis A viral infection causing fever, sore throat, and swollen lymph glands, especially in the neck.

mons pubis The prominence caused by a pad of fatty tissue over the symphysis pubis in the female.

mood disorder Refers to changes in emotions that a person experiences in life (e.g., happiness, depression, fear, and anxiety).

morals Social standards or customs; dealing with what is right or wrong in a practical sense.

Moro reflex A normal infant response elicited by a sudden loud noise. The infant flexes the legs, makes an embracing gesture with the arms, and usually gives a brief cry.

morphology The study of the physical shape and size of a specimen, plant, or animal.

motor neuron A neuron that innervates skeletal, smooth, or cardiac muscle fibers; also known as an interneuron.

mucin The chief ingredient in mucus.

mucosa Mucous membrane.

mucus The viscous, slippery secretion of mucous membranes and glands.

multifocal premature ventricular complex A premature ventricular complex that originates from multiple sites in the ventricles.

multigravida A woman who has had two or more pregnancies.

multipara A woman who has had two or more deliveries.

multiple gestation A pregnancy with more than one fetus.

multiple myeloma A malignant neoplasm of the bone marrow.

multiple organ dysfunction syndrome The progressive failure of two or more organ systems after a severe illness or injury.

multiple sclerosis A progressive disease of the central nervous system in which scattered patches of myelin in the brain and spinal cord are destroyed.

multiplex mode A communications mode with the ability to transmit two or more different types of information simultaneously, in either or both directions, over the same frequency.

mumps An acute viral disease characterized by swelling of the parotid glands.

Munchausen syndrome A factitious disorder in which the patient makes routine pleas for treatment and hospitalization for a symptomatic, but imaginary, acute illness.

Munchausen syndrome by proxy A factitious disorder in which a person injures or induces illness in others (usually children) in order to gain sympathy.

Murphy's sign Cessation of inspiration during right upper quadrant examination (may indicate acute cholecystitis).

muscarinic receptor A class of cholinergic receptor molecule specifically activated by muscarine in addition to acetylcholine.

muscle strain A slight tear in a muscle or tendon.

muscle tone The constant tension produced by muscles of the body for long periods of time.

muscular dystrophy An inherited muscle disorder of unknown cause marked by a slow but progressive degeneration of muscle fibers.

muscular system The body system responsible for execution of movement and postural maintenance.

muscular tissue A primary tissue type characterized by its contractile abilities.

musculoskeletal system The body system comprised of bones, muscles, tendons and ligaments, and articulating surfaces (e.g., joints, bursa, disks).

mutagenic Any chemical or physical environmental agent that induces a genetic mutation or increases the mutation rate.

mutual aid An agreement with neighboring emergency agencies to exchange equipment and personnel when necessary.

myalgia Diffuse muscle pain, usually accompanied by malaise; it occurs in many infectious diseases.

myasthenia Muscle weakness.

myasthenia gravis An autoimmune disorder in which muscles become weak and tire easily.

Mycobacterium leprae A genus of gram-positive bacteria that cause leprosy.

Mycobacterium tuberculosis A genus of gram-positive bacteria that cause tuberculosis.

Mycoplasma A genus of microscopic organisms lacking rigid cell walls; they are considered to be the smallest free-living organisms.

mycoplasmal pneumonia A type of atypical pneumonia. It is caused by the bacteria *M. pneumoniae.*

myelinated axon A nerve fiber having a myelin sheath.

myeloblast Bone marrow cell.

myocardial hypertrophy An abnormal increase in the size of cardiac muscle.

myocardial infarction Necrosis of a portion of cardiac muscle caused by obstruction in a coronary artery from atherosclerosis or an embolus.

myoclonic seizure A seizure that causes brief muscle contractions that usually occur at the same time and on both sides of the body.

myoclonus A condition characterized by rapid, uncontrollable muscular contractions or spasms of muscles that occur at rest or during movement.

myoepithelium Tissue made up of contractile epithelial cells.

myofibril A slender, striated strand of smooth muscle.

myofilament An extremely fine, molecular, threadlike structure that helps to form the myofibril of muscle; thick myofibrils are formed of myosin, and thin myofilaments are formed of actin.

myoglobinuria The presence of myoglobin in the urine.

myometrium The muscular wall of the uterus.

myosin A cardiac and skeletal muscle protein; it makes up about half of the proteins that occur in muscle tissue.

myositis A muscular disorder characterized by progressive muscle weakness and wasting; also known as *inclusive body myositis.*

myxedema A condition that results from a deficiency in thyroid hormone.

nail bed The end of a finger or toe covered by the nail; it is abundant in blood vessels.

nail body The visible part of the nail.

narcolepsy A syndrome characterized by sudden sleep attacks and visual or auditory hallucinations at the onset of sleep.

nares Nostrils.

narrative The portion of the patient care report that allows for a chronological description of the call.

nasal bone The bony partition that separates the nasal cavity into left and right parts; also known as the *nasal septum.*

nasal septum A partition that separates the right and left nasal cavities.

nasogastric decompression The management of gastric distention or emesis control by means of a nasogastric tube.

nasogastric tube Any tube passed into the stomach through the nose.

nasolacrimal duct A duct that leads from the lacrimal sac to the nasal cavity.

nasopharynx The uppermost portion of the pharynx just behind the nasal cavities.

nasotracheal Accessing the trachea through the nasal cavity.

natural immunity Non–antigen-specific immunity that is present at birth; also known as *innate immunity* or *nonspecific immunity.*

nature of the illness The principal characteristics and causes of an illness.

near-drowning Submersion with at least temporary survival.

near-fatal asthma Acute asthma associated with respiratory arrest, a drop in blood pressure, and reduced cardiac output.

nebulizer A device for producing a fine spray of medication for inhalation therapy.

necrosis Death of a cell or group of cells as the result of disease or injury.

necrotizing fasciitis A rare infection of the deep layers of the skin and subcutaneous tissues.

negative feedback mechanisms Any mechanism that tends to produce a response that balances a change in a system.

neglect The refusal or failure of the caregiver to fulfill obligations or duties to a person.

negligence Failure to use such care as a reasonably prudent emergency medical services provider would use in similar circumstances.

nematocyst A capsule containing threadlike, venomous stinging cells found in some coelenterates.

neonate An infant in the first 28 days of life.

neoplasia The new and abnormal development of cells, which may be benign or malignant.

neoplasm Abnormal growth; a malignant or benign tumor.

nephron The functional unit of the kidney.

nerve A bundle of nerve fibers and accompanying connective tissue located outside the central nervous system.

nerve tract Bundles of parallel axons with associated sheaths in the central nervous system.

nervous tissue A major tissue type characterized by its conductive abilities.

nervous tunic The retina.

neuralgia Pain along a nerve.

neurogenic hypotension Hypotension following spinal shock; caused by a loss of sympathetic tone to the vessels.

neurogenic shock Shock resulting from vasomotor paralysis below the level of injury; also known as *spinal cord shock.*

neuroglia Specialized connective tissue cells that protect and hold functioning neurons together.

neurohormone A junction hormone secreted by a neuron.

neuromuscular A specialized synapse between a motor neuron and a muscle fiber.

neuromuscular junction The area of contact between the ends of a large myelinated nerve fiber and a fiber of skeletal muscle.

neuron The functional unit of the nervous system, consisting of the nerve cell body, the dendrites, and the axon.

neuropathy A disease of the peripheral nerves.

neurosis Any faulty or inefficient way of coping with anxiety or inner conflict; it may ultimately lead to a neurotic disorder.

neurotransmitter A chemical that is released from one neuron at the presynaptic nerve fiber.

neutrophil A small, phagocytic white blood cell with a lobed nucleus and small granules in the cytoplasm.

newborn An infant in the first few hours of life.

Newton's first law of motion The principle that an object, whether at rest or in linear motion, remains in that state unless force is applied.

Newton's second law of motion The principle that force is equal to mass times acceleration or deceleration.

nicad batteries Nickel cadmium rechargeable batteries, which are used in portable radios.

nicotinic receptor A class of cholinergic receptor molecules that are activated specifically by nicotine and acetylcholine.

nit The egg of a parasitic insect, particularly a louse.

nitrogen narcosis An illness associated with scuba diving in which nitrogen becomes dissolved in solution as a result of greater than normal atmospheric pressure; also known as rapture of the deep.

nocturia Particularly excessive urination at night.

node of Ranvier The short interval in the myelin sheath of a nerve fiber between adjacent Schwann cells.

noncardiogenic pulmonary edema See *acute respiratory distress syndrome.*

noncompensatory pause The pause that occurs when the next expected P wave of the underlying cardiac rhythm appears earlier than it would have if the sinoatrial node had not been disturbed by a conduction abnormality.

noncompetitive antagonist An agent that combines with different parts of the receptor mechanism and inactivates the receptor so that the agonist cannot be effective regardless of its concentration.

nonconducted premature atrial complex A premature atrial complex blocked at the atrioventricular node.

nonelectrolyte A substance with no electrical charge.

nonepileptic seizure A seizure that stems from psychological causes rather than electrical disturbances in the brain.

Non-Hodgkin's lymphoma Cancer of the lymphoid tissue, which includes the lymph nodes, spleen, and other organs of the immune system.

nonproprietary name See *generic name.*

nonsteroid hormones Hormones that are synthesized chiefly from amino acids, including insulin, parathyroid hormone, and others.

Non-ST-elevation MI (NSTEMI) Myocardial infarction characterized by ischemic ST-segment depression equal to or greater than 0.5 mm (0.05 mV) or dynamic T-wave inversion with pain or discomfort. Nonpersistent or transient ST-segment elevation equal to or greater than 0.5 mm (0.05 mV) for more than 20 minutes is also included in this category.

nonstriated muscle See *smooth muscle.*

noradrenaline An adrenergic hormone produced by the adrenal medulla, similar in chemical and pharmacological properties to epinephrine. It acts to increase blood pressure by vasoconstriction but does not affect cardiac output; also known as norepinephrine.

nuchal rigidity Neck stiffness with flexion, suggesting meningeal irritation.

nuclear membrane A double membrane structure surrounding and enclosing the nucleus; also known as the *nuclear envelope.*

nucleic acids Extremely complex, long-chain compounds of high molecular weight that occur naturally in the cells of all living organisms; they form the genetic material of the cell and direct the synthesis of protein within the cell.

nucleolus Any one of the somewhat rounded, dense, well-defined nuclear bodies with no surrounding membrane; the nucleolus contains ribosomal RNA and protein.

nucleoplasm The protoplasm of the nucleus, as contrasted with that of the cell.

nucleus The central controlling body within a living cell.

nullipara A woman who has never borne a child.

nutrient Any substance that nourishes and aids the growth and development of the body.

nystagmus Involuntary rhythmic movements of the eyes.

obesity A condition in which a person is 30% above ideal body weight.

obligate Necessary; compulsory.

obsessive-compulsive disorder A psychiatric disorder in which the person feels stress or anxiety about thoughts or rituals over which he or she has little control.

obstructive apnea A form of sleep apnea involving a physical obstruction of the upper airways that can lead to pulmonary failure, chronic fatigue, and cardiac abnormalities.

obstructive shock Shock that results from obstruction to blood flow.

obtundation A state of being insensitive to unpleasant or painful stimulation associated with a reduced level of consciousness, such as by anesthesia or a strong narcotic analgesic.

obturator foramen A large opening on each side of the lower portion of the hipbone, formed posteriorly by the ischium, superiorly by the ilium, and anteriorly by the pubis.

occipital bone The cuplike bone at the back of the skull, marked by a large opening (the foramen magnum) that communicates with the vertebral canal.

occipital foramen A passage in the occipital bone through which the spinal cord enters the spinal column.

occipital lobe One of the five lobes of each cerebral hemisphere.

occiput posterior presentation An abnormal presentation in which the infant's head is delivered face up instead of face down.

occlusive stroke A stroke (CVA) caused by blockage of a cerebral blood vessel.

oculomotor nerve The third cranial nerve, which contains sensory and motor fibers; it provides for movement in most of the muscles of the eye, for constriction of the pupil, and for accommodation of the eye to light.

odontoid process The toothlike projection that rises perpendicularly from the upper surface of the body of the second cervical vertebra (also known as the *axis*), which serves as a pivot point for the rotation of the atlas.

official name The name of a drug that is followed by the initials USP (*United States Pharmacopeia*) or NF (*National Formulary*), denoting its listing in one of the official publications; usually the same as the generic name.

off-line (indirect) medical direction The establishment and monitoring of all medical components of an emergency medical services system, including protocols, standing orders, educational programs, and the quality and delivery of online (direct) medical direction.

olecranon fossa The depression in the posterior surface of the humerus that receives the olecranon of the ulna when the forearm is extended.

olecranon process The large bony process of the ulna; also known as the olecranon.

olfactory Of or pertaining to the sense of smell.

olfactory bulb The tissue that receives the olfactory nerves from the nasal cavity.

olfactory membranes Membranes that contain the receptors for the sense of smell; they are located in the roof of the nasal cavity.

olfactory recess The extreme superior region of the nasal cavity.

olfactory tract The nerve tract that projects from the olfactory bulb to the olfactory cortex.

oliguria A diminished capacity to form or pass urine.

omphalocele Congenital herniation of intraabdominal viscera through a defect in the abdominal wall around the umbilicus.

oncotic pressure See *blood colloid osmotic pressure*.

ongoing assessment A repeat of the initial assessment that is performed throughout the paramedic-patient encounter.

online (direct) medical direction The medical direction physician or designee who directly supervises prehospital care activities via radio or phone. Online (direct) medical direction may also be responsible for the activities of the emergency department staff and others at the medical direction hospital.

onset of action The interval between the time a drug is administered and the first sign of its effects; also known as the *latent period of drug action*.

oocyte An incompletely developed ovum.

open-angle glaucoma The most common type of glaucoma where structures of the eye appear normal, but fluid in the eye does not flow properly through the trabecular meshwork; also called *wide-angle glaucoma*.

open-ended questions Questions asked in a narrative form that cannot be answered with a "yes" or "no."

open pneumothorax A chest wall injury that exposes the pleural space to atmospheric pressure.

open vault fracture A fracture that results in direct communication between a scalp laceration and cerebral substance.

opening questions Questions that determine why the patient is seeking medical care or advice.

opiate A narcotic drug that contains opium, derivatives of opium, or any of several semisynthetic or synthetic drugs with opium-like activity.

opioid Any synthetic narcotic that has opiate-like activities but is not derived from opium.

opportunistic infections Infections that take advantage of weakness in the immune defenses.

opposition Movement of the thumb and little finger toward each other for the purpose of grasping objects.

optic nerve The nerve that carries visual signals from the eye to the crossing of the optic tracts.

oral candidiasis An infection of yeast fungi of the genus *Candida* on the mucous membranes of the mouth; also known as *thrush*.

orbital cellulitis An acute infection of the tissues immediately surrounding the eye, including the eyelids, eyebrow, and cheek.

orchitis Painful inflammation of the testicle.

organ A structure made up of two or more kinds of tissues organized to perform a more complex function than any one tissue alone.

organ of Corti The organ of hearing; it is located in the cochlea and filled with endolymph.

organelle Any one of various particles of living substance bound within most cells, such as the mitochondria, the Golgi apparatus, the endoplasmic reticulum, the lysosomes, and the centrioles.

oriented Aware of one's surroundings.

origin The less movable attachment point of a muscle.

orogastric decompression The management of gastric distention or emesis control by means of an orogastric tube.

oropharyngeolaryngeal axis The three axes of the mouth, pharynx, and trachea; a patient position used for direct visualization of the larynx.

oropharynx The portion of the pharynx located behind the mouth.

orotracheal Gaining access to the trachea through the oral cavity.

orphan drug A medication that has been developed specifically to treat a rare medical condition.

orthostatic hypotension Abnormally low blood pressure that occurs when an individual assumes the standing posture; also called postural hypotension.

osmolality The osmotic concentration of a solution.

osmosis Diffusion of solvent (water) through a membrane from a less concentrated solution to a more concentrated solution.

osmotic pressure The force required to prevent the movement of water across a selectively permeable membrane.

ossified To be changed or developed into bone.

osteoarthritis A form of arthritis in which one or many joints undergo degenerative changes.

osteomyelitis Local or generalized infection of bone and bone marrow, usually caused by bacteria introduced by trauma or surgery.

osteoporosis A disorder characterized by a reduction in bone density; it occurs most often in postmenopausal women.

ostomy An artificial opening into the urinary tract, gastrointestinal tract, or trachea; any surgical procedure in which an opening is created between two hollow organs or between a hollow viscus and the abdominal wall.

otitis media Infection or inflammation of the middle ear.

otorrhea Any discharge from the external ear.

ounce A unit of weight equal to ⅟₁₆ lb, or 28.349 g.

ovarian follicle The spherical cell aggregation in the ovary that contains an oocyte.

ovarian ligament The bundle of fibers that passes to the uterus from the ovary.

ovarian torsion Twisting of an ovary around its vascular pedicle.

ovary One of the pair of female gonads found on each side of the lower abdomen beside the uterus.

overflow incontinence An overflow of urine from the bladder.

overhydration Water excess or water intoxication.

ovulation The release of an ovum or secondary oocyte from the vesicular follicle.

oxyhemoglobin Oxygenated hemoglobin.

P wave The first complex of the electrocardiogram, representing depolarization of the atria.

pacemaker cell Certain myocardial cells capable of initiating an electrical impulse.

packaging See *patient packaging*.

Paget's disease A common, nonmetabolic disease of bone of unknown cause characterized by excessive bone destruction and unorganized bone repair.

paging equipment Equipment typically using tone activation with one-way transmission to receive-only units.

palate A structure that forms the roof of the mouth; it is divided into the hard and soft palates.

palatine bone One of a pair of bones of the skull forming the posterior part of the hard palate, part of the nasal cavity, and the floor of the orbit of the eye.

palatine tonsil One of two large oval masses of lymphoid tissue embedded in the lateral wall of the oropharynx.

palliative care A unique form of health care primarily directed at providing relief to terminally ill persons through symptom management and pain management; also known as *comfort care*.

palmar grasp A normal infant response. The infant curls the fingers in response to a touch on the palm of the hand.

palpation A technique in which an examiner uses the hands and fingers to gather information from a patient by touch.

pancreas A fish-shaped nodular gland located across the posterior abdominal wall in the epigastric region of the body; it secretes various substances, including digestive enzymes, insulin, and glucagon.

pancreatic juice The fluid secretion of the pancreas produced by the stimulation of food in the duodenum.

pancreatitis Inflammation of the pancreas, which causes severe epigastric pain.

pandemic An infectious disease outbreak that infects large numbers of people in a large geographic region and may occur worldwide.

panic disorder An anxiety disorder characterized by unexpected and repeated episodes of intense fear accompanied by physical symptoms that may include chest pain, heart palpitations, shortness of breath, dizziness, or abdominal distress.

papilledema Swelling of the head of the optic disc, caused by a rise in intracranial pressure (ICP).

para The number of past pregnancies that have remained viable to delivery.

parainfluenza virus One of a group of viruses isolated from patients with upper respiratory tract disease of varying severity in infants and young children; it may cause croup, tracheobronchitis, bronchiolitis, bronchopneumonia, pharyngitis, and the common cold.

paralytic ileus The decrease in or absence of intestinal peristalsis that may occur after abdominal surgery, illness, or injury; the most common cause of intestinal obstruction.

paramedic a person who has completed training consistent with the national EMS education standards, including advanced training in clinical decision making, patient assessment, cardiac rhythm interpretation, defibrillation, drug therapy, and airway management.

parametritis An inflammatory condition of tissue of the structures around the uterus.

paranoia A condition characterized by an elaborate, overly suspicious system of thinking.

paraphimosis The inability of an uncircumcised male to pull the retracted foreskin back over the head of the penis.

paraplegia A weakness or paralysis of both legs and sometimes part of the trunk.

parasagittal plane An imaginary vertical plane passing through the body parallel to the medial plane; it divides the body into left and right portions.

parasympathetic Of or pertaining to the craniosacral division of the autonomic nervous system.

parasympathetic nervous system The subdivision of the autonomic nervous system usually involved in activating vegetative functions such as digestion, defecation, and urination.

parasympatholytic agent Anticholinergic; producing effects resembling those of interruption or blockade of the parasympathetic nerve supply to effector organs or tissues.

parasympathomimetic agent An agent with effects that mimic those resulting from stimulation of parasympathetic nerves, especially the effects produced by acetylcholine.

parasystole An independent ectopic rhythm initiated at a site other than the normal pacemaker of the heart (i.e., the sinoatrial node); the ectopic focus cannot be activated by impulses of the dominant rhythm because it is surrounded by an area of depressed conduction.

parenchyma The essential or functional elements of an organ.

parens patriae A term that refers to the authority of the state to intervene over the objections of parents to protect children.

parenteral Of or pertaining to any medication route other than the alimentary canal.

paresthesia A sensation of numbness, tingling, or "pins and needles."

parietal Of or pertaining to the outer wall of a cavity or organ.

parietal bone One of a pair of bones that form the side of the cranium.

parietal lobe The portion of each cerebral hemisphere that occupies the parts of the lateral and medial surfaces covered by the parietal bone.

parietal pericardium The portion of serous pericardium lining the fibrous pericardium.

parietal peritoneum The layer of peritoneum lining the abdominal walls.

Parkinson's disease A disease caused by degeneration or damage (of unknown origin) to nerve cells within the basal ganglia in the brain.

parkinsonism A neurological disorder characterized by tremor, muscle rigidity, hypokinesia, a slow shuffling gait, and difficulty in chewing, swallowing, and speaking; it frequently occurs in patients treated with antipsychotic drugs.

paronychia A common skin infection that occurs around the nails that that allows for an invasion of bacteria, yeast, or fungus.

parotitis Inflammation or infection of one or both parotid salivary glands.

paroxysm A sudden attack or recurrence of symptoms of a disease.

paroxysmal nocturnal dyspnea An abnormal condition of the respiratory system characterized by sudden attacks of shortness of breath, profuse sweating, tachycardia, and wheezing that awaken a person from sleep; often associated with left ventricular failure and pulmonary edema.

paroxysmal supraventricular tachycardia An ectopic rhythm in excess of 100 beats per minute and usually faster than 170 beats per minute that begins abruptly with a premature atrial or junctional beat and is supported by an atrioventricular nodal reentry mechanism or by an atrioventricular reentry involving an accessory pathway.

partial antagonist An agent that has affinity and some efficacy but that may antagonize the action of other drugs that have greater efficacy.

partial pressure The pressure exerted by a single gas.

partial reabsorption The amount of drug reabsorbed from the renal tubule by passive diffusion.

partial seizure A seizure that originates from an identifiable cortical lesion.

partial-thickness burn A burn injury that extends through the epidermis to the dermis; considered a deep partial-thickness injury if it extends to the basal layers of the skin; also known as a *second-degree burn*.

parturition The process of giving birth.

passive glomerular filtration The renal process whereby fluid in the blood is filtered across the capillaries of the glomerulus and into the urinary space of Bowman's capsule.

passive immunity Immunity acquired by the transfer of antibodies from the mother by way placental transfer to the fetus; a form of acquired immunity in which antibodies against disease are acquired naturally.

past medical history A patient's medical background that may offer insight into the patient's current problem.

patella A flat, triangular bone at the front of the knee joint; the kneecap.

pathogen A disease-causing agent.

pathogenic microbes Microscopic pathogens such as bacteria, parasites, fungi, and viruses that can cause infection.

pathological fracture A bone fracture that results from trauma or a metabolic disease, such as osteoporosis or a bone tumor.

patient care report A document used in the prehospital setting to record all patient care activities and circumstances related to an emergency response.

patient management plan A plan of care that is based on principles and applications of findings in the patient assessment.

patient packaging Completion of emergency care procedures needed to transfer a patient from the scene to the emergency vehicle.

pattern recognition The process of comparing gathered information with the paramedic's knowledge base of medical illness and disease.

patterned injuries Injuries that result from an identifiable object.

peak expiratory flow rate A measurement of how fast a person can exhale air.

peak plasma level The highest plasma concentration attained from a dose.

pectoral girdle See *shoulder girdle*.

pectus deformity Malformation of the chest wall.

pediatric trauma score An injury severity index that grades six components commonly seen in pediatric trauma patients: size (weight), airway, central nervous system, systolic blood pressure, open wound, and skeletal injury.

pelvic cavity The area of the body enclosed by the bones of the pelvis.

pelvic girdle The encircling bony structure supporting the lower limbs.

pelvic inflammatory disease Any inflammatory condition of the female pelvic organs, especially one caused by bacterial infection.

penetrating trauma An injury produced by crushing and stretching forces of a penetrating object that results in some form of tissue disruption.

penetration The flow of a hazardous liquid chemical through zippers, stitched seams, pinholes, or other imperfections in a material.

penis The external reproductive organ of the male.

pepsin The principal digestive enzyme of gastric juice.

pepsinogen A proenzyme formed and secreted by certain cells of the gastric mucosa.

peptic ulcer A sharply circumscribed loss of the mucous membrane of the stomach, duodenum, or any other part of the gastrointestinal system.

peptic ulcer disease Illness that results from a complex pathological interaction among the acidic gastric juice and proteolytic enzymes and the mucosal barrier.

peptide bond A chemical bond between amino acids.

percussion A technique used to evaluate the presence of air or fluid in body tissues.

perforated tympanic membrane A hole or rupture in the eardrum, usually from trauma or infection.

perfusion The circulation of blood to the tissues.

periappendiceal abscess A cavity containing pus and inflamed tissue around the vermiform appendix.

pericardial cavity The area of the body that surrounds the heart.

pericardial fluid A viscous fluid contained within the pericardial cavity between the visceral and parietal pericardium; it serves as a lubricant.

pericardial friction rub A dry, grating sound heard with a stethoscope during auscultation; suggestive of pericarditis.

pericardial sac The sac that surrounds the heart.

pericardial tamponade Compression of the heart produced by the accumulation of fluid or blood in the pericardial sac.

pericardiocentesis A procedure for withdrawing fluid from the pericardial sac.

pericarditis Inflammation of the pericardium.

pericardium The membrane that surrounds the heart.

perilymph The fluid contained within the bony labyrinth.

perinatal Occurring at or near the time of birth.

perineum The pelvic floor and associated structures occupying the pelvic outlet, bounded anteriorly by the pubic symphysis, laterally by the ischial tuberosities, and posteriorly by the coccyx.

periodontal disease Disease that affects tissue that surround or support the teeth.

periodontal membrane The membrane that surrounds the root of the tooth.

periosteum Tough connective tissue that covers the bone.

periostitis Inflammation of the periosteum characterized by tenderness and swelling of the affected bone, pain, fever, and chills.

peripheral nervous system A subdivision of the nervous system consisting of nerves and ganglia.

peripheral neuropathy Diseases and disorders that affect the peripheral nervous system, including spinal nerve roots, cranial nerves, and peripheral nerves.

peripheral thermoreceptors Nerve endings sensitive to heat, located in the skin and some mucous membranes; they usually are categorized as cold or warm receptors.

peripheral vascular disease Any abnormal condition that affects the blood vessels outside the heart and lymphatic vessels.

peripheral vascular resistance The total resistance against which blood must be pumped; also known as *afterload*.

peristalsis The coordinated, rhythmic, and serial contraction of smooth muscle that forces food through the digestive tract, bile through the bile duct, and urine through the ureters.

peristaltic Pertaining to peristalsis.

peritoneal Pertaining to the peritoneum.

peritoneal cavity The potential space between the parietal and visceral layers of the peritoneum; the two layers normally are in contact.

peritoneal dialysis A dialysis procedure that uses the peritoneum as a diffusible membrane; performed to correct an imbalance of fluid or electrolytes in the blood or to remove toxins, drugs, or other wastes normally excreted by the kidney.

peritoneum The serous membrane that covers the abdominal wall of the body and is reflected over the contained viscera.

peritonitis Inflammation of the serous membrane that covers the abdominal wall.

peritonsillar abscess A collection of pus in and around one or both tonsils; often caused by tonsillitis.

peritubular capillary The capillary network located in the cortex of the kidney.

permeable A condition of being pervious so that fluids and other substances can pass through, as occurs in a semipermeable membrane.

permeation The process by which a hazardous liquid chemical moves through a material on a molecular level.

permissive hypotension A fluid resuscitation strategy that advocates withholding fluid and red cell products until after surgical control of bleeding is achieved.

pernicious anemia Anemia that results from a vitamin B_{12} deficiency.

PERRL Acronym for pupils that are equal, round, and react to light.

persistent generalized lymphadenopathy Enlarged lymph nodes involving two noncontiguous sites other than the inguinal nodes; a common feature in early human immunodeficiency virus infection.

personal protective equipment Clothing or specialized equipment that provides some protection to the wearer.

personality disorder A large group of conditions distinguished by a failure to learn from experience or to adapt appropriately to changes; results in personal distress and impairment of social functioning.

pertinent negative findings Findings that warrant no medical care or intervention but that, by seeking them, show evidence of the thoroughness of the examination and history of the event.

pertussis An acute, highly contagious respiratory disease characterized by paroxysmal coughing that ends in a loud, whooping inspiration; also known as *whooping cough.*

petit mal seizure An epileptic seizure characterized by a sudden, momentary loss of consciousness occasionally accompanied by minor muscle spasms of the neck or upper extremities.

pH An inverse logarithm of the hydrogen ion concentration.

phagocytic Pertaining to phagocytosis.

phagocytosis The process of ingestion by cells of solid substances such as other cells, bacteria, bits of necrosed tissue, and foreign particles.

phalanges Any bone of a finger or toe.

pharmaceutics The science of dispensing drugs.

pharmacodynamics The study of how a drug acts on a living organism.

pharmacokinetics The study of how the body handles a drug over a period of time, including the processes of absorption, distribution, biotransformation, and excretion.

pharmacology The science of drugs used to prevent, diagnose, and treat disease.

pharyngeal tonsil One of two collections of aggregated lymphoid nodules on the posterior wall of the nasopharynx.

pharyngitis Inflammation or infection of the pharynx.

phase 0 The rapid depolarization phase; it represents the rapid upstroke of the action potential that occurs when the cell membrane reaches the threshold potential (approximately -70 mV).

phase 1 The early rapid repolarization phase; the phase in which the fast sodium channels close, the flow of sodium ions into the cell terminates, and the loss of potassium from the cell continues.

phase 2 The plateau phase; the prolonged phase of slow repolarization of the action potential.

phase 3 The terminal phase of rapid repolarization; it results in the inside of the cell becoming considerably negative and the membrane potential returning to approximately -90 mV, or its resting level.

phase 4 The period between action potentials when the membrane has returned to its resting membrane potential.

phencyclidine psychosis A true psychiatric emergency with clinical syndromes ranging from a catatonic and unresponsive state to bizarre and violent behavior; it may occur after a single low-dose exposure to phencyclidine and may last several days to weeks.

phimosis Tightness of the prepuce (foreskin) of the penis of an uncircumcised male.

phlebitis Inflammation of a vein, often accompanied by formation of a clot; also known as *thrombophlebitis.*

phlebotomy The incision or puncture of a vein for allowing the collection of blood.

phobia An anxiety disorder characterized by an obsessive, irrational, and intense fear of a specific object or activity.

phonation The production of speech sounds.

phosgene A poisonous gas that appears as a grayish white cloud and smells of newly mowed hay.

phospholipid One of a class of compounds, widely distributed in living cells, that contains phosphoric acid, fatty acids, and a nitrogenous base.

photophobia Abnormal sensitivity to light.

phrenic nerve A nerve comprised mostly of motor nerve fibers that produce contractions of the diaphragm; also provides sensory innervation for many components of the mediastinum and pleura.

physical abuse The use of physical force that may result in bodily injury, physical pain, or impairment.

physical dependence An adaptive physiological state that occurs after prolonged use of many drugs; discontinuation causes withdrawal syndromes that are relieved by readministering the same drug or a pharmacologically related drug.

physical examination An assessment of a patient that includes examination techniques, measurement of vital signs, an assessment of height and weight, and the skillful use of examination equipment.

physiological dead space The sum of the anatomical dead space plus the volume of any nonfunctional alveoli.

pia mater The innermost layer of the meninges that directly covers the brain.

Pick's disease A rare neurodegenerative disease associated with the shrinking of the frontal and temporal anterior lobes of the brain.

pickwickian syndrome An abnormal condition characterized by obesity, decreased pulmonary function, somnolence, and polycythemia.

pigmented retina The pigmented portion of the retina.

piloerection Erection of the hairs of the skin in response to cold environment, emotional stimulus, or irritation of the skin.

pineal gland A cone-shaped structure in the brain that secretes the hormone melatonin.

pinna See *auricle*.

piriformis syndrome A neuromuscular disorder associated with irritation or compression of the sciatic nerve.

pitting edema Observable indentation of body tissues that persists after applying pressure to an area swollen from fluid accumulation.

pituitary gland A small gland attached to the hypothalamus; it supplies numerous hormones that govern many vital processes.

pivot joint A joint that consists of a relatively cylindrical bony process that rotates within a ring composed partly of bone and partly of ligament.

placards Four-sided, diamond-shaped signs displayed on hazardous materials containers that usually are yellow, orange, white, or green. They have a four-digit United Nations identification number and a legend to indicate the contents of the container.

placebo An inactive substance or a less than effective dose of a harmless substance; it is used in experimental drug studies to compare the effects of the inactive substance with those of the experimental drug.

placenta A highly vascular fetal-maternal organ through which the fetus absorbs oxygen, nutrients, and other substances and excretes carbon dioxide and other wastes.

placenta previa A condition of pregnancy in which the placenta is implanted abnormally in the uterus so that it impinges on or covers the internal os of the uterine cervix.

placental barrier A protective biological membrane that separates the blood vessels of the mother and the fetus.

plague A disease caused by the bacteria *Yersinia pestis,* found in rodents (e.g., chipmunks, prairie dogs, ground squirrels, and mice) and their fleas in many areas around the world.

plane joint A joint that consists of two opposed flat surfaces that are approximately equal in size; also known as a *gliding joint.*

plasma The fluid portion of blood.

plasma membrane The outer covering of a cell that contains the cellular cytoplasm; also known as the cell membrane.

plasma-protein binding A type of drug reservoir in which drugs attach to proteins, mainly albumin, and form a drug-protein complex.

plateau phase Prolongation of the depolarization phase of the cardiac muscle cell membrane; it results in a prolonged refractory period.

platelet A fragment of a cell; it contains granules in the central part and clear protoplasm peripherally but has no definite nucleus.

platelet plug A plug consisting of a mass of linked platelets that seals an injured vessel; part of the clotting cascade.

pleural cavity The area of the body that surrounds the lungs.

pleural fluid Serous fluid found in the pleural cavity; it helps to reduce friction when the pleural membranes rub together.

pleural friction rub A rubbing or grating sound that occurs as one layer of the pleural membrane slides over the other during breathing.

pleural lavage A rewarming technique that uses warm saline to irrigate the thorax; it is used to treat some patients with severe hypothermia.

pleural space The potential space between the visceral and parietal layers of the pleura.

pleurisy Inflammation of the parietal pleura of the lungs, characterized by dyspnea and stabbing chest pain.

plexus A network of intersecting nerves and blood vessels or lymphatic vessels.

pneumatic antishock garment A garment used to manage some forms of hypovolemia and to stabilize some fractures.

pneumococcus A gram-positive diplococcal bacterium of the species *Diplococcus pneumoniae;* the most common cause of bacterial pneumonia.

***Pneumocystis carinii* pneumonia** A bacterial pneumonia caused by infection with the parasite *Pneumocystis carinii;* it usually is seen in infants or debilitated or immunosuppressed persons and is characterized by fever, cough, tachypnea, and, frequently, cyanosis.

pneumohemothorax A collection of air and blood in the pleural space; also known as a *hemopneumothorax.*

pneumomediastinum The presence of air or gas in the mediastinal tissues.

pneumonia An acute inflammation of the lungs, usually caused by inhaled pneumococci of the species *Streptococcus pneumoniae.*

pneumopericardium The presence of air or gas in the pericardial cavity.

pneumoperitoneum The presence of air or gas within the peritoneal cavity of the abdomen.

pneumotaxic center A group of neurons in the pons that have an inhibitory effect on the inspiratory center.

pneumothorax A collection of air or gas in the pleural space that causes the lung to collapse.

poikilothermy Variation in body temperature according to the ambient temperature.

point of maximum impulse The location or area where the apical pulse is palpated the strongest, often in the fifth intercostal space of the thorax just medial to the left midclavicular line.

point-to-point movements Refers to methods used to evaluate a patient's coordination.

poison Any substance that produces harmful physiological or psychological effects.

polio See *poliomyelitis*.

poliomyelitis An infectious disease caused by one of three polio viruses; asymptomatic, mild, and paralytic forms of the disease occur.

poliovirus hominis The causative organism of poliomyelitis.

polyarthritis Inflammation of several joints.

polycythemia A condition characterized by an unusually large number of red cells in the blood as a result of their increased production by the bone marrow.

polydipsia Excessive thirst.

polymorphic Occurring in many forms.

polymyositis Slow, but progressive muscle weakness that affects skeletal muscle on both sides of the body.

polyp A small, tumorlike growth that projects from a mucous membrane surface.

polyphagia Excessive eating.

polysaccharide A carbohydrate that contains three or more molecules of simple carbohydrates.

polyuria Excessive secretion of urine.

pons The part of the brainstem between the medulla and the midbrain.

portal hypertension An increased venous pressure in the portal circulation caused by compression or by occlusion in the portal or hepatic vascular system.

portal of entry The means by which a pathogenic agent enters a new host.

portal of exit The method by which a pathogenic agent leaves one host to invade another.

portal vein A vein that ramifies like an artery in the liver and ends in capillary-like sinusoids that convey the blood to the inferior vena cava through the hepatic veins.

positive end-expiratory pressure Airway support that maintains a degree of positive pressure at the end of exhalation.

postcapillary sphincter The smooth muscle sphincter at the venous end of a capillary that regulates blood flow through the capillary.

posterior The back, or dorsal, surface.

posterior cerebral artery The artery that supplies the posterior portion of the cerebrum.

posterior chamber of the eye The chamber of the eye between the iris and the lens.

posterior communicating artery The artery that branches off each internal carotid artery and connects with the ipsilateral posterior cerebral artery.

posterior superior iliac spine One of two bony segments that form the iliac crest.

postictal phase The phase that usually follows a seizure in which the person is drowsy and lethargic.

postpartum The maternal period after delivery.

postpartum hemorrhage Blood loss of more than 500 mL after delivery of the newborn.

postrenal disease Refers to diseases that block the system that collects urine; usually caused by urinary tract obstruction.

postsynaptic neuron The membrane of a nerve that is in close association with a presynaptic terminal.

posttraumatic syndrome An anxiety reaction to a severe psychosocial event; also known as posttraumatic stress disorder.

postural maintenance The result of muscle tone responsible for keeping the back and legs straight, the head in an upright position, and the abdomen from bulging; also balances the distribution of body weight.

potassium ion The predominant intracellular cation; it helps to regulate neuromuscular excitability and muscle contraction.

potassium-sparing agent A group of medications that promote sodium and water loss without an accompanying loss of potassium.

potential difference The difference in electrical potential, measured as the charge difference across the cell membrane.

potentiation Enhancement of the effect of a drug, caused by concurrent administration of two drugs in which one drug increases the effect of the other.

pound A unit of measure equal to 16 oz, or 0.45359 kg.

P-R interval The time elapsing between the beginning of the P wave and the beginning of the QRS complex in the electrocardiogram.

precapillary sphincter The smooth muscle sphincter at the arterial end of a capillary that regulates blood flow through the capillary.

precipitous delivery A rapid, spontaneous delivery of less than 3 hours from onset of labor to birth; it results from overactive uterine contractions and little maternal soft tissue or bony resistance. Childbirth that occurs with such speed that usual preparations cannot be made.

precordial thump A cardiopulmonary resuscitation technique used to restore circulation in monitored ventricular fibrillation or unstable ventricular tachycardia.

preeclampsia An abnormal disease of pregnancy characterized by the onset of acute hypertension after 24 weeks' gestation.

pregravid Before pregnancy.

preload The amount of blood returning to the ventricle.

premature atrial complex A cardiac dysrhythmia characterized by an atrial beat occurring before the expected excitation and indicated on the electrocardiogram as an early P wave.

premature birth Refers to an infant who is born before 37 weeks' gestation.

premature junctional complex A cardiac dysrhythmia that occurs during sinus rhythm earlier than the next expected sinus beat and is caused by premature discharge of an ectopic focus in the atrioventricular junctional tissue.

premature rupture of membranes Rupture of the amniotic sac before the onset of labor, regardless of gestational age.

premature ventricular complex A cardiac dysrhythmia characterized by a ventricular beat preceding the expected electrical impulse and indicated on the electrocardiogram as an early, wide QRS complex without a preceding related P wave.

prenatal Existing or occurring before birth.

prepuce In males, the free fold of skin that covers the glans penis; the foreskin. In females, the external fold of the labia minora that covers the clitoris.

prerenal disease Refers to diseases that compromise renal perfusion.

preschooler A child 3 to 5 years of age.

present illness Identification of the chief complaint and a full, clear, chronological account of the symptoms.

presenting part The part of the fetus that lies closest to the internal os of the cervix.

presenting the patient The effective communication and transfer of patient information in the course of out-of-hospital and hospital care.

pressure gradient The force produced by differences between atmospheric pressure, intrapulmonic pressure, and intrathoracic pressure.

pressure ulcers Sores or ulcers in the skin over a bony prominence that occur most frequently on the sacrum, elbows, heels, outer ankles, inner knees, hips, and shoulder blades of high-risk patients, especially those who are obese, elderly, or suffering from chronic diseases, infections, injuries, or a poor nutritional state.

presynaptic neuron The nerve terminal that contains neurotransmitter vesicles.

presynaptic terminal The enlarged axon terminal.

preterm infant An infant born before 37 weeks' gestation.

priapism Painful, persistent erection of the penis.

primary bronchus One of the two tubes arising at the inferior end of the trachea; each primary bronchus extends into one of the lungs.

primary contamination Exposure to a hazardous substance that is harmful only to the person exposed and that poses little risk of exposure to others.

primary epilepsy Epilepsy for which the cause is unknown; also known as *idiopathic epilepsy.*

primary follicle The ovarian follicle that contains the primary oocyte.

primary injury prevention The practice of preventing the occurrence of an injury.

primary oocyte The oocyte before the first meiotic division.

primary polycythemia A rare disorder of the bone marrow where an increased production of RBCs causes the blood to thicken; also known as *polycythemia vera.*

primary pulmonary hypertension Abnormally high pressure within the pulmonary circulation.

primary survey A component of the patient assessment to recognize and manage all immediate life-threatening conditions.

primary tumor A malignant tumor in the original site where it first arose.

prime mover A muscle that plays a major role in accomplishing movement.

primigravida A woman who is pregnant for the first time.

primipara A woman who has given birth only one time.

Prinzmetal's angina An atypical form of angina that occurs at rest rather than with effort; it is associated with gross ST segment elevation in the electrocardiogram that disappears when the pain subsides.

priority patients Patients who need immediate care and transport.

private space A comfortable distance from the patient's body; usually about 4 to 5 feet or twice the patient's arm length away (also known as *personal space*).

proarrhythmia A new or worsened rhythm disturbance seemingly generated by antidysrhythmic therapy.

prodromal stage The early period of labor before uterine contractions become forceful and frequent enough to result in progressive dilation of the uterine cervix.

progesterone A steroid sex hormone prescribed to treat various menstrual disorders, functional uterine bleeding, and repeated spontaneous abortions.

progestin Any group of hormones secreted by the corpus luteum, placenta, or adrenal cortex that have a progesterone-like effect on the uterus.

prokaryote A cell without a true nucleus and with nuclear material scattered throughout the cytoplasm.

prolapsed umbilical cord An umbilical cord that protrudes beside or ahead of the presenting part of the fetus.

proliferative phase The time between the end of menses and ovulation characterized by rapid division of endometrial cells and the development of follicles in the ovary.

pronation Rotation of the forearm so that the anterior surface is down.

pronator drift test A test to evaluate balance and upper extremity weakness; performed by having the patient close the eyes and hold both arms out from the body.

prone The position in which the patient is lying on the stomach (face down).

proprietary name See *trade name.*

proprioception Information about the position of the body and its various parts.

prostaglandin A class of naturally occurring fatty acids that affect body functions such as vasodilation, stimulation and contraction of uterine smooth muscle, and promotion of inflammation and pain.

prostate gland The gland that lies just below the male bladder; it secretes one of the components of semen.

prostatic hypertrophy Hypertrophy or enlargement of the prostate gland.

prostatitis Acute or chronic inflammation of the prostate gland.

prosthesis An artificial replacement for a missing part of the body, such as an artificial limb.

protein Any of a large group of naturally occurring, complex, organic nitrogen compounds.

prothrombin A chemical that is part of the clotting cascade; the precursor of thrombin.

prothrombin activator A substance that combines with an enzyme to increase its catalytic activity; converts prothrombin to thrombin.

protoplasm The living substance of a cell.

protraction Movement in the anterior direction.

pseudoaneurysm A condition resembling an aneurysm, caused by enlargement and tortuosity of a vessel.

pseudogout Inflammation caused by calcium pyrophosphate (CPP) crystals; often clinically indistinguishable from gout.

pseudomembranous colitis A life-threatening form of diarrhea caused by *Clostridium difficile.*

psoas muscle A long muscle originating from the transverse processes of the lumbar vertebrae and the fibrocartilage and sides of the vertebral bodies of the lower thoracic vertebrae and the lumbar vertebrae.

psoriasis A common, chronic, inheritable skin disorder characterized by circumscribed red patches covered by thick, dry, adherent scales that result from excessive development of epithelial cells.

psychological dependence Emotional reliance on a drug; manifestations range from a mild desire for a drug to craving and drug-seeking behavior to repeated compulsive use of a drug for its subjectively satisfying or pleasurable effects.

psychology The science or study of behavior.

psychomotor seizure A seizure manifested by impaired consciousness of variable degree; the patient carries out a series of coordinated acts that are inappropriate, bizarre, and serve no useful purpose, about which the patient is amnesic.

psychosis Maladaptive behavior involving major distortions of reality.

puberty The period of life when the ability to reproduce begins.

pubic lice Tiny parasites that concentrate in the pubic area.

pubis One of a pair of pubic bones that, with the ischium and the ilium, form the hipbone and join the pubic bone from the opposite side at the pubic symphysis.

public duty doctrine or rule The provision that a public official is generally not liable to individuals for his or her negligence in discharging public duties.

public service answering point A communications center that coordinates the deployment of emergency personnel and other resources required for an emergence response.

pulmonary artery The artery that carries deoxygenated blood from the right ventricle into the lung.

pulmonary capacity The sum of two or more pulmonary volumes.

pulmonary contusion Bruising of the lung tissue that results in rupture of the alveoli and interstitial edema.

pulmonary edema The accumulation of extravascular fluid in lung tissues and alveoli.

pulmonary embolism The blockage of a pulmonary artery by foreign matter such as fat, air, tumor tissue, or a thrombus that usually arises from a peripheral vein.

pulmonary hypertension A condition of abnormally high pressure within the pulmonary circulation.

pulmonary overpressurization syndrome A condition that results from expansion of trapped air in the lungs; it may lead to alveolar rupture and extravasation of air into extraalveolar locations.

pulmonary respiration The exchange of gases between the cells of the body and the outside environment.

pulmonary semilunar valve A valve that guards the orifice between the right ventricle and the pulmonary artery.

pulmonary surfactant Certain lipoproteins that reduce the surface tension of pulmonary fluids, allowing the exchange of gases in the alveoli of the lungs and contributing to the elasticity of pulmonary tissue.

pulmonary trunk The large elastic artery that carries blood from the right ventricle of the heart to the right and left pulmonary arteries.

pulmonary vein Any vein that carries oxygenated blood from the lung to the left atrium.

pulmonary ventilation The movement of air in and out of the lungs. This process brings oxygen into the lungs and removes carbon dioxide.

pulmonic pressure Pressure generated by the right side of the heart.

pulp The soft, spongy chamber of the tooth.

pulse deficit A condition that exists when the radial pulse is less than the ventricular rate; it indicates a lack of peripheral perfusion.

pulse pressure The difference between the systolic and diastolic blood pressures.

pulsus paradoxus An abnormal decrease in systolic blood pressure that drops more than 10 to 15 mm Hg during inspiration compared with expiration.

punctate Spotted; marked with points of puncture.

punctum The opening of each lacrimal canal.

puncture wound An open injury that results from contact with a penetrating object.

pupil The opening in the center of the iris that regulates the amount of light entering the eye.

purified protein derivative A dried form of tuberculin used in testing for past or present infection with tubercle bacilli.

Purkinje fibers Myocardial fibers that are a continuation of the bundle of His and that extend into the muscle walls of the ventricles.

pustule A small, circumscribed elevation of skin containing fluid, which is usually purulent.

pyelolithotomy Removal of a stone from a kidney by surgical incision.

pyelonephritis An inflammation of the kidney parenchyma associated with microbial infection.

pyloric sphincter A thickened, muscular ring in the stomach that separates the pylorus from the duodenum.

pyorrhea Discharge of pus.

pyrogen Any substance or agent that tends to cause a rise in body temperature.

pyrogenic A substance or agent that produces fever.

pyruvate The end product of glycolysis; it may be metabolized to lactate or acetyl coenzyme A.

QRS complex The principal deflection in the electrocardiogram, representing ventricular depolarization.

Q-T interval The time elapsing from the beginning of the QRS complex to the end of the T wave, representing the total duration of electrical activity of the ventricles.

quadriplegia A weakness or paralysis of all four extremities and the trunk.

R prime A subsequent positive deflection in the QRS complex that extends above the baseline and that is taller than the first R wave.

rabies An acute, usually fatal viral disease of the central nervous system of animals; it is transmitted from animals to human beings by infected blood, tissue, or, most commonly, saliva.

raccoon's eyes Ecchymosis of one or both orbits caused by fracture of the base of the sphenoid sinus.

radial tuberosity A large, oblong elevation at the distal end of the radius.

radioulnar syndesmosis The articulation of the radius and ulna, consisting of a proximal articulation, a distal articulation, and three sets of ligaments.

radius One of the bones of the forearm, lying parallel to the ulna.

range The general perimeter of communications coverage, beyond which coverage is nonexistent or severely degraded to an unusable level; it is measured in miles.

rape Nonconsensual sex, or an attempt to force another person to have sex against his or her will; includes intercourse in the vagina, anus, or mouth.

rapid sequence intubation An airway management technique that involves the virtually simultaneous administration of a potent sedative agent and a neuromuscular blocking agent for the purpose of endotracheal intubation; it provides optimal intubation conditions while minimizing the risk of aspiration of gastric contents.

rappelling A method of descent that involves lowering oneself with a rope.

Raynaud's phenomenon A condition in which cold temperatures or strong emotions cause blood vessel spasms that block blood flow to the fingers, toes, ears, and nose.

reabsorption The process of absorbing again that occurs in the kidneys.

reactive airway disease An inflammatory airway condition that develops as a reaction to an antigen.

reactive hyperemia Increased blood flow associated with increased metabolic activity.

reactivity The ability of a chemical to interact with other chemicals and body tissue.

reassessment The ongoing assessment that follows the paramedic's initial evaluation of the patient.

rebound tenderness A sign of peritoneal inflammation in which pain is caused by the sudden release of fingertip pressure on the abdomen.

receptor molecule A reactive site on the cell surface or within the cell that combines with a drug molecule to produce a biological effect.

reciprocal socialization A term that refers to a child's temperament and the responses it obtains from adults and family members. This interaction forms the basis for early social interactions with others and with the child's environment.

reciprocity The practice of granting an individual licensure or certification/registration based on licensure or certification/registration by another state, agency, or association.

rectal abscess An infected pus-filled cavity near the anus.

rectum The segment of the large intestine continuous with the descending sigmoid colon just proximal to the anal canal.

rectus femoris muscle A muscle of the anterior thigh; one of the four parts of the quadriceps femoris.

red marrow Specialized soft tissue found in many bones of infants and children, in the spongy bone of the proximal epiphyses of the humerus and femur, and in the sternum, ribs, and vertebral bodies of adults. It is essential in the manufacture of red blood cells.

red measles See *rubeola*.

reentry The reactivation of tissue by a returning impulse; the sustaining mechanism in some cases of ventricular bigeminy or trigeminy, ventricular tachycardia, and paroxysmal supraventricular tachycardia.

referred pain Visceral pain felt at a site distant from its origin.

reflection on action A component of critical thinking (usually performed after the event) in which the examiner evaluates a patient care episode for possible improvement in similar future responses.

reflex An automatic response to a stimulus that occurs without conscious thought; produced by a reflex arc.

reflex arc The smallest portion of the nervous system capable of receiving a stimulus and producing a response.

refractory period The period after effective stimulation during which excitable tissue fails to respond to a stimulus of threshold intensity.

refractory shock Shock that is resistant to treatment but is still reversible.

relative hypovolemia Inadequate preload as a result of vasodilation.

relative refractory period The portion of the action potential after the absolute refractory period during which another action potential can be produced with a greater than threshold stimulus strength.

renal calculus Kidney stone.

renal calyx The first unit in the system of the ducts of the kidney carrying urine from the renal pyramid of the cortex to the renal pelvis for excretion through the ureters.

renal capsule The cortical substance that separates the renal pyramids.

renal corpuscle The glomerulus and its enclosing Bowman's capsule.

renal cortex The outer layer of the kidney, which contains approximately 1.25 million renal tubules, which remove body waste in the form of urine.

renal failure Inability of the kidneys to secrete wastes, concentrate urine, and conserve electrolytes; it may be chronic or acute.

renal medulla The inner layer of the kidney.

renal papilla The apex of the renal pyramid.

renal pelvis The funnel-shaped expansion of the upper end of the ureter that receives the calyces.

renal pyramid One of a number of pyramidal masses seen on longitudinal section of the kidney; it contains part of the loop of Henle and the collecting tubules.

renal tubule One of the collecting tubules in the kidney.

renin A proteolytic enzyme that surrounds each arteriole as it enters a glomerulus; it affects blood pressure by catalyzing the change of angiotensin I to angiotensin II.

renin-angiotensin-aldosterone mechanism Renin, released from the kidneys in response to low blood pressure, converts angiotensinogen to angiotensin I. Angiotensin I is converted by angiotensin-converting enzyme to angiotensin II, which causes vasoconstriction, resulting in increased blood pressure. Angiotensin II also increases aldosterone secretion, which increases blood pressure by increasing blood volume.

repolarization The phase of the action potential in which the membrane potential moves from its maximum degree of depolarization toward the value of the resting membrane potential.

reposition To move a structure to its original position.

reproductive maturity The time at which a person has attained the ability to reproduce.

rescue The act of delivery from danger or imprisonment.

reservoir Any person, animal, plant, soil, or substance in which an infectious agent normally lives and multiplies; typically harbors the infectious agent without injury to itself and serves as a source from which other individuals can be infected.

residual volume The volume of air remaining in the lungs after a maximum expiratory effort.

resistance The immune status of the host; the ability to ward off infection.

respiration The process of the molecular change of oxygen and carbon dioxide within the body's tissues.

respiratory acidosis An abnormal condition characterized by increased arterial PCO_2, excess carbonic acid, and increased plasma hydrogen ion concentration.

respiratory alkalosis An abnormal condition characterized by decreased PCO_2, decreased hydrogen ion concentration, and increased blood pH.

respiratory bronchiole The smallest bronchiole that connects the terminal bronchiole to the alveolar duct.

respiratory membrane The membrane in the lungs across which gas exchange occurs with the blood.

respiratory syncytial virus A single-strand virus that is a common cause of epidemics of acute bronchiolitis, bronchopneumonia, and the common cold in young children and sporadic acute bronchitis and mild upper respiratory tract infections in adults.

resting membrane potential The electrical charge difference inside a cell membrane measured relative to that just outside the cell membrane.

reticular activating system A functional system in the brain essential for wakefulness, attention, concentration, and introspection.

reticular Relating to a fine network of cells or collagen fibers.

reticular formation A small, thick cluster of neurons nestled within the brainstem that controls breathing, the heartbeat, blood pressure, level of consciousness, and other vital functions.

reticuloendothelial system Part of the immune system; it is composed of immune cells in the spleen, lymph nodes, liver, bone marrow, lungs, and intestines; stores mature B and T cells until the immune system is activated.

retina The nervous tunic of the eye; it is continuous with the optic nerve.

retinal detachment A separation of the light-sensitive retina from its supporting layers.

retinopathy A group of inflammatory eye disorders often caused by diabetes, hypertension, and atherosclerotic vascular disease.

retraction Movement in the posterior direction.

retrograde amnesia The loss of memory for events that occurred before the event that precipitated the amnesia.

retroperitoneal Of or pertaining to the organs closely attached to the abdominal wall and partly covered by peritoneum.

retroperitoneum Behind the peritoneum.

retrovirus Any of a family of viruses that converts genetic RNA to DNA after entering the host cell.

Revised Trauma Score An injury severity index that uses the Glasgow Coma Scale and measurements for systolic blood pressure and respiratory rate.

Reye's syndrome A combination of acute encephalopathy and fatty infiltration of the internal organs that may follow acute viral infections.

Rh factor An antigenic substance present in the erythrocytes of most persons; a person lacking the Rh factor is Rh negative.

rhabdomyolysis An acute, sometimes fatal disease characterized by destruction of skeletal muscle.

rheumatic fever An inflammatory disease that may develop as a delayed reaction to streptococcal infection of the upper respiratory tract.

rheumatoid arthritis A chronic, sometimes deforming destructive collagen disease that has an autoimmune component.

rheumatoid lungs Rheumatoid arthritis with emphasis on nonarticular changes; for example, pulmonary interstitial fibrosis, pleural effusion, and lung nodules.

rhinitis Inflammation of the mucous membranes of the nose.

rhinorrhea The free discharge of watery nasal fluid.

rhonchi Abnormal sounds heard on auscultation of a respiratory airway obstructed by thick secretions, muscular spasm, neoplasm, or external pressure.

rib One of the 12 pairs of elastic arches of bone forming a large part of the thoracic skeleton. The first seven ribs on each side are called *true ribs* because they articulate directly with the sternum. The remaining five ribs are called *false ribs;* the first three attach ventrally to the ribs, and the last two ribs are free at their ventral extremities and are called *floating ribs.*

ribonucleic acid A nucleic acid found in the nucleus and the cytoplasm of cells that transmits genetic instructions from the nucleus to the cytoplasm. In the cytoplasm, RNA functions in the assembly of proteins.

ribosome The "factory" of a cell where protein is synthesized.

ricin A potent protein cytotoxin derived from the beans of the castor plant *(Ricinus communis).*

right atrium One of the four chambers of the human heart; receives deoxygenated blood from the body through the vena cava and pumps it into the right ventricle.

right lymphatic duct A vessel that conveys lymph from the right upper quadrant of the body into the bloodstream in the neck at the junction of the right internal jugular and the right subclavian veins.

rigor mortis The rigid stiffening of skeletal and cardiac muscle shortly after death.

riot control agents Chemicals that can produce sensory irritation or disabling physical effects that disappear within a short time after termination of exposure.

Rocky Mountain spotted fever A serious tick-borne infectious disease characterized by chills, fever, severe headache, mental confusion, and rash.

rod A photoreceptor in the retina of the eye; it is responsible for noncolor vision in low-intensity light.

Romberg's test A test to evaluate stance and balance; performed by having the patient stand erect with the feet together and arms at the sides.

R-on-T phenomenon The occurrence of a ventricular depolarization during a vulnerable period of relative refractoriness.

root The lowest part of the tooth; it is covered by cementum.

rooting reflex A normal infant response elicited by touching or stroking the side of the cheek or mouth; this causes the infant to turn the head toward the stimulated side and to begin to suck.

rotation Movement of a structure about its axis.

rouleau formation An aggregation of red cells in what looks like a stack of coins or checkers.

round ligament The remains of the umbilical vein.

rubella A contagious viral disease characterized by fever, symptoms of mild upper respiratory tract infection, lymph node enlargement, and a diffuse, fine, red maculopapular rash; it is spread by droplet infection; also known as *German measles.*

rubeola An acute, highly contagious viral disease involving the respiratory tract; it is characterized by a spreading, maculopapular, cutaneous rash and occurs primarily in young children who have not been immunized; also known as *red measles.*

rule of nines A method to estimate burn injury that divides the total body surface area into segments that are multiples of 9%.

rupture of membranes Rupture of the amniotic sac; it usually occurs toward the end of the first stage of labor.

ruptured diaphragm A tear or break in the diaphragm, usually as a result of injury.

ruptured ovarian cyst A ruptured globular sac filled with fluid or semisolid material that develops in or on the ovary.

S prime A subsequent negative deflection in the QRS complex that extends below the baseline.

sacral bone A bone composed of the five segments of the vertebral column that are fused in the adult to form the sacrum; the segments are designated S1 to S5.

sacral promontory The projecting portion of the pelvis at the base of the sacrum.

sacral sparing The preservation of sensory or voluntary motor function of the perineum, buttocks, scrotum, or anus.

sacrum The large, triangular bone at the dorsal part of the pelvis; it is inserted like a wedge between the two hipbones.

saddle joint A joint that consists of two saddle-shaped articulating surfaces oriented at right angles to each other.

safe holding area An area away from the emergency scene that provides for safety.

sagittal plane An imaginary plane that runs vertically through the middle of the body, producing right and left sections.

salicylate Any one of several widely prescribed drugs derived from salicylic acid (e.g., aspirin).

salivary amylase A digestive enzyme found in saliva that begins the chemical digestion of carbohydrates.

salivary gland One of the three pairs of glands that empty their secretions into the mouth, thus aiding the digestive process.

salpingitis An inflammation or infection of the fallopian tube.

saltatory conduction Conduction in which action potentials jump from one node of Ranvier to the next node of Ranvier.

saphenous vein One of a pair of the longest veins in the body; it begins in the medial marginal vein in the dorsum of the foot and ends in the femoral vein.

sarcoidosis A chronic disorder of unknown origin characterized by the formation of lesions in the lung, spleen, liver, skin, and mucous membranes and in the lacrimal and salivary glands.

sarcolemma Part of a myofibril between adjacent Z lines.

sarcomere The contractile unit of skeletal muscle, which contains thick and thin myofilaments.

sarcoplasmic reticulum Endoplasmic reticulum of the muscle.

sarin A clear, colorless, and tasteless liquid that has no odor in its pure form; may be used as a nerve agent.

scabies A contagious parasitic skin infection characterized by superficial burrows and intense pruritus; caused by the mite *Sarcoptes scabiei.*

scanning A component of attention that refers to one's ability to review a large amount of sensory input rapidly. Different individuals have different capacities for scanning and may use various approaches and styles in their scanning.

scapula One of the pair of large, flat triangular bones that form the dorsal part of the shoulder girdle.

scene size-up An assessment of the scene to ensure scene safety for the paramedic crew, patient(s), and bystanders; a quick assessment to determine the resources needed to manage the scene adequately.

schizophrenia A group of disorders characterized by recurrent episodes of psychotic behavior.

school age Children 6 to 12 years of age.

Schwann cell A cell that forms a myelin sheath around each nerve fiber of the peripheral nervous system.

sciatic nerve A long nerve that originates in the sacral plexus and extends through the muscles of the thigh, leg, and foot with numerous branches.

sciatica Inflammation of the sciatic nerve.

sclera The opaque membrane covering the eyeball.

scleroderma A collagen vascular disease thought to result from the immune system stimulating certain cells (fibroblasts) that cause an increased production of collagen.

scoliosis A lateral curvature of the spine.

scrambling Movement over rough terrain that is not steep enough to require the use of a rope.

scrotum The sac of skin that contains the testes.

sebaceous gland A gland of the skin, usually associated with a hair follicle that produces sebum.

sebum The secretion of sebaceous glands; it prevents drying and protects against some bacteria.

second stage of labor The stage of labor measured from full dilation of the cervix to delivery of the newborn.

secondary assessment Consists of physical examination techniques, measurement of vital signs, an assessment of body systems, and the skillful use of examination equipment.

secondary bronchus A branch from a primary bronchus that conducts air to each lobe of the lungs.

secondary contamination Exposure to a hazardous substance whereby liquid and particulate substances are transferred easily to others by touching.

secondary epilepsy Epilepsy that can be traced to trauma, infection, a cerebrovascular disorder, or another illness that contributes to or causes the seizure disorder.

secondary follicle The follicle in which the secondary oocyte is surrounded by granulosa cells.

secondary polycythemia A condition of increased production of RBCs caused by reduced air pressure and low oxygen; may be a natural response to chronic hypoxia.

secondary tumor A malignant tumor that originates in one area of the body and spreads to another area of the body.

second-degree burn A burn injury that extends through the epidermis to the dermis (superficial partial thickness); it is considered a deep partial-thickness injury if it extends to the basal layers of the skin.

secretin The hormone that stimulates secretion of pancreatic juice.

secretion A general term for a substance produced inside a cell and released from the cell.

secretory phase The portion of the menstrual cycle extending from the time of formation of the corpus luteum after ovulation to the time when menstrual flow begins.

sedative-hypnotic A drug that reversibly depresses the activity of the central nervous system; these drugs are used chiefly to induce sleep and relieve anxiety.

seizure A temporary alteration in behavior or consciousness caused by abnormal electrical activity of one or more groups of neurons in the brain.

selectivity A component of attention that refers to a person's ability to pick or choose specific components of the sensory input that the person is reviewing and then focus on that input.

self-concept The accumulation of knowledge about one's self, including beliefs regarding personality traits, physical characteristics, abilities, values, goals, and roles.

self-contained breathing apparatus A respiratory protection device that provides an enclosed system of air.

self-esteem A person's overall evaluation or appraisal of his or her own worth.

self-neglect A type of elder abuse; behaviors of an older adult that intentionally threaten personal health or safety.

Sellick maneuver Cricoid cartilage pressure directed posteriorly to compress the trachea against the cervical vertebrae, thereby occluding the esophagus; this maneuver is useful for limiting the risk of aspiration during an intubation procedure.

semen Male reproductive fluid.

semicircular canal A structure located in the inner ear that generates a nerve impulse when the head moves.

semi-Fowler position An inclined position with the upper half of the body raised by elevating the head of the bed or stretcher about 30 degrees to prevent reflux of gastric contents.

semilunar valve A valve with a half-moon shape, such as the aortic valve and the pulmonary valve.

seminal vesicle One of two glandular structures that empty into the ejaculatory ducts; its secretion is one of the components of semen.

semipermeable membranes A membrane that allows some fluids and substances to pass through it but not others, usually depending on size, shape, electrical charge, or other chemical properties.

senile dementia An organic mental disorder of the aged resulting from generalized atrophy of the brain with no evidence of cerebrovascular disease.

sensitization An acquired reaction in which specific antibodies develop in response to an antigen.

sensory Pertaining to a part or all of the sensory nerve network of the body.

sensory layer The portion of the retina that contains rods and cones; also known as the *sensory retina*.

sensory neuron A neuron that transmits impulses to the spinal cord and brain from all parts of the body.

sensory retina See *sensory layer*.

separation anxiety A normal period during development in which a child experiences anxiety when separated from the primary caregiver.

sepsis Infection.

septic arthritis A condition that results from direct invasion of the joint space by various microorganisms; also known as *infectious arthritis*.

septic shock A form of shock that most often results from a serious systemic bacterial infection.

septicemia Systemic infection in which the pathogens are present in the bloodstream, having spread from an infection in any part of the body.

septum A thin wall dividing two cavities or masses of soft tissue.

serotonin A hormone and neurotransmitter released from platelets when blood vessel walls are damaged.

serotonin syndrome A potentially life-threatening drug reaction; most often occurs when two or more drugs that affect serotonin levels are taken together.

serous membrane One of the many thin sheets of tissue that line closed cavities of the body, such as the pleura lining the thoracic cavity, the peritoneum lining the abdominal cavity, and the pericardium lining the sac that encloses the heart.

serous pericardium The thin inner layer of the pericardium that surrounds the heart.

serum Blood plasma without its clotting factors.

sexual abuse Nonconsensual sexual contact of any kind.

sexual assault The forcible perpetration of an act of sexual contact on the body of another person, male or female, without his or her consent.

sexually transmitted disease Refers to a group infections that are passed from one person to another through sexual contact.

shaken baby syndrome A serious form of child abuse that describes injuries to infants that occur after being violently shaken.

shingles An acute infection caused by reactivation of the latent varicella-zoster virus; it is characterized by painful vesicular eruptions that follow the underlying route of cranial or spinal nerves inflamed by the virus; also known as *herpes zoster*.

shipping papers Descriptions of the hazardous materials that include the substance name, classification, and United Nations identification number.

shock An abnormal condition of inadequate blood flow to the body's peripheral tissues that is associated with life-threatening cellular dysfunction; also known as *hypoperfusion*.

short bones Bones that are approximately as broad as they are long, such as the carpal bones of the wrist and the tarsal bones of the ankle.

shoulder dystocia An obstacle to delivery that occurs when the fetal shoulders press against the maternal symphysis pubis, blocking shoulder delivery.

shoulder girdle The encircling bony structure that supports the upper limbs; also known as the *pectoral girdle*.

shoulder presentation The presentation that results when the long axis of the fetus lies perpendicular to that of the mother; also known as *transverse presentation*.

shunt A tube or device surgically implanted in the body to redirect body fluid from one cavity or vessel to another.

shunting The redirection of a flow of body fluid from one cavity or vessel to another.

sibling rivalry Jealousy or competitiveness between brothers and sisters.

sickle cell anemia An inherited blood disorder that affects red blood cells; the most common type of sickle cell disease.

sickle cell crisis An acute episodic condition that occurs in individuals with sickle cell anemia.

sickle cell disease A debilitating and unpredictable recessive genetic illness that produces an abnormal type of hemoglobin with an inferior oxygen-carrying capacity.

side effect An often unavoidable and undesirable effect of using therapeutic doses of a drug; actions or effects other than those for which the drug was originally given.

sighing An occasional deep, audible inspiration that usually is insignificant.

sigmoid colon The segment of the colon that extends from the end of the descending colon in the pelvis to the juncture with the rectum.

significant medical history A patient's medical background that may offer insight into the patient's current problem.

silicosis A lung disorder caused by continued long-term inhalation of the dust of an inorganic compound, silicon dioxide; the disorder is characterized by dyspnea and the development of nodular fibrosis in the lungs.

simplex mode A communications mode with the ability to transmit or receive in one direction at a time. Simultaneous transmission cannot occur.

sinoatrial node An area of specialized heart tissue that generates the cardiac electrical impulse.

sinus One of several cavities in the bones of the skull that connect to the nasal cavities by small channels.

sinus headache A headache characterized by pain in the forehead, nasal area, and eyes.

sinusitis Inflammation of one or more paranasal sinuses.

sinusoid A form of terminating blood channel, somewhat larger than a capillary, lined with reticuloendothelial cells.

six cardinal fields of gaze A test to evaluate extraocular muscle function; performed by having the patient visually track an object in six visual fields in an H pattern.

size-up See *scene size-up*.

skeletal muscle Muscle tissue that appears microscopically to consist of striped myofibrils; also known as *striated muscle* and *voluntary muscle*.

skeletal system The body system comprised of bones, muscles, tendons and ligaments, and articulating surfaces (e.g., joints, bursa, disks).

Skene's glands The largest of the glands that open into the urethra of women.

skin graft A portion of skin implanted to cover areas where skin has been lost through burns or injury or by surgical removal of diseased tissue.

slander Verbally making false statements to others about a person, knowing that the statements are false, and with malicious intent or reckless disregard for their falsity.

sleep apnea A sleep disorder characterized by periods in which attempts to breathe are absent.

slipped capital femoral epiphysis A separation of the ball of the hip joint from the femur at the upper, growing end (growth plate) of the bone.

slough To shed or cast off; tissue that has been shed.

slow reactive substance of anaphylaxis A bronchoconstrictor mediator released from mast cells; it increases the production of prostaglandins.

small intestine The longest portion of the digestive tract; it is divided into the duodenum, jejunum, and ileum.

smallpox A highly contagious viral disease characterized by fever, prostration, and a vesicular, pustular rash.

smooth muscle One of two kinds of muscle; it is composed of elongated, spindle-shaped cells in muscles not under voluntary control, such as smooth muscle of the intestines, stomach, and other visceral organs; also known as *visceral muscle, involuntary muscle,* and *nonstriated muscle.*

sniffing position The patient position used during orotracheal intubation in which the patient's neck is flexed at C5 and C6 and the head is extended at C1 and C2.

SOAP format A memory aid used to organize written and verbal patient reports; it includes subjective data, objective data, assessment data, and plan of patient management.

sodium bicarbonate An antacid, electrolyte, and urinary alkalinizing agent.

sodium ions Ions involved in acid-base balance, water balance, nerve impulse transmission, and muscle contraction.

sodium-potassium exchange pump The biochemical mechanism that uses energy derived from adenosine triphosphate to achieve the active transport of potassium ions opposite to that of sodium ions.

soft palate The posterior muscular portion of the palate, which forms an incomplete septum between the mouth and the oropharynx and between the oropharynx and the nasopharynx.

solutes Substances dissolved in solution.

soman A clear, colorless, tasteless liquid with a slight camphor odor; may be used as a nerve agent.

somatic nervous system The part of the nervous system composed of nerve fibers that send impulses from the central nervous system to skeletal muscle.

somatic pain Pain that arises from skeletal muscles, ligaments, vessels, or joints.

somatization disorder A condition in which an individual has complaints (lasting several years) of various physical problems for which no physical cause can be found.

somatoform disorder Any of a group of neurotic disorders characterized by symptoms suggesting physical illness or disease for which there are no organic or physiological causes.

somatomotor Referring to cranial nerves that control the skeletal muscles through motor neurons.

somatomotor nerves Motor nerves to the skeletal muscles.

somatomotor neurons Neurons that innervate skeletal muscles.

spasm An involuntary muscle contraction of sudden onset.

spastic colon Abnormally increased motility of the small and large intestines, generally associated with stress; also known as irritable bowel syndrome.

special emergency radio service A specific group of radio frequencies designated by the Federal Communications Commission for use by emergency agencies.

sperm See *spermatozoon*.

spermatic cord A structure that extends from the deep inguinal ring in the abdomen to the testes; each cord comprises arteries, veins, lymphatics, nerves, and the excretory duct of the testis.

spermatogenesis The process of development of spermatozoa.

spermatozoa See *spermatozoon.*

spermatozoon The male sex cell, composed of a head and tail; it contains genetic information transmitted by the male.

sphenoid bone The bone at the base of the skull anterior to the temporal bones and the basilar part of the occipital bone.

sphenoid sinus One of a pair of cavities in the sphenoid bone that are lined with mucous membrane continuous with that of the nasal cavity.

sphincter Ring-shaped muscle.

sphygmomanometer The device used to measure blood pressure.

spina bifida A congenital defect in which part of one or more vertebrae fail to develop completely, leaving a portion of the spinal cord exposed.

spinal cord shock See *neurogenic shock.*

spinal cord tumor A benign or malignant tumor that originates in the cells within or next to the spinal cord.

spinal ganglia The structures that contain the cell bodies of sensory neurons; also known as *dorsal root ganglia.*

spinal nerve One of 31 pairs of nerves formed by the joining of the dorsal and ventral routes that arise from the spinal cord.

spinal shock A temporary loss of all types of spinal cord function distal to a cord injury.

spinal stenosis Narrowing of the spinal canal.

spinous process A part of the vertebrae that projects backward from the vertebral arch, giving attachment to muscles of the back.

spleen A large, highly vascular lymphatic organ situated in the upper part of the abdominal cavity between the stomach and the diaphragm; it responds to foreign substances in the blood, destroys worn-out erythrocytes, and is a storage site for red blood cells.

splenomegaly An abnormal enlargement of the spleen.

spondylosis A condition of the spine characterized by fixation or stiffness of the vertebral joint.

spontaneous abortion An abortion that usually occurs before 12 weeks' gestation; the lay term is *miscarriage.*

spontaneous pneumothorax A condition that results when a subpleural bleb ruptures, allowing air to enter the pleural space from within the lung.

sprain A partial tearing of a ligament caused by a sudden twisting or stretching of a joint beyond its normal range of motion.

sputum Material coughed up from the lungs and expectorated from the mouth.

squelch A radio receiver circuit used to suppress the audio portion of unwanted radio signals or radio noises below a predetermined carrier strength level.

ST segment The early part of repolarization in the electrocardiogram of the right and left ventricles.

ST-segment elevation myocardial infarction (STEMI) Myocardial infarction characterized by ST-segment elevation greater than 1 mm (0.1 mV) in two or more adjacent limb leads or any two contiguous chest leads.

staging area A designated area where incident-assigned vehicles are directed and held until needed.

stance The position of the body while standing.

standing orders Specific treatment protocols used by prehospital emergency care providers in the absence of online (direct) medical direction when delay in treatment would harm the patient.

stapes The smallest of the three ossicles in the middle ear.

staphylococcal infection An infection caused by any one of several pathogenic species of *Staphylococcus,* commonly characterized by the formation of abscesses of the skin or other organs.

starch The principal molecule used for the storage of food energy in plants.

Starling hypothesis The concept that describes the movement of fluid back and forth across the capillary wall (net filtration).

Starling's law of the heart A rule that the force of the heartbeat is determined by the length of the fibers making up the myocardial walls.

stasis A disorder in which the normal flow of fluid through a vessel of the body is slowed or halted.

status asthmaticus A severe, prolonged asthma exacerbation that has not been terminated with repeated doses of bronchodilators.

status epilepticus Continuous seizure activity lasting 30 minutes or longer, or a recurrent seizure without an intervening period of consciousness.

stellate wound A star-shaped wound.

stenosis Abnormal constriction or narrowing of an opening or passageway in a body structure.

sternal angle The point at which the manubrium joins the body of the sternum; also known as the *angle of Louis.*

sternoclavicular joint The double gliding joint between the sternum and the clavicle.

sternomanubrial joint See *sternal angle.*

sternum The elongated, flattened bone forming the middle portion of the thorax.

steroid A member of a large family of lipids, including some reproductive hormones, vitamins, and cholesterol.

steroid hormones Hormones that are synthesized by endocrine cells from cholesterol, including cortisol, aldosterone, estrogen, progesterone, and testosterone.

stimulant A drug that enhances or increases body function or activity.

Stokes-Adams syndrome A condition characterized by sudden episodes of loss of consciousness caused by incomplete heart block; seizures may accompany the episodes.

stoma A surgically created artificial opening of an internal organ on the surface of the body.

stomach The major organ of digestion, located in the right upper quadrant of the abdomen.

strain An injury to the muscle or its tendon from overexertion or overextension.

stratum basale The innermost layer of the epidermis.

stratum corneum The most superficial layer of the epidermis.

stratum granulosum The layer of the epidermis that lies just beneath the stratum corneum except in the palms of the hands and soles of the feet, where it lies just beneath the stratum lucidum.

stratum lucidum The layer of the epidermis that lies just beneath the stratum corneum; it is present only in the thick skin of the palms of the hands and soles of the feet.

stratum spinosum The layer of the epidermis that lies on top of the stratum basale and beneath the stratum granulosum.

strep throat An infection of the throat caused by streptococcal bacteria.

streptococcal infection An infection caused by pathogenic bacteria from one of several species of the genus *Streptococcus* or their toxins.

stress A nonspecific mental or physical strain caused by any emotional, physical, social, economic, or other factor that initiates a physiological response.

stressor Any factor that causes wear and tear on the physical or mental resources of the body.

stretch mark See *stria*.

stria A streak or linear scar that often results from rapidly developing tension in the skin; also known as a *stretch mark*.

striated Having striped or parallel lines, as in skeletal muscle.

striated muscle See *skeletal muscle*.

stridor An abnormal, high-pitched musical sound caused by obstruction in the trachea or larynx.

stroke See *cerebrovascular accident*.

stroke volume The volume of blood ejected from one ventricle in a single heartbeat.

stupor A state of lethargy and unresponsiveness in which a person seems unaware of his or her surroundings.

stylet A thin metal probe for inserting into or passing through a needle, tube, or catheter; it sometimes is used to change the configuration of an endotracheal tube.

styloid process A bony projection.

subarachnoid hematoma A collection of blood or fluid in the subarachnoid space.

subarachnoid hemorrhage Bleeding within the subarachnoid space.

subarachnoid space The area below the arachnoid membrane but above the pia matter that contains cerebrospinal fluid.

subclavian vein The continuation of the axillary vein in the upper body; it extends from the lateral border of the first rib to the sternal end of the clavicle, where it joins the internal jugular to form the brachiocephalic vein.

subcutaneous emphysema The presence of air in the subcutaneous tissues.

subcutaneous injection The introduction of medicine through a hypodermic needle into the subcutaneous tissue beneath the skin.

subcutaneous tissue The adherent layer of adipose tissue just below the dermal layer; also known as the hypodermis.

subdural hematoma A collection of blood in the subdural space.

subdural space The space between the dura mater and arachnoid.

subendocardial infarction See *transmural infarction*.

subgaleal hematoma A collection of blood beneath the strong sheet of fibrous connective tissue that joins the frontal and occipitofrontal muscles.

sublingual route The route of medication administration in which the medication is placed under the tongue so that the tablet dissolves in salivary secretions.

subluxation A partial dislocation.

submersion An incident in which a person experiences some swimming-related distress that is sufficient to require support in the prehospital setting and transportation to a medical facility for further observation and treatment.

substrate A substance acted upon and changed by an enzyme in any chemical reaction.

sucking reflex A normal infant response in which touching the infant's lips with the nipple of a breast or bottle causes involuntary sucking movements.

sudden death A death that occurs within the first 2 hours after the onset of illness or injury.

sudden infant death syndrome The unexpected and sudden death of an apparently normal and healthy infant that occurs during sleep.

sudoriferous gland See *sweat gland*.

suicide The act of a human being intentionally causing his or her own death.

summation The combined effects of two drugs that equal the sum of the individual effects of each agent.

superficial burn A burn injury where only a superficial layer of epidermal cells is destroyed; also known as a *first-degree burn*.

superficial frostbite A cold injury with at least some minimal tissue loss; it usually involves the dermis and shallow subcutaneous layers.

superficial pain Pain that arises from the skin or mucous membrane.

superficial reflexes Reflexes elicited by sensory afferents from skin.

superior Situated above or higher than a point of reference in the anatomical position.

superior vena cava The vein that returns blood from the head and neck, upper limbs, and thorax to the right atrium.

supination Rotation of the forearm so that the anterior surface is up.

supine The position in which the patient is lying on the back (face up).

supine hypotension syndrome Hypotension that occurs in pregnant women who are in a supine position; it results when the uterus compresses the inferior vena cava, decreasing cardiac filling and cardiac output.

suprasternal notch The superior margin of the manubrium, which can be felt easily at the anterior base of the neck; also known as the *jugular notch.*

surface tension The tendency of the surface of a liquid to minimize the area of its surface by contracting.

surfactant Lipoproteins that reduce the surface tension of pulmonary fluids.

suspensory ligament The band of peritoneum that extends from the ovary to the body wall; it contains the ovarian vessels and nerves.

suture A border or joint between two bones of the cranium.

sweat gland A structure that produces sweat or viscus organic secretions; also known as a *sudoriferous gland.*

sympathetic nervous system A subdivision of the autonomic nervous system that usually is involved in preparing the body for physical activity.

sympatholytic Antiadrenergic; blocking transmission of impulses from the adrenergic postganglionic fibers to effector organs or tissues.

sympathomimetic A pharmacological agent that mimics the effects of sympathetic nervous system stimulation of organs and structures by acting as an agonist or by increasing the release of the neurotransmitter norepinephrine at postganglionic nerve endings.

sympathy The expression of one's feelings about another person's problem.

symphysis A cartilaginous joint.

symphysis pubis The slightly movable, interpubic joint of the pelvis; it consists of two bones separated by a disk of fibrocartilage and connected by two ligaments; also known as the pubic symphysis.

synapse Functional membrane-to-membrane contact of a nerve cell with another nerve cell, muscle cell, gland cell, or sensory receptor; it functions in transmitting action potentials from one cell to another.

synaptic cleft The space between the presynaptic and postsynaptic membranes.

synaptic vesicle A secretory vesicle in the presynaptic terminal that contains neurotransmitter substances.

synchondrosis A cartilaginous joint between two immovable bones, such as the symphysis pubis, the sternum, and the manubrium.

syncope A brief lapse in consciousness caused by transient cerebral hypoxia.

syncytium Cardiac muscle cells that are bound together so tightly and their membranes are so permeable to electrical impulse that they act as a mass of merged cells or a single cell.

syndesmosis A fibrous articulation in which two bones are connected by interosseous ligaments.

synergism The combined action of two drugs that is greater than the sum of each agent acting independently.

synergist A muscle that works with other muscles to cause movement.

synovial fluid A thin, lubricating film that allows considerable movement between articulating bones.

synovial joint See *joint.*

synovial membrane The inner layer of an articular capsule that surrounds a freely movable joint.

syphilis A sexually transmitted disease characterized by distinct stages of effects over a period of years; any organ system may be involved.

system Interconnected functions or organs in which a stimulus or an action in one area affects all other areas.

systemic circulation Blood flow from the left ventricle to all parts of the body and back to the right atrium.

systemic lupus erythematosus A chronic inflammatory disease that affects many systems of the body; it is characterized by severe vasculitis, renal involvement, and lesions of the skin and nervous system.

systemic pressure Pressure generated by the left side of the heart.

systolic blood pressure The blood pressure measured during the period of ventricular contraction.

T lymphocytes The lymphocytes responsible for cell-mediated immunity.

T tubule Tubelike invagination of the sarcolemma that conducts action potentials toward the center of the cylindrical muscle fibers.

T wave A deflection in the electrocardiogram after the QRS complex, representing ventricular repolarization.

tabes dorsalis An abnormal condition characterized by the slow degeneration of all or part of the spinal cord and the progressive loss of peripheral reflexes.

tabun A clear, colorless, tasteless liquid with a faint fruity odor; may be used as a nerve agent.

tachycardia A heart rate that exceeds 99 beats per minute.

tachyphylaxis A phenomenon in which the repeated administration of some drugs results in a significant decrease in their effectiveness.

tachypnea A persistent respiratory rate that exceeds 20 breaths per minute.

tactical EMS Emergency medical services provided by EMS personnel who are specially trained and equipped to provide prehospital emergency care in tactical environments.

tactical patient care Patient care activities that occur inside the scene perimeter, or hot zone, of a dangerous scene.

tactical retreat Leaving the scene when danger is observed or when violence or indicators of violence are displayed; requires immediate and decisive action.

talus The second largest tarsal bone; the ankle bone.

tardive dyskinesia An abnormal condition characterized by involuntary, repetitious movements of the muscles of the face, limbs, and trunk.

tarsal Pertaining to the area of articulation between the foot and the leg.

tarsal bones Bones of the ankle.

taste bud Any one of many peripheral taste organs distributed over the tongue and roof of the mouth.

TB disease Active tuberculosis.

teachable moment The time after an injury has occurred when the patient and observers remain acutely aware of what has happened and may be more receptive to being taught ways that the event or illness could have been prevented.

telecommunicator A person trained in public safety telecommunications; the term applies to call takers, dispatchers, radio operators, data terminal operators, or any combination of such functions in a public service answering point.

telemedicine Refers to technological communications that allow for the transmission of photographs, video, and other information to be sent directly from the scene to a hospital for physician evaluation and consultation.

telemetry The transmission and reception of physiological data by radio or telephone; for example, electrocardiograms.

temperament A person's style of behavior; the way the person interacts with the environment. It is the basis on which children develop relationships.

temporal bone One of a pair of large bones that form part of the lower cranium and that contain various cavities and recesses associated with the ear.

temporal lobe The lateral region of the cerebrum; it contains the center for smell and some association areas for memory and learning.

temporomandibular joint dysfunction Acute or chronic inflammation in the temporomandibular joint.

ten code (10 code) A code sometimes used in radio communications that uses the number 10 plus another number to relay a particular message.

tendon A band or cord of dense connective tissue that connects muscle to bone or other structures; it is characterized by strength and nonstretchability.

tendonitis An inflammatory condition of a tendon, usually caused by a sprain.

tenosynovitis Inflammation of a tendon sheath.

tension headache A headache caused by muscle contractions of the face, neck, and scalp.

tension pneumothorax An accumulation of air or gas in the pleural cavity that can lead to collapse of the lung.

teratogenic Any substance, agent, or process that interferes with normal prenatal development.

term A pregnancy that has reached 40 weeks' gestation.

terminal bronchiole The end of the conducting airway.

terminal drop A theory that a decline in intelligence in older adulthood may be caused by a person's conscious or unconscious perception of coming death.

terminally ill patients Patients with advanced stage of disease with an unfavorable prognosis and no known cure.

termination of action The point at which a drug effect is no longer seen.

tertiary segmental bronchus The bronchus that extends from the secondary bronchus and conducts air to each lobule of the lung.

testes The male gonads, which produce the male sex cells, or sperm.

testicular mass An enlargement or growth on one or both testicles.

testicular torsion A condition in which a testicle twists on its spermatic cord, disrupting its own blood supply.

testosterone The male sex hormone.

tetanus An acute, potentially fatal infection of the central nervous system caused by the tetanus bacillus *Clostridium tetani*; it is characterized by muscle spasms and convulsions.

tetany The involuntary contraction of skeletal muscles.

tetralogy of Fallot A congenital cardiac anomaly that consists of four defects: pulmonic stenosis, ventricular septal defect, malposition of the aorta so that it rises from the septal defect or the right ventricle, and right ventricular hypertrophy.

thalamus Tissue located just above the hypothalamus; it helps to produce sensations, associates sensations with emotions, and plays a part in arousal.

therapeutic abortion The legal termination of a pregnancy for reasons of maternal well-being.

therapeutic action The desired, intended action of a drug.

therapeutic communications A planned, deliberate, professional act that involves the use of communications techniques to achieve two purposes: (1) a positive relationship with a patient and (2) a shared understanding of information for desired patient care goals.

therapeutic index A measurement of the relative safety of a drug.

therapeutic range The range of plasma concentrations that is most likely to produce the desired drug effect with the least likelihood of toxicity; the range between minimal effective concentration and toxic level.

thermogenesis Production of heat, especially by the cells of the body.

thermolysis The dissipation of heat by means of radiation, evaporation, conduction, or convection.

thiazide A group of diuretics that are moderately effective in lowering blood pressure.

third stage of labor The stage of labor that begins with delivery of the infant and ends when the placenta has been expelled and the uterus has contracted.

third ventricle The ventricle located in the center of the diencephalon between the two halves of the thalamus.

third-degree burn A burn injury in which the entire thickness of the epidermis and dermis is destroyed.

thoracentesis Puncturing of pleural space.

thoracic aorta The large upper portion of the descending aorta; it supplies many parts of the body such as the heart, ribs, chest muscles, and stomach.

thoracic cavity The area of the body enclosed by the ribs.

thoracic duct The common trunk of all the lymphatic vessels of the body except those on the right side of the head and neck, the thorax, right upper limb, right lung, right side of the heart, and the diaphragmatic surface of the liver.

thoracic vertebrae The 12 bony segments of the spinal column of the upper back, designated T1 to T12.

thoroughfare channel The channel for blood through a capillary bed from an arteriole to a venule.

threatened abortion An abortion diagnosed when a patient has some uterine bleeding with an intrauterine pregnancy in which the internal cervical os is closed; it may stabilize and end in normal delivery or progress to an incomplete or complete abortion.

threshold potential The value of the membrane potential at which an action potential is produced as a result of depolarization in response to a stimulus.

thrill A fine vibration felt by an examiner's hands over the site of an aneurysm or on the pericardium.

thrombectomy The removal of a thrombus from a blood vessel.

thrombin An enzyme formed in plasma as part of the clotting process; it causes fibrinogen to change to fibrin, which is essential in the formation of a clot.

thrombocytes Cell fragments.

thrombocytopenia An abnormal hematological condition in which the number of platelets is reduced; the most common cause is a bleeding disorder.

thromboembolism A condition in which a blood vessel is blocked by an embolus carried in the bloodstream from the site of formation of the clot.

thrombogenesis Clot formation.

thrombolytic agent A drug that dissolves clots after their formation by promoting the digestion of fibrin.

thrombophlebitis See *phlebitis*.

thrombosis An abnormal formation of a thrombus within a blood vessel of the body.

thromboxanes Antagonistic prostaglandin derivatives that are synthesized and released by degranulating platelets, causing vasoconstriction and promoting the degranulation of other platelets.

thrombus An aggregation of platelets, fibrin, clotting factors, and the cellular elements of the blood attached to the interior wall of a vein or artery, which sometimes occludes the lumen of the vessel.

thymectomy Excision of the thymus.

thymus A single, unpaired gland located in the mediastinum; the primary central gland of the lymphatic system.

thyroid cartilage The largest laryngeal cartilage; it forms the laryngeal prominence, or Adam's apple.

thyroid membrane The fibrous membrane that joins the hyoid and the thyroid cartilages.

thyroid storm A life-threatening form of hyperthyroidism.

thyrotoxicosis A term that refers to any toxic condition that results from thyroid hyperfunction.

tibia The second longest bone of the skeleton; it is located on the medial side of the lower leg.

tibial tuberosity A large, oblong elevation at the proximal end of the tibia that attaches to the ligament of the patella.

tick paralysis A rare, progressive, reversible disorder caused by several species of ticks that release a neurotoxin that causes weakness, incoordination, and paralysis.

tidal volume The volume of gas inhaled or exhaled in a single, resting breath.

tinea A group of fungal skin diseases characterized by itching and scaling and sometimes by painful lesions.

tinnitus A ringing sound in the ears.

tissue binding A type of drug reservoir in which drug pooling occurs in fat tissue and bone.

toddler A child 1 to 3 years of age.

tolerance A physiological response that requires that a drug dosage be increased to produce the same effect formerly produced by a smaller dose.

tone The audio signal or carrier wave of controlled amplitude and frequency used for equipment control purposes or to selectively signal a receiver, such as activating a pager; tones are measured in hertz.

tonic-clonic seizure A generalized seizure involving the entire body; also known as *a grand mal seizure*.

tonsil A large collection of lymphatic tissue beneath the mucous membrane of the oral cavity and pharynx.

tonsillectomy Surgical removal of the tonsils.

tonsillitis Inflammation of the tonsils.

torr A measurement in millimeters of mercury.

torsades de pointes An unusual bidirectional ventricular tachycardia.

total body water All the water within the body, including intracellular and extracellular water and the water in the gastrointestinal and urinary tracts.

total lung capacity The sum of the inspiratory and expiratory reserve volumes plus the tidal volume and residual volume.

total pressure The combination of pressures exerted by all the gases in any mixture of gas.

Tourette's syndrome An abnormal condition characterized by facial grimaces, tics, and involuntary arm and shoulder movements.

toxic level The plasma concentration at which a drug is likely to produce serious adverse effects.

toxic shock syndrome A severe, acute disease caused by infection with strains of *Staphylococcus aureus*.

toxidromes Clinical syndromes grouped together for the successful recognition of poisoning patterns.

toxin A poison usually produced by or occurring in a plant or microorganism.

toxoid A toxin that has been treated with chemicals or with heat to reduce its toxic effects but that retains its antigenic power.

trachea A cylindrical tube in the neck composed of cartilage and membrane; it conveys air to the lungs.

tracheal stenosis Constriction of the trachea.

tracheitis A bacterial infection of the upper airway and subglottic trachea.

tracheostomy An opening through the neck into the trachea through which an indwelling tube may be inserted.

trade name The trademark name of a drug, designated by the drug company that sells the medication.

tragus A projection of the cartilage of the auricle at the opening of the external auditory meatus.

transceiver A combination transmitter and receiver with a switching circuit or duplexer to use a single antenna.

transcutaneous cardiac pacing The use of an artificial pacemaker to substitute for a natural pacemaker of the heart that is blocked or dysfunctional. In the prehospital setting a transcutaneous pacemaker is used to treat symptomatic bradycardia, heart block associated with reduced cardiac output that is unresponsive to atropine, pacemaker failure, and asystole.

transection A complete or incomplete lesion of the spinal cord.

transfusion hepatitis Hepatitis that results from a transfusion with infected blood.

transient dysphagia A temporary impairment of speech.

transient ischemic attack An acute episode of temporary neurological dysfunction resulting from focal cerebral ischemia; also called a "mini stroke."

translaryngeal cannula ventilation An advanced airway procedure that provides high-volume, high-pressure oxygenation of the lungs through cannulation of the trachea below the glottis; also known as needle percutaneous transtracheal ventilation and needle cricothyrotomy.

transmembrane potential The difference in electrical charge between inside and outside the plasma membrane.

transmitted nonspecific urethritis A sexually transmitted disease characterized by inflammation or infection of the urethra in which the cause is not defined; also known as nongonococcal urethritis.

transmural infarction A myocardial infarction that extends through the full thickness of the myocardium, including the endocardium and epicardium.

transudate A fluid passed through a membrane as a result of a difference in hydrostatic pressure.

transverse At right angles to the long axis of any common part.

transverse colon The segment of the colon that extends from the end of the ascending colon at the hepatic flexure on the right side across the midabdomen to the beginning of the descending colon at the splenic flexure on the left side.

transverse plane An imaginary plane that divides the body into top and bottom or superior and inferior sections; also known as the *horizontal plane.*

transverse presentation See *shoulder presentation.*

transverse process The bony segment that extends laterally from each side of the vertebral arch.

trauma An injury caused by a transfer of energy from some external source to the human body.

trauma index An early measurement that used a numerical injury rating system based on a patient's injured body region, type of injury, and cardiovascular, central nervous system, and respiratory status.

trauma score An injury severity index used to predict the outcome for patients with blunt or penetrating injuries.

traumatic asphyxia A severe crushing injury to the chest and abdomen that causes an increase in intrathoracic pressure. The increased pressure forces blood from the right side of the heart into the veins of the upper thorax, neck, and face.

traumatic hyphema See *hyphema.*

traumatic iridoplegia Traumatic dilation or, less commonly, constriction of the pupil.

treatment protocols Guidelines that define the scope of prehospital intervention practiced by emergency care providers.

Trendelenburg's position A position in which the head is low and the body and legs are on an inclined plane.

triage A method used to sort or categorize patients according to severity of injury.

triaxial reference system Three intersecting lines of reference used in standard limb leads.

trichomoniasis A vaginal infection caused by the protozoan *Trichomonas vaginalis;* it is characterized by itching, burning, and a frothy, pale yellow to green vaginal discharge.

tricuspid valve The valve located between the right atrium and ventricle.

trigeminal nerve Either of the largest pair of cranial nerves, which are essential for chewing and the general sensibility of the face.

trigeminal neuralgia Infection or disease of the trigeminal nerve (cranial nerve V); also known as *central pain syndrome.*

triglyceride A compound consisting of a fatty acid and glycerol.

trigone The triangular smooth area at the base of the bladder between the openings of two ureters and that of the urethra.

trimester One of three periods of approximately 3 months into which pregnancy is divided.

triphosphate bond Energy sources for the muscles, nerves, and overall function of the body; an example is adenosine triphosphate.

triplets Three premature ventricular contractions in a row.

trismus Muscle spasms of the jaw.

trochanter One of the two bony projections at the proximal end of the femur that serve as the attachment point for various muscles.

trochlea The medial aspect of the humerus; it articulates with the ulna.

trophoblast A cell layer that forms the outer layer of the blastocyst, which erodes the uterine mucosa during implantation; it contributes to the formation of the placenta.

true rib See *rib*.

true vocal cord See *vocal cord*.

truncal obesity Obesity that preferentially affects or is isolated in the trunk of the body rather than the extremities.

trunking system A radio system consisting of base stations on different channels connected to each other with small computers that work with special mobile and portable signaling to allow multiple simultaneous conversations.

tubal ligation One of several sterilization procedures in which both fallopian tubes are blocked to prevent conception..

tubercle A nodule or small eminence, such as that on a bone or that produced by infection from tubercle bacilli.

tuberculosis A chronic granulomatous infection caused by *Mycobacterium tuberculosis;* it usually affects the lungs and generally is transmitted by inhalation or ingestion of infected droplets.

tuberosities Elevations or protuberances, especially of bones.

tuboovarian abscess An abscess involving the ovary and fallopian tube.

tularemia A serious illness that is caused by the bacterium *Francisella tularensis* found in animals (especially rodents, rabbits, and hares).

tunic One of the enveloping layers of a part; one of the coats of a blood vessel; one of the coats of the eye; one of the coats of the digestive tract.

tunica adventitia The outermost fibrous coat of a vessel or an organ that is derived from the surrounding connective tissue.

tunica intima The innermost coat of a blood vessel.

tunica media The middle coat, usually muscular, of an artery or other tubular structure.

turbinate The concha nasalis.

turgor The normal resiliency of the skin caused by the outward pressure of the cells and interstitial fluid.

Turner's sign Bruising of the skin of the flanks or loin in acute hemorrhagic pancreatitis; also known as Grey Turner's sign.

Turner's syndrome A chromosomal anomaly characterized by the absence of one X chromosome and characterized by short stature, undifferentiated gonads, and various other abnormalities.

tympanic membrane See *eardrum*.

tympany A hollow drumlike sound produced when a gas-containing cavity is percussed.

type 1 diabetes Diabetes that is characterized by inadequate production of insulin by the pancreas. It may occur any time after birth; requires lifelong treatment with insulin.

type 2 diabetes Diabetes that usually is characterized by a decrease in the production of insulin by the pancreatic beta cells and diminished tissue sensitivity to insulin (*insulin resistance*).

type and crossmatch A test used to determine the patient's ABO group and Rh type.

U wave The gradual deviation from the T wave in the electrocardiogram; thought to represent the final stage of repolarization of the ventricles.

ulceration The formation of a craterlike lesion on the skin or mucous membranes.

ulcerative colitis An inflammatory condition of the large intestine characterized by severe diarrhea and ulceration of the mucosa of the intestine.

ulna One of the bones of the forearm.

ulnar nerve entrapment An injury that occurs when the ulnar nerve in the arm becomes compressed.

ultrahigh frequency Radio frequency between 300 and 3000 MHz; the 460-MHz range commonly is used for emergency medical services communications.

umbilical cord A flexible structure connecting the umbilicus with the placenta and giving passage to the umbilical arteries and vein.

umbilicus The point on the abdomen at which the umbilical cord joined the fetal abdomen.

uncompensated shock A stage of shock that occurs when the body is no longer able to maintain systemic blood pressure.

unethical Conduct that fails to conform to moral principles, values, or standards.

unifocal premature ventricular complex A premature ventricular complex that originates from a single ectopic pacemaker site.

unipolar lead A lead composed of a single positive electrode and a reference point.

universal donor A person with blood of type O, Rh factor negative.

universal precautions Infection control practices in health care that are observed with every patient and procedure and that prevent exposure to blood-borne pathogens.

universal recipient A person with blood type AB who can receive any of the four types of blood.

unmyelinated axon A nerve fiber lacking a myelin sheath.

untoward effects Side effects that prove harmful to the patient.

upper airway Airway structures above the glottis.

upper esophageal sphincter The ring of muscle located at the superior opening of the esophagus that regulates the passage of materials into the esophagus.

upper respiratory tract infection Infection of the upper airway, affecting the nose, throat, sinuses, and larynx.

urea A nitrogen-containing waste product.

uremia The presence of excessive amounts of urea and other nitrogenous wastes produced in the blood.

uremic frost A pale, frostlike deposit of white crystals on the skin caused by kidney failure and uremia.

ureter One of a pair of tubes that carry the urine from the kidney into the bladder.

urethra A small tubular structure that drains urine from the bladder; in men, it also serves as a passageway for semen during ejaculation.

urethritis An inflammatory condition of the urethra.

uric acid A product of the metabolism of protein present in the blood and excreted in the urine.

urinary bladder The muscular, membranous sac in the pelvis that stores urine for discharge through the urethra.

urinary calculi Solid particles in the urinary system; commonly known as "kidney stones."

urinary retention The inability to urinate.

urinary tract infection An infection of one or more structures of the urinary tract.

urogenital triangle The anterior portion of the perianal region; it contains the openings of the urethra and vagina in the female and the root structures of the penis in the male.

urosepsis Septic poisoning caused by retention and absorption of urinary products in the tissues.

urticaria A pruritic skin eruption characterized by transient wheals of various shapes and sizes with well-defined margins and pale centers; also known as *hives*.

uterine Pertaining to the uterus.

uterine inversion A rare event in which the uterus turns inside out after birth.

uterine prolapse The falling or sliding of the uterus from its normal position in the pelvic cavity into the vaginal canal.

uterine rupture A rare event in which the wall of the uterus ruptures when it is unable to withstand the strain placed on it.

uterine tube One of a pair of ducts opening at one end into the uterus and the other end into the peritoneal cavity, over the ovary; also known as a *fallopian tube*.

uterosacral ligament A primary ligament that holds the uterus in place.

uterus The hollow, pear-shaped internal female organ of reproduction.

uvula The cone-shaped process hanging down from the soft palate that helps prevent food and liquid from entering the nasal cavities.

vagina The part of the female genitalia that forms a canal from the orifice through the vestibule to the uterine cervix.

vaginal bleeding The loss of blood from the uterus, cervix, or vagina.

vaginitis An inflammation of the vaginal tissues.

vagus nerve Either of the longest pair of cranial nerves essential for speech, swallowing, and the sensibilities and functions of many parts of the body.

vallecula A furrow between the glossoepiglottic folds on each side of the posterior oropharynx.

Valsalva maneuver A vagal maneuver used to slow the heart and decrease the force of atrial contraction by stimulating postganglionic parasympathetic nerve fibers in the wall of the atria and specialized tissues of the sinoatrial and atrioventricular nodes via the vagus nerve.

varicella An acute, highly contagious viral disease caused by a herpesvirus, varicella-zoster virus; it occurs primarily in young children and is characterized by crops of pruritic vesicular eruptions on the skin; also known as *chickenpox.*

varicella-zoster virus A member of the herpesvirus family that causes the disease varicella (chickenpox) and herpes zoster (shingles).

varicocele An abnormal enlargement of the veins that drain the testicle.

vas deferens See *ductus deferens*.

vascular tunic The choroid, ciliary body, and iris.

vasoconstriction A narrowing of the lumen of any blood vessel.

vasodilation An increase in the diameter of a blood vessel caused by inhibition of its constrictor nerves or stimulation of dilator nerves.

vasomotor Of or pertaining to the nerves and muscles that control the diameter of the lumen of blood vessels.

vasopressin mechanism The mechanism by which antidiuretic hormone secretion increases when blood pressure drops or plasma osmolarity increases; it reduces urine production and stimulates vasoconstriction.

vastus lateralis muscle The largest of the four muscles of the quadriceps femoris; it is situated on the lateral side of the thigh.

vein A vessel that carries blood toward the heart.

venereal disease A contagious disease usually acquired by sexual intercourse or genital contact.

venostasis Retardation of venous flow in a part.

venous capillary The ends of capillaries closest to venules.

venous sinus One of many sinuses that collect blood from the dura mater and drain it into the internal jugular vein.

ventilation The mechanical movement of air into and out of the lungs; makes respiration possible.

ventral root The nerve that conveys efferent nerve processes away from the spinal cord.

ventricle A small cavity; it usually refers to the right or left ventricle of the heart.

ventricular bigeminy A cardiac rhythm disturbance characterized by two ventricular beats in rapid succession followed by a longer interval.

ventricular fibrillation A cardiac dysrhythmia marked by rapid, disorganized depolarization of the ventricular myocardium.

ventricular quadrigeminy A cardiac dysrhythmia that occurs when every fourth complex is a premature ventricular complex.

ventricular tachycardia A tachycardia that usually originates in the Purkinje fibers.

ventricular trigeminy A cardiac dysrhythmia characterized by three ventricular beats in rapid succession followed by a longer interval.

ventrogluteal muscle The muscle that overlies the iliac crest and the anterior-superior iliac spine.

venule Small blood vessels that collect blood from the capillaries and join to form veins.

vermiform appendix See *appendix*.

vertebra Any one of 33 bones of the spinal column.

vertebral arch The dorsal, bony arch of a vertebra composed of the laminae and pedicles; it protects the spinal cord.

vertebral artery Each of the two arteries branching from the subclavian arteries.

vertebral body A bony disk that serves as the weight-bearing portion of the vertebra.

vertex presentation See *cephalic presentation*.

vertigo A sensation of faintness or an inability to maintain normal balance in a standing or seated position.

very high frequency Radio frequencies between 30 and 300 MHz (usually in the 150-MHz range). The very high frequency spectrum is divided further into high and low bands.

vesicants Chemicals with severely irritating properties that produce fluid-filled pockets on the skin and damage to the eyes, lungs, and other mucous membranes.

vesicular Pertaining to a blisterlike condition.

vesicular follicle The secondary follicle in which the oocyte attains its full size; also known as the *graafian follicle*.

vesiculation The formation of vesicles.

vestibular fold One of two folds of mucous membrane that stretch across the laryngeal cavity; it helps close the glottis; also known as the *false vocal cord*.

vestibule The portion of the inner ear adjacent to the oval window between the semicircular canals and the cochlea.

vestibule of the ear The middle region of the middle ear.

vestibule of the vagina The space behind the labia minora that contains the opening of the vagina, the urethra, and the vestibular glands.

vesicular breath sounds Breath sounds heard over most of the lung fields; the major normal breath sound.

vestibulocochlear nerve The eighth cranial nerve, formed by the cochlear and vestibular nerves; it extends to the brain.

viral hemorrhagic fevers A group of illnesses caused by several distinct families of viruses that include arenaviruses, filoviruses, bunyaviruses, and flaviviruses.

viral meningitis A syndrome generally associated with an existing systemic viral disease (e.g., enteroviral infection, herpesvirus infection, mumps, and, less commonly, influenza); also known as *aseptic meningitis*.

viral pneumonia An inflammation of the lungs caused by viral infection.

virulence The relative strength of a pathogen.

virus A minute, parasitic microorganism without independent metabolic activity that can replicate only within a cell of a living plant or animal host.

visceral Pertaining to internal organs enclosed within a body cavity, primarily the abdominal organs.

visceral pain Deep pain that arises from smooth vasculature or organ systems.

visceral pericardium The portion of the serous pericardium that covers the heart surface; also known as the *epicardium*.

visceral peritoneum The layer of peritoneum that covers the abdominal organs.

viscosity The physical property of a liquid. It is characterized by the degree of friction between its component molecules.

vital capacity The volume of gas moved on deepest inspiration and expiration, or the sum of the inspiratory reserve volume, the tidal volume, and the expiratory reserve volume.

vitamin An organic compound essential in small quantities for normal physiological and metabolic functioning of the body.

vitamin D A fat-soluble vitamin essential for the normal formation of bones and teeth and for absorption of calcium and phosphorus from the gastrointestinal tract.

vitamin K A fat-soluble compound essential for the synthesis of several related proteins involved in the clotting of blood.

vitreous humor The transparent, jellylike material that fills the space between the lens and the retina.

vocal cord One of two folds of elastic ligaments covered by mucous membrane that stretch from the thyroid cartilage to the arytenoid cartilage; vibration of the vocal cords is responsible for voice production; also known as a *true vocal cord*.

Volkmann's contracture A serious, persistent flexion contraction of the forearm and hand caused by ischemia.

voluntary Action originated or accomplished by a person's free will or choice.

voluntary muscle A muscle that is controlled consciously; see *skeletal muscle*.

vomer bone The bone forming the posterior and inferior part of the nasal septum.

vulva The external genitalia of the female.

VX A thick, amber-colored, odorless liquid that resembles motor oil; may be used as a nerve agent.

wandering atrial pacemaker The passive transfer of pacemaker sites from the sinus node to other latent pacemaker sites in the atria and atrioventricular junction.

water vapor pressure The partial pressure exerted by water molecules after they have been converted into a gas.

watt The unit of measurement of a transmitter's power output.

weapons of mass destruction Large conventional biological, nuclear, incendiary, chemical, or explosive weapons (B-NICE).

Wenckebach heart block Type I second-degree atrioventricular block; a progressive, beat-to-beat prolongation of the P-R interval that finally results in a nonconducted P wave; at this point, the sequence recurs.

Wernicke-Korsakoff syndrome A disease that results from chronic thiamine deficiency combined with an inability to use thiamine because of a heritable disorder or because of a reduction in intestinal absorption and metabolism of thiamine by alcohol.

Wernicke's encephalopathy A stage of Wernicke-Korsakoff syndrome that usually develops suddenly with the clinical manifestations of ataxia, nystagmus, disturbances of speech and gait, signs of neuropathy, stupor, or coma.

West Nile virus A potentially serious mosquito-borne illness that affects the central nervous system.

wheals Small areas of swelling of the skin that result from an allergic reaction.

wheeze A form of rhonchus characterized by a high-pitched, musical quality; it is caused by high-velocity airflow through narrowed airways.

whole-bowel irrigation An in-hospital method of GI decontamination; involves the rapid administration of large amounts of a specially balanced fluid to flush the GI tract.

windchill chart An index developed to calculate the cooling effects of the ambient temperature based on thermometer readings and the wind speed.

withdrawal syndrome A predictable set of signs and symptoms that occurs after a decrease in the usual dose of a drug or its sudden cessation.

xiphoid process The smallest of three parts of the sternum; it articulates caudally with the body of the sternum and laterally with the seventh rib.

years of productive life The calculation obtained by subtracting the victim's age at death from 65 (the average age of retirement).

yellow fever An acute infection transmitted by mosquitoes; it is characterized by headache, fever, jaundice, vomiting, and bleeding.

yellow marrow Specialized soft tissue (mainly adipose) found in the compact bone of most adult epiphyses.

Z line The delicate, membrane-like structure found at either end of a sarcomere.

zone of coagulation In a burn wound, the central area that has sustained the most intense contact with the thermal source; in this area coagulation necrosis of the cells has occurred and the tissue is nonviable.

zone of hyperemia An area in which blood flow is increased as a result of the normal inflammatory response to injury; it lies at the periphery of the zone of stasis.

zone of stasis The area of burn tissue that surrounds the critically injured area; it consists of tissue that is potentially viable despite the serious thermal injury.

zygomatic bone One of a pair of bones that forms the prominence of the cheek, the lower part of the orbit of the eye, and parts of the temporal bone; also known as the *zygomatic process.*

zygomatic process See *zygomatic bone.*

zygote The developing ovum from the time it is fertilized until it is implanted in the uterus as a blastocyst.

Appendix: Advanced Practice Procedures for Critical Care Paramedics

*S*ome critically ill or injured patients require a level of care that is beyond the normal scope of the paramedic. For example, a patient may have special needs that require continuous medical supervision by one or more health professionals. These duties usually are provided by specialty personnel working in nursing, emergency medicine, respiratory care, and cardiovascular care. Supervision of the patient also can be provided by paramedics with advanced levels of training. This chapter addresses some of the advanced knowledge and patient care procedures that may be required of the paramedic who practices in critical care.

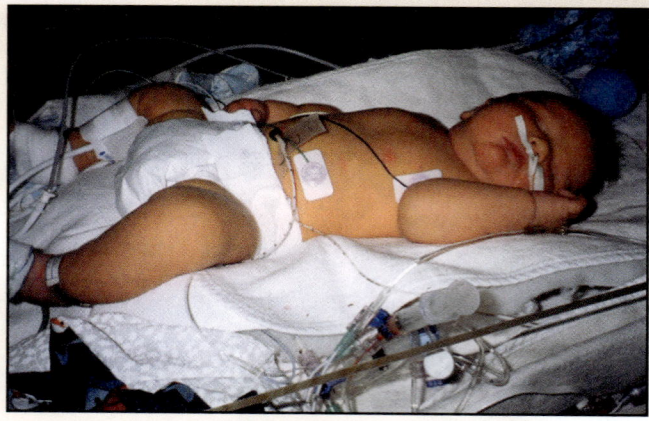

(Courtesy Keith and Margie Allen, O'Fallon, Mo.)

CRITICAL CARE AND CRITICAL CARE TRANSPORT

Critical care is a specialty within professional health care that deals with patients who have life-threatening illness or injury. Historically, this level of care has been provided primarily by physicians, physician assistants, specially trained registered nurses, respiratory therapists, clinical nurse specialists, and nurse practitioners. In recent years, providers of critical care have been expanded to include other health care professionals, including paramedics. Paramedics who practice in critical care settings (including critical care transport) have special training and advanced certifications. They also have additional experience working with critical care patients. Through this education, these paramedics are trained, credentialed, and become skilled in advanced practice procedures that may be performed infrequently by most other prehospital personnel.

Critical care transport (CCT) is also known as *specialty care transport* (SCT). The term is used to describe the delivery of medical services for a critically ill or injured patient during transport. Most paramedics who are members of a CCT team have completed a training program, such as Critical Care EMT-Paramedic (CCEMT-P), Critical Intensive Care Provider (CICP), and/or have other advanced certifications. These certification programs are focused on the most common and serious conditions that may require transport from a community hospital to a tertiary care facility.

SECTION ONE
Advanced Practice Procedures

Most educational programs for critical care include advanced training and skill procedures that are based on body systems (cardiac, respiratory, gastrointestinal, gastrourinary, renal, and neurologic), surgical airway management, and drug therapy. *It should be noted that the descriptions of the advanced practice procedures presented in this appendix are intended as an overview. All procedures carry significant complications and risks. In addition, all procedures require advanced training and authorization from the program's medical director. Any advanced procedures performed should have a written advanced protocol.* Advanced practice procedures that are described in this appendix include:

- Central venous cannulation
- Accessing the umbilical vein

- Arterial blood gas sampling
- Bladder catheterization
- Invasive hemodynamic monitoring
- Monitoring of an intraaortic balloon pump (IABP)
- Blood administration
- Use of IV infusion pumps
- Tube thoracostomy
- Pericardiocentesis

CENTRAL VENOUS CANNULATION

Central venous cannulation may be within the scope of paramedic practice in some critical care programs. Sites for central venous cannulation include the femoral vein, internal jugular vein, and subclavian vein (Figures 1 to 3). (Although the femoral vein is not truly a central vein, because the catheter is inserted in an area below the diaphragm, it is included in this section.)

The preparation for cannulation of the central vessels is similar to that for the peripheral veins (described in Chapter 14); however, attention to providing and maintaining a sterile field during placement is especially important. Several factors affect the success of central venous cannulation. Two of these factors are the position of the patient's body and the paramedic's knowledge of anatomy. The paramedic's familiarity with the procedure also is a key factor.

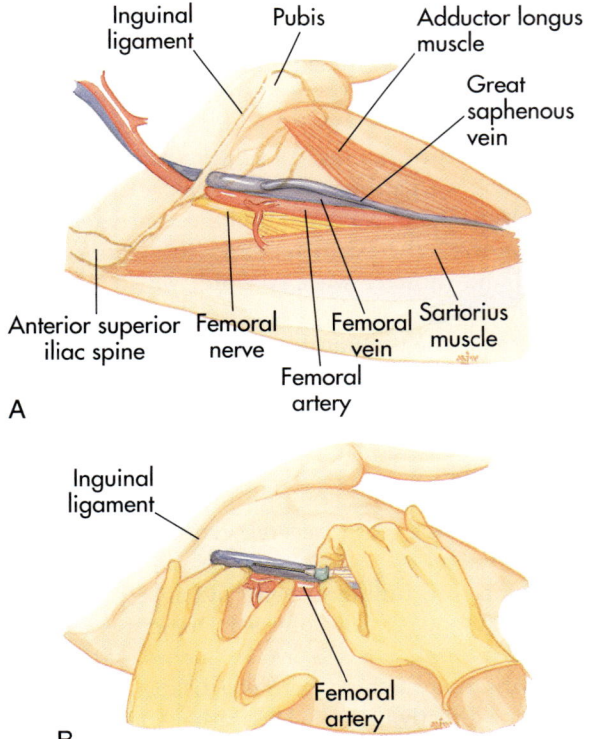

FIGURE 1 A, Anatomy of the femoral vein. **B,** Femoral venipuncture.

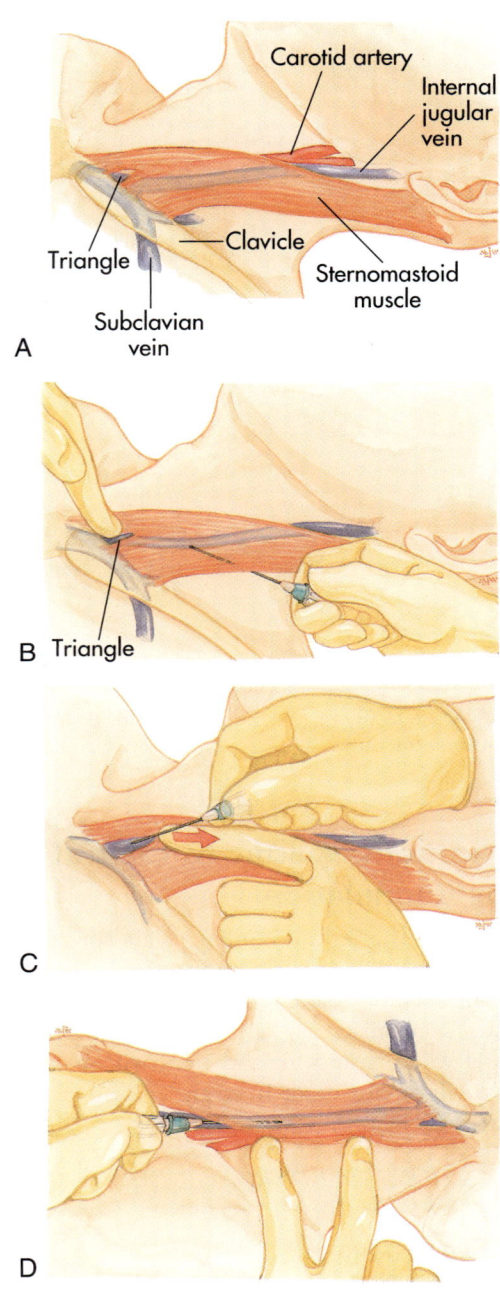

FIGURE 2 A, Anatomy of the internal jugular vein. **B,** Posterior approach for internal jugular venipuncture. **C,** Central approach for internal jugular venipuncture. **D,** Anterior approach for internal jugular venipuncture.

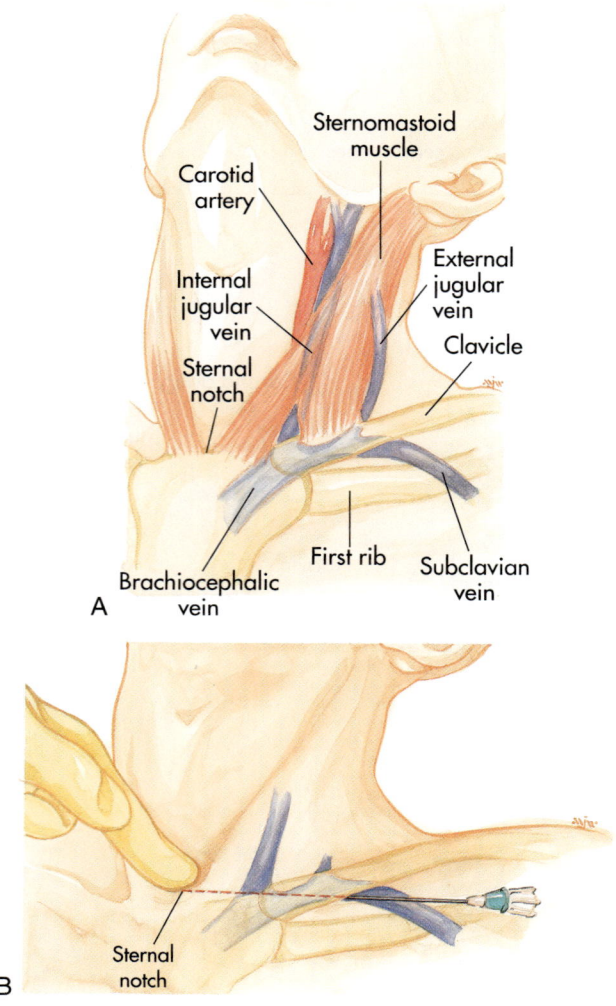

Sternomastoid muscle

Carotid artery

Internal jugular vein

Sternal notch

External jugular vein

Clavicle

Brachiocephalic vein

First rib

Subclavian vein

A

Sternal notch

B

FIGURE 3 A, Anatomy of the subclavian vein. **B,** Infraclavicular subclavian venipuncture.

Complications Specific to Central Venous Cannulation

Cannulation of the central veins presents specific dangers. These are in addition to the complications common to all intravenous techniques. The paramedic must be alert to these dangers because they can be fatal if unrecognized. It is essential when caring for a patient with a central vein catheter to eliminate all air from the tubing to reduce the risk of air embolism.

COMPLICATIONS OF INTERNAL JUGULAR AND SUBCLAVIAN VEIN CANNULATION

Local Complications
- Hematoma may occur, either from the vein itself or from an adjacent artery.
- Damage may occur to an adjacent artery, nerve, or lymphatic duct. Inadvertent puncture of the carotid artery is not uncommon when jugular vein cannulation is

attempted. If a hematoma occurs on one side of the neck, it is hazardous to attempt puncture on the opposite side. This could result in bilateral hematomas that severely compromise the airway.

Systemic Complications
- Pneumothorax is common.
- Hemothorax can occur.
- Air embolism can occur.
- Fluid may infiltrate into the mediastinum or the pleural cavity from an extruded catheter.

COMPLICATIONS OF FEMORAL VEIN CANNULATION

Local Complications
- Hematoma may occur, either from the vein itself or from the adjacent femoral artery.
- Thrombosis may extend to the deep veins and lead to edema of the leg.
- Phlebitis may extend to the deep veins.
- Use of the femoral vein frequently precludes subsequent use of the saphenous vein.
- Inadvertent arterial puncture may lead to excessive bleeding (including retroperitoneal bleeding) and can also lead to delayed aneurysm or pseudoaneurysm formation.

Systemic Complications
- Thrombosis or phlebitis may occur and extend to the iliac veins or even the inferior vena cava.

ACCESSING THE UMBILICAL VEIN

As described in Chapter 46, the umbilical cord contains three vessels: two arteries and one vein. The vein in the umbilical cord has a thin wall and is larger than the arteries. The arteries are thick walled and usually paired. To gain access to the umbilical vein, the paramedic should take the following steps (Figure 4):

1. Set up intravenous (IV) fluid (per protocol) and tubing with a three-way stopcock.
2. Select a 3.5 or 5 French umbilical catheter.
3. Connect the catheter to the stopcock and fill the catheter with IV fluid, which will remove any air.
4. Cleanse the umbilical stump and surrounding skin with antibacterial solution (per protocol).
5. Loosely tie umbilical tape around the cord near the body so that pressure can be applied to control bleeding.
6. Hold the umbilical stump firmly and trim (with a scalpel) the cord several centimeters above the abdomen.
7. Locate the umbilical vein and insert the catheter until blood is freely obtained. Do not insert the catheter more than 6 to 8 cm (2-3 inches). If the catheter is inserted farther, there is a risk of infusing solutions directly into the liver rather than the systemic circulation. Take care to avoid introduction of air emboli into the umbilical vein.
8. Draw blood for a sample, if needed.

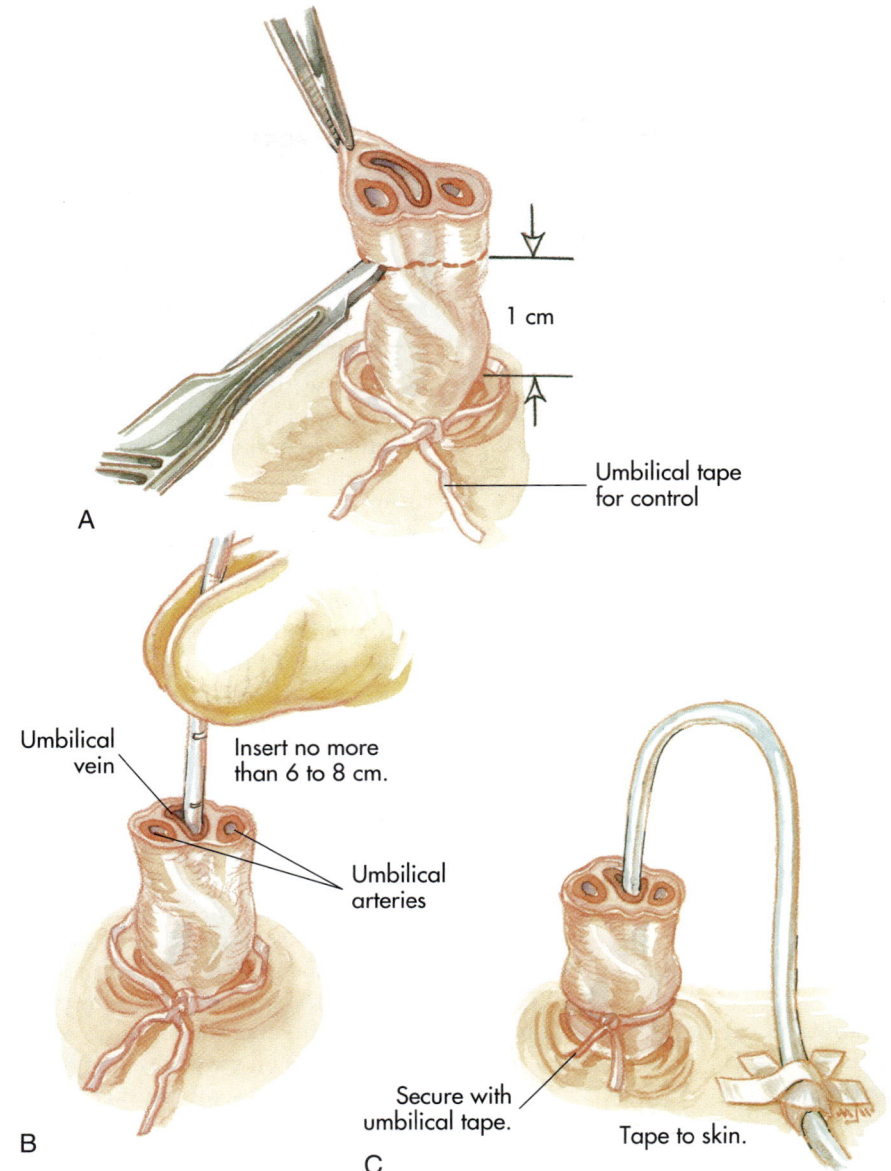

1 cm

Umbilical tape
for control

A

Umbilical
vein

Insert no more
than 6 to 8 cm.

Umbilical
arteries

Secure with
umbilical tape.

Tape to skin.

B

C

FIGURE 4 Umbilical vein cannulation procedure. **A,** Identify the umbilical vein after trimming the cord. **B,** Insert the umbilical catheter into the vein. **C,** Secure the base of the cord to hold the catheter in place and stabilize the catheter with tape.

9. Initiate the infusion and regulate the fluid flow per medical direction.
10. Secure the catheter in place with tape and cover with a sterile dressing.
11. Document the procedure.

The umbilical cord also may be cannulated by using a typical IV catheter. Insert the catheter-over-needle through the side of the proximal end of the cord into the vein and advance it upward through the translucent wall. Start the infusion, adjust the fluid flow per medical direction, and secure the catheter in place with tape.

ARTERIAL BLOOD GAS (ABG) SAMPLING

Arterial blood gas (ABG) measurements refer to the analyses of arterial blood to determine the pH (the negative log of the hydrogen ion concentration), the partial pressure of carbon dioxide, the partial pressure of oxygen, and the hemoglobin saturation of arterial blood. Pulse oximetry has made ABG measurement much less common. However, it is useful for measuring carbon dioxide and helps identify abnormal hemoglobin states such as carboxyhemoglobin and methemoglobin, although these can also be determined through venous blood gas analysis. The measurements often are used along with pulmonary function tests. The results of ABG sampling provide information about the diffusion of gas across the alveolar-capillary membrane. It also provides a measurement of the adequacy of tissue oxygenation. Patients with acid-base disturbances may require repeated ABG analysis to determine acid-base status and the adequacy of ventilation and oxygenation. The ABG sample that is tested should be less than 1 hour old.

LOOK AGAIN
See Chapter 11: General Principles of Pathophysiology, pp. 227-232.

Obtaining the ABG Sample

ABGs usually are drawn from the radial or femoral artery (or from an indwelling arterial catheter). To obtain an ABG sample, the paramedic should take the following steps:

Arterial Puncture of the Radial Artery

1. Collect the following equipment: (Commercial ABG kits are available)
   a. Heparinized 3-mL syringe
   b. 23-gauge or 25-gauge needle with safety guard
   c. Crushed ice for arterial blood sample
   d. Antiseptic wipes
   e. 2 × 2 gauze
   f. Air lock or cap for syringe
   g. Disposable gloves
   h. Tape
2. Verify the patient's name and explain the procedure.
3. Palpate the radial artery.
4. Perform Allen's Test (Figure 5)
   a. Have the patient make a tight fist
   b. Apply direct pressure to the radial and ulnar arteries
   c. Have the patient open fisted hand
   d. Release pressure over the ulnar artery; observe color of fingers, thumbs, and hands. If flushing occurs within 15 seconds, the test is positive and the puncture can proceed. If flushing does not occur within 15 seconds, the test is negative and the radial artery in that wrist should be avoided. Check opposite wrist.
5. Hyperextend the patient's wrist over a rolled towel.
6. Wash hands and don disposable gloves.
7. Cleanse the site in a circular motion with approved antiseptic wipes.
8. Flush heparin from the syringe, leaving heparin in the needle and hub.
9. While palpating the radial artery, insert the needle at a 45-degree angle while stabilizing the artery with your free hand (Figure 6).
10. Observe for pulsating blood into the syringe, indicating arterial puncture.
11. Withdraw 2 mL of blood.
12. Remove the needle and syringe from the artery and have a co-worker apply direct pressure to the puncture site with 2 × 2 gauze for approximately 3 to 5 minutes. Skin should remain warm, pink, and with good capillary refill (Figure 7). Reevaluate the puncture site for continued bleeding or hematoma formation. Assess arterial flow above and below the puncture site.
13. Expel any air and cap syringe. Rotate the syringe so that blood mixes with heparin to prevent clotting.
14. Place the syringe in crushed ice.
15. Label the specimen with the patient's name, body temperature, and the amount of inspired oxygen (if the patient is on oxygen therapy).
16. Immediately send the specimen to the laboratory (per policy).
17. Document and record the procedure in the patient care report.

FIGURE 5 Applying pressure to radial and ulnar arteries. (Perry AG, Potter PA: *Clinical nursing skills and techniques,* ed 7, St Louis, 2010, Mosby.)

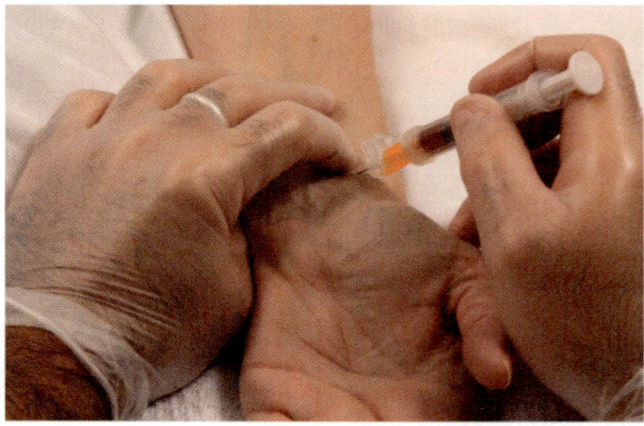

FIGURE 6 Blood flowing into syringe. (Perry AG, Potter PA: *Clinical nursing skills and techniques,* ed 7, St Louis, 2010, Mosby.)

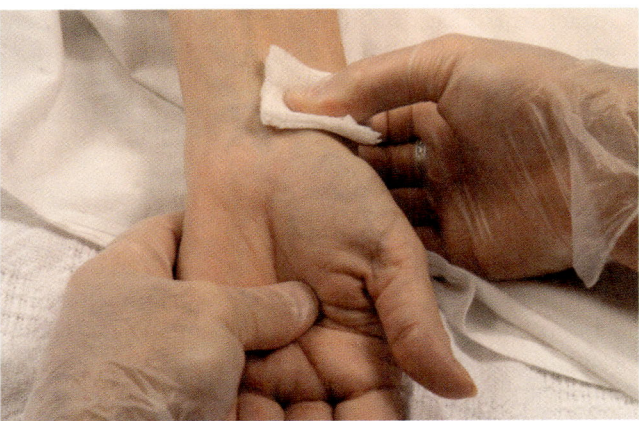

FIGURE 7 Applying firm pressure to arterial puncture site. (Perry AG, Potter PA: *Clinical nursing skills and techniques,* ed 7, St Louis, 2010, Mosby.)

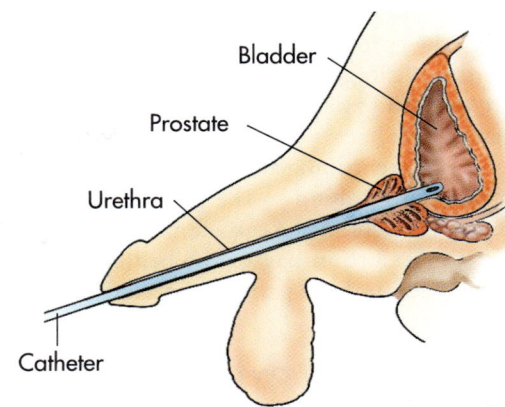

FIGURE 8 Male bladder catheterization.

BOX 1 Necessary Equipment for Bladder Catheterization

- Personal protective equipment
- Urinary catheterization set containing the following:
  - Sterile gloves
  - Antiseptic solution
  - Sterile cleansing sponges
  - Sterile drapes or towels
  - Syringe containing 5 mL sterile water
  - Connecting tubing and collection bag
  - Water-soluble sterile lubricant
- Urinary catheter with 5-mL Foley balloon
  - Catheter usually is a 16 Foley for males and a 14 Foley for females.
  - Standard length is 18 inches.

BLADDER CATHETERIZATION

As described in Chapter 52, bladder catheterization using a Foley catheter may be indicated to empty the bladder of a patient with urinary retention, to replace an indwelling urinary catheter that is not functioning, or to measure urine output in critical patients. Bladder catheterization is an invasive procedure. It carries some associated risks. These include the introduction of bacteria, which may lead to urinary tract infection, hematuria, and the creation of a false urethral passage, which may result in significant blood loss and the need for surgical repair.

Indwelling Foley Catheter Insertion

To insert a Foley catheter, the paramedic should prepare the required equipment (e.g., Foley catheter insertion set). The recommendations of the manufacturer should be closely followed (Box 1). Most patients will be anxious and frightened of the procedure. The paramedic should provide a full explanation of the procedure, reassure the patient, and make every effort to ensure privacy.

MALE CATHETERIZATION (FIGURE 8)

1. Explain the procedure to the patient.
2. Wash hands.
3. Place the patient in the supine position and remove the patient's pants and undergarments.
4. Wash hands.
5. Open the catheterization set using sterile technique.
6. Wash hands and don sterile gloves.
7. Place one sterile drape under the patient's penis and another above the penis to cover the abdomen.
8. Open a package of antiseptic solution and saturate sterile sponges (or cotton balls).
9. Attach the syringe to the catheter and test the balloon to make sure it inflates.
10. Open a package of water-soluble lubricant and lubricate the first several inches of the catheter.
11. Grasp the patient's penis with one hand and retract the foreskin (if present).
12. With the other hand, cleanse the glans with a sterile sponge (maintaining hand sterility) and then discard the sponge. Repeat the procedure.
13. Raise the shaft of the penis upright to straighten the penile urethra and pass the tip of the catheter through the meatus.
14. Continue passing the catheter with gentle, steady pressure, advancing the catheter 7 to 9 inches or until urine flows out the distal end of the catheter. Once urine appears, advance the catheter another 2 inches. If mild resistance is felt at the external sphincter, slightly increase traction on the penis and continue with steady, gentle pressure on the catheter. *If significant resistance is met, withdraw the catheter and consult with medical direction.*
15. Attach the syringe to the catheter and inflate the balloon with 3 to 5 mL of sterile saline.

16. Gently pull back on the catheter until the balloon rests against the prostatic urethra. (Resistance will be encountered.) Reposition the retracted foreskin of an uncircumcised patient. Attach the drainage bag to the catheter.

17. Run the catheter tubing along the patient's leg and tape the connecting tubing to the patient's thigh. Do not place any tension on the catheter.

18. Attach the collection bag to the bed or stretcher at a level below that of the patient to facilitate drainage by gravity.

FEMALE CATHETERIZATION (FIGURE 9)

1. Prepare the patient and equipment as described in steps 1 to 4 and 6 to 8 of the previous procedure. Female patients should be positioned with knees bent, hips flexed, and feet resting about 24 inches apart. The patient should be draped appropriately by placing one sterile drape just under the patient's buttocks; position the fenestrated drape over the perineum, exposing the labia.

2. With one hand, separate the patient's labia to expose the urethral meatus.

3. Cleanse the surrounding area with a sterile sponge or cotton ball (maintaining hand sterility) in downward strokes from anterior to posterior. Discard the sponge. Repeat the procedure.

4. Introduce the tip of the well-lubricated catheter into the urethra using aseptic technique. Continue to advance the catheter 2 to 3 inches with gentle, steady pressure until urine flows out of the distal end of the catheter. Once urine appears, advance the catheter another 2 inches.

5. Attach a syringe to the catheter. Inflate the balloon with 3 to 5 mL of sterile saline.

6. Gently pull on the catheter until resistance is encountered.

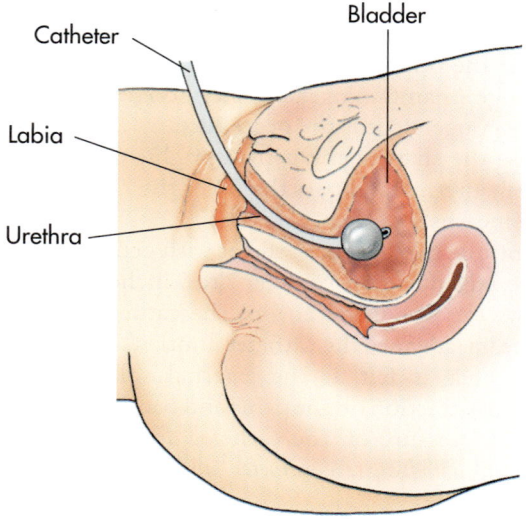

FIGURE 9 Female bladder catheterization.

7. Attach the collection tubing and bag to the catheter and secure the collection tubing to the patient's thigh as described above in steps 14 and 16 of the previous procedure. Position the collection bag to facilitate drainage.

INVASIVE HEMODYNAMIC MONITORING

Invasive hemodynamic monitoring is the measurement and interpretation of hemodynamic parameters. It requires placement of a catheter (central venous line, arterial line) in a vein, artery, or heart chamber. Knowledgeable health care personnel can obtain and interpret many different pieces of information from this tool, depending on the type of catheter used. Box 2 lists possible complications and risks associated with hemodynamic monitoring.

Hemodynamic monitoring is most useful for assessing and managing patients with hypertensive emergencies, shock, pulmonary edema, sepsis, and multiple organ failure. In particular, a pulmonary artery (PA) catheter can help distinguish among the various types of shock (cardiogenic, hypovolemic, obstructive, and distributive). Hemodynamic monitoring requires special equipment to produce visible waveforms on an oscilloscope and pressure monitor (Figure 10 and Box 3). These waveforms reflect the phases of the cardiac cycle and can be used to monitor systemic arterial pressure, right atrial pressure (central venous pressure), left atrial pressure, and pulmonary artery pressure (Figure 11).

Systemic Arterial Pressure Monitoring

Systemic arterial pressure monitoring is designed to measure systemic pressure as close to the heart as possible. This monitoring often implies continuous arterial pressure monitoring through the use of an arterial line. The placement of an arterial line in a peripheral artery allows for continuous and accurate measurement of arterial pressure. It may be indicated for monitoring drug therapy (e.g., titration of vasopressors, inotropics), blood pressure, or for frequent arterial blood gas sampling. Indwelling arterial catheters may be inserted into the radial, femoral, brachial,

---

BOX 2 Possible Complications and Risks Associated with Hemodynamic Monitoring

- Air embolism
- Arterial spasm
- Bleeding
- Dysrhythmias (with heart chamber catheterization)
- Hematoma
- Pneumothorax (with some insertion sites)
- Systemic infection
- Thrombosis
- Tissue and blood vessel injury

FIGURE 10 Hemodynamic monitoring equipment.

BOX 3 Troubleshooting Monitors

Most monitors used in patient care have a variety of alarms to alert a malfunction. A systematic method of troubleshooting the alarms is to begin with the patient first. Then, look at the equipment:

1. Check the patient.
2. Check the insertion site.
3. Check the tubing or lead wire.
4. Check connections to the monitor.
5. Check the monitor.
6. Check the electrical connection or power source.

---

the pressure in the right atrium, this is used to indirectly determine the volume of blood in the right atrium and thus the right ventricular preload. Common insertion sites for RAP monitoring are the internal jugular vein and the subclavian vein.

NOTE
RAP monitoring may reflect left ventricular preload but can be misleading, particularly in conditions in which there is right atrial or right ventricular dysfunction.

---

or dorsalis pedis artery. The radial or brachial artery is most commonly used for continuous pressure monitoring.

Right Atrial Pressure (RAP) Monitoring

Right atrial pressure monitoring may be used to assess right ventricular preload in critically ill patients. RAP monitoring (also known as *central venous pressure [CVP] monitoring*) allows direct measurement of pressure in the right atrium and *reflects* right ventricular pressure. It is used to monitor blood volume, right ventricular function, and central venous return. The vascular access device also can be used to administer IV fluids, medications, blood, and to obtain blood samples. Although monitoring RAP measures

Left Atrial Pressure (LAP) Monitoring

Left atrial pressure monitoring measures the pressure of the blood as it returns to the left side of the heart. It is normally measured indirectly by measuring the pulmonary capillary wedge pressure described later. LAP is a reliable indicator of left ventricular end-diastolic pressure, and therefore, of left ventricular function. (This is true except in cases of severe mitral stenosis if LAP is obtained using PCWP.) Short-term LAP monitoring is usually performed in the operating room during cardiac surgery, when a catheter is placed directly into the left atrium. In most other settings, LAP more often is indirectly monitored through a pulmonary artery catheter.

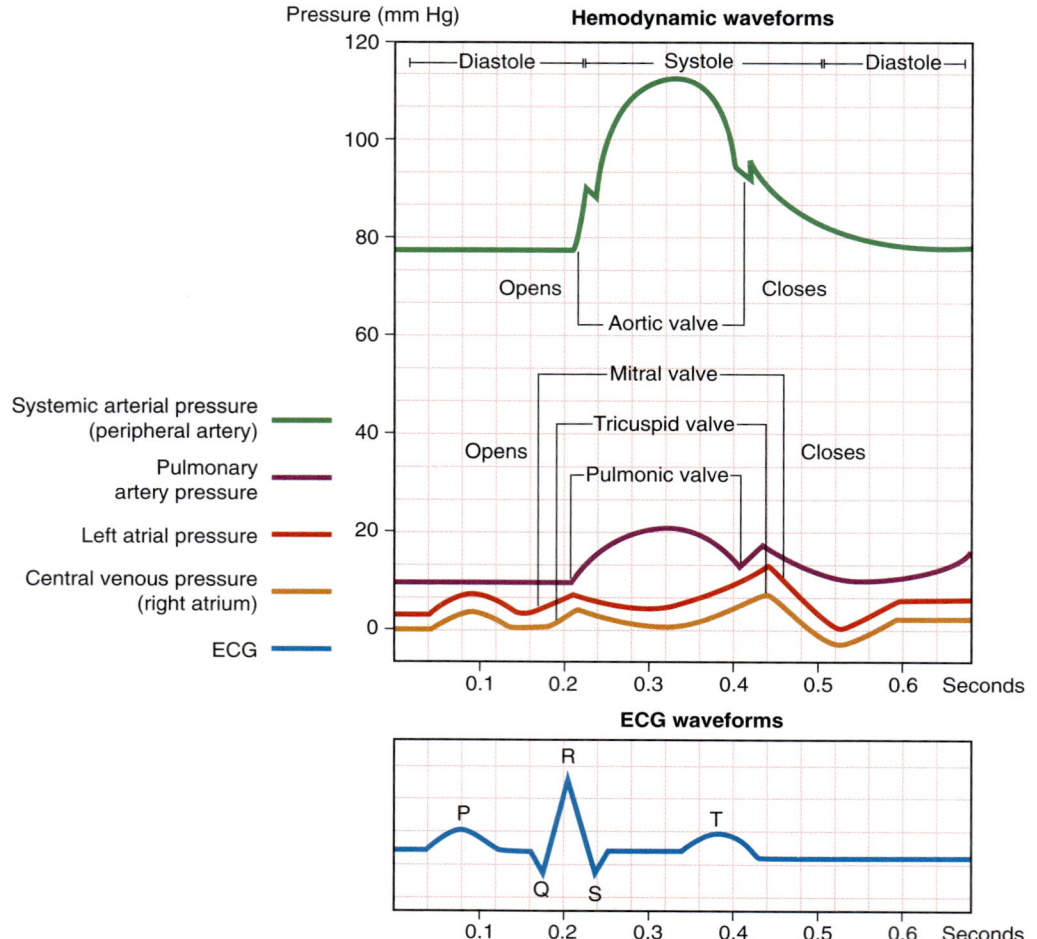

Pressure (mm Hg)

Hemodynamic waveforms

Systemic arterial pressure (peripheral artery)
Pulmonary artery pressure
Left atrial pressure
Central venous pressure (right atrium)
ECG

ECG waveforms

FIGURE 11 How hemodynamic waveforms reflect the cardiac cycle.

Pulmonary Artery Pressure (PAP) Monitoring

Pulmonary artery pressure monitoring provides an indirect measure of left ventricular function. The catheter used for PAP monitoring has four lumens (and sometimes a fifth proximal infusion port) that contain a balloon inflation port, proximal and distal injection ports, and a thermistor lumen for obtaining cardiac output measurements (Figure 12). Some PAP devices are also designed for transvenous pacing.

The catheter is usually inserted in the subclavian or internal jugular vein and is passed through the right atrium and right ventricle into the pulmonary artery. PAP monitoring is useful in treating shock, congestive heart failure (CHF), pulmonary edema, pulmonary embolism, and for monitoring patients who are undergoing cardiac surgery. The PAP reflects venous pressure in the lungs, the mean filling pressure for the left side of the heart, and indicates left ventricular end-diastolic pressure (in the absence of mitral valve disease). In addition to measuring pulmonary artery pressure, PAP monitoring provides a measurement

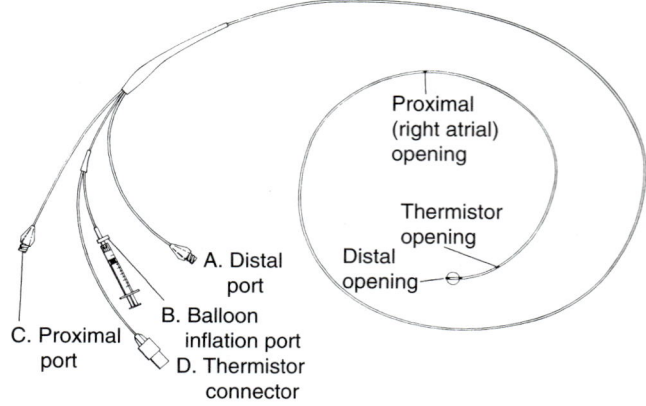

FIGURE 12 Number 7 French quadruple lumen, thermodilution pulmonary artery catheter. (Darovic GO: *Hemodynamic monitoring, invasive and noninvasive clinical application,* ed 3, Philadelphia, 2003, Saunders.)

of RAP during insertion, pulmonary capillary wedge pressure (PCWP), cardiac output, and mixed venous oxygen saturation.

PULMONARY CAPILLARY WEDGE PRESSURE

Pulmonary capillary wedge pressure (PCWP) (also known as *pulmonary artery wedge pressure [PAWP]*) helps to determine left ventricular function. It is measured when the pulmonary balloon of the PA catheter is inflated and occludes a pulmonary artery branch, allowing the distal lumen in front of the balloon to register left heart pressure. Once the measurement is obtained, the balloon is deflated and the catheter will float back into the pulmonary artery. (The balloon is only inflated for PCWP readings; it remains deflated for continuous PAP monitoring and during patient transports.) PCWP usually is measured every 4 hours.

CARDIAC OUTPUT

The **thermistor lumen** is a multilumen catheter device that measures cardiac output (CO) through a special computer. It does this by measuring the temperature of fluid in the body. It also aids in assessing left ventricular function and the function of heart valves. This measure is taken (as needed) by injecting a solution called *injectate* at a known temperature (iced or room temperature) into the proximal lumen port of the PA catheter or through a closed injectate delivery system. The solution then mixes with blood from the superior vena cava or the right atrium (depending on the location of the catheter), and lowers the temperature of the heart's blood. The thermistor detects the drop in temperature. The temperature change is analyzed by the computer, calculating cardiac output of the right and left ventricle. Continuous CO measurements can also be obtained by special catheters and equipment that change the temperature of the heart's blood at specific intervals without injectate, calculating CO over several minutes.

MIXED VENOUS OXYGEN SATURATION

Mixed venous oxygen saturation (SVO_2) is the direct measurement of the blended venous blood (from the inferior and superior vena cavae) usually sampled from the right atrium or ventricle. It reflects the balance between oxygen delivery and consumption in the tissues and can serve as an early indicator of low cardiac output. SVO_2 can be measured from a PA catheter when mixed venous blood from organs and tissues flows back to the lungs. This measurement can be taken intermittently by withdrawing blood from the port of a PA catheter, or continuously by using fiberoptic catheters and an oximetry system that assesses cardiac and pulmonary function.

INTRAAORTIC BALLOON PUMP

An **intraaortic balloon pump** (IABP) is a mechanical cardiac assist device that benefits patients with actual or potentially life-threatening circulatory problems. Indications for its use include patients:

- In cardiogenic shock as a bridge to reperfusion therapy
- With ventricular septal defect and acute mitral regurgitation
- Who are candidates for cardiac transplant
- Who are high-risk surgical patients
- Who are high risk and undergoing angiography or angioplasty
- Who have refractory ventricular dysrhythmias complicating AMI
- Who have recurrent postinfarction angina

The catheter with balloon usually is inserted in the patient's femoral artery and is advanced until the catheter lies in the aorta, just beyond the left subclavian artery. The balloon is at the distal end of the catheter, and when inflated by a computerized pump, it fills the patient's descending thoracic aorta. The balloon inflates during diastole, causing blood in the aorta to be forced back proximally into the coronary arteries, thus increasing coronary artery flow. This allows for increased perfusion of the myocardium, helping to relieve myocardial ischemia. Just before systole, the balloon deflates, causing a decrease of the pressure in the aorta, making it easier for the left ventricle to expel blood during contraction. This results in decreased workload for the left ventricle, and increases cardiac output and perfusion of vital organs. As a rule, the IABP is initially set to an inflation/deflation cycle for each cardiac cycle (1:1 ratio) and then is gradually reduced (2:1, 3:1 ratio), based on the patient's condition. Most IABP devices adapt the deflation automatically in the situation of ventricular ectopy or other dysrhythmias. If the timing is not correct, a number of physiologic changes can occur (Table 1) (Figure 13).

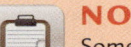

NOTE

Some manufacturers have adapters especially for transport in the event the transport team's pump is different than the one at the referring facility. These adapters allow interfacing between the different pumps.

TABLE 1 IABP Timing Errors

Timing Error	Effect
Early inflation	Premature closure of the aortic valve causing aortic regurgitation
Late inflation	Sub-optimal coronary perfusion
Early deflation	Retrograde coronary blood flow
Late deflation	Increases the resistance the balloon pumps against (afterload)

From ASTNA: *ASTNA patient transport: principles and practice,* ed 4, St Louis, 2009, Mosby.

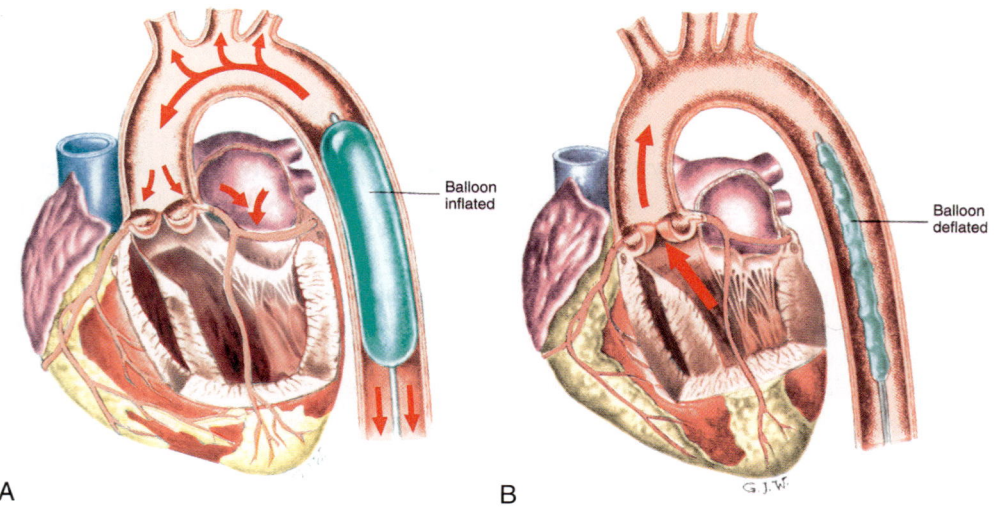

A   B

FIGURE 13 Mechanisms of action of the intraaortic balloon pump. **A,** Diastolic balloon inflation augments coronary blood flow. **B,** Systolic balloon deflation decreases afterload.

SHOW ME THE EVIDENCE

In this case series, researchers prospectively evaluated critical care paramedic transport of 29 patients transferred with IABP. Reports were evaluated to determine appropriateness of care and adverse events. During transport, there were 22 complications involving 11 patients. All were managed effectively by the paramedics. No life-threatening complications persisted, and no patient died during transfer. The authors conclude that specially trained paramedics can safely transfer IABP patients in their system.

From MacDonald R, Farquhar S: *Transfer of intra-aortic balloon pump-dependent patients by paramedics: a case-series,* 2009. Paper presented at the National Association of EMS Physicians, Naples, Fla. www.allacademic.com/one/www/www/index.php?cmd=www_search&offset=0&limit=5&multi_search_search_mode=publication&multi_search_publication_fulltext_mod=fulltext&textfield_submit=true&search_module=multi_search&search=Search&search_field=title_idx&fulltext_search=Transfer+of+intra-aortic+balloon+pump-dependent+patients+by+paramedics%3A++a+case-series.

INTRACRANIAL PRESSURE MONITORING

As described in Chapter 40, a rise in intracranial pressure (ICP) can decrease cerebral perfusion. ICP monitoring is often used in patients with brain lesions, head trauma with bleeding or edema, hydrocephalus, encephalitis, and those who have an overproduction and/or insufficient absorption of cerebrospinal fluid. ICP can be monitored using an intraventricular cannula (the most common method), an epidural catheter, a subdural or subarachnoid monitoring device, or by a fiberoptic transducer tipped probe (Figure 14). All devices must be placed by a physician, and all monitoring systems require calibration (Box 4).

LOOK AGAIN

See Chapter 40: Head, Face, and Neck Trauma, pp. 1166-1168.

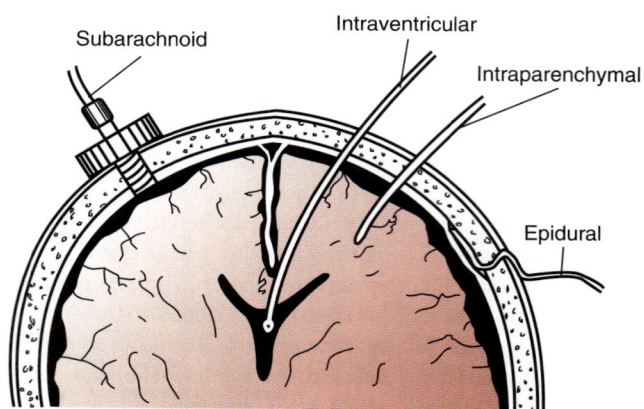

FIGURE 14 Intracranial pressure monitoring sites. (Kee JT: *Youman's neurological surgery,* ed 4, Philadelphia, 1996, Saunders.)

BOX 4 Important Considerations in ICP Monitoring

- Maintain sterile technique.
- Keep all stopcocks ports capped unless one must be opened to expel air or to balance the transducer.
- Expel all air from the tubing or stopcock ports before connecting the line to the patient.
- Never flush any fluid into the patient's cranial cavity. Doing so will raise ICP and invite infection.

ICP Waveforms

The normal range for ICP in an adult is 10 to 15 mm Hg or less, but this can vary by individual with position changes and activity level. For example, rotation of the head either to the right or left and head-down positions can increase ICP significantly in both normal patients as well as those with head injury or stroke.[1] For patients with head trauma, it is generally agreed that moderate (15° to 45°) head elevation significantly reduces ICP, whereas head elevation >45° may be dangerous because of a critical decrease in cerebral perfusion pressure (CPP).[2] Therapies that may be needed to control increasing ICP include:

- Maintaining oxygenation to improve gas exchange
- Avoiding hypoxia and/or hypercapnia
- Positioning the patient by moderately elevating the patient's head or the head of the stretcher to optimize cerebral perfusion pressure (CPP) and to lower ICP
- Avoiding maneuvers that might increase intrathoracic or intraabdominal pressure (e.g., coughing, Valsalva maneuver, patient movement, hip flexion)
- Preventing sudden variation in systemic blood pressure
- Administering osmotic diuretics and/or steroids to reduce cerebral edema and inflammation
- Restricting IV fluid therapy
- Providing sedation to prevent agitation
- Maintaining normal body temperature
- Avoiding seizure activity

BLOOD ADMINISTRATION

As described in Chapters 11 and 32, blood replacement therapy may be indicated when caring for patients who have suffered acute blood loss and in some patients who have symptomatic anemia or other disorders. Blood products that commonly are administered to critical patients include packed red blood cells, fresh frozen plasma, and platelets. (Whole blood is not commonly available, but it is still used occasionally.) Because of the risk of transfusion reactions and the possible transmission of infectious disease, blood products should be given only when specifically indicated. Before administering a blood transfusion:

1. The patient and blood product must be identified by two health care professionals.
2. Blood containing RBCs must be compared to the patient's ABO group and Rh type.
3. The name and identification number on the patient's wrist band must be compared to the slip on the blood bag.
4. The expiration date and time on the blood product must be identified. The blood bag should be turned upside down to gently mix it and inspect its contents for color and consistency.
5. The label must remain attached to the blood product until the transfusion is complete.

Blood and blood products can be safely administered through a peripheral IV line, Portacath, and most central lines. Optimally, the tubing of the administration set should be connected directly to the access line and should not be piggy-backed into an existing IV line (which can increase the risk of contamination). Peripheral IV access must be sufficient to maintain an adequate flow rate for the transfusion. Straight-type blood administration sets contain a standard filter in the tubing and are adequate for

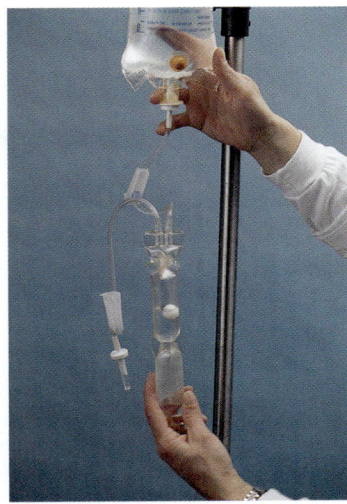

FIGURE 15 Blood administration set primed with normal saline. (Perry AG, Potter PA, Elkin MA: *Nursing interventions and clinical skills*, ed 5, St. Louis, 2012, Mosby.)

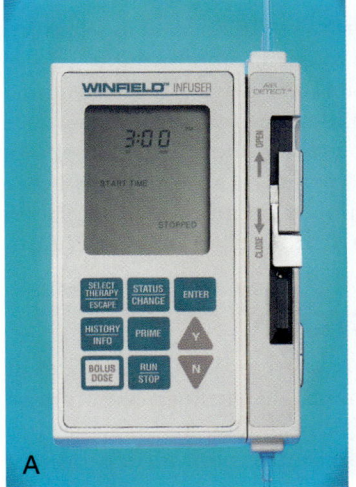 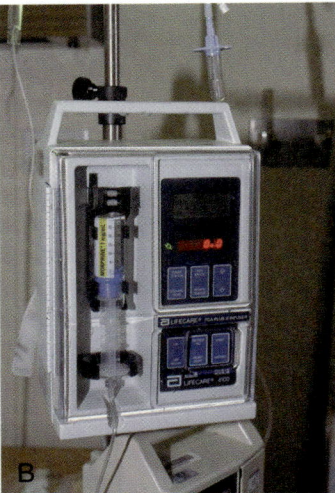

FIGURE 16 A, Electronic infusion device. **B,** Ambulatory infusion pump. (Perry AG, Potter PA, Elkin MA: *Nursing interventions and clinical skills*, ed 5, St. Louis, 2012, Mosby.)

the administration of most blood products (Figure 15). Y type blood/solution administration sets contain a standard filter in the tubing with a Y-tubing above the filter to permit a dual connection for a blood component (e.g., red blood cells) and saline.

IV INFUSION PUMPS

IV infusion pumps maintain a more accurate flow rate when providing fluid and medication therapy than the more common gravity systems. Many IV infusion pumps are available, and all require familiarity with the operating instructions for the specific device (Figure 16). Most models can be operated by battery as well as electric current. They incorporate warnings and alarms of low or high occlusion

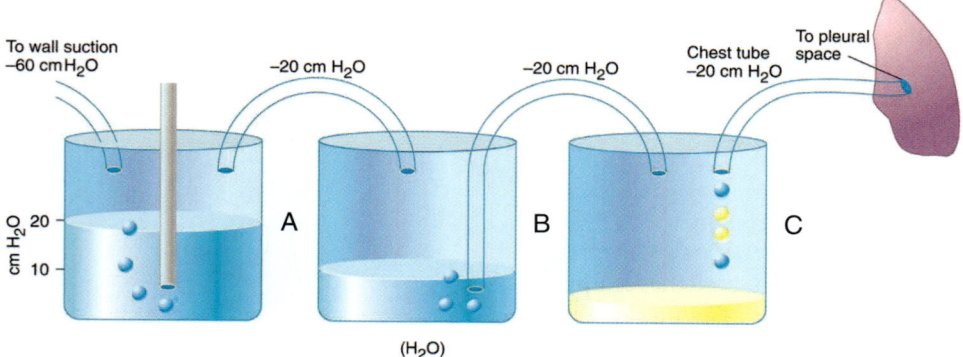

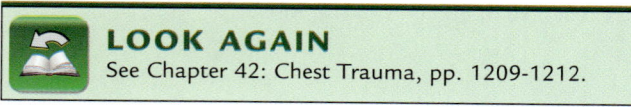

FIGURE 17 The standard three-bottle system is the basis for all commercial chest tube drainage systems. Pleural fluid and pleural air enter compartment C, which serves as a fluid collection trap so that the water-seal fluid volume will not rise (compartment B) and create resistance to air escaping the chest. Air cannot be inspired into the chest because of the water in compartment B. Open entrainment of room air through a submerged tube in compartment A buffers the amount of wall suction applied (-60 cm H_2O) to the height of the water column to standardize the pressure (-20 cm H_2O) transmitted to the chest. (Wilkins RL: *Egan's fundamentals of respiratory care*, ed 9, St Louis, 2009, Mosby.)

pressure, air in tubing, infusion complete, and low battery. All infusion pumps require frequent monitoring to ensure that they are accurately calibrated. During the infusion, a periodic assessment should include ensuring the flow rate corresponds to the rate displayed on the IV infusion pump, and that the infusion site is patent. If any problems occur during IV therapy, the paramedic should check all alarms (per the manufacturer's instructions), and stop the IV infusion if necessary.

TUBE THORACOSTOMY

As described in Chapter 42, chest wall injury can result in pneumothorax, hemothorax, or hemopneumothorax. These conditions can be life threatening and may need to be managed with pleural decompression. Pleural decompression can be achieved though needle thoracostomy (described in Chapter 42) or through tube thoracostomy.

LOOK AGAIN
See Chapter 42: Chest Trauma, pp. 1209-1212.

Tube thoracostomy involves the insertion of a catheter ("chest tube") through the chest wall into the pleural space. The tube is usually secured to the chest wall with sutures, and further secured with occlusive dressing and tape. It is then attached to suction to help with drainage. There are various chest wall drainage systems, but all work on the same principle as the original three-bottle system, described here for illustration (Figure 17). (Modern, rectangular plastic containers with three chambers have largely replaced the three-bottle system [Figure 18].) The first bottle collects the air, blood, or other fluid from the patient's pleural space through the chest tube. The second bottle or chamber is a

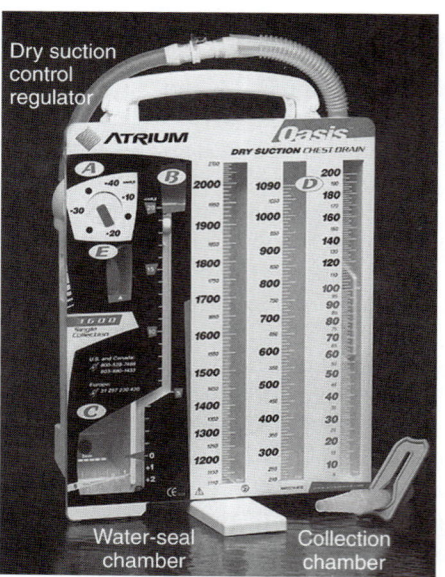

FIGURE 18 Chest tube drainage systems have three chambers: (1) collection chamber, (2) water-seal chamber, and (3) suction control chamber. Suction control chamber requires a connection to a wall suction source that is dialed up higher than the prescribed suction for the suction to work. (ENA: *Sheehy's emergency nursing: principles and practice*, ed 6, St Louis, 2010, Mosby.)

water seal bottle with a one-way valve that prevents air or fluid from moving backward into the first bottle. The third bottle contains water and is connected to suction. It controls the amount of suction either by a control valve or through a tube below the water surface. The higher the water level in the third bottle, the stronger the suction. (Some systems are waterless and contain a mechanical valve instead of water that allows drainage of blood or air.) The chest tube remains in place until all or most of the air or fluid has been drained from the pleural space (usually a few days). Tube thoracostomy also is helpful in collecting infected fluid (e.g., pus) that has accumulated in the pleural space from bacterial infection or tuberculosis. Components and management of chest drainage systems are outlined in Box 5.

Care Considerations

After a chest tube is inserted, all tubing connections should be taped to minimize the risk of disconnection. Occlusive Vaseline gauze often is placed at the insertion site to minimize the risk of air leak. The chest drainage unit should be kept below the level of the chest when moving the patient, and the water seal units should always be maintained in an upright position. Tubing must be monitored for accidental kinking. Initial chest tube drainage that is more than 1500 mL should be reported. During transport all equipment should be assessed for air leaks and tube patency. Air leaks may be related to the chest drainage system, the injury to the lung, esophageal or bronchial injury, or a chest tube that is improperly placed. Persistent air leaks should be suspected if constant bubbling in the water seal chamber is observed (Box 6).

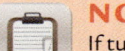

NOTE

If tube drainage stops suddenly, it is possible a clot has formed. If this occurs, the tube should be squeezed gently from its proximal to its distal end. Avoid clamping the chest tube during transport. With some injuries, this could lead to a tension pneumothorax. In some cases in which there is minimal drainage from the chest tube, a one-way valve may be attached to the tube during transport.[5]

BOX 5 Chest Drainage Systems: Components and Management[3,4]

Fluid Collection Chamber

Fluid drains from the patient through a long tube to a collection chamber, marked for assessment of drainage.

Water Seal Chamber

Allows air to pass out, via bubbles, through the bottom of the chamber. Often calibrated for measuring intrathoracic pressure and may have float valve to protect patient from high negativity. With the water seal chamber, during spontaneous respirations, the water level should rise during inhalation and fall during exhalation. This oscillation is called *tidaling* and is one indicator of a patent pleural chest tube.

Suction Control Chamber

Improves drainage and helps overcome the air leak. Keep suction control at −10 to −20 cm H_2O. Dry suction control systems provide many advantages: higher suction pressure levels can be achieved, set-up is easy, no continuous bubbling provides for quiet operation, and there is no fluid to evaporate, which would decrease the amount of suction applied to the patient. Instead of regulating the level of suction with a column of water, the dry suction units are controlled by a self-compensating regulator. Suction can be set at −10, −15, −20, −30, or −40 cm H_2O. The unit is preset at −20 cm H_2O when opened. Patient situations that may require higher suction pressures of −30 or −40 cm H_2O include a large air leak from the lung surface, empyema, a reduction in pulmonary compliance, or anticipated difficulty in expansion of the pulmonary tissue.

Nursing Responsibilities

Secure all connections. Monitor catheters to prevent kinking. Monitor drainage output. Assess for air leaks. Maintain unit in upright position.

Assessing for Air Leaks

Look at the underwater seal. Leaks may originate with the patient or the drainage system. (Check the patient history. Would you expect a patient air leak?). For a patient receiving mechanical ventilation with positive end-expiratory pressure (PEEP), leaking causes continuous bubbling. Note the pattern of the bubbling. If it fluctuates with respirations (i.e., occurs on exhalation in a patient breathing spontaneously), the most likely source is the lung. Momentarily clamp the chest tube at the dressing site with a toothless/padded clamp. Move the clamp incrementally toward the drainage unit—when you place the clamp between the source of the air leak, and the water seal/air leak meter chamber, the bubbling will stop. If bubbling stops the first time you clamp, the air leak must be at the chest tube insertion site or the lung. If bubbling continues, the leak is distal to the clamp. If bubbling stops before the end of the tubing, the leak is in the tube, so it must be replaced. If the unit is still bubbling when the very end of the tubing is clamped, the unit has the leak and should be changed. If the leak is at the insertion site, remove the chest tube dressing and inspect the site. Make sure the catheter eyelets have not pulled out beyond the chest wall. Replace the dressing. Notify the physician of any new, increased, or unexpected air leaks that are not corrected by the above actions.

Indications of Patency

The water level in the water seal should fluctuate with breathing, rising with inspiration and falling with expiration, and is an indicator of chest tube patency. If the patient is on mechanical ventilation, this pattern is reversed because breaths are delivered under positive pressure. Fluctuations stop when the lung is fully reexpanded or when the tube is kinked or compressed.

Milking/Stripping the Tube

Vigorous milking or stripping can create dangerously high negative pressures, placing the patient at risk for mediastinal trauma. Use extreme caution, and follow your hospital policy.

To Clamp or Not to Clamp?

Never clamp a chest tube during patient transport unless the chest drainage system becomes disrupted during patient movement, and then only if there is no air leak.

From Emergency Nurses Association: *Sheehy's emergency nursing: principles and practice,* ed 6, St Louis, 2009, Mosby.

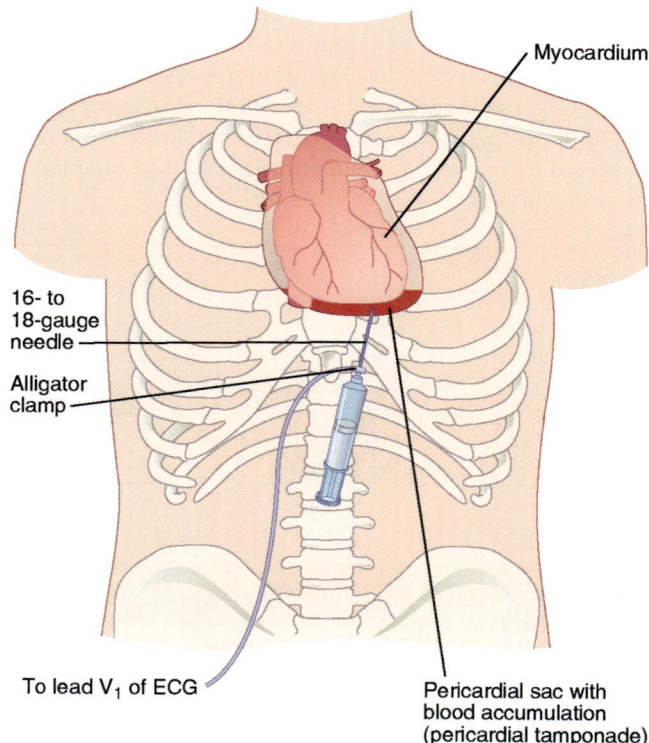

Myocardium

16- to 18-gauge needle

Alligator clamp

To lead V₁ of ECG

Pericardial sac with blood accumulation (pericardial tamponade)

FIGURE 19 Pericardiocentesis (Holleran RS: *Air and surface patient transport: principles and practice,* ed 3, St Louis, 2010, Mosby.)

BOX 6 Checking for Air Leaks in a Chest Drainage System

1. Occlude the chest or drainage tube intermittently along the length of the system.
2. Reinforce the chest dressing and all connections.
3. If the bubbling stops when you occlude the tubing close to the drainage unit, consider replacing the unit if possible.

PERICARDIOCENTESIS

Pericardiocentesis is an invasive procedure in which a needle is inserted in the pericardial sac to aspirate blood or fluid. The primary indication for pericardiocentesis is pericardial tamponade. Pericardiocentesis carries significant risk, including penetration through the surface of the heart. Other complications include laceration of a coronary artery, laceration of the lung or liver, cardiac dysrhythmias, and increased tamponade. Ultrasound-guided pericardiocentesis is commonly used today and is deemed to reduce the rate of complications. The procedure for pericardiocentesis that is not guided by ultrasound is as follows (Figure 19):

1. Using aseptic technique, insert a 3-inch, 16- or 18-gauge needle (attached to a 50-cc syringe) at the angle of the xiphoid cartilage and the seventh rib.
2. Advance the needle at a 45-degree angle to the skin toward the right or left midclavicular line while

aspirating the syringe with negative pressure. If the needle is advanced too far, a pulsation will be felt through the needle and syringe.

3. Aspirate as much fluid as possible. Fluid is usually encountered at a depth of 3 to 4 cm.(Removal of as little as 20 to 25 mL of blood from a distended pericardium may produce a dramatic blood pressure response.)
4. After withdrawing blood from the pericardia sac, attach a surgical clamp to the needle at the level of the skin to avoid accidental advancement of the needle.
5. If tamponade recurs, aspirate blood again if necessary.

SECTION TWO
Special Transport Considerations in Critical Care

Transporting patients with critical care needs can present special challenges for the paramedic. Most of the challenges are related to the unique equipment required for their care– equipment that is often unfamiliar to the EMS crew. Specific considerations that are discussed in this section are management of IV drug drips, transport ventilators, and extracorporeal membrane oxygenation (ECMO) support.

NOTE

Technical mishaps that are common in critical care transport include accidental extubation, ventilator disconnect, ECG monitor power failure, vasoactive drug interruption, and intravenous infiltration or disconnection.

DID YOU KNOW?
Flight Paramedics

Flight paramedics have played an important role in critical care transport since the 1970s. In 1986, these specialty care professionals united to form the National Flight Paramedic Association (NFPA). (The NFPA is now known as the International Association of Flight Paramedics [IAFP]). The NFPA prompted quality within the industry by serving as a founding member of the Commission on Accreditation of Air Medical Services (CAAMS) in 1990, now known as the Commission on Accreditation of Medical Transport Systems (CAMTS). Flight paramedics have special training and certification in critical care procedures and flight physiology (Certified Flight Paramedic [FP-C]). Today there are more than 1500 certified flight paramedics worldwide. (Figure 20). Air medical transport is further described in Chapter 53.

MANAGING IV DRUG DRIPS

There are a number of IV drugs that are administered via continuous infusion to critical care patients. Common drugs include *amiodarone*, *diltiazem*, *dobutamine*, *dopamine*,

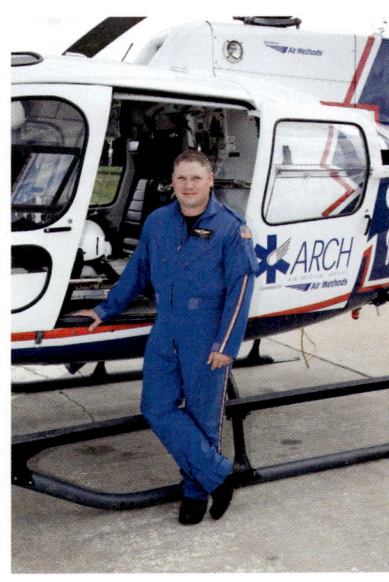

FIGURE 20 Flight paramedic.

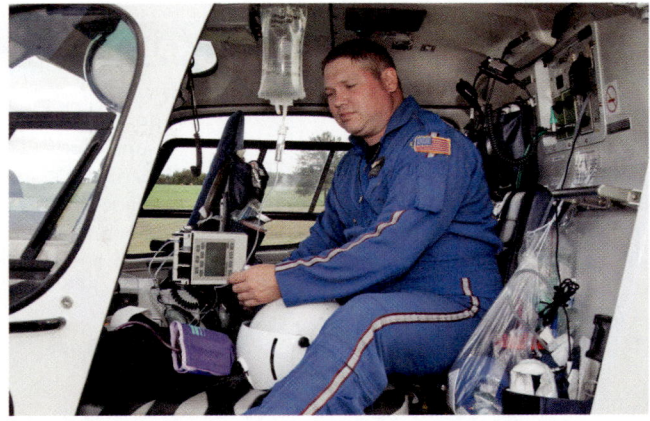

FIGURE 21 Drug infusion during critical care transport.

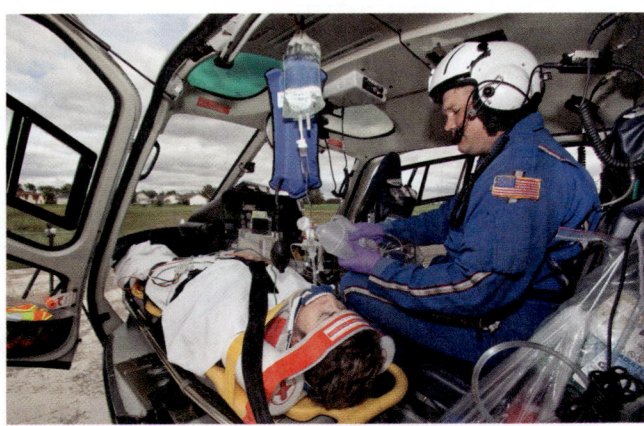

FIGURE 22 Transferring a patient with a transport ventilator.

fentanyl, *furosemide*, *midazolam*, *norepinephrine*, *vasopressin*, and others. (See the Emergency Drug Index.) When preparing to transport a patient who is receiving an IV infusion of a drug that is unfamiliar to the paramedic, the paramedic should:

1. Consult with the physician or nurse caring for the patient before transport.
2. Ensure that the prescribed drip rate is documented and clearly understood.
3. Ensure personal comfort with workings of the infusion equipment and any equipment alarms.
4. Ask about any suspected complications or possible adverse reactions associated with the drug.

Paramedics who are transporting a patient who is receiving an unfamiliar drug(s) should have ready access to an infusion drip chart or electronic drug dose information source (Figure 21) (Box 7).

MANAGING TRANSPORT VENTILATORS

Transitioning a patient from a hospital ventilator to a transport ventilator (and vice versa) is often a complicated procedure. It also can be a source of anxiety for the patient and the paramedic crew (Figure 22). Although there are many ventilator devices used in both in-hospital and prehospital care, guidelines for transition between the devices should be followed.[6] These include:

1. Prepare all necessary equipment and supplies.
2. Check that all equipment is functioning properly. Ensure sufficient oxygen is available for transport by calculating flow rate, and volume consumption versus the amount of available oxygen.
3. Ensure emergency airway equipment is readily available.
4. Assemble all equipment near the head of the stretcher.
5. Disconnect the patient from the mechanical ventilator and put the ventilator on standby.
6. During transition, ensure mechanical ventilation continues with 100% oxygen. The rate and depth of mechanical ventilation should closely simulate the rate and depth of what was provided by the ventilator.
7. Transition the patient to the transport ventilator and set the ventilation parameters as prescribed.
8. Closely observe the patent for tolerance of the change in mode of ventilation.

Ventilator Alarms

Ventilator alarms are set to warn of mechanical or physiologic problems. Therefore, continuous monitoring of the patient and alarm parameters is important. During transport, ventilator alarms may be difficult to hear. The alarms should be set to maximum volume, and the ventilator should be positioned so that flashing warning lights are visible. Table 2 provides guidelines for troubleshooting common ventilator alarms.

BOX 7 IV Drugs Used in Critical Care*

Abciximab	Esmolol	Milrinone
Alteplase	Fenoldopam	Nesiritide
Aminophylline	Haloperidol	Nicardipine
Amiodarone	Heparin	Nitroglycerin
Argatroban	Ibutilide	Nitroprusside
Atracurium	Immune globulin	Norepinephrine
Bivalirudin	Inamrinone	Octreotide
Cisatracurium	Infliximab	Pantoprazole
Conivaptan	Insulin	Phenylephrine
Dexmedetomidine	Isoproterenol	Potassium chloride
Diltiazem	Labetalol	Procainamide
Dobutamine	Lepirudin	Propofol
Dopamine	Lidocaine	Reteplase
Drotrecogin alfa	Lorazepam	Tenecteplase
Epinephrine	Magnesium sulfate	Tirofiban HCL
Eptifibatide	Midazolam	Vasopressin

From Algozzine G et al: *Critical care infusion drug handbook,* ed 3, St Louis, 2004, Mosby.
*All infusions should be verified through medical direction or written protocol.

TABLE 2 Troubleshooting Ventilator Alarms

1. Initial assessment:
   Airway: Is the endotracheal tube (ETT) in correct position? Check ETT insertion depth, check end tidal CO_2, check breath sounds.
   Breathing: Check breath sounds, look for chest excursion, check pulse oximetry, check patient color.
   Circulation: Check the pulse, electrocardiogram (ECG), and blood pressure.
2. Remove patient from the ventilator and manually use a resuscitation bag if any compromise is found.
   Alarm
   Cause
   Management
   Apnea
   Insufficient spontaneous breathing by patient in CPAP or pressure-support mode
3. Switch ventilator mode to one that provides set rate
   High airway pressure
   ETT obstruction: sputum, kink, biting
   Decreased compliance or increased resistance
   Circumferential burns
   Bronchospasm, lung collapse, pneumothorax, endobronchial intubation, worsening of lung process
   Anxiety/fear/pain/fighting of ventilator
   Suction airway
4. Treat cause of resistance
   Adjust mode or settings
   Rule out hypoxia before treating agitation
   CXR analysis
   Change ventilator mode to one that is better tolerated or provides sedation/analgesia
   Low airway pressure
   Ventilator disconnect
   Leak in ventilator system
   Cuff leak
   Inadvertent extubation
   Ensure that all connections are intact and tight
   Troubleshoot ETT cuff
   Bag-valve-mask if ETT was dislodged
   Oxygen pressure low
   Oxygen cylinder is empty
   Closed cylinder valve
   Unit not connected to wall terminal
   Aircraft/ambulance oxygen flow in off position
   Check wall and cylinder connections
   Bag-mask-ventilate until resolved

From ASTNA: *ASTNA patient transport: principles and practice,* ed 4, St Louis, 2009, Mosby.

EXTRACORPOREAL MEMBRANE OXYGENATION (ECMO) SUPPORT

Extracorporeal Membrane Oxygenation is temporary support of a patient's heart and lung function by partial cardiopulmonary bypass (up to 75% of cardiac output). It is often used for patients who have reversible cardiopulmonary failure from pulmonary, cardiac, or other disease, and is often used in infants. With ECMO, blood is drained from the patient to an external pump. The pump pushes the blood through a membrane gas exchanger (for oxygenation and CO_2 removal) and a warmer (Figure 23). The blood is then returned to the patient's circulation. ECMO requires anticoagulation of the patient usually with unfractionated **heparin**, guided by frequent measurements of activated clotting time (ACT). Various devices monitor the patient, and the pressures, flow, and temperature of the ECMO blood and gas circuits. ECMO can be either veno-arterial or veno-venous[7]:

- *Veno-arterial (VA)-ECMO,* can be central, in which blood is drained from the right atrium (via a right internal jugular venous catheter) and is returned to the thoracic aorta (via a right carotid arterial catheter). It may also be peripheral, in which the blood is often drained from a femoral artery and returned via a femoral vein approach into the inferior vena cava. VA-ECMO provides cardiac as well as pulmonary support.
- *Veno-venous (VV)-ECM* can also be central or peripheral. In central VV-ECMO blood is drained from right atrium (via side holes of a double lumen catheter) and returned to the right atrium through the end hole of the catheter, which is directed toward the tricuspid valve. Peripheral VV-ECMO may involve the femoral artery to femoral vein approach; femoral vein to femoral vein; or femoral vein to internal jugular vein if circulation is intact. VV-ECMO requires good cardiac function and avoids cannulation of the carotid artery. With improved ECMO technology, the less invasive approaches are most commonly used when possible.

The duration of ECMO treatment is usually limited to 7 to 10 days for neonatal respiratory diseases. Longer treatment may be needed for newborns with diaphragmatic hernia and cardiac disease, and in older children or adults. Complications of ECMO treatment include severe bleeding (gastrointestinal hemorrhage, intracranial bleeds), thromboembolism, air embolism, limb ischemia, acute renal failure, and oxygenator failure.[8]

Transport Considerations

Interfacility transport of ECMO patients is uncommon. This is because most institutions that initiate ECMO treatment are well-qualified to continue the patient's care. However, EMS transports do occur for reasons such as suboptimal cardiothoracic physician staffing, centers that are not capable of initiating ventricular assist device (VAD) therapies in the patient (described in Chapter 22), and institutions that do not have cardiac transplant capabilities. ECMO patients are extremely ill. Because of this and the complexity of the ECMO apparatus, most interfacility transports are provided by medical teams to ensure safe transport. Additional staff may include a cardiothoracic surgeon, a clinical perfusionist, and an anesthesiologist or nurse anesthetist. Often the EMS crew will only assist with safely moving the patient and equipment.

> **NOTE**
> It is critical that all devices placed in the ambulance be strapped in place to prevent inadvertent movement during transport. Additionally, all team members must have the ability to sit and be seat-belted while the vehicle is in motion.

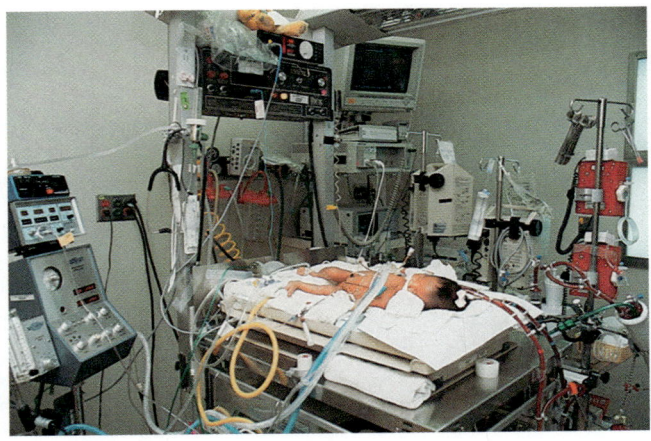

FIGURE 23 Extracorporeal membrane oxygenation. (Hockenberry MJ, Wilson D: *Wong's nursing care of infants and children,* ed 9, St. Louis, 2011, Mosby.)

As noted earlier, these patients are extremely ill. They often require multiple vasopressors and blood products to maintain adequate hemodynamics.[9] If possible, continuous IV infusions that are nonessential or that can be given IV push should be discontinued or switched to smaller IV pumps to preserve space in the ambulance. All IV lines and insertion sites should be labeled and secured. (Surgical and arterial sites should be evaluated often for bleeding and after each move.) These patients often require continuous monitoring of arterial and central venous pressures, end-tidal CO_2, ECG, blood pressure, and core temperature. Once completely prepared for movement, the patient should be moved to and from the EMS stretcher with as much assistance as possible.

REFERENCES

1. Grover V, et al: Changes in intracranial pressure in various positions of the head in anaesthetized patients, *Bahrain Med Bull* 25(4), 2003.
2. Schwartz S, et al: Effects of body position on intracranial pressure and cerebral perfusion in patients with large hemispheric stroke, *Stroke* 33(2):497-501, 2002.
3. Atrium Medical Corporation: Chest drainage competency manual, 2004. www.atriummed.com/PDF/CompetencyManual2004.pdf. Accessed June 14, 2008.
4. Baumann MH: What size chest tube? What drainage system is ideal? And other chest tube management questions, *Curr Opin Pulm Med* 9:276, 2003.
5. Emergency Nurses Association: *Trauma nurse core course,* ed 6, Park Ridge, Ill., 2007, Emergency Nurses Association.
6. Branson RD: Intrahospital transport of critically ill, mechanically ventilated patients, *Resp Care* 37:775-793, 1992.
7. Intensive Care Nursery House Staff Manual, UCSF Children's Hospital, Regents of the University of California, 2004.
8. Libby P: *Braunwald's heart disease: a textbook of cardiovascular medicine,* ed 8, Philadelphia, 2007, Saunders.
9. Ellenger F, et al: Interfacility care transport of a patient on ECMO. Critical transport issues, EMS Responder.com http://www.emsresponder.com/print/EMS-Magazine/Critical-Transport-Issues/1$10585, accessed 6-16-10.

BIBLIOGRAPHY

Dalton A, et al: *Advanced medical life support: a practical approach to adult medical emergencies*, ed 3, 2007, Brady/Prentice Hall.

Daly E, Schroeder J: *Techniques in bedside hemodynamic monitoring*, ed 5, St Louis, 1994, Mosby.

Darovic G: *Hemodynamic monitoring: invasive and noninvasive clinical application*, ed 3, Philadelphia, 2002, Saunders.

Holleran R, editor: *Air and surface care transport: principles and practice*, ed 3, St Louis, 2010, Mosby.

Marx J, editor: *Rosen's emergency medicine: concepts and clinical practice*, ed 7, St Louis, 2006, Mosby.

Sole M, et al: Introduction to critical care nursing, ed 3, Philadelphia, 2001, Saunders.

Index

Note: Page numbers followed by f indicate figures;
t, tables; and b, boxes.

1713